MODERN SURGICAL CARE

Physiologic Foundations & Clinical Applications

MODERN SURGICAL CARE

Physiologic Foundations & Clinical Applications

EDITED BY

Thomas A. Miller, M.D.

C. Rollins Hanlon Professor and Chairman, Department of Surgery,
Saint Louis University School of Medicine,
St. Louis, Missouri

SECOND EDITION

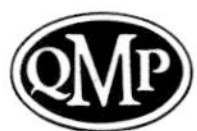

Quality Medical Publishing, Inc.

ST. LOUIS, MISSOURI
1998

Printed in the United States of America.

Previously published as *Physiologic Basis of Modern Surgical Care* in 1988 by The C.V. Mosby Company.

This book presents current scientific information and opinion pertinent to medical professionals. It does not provide advice concerning specific diagnosis and treatment of individual cases and is not intended for use by the layperson. The editor, authors, and publisher will not be responsible or liable for actions taken as a result of these opinions.

The Publisher has made every effort to trace the copyright holders for borrowed material. If any has been overlooked, the publisher will be pleased to make the necessary arrangements at the first opportunity.

PUBLISHER Karen Berger

PROJECT MANAGEMENT Top Graphics, Inc.

ASSISTANT EDITOR Esha Gupta

EDITORIAL ASSISTANT Kathy Jenkins

PRODUCTION Billie Forshee, Judy Bamert

BOOK DESIGN Diane M. Beasley Design, Susan Trail

COVER DESIGN Diane M. Beasley Design

Quality Medical Publishing, Inc.
11970 Borman Drive, Suite 222
St. Louis, Missouri 63146
Telephone: 1-800-348-7808
Web Site: http://qmp@qmp.com

LIBRARY OF CONGRESS CATALOGING-IN-PUBLICATION DATA

Modern surgical care : physiologic foundations & clinical applications / edited by Thomas A. Miller.—2nd ed.
p. cm.
Rev. ed. of: Physiologic basis of modern surgical care. 1988.
Includes bibliographical references and index.
ISBN 1-57626-060-7 (hard cover)
1. Physiology, Pathological. 2. Surgery. I. Miller, Thomas A. (Thomas Allen), 1944- . II. Physiologic basis of modern surgical care.
[DNLM: 1. Surgery. 2. Physiology. WO 102 M689 1998]
RB113.P47 1998
616.07—dc21
DNLM/DLC
for Library of Congress 97-50113
CIP

TG/WW/WW
5 4 3 2 1

Contributors

Carlos Alvarez, M.D.
Assistant Professor, Department of Surgery, University of Maryland, Baltimore, Maryland

Joseph F. Amaral, M.D.
Associate Professor of Surgery, Department of Surgery, Brown University/Rhode Island Hospital, Providence, Rhode Island

Dana K. Andersen, M.D.
Professor and Chief, Section of Surgical Gastroenterology, and Chief, General Surgery Service, Department of Surgery, Yale University School of Medicine, New Haven, Connecticut

Richard J. Andrassy, M.D.
A.G. McNeese Professor of Surgery and Chairman, Department of Surgery, University of Texas Medical School at Houston, Houston, Texas

Sheryl L. Artmann, M.D.
Assistant Professor, Department of Anesthesiology, University of Texas Medical School at Houston, Houston, Texas

Stanley W. Ashley, M.D.
Associate Professor of Surgery, Department of Surgery, Brigham and Women's Hospital, Harvard Medical School, Boston, Massachusetts

Dennis F. Bandyk, M.D.
Professor of Surgery, Department of Surgery, University of South Florida College of Medicine, Tampa, Florida

Lynn M. Bartl, M.D.
Chief Resident in Neurosurgery, Division of Neurosurgery, Department of Surgery, Saint Louis University School of Medicine, St. Louis, Missouri

Giacomo P. Basadonna, M.D., Ph.D.
Associate Professor of Surgery and Chief, Pancreas Transplantation Services, Section of Organ Donation and Transplantation, Department of Surgery, Yale University School of Medicine, New Haven, Connecticut

Barbara Lee Bass, M.D.
Professor, Department of Surgery, University of Maryland School of Medicine, Baltimore, Maryland

Donald P. Becker, M.D.
Professor and Chief, Department of Surgery/Neurosurgery, University of California–Los Angeles, Los Angeles, California

James M. Becker, M.D.
James Utley Professor and Chairman, Department of Surgery, Boston University School of Medicine, Boston, Massachusetts

George S. Benson, M.D.
Professor, Division of Urology, Department of Surgery, University of Texas Medical School at Houston, Houston, Texas

Karen Bitzer, O.T.R./L., C.H.T.
Musculoskeletal Division Coordinator, Department of Rehabilitation Services, University Hospitals of Cleveland, Cleveland, Ohio

Kirby I. Bland, M.D.
J. Murray Beardsley Professor and Chairman, Department of Surgery, Brown University School of Medicine, Providence, Rhode Island

Steven A. Blau, M.D.
Director of Surgical Critical Care, Hackensack University Medical Center, Hackensack, New Jersey

Edward L. Bove, M.D.
Professor of Surgery, Department of Pediatric Cardiovascular Surgery, University of Michigan Medical Center, Ann Arbor, Michigan

Robert E. Brolin, M.D.
Professor of Surgery, Department of Surgery, UMDNJ-Robert Wood Johnson Medical School, New Brunswick, New Jersey

Erica A. Brotschi, M.D.
Associate Professor of Surgery, Department of Surgery, Boston University School of Medicine, Boston, Massachusetts

Timothy G. Buchman, M.D., Ph.D.
Professor of Surgery, Anesthesiology, and Medicine, Departments of Surgery, Anesthesiology, and Medicine, Washington University School of Medicine, St. Louis, Missouri

Michael D. Caldwell, M.D., Ph.D.
Professor of Surgery and Biochemistry, Department of Surgery, University of Minnesota, Minneapolis, Minnesota

Thomas C. Chelimsky, M.D.
Assistant Professor of Neurology, Department of Neurology, Case Western Reserve University, Cleveland, Ohio

Laurence Y. Cheung, M.D.
Professor and Chairman, Department of Surgery, University of Kansas Medical Center, Kansas City, Kansas

G. Patrick Clagett, M.D.
Jan and Bob Pickens Professor of Medical Science and Chairman, Division of Vascular Surgery, Department of Surgery, University of Texas Southwestern Medical Center, Dallas, Texas

James H. Clark III, M.D.
Transplant Pathologist, Department of Pathology and Laboratory Medicine and Department of Surgery, University of Texas Medical School at Houston, Houston, Texas

Orlo H. Clark, M.D.
Professor and Vice Chairman, Department of Surgery, University of California–San Francisco, and Chief of Surgery, UCSF/Mount Zion Medical Center, San Francisco, California

Robert L. Conter, M.D.
Associate Professor of Surgery, Department of Surgery, Pennsylvania State University, Hershey, Pennsylvania

Edward M. Copeland III, M.D.
Edward R. Woodward Professor and Chairman, Department of Surgery, University of Florida College of Medicine; Director, University of Florida Shands Cancer Center, Gainesville, Florida

Joseph N. Corriere, Jr., M.D.
Professor of Surgery/Urology, Division of Urology, Department of Surgery, University of Texas Medical School at Houston, Houston, Texas

Charles S. Cox, Jr., M.D.
Assistant Professor of Surgery and Pediatrics, Division of Pediatric Surgery, Department of Surgery, University of Texas Medical School at Houston, Houston, Texas

Courtney Crim, M.D.
Associate Professor of Internal Medicine, Division of Pulmonology and Pulmonary Occupational Medicine, Department of Internal Medicine, Saint Louis University School of Medicine, St. Louis, Missouri

Peter F. Crookes, M.D.
Assistant Professor of Surgery, Department of Surgery, University of Southern California School of Medicine, Los Angeles, California

David Crooks, M.D.
Chief Resident, Department of Surgery, Stanford University School of Medicine, Stanford, California

Ronald L. Dalman, M.D.
Chief, Vascular Surgery Section, Surgical Service, VA Palo Alto Health Care System; Assistant Professor of Surgery, Division of Vascular Surgery, Department of Surgery, Stanford University School of Medicine, Stanford, California

John M. Daly, M.D.
Lewis Atterbury Stimson Professor and Chairman, Department of Surgery, Cornell University Medical College, New York, New York

Camelia A. Davtyan, M.D.
Assistant Professor of Clinical Medicine, Division of General Internal Medicine, Department of Internal Medicine, University of California–Los Angeles, Los Angeles, California

Haile T. Debas, M.D.
Professor of Surgery, Department of Surgery, and Dean, University of California–San Francisco School of Medicine, San Francisco, California

Reynolds M. Delgado III, M.D.
Assistant Medical Director, Heart Failure and Cardiac Transplantation Service, Texas Heart Institute, Houston, Texas

Tom R. DeMeester, M.D.
Professor and Chairman, Department of Surgery, University of Southern California School of Medicine, Los Angeles, California

Daniel T. Dempsey, M.D.
Professor of Surgery, Department of Surgery, Temple University School of Medicine, Philadelphia, Pennsylvania

Clifford W. Deveney, M.D.
Professor, Department of Surgery, Oregon Health Sciences University, Portland, Oregon

Philip E. Donahue, M.D.
Professor of Surgery, Department of General Surgery, University of Illinois at Chicago, Chicago, Illinois

Rodney M. Durham, M.D.
Associate Professor of Surgery, Department of Surgery, Saint Louis University School of Medicine, St. Louis, Missouri

Douglas B. Evans, M.D.
Associate Professor, Department of Surgical Oncology, University of Texas M.D. Anderson Cancer Center, Houston, Texas

Peter J. Fabri, M.D.
Professor of Surgery, Department of Surgery, University of South Florida, Tampa, Florida

Andrew C. Fiore, M.D.
Professor of Surgery, Division of Cardiothoracic Surgery, Department of Surgery, Saint Louis University School of Medicine, St. Louis, Missouri

R.Y. Declan Fleming, M.D.
Assistant Professor of Surgery, Department of Surgery, University of Texas Medical Branch at Galveston, Galveston, Texas

O. Howard Frazier, M.D.
Professor of Surgery, Department of Surgery, University of Texas Medical School at Houston; Chief, Cardiopulmonary Transplantation, and Director, Surgery Research, Cullen Cardiovascular Research Laboratories, Texas Heart Institute, Houston, Texas

Julie Ann Freischlag, M.D.
Professor of Surgery, Department of Surgery (Vascular Surgery), Medical College of Wisconsin, Milwaukee, Wisconsin

Francis Antony Frizelle, M.B., Ch.B., M. Med. Sci.
Consultant Colorectal Surgeon, Department of Surgery, Christchurch Hospital, Christchurch, New Zealand

Donald E. Fry, M.D.
Professor and Chairman, Department of Surgery, University of New Mexico School of Medicine, Albuquerque, New Mexico

David A. Fullerton, M.D.
Professor of Surgery, Division of Cardiothoracic Surgery, Department of Surgery, Northwestern University Medical School, Chicago, Illinois

Thomas R. Gadacz, M.D.
Professor and Chairman, Department of Surgery, Medical College of Georgia, Augusta, Georgia

Glenn W. Geelhoed, M.D., M.A., D.T.M.H., M.P.H.
Professor of Surgery and Professor of International Medical Education, George Washington University, Washington, D.C.

Bruce L. Gewertz, M.D.
Dallas B. Phemister Professor and Chairman, Department of Surgery, University of Chicago, Chicago, Illinois

Rafik M. Ghobrial, M.D., Ph.D.
Clinical Instructor in Surgery, Division of Liver Transplantation, Department of Surgery, University of California–Los Angeles, Los Angeles, California

Anita L. Giezentanner, M.D.
Assistant Professor, Department of Anesthesiology, University of Texas Medical School at Houston, Houston, Texas

Linda M. Graham, M.D.
Professor, Section of Vascular Surgery, Department of Surgery, University of Michigan Medical Center, Ann Arbor, Michigan

A. Gerson Greenburg, M.D., Ph.D.
Professor of Surgery, Department of Surgery, Brown University School of Medicine, Providence, Rhode Island

Marko R. Gudziak, M.D.
Assistant Professor and Director of Urodynamics, Department of Urology, Wayne State University, Detroit, Michigan

Ashish K. Gupta, M.D.
Department of Vascular Surgery, Vascular Institute of the Rockies, Denver, Colorado

Carl E. Haisch, M.D.
Professor, Department of Surgery, East Carolina University School of Medicine, Greenville, North Carolina

J. Michael Henderson, M.D.
Chairman, Department of General Surgery, The Cleveland Clinic Foundation, Cleveland, Ohio

Virginia M. Herrmann, M.D.
Professor of Surgery, Department of Surgery, Saint Louis University School of Medicine, St. Louis, Missouri

Martin C. Holland, M.D.
Assistant Clinical Professor, Department of Neurosurgery, University of California–San Francisco, San Francisco, California

Mark R. Jackson, M.D.
Assistant Professor, Division of Vascular Surgery, Department of Surgery, University of Texas Southwestern Medical Center, Dallas, Texas

Dawn Johnson, M.D.
Chief Resident, Department of Surgery (General Surgery), Medical College of Wisconsin, Milwaukee, Wisconsin

Barry D. Kahan, M.D., Ph.D.
Professor of Surgery, Department of Surgery, and Director, Division of Immunology and Organ Transplantation, University of Texas Medical School at Houston, Houston, Texas

Jeffrey Katz, M.D.
Professor and Chairman, Department of Anesthesiology, University of Texas Medical School at Houston, Houston, Texas

Gordon L. Kauffman, Jr., M.D.
Professor of Surgery and Cellular and Molecular Physiology; Vice-Chairman, Department of Surgery; Chief, Section of General Surgery, Penn State Geisinger Health System, The Milton S. Hershey Medical Center, Hershey, Pennsylvania

Kimberly S. Kirkwood, M.D.
Assistant Professor of Surgery, Department of Surgery, University of California–San Francisco, San Francisco, California

Mary E. Klingensmith, M.D.
Senior Surgical Resident, Department of Surgery, Brigham and Women's Hospital, Harvard Medical School, Boston, Massachusetts

Evan R. Kokoska, M.D.
Resident in Surgery, Department of Surgery, Saint Louis University School of Medicine, St. Louis, Missouri

Kara C. Kort, M.D.
Resident in Surgery, State University of New York Health Sciences Center at Syracuse, Syracuse, New York

Kevin P. Lally, M.D.
Professor and Chief of Pediatric Surgery, Department of Surgery, University of Texas Medical School at Houston, Houston, Texas

Jeffrey E. Lee, M.D.
Assistant Professor, Department of Surgical Oncology, University of Texas M.D. Anderson Cancer Center, Houston, Texas

Barry A. Levine, M.D.
New York, New York

Benjamin C. Ling, M.D.
Neurosurgery Resident, Department of Neurosurgery, University of Cincinnati, Cincinnati, Ohio

Alan H. Lockwood, M.D.
Professor of Neurology and Nuclear Medicine, VA Western New York Healthcare System, State University of New York at Buffalo, Buffalo, New York

Walter E. Longo, M.D.
Associate Professor of Surgery and Anatomy, Department of Surgery, Saint Louis University School of Medicine, St. Louis, Missouri

Marc I. Lorber, M.D.
Professor of Surgery and Chief, Organ Transplantation and Immunology, Department of Surgery, Yale University School of Medicine, New Haven, Connecticut

Michael P. Macris, M.D.
Clinical Assistant Professor, Department of Surgery, University of Texas Medical School at Houston, Houston, Texas

Gunwant Mallik, M.D.
Clinical Assistant Professor of Neurosurgery, Neurological Associates, Inc., and Ohio State University Hospitals, Columbus, Ohio

Robert G. Marvin, M.D.
Assistant Professor of Surgery, Department of Surgery, University of Texas Medical School at Houston, Houston, Texas

Stephen J. Mathes, M.D.
Professor of Surgery and Head, Division of Plastic and Reconstructive Surgery, Department of Surgery, University of California–San Francisco, San Francisco, California

James T. Mayes, M.D.
Department of General Surgery, The Cleveland Clinic Foundation, Cleveland, Ohio

John E. Mazuski, M.D., Ph.D.
Associate Professor of Surgery, Department of Surgery, Saint Louis University School of Medicine, St. Louis, Missouri

Stacey L. Mazzacco, M.D.
Chief Surgical Resident, Department of Surgery, Temple University School of Medicine, Philadelphia, Pennsylvania

David W. McFadden, M.D.
Professor and Chief, Division of General Surgery, Department of Surgery, University of California–Los Angeles, Los Angeles, California

James F. McKinsey, M.D.
Assistant Professor of Surgery, Department of Surgery, University of Chicago, Chicago, Illinois

Irvine G. McQuarrie, M.D.
Associate Professor of Neurosurgery and Neurosciences, Department of Surgery, School of Medicine, Case Western Reserve University; Cleveland VA Medical Center, Cleveland, Ohio

David W. Mercer, M.D.
Associate Professor, Department of Surgery, University of Texas Medical School at Houston, Houston, Texas

Ronald C. Merrell, M.D.
Lampman Professor and Chairman, Department of Surgery, Yale University School of Medicine, New Haven, Connecticut

Joseph E. Miller, M.D.
Chief Resident, General Surgery, Department of Surgery, University of Texas Health Sciences Center, San Antonio, Texas

Thomas A. Miller, M.D.
C. Rollins Hanlon Professor and Chairman, Department of Surgery, Saint Louis University School of Medicine, St. Louis, Missouri

Michael E. Miner, M.D., Ph.D.
Professor and Chairman, Division of Neurosurgery, Department of Surgery, Ohio State University, Columbus, Ohio

Ralph S. Mosca, M.D.
Assistant Professor of Surgery, Department of Pediatric Cardiovascular Surgery, University of Michigan Medical Center, Ann Arbor, Michigan

Michael W. Mulholland, M.D., Ph.D.
Professor and Head, Section of General Surgery, Department of Surgery, University of Michigan, Ann Arbor, Michigan

Stuart I. Myers, M.D.
Professor and Chairman, Department of Surgery, Temple University School of Medicine, Philadelphia, Pennsylvania

Attila Nakeeb, M.D.
Chief Resident in General Surgery, Department of Surgery, The Johns Hopkins Medical Institutions, Baltimore, Maryland

John E. Niederhuber, M.D.
Professor, Department of Surgery and Department of Oncology; Assistant Dean for Oncology; Director of Comprehensive Cancer Center, University of Wisconsin–Madison, Madison, Wisconsin

D.C.N.K. Nyam, M.B.B.S., M. Med. (Surgery)
Department of Colorectal Surgery, Singapore General Hospital, Singapore

Philip R. Orlander, M.D.
Professor of Medicine and Director, Division of Endocrinology and Metabolism, Department of Internal Medicine, University of Texas Health Medical School at Houston, Houston, Texas

Donald H. Parks, M.D.
Professor and Chief, Division of Plastic and Reconstructive Surgery, Department of Surgery, University of Texas Medical School at Houston, Houston, Texas

Steven M. Parnis, M.D.
Coordinator, Laboratory Research, Department of Cardiovascular Surgery Research, Texas Heart Institute, Houston, Texas

John H. Pemberton, M.D.
Professor of Surgery, Department of Colon and Rectal Surgery, Mayo Graduate School of Medicine, Rochester, Minnesota

Henry A. Pitt, M.D.
Professor and Chairman, Department of Surgery, Medical College of Wisconsin, Milwaukee, Wisconsin

Howard A. Reber, M.D.
Professor and Chief, Gastrointestinal Surgery, Department of Surgery, University of California–Los Angeles, Los Angeles, California

J. David Richardson, M.D.
Professor and Vice Chairman, Department of Surgery, University of Louisville, Louisville, Kentucky

Gardiner Roddey, M.D.
Gastroenterologist, Mecklenburg Medical Group, Charlotte, North Carolina

Anthony J. Rongione, M.D.
Chief Resident, Department of Surgery (General Surgery), University of California–Los Angeles, Los Angeles, California

Ronnie Ann Rosenthal, M.D.
Associate Professor and Chief, General Surgery (VA Connecticut), Department of Surgery, Yale University School of Medicine, New Haven, Connecticut

John Sayles, M.D.
Surgical Resident, Department of Surgery, Walter Reed Army Medical Center, Washington, D.C.

Henry J. Schiller, M.D.
Assistant Professor of Surgery and Director, William R. Clark Burn Unit, State University of New York Health Science Center at Syracuse, Syracuse, New York

Joseph H. Sellin, M.D.
Professor of Medicine and Integrative Biology, and Director, Division of Gastroenterology, Department of Internal Medicine, University of Texas Medical School at Houston, Houston, Texas

Richard M. Sherry, M.D.
Senior Investigator, Surgery Branch, National Cancer Institute, Bethesda, Maryland

Lelan F. Sillin, M.D.
Professor of Surgery, State University of New York Health Science Center at Syracuse, Syracuse, New York

H. Hank Simms, M.D.
Associate Professor of Surgery, Department of Surgery, Brown University School of Medicine, Providence, Rhode Island

Kenneth R. Sirinek, M.D., Ph.D.
Professor, Department of Surgery, University of Texas Health Sciences Center, San Antonio, Texas

David I. Soybel, M.D.
Associate Professor of Surgery, Department of Surgery, Harvard Medical School, Boston, Massachusetts

James C. Stanley, M.D.
Professor of Surgery and Head, Section of Vascular Surgery, Department of Surgery, University of Michigan Medical Center, Ann Arbor, Michigan

Heinrich Taegtmeyer, M.D., D.Phil.
Professor of Medicine, Division of Cardiology, Department of Internal Medicine, University of Texas Medical School at Houston, Houston, Texas

Alan S. Tonnesen, M.D.
Professor of Anesthesiology, Department of Anesthesiology, University of Texas Medical School at Houston, Houston, Texas

Mark T. Toyama, M.D.
Resident, Department of Surgery (General Surgery), University of California–Los Angeles School of Medicine, Los Angeles, California

Gage Van Horn, M.D.
Professor and Vice-Chairman, Department of Neurology, University of Texas Medical School at Houston, Houston, Texas

Anthony M. Vernava III, M.D.
Associate Professor of Surgery and Chief, Section of Colon and Rectal Surgery, Department of Surgery, Saint Louis University School of Medicine, St. Louis, Missouri

Kathryn M. Verbanac, Ph.D.
Associate Professor of Surgery, Division of Transplantation, Department of Surgery, East Carolina University School of Medicine, Greenville, North Carolina

Michael P. Vezeridis, M.D.
Professor of Surgery, Department of Surgery, Brown University School of Medicine, Providence, Rhode Island

David J. Wainwright, M.D.
Associate Professor of Surgery, Division of Plastic Surgery, Department of Surgery, University of Texas Medical School at Houston, Houston, Texas

Thomas R. Weber, M.D.
Professor and Director of Pediatric Surgery, Department of Surgery, Saint Louis University School of Medicine, St. Louis, Missouri

Andrew S. Wechsler, M.D.
Stuart McGuire Professor and Chairman, Department of Surgery, and Professor of Physiology, Medical College of Virginia/Virginia Commonwealth University, Richmond, Virginia

Glenn J.R. Whitman, M.D.
Professor of Surgery and Section Chief, Department of Cardiothoracic Surgery, Allegheny Medical College of Pennsylvania, Allegheny University of the Health Sciences, Philadelphia, Pennsylvania

R. Patrick Wood, M.D.
Professor of Surgery, Department of Surgery, University of Texas Medical School at Houston, Houston, Texas

Kong-Woo Yoon, M.D.
Associate Professor, Division of Neurosurgery, Department of Surgery, Saint Louis University School of Medicine, St. Louis, Missouri

David M. Young, M.D.
Assistant Professor-in-Residence, Department of Surgery, University of California–San Francisco Medical Center, San Francisco, California

Christopher K. Zarins, M.D.
Chidester Professor of Surgery, Department of Surgery, Stanford University Medical Center, Stanford, California

Barbara Ann Zehnbauer, Ph.D.
Research Associate Professor, Department of Pediatrics and Department of Pathology, Washington University School of Medicine, St. Louis, Missouri

To

Janet

for her unwavering
love, support, and friendship

I love you.

Preface

This volume is the second edition of a book originally published under the title *Physiologic Basis of Modern Surgical Care.* When released in 1988, the original edition was widely received by the surgical community as a unique book focused on the physiologic underpinnings of surgical care. During the decade since the publication of that book, I have received numerous comments regarding its role in surgical education, particularly in the training of surgical residents. A number of program directors adopted the book as essential reading and used it to prepare residents for various examinations, such as the annual in-service training examination in surgery and the certification examination in surgery following completion of residency training. Because of the wide acceptance of this book as an important vehicle to train house officers in the physiologic principles underlying normal bodily functions and the derangements that occur in surgical disease states, a second edition was considered to be appropriate and warranted.

The purpose of this second edition is the same as that of the first edition: to bridge the gap that exists between the fund of information about physiology learned in medical school during the basic science courses and the commonly encountered inability to apply this information to clinical care. Thus this book approaches surgical disease as a derangement in normal physiology. Accordingly, in diagnosing surgical disorders, signs and symptoms of disease are explained in terms of physiologic dysfunction and are correlated with the appropriate use of laboratory and radiologic modalities to define disease processes better. As emphasized in the first edition, this book is not meant to replace standard textbooks of surgery; nor is it a comprehensive discussion of all types of surgical diseases. Rather, its purpose is to emphasize that surgical disease is basically a derangement in normal physiology and that the best way to diagnose and treat it is to understand thoroughly this deviation from normal.

This edition has been completely updated. Each chapter has been revised, and many chapters have been totally rewritten. Several chapters in the first edition were deleted because their relevance was thought to be in question. More than 80 new authors have been involved in the preparation of this second edition. As with the first edition, in selecting contributors to this book, I recruited individuals who have not only made substantial clinical contributions in their respective fields but also are fully current on the physiologic processes pertinent to the topics that they have been asked to address. In addition, each contributor is aware of the tremendous importance of critically assessing current knowledge and physiologic processes within his or her given discipline and of applying that which is important to the given clinical situation.

As was true in the first edition, the physiologic information is primarily focused on the needs of the general surgeon. The book has been divided into nine parts, with the first part devoted to general information pertinent to the human body as a whole and the eight remaining ones focused specifically on various organs systems. Since the current practice of general surgery only rarely involves diseases affecting the reproductive organs, disorders of the head and neck (other than thyroid and parathyroid glands), and disorders of the musculoskeletal system, specific chapters dealing with these entities have not been included.

A criticism of the first edition was the title of the book, which was thought to overemphasize physiology to the exclusion of clinical care. This misrepresentation was never intended, and I apologize for misleading potential readers. To reflect the emphasis of this book more adequately, it is hoped that the title of this second edition more appropriately defines the purpose of this book.

I am extremely pleased that Quality Medical Publishing (QMP) enthusiastically agreed to publish this second edition. I am especially grateful to Karen Berger, President of QMP, who immediately recognized the need for a second edition and understood the important role that such a book could play in educating future surgeons and updating practicing surgeons on the important physiologic underpinnings of surgical disease. I have truly enjoyed working with Karen Berger in this exciting venture. Other individuals from QMP whose friendship I have valued during the completion of this work include Esha Gupta and Beth Campbell.

Thomas A. Miller

Contents

PART SIX

THE PERIPHERAL VASCULAR SYSTEM

PART SEVEN

THE ENDOCRINE SYSTEM

PART EIGHT

THE INTEGUMENT AND BODY WALL

PART NINE

SPECIAL PHYSIOLOGIC CONSIDERATIONS

PART ONE

GENERAL CONSIDERATIONS IN THE MANAGEMENT OF SURGICAL PATIENTS

1

Metabolic Response to Starvation, Stress, and Sepsis

Joseph F. Amaral and Michael D. Caldwell

The metabolic response to stress, starvation, and sepsis should be viewed as a complex series of neuroendocrine reflexes resulting in an integrated attempt by the organism to mobilize energy substrates, to preserve oxygen and substrate delivery, and to maintain essential body functions.[1] These alterations involve changes in the distribution and use of water, proteins, fats, and carbohydrates. As such, an understanding of normal body composition is essential to make discussion of the metabolic response meaningful.

BODY COMPOSITION

Body composition has been defined by Moore[2] as "the study of the total mass and volume of body components in relation to body size, body configuration, age, sex, disease, and concentration changes." It can be considered from several aspects, including tissue anatomy, chemical composition, or metabolic structure (Fig. 1-1), with the latter two being the most important with regard to energy stores and intermediary metabolism.

Chemical Composition

All living organisms may be considered as complex and organized arrangements of fats, proteins, carbohydrates, minerals, and electrolytes in an aqueous environment. Although the percentage of each of these chemical groups varies among and within species, by far the largest component of all living organisms is water.

Water

Water is an important substance involved in virtually all physiologic processes. Its physiochemical properties result largely from its electron structure. The hydrogen ions have a slightly positive charge, whereas the oxygen molecule, with its lone pair of electrons, has a negative charge. This difference allows extensive hydrogen bonding and a relatively high dipole moment[3] that causes the water molecules to orient themselves in an external electric field in such a way that they act as an electric buffer. When ionic substances are placed in water, a hydrational shell forms around the individual ions, reducing their electrochemical attraction and thus forming a solution.[3] Water thus keeps electrolytes and other polar molecules in solution and allows them independent motion, which is critical to nutrient transport.

The extensive hydrogen-bonding capacity of water molecules causes them to orient themselves in a highly organized structure similar to ice. This structure accounts for the relatively high boiling point of water, its relatively high freezing point, and its high specific heat (the energy required to raise the temperature of 1 g of a substance 1° C). This latter property allows water to exert a major role in temperature regulation, since a large amount of heat is lost as water evaporates (perspiration) and a large amount of heat is required to raise the temperature of water. The extensive hydrogen bonding of water also makes it important in establishing the tertiary structure of proteins and other molecules.

Total body water (TBW) is divisible into two components: intracellular water (ICW) and extracellular water (ECW). These two components are separated by cell membranes. Measurement of body fluid compartments uses dilution techniques based on the concept that a substance that distributes itself equally and exclusively throughout a given compartment (e.g., TBW) can be used to determine the volume of that compartment. This procedure is done by injecting a known amount of the substance and measuring its concentration at steady state, as well as measuring the amount excreted during the period of time required to reach steady state. Thus:

$$\text{Volume} = \frac{\text{Amount injected} - \text{Amount excreted}}{\text{Steady state concentration}}$$

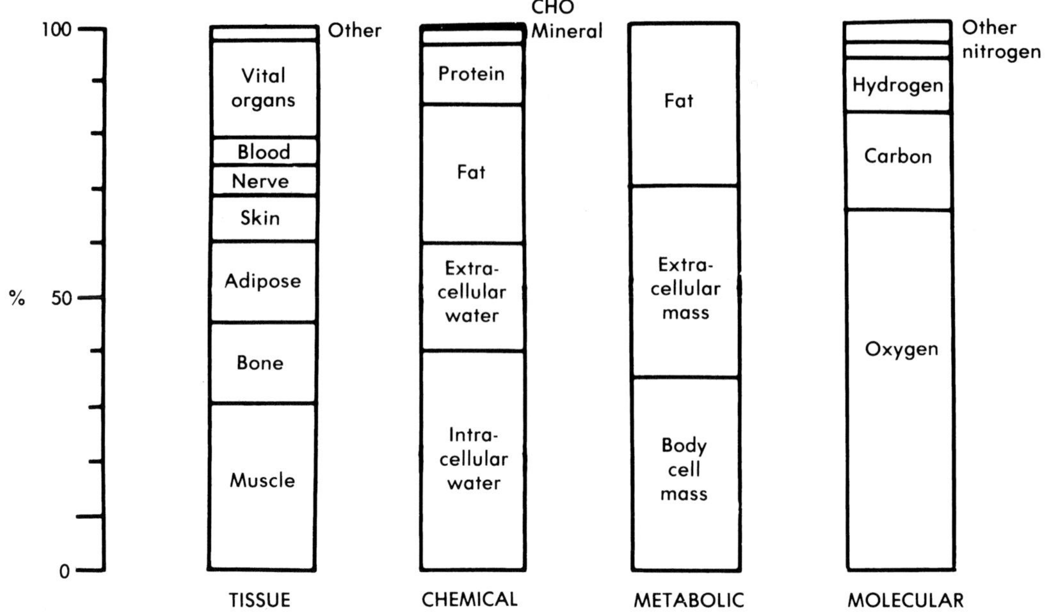

Fig. 1-1. Body composition in adult man. (From Shizgal HM. Body composition. In Fischer JE, ed. Surgical Nutrition. Boston: Little, Brown, 1983; Bell GH, Davidson JN, Emslie-Smith D. Textbook of Physiology and Biochemistry. London: Churchill Livingstone, 1972.)

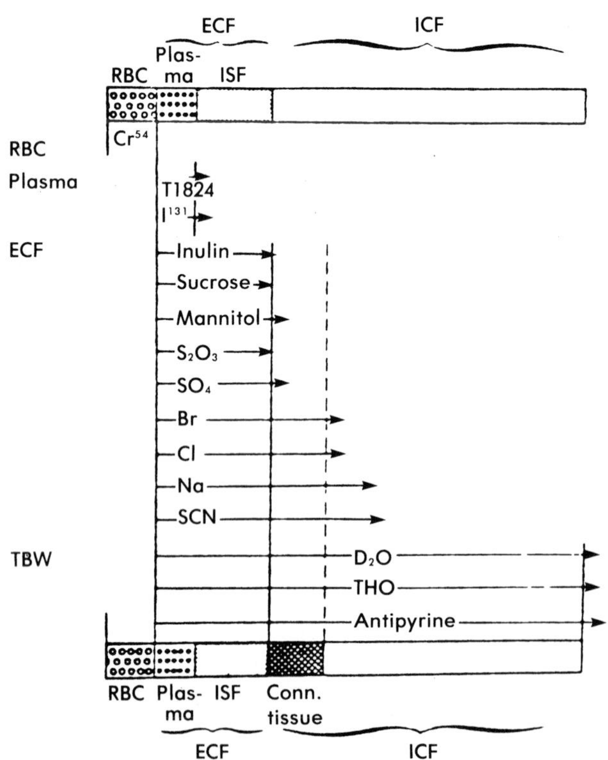

Fig. 1-2. Substances used to measure the body fluid compartments. *ECF,* Extracellular fluid; *ICF,* intracellular fluid; *ISF,* interstitial fluid; *RBC,* red blood cell; *TBW,* total body water; *THO,* titrated water. (From Winters RW. The Body Fluids in Pediatrics. Boston: Little, Brown, 1973.)

Since the amount lost is usually negligible, the convention is to use:

$$\text{Volume} = \frac{\text{Amount injected}}{\text{Steady state concentration}}$$

Numerous substances are available that allow measurement of various fluid compartments (Fig. 1-2). Generally, the TBW is the most accurately measured compartment. The TBW varies with age, sex, body build, physical activity, disease, and state of hydration. The TBW can be measured accurately using deuterium oxide or tritiated water. For a healthy man, TBW constitutes approximately 60% of total body weight, and for a healthy woman, it constitutes approximately 50% (Table 1-1). The differences in the proportion of TBW reflect the quantity of skeletal muscle and adipose tissue present in the two sexes. Adipose tissue contains little ICW, whereas skeletal muscle has one of the largest water contents of all tissues (Table 1-2). Women, with their larger adipose tissue stores and smaller skeletal muscle mass, have less TBW than men. Similarly, the TBW of young, lean athletes is greater than that of elderly, obese nonathletes.

The TBW as a percentage of body weight decreases steadily with age (see Table 1-1). Newborns have the highest percentage, with 75% to 80% of body weight representing water. This percentage decreases during the first few months after birth to approximately 65% of the body weight, where it remains for the remainder of infancy and childhood. This reduction in TBW is primarily the result of reduction in ECW (Fig. 1-3). Until the age of 12, no difference in TBW is noted between boys and girls. With

Table 1-1. Distribution of Total Body Water in Infants, Children, and Adults

Age	Total Body Water (%)	
	Men	Women
0-1 day	79	79
1-10 days	74	74
1-3 mo	72.3	72.3
3-6 mo	70.1	70.1
6-12 mo	60.4	60.4
1-2 yr	58.7	58.7
2-3 yr	63.5	63.5
3-5 yr	62.2	62.2
5-10 yr	61.5	61.5
10-16 yr	58.9	57.3
17-39 yr	60.6	50.2
40-59 yr	54.7	46.7
60 + yr	51.5	45.5

Modified from Maxwell MH, Kleeman CR. Clinical Disorders of Fluid and Electrolyte Metabolism, 3rd ed. New York: McGraw-Hill, 1979.

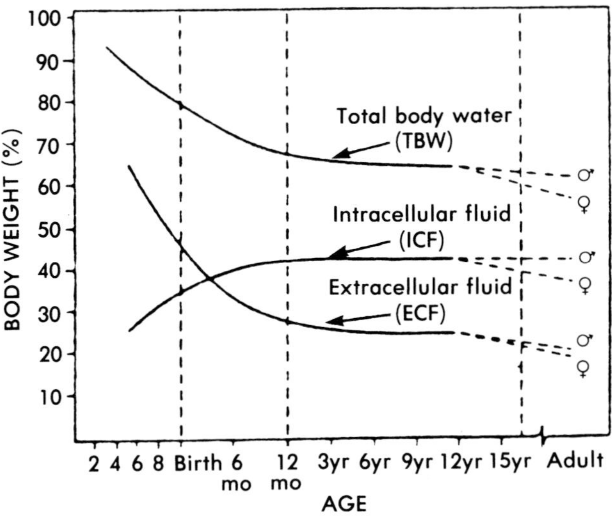

Fig. 1-3. Distribution of body fluids in children as a function of age and sex. (From Winters RW. The Body Fluids in Pediatrics. Boston: Little, Brown, 1973. Reproduced by permission of Pediatrics 28: 169, 1961.)

Table 1-2. Distribution of Water in the Various Tissues of a 70 kg Man

Tissue	Water (%)	Body Weight (%)	Liters of Water per 70 kg
Skin	72	18	9.07
Muscle	75.6	41.7	22.1
Skeleton	22	15.9	2.45
Brain	74.8	2	1.05
Liver	68.3	2.3	1.03
Heart	79.2	0.5	0.28
Lungs	79	0.7	0.39
Kidneys	82.7	0.4	0.25
Spleen	75.8	0.2	0.1
Blood	83	8	4.65
Intestine	74.5	1.8	0.94
Adipose tissue	10	± 10	0.7

From Skeleton H. Arch Int Med 40:140, 1927. Copyright © 1927, American Medical Association.

advancing age, TBW as a percentage of body weight decreases to a low of 52% and 47% in males and females, respectively.[2] This results primarily from a decrease in ICW, since ECW remains unchanged.[3] The size of the ECW space depends on the method used for determining it. Large molecules such as insulin, mannitol, or sucrose appear to underestimate the ECW compartment because of the slower diffusion of these larger molecules into noncellular spaces.[3] An ECW space of 15% to 16% of body weight is usually reported with these methods.[3] Assessment of the ECW with small molecules such as $^{35}SO_4$, ^{82}Br, and ^{24}Na appears to overestimate the ECW space because of the ability of these small ions to diffuse into cells. An ECW space of 21% to 27% of body weight is usually reported when these methods are used.[3]

In general, it is estimated that the ECW occupies 20% of the body weight (and therefore 30% to 40% of TBW). It is divided into plasma (5% of body weight) and interstitial fluid (15% of body weight). The interstitial fluid occupies a rapidly equilibrating functional space between cells and a slowly equilibrating (or nonequilibrating) space composed of epithelial cell secretions, connective tissue, joint space, and cerebrospinal fluids, the so-called transcellular space.[4] The functional interstitial fluid accounts for 90%, and the transcellular space accounts for 10% of the total interstitial fluid.

The transcellular space should not be equated with the "third space." The transcellular fluids are a normal component of the ECW and do not affect the functional volume of the extracellular space. The third space results from abnormalities in the permeability of cells such as those abnormalities seen after ischemia and those seen with inflammation that increases the size of the extracellular space but not, *a priori,* the volume of the ECW. Third space size is proportional to the severity of the injury. Since fluid and electrolytes in the third space are derived from functional extracellular fluid, the increase in size of the space reduces the functional extracellular volume.

Direct measurement of the ICW compartment is extremely difficult, since substances that equilibrate only in the intracellular space have not been defined. Consequently, the ICW space is estimated as the difference between TBW and ECW. The ICW space varies from individual to individual. In healthy normal adults it constitutes approximately 30% to 40% of body weight (55% of TBW). Since fat has little ICW and skeletal muscle has the

Table 1-3. Electrolyte Composition of the Body Fluid Compartments

Electrolytes	Serum (mEq/L)	Serum Water (mEq/L)	Interstitial Fluid (mEq/L)	Intracellular Fluid (Muscle) (mEq/kg of H_2O)
Cations				
Sodium (Na^+)	142	152.7	145	±10
Potassium (K^+)	4	4.3	4	156
Calcium (Ca^{++})	5	5.4		3.3
Magnesium (Mg^{++})	2	2.2		26
Total cations	153	165	149	195
Anions				
Chloride (Cl^-)	102	109.7	114	±2
Bicarbonate (HCO_3^{2-})	26	28	31	±8
Phosphate (HPO_4^{2-})	2	2.2		95
Sulfate (SO_4^{2-})	1	1.1		20
Organic acids	6	6.5		
Protein	16	17.2		55
Total anions	153	165	145	180+

From Maxwell MH, Kleeman CR. Clinical Disorders of Fluid and Electrolyte Metabolism, 3rd ed. New York: McGraw-Hill, 1979.

Table 1-4. Total and Exchangeable Amounts of Electrolytes in Fluid Compartments of Adult Man

Compartment	Sodium	Potassium	Magnesium	Chloride	Bicarbonate
	(mEq/kg of Body Weight)				
Total extracellular	52.8	2.5	21.8	27.8	6.8
Total intracellular	5.2	51.3	8.2	5.2	5.9
Total body	58	53.8	30	33	12.7
Total exchangeable	41	52.8	3.4, 4.9, 10*	33	12.7
Total body intracellular concentration (milliequivalent per liter intracellular water)	14.4	14.3	22.8	14.4	16.4

From Ruch TC, Patton HD. Physiology and Biophysics, vol 2. Philadelphia: WB Saunders, 1974.
*Equilibrated for 24, 48, and 89 hours, respectively. Total exchangeable magnesium is a function of time of equilibration.

Table 1-5. Mean Electrolyte Composition of Transcellular Fluids

Fluid	Na^- mEq/L	K^- mEq/L	Cl^- mEq/L	HCO_3^- mEq/L	H^+ mEq/L
Saliva	33	20	34	0	—
Gastric juice	60	10	130	0	90
Bile	149	5	101	45	—
Pancreatic juice	141	5	77	92	—
Ileal fluid	129	11	116	29	—
Cecal fluid	80	21	48	22	—
Cerebrospinal fluid	141	3	127	23	—
Sweat	45	5	58	0	—

Modified from Rose BD. Clinical Physiology of Acid-Base and Electrolyte Disorders. New York: McGraw-Hill, 1977.

Table 1-6. Body Composition of Infants and Children as Function of Age

Age (Months)	Body Weight (kg)	Whole Body (g/100 g) Water	Protein	Lipid	Other
Birth	3.5	75.1	11.4	11	2.5
4	7	60.2	11.4	26.3	2.1
12	10.5	59	14.6	23.9	2.5
24	13	61	15.7	20.6	2.7
36	15	62	16.4	18.3	3.3

From Fomon SJ. Infant Nutrition, 2nd ed. Philadelphia: WB Saunders, 1974.

highest percentage of ICW, athletic muscular individuals have a higher proportion of ICW; but women, the obese, and the elderly have a smaller muscle mass and therefore have a smaller percentage of their body weight as ICW.

The electrolyte composition of the various fluid compartments is noted in Table 1-3. The major cations are sodium and potassium, and the major anions are chloride and bicarbonate. The absolute amount of a particular ion can only be measured by cadaveric analyses, but the total exchangeable amount of an ion can be estimated by dilution with a labeled form of the compound. Total exchangeable sodium is not equivalent to total body sodium. A large amount, approximately 1000 mEq, is present in a nonexchangeable form in bone.[5] The total exchangeable potassium is more closely equivalent to the total body potassium (less than 0.5% is nonexchangeable).[5]

Sodium is the major extracellular cation, and potassium is the major intracellular cation (Table 1-4). The ECW space is approximated by the total body sodium, the ICW space by the total body potassium, and the TBW by the sum of total body sodium and total body potassium. Moore[5] has used this relationship to estimate TBW from total exchangeable sodium (Na_e) and potassium (K_e) using the formula below:

$$\text{TBW} = \frac{(Na_e + K_e) + 70}{163} \pm (2\text{ L})$$

The differing ionic compositions of the various fluid compartments are the result of variations in the permeabilities and active transport mechanisms present in the cell membranes separating these spaces. There is a great diversity among the transcellular fluids in this regard (Table 1-5).

Fat (Lipids)

Until the 1950s, lipids, the second largest chemical constituent of the body, were considered relatively inert substances that served as a source of protection and insulation. They now are recognized as essential components of energy metabolism (providing 9.3 kcal/g), hormonal synthesis (steroids), hormonal regulation and action (prostaglandins), and neural transmission (sphingomyelins). In addition, they are required for general cellular integrity and stability (cell membrane phospholipids and cholesterol). Many of the functions of lipids require fatty acids that cannot be synthesized by human beings. The three major essential fatty acids are arachidonic acid, linoleic acid, and linolenic acid. Total body fat (TBF) varies inversely with TBW in normal individuals. During the first 4 months of life, there is a decrease in the percentage of TBF, expressed as percent of total body weight (Table 1-6). After puberty the TBF content increases, with increase greater in girls than in boys. In healthy men TBF accounts for approximately 25% of body weight, and in healthy women fat accounts of approximately 35% of body weight. With age there is an increase in the percentage of body weight occupied by fat. However, it is of note that body weight often remains unchanged with age. Since total body weight equals body fat plus fat-free tissues, a decrease in fat-free tissue is thought to occur with aging.[6] The percentage of body weight occupied by fat is also inversely related to the level of physical activity. Muscular athletic individuals have a greater muscle mass and smaller percentage of body fat than sedentary individuals of similar body weight.[7] These changes are somewhat adaptive, however. For example, a long-distance swimmer benefits from the buoyancy and insulation provided by fat and often has a greater amount of fat than a long-distance runner of equivalent body build.[7] This presumably results from a difference in caloric intake between these two groups. Approximately 50% of the fat in human beings is located in the subcutaneous tissue, but the distribution of the subcutaneous tissue varies with age, sex, and physical activity.[6] Children have a large amount of subcutaneous tissue over their triceps but only a small amount of subcutaneous tissue in their abdominal walls. The distribution is reversed in adults. Changes in the body fat distribution occurring as a result of weight gain are not equally distributed.[6] For this reason, serial measurement of an isolated anthropometric index may not adequately reflect body composition changes in malnourished individuals who are being repleted. However, changes in the body fat distribution occurring as a result of weight loss are equally distributed. A 10% loss in triceps skinfold is accompanied by a concomitant 10% loss in the size of the subcutaneous tissues of other areas such as the hips, abdomen, thighs, and breasts.[6]

TBF is defined as the difference between total body weight and fat-free mass (see the following equation). Fat contains very little water and virtually no potassium. On the other hand, the total water content of fat-free tissue averages 73.2% of TBW,[8] and the potassium content of fat-free tissues averages 68.1 mEq/kg.[6] Consequently, fat-free tissue may be approximated from either TBW or total exchangeable potassium (K_e) and the TBF estimated by inference. Equations for these calculations are:

For TBW: $\text{TBF} = \text{BWt} - (\text{TBW}/0.732)$

and

$\%\text{TBF} = 1 - (\%\text{TBW}/0.732)$

For K_e: $\text{TBF} = \text{BWt} - (K_e)/68.1$

and

$\%\text{TBF} = [\text{BWt} - (K_e/68.1)]/\text{BWt}$

where BWt is body weight. It should be noted that these methods assume that the hydration and potassium content of that portion of the body that is fat free is constant. However, these assumptions are not always valid because the hydration of the fat-free tissue can vary considerably (e.g., greatest in edematous states and least in dehydrated states).

A third method used in calculating TBF involves the measurement of the specific gravity of the individual by underwater weighing procedure.[6,7,9,10] This method is based on the findings that normal human fat has a density of 0.9 g/ml and nonfat tissue has an average density of 1.1 g/ml at 37° C. At 37° C, the density of an average reference male containing 15.3% body fat is 1.064 g/ml.[11] With the use of these values the percentage fat in an individual can be determined by measuring the density (D) in water as indicated by the equation:

$$\%Fat = [(4.570/D) - 4.142] \times 100^{20}$$

Although the density of human fat changes only with temperature, the density of fat-free tissue changes with age, degree of obesity, and degree of hydration.[6] When estimates of TBF made by densitometric methods are compared to calculations of TBF made from TBW, the densitometric methods give a higher estimate of TBF.[7,9] Densitometric methods give a lower estimate of TBF when compared to calculations of TBF made from total exchangeable potassium.[9,12]

A fourth method used to calculate TBF involves the measurement of the uptake of an inert, highly fat-soluble gas such as cyclopropane or krypton.[13] The assumption made in this technique is that the gas will only go into fat cells. Thus it should yield a more accurate measurement of TBF than the other methods noted. When compared to measurements made by TBW determination, similar results are obtained.[14] When compared to total exchangeable potassium measurements or densitometric measurements, lower values are obtained.[15] However, no data are available comparing the inert gas method with cadaver analyses.

Proteins

Proteins are chains of amino acids. Proteins and amino acids form essential components of all living cells and are involved in virtually all body functions. These molecules serve as enzymes, hormones, neurotransmitters, immunoglobulins, and transport molecules. They are also essential components of all cell membranes and various cellular components, including receptors, transport systems, and contractile elements. As such, they are necessary for the metabolism, growth, regulation, replication, protection, repair, communication, and motion of individual cells and the coordinated function of the entire organism. Consequently, it is somewhat remarkable that total body proteins (TBPs) account for only 15% of the body weight in a healthy man and that over 80% of the TBP is present in skeletal muscle and connective tissue. Unlike fat, there are no storage depots for protein. All the body's protein is functional.

As a result of its numerous and varied functions, protein, unlike fat, undergoes considerable daily turnover. Approximately 2.5% of the TBP (250 g in a 70 kg man) is broken down and resynthesized each day.[15] More than half this turnover is accounted for by daily secretory processes, white cell turnover, hemoglobin turnover, muscle protein turnover, and plasma protein turnover. The total turnover rate of body protein diminishes progressively with age.[16] The protein synthesis rate per kilogram of body weight decreases from 25 g/kg/d in the neonate to 7 g in a 1-year-old infant. In the average man and woman, protein synthesis is 3.2 and 2.6 g/kg of body weight per day, respectively; in an elderly man and woman, it is 2.6 and 1.9 g, respectively.

The synthesis rate of transport protein, such as albumin, remains unchanged with increasing age, but the breakdown rate (and presumably synthesis rate) of skeletal muscle decreases (Table 1-7). If the total turnover rate of protein is expressed per lean body mass rather than body weight, an increase in turnover is noted with aging. Since the lean body mass decreases with aging as a result of a reduction in skeletal muscle mass and the synthesis rate of albumin is unchanged, it is apparent that the changes in protein turnover per kilogram of body weight are the result of a decrease in skeletal muscle mass.

TBP may be estimated by one of two methods: (1) measurement of total exchangeable potassium or (2) mea-

Table 1-7. Comparison of Whole Body Protein Breakdown With Estimates of Muscle Protein Breakdown and Albumin Synthesis in Young and Old Adult Human Beings

		Whole Body Protein Breakdown* (g/day)			Muscle Protein Breakdown† (g/day)			Albumin Synthesis‡ (g/day)		
Group	Mean Age (yr)	Per kg Body Weight	Per kg Body Cell Mass	Per g Creatinine	Per kg Body Weight	Per kg Body Cell Mass	Per g Creatinine	Per kg Body Weight	Per kg Body Cell Mass	Per g Creatinine
Males										
Young	22	2.94	6.7	115	0.76	1.74	30	0.19	0.39	7
Old	70	2.64	7.5	163	0.53	1.50	32	0.15	0.40	8.4
Females										
Young	20	2.35	6.1	103	0.64	1.69	28	—	—	—
Old	76	1.94	6.6	166	0.31	1.05	26	—	—	—

From Valgeirsdöttir K, Munro HN. Protein and amino acid metabolism. In Fischer JE, ed. Surgical Nutrition. Boston: Little, Brown, 1983, p 129.
*Measured by administration of ^{15}N-glycine.
†Measured as 3-methylhistidine output in urine and computed as muscle protein.
‡Measured by administration of ^{15}N-glycine.

surement of total body nitrogen (TBN) by neutron activation. TBN is linearly related to total exchangeable potassium in both normal and decreased conditions.[17,18] The average exchangeable potassium to nitrogen ratio in tissue is 3 mEq/g nitrogen.[5] Thus:

$$TBN = K_e/3$$

where K_e equals exchangeable potassium. TBP is directly proportional to TBN by a factor of approximately 6.25. Thus:

$$TBP = (6.25)\,(TBN) = (6.25)\,(K_e/3) = 2.08\ K_e$$

TBN can also be measured using neutron activation analysis.[17,19] When tissues are irradiated with neutrons from either a cyclotron or a plutonium source, gamma rays specific for a substance capturing the neutron are emitted. For nitrogen, gamma rays of 10.83 meV are emitted. Consequently, measurement of the gamma rays produced after neutron activation allows determination of TBN. In general, the results obtained with either method correlate well with each other.

Carbohydrates

Carbohydrates serve as the energy source of the body when energy is rapidly required, providing approximately 4 kcal/g. They also serve important roles in cell membrane function and stability (glycoproteins and glycolipids), in hormone function (glycoproteins), and as precursors of lipid and nonessential amino acid synthesis. In addition, the brain, RBCs, WBCs, and wounds are to a large extent glucose-dependent tissues. Of the three major sugars found in the human body (glucose, fructose, and galactose), glucose is the primary carbohydrate. In addition to ingested carbohydrates, glucose is readily available from pyruvate and lactate, gluconeogenic amino acids (alanine and glutamine), the glycerol moiety of lipids, and its storage form, glycogen.

Most of the body's glycogen is stored in the liver, skeletal muscle, and cardiac muscle. Muscle glycogen is used primarily by the muscle itself because muscle lacks glucose-6-phosphatase. In contrast, hepatic glycogen is primarily used in providing glucose to glucose-dependent tissues. Since little glycogen is stored in the liver, the hepatic stores of glycogen are rapidly depleted by an overnight fast. Cahill[20] has estimated the total hepatic glycogen content of a 70 kg man to be 75 g and the total muscle glycogen content to be 105 g.

The total carbohydrate content of the body is approximately 300 g.[21] Except by cadaver analysis, no method is available to measure total body carbohydrate. However, it is of note that the daily intake of carbohydrate approximates the total body stores.

Lean Body Mass and Body Cell Mass

Based on densitometric measurements, Behnke[9] and Behnke and Wilmore[7] proposed the division of total body weight into fat and lean body mass. The lean body mass was defined as that portion of the body mass with the least amount of essential body fat compatible with health. The essential body fat was thought to represent 2% to 10% of the total body weight. However, because the essential body fat cannot be differentiated from the nonessential body fat, most investigators have redefined lean body mass as the portion of body mass devoid of all fat, the so-called fat-free body.[6] Although "fat-free body" and "lean body mass" are often used interchangeably, there is a small (2% to 10%) difference between them (Table 1-8). This chapter subsequently refers only to the fat-free body, but it should be kept in mind that the same statements are generally true for lean body mass. Since the total body weight is equal to TBF plus the fat-free body, the size of the fat-free body can be determined by the same methods used to determine the size of the TBF.

The fat-free body is divisible into the extracellular mass, composed primarily of water, and the body cell mass (BCM), composed of all the metabolically active cells in the body.[2,5] The cells in the BCM are actively involved in energy exchange, protein synthesis, enzyme replication, and morphogenesis.[2] Therefore the BCM is composed of the skeletal muscle mass (60%), visceral cell mass (20%), and the peripheral cell mass (20%)[5] (see Table 1-8). The peripheral cell mass includes blood cells and connective tissue cells.

Although the BCM cannot be measured directly, it can be calculated from the exchangeable potassium, the exchangeable sodium, the TBN or the ICW. Since more than 98% of the total body potassium (TBK) is intracellular, a linear relationship exists between BCM, TBK, total exchangeable potassium, and ICW. Histochemical analysis has demonstrated that approximately one fourth of the wet weight of cells is protein.[22] Consequently:

$$BCM = (TBK)\,(4) = (2.08\ K_e)\,(4) = 8.33\ K_e$$
$$BCM = (TBN)\,(6.25)\,(4) = 25\,(TBN)$$

Since the average cell has 150 mEq of intracellular potassium per liter[5] and since each cell is composed of 25.8% solids (74.2% water),[22] BCM is also equivalent to:

$$K_e\,(1000/0.732)/150 = (K_e)\,(9.10)$$

or

$$ICW/0.742$$

Each of these methods yields a different value for the BCM of a given individual. This is most obvious when the two methods presented for total exchangeable potassium are used. However, any of these methods provide accurate estimates of sequential changes in an individual or differences among populations if the same method is used throughout the study.

Measurements of total exchangeable potassium by whole body ^{40}K counting or of TBN by neutron activation are difficult to perform and require equipment that is expensive and not readily available. To avoid these practical problems, Shizgal et al.[23] developed a method to estimate

Table 1-8. Comparison of Body Cell Mass, Lean Body Mass, and Fat-Free Body

	Body Cell Mass (BCM)	Lean Body Mass (LBM)	Fat-Free Body (FFB)
Anatomy	**All body cells** Protoplasm Nucleus Membrane $[ICK]_{AV} = 150\ mE/L_{ICW}$	**All body cells} BCM** Plus: Plasma, ECF, TCF } ECF Tendon, Fascia, Collagen, Elastin, Dermis, Skeleton } ECS ECF + ECS } ECT "2% = 10% essential lipid"} Fat	Same as LBM but no lipid at all
Function	**Cellular metabolism** Respiration Oxidation Synthesis Cretion Mitosis	**Cellular metabolism** Support Transport Circulation Protection Integument	Same as LBM
Composition	$[K_e - ECK] \times f = BCM$ f = 7.5 to 10 *or* $K_e \times 8.33 = BCM$ 70 kg man 3200 × 8.33 = 26.6 kg Calories 2.7 to 3.6 $kcal/hr/kg_{BCM}$	**Density = 1100** $\%\ LBM = 100 - \frac{495}{d} - 450$ 70 kg man Approx 50 kg Calories 110 $kcal/hr/kg_{LBM}$	$FFB = \frac{TBW}{f}$ f = 0.695 − 0.735 70 kg man $\frac{36.4}{0.732} = 49.7$ Calories (same as LBM)

From Moore FD. Energy and the maintenance of the body cell mass. JPEN 4: 227, 1980.
ECF, Extracellular fluid; *ECK,* extracellular potassium; *ECS,* extracellular supporting structure; *ECT,* total extracellular space; *f,* coefficient; *ICK,* intracellular potassium; *ICW,* intracellular water; K_e, exchangeable potassium; *TBW,* total body water; *TCF,* total cellular fluid.

total exchangeable potassium from isotope dilution measurements of TBW and total exchangeable sodium. As noted previously, TBW is approximately equal to the sum of the total exchangeable sodium and potassium. Thus:

$$Na_e + K_e/TBW = R$$

where R is constant. Total exchangeable sodium and TBW can be easily measured by isotope dilution with deuterium oxide or tritiated water and ^{22}Na. The constant, R, can be approximated by measurement of the sodium, potassium, and water of whole blood. Thus:

$$K_e = [(R)\ (TBW)] - Na_e$$

and

$$BCM = 8.33\ K_e \text{ or } 9.10\ K_e$$

As might be expected, BCM increases with age until the middle years of life. With advancing age, the percentage of body weight composed of the BCM decreases as a result of a decrease in skeletal muscle mass. In addition, men generally have a greater percentage of body weight composed of BCM than women, athletic individuals greater than sedentary individuals, and lean individuals greater than obese individuals. Thus the BCM varies from 20% of body weight in morbidly obese individuals to 54% in lean athletic men.[24]

A direct correlation exist between total energy expenditure and BCM, whereas other measurements of body composition such as total body mass and fat-free body demonstrate a variable or poor correlation.[25] Kinney et al.[25] have demonstrated an oxygen consumption of 8 to 10 ml oxygen per kilogram BCM and an energy expenditure of 2.7 to 3.6 kcal/kg/hr $_{BCM}$. As noted in Fig. 1-4, total exchangeable potassium (and therefore BCM) is linearly related to the total metabolic energy expenditure in healthy adults and surgical patients until 1800 cal/day are expended. However, when measurements of total metabolic energy expenditure greater than this are included, the relationship is parabolic. This relationship is believed to reflect the lower resting metabolic rate of skeletal muscles per milliequivalent intracellular potassium when compared to visceral tissues. Skeletal muscle, which provides approximately 50% of the TBK, accounts for only 15% of the body's resting energy expenditure. On the other hand, visceral tissues, such as brain, heart, and kidneys, which provide only 10% of the TBK, account for 70% of the body's resting energy expenditure.[26] Consequently, individuals with a small BCM have less skeletal muscle mass and a good correlation of total exchangeable potassium with total metabolic energy expenditure. In contrast, individuals with a large BCM have a smaller increase in total

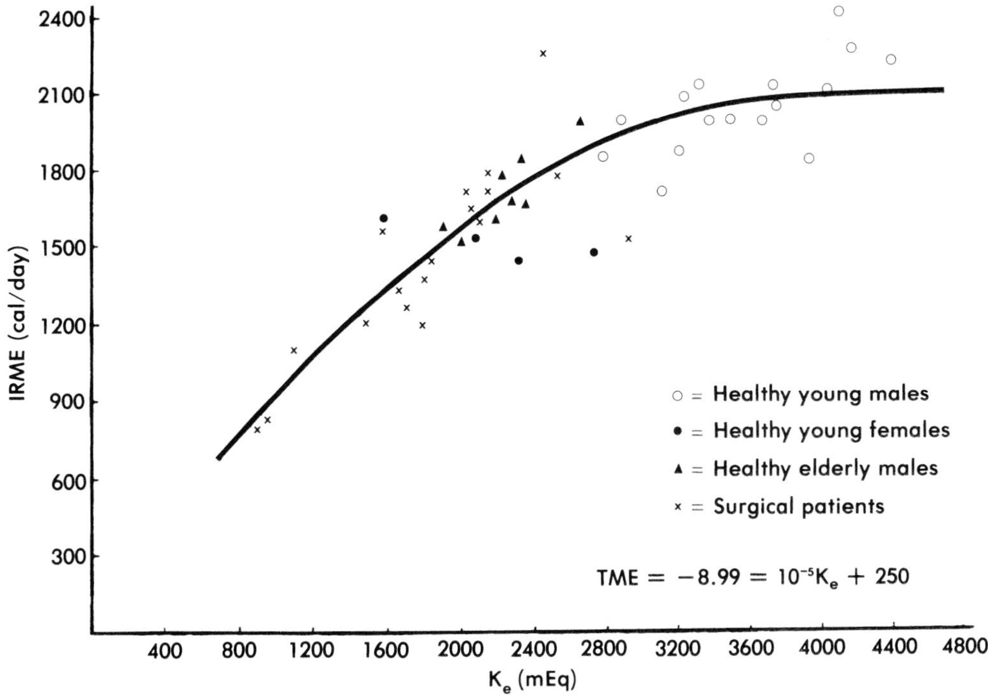

Fig. 1-4. Relationship of total body energy expenditure to the total exchangeable potassium (K_e). K_e, Exchangeable potassium; *IRME/TME,* total metabolized energy. (From Kinney JM, Lister J, Moore FD. Relationship of energy expenditure to total exchangeable potassium. Ann NY Acad Sci 110: 711, 1963.)

Table 1-9. Estimation of Total Body Water by Age, Sex, and Body Weight

Sex	Age (yr)	Total Body Water (Liters)	95% Conf. Limits (%)
Males	16-30	0.4 (BWt) + 13	±16
	31-60	0.4 (BWt) + 11	±17
	61-90	0.34 (BWt) + 12	±16
Females	16-30	0.31 (BWt) + 11.6	±13
	31-90	0.33 (BWt) + 8.84	±21

From Moore FD. Energy and the maintenance of the body cell mass. JPEN 4: 227, 1980.
BWt, Body weight.

Table 1-10. Estimation of Total Exchangeable Potassium by Age, Sex, and Body Weight

Sex	Age (yr)	Exchangeable Potassium (mEq)	95% Conf. Limits (%)
Males	16-30	38 (BWt) + 735	±23
	31-60	26 (BWt) + 1383	±20
	61-90	27 (BWt) + 723	±16
Females	16-30	18 (BWt) + 1250	±20
	31-90	17 (BWt) + 1176	±23
	61-90	18 (BWt) + 757	±29
By Total Body Water (TBW)			
Males and females	20-60	97.4 (TBW) − 409	±10
	61-84	2 + 77 (TBW)	±17

From Moore FD. Energy and the maintenance of the body cell mass. JPEN 4: 227, 1980.
BWt, Body weight.

metabolic energy expenditure when compared to total exchangeable potassium because skeletal muscle at rest contributes significantly to total exchangeable potassium but not to total metabolic energy expenditure.

Changes in Body Composition With Stress, Sepsis, and Starvation

The body composition of a human being at any given moment is influenced significantly by the individual's age, sex, physical activity, and previous nutritional status, as well as by concurrent infections, injuries, and disease processes. Changes produced by age, sex, and physical activity have been discussed at length. Tables 1-9 and 1-10 and the box on p. 10 provide a summary of the formulas derived from multiple body composition studies of normal individuals.[2,5] These formulas can be applied to any healthy adult under normal circumstances to estimate the components of body composition.

Ultimately, body composition is the net result of the total chemical constituents taken in minus the total chemical constituents used and excreted. Since carbohydrates

ESTIMATION OF BODY COMPOSITION BY SEX AND BODY WEIGHT

TBW = 0.7945 (BWt) − 0.0024 $(BWt)^2$ − 0.0015 (age) (BWt) (males)
TBW = 0.6981 (BWt) − 0.0026 $(BWt)^2$ − 0.0012 (age) (BWt) (females)
ICW = 0.623 (TBW) − 0.0016 (age) (TBW) (males)
ICW = 0.553 (TBW) − 0.0007 (age) (TBW) (females)
Fat = BWt − TBW/0.732
ECW = TBW − ICW
K_e = 150 (ICW) + 4 (ECW)
Na_e = 163.2 (TBW) − K_e − 69

From Moore FD. The Body Cell Mass and Its Supporting Environment. Philadelphia: WB Saunders, 1963.
BWt, Body weight; *ECW,* extracellular water; *ICW,* intracellular water; *K_e,* exchangeable potassium; *Na_e,* exchangeable sodium; *TBW,* total body water.

and lipids primarily serve as a source of calories, this relationship can be estimated by:

$$\Delta BC = [(C_{in} + N_{in} + WS_{in}) - (C_{out} + N_{out} + WS_{out})]$$

where Δ is change; BC is body composition; C is calories; N is nitrogen; W is water; and S is solutes (electrolytes and minerals). Under normal steady-state conditions, the quantities of these components taken in equal the quantities used or lost, and there is no net change in body composition (BC = 0). If the quantity of a component taken in is greater than the quantity used, this component either is stored (BC >0), thus changing body composition, or is lost (BC <0). For example, if caloric intake is greater than caloric loss or expenditure, energy is stored in the body in the form of lipids and carbohydrates. If water intake is greater than output, water is retained (e.g., edema). Fortunately, regulatory mechanisms exist that protect against an increase in body water (see Chapter 2) and other nutrients. Consequently, for a net increase to be seen in TBW, there must be a neuroendocrine alteration present as well. Such is the case after trauma and surgery when elevated secretion rates of aldosterone and vasopressin promote the retention of salt and water. On the other hand, excess nitrogen intake is not stored, and, as already noted, maximum rates of protein synthesis exist in each individual. When the intake of nitrogen exceeds the need, the excess nitrogen is converted into urea and is excreted.

There are five basic situations in which intake does not equal output—dehydration and the four catabolic stresses defined by Moore[2] as fasting, starvation, injury, and febrile illness. In dehydration, the loss of water exceeds the intake resulting in a reduction in TBW that is distributed throughout the ICW and ECW. In fasting and in starvation (prolonged fasting), caloric and nitrogen expenditures are the same or less than those of a normal individual, but the intake of these substrates is markedly reduced or absent. As a result there is a loss of total body lipids, carbohydrates, and nitrogen. In patients with injury or febrile illness, caloric and nitrogen expenditures are greater than those of the normal individual. The increase in energy expenditure produced by an injury or infection is in proportion to the severity of the insult. Burns are the most severe injury, and generalized sepsis is the most severe febrile illness (Fig. 1-5). A healthy adult undergoing an elective operation increases the resting energy expenditure by approximately 10%, but the same individual with a severe burn increases the resting energy expenditure by 40% to 120%, depending on the size and the degree of the burn injury.[27] A minor febrile illness or a minor febrile complication after an elective operation increases the resting energy expenditure by 13% for each degree Celsius of temperature elevation,[28] but generalized sepsis increases the resting energy expenditure by 15% to 50%.[27] The changes in body composition resulting from an increase in caloric and nitrogen expenditure during injury and febrile illness are frequently compounded by reductions in intake as a result of anorexia and ileus. However, if the increased measurements are adequately met by exogenous substrate sources (enteral or parenteral), little change in body composition occurs.[5,19,29,30]

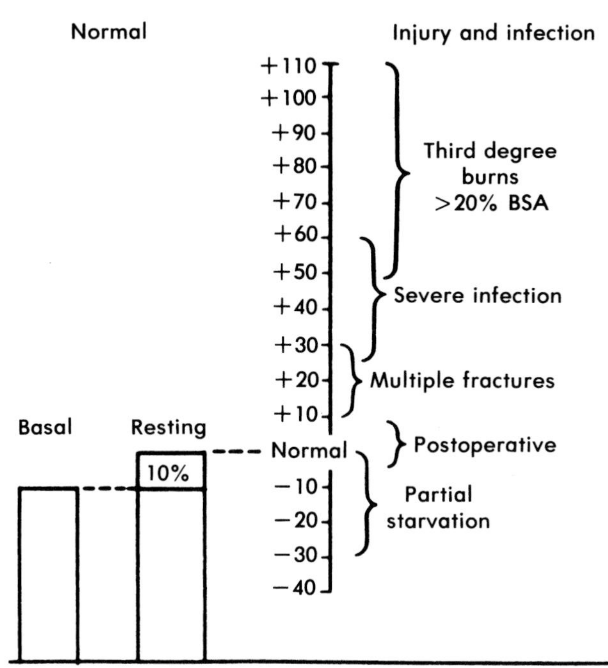

Fig. 1-5. Resting energy expenditure during injury and starvation in man. *BSA,* Body surface area. (From Kinney JM. The application of indirect calorimetry to clinical studies. In Kinney JM, ed. Assessment of Energy Metabolism in Health and Disease. Report of the First Ross Conference on Medical Research. Columbus, Ohio: Ross Laboratories, 1980, p 48.)

Table 1-11. Energy Released (G°′) During Hydrolysis of High-Energy Phosphate Compounds

Reaction	G°′ (Joules/Mol)
ATP + H_2O → ADP + Pi	−36,800
ADP + H_2O → AMP + Pi	−36,000
ATP + H_2O → AMP + PPi	−40,600
PPi + H_2O → 2Pi	−31,800
AMP + H_2O → A + Pi	−12,600

Based on data from Lehninger AL. Biochemistry: The Molecular Basis of Cell Structure and Function, 2nd ed. Menlo Park, Calif.: Worth Publishing, 1975.

A, Adenine; *ADP,* adenosine diphosphate; *AMP,* adenosine monophosphate; *ATP,* Adenosine triphosphate; *Pi,* inorganic phosphate; *PPI,* inorganic pyrophosphate.

NORMAL METABOLISM: INTERMEDIARY METABOLISM AND SUBSTRATE INTERACTIONS

Body composition remains in a steady state when four essential conditions are met: (1) energy is supplied in sufficient quantities to meet the metabolic demands of all the body's tissues; (2) carbohydrates are supplied in sufficient quantities to meet the requirements of glucose-dependent tissues, such as those of the brain, RBCs, and WBCs; (3) nitrogen is supplied in sufficient quantities to meet the obligatory synthesis of protein; and (4) water and solutes (electrolytes and minerals) are supplied in sufficient quantities to replace daily obligatory losses (water and electrolyte metabolism). In addition, these conditions must be met in the face of varying dietary intakes and varying daily energy requirements. This achievement is possible as a result of numerous substrate-to-substrate interactions (e.g., conversion of protein to carbohydrates) and the neuroendocrine regulation of intermediary metabolism.

Energy Metabolism

All metabolic processes in cells either produce energy (exergonic reactions) or use energy (endergonic reactions). The energy required for the operation of all biologic processes in mammalian cells is derived from the inherent energy present in the structure of organic molecules.[31] The chemical energy produced by the processing of these organic molecules is transferred to the phosphate bonds of purine nucleotides and other molecules with phosphate bonds such as phosphagens. As noted in Table 1-11, the hydrolysis of the phosphate bonds of adenosine triphosphate (ATP) or its precursors releases a considerable amount of energy that can be used to drive other biologic processes. The formation of these compounds with high-energy phosphate (HEP) group transfer potential is usually a result of the transfer of reducing equivalents from the substrate by reduction of nicotinamide adenine dinucleotide (oxidized form) (NAD^+), flavoproteins, and other coenzymes followed by coupled oxidative phosphorylation of adenosine diphosphate (ADP) in the mitochrondria.[32]

Although ATP serves as a carrier of chemical energy in all living cells, it is not a reservoir of energy.[31] The intracellular concentrations of ATP are small, highly regulated, and rapidly depleted. Reservoirs of energy (phosphagens), such as phosphocreatine, do exist in some cells.[31] These reservoirs accept HEP bonds when the intracellular concentration of ATP is high and transfer a phosphate group to ADP nucleotides when the availability of ATP is low.[31]

The intracellular concentrations of adenine nucleotides also provide the cell with a sensitive control mechanism for regulating energy-producing and energy-using processes in cells. Atkinson[33] has introduced the concept of energy charge to explain this regulatory mechanism. Adenylate energy charge (EC) represents the balance between energy-using processes and energy-producing processes. It is defined by the equation:

$$EC = (ATP + 0.5\,ADP)/(ATP + ADP + AMP)$$

A normal energy charge signals that energy-producing processes and energy-using processes are in balance. If the energy charge is increased, energy-producing processes are exceeding energy-using processes, and a resultant reduction of energy-producing processes occurs. If the energy charge is decreased, energy-using processes are exceeding energy-producing processes, resulting in a decrease in energy-using processes that may jeopardize cell survival.

The major energy-producing processes include the catabolism of carbohydrates, proteins, and lipids. Each of these substrate groups can provide part of the energy present in their structure through cytoplasmic catabolic reactions (e.g., glycolysis). The remainder of the available energy present in these substrates is released during oxidation of the remaining carbon fragments in the intramitochondrial tricarboxylic acid cycle (TCA). The final common pathway into the TCA cycle for carbohydrates, proteins, and lipids is through the formation of acetyl coenzyme A (CoA) (Figs. 1-6 through 1-8). For each molecule of acetyl-CoA completely oxidized in the TCA cycle, two molecules of carbon dioxide, three molecules of nicotinamide adenine dinucleotide (reduced form) (NADH), one molecule of flavin adenine dinucleotide (FADH), and one molecule of guanosine triphosphate (GTP) 190 are produced. In total, 12 HEPs are formed primarily by way of transfer of the reducing equivalents from NADH and FADH to oxygen in the electron transport system with the subsequent phosphorylation of ADP linked to this oxidative process (oxidative phosphorylation). Unlike carbohydrates and lipids, amino acids may directly enter the TCA cycle at one of the intermediate reactions (Fig. 1-6).

Carbohydrate Metabolism

In the cytoplasm of all cells, one molecule of glucose is catabolized to pyruvate through the Embden-Meyerhof pathway to yield two molecules of pyruvate, two molecules of ATP, and one molecule of NADH (Fig. 1-7). The completion of glycolysis (i.e., glucose to lactate) uses one

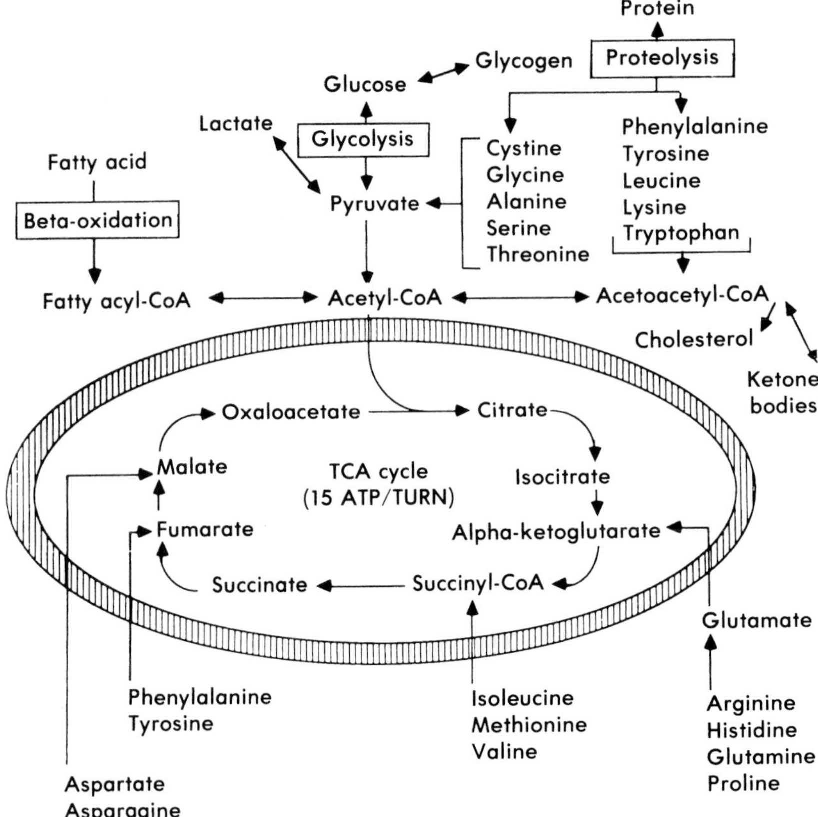

Fig. 1-6. Pathways for production and use of acetyl coenzyme A *(CoA)*. *TCA,* Tricarboxylic acid. (From Gann DS, Amaral JF, Caldwell MD. Metabolic response to injury, stress, and starvation. In Davis JH, et al. Clinical Surgery. St. Louis: Mosby, 1987.)

molecule of NADH in the conversion of pyruvate to lactate. Conversely, the conversion of pyruvate to acetyl-CoA produces one molecule of NADH. Since the oxidation of acetyl-CoA in the TCA cycle produces 15 HEPs, the complete oxidation of one molecule of glucose to carbon dioxide and water produces 26 HEPs [(2 × 12) + 2] and four molecules of NADH. The latter molecules produce 12 HEPs (three HEPs per molecule of NADH) through coupled oxidative phosphorylation. Consequently, the total energy produced in the complete oxidation of one molecule of glucose to carbon dioxide and water is equivalent to 38 HEPs. This result is in contrast to glycolysis where only two HEPs are produced in the conversion of glucose to lactate. As noted in Fig. 1-7 there are two nonreversible reactions in glycolysis: (1) the conversion of glucose to glucose 6-phosphate, catalyzed by hexokinase, and (2) the conversion of phosphoenolpyruvate to pyruvate, catalyzed by pyruvate kinase. These reactions are irreversible because they lose a considerable amount of energy as heat. It is the presence of these two nonreversible reactions that drives glucose to pyruvate. In addition, phosphofructokinase (PFK) and pyruvate kinase act as the major regulators of glycolysis.[34]

Once the catabolism of glucose has begun, it rapidly proceeds to pyruvate. Under aerobic conditions, most tissues oxidatively decarboxylate pyruvate to acetyl-CoA and then oxidize the acetyl-CoA in the TCA cycle. Under an aerobic condition, pyruvate cannot be decarboxylated, and it is converted instead to lactate. As a result, elevated tissue and plasma concentrations of lactate (and pyruvate) are characteristic of ischemia and anoxia. Some tissues with a paucity of mitochrondria, such as erythrocytes and leukocytes, are capable of glycolysis only. These cells lack the ability to oxidize pyruvate and acetyl-CoA even under aerobic conditions. Therefore they derive all their energy from conversion of glucose to pyruvate and lactate. Carbohydrates other than glucose can also be metabolized through glycolysis. For example, fructose, galactose, mannose, and triose sugars can enter glycolysis after modification by endergonic reactions. Similarly, pentose sugars may also enter the glycolytic pathway.

As noted earlier, the total carbohydrate stores of the human body are limited and are rapidly depleted.[22] In addition, RBCs, WBCs, and the brain are glucose-dependent tissues that are unable to use nonglucose energy substrates. Thus glucose must be made continuously available. The synthesis of glucose through a process called gluconeogenesis can proceed from lactate, pyruvate, and amino acids. Gluconeogenesis is not simply the reversal of glycolysis because the unidirectional reactions make glycoly-

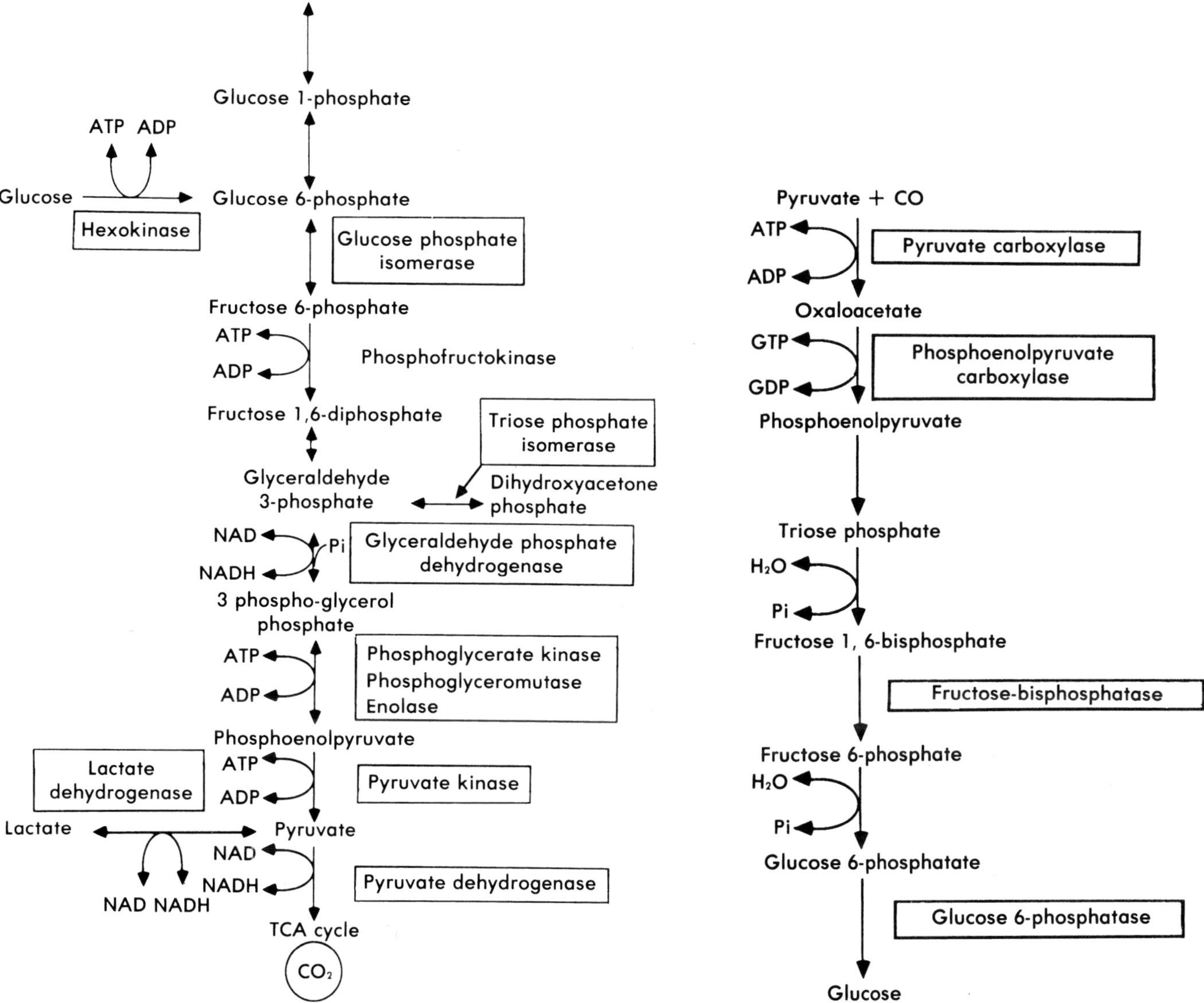

Fig. 1-7. Catabolism of glucose and major carbohydrate precursors. *ADP,* Adenosine diphosphate; *ATP,* adenosine triphosphate; *NAD,* nicotinamide adenine dinucleotide; *NADH,* reduced form of NAD; *Pi,* inorganic phosphate; *TCA,* tricarboxylic acid. (From Gann DS, Amaral JF, Caldwell MD. Metabolic response to injury, stress, and starvation. In Davis JH, et al. Clinical Surgery. St. Louis: Mosby, 1987.)

Fig. 1-8. Gluconeogenic pathway in the liver and the kidney. (From Gann DS, Amaral JF, Caldwell, MD. Metabolic response to injury, stress, and starvation. In Davis JH, et al. Clinical Surgery. St. Louis: Mosby, 1987.)

sis irreversible. However, gluconeogenic tissues, such as the liver and the kidney, contain four enzymes that essentially allow glycolysis to proceed in reverse fashion from pyruvate (and lactate) to glucose (Fig. 1-8). The first of these enzymes, pyruvate carboxylase, in the presence of ATP, carbon dioxide, and biotin, converts pyruvate to oxaloacetate in the mitochondria. (Although it does not act as a cofactor, acetyl-CoA must be present in excess for this reaction to proceed.[35]) Oxaloacetate is then converted to phosphoenolpyruvate by the cytoplasmic enzyme phosphoenolpyruvate carboxylase and GTP. Since the oxaloacetate is found in the mitochondria and phosphoenolypruvate carboxylase in the cytoplasm, oxaloacetate must cross the mitochondrial membranes into the cytoplasm. However, since the mitochondrial membranes are relatively impermeable to oxaloacetate, it is thought that oxaloacetate leaves the mitochondria as either malate or aspartate, which can be transported through the mitochondrial membranes and then reconverted to oxaloacetate in the cytoplasm.[36]

Once phosphoenolpyruvate is formed, glycolysis can easily proceed in reverse fashion to fructose-1,6-biphosphatase. The enzyme fructose-1,6-bisphosphatase is required to form fructose 6-phosphate. This enzyme is present in the liver and kidney and to a lesser extent in skeletal muscle. However, it is not present in adipose tissue, smooth muscle, or cardiac muscle.[37] Fructose 6-phosphate can then proceed to glucose 6-phosphate by the reversible glycolytic reaction catalyzed by glucose phosphate isomerase, but the conversion of glucose 6-phosphate to glucose requires the last of the gluconeogenic enzymes, glucose 6-phosphatase. This enzyme is present in the liver and kidney but not in skeletal, smooth, or cardiac muscle. Any glucose 6-phosphate that might be formed in skeletal muscle must either be converted to glycogen, be used in glycolysis, or be used in the hexose monophosphate shunt because skeletal muscle cannot release free glucose as a result of the absence of glucose 6-phosphatase. The glucose 6-phosphate formed in the liver and kidney can be converted to glucose and released into the circulation.

Since there is a constant production of lactate and pyruvate in aerobic glycolytic tissues, in all tissues during anaerobic conditions, and from the reticuloendothelial system during sepsis and locally inflamed tissues, a constant source of lactate and pyruvate is available to gluconeogenic tissues such as the liver and kidney. In the liver and kidney these substrates can be converted back to glucose and released into the circulation. The newly formed glucose is then available to glucose-dependent tissues for reconversion to lactate in the so-called Cori cycle (Fig. 1-9). However, it should be noted that this reconversion does not result in a net increase in glucose carbon, since lactate is itself derived from glucose.[38]

Protein and Amino Acid Metabolism

Energy and glucose can also be derived from the metabolism of amino acids. Although the partial catabolism and transformation of all α-amino acids to their α-keto acid derivatives can occur in most tissues, the complete oxidation of α-amino acids to urea and carbon dioxide occurs primarily in the liver and secondarily in the kidney.[39] In general, the catabolism of all amino acids (except lysine) involves the removal of the α-amino acid group from the carbon skeleton to form ammonia and an α-keto acid. This is followed by the conversion of ammonia to urea and by the conversion of the α-keto acids to TCA-cycle intermediates or precursors.[40,41]

Removal of the α-amino group can occur by one of three processes: (1) transamination; (2) oxidative deamination; and (3) nonoxidative deamination.[36,37] The most common mechanism is transamination. Transaminases (aminotransferases) interconvert a pair of amino acids and a pair of α-keto acids (Fig. 1-10). This process requires the presence of pyridoxal phosphate (vitamin B_6) for the transfer of the amino group. These reactions are freely reversible and function both in synthesis and in catabolism. At least 12 of the amino acids undergo transaminations, including the branched-chain amino acids, valine, leucine, and isoleucine. The most notable transaminases are glutamine-oxaloacetic transaminase (GOT or aspartate transaminase) and glutamic-pyruvic transaminase (GPT or alanine transaminase). Through the collective action of all the transaminases, the α-amino groups are usually collected in the form of glutamate or alanine. Since α-ketoglutarate can accept the α-amino group of all the amino acids that are transaminated, including alanine, it serves as the final common amino group acceptor to form glutamate.

Mallette et al.[42] have proposed and Felig[43] has expanded the concept of an alanine-glucose cycle similar to the Cori cycle (see Fig. 1-9). In peripheral tissues, amino acids are

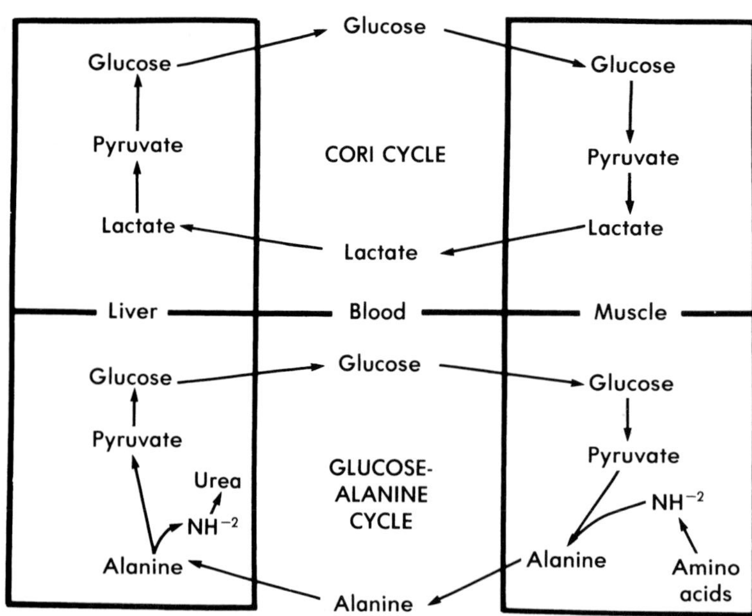

Fig. 1-9. Glucose-lactate (Cori) cycle and glucose-alanine cycle. (From Gann DS, Amaral JF. The pathophysiology of trauma and shock. In Zuidema GD, Rutherford WF, Ballinger WF, eds. The Management of Trauma. Philadelphia: WB Saunders, 1984.)

transaminated with pyruvate to form alanine and an α-keto acid. The alanine is then transported to the liver, where it is transaminated with α-ketoglutarate to form pyruvate and glutamate. The pyruvate can then be converted back to glucose and released into the circulation, where it may be taken up by peripheral tissues and converted to pyruvate and lactate.

The oxidative deamination of glutamate by glutamate dehydrogenase is an important mechanism in the liver for the removal of the amino group (see Fig. 1-10). Since α-ketoglutarate is the common acceptor for all transaminases,

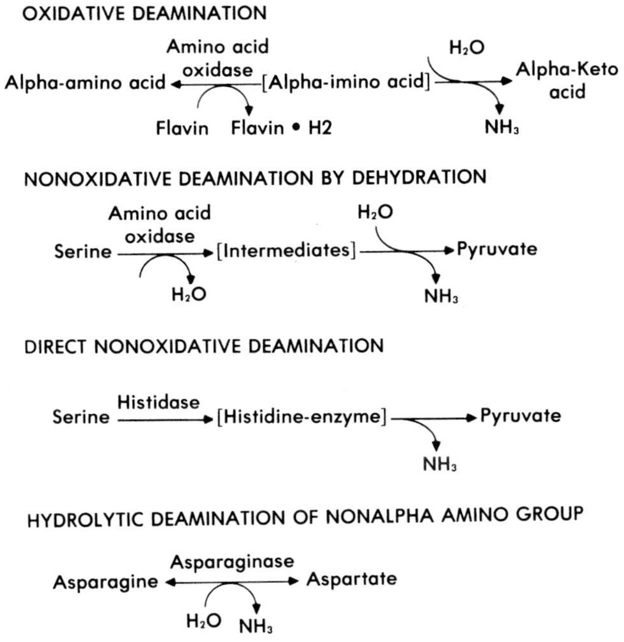

OXIDATIVE DEAMINATION

Amino acid oxidase
Alpha-amino acid ⟷ [Alpha-imino acid] → Alpha-Keto acid
Flavin Flavin • H2
H_2O
NH_3

NONOXIDATIVE DEAMINATION BY DEHYDRATION

Amino acid oxidase
Serine → [Intermediates] → Pyruvate
H_2O
H_2O
NH_3

DIRECT NONOXIDATIVE DEAMINATION

Histidase
Serine → [Histidine-enzyme] → Pyruvate
NH_3

HYDROLYTIC DEAMINATION OF NONALPHA AMINO GROUP

Asparaginase
Asparagine ⟷ Aspartate
H_2O NH_3

Fig. 1-10. Mechanisms for removal of the amino group. (From Gann DS, Amaral JF, Caldwell, MD. Metabolic response to injury, stress, and starvation. In Davis JH, et al. Clinical Surgery. St. Louis: Mosby, 1987.)

substantial amounts of glutamate are formed. Consequently, the oxidative deamination of glutamine allows for the regeneration of α-ketoglutarate and the removal of free ammonia. Oxidative deamination of other amino acids is also possible through the action of α-amino acid oxidases that are present in the liver and kidney. However, with the exception of glutamate dehydrogenase, these enzymes do not appear to exert a major physiologic role in humans.[39,41] Three amino acids, serine, threonine, and histidine, are primarily deaminated nonoxidatively[36] (see Fig. 1-10). The former two amino acids undergo nonoxidative deamination by dehydration, whereas histidine undergoes direct deamination. The non–α-amino groups of glutamine and asparagine are removed by hydrolytic deamination.[36]

Free ammonia, even in small concentrations, is poorly tolerated by cells. Four mechanisms exist to handle the free ammonia produced by oxidative or nonoxidative deamination, thereby keeping the intracellular (and extracellular) concentration of this substance low. Free ammonia can be added to glutamate by glutamine synthetase to form glutamine. This is the primary mechanism for the elimination of ammonia in brain cells and muscle cells. The free ammonia may also be added to α-ketoglutarate, forming glutamate in the freely reversible reaction catalyzed by glutamate dehydrogenase. The resulting glutamate may be used as an amino acid in protein, as a precursor in arginine and citrulline syntheses, or as an α-amino group donor in transaminase reactions. A third mechanism for ammonia elimination is through its excretion by the kidney. Two thirds of the ammonia excreted by the kidney is derived from the amide nitrogen of glutamine from renal arterial blood and one third from the α-amino nitrogen of renal arterial amino acids.[44]

Although these three mechanisms remove a substantial amount of the ammonia formed, most of it is cleared by the liver with subsequent entry into the urea cycle (Krebs-Henseleit cycle).[39] As noted in Fig. 1-11, the urea cycle

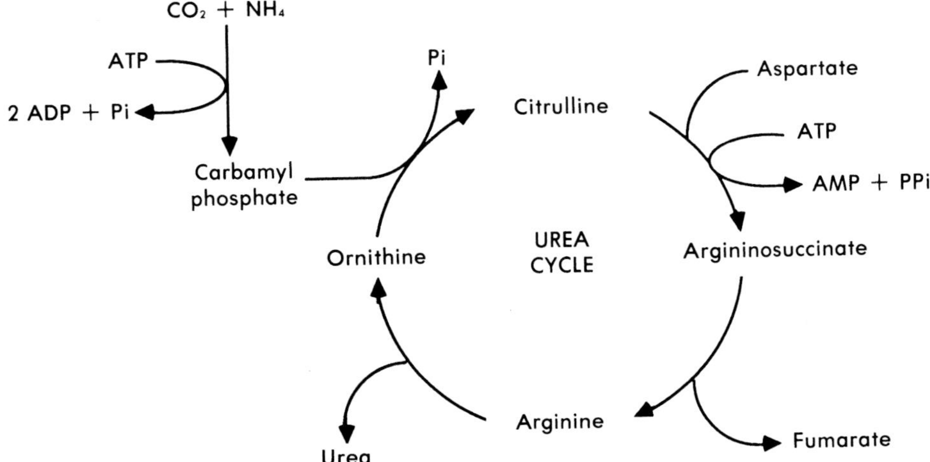

Fig. 1-11. Urea cycle. *ADP,* Adenosine diphosphate; *AMP,* adenosine monophosphate; *ATP,* adenosine triphosphate; *PPi,* inorganic pyrophosphate. (From Gann DS, Amaral JF, Caldwell MD. Metabolic response to injury, stress, and starvation. In Davis JH, et al. Clinical Surgery. St. Louis: Mosby, 1987.)

essentially involves the cleavage of a molecule of urea from arginine. The ammonia is first combined with carbon dioxide in the presence of ATP to form carbamylphosphate. Carbamylphosphate then condenses with ornithine to form citrulline, which, through a series of reactions, forms arginine. The arginine is then cleaved into urea and ornithine, thereby reestablishing the cycle. The net energy cost of this cycle is four HEPs derived from three molecules of ATP. Atkinson and Bourke[45] have suggested an important role for ureagenesis in the maintenance of pH homeostasis. Since the oxidation of amino acids yields both bicarbonate and ammonium ions, the urea cycle promotes the neutralization of the bicarbonate ion by the proton of the ammonium ion during the formation of carbonylphosphate.

The remaining carbon skeletons of amino acid deamination or transamination are converted either to intermediates of the TCA cycle or to precursors of acetyl-CoA, such as pyruvate and acetoacetate. Consequently, all the carbon skeletons of amino acids can be oxidized in the TCA cycle to carbon dioxide and water. The carbon skeletons of all the amino acids may also be converted to glucose or fat. As such, they may be classified as glucogenic, ketogenic, or glucogenic and ketogenic (see Table 1-10). Seven (alanine, serine, glycine, cysteine, cystine, proline, and hydroxyproline) of the 22 most common amino acids in proteins are converted to pyruvate. Depending on the redox state of the cell, the pyruvate can either be used for gluconeogenesis or converted to acetyl-CoA. Five amino acid carbon skeletons (phenylalanine, tyrosine, tryptophan, leucine, and lysine) form acetoacetate that may be converted to acetyl-CoA and either oxidized in the TCA cycle or used in fatty acid synthesis. In addition, in the process of producing acetoacetate, phenylalanine and tyrosine are also cleaved to fumarate, and tryptophan is cleaved to alanine. Thus phenylalanine tyrosine and tryptophan may be used both in glucogenesis and in ketogenesis. Lysine may also be used both in glucogenesis and ketogenesis, but its precursor for gluconeogenesis is not known. In contrast, leucine forms one molecule of acetyl-CoA and one molecule of acetoacetate. Since neither acetyl-CoA nor acetoacetate can be converted to pyruvate, the carbon skeleton of leucine can only be used for ketogenesis or oxidation.

It should be apparent that any compound that enters the TCA cycle as acetyl-CoA cannot be used as a precursor of glucose. This relates to the fact that by the time it reaches malate, the acetyl-CoA that entered the TCA cycle has been completely oxidized. However, the carbon skeletons of amino acids that are TCA-cycle intermediates can be used for gluconeogenesis. In addition to phenylalanine and tyrosine, which enter the TCA cycle as fumarate, three amino acids enter as succinyl-CoA (isoleucine, methionine, and valine), and two other amino acids enter as oxaloacetate (aspartate and asparagine) and give amino acids that enter as α-ketoglutarate (glutamate, glutamine, proline, histidine, and arginine) (Fig. 1-12). Consequently, all these amino acids may be used either in gluconeogenesis or oxidation. Quantitatively, in the isolated perfused liver, only alanine, serine, threonine, and glycine are used in significant amounts for gluconeogenesis.[46]

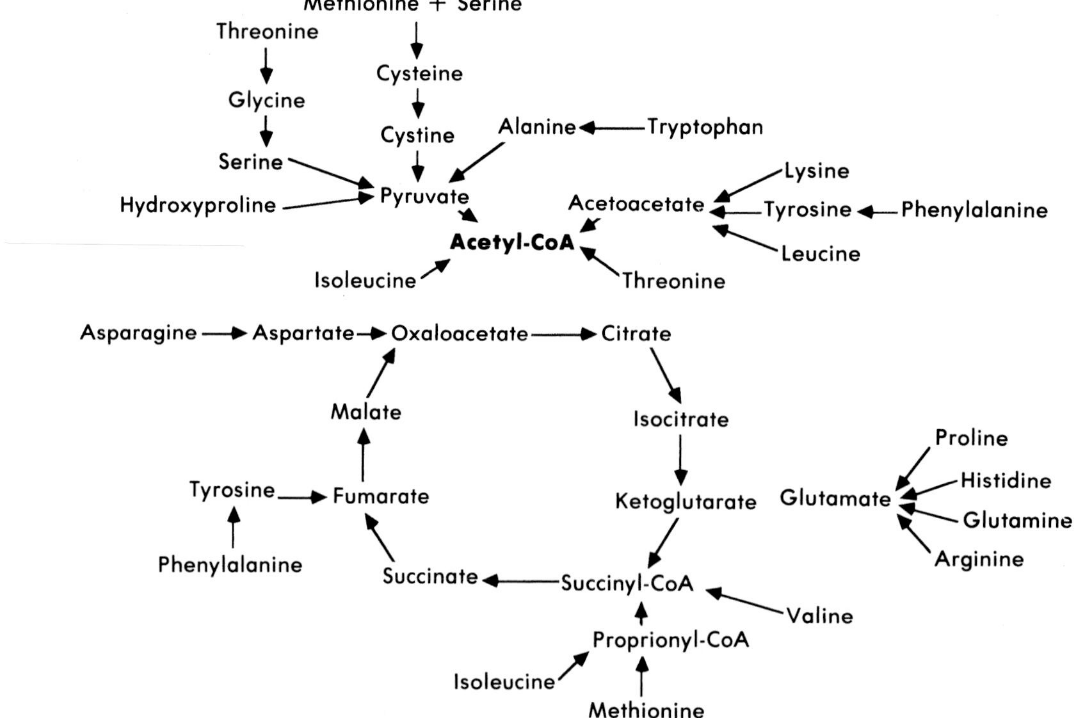

Fig. 1-12. Pathways through which the carbon skeletons of α-amino acids enter the tricarboxylic acid cycle.

As noted previously, excess nitrogen cannot be stored. When the protein intake is excessive, the amino acids resulting from proteolysis are catabolized to nitrogen and a carbon skeleton. The nitrogen is converted to urea, and the carbon skeleton is converted to either glucose, lipid, or carbon dioxide depending on the needs of the cell and the redox state present. Similarly, when glucose is needed but unavailable, excess ingested proteins or existing body proteins are degraded. Although it may be imperceptible, the use of existing body protein for energy or gluconeogenesis always results in the loss of some cellular function.

Lipid Metabolism

The final and greatest source of energy in the body is lipid. Stored in adipose tissues as triglycerides, lipids can be released on demand and transported to most tissues for use as an energy source. Tissues capable of using lipids include the liver, kidney, heart, and skeletal muscle; such use, however, must occur under aerobic conditions. Non–lipid-using tissues include erythrocytes, leukocytes, and nerve cells.

Triglycerides are composed of three fatty acid chains linked together by a glycerol molecule. During lipolysis, the fatty acids are sequentially cleaved off the glycerol moiety by lipases. The remaining glycerol moiety can then be used for glucose synthesis or converted to pyruvate (see Fig. 1-7). In contrast, fatty acids themselves cannot be used as substrate for gluconeogenesis, since they are ultimately broken down to acetyl-CoA.

The catabolism of fatty acids can be divided into two stages. These stages include β-oxidation in the outer mitochondrial membrane to produce molecules of acetyl-CoA and the processing of acetyl-CoA in the mitochondria to produce carbon dioxide and energy or ketone bodies[47,48] (Fig. 1-13). Only the first step in fatty acid catabolism requires energy. In this step the enzyme thiokinase adds CoA to a fatty acid, producing a fatty acetyl-CoA (see Fig. 1-13). After a sequence of reactions the final two carbons on the fatty acetyl-CoA are cleaved, resulting in the production of one molecule of acetyl-CoA and a new fatty acetyl-CoA that is two carbon atoms shorter than the parent fatty acetyl-CoA. This process of β-oxidation yields five HEPs per acetyl-CoA formed and, with even-numbered fatty acid chains, continues until the entire fatty acid has been cleaved to acetyl-CoA. In the case of odd-numbered fatty acid chains, β-oxidation continues until a

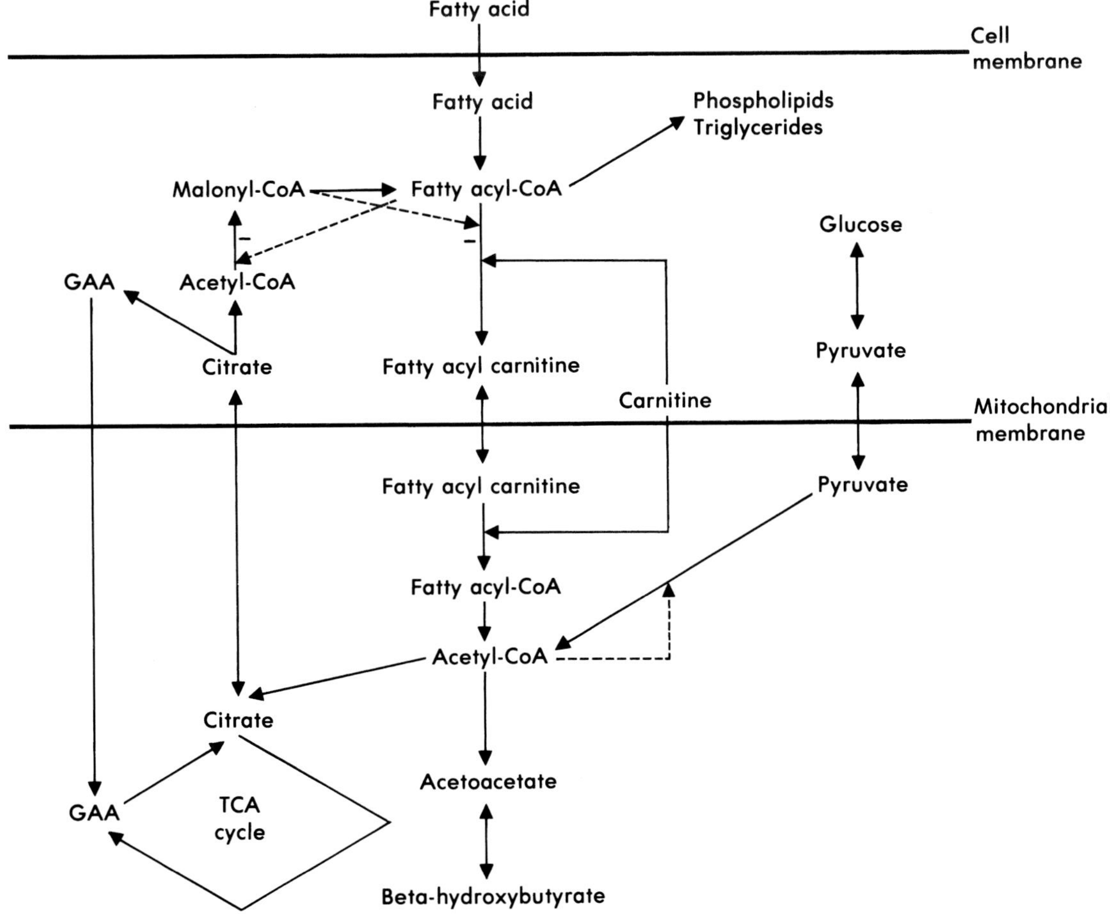

Fig. 1-13. Metabolic pathways of fatty acid metabolism in the liver. *GAA,* Gossypol acetic acid; *TCA,* tricarboxylic acid. (From Gann DS, Amaral JF. The pathophysiology of trauma and shock. In Zuidema GD, Rutherford WF, Ballinger WF, eds. The Management of Trauma. Philadelphia: WB Saunders, 1984.)

three-carbon fatty acetyl-CoA (propionyl-CoA) remains. The latter substance may then be converted to succinyl-CoA and enter the TCA cycle.

The acetyl-CoA that results from the oxidation of fatty acids can be used in one of three available pathways[47,49] (see Fig. 1-13). The first involves the intramitochondrial oxidation of acetyl-CoA through the TCA cycle to two molecules of carbon dioxide and 12 HEPs. Thus the total oxidation of a 20-carbon fatty acid, for example, yields:

$$169 \text{ HEPs} = [(10 \times 5) + (10 \times 12) - 1]$$

The second pathway involves the ketogenic pathway in the liver (Fig. 1-14). Through the action of the enzyme thiolase, two molecules of acetyl-CoA combine to form acetoacetyl-CoA in a freely reversible reaction. Acetoacetyl-CoA can then be converted to 3-hydroxy-3-methylglutaryl CoA, the precursor in cholesterol synthesis and ketone body formation. The three ketone bodies, acetoacetate, β-hydroxybutyrate, and acetone, are normally produced and released by the liver. Under conditions in which there is an abundance of hepatic glycogen, β-hydroxybutyrate predominates; under conditions in which the liver glycogen is low, acetoacetate predominates. The ketone bodies that are released by the liver can then be used by a variety of peripheral tissues, such as cardiac and skeletal muscle, as a source of energy by conversion back to acetyl-CoA.

The final pathway for use of acetyl-CoA is in the synthesis of fatty acids and triglycerides (see Fig. 1-13). This pathway is stimulated by neuroendocrine mechanisms and low cytoplasmic concentrations of fatty acids. Lipogenesis is a cytoplasmic process that requires malonyl-CoA. Malonyl-CoA is formed from acetyl-CoA by acetyl-CoA carboxylase. When fatty acid levels are low, the rate-limiting enzyme in malonyl-CoA formation, acetyl-CoA carboxylase, is stimulated, leading to increased intracellular concentrations of malonyl-CoA.[50] In turn the elevated concentration of malonyl-CoA inhibit carnitine acetyl transferase, the enzyme necessary for transport of acetyl-CoA into the mitrochondria,[51] resulting in an increased concentration of cytoplasmic acetyl-CoA that can then be used for malonyl-CoA synthesis and ultimately for the synthesis of triglycerides and other lipids. In contrast, when the intracellular concentrations of fatty acids are elevated, the rate-limiting enzyme in malonyl-CoA synthesis (acetyl-CoA carboxylase) is inhibited. Malonyl-CoA concentrations decrease, thereby stimulating carnitine acetyl transferase and increasing the transport of acetyl-CoA into the mitochondria for oxidation and ketogenesis.[51] The inhibition of acetyl-CoA carboxylase also results in the accumulation of cytoplasmic citrate that in turn inhibits glycolysis through inhibition of PFK, the so-called Randle effect.[34]

NEUROENDOCRINE REGULATORY MECHANISMS

Stimuli and Mechanism of Action of the Neuroendocrine System

The pathways of intermediary metabolism and substrate-to-substrate interactions noted previously are under the local control of substrate availability, cellular redox potential, and cellular energy availability. The integration of this control is governed by the neuroendocrine system. This system may be thought of as a reflex physiologic network in which alterations in homeostasis are perceived by specialized receptors that are located both peripherally and centrally. The receptors transmit their information to the CNS, where the afferent signals are processed and modu-

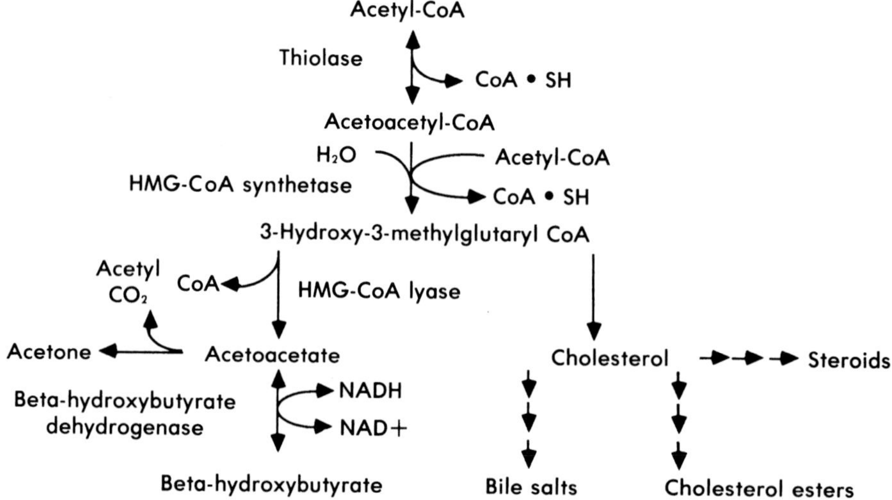

Fig. 1-14. Ketogenic pathway and cholesterol pathway in the liver. *CoA,* Coenzyme A; *HMG,* 3-hydroxy-3-methylglutaryl; *NADH,* reduced nicotinamide adenine dinucleotide. (From Gann DS, Amaral JF, Caldwell MD. Metabolic response to injury, stress, and starvation. In Davis JH, et al. Clinical Surgery. St. Louis: Mosby, 1987.)

lated, resulting in release or inhibition of numerous neuroendocrine effectors that produce physiologic changes aimed at correcting the alterations in homeostasis. In the absence of significant injury, sepsis, or starvation, alterations in homeostasis are small, and the responses of the neuroendocrine system to stimuli are directed at fine tuning and integrating the functioning of the organism. In the presence of significant injury, sepsis, or starvation, the stimuli are multiple and intensified, and the reflexes are directed at an integrated attempt by the organism to preserve oxygen delivery, mobilize energy substrates, and minimize pain[1] (Fig. 1-15). The major stimuli affecting neuroendocrine reflexes include (1) changes in the circulating body fluids; (2) changes in the oxygen, hydrogen ion, and carbon dioxide concentrations in tissues and blood; (3) changes in ambient and core temperature; (4) changes in substrate availability; (5) emotional arousal; (6) pain; and (7) infection.

Critical to the initiation of the neuroendocrine response is the perception of the stimulus. Paraplegics do not respond to stimuli below the level of cord transection. This lack of response is thought to be the result of the absence of afferent impulses reaching the brain.[52] However, conscious perception of the stimulus is not required. An individual responds to a stimulus in the presence of anesthesia, but the response may not be the same had anesthesia been absent.

Changes in the circulating body fluids may result from the direct loss of blood (as in hemorrhage), from the loss of plasma volume (as in third space losses and dehydration), or from the inability of the body fluids to circulate (as in cardiac failure or pulmonary embolism). The changes in circulating body fluids are sensed by high-pressure baroreceptors in the carotid arteries and aorta and by low-pressure stretch receptors in the right atrium. Under normal conditions the afferent signals from these receptors exert a tonic inhibition of the release of many hormones and of the activities of the CNS and autonomic nervous system.[53] When baroreceptor or stretch receptor activities decrease (e.g., a decrease in blood pressure or blood volume), the tonic inhibition is released, resulting in the increased secretion of adrenocorticotropic hormone (ACTH), vasopressin, β-endorphin, and growth hormone through central pathways and resulting n the increased secretion of epinephrine, norepinephrine, renin, and glucagon through peripheral autonomic neural pathways. These responses bring about further neuroendocrine changes such as the inhibition of insulin secretion by epinephrine[54] and the stimulation of aldosterone secretion by renin and ACTH.[55]

Changes in blood concentrations of oxygen, hydrogen ion, and carbon dioxide initiate neuroendocrine responses through the activation of peripheral chemoreceptors. The chemoreceptors, which are located in the aortic and carotid bodies, have an extremely high blood flow rate.[56] Under normal conditions, these receptors are not activated. However, changes primarily in oxygen and secondarily in carbon dioxide and in hydrogen ions are sensed by these receptors, which results in the activation of neuroendocrine pathways. Because of the high blood flow through the chemoreceptors, the partial pressure of oxygen (PO_2) of arterial blood, chemoreceptor tissue, and venous blood is nearly the same. However, a drop in blood flow increases the oxygen extraction by the chemoreceptor tissue, decreases the venous PO_2, and through an unknown mechanism, activates the chemoreceptor.[56] Consequently, a decrease in circulating volume or pressure not only inhibits baroreceptors and stretch receptors but also activates chemoreceptors.

Pain and emotion also activate the neuroendocrine system. The former acts through the projections of periph-

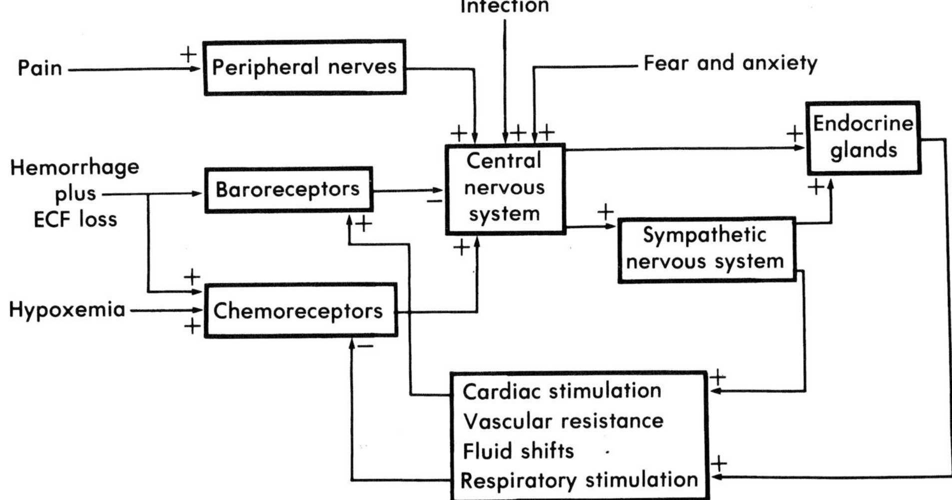

Fig. 1-15. Overview of the neuroendocrine reflexes induced by shock and trauma. *ECF,* Extracellular fluid. (From Gann DS, Amaral JF. The pathophysiology of trauma and shock. In Zuidema GD, Rutherford WF, Ballinger WF, eds. The Management of Trauma. Philadelphia: WB Saunders, 1984.)

eral nociceptive receptors to the CNS, and the latter acts through projections from the limbic areas of the brain to the hypothalamus and lower brain stem nuclei.[57] Through these pathways, pain and emotional arousal bring about increased hypothalamic, autonomic, adrenomedullary, and adrenocortical activities, the so-called fight-or-flight reaction of Cannon.[58]

Abnormalities in core and ambient temperatures, as well as infection, also stimulate neuroendocrine reflexes. Changes in the core temperature of the body are sensed in the preoptic area of the hypothalamus. These changes may result from alterations in ambient temperature, a loss of the normal insulating barrier of the skin (e.g., burns), or a reduction in hepatic thermogenesis produced by inadequate blood flow or substrate supply or in response to inadequate peripheral vasoconstriction or vasodilation. Infection may also decrease the core temperature through the action of endotoxin. Infection may further stimulate neuroendocrine reflexes through a direct action of endotoxin on the hypothalamus[59] or through secondary changes in blood volume, oxygen concentration, substrate concentrations, and pain.

The primary substrate alterations that activate the neuroendocrine system are those induced by changes in the plasma glucose concentration. Plasma glucose alterations are sensed by receptors in the hypothalamus and the pancreas. A decrease in plasma glucose concentration stimulates the release of catecholamines, cortisol, growth hormone, and vasopressin through central mechanisms and stimulates the release of glucagon both by central pathways (autonomic nervous system) and peripheral pathways (direct pancreatic activation).[60] In addition, the secretion of insulin is inhibited through central pathways (autonomic nervous system) and directly by the pancreas itself.[54]

All these stimuli are commonly produced by injury, sepsis, and starvation. Furthermore, these stimuli rarely occur singly. Generally, the individual perceives multiple stimuli that occur both simultaneously and sequentially. Thus the neuroendocrine response is the summation of all the stimuli the individual perceives and processes. According to classic endocrine feedback mechanisms, the elevation of serum cortisol resulting from one set of stimuli would be expected to inhibit the release of ACTH by a new set of stimuli. Following most injuries, this is not true. The secretion of ACTH is unchanged or increased (potentiated), and the secretion of cortisol may also increase. The mechanism of action of this physiologic facilitation is unknown, but it appears to take 60 to 90 minutes to be of sufficient magnitude to offset the inhibition and lasts for at least 24 hours.[61] Physiologic facilitation and potentiation have been demonstrated with sequential hemorrhages[62] and repeated operations,[63] in response to hypoxia and surgery,[64] with pain and hemorrhage,[12] and with elevated core temperature and hemorrhage.[65] Consequently, the response to an injury or an alteration in homeostasis may be modified by previous stimuli, and the response to a second set of stimuli may be different if they had occurred first.

The efferent limb of the neuroendocrine system arises from two primary areas, the hypothalamic-pituitary axis and the autonomic regions of the brain stem. The output from the former region involves the release of numerous pituitary hormones, and the output from the latter region involves changes in the neural activities of the sympathetic and parasympathetic nervous systems. Both sets of output either may cause direct changes in physiologic functions or may stimulate or inhibit the secretion of peripheral endocrine organs.

The hormones secreted by endocrine organs and the autacoids produced by tissues fall into one of five chemical classes. These include the fatty acid derivatives of cholesterol (cortisol, aldosterone) or arachidonic acid (prostaglandins), proteins (insulin, glucagon), glycoproteins (thyroid-stimulating hormone [TSH], corticotropin), small polypeptides (vasopressin, enkephalin), and the amines (catecholamines, serotonin). All these agents act on cellular receptors that are either on the surface of cell membranes or in the cytoplasm of the cell. These cellular receptors are neither fixed nor unchangeable. Instead, they are in a dynamic state in which the number of receptors on cells can be increased (up regulation) or decreased (down regulation) according to need. Furthermore, the affinity of these receptors for their specific hormone can also be changed.[66]

Steroid hormones (and possibly thyroxine), which are freely permeable to cell membranes, bind to cytosolic receptors in target cells.[67,68] The hormone-receptor complex migrates to the cell nuclei, where it interacts with DNA to modulate the transcription of messenger RNA and ultimately the synthesis of enzymatic, structural, and regulatory proteins[67] (Fig. 1-16, *A*). This may, in part, explain the 1- to 2-hour delay in the action of steroid hormones. In contrast, the action of most peptide and amine hormones, which generally bind to cell surface receptors, is faster and of shorter duration. In general, these hormones act either through alterations in the intracellular concentrations of cyclic adenosine monophosphate (cAMP) or calcium, the so-called second messengers,[69,70] or through other intermediates (growth hormone through somatomedins). The second messenger system of hormonal action operates primarily through the activation and inactivation of regulatory proteins and enzymes rather than through the synthesis of new proteins. This difference explains the faster onset of action and shorter duration of effect of hormones that operate through this system in contrast to those of steroid and other lipid-soluble hormones.

The adrenergic receptor system may be considered the prototype for examining the mechanisms of second messengers, since all the second messenger pathways known are represented in the four adrenergic receptors (α_1, α_2, β_1, and β_2) (Fig. 1-16, *B*). β_1- and β_2-receptors (differentiated on the basis of radioligand-binding affinity) both function through the activation of membrane-bound adenylate cyclase, which in turn leads to the production of cAMP.[69] The increased intracellular concentration of cAMP activates an inactive protein kinase by attaching to a binding protein on the protein kinase molecule. The attachment of cAMP to the regulatory subunit protein results in the release of an active protein kinase that in turn phosphorylates an inactive phosphorylase kinase to an active form. The active phosphorylase kinase then phosphorylates dephosphoregulatory enzymes, possibly resulting in the activation of the regulatory enzyme (e.g., glycogen phosphorylase) or in its inactivation (e.g., glycogen synthetase)[71] (Fig. 1-17). In addition, active protein kinase may directly act on dephosphoregulatory enzymes without the activation of phosphorylase kinase. In contrast, α_2-receptor activation inhibits membrane-bound adenylate cyclase, thereby decreasing the concentration of cAMP and active protein kinase. Activation of α_1-adrenergic recep-

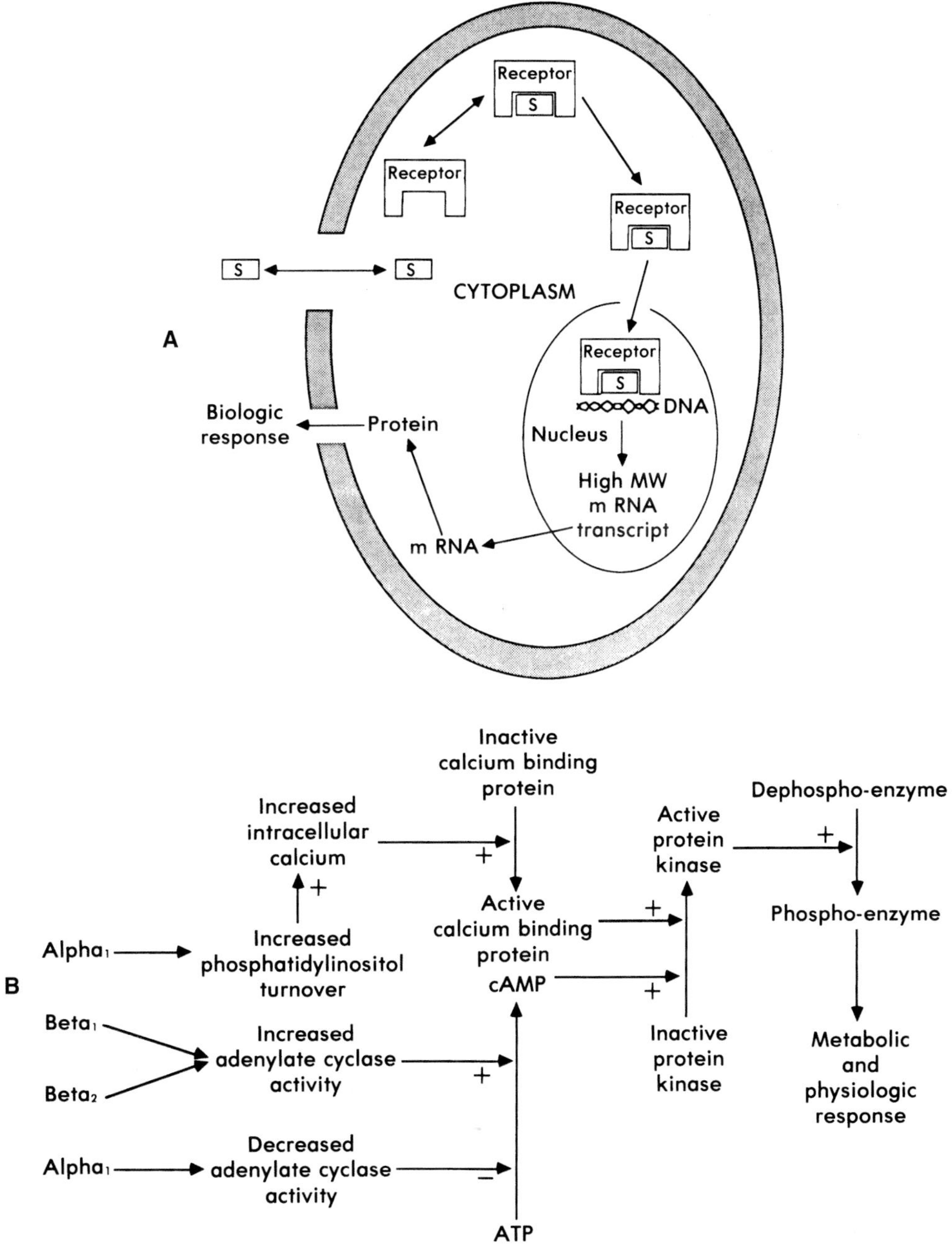

Fig. 1-16. A, Proposed mechanism of action of steroid hormones. **B,** Proposed mechanism of action of peptide hormones through the second messenger system. *ATP,* Adenosine triphosphate; *cAMP,* cyclic adenosine monophosphate; *m,* molecular; *MW,* molecular weight. (**A,** From Gann DS, Amaral JF, Caldwell MD. Neuroendocrine response to injury, stress, and starvation. In Davis JH, et al. Clinical Surgery. St. Louis: Mosby, 1987. **B,** From Gann DS, Amaral JF. The pathophysiology of trauma and shock. In Zuidema GD, Rutherford WF, Ballinger WF, eds. The Management of Trauma. Philadelphia: WB Saunders, 1984.)

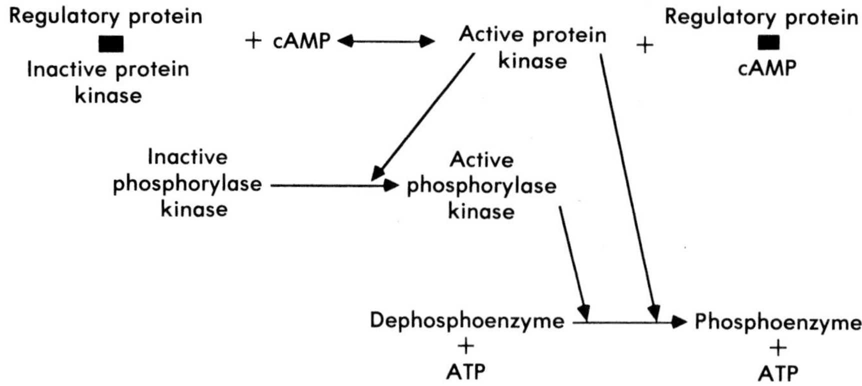

Fig. 1-17. Activation of protein kinase leading to enzymatic or physiologic response. Activation of the dephosphoenzyme by phosphorylation may be brought about either directly by the active protein kinase or indirectly through the activation of a phosphorylase kinase by the active protein kinase. *ATP,* Adenosine triophosphate; *cAMP,* cyclic adenosine monophosphate. (From Gann DS, Amaral JF, Caldwell MD. Neuroendocrine response to injury, stress, and starvation. In Davis JH, et al. Clinical Surgery. St. Louis: Mosby, 1987.)

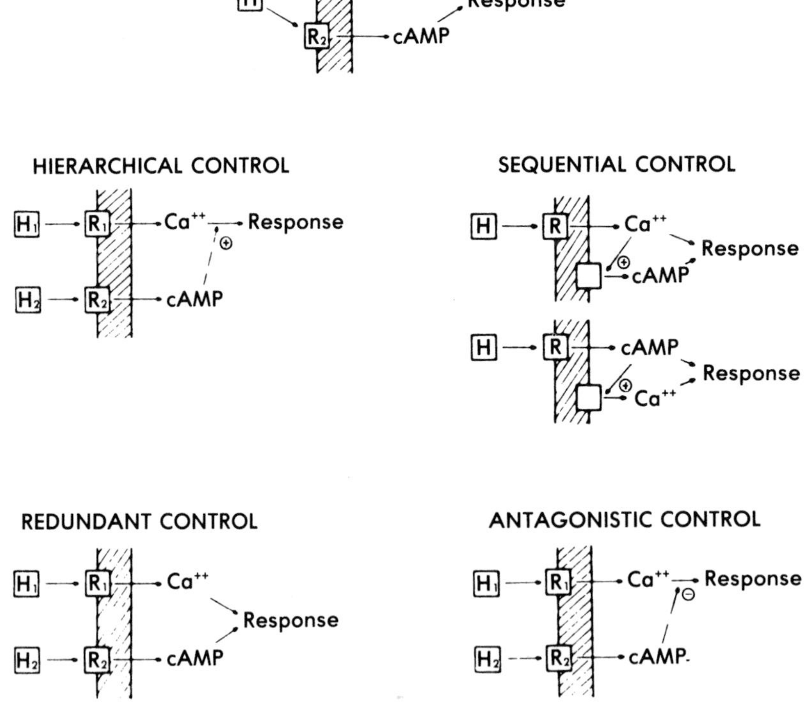

Fig. 1-18. Patterns of synarchic regulation by calcium and cyclic adenosine monophosphate. (From Rasmusen H. Calcium and cAMP as Synarchic Messengers. New York: John Wiley, 1981. Reprinted by permission of John Wiley & Sons, Inc.)

tors results in an increase in phosphatidylinositol turnover that then mediates an increase in intracellular calcium from intracellular and extracellular sources.[69,72] The increase in intracellular calcium activates a calcium-binding protein kinase or phosphorylase kinase (see Fig. 1-16, *B*).

The actions of intracellular cAMP and calcium in the coupling of receptor activation with hormonal action (stimulus-response coupling) are not independent. Instead, there is a duality to this system in which the actions of calcium and cAMP are highly interrelated, termed synarchic control by Rasmusen.[69] As noted in Fig. 1-18, and the boxed material, there are five basic patterns to the synar-

CALCIUM–CYCLIC AMP INTERACTIONS IN STIMULUS-RESPONSE COUPLING

1. Effects of calcium on cAMP messenger systems
   a. Stimulates cAMP production—brain, adrenal cortex, pancreatic islets, adrenal medulla, slime mold
   b. Stimulates cAMP hydrolysis—brain, heart, liver, kidney, fly salivary gland, many other tissues
   c. Activates phosphoprotein product of cAMP-dependent protein kinase, glycogenolysis in many tissues
2. Effects of cAMP on calcium messenger system
   a. Increases calcium entry across plasma membrane—heart, synapse
   b. Increases calcium release from mitochondria—kidney, liver, fly salivary gland, others
   c. Increases calcium uptake by microsomes—heart, uterus, liver, smooth muscles
   d. Increases calcium efflux across plasma membrane—smooth muscle, heart
   e. Decreases sensitivity of response elements to calcium—smooth muscle, heart
   f. Increases sensitivity of response element to calcium—phosphorylase beta kinase, liver, muscle
3. Interrelated activities
   a. cAMP-dependent and calcium-dependent protein kinases act upon same protein substrate—liver, brain, adrenal cortex
   b. Regulate sequential steps in metabolic or transport process—secretion in fly salivary gland, glycogenolysis

From Rasmusen H. Calcium and cAMP as Synarchic Messengers. New York: John Wiley, 1981. Reprinted by permission of John Wiley & Sons, Inc.

chic control of hormone-response coupling through cAMP and calcium. In coordinate control, a hormone activates both a calcium-activating receptor and a cAMP-activating receptor, either one of which may produce the response alone. In hierarchal control, separate stimuli activate independently the calcium and cAMP pathways that are both necessary for a given response. In sequential control, the activation of one of the two lines of the system leads to the activation of the other limb. Although the first limb can produce the response, activation of the second limb augments the response. In redundant control, two separate stimuli independently activate the two different limbs of the messenger system, either one of which can produce the response. Finally, in antagonist control, one stimulus activates one limb of the messenger system that leads to the response, and a second stimulus activates the second limb, which inhibits the ability of the first limb to produce the response. Although each of these control mechanisms can occasionally be found in cells in pure form, most of the presently known hormone-response coupling mechanisms involve mixed patterns.[69]

Hormonal Regulation of Metabolism

The neuroendocrine system is able to regulate metabolic reactions through three basic processes. First, it may increase substrate availability so that by simple stoichiometry (mass action), reactions proceed in a desired direction. This process can be brought about either by an increase in the plasma concentration of a substrate or by alterations in blood flow and its distribution. Second, the neuroendocrine effectors can alter the membrane transport properties of cells for a given substrate so that more or less of the substrate enters or leaves the cell. Third, the neuroendocrine effectors can alter the activity or synthesis of key regulatory enzymes that are necessary for reactions to proceed.

Most hormones operate through more than one of these processes. For example, insulin stimulates both glycogen synthetase and the transport of glucose into cells. In this manner, insulin not only activates the enzymatic mechanisms necessary for glycogenesis, it also increases the availability of the necessary substrates. It would be futile for a hormone to stimulate opposing processes in a given cell. If a hormone stimulated both glycogenesis and glycogenolysis, there would be no net effect. As a result, most hormones not only activate the enzymes necessary for one metabolic pathway, they also inhibit the enzymes necessary for the opposing process. Thus epinephrine, through an α-mechanism, activates glycogen phosphorylase and inactivates glycogen synthetase, whereas insulin inactivates glycogen phosphorylase and activates glycogen synthetase.

The coordinated control of metabolism also requires that a hormone not have opposing actions in different tissues. Thus by increasing amino acid uptake in skeletal muscle and decreasing amino acid degradation in the liver, insulin promotes the availability of an abundant substrate supply for the enzymes of protein synthesis it activates. Cortisol produces an inhibition of amino acid uptake in skeletal muscle, increases amino acid uptake by the liver, and stimulates hepatic gluconeogenic enzymes. These processes ensure that an abundant supply of amino acids are available to the liver for cortisol-stimulated gluconeogenesis.

The primary hormones involved in the regulation of metabolism include insulin, cortisol, epinephrine, glucagon, growth hormone, vasopressin, and somatostatin, Insulin is the primary anabolic hormone promoting the snythesis of glycogen, proteins, and lipids. Cortisol, epinephrine, glucagon, and vasopressin are the primary catabolic hormones promoting the breakdown of glycogen, proteins, and lipids and the synthesis of glucose from gluconeogenic amino acids, lactate, and pyruvate. In contrast, the actions of growth hormone initially are anabolic, but its late effects are primarily catabolic.

Insulin, Glucagon, and Somatostatin

Insulin, composed of two polypeptide chains, one containing 21 amino acids and the other 30 amino acids, and glucagon, a 29–amino acid polypeptide, are produced and secreted by the pancreatic B cells (beta islets of Langerhans) and A cells (alpha islets of Langerhans), respectively. The secretion of both of these hormones is under the control of at least three mechanisms: (1) circulating substrates (glucose, amino acids, and free fatty acids); (2) the autonomic nervous system; and (3) other circulating hormones.

Under normal physiologic conditions, glucose is the most important regulator of insulin and glucagon secretion. When the plasma concentration of glucose increases, the secretion of insulin increases, and the secretion of glucagon decreases. When the plasma concentration of glucose decreases, the secretion of insulin decreases, and the secretion of glucagon increases. These changes are probably the result of a direct action of glucose on pancreatic islet cells and not a result of neuroendocrine modulation of the pancreas by other neuroendocrine effectors.[73] The direct action of glucose on islet cell function may be mediated either through a glucoreceptor on the surface of the islet cell or through the intracellular metabolism of glucose in the islet cells.[74]

Elevations in the plasma concentration of amino acids stimulate the release of both insulin and glucagon. Most, if not all, of the amino acids increase insulin secretion, but the potency of amino acids in stimulating glucagon secretion is variable.[75] In general, the more gluconeogenic amino acids appear to stimulate glucagon secretion.[75]

High concentrations of fatty acids stimulate the secretion of insulin and inhibit the secretion of glucagon. Conversely, low concentrations of free fatty acids inhibit the secretion of insulin and stimulate the secretion of glucagon. The potency of fatty acids in regulating insulin and glucagon secretion is substantially less than that of glucose.[75]

The stimulation of insulin secretion and the inhibition of glucagon secretion after the administration of an oral glucose load is greater than that following the intravenous administration of glucose.[76] Similarly, the stimulation of both insulin and glucagon secretion is greater after an oral protein or amino acid load than it is after the intravenous administration of amino acids and protein.[77] This effect is thought to be the result of the higher concentrations of substrate in the pancreas, the potentiation by gastrointestinal hormones of the substrate effect on the pancreas, and the effect of neural input to the pancreas that has been stimulated by eating.[75] The gastrointestinal hormones, cholecystokinin, gastrin, vasoactive intestinal peptide (VIP), substance P, neurotensin, and gastric inhibitory peptide (GIP), increase the secretion of both insulin and glucagon in pharmacologic concentrations.[75,78] Although gastrin does appear to potentiate the release of glucagon and insulin induced by amino acids and GIP in physiologic concentrations appears to augment the release of insulin by glucose,[75] the physiologic role of gastrointestinal hormones is not certain.

The pancreatic A cells and B cells both have α- and β-adrenergic receptors that alter the secretion of insulin and glucagon. α-Adrenergic stimulation of the pancreas inhibits the secretion of both insulin and glucagon, whereas β-adrenergic stimulation of the pancreas stimulates the secretion of both insulin and glucagon.[79,80] However, the α- and β-adrenergic receptor density of A cells and B cells is not the same. The β-adrenergic receptor density of A cells is greater than that of B cells.[80] As a result, increased sympathetic stimulation of the pancreas or increased circulating concentrations of epinephrine or norepinephrine increase the secretion of glucagon but decrease the secretion of insulin.[79,80] In contrast, isoproterenol infusion increases the secretion of both insulin and glucagon.[80] In addition to sympathetic stimulation, the parasympathetic limb of the autonomic nervous system alters pancreatic hormone secretion. Both acetylcholine infusion and direct parasympathetic stimulation of the pancreas increase the secretion of both insulin and glucagon.[75]

In addition to the gastrointestinal hormones and the autonomic nervous system, other hormones alter the secretion of insulin and glucagon. β-Endorphin appears to directly increase the secretion of insulin and glucagon,[81] insulin inhibits the release of insulin and stimulates the release of glucagon,[75] and glucagon inhibits the release of glucagon and stimulates the release of insulin.[75,82] Insulin and glucagon appear to exert their action both directly on islet cells and by the alterations they produce in circulating substrates.[75] Cortisol stimulates the release of insulin and glucagon, but it appears to have no direct activity on the secretory ability of A cells and B cells. Instead, cortisol is believed to increase glucagon secretion through an increase in plasma amino acids and to increase insulin secretion by an increase in plasma glucose. In this regard, both cortisol and epinephrine are able to inhibit the peripheral actions of insulin, and both are thought to exert a major role in insulin resistance.[83,84]

Somatostatin, a tetradecapeptide, is a potent inhibitor of both insulin and glucagon secretion.[78,85] In addition to its location in pancreatic D cells, somatostatin is found in the hypothalamus, limbic system, brain stem, spinal cord, other neural tissue, salivary glands, parafollicular thyroid cells, kidneys, and gastrointestinal tissue.[78] Although somatostatin was originally named for its ability to inhibit growth hormone secretion, somatostatin is now recognized to inhibit the secretion of TSH, renin, calcitonin, gastrin, secretion, cholecystokinin, insulin, and glucagon.[78] In addition, somatostatinergic nerve fibers are involved in the projection of impulses from peripheral sensory organs to the neuroaxis.[78]

The role somatostatin exerts in the physiologic regulation of insulin and glucagon secretion is not known precisely. The A, B, and D cells have somatostatin receptors that, when activated, inhibit the secretion of glucagon, insulin, and somatostatin, respectively. Although the mechanism of action of somatostatin is thought to be mediated primarily by the local diffusion of somatostatin from D cells to A cells and B cells,[78,85] recent evidence suggests that somatostatin reaching the pancreas through the blood stream may be more important.[86] The effects of somatostatin on A cells are transient, but the effects on B cells are persistent.[85] This persistence may account for the relative hyperglycemia that occurs in patients with somatostatinomas or after the long-term administration of somatostatin.[85]

The physiologic actions of glucagon occur primarily in the liver and are mediated through an increase in intracellular cAMP. The activation of glycogen phosphorylase and the inhibition of glycogen synthetase by glucagon promotes the breakdown of glycogen to glucose (glycogenolysis).[34] In addition, glucagon stimulates gluconeogenesis through the stimulation of phosphoenolpyruvate carboxykinase, amino acid transport, and amino acid transamination.[34,87] The net result is an increase in hepatic production and release of glucose that under basal conditions accounts for 75% of the glucose produced by the liver.[88]

Glucagon also exerts an important influence over hepatic lipid metabolism. In addition to stimulating lipolysis in adipose tissue and the liver, glucagon inhibits acetyl-CoA carboxylase, the enzyme that converts acetyl-CoA to malonyl-CoA.[75] In turn, the reduction in malonyl-CoA produces inhibition of triglyceride synthesis and activation of carnitine acyl transferase. The latter increases fatty acid transfer to the mitochondria and therefore increases the oxidation of acetyl-CoA and ketogenesis.[47,75]

Peripheral actions of glucagon include the stimulation of lipolysis in adipose tissue, of glycogenolysis in skeletal muscle, and of myocardial contractility.[89-91] However, these actions do not appear to be of physiologic significance in human beings.[89-91]

As a result of glucagon's ability to increase hepatic glucose production, mobilize fat, and increase ketogenesis, glucagon is important in normal metabolism and more so in the metabolism of altered states. However, the effects of glucagon are evanescent.[92] After 30 to 60 minutes, the activity assigned to glucagon decreases even if plasma glucagon concentrations remain elevated. Therefore it appears that an increase in glucagon concentration rather than the absolute amount of glucagon present is a key determinant of glucagon activity.[92] This effect also appears to be true of other cAMP-mediated hormones (the burst effect).

The physiologic activity of insulin is primarily in the liver, skeletal muscle, and adipose tissue, but insulin does affect many other peripheral tissues. Notable exceptions include erythrocytes and wounded tissue. Insulin promotes the entry of glucose into cells by stimulating the membrane transport of glucose. The increased intracellular concentrations of glucose are used in glycogen synthesis (stimulation of glycogen synthetase and inhibition of glycogen phosphorylase) and in glycolysis (stimulation of glucokinase, PFK, and pyruvate kinase) to produce energy.[34] In addition, insulin inhibits gluconeogenesis through the inhibition of phosphoenolpyruvate carboxylase and the stimulation of PFK and pyruvate kinase.[34]

Insulin also increases the membrane transport of amino acids into the liver and peripheral tissues. The increased intracellular concentrations of amino acids are used in protein synthesis (stimulation of protein synthesis and inhibition of proteolysis). By inhibiting gluconeogenesis and amino acid oxidation, insulin further directs the intracellular amino acids to protein synthesis.[87]

In adipose tissue, insulin stimulates lipogenesis and inhibits lipolysis, as it does in the liver. By stimulating lipoprotein lipase, insulin also makes triglycerides more available for uptake from the plasma by adipose tissue. Glycerol synthesis and the action of the pentose-phosphate shunt also are increased by insulin in adipose tissue and the liver. Thus insulin is the primary anabolic hormone promoting the storage of lipid, glucose, and protein.

Although insulin and glucagon oppose each other in the metabolic processes each stimulates, a bihormonal response is necessary for maintenance of glucose homeostasis after a protein meal.[78] If insulin were secreted alone in response to a protein meal, the increase in protein synthesis and decrease in hepatic glucose production would result in hypoglycemia. Conversely, if glucagon were secreted alone, the decrease in protein synthesis and the increase in hepatic gluconeogenesis would result in hyperglycemia. However, when a rise in glucagon is accompanied by an increase in insulin, hepatic glucose production remains unchanged and euglycemia is maintained. In this regard, Unger[93] has proposed the insulin/glucagon (I/G) ratio as a quantitative measure of hepatic glucose balance. When the I/G ratio is greater than 5, anabolism and protein synthesis are favored. When the I/G ratio is less than 3, glycogenolysis, gluconeogenesis, and lipolysis are favored. However, the validity of this relationship has been questioned.[74]

ACTH, Cortisol, and Epinephrine

The primary hormones released in response to any physiologic or psychologic stress are the glucocorticoids and catecholamines. These hormones are in large part responsible for the "fight-or-flight reaction." The release of cortisol is under the control of ACTH, a 39–amino acid polypeptide released from the chromophobe cells in the anterior pituitary gland. In turn the release of ACTH is itself under the inhibitory influence of cortisol and the stimulatory influence of corticotropin-releasing factor (CRF) produced by the hypothalamus. The release of CRF (and ACTH-cortisol) is stimulated by all the stimuli noted previously and is potentiated by vasopressin, oxytocin, and angiotensin II.[94,95] ACTH acts directly on cells of the adrenal zona fasciculata, stimulating the production and release of cortisol through a cAMP-mediated conversion of cholesterol to pregnenolone.[96]

The catecholamines (epinephrine, norepinephrine, and dopamine) are the prototypical neuroendocrine effectors that act as neurotransmitters and hormones.[97] Epinephrine, produced almost exclusively by the adrenal medulla, functions primarily as a hormone, whereas norepinephrine and dopamine function primarily as neurotransmitters.[97] Although the adrenal medulla may be viewed as a collection of postganglionic sympathetic neurons without axons that release their neurotransmitters into the general circulation, the activation of the sympathetic nervous system does not occur in an all-or-none fashion, and it is not synonymous with adrenomedullary secretion.[98] Similarly, adrenomedullary stimulation is not synonymous with the complete activation of the sympathetic nervous system. Numerous stimuli have been identified that lead to increased secretion of catecholamines from the adrenal medulla (e.g., hypotension, hypoxia, hypoglycemia, pain, and fear), but the exact mechanisms involved in adrenomedullary control remain poorly understood.[98]

Both cortisol and epinephrine function as "counterregulatory" hormones, mediating catabolic processes throughout the body. In the liver, cortisol inhibits several key glycolytic enzymes (glucokinase, PFK, and pyruvate kinase), the pentose-phosphate shunt, and the actions of insulin.[34,96] In addition, cortisol stimulates the hepatic uptake of amino acids, transaminases, and several gluconeogenic enzymes (pyruvate carboxylase, phosphoenolpyruvate carboxykinase, and glucose 6-phosphatase), as well as potentiating the actions of glucagon and epinephrine.[34,83,99] As a result, the production of glucose, lactate, and pyruvate by the liver is increased.

The metabolic effects of epinephrine are similar to those of glucagon but are more widespread, affecting peripheral tissues and the liver. In the liver, epinephrine stimulates glycogenolysis (α_1-mediated stimulation of glycogen phosphorylase and inhibition of glycogen synthetase),[69] lipolysis (β_1-mediated activation of triacylglycerol lipase),[100] ketogenesis (β_1-mediated inhibition of acetyl-CoA carboxylase leading to decreased malonyl-CoA and increased carnitine acyl transferase),[57] and gluconeogenesis (β_1-mediated inhibition of PFK and hexokinase by the products of glycolysis and glycogenolysis).[101] Thus epinephrine serves to increase hepatic glucose production and lipid breakdown.

Although both glucagon and epinephrine increase glucose production by the liver, glucose use by peripheral tissues is not the same in the presence of epinephrine as it is in the presence of glucagon.[87] Glucagon promotes the use of glucose by peripheral tissues through the stimulation of insulin secretion. In contract, epinephrine inhibits both the release and the action of insulin, thereby decreasing glucose use in insulin-dependent peripheral tissues. However, epinephrine serves to increase glucose availability to insulin-insensitive tissues such as the brain, whereas glucagon does not shunt glucose to insulin-insensitive tissues.[87]

In adipose tissue, epinephrine increases lipolysis (β-mediated activation of triacylglycerol lipase). In peripheral tissues, epinephrine stimulates glycogenolysis (α_1) and inhibits stimulated glucose uptake through a β_2- and α_1-mechanism.[102,103] As a result of increased substrate availability, glycolysis is increased in skeletal muscle, and large amounts of lactate are produced and released into the circulation. The lactate can then be taken up by the liver for subsequent gluconeogenesis (Cori cycle). Therefore during stressful conditions, epinephrine and cortisol both promote a rise in blood glucose and make glucose more available to glucose-dependent tissues. Both of these hormones also promote the breakdown of lipid and thereby its use as a source of fuel. Whereas the actions of epinephrine are direct, many of the actions of cortisol occur as a result of the potentiation or inhibition of other hormones, the so-called permissive action of cortisol.

Growth Hormone and Vasopressin

Growth hormone is a 191–amino acid polypeptide that is released from acidophilic cells in the anterior pituitary gland. Its secretion is under the control of a releasing factor (growth hormone–releasing factor) and by an inhibiting factor (somatostatin).[104] Elevation of blood glucose or free fatty acids stimulates the release of growth hormone.[104] In addition, the release of growth hormone is stimulated by vasopressin, ACTH, α-melanocyte-stimulating hormone, and estrogen; release of growth hormone is inhibited by cortisol, thyroxine, and growth hormone itself.

In addition to its ability to promote protein synthesis and RNA synthesis and to increase in linear growth, growth hormone exhibits an important role in the regulation of metabolic processes. Its effects are biphasic, composed of early effects of 3 to 4 hours' duration and late effects of longer duration.[104] In muscle and liver, growth hormone increases amino acid uptake and protein synthesis.[105] In addition, growth hormone stimulates glucose uptake in skeletal muscle and antagonizes the lipolytic effects of catecholamines in adipose tissue while increasing protein synthesis.[105] Therefore the early effects of growth hormone are similar to insulin. In fact, growth hormone directly stimulates the secretion of insulin by pancreatic B cells during its early phase.[55] The late effects of growth hormone include an increased mobilization of fatty acids and ketone bodies by adipose tissue as a result of increased lipolysis. This action of growth hormone occurs only in the presence of cortisol.[106] In addition, growth hormone inhibits insulin stimulated glucose uptake and use, thereby producing a profound stimulation of insulin release by hyperglycemia.[55]

Arginine vasopressin (antidiuretic hormone) is a nonapeptide that is released by the posterior pituitary gland. Although released primarily in response to an increase in plasma osmolality and to a reduction in effective circulating volume,[86,107] vasopressin release is also stimulated by hypoglycemia through nonosmotic pathways.[108] Vasopressin is a powerful stimulator of hepatic glycogenolysis (α-receptor) and also stimulates hepatic gluconeogenesis.[109,110] As such, it may exert an important role in elevating the blood glucose after injury and during hypoglycemia.

METABOLIC RESPONSE IN STARVATION, INJURY, AND SEPSIS

Fasting and Starvation

In the absence of food, fasting humans must supply the energy required for daily activities, glucose for glucose-dependent tissue, essential amino acids (Table 1-12), and

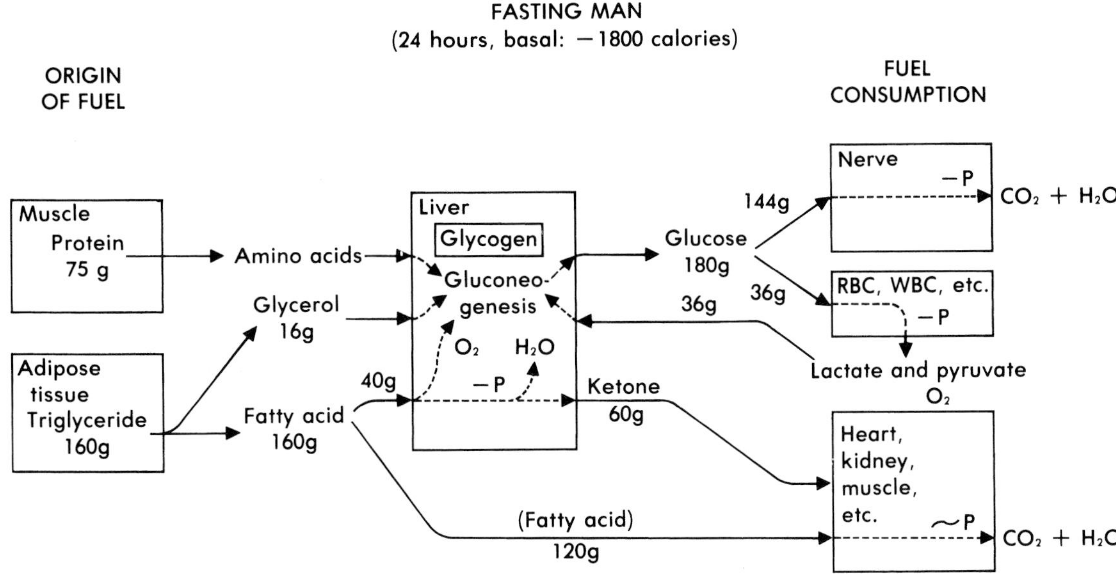

Fig. 1-19. Flow diagram of fuel metabolism in normal fasted man. (From Cahill GF. Starvation in man. N Engl J Med 282:669, 1970.)

Table 1-12. Pathways for the Use of Amino Acid Carbon Fragments

Gluconeogenesis	Ketogenesis	Gluconeogenesis and Ketogenesis
Alanine	Leucine	Isoleucine
Arginine		Lysine
Aspartic acid		Phenylalanine
Aspargine		Tyrosine
Cystine		Tryptophan
Glutamic acid		
Glycine		
Histidine		
Hydroxyproline		
Methionine		
Proline		
Serine		
Threonine		
Valine		

Table 1-13. Fuel Composition of Normal Humans

Fuel	Weight (kg)	Calories
Tissues		
Fat (adipose triglyceride)	15	141,000
Protein (mainly muscle)	6	24,000
Glycogen (muscle)	0.15	600
Glycogen (liver)	0.075	300
TOTAL		165,900
Circulating Fuels		
Glucose (extracellular fluid)	0.02	80
Free fatty acids (plasma)	0.0003	3
Triglycerides (plasma)	0.003	30
TOTAL		113

From Cahill GF. Starvation in man. N Engl J Med 282:668, 1970.

essential fatty acids from existing body stores. Cahill[20] has estimated that the average resting 70 kg man using 1800 kcal of energy per day requires 180 g of glucose daily—for the metabolism of nervous tissue (144 g) and for other glycolytic tissue (RBCs, WBCs, and the renal medulla) (36 g) (Fig. 1-19). Since the available glycogen in the liver is only 75 g (Table 1-13), this amount will not suffice for either the energy requirements or the glucose needs of a fasting man. Although an additional 150 g of glucose is in skeletal muscle as glycogen, as noted previously, it cannot be released from skeletal muscle as free glucose as a result of the absence of glucose 6-phosphatase. There it is apparent that the energy requirements and glucose requirements of fasting human beings must be supplied from noncarbohydrate sources and by gluconeogenesis.

The daily energy requirements can be met by the mobilization of approximately 160 g of triglycerides from adipose tissue in the form of free fatty acids.[11] The free fatty acids, as well as ketone bodies produced by the liver, are used throughout the body by nonglycolytic tissues such as the heart, kidney, muscle, and liver. In the liver, energy derived from β-oxidation of fat and from oxidation of acetyl-CoA is used to drive the necessary gluconeogenic processes. Gluconeogenic substrates are available

Table 1-14. Amount of Glucose Produced From Lactate, Glycerol, and Amino Acids During Starvation

Glucose Precursor	Grams of Glucose Produced per Day	
	3 or 4 Days of Starvation	Several Weeks of Starvation
Glycerol*	19	19
Lactate + pyruvate†	39	39
Amino acids‡	41	16
Total glucose produced from above precursors by liver and kidney cortex§	99	74
Maximum glucose available for oxidation by the brain (i.e., glycerol and amino acid as precursors)‖	60	35
Fuel requirement of brain (glucose equivalents)¶	120	120
Suggested alternative fuel to glucose for brain#	Ketone bodies	Ketone bodies

From Newsholme EA, Start C. Regulation in Metabolism. New York: John Wiley, 1975. Reprinted by permission of John Wiley & Sons, Inc.

*Amount of glucose produced from glycerol is estimated from the amount of triglyceride hydrolyzed per day. In starvation, 190 g of triglyceride is required to satisfy the caloric needs of the subject. Since glycerol represents 10% of triglyceride, it can provide 19 g of glucose per day. This amount is confirmed by measurement of glycerol uptake by liver and kidney using catheterization techniques.

†Amount calculated from glucose 1-C turnover studies in man that gives values between 27 and 58 g/day, and this is *not* affected by the dietary state. Also the measurement of lactate and pyruvate uptake by the liver and kidney in man by catheterization techniques estimates glucose formation as 39 g/day.

‡Amount calculated from nitrogen excreted in urine (100 g protein produces 57 g glucose; 1 g nitrogen is equivalent to 6 to 25 g protein). In early stages of starvation approximately 12 g nitrogen is excreted per day, but this is decreased in prolonged starvation to 4 to 7 g/day. Catheterization studies in subjects undergoing prolonged starvation indicate an uptake of amino acids by liver and kidney that could theoretically produce 26 g glucose per day.

§In prolonged starvation the hepatic-renal glucose production as measured by catheterization techniques provides an estimate of 86 g glucose per day, which is in good agreement with the 74 g obtained in this calculation.

‖Catheterization techniques have been used to measure the A-V differences across the brain. In prolonged starvation, glucose oxidation by the brain (excluding glucose converted to lactate, which is converted back to glucose in the liver and kidney) is estimated as 24 g/day.

¶Oxygen uptake or total fuel use is measured by catheterization techniques.

#The rate of ketone body uptake by the brain has been estimated from A-V differences using catheterization techniques. These studies strongly suggest that ketone bodies are the alternative fuel to glucose during starvation.

from three sources (Table 1-14). First, the lipolysis of 160 g of triglycerides releases 16 g of glycerol that can be converted by the liver to glucose. Second, some glucose-dependent tissue (i.e., RBCs and WBCs) converts glucose to lactate and pyruvate that may then be reused in the liver by the Cori cycle to produce new glucose. In addition to the 36 g of lactate and pyruvate produced in this manner, skeletal muscle can also release lactate and pyruvate by the breakdown of glycogen and glucose. Third, approximately 75 g of skeletal muscle protein is degraded daily during starvation, and the resulting amino acids are used in the liver for gluconeogenesis. Consequently, the energy required during brief fasting is derived primarily from adipose tissue. In contrast, the glucose required is supplied from lactate, pyruvate, glycogen, and amino acids.

During the first 2 to 4 days of fasting, there is a rapid increase in the urinary nitrogen excretion from 5 to 7 g/day to approximately 8 to 11 g/day.[112] This increase is associated with the previously noted breakdown of 50 to 75 g of protein per day. The rapid proteolysis of skeletal muscle protein does not continue during more prolonged fasting. During the next 20 to 40 days of fasting, the urinary nitrogen excretion begins gradually to decline and eventually reaches its nadir of 2 to 4 g of nitrogen per day.[112] This decline is the result of ketoadaptation to starvation. In this process, the brain, which does not normally use ketone bodies for fuel, adapts its metabolism and transport systems to use ketone bodies.[113] This adaptation results in a significant reduction in the amount of glucose needed by this glucose-dependent tissue and consequently in the amount of amino acid substrate necessary for gluconeogenesis (Fig. 1-20). Protein conservation follows with only 20 to 30 g of protein catabolized per day.[20]

Concurrent with these adaptations to starvation is a reduction in the resting energy expenditure by as much as 31%.[108] In part, the reduction in resting energy expenditure is the result of a reduction in BCM produced by the breakdown of muscle and other proteins. However, the reduction in body size is less than the reduction in resting energy expenditure.[108,114] Other factors that may contribute to the reduction in resting energy expenditure include a reduction in voluntary work, a decrease in body temperature, a decrease in cardiac work, a decrease in sympathetic nervous system activity, and a decrease in muscle activity.

The changes in metabolism accompanying fasting and starvation are primarily regulated by decreased concentrations of insulin and increased concentrations of glucagon in response to decreasing glucose concentrations.[20,47,112] The decreased insulin concentrations promote an increase in lipolysis in adipose tissue and a decrease in glucose uptake in insulin-dependent tissues. The increased concentrations of glucagon promote hepatic gluconeogenesis. These changes (including the decreased secretion of insulin and increased secretion of glucagon) may be further augmented by slight increases in the concentrations of epinephrine, ACTH, cortisol, and growth hormone.[91,115]

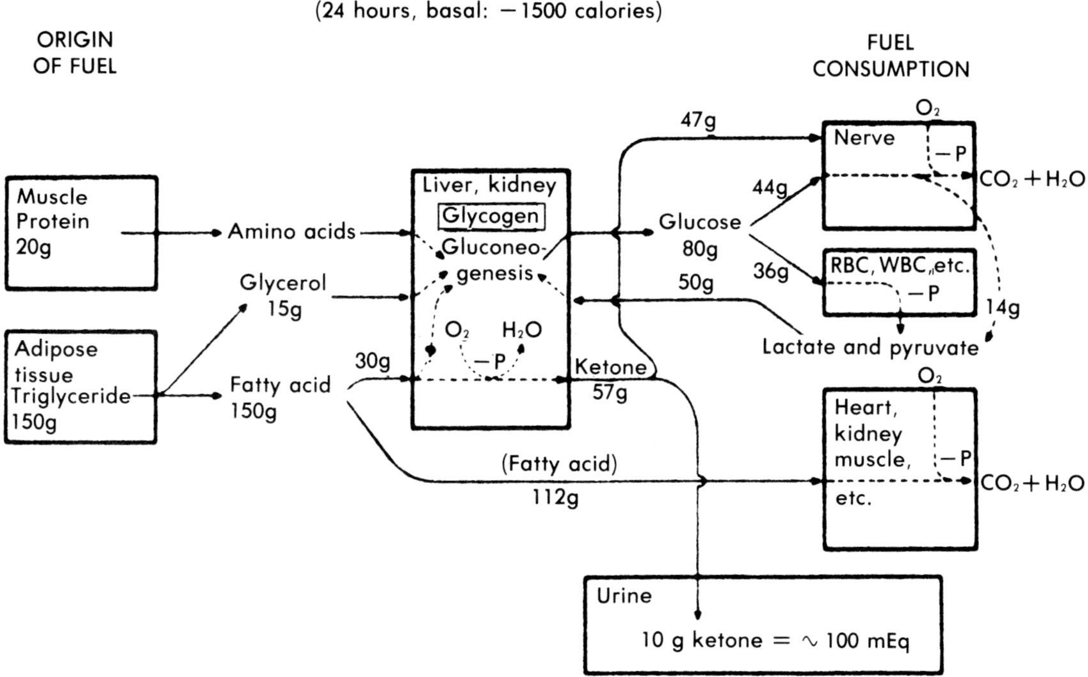

Fig. 1-20. Flow diagram of fuel metabolism in starved man after adaptation. (From Cahill GF. Starvation in man. N Engl J Med 282: 672, 1970. Copyright © 1970 Massachusetts Medical Society. All rights reserved.)

However, an actual increase in these hormones is not necessary, since basal concentrations of the counterregulatory hormones are unopposed by the reduced secretion of insulin that is stimulated by hypoglycemia.

Thus through four major adaptive mechanisms, a reduction in resting energy expenditure, the use of protein for gluconeogenesis, the use of fat for energy, and ketoadaptation of the brain, a human is able to survive for prolonged periods of time without food. As a result of the decreased excretion of urea and nitrogen during prolonged starvation, water intake is also reduced. However, it is apparent that this condition cannot be maintained indefinitely. In the average 70 kg man, there are approximately 170,000 calories and 6000 g of protein (see Table 1-13). If it could all be used, starvation for up to 100 days would be tolerated. However, this is not possible because of the loss of essential body functions as body protein is consumed and not replenished. In fact, acute weight losses of 30% to 40% of body weight are usually fatal and associated with a rapid increase in urinary nitrogen excretion and a rapid decline in plasma glucose.[112,116,117]

Injury and Sepsis

Cuthbertson,[118,119] in his classic studies of the metabolic response to long-bone fractures, defined two phases of the metabolic response to injury—an ebb or shock phase and a flow phase. Moore[120] subsequently divided the flow phase into catabolic and anabolic stages. The ebb phase, constituting the first several hours after injury, is characterized by hyperglycemia and the restoration of circulatory volume and tissue perfusion. Once perfusion is restored, the flow phase begins. It is characterized by generalized catabolism, negative nitrogen balance, hyperglycemia, and heat production. The flow phase is the best-studied phase and may last from days to weeks depending on the severity of the injury, the previous health of the individual, and medical intervention. Finally, once volume deficits have been corrected, pain has been eliminated, wounds have been closed, infection has been controlled, and complete oxygenation has been restored, the anabolic phase begins.[1] This phase can be divided into a slow but progressive reaccumulation of protein, followed by the reaccumulation of body fat. Since protein synthesis cannot exceed 3 to 5 g of nitrogen per day, the protein repletion phase may be considerably longer than the catabolic phase in which protein is broken down.

The posttraumatic state is characterized by starvation, immobilization, and repair. Although starvation and immobilization are both associated with decreased energy requirements, reparative processes increase energy needs. As a result, the overall energy requirements of traumatized and septic individuals are increased. The increase in energy need varies directly with the severity of injury and the complications that develop. In this regard, the most severe injury is the burn, the most severe complication is sepsis (see Fig. 1-5). Despite the use of protein and carbohydrate for calories, most of the energy used after trauma and after sepsis is derived from fat. This use is reflected in the low respiratory quotients noted after injury and sepsis. For example, Wilmore et al.[121] found respiratory quotients of 0.70 to 0.76 after severe burns. In addition, septic injury appears to have a greater lipid dependence for energy than nonseptic injury.[88,122]

Increased lipolysis is seen in both the ebb phase and the flow phase of the metabolic response to injury. During the ebb phase, elevated concentrations of cortisol, catecholamines, glucagon, growth hormone, ACTH, increased sympathetic nervous system activity, and depressed concentrations of insulin favor lipolysis. The presence of cortisol appears to be necessary for the remainder of the hormonal agents to be effective.[123,124] Elevated concentrations of glycerol and free fatty acids during the ebb phase are well documented.[125-127] However, Kovach et al.[128] have noted that elevation of plasma free fatty acids may not occur after severe hemorrhage as a result of intense vasoconstriction in adipose tissue, producing minimum blood flow.

During the flow phase, net lipolysis persists despite an increase in the concentration of insulin. Increased free fatty acids have been documented after trauma, burns, and sepsis.[88,120,129-133] The fatty acids are used throughout the body for energy. In both the ebb and flow phases, the high concentration of intracellular fatty acids and the elevated concentration of glucagon inhibit acetyl-CoA carboxylase, thereby decreasing malonyl-CoA concentrations and fatty acid synthesis. In hepatocytes, the decreased concentration of malonyl-CoA also stimulates carnitine acyl transferase, thereby increasing the transport of acetyl-CoA into the mitrochondria for oxidation and ketogenesis. However, the activity of ketogenesis after shock, injury, and sepsis is variable and correlates with the severity of injury.[131-133] After major injury and sepsis, ketogenesis is low or absent; whereas after minor injury and sepsis, it is increased but to a lesser extent than is seen during nonstressed starvation.[129,134] During starvation, the inhibition of acetyl-CoA carboxylase also results in the accumulation of cytoplasmic citrate that in turn inhibits glycolysis through PFK inhibition (Randle effect).[34] However, after shock and major injury, citrate does not accumulate.[135,136] This lack of accumulation may play a role in the persistence of glycolysis after injury.

Unlike fasting and starvation, hyperglycemia is a hallmark of the response to injury, sepsis, and stress. An increase in blood glucose occurs during both the ebb and flow phases and is proportional to the severity of the injury.[137,138] There is also an increased concentration of lactate, pyruvate, organic phosphates, total amino acids, glycerol, and free fatty acids. Changes in lactate, pyruvate, and alanine have also been found to correlate with the severity of injury.[131] The rise in the concentrations of glucose and other solutes contributes to an elevated plasma osmolality after hemorrhage and injury that is thought to be critical in the complete restitution of blood volume and plasma proteins.[107,139-142] The hyperosmolality appears to augment the transcapillary refill phase and the plasma protein restoration phase of blood volume restitution by mediating the movement of water from cells to the interstitium and ultimately to the plasma.[140-142]

The metabolic changes in carbohydrate metabolism arise primarily as the result of the actions and interactions of catecholamines, cortisol, glycogen, insulin, growth hormone, and somatostatin.* It is apparent that the elevated blood glucose concentration results from increased hepatic production and from impaired peripheral uptake that are under endocrine control. Both the ebb and the flow phases are associated with hyperglycemia, increased gluconeogenesis, and hepatic and peripheral insulin resistance. However, the mechanisms involved in these carbohydrate "abnormalities" are different. During the ebb phase, plasma insulin is clearly depressed in relationship to the degree of hyperglycemia.[99,137,145,146] This results from decreased B-cell sensitivity to glucose that is secondary to catecholamines, somatostatin, reduced pancreatic blood flow, and the increased activity of the sympathetic nervous system.[80,103,126,147-149] However, during the flow phase, B-cell sensitivity returns to normal, and insulin concentrations rise to more appropriate values. Nevertheless, hyperglycemia persists.[99,150]

In both the ebb and the flow phases, there is a delayed rate of assimilation of a glucose load, glucosuria, and a resistance to exogenously administered insulin.[143,147,151] Despite this "diabetes of injury," glucose uptake and use by peripheral tissues in both the ebb and the flow phases have been demonstrated consistently to be greater than under normal circumstances.[99,152-156] The resistance to insulin is manifested in a decreased glucose clearance. Consequently, the high plasma glucose concentration and the attendant increase in plasma-tissue glucose concentration gradient appear to overcome the resistance of peripheral tissues to glucose entry. The insulin resistance that develops appears to result from the action of catecholamines, cortisol, and other factors.[54,83,84,103,144]

Hepatic carbohydrate metabolism is also affected by insulin resistance. During the ebb phase, elevated concentration of catecholamines, cortisol, and glucagon and a decreased concentration of insulin result in rapid glycogenolysis and an outpouring of glucose from the liver. In addition, these hormonal alterations stimulate gluconeogenesis from alanine, lactate, and pyruvate. Growth hormone also is involved in these processes by inhibiting glucose uptake through inhibition of glucokinase. During the flow phase, gluconeogenesis persists despite near-normal concentrations of insulin. This persistence appears to result from insulin resistance and produces a continued flow of glucose from the liver. Therefore the hyperglycemia that results after injury results from a combination of increased glucose production and glucose release

*References 54, 83, 84, 137, 143, 144.

and from a peripheral resistance to the entrance of glucose.

After injury and during sepsis, glucose must be provided not only to RBCs, WBCs, renal medulla, and neural tissues, but also to wounded tissue.[149,157,158] Glucose uptake in wounded tissue is increased by up to 100%. Wounds demonstrate a lack of insulin sensitivity and do not increase their glucose uptake or glycogenesis in response to insulin.[49,159,160] The accelerated glucose uptake in wounded tissue and possibly in septic tissue appears to correlate with the degree of inflammatory cellular infiltrate.[158] In addition, it has recently been demonstrated that the accelerated glycolysis of wounded tissue may be aerobic and not anaerobic as thought previously.[157] In aerobic glycolysis, glycolysis proceeds to lactate in the presence of adequate oxygen. Thus oxygen consumption and carbon dioxide production are normal, but lactate production is accelerated. Increased lactate production may be related to an inability of the NADH shuttle to transfer reducing equivalents from the cytoplasm to the mitrochondrion.[73,161] Metabolic derangements suggestive of aerobic glycolysis have also been seen in septic tissue.[162] In this regard, it is of note that aerobic glycolysis is characteristic of the cellular infiltrate.[163]

As one might expect, negative nitrogen balance and net proteolysis are characteristic of the posttraumatic and the septic states.[164,165] However, only 20% of the protein broken down is used for calories.[60] The remainder is used in gluconeogenesis. As noted previously, the production of lactate in the presence of oxygen primarily results from the actions of cortisol, glucagon, catecholamines, and the decreased effectiveness of insulin.

The rise in urinary nitrogen is associated with an increased excretion of urea, sulfur, phosphorus, potassium, magnesium, and creatinine, suggesting the breakdown of intracellular material.[118,166] Isotope dilution studies suggest that this loss of protein results from the loss of cell mass rather than cell number.[118] The nitrogen-to-sulfur and nitrogen-to-potassium ratios suggest that this loss occurs mainly from muscle.[118] The marked increase in the urinary excretion of 3-methylhistidine during trauma, sepsis, and burns also suggests the importance of skeletal muscle in this response.[167-169] Analysis of the protein content and the incorporation of radiolabeled amino acids in visceral tissues and skeletal muscle confirm that it is skeletal muscle that is depleted and visceral tissue (liver, kidney) is spared.[170] This is the opposite of nonstressed starvation in which visceral protein is used before muscle protein and has been termed visceral translocation of protein.[27,170]

The alterations in plasma amino acids are not well defined during the ebb and flow phases. During the ebb phase, little change in total amino acid concentrations were noted by Elwyn et al.[171] until the late phases of shock. In addition, it appears that these changes result primarily from a decreased hepatic uptake[171] and not an increased peripheral release as was thought previously.[172] During the flow phase, alterations in plasma amino acids appear to be related to the severity of injury and the specific type of injury.[109,173-175] Alanine, the major gluconeogenic amino acid, appears to be released from peripheral tissues and taken up by the liver for gluconeogenesis. Early in the flow phase, the concentration of alanine in plasma is increased; but as the injury persists, serum alanine decreases, presumably as a result of its lack of availability in peripheral tissues and its continued hepatic uptake. Branched-chain amino acids and aspartate and asparagine are transaminated in peripheral tissues, and their remaining carbon fragments are used in the TCA cycle. Nonetheless, muscle concentrations of amino acids generally reveal normal or elevated concentrations of all amino acids except alanine, glutamine, and arginine.[176]

The net catabolism of protein can result from either increased catabolism, decreased synthesis, or a combination of the two. Available data on TBP turnover suggest that after injury the net changes in catabolism and synthesis depend on the severity of the injury.[177] Elective operations and minor injury appear to result in a decreased rate of synthesis with a normal rate of protein catabolism.[106,127] Severe trauma, burns, and sepsis appear to be associated with increases in both synthesis and catabolism but with a greater increase in the latter, resulting in net catabolism.[110,168,177,178] In this regard, it is important to note that accelerated proteolysis and a high rate of gluconeogenesis persist after injury and during sepsis.[173,179] This persistence appears to result from an inhibition of ketoadaptation after injury and sepsis. Unlike starvation, ketogenesis is not prominent, and it does not fuel the brain in significant amounts. Therefore a high requirement for glucose and therefore gluconeogenesis persists. The mechanism for this inhibition of ketoadaptation is not understood presently. Clowes et al.[180] have recently presented evidence suggesting the involvement of a circulating peptide containing 33 amino acids in this response. In addition, Baracos et al.[181] have proposed that interleukin-1 (a human leukocyte pyrogen) may be responsible for the accelerated proteolysis that accompanies fever and sepsis.

The net catabolism of protein that occurs after any injury is dependent on the prior nutritional status and intake, sex and age of the individual, and the severity of the injury. Young healthy males lose more protein in response to an injury than do women or the elderly.[30] In addition, the urinary excretion of nitrogen is less after a second operation if it closely follows the first.[132,165] This decline is presumably the result of a reduction in available protein stores. Finally, negative nitrogen balance can be reduced or virtually eliminated by high caloric and nitrogen supplementation.[25,143,178,182,183] Together, these facts suggest that the loss of protein that occurs after injury is not entirely obligatory to the injury but is also a manifestation of acute starvation.[133]

Local Wound Metabolism

Injury is associated with a negative bodily balance of many substrates.[184-187] Despite injury-induced abnormalities in cofactors and substrates known to be important in wound healing, most wounds heal after injury.[187-189] The ability of the wound to heal in the face of varying hormone and substrate supply suggests that the wound has a biologic priority over the host. This concept of biologic priority of healing wounds was described by Moore and Brennan,[190] who stated that 75% of wounds or surgical incisions healed to the point of tensile integrity during a period of negative energy and nitrogen balance. The other 25% healed in patients who returned to eating so rapidly that the period of negative balance was of minimal duration.[190] It is therefore evident that during a period of postinjury hormonal alterations and general catabolism, the wound has a favored status. This concept suggests that the metabolic and functional determinants of normal wound repair are inherent within the local wound environment. This further suggests that the local wound environment is differently sensitive to substrate and hormonal alterations than are other organ systems.

Cellular Infiltrate as a Determinant of Biologic Priority

Following injury, there is a local ordered infiltration of inflammatory cells and a characteristic pattern of cellular predominance within the wound over time. This ordered sequence of cellular predominance leads to every characteristic alterations in extracellular substrate concentrations, temporal effects of wound fluid on wound cell function, an altered sequence of expression for peptide growth factors, and degradation of classical peptide hormones.

It appears that the metabolism of the wound is determined by the cellular infiltrate and is independent of systemic hormonal and substrate alterations. This is supported by the following findings:

1. A direct relationship exists between DNA content of wounded tissue and the cellular infiltrate.[191]
2. Wounded tissue metabolizes glucose rapidly through aerobic glycolysis. This unusual form of glycolysis is characteristic of the leukocytes that comprise the cellular infiltrate.[192]
3. A time course for glucose uptake and lactate production by wounded tissue appears to correlate with the development of the cellular infiltrate.[191]
4. Autoradiographic studies using [^{3}H]-2-deoxyglucose reveal that the majority of the glucose uptake in wounded tissue occurs in the cellular infiltrate.[193]
5. Both wounded tissue and macrophages increase their glucose uptake in response to increasing glucose concentrations in the environment, and this glucose clearance is concentration independent. Thus the lack of saturation of glucose uptake of wounded tissue appears to be determined by the macrophages in the cellular infiltrate.[194]
6. A high PFK activity of wounded tissue can be explained by the PFK activity of the cellular infiltrate as measured by 5-[^{3}H]-glucose.[193]
7. Macrophage glucose uptake and lactate production are independent of local epinephrine concentrations.[195]
8. Macrophages have a stimulatory effect on the HEP content of resident host tissue.[196]
9. A decreased HEP content of wounded tissue appears to be secondary to the dilutional effect of the cellular infiltrate.[197]
10. The presence of macrophages seems to explain the pattern of purine release from wounded muscle.[198]
11. Glutamine utilization by the cellular infiltrate appears to explain the decrease in glutamine content of wounded tissue.[199]
12. In the isolated perfused system, hormone and substrate profiles similar to those found following injury do not affect wound metabolism.
13. A prior adrenalectomy does not affect wound metabolism despite substantial effects on noninjured tissue.

In addition, other investigators have shown a lack of effect of exogenous insulin on local wound metabolism in an incubated system.[200] Thus there are substantial data to support the position of the wound as independent of circulating hormone and substrate concentrations. Yet it is known that several of the more common clinical examples of impaired wound healing involve systemic hormonal and substrate changes. Specifically, diabetes mellitus,[201-204] steroid therapy,[205-207] amino acid deprivation,[208,209] an hypophysectomy[210] have been shown to impair wound healing.

In summary, generalized catabolism, hyperglycemia, persistent gluconeogenesis, protein wasting, negative nitrogen balance, heat production, and loss of the body mass that parallel the severity of the injury are characteristic after trauma and during sepsis. Most of the energy necessary for biologic processes to proceed is derived from fat. The net catabolism of 300 to 500 g of lean body mass per day is apparently required as a source of amino acids for gluconeogenesis. The persistence of the injury, particularly sepsis, through unknown mechanisms produces inhibition of the usual adaptive mechanisms that occur in starvation, resulting in the persistence of a highly catabolic state. This state in turn leads to protein wasting and malnutrition and ultimately in multiple organ failure[211] and in death if the stimuli are not eliminated.

SUMMARY

Starvation, stress from injury or surgical procedures, and sepsis induce a series of metabolic changes that are regulated by neuroendocrine reflexes and result in mobilization of substrates from endogenous tissue stores. These metabolic changes ensure that energy is available for vital functions, that oxygen delivery is maintained, and that reparative processes take place. An understanding of these complex metabolic interactions depends on an appreciation of normal homeostasis and the distribution of body water, proteins, fat, and carbohydrates. The role of each component of body tissue is important in periods of starvation, stress, and sepsis, especially when the ability to replenish endogenous food stores is impaired as a result of either the inability to consume adequate nutrients or the excessive consumption of tissue stores. The mechanisms described in this chapter illustrate the complexity of the metabolic response to stress, the interrelationships between the neuroendocrine responses and substrate mobilization and use, and the importance of adequate energy and tissue stores for survival and repair of the organisms under conditions of nutrient deprivation.

REFERENCES

1. Gann DS, Amaral JF. The pathology of trauma and shock. In Fridema GD, Rutherford WF, Bullinger WF, eds. The Management of Trauma. Philadelphia: WB Saunders, 1984.
2. Moore FD. The Body Cell Mass and its Supporting Environment. Philadelphia: WB Saunders, 1963.
3. Maxwell MH, Kleeman CR. Dynamics of body water and electrolytes. In Clinical Disorders of Fluid and Electrolyte Metabolism. 4th ed. New York: McGraw-Hill, 1987.
4. Edelman IS, Leibman J. Anatomy of body water and electrolytes. Am J Med 27:256, 1959.
5. Moore FD. Energy and the maintenance of the body cell mass. JPEN 4:228, 1980.
6. Grande F, Keys A. Body weight, body composition, and calorie status. In Goodhart RS, Shihs ME, eds. Modern Nutrition in Health and Disease. Philadelphia: Lea & Febiger, 1980.
7. Behnke AR, Wilmore JH. Evaluation and Regulation of Body Build and Composition. Englewood Cliffs, N.J.: Prentice Hall, 1974.
8. Pace H, Rathbun EN. Studies in body composition. III. The body water and chemically combined nitrogen content in relation to fat content. J Biol Chem 158:685, 1945.
9. Behnke AR. Physiologic studies pertaining to deep sea diving and aviation, especially in relation to the fat content and composition of the body. Harvey Lect 37:198, 1941.
10. Brozek J, et al. Densitometric analysis of body composition: Revision of some quantitative assumptions. Ann NY Acad Sci 110:113, 1963.
11. Baylis PH, Zerbe RL, Robertson GL. Arginine vasopressin response to insulin-induced hypoglycemia in man. J Clin Endocrinol Metab 53:935, 1981.
12. Bereiter DA, Plotsky PM, Gann DS. Tooth pulp stimulation potentiates the ACTH response to hemorrhage in cats. Endocrinology 111:1127, 1982.
13. Lesser GT, Deutsch S, Markofsy T. Use of independent measurement of body fat to evaluate overweight and underweight. Metabolism 20:792, 1971.
14. Norris AH, Lundry T, Shock NW. Trends in selected indices of body composition in men between the ages 30 and 80 years. Ann NY Acad Sci 110:623, 1963.
15. Vaglcirsdottir K, Munro HN. Protein and amino acid metabolism. In Fischer JE, ed. Surgical Nutrition. Boston: Little Brown, 1983.
16. Munro HN, Young VR. Protein metabolism in the elderly: Observations relating to dietary needs. Postgrad Med 63:143, 1978.
17. Harvey TC, et al. Measurement of whole body nitrogen by neutron activation analysis. Lancet 2:359, 1973.
18. Tarso PJ, Spafford MS, Blaw M. The metabolism of water and electrolytes in congestive heart failure. J Lab Clin Med 41:280, 1953.
19. Hill GL, et al. Multi-element analysis of the living body by neutron activation analysis—Application to critically ill patients receiving intravenous nutrition. Br J Surg 66:868, 1979.
20. Cahill GF. Starvation in man. N Engl J Med 668:282, 1970.
21. Kinney JM, Gump FE. The metabolic response to injury. In American College of Surgeons, eds. Manual of Pre and Post Operative Care. Philadelphia: WB Saunders, 1983.
22. Hastings AB. The electrolytes of tissue and body fluids. Harvey Lect 36:91, 1940-1941.
23. Shizgal HM, et al. The indirect measurement of total exchangeable potassium. Am J Physiol 233:F253, 1977.
24. Randall HT. Water, electrolytes and acid base balance. In Goodhart RS, Shils ME, eds. Modern Nutrition in Health and Disease. Philadelphia: Lea & Febiger, 1980.
25. Kinney JM, Lister J, Moore FD. Relationship of energy expenditure to total exchangeable potassium. Ann NY Acad Sci 110:711, 1963.
26. Drabkin DL. The distribution of the chromoproteins, hemoglobin, myoglobin and cytochrome C, in the tissue of different species, and the relationship to the total content of each chromoprotein to body mass. J Biol Chem 182:317, 1950.
27. Kinney JM. Energy requirements in injury and sepsis. Acta Anaesthesiol Scand 55:15, 1974.
28. Dubois EF. The Mechanism of Heat Loss and Temperature Regulation. Lane Medical Lectures. Stanford University Press, 1937.
29. Clowes GHA, Randall H, Cha C. Effects of parenteral alimentation on metabolism in septic patients. Surgery 88:531, 1980.
30. Shizgal HM, Milne CA, Spainer HA. The effect of nitrogen-sparing intravenously administered fluids on postoperative body composition. Surgery 86:60, 1979.
31. Lehninger AL. Biochemistry: The Molecular Basis of Cell Structure and Function. 2nd ed. New York: Worth Publishing, 1975.
32. Lehninger AL. Bioenergetics, 2nd ed. Menlo Park, Calif.: Benjamin/Cummings Publishing, 1972.
33. Atkinson DE. The energy charge of the adenylate pool as a regulator parameter interaction with feedback modifiers. Biochemistry 7:4030, 1966.
34. Newsholme EA, Start C. Regulation in Metabolism. New York: John Wiley, 1973.
35. Bie P. Osmoreceptors, vasopressin, and control of renal water excretion. Physiol Rev 60:961, 1980.
36. McGilvery RW. Biochemistry—A Functional Approach. Philadelphia: WB Saunders, 1970.
37. Harper HA, Rodwell VW, Mayes PA. Review of physiological chemistry, 16th ed. Los Altos, Calif.: Lange Medical Publications, 1977.
38. Exton JH. Gluconeogenesis, Metabolism 21:945, 1972.
39. Krebs HA. The metabolic fate of amino acids. In Munroe HN, Allison JB, eds. Mammalian Protein Metabolism. New York: Academic Press, 1964.
40. Munro HN. Biochemical aspects of protein metabolism. In Munro HN, Allison JB, eds. Mammalian Protein Metabolism. New York: Academic Press, 1964.
41. Munro HN, Crim MC. The proteins and amino acids. In Goodhart RS, Shils ME, eds. Modern Nutrition in Health and Disease. Philadelphia: Lea & Febiger, 1980.
42. Mallette LE, Exton JH, Park CR. Control of gluconeogenesis from amino acids in the perfused rat liver. J Biol Chem 244:5713, 1969.
43. Felig P. The glucose-alanine cycle. Metabolism 22:179, 1973.
44. White A, Handler P, Smith EL. Principles of Biochemistry. New York: McGraw-Hill, 1973.
45. Atkinson DE, Bourke E. The role of ureagenesis in pH homeostasis. Trends Biochem Sci 9:297, 1984.
46. Ross BD, Hems R, Krebs HA. The rate of gluconeogenesis from various precursors in the perfused rat liver. Biochem J 102:942, 1967.
47. Cahill GF. Ketosis. JPEN 5:281, 1981.
48. Masoro EJ. Lipids and lipid metabolism. Annu Rev Physiol 39:301, 1977.
49. Nelson KM, Turinsky J. Analysis of postburn insulin unresponsiveness in skeletal muscle. J Surg Res 31:404, 1981.

50. Korchak HM, Masoro EJ. Changes in the level of the fatty acids synthesizing enzymes during starvation. Biochem Biophys Acta 58:354, 1962.
51. McGarry JD, Foster DW. Hormonal control of ketogenesis: Biochemical considerations. Arch Intern Med 137:495, 1977.
52. Egdahl RH. Pituitary-adrenal response following trauma to the isolated leg. Surgery 46:9, 1959.
53. Gann DS, Ward DG, Carlson DE. Neural control of ACTH: A hemostatic reflex. Recent Prog Horm Res 35:357, 1978.
54. Rizza RA, et al. Adrenergic mechanism for the effect of epinephrine on glucose production and clearance in man. J Clin Invest 65:682, 1980.
55. Kaplan NM, Bartter FC. The effect of ACTH, renin angiotensin II and various precursors on biosynthesis of aldosterone by adrenal slices. J Clin Invest 41:715, 1962.
56. Guyton AC. Textbook of Medical Physiology, 6th ed. Philadelphia: WB Saunders, 1981.
57. Gann DS, Dallman MF, Engeland WC. Reflex control and modulation of ACTH and corticosteroids. In McCann SM, ed. Endocrinology Physiology. III. International Review of Physiology, vol. 24, Baltimore: University Park Press, 1981.
58. Cannon WB. The Wisdom of the Body. New York: WW Norton, 1939.
59. Egdabl RH. The differential response of the adrenal cortex and medulla to bacterial endotoxin. J Clin Invest 38:1120, 1959.
60. Duke JH, et al. Contribution of protein to caloric expenditure following injury. Surgery 68:168, 1970.
61. Gann DS, Cryer GL, Pirkle JC Jr. Physiological inhibition and facilitation of adrenocortical response to hemorrhage. Am J Physiol 232:R5, 1977.
62. Lilly MP, Engeland WC, Gann DS. Adrenal response to repeated hemorrhage: Implications for studies of trauma. J Trauma 22:809, 1982.
63. Lilly MP, Gann DS. The effect of repeated operation on the response of the adrenal cortex to infused ACTH. Surg Forum 33:10, 1982.
64. Raff H, Shinsako J, Dallman MF. Surgery potentiates adrenocortical responses to hypoxia in dogs. Proc Soc Exp Biol Med 172:400, 1983.
65. Wood CE, et al. Hormonal and hemodynamic responses to 15 ml/kg hemorrhage in conscious dogs: Responses correlate to body temperature. Proc Soc Exp Biol Med 167:15, 1981.
66. Roth J, Grunfeld C. Endocrine systems: Mechanisms of disease, target cells, and receptors. In William RH, ed. Textbook of Endocrinology. Philadelphia: WB Saunders, 1981.
67. O'Malley BW, Schrader WT. The receptors of steroid hormones. Sci Am 234:32, 1976.
68. Oppenheimer JH. Thyroid hormone action at the cellular level. Science 203:971, 1979.
69. Rasmusen H. Calcium and cAMP as Synarchic Messengers. New York: John Wiley, 1981.
70. Sutherland EW. Studies on the mechanism of hormone action. Science 177:401, 1972.
71. Greengard P. Phosphorylated proteins as physiological effectors. Science 199:146, 1978.
72. Fain JN. Involvement of phosphatidylinositol breakdown in elevation of cytosol Ca^{2+} by hormones and relationship to prostaglandin formation. In Kohn LD, ed. Hormone Receptors, vol. 6. New York: John Wiley, 1982.
73. Needham AE. Regeneration of wound healing. In Albercrombie M, ed. Methuen's Monographs on Geological Subjects. New York: John Wiley, 1952.
74. Felig P. The endocrine pancreas: Diabetes mellitus. In Felig P, et al., eds. Endocrinology and Metabolism. New York: McGraw-Hill, p 761.
75. Porte D Jr, Halter JB. The endocrine pancreas and diabetes mellitus. In Williams RH, ed. Textbook of Endocrinology. Philadelphia: WB Saunders, 1981.
76. McIntyre N, Holdsworth CD, Turner DS. Intestinal factors in the control of insulin secretion. J Clin Endocrinol Metab 25:1317, 1965.
77. Raptis S, et al. Differences in insulin, growth hormone, and pancreatic enzyme secretion after intravenous and intraduodenal administration of mixed amino acids in man. N Engl J Med 288:1199, 1973.
78. Reichlin S. Somatostatin. N Engl J Med 309:1495, 1983.
79. Kaneto A, Kajinuma H, Kosaka K. Effect of splanchnic nerve stimulation on glucagon and insulin output in the dog. Endocrinology 96:143, 1975.
80. Porte D Jr, Smith PH, Ensinick JW. Neurohumoral regulation of the pancreatic islet A and B cells. Metabolism 25:1453, 1976.
81. Feldman M, et al. Beta-endorphin and the endocrine pancreas. N Engl J Med 208:350, 1983.
82. Felig P, Wahren J, Hendler R. Influence of physiologic hyperglucagonemia on basal and insulin inhibited splanchnic glucose output in normal man. J Clin Invest 58:961, 1976.
83. Eigler N, Sacca L, Sherwin RS. Synergistic interactions of physiologic increments of glucagon, epinephrine, and cortisol in the dog. J Clin Invest 63:114, 1979.
84. Felig P, et al. Hormonal interactions in the regulation of blood glucose. Recent Prog Horm Res 35:501, 1979.
85. Unger RH, Dobbs RE, Orci L. Insulin, glucagon, and somatostatin secretion in the regulation of metabolism. Ann Rev Physiol 40:307, 1978.
86. Kawai K, et al. Circulating somatostatin acts on the islet of Langerhans by way of a somatostatin poor compartment. Science 218:417, 1982.
87. Kraus-Friedmann H. Hormonal regulation of hepatic gluconeogenesis. Physiol Rev 64:170, 1984.
88. Nanni G, et al. Increased lipid fuel dependence in the critically ill septic patient. J Trauma 24:14, 1983.
89. Parmley WW, Glick G, Sonnenblick EH. Cardiovascular effects of glucagon in man. N Engl J Med 12:279, 1968.
90. Posefsky T, et al. Metabolism of forearm tissues in man: Studies with glucagon. Diabetes 25:128, 1976.
91. Unger RH, Orci L. Glucagon and the A cell: Physiology and pathophysiology. N Engl J Med 304:1518, 1981.
92. Fradkin J, et al. Evidence for an important role of changes in relative rather than absolute concentrations of glucagon in the regulation of glucose production in humans. J Clin Endocrinol Metab 50:698, 1980.
93. Unger RH. Diabetes and the alpha cell. Diabetes 25:136, 1976.
94. Gibbs DM. Measurement of hypothalamic corticotropin-releasing factors in hypophyseal-portal blood. Federat Proc 44(1, Pt 2):203, 1985.
95. Makara G. Pathways by which stressful stimuli activate the pituitary-adrenal system. Regul Pept (in press).
96. Yates FE, Marsh DJ, Maran JW. The adrenal cortex. In Mountcastle VB, ed. Medical Physiology, 14th ed. St. Louis: Mosby, 1980.
97. Cryer PE. Physiology and pathophysiology of the human sympathoadrenal neuroendocrine system. N Engl J Med 303:436, 1980.
98. Gann DS, Lilly MP. The neuroendocrine response to multiple trauma. World J Surg 7:101, 1983.
99. Wilmore DW, Mason AD, Pruitt BA. Insulin response to glucose in hypermetabolic burn patients. Ann Surg 183:314, 1976.
100. Fain JN, Garcia-Sainz JA. Adrenergic regulation of adipocyte metabolism. J Lipid Res 24:945, 1983.
101. Altszuler N, et al. Glucose metabolism and plasma insulin level during epinephrine infusion in the dog. Am J Physiol 212:677, 1967.

102. Chaisson JL, et al. Inhibitory effect of epinephrine on insulin stimulated glucose uptake by rat skeletal muscle. J Clin Invest 68:706, 1981.
103. Palmer BQ, et al. Epinephrine acutely mediates skeletal muscle insulin resistance. Surgery 94:172, 1983.
104. Goodman HM. The pituitary gland. In Mountcastle VB, ed. Medical Physiology, 14th ed. St. Louis: Mosby, 1980.
105. Frohman LA. Diseases of the anterior pituitary. In Felig P, et al., eds. Endocrinology and Metabolism. New York: McGraw-Hill, 1981.
106. Crane CW, et al. Protein turnover in patients before and after elective orthopedic operations. Br J Surg 64:129, 1977.
107. Kenney PR, Allen-Rowlands CF, Gann DS. Glucose and osmolality as predictors of injury severity. J Trauma 23:712, 1983.
108. Keys A, et al. The Biology of Human Starvation. Minneapolis: University of Minnesota Press, 1950.
109. Freund HR, Ryan JA, Fischer JE. Amino acid derangements in patients with sepsis: Treatment with branched chain amino acid rich infusions. Ann Surg 188:423, 1978.
110. Kien CL, et al. Increased rates of whole body protein synthesis and breakdown in children recovering from burns. Ann Surg 187:383, 1978.
111. Browne JSL, Schenker V. Conferences on Metabolic Aspects of Convalescence Including Bone and Wound Healing: Transactions of the Third Meeting. New York: Joshiah Macy, 1943.
112. Moore FD, Brennan MF. Surgical injury: Body composition, protein metabolism and neuroendocrinology. In Ballinger WF, et al., eds. Manual of Surgical Nutrition. Philadelphia: WB Saunders, 1975.
113. Owen OE, et al. Brain metabolism during fasting. J Clin Invest 46:1589, 1967.
114. Crowley CV, et al. Effects of environmental temperature and femoral fracture on wound healing in rats. J Trauma 17:436, 1977.
115. Palmblad J, et al. Effect of total energy withdrawal (fasting) on the levels of growth hormone, thyrotropin, cortisol, adrenaline, norepinephrine, T4, T3 and rT3 in healthy males. Acta Med Scand 201:15, 1977.
116. Levenson SM, Seifter E. Starvation. In Fischer JE, ed. Metabolic and Physiologic Responses. Boston: Little, Brown, 1982.
117. Studley HO. Percentage of weight loss, a basic indicator of surgical risk. JAMA 106:458, 1936.
118. Cuthbertson DP. Observations on the disturbance of metabolism by injury to the limbs. Q J Med 1:233, 1932.
119. Cuthbertson DP. Further observations on the disturbance of metabolism caused by injury, with particular reference to the dietary requirements of fracture cases. Br J Surg 23:505, 1936.
120. Moore FD. Bodily changes in surgical convalescence. Ann Surg 137:289, 1953.
121. Wilmore DW, et al. Effect of injury and infection on visceral metabolism and circulation. Ann Surg 192:491, 1980.
122. Askanazi J, et al. Respiratory distress secondary to a high carbohydrate load. Surgery 86:596, 1980.
123. Fain JN, Kovacev VP, Scow RO. Effect of growth hormone and dexamethasone on lipolysis and metabolism in isolated fat cells of the rat. J Biol Chem 240:3522, 1965.
124. Shafnr E, Steinberg D. The essential role of the adrenal cortex in the response of plasma free fatty acids, cholesterol, and phospholipids to epinephrine injection. J Clin Invest 39:310, 1960.
125. Coran AG, et al. Fat and carbohydrate metabolism during hemorrhagic shock in the unanesthetized baboon. Surg Forum 9:10, 1971.
126. Halmagyi DFJ, Irving MH, Varga D. Effect of adrenergic blockade on the metabolic response to hemorrhagic shock. J Appl Physiol 25:384, 1968.
127. O'Keefe SJD, Sender PM, James WPT. Catabolic loss of body nitrogen in response to surgery. Lancet 2:1035, 1974.
128. Kovach AGB, et al. Blood flow, oxygen consumption, and free fatty acid release in subcutaneous adipose tissue during hemorrhagic shock in control and phenoxybenzamine-treated dogs. Circ Res 26:733, 1970.
129. Birkhain RH, et al. A comparison of the effects of skeletal trauma and surgery on the ketosis of starvation in man. J Trauma 21:513, 1981.
130. Mays ET. The effect of surgical stress on plasma-free fatty acids. J Surg Res 10:315, 1970.
131. Oppenheim W, Williamson D, Smith R. Early biochemical changes and severity of injury in man. J Trauma 20:135, 1980.
132. Smith R, et al. Initial effect of injury on ketone bodies and other blood metabolites. Lancet 1:1, 1975.
133. Stoner HB, et al. The relationships between plasma substrates and hormones and the severity of injury in 277 recently injured patients. Clin Sci 56:563, 1979.
134. Miller JDB, Bistran BR, Blackburn GL. Failure of postoperative infection to increase nitrogen excretion in patients maintained on peripheral amino acids. Am J Clin Nutr 30:1523, 1977.
135. Drucker WR, et al. Citrate metabolism during surgery. Arch Surg 85:557, 1962.
136. Morris AS, et al. The role of effectors of phosphofructokinase on the regulation of aerobic glycolysis in a A-carrageenan wounded muscle. Metabolism (in press).
137. Carey LC, Lowery BD, Cloutier CT. Blood sugar and insulin response in human shock. Ann Surg 172:342, 1970.
138. Meguid MM, et al. Hormone-substrate interrelationships following trauma. Arch Surg 109:776, 1974.
139. Byrnes GJ, Pirkle JC Jr, Gann DS. Cardiovascular stabilization after hemorrhage depends upon restitution of blood volume. J Trauma 18:623, 1978.
140. Drucker WR, Chadwick CDJ, Gann DS. Transcapillary refill in hemorrhage and shock. Arch Surg 116:1344, 1981.
141. Gann DS. Endocrine control of plasma protein and volume. Surg Clin North Am 56:1135, 1976.
142. Gann DS, et al. Role of solute in the early restitution of blood volume after hemorrhage. Surgery 94:439, 1983.
143. Carey LC, Cloutier CT, Lowery BD. Growth hormone and adrenal cortisol response to shock and trauma in the human. Ann Surg 174:451, 1971.
144. Rizza RA, Mandarino LJ, Gerich JE. Cortisol induced insulin resistance in man: Impaired suppression of glucose production and stimulation of glucose utilization due to a postreceptor defect of insulin action. J Clin Endocrinol Metab 54:131, 1982.
145. Cryer PE, Herman CM, Sode J. Carbohydrate metabolism in the baboon subjected to gram-negative septicemia. I. Hyperglycemia with depressed plasma insulin concentrations. J Lab Clin Med 79:622, 1972.
146. Moss GS, et al. Serum insulin response in hemorrhagic shock in baboons. Surgery 68:34, 1970.
147. Black PR, et al. Mechanisms of insulin resistance following injury. Ann Surg 196:420, 1982.
148. Drucker WR, et al. The effect of persisting hypovolemic shock on pancreatic output of insulin. In Kovach AGB, Stoner HB, Spitzer JJ, eds. Neurohumoral and Metabolic Response to Injury. New York: Plenum Publishing, 1978.
149. Hiebert JM, et al. Insulin response to hemorrhagic shock in the intact and adrenalectomized primate. Am J Surg 125:501, 1973.
150. Kahn CR. Insulin resistance, insulin insensitivity and insulin unresponsiveness: A necessary definition. Metabolism 27:1893, 1973.
151. Allison SP, Hinton P, Chamberlain JJ. Intravenous glucose tolerance insulin and free fatty acid levels in burn patients. Lancet 2:1116, 1968.
152. Drucker WR, Dekieweit JC. Glucose uptake by diaphragm from rats subjected to hemorrhagic shock. Am J Physiol 206:317, 1964.

153. Long CL, et al. Carbohydrate metabolism in men: Effect of elective operations and major injury. J Appl Physiol 31:110, 1971.
154. Randle PJ, Smith GH. Regulation of glucose uptake by muscle. I. The effect of insulin, anaerobosis and cell poisons on the uptake of glucose and release of potassium by isolated rat diaphragm. Biochem J 70:409, 1958.
155. Russel JA, Long CNH, Engel FL. Biochemical studies of shock: Peripheral tissues on the metabolism of protein and carbohydrate during hemorrhagic shock in the rat. J Exp Med 79:1, 1944.
156. Swerlick RA, Drucker NA, McCoy S. Insulin effectiveness in hypovolemic dogs. J Trauma 21:1013, 1981.
157. Caldwell MD, et al. Evidence for aerobic glycolysis in A-carrageenan wounded skeletal muscle. J Surg Res 37:63, 1984.
158. Turinsky J. Glucose metabolism in the region recovering from burn injury. Endocrinology 113:1370, 1983.
159. Nelson KM, Turinsky J. Local effect of burn on skeletal muscle insulin responsiveness. J Surg Res 31:288, 1981.
160. Wilmore DW, et al. Influence of the burn wound on local and systemic responses to injury. Ann Surg 186:444, 1977.
161. Hochachka PN. Living without Oxygen. Cambridge, Mass: Harvard University Press, 1980.
162. Romanosky AJ, et al. Increased muscle glucose uptake and lactate release after endotoxin administration. Am J Physiol 239:E311, 1980.
163. Ross R. The fibroblast and wound repair. Biol Rev 43:51, 1968.
164. Abbott WE, Anderson K. The effect of starvation, infection, and injury on the metabolic processes and body composition. Ann NY Acad Sci 110:941, 1963.
165. Siegel JH, et al. Physiological and metabolic correlations in human sepsis. Surgery 86:163, 1979.
166. Frawley JP, Artz CP, Howard JM. Muscle metabolism and catabolism in combat casualties. Arch Surg 71:612, 1955.
167. Bilmazer C, et al. Quantitative contribution by skeletal muscle to elevated rates of whole-body protein breakdown in burned children as measured by 3-MEH output. Metabolism 27:671, 1978.
168. Long CL, et al. Muscle protein catabolism in the septic patient as measured by 3-methyl histidine excretion. Am J Clin Nutr 30:1349, 1977.
169. Williamson OH, et al. Muscle-protein catabolism after injury in man, as measured by urinary excretion of 3-methyl histidine. Clin Sci Mol Med 52:527, 1977.
170. Ryan NT. Metabolic adaptations for energy production during trauma and sepsis. Surg Clin North Am S6:1073, 1976.
171. Elwyn DH, et al. Interorgan transport of amino acids in hemorrhagic shock. Am J Physiol 231:377, 1976.
172. Engel FL. The significance of the metabolic changes during shock. Ann NY Acad Sci 55:383, 1956.
173. Clowes GHA, Randall H, Cha C. Amino acid and energy metabolism in septic and traumatized patients. JPEN 4:195, 1980.
174. Dale G, et al. The effect of surgical operation on venous plasma free amino acids. Surgery 81:295, 1977.
175. Woolfe LI, Groves AC, Moore JP. Arterial plasma amino acids in patients with serious postoperative infections and in patients with major fractures. Surgery 79:283, 1976.
176. Askanazi J, et al. Muscle and plasma amino acids following injury. Ann Surg 192:78, 1980.
177. Birkhain RH, et al. Effects of major skeletal trauma on whole body protein turnover in man measured by L-[1,14C]-leucine. Surgery 88:294, 1980.
178. Stein TP, et al. Changes in protein synthesis after trauma: Importance of nutrition. Am J Physiol 233:E348, 1977.
179. O'Donnell TF, et al. Proteolysis associated with a deficit of peripheral energy fuel substrates in septic man. Surgery 80:192, 1976.
180. Clowes GHA, et al. Muscle proteolysis induced by a circulating peptide in patients with sepsis or trauma. N Engl J Med 308:545, 1983.
181. Baracos V, et al. Stimulation of muscle protein degradation and prostaglandin E_2 release by leukocyte pyrogen (interleukin-1). N Engl J Med 308:553, 1983.
182. Schrier RW, Berl WT, Anderson RJ. Osmotic and nonosmotic control of vasopressin release. Am J Physiol 236:F321, 1979.
183. Stephens RV, Randall HT. Use of a concentrated, balanced, liquid elemental diet for nutritional management of catabolic states. Ann Surg 170:642, 1969.
184. Levenson SM, Green RW, Taylor FH. Ascorbic acid, riboflavin, thiamine and nicotinic acid in relation to severe injury, hemorrhage and infection in the human. Ann Surg 124:840, 1946.
185. Lund CC, Levenson SM, Green RW. Ascorbic acid, thiamine, riboflavin and nicotinic acid in relation to acute burns in man. Arch Surg 55:557, 1947.
186. Cuthbertson DP. Interrelationships of metabolic changes consequent to injury. Br Med Bull 10:33-37, 1954.
187. Moore FD. Metabolic Care of the Surgical Patient. Philadelphia: WB Saunders, 1959.
188. Hunt TK, VanWinkle W. In Hunt TK, Dunphy JE, eds. Fundamentals of Wound Management. New York: Appleton-Century-Crofts, 1979, p 2.
189. Levenson SM, Seifter E, VanWinkle W. In Hunt TK, Dunphy JE, eds. Fundamentals of Wound Management. New York: Appleton-Century-Crofts, 1979, p 286.
190. Moore FD, Brennan MF. Manual of Surgical Nutrition, by the Committee on Pre- and Post-operative Care of the American College of Surgeons. Philadelphia: 1975, WB Saunders, p 169.
191. Daley JM, et al. Does wounded tissue regulate hepatic glucose production. Surg Forum 38:23, 1987.
192. Caldwell MD, et al. Evidence for aerobic glycolysis in lambda-carrageenan wounded skeletal muscle. J Surg Res 37:63, 1984.
193. Forster J, et al. Glucose uptake and flux through phosphofructokinase in wounded rate skeletal muscle. Am J Physiol (Endocrinol Metab 19) 256:E788, 1989.
194. Caldwell MD. Carbohydrate and energy metabolism in healing wounds. In Barbul A, et al. Growth Factors and Other Aspects of Wound Healing: Biological and Clinical Implications. New York: Alan R Liss, 1988, p 183.
195. Forster J, et al. Glucose uptake and flux through phosphofructokinase in wounded rat skeletal muscle. Am J Physiol 256(6):E788, 1989.
196. Morris A, et al. A macrophage-mediated factor that increases the high energy phosphate content of skeletal muscle. J Surg Res 38:373, 1985.
197. Morris A, et al. Macrophage interaction with skeletal muscle: Potential role of macrophages in determining the energy state of healing wounds. J Trauma 25(8):751, 1985.
198. Morris AS, et al. The role of purine metabolism in the macrophage mediated increase in high energy phosphates in skeletal muscle. J Surg Res 41:339, 1986.
199. Caldwell MD. Local glutamine metabolism in wounds and inflammation. Metabolism 38(Suppl 1):34, 1989.
200. Turinksy J. Glucose metabolism in the region recovering from burn injury: Effect of insulin on 2-deoxyglucose uptake in vivo. Endocrinology 13:1370, 1983.
201. Goodson WH, Hunt TK. Studies of wound healing in experimental diabetes mellitus. J Surg Res 22:221, 1977.
202. Spanheimer RG, Umpierrez GE, Stumpf V. Decreased collagen production in diabetic rats. Diabetes 37:371, 1988.
203. Yue EK, et al. Effects of experimental diabetes, uremia, and malnutrition on wound healing. Diabetes 36:295, 1987.
204. Rosenberg CS. Wound healing in the patient with diabetes mellitus. Nurs Clin North Am 25:247, 1990.
205. Ehrlich HP, Hunt TK. Effects of cortisone and vitamin A on wound healing. Ann Surg 167:324, 1968.

206. Hunt TK, et al. Effects of vitamin A on reversing the inhibitory effect of cortisone on healing of open wounds in animal and man. Ann Surg 170:633, 1969.
207. Salmela K, et al. The effect of local methylprednisolone on granulation tissue formation. Acta Chir Scand 146:541, 1980.
208. Seifter E, et al. Arginine: An essential amino acid for injured rats. Surgery 84:224, 1978.
209. Barbul A. Arginine: Biochemistry, physiology and therapeutic implications. J Parenter Enter Nutr 10:227, 1986.
210. Skottner A, et al. Anabolic and tissue repair functions of recombinant insulin-like growth factor 1. Acta Paediatr Scand (Suppl) 367:63, 1990.
211. Hassett J, Border JR. The metabolic response to trauma and sepsis, World J Surg 7:125, 1983.

2

Fluid and Electrolyte Physiology and Pathophysiology

Peter J. Fabri

The human body can be likened to a sac of electrolyte-rich fluids in which is suspended or dissolved a complex network of solids known collectively as "organs." The common medium of these fluids is water; the electrolytes are a mixture of primarily monovalent and divalent ions. The total volume of water, known as total body water, accounts for approximately 60% of total body mass. Substances are continually added to and excreted from this aqueous environment, and only through a system of homeostatic, protective mechanisms is the composition and distribution of this fluid-based system maintained. Disease, pharmaceuticals, and medical interventions have the potential to disrupt the balance of this fluid medium and result in clinically evident fluid and electrolyte disturbances. To achieve the desired goal of preventing or treating such disturbances, the nature, composition, and interrelationships of these fluids and the homeostatic mechanisms that maintain them must be clearly understood.

MAINTENANCE OF THE INTERNAL MILIEU: TOTAL BODY WATER

Water is the universal solvent of the human body. The total volume of this substance is subdivided into discrete parts known as intracellular, extracellular, and transcellular water (Fig. 2-1). These parts are separated by semipermeable membranes equipped with energy-consuming, work-producing pumps that are usually based on an adenosine-triphoshatase (ATPase) enzyme system. These pumps are able to maintain electrochemical and concentration gradients across membranes that result in a marked difference in composition between the intracellular and extracellular spaces. Water, on the other hand, passively follows the laws of osmotic and ionic equilibrium. It traverses these membranes freely to maintain an equal number of solute molecules (osmolality) and ionic particles (tonicity) per unit volume on each side of such semipermeable membranes. This difference between the control of solute/ions and that of water results in marked differences in volume and electrolyte composition of the two spaces. The normal balance can be disturbed by changing the number of solute molecules on either side of the membrane (e.g., hypoalbuminemia, hyperglycemia) or by disrupting its enzyme-based pumps (e.g., shock, digitalis).

The extracellular space can be considered an open system in that the alimentary tract serves as a mode of entrance and exit of water and solute as shown in Fig. 2-1. Similarly, the lungs, kidneys, and skin also serve as excretory conduits. Entrance and excretion of water and solute are controlled by active systems that are under homeostatic (nervous or hormonal) control. Thus the composition of this open, extracellular system can be maintained within relatively tight limits.[1] Nonstandard entrance routes, such as the administration of fluids intravenously, bypass the normal entry control mechanisms and directly add water and solute to the extracellular space. In this circumstance the *intrinsic* ability of the excretory systems to maintain osmotic and ionic stability becomes the limiting factor in maintaining ionic stability and composition of the extracellular space. Failure of these excretory control mechanisms, either by inability to conserve or increase loss, threatens the chemical stability of the extracellular fluids.

The intracellular space, on the other hand, is a closed space and is represented by the numerous cells floating within the extracellular water in Fig. 2-1. The only route of entrance and exit is across the semipermeable cellular membrane and its contained enzyme systems. Therefore extracellular space can be thought of as a conduit and the buffer zone to the intracellular space. Only by transfer from or to the extracellular water can intracellular composition be changed. This complex system, richly furnished with active transport mechanisms and buffer zones, rigidly protects the stability of the body fluids and maintains constancy of the internal milieu. Although not depicted accurately in our model, two thirds of the total body water

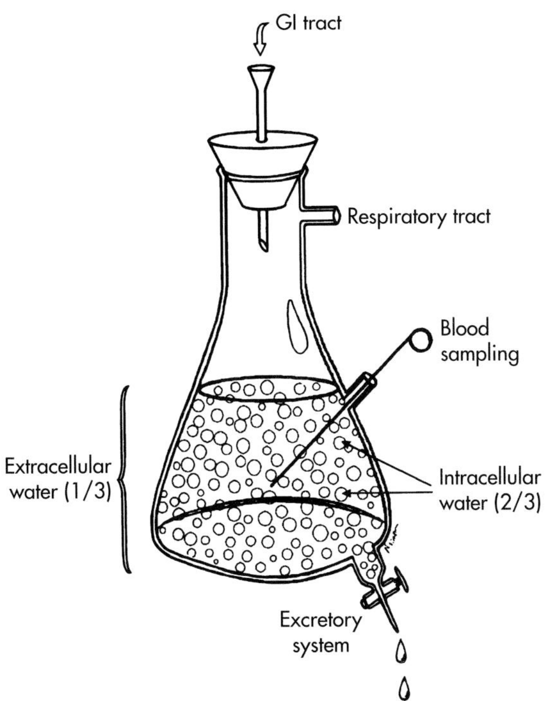

Fig. 2-1. Conceptualized model of the human body. Note that everything enters into, is excreted from, and is sampled in extracellular water.

Table 2-1. Normal Distribution of Body Water as Percent of Body Weight

	Men (%)	Women* (%)
Total body water	60	55
Extracellular water	15	15
Intracellular water	45	40

*Values are less than equivalent for men because women have a relatively greater amount of adipose tissue.

is intracellular, and one third is extracellular. This translates to about 40% and 20% of total body weight for the intracellular and extracellular compartments, respectively (Table 2-1).

Extracellular Water

The extracellular space is composed of the intravascular space (blood cells plus plasma) (comprising about 8% of total body weight) and the extravascular space (interstitial fluid and lymph). Cerebrospinal fluid is a specialized subspace of extracellular fluid. The vascular and extravascular spaces are in relative continuity, separated only by the rather permeable basement membranes of the blood vessel walls. When these vessels are intact, the formed, cellular elements of the blood remain contained in the intravascular space, whereas the aqueous, noncellular plasma undergoes continuous "filtration" through the relatively leaky vessel walls into the extravascular space. The extravascular space, however, is continuously "drained" by a system of lymphatic channels that return protein-rich extracellular fluid to the vascular space through the lymphatic ducts. This continuous-cycle system results in moment-to-moment renewing of the interstitial, pericellular space, bringing fresh nutrients from and carrying waste products to the vascular space, which is in direct continuity with normal routes of incretion and excretion.

The volume of intravascular fluid (blood) is determined by the oncotic effect of blood cells and large molecules such as albumin, as well as the rate of return of lymph. The volume of the extravascular fluid space depends on the balance between "filtration" of plasma and "drainage" of lymph. Plasma is continuously filtered across the vascular pores, particularly at the capillary level. The rate of filtration is governed by Starling's law, which takes into account net hydrostatic pressure, net oncotic pressure, and pore size (reflectance and permeability). Fluid shifts across the vascular membrane are controlled by the summed effect of hydrostatic and oncotic pressures. Hydrostatic pressure exists in both the vessel (mean capillary pressure) and the tissue (mean tissue pressure). The difference results in a vector force that typically acts to drive fluid into the extravascular space. Simultaneously, this vector is offset by an oncotic pressure vector, which is the net difference between plasma oncotic pressure and tissue oncotic pressure adjusted for a permeability factor (reflectance) that varies as the "size" of the pores changes. On the average, these vectors tend to cancel, and there is only a small flux of fluid across the membrane. However, alteration in any of the main forces can lead to marked derangement in fluid distribution and the development of increased interstitial fluid recognized as clinical edema. The balanced forces in Starling's equation result in the passage of fluid across the vascular membrane into the interstitial (extravascular) space. Not yet considered is the "drainage" effect of the lymphatic system that tends to remove filtered plasma from the interstitium. Obstruction of lymphatics by complications such as tumor and infection can further impair fluid clearance and result in localized edema or lymphedema.

Osmolality and Tonicity

The composition of extracellular water is reflected by the concentration of solutes. Ordinarily, extracellular composition is maintained within tight boundaries by accurate renal control mechanisms (e.g., antidiuretic hormone [ADH] and aldosterone). These control mechanisms, however, tend to respond to the concentration of a given substance rather than to the total amount of all substances. Concentration represents the combined effect of the amount of a given substance (numerator) dissolved in a given amount of water (denominator). Thus abnormalities in concentration may represent changes in the amount of solute, amount of water, or both. The concentration of total solute of a given substance is most easily measured by plasma osmolality (mOsm/kg). This value indicates the ratio of solute to water in the plasma and in the extravascular space. Since extracellular water is in equilibrium with intracellular water, shifts of membrane-permeable water result in maintenance of osmotic equality throughout total body water. In other words, accumulation of intracellular solute is compensated by a shift in water from the extracellular space to the intracellular space until osmolality is equal.

The concentration of total ions, indicating ionic strength, is approximated by assessing the concentration of the principal extracellular cation, sodium. Changes in sodium concentration represent changes in *tonicity,* a term related to but not synonymous with osmolality. Typically, tonicity and osmolality change together, and hyperosmolality usually includes hypertonicity.[2] However, any substance that has a low molecular weight and a sizable concentration contributes to serum osmolality. Thus conditions such as hyperglycemia, azotemia, hyperlactacidemia, and accumulation of ethanol raise osmolality without a change in tonicity.

The contributing factors to osmolality can be understood more clearly by determining the osmolal gradient. This represents the difference between calculated (Osm[c]) and measured (Osm[m]) osmolality. Calculated osmolality is estimated by the formula:

$$\text{Osm(c)} = 1.86(\text{Na}) + \text{Glu}/18 + \text{BUN}/2.8$$

where Na is serum sodium concentration in mEq/L, Glu is serum glucose in mg/100 ml, and BUN is blood urea nitrogen in mg/100 ml (1.86 is twice the osmotic activity coefficient of a monovalent ion; 18 is the molecular weight of glucose divided by 10; [a correction factor to convert mg/dl to mg/mEq/L 2.8 is the molecular weight of urea nitrogen divided again by the correction factor 10). Ordinarily, the osmolal gradient is less than 10 mOsm/kg where:

$$\text{Osmolal gradient} = \text{Osm(m)} - \text{Osm(c)}$$

A gradient greater than 10 mOsm/kg represents the accumulation of some unmeasured, osmotically active (low molecular weight) substance such as lactate, ethanol, and mannitol. A common error in clinical practice is to assume that a change in measured osmolality represents an increase or decrease in water. As might be anticipated, *osmolality* is a concentration term and therefore can be disrupted by a change in amount of solute (e.g., azotemia) or amount of water (e.g., dehydration) or both (e.g., hyperosmolar coma). Since measured osmolality equals the ratio of solute molecules to water:

$$\text{Osm} = \text{Solute}/\text{Water}$$

by rearrangement solute must equal osmolality multiplied by total body water (which can be estimated as 60% of total body weight), as shown by the formula:

$$\text{Solute} = \text{Osm} \times 0.6 \times \text{wt}$$

Estimation of this compound variable allows assessment of changes in total body solute, and by inference permits an appraisal of changes in body water.

Table 2-2. Electrolyte Composition

	Na	K	Cl	Ca	Mg
Total body content (mEq/kg)	67	58	42	940	32
Exchangeable content (mEq/kg)	41	44	30	—	—
Intracellular concentration (mEq/L)	10	160	3	2	26
Plasma water concentration (mEq/L)	152	5	110	5	3
Serum concentration (mEq/L)	142	5	103	5	—

Electrolyte Composition

As previously indicated, intracellular and extracellular fluids vary in concentration of electrolytes. The total body content of each electrolyte[3] has been estimated by direct assay[4] and by radionuclide exchange (exchangeable ion).[5-7] The distribution of these electrolytes is unequal and results in marked concentration differences throughout the body (Table 2-2).

Most of the difference between total body content (gravimetric) and exchangeable content is accounted for as substance in bone. As a glance at Table 2-2 confirms and contrary to the impression gained from evaluating serum electrolytes, the content of total exchangeable sodium (Na) is roughly equal to the content of total exchangeable potassium (K). The sum of these ions (exchangeable Na + K) validly estimates total body exchangeable cations that are roughly equally divided between intracellular and extracellular water. Accordingly, the serum sodium concentration (or conversely the intracellular potassium concentration) represents the ratio of total body cations to total body water, as shown below:

$$\text{Na (Serum)} = (\text{Na} + \text{K})/(0.6 \times \text{wt})$$

By a process analogous to osmolality, cross-multiplying serum sodium concentration by an estimate of total body water yields total body exchangeable cations. An estimate therefore of total body water, total body solute, and total body cations allows serial assessment of fluid and electrolyte balance for patients in whom derangements are suspected.

HOMEOSTATIC CONTROL MECHANISMS

General Concepts

The kidney is the cornerstone of the homeostatic mechanisms controlling fluid and electrolyte balance. Although it is true that fluid losses from the skin, lungs, and gastrointestinal tract may be impressive, the kidney is the only part of the system that is able to "control" its output. Accepting that fact, it is helpful to think of renal homeostasis as "throwing the baby out with the bath water, and catching the baby before it goes down the drain." In other words, glomerular filtration, the frontline initiator of renal excretion, is relatively nonspecific. It only limits excretion of substances that are associated with large proteins and therefore too big to pass through the renal vascular pores. Glomerular filtrate therefore is an ultrafiltrate of plasma. This ultrafiltrate passes through the proximal tubule where approximately 95% of most solute and most of the water are reabsorbed. In effect, control of absorption to this point is really a question of "what isn't reabsorbed." Final modification of urinary composition takes place in the distal tubule and collecting duct,[8] where sodium is, in a manner of speaking, "exchanged" for hydrogen or potassium[9] and the remaining water either is or is not reabsorbed.[10]

Sodium and Water Homeostasis

Intracellular water is in equilibrium with extracellular water through osmotic and ionic neutrality. A small gradient is accounted for by anion proteins, which results in a concentration inequality referred to as the Gibbs-Donnan equilibrium (distribution). Extracellular water is controlled largely by plasma volume and serum sodium concentration.

Sodium and water conservation must be considered together, since their control mechanisms are inseparable. Water deficits or excesses are compensated by changes in ADH release from the pituitary gland and its effect within the renal collecting duct.[11] Changes in sodium homeostasis are accompanied by both ADH and mineralocorticoid responses. A decrease in plasma volume stimulates baroreceptors located in sites such as the right atrium and carotid body, as well as in the juxtaglomerular apparatus and macula densa of the kidney.[12] The baroreceptor response results in an increase in ADH release from the posterior pituitary gland and causes decreased loss of solute-free water in the collecting duct of the kidney. Conversely, as the serum sodium concentration falls, ADH release is inhibited and further water conservation is blunted. The simultaneous effects of decreased glomerular filtration leading to decreased sodium delivery to the juxtaglomerular apparatus results in renin release, which subsequently causes cleavage of angiotensinogen into the decapeptide angiotensin I. This latter substance is converted in the lung to the octapeptide angiotensin II by the angiotensin-converting enzyme (ACE). Angiotensin II is a very potent vasoconstrictor substance that also directly stimulates aldosterone release from the zona glomerulosa of the adrenal cortex. The resultant increase in circulating aldosterone increases sodium reabsorption in the distal tubule of the kidney in exchange for potassium and/or hydrogen ions.

As serum sodium concentration changes, release of ADH from the posterior pituitary gland is altered by osmoreceptors in the hypothalamus. Very small changes (2 mOsm) can predictably result in a measurable change in plasma ADH levels. Corresponding changes in thirst perception and the permeability of the collecting duct of the kidney to water also occur. In the case of hypernatremia, thirst increases, and maximum concentration of solute-free water occurs in the kidney. This can be corroborated by a high measured urine osmolality (usually >500 mOsm). During hyponatremia, ADH release is inhibited, the stimulus for water conservation in the collecting duct ceases, and solute-free water ("free water") is excreted, resulting in a hypotonic (<280 mOsm/kg) urine and a return of serum sodium to normal. In addition, the zona glomerulosa of the adrenal gland appears to be sensitive to changes in serum sodium concentration, resulting in feedback control of aldosterone release.

Potassium Homeostasis

Control of serum potassium levels is quite unlike sodium. Potassium is primarily an intracellular ion, with concentration many fold greater than plasma. Yet the extracellular concentration is extremely important in maintaining electrochemical gradients across cell membranes that facilitate depolarization of electrically active cells such as cardiac muscle and specialized conduction cells. Therefore control of extracellular potassium is important. Typically, mammalian diets contain large amounts of potassium, such that conservation of potassium is not usually a problem unless losses are excessive (diuretics, diarrhea) or renal mechanisms are abnormal (hyperaldosteronism).

Potassium conservation and excretion tends to be a direct contrast to sodium conservation. Excess potassium, for example, stimulates the release of aldosterone from the adrenal glands, whereas too little sodium would result in the same response.[13] Although the majority of potassium reabsorption (like sodium) occurs in the proximal tubule, it is excreted in the distal tubule in response to the aldosterone stimulus. Sodium can be reabsorbed almost entirely within the nephron, wheres potassium conservation is less complete until profound body deficits occur. Distal tubular flow rate is also a major factor in potassium homeostasis. As flow rates increase, potassium excretion becomes inappropriately high. Although total body potassium distribution is affected by renal mechanisms, it is also subject to exchange mechanisms at the cell surface of all cells such that, as sodium (or hydrogen) is transported out, potassium reenters the intracellular fluid (probably insulin dependent). Likewise, in severe acidosis or alkalosis, plasma potassium levels may change as a result of the fluxes of potassium that are consequent to the hydrogen ion shifts.

Acid-Base Conservation

With the exception of several specialized body fluids, the pH of body water is very closely guarded in a narrow range. Normal plasma pH (7.4 ± 0.05) generally is representative of the pH of total body water, although the pH of fluids such as cerebrospinal fluid and intracellular fluid may transiently diverge from that of plasma because of differing controlling factors and influences. For practical purposes, however, the pH of all compartments of body water can be assumed to be equal.

To appreciate the intricacies of acid-base balance, a

solid understanding of the basic chemical concepts of acids, bases, and dissociation is essential. Acids are substances that have the capability of donating protons (hydrogen ions; hydronium ions). Bases, conversely, are substances that have the ability to accept protons during chemical reactions. Both acids and bases are ionic compounds that, when dissolved in water, have the ability to dissociate into cationic and anionic species. For most organic acids and bases in the body dissociation is only partial, and the ratio of dissociated to nondissociated chemicals is determined by the dissociation constant. Acids, when dissociated, contribute hydrogen ions (H^+) and a corresponding anion (An^-) to the total ionic composition of the solution. Bases typically contribute a cation and a hydroxyl (OH^-) ion.

A typical acid (or base) dissociation can be described by the chemical reaction:

$$HAn = H^+ + An^-$$

The dissociation constant is determined by the ratio of products to reactants; therefore:

$$K = [H^+][An^-]/[HAn]$$

where the brackets represent concentration in solution. Taking the logarithm of both sides of this equation results in a useful and familiar form of the dissociation equation:

$$\log K = \log H^+ + \log([An^-]/[HAn])$$
$$pK = pH - \log([An^-]/[HAn])$$
$$pH = pK + \log([An^-]/[HAn])$$

The dissociation constant (and consequently the pK) takes into account the simultaneous equilibrium of water.

In the human, many acid-base pairs (buffer pairs) exist in simultaneous equilibrium. This means that the ambient pH of the body determines the ratio of anion to dissociated acid for a number of acids present in the body. Although substances such as phosphoric acid, proteins, and amino acids are present in abundance and could be used as estimates of acid-base status, the carbonic acid-bicarbonate buffer system is most commonly used for this purpose. The reason for using this buffer system is clear. The major homeostatic mechanisms of acid-base control are pulmonary (the excretion of carbon dioxide) and renal (the conservation of bicarbonate and excretion of hydrogen ions). Consequently, this buffer pair reflects the efficacy of the homeostatic mechanisms that are operative in compensating for changes in acid or base gain or loss. In addition, bicarbonate and carbon dioxide (P_{CO_2}) are easily measured in plasma.

The general dissociation equation, when applied to the bicarbonate-carbonic acid buffer system, is known as the Henderson-Hasselbalch equation:

$$pH = 6.1 + \log([HCO_3^-]/[H_2CO_3])$$

where HCO_3^- is the concentration of bicarbonate and H_2CO_3 is the concentration of carbonic acid. Since the concentration of carbonic acid is determined by the partial pressure of carbon dioxide and the solubility of carbon dioxide in water is 0.03:

$$pH = 6.1 + \log([HCO_3^-]0.03\ P_{CO_2})$$

and

$$[H^+] = 24\ (P_{CO_2}/[HCO_3^-])$$

Current technology allows the direct measurement of pH and P_{CO_2} in arterial (or venous) blood, enabling the estimation of bicarbonate concentration by the above equation. Alternatively, measurement of bicarbonate concentration and pH would enable calculation of P_{CO_2}. In normal circumstances the ratio of $HCO_3^-/0.03\ P_{CO_2}$ is 20/1.

Other electrolytes enter the body pool only by ingestion (or injection), but acids (and bases) are rarely present in the diet. Acid is a product of metabolism of other substances and is added to total body water as a function of the rate of metabolism and the fractional use of acid-producing metabolites (Table 2-3).

In general, net acid production is approximately 1 mEq/kg/day (2 to 3 mEq/kg/day in infants) and is primarily caused by the production of sulfuric acid from metabolism of thiols; phosphoric acid from metabolism of organic phosphates; and other organic acids from the metabolism of proteins, carbohydrates, and fats. Any addition of base (e.g., antacids) or compounds that generate base (e.g., citrate, lactate) tend to offset the daily endogenous acid load.

To maintain acid-base equilibrium, the body must excrete a quantity of acid equal to endogenous production (plus any exogenous acid and minus any exogenous base). This is accomplished primarily by renal excretion of fixed acid in the form of phosphates and ammonia. Ammonia is actively produced by metabolism of glutamine in the kidney and subsequently excreted into the renal tubular lumen. Simultaneously, monohydrogen phosphate is filtered at the glomerulus. Hydrogen ions, filtered or secreted, are trapped by the buffering capability of these two proton acceptors and excreted. In addition, through a carbonic anhydrase-dependent system, the tubular epithelial cell is capable of generating a hydrogen and a bicarbonate ion from carbonic acid (dissolved carbon dioxide) and reabsorbing the bicarbonate while the hydrogen ion is excreted. This regenerates the bicarbonate pool and facilitates acid-base

Table 2-3. Physiologic Factors Affecting Plasma Acidity

Through Plasma Bicarbonate Changes	Through Plasma P_{CO_2}
Rate of hydrogen ion input	Rate of carbon dioxide production
Rate of hydrogen ion or bicarbonate loss (gastrointestinal)	Rate of alveolar ventilation
Availability of buffers	
Bicarbonate space of distribution	
Rate of net renal acid excretion	

stability. If the bicarbonate pool becomes excessive, renal excretion of bicarbonate is increased by a complex mechanism dependent on the decreased hydrogen ion in the tubular fluid. In effect, the kidney is able to directly influence acid excretion by three mechanisms: excretion of phosphate (affected by glomerular filtration and parathyroid hormone), synthesis of ammonia, and control of the directional flow of bicarbonate.

The last of the three mechanisms just enumerated requires further comment. Because of the ready availability of carbon dioxide and water (and consequently carbonic acid), the kidney, through carbonic anhydrase, can control the abundance of hydrogen ions and bicarbonate. By directing the excretion of hydrogen ions into the tubular lumen and the return of bicarbonate to plasma, the kidney has a great capacity to excrete acid and control base. Only when the renal mechanisms responsible for reabsorption of base or excretion of acid are compromised does the renal contribution to acid-base balance become limited. In normal circumstances the rate at which the kidney returns bicarbonate to the body is equivalent to the rate of sodium-hydrogen exchange in the distal tubule. Although the proximal tubule is quantitatively the most important site of bicarbonate reabsorption in the kidney, with a small contribution from the loop of Henle, the distal segment is capable of "fine tuning" the acid-base excretory balance.

As indicated, carbon dioxide (and its hydrated form, carbonic acid) plays a central role in maintenance of acid-base homeostasis. The major parameter of carbon dioxide concentration in the blood is its partial gas pressure (P_{CO_2}). The P_{CO_2} of arterial blood (venous blood has increased P_{CO_2} caused by addition of carbon dioxide from tissue metabolism) is determined by the balance between the amount of alveolar (effective) ventilation ($\dot{V}_A$) in the lung and the amount of carbon dioxide produced per minute ($\dot{V}_{CO_2}$). Further stated, the arterial P_{CO_2} is actually proportional to the ratio of carbon dioxide production to alveolar ventilation. Normal metabolism consumes oxygen and a fuel substrate (carbohydrate, protein, fat), with the subsequent production of carbon dioxide to be excreted by ventilation. The amount of carbon dioxide produced per volume of oxygen consumed is determined by the "mix" of fuel and is known as the *respiratory quotient* (RQ). At a higher respiratory quotient (e.g., during pure carbohydrate metabolism when 1 mol of carbon dioxide is produced for each mole of oxygen consumed [RQ = 1]), even though metabolic rate is constant, more carbon dioxide is produced than during metabolism of pure fat (RQ = 0.7). Both an increase in metabolic rate and an increase in respiratory quotient increase carbon dioxide production. Total minute ventilation is the sum of alveolar ventilation (effective breathing) and dead space ventilation (ineffective, wasted breathing). The product of the alveolar ventilation and respiratory rate is the minute alveolar ventilation and is the portion of breathing that is effective in eliminating carbon dioxide and absorbing oxygen. Conversely, dead space ventilation is air that must be moved into and out of the lungs but does not contribute to gas exchange. Dead space ventilation can be anatomic (trachea, large bronchi, cysts) or physiologic. Physiologic dead space commonly increases during diseases involving the lung and leads to a smaller percentage of each breath that contributes to gas exchange. The amount of alveolar ventilation determines the adequacy of carbon dioxide elimination. When alveolar ventilation increases without an increase in carbon dioxide production, P_{CO_2} falls, resulting in decreased H_2CO_3 and respiratory alkalosis. Alternatively, a decrease in alveolar ventilation relative to carbon dioxide production causes increased P_{CO_2} with resulting increased H_2CO_3 and respiratory acidosis.

PATHOPHYSIOLOGY AND TREATMENT OF SPECIFIC ELECTROLYTE AND ACID-BASE ABNORMALITIES

To understand abnormalities of electrolyte homeostasis, some attention must be given to normal daily requirements (Table 2-4). Although it is true that a state of electrolyte balance requires that intake is equal to losses (and losses can be minimized), realistically daily excretion of electrolytes is fairly predictable, allowing a range of estimated daily needs. Under normal conditions, losses are primarily through urinary excretion and water losses secondary to evaporation from the skin and water losses through the lungs. These latter two sources are referred to as insensible losses because they are not visible or readily measurable and amount to 500 to 800 ml of water daily with almost negligible amounts of sodium and chloride. Urine is the major sensible loss (one that is visible and measurable) and averages between 1200 and 1500 ml of water daily with 10 to 30 mEq of sodium and 20 to 60 mEq of potassium. Another sensible loss is water loss through the feces, which is usually quite minimal. Losses greater than those routinely encountered (e.g., diarrhea) result in corresponding increases in requirements; decreases in normal excretion rates (e.g., renal failure) necessitate a reduction in intake.

Table 2-4. Adult Daily Requirements

	Normal	Minimal
Water (total)	1500 ml/m^2	(870 ml/m^2)
Water (insensible)	500 ml/m^2	—
Sodium	0.7-3.6 mEq/kg	(0.3 mEq/kg)
Potassium	0.7-2.1 mEq/kg	0.3-0.5 mEq/kg)
Chloride	0.7-3.6 mEq/kg	(0.3 mEq/kg)
Calcium	0.4-1.1 mEq/kg	(0.2 mEq/kg)
Magnesium	0.3-0.7 mEq/kg	(0.2-0.4 mEq/kg)

Modified from Goodenough RD, Burke JF. Fluid, electrolyte, and acid-base homeostasis in surgery. In Burke JF. Surgical Physiology. Philadelphia: WB Saunders, 1983.

Abnormalities of Water Balance

Disturbances in the amount of distribution of total body water are common in clinical practice. Since water distributes throughout the body, restricted in its movement only by osmotic and ionic barriers, abnormalities in amount with maintenance of normal electrolyte concentrations are frequent. An isotonic increase in total body water results in edema, whereas an isotonic decrease produces clinical dehydration. Since electrolyte conservatory mechanisms are extremely efficient, deviation from isotonicity is uncommon except at the extremes of age when compensatory mechanisms are less adequate or access to water or salt is restricted. In infants and the elderly therefore hypertonic (sodium >145) and hypotonic (sodium >135 mEq/L) abnormalities are more common and require attention be given to the volume and the concentration problems. It is important, however, to realize that isotonic abnormalities in total body water are more prevalent in adults than other fluid derangements only because compensatory mechanisms maintain the concentration of important solutes. In circumstances in which a coexistent problem compromises these compensatory mechanisms (e.g., renal disease, inappropriate ADH secretion, diuretic use, adrenal insufficiency), a superimposed fluid loss or gain may very well not be isotonic.

Dehydration is an absolute decrease in total body water and usually represents a balanced loss between intracellular and extracellular volume. Dehydration can be assessed on clinical grounds alone, and in fact there is no readily available "test" that identifies it unless there is a coexistent abnormality of concentration. Blood urea nitrogen and consequently osmolality are frequently elevated, however, and may be supportive of the diagnosis when the creatinine concentration is normal and the blood urea nitrogen-creatinine ratio >20. Up to a 5% decrease in total body water can escape clinical detection without appropriate suspicion by history. Thirst is usually present, however, and is an accurate sign of water deficit. Losses greater than 5% usually lead to conditions such as sunken eyes, loss of skin turgor with tenting of presternal skin, and dry mucous membranes. Greater than 10% dehydration commonly demonstrates hemodynamic changes with tachycardia and postural hypotension.

Treatment of dehydration requires an understanding of the composition of the fluid deficits. Isotonic dehydration reflects a loss of all fluid compartments (and their contained electrolytes) and is corrected by infusing intravenously a balanced salt solution such as lactated Ringer's solution (Table 2-5). Concomitant abnormalities in concentration or tonicity are best assessed by the serum sodium concentration; such electrolyte abnormalities should be treated simultaneously with management of the volume deficit. For example, in hypernatremic dehydration (see Table 2-5), water alone as 5% dextrose in water is used for replacement of the water deficit and a balanced salt solution for volume restoration. The appropriate intravenous fluid should be administered to correct one half of the estimated abnormality during a period of 24 hours. This approach is used, since most deficits develop over a period of days or weeks and the patient has usually adjusted to them. Rapid replacement of losses may actually impose a greater risk than the deficit itself.

Edema can be related to an underlying disease (cardiac, renal, hepatic) or, as is more common in modern practice, abundant or excessive intravenous fluid administration. Excesses in extracellular fluid typically are susceptible to gravity and hence are most pronounced in dependent areas. Conditions such as pretibial and ankle edema are common in the upright patient. Presacral edema or pitting of the skin overlying the iliac crest is more likely in the recumbent patient.

Water intoxication represents a specific abnormality of water balance. Ordinarily, large amounts of ingested or administered water can be excreted quantitatively without resultant volume excess or ionic dilution. Very marked amounts, however, particularly in a setting of compromised homeostatic mechanisms, can result in edema, hyponatremia, and dilution of other electrolytes as well. (For a further discussion, see Hyponatremia.)

Treatment of fluid excess requires an understanding of cause and an assessment of the integrity of homeostatic mechanisms, particularly renal, hepatic, and CNS function. In the setting of normal compensation, simple fluid restriction or decreased administration is likely to be effective. When simultaneous abnormalities in renal, hepatic, adrenal, or cardiac physiology exist, careful attention to intake and output (an "accountant" approach) is indicated. Only by specific accounting of all volumes, concentrations, and amounts can aggravation or creation of abnormalities be prevented.

Table 2-5. Composition of Common Solutions Used for Intravenous Therapy

Solutions	Glucose (g/L)	Na (mEq/L)	Cl (mEq/L)	HCO_3^- (mEq/L)	K (mEq/L)	Ca (mEq/L)
5% Dextrose and water	50	—	—	—	—	—
0.9% Sodium chloride (normal saline)	—	154	154	—	—	—
0.45% Sodium chloride (half-normal saline)	—	77	77	—	—	—
3% Sodium chloride (hypertonic saline)	—	513	513	—	—	—
Lactated Ringer's solution	—	130	109	28*	4	2.7

*Exists in solution as lactate and is ultimately metabolized to bicarbonate (HCO_3^-).

Abnormalities of Sodium

Since sodium is the major cation within extracellular water and is regularly analyzed in the laboratory, it is surprising that abnormalities in sodium concentration are not more frequent. Although hypernatremia and hyponatremia are seen, they are rigorously prevented by compensatory mechanisms within the kidney. In fact, very small changes in sodium concentration (and subsequently osmolality) result in a measurable change in ADH release in the same direction.

When renal concentrating mechanisms are defective[14] (e.g., washout of renal medullary concentration gradient as with diuretics, partial tubular dysfunction from incipient or resolving acute tubular necrosis, or massive sodium loss in interstitial nephritis), abnormalities in serum sodium are more common.

Hyponatremia

Virtually all acute, stressful situations (e.g., infection, anesthesia, and surgery) are accompanied by release of ADH and conservation of free water.[15] This homeostatic mechanism is very effective in preserving extracellular volume when combined with sodium conservation, which depends on a decrease in delivered sodium or perfusion pressure at the juxtaglomerular apparatus.[12,16] Consequently, hyponatremia in adult patients at the time of admission for elective surgery is distinctly uncommon. However, once a patient has received intravenous administration of hypotonic fluids (e.g., 0.45% saline), the inability to excrete the "free" water due to an obligatory ADH release frequently results in a dilutional decrease in serum sodium to some degree.

When hyponatremia is present, spurious causes must be excluded. This is accomplished most simply by evaluating the serum osmolality. Since osmolality measures the amount of solute per *mass* of water instead of volume, it is independent of the amount of water in a volume of serum. Normally, serum is 94% water. Increases in protein or lipid concentrations can, however, alter the amount of water and lead to an analytic error in sodium determination. Osmolality is not so affected. Consequently, hyponatremia in the setting of normal osmolality would raise the suspicion of paraproteinemia (e.g., multiple myeloma, macroglobulinemia) or hyperlipidemia.

Alternatively, an increase in an extracellular solute such as glucose (or mannitol) causes a shift in water from the intracellular to extracellular space to conserve osmotic equality. This results in a subsequent "dilution" of extracellular sodium but a maintained osmolality because of the presence of another osmotically active substance, glucose. Confirmation of hyperglycemia in the setting of normal osmolality justifies a fall in sodium of approximately 1.6 mEq/L for each 100 mg/100 ml rise in blood glucose above normal.

When true hyponatremia does occur (low sodium plus low osmolality), evaluating how the kidney is behaving allows a rational interpretation of the probable pathophysiology. A careful assessment of overall fluid and electrolyte status (weight change, input and output summaries, presence or absence of edema) is essential.[17] Characterizing the patient as ahead or behind in volume allows appropriate interpretation of the renal response, which is best ascertained by measuring the urinary osmolality and sodium concentration.

During active sodium conservation, urinary sodium is typically low (<5 mEq/L). This indicates either that there is a true deficit in sodium or that the kidney "thinks" there is one. The latter occurs when circulating substances (e.g., aldosterone) are inappropriately present in edematous states such as cirrhosis and chronic congestive heart failure. In each of these settings, however, the patient is both edematous and has ascites. In the absence of either of these findings, true sodium depletion is probably present. Sodium administration should be guided by an estimate of the deficit, which must be considered independently of (added to) volume deficits that are isotonic (Na = 140 mEq/L). The sodium deficit approximates 0.6 mEq/kg per milliequivalent fall in serum sodium. Unless neurologic symptoms are present, which would mandate urgent treatment, the sodium replacement should take 24 to 48 hours. After one half of the deficit has been replaced, serum electrolyte levels should be rechecked.

When urinary sodium is increased (>20 mEq/L), simple sodium depletion can be excluded. Sodium conservation either will not or cannot take place. This occurs in the setting of abnormal ADH release, adrenal insufficiency, severe hyperthyroidism, recent use of diuretics, or intrinsic renal tubular dysfunction as in renal failure or interstitial nephritis. This can be clarified by measuring urinary osmolality.

Since the normal response to hyponatremia and hypoosmolality is excretion of solute-free water (and dilute urine), the finding of a urine osmolality above that of serum plus hyponatremia indicates an abnormal ADH response.[15,18] This implies a continued release of ADH in spite of a hypoosmolar state. If this is present at the time of admission or in the absence of intravenous fluids, it implies a CNS abnormality (e.g., head trauma, intracranial tumor) or an ectopic site of production (e.g., bronchogenic carcinoma). In the patient receiving hypotonic fluids, this finding more commonly reflects the release of ADH associated with a central "acute phase response" or "systemic inflammatory response" to stress or illness. In either event, fluid balance will be "ahead," as is the total amount of sodium in the body. The hyponatremia means that water is "more ahead" than sodium. This paradoxic increased sodium in the face of decreased serum sodium concentration results in a high urinary sodium excretion (>20 mEq/L) and a high salt excretion fraction (>5%).[19]

The finding of isosthenuria (urine osmolality equals serum osmolality) implies intrinsic renal dysfunction or pharmacologic dysfunction from diuretics. The finding of low urine osmolality and high urine sodium, however, suggests that ADH release is appropriately terminated but that sodium is not being conserved. This situation is seen in mineralocorticoid insufficiency.

Laboratory evaluation of the renal response to hyponatremia can be enlightening but does not replace clinical assessment. Since hyponatremia means either a decrease in sodium or an increase in water, appropriate interpretation of readily available data should allow discrimination. A decrease in sodium requires the presence of a route of loss and usually is associated with weight loss. Alternatively, an increase in water should be manifested by a gain in weight and excess fluid intake over output.

In the patient who is not receiving intravenous fluids, a serum sodium below 135 mEq/L constitutes hyponatremia and deserves investigation. In the patient who is receiving hypotonic fluids, however, mild hyponatremia is common enough to be almost expected. Although it is not normal, mild hyponatremia down to 130 mEq/L can probably be ignored. A sodium level of 125 to 130 mEq/L justifies vigorous diagnostic efforts to identify the cause. A serum sodium level of 120 to 125 mEq/L necessitates vigorous institution of appropriate therapy. A sodium level of <120 mEq/L is a medical emergency and frequently requires careful administration of hypertonic saline for correction. It is not the low sodium per se that is detrimental, but rather the increase in the intracellular fluid compartment that accompanies this circumstance. This intracellular volume increase is especially detrimental to brain cells, since the brain is contained within a fixed space with little or no room for expansion. When brain cells swell, an increase in intracranial pressure ultimately develops and presents clinically by a variety of manifestations, including apathy, confusion, weakness, nausea, and occasionally vomiting. If this water intoxication is not corrected, it will ultimately lead to convulsions, stupor, and possibly even death.

Hypernatremia

The body rigorously defends itself against hyperosmolality. Even a small rise results in increased ADH release and subsequent free water retention by the kidney, unless, of course, ADH release cannot occur (diabetes insipidus), ADH is ineffective (nephrogenic diabetes insipidus), or the patient is prevented from access to water (infants, geriatric patients, unconscious or restrained patients). A simple review of the clinical situation often identifies the cause. Since hypernatremia implies either an increase in sodium or a decrease in water, both must be considered. An increase in sodium can result from vigorous administration of normal saline or sodium bicarbonate. A decrease in water can occur by renal or extrarenal mechanisms. Nonrenal causes should be clinically apparent and include such symptoms as diarrhea and excessive sweating. In addition to the forms of diabetes insipidus (pituitary dysfunction or nephrogenic), renal sources must include osmotic diuresis with obligatory "free" water loss. In all cases, treatment is simple. Administration of hypotonic solutions restores sodium concentration; when sodium excess is a component, judicious diuretic use hastens sodium excretion.

Care in treating hypernatremia must be exercised, however, since a rapid change in sodium concentration is of greater clinical importance than the actual sodium concentration.[16] Too rapid correction of sodium abnormalities can result in dramatic CNS effects, including seizures secondary to rapid changes in intracellular volume. Accordingly, treatment should be planned to correct one half of the estimated deficit during a period of 24 hours. In the case of hypernatremia, this usually translates into the administration of 2 ml of free water per kilogram during a period of 24 hours for each milliequivalent of planned decrease in serum sodium concentration.

In the patient with head injury or recent neurosurgical intervention with accompanying diabetes insipidus, unless actual hypophysectomy has been performed, early administration of ADH should be avoided. Careful replacement of losses maintains fluid and electrolyte balance until the usually transient abnormality resolves. Accordingly, hypernatremia should be avoidable. If permanent diabetes insipidus is anticipated, however, administration of ADH or its synthetic analog, desmopressin acetate (DDAVP), should be instituted. Serious complications of diabetes insipidus (or inappropriate ADH secretion) are not a function of difficulty in treatment but rather failure of recognition. Anticipation of such problems greatly simplifies their subsequent management.

Abnormalities of Potassium

Since mammals usually ingest large amounts of potassium, it is not surprising that most abnormalities in potassium balance are the result not of intake but of excretion. Further, the very narrow range of normal potassium concentration in plasma and the relatively massive adjacent intracellular pool[5] (with exchange influenced by variables such as pH and drugs) make control of serum potassium both important and tenuous. This importance is underscored by the critical nature of severe potassium abnormalities on the cardiac, neural, and muscular systems and evidenced by the diligent monitoring of potassium concentrations that occurs in operating suites and intensive care units. An understanding of the common circumstances leading to potassium abnormalities facilitates maintenance of normal homeostasis and simplifies treatment of abnormalities.[20]

Hyperkalemia

Since the kidney is the major site of potassium excretion, compromised renal function is almost always a component of hyperkalemia.[21,22] Although increased potassium levels can occur from either excess intake or decreased excretion, the former is quite rare and is usually iatrogenic and occurs in the setting or administering massive intravenous doses of potassium (or potassium-containing drugs such as penicillin) or giving potassium to a patient receiving a drug that inhibits potassium excretion (spironolactone, triamterene). Abnormalities of excretion are common and can be caused by intrinsic abnormalities of renal function (acute, oliguric renal failure), disturbances in hormonal control of potassium exchange (hypoaldosteronism, adrenal insufficiency), or alterations in the potassium exchange mechanism per se (drugs, acidosis). Occasionally, serum potassium factitiously is elevated (compared to plasma potassium) because of K^+ release from platelets in thrombocytosis.[23]

Hyperkalemia produces predictable clinical consequences that affect neuromuscular function (weakness, irritability) and cardiac conduction (peaking of T waves, prolongation of PR and QT intervals, widening of QRS complexes, and heart block). Monitoring of the electrocardiogram provides a simple, noninvasive method of assessing change in the hyperkalemic or potentially hyperkalemic patient. Predictable changes, beginning with T-wave peaking, are the harbingers of subsequent complications, which are evidenced by alterations in the shape and duration of the major electrocardiogram complexes.

Since hyperkalemia poses a life-threatening problem, urgent and definitive correction is imperative.[24] Transient decrease in serum potassium can be accomplished by translocating extracellular potassium back into cells with glucose and insulin, and the membrane effects of hyperkalemia can be offset by the administration of calcium. In the rare patient with reasonable renal function, potassium diuresis can be induced by use of loop-active diuretics. More commonly, potassium is removed from the body by the use of potassium-exchanging resins (sodium polystyrene sulfonate [Kayexalate]) that can be given by mouth or rectum and predictably lower potassium. This is accomplished, however, through exchange with sodium and may alter fluid and sodium balance. Institution of peritoneal dialysis or hemodialysis is clearly the most effective, long-term approach to potassium control in the patient with renal compromise. It is important to remember, however, that continued administration of hypertonic glucose, as in parenteral nutrition support, results in a predictable and sustained fall in serum potassium as the egress of potassium associated with catabolism is prevented.

Hypokalemia

Hypokalemia is a common electrolyte abnormality in both hospitalized and ambulatory patients.[13,25] Although it may be precipitated by an underlying disease (mineralocorticoid excess as in Cushing's syndrome, potassium loss from colonic villous adenoma, potassium wasting in renal disease) or by decreased potassium intake (low-potassium diet), most hypokalemia is iatrogenic in that it is induced pharmacologically by agents having potassium wasting as a side effect.[26] Most notable are the diuretic agents currently used in the management of hypertension and fluid overload. The loop-acting agents in particular are associated with a substantial potassium loss in the urine. Other classes of drugs, however, also induce hypokalemia.[27,28] Recent increased use of amphotericin B in the treatment of immunocompromised patients has uncovered a profound and difficult-to-manage hypokalemia.[29] Use of newer synthetic penicillins in ultrahigh concentration is also associated with increased renal potassium loss and subsequent hypokalemia.

Hypokalemia may manifest itself in various ways (e.g., muscle weakness, paralysis). More frequently, however, hypokalemia produces myocardial irritability and subsequent arrhythmias such as frequent premature contractions, sustained tachycardias, and potentiation of digitalis toxicity. Although these complications are more feared than common, they are serious complications and justify both respect and careful monitoring. Treatment is simple. Administration of potassium as the chloride salt corrects the usual associated chloride-dependent alkalosis, decreases renal potassium loss, and corrects the hypokalemia. Beware, however, since the degree of hypokalemia is very poorly correlated to the magnitude of potassium deficit. Therefore strict guidelines for replacement are dangerous. Since the hazards of hypokalemia appear to be virtually eliminated by institution of treatment rather than total correction, the identification of the abnormality and institution of treatment are more important than the rapidity of treatment. Frequently, discontinuation of the offending drug or control of the underlying disease is necessary for long-term potassium control.

Abnormalities of Chloride

Since chloride is the most abundant anion in plasma and extracellular water, it is not surprising that its range of variation is large and its mechanism of variation somewhat passive. The high concentration of chloride in gastric juice accounts for the hypochloremia that accompanies the metabolic alkalosis of conditions such as gastric outlet obstruction, repetitive vomiting, and pyloric stenosis. Chloride is absorbed in large quantities from the gut, and its level is controlled by urinary excretion. Most reabsorption of chloride occurs in the proximal tubule of the kidney in association with sodium absorption. A considerable component is also actively reabsorbed in Henle's limb.[30] Alterations in proximal tubule absorption (osmotic diuretics) or Henle's limb (loop-active diuretics) can lead to hypochloremia and metabolic alkalosis. In addition, in the presence of "hormone-dependent" (e.g., aldosterone) alkalosis, the fraction of chloride that is reabsorbed is decreased. This interaction of chloride and bicarbonate is important in the evaluation of the patient with metabolic alkalosis.

Chloride is present in abundance in gastrointestinal secretions. Substantial chloride loss can result from gastrointestinal fluid losses from the upper tract (e.g., gastric outlet obstruction) or lower tract (e.g., diarrhea). Assessment of the chloride deficit provides complementary information in the evaluation of volume depletion secondary to gastrointestinal losses.

Isolated Acid-Base Abnormalities

The availability of routine measurement of "arterial blood gases" has resulted in a much clearer understanding of the nature and treatment of acid-base disturbances in clinical practice. On the basis of the normal physiologic determinants previously described and the pathophysiologic mechanisms enumerated later in this chapter, acid-base disturbances can be classified into acidosis or alkalosis. Both of these categories can be further subdivided into metabolic and respiratory, as well as combined metabolic-respiratory. Tables, nomograms, and algorithms have been developed for the assessment of the excess or deficit of acid (or base) to assist the clinician in management. Unfortunately, all these aids are of only limited practical value because of the concurrent and efficient efforts of the compensatory mechanisms of the body to correct the acid-base disturbance. In other words, the onset of a disturbance in pH (by change in either HCO_3^- or PCO_2) results in very rapid initiation of respiratory and metabolic compensatory mechanisms to partially correct the pH. It is essential in planning treatment of acid-base disturbances to keep this compensation in mind, lest overaggressive management results in new, iatrogenic acid-base disturbances in the opposite direction.

Acidosis

As described previously, acidosis can occur by the absolute gain in acid or loss of base from the body. Since the buffering system of the body is "open" in the sense that the CO_2-HCO_3^- system uses both respiratory and renal control systems, all but the most acute form of acidosis are combined with compensatory adjustments. Consequently, all respiratory disturbances have a metabolic compensatory component, and metabolic imbalance stimulates respiratory compensation. Frequently, the pH is remarkably well corrected, and only a careful review of the historical facts associated with the illness allows a clear analysis of the inciting cause. Occasionally, the cause is so elusive that only by disturbing the system with exogenous alkali and observing the respiratory response (or lack thereof) does the primary problem become apparent.

Respiratory acidosis. Pure respiratory acidosis is the simplest of the acid-base disturbances conceptually because it results from a decrease in effective alveolar ventilation (relative to carbon dioxide production). Normal carbon dioxide production from metabolic processes is approximately 450 L/day (20,000 mmol). When carbon dioxide elimination lags behind production, respiratory acidosis ensues. The consequent laboratory abnormalities include a decrease in pH and an increase in PCO_2. It is important to look at the pH first, since compensatory hypercapnea (increase in serum PCO_2) in the setting of profound metabolic alkalosis is not uncommon, particularly in patients receiving mechanical ventilation by an intermittent (intermittent mandatory ventilation, intermittent demand ventilation, pressure support ventilation) modality. Once respiratory acidosis is identified, a differential consideration of causes must include central respiratory depression (e.g., narcotics, intrinsic CNS disease), mechanical causes of decreased ventilation and/or increased dead space (e.g., tension pneumothorax, hemothorax, massive pleural effusions), or pathophysiologic causes of increased carbon dioxide production. The common causes of acute or chronic respiratory acidosis are summarized as follows:

Airway obstruction
Respiratory center depression
Neuromuscular defects
Restrictive lung diseases
Smoke inhalation
Inadequate mechanical ventilation

Appropriate treatment logically follows an identification of the underlying mechanism and may include ventilatory assistance to enhance alveolar ventilation to eliminate the retained carbon dioxide and thereby correct the acidic pH.

Metabolic acidosis. In marked contradistinction to respiratory acidosis, metabolic acidosis can result from a variety of causes that include gain of metabolic acids above excretion rates and loss of bicarbonate greater than its rate of regeneration.[10,31-33] Again, clinical evaluation and elucidation of the underlying mechanism greatly simplifies the task of evaluating the data. Also, it is important to avoid jumping to a conclusion of acidosis on the basis of only a decrease in the bicarbonate concentration of the serum, since this finding may also represent metabolic compensation for a respiratory alkalosis.

As is true with all biologic systems, electric neutrality is maintained in all fluid compartments throughout the body by balancing the total number of cations with the total number of anions. In the extracellular compartment under normal conditions, the concentration of the cation sodium roughly equals the sum of the concentrations of the anions, chloride, and bicarbonate, except for a small anion gap of 8 ± 2 mEq/L. An increase in this gap can give an important clue concerning the cause of the acidosis. Thus it is helpful to subdivide metabolic acidosis into those categories that manifest an increase in unmeasured anions (increased anion gap) and those that do not and that subsequently have a normal anion gap (nonanionic gap). As a generality, metabolic acidosis associated with the accumulation of organic acid has an associated increased anion gap, whereas that caused by a loss of bicarbonate has a normal anion gap. The distinction is important. Although both causes may require replacement of bicarbonate to correct the acidosis, the former group requires correction of an associated metabolic abnormality, and the latter requires attention to the site of bicarbonate loss (e.g., fistula).

Increased gap acidosis. Any metabolic acidosis that is caused by the accumulation of organic acid (and therefore not measured by routine electrolyte analysis) has a calculated anion gap that is greater than normal (uremia, diabetic ketoacidosis, lactic acidosis, and drug ingestion). In some circumstances (e.g., diabetic ketoacidosis), combined mechanisms are operative, and the component caused by ketoacids is proportional to the anion gap. The presence of an acidosis with an anion gap >14 mEq/L implies either an ingestion of an organic substance or an endogenous metabolic abnormality. Of the four commonly ingested "organic toxins" (methanol, ethylene glycol, ethanol, and isopropanol), only methanol (formic acid) and ethylene glycol (oxalic acid) produce a metabolic acidosis. Ethylene glycol also produces oxaluria, whereas methanol ingestion usually produces rapid retinal blindness. Acetylsalicylic acid (aspirin) and paraldehyde can also produce metabolic acidosis if ingested in large amounts.

Endogenous production of organic acid in excess of excretory capacity is seen in uremia, diabetic ketoacidosis, and lactic acidosis. Each is usually identifiable by the company it keeps: acidosis caused by renal failure is associated with the clinical and metabolic abnormalities of uremia; diabetic ketoacidosis is usually seen in known diabetic individuals and is associated with hyperglycemia, dehydration, and ketosis in urine and serum[34]; lactic acidosis can be caused by a variety of clinical states but usually represents some form of hypoperfusion such as sepsis or trauma.[35] Lactic acidosis is associated with an increase in lactate in the blood (>4 mEq/L) and an altered ratio of lactate to pyruvate (>30:1) and other oxidation-reduction pairs (e.g., acetoacetate/β-hydroxybutric acid, nicotinamide adenine dinucleotide/reduced form of nicotinamide adenine dinucleotide [NAD/NADH]). It is also important to recognize that lactic acid may represent a component of the metabolic acidosis caused by diabetic ketoacidosis, methanol poisoning, and salicylate intoxication.

Treatment of all forms of anion gap acidosis is both supportive (restore circulation, correct acidosis with bicarbonate) and specific (correct underlying abnormality). Bicarbonate should be given in adequate quantities to keep the pH above 7.2 and/or the bicarbonate level above 15 mEq/L. Situations with ongoing tissue hypoxia may require substantial replacement, whereas transient problems such as postictal lactic acidosis usually correct themselves spontaneously. When bicarbonate is required, the bicarbonate deficit can be determined by a variety of formulas. An easy-to-remember fact is that the bicarbonate space corresponds roughly to one half of total body water (approximately 30% of total body weight in kilograms). Thus:

$$HCO_3^- \text{ deficit} = 0.3 \times \text{wt} \times (24 - HCO_3^-)$$

Usually one half of the calculated deficit is replaced to avoid overcorrection, following which blood gases are repeated before infusing additional bicarbonate. In patients with compromised renal function and metabolic acidosis, it is important to remember that disorders of potassium, magnesium, and phosphate are commonly found and should be sought.

Nonanion gap acidosis (hyperchloremic). Causes of metabolic acidosis with a normal anion gap include bicarbonate loss, inability to excrete hydrogen ion, or administration of exogenous HCl, NH_4Cl. Most commonly there is either a perceived source of bicarbonate loss or an abnormality in the kidney (or adrenal). Recognized bicarbonate loss is usually from the gastrointestinal tract distal to the pylorus and may include duodenal fistula, biliary drainage, pancreatic fistula, small intestinal fistula, ureterosigmoidostomy, and diarrhea. Intrinsic renal losses of bicarbonate include interstitial nephritis, renal tubular acidosis,[30,36,37] adrenal insufficiency, hypoaldosteronism,[38] and acetazolamide administration.

Treatment of nonanion gap acidosis requires correction of the existing acidosis plus routine administration of bicarbonate on a regular basis. The dosage of bicarbonate required depends on the underlying disease, its magnitude, and the need for dialysis. Guidelines for acute correction are the same as for anion gap acidosis: calculate bicarbonate deficit (base deficit), estimate bicarbonate space, and administer only as much as should correct one half of the predicted deficit over a period of 24 hours.

As indicated previously, compensation for metabolic acidosis is usual and is manifested as hyperpnea, tachypnea, nasal flaring, or even Kussmaul's respiration. The degree of compensatory hyperventilation in a stable, chronic metabolic acidosis (as opposed to the acute changes seen in conditions such as sepsis and hypovolemia) can be predicted[31] by the following formula:

$$P\text{CO}_2 = 1.5\ (HCO_3^-) + \Delta$$

where HCO_3^- is the milliequivalent of HCO_3^- and Δ is 8 ± 2 mEq/L. Recognition of this compensatory phenomenon assists in preventing iatrogenic metabolic alkalosis from overtreatment with bicarbonate.

Alkalosis

As is the case with acidosis, alkalosis may be either respiratory or metabolic in origin. In contradistinction to acidosis, it is the metabolic component that is rather simple to define and correct, whereas respiratory alkalosis may have a myriad of causes.

Respiratory alkalosis. Respiratory alkalosis is probably the most common acid-base disturbance in clinical medicine and can be induced by a multitude of underlying conditions. The pathophysiologic mechanism is excess alveolar ventilation above the requirements of carbon dioxide production. This abnormality typically represents some form of CNS overstimulation but may include as causes those factors summarized as follows:

- Anxiety
- Fever
- Salicylate intoxication
- CNS disorders
- Intrathoracic processes
- Hypoxemia
- Hepatic insufficiency
- Gram-negative septicemia
- Pregnancy
- Mechanical hyperventilation

Treatment of respiratory alkalosis must be directed at correcting the underlying cause (e.g., correct fever with antipyretics). In patients requiring assisted ventilation, use of intermittent demand systems tends to minimize the typical overventilation that is seen with controlled or assist/

control mode ventilation. Other attempts at increasing P_{CO_2} such as inspired carbon dioxide, rebreathing devices, and added mechanical dead space are relatively ineffective.

Metabolic alkalosis. The fundamental abnormality in pure metabolic alkalosis is an absolute or relative excess of base (primarily bicarbonate) in extracellular fluid.[25,32,39] This excess tends to be offset by a compensatory decrease in minute alveolar ventilation with subsequent hypercarbia. The mechanisms underlying metabolic alkalosis are the loss of hydrogen (with chloride), gain of exogenous base, or extracellular fluid-volume contraction. Identification of the latter two mechanisms should be straightforward, although gain of exogenous base may be masked as in blood or fresh frozen plasma transfusions (citrate) or intravenous infusions of fresh frozen plasma (citrate) or inappropriate infusion of lactated Ringer's solution.

The most common clinically important form of metabolic alkalosis is a result of loss of hydrogen ion and chloride from the stomach or the kidney. These two varieties can be separated by attention to the amount of urinary chloride. Low urinary chloride (<10 mEq/L) reflects a "chloride responsive" alkalosis that corrects itself by the appropriate administration of saline[40] (usually with some potassium). This variety is typically related to volume contraction, gastric losses, or base administration. High urinary chloride (>10 mEq/L) indicates a "chloride-resistant" alkalosis[41] (caused by hyperaldosteronism, increased plasma desoxycorticosterone, exogenous corticosteroids, licorice ingestion or carbenoxolone therapy, and chloruretic diuretics) and suggests a renal origin, more specifically a "hormone" or drug-related effect on tubular function causing a change in tubular resorption of bicarbonate and increased excretion of H^+ and K^+.[42,43] This latter variety is dependent on (although not initiated by) hypokalemia,[27,44] and correction of the potassium deficit is essential to restoration of acid-base balance.[13] Active reabsorption of potassium in the distal renal tubule in "exchange" for H^+ leads to the paradox of acid urine (paradoxic aciduria) associated with hypokalemic alkalosis. Occasionally, massive doses of potassium are required to achieve equilibrium. When clinically significant hypoventilation develops as compensation for metabolic alkalosis, more rapid treatment may be needed.[45] Two approaches are described, including administration of acid or inducing renal tubular acidosis with acetazolamide. Recent experience with 0.1 normal (N) HCl infusions (or as high as 0.2 N) has shown this form of treatment to be quite safe if administered through a central venous line. The dose of H^+ should be calculated by determining base excess (or increase in bicarbonate above 25 mEq/L), and multiplying it by one half of estimated total body water (0.3 × weight). One half of this calculated amount is then administered during a period of 24 hours. Although anecdotal experience suggests that acetazolamide administration is effective, no controlled studies exist to confirm this contention.

Combined Acid-Base Disorders

It is crucial to realize that acid-base disorders are in no way limited to a single pathophysiologic derangement at a time. Consequently, combinations of abnormalities are common. To distinguish single from combined disturbances, an objective approach is essential. Most standard texts contain graphs that indicate the 95% probability range for single acid-base disorders (i.e., the laboratory values that are 95% likely to represent a single pathophysiologic abnormality). In addition, numerous empiric equations have been developed to identify compensatory changes as opposed to coexistent abnormalities. Characteristics of isolated acid-base disturbances are listed in Table 2-6.

Certain combinations of acid-base disturbances are encountered commonly enough clinically to also justify listing. The components of these combinations and the clinical settings in which they are likely to occur are summarized as follows:

1. *Respiratory acidosis and metabolic alkalosis* occur in patients with chronic respiratory acidosis with superimposed congestive heart failure requiring diuretics.
2. *Respiratory acidosis and metabolic acidosis* occur in patients with cardiopulmonary arrest, chronic lung disease in shock, and chronic renal failure with respiratory insufficiency.
3. *Respiratory alkalosis and metabolic acidosis* occur in patients with hepatic failure caused by central hyperventilation plus hepatic or renal insufficiency.
4. *Respiratory alkalosis and metabolic alkalosis* occur in patients with hepatic cirrhosis with hyperventilation associated with vomiting or in patients with chronic respiratory failure following institution of vigorous mechanical ventilation.
5. *Metabolic acidosis and metabolic alkalosis* are actually sequential rather than simultaneous abnormalities. The

Table 2-6. Identification of Isolated Acid-Base Disturbances

Disturbance	Effect
Metabolic acidosis	P_{CO_2} should fall by 1 to 1.5 times the fall in HCO_3^-
Metabolic alkalosis	P_{CO_2} should rise by 0.5 to 1 times the rise in HCO_3^-
Respiratory acidosis (acute)	Plasma HCO_3^- should be <30 mEq/L
Respiratory acidosis (chronic)	Plasma HCO_3^- should rise by 4 mmol/10 mm Hg rise in P_{CO_2}
Respiratory alkalosis (acute)	Plasma HCO_3^- should fall by 2.5 mmol/10 mm Hg fall in P_{CO_2} (usually >18 mEq/L)
Respiratory alkalosis (chronic)	Plasma HCO_3^- should fall at least as much as acute but not <15 mEq/L

Modified from Schrier RW, ed. Renal and Electrolyte Disorders. Boston: Little, Brown, 1980.
HCO_3^-, Bicarbonate; *P_{CO_2}*, carbon dioxide partial pressure.

combination is identified when the anion gap is greater than the HCO_3^- deficit and occurs with progressive contraction alkalosis caused by vomiting when hypotension develops.

PRINCIPLES OF FLUID THERAPY

In any patient requiring intravenous fluid therapy, three categories of fluid loss must be taken into consideration. These include losses related to normal body maintenance, losses resulting from the patient's underlying disease, and any preexisting fluid deficits. As indicated in an earlier section of this chapter, all patients have normal maintenance requirements related to daily sensible and insensible losses. These losses vary somewhat depending on the person's age, body build, and sex but generally average between 2000 and 2500 ml of fluid every 24 hours. The major sensible loss is urine, and the major insensible loss is related to evaporative losses from the skin and water losses through the lungs. All of these losses are primarily water losses containing only minimal amounts of electrolytes. If an individual patient requires intravenous therapy for only short periods of time, replacement of electrolyte losses is generally unnecessary, and maintenance volume losses can be replaced with solutions of 5% dextrose and water (see Table 2-5). If prolonged intravenous therapy is expected, the small but consistent daily electrolyte losses need to be taken into account and can generally be managed by giving 1 mEq/kg of body weight of sodium, chloride, and potassium daily. Thus if a patient requires 2500 ml of fluid to meet normal maintenance needs, 1500 ml could be provided as dextrose and water, and the remaining 1000 ml could be given as half normal saline with the addition of appropriate amounts of potassium chloride (see Table 2-5).

Losses arising from the patient's underlying disease must also be replaced. In surgical patients these losses are almost always from some portion of the gastrointestinal tract. As a general rule, intestinal secretions, bile, or pancreatic juice can be replaced on a volume-to-volume basis with a balanced salt solution such as lactated Ringer's solution or normal saline, whereas losses from an actively secreting stomach are replaced with half normal saline solution (see Table 2-5). In addition, each of these secretions contains varying amounts of potassium. Generally, gastric secretions contain about twice the amount of potassium as exists in secretions from the small intestine, bile, or pancreas (Table 2-7). To prevent the development of problems with hypokalemia, 10 to 20 mEq of potassium for every liter of fluid loss from any of these sites should be administered. If long-term intravenous therapy is required, these requirements may increase and should be monitored by the determination of serum electrolyte values every 2 to 3 days.

Another source of abnormal losses is an increased evaporative loss from the skin and respiratory tract in patients who are septic. Loss of as much as 1000 ml daily may occur over and above normal insensible losses if the body temperature is markedly elevated. In patients with persistent temperature elevations above 101° F (38.4° C), 500 to 1000 ml of additional fluid may be required daily. Since such fluid loss is primarily water, it can generally be replaced with a dextrose and water intravenous solution.

Finally, preexisting solute or volume deficits must also be corrected. Again, such deficits generally arise from the gastrointestinal tract and are the result of such problems as vomiting, diarrhea, or sequestration of fluid as may occur in patients with bowel obstruction. A correct estimate of these losses is often difficult, but careful attention to physical findings and important historical information from the patient summarizing the duration of disease and the frequency and amount of fluid losses (e.g., through vomiting or diarrhea) are usually helpful in deriving an appropriate estimate of the magnitude of underlying deficits. As emphasized previously, only one half of this calculated estimate should be replaced in a given 24-hour period, and the patient should be reassessed clinically and with supporting laboratory data before attempting any further deficit replacement.

If the principles just enumerated are followed, the large majority of patients requiring intravenous therapy can be managed without difficulty. Especially pertinent in such management is frequent reassessment of the patient clinically and daily review of the patient's input and output records to ensure that the proper amount and type of fluid is being given. Daily weights are especially helpful in this regard and can give valuable clues as to whether abrupt or even subtle changes in fluid balance (either fluid overload or fluid deficit) are occurring. Further, attention to such detail helps prevent the development of any major imbalances that may occur insidiously before they become clinically obvious.

SUMMARY

The plasma is a subset of the total fluid (extracellular fluid) that bathes the cells. As such, when sampled it allows an in-

Table 2-7. Composition of Gastrointestinal Secretions

	Volume (ml/24 hr)	Na (mEq/L)	K (mEq/L)	Cl (mEq/L)	HCO_3^- (mEq/L)
Stomach	1000-2000	60-100	10-20	100-130	—
Pancreas	300-800	135-145	5-10	70-90	95-120
Bile	300-600	135-145	5-10	90-130	30-40
Intestine (primarily small)	2000-4000	120-140	5-10	90-140	30-40

direct look at cellular events and the interaction between the cells and the extracellular fluid. Fluid and electrolyte disorders are legion and commonplace. The correct, critical interpretation of laboratory parameters to identify the pathophysiologic mechanisms underlying these abnormalities requires a willingness to go beyond the obvious. A logical, analytic approach to the meaning of the observed laboratory disturbances should lead to an insight into the significance of the observation. A cookbook approach to "correct" the abnormal test result may actually worsen the situation.

It is critical to appreciate that a concentration actually represents a ratio of the amount of a substance to the amount of fluid in which it is dissolved or suspended. Abnormalities in concentration can be caused by a change in either component. Attention to a variety of clinical factors (weight changes, vital signs, nursing notes, even history and physical examination) often provides the insight necessary to identify the true problem and chart its solution.

REFERENCES

1. Pitts RF. Physiology of the Kidney and Body Fluids: Volume and Composition of the Body Fluids. Chicago: Year Book Medical Publishers, 1968.
2. Loeb JN. The hyperosmolar state. N Engl J Med 290:1184, 1984.
3. Gruber UF, Allgower M. Water and electrolyte balance. In Diem K, ed. Documenta Geigy, Scientific Tables. Ardsley, N.Y.: Geigy Pharmaceuticals, 1970.
4. Forbes RM, Mitchell HH, Cooper AR. Further studies on the gross composition and mineral elements of the adult human body. J Biol Chem 223:969, 1956.
5. Corsa L, et al. Measurement of exchangeable potassium in man by isotope dilution. J Clin Invest 29:1280, 1950.
6. Moore FD. Determination of total body water and solids with isotopes. Science 104:157, 1946.
7. Moore FD, et al. Body composition: Total body water and electrolytes: Intravascular and extravascular phase volumes. Metabolism 5:447, 1956.
8. Kunau RT, Webb HL, Borman SC. Characteristics of sodium reabsorption in the loop of Henle and distal tubule. Am J Physiol 227:1181, 1974.
9. Jorgensen PL. Sodium and potassium ion pumps in kidney tubules. Physiol Rev 60:864, 1980.
10. Handler JS, Orlof J. Antidiuretic hormone. Annu Rev Physiol 43:611, 1981.
11. Bie P. Osmoreceptors, vasopressin, and control of renal water excretion. Physiol Rev 60:961, 1980.
12. Davis JO, Freeman RH. Mechanisms regulating renin release. Physiol Rev 56:1, 1976.
13. Boyd JE, Mulrow TJ. Further studies of the influence of potassium on aldosterone production in the rat. Endocrinol 90:299, 1972.
14. Imai M, Kokko J. Sodium urea and water transport in the thin ascending limb of Henle: Generation of osmotic gradients by passive diffusion of solutes. J Clin Invest 53:393, 1974.
15. Hays RM. Antidiuretic hormone. N Engl J Med 295:659, 1976.
16. Oh MS, Carroll HJ. Disorders of sodium metabolism: Hypernatremia and hyponatremia. Crit Care Med 20:94, 1992.
17. Oh MS, Carroll HJ. Decreased anion gap and hyponatremia. N Engl J Med 298:111, 1978.
18. Cooke CR, Turin MD, Walker WG. The syndrome of inappropriate antidiuretic hormone secretion (SIADH): Pathophysiologic mechanisms in solute and volume regulation. Medicine 58:240, 1979.
19. Espinel CH. The FeNa test. JAMA 6:579, 1976.
20. Kunau RT, Stein JH. Disorders of hypo- and hyperkalemia. Clin Nephrol 7:173, 1977.
21. Gennari FJ, Cohen JJ. Role of the kidney in potassium homeostasis: Lessons from acid base disturbances (editorial). Kidney Int 8:1, 1975.
22. Schultze RG. Recent advances in the physiology and pathophysiology of potassium excretion. Arch Intern Med 131:885, 1973.
23. Harmann RC, Mellinkoff SM. The relationship of platelets to the serum potassium concentration. J Clin Invest 34:938, 1955.
24. Williams ME. Hyperkalemia. Crit Care Clin 7:155, 1991.
25. Hodgkin JE, Soeprono FF, Chan DM. Incidence of metabolic alkalemia in hospitalized patients. Crit Care Med 8:725, 1980.
26. Knochel JP. Role of glucoregulatory hormones in potassium homeostasis. Kidney Int 11:443, 1977.
27. Roscoe JM, et al. Effect of amphotericin-B on urine acidification in rats: Implications for the pathogenesis of distal renal tubular acidosis. J Lab Clin Med 89:463, 1977.
28. Sebastian A, Morris RC Jr. Renal tubular acidosis. Clin Nephrol 7:216, 1977.
29. Lipner HI, et al. The behavior of carbenicillin as a nonreabsorbable anion. J Lab Clin Med 290:1184, 1974.
30. Rocha AS, Kokko JP. Sodium chloride and water transport in the medullary thick ascending limb of Henle: Evidence for active chloride transport. J Clin Invest 52:612, 1973.
31. Albert MD, Dell RB, Winters RW. Quantitative displacement of acid base equilibrium in metabolic acidosis. Ann Intern Med 66:312, 1967.
32. Arruda JAL, Kurtzman NA. Metabolic acidosis and alkalosis. Clin Nephrol 7:201, 1977.
33. Emmett M, et al. The pathophysiology of acid-base changes in chronically phosphate-depleted rats. J Clin Invest 59:291, 1977.
34. Felig P. Diabetic ketoacidosis. N Engl J Med 290:1360, 1974.
35. Olivja PB. Lactic acidosis. Am J Med 48:209, 1970.
36. Halperin ML, et al. Studies on the pathogenesis of type 1 (distal) renal tubular acidosis as revealed by the urinary P_{CO_2} tensions. J Clin Invest 53:669, 1974.
37. Sebastian A, McSherry E, Morris RC Jr. Renal potassium wasting in renal tubular acidosis. J Clin Invest 50:667, 1971.
38. Szylman P, et al. Role of hyperkalemia in the metabolic acidosis of isolated hypoaldosteronism. N Engl J Med 294:361, 1976.
39. Madias NE, Ayus JC, Adroque HJ. Increased anion gap in metabolic alkalosis: The role of plasma-protein equivalency. N Engl J Med 300:1421, 1979.
40. Kassirer JP, et al. The critical role of chloride in the correction of hypokalemic alkalosis in man. Am J Med 38:172, 1965.
41. Garella S, Chazan JA, Cohen JJ. Saline resistant metabolic alkalosis or "chloride-wasting nephropathy." Report of four cases with severe potassium depletion. Ann Intern Med 73:31, 1970.
42. Fanestil DO, Park CS. Steroid hormones and the kidney. Annu Rev Physiol 43:637, 1981.
43. Gill JR, Bartter FC. Evidence for a prostaglandin-independent defect in chloride reabsorption in the loop of Henle as a proximal cause of Bartter's syndrome. Am J Med 65:766, 1978.
44. Seldin DW, Rector RC Jr. The generation and maintenance of metabolic alkalosis. Kidney Int 1:306, 1972.
45. Shear L, Brandman IS. Hypoxia and hypercapnia caused by respiratory compensation for metabolic alkalosis. Am Rev Respir Dis 107:836, 1973.

SUGGESTED READINGS

Brenner BM, Stein JH, eds. Contemporary Issues in Nephrology, vol 2. Acid-base and Potassium Homeostasis. New York: Churchill Livingstone, 1978.

Diem K, ed. Water and electrolyte balance. In Documenta Geigy, Scientific Tables. Ardsley, N.Y.: Geigy Pharmaceuticals, 1962.

Goodenough RD, Burke JF. Fluid, electrolyte and acid-base homeostasis in surgery. In Burke JF, ed. Surgical Physiology. Philadelphia: WB Saunders, 1983.

Maxwell MH, Kleeman CR, Narins RG, eds. Clinical Disorders of Fluid and Electrolyte Metabolism, 4th ed. New York: McGraw-Hill, 1987.

Murphy JE, Preuss HG, Henry JB. Evaluation of renal function and water, electrolyte, and acid-base balance. In Henry JB, ed. Clinical Diagnosis and Management by Laboratory Methods. Philadelphia: WB Saunders, 1984.

Narins RG, et al. Diagnostic strategies in disorders of fluid, electrolyte, and acid-base homeostasis. Am J Med 72:496, 1982.

Schrier RW, ed. Renal and Electrolyte Disorders. Boston: Little, Brown, 1980.

Shoemaker WC. Fluids and electrolytes in the adult. In Shoemaker WC, Thompson WL, eds. Critical Care—State of the Art, vol 3. Fullerton, Calif.: Society of Critical Care Medicine, 1982.

Vanatta JC, Gogelman MJ. Moyer's Fluid Balance. Chicago: Year Book Medical Publishers, 1976.

3

Surgical Nutrition

Virginia M. Herrmann and John M. Daly

For centuries, physicians have been aware of the effect of various disease states on body composition and the importance of nutrition in maintaining health. More recently, protein-calorie undernutrition has become recognized as contributing significantly to morbidity and mortality in hospitalized patients. During the past two decades, biochemical indexes and anthropometric studies demonstrated that significant malnutrition occurs in up to 50% of surgical patients[1] and identified factors that render the patient at increased nutritional risk and provide warning signs of impending development of malnutrition[2,3] (see box, p. 55). Butterworth[4] described the prevalence of malnutrition in patients as the "skeleton in the hospital closet," and others confirmed the presence of mild-to-severe malnutrition in many hospitalized patients.[5] The provision of enteral and parenteral nutrition support strategies for malnourished patients has also developed concomitantly during the past two decades and currently demands a sophisticated understanding of the metabolic alterations that occur in starvation, mild stress, or multisystem organ failure. The generalized provision of enteral or intravenous nutrition to prevent malnutrition has been enhanced by our ability to use specific nutritional substrates or manipulations to alter immune function and the response to sepsis or injury. Despite the lack of documented efficacy of nutrition support favorably impacting morbidity or mortality in many disease states, the prevalence of malnutrition in hospitalized patients and the association between malnutrition and mortality and morbidity suggest that maintaining or repleting nutritional status should favorably alter outcome.[6,7]

Protein-calorie malnutrition occurs as one of three clinical entities: marasmus, kwashiorkor, and a mixture of the two. Marasmus is simple starvation resulting from prolonged inadequate intake of all nutrients. Cahill[8] described the adaptive processes to starvation, which include use of available endogenous energy stores, predominantly fat. The initial, relatively high urinary loss of protein decreases as the body adapts to a lipid source of calories. Prolonged starvation leads to continued reduction of protein stores. Clinically, patients with marasmus exhibit loss of subcutaneous fat, diminution of muscle mass, and weight loss. Biochemical markers of visceral protein status may be relatively normal. Kwashiorkor occurs as a result of diets lacking in protein but with sufficient calories. Patients with this entity exhibit signs of protein loss, including reduction of visceral mass and muscle bulk, edema, and hair loss. The degree of weight loss is variable because of adequate calorie intake. Laboratory biochemical markers are usually abnormal with low serum concentrations of albumin, transferrin, and prealbumin. Cellular immunity is depressed and may be demonstrated by anergy to skin test antigens and depression of the total lymphocyte count. The third kind of protein-calorie malnutrition, a mixed marasmus-kwashiorkor type, is most common in hospitalized patients. Underlying malnutrition is enhanced by stress resulting from a given disease, its treatment, or its complications. These patients are at high risk for increased morbidity and mortality.

The changes in nitrogen balance associated with significant protein undernutrition are reflected in a loss in lean body mass and muscle protein content. Protein malnutrition in surgical patients is associated with decreased immune function,[9] diminished respiratory mechanics,[10] and intestinal atrophy.[11] Understanding the pathophysiology of these effects and designing management strategies to ensure their prevention is paramount to good surgical practice.

ENERGY STORAGE AND STARVATION

Starvation in humans results in a reliance on endogenous fuel reserves to satisfy energy and protein requirements. Endogenous stores are in three forms, including carbohydrate, protein, and fat. Carbohydrate, along with water, is stored as glycogen intracellularly. The amount of stored glycogen is limited, and it is a relatively inefficient fuel on a per weight basis. Total liver and muscle glycogen stores provide approximately 900 calories in healthy humans

NUTRITIONALLY HIGH-RISK PATIENT—FOR HOSPITAL-ASSOCIATED MORBIDITY AND MORTALITY

Gross underweight: Weight-for-height below 80% of standard
Gross overweight: Weight-for-height above 120% of standard
Recent loss of 10% or more of usual body weight
Alcoholism
No oral intake for more than 10 days receiving simple intravenous solutions
Protracted nutrient losses
- Malabsorption syndromes
- Short gut syndromes/fistulas
- Renal dialysis
- Draining abscesses, wounds

Increased metabolic needs
- Extensive burns, infection, trauma
- Protracted fever

Intake of drugs with antinutrient or catabolic properties: steroids, immunosuppressants, antitumor agents.

Modified from Butterworth CE. Malnutrition in hospital patients: Assessment and treatment. In Goodhart RS, Shils ME, eds. Modern Nutrition in Health and Disease. Philadelphia: Lea & Febiger, 1980.

Table 3-1. Tissue Fuel Composition of Normal Man

Fuel*	Kg	Calories
Fat (adipose triglyceride)	15	141,000
Protein (mainly muscle)	6	24,000
Glycogen (muscle)	0.15	600
Glycogen (liver)	0.075	300
TOTAL		165,900

Modified from Cahill GF. Starvation in man. N Engl J Med 282:668, 1970.
*Total available carbohydrate fuel is approximately 900 calories.

(Table 3-1).[8] Protein is stored predominantly in lean body mass intracellularly in an aqueous environment. Approximately 24,000 calories are potentially available in healthy humans from protein. In addition to its role as an energy source, protein also serves other essential functions in tissue repair and homeostasis. Fat is stored intracellularly in a nonaqueous environment[8] and constitutes the major fuel source with over 140,000 calories potentially available in healthy humans. Although fat stores also provide insulation, their major role is energy provision.

During brief starvation, body reserves are used for nutritional requirements. Following a 24-hour fast, resting energy expenditures, approximately 1800 calories in a healthy person, are derived from glycogen, protein, and fat. Glycogen stores are inadequate to meet these requirements, necessitating the use of other fuel reserves. Starvation initially results in increased production of urinary urea, reflecting mobilization of endogenous protein reserves to meet energy requirements. Increased urea production in the liver is a consequence of an increased release of NH_2 moieties for gluconeogenesis from amino acid precursors. Alanine and glutamine are released from muscle breakdown, and additional alanine is released from the gut proportionate to glutamine uptake by the splanchnic bed. The resulting production of hepatic glucose is used by the brain and other glycolytic tissues such as red blood cells. Red blood cells convert glucose into lactate and pyruvate that are transported back to the liver and act as gluconeogenic precursors. This energy requiring activity is called the Cori cycle.

Energy for these activities is derived from the oxidation of fat.[12] The fall in plasma glucose concentrations during starvation is reflected by a corresponding fall in plasma insulin and a rise in plasma glucagon concentrations, resulting in an increase in lipolysis with corresponding increased free fatty acid levels. Fatty acids may be used for energy by certain tissues or may be oxidized to ketone bodies by the liver; they may then be used for energy by the liver and other tissues.

Prolonged starvation is characterized by the conversion from a glucose to a lipid system of energy use. Continued reliance on glucose would require continued skeletal muscle breakdown for gluconeogenesis precursors. This would severely compromise other important functions of proteins, including enzymatic, structural, and transport requirements. Continued use of fat for energy is characterized by a fall in urinary urea, reflecting decreased amino acid efflux from skeletal muscle, and by a corresponding increase in plasma concentrations of free fatty acids and ketone bodies. The brain converts to the use of ketone bodies for energy. Prolonged starvation may be tolerated for approximately 50 days because of the size of normal fat reserves in humans.

STARVATION IN STRESS OR ILLNESS (STRESSED STARVATION)

The addition of stress or illness (e.g., sepsis, traumatic injury, burns, major elective surgery) complicates the picture of simple starvation. The hormonal response to severe stress or injury is associated with increased adrenocorticotropic hormone (ACTH), epinephrine, glucagon, and cortisol production and significantly alters carbohydrate, protein, and fat metabolism, as well as metabolic rate. Stressed starvation is therefore characterized by increased energy and protein requirements without the usual adaptive protein-conserving mechanisms present in simple starvation. Cytokines released with injury or illness mediate the inflammatory response, increase temperature and metabolic rate, produce anorexia, and further complicate starvation in this patient subset.

During starvation in the patient with associated stress or illness, increased mobilization of amino acids from skeletal muscle (primarily alanine) occurs to promote hepatic gluconeogenesis. Amino acids are also released to enable wound repair and immune function. Cori cycle activity, or recycling 3-carbon precursors (e.g., lactate, pyruvate) to form hepatic glucose, increases in stressed starvation. Cori cycle activity is energy wasting and associated with mild-to-moderate lactic acidosis and thus further compromises the stressed individual who is starving. As a result of increased Cori cycle activity, lipolysis is enhanced without a corresponding fall in skeletal muscle breakdown. The magnitude of injury or stress is the major determinant of urinary urea nitrogen losses.

The goals of nutrition support in the starved patient, with or without stress or associated illness, is to meet the requirements of energy, protein, fat, trace minerals, and vitamins exogenously, using the appropriate route of administration. The ability to preserve body mass and function by nutrition support is discussed in the following sections.

NUTRITIONAL ASSESSMENT

In surgical patients, malnutrition is associated with delayed wound healing, decreased resistance to infection, and other potential complications.[13] Implementation of perioperative nutritional intervention results in the reversal of markers associated with malnutrition such as improvement in short half-life serum protein concentrations and reversal of skin test anergy and in turn is associated with reduced postoperative morbidity and mortality.[14] Assessment of operative risk requires qualitative and quantitative methods of nutritional assessment. Nutritional assessment techniques correlate physiologic and body compositional aberrations with useful clinical markers that are associated with malnutrition. Standard methods for assessing nutritional status include a history and physical examination, anthropometric measurements, laboratory determinations, and measurement of immune competence.

Nutritional assessment should be undertaken in all patients under consideration for nutrition support and should be used as a guideline to quantitate the degree of malnutrition.

Impact of Malnutrition

Complete assessment includes the identification of both undernourishment or overnourishment secondary to specific nutrient deficits or excesses. During the past 10 to 15 years, the impact of malnutrition on various organ systems at the cellular and subcellular level has been examined.[15] This broader definition of assessment provides for the identification of specific nutrients or substrates in an effort to reduce the morbidity associated with malnutrition. The adverse effects of malnutrition in hospitalized patients has been well documented,[16,17] as have been studies demonstrating that adequate nutritional repletion may reduce otherwise commonly encountered complications.[14,18] Accurate nutritional assessment allows the surgeon to classify malnutrition into specific diagnostic categories specified by ICDA codes. With this coding system, marasmus (ICDA Code 268.0) is defined as chronic protein-calorie undernutrition associated with a decrease in body cell mass and altered anthropometric measurements, weight loss, significant wasting of skeletal muscle and loss of body fat, and immune incompetence. Kwashiorkor (ICDA Code 267.0) identifies patients who have been receiving adequate calories but inadequate protein. Obesity and peripheral edema are common, although skeletal muscle mass and immune competence may be preserved. Since most hospitalized patients who are malnourished exhibit mixed malnutrition (ICDA Code 269.9), a wide variety of specific nutritional deficiencies have been identified and can be defined by ICDA codes in an attempt to categorize the assessment.

History and Physical Examination

The importance of a thorough history and physical examination to provide accurate nutritional assessment should be emphasized, despite the sophisticated biochemical testing that has been developed.

Nutritional deficiencies may be generalized or may involve only specific nutrients. Certain clinical entities are associated with generalized nutritional deficiencies (e.g., alcoholism is associated with protein-calorie malnutrition and deficits of various vitamins and minerals, including niacin and zinc). Specific operative procedures may be responsible for individual vitamin and mineral deficiencies. Ileal resection or diversion may result in steatorrhea with deficiencies in fat-soluble vitamins and magnesium.

A complete dietary history may give clues to underlying deficiencies, including a history of recent weight loss or use of fad diets.[19] The medical history should evaluate prior operations or conditions that may have resulted in nutritional deficits (e.g., folate deficiency as a result of a prior gastrectomy or a history of chronic illness such as pancreatic insufficiency may indicate deficiencies of the fat-soluble vitamins). The social history may help explain underlying deficiencies. Poverty, alcoholism, and fad diets have been implicated in malnutrition. Finally, a careful systems review should uncover symptoms associated with anorexia and weight loss. The presence of nausea and vomiting, diarrhea, melena, abdominal pain, dysphagia, peripheral edema, and fever are often present in disease states that are associated with protein-calorie malnutrition, as shown in Table 3-2.

A careful physical examination identifies most patients with malnutrition (see box, p. 58). Overall patient appearance should be noted. Although most patients are not obviously emaciated, the presence of pallor, edema, skin lesions, and muscle wasting often provides specific and general signs of nutritional deficiency states. Loss of hair is associated with protein deficiency. Loss of subcutaneous fat may be associated with calorie depletion. Iron deficiency may be the cause of spoon-shaped nails. Niacin deficiency,

Table 3-2. Nutritional Deficiencies Commonly Associated With Disease States

Nutrient	Clinical State
Protein	Burns, nephrosis, alcoholism, surgery, protein-losing enteropathy
Fat	Gluten-induced enteropathy, blind loop syndrome, tropical sprue, pancreatic insufficiency, ileal resection, gastrectomy, short bowel syndrome
Potassium	Surgery, intestinal bypass
Calcium	Chronic renal failure, gastrectomy, intestinal bypass
Iron	Hemorrhage, gastrectomy
Magnesium	Alcoholism, intestinal bypass surgery, malabsorption syndromes, intestinal and biliary fistulas, acute pancreatitis, diabetes, parathyroid disease, renal disease, diuretic therapy
Zinc	Alcoholism, surgery
Vitamin A	Chronic obstructive lung disease, congestive heart failure, pancreatic insufficiency, fever, thyrotoxicosis, gastrectomy, bile salt depletion, sprue, cystic fibrosis
Vitamin D	Gastrectomy, cirrhosis, pancreatic insufficiency
Vitamin K	Pancreatic insufficiency, obstructive jaundice, cholestyramine ingestion, prolonged antibiotic therapy
Vitamin E	Pancreatitis, cystic fibrosis, steatorrhea, gastrectomy
Thiamine	Wernicke encephalopathy, beriberi, thyrotoxicosis, fever, diuresis, prolonged antacid therapy
Riboflavin	Alcoholism, fever
Niacin	Alcoholism
Pyridoxine	Thyrotoxicosis, alcoholism
Folate	Alcoholism, psoriasis, rheumatoid arthritis, fever, liver disease, sickle cell disease, leukemia, thyrotoxicosis, gastrectomy, macrocytic anemia, gluten-induced enteropathy, malignancy
Vitamin B_{12}	Ileal resection, pernicious anemia, regional enteritis, blind loop syndrome, thyrotoxicosis, alcoholism, gastrectomy
Vitamin C	Drug addiction, fever, rheumatoid arthritis, alcoholism, thyrotoxicosis, congestive heart failure, peptic ulcer disease

Modified from Grant JP, Custer PB, Thurlow J. Current techniques of nutritional assessment. J Surg Clin North Am 61:437, 1981.

pellagra, may result in a symmetric, hyperpigmented skin rash over body parts exposed to sunlight.

The oral cavity is commonly affected in malnutrition. The absence of teeth or the presence of caries may contribute to the underlying deficiency. Glossitis is associated with vitamin B deficiency; and swollen, bleeding gums are associated with vitamin C deficiency.

Muscle wasting is the most recognizable sign of protein-calorie malnutrition. It may be associated with peripheral edema. All muscle groups may be affected, although signs may be more obvious in the small muscles of the hand and in the muscles of facial expression.

Anthropometric Measurements

Anthropometry is the science that deals with the measurement of the size, weight, and proportions of the human body. Body proportions or composition may be assessed using analytic methods to determine total body nitrogen, potassium, and water. These standardized anthropometric measurements have been compared with direct body composition analyses; they may be helpful in determining nutritional status, although this appears to be more likely in groups rather than in individuals.

The body can be divided into six compartments: fat, skin and skeleton, extracellular mass, plasma protein, visceral protein, and somatic protein mass.[19] Assessment of the various compartments is useful in quantifying the type and degree of deficits present (Fig. 3-1). Assessing compartment losses is important not only for determining nutrient needs but also for determining individual deficits.

Somatic Protein Mass

Anthropometric measurements of somatic protein mass (skeletal muscle) are body weight and mid-upper arm muscle circumference.

Body weight. Body weight should be measured at the time of hospital admission in all surgical patients. Body weight with respect to one's height is essential to initial assessment, and daily or frequent body weight measurement is essential to assess the adequacy of repletion in patients receiving nutrition support.[20] Normal or "ideal" body weight is usually determined by standards produced by the Metropolitan Life Insurance Company, and statistics are available in actuarial charts that average information about individuals who apply for life insurance.

However, a comparison of actual to ideal body weight may have little clinical application because of the wide range of weights for any given frame size. In addition, obesity is prevalent in our society so that actual weight may be greater than ideal weight. Substantial recent weight loss may have occurred in a given patient, also obscuring the meaning of actual weight measurements. Insufficient caloric intake results in increased use of endogenous fat and protein stores for caloric needs, resulting in weight loss. Extracellular sodium and water may be retained in protein-depleted patients, causing an underestimation of malnutrition when determined by body weight. However, loss of weight over a prolonged period (weeks) is usually specific for decreased energy intake in relation to energy needs.

Although "ideal body weight" is important, changes in body weight that occur in hospitalized patients when compared to *usual* body weight are more significant than comparisons to a patient's *ideal* weight. Body weight should be measured in a consistent and precise manner as clinical decisions based on any single weight are problematic.[21]

Recent data from the First and Second Health and Nu-

PHYSICAL SIGNS ASSOCIATED WITH MALNUTRITION

Dietary Obesity

Excess weight
Excessive weight
Excessive skinfolds
Excessive abdominal girth

Undernutrition

Lethargy, mental and physical
Low weight in relation to height
Diminished skinfolds
Exaggerated skeletal prominences
Loss of elasticity of skin

Protein-Calorie Deficiency Disease

Edema
Muscle wasting
Low body weight
Psychomotor change
Dyspigmentation of the hair
Thin, sparse hair
Moon face
Flaky pain dermatosis
Areas of hyperpigmentation

Vitamin A Deficiency

Xerosis of skin
Follicular hyperkeratosis
Xerosis conjunctivae
Keratomalacia
Bitot's spots

Riboflavin Deficiency

Angular stomatitis
Cheilosis
Magenta tongue
Central atrophy of lingual papillae
Nasolabial dyssebacia
Angular palpebritis
Scrotal and vulval dermatosis
Corneal vascularization

Thiamin Deficiency

Loss of ankle jerks
Sensory loss and motor weakness
Calf-muscle tenderness
Cardiovascular dysfunction
Edema

Niacin Deficiency

Pellagrous dermatosis
Scarlet and raw tongue
Tongue fissuring
Atrophic lingual papillae
Malar and supraorbital pigmentation

Vitamin C Deficiency

Spongy and bleeding gums
Folliculosis
Petechiae
Ecchymoses
Intramuscular or subperiosteal hematoma
Epiphyseal enlargement (painful)

Vitamin D Deficiency

Active rickets (in children)
Epiphyseal enlargement (older than 6 months of age, painless)
Beading of ribs
Craniotabes (younger than 1 year of age)
Muscular hypotonia
Healed rickets (in children or adults)
Frontal and parietal bossing
Knock-knees or bow legs
Deformities of thorax
Osteomalacia (in adults)
Local or generalized skeletal deformities

Iron Deficiency

Pallor of mucous membranes
Koilonychia
Atrophic lingual papillae

Modified from Scrimshaw NS. Cecil Textbook of Medicine. Philadelphia: WB Saunders, 1979.

trition Surveys (Hanes I and Hanes II) include height and weight and various other anthropometric measurements. These data provide information on weight and anthropometric standards by height, sex, and frame size for all races. The data have been divided into two groups, consisting of adults between ages 25 and 54 years and those between ages 55 and 74 years. These tables can be used to establish new criteria identifying patients by age group at risk for malnutrition.[22]

Accurate determination of weight loss is essential in patients requiring specialized support. The accuracy of determining weight loss is dependent on the precision of initial hospital weight and subsequent measurements. Body weight fluctuates throughout a 24-hour period secondary to intake and output and insensible loss. Surgical patients should be weighed at the same time or as near to the same time each day and on the same scale. Weight gain or loss following operative procedures or the loss of fluid in patients with traumatic injury or sepsis may be suggested by wide fluctuation in the daily weight of these patients. Data suggest that weight loss is an important indicator of operative risk and an accurate predictor of morbidity in surgical patients.[23]

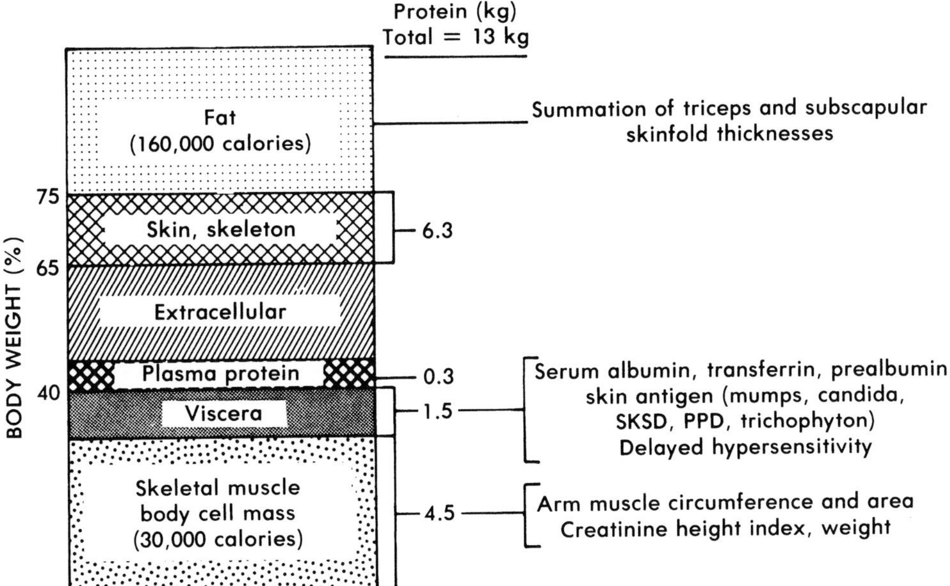

Fig. 3-1. Body composition components and corresponding nutritional assessment methods. *PPD,* Purified protein derivative; *SKSD,* streptokinase-streptodornase. (Modified from Blackburn GL, Bothe A. Assessment of malnutrition in cancer patients. Cancer Bull 30:88, 1978.)

Arm circumference measurement. The mid-upper arm circumference has been found to be a simple anthropometric estimate of skeletal muscle mass. The mid-upper arm is defined as the midpoint between the olecranon and the acromial process. The circumference of the arm muscle at this point calculated with the use of the triceps skinfold thickness is compared with results in standard tables. Less than 60% of standard is considered abnormal.

Body Fat Mass

Depletion of body fat is an indicator of inadequate caloric intake relative to energy needs. Body fat is also determined anthropometrically by measurement of skinfold thickness. This method is justified because subcutaneous fat accounts for approximately 50% of total body fat. Various sites can be used for measurement of skinfold thickness, including thigh, calf, biceps, suprailiac, and chin. The summation of measurements taken at three or four different sites (Durnin's equation) may also be used. However, the most common method for assessing subcutaneous fat has been the use of triceps and subscapular skinfolds. Triceps and subscapular skinfolds are easier to measure, and the measurements tend to be more accurate than that of other skinfolds in edematous patients.

It must be emphasized, however, that these anthropometric measurements have serious limitations in hospitalized patients.[24] They are of little value in assessing short-term changes in energy or nitrogen balance or body composition. Further, these measurements are of limited usefulness as they provide static information about body composition, and the effectiveness of nutritional repletion is better determined by dynamic assessment of tissue and organ function. These measurements also lack both sensitivity and specificity in accurately assessing alterations in body composition and are unreliable in obese patients. Despite these limitations, anthropometric measurements, when meticulously performed in select patient groups, may allow a more complete nutritional assessment but should be used in conjunction with other means of determining nutritional status.

Laboratory Determinations

Estimation of somatic and visceral protein mass can be obtained by laboratory tests. Depletion of somatic mass can be determined by measurement of 24-hour urinary creatinine excretion in the presence of normal renal function. Creatinine is the breakdown product of creatine, a liver-synthesized energy molecule that is stored in skeletal muscle. By measurement of the 24-hour urinary creatinine excretion in the absence of renal impairment, skeletal muscle mass is assessed indirectly. Known 24-hour urinary creatinine levels for normal adults of similar sex and height can be compared to an actual patient measurement. The ratio of the patient's 24-hour urinary creatinine excretion to normal values, expressed as a percentage, is called the creatinine-height index (CHI). A CHI of 100% indicates normal lean body mass. Depletion of lean body mass should result in a CHI of less than 80%.[25] Nevertheless, this methodology suffers from the use of "ideal" values found in tables and from the difficulties encountered in obtaining accurate 24-hour urine collections.

Nitrogen balance is another means of assessing protein

mass in hospitalized patients. Knowledge of urinary urea kinetics allows this estimation, even in patients with poor renal function.[26] Total nitrogen excretion has been replaced by the 24-hour urinary nitrogen excretion, adjusted for nonurinary nitrogen losses (skin and feces) and nonurea nitrogen losses (creatinine or ammonia). Nitrogen balance in surgical patients can be determined in the following manner:

$$N_{Bal} = \frac{\text{Protein intake}}{6.25} - (\text{Urinary urea nitrogen} + 4)$$

$$6.25 = \text{Conversion factor for protein intake to nitrogen intake (g/24 hr)}$$

and

$$4 = \text{Nonurinary nitrogen loss adjustment (g/24 hr)}$$

Because determination of 24-hour urinary urea excretion is difficult to obtain in hospitalized patients, the validity of using shorter collection times has been studied and compared to 24-hour collection times in critically ill adult patients.[27] Twelve-hour collection times are a satisfactory estimate of 24-hour nitrogen excretion times, but shorter collection times (e.g., 4-hour and 8-hour determinations) are not representative of 24-hour excretion. A 12-hour determination provides results that can be used to accurately estimate 24-hour urea urinary nitrogen excretion and is more rapidly available and easier to perform in the hospital setting. The 12-hour determination requires less nursing time and is associated with fewer errors caused by inaccurate or lost specimens.

Visceral protein mass is estimated by measurement of plasma transport protein concentrations. The ideal measurable plasma protein should have a short half-life (high rate of synthesis and catabolism) with few factors altering catabolism.[28] Current laboratory methods measure plasma levels of albumin, transferrin, prealbumin, and retinol-binding protein.

Serum albumin concentration has been one of the more widely used indexes of nutritional assessment. Hypoalbuminemia is often seen in patients with malnutrition and is associated with increased morbidity and mortality in both medical and surgical hospitalized patients.[29,30] The effect of low body weight and low serum albumin levels are additive on mortality rate.[31] Yet serum albumin level has been criticized as an accurate predictor of nutritional depletion and is not an ideal transport protein for estimation of visceral protein mass. Normal albumin synthesis in humans ranges between 120 and 220 mg/kg/day and is significantly affected by dietary intake, illness, traumatic injury, stress, and liver function. Forty percent of total body albumin is located in the intravascular space, providing a normal albumin level between 3 and 5 g/kg. Body albumin is also present to a great extent in the extravascular space. The metabolic half-life of albumin is approximately 20 days, and serum albumin levels may be greatly altered by hydrational changes, stress, catabolic illness, and starvation. Significant thermal injury or traumatic injury may result in abnormally large losses of albumin. Similar losses are noted in patients with renal disease, nephrotic syndrome, severe diarrhea, or protein-losing enteropathy. Albumin levels are very sensitive to changes in body hydration or changes in the distribution of body fluid. Albumin can be mobilized from the extravascular pool into the vascular space; conversely, albumin has been shown to leave the intravascular space and diffuse into other body compartments. Thus serum concentrations of albumin may not adequately assess visceral protein mass, particularly in the acute setting. Nevertheless, depressed serum albumin concentrations are associated with chronic visceral protein depletion, particularly when levels fall below 3.0 g/ml.

Plasma transferrin concentration may be a better estimate of visceral protein mass than serum albumin. Plasma transferrin has a half-life of 8 days and a smaller total body pool. This shorter half-life allows transferrin to be a more useful and practical indicator of nutritional repletion. Serum transferrin values have been demonstrated to significantly correlate with body cell mass and nutritional state. Nonetheless, hepatic transferrin synthesis rates may be affected by different nutrient deficiencies (e.g., iron deficiency) that have marked underlying protein depletion. Thus although better than albumin as a marker of nutritional assessment, serum transferrin should never be the sole indicator of the adequacy of nutrition or estimate of nutritional repletion.[32]

Finally, short half-life proteins such as prealbumin and retinol-binding protein have also been used for estimation of visceral protein mass. Prealbumin is involved in the transport of thyroid hormone. It has a metabolic half-life of 2 days. However, it is rapidly depressed in nonmalnourished patients with traumatic injuries or sepsis.[19] Retinol-binding protein has a metabolic half-life of 12 hours. This serum protein is considered unreliable in patients with renal failure because it is cleared by the kidneys. In addition, it is very sensitive to other factors, including stress, which has limited its clinical use.

Immune Competence

Anergy to skin test antigens has been shown to be a predictor of septic complications.[33] Although delayed cutaneous hypersensitivity is usually considered a test specifically for cell-mediated immunity, both cell-mediated and humoral immune responses are interrelated. Specifically, subsets of T lymphocytes, T-helper and T-suppressor cells, interact with B cells, allowing and controlling the ability of B cells to produce antibodies. Therefore depression of T-cell function as measured by anergy to skin test antigens helps assess the ability of the patient to mount an immune response to injury and infection. Various skin test antigens used include mumps, tuberculin, and *Candida* species. A positive response has a diameter of induration greater than 5 mm. A patient is considered anergic if induration fails to form to all skin test antigens, although a graded system of immune responsiveness may be used.

The immune system may be depressed in old age and by

trauma, inhalation anesthetic agents, drugs, malignancy, and oncologic therapy.[34,35] Malnutrition is also associated with impairment of the immune response.[36] Reversal of skin test anergy in malnourished patients has been demonstrated following nutritional repletion.[37] This supports the belief that nutritional intervention is useful in immune-suppressed patients. Nevertheless, because of the complexity of the immune system, as well as the ability of various factors to alter the immune response, delayed cutaneous hypersensitivity skin testing should be considered complementary to other means of assessing nutritional status (Fig. 3-2).

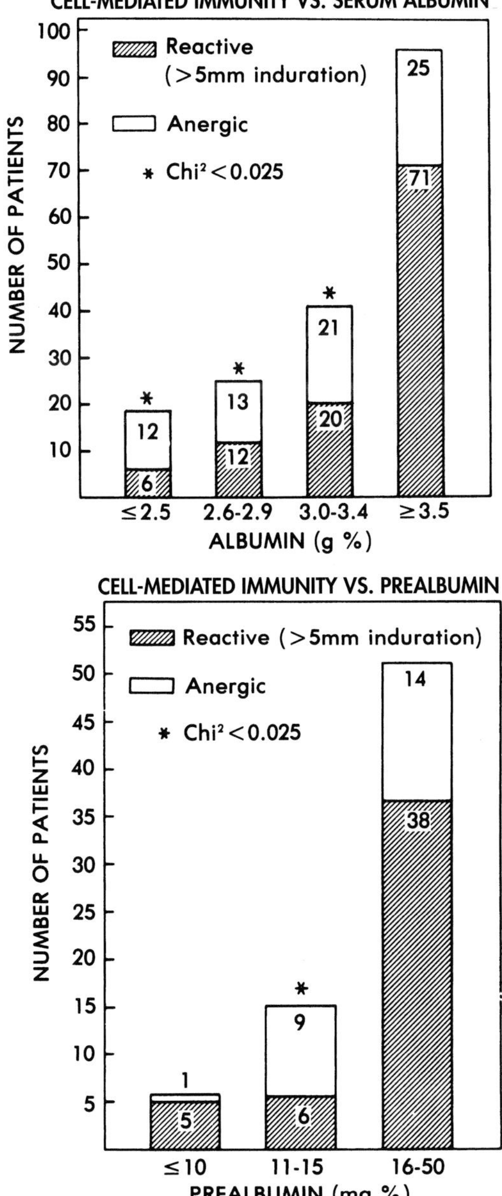

Fig. 3-2. Correlation of cell-mediated immunity with laboratory markers of nutritional status. (Modified from Grant JP, Custer PB, Thurlow J. Current techniques of nutritional assessment. Surg Clin North Am 61:437, 1981.)

Accuracy of Nutritional Assessment

There is no complete agreement on the accuracy and usefulness of the various techniques used to determine nutritional status because of the lack of one specific, accurate test to which the other techniques of nutritional assessment may be compared. The prognostic nutritional index (PNI) is an attempt to correlate various methods of nutritional assessment with the occurrence of postoperative morbidity and mortality through stepwise regression analyses[38] as shown below:

$$\text{PNI}(\%) = 158 - 16.6(\text{ALB}) - 0.78(\text{TSF}) - 0.20(\text{TFN}) - 5.8(\text{DH})$$

where PNI is an estimate of the risk of a complication occurring in an individual patient; ALB is the serum albumin concentration (g/100 ml); TSF is the triceps skinfold thickness (mm); TFN is the serum transferrin concentration (mg/100 ml); and DH is delayed hypersensitivity reactivity to any of three recall antigens (0 = nonreactive, 1 = <5 mm induration, 2 = > 5 mm induration). The PNI has been shown to be accurate in predicting which surgical patients were at a high risk for postoperative morbidity and mortality. Application of perioperative nutrition support to patients considered to be high risk reduced postoperative morbidity and mortality in a retrospective study.[14] However, other investigators have questioned the ability of preoperative nutritional assessment to predict postoperative morbidity and mortality.[39]

The history and physical examination have been prospectively compared to anthropometric data, laboratory data, delayed cutaneous hypersensitivity, and highly sophisticated direct body composition analyses as a method of nutritional assessment.[17] Two clinicians trained in nutritional assessment techniques independently examined 59 patients and categorized them into one of three groups: normal, mild malnutrition, and severe malnutrition. The two examiners agreed on the classification in 48 of the 59 patients (81%). Furthermore, the clinical evaluation of nutritional status was then compared to the objective measurements. There was a significant correlation in all tests with the clinical status, except for total lymphocyte count. The clinical status was also able to separate the patients into groups with significantly different mean values for six of the nine objective measurements.

Finally, the investigators demonstrated that the morbidity of these patients correlated with the clinical nutritional status. They concluded that

> general clinical assessment is a reproducible and valid technique for evaluating nutritional status before surgery. Unless further studies show that laboratory measurements of nutritional status are more accurate than clinical evaluation or provide better prognostic information, we suggest that carefully performed history-taking and physical examinations are sufficient for nutritional assessment.[17]

Researchers have suggested that carefully performed history and physical examinations are sufficient for nutritional assessment ("subjective global assessment"). Subjective global assessment has been compared to single objective measurements, such as serum albumin, transferrin level, delayed cutaneous hypersensitivity, anthropometrics, and PNI. Subjective global assessment alone, or in combination with any single objective measurement, was the most sensitive and specific tool of nutritional assessment in predicting outcome. The wide variation in accuracy of nutritional assessment tools in predicting outcome suggests that no single tool should be used as a sole indicator of nutritional status or repletion or as a predictor of outcome.

However, it should also be noted that objective evaluation of nutritional status also correlated with clinical outcome and allowed a means to quantitate nutritional status changes with supplementation. These evaluations, however, are adjuncts to and not replacements for a thorough medical history and a complete physical examination.

ENTERAL NUTRITION

Use of an intact gastrointestinal tract for nutrition support should be the initial step in alimentation. The concept of enteral alimentation is not new; in patients unable to eat, ancient Egyptians and Greeks attempted artificial alimentation through the use of nutrient enemas and clysters. The use of large-bore tubes with bolus "home-style" feeding was used in past years but was not well accepted because of patient discomfort with this technique. Recent technical advances, however, have improved the quality of the equipment and the method of delivery and have increased the spectrum of available nutrient formulas.

An understanding of intestinal physiology is important to a discussion of enteral nutrition because of the variety of dietary formulas and gastrointestinal abnormalities encountered in clinical situations. The reader should refer to discussions elsewhere in this book on intestinal physiology, digestion, and absorption.

Indications for Enteral Nutrition

Malnourished patients with an intact gastrointestinal tract should initially be given enteral nutrition support. The specific disease processes affecting oral nutrition are diverse. In general, patients who are unable or unwilling to eat or unable or unwilling to eat enough should be considered for enteral nutrition support.

Patients with upper gastrointestinal or oral malignancies commonly develop problems resulting in an inability to eat. Many patients develop difficulty in chewing or swallowing as a result of their underlying disease process. In addition, radiation or chemotherapy treatment for various malignancies may result in stomatitis, mucositis, or nausea, which may affect oral intake. Finally, some patients may have a functional intestinal tract but be unable to eat as a result of proximal atrophy, obstruction, or fistula. These patients may receive enteral support through various enteric catheters.

Patients may be able to eat but often are unwilling to do so either because of a lack of desire to eat or because of unwanted side effects from eating. Patients with anorexia nervosa and cancer are commonly encountered in this category. Unwillingness to eat is probably the single most important cause of malnutrition in cancer patients.

Patients with substantially increased energy expenditures and catabolism often are unable or unwilling to eat enough to meet their requirements. Patients with major skeletal trauma or sepsis may have a 40% increase in energy expenditures, whereas those with major burns may have increases of 60% to 100% above normal levels. Such patients commonly require nutrition support.

Finally, patients may have difficulty in digestion or absorption of various nutrients because of anatomic or physiologic lesions (e.g., following total pancreatectomy there may be impaired digestion of fats, even with supplemental oral pancreatic enzymes). Patients undergoing abdominal radiation commonly develop inadequate terminal digestion and absorption of various nutrients.

Role of Enteral Nutrition in the Septic State

The gastrointestinal tract serves as both an absorptive surface and a protective barrier. The barrier function relies on a system of immunologic, physiologic, and mechanical defenses. The immunologic mechanisms of the intestinal tract are complex. The lamina propria contains a cellular immune system, including lymphocytes, eosinophils, and macrophages. Immunoglobulins (IgA, IgM, IgG, and IgE) are present within the lamina propria of the small intestine. The presence of IgA is particularly crucial in gut barrier function. IgA binds and "detoxifies" bacteria in the gut lumen. IgA is present in saliva, bile, and gastric and intestinal secretions and in the mucin produced by gastrointestinal mucosal cells. Malnutrition is associated with decreased mucin production and decreased IgA production in the enteric secretions. IgA production has been shown to decrease significantly in patients receiving parenteral nutrition, whereas levels are maintained in patients receiving enteral feedings.[40,41]

Altered intestinal permeability has also received much attention recently as playing an important role in the development of systemic inflammatory changes.[42] Increased intestinal permeability has been noted experimentally after delivery of intravenous endotoxin.[43] Ziegler et al.[44] used the absorption of lactulose as marker of intestinal permeability in burn patients. Permeability was increased in burn patients who were infected, compared with noninfected patients or nonburn controls. Starvation and hypocaloric diets have not consistently been shown to alter intestinal permeability in humans. It has been suggested therefore that the incidence of intestinal permeability is increased when starvation is associated with a secondary or additional insult. Data also exist suggesting that bacteria translocation across the gut wall and enhanced intestinal permeability may play important roles in the mediation of systemic sepsis in critically ill and injured patients, implicating disruption of the intestinal barrier as being responsible for these events.[45] It has been further postulated that

Table 3-3. Indications and Route for Nutritional Supplementation With Normal Gastrointestinal Function

Oral	Nasoenteric	Gastrostomy or Jejunostomy
Normal nutritional status with increased nutritional needs	Difficulties in swallowing	Oral or upper gastrointestinal Obstruction Dysfunction Fistula
Mild protein-calorie malnutrition with normal or increased nutritional requirements	Increased nutritional needs Moderate-to-severe protein-calorie malnutrition Anorexia	Chronic enteral nutritional support

Modified from Hearne BE, Daly JM. Enteral nutrition. In Kirkpatrick J, ed. Nutrition and Metabolism in the Surgical Patient. Mt. Kisco, N.Y.: Futura Publishing, 1983.

the provision of enteral nutrition preserves the intestinal barrier and decreases intestinal permeability.[45-47] Experimentally, the lack of intraluminal nutrients leads to intestinal villous atrophy in parenterally fed animals and negatively impacts the gut barrier and immune function. Further, parenteral nutrition is associated with decreased intestinal IgA levels, increased bacterial overgrowth, and may increase intestinal permeability. Studies in humans with systemic illness show that septic morbidity is decreased in patients who are fed enterally early in the course of their illness.[45-47] Other studies in critically ill surgical patients and patients with traumatic injuries confirm a marked decrease in infectious complications when fed enterally.[45-47] Finally, early enteral nutrition has been successfully used in patients undergoing solid organ transplantation as a means of decreasing septic complications.[48] Nitrogen balance is improved and infectious complications appear to be lower in patients fed enterally, compared to parenterally fed counterparts.[46-48]

Selection of Enteral Nutrient Delivery

Patients who require enteral nutritional supplementation may be supported through various routes of administration. These are either oral, nasoenteric, or enteric (gastrostomy or jejunostomy) (Table 3-3). The selection of the route of administration should parallel the underlying indication for nutrition support. In general, patients with only moderately insufficient oral intake may be supplemented orally with aggressive dietary counseling. Patients with more severe deficiencies of higher nutrient needs commonly require tube feedings (see Table 3-3).[49]

Use of silicone rubber or polyurethane small-bore feeding tubes has significantly reduced patient discomfort caused by older, large-bore, inflexible nasogastric tubes. Longer catheters with mercury-weighted ends may be used for nasoduodenal feedings. For patients who require long-term enteral support, surgically placed gastrostomy or jejunostomy catheters are more direct routes for feedings. These feeding enterostomies have been considered a routine part of complicated surgical procedures by some surgeons.[50]

Table 3-4. Jejunostomy Feeding Schedule*

Day	Strength	Dosage (ml/hr)
1	¼	50
2	½	75
3	½	100
4	¾	100
5	Full	100

*Volume increase precedes concentration increase in jejunostomy feeding schedule.

Gastric feedings are advantageous in some patients. Osmolality of the feeding formula is rarely of significant consideration because of the ability of the stomach to dilute hyperosmolar solutions. In addition, bolus feedings may be used and thereby reduce patient care time. However, gastric outlet obstruction, obtundation, or laryngeal incompetence are contraindications for this mode of feedings because of the high incidence of aspiration.[51]

Jejunal feedings require continuous pump infusions. Diarrhea is more commonly encountered than in gastric feedings because of the delivery of hyperosmolar feedings into the small intestine. The presence of hyperosmolar solutions in the intestine results in diffusion of water into the intestinal lumen. To reduce the incidence of diarrhea, jejunal feedings should be started with dilute solutions, and the concentration of feedings should be increased only after the patient is tolerating adequate volumes (Table 3-4). If diarrhea persists, antiperistaltic agents may be added to the feeding formula, or the delivery rate may be decreased.

Dietary Formulations

Currently available dietary formulations may be divided among blenderized formulas, nutritionally complete commercial formulas, chemically defined formulas, and modular formulas.

Blenderized tube feedings may be composed of any food that can be blenderized. These may be prepared at home or may be commercial preparations. Caloric distribution of these formulas should parallel a normal diet. Blenderized formulas are indicated most often in patients with feeding gastrostomies unable to eat by mouth.

Nutritionally complete commercial formulas vary in protein, carbohydrate, and fat composition. Several are flavored and are considered suitable for oral supplementation. Several formulas use sucrose or glucose as carbohydrate sources and are suitable for lactose-deficient patients. Commercial formulas are convenient, sterile, and low in cost; they are the most frequently used diet for patients requiring tube feedings.

Chemically defined formulas are commonly called elemental diets. The nutrients are provided in a predigested and readily absorbed form. These diets are not often used in oral feedings, since the presence of amino acids in the formula markedly reduces its palatability. They are useful in patients with digestive disturbances (e.g., in patients with radiation enteritis or pancreatic insufficiency). However, they are more expensive than nutritionally complete commercial formulas and are hyperosmolar, which may cause cramping and diarrhea.

Modular formulations include special formulas used for specific nutrient needs or because of organ dysfunction. Single-nutrient formulas are used to modify other enteral formulas, tailoring them for special needs. Patients with renal or hepatic failure may require specialized modular formulas that take into account underlying fluid and amino acid abnormalities.

Role of Gut-Specific Substrates

During the last decade, nutrition support has focused on the use of specific substrates or nutrients to alter the metabolic response to severe injury or illness and to enhance immune function.[52,53] A number of gut-specific nutrients have been employed in an attempt to maintain gut barrier function and attenuate the inflammatory response. A brief review follows.

Glutamine. Although classified as a nonessential amino acid, glutamine is the crucial respiratory fuel for the gastrointestinal mucosal cell, or enterocyte. Glutamine is metabolized in the small intestine to ammonia, citrulline, alanine, and proline, and the carbon skeleton then serves as an energy precursor for the enterocyte. Glutamine uptake by the intestinal tract increases dramatically in periods of stress or sepsis. Glutamine-supplemented enteral formulas (glutamine can also be given parenterally) prevent the decrease in plasma and muscle glutamine noted in stress and maintain intestinal cell integrity, villous height, and mucosal DNA activity.[54] Glutamine-supplemented enteral diets, compared with controls, have been associated with a lower incidence of translocation from the intestine in transfused and burned mice.[55] Glutamine supplementation allows more rapid recovery of mucosa and lower mortality in animals and humans challenged with chemotherapy. The decrease in bacterial translocation noted with glutamine supplementation may be due in part to restoring IgA levels and decreasing bacterial adherence to the intestinal wall. Glutamine-supplemented nutrition also reduces the decrease in T- and B-cell lymphocytes seen with standard formulas and may improve neutrophil and macrophage function in burn patients.[56] A study using glutamine with epidermal growth factor shows that this combination may further improve nitrogen retention, intestinal cell integrity, and DNA and protein content of mucosal cells.[57] Prospective, randomized trials using glutamine-supplemented parenteral nutrition demonstrated a reduced incidence of infection and shortened hospital stay in bone marrow transplant patients.[58] Although the glutamine was given parenterally, preliminary data suggest that the enteral route would be as effective if patients were given this substrate enterally. Glutamine-supplemented enteral diets are commercially available.

Arginine. Arginine-supplemented enteral formulas have been shown to improve nitrogen balance, improve wound healing, stimulate T-cell response, and reduce infectious complications.[59] Arginine stimulates T-cell proliferation in humans and increases albumin synthesis. The effects of arginine on T cells are important in facilitating gut barrier function. Enteral nutrition supplemented with arginine has been shown to improve nitrogen balance and T-helper cell response.[59,60] Further, arginine supplementation decreases infection after burn injury and abdominal sepsis.[61] Arginine-enriched diets have also been shown to improve both T-cell immunity and wound healing in humans[62] and slow the growth of cancer in experimental animals.[63] This effect of arginine on improved immune function and resistance to infection appears to be at least partially related to nitric oxide, as administration of nitric oxide synthetase inhibitors blocks the beneficial effect of arginine.[61]

Omega-3 fatty acids. Nutrition support may preserve the gut mucosal barrier by indirect effects, that is, by altering the systemic response to stress or sepsis. Endogenous mediators, such as interleukins (IL-1, IL-6) and tumor necrosis factor (TNF), directly affect cell membrane activity. Dietary fats are the sole precursors to eicosanoid production and, as such, are potent immunomodulators. Linolenic acid is lengthened and desaturated to arachidonic acid, which is a precursor to prostanoids, which mediate the inflammatory response (e.g., PGE_2 and TXA_2), and to leukotrienes, which also mediate this response (LTB_4). PGE_2 suppresses T-cell function by diminishing the T-cell response to mitogens and antigens. The fat derivatives just described belong to the ω-6 family and are found in most meats (particularly red meats). In contrast, the ω-3 fatty acid family is found in fish and marine products. The addition of ω-3 polyunsaturated fatty acids to diets alters cytokine function by suppressing both IL-1 and TNF production in both animals and humans. The use of ω-3 fatty acids may decrease the inflammatory response observed with standard ω-6 formulas. As ω-6 fatty acids are the mediators of the inflammatory response, reducing the production of cytokines may indirectly preserve the gut mucosal barrier and lessen the systemic inflammatory response.

The ω-3 and ω-6 dietary lipids have been extensively studied in surgical patients receiving solid organ transplants. ω-3 fatty acid supplementation has been associated with a reduction in cyclosporine-induced nephrotoxicity and lowers the production of TXA_2 which appears to play a role in this process.[64,65] More recent data have demonstrated that ω-3 fatty acid supplementation in patients receiving cyclosporine for renal transplantation reduced the incidence of rejection and improved glomerular filtration rates.[66] Other studies have shown that high doses of ω-3 fatty acids had deleterious effects on metabolism and immunity in thermal injury and may, in fact, inhibit wound tensile strength.[67,68] In contrast, a study in surgical patients at risk for sepsis found that the addition of ω-3 fatty acids to enteral formulas is well tolerated and may reduce infectious complications.[69] The response to ω-3 and ω-6 fatty acids cannot be entirely explained by effects on eicosanoid metabolism. The varying dose-associated responses that are observed with both types of fatty acids make precise outcomes difficult to predict. There is no doubt, however, that provision of specific amounts of ω-3 and ω-6 fatty acids may alter the inflammatory response and alter survival in sepsis either for good or bad.[69]

In summary, the influence of specific amounts of ω-3 and o-6 fatty acids may be determined by specific disease states. Lipid emulsions are composed entirely of ω-6 fatty acids. In general, the ω-6 fatty acids are associated with eicosanoid and prostaglandin function that more profoundly stimulates the inflammatory response. Critically ill patients who are septic should probably receive no more than 15% to 20% of their energy as lipid. An effort to provide equal amounts of ω-3 and ω-6 fatty acids is reasonable in patients fed enterally. Patients who are not septic may easily tolerate 30% of their energy provided as fatty acids.

Short-chain fatty acids. Short-chain fatty acids (SCFAs), or volatile fatty acids, are produced in the large intestine by anaerobic fermentation of nonabsorbable carbohydrates (fiber). These SCFAs include acetate, propionate, and butyrate and are readily absorbed by the bowel and metabolized, supplying ketone products and glutamine, which are the preferred oxidated fuels for the enterocyte. Experimentally, SCFAs stimulate mucosal proliferation in both the small intestine and colon, improve integrity of intestinal anastomoses, stimulate intestinal adaptation after small bowel resection, and reduce the incidence of bacterial translocation.[52,70] Whether SCFAs will prove useful in modulating these processes in humans must await further study.

Complications of Enteral Nutrition

Complications of enteral nutrition may be considered mechanical, gastrointestinal, or metabolic (Table 3-5). Mechanical problems relate to the placement and care of tubes used for feedings. In general, placement of the tubes should be followed by radiologic verification of proper intraluminal positioning.

Some of the more serious mechanical complications associated with the placement and maintenance of enteral feeding tubes are related to malposition or malplacement of the tube. A number of immediate complications have been associated with placement of both nasogastric and nasoenteric tubes. The most common problems include

Table 3-5. Potential Complications of Enteral Nutrition and Associated Preventive Measures

Complication	Prevention
Mechanical	
Regurgitation and aspiration	Elevate patient to 30-degree angle
Tube or ostomy leak or malfunction	Use careful surgical technique and local care
Erosion of external nares	Tape tube to prevent contact with nares
Erosion of tube lumen	Use small diameter silicone rubber or polyurethane tubes
Clogging of tube lumen	Irrigate before and after feeding with 50 ml tepid water; use appropriate bore tube with formula and mode of administration
Otitis media	Use small-bore, soft feeding tube
Gastrointestinal	
Nausea, vomiting, or bloating	Reduce flow rate; increase time interval between intermittent feedings
Diarrhea or cramping	Reduce flow rate; reduce formula concentration; appropriate formula selection
Metabolic	
Hyperglycemia and glycosuria, osmotic diuresis, and hyperosmotic dehydration	Monitor urine for glucose and acetone, blood glucose, serum electrolytes
Edema	Monitor body weight, fluid and salt requirements, intake and output
Prerenal azotemia	Monitor blood urea nitrogen and creatinine

Modified from Hearne BE, Daly JM. Enteral nutrition. In Kirkpatrick J, ed. Nutrition and Metabolism in the Surgical Patient. Mt. Kisco, N.Y.: Futura Publishing, 1983.

initial tube malposition, with placement of the tube into the bronchus or pulmonary tract. This may occur initially in as many as 5% of cases. Patients with decreased consciousness, impaired gag reflex, or who have undergone endotracheal intubation are at increased risks, as are those who have malformation of the upper gastrointestinal tract or nasopharyngeal area. Radiographs obtained after insertion have shown that tube displacement is more commonly observed after insertion of small-bore tubes. As many as 15% of small-bore tubes may be displaced compared with larger tubes. Pulmonary aspiration is a frequent and often-discussed complication associated with enteral feeding. Gastroesophageal reflux is common in many critically ill patients and is dependent on gastric emptying time, gastric secretory rate, patient position, lower esophageal sphincter competence, and esophageal motility. The size of the nasogastric tube has been associated with an increased risk of pulmonary aspirations as well, with a smaller bore tube being somewhat more successful.[71] pH testing of feeding tube aspirates has also been used to determine successful placement.[72]

Intraoperative placement of a jejunostomy can be verified by the installation of saline into the catheter while the jejunum is compressed immediately distal to the catheter. Placement of small-bore nasogastric tubes should always be verified radiologically before initiation of feedings, particularly if they are placed in obtunded patients or patients with a poor cough reflex. The presence of symptoms of peritoneal irritation in patients being fed through a jejunostomy tube warrants further evaluation to ensure that dislodgment of the catheter has not resulted in the intraperitoneal delivery of feedings. Attachment of the stomach or small bowel to the anterior abdominal wall reduces the chance of accidental intraperitoneal catheter dislodgment.

Permanently placed gastrostomy and jejunostomy tubes are associated with many of the same complications associated with nasoenteric tubes. However, some complications are unique to this method of placement. Because these tubes require surgical placement, they are associated with the usual risk of anesthesia to include infection, bleeding, hypotension, and wound infection. Tube exit site problems, including cellulitis, infection, and fistula formation, are troublesome and should be avoided by meticulous care during the time of insertion and during the postoperative period. Dislodgment of a surgically placed gastrostomy or jejunostomy tube in the immediate postoperative period is associated with peritonitis and possible enteroabdominal abscess formation. In the case of gastrostomy tubes, the use of both internal and external bolsters or bumpers has helped to avoid tube displacement, keeps the stomach adherent to the intra-abdominal wall, and prevents migration of the tube toward the pylorus. If surgically placed gastrostomy tubes become dislodged, they have the capability of inducing gastric obstruction, usually occurring at the level of the pylorus.

In recent years the use of percutaneous endoscopic gastrostomy (PEG) has become the most common method of long-term enteral access. The common complications associated with immediate PEG placement include tube dislodgment or displacement and bleeding. Organ perforation during the time of PEG placement is relatively rare. Leakage of enteral contents into the abdomen or around the site of the tube is somewhat more frequent and may be associated with significant peritonitis. One of the more common and aggravating complications of PEG placement is necrosis around the tube exit site, which may be associated with significant cellulitis, fistula formation, and in severe cases fasciitis. This complication is usually due to excessive tension placed on the tube, which then necroses the abdominal wall between the internal and external bolster or bumper. Careful attention to detail immediately following tube placement and in the postoperative period should avoid this complication.

Further reported complications associated with PEG placement include gastrocolic fistula and separation of the gastrostomy tube from the abdominal wall. Nevertheless, skin erosion or excoriation remains a very common and frequent problem and can be avoided by meticulous attention to detail. A number of comparisons between the different techniques ("push," "pull," or "introducer") have been undertaken, with little difference in complications between these techniques. Infectious complications remain the most frequent and include minor skin infection, erosion, or excoriation. The addition of antibiotics prophylactically and the cleansing of the mouth with antibiotic solution prior to the procedure has reduced the effect of oral flora in causing peritubular skin infections.[73] Transillumination of the stomach during the performance of the procedure should prevent puncture of adjacent organs. Pneumoperitoneum is a very common and frequent occurrence following PEG placement and is of no significance, with the intra-abdominal air being absorbed in approximately 1 week.

Gastrointestinal side effects of enteral feedings are common. These include abdominal distention, diarrhea, and vomiting. Gastric feedings usually are better tolerated by bolus infusion. However, the presence of 200 ml or more residual volume may indicate gastric atony or distal obstruction. Feedings should be stopped in patients with this quantity of residual volume. Proper monitoring of residual volume reduces the incidence of vomiting. Patients being fed intragastrically should first receive small amounts of full-strength formulas, with gradually increasing volumes as tolerated.

Patients being fed through a jejunostomy tube are more likely to develop diarrhea than when other delivery routes are used. The presence of the hyperosmolar feeding in the proximal small intestine results in a passive diffusion of water into the lumen to render the intraluminal contents isotonic. If the infusion rate is too rapid for a given osmolality, diarrhea occurs. Therefore patients with jejunostomies should be able to tolerate a sufficient volume of the infusate before the concentration is increased. If diarrhea occurs, either an antiperistaltic agent should be added to the infusate or its rate of delivery decreased until symptoms abate. Finally, each patient should be matched to a defined formula. This should reduce the incidence of gastrointestinal side effects in patients with lactose intolerance caused by infusion of a lactose-based carbohydrate source. Additionally, patients not demonstrating a specific need for elemental diets could be fed other nutritionally balanced commercial formulas that may be less hyperosmolar and less expensive.

Occasionally, the diarrhea associated with enteral feeding is more aggravating and does not respond to the measures enumerated above. In this circumstance the cause of the diarrhea must be adequately determined if it is to be treated appropriately. Since diarrhea may be either osmotic or secretory, it can occur by either ineffective water absorption or an increase in secretion of water by the colon. As already noted, osmotic diarrhea is associated with the presence of osmotic products in the gastrointestinal tract and is the most common diarrhea that occurs with enteral feeding. Secretory diarrhea is more likely if the diarrhea occurs for longer than 1 or 2 days and continues after enteral feeding has been discontinued. The diarrhea associated with *Colostridium difficile* and other enteric pathogens is typically secretory in nature. Differentiation between secretory and osmotic diarrhea can be determined by calculating the osmotic gap between the concentration of ions in the colonic fluid and the fecal osmolality. Patients with osmotic diarrhea have an osmotic gap of 160 mOsm/L or more. Patients with secretory diarrhea have a very minimal or negative osmotic gap. Patients with short bowel syndrome often have diarrhea that increases when enteral feeding is initiated. Treatment of the underlying disease should be undertaken in an effort to minimize diarrhea associated with enteral feeding. *C. difficile* is commonly observed in critically ill patients and associated with frequent watery stools. These patients respond briskly to identification and treatment of *C. difficile.* A stool culture, as well as testing for *C. difficile* toxin, should identify this problem. Antidiarrheal medications may be used once stool cultures have been obtained and results are negative for *C. difficile.*

Metabolic complications can also occur with enteral feedings. Glucose intolerance can result from the relative infusion of too much glucose. Patients receiving tube feedings, particularly those with constant infusions, should be monitored serially for blood and urine glucose levels. Diabetic patients may require exogenous insulin or a lower rate of nutrient delivery. Hypertonic dehydration can result from the intraluminal loss of free water. Free water can be given to reduce the chance of this occurring. Infusion rates can also be reduced if the problem develops.

Tube feedings may be contraindicated in situations of severe gastrointestinal dysfunction, upper gastrointestinal bleeding, and intractable vomiting and diarrhea. Nasogastric feedings are especially contraindicated in obtunded patients.

Clinical Trials of Enteral Nutrition

Enteral nutrition has been favorably compared to parenteral nutrition in several clinical trials. Rombeau and Barot[51] compared 10 seriously ill patients fed enterally with 10 similar patients given total parenteral nutrition (TPN) and demonstrated that the patients given enteral nutrition achieved better nitrogen balances. Other studies have consistently demonstrated that patients receiving enteral nutrition achieve at least similar nutritional gains when compared to patients on TPN.[74,75]

McArdle et al.[76] compared nutritional benefits in patients randomized to receive enteral or parenteral nutrition. Although the nitrogen balances from both groups were similar, the patients on parenteral nutrition demonstrated high levels of blood cortisol and plasma insulin concentrations compared to those patients on enteral nutrition. In addition, patients receiving parenteral alimentation also demonstrated a significant decrease in free fatty acid levels compared to the other group. This was presumably the result of decreased lipolysis as a result of increased circulating insulin levels present in the group receiving parenteral nutrition. Other benefits of enteral nutrition included decreased cost, ease of solution handling, and decreased septic complications.

Others have demonstrated the beneficial effects of enteral compared with parenteral nutrition.[46,47] Recent studies have examined the effects of combining a number of gut-specific nutrients and outcome. Enteral feeding formulas supplemented with arginine, ω-3 fatty acids, and nucleic acids are now available. Supplemented enteral feedings of this type have been shown to improve immune function, decrease PGE_2 production, and reduce the incidence of postoperative infectious wound complications. Recently, earlier enteral feedings supplemented with arginine, nucleotides, and ω-3 fatty acids in critically ill patients demonstrated a reduction in hospital length of stay and nosocomial acquired infections.[77] In summary, nutritional immunomodulation by supplying varying substrates in enteral nutrition may reduce morbidity and improve outcome. The results of these specialized enteral formulas are still preliminary, and further trials are necessary to fully elucidate the role of these carefully configured diets in the management of patients requiring nutrition support.

PARENTERAL NUTRITION

The ability to provide complete, intravenous feedings to patients in a clinically practical manner has been appreciated since the late 1960s.[78] The application of TPN as an adjunct or as primary therapy to a variety of clinical situations has resulted in its general acceptance as a safe, clinically useful technique. Although relatively few major advances in the delivery techniques of TPN have been made since 1968, widespread application of TPN has resulted in a greater understanding of underlying physiologic principles. In turn this has allowed a standardization of methodology with a resultant decrease in complications associated with TPN.

Indications

The initial application of TPN was as supportive care in critically ill patients with severe nutritional deficiencies. The technique of feeding these patients parenterally was initially referred to as hyperalimentation. However, more recent studies demonstrated its usefulness in patients who were not nutritionally depleted but who required only maintenance of their nutritional state. Although the ability to improve clinical outcome through the judicious application of TPN has been demonstrated in several disease states such as in enterocutaneous fistulae, in other situations the evidence of improved clinical outcome has been indirect. For example, for a variety of reasons it has been difficult to demonstrate improved clinical outcome by the addition of TPN in patients with cancer undergoing chemotherapy, although cellular immunity and nutritional status may be improved. The greatest difficulty in conducting these clinical trials in a randomized prospective fashion is the ethical dilemma of not feeding patients who are severely malnourished. Therefore the evidence for improved clinical outcome in these situations may continue to be indirect.

TPN should be initiated in patients who fulfill the following three criteria: (1) patients who are malnourished or as a result of their medical care are unable to maintain their current nutritional state; (2) patients who cannot maintain an adequate enteral intake or who do not have a functional gastrointestinal tract; and (3) patients whose clinical outcome is improved by the application of TPN.

Techniques

The provision of hypertonic nutrient solutions necessitates the use of a large-bore, high-flow vein, to decrease the possibility of thrombophlebitis. These criteria are met by delivery of these solutions into the superior vena cava. Infraclavicular percutaneous subclavian venous catheterization has been a safe and effective method since its use for delivery of TPN was initiated by Dudrick et al.[78] Although delivery of TPN into the superior vena cava may be accomplished by other methods of catheter introduction by way of the saphenous, basilic, or jugular (external and internal) veins, the higher incidence of infection and thrombophlebitis with these techniques precludes their use except when subclavian vein catheterization is contraindicated.[79]

After the patient has been reassured and the procedure explained, insertion of the subclavian catheter is best accomplished with the patient in a slight Trendelenburg position, with a sheet roll placed longitudinally under the spine. The skin of the shoulder, neck, and chest is shaved, defatted with acetone, and covered with a povidone-iodine solution. The infraclavicular area is draped, and local anesthesia is infiltrated into the skin and periosteum of the inferior portion of the clavicle at its midpoint. Venipuncture is accomplished by introduction of a large-bore needle attached to a syringe into the area anesthetized and advancement of the needle paralleled to the floor, aiming at the supersternal notch. A flashback of venous blood signals successful venipuncture. The patient is asked to perform the Valsalva maneuver as the syringe is removed, and the catheter is introduced without forcing. The needle is withdrawn, the catheter at its entrance site anchored to the skin with a suture, and its end attached to the intravenous tubing. The bottle of intravenous fluid is lowered to ensure venous return into the tubing. A sterile, secure dressing is then placed over the introduction site, and a chest x-ray film is taken to ensure accurate placement of the catheter tip without pneumothorax.

TPN may be initiated after the chest x-ray film confirms correct positioning of the catheter. Although many patients are able to tolerate their calculated caloric requirements initially, a gradual increase in caloric loads until requirement levels are reached is preferable. The solutions may be prepared with lower amounts of dextrose initially and increased gradually, with full amounts of nitrogen, trace minerals, vitamins, and fluids provided daily. Full-strength solutions may also be prepared initially but delivered at lower rates, which are gradually increased as tolerated by the patient. In either instance, similar guidelines for patient management should be followed. Body weight should be measured daily, vital signs should be taken at least every 4 hours, and fluid balance observed every 8 hours. Urinary sugar and acetone should be measured every 6 hours; whereas serum electrolyte concentrations, blood urea nitrogen, and blood glucose should be measured at least daily until stable and twice weekly thereafter. Liver function studies, serum albumin, calcium, and phosphorus should be determined weekly.

Complications

Potential complications of TPN may be divided into technical, infectious, and metabolic.

Although subclavian vein catheterization is widely used, it is not free of potential complications. These complications can be minimized by rigid adherence to the previously described techniques. If catheterization is performed by those who have performed few catheterizations, adequate supervision can further reduce the incidence of complications. A list of potential complications associated with catheterization of the superior vena cava is summarized in the box on p. 69. Arterial puncture during catheterization is indicated by the filling of a syringe with bright red blood. The needle should be withdrawn, and firm pressure applied for several minutes. Pneumothorax is the most common technical complication. This may be suggested if air is aspirated into the syringe during insertion. The needle should be withdrawn, and the patient observed for signs of respiratory distress. A chest x-ray film should be obtained to rule out pneumothorax and to check the catheter position after all insertions. TPN should not be initiated until the chest x-ray film is reviewed. This reduces the incidence of hydrothorax. Catheter embolism is an iatrogenic complication that may occur when the catheter is withdrawn through the needle used for inser-

COMPLICATIONS OF CENTRAL VENOUS CATHETERIZATION

Pleural space
- Pneumothorax
- Tension pneumothorax
- Hemothorax
- Hydrothorax (intrapleural infusion)

Mediastinum
- Hemomediastinum
- Hydromediastinum
- Superior vena cava syndrome

Neck
- Subcutaneous emphysema
- Arterial injury (hematoma, arteriovenous malformation, false aneurysm, stenosis)
  - Subclavian artery
  - Carotid artery
  - Cervical and thoracic arteries
- Nerve injury
  - Phrenic nerve
  - Vagus nerve
  - Recurrent laryngeal nerve
  - Brachial plexus
- Lymphatic injury to the thoracic duct
- Tracheal injury

Veins
- Laceration with hemorrhage
- Air embolism
- Catheter embolism (paradoxic embolism)
- Cardiac arrhythmia
- Myocardial perforation (hydropericardium, tamponade)
- Coronary sinus block (tamponade)
- Venobronchial fistula
- Hepatic vein thrombosis
- Superior vena cava thrombosis (pulmonary embolism)
- Catheter sepsis

Modified from Ryan JA. Complications of total parenteral nutrition. In Fischer JE, ed. Total Parenteral Nutrition. Boston: Little, Brown, 1976.

tion, either for repositioning of the catheter or after a failed venipuncture. Joint withdrawal of the catheter and needle should eliminate this complication.

Infectious complications associated with TPN are potentially serious. Contamination may occur as a result of faulty techniques of catheter insertion or maintenance, infusion of contaminated solutions, or use of the subclavian catheter for other purposes such as infusion of medications. Most patients receiving TPN are predisposed to infectious complications because of the nature of the underlying disease, their nutritional state, and interference of host defense mechanisms from treatment.[80]

Management of patients who become febrile while receiving TPN requires a methodic approach because of the potential seriousness of catheter sepsis. A diligent examination and fever workup should be instituted to rule out other potential sources of the fever. Failure to demonstrate another cause requires removal of the nutrient solution and tubing. Cultures of the solution, peripheral blood, and central venous blood should be taken. Positive culture results, cardiovascular instability, or persistent fever require replacement of the indwelling catheter. To avoid complications associated with catheter reinsertion, the catheter may be changed over a guide wire. The tip of the removed catheter should be cultured, and broad-spectrum antibiotics initiated if blood culture results continue to remain positive.

Table 3-6 reviews common potential metabolic complications of TPN. Infusions of hypercaloric solutions may result in glucose intolerance. A normal adult can use 0.5 g of glucose per kilogram per hour. For a 70 kg person, this extrapolates to the use of 3500 calories per day. Patients who are severely catabolic, as is often the case in burns, polytrauma, and severe sepsis, may use up to 6000 calories per day. However, glucose tolerance is often unpredictable. In addition, many patients are either frankly diabetic or may have underlying disease that renders them relatively glucose intolerant, as may be the case in severe sepsis or trauma. Therefore these patients may exceed the glucose renal threshold with resultant hyperglycemia and glucosuria. Diligent monitoring of urinary sugar and blood glucose levels is necessary to prevent potentially severe complications from occurring.

The ability of patients to metabolize large glucose loads is directly related to their ability to mount an insulin response to the infused glucose. Studies conducted on the insulin response in nondiabetic patients receiving TPN have demonstrated several points: (1) abrupt initiation of hypercaloric feedings results in insulin levels four to six times basal levels by 6 hours; (2) continued infusion is associated with lowering of both the insulin and glucose levels; (3) the glucose tolerance test was normal during TPN, demonstrating the ability of the normal pancreas to increase insulin production if faced with increasing glucose load; and (4) cessation of TPN does not usually result in rebound hypoglycemia.[81] Diabetic patients cannot mount an insulin response, or their hormonal response may be inadequate. Other patients with severe sepsis or polytrauma may have diminished ability to produce sufficient insulin relative to the hyperglycemic state (Fig. 3-3). In addition, increased adrenal stimulation with resultant increased production of glucocorticoids also influences glucose tolerance in these patients. Finally, although rebound hypoglycemia is usually not a complication of TPN cessation in normal patients, a gradual reduction of TPN or use of a hypocaloric dextrose infusion after TPN is stopped is recommended.

To avoid osmotic diuresis, TPN is maintained at a rate that results in blood glucose levels below 225 mg/100 ml and urinary glucose levels below 2 g/100 ml. Patients with diabetes mellitus or persistent glycosuria require exogenous administration of crystalline insulin, which may be

Table 3-6. Metabolic Complications and Possible Causes Associated With Total Parenteral Nutrition

Complication	Possible Cause
Carbohydrate Metabolism	
Hyperglycemia	Excessive rate of infusion of glucose Insufficient endogenous insulin secretion Sepsis
Hyperosmolar nonketotic dehydration (hyperosmolar syndrome)	Glucocorticoids Persistent hyperglycemia Osmotic diuresis Dehydration
Hypoglycemia	Abrupt interruption of TPN infusion Excessive insulin
Amino Acid Metabolism	
Elevated blood urea nitrogen	Intrinsic renal disease Dehydration Excessive rate of infusion of amino acids Low caloric nitrogen ratio of TPN solution
Hyperammonemia	Intrinsic liver disease
Electrolyte and Mineral Metabolism	
Hypokalemia	Insufficient potassium intake relative to losses and anabolic requirements
Hypophosphatemia	Insufficient phosphate intake relative to losses and anabolic requirements
Hypomagnesemia	Insufficient magnesium intake relative to losses and anabolic requirements

Modified from Reinhardt GF, De Orio AJ, Kaminski MV Jr. Total parenteral nutrition. Surg Clin North Am 57:1283, 1977.
TPN, Total parenteral nutrition.

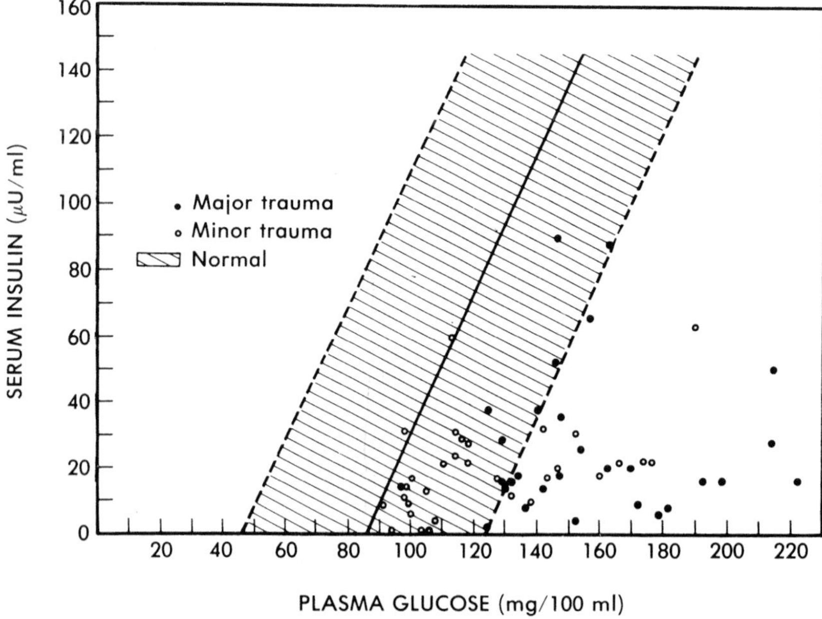

Fig. 3-3. Demonstration of elevated plasma glucose concentrations with inappropriately low insulin levels in patients with minor and major trauma. Normal levels are represented by the heavy line with two standard deviations. (Modified from Meguid MM, et al. Hormone-substrate interrelationships following trauma. Arch Surg 109:776, 1974. Copyright 1974, American Medical Association.)

added to the nutrient solution in dosages up to 60 U/1000 calories to achieve a reduction in blood glucose concentration. This protocol should prevent the development of nonketotic hyperosmolar coma that occurs when the rate of glucose infusion far exceeds the ability of the cells to metabolize glucose leading to hyperglycemia, glycosuria, and osmotic diuresis. Dehydration and coma may ensue and should be treated along the same lines as the management of diabetic coma by stopping the hypertonic carbohydrate infusion and giving intravenous fluids, electrolytes, and insulin to normalize hydration, acid-base balance, and blood glucose. Patients at risk include those with sepsis, burns, polytrauma, or diabetes mellitus. Treatment consists of infusion of dextrose solutions with isotonic or half-strength saline plus insulin. Measurement of serum electrolytes and blood glucose levels, as well as clinical assessment, allows appropriate rehydration.

Infusion of amino acid solutions is also associated with potential complications. A rising blood urea nitrogen level may be indicative of excess provision of amino acids, prerenal azotemia, renal disease, or a combination of all three. Reduction of the amino acid load and appropriate hydration is the treatment of choice. Hyperammonemia primarily occurs in patients with hepatic disease. Although it may be related to free ammonia infused in protein hydrolysates, this entity can occur with infusions of crystalline amino acids that contain essentially no free ammonia.[82]

Hyperchloremic metabolic acidosis can occur with infusions of crystalline amino acids because of the liberation of hydrochloric acid as the amino acids are used. Reducing the chloride intake decreases the incidence of metabolic acidosis. This reduction may be accomplished by providing potassium and sodium as their acetate salts.[82]

Serum electrolyte and trace metal abnormalities are a common complication of TPN. These deficiencies can be the result of inadequate intake to compensate for losses or because of the increased requirements during continued anabolism. These ions include potassium, phosphorus, calcium, and magnesium. Potassium may be further depleted as a result of the intracellular influx of potassium secondary to the infusion of dextrose and increased serum insulin levels.

Refeeding syndrome is commonly observed in patients receiving parenteral nutrition who are either receiving excessive total calories (glucose and fat) or receiving excessive carbohydrate calories. Overfeeding can result in significant hypophosphatemia, characterized by malaise, lethargy, perioral paresthesias, tremors, and dysarthrias. Progression can lead to coma and death. Phosphorus is an essential intracellular anion involved in protein synthesis. Overfeeding with carbohydrate calories depletes plasma levels of phosphate. Cellular effects include increased affinity for hemoglobin to oxygen and therefore decreased oxygen availability at the periphery and diminished neutrophil function. Phagocytosis has been noted to decline in patients with significant hypophosphatemia. Phosphorus should be added to parenteral solutions in doses of 15 to 30 mEq/L in ordinary circumstances. Severely malnourished patients may need additional parenteral phosphate supplementation, particularly during periods of refeeding. In this latter circumstance as much as 30 to 50 mEq/L may be required.

TPN can result in significant hypophosphatemia, characterized by malaise, lethargy, perioral paresthesias, tremors, and dysarthrias. Progression can lead to coma and death. Phosphorus is an essential intracellular anion involved in protein synthesis. Trapping of the ion in protein synthesis may result in hypophosphatemia. Phosphorus should be added to TPN in doses of 15 to 30 mEq/L in ordinary circumstances and 30 to 50 mEq/L in severely malnourished patients.

Calcium and magnesium are also required for the anabolic process. Calcium should be added to TPN in amounts of 4.5 to 9 mEq daily. In pediatric patients, 4 mEq/kg of body weight should be added daily. Approximately 24 mEq of magnesium daily is required for normal adults. These levels may be increased in severely malnourished patients who may also manifest evidence of zinc and selenium deficiencies. Renal function should be observed closely because requirements for electrolytes and minerals may be reduced.

Essential fatty acid deficiency may result in patients requiring infusion with fat-free dextrose and amino acid solutions. This is reflected in the lowered serum levels of linoleic and arachidonic acids and increased serum eicosanoic acid. The deficiency may be corrected by the infusion of a fat emulsion in amounts of about 10% of nonprotein calories. Currently, fat emulsions are available in concentrations of 10% or 20%.

Other metabolic complications, including fluid overload, vitamin abnormalities, and trace element deficiencies, are usually iatrogenic and may be easily corrected by provision of daily vitamin and mineral supplements to replenish deficiencies and replace ongoing losses (Table 3-7).

Glucose vs. Fat

The use of fat emulsions as a calorie source for parenteral feedings in patients has been investigated for many years. The ability to provide nitrogen parenterally by infusion of protein hydrolysates has been available since the 1930s but was not used clinically because of the absence of a feasible means to provide calories. In the late 1960s, Dudrick et al.[78] were able to demonstrate normal growth in puppies and infants through the use of amino acid solutions and hypertonic dextrose infused into the superior vena cava. Consequently, dextrose was the preferred caloric source. Further modifications in preparation techniques of parenteral fat emulsions reduced many of the complications associated with their early use, including fever and infection.

Parenteral fat emulsions contain soybean oil as a source of fatty acids, an emulsifier (egg yolk phospholipid in Intralipid), and other agents to obtain isotonicity such as glycerol. Administration of a fat emulsion as a calorie source has theoretic advantages. Because of the higher

Table 3-7. Fluid and Nutritional Deficiencies During Total Parenteral Nutrition

Deficiency	Supplemental Feeding Technique
Water	Decrease rate of TPN infusion Administer 5% dextrose in water intravenously Replace using enteral feedings, water, or dilute nutritional solution
Iron	Use appropriate dosage of intramuscular iron preparation
Trace elements (copper, zinc, manganese, chromium, cobalt, fluoride)	Present in variable and usually insufficient amounts as contaminants in TPN solutions; present to some degree in blood and blood products Replace using enteral feedings, trace element concentrates, or deliver individual trace element
Essential fatty acids	Replace using enteral feedings, intravenous fat preparations

Modified from Reinhardt GF, De Orio AJ, Kaminski MV Jr. Total parenteral nutrition. Surg Clin North Am 57:1283, 1977.
TPN, Total parenteral nutrition.

caloric value of fats compared to glucose, more total calories can be provided by fat emulsions than by glucose if equal amounts are given. In addition, fat emulsions are isotonic and therefore may be delivered by way of peripheral veins. For these reasons, parenteral fat emulsions have distinct advantages in certain types of peripheral parenteral nutrition that are discussed later in this chapter.

The use of fat emulsions eliminates the potential complication of essential fatty acid deficiency that may result from fat-free TPN. Fatty acids are required for several important functions, including prostaglandin synthesis and cholesterol metabolism. The most important fatty acids appear to be linoleic, linolenic, and arachidonic acid, of which only linoleic is considered essential.

The absence of fatty acid intake in long-term TPN is associated with fatty acid deficiency.[83] Levels of linoleic acid and arachidonic acids are decreased. As the level of linoleic acid decreases, serum levels of oleic acid, an endogenous fatty acid, increase. In turn elongation and desaturation of oleic acid lead to increases of eicosatrienoic acid, a fatty acid that is considered unique to essential fatty acid deficiency. Depletion of essential fatty acids may lead to an impaired immune response, impaired wound healing, and platelet dysfunction. Clinically, the presence of dry scaly skin, hair loss, and delayed wound healing may be related to an essential fatty acid deficiency.

The use of fat emulsions has been investigated in several clinical trials. Jeejeebhoy and associates[84] compared nitrogen balances in two groups of patients with gastrointestinal disease. Both groups received equal amounts of amino acids, minerals, and vitamins daily. Nonprotein calories were provided as 100% dextrose in one group and as 17% dextrose/83% lipid in the other group. There was no significant difference in nitrogen balance between the two groups. In the lipid-based group, there was a rise in free fatty acids and ketone bodies with concomitant lower insulin levels, demonstrating that lipid had become the major energy source. Other investigators compared the effects of different levels of dextrose and lipid intake on protein metabolism and demonstrated no disadvantage as long as significant amounts of fat calories were provided.[85,86]

The infusion of lipid-based TPN to critically ill patients remains controversial. The use of lipid-based TPN eliminates the incidence of essential fatty acid deficiency, which may be more prevalent in patients with increased requirements for fatty acids. In addition, many of these patients have concurrent respiratory problems and may require ventilatory support. The use of hypercaloric dextrose infusions in these patients theoretically results in increased glucose oxidation with resultant increased carbon dioxide production. This may increase ventilatory demands and may result in respiratory and acid-base complications.[87] However, Long et al.[88] studied the use of fat emulsions in injured patients and demonstrated that nitrogen conservation is accomplished if dextrose calories are infused at levels corresponding to other resting metabolic rates. The provision of fat calories did not correlate with nitrogen-sparing efficacy of TPN.

Because of the relatively cheaper costs associated with dextrose-based regimens compared to lipid-based regimens, the use of fat as the major caloric source may be justified only in patients with respiratory difficulties, glucose intolerance, and subclavian vein thrombosis (preventing infusion of hypercaloric dextrose infusions centrally). The clearest indication for the infusion of fat emulsions is in the prevention of essential fatty acid deficiency and as a supplemental source of parenteral calories.

Peripheral Parenteral Nutrition

The parenteral solution most widely used perioperatively to reduce protein catabolism is hypocaloric dextrose. A 1 L amount of a 5% dextrose solution yields 50 g of carbohydrate. This is obviously insufficient to meet the patient's energy requirements at an average level of total fluid intake. However, nitrogen balance is improved in patients receiving a hypocaloric dextrose solution when compared with patients receiving saline solutions without dextrose. Theoretically, the carbohydrate calorie intake in hypocaloric dextrose infusions is used for endogenous caloric needs. This in turn reduces the caloric requirements to be provided by gluconeogenesis. Substrates for hepatic gluconeogenesis are derived from the catabolism of peripheral muscle, providing amino acids (predominantly alanine) as a carbon skeleton source for the endogenous conversion to glucose. By providing at least some calories exogenously, the rate of gluconeogenesis and in turn protein catabolism is reduced. However, infusion of dextrose alone does not eliminate the requirements for amino acids other than as an energy source.

To reduce protein losses further, Blackburn et al.[89] proposed infusions of amino acid solutions to patients without a caloric source. They demonstrated that, in contrast to hypocaloric dextrose solutions, infusions of amino acids alone would result in nitrogen balance in surgical patients. It was theorized that the provision of amino acids reduced the requirements of endogenous protein as a calorie source (through hepatic gluconeogenesis) and as visceral and transport substrates. Caloric requirements would be met partially by the hepatic conversion of endogenous and exogenous amino acids to glucose. Most of the caloric requirements in other tissues were provided by endogenous fat stores that were mobilized as a result of decreased insulin levels. Increased lipolysis was reflected by increased serum levels of free fatty acids and ketone bodies.

Other investigators were also able to demonstrate improved nitrogen balance in patients receiving amino acid solutions compared to patients receiving only hypocaloric dextrose.[90] However, the advantage of infusing only amino acid solutions as opposed to amino acids plus hypocaloric dextrose has been disputed by others.[91] These latter investigators were able to demonstrate improvement in nitrogen balance when hypocaloric dextrose was added to the amino acid infusions. It was speculated that the advantages of low insulin and glucose levels were overstated and that infusions of hypocaloric glucose simply allow adjustments to be made of how much fat is actually mobilized to meet caloric requirements.[92]

The use of protein-sparing solutions has been compared to TPN and hypocaloric dextrose infusions in surgical patients.[90] Although nitrogen balance was improved when either TPN or amino acid solutions were infused postoperatively, there was no difference in clinical outcome between those patients receiving hypocaloric dextrose and those receiving amino acids. Indeed, only patients receiving TPN were able to demonstrate clinical improvement. It seems clear that TPN is preferable in patients who require more nutrition support than can be provided by hypocaloric dextrose.

Because of the increased costs of protein-sparing amino acid solutions and the inability to improve clinical outcome, their routine perioperative use is contraindicated. It appears that they can be best used in those patients (e.g., obese patients) who may benefit from a nitrogen-sparing diet without actual anabolism. Finally, this regimen is useful in those patients who require nutrition support but in whom subclavian vein catheterization is contraindicated. In the latter group of patients, caloric requirements may be met by peripheral infusions of isotonic fat emulsions.

Specialized Amino Acid Solutions

The ability to modify calorie sources, calorie and nitrogen quantities, trace minerals, vitamins, and fluid volumes allows the physician to tailor nutrients to suit the specific needs of the patient. Certain clinical situations may require different proportions or elimination of certain amino acids. Three specific clinical settings have created roles for specialized amino acid formulations.

Renal Insufficiency

Renal insufficiency, whether functional or organic, is a common complication in patients following multiple trauma or sepsis. Acute renal failure that occurs in this setting is often reversible and is characterized by increased protein catabolism combined with an inability to excrete protein breakdown products. The result is an increase in blood urea nitrogen with concurrent loss of body cell mass. Nutritional intervention in this setting is complicated by the patient's inability to tolerate normal nitrogen or fluid volumes in standard TPN regimens.

Patients with oliguric renal insufficiency should be given sufficient fluid to compensate for insensible and measurable losses. Additional fluid may be deleterious. Therefore protein and calorie administration must be tailored for these limitations. Guidelines for fluid intake may be liberalized in patients undergoing peritoneal dialysis and hemodialysis.

An obvious limiting factor in the provision of protein is the contribution of that protein to the underlying azotemia. Protein catabolism can be reduced by provision of adequate calories, as in other catabolic states. Nevertheless, positive nitrogen balance cannot be achieved by high calorie intake only; protein must be given concurrently. Protein catabolism results in amino acids entering into a metabolic pool from which the individual amino acids are either reused for protein synthesis or further deaminated with resultant urea production. The goal of nutritional intervention in patients with renal failure should be to provide sufficient protein to meet demands for protein synthesis with a reduction in protein catabolism.[93] Nutritional therapy with the use of high-calorie, low-protein diets in a setting of renal failure has resulted in improved nitrogen balance, weight gain, and reduction of blood urea nitrogen concentration.[94]

Provision of high-quality protein or essential amino acids alone allows use of available urea for production of nonessential amino acids, reduction of the nitrogen load and blood urea nitrogen levels, and achievement of positive nitrogen balance. Dietary therapy in the surgical patient with renal insufficiency is often hindered by gastrointestinal dysfunction resulting from the underlying pathology, operative treatment, hypermetabolic states, and renal insufficiency itself. The efficacy of parenteral administration of essential amino acids and hypertonic dextrose was demonstrated by Dudrick et al.,[95] who showed improvement of nitrogen balance and weight gain with concomitant maintenance or reduction in blood urea nitrogen levels.

Controversy exists as to the proper amino acid mixture to use in renal failure patients. Caloric intake should be high with concomitant fluid and nitrogen restriction. Whether nitrogen sources of only essential amino acids or a combination of essential and nonessential amino acids are more efficacious remains debatable. Some investigators have reasoned that, since these patients are hypercatabolic, perhaps a mixture of essential and nonessential amino acids can more adequately provide nitrogen requirements.[96] Others have reasoned that, because of the catabolic nature of these patients, there is an increased requirement of essential amino acids.[97]

In a prospective controlled trial, Abel et al.[98] randomized 53 patients to receive either hypertonic dextrose or hypertonic dextrose plus essential amino acids. Both groups received similar quantities of nonprotein calories. They demonstrated a significantly higher recovery from renal failure in those patients receiving the essential amino acids plus hypertonic dextrose. The improved outcome was reflected by improvement in the underlying renal failure as a result of nutrition support (Fig. 3-4). Freund et al.[97] studied patients with renal insufficiency and infused a balanced amino acid solution containing both essential and nonessential amino acids plus hypertonic dextrose. They demonstrated significantly increased mortality in patients receiving the balanced amino acid solution when compared with patients treated with only essential amino acids plus the hypertonic dextrose previously studied.[98] However, studies by Leonard et al.[99] and Feinstein et al.[100] demonstrated no significant improvement in patients with renal failure given an essential amino acid solution compared with patients with renal failure receiving essential and nonessential amino acids. Both groups included patients undergoing dialysis during the course of their treatment. Although nitrogen requirements are higher in patients undergoing dialysis, the use of dialysis allows more liberalization of fluid and nitrogen intake and may negate any advantage of a solution containing only essential amino acids. Further prospective, randomized clinical trials are required before the role of essential amino acid solutions in acute and chronic renal failure can be completely assessed.

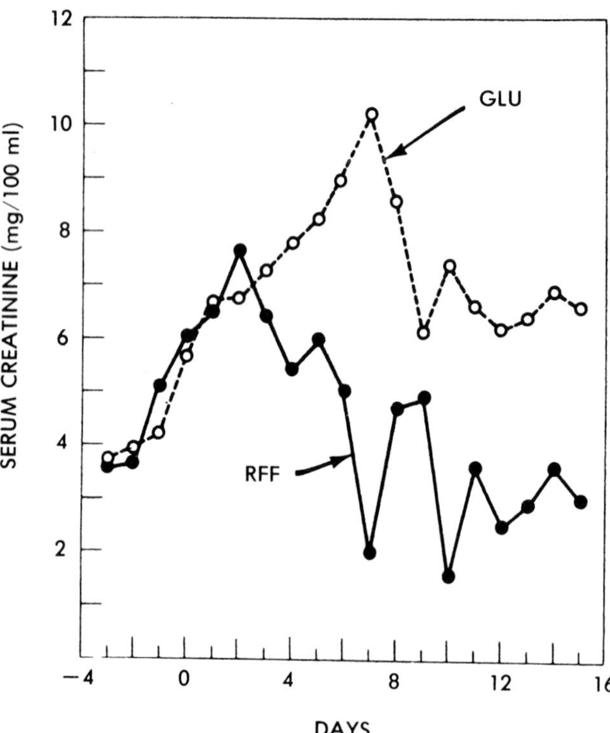

Fig. 3-4. Reduction of mean serum creatinine with infusion of renal failure formula *(RFF)* compared to patients receiving glucose *(GLU)*. (Modified from Abel RM, et al. Improved survival from acute renal failure after treatment with intravenous essential L-amino acids and glucose. N Engl J Med 288:695, 1973. Copyright © 1973 Massachusetts Medical Society. All rights reserved.)

Hepatic Encephalopathy

Numerous metabolic alterations occur in patients with hepatic failure. These alterations, singly or in combination, have been proposed as causative agents in hepatic encephalopathy, a condition consisting of various neuropsychiatric abnormalities that may be manifested in patients with hepatic failure. In recent years, attention has focused on neurotransmitted precursor concentrations and toxic metabolites as important causative agents in hepatic encephalopathy (Fig. 3-5).

Several investigators have reported plasma and urine amino acid abnormalities that occur in patients with encephalopathy.[101] Plasma aminograms in patients with encephalopathy typically demonstrate abnormally low levels of the branched-chain amino acids (BCAAs) with corresponding high levels of the aromatic amino acids, tyrosine, phenylalanine, and free tryptophan, as well as methionine.[102] Morgan et al.[103] compared the levels of plasma leucine plus isoleucine plus valine to phenylalanine plus tyrosine and demonstrated a correlation between this ratio and the severity of liver disease. BCAAs are primarily metabolized in skeletal muscle, whereas aromatic amino acids and methionine are primarily metabolized in the liver. Severe hepatic dysfunction that occurs in the setting of hypercatabolism results in the typical plasma amino acid patterns of low BCAAs/aromatic amino acids (Fig. 3-6).

Transport of amino acids across the blood-brain barrier appears to be regulated by plasma amino acid concentrations. Several amino acids competitively share the same transport mechanisms. Increased plasma concentrations of aromatic amino acids with lowered BCAA concentrations allow greater entry of the aromatic amino acids into the brain.[104] Fischer and Baldessarini[105] proposed that abnormal plasma acid levels may alter brain amino acid patterns and in turn brain neurotransmitter levels, with resultant encephalopathy. Abnormal plasma ratios of BCAAs to aromatic amino acids would preferentially allow increased transportation of aromatic amino acids across the blood-brain barrier.

Increased plasma levels of phenylalanine contribute to

already elevated levels of brain tyrosine. Accumulation of phenylalanine and tyrosine in the brain results in increased levels of β-hydroxylated phenyldothylamines including octopamine by way of increased levels of brain tyramine. Increased brain phenylalanine may also interfere with normal tyrosine metabolism. Elevated urinary and plasma levels of octopamine have been demonstrated in patients with hepatic encephalopathy.[106] Intestinal bacteria enzymes can directly metabolize dietary proteins, also resulting in increased levels of plasma tyramine. These substances are weak neurotransmitters, but with substantial brain accumulation they can replace normal neurotransmitters in neural synapses.

Elevated levels of plasma-free tryptophan readily cross the blood-brain barrier and are implicated in abnormal brain serotonin production.[107] Additionally, elevated

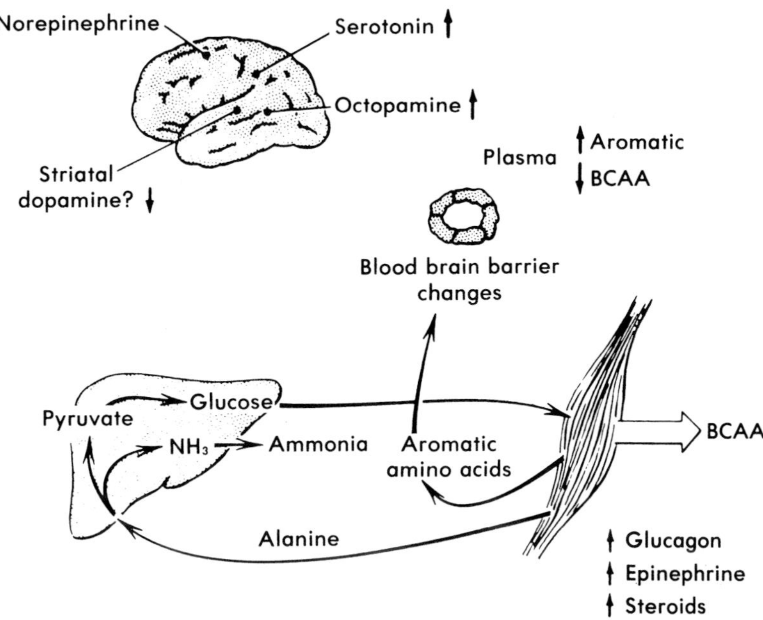

Fig. 3-5. Overall metabolic scheme leading to hepatic coma. *BCAA,* Branched-chain amino acid. (Modified from Fischer JE, Bower RH. Nutritional support in liver disease. Surg Clin North Am 61:653, 1981.)

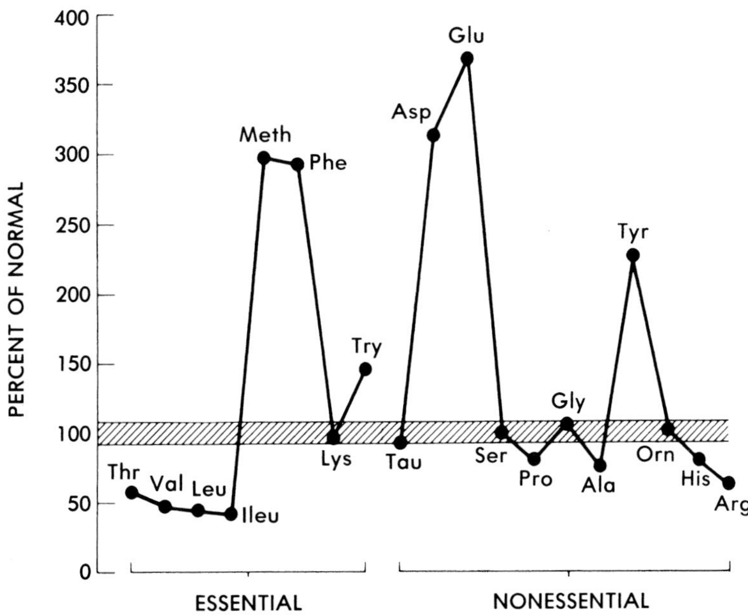

Fig. 3-6. Abnormal plasma amino acid pattern in patients with chronic liver disease expressed as percent of normal. (Reprinted with permission from Rosen HM, et al. Plasma amino acid patterns in hepatic encephalopathy of differing etiology. Gastroenterology 72:483, 1977. Copyright © Williams & Wilkins.)

plasma-free tryptophan levels have been implicated in sleep disorders.[108] Plasma and brain methionine have also been implicated in encephalopathy.

Patients with hepatic failure manifest unique biochemical and physiologic alterations. In addition, these patients are often malnourished, requiring nutritional intervention during treatment. Studies in animals with experimentally induced encephalopathy demonstrated that administration of amino acid solutions containing a greater proportion of the BCAAs and a reduced proportion of methionine and the aromatic amino acids resulted in amelioration of encephalopathy and a normalization of the plasma amino acid patterns.[109]

Clinical studies have been conducted to evaluate solutions containing a greater proportion of BCAAs and a reduced proportion of aromatic amino acids and methionine. A study of 63 patients by Freund et al.[110] demonstrated that improved nutrition support with positive nitrogen balance could be achieved by BCAA-enriched solutions in patients with hepatic insufficiency and protein intolerance. These patients maintained or improved their hepatic encephalopathy in response to increased nutritional intake. Other controlled studies comparing high BCAA solutions with standard types of therapy in hepatic encephalopathy demonstrated significant improvement in encephalopathy and concurrent improvement in nutritional status in patients receiving specialized amino acid formulas.[111-113]

Other studies have not demonstrated similar results in encephalopathic patients receiving specialized amino acid formulas.[114] Encephalopathy occurs as a combination of several metabolic disturbances, including increased levels of SCFAs and ammonia. Other concurrent complications such as hypovolemia, hepatorenal syndrome, or gastrointestinal bleeding may prohibit improvement in mental status with nutritional supplementation. In addition, nutritional intervention with specialized formulas in hepatic failure of different causes other than alcoholic cirrhosis have not yet been adequately studied. Nevertheless, it would appear that specialized nutritional formulas may improve amino acid tolerance and nutritional status in patients with hepatic encephalopathy.

STRESS AND SEPSIS

Increased energy expenditure and skeletal muscle catabolism are characteristic features of sepsis and multiple trauma.[115] Energy- and nitrogen-conserving mechanisms used by the body in simple starvation are altered in this setting, leading to rapid depletion of lean body mass.

Skeletal muscle preferentially uses the BCAAs, leucine, isoleucine, and valine for energy production. The individual BCAA is deaminated to its individual keto acid and an amino group. The keto acids are further metabolized and decarboxylated, resulting in adenosine triphosphate (ATP) production.[116] The donation of the amino group contributes to the production of alanine and glutamine by combining with pyruvate and glutamate, respectively.[117] In addition, the carbon skeletons of valine and isoleucine may be converted to glutamine by way of the tricarboxylic acid cycle.[118] Alanine and glutamine are released by skeletal muscle and are used by the liver for glucose production.[119]

The role of BCAAs in skeletal muscle protein turnover has been studied by various investigators. In vitro studies demonstrated that the BCAAs were able to promote protein synthesis and inhibit protein degradation.[120,121] It was postulated that the BCAAs may play important roles in the muscle protein-sparing effect of amino acid solutions.

Studies in catabolic patients paralleled these results. Plasma aminograms in septic patients demonstrated decreased concentrations of BCAAs and increased concentrations of other amino acids not catabolized by skeletal muscle.[116] Increased muscle proteolysis in traumatized patients are postulated as resulting directly in the increased glucose turnover and the amino acid abnormalities present in these patients.[122] Catabolic clinical settings have been demonstrated to cause increased protein catabolism and decreased protein synthesis[123,124] (Fig. 3-7).

As a result of these findings, it is hypothesized that amino acid solutions enriched with the BCAAs may be more nitrogen sparing in hypermetabolic patients than standard amino acid solutions. Studies in animals suggested that infusion of BCAAs may result in improved nitrogen sparing.[125] Studies in patients following surgery demonstrated that infusion of BCAA-enriched solutions improved nitrogen balance on peak "stress" days.[126] These investigators further postulated that the nitrogen-sparing effect of BCAAs was related to the amount of BCAAs present in the solutions.[127] However, studies in patients following surgery demonstrated no improvement on nitrogen balance by BCAA-enriched solutions, although these solutions did result in increased uptake of BCAAs across skeletal muscle.[128] Subsequent clinical studies demonstrated that solutions enriched with BCAAs but relatively lower in leucine than standard amino acid solutions resulted in lower nitrogen balance and increased whole body protein catabolism in the postoperative patients receiving the BCAA-enriched solutions. Correction of the leucine imbalance improved nitrogen balance and decreased whole body protein catabolism but was not significantly different compared with the standard amino acid solution.[129]

Conclusive evidence of improved nitrogen sparing as a result of BCAA-enriched solutions in stressed patients has not been demonstrated. The level of the BCAAs present in standard amino acid solutions may be sufficient to optimize nitrogen-sparing mechanisms in a variety of stressed conditions. BCAA-enriched solutions may be more beneficial in a severely stressed population such as in severe, prolonged sepsis. The difficulty in conducting randomized, prospective studies in these patients has handicapped attempts at answering this important question. Additionally, the identification of the patient population that may benefit from BCAA-enriched solutions is unknown and may actually be relatively small. These important questions must be answered by well-conducted, prospective,

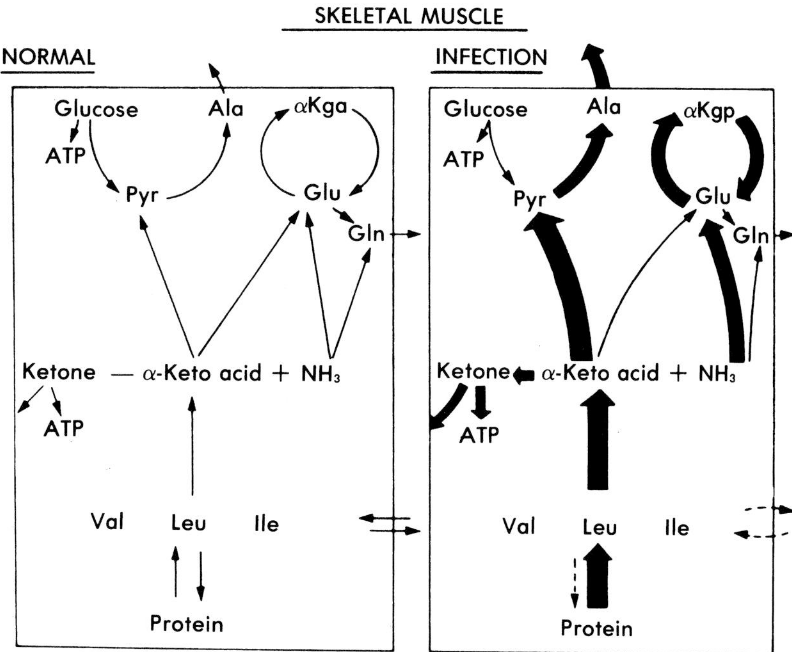

Fig. 3-7. The role of branched-chain amino acids in response to infection. *Ala,* Alanine; *ATP,* adenosine triphosphate; *Gln,* glutamine; *Glu,* glucose; *Ile,* isoleucine; α*Kga,* α-ketoglutaric acid; *Leu,* leucine; *Pyr,* pyruvate; *Val,* valine. (Modified from Wannemacher RW Jr. Key role of various individual amino acids in host response to infection. Am J Clin Nutr 30:1269, 1977. Copyright © American Society for Clinical Nutrition.)

randomized trials before the widespread use of BCAA-enriched solutions can be justified.

Glutamine has also been studied as an additive to parenteral nutrition. Although unstable for long periods of time in parenteral solutions, glutamine dipeptide–supplemented parenteral nutrition has been shown to maintain intestinal function in the critically ill patient.[130] Glutamine dipeptide–containing parenteral nutrition has been demonstrated to prevent intestinal atrophy and reduce the incidence of increased intestinal permeability associated with glutamine-free solutions.[130] Others have shown the benefits of glutamine-supplemented parenteral nutrition in patients undergoing bone marrow transplantation.[58] There is no doubt that, as our knowledge of molecular biology grows, immunomodulation with parenteral nutrition will become more sophisticated.

NUTRITION AND CANCER

The association between weight loss, malnutrition, and cancer has been well established. Nutrition support of cancer patients has gained increased acceptance as a valuable adjuvant for several reasons. The successful use of nutrition support has been demonstrated in clinical trials involving noncancer patients, suggesting that similar results may be possible in cancer patients. In addition, aggressive, multimodality treatment regimens that have been credited with improving survival rates for various types of malignancies are also associated with systemic, toxic effects that may impair the ability of the patient to maintain an adequate intake of nutrients. Often this occurs in patients with existing nutritional deficits. Finally, improvements in delivery and composition of nutrition support have resulted in a greater acceptance of this modality as a viable tool in the management of cancer patients.

Anorexia, a common symptom in malignancies, results in diminished nutrient intake and weight loss. Host and tumor requirements for energy and protein may be greater than nutrient intake in cancer patients with anorexia, which results in a greater use of endogenous fuel reserves. Patients with gastrointestinal malignancies may have reduced nutrient intake because of the mechanical obstruction of the tumor. Compounding the effects of the tumor on nutrient availability to the host are the nutritionally debilitating effects of surgery, radiation therapy, or chemotherapy. The resulting weight loss has been previously documented in various types of malignancies using different criteria.[131,132]

Malnutrition in cancer patients often is characterized as "cancer cachexia," which is a sign and symptom complex, including inanition, anorexia, weakness, wasting, and organ dysfunction. Cachexia may be present in patients with advanced metastatic or localized disease, demonstrating an inconsistent relationship between tumor burden, stage, and histologic characteristics of the malignancy. The true cause of cancer cachexia is often unclear. Nevertheless, a variety of etiologic factors, involving decreased nutrient uptake and increased or deranged nutrient requirements, is usually present (Fig. 3-8), leading to altered substrate metabolism associated with cancer (see box, p. 78).

Cancer patients may have decreased nutrient intake for a variety of reasons and often do not demonstrate the nor-

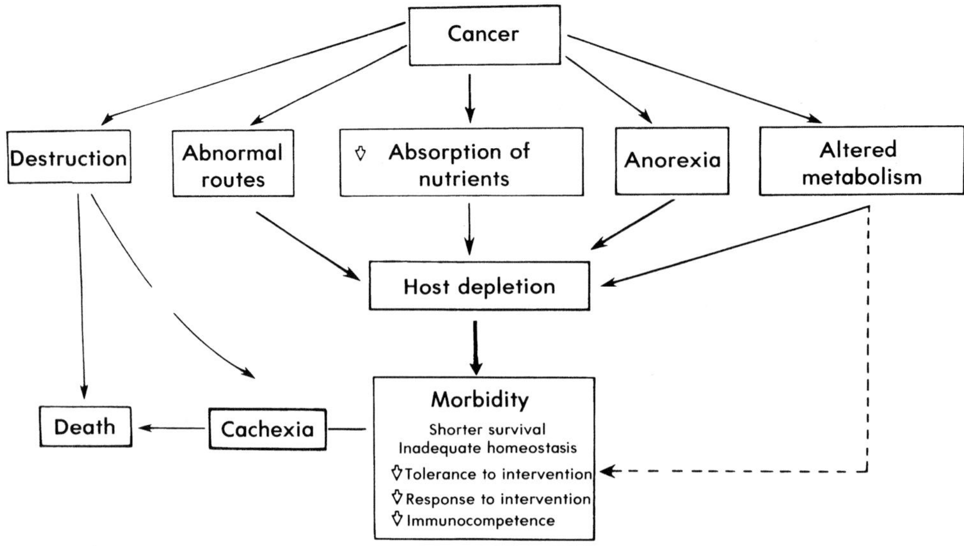

Fig. 3-8. Mechanisms leading to host depletion and morbidity in patients with cancer. (Modified from Costa G. Cachexia, the metabolic component of neoplastic diseases [review]. Cancer Res 37:2327, 1977.)

ALTERED SUBSTRATE METABOLISM IN PATIENTS WITH CANCER

Carbohydrate Metabolism

Abnormal response to glucose tolerance test
Increased insulin resistance (hepatic and peripheral)
Increased gluconeogenesis from alanine and lactate
Increased Cori cycle activity

Protein Metabolism

"Nitrogen trapping" by the tumor
Increased protein turnover
Impaired muscle protein synthesis

Fat Metabolism

Increased neutral fat breakdown and fatty acid use for energy

Energy Expenditure

Increased energy expenditure
Inefficient energy expenditure

mal response to starvation by the conservation of endogenous nutrient stores. Malnutrition in cancer patients may contribute to a number of severe sequelae. Protein-calorie malnutrition may result in weight loss and a compromise of visceral and somatic protein compartments that are vital to enzymatic, structural, and mechanical function. Immunocompetence may be compromised with resultant increased suspectibility to infection.[133] Treatment regimens involving radiation, chemotherapy, and surgery may also contribute to impaired immunity. In addition, poor wound healing, prolonged ileus, and increased morbidity and mortality following surgical procedures have been linked to poor nutritional status in cancer patients. Review of autopsy reports in cancer patients has demonstrated that malnutrition is implicated in at least 22% of cancer deaths.[134] Therefore patients with cancer who are malnourished and who are undergoing or will undergo treatment for their malignancy may benefit from nutrition support.

The selection of the route for administration of nutrition support in cancer patients does not differ from that in noncancer patients. If gastrointestinal function is adequate, oral supplementation should be the initial form of support. However, an unwillingness or an inability of the patient to tolerate oral feedings should be followed by an attempt at tube feeding. Nevertheless, patients with cancer often have inadequate gastrointestinal function. In these patients, parenteral feedings usually offer the best alternative for nutrition support.

The use of nutrition support in cancer patients previously was discouraged because of fear of enhanced tumor growth. Various animal studies have demonstrated that tumor growth may be enhanced by dietary manipulations. However, interpretations of animal studies should be tempered with caution. In rats, tumor burdens are disproportionately large, and tumor growth rates are very high in contrast to patients with cancer. In addition, in contrast to animals, patients with cancer receiving nutrition support usually receive concurrent antineoplastic therapy in these studies. Indeed, various investigators have been unable to demonstrate increased tumor growth in patients receiving antineoplastic therapy and nutrition support.[135,136]

The use of nutrition support in patients with cancer remains a controversial subject. Malnourished cancer patients receiving antineoplastic therapy usually receive nutrition support. The benefits of nutrition support in these patients were demonstrated by retrospective studies.

Prospective, randomized trials involving malnourished patients with cancer are difficult to conduct, and most physicians are unwilling to withhold nutrition support in these patients if they are to receive concurrent treatment. Prospective randomized trials of TPN in cancer patients undergoing treatment have been conducted and recently reviewed.[135] The results of these studies are inconclusive and somewhat conflicting. The majority of these studies failed to demonstrate a significant increase in tumor response in patients receiving TPN. However, many of the series contained a limited number of patients, and most were not malnourished. In addition, benefits of TPN were demonstrated in several of the studies, particularly in patients undergoing surgery for gastrointestinal neoplasms.[137]

Drawing solid conclusions from these trials is difficult. Trials in patients with malignancies that carry a dismal prognosis may fail to demonstrate statistical improvement when receiving TPN as a result of the low number of these patients that respond to any treatment. Nevertheless, retrospective data do indicate that an improvement in nutritional status in cancer patients may be advantageous. Ultimately, the implementation of nutrition support in these patients should be based on several principles. First, malnutrition should not be allowed to interfere with required cancer therapy by diminishing the ability of the patient to withstand therapeutic procedures. Second, no patient should be allowed to develop malnutrition as a result of necessary treatment. Finally, only those patients with a hope of a meaningful therapeutic response should be considered for nutrition support.

Recent review of studies on the role of nutrition support in the patient with cancer demonstrates that the routine use of short-term TPN does not decrease mortality or complications in patients receiving chemotherapy or radiation therapy. However, many of these trials have serious limitations in study design that may limit their usefulness in drawing meaningful conclusions.[138] In contrast, long-term TPN may be beneficial in maintaining hydration, providing nutrients, and improving quality of life.

LONG-TERM NUTRITION SUPPORT

Nutritional intervention has been found to be efficacious in a variety of clinical settings. Increased use of this treatment modality has resulted in a reduction of associated complications with associated greater efficiency of delivery systems. Technical advances have allowed application of nutrition support for nonhospitalized patients.[139] Patients who would otherwise have little hope for life because of refractory malnutrition, either from their underlying disease or its treatment, can maintain adequate nutrient intake from home parenteral and home enteral nutrition.

Home Parenteral and Enteral Nutrition

Home parenteral nutrition (HPN) is indicated in patients who are unable to eat and absorb enough nutrients for maintenance. The specific diseases and/or subsequent treatments that create a need for HPN in patients are varied. The majority of patients currently receiving HPN are patients with short bowel syndromes. These patients usually suffer from extensive Crohn's disease, mesenteric infarction, or severe abdominal trauma.[140] Other reported cases include patients with severe intestinal obstruction, radiation enteritis, cancer, necrotizing enterocolitis, or congenital short bowel syndrome.[141]

The majority of these patients cannot receive adequate nutrition enterally, although compensatory mucosal growth with resultant increased efficiency of absorption can occur in some patients and may either reduce or remove the need for continued HPN. Other categories of patients requiring HPN include those with malabsorption syndromes, intestinal pseudo-obstruction, radiation enteritis, and severe anorexia nervosa.[141]

Complications of HPN parallel those of in-hospital TPN. Patients with proximal gastrointestinal tract obstruction or diversion may receive their nutrition at home enterally, by way of gastrostomy or jejunostomy. Debilitated patients have been fed for many years through nasoenteric feeding tubes, the more recently developed Silastic tubes being considerably more comfortable than earlier examples. Advantages to home enteral nutrition parallel those of in-hospital programs: lower cost, ease of administration, and fewer complications.[142]

SUMMARY

Subclinical and clinical malnutrition have become increasingly recognized in hospitalized surgical patients and have been shown to be associated with increased morbidity and mortality. The metabolic response to starvation and surgical stress (e.g., trauma, operative procedures, and infection) leads to an erosion of lean body mass and endogenous fat stores, which, if allowed to persist, ultimately leads to organ failure and death. The development of techniques of nutrition support by way of enteral or parenteral routes on the basis of sound physiologic principles has allowed the provision of optimal nutritional therapy to all patients at all times and has minimized the devastating effects that nutritional failure may have on patient outcome and survival.

REFERENCES

1. Bistrian BR, et al. Protein status of general surgical patients. JAMA 230:858, 1974.
2. Butterworth CE, Weinsier RL. Malnutrition in hospital patients: Assessment and treatment. In Goodhart RS, Shils ME, eds. Modern Nutrition in Health and Disease. Philadelphia: Lea & Febiger, 1980.
3. Larson J, et al. Impact of nutritional state on quality of life in surgical patient. Nutrition 2:217, 1995.
4. Butterworth CE. Skeleton in the hospital closet. Nutrition Today 9:4, 1976.
5. Hill GL, et al. Malnutrition in surgical patients: An unrecognized problem. Lancet 1:689, 1977.
6. Souba WW. Nutritional support. N Engl J Med 336:41, 1997.
7. Stein TP. Protein metabolism. In Torosian M, ed. Nutrition for the Hospitalized Patient. New York: Marcel Dekker, 1995, p 19.
8. Cahill GF. Starvation in man. N Engl J Med 282:668, 1970.

9. Cunningham RS. Effects of nutritional status on immune function. Am J Clin Nutr 35:1202, 1982.
10. Askenazi JA, et al. Nutrition and the respiratory system. Crit Care Med 10:163, 1982.
11. Smith RJ, Wilmore DW. Glutamine nutrition and requirements. J Parenter Enter Nutr 14:945, 1990.
12. Meguid MM, Collier MD, Howard LJ. Uncomplicated and stressed starvation. Surg Clin North Am 61:529, 1981.
13. Mullen JL, et al. Implications of malnutrition in the surgical patient. Arch Surg 114:121, 1979.
14. Mullen JL, et al. Reduction of operative morbidity and mortality by combined preoperative and postoperative nutritional support. Ann Surg 192:604, 1980.
15. Grant JP. Nutritional assessment in clinical practice. Nutr Clin Pract 1:3, 1986.
16. Aselgren KN, et al. Comparison of nutritional indices and outcome in critically ill patients. Crit Care Med 10:305, 1988.
17. Baker JP, et al. Nutritional assessment: A comparison of clinical judgement and objective measurements. N Engl J Med 306:969, 1982.
18. Starker PM, et al. The influence of preoperative total parenteral nutrition upon morbidity and mortality. Surg Gynecol Obstet 162:569, 1986.
19. Grant JP, Custer PB, Thurlow J. Current techniques of nutritional assessment. Surg Clin North Am 61:437, 1981.
20. Hill GL. Nutritional assessment. In Fisher JE, ed. Total Parenteral Nutrition. Boston: Little, Brown, 1991, p 139.
21. Morgan DB, Hill GL, Buckinshow L. The assessment of weight loss from a single measurement of body weight: The problems and limitations. Am J Clin Nutr 33:2101, 1980.
22. Hill GL, Beddoe AH. Dimensions of the human body and its compartments. In Kinney JR, Jeejeebhoy KN, Hill GL, Owen OE, eds. Nutrition and Metabolism in Patient Care. Philadelphia: WB Saunders, 1988.
23. Pettigrew RA, Hill GL. Indicators of surgical risk and clinical judgment: A prospective comparative study. Br J Surg 73:47, 1986.
24. Heymfield SB, Casper K. Anthropometric assessment of the adult hospitalized patient. J Parenter Enter Nutr 11:365, 1987.
25. Bistrian BR, et al. Therapeutic index of nutritional depletion in hospitalized patients. Surg Gynecol Obstet 141:512, 1975.
26. Kosonovich JM, Dumur F, Horst M. Use of urea kinetics in the nutritional care of the acutely ill patient. J Parenter Enter Nutr 9:165, 1985.
27. Candio JA, Hoffman MJ, Lucke JF. Estimation of nitrogen excretion based on abbreviated urinary collections in patients on continuous parenteral nutrition. J Parenter Enter Nutr 15:148, 1991.
28. Fischer JE. Nutritional assessment before surgery. Am J Clin Nutr 35:1128, 1982.
29. Rheinhardt GF, Myscofski JW, Wikens DB. Incidence and mortality of hypoalbuminemic patients in hospitalized veterans. J Parenter Enter Nutr 4:357, 1980.
30. Hickman DM, et al. Serum albumin and body weight as predictors of postoperative course in colorectal cancer. J Parenter Enter Nutr 4:314, 1980.
31. Starker DM, et al. Serum albumin levels as an index of nutritional support. Surgery 91:194, 1982.
32. Roza AM, Tritt D, Shizzal HM. Transferrin—A poor measure of nutritional status. J Parenter Enter Nutr 8:523, 1984.
33. MacLean LD, et al. Host resistance in sepsis and trauma. Ann Surg 182:207, 1975.
34. Haffejee AA, Angorn IB. Nutritional status and the nonspecific cellular and humoral immune response in esophageal carcinoma. Ann Surg 189:475, 1979.
35. McIrvine AJ, Mannick JA. Lymphocyte function in the critically ill surgical patient. Surg Clin North Am 63:245, 1983.
36. Lloyd AVC. Tuberculin test in children with malnutrition. Br Med J 3:529, 1968.
37. Daly JM, Dudrick SJ, Copeland EM III. Intravenous hyperalimentation: Effect on delayed cutaneous hypersensitivity in cancer patients. Ann Surg 192:587, 1980.
38. Mullen JL, et al. Prediction of operative morbidity and mortality by preoperative nutritional assessment. Surg Forum 30:80, 1979.
39. Ryan JA, Taft DA. Preoperative nutritional assessment does not predict morbidity and mortality in abdominal operations. Surg Forum 31:96, 1980.
40. Alverdy JC, Aoys E, Moss GS. Total parenteral nutrition promotes translocation of bacteria from the gut. Surgery 104:185, 1988.
41. Alverdy JC, Chi HS, Sheldon GF. The effect of parenteral nutrition on gastrointestinal immunity: The importance of enteral stimulation. Ann Surg 202:681-684, 1985.
42. Deitch EA, et al. The gut as a portal of entry for bacteremia: Role of protein malnutrition. Ann Surg 205:681-692, 1987.
43. O'Dwyer ST, et al. A single dose of endotoxin increases intestinal permeability in healthy humans. Arch Surg 123:1459, 1988.
44. Ziegler TR, et al. Increased intestinal permeability associated with infection in burn patients. Arch Surg 123:1313, 1988.
45. Steinmetz OK, Meakins, JL. Translocation of bacteria from the gut: Clinically relevant? In Fry DE, ed. Multiple System Organ Failure. St. Louis: Mosby 1992, p 373.
46. Moore FA, et al. TEN versus TPN following major abdominal trauma. J Trauma 26:874, 1986.
47. Kudsk KA, et al. Enteral vs. parenteral feeding effects on septic morbidity after blunt and penetrating abdominal trauma. Ann Surg 215:503, 1992.
48. Hasse JM, et al. Early enteral nutrition support in patients undergoing liver transplantation. J Parenter Enter Nutr 19:437, 1995.
49. Hearne BE, Daly JM. Enteral nutrition. In Kirkpatrick J, ed. Nutrition and Metabolism in the Surgical Patient. Mt. Kisco, N.Y.: Futura Publishing, 1983.
50. Freeman JB, Fairfull-Smith RJ. Current concepts of enteral feeding. Adv Surg 16:75, 1983.
51. Rombeau JL, Barot LR. Enteral nutritional therapy. Surg Clin North Am 61:605, 1981.
52. Alexander JW. Specific nutrients and the immune response. Nutrition 11:229, 1995.
53. Barton RG. Immune enhancing enteral formulas: Are they beneficial in critically ill patients? Nutr Clin Pract 12:51, 1997.
54. Alverdy JC. Effects of glutamine supplemented diets on immunology of the gut. J Parenter Enter Nutr 14:1095, 1990.
55. Gianotti L, et al. Oral glutamine decreases bacterial translocation and improves survival in experimental gut origin sepsis. J Parenter Enter Nutr 19:69, 1995.
56. Ogle CK, et al. Effect of glutamine on phagocytosis and bacterial killing by normal and pediatric burn patient neutrophils. J Parenter Enter Nutr 18:128, 1994.
57. Jacobs DO, et al. Combined effects of glutamine and EGF on the rat intestine. Surgery 1044:358, 1988.
58. Ziegler TR, et al. Clinical and metabolic efficacy of glutamine supplemented parenteral nutrition after bone marrow transplantation. Ann Int Med 116:832, 1992.
59. Daly JM, et al. Immune and metabolic effects of arginine in the surgical patient. Ann Surg 208:512, 1988.
60. Barbul D. Arginine: Biochemistry, physiology and therapeutic implication. J Parenter Enter Nutr 10:227, 1986.
61. Gianotti L, et al. Arginine supplemented diets improve survival in gut-derived sepsis and peritonitis by modulating bacterial clearance: The role of nitric oxide. Ann Surg 217:644, 1993.
62. Kirk SJ, et al. Arginine stimulates wound healing and immune function in elderly human beings. Surgery 114:155, 1993.
63. Reynold JS, et al. Immunologic effects of arginine supplementation in tumor bearing and non-tumor bearing hosts. Ann Surg 211:202, 1990.
64. Endreo S, et al. The effect of dietary supplementation with omega-3 polyunsaturated fatty acids on the synthesis of interleukin-1 and tumor necrosis factor by mononuclear cells. N Engl J Med 320:265, 1985.

65. Kelley JE, et al. Enhancement of immunosuppression by substitution of fish oil for olive oil as a vehicle for cyclosporine. Transplantation 48:98, 1989.
66. van der Heide JJH, et al. Effect of dietary fish oil on renal function and rejection in cyclosporine-treated recipients of renal transplants. N Engl J Med 329:769, 1993.
67. Trocki O, et al. Effects of fish oil on postburn metabolism and immunity. J Parenter Enter Nutr 11:521, 1987.
68. Albina JE, Gladden P, Walsh WR. Detrimental effects of an omega-3 fatty acid enriched diet on wound healing. J Parenter Enter Nutr 17:519, 1993.
69. Johnson JA III, Griswold JA, Muakkassa FF. Essential fatty acids influence survival in sepsis. J Trauma 35:128, 1993.
70. Rolandelli RH, et al. Effect of intraluminal short chain fatty acids on healing of colonic anastomosis in the rat. Surgery 100:198, 1986.
71. Cohen RM, et al. Gastroesophageal reflux during gastrostomy feeding. Gastroenterology 106:13, 1994.
72. Metheny NA, et al. pH testing of feeding tube aspirates to determine placement. Nutr Clin Pract 9:185, 1994.
73. Ponsky, JL, Gauderer MWL, Stellato TA. Percutaneous endoscopic gastrostomy: Indications, limitations, techniques and results. World J Surg 13:165, 1989.
74. Allardyce DB, Groves AC. A comparison of nutritional gains resulting from intravenous and enteral feeding. Surg Gynecol Obstet 139:179, 1974.
75. Burt ME, Gorschboth CM, Brennan MF. A controlled, prospective, randomized trial evaluating the metabolic effects of enteral and parenteral nutrition in the cancer patient. Cancer 49:1092, 1982.
76. McArdle AH, et al. A rationale for enteral feeding as the preferable route for hyperalimentation. Surgery 90:616, 1981.
77. Bowen RH, et al. Early enteral administration of a formula supplemented with arginine, nucleotides and fish oil in intensive care unit patients: Results of a multicenter prospective randomized clinical trial. Crit Care Med 23:436, 1995.
78. Dudrick SJ, et al. Long-term parenteral nutrition with growth, development, and positive nitrogen balance. Surgery 64:134, 1968.
79. Daly JM, Long JM. Intravenous hyperalimentation: Techniques and potential complications. Surg Clin North Am 61:583, 1981.
80. Sanderson I, Deitel M. Intravenous hyperalimentation without sepsis. Surg Gynecol Obstet 136:577, 1973.
81. Sanderson I. Insulin response in patients receiving concentrated infusions of glucose and casein hydrolysates for complete parenteral nutrition. Ann Surg 179:387, 1974.
82. Heird WC, et al. Hyperammonemia resulting from intravenous alimentation using a mixture of synthetic L-amino acids. J Pediatr 81:162, 1972.
83. McCarthy MC, Cottam GL, Turner WW. Essential fatty acid deficiency in critically ill surgical patients. Am J Surg 142:747, 1981.
84. Jeejeebhoy KN, et al. Metabolic studies in total parenteral nutrition with lipid in man: Comparison with glucose. J Clin Invest 57:125, 1976.
85. Baker JP, et al. Randomized trial of total parenteral nutrition in critically ill patients: Metabolic effects of varying glucose-lipid ratios as the energy source. Gastroenterology 87:53, 1984.
86. Macfie J, Smith RC, Hill GL. Glucose or fat as a nonprotein source? A controlled clinical trial in gastroenterological patients requiring intravenous nutrition. Gastroenterology 80:103, 1981.
87. Burke JF, et al. Glucose requirements following burn injury, parameters of optimal glucose infusion and possible hepatic and respiratory abnormalities following excessive glucose intake. Ann Surg 190:274, 1979.
88. Long JM, et al. Effect of carbohydrate and fat intake on nitrogen excretion during total intravenous feeding. Ann Surg 185:417, 1977.
89. Blackburn GL, et al. Protein sparing therapy during periods of starvation with sepsis or trauma. Ann Surg 177:589, 1973.
90. Collins JP, Oxby CB, Hill GL. Intravenous amino acids and intravenous hyperalimentation as protein-sparing therapy after major surgery: A controlled clinical trial. Lancet 1:788, 1978.
91. Elwyn DJ, et al. Protein and energy sparing of glucose added in hypocaloric amounts to peripheral infusions of amino acids. Metabolism 27:325, 1978.
92. Watters JM, Freeman JB. Parenteral nutrition by peripheral vein. Surg Clin North Am 61:593, 1981.
93. Jeejeebhoy, KN. Nutritional support of the azotemic patient. Urol Clin North Am 1:345, 1974.
94. Giovannetti S, Maggiore Q. A low-nitrogen diet with proteins of high biologic value for severe chronic uraemia. Lancet 1:1000, 1964.
95. Dudrick SJ, Steiger E, Long JM. Renal failure in surgical patients: Treatment with intravenous essential amino acids and hypertonic glucose. Surgery 68:180, 1970.
96. Bergstrom J, Furst P, Josephson B. Factors affecting the nitrogen balance in chronic uremic patients receiving essential amino acid intravenously or by mouth. Nutr Metab 14(Suppl):162, 1972.
97. Freund H, Atamian S, Fischer JE. Comparative study of parenteral nutrition in renal failure using essential and nonessential amino acid containing solutions. Surg Gynecol Obstet 151:652, 1980.
98. Abel RM, et al. Improved survival from acute renal failure after treatment with intravenous essential L-amino acids and glucose. N Engl J Med 288:695, 1973.
99. Leonard CD, Luke RG, Sieger RR: Parenteral essential amino acids in acute renal failure. Urology 6:154, 1975.
100. Feinstein EI, et al. Clinical and metabolic responses to parenteral nutrition in acute renal failure. Medicine 60:124, 1981.
101. Cascino A, et al. Plasma amino acids imbalance in patients with liver disease. Dig Dis Sci 23:591, 1978.
102. Fischer JE, et al. The role of plasma amino acids in hepatic encephalopathy. Surgery 78:276, 1975.
103. Morgan MY, Milsom JP, Sherlock S. Plasma ration of valine, leucine, and isoleucine to phenylalanine and tyrosine in liver disease. Gut 19:1068, 1978.
104. Oldendorf WH, Szabo J. Amino acid assignment to one of three blood-brain barrier amino acid carriers. Am J Physiol 230:94, 1976.
105. Fischer JE, Baldessarini RJ. False neurotransmitters and hepatic failure. Lancet 2:75, 1971.
106. Manghani KK, et al. Urinary and serum octopamine in patients with portal-systemic encephalopathy, Lancet 2:943, 1975.
107. Knell AJ, et al. Dopamine and serotonin metabolism in hepatic encephalopathy. Br Med J 23:549, 1974.
108. James JH, et al. Brain tryptophan, plasma free tryptophan and distribution of plasma neutral amino acids. Metabolism 25:471, 1976.
109. Rosen HM, et al. Influences of exogenous intake and nitrogen balance on plasma and brain aromatic amino acid concentrations. Metabolism 27:393, 1978.
110. Freund H, et al. Infusion of branched chain enriched amino acid solution in patient with hepatic encephalopathy. Ann Surg 196:209, 1982.
111. Cerra FB, et al. Cirrhosis, encephalopathy, and improved results with metabolic support. Surgery 94:612, 1983.
112. Horst D, et al. Comparison of dietary protein with an oral, branched chain enriched amino acid supplement in chronic portal-systemic encephalopathy: A randomized controlled trial. Hepatology 4:279, 1984.
113. Rossi-Fanelli F, et al. Branched chain amino acids vs. lactulose in the treatment of hepatic coma. Dig Dis Sci 27:929, 1982.
114. Millikan WJ, et al. Total parenteral nutrition with F080 in cirrhotics with subclinical encephalopathy. Ann Surg 197:294, 1983.
115. Cerra FB, et al. Correlations between metabolic and cardiopulmonary measurements in patients after trauma, general surgery, and sepsis. J Trauma 19:621, 1979.
116. Wannemacher RW. Key role of various individual amino acids in host response to infection, J Biochem 249:5500, 1974.

117. Ruderman NB, Berger M. The formation of glutamine and alanine in skeletal muscle. J Biochem 249:5500, 1974.
118. Goldberg AL, Chang, TW. Regulation and significance of amino acid metabolism in skeletal muscle. Fed Proc 37:2301, 1978.
119. Odessy R, Khairallah EA, Goldberg AL. Origin and possible significance of alanine production by skeletal muscle. J Biochem 249:7323, 1974.
120. Buse MG, Reid SS. Leucine: A possible regulator of protein turnover in muscle. J Clin Invest 56:1250, 1975.
121. Fulks, RM, Li JB, Goldberg AL. Effects of insulin, glucose, and amino acids on protein turnover in rat diaphragm. J Biochem 250:290, 1975.
122. Clowes GHA, Randall HT, Cha CJ. Amino acid and energy metabolism in septic and traumatized patients. JPEN 4:195, 1980.
123. Birkhahn RH, et al. Effects of major skeletal trauma on whole body protein turnover in man measured by L-(1,14C)-leucine. Surgery 88:294, 1980.
124. O'Keefe SJD, Sender PM, James WPT. "Catabolic" loss of body nitrogen in response to surgery. Lancet 2:1035, 1974.
125. Blackburn GL, et al. Branched chain amino acid administration and metabolism during starvation, injury, and infection. Surgery 86:307, 1979.
126. Kern KA, et al. The effect of a new branched chain enriched amino acid solution on postoperative catabolism. Surgery 92:780, 1982.
127. Cerra FB, et al. Nitrogen retention in critically ill patients is proportional to the branched chain amino acid load. Crit Care Med 11:775, 1983.
128. Daly JM, et al. Effects of postoperative infusion of branched chain amino acids on nitrogen balance and forearm muscle substrate flux. Surgery 94:151, 1983.
129. Bonau RA, et al. High branched amino acid solutions: Relationship of composition to efficacy. JPEN 8:622, 1984.
130. Tremel H, et al. Glutamine dipeptide supplemented parenteral nutrition maintains intestinal function in the critically ill. Gastroenterology 107:1595, 1994.
131. DeWys WD, et al. Prognostic effect of weight loss prior to chemotherapy in cancer patients. Am J Med 69:491, 1980.
132. Nixon DW, et al. Protein calorie undernutrition in hospitalized cancer patients. Am J Med 68:683, 1980.
133. Daly JM, Dudrick SJ, Copeland EM III. Effects of protein depletion and repletion on cell-mediated immunity in experimental animals. Ann Surg 188:791, 1978.
134. Mullen JL, et al. Protein synthesis dynamics in human gastrointestinal malignancies. Surgery 87:331, 1980.
135. Brennan MF: Total parenteral nutrition in the cancer patient. N Engl J Med 305:375, 1981.
136. Copeland EM III, Daly JM, Dudrick SJ. Nutrition and cancer. Int Adv Surg Oncol 4:1, 1981.
137. Daly JM, et al. Enteral nutrition during multimodality therapy in upper gastrointestinal cancer patients. Ann Surg 221:327, 1995.
138. Klein S, et al. Nutrition support in clinical practice: A review of published data and recommendations for future research directions. J Parenter Enter Nutr 21:133, 1997.
139. Dudrick SJ, et al: Update on ambulatory home hyperalimentation. Nutr Sup Ser 1:18, 1981.
140. Fleming CR, et al. Home parenteral nutrition for management of the severely malnourished adult patient. Gastroenterology 79:18, 1980.
141. Wolfe BM, et al. Experience with home parenteral nutrition. Am J Surg 146:7, 1983.
142. Chrysomilides SA, Kaminski MV. Home enteral and parenteral nutritional support: A comparison. Am J Clin Nutr 34:2271, 1981.

4

Immunity and the Immunocompromised Patient

Carl E. Haisch and Kathryn M. Verbanac

The immune system functions to protect the body's internal environment from a variety of potential insults such as foreign proteins, potentially adverse cells, microorganisms, and other noxious substances. Since immune competence plays such an important role in the insurance of good health and the response of a patient to surgical intervention, alterations in the immune system can greatly affect the outcome of an operation both in terms of morbidity and mortality.

Immune competence reflects the highly integrated, carefully orchestrated homeostatic interplay of a number of physiologic processes whose primary function is to discriminate between substances that are a part of the body's own makeup ("self") and those that are foreign to it ("no self"). The purpose of this chapter is to review the components of this immune system, how they interrelate, how this recognition between self and nonself occurs, and the impact that alterations in these processes can have on the surgical patient.

OVERVIEW OF THE IMMUNE SYSTEM

In this section, we introduce the cellular components of the immune system, describe the initiation and effector stages of the humoral and cellular immune response, and discuss clinical assessment of immune function. This section is to serve as a general introduction and review and to provide a basis for the clinical considerations that follow. There are several excellent immunology textbooks that should be referred to for a more comprehensive description of the immune system.[1-4] In addition, we have cited key articles within each section that provide current reviews and references of the primary literature.

Cellular Components

Leukocytes, the white blood cells that participate in the immune response, are derived from a common pluripotent stem cell in the bone marrow (Fig. 4-1). The mature cellular components of the immune system are distinguished on the basis of function and phenotype. Lymphocytes are distinguished from the other cells of the immune system because only lymphocytes exhibit diversity, specificity, memory, and self/nonself recognition.

The cellular phenotype is principally defined by cell surface markers, the majority of which are designated as cluster of differentiation (CD) antigens and are identified by monoclonal antibodies. Monoclonal antibodies serve as important immunologic reagents for both the identification and quantitation of leukocyte and lymphocyte subpopulations that express these markers. There are currently 166 CD antigens that have been designated by the International Workshops on Leukocyte Differentiation Antigens.[5] Since the expression of cell surface antigens varies qualitatively and quantitatively with both the maturation stage and activation state of the cell, monoclonal antibodies are also valuable for monitoring the phenotype of a specific leukocyte subpopulation (Table 4-1). Many of the cell surface antigens serve as specific receptors for ligands,

Table 4-1. Characteristic Leukocyte Cell Surface Markers*

Cell	Marker
B cell	**CD19, CD20,** CD21, **slg,** CD45RB, CD40, CD80/CD86 (B7-1/B7-2)
T cell	CD2, **CD3, TCR,** CD28, **CD154** (CD40L)
T helper	**CD4**
T cytotoxic	**CD8**
Natural killer cell	CD2, CD16a, (FcγRIII), **CD56,** CD11b (iC3bR), CD11c
Monocyte/macrophage	CD11b, CD11c, CD16a, CD32 (FcγRII), **CD64** (FcγRI)
Granulocytes	CD10 (CALLA), CD11b, CD11c, **CD15**, CD16b, CD32

*This list is not comprehensive. The cell surface antigens **unique** to the cell type are in bold type. The combination of coexpressed antigens is often most characteristic of a cell type.

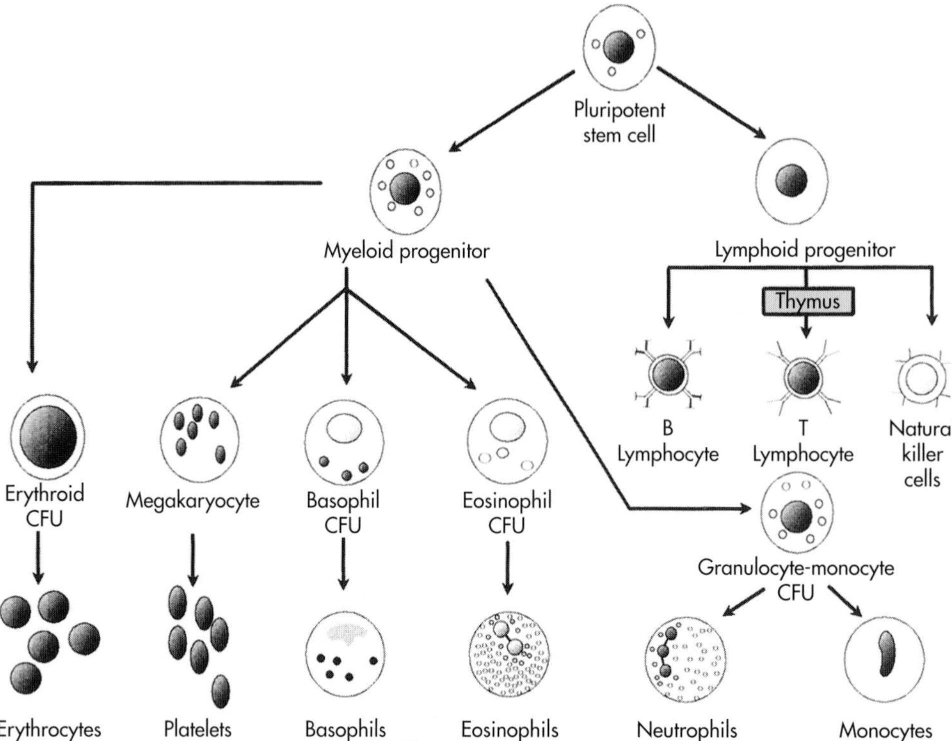

Fig. 4-1. Maturation of blood cells from the pluripotent stem cell in bone marrow. *CFU,* Colony-forming unit. (From Abbas AK, Lichtman AH, Pober JS. Cellular and Molecular Immunology, 3rd ed. Philadelphia: WB Saunders, 1997, p 25.)

thus ligand binding and receptor engagement have important immunologic consequences. These ligands include immunoglobulins, complement, cytokines, viruses, and bacterial products.

B Lymphocytes

A schematic diagram of an immunoglobulin is presented in Fig. 4-2. The development of the B lymphocyte occurs predominantly in the bone marrow of mammals and is centered around the expression of membrane-bound immunoglobulin. Membrane-bound antibody comprises the ligand-binding portion of the B-cell antigen receptor; since the antigen-binding variable region of the protein is extracellular, this region readily binds to soluble antigen. The expression of surface immunoglobulin (gIg) imbues the B lymphocyte with both antigen specificity and memory. Recent studies have shown that, after antigen binding, signal transduction is mediated by another component of the B-cell receptor. This function is carried out by a disulfide-bonded heterodimer that is noncovalently complexed with surface immunoglobulin and has been designated Ig-α/Ig-β or CD79a/CD79b.[6]

The DNA encoding antibody heavy chains, κ light chains and λ light chains are located on different chromosomes. Within each chromosome, immunoglobulin sequences are present in germline DNA as multigene families that contain numerous gene segments (Fig. 4-3). In progenitor and precursor B cells the variable region-diversity region-joining region (V-D-J) gene segments that comprise the variable region of the heavy chain undergo random gene rearrangement to form a functional Ig heavy chain.[7] This is followed by light chain gene rearrangements that result in the expression of membrane-bound IgM. These rearrangements are regulated so that only one of the allelic forms of the immunoglobulin is expressed, that is, DNA from only one of the parental chromosomes is rearranged. This is referred to as allelic exclusion and ensures that immunoglobulin with a single antigenic specificity is expressed by a given B cell.

B cells at this developmental stage are released from the bone marrow into the blood. Most B cells encounter antigen in regional lymph nodes or in the spleen, where they undergo antigen-dependent stages of differentiation. In the absence of antigen activation, peripheral B cells die within several days. If the membrane-bound antibody present on the surface of the B cell encounters specific antigen, these cells undergo class switching by additional gene rearrangements of the constant region of the heavy chain and by changes in RNA processing. These class switching events lead to different clones of B cells that express different isotypes or classes of antibody with the same antigenic specificity. Different antibody isotypes have different effector functions, thus the range and type of immune response is broadened. (Table 4-2).

At this stage, some B cells clonally expand and differentiate into plasma cells that secrete various isotypes. Other

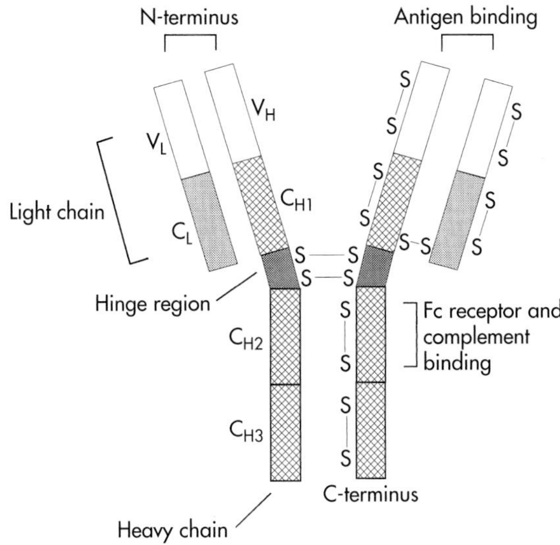

Fig. 4-2. Schematic diagram of an immunoglobulin molecule. Each heavy *(H)* and light *(L)* chain contains an amino-terminal variable *(V)* region that is unique to each B-cell clone; together they form the antigen-binding site. The constant *(C)* domains exhibit limited variation and define the immunoglobulin isotype and effector functions. Intrachain and interchain disulfide bonds play a major role in the folding of the protein domains and in the formation of the polypeptide chain tetramer. The γ, δ, α heavy chains contain a hinge region, and the μ and ϵ heavy chains contain a fourth central C_H domain.

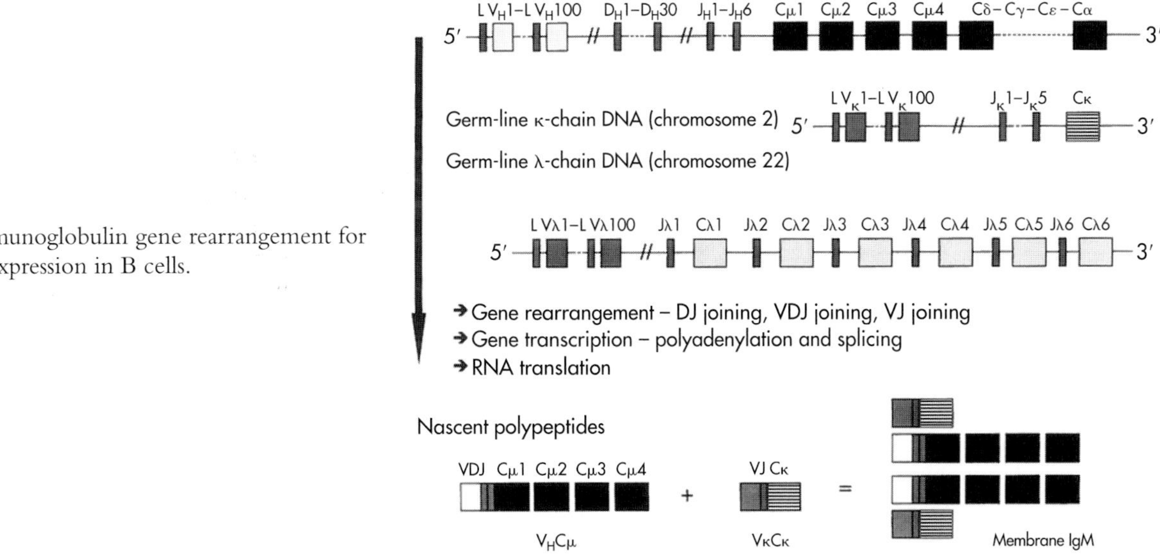

Fig. 4-3. Immunoglobulin gene rearrangement for surface IgM expression in B cells.

Table 4-2. Properties and Biologic Activities* of Classes and Subclasses of Serum Immunoglobulins

Property/Activity	IgG1	IgG2	IgG3	IgG4	IgA1	IgA2	IgM‡	IgE	IgD
Molecular weight† (KDa)	150	150	150	150	150-600	150-600	900	190	150
Heavy-chain component	γ1	γ2	γ3	γ4	α1	α2	μ	ϵ	δ
Normal serum level (mg/ml)	9	3	1	0.5	3	0.5	1.5	0.0003	0.03
In vivo serum half-life (days)	23	23	8	23	6	6	5	2.5	3
Activates classical complement pathway	+	+/−	++	−	−	−	+++	−	−
Crosses placenta	+	+/−	+	+	−	−	−	−	−
Present on membrane of mature B cells	−	−	−	−	−	−	+	−	+
Binds to macrophage Fc receptors	++	+/−	++	+	−	−	+	−	−
Present in secretions	−	−	−	−	++	++	+	−	−
Induces mast-cell degranulation	−	−	−	−	−	−	−	+	−

From Kuby J. Immunology, 3rd ed. New York: WH Freeman, 1997. Used with permission.
*Activity levels indicated as follows: ++, high; +, moderate; +/−, minimal; and −, none.
†IgG, IgE, and IgD always exist as monomers, IgA can exist as a monomer, dimer, trimer, or tetramer. Membrane-bound IgM is a monomer, but secreted IgM in serum is a pentamer.
‡IgM is the first isotype produced by the neonate and during a primary immune response.

B cells differentiate into memory B cells that have a longer life span and express membrane-bound immunoglobulin of different isotypes. Memory B cells are able to undergo somatic mutation to generate higher affinity antibodies, that is, antibodies with a greater binding strength or association constant but of the same specificity. This process is termed affinity maturation. All these mechanisms contribute to the generation of a high degree of antibody diversity; it is estimated that humans can produce antibodies that have 10^8 to 10^{11} different specificities.

T Lymphocytes

T lymphocytes are termed thymus dependent because the lymphoid stem cell migrates from the bone marrow to the thymus, where it differentiates and matures during normal fetal development. It is in the thymus that T-cell receptor (TCR) rearrangement occurs to generate the diverse repertoire of antigen specificities exhibited by T-cell clones in the periphery. During thymic education, negative and positive selection processes result in the death of self-reactive T cells and the survival of a large number of T-lymphocyte clones, "each bearing a different antigen receptor to match the enormous variety of antigens present in the microbial world."[8]

The TCR is the antigen-binding receptor on the surface of T cells. It is expressed as either an α/β or γ/δ heterodimer and is associated on the membrane with the multiple components of CD3 (Fig. 4-4). The CD3 components are critical for the signal transduction events that occur after antigen binding. The initial activation of protein tyrosine kinases is followed by many diverse intracellular signals whose key outcome is to affect the expression of cytokine genes.[9]

Although the TCR is the unique distinguishing marker of the T cell today, T cells were historically distinguished from B cells on the basis of the so-called E rosette receptor, now designated CD2. T cells have been subdivided into two subtypes, those with helper/inducer function (primarily $CD4^+$) and those with cytotoxic/suppressor function (primarily $CD8^+$). In the thymus, $CD4^-$ $CD8^-$ bone marrow progenitors go through sequential developmental changes before the so-called "single positive" T cells expressing either CD4 or CD8 and the αβTCR are produced. Although these latter cells comprise the vast majority of peripheral T cells, it has recently been discovered that a small number of T cells expressing the γδTCR are present in adult epithelial tissues.

The majority of $\alpha\beta TCR^+$ T cells in the periphery are naive or precursor T cells that have not yet encountered antigen and are in the G_o (resting) stage of the cell cycle. Once these cells are antigen-activated (as discussed below), they become effectors that perform helper, cytotoxic, and delayed-type hypersensitivity (DTH) functions. Memory T cells are also generated during a primary response to antigen and recirculate in the blood and lymph as extremely long-lived resting cells with less stringent requirements for activation.

T-helper (Th) cells have been classified into Th0, Th1,

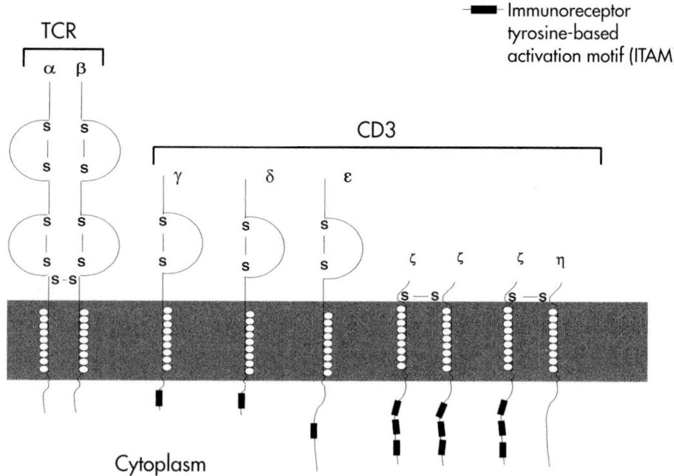

Fig. 4-4. Schematic diagram of the T-cell receptor–CD3 complex. The polypeptide chains of CD3 noncovalently associate with the TCR-α/β chains and with each other as γε, δε, ζζ, and ζη heterodimers, as well as ηη homodimers. The extracellular disulfide-bonded domains are homologous to the immunoglobulin fold structure. The ITAM is a conserved sequence located in the cytoplasmic domains; it includes tyrosine phosphorylation sites and functions in signal transduction.

and Th2 cells, on the basis of the distinct, mutually exclusive cytokines they secrete and on the functional effects of these cytokines.[10] The cytokines were originally discovered in mice; however, it is now certain that T cells with definite Th1 and Th2 patterns of cytokine "help" exist in humans as well. Th0 cells comprise the majority of T cells in the human circulation. They are thought to be precursors of Th1 and Th2 cells and exhibit an intermediate phenotype; they synthesize cytokines characteristic of both Th1 and Th2 cells.

On antigenic stimulation, Th1 cells secrete interleukin-2 (IL-2), interferon-gamma (INF-γ), and tumor necrosis factor (TNF-β), which serve to channel the immune system toward cell-mediated immunity, including macrophage activation and DTH responses. Th1 cells are thus effective in the defense against intracellular pathogens (e.g. Leishmania) and are thought to be involved in the pathogenesis of acute allograft rejection, organ-specific autoimmune disorders, contact dermatitis, and certain chronic inflammatory diseases.

In contrast, Th2 cells secrete Il-4, Il-5, IL-6, and IL-10; induce humoral and allergic responses; and are most effective against extracellular microorganisms and soluble toxins. Studies of Th2 cells have concentrated on IgE responses to helminth antigens and allergens. Th2 cytokines generally exert anti-inflammatory immunosuppressive effects, and Th2 responses have been associated with transplantation tolerance, the immunopathology of chronic graft-versus-host disease, and systemic autoimmune disease. It is clear that reciprocal regulation occurs between the Th1 and Th2 subsets, mediated by specific cytokine effects on differentiation and on effector functions.

There has not been a similar functional division of

$CD8^+$ T-cell subpopulations. Although CD8 originally characterized suppressor and cytotoxic cells, a definitive suppressor cell has been elusive and has not been isolated or cloned. Therefore most contemporary immunologists view the suppressor cell as a functional designation rather than the definition of a separate subpopulation. The classic $CD8^+$ T lymphocyte is the cytotoxic T lymphocyte (CTL). CTLs are major histocompatibility complex (MHC) class I–restricted cells that recognize and eliminate "altered self" target cells. Target cells include virally infected cells, malignant cells, and allogeneic cells. The primary mechanism of CTL-mediated killing involves degranulation and release of a pore-forming protein (perforin) and a battery of serine proteases (granzymes) that rapidly induce target cell lysis.[11] CTLs have also been recently shown to induce apoptosis, or programmed cell death, of target cells.

Natural Killer Cells

Although their developmental pathway is not fully understood, natural killer (NK) cells, like T and B lymphocytes, arise from $CD34^+$ lymphoid stem cells in the bone marrow. NK cells make up 5% to 10% of human peripheral blood mononuclear cells (PBMCs). NK cells are termed null cells because they do not express the distinct cell membrane markers that would characterize them as T or B cells, including the T-cell and B-cell antigen-binding receptors. NK cells and T cells are both $CD2^+$ and are thought to share a common thymic developmental precursor. Unlike CTLs, NK cells typically express the phenotype CD16 and CD56 and do not typically express CD3 or CD8. It should be noted, however, that distinct subpopulations of NK cells with atypical phenotypes have been observed at very low levels in healthy individuals and at significant levels in recovering bone marrow transplantation recipients.

NK cells were originally referred to as large granular lymphocytes (LGL) and discovered on the basis of their tumoricidal activity. The adjective *natural* refers to the important fact that NK cell effector activity does not require antigen activation or sensitization and thus provides "natural immunity" or "innate" antiviral and antitumor protection. This immunity is critical in the early days of exposure, before CTL precursor cells can become activated, proliferate, and differentiate into mature CTLs. Unlike CTLs, NK cells do not express antigen receptors, hence they do not exhibit immunologic specificity or memory.

There are two methods by which NK cells can identify an appropriate target cell. It has been shown experimentally for some time that NK cells detect the "absence of self" on target cells, and the specific NK receptors that mediate this recognition have recently been identified.[12] These so-called NK "inhibitory" receptors are specific for MHC class I on potential target cells. If the receptors are engaged, NK cell activity is inhibited and the cognate cell is released. If no "self" MHC class I is detected on the potential target cell, there is no receptor engagement and no inhibitory signal. In this scenario, NK lytic effector mechanisms are triggered. A single NK cell may carry multiple inhibitory receptors specific for human leukocyte antigens (HLA)-A, -B, and -C (MHC class I antigens).

The second means of identifying a target cell involves antibody-dependent cell-mediated cytotoxicity (ADCC), which is described in detail later in this chapter. In short, NK cells express CD16, which can bind to the Fc region of IgG that is bound to target cell membranes. CD16 engagement activates the NK cell, inducing the lytic mechanism and cytokine production.

NK cells appear to kill target tumor cells and virally infected cells by mechanisms similar to those described for CTLs, namely the release of lytic granules. NK cells have also been recently shown to induce apoptosis via direct target cell killing or in ADCC. These two mechanisms are probably not mutually exclusive, and some studies suggest that perforin and granzymes may synergistically trigger apoptosis.

Monocytes and Macrophages

The remainder of the cellular components to be described develop from the same pluripotent hematopoietic stem cell in the bone marrow but along the myeloid lineage rather than the lymphoid lineage. These cells differ significantly from lymphocytes; they lack antigen specificity, and they lack memory. The monocyte is a phagocytic mononuclear myeloid cell that circulates briefly before migrating into tissue where it differentiates into a macrophage. The macrophage can take up permanent residence in particular tissues or remain motile. The primary function of the monocyte and macrophage is to phagocytose and eliminate antigen.[13,14] Their digestive granules contain lytic enzymes, reactive oxygen and nitrogen intermediates and TNF. Macrophages can ingest and digest whole microorganisms, as well as injured and dead cells, cellular debris, and activated clotting factors. The macrophage also digests internalized proteins and presents peptides in association with MHC class II on its surface. It plays a critical role in T-helper cell activation, both as an antigen-presenting cell (APC) and as a source of IL-1. The T-helper cell in turn promotes macrophage activation, by secretion of IFN-γ. Activated macrophages have increased phagocytic activity and increased microbicidal activity and secrete many factors that promote the inflammatory response. Finally, monocytes and macrophages express all three forms of the receptor for the Fc region of IgG (FcγR) (CD16, CD32, and CD64) and thus can participate in ADCC.

Granulocytes

Granulocyte is a general term for motile cells that contain cytoplasmic granules. These cells are categorized into basophils, eosinophils, and neutrophils on the basis of cell morphology and cytoplasmic staining properties. Granulocytes characteristically play a major role in the inflammatory response, which can be beneficial in host defenses and detrimental in inflammatory disease.[15]

Neutrophils are also referred to as "polys" or polymorphonuclear neutrophil leukocytes (PMNs) and constitute

50% to 70% of the circulating white blood cells in humans. Neutrophils are active phagocytic scavengers of the immune system and are usually the first cells to arrive at an inflammatory site. Their granules contain lytic enzymes, bactericidal defensin peptides, and reactive oxygen and nitrogen intermediates; however, unlike macrophages, they do not contain TNF.

Eosinophils are also phagocytic and function primarily against parasites via ADCC. The nonphagocytic basophils play a major role in allergic responses when they release their granules of pharmacologic agents, including histamine.

Immune Response

The interaction of a T-helper cell with an APC is the central event that initiates virtually all immune responses, for generation of both cell-mediated immunity (CMI) and antibody-mediated immunity (humoral). The T cell and APC interact primarily in the secondary lymphoid organs—the lymph nodes and the spleen. Antigen can be transported to these organs as soluble antigen, as antigen-antibody complexes, or via mobile APC (including certain dendritic cells and macrophages). After recognition of a peptide–MHC class II complex on an APC, T-helper cells are activated and proliferate extensively. The T-helper cell progeny secrete cytokine "help" and play a central role in the activation of B cells, CTLs, and macrophages.

T Cell–Antigen-Presenting Cell Interactions

The T cell–APC association is based on specific antigen recognition and is mediated by the requisite binding of two cell surface molecules, the TCR of the T-helper cell with the MHC-peptide complex of the APC. MHC molecules are cell surface molecules encoded by the MHC gene complex that control the ability of an animal to respond immunologically to a given antigen. The multiple alleles (estimated at >100) within a given MHC locus encode highly polymorphic gene products that vary in their individual ability to bind a specific peptide. The inherited polymorphisms provide a large repertoire of specificities for antigen-derived peptides and thus provide the host with the ability to respond immunologically to a large range of different antigens.

Many cell types can present antigen to T cells, that is, they can degrade and present antigen-derived peptides via their MHC class I and class II molecules. The so-called professional APCs are those cells that constitutively express MHC class II and in humans include dendritic cells, macrophages, B cells, and vascular endothelial cells. These cell types can vary in the effectiveness with which they present antigen and stimulate an immune response in vitro. The dendritic cell appears to be one of the most potent APC in vitro, expressing high levels of MHC class II and possessing long dendritelike membrane processes that provide a large surface area for cell-to-cell interactions. The concentration of antigen, as well as other variables, may determine which cell type is the operative APC in vivo. Since a B cell recognizes an antigen specifically via its surface immunoglobulin, it can present antigenic peptides effectively even at low antigen concentrations.

After intracellular degradation of foreign proteins, the MHC class I and class II molecules of the APC bind certain processed peptides within a groove formed by the polymorphic residues of the MHC. The TCR thus recognizes the specific amino acid sequence of a peptide (processed antigen) in association with self-MHC. This interaction is termed self-MHC restriction or associative recognition. APCs generally "present" processed foreign antigen in association with MHC class II to CD4 T cells, or in association with MHC class I to CD8 T cells (Fig. 4-5). CD4 and CD8 specifically recognize residues within the monomorphic conserved domains of MHC class II and class I antigens, respectively; thus CD4 and CD8 cells are termed MHC class II–and MHC class I–restricted, respectively.

There are additional accessory cell surface proteins that play important roles in the T cell–APC interaction. Some act as adhesion molecules to stabilize or increase the strength of T cell–APC interactions. Examples of such T cell–APC ligand pairs include CD2–leukocyte function–associated antigen-3 (LFA-3); LFA-1– intercellular adhesion molecule 1 (ICAM-1) or ICAM-2; CD4–MHC class II; and CD8–MHC class I. Some ligand pair interactions provide signals to enhance T-cell activation; many ligands have cytoplasmic domains possessing enzymatic activity, usually kinase activity (phosphorylating enzymes). Such ligands are often called signal transducers because they send a signal from outside the cell to the inside. CD4 and CD8 molecules are associated with intracellular T-cell protein tyrosine kinases, which appear to be activated by CD4 or CD8 binding to the monomorphic domains of MHC molecules.

There is compelling evidence that certain ligand pair interactions provide critical "second signals" required for T-cell activation after the antigenic "signal 1" is delivered via TCR ligation to MHC-peptide. The most significant ligand-receptor pairs that have been identified on T cells and APCs, respectively, are CD40L-CD40, CD28-CD80, and CTLA-4–CD86.[16,17] In the current working model of Th-cell activation[18,19] (Fig. 4-6), CD40L expression is

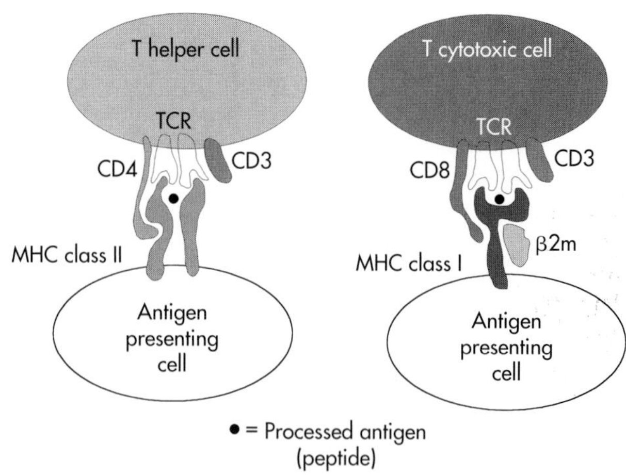

Fig. 4-5. Antigen presentation and recognition. *MHC,* Major histocompatibility complex; *TCR,* T-cell receptor.

upregulated by T cells that have received signal 1 (ligation of the TCR with MHC-antigen). CD40L can then engage CD40, its cognate ligand on the APC, which in turn triggers the APC to express CD80 and CD86 (originally named B7.1 and B7.2). CD80 binding to CD28, which are constitutively expressed on T cells, results in full T-cell activation. It now appears that the T-cell surface protein, CTLA-4, although homologous to CD28, may be a negative regulator of T-cell activation. It is important to note that APC activation is usually a corollary to these interactions and is also dependent on CD40-CD40L engagement. Activated B cells, macrophages, and dendritic cells are key players in the effector phase of an immune response. Soluble cytokines are also involved in mediating this "cross-talk" and include T cell–derived IL-4, as well as IL-1, IL-6, and IL-12, which are secreted by specific APC cell types.

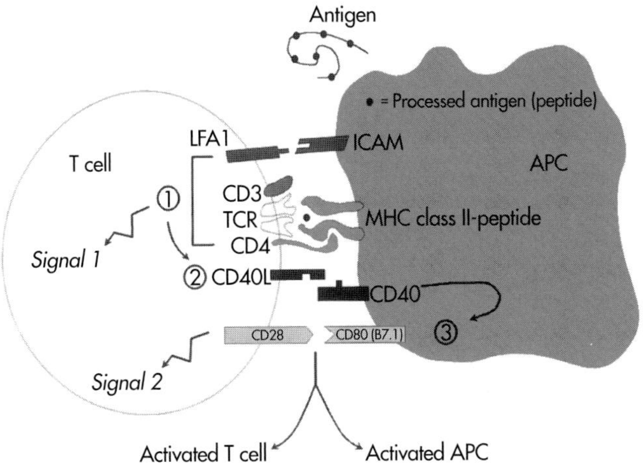

Fig. 4-6. Th-cell activation. *APC,* Antigen-presenting cell; *ICAM,* intracellular-antigen mediated; *LFA,* leukocyte function associated; *TCR,* T-cell receptor.

The central role of the Th cell in the immune response is presented in Fig. 4-7. Once the Th cell is activated by productive engagement of the appropriate receptor ligand pairs and after receipt of the appropriate signals, it produces IL-2 "help," which functions in an autocrine manner to induce proliferation and clonal expansion. This Th progeny can now produce cytokines that "help" B cells, macrophages, and CTLs differentiate and perform their full effector functions.

Humoral Immune Response

It is clear that B cells, T cells, and macrophages are required for the generation of most humoral immune responses. As described above, the B-cell antigen receptor is a multicomponent receptor, consisting of surface immunoglobulin noncovalently associated with two other distinct trans-

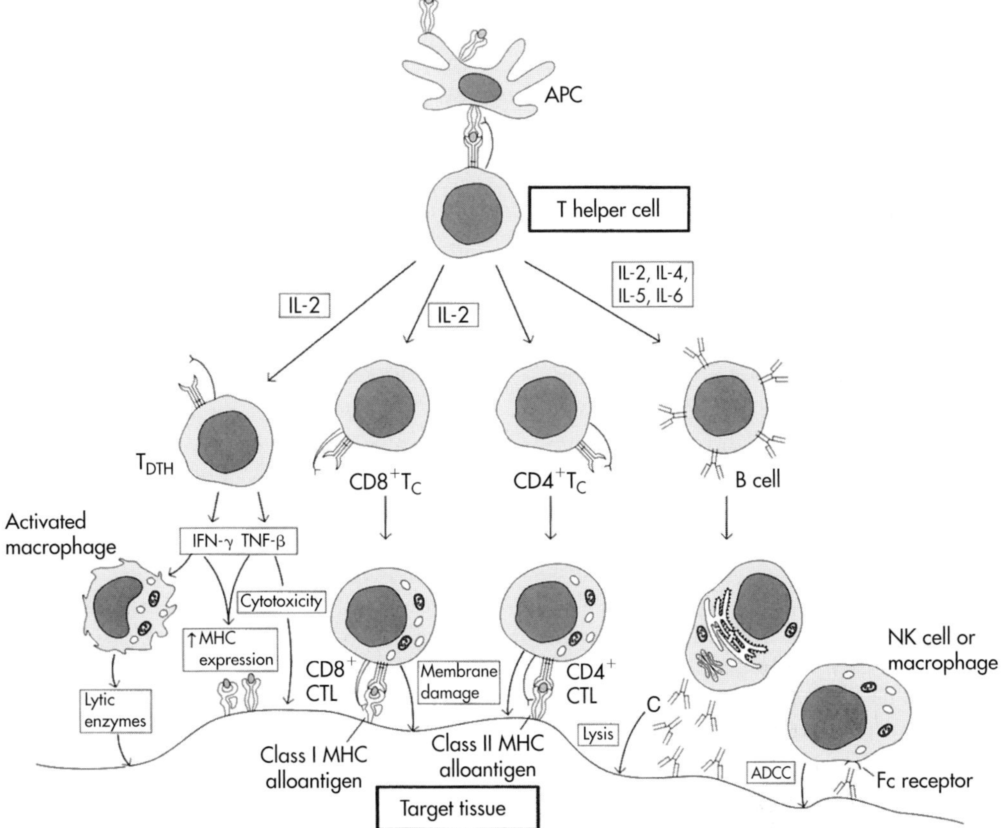

Fig. 4-7. Schematic of the central role of the Th cell in the effector mechanisms of the immune response. *ADCC,* Antibody-dependent cell-mediated cytotoxicity; *APC,* antigen-presenting cell; *C,* complement; *CTL,* cytotoxic T lymphocyte; *DTH,* delayed-type hypersensitivity; *MHC,* major histocompatibility complex; *TNF,* tissue necrosis factor. (Modified from Kuby J. Immunology, 3rd ed. New York: WH Freeman, 1997. Used with permission.)

membrane proteins. The surface antibody mediates the internalization of specific antigen via receptor-mediated endocytosis. In the B-cell endosome, newly synthesized MHC class II antigens encounter peptides derived from antigen proteolysis and present certain peptides on the surface of the B cell.

These "antigen-primed" B cells act as APCs to interact with activated T-helper cells (which are antigen specific on the basis of their TCR) and form specific B–T-helper cell conjugates. Antigen-specific conjugate formation appears to actually cause redistribution of the TCR, LFA-1, and CD4 molecules within the T cell at the interface of the cell-to-cell contact. Conjugate formation induces T-cell expression of CD40L, which then engages CD40 on the B-cell surface, as described above. The B-cell receptor itself is associated with cytoplasmic *src*-family tyrosine protein kinases, which are activated on antigen binding and initiate an intracellular signaling cascade that leads to many cellular responses, including cytokine production. B-cell activation ensues, triggered by a combination of membrane events and cytokine signaling.

T-helper cytokines play predominant roles as costimulatory signals in B-cell activation. The activated B cell is driven into the S (or DNA synthesis) phase of the cell cycle by IL-2, IL-4, and IL-5. As discussed earlier, IgM is the first isotype expressed by plasma cells during a primary immune response. Numerous Th1 and/or Th2 cytokines (including IL-2, IL-4, IL-5, IFN-γ, and transforming growth factor-β [TGF-β]) induce differentiation into plasma cells producing different immunoglobulin isotypes. The changes in the activation and maturation stage of the cells are both caused by and marked by changes in gene expression.

"T-dependent" antigens exist that can directly stimulate B cells and elicit antibody responses without the assistance of T-helper cells.[20] This type of antigen, usually carbohydrate in nature and comprised of repeating epitopes, is best exemplified by bacterial polysaccharides.

Complement-mediated cytolysis is the major effector mechanism of the humoral immune response. Complement refers to a group of at least 20 distinct serum proteins that participate in a highly regulated enzymatic cascade.[21] There are two pathways of complement activation, the classic and the alternative pathways. Both pathways generate a membrane attack complex (MAC) that forms pores in cell membranes and causes cell lysis. A conformational change occurs when an antibody binds to its antigen, such that a binding site on the Fc portion of the molecule is exposed. Binding of the C1 component of the complement system to the Fc sites exposed on two adjacent antibody molecules activates the classic pathway. In humans, IgM and certain subclasses of IgG (IgG1, IgG2, and IgG3) are capable of "fixing" complement in this manner. The alternative pathway is usually initiated by bacteria, yeast, and certain viruses in an antibody-independent fashion. Complement reaction products cause vasodilation and chemotaxis to promote a localized inflammatory response and also act as opsonins to promote phagocytosis of antigen.

Anaphylaxis is an immediate hypersensitivity reaction that is triggered by IgE-mediated mast cell or basophil degranulation and is initiated within 2 to 30 minutes of antigen exposure. Anaphylaxis can be localized to a specific target tissue or can occur throughout the organism, inducing systemic effects that can be fatal. On primary exposure to parasitic antigens or allergens, B cells are activated to become IgE-secreting plasma cells. IgE binds to the cell surface of mast cells and basophils via the high-affinity FcεRI, thus increasing the half-life of IgE from days to weeks. Mast cells are bone marrow–derived cells that differentiate in connective tissues where they reside. On secondary exposure to antigen, the IgE on these sensitized cells is cross-linked, which triggers degranulation and the release of pharmacologically active mediators. These mediators include histamine and serotonin, which cause increased vascular permeability and smooth muscle contraction, as well as granulocyte chemotactic factors and proteases, which mediate tissue destruction. Additional secondary mediators such as leukotrienes, are generated by the breakdown of the mast cell membrane phospholipids after degranulation. Eosinophils are also attracted to the site and can bind directly to antibody-coated antigen. They in turn are activated, degranulate, and release inflammatory mediators.

Opsonization refers to the deposition of molecules on an antigen (including a microorganism) that promotes contact with an appropriate phagocytic cell. Such molecules, or opsonins, are usually antibodies or components of complement. Since macrophages and granulocytes express receptors for both antibody and complement on their cell surfaces, opsonization increases antigen binding by these phagocytes. Opsonins thus serve as a bridge between antigen and the effector cell. The enhanced antigen binding results in a significant increase in the rate of phagocytosis.

Antibody-Dependent Cell-Mediated Cytotoxicity

ADCC is the complement-independent process in which antibodies can affect cell-mediated responses to foreign cells. In this scenario, antibody serves as a bridge connecting a foreign target cell to an immune effector cell and thus provides antigen specificity to a nonspecific cytotoxic cell. NK cells, neutrophils, macrophages, and eosinophils express Fc receptors on their cell surfaces. These receptors can thus recognize the carboxy terminal region of an immunoglobulin molecule that is itself bound to foreign cells via its amino-terminal antigen-binding hypervariable domains. This binding stimulates the cytotoxic cells to increase the lytic components in their cytoplasmic granules (including enzymes, TNF, perforin) and then to release the granule contents, culminating in destruction of the target cell.

Cytotoxic T Lymphocyte–Mediated Cytotoxicity

The CTL-mediated immune response is initiated by the activation and differentiation of precursor CTL (CTLp) into functional effectors. The interaction of the TCR of a resting CTLp with the MHC class I–peptide complex of its target cell induces the expression of T-cell IL-2 receptors. As described earlier, IL-2 "help" is produced as a result of a similar interaction between $CD4^+$ Th and MHC class II^+ APC. This IL-2 provides the principal "second signal" required by CTLp for activation, triggering its clonal proliferation and differentiation into a mature CTL effector. As discussed earlier, other ligands interactions also supply strong costimulatory signals, particularly the B7/CD28 interaction.

The CTL progeny, mature effectors, are now able to form conjugates with target cells that bear the appropriate MHC class I–peptide complexes. Exocytosis of cytoplasmic granules at the interface of cell-to-cell contact releases lytic molecules, which damage the membrane of the target cell and cause death, as described previously. Secondary to antigen recognition, the LFA-1–ICAM interaction between T cell and target cell appears to be critical for both conjugate formation and subsequent dissociation of the CTL from the target cell.

Delayed-Type Hypersensitivity Reactions

DTH responses refer to an increased reactivity to a specific antigen that is T cell mediated. The increased reactivity is a function of previous antigen sensitization (via APC–T cell interactions described previously) that has induced T cells to proliferate and differentiate into a subset of T (usually $CD4^+$ Th1) cells, designated T_{DTH} cells. Following the second exposure to an antigen, T_{DTH} cells secrete a myriad of cytokines that induce a localized inflammatory reaction (DTH). The macrophage is the major effector cell that is attracted by these cytokines and activated. The DTH response usually peaks 48 to 72 hours after secondary contact. This response is important and generally effective in the defense against intracellular pathogens and contact antigens.

Mediators of Immune Function

We have already discussed the critical roles that the major cytokines play in immune function and regulation. Cytokines are regulatory peptides that have pleiotropic effects on cells that participate in host defense and repair processes. Their main function is to "maintain the integrity of the host by mediating the differentiation between self and nonself, through damage control and by promotion of repair processes."[23]

Originally termed lymphokines, the cytokine terminology evolved to indicate that these factors can be nonlymphocyte derived and can also have nonlymphoid targets. The current "interleukin" terminology was born at the 1978 Second International Lymphocyte Workshop and incorporates the concept of bidirectional, intercellular signaling between somatic, myeloid, and lymphoid cells. At this writing, 16 cytokines have been officially designated as interleukins; lymphocyte chemoattractant factor (LCF) is the most recent cytokine named by the IUIS/WHO Standing Committee on Interleukin Designation as interleukin-16.[24]

Cytokines typically are very potent. They act at pg-ng levels and exert paracrine and autocrine effects. The expression of cytokines is inducible, triggered by diverse stimuli from diverse cellular sources. Cytokines operate in a network that can be overlapping, redundant, synergistic, additive, and/or antagonistic. Cytokines are grouped into families based on structural homologies and are also classified by function (Table 4-3). Finally, they act by binding to high-affinity receptors that are transmembrane proteins, many possessing kinase activity or enzymatic activities that activate the kinases that effect signal transduction. Further comprehensive descriptions of the cytokines are beyond the scope of this chapter and can be found elsewhere.[25,26]

Clinical Assessment of Immune Function

Clinical assessment of human immune function can help define defects in local and systemic defense mechanisms. This is true for both patients with primary hereditary immunodeficiencies and for those with acquired immunodeficiencies. Although some of the tests described below are not routinely conducted clinically, they are available at most tertiary care centers and can be valuable for the identification of the immunocompromised patient at increased risk for local and systemic infections. A summary of laboratory tests used to detect immunodeficiencies is found in Table 4-4.

An obvious key to the successful treatment of infection in the immunocompromised host is early diagnosis of infection. Discussion of these detection techniques is beyond the scope of this review; however, it should be noted that advances in molecular biology have brought innovations to these analyses. Molecular techniques include the use of chemiluminescent-labeled DNA probes that hybridize to DNA of specific bacteria and viruses, as well as virus- and bacteria-specific DNA primers that have been developed for DNA amplification in the polymerase chain reaction. In this section, we briefly discuss some of the clinical predictors and laboratory tests that are valuable.

Leukocyte Enumeration and Subsets

Quantitative determinations of circulating leukocytes are routinely determined by critical blood count (CBC) and differential analysis (Table 4-5). This detects gross changes in cells that might occur in conditions such as leukemia or in certain immunodeficiency diseases. For example, the absolute neutrophil count is very important in patients with cancer; a level lower than 1000 cells/μl strongly correlates with an increased incidence of sepsis, a level lower than 500 cells/μl, if not corrected, is associated with an increased incidence of death.

Enumeration of lymphocyte subsets can be performed by flow cytometric analysis, and characteristic markers have been described in the previous sections. There is a marked reduction of both T- and B-cell counts in severe combined immunodeficiency (SCID). Although lympho-

Table 4-3. General Cytokine Classification by Function

Hematopoietic	IL-3, IL-11, colony-stimulating factors, stem cell factor, erythropoietin
B cell growth	IL-4, IL-5, IL-6, IL-14, IL-15
T cell growth	IL-2, IL-4, IL-7, IL-9, IL-12, IL-15, IL-16
Antiviral	Interferon family (α/β/γ/ω)
Inflammatory	TNF family (TNF-α/β, lymphotoxin), (IL-1 family IL-1 α/β, IL-1RA), IL-6, IL-8)
Chemotactic	IL-8, MCP-1, MIP-1, MIF, MGSA, RANTES, IL-16
Antimitotic	TNF family
Immunosuppressive	IL-4, IL-10, IL-13, TGF-β

Adapted from Aggarwal BB, Puri RK, eds. Human Cytokines: Their Role in Disease and Therapy. Cambridge, Mass.: Blackwell Science, 1995, p 736. *IL,* Interleukin; *MCP,* macrophage chemotactic protein; *MGSA,* melanocyte growth-stimulatory activity; *MIF,* migration inhibiting factor; *MIP,* macrophage inhibitory protein; *TGF,* transforming growth factor; *TNF,* tumor necrosis factor.

Table 4-4. Laboratory Evaluation of Possible Immunodeficiency

Type of Deficiency	Screening Test	Definitive Tests
Antibody deficiency	Immunoelectrophoresis Schick test Isoagglutinin titers	Quantitative immunoglobulin determination Enumeration of B lymphocytes Secretory immunoglobulins and antibodies Rectal or lymph node biopsy Lateral pharyngeal x-ray study Preexistent antibodies to polio, tetanus, etc. Antibody response to injected antigens Immunoglobulin kinetics IgG subclass determination
Cell-mediated immunity deficiency	Lymphocyte count and morphology Thymic x-ray study Skin tests with battery of skin test antigens (candida, mumps, etc.)	Enumeration of T lymphocytes Dinitrochlorobenzene challenge Lymphokine and blastogenic response in vitro Lymph node biopsy
Phagocytic deficiency	White blood cell count, differential, and morphology	Nitroblue tetrazolium assay Assays of chemotactic responsiveness, random migration, phagocytosis, bactericidal activity Enumeration of granulocytes Splenic scan
Complement and opsonic deficiency	Total hemolytic complement (CH_{50}), C3 level	Assay of specific complement components Generation of chemotactic factors Opsonic assay

Adapted from Rubin RH, Cosimi AB. Infections in the immunocompromised host. In Howard RJ, Simmons RL, eds. Surgical Infectious Disease. Norwalk, Conn.: Appleton & Lange, 1995, p 1309.

Table 4-5. Normal Adult Circulating White Blood Cell Populations

Cell Type	Absolute Count*	Percentage
White Blood Cells	4.5-11	
Lymphocytes	1-4.8	25-30% of white blood cells
T cells	—	~70% of lymphocytes
B cells	—	15-25% of lymphocytes
NK cells	—	5-15% of lymphocytes
Monocytes	0-0.8	
Granulocytes	1.8-8.4	
Neutrophils	1.8-7.7	50-70% of white blood cells
Eosinophils	0-0.5	
Basophils	0-0.2	

*(10^3 cells mm^{-3}).

cytes comprise about 25% of the mononuclear cells in the human circulation, the blood actually contains a small proportion (about 2%) of the body's total T- and B-lymphocyte pool.[27] The majority of the lymphocytes are concentrated in the lymph nodes and the spleen. However, because of the dynamic nature of lymphocyte traffic, it is estimated that about 500 × 10^9 lymphocytes travel through the blood compartment each day.

The CD4:CD8 ratio in peripheral blood cells is approximately 2:1 in healthy individuals, and deviations from this ratio can be prognostic indicators of immune dysfunction, especially of immunodeficiency and autoimmune diseases. This ratio is monitored closely clinically in conditions such as AIDS. However, the blood does not always mirror lymphocyte alterations in other tissue, and inferences about pathologic changes in other organs must be made judiciously. As a further caution, it is now known that CD4 and CD8 are not absolute indicators of cell function. For example, $CD4^+$ T cells have been described that are cytotoxic, and some $CD8^+$ cells can generate their own "help."

Flow cytometry can also analyze cell surface antigens that are unique to cells at different stages of differentiation, as described earlier for surface immunoglobulin isotypes in B-cell development. Activation markers, indicative of an ongoing immune response, can also be monitored within different subpopulations by dual parameter flow cytometry. For example, HLA-DR expression on peripheral blood monocytes strongly correlates with infection in many clinical scenarios, particularly in the traumatized patient.[28] Bone marrow and lymph nodes may also be examined in addition to blood to determine if the immune cell distributions are normal.

The number of plasma cells can be determined by the Jerne hemolytic plaque-forming assay or by the recently developed ELISPOT method. In both these methods, PBMC are cultured in vitro, and the halo of antibody secreted by plasma cells is detected, enabling enumeration of each plasma cell. The frequency of antigen-specific CTL, T-helper cells, and their precursors can be measured in peripheral blood by in vitro limiting dilution analysis (LDA) of PBMC. It must be noted that although these latter assays are not routinely available in clinical laboratories, they are standard immunologic methods in many laboratories.

Serum Components

Serum immunoglobulin levels can be determined electrophoretically and by enzyme-linked immunosorbent assay (ELISA). In humoral immunodeficiency diseases, serum immunoglobulins may be totally absent, as occurs in X-linked agammaglobulinemia, or decreased, as occurs in common variable hypergammaglobulinemia. There may also be selective increases or decreases in certain classes of immunoglobulins in the immunocompromised patient.

Complement components can also be accurately measured in serum,[29] most typically by the CH50 test, which simply measures the amount of serum required to lyse 50% of antibody-coated sheep red blood cells. If results are abnormal, this test is followed by analysis of individual complement components, usually C3 and C4. Although not commonly occurring in the homozygous state in humans, genetic deficiencies have been identified in each of the complement components except factor B and are associated with increased susceptibility to bacterial infections and/or immune complex diseases, including systemic lupus erythematosus and glomerulonephritis. Interestingly, an inherited deficiency in C1 inhibitor, a complement regulatory protein, occurs more frequently and results in hereditary angioedema.

The functional activity of lymphoid cells can be evaluated on the basis of the cytokines they secrete. As described previously, the different populations and subpopulations of leukocytes secrete distinct cytokines, and all the major human cytokines can be measured by ELISA or bioassay. However, accurate methods are still lacking for the standard quantitation of many immune mediators in biologic fluids and cells.[30] For many cytokines, serum levels have not proved to be consistent indicators of immune status. This is partly due to their short half-lives and the fact that many cytokines are associated with protein carriers in the serum or are predominantly present in latent, inactive forms. In addition, cytokines typically act locally in an autocrine or paracrine manner and are not usually systemic effectors. Cytokine production is thus often measured after the isolation of leukocytes from an individual and subsequent in vitro culture with antigen.

Bacterial septic shock provides the most dramatic exception to this rule. In this condition, bacterial cell wall endotoxins stimulate macrophages to overproduce IL-1 and TNF-α. These cytokines mediate drastic systemic effects that can be fatal, including a drop in blood pressure, fever, diarrhea, and extensive blood clotting.

Although not routinely analyzed clinically, other regulatory molecules circulate in serum in soluble form and may modulate the immune response. Many of these are cell surface antigens that can be synthesized in a soluble form by alternative mRNA splicing or can be "shed" or generated via proteolytic cleavage from the cell surface. Soluble forms of these antigens are frequently produced by activated cells, thus elevations may indicate an ongoing immune response. For example, significant increases in serum HLA class I antigens have been observed in humans during the course of viral infections (including cytomegalovirus (CMV), hepatitis B and C, and HIV-1) and in allograft recipients undergoing acute rejection episodes. Another example of soluble immunomodulatory molecules are membrane-released Fc receptors, which have been reported to promote the differentiation of normal and leukemic hematopoietic progenitor and precursor cells and regulate antibody production. Finally, many cytokine receptors exist as secreted soluble proteins,[31] and some of these appear to serve as markers of immune suppression (IL-2R) and sepsis (TNFR).

Leukocyte Function

Analyses can also be conducted to determine if the leukocytes that are present in a patient exhibit normal functional activities. PBMC are generally isolated by density gradient centrifugation prior to analysis in one of the following tests.

Mitogenic proliferation. Mitogens are substances that induce DNA synthesis and cell division. Mitogens are often termed polyclonal activators because they activate cells without regard to their clonal antigenic specificities. Many mitogens are plant proteins termed lectins, that have affinities for specific carbohydrate moieties on cell surface glycoproteins and glycolipids. Some mitogens are T cell specific (such as concanavalin A [ConA] and phytohemagglutinin [PHA]), some are B cell specific (such as the lipopolysaccharide of gram negative bacteria), and some mitogens activate both T and B cells (such as pokeweed mitogen). Proliferation is generally measured in the laboratory by incorporation of ^{3}H-thymidine into DNA. Finally, many superantigens are potent activators of T cells (e.g., staphylococcal enterotoxin A) and B cells (e.g., staphylococcal protein A).

Mixed lymphocyte reaction. The mixed lymphocyte reaction (MLR) is an assay in which lymphocytes from different individuals are cultured together and proliferate in response to allogeneic antigens. In the typical one-way MLR, cells from the individual to be tested (the responder cells) are mixed with different allogeneic stimulator cells that have been irradiated to prevent proliferation. This assay can also be used to test the ability of the stimulator lymphocytes (the APC) to present antigen. The amount of ^{3}H-thymidine incorporated into DNA is determined after 4 days of culture and is proportional to the proliferative response. The MLR primarily measures the proliferation of T-helper cells and thus is a strong indicator of differences in the MHC class II antigens of responder and stimulator cells. However, MHC class I antigens and minor transplantation antigens have also been reported to contribute to this response.

Cell-mediated lympholysis. Cell-mediated lympholysis (CML) is an analogous assay to the MLR but analyzes the activity of $CD8^{+}$ CTL instead of $CD4^{+}$ T-helper cells. This assay can evaluate in vivo–generated CTLs (isolated from the circulation) or CTLs that are induced in vitro by MLR. In either case, effector function is measured by the ability of these cells to lyse target cells. Target cells are generally allogeneic or virally infected syngeneic cells. Target cells are genetically identical to the cells injected or transplanted in vivo or identical to the stimulator cells for in vitro MLR-induced CML assays. Target cells are prelabeled intracellularly with ^{51}chromium or a dye that on lysis is released from the cell into solution at a level proportional to the level of cell-mediated cytotoxicity. When conducted as an MLR-induced CML, this assay can also be used to evaluate the functional ability of T-helper cells to induce CTL effectors.

In Vivo Tests

DTH is the most common in vivo assay of *cell-mediated* immune status in humans. A recent retrospective study of surgical intensive care/trauma patients found that a reduced result from a DTH test is a statistically significant predictor of septic mortality.[32] The presence of a DTH reaction can be measured in vivo by injecting the antigen intradermally. A characteristic skin lesion, caused by erythema at the injection site, indicates a positive reaction and is evident 48 to 72 hours after antigen application. The prototype of this test in humans is the administration of the purified protein derivative (PPD) extracted from the cell wall of the *Mycobacterium tuberculosis;* however, other test antigens from histoplasmosis, candidiasis, and nocardiosis are also used. The DTH test is usually given to determine if an individual has been previously exposed to the bacteria (either through injection or prior immunization).

DTH can be used to assess cellular immune function by evaluating the response of an individual to recall antigens, antigens to which the patient presumably has been previously exposed. The CMI-multitest includes eight recall antigens. Dinitrochlorobenzene (DNCB) has also been used as an antigen to test for cellular immune function, and patient response to *de novo* antigen challenge is measured 2 weeks after the initial DNCB skin contact.

The status of *humoral* immune function can be tested in vivo by testing antibody titers to recall antigens such as diphtheria and tetanus toxin. If titers are low, antibody responses to these antigens can also be tested 2 weeks after antigen boost or after active vaccination. Pneumococcal vaccine has been used in this manner to test human antibody responses to carbohydrate antigens. B-cell function can also be tested by analyzing serum for appropriate isohemagglutinin titers (antibodies against the A or B blood group antigens). In addition, if the patient has experienced a documented infection, the current antibody titer against the specific organism can be informative.

Finally, the function of circulating neutrophils and monocytes can be evaluated by the nitroblue tetrazolium (NBT) test. NBT is reduced during the normal respiratory oxidative burst and can provide both qualitative and quantitative data on freshly isolated cells.

THE IMMUNOCOMPROMISED SURGICAL PATIENT

Immunodeficiency Clinical States

Primary Immunodeficiency

There are more than 70 primary immunodeficiency diseases (Table 4-6). Some are manifest from birth, whereas others are not identified until much later in life. The World Health Organization has categorized primary immunodeficiencies into six basic groups: (1) combined deficiencies, (2) predominantly antibody deficiencies, (3) other well-defined immunodeficiency syndromes, (4) immunodeficiencies associated with other diseases, (5) complement deficiencies, and (6) defects of phagocytic func-

Table 4-6. Primary Immunodeficiency Diseases

Disorder	Defective Component or Function	Probable Pathogenesis
Predominantly B-cell defect		
X-linked agammaglobulinemia	All immunoglobulin classes	Impaired maturation of B cells
Autosomal recessive agammaglobulinemia	All immunoglobulin classes	Impaired maturation of B cells
Immunoglobulin deficiency with increased IgM	IgG	Impaired maturation of B cells
Selective IgA deficiency	IgA	Immature IgA B cells
IgG subclass deficiencies	IgG subclasses	?
IgM deficiency	IgM	?
Common variable agammaglobulinemia	All immunoglobulin classes	Impaired differentiation of plasma cells, presence of autoantibodies, imbalance in regulatory T cells
Predominantly T-cell defect		
Severe combine immunodeficiency	Antibodies and T cells	?
Thymic hypoplasia	T cells	Abnormal embryologic development
Cellular immunodeficiency with thymoma	T cells and B cells	?
Wiskott-Aldrich syndrome	Antibodies and T cells	?
Ataxia-telangiectasia	Antibodies and T cells	Impaired maturation of T cells
Chronic mucocutaneous candidiasis	T cells	?
Predominantly neutrophil defect		
Neutrophil dysfunction with high IgE levels	Chemotaxis	?
Actin dysfunction	Phagocyte motility	Actin dysfunction
Glycoprotein deficiency	Phagocyte motility	Glycoprotein deficiency
Chronic granulomatous disease	Microbicidal activity	Enzyme deficiency
Glucose-6-phosphate dehydrogenase deficiency	Microbicidal activity	Enzyme deficiency
Myeloperoxidase deficiency	Microbicidal activity	Enzyme deficiency
Chédiak-Higashi syndrome	Microbicidal activity	Lysosomal defect
Complement defect		
Deficiency of complement components	Complement function	?
Dysfunction of C1 inhibitor, C3 inactivator, or C5	Complement function	?

From Nohr C. Host defenses. In Meakins JL, ed. Surgical Infections: Diagnosis and Treatment. New York: Scientific American, 1994, p 24. Reprinted with permission.

tion.[33] The major complication of primary immunodeficiencies is an increased susceptibility to viral or bacterial infection, although there are increases in certain types of cancer.

Patients with severe T- or B-cell immune defects have an increased incidence of cancer. The type of immunodeficiency can determine the type of cancer that develops. In those patients with combined immunodeficiencies, non-Hodgkin's lymphomas represent the major type of tumor reported. This was the case even though almost half the patients had received some therapy aimed at immunoreconstitution.[34] In patients with SCID, the major cause of death is infection.

Those patients with primary antibody deficiencies have an increased propensity to recurrent and chronic pyogenic infections, usually involving the respiratory tract. The usual tumor is a lymphoma with gastrointestinal carcinomas following. Compared to immunodeficiency states, central nervous system lymphomas are less common. The incidence of gastric carcinoma may be related to the gastric atrophy, achlorhydria, and decreased acid secretions. Many of these patients have low IgA levels and may be at increased risk of *Helicobacter* or related infections.[35]

Those patients with well-characterized immunodeficiencies such as Wiskott-Aldrich syndrome also have an increased risk of malignant tumors. This risk is almost 100% by age 30 in Wiskott-Aldrich syndrome, with the most common site being the brain.[36] Respiratory infections are common in ataxia-telangiectasia. Non-Hodgkin's lymphomas account for almost half the malignancies in this group of patients; however, almost a quarter of the patients develop leukemia. As with other immunodeficiencies, these patients have not done well with single-drug chemotherapy. Recently, however, there have been some patients who have been helped using certain combinations of chemotherapy.

Patients who have a primary immunodeficiency and those who develop a secondary immunodeficiency develop a high proportion of lymphoproliferative disorders. In a review of the incidence of cancer in patients with primary immunodeficiencies, the incidence was approximately 1% to 4%.[37] It must be remembered that this apparently low figure is for all patients with immunodeficiencies and that there are specific immunodeficiencies that have a high incidence of cancer. This level is compared to the incidence of cancer in recipients of an organ transplantation, which is approximately 1% to 5%.[38] In recipients of heart transplants, the risk for posttransplant B-cell lymphoproliferative disease is 5% to 65% of patients. This is believed to be due to the high immunosuppressive drug doses that recipients of heart transplants receive.[39] These data would lead to the conclusion that there may be a common mechanism to explain the incidence of solid cancer in the patients who have been immunosuppressed to maintain an organ transplantation and those patients suffering from primary immunodeficiencies.

Tumors in Transplantation Recipients as Secondary Immunodeficiency Patients

The interval between transplantation and the onset of cancer after transplantation (approximately 32 months) is much shorter than that of the average person who has been exposed to a carcinogen (5 to 20 years).[40] The incidence of the most common cancers (lung, breast, prostate, colon, and invasive uterine cancer) is the same in the general population as it is for transplantation recipients. However, squamous cell carcinomas are markedly increased. A variety of tumors in transplantation recipients compared to the general population are as follows: lymphomas 23% vs. 5%; lip cancers 7% vs. 0.3%; Kaposi's sarcoma 6% vs. minimal; carcinoma of the kidney 5% vs. 2%; and sarcomas 1.7% vs. 0.5%, respectively.[41] Thus in certain tumors the incidence in transplant recipients is markedly different from that of the general population.

Viral infections have been postulated to play a role in cancer development in these immunoincompetent patients. Epstein-Barr virus (EBV) has been closely linked with lymphomas in certain animal models. It has been associated with Burkitt's lymphoma and Hodgkin's disease in the general population. Approximately 30% to 60% of patients with primary disorders are EBV positive. The postulated mechanism is that the virus infects B cells and stimulates a polyclonal B-cell proliferation.[42] This proliferation is abated in normal patients by CTLs, but in immunocompromised individuals the proliferation continues unchecked. This proliferation of multiple B cells is occasionally interrupted by an unknown event that results in the emergence of a monoclonal tumor, thus explaining the incidence of EVB-DNA–specific sequences in tumor specimens of patients who have received a transplant, are congenitally immunodeficient, or have AIDS.[43,44]

It is not clear why patients with primary immunodeficiency or transplants develop disturbances in immunity that result in cancer. Several theories exist but are open to discussion. The first theory is that the patients have a defective surveillance system. If this were the case, then one would expect a higher percentage of cancers of all types and not an increase in certain cancers that have been described. Indeed, when immunosuppression is withdrawn from patients who develop a non-Hodgkin's lymphoma or a Kaposi's sarcoma, a regression of the tumor often occurs. Thus the innate immune response can be effective.

Another popular theory is that patients have chronic antigenic stimulation. Animal models have shown that continuous stimulation with a foreign antigen can give a high yield of lymphomas.[41] Patients with AIDS have chronic infections that could result in continued immunologic stimulation. Transplant recipients have a chronic source of antigenic stimulation from the transplant that could thereby result in the development of lymphomas.

Transplant recipients may also develop cancer because of the carcinogenic effects of the immunosuppressive agents they receive. Azathioprine, cyclophosphamide, and cyclosporine may directly damage DNA and cause malignant changes.[41] However, most animal models require these drugs in combination with another chemical or physical agent to develop cancer. For example, mice treated with azathioprine, cyclophosphamide, cyclosporine, and prednisolone develop cancer when exposed to ultraviolet light in the presence of azathioprine and cyclophosphamide[41] (Table 4-7). There is also an established incidence of skin cancer in patients who reside in climates with sun exposure such as the southwestern United States or Australia.

The most fascinating question of cancer development in immunocompromised patients is why such a small percentage of patients develop cancer. There may be a genetic predisposition, an increased susceptibility to viral

Table 4-7. Effects of Major Immunosuppressive Agents

	Cyclosporine	Corticosteroids	Azathioprine	Cyclophosphamide
Cytotoxicity	–	–	*	*
Myelosuppression	–	–	*	*
Cell specificity	*	–	–	–
Delayed wound healing	–	*	–	–
Impaired microbial defense	+	*	+	+
Organotoxicity	*	–	*	*
Tumorigenesis	*	–	*	*
Diabetogenicity	–	*	–	–
Therapeutic monitoring possible	Yes	No	No	Yes

From Flye MW, ed. Immunosuppressive therapy. In Principles of Organ Transplantation. Philadelphia: WB Saunders, 1989, p 165.
–, No effect; +, small, variable effect; *, significant effect.

functions, or malignancies. For example, several studies link HLA types to susceptibility or resistance to Kaposi's sarcoma.

Specific Problems

Malnutrition

General considerations. Malnutrition is an important problem in surgical patients. In fact, it is the most common cause of acquired immunodeficiency in the world. Malnutrition is not uncommon in patients who have cancer, fistulas, burns, and trauma and predisposes to sepsis and infection.

A consistent finding in malnutrition is the lack of maturation of T lymphocytes in the thymic environment. This is caused by decreased amounts of thymic hormones and a defect in the thymic epithelium and results in the release of immature cells to the periphery.[45] The decrease in mature T lymphocytes is manifested by in vivo abnormalities such as lack of impaired DTH skin responses. In vitro this is detected as a decrease in mitogen and antigen lymphocyte proliferative responses.[46] Malnourished patients exhibit many abnormal T-cell responses that lead to additional host abnormalities in those processes that are dependent on the T-cell response. These include macrophage activation, T cell–dependent antibody production and T cell–mediated cytotoxic responses to viruses.

Patients who are both malnourished and vitamin A deficient have depressed CMI. These individuals also exhibit decreases in antibody response and may have defects in B-cell clonal expansion. Studies[47,48] have shown that immunoglobulin levels are normal or even high in these malnourished patients. Even with the above changes, the use of live vaccines in malnourished children is generally safe.

The complement cascade is very important in the defense against infection. Malnutrition results in decreased serum levels of most complement components, particularly C3. In addition, the normal increase in complement levels, seen in stress situations, is blunted. In malnourished children, complement activation by both pathways appears to be intact but diminished (particularly the alternative pathway). This may be a major predisposing factor to the increased susceptibility of malnourished patients to gram negative sepsis.[49]

Clinically malnourished patients tend to fare poorly and are found to have prolonged infections or infections of greater severity than patients with normal nutritional levels. Malnutrition and infection can become part of a vicious cycle with infection causing increased malnutrition, which in turn causes prolonged or exacerbated infection. Malnutrition is a major predisposing factor for postoperative complications. It is associated with decreased wound healing, an increased complication rate, and an increased death rate.[50]

The route of nutritional support has also been determined to be of importance in the posttraumatic care of patients. Moore et al.[51] have shown that among patients with abdominal trauma, those who received early enteral feedings had significantly fewer intra-abdominal abscesses and lower rates of pneumonia compared to patients who received delayed total parenteral nutrition (TPN). These findings were confirmed by Kudsk et al.[52] who found a decreased incidence of intra-abdominal abscesses, pneumonia, and number of infections in patients who received enteral feeding. Interestingly, these findings are opposite to those found by authors who reviewed enteral and parenteral nutrition in patients with severe head injuries, who showed that parenteral feedings were more favorable.[53] Thus one must evaluate a patient carefully and make sure there are no contraindications for a particular form of nutrition.

Nutritional supplements. An increasing number of nutritional supplements have been identified in nutritional support. Some agents have been shown to have clinical utility, and others are still experimental. The agents that have been evaluated include vitamins, prostaglandins, lipids, and amino acids. Vitamins that have been studied include A, D, E, and K. Vitamin A deficiency has been shown to have a markedly favorable influence on the survival of children who have measles and in patients with bacterial, protozoal, and viral infections. Vitamin A levels are markedly decreased in patients after an operation or a major burn. In these groups of patients, vitamin A supplementation is crucial and can reverse the postinjury immunosuppression.[54] Other fat-soluble vitamins such as D, E, and K are important in immune function. Vitamin E has a major influence on immune function, and its deficiency results in a decrease in T cell–mediated antibody response. Studies in a mouse model using vitamin E showed an increase in IL-2 formation.[55]

Fatty acids also have an influence on immune function. Linoleic acid can prolong graft survival in mice, whereas a deficiency in the same fatty acid decreases allograft survival in the same model. These results indicate the importance of linoleic acid in immunomodulation.[56] Diets high in soybean, corn, sunflower, and safflower oil suppress the response of splenocytes and T cells to mitogens in mice and guinea pigs. These same sources of fatty acids also result in decreased immune competence.

Large amounts of prostaglandin E_2 (PGE_2) are produced by suppressor cells in chronic inflammatory conditions such as multiple sclerosis, rheumatoid arthritis, and infections.[57] PGE_2 is produced by monocytes and macrophages and can modulate the responses of immune cells. The importance of PGE_2 has been studied in patients with chronic infections, who have abnormally high circulating levels of PGE_2. Patients who experience a suppressed immune function postoperatively have a marked increase in PGE_2 synthesis.[58] Tumor cells can stimulate large amounts of PGE_2 released by macrophages. PGE_2 causes an overall decrease in immune surveillance and may be one mechanism by which tumor cells escape normal immune surveillance.[58] Patients with Hodgkin's disease produce four times the normal amount of PGE_2. This suppresses the immune response by inhibiting the production of lymphokines necessary for lymphocyte function. Patients with cancer macrophages appear to be the major source of PGE_2 and can suppress NK cells, T-cell proliferation, and CTLs. The macrophages seem to produce PGE_2 in an uncontrolled fashion and are not subject to the normal feedback mechanism. Prostaglandin synthetase inhibitors have been shown in some models to improve immune function and inhibit tumor growth.[58]

An amino acid that has been shown to be of major importance in a stress situation is arginine. This semiessential amino acid is required for optimal nitrogen balance in young growing rats and has been shown to be necessary for the survival of mildly injured rats.[59] In humans it has been shown to cause a marked increase in human growth hormone secretion.[60] In vivo arginine has been shown to increase the thymic weight of uninjured rats and mice and minimizes the thymic weight involution that occurs with injury.[61] Additional data have shown that arginine increases the activity of existing T cells and that it can induce formation and maturation of T cells.[62]

In studies in humans, arginine given orally significantly increased peripheral blood lymphocyte blastogenesis in response to ConA and PHA. This change begins within 3 days of supplementation. This supplementation has also been studied in a clinical setting of patients receiving TPN with and without arginine. Those patients who received arginine showed an increased response of both PHA and ConA stimulation at days 3 and 7 after surgery compared to those patients who did not receive arginine.[63] The same author completed a study of patients with HIV and a Th/Ts (T-helper/T-suppressor cell) ratio of 0.8 or less (normal = 2). These patients received supplementation with 20 g of arginine daily for at least 2 weeks. There were no changes in the Th/Ts ratio, but there was a significant increase in mitogenic responses to ConA and PHA in the patients tested. Arginine has also been used postoperatively in surgical patients and has been shown to give an increased T-cell response to ConA and PHA and increased T-helper cell numbers. There was no change in other T-cell subsets.[64]

Cerra et al.[65] reported use of arginine, RNA precursors, purines, pyrimidines, and n-3 polyunsaturated fatty acids (PUFAs), a major component of the cell membrane, in a group of ICU patients. Use of these three agents in combination was associated with an improvement in the in vitro responses to ConA, PHA, and tetanus antigen. This study showed that nutritional supplementation must not only supply calories but must also supply elements that are essential to the improvement of immune parameters.[65]

There are several innovations in dietary treatments of the immunocompromised state. Babineau et al.[66] reported that PGG-glucan, a glucose polymer that stimulates and enhances humoral and cellular responses in infectious challenge, is useful in decreasing infections in high-risk surgical patients who received the high dose of the drug. At low drug dosage the number of patients who developed an infection was comparable between the placebo and the low-dose experimental group.[66]

Granulocyte-macrophage colony-stimulating factor (GM-CSF) has been shown to decrease infection in a mouse model. Mice were given a control diet or protein-free diet. Those animals receiving the protein-free diet either received GM-CSF or saline by subcutaneous injection. On day 7 both groups received *Candida albicans* by tail vein injection. Those animals who were given the protein-free diet and GM-CSF had survival rates comparable to control animals. These data show the importance of GM-CSF as an immunomodulatory agent in protein malnutrition.[67]

Trauma, Burns, and Surgery

Trauma and surgery. The importance of immune consequences during trauma, burns, or surgery is becoming better understood. Much of the data that have been discovered are now being used as a basis for intervention and treatment to prevent further morbidity after the traumatic event. These immune changes may occur secondary to blood transfusions, tissue injury, or the neuroendocrine changes that have occurred (Table 4-8).

Even in the individual who has undergone uncomplicated surgery, postoperative changes in the immune system include a depression of both T and B lymphocytes. There is also a decrease in the response to a number of agents that cause a blastogenic response, including PPD, *Staphylococcus aureus* and *Escherichia coli,* pokeweed mitogen, and PHA. Even with uncomplicated surgery there can be major depression in these blastogenic responses. The major change occurs on day 3 and returns to normal by day 9.[68]

In patients who were judged to have moderate-to-severe injuries, creatinine phosphokinase (CPD), cortisol, and white blood cell and T- and B-cell counts were performed. There were depressions in the total number of T and B lymphocytes and in the white blood cell by injury day 1, which returned to normal within approximately 5 days. During these changes in lymphocyte levels, the serum cortisol and CPK levels also increased markedly and returned to normal within 5 to 7 days.[69]

The realization that major trauma caused a change in immune status provided impetus to examine other measures of immune reactivity. Keane et al.[70] studied 31 injured patients and studied lymphocyte responsiveness for up to 20 days after injury, comparing patients who became septic with those who did not. When compared to normals the immune responses in traumatized patients were depressed for more than 20 days. In addition, the immune responses studied were significantly worse in the septic compared to the nonseptic patients. After injury, responses to streptokinase, streptodornase, mumps antigen, ConA, and PHA were depressed and did not return to normal levels even after 20 days. In addition, the mixed lymphocyte culture was also abnormally depressed. Those patients were severely injured as indicated by the number of units of blood required and by the number of organ systems injured. Blood transfusions may have contributed to the observed immune depression.[70]

Table 4-8. Effect of Illness, Injury, or Treatment on Host Defense Mechanisms

Condition	Local Immunity	T-Cell Function	B-Cell Function	Phagocytic Function	Complement
Primary immunodeficiencies	↓	↓	↓	↓	↓
Secondary (acquired) Immunodeficiencies					
Age	NC	↓	↓	NC	NC
Malnutrition	NC	↓	↑ or ↓	↓	↓
Malignancy	NC	↓	↓	NC	NC
Burns	↓	↓	↓	↓	↓
Infection	↓	↓	?	↓	?
Trauma or surgery	↓	↓	?	↓	?
Anesthesia	NC	↓	?	↓	?
Blood transfusion	NC	↓	?	?	?
Diabetes mellitus	↓	↓	?	↓	?
Renal failure	NC	↓	NC or ↓	↓	?
Liver disease	NC	↓	↓	?	?
Splenectomy	NC	NC	↓	↓	?
Radiation	↓	?	?	?	?
Protein-losing diseases	NC	↓	↓	NC	?
Foreign bodies	↓	NC	NC	NC	?
Drugs	NC	↓	↑ or ↓	↓	?

From Nohr C. Host defenses. In Meakins JL, ed. Surgical Infections: Diagnosis and Treatment. New York: Scientific American, 1994, p 25. Reprinted with permission.
NC, No change; ↑, increased; ↓, decreased, *?,* unknown.

Another study[71] reviewed cellular immune depression after multiple trauma in patients who did not become septic during their hospital course. Significant suppression of lymphocyte responses to mitogens was noted, and there was a reversal of the T-helper to T-suppressor cell ratio (normal 2.0:1 vs. patients at 0.96:1). Suppressor cell functional activity was also detected early after trauma. This suppressor cell activity decreased but persisted in three patients, who developed sepsis (one of whom died). These data indicate that lymphocyte abnormalities exist after major trauma and some of these depressions can be associated with ultimate sepsis.[71] This depression in cellular immunity is also reflected in antibody production in surgical patients. Nohr et al.[72] have shown that in vivo and in vitro antibody production are decreased in all surgical patients and are most depressed in those patients who have demonstrated reduced DTH responses.[72]

The studies outlined above have basically examined lymphocyte function. There are abnormalities in the PMNs in these seriously injured patients. Defects in the adherence and killing ability of PMNs have been reported along with migration abnormalities.[73-75] These latter patients showed marked depression of both serum and cell-mediated migration, which was proportional to the degree of trauma suffered.

The macrophage is a pivotal cell in the immune response—exerting both helper and suppressive effects—and may play a major role in the immunosuppressive effects of trauma. In one study, macrophage function was measured in a group of traumatized patients with a mean injury severity score (TSS) of 38 (25 to 40 gives approximately 50% mortality). The number of macrophages increased almost threefold from day 3 to day 14, and the number of T-helper cells markedly decreased. During this same period, the level of PGE_2 synthesis in vitro of isolated monocytes was also found to be highly elevated and in fact correlated with the level of injury reflected by the injury severity score. The level of IL-2 generated in an in vitro assay was also decreased, which would lead to decreased clonal expansion of T cells.[76] As discussed previously, monocytes and macrophages show markedly increased secretion of PGE_2 following injury and burns. In addition, PGE_2 can be shown to be secreted from suppressor cells following injury.[77]

Changes in the surface expression of MHC antigens on monocytes and T cells can be detected postoperatively. Since these molecules are critical for antigen presentation, their expression is central to the specific immune response an individual can mount to a unique antigen. Wakefield et al.[78] detected changes in MHC class II expression in a group of patients after surgery. HLA-DR expression on monocytes declined in all postoperative patients, with a more marked decline in those who developed sepsis. All postoperative patients had a marked increase in the number of T cells that expressed DR, with a larger increase in those patients who did not develop sepsis.[78] The exact mechanism of these changes is not known, but it appears that the patients who developed sepsis were unable to mount an appropriate immune response and had a major defect in antigen presentation and T-cell activation. INF-

γ production has been reported to be decreased after trauma, and it has been suggested that exogenous administration of INF-γ may be effective in reducing infection in traumatized patients. This effect may be related to effects on DR expression.[79] Other cytokines also appear to act by this mechanism; GM-CSF is known to increase the DR expression of monocytes and thus their antigen-presenting capacity.[80] It may be possible to predict the potential for infection in patients based on postoperative levels of DR expression on monocytes or T cells.

Polk et al.[81] have tested the hypothesis that increased MHC class II expression may make a difference in survival of patients after use of recombinant TNF-γ. In a randomized, prospective trial, the authors were able to show that those traumatized patients who received INF-γ for 10 days had an increased level of DR expression on their monocytes compared to those patients who received placebo only. Although there was no significant difference in mortality between the two groups of patients, there was a suggestion that the treated patients had a decreased mortality compared to those patients who received placebo only. There were also fewer severe infections in the treatment group that required reoperation or CT scan guided drainage. The authors believed that a larger trial or a longer treatment period would be useful to determine the utility of INF-γ in these patients.[81]

IL-4 and IL-10, two cytokines associated with the T2 lymphocyte subset, have also been implicated in the occurrence of sepsis after surgery. These cytokines are generally considered immunosuppressive. In a posthemorrhage mouse model, splenocytes and T cells showed increased levels of IL-10 release compared to macrophages. PGE_2 was shown to stimulate the release of IL-10, suggesting that IL-10 may be the ultimate effector of posttrauma PGE_2.[82] Mack et al.[83] have used a mouse model in which the animals received a femur fracture and hemorrhage to show that the cytokine pattern in splenocytes after injury was consistent with T2. This pattern may explain some of the changes in cellular immune response after injury.[83] IL-4 activity has been studied in a group of traumatized patients with an ISS greater than 25. Plasma IL-4 was found to be higher in those, who when admitted to the hospital, had greater severity of injury, younger age (30 years or younger), and hypotension. Those patients who had high levels of IL-4 on admission had a lower incidence of nosocomial infection compared to those patients with a lower IL-4 level. However, if the IL-4 increased during the ICU stay, the patients had a greater incidence of sepsis, pneumonia, or renal dysfunction, even if they had low IL-4 levels on admission. Whether IL-4 has a role in sepsis must be clarified.[84]

In studying the interrelationship between T1 and T2 cells in trauma and burns, O'Sullivan et al.[85] studied the occurrence of IL-2 and INF-γ (T1 cytokines) and IL-4 (T2 cytokine). After trauma (ISS >25) in human subjects, the authors showed a markedly decreased level of IL-2 when compared to normal control subjects. However, the production of IL-4 was markedly increased. The same pattern was observed in a murine burn model. When IL-12 was given to the burned animals after cecal puncture and ligation, a significant decrease in death from sepsis resulted. This study suggests that there may be a shift away from T1 cells toward T2 cells and this may result in an increased susceptibility to sepsis after trauma.[85]

Burns. Those patients who have undergone a severe burn injury also have major changes in immune status. In addition to nonspecific loss of the skin barrier, they have other immune defects. The total number of lymphocytes are reduced, as in severe nonburn trauma, and there is a decrease in the number of both T-helper cells and T-suppressor cells. Lymphocytes from severely burned patients exhibit decreased expression of HLA-DR and IL-2 receptor, both markers of T-cell activation. Serum from burned mice has been shown to inhibit lymphocyte proliferation and surface antigen expression in vitro. This may be due to PGE_2 effects. Patients who have experienced large burns can be shown to have increased PGE_2. This release may be in the range of 5 to 10 times normal and results in a concomitant suppression of the T-lymphocyte response. The lymphocyte response can be restored when PGE_2 synthesis is blocked.[86,87]

Burned patients have a decreased level of IL-2. This may provide a molecular explanation for the immunosuppression seen in burned patients. IL-2 plays a central role in immunoregulation supporting lymphocyte proliferation, increasing T-helper cell proliferation, and causing CTLs to differentiate into cytotoxic T cells.[88]

In conclusion, surgery and other trauma can result in marked changes in the immune system. These changes are being studied and defined, and various measures are being designed for intervention. It is hoped that these interventions will result in decreased morbidity and mortality.

Aging

Surgery in the aged patient is fraught with many physiologic concerns such as cardiac and pulmonary disease. The mortality rate increases with age after major surgery and after major trauma. In the aged patient, the natural barriers against infection are impaired. The skin becomes thinner, and there is a loss of Langerhans' cells. There is also a decrease in blood supply to the skin. There is loss of bacteriostatic effects of urine and decline of renal function, leading to less acidification of the urine and a propensity to urinary tract infection. The pulmonary tree is also compromised by decreased ventilation and decreased saliva.

Also immunologic changes occur with aging that influence the susceptibility to infection in these patients. A study by Charpentier et al.[89] found that when T-cell levels, PHA stimulation, and allogeneic responses were compared, there were no significant differences in T-cell function between young patients and those older than 70 years. However, if low levels of mitogens were used, lower levels of stimulation were observed in the older patients.[89] Age-related changes have also been detected in B-cell function. A Japanese group showed that there was a decrease in IgG antibody synthesis after tetanus toxic in aged patients.[90]

Most T and B cells decrease in number with age; however, the changes in NK cells are less straightforward. Some high-affinity NK cells actually increase with age in humans. This is in contrast to NK cells that are considered low affinity and are stable with increasing age.[91] The activity of NK cells in different compartments of the body may provide insights to the reason for increased neoplasms in the elderly. NK cells isolated from murine spleen and lymph nodes exhibited markedly decreased NK activity. This is in contrast to those NK cells isolated from human PBMCs, which showed normal activity. Thus, NK cells in solid organs that could prevent neoplastic formation may be lacking effective activity.[92]

Specific immune factors are also decreased during aging. As mentioned previously, there is an in vivo decrease of delayed hypersensitivity to common antigen skin tests. This decrease may also be due to decreased production of IL-2 by stimulated cells and therefore a decrease in the number of T-helper cells and T-suppressor cells. This decrease may be due to a decrease in the level of thymic hormones.[93] During the aging process, there are markedly decreased levels of natural antibodies and a decrease in the primary immune response to an antigen. It has been postulated that the immunosuppression of old age is due to the development of a greater sensitivity to PGE_2, which would cause increased activation of T-suppressor cells by PGE_2.[58]

These changes in delayed cellular immunity increase the individual's susceptibility to all infectious agents. This can result in an increase in colonization and frank infection and increased incidence of bacteremia, septicemia, and infections that are spread via the hematogenous route. Because of these changes, care must be taken to make certain the aged patient is as well physiologically as possible prior to elective surgery. Adequate nutrition is required. Underlying diseases must be controlled prior to any invasive procedures. Vaccinations also decrease morbidity and mortality in these patients.

Splenectomy, Hemophilia, and Blood Transfusion

Splenectomy. The incidence of overwhelming sepsis after splenectomy is increased compared to that of patients with an intact spleen. The important phagocytic and antibody production capabilities of the spleen are lost after splenectomy. The greatest risk for sepsis is to encapsulated organisms and appears to be the greatest within the early postsplenectomy period; however, this risk remains lifelong. In a study in adult patients who had either underlying malignancy or trauma as the reason for splenectomy, lethal sepsis occurred in 2.7% of adult patients approximately 2 years after splenectomy.[94] The highest risk was in those patients who had an underlying malignancy. A 1983 study[95] indicated the incidence of sepsis in patients who lost their spleen secondary to trauma was 2.5% at 2 years, but there were no fatalities. In this study, the most common organism involved was *Streptococcus pneumonia.* Splenectomy is also known to be associated with sepsis from gram negative rods, *Neisseria menigitidis, E. coli,* and *Haemophilus influenzae.* Less common problems include babesiosis, histoplasmosis, and malaria.

Splenectomy decreases a major protective mechanism in the body. Splenectomy in animals has been shown to decrease the removal of bacteria from the blood stream. The liver can remove organisms that are well opsonized, but the spleen can remove those organisms that are not well opsonized.[96] Since the spleen is a major site of antigen presentation to B cells, splenic removal of an organism not only removes the organism but also promotes an antibody response in which the spleen plays a pivotal role. The spleen is the first site in which antibody to an organism is detected after exposure to the offending agent. Consistent with this observation, splenectomy also causes IgM levels to decrease.

Strategies for prophylaxis include prophylactic antibiotics or starting prescribed antibiotics at the first sign of infection. Pneumococcal vaccine is ideally given to patients after splenectomy. Those patients who have had splenectomy for malignancy show a poor antibody response to the vaccine. Those who have had splenectomy for trauma apparently have a better response, but the response is less than that of normal control subjects in terms of absolute titer, relative rise, and rate of rise. Those patients who receive meningococcal and *H. influenzae* vaccine show similar titers to those who receive pneumococcal vaccine. Clearly patients subjected to splenectomy must be educated about the risks, have a supply of antibiotics, and be given the vaccines. Some physicians recommend repeating pneumococcal vaccination at 5- to 10-year intervals or in the face of a falling titer.

Hemophilia. Patients with hemophilia receive blood and factor VIII transfusions and thus are at high risk for HIV infection compared to the rest of the population. However, these patients experience a number of immunologic abnormalities that are not related to infection with HIV. The most common abnormality is a lowering of the CD4 count, a decrease in the CD8 count, and an overall lowering of the CD4:CD8 ratio. There is also decreased NK cell activity in HIV-negative patients with hemophilia.[97] Hypergammaglobulinemia is seen in patients who are HIV negative. There are increased numbers of activated B cells in these patients, which is evidence for continued stimulation of B cells.

In spite of these abnormalities in HIV-negative patients with hemophilia, there is little evidence for clinically significant immunosuppression. Infections were the cause of death in 3.3% of patients with hemophilia compared to 0.9% of patients without hemophilia. The incidence of cancer in these patients is approximately 25% of that in the general population.[98] In a report of wound infection rate after surgery, there were no significant differences between patients with hemophilia and the general population. There is one notable exception to these findings, namely a report from the United Kingdom in which 38% of boys with hemophilia developed active tuberculosis after exposure to a single patient with active tuberculosis. This is similar to the incidence of the disease in patients who are severely immunosuppressed. Patients who developed tuberculosis had a higher incidence of blood usage including factor VIII, factor IX, and cryoprecipitate.[99]

Blood transfusion and hemorrhage. Unfortunately, blood transfusions are given with little thought of the potential immunologic consequences. The obvious hazards of passing hepatitis B and C, HIV, and CMV are common concerns along with the hazards of transfusion reactions, but little thought is given to the other effects that blood may have on a given patient. Hemorrhage itself can have an effect on the immune response. Experimentally many changes have been documented in animal models. In a rat model of hemorrhage one can show that there is a marked decline in the mitogen-induced response of lymphocytes and a decrease in the production of IL-2, which is necessary for the differentiation of T cells into helper and cytotoxic cells. However, this response did return to normal within 48 hours after hemorrhage without resuscitation.[100] The serum from these animals depresses the mitogen response of lymphocytes from normal animals.

The preceding results were confirmed using a mouse model.[101] In addition, although there was no change in the relative numbers of T and B cells, there was still the depression of mitogen response of splenocytes. An additional murine study added resuscitation after the hemorrhage. This model also showed the same impairment in mitogenic responses, which were evident up to day 10, at which time they returned to normal. The production of IL-2 was also depressed during this time course.[101]

Additional studies confirmed the finding that murine splenocyte IL-2 was depressed after hemorrhage but also showed that IL-3, IL-6, and IFN-γ were depressed. The depression of IFN-γ might result in the marked decline of macrophage function, depression of NK cell function, and decreased activation of CTL.[102] The lack of IL-6 production may result in depressed humoral function because this cytokine is heavily involved in B-cell activation.[103] Humoral immunity can also be shown to be depressed after hemorrhage in a murine model.

The cause of nonspecific immune dysfunction after hemorrhage is unknown. There are data to indicate that this depression may be due to macrophage dysfunction. The macrophage is also key to antigen presentation in a shock state. In a murine model Stephan et al.[104] demonstrated that antigen presentation was markedly depressed in animals subjected to hemorrhage and then resuscitation 1 hour later. The length of this depression is at least 120 hours, with onset as early as 15 minutes, with a blood pressure of 35 mm Hg. Thus this change in antigen presentation in a murine model can be early and prolonged even in the face of adequate resuscitation. Additional studies using Kupffer's cells have shown similar findings.

The cause of the changes in immune function after hemorrhage are yet to be clearly elucidated. The agent which is most widely implicated is endotoxin, believed to come from the gastrointestinal tract. The poor oxygen and nutrient delivery during severe hemorrhage may also cause immune suppression. Hemorrhage is also a major stimulator of catecholamine release. Epinephrine has been shown in humans to result in altered mitogen-induced proliferation of lymphocytes and changes in the ratios of different subsets of lymphocytes.[105] Catecholamines can also suppress phagocyte function and B-cell function.[106] These changes may be addressed by various specific pharmacologic interventions.

Hemorrhage plus injury has an additive detrimental effect on immune function. Wichmann et al.[107] have shown in a murine model that hemorrhage caused a depression in splenic and macrophage function; however, the addition of a femur fracture caused an even deeper depression in these parameters. Thus traumatized patients may be experiencing an immune depression secondary to both the blood loss and shock, as well as to the injury.[107]

Blood transfusions are believed to have some deleterious effects on the immune system in those patients who have cancer. These changes have been studied in a number of types of cancer. In those patients with colorectal cancer, cancer recurrence was increased in those patients who received blood. The results of this retrospective study took into account the complexity of the surgery.[108] Foster et al.[109] confirmed these findings showing that those patients who did not receive any blood during their hospitalization did significantly better than those who received blood transfusions.

In evaluating those patients who underwent surgery for lung cancer, similar findings have been discovered. Hyman et al.[110] reported that a group of patients who underwent transfusion in conjunction with resection for non–small cell carcinoma of the lung showed a significantly worse 5-year survival rate than those patients who underwent resection without transfusion. The same sort of association between blood transfusion and long-term survival has been identified for patients suffering from soft tissue sarcomas. Those patients who received blood transfusions had a 20% decrease in 5-year survival.[111]

The three major cancer groups just examined are in contrast to breast cancer, renal cell carcinoma, and head and neck cancers. Patients who had invasive breast cancer and either a total or partial mastectomy showed no effect of blood transfusion on long-term survival.[112] Likewise, no effects of blood transfusion on long-term survival can be found in those patients with renal cell carcinoma and those with head and neck cancer.[113,114] Why blood causes decreased survival in patients with certain types of cancer is unknown.

The mechanism for the selective immunosuppressive effect with blood transfusion is still unknown. This immunosuppressive effect is clearly seen in those patients who have received a kidney transplantation. Early in the history of transplantation, blood transfusions to the recipient were largely avoided; however, in 1973 Opelz et al.[115]

reported a beneficial effect of transfusions on graft survival. The major reason for this effect was believed to be the immunosuppressive action of blood.[115] This finding could not be replicated in those patients who received frozen packed red blood cells. Fischer et al.[116] showed that transfusion with 1 to 3 U of blood caused suppression of cellular immunity defined by a mixed lymphocyte response. When they compared the effects to autologous units, there was no depression in cellular immunity.[116] One of the theories put forth to explain this finding was that suppressor cells might be activated. This theory was confirmed when Smith et al.[117] found that patients who had received hemodialysis and blood transfusions had evidence of T-suppressor cell activity. These changes were found to last approximately 5 months.

Matsumoto et al.[118] studied MLR in patients who had undergone donor-specific transfusions while being readied for transplantation. They found both suppressor cells and antibodies, which they thought were anti-idiotypic antibodies. This latter finding was confirmed by Singal et al.,[119] who showed that sera from transfused patients resulted in depression of MLR whereas sera from nontransfused patients did not give the same depression. Animal studies suggested that PGE_2 may be a mediator of these changes.[120]

The effects of blood transfusion in patients is still being investigated; however, there is no doubt that it has a major influence in the immune system. Some of these immunosuppressive effects may be desirable, as in the case of transplantation, in which transfusion improves graft survival. Transfusion and hemorrhage may be undesirable, as in the case of patients with certain types of cancer. The use of transfusion is always worth careful evaluation in the individual patient.

Renal Failure

Infections are common in patients with renal failure and are a major cause of death in patients with end-stage renal disease. One would expect major changes in the immune system of these patients; in fact, patients with end-stage renal disease show defects in specific and nonspecific immunity. Cellular immunity is markedly abnormal in these patients. Damin et al.[121] found that skin graft survival was prolonged in uremic patients. This clinical finding has been confirmed in various ways by showing that these patients also have a markedly decreased response to cutaneous injection of various antigens.[122,123] Hepatitis B vaccination in chronic renal failure patients receiving dialysis treatment resulted in a very low rate of seroconversion after vaccination compared to the general population.[124] This was in the face of the normal levels of immunoglobulin in the patient receiving dialysis treatment. Lymphocyte counts have been shown to be decreased in these patients; however, the CD4:CD8 ratios are reported to be normal.[125] The above findings of Damin et al.[121] have been confirmed using in vitro studies that show that uremic patients have impaired responses to mitogens and allogeneic lymphocytes. Since these findings are marked in the presence of uremic serum, there may be a soluble factor that causes this depression.[126] Because these changes were seen in patients receiving dialysis treatment, the substance is not dialyzable. There were indications that the TCR/CD3 antigen complex in the uremic patient may be downregulated. This finding may be due to a combination of uremia, hyperparathyroidism, and dialysis itself.[127]

B cells and NK cells are also affected in uremia. Uremic patients show normal to supranormal levels of IgG and IgM. The actual mechanism for this finding is not well delineated.[128] There is recent evidence that monocytes may be defective in uremic patients.[129] This defect also influences how the monocytes present antigens. Thus the defects that are seen may be a combination of both T-cell and APC deficiencies.

The disturbances just outlined undoubtedly have an influence on the decreased ability of these patients to handle both bacterial and viral infectious challenges. Vigilance for infection is necessary in these patients. This concern is heightened for the large number of dialysis patients who are diabetic. Patients who are diabetic and receiving dialysis treatment appear to be at an especially high risk for developing infections.

Diabetes Mellitus

Although most of the deaths in patients with diabetes mellitus can be attributed to cardiovascular disease, infection is a major cause of morbidity and at times also death. Early studies indicated that patients with diabetes had a greater number of infections than did control subjects. For example, one early study reported a 2.4% incidence of limb infection in diabetic patients compared to 0.5% in nondiabetic subjects.[130] In addition, those patients with diabetes for longer than 20 years were found to have a prevalence of bacteriuria (19% compared to 8% in control subjects).[131] Most clinicians agree that diabetic patients have more severe infections and a more protracted clinical course than nondiabetic individuals. The World Health Organization classifies diabetes as a secondary immunodeficiency disease.

The ability of patients to fight infection can be shown to be altered in diabetic individuals. Polymorphonuclear granulocytes have several functional abnormalities. These cells can be shown to have decreased migration characteristics, especially in those patients with poorly controlled serum glucose levels.[132] Phagocytosis is defective in diabetic persons, especially when the glucose level is elevated.[133] However, following normalization of glucose levels, these abnormalities disappear.

Lymphocyte subsets can be altered in diabetic individuals. A study of persons with type 1 diabetes reported a decrease in circulating CD4 cells, which results in a decrease of the CD4:CD8 ratio.[134] This change may be due to decreased levels of insulin or decreased insulin activity. As was found with neutrophil function, normalization of insulin levels results in normal lymphocyte transformation on stimulation, as well as normalization of lymphocyte levels.[135] However, the report that approximately 50% of the diabetic patients who received hepatitis B vaccine responded poorly indicates that there may be additional immunosuppressive factors operative in these patients. Specific infections can be more fatal in diabetic patients compared to normal patients. Patients who have a well-controlled glucose level do not have a higher susceptibility to *Staphylococcus* infections. However, in older patients the risk of bacteremia is higher. Those patients who are diabetic and develop bacteremia have a higher mortality rate than those without diabetes.[136] *Candida* infections are more prevalent in diabetic patients compared to the normal population and are particularly more common in those patients whose glucose levels are poorly controlled. However, this was not the case with other fungal infections.[137] The treatment of fungal and bacterial infections requires the initiation of good glucose control and appropriate antibiotic or antifungal therapy.

Major factors that lead to increased infections in diabetic patients in addition to poor glucose control include underlying vascular disease and nerve damage. Poor blood supply results in inadequate oxygen, which leads to anaerobic infection and also limits host defense mechanisms. If a patient has a peripheral neuropathy, the result can be an ulcer, which can become secondarily infected.

The key to prevention of infection in the diabetic patient includes control of hyperglycemia; if one reduces the glucose to normal levels, the incidence of infections decreases. Complications that lead to increased levels of insulin must be avoided. One must also aggressively look for infection and treat those conditions that can result in infection becoming widespread or locally uncontrollable.

Prevention and Therapy

Clinical Guidelines

Prevention of infection in the immunocompromised patient calls for an awareness of the possible infections these patients can develop and an approach to deal with the problem. One must also be aware that patients with certain immune defects can develop cancer. When these patients are examined, one must check for the presence of lymph nodes and also carefully examine the skin to look for suspicious lesions.

The risk of infection in these patients is dependent on both the immunosuppressive status of the patient and environmental factors. The amount of immunosuppression is dependent on the level of nutrition, the state of the various portions of the immune system, defects in the skin or mucous membranes, and any invasive lines or procedures that have been undertaken. The importance of environmental factors is illustrated by the realization that one can infect even an immunocompetent patient if he or she comes in contact with a large enough inoculum of an infectious agent. Thus a patient who is immunosuppressed can become infected with a proportionately smaller number of infectious agents, depending on the patient's overall immune status.

In caring for these patients one must apply the principles outlined in the accompanying box. Hand washing is particularly critical in these patients. This will prevent patient to patient transmission of infection. Deep lines such as subclavian and internal jugular lines and Swan-Ganz catheters must be watched particularly carefully. In immunosuppressed patients there is no evidence of infection; therefore changing lines or making sure they are absolutely necessary is imperative. Nutritional support bolsters the immune system and prevents a catabolic state in the immunocompromised patient. One must also be certain that the integument is intact and that the skin does not become a site for entrance of bacteria.

Immunocompromised patients can develop infections in a number of places. These infections can include skin, respiratory, gastrointestinal, or central nervous system. Sus-

PRINCIPLES OF INFECTION PREVENTION IN THE COMPROMISED HOST

- Reduce acquisition of ambient organisms from hospital environment
  - Avoid hospitalization
  - Segregate patients with potentially communicable diseases
  - Avoid overcrowding in wards and intensive care units
  - Enforce strict hygiene, particularly hand washing, among physicians, nurses, and aides
- Avoid invasive procedures whenever possible
  - Employ indwelling intravenous and urinary catheters only if absolutely necessary
  - Change scalp vein needles, tubing, and intravenous bottles daily
  - Use respiratory assistance devices, particularly those requiring intubation, with great care and with close monitoring to ensure that they are adequately decontaminated
- Reduce number of colonizing organisms
  - Remove or reduce sites of prior infection
  - Consider the use of isoniazid prophylaxis in patients with histories, positive skin tests, or chest x-ray findings of old tuberculosis
  - Closely monitor serologic tests and clinical course in patients with evidence of old coccidioidomycosis or histoplasmosis who have now become immunosuppressed
- Bolster host defense mechanisms
  - Successfully treat the underlying disease
  - Prescribe adequate nutrition and exercise
  - Improve respiratory toilet
  - Control diabetes mellitus, congestive heart failure, or respiratory insufficiency
  - Reduce local obstruction caused by tumor
  - Protect the integrity of oral and anorectal mucosae
  - When appropriate, prescribe immunotherapy with vaccines and/or immunoglobulin preparation

From Rubin RH, Cosimi AB. In Infections in the immunocompromised host. In Howard RJ, Simmons RL, eds., Surgical Infectious Diseases. Norwalk, Conn.: Appleton & Lange, 1995, p 1311. Reprinted with permission.

picious skin lesions should be tested by biopsy, aspiration, or culture.

The neutropenic patient who develops a fever requires careful evaluation. Approximately 40% of patients who are neutropenic and develop a fever have a documented infection.[138] Only 20% of fevers in these patients are due to the underlying disease or to other noninfectious causes. The remaining 40% are due to possible but nonproven infections.

The classic signs of infection in these patients frequently are missing. They do not exhibit fluctuance, calor, rubor, or lymphadenopathy as commonly as in patients with normal neutrophil count. The physical examination should focus on skin, mucosa, and perianal areas. The therapy early on should include broad-spectrum antibiotics after adequate cultures have been obtained. The optimal drug choice is still debated. Antibiotics are useful in these patients, but other methods of stimulating the immune response are being sought.

Biologic Response Modifiers

Biologic response modifiers (BRMs) are being explored in hopes of increasing the activity of specific groups of cells in the body. BRMs include cytokines, colony-stimulating factors, interferons, and tumor necrosis factors. Most were named based on a primary property, but these agents have a large amount of overlap in their individual effects and have many diverse effects.

IL-1 is a product of monocytes and has a myriad of effects. These include activation of T, B, and NK cells, activation of vascular endothelium, fibroblast proliferation, and activity against human tumors. It has also been shown to have anti-infective properties and to offer protection against IL-2 toxicity. In mice it has been shown to be protective in bacterial infections.[139] IL-1 has also been used in patients with cancers and has been shown to increase the white blood cell count and the cellularity in bone marrow but does not carry the risk of inducing major hypotension after use.[140] IL-2 is produced primarily by T1 cells. Treatment of NK cells with IL-2 results in their differentiation into LAK cells, which appear to home to the site of viral infection. Because of these promising results, IL-2 was the first BRM used in clinical trials. The cytokine has been shown to be effective in a number of animal models, yet its use in clinical trials has been disappointing. Surprisingly, its use in patients with AIDS was shown to decrease some immune functions such as that of NK cells. Because of its general effectiveness in increasing the activity of NK cells, IL-2 is still used in patients with cancer. It is used at the maximal tolerated dose with the major side effects being cardiovascular.

CSFs are commonly used in cancer chemotherapy. The major interest in these agents is because they can reverse the severe neutropenia after chemotherapy that can lead to severe bacterial infections. Granulocyte colony-stimulating factor (G-CSF) is produced by a number of cells in the body including endothelial cells, fibroblasts, and macrophages. The agent has been used in cancer chemotherapy to prevent the periods of severe neutropenia associated with such management.[141] This CSF has minimal toxicities which include mild bone pain and cellulitis at the injection site. G-CSF is not useful in patients who have an established infection but is only useful in preventing the neutropenia associated with cancer chemotherapy.[142]

GM-CSF has an effect on both stem cells and megakaryocytes. It, like G-CSF, is produced by endothelial cells, fibroblasts, and T lymphocytes. It has been used in patients with aplastic anemia and those who have undergone bone marrow transplantation. It has also found clinical application in patients with acute and chronic leukemia, Hodgkin's and non-Hodgkin's lymphomas, and treatment-related cytopenias from chemotherapy in solid tumors.[143,144] It has also been used in AIDS-related neutropenia.[145] The functional capabilities of the induced cells are normal. The therapy results in increased numbers of leukocytes in peripheral blood. The toxicity is mild when used in small doses; however, there is marked toxicity in large doses including fever, capillary leak syndrome, and pericarditis.

The interferons were among the first BRMs discovered to have clinical application. INF-α has shown clinical use in hairy cell leukemia, condyloma acuminatum, and AIDS-associated Kaposi's sarcoma.[146-148] The side effects are primarily a flulike syndrome including fever, headache, nausea, and vomiting. In most patients these symptoms abate, and therapy is not limited. INF-γ is important in macrophage activation and B- and T-cell responses.[149,150] INF-α has been used to treat hepatitis B. INF-α has been shown to give a seroconversion rate of approximately 25% to 40%.[151] Hepatitis C has been especially prominent in the patients requiring dialysis and is associated with a chronic carrier state. Treatment with INF-α for approximately 6 months has been shown to give a response rate of approximately 50%, but about half of those who respond relapse.[152]

The last group of BRMs to be discussed are tumor necrosis factors. This group of agents was discovered when it was shown that certain bacterial products could reduce the size of tumors.[153] TNF-α is released by macrophages. It has many biologic effects including proliferation of T cells and NK cells, adherence of neutrophils to endothelium, increased cytolytic activity of T cells and NK cells, and stimulation of other BRMs such as IL-1 and IL-6. It has been proved useful in hairy cell leukemia and in Kaposi's sarcoma.[146,154] During clinical use the side effects of TNF-α are quite mild including fever, headache, nausea, and vomiting. TNF-β carries some similarity to TNF-α and is produced by T, B, and NK cells. It causes the biologic response to microbial infections. The agent has been used in an attempt to improve outcomes in infection in an animal model.[155] Antibodies to TNF have been used in septic patients; however, there was no survival benefit noted in this group of patients.[156]

The use of these agents in the treatment of human disease is still being explored. The importance of these agents is now being realized, as is the complexity of their interactions. Much additional work must be completed before their potential for therapy can be realized.

SUMMARY

The causes of immunosuppression in surgical patients have been outlined. These include malnutrition, trauma, burns, surgery, aging, splenectomy, hemophilia, blood transfusions, sepsis, renal failure, diabetes mellitus, and cancer. Each of these causes can be evaluated and the individual problem corrected if possible. The individual patient with severe neutropenia must be evaluated very carefully and steps taken to prevent infection. The place of BRMs has been defined in neutropenia in certain disease states but additional uses still are to be defined.

ACKNOWLEDGMENTS

The authors wish to acknowledge Mr. Dorian Araneda for his preparation of Figs. 4-1 and 4-4.

REFERENCES

1. Paul WE, ed. Fundamental Immunology, 3rd ed. New York: Raven Press, 1993, p 1497.
2. Kuby J. Immunology, 3rd ed. New York: WH Freeman, 1997, p 660.
3. Janeway C, Travers P. Immunobiology: The Immune System in Health and Disease, 3rd ed. New York: Garland Publishers, 1997.
4. Abbas AK, Lichtman AH, Pober JS. Cellular and Molecular Immunology. 3rd ed. Philadelphia: WB Saunders, 1997.
5. Kishimoto T, et al., eds. Leucocyte Typing VI: White Cell Differentiation Antigens. New York: Garland Publishers, 1997.
6. Pleiman CM, D'Ambrosio D, Cambier JC. The B-cell antigen receptor complex: Structure and signal transduction. Immunol Today 15:393, 1994.
7. Chen J, Alt FW. Gene rearrangement and B-cell development. Curr Opin Immunol 5:194, 1993.
8. Mondino A, Khoruts A, Jenkins MK. The anatomy of T-cell activation and tolerance. Proc Natl Acad Sci USA 93:2245, 1996.
9. Cantrell D. T cell antigen receptor signal transduction pathways. Annu Rev Immunol 14:259, 1996.
10. Romagnani S. Lymphokine production by human T cells in disease states. Annu Rev Immunol 12:227, 1994.
11. Lowin B, Peitsch MC, Tschopp J. Perforin and granzymes: Crucial effector molecules in cytolytic T lymphocyte and natural killer cell–mediated cytotoxicity. Curr Top Microbiol Immunol 198:1, 1995.
12. Parham P, ed. NK cells, MHC class I antigens and missing self. Immunol Rev 155:221, 1997.
13. Tapper H. The secretion of preformed granules by macrophages and neutrophils. J Leukocyte Biol 59:613, 1996.
14. van Rooijen N, Wijburg OL, van den Dobbelsteen GP, Sanders A. Macrophages in host defense mechanisms. Curr Top Microbiol Immunol 210:159, 1996.
15. Nourshargh S, Williams TJ. Molecular and cellular interactions mediating granulocyte accumulation in vivo. Semin Cell Biol 6:316, 1995.
16. Banchereau J, et al. The CD40 antigen and its ligand. Annu Rev Immunol 12:881, 1994.
17. Ward SG. CD28: A signalling perspective. Biochem J 318:361, 1996.
18. Grewal IS, Flavell RA. A central role of CD40 ligand in the regulation of $CD4^+$ T-cell responses. Immunol Today 17:410, 1996.
19. Durie FH, et al. The role of CD40 in the regulation of humoral and cell-mediated immunity. Immunol Today 15:406, 1994.
20. Mond JJ, Lees A. Snapper CM. T cell–independent antigens type 2. Annu Rev Immunol 13:655, 1995.
21. Morgan BP. Physiology and pathophysiology of complement: Progress and trends. Crit Rev Clin Lab Sci 32:265, 1995.
22. van de Winkle JP, Capel PJ. Human IgG Fc receptor heterogeneity: Molecular aspects and clinical implications. Immunol Today 14:215, 1993.
23. Oppenheim JJ. Forward. In Thomson A, ed. The Cytokine Handbook, 2nd ed. San Diego, Calif.: Academic Press, 1994, p xvii.
24. Kazatchkine MD. Interleukin 16 (IL-16). Bull WHO 74:451, 1996.
25. Thomson A, ed. The Cytokine Handbook, 2nd ed. San Diego, Calif.: Academic Press, 1994, p 615.
26. Aggarwal BB, Puri RK, eds. Human Cytokines: Their Role in Disease and Therapy. Cambridge, Mass.: Blackwell Science, 1995, p 736.
27. Westermann J, Pabst R. Distribution of lymphocyte subsets and natural killer cells in the human body. Clinical Investigator 70:539, 1992.
28. Cheadle WG. The human leukocyte antigens and their relationship to infection. Am J Surg 165:75S, 1993.
29. Ahmed AE, Peter JB. Clinical utility of complement assessment. Clin Diag Lab Immunol 2:509, 1995.
30. Patarca R, et al. Assessment of immune mediator expression levels in biological fluids and cells: A critical appraisal. Crit Rev Oncog 6:117, 1995.
31. Heaney ML, Golde DW. Soluble cytokine receptors. Blood 87:847, 1996.
32. Christou NV, et al. The delayed hypersensitivity response and host resistance in surgical patients: 20 years later. Ann Surg 222:534, 1995.
33. Scientific Group on Immunodeficiency. Primary immunodeficiency diseases. Immunodeficiency Rev 1:173, 1989.
34. Kersey JH, et al. Lymphoma after thymus transplantation [letter to the editor]. N Engl J Med 302:301, 1980.
35. Den Gartog G, et al. Decreased gastrin secretion in patients with late onset hypogammaglobulinemia. N Engl J Med 318:1563, 1988.
36. Perry GS III, et al. The Wiskott-Aldrich syndrome in the United States and Canada (1892-1979). J Pediatr 97:72, 1980.
37. Fasth A. Primary immunodeficiency disorders in Sweden: Cases among children 1974-1979. J Clin Immunol 2:86, 1982.
38. Hoover R, Fraumeni JF Jr. Risk of cancer in renal transplant recipients. Lancet 3:55, 1973.
39. Brumbaugh J, Baldwin JC, Stinson EB. Quantitative analysis of immunosuppression in cyclosporin-treated heart transplant patients with lymphoma. J Heart Transplant 4:307, 1985.
40. Penn I. The changing patterns of posttransplant malignancies. Transplant Proc 23:1101, 1993.
41. Penn I. Why do immunosuppressed patients develop cancer? Crit Rev Oncog 1:27, 1989.
42. Nalasnik MA, Makowka L, Starzl TE. The diagnosis and treatment of post-transplant lymphoproliferative disorders. Curr Probl Surg 25:371, 1988.
43. Penn I. Depressed immunity and the development of cancer. Cancer Detect Prev 18:241, 1994.
44. Filipovich AH, et al. Lymphomas in persons with naturally occurring immunodeficiency disorders. In McGrath IT, O'Conor GR, Ramot B, eds. Pathogenesis of Leukemias and Lymphomas: Environmental Influences. New York: Raven Press, 1984, p 225.
45. Gershwin ME, Beach RS, Hurley LS. Nutrition and immunity. New York: Academic Press, 1985.
46. Nohr CW, et al. Malnutrition and humoral immunity: Short-term acute nutritional deprivation. Surgery 98:769, 1985.
47. West KP Jr, Howard GR, Sommer A. Vitamin A and infection: Public health implications. Annu Rev Nutr 9:63, 1989.
48. Stiehm ER. Humoral immunity in malnutrition. Fed Proc 39:3093, 1980.

49. Keusch GT, et al. Impairment of hemolytic complement activation by both classical and alternative pathways in serum from patients with kwashiorkor. J Pediatr 105:434, 1984.
50. Keusch GT. Nutrition and infection. Curr Clin Top Infect Dis 5:106, 1984.
51. Moore FA, et al. TEN vs TPN following major abdominal trauma: Reduced septic morbidity. J Trauma 29:916, 1989.
52. Kudsk KA, et al. Enteral vs parenteral feeding: Effects on septic morbidity following blunt and penetrating abdominal trauma. Ann Surg 215:503, 1992.
53. Rapp RP, et al. The favorable effect of early parenteral feeding on survival in head-injured patients. J Neurosurg 58:906, 1983.
54. Cohen BE, et al. Reversal of postoperative immunosuppression in man by vitamin A. Surg Gynecol Obstet 149:658, 1979.
55. Meydani SN, et al. Fish oil and tocopherol-induced changes in natural killer cell mediated cytotoxicity and PGE_2 synthesis in young and old mice. J Nutr 118:1245, 1988.
56. Mead CJ, Mertin J. Fatty acid and immunity. Adv Lipid Res 16:127, 1988.
57. Lands WEM. Essential fatty acids revisited. Nutr Rev 44:189, 1986.
58. Goodwin JS. Prostaglandins and immunity. Boston, Mass: Martinus Nijhoff Publishing, 1985.
59. Seifter E, et al. Arginine: An essential amino acid for injured rats. Surgery 84:224, 1978.
60. Merimee TJ, Tabinowitz D, Riggs L. Plasma growth hormone after arginine infusion: Clinical experiences. N Engl J Med 276:434, 1967.
61. Barbul A, et al. Arginine: Thymotropic and wound healing promoting agent. Surg Forum 29:101, 1977.
62. Barbul A, Efron JE, Shawe T. Arginine increases the number of T-lymphocytes in nude mice [abstract 14]. JPEN 13:7S, 1989.
63. Barbul A. Arginine and immune function. Nutrition 6:53, 1990.
64. Daly JM, et al. Effect of dietary protein and amino acids on immune function. Crit Care Med 18:S86, 1990.
65. Cerra FB, et al. Effect of enteral nutrient on in vitro tests of immune function in ICU patients: A preliminary report. Nutrition 6:84, 1990.
66. Babineau TJ, et al. A phase II multicenter, double-blind, randomized, placebo-controlled study of three dosages of an immunomodulator (PGG-glucan) in high-risk surgical patients. Arch Surg 129:1204, 1994.
67. Hill ADK, et al. Antimicrobial effects of granulocyte-macrophage colony-stimulating factor in protein-energy malnutrition. Arch Surg 130:1273, 1995.
68. Kehlet H, et al. Postoperative depression of lymphocyte transformation response to microbial antigens. Br J Surg 64:890, 1977.
69. Bauer AR, et al. The depression of T lymphocytes after trauma. Am J Surg 136:674, 1978.
70. Keane RM, et al. Prediction of sepsis in the multitraumatic patient by assays of lymphocyte responsiveness. SG&O 156:163, 1983.
71. O'Mahony JB, et al. Depression of cellular immunity after multiple trauma in the absence of sepsis. J Trauma 24:869, 1984.
72. Nohr CW, et al. In vivo and in vitro humoral immunity in surgical patients. Ann Surg 200: 373, 1984.
73. Alexander JW, Hegg M, Altemeier WA. Neutrophil function in selected surgical disorders. Ann Surg 168:447, 1968.
74. Christou NV, Meakins JL. Neutrophil function in surgical patients: Two inhibitors of granulocyte chemotaxis associated with sepsis. J Surg Res 26:355, 1979.
75. Maderazo EG, et al. Polymorphonuclear leukocyte migration abnormalities and their significance in seriously traumatized patients. Ann Surg 198:736, 1983.
76. Faist E, et al. Alteration of monocyte function following major injury. Arch Surg 123:287, 1988.
77. Miller-Graziano C, et al. Mechanisms of altered monocyte PGE_1 production in severely injured patients. Arch Surg 123:293, 1988.
78. Wakefield CH, et al. Changes in major histocompatibility complex class II expression in monocytes and T cells of patients developing infection after surgery. Br J Surg 80:205, 1993.
79. Hershman MJ, et al. Interferon-gamma treatment increases HLA-DR expression on monocytes in severely injured patients. Clin Exp Immunol 77:67, 1989.
80. Morrissey PH, et al. Granulocyte-macrophage colony-stimulating factor augments the primary antibody response by enhancing the function of antigen-presenting cells. J Immunol 137:1113, 1987.
81. Polk HC Jr, et al. A randomized prospective clinical trial to determine the efficacy of interferon-gamma in severely injured patients. Am J Surg 163:191, 1992.
82. Ayala A, et al. Mechanism of enhanced susceptibility to sepsis following hemorrhage: Interleukin-10 suppression of T-cell response is mediated by eicosanoid-induced interleukin-4 release. Arch Surg 129:1172, 1994.
83. Mack VE, et al. Dominance of T-helper 2-type cytokines after severe injury. Arch Surg 131:1303, 1996.
84. DiPiro JT, et al. Association of interleukin-4 plasma levels with traumatic injury and clinical course. Arch Surg 130:1159, 1995.
85. O'Sullivan ST, et al. Major injury leads to predominance of the T helper-2 lymphocyte phenotype and diminished interleukin-12 production associated with decreased resistance to infection. Ann Surg 222:482, 1995.
86. Ninnemann JL, Stockland AE. Participation of PGE_2 in immunosuppression following thermal injury. J Trauma 24:201, 1984.
87. Freeman TR, Shelby J. Effects of anti-PGE antibody on cell mediated immune response in thermally injured mice. J Trauma 28:190, 1988.
88. Horgan AF, et al. Altered gene transcription after burn injury results in depressed T-lymphocyte activation. Ann Surg 220:342, 1994.
89. Charpentier B, et al. Immunological studies in human aging. I. In vitro functions of T cells and polymorphs. J Clin Lab Immunol 5:87, 1981.
90. Kishimoto S, et al. Age-related decline in the in vitro and in vivo synthesis of anti-tetanus toxoid antibody in humans. J Immunol 125:2347, 1980.
91. Franceschi C, et al. The immunology of exceptional individuals: The lesson of centenarians. Immunol Today 16:12, 1995.
92. Miller R. The aging immune system: Primer and prospectus. Science 273:70, 1996.
93. Leary J, Hallgren H. Aging and lymphocyte function: A model for testing gerontologic hypothesis of aging in man. Arch Gerontol Geriatr 112:199, 1991.
94. O'Neal BJ, McDonald JC. The risk of sepsis in the asplenic adult. Ann Surg 194:775, 1981.
95. Sekikawa T, Shatney CH. Septic sequelae after splenectomy for trauma in adults. Am J Surg 143:545, 1983.
96. Bohnsack JF, Brown EJ. The role of the spleen in resistance to infection. Ann Rev Med 37:49, 1986.
97. Matheson DS, et al. Natural killer cell activity from hemophiliacs exhibits differential response to various forms of interferon. Blood 67:164, 1986.
98. Aronson DL. Cause of death in hemophilia A patients in the United States from 1968 to 1979. Am J Hematol 27:7, 1988.
99. Beddal AC, et al. Unusually high incidence of tuberculosis among boys with hemophilia during an outbreak of the disease in hospital. J Clin Pathol 38:1163, 1985.
100. Abraham E, Chang YH. Cellular and humoral bases of hemorrhage-induced depression of lymphocyte function. Crit Care Med 14:81, 1986.
101. Stephan RN, et al. Hemorrhage without tissue trauma produces immunosuppression and enhances susceptibility to sepsis. Arch Surg 122:62, 1987.
102. Vilcek J, et al. Structure and function of human interferon-gamma. In Ford RJ, Maizel AL, eds. Mediators in Cell Growth and Differentiation. New York: Raven Press, 1985, p 299.

103. Meldrum DR, et al. Diltiazem restores IL-2, IL-3, IL-6, and IFN gamma synthesis and decreases host susceptibility to sepsis following hemorrhage. J Surg Res 51:158, 1991.
104. Stephan RN, et al. Mechanism of immunosuppression following hemorrhage: Defective antigen presentation by macrophages. J Surg Res 46:553, 1989.
105. Crary B, et al. Decrease in mitogen responsiveness of mononuclear cells from peripheral blood after epinephrine administration in humans. J Immunol 130:694, 1983.
106. Abrass CK, et al. Characterization of the beta-adrenergic receptor of the rat peritoneal macrophage. J Immunol 135:1338, 1985.
107. Wichmann MW, et al. Immune function is more compromised after closed bone fracture and hemorrhage shock than hemorrhage alone. Arch Surg 131:995, 1996.
108. Agarwal M, Blumberg N. Colon cancer patients transfused perioperatively have an increased incidence of recurrence. Transfusion 23(Suppl 56):421, 1983.
109. Foster RS Jr, et al. Adverse relationship between blood transfusions and survival after colectomy for colon cancer. Cancer 55:1195, 1985.
110. Hyman NH, et al. Blood transfusions and survival after lung cancer resection. Am J Surg 149:502, 1985.
111. Rosenberg SA, et al. Perioperative blood transfusions are associated with increased rates of recurrence and decreased survival in patients with high-grade soft tissue sarcomas of the extremities. J Clin Oncol 3:698, 1985.
112. Foster RS Jr, Foster JC, Costanza MC. Blood transfusions and survival after surgery for breast cancer. Arch Surg 119:1138, 1984.
113. Desmyter J, Reyndes M, Goubau P. Renal cell carcinoma: Blood transfusion and survival. Br Med J 293:537, 1986.
114. Johnson JT, Taylor FH, Thearle PB. Blood transfusion and outcome in stage III head and neck carcinoma. Ann Otolaryngol Head Neck Surg 113:307, 1987.
115. Opelz G, et al. Effect of blood transfusions on subsequent kidney transplants. Transplant Proc 5:253, 1973.
116. Fischer E, et al. Blood transfusion induced suppression of cellular immunity in man. Hum Immunol 1:187, 1980.
117. Smith MD, et al. The effect of blood transfusion on T-suppressor cells in renal dialysis patients. Transplant Proc 13:181, 1981.
118. Matsumoto T, Sakagami K, Orita K. Role of donor specific blood transfusions in prolongation of kidney graft survival. Transplant Proc 19:2264, 1983.
119. Singal DO, Fagnilli L, Joseph S. Blood transfusions induce anti-idiotypic antibodies in renal transplant patients. Transplant Proc 15:1005, 1983.
120. Waymack JP, et al. Effect of blood transfusions on macrophage-lymphocyte interaction in an animal model. Ann Surg 204:681, 1986.
121. Damin GJ, Couch NP, Murray JE. Prolonged survival skin homografts in uremic patients. Ann NY Acad Sci 64:967, 1957.
122. Boulton-Jones JM, et al. Immune responses in uremia. Clin Nephrol 1:351, 1973.
123. Selroos O, Pasternack A, Virolainen M. Skin test sensitivity and antigen-induced lymphocyte transformation in uremia. Clin Exp Immunol 14:365, 1973.
124. Stevens CE, et al. Hepatitis B vaccine in patients receiving hemodialysis: Immunogenicity and efficacy. N Engl J Med 311:496, 1984.
125. Donati D, et al. Immune deficiency in uremia: Interleukin-2 production and responsiveness and interleukin-2 receptor expression and release. Nephron 58:268, 1991.
126. Chatenaud L, et al. Immune deficiency of the uremic patient. Adv Nephrol 19:259, 1990.
127. Touraine JL, et al. T-lymphocytes and serum inhibitors of cell mediated immunity in renal insufficiency. Nephron 14:195, 1975.
128. Badger AM, et al. Depressed spontaneous cellular cytotoxicity associated with normal or enhanced antibody-dependent cellular cytotoxicity in patients on chronic hemodialysis. Clin Exp Immunol 45:568, 1981.
129. Gibbons RAS, Marinex OM, Garovoy MR. Altered monocyte function in uremia. Clin Immunol Immunopathol 56:66, 1990.
130. Robbins SL, Rucker AW Jr. The cause of death in diabetics. A report of 307 autopsied cases. N Engl J Med 231:865, 1944.
131. Vejilsgaard R. Studies on urinary infection in diabetes. Bacteria in patients with diabetes mellitus and in control subjects. Acta Med Scand 179:173, 1966.
132. Moutschen MP, Scheen AJ, Lefebvre PF. Impaired immune responses in diabetes mellitus: Analysis of the factors involved. Relevance to the increased susceptibility of diabetic patients to specific infections. Diabetes Metab 18:187, 1992.
133. Wilson RM, Reeves WG. Neutrophil function in diabetes. In Nattrass M, ed. Recent Advances in Type 2 Diabetes. London: Churchill Livingstone, 1986, p 127.
134. Rodier M, et al. Peripheral blood T cell subsets studies by monoclonal antibodies in type 1 (insulin-dependent) diabetes: Effect of blood glucose control. Diabetologia 27:136, 1984.
135. Visalli N, Signore A, Pozzilli P. Immunodeficiency in long-standing diabetes: Evidence and approaches to prevention. In Andreani D, Kolb H, Pozzilli P, eds. Immunotherapy of Type 1 Diabetes. Chichester: Wiley, 1989, p 185.
136. Cluff LE, Reynolds RC, Page DL. Staphylococcal bacteremia: Demographic, clinical and microbiological features of 185 cases. Trans Am Clin Climatol Assoc 79:905, 1968.
137. Alteras I, Saryt E. Prevalence of pathogenic fungi in the toe-webs and toe nails of diabetic patients. Mycopathologia 67:157, 1979.
138. The International Antimicrobial Therapy Project Group of the European Organization for Research and Treatment of Cancer. Combination of amikacin and carbenicillin with or without cefazolin as empirical treatment of febrile neutropenic patients. J Clin Oncol 1:597, 1983.
139. Ozaki Y, et al. Enhanced resistance of mice to bacterial infection induced by recombinant human interleukin-1 alpha. Infect Immunol 55:1436, 1987.
140. Smith JW, et al. The toxic and hematologic effects of interleukin-1 alpha administration in phase I trial to patients with advanced malignancies. J Clin Oncol 10:1141, 1992.
141. Sarosy G, et al. Phase I study of taxol and granulocyte colony-stimulating factor in patients with refractory ovarian cancer. J Clin Oncol 10:1165, 1992.
142. Linch DC, et al. Randomized vehicle-controlled dose-finding study of glycosylated recombinant human granulocyte colony-stimulating factor after bone marrow transplantation. Bone Marrow Transplant 11:307, 1993.
143. Fan D, et al. Granulocyte-macrophage colony-stimulating factor (GM-CSF) in the management of cancer. In Vivo 5:571, 1991.
144. Peters WP, et al. Comparative effects of granulocyte-macrophage colony-stimulating factor (GM-CSF) and granulocyte colony-stimulating factor (G-CSF) on priming peripheral blood progenitor cells for use with autologous bone marrow after high-dose chemotherapy. Blood 81:1709, 1993.
145. Baldwin GC, et al. Granulocyte-macrophage colony-stimulating factor enhances neutrophil function in acquired immunodeficiency syndrome patients. Proc Natl Acad Sci USA 85:2763, 1988.
146. Quesada JR, et al. Alpha interferon for induction of remission in hairy-cell leukemia. N Engl J Med 310:15, 1984.
147. Tyring SK. Treatment of condyloma acuminata with interferon. Semin Oncol 15(Suppl 5):35, 1988.
148. Groopman JE, Scadden DT. Interferon therapy for Kaposi's sarcoma associated with the acquired immunodeficiency syndrome (AIDS). Ann Intern Med 110:335, 1989.

149. Rothermel CD, Rubin BY, Murry H. Gamma interferon is the factor in lymphokine that activate human macrophages to inhibit intracellular *Chlamydia psittaci* replication. J Immunol 131:2542, 1983.
150. Siegel JP. Effects of human interferon-gamma on the activation of human T lymphocytes. Cell Immunol 111:461, 1988.
151. Wong DKH, et al. Effect of alpha-interferon treatment in patients with hepatitis B e antigen-positive chronic hepatitis B. Ann Intern Med 118:312, 1993.
152. Kleter GEM, et al. Detection of hepatitis C virus RNA in patients with chronic hepatitis C virus infections during and after therapy with alpha interferon. Antimicrob Agents Chemother 37:595, 1993.
153. Carswell EA, et al. An endotoxin induced serum factor which causes necrosis of tumors. Proc Natl Acad Sci USA 72:3666, 1975.
154. Lane HC, et al. Anti-retroviral effects of interferon-alpha in AIDS-associated Kaposi's sarcoma. Lancet 2:1218, 1988.
155. Sheppard BC, Fraker DL, Norton JA. Prevention and treatment of endotoxin and sepsis lethality with recombinant human tumor necrosis factor. Surgery 106:156, 1989.
156. Fisher CJ, et al. Influence of an anti-tumor necrosis factor monoclonal antibody on cytokine levels in patients with sepsis. Crit Care Med 21:318, 1993.

5

Physiologic Basis of Transplantation

Rafik M. Ghobrial and Barry D. Kahan

Successful clinical transplantation is limited not by technical pitfalls but rather by the immune process that mediates rejection of the transplanted tissue or organ.[1] Thus an understanding of the physiologic basis of transplantation rests on an understanding of the immunologic rejection process. The goal of the transplant surgeon is to manipulate either the host (the recipient of the transplanted organ or tissue) or the allograft (the organ or tissue being transplanted from a donor within the same species) to avert, minimize, or reduce this physiologic process. Immunologic events leading to allograft rejection are classified as afferent, central, and efferent limbs: the afferent limb includes presentation and T-lymphocyte recognition of foreign histocompatibility antigens; the central limb includes proliferation, differentiation, and production of lymphokines by T cells and of humoral antibody by B cells; and the efferent limb includes the action of the immune mediators to destroy the graft.

ALLOGRAFT REJECTION

Afferent Limb: Presentation and Antigen Recognition

Major Histocompatibility Antigens

Major histocompatibility complex (MHC). The antigen disparity between the host and the graft initiates the immune response and ultimately the rejection process. Early experiments in clinical transplantation revealed the presence of a single, strong antigenic system controlling the outcome of transplantation in every species. The human MHC encodes the human leukocyte (HLA) antigens, including class I, class II, class III and many other genes that encode proteins of unknown function. The MHC spans 3.5 million DNA base pairs, approximately 2% of the genetic material in autosomal chromosome 6 (Fig. 5-1). The class II genes are located closest to the centromere in the order DP, DQ, and DR. The class III region encodes components of the complement system (C2, C4a, C4b and factor B), as well as the enzyme steroid 21-hydroxylase. The genes for heat shock proteins (HSPs), tumor necrosis factor (TNF), lymphotoxin (LT), and LTβ lie between the complement and class I genes. The most telomeric portion of the MHC contains the class I α-chain genes in the sequence B, C, and A. Nonpolymorphic class I–like genes and pseudogenes, located in the large space between the C and A genes and telomeric to HLA-A, occupy 11 centimorgans. The function of the class I–like genes remains largely unknown. However, these genes may serve as a repository for alternative nucleic acid sequences used for generating polymorphism in the true class I molecules by the process of gene conversion (incorporation of variant sequences in the class I or class II genes without reciprocal crossing over). Located within the class II region are the genes encoding multiple subunits of a cytosolic protease termed *proteasome,* which is involved in the generation of peptide fragments from intracellular endogenous cytosolic proteins. The transporter in antigen processing (TAP)–1 and –2 genes are located next to the proteasome complex in the class II region. Such TAP genes encode subunits of a heterodimeric pump protein that transports the endogenous peptide fragments into the endoplasmic reticulum (ER), where such peptides bind to class I but not class II molecules. Class I and class II glycoproteins serve as scaffolds for the presentation of processed antigenic peptides to T cells; class I molecules present peptides from endogenous proteins to $CD8^+$ T cells, whereas class II molecules present peptides from exogenous antigens to $CD4^+$ T cells. The polymorphism, and therefore antigenicity, of the MHC class I and class II transplantation antigens is the result of amino acid sequence differences between donor and recipient MHC molecules.

Characteristics of class I MHC antigens

Structure. The class I MHC antigens are expressed as complexes of a membrane-bound glycoprotein heavy chain polypeptide (45 kd) that is noncovalently associated with a non–MHC-encoded β_2-microglobulin (β_2m; 12 kd) light chain (Fig. 5-2, *A*). Crystallographic analysis of human HLA-A2,[2] HLA-B27, HLA-Aw68, and mouse H-$2D^b$ class I molecules reveal similar molecular configurations. The membrane-distal polymorphic α_1 (90 amino

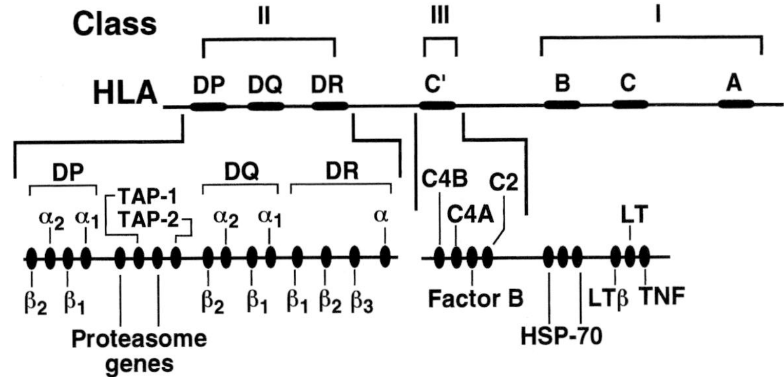

Fig. 5-1. Chromosomal map of the human major histocompatibility complex. The MHC locus encodes HLA class I (A, B, and C), class II (DP, DQ, and DR) and class III, including the complement (C′) locus. Proteasome and transporter (TAP-1, TAP-2) genes are located in the class II region. Genes encoding HSP and TNF/LT family of cytokines (LT-β, LT, TNF) sit in a telomeric position to class III loci. Class I–like genes and multiple pseuodogenes are located between the C and A loci.

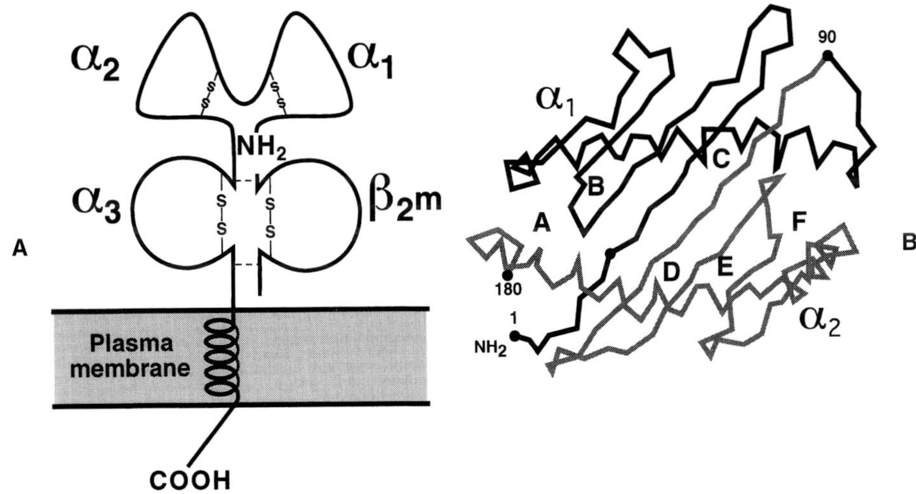

Fig. 5-2. MHC class I antigen. **A,** Schematic illustration of the heavy chain, including α_1, α_2, α_3, transmembrane, and intracytoplasmic domains. The heavy chain is noncovalently associated with the light chain (β_2m). **B,** Schematic illustration of the peptide-binding cleft formed by the α_1 and α_2 domains, each contributing an α helix and four β strands. Both domains are in continuity with one another (180 amino acids) to provide a peptide-binding groove with closed ends. *A* through *F* denote peptide-binding pockets formed by polymorphic amino acid residues in the cleft. NH_2 and COOH are the aminoterminal and carboxyterminal ends of the protein.

acids [aa]) and α_2 (92 aa) domains bear eight antiparallel β-pleated strands bordered by two α-helical regions (the first from the α_1 and the second from the α_2 domain), which jointly form the peptide-binding cleft (Fig. 5-2, *B*). The α_2 domain is attached to a less-polymorphic, immunoglobulin (Ig)–like, membrane-proximal α_3 (92 aa) domain, which is followed by conserved transmembrane (25 aa) and intracytoplasmic (30 aa) segments. The α_3 domain contains the binding sites for the CD8 molecule. The β_2m forms an Ig-like domain that is noncovalently associated with the extracellular portion of the heavy chain and appears to be critical in maintaining the native conformation of class I molecules.

Antigen presentation. Class I molecules present peptides derived from proteins in the cytosol to $CD8^+$-bearing T cells. T cells recognize both the MHC molecule and the associated peptide presented in the peptide-binding groove. Six pockets (A, B, C, D, E, and F) present within the groove (Fig. 5-2, *B*) provide specificity for interactions with the peptide side chains. The closed ends of the groove result in a strong bias for stable binding of short peptides in the range of 8 to 10 residues.[3] A broad peptide-binding capacity arises from hydrogen bonding between the amino (NH_2) and carboxyl (COOH) groups of the peptide and the residues at the end of the groove (A and F pockets). A second, more specific, bonding links the

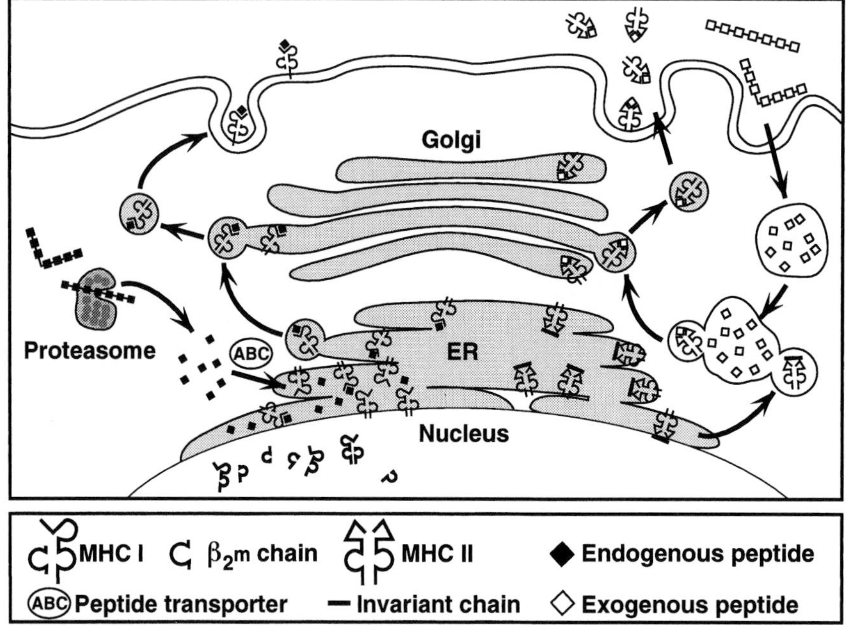

Fig. 5-3. Schematic illustration of antigen processing and presentation by class I or class II molecules. Endogenously generated proteins (■—■—■) are degraded in the cytoplasm by the action of a macromolecular proteasome complex. Endogenous peptides (■) are transported into the endoplasmic reticulum *(ER)* by the ATP-binding cassette (ABC)-peptide transporters, where they bind to class I molecules. The assembled trimolecular complex (peptide, heavy, and β chains) are transported through the Golgi complex to the plasma membranes for surface expression. Exogenous proteins (□—□—□) are degraded in the lysosomal compartments into peptides (□), which replace the invariant chain (—) on the peptide-binding surface of class II molecules prior to vesicular surface transport.

polymorphic residues in the pockets B through E to specific peptide side chains (anchor residues). Such anchor peptide residues that fit optimally into the pockets of the peptide-binding groove stipulate the repertoire of peptides that associate with a particular class I molecule. For example, HLA-A0201 binds peptides exhibiting leucine at position 2 and valine at position 9. Such peptide motifs have been defined for HLA-A0205 and HLA-B 27, as well as many mouse class I molecules. Thus each class I allelic product selects its bound peptides according to specific motifs characterized by an allele-specific length and positions of anchor peptide residues.

Assembly and expression. Short nanomeric peptides produced from intracellular antigens, possible by the function of a macromolecular proteasome complex, are translocated by the MHC-encoded ATP-binding cassette (ABC) transporters from the cytosol to the endoplasmic reticulum (ER) to stabilize the assembly between class I heavy chain and β_2m (Fig. 5-3). The assembled trimolecular complexes (peptide, heavy chain, and β chain) then pass through the Golgi apparatus, followed by vesicular transport to the plasma membrane for surface expression as membrane-bound glycoproteins.[4] The 90 kd membrane-bound chaperone of the ER termed *calnexin* (p88, IP90) may contribute to the efficient intracellular formation of class I–peptide complexes by retarding the intracellular transport of the peptide-deficient heavy chain-β_2m heterodimers.[5] Class I antigens are expressed on almost all cells of the body, although levels of expression may vary and are typically highest on hematopoietic elements.

Characteristics of class II MHC antigens

Structure and antigen presentation. Class II MHC antigens are composed of a heterodimer of two transmembrane α (33kd) and β (29 kd) molecular chains, each bearing one peptide binding-domain (α_1 or β_1) and one immunoglobulin domain (α_2 or β_2; Fig. 5-4, *A*). Crystallographic analysis of the class II HLA-DR1 revealed a three-dimensional structure similar to that of class I molecules.[6] Similar to class I molecules, class II polymorphic residues are concentrated in the α helical sides or the β strands of the peptide-binding cleft, which bear allele-specific motifs that interact with the peptide anchor residues at five binding pockets. In contrast to that of class I molecules, the peptide binding site of class II molecules includes two noncovalently associated halves (α_1 and β_1), with one α helix and four β strands (90 aa) contributed by each chain (Fig. 5-4, *B*) to form an open peptide-binding groove (Fig. 5-5). In addition, class II molecules form conserved bonds with the main chains atoms of the peptide, not the terminal groups, thus allowing the ends of the peptides to ex-

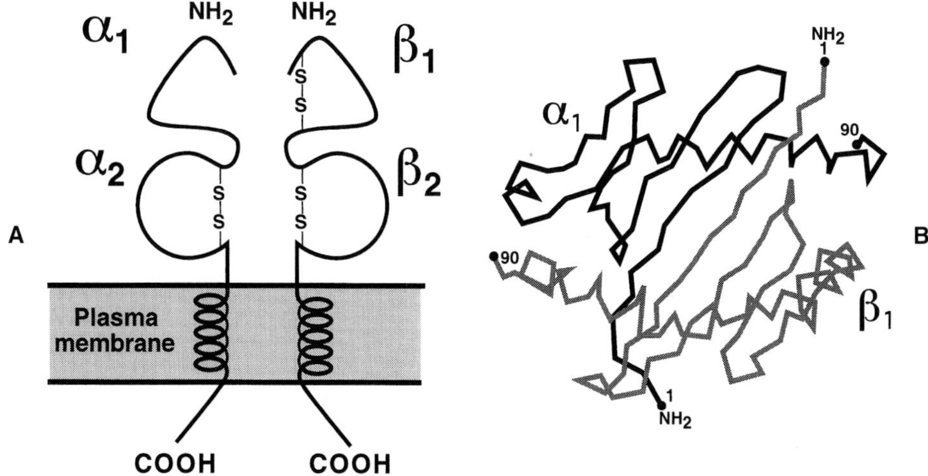

Fig. 5-4. Class II MHC antigen. **A,** Schematic illustration of the α and β chains; each contains membrane-distal α_1 and β_1 domains that form the peptide-binding cleft and membrane-proximal α_2 and β_2 domains. Each is followed by a transmembrane and an intracytoplasmic domain. **B,** Schematic illustration of the peptide-binding cleft formed by two separate α_1 and β_1 domains, each containing approximately 90 amino acids. One α helix and four β strands are contributed by each domain. NH_2 and *COOH* are aminoterminal and carboxyterminal ends, respectively.

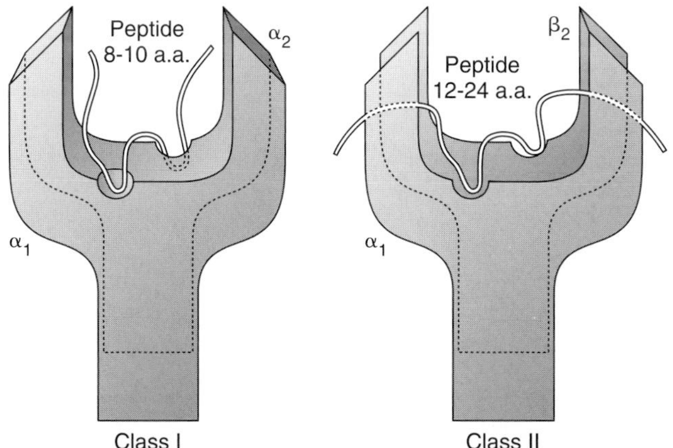

Fig. 5-5. Schematic illustration of peptide binding to class I or class II molecules. The continuity between α_1 and α_2 domains of the class I molecules provides a *closed* peptide-binding groove that limits binding to peptides 8 to 10 amino acids long. Class II molecules exhibit an *open* peptide-binding groove formed by two separate α_1 and β_1 domains, thus allowing longer peptides (12 to 24 amino acids) to bind and protrude beyond the peptide-binding groove.

tend out of the binding groove.[6] Thus class II–associated peptides exhibit a broader range of lengths, typically 12 to 24 residues (see Fig. 5-5). Class II molecules may even bind whole proteins.

Assembly and expression. Whereas class I molecules present peptides derived primarily from proteins synthesized within the cell, such as viral antigens, class II molecules bind to foreign peptides introduced into the cell through the endocytic pathway (exogenous antigens). These differences result from distinct intracellular trafficking and assembly pathways of class I and class II molecules (see Fig. 5-3). In contradistinction to the endogenous pathway used by class I molecules, an exogenous assembly pathway links class II molecules to the antigenic peptides generated after endocytosis and endosomal digestion of antigens.[7] The class II chains synthesized intracellularly associate in the ER with a nonpolymorphic, non–MHC-encoded chain termed *invariant chain* (li 30 kd). Three invariant chains combine to form a homotrimer, with each subunit binding to a newly synthesized class II α/β heterodimer to form a nine-chain complex. The invariant chain serves to make the class II α/β heterodimers more compact and reduces the binding of the class II molecules to endogenous peptides in the ER. The invariant chain then guides the class II complexes to the lysosomal compartments of the exogenous pathway, which contain the proteolytically cleaved, exogenous antigenic peptides. The acidic environment of the endosomes allows the dissociation of the invariant chain from class II molecules, followed by the association of the peptides with the α/β heterodimers. Vesicularly transported class II α/β-peptide complexes are then expressed on the cell surface for antigen presentation. Class II molecules exhibit limited distribution to vascular endothelium and cells of lymphoreticular origin, specifically B lymphocytes, monocytes, antigen-presenting cells (APCs; including macrophages, B cells, dendritic cells, and Langerhans' epidermal cells), and immune-activated T lymphocytes.

Blood Group Antigens

Red blood cell carbohydrate antigens vary in their tissue distribution and degree of expression. Rh antigens are found exclusively on red cells, whereas ABO antigens are widely distributed on other tissues and body fluids. The ABO system of blood typing is the only non-HLA–histocompatibility system that has been identified to mediate rejection in humans.[8] Renal transplantation across an ABO incompatibility is almost always unsuccessful.[9] The recipient responds as a presensitized host because he or she bears circulating isoantibodies toward foreign blood group antigens, resulting in hyperacute rejection. Renal function ceases within minutes to hours. Recently, the development of techniques for removal of anti-A and anti-B isoantibodies by plasmapheresis renewed some interest in ABO-incompatible kidney transplants. Alexandre et al.[10] reported on a series of successful ABO-incompatible living related and unrelated kidney transplants. Interestingly, after treatment the isoagglutinin titers nearly returned to preoperative levels, even in successful grafts. Successful outcome of cadaveric renal transplantation from blood group A_2 donors to O recipients has been reported, a success attributed to the lower density of the A_2 form of antigen expressed on the donor kidney.

Lewis (Le) antigens, which are blood group-related complex-carbohydrate antigens consisting of 1, 3 fucosylated *N*-acetylglucosamine groups within repeating lactosamine subunits, may also influence renal allograft survival. They result from a complex interaction between gene products of ABO, Rh, secretor, and Le loci. The Le antigens exist in a soluble form in the serum (Le^a, Le^b) and body fluids, but not on erythrocytes. Oriol et al.[11] implicated incompatible Le antigens as the cause of renal allograft failure in presensitized hosts bearing anti-Le antibodies after multiple blood transfusions. Although Le and HLA antigen disparities display negative additive effects on transplant survival, HLA identity cannot override the deleterious influence of a Lewis antigen mismatch. Le antigens are expressed on lymphocytes and on epithelial cells of both the distal convoluted tubules and collecting ducts. Spitalnik et al.[12] reported that eight Le-negative persons with circulating anti-Le antibodies who received Le-incompatible grafts all displayed allograft rejection. In contrast, Rh incompatibility in renal transplantation plays a minor role in allograft survival, except possibly in a presensitized Rh-negative recipient.[8] Currently, ABO incompatibility between donor and recipient is routinely avoided by blood grouping, but Le mismatches are only sought when there has been an extensive recipient transfusion history.

T Lymphocytes

T-cell receptor (TcR). There are two forms of TcR; the α/β heterodimers that are expressed on most mature peripheral blood T cells and the γ/δ heterodimers expressed on 10% of intestinal T cells and 5% of peripheral blood T cells. The α/β TcR recognizes processed peptides presented by classical polymorphic class I or class II MHC molecules to activate a wide variety of T cell–mediated immune mechanisms, including the alloimmune response. Activation of α/β T cells is thus restricted by the recognition of the appropriate MHC antigens. T cells expressing the γ/δ TcR are not restricted by the conventional polymorphic self MHC but may recognize the nonpolymorphic MHC-like molecules. The function of the γ/δ T cells is largely unknown; they may play a role in the initiation of the immune response to some commonly encountered microbial antigens at the epithelial boundaries.

The α/β TcR consists of two polypeptide chains (Fig. 5-6). The α chain (40 to 50 kd) and the β chain (40 to 45 kd) bear striking similarities to Ig. Both chains have variable (V) and constant (C) domains with appropriately spaced cysteine residues to allow the formation of an interchain disulfide-bonded loops similar to Ig V and C domains. Thus the TcR and many other membrane proteins structurally homologous to Ig domains are referred to as the *Ig superfamily,* and the genes encoding these molecules are termed the *Ig gene superfamily* (see box on p. 115). The C-terminal end of the V region in both chains (the junction between the V and C domains) is encoded by a joining (J) segment gene, and in case of the β chain only by an additional diversity (D) segment gene. The presence of V, D, J, and C regions is also characteristic of Ig. The similarity between the TcR and Ig may reflect the common

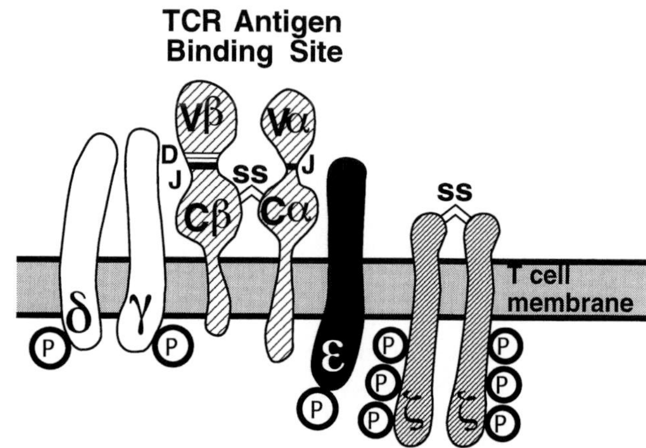

Fig. 5-6. Schematic illustration of the TcR complex. The TcR consists of two chains, α and β, each containing an Ig-like variable *(V)* and constant *(C)* domains. Each chain has a transmembrane and a short intracytoplasmic segment. Diversity *(D)* and joining *(J)* segments are present at the junction of the V and C regions in the β chain, whereas the α chain exhibits only a J segment. The TcR-associated proteins consist of the CD3 complex γ, δ, and ϵ chains associated with ζ-ζ chain homodimer. On 10% of T cells, the ζ-ζ homodimer is replaced by an η-ζ heterodimer. The transmembrane segments of the TcR α and β chains exhibit positively charged side chains *(+)* that interact with the negatively charged residues *(-)* in the transmembrane portions of the γ,δ, ϵ, and ζ chains. Antigen recognition activation motifs containing sites for tyrosine phosphorylation (P) are present in the cytoplasmic tails of the γ, δ, ϵ, and ζ chains.

function of both structures to detect foreign antigens. The Ig domain of the C region of both chains is followed by a hinge region that forms a disulfide linkage between the two chains. The transmembrane segments exhibit positively charged side chains that interact with the negatively charged residues in the CD3 polypeptides. The carboxyterminus of the C regions of both the α and β chains forms a 5 to 12 aa intracytoplasmic tail that is too short for signal transduction; rather, this function is performed by the TcR-associated CD3 complex.

TcR-associated proteins. Foreign transplantation antigens binding to host TcR perturb the TcR-associated protein complex by means of noncovalent salt bridges. The CD3 complex contains three peptide products (γ, δ, ϵ). The γ, δ, and ϵ chains, encoded on chromosome 11, are nonpolymorphic, highly homologous peptides (see Fig. 5-6). Each chain exhibits an Ig-like exrtracellular domain, a transmembrane segment containing a negatively charged aspartic acid residue important for association with the TcR, and a cytoplasmic domain ranging from 44 to 80 aa. The η and ζ chains are encoded by the same gene, by means of alternative splicing, on chromosome 1. Long cytoplasmic tails (113 to 155 aa) characterize the η and ζ chains in addition to their negatively charged transmembrane domains. The cytoplasmic tails of the CD3 complex chains, essential for the TcR signal transduction, exhibit the *antigen recognition activation motif,* which consists of 17 aa residues containing tyrosine-X-X-tyrosine, where *X* is any amino acid. The tyrosine residues undergo phosphoryolation during TcR activation. This motif occurs once in the tails of γ, δ, and ϵ chains and thrice on the tail of the ζ chain. The CD3 chains are expressed as a monomer of γ, δ, and ϵ chains, which is associated with ζ-ζ homodimers on 90% of T cells or with η-ζ heterodimers on the rest of the T cells. Thus, the most common TcR bears a $\alpha\beta{:}\gamma\delta\epsilon\zeta_2$ configuration. A major function of the CD3, ζ, and η proteins is to facilitate the expression of the entire TcR complex.

Rearrangement and expression of TcR α and β genes. Genomic sequences encoding the β chain are located on chromosome 7 (Fig. 5-7). Each C_β gene is associated with a 5′ cluster of six J_β genes and one D_β gene. V_β segments (75 to 100) are located 5′ of the DJC clusters. The α chain sequences on chromosome 14 contain a single C_α gene associated with at least 60 different J_α genes and 75 V_α gene segments grouped in 12 different families (Fig. 7-5). The assembly of the multiple units of the V, D, and J segments (somatic recombination) is mediated by the products of the recombination activator genes RAG-1 and RAG-2,[13] found only in the immature T and B cells. The multiple combinatorial associations of different V, D, and J segments during TcR rearrangement allows a broad TcR diversity. Further, the *N-region diversification,* involving the random addition of nucleotides that are not a part of the genomic sequences at the VJ, VD, and DJ junctions, and the pairing of α/β chains serve to multiply the diversity of the TcR. Thus the potential size of the generated T-cell repertoire may exceed 10^{15} specificities.

IMMUNOGLOBULIN SUPERFAMILY MEMBERS

Immunoglobulin (IgG)
MHC antigens (class I, class II)
TcR
CD3(γ, δ, ϵ)
Invariant chain (li)
CD4, CD8
Thy-1
CD2 (LFA-2)
ICAM-1, ICAM-2
VCAM-1
CD28, CTLA-4, B7/BB1, B7.2
IL-1R

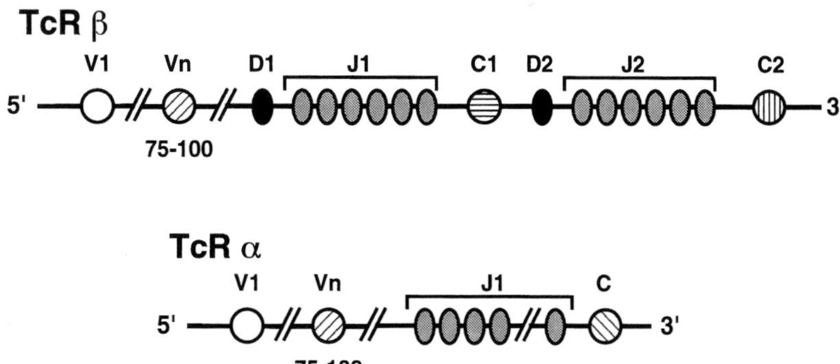

Fig. 5-7. Genomic sequences encoding the TcR α and β chains. V_β segments are located 5′ of the DJC clusters, whereas each C_β gene is associated with a 5′ cluster of six J_β genes and one 3′ D_β gene. The α chain sequences contain a single C_α gene associated with multiple J_α and V_α gene segments. The assembly of different V, D, and J segments with the C gene segments results in multiple genomic sequences encoding α and β chains with different specificities.

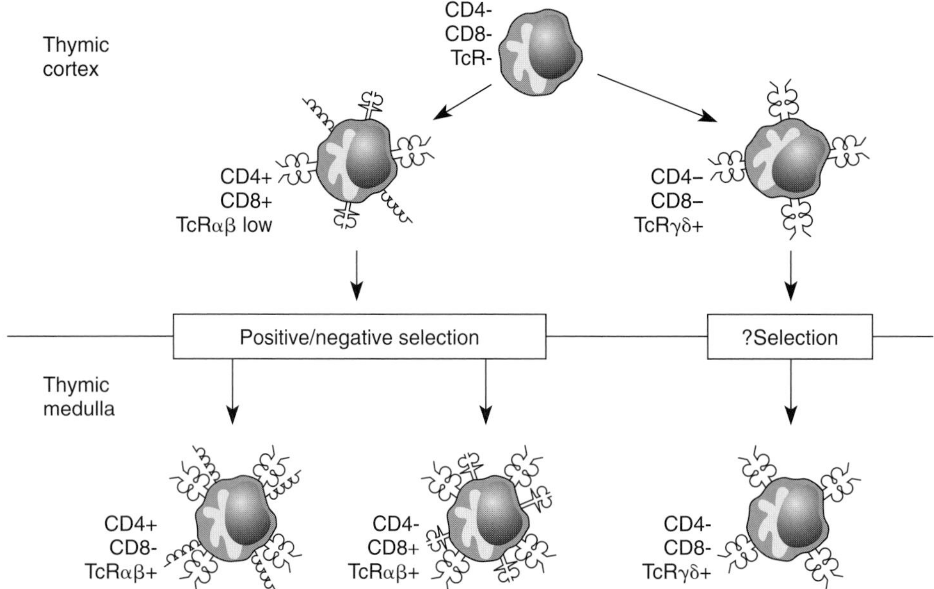

Fig. 5-8. T-cell maturation in the thymus. In the α/β T-cell lineage, double-negative ($CD4^-CD8^-$) thymocytes develop into $CD4^+CD8^+$ (double-positive). The majority of double-positive thymocytes die in vivo, and the remaining minority ultimately gives rise to the $CD4^+$ TcR α/β^+ or $CD8^+$ TCRα/β^+ self-MHC–restricted (single-positive) mature T cells that recognize foreign antigen in association with self-MHC. Positive selection allows thymocytes with TcR that recognize self-MHC molecules to survive and eliminates all non-self-MHC–reactive cells. Negative selection eliminates all T cells that recognize self-antigens in association with self-MHC. A small population of double-negative thymocytes expresses the γ/δ TcR and develops into $CD4^-CD8^-$ non–MHC-restricted T cells.

Maturation and MHC restriction. After migration from the bone marrow, T cells mature in the thymus, where rearrangement and expression of the TcR genes occur. The CD4 and CD8 molecules expressed on mature T cell subsets are commonly used as markers for thymocyte maturation. Most immature cells in the thymic cortex are rapidly dividing thymocytes that lack CD4 and CD8 molecules ($CD4^-CD8^-$, double-negative) but are actively rearranging the α and β TcR genes (Fig. 5-8). Most of the double-negative cells (80%) begin to express CD4 and CD8, thus developing into $CD4^+CD8^+$ (double-positive). The vast majority of double-negative cells die in vivo, and only 20% of such cells develop into $CD4^+$TcRα/β^+ or $CD8^+$TcRα/β^+ MHC-restricted (single-positive) mature T cells, which are predominantly detected in the medulla. These single-positive T cells constitute the vast majority of the T cells in the peripheral circulation. A small proportion of double-negative T cells will never express CD4 or CD8 and rearrange the γ/δ but not the α/β TcR genes, giving rise to the γ/δ TcR-expressing T cells that are not restricted by the conventional polymorphic self-MHC.

T cells maturing in the thymus exhibit a broad range of specificities, including clones potentially reactive to self-antigens. Thus the second important event in the thymic T cell maturation is the selection of T cells that are tolerant to self-antigens yet reactive to foreign antigens. On the one hand, there is selection of T cells with receptors recognizing foreign antigens in association with self-MHC molecules (positive selection).[14] On the other hand, there is selective elimination of T cells (negative selection)[15,16] that bind with high affinity to self-antigens in association with self-MHC. Such self-reacting T-cells clones undergo clonal deletion by a Ca^{2+} dependent process of cell death or apoptosis.[17] Thus thymic selection results in a T-cell repertoire recognizing foreign antigens, including alloantigens, in the context of self-MHC.

Accessory molecules. The binding of the peptide-histocompatibility antigen assembly to the TcR is complemented by a set of independent, accessory receptor-ligand interactions: CD4 to class II MHC molecules (Fig. 5-9, *A*) or CD8 markers to class I (Fig. 5-9, *B*); leukocyte function–associated antigen-1 (LFA-1) of the integrin gene family to intercellular adhesion molecules (ICAM-1 or ICAM-2), two members of the Ig gene superfamily; CD2 (LFA-2) to LFA-3 (CD58); and Ig gene superfamily B7-1/BB1 and B7-2 to CD28 and CTLA-4. Although the TcR-CD3 complexes are the key molecules in the antigen-specific recognition of the MHC-peptide complex and T-cell activation, binding of the accessory molecules is necessary for modulation of signal transduction, as well as to increase the affinity of cellular interactions with T cells, as evidenced by the capacity of antibodies directed against accessory molecules to inhibit T-cell activation.

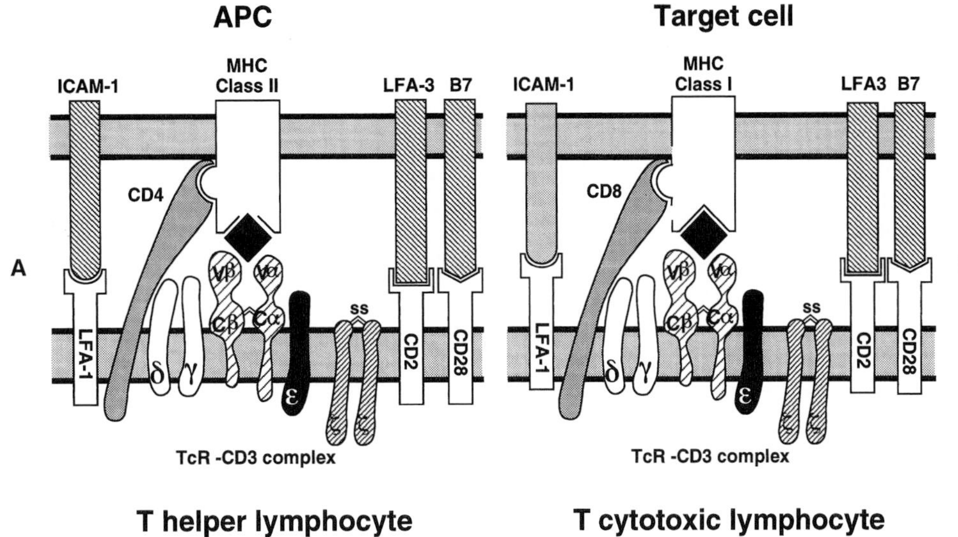

Fig. 5-9. Interaction of TcR complex and accessory molecules with target ligands. **A,** Interaction of $CD4^+$ Th cell with APC. **B,** Interaction of $CD8^+$ Tc cell with target cell. LFA-1 binds to ICAM-1, CD2 to LFA-3, and CD28 to B7. The antigen-binding site of the TcR complex interacts with both the peptide and the peptide-binding groove of the MHC molecule. CD4 and CD8 molecules bind to MHC class II or class I, respectively.

Coreceptor molecules, CD4 and CD8. These nonpolymorphic transmembrane glycoproteins members of the Ig gene superfamily (Fig. 5-10) are expressed in a mutually exclusive fashion on mature T cells subsets that are either $CD4^+$ or $CD8^+$. The CD4 (T4, L3T4) molecule (55kd), encoded on chromosome 12, contains four extracellular Ig-like domains, a transmembrane domain, and an intracytoplasmic tail. The two amino terminal Ig-like domains only bind to the β_2 domain of class II MHC, thus imposing a restriction of $CD4^+$ T-cell interactions to class II MHC–bearing cells such as APCs. The intracytoplasmic tail is physically associated with a lymphocyte-specific protein tyrosine kinase of the *src* oncogene family $p56^{lck}$. Rapid phosphorylation of the serine residues in the cytoplasmic tail upon antigen-specific stimulation of the T cell (MCH-peptide complex interaction with TcR) underlines the role of CD4 in signal transduction. Binding of the CD4 coreceptor to the lateral surface of the MHC molecule augments signaling by means of the TcR as much as 100 times. However, ligation of the CD4 molecules alone, without TcR activation, inhibits T-cell activation.[18] These dual opposing behaviors presumably reflect an interplay between $p56^{lck}$ and the cytoplasmic tails of the CD3 ζ chains. The major function of $CD4^+$ T cells (65% of the α/β mature T cells) after antigen-specific stimulation is the secretion of cytokines that act on other T cells, B cells, macrophages, neutrophils, and vascular endothelium. These cells are thus designated *helper-inducer T cells (Th).* The Th population has been subdivided on the basis of the cellular pattern of cytokine production.[19] $CD4^+$ Th cells produce either interleukin (IL)–2, interferon (IFN)–γ, and

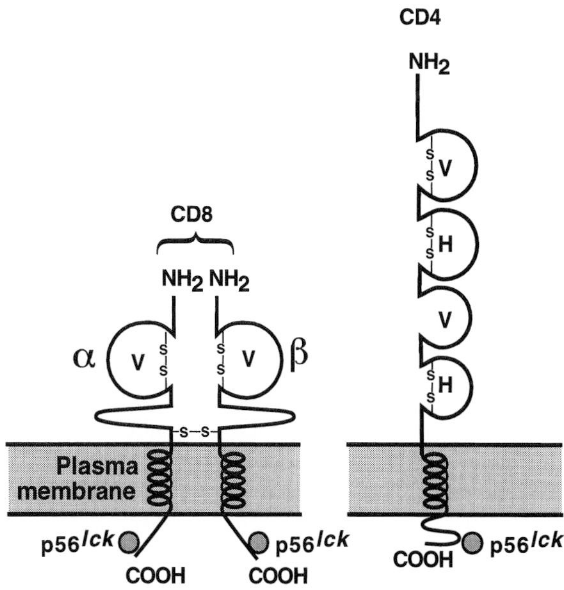

Fig. 5-10. Schematic illustration of coreceptor molecules. The CD4 molecule (55 kd) is expressed on cellular membranes as a monomer that consists of four extracellular Ig-like domains, a transmembrane domain, and an intracytoplasmic tail. The two membrane-distal domains contain the binding sites for class II MHC β_2 domain, whereas the intracytoplasmic domain is associated with $p56^{lck}$ protein kinase. The CD8 molecule is mostly expressed as a heterodimer of α (34 kd) and β (34 kd) chains that contain the class I MHC binding domain in the extracellular domains. Similar to CD4, the CD8 intracytoplasmic domain is associated with $p56^{lck}$.

TNF-β (Th_1) or IL-4, IL-5, IL-6, IL-10, and IL-13 (Th_2) as their unique products. Accordingly, Th_1 responses are characterized by cell-mediated activation of T cells and macrophages resulting in potent immunity and allograft destruction. In contrast, Th_2 cells are predisposed to help B cells in the development of antibody production. Nevertheless, both subsets influence each other's function. Recent reports suggest that prolongation of allograft survival is associated with selective activation of the IL-4 and IL-10 Th_2 helper cells but not the IL-2- and IFN-γ-producing Th_1 cells.[20]

The CD8 (T8, Lyt-2) molecule exists in two forms: either as a homodimer of CD8α chain (34 kd) or a heterodimer of CD8α and CD8β (34 kd) chains (see Fig. 5-10) encoded by genes located on chromosome 2. The extracellular domains contain the binding sites to MHC class I α_3 domain, resulting in restricted interaction of $CD8^+$ T cells (35% of the α/β T cells) with class I MHC–bearing cells. Similar to the CD4 molecules, the intracytoplasmic domains of CD8 undergo serine phosphorylation after antigen-specific stimulation of $CD8^+$ T cells as a result of the physical association of $p56^{lck}$. The CD8 marker is expressed on killer or cytotoxic T lymphocytes (CTL; Tc), which constitute the effector T-cell population that ultimately contributes to allograft destruction. Cytokines involved in the differentiation and induction of CTLs including IL-2, IFN-γ, and IL-6. The division of T cells into Th or CTL populations on the basis of the expression of CD4 or CD8 molecules, although convenient, is not exclusive. Cytotoxic activity has been shown to be mediated by $CD4^+$ T cells, and helper activity can be provided by CD8 cells. Animal studies with antibodies directed against CD8 and CD4 have demonstrated that rejection of class I allodisparate grafts is primarily mediated by $CD8^+$ cells, whereas $CD4^+$ cells are responsible for rejection of class II disparate allografts.[21] However, CD4 and CD8 cells cooperate in nearly all episodes of clinical graft rejection.

Adhesion molecules. Specific cell-cell adhesion mechanisms represent basic components of interactions mediating multiple biologic processes including alloantigen recognition, cell migration, homing, extravasation of alloantigen specific and nonspecific elements to mediate graft rejection or inflammatory responses, wound healing, embryogenesis, and metastasis. Adhesion molecules are categorized into Ig, integrin, selectin, cadaherin, and cartilage link gene families. Members of the Ig, selectin, and integrin families are involved in the specific and nonspecific immune responses.

IG GENE SUPERFAMILY. Members of this family (see Box) are characterized by the presence of Ig domains, namely, regions of 70 to 110 aa homologous to the Ig V (variable) or Ig C (constant) domains. The Ig domain contains conserved residues that allow the protein to assume a globular tertiary structure (Ig homology unit) composed of two β sheets contained in a loop stabilized by a disulfide-bond contributed by conserved cysteine residues. Although members of a superfamily contain homologous structural units that are evolutionarily related, they may not necessarily share similar functional properties or genomic proximity. Through evolutionary divergence and the addition of other protein domains, members of a single superfamily may gain characteristics of other protein superfamilies. The members of the Ig superfamily that serve as adhesion molecules include ICAM-1, ICAM-2, vascular cell adhesion molecule (VCAM)–1, CD2, CD28, CTLA-4, and B7 (Fig. 5-11).

ICAM-1 (114kd) contains five Ig-like extracellular domains and is expressed on T and B cells, fibroblasts, and endothelial cells. ICAM-1 contains the binding sites for the adhesion molecules leukocyte function-associated antigen (LFA)–1 and macrophage adhesion complex (MAC)-1, both members of the β_2 integrin family. The binding of LFA-1 to ICAM-1 may deliver a costimulatory signal to T cells, thus enhancing the TcR-mediated signal for T-cell activation. ICAM-2 bears only two Ig-like extracellular domains and can only bind to LFA-1. CD2 (T11, LFA-2, Tp50, sheep red blood cell receptor; 50 kd) is expressed on mature T cells, on 50% of thymocytes, and on natural killer (NK) cells. CD2 binds to a molecule that is structurally similar to itself LFA-3 (CD58, 55kd), which is expressed on a wide variety of hematopoietic cells. CD2 binding to LFA-3 is important for the binding of Th cells

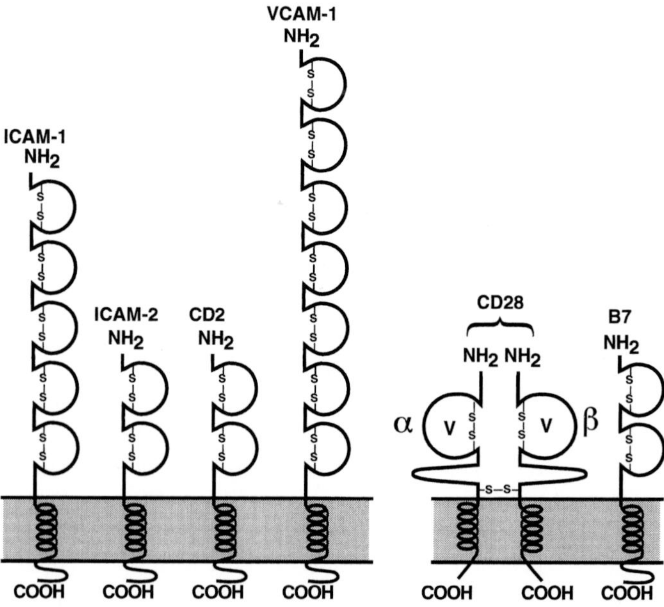

Fig. 5-11. Adhesion molecules of the Ig gene superfamily. These are characterized by the presence of the Ig homology unit, demonstrated schematically as a loop stabilized by a disulfide-bond *(-S-S-)* contributed by conserved cysteine residues. Members of this family include ICAM-1, ICAM-2, CD-2, VCAM-1, CD28, and B7 molecules. Each molecule contains multiple Ig-like domains, a transmembrane region, and an intracytoplasmic segment. *NH_2* and *COOH* are the aminoterminal and carboxyterminal ends, respectively.

to APCs or CTLs to their targets. In addition to its adhesive function, CD2 plays an important role in T-cell activation, as evidenced by the ability of some anti-CD2 antibodies to stimulate T-cell proliferation and cytokine production. This has led to the hypothesis that CD2 may mediate an alternate pathway for T-cell activation, independent of the TcR. VCAM-1 expressed on activated endothelial cells, contains seven Ig-like extracelluar domains. VCAM-1 is the ligand for very late activation molecule (VLA)–4 (β_1 integrin) expressed on T cells. The VCAM-1/VLA-4 interaction is critical for T-cell migration from the bloodstream into the sites of inflammation and may further provide a costimulatory signal for T-cell activation. The CD28 molecule (44kd) is expressed as a homodimer on naive T cells and is closely linked to CTLA-4, which is encoded by an adjacent highly homologous gene. CTLA-4 is expressed on activated or antigen-stimulated, but not naive, CD4 T cells. Both molecules bind to B7/BB1 (60 kd), which is constitutively expressed on dendritic cells and may be induced on B cells. A newly identified ligand for CD28 is the inducible B7.2 molecule. The CD28, CTLA-4/B7, B7.2 interaction mediates a costimulatory signal critical for T-cell activation.

SELECTINS (LECTIN ADHESION MOLECULES; LEC-AM). A family of three closely related proteins L-, E-, and P-selectin, provide calcium-dependent specific recognition signals on interaction with carbohydrate[22] but not protein, leading primarily to adhesion of leukocytes to endothelial cells. All three selectins are single-chain transmembrane glycoproteins that share similar structural features (Fig. 5-12, *A*): first, a lectin-binding domain at the aminoterminus, then an epidermal growth factor–like domain and a number of tandemly repeated domains homologous to the complement regulatory proteins, followed by a transmembrane domain and a short intracytoplasmic tail. The L-selectin (CD62L, MEL-14, LAM-1; 90kd) expressed on leukocytes serves as a homing receptor for lymphocytes to attach to lymph node high endothelial venules. It also binds leukocytes to cytokine (TNF, IL-1, IFN-γ)–activated endothelial cells at the site of inflammation. E-selectin (CD62E, ELAM-1; 110 kd) is exclusively expressed by cytokine-activated endothelial cells. Its ligand is a complex, sialylated carbohydrate group related to Le^x antigens. P-selectin (CD62P, PADGEM, GMP-140; 140 kd) is present in the secretory granules of platelets and endothelial cells. On activation of endothelial cells, P-selectins are rapidly distributed to the cell surface to bind circulating monocytes and neutrophils. P- and E-selectins recognize similar ligands.

INTEGRIN SUPERFAMILY. All integrin are heterodimeric cell-surface proteins composed of two noncovalently associated α (120 to 200 kd) and β chains (90 to 110 kda[23]; Fig. 5-12, *B*). The integrin β chains contain tandem-repeats of a cysteine-rich domain. The globular heads of the α chains contain a series of divalent-cation–binding regions important for receptor function because many integrins have been shown to require divalent cations for ligand binding. The extracellular domains of the two chains bind to a wide variety of ligands, including extracellular matrix glycoproteins fibronectin and vitronectin, other cell surface proteins, and complement components. The three original integrin subfamilies were defined on the basis of three β subunits (β_{1-3}), which were believed to bind several distinct nonoverlapping sets of α chains. Recently, at least

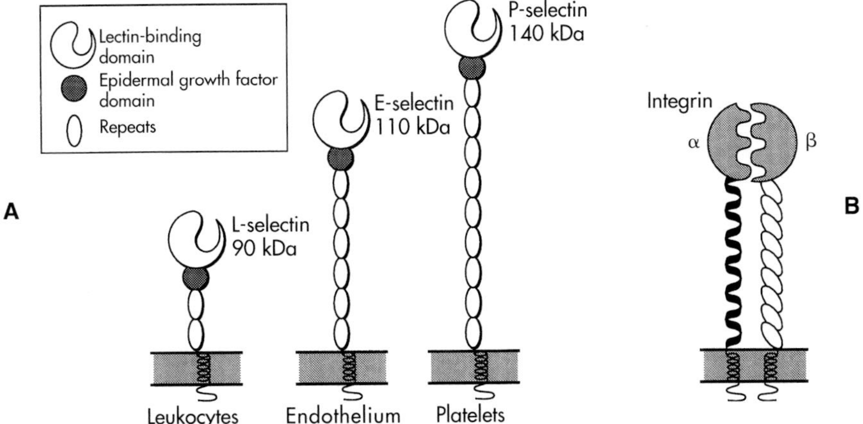

Fig. 5-12. Schematic illustration of selectins and integrins. **A,** The extracellular regions of L-, E- and P-selectin consist of the characteristic lectin-binding domain, an epidermal growth factor–like domain followed by a variable number of short consensus repeats similar to the complement regulatory proteins. Each molecule contains transmembrane and short intracytoplasmic domains. **B,** Integrins are heterodimeric complexes of noncovalently-associated α and β chains with characteristic globular heads that contribute to interchain linkage and ligand interactions. Stalks extend from the heads to the cellular membrane, followed by transmembranous and cytoplasmic segments.

eight forms of the β chain have been identified; furthermore, several α chains have been shown to pair with more than one β subunit.

The VLA molecules or β_1 integrins (CD49a-f linked to CD29) display six different α chains (CD49a-f) that bind to the same β_1 chain (CD29). VLA-4 ($\alpha_4\beta_1$, CD49d CD29) mediates adhesion of T cells to endothelial cells by binding to VCAM-1. In addition, VLA-4 and VLA-5 ($\alpha_5\beta_1$, CD49e CD29) bind to fibronectin and VLA-6 ($\alpha_6\beta_1$, CD49f CD29) binds to laminin in the extracellular matrix. Such interactions may be important for the retention of T cells in the tissues after extravasation from the intravascular compartment. Further, the binding of VLA-4 to VCAM-1 and extracellular matrix proteins can provide costimulatory signals for T-cell activation.

The three β_2 integrins, LFA-1 (CD11a CD18), Mac-1 (CR3; CD11b CD18) and p150,95 (CR4; CD11c CD18); share the same β_2 subunit (CD18) that combines with three different α chains (CD11a, CD11b, CD11c). These molecules play an important role in the adhesion of lymphocytes to other cells, such as the APCs and vascular endothelium. Ligands for LFA-1 include ICAM-1 and ICAM-2 (members of the Ig gene superfamily). Mac-1 also binds to ICAM-1. Anti-LFA-1 antibodies inhibit a wide variety of lymphocyte functions, including APC-induced Th-cell activation and CTL target cell lysis. This is presumably caused by inhibition of the conjugate formation between the involved cells. TcR-specific stimulation results in functional modulation of integrins, resulting in an increase in their binding affinity to their corresponding ligands. The increased affinity may be caused by phosphorylation of the integrin intracytoplasmic tails. In addition, after ligand binding, integrins deliver stimulatory signals to cells. The critical role of the integrin function is demonstrated in the familial disease leukocyte deficiency–type 1, which occurs as a result of genetic mutation of the β chain (CD18). Afflicted individuals display a deficiency in all β_2 integrins, leading to recurrent bacterial and fungal infections as a result of lack of polymorphonuclear leukocyte accumulation and adhesion-dependent lymphocyte function.

Adhesion molecules play an important role in the migration of cells from the vascular compartment to the sites of inflammation.[24] Inflammatory cytokines (mainly TNF) induce this complex process leading to activation of endothelial cells that regulate the extravasation of neutrophils, monocytes, and T cells. Endothelial cells release vasodilators such as prostacyclin (PGI_2) and nitric oxide (NO), which increase blood flow at the inflammatory site. TNF production enhances PGI_2 synthesis, increases NO, production and induces endothelial cell surface E-selectin expression. E-selectin–mediated interaction with neutrophils results in slowing and *rolling* of cells (Fig. 5-13). Endothelial cell expression of VCAM-1 and ICAM-1, which occurs approximately 4 to 6 hours after the initiation of the inflammatory response, is critical for the *attachment* of leukocytes. The T-cell ligand for ICAM-1 is LFA-1 and that for VCAM-1 is VLA-4, whereas neutrophils engage ICAM-1 through Mac-1. Chemokines, secreted by the endothelial cells under the effect of TNF-α, such as IL-8 and monocyte chemotactic protein (MCP)–1 induce leukocyte flattening and cell locomotion. TNF-α and IFN-γ cause endothelial basement membrane changes that allow *migration* and extravasation of cells, as well as other macromolecules such as fibrinogen. Once leukocytes enter the tissues, VLA-4, VLA-5, and VLA-6 encourage cell binding to the extracellular matrix proteins.

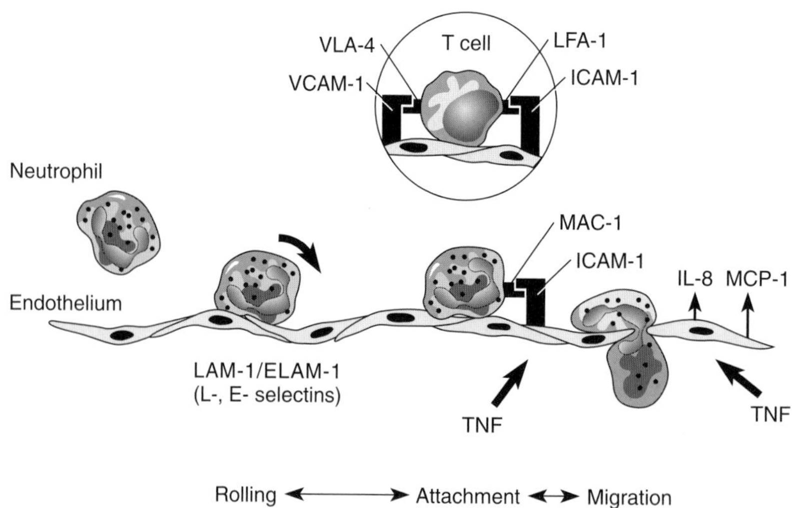

Fig. 5-13. Transendothelial migration of leukocytes. *1,* Rolling: inflammatory cytokines *(TNF)* induce the expression of L- and E-selectins on endothelial cells, which initiate rolling of leukocytes. *2,* Attachment: ICAM-1 expressed on endothelial cell surfaces binds to MAC-1 on neutrophils or LFA-1 on T cells. VCAM-1 engages VLA-4 on T cells. IL-8 and MCP-1 induce leukocyte conformational changes. *3,* Migration: attached leukocytes migrate into the interstitial space.

The extravasation of neutrophils and monocytes accompanied by the deposition of fibrin results in induration at the site of inflammation or graft rejection. Such induration is characteristic of a *delayed-type hypersensitivity (DTH)* reaction, which is apparent by 18 hours after the deposition of antigen eliciting the inflammatory response and reaches a maximum at 24 to 48 hours. Antigen-activated $CD8^+$ or $CD4^+$ T cells can adoptively transfer DTH-like reactions. Monocytes deposited in the tissues differentiate into macrophages, which are the main effector cells in DTH. IFN-γ is the main cytokine in DTH because of its macrophage-activating capacity. IFN-γ augments the phagocytic activity of macrophages and increases the expression of the high-affinity receptors for the Fc portion of Ig molecules, thereby enhancing phagocytosis of opsonized bacteria. Activated macrophages display more efficient APC function, express higher levels of class II, ICAM-1, and LFA-3, and release platelet-activating factor, prostaglandins, thrombin, transforming growth factor (TGF)–β, fibroblast growth factor (FGF), tissue factors that initiate the extrinsic clotting cascade, and other inflammatory mediators. DTH results in tissue destruction (necrosis) followed by angiogenesis and fibrosis when the antigen is eliminated.

T-cell activation

Two-signal hypothesis for T-cell activation. Activation of naive CD4 T cells may be the most important initial event in induction of alloimmunity. Activated CD4 Th cells secrete cytokines that act on a wide variety of cells and induce cytokine-mediated activation of CD8 cells, macrophages, and B cells. It is now widely believed that naive CD4 T cells require two distinct signals to proliferate and differentiate into a cytokine-producing effector cell.[18] The first signal is the alloantigen-specific stimulation provided by the MHC-peptide complexes and delivered by the TcR. The second signal, which is not antigen-specific, is termed a *costimulatory signal* because, although essential, it is not sufficient by itself to induce a T-cell response. When a T cell has its receptor ligated and receives a costimulatory signal, it will proliferate and differentiate into an effector cell. In contrast, T cells that bind antigen but do not receive a costimulatory signal are thought to die or become anergic (antigen-specific unresponsiveness). Thus the outcome of antigen/TcR interaction is dependent on the delivery of costimulatory signals.

CD28-mediated signaling provides costimulatory signals that prevent anergy induction of T cells[25] and induce T-cell proliferation when TcR binds antigen. Such characteristics provide an important distinction from other molecules, such as cell adhesion molecules or the coreceptor CD4 and CD8 molecules, which promote signaling through the TcR. The ligand for CD28 expressed on naive T cells is the B7.1 molecule present on APCs (Fig. 5-9). Thus B7.1 is a candidate costimulatory molecule. CTLA-4 is closely related to CD28 and binds B7.1 with a higher affinity than CD28. However, CTLA-4 is not expressed on naive T cells and therfore may not mediate naive T-cell activation but rather augment the activation process. The second ligand for CTLA-4/CD28 is the B7.2 molecule, which is readily expressed on the surface of APCs within minutes after activation, in contrast to B7.1, which is detected on the cell surfaces 24 hours after activation. Thus B7.2 may be the more important costimulator in naive T-cell activation. Multiple in vitro and in vivo data strongly support the costimulator role of the CD28/B7 system for both CD4 and CD8 cells. Anti-CD3 and anti-CD28 synergistically activate *c-jun* kinase, which in turn activates cytosolic components of the AP-1 transcription factor that is required for initiation of T-cell growth. Further, concurrent activation of TcR and CD28 enhances IL-2 transcription and stabilizes IL-2 messenger RNA (mRNA), thus increasing IL-2 production 100 times.[26] A sequence in the 5′ regulatory sequence of the IL-2 gene has been identified as a response element for CD28-mediated signaling, which presumably binds a transcription factor generated in response to those signals.

The heat-stable antigen (HSA), which is phosphoinositol-glycolipid linked glycoprotein, is a second molecule that meets both criteria for a costimulator. Although little it known about this molecule, anti-HSA blocks the proliferation of CD4 T cells and induces T cell anergy in vitro. The receptor for HSA on T cells remains unknown.

T-cell activation is facilitated by a number of other molecules, such as cytokines, coreceptor molecules (CD4, CD8), and adhesion molecules such as VCAM-1, ICAM-1, and LFA-3, which bind to VLA-4, LFA-1, and CD2, respectively, on T cells (see Fig. 5-9). Thus it is becoming clear that the two-signal hypothesis may be an oversimplification and that the TcR is not a simple on-off switch. T-cell activation may be regarded as a semiotic process in which the lymphocyte interprets signals delivered through the TcR in terms of the microenvironment generated by the presented peptide, costimulatory molecules, adhesion molecules, coreceptors, and cytokines.

Biochemical basis of T-cell activation. Within seconds of antigen recognition by T cells,[27] the tyrosine components in the antigen recognition activation motif of the CD3 complex are phosphorylated, which leads to the activtion of the enzyme *phosphatidylinositol phospholipase C-γ1 (PI-PLC-γ1).* Members of the *src* family of phosphotyrosine kinases such as *fyn* and *lck,* which are associated with CD4 and CD8 coreceptor molecules, or the CD3 ζ–associated protein (ZAP) kinase, have been implicated in the PI-PLC-γ1 phosphorylation (Fig. 5-14). PI-PLC-γ1 catalyses the hydrolysis of the plasma membrane phospholipid *phosphatidyl inositol 4,5-biphosphate ($PtInsP_2$, PIP_2)* leading to an increase in cytoplasmic levels of $PtdInsP_2$ breakdown products: *inositol 1,4,5-triphosphate (IP3)* and *diacylglycerol (DAG).* IP_3 causes a rapid rise of Ca^{2+} as a result of release of sequestered intracytoplasmic stores accompanying the influx of extracellular Ca^{2+}. Ca^{2+} combines with the ubiquitous calcium-dependent regulatory protein calmodulin (CaM) to form complexes that activate kinases and phosphatases such as calcineurin

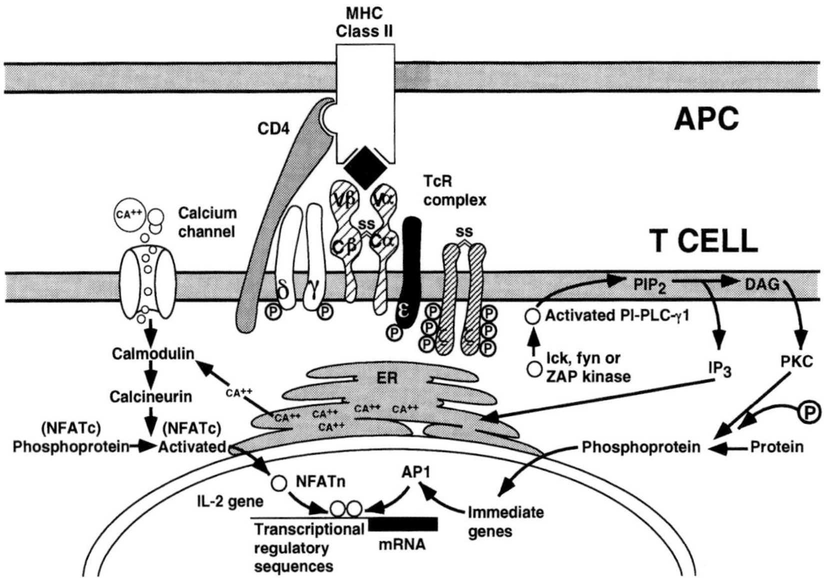

Fig. 5-14. Biochemical T-cell activation. After T-cell antigen recognition, phosphatidylinositol phospholipase C-γ_1 (○; PI-PLC-γ_1) is phosphorylated by the CD3ζ-associated protein (ZAP) kinase or by members of the *src* family of phosphotyrosine kinases (*lck* or *fyn*) associated with CD4 and CD8. Activated PI-PLC-γ_1 induces phosphatidyl inositol 4,5-biphosphate (PIP_2) hydrolysis to generate inositol 1,4,5-triphosphate (IP_3) and DAG. IP_3 causes a rapid rise of intracellular Ca^{2+} in addition to Ca^{2+} influx. Ca^{2+} combines with CaM to activate kinases and phosphatases. DAG and Ca^{2+} independently activate PKC, which rapidly phosphorylates multiple membrane and cytoplasmic proteins. Activated regulatory proteins such as the nuclear factor of activated T cells *(NFAT),* AP-1, and others induce the transcription of multiple genes encoding proto-oncogenes, cytokines, cytokine receptors, MHC products, and adhesion molecules. *APC,* Activated protein.

(CaN). The increase in Ca^{2+} and DAG independently activates *protein kinase C (PKC).*

Within minutes of antigen recognition, de novo transcription of more than 70 genes occurs. These are categorized as immediate, early, and late according to the time of activation during the T-cell response. The cellular protooncogenes *c-fos* and *c-myc* are in the immediate gene category. Their products act as trans-acting regulator proteins: *c-fos* combines with *c-jun* (which is induced by IL-1) to form the transcription activating protein AP-1. Cytokine gene transcripts appear within 4 hours after stimulation and are therfore classified in the early gene category. The most important cytokine is IL-2, which is essential for the mitotic activity of the T cell. The late gene category involves the transcription and expression of MHC products and adhesion molecules.

Alloimmune Recognition

Vigorous T-cell responses initiated by multiple T-cell clones expressing a wide variety of receptor genes in response to alloantigen is the essential component of graft rejection. In contrast to the low frequency of T cells (less than 0.1%) responding to other nominal antigens, as many as 10% of host T cells can respond to alloantigen. The molecular analysis of allorecognition included the dissection of the polymorphic MHC antigens that initiate the alloimmune response and the mechanisms of TcR recognition.[28]

Molecular basis of allorecognition. Immune induction requires the recognition of foreign donor antigens by responding host lymphocytes. The amino acid sequence variation between donor and recipient polymorphic class I or class II MHC alloantigens induces rejection. This variability is mainly confined to amino acids present on the top, sides, and floor of the peptide-binding groove of MHC molecules[2] (Fig. 5-15, *A*). Polymorphic amino acid residues within the peptide-binding groove serve as sites for peptide binding or TcR recognition, with the TcR recognizing a complex formed of a peptide anchored in the peptide-binding groove[29] (Fig. 5-15, *A*). Normally, thymic selection allows a T-cell repertoire that is tolerant to self-peptides presented on self-MHC (Fig. 5-15, *B, panel 1)* but is induced by foreign peptides presented on self-MHC molecules (Fig. 5-15, *B, panel 2).* Thus MHC-peptide complexes that exhibit amino acid differences from self-peptide-MHC complexes trigger the alloimmune response.[28]

T cells recognize alloantigens either as intact molecules expressed on the graft *(direct recognition)* or as processed allopeptides presented by the self-MHC *(indirect recognition).* Acute allograft rejection is conventionally thought to be mediated largely by direct recognition of allo–MHC-pep-

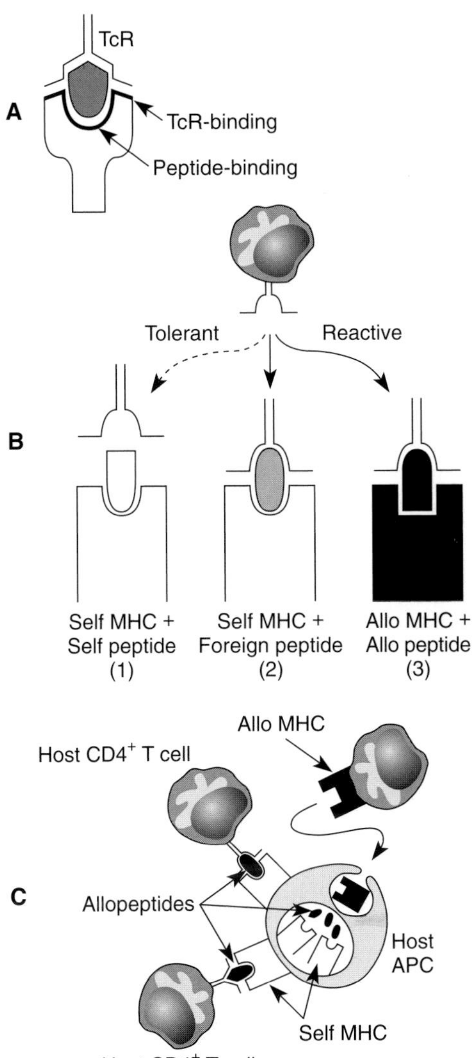

Fig. 5-15. Molecular basis of allorecognition. **A,** TcR recognition sites. Polymorphic amino acids present in the MHC peptide-binding groove (—) serve as sites for peptide and TcR binding. The TcR binds to amino acids present in both the peptide- and the MHC-binding grooves. **B,** Direct recognition. Host TcRs are tolerant of self-MHC molecules presenting self-peptides *(panel 1)* but are reactive to self-MHC molecules presenting foreign peptides *(panel 2)* or allo-MHC-peptide complexes that resemble foreign-peptide–self-MHC complexes *(panel 3).* **C,** Indirect recognition. MHC alloantigens are processed and presented as allopeptides on self-MHC molecules to stimulate host T cells.

tide complexes. However, recent evidence suggests that indirect recognition plays an important role in both the initiation and amplification of the rejection process.[30,31] In the model of direct recognition (Fig. 5-15, *B*), it is belived that the three-dimensional surface determinant formed by allo-MHC-peptide complex (Fig. 5-15, *B, panel 3)* resembles that of a foreign-peptide bound to self-MHC (Fig. 5-15, *B, panel 2),* which optimally binds to and activates host TcR, but differs from the self-MHC-peptide complex to which the T cell is tolerant (Fig. 5-15, *B, panel 1).* Thus direct recognition of alloantigens represents cross-reactivity for a TcR selected to recognize foreign antigen in the context of self-MHC. The presence of multiple amino acid differences between allo–MHC-peptide and self–MHC-peptide complexes generates numerous determinants that trigger multiple cross-reactive T-cell clones. An important concept arising from the direct recognition model is that alloreactive T cells are the same cells involved in foreign antigen recognition. Thus the allospecific and antigen-specific T-cell repertoires are one and the same.

In the indirect recognition model, class I or class II MHC alloantigens undergo cellular digestion, processing, and presentation as allopeptides by host APCs (Fig. 5-15, *C*) in a similar fashion to foreign antigens. Thus peptides derived from MHC alloantigens trigger the alloimmune response when presented on self class II. A single alloantigen may produce multiple peptides exhibiting variable lengths and amino acid composition. Each cell can display as many as 10^4 copies of an individual peptide and as many as 10^2 to 10^3 different peptides bound to the same MHC molecule.[28] Further, each peptide may specifically bind to different MHC molecules. It is estimated that a heterozygous individual can express 10 to 20 different class II and six different class I molecules per cell. Thus binding of numerous self-peptides to allo-MHC molecules, or conversely processing and presentation of multiple allopeptides derived from allo-MHC molecules on self-MHC molecules, results in a vast diversity of MHC-peptide complexes that differ from self-MHC-peptide complexes. This diversity accounts for the large number of T-cell clones responding to a single alloantigen. Nevertheless, several reports have observed that one or several Vβ segments of the responding TcRs recur with a high frequency,[32] suggesting the dominance of some epitopes displayed by the MHC-peptide complexes in triggering the alloimmune reaction. The model of indirect alloantigen recognition is currently under intense investigation because recent evidence suggests that modified MHC-derived allopeptides may deliver an inhibitory[33] rather than an immunogenic signal to the TcR that results in tolerance rather than rejection[34,35] of allografts.

Cellular basis of allorecognition. A unifying perspective in the alloimmune response is that rejection is initiated by disparate histocompatibility antigens (class I, class II, or both) that activate cytokine-producing Th cells and is executed by cytokine-dependent CTL, although many phenotypes of cells may participate. The mixed lymphocyte culture (MLC) reaction (Fig. 5-16) seems to provide an in vitro correlate of the in vivo rejection response to dissect the contribution of individual elements.

MLC reaction. A "two-way" allogeneic MLC is induced by culturing mononuclear leukocytes (T cells, B cells, mononuclear phagocytes, and dendritic cells) obtained from peripheral blood of one individual (donor cells) with a similar population of cells from another individual (recipient cells). These cultures display proliferation

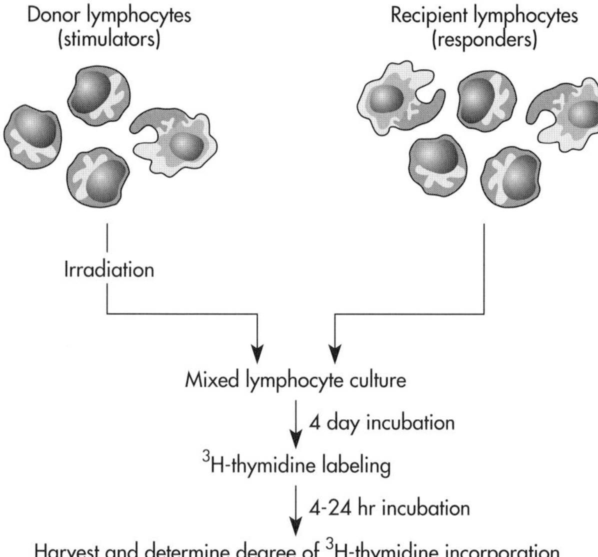

Fig. 5-16. Mixed lymphocyte culture (MLC) reaction. The MLC is an in vivo determination of histoincompatibility. Proliferative responses of responder lymphocytes toward donor stimulators are determined by tritiated-thymidine (^{3}H) incorporation.

of both cell populations if there are allelic differences at MHC loci. In a "one-way" MLC, donor lymphocytes are γ-irradiated to inhibit their proliferation, thereby allowing one to selectively measure the proliferative response of responder host cells (measured by tritiated thymidine incorporation) toward stimulator donor cells. Two major populations of alloreactive T cells emerge during the MLC. The first is IL-2-producing CD4$^+$ T cells specific for allogeneic class II molecules (HLA-DR, DP, and DQ), which undergo the proliferative response. In practice, HLA-D disparity is detected by the proliferative response of recipient to donor cells. The magnitude of the proliferative response seems to correlate well with the length of graft survival: living related donor-recipient combinations producing high MLC stimulation indicative of a significant class II antigen mismatch have a lower 1-year survival rate than do low MLC responders.[36] However, treatment with cyclosporine and prednisone resulted in excellent graft survival in MLC high-responder living related recipients.[36] The second cell type, CD8$^+$ T cells, functions as CTLs recognizing foreign class I MHC product, namely HLA-A, B, or C. Each individual CTL is specific for only one class I MHC gene product. However, the bulk population contains CTLs directed against most class I differences between the stimulators and responders. CTLs produce IL-2, IFN-γ, TNF-α, and LT. It is the cooperation between these two distinct cell populations that ultimately leads to allograft destruction. It is emphasized that the functional subdivision of alloreactive T cells into CD4$^+$ Th cells and CD8$^+$ CTLs is not absolute; both CD4$^+$ CTLs and CD8$^+$ Th cells have been identified as participating in MLC response.

Central Limb: Proliferation and Differentiation

Cytokine Network

Cytokines are a diverse group of proteins that regulate both the specific and nonspecific phases of the immune response. They are produced by a variety of cells and act on target cells in an autocrine (same secreting cell), paracrine (nearby cell), or endocrine (distant cell) fashion. Their short-lived effects are mediated by binding to high-affinity receptors on a wide variety of cells. Most cytokines are pleiotropic; that is, a single cytokine exhibits a wide range of biologic effects on various tissues and cells. Conversely, a single cell has different receptors for multiple cytokines and can interact with more than one cytokine. Cytokines also function in a redundant fashion; different cytokines act on the same cell to produce similar effects. This complex intercellular cytokine network allows T, B, or hemopoietic cells to be differentially activated and to produce varied responses.

According to origin, sequence of discovery, and chromosome location, cytokines have been subdivided as ILs, IFNs, colony-stimulating factors (CSFs), tumor necrosis factors (TNFs), TGFs, chemokines, and other growth factors[37] (Table 5-1). Structurally, cytokines may be grouped into large famiies that share conserved motifs or sequence homologies. For example hematopoietins comprise the set of molecules IL-2, IL-3, IL-4, IL-5, IL-6, IL-7, IL-9, and IL-12; granulocyte macrophage–CSF (GM-CSF); granulocyte-CSF (G-CSF); and erythropoietin. These molecules contain a four α-helix bundle motif that is also shared by growth hormone (GH), prolactin (PRL), and ciliary neurotrophic factor.[38] Similarly, IL-1α, IL-1β, FGF, and keratinocyte growth factor exhibit a β-trefoil motif, whereas nerve growth factor (NGF), TGF-β, and platelet-derived growth factor (PDGF) assume a cysteine knot motif (two pairs of antiparallel β strands anchored by three cysteine bridges).[39] Table 5-2 illustrates the most important cytokines and their prominent features. Functionally, cytokines may be organized into three broad, overlapping categories: cytokines that influence T- and B-cell activation, cytokines that mediate nonspecific immunity and inflammation, and cytokines that stimulate hematopoiesis.[40]

Cytokines that influence T- and B-cell activation

IL-2. IL-2, originally identified as a T-cell growth factor, is a 14 to 17 kd glycoprotein encoded by a single gene on chromosome 4. This molecule assumes a four α-helical structure and plays a key role in the development of T cells in the thymus as well as in the regulation of immune responses by promoting activation, autocrine growth, and paracrine growth of T cells. IL-2 also promotes B cell growth and antibody production and enhances the cytolytic activity of NK cells to produce the lymphocyte-activated killer (LAK) cells. IL-2 is transcribed, synthesized, and secreted by T cells upon antigenic stimulation, with a peak production at 24 hours after stimulation. Further, it stimulates the production of other T-cell cytokines such as IFN-γ and LT (TNF-β).

Table 5-1. Cytokine Families

Interleukins	Interferons	CSFs and TNFs	TGF-β	Chemokines	Growth Factors
IL-1 α, β	IFN-α	GM-CSF	TGF-β1	IL-8	EGF
IL-2	IFN-β	G-CSF	TGF-β2	MCP-1	TGF-α
IL-3	IFN-γ	M-CSF	TGF-β3		FGF
IL-4		EPO	TGF-β4		KGF
IL-5		TNF-α	TGF-β5		PDGF
IL-6		LT (TNF-β)	Activins		NGF
IL-7		LT-β	Inhibins		
IL-9			BMPs		
IL-10					
IL-11					
IL-12					

EPO, Erythropoietin; *BMP,* bone morphogenic protein; *EGF,* epidermal GF; *KGF,* keratinocyte GF.

Table 5-2. Major Cytokines and Their Features

Cytokine	Gene Number	Cell Source	Function
IL-1 (17 kd) Monomer	2 (IL-1α, IL-1β)	Macrophages, APCs	Facilitates activation of Th cells, acute-phase reactants
IL-2 (17 kd) Monomer	1	$CD4^+$ T cells	Autocrine and paracrine T-cell growth and differentiation, activation of NK and B cells
IL-3 (26 kd) Monomer	1	$CD4^+$ T cells	Growth and differentiation of hematopoietic stem cells
IL-4 (20 kd) Monomer	1	$CD4^+$ T cells	B-cell differentiation, IgE production, mast cell growth
IL-5 (20 kd) Homodimer	1	T cells	B-cell and eosinophil differentiation, IgA production
IL-6 (26 kd) Monomer	1	Macrophages, Th cells	B-cell differentiation, acute-phase reactants
IL-7 (25 kd) Monomer	1	Bone marrow, stromal cells	Growth and differentiation of B-cell progenitors
IL-10 (18 kd) Homodimer	1	T cells	Inhibit TNF, IL-1 production by macrophages, B-cell activation
IL-12 (40 kd) Heterodimer	2	Macrophages	Activation of NK cells, CTL activation, Th1 differentiation
Type I IFN (α, β) (18 kd) Monomer	20 IFN-α 1 IFN-β	Macrophages α, fibroblasts β	Inhibit viral replication, cell proliferation, increase class I expression and NK activity
Type II, IFN (IFN-γ) (24 kd) Homodimer	1	T cells	Activation of macrophages and T, B, NK, and endothelial cells; increase class I and class II expression, antiviral activity
TGF-β (14 kd) Homodimer	Multiple	Macrophages, T cells	Inhibition of macrophages and T cells
Chemokines (8 to 10 kd) Monomer	Multiple	Endothelial cells, T cells, phagocytes, fibroblasts	Leukocyte chemotaxis, activation
TNF (17 kd) Homotrimer	1	Macrophages, T cells	Activation of neutrophils, endothelial cells, fever acute-phase reactants, cachexia T- and B-cell stimulator
LT (TNF-β) (24 kd) Monomer	1	Activated T cells	Similar to TNF
GM-CSF (22 kd) Homodimer	1	Endothelial cells, T cells, phagocytes, fibroblasts	Acts on marrow progenitors for growth and differentiation of granulocytes and mononuclear phagocytes, granulocyte activation
M-CSF (40 kd)	1	Phagocytes, fibroblasts, endothelial cells	Differentiation to mononuclear phagocytes
G-CSF (19kd)	1	Phagocytes, fibroblasts, endothelial cells	Differentiation granulocytes

Mononuclear phagocytes include monocytes and macrophages; granulocytes include esinophils, basophils, and neutrophils.

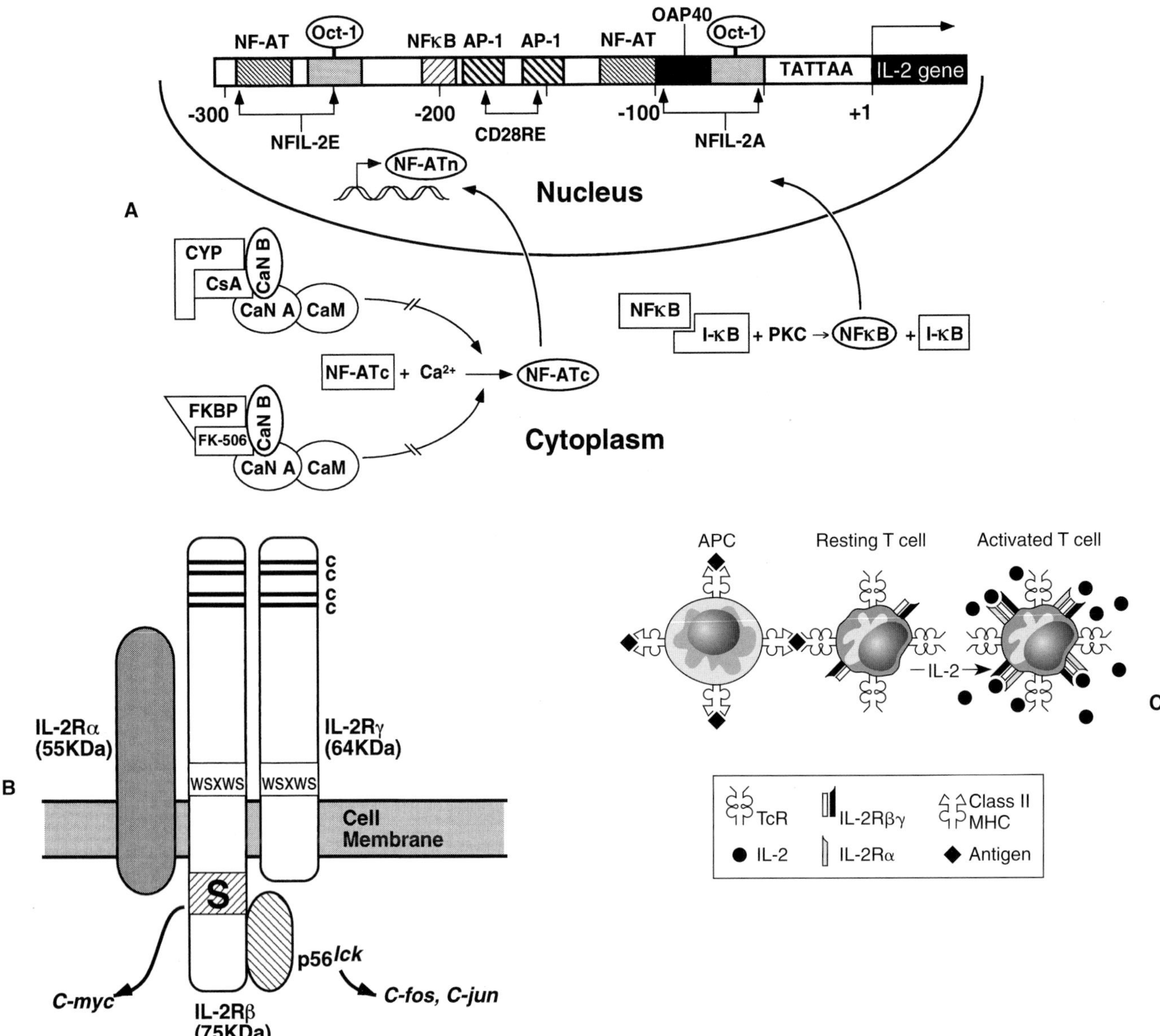

Fig. 5-17. Regulation of T-cell activation by the IL-2/IL-2R system. **A,** Regulatory sequences of the IL-2 gene. The promoter region of the IL-2 gene contains binding sites for the Oct-1, AP-1, OCT-1-activating protein (OAP), and NF-κB DNA-regulatory proteins. NFIL-2A and NFIL-2E sites bind Oct-1/OAP and NF-AT proteins, respectively. The pentameric complexes CaN A-CaN B-Ca^{2+}-CaM-CsA-CYP or CaN A-CaN B-Ca^{2+}-CaM-FK506-CYP prevent activation and nuclear migration of NF-ATc, which normally binds to NF-ATn to induce activation of the IL-2 promoter at the NFIL-2E site. **B,** IL-2R system. Three distinct chains (α, β, and γ) combine to form a high-affinity IL-2R. The IL-2Rβ and γ chains exhibit four membrane-distal conserved cysteine residues *(C)* and the membrane-proximal WSXWS (tryptophan-serine-X-tryptophan-serine) motif characteristic of type I cytokine receptors. *S,* Serine rich. **C,** IL-2R expression on T cells. Activation of T cells induces the expression of IL-2Rα in addition to IL-2Rβγ chains normally present on resting T cells.

IL-2 production after TcR-antigen recognition represents the paradigm of DNA regulatory proteins controlling critical growth events. Induction of IL-2 gene transcription is mediated by a regulatory region extending 300 base pairs upstream from the transcription start site (Fig. 5-17, *A*). This region contains DNA-binding sites for a number of nuclear proteins common to other promoters such as Oct-1, AP-1, and NF-κB. Oct-1 is a ubiquitous, non–T-cell–specific, constitutively expressed DNA-binding protein. AP-1 is composed of *c-jun* and *c-fos,* both of which are products of cellular proto-oncogenes. NF-κB is a nuclear protein necessary for the constitutive expression of the Ig κ light chain in B cells. After phosphorylation of its inhibitory protein (IκB) by PKC, NF-κB is activated, dimerized, and translocated into the nucleus to bind homologous DNA sequence elements. Two sequences in the IL-2 promoter appear to be particularly sensitive to the immunosuppressive drugs cyclosporine (CsA) and FK-506, the NFIL-2A site, which binds both Oct-1 and the inducible T-cell–specific protein called Oct-1–activating protein (see Fig. 5-17, *A*), and the NFIL-2E site, which binds the nuclear factor of activated T cells (NF-AT; Fig. 5-17, *A*). NF-AT is composed of nuclear (NF-ATn) and cytoplasmic (NF-ATc) subunits. On T-cell activation PKC phosphorylation allows de novo synthesis of NF-ATn subunit and a rise in intracellular Ca^{2+} allows activation of the preexisting NF-ATc component, followed by its translocation to the nucleus. In the nucleus both components form the active NF-AT-1 that binds the NFIL-2E site. Finally, a CD28-responsive element (CD28RE) has been identified. However, the nuclear factors modulating the function of the CD28RE are not well defined.

CsA and FK-506 bind to cytoplasmic proteins (*cis-trans* peptidyl-propyl isomerases; immunophilins) termed cyclophilin (CYP) and FK-binding protein (FKBP). These complexes bind to and inhibit cytoplasmic Ca^{2+} CaM–dependent serine-threonine phosphatases, CaNs A and B, that are necessary for dephosphorylation and activation of NF-ATc (Fig. 5-17, *A*). In addition, both CsA and FK-506 abolish transcription activation from the NFIL-2A (Oct-1) and NFIL-2E (NF-AT) sites, which are totally dependent on Ca^{2+}. Transcription driven by NF-κB is partially inactivated, whereas AP-1 effect is totally resistant to the drugs.[41] This demonstrates a striking relationship between Ca^{2+} mobilization and the effect of the drugs.

The effects of IL-2 on target cells are mediated by binding to the IL-2 receptor (IL-2R), which is made up of at least three distinct membrane components[42]: α chain (IL-2Rα, CD25, TAC, p55; 55 kd), β chain (IL-2Rβ, p75; 75 kd), and γ chain (IL-2Rγ; 65 kd; Fig. 5-17, *B*). The IL-2Rα is a low-affinity receptor that binds IL-2 with a K_a of 10^{-8}mol/L. It is not detected in resting T cells but is efficiently induced after T-cell stimulation. In contrast, the IL-2Rβ (K_d of 10^{-7} mol/L) is constitutively expressed on $CD8^+$ T-cells and is induced in $CD4^+$ Th cells on TcR activation. The IL-2Rγ is constitutively expressed by all lymphoid cells. The IL-2Rβ and γ are coordinately expressed to form a complex designated IL-2Rβγ. Both IL2Rβ and γ but not IL-2Rα, belong to the superfamily of type I cytokine receptors that share the WSXWS motif (tryptophan-serine-X-tryptophan-serine, where *X* is any amino acid). The IL-2Rβ component has a long cytoplasmic domain (286 aa) that contains a serine-rich region essential for induction of *c-myc* by IL-2. IL-2Rβ also interacts with the cytoplasmic tyrosine kinase $p56^{lck}$ of the *src* family, which links IL-2 activation with *c-jun* and *c-fos* (Fig. 5-17, *B*). IL-2Rα and β but not IL-2Rγ subunits bind IL-2. The heterotrimeric (α, β, γ) IL-2R complex triggers the activation of protein tyrosine kinases of the *src* family, including the $p56^{lck}$ and $p59^{fyn}$. When $p59^{fyn}$ is phosphorylated, it acquires a binding domain for the novel phosphatidyl inositol 3–kinase, which inserts a phosphate at the 3 position of inositol ring, thereby generating 3-phosphorylated phosphoinositides (PI-3-P, PI-3,4-P_2, and PI-3,4,5-P_3) that function as growth and division signals and may activate the ubiquitous c-Raf serine-threonine kinase.

In humans, expression of different combinations of α, β, and γ components of the IL-2R yields different IL-2R isoforms with different binding affinities for IL-2 (Table 5-3). The combination of γ and β chains is required for IL-2R signal transduction after binding to IL-2; addition of the α chain is required to produce a receptor with a high IL-2 binding affinity. It is believed that in activated T cells binding of the newly expressed IL-2Rα with IL-2Rβγ increases the affinity of the complex for IL-2 to K_d of 10^{-11} mol/L, thus producing signal transduction at extremely low IL-2 concentrations (Fig. 5-17, *C*), whereas resting T cells expressing only the IL-2Rβγ complex require higher amounts of IL-2.

IL-4, IL-5, and IL-10. IL-4 (20 kd), originally described as a B-cell growth and differentiation factor, is produced by the Th_2 subset of CD4 T cells. It is the principal cytokine that promotes the switching of Bμ (IgM)– to $B\gamma_1$ (IgG_1)– or Bε (IgE)–producing B cells and induces mast cell proliferation. Thus IL-4 plays a critical role in the induction of immediate hypersensitivity reactions including anaphylaxis, hay fever, asthma, and eczema, and it is abnormally elevated in individuals affected by atopy. In addition, IL-4 inhibits switching to IgG_{2a}, thus opposing the

Table 5-3. Avidity of IL-2 Binding to IL-2R Subunits

Subunit	IL-2 Binding (kd mol/L)	IL-2 Signal
α	10^{-8}m	–
β	10^{-7}m	–
αβ	10^{-10}m	–
γ	—	–
αγ	10^{-8}m	–
βγ	10^{-9}m	+
αβγ	10^{-11}m	+

effect of IFN-γ, which augments the production of IgG_{2a}. It is the primary cytokine that preferentially promotes the development of naive T cells into Th_2 cells. IL-4 also inhibits macrophage activation and antagonizes most of the effects of IFN-γ. IL-5 is a 40 kd homodimer produced by the Th_2 subset that stimulates the growth and differentiation of eosinophils, thus playing an important role in host defense against helminthic infections. IL-5 complements the activities of IL-4 and IL-10 to promote IgE and IgG_4 switching, respectively. IL-10 (18 kd), which is produced by Th_2 cells, functions as a switching factor for B cells to produce IgG_4 and as an inhibitor of T-cell–mediated immune responses. It inhibits production of TNF, IL-1, IL-12, IL-2, and IFN-γ and reduces class II and B7 expression, thereby inhibiting the APC function of macrophages.

IL-12. IL-12, a 70 kd heterodimer produced by many cell types including T and B cells, monocytes, and NK cells, stimulates the differentiation of naive T cells into the Th_1 subset. It is the most potent stimulator of NK cells and enhances the differentiation of $CD8^+$ T cells into mature CTLs.

The study of murine T-cell clones has yielded the presently popular paradigm of lymphokine biology (Fig. 5-18), which subdivides the Th cell population into Th_1 or Th_2. Th_1 clones tend to produce IFN-γ, IL-2, and TNF-β, whereas the Th_2 subsets produce IL-4, IL-5, IL-6, IL-10, and IL-13.[43] Cytokine priming in vitro causes precursor Th (pTh) cells to differentiate into Th_1 or Th_2 elements. Th_2 cells could be generated if both IL-2 and IL-4 are used for priming. In the absence of IL-4, pTh clones are driven by IL-12 into the Th_1 pathway. Further, IL-12 and IL-14 can block the Th_2 and Th_1 differentiation pathways, respectively. However, cytokine profiles are not mutually exclusive; some clones produce IL-2, IFN-γ, and IL-4. These cells have been designated *pTho* and are thought to be mulipotential elements that may represent an intermediate step in the differentiation of pTh cells into Th_1 or Th_2 lineages. Recent reports have documented such functional dichotomy in vivo.

TGF-β. A family of closely related molecules encoded by distinct genes are designated TGF-β. At least five isoforms (TGF-β1 through TGF-β5) display similar effects on a wide variety of cells. Cells of the immune system primarily synthesize TGF-β1, a 28 kd homodimeric protein that acts mainly as an inhibitory cytokine on T-cell proliferation, CTLs, macrophages, and polymorphonuclear leukocytes, therby counteracting the effects of proinflammatory cytokines (IFN-γ, IL-2). Thus TGF-β may provide a signal for shutting off the immune response.

Cytokines mediating non-specific immunity and inflammation

IFNs

TYPE I IFNs. These include two distinct groups of proteins. The first includes 20 structurally related polypeptides (18 kd) encoded by separate genes and collectively known as IFN-α. The second group, IFN-β, consists of a single 20 kd glycoprotein gene product. IFN-α is produced by mononuclear phagocytes, whereas fibroblasts are the major cell source for IFN-β. Type I interferons inhibit viral replication and increase the lytic potential of NK cells targeting virally infected cells. Both IFN-α and IFN-β induce class I but not class II MHC expression, thereby enhancing the efficiency of CTL-mediated killing.

TYPE II (IMMUNE OR GAMMA) IFN. IFN-γ, a 24 kd homodimer glycoprotein produced by CD4 (Th_1) and CD8 T cells, exhibits all the antiviral effects of type I IFNs. In addition, IFN-γ is the major macrophage-activating factor and provides the means by which T cells induce macrophages. It augments the phagocytic activity of mononuclear phagocytes by enhancing the synthesis of enzymes mediating the respiratory burst. IFN-γ increase

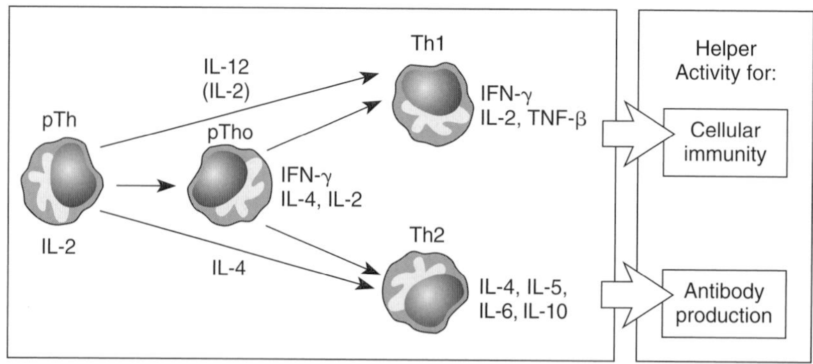

Fig. 5-18. Cytokine-induced differentiation of pT helper cell clones. pTho clones produce IL-2, IFN-γ, and IL-4. Th1 clones secrete IL-2, IFN-γ, and TNF-β to induce cellular immunity. Th2 clones mediate help for humoral immunity by the predominant production of IL-4, IL-5, IL-6, and IL-10. IL-4 induces Th2; IL-12 and IL-2 induce Th1 differentiation from pTh precursors. The multipotential pTho populations may represent an intermediate step in the development of Th1 and Th2 from pTh cells.

both class I and class II MHC expression on a wide variety of cells, promotes the differentiation of T and B cells, augments the production of IgG_{2a} and inhibits isotype switching to IgE, and activates neutrophils, NKs, and vascular endothelial cells.

TNF. TNF, often referred to as *TNF-α,* is initially synthesized as a 25 kd transmembrane protein with the amino-terminus oriented intracellularly and the carboxy-terminus oriented extracellularly. A 17 kd fragment is proteolytically cleaved from plasma membranes of mononuclear phagocytes to form stable "secreted" 51 kd homotrimers that bind cell-surface TNF receptors. TNF binds to two distinct 55 and 57 kd receptors that are present on almost every cell examined.

TNF is the principal mediator of the host response to gram-negative sepsis. Increasing evidence implicate the lipid A component of the lipopolysaccharide (LPS) endotoxin derived from the gram-negative bacterial cell wall as the active inducer of sepsis. The effects of TNF, like those of LPS, are best understood as a function of quantity. LPS at low concentrations induces nonspecific polyclonal B-cell proliferation and enhances mononuclear phagocytosis, contributing to elimination of the invading bacteria. At high concentrations, however, LPS precipitates tissue injury, disseminated intravascular coagulopathy (DIC), shock, and even death. At low quantities (10^{-9} mol/L), TNF acts *locally* on leukocytes and endothelial cells to enhance elimination of invading pathogens. It stimulates the expression of adhesion molecules on neutrophils, monocytes, lymphocytes, and endothelial cells, resulting in extravasation of cells to the sites of inflammation. It is a potent activator of neutrophils and induces IL-1, IL-6, TNF, and chemokine production. Further, it increases class I expression, thus enhancing CTL-mediated lysis of target cells. With increasing TNF production, it enters the circulation where it acts *systemically* in an endocrine fashion to induce fever, elevate serum levels of IL-1 and IL-6, and initiate metabolic wasting (cachexia). Fever results from prostaglandin synthesis by cytokine-driven hypothalamic cells and is therefore blocked by prostaglandin synthesis inhibitors such as aspirin. TNF acts on hepatocytes to produce the *acute-phase response* characterized by increased synthesis of C-reactive protein, α_2 macroglobulin, amyloid A, and fibrinogen while decreasing the production of albumin and transferrin. In gram-negative sepsis, massive quantities of TNF (10^{-7} mol/L) result in DIC, reduced tissue perfusion, hypoglycemia, vasodilatation, and circulatory collapse. TNF induces the NO synthetase present in myocardial and endothelial cells that converts arginine into citrulline and NO resulting in myocardial suppression and vascular smooth muscle dilatation.

LT. LT (TNF-β), a 24 kd glycoprotein, is 30% homologous to TNF and competes with TNF for binding to the same cell surface receptors. LT exhibits similar biologic effects to TNF. It is a potent activator of neutrophils and vascular endothelial cells, causing increased leukocyte adhesion, cytokine production, and leukocyte extravasation. Unlike TNF, LT acts locally in a paracrine fashion, does not mediate systemic tissue injury, and is produced exclusively by activated T cells. Recently, a third member of TNF/LT family, termed *LT*-β, has been described. It appears to have similar characteristics to LT.

IL-1. The IL-1 family includes two separate polypeptide products, IL-1α and IL-1β, encoded by two separate genes. Although the two forms are only 30% homologous, they bind to the same cell-surface receptors and mediate similar biologic functions. Both polypeptides are produced as 33 kd precursors that are proteolytically cleaved to mature 17 kd products. IL-1 was originally described as a co-stimulator of T cells derived from macrophages. It is now clear, however, that the principal function of IL-1 is to act as a mediator of inflammation in a similar fashion to TNF. Like TNF, IL-1 is produced by activated mononuclear phagocytes triggered by lipopolysaccharide, TNF, or IL-1 itself. At low concentrations it exhibits the local inflammatory properties of TNF. IL-1 does not activate neutrophils, however, but induces the production of chemokines by macrophages and endothelial cells. At high concentrations, it enters the circulation to induce manifestations similar to those of TNF.

IL-1 is the only cytokine that exhibits naturally occurring inhibitors. The biologically inactive IL-1 receptor antagonist (IL-1Ra), which is structurally homologous to IL-1, is secreted by activated mononuclear phagocytes to compete with binding of IL-1 to its receptors, thereby downregulating the biologic response to IL-1. The use of such antagonists may be clinically beneficial in diseased states characterized by overactivity of cytokines, such as septic shock.

IL-6. IL-6, a 26 kd protein, is produced by activated mononuclear phagocytes, fibroblasts, T cells, and vascular endothelial cells. IL-6 may be secreted in the circulation during gram-negative sepsis in response to IL-1 and TNF stimulation, rather than to lipopolysaccharide. Unlike TNF and IL-1, IL-6 does not cause tissue injury but induces the synthesis of acute phase proteins by hepatocytes. IL-6 functions as a major B-cell growth and differentiation factor.

Chemokines. A recently identified large family of structurally related homologous cytokines (8 to 10 kd), chemokines stimulate leukocyte movement (chemokinesis) or directed leukocyte trafficking (chemotaxis). Two subfamilies are identified according to whether the amino-terminal cysteine residues are in close proximity (cys-cys motif) or are separated (cys-X-cys motif). IL-8 is the best characterized member of the first subfamily, whereas MCP-1 belongs to the second family. Chemokines are secreted by mononuclear phagocytes, endothelial cells, fibroblasts, and activated T cells. They bind to heparan sulfate proteoglycans on the endothelial cell surfaces to stimulate chemokinesis of leukocytes that bind to cytokine-activated endothelium through adhesion molecules (see Fig. 5-13).

Cytokines stimulating hematopoiesis

IL-3, IL-7, IL-9, and IL-11. IL-3 (20 to 26 kd) is a multilineage CSF produced by both Th_1 and Th_2 subsets of CD4 T cells that acts on most immature bone marrow progenitors to stimulate differentiation into all mature hematopoietic cell types. IL-7 (25 kd) is a cytokine produced by bone marrow stromal cells that acts on hematopoeitic progenitors committed to the B-cell lineage. It may also stimulate the growth and differentiation of $CD4^-$ $CD8^-$ T-cell precursors in the thymus. IL-9 supports the growth of T- and mast-cell progenitors. IL-11 is a 20 kd protein produced by bone marrow stromal cells that stimulates megakaryopoiesis. It is being examined for its therapeutic benefits in platelet deficiency disorders.

CSFs. GM-CSF (22 kd) is produced by activated T cells, mononuclear phagocytes, fibroblasts, and endothelial cells. GM-CSF acts on marrow progenitors already committed to leukocyte lineages and therefore may act at a later stage than IL-3. In peripheral tissues GM-CSF mainly functions as an activator of mature leukocytes at inflammatory sites. Therapeutically, recombinant GM-CSF has been used to stimulate hematopoiesis after chemotherapy or bone marrow transplantation. Monocyte-macrophage CSF (M-CSF; 40 kd) and G-CSF (19 kd) promote the differentiation of progenitors committed to develop into monocytes and granulocytes, respectively.

Cytokine Receptors

Cytokine receptor families. Most cytokine receptors consist of multichain complexes, including a private ligand-specific receptor and a public class-specific transducer.[38] Sequence analysis of ligand-specific cytokine receptor chains has revealed that all receptors are integral membrane glycoproteins oriented with the amino terminus facing outside the cell, followed by a transmembrane segment. The ligand-specific receptor chains have been classified into five large families on the basis of the presence of conserved motifs and sequence homologies among their extracellular domains.

Type I cytokine receptors—Hemopoietic growth factor receptors. Hematopoietins, including IL-2, IL-3, IL-4, IL-5, IL-6, IL-7, IL-9, IL-12, GM-CSF, G-CSF, erythropoietin, PRL, and GH, all share a similar four α-helical bundle motif in which the first and second helices run parallel and the third and fourth parallel helices are antiparallel to the first pair (four α-helical bundle with two crossovers). In addition, they all bind to ligand-specific receptor chains that exhibit a common structural motif (Fig. 5-19). The membrane-distal domain contains a set of four spaced cysteines, whereas the membrane-proximal domain contains a conserved sequence of five amino acid residues, tryptophan-serine-X-tryptophan-serine (WSXWS), where *X* is any amino acid. The IL-6R exhibits an Ig-like domain in the membrane-distal domain in addition to the sequence characteristic of type I receptors. Most of the hematopoietins induce protein tyrosine phosphorylation on receptor binding. However, none of their ligand-specific receptors exhibit tyrosine kinase in their cytoplasmic domains, suggesting the association of their receptors with other components for signal transduction.

Type II cytokine receptors—IFN receptors (IFNRs). IFN-α and IFN-β share a common receptor that does not exhibit sequence homology with the IFN-γR. However, a conserved motif was identified in a segment of approximately 200 amino acids. The IFN-α/βR has two of such domains, whereas IFN-γR has one (see Fig. 5-19). These consensus domains contain conserved four cysteine residues clustered in **C**-X-N-X_3-T-X-**C**-X-Y and Y-**C**-K-X_2-A-X_{10}-V-X-S-X_3-**C**-X_2-T, where *X* is a nonconserved amino acid. The IFNRs appear to be evolutionarily related to type I receptors. Both the IFN-α/βR and the IFN-γR require association with other subunits for signal transduction.

Type III cytokine receptors—TNF receptors (TNFRs). TNF-α and TNF-β exhibit highly similar overall structures, despite their relatively low sequence homology

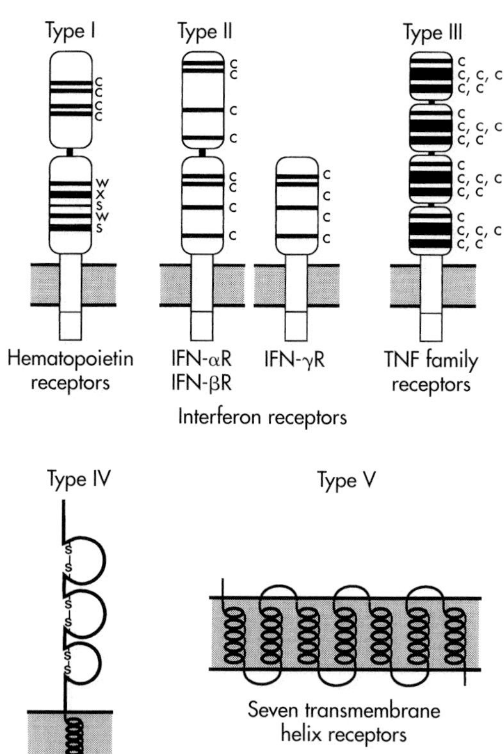

Fig. 5-19. Cytokine receptor families. Hematopoietins (IL-2, IL-3, IL-4, IL-5, IL-6, IL-7, IL-9, IL-12, GM-CSF G-CSF, erythropoietin, PRL, and GH) bind to type I ligand-specific receptors characterized by four cysteines in the membrane-distal domain and the WSXWS (tryptophan-serine-X-tryptophan-serine) motif in the membrane-proximal domain. Type II interferon receptors include consensus domains characterized by four cysteine residue clusters. Two consensus domains are present in IFN-αR and IFN-βR, whereas IFN-γR contains one consensus domain. TNF-α and TNF-β bind to type III TNF receptors that display a characteristic 6-cysteine consensus motif repeated four times. Type IV Ig-like receptors contain multiple Ig domains. Type V receptors consists of seven transmembrane α-helical structures. *C*, Conserved cysteines.

(33%). However, both cytokines compete for binding to two receptors, TNF-R55 and TNF-R75, that have clear sequence similarities in the extracellular binding domains (see Fig. 5-19). Both receptors contain a characteristic 6-cysteine consensus motif repeated four times.[44] The TN-FRs are homologous to the CD40 antigen of B cell and NGF receptor (NGFR).

Type IV cytokine receptors—Ig-like receptors. Typical receptors of this family are the IL-1Rs. Two types of IL-1R have been identified; the first is expressed on T cells and has a slightly higher affinity for IL-1β, while the second is present on B cells and exhibits a slightly greater affinity for IL-1α. Both types of receptors contain Ig domains (Fig. 5-19) and can bind to IL-1α and IL-1β. This Ig-like motif is also present on PDGF receptor (PDGFR) and FGF receptor (FGFR).

Type V cytokine receptors—Seven transmembrane helical receptors. This seven transmembrane spanning α-helical structure is displayed by chemokine receptors (see Fig. 5-19). This motif was originally described for β-adrenergic receptors and rhodopsin and is widely shared by receptors that are coupled to guanosine triphosphate (GTP)–binding proteins.

Pleiotropy and redundancy. The functional pleiotropy and redundancy of the various cytokines may be explained by sharing of common signal transducer chains by different receptor complexes. The IL-6 ligand-specific receptor (80 kd) exhibits two distinct segments, an Ig-like structure linked to a type I cytokine receptor. On binding to IL-6, the 80 kd IL-6R chain associates with a 130 kd membrane glycoprotein, gp130, that provides signal transduction.[37] Oncostatin, leukemia inhibitory factor, and IL-11, which share functional similarities with IL-6 including induction of acute-phase proteins in hepatocytes, osteoclast activation, and induction of megakaryocytes and platelet formation, were found to use gp130 for signal transduction. Similarly, the functions of IL-3 and GM-CSF overlap in various hematopoietic cells: both induce GM colonies, activate monocytes, and stimulate eosinophil colonies, with the last effect being shared by IL-5. These experimental observations can be explained by the fact that IL-3, IL-5, and GM-CSF receptors all use a common signal transducer termed *KH97* in humans. The IL-2 receptor system consists of α, β, and γ chains (see Fig. 5-17, *B*). The IL-2R β and γ subunits are members of the type I cytokine receptors, whereas the α chain is structurally unrelated to any identified receptor family. The IL-2R γ chain, which is important for cytokine signal transduction, has been shown to participate in the formation of a high-affinity IL-4R complex and in IL-4 signal transduction.[38] The sharing of the IL-2R γ chain by IL-2R and IL-4R systems may explain the redundant function of both cytokines on T cells.

Efferent Limb: Immune Mediators and Graft Destruction

The rejection process (Table 5-4), which is initiated by antigen recognition and lymphocyte activation, is ultimately effected by (1) antigen-specific cytotoxic T cells reacting specifically with class I antigen-bearing cells; (2) non–antigen-specific effector cells activated by a lymphokine mechanism;[45] or (3) humoral antibodies, including a variety of complement-dependent and lymphocyte-dependent moieties. Clinically, graft rejection is classified on the basis of its timing as *hyperacute, accelerated, acute, or chronic.*

Hyperacute Rejection

Hyperacute rejection is characterized by cessation of graft function minutes to hours after graft revascularization. This form of rejection is thought to be secondary to host presensitization; that is, to the presence of host preformed an-

Table 5-4. Summary of Rejection Process

Rejection	Time Course	Clinical Signs and Symptoms	Mechanism	Pathology	Response to Therapy
Hyperacute	Sudden onset, minutes or hours after vascularization	Abrupt loss of function; no perfusion	Humoral with preformed anti-HLA antibodies	Fibrin thrombi within arterioles, endothelial sloughing, platelet aggregation	− Irreversible
Accelerated	Rapid loss of function 72 to 100 hr after transplantation	Abrupt loss of function; tender, swollen graft	Cellular presensitization, destruction by specific Tc cells or ADCC	Interstitial hemorrhage, fibrinoid necrosis of small arterial vessels	±
Acute	First 3 months after transplantation	Graft swelling, fever, and oliguria	Cellular; Tc cells and DTH mechanism	Interstitial and perivascular mononuclear infiltration, tubulitis, and interstitial edema	+ Reversible
Chronic	Gradual decline in graft function	Progressive loss of function, hypertension, glomerulopathy	Humoral	Obliterative vascular changes, interstitial fibrosis	− Irreversible

ADDC, Antibody-dependent cell-mediated cytotoxicity.

tidonor antibodies. Further, it is not amenable to any form of pharmacologic immunosuppressive agents. A classic setting for hyperacute rejection is ABO incompatibility, wherein circulating antidonor hemagglutinins rapidly thrombose the graft after binding to endothelial cells and through the Fc tails activate complement. Damaged endothelial cells secrete high-molecular weight forms of von Willebrand factor, which mediates platelet adhesion, platelet aggregation, and granulocyte activation. Although anti-ABO antibodies do not present a clinical problem because of pretransplant ABO typing, preformed antibodies toward HLA or endothelial E-M antigens are the more usual causes of hyperacute rejection. These antibodies may be induced by prior transplants, blood transfusion, or pregnancy. Correlation between a positive pretransplant microcytotoxicity crossmatch (an assay for detection of recipient antidonor antibodies) and the occurrence of hyperacute rejection is well documented.[46] Pretransplant testing of recipients for antidonor antibodies has markedly reduced the incidence of hyperacute rejection in clinical allotransplantation. On the one hand, renal and heart transplants are particularly susceptible to hyperacute rejection. Thus a negative T-cell crossmatch and ABO compatibility are usual prerequisites. On the other hand, the liver is less susceptible to hyperacute rejection, and liver transplants have been performed in the face of ABO incompatibility and positive crossmatches.

Microscopically, hyperacutely rejected transplants show fibrin thrombi within the small arteries and arterioles, capillary dilation, endothelial cell sloughing, platelet aggregation, and adhesion of polymorphonuclear leukocytes. Both animal and human renal allograft studies suggest that rejection is initiated by a primary immune injury to the vascular endothelium. Circulating antibodies bind specifically to the class I histocompatibility antigens exposed on the vascular endothelial cell surface and activate complement. Platelet aggregation and subsequent release of platelet factors and vasoactive substances occur at the site of injury. The initial vasoconstrictive response progresses to thrombosis after aggregation of platelets, red blood cells, and polymorphonuclear leukocytes, followed by fibrin deposition. The ischemic cascade obviates perfusion to the transplanted organ. Sometimes the reaction is not immediate, but rather occurs 24 to 48 hours after transplantation, in which case it is referred to *delayed hyperacute rejection*. Presumably these cases reflect initial low titers of antibodies with a prompt secondary response. Thus delayed hyperacute rejection appears to be the result of a qualitatively weaker immune response than that which causes hyperacute rejection.

Accelerated Rejection

Accelerated rejection frequently produces rapid loss of graft function; in many cases, it is refractory to antirejection therapy. The graft usually functions satisfactorily for 72 to 100 hours before graft function declines precipitously. Histologically, there are vascular lesions of capillary disruption with interstitial hemorrhage, hemorrhagic infarcts, and fibrinoid necrosis of small arterial vessels. Two pathogenic mechanisms appear to mediate the response: cellular presensitization with rapid graft destruction by specific CTLs or a secondary antibody production of a moiety that depends on lymphocytes to execute cytotoxicity (antibody-dependent cell-mediated cytotoxicity). In such a reaction, antibody acts as a bridge between donor tissue and CTLs, an interaction that results in activation of the lytic mechanism of the CTL with subsequent tissue destruction.

Acute Rejection

Acute rejection, unlike the accelerated or hyperacute mechanisms, tends to be reversible with therapy. Acute rejection episodes ar the most common type, affecting 30% of renal allografts and usually occurring during the first 3 months after surgery, with a peak incidence at 5 weeks. Acute rejection is uncommon after the first year unless there is lack of compliance with the drug regimen by the patient or inappropriate reduction of immunotherapy by the physician.

The clinical features of cell-mediated renal allograft rejection, including graft swelling and tenderness, fever, oliguria, and hypertension, are rarely obscured in the CsA era. Laboratory assessment reveals an increased serum creatinine level, and the diagnosis may be confirmed by percutaneous needle biopsy. However, attenuation of the clinical picture by CsA therapy has led to greater reliance on laboratory data and imaging studies. The greatest dilemma is the differentiation between acute rejection and CsA-induced nephrotoxicity. Further, anuria secondary to acute tubular necrosis (ATN) may occur immediately after operation or within the first few weeks after transplantation. In general, a 25% rise in serum creatinine level demands immediate evaluation.[47] Imaging studies include the evaluation of the physiologic status of the allograft by nuclear renograms or ultrasonographic examination enhanced by color-flow Doppler (CFD) measurement. Nuclear renograms include three phases that use two radiolabeled compounds (^{99m}Tc-labeled diethylenetriaminepentaacetic acid (DTPA) and ^{99m}Tc-labeled mercaptoacetyltriglygine (MAG3). The first phase evaluates *renal perfusion,* which should be evident within 4 seconds of the aortic blush after the administration of ^{99m}Tc-DTPA. The second phase quantitates *graft flow* by the interval between injection and the appearance of parenchymal activity. The third phase evaluates the *excretory function* by comparing the amount of the isotope in the bladder relative to that in the graft. In acute rejection, there is decreased perfusion, poor parenchyma uptake, and poor excretion. Good perfusion with impaired parenchymal uptake is common in ATN. The findings in early CsA toxicity are similar to those of ATN. In severe CsA toxicity, altered perfusion may be present as a result of the α-agonist effect of CsA. Thus the diagnosis of CsA toxicity is tentative until rejection and ATN have been ruled out. Ultrasonographic examination with CFD accurately detects allograft swelling common to both ATN and rejection, but it is less helpful than nuclear scans in differentiating the entities. It also demonstrates ureteric or renal pelvic dilatation caused by obstruction or accumulation of perinephric fluid collections that contribute to the declining renal allograft function. CFD sensitively detects the increase in vascular resistance associated with rejection but not an early feature of CsA toxicity. CFD is operator dependent, however, and the evaluation of acute rejection often demands histopathologic examination.

Histologic features of acute rejection include prominent interstitial and perivascular mononuclear infiltrates with interstitial edema and tubulitis (Fig. 5-20, *A*). Macrophages and T lymphocytes, specifically CTLs, are the predominant infiltrating cell types. In addition, CD4 helper cells mediating delayed-type hypersensitivity mechanisms are important contributors. Significant interstitial cellular infiltration with moderate tubulitis (>4 mononuclear cells/tubular cross-section) constitute grade I, or mild, acute rejection. Grade II, or moderate, rejection demonstrates significant interstitial infiltration, severe tubulitis, and/or intimal arteritis, whereas severe, or grade II, rejection involves transmural arteritis, medial smooth muscle necrosis, and/or focal infarction and interstitial hemorrhage. In mild-to-moderate cellular rejection, two cell types predominate within the interstitial cellular infiltrates[48]: macrophages comprising 40% to 50%, and T lymphocytes comprising 30% to 40%. Microscopically, infiltrating T cells include CTLs bearing the CD8 cell surface marker and Th CD4 cells. In severe cellular rejection, the cellular infiltrate is composed of 60% macrophages, 20% to 30% polymorphonuclear leukocytes, and 15% T lymphocytes, most of which are Tc cells. Although there are no classic histologic changes of acute CsA toxicity, inclusion bodies, peritubular capillary congestion, tubular vacuolization, microcalcifications, and thrombotic microangiopathy have been described. ATN is a difficult histologic diagnosis, although swelling of tubular cells and disrupted tubulues in the absence of signs of rejection or drug toxicity are helpful observations.

A

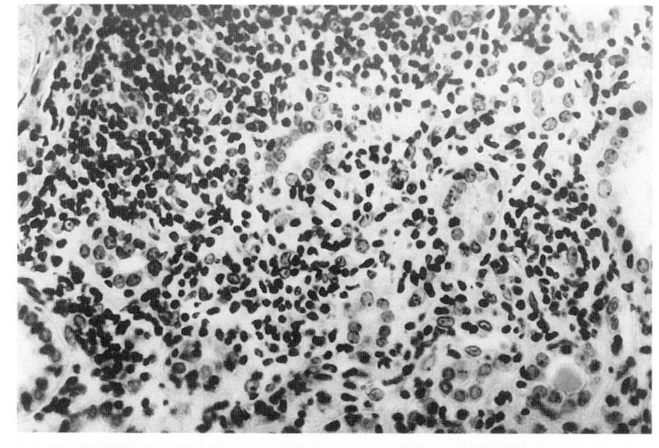

B

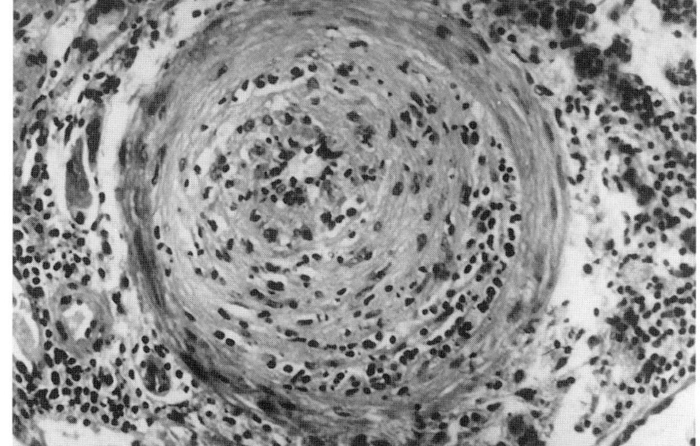

Fig. 5-20. Renal allograft rejection. **A,** Acute rejection demonstrating prominent interstitial and perivascular mononuclear infiltrates with interstitial edema. **B,** Chronic rejection characterized by interstitial fibrosis and obliterative vascular changes.

After activation of CD4 and CD8 lymphocytes, circulating immune cells recognize the allograft at the periphery. The CD4 cells play a critical role by releasing lynphokines that recruit and activate immunologically incompetent lymphocytes and macrophages toward the allograft through a delayed-type hypersensitivity mechanism. This mechanism is specific, although the target cytotoxic cell activated by lymphokines is not. On the one hand, the delayed-type hypersensitivity effector CD4 cell does not directly mediate allograft damage but secretes LTs responsible for cellular destruction and lymphokines that attract and activate macrophages, lymphocytes, and NK cells to produce cellular necrosis. On the other hand, Tc CD8 lymphocytes display specific activity against class I alloantigen on the graft, thereby participating in the tissue destruction. Although the CD8 Tc cell is the predominant specific lymphocyte involved in cellular rejection, the CD4 Th cell is an important component of the process because of its ability to magnify the cellular response by recruitment of other immune elements. In summary, CTLs specifically react with the class I alloantigen disparity, whereas the delayed-type hypersensitivity mechanism of CD4 Th cells causes a nonspecific response in recognition of the class II aloantigen disparity.

Acute rejection episodes may be precipitated by viral syndromes[49] that are caused by the following:

1. Direct viral damage, as in mumps or influenza viral syndromes, releasing increased amounts of histocompatibility antigens from the graft.
2. Viral antigens expressed during a clinical infection may cross-react with donor histocompatibility antigens. Thus the immune response directed against the virus can potentially result in graft rejection.
3. The virus may augment the host's immune system by acting as an adjuvant, making the host more susceptible to an acute rejection episode; although in most cases, particularly with cytomegalovirus, the infection tends to induce immunodepression.

From the opposite standpoint, allograft rejection sometimes produces activation of a latent viral infection, caused either by viral transformation of lymphocytes or by release of virus from damaged donor kidney cells.

Chronic Rejection

Chronic rejection is characterized by a gradual decline in graft function and tends to be unresponsive to steroid antirejection therapy and to end in transplant failure. Although CsA has reduced the incidence of acute renal allograft rejection, it has failed to reduce the incidence of chronic rejection.[47] The clinical syndrome of progressive deterioration of graft function after renal transplantation included hypertension and glomerulopathy with hematuria or proteinuria. Graft damage has been ascribed to a humoral process on the basis of detection of donor-specific circulating antibodies in recipient sera. Deposition of immunoglobulins and complement on glomerular capillary walls and low serum complement levels suggest that the humoral antibodies mediate a glomerular lesion. The immunoglobulin deposits appear to produce obliterative vascular changes (Fig. 5-20, *B*) eventuating in interstitial fibrosis.[46] Chronic rejection tends to be a separate pathologic and clinical entity, reflecting an alloantibody response frequently triggered but not caused by recurrent acute rejection episodes.

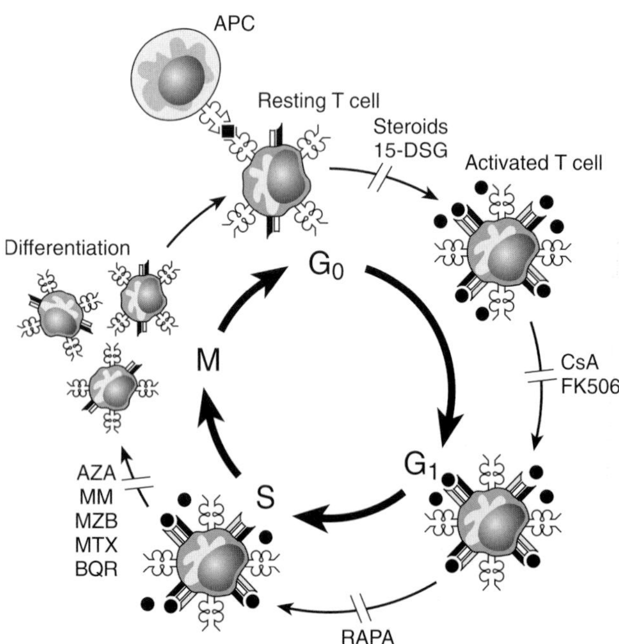

Fig. 5-21. Sites of action of immunosuppressive drugs in relation to the cell cycle. Steroids and 15-DSG block initial activation events at the G_0 phase. CsA and FK506 inhibits G_0 to G_1 progression by inhibiting IL-2 transcription. RAPA acts during the late G_1 phase by blocking cytokine signal transduction. Aza, MM, MTX, and MZB inhibit purine, whereas BQR inhibits pyrimidine synthesis at the S phase.

IMMUNOSUPPRESSIVE THERAPY

The ultimate goal in organ transplantation is to achieve immunologic tolerance of the host for his graft, thereby obviating any rejection process. Although there have been important experimental leads toward the goal of decreasing graft immunogenicity, only the recipient immunosuppressive approach has proven clinical efficacy. The ideal immunosuppressive regimen would specifically dampen host responses toward donor but not toward third-party transplants. Currently, the immunosuppressive modalities used for organ transplantation are nonspecific, altering host responses not only toward histocompatibility but also toward an array of other antigens. In general, two types of agents are used in clinical practice: pharmacologic agents exemplified by corticosteroids, CsA, and antiproliferative agents, and biologic agents such as antilymphocyte sera and monoclonal antibodies. Irradiation, although used in the early days of clinical transplantation, has no current applications.

Mechanisms of Pharmacologic Agents

Current clinical and experimental immunosuppressive agents[50] seek to inhibit the recognition of alloantigens, destroy alloreactive T cells, or alter the regulatory events leading to maturation and differentiation of mature alloreactive elements (Fig. 5-21).

Inhibition of Antigen Recognition, Processing, and Presentation

Corticosteroids. The first step in the development of transplant rejection is the generation of costimulatory activity by APCs, an event necessary for T-cell activation. Corticosteroids impair transcription of the IL-1β gene, cause rapid degradation of IL-1 mRNA, and reduce IL-6 transcription, thereby inhibiting the generation of the costimulatory signal.[51] Moreover, steroids also inhibit the gene transcription and expression of IL-2, TNF, and IFN-γ. These compounds diffuse intracellularly and bind to cytoplasmic receptors that exist in association with the 90 kd HSP. Steroid binding induces the dissociation of the HSP from the complex and translocation of the ligand-receptor complex into the nucleus. The activated complex reversibly binds to DNA sites collectively called *glucocorticoid response elements* (GREs), that exhibit the TGTTCT DNA motif and are present on multiple promoter regions of several cytokine genes, including the IL-2 promoter. Recent evidence suggests that the activated ligand-receptor complex impedes the activation but not binding effects of AP-1 and NFAT DNA-binding proteins on the IL-2 gene promoter region. Because of their tendency to inhibit nonspecific resistance more intensively than specific resistance (low immunosuppressive index) and their pleiotropic toxicities as a result of widespread use of GREs in other gene transcription units (an unfavorable therapeutic index), steroids are the weakest link in present clinical regimens.

Steroid therapy may produce multiple, severe side effects of hypertension, cushingoid syndrome, steroid-induced diabetes, osteoporosis, avascular necrosis of bones, weight gain, growth retardation, poor wound healing, cataracts, pancreatitis, peptic ulceration, colonic perforation, gastrointestinal bleeding, and psychosis.

15-Deoxyspergualin (15-DSG). DSG (0.5 kd),[52] an analog of an antitumor antibiotic, is currently under experimental evaluation for its clinical efficacy. It binds the intracellular HSP40 and 90 molecules that are involved in peptide loading onto and intracellular transport of MHC proteins. DSG inhibits antigen-specific but not mitogen-driven T-cell proliferation by inhibiting class II MHC expression and APC processing and presentation without affecting IL-1 or IL-6 synthesis, and it is a weak inhibitor of IL-2 synthesis. Preliminary clinical trials of DSG demonstrate modest clinical activity for treatment of or prophylaxis against acute rejection. However, only short courses of therapy are currently recommended because of the toxicities of leukopenia, thrombocytopenia, nausea, vomiting, anorexia, and headache. A randomized trial with OKT3 or DSG against steroid-resistant acute rejection showed a reversal of rejection in 58% of patients treated with DSG compared with 61% with OKT3 therapy.[53]

Lymphokine Synthesis Inhibitors

Cyclosporine (CsA, Sandimmune). CsA[54] is a cyclic endecapeptide extracted from the soil fungus *Tolypocladium inflatum gams* that exhibits a hydrophobic exterior and a hydrophilic center shielded in the interior of the structure. CsA binds to a cytoplasmic protein, cyclophilin (CYP; see Fig. 5-17, *A*), which displays *cis-trans* peptidyl-propyl-isomerase activity, which everts the hydrophilic CsA site from the interior to the exterior of the molecule, presumably converting the prodrug into the active moiety. CsA inhibits processes dependent on an increased cytoplasmic calcium burst. CsA binding to CYP changes the substrate affinity of the isomerase such that it complexes with and inhibits CaNs A and B, serine-threonine phosphatases associated with Ca^{2+}, and CaM. The formation of the complex CaN A-CaN B-Ca^{2+}-CaM-CsA-CYP prevents the dephosphorylation, activation, and nuclear translocation of NF-ATc, the first regulatory protein controlling the enhancer region of the IL-2 gene.[41] CsA inhibits T-cell synthesis of not only IL-2 but also IL-3, IFN-γ, IL-6, and IL-7. IL-1 synthesis and IL-2R generation appear to be calcium independent and therefore CsA resistant. Th and Tc cell functions are downregulated by CsA, in addition to the generation of regulatory T-suppressor cells that appear to enhance allograft survival in animal models.[54] The lack of inhibitory effects of CsA on the generation, proliferation, or function of nonspecific host resistance elements produces a high immunosuppressive index.

CsA exhibits a variety of side effects that include nephrotoxicity, hypertension, hyperkalemia, hyperuricemia, hypercholestrolemia, hypertriglyceridemia, hyperglycemia, hemolytic uremic syndrome, hepatotoxicity, and such mild neurologic symptoms as insomnia, hyperactivity tremors, and depression. Further, the concentration of CsA is affected by several drugs that enhance or inhibit CsA metabolism through the cytochrome P-4503A enzyme system. Rifampin, phenobarbital, phenytoin, and valproic acid increase CsA metabolism, whereas erythromycin, verapamil, and ketoconazole reduce it.

It has been difficult to optimize CsA therapy because of the agent's marked interindividual variations in pharmacokinetics and pharmacodynamics. Among renal transplant recipients there is a sixfold span of drug clearance rates and a ninefold span of relative oral bioavailability. Thus CsA doses are based on measured drug levels or calculated pharmacokinetic parameters, rather than on either fixed weight- or surface area-adjusted amounts.

CsA whole-blood levels are more reproducible than plasma levels. CsA levels are measured by fluorescence or radioimmunoassays that measure primarily the parent compound and about 15% of its metabolites or by high-performance liquid chromatography, which measures only the parent compound. Some centers tailor CsA therapy on the basis of trough levels (175 to 225 ng/ml for renal and 350 to 450 ng/ml for hepatic transplants). However, clinically obtained trough levels do not show a good correlation with areas under the concentration curve (AUC).[55] In response to Greenblatt's recommended strategy for drugs that display marked interindividual variations, our CsA concentration control regimen is based on serial pharmacokinetic profiling,[56] beginning with pretransplant studies conducted after administration of "test" intravenous and oral CsA doses. In 73% of patients, drug clearance rates calculated after administration of the intravenous "test" dose (3 mg/kg CsA delivered over 3 hours) predicted individualized drug doses that produced target steady-state concentrations of 400 $\pm$ 40 ng/ml. The excessive initial CsA levels that predispose patients toward nephrotoxicity, or contrariwise the low levels that are insufficient for immunosuppression, are avoided by use of this method. However, in only 40% of renal transplant recipients does the relative bioavailability calculated from the oral "test" dose yield the correct prediction for the initial oral dose to achieve the target average concentration (AUC/dosing interval = 550 $\pm$ 50 ng/ml), most likely as a result of the alterations in postoperative drug absorption. Our recent strategy refines the dose prediction by using the AUC measured during the absorption test after administration of the predicted oral dose during the intravenous CsA infusion to obtain a revised, predicted dose. Use of the new glycol-furan microemulsion formulation of CsA (Neoral) may also facilitate the dose prediction. Neoral absorption appears to be independent of bile and food composition.

Long-term dose adjustment that is based on serial pharmacokinetic profiles rather than on random blood levels appears to minimize the chronic renal injury attributed to CsA. Although pharmacokinetic control of drug dosing has eliminated excessive immunodepression from CsA therapy, there remain two major pharmacodynamic limitations to CsA treatment; the existence of Ca^{2+}-independent lymphocyte activation pathways, particularly in cases of black and presensitized patients, and apparently concentration-independent, drug-induced renal injury.

Tacrolimus (Prograf, FK506). FK506 is a polycyclic macrolide antibiotic produced by *Streptomyces tsukubaensis* that inhibits T-cell production of IL-2, IL-3, IL-4, and IFN-γ 10 to 100 times more potently than does CsA. Further, it blocks the expression of IL-2R and inhibits the synthesis of TNF-α, GM-CSF, and *c-myc.* Tacrolimus, like CsA, inhibits Ca^{2+}-dependent intracellular pathways mediated by interactions with an intracellular binding protein (FKBP; see Fig. 5-17, *A*), which like CYP is a member of the *cis-trans* propyl isomerase "immunophilin" family. This interaction ultimately results in inhibition of IL-2 production.[41] Tacrolimus and CsA exhibit in vitro and in vivo antagonism, which may be explained by the fact that they share a common intracellular pathway. The two drugs, however, do not act by precisely the same mechanism. Tacrolimus inhibits and CsA facilitates the induction of suppressive cells. Further, tacrolimus appears to exhibit a narrower therapeutic window and more severe side effects than does CsA.

In experimental models, tacrolimus has been shown to prolong skin and vascularized organ allografts in rodents and in primates. However, tacrolimus has not improved the outcome in clinical kidney or liver transplantation when compared with CsA. Tacrolimus absorption after oral administration is less bile-dependent than CsA. This may be beneficial during the biliary diversion with T-tube drainage after hepatic transplantation. Tacrolimus shows potency equal to but not greater than that of CsA in dual-drug regimens with prednisone for primary immunosuppression of liver transplant recipients. Although some studies have suggested that tacrolimus therapy allows steroid withdrawal, particularly in pediatric cardiac transplant recipients, CsA-based regimens routinely permit successful steroid withdrawal. Further, long-term immunosuppression with CsA allows withdrawal of steroids in hepatic transplant recipients at a rate equal to that suggested by tacrolimus studies.

Tacrolimus therapy is associated with nephrotoxicity caused by decreased renal cortical blood flow and reduced glomerular filtration rates, drug-induced hyperkalemia, and hypertension, findings previously reported with CsA therapy. Current tacrolimus protocols use excessively high doses, causing 34% of patients to experience severe neurotoxicity, which includes expressive aphasia, coma, and seizures, 68% to experience nephrotoxicity, 20% to experience new-onset diabetes mellitus, and 1.6% to experience lymphoproliferative disorders. This apparent narrow therapeutic window of tacrolimus probably results from treatment regimens that seek to maximize therapeutic activity at the penalty of heightened toxicity.

Thus tacrolimus appears to have about an equal immunosuppressive index to that of CsA but a lower therapeutic index. Advances in defining the therapeutic utility of tacrolimus in clinical transplantation will accompany the development of a clinically applicable, accurate drug measurement technique to be used in a concentration-control strategy.

Cytokine Signal Transduction Inhibitors

Sirolimus (Rapamune, Rapamycin, RAPA, AY22). RAPA,[57] a macrolide antibiotic produced by the actinomycete *Streptomyces hygroscopicus,* is structurally related to FK506. Unlike CsA and tacrolimus, which influence the G_0 to G_1 progression, Sirolimus does not affect lymphokine synthesis but rather inhibits their effects on the G_1 build-up phase (see Fig. 5-21). Thus RAPA inhibits a broad array of calcium-independent activation events mediated by CD28, protein kinase C, and lymphokine stimulation. Although Sirolimus binds to FKBP to form RAPA-FKBP complex, the target of its inhibitory effects on isolated lymphocytes is unknown. Various authors report retarded endocytosis of receptor complexes or inhibited PI-3-kinase activity necessary to generate the 3-phosphorylated phosphoinositides (PI-3-P, PI-3,4-P_2 and PI-3,4,5-P_3) that function as growth and division signals. RAPA also inhibits the IL-2–stimulated T-cell S-phase entry[58] by blocking $p70^{S6}$ or the $p34^{cdc2}$ kinases, thereby blocking the proliferative but not the differentiation events induced by IL-2.

Sirolimus prolongs the survival of rat heart, kidney, small-bowel, and pancreaticoduodenal allografts in dose-dependent fashion.[50] The humoral arm of the immune response is also potently inhibited by Sirolimus. Further, it also inhibits transduction of all cytokine signals tested to date. It offers the promise of clinical use because of its synergistic immunosuppressive effect with CsA. Thus the combination of RAPA and CsA may allow the use of both drugs at extremely low doses to produce a high immunosuppressive index with a low toxic profile.

Other agents. Leflunomide (HWA 486) is believed to inhibit the *lck* and *fyn* families of tyrosine kinases, enzymes that are associated with transduction of many growth factor receptor signals, including IL-2, IL-3, and TNF-α. In experimental animals, the drug inhibits murine graft-versus-host reactions and prolongs allograft survival. However, its propensity for gastric toxicity, emaciation, and anemia, combined with its embryotoxicity, has beclouded clinical evaluation.

Recombinant gene technology has yielded soluble extramembrane constructs of IL-1R and IL-4R. Initial results suggest that these constructs modestly prolong allografts in experimental animal models.

Nucleoside Synthesis Inhibitors

Azathioprine (Aza). Aza, a purine analog, is a nitroimidazole derivative 6-mercaptopurine (6-MP). It was first used at the Peter Bent Brigham Hospital in Boston and rapidly became the cornerstone of chemical immunosuppression in the 1960s. Aza must be metabolized in the liver through conversion to 6-MP and then to its active metabolite 6-thioinosinic acid. It exerts its immunosuppressive effect by broadly inhibiting DNA and RNA synthesis by preventing the synthesis of adenosine monophosphate (AMP) and guanosine monophosphate (GMP) from inosinc acid (*de novo* purine synthesis pathway) and blocking the interconversion among the precursors of purine nucleotides (*salvage* pathway). However, Aza exhibits multiple limitations. Because Aza can be incorporated into DNA as a fraudulent base, it carries an increased proclivity toward malignancy and papillomatosis. Aza also produces a hepatotoxicity that can potentiate the CsA injury. Because Aza acts as a *competitive* enzyme inhibitor of both de novo and salvage pathways, it must be used at high concentrations, resulting in bone marrow depression to a greater degree than its immunosuppressive effect.

Although it still tends to be used as a third agent with the CsA-steroid regimen, Aza has no demonstrable synergistic effect with CsA immunosuppression. Further, Aza-steroid regimens display a low therapeutic index, with 90% of renal allograft recipients experiencing rejection episodes and only 50% 1-year graft survival. The limitations of Aza as an immunosuppressive drug led to an urgent need to identify new nucleoside synthesis inhibitors that acted *noncompetitively* to inhibit synthesis of either purines (Mizorbine and mycophenolate mofetil [MM]) or pyrimidines (Brequinar [BQR]), were not incorporated into DNA, showed reduced myelotoxicity, and displayed synergistic interactions with CsA.

Mizorbine (MZB; Bredinin). MZB, an imidazole nucleoside antibiotic isolated from *Eupenicillum brefeldianum,* is converted to its active monophosphate form by adenosine kinase. It has been used experimentally and to a limited extent clinically in Japan as an immunosuppressive agent. MZB noncompetitively inhibits inosine monophosphate (IMP) dehydrogenase (IMPDH), which converts IMP to xanthine monophosphate, an intermediate compound in the synthesis of GMP. Thus, like Aza and MM, MZB progressively depletes intracellular GMP stores. Its immunosuppressive capacity is estimated to be comparable to that of Aza, whereas associated marrow depression is less prominent. The drug is not metabolized in the liver and demonstrates no significant hepatotoxicity. Its use has been associated with significant anorexia and subsequent weight loss in the canine model. As yet, no clinical trials have been published outside Japan, and worldwide distribution of the drug is not anticipated.

MM (Cellcept, RS-61443). MM is a semisynthetic morpholinoethyl ester of mycophenolic acid, which is produced by the fungus *Penicillin glaucum.* Like MZB, MM noncompetitively inhibits IMPDH, the crucial enzyme in the *de novo* pathway that is predominantly used by T and B lymphocytes for purine synthesis. MM prolongs the survival of allografts and xenografts in animal models. Initial reports suggested that MM does not produce significant hepatotoxicity or nephrotoxicity, but it does cause mild myelosuppression and gastrointestinal toxicity.[59] In contrast to other purine synthesis inhibitors, MM seems to have a favorable therapeutic index but only an additive effect in combination with CsA. The drug is now undergoing multicenter phase III investigations in renal transplantation.

BQR. BQR, a synthetic difluoroquinoline carboxylic acid derivative, was originally developed as an antineoplastic drug. It reversibly inhibits the mitochondrial enzyme dihydro-orotate dehydrogenase, the fourth enzyme in the de novo pyrimidine biosynthesis pathway. The greater potency of BQR than MM, MZB, or Aza is probably due to the 100 times lower concentration of pyrimidine than of purine precursors.

Oral drug administration prolongs the survival of heart, kidney, and liver grafts in rat models.[60] BQR exhibits synergistic interaction with CsA, both in vitro and in vivo. Although high-dose BQR therapy in patients with cancer produced gastric toxicity, phase I study only showed thrombocytopenia, which can be avoided by the use of lower drug doses. Phase II trials to further assess the efficacy of BQR are currently pending.

Methotrexate (MTX). MTX is an antimetabolite that antagonizes folic acid metabolism by binding dihydrofolate reductase, thereby inhibiting DNA synthesis.[61] Its immunosuppressive effects have been attributed to inhibition of macrophage migration as a result of decreased IL-1 production and to reduced accumulation of inflammatory cells or immune mediators. Combined low-dose treatment with MTX and CsA downregulates the transcription of some gene products that mediate cytotoxicity, including TNF-α, LT, and some serine proteases, thereby prolonging graft survival. Low-dose administration of MTX has recently been used to control persistent mild cardiac allograft rejection in humans.

Biologic Agents

Polyclonal Antibodies

Potent, nonspecific, immunosuppressive antibodies can be produced by immunizing a xenogeneic host (a species-divergent host) with human lymphocytes. These sera contain polyclonal antibodies that opsonize the corresponding peripheral blood cellular elements, including T cells, leading to their autodestruction in the liver and spleen. In addition, antibody binding onto lymphocytes may "blind" them to antigenic stimuli. The resulting in vivo depletion or inactivation of T lymphocytes interferes with T-cell–mediated reactions, including allograft rejection, DTH, and graft-versus-host reactions. Immunosuppression with antilymphocyte sera (ALS) or purified globulin fraction (ALG) has been demonstrated in experimental animal trials to prevent skin allograft rejection in mice, rats, and primates and to prevent rejection of vascularized allografts in experimental canine renal and hepatic transplantation.

ALG has been used for *prophylactic* therapy during the first week after transplantation to reduce the frequency and severity of early rejection episodes. However, clinical studies have not yielded unequivocal evidence supporting the use of ALS prophylactically. Some centers demonstrated improved graft survival and fewer rejection episodes, with a relative paucity of the reported side effects of serum sickness, anaphylactoid reactions, vascular thrombosis, or infection. On the other hand, other well-controlled studies suggest no therapeutic benefit from prophylactic ALG, but rather a significant risk of fatal infections. Alternatively, ALG can be used for *therapy* of acute renal allograft rejection episodes. The use of ALG in conjunction with high-dose steroids to reverse acute renal allograft rejection episodes produces a 13% increased incidence of viral sepsis and a 13% incidence of serum sickness, but an improved 1-year allograft survival. Therefore sequential rather than simultaneous use of ALS and high-dose steroids is recommended for rejection therapy.

The methods of production of ALS are varied. The most common method immunizes heterologous equine or rabbit hosts with either thymic T or cultured B-blastoid lymphocytes to yield a polyclonal product containing a heterogeneous array of antibodies reactive with T cells, as well as a range of other normal lymphoid elements. In addition to requiring central venous access for administration, there are several disadvantages of the product. First, only 5% to 10% of the total antithymocyte globulin dose is responsible for the therapeutic effect. Second, there is appreciable batch-to-batch variability. Third, side effects, including serum sickness and increased cytomegalovirus infections, are prominent.

Monoclonal Antibodies

A second class of biologic agents that disrupt early activation events are monoclonal antibodies (MAbs) directed toward surface-receptor (α/βTcR, CD3) or coreceptor (CD4) epitopes present on T cells or on APCs, such as B7, LFA-1, or ICAM-1. Immunosuppressive therapy with MAb reagents inactivates cell-surface epitopes that mediate alloreactivity. Hybridoma technology, which was initially reported by Kohler and Milstein,[62] yields readily standardized, specific xenogeneic murine MAbs of greater purity and molecular specificity than polyclonal reagents. OKT3 is a murine IgG_{2a} MAb that dampens alloantigen recognition and cytolytic function of T cells by modulating or "blinding" cell-surface CD3 epitopes, thereby reversing allorejection episodes. However, OKT3 therapy may evoke the production of human antimouse antibodies (HAMAs), including anti-idiotypic and anti-isotypic varieties[63] that preclude retreatment with mouse antibodies. Further, the administration of OKT3 may be associated with fever, chills, diarrhea, headache, pulmonary edema, wheezing, hypotension, aseptic meningitis, seizures, or even coma as a result of the release of IFN-γ, IL-1, and TNF. In addition to the acute cytokine-release reactions, excessive OKT3 therapy predisposes toward cytomegalovirus (CMV) infections and posttransplant lymphoproliferative diseases (PTLDs). Second-generation MAbs seek to avoid the severe systemic reactions caused by the cytokine release that follows OKT3 administration and the proclivity toward lymphoma development. $T_{10}B_9$ and BMA 031 are two MAbs that are putatively directed against the α/βTcR, which represents the initial site of T-cell recognition. Both antibodies are currently under clinical evaluation, the former for use in acute rejection episodes and the latter for prophylaxis against rejection. A major limitation of treatment with anti-TcR antibodies is the rapid development of HAMAs.

Alternate approaches seek to use MAbs directed against accessory T-cell molecules. OKT-4A IgG_{2a} MAb, which reacts with the CD4 coreceptor of Th cells, appears to provoke fewer side effects than does OKT3.[64] Unfortunately, OKT-4A also generates strong HAMAs. The lack of efficacy of the original murine antibody seems to be overcome with the humanized variant of OKT-4A. A second target is the molecular pair LFA-1 on T cells and ICAM-1 (CD54) on monocytes. A phase I clinical trial of anti-CD54 MAb-induction therapy in "high-risk recipients" demonstrated a 78% renal allograft survival, in contrast to 56% with conventional immunosuppression.[65] Anti-LFA-1 MAb successfully reversed steroid-resistant acute graft-versus-host reactions in humans. Further, in murine experimental models, the combination of anti–ICAM-1 and anti–LFA-1 MAbs produced tolerance to cardiac allografts.[66] These promising results with MAbs directed against T-cell/monocyte coreceptors await confirmation in controlled clinical trials. The rat (33B3.1) or murine (LO-Tact-1, BT 563) anti-IL-2R MAbs were successfully utilized for immunoprophylaxis induction protocols. However, their clinical effectiveness were limited by a short half-life and the development of host anti-MAb responses.

Two innovations have been adopted to avoid the production of HAMAs after administration of mouse MAbs. Chimeric antibodies combine the variable regions of mouse antibodies with human antibody constant regions and therefore present fewer foreign amino acid sequences to the host. However, one-third of the structure is still of mouse origin, which may stimulate the production of anti-idiotypic antibodies. Humanized antibodies combine only the smallest part of a mouse antibody required for target recognition, the distinctive complementarity-determining regions, with human variable and constant region frameworks (Fig. 5-22). However, humanized antibodies may exhibit reduced affinity to antigen epitopes. Moreover, a recent study in primates demonstrated that humanized OKT4A still causes a nonhuman primate antimurine response. Neverthless, the beneficial effects of chimeric and humanized variants of mouse MAbs will be clarified only by randomized clinical trials.

Irradiation

The immunosuppressive effect of irradiation is caused by the inhibition of DNA synthesis and cellular replication.

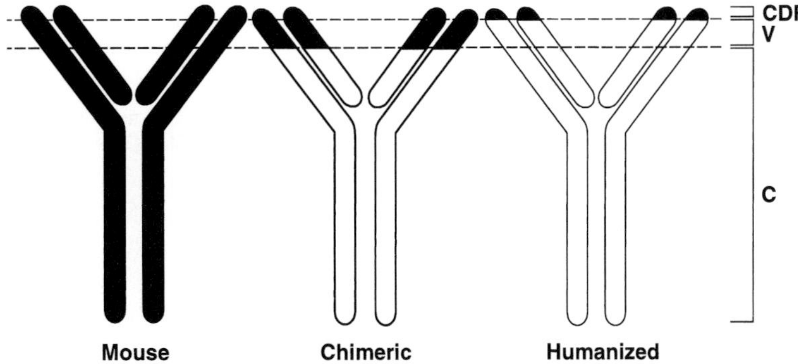

Fig. 5-22. Schematic illustration of chimeric and humanized antibodies. The murine portion of the antibody is shown in black and the human portion in white. *CDR,* Complementarity-determining region; *V,* variable region; *C,* constant region.

Total-body irradiation of renal transplant recipients was used in the early days of clinical transplantation with limited but unequivocal success. However, total-body irradiation was abandoned in favor of local graft radiotherapy because of its associated toxicity, including severe bone marrow depression and fatal infections. Subsequent clinical trials demonstrated that local graft irradiation increased the rate of reversal of allograft rejection but adversely affected the ultimate fate of the graft when used in combination with steroids. These findings, coupled with the superiority of other emerging immunologic strategies for managing graft rejection, resulted in limited clinical application of local graft irradiation, which was ultimately abandoned.

Because of the potent immunodepressive effect of radiotherapy and the need to minimize other organ toxicity, a regimen called total lymphoid irradiation (TLI) that focuses on cervical, axillary, mediastinal, para-aortic, splenic, and ilioinguinal nodes was devised and first applied for treatment of Hodgkin's disease. After therapy, hosts displayed a state of immunosuppression characterized by T lymphocytopenia, decreased alloreactivity, and induction of nonspecific T-suppressor cells. A decreased number and function of T cells were documented for years after therapy. Although TLI decreases cell-mediated immunity and prolongs allograft survival in mice, success in large-mammal models has not been consistent. Even if the logistic issue that TLI must be performed before transplantation is ignored, the complications associated with its administration (nausea, vomiting, possible increased incidence of lymphoma, and opportunistic infections) have limited its application in the clinical arena.

Risks of Immunosuppression

Neoplasia

Immunodeficiency states predispose toward the development of de novo cancers. The incidence of neoplasms in renal allograft recipients varies between 1% and 16%, far greater than in the general population matched for age.[67] Nonmelanotic skin and lip cancers, PTLDs, and cervical carcinomas account for 60% of the total cancers.[68] Conversely, the malignancies that are most commonly encountered in the general population, namely, carcinoma of the breast, lung, prostate, and colon, are relatively uncommon in transplant recipients. There is an increased incidence of de novo skin and lip cancers in transplant recipients, 39% of which are squamous cell and basal cell carcinomas. Melanomas, which comprise only about 5% of skin cancers, behave in a similar fashion to those in the general population. OKT3 treatment poses a particularly high risk for PTLD, which encompasses a wide morphologic spectrum of Epstein-Barr virus (EBV)–induced B-cell diseases ranging from reactive, polyclonal hyperplasia to true monoclonal malignant lymphoma. A common picture in renal allograft recipients[67] shows non-Hodgkin lymphomas containing TcR-β gene rearrangements consistent with monoclonal T-cell proliferation. Treatment with azathioprine, prednisone, or methotrexate, as well as the high frequency of herpes simplex virus (HSV) infection, predisposes recipients toward cervical dysplasia and carcinoma in 21% of women who have posttransplant cancers. Treatment is based on surgical extirpation of the tumors if possible, together with reduction of immunosuppressive therapy.

Conflicting data suggest that immunosuppression potentiates the growth of existing cancers. On the basis of recurrence rates of neoplasms after transplantation, a 2-year waiting period between treatment of cancers and transplantation is justified for most neoplasms, except incidentally discovered renal carcinomas, in situ carcinomas, low-greade bladder cancers, and basal cell skin cancers.

Infections

More than 80% of transplant recipients acquire at least one infection after transplantation, and 40% of deaths are caused by infectious complications occurring alone or after rejection and treatment. About 55% of posttransplant infections are caused by bacterial agents, 30% by viral agents, and 15% by fungal agents.[69] Most bacterial infections arise in the urinary tract, plastic venous catheters, the surgical wound, or intraabdominal sites from a spectrum of gram-negative and gram-positive agents akin to those occurring in other surgical patients.

The most common viral infections after transplantation are caused by DNA viruses of the herpesvirus family including CMV, EBV, HSV, and varicella zoster virus (VZV). Viral infections tend to be latent but are potentially oncogenic. Symptomatic CMV is associated with intense immunosuppression, particularly the use of ATG or OKT3, exhibiting a peak incidence at 6 weeks after transplantation. In addition, CMV constitutes a risk factor for subsequent rejection episodes and bacterial, fungal, and parasitic (particularly *Pneumocystis carinii*) superinfections. The reduced incidence of such infections under CsA rather than Aza therapy may reflect both the less frequent rejection episodes requiring MAb or polyclonal antibody intervention[70] as well as CsA's capacity to spare nonspecific immune elements.

Candida albicans is the most common fungal infection, although *Candida globrata* is seen with increasing frequency. *Aspergillus fumigates* and *Aspergillus flavus* are the second most common fungal infections and present as pulmonary infiltrates. Other less common agents include *Coccidioides immitis, Histoplasma capsulatum,* and *Nocardia asteroides.* The protozoan parasite *P. carinii* has become an important cause of pneumonia in the immunocompromised patient. However, prophylaxis with trimethoprim-sulfamethoxasole has nearly eliminated these infections in transplant recipients.

Clinical Application

Unfortunately, current clinical practices are based on empiric rather than scientific foundations. Despite the widely disparate intrinsic immunogenicity of various organs, the various degrees of donor-recipient incompatibility, and the well-recognized interindividual variations in host immunosuppressiveness, transplant centers tend to use uniform initial induction and early maintenance immunosuppressive regimens.

Induction Immunosuppression

The first 2 weeks after transplantation pose the greatest challenge because of the requirement to promptly establish adequate immunosuppression to avert an acute allograft rejection episode. Many clinicians initiate CsA therapy either prior to or immediately after the transplantation procedure because experimental data suggest that CsA exerts maximal benefit at the time of antigen presentation. Others cite the proclivity of CsA to produce renal or hepatic dysfunction as the basis for delayed CsA administration, preferring sequential initiation protocols with antilymphocyte antibodies that provide rapid T-cell depletion with significant effects on granulocytes and platelets. Selective effects on T cells may be achieved by OKT3, although its early administration carries the risk of development of HAMAs that preclude its subsequent administration. Most workers therefore prefer the polyclonal reagents for the initial induction and reserve the use of the MAbs for subsequent acute rejection episodes. Antilymphocyte induction protocols carry several penalties: delayed hospital discharge as a result of postponing optimization of CsA regimen, delayed onset (but not reduced incidence) of acute rejection episodes, and proclivity for viral infections and PTLD.

Short-Term Maintenance Immunosuppression

The short-term immunosuppressive regimen uses the dual drug combination of CsA and steroids to avert allograft rejection during the first 90 days after transplantation. The most popular strategy starts with an 8 to 10 mg/kd dose of CsA divided as a twice a day regimen. The dose is adjusted according to measured trough levels. Most clinicians strive for whole-blood parent CsA compound concentration of 175 to 350 ng/ml. The major disadvantage of this strategy is that the tremendous 54-fold interindividual variation in CsA pharmacokinetics poses appreciable obstacles to the dose-finding endeavor. Furthermore, there is poor correlation between CsA trough levels and the AUC, a measure of drug exposure during the dosing interval.[55] One approach to protect the patient from acute rejection episodes during the delay to achieve target CsA levels adds Aza to the CsA-prednisone regimen, although there is no evidence that this strategy improves outcome. We have adopted a pharmacokinetic strategy that uses parameters measured both before and after transplantation to determine the appropriate CsA doses for intravenous induction and oral maintenance therapy.[56] This pharmacokinetic approach is rewarded by early hospital discharge, avoidance of concomitant Aza, and reduced incidence of acute rejection episodes compared with the empiric dose-finding strategies.

The combination of corticosteroids with CsA is based on both clinical and experimental data that suggest a synergistic effect. Almost all steroid regimens include a massive (250 to 1000 mg) intraoperative dose of methylprednisolone to dampen graft tissue injury and reduce T-cell activation. During the immediate postoperative period, steroid doses are rapidly tapered from 200 mg to 20 to 30 mg by day 7, followed by a more gradual taper to 15 mg between 30 and 90 days.

Antirejection Immunosuppression

The principles of treatment for rejection episodes are relatively uniform across organs and among transplant centers. Most centers demand histopathologic evidence of rejection, because of the significant penalties for excessive treatment of an adequately immunosuppressed patient. Steroid regimens combine large intravenous doses of methylprednisolone with an oral prednisone taper. Delivery of intravenous steroids achieves high plasma concentrations and rapid reversal of symptoms. The risks of therapy include exacerbating or inducing diabetes mellitus, gastrointestinal irritation or perforation, and triggering psychosis. Administration of more than 7 g methylprednisolone within the first 30 days after transplantation constitutes a risk factor for survival because of the pronounced depression of the nonspecific immune resistance of the host. It is important to reduce the level of steroids to the pretherapy dose within 1 month because long-term administration of high doses predisposes toward gastrointestinal bleeding, myopathy, osteoporosis, bacterial and fugal infections, and hypertension. The advantages of steroid treatment are the low medication costs and the 90% efficacy rate.

After 3 to 5 days of steroid treatment, most centers assess the success according to remission of symptoms and improved graft function. However, this assessment is not clinically easy. On the one hand, blood chemistry values that reflect tissue damage end points slowly reverse even after control of the immune process; on the other hand, delay in the delivery of adequate immunosuppression may result in graft failure or severe permanent impairment. If the response to steroids is deemed inadequate and if the graft biopsy documents persistent rejection, the physician proceeds with the administration of an antilymphocyte preparation. Most workers use OKT3 rather than polyclonal sera. To minimize the toxicity of OKT3 due to cytokine release, our regimen employs a split-dose approach, delivering 1, 2, and 2 mg intravenously every 8 hours for the first day, followed by 2.5 mg every 12 hours on the second day and 5 mg per day therafter. Each dose is administered with an anti-inflammatory pretreatment cocktail of 100 mg hydrocortisone, 50 mg diphenhydramine (Benadryl), and 120 mg acetaminophen. An intermediate point for the efficacy of OKT3 therapy is the reduction of T cells bearing the CD3 marker from about 65% to <10%, determined by flow cytometric analysis of whole-blood samples with a fluoresceinated OKT3 reagent. Unfortunately, there are no secure algorithms for the length of OKT3 therapy because there is a delay in the therapeutic effect by 7 to 10 days and in the toxic effects by 14 to 30 days.

Long-Term Maintenance Immunosuppression

Although CsA has reduced the incidence and severity of graft rejection episodes, it has had little impact on the 10% incidence of chronic rejection observed under Aza-prednisone therapy. Although it is possible that the failure represents inadequate CsA therapy as a result of suboptimal dose adjustments, it is more likely that host B-cell responses are less CsA-sensitive than are T-cell responses. Long-term management schemes show more variation than do short-term regimens; there are advocates for CsA only, CsA-prednisone, CsA-Aza, and Aza-prednisone strategies. Although no data suggest differences in outcome, there have been no truly randomized trials.

CLINICAL TRANSPLANTATION OUTCOMES

The modern era of organ transplantation began with the first successful grafting of a kidney between identical twins in 1954.[71] Subsequent advances in knowledge concerning the pathogenesis of rejection and the ability to manipulate this immune response by various therapeutic strategies have allowed transplantation to proceed to a point where many diseased organs can now be replaced with a minimum of difficulty. Kidney transplantation is relatively commonplace throughout the United States and many other countries, and organs such as the liver and the heart are now being transplanted with increasing frequency. Although allograft rejection continues to be an important problem, CsA has done much to improve graft survival rate. Thus for many organs the availability of donors has posed more of a problem than have the potential difficulties surrounding the rejection process. To gain insight into the advances that have been made in organ transplantation during the last three decades, this section will briefly review the current status of organs that are transplantable. For purposes of discussion, three types of donor grafts should be recognized. These include (1) grafting between twins, in which the immunologic match is identical between host and donor, (2) living-related grafts, in which there is considerable immunologic similarity between the host and donor but not to the same degree as with twins, and (3) cadaveric grafts obtained from unrelated individuals (subjects who are brain dead but in whom function of the organ to be potentially transplanted is normal), in which immunologic matching between host and donor may be quite dissimilar even though every attempt is made before transplantation to optimize this match as much as possible. For renal transplantation, all three types of grafts have been used. For transplantation of organs such as the liver and heart, it is obvious that only cadaver grafts can be used.

Renal Transplantation

Approximately 6000 to 10,000 new patients annually acquire end-stage renal disease in the United States, necessitating treatment with either long-term dialysis or renal transplantation. For patients 70 years old or younger, renal transplantation has emerged as the treatment of choice. This relates to the recent advances in immunosuppression, particularly the discovery of CsA, which has drastically improved both renal allograft and patient survival.[47] Before the availability of CsA, survival rates for patients receiving cadaveric allografts approached 90%, whereas graft survivals approximated 50%. With the advent of CsA, graft and patient 1-year survival rates of 80% and 95%, respectively, have been routinely achieved for cadaveric transplantation. Similar results have been obtained with patients receiving living-related donor kidneys. With HLA-identical grafts, graft survival has approached 90% to 95%, and for all other living-related grafts 75% to 85% graft survival has been obtained.

Historically, patient survival after renal transplantation with a kidney from a living-related donor has always exceeded that achieved with hemodialysis. In contrast, patient survival after cadaveric transplantation generally paralleled that associated with hemodialysis. With the use of CsA, however, a clear improvement in patient survival after cadaveric transplantation has been observed with respect to hemodialysis. In addition, renal transplant recipients demonstrated a significantly improved rehabilitation rate. Without question, both the longevity and quality of life

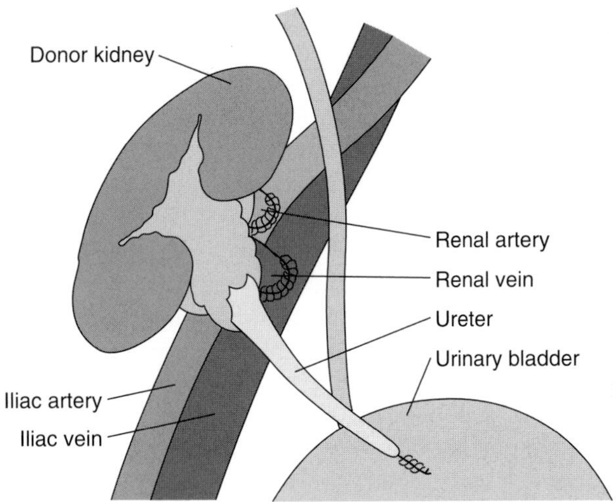

Fig. 5-23. Renal transplantation. The donor kidney is placed in the retroperitonium of the iliac fossa. The donor renal artery and vein are anastomosed to the recipient iliac artery and vein, respectively, in an end-to-side fashion. Ureteroneocystostomy establishes urinary continuity.

have been clearly improved with this therapeutic modality.

The transplanted kidney is usually placed in the retroperitonium of the iliac fossa through a lower abdominal incision (Fig. 5-23). Generally, the blood supply is assured by anastomosing the renal artery to the external iliac artery in an end-to-side fashion or to the hypogastric artery in an end-to-end fashion. The renal vein is anastomosed to the iliac vein end-to-side. Urinary tract continuity is usually established by a ureteroneocystostomy by placing the ureter either through a submucosal tunnel or by a direct implantation that prevents the subsequent development of reflux. The success of this surgical approach has been clearly demonstrated in the thousands of kidneys that have been transplanted during the last 30 years.

Cardiac Transplantation

Since the performance of the first human cardiac transplant by Dr. Christian Barnard in December 1967, several hundred heart transplants have been performed to prolong the life expectancy of patients with end-stage cardiac disease. Although enthusiasm for cardiac transplantation has waxed and waned during the last two decades, the use of CsA to treat rejection has clearly improved the clinical outcome and rejuvenated interest in this procedure. The impact of CsA is evidenced by the worldwide increase in cardiac transplantation centers. In 1989 there were 236 centers performing cardiac transplants, compared with 17 in 1980.

Patients considered suitable candidates for cardiac transplantation are those with end-stage heart disease provided that they have no other disease condition that potentially affects long-term survival. Priority is given to hospitalized candidates undergoing maximal medical or mechanical circulatory support and to patients who are at a risk for sudden death due to malignant arrhythmias. Generally, candidates for cardiac transplantation should be younger than 65 years and without an underlying malignant disease, insulin-dependent diabetes mellitus, severe peripheral vascular disease, morbid obesity, or an active infectious process. In addition, a high fixed pulmonary vascular resistance is gnenerally considered a contraindication for this procedure.

Cardiac allotransplantation[72] is usually performed orthotopically. The recipient heart is removed, leaving a remnant of the right and left atria posteriorly. The atria, pulmonary artery, and aorta from the donor heart are then anastomosed primarily. Heterotopic cardiac transplantation has also been performed, in which the allograft is connected in parallel with the native heart. The theoretic advantage of this latter procedure is the maintenance of the native myocardium to sustain the recipient for reimplantation if the organ comes from a suboptimal donor or if it undergoes acute irreversible rejection.

The current overall survival rate is 77% at 1 year and 58.4% at 5 years. Regularly scheduled right endocardial biopsies in conjunction with cardiac catheterization and coronary angiography are used to evaluate the status of the transplanted heart. Although fever, hemodynamic instability, signs of congestive heart failure, arrhythmias, and electrocardiographic alterations are clinical indexes suggesting rejection, histologic evaluation of the endocardium is usually necessary to rule out a rejection episode. Although rejection may occur at any time after transplantation, late graft failure is often associated with atherosclerotic coronary artery disease of the transplanted heart. To minimize the likelihood of this problem, most patients are treated prophylactically with antithrombogenic agents.

Hepatic Transplantation

Liver transplantation is now considered an accepted therapeutic modality for a number of hepatic disorders, and for certain conditions it is the treatment of choice. As with heart transplantation, the general acceptance of this procedure has paralleled the significant improvement in survival resulting from the use of CsA. Before the use of CsA, Starzl et al.,[73] pioneers in clinical hepatic transplantation, reported 1- and 5-year survival rates of 30% and 20%, respectively, between 1963 and 1980. Immunosuppression with CsA has drastically improved these results, with the actuarial survival rates at 1 and 5 years now being 75% and 70%, respectively. When liver transplantation is carried out to improve the quality-of-life for noncritically ill patients, the 1-year survival is in excess of 90%.[74]

Indications for liver transplantation are only now becoming clearly defined. In the pediatric population, biliary atresia is the most common clinical condition in which this procedure is used. The 1- and 5-year actuarial survival rates for this population of patients are 76.2% and 73.7%, respectively. Because clinical success with hepatic transplantation has exceeded that of the Kasai procedure for biliary atresia, it is now considered the treatment of choice for this pediatric disease. Other pediatric conditions in which hepatic transplantation offers a therapeutic alternative include various inborn errors of metabolism, such as Wilson's disease, tyrosinemia, glycogen storage disease, and the α_1-antitrypsin deficiency. However, the severe shortage of pediatric liver donors has limited the expansion of liver transplantation in the pediatric population. New surgical approaches including reduced-size liver transplantation, split-liver transplantation, and use of living-related donors are currently under evaluation to increase the supply of organs.

Alcohol-related liver disease (Laënnec's cirrhosis) is now the most common indication for liver transplantation in adults in the United States. This is in sharp contrast to earlier reports that alcoholics accounted for fewer than 10% of patients coming to transplantation. Other indications include end-stage cryptogenic and primary biliary cirrhosis, sclerosing cholangitis, hepatitis C, fulminant hepatic failure, and chronic active hepatitis. Those patients with a positive antigen for hepatitis B are usually not accepted as suitable candidates for transplantation because of the significant risk of recurrence of hepatitis. Similarly, patients older than 70 years, those with significant cardiopulmonary disease, advanced alcoholic disease, or sepsis, and those deemed psychologically unfit for transplantation because of potential difficulty with immunologic drug compliance are also eliminated as acceptable transplant candidates. The role of hepatic transplantation in malignant disease remains uncertain. Although the literature is replete with examples of transplantation in patients with a variety of malignant disorders, including hepatocellular carcinoma, cholangiocarcinoma, and hemangioendothelioma, the relatively high recurrence rate among patients with neoplastic disease has called into question the value of this procedure for this patient population. As a general rule, patients with hepatic malignancy from an extrahepatic source are no longer considered acceptable candidates for liver transplantation. If the malignancy is primary and confined to the liver parenchyma, hepatic transplantation is still considered an acceptable therapeutic modality for selected patients.[75]

Liver transplantation (Fig. 5-24) is a formidable procedure conducted in three phases. The first phase involves dissection and removal of the recipient liver through a bilateral subcostal incision with an upper midline extension. During the second anhepatic phase, the venovenous bypass employed by most centers decompresses the splanchnic bed, lower extremities, and kidneys by establishing venous flow from the portal vein and inferior vena cava to the axillary vein with a centrifugal pump. The third phase of hepatic implantation involves four vascular anastomoses: the inferior vena cava above and below the liver, the portal vein, and the hepatic artery. The most common biliary reconstruction is a choledochocholedochostomy followed

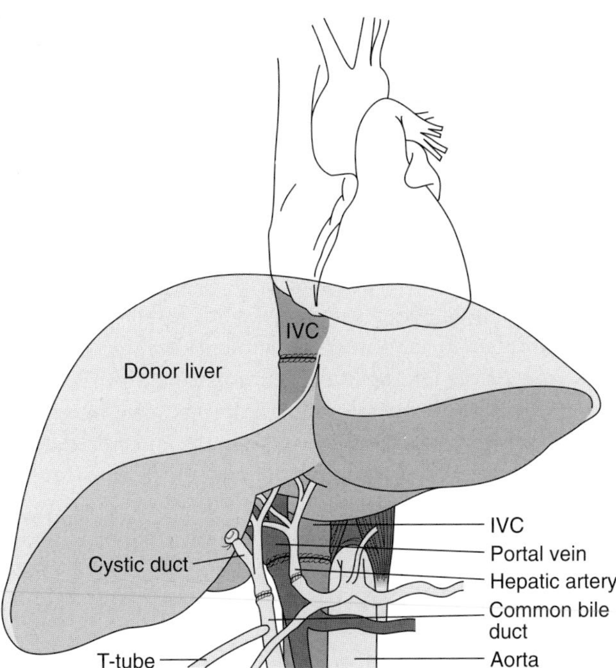

Fig. 5-24. Hepatic transplantation. Vascular continuity is established through four anastomoses that include the inferior vena cava *(IVC)* above and below the liver, the portal vein, and the hepatic artery. Biliary tract reconstruction is obtained by a choledochocholedochostomy performed over a T-tube.

by a choledochoenteric anastomosis with a standard Roux-en-Y choledochojejunostomy. Reported complications after liver transplantation range from 14% to 55%. These include postoperative hemorrhage, vascular thrombosis, biliary leaks and obstructions, bowel obstruction and perforation, gastrointestinal bleeding, and wound complications.[76]

In deciding whether a patient is a suitable candidate for hepatic transplantation, the most important determinants are clearly the extent to which the patient's underlying disease is interfering with quality of life and how transplantation will ultimately influence the long-term prognosis of the disease.

Lung Transplantation

Transplantation of the lung can be performed either by itself or as an en bloc heart-lung combination. Clinical experience with solitary lung transplants has been fraught with considerable problems, including infection, hemorrhagic consolidation, and severe rejection, although this latter problem appears to be less noteworthy with the availability of CsA. Most centers in which solitary transplants have been performed have had few survivors beyond 1 month. For this reason the heart-lung combination transplant has gained in popularity. Not only does the combined graft ensure a better blood supply to the transplanted bronchus, which has historically been a major problem with solitary pulmonary transplants in which anastomotic dehiscence of the bronchus has frequently occurred, but the operation is also technically more feasible than is the solitary transplant and provides a maximum amount of lung parenchyma to optimize function of the allograft. Currently, heart-lung grafting boasts 1- and 2-year survival rates approaching 70% and 60%, respectively. As with other transplants, the use of CsA has contributed greatly to this success.

Although clinical experience with lung transplantation has been limited when compared with kidney, heart, or liver transplantation, potential recipients include patients with irreversible and terminal pulmonary failure. Among those who have received lung transplants have been patients with end-stage pulmonary vascular disease, such as primary pulmonary hypertension, and those with severe parenchymal disease, including chronic obstructive pulmonary disease, respiratory burns, pulmonary fibrosis, toxic pneumonitis, and bronchiectasis.

Pancreas Transplantation

More than 1 million patients in the United States currently are affected by insulin-dependent diabetes mellitus. An additional 10,000 to 15,000 new cases can be expected each year. Despite exacting control of the serum glucose level by exogenously administered insulin, serious complications are associated with this disease. The microangioplastic lesions resulting from aberrant diabetic carbohydrate metabolism produce severe retinopathy that may ultimately lead to blindness, nephropathy eventuating in renal failure, and peripheral vascular disease that is commonly associated with neuropathy and limb loss. Pancreatic transplantation in rodent models has successfully prevented and in some cases halted the progression of these microangiopathic lesions; it is thus not surprising that enormous efforts have been made to develop a successful means of transplanting pancreatic tissue in humans.

The first pancreatic transplant was performed by Kelly and Lillekei at the University of Minnesota in 1996.[77] The 1-year survival for all pancreas transplants between 1966 and 1980 was 21%, with the outcome being influenced greatly by the magnitude of the rejection process. With the advent of CsA, there is renewed interest in this endeavor. Although segmental pancreatic grafting encompassing transplantation of the body and tail of the pancreas with the use of the splenic artery and vein to reestablish vascularization is technically less complex, control of pancreatic duct drainage has been a major technical difficulty. Attempts at intraperitoneal transplantation with intra-abdominal pancreatic drainage, although successful in large-animal models, have been abandoned clinically because of the high complication rate encountered in patients. Other approaches have included duct ligation or duct obliteration by the intraductal injection of synthetic polymers in an attempt to reduce the quantity of pancreatic exocrine secretion. Unfortunately, blockage of exocrine function may lead to sclerosis of the pancreas and the eventual failure of its endocrine function.

Whole-organ pancreatic transplants[78] include en bloc placement of the pancreas and a portion of duodenum surrounding the papilla of Vater to the urinary bladder to provide a means of exocrine drainage (Fig. 5-25). The splenic artery and vein are then anastomosed to the hypogastric artery and external iliac vein, respectively, to reestablish blood supply. The most recent data on all pancreas transplants performed in the United States between 1987 and 1993 demonstrated a 1-year graft survival of 72% and a 1-year patient survival of 91%. However, these patients have a much higher morbidity rate than do renal transplant recipients.

In addition to the vascularized pancreatic allograft, treatment of diabetes has also been attempted with transplantation of isolated pancreatic islet cells. It is estimated that approximately 500,000 islets are required normal carbohydrate metabolism. For this procedure, the pancreas is mechanically and enzymatically disrupted to harvest the islet cells. These cells are then transferred to the recipient. A variety of recipient sites have been used, including the testes, peritoneal cavity, beneath the renal capsule, spleen, and portal vein with the last being used the most often. Although this technique has been quite successful experimentally in preventing or halting the metabolic consequences of diabetes in various animal models, clinical trials to date in human subjects with diabetes failed to abrogate the need for insulin, although some groups reported temporary total insulin independence. Thus, despite its potential advantage, islet transplantation is still in its infancy.

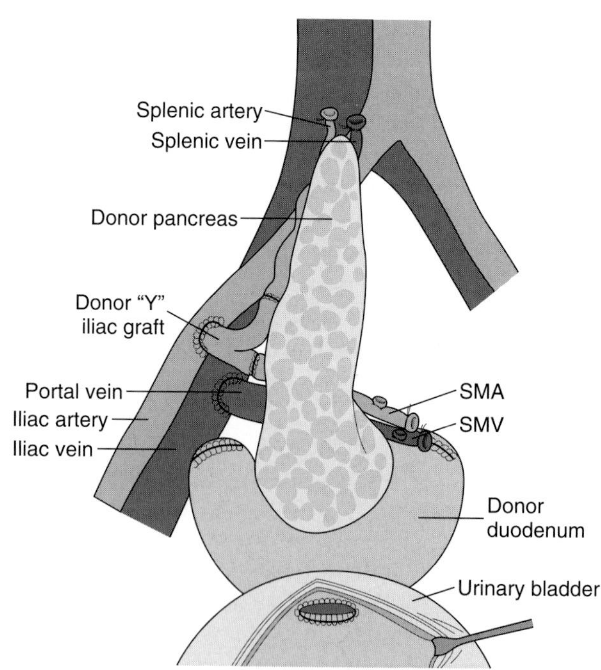

Fig. 5-25. Pancreas transplantation. Donor portal vein is anastomosed to the recipient iliac vein. Donor iliac Y graft connects donor superior mesenteric artery *(SMA)* and donor splenic artery to recipient iliac artery. The duodenal segment is anastomosed to the recipient urinary bladder. *SMV*, Superior mesenteric vein.

Small Bowel Transplantation

Thousands of patients annually are affected by the short-gut syndrome, usually as a result of thrombosis or embolization of the superior mesenteric artery necessitating massive intestinal resection. The minimal digestive absorptive capacity with which these patients is left is often inadequate to maintain a normal nutritional status, requiring the use of long-term parenteral alimentation for survival. Obviously, replacement of this missing intestine with a small bowel transplant would be highly desirable.

Experimentally, small bowel transplantation (SBT) has been successfully performed in animals since 1959. Lillehei, Goott, and Miller[79] were the first to describe this technique in a canine model. Continuing experimental refinements have made the technique of SBT quite feasible from a technical standpoint. As with other organ transplants, the major problem in making SBT a clinically useful modality concerns the control of rejection. The magnitude of this problem directly relates to the length of intestine transplanted. Large segments of small intestine have resulted experimentally in a graft-versus-host disease reaction because of the large amount of lymphoid tissue contained in intestinal mesenteric lymph nodes, Peyer's patches, and lamina propria that are capable mounting an immune response against the host. In humans, the typical erythematous rash of graft-versus-host disease develops concurrently with the appearance of donor lymphocytes in the recipient's peripheral circulation. When small segments of intestine are transplanted, this is less of a problem but the allograft still undergoes the standard rejection process. Immunospupressive regimens that have recently been successful in preventing the rejection process and graft-versus-host disease in various experimental models include CsA or FK506 administration, donor organ irradiation, and microsurgical excision of mesenteric lymph nodes.

In the 1960s, several clinical attempts were made to transplant human intestine. However, all patients died because of technical difficulties associated with the operation, sepsis, graft rejection, or a combination of these factors. Interest in SBT in the 1970s faded with the advent of total parenteral nutrition (TPN). In the 1980s, interest in SBT was renewed after realization of TPN limitations and the success of CsA in prolonging SBT survival in experimental animals. Current attempts of isolated SBT or combined liver/small-bowel transplantation have used high doses of FK506 and prostaglandin E_1, with a 70% actuarial graft and patient survival rate.[80] However, this is associated with a 90% incidence of bacterial infections, a 43% incidence of viral infections, and an increased rate of lymphoproliferative disorders. Until these formidable problems are more effectively managed, human intestinal transplantation must be viewed as an experimental procedure.

Bone Marrow Transplantation

The indications for bone marrow transplantation include severe inherited immune deficiency disorders, bone marrow failure, and certain malignancies. The potentially fatal inherited diseases for which bone marrow transplantation has been used include various hemoglobinopathies such as thalassemia and sickle-cell disease, immunodeficiency states, and such enzymatic disorders as mucopolysaccharoidosis, osteopetrosis, chronic granulomatous disease, adenosine deaminase deficiency, and Diamond-Blackfan anemia. Acquired disorders of marrow failure responding to bone marrow transplantation have included aplastic anemia and such malignancies as acute lymphocytic leukemia, acute nonlymphocytic leukemia, chronic myelogenous leukemia, hairy-cell leukemia, Hodgkin's disease, non-Hodgkin's lymphoma, neuroblastoma, multiple myeloma, and acute myelofibrosis. Marrow transplantation has also been used in selected cases of marrow failure resulting from toxic chemotherapeutic agents.

Human bone marrow transplantation has stressed the use of HLA-histocompatible marrow between donor and recipient, as determined by serologic typing for the alleles of HLA-A, HLA-B, HLA-DR, and HLA-D loci and nonreactive MLC. Bone marrow for transplantation has been obtained from syngeneic, allogeneic, and autologous sources. Whereas syngeneic marrow transplantation is a transfer of bone marrow between genetically identical twins, allogeneic marrow transplantation is usually accomplished between HLA-identical siblings who inherited the same haplotype of chromosome 6 from each parent. The chances of HLA-identity between siblings is 1:4. Recipients of allogeneic or syngeneic marrow are pretreated with immunosuppressive agents and myeloablative drugs if the underlying cause of marrow failure is a malignancy. In autologous transplantation, marrow is harvested from the patient during remission and cryopreserved. The marrow is then replanted after myeloablative antineoplastic therapy to eliminate residual malignant cells. Of interest, autologous transplantation has been as effective in treating acute nonlymphocytic and chronic myelogenous leukemia as has allogeneic or syngeneic marrow transplantation.

The major complications associated with bone marrow transplantation have included rejection of the grafted marrow, graft-versus-host disease, and potentially lethal infections. If the transplanted marrow functions only briefly and a marrow biopsy sample reveals the absence of marrow elements, this indicates that the recipient has rejected the donor marrow because of presensitization, usually resulting from prior blood transfusions. Graft-versus-host disease results from the transplanted T cells reacting to the genetically different host cells. The lymphohematopoietic system, including the skin, liver, and gastrointestinal tract, are primarily affected by the graft-versus-host response, which manifests clinically as dermatitis, diarrhea, alterations in liver function, weight loss, and high susceptibility to infection. Graft-versus-host disease occurs in 30% to 70% of allogeneic marrow transplant recipients and results in the deaths of 20% to 40% of those individuals affected.

The infectious complications after bone marrow transplantation usually occur within the first several weeks before the production of granulocytes by the grafted marrow. The recipient is susceptible to all types of infections, including bacterial, fungal, and HSV infections. Beyond the first month after grafting, the increase in the peripheral white blood cell count suggests the engraftment of the donor marrow. Subsequent infections include CMV and *P. carinii* infections, both of which usually manifest as interstitial pneumonias. The use of prophylactic trimethoprim-sulfamethoxazole has greatly reduced the incidence of interstitial pneumonia caused by *Pneumocystis.* Those patients with CMV as the offending organism are much less fortunate, and many of these individuals die because no current effective treatment exists. Thus, to prevent cytomegalovirus infections, hyperimmune globulin is usually administered prophylactically early after transplantation.

Corneal Transplantation

Corneal transplantation, also referred to as *corneal grafting* or *penetrating keratoplasty,* is performed in the United States at a rate of approximately 10,000 operations per year. The success of this procedure is limited only by the technical skills of the surgeon, not by the immune response. This is because the cornea is an immunologically privileged structure in which oxygen is derived from the oxygen content of the internal aqueous humor, rather than from specific blood vessels. Consequently, circulating antibodies are isolated from the transplanted cornea. When they occur, rejection episodes are usually mild and develop at a rate of only 10% to 12%. If rejection becomes a problem, it is usually ablated by the use of topical steroids. In more than 90% of operations performed, corneal transplantation proves successful. Currently, corneal transplantation is the procedure of choice for all patients with opaque corneas. It is limited only by the availability of donor corneas.

The persistence of the immunologically privileged status of the transplanted cornea depends on the vascularity of the graft. Scarring of the cornea results in an increased vascularity, and consequently an increased risk of rejection. Under this circumstance the cornea has a 25% incidence of irreversible rejection. Rejection occurs primarily through a cellular immune response. Previous corneal grafting resulting in corneal scarring and increased vascularity have been associated with graft failure. Histocompatibility matching is not routinely necessary, but it is beneficial in the presence of heavily vascularized corneas.

SUMMARY

Successful transplantation of organs or tissues rests on an understanding of the immunologic rejection process. The events leading to allograft rejection consist of afferent, central, and efferent limbs. The presentation and recognition of foreign antigens are manifestations of the afferent limb. The central limb encompasses the proliferation, differentiation, and production of lymphokines by T cells and of humoral antibody by B cells, whereas the efferent limb represents the activation of various cell populations that ultimately lead to the rejection of the transplanted tissue or organ. Clinically, allograft rejection is classified as hyperacute, accelerated, acute, or chronic.

A variety of immunologic strategies have been used to avert, minimize, or reduce the rejection response of the host or the immunogenicity of the allograft. The latter approach has had only limited success experimentally with nonvascularized grafts. Host immunosuppression by means of chemical substances (corticosteroids, CsA, Aza, FK506, and MM) nonspecifically diminishes the immune response. Biologic agents (polyclonal sera and MAbs) provide both generalized and specific immunosuppressive effects. Polyclonal sera nonspecifically deplete the host of lymphoid cells, whereas MAbs delete a specific T-cell subset. To date, immunologic manipulation to achieve transplantation tolerance has not progressed to a level satisfactory for clinical use. Continued research in basic immunology provides foundations for further advances in immunosuppressive manipulations. The next era of transplantation will witness progress from the nonspecific immunosuppressive strategy associated with a high morbidity to a strategy that seeks to alter regulation of the immune response to selectively downregulate antidonor responses to achieve immunologic tolerance, the ideal state of immunosuppression.

REFERENCES

1. Kahan BD. Transplantation timeline. Transplantation 51:1, 1991.
2. Bjorkman PF, Parham P. Structure, function, and diversity of class I major histocompatibility complex molecules. Annu Rev Biochem 59:253, 1990.
3. Rammensee HG, Falk K, Rotzschke O. Peptides naturally presented by MHC class I molecules. Annu Rev Immunol 11:213, 1993.
4. Brodsky FM, Guagliardi LE. The cell biology of antigen presentation. Annu Rev Immunol 9:707, 1991.
5. Jackson MR, et al. Regulation of MHC class I transport by the molecular chaperone, calnexin (p88, IP90). Science 263:384, 1994.
6. Brown JH, et al. The three dimensional structure of the human class II histocompatibility antigen HLA-DL1. Nature 364:33, 1993.
7. Germain RN. MCH-dependent antigen processing and peptide presentation: providing ligands for T lymphocyte activation. Cell 76:287, 1994.
8. Flye MW. Immunohematology. In Flye MW, ed. Principles of Organ Transplantation. Philadelphia: WB Saunders, 1989, p 236.
9. Sheil AGR, et al. ABO blood group incompatibility in renal transplantation. Transplantation 8:299, 1969.
10. Alexandre GPJ, et al. Present experiences in a series of 26 ABO-incompatible living donor renal allografts. Transplant Proc 19:4835, 1987.
11. Oriol R, et al. The Lewis system: new histocompatibility antigens in renal transplanting. Lancet 1(2):574, 1978.
12. Spitalnik S, et al. Correlation of humoral immunity to Lewis blood group antigens with renal transplant rejection. Transplantation 37:265, 1984.
13. Weei-Chin L, Desiderio S. Regulation of V(D)J recombination activator protein RAG-2 by phosphorylation. Science 260:953, 1993.
14. Benoist C, Mathis D. Positive selection of the T cell repertoire: where and when does it occur? Cell 58:1027, 1989.
15. Kappler J, Roehm N, Marrack P. T cell tolerance by clonal elimination in the thymus. Cell 49:273, 1987.
16. Nossal GJV. Negative selection of lymphocytes. Cell 76:229, 1994.
17. Finkel TH, Kubo RT, Cambier JC. T-cell development and transmembrane signaling: changing biological responses through an unchanging receptor, Immunol Today 12:79, 1991.

18. Janeway CA. Signals and signs for lymphocyte responses. Cell 76:275, 1994.
19. Mosmann TR, Cofman RL. Th1 and Th2 cells: different patterns of lymphokine secretion lead to different functional properties. Annu Rev Immunol 7:145, 1989.
20. Dallman MJ, et al. Cytokines and peripheral tolerance to alloantigens. Immunol Rev 133:5, 1993.
21. Auchincloss H Jr, et al. T cell subsets, b^{m} mutants, and the mechanism of allogeneic skin graft rejection. Immunol Res 8:149, 1989.
22. Tiemeyer M, et al. Carbohydrate ligands for endothelial-leukocyte adhesion molecule. Proc Natl Acad Sci U S A 88:1138, 1991.
23. Springer TA. Adhesion receptors of the immune system. Nature 346:425, 1990.
24. Springer TA. Traffic signals for lymphocyte recirculation and leukocyte emigration: the multistep paradigm. Cell 76:301, 1994.
25. Harding FA, et al. CD28-mediated signaling co-stimulates murine T cells and prevents induction of anergy in T cell clones. Nature 356:607, 1992.
26. Shwartz RH. Costimulation of T lymphocytes: the role of CD28, CTLA-4, and B7/BB1 in interleukin-2 production and immunotherapy. Cell 71:1065, 1992.
27. Weiss A, Littman DR. Signal transduction by lymphocyte antigen receptors. Cell 76:263, 1994.
28. Sherman LA, Chattopadhyay S. The molecular basis of allorecognition. Annu Rev Immunol 11:385, 1993.
29. Chien Y, Davis MM. How αβ T-cell receptors 'see' peptide/MHC complexes. Immunol Today 14:597, 1993.
30. Ghobrial R, et al. Membrane-bound or soluble truncated RT1.A^{a} rat class I major histocompatibility antigens induce specific alloimmunity. Transplantation 60:602, 1995.
31. Shokes DA, Wood KJ. Indirect presentation of MHC antigens in transplantation. Immunol Today 15:32, 1994.
32. Shirwan H, et al. Lymphocytes infiltrating rat cardiac allografts express a limited repertoire of T cell receptor Vβ genes. J Immunol 151:5228, 1993.
33. Evavold BD, et al. Tickling the TCR: Selective T-cell functions stimulated by altered peptide ligands. Immunol Today 14:602, 1993.
34. Ghobrial R, et al. Induction of transplantation tolerance by perioperative injection of "quasi-self" chimeric class I MHC antigen combined with a short cyclosporine course. Transplant Proc 27:239, 1995.
35. Nisco S, et al. Induction of allograft tolerance by an HLA class-I-derived peptide and cyclosporine A. J Immunol 152:3786, 1994.
36. Kerman RH. Relevance of histocompatibility testing in clinical transplantation. Surg Clin North Am 74:1015, 1994.
37. Miyajima A, et al. Cytokine receptors and signal transduction. Annu Rev Immunol 10:295, 1992.
38. Kishimoto T, Taga T, Akira S. Cytokine signal transduction. Cell 76:253, 1994.
39. McDonald NG, Hendrickson WA. A structural superfamily of growth factors containing a cysteine knot motif. Cell 73:421, 1994.
40. Abbas AK, Lichtman AH, Pober JS. Cytokines. In Abbas AK, Lichtman AH, Pober JS, eds. Cellular and Molecular Immunology, 2nd ed. Philadelphia: WB Saunders, 1994, p 240.
41. Sigal NH, Dumont FJ. Cyclosporine A, FK-506, and rapamycin: pharmacologic probes of lymphocyte signal transduction. Annu Rev Immunol 10:519, 1992.
42. Taniguchi T, Minami Y. The IL-2/IL-2 receptor system: a current overview. Cell 73:5, 1993.
43. Paul WE, Seder RA. Lymphocyte responses and cytokines. Cell 76:241, 1994.
44. Banner DW, et al. Crystal structure of the soluble human 55 kd TNF receptor-human TNFβ complex: implications for TNF receptor activation. Cell 73:431, 1993.
45. Rosenberg AS, Singer A. Cellular basis of skin allograft rejection: an in vivo model of immune-mediated tissue destruction. Annu Rev Immunol 10:333, 1992.
46. Jeannet M, et al. Humoral antibodies in renal allotransplantation in man. N Engl J Med 282:111, 1970.
47. Browne BJ, Kahan BD. Renal transplantation. Surg Clin North Am 74:1097, 1994.
48. Hancock WW. Analysis of intragraft effector mechanisms associated with human renal allograft rejection: immunohistological studies with monoclonal Abs. Immunol Rev 77:61, 1984.
49. Lopez C, et al. Association of renal allograft rejection with viral infections. Am J Med 56:280, 1974.
50. Kahan BD, Ghobrial R. Immunosuppressive agents. Surg Clin North Am 74:1029, 1994.
51. Hricik DE, Almawi WY, Strom TB. Trends in the use of glucocorticoids in renal transplantation. Transplantation 57:979, 1994.
52. Yuh DD, Morris RE. The immunopharmacology of immunosuppression by 15-deoxyspergualin. Transplantation 55:578, 1993.
53. Okubo M, et al. 15-Deoxyspergualin "rescue therapy" for methylprednisolone-resistant rejection of renal transplants as compared with anti-T cell monoclonal antibody (OKT3). Transplantation 55:505, 1993.
54. Kahan BD. Drug therapy: cyclosporine. N Engl J Med 321:1725, 1989.
55. Linholm A, Kahan BD. Influence of cyclosporine pharmacokinetic parameters, trough concentrations and AUC monitoring on outcome after kidney transplantation. Clin Pharmacol Ther 54:205, 1993.
56. Kahan BD, et al. The ability of pretransplant test-dose pharmacokinetic profiles to reduce early adverse events after renal transplantation. Transplantation 53:345, 1992.
57. Kahan BD, Chang JY, Seghal SN. Preclinical evaluation of a new potent immunosuppressive agent, rapamycin. Transplantation 52:185, 1991.
58. Kuo CJ, et al. Rapamycin selectively inhibits interleukin-2 activation of p70 S6 kinase, Nature 358:70, 1992.
59. Sollinger HW, et al. RS61443: A phase I clinical trial and pilot rescue study. Transplantation 53:428, 1992.
60. Cramer DV, et al. The effect of a new immunosuppressive drug, brequinar sodium, on heart, liver and kidney allograft rejection in the rat. Transplantation 53:303, 1992.
61. Jolivet J, et al. The pharmacology and clinical use of methotrexate. N Engl J Med 309:1094, 1983.
62. Kohler G, Milstein C. Continuous cultures of fused cells secreting antibody or predefined specificity. Nature 256:495, 1975.
63. Jaffers G, et al. Monoclonal antibody therapy, anti-idiotypic and anti-isotypic antibodies to OKT3 arising despite intense immunosuppression. Transplantation 41:572, 1986.
64. Wee SL, et al. The effects of OKT4A monoclonal antibody on cellular immunity of nonhuman primate renal allograft recipients. Transplantation 53:501, 1992.
65. Haug CE, et al. A phase I trial of immunosuppression with anti-ICAM-1 (CD54) mAB in renal allograft recipients. Transplantation 55:766, 1993.
66. Isobe M, et al. Specific acceptance of cardiac allograft after treatment with antibodies to ICAM-1 and LFA-1. Science 255:1125, 1992.
67. Hanto DW, Shelton MW, Simmons RI. Cancer in recipients of organ allografts. In Williams GM, Burdick J, Solez K, eds. Kidney Transplant Rejection: Diagnosis and Treatment, 2nd ed. New York: Marcel Dekker, 1991, p 649.
68. Penn I. Development of new tumors after transplantation. In Cerelli GJ, ed. Organ Transplantation and Replacement. Philadelphia: JB Lippincott, 1988, p 439.
69. Rubin RH, Young LS, eds. Clinical Approach to Infection in the Compromised Host, 2nd ed. New York: Plenum, 1988.
70. Johnson M, Flye MW. Infectious complications in renal transplant patients. In Flye MW, ed. Principles of Organ Transplantation. Philadelphia: WB Saunders, 1989, p 294.
71. Merrill JP, et al. Successful homotransplantation of human kidney between identical twins. JAMA 160:277, 1956.

72. Frazier OH, Macris MP. Progress in cardiac transplantation. Surg Clin North Am 74:1169, 1994.
73. Starzl TE, Iwatsuki S, Van Thiel DH. Evolution of orthotopic liver transplantation. Hepatology 2:613, 1982.
74. Wood RP, et al. Liver transplantation. Surg Clin North Am 74:1133, 1994.
75. Farmer DG, et al. Current and future treatment modalities for hepatocellular carcinoma. Clinics in Liver Disease 1:361, 1997.
76. Ozaki CF, et al. Surgical complications of liver transplantation, Surg Clin North Am 74:1155, 1994.
77. Kelly WD, et al. Allotransplantation of the pancreas and the duodenum along with the kidney in diabetic nephropathy. Surgery 61:827, 1967.
78. Sollinger HW, Geffner SR. Pancreas transplantation. Surg Clin North Am 74:1183, 1994.
79. Lillehei RC, Goott B, Miller FA. The physiologic response of the small bowel of the dog to ischemia including prolonged in vitro preservation of the bowel with successful replacement and survival. Annals of Surgery 150:543, 1959.
80. Asfar S, Zhong R, Grant D. Small bowel transplantation. Surg Clin North Am 74:1197, 1994.

6

Surgical Infection: Principles of Management and Antibiotic Usage

Rodney M. Durham and John E. Mazuski

The prevention and treatment of microbial infections is an important component of the surgeon's clinical practice. Patients may first present to a surgeon because of an infection requiring drainage or some other form of surgical treatment. In addition, postoperative infections are among the most common complications of surgical therapy, even in patients whose original problem was noninfectious in nature. For these reasons, it is important for the surgeon to have an understanding of the basic pathophysiology of infection, as well as the fundamental principles of management, including antibiotic therapy.

PATHOPHYSIOLOGY OF SURGICAL INFECTIONS

Infections result when the balance between pathogenic organisms and the host's defense mechanisms is disrupted. Large numbers of bacteria and other microorganisms colonize many of the epithelial surfaces of the body, including the skin, most portions of the upper aerodigestive tract, the gastrointestinal tract below the duodenum, the vagina, and the lower genitourinary tract. Overall, approximately 10^{14} bacteria colonize the human body, or about 10 bacteria for every eucaryotic cell.[1] Anaerobic bacteria predominate over aerobic bacteria by a 10:1 ratio, and this ratio may be even higher in the lower GI tract. These endogenous microorganisms prevent colonization of these epithelial surfaces by more pathogenic organisms, but can themselves be pathogenic under appropriate circumstances. Further, the endogenous flora is responsible for most of the infections observed in surgical patients.

The virulence of a particular microbe is related to many different properties. Specific molecules on the microbial surface may allow an organism to adhere to an epithelial surface, thereby initiating an infection. For instance, *Escherichia coli* strains bearing specific types of fimbriae can attach to the urinary epithelium; these strains are much more likely to produce clinical urinary tract infections than strains not bearing those structures. Other microbial products may facilitate invasion of the host tissues. Streptokinase, hyaluronidase, and collagenase are enzymes secreted by some types of bacteria that allow spreading infections to occur. Finally, many microorganisms have mechanisms that allow them to escape the host defenses. Thus microbial proteins have been identified that disrupt chemotaxis by white blood cells, interfere with phagocytosis, or prevent intracellular killing. Thus certain intracellular pathogens, such as *Listeria,* actually survive within the phagocyte.

Various exotoxins and endotoxins may be responsible for many of the deleterious effects of microbial infections. Many times, the actual infection itself is of little consequence, but the potent toxins released result in fulminate disease. Examples of such infections are those produced by diphtheria, cholera, and tetanus bacteria. Microbial toxins produce a variety of effects on the host. Some exotoxins are cytotoxic for eucaryotic cells, such as the exotoxins produced by *Clostridium difficile.* Other toxins trigger an overwhelming host response, and it is the host response rather than the actual infection that results in damage to distant tissues. For instance, many of the pathogenic effects of lipopolysaccharide, the complex endotoxin of gram-negative bacteria, are thought to be mediated by this overwhelming host response.

There are numerous mechanisms by which the host prevents these pathogenic microorganisms from producing frank infection. The intact epitheluim of the skin or mucosal surface presents the initial barrier against microbial invasion. Both physical and chemical components contribute to this barrier function. Tight junctions and other components of the intercellular adhesion complex prevent microorganisms from gaining access to internal tissues. Mucosal surfaces are protected by a surface layer of mucus, which prevents bacterial attachment, and the dry, somewhat acidic, keratinized surface of the skin inhibits bacterial proliferation. In addition, epithelial cells secrete a number of substances, such as lysozyme, which are also inhibitory for microbial growth. Finally, some epithelial surfaces have mechanical mechanisms by which to directly remove microorganisms, as is seen with the mucociliary apparatus of the respiratory epithelium.

Microbial organisms that breach the epithelial barrier or otherwise gain access to interior tissues have to face both nonspecific and specific humoral and cellular defense mechanisms. Nonspecific humoral components of the inflammatory response, such as the complement cascade, the kallikrein-kinin system, and the coagulation system, are activated. This activation helps to localize the invading microorganisms and also signals for the recruitment of phagocytic cells, such as neutrophils and macrophages, to the site of invasion. The nonspecific inflammatory response is accompanied by the development of the specific immune response. The humoral arm of the immune response is represented by the various immunoglobulin molecules produced by B lymphocytes and plasma cells, and the cellular arm by specific cytotoxic T lymphocytes and natural killer cells, among others.

Many aspects of surgical treatment interfere with these host defense mechanisms. The most obvious of these is the surgical incision through intact skin or mucosa. The placement of intravenous and other vascular access catheters also breaks the intact skin barrier. Other devices, such as endotracheal tubes and indwelling urinary catheters, provide microorganisms with direct access from sites of heavy colonization to normally sterile areas. Ischemic and devitalized tissues produced as a result of a surgical procedure provide a haven for the growth of bacteria, since they may be inaccessible to phagocytic cells. In addition, the presence of blood in areas of damage provides essential nutrients for bacterial growth. The use of prophylatic antibiotics for many operative procedures, while undeniably reducing the risk of wound infections, may also change the resident microbial flora, allowing a pathogen to proliferate. This has been well demonstrated in the development of antibiotic-associated colitis.

The patient's preexisting medical condition can also interfere with host defense mechanisms. For instance, the presence of diabetes mellitus or the prior use of corticosteroid or immunosuppressive medications may impair the development of an adequate inflammatory or immunologic response. Severe malnutrition is also associated with an increased risk of postoperative infections.

Finally, the pathologic process that has necessitated the surgical procedure may increase the risk of a significant infection. There is a high likelihood of developing an intra-abdominal abscess or surgical wound infection when massive peritoneal contamination, for instance, from a free colonic perforation, has occurred. Shock and hypothermia also result in a generalized impairment in the function of phagocytic cells, as well as in the cellular immune responses, and predispose patients to postoperative infections.

SYSTEMIC INFLAMMATORY RESPONSE

The local inflammatory response generated as a result of an infection is usually accompanied by a systemic response of the organism. This systemic response to a proinflammatory stimulus, whether infectious or noninfectious, is

DEFINITIONS

Infection: Microbial phenomenon characterized by an inflammatory response to the presence of microorganisms or the invasion of normally sterile host tissue by those organisms.

Bacteremia: The presence of viable bacteria in the blood.

Systemic inflammatory response syndrome (SIRS): The systemic inflammatory response to a variety of severe clinical insults. The response is manifested by two or more of the following conditions:
Temperature >38° C or <36° C
Heart rate >90 beats/min
Respiratory rate >20 breaths/min or $Pa\text{CO}_2$ <32 torr (<4.3 kPa)
WBC > 12,000 cells/mm^3, <4000 cells/mm^3, or >10% immature (band) forms

Sepsis: The systemic response to infection. This systemic response is manifested by two or more of the following conditions as a result of infection:
Temperature >38° C or <36° C
Heart rate >90 beats/min
Respiratory rate >20 breaths/min or $Pa\text{CO}_2$ <3 torr (<4.3 kPa)
WBC >12,000 cells/mm^3, <4000 cells/mm^3, or >10% immature (band) forms

Severe sepsis: Sepsis associated with organ dysfunction, hypoperfusion, or hypotension. Hypoperfusion and perfusion abnormalities may include, but are not limited to lactic acidosis, oliguria, or an acute alteration in mental status.

Septic shock: Sepsis with hypotension, despite adequate fluid resuscitation, along with the presence of perfusion abnormalities that may include, but are not limited to, lactic acidosis, oliguria, or an acute alteration in mental status. Patients who are receiving inotropic or vasopressor agents may not be hypotensive at the time that perfusion abnormalities are measured.

Hypotension: A systolic blood pressure of <90 mm Hg or a reduction of <40 mm Hg from baseline in the absence of other causes for hypotension.

Multiple-organ dysfunction syndrome (MODS): Presence of altered organ function in an acutely ill patient such that homeostasis cannot be maintained without intervention.

Modified from Members of the American College of Chest Physicians/Society of Critical Care Medicine Consensus Conference Committee: American College of Chest Physicians/Society of Critical Care Medicine Consensus Conference. Definitions for sepsis and organ failure and guidelines for the use of innovative therapies in sepsis. Crit Care Med 20: 864, 1992.

now referred to as the systemic inflammatory response syndrome (SIRS).[2] SIRS is considered to be present if a patient has two or more abnormalities in temperature, heart rate, respiratory function, or white blood cell count (see box on p. 150). When an infection is the cause of SIRS, sepsis is considered to be present.

Although alterations in these four parameters suffice to define the clinical syndrome of SIRS, the systemic response to infection involves changes in many more physiologic parameters. In general, this systemic response includes the development of a hyperdynamic cardiovascular state characterized by increased cardiac output and decreased systemic vascular resistance and a hypermetabolic state characterized by increased oxygen consumption and carbon dioxide production, production and utilization of glucose, mobilization of free fatty acids, and breakdown of the body's muscle protein stores.[3] This overall systemic response is probably important in ensuring the organism's survival during an infectious episode. Indeed, in experimental settings it has been shown that the development of fever is associated with increased survival following a normally lethal bacterial challenge.[4] It has also been observed in clinical studies that the inability to develop an adequate cardiovascular or metabolic response has an adverse impact on patient survival during sepsis.[5,6]

The mechanisms by which the systemic inflammatory response is generated have been extensively investigated in recent years. It is apparent that a large number of endogenous mediators are involved in this response. Such mediators include neurotransmitters and hormones (such as catecholamines, glucagon, and glucocorticoids), various proinflammatory mediators (including lipid-derived mediators such as eicosanoids and platelet-activating factor), and polypeptide mediators (such as activated components of the complement system). Of particular importance in triggering the systemic response to infections are certain peptide regulatory factors referred to as cytokines. Cytokines that may be especially important in the development of this response include tumor necrosis factor (TNF), lymphotoxin, colony-stimulating factors, and various interleukins (particularly interleukin-1 (IL-1), interleukin-6 (IL-6), and interleukin-8 (IL-8), and interferon-α, -β and -γ.[7]

The importance of these agents has been demonstrated in experimental studies in which endotoxin was infused into laboratory animals or human volunteers. Endotoxin infusion was found to be followed by the sequential release of TNF, IL-1, and IL-6.[8] Inhibition of TNF using a neutralizing antibody abrogated the release of the other cytokines and also suppressed many of the physiologic changes typical of the systemic inflammatory response.[9] In clinical studies, however, circulating levels of IL-6 rather than TNF have been found to correlate most closely with an adverse clinical outcome, but the combined inflammatory score based on circulating concentrations of endotoxin, TNF, IL-1, and IL-6 appeared to be the best predictor of outcome in patients with the sepsis syndrome.[10]

Given the importance of these proinflammatory mediators in the development of the clinical manifestations of infections, it is not surprising that antagonists of these cytokines have been developed and subjected to clinical trials. In general, however, the use of antiendotoxin antibodies, anti-TNF antibodies, and an IL-1 receptor antagonist has not proved beneficial. There are several potential reasons why these agents have not been useful clinically. First of all, although the experimental infusion of endotoxin produces an orderly release of cytokines with TNF playing a primary role, most clinical infections, even those due to gram-negative organisms, are likely to involve a much more complicated pattern of mediator release. Second, the therapeutic use of cytokine antagonists may occur too late, since much of the initial wave of cytokine release occurs within a few hours of the infusion of bacteria or endotoxin. It is only under very special circumstances, in which an antagonist can be given prior to the expected release of the mediators, that anticytokine therapy has proved beneficial.[11] Finally, from the biologic viewpoint, it should be noted that the systemic inflammatory response has evolved in vertebrates as a mechanism in which to counteract infectious and other damaging stimuli. Thus this reaction should ultimately be advantageous for survival, even though acutely it increases the physiologic demands placed on the organism. Thus it is certainly possible that counteracting this response may not benefit the patient.

DEFINITIONS OF SURGICAL INFECTIONS

In 1992 the Centers for Disease Control and Prevention revised its definition of surgical wound infections. At this time it was proposed to change the terminology from *wound infection* to *surgical site infections.*[12] This latter terminology was designed to take into account both incisional (superficial and deep) infections and infections of organs or body spaces (e.g., subphrenic abscesses). More distant infections (e.g., postoperative pneumonia), excluding blood infections directly related to surgical site infection, are classified as postoperative complications. Superficial incisional infections involve only the skin and subcutaneous tissues. Deep incisional infections involve the fascial and muscle layers, and organ/space infections involve any organs or body cavities that were manipulated during the surgical procedure. To be considered a surgical site infection, the infection must occur within 30 days of the procedure, unless an implant is in place, in which case the time period is lengthened to 1 year. Characteristics of the different types of infection are listed in the box on p. 152.

Infections that arise in tissues begin as a *cellulitis.* This is manifested clinically by local tenderness, heat, swelling, redness, and pain. Because this type of infection has no localized areas of pus formation, it does not lend itself to drainage and can often be managed by rest, application of local heat, antibiotic therapy, and elevation if an extremity is involved. If left untreated, cellulitis may spread through adjacent tissue planes (as occurs with β-hemolytic streptococcus) or remain localized to form an abscess (as may

CHARACTERISTICS OF SURGICAL SITE INFECTIONS

Superficial Incisional SSIs

1. Purulent drainage from the superficial incision.
2. Organisms isolated from an aseptically obtained culture of fluid or tissue from the superficial incision.
3. At least one of the following signs or symptoms of infection: Pain or tenderness, localized swelling, redness, or heat and superficial incision is deliberately opened by surgeon, unless culture result of incision is negative.
4. Diagnosis of superficial incisional SSI by the surgeon or attending physician.

The following are not reported as superficial incisional SSIs: (1) stitch abscess (minimal inflammation and discharge confined to the points of suture penetration), (2) infection of an episiotomy or a neonate's circumcision site (episiotomy and circumcision are not considered National Nosocomial Infection Surveillance System [NNISS] operative procedures), (3) infected burn wound, and (4) incisional SSI that extends into the fascial and muscle layers (see deep incisional SSIs).

Deep Incisional SSIs

1. Purulent drainage from the deep incision but not from the organ/space component of the surgical site.
2. A deep incision spontaneously dehisces or is deliberately opened by a surgeon when the patient has at least one of the following signs or symptoms: Fever (higher than 38° C), localized pain, or tenderness, unless culture result of the incision is negative.
3. An abscess or other evidence of infection involving the deep incision is found on direct examination, during reoperation, or by histopathologic or radiologic examination.
4. Diagnosis of a deep incisional SSI by a surgeon or attending physician.

Organ/Space SSIs

1. Purulent drainage from a drain placed through a stab wound into an organ/space.
2. Organisms isolated from an aseptically obtained culture or fluid or tissue in the organ/space.
3. An abscess or other evidence of infection involving the organ/space on direct examination, during reoperation, or by histopathologic or radiologic examination.
4. Diagnosis of an organ/space SSI by a surgeon or attending physician.

For an SSI involving more than one specific site, the following criteria must be met:

1. Infection that involves both superficial and deep incision sites is classified as deep incisional SSI.
2. Occasionally, an organ/space infection drains through the incision. Such infection generally does not involve reoperation and is considered a complication of the incision. It is therefore classified as a deep incisional SSI.

A surgeon's or physician's diagnosis of infection is an accepted criterion of an SSI unless there is compelling evidence to the contrary.

Modified from Horan T, et al. CDC definitions of nosocomial surgical site infections, 1992: A modification of CDC definitions of surgical wound infections. Infect Control Hosp Epidemiol 13:606, 1992.
SSI, Surgical site infection.

occur with staphylococcus). In contrast to cellulitis, an *abscess* denotes a local collection of necrotic tissue, white blood cells, and bacteria designated clinically as pus. The increased osmotic pressure that exists within a walled-off abscess can lead to movement of water into the area from adjacent tissues, resulting in pressure that is seen clinically as severe pain and tenderness. All abscesses should be drained to prevent the risk of bacterial spread along adjacent tissue planes or through the blood or lymphatic vessels and to provide symptomatic relief. Adjunctive antibiotic therapy is indicated to treat associated areas of cellulitis and to control any bacteria that may have entered the lymph or blood during the drainage process.

Not uncommonly, products of infection from areas of cellulitis or abscess formation gain access to the blood and lymph systems. Occasionally, during the spread of infection, lymph channels may become infected and are seen clinically as hyperemic streaks. This condition is *acute lymphangitis,* colloquially referred to as blood poisoning. If this infection is not controlled, the involved lymph nodes may later abscess and progress to a more severe state of infection known as *suppurative lymphangitis.* Invasion of vascular channels by bacteria is referred to as *bacteremia.* Because of the direct consequences that may result from bacterial spread both lymphatically and through the vascular system, aggressive treatment including appropriate antibiotic therapy and local management of the source of infection with drainage of any abscesses is indicated.

Approximately 30% of surgical patients either enter the hospital with an infection or subsequently develop one during the course of their postoperative care. Operative intervention is usually required in patients who are admitted to surgical services with evidence of infection. Infections of this nature include such diseases as appendicitis, cholecystitis, diverticular abscess, and gangrene of the leg. Although antibiotics are used as an adjunct to surgery in these patients, antibiotics by themselves are usually not efficacious in controlling the infectious process. The most frequent types of infection encountered in surgical patients are postoperative infections. In general, this classification implies a hospital-acquired infection, commonly referred to as a *nosocomial infection*. Of all nosocomial infections, as many as 70% occur in surgical patients.[13] Approximately 40% of these infections occur at the surgical site, 42% originate in the urinary tract, 14% are respiratory, and 4% are blood stream infections. As discussed in the preceding section, nosocomial infections are most commonly caused by the patient's normal endogenous flora and are a consequence of breaches in the patient's host defenses from the surgical procedure itself or secondary to other invasive procedures such as the placement of intravenous cathethers. However, if the patient has been hospitalized for a period of time, colonization of the patient with hospital-acquired organisms occurs and may result in infections that are resistant to multiple antibiotics.[14] Nosocomial infections are less frequently caused by organisms acquired directly from the hospital environment. Examples include infections derived from contaminated respiratory equipment resulting in pneumonia, intravenous fluid contamination resulting in sepsis, and the infrequent situation in which hospital personnel may be the source of infection.

EVALUATION OF SUSPECTED INFECTION IN THE SURGICAL PATIENT

An understanding of the clinical manifestations and types of infection that develop postoperatively assists greatly in expediting the diagnosis and in instituting appropriate therapy for the infectious process. Normal body temperature is maintained by the thermoregulatory center in the hypothalamus within narrow limits (98.6° ± 0.9° F) and varies only slightly throughout a given 24-hour period. An elevation in temperature above normal daily fluctuations represents the presence of fever. Although fever in the postoperative period may be due to numerous causes (see accompanying box), the presence of fever should be assumed to be due to infection until proved otherwise. The timing of the onset of fever is a classic aid in determining the possible cause of these infections. A temperature elevation in the first day or two following surgery is usually related to atelectasis involving one or both lungs. In the next 24 to 48 hours, urinary tract manifestations may become apparent. Under most conditions, wound infections do not cause fever until 4 to 6 days postoperatively, although streptococcal and clostridial wound infections can be seen as early as 24 hours after surgery. Thrombophlebitis almost never occurs before the third postoperative day and usually does not become apparent until a week to 10 days following surgery. Venous disorders involving the lower extremities as a cause of postoperative fever are generally less commonly encountered than those associated with phlebitis secondary to upper-extremity venous catheter placement (i.e., intravenous lines). A mnemonic to assist in remembering this sequence of fever onset is *wind* (pulmonary), *water* (urinary), *wound,* and *walking* (phlebitis). Despite the convenience of these guidelines, they should not preclude careful examination of other potential sources for infection. Furthermore, exceptions to the timing of these guidelines and fever patterns are legion so that the rational assessment of postoperative fever should begin with an organized approach to diagnosis (Fig. 6-1).

CAUSES OF POSTOPERATIVE FEVER

- Respiratory tract infections
  - Atelectasis
  - Pneumonia
- Urinary tract infections
- Wound infections
  - Early wound infections
  - *Streptococcus* species
  - *Clostridium* species
- Late wound infections
  - *Staphylococcus* species
  - Mixed aeobic-anaerobic organisms
- Thrombophlebitis
  - Upper extremity (almost always catheter-related infections)
  - Lower extremity (usually related to venous stasis and not infected)
- Intra-abdominal causes
  - Peritonitis
  - Abscess
- Miscellaneous causes (considerably less common)
  - Gastrointestinal infections
  - Blood transfusion reaction
  - Allergies
  - Dehydration
  - Undrained sterile fluids (e.g., pleural fluid, hematoma)
  - Pancreatitis
  - Blood transfusion–related infections (e.g., non-A hepatitis, non-B hepatitis, cytomegalovirus)

In addition to elicitation of the patient's history, a careful physical examination focusing on likely sources of infection is mandatory. Wounds and drain sites must be inspected carefully. Patients with urinary bladder catheters should be examined for signs of urinary tract infection (e.g., flank pain and cloudy urine). Intravenous catheter sites may be a source of serious infection even though the evidence for inflammation at the catheter site may be subtle. Swelling in the arm distal to a subclavian catheter might indicate septic thrombophlebitis. The skin should be carefully examined for rashes, which may be allergic or infectious in origin. Infections lesions should be uncapped, and a Gram stain and culture of the pustular contents should be performed. Careful assessment of the lung and chest tube sites, if present, is mandatory to exclude pneumonitis and other pulmonary infections such as empyema. Evaluation of the abdomen may disclose peritonitis or a suspected subphrenic or other deep abscess. Evaluation of the abdomen may disclose peritonitis or a suspected subphrenic or other deep abscess. The rectal and pelvic examinations must not be excluded; otherwise, perirectal and

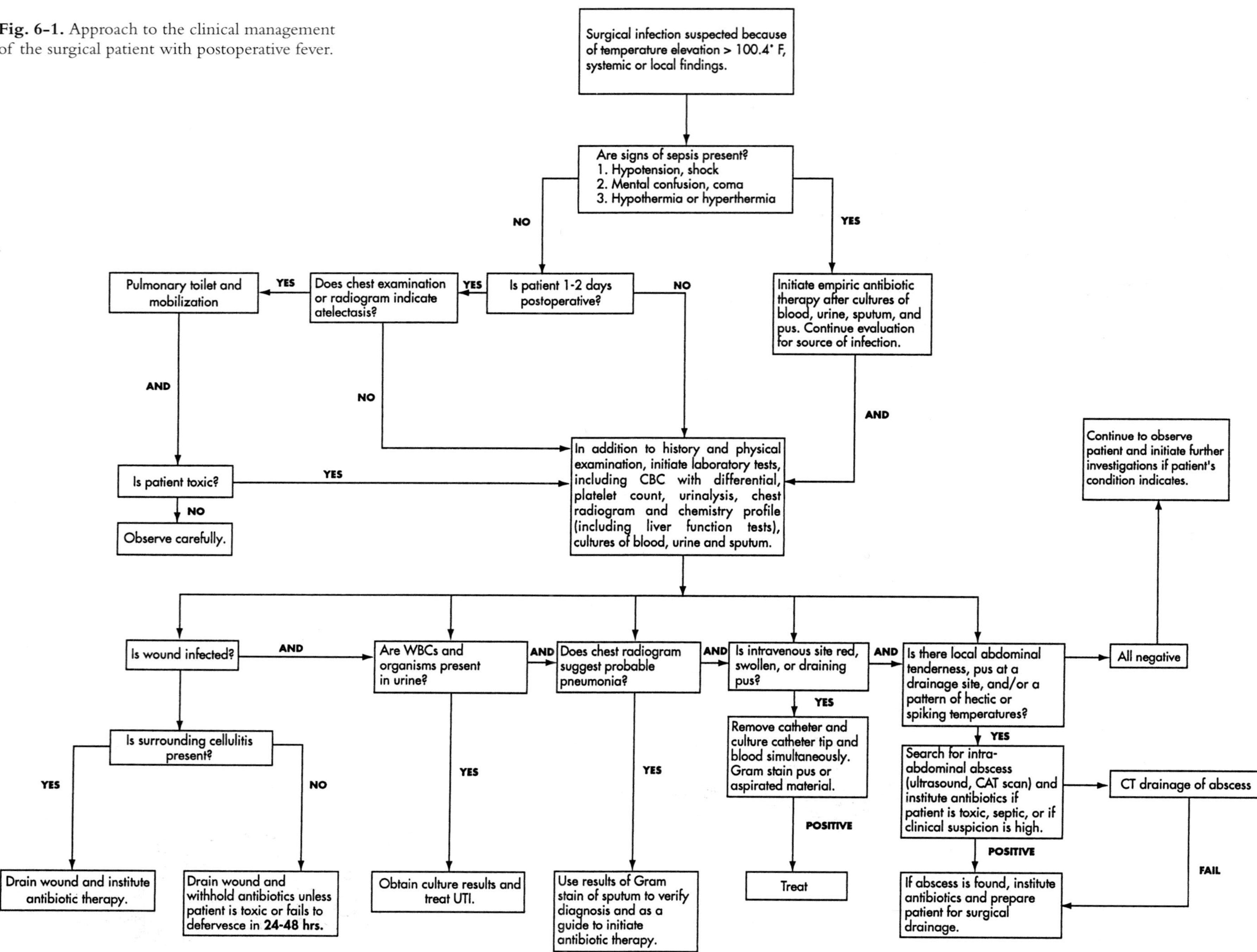

Fig. 6-1. Approach to the clinical management of the surgical patient with postoperative fever.

pelvic abscesses might be missed. Appropriate laboratory and radiologic studies are obtained based on the clinical findings after completion of the history and physical examination.

ROLE OF THE LABORATORY IN INFECTION DIAGNOSIS

Stress caused by trauma, burns, or infections results in a nonspecific host response that has been referred to as the acute phase response.[15,16] This response occurs within hours to days after tissue injury and may last indefinitely depending on the persistence of the disease. This response results in metabolic changes in numerous organ systems (hepatic, hematologic, endocrine, and neurologic systems), some of which may be detected by laboratory tests. One of the more sensitive indicators of the acute phase response is an increase in the number and a decrease in the maturity of circulating neutrophils. Many surgical infections are characterized by leukocytosis with a left shift in the differential count. However, white blood cell counts by themselves can be misleading. As noted in the definitions of sepsis discussed in the box on p. 150, a low white blood cell count, especially in the elderly or compromised host, may be associated with particularly severe episodes of sepsis. A number of other nonspecific laboratory tests may also be indicative of infection. An increase in hepatic protein synthesis results in elevated levels of C-reactive protein and an increase in the erythrocyte sedimentation rate during the acute phase response. In addition, abnormalities of glucose metabolism during sepsis can lead to both hypoglycemia and hyperglycemia.[17,18]

Laboratory tests may also support the presence of specific disease processes. Liver function studies including bilirubin and alkaline phosphatase may be elevated secondary to infections of the liver such as ascending cholangitis, cholecystitis, liver abscess, or hepatitis. However the range of overlap in liver function derangements in fundamentally different disease states is so high that these tests may be difficult to interpret clinically. For example, exceedingly high aminotransferase levels (i.e., in the thousands) are virtually diagnostic of hepatitis (usually A, B, or non-A/non-B), but lower levels (i.e., in the hundreds) can be seen in hepatitis caused by cytomegalovirus infections, Epstein-Barr viral disease, syphilis, and toxoplasmosis. These lower levels can be seen in alcoholic hepatitis, liver abscess, and occasionally gallbladder disease, among other disease states. If hepatitis is considered a possibility, more specific serum tests, such as hepatitis B surface antigen and cytomegalovirus titers, should be obtained.

Although the history, physical examination, radiographic tests, and nonspecific laboratory tests are valuable in establishing the presence and defining the focus of infection, identifying the offending organism depends on obtaining stains and cultures of relevant material. Care must be taken to ensure appropriate collection of these specimens.[19] Many surgical infections occur adjacent to mucous membranes or other areas where *colonizing* flora may be confused with *causal* flora. Classic examples of inappropriate and irrelevant cultures are as follows: culturing sputum for anaerobes in necrotizing pneumonia; culturing chest tube contents rather than percutaneously obtained pleural space material when empyema is suspected; swabbing wounds for culture rather than aspirating underlying abscesses through intact skin or cellulitic areas; and culturing sinus tracts rather than obtaining bone biopsies without contamination from the tract when osteomyelitis is suspected.

Direct examination of a specimen either as a wet mount or stained specimen is often useful in the diagnosis of infection. Wet mounts examined with an ordinary light microscope are useful in the identification of protozoa and fungi.[20] Gram's stain is the most widely used procedure for the direct examination of a specimen. Stained smears can demonstrate the presence of inflammatory cells and bacteria. The presence of inflammatory cells may be useful in determining the adequacy of a specimen particularly in Gram's stains of sputum in which the presence of inflammatory cells suggests pneumonia, whereas a stain demonstrating squamous epithelial cells and a wide variety of organisms suggests that the specimen has been contaminated with saliva.[21] With experience, many causative agents can be predicted, and the Gram's stain result can guide empiric therapy. For instance, clumps of staphylococci are clearly different from chains of streptococci. Clostridial species have a characteristic appearance of plump, gram-positive rods. Among surgical infections, mixed anaerobic-aerobic infections are common; the Gram's stain result may be the only clue to the presence of an anaerobe that may fail to grow in culture.

Traditionally, urine, sputum, and blood cultures in addition to cultures of any infected material obtained from debridement or aspiration have been used to evaluate patients suspected of having a postoperative infection. However, if negative urinalysis results are obtained and the patient has no symptoms relating to the urinary tract, urine cultures may be omitted. In addition, routine culturing of the patient need not include a sputum sample if there is no realistic concern for pulmonary infection (i.e., no cough, no rales during pulmonary auscultation, and a normal chest radiogram). Finally, the utility of routine culturing of the blood in patients with postoperative fevers in the absence of clinical signs of sepsis or neutropenia has been questioned. Theuer et al.[22] found the yield of positive blood cultures per patient febrile event was only 5% when routine blood cultures were obtained. Of interest, bacterial cultures in patients receiving broad-spectrum antibiotics were uniformly negative. Since many patients were begun on antibiotic coverage after obtaining one set of cultures, reculturing the patient was not productive if initial cultures did not reveal the source of fever. As a result, appropriateness of antibiotic therapy could not be evaluated in these patients. Therefore it has been suggested that antibiotic therapy be withheld until there is a defined bacterial source of infection in patients who are not neutropenic or septic. Empiric antibiotic therapy can and should be initiated in these patients if clinical deterioration occurs.

The approach outlined above is designed to have an organism available in the laboratory so that tests can be performed on it to verify that the correct antibiotics have been chosen and to allow for appropriate changes in antibiotic coverage if the organism proves to be resistant. To predict antibiotic susceptibility of an organism, most microbiology laboratories use the disk diffusion test in which an antibiotic impregnated in a paper disk diffuses into the Mueller-Hinton agar plate on which bacteria are plated.[23,24] The utility of this test is limited to organisms that grow rapidly on this agar (staphylococci, *Enterobacteriaceae,* pseudomonads, *Haemophilus influenzae*). This method is not reliable for determining susceptibility of anaerobic bacteria. In 24 hours a sizable clear zone (no growth) around the disk indicates that the organism is susceptible to that antibiotic. It must be noted, however, that the amount of antibiotic in a disk has been chosen so that the result of the test predicts that an organism *in the blood stream* can be killed or its growth inhibited by concentrations of antibiotic achievable in the blood stream. The minimum inhibitory concentration (MIC) must be *exceeded* in the blood stream to penetrate an abscess and kill susceptible organisms. Conversely, a urinary tract infection caused by an "antibiotic-resistant" organism may actually be cured by that antibiotic because the antibiotic is excreted, and thereby concentrated, in the urine. The apparent susceptibilities of certain organisms are also subject to the exact number of organisms placed on the agar plate (i.e., inoculum effect). Susceptibilities of organisms such as *Pseudomonas aeruginosa* are very dependent on control of the cationic content of the media. Finally, a slow-growing organism may appear falsely susceptible to antibiotic therapy by disk diffusion testing.

Additional information about antibiotic susceptibility can be obtained by dilution susceptibility testing, which may be performed in agar or broth. A highly controlled inoculum (often in serum to control the effects of protein binding) is exposed to specific antibiotics in twofold dilutions. The MIC and minimum bactericidal concentration (MBC) of the antibiotic can then be defined and related to the measured or anticipated concentration of antibiotic achieved or achievable in target tissues.[25,26] This kind of data is useful for testing of slow-growing bacteria, when the duration of antibiotic therapy is long (i.e., osteomyelitis, endocarditis), or if another antibiotic must be substituted because of the development of adverse reactions. Automated systems using both the disk diffusion and the dilution method can produce susceptibility results in 3 to 7 hours. However, results for important isolates should be confirmed by conventional methods, which require 24 to 48 hours to perform.

Most surgical infections can be well managed by using standard antibiotic susceptibility data. One very important exception to this rule is the apparent susceptibility of methicillin-resistant *Staphylococcus aureus* (MRSA) to cephalosporins when tested by the disk diffusion method.[27] MRSA may appear to be susceptible, but when checked by dilution susceptibility testing, the MICs are found to be high. Consequently, clinical failures can occur when MRSA is treated with even high doses of cephalosporins. For this reason, many laboratories no longer report the cephalosporin susceptibility of MRSA.

TYPES OF POSTOPERATIVE INFECTIONS

Respiratory Infections

Pneumonia is the second most common nosocomial infection after urinary tract infections but is the leading infectious cause of morbidity and mortality in hospitals in the United States. Nosocomial pneumonias related to surgery have been noted to occur in 5.4 to 11.2 cases per 1000 discharges depending on the type of operation performed.[28] A number of factors predispose surgical patients to the development of respiratory infections. These include suppression of the immune system that occurs after surgical or accidental trauma, infections occurring at surgical sites remote from the lung that may lead adult respiratory distress syndrome (ARDS), and mechanical interference with lung function secondary to operative procedures. Thoracic and upper abdominal incisions are particularly likely to impair respiratory function. Pain and splinting from these incisions lead to postoperative hypoventilation and bronchiolar construction, resulting in atelectasis and a reduction in the functional residual capacity (FRC) of the lung. The extent of the decrease in FRC depends on the type of incision used. Thoracic incisions have been shown to decrease FRC by as much as 65%. Upper abdominal incisions decrease FRC by about 35%, while lower abdominal incisions decrease FRC by as little as 7%.[29] Atelectasis, defined as areas of alveolar collapse, result in retention of bronchial secretions and the entrapment of bacteria. As alveolar macrophages and systemically recruited neutrophils attempt to eradicate these bacteria, fever ensues. Since atelectasis is a common inciting event leading to the development of postoperative pneumonia, every effort should be directed at preventing or reexpanding collapsed alveoli. This goal may be accomplished through early ambulation, frequent coughing and deep breathing, frequent changes in position when in bed, and the use of incentive spirometry to improve pulmonary expansion.

Patient-related risk factors for the development of postoperative pulmonary complications include advanced age, comorbid illnesses (e.g., chronic obstructive lung disease, diabetes, alcoholism), malnutrition, decreased mental status, and cigarette smoking.[30,31] In addition, microaspiration of small volumes of gastric and oropharyngeal secretions colonized with pathogenic bacteria is a common precursor of pneumonia. While microaspiration may occur in up to 45% of normal volunteers, it does not usually lead to pneumonia in the absence of colonization by pathogenic bacteria. As many as 35% of moderately ill patients and about 75% of critically ill patients develop oropharyngeal colonization with pathogenic bacteria, primarily gram-negative enteric organisms, during the course of hospitalization.[32] Colonization of gastric secretions is particularly likely in patients receiving acid-reducing therapy for the prophylaxis of stress gastritis. Aspiration of these secretions may lead to pneumonia. Endotracheal intubation and mechanical ventilation also predispose the patient to develop pneumonia by interfering with lung defenses and by allowing direct access of bacteria to the bronchial tree. Efforts to minimize the likelihood of aspiration of oropharyngeal and gastric contents are equally important in the prevention of postoperative pneumonia. Thus removal of tubes that alter the normal function of the gastroesophageal (i.e., a nasogastric tube) and pharyngoesophageal sphincters (i.e., an endotracheal tube) and discontinuation of drugs that depress the central nervous system should be effected as early as is safely possible.

Clinically, the diagnosis of pneumonia is made by the demonstration of an infiltrate on a chest x-ray examination and the presence of purulent sputum, fever, and leucocytosis.[21] If a pleural effusion is identified on chest x-ray examination, a diagnostic thoracentesis should be performed. CT scans of the chest are not used routinely but may be useful to identify empyemas, lung abscesses, and other pulmonary pathology in patients who are not responding to therapy. Blood cultures should be obtained and have been shown to isolate the etiologic pathogen in 8% to 20% of cases.[33] Gram's stains and cultures of purulent sputum should be obtained. However, it should be recognized that the utility of sputum cultures in patients with hospital-acquired pneumonia is limited and that the interpretation of culture results is based on how the specimen was collected. Cultures of expectorated sputum are neither sensitive nor specific for identifying the infecting pathogen and are primarily useful to establish sensitivity patterns when resistant organisms are suspected.[32] In patients who are intubated, routine nonquantitative cultures are a sensitive but not specific method of identifying possible pathogens because critically ill patients often have colonization of the lower respiratory tract with pathogenic organisms. The simple recovery of a pathogenic organism in these patients does not establish that organism as the cause of infection. However, these culture results have a significant negative predictive value so that antibiotic regimens may be modified once culture results are available. Quantitative and semiquantitative cultures obtained using fiber-optic bronchoscopy may be useful in some intubated patients. Organisms for culture are obtained by use of a protected specimen brush (PSB) or by bronchoalveolar lavage (BAL). The etiologic pathogen is defined by the recovery of bacteria above a predetermined threshold (PSB $>10^3$, BAL $>10^4$ or 10^5 colony-forming units per milliliter). However, the role of quantitative culture techniques in the diagnosis of hospital-acquired pneumonia remains controversial, and the techniques for obtaining the cultures and concentration of bacteria that establish the presence of infection have not been standardized.

The choice of antibiotics for the treatment of nosocomial pneumonias is based on likely pathogens and the spectrum of activity, pharmacodynamic profile, and adverse reactions associated with individual drugs.[34] Likely pathogens may be deduced from the timing of the onset and the severity of the pneumonia, as well as from the presence of patient-associated risk factors. The choice of antibiotic is also influenced by the concentrations of the agent attainable in respiratory secretions. Quinolones attain concentrations in respiratory secretions close to those attained in serum. On the other hand, aminoglycosides penetrate respiratory secretions poorly and should not be used alone to treat gram negative respiratory infections.[35] Clinical improvement should be used as the ultimate end point of therapy. In general, clinical impovement does not occur before 48 to 72 hours after the initiation of therapy. Changes in antibiotics during this period should not be undertaken unless progressive deterioration of the patient's clinical status is apparent. Every effort should be made to determine the reason for failure in patients who are unresponsive to therapy after this time period.[36] The optimal duration of treatment for nosocomial pneumonias has not been established. For gram-negative pneumonias, which are associated with high rates of treatment failure, relapse, and death, 14 to 21 days of treatment have been recommended. Other less virulent organisms may be adequately treated with a 7- to 10-day course of antibiotics. For a further discussion of pneumonia, see Chapter 36.

Urinary Tract Infections

The largest percentage of infections that occur on surgery services arise in the urinary tract (approximately 13.3 cases per 1000 hospital discharges).[37] This circumstance is a simple consequence of the placement of urinary bladder catheters. Although serious infectious problems may ensue from the catheterization of the elderly male with an unrecognized prostate infection or obstruction, most urinary tract problems occur because closed urinary drainage systems eventually become colonized by enteric bacteria such as *Escherichia* from which the patient may become infected. No measure is particularly effective in preventing these catheter-related infections, although a number of approaches have been tried including the administration of antibiotics (both systemic and local), the use of special tubes with irrigants, and various regimens of catheter care.[38] Use of prophylactic antibiotics encourages infection by resistant bacteria or the fungus *Candida* (especially in diabetic patients). Frequent catether care with cleansing of the urethral meatus leads to an increased frequency of urinary tract infections so that only daily (rather than more frequent) catheter care has become standard practice. The best prevention of urinary tract infections is to avoid prolonged catheterization and to use alternatives such as intermittent catheterization or, in the case of men, condom catheters whenever possible. Regardless of the technique of drainage, patients should be kept well hydrated so that the bladder is constantly flushed, thereby decreasing the number of potentially infecting bacteria.

Many physicians overreact to the presence of more than 10^5 organisms in the patient's urine without first obtaining a urinalysis to prove the presence (or absence) of pyuria. Colonization without pyuria can usually be resolved without the use of antibiotics simply by removing the patient's catheter and maintaining adequate hydration. In the patient with significant bacteriuria and pyuria in combination and a high temperature elevation in the range of 103° to 104° F, a source of infection other than the bladder should be sought. Pyelonephritis with its attendant high frequency of bacteremia may be present under these circumstances and require aggressive antibiotic therapy; simple cystitis rarely causes high fever.[39] The majority of catheterized patients with bacteriuria and pyuria have a low-grade fever secondary to a simple catheter-related cystitis. The principles of management in this latter circumstance include removal of the catheter, if possible, and in most instances a single dose of an antimicrobial agent that is excreted in the urine. For those patients in whom catheter placement must remain in the presence of pyuria, the use of a brief course of an antibiotic is warranted to prevent the bladder from becoming a nidus for systemic infection. This latter condition is most likely to occur if the catheter becomes obstructed.

Although most postoperative urinary tract infections occur in association with indwelling urethral catheters, occasionally such infections develop in the early postoperative period secondary to urinary statis and necessitate catheter placement as a therapeutic measure. Patients at risk for this problem include those with prostatic hypertrophy, various neuromuscular disorders such as multiple sclerosis, and previous anorectal procedures that have resulted in ineffective postoperative voiding and those individuals in whom a spinal anesthetic was used. Under most circumstances, a urinary catheter should be prophylactically placed in such patients before surgery to prevent these stasis problems and should be removed as soon as normal voiding can be ensured. If a catheter-associated infection develops, the principles of treatment outlined previously should be followed.

Wound and Soft Tissue Infection

The development of surgical site infections, usually in the skin and subcutaneous tissues of the operative side, is a common postoperative problem. Overall, it is estimated that 4% to 7% of surgical patients develop these infections postoperatively. These infections contribute to postoperative morbidity and increased length of stay, with attendant increased costs of medical care.

Both local factors, such as the degree of contamination of the wound, and systemic factors, such as the overall condition of the patient, influence the rates of wound infections. The degree of contamination of the surgical wound has traditionally been assessed according to the National Research Council (NRC) wound classification scheme. In this system, wounds are classified as clean, clean contaminated, contaminated, or dirty (Table 6-1). The NRC wound classification does not, however, take into consideration any other risk factors for wound infection.

Additional risk factors for wound infection have been defined. In one prospective study involving nearly 24,000 patients, advanced age; the presence of diabetes, obesity, or malnutrition; and a perioperative hospital stay of greater than 2 weeks were identified as risk factors.[40] In other studies, malignancy, alcoholism, recent cigarette smoking, hypoxemia, remote infection, chronic inflammation, prior surgical site irradiation, recent operation, prior use of antibiotics, and recent use of corticosteroids or cytotoxic agents have also been associated with an increased risk of postoperative infection.[41,42]

The interaction between these and other factors and the NRC wound classification was investigated in two very large epidemiologic evaluations. One of these took place during the Study on the Efficacy of Nosocomial Infection Control (SENIC) project.[43] This analysis of nearly 60,000 patients undergoing surgical procedures identified

Table 6-1. National Research Council (NRC) Wound Classification Criteria

Classification	Criteria
Clean (<2%*)	Elective (not urgent or emergency), primarily closed; no acute inflammation or transection of gastrointestinal, oropharyngeal, genitourinary, biliary, or tracheobronchial tracts; no technique break (e.g., elective inguinal herniorrhaphy)
Clean contaminated (<10%*)	Urgent or emergency case that is otherwise "clean"; elective, controlled opening of gastrointestinal, oropharyngeal, biliary, or tracheobronchial tracts; minimal spillage and/or minor technique break; reoperation via "clean" incision within 7 days; blunt trauma, intact skin, negative exploration (e.g., vagotomy and pyloroplasty)
Contaminated (20%*)	Acute, nonpurulent inflammation (note absence of purulence); major technique break or major spill from hollow organ; penetrating trauma <4 hr old; chronic open wounds to be gratted or covered (e.g., acute, nonperforated, nongangrenous appendicitis)
Dirty (40%*)	Purulence or abscess: e.g., preoperative perforation of gastrointestinal, oropharyngeal, biliary, or tracheobronchial tracts; penetrating trauma >4 hr old (e.g., perforated appendicitis with abscess)

Adapted from Page C, et al. Antimicrobial prophylaxis for surgical wounds: Guidelines for clinical care. Arch Surg 128:79, 1993.
*Wound infection rate after Cruse et al. Arch Surg 107: 2061, 1973.

four factors of nearly equal weight in predicting postoperative wound infection: an abdominal operation, an operation that took longer than 2 hours, a wound classified as either contaminated or dirty, and the presence of three or more diagnoses at the time of discharge. The surgical wound infection rates in patients ranged from 1.0% in patients with no risk factors to 27.0% in patients with four risk factors (Table 6-2). Even in patients with clean wounds, the postoperative wound infection rate ranged from 1.1% to 15.8% as the number of risk factors increased from zero to three.

The second large study involved patients evaluated as part of the National Nosocomial Infection Surveillance System (NNISS) sponsored by the Centers for Disease Control and Prevention.[44] In this survey of nearly 85,000 operations, three risk factors were identified: a patient having an American Society of Anesthesiologists (ASA) score of 3, 4, or 5; an operation considered contaminated or dirty-infected; and an operation that took longer than T hours, when the value of T depended on the actual operative procedure, and ranged from 1 hour for a simple procedure such as appendectomy to 4 hours for complex procedures on the liver, bile ducts, or pancreas. The risk of a surgical wound infection varied from 1.5% to 13% as the number of risk factors increased from zero to three (Fig. 6-2). In patients with clean wounds, the infection rates varied from 1% to 5.4% as the number of risk factors increased from zero to two. The NNISS data also showed that there was an increased risk of other nosocomial infections, including pneumonias, blood stream infections, and urinary tract infections as the number of risk factors increased.

Thus the inclusion of additional factors along with the NRC wound classification predicted the risk of surgical wound infection better than did the NRC wound classification scheme alone. Although the variables identified in these two large prospective studies were different, it is apparent that the length of the procedure and the patient's premorbid condition, as assessed in the SENIC study by number of discharge diagnoses and in the NNISS study by the ASA classification have as much bearing on wound infection rates as the NRC wound classification category.

Rational interventions designed to decrease the risk of surgical wound infection can be developed on the basis of this risk factor data. Currently, one of the most commonly used interventions is the use of perioperative prophylactic antibiotics. Because of the low rate of infections (approximately 1% to 3%) usually observed in patients classified as having clean wounds, it had been argued that prophylactic antibiotics were not needed in that group of patients. However, both the SENIC and the NNISS studies indicate that there are patients with clean wounds who have a much higher risk of wound infection. Thus selected patients having clean operations might warrant prophylaxis. The use of perioperative antibiotics is discussed more fully later in this chapter.

Other factors might also be subject to modification. The length of the surgical procedure was identified in both studies as a risk factor for the development of surgical wound infection. This might suggest that efforts made by the surgeon to increase the speed of the operation would result in decreased infectious complications. However, it is unclear from these studies if the length of the surgical procedure was actually a surrogate end point for surgical skill or was rather related to the difficulty of the particular procedure as determined by the complexity of the patient's pathologic condition. Thus if the latter were true, it is unlikely that efforts designed to increase the ra-

Table 6-2. Distribution of Patients and Infections by the Study on the Efficacy of Nosocomial Infection Control (SENIC) Risk Factors and National Research Council (NRC) Wound Classification

SENIC Risk Factors	% Infection by NRC Wound Classification: Clean	Clean Contaminated	Contaminated	Dirty	SENIC, % of All Patients	SENIC, % of Patients with Infection	SENIC, % of Group with Infection
0	1.1	0.6	N/A	N/A	46‖	10¶	1#
1	3.9	2.8	4.5	6.7	32	29	3.6
2	8.4	8.4	8.3	10.9	16	35	8.9
3	15.8	17.7	11.0	18.8	5	20	17.2
4	N/A	N/A	23.9	27.4	1	6	26.7
NRC, % of all patients	55†	36	2	7	100	—	—
NRC, % of patients with infection	39‡	35	4	22	—	100	—
NRC, % of group with infection	2.9§	3.9	8.5	12.6	—	—	4.1

Adapted from Haley RW, et al. Antimicrobial prophylaxis for surgical wounds: Guidelines for clinical care. Am J Epidemiol 121:206, 1985.
Example statements indicating how to read this table: The NRC clean wounds accounted for 55% (†) of all patients and 39% (‡) of all infected patients. The infection rate for patients with NRC clean wounds was 2.9%(§). Patients with 0 SENIC risk factors accounted for 46% (‖) of all patients and 10% (¶) of all infected patients. The infection rate for patients with 0 SENIC risk factors was 1% (#). SENIC risk factors include abdominal operations, operations longer than 2 hours, three or more associated diagnoses, and NRC wound classification dirty or contaminated. Patients with contaminated or dirty wounds cannot have 0 SENIC risk factors. Patients with clean or clean-contaminated wounds cannot have four SENIC risk factors.

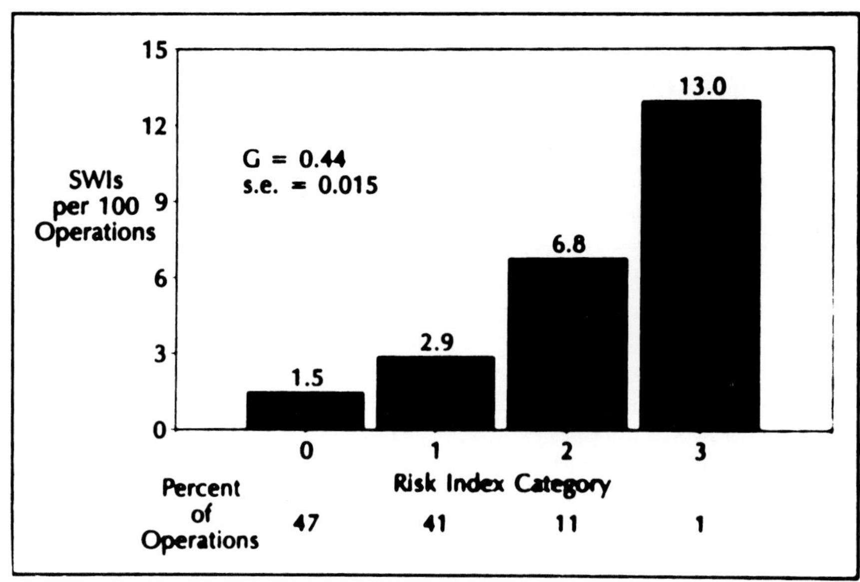

Fig. 6-2. Surgical wound infection *(SWI)* rates within categories of the surgical patient risk index. *G,* Goodman-Kruskal correlation coefficient; *s.e.,* standard error. (From Culver D, et al. Surgical wound infection rates by wound class, operative procedure, and patient risk index. Am J Med 91:1525, 1991. Reprinted by permission of the publisher. Copyright © by Excerpta Medica, Inc.)

pidity with which an operative procedure is carried out would have a significant effect on postoperative infections.

From additional studies, it does appear that the prevention of intraoperative hypothermia reduces the likelihood of surgical wound infections. In a recent prospective, randomized study, the maintenance of normothermia during elective colorectal surgery decreased the rate of wound infections threefold.[45] It was speculated that hypothermia interfered with blood flow to the surgical wound by triggering vasoconstriction or in some other way impaired the immunologic response in those areas.

Many of the risk factors related to the patient's pathologic process and underlying physiologic reserves cannot be readily controlled. However, several factors related directly or indirectly to nutritional status. Thus interventions designed to improve the patient's nutritional status, particularly the use of parenteral nutrition, have been proposed as a means of reducing postoperative infectious morbidity. However, preoperative parenteral nutritional support has not been found to benefit the majority of patients and may even contribute to postoperative infections. In the Veterans Affairs Total Parenteral Nutrition Cooperative Study, only the patients with severe malnutrition had a slight benefit from preoperative nutritional support.[46] In the remainder of the patients, who had mild-to-moderate malnutrition, preoperative therapy may actually have been detrimental. This investigation did not examine the potential role of oral or enteral nutrition preoperatively, and there is no reason to discourage adequate nutrition during the preoperative period if it does not unnecessarily delay a needed procedure. However, exhaustive efforts to improve nutritional intake, particularly using parenteral nutrition, are unlikely to be useful except in the most severely malnourished patients.

One final intervention that appears useful in reducing global rates of surgical wound infections is an effective infection control program.[47] This intervention has been estimated to provide reductions in wound infection rates of 20% to 38%. Effective programs should include wound surveillance, both in the inpatient and outpatient setting, to detect the presence of surgical wound infections. However, of greater importance is feedback to individual practitioners with regard to their own wound infection rates and an effective program for policy development and teaching that allows individual practitioners to adapt effective techniques in controlling wound infection rates.

Phlebitis

Although phlebitis of the lower extremities may develop in any patient following surgery (see Chapter 54 about venous disorders) and result in postoperative fever, it seldom has a bacterial cause. In contrast, catheter-related phlebitis is a true infection. Bacteremias secondary to intravascular devices occur in as many as 25,000 to 50,000 patients per year in the United States.[48]

An intravenous catheter breaches local skin defenses and allows several portals of entry for bacteria. The most common portal of entry is along the skin tract on the outside of the catheter. The predominant organisms that gain entry by this route are skin flora (e.g., *Staphylococcus aureus,* but also, with increasing recognition, *Staphylococcus epidermidis*). Contamination of the catheter hub infusion junction has also been implicated as a cause of bacteremia in patients with central venous lines. Again skin flora are the most common organisms. Rarely, bacteremias may occur from the infusion of contaminated solutions. These infections are most commonly due to gram negative organisms (e.g., pseudomonas, *Enterobacteriaceae*).

Definitive diagnosis of a catheter-related infection can only be made if there is purulence or inflammation at the insertion site with recovery of a pathogen on culture or if blood culture results and culture results from of the catheter tip are positive for the same organism and there is no other identifiable source of bacteremia. The diagnosis is considered probable if (1) there is purulence at the insertion site but no pathogen is recovered, (2) blood and catheter tip culture results are positive for the same organism and a separate identifiable source of bacteremia is present, or (3) bacteremia is present without an identifiable source and the catheter tip and insertion site were not cultured. Catheter tip cultures are obtained when a blood stream infection is thought to be related to contamination of the catheter. Under these circumstances the tip of the catheter is cut off with sterile scissors and placed in a sterile container so that semiquantitative cultures can be obtained. Maki et al.[49] reported that these cultures have a 76% to 96% specificity and a positive predictive value of 16% to 31% for identifying the presence of a catheter-related infection.

Prevention of infection requires careful use of sterile technique for the placement of all intravascular catheters and particularly for central venous lines. In addition, the insertion site must be dressed appropriately. A recent meta-analysis[50] found a significantly increased risk of catheter colonization when transparent semipermeable dressings were used compared with gauze dressings. This study also found a trend toward an increase in bacteremia with the use of transparent dressings, but this difference was not statistically significant. Frequent catheter changes (every 72 to 96 hours) may be necessary in patients with clinical signs of infection. This is especially true if the catheters are being frequently manipulated to administer medications or to draw blood samples. In the absence of clinical signs of infection and particularly if the catheter is dedicated for a single purpose (i.e., total parenteral nutrition [TPN] administration), the catheters may be left in place indefinitely. Exchange over a guide wire should not be used if a device infection is suspected.[51]

Three therapeutic decisions involving intravenous catheters are particularly controversial. The first is bacteremia caused by *S. aureus,* which may be secondary to infected intravenous catheters. *S. aureus* is notorious for persisting within leukocytes and disseminating widely throughout the body.[52] A body of data has suggested that if the focus of infection is removable (e.g., an intravenous catheter that can be removed or a furuncle that can be rapidly drained), the patient can be treated with a relatively short course of antibiotics, specifically, 2 weeks. Conflicting evidence reveals the occasional case of endocarditis that develop despite adherence to appropriate principles of short-course antistaphylococcal therapy.[53] This has led some infectious disease experts to recommend a long (4- to 6-week) course of antibiotics, particularly if the patient is immunocompromised or if the patient has persistent staphylococcal bacteremia.

A second and relatively common therapeutic dilemma is the approach to *C. albicans* fungemia related to an infected intravenous catheter site. Until recently the usual approach was to remove the catheter and, because *C. albicans* is an avirulent pathogen, to rely on host defenses to clear the infection. With the introduction of less toxic antifungal agents, therapy is commonly administered to almost all patients with fungemia. Recent data have documented that fluconazole can replace amphotericin B for the treatment of susceptible fungi in patients without neutropenia.[54] Fluconazole should not be used to treat *Candida krusei, Torulopsis glabrata,* and *C. lusitaniae* because of the high incidence of resistance of these organisms to triazoles. In patients with obvious host deficits (e.g., neutropenia, immunosuppressive drugs), the current recommendation is removal of the catheter followed by a short course (7 to 10 days)of amphotericin B.

The third difficulty in the treatment of infected intravenous catheter sites arises when thrombophlebitis supervenes. If a central vein is thrombosed and infected, high-dose antimicrobial therapy often suffices. The incidence of pulmonary embolism in this setting is probably higher than previously thought, and the use of heparin may be appropriate for selected patients.[55] When a peripheral vein is thrombosed, as evidenced by a palpable venous cord, and is believed to be a source of continuing infection, efforts to aspirate the vein are usually unrevealing but worth attempting. In general, treatment consists of a conventional course of antibiotics for approximately 10 days. If the patient does not exhibit a clinical response to antibiotic therapy, excision of the vein may be necessary. It should be recognized that veins that appear grossly normal at the time of surgery may in fact contain multiple microabscesses in their walls when they are examined microscopically.

Intra-abdominal Infections

Intra-abdominal infections may occur with or without contamination of the peritoneal cavity. Infections (e.g., appendicitis, simple cholecystitis) confined to a diseased organ that is resectable are usually easily cured surgically, may not require prolonged antibiotic therapy, and are not associated with diffuse peritonitis. Peritonitis is defined as inflammation of the peritoneum from any cause, with the most common cause being intra-abdominal infection secondary to bacteria or other microorganisms. Bacterial peritonitis has been classified into primary, secondary, and tertiary peritonitis. Primary peritonitis occurs because of seeding of the peritoneum with bacteria from the blood stream or the lymphatic system and occurs most commonly in cirrhotic patients with ascites. It accounts for less than 1% of peritonitis and treatment is primarily medical with antibiotic therapy.[56] Tertiary peritonitis is a peritonitis-like syndrome occurring after a patient has had persistent intra-abdominal infection. Organisms causing tertiary peritonitis are generally nosocomial pathogens such as multiply resistant bacteria or fungi. Most of these patients have been on multiple antibiotics and have had numerous abdominal procedures performed. Secondary peritonitis is the most common form of peritonitis encountered by the surgeon and occurs because of a loss of integrity of the gastrointestinal tract with resultant contamination of the peritoneal cavity by gastrointestinal contents.[57]

The natural history of secondary peritonitis has been demonstrated in animal experiments. In these studies, a two-stage process was noted to occur.[58,59] The first stage, lasting approximately 5 days, was a generalized peritonitis in which gram-negative enteric aerobes were the predominate organism. *E. coli* bacteremia was common, and a mortality rate of 43% occurred during this stage without treatment. The second stage occurred after 5 days as the peritoneal defenses attempted to wall off the infection. This resulted in multiple intra-abdominal abscesses with grossly purulent material contained within a collagen wall. The predominant organism within these abscesses was *Bacteroides fragilis.* Antibiotic therapy (e.g., aminoglycosides) directed toward aerobic enteric organisms decreased early mortality and the incidence of *E. coli* bacteremia but did not prevent abscess formation. Conversely, treatment directed against anaerobic organisms (metronidazole, clindamycin) did not affect early mortality but prevented the formation of abscesses. Other studies have demonstrated that mortality rates are directly correlated with the *E. coli* inoculum size. In addition, large inoculums of bacteria within an abscess cavity inactivate antimicrobial agents at a rate proportional to bacterial density and to the individual inactivating ability. Dead bacteria and debris within the abscess cavity can bind to and inactivate antimicrobial agents. Finally inactivation of antibiotics, particularly clindamycin and aminoglycosides, occurs because of the acidic conditions within the abscess.

The diagnosis of secondary peritonitis in an alert patient may be made by physical examination, which characteristically demonstrates diffuse tenderness, rebound tenderness, involuntary muscle guarding, and abdominal wall rigidity. The presence of these signs of generalized peritonitis should lead to prompt operation without further diagnostic studies. However, the physical examination may be difficult to interpret in critically ill patients, patients with altered mental status, postoperative patients, and patients with intra-abdominal abscesses. In addition, elderly patients and patients who are immunosuppressed may not exhibit signs of peritonitis even in the face of generalized infection. Ancillary diagnostic tests may be necessary in these patients.[60] Plain films may be of use in detecting a perforated viscus if free peritoneal air is demonstrated. In the absence of significant findings on plain films, ultrasonography has been used as the initial procedure to diagnose intra-abdominal infection in some studies. It offers the advantage of the ability to perform the test at the bedside in critically ill patients, low cost, and rapid results. However, interpretation of the scans may be limited by wounds, dressings, ostomies, obesity, and air-filled bowel loops. Ultrasound may be most useful for detecting infections originating in the liver or biliary tree. Overall sensitivity of ultrasound for the detection of intra-abdominal infection is between 75% and 82%. For the majority of patients, CT scan is the most appropriate initial study. Although CT scan is more costly than ultrasound, it has a sensitivity of 78% to 100% for the detection of intra-abdominal infection. Suspicious fluid collections identified on CT scan should be aspirated for gram's stain and culture. When aspiration is used in conjunction with CT scans, specificity for the identification of intra-abdominal abscesses is 98%.[58]

Optimal management of intra-abdominal infection requires physiologic support of the patient, resection or repair of the source of infection, drainage of any established abscesses, and elimination of residual contamination with antimicrobial therapy.[61] Patients with diffuse peritonitis exhibit marked sequestration of extracellular fluid within the inflamed peritoneal cavity, and the intestine and may require large amounts of volume resuscitation. In addition, these patients may develop multiple-organ dysfunction syndrome (MODS) secondary to intra-abdominal sepsis and require support of other organ systems (i.e., mechanical ventilation, dialysis) while the primary focus of sepsis is being addressed. Operation is usually necessary to control the source of infection. When frank perforation of the gastrointestinal tract is the source of infection, the operation may involve resection or repair of the intestine with or without anastomoses or exteriorization of the intestine.

Established abscesses should be drained to reduce the bacterial inoculum. This may be accomplished by CT-guided percutaneous drainage or by operative drainage.[62-64] A safe percutaneous drainage route that avoids puncturing solid or hollow viscera can be identified in 85% to 90% of patients. After successful drainage, there should be prompt clinical improvement within 48 to 72 hours. Failure to improve within this time frame requires a repeat CT scanning. If residual fluid cannot be evacuated with the placement of additional drains, surgical drainage should be performed. The success of percutaneous drainage of well-defined unilocular abscesses ranges from 80% to 90%, and CT-guided drainage has become the procedure of choice for these abscesses.[58,65] Percutaneous drainage of complex abscesses (i.e., loculated, pancreatic, interloop, multiple, or abscesses associated with enteric fistula) has been less successful and may require surgery.

Based on the experimental data just discussed, antibiotic therapy should be directed toward both aerobic and anaerobic enteric organisms to prevent early mortality and subsequent abscess formation.[59] This may be accomplished with combination therapy or with broad-spectrum single-agent therapy. The requirement for treatment of enterococcus and candida recovered from intra-abdominal infections continues to be an area of controversy. In animal studies and in past clinical experience, successful treatment of intra-abdominal infection has been accomplished with agents that have no activity against these organisms. However, both organisms are commonly found in the gastrointestinal tract and have become major nosocomial pathogens over the last 15 to 20 years. Currently, recommendations are that these organisms do not require antibiotic coverage if they are a part of a polymicrobial infection. However, if these organisms are isolated in pure culture or are recovered from the blood stream or in the case of candida if disseminated infection is present, treatment of these organisms should be initiated. A complete discussion of antibiotic therapy in the treatment of intra-abdominal infection is beyond the scope of this chapter but may be found in a consensus statement by the Surgical Infection Society.[66]

Miscellaneous Infections

Although the foregoing discussion has considered the usual causes of postoperative infection, in reality many other causes can exist. For this reason, the surgeon must always maintain an open mind and frequently reexamine the patient to look for the underlying source of infection if the patient continues to exhibit clinical signs of infection. An unexplained heart murmur may lead to a diagnosis of endocarditis on echocardiogram, whereas unusual obtundation may be secondary to undiagnosed meningitis or brain abscess. In traumatized patients with facial fractures, sinusitis may occur, particularly in patients who are nasotracheally intubated. Parotitis from an obstructed salivary gland duct may also be an incipient source of infection. Conversely, in some patients fever may not be related to infection at all, but may be secondary to a drug reaction or may be an allergic reaction to a blood transfusion.

Finally, an additional type of infectious process is the intrinsic infections of the gastrointestinal tract that may occasionally occur following surgery. The most common manifestations of these infections are fever and diarrhea. However, these are nonspecific findings and in some patients diarrhea may be related to enteral feedings and have nothing to do with the fever. Of more concern to the surgeon is the patient who has received antibiotic therapy and then has developed diarrhea. In many instances, this diarrhea is caused by an overgrowth of *C. difficile,* which produces a cytotoxin.[67,68] Antibiotics that are notably linked with antibiotic-associated colitis (AAC) include ampicillin, cephalosporins, and clindamycin, but the syndrome may occur with the administration of almost any antibiotic. AAC may be accompanied by fever and toxicity and is frequently overlooked as the potential source of postoperative fever. Diagnosis includes an assessment of stool for the presence of *C. difficile* toxin. The fecal leukocyte examination results may be positive, but negative results do not exclude AAC. The diagnosis may also be made by sigmoidoscopy if the typical pseudomembranous lesions associated with this entity are seen. After diagnosis, therapy is oral vancomycin—125 mg four times daily for 10 days. Parenteral vancomycin is not recommended because the object of therapy is to obtain intraluminal levels of antibiotic, which intravenous vancomycin does not provide. An alternative therapeutic option is oral (250 mg four times daily) or intravenous metronidazole, since both routes of administration of metronidazole are effective. Because *Clostridium* spores may survive a course of vancomycin or metronidazole, relapses of AAC may occur. These are treated by an additional course of the same antimicrobial agent.

PATHOGENS RESPONSIBLE FOR SURGICAL INFECTION

A common approach to characterizing surgical infection is to list the microbial agents that cause such infections. Considering the phenomenal number of organisms that can infect compromised hosts, a list of "surgical microbes" becomes merely a weak attempt at a review of the entire field of microbiology. Equally inappropriate are lists of microbes and the preferred antimicrobial agents to treat them. Memorizing such lists is a relatively fruitless exercise because many surgical infections are polymicrobic; thus the surgeon must more realistically design an empiric therapy wiht a broad-spectrum agent or a combination of agents. The rational approach to surgical microbiology is to learn those microbes that can singly cause important infections and that may have classic clinical presentations. Also the surgeon must learn the combinations of microbes that are frequently encountered in surgical situations so that empiric therapy can be instituted until the results of appropriate Gram's stains and cultures are available. Table 6-3 lists the most common pathogens identified by the National Nosocomial Infections Surveillance System from 1986 to 1989.[69]

Among the fungi, *C. albicans* is the most important and is not infrequently involved in intravenous catheter-related fungemia. A recent multicenter study has documented the efficacy of fluconazole in the treatment of candidemia in nonneutropenic patients.[54] In compromised hosts, however, amphotericin B should be used until further data are available. Two new lipophilic preparations of amphotericin B may reduce the toxicity of this agent.[70] The easiest way to control *Candida* infections in routine surgical practice is to prevent their occurrence by choosing the most narrow-spectrum antibiotic or combination of antibiotics and using them for the briefest duration consistent with guaranteed clinical success.[71] Other fungal pathogens, including *Aspergillus* and *Mucor,* are still occasionally problems for the surgeon and may cause systemic infections in debilitated patients. The source of these infections (e.g., the burn wound or diabetic abscess) requires aggressive surgical excision in conjunction with high-dose (as much as 1 mg/kg/day for the first week) amphotericin B if effective treatment is to be rendered.[72]

The role of viruses in surgical infection is poorly studied except for the blood-borne hepatitides such as hepati-

Table 6-3. Pathogen Distribution for Major Sites of Nosocomial Infection, National Nosocomial Infection Surveillance System (NNISS), 1986-1989

Pathogen	Urinary Tract Infection	Wound	Pneumonia	Blood Stream	Total
E. coli	11,135 (26)*	1,951 (10)	946 (6)	733 (6)	14,765 (16)
Enterococci	6,720 (16)	2,645 (13)	342 (2)	1,037 (8)	10,744 (12)
P. aeruginosa	5,127 (12)	1,668 (8)	2,598 (17)	543 (4)	9,936 (11)
S. aureus	823 (2)	3,439 (17)	2,401 (16)	1,984 (16)	8,647 (10)
Coagulase-negative staphylococci	1,634 (4)	2,472 (12)	293 (2)	3,384 (27)	7,783 (9)
Enterobacter sp.	2,339 (6)	1,529 (8)	1,625 (11)	610 (5)	6,103 (7)
K. pneumoniae	2,664 (6)	618 (3)	1,042 (7)	548 (4)	4,872 (5)
C. albicans	2,978 (7)	481 (2)	615 (4)	617 (5)	4,691 (5)
P. mirabilis	2,312 (5)	712 (4)	503 (3)	105 (1)	3,632 (4)
Streptococcal species	207 (0)	539 (3)	231 (1)	465 (4)	1,442 (2)
Citrobacter sp.	812 (2)	321 (2)	226 (1)	82 (1)	1,441 (2)
Candida sp.	853 (2)	81 (0)	109 (1)	330 (3)	1,373 (2)
S. marcescens	367 (1)	271 (1)	579 (4)	152 (1)	1,369 (2)

From Schaberg D, Culver D, Gaynes R. Major trends in the microbial etiology of nosocomial infection. Am J Med 91: 3B, 1991.
*Number (percent). Note: a site may have up to four pathogens.

tis B and C and cytomegalovirus. Cytomegalovirus is a common problem in transplantation recipients. Presently no effective therapy exists for cytomegalovirus, but new agents are being tested. HIV is an uncommon cause of postoperative infection in surgical patients; however, most surgeons will be called on to treat patients with HIV infections. Although occupational risks for the infection of health care workers is low, all surgeons should be aware of preventive strategies to limit transmission of this disease.[73,74] In addition, a number of parasites that are not commonly seen, including *Pneumocystis carinii* and *Toxoplasma gondii,* are encountered routinely in AIDS patients, obliging all physicians, including surgeons, to become reacquainted with their clinical presentations.

Knowledge of other parasitic infections may also be relevant to surgical practice. The classic example is the huge solitary liver abscess in the right lobe of the liver. In such cases amebic disease must be suspected and confirmed by an ameba serology test. Metronidazole is the antibiotic of choice for these infections. Unless such abscesses threaten to rupture, they are usually managed with antimicrobial agents alone, and surgery or percutaneous drainage is generally not necessary.[75] When hydatid disease is suspected, it should be confirmed serologically, and serious consideration should be given to treating the patient with benzimidazole compounds (mebendazole, albendazole) before surgery.[76]

ANTIBIOTICS IN THE MANAGEMENT OF INFECTION

It is beyond the scope of this chapter to discuss the use of antibiotics in the treatment of infection in a comprehensive fashion. Therefore a brief discussion of the mechanisms of antibiotic action, antibiotic prophylaxis, and the therapeutic use of antibiotics is presented.

Mechanisms of Action

Differing modes of action are responsible for the efficacy of individual antibiotics against various microorganisms (Table 6-4). The extent to which these antibiotic effects prevent bacterial growth often influences the efficacy of an antibiotic under a given set of clinical conditions. A bactericidal antibiotic is often preferable to a bacteriostatic antibiotic, which inhibits growth or multiplication of bacteria and allows normal host defenses to actually effect bacterial destruction. In an immunocompromised patient in whom host defenses may be severely depleted, use of a bactericidal drug is even more important. In the same way that antibiotics differ in their modes of action, microorganisms develop bacterial resistance in a variety of ways. These ways may include mutation to a resistant strain or the production of an enzyme such as penicillinase or β-lactamase that can destroy the antibiotic effects of penicillins and cephalosporins, respectively. In addition, a given pathogen may activate a latent biochemical process or acquire by transfer a chromosome-like factor, known as a resistance factor, that may block the mode of action of a particular antibiotic. It is for these reasons that an antibiotic, although once effective therapeutically against a specific pathogen, may lose its efficacy.

Antimicrobials containing the β-lactam ring (penicillins, cephalosporins, carbapenems, monobactams) characteristically inhibit cell wall synthesis by preventing normal cross-linkage of peptidoglycans or by interfering with the biosynthesis of peptidoglycans.[77] Inhibition of cell wall synthesis allows water from isotonic body fluids to move freely into bacteria, creating a bursting effect. Resistance to β-lactam antibiotics occurs through one or a combination of three mechanisms: production of a β-lactamase, which inactivates the β-lactam ring; alteration of the target penicillin-binding protein of the cell surface; or

Table 6-4. Mechanisms of Action Responsible for Efficacy of Antibiotics Against Different Microorganisms

Antibiotic	Mechanism of Action	Bacteriostatic/ Bactericidal
Aminoglycoside	Inhibit protein synthesis by binding to 30S ribosome	Bactericidal
β-Lactams	Inhibit cell wall synthesis by interleukin with the production or cross-linking of peptidoglycans	Bactericidal
Clindamycin	Binds to 50S ribosomes subunit and inhibits peptide bond formation	Bactericidal
Macrolides	Binds to 50S ribosome subunit and inhibits protein synthesis	Bacteriostatic
Metronidazole	Redox reaction produces toxic metabolites that damage bacterial DNA, inhibits DNA gyrase	Bactericidal
Quinolones	Interfering with DNA replication and repair	Bactericidal
Rifampin	Blocks RNA synthesis by inhibiting DNA dependent RNA polymerase	Bactericidal
Sulfonamides/trimethoprim	Blocks folic acid synthesis; binds to 30S ribosomal subunit and inhibits protein synthesis	Bacteriostatic
Tetracyclines	Interfering with production of purine and pyrimidine, blocks dihydrofolate reductase	Bacteriostatic
Vancomycin	Inhibits all well synthesis by interfering with peptidoglycan production at a different site from penicillins; also may alter membrane permeability and inhibit RNA synthesis	Bactericidal

interference with the antibiotic's ability to reach the protein target. The problem with resistance to β-lactam antibiotics has been partially addressed by the introduction of a number of β-lactamase inhibitors. These inhibitors are most effective against plasmid encoded β-lactamases. *Enterobacteriaceae* produce chromosomal β-lactamases that are only weakly inhibited. Currently, three β-lactamase inhibitors are commercially available: clavulanate, sulbactam, and tazobactam. Although there are some minor pharmacologic differences in these compounds, therapeutic efficacy is similar. These products are only available in fixed combinations with certain β-lactam antibiotics in which the antibacterial activity of the combination is determined by the spectrum of the antibiotic.

The aminoglycosides inhibit protein synthesis by irreversibly binding to the 30S subunit of bacterial ribosomes.[78] This results in the misreading of mRNA and the subsequent intereference with amino acid replication. Bacteria become resistant to aminoglycosides by a combination of three mechanisms: prevention of uptake of the antibiotic into the cell, synthesis of enzymes that modify the antibiotic, or by change of the ribosomal binding sites. Unlike third-generation cephalosporins in which resistance may emerge during a 2- to 3-week course of therapy, resistance to aminoglycosides appears to require long periods of exposure or a large inoculum of bacteria as is found in cystic fibrosis or burned patients.

Quinolones inhibit DNA gyrase, an enzyme that is involved in bacterial DNA replication, recombination and repair.[79] Bacterial resistance to quinolones occurs by spontaneous mutations of the chromosomes that alter DNA gyrase or which alter cell permeability of the drug. Despite their relatively recent introduction into clinical use, the development of resistance has already become a problem. *Pseudomonas* organisms and *S. aureus* are particularly likely to develop resistance to quinolones during the course of therapy. Vancomycin inhibits cell wall formation by interfering with peptidoglycan synthesis by binding to a cell surface receptor. Vancomycin may also injure protoplasts by affecting cytoplasmic permeability and by interfering with RNA synthesis. Resistance to vancomycin occurs primarily because of a plasmid-mediated change in the target protein on the cell surface.[80] However, because of its multiple sites of action, resistance to vancomycin has been slow to emerge. This has led to vancomycin being widely used in the prophylaxis and treatment of infections caused by MRSA. As a result, vancomycin use increased 20-fold at one teaching hospital in the 10-year period from 1981 until 1991.[81] With the increase in use of vancomycin, isolated reports of vancomycin resistance in enterococci began to surface in the mid-1980s. Since this time vancomycin-resistant enterococci (VRE) have become a major problem in the United States. Data from the Centers of Disease Control and Prevention indicate that the incidence of vancomycin resistance in nosocomial isolates of enterococci has risen from 0.5% in 1989 to 10% in 1995, with mortality rates secondary to VRE bacteremia approaching 50%.[82]

The emergence of VRE is just one example of the increasing emergence of antimicrobial resistance that is rapidly becoming a worldwide crisis. A recent consensus statement sponsored by the Centers for Disease Control and Prevention and the National Foundation for Infectious Diseases identified excessive and inappropriate prescribing of antimicrobials and the failure to use basic infection control techniques as the primary causes of this crisis. These problems must be resolved to prevent the further spread of multi–drug-resistant organisms.[83]

Clinical Use of Antibiotics

An antibiotic may be administered prophylactically to prevent the subsequent development of an infection, empirically to treat presumed infection in a critically ill or neutropenic patient, or therapeutically to treat an infection when it has actually occurred. The following discussion outlines a rational approach to each of these types of antibiotic usage.

Prophylaxis

Prophylaxis in the strictest sense refers to the administration of antibiotics prior to the occurrence of contamination. However, this term is also commonly applied to instances in which surgery is the primary treatment for a patient with presumed contamination or with a possible infection (e.g., penetrating abdominal trauma treated within 6 hours, simple acute appendicitis, or cholecystitis). Under these circumstances antibiotic coverage is limited to 24 to 48 hours. This prophylactic use of antibiotics to prevent wound infections is currently the most common reason for administration of antibiotics in surgical patients. Surgical wound infections significantly prolong hospital stay, increase cost, and can result in systemic sepsis and death in some patients. Appropriate use of prophylactic antibiotics has been shown to reduce infectious morbidity and hospital costs. However, indiscriminate use of antibiotics does not further decrease the incidence of wound infections and may result in increased costs and the emergence of resistant infections.

An approach to prophylaxis is outlined in Table 6-5. The use of prophylactic antibiotics is recommended in high-risk patients or in high-risk surgical procedures. Pa-

Table 6-5. Recommendations for Prophylactic Antibiotic Agents by Site

Operations	Bacteria	Intravenous Administration of Antimicrobial	Dose*
Cardiac: all with sternotomy, cadiopulmonary bypass	*Staphylococcus aureus, Staphylococcus epidermidis,* diphtheroids, gram-negative enterics	Cefazolin (Vancomycin)	1-2g (1 g slowly) preinduction, 1-2 g every 8 hr for 48 hr
Noncardiac vascular: aortic resection and prosthetic bypass	*S. aureus, S. epidermidis,* diphtheroids, gram-negative enterics	Cefazolin (Vancomycin)	1 g (1 g slowly) preinduction, 2 postoperative doses
Orthopedic: insertion of prosthetic joints, open operations	*S. aureus, S. epidermidis*	Cefazolin (Vancomycin)	1 g (1 g slowly) preinduction
Neurosurgery	*S. aureus, S. epidermidis*	Cefazolin (Vancomycin)	1 g (1 g slowly) preinduction
Head and neck: operations involving the mucous membranes and deep tissue	Oral aerobes and anaerobes, *S. aureus,* streptococci	Cefazolin	2 g preinduction
General thoracic: pulmonary and esophageal	Oral anaerobes, *S. aureus,* streptococci, gram-negative enterics	Cefazolin	1-2 g preinduction
Gastroduodenal: bariatric, ulcer patients treated with H_2 blockers, bleeding duodenal ulcer, genitourinary or gastric cancer	Oropharyngeal flora and gram-negative enterics, *S. aureus*	Cefazolin	1-2 g preinduction
Biliary: all open and laparoscopic procedures (chronically intubated biliary tract)	Gram-negative enterics, *S. aureus, Enterococcus fecalis,* clostridia (above plus *Pseudomonas* species)	Cefazolin (culture-based selection)	1-2 g preinduction (preinduction dose and repeat interval based on drug kinetics)
Colorectal: operations that open the colon and/or rectum	Enteric aerobes and anaerobes	Oral neomycin/erythromycin (cefoxitin or cefotetan or cefmetazole)	Operating room day 1:1 g at 1, 2 and 11 PM (1 g preinduction)
Appendectomy: simple appendicitis (antibiotics are empiric or definitive for complicated appendicitis)	Enteric aerobes and anaerobes	Cefoxitin or cefotetan or cefmetazole	1 g preinduction
Cesarean section	Enteric aerobes and anaerobes, *E. fecalis,* group B streptococci	Cefazolin	1 g after umbilical cord is clamped
Hysterectomy	Enteric aerobes and anaerobes, *E. fecalis,* group B streptococci	Cefazolin	1 g preinduction
Abdominal trauma	Enteric aerobes and anaerobes	Cefoxin	2 g preinduction

From Haley RW, et al. Antimicrobial prophylaxis for surgical wounds: Guidelines for clinical care. Am J Epidemiol 121:206, 1985.
*Parenthetic text refers to alternate antibiotic or situation. Current data suggest repeat dosing for operations lasting longer than the serum half-life. Preinduction indicates in operating room before initiating anesthesia.

tient-related risks include such factors as extremes of age, malnutrition, chronic illnesses (diabetes, chronic obstructive pulmonary disease [COPD]), remote infections, immunosuppression, recent operations, and prior irradiation of the surgical site. Risks have been classified by two scoring systems as previously discussed. In general, the use of the SENIC classification is preferred because it incorporates both wound and patient factors. Patients with clean wounds by the NRC wound classification who have two or more patient-related risk factors as defined by the SENIC classification have an 8% to 15% incidence of wound infection[84,85] (see Tables 6-1 and 6-2). This is similar to the incidence found with clean contaminated wounds using the NRC wound classification and qualifies these patients for the administration of prophylactic antibiotics. This approach also addresses questions that have been raised by Platt et al.[86] concerning the use of prophylactic antibiotics in clean operations. These investigators found a trend toward a decrease in rates of infection in patients undergoing clean operations (breast and hernia) with the use of prophylactic cefonicid. However, this study has been criticized because patient-related risk factors were not evaluated, all infectious complications (wound, pneumonias, urinary tract) were included in the analysis, and a higher incidence of infection was found with breast operations in this study than has been reported in other studies.[87] At the present time chemoprophylaxis is not recommended in clean operations unless two or more patient-related risk factors are present as defined by SENIC or prosthetic materal such as cardiac valves, prosthetic joints, or vascular grafts are being implanted. Although the risk of infections is low in these operations, the use of prophylactic antibiotics is justified because the consequences of infection in terms of morbidity and mortality are great. In addition, although definitive evidence to support the use of chemoprophylaxis is not available, prophylaxis is commonly used in cardiac and neurosurgical procedures even when prosthetic materials are not inserted because of the morbidity of sternal or skull infections.[88]

The choice of a specific antibiotic agent depends on the operation to be performed, the spectrum of coverage, toxicity, and lastly cost. Antimicrobial prophylaxis should be directed toward common bacterial flora encountered in the course of a specific operation and most importantly toward the most common pathogens responsible for infection after a given procedure. Therapy should be tailored to flora endemic to individual hospitals as patterns of antibiotic use may result in the emergence of resistant organisms. If MRSA or methicillin-resistant *S. epidermidis* is a common colonizer in a given hospital setting, methicillin would obviously be contraindicated and another prophylactic antibiotic such as vancomycin should be substituted.[89-91] Prophylaxis should be limited to common pathogens, as use of antibiotics with an unnecessarily wide spectrum also leads to the development of resistant strains of bacteria and to the occurrence of difficult-to-treat infections. The least toxic antibiotic that has an appropriate spectrum of activity should be chosen. In general, in the absence of allergies β-lactam antibiotics (particularly cephalosporins) have acceptable safety profiles. Although the use of aminoglycosides for less than 48 hours rarely results in major toxicity, the potential for both renal and ototoxicity is present and these drugs are best reserved for therapeutic regimens.

The timing and duration of antibiotic therapy is critical and successful prophylaxis. Antibiotics are most effective in preventing infection when adequate tissue levels are present at the time of bacterial contamination.[92] Parenteral administration is necessary to reliably attain adequate tissue levels. Administration of the antibiotic at intervals greater than 1 hour prior to operation have been associated with falling antibiotic tissue levels and an increased incidence of infection.[93] In most cases antibiotics should be administered in the operating room no greater than 30 minutes prior to making the incision.[89] This approach ensures adequate tissue levels at the time of operation. When administration prior to contamination is not possible (i.e., penetrating abdominal trauma, ruptured viscus) antibiotics should be administered as soon as possible after contamination. Adequate tissue levels should be maintained throughout the procedure. This requires frequent dosing at intervals of two times the plasma half-life for drugs that are rapidly cleared from the circulation.[92] For many cephalosporins, dosing at 2- to 3-hour intervals during a procedure may be necessary. Postoperatively, the shortest effective course of antibiotics limits costs, toxicity, and the development of resistant infections. Several studies have demonstrated the efficacy of single-dose prophylaxis in operations (gastrointestinal, gynecologic, orthopedic) lasting less than 2 to 3 hours.[41,89] The need for prophylaxis longer than 24 to 48 hours is extremely rare even in cases of preexistent contamination as in penetrating abdominal trauma or open fractures.[94-96] Finally, it should be remembered that antibiotics are an adjunctive measure for decreasing the incidence of wound infection and do not replace adequate patient preparation, infection control protocols, and the use of meticulous surgical technique.

Other methods of prophylaxis. Mechanical means to decrease the concentration of infective organisms in the wound should be used whenever possible. For example, in operations involving the large bowel, a period of mechanical cleaning through the use of cathartics and/or enemas before surgery decreases the enteric bacterial count and thereby lessens the risk of infection. In such clean contaminated cases involving the colon, oral antibiotics (neomycin and erythromycin base) administered on the day prior to operation reduce the concentration of bacteria within the colon and provide a significant reduction in the incidence of wound infection with or without the use of systemic antibiotics.[97]

Topical antibiotic prophylaxis has been most successfully applied to burn wound sepsis.[98] The goal with such therapy is not to prevent colonization of the wound but to control bacterial proliferation. The ideal agent possesses a broad spectrum of activity against bacterial and fungal pathogens, penetrates the burn eschar, has limited systemic toxicity, is inexpensive, and is easy to apply and remove. Although none of the available agents meets all these criteria, the most commonly used agents are silver sulfadiazine, silver nitrate, and mafenide acetate.

Empiric Use

Empiric antibiotic therapy differs from the therapeutic use of antibiotics in that antibiotics are administered early to treat presumptive infections. Antibiotics have been used in this fashion primarily in immunocompromised patients or in patients with presumed septic shock in an attempt to prevent death during the early phases of an infection before the infecting organism or the source of infection has been identified.[34,99-102] In general, broad-spectrum therapy is used to cover the most likely pathogens. This therapy is then tailored to the specific infection, usually after 72 hours when the culture results are available. In neutropenic patients (granulocyte counts <500 mm^3) prior to the institution of empiric therapy in the 1970s, mortality secondary to gram negative bacteremias approached 90%. With the early use of antibiotics, mortality has decreased to about 10% currently. The classic organisms associated with infections in neutropenic patients has been the *Enterobacteriaceae,* specifically *Pseudomonas,* and more recently *Enterobacter* species. However, in the 1980s an increasing incidence of gram-positive organisms, including *S. aureus, S. epidermidis,* and α-hemolytic streptococci, has been observed.[101] In addition, with more prolonged hospitalization, the frequent use of immunosuppressive agents in transplantation recipients and the frequent occurrence of previous antibiotic usage, fungal infections, particularly with *Candida* and *Aspergillus* organisms, are becoming more common. In patient populations with other disease processes such as AIDS, *P. carinii* and *Mycobacterium tuberculosis* are the most common pathogens.

Choices for empiric antibiotic therapy fall into three basic categories: (1) the classic approach of a broad-spectrum β-lactam antibiotic in combination with an aminoglycoside, (2) the use of two β-lactam antibiotics, and (3) broad-spectrum monotherapy with or without additional gram positive (i.e., vancomycin) or anaerobic coverage (i.e., clindamycin or metronidazole). Data exist to support each regimen. The first regimen provides broad-spectrum coverage and rapid bactericidal activity and has the advantage of synergy between the β-lactam and the aminoglycoside, thereby limiting the emergence of resistant organisms. Under most circumstances an antipseudomonal penicillin with an aminoglycoside has been demonstrated to be the best combination. The primary disadvantage of this regimen is the potential toxicity from the use of aminoglycosides. The combination of two β-lactam antibiotics has also been demonstrated to be effective empiric therapy. The primary disadvantage with this regimen is the selection of organisms resistant to β-lactams. Monotherapy with a number of different agents (extended-spectrum penicillins, third-generation cephalosporins, penicillins, or cephalosporins plus β-lactamase inhibitors, carbapenems, or quinolones) has been used with success. The most extensively studied regimens in neutropenic patients have used imipenem or ceftazidime.[99] These regimens have the advantage of ease of administration, lower cost, and toxicity, but again the occurrence of resistance is the major disadvantage. Regardless of the inital regimen, additions and modifications are frequently necessary when culture results become available. In addition, overall clinical response should be evaluated at 72 hours to determine the effectiveness of the regimen. Patients with documented infections and patients remaining neutropenic after 7 to 10 days of therapy are most likely to require changes in antibiotics.[101] For the latter patients, infections with nonbacterial pathogens, particularly viruses and fungal agents, should be considered.

Debate continues about the inclusion of vancomycin in the initial empiric regimen. Several randomized studies have demonstrated no survival advantage when all neutropenic patients are considered. However, vancomycin should be included initially in hospitals in which MRSA is endemic. In addition, vancomycin should be added in severely septic patients and in patients in whom MRSA is a likely pathogen (i.e., patients suspected of intravenous line sepsis). In such cases vancomycin may be deleted after 72 hours if culture results are negative for gram positive organisms. The optimal duration of antibiotic therapy has also been debated. For patients with negative culture results in whom the neutropenia resolves, antibiotics may be discontinued after 7 days. Antibiotics may be discontinued earlier in nonneutropenic patients with negative culture results, usually after 3 days. A reasonable approach in patients who remain neutropenic is to continue antibiotics for 14 days or for 7 days after they become afebrile. About one third of these patients become febrile again and require additional therapy. Patients with severe neutropenia (<100 mm^3) may require therapy until granulocyte counts increase above 500 mm^3.

In conclusion, the regimen chosen must be adapted to the individual patient and the profile of common pathogens in a given institution. Regardless of the initial regimen chosen, the clinician must recognize the need for and the indications to modify initial therapy based on culture results and the patient's clinical response.

Therapeutic Use

A complete listing of suggested therapy for surgical infections and recommendations for antibiotic therapy of the various pathogens is beyond the scope of this chapter but may be found in standard infectious disease texts. Several aspects of the basic principles governing the therapeutic use of antibiotics to treat established infections are discussed in the box on p. 169. Essential to these principles is a knowledge of the pharmacodynamic effects of antimicrobial agents.[103,104] These effects are determined by the drug interaction with the microorganism, as well as by host factors. Bactericidal antimicrobials can be classified as having concentration-dependent or concentration-independent bacterial killing. Overlap exists with many antibiotics demonstrating both types of behavior depending on the microorganism targeted. In general, aminoglycoside antibiotics are noted for having concentration-dependent killing. Although conflicting data have been reported regarding the usefulness of serum concentrations to titrate therapy, most investigators have found a relationship between serum concentrations and the efficacy, as well as the toxicity, of aminoglycosides.[105] Traditionally, for life-threatening infections, peak serum concentrations of 8 to 10 mg/dl and trough concentrations of 1 to 2 mg/dl have been used. More recently, the ratio of peak serum concentration to the MIC, defined as the lowest serum concentration that inhibits bacterial growth, has been directly related to the bacterial killing rate. This increase in bacterial killing is seen up to peak/MIC ratios of about 10 to 12. Early achievement of these therapeutic levels has been associated with improved outcome in patients with intra-abdominal infections.[66,103] The relationship of serum levels to toxicity is less well defined. Some investigators have reported that both nephrotoxicity and ototoxicity are associated with peak serum concentrations of gentamicin greater than 12 to 14 mg/dl and trough concentrations greater than 2 mg/dl. However, toxicity may occur with therapeutic serum concentrations, and in some patients it may be difficult to determine if increased serum levels of aminoglycosides are the cause or the result of decreased renal function.

To maintain therapeutic aminoglycoside levels, it is important to recognize that critically ill patients have marked interpatient variability in pharmacodynamics, particularly with respect to volume of distribution (Vd) and clearance of the antibiotic. The major factor associated with the increase in Vd in critically ill surgery patients is volume replacement resulting in intracellular fluid shifts. Other factors involved include fever, ascites, peritonitis, vasodilator therapy, and parenteral nutrition. In addition to increased Vd, critically ill patients have been demonstrated to have lower elimination constants and lower total body clearance of aminoglycosides compared to noncritically ill patients. The increase in Vd and decrease in clearance of the drug results in the need to increase the dose and interval of administration of aminoglycosides in these patients compared to conventional regimens.[78,105] Chelluri and Jastremski[106,107] demonstrated that a loading dose of 3 mg/kg of tobramycin or gentamicin was necessary to achieve a peak serum concentration greater than 8 mg/dl in 11 of 14 critically ill patients. In addition, it has been recommended that the dose be increased to 7 mg/kg/day given in divided doses (i.e., every 12 hours) or as a single daily dose. Once-daily dosing is possible in these patients because of the pharmacodynamics and because aminoglycosides exhibit a relatively long postantibiotic effect (PAE).[108] The PAE is manifested by the ability of some antimicrobials to suppress bacterial growth despite serum concen-

PRINCIPLES OF ANTIBIOTIC THERAPY

1. The organism should be sensitive to the antibiotic chosen. Obtain an appropriate culture with susceptibility testing to guide possible changes in antibiotic coverage. Recall in vitro/in vivo disparity in susceptibility of some organisms (e.g., cephalosporins are not effective in vivo against methicillin-resistant *Staphylococcus aureus* [MRSA]).
2. Antibiotics should be in doses that ensure adequate peak concentrations and tissue penetration. Blood levels should exceed minimum inhibitory concentration by two to three times to ensure penetration of infected tissues.
3. Host factors must be taken into consideration (preexisting diseases, allergies, age, immunosuppression, remote infections, etc.).
4. The antibiotic must come in contact with the organism. The blood-brain, prostatic, obstructed bile, and other barriers prevent penetration of some antibiotics.
5. Frequency of administration is based on the half-life and the route of elimination of the antibiotic. Inadequate antibiotic serum concentrations at the end of a dosing interval may lead to "break-through" bacteremia. With developing renal or hepatic dysfunction, the dosing interval is lengthened and, as function improves, is shortened again.
6. Choose a bactericidal antibiotic when appropriate. Endocarditis, osteomyelitis, and the infected compromised host with neutropenia require bactericidal antibiotics.
7. Use synergistic therapy when appropriate. *Pseudomonas* infections (especially compromised host), serious enterococcal infection, *Staphylococcus epidermidis* endocarditis, or ventriculoperitoneal shunt infections deserve synergistic therapy.
8. Avoid antagonistic combinations of antibiotics. Antagonism is most likely when two "bacteriostatic" antibiotics are used together.
9. Choose the most narrow-spectrum antibiotic. Superinfection is minimized. Often cost is less.
10. Avoid side effects when possible. Decreasing the side effects should dictate choice of antibiotic more than cost or convenience of administration. Many antibiotics may interact adversely with other drugs (e.g., metronidazole with ethanol).
11. Control potential interfering conditions or substances. Acidic pus may render an antibiotic useless; therefore drain pus. Organisms may survive an antibiotic when a foreign body is present; therefore remove the foreign body.
12. Ensure the proper duration of therapy. For many surgical infections, continuing antibiotics 3 or 4 days past the day of afebrility suffices; however, undrained pus may require long therapy, and an unremoved foreign body (e.g., infected vascular graft) may require therapy for life. Clinical response is the most important factor in determining efficacy and duration of treatment.

trations well below MIC. Several clinical trials have demonstrated efficacy with some decrease in toxicity with once-daily dosing of aminoglycosides. However, the benefits of once-daily dosing have not been conclusively demonstrated, particularly in neutropenic patients. Regardless of the dosing interval, serum concentrations should be followed to maximize efficacy.

In contrast to aminoglycosides, most β-lactam antibiotics exhibit concentration-independent bacterial killing.[103] For these antimicrobials the length of time that serum levels remain above MIC, rather than peak concentrations, appears to be the primary determinant of bacterial killing. These characteristics support the use of frequent dosing intervals, with lower doses or alternatively continuous infusions of β-lactam antibiotics, to ensure that serum concentrations remain above MIC for prolonged periods of time. Although several animal and human studies have been carried out, it is difficult to demonstrate a definite benefit of continuous dosing over intermittent dosing at the present time. However, if continuous dosing is used, a loading dose should be given to ensure that the MIC is rapidly exceeded.

As with empiric therapy, there has been a recent trend toward the use of single broad-spectrum β-lactam antibiotics as substitutes for combination therapy with aminoglycosides to treat established infections caused by aerobic gram negative bacilli. These organisms are usually a part of a mixed aerobic-anaerobic flora causing intra-abdominal infections. Current recommendations are that all regimens for intra-abdominal infections cover both aerobic gram negative organisms and anaerobic organisms. No clear benefit of combination therapy over monotherapy with broad-spectrum β-lactams has been demonstrated overall. However, combination therapy should be strongly considered in neutropenic patients with gram negative bacteremia and in patients with infections secondary to bacteria that are known to develop resistance to β-lactam antibiotics.[66,102,109,110]

Finally, it cannot be emphasized too strongly that the use of antibiotics in most surgical infections is an adjunct to the proper management of the locus of infection. Thus abscesses must be drained, devitalized tissue must be debrided, and grossly contaminated wounds must be packed and left open to heal by secondary intention. Equally important is the maintenance of the immune system through nutritional support of the infected patient. It is not uncommon for a patient with surgical infection to be grossly malnourished with subsequent compromise of the immune system. In providing optimum care, surgical management of infection and maintenance of metabolic homeostasis are the primary components of therapy and are supported by the adjunctive use of antibiotics.

SUMMARY

Despite advances in surgical management and antibiotic therapy, infection continues to be the most important cause of morbidiy and mortality in postoperative surgical patients. The most common surgical infections are hospital acquired, and the responsible microorganisms are usually endogenous. If the development of such infections is to be minimized, efforts at preventing derangements in host-defense mechanisms must be ensured, and meticulous surgical techniques must be employed. When infections do occur, rational treatment should stress the importance of accurate identification of the responsible microorganism, logical investigation of the underlying source of infection, and adherence to sound principles governing antibiotic prophylaxis and treatment. The application of these guidelines to the clinical management of the surgical patient should lead to substantial improvements in the outcome of surgical disorders that are complicated by infection in terms of both a reduction in complications and an enhancement of survival.

REFERENCES

1. Wells C, Howard R. Overview of etiologic agents of surgical infections. In Surgical Infectious Diseases, 3rd ed. Howard R, Simmons R, eds. Norwalk, Conn.: Appleton & Lange, 1995.
2. Members of the American College of Chest Physicians/Society of Critical Care Medicine Consensus Conference Committee: American College of Chest Physicians/Society of Critical Care Medicine Consensus Conference. Definitions for sepsis and organ failure and guidelines for the use of innovative therapies in sepsis. Crit Care Med 20:864, 1992.
3. Cerra F. Hypermetabolism—Organ failure syndrome: A metabolic response to injury. Crit Care Clin 5:229, 1989.
4. Kluger M, Ringler D, Anver M. Fever and survival. Science 188:166, 1975.
5. Clowes G, Vucinic M, Weidner M. Circulatory and metabolic alterations associated with survival or death in peritonitis: Clinical analysis of 25 cases. Ann Surg 163:866, 1966.
6. Shoemaker W, et al. Physiologic patterns in surviving and nonsurviving shock patients: Use of sequential cardiorespiratory variables in defining criteria for therapeutic goals and early warning of death. Arch Surg 106:630, 1973.
7. Lowry S. Cytokine mediators of immunity and inflammation. Arch Surg 128:1235, 1993.
8. Hesse D, et al. Cytokine appearance in human endotoxemia and primate bacteremia. Surg Gynecol Obstet 166:147, 1988.
9. Fong Y, et al. Antibodies to cachectin/tumor necrosis factor reduce interleukin 1β and interleukin 6 appearance during lethal bacteremia. J Exp Med 170:1627, 1989.
10. Casey L, Balk R, Bone R. Plasma cytokine and endotoxin levels correlate with survival in patients with the sepsis syndrome. Ann Intern Med 119:771, 1993.
11. Fekade D, et al. Prevention of Jarisch-Hexheimer reactions by treatment with antibodies against tumor necrosis factor alpha. N Engl J Med 335:311, 1996.
12. Horan T, et al. CDC definitions of nosocomial surgical site infections, 1992: A modification of CDC definitions of surgical wound infections. Infect Control Hosp Epidemiol 13:606, 1992.
13. Tetteroo G, Wagenvoort, J, Bruining H. Role of selective decontamination in surgery. Br J Surg 79:300, 1992.
14. Martin M: Nosocomial infections in intensive care units: An overview of their epidemiology, outcome, and prevention. New Horizons 2:162, 1993.
15. Dinarello C. Interleukin-1 and the pathogensis of the acute phase response. N Engl J Med 311:1413, 1984.
16. Pannen B, Robotham J: The acute-phase response. New Horizons 3:183, 1995.

17. Baker C, Huynh T. Sepsis in the critically ill patient. In Wells S, ed. Current problems in Surgery. Chapel Hill, N.C.: Mosby, 1995, p 1015.
18. Parrillo J. Pathogenetic mechanisms of septic shock. N Engl J Med 328:1471, 1993.
19. Isenberg H, et al. Specimen collection and handling. In Balows A, et al., eds. Manual of Clinical Microbiology. Washington, D.C.: American Society for Microbiology, 1991, p 15.
20. Balows A, et al., eds. Manual of Clinical Microbiology, 5th ed. Washington, D.C.: American Society for Microbiology, 1991.
21. Bonten MJM, et al. Problems in diagnosing nosocomial pneumonia in mechanically ventilated patients: A review. Crit Care Med 22:1683, 1994.
22. Theuer C, Bongard F, Klein S. Are blood cultures effective in the evaluation of fever in perioperative patients? Am J Surg 162:615, 1991.
23. National Committee for Clinical Laboratory Standards. Performance Standard for Antimicrobial Susceptibility Testing. Vol Fourth Informational Supplement. Villanova, Pa.: NCCLS, 1992.
24. National Commitee for Clinical Laboratory Standards. Performance Standards for Antimicrobial Disk Susceptibility Tests. Villanova, Pa.: NCCLS, 1993.
25. National Committee for Clinical Laboratory Standards. Methods for Determining Bactericidal Activity of Antimicrobial Agents: Tentative Guideline. Vol Document M26-T. Villanova, Pa.: NCCLS, 1992.
26. National Committee for Clinical Laboratory Standards. Dilution Procedures for Susceptibility Testing of Aerobic Bacteria. Vol Publication M7-A3. Villanova, Pa.: NCCLS, 1993.
27. Benner E, Morthland V. Methicillin-resistant *Staphylococcus aureus:* Antimicrobial susceptibility. N Engl J Med 277:678, 1967.
28. Horan T, White J, Jarvis W. Nosocomial infection surveillance, 1984. MMWR 35(1SS):17SS, 1986.
29. Clevenger F. Postoperative pneumonia. In Fry D, ed. Surgical Infections. Boston: Little Brown, 1995, p 327.
30. Bergogne-Berezin E. Treatment and prevention of nosocomial pneumonia. Chest 108:26S, 1995.
31. Broughton W, Fones B, Bass JJ. Nosocomial pneumonia—Trying to make sense of the literature. Postgrad Med 99:221, 1996.
32. American Thoracic Society: Hospital-acquired pneumonia in adults: Diagnosis, assessment of severity, initial antimicrobial therapy, and preventative strategies. Am J Respir Crit Care Med 153:1711, 1995.
33. Bryan C, Reynolds K. Bacteremic nosocomial pneumonia. Am Rev Respir Dis 129:668, 1984.
34. Cunha B. Antibiotic treatment of sepsis. Med Clin North Am 79:551, 1995.
35. Honeybourne D. Antibiotic penetration into lung tissue. Thorax 49:104, 1994.
36. Fein A, et al. When the pneumonia doesn't get better. Clin Chest Med 8:529, 1987.
37. Haley R, et al. Nosocomial infections in U.S. hospitals, 1975-1976. Am J Med 70:947, 1981.
38. Stamm W, Hooton T. Management of urinary tract infections in adults. N Engl J Med 329:1328, 1993.
39. Wilkie M, Almond M, Marsh F. Diagnosis and management of urinary tract infection in adults. BMJ 305:1137, 1992.
40. Cruse P, Foord R. A five-year prospective study of 23,649 surgical wounds. Arch Surg 107:206, 1973.
41. Page C, et al. Antimicrobial prophylaxis for surgical wounds: Guidelines for clinical care. Arch Surg 128:79, 1993.
42. Cruse G. Life-threatening surgical infection: Its detection and prevention. Ann R Coll Surg Engl 60:92, 1978.
43. Haley R. Nosocomial infections in surgical patients: Developing valid measures of intrinsic patient risk. Am J Med 91:1453, 1991.
44. Culver D, et al. Surgical wound infection rates by wound class, operative procedure, and patient risk index. Am J Med 91:1525, 1991.
45. Kurz A, Sessler D, Lenhardt R. Perioperative normothermia to reduce the incidence of surgical wound infection and shorten hospitalization. N Engl J Med 334:1209, 1992.
46. Group VACS. Perioperative total parenteral nutrition in surgical patients. N Engl J Med 325:525, 1991.
47. Condon R, et al. Does infection control, control infection? Arch Surg 123:250, 1988.
48. Maki D. Infection due to infusion therapy. In Bennett J, Brachman P, eds. Hospital Infections. Boston: Little, Brown, 1986, p 561.
49. Maki D, Weise C, Sarafin H. A semi-quantitative method for identifying intravenous catheter-related infection. N Engl J Med 296:1305, 1977.
50. Hoffman K, Weber D, Samsa G. Transparent polyurethane film as an intravenous catheter dressing: A meta-analysis of the infection risks. JAMA 267:2072, 1992.
51. Cobb D, et al. A controlled trial of scheduled replacement of central venous and pulmonary artery catheters. N Engl J Med 327:1062, 1992.
52. Melly M, Thomison J, Rogers D. Fate of staphylococci within human leukocytes. J Exp Med 112:1121, 1960.
53. Libman H, Arbeit R. Complications associated with *Staphylococcus aureus* bacteremia. Arch Intern Med 144:541, 1984.
54. Rex J, et al. A randomized trial comparing fluconazole with amphotericin B for the treatment of candidemia in patients without neutropenia. N Engl J Med 331:1325, 1994.
55. Harley D, et al. Pulmonary embolism secondary to venous thrombosis of the arm. Am J Surg 147:221, 1984.
56. Joefs J, Runyon B. Spontaneous bacterial peritonitis. Dis Mon 31:1, 1984.
57. Wittmann D, Schein M, Condon R. Management of secondary peritonitis. Ann Surg 224:10, 1996.
58. McClean K, Sheehan G, Harding G. Intraabdominal infection: A review. Clin Infect Dis 19:100, 1994.
59. Bartlett J: Intra-abdominal sepsis. Med Clin North Am 79:599, 1995.
60. McDowell R, Dawson S. Evaluation of the abdomen in sepsis of unknown origin. Radiol Clin North Am 34:177, 1996.
61. Nathens A, Rotstein O. Therapeutic options in peritonitis. Surg Clin North Am 74:677, 1994.
62. Dondelinger R, Kurdziel J, Boverie J. Percutaneous management of intraperitoneal, hepatic and other fluid collections. Baillieres Clin Gastroenterol 6:273, 1992.
63. Lambiase R, et al. Percutaneous drainage of 336 consecutive abscesses: Results of primary drainage with 1-year follow-up. Radiology 184:167, 1992.
64. Scheckter S, et al. Computerized tomographic scan-guided drainage of intra-abdominal abscesses. Dis Colon Rectum 37:984, 1994.
65. Malangoni M, et al. Factors influencing the treatment of intra-abdominal abscesses. Am J Surg 159:167, 1990.
66. Bohnen J, et al. Guidelines for clinical care: Anti-infective agents for intra-abdominal infections. Arch Surg 127:83, 1992.
67. Fekety R, Shah A. Diagnosis and treatment of *Clostridium difficile* colitis. JAMA 269:71, 1993.
68. Kelly C, Pothoulakis C, LaMont J. *Clostridium difficile* colitis. N Engl J Med 330:257, 1994.
69. Schaberg D, Culver D, Gaynes R. Major trends in the microbial etiology of nosocomial infection. Am J Med 91:3B, 1991.
70. Carlson M, Condon R. Nephrotoxicity of amphotericin B. J Am Coll Surg 179:361, 1994.
71. Solomkin J. Pathogenesis and management of *Candida* infection syndromes in nonneutropenic patients. New Horizons 1:202, 1993.
72. Anaissie E, Solomkin J. Fungal infection. In Willmore B, et al., eds. Care of the Surgical Patient. New York: Scientific American, 1994.
73. Davis J, et al. The Surgical Infection Society's policy on human immunodeficiency virus and hepatitis B and C infection. Arch Surg 127:218, 1992.

74. Courington K, Patterson S, Howard R. Universal precautions are not universally followed. Arch Surg 126:154, 1991.
75. Katzenstein D, Rickerson V, Brande A. New concepts of amebic liver abscess derived from hepatic imaging serodiagnosis and hepatic enzymes in 67 consecutive cases in San Diego. Medicine 61:237, 1982.
76. Kammerer W, Schantz P. Echinococcal disease. Infect Dis Clin North Am 7:605, 1993.
77. Solomkin J. Use of new beta lactam antibiotics for surgical infections. Surg Clin North Am 68:1, 1988.
78. Lortholary O, et al. Aminoglycosides. Med Clin North Am 79:761, 1995.
79. Hooper D, Wolfson J. Mechanisms of quinolone action and bacterial killing. In Hooper D, Wolfson J, eds. Quionlone Antimicrobial Agents. Washington, D.C.: American Society for Microbiology, 1993, p 53.
80. Neu H. Emergence and mechanisms of bacterial resistance in surgical infections. Am J Surg 169:13S, 1995.
81. Gold H, Moellering RJ. Antimicrobial-drug resistance. N Engl J Med 335:1445, 1996.
82. Centers for Disease Control and Prevention. Nosocomial enterococci resistance to vancomycin: United States 1989-1993. MMWR Morb Mortal Wkly Rep 42:597, 1993.
83. Goldman D, et al. Strategies to prevent and control the emergence and spread of antimicrobial-resistant microorganisms in hospitals. JAMA 275:234, 1996.
84. Haley R, et al. Identifying patients at high risk of surgical wound infection. A simple multivariate index of patient susceptibility and wound contamination. Am J Epidemiol 121:206, 1985.
85. National Academy of Sciences, National Research Council, Division of Medical Sciences, Ad Hoc Committee on Trauma. Postoperative wound infections: The influence of ultraviolet irradiation on the operating room and of various other factors. Ann Surg 160(Suppl 2):1, 1964.
86. Platt R, et al. Perioperative antibiotic prophylaxis for herniorrhaphy and breast surgery. N Engl J Med 322:153, 1990.
87. Ranaboldo CJ, et al. Antimicrobial prophylaxis in 'clean' surgery: Hernia repair. J Antimicrob Chemother 31:35, 1993.
88. Waddell TK, Rotstein OD. Antimicrobial prophylaxis in surgery. Committee on Antimicrobial. Agents, Canadian Infectious Disease Society. Can Med Assoc J 151:925, 1994.
89. Nichols R. Surgical antibiotic prophylaxis. Med Clin North Am 79:509, 1995.
90. Paluzzi R. Antimicrobial prophylaxis for surgery. Med Clin North Am 77:427, 1993.
91. Leaper D. Prophylactic and therapeutic role of antibiotics in wound care. Am J Surg 167:15S, 1994.
92. Bergamini T, Polk HJ. Pharmacodynamics of antibiotic penetration of tissue and surgical prophylaxis. Surg Gynecol Obstet 168:283, 1989.
93. Galandiuk S. Re-emphasis of priorities in surgical antibiotic prophylaxis. Surg Gynecol Obstet 169:223, 1989.
94. Gustilo RB, Merkow RL, Templeman D. The management of open fractures. J Bone Joint Surg 72-A:299, 1990.
95. Fabian T, et al. Duration of antibiotic therapy for penetrating abdominal trauma: A prospective trial. Surgery 112:788, 1992.
96. Dellinger E. Antibiotic prophylaxis in trauma: Penetrating abdominal injuries and open fractures. Rev Infect Dis 13:S847, 1991.
97. Gorbach S. Antimicrobial prophylaxis for appendectomy and colorectal surgery. Rev Infect Dis 13(Suppl 10):S815, 1991.
98. Pruitt B, McManus A. The changing epidemiology of infection in burn patients. World J Surg 16:57, 1992.
99. Pizzo PA. Drug therapy—Management of fever in patients with cancer and treatment-induced neutropenia. N Engl J Med 238:1323, 1993.
100. Shands JJ. Empiric antibiotic therapy of abdominal sepsis and serious perioperative infections. Surg Clin North Am 73:291, 1993.
101. Giamarellou H. Empiric therapy for infections in the febrile, neutropenic, compromised host. Med Clin North Am 79:559, 1995.
102. Dunn DL. Gram-negative bacterial sepsis and sepsis syndrome [review]. Surg Clin North Am 74:621, 1994.
103. DiPiro J, Edmiston C. Pharmacodynamics of antimicrobial therapy in surgery. Am J Surg 171:615, 1996.
104. Solomkin JS, Miyagawa CI. Principles of antibiotic therapy [review]. Surg Clin North Am 74:497, 1994.
105. Miyagawa C. Aminoglycosides in the intensive care unit: An old drug in a dynamic environment. New Horizons 2:172, 1993.
106. Chelluri L, Jastremski M. Inadequacy of standard aminoglycoside pharmacokinetics in critically ill surgical patients. Crit Care Med 15:1143, 1987.
107. Chelluri L, Warren J, Jastremski M. Pharmacokinetics of a 3 mg/kg body weight loading dose of gentamicin or tobramycin in critically ill patients. Chest 95:1295, 1989.
108. Perriols-Lisart R, Alos-Alminana M. Effectiveness and safety of once-daily aminoglycosides: A meta-analysis. Am J Health Syst Pharm 53:1141, 1995.
109. DiPiro JT, Forston N. Combination antibiotic therapy in the management of intra-abdominal infection. Am J Surg 165:82S, 1993.
110. Shands JW Jr. Empiric antibiotic therapy of abdominal sepsis and serious perioperative infections. Surg Clin North Am 73:291, 1993.

7

Hemostasis and Thrombosis in the Surgical Patient

Mark R. Jackson and G. Patrick Clagett

The safe practice of surgery requires a fundamental understanding of the concepts of hemostasis. Traditionally, standard textbooks of surgery have focused on the basics of the coagulation pathways and platelet function, with an overview of inherited and acquired defects of these mechanisms. In organizing this chapter we have sought to summarize these basic concepts and provide additional information on more recent developments that have enhanced our understanding of hemostasis in vivo. The central roles of the tissue factor pathway and thrombin in the coagulation cascade, for example, are emphasized. In addition, newer information on the hypercoagulable syndromes and their role in thrombotic disorders are also presented. Developments in molecular biology are providing unprecedented insight and fundamental understanding of the genetics of inherited bleeding and hypercoagulable disorders that have translated into improved diagnostic testing, such as with resistance to activated protein C and hyperhomocystinemia. Similarly, as the molecular mechanisms of hemostasis are increasingly understood, potent antiplatelet and antithrombotic agents are being developed and made available for clinical use. An appreciation of their therapeutic potential and challenge to surgical hemostasis requires a basic understanding of their mechanisms of action.

MECHANISMS OF HEMOSTASIS

Platelets

Platelets are anucleate cells produced in the bone marrow by fragmentation of megakaryocytes. The megakaryocytes are located in the subendothelial space of bone marrow vascular sinuses, where proliferation and maturation is regulated. Platelet production is stimulated by thrombopoietin, interleukin-3 (IL-3), and IL-6.[1] Factors that inhibit this process include platelet factor 4 (PF4), transforming growth factor-β, and interferon-α.[2,3,4] Thrombopoiesis is also influenced by circulating platelet mass. The identification, purification, and cloning of thrombopoietin, or the c-Mpl ligand, followed characterization of the *c-mpl* gene that encodes for a cell surface receptor present on megakaryocytes and platelets.[5] Thrombopoietin bound to *c-mpl* on megakaryocytes stimulates all stages of megakaryocyte maturation, thus leading to platelet production. Thrombopoietin bound to platelet *c-mpl* aids in its removal from the circulation, a possible mechanism by which platelet mass regulates the plasma concentration of thrombopoietin.

Once released into the circulation, platelet hemostatic function is initiated with adhesion of the platelet to the subendothelial matrix of the injured blood vessel. Platelet activation is followed by platelet aggregation and secretion, the end result of which is a hemostatic plug. The two most potent agonists for platelet aggregation are collagen and thrombin. Once platelet activation is initiated, the platelet changes shape from discoid to spherical and develops pseudopods as a result of changes in the platelet cytoskeleton. Thromboxane A_2 is then produced through the cyclooxygenase pathway of arachidonic acid metabolism and further stimulates platelet aggregation.

Platelets contain numerous intracellular and membrane components that contribute to their hemostatic function. Platelet activation is initiated following binding of thrombin or other agonists to the extracellular domain of specific membrane receptors[6] (Fig. 7-1). As in other cells, platelet receptors for agonists and inhibitors are transmembrane proteins with cell surface and cytoplasmic components. The signal, initiated by receptor occupancy, is then transmitted by the cytoplasmic domain of the receptor through guanosine triphosphate–binding regulatory proteins (G proteins) to membrane-bound, signal-generating enzymes such as phospholipase C (Fig. 7-2).[7] Activation of these enzymes induces generation of second-messenger molecules such as inositol 1,4,5-triphosphate (IP_3) and diacylglycerol (DAG). Inositol triphosphate induces calcium release from the platelet-dense tubular system. A rise in free calcium in the cytosol is a critically important aspect of platelet activation. DAG activates protein kinase C, which in turn promotes protein phosphorylation and

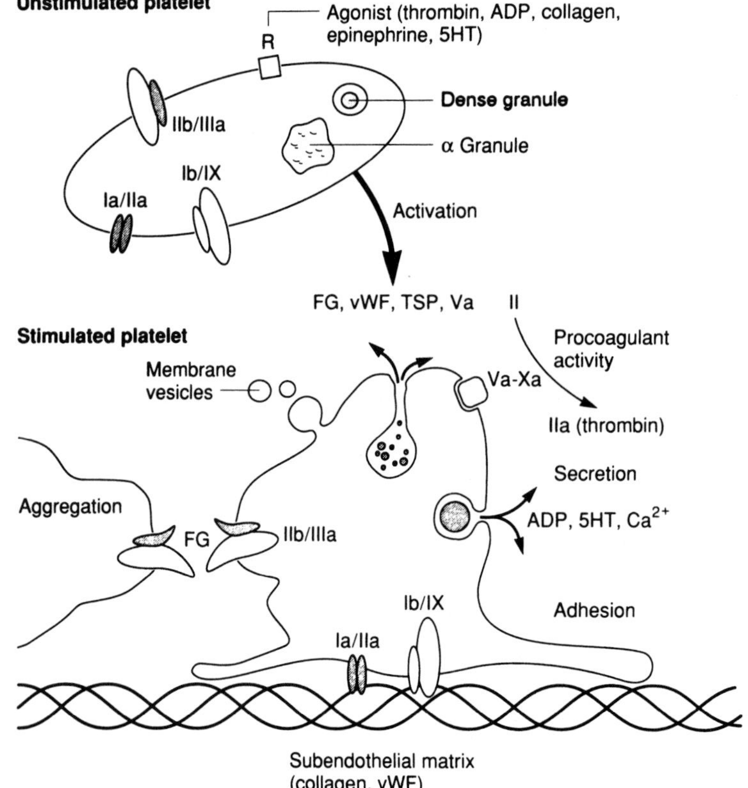

Fig. 7-1. The receptor-mediated events of platelet activation, adhesion, secretion, and aggregation. *R,* Receptor; *ADP,* adenosine diphosphate; *5HT,* serotinin; *FG,* fibrinogen; *vWF,* von Willebrand factor; *TSP,* thrombospondin. (From Clagett GP Jr. Occlusive disease: Thrombosis. In Greenfield LJ, et al., eds. Surgery: Scientific Principles and Practice, 2nd ed. Philadelphia: Lippincott-Raven, 1997, p 1612. Reproduced with permission.)

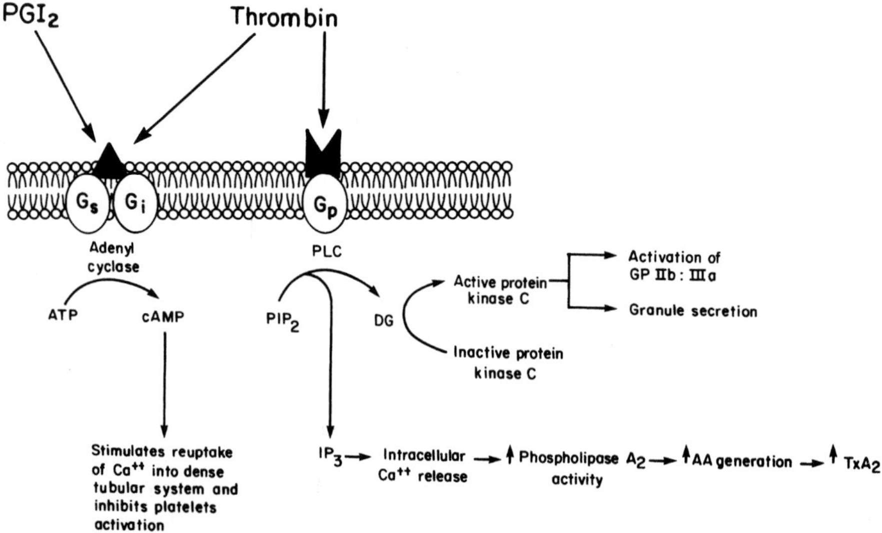

Fig. 7-2. Agonists of platelet activation bind to membrane receptors that activate a G protein *(Gp0),* which activates phospholipase C *(PLC),* which in turn stimulates the phosphoinositide pathway. The second messengers, diacylglycerol *(DAG),* and inositol triphosphate *(IP_3)* lead to exposure of the GPIIb:IIIa complex, platelet secretion, and thromboxane A_2 *(TXA_2)* generation. This signal transduction system also regulates intraplatelet cyclic AMP *(cAMP)* formation. Thrombin stimulates an inhibitory G protein *(G_i)* that inhibits adenylate cyclase and prevents cAMP formation. In contrast, prostacyclin *(PGI_2)* interacts with a stimulatory G protein *(G_s)* that stimulates adenylate cyclase activity in the formation of cAMP. cAMP lowers intracellular calcium levels and inhibits platelet activation.

causes platelet secretion and the expression of the fibrinogen receptor (GPIIb/IIIa) on the platelet surface that leads to platelet aggregation.

Platelets contain two major types of secretory granules, the most predominate of which is the α-granule. Contents of the α-granule include PF4, transforming growth factor-β, platelet-derived growth factor (PGDF), coagulation factor V, and β-thromboglobulin. The dense granules contain serotonin, adenosine triphosphate, adenosine diphosphate, and calcium. Release of these biologically active substances occurs by exocytosis during platelet aggregation and results in platelet recruitment to the site of injury, vasoconstriction, and other hemostatic and vascular responses.

The platelet membrane contains a number of glycoprotein receptors that bind various ligands during platelet activation and thereby promote adhesion and aggregation. GPIb/IX functions as a receptor for von Willebrand factor (vWF) at high shear rates, such as during arterial injury, and allows vWF to bridge the platelet to the subendothelial matrix at the site of arterial injury.[8] GPIIb/IIIa is the platelet membrane receptor for fibrinogen and is essential for aggregation. GPIIb/IIIa binds fibrinogen only after undergoing a conformational change mediated by the platelet cytoskeleton and actin, its major contractile protein. Deficiency of GPIIb/IIIa results in Glanzmann's thrombasthenia, an autosomal recessive bleeding disorder characterized by absence of platelet aggregation and clot retraction. Under conditions of low shear stress, such as with venous injury and thrombosis, platelet adherence to subendothelial collagen occurs through the action of receptors GPIa/IIa and GPIb.

Another function of the platelet is to provide a surface for activation of clotting factors. Many of the reactions in the coagulation cascade are greatly enhanced by the phospholipid surface of the platelet membrane. This enhancement of coagulation by platelets is termed "platelet coagulant activity" and is an important factor during thrombogenesis.[9] Since platelets adhere to the site of vascular injury where bleeding occurs, this allows an increased local concentration of clotting factors. Activated factor X (factor Xa) is a pivotal enzyme in the coagulation cascade; when bound to platelet factor Va, its efficiency in thrombin generation is dramatically increased. In addition, factor Xa bound to activated platelets is protected from inactivation by the heparin/antithrombin III (AT-III) complex.

Coagulation Cascade

In vivo, the primary role in the activation of the coagulation cascade involves the tissue factor/factor VIIa (TF/VIIa) complex (Fig. 7-3).[10,11] Tissue factor is a 45 kd transmembrane protein present in the subendothelium and endothelial cells that have been exposed to thrombin or endotoxin. Following vascular injury, factor VII binds to tissue factor and activates small amounts of factor X, which in turn activates additional factor VII. The TF/VIIa complex then activates additional factor X, either directly or through the activation of factor IX. Under basal conditions, the TF/VIIa complex is the primary activator of factors IX and X (see Fig. 7-3).[12,13] Sustained generation of factor Xa requires the factor IXa/factor VIIIa complex. The VIIIa-IXa-X-Ca^{2+} assembly is known as the Xase ("tenase") complex that leads to the rapid conversion of factor X to Xa. Similarly, while TF/VIIa is the primary activator of factor IX, factor XIa is required for sustained generation of factor IXa. Factor XI is autoactivated, as well as activated by thrombin in vivo; therefore the contact activation system, or intrinsic pathway, is not required for hemostasis in vivo.

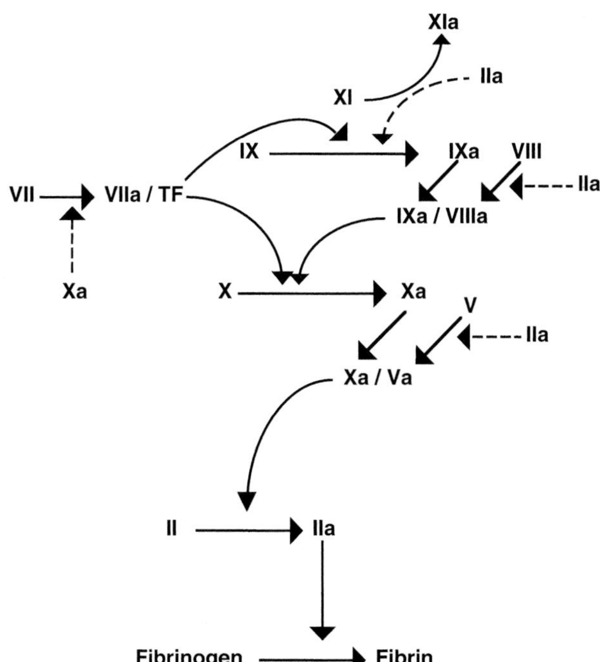

Fig. 7-3. Proposed coagulation pathway under in vivo conditions. Coagulation is initiated by the tissue factor/factor VII complex, which can activate factor X directly or through activation of factor IX. Thrombin can reciprocally activate factors XI, V, and VIII. Factor Xa can promote activation of factor VII. The contact system appears to play no role in hemostasis in vivo. (Modified from American College of Physicians. Medical Knowledge Self-Assessment Program in the Subspecialty of Hematology. Philadelphia: American College of Physicians, 1994, p 201.)

Initiation of the intrinsic pathway (termed "contact activation") involves a complex interaction in which factor XII undergoes a conformational change following exposure to nonendothelialized surfaces. The activation of factor XII occurs principally through the action of kallikrein, with high-molecular-weight kininogen acting as a necessary cofactor. This complicated surface-mediated series of reactions can lead not only to clotting but also to kinin formation, complement activation, and fibrinolysis. In fact, the higher reactions in the intrinsic coagulation cascade are probably more important in triggering inflammatory responses and other defense reactions than they are in hemostasis. Patients with factor XII (Hageman factor) deficiency have no bleeding diathesis, and patients with factor XI deficiency generally have only mild bleeding.

The tissue factor pathway is also referred to as the extrinsic pathway and is the dominant system of the coagulation cascade in vivo. Factor Xa then binds with factor Va to convert prothrombin to thrombin. Assembly of the Va-Xa-II-Ca^{2+} complex occurs on the platelet membrane where Va is located and this thrombin-generating unit is known as the IIase ("prothrombinase") complex. Thrombin generation results in the cleavage of prothrombin fragment F1.2, which has been used as a sensitive marker of thrombin generation and hemostatic activation.[14] Thrombin then converts fibrinogen to fibrin monomers, which are subsequently cross-linked by factor XIII. The cross-linked fibrin clot is comparatively stable and more resistant to lysis because it incorporates α_2-antiplasmin into the clot. The central role of thrombin in the coagulation cascade is demonstrated through its other multiple procoagulant functions, which include the activation of factors V, XI, VIII, and XIII, as well as its potent effect as an inducer of platelet aggregation.

REGULATION OF HEMOSTASIS

Endothelium

Vascular endothelium is interposed between blood and tissue, and in this pivotal position, it carries out multiple regulatory functions that protects against vascular injury and maintains blood fluidity.[15] Endothelium releases prostacyclin (PGI_2) and nitric oxide (NO), potent inhibitors of platelets and vasodilators, and secretes plasminogen activator, which activates the fibrinolytic system. Normal endothelium expresses thrombomodulin, which serves as a binding site for thrombin to activate protein C; heparin-like molecules that can activate At-III; and ectoadenosine diphosphatase, that inhibits platelet aggregation by degrading adenosine diphosphate. Endothelium also produces vWF and releases it into subendothelial matrix, where it mediates platelet adhesions when endothelium is lost. Endothelial injury is accompanied by loss of antithrombotic, protective molecules and expression of procoagulant properties, white blood cell adhesion molecules, and mitogenic activities that can engender thrombosis, smooth muscle cell migration and proliferation, and atherosclerosis. These multiple endothelial functions and their regulatory effects on platelets, coagulation proteins, and the fibrinolytic system are illustrated in Fig. 7-4.

Tissue Factor Pathway Inhibitor

The primary regulator of the tissue factor/factor VIIa complex in hemostasis is the tissue factor pathway inhibitor (TFPI).[11] TFPI is present in circulating form and bound to endothelium (see Fig. 7-4). The inhibitory

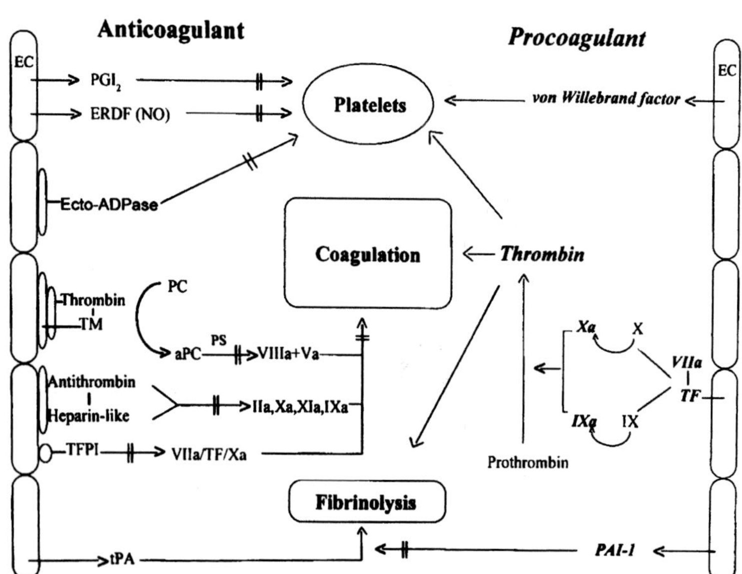

Fig. 7-4. Vasoprotective and procoagulant properties of endothelial cells *(EC)*. On the left, inhibition of platelet function and coagulation by several endothelial molecules and factors and the targeted coagulation factors are shown. In addition, activation of fibrinolysis of EC tissue plasminogen activator *(tPA)* and its inhibition by plasminogen activator *(PAI-1)* is depicted. Thrombomodulin *(TM)* is a surface molecule that binds thrombin, thereby activating protein C *(PC)* to activated protein C (aPC), which in the presence of protein S *(PS)* degrades factor Va and VIIIa-heparin-like molecules expressed on endothelial surface serve as a cofactor for antithrombin III, thereby inactivating thrombin *(ILa)* and several other activated coagulation factors shown. On the right, tisue factor *(TF)* expressed on EC surface during activation serves as a cofactor factor VIIa to activate X and IX respectively. Generated thrombin activates platelets, coagulation, and fibrinolysis. (From Wu KK. Role of endothelium in thrombosis and hemostasis. Annu Rev Med 47:315, 1996. Reprinted with permission of the Annual Review of Medicine. Copyright © 1996 by Annual Reviews, Inc.)

process of TFPI involves two steps.[16] First, TFPI inactivates factor Xa by forming a TFPI/Xa complex. This complex then binds the TF/factor VIIa complex, forming a quaternary Xa/TFPI/VIIa/TF complex, which lacks TF/VIIa activity. Heparin causes the release of TFPI from endothelial stores bound to heparin sulfate or other glycosaminoglycans.[17] More TFPI is available from the endothelial source than that circulating in plasma.

Activated Protein C and Protein S

Endothelium possesses a thrombin receptor, thrombomodulin, that serves as a cofactor together with thrombin for the activation of circulating protein C. Protein S is the cofactor for protein C, which are both vitamin K–dependent proteins. Activated protein C is the major inhibitor of factors Va and VIIIa (see Fig. 7-4).[18] Thrombin bound to thrombomodulin cannot activate factors V, VIII, XIII, fibrinogen, or platelets.[19] The expression of thrombomodulin is downregulated by endotoxin, tumor necrosis factor (TNF), and IL-1.[19]

Antithrombin III

AT-III is a 58 kd glycoprotein that is synthesized in the liver and is the major inhibitor of thrombin and factor Xa.[20] AT-III also inactivates factors XIIa, XIa, and IXa. Heparin accelerates the activity of AT-III by 1000-fold.[21] Heparin dissociates from AT-III once covalent bonds are formed between AT-III and thrombin or other factors, and is then able to activate additional AT-III. AT-III activity is also accelerated by heparin sulfate present on endothelium (see Fig. 7-4).

Fibrinolytic System

Fibrinolysis is stimulated by vascular injury and release of plasminogen activator from endothelial cells (see Fig. 7-4). By the action of tissue-type plasminogen activator (t-PA) or urokinase, the inactive plasma precursor molecule plasminogen is converted to the proteolytic enzyme plasmin, which can digest fibrin and fibrinogen. There are two major forms of circulating plasminogen, lys-plasminogen and glu-plasminogen.[22] Lys-plasminogen selectively binds to fibrin during clotting and is more easily converted to plasmin than is gluplasminogen. Selective incorporation of lys-plasminogen into thrombus also protects the subsequent conversion product plasmin from the natural inhibitor α_2-antiplasmin, which efficiently neutralizes plasmin in the fluid phase only. Thus the action of plasmin is localized to the site of clotting or thrombus formation, where fibrin is digested. Free plasmin is thus prevented from escaping into the general circulation. Small amounts of plasmin that leak into the circulation or are generated in flowing blood are rapidly inactivated by the action of α_2-antiplasmin and other inhibitors.

t-PA is inactivated by plasminogen activator inhibitor (PAI-1), a 52 kd protein synthesized in the endothelial cell (see Fig. 7-4). PAI-1 is the primary regulator of endogenous t-PA activity.[22] α_2-Antiplasmin is a specific inhibitor of plasminogen and is incorporated into the fibrin clot, thereby rendering it resistant to lysis by plasmin.[23] Plasma levels of α_2-antiplasmin are less than those of plasminogen, so that depletion of α_2-antiplasmin, such as during disseminated intravascular coagulation (DIC), can result in uninhibited plasmin activity and worsening of the coagulopathy.

Nitric Oxide

NO is a free radical produced from the amino acid L-arginine (L-Arg) and has a half-life of 3 to 5 seconds.[24] NO is produced by the action of NO synthase (NOS), which converts the terminal guanidine group of L-Arg to NO. Two forms of NOS have been identified, an inducible form (INOS), found primarily in macrophages, and a constitutive form (CNOS), found in neuronal tissue, platelets, and vascular endothelium. In addition to its potent vasodilator function, NO interacts with platelets, inhibiting both adhesion and aggregation by increasing intracellular cyclic guanosine monophosphate (cGMP). Platelets can also release NO, which acts in an autocrine fashion to prevent aggregation. In vivo, platelet deposition at the site of endothelial injury is increased by cell-free hemoglobin, an NO inhibitor. This augmented platelet deposition can be blocked by L-Arg, but not by aspirin.[25]

Prostacyclin

Endothelial cells synthesize PGI_2, which inhibits platelet aggregation and causes smooth muscle relaxation and vasodilation. Released endothelial cell PGI_2 can react with the platelet surface domain of a specific receptor, thereby initiating a signal transduction pathway that is G protein linked and of the type described for activation of phospholipase C. In this case, the signal generating enzyme is adenylate cyclase, which catalyzes formation of the second-messenger cyclic adenosine monophosphate (cAMP) from adenosine triphosphate, resulting in inhibition of platelet function. Through a process of transcellular metabolism between platelets and endothelial cells, prostaglandin intermediates produced by activated platelets are shunted to endothelial cells, which in turn process these intermediates into PGI_2. The resulting negative feedback serves to limit platelet thrombogenesis. Continuous, basal endothelial PGI_2 production occurs in vivo, and marked increases are seen in response to increases in shear stress, local thrombin generation, and cytokines. Another product of endothelial prostaglandin metabolism includes lipoxygenase products that inhibit platelet adhesion. By reducing platelet adhesion, inhibiting platelet aggregation, and causing vasodilation, PGI_2 can lead to local increases in blood flow that help to wash away any thrombi that may be forming.

INHERITED DISORDERS OF COAGULATION

Inherited disorders of hemostasis are generally characterized by a history of prior bleeding episodes, particularly hemarthrosis, which can result in significant joint damage. Surgical treatment in these individuals is best provided at a center where the expertise of a hematologist and others

Table 7-1. Genetics, Epidemiology, and Therapy of Inherited Coagulation Protein Deficiencies

Coagulation Protein Deficiency	Inheritance Pattern	Prevalence	Minimum Desired Level to Control Active Bleeding or Prevent Surgical Bleeding	Replacement Sources
Factor I (fibrinogen)				
Afibrinogenemia	Autosomal recessive	Rare (<200 families reported)	100 mg/dl	Cryoprecipitate/fresh frozen plasma
Hypofibrinogenemia	Autosomal dominant or recessive	Extremely rare		
Dysfibrinogenemia	Autosomal dominant or recessive	Rare (>200 types described)		
Factor II (prothrombin)	Autosomal dominant or recessive	Extremely rare (approximately 25 kindreds)	30% of normal	Fresh-frozen plasma/factor IX complex concentrates
Factor V (labile factor)	Autosomal recessive	1 per million births	25% of normal	Fresh frozen plasma
Factor VII	Autosomal recessive	1 per 500,000 births	25% of normal	Fresh frozen plasma/factor IX complex concentrates
Factor VIII (antihemophilia factor) Hemophilia A	X-linked recessive	1 per 10,000 births 1 per 5000 male births	80% to 100% of normal for life-threatening bleeding, 50% of normal for significant bleeding, 30% of normal for minor bleeding	Factor VIII concentrates; desmopressin for mild to moderate disease
vWf	Usually autosomal dominant	Approximately 1 per 100 births	Total or partial correction of bleeding time and raising vWF activity to 50% of normal	Desmopressin for mild to moderate vWD (except IIB) (variable responses in IIA); cryprecipitate; Intermediate-purity factor concentrates containing a full complement of vWF multimers
Type III	Severe type III disease usually recessive	1 per million births		
Factor IX Hemophilia B Christmas Disease	X-linked recessive	1 per 30,000 male births	25-50% of normal depending on extent of surgery or bleeding	Factor IX complex concentrates, or factor IX (human) concentrates
Factor X	Autosomal recessive	1 per 500,000 births	10-25% of normal	Fresh frozen plasma or factor IX complex concentrates
Factor XI	Autosomal dominant; severe type homozygous	Approximately 4% of Ashkenazi Jews	20-40% of normal	Fresh frozen plasma
Factor XII	Autosomal recessive	Extremely rare		No replacement therapy required
Prekallikrein (Fletcher factor)	Autosomal recessive	Extremely rare		No replacement therapy required
High-molecular-weight fibrinogen (Williams, Flaujeac, or Fitzgerald factor)	Autosomal recessive	Extremely rare		No replacement therapy required
Factor XIII	Autosomal recessive	1 per several million births	5% of normal	Fresh frozen plasma or cryoprecipitate

From American College of Physicians. Medical Knowledge Self-Assessment Program in the Subspecialty of Hematology. Philadelphia: American College of Physicians, 1994, p 204.

vWD, von Willebrand disease; *vWF,* von Willebrand factor.

Table 7-2. Recombinant and Immunoaffinity-Purified Factor VIII Products

	Product Name	Manufacturer	Cell of Origin	Method of Viral Inactivation	Specific Activity (U/mg) Final	Specific Activity (U/mg) Discounting Albumin
Recombinant*	Recombinate	Baxter-Hyland Genetics Institute	Chinese hamster ovary		2.2-5	4000+
	Kogenate	Miles-Cutter	Baby hamster kidney		8-30	4000-6000
Immunoaffinity-purified†	Monoclate P	Armour		Pasteurized (60° C, 10 hr)	5-10	3000+
	Hemofil M	Baxter-Hyland		Solvent detergent (TNBP/Triton X-100, 25° C, ≥10 hr)	2-11	3000+
	Coagulation FVIII, M method	Baxter-Hyland‡		Solvent detergent (TNBP/Triton X-100, 25° C, ≥10 hr)	2-11	3000+

From American College of Physicians. Medical knowledge self-assessment program in the subspecialty of hematology. Philadelphia: American College of Physicians, 1994, p 205.
TNBP, Tri-(n-butyl) phosphate.
*Genetically engineered.
†Derived from human plasma.
‡Manufactured for the American Red Cross.

skilled at providing care for these patients is available. A summary of these deficiencies and their inheritance patterns and treatment is provided in Table 7-1.

Hemophilia A (Factor VIII Deficiency)

Hemophilia A is an X-linked disorder and has an incidence of 10 to 20 cases per 100,000 live births.[8] As many as 30% of new cases are not associated with a family history, thereby suggesting that the factor VIII gene undergoes frequent mutation. Hemophilia A is suspected in any male with a history of excessive bleeding following trauma or spontaneous hemarthrosis. The severity of hemophilia A is correlated with the level of factor VIII. Patients with factor VIII levels greater than 5% have mild hemophilia and are at reduced risk for spontaneous bleeding but are at increased risk for bleeding following surgery or trauma. Patients with factor VIII levels between 1% and 4% have moderate hemophilia. Patients with factor VIII levels less than 1% have severe hemophilia and are at risk for spontaneous bleeding.

Laboratory abnormalities in hemophilia A, other than reduced factor VIII levels, can include a variable prolongation of the activated partial thrompoplastin time (aPTT). Carrier and prenatal testing can be performed by analyzing the DNA from blood samples following amplification using the polymerase chain reaction and then using restriction enzymes that recognize and cleave specific DNA base sequences. The DNA is then analyzed using gel electrophoresis and compared with known patterns of abnormal DNA polymorphism.

Treatment of hemophilia A depends on the severity of the disease and the indication (see Table 7-1). For example, patients with mild hemophilia undergoing dental procedures can be effectively treated with desmopressin (DDAVP, 0.3 μg/kg intravenously), which releases stores of factor VIII and vWF and will increase factor VIII to a median level of 62%. DDAVP cannot be used in patients with severe hemophilia A, since they have no stored form of factor VIII.

Patients with hemophilia A who are undergoing surgery should be treated with factor VIII concentrates (Table 7-2). Since 1985, all factor VIII concentrates in the United States have undergone viral inactivation using heat or solvent-detergent treatment, which has essentially eliminated the risk of transmitting HIV or hepatitis B and C. Commercial factor VIII concentrates are available in a range of purity and specific activity, depending on their source and methods of purification. The half-life of factor VIII is approximately 12 hours, so replacement therapy should be given at 8- to 12-hour intervals during periods of increased bleeding risk. Recombinant factor VIII from genetically engineered mammalian cells has been approved by the FDA.

Hemophilia B (Factor IX Deficiency)

Hemophilia B is inherited in an X-linked fashion and has a clinical presentation similar to hemophilia A.[8] The incidence of hemophilia B is approximately 10-fold lower. As with hemophilia A, spontaneous mutations of the factor IX gene can cause the disorder without a prior family history. Hemophilia B is a heterogenous disorder characterized by a number of point mutations and deletions of the factor IX gene on the X chromosome. The degree of severity of hemophilia B is categorized as with hemophilia A based on the factor IX levels: severe is less than 1% of normal, moderate is 1% to 5%, and mild is 6% to 60% of normal.

Treatment principles for factor IX replacement are similar to those with hemophilia A (see Table 7-1). For major surgery or active bleeding, a factor IX level of 50% to 100% should be achieved using factor IX concentrates. A level of 30% may be adequate for prophylaxis or minor bleeding. The biologic half-life of factor IX is 18 to 30 hours, so concentrates should be readministered at 12- to 24-hour intervals during periods of increased bleeding risk. Replacement therapy for factor IX and VIII can also be guided by periodic assessment of factor levels. The aPTT is inadequate for monitoring factor replacement therapy, since some factor IX products also contain activated clotting factors. The availability of high-purity, virally inactivated factor IX concentrates since 1991 has essentially eliminated the risks of viral transmission and thrombogenicity (Table 7-3). Approximately 50% of patients exposed to factor IX concentrates before the introduction of virus attenuation procedures in 1985 are HIV positive, and virtually all are seropositive for hepatitis C.

von Willebrand Disease

The functions of vWF during normal hemostasis are to promote platelet adhesion in conditions of high shear stress (such as in arterial injury) by binding of the subendothelial vWF to the platelet GPIb receptor and the promotion of platelet aggregation by binding of vWF and fibrinogen to the platelet GPIIb/IIIa receptor. vWF is synthesized in the megakaryocyte and in endothelial cells and is then stored in the Weibel-Palade bodies of the endothelial cell and the α-granules of the platelet.

von Willebrand disease (vWD) results from a quantitative or qualitative deficiency of vWF and has an estimated prevalence of 0.8%, making this the most common inherited bleeding disorder.[26] It is usually transmitted as an autosomal dominant trait with variable expression. However, there is considerable heterogeneity in the spectrum of this disorder, with at least 20 distinct subtypes.[27] Clinically, vWD is characterized by easy bruisability, mucosal bleeding, and potentially heavy bleeding during surgery or from trauma. The laboratory diagnosis includes measurement of vWF activity and antigen. The bleeding time is frequently abnormal as is the aPTT.

There are at least three main types of vWD, each with subtypes. The types are categorized based on a quantitative or qualitative deficiency of vWF. Types I and III are due to quantitative deficiencies, and type II (and other variants) results from a qualitative deficiency in vWF. Type I is most common and is responsible for 70% to 85% of all forms of vWD. Type I vWD results from a quantitative deficiency of vWF of 50% or less of normal. In type IIB, thrombocytopenia can result from treatment with DDAVP because the release of additional abnormal vWF can cause platelet agglutination. Type III vWD is the most severe and results from greatly reduced levels of vWF caused either by an autosomal recessive homozygous state or double heterozygote with an autosomal dominant mode of inheritance. In addition, a platelet type of vWD is caused by an abnormal platelet GPIb receptor, which has an increased affinity for normal vWF, and is associated with platelet agglutination when more vWF is administered.

Patients with type I vWD generally respond well to DDAVP with adequately increased vWF levels for 4 to 8 hours. This effect is presumably mediated through release

Table 7-3. Factor IX Products

	Product Name	Manufacturer	Method of Virus Inactivation	Specific Activity (U/mg)
Coagulation products	AlphaNine	Alpha Therapeutic	Heated in N-heptane solution, 60° C, 20 hr	84
	AlphaNine SD	Alpha Therapeutic	TNBP and polysorbate 80, 24-30° C, >24 hr	190
	Mononine	Armour	Sodium thiocyanate, ultrafiltration	160+
Complex concentrates	Konyne 80	Miles-Cutter	Dry heat, 80° C, 72 hr	1.3
	Proplex T	Baxter-Hyland	Dry heat, 68° C, 144 hr	47
	Profilnine HT (wet method)	Alpha Therapeutic	Heated in N-heptane solution 60° C, 20 hr	4.5
	Bebulin	Immuno	Vapor heated (10 hr, 60° C, 1190 mb pressure plus 1 h, 80° C, 1375 mb)	2
Activated complex concentrates	Autoplex T	Baxter-Hyland	Dry heat, 68° C, 144 hr	5
	FEIBA VH	Immuno-U.S.	Vapor heated (10 hr 60° C, 1190 mb plus 1 hr, 80° C, 1375 mb)	0.8

From American College of Physicians. Medical Knowledge Self-Assessment Program in the Subspecialty of Hematology. Philadelphia: American College of Physicians, 1994, p 207.
mb, Millibar; *TNBP,* tri in butyl phosphate.

of endogenous vWF from the endothelium, although the mechanism for this is not completely understood. For patients with type IIA vWD response to DDAVP is unpredictable and should be tested in advance. Use of DDAVP in type IIB and platelet type vWD is contraindicated due to resulting thrombocytopenia. For patients in whom DDAVP is not effective or contraindicated, replacement therapy using cryoprecipitate or intermediate-purity factor VIII concentrates that contain functional vWF is indicated. A retrospective review of the use of cryoprecipitate and factor VIII concentrates in vWD unresponsive to DDAVP in 21 treatment centers showed equivalent efficacy.[28] since factor VIII concentrates are virally inactivated and cryoprecipitate is not, and since there appears to be no advantage to the use of cryoprecipitate, factor VIII concentrates should be considered the treatment of choice in vWD when DDAVP cannot be used.

INHERITED QUALITATIVE PLATELET DISORDERS

Glanzmann's Thrombasthenia

Glanzmann's thrombasthenia results from a congenital absence of functional platelet GPIIb/IIIa receptor to bind fibrinogen and participate in clot retraction, which is mediated by interaction of GPIIb/IIa with the platelet cytoskeleton.[29] The genetic defects that result in Glanzmann's thrombasthenia are remarkably heterogenous, can result in abnormal GPIIIa or GPIIb, and are generally inherited in an autosomal recessive pattern.[30] A deficiency in either glycoprotein causes a functional abnormality of GPIIb/IIIa. Clinically, the disorder is characterized by a history of excessive bleeding at an early age, easy bruisability, and menorrhagia. Hemarthroses are rare. Laboratory diagnosis is established by the absence of the GPIIb/IIIa receptor by flow cytometry or gel electrophoresis. The platelet count and morphology are normal. Platelet aggregometry reveals agglutination of Glanzmann's platelets with ristocetin, but not with adenosine diphosphate (ADP), epinephrine, thrombin, or collagen.

Treatment of Glanzmann's thrombasthenia requires antifibrinolytic agents, either ϵ-aminocaproic acid (EACA) or tranexamic acid, for epistaxis, dental surgery, or minor bleeding.[8] Oral contraceptives are effective in treating menorrhagia. Platelet transfusions, preferably human leukocyte (HLA)-matched, are required for surgery. Development of alloimmunization or antibodies to GPIIb/IIIa limits the usefulness of platelet transfusion, so this should be used only when serious bleeding occurs or is likely. DDAVP does not prevent bleeding with this disorder.

Although Glanzmann's thrombasthenia is a rare disorder, the understanding of its molecular basis has led to advances in antiplatelet therapy. Antibody inhibitors of the GPIIb/IIIa receptor are now used as antiplatelet agents and are discussed in a subsequent section.

Bernard-Soulier Disease (Syndrome)

Bernard-Soulier disease (syndrome) results from congenital absence of platelet GPIb/IX, the receptor for vWF.[31] This is a rare disorder, with only approximately 100 reported cases. The pattern of inheritance is usually autosomal recessive, although an autosomal dominant form has been described. These patients have a similar clinical presentation to that of Glanzmann's thrombasthenia but have thrombocytopenia and large platelets.[8] The thrombocytopenia can be as low as 20,000/μl. Since the interaction with vWF is affected, platelets do not aggregate in high shear conditions, such as with arterial injury. Platelet aggregometry reveals agglutination in the presence of ADP, collagen, and epinephrine but not to ristocetin. Aggregation response to thrombin is dose dependent. Treatment principles using oral contraceptives, antifibrinolytic agents, and platelet transfusion are as for Glanzmann's thrombasthenia. Similarly, DDAVP is not considered effective.

ACQUIRED DISORDERS OF HEMOSTASIS

Disseminated Intravascular Coagulation

Disseminated intravascular coagulation (DIC) is a hemorrhagic and thrombotic disorder that is triggered by a variety of underlying illnesses and results in generation of tissue factor with consequent activation of coagulation. The disorder is characterized by excess thrombin generation and fibrinolysis. Microvascular thrombosis occurs and can exacerbate underlying tissue and organ injury.

In surgical patients, multiple clinical settings are associated with DIC and intraoperative coagulopathy. Severe bacterial infections with septicemia and endotoxemia, particularly from gram-negative enteric organisms, can trigger DIC. Gram-positive bacterial infections also can be etiologic. Massive tissue trauma, especially when associated with shock, can flood the circulation with thromboplastic and procoagulant substances and lead to acute consumption of hemostatic elements sufficient to incite bleeding. Localized trauma in the form of brain injury (usually severe and penetrating) and long bone fractures can trigger DIC by similar mechanisms. Malignancy can be associated with acute or chronic DIC. Similarly, chronic partially compensated DIC can occur with aortic aneurysms. A review of 34 such cases has been recently reported.[32]

A major transfusion reaction can cause DIC and should be suspected when sudden intraoperative bleeding occurs in the absence of a surgical source during blood transfusion. This can occur with the infusion of as little as 25 ml of mismatched blood. The clinical manifestations of shaking chills, fever, and back pain can be obscured by general anesthesia. Hypotension, diffuse bleeding, and darkening of the urine may be the only clues of intraoperative transfusion reaction. Treatment is directed at (1) stopping transfusion, (2) restoring normal blood pressure and volume with crystalloid and appropriate pharmacologic support, (3) attaining alkalinization with sodium bicarbonate, and (4) administering mannitol to protect against renal tubular necrosis. Fortunately, the DIC that attends a major transfusion reaction is transient and usually requires no treatment once the causative agent has been stopped.

The laboratory diagnosis of DIC is demonstrated by

evidence of platelet and fibrinogen consumption, as well as fibrinolysis. Fibrinogen levels can, however, be normal in up to 57% of patients with DIC.[33] The prothrombin time and thrombin times are elevated in DIC. The aPTT is variable depending on the level of factor VIII activation. Elevated levels of fibrinopeptide A indicate conversion of fibrinogen to fibrin. Elevated prothrombin fragment F1.2 indicates thrombin generation from the action of factor Xa on prothrombin. D-Dimer is generated by lysis of cross-linked fibrin and forms the basis of a sensitive laboratory test.[34] Elevation of D-dimer is typically seen in DIC but can occur in other conditions where there is physiologic fibrinolysis.

The treatment of all forms of DIC occurring intraoperatively is aimed primarily at supporting normal blood volume and pressure and expeditious removal of the stimulus for DIC. Specific therapies directed against DIC, such as heparinization, have no place in an acutely bleeding patient and are contraindicated in this setting. Heparin may be used in conditions where DIC is not associated with bleeding, such as sepsis or chronic DIC with an intact aortic aneurysm. Likewise, antifibrinolytic agents are not advised because a degree of fibrinolysis protects against occlusive thrombosis of capillaries and prevents organ ischemia. Most authorities believe that EACA should not be used for DIC unless the patient is heparinized. In a patient with DIC undergoing operation, control of bleeding must by necessity be effected by infusion of fresh frozen plasma (FFP), cryoprecipitate, and platelets. The fear of "fueling the fire" and making the process worse has been overemphasized in the past. Component therapy can be lifesaving in this difficult clinical circumstance.

ACQUIRED DISORDERS OF PLATELET FUNCTION

Of the long list of substances that have been shown to inhibit platelet function (Table 7-4), only aspirin has been clearly documented to increase the clinical risk of bleeding. Aspirin irreversibly inactivates cyclooxygenase, thereby preventing the production of thromboxane A_2 from arachidonic acid.[35] One 80 to 100 mg dose of aspirin can totally inhibit thromboxane production for the 10-day lifespan of the platelet.[36]

The true impact of aspirin on intraoperative bleeding is difficult to determine. Several trials have shown an increased amount of surgical bleeding in aspirin-treated patients undergoing coronary artery bypass grafting,[37-39] but other studies in this clinical setting have shown no increased risk of bleeding.[36,40,41] Results of the Physician's Health Study on the efficacy of aspirin for primary prevention of myocardial infarction showed an increased risk of bleeding episodes compared to subjects taking placebo (27% vs. 20%).[42] The ubiquitous use of aspirin is reflected in a study that reported that approximately one half of patients undergoing unexpected surgery had taken aspirin within the previous 72 hours.[43] In this study, however, there was no increased risk of bleeding or increased use of blood transfusions. However, aspirin can increase bleeding in surgical patients who have other hemostatic problems such as those induced by cardiopulmonary bypass and anticoagulant (e.g., heparin, warfarin) use and should be used with caution in these settings.

Table 7-4. Acquired Platelet Dysfunction

Associated With Medication	Associated With Medical Conditions
Aspirin	Chronic renal failure
NSAIDs	Cardiopulmonary bypass
Cephalosporin antibiotics	Disseminated intravascular coagulation
Penicillins	Chronic hepatic disease
Thrombolytic agents	Multiple myeloma
Dextran	Collagen vascular diseases, particularly SLE
Prostacyclin (Iloprost)	Chronic myeloproliferative disorders
β-Blockers	Myelodysplastic syndromes
Calcium channel blockers	
Nifedipine, verapamil, diltiazem	
Nitroprusside	
Nitroglycerin	
Quinidine	
Tricyclic antidepressants or antipsychotics	
Antihistamines	
Eicosapentanoic acid (ω-3 fatty acids)	
Ticlopidine	

From American College of Physicians. Medical Knowledge Self-Assessment Program in the Subspecialty of Hematology. Philadelphia: American College of Physicians, 1994, p 212.
NSAIDs, Nonsteroidal anti-inflammatory drugs; *SLE,* systemic lupus erythematosus.

Although other nonsteroidal anti-inflammatory drugs inhibit platelet function, they do so reversibly and have not been shown to cause clinically important bleeding. Antibiotics that have the β-lactam structure interfere with platelet function by inhibition of platelet surface receptor functions.[44]

Laboratory tests of platelet function as used by the clinician are the bleeding time and platelet aggregation studies. Platelet aggregometry measures the change in optical density over time in a sample of platelet-rich plasma to which an agonist of platelet aggregation has been added. The optical density decreases as the platelets in suspension cluster into aggregates. Although most acquired disorders of platelet function are associated with abnormal platelet aggregometry, the clinical usefulness of these studies are limited.[44] Normal criteria are specific only for individual laboratories.[45] Furthermore, abnormalities in platelet aggregometry assays have not always correlated with risk of bleeding.[46]

Measurement of the forearm template bleeding time is probably the most commonly used laboratory measure of platelet function. The test is performed by making a standard skin incision on the medial aspect of the forearm using a template blade, blotting the incision every 30 seconds, and measuring the time until bleeding stops. While antiplatelet agents generally prolong the bleeding time, a review of the literature shows no clear evidence that a prolonged bleeding time predicts excessive bleeding during surgery.[47,48]

Systemic disorders such as uremia may also inhibit platelet function. The many reports of serious bleeding complications in uremic patients may have more to do with underlying gastrointestinal lesions and heparin treatment (during dialysis) than with the platelet inhibition per se.[46] Platelet function abnormalities can be improved following dialysis.[49] DDAVP has been used to correct qualitative platelet dysfunction due to uremia and other causes.[50]

BLEEDING IN THE SURGICAL PATIENT

Preoperative Assessment

The most important element in the preoperative evaluation of risk of bleeding is the history and physical examination. The history should elicit whether the patient bleeds unusually in response to minor trauma or spontaneously in the absence of trauma (see accompanying box). The responses to major and minor surgery and to dental extractions are particularly helpful. A patient who has recently undergone surgery without bleeding complications has had a far better "stress test" of hemostasis than any laboratory can provide. The manifestations of abnormal bleeding can provide clues to the nature of the underlying hemostatic defect. Easy bruisability, ecchymoses, petechial hemorrhages, nosebleeds, and oral mucosal and gingival bleeding generally indicate thrombocytopenia or a qualitative platelet disorder, whereas joint hemorrhages, deep muscular hematomas, and retroperitoneal bleeding are usually signs of a coagulation defect (congenital factor deficiency or anticoagulant use). These distinctions are not specific, however, and the presence of any of these abnormalities should prompt a more thorough laboratory evaluation for an underlying hemostatic deficit. The family history is relevant and a pedigree chart of a familial bleeding tendency may provide important clues. The family history is not always positive with the "inherited" clotting disorders. Up to 30% of new cases of hemophilia A are not associated with a positive family history and are thought to represent spontaneous mutation.[57]

The routine use of preoperative laboratory screening tests is unnecessary when an underlying coagulation disorder is not clinically suspected. The inability of the bleeding time to predict surgical bleeding has been described previously. Similarly, preoperative assessment of the prothrombin time and the aPTT in the absence of a clinically suspected clotting disorder has been shown not to predict surgical bleeding complications.[52,54] When evaluating a patient for a major operation that has greater potential to impair clotting mechanisms, such as coronary artery bypass or major vascular reconstruction, or where the consequences of excessive bleeding are particularly hazardous, such as with neurologic surgery or tissue flaps, it is reasonable to routinely perform basic coagulation tests such as a platelet count, prothrombin time, and partial thromboplastin time. This recommendation should not be viewed as a substitute for a proper clinical assessment.

BLEEDING HISTORY

Hemostatic Response to Surgery and Trauma

1. What operations have you had, including minor ones, such as tonsillectomy, circumcision, or biopsies? Was bleeding after surgery hard to stop? Have you ever developed unusual bruising in the skin around an area of surgery?
2. Have you ever required a blood transfusion?
3. Have you ever bled for a long time or developed a swollen tongue or mouth after cutting or biting your tongue, cheek or lip? What was the longest time it took to stop bleeding from cuts or scrapes? Has bleeding from a cut or scrape ever restarted after stopping completely?
4. How many times have you had teeth pulled and what was the longest time that you bled afterward? Has bleeding ever restarted the day after extraction?

Spontaneous Bleeding

1. Do you develop bruises larger than a silver dollar without remembering when or how you injured yourself? If so, how big was the largest of these bruises?
2. Do you ever have nose bleeds?
3. Do your gums bleed easily?
4. Do you ever have abnormally heavy menstrual periods or spotting between periods?
5. Do you have blood in your urine or stool? Do you ever have black, tarry stools?
6. Have you ever had bleeding into joints or muscles?

Medication History

1. What medication, including aspirin or any other pills or powders for headaches, colds, menstrual cramps, arthritis, joint pains, back aches, or other pains, have you taken within the last week?
2. Do you take medicine to thin the blood or to prevent blood clots?
3. Have you had a medical problem within the past 5 years requiring a doctor's care? If so, what is its nature?

Family History

1. Are there any bleeders in the family?
2. Has any blood relative had a problem with unusual bleeding or bruising after surgery? Were blood transfusions required to control this bleeding?

Intraoperative and Postoperative Bleeding

The most common cause of significant intraoperative bleeding is inadequate surgical hemostasis, the so-called "silk deficiency." There are no pharmacologic or blood bank substitutes for a careful dissection and attention to technical detail. Even what seems like trivial bleeding from skin edges and subcutaneous tissue can add up, and such bleeding can account for up to 100 to 200 ml of blood loss if unattended.[55] Dissection using electrocautery rather than a scalpel has been shown to reduce blood loss.[57,57]

Intraoperative disorders of hemostasis can be acquired for a number of reasons. Coagulopathy in vascular disorders and trauma has been shown to be related more to hypotension and hypoperfusion than to dilutional factors.[58] Tissue hypoxia can cause release of plasminogen activators, thereby stimulating fibrinolysis. Hypothermia may be another contributing factor, particularly in the traumatized patient.

Dilutional thrombocytopenia may occur in the massively transfused patient, particularly following 20 or more units of banked or cell salvage blood.[59] In a prospective, randomized clinical trial evaluating the efficacy of prophylactic transfusion of either 6 U of platelets or 2 U of FFP given after transfusion of every 12 U of blood, there was no difference in platelet counts or microvascular bleeding (18% in platelet group, 19% in FFP group) between groups, leading the authors to conclude that prophylactic platelet transfusion is unnecessary in the massively transfused patient.[60] Of the six patients who developed microvascular bleeding, however, four subsequently required platelet transfusions to correct persistent thrombocytopenia and oozing. This study also illustrates that measured platelet counts are significantly higher following massive transfusion than would be predicted on the basis of dilution alone, indicating that endogenous release of platelets, presumably from the spleen, is responsible for continued release of platelets into the circulation in such patients. Since there was not a control group that did not receive prophylactic FFP transfusion, the issue of prophylactic repletion of labile clotting factors was not addressed. Prophylactic treatment with DDAVP did not decrease blood loss and transfusion requirements in a randomized study in patients undergoing aortic surgery.[61]; however, DDAVP can be useful in patients undergoing complex cardiac operations with prolonged cardiopulmonary bypass.[62]

Recommendations for platelet and labile clotting factor replacement during surgery are best guided by specific laboratory measurement of coagulation deficiency rather than an arbitrary formula.[63] The time delay from when the intraoperative microvascular bleeding is first noticed until laboratory measurements to document the particular coagulation disorder are complete can be problematic. If the surgeon's clinical judgment is confirmed by the laboratory test, additional blood loss and factor depletion has occurred before the appropriate factor replacement products can be made available. A potential solution to this problem would involve improved near-site monitoring of coagulation function.

Despite appropriate factor replacement for acquired and congenital coagulation disorders, nonsurgical bleeding can persist and be difficult to treat. A variety of commercially available topical hemostatic agents have been used in this situation. These topical agents are generally derived from bovine collagen or gelatin, or oxidized cellulose. Although these products create a mechanical template on which clot can form, they are limited by a lack of any inherent coagulation mechanism. Fibrin sealant is a potential alternative topical hemostatic agent. Fibrin sealant mimics the final step in the coagulation cascade by combining thrombin and fibrinogen (generally in liquid form) and can be applied directly to a surgical wound or a vascular anastomosis.[64,65] Fibrin sealant can be made in the operating room by combining equal volumes of bovine thrombin (with calcium chloride) and cryoprecipitated plasma using separate syringes for each. Commercially prepared fibrin sealant is made of purified, virally inactivated human thrombin and fibrinogen, is available in Europe, and is undergoing clinical trials in the United States.[66]

CONGENITAL DISORDERS OF HYPERCOAGULABILITY

Resistance to Activated Protein C

Resistance to activated protein C is the most common inherited hypercoagulable disorder, affecting approximately 3% to 5% of populations of Western European origin. It is inherited in an autosomal dominant fashion and is due to a single point mutation in the gene coding for factor V, resulting in an Arg506 to Gln amino acid substitution, rendering it "resistant" to inactivation by protein C. Resistance to activated protein C is common in patient who have venous thrombosis, with a prevalence in this group of 20% to 60%.[67-69] Activated protein C resistance is the most common abnormality associated with deep venous thrombosis during pregnancy, and the diagnosis should be diligently sought in this setting. This disorder is also commonly found among patients with recurrent venous thromboembolism.[70]

The diagnosis can be made using either a plasma-based clotting assay or a DNA assay. The clotting assay is an aPTT with a mixture of patient plasma and factor V–deficient plasma in the presence and absence of added activated protein C. When the added activated protein C does not prolong the aPTT adequately, resistance is suggested. In the DNA-based assay, DNA is extracted from the patient's blood and amplified using the polymerase chain reaction. A restriction enzyme that recognizes only the normal factor V DNA is added. Normal and abnormal genotypes can then be determined by examination of the DNA electrophoretic bands.

The effect of anticoagulants on the results of hypercoagulability testing can present a point of confusion. The potential for interference with laboratory assays because of therapeutic anticoagulation is generally only an issue for protein C and protein S, the levels of which are decreased by warfarin, since they are vitamin K–dependent proteins. Since a DNA assay is available for resistance to activated protein C, anticoagulation does not interfere with the results. Generally, all factors can be tested for in the presence of heparin, although AT-III levels may be decreased (Fig. 7-5).

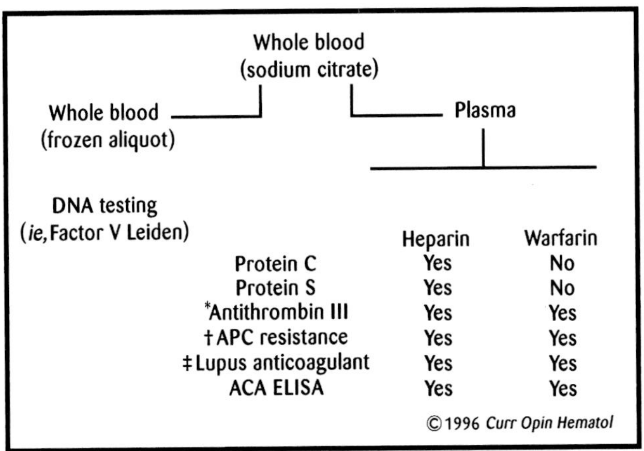

Fig. 7-5. Laboratory testing for hypercoagulability. Antithrombin III may be decreased in vivo in patients receiving heparin. Test of APC resistance can be performed if heparin is removed; test plasma should be mixed with factor V–deficient plasma. In an assay for lupus anticoagulant, heparin removed or heparin-insensitive assay should be used. Test is performed with 1:1 mixture of patients and normal plasma. *ACA,* Anticardiolipin antibody; *APC,* activated protein C; *AT-III,* antithrombin III. (From Jones MP, Alving B. Laboratory testing for hypercoagulable disorders. Curr Opin Hematol 3:365, 1996.)

The role of resistance to activated protein C in arterial thrombosis has not been determined. In a cohort study of men in the Physician's Health Study, resistance to activated protein C was found to be a risk factor for venous thrombosis but not for myocardial infarction or stroke.[71] Another recent study, however, suggests that resistance to activated protein C might be a risk factor for failure of infrainguinal bypass grafts.[72]

Protein S Deficiency

Protein S, the vitamin K–dependent cofactor of activated protein C, is also associated with thromboembolic disease when deficiency states exist. The deficiency is generally inherited as an autosomal dominant trait; however, several point mutations have been identified.[73] The clinical manifestations are similar to those seen with deficiency of protein C and AT-III, primarily venous thrombotic events. Arterial thrombotic events can also occur but less commonly than venous thrombosis.

About 60% of protein S circulates in inactive form bound to C4b-binding protein.[74] The remaining 40% is free and is the active form. Increased plasma levels of C4b-binding protein decrease the levels of free protein S and can influence thrombotic events.[75] Since C4b-binding protein is an acute phase reactant that increases during inflammatory states and the postoperative period, relative decreases in free protein S may result, predisposing to thrombotic complications. Levels of total protein S in deficient heterozygotes range from 30% to 65% and levels of free protein S range from 15% to50% of normal.[75] Inherited deficiency states characterized by normal total protein S antigen level, normal or reduced free protein S levels, and diminished protein S activity have also been reported.[76,77] Patients with protein S deficiency who have sustained thromboembolic episodes are best managed with lifelong anticoagulation.

Protein C Deficiency

Protein C is a vitamin K–dependent enzyme that when activated inhibits factors Va and VIIIa. Protein C deficiency is inherited as an autosomal dominant trait with heterozygotes suffering recurrent venous thromboembolism. The initial thrombotic episode occurs spontaneously in approximately 70% of affected individuals. As with protein S deficiency, the relationship to arterial thrombotic events is unknown. Homozygous infants can develop neonatal purpura fulminans. Interestingly, the heterozygote parents infrequently have thrombotic events, suggesting other factors are involved that modulate phenotypic expression. As with protein S deficiency states, a number of genetic point mutations have been recognized, which might account for the clinical heterogeneity of this disorder.[78] Laboratory testing is done using a functional assay that measures the ability of activated protein C to inhibit factors Va and VIIIa in a modified aPTT using protein C–deficient plasma that provides the other factors.[79] As with protein S, protein C is a vitamin K–dependent protein, so testing should not be performed while the patient is receiving warfarin therapy. These assays are not influenced by heparin (see Fig. 7-5).

Warfarin-induced skin necrosis has occurred in some patients with protein C or protein S deficiency. The clinical and pathologic manifestations are similar to those seen with neonatal purpura fulminans caused by severe protein C deficiency, with skin lesions on the extremities, breasts, trunk, and penis occurring during the first few days of warfarin therapy. The mechanism is thought to be due to a transient hypercoagulable state in which protein C levels decrease faster than factor X levels, as well as a greater effect on hemostatic function from protein C reduction than from factor VII reduction. Since only about one third of patients with warfarin-induced skin necrosis have an underlying inherited deficiency of protein C,[80] heparin is generally administered with warfarin until there is an increase in the prothrombin time. Patients with protein C deficiency who have sustained thromboembolic episodes are best managed with lifelong anticoagulation.

Antithrombin-III Deficiency

Congenital deficiency of AT-III, first described in 1965,[81] has a prevalence of one per 2000 to 5000 and is one of the uncommon hypercoagulable syndromes. Deficiency of AT-III is inherited as an autosomal dominant trait and clinically is characterized by venous thrombosis occurring at an early age. Two thirds of affected patients have a venous thrombosis by age 35. In the most common form of AT-III deficiency (type I), both the functional and antigenic levels of AT-III are reduced, resulting from any one of a number of identified mutations.[82,83] Two other types have been identified where the antigenic level of AT-III is normal, but the functional activity is reduced, either because of a defect in the thrombin-binding site (type II) or in the heparin-binding site (type III). Patients with type III AT-III deficiency do not appear to be at increased thrombotic risk unless they are homozygous.[79]

Patients with AT-III deficiency who have sustained thrombotic episodes re generally treated with lifelong warfarin anticoagulation. Although these patients are often considered to be "heparin resistant," heparin anticoagulation can be achieved when necessary to acutely treat a thrombotic event. More importantly, AT-III deficiency is the only inherited hypercoagulable disorder for which replacement therapy, comprised of concentrates of purified human AT-III, has been approved by the FDA. The concentrates are pasteurized for viral inactivation.[84,85] Perioperative replacement therapy with AT-III concentrate is recommended, since 17% to 24% of AT-III–deficient patients undergoing surgery without receiving concentrates develop deep venous thrombosis, even when other forms of prophylaxis are used.[86,87] Despite the commercial availability of the concentrates in the United States since 1990, clinical experience with their perioperative use in conjunction with anticoagulation has been limited. Successful perioperative use of AT-III concentrates for venous surgery in deficient patients has been described.[88]

Hyperhomocysteinemia

Homocysteine is an amino acid formed in the metabolism of methionine. Elevated plasma levels of homocysteine can result when there is a deficiency in either one of two enzymes that are involved in cysteine metabolism. A deficiency of cystathione β-synthase prevents adequate transsulfuration of homocysteine. A deficiency of methylenetetrahydrofolate reductase (MTHFR) prevents remethylation of homocysteine to methionine. A number of studies have linked elevated plasma homocysteine levels to an increased risk of premature atherosclerosis and thrombosis.[89-93] In the past, much ambiguity has resulted when studies using plasma homocysteine levels as an end point have shown conflicting results regarding the association of homocysteine levels and atherosclerotic risk.[94]

Recent work has identified a common point mutation in the gene coding for the MTHFR enzyme rendering it thermolabile, resulting in elevated plasma homocysteine levels.[95-97] Both homozygotes and heterozygotes have diminished enzyme activity compared to normal, at 30% and 65%, respectively.[98] The genomic region of DNA can be amplified using the polymerase chain reaction and then subjected to restriction enzyme analysis so that genotype can be definitively determined. Populations of Northern European descent have a high prevalence of this mutation, with approximately 10% homozygosity and 40% heterozygosity. It appears that dietary supplementation with folic acid can reduce plasma homocysteine levels in both heterozygotes and homozygotes, which promises a simple and effective therapy for this disorder.[97,98] Future studies using these molecular techniques should yield additional insight regarding the role of hyperhomocysteinemia in atherosclerosis and thrombosis, as well as for the potential role of folic acid as a therapeutic agent.

ACQUIRED HYPERCOAGULABLE DISORDERS

Antiphospholipid Antibody Syndrome

Lupus anticoagulants are antiphospholipid antibodies that have in vitro anticoagulant activity yet are clinically associated with arterial and venous thrombosis. The constellation of any one of the following clinical manifestations (arterial or venous thrombosis, recurrent abortion, or thrombocytopenia) in the presence of antiphospholid antibodies has been described as the antiphospholipid syndrome.[99] When the syndrome occurs in the absence of lupus or other connective tissue disorders, it is referred to as primary antiphospholipid syndrome, and secondary antiphospholid antibody syndrome when in the presence of lupus or other connective tissue disorders. Antiphospholipid antibodies can also be caused by drugs such as procainamide, hydralazine, chlorpromazine, quinidine, isoniazid, and methyldopa, with procainamide being most common in the United States.[99] When the condition is drug associated, however, there does not appear to be a significant thrombotic risk.

The pathogenesis of thrombosis with antiphospholipid antibodies is not completely understood. Proposed mechanisms include platelet activation, inhibition of PGI_2 production, vascular injury, and interference with protein C.[99] Alternatively, it is possible that antiphospholipid antibodies are a marker for some other process that is more closely linked with thrombosis. The almost equal tendency for arterial and venous thrombosis with antiphospholipid syndrome distinguishes this disorder from the inherited hypercoagulable conditions where venous thrombosis predominates.

Several enzyme-linked immunosorbent assays (ELISAs) for IgG and IgM antiphospholipid antibodies are now commercially available and have been standardized.[100] The diagnosis of antiphospholipid antibody syndrome can only be confirmed after appropriate laboratory testing on two separate occasions separated by at least 12 weeks.[79] Patients who develop thrombotic complications are generally treated with long-term anticoagulation. Treatment regimens when associated with cerebrovascular thrombosis can also include antiplatelet agents and steroids, although this has not been standardized.[99]

Heparin-Induced Thrombocytopenia (With or Without Thrombosis)

Heparin-induced thrombocytopenia (HIT) with or without thrombosis, first recognized in 1973,[101] is associated with morbidity and mortality especially in patients with atherosclerosis, sepsis, and recent surgery.[102-104] Recent studies have documented that patients with HIT have antibodies that are directed against a complex of heparin and PF4, a protein which has extremely high affinity for heparin.[105-108] The major factor in the development of HIT (with or without thrombosis) is the formation of antibodies, usually of IgG isotope against the heparin/PF4 complex, which may be localized to the platelet membrane or to other phospholipid surfaces such as heparin sulfates on the endothelial cells. Binding of these antibodies to the complex of heparin and PF4 allows the Fc portion of the IgG molecule to activate platelets through the platelet Fc receptor (Fig. 7-6). Receptor expression can be elevated threefold to fivefold during sepsis or other acute illnesses and returns to normal as the inflammatory process resolves.[109] Patients with high levels of receptor expression appear to have the most severe forms of thrombosis with HIT.[109] This process then initiates thrombosis, which is characteristically rich in platelets, hence the name "white clot syndrome."

The standard diagnostic test for HIT in most laboratories is the platelet aggregation test. Although this test is simple and quickly performed, its sensitivity has been questioned. Depending on the reactivity to donor platelets and heparin concentration used in the aggregation test, the sensitivity can range from 29% to 88%.[110] A more sensitive test appears to be the ^{14}C serotonin release assay.[107,111] In this test the release of ^{14}C serotonin from the platelets is measured rather than the ability of platelets to aggregate, since immune complexes can induce release without causing aggregation. Several laboratories have now developed ELISAs that use heparin/PF4 to detect IgG or IgM antibodies in sera from patients suspected of having HIT.[106,112] The ELISA for detection of anti–heparin/PF4 antibodies appears to be more sensitive than the ^{14}C serotonin release assay and the platelet aggregation test and has been used clinically to document heparin-induced antibodies.[113]

The clinical management of HIT poses many dilemmas, particularly when continued anticoagulation is necessary or desired. Although heparin must be discontinued, few alternatives are readily available. Ideal agents are thrombin-specific inhibitors such as argatroban, hirudin, or its analog hirulog; however, these agents are not yet widely available. Hirudin[114] and argatroban[115] have been used successfully as alternate anticoagulation in patients with HIT. Low-molecular-weight heparin (LMWH) is now available and seems to be less immunogenic than unfractionated heparin. However, 90% of patients with HIT have antibodies that cross-react with LMWH,[116] making this a poor alternative when continued anticoagulation is necessary. Heparinoid has been used successfully on a compassionate basis to treat HIT.[117] Success has also been

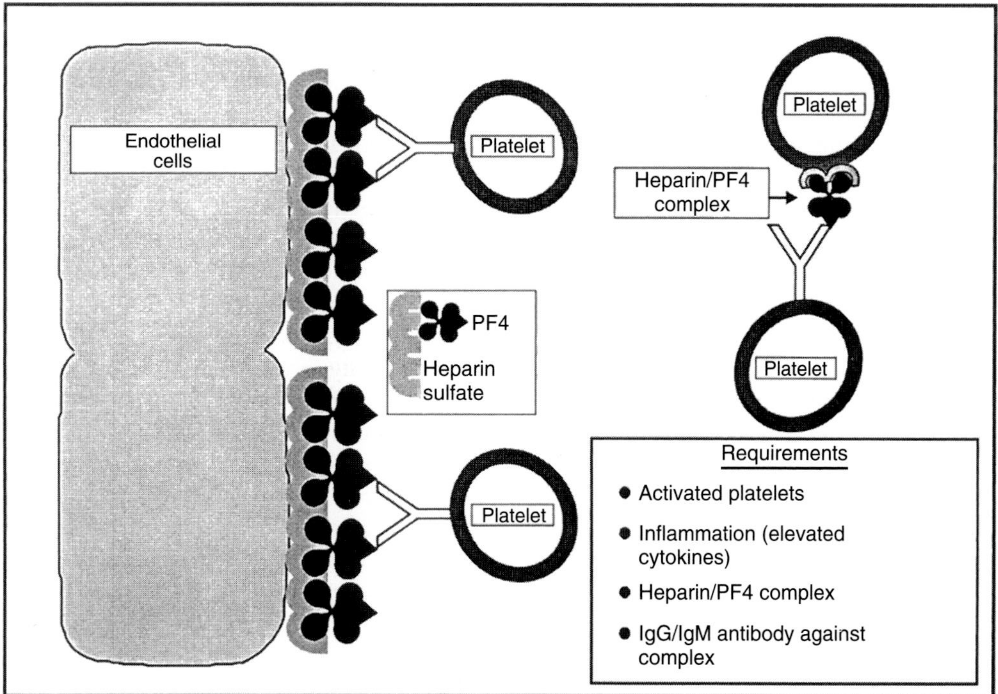

Fig. 7-6. Proposed mechanisms by which heparin-induced thrombocytopenia with or without thrombosis occurs. Platelets are activated by thrombin or other agonists and release platelet factor 4 (PF4) from their α-granules. PF4 complexes with heparin on the surface of the platelet. The complex is immunogenic and induces formation of both IgC and IgM antibodies. The Fc portion of IgG antibodies binds to FcII receptors on platelets and induces further activation and throbocytopenia. FcII receptors are increased by interleukin-6 and are therefore upregulated in patients with ongoing inflammation. PF4 released from platelets can also bind to heparin sulfate on endothelial cells. IgG or IgM antibodies directed against this complex may cause endothelial cell damage and promote venous or arterial thrombosis. (From Jackson MR, et al. Diagnosis of heparin-induced thrombocytopenia in the vascular surgery patient. Surgery 131:419, 1997.)

reported with the use of ancrod, a rapid-acting defibrinating agent. In patients who have venous thromboembolism as a complication of heparin therapy, placement of a Greenfield filter, thrombolytic therapy, and warfarin treatment are useful.

In the absence of alternative parenteral anticoagulants, heparin can be considered for use in the HIT patient but only after repeat test results for the antibody are negative. Heparin has been given successfully to patients with a history of HIT and thrombosis who required cardiac bypass.[118] In these patients, the interval between the initial and second exposure has usually been 1 to 2 months, and heparin has been administered only during surgery, either alone or in the presence of antiplatelet agents such as aspirin. In those situations where heparin absolutely cannot be used, argatroban or heparinoid should be considered under compassionate use.

Malignancy

The incidence of thrombosis in patients with malignancy generally ranges between 5% and 15% but may be as high as 50% with some tumors, notably pancreatic carcinoma.[119] The highest incidence of thrombotic manifestations is found in patients with acute promyelocytic leukemia, myeloproliferative disorders, primary brain tumors, and mucin-secreting adenocarcinomas of the pancreas, gastrointestinal tract, lung, and ovary. Episodes of thrombosis, particularly migratory superficial thrombophlebitis, may antedate by months the clinical diagnosis of cancer in some patients and may be the first indication of an underlying malignancy. In addition to venous thrombosis, arterial thromboembolism from nonbacterial thrombotic endocarditis may occur.

Multiple coagulation abnormalities predisposing to thrombosis have been identified in patients with malignancy. These include thrombocytosis, shortening of the prothrombin time and aPTTs, elevation of plasma coagulation factors (fibrinogen, factors V, VIII, IX, and XI) and fibrinogen-fibrin degradation products, shortened platelet survival, decreased AT-III levels, and increased PAI-1 activity. Many of these changes reflect generalized activation of the clotting system resulting in chronic, partially compensated DIC. In addition, tissue factor can be expressed by macrophages and endothelial cells stimulated by tumor cytokines. Cytotoxic chemotherapy can also cause release of thromboplastic substances from tumor cells. In some cases, the chemotherapeutic agents themselves may contribute to thrombosis.

ANTITHROMBOTIC THERAPY

General Considerations

Because of its dependency on coagulation reactions resulting in fibrin formation, venous thrombosis is best treated with the anticoagulants heparin and warfarin. Heparin, heparin-like compounds, and warfarin, given in small doses, prevent the onset of venous thrombosis and can therefore be used successfully as prophylaxis of postoperative deep venous thrombosis in high-risk surgical patients.[120] Agents that are pure inhibitors of platelet function, such as aspirin, are much less successful in prophylaxis of postoperative venous thrombosis. Methods that prevent venous pooling and stasis of blood in the lower extremities are also beneficial in preventing deep vein thrombosis; augmentation of venous emptying by application of intermittent pneumatic compression boots is as effective as anticoagulants.

In addition to preventing the onset of venous thrombosis, anticoagulants inhibit the growth, propagation, and embolization of established thrombi. In doing so, these agents are the mainstay of therapy for patients with active venous thrombosis in those who are at risk for pulmonary embolism. Aspirin and other antiplatelet agents are not effective in the treatment of active venous thrombosis.

Intracardiac thromboemboli are also responsive to anticoagulant therapy. These thrombi are fibrin rich and form under the relatively static flow conditions of dilated chambers, obstructed valve orifices, areas of low shear associated with prosthetic valves, ventricular aneurysm formation, and poor pumping action with impaired chamber emptying secondary to cardiac failure of dysrhythmia. Acute treatment with heparin and long-term treatment with warfarin reduces the incidence of symptomatic emboli stemming from intracardiac thrombi.

Antiplatelet agents are effective in preventing thrombogenesis in areas of high shear and disturbed flow in the arterial circulation. this most commonly involves the surface irregularity or stenoses caused by atherosclerotic plaque. Aspirin is the antiplatelet agent in widest use and has been found to be effective in preventing myocardial infarction in patients with unstable angina and stable coronary disease[121]; stroke and transient ischemic attacks in patients with cerebral vascular arteriosclerosis, or after carotid endarterectomy; vein graft thrombosis after coronary artery bypass; and prosthetic bypass thrombosis in patients with femoropopliteal reconstruction. Dipyridamole, often combined with aspirin, had generally been found to be ineffective in rigorous clinical trials. There is no indication to use this drug, alone or in combination with aspirin, to prevent arterial thrombosis. Although aspirin retards platelet thrombogenesis on the surface of atherosclerotic plaque, there is no evidence that it prevents plaque formation. Ticlopidine is another antiplatelet agent that is effective in preventing platelet-dependent arterial thromboembolism.

Fibrinolytic agents include streptokinase, recombinant t-PA, and urokinase; all act by accelerating the conversion of plasminogen to plasmin. These substances can be given systemically or regionally by means of selective infusion through an intra-arterial catheter and have been found to be most effective in treating patients with acute myocardial infarction. Clinical trials have demonstrated a reduction in infarct size, preservation of ventricular function, and a reduction in mortality. Clinical benefit has been noted less consistently in venous thromboembolism, acute stroke, arterial bypass graft, peripheral arterial bypass graft thrombosis, and peripheral arterial thrombosis. Because fibrinolytic agents dissolve hemostatic clots along with pathologic clots, they are associated with a much higher incidence of bleeding complications than anticoagulants.

THERAPEUTIC AGENTS

Anticoagulants

Heparin

Heparin is a highly sulfated glycosaminoglycan that exhibits an anticoagulant effect through its interaction with AT-III, which then inhibits thrombin and the activated forms of factors XII, XI, X, and IX. The anticoagulant effect of heparin was first described in 1922 and so named because of its hepatic derivation.[122] Mast cell synthesis of heparin results in many structurally diverse polysaccharide chains and variable degrees of sulfation.[123] Commercially prepared heparin is a heterogenous mixture of heparin chains and is obtained from porcine intestinal mucosa or bovine lung.

Heparin is not absorbed orally and must be administered parenterally or subcutaneously. Heparin action is immediate following intravenous administration and is delayed 20 to 60 minutes after subcutaneous administration. Following intravenous administration the average half-life is about 90 minutes and can range from 30 to 360 minutes. Clearance is primarily hepatic, with a small potion excreted intact by the kidneys. Recommended dosing uses an initial intravenous bolus (75 U/kg) to ensure rapid anticoagulation, followed by continuous intravenous infusion (10 to 25 U/kg/hr). Heparin does not cross the placenta and is considered the drug of choice for long-term anticoagulation during pregnancy.

Monitoring of heparin administration is most commonly performed using the aPTT. For active thrombosis (venous or arterial) a range of 1.5 to 2.5 times the normal control value is considered therapeutic. Caution is advised when following therapeutic nomograms and algorithms because of the variability of heparin products and individual response. The aPTT should be checked every 4 to 6 hours until a steady state infusion dose can be determined.

The most common complication of heparin use is bleeding, the incidence of which ranges form 1% to 7% with continuous infusion and 8% to 14% with intermittent bolus.[123] Heparin can be reversed using protamine sulfate. One milligram of protamine sulfate neutralizes 100 U of heparin. Another significant potential complication is heparin-induced thrombocytopenia, with or without thrombosis, which was discussed in a previous section. Other complications include osteoporosis from prolonged heparin use and, rarely, allergic reactions.

Warfarin

Warfarin is a vitamin K antagonist that exerts its anticoagulant effect through inhibition of synthesis of the vitamin K–dependent factors, prothrombin (II), VII, IX, and X. The name *warfarin* is an acronym for the patent holder, Wisconsin Alumni Research Foundation, and "arin" for the chemical structure of the 4-hydroxycoumarin ring. Warfarin inhibits the vitamin K–dependent ribosomal posttranslational modification of the precursor proteins of the affected clotting factors and proteins C and S. Under normal circumstances, 10 or more glutamic acid residues near the amino-terminus of each precursor protein must be carboxylated, resulting in the formation of the unique amino acid γ-carboxyglutamate, which allows the clotting factor proteins to bind calcium during the coagulation cascade (Fig. 7-7).[123] Warfarin induces hepatic production of partially carboxylated and decarboxylated proteins. Prothrombin molecules with fewer than six γ-carboxyglutamic acid residues have markedly reduced activity.

Warfarin action is not immediate, since it has no effect on the existing circulating factors. Plasma warfarin is 98% to 99% protein bound to albumin. It is the remaining 1% to 2% free warfarin that exerts the anticoagulant effect. Metabolized warfarin is excreted in the bile, with a plasma half-life that ranges from 20 to 60 hours. Warfarin is administered orally, where it is more than 95% absorbed through the gastrointestinal tract. Dosage is generally initiated at 5 to 10 mg/day until a steady state is reached, at which time a lower dose can be maintained.

Monitoring of warfarin therapy has presented problems because of the significant variability in activity of the numerous available thromboplastins available for prothrombin

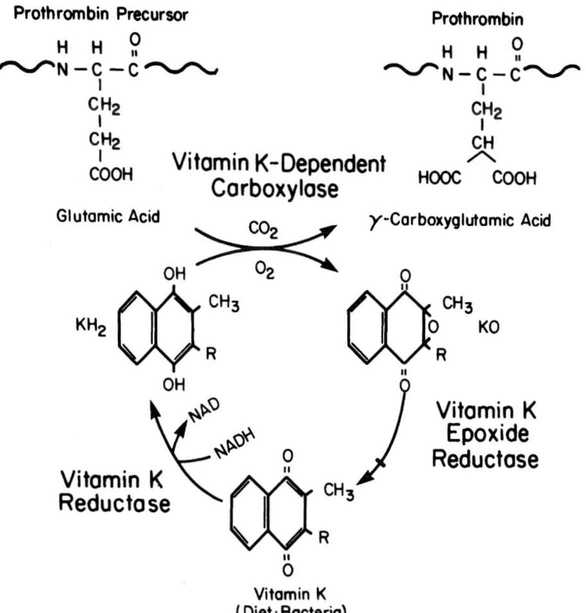

Fig. 7-7. Vitamin K metabolism and the mechanism of action of warfarin. Vitamin KH_2 serves as a cofactor for a vitamin K–dependent carboxylase that converts glutamic acid residues in precursor coagulation factors to γ-carboxyglutamic acid residues. In addition to vitamin KH_2, molecular oxygen and carbon dioxide are required. Vitamin KH_2 is oxidized to vitamin K epoxide *(KO),* which is then converted to vitamin K by vitamin K epoxide reductase. Vitamin K reductase reduces vitamin K to its reduced form, vitamin KH_2. Warfarin inhibits vitamin K epoxide reductase and possibly vitamin K reductase. The decrease in vitamin KH_2 limits γ-carboxylation of the vitamin K–dependent proteins and interferes with their function. (From Hirsh J, Ginsberg JS, Marder VJ. Anticoagulant therapy with coumarin agents. In Coman RW, et al., eds. Hemostasis and Thrombosis: Basic Principles and Clinical Practice, 3rd ed. Philadelphia: Lippincott-Raven, 1994, p 1568.)

time measurement. This problem with nonstandardized thromboplastins is a particular issue in North America. So that warfarin dosage can be standardized in the presence of the many thromboplastins used in the prothrombin time (PT), most laboratories report prothrombin time results as the international normalized ratio (INR). The system is based on a standardized thromboplastin preparation referred to as the World Health Organization (WHO) primary international preparation of thromboplastin. This system has been accepted as an international standard for clinical use by most western countries. The INR is calculated as follows:

$$INR = (\text{Observed PT}/\text{Control PT})^{ISI}$$

where the ISI is the international sensitivity index and is a measure of the responsiveness of any given lot of a thromboplastin preparation to that of a standard thromboplastin. For most commercial thromboplastins used in North America, the ISI ranges from 2 to 2.8. the relationship between the prothrombin time ratio with different thromboplastins and the INR is illustrated with the nomogram in Fig. 7-8. the recommended therapeutic range of the INR for given clinical indications is listed in Table 7-5. Portable devices the size of a glucometer are available that can measure the prothrombin time and calculate the INR in seconds using a drop of whole blood.

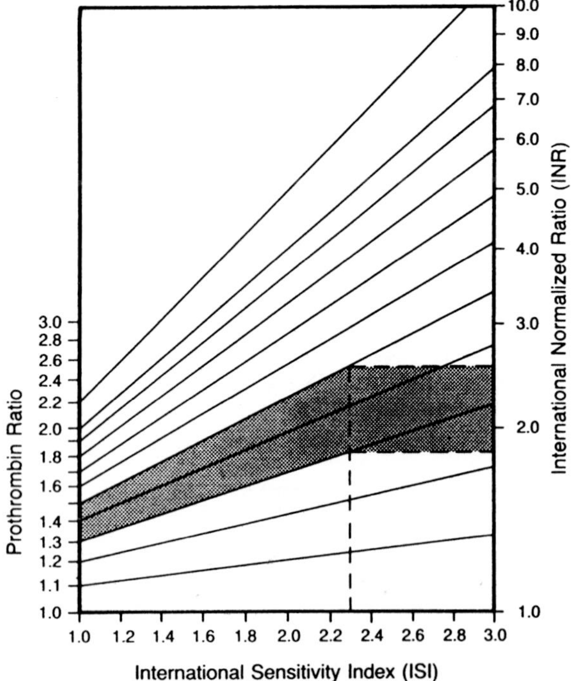

Fig. 7-8. Relation between the prothrombin time *(PT)* ratio and the international normalized ratio *(INR)* for thromboplastin reagents over a range of international sensitivity index *(ISI)* values. The example shown is for a PT ratio of 1.3 to 11.5 for a thromboplastin preparation with an ISI of 2.3. (From Hirsh J, et al. Drug therapy: Oral anticoagulant drugs. N Engl J Med 324:1865, 1991. Copyright © 1991 Massachusetts Medical Society. All rights reserved.)

As with heparin, the major complication with warfarin is bleeding. The frequency of this complication can vary considerably and is likely related to the degree and duration of desired anticoagulation, underlying illness, concomitant medications, and patient compliance. The risk of major bleeding is generally in the range of 4% to 5% per treatment year, with major bleeding events occurring at 1% to 2% per year.[123] Warfarin-induced skin necrosis can occur and is characterized by skin lesions similar to those of neonatal purpura fulminans. This condition is classically associated with homozygous protein C deficiency, as was previously discussed earlier in that section. Warfarin crosses the placenta, where it can cause an embryopathy or fetal bleeding, and therefore should not be used during pregnancy.

Low-Molecular-Weight Heparin

LMWH is produced by chemical or enzymatic depolymerization of heparin molecules and has a molecular weight of 3000 to 6000. Unlike heparin, neither LMWH no heparinoid are fully reversed by protamine. The anticoagulant effect of LMWH is primarily directed against factor Xa. To neutralize thrombin, heparin must interact with and combine to both AT-III and thrombin.[124]

Table 7-5. Effectiveness of Oral Anticoagulant Therapy

	International Normalized Ratio (INR)*	
Condition	**Minimal Effective**	**Recommended**
Deep vein thrombosis		
Prevention	1.5-2.5	2.0-3.0†
Treatment	2.0-2.3	2.0-3.0
Acute myocardial infarction		
Prevention of stroke	2.0	2.0-3.0
Prevention of recurrence	2.7-4.5	3.0-4.5†
Reduction of mortality	2.7-4.5	3.0-4.5†
Atrial fibrillation		
Prevention of systemic embolism	1.5-2.5	2.0-3.0†
Cardiac valve replacement		
Tissue valves	2.0-2.3	2.0-3.0
Mechanical valves	1.9-3.6	3.0-4.5
Cerebral embolism	Not evaluated	
Native valvular heart disease	Not evaluated	

Modified from Hirsh J, et al. Oral anticoagulant drugs. N Engl J Med 324:1865, 1991. Reprinted with permission.

*For thromboplastin with an ISI of 2.3 the INRs and the corresponding prothrombin time ratios follow:

INR	1.5	2.0	2.5	3.0	3.5	4.0	4.5	5.0
Prothrombin time ratio	1.20	1.35	1.49	1.61	1.72	1.83	1.92	2.01

†A lower range might be effective.

LMWH is unable to bind thrombin and AT-III simultaneously and therefore cannot accelerate the inactivation of thrombin. The combination of LMWH and AT-III can, however, inactivate factor Xa. The low molecular weight heparins produce less prolongation of the aPTT than does standard heparin because this clotting test depends more on the antithrombin effect than the anti–factor Xa effect.

There are several advantages of LMWH over conventional heparin. Bioavailability of LMWH is greater due to lack of binding of LMWH to plasma proteins and endothelial cells. Also, LMWH is not inactivated by P4, as is heparin. LMWH has a longer half-life and a more predictable dose response than heparin, allowing for more convenient outpatient treatment of venous thrombosis using a once- or twice-daily subcutaneous dosage. LMWH also appears to be less immunogenic than conventional heparin. In a recent prospective study of the incidence of HIT with unfractionated heparin and LMWH used as prophylaxis during hip surgery in 655 patients, HIT occurred n 2.7% of recipients of unfractionated heparin and in none of the patients receiving LMWH.[125] However, as previously discussed, 90% of HIT patients have antibodies that cross-react with LMWH, making this a poor alternative when continued anticoagulation is necessary in patients with an established diagnosis of HIT.

Heparinoid

Heparinoids are nonheparin glycosaminoglycans obtained as a by-product of heparin production from porcine intestinal mucosa.[126] The anticoagulant effect of heparinoid is directed primarily against factor Xa. Heparinoid is composed of a mixture of dermatan, heparin, and chondroitin sulfates; heparinoid has a very low degree of sulfation and a reduced molecular weight compared to unfractionated heparin. Heparinoid is less likely to bind to platelets[127] or to be immunogenic. In the United States, heparinoid has been obtained for compassionate use from Organon, Inc., in West Orange, New Jersey. Since heparinoid contains a small amount of heparin-like substance that would have the capacity to cause HIT, a test for antibody cross-reactivity should be done before substitution of the heparinoid for heparin.[128,129] In a recent review of 230 patients who received heparinoid for HIT, 93% of the recipients were judged to have responded in a satisfactory manner.[129] Only 10% of the sera obtained from patients with HIT showed cross-reactivity with heparinoid, whereas 90% showed cross-reactivity with LMWH.

Argatroban

Argatroban, a synthetic derivative of L-Arg, is a reversible, direct thrombin inhibitor with a half-life of approximately 20 to 25 minutes. There is no antidote for argatroban. In a phase I trial argatroban was shown to prolong the aPTT and thrombin time in a dose-dependent fashion.[130] In a more recent phase I dose-ranging clinical trial, argatroban was administered to patients with unstable angina.[131] Although there were no significant bleeding complications, there was a rebound effect with recurrence of angina following cessation of argatroban. Argatroban has been used successfully as an alternative anticoagulant in patients with HIT, and its use for this indication is currently under investigation.[132] Given its short half-life and direct thrombin inhibition, its potential as an alternative to heparin in patients with HIT is encouraging.

Hirudin and Its Analogs

Hirudin is an anticoagulant derived from the saliva of the medicinal leech and directly inhibits thrombin. Interest in hirudin as an anticoagulant has increased since its gene was cloned in 1986 with subsequent production by recombinant techniques.[133-135] Hirulog is a 20–amino acid polypeptide that consists of three components: an inhibitor of the active site of thrombin, an inhibitor of the fibrinogen-binding site, and a polyglycine spacer that links the other two segments. In normal human volunteers, hirulog has a half-life of 36 minutes. There is no known inhibitor for use as an antidote for hirudin or hirulog. Unlike the heparin/AT-III complex, hirudin and hirulog inhibit clot-bound thrombin[136] and do not induce thrombocytopenia.

The anticoagulant effects and safety of hirulog have been studied in healthy human volunteers.[137] There were no significant bleeding complications. No antihirulog antibodies were noted at 7 and 14 days. In addition to use in animal thrombosis models[138,139] hirulog is being tested in clinical trials and has been used successfully in 291 patients undergoing elective coronary angioplasty.[140] Hirulog has been used successfully as an anticoagulant in an animal model of carotid endarterectomy in a dose that allowed inhibition of fibrin deposition without significant bleeding.[141] Hirudin has been used as an anticoagulant during coronary artery bypass surgery.[142]

Ancrod

Another antithrombotic strategy is to deplete fibrinogen concentration and thus impair fibrin formation. This may be achieved by using a number of snake venom enzymes of which only ancrod (extracted from the Malayan pit viper, Agkistrodon rhodostoma) has been used clinically. Ancrod cleaves fibrinopeptide A but not fibrinopeptide B from fibrinogen to produce fibrin that is very sensitive to endogenous fibrinolysis. The fibrin formed by the action of ancrod is deposited in the microcirculation, where it is rapidly lysed by endothelial fibrinolytic mechanisms. Ancrod may be given intravenously, subcutaneously, or intramuscularly. Within hours, marked defibrination occurs and is accompanied by a delayed but striking rise in fibrinogen-fibrin degradation products. Hypofibrinogenemia is sustained by daily administration; however, resistance develops because of the elaboration of neutralizing antibodies when repeated injections are given. A potentially important indication for ancrod use may be HIT, for which there is no established treatment at present.

Antiplatelet Agents

Aspirin

Aspirin acts by acetylating and inhibiting platelet cyclooxygenase, the enzyme that converts arachidonic acid to the endoperoxide intermediates PGG_2 and PGH_2.[143] This process inhibits formation of thromboxane A_2, and because platelets are anucleate and incapable of replenishing cyclooxygenase, platelets exposed to aspirin are permanently affected. Because of differential effects on platelets and endothelial cells (platelets being more sensitive), a great deal of effort has been devoted to finding the lowest possible dose of aspirin that inhibits platelet thromboxane A_2 production and that allows endothelial PTI_2 synthesis to continue. There appears to be no difference in the antiplatelet effectiveness between high- and low-dose aspirin.[144] A dose as low as 40 mg daily completely inhibits cyclooxygenase activity and has been shown to reduce the incidence of fatal and nonfatal myocardial infarction in patients with unstable angina.[145] Whether this dose provides adequate antiplatelet activity in all patients and for a wide spectrum of indications, however, remains uncertain. Another advantage of a lower aspirin dose appears to be less gastrointestinal bleeding, although this advantage might be realized with enteric-coated preparations.

Aspirin is rapidly absorbed in the stomach and upper intestine, with peak plasma levels occurring 15 to 20 minutes after ingestion. Absorption from enteric-coated tablets may be delayed; however, reliable and sustained antiplatelet effects are observed after multiple daily doses of such tablets.[146] Although aspirin is moderately effective in preventing arterial thromboembolic complications, it is not helpful in halting the progression of atherosclerosis and the development of intimal hyperplasia.[147] Aspirin does not prevent platelet adhesion to collagen and subendothelial vWF, and it does not inhibit α-granule secretion in response to platelet agonists.[148] Therefore release of growth factors from the α-granule, such as PGDF and transforming growth factor-β, are unaffected by cyclooxygenase inhibitors.

Ticlopidine

Ticlopidine inhibits platelet aggregation by altering the platelet membrane and interfering with the membrane-fibrinogen interaction, thereby blocking the platelet GPIIv/IIIa receptor.[149] Unlike aspirin, ticlopidine does not interfere with the cyclooxygenase pathway. The antiplatelet effect of ticlopidine is maximal at 24 to 48 hours and is not reversible. It prolongs the bleeding time and has no effect on coagulation assays. In trials studying cerebrovascular disease, ticlopidine appears to be marginally superior to aspirin in preventing stroke and transient ischemic attacks.[150,151] The use of ticlopidine during coronary artery stenting appears to be associated with fewer thrombotic complications than aspirin.[152] The only known serious adverse effect of ticlopidine appears to be neutropenia, which occurs in less than 1% of patients taking the drug. This condition appears during the first months of therapy and reverses when the drug is discontinued. It is therefore recommended that white blood cell counts be monitored during the first months of treatment. Other adverse effects include diarrhea and skin rash, which may occur in up to 20% of patients. Because of these side effects, a ticlopidine analog, clopidogrel, is being developed.

Dextran

Dextran is a polysaccharide that is hydrolyzed and fractionated into polymers of variable molecular weight. The preparations most commonly used as an antiplatelet agent has an average molecular mass of 40,00 kd (dextran 40). Although the drug was first used as a volume expander, it was subsequently found to have an effect on hemostasis and thrombosis. The principal antithrombotic properties are (1) antiplatelet activity through the reduction of plasma vWF and resulting in a mild defect in platelet adhesion,[153] (2) defective fibrin polymerization and increased clot lysis,[154] and (3) increased blood flow through volume expansion. Dextran has been shown to be useful in prevention of venous thromboembolism, but it is rarely used for this purpose because it must be administered intravenously and its use is cumbersome.[155,156] The use of dextran 40 has also been shown to improve early patency following infrainguinal arterial reconstruction.[157] Adverse reactions include pulmonary edema from volume expansion, allergic reactions, and rarely anaphylactic reactions.

c7E3 Fab

A new class of potent antiplatelet agents inhibit platelet aggregation by binding the GPIIb/IIIa fibrinogen receptor, causing a defect similar to that found in Glanzmann's thrombasthenia. One of the most promising of such agents is a monoclonal fragment antigen-binding (Fab) fragment of an IgG antibody, chimeric 7E3 (c7E3), that contains the mouse variable regions and the human constant regions.[158] The generic name of c7E3 is abciximab and the trade name is ReoPro. Platelet aggregation is profoundly inhibited by c7E3, both in vitro and in vivo.[159] In a study evaluating c7E3 with aspirin and heparin during high-risk coronary angioplasty, there was a significant decrease in thrombotic events compared to the use of aspirin and heparin alone.[160] Patients treated with c7E3 had a twofold increase in bleeding complications, but no increase in cerebral hemorrhage or bleeding-related mortality. Antibody formation against the murine component of c7E3 occurred in 6.5%, but there were no allergic or anaphylactic reactions. The FDA has approved c7E3 for use during high-risk coronary angioplasty and atherectomy. The activating clotting time is prolonged with the use of c7E3,[161] and specific assays to monitor dosage are being developed. The results of additional trials defining the optimal dosage of heparin when administered with c7E3 and evaluating the role of c7E3 in the treatment of other thrombotic disorders, are eagerly awaited.[162]

Because increasing numbers of routine and complex

operations are being performed on patients who have diseases that alter hemostasis, the frequency of abnormal bleeding in surgical patients can be expected to increase. Knowledge of the physiologic principles underlying hemostasis and of derangements that precipitate bleeding is important in modern surgical care. Hemostasis depends on interactions among circulating proteins (coagulation factors and inhibitors), cellular elements (platelets and white blood cells), and vascular endothelium and smooth muscle. In the early stages of hemostasis, platelets rapidly adhere and aggregate at the site of vascular injury and form a platelet plug that temporarily stops blood flow. At the same time, the intrinsic and extrinsic coagulation pathways reactivated, resulting in a fibrin network that fortifies the platelet plug and provides a frame for fibroblastic ingrowth and ultimate healing of the injury. The hemostatic response is finely regulated to limit clotting to the site of injury and thereby to maintain vascular patency. Inhibitory mechanisms include the fibrinolytic system, plasma serine protease inhibitors (the most important of which is AT-III), and the antithrombotic properties and functions of endothelial cells. Derangements in hemostatic mechanisms can be both congenital and acquired. In surgical patients, acquired bleeding disorders are far more common than congenital ones. To diagnose and treat such disorders adequately, preoperative assessment of hemostatic competence is mandatory in all surgical problems. The keystone to preoperative evaluation for all bleeding disorders is through history and physical examination.

REFERENCES

1. Mazur EM, et al. Human serum megakaryocyte colony-stimulating activity appears to be distinct from interleuken-3, granulocyte-macrophage colony-stimulating factor, and lymphocyte-conditioned medium. Blood 76:290, 1990.
2. Gewirtz AM, et al. Inhibition of human megakaryocytopoiesis in vitro by platelet factor 4 (PF4) and a synthetic COOH-terminal PF4 peptide. J Clin Invest 83:1477, 1989.
3. Mitjavila MT, et al. Human platelet alpha granules contain a nonspecific inhibitor of megakaryocyte colony formation: its relationship to type β transforming growth factor (TGF-β). J Cell Physiol 134:93, 1988.
4. Chott A, et al. Interferon-alpha–induced morphologic changes of megakaryocytes: A histomorphometrical study on bone marrow biopsies in chronic myeloproliferative disorders with excessive thrombocytosis. Br J Haematol 74:10, 1990.
5. Kaushansky K. Thrombopoietin: The primary regulator of platelet production. Blood 86:419, 1995.
6. Siess W. Molecular mechanisms of platelet activation. Physiol Rev 69:58, 1989.
7. Hawiger J, Brass LF, Salzman EW. Signal transduction and intracellular regulatory processes in platelets. In Coleman RW, et al., eds. Hemostasis and Thrombosis: Basic Principles and Clinical Practice, 3rd ed. Philadelphia: JB Lippincott, 1994, p 603.
8. Lessin LS, et al., eds. Hemostasis and thrombosis: I. Hemostasis. In Medical Knowledge Self-Assessment Program in the Subspecialty of Hematology. Philadelphia: American College of Physicians, 1994, p 194.
9. Walsh PN. Platelet-coagulant protein interactions. In Coleman RW, et al., eds. Hemostasis and Thrombosis: Basic Principles and Clinical Practice, 3rd ed. Philadelphia: JB Lippincott, 1994, p 629.
10. Weiss HJ, et al. Evidence for the presence of tissue factor activity on subendothelium. Blood 73:968, 1989.
11. Rapaport SI, Rao LVM. The tissue factor pathway: How it has become a "prima ballerina." Thromb Haemost 74:7, 1995.
12. Bauer KA, et al. Detection of factor X activation in humans. Blood 74:2007, 1989.
13. Bauer KA, et al. Factor IX is activated in vivo by the tissue factor mechanism. Blood 76:731, 1990.
14. Bauer KA, Rosenberg RD. The pathophysiology of the prethrombotic state in humans: Insights gained from studies using markers of hemostatic system activation. Blood 70:343, 1987.
15. Wu KK, Thiagarajan P. Role of endothelium in thrombosis and hemostasis. Annu Rev Med 47:315, 1996.
16. Wam-Cramer BJ, et al. Modifications of the extrinsic pathway inhibitor (EPI) and factor Xa that affect their ability to interact and to inhibit factor VIIa/tissue factor: Evidence for a two-step model of inhibition. Thromb Haemost 60:453, 1988.
17. Sandset PM, Abilegaard U, Larsen ML. Heparin induces release of extrinsic coagulation pathway inhibitor (EPI). Thromb Res 40:803, 1988.
18. Solymoss S, Tucker MM, Tracy P. Kinetics of inactivation of membrane-bound factor Va by activated protein C. J Biol Chem 263:14884, 1988.
19. Mulvey KP, Lucas DL, Alving BM. Hemostasis. In Anderson KC, Ness PM, eds. Scientific Basis of Transfusion Medicine: Implications for Clinical Practice. Philadelphia: WB Saunders Co, 1994, p 330.
20. Bauer KA, Rosenberg RD. Role of antithrombin III as a regulator of in vivo coagulation. Semin Hematol 28:10, 1991.
21. Jordan RE, et al. The kinetics of hemostatic enzyme-antithrombin interactions in the presence of low molecular weight heparin. J Biol Chem 255:10081, 1980.
22. Ouimet H, Loscalzo J. Fibrinolysis. In Loscalzo J, Schafer AI, eds. Thrombosis and Hemorrhage. Boston: Blackwell Scientific Publications, 1994, p 127.
23. Aoki N. Natural inhibitors of fibrinolysis. Prog Cardiovasc Dis 21:267, 1979.
24. Rodeberg DA, et al. Nitric oxide: An overview. Am J Surg 170:292, 1995.
25. Olsen SB, et al. Enhancement of platelet deposition by cross-linked hemoglobin in a rat carotid endarterectomy model. Circulation 93:327, 1996.
26. Rodeghiero F, Castaman G, Dini E. Epidemiological investigation of the prevalence of von Willebrand's disease. Blood 69:454, 1987.
27. Cooney KA, Ginsburg D, Ruggeri ZM. Von Willebrand disease. In Loscalzo J, Schafer Al, eds. Thrombosis and Hemorrhage. Boston: Blackwell Scientific Publications, 1994, p 657.
28. Foster PA. A perspective on the use of FVIII concentrates and cryoprecipitate prophylactically in surgery or therapeutically in severe bleeds in patients with von Willebrand disease unresponsive to DDAVP: Results of an international survey. Thromb Haemost 74:1370, 1995.
29. Coller BS. Platelets and their disorders. In Ratnoff OD, Forbes CD, eds. Disorders of Hemostasis. Orlando, Fla.: Grune & Stratton, 1984, p 73.
30. Caen JP. Glanzmann's thrombasthenia. Baillieres Clin Haematol 2:609, 1989.
31. Clemetson KJ, et al. Characterization of the platelet membrane glycoprotein abnormalities in Bernard-Soulier syndrome and comparison with normal by surface-labeling techniques and high-resolution two-dimensional gel electrophoresis. J Clin Invest 70:304, 1982.
32. Aboulafia DM, Aboulafia ED. Aortic aneurysm-induced disseminated intravascular coagulation. Ann Vasc Surg 10:396, 1996.
33. Spero JA, Lewis JH, Hasiba U. DIC: Findings in 346 patients. Thromb Haemost 43:28, 1980.
34. Bick RL, Baker W. Diagnostic efficacy of the D-dimer assay in DIC and related disorders. Thromb Res 65:785, 1992.

35. Roth GJ, Siok CJ. Acetylation of the NH_2-terminal serine of prostaglandin synthetase by aspirin. J Biol Chem 253:3782, 1978.
36. Weksler BB, et al. Differential inhibition by aspirin of vascular and platelet prostaglandin synthesis in atherosclerotic patients. N Engl J Med 308:800, 1983.
37. Goldman S, et al. Improvement in early saphenous vein graft patency after coronary artery bypass surgery with antiplatelet therapy: Results of a Veteran's Administration Cooperative Study. Circulation 77(6):1324, 1988.
38. Taggart DP, Siddiqui A, Wheatley DJ. Low-dose preoperative aspirin therapy, postoperative blood loss, and transfusion requirements. Ann Thorac Surg 50:424, 1990.
39. Ferraris VA, et al. Preoperative aspirin ingestion increases operative blood loss after coronary artery bypass grafting. Ann Thorac Surg 45:71, 1988.
40. Rajah SM, et al. Acetylsalicylic acid and dipyrimadole improve the early patency of aorta-coronary bypass grafts: A double-blind, placebo-controlled, randomized trial. J Thorac Cardiovasc Surg 90:373, 1985.
41. Karwande SV, et al. Effect of preoperative antiplatelet drugs on vascular prostacyclin synthesis. Ann Thorac Surg 43:318, 1987.
42. Steering Committee of the Physician's Health Study Research Group. Final report of the aspirin component of the ongoing Physician's Health Study. N Engl J Med 321:129, 1989.
43. Ferraris VA, Swanson E. Aspirin usage and perioperative blood loss in patients undergoing unexpected operations. Surg Gynecol Obstet 156:439, 1983.
44. George JN, Shattil SJ. The clinical importance of acquired abnormalities of platelet function. N Engl J Med 324:27, 1991.
45. Coller BS. Platelet aggregation by ADP, collagen, and ristocetin: A critical review of methodology and analysis. In Schmidt RM, ed. CRC Handbook Series in Clinical Laboratory Sciences. Section I: Hematology. Boca Raton, Fla.: CRC Press 1979, p 381.
46. George JN, Caen JP, Nurden AT. Glanzmann's thrombasthenia: The spectrum of clinical disease. Blood 75:1383, 1990.
47. Lind SE. The bleeding time does not predict surgical bleeding. Blood 77:2547, 1991.
48. Rodgers RPC, Levin J. A critical reappraisal of the bleeding time. Semin Thromb Hemost 16:1, 1990.
49. Stewart JH, Castaldi PA. Uraemic bleeding: A reversible platelet defect corrected by dialysis. Q J Med 36:409, 1967.
50. Bolan CD, Alving BM. Pharmacologic agents in the management of bleeding disorders. Transfusion 30:541, 1990.
51. Barrai I, et al. The effect of parental age on rates of mutation for hemophilia and evidence for differing mutation rates for hemophilia A and B. Am J Hum Genet 20:175, 1968.
52. Robbins JA, Rose SD. Partial thrombloplastin time as a screening test. Ann Intern Med 90:796, 1979.
53. Eisenberg JM, Clarke JR, Sussman SA. Prothrombin and partial thromboplastin times as preoperative screening tests. Arch Surg 117:48, 1982.
54. Suchman AL, Mushlin AI. How well does the activated partial thromboplastin time predict postoperative hemorrhage? JAMA 256:750, 1986.
55. Spence RK. Bleeding and the vascular surgery patient. Semin Vasc Surg 7:104, 1994.
56. Miller E, et al. Scalpel versus electrocautery in modified radical mastectomy. Am Surg 54:284, 1988.
57. Pearlman NW, et al. A prospective study of incisional time, blood loss, pain and healing with carbon dioxide laser, scalpel and electrosurgery. Arch Surg 126:1018, 1991.
58. Collins JA. Recent developments in the area of massive transfusion. World J Surg 11:75, 1987.
59. Leslie S, Toy P. Laboratory hemostatic abnormalities in massively transfused patients given red blood cells and crystalloid. AJCP 96:770, 1991.
60. Reed RL, et al. Prophylactic platelet administration during massive transfusion. Ann Surg 203:40, 1986.
61. Clagett GP, et al. Does desmopressin improve hemostasis and reduce blood loss from aortic surgery? A randomized, double-blind study. J Vasc Surg 22:223, 1995.
62. Clagett GP. Desmopressin, hemostasis, and vascular surgery. Semin Vasc Surg 9(4):340, 1996.
63. Contreras M, et al. Guidelines for the use of fresh frozen plasma. British Committee for Standards in Haematology, Working Party for the Blood Transfusion Task Force. Transfus Med 2:57, 1992.
64. Rousou J, et al. Randomized clinical trial of fibrin sealant in patients undergoing resternotomy or reoperation after cardiac operations. A multicenter study. J Thorac Cardiovasc Surg 97:194, 1989.
65. Milne AA, et al. Fibrin sealant reduces suture line bleeding during carotid endarterectomy: A randomized trial. Eur J Vasc Endovasc Surg 10:91, 1995.
66. Jackson MR. Tissue sealants: Current status, future potential. Nature Med 2:637, 1996.
67. Griffin JH, et al. Anticoagulant protein C pathway defective in majority of thrombophilic patients. Blood 82:1989, 1993.
68. Svensson PJ, Dahlback B. Resistance to activated protein C as a basis for venous thrombosis. N Engl J Med 330:517, 1994.
69. Gillespie DL, et al. Resistance to activated protein C: A common inherited cause of venous thrombosis. Ann Vasc Surg 10:174, 1996.
70. Simioni P, et al. The risk of recurrent venous thromboembolism in patients with an $Arg^{506} \rightarrow Gln$ mutation in the gene for factor V (factor V Leiden). N Engl J Med 336:399, 1997.
71. Ridker PM, et al. Mutation in the gene coding for coagulation factor V and the risk of myocardial infarction, stroke, and venous thrombosis in apparently healthy men. N Engl J Med 333:880, 1995.
72. Ouriel K, et al. Activated protein C resistance: Prevalence and implications in peripheral vascular disease. J Vasc Surg 23:46, 1996.
73. Gomez E, et al. Identification of eight point mutations in protein S deficiency type I: Analysis of 15 pedigrees. Thromb Haemost 73:750, 1995.
74. Comp PC. Hereditary disorders predisposing to thrombosis. Prog Hemost Thromb 8:71, 1986.
75. Esmon CT. The protein C anticoagulant pathway. Arterioscler Thromb 12:135, 1992.
76. Bauer KA. Inherited hypercoagulable states. In Loscalzo J, Schafer AI, eds. Thrombosis and Hemorrhage. Boston: Blackwell Scientific Publications, 1994, p 809.
77. Mannucci P, et al. Familial dysfunction of protein S. Thromb Haemost 62:736, 1989.
78. Reitsma PH, et al. Protein C deficiency: A database of mutations, 1995 update. Thromb Haemost 73:876, 1995.
79. Jones MP, Alving BA. Laboratory testing for hypercoagulable disorders. Curr Opin Hematol 3:365, 1996.
80. Broekmans AW, et al. Protein C (PC) and coumarin-induced skin necrosis. Thromb Res 6:137, 1986.
81. Egeberg O. Inherited antithrombin deficiency causing thrombophilia. Thromb Diath Haemorrh 13:516, 1965.
82. Bock SC, Prochownik EV. Molecular genetic survey of 16 kindreds with hereditary antithrombin III deficiency. Blood 70:1272, 1987.
83. Olds RJ, et al. Novel point mutations leading to type I antithrombin deficiency and thrombosis. Br J Haematol 78:408, 1991.
84. Nunez H, Drohan WD. Purification of antithrombin III (human). Semin Hematol 28:24, 1991.
85. Einarsson M, et al. Heat inactivation of human immunodeficiency virus in solutions of antithrombin III. Transfusion 29:148, 1989.
86. Tengborn L, Bergvist D. Surgery in patients with congenital antithrombin III deficiency. Acta Chir Scand 154:179, 1988.
87. De Stefano V, et al. Thrombosis during pregnancy and surgery in patients with congenital deficiency of antithrombin III, protein C, protein S [letter]. Thromb Haemost 71:799, 1994.

88. Jackson MR, et al. Use of antithrombin III concentrates to correct antithrombin III deficiency during vascular surgery. J Vasc Surg 22:804, 1995.
89. Clarke R, et al. Hyperhomocysteinemia: An independent risk factor for vascular disease. N Engl J Med 324:1149, 1991.
90. Fermo I, et al. Prevalence of moderate hyperhomocysteinemia in patients with early-onset venous and arterial occlusive disease. Ann Intern Med 123:747, 1995.
91. Selhub J, et al. Association between homocysteine concentrations and extracranial carotid-artery stenosis. N Engl J Med 332:286, 1995.
92. den Heijer M, et al. Is hyperhomocysteinemia a risk factor for recurrent venous thrombosis? Lancet 345:882, 1995.
93. Simione P, et al. Hyperhomocysteinemia and deep-vein thrombosis: A case-control study. Thromb Haemost 76:883, 1996.
94. Valentine RJ, et al. Lipoprotein (a), homocysteine, and hypercoagulable states in young men with premature peripheral atherosclerosis: A prospective, controlled analysis. J Vasc Surg 23:53, 1996.
95. Goyette P, et al. Human methylenetetrahydrofolate reductase: Isolation of cDNA, mapping and mutation identification. Nature Genet 7:195, 1994.
96. Frosst P, et al. A candidate genetic risk factor for vascular disease: A common mutation in methylenetetrahydrofolate reductase. Nature Genet 10:111, 1995.
97. Jacques PF, et al. Relation between folate status, a common mutation in methylenetetrahydrofolate reductase, and plasma homocysteine concentrations. Circulation 93:7, 1996.
98. Boushey CJ, et al. A quantitative assessment of plasma homocysteine as a risk factor for vascular disease: Probable benefits of increasing folic acid intakes. JAMA 274:1049, 1995.
99. Alving BM. Lupus anticoagulants, anticardiolipin antibodies, and the antiphospholipid syndrome. In Loscalzo J, Schafer AI, eds. Thrombosis and Hemorrhage. Boston: Blackwell Scientific Publications, 1994, p 749.
100. Harris EN, Pierangeli S, Birch D. Anticardiolipin wet workshop report. Fifth International Symposium on Antiphospholipid Antibodies. Am J Clin Pathol 101:616, 1994.
101. Rhodes GR, Dixon RH, Silver D. Heparin induced thrombocytopenia with thrombotic and hemorrhagic manifestations. Surg Gynecol Obstet 136:409, 1973.
102. Silver D, Kapsch DN, Tsoi EKM. Heparin-induced thrombocytopenia, thrombosis, and hemorrhage. Ann Surg 198:301, 1983.
103. Laster J, et al. The heparin-induced thrombocytopenia syndrome: An update. Surgery 102:763, 1987.
104. Boshkov LK, et al. Heparin-induced thrombocytopenia and thrombosis: Clinical and laboratory studies. Br J Haematol 84:322, 1993.
105. Visentin GP, et al. Antibodies from patients with heparin-induced thrombocytopenia/thrombosis are specific for platelet factor 4 complexed with heparin or bound to endothelial cells. J Clin Invest 93:81, 1994.
106. Amiral J, et al. Platelet factor 4 complexed to heparin is the target for antibodies generated in heparin-induced thrombocytopenia [letter]. Thromb Haemost 68:95, 1992.
107. Greinacher A, et al. Heparin-associated thrombocytopenia: Isolation of the antibody and characterization of a multimolecular PF4-heparin complex as the major antigen. Thromb Haemost 71:247, 1994.
108. Kelton JG, et al. Immunoglobulin G from patients with thrombocytopenia binds to a complex of heparin and platelet factor 4. Blood 83:3232, 1994.
109. Amiral JA, et al. Pathogenicity of IgA and/or IgM antibodies to heparin-PF4 complexes in patients with heparin-induced thrombocytopenia. Br J Haematol 92:954, 1995.
110. Chong BH, Burgess J, Ismail F. The clinical usefulness of the platelet aggregation test for the diagnosis of heparin-induced thrombocytopenia. Thromb Haemost 69:344, 1993.
111. Sheridan D, Carter C, Kelton JG. A diagnostic test for heparin-induced thrombocytopenia. Blood 67:27, 1986.
112. Aylesworth CL, et al. ELISA for detection of antibodies against the platelet factor 4 (PF4)/heparin complex: Methods for standardization. Blood 86:865a, 1995.
113. Jackson MR, et al. Diagnosis of heparin-induced thrombocytopenia in the vascular surgery patient. Surgery 131:419, 1997.
114. Cummins D, Halil O, Amin S. Which patients undergoing cardiopulmonary bypass should be assessed for development of heparin-induced thrombocytopenia? Thromb Haemost 73:890, 1995.
115. Nand S. Hirudin therapy for heparin-associated thrombocytopenia and deep vein thrombosis. Am J Hematol 43:312, 1993.
116. Magnani HN. Heparin-induced thrombocytopenia (HIT): An overview of 230 patients treated with orgaran (Org 10172). Thromb Haemost 70:554, 1993.
117. Ortel TL, et al. Parenteral anticoagulation with the heparinoid Lomoparan (Org 10172) in patients with heparin induced thrombocytopenia and thrombosis. Thromb Haemost 67:292, 1992.
118. Olinger GN, et al. Cardiopulmonary bypass for patients with previously documented heparin-induced platelet aggregation. J Thorac Cardiovasc Surg 87:673, 1984.
119. Dvorak HF. Abnormalities of hemostasis in malignant disease. In Coleman RW, et al., eds. Hemostasis and Thrombosis: Basic Principles and Clinical Practice, 3rd ed. Philadelphia: JB Lippincott, 1994, p 1238.
120. Clagett GP, et al. Prevention of venous thromboembolism. Chest 108(4):312S, 1995.
121. Cairns JA, et al. Antithrombotic agents in coronary artery disease. Chest 108(4):380S, 1995.
122. Howell WH. Heparin, an anticoagulant: Preliminary communication. Am J Physiol 63:434, 1922.
123. Freedman JE, Adelman B. Pharmacology of heparin and oral anticoagulants. In Loscalzo J, Schafer AI, eds. Thrombosis and Hemorrhage. Boston: Blackwell Scientific Publications, 1994, p 1155.
124. Scharfstein J, Loscalzo J. Molecular approaches to antithrombotic therapy. Hosp Pract 27(5):41, 1992.
125. Warketin TE, et al. Heparin-induced thrombocytopenia in patients treated with low-molecular-weight heparin or unfractionated heparin. N Engl J Med 332:1330, 1995.
126. Doherty DC, et al. "Heparin-free" cardiopulmonary bypass: First reported use of heparinoid (Org 10172) to provide anticoagulation for cardiopulmonary bypass. Anesthesiology 73:562, 1990.
127. Greinacher A, et al. Heparin-associated thrombocytopenia: Immune complexes are attached to the platelet membrane by the negative charge of highly sulphated oligosaccharides. Br J Haematol 84:711, 1993.
128. Ortel TL, et al. Parenteral anticoagulation with the heparinoid Lomoparan (Org 10172) in patients with heparin induced thrombocytopenia and thrombosis. Thromb Haemost 67:292, 1992.
129. Magnani HN. Heparin-induced thrombocytopenia (HIT): An overview of 230 patients treated with orgaran (Org 10172). Thromb Haemost 70:554, 1993.
130. Clarke RJ, et al. Combined administration of aspirin and a specific thrombin inhibitor in man. Circulation 83:1510, 1991.
131. Gold HK, et al. Evidence for a rebound coagulation phenomenon after cessation of a 4-hour infusion of a specific thrombin inhibitor in patients with unstable angina pectoris. J Am Coll Cardiol 21:1039, 1993.
132. Matsuo T, et al. Treatment of heparin-induced thrombocytopenia by use of argatroban, a synthetic thrombin inhibitor. Br J Haematol 82:627, 1992.
133. Sawyer RT. Thrombolytics and anticoagulants from leeches. Biotechnology 9:513, 1991.
134. Maraganore JM, et al. Anticoagulant activity of synthetic hirudin peptides. J Biol Chem 264(15):8692, 1989.
135. Maraganore JM, et al. Design and characterization of hirulogs: A novel class of bivalent peptide inhibitors of thrombin. Bichem 29:7095, 1990.

136. Weitz JI, et al. Clot-bound thrombin is protected from inhibition by heparin-antithrombin III but is susceptible to inactivation by antithrombin III-independent inhibitors. J Clin Invest 86:385, 1990.
137. Fox I, et al. Anticoagulant activity of HirulogTM, a direct thrombin inhibitor, in humans. Thromb Haemost 69:157, 1993.
138. Yao SK, et al. Thrombin inhibition enhances tissue-type plasminogen activator-induced thrombolysis and delays reocclusion. (Part 2). Am J Physiol 262(2):H374, 1992.
139. Klement P, et al. Effects of heparin and hirulog on t-PA induced thrombolysis in a rat model. Fibrinolysis 4(Suppl 3):9, 1990.
140. Topol EJ, et al. Use of a direct antithrombin, Hirulog, in place of heparin during coronary angioplasty. Circulation 87:1622, 1993.
141. Jackson MR, et al. Antithrombotic effects o hirulog in a microsurgical carotid endarterectomy model. J Surg Res 60:15, 1996.
142. Riess FC, Potzsch B, Bader R. A case report on the use of recombinant hirudin as an anticoagulant for cardiopulmonary bypass in open heart surgery. Eur J Cardiothorac Surg 10:386, 1996.
143. FitzGerald GA. Mechanisms of platelet activation: Thromboxane A_2 as an amplifying signal for other agonists. Am J Cardiol 68:11B, 1991.
144. Hirsh J, et al. Aspirin and other platelet-active drugs. The relationship between dose, effectiveness, and side effects. Chest 108:247S, 1995.
145. Barnett HJM, Eliasziw M, Meldrum HE. Drugs and surgery in the prevention of ischemic stroke. N Engl J Med 332:238, 1995.
146. Jakubowski JA, et al. Cumulative anti-platelet effect of low-dose enteric-coated aspirin. Br J Haematol 60:635, 1985.
147. Clagett GP, Krupski WC. Antithrombotic therapy in peripheral arterial occlusive disease. Chest 108(4):431S, 1995.
148. Rinder CS, et al. Aspirin does not inhibit adenosine diphosphate-induced platelet α-granule release. Blood 32:505, 1993.
149. Di Minno G, et al. Functionally thrombasthenic state in normal platelets following the administration of ticlopidine. J Clin Invest 75:328, 1985.
150. Hass EK, et al. A randomized trial comparing ticlopidine hydrochloride with aspirin for the prevention of stroke in high-risk patients. N Engl J Med 321:501, 1989.
151. Gent M, et al. The Canadian American Ticlopidine Study (CATS) in thromboembolic stroke. Lancet 1:1215, 1989.
152. Goods CM, et al. Comparison of aspirin alone versus aspirin plus ticlopidine after coronary artery stenting. Am J Cardiol 78:1042, 1996.
153. Aberg M, Hedner U, Bergentz SE. Effect of dextran on factor VIII (antihemophilic factor) and platelet function. Ann Surg 189:182, 1979.
154. Aberg M, Bergentz SE, Hedner U. The effect of dextran on the lysability of ex vivo thrombi. Ann Surg 181:342, 1975.
155. Harris WH, et al. Prevention of venous thromboembolism following total hip replacement: Warfarin vs dextran 40. JAMA 220:1319, 1972.
156. Clagett GP, Reisch JS. Prevention of venous thromboembolism in general surgical patients. Results of meta-analysis. Ann Surg 208(2):227, 1988.
157. Rutherford RB, et al. The efficacy of dextran 40 in preventing early postoperative thrombus following difficult lower extremity bypass. J Vasc Surg 1:765, 1984.
158. Tcheng JE, et al. Pharmacodynamics of chimeric glycoprotein Iib/IIIa integrin antiplatelet antibody Fab 7E3 in high-risk coronary angioplasty. Circulation 90:1757, 1994.
159. Coller BS, Anderson K, Weisman HF. New antiplatelet agents: Platelet GPIIb/IIIa antagonists. Thromb Haemost 74:302, 1995.
160. The EPIC investigators. Use of a monoclonal antibody directed against the platelet glycoprotein IIb/IIIa receptor in high-risk coronary angioplasty. N Engl J Med 330:956, 1994.
161. Moliterno DJ, et al. Effect of platelet glycoprotein IIb/IIIa integrin blockade on activated clotting time during percutaneous transluminal coronary angioplasty or directional atherectomy (the EPIC trial). Evaluation of c7E3 Fab in the Prevention of Ischemic Complications Trial. Am J Cardiol 75:559, 1995.
162. Faulds D. Sorkin EM. Abciximab (c7E3 Fab). A review of its pharmacology and therapeutic potential in ischemic heart disease. Drugs 48:583, 1994.

8

Pathophysiology of Shock

A. Gerson Greenburg and H. Hank Simms

"Shock" is defined as a state of altered tissue perfusion severe enough to induce derangements in normal cellular metabolic function. It occurs when the blood flow to organs and tissues is insufficient to provide necessary nutrients and oxygen and to remove the waste products resulting from their metabolism. If left untreated, the cellular dysfunction that attends shock ultimately leads to death. Since shock represents the end result of circulatory failure, an understanding of its clinical presentation is mandatory if aggressive and expeditious treatment is to be rendered. It is not unusual for a patient in shock to require rapid restoration of an effective circulating blood volume within a short period of time (often within minutes) if there is to be any hope of survival. This treatment involves both a thorough understanding of the pathophysiologic derangements associated with shock and the distinguishing characteristics of the various etiologic factors responsible for its development.

TYPES OF SHOCK

Although shock has been classified in a number of ways, from an etiologic standpoint, four types of shock have been recognized and described (Table 8-1). These are hypovolemic shock, septic shock, cardiogenic shock, and neurogenic shock. It is important to remember, however, that a given patient may not fit conveniently into one of these four categories but rather may have components of more than one category contributing to the shocklike state. For example, a patient with compromised cardiac reserve from atherosclerotic heart disease is commonly a victim of an automobile accident in which there is blood loss from a ruptured spleen and/or a long bone fracture. Although the initial presentation to the emergency suite may be primarily one of hypovolemic shock, the compromised cardiac reserve may result in myocardial failure, in which case cardiogenic shock would also be a major factor contributing to the patient's shock state. Realizing the potential interplay of the various etiologic factors in a given patient is crucial if effective treatment is to be instituted. Further, it cannot be stressed too strongly that, independent of etiologic factors, altered tissue perfusion with impaired oxygen delivery and/or oxygen use is common to all forms of shock.[1-3] A more physiologically oriented schema for classifying shock is detailed in Table 8-2. By considering the physiologic derangements that occur in shock, one can direct treatment at correcting these perturbations with appropriate interventions.

Hypovolemic Shock

Hypovolemic shock is the circulatory failure that results from a decrease in intravascular blood volume. This decrease in "effective circulation" results in a corresponding decrease in both the cardiac output and tissue perfusion. This form of shock may be caused by the loss of blood or plasma volume or both from the circulation. Hemorrhage (e.g., from the gastrointestinal tract, injuries), vomiting, diarrhea, and sequestration of fluid (as may occur intraluminally in bowel obstruction, intraperitoneally in pancreatitis or peritonitis, and interstitially in burns) may each lead to a decrease in intravascular volume.

In the early stages of hypovolemic shock, blood is diverted from the skin so that perfusion to such organs as the liver, kidneys, brain, and heart is maintained. Generally, the only clinical findings include a postural increase in the patient's pulse and *decrease in* blood pressure in the sitting or standing position, compared with the supine posture. In addition, the skin may be pale and cool, and the neck veins may be flat. If the hypovolemia continues, further redistribution of blood flow occurs from such organs as the kidneys and gut to ensure adequate flow to the heart and brain. At this stage in shock development, the patient is usually thirsty, the urine becomes concentrated, and its volume decreases. A tachycardia is usually present, and the blood pressure is more labile. If hypovolemia worsens further, blood flow to the brain and heart becomes compromised. This circumstance is characterized clinically by restlessness, agitation, confusion, and occasionally even obtundation. The measurable blood pressure is lower, and the pulse becomes more rapid, weak, and often irregular. Respiration is also compromised and is characterized by deep,

Table 8-1. Etiologic Classification of Shock

Type of Shock	Primary Etiology
Hypovolemic	Hemorrhage, vomiting, diarrhea, intraperitoneal fluid sequestration (e.g., pancreatitis), intraluminal fluid sequestration (e.g., bowel obstruction), interstitial fluid sequestration (e.g., burns and traumatized tissues)
Septic	Bacterial, viral, or fungal sepsis; endotoxin from bacterial wall breakdown
Cardiogenic	Intrinsic to the heart: myocardial infarction, myocarditis, ventricular aneurysms, valve prolapse, arrhythmias Extrinsic to the heart: pericardial tamponade, pericarditis, tension pneumothorax, pulmonary embolus
Neurogenic	Spinal cord trauma, gastric dilation, spinal anesthesia

Table 8-2. Physiologic Classification of Shock

Type of Shock	Primary Etiology
Hypovolemic	
Exogenous losses	Diarrhea, vomiting, dehydration, burns, and hemorrhage (i.e., blood, plasma, or water losses)
Endogenous losses	Inflammation, trauma, tourniquet
Cardiogenic	
Focal power failure	Myocardial infarction, ventricular aneurysm, cardiac valve prolapse
Generalized power failure	Viral, drug, or chemical myocarditis
Distributive	
Normal or high peripheral vascular resistance	Sepsis, endotoxin
Low peripheral vascular resistance	Sepsis, central nervous system/spinal cord injury, anaphylaxis, spinal anesthesia

rapid breathing. Ultimately, cardiac arrest and death ensue if this sequence of events is not reversed. A summary of the clinical signs associated with a form of hypovolemic shock (e.g., hemorrhage), based on the magnitude of blood volume loss, is detailed in Table 8-3.

Since hypovolemic shock represents a deficit in circulating blood volume, the goals in treatment should include identification of the source of the plasma or blood loss, an attempt at controlling this loss, and efforts to restore the volume of effective circulation. As discussed later in this chapter, this volume restoration includes infusion of balanced salt solutions and blood if hemorrhage is present.

Septic Shock

Septic shock usually occurs under conditions of severe infection and is characterized by a decrease in peripheral vas-

Table 8-3. Clinical Signs Related to Magnitude of Blood Volume Lost

Decrease in Blood Volume (%)	Approximate Blood Loss (ml)	Signs
0–10	0–500	None; slight tachycardia
10–20	500–1200	Slight tachycardia, decreased blood pressure, peripheral vasoconstriction
20–30	1200–1800	Tachycardia (>120 beats/min), hypotension, vasoconstriction, diaphoresis, postural hypotension, anxiety, restlessness, oliguria
30+	1800–3000	Hypotension (blood pressure <70 systolic), diaphoresis, obtundation, anuria

cular resistance and a hyperdynamic circulatory state. Although the exact sequence of events responsible for these findings remains to be defined, the pathogenetic organisms associated with this form of shock appear to increase the circulation at the site of the infectious process. Organisms commonly involved include gram negative pathogens such as *Escherichia coli, Klebsiella pneumoniae, Aerobacter aerogenes, Pseudomonas aeruginosa,* and at times *Proteus* organisms and *Bacteroides* species. On occasion, gram-positive organisms such as *Staphylococcus aureus* and fungal agents such as *Candida albicans* may also be implicated. In addition to the direct effects that bacteria may have on the cardiovascular system and cellular metabolism, endotoxin, a lipopolysaccharide component of cell walls of gram negative bacteria, apparently activates the complement system, releasing biologically active amines that regulate release of vasoactive and cardiotonic factors. This outpouring of vasoactive and metabolically inhibiting factors leads to a hyperdynamic state, resulting in peripheral vasodilation and increased cardiac output. Oxygen use is blocked at the subcellular level with accumulation of lactic acid, despite the adequacy of oxygen delivery to cells and the high blood flow state that usually exists. Clinically, such patients have fever; a rapid, bounding pulse; and usually a normal blood pressure. The respiration rate is often rapid, and the neck veins are normal. Because of the enhanced blood flow peripherally, the skin is warm and usually somewhat flushed. If this *hyperdynamic state* continues and is maintained, the urine output is usually adequate. As the septic process continues, however, fluid is lost from the intravascular space into the interstitial and cellular spaces and ultimately gives rise to *hypodynamic septic shock.* When this form of septic shock occurs, it appears clinically much like hypovolemic shock. Thus the skin becomes cold and clammy, the neck veins are flat, the pulse continues to be rapid but now becomes weak, the blood pressure lowers, and the urinary output decreases. If this shock is not successfully treated, confusion followed by obtundation, coma, and death eventually supervenes.

The treatment of this form of shock almost always requires identification of the septic focus with appropriate antibiotic coverage and definitive surgical drainage. Until drainage of the septic focus has been accomplished, therapy is at best supportive and symptomatic. Beside broad-spectrum antimicrobial coverage, this includes fluid replacement and inotropic drugs to maintain ventricular function so that adequate tissue perfusion is ensured.

A variant of the septic shock presentation is associated with release of vasoactive agents and cytokines. This "systemic inflammatory response syndrome" (SIRS) can mimic the various phases of septic shock and requires the patient be treated in a similar manner. Failure to identify a causative bacterial or viral agent is no reason to delay supportive therapeutic interventions.

Cardiogenic Shock

Cardiogenic shock occurs when tissue perfusion is impaired because of underlying heart failure. Conditions leading to this form of shock include compromised ventricular function secondary to atherosclerotic coronary artery disease, myocardial infarction, mechanical obstruction of venous return (as occurs in pericardial tamponade or tension pneumothorax), ineffective cardiac contraction (as may occur in various arrhythmic states), and pulmonary embolism. Clinically, these patients appear much like those with hypovolemic shock. The pulse is usually rapid and weak, the blood pressure is low, the skin is cold and clammy, and the respiration rate is rapid. Urinary output is also low; but unlike the case in other forms of shock, the neck veins are distended. If the shock is secondary to pericardial tamponade, a paradoxical pulse may also be present. If a tension pneumothorax is responsible for this shock, the trachea may be shifted away from the involved side with hyperresonance on percussion of that side.

Treatment of this form of shock consists of supporting the failing circulation with an adequate circulating blood volume through the administration of intravenous fluids and providing appropriate cardiotonic agents to support the failing heart. If cardiac tamponade is responsible for the shock, pericardiocentesis is indicated. Similarly, chest tube placement is necessary in a tension pneumothorax. If pulmonary embolism is the underlying cause, a surgical embolectomy may become necessary. For a more in-depth discussion of this form of shock, see Chapter 54.

Neurogenic Shock

Neurogenic shock is the result of a reduction in vasomotor tone from a loss of sympathetic innervation. This form of shock is most commonly encountered from some impairment of the central nervous system, usually spinal cord trauma. It also can occur following the administration of a high spinal anesthetic and on occasion secondary to acute gastric dilation. Although severe forms of neurogenic shock may result in inadequate cardiac output and poor tissue perfusion, as noted in other forms of shock, the clinical picture with this entity is usually appreciably different. Although the pulse rate may be rapid and the blood pressure may be low, the common clinical picture is one of a slow pulse rate; a warm, dry skin; and only mild hypotension. In addition, the mental status is usually normal, respiratory function is undisturbed, and the neck veins are flat. Often, elevating the legs for a short period of time may be all that is needed to correct this problem, particularly if it has been induced from a spinal anesthetic. If neurogenic shock is secondary to spinal cord injury, increasing an effective circulating blood volume with a balanced salt solution generally proves to be sufficient treatment. On rare occasions, vasoconstrictive agents may be needed to increase the vasomotor tone.

PATHOPHYSIOLOGIC RESPONSE TO SHOCK

Since shock indicates a state of tissue perfusion inadequate to maintain nutrition of cells and remove metabolic waste products, it is not surprising that a common pathophysiologic response occurs in all shock states to avert these derangements. The components of this response may differ somewhat depending on the form of shock encountered, but the compensatory mechanisms called into play are virtually identical. It is primarily the magnitude of these mechanisms that differs among the various forms of shock. In hypovolemic shock, for example, these mechanisms are quite pronounced because tissue perfusion is severely compromised in this state, whereas in neurogenic shock they may be minimal or absent because impairment of tissue perfusion is only mildly affected. Because the overall pathophysiologic response to shock is similar for all etiologic factors, an understanding of this response is paramount if appropriate treatment is to be rendered.

Neuroendocrine Response

A complex neuroendocrine response is triggered to various degrees in the different shock states to assuage the ineffective circulating blood volume[4–8] (Fig. 8-1). The decrease in circulating volume is sensed by low-pressure stretch receptors in the right atrium and by high-pressure baroreceptors in the aorta and the carotid arteries. As blood volume, venous return, and cardiac output decrease, baroreceptor activity is also attenuated, resulting in loss of the tonic inhibition of the central and sympathetic nervous systems. Such a loss triggers increased secretion of adrenocorticotropic hormone (ACTH), antidiuretic hormone (ADH), and growth hormone by the pituitary gland through central hypothalamic pathways, and of epinephrine and norepinephrine secretion by the adrenal medulla through peripheral sympathetic pathways. Additional hormonal interactions arising from the adrenal cortex include stimulation of cortisol release by ACTH and aldosterone release by both ACTH and by way of the renin-angiotensin system secondary to decreased renal perfusion. Glucagon and insulin are also released by the pancreas in shock; but because of the antagonism of epinephrine, cortisol, and glucagon against the metabolic effects of insulin, a relative insulin deficiency is usually present. Fear or anxiety augments this neuroendocrine response through stimulation of the limbic areas of the brain. Limbic system projections to the hypothalamus and lower brain stem nuclei lead to increased hy-

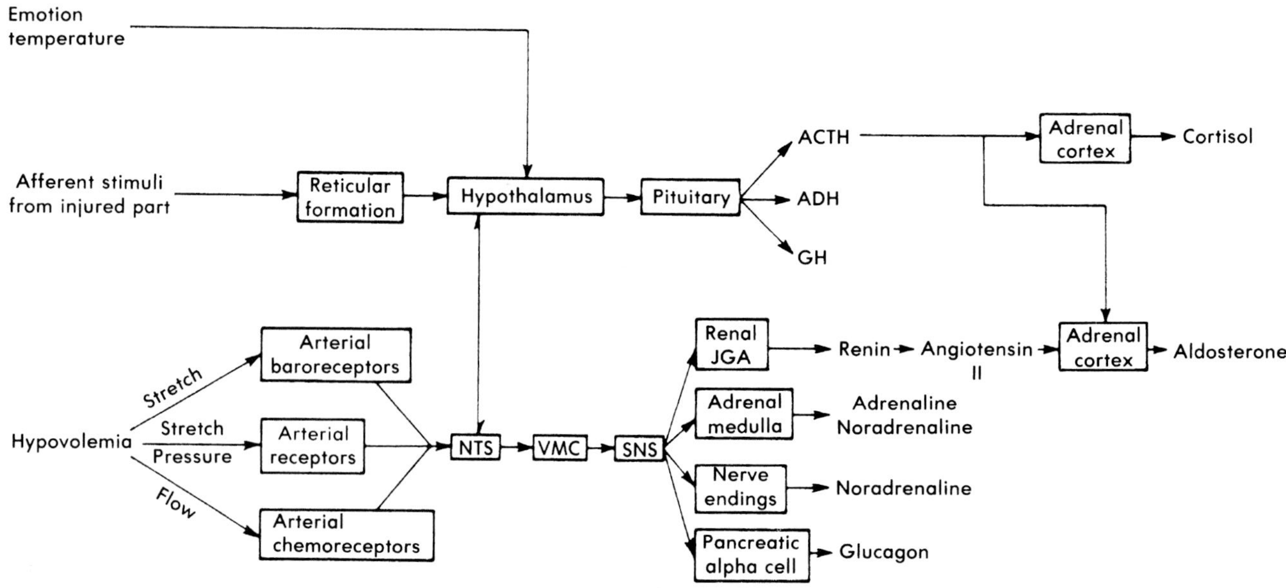

Fig. 8-1. Schematic representation of the neuroendocrine response to ineffective circulating blood volume, as seen in hypovolemic shock. *ACTH,* Adrenocorticotropic hormone; *ADH,* antidiuretic hormone; *GH,* growth hormone; *JGA,* juxtaglomerular apparatus; *NTS,* nuclei of the solitary tract; *SNS,* sympathetic nervous system; *VMC,* vasomotor center. (From Pardy BJ. Trauma and shock. In Burnett W, ed. Clinical Science for Surgeons. Boston: Butterworth Publishers, 1981.)

pothalamic, adrenomedullary, and adrenocortical activity (see Fig. 8-1). Abnormalities in both body and ambient temperatures produce similar changes along identical pathways. An additional entry into this response pathway includes stimulation of chemoreceptors located in the aortic and carotid bodies. Changes in the concentration of oxygen, hydrogen ion, or carbon dioxide in the blood result in further neuroendocrine perturbations. The net result of this interplay of hormonal interactions is arteriolar vasoconstriction (i.e., increased peripheral vascular resistance), renal conservation of both water and salt, and the provision of circulating glucose adequate to maintain the nutritional needs of such vital organs as the heart and brain.

Hemodynamic Perturbations

The primary function of the neuroendocrine response to shock is to correct inadequate tissue perfusion. This response is particularly pronounced in patients with hypovolemic shock and those with the hypodynamic form of septic shock. It is directed at all elements of the circulation, including the heart, peripheral vasculature, and blood volume. Mechanisms responsible for restoring cardiovascular homeostasis include (1) augmentation of cardiac output, (2) redistribution of blood flow, and (3) restoration of intravascular volume.

Cardiac output, the principal determinant of tissue perfusion, is directly proportional to venous return.[9-13] The increase in the end-diastolic stretch of ventricular muscle fibers (preload) results in a stronger contraction during systole and therefore an increased ejection of blood. The compensatory mechanism by which venous return is increased in shock—with a corresponding preload increase—is through decreasing venous capacitance, which restores an effective circulating blood volume. Decreased venous capacitance occurs secondary to specific organ vasoconstriction. The vasoconstriction is mediated by sympathetic nerves, circulating catecholamines, angiotensin II (via the renin-angiotensin system), and ADH (also called vasopressin). Blood flow to the heart, brain, and adrenal and pituitary glands is protected by vasodilation of their vessels. Blood flow to skin, skeletal muscles, and the splanchnic circulation is decreased, with the degree of vasoconstriction being proportional to the deficit in circulating blood volume. These alterations are particularly pronounced in hemorrhage, with changes in hepatic and renal blood flow varying in direct proportion with the degree of hemorrhage. For example, following mild hemorrhage, portal blood flow decreases secondary to vasoconstriction of the splanchnic circulation. The hepatic arteries initially dilate, but total hepatic blood flow is decreased following even minor blood loss. In cases of moderate-to-severe hemorrhage, this arterial autoregulation is lost, and the hepatic arteries actually vasoconstrict. Renal blood flow is only compromised following loss of a large volume of blood. With continued blood loss, the mechanisms responsible for maintaining blood flow to the heart and brain are also compromised and eventually fail.

Systemic arterial resistance increases secondary to arteriolar constriction and is also mediated by sympathetic nerves, circulating catecholamines, angiotensin II, and ADH.[4-8] This increase in afterload results in a net decrease in cardiac output. However, blood flow to the heart and lung is maintained at near-normal levels through redistri-

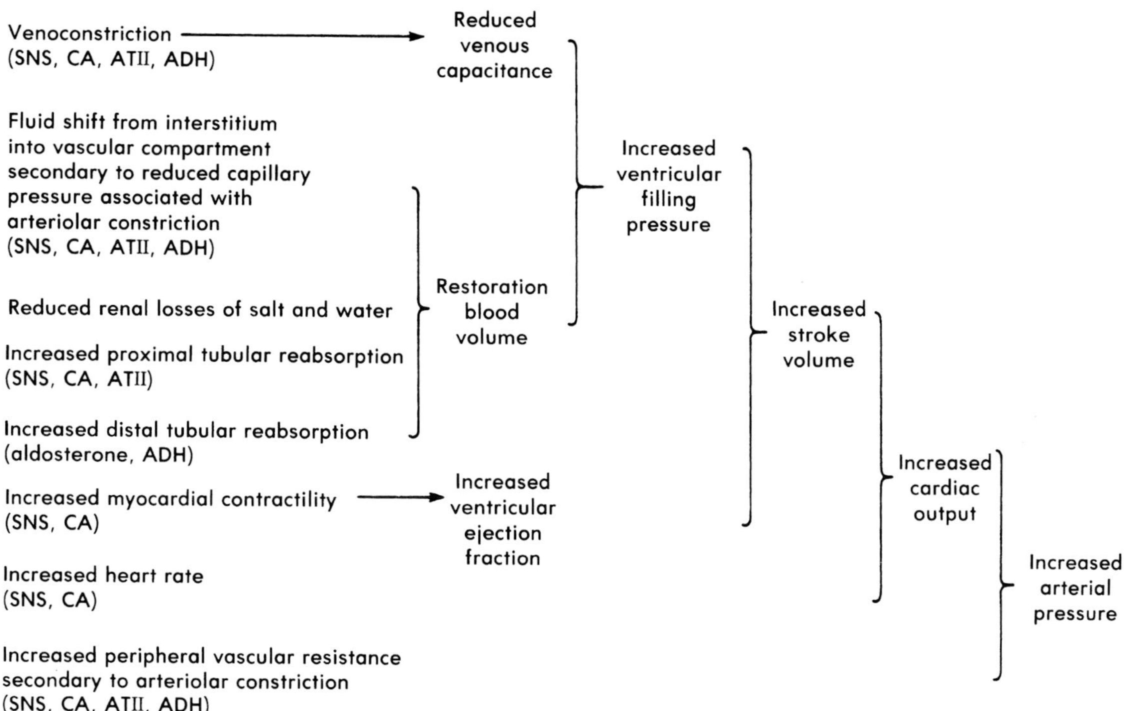

Fig. 8-2. Hemodynamic responses to ineffective circulating blood volume, as seen in hypovolemic shock. *ADH,* Antidiuretic hormone; *AT II,* angiotensin II; *CA,* catecholamines; *SNS,* sympathetic nervous system. (From Pardy BJ. Trauma and shock. In Burnett W, ed. Clinical Science for Surgeons. Boston: Butterworth Publishers, 1981.)

bution of available cardiac output to these critical, nonconstricted areas of the circulation. The increase in systemic arterial resistance is most pronounced in hypovolemic shock. It is also seen in cardiogenic shock and the hypodynamic phase of septic shock. In contrast, in the early, hyperdynamic phase of septic shock, a decrease in peripheral arterial resistance is seen. This is probably related to the direct effects of bacteria and endotoxin on the cardiovascular system and cellular metabolism.

The other determinants of cardiac output are contractility and heart rate. Increases in contractility result in direct increases in cardiac output. Increased heart rate also increases cardiac output, but the response to this mechanism is limited. A heart rate beyond 180 beats/min is associated with a decreased cardiac output secondary to a reduced diastolic filling time. Increases in both contractility and heart rate occur secondary to stimulation of cardiac sympathetic nerves and by the action of circulating catecholamines. Other vasoactive substances that are known to circulate in shock include enkephalins, endorphins, arachidonic acid metabolites, serotonin, kinins, and histamine; but the physiologic importance of these substances in mediating the hemodynamic response to shock remains to be determined. The overall hemodynamic perturbations are summarized in Fig. 8-2.

Restitution of an effective circulating blood volume, in addition to the compensatory changes already noted, is important in preventing the deleterious effects of shock (i.e., tissue ischemia and death). According to Gann and Amaral,[9] this blood volume restoration occurs in two phases: an initial transcapillary refill phase and a plasma protein restitution phase. These responses are particularly pronounced in patients with hypovolemic shock secondary to hemorrhage. Acute blood loss, for example, results in a decrease in capillary pressure initiated by hypotension and augmented by sympathetically mediated precapillary arteriolar constriction. The resultant decrease in capillary hydrostatic pressure promotes movement of fluid from the interstitial space into the capillary bed. This extracellular fluid shift to the vascular compartment may restore up to 50% of the lost blood volume.

The second phase of vascular restitution begins with increases in the serum osmolality. The liver is the primary source of the solutes contributing to this hyperosmolality, which include glucose, phosphate, lactate, pyruvate, amino acids, and urea. The elevation in serum osmolality is proportional to both the degree and the rate of hemorrhage. The rise in plasma osmolality results in an increase in osmolality in the interstitial space. Interstitial hyperosmolality leads to an osmotic gradient, with a resultant movement of water from the cells. The increased interstitial volume results in an increase in interstitial pressure, promoting a transcapillary movement of albumin from the interstitial space to the intravascular compartment. Complete restoration of blood volume depends on this restitution of plasma protein.

Metabolic Perturbations

The ineffective circulating blood volume that occurs in shock and the corresponding reduction in cardiac output result in an increased extraction of oxygen by the tissues from arterial blood. The cellular hypoperfusion and hypoxia result in a shift to anaerobic glycolysis. Instead of entering the citric acid cycle through coenzyme A, pyruvate is converted to lactic acid. This cellular acidosis is transmitted to the circulation, as reflected in the increased blood lactic acid levels that are commonly observed in patients in shock. Each mole of lactic acid releases 1 mol of hydrogen ion to body fluids, with a corresponding reduction of buffering capacity and a resultant systemic acidosis. If not treated, this acidosis offsets the normal hemodynamic responses and leads to irreversible shock and death.

Hyperglycemia also occurs in response to shock. Changes in carbohydrate metabolism arise secondary to the action of catecholamines, cortisol, glucagon, and growth hormone. Although insulin secretion is also increased in shock, its anabolic effects—at least acutely—are antagonized by these substances so that a state of catabolism ensues.[10] The hyperglycemic response is mediated by these various agents and is secondary to increased hepatic production of glucose through (1) glycogen breakdown, (2) stimulation of gluconeogenesis from breakdown of skeletal muscle protein into amino acids and the conversion of these amino acids in the liver into glucose, and (3) impaired peripheral uptake of glucose by tissues. Further, epinephrine selectively inhibits insulin secretion. This metabolic response is primarily invoked to provide glucose to the cerebral circulation, since this substance is the only metabolic fuel that can be used effectively by brain tissue.

In addition to the alterations in glucose metabolism that occur in shock, cortisol and glucagon, in conjunction with catecholamines, stimulate lipolysis and thereby increase plasma concentrations of free fatty acids. This lipolytic action, which is also antagonistic to the effects of insulin, is another mechanism by which additional fuel and energy substrate are provided at a time of increased metabolic demand.

Other metabolically and hemodynamically active agents are released in various shock states. The known elevation in blood levels of endorphins, opiate-like agents, may contribute to the hypotension and myocardial depression seen in those forms of shock in which hypovolemia is not a major underlying etiologic factor.[14] Elevations of arachidonic acid metabolites, particularly thromboxane A_2 and prostacyclin, have also been observed in both clinical and experimental shock.[15] Since these agents have opposite physiologic effects (thromboxane A_2 aggregates platelets and is a vasoconstrictor, whereas prostacyclin inhibits platelet aggregation and is a vasodilator), and since both are generally elevated in shock, the net effect depends on which one dominates. In addition, since both agents have relatively short half-lives, their importance probably lies in regulating the microcirculatory alterations that occur in shock (see the next section).

Other hormones may also play a role in shock, but experimental information to date is too meager to allow any meaningful conclusions. In particular, the thyroid and parathyroid glands do not receive much basal blood flow, and in shock they could undergo further compromise, leading to tissue hypoxia and cell damage. Since thyroxin plays an important role in regulating oxygen consumption of tissues, a deficit of this hormone could contribute to the impaired oxygen utilization seen in some shock states. Similarly, alterations in calcium metabolism, caused by changes in the synthesis and/or release of parathormone or thyrocalcitonin, may impair important metabolic functions necessary for cellular viability.[16]

Effects of Shock at the Cellular Level

The Microcirculation

The microcirculation is that component of the vasculature that provides nutrient blood flow directly to tissues and is involved with the removal of metabolic waste products. Although much more must be learned about the physiology of the microcirculation and what derangements actually exist in the various shock states, considerable useful pathophysiologic information has been obtained in recent years from the study of various laboratory animals under normal and shock conditions. Just as the neurohumoral response to shock produces changes in various hemodynamic parameters (e.g., tachycardia, altered peripheral resistance) that are potentially detrimental to some organs (e.g., kidney and gut) and protective of others (e.g., heart and brain), corresponding changes also occur in the microcirculation that may be either protective or detrimental.

Various vascular mediators released during shock (i.e., angiotensin II, arachidonic acid metabolites, kinins) appear to act selectively at the level of afferent arterioles or efferent venules. These agents may induce arteriovenous shunting, occlusion of capillary beds, and altered pressure-flow relationships in oxygen delivery to cells. Such vascular aberrations, coupled with the low flow state induced by hypovolemia or cardiac failure, often lead to platelet aggregation and thrombus formation. A variety of vasoactive substances (e.g., prostanoids, serotonin) are then liberated as the clot forms. These agents, together with the resulting anoxia, produce endothelial damage and increased capillary permeability, which then result in the formation of edema and further restriction and redistribution of blood flow.

Although it is uncertain which of these precipitating events is most important, it is known that anoxia has a direct effect on vascular endothelium and may indeed be the mechanism responsible for the increased capillary permeability.[17] Like other cells, endothelium appears to require oxygen to function; when the endothelium is oxygen deprived, a leaky capillary membrane ensues. The leak results from a widening of cell-to-cell junctions, with aggressive fluid movement into the interstitium. This effective increase in interstitial fluid is noticeable in a number of organs but can be especially pronounced in the lungs, particularly during septic shock. In fact, monitoring lung water has proved helpful in assessing the presence and magnitude of this capillary leak, independent of the underlying cause of shock.[18] Other investigators have suggested that this capillary leak may not be caused by the anoxia per se but rather may be related to the release of oxygen-derived free radicals associated with rapid volume expansion and oxygen delivery during shock resuscitation. It is known, for example, that the superoxide anion, a major component of this oxygen radical system, directly damages cells and cell membranes. If oxygen radicals are ultimately shown to play a major role in the microcirculatory events during shock and its resuscitation, future pharmacologic therapy may include measures directed at attenuating or eliminating the effects of these toxic anions.[19,20]

Nitric oxide. The free radical nitric oxide (NO) is formed from the guanidino group of L-arginine by a family of enzymes termed NO synthase (NOS). The constitutive form of NOS derived from endothelial cells (ecNOS) maintains active vasodilation and reduces platelet and polymorphonuclear neutrophil leukocytes (PMN) adhesion to endothelial surfaces. The inducible form of NOS (iNOS) is expressed in response to inflammatory stimuli (proinflammatory cytokines and lipopolysaccharide [LPS]) and is Ca^{++} independent. In contrast, ecNOS is regulated both by calmodulin and intracellular Ca^{++}.[21]

NO is a labile compound produced by endothelial cells activated by vasorelaxant agents that include acetylcholine, bradykinin, histamine, and serotinin. Since the half-life of NO is measured in seconds, NO exerts its effects in a paracrine fashion.

Vascular endothelium continually produces NO, promoting a vasorelaxant effect on arterial smooth muscle.[22] Inhibition of NO production with N^G monomethyl L-arginine (NMA), methylene blue, or hemoglibin is associated with reduced formation of cyclic guanosine monophosphate (cGMP) by muscle cells.[23]

A potential role for NO in the pathophysiology of sepsis is suggested by the fact that inhibitors of NO synthesis by L-arginine analogs increases blood pressure and systemic vascular resistance in multiple animal species including rabbits, guinea pigs, and dogs.[24] NO synthesis may be increased during sepsis; bovine aortic endothelial cells, release NO after 1 minute of incubation with *E. coli* LPS. Further, the contractile impairment observed in vascular rings from endotoxin-treated animals can be reversed by inhibiting NO synthesis.[25] In vivo support for the concept that NO contributes to the hemodynamic changes seen during sepsis was recently seen in a sheep model using the intravenous infusion of live *E. coli*.[26] An inhibitor of NO production, N^g-nitro L-arginine significantly increased both blood pressure and systemic vascular resistance. Pretreatment of septic sheep with L-arginine totally abolished the increases in systemic and pulmonary vascular resistances induced by N^g-nitro L-arginine. *Treatment after sepsis is established is also beneficial.*[8]

Many of the biologic actions of NO are mediated via the guanylyl cyclase/cGMP system. Local concentrations of NO can be increased via NO donors (glyceryl trinitrate, sodium nitroprusside) or reduced by inhibiting NOS activity (N^g-monomethyl-L-arginine).

In animal models of endotoxic shock, endotoxin produces an acute release of NO in multiple organs. In contrast, prolonged periods of endotoxemia are also associated with impairment of endothelium-dependent relaxations.[27] iNOS activity in vivo is mediated by secondary cytokines (TNF, interferon-γ [INF-γ], IL-1); this concept is supported by the fact that (1) these cytokines are released in response to endotoxin, (2) administration of these agents to normal animals mimics the effects of NO by inducing iNOS formation, and (3) neutralizing these cytokines can prevent the endotoxin-induced alterations in NO biosynthesis.[28,29]

Hemorrhagic shock results in the impairment of the biosynthesis of NO from L-arginine by ecNOS in the vascular endothelium. Diminution of the endothelium-dependent retardation during hemorrhagic shock is due to an impairment of agonist-stimulated biosynthesis of NO by ecNOS.[30] This impairment of NO synthesis is thought to contribute to the decreased cerebral, renal, and cardiac performance seen during hemorrhagic shock. Possible mechanisms underlying this endothelium dysfunction (i.e., reduced NO formation from L-arginine by ecNOS) include platelet activating factor (PAF), PMN activation, and increasing the degradation of mRNA for ecNOS induced by TNF. Importantly, infusion of the NO donor S-nitroso N-acetyl penicillamine reduces PMN infiltration and prevents endothelium dysfunction in the splanchnic circulation of rats subjected to hemorrhagic shock.[31]

Evidence also exists for the enhanced formation of NO in hemorrhagic shock. Significant increases in NO-hemoglobin complexes detected by electron spin resonance have been detected 2 to 6 hours after hemorrhage. Enhanced formation of NO during early hemorrhagic shock is due to activation of ecNOS, as dexamethasone (an inhibitor of iNOS induction) only delays the onset of vascular hyporeactivity during hemorrhage and iNOS activity is not detectable in multiple organs 60 minutes after hemorrhage.[28-33] Prolonged periods of hemorrhagic shock are associated with vascular decompensation caused by enhanced formation of NO by iNOS. This statement is supported by the fact that (1) calcium-independent iNOS activity appears in several organs at the same time decompensation occurs, (2) inhibition of NOS activity with L-[NAME] attenuates this vascular decompensation, and (3) inhibition of iNOS formation with dexamethasone prevents the vascular decompensation associated with prolonged hemorrhagic shock.

The induction of iNOS during hemorrhagic shock is likely to be due to cytokines such as TNF-α and IL-1α because intravenous administration of TNF-α or IL-1β increases NO production and anti–TNF-α antibodies prevent NO-mediated vascular hyporeactivity ex vivo.[34] On a cellular level, local formation of NO in large amounts leads to autoinhibition of cellular respiration. This is accompanied by increased lactate production, inability to use oxygen, and a reduction in the arteriovenous oxygen differences.[35] Thus, ample evidence exists that NO plays an important role in the pathophysiologic changes seen during shock, particularly those associated with hemorrhage.

Cytokines. Proinflammatory, cytokines such as TNF-α and IL-1 are released from a variety of cells in response to bacterial endotoxin or other microbial products. These compounds promote the release of additional cytokines including IL-6, IL-8, and prostaglandin E_2 (PGE_2).

A recent study has demonstrated that mortality rates of critically ill septic patients correlates with levels of both LPS and the cytokines TNF-α, IL-1, and IL-6.[36]

Human TNF-α is a 17 kd polypeptide cytokine composed of 157 amino acids. When infused into various animal models, hypotension, tachycardia, tachypnea, and profound metabolic acidosis ensue.[37] TNF-α is also capable of causing the development of a systemic capillary leak with depressed cardiac output. The relevant role of TNF-α in mediating the pathophysiologic changes seen during septic shock was confirmed by Hinshaw et al.,[38] who demonstrated a protective effect of anti–TNF-α monoclonal antibodies on survival in a baboon model even after intravenous infusion of *E. coli*. Like IL-1β, TNF-α augments the procoagulant properties of endothelial cells. Unlike IL-1β, however, TNF-α has been shown to induce H_2O_2 production in neutrophils with subsequent endothelial cell monolayer disruption.[39] The toxicity of TNF-α appears to be species dependent; although TNF-α by itself has little toxicity in mice, TNF-α decreases arterial blood pressure and left ventricular ejection fractions in dogs. In sheep, infusion of TNF-α causes a syndrome very similar to adult respiratory distress syndrome (ARDS). Lastly, in humans, a simple injection of TNF-α causes fever and the sustained activation of the extrinsic pathway of coagulation.[40]

PAF (1-aklyl-2 acetyl-sn-glycero-3 phopho) is an important lipid mediator in the pathogenesis of shock. PAF is induced by a variety of cell lines including endothelial cells, type II pneumocytes, neutrophils, and platelets.[5,41] PAF production is regulated, in part, by phospholipase A_2 (PLA_2). PLA_2 converts membrane phospholipid to lyso-PAF (inactive). Lyso-PAF is then acetylated to biologically active PAF by acetyltransferase. Experimental data have demonstrated that TNF-α can promote PLA_2 activation, PAF generation, and eicosanoid production. This process may be amplified by the concomitant presence of IL-1β.[42]

IL-1β is a 17.5 kd protein produced by a variety of cells including macrophages and endothelial cells. Endotoxin, TNF-α, and IL-1 itself can induce the production and secretion of IL-1β. IL-1 has been reported to induce hemorrhagic shock in rabbits and importantly enhances in a synergistic fashion the toxicity of TNF-α in multiple animal models.[43]

IL-1 profoundly affects the endothelial cell and induces a prothrombotic state; IL-1β induces the expression of E-selectin to facilitate PMN-endothelial cell adherence. IL-1β increases the production of tissue factor, decreases thrombomodulin, and increases production of plasminogen activation inhibitors. These changes may contribute to the development of disseminated intravascular coagulation (DIC) and overall decreased tissue perfusion.[44] Lastly, IL-1β induces the synthesis of prostacyclin, which contributes to the hypotension seen during shock by inducing vascular smooth muscle relaxation.

INF-γ is a 17 kd glycoprotein produced primarily by lymphocytes; the role of INF-α in the pathophysiology of shock resides in its ability to synergize with other cytokines. INF-α treatment of macrophages results in the production of TNF-α, H_2O_2, and PAF.[45] Unlike TNF-α, INF-α has little acute in vivo toxicity in animal models by itself; however, when given to mice in sensitizing doses followed by either endotoxin or LPS a lethal generalized Shwartzman-type reaction results. Further, in mice given neutralizing monoclonal anti–INF-γ antibody, lethal endotoxic shock was prevented, as was the generalized Shwartzman reaction. In mice who received these antibodies, markedly reduced levels of TNF-α were seen in their circulation.[46] Thus cytokines contribute to the pathophysiologic changes of septic shock by influencing inflammatory cell–endothelial cell interaction and subsequently whole organ function primarily in a paracrine fashion. The clinical and therapeutic implications of this information are not yet appreciated.

Ischemia-reperfusion. Episodes of hypoxemia with or without reoxygenation are associated with a variety of pathologic conditions that result in profound physiologic changes. Intestinal ischemia-reperfusion and the sepsis syndrome have been associated with regional reduction in blood flow and associated oxygen debt.[47,48] Further, improving regional blood flow and global oxygen delivery with pressor therapy has been shown to reduce morbidity in critically ill patients.[49-51] Recent data have implicated the PMN as an important component of both local and systemic tissue damage following hypoxemia with or without reoxygenation.

The initial phase of PMN-induced tissue injury following hypoxemia with or without reoxygenation involves PMN-endothelial cell interactions. This process appears to involve three phases. First, endothelial cells are stimulated by cytokines at sites of inflammation to produce endothelial leukocyte adherence molecules-1 (ELAM-1) and intercellular cell adherence molecule-1 (ICAM-1).[52] Simultaneously, adhesive molecules called LECAM-1 present themselves on the PMN surface and induce PMN rolling and reversible sticking to the endothelial cell. Second, in the presence of chemoattractants or cytokines there is a rapid shedding of surface LECAM-1 and upregulation of PMN CD11b/CD18 (Mac-1).[53] This results in CD11b/CD18–ICAM-1 binding and tight adhesiveness of the PMN to the endothelial cell. Finally, chemoattractants (particularly endothelial produced IL-8) induce directed motility through three-dimensional matrixes and migration of PMN into tissue stroma.[54] It is important to note that this process of PMN-endothelial cell adherence can be elicited from hypoxemia with or without reoxygenation itself and appears to be mediated by both CD11a/CD18– and CD11a/CD18–dependent interactions with ICAM-1.[55] Recent data demonstrate that hypoxemia alone is capable of inducing PMN CD18–dependent adherence to fibronectin.[56] Hypoxemia with or without reoxygenation has also upregulated PMN phagocytosis and chemotaxis.[57]

The key physiologic relevance of hypoxemia with or without reoxygenation is the fact that following PMN endothelial cell or interstitial matrix protein adherence, PMN can induce tissue injury. Several lines of data support this concept. A monoclonal antibody (R17) directed against CD11b/CD18 was recently shown to reduce lung and liver injury after intestinal ischemia-reperfusion.[58] Second, phospholipase A_2 inhibition reduces lung injury following intestinal ischemia-reperfusion.[59] Most importantly, the use of antioxidants has been shown to reduce organ system injury in various experimental models.[60] Use of antioxidants, however, is predicated on an understanding of the PMN oxidative cascade. The critical enzyme in this pathway is NADPH oxidase. Activation of this enzyme involves guanosine diphosphate (GTP)-binding proteins of the Ras superfamily. A cytosolic GTP-binding protein (G_{ox}) regulates NADPH oxidase in human neutrophils; in addition, NADPH oxidase is associated with GDP/cytidine triphosphate (CTP) recycline, which is mediated by Rac 2 and rap 1A (GTP-binding proteins). Ultimately, gp^{91}-phox and p22 phox subunits of cytochrome b_{558} are activated with eventual production of molecular oxygen products (superoxide anion, etc.).[61,62]

Oxygen-derived free radicals, especially the hydroxyl radical, interact with membrane polyunsaturated fatty acids, leading to lipid peroxidation and cell death. Vitamin E, by protecting the conjugated double bonds of β-carotene from oxidation, has been shown to reduce DIC, decrease the incidence of lipid peroxidation, and improve survival in mice after endotoxin administration.[63] *N*-acetyl cysteine, which directly scavenges hydrogen peroxide and reacts with hydroxyl radicals, reduced lung microvascular permeability and intracellular coagulation in endotoxemic mice.[64] In man, a marked reduction in mortality was observed in sepsis-related ARDS when patients were given selenium (a constituent of glutathione reductase), ascorbic acid (direct cytosolic antioxidant), and *N*-acetyl cysteine.[65] Additional studies are required for confirmation prior to generalized use.

Taken together, these new findings demonstrate that following periods of ischemia-reperfusion and/or hypoxemia with or without reoxygenation, tissue injury is mediated in large part by activated PMN. This involves both PMN-endothelial cell adherence and subsequent migration into interstitial tissues. Tissue damage is caused in large part by toxic reactive oxygen metabolites derived from PMN.

The Cell

The primary pathophysiology of shock at the cellular level is a change in metabolism affecting energy production and function. Crucial to cell function is the need for oxygen as basic fuel. Aerobic metabolism more efficiently replenishes the high-energy phosphates required for ongoing metabolism. Under low flow, poor perfusion states, less oxygen is delivered, and the cells are forced into a state of anaerobic metabolism. In this situation, fewer high-energy bonds are created, and cellular efficiency is reduced as the acidosis generated anaerobically alters normal enzyme kinetics.[12,13,66] This observation serves as the basis for ATP-n-$MgCl_2$ therapy, *an approach that has not attained clinical implementation.*

The major protective mechanism of a cell is its membrane.[4] This bi-lipid layer, which is composed of fatty acids, is responsible for the ionic differential that exists between the cell and its surrounding environment and maintains the high-potassium and low-sodium intracellular concentrations. Malfunction of this membrane ultimately sets the stage for cellular death. When this occurs, sodium moves into the cell, drawing with it a volume of water appropriate to maintain osmotic equilibrium with the surrounding interstitial space. The resulting cellular edema ultimately impairs normal intracellular metabolism, causing cell death. Cell membrane damage may be the result of a primary insult from endotoxin, complement, or some other unidentified agent that may accumulate during shock. Membrane injury may also occur secondarily from deranged intracellular metabolism that fails to regulate the sodium/potassium ratio within the cell or its corresponding concentration of calcium, a substance necessary for normal enzyme function. Failure of mitochondrial oxidative phosphorylation and the accumulation of lactic acid and other anions within the cell, also produce intracellular and membrane damage. In general, the accumulation of hydrogen ion in the cell results in intracellular acidosis and is detrimental to all cellular organelle function. In addition to the ion and water changes that may occur within the cell when its membrane loses its integrity, such disruption may also alter normal responses to various circulating agents such as catecholamines, corticosteroids, insulin, and glucagon, substances that play important roles in normal cellular metabolism. Thus an "expected response" may be attenuated or exaggerated, depending on the state of cellular enzymes at the time of the shock injury.

Although the cell and microcirculation have been considered separately in this discussion, it must be remembered that any perturbations in their function secondary to shock are intimately related. Thus alterations in the microcirculation secondary to a low flow state generally result in derangements in normal cellular metabolism because of the absence of adequate oxygen and nutrients to maintain cell function. Similarly, aberrations in cellular physiology alter the surrounding microcirculation secondary to the accumulation of hydrogen ion and the release of such lysosomal enzymes as acid phosphatases and dehydrogenases.

Organ Failure in Shock

With the exception of neurogenic shock, which is usually mild and easily controlled, all forms of shock, if severe enough, can result in major organ dysfunction. The pattern of this dysfunction relates to (1) the various abilities of organs to withstand hypoxia and low flow, (2) the type of shock insult (hypovolemic vs. septic), and (3) the underlying basic metabolic rate. This dysfunction is further influenced by the degree of "organ reserve" and the innate ability of a particular organ to withstand a metabolic insult. If preexisting or intercurrent disease is present, the ability of a given organ to withstand the detrimental effects of low flow and hypoxia are further compromised.

The *kidney* is a flow-sensitive organ that, as previously noted, is involved in the basic compensatory response to shock, acting to conserve sodium and water. The mechanisms responsible for this action include the renin-angiotensin system, release of ADH from the pituitary gland, and intrinsic regulatory alterations within the kidney tubules themselves. If shock is severe enough, a considerable redistribution of blood flow away from the kidney may occur to provide a more effective circulation to other organs, such as the heart and brain. In this circumstance, the kidney may sustain an ischemic insult as a result of the accompanying poor perfusion. Sepsis and other factors (e.g., nephrotoxic drugs) may further aggravate this insult. When renal function is impaired secondary to shock, one of two responses may occur: oliguric renal failure or high-output (i.e., nonoliguric) renal failure. These two clinical presentations probably represent different points on a continuum of acute renal failure. The exact mechanisms underlying these different presentations are not known; but it is generally accepted that in oliguric failure, poor perfusion and anoxia alter glomerular function, which is reflected in a lower glomerular filtration rate and a decrease in urine output. In nonoliguric renal failure, a diuretic form of renal dysfunction occurs, presumably from a lesser insult to the glomerulus and renal tubules.

The *liver* has a high metabolic rate and plays a prominent role in protein synthesis, among other functions. The liver depends on an adequate blood flow; under normal conditions approximately 30% of the cardiac output is directed to this organ by way of the hepatic artery (systemic circulation) and portal vein (splanchnic circulation). In hypovolemic states, the liver "autotransfuses" its vascular contents by mechanically shunting inflow to the hepatic sinusoids. In moderate-to-severe states of shock, the splanchnic blood flow may decrease significantly (by as much as 40% to 50%), resulting in a corresponding decrease in flow to the hepatic Kupffer cells, the name given to the hepatic reticuloendothelial system. As a consequence of this event, the filtration of debris and bacteria by the liver is impaired, allowing toxic material to pass through it to the lungs. Although significant morphologic damage can be detected in the liver soon after shock—particularly shock occurring after hemorrhage—clinical evidence of hepatic dysfunction is often absent. Generally, only a modest increase in serum bilirubin concentration is noted, whereas other indexes of liver function remain normal or show only modest abnormalities. Thus if a patient is successfully resuscitated from shock, liver dysfunction is only minor in terms of clinical significance. In shock patients in whom sepsis is a major underlying etiologic factor, pronounced liver failure may occur, with serum bilirubin concentrations reaching levels as high as 15 to 20 mg/100 ml. Histologic examination of such livers has usually revealed fatty infiltration. Although impaired perfusion probably plays a role in the pathogenesis of this failure, the exact mechanisms responsible for it remain ill defined. Interestingly, in septic and/or endotoxin-infused animal models simulating septic shock, hepatic lactate use is diminished. Thus the use of a lactated Ringer's solution in patients with septic shock is probably contraindicated; an acetate-based solution should be used in its place.[6]

The *pancreas* and *gastrointestinal tract,* other organs that are very active metabolically, may also be adversely affected in shock. The changes in insulin and glucagon release that occur during sepsis and hypovolemia indicate that the pancreas is influenced by the shock state. Whether these responses are primarily protective mechanisms to assist the body in meeting its metabolic demands, or whether they occur because of impaired perfusion to the pancreas, remains to be determined. There is some evidence that the pancreas releases a myocardial depressant factor during shock that is directly related to impaired blood flow to this organ.

In contrast to the uncertain effects of shock on the pancreas, both sepsis and hypovolemia have been shown to have adverse effects on the gastric mucosa through impaired blood flow. The resulting erosive gastritis may produce profound hemorrhage that by itself is life threatening. It is now known that buffering gastric acid with topical antacids and antisecretory agents such as cimetidine can significantly lessen this risk. The potentially adverse effect of shock on blood flow to the intestinal mucosa is less certain. Since this epithelial surface forms a barrier to protect the host from its luminal environment, it seems likely that its breakdown in response to ischemia could allow a sudden influx of bacteria and toxins to cross the intestinal wall and translocate to other organs. There is some experimental evidence to suggest that such a breakdown can occur in severe states of shock (particularly hemorrhagic) and can be responsible for the delayed sepsis that can occur following initial resuscitation.[25]

The response of the *lungs* to shock has been studied extensively. Critical for survival following any shock insult is the lungs' basic function of oxygenation. It is now clearly recognized that the lung may suffer profoundly adverse effects from shock and its resuscitation and that pulmonary failure is a major complication contributing to mortality and morbidity in shock. This relates to the lung's function as a natural filter for intravenous debris, cellular aggregates, lipids, and bone marrow particles. When these materials lodge deep in the pulmonary capillaries, they initiate an

Table 8-5. Basic Hemodynamic and Metabolic Abnormalities Seen in Shock

Indicator	Hypovolemic	Cardiogenic	Hyperdynamic	Hypodynamic
Blood pressure	−	−/N/+	−	− −
Pulse rate	++	+	+++	+
Central venous pressure	− −	N/+	N/+	−
Respiration rate	+	++	++++	++
Urinary output	−	−	+/−	−
Cardiac index	−	− −	++	−
Pulmonary capillary wedge pressure	− −	++	−/N	−/N
Peripheral resistance	+++	+	− − −	− −
Arteriovenous oxygen difference	++	+	− −	−
PO_2	−	−	−	−
PCO_2	−	+/−	−/+	++
Arterial pH	−	−	−/N	−
Arterial lactate	++	+	−/N	+/−
Response to volume load*	+++	−	+	− −
Skin temperature	Cold	Cold	Warm	Cold
Skin sensation to touch	Clammy	Clammy	Dry	Clammy

Symbols: −, decreased, +, increased, *N*, normal. The relative magnitude of change is shown by multiple plus or minus signs.
*Usually 250 to 500 ml of balanced salt solution; this will increase blood pressure, decrease heart rate, and increase cardiac output.

INDICATIONS FOR INTUBATION AND VENTILATORY SUPPORT

Respiration rate of 30 breaths/min or greater
PCO_2 greater than 45 mm Hg with metabolic acidosis
PCO_2 greater than 50 mm Hg with normal bicarbonate levels
PO_2 less than 60 mm Hg on 40% O_2
Tidal volume less than 5 ml/kg
Vital capacity less than 10 ml/kg
Minute ventilation less than 8 L/min
Excessive ventilatory effort

states. A normal sensorium generally indicates adequate tissue perfusion.

Treatment Considerations

Ventilation

Failure of respiratory gas exchange is one of the most frequent causes of death in patients with shock. Thus the first priority in treating shock is to ensure effective ventilation. Maintenance of adequate oxygen and carbon dioxide exchange is essential to survival. In the traumatized, septic, or hypovolemic patient, there is a significantly higher oxygen demand that often reaches twice normal. Under most circumstances, hyperventilation provides an effective means of increasing oxygen delivery when needed. The shock patient, however, has difficulty exerting this additional effort and rapidly develops signs of respiratory failure together with respiratory acidosis. Depending on the magnitude of shock, supplemental oxygen may help to maintain efficient oxygen delivery. In more severe situations, endotracheal intubation and ventilatory assistance may be warranted, as discussed elsewhere in this book and summarized in the accompanying box. Critically ill patients (especially comatose and lethargic patients) must be intubated early to avoid respiratory failure.

The goals of ventilator therapy, when it is needed, are relatively specific. Respiratory alkalosis must be avoided. Adjusting the respiratory rate to ensure a PCO_2 of 35 to 40 mm Hg maintains cerebral perfusion and avoids a left shift of the oxyhemoglobin dissociation curve, which results in an increased affinity of oxygen for hemoglobin (see Chapter 33). Such a left shift represents a significant decrease in oxygen availability to tissues and requires a hemodynamic compensation by way of increased cardiac output to maintain adequate tissue oxygenation. Generally, the arterial PO_2 is maintained at 80 to 100 mm Hg through provision of an inspired oxygen concentration that is as low as possible. Failure to achieve this goal requires additional inspired oxygen or the use of end-expiratory pressure to improve oxygenation by increasing the functional residual capacity of the lungs. Peak inspiratory pressure is minimized to avoid barotrauma (i.e., pneumothorax), pressures less than 20 to 22 cm of water being desirable. A tidal volume of 9 to 13 ml/kg of body weight, which exceeds normal by 50% or more, is generally needed to respond to the increased metabolic and oxygenation demands in shock patients.

Perfusion

After adequate ventilation is assured, aggressive restoration of an "effective" circulating blood volume becomes the central focus of therapy. Volume resuscitation brings about a rapid improvement in circulatory status and oxygen delivery.[2,70] At the same time that fluid is being administered to restore blood volume, pharmacologic intervention may prove useful. There is mounting evidence that many of the hemodynamic aberrations induced by shock are amenable to pharmacologic manipulation.

The improved cardiac output that follows such maneuvers enhances oxygen delivery and tissue perfusion, as described by the relationship between cardiac output (CO), arterial oxygen content (CaO_2), and oxygen delivery:

$$\text{Oxygen delivery} = \text{CO (ml/min)} \times CaO_2 \text{ (ml of } O_2 \text{ per 100 ml of blood)}$$

Oxygen content is described in terms of hemoglobin (Hb) concentration, oxygen saturation (SO_2), and arterial oxygen pressure (PO_2) by the relation:

$$CaO_2 = Hb \times SO_2 \times 1.34 + Hb \times 0.00034\ PO_2$$

Both saturation and PO_2 depend at least partially on the inspired oxygen content (FIO_2) and the pulmonary status of a patient in terms of gas exchange. Increases in oxygen content (by way of blood transfusion or supplemental oxygen administration) and/or flow (cardiac output) enhance oxygen delivery. The rapid restoration of vascular volume in the hypovolemic patient increases cardiac output and thus oxygen delivery. Increasing the volume of a hypovolemic patient by 25% to 35% frequently increases cardiac output by more than 100%. In response to this enhanced output, normalization of oxygen consumption occurs, which indicates restoration of tissue perfusion.[3]

Resuscitation fluids. Balanced salt solutions are effective volume expanders for the initial resuscitation of patients from shock. If hypovolemia from the loss of fluid (e.g., diarrhea) or blood (e.g., gastrointestinal hemorrhage) is the underlying cause of the shock, a volume of solution in excess of measured losses is generally required to effect improved function and survival.[7,38] The additional fluid, 1 to 1.5 times the fluid lost, replaces the extracellular fluid deficit that results from the rapid equilibration of plasma volume with interstitial fluid (Table 8-6). For most patients, lactated Ringer's solution is the preferred resuscitation solution. The lactate ion acts as a buffer, eventually being metabolized to carbon dioxide and water. Septic patients and those with significant hepatic dysfunction, do not metabolize lactate well.[6] For these individuals, balanced salt solutions with acetate as the major anion are preferred.

Initially, the hypovolemic patient is given 2 to 3 L of crystalloid, and the response of pulse rate, blood pressure, and urinary output is observed. If this therapy fails to correct hemodynamic abnormalities, as may occur in patients sustaining significant blood losses, additional crystalloid followed by type-specific blood is indicated, especially if an urgent operation is anticipated to control the blood loss. It must be remembered that crystalloids in large quantities ultimately provoke a dilutional effect that can significantly decrease the blood's oxygen-carrying capacity. *Large-volume crystalloid resuscitation has been shown detrimental in certain experimental models that include uncontrolled hemorrhage as a component. These models may more closely approximate clinical situations and thus have relevance to clinical resuscitation.*[71-73] Even in this setting, delivery of oxygen to tissues may be improved because of the restored vascular volume and the accompanying increase in cardiac output through the mechanisms discussed earlier (see Perfusion). Nevertheless, even though a young, nondiseased heart can mount a sustained increase in cardiac output in response to this excess fluid, an older patient with coronary arteriosclerotic disease is generally unable to do so and may develop myocardial failure or infarction from this added stress. In these older patients, red-cell blood transfusions should be given early in the resuscitation to obviate this problem.

Table 8-6. Endogenous Response to Loss of Circulating Blood Volume

Mechanism	Time Frame (With No Therapeutic Intervention)
Restoration/maintenance of hemodynamic stability; redistribution of flow	Seconds to minutes
Restoration of vascular volume; transcapillary refill, primarily from interstitial fluid compartment	3-4 hr
Restoration of vascular volume with albumin stores	18-24 hr
Addition of new (i.e., synthesized) albumin	24-36 hr
Replacement of lost red-cell mass	3-5 wk

The sequence of events assumes that the loss of blood volume was mild to moderate and that survival does not depend on therapeutic intervention.

Although crystalloids are the preferred solution for resuscitation in shock, with the use of red cells as indicated for massive or ongoing blood losses, colloid solutions such as albumin have also been advocated in shock treatment. Colloid solutions, however, are expensive and have no apparent advantage over crystalloids, provided similar physiologic end points are measured. In addition, there is some evidence that colloids may be detrimental in treating shock.[74,75] When given to equivalent cardiac filling pressures during elective surgical procedures, for example, these solutions are effective for volume replacement, and no apparent differences in pulmonary function— presumably from increased lung water—can be detected. However, such resuscitation is actually controlled volume replacement, a model not really comparable to the hypovolemia and ischemia that occur in shock. Real differences are apparent, though, in septic patients in whom the leak of proteins across a damaged pulmonary membrane can be demonstrated with colloids. Albumin, for example, produces a significant oncotic effect, drawing and holding water in the alveoli and impairing cellular function. On the other hand, there are no firm data to support the idea of a decrease in oncotic pressure being detrimental in the shock state, provided the vascular pressures are not allowed to exceed acceptable levels. It may be that a difference in the hydrostatic and oncotic pressures is more important for fluid flux into the lungs or other tissues than is an absolute level of either. Based on these considerations, colloids are not recommended as being of any major importance in the treatment of shock.[73]

The role of hypertonic salt resuscitation in shock management remains undefined. This form of treatment has been tested in patients undergoing elective major vascular surgery, and it appears effective.[76] *Results in trauma resuscitation have been equivocal at best. An attractive concept, low-volume resuscitation could obviate additional hemorrhage and thus conserve red-cell volume. When coupled with aggressive prehospital systems, benefits may arise for specific subsets of patients.*[11,22,77] The concept of hypertonic resuscitation is based on the aim of refilling the intravascular space with interstitial fluid by drawing on the body's reserves to augment intravascular volume.[78,79] In elective surgery in well-hydrated patients, this aim may be valid. In hypotensive, hypovolemic patients, it may not achieve the desired results because the interstitial space is already contracted and cannot serve as a reserve.

Starches can also be used for volume expansion and have been employed successfully in the treatment of shock. These agents are nonprotein plant derivatives that have little antigenicity. On the basis of molecular size and weight, they increase oncotic pressure by binding plasma water or by drawing interstitial fluid into the vascular space and thus rearranging water distribution in much the same way that hypertonic saline does. Two particular starches, dextran and hydroxyethyl starch (HES), have been shown to improve capillary perfusion by augmentation of cardiac output and flow and also by lowering viscosity. HES has fewer problems than dextran in the clinical setting and is an effective and safe volume expander and resuscitative agent.[80] Despite their ability to resuscitate shock patients, there is no evidence that starch solutions are more effective than crystalloids in this regard, and the starches are considerably more expensive.

Transfusion of blood and blood products

General principles. Although intravenous infusion of balanced salt solutions is an appropriate therapeutic modality in the early treatment of shock, transfusion of blood and/or blood products is eventually required in hypovolemic shock secondary to hemorrhage.[70] Because of the many physiologic functions of blood, its importance in the treatment of hemorrhagic shock cannot be overemphasized. Unlike salt solutions, whose primary role in shock is to re-establish an effective circulating blood volume, blood, in addition to this function, possesses the unique ability to transport oxygen and also provides coagulation factors that ultimately become depleted if hemorrhage continues.

Since so much of the body's physiology depends on oxygen delivery, this function must be supported to avoid any significant hemodynamic or respiratory compromise in already stressed patients. Maintenance of near-normal levels of hemoglobin may have a benefit in providing reserve when an additional stress is encountered. The intimate relationship between hemoglobin concentration and the adequacy of oxygen consumption at the tissue level is well established[81] and underscores the importance of maintaining normal levels of hemoglobin in circulating blood. Since increases in oxygen availability can be provided only by increasing blood flow to tissues or by enhancing the blood's oxygen-carrying capacity, red-cell transfusions are particularly useful in this subset of shock patients. In hemorrhagic shock, excessive loss of blood or massive ongoing losses (i.e., 100 ml/min) often occur. In such patients, it is desirable to maintain hemoglobin concentrations at 10 g/100 ml *and global oxygen delivery as normal* to provide some reserve in the oxygen delivery system while preparations are being made to control the etiologic factor(s) responsible for the blood loss.

In the past, whole-blood transfusions were fashionable in the treatment of hemorrhagic shock; in contrast, only red-cell transfusions are recommended today to provide an adequate hemoglobin concentration, with concurrent supplementation of crystalloid solutions to maintain an adequate circulating blood volume. The other blood components can then be used to benefit patients who do not require red cells but who have a particular need for a specific component to treat an underlying physiologic deficit, such as a clotting deficiency. Table 8-7 gives the primary components of blood, their forms and storage modalities, and the defects corrected by their administration.

Because of the rapidity of blood loss in hemorrhagic shock and the need to correct the diminished oxygen-carrying capacity quickly, *stored* red cells are generally transfused. Depending on the age of these cells, optimal oxygen delivery to tissues may not be as ideal as one wishes, since stored red cells develop a specific defect in energy metabolism (i.e., a loss of 2,3-diphosphoglyceric acid and adenosine triphosphate [ATP]) that results in an increased affinity of oxygen for hemoglobin and an accompanying shift in the oxyhemoglobin dissociation curve to the left (see Chapter 33). If this shift is significant, a hemodynamic compensation (i.e., increased cardiac output) may be required to ensure adequate oxygen delivery to ischemic tissues. In such blood, there is sufficient oxygen present, but it is not "available" because of the tight binding of oxygen to hemoglobin. Large quantities of old, banked red cells can induce this effect, which usually corrects itself within 24 hours of infusion. The exact physiologic impact of high-oxygen-affinity blood remains controversial. By itself the effect may be minimal; but when coupled with existing hemodynamic, metabolic, and cardiac abnormalities, it may be significant.[2,82] Newer blood preservation techniques have addressed the issue of red-cell energy loss so that shelf storage can be enhanced and prolonged without compromising patient care. Older blood is usually used during the period of ongoing blood loss, despite the potential metabolic defect. Fresher red cells are preferred once the blood loss has been controlled, as these cells last longer and provide more efficient oxygen delivery.

In a number of trauma centers, autologous blood has been used to replace ongoing blood losses in shock patients, together with attempts at operative correction of the bleeding site. This autotransfusion of lost blood has

Table 8-7. Blood Components

Component	Volume (ml) Administered	Expected Increase (70 kg Patient)	Deficit Corrected
Oxygen carriers			
Whole blood	500	2-3%, Hematocrit	Anemia, plasma volume
Red cells, packed	250-300	3-4%, Hematocrit	Anemia
Frozen	200	2-3%, Hematocrit	Anemia
WBC poor	200	2-3%, Hematocrit	Anemia
Coagulation factors			
Platelets	35-50	5-10,000/U of platelets	Thrombocytopenia (absolute, functional)
Fresh frozen plasma	210-250	3-4%, Factor VIII	Coagulation factors; fibrinogen
Cryoprecipitate	10-25	2-3%, Factor VIII; 10-30 mg fibronectin	Coagulation factors; fibrinogen; factor VIII; fibronectin
Oncotic agents			
Albumin			
Standard	250	—	Plasma volume expansion
Salt poor	25	—	Plasma volume expansion
Plasma protein factor	250	—	Plasma volume expansion
Other			
Granulocyte	50-75	2-500/unit	Leukopenia
Gamma globulin	100-300	3-5%/unit	Compromised immune system

proved to be an effective and useful therapeutic tool in selected cases of hemorrhagic shock. Although the risk of transfusion reactions is virtually eliminated with this approach, contamination is a potentially serious problem, since the collected blood is often mixed with other body secretions and thus requires careful filtering before its infusion.

Although the ideal in transfusion therapy is the use of fresh frozen blood, its availability is often limited. Further, the time required to thaw and prepare it for infusion often limits its usefulness in a patient who requires blood quickly.[83] Finally, once thawed, fresh frozen blood has a shelf life of only 24 hours. Thus in most situations this form of blood is not applicable for treatment in the majority of shock patients requiring urgent transfusion.

Unless life-threatening blood loss is encountered, blood should not be administered until definitive typing and crossmatching have been done. Only if resuscitation with salt solutions is not efficacious should emergency blood transfusions be given. In this circumstance, type-specific blood may prove to be lifesaving until the crossmatch has been completed.

Consequences of transfusion therapy. Although blood transfusions are necessary in the treatment of most patients sustaining hemorrhagic shock (unless the bleeding is mild and stops spontaneously), it must be remembered that transfusion therapy is not without risks. Thus in deciding to transfuse a patient, one must be fully aware of the potential complications and be prepared to manage them should they occur. The morbidity and mortality associated with transfusion therapy are directly related to the volume of blood infused (i.e., the greater the volume infused, the greater the risk). Posttransfusion fatalities generally result from clerical errors and are usually associated with a single-unit transfusion that is not compatible with the patient's own blood type. Despite occasional human error during infusion of blood, transfusion reactions are relatively rare (less than 0.05%). The transmission of disease by infused blood, once thought to be 10% to 12%, is probably less but is clearly related to the donor population. *The risk per unit of transfused red cell or blood product for the common problems is shown in Table 8-8.*

Citrate toxicity and hypothermia are rate related. The infusion of stored blood, unwarmed, at a rate in excess of 100 ml/min results in the binding of ionized serum calcium, which produces myocardial depression and dysrhythmias. High levels of citrate, seen with rapid infusion, sensitize the myocardium to the effects of potassium. Each unit of old, banked blood or red cells contains 10 to 20 mEq or more of potassium. In the presence of excess citrate, the myocardium is in peril. Calcium chloride, 2.5 mEq/U, is given when the rate of infusion exceeds 100 ml/min. Hypothermia likewise ensues when cold blood is infused too rapidly. Hypothermia also induces a sensitive myocardium, which in the face of altered calcium and potassium concentrations, may precipitate arrhythmias with untoward hemodynamic consequences.

A dilutional coagulopathy can be seen after massive blood transfusions.[84] This is primarily a thrombocytopenia and is corrected with infusion of platelets once the major bleeding site is controlled. One unit of platelets raises the peripheral platelet count by 5000 to 10,000 cells. Therapy for counts over 60,000 is usually not necessary.

Various diseases can also be transmitted by blood (e.g., hepatitis, AIDS, parasites). There is likewise the possibility of infusing bacteria or contaminated blood products, resulting in septicemia. Emboli to the lungs (i.e., air and microembolic debris) are similarly possible during blood

Table 8-8. Transfusion-Related Complications Risk per Unit Transfused, United States-1994

	Rate	Incidence (% per unit)
Minor allergic reaction	1:100	(1)
Viral hepatitis, overall	1:5,000	(0.02)
90%—Hepatitis C		
2%—Hepatitis B		
Hemolytic reaction	1:6,000	(0.02)
Fatal hemolytic reaction	1:600,000	(0.0002)
HIV infection	1:420,000	(0.0002)
Human T-cell leukemia (HTLV) I/II	1:200,000	(0.0005)

From Greenburg AG. Benefits and risks of blood transfusion in surgical patients. World J Surg 20:1189, 1996. Reprinted by permission of The Western Journal of Medicine.

transfusion, with a potentially dire outcome. This latter complication is considered a technical problem during administration and should be preventable if appropriate care is exercised.

Immunologically modulated transfusion reactions can be immediate or delayed and have been traced to virtually every component of blood. Immediate hemolytic reactions are almost always the result of a clerical error in which mismatched blood is infused. Bleeding, fever, hypotension, pain in the back (referred from kidneys), and a constricting feeling in the chest are possible clinical signs of a transfusion reaction. The patient in the operating room and asleep may manifest only a slight coagulopathy; the hemolysis resulting from such a reaction may be fatal. If the reaction occurs, the transfusion should be stopped immediately, all clerical information should be rechecked, and the typing and crossmatch should be repeated. Specific therapy includes maintaining adequate renal blood flow and treatment of any hypotension, both with intravenous crystalloid solutions. A diuretic can be added to aid in the renal clearance of toxins developing from the transfusion reactions. In terms of renal damage, the red-cell stroma (i.e., cell wall), not the hemoglobin, is the primary offending agent. If renal failure ensues, prompt dialysis is indicated.

White cells, platelets, and proteins can also induce immediate or delayed immunologic reactions, all modulated by the immune system. Graft-vs.-host disease, a rare complication of blood transfusion, is seen primarily in immunosuppressed patients.

Blockade of the host-defense system and immune mechanisms may also be a consequence of transfusion therapy. In the severely ill patient, it is unwise to compromise this important system. Debris from red-cell transfusions can lodge in the pulmonary circuit, producing local inflammation and infiltrates. The exact effects are not usually apparent in terms of altered clinical function; this probably reflects our lack of sensitivity in detecting such abnormalities.

Pharmacologic Interventions

In the historical development of recommended treatment modalities for shock, both vasoconstrictive and vasodilatory drugs have been in vogue at different times as potentially useful agents. It was thought that vasoconstrictor drugs could assist in increasing blood pressure until effective circulating blood volume was restored. It is now known that the already compromised tissue perfusion is further aggravated by such vasoconstriction, which therefore actually compounds the shock state rather than assisting in its control. Similarly, vasodilator drugs were thought advantageous in improving flow to tissues at the microcirculatory level. Despite the logic of this concept, the clinical use of these agents did not bring improvement and actually resulted in peripheral pooling of blood, with adverse effects on cardiac output. As the pathophysiology of shock has become more clearly understood, both of these treatment approaches have been abandoned.

The major role of vasoactive drugs in modern shock treatment relates to their potentially useful inotropic and chronotropic effects on the heart. Since an appropriate cardiac output is desirable in patients with shock, factors that govern heart rate and stroke volume can be manipulated to improve peripheral blood flow. Although such therapy cannot be justified as appropriate routine treatment, it may prove efficacious in patients with compromised cardiac reserve.

As discussed in more detail in Chapter 37, stroke volume is governed by ventricular preload, afterload, and contractility. Although preload is primarily influenced by the volume of circulating blood, both afterload and contractility can be manipulated by a number of pharmacologic agents. Afterload reduction may prove efficacious in the patient who has a relatively normal or slightly depressed arterial blood pressure, but in whom the cardiac output is low and the pulmonary arterial wedge pressure is high (>18 mm Hg). Nitroprusside is especially useful for this circumstance and has balanced vasodilating effects on both the arterial and venous circulations, so that adverse affects on arterial blood pressure are minimized. Nitroglycerin has also been used for this purpose, but its action is primarily to dilate the venous capacitance vessels—specifically the pulmonary vasculature—and it has only minimal effects on systemic vasodilation. Recent studies have also suggested that PGE_2 may be an effective reducer of cardiac afterload, but the precise effects of this agent, which appear to be directed primarily on the pulmonary circulation, require further investigation.[15] Ganglionic blocking agents have also been employed to reduce afterload, but, since their effects are primarily on the arterioles, systemic hypotension has been a major side effect. If used appropriately, afterload reduction—particularly with an easy-to-titrate agent such as nitroprusside—should result in an effective increase in cardiac output, with little or no change in arterial blood pressure.

A number of agents have been shown to effectively improve cardiac contractility by their inotropic effects.[3] The major agents used for this purpose today are dopamine, dobutamine, isoproterenol, and digoxin. Each of these agents has specific properties that can prove useful in altering hemodynamics to obtain the desired therapeutic effect. Dopamine, for example, effectively increases both blood pressure and cardiac output and thus improves oxygen delivery to tissues. Dopamine appears to have specific effects on renal blood flow (presumably through dopamine receptors) and thus can be especially beneficial when the clinical situation suggests that renal perfusion is a problem. Dopamine has been used effectively in the treatment of both cardiogenic and hypovolemic shock, with minimal side effects. Its use in septic shock has been less impressive. Failure to respond to dopamine is most likely the result of inadequate cyclic adenosine monophosphate (cAMP) in tissues (which is necessary for membrane function and receptor integrity) or to the presence of alkalosis. Both conditions are frequently seen in septic patients. Dobutamine is similar to dopamine in its inotropic effects and has proved useful in situations in which dopamine has not been effective.

Isoproterenol and epinephrine have also been shown to be effective inotropic agents. Isoproterenol not only improves ventricular contraction but increases the heart rate as well. Because it also decreases peripheral resistance, it is a very useful agent when this effect is desired in combination with the drug's cardiac effects. Epinephrine is likewise an effective inotropic and chronotropic agent, but it can cause increases in peripheral resistance and ventricular irritability. Thus it must be administered more cautiously than isoproterenol and is probably contraindicated in hypovolemic patients. Norepinephrine also has both inotropic and chronotropic effects, but unfortunately its peripheral effects of increased vascular resistance and increased afterload augment and exaggerate its potentially beneficial effects on cardiac contraction. Some investigators have proposed that an α-adrenergic blocking agent be used in combination with norepinephrine to enhance its cardiac effects; but with the availability of other agents, this is generally considered inappropriate and potentially dangerous.

Although digitalis compounds, and particularly digoxin, are the mainstay of drugs used to enhance cardiac contractility, their use in acute situations such as shock is limited because it takes considerable time for even the more rapid-acting compounds to have an effect. Consequently, another inotropic drug is usually required if cardiac support must be assured more expeditiously. In less acute situations, digoxin is the most appropriate drug and is quite effective when there is a need for a prolonged increase in cardiac contractility.

Occasionally, the blood-ionized calcium levels may be low in patients in shock, particularly those in whom a septic component is present. This calcium depletion may have adverse effects on cardiac hemodynamics. In patients in septic shock with low calcium levels, cautious infusion of ionized calcium is effective in enhancing cardiac output.

Glucagon also has inotropic effects, but compared with the agents discussed previously, its action is weak. Its effects are most likely mediated through mobilization of stored glycogen. In addition, glucagon also has slight direct vasoconstrictor activity. As a routine inotropic drug, glucagon has no advantage over other agents and thus is not recommended by most clinicians.

Over the years, steroids have been intermittently recommended as an effective adjunctive measure in the treatment of shock, particularly in patients with septic shock. The physiologic basis for using steroids stems from experimental observations in various animal models in which these agents have been shown to have a protective effective against gram negative organisms and/or their endotoxins, presumably through membrane and lysosomal stabilization. Since experimental evidence suggests that the most opportune time to give steroids is early in the pathogenesis of septic shock, at a time when the glucocorticoid and mineralocorticoid response to shock is maximal, it is unlikely that exogenous administration of these agents would offer any additional benefit. In those studies that have addressed this issue in some systematic fashion, there has been virtually no evidence to support the claim that steroids should be used in the treatment of shock.

The use of antibiotics in the treatment of shock depends on the underlying etiologic factor. For most forms of hypovolemic and cardiogenic shock, antibiotic coverage cannot be justified. If tissue injury produces the shock, as may occur from vascular disruption secondary to penetrating trauma, antibiotics may prove efficacious in preventing the subsequent development of wound infections and/or abscesses. In this circumstance, a broad-spectrum antibiotic should be administered as early as possible after wounding and should be continued for 2 or 3 days thereafter. In contrast to their relative significance in hypovolemic or cardiogenic shock, antibiotics form an important component of therapy in the management of patients with septic shock. In fact, the antibiotic selected for the patient with sepsis is the most important determinant of subsequent morbidity and mortality. Thus every effort must be made to select an antibiotic against the organism that seems most likely to be responsible for the underlying infection. In general, the antibiotic should have broad-spectrum properties and should be administered intravenously to ensure adequate blood levels. Frequently a combination of antibiotics are needed. For gram-negative infections, an aminoglycoside is an appropriate first-line defense agent. If the infection is thought to be gram positive in origin, particularly if cocci are involved, intravenous penicillin should be administered. When the antibiotic sensitivities have been determined from the cultured sources thought to be responsible for the infection, appropriate alterations in antibiotic coverage can be instituted as needed. Since surgical drainage is ultimately necessary in most patients to eradicate the source of infection, it is important that high blood levels of antibiotics be established before operative intervention and continued for a reasonable period of time thereafter (usually 7 to 10 days).

MAST Trousers

MAST trousers, or the MAST suit, is a pneumatic antishock garment that is placed on a patient much as a pair of pants would be and then is filled with air to a predetermined pressure. First introduced during the Vietnam war, its purpose is to maintain effective circulating blood volume by reducing perfusion to the lower half of the body and increasing peripheral resistance so that blood flow is directed centrally to maintain flow to oxygen-sensitive organs such as the heart and brain. Although the logic underlying its use is quite simple, its effect on prolonging survival in seriously ill patients in hypovolemic shock remains to be determined. Its major use in most trauma centers has been in stabilizing pelvic and long bone fractures to reduce the severe blood loss accompanying these disorders until other resuscitative efforts can be effectively administered. Problems relating to its use include restriction of rib cage motion by the abdominal portion of the garment because of the compression of the abdominal contents and elevation of the diaphragm. Such restriction can markedly reduce the vital capacity of the lungs. In addition, the increased blood pressure that often occurs following application of this garment may lead to increased bleeding above the level of the trousers. Since most reports summarizing the efficacy of MAST trousers in the treatment of hypovolemic shock are based on anecdotal accounts, its role in shock treatment must await further studies.

Future Therapeutic Modalities

Blood substitutes

Red-cell substitutes. Since the major function of red blood cells in the treatment of shock relates to their oxygen-carrying capacity, considerable interest has been generated in recent years in developing red-cell substitutes.[85] One approach has used enzymatic cleavage of specific blood-type antigens from the surface of red cells, creating in effect a universal blood donor. The merit of this approach is that it eliminates the need to type and crossmatch blood before infusion. Experimental work so far has demonstrated that cells modified in this fashion have altered function and a markedly decreased half-life.

Another approach has used the oxygen-carrying capacity of fluorocarbons.[86] These substances are dense organic chemicals that carry oxygen in proportion to ambient oxygen pressure that varies from one fluorocarbon to another, depending on the underlying molecular structure. Unfortunately, fluorocarbons are toxic in their pure form, primarily because of an accompanying vapor pressure, and are also insoluble in water. Even though oxygen is more soluble in fluorocarbons than in water by a factor of 10 to 20 times, the oxygen-carrying capacity of a fluorocarbon emulsion equals that of blood only at 100% inspired oxygen, an undesirable therapeutic modality. The emulsification that is necessary to reduce the toxicity of fluorocarbons before their infusion contributes to a limited circulating half-time that is generally on the order of hours to days. Since the clearance of fluorocarbons from the blood stream is primarily by way of the reticuloendothelial system (RES) and since dwell time in this system may be months or longer, a long-term toxicity problem is potentially posed, the significance of which remains unknown. Further, RES clearance introduces another major problem because this system is also stressed and impaired in septic and hypovolemic shock. The fact that it does not seem wise to further impair this vital system, coupled with the observation that fluorocarbons are not biologically inert in either their native or emulsified form, makes it questionable whether they will ever be clinically useful in the treatment of shock.

Interestingly, the efficacy of a 20% fluorocarbon emulsion in carrying oxygen has been reported in a small population of patients.[56] At best, the solution proved to be a moderate volume expander, but its ability to carry oxygen and to effect an improvement in tissue perfusion in ischemic or low flow states was far from convincingly documented. In another study, involving seven severely anemic patients, it was noted that at ambient oxygen tensions, fluorocarbon acted primarily as a volume expander, whereas only at higher inspired oxygen tensions (>300 mm Hg) did it contribute substantially to effective oxygen delivery.[87]

In animal studies evaluating fluorocarbons, adequate hemodynamic resuscitation following shock has been demonstrated, but the complication of coagulation problems, particularly thrombocytopenia, has been noted.[85] Other abnormalities at the microcirculatory level have been encountered, including white-cell clumping and platelet aggregation. Further, in baboons with hematocrits as low as zero, fluorocarbons were shown to have no clear advantage over stroma-free hemoglobin in terms of oxygen delivery characteristics (see following paragraph). Thus despite the initial enthusiasm for the use of fluorocarbons as red-cell substitutes, these animal studies, as well as available human data, have failed to substantiate any significant clinical role for these agents.[88]

Stroma-free hemoglobin. In contrast to other red-cell substitutes, which to date have not demonstrated features that would allow them to be used clinically, *chemically modified* stroma-free hemoglobin (SFH) possesses many properties that are desirable in a blood substitute. It carries and releases oxygen in a cooperative fashion, has virtually no antigenic properties, is not nephrotoxic, and is oncotically active. When properly prepared it is neither an anticoagulant nor a procoagulant, and it can be stored for reasonable periods of time. Finally, at ambient Po_2 it has been shown to preserve life function as an efficient and effective resuscitation fluid in total blood exchange and hemorrhagic shock animal models. Further, SFH effects an excellent hemodynamic resuscitation and affords improved tissue oxygenation as measured by hepatic mitochondrial function during the postresuscitation period.[85] Despite these desirable characteristics, two major problems have kept SFH in the laboratory and have detained clinical study. These were (1) a profound affinity for oxygen by SFH and (2) the perception on the part of potential users of this agent clinically that its intravascular persistence is too short to be of therapeutic usefulness. *Moreover, the perception of a hemoglobin-induced nephrotoxicity remains despite clear evidence of safety when infused clinically.*

An appreciation of hemoglobin biophysics and the basic structure-function relationships that determine the metabolic fate of free hemoglobin led to attempts to modify SFH to solve these problems. Both intermolecular and intramolecular chemical modifications of SFH have been attempted. Polymerizing SFH (i.e., intermolecular modification) to increase its molecular weight has been reported to improve its intravascular persistence (for 2 to 3 days) and to maintain near normal oxyhemoglobin affinity.[85] Although most SFH is excreted by the kidneys, no one can predict the impact that these larger molecules may have on the RES.[89] These polyhemoglobins may follow different metabolic pathways and excretory routes that could be detrimental and might result in RES blockade, a particularly undesirable side effect in the polytraumatized patient. *There are no data to support compromise of the RES or coagulation systems with the use of polymerized hemoglobin solutions.*[32,90]

Intramolecular modifications of SFH have also been undertaken to improve intravascular persistence without increasing oxyhemoglobin affinity. These chemical modifications have used various phosphate analogs to bind to various sites on the β chains of the hemoglobin molecule, normally occupied by 2,3-diphosphoglycerate, the key intracellular phosphate in hemoglobin that is involved intimately with oxyhemoglobin affinity. SFH chemically modified with a number of phosphorylated dialdehydes has been shown in dogs to persist intravascularly for as long as 12 hours (a sixfold increase over unmodified SFH), with maintenance of normal oxyhemoglobin affinity.[85] Moreover, resuscitation with these modified SFHs has demonstrated a beneficial effect. Further, this intramolecularly modified SFH is not a polyhemoglobin and thus may be less of a problem to the RES. In one study of hemorrhagic shock resuscitation followed 5 days later by septic challenge, modified-SFH animals did not demonstrate any impairment in defense mechanisms.

The concept of a neohemocyte is also being evaluated. The idea underlying this approach is to encapsulate SFH with a modifier to improve its functional capacity. Although this appears technically feasible, how these artificial cells will react in the circulation remains unknown. What little information is available indicates that these artificial cells would function as a foreign body and probably would be cleared rapidly by the RES. Consequently, only with repeated infusions of neohemocytes would a sufficient concentration be obtained in the blood to afford effective oxygen delivery.[91,92]

On the basis of current knowledge, chemically modified SFH continues to evolve as the most useful of the potential red-cell substitutes.[93,94] Although considerable clinical testing must be undertaken to ensure the safety and efficacy of modified SFH, research to date has been most encouraging. As an oxygen-carrying colloid suspended in a balanced salt solution, it may very well prove to be the ultimate resuscitation fluid.

Metabolic Manipulations

As additional information is obtained concerning the altered mechanisms that underlie the various shock states, more specific metabolic manipulations to prevent these derangements can be anticipated. A more beneficial outcome is likely to result from either blocking the detrimental aspects of these processes or augmenting those responses that are clearly protective. In this regard, several investigative observations have been noted in recent years that may directly influence shock management in the near future. For example, the endogenous opiate, β-endorphin appears to be involved in the hypotension and impaired tissue perfusion that commonly occur in both hypovolemic and septic shock states; elevations in this substance can be demonstrated at the time these physiologic aberrations occur.[14]

Naloxone, an inhibitor of endorphin activity, has been studied as a possible agent to prevent these alterations. Although it has no effect on the cardiovascular system under normal circumstances, naloxone has been shown in animal studies to elevate blood pressure and cardiac output and to significantly improve survival in septic, endotoxic, and hemorrhagic shock models.[14] Early clinical studies with this agent in patients in shock have also demonstrated its potential efficacy as a therapeutic tool.[57] More detailed studies have failed to demonstrate efficacy.

Another approach to shock management has involved the use of various metabolic substrates to improve cell function. A clear relationship exists between ATP depletion and organ dysfunction in shock and ischemia; intravenous infusion of ATP complexed with $MgCl_2$ can promote "survival" in both hemorrhagic and septic animal shock models.[4,95] Derangements in hepatic metabolism secondary to shock have been especially responsive to ATP-n-$MgCl_2$.[7] Beneficial effects have also been achieved in various shock models by providing substrates such as pyruvate, inosine, adenosine, and creatine phosphate.[8] These moieties presumably provide the substrate for synthesis of high-energy phosphates. Solutions of glucose, insulin, and potassium have also been shown to be efficacious.[96] None of these approaches *have gained sufficient credibility to achieve broad clinical application.*

cAMP, the "second messenger" that instructs the cell to respond to a stimulus when its membrane is activated by a specific hormone, is depleted in septic and hemorrhagic shock.[33] Defects in cAMP metabolism produce dysfunctional cells and thereby impair normal beneficial homeostatic responses. Administration of cAMP to experimental animals has yielded varied beneficial results.

Many of the cellular deficits in various shock states result from increased cell membrane permeability.[1] In shock, control of the large and small channels within cell membranes directly relates to cell viability. If membrane integrity is preserved, intracellular homeostasis is maintained. Future therapy for shock may involve pharmacologic manipulation of calcium, sodium, and potassium flux as a means of preserving cellular function and structure in the face of the shock insult.

Alterations in the metabolism of prostaglandins in shock have been recently recognized. These ubiquitous, vasoactive lipids with short half-lives may play a role in the pathophysiology of shock. In addition, prostaglandins probably play a role in coagulation and regulation of white cells by preventing them from releasing toxic or vasoactive substances.[9] The therapeutic role of prostaglandins in shock management is not yet defined. The previous discussion covers many of the possibilities that arise from current efforts.

SUMMARY

"Shock" is a state of altered tissue perfusion that occurs when the cardiac output is inadequate to maintain effective blood flow to organs and tissues sufficient to provide necessary nutrients and oxygen and the removal of waste products resulting from their metabolism. Etiologically, four types of shock have been recognized: hypovolemic, septic, cardiogenic, and neurogenic. Despite the underlying cause of shock, a basic neuroendocrine response is evoked when shock occurs that results in redistribution of the body's blood flow to ensure adequate perfusion to such vital organs as the heart and brain. In addition, a number of metabolic aberrations ensure adequate nutrients (e.g., glucose) to maintain normal cellular function. The magnitude of these responses depends on the severity of shock, but they can be particularly pronounced in those forms of shock secondary to hypovolemia and/or sepsis.

The successful treatment of shock involves a thorough understanding of these pathophysiologic derangements and the distinguishing characteristics of the various etiologic factors that can give rise to its development. By careful hemodynamic monitoring and the reestablishment of an effective circulating blood volume (through the infusion of intravenous fluids and/or blood and by various pharmacologic manipulations), adequate tissue perfusion and oxygen-carrying capacity of blood can be assured under most shock conditions. Metabolic abnormalities usually are not treated directly, but rather tend to resolve when the underlying source of shock is corrected. With such physiologically directed therapy, many more patients survive their shock insult today than did as recently as 5 or 10 years ago. As knowledge in this area continues to improve, we can expect even greater advances.

REFERENCES

1. Gould SA, Rice CL, Moss GS. The physiologic basis of the use of blood and blood products. Surg Ann 16:13, 1984.
2. Shoemaker, WC, Paul PL, Krass MD. Hemodynamic and oxygen transport responses in survivors and non-survivors of high risk surgery. Crit Care Med 21:977, 1993.
3. Sibbald WJ, et al. Concepts in the pharmacologic and nonpharmacologic support of cardiovascular function in critically ill patients. Surg. Clin North Am 63:455, 1983.
4. Chaudry IH, Sayeed MM, Baue AE. Effect of adenosine triphosphate-magnesium chloride administration in shock. Surgery 75:220, 1974.
5. Fracescangeli E, Goracci G. The de novo biosynthesis of platelet-activating factor in rat brain. Biochem Biophys Res Commun 161:107, 1989.
6. Greenburg AG, Peskin GW. Blood, salt and water: Recent advances. In Bartlett RH, Whitehouse WM, Turcotte JG, eds. Life Support Systems in Intensive Care. Chicago: Year Book,1984.
7. Hirasawa H, et al. Improved survival and reticuloendothelial function with intravenous ATP-$MgCl_2$ following hemorrhagic shock. Circ Shock 11:141, 1983.
8. Kim HW, et al. Nitric oxide scavenging: An alternative therapeutic approach to nitric oxide synthesis inhibition in nitric oxide mediated hypotension of sepsis. Surg Forum 45:67, 1994.
9. Gann DS, Amaral JF. Pathophysiology of trauma and shock. In Zuidema GD, Rutherford RD, Ballinger WF, eds. The Management of Trauma. Philadelphia: WB Saunders, 1985.
10. Gump FE. Whole body metabolism. In Altura BM, et al., eds. Handbook of Shock and Trauma, vol 1. Basic Sciences. New York: Raven Press, 1983.
11. Mattox KM, Maningas PA, Moore EE. Pre-hospital hypertonic saline/dextrose infusion for post-traumatic hypotension. The USA results center study. Ann Surg 213:482, 1991.
12. Shires GT, Carrico CJ, Canizaro PC. Shock. Philadelphia: WB Saunders, 1973.
13. Trachte GJ. Endocrinology of shock. In Altura BM, Lefer AM, Schumer W, eds. Handbook of Shock and Trauma, vol 1. Basic Science. New York: Raven Press, 1983.
14. Bone RC, et al. Endorphins in endotoxin shock. Microcirculation 1:265, 1981.
15. Hechtman HB, et al. Prostaglandin and thromboxane mediation of cardiopulmonary failure. Surg Clin North Am 63:263, 1983.
16. Trunkey DD, Dolcroft J, Carpenter MA. Calcium flux during hemorrhagic shock in baboons. J Trauma 16:633, 1976.
17. Shires GT, Williams J, Brown F. Acute change in extracellular fluids associated with major surgical procedures. Ann Surg 154:803, 1961.
18. Tranbaugh RF, et al. Lung water changes after thermal injury: The effects of crystalloid resuscitation and sepsis. Ann Surg 192:479, 1980.
19. Del Maestro RF, Bjork J, Arfars KE. Free radicals and microvascular permeability. In Autar AP, ed. Pathology of Oxygen. New York: Academic Press, 1982.
20. Halliwell B. Oxygen is poisonous: The nature and medical importance of oxygen radicals. Med Lab Sci 4:157, 1984.
21. Stuehr DJ, Griffith OW. Mammalian nitric oxide synthesis. Adv Enzymol Mol Biol 65:287, 1993.
22. Bickell WH, et al. Immediate versus delayed fluid resuscitation for hypotensive patients with penetrating torso injuries. N Engl J Med 331:1105, 1994.

23. Gold ME, et al. Ng-Methyl-L-arginine causes endothelium-dependent contraction and inhibition of cyclic GMP formation in artery and vein. Proc Natl Acad Sci USA 87:4430, 1990.
24. Rees DD, et al. A specific inhibitor of nitric oxide formation form L-arginine attenuates endothelium-dependent relaxation. Br J Pharmacol 96:418, 1989.
25. Carrico CJ, et al. Multiple-organ-failure syndrome. Arch Surg 121:196, 1986.
26. Lorente JA, et al. Role of nitric oxide in the hemodynamic changes of sepsis. Crit Care Med 21(5):759, 1993.
27. Parker JL, Adams HR. Selective inhibition of endothelium-dependent vasodilator capacity by *Eschericia-coli* endotoxaemia. Circ Res 72:539, 1993.
28. Greenberg SS, et al. Tumor necrosis factor-alpha inhibits endothelium-dependent relaxation. J Appl Physiol 74:2394, 1993.
29. Xie J, et al. Tumor necrosis factor inhibits stimulated but not basal release of nitric oxide. Am Rev Respir Dis 148:627, 1993.
30. Szabo C, et al. Hemorrhagic hypotension impairs endothelium-dependent relaxations in the renal artery of the cat. Circ Shock 36:238, 1992.
31. Symington PA, Ma XL, Lefer AM. Protective actions of S-nitroso-N-acetylpenicillamine (SNAP) in a rat model of hemorrhagic shock. Meth Find Exp Clin Pharmacol 14:789, 1992.
32. Miller VM, Vanhoutte PM. Endothelium-dependent responses and their potential relevance to the distribution of blood flow during hemorrhagic shock. Resuscitation 18:165, 1989.
33. Thiemermann C, et al. Vascular hyporeactivity to vasoconstrictor agents and haemodynamic decompensation in hemorrhagic shock is mediated by nitric oxide. Proc Natl Acad Sci U S A 90:267, 1993.
34. Zingarelli B, Squadrito F, Caputi AP. Tumor necrosis factor induces NO synthase in acute hypovolemic shock in the rat. Endothelium 1:S83, 1993.
35. Geng Y, Hansson GK, Holme E. Interferon-γ and tumor necrosis factor synergize to induce nitric oxide production and inhibit mitochondrial respiration in vascular smooth muscle cells. Cir Res 71:1268, 1992.
36. Casey LC, Balk RA, Bone RC. Plasma cytokine and endotoxin levels correlate with survival in patients with the sepsis syndrome. Ann Intern Med 119:771, 1993.
37. Tracey KJ, et al. Shock and tissue injury induced by recombinant human cachectin. Science 234:470, 1986.
38. Hinshaw L, Olson P, Kuo G. Efficacy of post-treatment with anti-TNF monoclonal antibody in preventing the pathophysiology and lethality of sepsis in the baboon. Circ Shock 27:362, 1989.
39. Shalaby MR, et al. Receptor binding and activation of polymorphonuclear neutrophils by tumor necrosis factor-alpha. J Leukocyte Biol 41:196, 1987.
40. van der Poll T, et al. Activation of coagulation after administration of tumor necrosis factor to normal subjects. N Engl J Med 322:1622, 1990.
41. Lagente V, et al. PAF-acether and endotoxin display similar effects on rat mesenteric microvessels. Inhibition by specific antagonists. J Pharmacol Exp Ther 247:254, 1988.
42. Blank ML, et al. A specific acetyl-hydrolase for 1-alkyl-2-acetyl-sn-glycero-3-phosphocholine (a hypotensive platelet-activating lipid). J Biol Chem 256:175, 1981.
43. Pfeilschifter J, et al. Cyclic AMP mimics, but does not mediate, interleukin-1 and tumor necrosis factor–stimulated phospholipase A_2 secretion from rat renal mesangial cells. Biochem J 273:199, 1991.
44. Bevilacqua MP, et al. Interleukin 1 induces biosynthesis and cell surface expression of proagulant activity in human vascular endothelial cells. J Exp Med 160:618, 1984.
45. Bevilacqua MP, et al. Identification of an inducible endothelial-leukocyte adhesion molecule. Proc Natl Acad Sci USA 84:923, 1987.
46. Heremans H, et al. Interferon-γ antibody protects mice against the generalized Schwartzman reaction. J Exp Med 171:1853, 1990.
47. Ruokonen E, et al. Regional blood flow and oxygen transport in septic shock. Crit Care Med 21(9):1296, 1993.
48. Schoenberg MH, Berger HG. Reperfusion injury after ischemia. Crit Care Med 21(0):1376, 1993.
49. Russel J, et al. Oxygen delivery and consumption and ventricular preload are greater in the survivors than in non-survivors of the adult respiratory distress syndrome. Am Rev Respir Dis 141:659, 1990.
50. Shoemaker WC, et al. Prospective trial of supranormal values as therapeutic goals in high-risk surgical patients. Chest 94:1176, 1988.
51. Tuchschmidt J, et al. Elevation of cardiac output and oxygen delivery improves outcome in septic shock. Chest 102(1):216, 1992.
52. Springer TA, Lasky LA. Cell adhesion: Sticky sugars for selection. Nature 349:191, 1991.
53. Spertini O, et al. Regulation of leukocyte migration by activation of the leukocyte adhesion molecule-1 (LAM-1) selectin. Nature 349:691, 1991.
54. Huber AR, et al. Regulation of transendothelial neutrophil migration by endogenous interleukin-8. Science 254:99, 1991.
55. Wiles ME, et al. Hypoxia reoxygenation-induced injury of cultured pulmonary microvessel endothelial cells. J Leukocyte Biol 53:490, 1993.
56. Pietersma A, et al. Studies on the interaction of leucocytes and the myocardial vasculature. Mol Cell Biochem 116:197, 1992.
57. Peters WP, et al. Pressor effect of naloxone in septic shock. Lancet 2:529, 1981.
58. Freischlag JA, Hanna D. Neutrophil (PMN) phagocytosis and chemotaxis after 2 hours of ischemia. J Surg Res 50:648, 1991.
59. Hill J, et al. A Mac-1 antibody reduces liver and lung injury but not neutrophil sequestration after intestinal ischemia-reperfusion. Surgery 112(2):166, 1992.
60. Boros M, et al. Reperfusion mucosal damage after complete intestinal ischemia in the dog: The effect of antioxidant and phospholipase A_2 inhibitor therapy. Surgery 113(2):184, 1993.
61. Baggiolini M, et al. Activation of neutrophil leukocytes: Chemoattractant receptors and respiratory burst. FASEB J 7:1004, 1993.
62. Youn YK, LaLonde C, Demling R. Trends in shock research: Use of antioxidant therapy in shock and trauma. Circ Shock 35:245, 1991.
63. Ingold KU, et al. Vitamin E remains the major lipid soluble chain-breaking antioxidant in human plasma even in individuals suffering from severe vitamin E deficiency. Arch Biochem Biophys 259:224, 1987.
64. McKechni K, Furman BL, Parrat JR. Modification by oxygen free radical scavengers of the metabolic and cardiovascular effect of endotoxin infusion in conscious rats. Circ Shock 19:429, 1986.
65. Jepsen S, et al. Antioxidant treatment with *N*-acetyl cysteine during adult respiratory distress syndrome. A prospective randomized, placebo-controlled study. Crit Care Med 20:918, 1992.
66. Rhodes RS, DePalma RG. Mitochondrial dysfunction of the liver and hypoglycemia in hemorrhagic shock. Surg Gynecol Obstet 150:347, 1980.
67. Christou NV, Meakins JL, Superina R. Host defenses, sepsis and the critically ill patient. In Bartlet RH, Whitehouse WM, Turcotte JC, eds. Life Support Systems in Intensive Care. Chicago: Year Book, 1984.
68. Mosher DF. Physiology of fibronectin. Annu Rev Med 35:361, 1984.
69. Shoemaker WC, Czer LSC. Evaluation of the biologic importance of various hemodynamic and oxygen transport variables. Crit Care Med 7:424, 1979.
70. Greenburg AG. Indications for red cell transfusion. In Wilmore DW, ed. Scientific American Surgery, New York: Scientific American Library, 1988.
71. Stern SA. Effect of blood pressure on hemorrhage volume and survival in a near fatal hemorrhage model incorporating a vascular injury. Ann Emerg Med 22:155, 1993.

72. Vasser MJ, Perry CI, Holcroft JW. Hypertonic/hyperoncotic resuscitation and improvement in predicted outcome for trauma patients. Circ SHR 37:1309, 1992.
73. Velanovich V. Crystalloid versus colloid fluid resuscitation: A meta-analysis of mortality. Surgery 105:65, 1989.
74. Poole GU, et al. Comparison of colloids and crystalloids in resuscitation from hemorrhagic shock. Surg Gynecol Obstet 154:577, 1982.
75. Virgilio RW, et al. Crystalloid versus colloid resuscitation: Is one better? Surgery 85:129, 1979.
76. Sibbald WJ, et al. Variations in plasma levels of adenosine 3′5′ monophosphate during clinical sepsis. Surg Gynecol Obstet 144:199, 1977.
77. Krauz MM. Controversies in shock research: Hypertonic resuscitation—Pros & cons. Shock 3:69, 1995.
78. Velasco IT, et al. Hyperosmotic NaCl and severe hemorrhagic shock. Am J Physiol 239(Heart Circ Physiol 8):H664, 1980.
79. Shackford SR, et al. Hypertonic sodium lactate versus lactated Ringer's solution for intravenous fluid therapy in operations on the abdominal aorta. Surgery 94:41, 1983.
80. Shatney CH, et al. Efficacy of hetastarch in the resuscitation of patients with multisystem trauma and shock. Arch Surg 118:804, 1983.
81. Schneider AJ, Stockman JA, Oski FA. Transfusion nomogram: An application of physiology to clinical decisions regarding the use of blood. Crit Care Med 9:469, 1981.
82. Woodson RD. Hemoglobin structure and oxygen transport. In Ressi EC, Simon TL, Moss GS, eds. Principles of Transfusion Medicine, 3rd ed. Baltimore: Williams & Wilkins, 1991, p 23.
83. Valeri CR, Zarvoulis CG. Rejuvenation and freezing of outdated stored human red cells. N Engl J Med 287:1307, 1972.
84. Counts RB, et al. Hemostasis in massively transfused trauma patients. Ann Surg 190:91, 1979.
85. Greenburg AG. Alternatives to conventional use of blood products. State of the Art 14:325, 1992.
86. Mitsuno T, Ohyanogi H, Naito R. Clinical studies of a perfluorocarbon whole blood substitute: Fluosol DA-20. Ann Surg 195:60, 1982.
87. Tremper KK, et al. The preoperative treatment of severely anemic patients with a perfluorochemical oxygen transport fluid, Fluosol-DA. N Engl J Med 307:277, 1982.
88. Goodin TH, et al. A perfluoro chemical emulsion for pre-hospital resuscitation of experimental hemorrhage shock: A prospective, randomized controlled study. Crit Care Med 22:686, 1994.
89. Kim HW, Chen F, Greenburg AG. A double (exchange transfusion–carbon clearance) model for testing post-resuscitation reticuloendothelial function. Biomat Art Cells Art Org 20:777, 1992.
90. Kim HW, et al. Hepatic RE function following resuscitation with hemoglobin solutions. In Chang TMS, ed. Blood Substitutes and Oxygen Carriers. New York: Marcel Dekker, 1993, p 789.
91. Rudolph AS. Encapsulated hemoglobin. Curr Iss Fut Goals, Art Cells Blood Subs Immob Biotech 22:347, 1994.
92. Rudolph AS, et al. Circulation persistance and biodistribution of lyophilized liposome-encapsulated hemoglobin: An oxygen-carrying resuscitative fluid. Crit Care Med 22:142, 1994.
93. Schultz SC, Hamilton IN, Malcola DS. Use of base deficit to compare resuscitation with lactated Ringer's solution, haemacel, whole blood, and diaspirin cross-linked hemoglobin following hemorrhage in rats. J Trauma 35:619, 1993.
94. Schultz SC, et al. The efficacy of diaspirin cross linked hemoglobin solution resuscitation in a model of uncontrolled hemorrhage. J Trauma 37:408, 1994.
95. Chaudry IH, Clemens MG, Baue AE. Alterations in cell function with ischemia and shock and their correction. Arch Surg 116:1309, 1981.
96. Bronsveld W, et al. Effects of glucose-insulin-potassium (GIK) on myocardial blood flow metabolism in canine endotoxin shock. Circ Shock 13:325, 1984.

9

Neoplastic Disease: Pathophysiology and Rationale for Treatment

John E. Niederhuber and David Crooks

Our understanding of both the cellular and molecular aspects of neoplasia has been significantly enhanced by studies of clonogenic tumor cells in tissue culture and by the processes associated with the expression of oncogenes, tumor suppressor genes, genes coding for DNA repair enzymes, and cell-cycle regulators. Cancer growth can be regarded as a mixture of dying cells and cells that have the capacity to renew themselves ("stem cells"), thus maintaining tumor survival. Dying cells occur within a tumor when tumor growth exceeds vascular support (causing tumor cells to undergo necrosis) and as a result of programmed cell death (apoptosis). Host immune reaction against tumor and, of course, external intervention such as chemotherapy or radiation can increase the number of dying cells within a tumor either by inducing tumor cell necrosis or apoptosis of tumor cells. Following a discussion of these basic concepts of cell biology, this chapter attempts to relate the genetic events of growth (both normal and abnormal) to the development of tumorigenesis, metastasis, and finally to the relationship of therapy to these cell processes.

Advances in our understanding of cell proliferation, both normal and abnormal, and our understanding of the transformation of normal cells has great importance in the design of treatment using multiple therapeutic modalities. The timing, dosage, and implementation of all forms of treatment for cancer growth are significantly enhanced by understanding and using the fundamental concepts of tumor cell biology. The basis for such knowledge begins with a study of cell growth, cell cycle kinetics, and apoptosis (programmed cell death).

BASIC CONCEPTS OF CELL BIOLOGY

Cell Growth and Cell Cycle Kinetics

In normal tissue, new cells are generated from a subset of cells that have a high capacity to divide and replace themselves ("stem cells"), but their actual rate of cell division is quite low unless there is tissue injury or system/organ demand.[1] During the growth of a cancer, the rate of cell division and replacement exceeds cell loss as a consequence of the deregulation of normal growth. Both normal cells and tumor cells proliferate by an identical process termed the cell division cycle.[2] The classic cycle of cell division can be divided into four ordered and strictly regulated stages: G_1 (gap 1), S (DNA synthesis), G_2 (gap 2), and M (mitosis/meiosis) (Fig. 9-1).[3-6] G_1 is the variable "gap" (growth phase) between the completion of cell division and the beginning of DNA synthesis (S phase). Daughter cells generated by mitosis reside in either G_1 or G_0 (resting or quiescent state) and retain a diploid (2N) set of chromosomes.

Cells residing in G_1, S, G_2, or M are said to be in the proliferative fraction, the growth fraction, or the growth compartment. This fraction of cells can be measured by DNA flow cytometry. In contrast, cells in prolonged G_0 are in the nonproliferative fraction. This nonproliferative compartment may on occasion contain cells that have been arrested in S phase (S_0) or in G_2.

A specific control event (the restriction point) exists within G_1, and this control point determines whether a cell can progress (i.e., become committed) to DNA synthesis (the S phase). The restriction point (R) divides G_1 into two stages: prerestriction point (growth factor dependent) and postrestriction point (growth factor independent).[4] The growth factors required for prerestriction point G_1 progression are cell type specific.[7] Platelet-derived growth factor (PDGF), epidermal growth factor (EGF), insulin, insulin-like growth factor (IGF-1), and colony-stimulating factor (CSF) are a few examples of known extracellular stimuli required during the first part of the G_1 phase. These factors and their receptors are of primary importance in bringing the cell to the "R" point and in controlling cell growth. Once the restriction point is triggered, the remaining phases of the cell cycle are es-

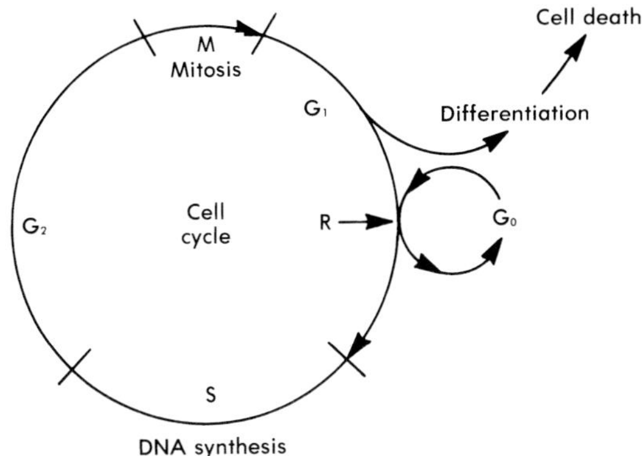

Fig. 9-1. The cell cycle division is divided into two parts: interphase and mitosis *(M)*. Interphase can be divided into three parts: gap 1 *(G_1)*, phase of DNA synthesis *(S)*, and gap 2 *(G_2)*. A point, restriction point *(R)*, exists in G_1 and determines whether a cell can progress to S. If a cell is not triggered to DNA synthesis, it may be shunted to a resting place *(G_0)*. The amount of time that is spent in each phase of the cycle is unique to the particular cell type.

sentially independent of extracellular factors. If the mammalian cell is not triggered to DNA synthesis (i.e., the restriction point is not triggered), the cell will be shunted into a G_0 state.

During the S phase, cells synthesize DNA and chromosomal replication begins.[8] On completion of DNA synthesis the cell has two diploid sets of chromosomes. The S phase is followed by a second gap (growth phase) termed G_2. Throughout G_1, S, and G_2, the interphase of the cell cycle, RNA and protein synthesis are steadily increasing with duplication of all organelles. Mitosis represents the culmination of cell growth that has occurred during G_1, S, and G_2 and is the process by which a cell distributes two sets of chromosomes to the two daughter cells. Mitosis is dependent on prior completion of DNA replication. Studies of the cell cycle have established that two similar mechanisms control the progression from G_1 to S and from G_2 to M. These have been termed checkpoint control genes.[9]

Checkpoints are events in the cell cycle that ensure the integrity of DNA replication and the accuracy of chromosomal segregation.[9] Checkpoint controls operate as a positive or negative switch determining the cells readiness to progress to the next phase of the cell cycle and ensure the necessary editing and repair of defective genetic information. At least two checkpoints are known, and they detect DNA damage at the G_1/S transition and the G_2/M transition. Loss of the G_1/S checkpoint can lead to genomic instability and the evolution of cells toward a malignant phenotype.[9,10] Studies of mammalian cells undergoing G_1/S arrest indicate a primary role for the *p53* gene, a transcriptional activator.[11-13] Mammalian cells treated with γ-irradiation show increased levels of *p53* protein, whereas cells with mutant *p53* alleles fail to undergo G_1/S arrest when γ-irradiated.[11,14] The *GADD45* gene can be shown to be induced when DNA damage and G_1/S arrest occur. The *GADD45* gene contains a DNA sequence that binds the *p53* gene transcriptional activator. Thus activation of *GADD45* and other genes as yet unknown act to hold cells at the G_1/S checkpoint in response to damaged DNA.

At the G_2/M checkpoint, cells may be held in G_2 again to repair their DNA before allowing the cells to proceed with chromosome segregation. Several genes have been shown to be involved in the G_2/M checkpoint process. Examples are *rad9* (a gene sensitive to DNA-damaging agents such as γ-irradiation) and *RCC1* (a repressor of chromosome condensation). The *RCC1* gene product functions by classic signal transduction mechanisms inhibiting guanosine triphosphatase (GTPase) activity of the RAN protein.

In addition to the DNA repair enzymes operating at known checkpoints, cell cycle progression is also controlled, in part, by regulators termed cyclins and cyclin-dependent kinases (CDKs) that associate with one another to form an active complex (Fig. 9-2). The first cell cycle protein kinase gene to be identified was *cdc2*.[15-17] It is involved in the regulation of the G_1/S and G_2/M phase transitions. The activities of CDKs are controlled by cyclin binding, phosphorylation, and inhibition by cyclin kinase inhibitors (CKIs). Changes in the cyclin-CDK complexes help drive the cell from one stage to another. Cell cycle progression and its integrity are achieved by the complex coordinated activities of checkpoint controls (CDKs) and repair pathway processes.[18] Cyclins associated with CDKs are generally divided into two functional groups. The first group acts at the G_2/M boundary (cyclins B1 and B2). The second group acts at the G_1/S boundary (D, E). Cyclin A is the exception. It is present, and thought to be functioning, from the S phase through the M phase.[19]

The complexity of the process of simple cell duplication is impressive and readily leads one to understand how defects in the myriad of cell cycle controls can lead to genomic instability and progression to a malignant phenotype. Various human cancers (e.g., lymphomas, breast, esophageal, and pancreatic adenocarcinomas) occur when G_1 cyclins are overexpressed as a consequence of genetic rearrangement, deletions, or mutations.

The growth of both normal and transformed cells depends on the presence of specific growth factors and cell surface protein receptors. Genes that code for these factors, their receptors, and the intracellular proteins involved in signal transmissions to the nucleus are critical to orderly cell proliferation. Abnormalities in these genes influence the controls of the cell cycle, cell proliferation, and apoptosis and ultimately predispose the cell toward generation of the malignant phenotype.

Apoptosis

The intracellular mechanisms involved in cell death are as complex as the regulatory elements involved in cellular proliferation. Apoptosis, or programmed cell death, is an

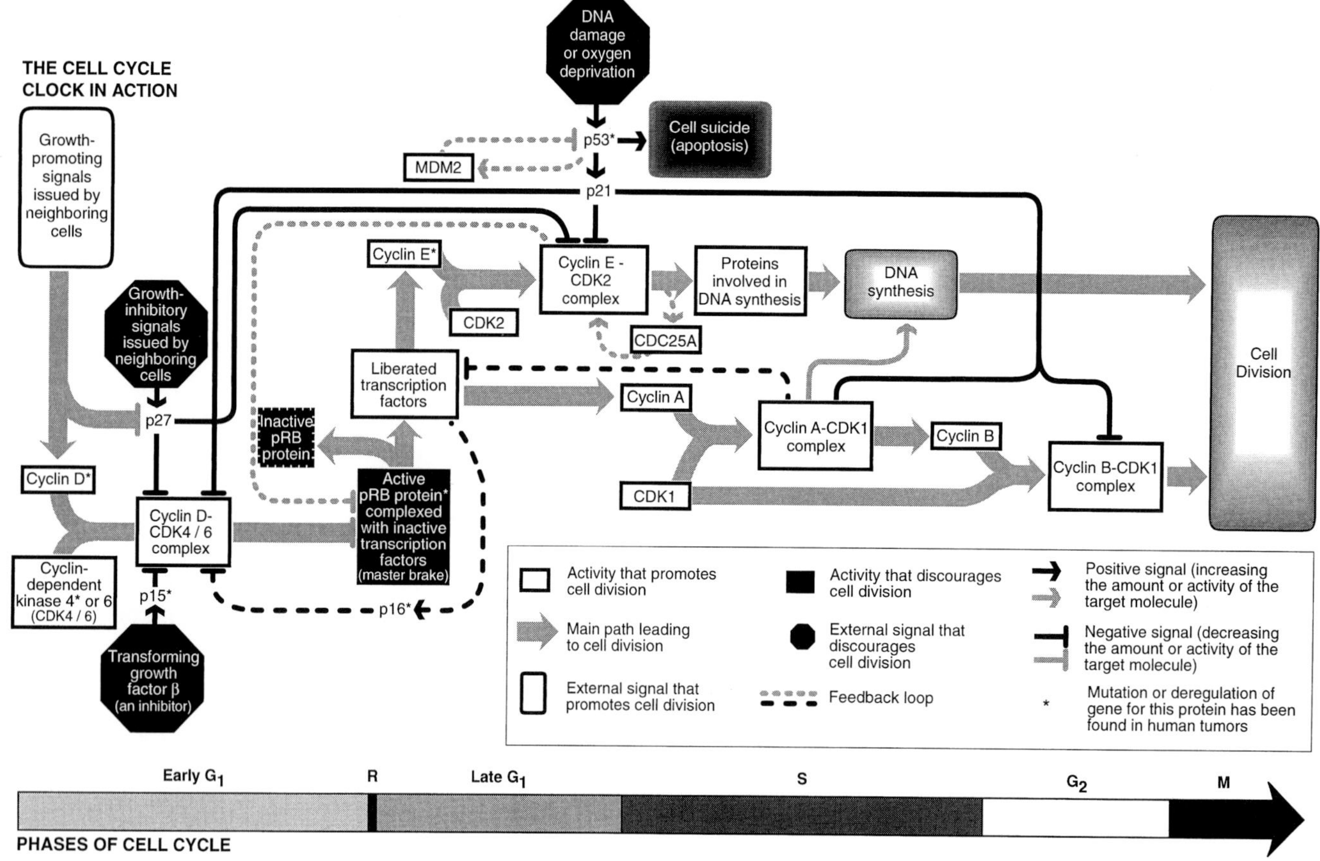

Fig. 9-2. The cell cycle clock in action. *G_1*, Gap 1; *G_2*, gap 2; *M*, mitosis; *R*, restriction point; *S*, synthesis. (Modified from Weinberg RA. How cancer arises. Scientific American 275: 62, 1996. Reproduced with permission.)

evolutionarily conserved, morphologically distinct process of internally encoded cell elimination in which cells die in a controlled manner.[20,21] Apoptosis occurs in all organ systems from fetal development onward, first appearing during embryogenesis, cellular differentiation, and metamorphosis. Apoptosis is also a part of normal tissue turnover and is involved in the regulation of the immune system. Recently, it has become apparent that apoptosis is also an important component of abnormal cell growth and therefore tumor progression.[22] Thus apoptosis is of central importance in the regulatory mechanisms involved in homeostasis of all multicellular organisms.

Apoptotic cell death is distinguished from necrotic cell death by characteristic morphologic and biochemical changes. Activation of apoptosis is regulated by many different signals that originate from both the intracellular and extracellular environment.[23,24] Necrotic cell death, in contrast to apoptosis, is a pathologic form of cell killing that results from acute cellular injury leading to rapid cell swelling and membrane lysis.

Another unique and important aspect of apoptotic cell death is characterized by controlled autodigestion of the cell, which prevents an inflammatory response. Apoptotic cells undergo cytoplasmic, nuclear condensation, and fragmentation, setting the stage for engulfment and phagocytosis. Cellular shrinkage and membrane blebbing occur with maintenance of plasma membrane integrity. These events are tightly controlled by a series of genetic signals within the cell and act to prevent an inflammatory response that would be caused by leakage of the apoptotic cellular contents. Phagocytosis and intracellular degradation by lysosomes occur expeditiously by macrophages and other neighboring cells. As a result, the phagocyte that ingests an apoptotic cell does not become activated.[22,24,25]

Alterations in the control of cell survival are important in the development of various human illnesses. Cells failing to undergo a normal apoptotic pathway contribute to the pathogenesis of human disease, including cancer, autoimmune diseases, and viral infections. The process of apoptosis is responsible for the normal elimination of cells and cells containing damaged DNA. Cells unable to undergo apoptosis in response to DNA damage survive longer and are more prone to genetic mutations and genomic instability, with eventual propagation toward a malignant phenotype. Various malignant cells are known to demonstrate a decreased ability to undergo cellular apoptosis.[22,24,25]

The trigger to initiate apoptotic cell death and the mechanism operative in this signaling pathway is still largely unknown. It has been postulated that apoptosis rep-

Table 9-1. Retroviral Oncogenes and Tumors

v-onc Gene	RNA Tumor Virus	Species of Origin	Major Disease
Growth factor family			
v-sis	SSV	Wooly monkey	Glioma/sarcoma
	PI-FeSV	Cat	Sarcoma
Integral membrane tyrosine kinases			
v-fms	SM-FeSV	Cat	Sarcoma
v-erbB	AEV-H, AEV-	Chicken	Erythroleukemia, sarcoma
v-kit	ES4	Cat	Sarcoma
v-ros	HZ4-FeSV	Chicken	Sarcoma
	UR2		
Membrane-associated tyrosine kinases			
v-src	RSV	Chicken	Sarcoma
v-fgr	Gr-FeSV	Cat	Sarcoma
v-yes	Y73/ESV	Chicken	Sarcoma
v-fps	FuSV/PRCII	Chicken	Sarcoma
v-abl	Ab-MLV	Mouse	Leukemia
v-abl	HZ2-FeSV	Cat	Sarcoma
Serine-threonine kinases			
v-mos	Mo-MSV	Mouse	Sarcoma
v-raf	MSV-3611	Mouse	Sarcoma
RAS family			
v-H-ras	Ha-MSV	Rat	Sarcoma
v-K-ras	Ki-MSV	Rat	Sarcoma
Nuclear proteins			
v-myc	MC29	Chicken	Carcinoma, myeloid leukemia
v-myb	E26	Chicken	Erythroleukemia
v-fos	FBJ-MSV	Mouse	Osteosarcoma
v-ski	SKV770	Chicken	Carcinoma
v-rel	REV-T	Turkey	Lymphatic leukemia
v-ets	E26	Chicken	Erythroleukemia
v-erba	AEV-ES4	Chicken	Erythroblastosis

From Weinburg RA. Oncogenes and tumor suppressor genes. CA Cancer J Clin Oncol 44: 160, 1994.

resents a mechanism for protecting an organism from cells that have acquired genetic alterations that predispose them to cell proliferation. Ultimately, multiple factors may contribute to programmed cell death. Even within the cell, different compartments may have considerable autonomy in undergoing structural changes during this process. Studies of the structures involved have clearly identified several genes and proteins that are critical in the regulation and susceptibility of cells undergoing apoptosis.[24,26] These regulatory genes and proteins are discussed in the following sections dealing with the deregulation of cell growth.

Numerous overall similarities between apoptosis and the cell cycle have been identified. It has been suggested that apoptosis and mitosis may have closely related mechanisms (albeit very different results). Further elucidation of the relationship between the cell cycle and apoptosis is warranted, as it provides powerful insight into the mechanisms of cellular growth and stability.

MOLECULAR BASIS OF NEOPLASIA

Viral and Proto-oncogenes

The supposition that tumorigenesis could occur on a genetic level was first suggested in 1866 by Broca, who described a family with a high prevalence of breast cancer and liver cancer.[27] It was not, however, until 1911 that Peyton Rous made the seminal discovery regarding the pathogenesis of cancer.[28] He observed that sarcoma could be induced in healthy chickens by introducing cell-free extracts obtained from chicken sarcomas. Not much was made of Rous's initial observation until the mid-1960s, when several investigators were able to demonstrate that other viruses besides the "Rous sarcoma virus" could induce cancers in animals. These experiments not only proposed the theory that viruses were directly linked with cancer initiation but led to the hypothesis that cancer developed in part from the introduction of specific genetic elements into the cell.

These initial concepts concerning the cause of malignancy were revolutionized by the recognition that certain viruses contained specific nucleic acid sequences (genes) responsible for transforming the infected cell.[28,29-31] The transforming nucleic acid sequences were termed retroviral oncogenes (*v-onc* genes)(Table 9-1).

Initially, retroviral oncogenes were thought to be of viral origin and to be required for some purpose important to the life cycle of the virus. However, this model did not easily explain why some retroviruses lacked oncogenes yet were able to propagate in a satisfactory manner. A major breakthrough was achieved with the discovery that genes very similar to the viral oncogenes were already present in tissues of normal, uninfected animals.[29,32] This discovery led to the concept that viral oncogenes were actually "abducted" by viruses early in evolution from their host cells.

Thus for each of the viral oncogenes *(v-onc)* there is a corresponding gene in the normal cells of vertebrates *(c-onc)*. In fact, some of these genes have been found in all species examined. The cellular genes homologous to the viral oncogenes are designated proto-oncogenes (or cellular oncogenes/*c-onc*).[30,31,33] In some instances proto-oncogenes are essentially identical in structure to the corresponding viral oncogenes; in other cases there has been some divergence in structure between viral and animal genes during the course of evolution.

Proto-oncogenes are phylogenetically ancient; related genes are even found in invertebrates such as *Drosophila* and in the primitive nucleated cells of yeast.[34] Preservation of proto-oncogenes through phylogeny with relatively little structural change suggested to investigators that these genes coded for essential cellular proteins.[35] Years of study have proved this to be the case with each proto-oncogene residing in our genome having an essential role in the life and function of the cell where it is expressed.

Of course, proto-oncogenes have such a critical function that they are prime candidates for mutations, which alter their expression, resulting in abnormal cell growth. Such mutations may occur spontaneously during the process of cell duplication or may be induced by carcinogenic agents in our environment. Because proto-oncogenes are critical to normal cell function, evolution has selected a limited number. Even so, over 50 have been found in a mutant form in human tumors (Table 9-2).

Having established that proto-oncogenes are important regulators of cell growth and function when normally expressed, it remains to be determined how a specific mutation(s) alters their normal structure and/or expression pattern generating a tumorigenic variant with abnormal function. Such oncogenic alleles have been termed gain-of-function mutations, since they act in a positive way in changing cell growth. As is described later in the chapter, more information regarding specific mutant variants is being discovered as these investigations proceed in numerous laboratories.

To briefly review, there are four key attributes of oncogenes:

Table 9-2. Representative Proto-oncogenes

Gene	Activation Mechanism	Protein Properties	Tumor Type
K-RAS	Point mutation	p21 GTPase	Pancreatic, colorectal, lung (adeno) and other cancers, leukemia
N-RAS	Point mutation	p21 GTPase	Myeloid leukemia
H-RAS	Point mutation	p21 GTPase	Bladder and other cancers
EGFR (ERBB)	Amplification, rearrangement	Growth factor receptor	Gliomas, carcinomas
NEU (ERBB2)	Amplification	Growth factor receptor	Breast, ovarian, and other carcinomas
MYC	Chromosome translocation amplification	Transcription factor	Burkitt's lymphoma; SCLC; other cancers
N-MYC	Amplification	Transcription factor	Neuroblastoma, SCLC
L-MYC	Amplification	Transcription factor	SCLC
BCL-2	Chromosome translocation	Anti-apoptosis protein	B-cell lymphoma (follicular type)
CYCD1	Amplification, chromosome translocation	Cyclin D (G_1 phase?)	Breast cancer, B-cell lymphoma, various carcinomas
BCR-ABL	Chromosome translocation	Chimeric nonreceptor tyrosine kinase	CML, ALL (T cell)
RET	Rearrangement	Chimeric receptor tyrosine kinase	Thyroid cancer (papillary)
TRK	Rearrangement	Chimeric receptor tyrosine kinase	Colorectal cancer
HST	Amplification	Growth factor (FGF-like)	Gastric cancer
APL-RARA	Chromosome translocation	Chimeric transcription factor	Acute promyelocytic leukemia
E2A-PBX1	Chromosome translocation	Chimeric transcription factor	Pre-B-ALL
MDM-2	Amplification	p53 binding protein (nuclear)	Sarcomas
GL1	Amplification	Transcription factor	Sarcomas, gliomas
TTG	Chromosome translocation	Transcription factor	T-ALL
CDK4	Amplification	Cyclin-dependent kinase	Sarcomas, gliomas

From Fearon ER. Oncogenes and tumor suppressor genes. In Abeloff MA, et al., eds. Clinical Oncology. New York: Churchill Livingstone, 1995. Reproduced with permission.

ALL, Acute lymphoid leukemia; *CML,* chronic myeloid leukemia; *FGF,* fibroblast growth factor; *GTPase,* guanosine triphosphatase; *SCLC,* small cell lung cancer.

1. Genes of this class are found in many different species of vertebrates and invertebrates. In fact, the *RAS* oncogene (an acronym for *rat*sarcoma, the source of the prototypic viral gene), was conserved by evolution in organisms as distinctly different from humans as yeast.
2. These genes are activated in common, nonviral cancers affecting humans.
3. The effects of activated oncogenes on cells are dominant. There is a positive effect on growth even in the presence of the normal (or inactivated) version of the same gene.
4. Each oncogene encodes a protein that is implicated in signal transduction (the transmission of growth regulatory messages from outside the cell to the processes controlling replication inside the cell's nucleus). Thus it has been shown that the mutation of cellular signal transduction genes (proto-oncogenes) can permanently activate (gain-of-function) a message to make cells keep dividing.[32]

Before discussing in greater detail the specific examples of proto-oncogenes and how their activation or alteration of function as oncogenes is involved in the process of oncogenesis, it is necessary to introduce a second group of genes termed *tumor suppressor genes.*

Tumor Suppressor Genes

As evidence accumulated that multiple genetic events were required for the generation of a metastasizing cancer, investigators discovered that activation (gain of function), which occurs in the proto-oncogene, is almost always inhibited by genes known as tumor suppressor genes.[36] The concept of tumor suppressor genes was introduced through studies by Harris.[37] He observed that cell hybrids generated from fusion of murine tumor cells with nontumorigenic murine cells were frequently incapable of inducing a tumor when injected into the appropriate host. The inability of these hybrid cells to induce a tumor when injected occurred even when activated oncogenes such as mutated *RAS* genes were present in the hybrid cells.[38]

When these nontumorigenic hybrid cells were passaged multiple times, they occasionally reverted to being once again fully capable of inducing tumor growth. Such cells were called revertants. When the revertants were analyzed carefully, they were found to have specific chromosome losses. Hybrids containing both chromosome alleles were suppressed and failed to form tumors, whereas those with even only one allele lost were tumorigenic.

Additional evidence for the existence of tumor suppressor genes came from experiments in which a single chromosome was microinjected into a cell and shown to suppress tumorigenicity.[39-41] Often not all the tumorigenic capacity of the parental cell was suppressed by the injection of a single chromosome, leading to the hypothesis that more than one tumor suppressor gene was involved with a given tumor.

Much of our knowledge of tumor suppressor genes originally came from the study of a fairly rare cancer, retinoblastoma (1 in 30,000 live births), which occurs in children up to the age of 7. Knudsen[42,43] observed that 40% of these cancers occur in infants with a mean age of 14 months. In this group, the tumors observed were most commonly multiple (±3) and bilateral. This group was also prone to develop osteogenic sarcoma later in life (~20 to 30 years of age). Some of the patients had a family history of these types of tumors, which indicated an inherited disposition. The remaining 60% of cases did not fit into the same pattern. They usually occurred in older children (~30 months of age), and no family history could be distinguished. Tumors in this group were most commonly singular, unilateral tumors.

Knudsen then proposed that two distinct mutagenic events were necessary for the development of retinoblastoma in both classes of patients. Knudsen's hypothesis is often termed the "two-hit hypothesis." Knudsen proposed that patients with the inherited form of the disease had one mutation present in the germline and subsequently, in all cells of the body. A second mutational event in any of the developing retinoblasts would subsequently cause a retinoblastoma. A patient with the inherited form of the disease would be expected to develop multiple tumors depending on the frequency of second mutations.

With this model, Knudsen could also account for the absence of disease in some patients known to have the predisposing mutation. In the second group, the patient has two normal (wild-type *RB*) alleles. Very rarely, two independent mutations occur in the same gene in the same retinoblast. When this does occur, the *RB* gene becomes inactivated, and a tumor forms. Therefore a single hypothesis can explain two different epidemiologic patterns in this cancer.

The *RB* gene has now been isolated by molecular cloning and shown to reside in 200 kb of DNA on chromosome 13.[44] Thus the Knudsen hypothesis was proved correct. Formal proof that a gene and its protein act as a tumor suppressor comes from an experiment in which the wild-type allele is reintroduced into a tumorigenic cancer lacking the gene. If the resultant cell line is no longer able to induce tumor formation, the gene can be properly classified as a tumor suppressor gene.[45]

Genes classified as tumor suppressor genes must act to regulate growth in a negative manner and must be shown to be inactivated by inherited or by somatic mutations in active cancer cells. In many instances, the protein products of those tumor suppressor genes have been shown to physically interact with an oncogene product. In fact, the protein product of one tumor suppressor gene may be capable of interacting with several oncogene products present in different tumors.

DNA Damage Repair

DNA damage can result from spontaneous alterations or from the interaction of various chemical and physical agents within the structure of the DNA molecule. Spontaneous lesions occur during normal cellular processes (i.e., DNA replication, gene rearrangement) or through chemical alteration of the DNA molecule itself as a result of hydrolysis, oxidation, or methylation. Interaction of DNA with physical agents (i.e., ionizing radiation, ultraviolet light) can lead to single- or double-strand breaks of the DNA molecule. The ability to repair these defects is fundamental to all biologic processes, given that damaged sites can be converted to permanent mutations during DNA replication. Susceptibility to carcinogenesis is related to the ability of a cell to repair this damaged DNA.[46-49]

There are several mechanisms for repairing damaged DNA. The most common form of repair is DNA excision repair, which removes DNA lesions and reconstructs original DNA structure using a multistep enzymatic process.[46,48] This process of DNA repair is often referred to as "cut and patch." Another mechanism is DNA mismatch repair. In mismatch repair, a pair of incorrect bases is recognized, and one member of the mismatched pair is removed. The resulting gap is filled in by DNA polymerase, and the final seal is made by DNA ligase. Postreplication repair, or recombinational repair, often occurs after DNA replication and is useful for lesions that block DNA synthesis. Another component of the repair process is the delay of the damaged cell's progress through the cell cycle. These delays provide more time for DNA repair processes to remove DNA damage.[46-49]

Deregulation of Cell Growth

A great deal of the recent progress in understanding the cell cycle and apoptosis has been a direct result of a desire to know how oncogenes, tumor suppressor genes, and DNA damage recognition and repair enzymes deregulate normal cell growth. It is widely recognized that cancer results from mutations occurring in the otherwise normal genome of a cell. These mutational changes are the result of the activation or deactivation of key regulatory genes that encode products that profoundly effect cell growth and differentiation. Information accumulated from the early studies of viral oncogenesis greatly contributed to the understanding of the transformation process.

Although there are multiple events in the process of oncogenesis, as previously stated, it is now known that activation (gain of function), which occurs in the proto-oncogene, is generally inhibited by genes known as tumor suppressor genes.[36] As indicated above, inactivation of tumor suppressor genes (loss of function) plays a significant role in tumorigenesis, perhaps as important as the effect of the oncogene. The number of tumor suppressor genes discovered to date is still small; however, these genes are clearly important factors in human cancer formation.

As mentioned earlier, certain oncogenes have a significant role in the cell cycle in that they inhibit a cell's ability to destroy itself when necessary (apoptosis). Three oncogenes are specifically implicated: *BCL-2* (proto-oncogene), *MYC* (proto-oncogene), and *p53* (tumor suppressor gene). Overexpression of *BCL-2* specifically inhibits a cell from initiating apoptosis in response to appropriate stimuli.[22,50] The *BCL-2* protein has been localized to the nuclear envelope, parts of the endoplasmic reticulum, and outer mitochondral membrane.[50] Despite the intensive study of *BCL-2,* the specific biochemical activity of the *BCL-2* protein remains relatively undefined. The introduction of genes that inhibit *BCL-2* can induce apoptosis in a number of different tumors that seem to rely on *BCL-2* to prevent cell death. *BCL-2* expression has been associated with a poor prognosis in prostate cancer, colon cancer, and neuroblastoma.[22]

MYC encodes for nuclear phospholipids that function as transcriptional regulators by binding to specific DNA sequences following dimerization with the protein MAX.[51-53] Expression of *MYC* is required for cell growth and entry into the S phase of the cell cycle. An apoptotic response induced by *MYC* requires the presence of wild-type *p53*. Thus a deregulated expression of *MYC* and loss of wild-type *p53* function are common findings in various human tumors including small cell lung cancer, breast cancer, and colorectal cancer.[54,55]

The *p53* protein has a number of functions, but in relation to the cell cycle it has been shown to be a transcriptional regulatory protein. It plays a key role in the positive regulation of several genes that are critical in the cell cycle including the *WAF1/CIPI/p21* gene, which regulates CDK activity and the *GADD45* (growth arrest DNA damage inducible) gene.[56,57] In certain situations, *p53* acts as a G_1/S checkpoint and controls the cell's decision to synthesize DNA. The *p53* gene represents one member of a class of genes that participate in cell cycle regulation and DNA repair.[58,59] Cells with intact wild-type *p53* function have been shown to arrest cell growth in the G_1 phase of the cell cycle in response to DNA damage and facilitate repair of the damage before allowing DNA synthesis. Cells that do not have functional *p53* fail to arrest and therefore allow replication of the damaged DNA. It can therefore be concluded that loss of *p53* function leads to increased genomic instability in tumor cells. In addition, studies have shown that when a cell regains wild-type *p53* functionality (i.e., following gene transfer), such cells have a greater sensitivity to radiation and some forms of chemotherapy (i.e., cisplatin) than do cells that have no *p53* function.[60]

There is now a large body of evidence to suggest that failures in the function of a number of DNA repair enzymes (including *p53*) are intimately involved in the promotion of tumorigenesis.[61] The importance of the protection of appropriate DNA cellular repair is best illustrated by the severe effects of sunlight in individuals who are deficient in DNA repair enzymes.[62,63] Several rare inherited diseases exhibit altered cellular response to DNA damage including xeroderma pigmentosum (XP), ataxia-telangiectasia (AT), Bloom syndrome, and Fanconi's anemia.[63-65]

A dramatic example of how oncogene activation (and tumor suppressor gene inactivation) leads to carcinogenesis was described by Vogelstein et al.[66] They identified four

Table 9-3. Tumor Suppressor Gene Alterations in Selected Human Tumor Types or Tumor Syndromes

Tumor Type/ Tumor Syndrome	Chromosomal Region	Evidence
Retinoblastoma	13q14	LA, LOH, RB1 mutation
Osteosarcoma	13q14	LA, LOH, RB1 mutation
	17p13	LA, LOH, p53 mutation
Wilms' tumor	11p13	LA, LOH, WT1 mutation
	11p15	LA, LOH
	16q	LOH
	Other(s)	LA
Rhabdomyosarcoma	17p13	LA, LOH, p53 mutation
	11p15	LOH
Hepatoblastoma	11p15	LOH
Colorectal	1p	LOH
	5q21	LA, LOH, APC mutation
	8p	LOH
	17p13	LOH, p53 mutation
	18q21	LOH, DCC mutation
	Others	LOH
Breast	17p13	LA, LOH, p53 mutation
	17q	LA, LOH, BRCA1 mutation
	16q	LOH, E-cadherin mutation
	11p15	LOH
	11q	LOH
	13q	LA (BRCA2)
	13q	LOH
	13q	RB1 mutation
	Others	LOH
Lung (small cell)	3p	LOH
	13q14	LOH, RB1 mutation
	17p13	LOH, p53 mutation
	Others	LOH
Lung (non–small cell)	3p	LOH
	17p13	LOH, p53 mutation
	Others	LOH
Bladder (transitional cell)	9p21	LOH, p16 (CDKN2) mutation
	9q	LOH
	11p15	LOH
	17p13	LOH, p53 mutation
	Others	LOH
Kidney (renal cell)	3p	LA, LOH, VHL mutation
	17p13	LOH, p53 mutation
	Others	LOH
Glioblastoma	9p21	LOH, p16 (CDKN2) mutation
	10q	LOH
	17p13	LOH, p53 mutation
	Others	LOH
Melanoma	9p21	LA, LOH, p16 (CDKN2) mutation
	17q	NF1 mutation
	Others	LOH
Neurofibromatosis type 1	17q	LA, LOH, NF1 mutation
Neurofibromatosis type 2	22q	LA, LOH, NF2 mutation
Meningioma	22q	LOH, NF2 mutation

From Fearon ER. Oncogenes and tumor suppressor genes. In Abeloff MA, et al., eds. Clinical Oncology. New York: Churchill Livingstone, 1995. Reproduced with permission.

APC, Adenomatous polyposis; *DCC,* deleted in colon cancer; *LA,* linkage analysis; *LOH,* loss of heterozygosity; *VHL,* von Hippel-Landau. Genes (other than E-cadherin) are described in the text.

genes implicated in colon carcinogenesis, *RAS, FAP* (a.k.a., *APC*), *DCC,* and *p53.* A decade of study has shown that the *RAS* oncogene is a growth-promoting gene in its normal cellular state[67], but at least a third of tumors contain mutated *RAS* genes that affect the control of tumor growth.[68] The *K-RAS* gene has been found to be a more frequent target for mutation than either the *H-RAS* or the *N-RAS* gene. Activated *RAS* genes seem to ignore the normal regulatory pathways of cell growth by failing to hydrolyze guanosine triphosphate (GTP) to guanosine diphosphate. The resulting effect is that the *RAS* protein remains in the GTP-bound or "active" state.

The three remaining genes (*FAP, APC,* and *p53*) identified by Vogelstein et al. belong to the class of tumor suppressor genes described earlier in this chapter. The Vogelstein team found that *RAS* mutations occurred in approximately 50% of colorectal carcinomas. However, the most interesting observation was that *RAS* mutations were common not only in malignant lesions but also in lesions with reduced metastatic potential or premalignant lesions (i.e., hyperplastic polyps). It was thus hypothesized that the progression toward tumorigenicity was aided by the shedding of the other three genes (*FAP, DCC,* and *p53*), which normally acted to constrain or suppress cell growth.[66]

Study of this phenomenon was also taken up by Harris et al.[69] In their experiments, a mutated cell, which was shown to cause the formation of a tumor in an animal, was fused with a nontumorigenic normal cell. The hybrid cells retained many of the phenotypes of the cancerous parent cell, but these cells no longer produced tumors in the laboratory animals. The hybrid between a tumorigenic and nontumorigenic cell was nontumorigenic, suggesting that a gene or genes from the normal cell were dominant and suppressed the tumorigenic potential of cancer cells.

As various studies were undertaken, it was noted that occasionally the hybrid cell line would cause tumor formation in animals. On studying the cells found in these tumors, it became evident that the tumorigenic cells had lost one or more chromosomes supplied by the normal parent cell. Thus chromosomes that apparently carried the tumor suppressor genes and conferred the normal phenotype to the hybrid cell could be identified as deletions from these cells. Experiments using advanced somatic cell fusion techniques using a single normal human chromosome and a cancerous cell were conducted.[70] Several of the resultant hybrid cells that did not show tumor formation in animals were identified. Based on these experiments, several different chromosomes from normal human cells were shown to carry putative tumor suppressor genes believed to block tumor formation (Table 9-3).

p53 has become something of a celebrity. In 1993, *Science* magazine named it "Molecule of the Year."[71] Researchers have documented more than 51 types of human tumors that carry *p53* mutations.[72] As mentioned earlier, *p53* is unique in its role both as a tumor suppressor and in the cell cycle, as it has been shown to be crucial in the apoptotic pathway induced by DNA damage.[58,59,61,73] As described previously, both copies of a gene like the *RB* suppressor gene must be inactivated before the cell functions abnormally. However, in the case of *p53,* a similar end result can be reached if the initially mutated gene copy loses growth-suppressing function and simultaneously acquires the ability to actively interfere with the function of the remaining copy. This represents what has been termed a "dominant negative" mode of action (in contrast, the *RB* gene acts as a "simple recessive" allele).[36,74]

There are a number of other tumor suppressor genes that fulfill the criteria of having both alleles lost or selected against in cancerous tissues (adenomatous polyposis *[APC];* deleted in colon cancer *[DCC]*) or in which mutation contributes to an inherited predisposition to a specific cancer in a dominant fashion *(WT1, NF1, APC).* These are listed in Table 9-4.

A number of contrasts can be made between oncogenes and tumor suppressor genes (Table 9-5). While oncogenes had a monopoly of the limelight for many years, the study of tumor suppressor genes provided a clearer understanding of the inherited predispositions to cancer, the cell type or tissue specificity associated with some abnormal genes and their products, and the reproducible karyotypic abnormalities of certain cancers.

Characteristics of Tumor Growth, Invasion, and Metastasis

Growth Factors and Receptors

Cells within normal tissue are regulated by processes of growth and differentiation based on signals received from other cells in the tissue or organism. The molecules that regulate this process are found in the extracellular environment and are termed growth factors. Studies of various cultured normal and transformed cells have demonstrated significant growth pattern differences between them. Normal cells in culture have a limited growth potential and show a density-dependent inhibition of growth. Normal cells do not grow across one another but arrange in an even monolayer (i.e., contact inhibited), with cessation of cell division and DNA synthesis.[75] Normal cells are also much more dependent than tumor cells on exogenous growth factors (survival signals).

Tumor cells often appear to produce their own growth factors, creating autocrine stimulation. As a result, transformed cells show loss of contact inhibition by growing across one another and forming dense, piled-up colonies with unlimited growth potential. Frequently, transformed cells lose their requirement for surface attachment (loss of anchorage) and grow in suspension or in soft agar.[76] Loss of adhesiveness by transformed cells is generally associated with a number of phenotypic changes. These phenotypic changes (especially loss of anchorage) are more likely to facilitate in vivo tumor formation.

The idea that cell transformation might be due, at least in part, to these extracellular components was first proposed in 1978, when reports were published that factors produced by transformed or tumor cells were capable of

Table 9-4. Cloned Tumor Suppressor Genes

Syndrome (or Tumor)	Name of Gene	Types of Tumor(s)	Cellular Location of Gene Product	Chromosome Localization
(Colon carcinomas)	*DCC*	Colon carcinomas	Cytoplasm	18q
Familial adenomatous polyposis	*APC*	Colon carcinomas	Cytoplasm	5q
Li-Fraumeni	*p53*	Carcinomas, leukemias	Nucleus	17p
Neurofibromatosis type 1	*NF1*	Neurofibromas	Cytoplasm	17q
Neurofibromatosis type 2	*NF2*	Schwannomas, Meningiomas	Cytoplasm	22q
Retinoblastoma	*RB*	Retinoblastomas, small cell lung carcinomas, osteosarcomas	Nucleus	13q
Wilms' tumor	*WT1*	Renal cell carcinomas	Nucleus	11p

From Weinberg RA. Oncogenes and tumor suppressor genes. CA Cancer J Clin Oncol 44: 160, 1994. Reproduced with permission.

Table 9-5. Properties of Oncogenes and Tumor Suppressor Genes

Property	Proto-oncogenes	Tumor Suppressor Genes
Number of mutational events required to contribute to the cancer	One	Two
Function of the mutant allele	Gain of function, acts in a dominant fashion	Loss of function, acts in a recessive fashion
Mutant allele may be inherited through the germ line	No examples at this time	Frequently has an inherited form
Somatic mutation contributes to cancer	Yes	Yes
Tissue specificity of mutational event	Some, but can act in many tissues	Inherited form commonly has a tissue preference

From Levine AJ. Tumor suppressor genes. In Mendelsohn J, et al., eds. The Molecular Basis of Cancer. Philadelphia: WB Saunders, 1995. Reproduced with permission.

inducing transformation transiently in cultured cells.[77,78] It was shown that unregulated production of growth factors or production of mutant growth factors might affect the producer cell itself (autocrine stimulation), adjacent cells (paracrine), or distant cells (endocrine).

Several efforts to purify and sequence growth factors led to the discovery that the sequence of the PDGF B chain matched the predicted product of the transforming gene of simian sarcoma virus, designated *v-sis*.[79,80] It was then found that the *v-erbB* product of avian erythroblastosis virus, predicted to encode a *v-src* related protein tyrosine kinase, actually represented a truncated form of the EGF receptor.[81] Subsequent evidence demonstrated that EGF triggering of its receptor resulted in tyrosine kinase autophosphorylation.[82] Protein phosphorylation and dephosphorylation serves as rapid reversible mechanisms mediating growth factor activity. Protein phosphorylation regulates protein-to-protein interactions, and protein activity ultimately affects gene expression.[83] Thus a direct link between growth factors, receptors with tyrosine kinase activity, and oncogenes was formulated. Current evidence indicates that the constitutive activation of growth factor signaling pathways through genetic alterations affecting these genes contributes to the development and subsequent progression of most, if not all, human cancers.[84]

A number of other secretory polypeptides have been strongly or weakly implicated as oncoproteins (Table 9-6). Some of these were first discovered as products of oncogenes and thought to be secretory proteins through sequence analysis or protein biochemistry. Others were first recognized as growth or differentiation factors that have subsequently been tested for oncogenic activity.

This expanding field of knowledge concerning growth factor–mediated mitogenic signaling pathways holds promise for the development of new cancer treatments. In considering the events that lead to the onset of growth factor–induced cell proliferation, the point at which therapy would be most effective is obviously during the initial interaction between the growth factor and its cognate receptor at the cell surface of tumor cells whose growth is dependent on autocrine or paracrine mechanisms.[84] Other suggested approaches include the production of specific monoclonal antibodies that would specifically neutralize the activities of growth factors. Some promising findings have been reported by investigators using experimental animal models in which administration of monoclonal receptor antibodies induced receptor down regulation and impairment of tumor cell proliferation.[85,86]

Table 9-6. Some Frequently Studied Growth Factors (GFs)

Acronym(s)	Name	Sources	Typical Targets
EGF	Epidermal GF	Embryos Submaxillary gland	Epithelia
TGF-α	Tumor GF-α	Embryos Oncogene-transformed cells	Epithelia
PDGF-A, -B	Platelet-derived GF	Platelets, tumor cells	Mesenchymal cells
aFGF	Acidic fibroblast GF	Brain, pituitary	Mesenchymal cells
bFGF	Basic fibroblast GF	Brain, pituitary	Mesenchymal cells
TGF-β 1, 2, 3	Tumor GF-β	Oncogene-transformed cells	Wide spectrum
GM-CSF (CSF-2) (CSF-α)	Granulocyte-macrophage colony-stimulating factor	T lymphocytes Fibroblasts	Mixed granulocyte-macrophage colonies
M-CSF (CSF-1)	Macrophage colony-stimulating factor	Fibroblasts	Macrophages
G-CSF (CSFβ)	Granulocyte colony-stimulating factor	Monocytes	Granulocytes
Multi-CSF (IL-3)	Multipotential GF	T lymphocytes	Multipotential progenitors
IGF-I, -II	Insulin-like GF	Extra-embryonic membranes, fetal serum	Mesenchymal, epithelial cells
NGF	Nerve growth factor	Submaxillary gland	Neuronal cells
TCGF (IL-2)	T-cell GF	T lymphocytes	B, T lymphocytes
IL-1	Interleukin-1	Leukemia cells	B, T lymphocytes, neutrophils
EPO	Erythropoietin	Kidney cells	Erythroid precursors

From Weinberg RA. Oncogenes and the Molecular Basis of Cancer. Cold Spring Harbor: Cold Spring Harbor Press, 1989. Reproduced with permission.

Tumor Growth Kinetics

Tumors appear to grow exponentially. However, with increasing size the doubling time also increases.[87,88] This relationship, in which the rate of growth decreases as the tumor grows, is described mathematically as a Gompertzian function.[89,90] The decreasing growth rate with increasing tumor size prohibits determining the date of tumor origin from a simple extrapolation of metastatic tumor doubling time. But despite the Gompertzian growth curve, useful information is obtained from knowledge of the doubling time of measurable tumor. For most human tumors, such predicted growth rates are only an approximation because they cannot accurately account for tumor cell loss caused by cell death and exfoliation. The growth of human tumors results in increased size, leading to areas of inadequate tumor blood supply and partial necrosis. Thus the rate of cell proliferation may vary considerably even within the tumor.

Prehn[88] suggested that a tumor behaves more like an integrated organ in its pattern of growth than a collection of independently growing cells. He stated that tumors appear to undergo a "compensatory hyperplasia" when a portion is removed or destroyed (similar to the regenerative processes seen in resected liver tissue). This compensatory growth may account for otherwise inexplicable clinical observations. He admitted that definitive figures are not available but suggested there is a prevalent impression that patient survival is, in many cases, benefited little, if at all, by therapies that reduce the tumor burden. This conclusion is based, in part, on the notion that tumor growth starts again at the beginning of the Gompertzian growth curve when the size of the tumor is reduced. Thus an appropriate mode of therapy might include inducing a tumor into behaving as though it has a greater mass. In such a case, the tumor might stop growing. The author admitted that therapy based on this idea must await the identification and synthesis of the putative organ-specific (or tumor-specific) control entities.

Invasion and Metastasis

Despite phenomenal advances in cancer screening, adjuvant and local treatments, and the surgical management of cancer, the process of invasion and metastasis continues to be the greatest obstacle to successful cancer management. The fearsome stigma of a cancer diagnosis is closely associated with the process of metastasis, and there is no question that this stigma is justified, as most cancer deaths result from the relentless progression of metastatic disease. In nearly 50% of cancer patients, surgical excision of the primary neoplasm is not curative because metastasis has already occurred by the time the surgery is carried out.[91,92]

A remarkable series of interrelated steps is required for the transition of in situ tumor growth to metastatic disease. These steps are outlined in the box on p. 231 and further elucidated by Fig. 9-3. It is interesting to note that although the balance of these interactions vary based on properties of the tumor cells themselves and their host environment, the steps or events in the pathogenesis of a metastasis are similar in all tumors.[91,92]

STEPS IN THE PATHOGENESIS OF METASTASIS

1. *Transformation of normal cells into tumor cells and growth:* After the initial transforming event, the growth of neoplastic cells must be progressive, with nutrients for the expanding tumor mass initially supplied by simple diffusion.
2. *Extensive vascularization:* This step is necessary if a tumor mass is to exceed 1 to 2 mm in diameter. The synthesis and secretion of angiogenesis factors are key to establishing a capillary network from the surrounding host tissue.
3. *Local invasion:* Several parallel mechanisms lead to local invasion of the host stroma by some tumor cells. Thin-walled venules, like lymphatic channels, offer very little resistance to penetration by tumor cells and provide the most common pathways for tumor cell entry into the circulation.
4. *Detachment and embolization:* Single tumor cells or aggregates detach and embolize, with the vast majority of circulating tumor cells rapidly destroyed.
5. *Survival:* The tumor cells survive the circulation.
6. *Arrest:* The tumor cells arrest in the capillary beds of distant organs, by adhering either to capillary endothelial cells or to subendothelial basement membrane, which may exposed.
7. *Extravasation:* This step probably occurs through mechanisms similar to those operative during invasion.
8. *Proliferation:* Within the organ parenchyma, proliferation completes the metastatic process. To continue growing, the micrometastasis must develop a vascular network and evade destruction by host defenses. The cells can then invade blood vessels, enter the circulation, and produce additional metastases.

From Fidler IJ. Invasion and metastasis. In Abeloff MA, et al., eds. Clinical Oncology. New York: Churchill Livingstone, 1995. Reproduced with permission.

Angiogenesis. A critical event in the history of a tumor and what may separate a slow-growing (almost dormant) in situ cancer from an invasive neoplasm is the process of neovascularization or angiogenesis. This process refers to the growth of new vessels toward and within the tumor. The vascularization of the tumor, stimulated by a specific factor(s), results in increased tumor growth, leading to compression of surrounding tissues, invasion through the basement membrane, and distant seeding (metastases) of tumor cells in other body tissues. Studies show that if angiogenesis does not occur, cell proliferation reaches a steady state, and the tumor grows no larger than about 2 mm in greatest diameter.[93] Also for tumor cells to metastasize, they must gain access to the vascularization from the primary tumor, survive the circulation, localize in the target organ, and induce angiogenesis in that organ.[93]

Experimental and clinical evidence has been developed that postulates that neovascularization of a tumor requires that a critical number of its cells have switched to the angiogenic phenotype.[94,95] There are two general categories of mechanisms by which tumor cells become angiogenic: (1) angiogenic activity arises from the tumor cell itself in the form of the release of angiogenic molecules (e.g., the basic fibroblast growth factor); (2) angiogenic activity may also arise from host cells recruited by the tumor (e.g., macrophages), may be mobilized by the extracellular matrix, or possibly may even require a concomitant loss of physiologic inhibition of endothelial cell proliferation. Evidence has begun to suggest that for most tumors, the process of acquiring an angiogenic phenotype depends on the outcome of a balance between angiogenic stimulators and angiogenic inhibitors, both of which may be produced by tumor cells and possibly even by certain host cells.[94-96]

The synthesis of specific angiogenesis inhibitor genes shows great promise as a new therapeutic approach designed to suppress angiogenesis, thereby reducing the metastatic potential of a given tumor.[94,96-101] Several studies have demonstrated that the removal of certain tumors (i.e., breast, colon, and osteogenic sarcomas) is related to a higher incidence of secondary tumors and metastasis.[94,96-101] O'Reilly et al.[102] suggested a possible hypothesis to explain this phenomenon. They proposed that a primary tumor initiates its own neovascularization by generating angiogenic stimulators in excess of appropriate angiogenic inhibitors. However, the angiogenesis inhibitor, by virtue of its longer half-life in the circulation, reaches the vascular bed of a secondary tumor in excess of angiogenic stimulator escaping from the primary tumor or generated by the secondary tumor. Therefore there is an inhibition of the growth of the metastasis or secondary tumor.[102] In experimental animal models the angiogenesis inhibitor associated with murine Lewis lung tumor, angiostatin, has been shown to effectively inhibit metastases.[96] There are a number of ongoing studies that have attempted to isolate specific angiogenesis inhibitors in human tumors.

Tumor cell invasion. Angiogenesis occurs in parallel with the transition to tumor cell invasion and provides a vascular entry portal for dissemination, which may take place long before primary tumor growth can be detected. Invasion is the active translocation of cancer cells across adjacent tissue boundaries and through host cellular and extracellular matrix barriers.[92,103-105] The invasion process occurs as an interaction with the basement membrane, which consists of attachment, matrix dissolution, motility, and penetration.[92] Cellular invasion is dependent on the coordinated activity of a series of interacting proteins extending from inside the cell, through the plasma membrane, to the cell surface, and into the pericellular microenvironment.[104]

The basement membrane and interstitial stroma play an important role in the process of tumor invasion. Basement

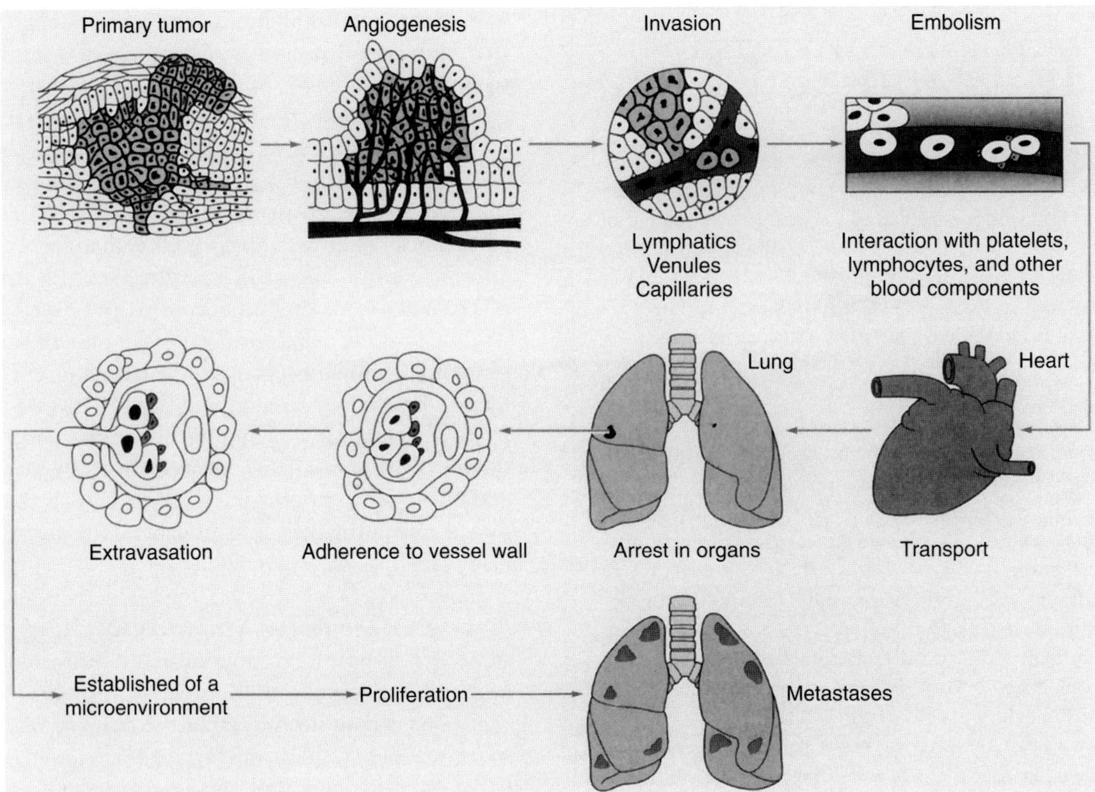

Fig. 9-3. The process of metastasis. Metastatic cells must complete all sequentially linked steps if a clinically relevant lesion is to develop. If a disseminating tumor cell fails to survive any of these steps, it does not produce a metastasis. (From Fidler IJ. Invasion and metastasis. In Abeloff MA, et al., eds. Clinical Oncology. New York: Churchill Livingstone, 1995. Reproduced with permission.)

membranes can be considered the barriers that confine the movement of cells to specific tissue compartments. It is now widely known that one way to regulate the integrity of the basement membrane is by maintaining the balance between metalloproteinases and metalloproteinase inhibitors (TIMPs).[106-108] With this hypothesis in mind, agents or treatments that are derived to maintain the integrity of the basement membrane may be an excellent approach to slow or possibly halt the process of invasion and angiogenesis. A family of TIMPs has been shown to halt the formation of new blood vessels required to nourish growing metastases in several laboratory studies.[104,109-112]

It should also be noted that a tumor cell must be motile to invade host stroma.[113-116] It should therefore follow that inhibition of cell motility would also be a possible limiting factor in tumor cell invasion and metastases. Unfortunately, the inhibition of cell motility can only prevent invasion by some tumors.[117,118] In fact, some normal cells are known to migrate extensively (i.e., lymphocytes).

Drugs that have been synthesized to combat angiogenesis, including TIMPs, motility inhibitors, and signaling inhibitors, have been shown to reduce tumor cell proliferation and invasion to varying degrees. Agents of this type have what has been termed a "cytostatic" rather than "cytotoxic" action. Current cytotoxic treatment regimens, although they do measurably reduce tumor burden, do not produce true cures in a high percentage of patients with metastatic cancer. The goal of the cytostatic paradigm of intervention is to prevent the onset of metastatic disease, slow or halt proliferation once the metastatic cascade has begun, and finally generate a period of disease stabilization. Subsequently, under the paradigm of cytostasis, new views of clinical strategies must be developed, which include consideration of time to progression, quality of life, and survival. It will also be important to develop new methods of detection and monitoring of tumor cytostasis in cancer patients.[104]

Metastasis. It is now widely accepted that neoplastic cells within a tumor are heterogeneous and contain subpopulations of tumor cells with different metastatic propensities.[92,119-122] Models for metastases of human neoplasms have shown it to be a highly selective process regulated by a number of different mechanisms. The evolution and progression to heterogeneity occurs not only in the primary tumor but in metastases as well (giving rise to metastases of metastases). Progression is characterized by a series of definitive irreversible changes that occur in each distinct subpopulation of cells.[123,124]

The ability of a metastasis to grow and develop is also believed to be largely dependent on the environment where it is located. In 1889, Paget[125] described the "seed and soil" hypothesis that site-specific metastasis was related to the existence of an environment (the "soil") in which compatible tumor cells (the "seed") could proliferate. Paget studied the autopsy reports of 735 women with breast cancer. The decisive pattern of visceral metastasis suggested to him that certain tumor cells had an affinity for certain organs. Paget suggested that metastases resulted only when the seed and the soil were matched.[125] Fidler and Balch[123] have defined three modern principles of the seed and soil hypothesis: (1) neoplasms are heterogeneous for biologic and metastatic properties; (2) the process of metastasis is not random; (3) the outcome of metastasis depends on the interaction of metastatic cells with different organ environments.

Recent studies have corroborated that both the seed and the soil are key in determining where metastatic deposits flourish.[126-128] Togo et al.[127,128] recently reported that the seed to soil hypothesis is reversible in metastasis. In other words, a tumor can spread in either direction. Intrahepatically transplanted Co-3 human colon tumor tissue reversely metastasized to the orthotopic site and secondarily spread into the abdominal cavity in the nude mice studied.[128] These results indicate that the seed to soil hypothesis is still a relevant model to explain and further investigate the process of metastasis.

Evans[126] suggested that although it is true that cells within a tumor are heterogeneous (the "seeds"), it is also true that the patients themselves (the "soil") are heterogeneous in regard to metastatic propensity. Patients who develop distant metastases early in their course of disease are like fertile soil, whereas patients who resist the development of distant metastases are like barren soil. He points to this hypothesis in support of preservation surgery in the treatment of breast cancer and other solid tumors.[126]

A potential metastasis suppressor protein, nm23, was first identified by Steeg et al.[129] while screening for differences in genetic activity between metastatic and nonmetastatic mouse cells. Clinical studies of patients with primary breast cancers reported that high levels of nm23 correlated with the absence of metastasis and a very favorable prognosis for patients, while low levels of *nm23* were associated with metastasis and poor survival.[130] Alterations in this protein correlate strongly with the transition to invasion and metastasis. Measurements of *nm23* could theoretically have important clinical value in terms of identifying those patients who are most at risk for hidden metastasis and treating them accordingly.[131] There is speculation relating to the theory that the introduction of nm23 into tumor cells of the body could halt the metastatic process.[130,131]

TUMOR IMMUNITY IN HOST RESISTANCE

In the early 1900s it was postulated that tumors expressed surface antigens that distinguished these tumor cells from normal cells.[132-135] This was based on experiments that demonstrated the rejection of tumors transplanted between outbred mice and clinical studies, suggesting the host development of anticancer serum globulins. Soon, however, it was recognized that this rejection of tumors transplanted in outbred mice was actually the result of immune recognition of normal transplantation antigens present on normal, as well as tumor, cells.[135,136]

In 1943 Gross demonstrated immunity to a methylcholanthrene-induced sarcoma in inbred mice.[137] These tumors could be transplanted to mice of the same inbred strain, where they would grow without difficulty. However, if the transplanted tumor was excised and then reinjected into the same mouse, the newly injected cells would almost always fail to grow.[138] These experiments provided the first evidence that tumors carry specific transplantation antigens that could cause their rejection in properly immunized hosts.

In the intervening years, tumor-specific antigens, or, as they are more commonly termed today, tumor-rejection antigens (TRAs), have been demonstrated to be a feature of most, if not all, cancers.[138-145] TRAs are unique to tumor cells and are not found associated with normal cells. TRAs probably occur as a result of two mechanisms. First, if point mutations occur in genes of the cell that are ubiquitously expressed, they may generate new antigenic peptides. Second, the activation of otherwise silent genes may produce novel antigenic peptides.[146] Their recognition by the immune system of the host can lead to tumor cell destruction by mechanisms identical to those of classic allograft rejection.[147,148]

An additional class of tumor antigens, the tumor-associated antigens (TAAs), can also be identified in tumor cells. TAAs in contrast to TRAs are also found on normal cells. These antigens may be expressed at different times during cell development or at different levels and appear to induce a state of immune tolerance. Although their reexpression in a tumor, or enhanced expression, may result in an immune response by the host, this is probably not a common or significant aspect of tumor immunogenicity. More commonly, such antigens serve simply as tumor markers, especially for recurrent metastatic disease.[149,150]

The uniqueness of TRAs or the degree to which these neotumor structures are more "nonself" than "self" is the basis by which the body's immune system responds to tumors. In experimental animal models, TRAs can stimulate an immune response that results in resistance to tumor growth. This protection against tumor growth can be adoptively transferred to syngeneic animals to afford similar protection. Although TRAs associated with oncogenic transforming viruses or with ultraviolet light exposure in animal models generate strong immune response. In contrast, chemically induced tumors generally produce weaker immune responses, and tumors that arise spontaneously produce little or no detectable immunity.[151]

From 1985 through 1997, clinical studies based solely on the manipulation of the immune system have greatly strengthened the confidence of scientists that what they have been observing in animal models is applicable to human cancers. For example, the numerous clinical trials using interleukin-2 (IL-2), a T-cell growth factor of central importance to the immune response, have consistently shown an ability to alter the growth of established metastases of melanoma and renal cell carcinoma.[152,153] In addition, the adoptive transfer of large numbers of in vitro expanded autologous tumor-infiltrating T lymphocytes (TILs) has also been shown to alter tumor growth in humans.[154,155]

Thus the conclusion of many such studies has been that most, and probably all, tumors bear antigens that can be targets for specific immune responses. They may, however, require manipulation to be recognized and to function optimally in generating an effective immune response. For example, adding new antigens to the tumor cell by gene transfection can confer on these tumor cells the ability to stimulate immune protection in the host against the original tumor.[156,157] In other experiments, tumor cells that had undergone appropriate mutations could be shown to be rapidly rejected because they expressed very strong new antigens.[158-160]

Very significant increases in tumor immunogenicity have also been obtained by transfecting tumor cells in vitro with various interleukin genes, for example IL-2, prior to reinjecting the cells into the host animal.[161,162] Transfections with IL-4, IL-7, interferon-γ (INF-γ), B7 (the co-stimulatory molecule that binds the ligand CD28 on T cells), and granulocyte-macrophage colony-stimulating factor (GM-CSF) have demonstrated the ability to convert tumors devoid of immunogenicity or tumors weakly immunogenic into tumors capable of generating a strong immune response in experimental animal models.[163-171]

As noted previously, the immune response to tumors is very similar to that of allograft rejection and, as in allograft rejection, the crucial cell is the T cell.[172] The various members of the T-lymphocyte family are responsible for secreting critical lymphokines necessary for differentiation and proliferation of eventual T-effector cells and for the generation of T cells that carry long-term memory to the tumor antigens. These T cells recognize not only the TRAs that are responsible for the rejection process but, in humans, must also recognize syngeneic molecules in the process of T-cell activation.[173,174]

The characterization of the T-cell receptor and the discovery that T cells recognize antigen in the context of class I and class II major histocompatibility (MHC) antigens are two of the most significant recent advances in the field of immunology.[175-179] This process of antigen recognition and T-cell triggering is completely different from the process used by antibody-producing B lymphocytes, where the antigen receptor is a surface immunoglobulin of the appropriate idiotype.

Studies of the T-cell receptor and of T-cell activation show that it is the CD8-bearing T cell that recognizes the MHC class I structure on the surface of the tumor cell when this MHC molecule contains a specific antigen peptide in its cleft, and it is the molecule associated with the T-cell receptor that binds to the α-domain of the MHC I determinant located on the tumor cell surface.[180] Fig. 9-4 illustrates the presentation of TRAs to a CD8$^+$ cytotoxic T lymphocyte (CTL). It appears that the TRA peptides binding to the MHC class I molecule are 8 to 10 amino acids in length and are derived from intracellular proteins that have undergone degradation.[181,182]

TRAs may also be presented by MHC class II molecules (human leukocyte [HLA]-DP, -DQ, -DR in humans); but since most of the class II determinants are present in the endoplasmic reticulum and traverse the endocytic compartments of the phagocytic antigen presenting cells, they are responsible for binding and presenting peptides produced from endocytosed exogenous molecules.[182,183] CD4$^+$ T cells are the subgroup that recognize class II bound peptides. Although the predominant presentation by class II MHC is for exogenous molecules, evidence exists to show that peptides synthesized within the antigen-presenting cell can sometimes be presented by class II molecules.[184-186]

The real significance of the elucidation of the T-cell receptor structure is the realization that T cells cannot only recognize cell surface antigens, as previously thought, but have the potential of recognizing all the proteins produced within the cell. Thus when mutations occur within the DNA coding for a cellular protein, the result is a new antigenic peptide; the novel peptide can be presented on class I molecules to the T-cell receptor.[69,173,178,187-189] In addition, by using the MHC class I molecule to transport the peptide to the cell surface for T-cell receptor recognition, a second important regulatory mechanism is introduced.

This second very important component of the presentation of TRAs is termed MHC restriction. More precisely, class I molecules encoded by different alleles do not bind and present the same peptides. For example, a tumor-specific peptide may be bound to the HLA-A MHC molecule in patients having the A1 allele but not be bound to the HLA-A2 molecule.[152,178] The phenomenon of MHC restriction therefore plays a very important role in designing potential immune therapies.

Two different approaches have been used to identify cancer rejection antigens. Boon[190] and van der Bruggen et al.[191] have used T cells derived from peripheral blood lymphocytes (PBLs) and from TILs to first clone CTLs specific for the tumor.[190,191] For example, when melanoma metastases are put into culture and supplemented with IL-2, the CD8$^+$ T cells present in the tumor are stimulated to proliferate.[192] These CTLs can be shown to have specific lytic activity against the autologous tumor but lack activity against other tumor cell targets and control targets.

Such CD8$^+$ CTL clones were then used to select resident variants from the melanoma cell line MZ2-MEL.[191] In this fashion, these investigators were able to identify sev-

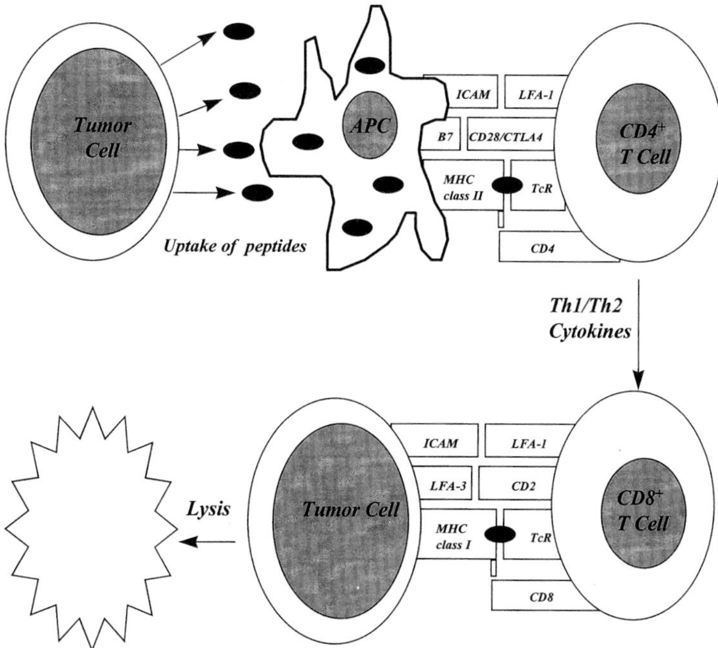

Fig. 9-4. Schematic representation of a cellular antitumor immune response. *ICAM,* Intracellular-antigen mediated; *MHC,* major histocompatibility complex; *TcR,* T-cell receptor.

eral different potential tumor rejection antigens for this melanoma tumor cell line. They termed these resistant cell lines antigen-loss variants and selected one as MZ2-MEL.E$^-$. They then transfected this cell line with DNA library from the original MZ2-MEL cells and identified transfectant cells expressing the new antigen MZ2-E. From these transfectants they were thus able to isolate the gene MAGE-1, which codes for MZ2.E. Further studies identified MZ2-E as a nonapeptide of the MAGE-1 protein and showed that it was presented to the T cell by the HLA-A1 molecule on the tumor cell.[191]

The Rosenberg group[144,155] at the National Cancer Institute has taken a different approach to identify novel TRAs. These investigators focused on selecting TILs that would recognize HLA-A2–bearing melanoma tumor cells (HLA-A2 is the most frequently expressed allele, being present in 49% of caucasians). They found that TILs from HLA-A2$^+$ tumors recognized almost all melanoma tumors that shared the HLA-A2 allele but failed to lyse cells that were HLA-A2 negative. They then very elegantly transfected HLA-A2$^-$ tumor cells with the gene encoding the HLA-A2 allele and showed that these cells could now be recognized and killed by HLA-A2$^+$ TILs, once again providing strong evidence for a common TRA.[144,155]

Rosenberg and his colleagues[155,157] have used TILs from patients that have shown good tumor regression to identify a series of genes encoding TRAs. They did this by preparing a cDNA library from the melanoma cell line and transfecting the library into an HLA-A2$^+$ breast cancer cell line.[193-197] Transfected cells derived from a single cell were cloned and expanded. HLA-A2$^+$ TIL from patients showing a good response to their TIL/Il-2 therapy were then used to select targets and the transfected genes in these individual cell clones were isolated and characterized.[144,155]

In another approach, COS-7 cells, a highly transfectable cell line, were transfected with the appropriate HLA restriction element (HLA-A2 or HLA-A24). The transfected cells were then transfected again, this time with pools of cDNA prepared from melanoma cells. These transfected COS-7 cells were screened with a specific TIL clone, which had caused complete regression of tumor in an HLA-A24 patient. In this manner, the specific TIL identified a subclone bearing the HLA-A24 class I MHC determinant and an appropriate TRA. This approach resulted in the identification of several melanoma TRAs. MART-1 and gp100 antigens were the first identified and later tyrosinase, p15, and gp75 were discovered. All five antigens have been associated with in vivo tumor response.[144,155]

By studying the tertiary structure of the HLA class I molecule, it was determined that the extracytoplasmic portion of the molecule contained a groove consisting of a β-pleated sheet surrounded by α-helixes. The amino acids in the base of this groove determine the specific three-dimensional structure of the groove and therefore predict which residues must be present in an antigen peptide nonamer to bind to that specific HLA molecule. Thus for each TRA of known structure it is possible to predict the 9 and 10 amino acid peptides most likely to bind to a specific HLA molecule. For example, 22 different peptides are potentially present in the MART-1 protein with the correct sequence for binding in the groove of the HLA-A2 molecule.[144,155]

These elegant new approaches for the very first time promise to provide critical information regarding TRAs for other solid tumors. Hopefully, the identification of such specific TRAs will provide new options for enhancing the immune response to these tumors and new vaccine therapies.

Potential for New Therapies

The characterization of specific TRAs and their encoding genes provides many new opportunities to enhance the patient's immune response. Whether the patient's tumor contains the respective TRA can be readily determined from a tumor sample by subjecting it to reverse transcriptase–polymerase chain reaction (PCR) analysis. Thus the appropriate protein or peptide antigen, produced in large scale, could then be used for direct patient immunization.[144,155,198]

For example, such peptide antigens could be used to pulse a patient's own antigen-presenting cells in vitro, and the pulsed cells could be reinfused. It should also be possible to transfect the patient's antigen-presenting cells with genes coding for the critical antigenic peptide. Perhaps it will also be possible to treat patients with recombinant BCG carrying the genetic information coding for the antigenic peptide or a bacterium such as *Salmonella* carrying the gene for an antigenic peptide.[198]

The difficulties to be overcome, of course, reside mainly in a lack of complete tumor specificity for many TRAs. This is certainly the case for MAGE genes and for tyrosinase. Immunization with such TRAs could cause damage to normal tissues. In addition, it may be difficult to generate highly effective CTLs against such antigens because of natural tolerance.[144,155,198]

A further concern is the development of antigen-loss variants within the tumor or HLA-loss variants. The effectiveness of the CTL would depend greatly on the extent to which these variants developed within a patient's tumor. These variants, especially the HLA-loss variants, would perhaps be selected for. Of course, natural killer (NK) cells are especially effective against tumor cells lacking HLA, and therefore effective immune therapies will certainly need to involve multiple cellular and cytokine approaches and perhaps chemotherapeutic approaches to maximize a chance for successful, complete elimination of tumor.[198]

Although a number of viral vectors have been developed to enable gene transfer, the success of immunotherapy of cancer will be heavily dependent on vectors that will be highly efficient, nonimmunogenic, and ideally controllable once placed within the patient. Other nonviral methods of gene delivery may also prove useful, and research in both areas is vitally important. In addition to vector research, much more information is needed regarding the mechanisms of the immune response to TRAs, especially regarding the breaking of immune tolerance to TRAs that are derived from normally occurring antigenic proteins.

Monoclonal Antibodies

A review of immunotherapy of cancer would not be complete without a discussion of the role of monoclonal antibodies. Monoclonal antibodies (mAb) specifically bound to tumor cells can initiate an antitumor response using complement-dependent cytotoxicity (CDC) and antibody-dependent cell-mediated cytotoxicity (ADCC) involving monocytes, macrophages, granulocytes, and lymphocytes with receptors to the Fc portion of the immunoglobulin molecule. Antibodies bound to tumor cells may cause a direct antiproliferative effect via inhibition of growth factors and growth factor receptors. Such antibodies, when bound to a cellular determinant, may induce an inhibitory growth pathway within the cell or have a direct catalytic effect (i.e., may induce hydrolysis of cell membrane). mAb when used in humans, may create an idiotype/anti-idiotype network against the tumor cells.[199]

Historically, one of the first examples of an antibody response against a human cancer occurred in a patient with a gastric cancer and was documented to be against an aberrantly expressed blood group antigen. The patient had received an incompatible blood transfusion that resulted in antibodies directed against the P1 antigen. The patient's tumor was shown to express P1 and the tumor completely regressed. The patient remained tumor free for 25 years.[200] Subsequently, a number of examples of antibodies reactive with expressed antigens on tumors have been implicated in tumor regressions, but treatment attempts with blood serum or plasma thought to contain anticancer antibodies have not shown any clear therapeutic benefit.[201-205]

A resurgence of interest in using antibodies to target therapy against tumors has evolved from the landmark work of Kohler and Milstein[206] in 1975, who developed a technique for generating a monoclonal antibody from a B-cell hybridoma. The technology for generating B-cell hybridomas has been further amplified by the tremendously powerful tool of recombinant DNA technology. These advances in molecular genetics have facilitated an understanding of antibody structure and the mechanisms underlying the extensive diversity of the antibody repertoire.

The B cell accomplishes the extensive diversity using a small number of germline DNA segments. If this were not the case and each immunoglobulin light and heavy chain were the product of a single different gene, more than one half of the B cell's genome would be required for the diversity that exists in humans. To accomplish this diversity, each heavy and light chain gene results from the joining of the variable (V), diversity (D), and joining (J) gene segments that exist as amplified families within the immunoglobulin DNA loci. Immunoglobulin gene rearrangement is further enhanced by a process termed junctional diversity. Junctional diversity is the method by which the cell introduces variation in the exact joining position for each of the V, D, and J segments. This process is a special type of rearrangement apparently unique to immunoglobulin genes and is controlled by a series of specific recombinase enzymes that function only during early B-cell development.[207]

The understanding of the steps and mechanisms involved in immunoglobulin-gene rearrangement has been used to generate specific immunoglobulin binding sites by a process of *repertoire cloning*. Specific immunoglobulin variable region genes are amplified by PCR and cloned into appropriate expression vectors. It has also been possible to produce a primary cDNA library of variable region genes from immunocompetent B cells; the library is then cloned and expressed on bacteriophage. Antigen is then used to select appropriate antibody-bearing phage and the specific variable region genes are rescued from the phage.[208-210] The specific variable region selected in this fashion is then mutated using PCR and cloned back into the phage vector to produce a secondary library. It is thus possible to generate and select over several rounds of subcloning very high-affinity variable-region binding sites.[211-215]

The structure of the immunoglobulin molecule facilitates genetic engineering of molecules that have a markedly reduced capacity to be recognized as foreign, a distinct advantage over monoclonal antibodies that are almost uniformly of murine background. It is also possible to alter the molecule so that it is processed within the body in a manner that decreases clearance and improves penetration of the tumor.[216,217]

Finally, these new techniques offer a variety of opportunities for creating special antitumor agents by coupling desired toxins, radionucleotides, or cytotoxic drugs. What is clear today is the realization that recent advances in molecular genetics have had a major impact on research in immunology. The result has been a much greater knowledge of cellular function, including antigen processing, T-cell recognition of antigen, T- and B-cell interaction, and the generation of antigen recognition site diversity. These advances in immunology as a science have created a rebirth of interest in the immune system as a potential therapy for cancer. Clearly, there is a delicate balance between immune tolerance to neotumor antigens and the destruction/rejection of the same.

BIOLOGIC RATIONALE FOR THERAPY

Chemotherapy

General Considerations

The ability to identify antitumor agents has been enhanced by insight into the patterns of growth of normal and neoplastic cells. The most fully characterized portions of the normal cell cycle are the S phase and mitosis. Most of the active chemotherapeutic agents are designed to inhibit processes occurring during these two phases of the cell cycle, and these drugs are in general more effective against rapidly dividing cells (in which a larger fraction of each cycle is devoted to DNA synthesis and mitosis) than slowly dividing cells. Although many classic anticancer treatments, such as the alkylating agents, are currently directed at nuclear targets, DNA is also the target for many new anticancer drugs.

The synthesis of DNA is a multistep process, using various enzyme pathways. Agents have been developed that, when combined, can inhibit the process at several points simultaneously, thereby enhancing the cytocidal effect. A variety of general strategies can be used, including sequential blockade of different steps in the same biosynthetic pathway, concurrent blockade of different pathways for the synthesis of necessary components, complementary inhibition of biochemical processes (whereby repair processes that circumvent chemotherapeutic damage are inhibited), metabolic sensitization of intracellular constituents to chemotherapeutic effects, and the utilization of combined chemotherapy and radiotherapy. Examples of each of these approaches have been described.[218-221]

Other considerations in the use of chemotherapeutic agents and the design of chemotherapy regimens include the emergence of drug-resistant cells (either by selection of insensitive clones or by the induction of cellular changes that result in drug resistance). The presence of sites that are inaccessible to drug effect on a physiologic or anatomic basis and the relative distribution of biologically effective drug between tumor cells and normal tissues determine the balance between toxic and therapeutic drug effects.

There have been many studies related to the origins of chemotherapeutic resistance.[222-225] Many patients manifest a resistance to a wide array of structurally unrelated antineoplastic agents, hence the term multidrug resistance (MDR). In vitro studies in cell culture indicate that this phenomenon is associated with amplification or overexpression of the MDR1 gene. The MDR1 gene codes for the expression of a cell surface protein, P-glycoprotein (P-gp), which acts as an energy-dependent efflux pump to transport drugs associated with MDR out of the cell before cytotoxic effects occur. Although this protein has been found in tumor samples from patients with acute leukemia, multiple myeloma, lymphomas, and a variety of solid tumors, it is also expressed in normal tissue, where it is thought to serve as an excretory pathway for xenobiotic drugs and toxins.

A number of drugs are able to reverse MDR, including calcium channel blockers, phenothiazines, quinidine, antimalarial agents, antiestrogenic and other steroids, and cyclosporine. Limited results from clinical trials suggest that the addition of verapamil, diltiazem, quinine, trifluoperazine, or cyclosporine to chemotherapeutic regimens has the potential to reverse MDR. Unfortunately, toxicities have limited their clinical usefulness. A great deal more research in this area is necessary to identify active modulators of MDR that are less toxic.[222-225]

Combination Chemotherapy

Optimal chemotherapy requires the use of combinations of drugs because with rare exceptions single agents do not cure cancer. Combination chemotherapy is now the standard for treatment of many disseminated or metastatic cancers and is curative in some.[226] A series of accepted guidelines for combination chemotherapy has been recognized for a number of years:

1. Select drugs that have been proven effective.
2. Select drugs that have different mechanisms of action.
3. Select drugs that have different spectrums of toxicity.
4. Each drug should be used at maximal dose.
5. Agents with similar dose-limiting toxicities can only be combined safely by reducing doses, resulting in decreased effects.
6. Drug combinations should be administered in the shortest interval between therapy cycles to allow for recovery of normal tissue.[227]

If these guidelines are followed, dosages that are close to the maximally tolerable dosages for each drug can be used in an intermittent drug treatment schedule designed to optimize the cytotoxic effect of each drug. In the case of hematologic toxicity, especially neutropenia, it is often possible to maintain the dosing schedule and to shorten the period of granulocytopenia by the use of hematopoietic growth factors G-CSF and GM-CSF.[228] The use of dosage modifications or the use of growth factors should be considered with the therapeutic goals of therapy in mind. If the regimen has potential for cure, every effort should be made to maintain dose and schedule. If palliation is the goal, dose reductions and lengthening of the interval between doses should be considered.

Adjuvant and Neoadjuvant Chemotherapy

The use of drugs as adjuvants to surgery or irradiation has led to significant advances in the chemotherapy of cancer.[227-230] In many instances, the primary localized tumor mass can be removed by surgery or destroyed by irradiation; but even if the diagnosis has been made relatively early, with certain tumors it is quite probable that small, clinically undetectable metastases have already occurred. Even with the considerable advances made in diagnostic techniques, the most common solid tumors (breast, lung, and colon carcinomas) are usually not detectable until the tumor attains a mass of 1 cm in diameter. By this time about 10^9 cells are present, and the tumor has already doubled in mass about 30 times. Since the chance for cell shedding into the lymphatic system or the blood stream increases with each doubling in tumor mass, there is a significant chance that cells have already metastasized by the time a tumor can be detected. Thus in many cases, patients have metastatic or micrometastatic disease at the time of diagnosis of the primary tumor. It is not usually practical to eliminate small metastatic foci by surgery or irradiation; thus chemotherapy is usually the treatment of choice in patients at risk for occult metastatic disease.

The principles for the use of drugs with surgery or radiotherapy are similar to those for the use of drugs in combination regimens. In general, drugs without a demonstrable activity against advanced tumor when used alone should not be used in adjuvant trials. A single drug with a demonstrated activity against advanced disease may actually have an enhanced antitumor effect after surgery or irradiation has produced a large decrease in total tumor bulk (debulking). If combinations of drugs have been shown to be effective in patients with advanced disease, they may also be used in adjuvant therapy. Another important consideration is that the drug or the drug combination must be relatively low in general toxicity. Since a significant number of patients may remain free of disease with surgery or radiotherapy alone, the added risk of drug toxicity (and in some cases the induction of secondary malignancies such as leukemia) must be carefully weighed against the potential benefit.

A second strategy that is used to treat the presence of micrometastatic disease at the time of diagnosis is neoadjuvant chemotherapy.[230] Neoadjuvant therapy is chemotherapy implemented before surgery in patients with apparently localized disease. The approach has several advantages over the more conventional postoperative adjuvant chemotherapy. It exposes the potential micrometastases to chemotherapy at an earlier stage, it is indicative of tumor response (based on in vivo response of the tumor itself), and it may cause significant regression of the primary tumor and perhaps allow for a more conservative surgical procedure (organ/function sparing). The dangers, of course, include ineffectiveness of chemotherapeutic regimens, which may in some cases obscure proper staging of disease or even render a primary tumor unresectable. Some tumors that have been effectively managed using neoadjuvant chemotherapy are soft tissue sarcoma, osteosarcoma, anal cancer, bladder cancer, larynx cancer, esophageal cancer, and locally advanced breast cancer.[229]

Another promising method that has matured greatly in recent years is the chemoprevention of cancer. Since the early 1990s, agents have shown significant activity in clinical trials in reversing oral, colon, and cervical premalignancy, as well as preventing primary skin and stomach cancer.[231] Agents that seem to have chemopreventive roles include retinoids, β-carotene, and α-tacopherol for oral and lung cancer; calcium and fiber for colon cancer; selenium for skin cancer; tamoxifen and fenretinide for breast cancer; and finasteride for prostate cancer. Chemoprevention is still being evaluated for efficacy, but it is hoped that it will be integrated with standard therapies in the near future.[231]

Radiation Therapy

General Considerations

Therapeutic radiation is ionizing; it ejects electrons from atoms or molecules with which it interacts. The energy transfer from radiation to tissue by this ionization is immediate. There is now a great deal of evidence that suggests that DNA is the target of this ionizing process and the cytotoxic effects of radiation.[232-234] The specific lesion believed to be responsible for most radiation-induced cellular death is known as the "double-strand break." Differences in cellular sensitivity to radiation may be a reflection of the cell's ability to repair this type of breakage.

Not all DNA is equally vulnerable to damage. DNA is associated with proteins in a complex three-dimensional structure called chromatin. The influence of DNA packaging into chromatin is evidenced by the fact that naked DNA (DNA removed from the cell and disassociated from its chromatin) is 50 times more susceptible to radiation-induced strand breakage than intact DNA.[235] Uncoiled DNA is also more susceptible to radiation damage, which means that cells in early synthesis (S phase) are more sensitive to radiation. Experimental data show that cells are more sensitive in early S phase and mitosis than in the late S phase and G_2.[236]

The radiosensitivity of a large variety of tissues, both normal and malignant, has been studied extensively. When surviving irradiated cells are plotted against dose along an x/y axis, a very typical mammalian cell survival curve results. To date, more than 20 different models have emerged.[237] The single-hit, multitarget model has a very typical mammalian cell survival curve result (Fig. 9-5).[238] Data are derived from the exposure of clonogenic cells to single radiation doses. The curve consists of two portions: an initial "shoulder," which is thought to represent a dosage range in which repair of sublethal injury takes place, and an experimental portion, in which a given dose of radiation kills a constant proportion of cells. The slope of the experimental portion of the curve is $1/D_0$, where D_0 is the dose of radiation that reduces the surviving fraction of irradiated cells to 37% of its former value, and "n" is the "extrapolation number" or the value obtained when the experimental portion of the curve is extrapolated back to the ordinate. Unfortunately, this model appears to underestimate the cell kill that takes place at relatively low doses.[239]

Today, the most commonly referred to model is the linear quadratic (LQ) formula. This model assumes two different types of radiation damage. It consists of an α-component, which is most important at low dose (related linearly to dose) representing irreparable damage, and a β-component, which assumes greater importance at a higher dose (dose squared term) representing repairable damage.[240,241] The early portion of the survival curve is a balance between the α- and β-component (Fig. 9-6). It is illustrated in the following equation, with survival denoted as S and dose of radiation represented as D:

$$\text{Log}_e S = \alpha D + \beta D^2$$

The linear quadratic equation has gained popularity because it can be used to determine the ratio of α- and β-components of cell kill (called the α/β ratio) to help predict the response of tumor and normal tissues to changes in the size of each radiation fraction.

Differences in the radioresponsiveness of various tumors and in the number of tumor vs. normal cells killed must be explained in terms other than those of inherent

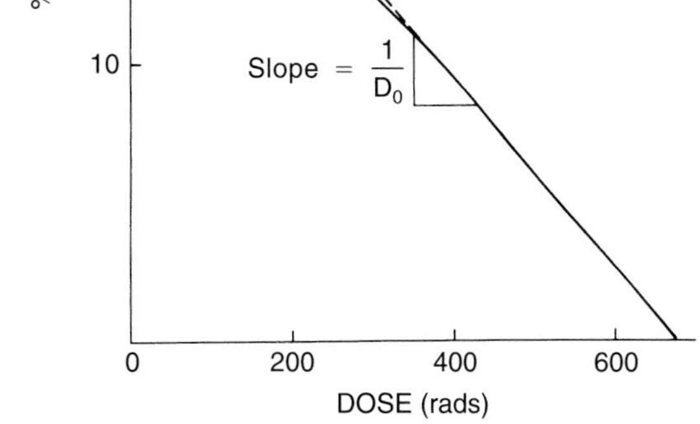

Fig. 9-5. Theoretic cell survival curve for mammalian cells exposed to a single dose of radiation. D_q denotes the quasi-threshold dose. D_0 represents the dose of radiation that reduces the surviving fraction of irradiated cells to 37% of its former value, or the extrapolation number, $L_n n$, the natural logarithm of n, D the dose of radiation, and S the surviving fraction.

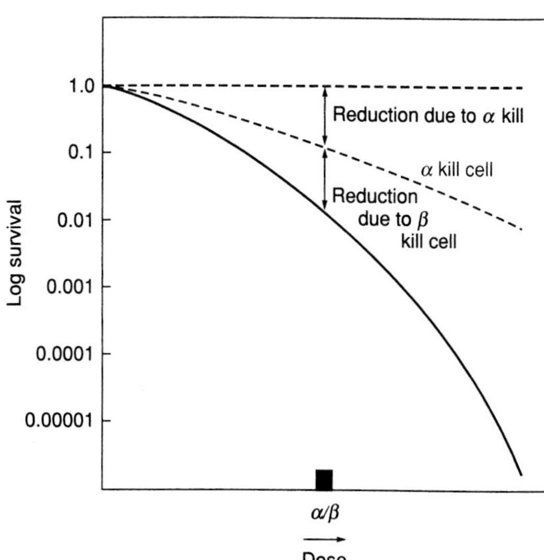

Fig. 9-6. The α/β ratio can be derived from the cell survival curve. Cell killing is made up of two components. α-Cell kill is irreparable, whereas β-cell kill can be repaired. The point at which the reduction in cell survival from α- and β-cell kill is equal represents the α/β ratio. It is expressed in units of dose. (From Lichter AL. Radiation therapy. In Abeloff MA, et al., eds. Clinical Oncology. New York: Churchill Livingstone, 1995. Reproduced with permission.)

radiosensitivity. The phenomena of repair, reoxygenation, repopulation, and redistribution are among the mechanisms invoked to account for these differences. If radiotherapy is given in one dose but in two or more fractions, repair of sublethal damage takes place between radiation treatments. The total dosage required for a given level of cell kill after fractionated radiotherapy is greater than that required when radiation is delivered in a single treatment. The strategy of treating tumors with multiple fractions of radiation is based on the supposition that sublethal radiation injury is repaired more effectively in normal tissue than in tumors.

Selection of an optimal time-dosage pattern for treating tumors is a complex problem. It is unlikely that one-time dosage prescription is optimal for a wide variety of kinetically different tumors located in different anatomic areas. The determination of fraction size, overall treatment time, and total dosage that is best for the control of various tumors constitutes a major, continuing research effort. It is based on several factors such as the inherent radiosensitivity of the tumor and surrounding normal tissues, tumor blood supply, and use of concomitant adjuvant therapy.

Although tumor type has limited effect on inherent radiosensitivity, oxygen has a profound influence on radiation response. It has been known for quite some time that radiation delivered in the presence of oxygen has a more potent biologic effect than in hypoxic conditions.[242] Hypoxic cells are 2.5 to 3 times more resistant to radiation than are well-oxygenated cells. There have been many attempts to overcome the hypoxic cell problem, including the use of hyperbaric oxygen, electron affinity compounds that selectively sensitize hypoxic cells, densely ionizing or high-energy transfer radiation such as neutrons or pi-mesons, optimization of the time-dosage schedule to increase reoxygenation between radiation doses, and hyperthermia.[243,244] Although the exact mechanism of the effect of oxygen is still speculative, it was noted that other compounds capable of accepting an electron can substitute for oxygen and restore sensitivity to hypoxic cells. These drugs include two thymidine analogs, iododeoxyuridine and bromodoeoxyuridinea, which increase cellular sensitivity to radiation in direct proportion to their incorporation into DNA by increasing radiation-induced DNA damage and decreasing its repair.

Radiation Oncology

Radiotherapy has three major roles in cancer treatment. It may be used singly as the primary curative method. It may be used as adjuvant therapy with surgery (either before or after operation) or with chemotherapy or both. Finally, radiation serves to palliate the symptoms of locally advanced or metastatic disease.

As a single method of treatment undertaken with curative intent, radiotherapy is a local or regional form of therapy that is often competitive with surgery. If the probability of cure is equivalent for the two methods, a choice between them is often made on the basis of which carries the lower risk of morbidity. In the case of large tumors, surgery usually has a higher likelihood of tumor cure. However, primary radiotherapy is often used in neoplasms that are technically unresectable or that require excessively mutilating surgery.

There is a growing trend toward combining radiotherapy with chemotherapy to manage a number of different types of cancer.[245-250] Combining these two modalities often allows for more conservative management of disease with the supplementation of local therapy with systemic therapy. Radiotherapy may be used in conjunction with surgery or as an alternative to surgery to treat the primary tumor bed, whereas chemotherapy is used to treat the patient systemically. Adjuvant radiotherapy is of value for the treatment of subclinical disease in "sanctuary" sites not usually accessible to systemic chemotherapy. The best example of this arose from the treatment of acute lymphoblastic leukemia in children. It was clear that, although the disease could be controlled in most parts of the body, relapse in the CNS was a particular risk. This problem was largely overcome by the addition of prophylactic irradiation that eradicated foci of the disease in the CNS that were not accessible to chemotherapy.[251]

Treatment of cancer of the anal canal is another excellent example of the clinical benefit of combined chemotherapy and radiotherapy. In fact, it was in the treatment of anal canal squamous cell carcinoma that the use of combined radiotherapy and chemotherapy was first shown to be effective. Standard surgical management of anal canal carcinoma historically involved an abdominoperineal resection, but when local control was achieved with chemoradiotherapy, a conservative local approach, with sphincter preservation, was adopted. With long-term follow-up it has been confirmed that chemoradiation is the preferred therapy for epidermoid carcinoma of the anal canal.[252,253] Uses of combined chemotherapy and radiotherapy are listed in Table 9-7.

Radiotherapy, chemotherapy, and surgery should be viewed as complementary and not competitive methods of cancer management. New investigative approaches in radiotherapeutic trials aimed at improving disease control have increased dramatically. It is to be hoped that intelligent integration of improved radiotherapy, along with chemotherapy and surgery, will prove beneficial in the treatment of cancer.

Surgical Oncology

Surgery is generally recognized as the original cancer therapy and for many years offered the only opportunity for cure. During the past few decades, however, there has been a tremendous advancement in the development of effective nonsurgical methods of treating cancer, and this has greatly changed the role of surgery. Perhaps, one of the most important advances in cancer surgery has been related to an understanding of the biology of cancer growth and metastases. The original concept of a local tumor spreading contiguously to surrounding tissues and to re-

Table 9-7. Use of Combined Chemotherapy/Radiotherapy in Clinical Practice

Site	Comments
Breast cancer	Neoadjuvant chemotherapy plus radiotherapy may render inoperable tumours operable Adjuvant chemotherapy improves both local control and survival
Rectal cancer	Combined chemotherapy plus radiotherapy may improve survival in certain patients
Anal canal cancer	Very high local control rates with combined chemotherapy/radiotherapy plus sphincter conserving surgery reported
Non–small cell lung cancer	Possible role for chemotherapy plus radiotherapy emerging
Small cell lung cancer	Prophylactic cranial irradiation reduces the incidence of cerebral metastases after chemotherapy
Limb sarcoma	Very high local control rates reported for intra-arterial chemotherapy plus radiotherapy and limb-conserving surgery
Lymphoma	Addition of radiotherapy to chemotherapy improves local control and possibly survival in Hodgkin's disease and some non-Hodgkin's lymphomas

From Mason M. Combined radiotherapy and chemotherapy: Twice the benefit, or double the trouble? Eur J Surg Oncol 20: 597, 1994. Reproduced with permission.

gional lymph nodes led to more and more radical operations. It is now recognized that at the time of cancer diagnosis some 70% of all solid tumors are already systemic. This understanding of the cancer process has helped the surgeon rethink the role of primary surgery and better define realistic therapeutic goals based on a multimodality approach to treatment.

The surgeon is most often the primary physician conducting the evaluation of the patient suspected of having cancer. As the primary physician, the surgeon must assume the responsibility for identifying which patients can be potentially cured by local resection alone and those who should have adjuvant multimodality treatment. The surgeon must also decide the extent of resectional therapy, balancing the potential for cure through local control with the morbidity of extensive tissue resection. Today, the use of surgery as the sole treatment for a given cancer is rare. Thus the surgeon has a critical role in coordinating a patient's care and interacting with other specialists.

The surgeon is frequently involved in treating patients with large, extensive tumors and patients with metastatic disease. The decision to resect isolated metastases or to attempt debulking of large tumor masses is always difficult. Although the resection of certain metastatic tumors may in fact extend the life of an individual patient, there is the possibility that overall survival may not be changed. The decision to attempt such procedures depends largely on the safety of the procedure to be undertaken and the availability of other effective treatment modalities for the tumor in question.

In recent years, the placement of short-term and long-term indwelling central venous catheters has become a relatively common procedure performed on patients with cancer. This provides chronic vascular access for administration of chemotherapy, hematologic support, and occasionally nutritional support. The implementation of chronic vascular access has allowed the use of more aggressive treatment involving multiple drugs given over complicated schedules. To meet this need, a number of new implantable catheter systems and drug delivery pumps have been developed. Important developments relating to implantation technique and design have decreased the operative time required to place these devices, and it can usually be done as an outpatient procedure.

The surgeon is also called on to handle a variety of surgical emergencies related to the advancing cancer or the use of aggressive therapy. Hemorrhage, sepsis, perforation of viscera, and obstruction of the gastrointestinal tract are examples of problems requiring surgical intervention. These emergencies require a thoughtful and caring physician who understands not only the need to solve the problem at hand but also the delicate balance between helping and not helping.

The role of the surgical oncologist, or cancer specialist involved in cancer diagnosis and treatment, continues to expand and includes an understanding of the biology of the cancer process, the natural history of specific tumors, the current status of integrated treatment options for each tumor, and the investigative options that may be important to the patient. The role of the surgeon assuming these responsibilities is best defined as that of a member of a multidisciplinary oncology team, skilled in various treatment modalities and dedicated to experimental research that can lead to new diagnostic and treatment options.[254,255]

Biologic Therapy

In 1992, Steven A. Rosenberg, M.D., stated, "In the last decade biologic therapy has emerged as a mode of treatment capable of mediating the regression of cancer. . . ."[256] Biologic therapy produces antitumor activity primarily through the action of natural host-defense mechanisms augmented by the administration of immunologically active substances.[257] Virtually any agent capable of altering the host-tumor relationship in favor of the host can be considered a biologic response modifier. In vivo studies

PROPERTIES OF SELECTED INTERLEUKINS

Interleukin-1

1. Monokine that has many roles in the inflammatory and the immune response
2. Secreted by mononuclear phagocytes following ingestion of antigen-antibody complex or lipopolysaccharide or following contact with T cells during antigen presentation
3. May also be synthesized by NK cells and B cells
4. IL-1 secretion is enhanced by IFN-α and -γ
5. Induces secretion of IL-2, which promotes the growth of T lymphocytes after antigen presentation
6. Endogenous pyrogen is identical to IL-1

Interleukin-2

1. Secreted mainly by helper T cells following stimulation by IL-1 and binding of antigen to the T-cell receptor
2. Promotes growth and proliferation of T cells
3. Promotes enhanced secretion by lymphokines, increased expression of membrane receptors for other growth factors, and increased expression of class II MHC molecules
4. Almost all T lymphocyte clones are dependent on IL-2 for growth in culture
5. Enhances the function of NK cells

Interleukin-4

1. Secreted by T-helper cells
2. Promotes antibody class switching (in mice)
3. Induces expression of class II MHC in B lymphocyte therapy promoting T-B-cell interaction
4. Promotes growth of T lymphocytes; some T-cell clones are IL-4 dependent
5. Its effect on B cells is antagonized by IFN

Interleukin-6

1. Secreted by mononuclear phagocytes, activated T lymphocytes, as well as some nonlymphoid cells
2. May promote secretion of immunoglobulin by activated B cells during T-B-cell interaction
3. A growth factor for hybridomas and plasmacytomas
4. Promotes release of acute-phase reactants from liver cells
5. Promotes differentiation of hematopoietic stem cells and nerve cells

From Gaynor ER, Fisher RI. Biologic therapy. In Abeloff MA, et al., eds. Clinical Oncology. New York: Churchill Livingstone, 1995. Reproduced with permission.

have demonstrated the efficacy of inducing tumor rejection by using immunomodulatory cytokines.[258] Bacterial products have also been used to stimulate the immune system to produce an antitumorigenic response in certain types of tumors.[257]

Interferons

Interferons (IFNs) were initially reported in 1957 as biologic agents interfering with virus replication.[259] They belong to a family of proteins that naturally occur in response to viruses, double-stranded RNA, and mitogens, and can be classified as cytokines.[260]

IFNs produced by recombinant DNA technology began phase I trials in the late 1970s. The biologic properties for these molecules include antimicrobial, immunomodulatory, antiproliferative, and differentiation-inducing effects.[261-263] They are classified according to biochemical characteristics as IFN-α, -β, or -γ. IFN-α has been the most extensively studied agent of the three. Reports suggest that it may act as a tumor suppressor gene or may augment the activity of these genes. Various combinations of retinoids and IFNs have demonstrated synergistic antiproliferative, differentiating, and antiangiogenic activity in some hematologic malignancies and solid tumors. This synergistic activity may be due to enhanced gene expression.[264,265]

IFN-α has demonstrated efficacy in treating a variety of cancers including hairy cell leukemia, chronic myeloid leukemia, non-Hodgkin's lymphoma, and multiple myelomas. It has also been studied as a single-agent therapy in a variety of solid tumors including renal cell carcinoma, Kaposi's sarcoma, and gastrointestinal endocrine tumors. However, unlike chemotherapy, tumor response to IFN therapy may be slow. IFN has shown more positive results in patients with a lower tumor burden without a history of prior therapy. Recent evidence suggests that a combination of IFN-α and chemotherapy may yield a higher response rate than chemotherapy alone.[249,264]

Interleukins

Interleukins are hormone-like substances, produced mainly by leukocytes, which have diverse activities on both immunologic and nonimmunologic targets.[266] Interleukins are produced by several types of leukocytes, which include T cells, B cells, NK cells, macrophages/monocytes, and mast cells. They may also be synthesized by fibroblasts, endothelial cells, dendritic cells, astrocytes, and bone marrow stomal cells.[266]

There are at least twelve well-defined interleukins, and ongoing research has detected several others.[267] Properties of selected interleukins are outlined in the accompanying box. The only FDA-approved interleukin is IL-2; others are in clinical trials and the final stages of preclinical investigation. The use of IL-2 to generate in vitro autologous cells with antitumor activity opened the way for the successful use of adoptive immunotherapy in humans. IL-2 stimulates the growth and activities of a wide range of cells including natural killer (NK) cells, lymphokine-activated killer cells (LAK), CTLs, and TILs. A large number of clinical trials have evaluated the administration of IL-2 alone or in combination with LAKs and TILs.[221,249,268] Objective and long-lived responses have been documented in a large proportion of cases, particularly renal cell carcinoma, melanoma, and acute myeloid leukemia.[269] Several toxicities associated with IL-2 are generally short lived and resolve within 24 hours of discontinuation. However, studies indicate that the rate of drug-related acute mortality is 4% to 5%.[266] Use of IL-2 should be restricted to those who are familiar with administration and toxicity. Ongoing trials of the remaining interleukins are underway to determine their value in clinical practice.[270]

G-CSF, GM-CSF, and Erythropoietin

There are currently three recombinant hematopoietic growth factors available for clinical use in the United States. These include granulocyte colony-stimulating factor (G-CSF), granulocyte-macrophage colony-stimulating factor (GM-CSF), and erythropoietin.[271] G-CSF and GM-CSF have shown clinical promise in the prevention of myelosuppression associated with conventional chemotherapy. In chemotherapy regimens of moderate intensity, high-dose chemotherapy and bone marrow transplantation studies have reported a reduction in the days patients experience neutropenia and require antibiotic therapy and a decrease in hospital stay.[272-275]

Research is being carried out to study other possible functions for hematopoietic growth factors in addition to the current indications for use in patients undergoing chemotherapy to reduce infection, neutropenia, and anemia. G-CSF and GM-CSF have been shown to increase circulating progenitors available for transplantation. Large scale ex vivo expansion of progenitor cells is an area of intense investigation.[276]

Tumor Necrosis Factor

Tumor necrosis factor (TNF) was originally described as a monocyte/macrophage-derived cytokine that exerts cytotoxic and cytostatic effects on certain neoplastic cells both in vivo and in vitro. It was characterized by its effect in vivo to induce hemorrhagic necrosis in a variety of transplantable murine tumors.[277] TNF acts by stimulating endothelial cells to synthesize cell surface molecules, which increases the adhesion of leukocytes to the surface of the endothelium. It also stimulates cell surface procoagulant activity, the expression of MHC class I molecules, and secretion of IL-1 by endothelial cells. All these elements contribute to an enhanced inflammatory response and intravascular coagulation resulting in hemorrhagic necrosis. TNF also has the ability to directly destroy a wide range of tumor cell lines in vitro. It can also increase and even activate the tumor-directed cytotoxicity of monocytes, macrophages, polymorphonuclear granulocytes, and NK cells.[267]

Several studies have confirmed that TNF exhibits antitumor effects in mice and rats with syngeneic tumors such as sarcoma, melanoma, colon adenocarcinoma, lung carcinoma, hepatoma, and plasmacytoma.[277-280] Reports also suggest that human tumors (melanoma, lung carcinoma, and neuroblastoma) transplanted in congenitally athymic nu/nu mice may be significantly inhibited by TNF.[280] Unfortunately, these encouraging preclinical results did not translate into promising clinical results. Several phase I clinical studies in humans from 1987 to 1989 revealed that an overall response rate in cancer patients to systemic infusion of TNF was only 4%.[281] However, local administration of TNF has proved promising for melanoma and sarcoma in the extremities when the therapy is combined with IFN-γ and cytostatics with response rates reaching up to 100%.[282-284]

• • •

The 1980s and early 1990s have witnessed exciting advances in cell biology and molecular genetics. These new developments in modern biomedical research have shed new light on the processes involved in transformation of normal cells into neoplastic cells, tumor cell proliferation, and the biology of tumor metastasis. Today's surgeon must have a thorough understanding of these processes and their relationship to therapy to participate as a key member of an integrated, multidisciplinary, oncology research and treatment program. This chapter reviews and highlights the genetic regulation of abnormal cell growth, the development of metastases, the host response, and the rationale for the integration of treatment options on the basis of our current understanding of those mechanisms responsible for oncogenesis.

REFERENCES

1. Mackillop WJ, et al. A stem cell model of human tumor growth; Implications for tumor cell clonogenic assays. J Natl Cancer Inst 70:9, 1983.
2. Howard A, Pelc S. Nuclear incorporation of ^{32}P as demonstrated by autoradiographs. Exp Cell Res 2:178, 1951.
3. Mitchison JM. The Biology of the Cell Cycle. London: Cambridge University Press, 1971.
4. Reddy GP. Cell cycle: Regulatory events in G_1-S transition of mammalian cells. J Cell Biochem 54:379, 1994.
5. Stanners CP, Till JE. DNA synthesis in individual L strain mouse cell. Biochem Biophys Acta 37:406, 1960.
6. Zetterberg A. Nuclear and cytoplasmic growth during interphase and mammalian cells. Adv Cell Biol 1:211, 1970.
7. Sherr CJ. G_1 phase progression: Cycling on cue. Cell 79:551, 1994.
8. Howard A, Pelc S. Synthesis of DNA in normal and irradiated cells and its relation to chromosome breakage. Heredity 6:261, 1953.
9. Murray A. Cell cycle checkpoints. Curr Opin Cell Biol 6:872, 1994.
10. Hoffman I, Karsenti E. The role of cdc25 in checkpoints and feedback controls in the eukaryotic cell cycle. J Cell Science 18:75, 1994.
11. Levine AJ. p53, the cellular gatekeeper for growth and division. Cell 88:323, 1997.
12. Prives C. Doing the right thing: Feedback control and p53. Curr Opin Cell Biol 5:214, 1993.
13. Zambetti GP, et al. Wild type p53 mediates positive regulation of gene expression through a specific DNA sequence element. Genes Dev 6:1143, 1992.

14. Kastan MB, et al. Participation of p53 protein in the cellular response to DNA damage. Cancer Res 51:6304, 1991.
15. Nurse P, Bissett Y. Gene required in G1 for commitment to cell cycle and in G2 for control of mitosis in fission yeast. Nature 292:558, 1981.
16. Piggot JR, Rae R, Carter BLA. A bifunctional gene product involved in two phases of the yeast cell cycle. Nature 298:391, 1982.
17. Simanis V, Nurse P. The cell cycle control gene cdc2+ of fission yeast encodes a protein kinase potentially regulated by phosporylation. Cell 45:261, 1986.
18. Hartwell LH, Kastan MB. Cell cycle control and cancer. Science 266:1821, 1994.
19. Murakami MS, Strobel MC, Vande Woude GF. Cell cycle regulation, oncogenes, and antineoplastic drugs. In Mendelsohn J, et al., eds. The Molecular Basis of Cancer. Philadelphia: WB Saunders, 1995.
20. Meikrantz W, Schlegel R. Apoptosis and the cell cycle. J Cell Biochem 58:160, 1995.
21. Singh N, Anand S. Cell death by apoptosis. Indian J Exp Biol 32:843, 1994.
22. Thompson CB. Apoptosis in the pathogenesis and treatment of disease. Science 267:1456, 1995.
23. King KL, Cilowski JA. Cell cycle and apoptosis: Common pathways to life and death. J Cell Biochem 58:175, 1995.
24. Steller H. Mechanisms and genes of cellular suicide. Science 267:1445, 1995.
25. D'Amico AV, McKenna WG. Apoptosis and a re-investigation of the biologic basis for cancer therapy. Radiother Oncol 33:3, 1994.
26. Nagata S. Apoptosis by death factor. Cell 88:355, 1997.
27. Broca PP. Traite de tumeurs. Paris: Asselin, 1866.
28. Rous P. A sarcoma of the fowl transmissable by an agent separable from the tumor cells. J Exp Med 13:397, 1911.
29. Stechlin D, et al. DNA related to transforming gene(s) of avian sarcoma viruses is present in normal avian DNA. Nature 260:170, 1976.
30. Varmus H, Weinberg RA. Genes and the Biology of Cancer. New York: Scientific American Library, 1993.
31. Weinberg RA. Oncogenes and the Molecular Basis of Cancer. Cold Spring Harbor, N.Y.: Cold Spring Harbor Laboratory Press, 1989.
32. Krontiris TG: Molecular medicine—Oncogenes. N Engl J Med 333:303, 1995.
33. Duesberg PH. Retroviral transforming genes in normal cells? Nature 304:219, 1983.
34. Shilo BZ, Weinberg RA. DNA sequences homologous to vertebrate oncogenes are concerved in *Drosophila melenogaster.* Proc Natl Acad Sci USA 78:789, 1982.
35. Goyette M, et al. Expression of a cellular oncogene during liver regeneration. Science 219:510, 1983.
36. Weinberg RA. Oncogenes and tumor suppressor genes. CA Cancer J Clin 44:160, 1994.
37. Harris H. The analysis of malignancy by cell fusion: The position in 1988. Cancer Res 48:3302, 1988.
38. Stanbridge EJ, Cavanee WK. Heritable cancer and tumor suppressor genes: A tentative connection. In Weinberg RA, ed. Oncogenes and the Molecular Origins of Cancer. Cold Spring Harbor, N.Y.: Cold Spring Harbor Laboratory Press, 1989.
39. Oshimura M, et al. Transfer of human chromosome 11 suppresses tumorigenicity of some but not all tumor cell lines. J Cell Biochem 42:135, 1990.
40. Trent JM, et al. Tumorigenicity in human melanoma cell lines controlled by introduction of human chromosome 6. Science 247:568, 1990.
41. Weissman BE, et al. Introduction of a normal human chromosome 11 into a Wilm's tumor cell line controls its tumorigenic expression. Science 236:175, 1987.
42. Knudsen AG Jr. Hereditary cancer, oncogenes, and anti-oncogenes. Cancer Res 45:137, 1985.
43. Knudsen AG Jr. Mutation and cancer. Statistical study of retinoblastoma. Proc Natl Acad Sci USA 68:820, 1971.
44. Friend SH, et al. A human DNA segment with properties of the gene that predisposes to retinoblastoma and osteosarcoma. Nature 323:643, 1986.
45. Huang HJ, et al. Suppression of the neoplastic phenotype by replacement of the Rb gene in human cancer cells. Science 242:1563, 1988.
46. Cleaver JE. It was a very good year for DNA repair. Cell 76:1, 1994.
47. Coleman WB, Tsongalis GJ. Multiple mechanisms account for genomic instability and molecular mutation in neoplastic transformation. Clin Chem 5:644, 1995.
48. Hanawalt PC. DNA repair. In Freifelder D, Malacinski GM, eds. Essentials of Molecular Biology. Boston: Jones and Bartlett Publishers, 1993.
49. Kaufmann WK, Kaufman DG. Cell cycle control, DNA repair, and initiation of carcinogenesis. FASEB J 7:1188, 1993.
50. Reed JC. Bcl-2 and the regulation of programmed cell death. J Cell Biol 124:1, 1994.
51. Blackwood EM, Eisenman RN. Max: A helix-loop-helix-zipper protein that forms a sequence-specific DNA binding complex with Myc. Science 251:1211, 1991.
52. Kato GJ, Dang CV. Function of the c-myc oncoprotein. FASEB J 6:3065, 1992.
53. Marcu KB, Bossone SA, Patel AJ. myc function and regulation. Annu Rev Biochem 61:809, 1992.
54. Hanson KD, et al. Effects of c-myc expression on cell cycle progression. Mol Cell Biol 14:5748, 1994.
55. Hermeking H, Eick D. Mediation of c-myc induced apoptosis by p53. Science 265:2091, 1994.
56. El-Deiry WS, et al. *WAF1,* a potential mediator of *p53* tumor suppression. Cell 75:817, 1993.
57. Kastan MB, et al. A mammalian cell cycle checkpoint pathway utilizing *p53* and *GADD45* is defective in ataxia telangiectasia. Cell 71:587, 1992.
58. Griffiths SD, et al. Absence of p53 permits propagation of mutant cells following genotoxic damage. Oncogene 14:523, 1997.
59. Mueller H, Eppenberger U. The dual role of mutant p53 protein in chemosensitivity of human cancers. Anticancer Res 16:3845, 1996.
60. Fujiwara T, et al. Induction of chemosensitivity in human lung cancer cells in vivo by adenovirus-mediated transfer of the wild-type *p53* gene. Cancer Res 54:2287, 1994.
61. Pellegata NS, et al. DNA damage and p53-mediated cell cycle arrest: A re-evaluation. Proc Natl Acad Sci USA 93:15209, 1996.
62. Kraemer KH, Slor H. Xeroderma pigmentosa. Clin Dematol 3:33, 1985.
63. Strickland P, Kensler TW. Chemical and physical agents in our environment. In Abeloff MA, et al., eds. Clinical Oncology. New York: Churchill Livingstone, 1995.
64. Friedberg EC. DNA repair. New York: WH Freeman, 1994.
65. Tolbert DM, Kantor GJ. Definition of DNA repair domain in the genomic region containing the human p53 gene. Cancer Res 56:3324, 1996.
66. Vogelstein B, et al. Genetic alterations during colorectal-tumor development. N Engl J Med 319:525, 1988.
67. Weinberg RA. The molecular basis of oncogenes and tumor suppressor genes. Ann NY Acad Sci 758:331, 1995.
68. Fearon ER. Oncogenes and tumor suppressor genes. In Abeloff MA, et al., eds. Clinical Oncology. New York: Churchill Livingstone, 1995.

69. De Plaen E, et al. Immunogenic (tum-) variants of mouse tumor P815: Cloning of the gene of tum- antigen P91A and identification of the tum- mutation. Proc Natl Acad Sci USA 85:2274, 1988.
70. Saxon PJ, Srivatsan ES, Stanbridge EJ. Introduction of chromosome 11 via microcell transfer controls tumorigenic expression of HeLa cells. EMBO J 5:3461, 1986.
71. Culotta E, Koshland DE Jr. Molecule of the year: p53 sweeps through cancer research. Science 262:1958, 1993.
72. Harris CC, Hollstein M. Clinical implications of the p53 tumor suppressor gene. N Engl J Med 329:1318, 1993.
73. Chen P-L, et al. Genetic mechanisms of tumor suppression by the human p53 gene. Science 250:1576, 1990.
74. Perry ME, Levine AJ. Tumor suppressor p53 and the cell cycle. Curr Opin Genet Dev 3:50, 1993.
75. Abercrombie M. Contact inhibition and malignancy. Nature 281:259, 1979.
76. Skehan P, Friedman SJ. Malignant transformation. In vitro methods and in vivo correlates. In Cameron IL, Pool TB, eds. The Transformed Cell. New York: Academic Press, 1981.
77. Delarco JE, Todaro GJ. Growth factors from murine sarcoma virus-transformed cells. Proc Natl Acad Sci USA 75:4001, 1978.
78. Sporn MB, Roberts AB. Autocrine growth factors and cancer. Nature 313:745, 1985.
79. Doolittle RF, et al. Simian sarcoma virus onc gene, v-sis, is derived from the gene (or genes) encoding a platelet-derived growth factor. Science 221:275, 1983.
80. Waterfield MD, et al. Platelet-derived growth factor is structurally related to the putative transforming protein p28sis of simian sarcoma virus. Nature 304:35, 1983.
81. Downward J, et al. Close similarity of epidermal growth factor receptor and v-erb-B oncogene protein sequences. Nature 307:521, 1984.
82. Carpenter G, Cohen S. Epidermal growth factor. J Biol Chem 265:7709, 1990.
83. Sumantran VN, Wicha M. Regulation of tumor cell growth. In Abeloff MA, et al., eds. Clinical Oncology. New York: Churchill Livingstone, 1995.
84. Tronick SR, Aaronson SA. Growth factors and signal transduction. In Mendelsohn J, et al., eds. The Molecular Basis of Cancer. Philadelphia: WB Saunders, 1995.
85. Arteaga CL. Interference of the IGF system as a strategy to inhibit breast cancer growth. Breast Cancer Res Treat 22:101, 1992.
86. Kumar R, Shephad HM, Mendelsohn J. Regulation of phosporylation of the c-erbB-2/HER2 gene product by a monoclonal antibody and serum growth factor(s) in human mammary carcinoma cells. Mol Cell Biol 11:979, 1991.
87. Collins VP, Leoffler RK, Twey H. Observation on growth rates of human tumors. AJR 76:988, 1956.
88. Prehn RT. The inhibition of tumor growth by tumor mass. Cancer Res 51:2, 1991.
89. Laird AK. Dynamics of tumour growth: Comparison of growth rates and extrapolation of growth curve to one cell. Br J Cancer 29:278, 1965.
90. Laird AK. The dynamics of tumour growth. Br J Cancer 28:490, 1966.
91. Fidler IJ. Critical factors in the biology of human cancer metastasis: 28th G.H.A. Clowes Memorial Award Lecture. Cancer Res 50:6130, 1990.
92. Fidler IJ. Invasion and metastasis. In Abeloff MA, et al., eds. Clinical Oncology. New York: Churchill Livingstone, 1995.
93. Weidner N. Tumor angiogenesis: Review of current applications in tumor prognostication. Semin Diag Pathol 10:302, 1993.
94. Fidler IJ, Ellis LM. The implications of angiogenesis for the biology and therapy of cancer metastasis. Cell 79:185, 1994.
95. Folkman J. The role of angiogenesis in tumor growth. Semin Cancer Biol 3:65, 1992.
96. O'Reilly MS, et al. Angiostatin: A novel angiogenesis inhibitor that mediates the suppression of metastases by a Lewis lung carcinoma. Cell 79:315, 1994.
97. Clark WH Jr, et al. Model predicting survival in stage I melanoma based on tumor progression. J Natl Cancer Inst 81:1893, 1989.
98. Sugarbaker EV, Thornthwaite J, Ketcham AS. Inhibitory effect of a primary tumor on metastasis. In Day SB, et al, eds. Progress in Cancer Research and Therapy. New York: Raven Press, 1977.
99. Warren BA, Chauvin WJ, Philips J. Blood-borne tumor emboli and their adherence to vessel walls. In Day SB, et al., eds. Progress in Cancer Research and Therapy. New York: Raven Press, 1977.
100. Woodruff M. Cellular Variation and Adaptation in Cancer. New York: Oxford University Press, 1990.
101. Woodruff M. The Interactions of Cancer and the Host. New York: Grune & Stratton, 1980.
102. O'Reilly MS, et al. The suppression of tumor metastases by a primary tumor. Surg Forum 44:474, 1993.
103. Folkman J, Klagsbrun M. Angiogenic factors. Science 235:442, 1987.
104. Kohn EC, Liotta L. Molecular insights into cancer invasion: Strategies for prevention and intervention. Cancer Res 55:1856, 1995.
105. Liotta LA. Cancer cell invasion and metastasis. Sci Am 266:54, 1992.
106. Barsky SH, et al. Loss of basement membrane components by invasive tumors but not by their benign counterparts. Lab Invest 49:140, 1983.
107. Liotta LA, et al. Metastatic potential correlates with enzymatic degradation of basement membrane collagen. Nature 284:67, 1980.
108. Talhouk RS, Bisell MJ, Werb Z. Coordinated expression of extracellular matrix degrading proteinases and their inhibitors regulates mammary epithelial function during involution. J Cell Biol 118:1271, 1992.
109. Baker T, Tickle S, Wasan H. Serum metalloproteinases and their inhibitors: Markers for malignant potential. Br J Cancer 70:506, 1994.
110. Khokha R. Suppression of tumorigenic and metastatic abilities of murine B16-F10 melanoma cells in vivo by the overexpression of the tissue inhibitor of metalloproteinase-1. J Natl Cancer Inst 86:299, 1994.
111. Mueller BM. Different roles for plasminogen activators and metalloproteinases in melanoma metastasis. Curr Top Micro Immunol 213:65, 1996.
112. Tanaka K, Iwamoto Y, Ito Y. Cyclic AMP-regulated synthesis of the tissue inhibitors of metalloproteinases suppresses the invasive potential of the human fibrosarcoma cell line HT1080. Cancer Res 55:2927, 1995.
113. Doyle GM, Sharief Y, Mohler JL. Prediction of metastatic potential by cancer cell motility in the Dunning R-3327 prostatic adenocarcinoma in vivo model. J Urol 147:514, 1992.
114. Gabbert H. Mechanisms of tumor invasion: Evidence of in vivo observation. Cancer Metastasis Rev 4:283, 1985.
115. Strauli P, Haemmerli O. The role of cancer cell motility in invasion. Cancer Metastasis Rev 3:127, 1984.
116. Volk T, Geiger B, Raz A. Motility and adhesive properties of high and low-metastatic murine neoplastic cells. Cancer Res 44:811, 1984.
117. Lotan R. Retinoids and modulators of tumor cell invasion and metastasis. Semin Cancer Biol 2:197, 1991.
118. Lotan R, et al. Suppression of motility factor receptor expression by retinoic acid. Cancer Res 52:4878, 1992.
119. Fidler IJ, Gersten DM, Hart IR. The biology of cancer invasion and metastasis. Adv Cancer Res 28:149, 1978.
120. Fidler IJ. Tumor heterogeneity and the biology of cancer invasion and metastasis. Cancer Res 38:2651, 1978.
121. Poste G, Fidler IJ. The pathogenesis of cancer metastasis. Nature 283:139, 1979.

122. Sugarbaker EV. Cancer metastasis: A product of tumor-host interactions. Curr Probl Cancer 3:1, 1979.
123. Fidler IJ, Balch CM. The biology of cancer metastasis and implications for therapy. Curr Probl Surg 24:129, 1987.
124. Killion JJ, Fidler IJ. The biology of tumor metastasis. Semin Oncol 16:106, 1989.
125. Paget S. The distribution of secondary growths in cancer of the breast. Lancet 571, 1889.
126. Evans RA. The "seed and soil" hypothesis and the decline of radical surgery: A surgeon's opinion. Tex Med J 86:85, 1990.
127. Togo S, et al. "Seed" to "soil" is a return trip in metastasis. Anticancer Res 15:791, 1995.
128. Togo S, et al. Cancer seed and soil can be highly selective: Human-patient colon tumor lung metastasis grows in nude mouse lung but not colon or subcutis. Anticancer Res 15:795, 1995.
129. Steeg P, et al. Evidence for a novel gene associated with low tumor metastatic potential. J Natl Cancer Inst 80:200, 1988.
130. Steeg P, et al. *Nm23* and breast cancer metastasis. Breast Cancer Res Treat 25:175, 1993.
131. McDonald NJ, de la Rosa A, Steep P. The potential roles of nm23 in cancer metastasis and cellular differentiation. Eur J Cancer 31:1096, 1995.
132. Berkeley WN. Results of three years' observations on a new form of cancer treatment. Am J Obstet 69:1060, 1914.
133. Ehrlich P. Ueber den jetzigen Stand der Karzinomforschung. (Part 1). Ned Tijdschr Geneeskd 5:273, 1909.
134. Vaughan JW. Cancer vaccine and anticancer globulin as an aid in the surgical treatment of malignancy. JAMA 63:1250, 1914.
135. Woglom WH. Immunity to transplantable tumors. Cancer Rev 4:129, 1929.
136. Andervont HB. The use of pure strain animals in studies on natural resistance to transplantable tumors. Pub Health Rep 52:1885, 1937.
137. Gross L. Intradermal immunization of C3H mice against a sarcoma that originated in an animal of the same line. Cancer Res 3:326, 1943.
138. Sjogren HO, et al. Resistance of polyoma virus immunized mice to transplantation of established polyoma tumor. Exp Cell Res 23:204, 1961.
139. Baldwin RW. Immunity to methylcholanthrene-induced tumors in inbred rats following implantation and regression of implanted tumors. Br J Cancer 9:652, 1955.
140. Campbell FA, Redmond HP, Bouchier-Hayes D. The role of tumor rejection antigens in host antitumor defense mechanisms. Cancer 75:2649, 1995.
141. Habel K. Resistance of polyoma virus immune animals to transplanted polyoma tumors. Proc Soc Exp Biol Med 106:772, 1961.
142. Hakomori S. Tumor-associated carbohydrate antigens. Annu Rev Immunol 2:103, 1984.
143. Prehn RT, Main JM. Immunity to methylcholanthrene-induced sarcomas. J Natl Cancer Inst 18:769, 1957.
144. Rosenberg SA. The development of new cancer therapies based on the molecular identification of cancer rejection antigens. Cancer J 1:90, 1995.
145. van der Bruggen P. The long-standing quest for tumor rejection antigens. Clin Immunol Immunopath 71:248, 1994.
146. Boon T. Tumor antigens and perspectives for cancer immunotherapy. Immunologist 3:262, 1995.
147. Old LJ, et al. Antigenic properties of chemically-induced tumors. Ann NY Acad Sci USA 101:80, 1962.
148. Rouse BT, Rollinghoff M, Warner NL. Antiserum-induced suppression of the cellular transfer of tumor-specific immunity to syngenesis plasma cell tumour. Natl New Biol 238:116, 1972.
149. Alpert ME. Alphafetoglobulins in the diagnosis of human hepatoma. N Engl J Med 278:984, 1968.
150. Gold P, Freedman SO. Specific carcinoembryonic antigens in the human digestive system. J Exp Med 22:467, 1965.
151. Gorelik E. Concomitant tumor immunity and the resistance to a second tumor challenge. Adv Cancer Res 39:71, 1983.
152. Linehan DC, Goedegebuure PS, Eberlein TJ. Vaccine therapy for cancer. Ann Surg Oncol 3:219, 1996.
153. Rosenberg SA, et al. Treatment of 283 consecutive patients with metastatic melanoma or renal cell cancer using high-dose bolus interleukin-2. JAMA 271:907, 1994.
154. Topalian SL, et al. Expansion of human tumor infiltrating lymphocytes for use in immunotherapy trials. J Immunol Methods 102:127, 1987.
155. Wang RF, Rosenberg SA. Human tumor antigens recognized by T lymphocytes: Implications for cancer therapy. J Leukocyte Biol 60:296, 1996.
156. Robbins PF, Kawakami Y. Human tumor antigens recognized by T cells. Curr Opin Immunol 8:628, 1996.
157. Rosenberg SA, et al. Identification of the genes encoding cancer antigens: Implications for cancer immunotherapy. Adv Cancer Res 70:145, 1996.
158. Nabel GJ, et al. Direct gene transfer for treatment of human cancer. Ann NY Acad Sci 772:227, 1995.
159. Rosenberg SA, et al. Treatment of patients with metastastic melanoma using autologous tumor-infiltrating lymphocytes and interleukin-2. J Natl Cancer Inst 86:1159, 1994.
160. Rosenfeld ME, Curiel DT. Gene therapy strategies for novel cancer therapeutics. Curr Opin Oncol 8:72, 1996.
161. Cavallo F, et al. Role of neutrophils and CD4+ T lymphocytes in the primary and memory response to non-immunogenic by IL-2 gene. J Immunol 149:3627, 1992.
162. Fearon ER, et al. Interleukin-2 production by tumor cells bypasses T helper function in the generation of an anti-tumor response. Cell 60:397, 1990.
163. Armstrong CA, et al. Antitumor effects of granulocyte-macrophage colony-stimulating factor production by melanoma cells. Cancer Res 56:2191, 1996.
164. Chen L. Costimulation of antitumor immunity by the B7 counter-receptor for the T lymphocyte molecules CD28 and CTLA-4. Cell 71:1093, 1992.
165. Dranoff G, et al. Vaccination with irradiated tumor cells engineered to secrete murine granulocyte-macrophage colony-stimulating factor stimulates potent, specific, and long-lasting anti-tumor immunity. Proc Natl Acad Sci USA 90:3539, 1993.
166. Golumbek PT, et al. Treatment of established renal cell cancer by tumor cells engineered to secrete interleukin-4. Science 254:713, 1991.
167. Hock H, et al. Mechanisms of rejection induced by tumor cell-targeted gene transfer of interleukin-2, interleukin-4, interleukin-7, tumor necrosis factor, or interferon gamma, Proc Natl Acad Sci USA 90:2774, 1993.
168. Lattime EC, et al. In situ cytokine gene transfection using vaccinia virus vectors. Semin Oncol 23:88, 1996.
169. Restifo NP, et al. A nonimmunogenic sarcoma transduced with the CDNA for interferon gamma elicits CD8+ T cells against the wild-type tumor: Correlation with antigen presentation capability. J Exp Med 175:1423, 1992.
170. Townsend JE, Allison JP. Tumor rejection after direct costimulation of CD8+ T cells by B7-transfected melanoma cells. Science 259:368, 1993.
171. Watanabe Y, et al. Exogenous expression of mouse interfereon gamma with DNA in mouse neuroblastoma C1300 cells results in reduced tumorigenicity by augmented anti-tumor immunity. Proc Natl Acad Sci USA 86:9456, 1989.
172. Anichini A, Fossati G, Parmiani G. Clonal analysis of the cytolytic T-cell response to human tumors. Immunol Today 8:385, 1987.
173. Bjorkman PJ, et al. The foreign antigen binding site and T cell recognition regions of class I histocompatibility antigens. Nature 329:512, 1987.
174. Townsend AR, et al. Cytotoxic T lymphocytes recognize influenza hemagglutinin that lacks a signal sequence. Nature 324:575, 1986.

175. Bjorkman PJ, et al. Structure of the human class I histocompatibility antigen HLA-A2. Nature 329:506, 1987.
176. Boniface JJ, Davis MM. T-cell recognition of antigen. A process controlled by transient intermolecular interactions. Ann NY Acad Sci 766:62, 1995.
177. Brown JH, et al. Three-dimensional structure of the human class II histocompatibility antigen HLA-DR1. Nature 364:33,1993.
178. Germain RN. MHC-dependent antigen processing and peptide presentation: Providing ligands for T lymphocyte activation. Cell 76:287, 1994.
179. Madden DR, et al. The three-dimensional structure of HLA-B27 at 2.1 a resolution suggests a general mechanism for tight peptide binding to MHC. Cell 70:1035, 1992.
180. Salter RD, et al. A binding site for the T-cell co-receptor CD8 on the alpha 3 domain of HLA-A2. Nature 345:41, 1990.
181. Falk K, Rotzschke O, Rammensee HG. Cellular peptide composition governed by major histocompatibility complex class I molecules. Nature 348:248, 1990.
182. Rothbard JB, Grafter ML. Interactions between immunogenic peptides and MHC proteins. Annu Rev Immunol 9:527, 1991.
183. Hunt DF, et al. Peptides presented to the immune system by murine class II histocompatibility complex I-A^d. Science 256:1817, 1992.
184. Brooks A, et al. Class II-restricted presentation of an endogenously derived immunodominant T-cell determinant of hen egg lysozyme. Proc Natl Acad Sci USA 88:3290, 1991.
185. Carreno BM, et al. Overlapping epitopes that are recognized by CD8+ HLA class 1–restricted and CD4+ class II–restricted cytotoxic T lymphocytes are contained within an influenza nucleoprotein peptide. J Immunol 148:894, 1992.
186. Nuchtern JG, Biddeson WE, Klausner RD. Class II MHC molecules can use the endogenous pathway antigen presentation. Nature 343:74, 1990.
187. Fossum B, et al. A k-*ras* 13 Gly > Asp mutation is recognized by HLA-DQ7 restricted T cells in a patient with colorectal cancer: Modifying effect of DQ7 on established cancers harboring this mutation. Int J Cancer 58:506, 1994.
188. Kelly A, et al. Assembly and function of the two ABC transporter proteins encoded in the human major histocompatibility complex. Nature 355:641, 1992.
189. Spiest T, et al. Presentation of viral antigen by MHC class I molecules is dependent on a putative peptide transporter heterodimer. Nature 355:644, 1992.
190. Boon T. Tumor antigens recognized by cytoloytic T lymphocytes: Present perspectives for specific immunotherapy. Int J Cancer 54:177, 1993.
191. van der Bruggen P, et al. A gene encoding an antigen recognized by cytolytic T lymphocytes on a human melanoma. Science 254:1643, 1991.
192. Greenberg PD, et al. Therapy of disseminated tumors by adoptive transfer of specifically immune T cells. Prog Exp Tumor Res 32:104, 1988.
193. Kawakami Y, et al. Cloning of the gene coding for a shared human melanoma antigen recognized by autologous T cells infiltrating into tumor. Proc Natl Acad Sci USA 91:3515, 1994.
194. Kawakami Y, et al. Cloning of the gene coding for a shared human melanoma antigen recognized by tumor infiltrating lymphocytes associated with in vivo tumor rejection. Proc Natl Acad Sci USA 91:6458, 1994.
195. Robbins PF, et al. Cloning of a new gene recognized by melanoma-specific HLA-A24 restricted tumor infiltrating lymphocytes. J Immunol 154:5944, 1995.
196. Robbins PF, et al. Recognition of tyrosinase by tumor infiltrating lymphocyte from a patient responding to immunotherapy. Cancer Res 54:3124, 1994.
197. Wang RF, et al. Identification of a gene encoding a melanoma tumor antigen recognized by HLA-A31-restricted tumor infiltrating lymphocytes. J Exp Med 181:799, 1995.
198. Rosenberg SA. The immunotherapy of solid cancers based on cloning the genes encoding tumor-rejection antigens. Annu Rev Med 47:481, 1996.
199. Bodey B, Siegel SE, Kaiser HE. Human cancer detection and immunotherapy with conjugated and non-conjugated monoclonal antibodies. Anticancer Res 16:661, 1996.
200. Levine P, et al. Isoimmunization by a new blood factor in tumor cells. Proc Soc Exp Biol Med 77:403, 1951.
201. Fass L. Evaluation of the effect of remission plasma on untreated patients with Burkitt's lymphoma. J Natl Cancer Inst 44:145, 1970.
202. Horn L, Horn HL. An immunological approach to the therapy of cancer. Lancet 2:466, 1971.
203. Shurkovich SV, et al. Treatment of children with acute leukemia by passive cyclic immunization with autologous and autoleukocytes operated during the remission period. Blood 33:186, 1969.
204. Summer WC, Foraker AG. Spontaneous regression of human melanoma: Clinical and experimental studies. Cancer 13:79, 1960.
205. Teimouraian B, McCune WS. Surgical management of malignant melanoma. Am Surg 29:515, 1963.
206. Kohler G, Milstein C. Continuous culture of fused cells secreting antibody of predefined specificity. Nature 236:495, 1975.
207. Maloney DG, Levy R, Campbell MJ. Monoclonal antibody therapy. In Mendelsohn J, et al., eds. The Molecular Basis of Cancer. Philadelphia: WB Saunders, 1995.
208. McCafferty J, et al. Phage antibodies: Filamentous phage displaying antibody variable domains. Nature 348:552, 1990.
209. Kang AS. Linkage of recognition and replication functions by assembling combinatorial antibody Fab libraries along phage surfaces. Proc Natl Acad Sci USA 88:4363, 1991.
210. Huse WD, et al. Generation of a large combinatorial library of the immunoglobulins repertoire in phage lambda. Science 246:1275, 1989.
211. Caton AJ, Koprowski H. Influenza virus hemagglutinin-specific antibodies isolated from a combinatorial expression library are closely related to the immune response of the donor. Proc Natl Acad Sci USA 87:6450, 1990.
212. Clackson T, et al. Making antibody fragments using phage display libraries. Nature 352:624, 1991.
213. Hawkins RE, et al. Cell selection strategies for making antibodies from variable gene libraries: Trapping the memory pool. Eur J Immunol 22:867, 1992.
214. Mullinax RL, et al. Identification of human antibody fragment clones specific for tetanus toxoid in a bacteriophage γ immunoexpression library. Proc Natl Acad Sci USA 87:8095, 1990.
215. Persson MA, et al. Generation of diverse high-affinity human monoclonal antibodies by repertoire cloning. Proc Natl Acad Sci USA 88:2432, 1991.
216. Caron PC, et al. Engineered humanized chimeric forms of IgG are more effective antibodies. J Exp Med 176:950, 1992.
217. Zhang H, et al. A human monoclonal antibody single-chain Fv antibody derived from tumor-infiltrating lymphocytes. Cancer Res 55:3584, 1995.
218. Abeloff MA, et al., eds. Clinical Oncology. New York: Churchill Livingstone, 1995.
219. Carmichael J. Cancer chemotherapy: Identifying novel anticancer drugs. Br Med J 308:1288, 1994.
220. DeVita VT, Hellman S, Rosenberg SA. Cancer: Principles and Practice of Oncology. Philadelphia: JB Lippincott, 1989.
221. Vokes EE. The promise of biochemical modulation in combined modality therapy. Semin Oncol 21:29, 1994.
222. Bellamy WT, Dalton WS. Multidrug resistance in the laboratory and clinic. Adv Clin Chem 31:1, 1994.
223. Childs S, Ling V. The MDR superfamily of genes and its biological implications. Imp Adv Oncol 1994, p 21.
224. Lum BL, et al. Molecular targets in oncology: Implications of the multidrug resistance gene. Pharmacotherapy 13:88, 1993.
225. Patel NH, Rothenberg ML. Multidrug resistance in cancer chemotherapy. Invest New Drugs 12:1, 1994.

226. Friedland M. Combination chemotherapy. In Perry MC. Chemotherapy Sourcebook. Baltimore: Williams & Wilkins, 1992.
227. DeVita VT, Schein PS. The use of drugs in combination for the treatment of patients with cancer. Rationale and results. N Engl J Med 288:998, 1973.
228. American Society of Clinical Oncology. Recommendations for the use of hematopoietic colony-stimulating factors: evidence-based, clinical practice guidelines, J Clin Oncol 12:2471, 1994.
229. Donehower RC, Abeloff MA, Perry MC. Chemotherapy. In Abeloff MA, et al., eds. Clinical Oncology. New York: Churchill Livingstone, 1995.
230. Frei E III, Clark JR, Miller D. The concept of neoadjuvant chemotherapy. In Salman SE. Adjuvant Therapy of Cancer, vol V. Orlando, Fla.: Grune & Stratton, 1987.
231. Lippman SM, Benner SE, Hong WK. Cancer chemoprevention. J Clin Oncol 12:851, 1994.
232. Elkind MM. DNA damage and cell killing: Cause and effect? Cancer 56:2351, 1985.
233. Frankenberg D, et al. Evidence for double-strand breaks as the critical lesion in yeast cells irradiated with sparsely or densely ionizing radiation under oxic or anoxic conditions. Radiat Res 88:524, 1981.
234. Iliakis G, Mehta R, Jackson M. Level of DNA double strand break rejoining in Chinese hamster xrs-5 cells is dose-dependent: Implications for the mechanism of radiosensitivity. Int J Radiol Biol 61:315, 1992.
235. Warters RL, Lyons BW. Variation in radiation-induced formation of DNA double-strand breaks as a function of chromatin structure. Radiat Res 130:309, 1992.
236. McMillan TJ. Residual DNA damage: What is left over and how does this determine cell fate? Eur J Cancer 28:267, 1992.
237. Alper T. Keynote address: Survival curve models. In Meyn RE, Withers HR. Radiation Biology in Cancer Research. New York: Raven Press, 1980.
238. Phillips TL. Principles of radiology and radiation. In Carter SK, Glatstein E, Livingston RB. Principles of Cancer Treatment. New York: McGraw-Hill, 1982.
239. Curtis SB. Lethal and potentially lethal lesions induced by radiation—A unified repair model. Radiat Res 106:252, 1986.
240. Fowler JF. The first James Kirk memorial lecture. What next in fractionated radiotherapy? Br J Cancer 6:285, 1984.
241. Lichter AL. Radiation therapy. In Abeloff MA, et al., eds. Clinical Oncology. New York: Churchill Livingstone, 1995.
242. Mottram JC. Factors of importance in radiosensitivity of tumors. Br J Radiol 9:606, 1936.
243. Castro JR. Particle radiation therapy: The first forty years. Semin Oncol 8:103, 1981.
244. Chapman JD. Hypoxic sensitizers-implications for radiation therapy. N Engl J Med 301:1429, 1979.
245. Aisner J, et al. Chemoradiotherapy for the treatment of regionally advanced head and neck cancers. Semin Oncol 21:35, 1994.
246. Hortobagyi GN. Multidisciplinary management of advanced primary and metastatic breast cancer. Cancer 74:416, 1994.
247. Sause WT. Combination chemotherapy and radiation therapy in lung cancer. Semin Oncol 21:72, 1994.
248. Rosenberg SA. Modern combined modality management of Hodgkin's disease. Curr Opin Oncol 6:470, 1994.
249. Sumiyoshi Y, et al. Neoadjuvant intra-arterial doxorubicin chemotherapy in combination with low dose radiotherapy for the treatment of locally advanced transition cell carcinoma of the bladder. J Urol 152:362, 1994.
250. Tepper JE. Combined radiotherapy and chemotherapy in the treatment of gastrointestinal malignancies. Semin Oncol 19:96, 1992.
251. Bleyer WA, Poplack DF. Prophylaxis and treatment of leukaemia in the central nervous system and other sanctuaries. Semin Oncol 12:131, 1985.
252. Beck DE, Karulf RE. Combination therapy for epidermoid carcinoma of the anal canal. Dis Colon Rectum 37:1118, 1994.
253. Mason M. Combined radiotherapy and chemotherapy: Twice the benefit, or double the trouble? Eur J Surg Oncol 20:597, 1994.
254. Balch CM. Surgical oncology in the 21st century. Presidential address. Arch Surg 127:1272, 1992.
255. Balch CM, et al. What is a surgical oncologist? [editorial]. Ann Surg Oncol 1:2, 1994.
256. Rosenberg SA. The immunotherapy and gene therapy of cancer. J Clin Oncol 10:180, 1992.
257. Gaynor ER, Fisher RI. Biologic therapy. In Abeloff MA, et al., eds. Clinical Oncology. New York: Churchill Livingstone, 1995.
258. Hermann F. Cancer gene therapy: Principles, problems, and perspectives. J Mol Med 73:157, 1995.
259. Isaacs A, Lindenmann J. Virus interference. I. The interferons. II. Some properties of interferons. Proc Roy Soc Lond Biol Sci 147:258, 1957.
260. Sen GC, Lengyell P. The interferon system: A bird's eye view of its biochemistry. Biol Chem 267:5017, 1992.
261. Dorr RT. Interferon-alpha in malignant and viral diseases. A review. Drugs 45:177, 1993.
262. Hansen RM, Borden EC. Current status of interferons in the treatment of cancer. Oncology 6:19, 1992.
263. Stuart-Harris RC, Lauchlan R, Day R. The clinical application of the interferons: A review. Med J Aust 156:869, 1992.
264. Bollag W, Majewski S, Jablonska S. Cancer combination chemotherapy with retinoids: Experimental rationale. Leukemia 8:1453, 1994.
265. Moore DM, Kalvakolanu DV, Lippman SM. Retinoic acid and interferon in human cancer: Mechanistic and clinical studies. Semin Hematol 31:31, 1994.
266. Holcombe RF. Clinical applications of the interleukins: Present and future. J LA State Med Soc 146:479, 1994.
267. Bubenik J. Cytokine gene-modified vaccines in the therapy of cancer. Pharmacol Ther 69:1, 1996.
268. Vujanovic NL, et al. Antitumor activity of human IL-2-activated natural killer (A-NK) cells in solid tumor tissue. Proc Ann Meet Am Assoc Cancer Res 35:A2934, 1994.
269. Foa R, Guarini A, Gansbacher B. IL2 treatment for cancer: From biology to gene therapy. Br J Cancer 66:992, 1992.
270. Aulitzy WE, et al. Interleukins: Clinical pharmacology and therapeutic use. Drugs 48:667, 1994.
271. Vose JM, Armitage JO. Clinical applications of hematopoietic growth factors. J Clin Oncol 13:1023, 1995.
272. Gerhartz HH, et al. Randomized, double-blind, placebo-controlled, phase III study of recombinant human granulocyte-macrophage colony-stimulating factor as adjunct to induction treatment of high grade malignant non-Hodgkin's lymphomas. Blood 82:2329, 1993.
273. Linch DC, et al. A randomized vehicle controlled dose finding study of glycosylated recombinant human granulocyte colony-stimulating factor after bone marrow transplantation. Bone Marrow Transplant 11:307, 1993.
274. Nemunatis J. Phase II trial of recombinant human granulocyte-macrophage colony-stimulating factor in patients undergoing allogenic bone marrow transplantation from unrelated donors. Blood 79:2572, 1992.
275. Pettengell R, et al. Granulocyte colony-stimulating factor to prevent dose-limiting neutropenia in non-Hodgkin's lymphoma: A randomized controlled trial. Blood 80:1430, 1992.
276. Koller MR, Emerson SG, Palsson BO. Large-scale expansion of human stem and progenitor cells from bone marrow mononuclear cell in continuous perfusion cultures. Blood 82:378, 1993.
277. Carswell EA, et al. An endotoxin-induced serum factor that causes necrosis of tumors. Proc Natl Acad Sci USA 72:3666, 1975.
278. Hieber U, Heim ME. Tumor necrosis factor for the treatment of malignancies. Oncology 51:142, 1994.
279. Sheppard BC, et al. Prolonged survival of tumor-bearing rats with repetitive low-dose recombinant tumor necrosis factor. Cancer Res 50:3928, 1990.

280. Sohmura Y, et al. Recombinant human tumor necrosis factor II. Antitumor effect on murine and human tumor transplanted into mice. Immunopharmacology 8:357, 1986.
281. Alexander RB, Rosenberg SA. Tumor necrosis factor: Clinical applications. In DeVita VT, et al., eds. Biologic Therapy of Cancer. Philadelphia: JB Lippincott, 1991.
282. Eggermont AM, Manusama ER, ten Hagen TL. Regional application of TNF-α in the treatment of cancer: A preclinical-clinical interactive program. J Inflam 47:104,1996.
283. Lienard D, et al. High dose recombinant tumor necrosis factor alpha in combination with interferon-gamma and melphalan in isolation perfusion of the limbs for melanoma and sarcoma. J Clin Oncol 10:52, 1992.
284. Yang JC, et al. Isolation perfusion with tumor necrosis factor-α, interferon-γ, and hyperthermia in the treatment of localized and metastatic cancer. Rec Res Cancer Res 138:161, 1995.

10

Physiology of Anesthesia and Pain

Sheryl L. Artmann, Anita L. Giezentanner, and Jeffrey Katz

Physiology of Anesthesia

Sheryl L. Artmann, Anita L. Giezentanner, and Jeffrey Katz

Since Horace Wells demonstrated in 1844 that teeth could be pulled painlessly if the patient inhaled nitrous oxide, anesthesiologists have been dedicated to improving surgical care from the perspectives of both patient and surgeon. A direct translation of *anesthesia,* which is Greek in origin, is "without feeling"; this is one of the four basic requirements for a general anesthetic. The other three are *amnesia, relaxation,* and *loss of consciousness.*

Numerous agents provide varying degrees of anesthesia when inhaled. Nitrous oxide was the first to be administered clinically. William T. G. Morton demonstrated the amazing effects of inhaled ether to a meeting of the Massachusetts General Hospital on October 16, 1846, when a tumor was removed painlessly from a patient's jaw. The next inhalation agent introduced was chloroform, and many others followed. Not until 1934 did J. S. Lundy of the Mayo Clinic introduce thiopental, the first anesthetic agent that could be injected intravenously.

Currently, anesthetic techniques are broadly classified into two areas. These include *conduction* and *general anesthesia.*

1. *Conduction anesthesia* includes both local and regional anesthesia. With this approach, chemicals that temporarily block normal nerve function are injected into the area immediately surrounding the nerve, where they induce anesthesia for a limited time.
2. *General anesthesia,* on the other hand, involves anesthesia administered by inhalational and intravenous routes. Inhalational anesthetics induce anesthesia with varying degrees of amnesia, relaxation, and loss of consciousness when a vapor is inhaled along with oxygen. Intravenous anesthesia, also called *balanced anesthesia,* provides the four basic anesthetic requirements through a combination of drugs especially used for those purposes (e.g., vecuronium for relaxation [paralysis], thiopental or the newer agent propofol for loss of consciousness, a narcotic for analgesia, and nitrous oxide, which enhances the analgesia and provides unconsciousness and amnesia).

This section reviews in detail these various approaches to anesthesia, the physiologic principles underlying the use of anesthetics, and the various clinical settings in which each approach is used.

ANESTHETIC TECHNIQUES

Local Anesthesia

Local anesthesia is administered by injecting an anesthetic solution into the tissues immediately surrounding a peripheral nerve or group of peripheral nerves so that the area supplied by these nerves is rendered totally insensate. Any interruption in function along a nerve from where an impulse is initiated to where it is perceived (the brain) is a form of local anesthesia.

Physiology of Nerve Conduction

The single most important structure in the propagation of neural impulses is the cell membrane of the neuron. The bimolecular membrane layer, the myelin sheath, and the nodes of Ranvier all play a role in setting up an electric gradient between the axoplasm within the cell and the extracellular environment. The arrival of an action potential along a nerve fiber changes the permeability of the cell membrane to sodium ions. These ions then move down a concentration gradient into the cell, which in turn changes the voltage difference across the cell membrane from a negative to a positive charge. It is now widely believed that the sodium ions pass through the cell membrane by traversing small pores called *sodium channels.* It is also accepted that some kind of structural gate to this passage exists and that this gate is opened by the arrival of an action potential.

Pharmacology of Blocking Agents

A local anesthetic's action must be totally reversible within a predictable period. Local anesthetics temporarily block neuronal function by interfering with the movement of sodium ions through the fast sodium channels.

Local anesthetics are all tertiary amines; that is, they are ammonia molecules with each of the three hydrogen atoms replaced by an organic group. The general configuration of the molecule comprises two structural components. The *lipophilic component,* which imparts lipid solubility, comprises the largest part of the molecule. Its aromatic structure is commonly derived from benzoic acid or aniline. The *hydrophilic component,* which imparts water solubility, is an amino derivative of either ethyl alcohol or acetic acid. These two components are joined by an intermediate hydrocarbon chain that is either an amide or an ester (Fig. 10-1). The drugs are therefore characterized as either *amides* or *esters.* Commonly used drugs within each group are the following:

Esters	Amides
Cocaine	Lidocaine
Procaine	Bupivacaine
2-Chloroprocaine	Prilocaine
Tetracaine	Mepivacaine
	Etidocaine

Toxic and Allergic Reactions

One significant difference between the amide and ester anesthetic agents is their potential to cause allergic responses. All esters are broken down into para-aminobenzoic acid, which is highly allergenic in humans, but the amides are rarely implicated in allergic reactions. Toxic reactions to local anesthetics occur when the blood concentration rises above the toxic threshold for a given patient. Local anesthetics enter the intravascular compartment by vascular absorption from infiltration sites or by being erroneously injected directly into vessels. Although maximum doses for various agents have been calculated,[1] responses vary widely from patient to patient, and extreme conservatism appears to be the wisest path.

Initial signs of local anesthetic toxicity are auditory hallucinations and vague paresthesias around the mouth. At higher doses, convulsions are typical; left untreated, and with blood levels of the drug remaining high, stupor, coma, and respiratory arrest follow. Central nervous system signs occur at lower doses; cardiovascular symptoms occur at higher doses. Hypotension from peripheral circulatory collapse is followed by direct myocardial depression and arrhythmias resulting from conduction aberrations. Deaths from local anesthetic toxicity are rare but have been reported.[1] The clinical manifestations of local anesthetic toxicity are caused by the ability of these drugs to depress the central nervous system. Although the earlier signs of toxicity (hallucinations and seizures) appear excitatory in nature, they are related to early depression of inhibitory pathways in the brain. As the blood level rises, more pathways are depressed, until coma and respiratory arrest result. In the heart, the local anesthetics are highly protein bound, and the contractile proteins appear to be no exception. Consequently, these contractile proteins do not perform normally, and myocardial depression and hypotension result (see Table 10-1).

Most important in the successful treatment of toxicity is that the patient be adequately ventilated. This may entail controlling seizures with barbiturates, benzodiazepines, or a muscle relaxant such as succinylcholine. Once seizures have been controlled, the airway is cleared and ventilation is supported; a paralyzed patient almost always needs intubation (see accompanying box). Cardiovascular collapse is treated with appropriate inotropic and chronotropic agents to maintain optimal cardiac function. In these situations, large doses of epinephrine are frequently required, and ventricular dysrhythmias are probably best converted with DC cardioversion or bretylium rather than lidocaine.[2]

Local anesthetic toxicity is more likely to occur when drugs are injected into highly vascular areas, such as the head and neck or the epidural space. The addition of dilute epinephrine to the local anesthetic solution slows the onset of action and the absorption of the anesthetic from the tissues; however, it also increases the duration of action. Care should be exercised when using epinephrine in patients with hypertensive or ischemic heart disease.

Lipophilic part	Linkage	Hydrophilic part
Benzoic acid	COO--R (Ester)	CN (Amino alcohol)
Aniline	NH--COR (Amide)	CN (Amino acid)

Fig. 10-1 Basic structures of two types of local anesthetics in clinical use. Ester structure is shown *above* and amide *below.*

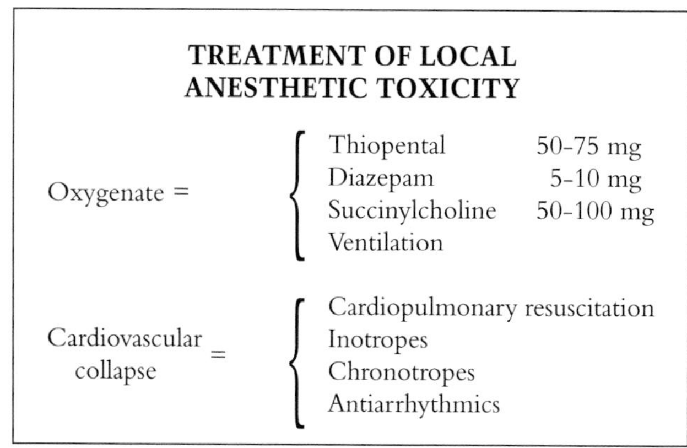

TREATMENT OF LOCAL ANESTHETIC TOXICITY

Oxygenate =	Thiopental	50-75 mg
	Diazepam	5-10 mg
	Succinylcholine	50-100 mg
	Ventilation	
Cardiovascular collapse =	Cardiopulmonary resuscitation	
	Inotropes	
	Chronotropes	
	Antiarrhythmics	

Table 10-1. Symptoms of Local Anesthetic Toxicity

Level	Symptoms
High ↑	Cardiovascular collapse
	Hypotension
	Respiratory arrest
Local	Coma
anesthetic	Stupor
blood	Grand mal convulsion
level	Localized seizure activity
	Auditory hallucinations (tinnitus)
	Confusion, anxiety
Low	Circumoral tongue parasthesias

Table 10-2. Order of Differential Blockade in Local Anesthesia

Conduction Speed	Nerve Function	Dose
Fast ↑	Motor	High ↑
	Touch/pressure	
	Proprioception	
	Pain (fast)/temperature	
	Pain (slow)/temperature	
	Autonomic/preganglionic (sympathetic)	
Slow	Autonomic postganglionic	Low

Regional Anesthesia

A local anesthetic affects a peripheral nerve or group of nerves; in contrast, regional anesthesia requires that a local anesthetic solution be injected into the vicinity of a nerve trunk that supplies an entire anatomic region (e.g., a brachial plexus block for anesthesia of the upper limb). The two most commonly used regional techniques are (1) spinal anesthesia, which blocks the lower part of the trunk and the legs, and (2) epidural anesthesia, which blocks a similar region but is more flexible because a catheter can be left at the site of action so that additional doses of anesthetic can be given.

Spinal Anesthesia

Spinal anesthesia refers to the block obtained when local anesthetics are injected through a lumbar puncture needle into the cerebrospinal fluid. The drug acts on the nerve roots as they leave the spinal cord, before they enter the foramina. There is evidence that when local anesthetics are injected directly into nerve tissues, significant irreversible damage can occur. Before drugs are injected, therefore, cerebrospinal fluid must be easily aspirated through the spinal needle. The extent of the spinal block (the level of the blockade) and its duration are related to the type of anesthetic agent used, the dose administered, and the positioning of the patient.

Although spinal anesthetics are safe and relatively easy to administer, careful patient selection is necessary. Patients with obvious infection in the area, documented clotting problems, and previous back problems may not be appropriate candidates for spinal anesthesia. Additionally, certain cardiac conditions (such as stenotic lesions) cause poor tolerance of regional anesthesia. In these situations, if regional anesthesia is to be used, it is probably best to proceed with an epidural rather than spinal anesthetic. Epidural anesthesia allows the level of sympathetic blockade and hemodynamic changes to be more slowly titrated to the patient's tolerance. Patients with heart disease also frequently require invasive monitoring for judicious fluid loading.

Different populations of nerve fibers blocked during spinal anesthesia have different sensitivities to local anesthetics. The order of differential blockage appears consistent, as shown in Table 10-2. Unmyelinated autonomic fibers are blocked at the lowest concentration of local anesthetic. Therefore, even though a local anesthetic is injected at a specific level and lack of sensation can be detected up to that level, sympathetic blockade can occur as much as four vertebral levels higher. If a spinal anesthetic provides loss of sensation as high as T4, the sympathetic fibers of levels T1 through T3 may also be blocked. This would constitute a total sympathectomy (sympathetic fibers come off spinal cord levels T1 through L5), which would remove the patient's ability to control blood pressure by changing the tone of the peripheral vasculature. Thus, one of the most severe problems associated with spinal anesthesia is profound hypotension. Patients should therefore receive at least 1 L crystalloid solution intravenously before receiving a spinal anesthetic if significant sympathectomy is anticipated.

Epidural Anesthesia

Epidural anesthesia, in which the anesthetic solution is injected into the epidural space, may be performed at any level along the spine. The injection may be a single shot, or a thin plastic catheter may be left in place for continuous infusion or intermittent bolus injection. The site of action for these techniques is at the nerve roots as they cross the epidural space.

Although the physiologic processes of epidural and spinal anesthesia are similar, certain basic differences are relevant to this discussion. The epidural space is potentially large and contains many blood vessels that can absorb anesthetic solution. Further, the dosage of anesthetics and the volume of drug injected are much larger than those for spinal anesthesia. Finally, because the dosage of anesthetic is so much larger, the potential for high blood levels, and thus for local anesthetic toxicity, is much greater.

The popularity of epidural anesthesia is related to its ability to provide continuous anesthesia for as long as the situation demands. Continuous lumbar epidural anesthesia is frequently used in obstetric practice; anesthesia can be provided during labor and the dosage can be increased to cover the pelvic area during the delivery. Caudal anesthesia has found popularity as a single injection for postoperative pain relief after many pediatric procedures. Thoracic and cervical epidural blocks are frequently placed for postoperative pain control and for treatment of chronic pain syndromes.

General Anesthesia

Although many interesting facts concerning the mode and site of action of general anesthetics are known,[3] the ultimate mechanism whereby patients lose consciousness and enter an analgesic state remains unclear. Two helpful facts have emerged in studies of this question. The first is that high barometric pressures (50 to 100 atm)[4] can reverse the effects of general anesthesia in certain animal models, probably because of the effects of pressure on molecular configuration. Second, in 1969 Eger and Saidman[5] showed that multiplication of the oil/gas partition coefficient by the minimum alveolar concentration of any inhalation agent consistently gave a product of 2.1. The *oil/gas partition coefficient* is a measure of the distribution of the inhalation agent between two phases, in this case the inhalation gases in the lung and the fatty component of the brain. *Minimum alveolar concentration,* a measure of potency, is the anesthetic concentration at which 50% of patients do not move in response to a noxious stimulus. Basically, Eger and Saidman's description[5] relates anesthetic potency to an agent's solubility in fat.

Preoperative Considerations

An understanding of the patient's reports and symptoms, the surgical diagnosis, and the intended procedure are essential components of a thorough anesthetic plan. Preparing the patient for what is to come can be achieved only when an intelligent plan has been made. Most important are the patient's histories of previous anesthesia and of current and past drug intake. Potential problems, such as difficulty with airway management, sensitivity to drugs, and anatomic problems in placing needles and endotracheal tubes, can be detected during a preoperative visit. Familial history of anesthetic complications can also be assessed.

Airway Management

Most anesthetic complications are associated with airway mishaps. Proper placement of an artificial airway, such as an endotracheal tube or tracheostomy tube, depends on knowledge of the anatomy of the mouth, nasopharynx, esophagus, and larynx. Essential to competent airway control is the ability to ventilate the patient with a reservoir bag and mask, because many patients do not require endotracheal intubation.

Airway management begins with the preoperative interview. It is during initial physical assessment that clues to the potential difficulty of intubation are obtained. Some obstacles to intubation may be obvious, such as burns or contractures, cervical spine instability, morbid obesity, severe arthritis, facial fractures involving the mandible, or congenital malformations. Other patients may have more subtle signs, and difficulty of intubation is heralded by the classification of Mallampati et al.[6] of temporomandibular joint mobility and the measurement of the distance between the lower border of the mandible and the thyroid notch. No assessment profile is completely accurate, but at least it may allow appropriate preparation. The patient's history of prior intubations is also a relevant factor. Airway management is closely related to the anesthetic technique chosen. Administration of general anesthesia includes three phases: *induction, maintenance,* and *emergence/recovery.* Induction includes the establishment of a secure airway. Anesthesia is commonly induced with a rapid-acting, potent intravenous barbiturate, such as thiopental. Another agent that is now commonly used is propofol. After the patient loses consciousness, control of the airway is the first priority. This may be accomplished with the traditional face mask, endotracheal intubation, or, in some cases, the newly available laryngeal mask. The laryngeal mask, a new device for airway management,[7,8] is a tube attached to an elliptic cuff that resembles a miniature face mask. It is intermediate between the use of a face mask and endotracheal intubation, and it may be put in place on patients who are under general anesthesia or awake with adequate topical coverage. Laryngeal mask airways have proved useful in the management of difficult airways. The laryngeal mask does not provide an airtight seal of the airway; thus, it should not be used when there is a likelihood of gastric regurgitation or when controlled ventilation with inflation pressure greater than 20 cm H_2O could be required.[9] Maintenance of anesthesia can be provided either by allowing the patient to inhale anesthetic agents mixed with oxygen or by injecting selected intravenous agents that are tailored to the patient's requirements. Most patients are ventilated with oxygen–nitrous oxide mixtures that are combined with either intravenous or inhalational agents as required.

Mechanisms and Stages of General Anesthesia

Although theories on the mechanism of action of general anesthetics abound, this burning question remains unanswered. It is not even clear whether various anesthetic agents, whose structures vary considerably, are in fact bringing about the same state, although they are all recognized under the term *general anesthesia.* It is understood that narcotics create analgesia by occupying specific receptors in the brain and spinal cord and that benzodiazepines induce their effects by reacting with central nervous system receptors. These individual effects, however, provide only components of general anesthesia. Further, receptor antagonists that reverse the effects of these drugs do not reverse general anesthetics.

However, anesthesiologists do not differ with respect to what constitutes general anesthesia and at what point patients are suitably anesthetized for surgery to take place. General anesthetics exert their main action (which is depressant, producing unconsciousness and abolishing reflexes) on the central nervous system, and through this action, they modify every system. By their action on the various centers (e.g., the respiratory center) and reflexes, various phenomena are produced. The study of these phenomena enables a competent anesthesiologist to accurately judge at any moment the depth of anesthesia. From commencement of induction to the point of death, anesthesia is divided into four stages:

1. *Stage 1:* This is the stage of analgesia, characterized by a progressive decrease in response to painful stimuli and progressive loss of consciousness.
2. *Stage 2:* During this phase, delirium becomes manifest, with incoherent talking and struggling. Patients are unconscious and amnesic. Respiration is irregular, and reflexes are inclined to be exaggerated.
3. *Stage 3:* This stage is heralded by muscular depression sufficient to prevent the patient from moving his or her limbs in response to stimuli. Surgical anesthesia is indicated by (1) the onset of automatic respiration and (2) the loss of eyelid reflex. Stage 3 is subdivided into four planes:
   a. *Plane 1:* There is progressive decrease in the range and rapidity of eyeball movement.
   b. *Plane 2:* The eye is in a central position, and the intercostal muscles and diaphragm retain function.
   c. *Plane 3:* Thoracic movement is depressed until only diaphragmatic function remains.
   d. *Plane 4:* Respiratory effort is absent.
4. *Stage 4:* The heart beats, and the patient remains alive if blood is oxygenated. As depth increases, pupils become dilated and irregular. This is an overdose.

Plane 3 of stage 3 is commonly thought to represent the ideal anesthetic state for most surgery.

CHOICE OF AN ANESTHETIC

Two important decisions face the anesthesiologist confronted with a new patient. One is what type of anesthetic technique to use (general, regional, or local), and the other concerns which pharmacologic agents to use.

Several factors play a part in the first decision. Frequently, if the surgery is to be performed on a small, localized part of the body that is amenable to neural blockade, local anesthesia seems appropriate. Other indications for local anesthesia include patient preference and illnesses that could make a more invasive technique dangerous. In situations in which multiple techniques are equally suitable, the anesthesiologist considers patient preference, his or her own familiarity with the regional technique, the surgeon's preference, the need to discuss the pathology during the operation, and whether intraoperative teaching will take place. Even when all other factors indicate that a regional technique is best, however, the degree of familiarity of the anesthesiologist with that technique should play an important role in the decision.

There are persuasive arguments for general anesthesia in some situations. (1) When a skin or bone graft from a location removed from the primary surgical site is planned, two regional injections would be needed. (2) The sound of some procedures, such as heavy orthopedic manipulations of sawing or chiseling, may be disturbing to an awake patient.

In patients with potentially difficult airways to manage, regional anesthesia is often recommended. However, it is wise to remember that the difficult airway is best managed electively. If a spinal block were to ascend too high or a cervical block were to paralyze the vocal cords, that difficult airway might have to be managed in an emergency situation. In patients expected to need blood transfusions, perhaps under pressure, general anesthesia is preferred because injecting blood intravenously under pressure can be uncomfortable and painful for the patient.

In conclusion, many factors play a role in the anesthesiologist's choice of technique. Sometimes the need to teach a particular technique dictates its use, especially if there are no reasons to avoid that technique. What is important is that these decisions be made in full harmony with the surgeon and the patient, so that all are happy with the way things are progressing.

The second decision, regarding the anesthetic agent to be used, depends more heavily on the preexisting medical and surgical conditions found in the patient; it is more fully discussed in a subsequent section of this chapter. Briefly, an important consideration in the selection of anesthetic agents is the route by which they are metabolized and excreted. Although most drugs are metabolized in the liver and excreted in the urine, some are degraded to active or toxic products. It is now believed that halothane hepatitis is related to the toxic metabolites of nonoxidative degradation of halothane in the liver. Care should also be taken to avoid agents that produce distortion or mask valuable signs. For example, it is well known that nitrous oxide expands gas-containing cavities; thereby distorting anatomy by massive dilation. Similarly, sedatives interfere with neurologic assessments, narcotics cause spasm of Oddi's sphincter, and general anesthesia can mask intra-abdominal pain after viscus perforation. With few exceptions, general anesthetics are regarded as myocardial depressants. Careful selection of anesthetic technique is therefore necessary when dealing with patients who have a history of heart disease.

Most anesthetic complications occur during induction and emergence; thus, airway management is as important during emergence and recovery as it is at the beginning of a procedure. Other potential postoperative problems related to anesthetics include arrhythmias, bleeding problems, renal failure, clotting of vascular grafts, malignant hyperthermia, and changes in the level of consciousness.

PATIENT MONITORING

As computers have become smaller and more widely available, many automated systems have been developed for patient monitoring during anesthesia. Nevertheless, there is no substitute for careful hands-on monitoring of surgical patients. Certain techniques have become standard and are considered minimum requirements for good patient care. These include monitoring blood pressure, heart rate, cardiac electric activity, temperature, breath sounds, heart sounds, inspired oxygen concentration, and pulse oximetry. Additionally, quantitative monitoring of the carbon dioxide content of exhaled gases or volume of expired gas is encouraged. Carbon dioxide detection and measurement are used both as an indication of successful endotracheal intubation and an assessment of the adequacy of ventilation.

Direct monitoring of blood pressure from an arterial catheter allows continuous evaluation of mean arterial, systolic, or diastolic pressure and makes arterial blood easily available for measuring arterial blood gases. If large changes in central blood volume are expected, central venous pressure monitoring may be indicated. Although urinary output, heart rate, and blood pressure give relevant information, central venous pressure allows the anesthesiologist to closely follow changes in volume and observe the effect of volume infusions. However, central venous pressure most accurately reflects the volume and compliance of the right side of the heart. If systemic blood volume and left ventricular function measurements are required, a pulmonary artery catheter is the only currently available device that provides measurement of central venous pressure, pulmonary artery pressure, and pulmonary capillary wedge pressure. This catheter also allows sampling of mixed venous blood, thermodilution measurement of cardiac output, and monitoring of cardiac electric activity or pacing of the heart. Pulmonary capillary wedge pressure reflects left atrial pressure, which in turn reflects left ventricular filling pressure and volume. Further, a ventricular function curve can be constructed through the Starling principle that allows optimal volume loading, of special value in the patient with a compromised left ventricle.

Two-dimensional transesophageal echocardiography is now available in some centers for intraoperative monitoring of cardiac function. Its intraoperative indications include assessment of valvular function, intracardiac volumes, and contractility.[10] Furthermore, transesophageal echocardiography has proved useful in early detection of venous air embolism.[11] Two-dimensional transesophageal echocardiography can allow early detection of myocardial ischemia by detection of regional wall motion abnormalities. It appears to be more sensitive than either electrocardiography or pulmonary capillary wedge pressure. Lack of equipment availability and training in correct interpretation of the findings, however, have somewhat hampered widespread use. Furthermore, such conditions as esophageal varices or strictures contraindicate its use.

A pulmonary artery catheter is recommended for the patient undergoing cardiac surgery, or for any patient with severe heart disease undergoing other types of surgery. Additional indications for pulmonary artery catheterization are (1) major surgery involving massive blood and fluid replacement and (2) any procedure associated with circulatory instability (e.g., massive trauma, extensive burns, hypotensive shock, severe sepsis, aortic surgery requiring clamping, pulmonary embolus, major portal surgery).

Pulse oximetry is a standard of care for monitoring oxygenation during anesthesia. This monitor has also found widespread use in all areas of patient care whenever either continuous or intermittent evaluation of oxygenation is needed. Although controlled trials have never been performed, there appears to have been a great improvement in safety of anesthetics, perhaps partially as a result of pulse oximetry.[12]

Pulse oximetry combines plethysmography and spectrophotometric analysis to evaluate the ratio of oxyhemoglobin to reduced hemoglobin. Thus, it is able to calculate oxygen saturation of hemoglobin in a vascular bed. Many factors, including temperature, perfusion pressure, motion, extraneous light sources, and nail polish, affect accuracy. Additionally, it may be inaccurate in the presence of methylene blue or increased carboxyhemoglobin concentration. Nevertheless, pulse oximetry is an extremely useful monitor for assessment of the patient at all perioperative stages.

Monitoring and quantification of expired gases have also evolved dramatically. Initially a research tool that first found clinical use in neurosurgical cases, end-expired carbon dioxide tension (PCO_2) measurement has now become virtually a standard of care in all operating rooms. Its use is not absolutely required but is encouraged by the American Society of Anesthesiologists standards. In addition to carbon dioxide analysis, the other gases that may be used during anesthesia may also be measured. The benefit of this is an increase in patient safety by measuring the concentrations of the gases. In addition, the expired carbon dioxide waveform may be diagnostic of many pathologic conditions. The end-expired PCO_2 is a measurement that is used extensively in neurosurgical procedures. Apart from the early detection of significant occlusion of pulmonary artery outflow caused by air embolism evidenced by any drop in end-expired PCO_2, the end-expired PCO_2 is also an indication of cardiac output. Computer technology has made it possible to measure the somatosensory-evoked potential that accurately indicates spinal cord function during surgery when spinal cord integrity might be threatened.

Electroencephalograph is a measure of adequacy of cerebral perfusion and oxygenation. It is now commonly used in the operating room during procedures in which cerebral blood flow could be compromised.

DISEASE-RELATED CONSIDERATIONS IN ANESTHETIC PRACTICE

Trauma

Anesthetic management of patients with trauma is primarily directed toward airway control and maintenance of

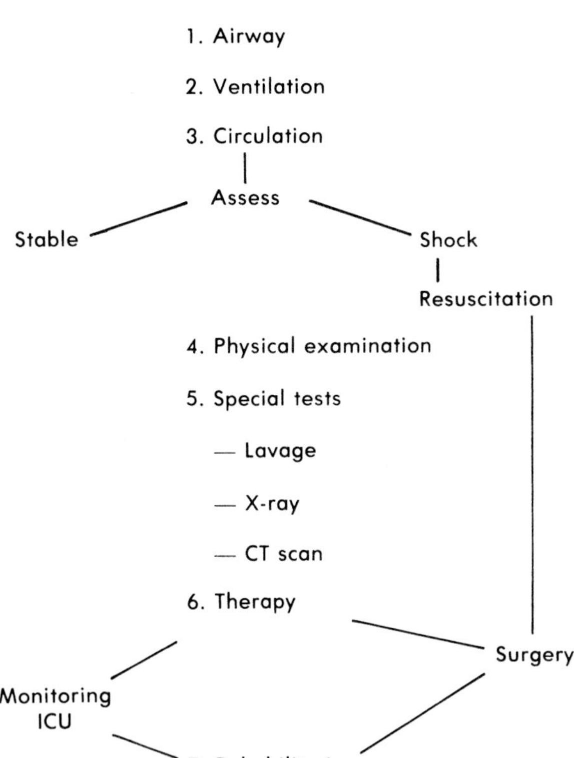

Fig. 10-2. Order of management of patient with trauma.

cardiovascular stability until bleeding has been controlled and blood loss has been replaced. Patients with trauma are often young and are therefore more likely than the usual surgical population to have normal cardiovascular systems. Therapeutic priorities in these patients are delineated in Fig. 10-2.

Special Problems

A number of unique constraints affect the treatment of victims of severe trauma:

- Frequently, they are unable to give any history regarding their medical status or their drug intake.
- Because of the high incidence of occult cervical vertebral fractures associated with traumatic head injury, the neck must be treated as fractured until radiologic evidence to the contrary is available.
- All patients with trauma are considered to have full stomachs, which affects airway management. Many are under the influence of alcohol or drugs.
- Patients with trauma are often bleeding actively, and all must be assumed to be in hemorrhagic, hypovolemic shock.
- Patients with trauma are inclined to be maximally sympathetically stimulated and thus peripherally vasoconstricted. This makes intravenous access difficult, especially when the patient is also hypothermic.

EFFECTS OF HYPOTHERMIA

1. Reduced oxygen consumption and basal metabolic rate
2. Central nervous system depression leading to coma
3. Arrhythmias: premature ventricular contractions (30° C, 86° F), ventricular fibrillation (28° C, 82° F)
4. Oxygen dissociation curve shift to left
5. Coagulopathy (28° C, 82° F)
6. Shivering (32° to 24° C, 89.6° to 75.2° F) and increased oxygen consumption
7. Increased blood viscosity (28° C, 82° F)
8. Respiratory depression—apnea at 23° C (73.4° F)
9. Hyperglycemia
10. Metabolic acidosis
11. Slow drug biotransformation
12. Depressed renal function—ceases at 20° C (68° F)
13. Arteriolar paralysis at 32° C (89.6° F)

Anesthetic Management

Hypothermia is common among patients with trauma, especially in areas of the country that have severe winters. Efforts must be made to warm these patients as rapidly as is physiologically safe. Although hypothermia may impart some cerebral protection from hypoxia, it is associated with a number of physiologic aberrations.

During periods of decreased cardiovascular function, hypothermia could be beneficial because metabolic activity is decreased, in turn lessening oxygen requirements at the same time that oxygen delivery is reduced. This is especially true of the brain, which can survive a much longer period of ischemia if it is cooled first. However, at 30° C (86° F), premature ventricular contractions become manifest and further degenerate to ventricular fibrillation at 28° C (82° F) or below. Further, with oxygen delivery threatened, blood viscosity increases with decreasing temperature, and shivering increases oxygen demand by as much as 300%. Despite the fact that induced hypothermia has been used with some success clinically, uncontrolled hypothermia is detrimental because most body functions become depressed as temperature drops (see accompanying box).

Gastric emptying stops as soon as sympathetic activity is stimulated by the occurrence of an accident. Therefore, the stomach is assumed to be full, no matter when the trauma occurred, and the airway must receive maximal protection from the possibility of aspiration of gastric contents. If general anesthesia is undertaken, induction should follow a definite sequence designed to minimize the chances of aspiration, as shown in Table 10-3.

Trunkey[13] stated that 99% of trauma victims may be intubated orally. In an emergency, cricothyrotomy[14] can be temporarily lifesaving until a more permanent artificial air-

Table 10-3. Rapid-Sequence Induction (Airway Protection)

Preparation	Suction Laryngoscopes (two blades) Tubes (three sizes) Preoxygenation (3 min) Precurarization (vecuronium 0.01/mg/kg)	
Induction	Thiopental (3-5 mg/kg) Succinylcholine (1-1.5 mg/kg)	Cricoid pressure
Airway	Intubate Ventilate (check right and left) $ETCO_2$ Secure tube well	Cricoid pressure

way can be established. If the anesthesiologist believes that intubation could be difficult, the patient should not be anesthetized until the airway has been secured,[15] because induction of general anesthesia and the resulting paralysis can simultaneously impair the reflexes that protect the airway and eliminate all respiratory effort. In cases where the intubation may be difficult because of anatomic factors concern regarding cervical spine stability, awake intubation is frequently employed. This may use either a blind nasal technique after adequate topical anesthesia or fiberoptic bronchoscopic assistance for oral or nasal awake intubation. Patients may be judiciously sedated for these procedures, to maximize their cooperation and comfort. Frequently, combinations of agents, such as narcotics (fentanyl) and benzodiazepenes (midazolam), are used, and they should be carefully titrated to the desired effect. These medications will render the patient comfortable yet conscious and cooperative. Both agents have antagonists available in case overdose should occur. Naloxone is a specific narcotic antagonist, and flumazenil[16] is newly available for benzodiazepene antagonism. By employing these techniques, safe control of the airway is achieved prior to induction of anesthesia.

Maintenance of anesthesia should be directed toward providing good operating conditions while maintaining cardiovascular stability, so that vital organ perfusion is ensured. After induction, anesthesia is maintained with agents that minimize cardiovascular depression. Frequently, paralysis is provided with intravenous pancuronium while the patient is ventilated with 100% oxygen. Analgesia is provided with intravenous narcotics that are titrated against the patient's blood pressure. Because as many as 40% of patients with trauma are awake during trauma surgery,[17] an amnestic sedative without cardiac depressive effects (e.g., midazolam) should be considered.

Monitoring should include use of a central venous pressure catheter, an electrocardiogram, an arterial line, pulse oximetry, end-tidal P_{CO_2} and gas monitoring, urinary catheter, and temperature and cuff blood pressure monitoring. Blood should be replaced as quickly as possible through blood warmers to minimize hypothermia, and microfilters should be used to lessen particulate matter trapped in the lung, which appears to be a major factor in the development of the adult respiratory distress syndrome after multiple transfusions.

Cardiothoracic Disease

During the past two decades, the number of open-heart procedures has increased markedly. The pulmonary artery catheter has revolutionized the management of patients with cardiovascular disease by allowing the anesthesiologist to optimally manipulate preload and afterload so that the myocardium is allowed to work at maximum efficiency within the constraints of its oxygen supply.

Preoperative Evaluation

Simple questions can establish the patient's exercise tolerance, the presence of orthopnea, and the frequency of chest pain. Histories of hypertension, rheumatic fever, diabetes mellitus, smoking, obesity, inactivity, and family cardiac disease all tend to increase the patient's chances of myocardial infarction during surgery. It is important to determine what drugs the patient takes (e.g., digitalis), their effects, and serum drug levels. It is particularly important for patients with heart disease to come to the operating room relaxed, free of pain, and with supplemental oxygen if necessary. They should be sedated enough to comfortably tolerate the placement of intra-arterial, pulmonary arterial, and peripheral intravenous catheters while awake.

Anesthetic Management

As the drive for the ideal cardiac anesthetic technique has progressed, two approaches have emerged. The first is related to the fact that inhalational agents are generally profound vasodilators that therefore routinely decrease afterload. Because they are also significant myocardial depressants, they act maximally to decrease cardiac work and thus oxygen consumption.[18] The problem with these agents is that they can cause hypotension so severe that coronary artery perfusion is inadequate for myocardial requirements. The second approach depends on the synthetic narcotic fentanyl, which has minimal cardiac depressant activity.[19] In extremely high doses[20] (50 to 100 μg/kg vs 3 to 5 μg/kg in balanced anesthesia), fentanyl is currently the anesthetic of choice for cardiac surgery. Alternative narcotic choices for the primary anesthetic are the newer agents sufentanil (10 to 20 μg/kg) and alfentanil (50 to 150 μg/kg). They may be associated with equal hemodynamic stability but faster emergence and therefore more rapid extubation. High-dose narcotics have been associated with bradycardia. Pancuronium is frequently chosen as the relaxant because of its sympathomimetic side effects. If an increase in heart rate is not desired, a relaxant without cardiovascular side effects, such as vecuronium or the newer agents pipecuronium and doxacurium, should be selected.[21,22] Abdominal and chest wall rigidity can also occur and may be quite severe. Patients usually receive a low dose of a nondepolarizing muscle relaxant prior to high-dose opioid administration to combat this problem.

Benzodiazepines are frequently added, and inhalational agents may be titrated to tolerance. Both of these agent types work to eliminate the awareness under anesthesia and hypertension in response to surgical stimuli that sometimes accompany anesthesia with narcotics only.

Hypotension and hypertension are frequently seen on weaning from cardiopulmonary bypass. The anesthesiologist should be prepared to vasodilate, vasoconstrict, stimulate heart rate, slow heart rate, or manipulate all cardiac performance indices to promote an adequate oxygen supply/demand ratio with satisfactory cardiac output. Invasive monitoring and the pulmonary artery catheter have enabled anesthesiologists to accurately determine all indices of cardiac performance and to tailor anesthetic management to protect the ailing myocardium from ischemic assault.

Chronic Pulmonary Disease

Much controversy surrounds the anesthetic management of patients with advanced lung diseases. Should they have regional anesthetics when possible? Should intubation be avoided? Should they be paralyzed? In general, these patients remain in stable condition as long as no change occurs. Typical changes are simple upper respiratory tract infection, the onset of an unrelated disease process, or a significant change in climate.

Preoperative Evaluation

Determining exercise tolerance in these patients is of great importance because incapacitated patients are more likely to have problems after the operation. The cessation of smoking before surgery[23,24] is of benefit in terms of both oxygen delivery and postoperative morbidity. Because the long-term smoker's airway is more reactive, however, attempts should still be made to avoid airway irritation. Dependence on bronchodilators is also associated with postoperative difficulties. Patients taking theophylline derivatives should have serum levels of these drugs within therapeutic ranges at all times. Dependence on steroids to control bronchospasm dictates the additional use of steroids during the stressful perioperative period.

If surgery is imminent, pulmonary function tests are more valuable in predicting postoperative problems than as aids in planning anesthetic technique. If there is time to act on pulmonary function test data, bronchodilators or chest physiotherapy can be prescribed as the situation demands. The most commonly used indicator of pulmonary function is the measurement of forced expiratory volume in 1 second (FEV_1). This test places patients with obstructive disease in one of three groups. (1) Because of their considerable pulmonary reserve, patients with FEV_1 greater than 50% of that predicted and normal arterial blood gases do not have an increased risk of perioperative problems. (2) Patients with FEV_1 25% to 50% of that predicted are at significant risk for postoperative morbidity and should be evaluated with a view to achieving the best possible preoperative condition. (3) Patients with FEV_1 less than 25% of predicted are hypoxemic, are at high risk, and should undergo surgery only for life-threatening conditions.[25]

Anesthetic Management

General anesthesia for patients with chronic pulmonary disease is associated with decreased clearing of pulmonary secretions, increased alveolar atelectasis, increased intrapulmonary shunting, and significant changes in the ventilation/perfusion ratio.[26] Furthermore, paralysis is associated with increased ventilation/perfusion mismatching.

Studies on patients with normal pulmonary function[27] have failed to demonstrate any positive correlation between anesthetic technique and incidence of postoperative pulmonary complications. Similar studies on patients with chronic obstructive pulmonary disease have shown a much higher incidence of postoperative respiratory failure among patients receiving general anesthesia[28] than among those receiving regional anesthesia. Ventilatory impairment is related to the anatomic site of surgery in patients with and without pulmonary disease. Upper abdominal and thoracic procedures are associated with significant degrees of impairment in vital capacity.[29]

When general anesthesia is used in patients with pulmonary disease, it should be tailored to compensate as much as possible for the abnormal airway architecture, the disturbed ventilation/perfusion ratios, the increased sensitivity to ventilatory depressants, the limited ability to mobilize secretions over a poorly functioning mucociliary escalator, and the restricted potential for humidifying inspired gases. Arterial blood gases should be monitored frequently to ensure adequate gas exchange. Finally, inhaled gases should be humidified to prevent the extreme drying of airways that follows prolonged ventilation with dry gases. When a general anesthetic technique is used, the specific pharmacologic agents administered do not appear to affect the outcome.

Efforts should be directed toward extubating patients as soon as possible after surgery. There is a tendency to leave these patients in surgical intensive care units for prolonged periods while they are being weaned from ventilators. The longer they depend on assisted ventilation, however, the greater their morbidity.

Liver Disease

There are four important considerations in managing surgical patients with liver disease. These are (1) worsening of the liver disease, (2) extrahepatic complications, (3) impairment of liver synthetic activity, and (4) alteration of drug disposition.

Anesthetic Risk Factors

Although hard evidence does not exist, it is intuitively clear that surgery and anesthesia are likely to worsen preexisting liver disease.[30] The liver is exquisitely sensitive to oxygen deprivations; thus, it is not surprising that postoperative morbidity and mortality are quite high among patients with advanced hepatic disease.[31,32] All anesthetics, especially inhalational agents, reduce hepatic blood flow. Surgical intervention alone and the natural physical and hormonal response to stress also reduce blood flow to the liver. The interplay of these factors is extremely difficult to differentiate, although the amount of blood flow reduction caused by surgical intervention seems to be related to the proximity of the manipulation to the organ itself.[33] Anesthetic agent effects may arise either directly from toxicity of the agent or its metabolite or indirectly from decreased blood flow, and thus oxygen supply, to the liver. Regional anesthesia is not a panacea; it too causes a reduction in hepatic blood flow, especially if hypotension develops. Moreover, concurrent coagulopathy frequently precludes the use of regional anesthesia. Studies have shown that spinal anesthesia, cyclopropane, and ether anesthesia are all associated with the same degree of postoperative hepatic dysfunction in patients with liver disease.[34] Hepatotoxicity from halothane is well reported, although the exact etiology is unclear. It would seem prudent when selecting a halogenated agent to select one that undergoes minimal hepatic metabolism, such as enflurane or isoflurane. Neither of the new inhalational agents desflurane and sevoflurane appears to injure the liver.[35]

Preoperative assessment and optimization of physical status is critical in the patient with hepatic failure. Extrahepatic complications include encephalopathy, which lowers anesthetic requirements; esophageal varices; predisposition toward renal failure; and ascites. Patients with severe liver parenchymal disease have a high tendency toward development of renal failure, either hepatorenal syndrome or acute tubular narcosis. Every attempt should be made to maintain urinary output during surgery. Such metabolic disturbances as sodium retention and hypokalemia are common. Hypokalemia should be addressed in particular, because it is implicated in worsening the potential for renal failure and hepatic encephalopathy. Serum electrolytes should be monitored during operation. Bleeding esophageal varices represent the most serious anesthetic risk factor in patients with liver disease because of the dual threats of aspiration of blood and hypovolemia. Many of the principles of trauma management apply equally well to this type of surgical emergency.

Hypoxemia is common in patients with portal hypertension and ascites. These patients frequently have pulmonic shunts and coexisting lung disease. Ascites reduces diaphragmatic excursion, compresses the lungs, and decreases the ventilation perfusion ratio in basilar sections of the lungs. Because of vena caval compression, ascites can also impair venous return to the heart, causing hypotension, which further complicates the hypovolemia of bleeding varices. Finally, ascites increases the volume of distribution of anesthetic drugs. Ascitic fluid is isolated from the circulation and can serve as a sink for drugs, delaying their onset and prolonging the duration of their action.

Anesthetic Management

Destruction of liver cells can impair the ability of the liver to synthesize such compounds as plasma proteins, plasma pseudocholinesterase, and clotting factors, which are vital to anesthetic management. Because a number of drugs used for anesthesia are significantly bound to plasma proteins, decreased levels of these proteins can cause altered pharmacokinetics and dynamics. Pseudocholinesterase is the enzyme responsible for metabolizing succinylcholine and all ester local anesthetics. Although significant hepatic destruction must be present before the metabolism of these drugs is affected, the duration of action of succinylcholine, an ultrashort-acting relaxant, can be significantly prolonged in patients with substantial liver disease. In such a setting of reduced plasma pseudocholinesterase activity, neuromuscular function could take hours to return to normal, rather than the expected 5 minutes. Finally, the decreased production of clotting factors that occurs in liver disease could also pose significant problems in anesthetic management, particularly in the patient who is hypovolemic from bleeding varices.

Many factors interact to alter the half-lives of drugs used in anesthetic practice. These include altered synthesis of plasma proteins, with changes in albumin/globulin ratio; decreased hepatic biotransformation; decreased hepatic blood flow; and changes in the volume of distribution. Furthermore, anesthesia itself may decrease hepatic blood flow and can inhibit the action of hepatic microsomal oxidative enzymes.

Local anesthetics of the amide type, which depend on liver metabolism for their breakdown, are likely inclined to clear the blood in patients with liver disease less rapidly than in healthy patients. Thus, the tendency toward local anesthetic toxicity with these agents is increased, and caution should therefore be exercised when using them.

Diabetes Mellitus

Infection is the leading cause of death in surgical patients with diabetes. In the past, it was thought that patients would remain in stable condition if they were hyperglycemic but not ketotic during surgery. Although short durations of hyperglycemia at levels of 400 to 600 mg/100 ml are not harmful to patients with diabetes, hypoglycemia of similar duration can cause severe and irreversible brain damage.

It is obvious that hypoglycemia would be difficult to detect clinically during administration of general anesthesia. Therefore, the tendency toward inducing hyperglycemia grew in popularity. Recent evidence, however, indicates that patients with diabetes in whom normal blood glucose levels are maintained have a lower incidence of morbidity.[36]

Preoperative Evaluation

Evaluation of the patient with diabetes before surgery must include consideration of the duration and severity of the illness and of current medications. Patients with juvenile-onset diabetes have lower circulating insulin levels and are more difficult to control perioperatively. The patient with maturity-onset diabetes is more likely to have a decreased fasting blood sugar without ketosis when starved before operation. The hypoglycemic agent prescribed, its dosage, and the frequency of administration predict both peak effect and potential for hypoglycemia in the patient. Long-acting insulins or oral agents such as chlorpropamide can still have an effect on the morning of surgery, even when the last dose was given 24 hours before the operation. A morning fasting glucose level should always be drawn before induction of anesthesia.

Anesthetic Management

In the interest of maintaining nearly normal glucose levels during the operation, many protocols have been developed. The desire to avoid hypoglycemia led to an approach based on minimal interference during the operation. No glucose or insulin was given on the day of surgery, and insulin was used only to treat severe hyperglycemia or ketosis.[37] More recently, a partial dose of the normal insulin requirement was given on the morning of surgery. Blood sugar levels were measured during the operation and treated appropriately, and glucose was added as necessary until the patient tolerated postoperative tube or oral feeding. Currently, intravenous insulin, administered either by injection or by continuous intravenous infusion, is given with intravenous dextrose during surgery. The insulin dose is either adjusted to the glucose infusion rate or titrated by frequent blood glucose measurements.[38] No single protocol can be expected to work adequately for all patients with diabetes. Frequent blood analysis with appropriate insulin therapy is probably the most reliable method available.

Inhalation anesthetics tend to increase blood sugar.[39] An anesthetic for patients with diabetes is tailored more toward the manifestations of the disease (e.g., renal failure) than toward the disease itself. If neuropathy or infection is present, spinal or epidural anesthesia is relatively contraindicated. Because of the need for repeated venous blood samples, monitoring of intraoperative blood sugar levels is easier in unconscious patients than in awake patients. Adherence to the concepts described here should allow any general anesthetic technique to be used safely.

Renal Failure

Acute renal failure is the abrupt impairment of renal function, whereas *chronic* renal failure implies a more permanent functional impairment that has profound systemic effects such that if there were no method of clearing the blood of toxic metabolites, death would surely follow. The anesthesiologist may prevent or attenuate postoperative renal dysfunction by preoperative identification of patients at risk and optimization of perioperative volume status and hemodynamic parameters.[40]

Medical Complications

Infection and sepsis are the leading causes of mortality in patients with renal impairment. These problems are aggravated in transplant recipients who are receiving immunosuppressive drugs, such as steroids.[41] Meticulous sterile technique should be used whenever catheters are placed. Invasive monitoring techniques should be used sparingly because the incidence of thrombophlebitis is high. For patients who depend on flow through arteriovenous shunts for dialysis, strict criteria for inserting arterial catheters should be developed.

Patients with renal failure have a high incidence of cardiovascular disease. Hypertension is common, and signs of left ventricular hypertrophy are frequent. The murmurs of aortic and mitral insufficiency occur as a result of hypertension, anemia, and fluid overload. However, these murmurs often resolve with dialysis. Uremia is also associated with cardiomyopathy and pericardial effusions. Hypertension is related either to fluid overload or to increased plasma renin levels. Although functionally overloaded, patients with renal impairment behave as though they are volume depleted during anesthesia. Hypotension can occur with minimal blood loss or vasodilation. The temptation to fill up the dilated vascular bed can cause severe hypertension after surgery and tends to push the patient into volume overload. The management of fluids in these patients is extremely precarious. Although the tendency is to err on the side of hypovolemia, hypotension should be treated early.

Dialysis is associated with several problems that can affect anesthesia. Patients may be placed on the dialysis machine in fluid overload and a hypertensive state, yet they come off in a hypovolemic, hypotensive state. The date of the most recent dialysis, postdialysis laboratory values, and weight loss must be determined before surgery. Dialysis is associated with anemia in patients with renal failure, with typical hematocrits ranging between 20% and 25%. Although this anemia is well tolerated, there are acceptable limits to its severity before anesthesia. These limits have not been definitively established, but hematocrits of 20% to 25% represent an oxygen-carrying capacity that is 50% or less of normal. Cardiac output is usually increased to compensate for this decreased oxygen-carrying capacity.

Anesthetic Management

It is best to avoid anesthetic agents that depend on renal function for elimination. Thiopental tends to have a longer duration of action in patients with uremia. Narcotics also appear to have prolonged effects. Atracurium besylate is a short-acting, nondepolarizing relaxant that is eliminated from the body by processes not requiring intact renal function. This drug is popular for patients with chronic renal failure. Caution must be exercised in the use of succinylcholine because it transiently increases the serum. Potassium level inhalational induction is the safest technique, because inhalant drugs are only minimally metabolized and do not depend on renal excretion for cessation of their action.

Pediatric Diseases

Two primary differences between children and adults influence the treatment of pediatric patients. First, although the child's surface area is one twentieth that of the adult, the child's surface-to-volume ratio is 70 times greater.[42] The most obvious effect of this circumstance is the increase in heat loss that children undergo and the increased caloric requirements therefore needed to maintain body temperature. The other important difference is that children usually have no insight into their problems, do not cooperate, and feel threatened and alienated, especially when coming to the operating room.

Physiologic Considerations

Basic differences in cardiovascular function do exist, but they are not so significant that the principles of safe management change. Infants 6 months old or younger tend to have right ventricular hypertrophy as a legacy of the fetal circulation. To compensate for the lower oxygen-carrying capacity of fetal hemoglobin, the infants have a cardiac output that is 30% to 50% greater than in adults. Arterial pressure also varies with age. Neonates tend to have systolic pressures around 60 to 70 mm Hg, which increase to systolic pressures of approximately 100 mm Hg by the age of 12 years. Finally, children also have an increased blood volume. During the first month of life, blood volume is approximately 85 ml/kg.[43] By the age of 2 years, it has decreased to 68 to 75 ml/kg.

For anatomic reasons, atelectasis is more likely to occur in infants. Their alveoli are smaller, and their chest wall is highly compliant. A term neonate has a wasted ventilation of 40%, which decreases to adult levels of 30% by 1 month. Oxygen requirements in children may exceed 6 ml/kg/min, more than twice that of adults.[44] When combined with the extremely small vital capacity of infants, this high oxygen requirement can rapidly lead to hypoxia and cyanosis during oxygen deprivation.

Renal function is poorly developed in neonates, but it is adequate to meet their metabolic needs. Infants have difficulty reabsorbing bicarbonate from their urine and in effect have renal tubular acidosis.[45] Only when their protein intake increases are they able to secrete hydrogen ions and ammonia. Neonates are unable to concentrate their urine as well as adults, although this ability can increase when stressed.

One significant difference between neonates and adults is how they maintain body temperature. Infants metabolize brown fat, which is located between the scapulae, around the heart, and around vital structures in the neck, as a source of calories.[46] Neonates are unable to shiver. Because of their enormous surface area-to-body weight ratio, they have a tendency to lose temperature to the environment, especially when uncovered or wet.[47] Cold operating rooms, hypoglycemia, exposure of abdominal and thoracic contents, and ventilation with cold, dry gases compound this problem. Temperature must therefore be carefully monitored in children.

Anesthetic Management

Most children come to the operating room without intravenous access. Preoperative sedation, especially with sedatives that do not involve invasive routes of administration, has become standard in many centers. Many options now exist for sublingual, oral, or intranasal administration of sedative drugs. The current technique used in pediatric anesthesia is inhalational induction followed by placement of an intravenous line as soon as the patient has lost consciousness. Once this access has been secured, the anesthetic management is similar to that used in the adult.

The pediatric larynx is somewhat different from that of the adult. The narrowest part of the larynx in the adult is the glottis, whereas the cricoid ring is the limiting factor in the child. The larynx is somewhat higher in the neck (C2, as opposed to C3 to C6 in the adult). Children are generally easier to intubate with a straight laryngoscope blade than with a curved one. No cuffs are needed on pediatric tubes because the cricoid ring seals the tube in the larynx.

Finally, children tend to emerge rapidly from anesthesia, and they need early support and encouragement until they are reunited with their parents.

ANESTHETIC EMERGENCIES

Cardiac Arrest

Three main groups of etiologic factors are associated with cardiac arrest.[48] (1) Impairment of cardiac electrical activity is usually manifested by some arrhythmia; the most common of these is ventricular fibrillation, but ventricular tachycardia, asystole, and complete heart block are also seen. (2) Disorders of myocardial contractility are caused by hypoxia, myocardial infarction, cardiac failure, acidosis, electrolyte abnormalities, or drug effects. (3) Entities associated with decreased venous return include hypovolemia, tamponade, pulmonary embolus, myocardial rupture, dissecting aneurysm, and vena caval compression. During anesthesia, all cardiac arrests are viewed as hypoxic until proved otherwise. By far the most prevalent of anesthetic accidents is the disconnection of the patient from the ventilatory source, resulting in hypoxic cardiac arrest.

Although the overall treatment of cardiac arrest is aimed at correcting the cause, the initial phases of cardiopulmonary resuscitation are similar for all arrests. All patients should be ventilated with 100% oxygen. A 5 to 10 ml amount of epinephrine administered intravenously at a ratio of 1:10,000 can elevate perfusion pressure, change fine to coarse fibrillation, which is more responsive to defibrillation, and stimulate spontaneous or more forceful cardiac contraction. Sodium bicarbonate is given intravenously in initial doses of 1 mEq/kg to combat metabolic acidosis. A dosage of 5 to 7 mg/kg 10% calcium chloride, infused intravenously, is also a reliable inotropic agent. Lidocaine can be given intravenously to suppress ventricular ectopy in doses of 1 mg/kg. Atropine in 0.5 mg doses repeated to a desired effect is used to accelerate heart rate in third-degree heart block and asystole. Isoproterenol can be infused to treat third-degree block or electromechanical dissociation.

Cardiac arrest that occurs in the operating room usually responds to this sequence of therapy. If arrest occurs during induction and the patient is successfully resuscitated, surgery should be postponed. If it occurs during the operation and is reversed, every effort should be made to end the procedure as soon as possible.

Pneumothorax

One of the complications of positive-pressure ventilation is the development of pulmonary interstitial emphysema. Pulmonary interstitial emphysema may be accompanied by pneumothorax.[49] Several surgical factors increase the chances of pneumothorax: (1) surgery deep in the flank in the kidney position, (2) any trauma surgery in which projectiles have passed through the diaphragm, and (3) any type of surgery performed near the diaphragm.

Although pneumothorax may not itself necessarily lead to an anesthetic emergency, the onset of tension pneumothorax is a potentially fatal emergency if not swiftly relieved. Tension pneumothorax occurs when a one-way valve effect is set up, allowing air to enter the pleural space but not to leave. If gases are being driven into the chest under pressure, as occurs with mechanical ventilation, the potential for disaster is large. Signs of pneumothorax include high inflation pressures, sudden shift of the mediastinum to the opposite side, circulatory collapse, subcutaneous emphysema, and coughing of serosanguinous material. In these situations, immediate decompression of the pleural space is required and can be accomplished by inserting a large-bore needle or chest tube into the pleural space.

The use of nitrous oxide further complicates the entrapment of air in any cavity such as the chest. Nitrous oxide expands these cavities relatively quickly and increases the circulatory and respiratory compromise caused by pneumothorax.[5]

Tension pneumothorax can occur spontaneously. When hypotension occurs and no obvious cause is seen, suspicion of tension pneumothorax may save a life that would otherwise have been lost.

Malignant Hyperthermia

Malignant hyperthermia is a disease of muscle tissue that, when triggered by various anesthetic agents, sets off a chain of events leading to uncontrollable muscle hypermetabolism, rampant metabolic acidosis, and severe hypoxia. It is a genetically determined disease, more common in children and young adults. The incidence of malignant hyperthermia among children is estimated to be about 1:14,000 anesthetic uses. It is more common in individuals with such muscular abnormalities as joint hypermobility, kyphoscoliosis, ptosis, squint, clubbed feet, and history of muscle cramps. The mortality rate associated with malignant hyperthermia approaches 50%.

The disease is usually reported to be initiated by the administration of either halothane or succinylcholine.[50] Failure of the jaw to relax after succinylcholine administration is associated with the disease.[51] Other early clinical signs include tachycardia and metabolic acidosis. Fever is a later finding, and the disorder is severe when it occurs. Arrhythmias, tachypnea, and an increase in tidal volume indicate the tremendously high Pco_2 manifested by these patients. The skin becomes mottled, and the tissues of the wound and viscera may feel hot. Profound sweating may occur. Pco_2 is usually extremely high, often higher than 100 mm Hg. Hypoxia may be present. Disseminated intravascular coagulopathy may follow. An elevated creatine kinase level is present in the serum in 70% of patients with this condition.[52] To make the diagnosis in susceptible patients, a muscle biopsy procedure that includes evaluation of caffeine-induced contractures with and without halothane is the most useful test.[53]

A protocol for the management of this condition should be written in summary form and taped to every anesthetic machine. A separate box and cart labeled "hyperthermia emergency kit" should be available in all operating room suites. Dantrolene, the current specific treatment for this disease, probably works by decreasing the amount of transmitter released by the excitation-contraction coupling process within muscle, thus indirectly re-

TREATMENT OF MALIGNANT HYPERTHERMIA

1. Stop administration of all anesthetics and end surgery as soon as possible.
2. Send for help.
3. Replace the anesthesia machine with a nonrebreathing circuit, free of anesthetic vapors.
4. Begin mixing dantrolene sodium (20 mg/60 ml water) and give 1 to 2 mg/kg intravenously.
5. Treat acidosis with sodium bicarbonate according to formula:
   Base deficit = 0.3 × weight (kg) × base excess (mEq/L)
6. Treat hypotension by correcting pH and giving cold crystalloid loading.
7. External cooling should be vigorous. Cool room and bathe patient in ice packs and wet towels soaked in alcohol.
8. Monitor all laboratory values. Treat hyperkalemia with glucose and insulin if necessary.
9. Admit patient to an intensive care unit and continue dantrolene and other therapy.

ducing the amount of calcium released. The sequence of treatment in this disease is shown in the box on p. 262.

Late complications of the disease include renal failure, myoglobinuria, and hypotension (prerenal failure); consumption coagulopathies, treated with fresh-frozen plasma and platelets; and central nervous system damage, which may become apparent only later.

Venous Air Embolism

Although the pathophysiologies of the various types of pulmonary venous emboli are similar, air embolism can occur rapidly and without warning in the operating room. The entry of air into the venous system occurs regularly when bubbles enter the veins through intravenous infusions. However, these small volumes are usually filtered out[54] or absorbed without causing any sequelae. In any procedure in which the wound is higher than the right atrium, a gravity gradient exists between the wound site and the right atrium, permitting entrainment of air. This complication is most commonly seen in neurosurgical procedures performed with the patient in the sitting position, but it has been reported after head and neck surgery,[55] dilation and curettage, hysterectomy,[56] and placement of subclavian central venous catheters.[57]

Once air has entered the venous system, it is carried to the right atrium. As the volume of gas increases, the bubbles move to the right ventricle and then to the pulmonary artery. There they block the pulmonary artery outflow tract, inducing acute right ventricular failure.

When surgical patients must be in positions in which air embolism is a possible complication, certain preparations can aid the diagnosis and treatment of this condition. Initially, a right atrial central catheter can be placed to monitor central venous pressure; it must be located so that air bubbles can be aspirated conveniently. Bubbles in the blood cause turbulence as they pass through the heart. As little as 0.5 ml air can be detected with an ultrasonographic chest Doppler scanner placed over the right atrium. When any type of pulmonary embolism occurs, some degree of occlusion of the pulmonary outflow tract is usually present. Perfusion of the lung by venous blood is therefore decreased, and the blood retains carbon dioxide that would have been eliminated in the alveoli. The arterial P_{CO_2} increases, whereas the end-expiratory P_{CO_2} decreases. These changes can be monitored on a capnograph, which is a reliable form of monitoring for pulmonary venous embolism. Treatment is described in the accompanying box.

TREATMENT OF VENOUS AIR EMBOLISM

1. Inform surgeon, who can cover wound with saline solution-soaked sponges and prevent further air entrainment.
2. Send for help.
3. Discontinue nitrous oxide.
4. Aspirate right atrial catheter.
5. Change height of wound with respect to the right atrium if possible.
6. Treat cardiovascular depression supportively.

Electrolyte Disturbances

Calcium and potassium ions are intimately involved with the generation of action potentials in the excitable tissue of the heart. The presence of these electrolytes in abnormal concentrations is thus reflected in abnormal electrocardiograms and arrhythmias, some of which may herald the onset of critical conduction defects.

Hypocalcemia

Normal serum calcium levels are between 8 and 10.5 mEq/L. Membrane function, neuromuscular function, and myocardial contractility depend on the amount of ionized calcium in extracellular fluid. The ionized portion of the serum calcium in turn depends on the pH (decreasing pH increases ionized calcium) and plasma proteins (decreased protein decreases ionized calcium). The causes of acute severe hypocalcemia are massive transfusion (citrate intoxication), severe alkalosis, and parathyroidectomy. Severe respiratory alkalosis may be the cause of true tetanic muscle spasms similar to those seen in hypocalcemic tetany after parathyroidectomy. In the operating room, hypocalcemia is associated with hypotension, electrocardiographic abnormalities (Fig. 10-3, *A*), and cardiac arrest in diastole if

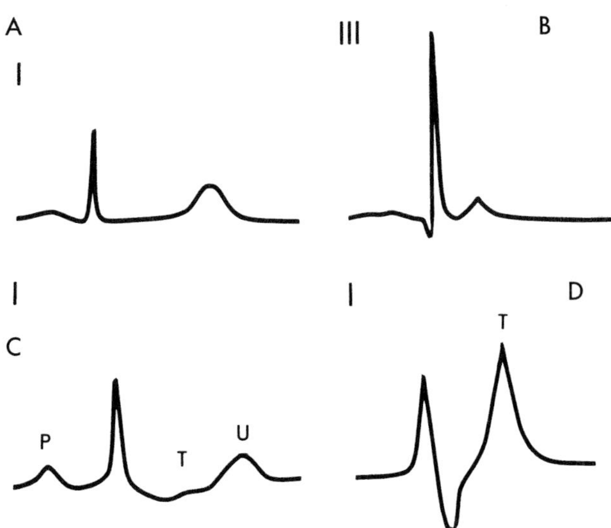

Fig. 10-3. Electrocardiographic changes in various electrolyte abnormalities. **A,** Hypocalcemia: Most obvious feature is prolonged QT interval and late T wave. Lead I. **B,** Hypercalcemia: Note shortened QT interval and shortened ST segment. Lead III. **C,** Hypokalemia: Exaggeration of U wave, depression of ST segment, and fusion of T wave with U wave. Lead I. **D,** Hyperkalemia: Peaked and tall T waves, widening of QRS, and decreased QT interval. Lead I.

calcium levels drop too low. Severe hypocalcemia is best treated with 1 g calcium chloride as a slow intravenous infusion for several minutes.

Hypercalcemia

Hypercalcemia is a much rarer phenomenon that results in calcium levels of 17 to 20 mg/100 ml or even higher, a severe and sometimes fatal problem. These levels are usually seen only in patients with severe hyperparathyroidism or metastatic bone cancer. Extracellular fluid expansion, chelating agents, steroids, and dialysis sometimes fail to control hypercalcemia. Electrocardiographic aberrations are seen, with cardiac arrest occurring in systole (Fig. 10-3, *B*).

Hypokalemia

Normal extracellular fluid potassium levels vary between 4 and 5 mEq/L. This accounts for 2% of total body potassium, the rest of which is intracellular (150 mEq/L). Potassium is shifted intracellularly by alkalosis, hyperventilation, and glucose-insulin therapy. The three most common causes of hypokalemia among surgical patients include excessive renal losses, unreplaced losses from gastrointestinal secretions, and movement of potassium ions into the cells. Most of the commonly used diuretics, especially the thiazides, are associated with increased potassium loss through the urine.

Hypokalemia results in poor contractile strength in skeletal, smooth, and cardiac muscle. It is recommended that anesthesia not be administered when potassium levels are below 3 mEq/L.[58] In surgical emergencies, potassium can be replaced at a rate not exceeding 0.5 mEq/kg/hour. Cardiac electrical activity and urinary output should be monitored during replacement, and levels should be checked frequently. During anesthesia, hyperventilation, which reduces potassium levels even further, should be avoided. Electrocardiographic changes are shown in Fig. 10-3, *C*.

Hyperkalemia

Arrhythmias, resistance to digitalis, and high-peaked T waves on electrocardiograms are the typical cardiac effects of hyperkalemia (Fig. 10-3, *D*). Usual causes include impaired excretion of potassium in renal failure and massive blood transfusions. Anesthesia should be postponed if potassium levels are greater than 6 mEq/L. The combination of hyperkalemia with arrhythmogenic anesthetics such as halothane is unwise. Potentially fatal hyperkalemia can occur after the administration of succinylcholine in certain conditions, including major burns, massive trauma, and neurologic injury.[59] Peak potassium levels of 10 to 15 mEq/L are associated with dangerous arrhythmias, including ventricular tachycardia and ventricular fibrillation.

RECENT ADVANCES AND FUTURE CONSIDERATIONS

Laparoscopic Surgery

Laparoscopic techniques have revolutionized the manner in which a myriad of operations are performed. These techniques can be used for peripheral procedures, such as orthopedic surgery, and for central procedures, such as cholecystectomy, appendectomy, fundoplication, nephrectomy, tubal ligation, laparoscopically assisted vaginal hysterectomy, and bowel resection or loop colostomy. The peripheral procedures do not specifically entail different anesthetic techniques, but the abdominal procedures require pneumoperitoneum, with its attendant anesthetic challenges. These are detailed in an extensive review by Cunningham and Brull.[60] Laparoscopic techniques have become quite widespread, and in some cases they are replacing the more traditional open approach. The numerous advantages include shorter hospital stay, faster recovery, decreased postoperative pain, and smaller scars. All things considered, they may be less expensive. The primary considerations for the anesthesiologist are patient positioning, pneumoperitoneum, necessity for urinary and gastric catheters, and the controversy surrounding the use of nitrous oxide.[61] General anesthesia is almost always required, although the use of regional techniques has been reported.[62]

Laparoscopic surgery is generally considered to cause less significant hemodynamic changes because of the less invasive nature of the procedures; however, the requirement for pneumoperitoneum and a steep Trendelenburg posture have sometimes caused severe hemodynamic and respiratory compromise. Some patients do not tolerate these changes, and these operative procedures should not be viewed as a panacea for the sick patient who would not otherwise be a good candidate for surgery. With this proviso, the rapid recovery and decreased need for narcotics, with their potential for respiratory compromise, make laparoscopy a useful technique for patients whose well-being may depend on their ability to mobilize quickly in the postoperative period.[63]

Anesthetic requirements include nasogastric and urinary catheters to decompress the stomach and bladder and prevent their injury during trochar insertion. Good muscle relaxation is a necessity to allow adequate insufflation of the abdomen. The patient may be placed supine or in the lithotomy orientation, and one or both arms are usually tucked. Depending on the procedure and the surgeon's preference, patients may be in the Trendelenburg or reverse-Trendelenburg position.

The problems associated with pneumoperitoneum include increased propensity toward main stem bronchial intubation as the carina moves upward with insufflation and potential for pneumothorax, pneumomediastinum, subcutaneous emphysema, or gas embolism.[64] Other potential complications are absorption of inflating gas, with possible hypercarbia if carbon dioxide is used; potential for bowel burns in presence of nitrous oxide; and hemodynamic compromise, especially if inflating pressures exceed the recommended 15 to 20 cm H_2O. The gas absorption and respiratory compromise of insufflation and Trendelenburg position can usually be countered by increasing the volume of ventilation by 20% to 30%.[65]

The common hemodynamic effects are primarily related to inflation pressures, patient positioning, and vagal reflexes for manipulation of intra-abdominal tissues. If the intra-abdominal pressure is allowed to rise too high, a decrease in venous return with peripheral pooling may occur. In one study by Joris et al.[66] patients in the head-up position demonstrated a 50% decrease in cardiac index after abdominal insufflation.

Nitrous oxide has been used both as the insufflating gas and as an anesthetic adjunct during general anesthesia. Carbon dioxide has replaced nitrous oxide as the insufflating gas in most centers because nitrous oxide supports combustion. When nitrous oxide is used as an anesthetic adjunct, it causes no discernible differences in bowel distention[61] but does diffuse into the carbon dioxide insufflating gas, once again raising the potential for combustion.[67] For this reason, its use cannot be recommended.

For the safety of operating room personnel, the pneumoperitoneal gas should be scavenged rather than vented to operating room air. The burning of tissue in the hypoxic environment of the abdomen can produce levels of carbon monoxide that exceed safe levels set by the Environmental Protection Agency. Blood levels of carboxyhemoglobin do not rise.[68]

Laparoscopic surgery can be a safe and attractive method for a number of surgical procedures. As we move into a new era of medicine, with emphasis on same-day surgery and shorter hospital stays, its use is sure to expand. The risks and potential for such serious consequences as hemodynamic and respiratory compromise must, however, not be minimized.

Monitoring

The future thrust in monitoring technology will be in the area of noninvasive techniques. Computer miniaturization has permitted the development of sophisticated equipment for operating room use. Mass spectrometry allows monitoring of concentrations of multiple anesthetic and physiologic gases. Equipment now available enables one observer at a central console in the operating room to monitor the expired gas concentrations of six to 12 rooms concurrently. Problems such as hypercarbia, hypoxia, and anesthetic overdose can be detected rapidly with the use of this system. The equipment is extremely sensitive in detecting air embolism. Further, anesthetic gas concentrations can be monitored, and dangerous errors can be corrected.

Agents

In these times of cost-containment, and with the attendant push toward minimizing hospital stays, new faster and shorter-acting agents are becoming more popular. The new ultrapotent narcotic agents alfentanil and sufentanil are already ingrained in many practices. Propofol is a new intravenous anesthetic agent from the series of alkyl phenols.[69] It may be used solely as the induction agent or to provide total anesthesia, especially in short cases. It provides rapid onset and has an extremely short duration of action. Propofol also possesses antiemetic properties. These qualities make it an attractive alternative, especially for same-day surgery. The respiratory and cardiovascular depressant properties of propofol are similar to those of thiopental; thus, it must be used with caution in elderly persons and those with cardiovascular compromise. Propofol has gained widespread acceptance, and its use has become a mainstay in many anesthetic practices. New short-acting muscle relaxants with faster onset, such as mivacurium[70] and rocuronium,[71] are being introduced.

The search for the "perfect" inhalational agent continues. Desflurane and sevoflurane are currently being evaluated. They may provide more precise control of anesthetic depth and more rapid recovery.[35]

Flumazenil, a newly available benzodiazepine antagonist, may be used to hasten recovery after sedation, especially if high doses of a benzodiazepene have been used. However, the potential for resedation must be considered in the outpatient setting.[16,72]

A common concern, especially in the outpatient setting, is prolonged postoperative nausea and vomiting, which can lead to an otherwise unnecessary hospitalization. Ondansetron (Zofran) is a new serotonin antagonist that appears to be quite effective in both prevention and treatment of nausea and vomiting.[73,74]

One area currently undergoing a resurgence of interest is patients' awareness while under anesthesia. The psychologic sequelae of auditory perception during general anesthesia is being investigated and is certainly an area of concern.[75] The highest incidence remains during cardiac surgery and cesarean section, but with the push toward "lighter" anesthesia and quicker recovery, we may expect to see the incidence rise. There have been estimates that as many as 1% to 3.8% of patients have some psychologic manifestation of memory or recall during anesthesia.[76,77] Prudence in operating room discussion is therefore recommended.

SUMMARY

An important component of surgical care relates to the ability to adequately anesthetize the portion of the body being subjected to operation. Currently, two broad categories of anesthetic technique are recognized: *conduction anesthesia,* in which chemicals are injected to areas immediately surrounding nerves to temporarily block their normal function, and *general anesthesia,* in which inhalant and intravenous substances elicit an anesthetic state by inducing varying degrees of amnesia, relaxation, and loss of consciousness. In choosing an anesthetic for a given patient, the anesthesiologist is confronted with two important decisions, (1) what type of technique to use and (2) what pharmacologic agent to use to induce anesthesia once the technique has been determined. Factors affecting these decisions include the part of the body being subjected to operation, the type of underlying illness that a given patient has, the patient's particular preference, and the expertise and familiarity of the anesthesiologist with a given technique in a particular situation. In all cases, flexibility should be the rule, and the advantages and disadvantages of each anesthetic in the specific clinical setting should be thoroughly considered in choosing the optimal approach for each patient. Such care will minimize the incidence of both intraoperative and postoperative problems.

Physiology of Pain

Sheryl L. Artmann and Anita L. Giezentanner

Despite the fact that current pharmacologic and technologic advances allow us to deal effectively with the problem of postoperative pain, a relatively large percentage of surgical patients remain undertreated for their pain. To a large extent, this is a result of a lack of teaching about the physiology, anatomy, and pharmacology of pain and pain management, beginning in medical school and extending into the postgraduate years of residency. Because of this lack of formal education in the field of pain management, students must rely on the "apprenticeship principle" of medical education, a system that tends to propagate misunderstanding and results in poor therapy.[78] In this section, the neurophysiologic pathways involved in the nociceptive process are discussed, followed by suggestions for a rational approach to the treatment of postoperative pain on the basis of this physiologic model.

NOCICEPTION

The International Association for the Study of Pain defines pain as "an unpleasant sensory and emotional experience associated with actual or potential tissue damage, or described in terms of such damage."[79] This definition encompasses not only the physical aspects associated with pain, defined by specific neural pathways, but also the psychologic and emotional importance assigned to the pain experience by the individual patient.

The four physiologic processes involved in the nociceptive process are transduction, transmission, modulation, and perception.[80]

Transduction may be defined as the process by which noxious stimuli are encoded into electric activity at the sensory nerve ending. *Transmission* is the process through which these transduced electrical impulses are propagated throughout the sensory nervous system. *Modulation* is the process through which endogenous analgesic systems are able to modify nociceptive transmission. These endogenous systems, which include opioid, serotonergic, and noradrenergic systems, exert their inhibitory influence at the level of the dorsal horn of the spinal cord. *Perception* is the final common pathway in which transduction, transmission, and modulation interact with the unique psychologic makeup of the individual to create the final subjective and emotional experience of pain.

Transduction

Nociceptors are primary afferent neurons that respond to noxious chemical, thermal, or mechanical stimuli. These nociceptors function to convert energy generated by the noxious stimulation into a train of neural impulses.

There are two major types of nociceptors, A δ and C fibers. Both are sensitive to thermal and mechanical noxious stimulation. C fibers additionally respond to noxious chemical stimulation, and they are therefore referred to as *C polymodal nociceptors.*

Repetitive stimulation of nociceptors results in sensitization (a lowering of their threshold for response). This process is accomplished through release of chemical mediators, which may leak from damaged cells, be synthesized locally, or be released by nociceptors themselves. Examples of chemicals that leak from damaged cells include potassium, histamine, acetylcholine, serotonin, and adenosine triphosphate. Those synthesized locally include bradykinin, serotonin, cholecystokinin, prostaglandins, and leukotrienes. Substance P is released by nociceptors themselves.

Transmission

Primary sensory afferent neurons involved in nociception carry information from the periphery to the spinal cord. Functional aspects of peripheral nerves may be determined by analyzing the compositions of their constituent axons. The most numerous axons found in peripheral nerves are A α, A δ, and C fibers, with smaller amounts of A β and A γ fibers. As previously noted, A δ and C fibers are primarily concerned with nociceptive transmission.

A δ fibers are small-diameter, myelinated fibers with conduction speeds faster than 100 m/sec. A α and A β fibers function in fine somatosensory discrimination. C fibers are the most numerous in peripheral nerves. They are small-diameter, unmyelinated, slowly conducting fibers. Most C fibers are primary sensory afferent fibers; however, 20% are sympathetic postganglionic efferents.[81]

Nociceptive information is carried by small-diameter, myelinated A δ fibers and unmyelinated C fibers. Activation of A δ fibers results in sharply localized pricking pain of short duration, whereas activation of only C fibers produces a poorly localized burning sensation of longer duration.[82]

As nociceptive A δ and C fibers approach the spinal cord, they enter the dorsal horn through the dorsal root. Here they occupy a dorsolateral position. Larger A α and A β fibers occupy a more medial position and continue as the dorsal columns. Collaterals of these A α fibers synapse within the dorsal horn and are important in diminishing nociceptive transmission. Nociceptive A δ and C fibers ascend or descend in Lissauer's tract prior to entering the spinal gray matter.[83]

Rexed[84] described the cytoarchitectural organization of the spinal gray matter as a series of layers, or *laminae.* A complete description of Rexed's laminae is beyond the scope of this text. The dorsal horn contains laminae I through VI. Nociceptive A δ and C fibers make synaptic termination in laminae I, II, and V.[84]

From laminae I, II, and V, projecting axons carrying nociceptive information coalesce to form the spinothalamic tract, which occupies the anterolateral quadrant of the spinal cord. Spinothalamic neurons divide into medial and lateral divisions, which terminate in specific thalamic areas. Neurons that form the lateral division of the spinothalamic tract project strictly to the somatosensory cortex. In contrast, those located medially are derived from deeper lamina (laminae VI, VII, and VIII) and make synaptic connections in the brain stem reticular formation. Because they project from the brain stem reticular formation, they are termed the *spinoreticular pathway.* This pathway projects widely to the basal ganglia, prefrontal, and motor cortex, as well as to the somatosensory and visual cortical areas.[80]

Modulation

Descending systems that modulate afferent activity at the level of the dorsal horn have been elucidated. When stimulated, cells in the periaqueductal gray matter, dorsolateral tegmentum of the pons, and rostroventral medulla increase the activity of a descending neural pathway termed the *dorsolateral funiculus.* The terminations of axons in this pathway are most concentrated in laminae I, II, and V, the same laminae in which primary sensory afferents (peripheral nociceptive fibers) make synaptic connection with cell bodies of the spinothalamic tract. Electric stimuli to the dorsolateral pontine tegmentum and rostroventral medulla result in release of norepinephrine and serotonin, respectively. Norepinephrine and serotonin result in the production of analgesia and inhibition of dorsal horn neuronal transmission.[82]

An endogenous opioid system that contributes to descending modulation of pain transmission has also been elucidated. Enkephalins are the primary mediators of descending inhibition. They are derived from the precursor molecules met-enkephalin and leu-enkephalin, which are derived from pro-enkephalin A. Enkephalins are found in the gastrointestinal tract, sympathetic nervous system, and adrenal medulla, as well as in areas important in nociceptive transmission, the periaqueductal gray, rostroventral medulla, and laminae I, II, V, and X. Pharmacologically, enkephalins are like opioids in their ability to produce analgesia, cross-tolerance to morphine, and reversal by naloxone.[85]

β-Endorphin is another endogenous opiate derived from pro-opiomelanocortin. Adrenocorticotropic hormone is also derived from this precursor molecule and is produced on a one-to-one molar basis with β-endorphin. β-endorphin, which is more potent than the enkephalins, is found in the hypothalamus, periaqueductal gray, and locus ceruleus.[85,86]

The injection of small amounts of opioids into areas with high concentrations of endogenous opioids results in the production of intense analgesia in experimental animals, leading to the belief that systemic or perispinal administration of exogenous opioids produces analgesia by activating endogenous opiate receptors.[85] Endogenous opiate receptor subtypes have been determined by binding studies. μ_1-Opioid receptors mediate supraspinal analgesia. μ_2-Opioid receptors mediate the respiratory depression and cardiovascular effects associated with opioid administration. δ-Opioid receptors mediate spinal analgesia. κ-Opioid receptors mediate spinal analgesia and sedation. σ-Opioid receptors are associated with psychotomimetic effects.[85,87] The analgesic effects of the opioids are mediated through complex interaction with μ-, κ- and δ-opioid receptors.

GATE CONTROL THEORY OF PAIN

The three main physiologic processes involved in nociception (transduction, transmission, and modulation) converge on nociceptive neurons in the dorsal horn of the spinal cord. The dorsal horn may therefore be conceptualized as a gate for the integration and modulation of the nociceptive process. Melzack and Wall[88] originally developed the "gate control" theory of pain, in which they attributed nociceptive transmission through the dorsal horn to the interplay between myelinated and unmyelinated inputs. Although the gate control theory of pain remains unproven, the concept of the dorsal horn as a gate that may be closed by specific pharmacologic maneuvers serves well as the basis for postoperative pain management.[80]

POSTOPERATIVE PAIN MANAGEMENT

The nociceptive process is complex. As previously described, there are three main physiologic processes involved: transduction, transmission, and modulation. Manipulation at any level affects the perception of pain. Intervention at multiple levels forms the physiologic basis of balanced analgesia, the combination of analgesic modalities to provide maximal pain relief with minimal side effects.[85]

Transduction

As established previously, the release of chemical mediators at the terminals of peripheral nociceptors can enhance transduction. It follows that blocking the effects of these mediators, either at their site of action or by preventing their release, results in inhibition of transduction. Prostaglandins are an example of this type of mediator, and their production may be inhibited by the administration of cyclo-oxygenase inhibitors, such as the nonsteroidal anti-inflammatory drugs (NSAIDs). Note that the NSAIDs only inhibit *production* of prostaglandins; therefore, any prostaglandins synthesized prior to the administration of the NSAID will continue to exert an effect on the transduction process.

Transmission

Neural blockade with local anesthetic agents inhibits axonal transmission by binding to sodium ionic channels. This may be accomplished at peripheral nerves with a single injection of local anesthetic agent, at the plexus level (with either a single injection or continuous infusion by catheter), or more centrally, at the epidural or intrathecal level.[89]

Use of local anesthetics as single agents for the control of postoperative pain poses some problems with respect to the side effects of motor blockade and cardiovascular instability associated with their use in high doses. However, dilute concentrations of local anesthetics in combination with opioids can provide prolonged periods of analgesia while avoiding motor blockade or cardiovascular instability.[85]

Modulation

Exogenous opioids may be administered systemically (through the oral, transdermal, subcutaneous, intramuscular, and intravenous routes) to provide postoperative analgesia. They produce profound analgesia but are associated with multiple side effects that may limit their effectiveness, including nausea and vomiting, respiratory depression, decreased gastrointestinal motility, altered mental status, and urinary retention.[90]

When administered epidurally or intrathecally, much smaller doses of opioids are required to produce profound analgesia, with a lower incidence of side effects than that associated with systemic opioids and without the autonomic and motor blockade associated with the use of local anesthetic agents. Tiny doses of opioids are effective by these routes because of close proximity to their site of action, the dorsal horn.[91]

PAIN MEASUREMENT

To effectively treat postoperative pain, accurate assessments must be made of the amount of pain felt by the patient. The subjective nature of the pain experience makes it extremely difficult for an observer to accurately assess the amount of pain felt by a particular patient. In assessing the amount of postsurgical pain, we must therefore rely heavily on patient report. As with other charted vital signs, for pain assessment to be meaningful, it must be assessed according to a systematic scale, reassessed at frequent intervals, and charted in an easily accessed area of the patient's medical record.

A number of different pain scales have been created in an attempt to quantify the intensity of pain felt by an individual patient.[92-94] In the most simple type of scale, the patient is asked to rank the pain as no pain, mild pain, moderate pain, or severe pain. A slightly more complex scale involves having the patient attach a number to his or her pain level, ranging from 0 (no pain) to 10 or 100 (the worst pain imaginable). This type of verbal-analog pain scale is easily assessed at the bedside and requires minimal training of nursing personnel in its application. For research purposes, a visual-analog pain scale may be employed, in which the patient is asked to place a mark on a 10 cm line anchored with the qualifiers "no pain" and "the worst pain imaginable." After the patient places a mark ranking his or her pain, the investigator measures the amount of pain indicated on the scale and assigns a numeric rating to it.

The type of pain scale used for pain measurement is not as important as its consistent application. Because many patients may be reluctant to "complain about" pain, nursing staff should be educated to inquire about pain levels at the same time that blood pressure, pulse, and respiratory rate are assessed. This assessment of pain intensity should then be recorded along with other vital signs in such a way that the clinician can quickly evaluate the adequacy of current analgesic therapy. Pain levels should also be assessed immediately before and after analgesic therapy is administered. In our institution, for example, a pain score of 3 of 10 is considered to be an unacceptably high level of pain. Should a patient report this (or a higher) amount of pain, the nurse offers an analgesic intervention. After the administration of pain medication, the nurse asks the patient to rate the pain once more. Both preanalgesic and postanalgesic pain scores are then recorded in the patient's chart. If the analgesic agents ordered in the chart fail to adequately relieve the patient's pain, the physician is notified.

Patients, as well as nurses and physicians, must be educated regarding the value of adequate analgesia. Patients may tend to underreport their pain experience to hospital staff. Some reasons for this are fear of addiction to narcotic agents, fear of side effects associated with pain medication, and the expectation that surgery is necessarily accompanied by pain. It is therefore important to emphasize to the patient that adequate analgesia will actually aid in the recovery process.

TREATMENT OF SURGICALLY INDUCED PAIN

Accurately diagnosing the source of pain is important. Sources of surgically induced pain include incisional pain, localized muscle spasm, pain resulting from inappropriate positioning during surgery, and deep (visceral) pain.[92]

Incisional pain is typically sharp and well localized. It results from the release of algogenic agents, as well as from the recruitment of the sympathetic nervous system. Incisional pain is responsive to narcotic agents, NSAIDs, and local anesthetic blockade.

Localized muscle spasms are the involuntary muscular contractions that occur in response to tissue injury. In teleological terms, this response tends to reduce continued nociception through reduction of noxious stimulus. For example, in the patient with multiple rib fractures, contraction of the chest wall musculature serves to provide a form of stabilization to the ribs. These muscular spasms are commonly contributory to nociception seen in intrathoracic and intra-abdominal surgery. When frank spasms occur, these spasmodic, uncontrolled muscular contractions may become so intense as to overshadow the incisional nociception and may be refractory to narcotic therapy. Muscle spasms also prevent the patient from effectively coughing, turning, clearing secretions, and ambulating, thereby increasing the risk of postoperative pulmonary complications and deep venous thrombosis. Therapy must be directed toward breaking the spasm-pain-spasm cycle. This may be accomplished by combining muscular relaxants with opioid therapy.

Patient positioning during the operation and in the immediate postoperative period may tend to aggravate muscle spasm pain. This can usually be overcome by repositioning the patient or massaging the affected muscle group. Poor intraoperative positioning during prolonged procedures may result in some element of ischemia to the skin and underlying soft tissues, which are compressed against bone. This type of pain generally resolves with gentle decompression and repositioning of the patient. Of greater concern are neural deficits associated with improper positioning. This type of deficit may be caused by localized pressure on nerves as they pass between bone and hard surfaces or may result from incorrect positioning of the extremities, which places a stretch on delicate neural tissue. It is best to prevent this type of injury with proper positioning, rather than attempting to treat it after the fact. If such an injury occurs, however, the affected limb should be protected from further injury and sensory and motor deficits should be carefully documented. Neuritic pain is poorly responsive to opioid agents and may necessitate treatment with tricyclic antidepressant agents or anticonvulsants. Prior to institution of therapy, a neurologic consultation should be obtained.

The visceral pain that occurs after an operation is markedly different from the somatic pain associated with incisional and musculoskeletal pain. Visceral pain is usually ill defined spatially and characterized by an "achy, burning, or crampy" quality. It may radiate or be referred to another part of the body entirely (as with infrascapular pain resulting from diaphragmatic irritation or left arm pain associated with myocardial infarction); it therefore may be diagnosed and treated incorrectly. Visceral pain is commonly encountered after abdominal or thoracic surgery because of widespread peritoneal irritation and the poorly defined and nonsegmental nature of innervation of the peritonealized structures and the pleura. Visceral pain may also result from distention of a hollow viscus, such as the bowel or the bladder. This type of pain may be treated with decompression (nasogastric tube or Foley catheter) or with opioids.

As discussed previously, when assessing postoperative pain, one must question the patient regarding the location, quality, and severity of the pain. Other important issues to evaluate include the patient's level of consciousness and responses to drug therapy. For example, a patient who has been receiving long-term opioid therapy prior to surgery will require a higher dosage of opioids to obtain analgesia than will the narcotic-naive patient. It is also important to assess the patient's need to ambulate or perform physical therapy, especially when considering the use of regional techniques for pain control.

SIMPLE TREATMENT STRATEGIES

Postoperative pain has traditionally been treated with intramuscular opioids administered on an as-needed basis. The "conventional" postoperative pain medication order has been "meperidine (Demerol) 50 to 100 mg intramuscularly every 3 to 4 hours as needed." Prescribing pain medication in this manner, without regard to surgical site (e.g., open cholecystectomy vs simple appendectomy) or patient characteristics (age, history of narcotic use, weight), hedges every pharmacologic bet imaginable. Dosage as well as dosing interval are left up to nursing personnel to determine. The amount of pain medication that the patient actually receives is therefore based on the nurse's perception of the patient's need.

Nurses did not traditionally assess patients' pain intensity as part of routine vital signs. Rather, they were instructed to wait until the patient requested pain medication to administer opioids. This system results in a variable delay after the patient's request for medication, during which plasma opioid levels decline and the patient feels unnecessary levels of pain. To illustrate, consider the following scenario. The patient reports pain. The nurse must then locate the patient's chart, determine the pain medication ordered and the length of time since the last medication was received, locate the key to the narcotic cabinet, draw up the medication, and, finally, administer the ordered opioid medication. By the time that the dosage administered has been absorbed, it is unlikely that the patient will have adequate pain relief, because by this time the pain has likely escalated beyond the level that would be expected to respond to the dosage of opioid ordered. In addition, the dosages that nurses actually administer have traditionally been at the lower end of the suggested dosing range, probably as a result of documentable fears of overdosage and iatrogenic addiction.[93,95]

This method of "as needed, depot therapy" has persisted despite the information that was introduced almost 15 years ago—namely, that there exists a threshold in drug concentration below which little analgesia is produced, the *minimum effective analgesic concentration* (MEAC).[96] Analgesia is achieved when the plasma opioid concentration reaches a particular level, the MEAC, which depends on the individual patient. Increases in plasma concentration above the MEAC result in no increase in analgesic effect but may result in a greater incidence of unwanted side effects. Small decreases in plasma concentration below the MEAC result in rapid decline in analgesia. With traditional "as needed" therapy, the patient's plasma level of opioid must drop below the MEAC before the patient requests intervention. As illustrated in the scenario, by the time the medication administered has been absorbed, achievement of the MEAC is highly unlikely.

To be most effective, opioid medications should be administered before the patient feels severe pain, in dosages sufficient to achieve the MEAC, and by a route that is rapidly and predictably absorbed. A simple strategy for obtaining and maintaining pain relief is to achieve analgesia by perioperative front-loading with narcotic agent followed by maintenance of plasma levels either orally or through intermittent intramuscular or subcutaneous deposition of analgesic medication. The depot drugs will be slowly absorbed, and if the repeated injections are properly timed, their absorption should approximate the clearance of the drug from the bloodstream and leave minimal variances in blood analgesic level. Two principles must be followed when using this treatment strategy. First, do not begin therapy until analgesia has been achieved by intravenous front-loading. Second, do not begin maintenance therapy until circulatory physiology is normal at the depot site.

Suggested doses for commonly used narcotic agents are listed in Tables 10-4 and 10-5. Doses should be reduced in patients who are at the extremes of age, have significant impairment of renal or hepatic function, or display significant cardiovascular or pulmonary dysfunction. It is extremely important when front-loading narcotics to titrate to the desired effect. Titration of small doses of narcotic, combined with careful assessment of level of sedation, respiratory pattern and rate, and amount of pain relief obtained, allows accurate calculation of the dosage required for pain control, thereby minimizing the risk of serious side effects (Tables 10-4 and 10-5).[79,97]

Meperidine is not recommended for patients with impaired renal function because its metabolite, normeperidine, may accumulate. Accumulation of this active metabolite may result in agitation, myoclonic jerks, and frank seizure activity. Even in patients with normal renal function, it is best to keep the meperidine dosage below 1 g in a 24-hour period.

Table 10-4. Guidelines for Front-Loading Intravenous Analgesics

Drug	Front Load (mg/kg)	Incremental Dose
Morphine	0.08-0.15	0.03 mg/kg every 10 minutes
Meperidine (Demerol)	1.0-2.0	0.30 mg/kg every 10 minutes
Hydromorphone (Dilaudid)	0.02	2550 μg/kg every 10 minutes

Adapted from Stevens DS, Edwards WT. Management of pain in intensive care settings. Anesth Clin North Am 10:408, 1992.

Table 10-5. Suggested Maintenance Dosages of Systemic Opioids

Drug	Route	Maintenance Dose (mg/kg)	Frequency (hours)
Morphine	SC/IM	0.1-0.2	3-4
Meperidine	IV	0.01-0.04/hr	Continuous
(Demerol)	SC/IM	1.0-1.5	3-4
Hydromorphone	IV	0.3-0.6/hr	Continuous
(Dilaudid)	SC/IM	0.03-0.06	3
	IV	0.01/hr	Continuous

Adapted from Ready LB, Edwards WT, eds. Management of Acute Pain: A Practical Guide. Seattle: IASP Publications, 1992.
SC, Subcutaneous; *IM,* intramuscular; *IV,* intravenous.

Continuous Infusion Therapy

Continuous infusion of opioid is another relatively simple technique. It may be preferable to intermittent intramuscular or subcutaneous dosing, especially in the patient requiring intensive postoperative care. After front-loading, a therapeutic blood level of opioid can be maintained by continuous infusion. The rate of infusion can be determined with a fairly simple calculation.[92] Because most opioid drugs have an elimination half-life of 3 hours, the dosage required every 3 hours to maintain the level of analgesia achieved during front-loading is half the dose required during the front-loading to produce that level of analgesia. For example, a patient requires 6 mg intravenous morphine to obtain analgesia after repair of a ventral hernia. A continuous infusion is to be used: 6 mg/2, or 3 mg, is eliminated every 3 hours, meaning that 3 mg/3 hr, or 1 mg/hr, is required. This approximation tends to underestimate the hourly requirement somewhat, because the elimination half-life is actually less than 3 hours.

Patient-Controlled Analgesia Therapy

Continuous intravenous infusions improve control of postoperative pain by eliminating wide fluctuations in opioid concentrations, but they respond poorly to rapid changes in nociceptive input. For example, the natural history of postoperative pain is that of progressive remission. As pain levels decline, frequent adjustment in infusion rate is required to prevent respiratory depression. It is also reasonable to expect that the amount of postoperative pain will fluctuate with activity levels in the immediate postoperative period. To address these issues, patient-controlled analgesia (PCA) therapy has been developed. In this technique, small doses of opioid medication are administered on a demand basis.

PCA therapy requires administration of analgesic agent on immediate patient demand in plentiful quantities. It does not necessarily require the presence of a sophisticated infusion device for this administration, but in most instances this type of pump is used. The remainder of this discussion centers on traditional intravenous PCA therapy with a microprocessor-driven infusion pump.[98]

Currently available PCA infusion pumps allow the physician to determine the type and dosage of opioid to be administered (demand dose), as well as the "lockout interval," or absolute period between patient demands during which the infusion pump will not administer analgesics. Many pumps also allow the physician to set an absolute 1- or 4-hour limit on the total amount of analgesic administered during that period. A background, constant-rate infusion can also be used to supplement patient demand (constant rate infusion plus demand dosing).

When establishing an upper limit for PCA it is best to take into account as much as a fivefold increase in need during the early postoperative period.[99,100] Therefore, if one predicts on the basis of intravenous front-loading that 1 mg/hr should be infused to maintain the MEAC for morphine in a particular patient, the 1-hour limit should be set at 5 mg/hr. Intermittent (demand) doses should generally not exceed 0.03 mg/kg morphine (or its equivalent), or 2 mg morphine per dose in most adult patients. Lockout intervals of 5 to 10 minutes are the norm; they are used to take into account the time required for a new concentration to be established at the active site before another dose can be given.[97]

Overdose is a low-risk problem with PCA therapy because patients tend to titrate the concentration into the therapeutic range and out of the toxic range. A negative-feedback loop is incorporated into this type of therapy; if the demand dosage is overestimated, the patient becomes sleepy and does not request additional medication, allowing the serum level of analgesic to decline. If a continuous, background infusion is added to demand therapy, the risk of overdose increases because accumulation may occur if the background infusion rate is set too high.

Lack of adequate analgesia with PCA can result from an inadequate demand dose, poor patient understanding of the technique, equipment malfunction, or programming errors. Overdose can also occur because of equipment malfunction, programming error, or administration of medication by someone other than the patient. Effective PCA therapy requires that patients be awake, cooperative, and able to dose themselves on demand. Unconscious, drowsy, uncooperative, or cognitively impaired patients make poor subjects for this type of pain management.[97]

Other, more complicated methods of pain control include neuraxial narcotics, continuous epidural infusion, and multiple methods of regional anesthetic blockade of the extremities. These types of therapy can be useful for selected patients but should be managed by physicians specializing in the management of postoperative pain and are therefore not discussed here.

SUMMARY

Because of the complexity of the nociceptive process, it may be negatively affected at a variety of levels, with resultant analgesia. A brief overview of the physiologic processes involved in nociception was presented here. Effective pain management requires an understanding of these physiologic processes, combined with frequent assessments of pain severity followed by prompt intervention. A simple approach to the management of postoperative pain was discussed here. Patients requiring more technically advanced methods of pain control may best be served by referral to a physician specializing in the management of postoperative pain.

REFERENCES

1. Munson ES, et al. Etidocaine, bupivacaine, and lidocaine seizure thresholds in monkeys. Anesthesiology 42:471, 1975.
2. Carpenter RL, McKey DC. Local anesthetics. In Barash PG, Cullen BF, Stoelting, RK, eds. Clinical Anesthesia, Philadelphia: JB Lippincott, 1992, p 509.
3. Halsey MJ. Mechanisms of general anesthesia. In Eger EI 2nd, ed. Anesthetic Uptake and Action, Baltimore: Williams & Wilkins, 1974.
4. Halsey MJ, Wardley-Smith B, Green CJ. Pressure reversal of general anesthesia: a multi-site expansion hypothesis. Br J Anaesth 50:1091, 1978.
5. Eger EI 2nd, Saidman LJ. Hazards of nitrous oxide anesthesia in bowel obstruction and pneumothorax. Anesthesiology 26:61, 1965.
6. Mallampati SR, et al. A clinical sign to predict difficult tracheal intubation: A prospective study. Can Anaesth Soc J 32:429, 1985.
7. Brodrick PM, Webster NR, Nunn JF. The laryngeal mask airway: A study of 100 patients during spontaneous breathing. Anaesthesia 44:238, 1989.
8. Maltby JR, Loren RG, Watson NC. The laryngeal mask airway: Clinical appraisal in 250 patients. Can J Anaesth 37:509, 1990.
9. Griffin RM, Hatcher JS. Aspiration pneumonia and the laryngeal mask airway. Anaesthesia 45:1039, 1990.
10. Goldman ME, et al. Intraoperative contrast two dimensional echocardiography to assess mitral valve operations. J Am Coll Cardiol 4:1035, 1984.
11. Cucchiara RF, et al. Air embolism in upright neurosurgical patients: detection and localization by two dimensional transesophageal echocardiography. Anesthesiology 60:353, 1984.
12. Duncan PG, Cohen MM. Pulse oximetry and capnography in anesthetic practice: An epidemiological appraisal. Can J Anaesth 38:5, 1991.
13. Trunkey DD. Resuscitation of the trauma victim. Surg Profiles Feb, 1982.
14. Sauderi PE, McLeskey CH, Comer PB. Emergency percutaneous transtracheal ventilation during anesthesia using readily available equipment. Anesth Analg 61:867, 1982.
15. Burtner DD, Goodman M. Anesthetic and operative management of potential upper airway obstruction. Arch Otolaryngol 104:657, 1978.
16. Hoffman EJ, Warren EW. Flumazenil: A benzodiazepine antagonist. Clin Pharm 12:9, 1993.
17. Bogetz MS, Katz JA. Recall of surgery in victims of major trauma: Effect of anesthetic dose. Anesthesiology 57:A331, 1982.
18. Sykes LA, Bowe EA. Cardiorespiratory Effects of Anesthesia. Clin Chest Med 14:2, 1993.
19. Stanley TH, Webster CR. Anesthetic requirements and cardiovascular effects of fentanyl-oxygen and fentanyl-diazepam-oxygen anesthesia in man. Anesth Analg 57:411, 1978.
20. Bovill JG, Sebel PS. Pharmacokinetics of high-dose fentanyl: A study in patients undergoing cardiac surgery. Br J Anaesth 52:795, 1980.
21. Stoops CM, et al. Hemodynamic effects of doxacurium chloride in patients receiving oxygen sufentanil anesthesia for coronary artery bypass grafting or valve replacement. Anesthesiology 69:365, 1988.
22. Wierda JM, et al. Pharmacokinetics and cardiovascular dynamics of pipecuronium bromide during coronary artery surgery. Can J Anaesth 37:183, 1990.
23. Pearce AC, Jones RM. Smoking and anesthesia: Preoperative abstinence and perioperative morbidity. Anesthesiology 61:576, 1984.
24. Warner MA, Tinker JH, Divertie MB. Preoperative cessation of smoking and pulmonary complications in pulmonary dysfunction. Anesthesiology 59:A60, 1983.
25. Hensley MJ, Fencl V. Lungs and respiration. In Vandam LD. To Make the Patient Ready for Anesthesia: Medical Care of the Surgical Patient. Menlo Park, Calif.: Addison-Wesley, 1980.
26. Nunn JF. Effects of anaesthesia on respiration. Br J Anaesth 65:54, 1990.
27. Egbert LD, Laver MB, Bendixen HH. The effect of site of operation and type of anesthesia upon the ability to cough in the postoperative period. Surg Gynecol Obstet 115:295, 1962.

28. Tarhan S, et al. Risk of anesthesia and surgery in patients with chronic bronchitis and chronic obstructive pulmonary disease. Surgery 74:720, 1973.
29. Diament ML, Palmer KNV. Postoperative changes in gas tensions of arterial blood and in ventilatory function. Lancet 2:180, 1966.
30. Gelman S. General Anesthesia and hepatic circulation. Can J Physiol Pharmacol 65:1762, 1987.
31. Aranha GV, Greenlee HB. Intraabdominal surgery in patients with advanced cirrhosis. Arch Surg 121:275, 1986.
32. Powell-Jackson P, Greenway B, Williams R. Adverse effects of exploratory laparotomy in patients with suspected liver disease. Br J Surg 69:449, 1982.
33. Gelman S. Disturbances in hepatic blood flow during anesthesia and surgery. Arch Surg 111:881, 1976.
34. French AB, et al. Metabolic effects of anesthesia in man. A comparison of the effects of ether and cyclopropane anesthesia on the abnormal liver. Ann Surg 135:145, 1952.
35. Eger EI. New inhaled anesthetics. Anesthesiology 80:906, 1994.
36. Davidson MB. The case for control in diabetes mellitus. West J Med 129:193, 1978.
37. Crawley BE, Seager R. Monitoring of blood sugar during surgery. Anaesthesia 25:73, 1970.
38. Hirsch IB, McGill JB. Role of insulin in management of surgical patients with diabetes mellitus. Diabetes Care 13:980, 1990.
39. Green NM. Insulin and anesthesia. Anesthesiology 41:75, 1974.
40. Byrick RJ, Rose DK. Pathophysiology and prevention of acute renal failure: The role of the anesthetist. Can J Anaesth 37:457, 1990.
41. Tapia HR, et al. Causes of death after renal transplantation. Arch Intern Med 131:204, 1973.
42. Gregory GA. Pediatric anesthesia. In Miller RD, ed. Anesthesia. New York: Churchill Livingstone, 1981.
43. Linderkamp O, et al. Estimation and prediction of blood volume in infants and children. Eur J Pediatr 125:227, 1977.
44. Lister G, Hoffman JIE, Rudolph AM. Oxygen uptake in infants and children: A simple method for measurement. Pediatrics 53:656, 1974.
45. Edelman CM Jr, et al. Renal bicarbonate reabsorption and hydrogen ion excretion in normal infants. J Clin Invest 46:1309, 1967.
46. Sinclair JC. Heat production and thermoregulation in small infants. Pediatr Clin North Am 17:147, 1970.
47. Silverman WA, Sinclair JC. Temperature regulation in the newborn. N Engl J Med 274:92, 1966.
48. Donegan JH. Cardiopulmonary resuscitation. In Miller RD, Anesthesia. New York: Churchill Livingstone, 1994, p 2537.
49. Lenaghan R, Silva YJ, Walt AJ. Hemodynamic alterations associated with expansion rupture of the lung. Arch Surg 99:339, 1969.
50. Goron RA, Britt BA, Kalow W. International Symposium on Malignant Hyperthermia. Springfield, Ill.: Charles C Thomas, 1973.
51. Ellis FR, Halball PJ. Suxemethonium spasm: A differential diagnosis conundrum. Br J Anaesth 567:381, 1984.
52. Isaacs H, Barlow MB. Malignant hyperpyrexia: Further muscle studies in asymptomatic carriers identified by creatinine phosphokinase screening. J Neurol Neurosurg Psychiatry 36:228, 1973.
53. Harrison GG. A pharmacological in vitro model of hyperpyrexia. S Afr Med J 47:774, 1973.
54. Butler BD, Hills BA. The lung as a filter for microbubbles. J Appl Physiol 47:537, 1978.
55. Amussat JZ. Recherches sur l'Introduction Accidentelle de l'Air dans les Veins. Paris: Germer Bailliere, 1839.
56. Lembke W. Ueber erfolgreiche Behandlung einer schweren Luftembolie durch Herzkammerpunktion. Chirurg 17-18:31, 1946.
57. Ordivay CG. Air embolus via CVP catheter without positive pressure: Presentation of a case and review. Ann Surg 179:479, 1974.
58. Goldstein G. Serum potassium levels and anesthesia. Curr Rev Clin Anesth 1(21):169, 1981.
59. Gronert G, Theye RA. Pathophysiology of hyperkalemia induced by succinylcholine. Anesthesiology 43:89, 1975.
60. Cunningham AA, Brull SJ. Laparoscopic cholecystectomy: anesthetic implications. Anesth Analg 76:1120, 1993.
61. Taylor E, et al. Anesthesia for laparoscopic cholecystectomy: Is nitrous oxide contraindicated? Anesthesiology 76:541, 1992.
62. Edelman DS. Laparoscopic cholecystectomy under continuous epidural anesthesia in a patient with cystic fibrosis. Am J Dis Child 145:723, 1991.
63. Frazee RC, et al. Open versus laparoscopic cholecystectomy: A comparison of postoperative pulmonary function. Ann Surg 213:651, 1991.
64. Greeville AC, et al. Pulmonary air embolism during laparoscopic laser cholecystectomy. Anaesthesia 46:113, 1991.
65. Tan PL, Lee TL, Tweed WA. Carbon dioxide absorption and gas exchange during pelvic laparoscopy. Can J Anaesth 39:677, 1992.
66. Joris JL, et al. Hemodynamic changes during laparoscopic cholecystectomy. Anesth Analg 76:1067, 1993.
67. Neuman GG, et al. Laparoscopy explosion hazards with nitrous oxide. Anesthesiology 18:875, 1993.
68. Beebe DS, et al. High levels of carbon monoxide are produced by electro-cantery during laparoscopic cholecystectomy. Anesth Analg 77:338, 1993.
69. Sebel PS, Lowdon JD. Propofol: A new intravenous anesthetic. Anesthesiology 71:260, 1989.
70. Basta SJ. Clinical pharmacology of mivacurium chloride: A review. J Clin Anesth 4:153, 1992.
71. Wierda JMKH, et al. Clinical observations on the neuromuscular blocking action of ORG 9426, a new steroidal non-depolarizing agent. Br J Anaesth 64:521, 1990.
72. Ghouri AF, Ruiz MAR, White PF. Effect of flumazenil or recovery after midazolam and propofol sedation. Anesthesiology 81:333, 1994.
73. Chaffee BJ, Tankanow RM. Ondansetron—The first of a new class of antiemetic agents. Clin Pharm 10:430, 1991.
74. Russell D, Kenny GNC. 5-Ht_3 antagonists in postoperative nausea and vomiting. Br J Anaesth 69:635, 1992.
75. Jelicic M, Bonke B. Auditory perception during general anesthesia. South Med J 82:1220, 1989.
76. Breckenridge JL, Aitkenhead AR. Awareness during anesthesia: A review. Ann R Coll Surg 65:93, 1983.
77. Mummaneni N, Rao TLK, Martoya A. Awareness and recall with high-dose fentanyl-oxygen anesthesia. Anesth Analg 59:948, 1980.
78. Oden RV: Acute postoperative pain: Incidence, severity, and the etiology of inadequate treatment. Anesth Clin North Am 7:1, 1989.
79. Ready LB, Edwards WT, eds. Management of acute pain: A practical guide. In Task Force on Acute Pain. Seattle: IASP Publications, 1992.
80. Katz N, Ferrante FM. Nociceptin. In Ferrante FM, VadeBoncouer TR, eds. Postoperative Pain Management. New York: Churchill Livingstone, 1993, p 17.
81. Price DD, Dubner R. Neurons that subserve the sensory-discriminative aspects of pain. Pain 3:307, 1977.
82. Sorkin LS. Pain pathways and spinal modulation. Anesth Clin North Am 7:17, 1989.
83. Sosnowski M. Receptors, neuropathways, and mechanisms. Anesth Clin North Am 10:211, 1992.
84. Rexed B. The cytoarchitectonic organization of the spinal cord in the cat. J Comp Neurol 96:415, 1952.
85. Ferrante FM, VadeBoncouer TR. Epidural analgesia with combinations of local anesthetics and opioids. In Ferrante FM, VadeBoncouer TR, eds. Postoperative Pain Management. New York: Churchill Livingstone, 1993, p 305.
86. Pasternak GW. Multiple morphine and enkephalin receptors and the relief of pain. JAMA 259:1362, 1988.
87. Sabbe MB, Yaksh TL. Pharmacology of spinal opioids. J Pain Symptom Manage 5:191, 1990.

88. Melzack R, Wall PD. Pain mechanisms: A new theory science. Pain 150:971, 1965.
89. Panos L, Panos A. Regional and local block of acute pain. Anesth Clin North Am 10:339, 1992.
90. Etches R. Complications of acute pain management. Anesth Clin North Am 10:417, 1992.
91. Badner N. Epidural agents for postoperative analgesia. Anesth Clin North Am 10:321, 1992.
92. Edwards WT, Breed RJ. The treatment of acute postoperative pain in the postanesthesia care unit. Anesth Clin North Am 8:235, 1990.
93. Edwards WT. Optimizing opioid treatment of postoperative pain. J Pain Symptom Manage 5:S24, 1990.
94. Jamison RN. Clinical measurement of pain. In Ferrante FM, VadeBoncouer TR, eds. Postoperative Pain Management. New York: Churchill Livingstone, 1993, p 119.
95. Chapman PJ, et al. Attitudes and knowledge of nursing staff in relation to management of postoperative pain. Aust N Z J Surg 57:447, 1987.
96. Austin KL, Stapleton JV, Mather LE. Multiple intramuscular injections: A major source of variability in analgesic response to meperidien. Pain 8:47, 1980.
97. Stevens DS, Edwards WT. Management of pain in intensive care settings. Anesth Clin North Am 10:395, 1992.
98. Ferrante FM: Patient-controlled analgesia. Anesth Clin North Am 10:287, 1992.
99. Mather LE, Phillips GB. Opioids and adjuvants: Principles of use. In Cousins MJ, Phillips GD, eds. Acute Pain Management. New York: Churchill Livingstone, 1986, p 77.
100. White PF. Patient-controlled analgesia: A new approach to the management of postoperative pain. Semin Anesth 4:255, 1985.

11

Sepsis and the Syndrome of Multiple Organ Failure

Donald E. Fry

Infection is the process where active bacterial growth and proliferation in tissues result in activation of the host inflammatory response. Soft tissue infections of either surgical or traumatic wounds are characterized in descriptive terms of inflammation; hence rubor, color, dolor, and tumor. The inflammatory characteristics of the soft tissue infection are the same processes that can be identified with tissue injury or trauma from any source. A traumatic injury is a temporally short event; inflammation is activated but then progressively subsides. The difference between traumatic injury and soft tissue infection is that the inciting event in infection of bacterial proliferation is sustained over time.

Soft tissue infection is ultimately contained by inflammation in concert with other elements of nonspecific host defenses in most instances. However, there are events where the proliferation of bacteria may exceed local host defenses, and a systemic response to the infection is elicited. Although fever and leukocytosis are biologically appropriate systemic responses even to well-contained inflammatory events, progression of infection beyond a critical threshold provokes a systemic response that is associated with a poor outcome.

The infected host with systemic infection has marked tachycardia, tachypnea, palpitations, diaphoresis, and anxiety. Shock may ensue. When supported by current health care technology, the sustained systemic response then becomes identified with the progressive loss of critical organ system functions. Clinicians use the term *sepsis* to describe the physiologic response when infection passes beyond the threshold of local containment. Unfortunately, sepsis as a pathophysiologic event is equated to uncontrolled infection. Like local blunt tissue trauma, biologic insults that do not have microbes nor clinical infection can systemically activate the host response known as sepsis (e.g., severe acute pancreatitis).

The premise of the subsequent discussion is that "sepsis" is the activation of the normally salutary local inflammatory response, but with that activation being systemic in domain. Sepsis, the systemic inflammatory response syndrome, is commonly activated by microbes and clinical infection but can be activated by noninfectious, proinflammatory events. The mediator and effector systems of benefit in local inflammation are the same mediator and effector systems responsible for human sepsis, septic shock, and multiple organ failure.

DEFINITION OF SEPSIS

A clear clinical definition of sepsis has remained elusive. Because terms such as *sepsis, septicemia,* and *septic syndrome* have been indiscriminately used in clinical parlance and in the written literature, a consensus conference was convened to provide better definition to these terms. From this conference, the term *systemic inflammatory response syndrome (SIRS)* emerged.[1] The elements of SIRS are presented in the box on p. 275. SIRS represents the clinical events seen when the scope of inflammation has become systemically activated. *SIRS* is a nonspecific term and may be activated by any of a number of biologic stimuli. "Sepsis" specifically refers to the activation of SIRS by invasive infection.

SIRS can be activated by noninfectious events, such as fulminant acute pancreatitis or large thermal injuries. Thus when a patient fulfills the criteria of SIRS, a difficult dilemma emerges for the clinician in discerning whether infection or some other biologic stimulus is responsible for the syndrome.

Although the concept of SIRS has been useful in providing a conceptual framework for defining sepsis, it really has not been clinically practical. Virtually every child with otitis media and every adult with a severe upper respiratory tract infection fulfills the criteria of SIRS. The vast majority of patients in the intensive care unit have SIRS and may have evidence of invasive infection, but they are not at risk for eminent septic death. The definition of SIRS is far too inclusive to be clinically useful in the care of surgical patients.

A meaningful classification system has been developed for the septic patient that uses physiologic and biochemical changes of the septic state[2] (Fig. 11-1). State A is the physiologic response to stress that is seen in many surgical patients. The patients have a modestly elevated cardiac output and a modestly reduced systemic vascular resistance, but have a normal arteriovenous oxygen content difference. Systemic oxygen consumption is elevated commensurate with the increase in cardiac output. The patients are euglycemic or may have a mild "stress" hyperglycemia. Blood lactate concentrations are normal. The patients usually have a mild leukocytosis and mild fever. They have normal urine output and clear mentation. State A is the commonly seen physiologic state identified after multiple trauma or major surgical procedures.

State B represents the exaggerated stress response and is the true septic or systemic inflammatory response. Cardiac output is dramatically elevated as a direct response of the dramatic reduction in systemic vascular resistance. When maximal preload to the heart is achieved, arteriovenous oxygen differences are diminished and *reflect a peripheral de-*

DEFINITIONS FOR CRITICAL TERMINOLOGY USED IN THE DESCRIPTION AND MANAGEMENT OF PATIENTS WITH SEVERE INFECTION AND SUBSEQUENT CLINICAL SEQUELAE

Infection: Microbial phenomenon characterized by an inflammatory response to the presence of microorganisms or the invasion of normally sterile host tissue by those organisms

Bacteremia: The presence of viable bacteria in the blood

Systemic inflammatory response syndrome: The systemic inflammatory response to a variety of severe clinical insults. The response is manifested by two or more of the following conditions:

1. Temperature >38° C or <36° C
2. Heart rate >90 beats/min
3. Respiratory rate >20 breaths/min or $Paco_2$ <32 torr (<4.3 kPa)
4. White blood cell count >12,000 cells/mm^3, <4000 cells/mm^3, or >10% immature (band) forms

Sepsis: The systemic response to infection. This sytemic response is manifested by two or more of the following conditions as a result of infection:

1. Temperature >38° C or <36° C
2. Heart rate >90 beats/min
3. Respiratory rate >20 breaths/min or $Paco_2$ <32 torr (<4.3 kPa)
4. White blood cell count >12,000 cells/mm^3, <4000 cells/mm^3, or >10% immature (band) forms

Severe sepsis: Sepsis associated with organ dysfunction, hypoperfusion, or hypotension. Hypoperfusion and perfusion abnormalities may include, but are not limited to lactic acidosis, oliguria, or an acute alteration in mental status

Septic shock: Sepsis with hypotension, despite adequate fluid resuscitation, along with the presence of perfusion abnormalities that may include, but are not limited to, lactic acidosis, oliguria, or an acute alteration in mental status. Patients who receive inotropic or vasopressor agents may not be hypotensive at the time that perfusion abnormalities are measured

Hypotension: A systolic blood pressure of <90 mm Hg or a reduction of >40 mm Hg from baseline in the absence of other causes for hypotension

Multiple organ dysfunction syndrome: Presence of altered organ function in an acutely ill patient such that homeostasis cannot be maintained without intervention

From American College of Chest Physicians/Society of Critical Care Medicine Consensus Conference. Definition for sepsis and organ failure and guidelines for the use of innovative therapies in sepsis. Crit Care Med 20:864, 1992.

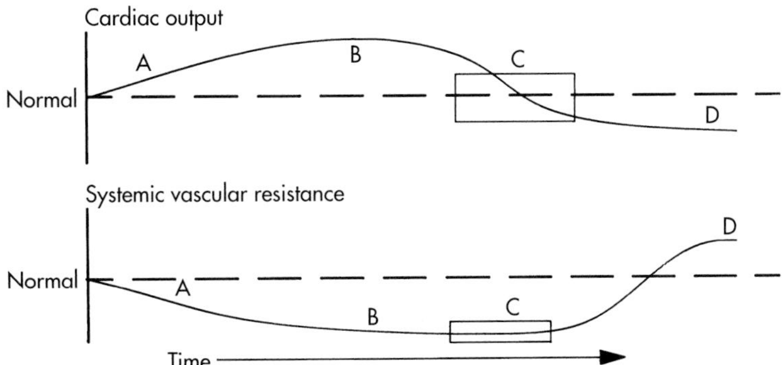

Fig. 11-1. Relationships of cardiac output with systemic vascular resistance in patients with each of the different states in human response to sepsis. Refer to text for more details.

fect in oxygen extraction. The patients have an elevated blood lactate concentration but do not have lactic acidemia. Fever and leukocytosis are present. Hyperglycemia is present in varying degrees, depending on nutritional support strategies and the patient's preseptic glucose tolerance. Confusion and lethargy are commonly seen. Urine output is usually normal and may even be inappropriately increased because of osmotic considerations (e.g., hyperglycemia) or the loss of the countercurrent concentrating mechanism of the kidney. State B is the physiologic condition of the patient with severe peritonitis, which has been managed with successful and appropriate expansion of the intravascular volume.

State C represents the disordered relationships between cardiac output and peripheral vascular resistance. The profound loss of systemic vascular resistance cannot be compensated by cardiac output, which leads to systemic hypotension and "septic shock." However, cardiac output is still considered "normal" or even elevated, which leads to the clinical interpretation that many of these patients are in "hot" shock. The loss of systemic perfusion pressure combined with the peripheral extraction defect for oxygen results in profound lactic acidemia and acidosis. Oxygen consumption is grossly inadequate. The patients are oliguric to anuric. Profound mental changes are seen, approaching coma for many patients.

State D represents the secondary evolution of cardiac failure on the fundamental septic process. The cardiac output is totally inadequate. Like patients with cardiac failure in other settings, patients in state D develop an increase in systemic vascular resistance in a physiologic attempt to preserve perfusion pressure. These patients have the appearance of "cold" shock, with cool and cyanotic extremities. The patients have severe lactic acidosis because of the defect of oxygen extraction, low cardiac output, and peripheral vasoconstriction. State D is a rapidly fatal condition, unless dramatic and aggressive support methods are rapidly and successfully implemented. It is still viewed by many knowledgeable clinicians as a preterminal state.

This classification methodology represents a convenient means to understand the natural history of the septic process. It must be emphasized that every patient who dies of sepsis does not proceed in an orderly fashion through each state. First, the presumption of the classification system is that the patient is receiving optimal therapy. A patient in state B who has an inadequate intravascular volume to support the elevated cardiac output and the increased vascular capacitance of the septic condition will lapse into systemic hypotension, which is inappropriate for the patient's actual physiologic circumstance. Patients may actually appear to pass from state A to state D with an acute septic event without adequate preload. Second, the classification system presumes normal cardiac reserve. Patients with underlying cardiac disease are not able to meet the demands of state B and commonly progress in rapid fashion from state A to state C or D because the impaired left ventricle cannot generate the cardiac output necessary to sustain blood pressure with the loss of afterload.

Thus sepsis is the systemic response of the host when infection activates the *SIRS*. The physiologic hallmark of sepsis is the loss of vascular resistance and the accompanying increase in vascular resistance. The seminal metabolic feature of sepsis is the peripheral defect in oxygen extraction that becomes most clearly recognized in the accumulation of lactate species in the blood of these patients well before any clinical evidence of hypotension is present. The rapid progression of the untreated septic state is septic shock and death. Vigorous clinical support of the septic host without eradication of the driving infectious focus may actually result in the sustained state B, where multiple organ failure emerges as the contemporary expression of sepsis in the intensive care unit.

SEPSIS AND MULTIPLE ORGAN FAILURE

Multiple organ failure (MOF) is now recognized as an associated event in patients with severe SIRS. MOF is the concurrent or sequential failure of critical organ functions that occurs in critically injured patients. More recently referred to as multiple-organ dysfunction syndrome (MODS),[1] the syndrome of MOF usually encompasses the failure of the lung, liver, kidney, and ultimately the heart. Gastrointestinal failure in the form of stress mucosal ulceration with or without clinical upper gastrointestinal bleeding is a well-recognized component of this syndrome. Metabolic failure can be identified where exogenous protein and caloric support does not downregulate the progessive proteolysis of muscle protein used to fuel hepatic gluconeogenesis.[3] Disseminated intravascular coagulation (i.e., coagulation failure) is also recognized as another feature of MOF in many patients.

The syndrome became conceptualized from numerous clinical observations. Skillman et al.[4] identified a temporal relationship between the emergence of pulmonary failure and stress gastrointestinal bleeding in septic patients. Tilney et al.[5] reported that following acutely successful surgical management of ruptured abdominal aortic aneurysms a number of patients developed sequential organ failure and late death. In a landmark editorial, Baue[6] really coined the term *multiple organ failure* and addressed the historical evolution and potential clinical causes of this new clinical entity. Eiseman et al.[7] reported on a series of patients with MOF and emphasized the common theme that invasive infection was an important feature. Polk and Shields[8] noted the reversal of organ failure syndromes when successful surgical interventions resulted in the drainage of abscess.

In an effort to define the frequency, clinical associations, and consequences of MOF, we studied a group of trauma and general surgical emergency patients.[9] Lung failure, hepatic failure, kidney failure, and gastrointestinal stress bleeding were the specific organ systems studied, and defined mortality rates for each failure complex were identified. The overall mortality for this group of patients was 10%, which underscored the significant outcome consequences when each of these organ functions failed.

A more significant observation was the number of organs that failed among these patients. Fig. 11-2 illustrates a nearly linear relationship between the number of involved organ systems and the probability of a fatal outcome. A prototypical sequence of organ failure was seen, with pulmonary failure occurring first in the sequence and renal failure occurring last. Our studies and those of others have confirmed the accumulative fatal consequences of each organ system involvement on patient outcome.

In an attempt to identify clinical associations with the development of the MOF syndrome, we examined numerous variables in these patients. Our initial evaluation showed that hemorrhagic shock, massive blood resuscitation, massive crystalloid resuscitation, multiple-system injury, and septicemia were statistically significant in association with patients who developed failure of two or more organ systems (Table 11-1). Since 34 of 38 patients with MOF met the criteria of "sepsis," we performed some sequential statistical analyses, which showed that when the septic group was deleted from the patient population, all other significant variables became insignificant. However, deletion of hemorrhagic shock, massive resuscitation, etc., sequentially did not change the statistical significance of sepsis. We concluded that uncontrolled infection was the strongest clinical association with the development of MOF. Shock, resuscitation, and severe injury appeared to have a statistical association in defining the patient population most likely to develop sepsis.

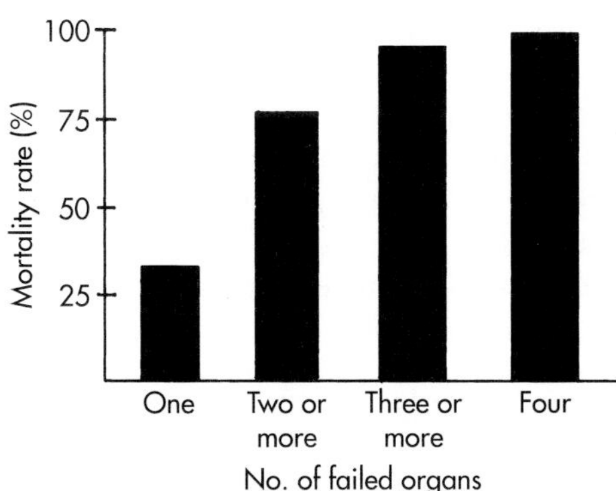

Fig. 11-2. Mortality rates of patients with organ failure syndromes. For those patients with multiple organ failure (two or more organ systems), the mortality rate is in excess of 70%.

It is now apparent that the patients who were interpreted as being septic because of infection were in fact patients with severe SIRS. The patients had clinical evidence of infection (e.g., fever and leukocytosis) but had the septic syndrome without necessarily having documented invasive infection. Severe SIRS, or the septic response, is the associated variable with the development of MOF and not only invasive infection. Furthermore, it was evident from these observations that patients with septic shock and MOF were really subpopulations of patients from the total SIRS patient population. Rapidly evolving SIRS became septic shock, while the more indolent SIRS patient usually under intense clinical management developed MOF. Sepsis, septic shock, and MOF all appeared to be part of the same clinical process.

MECHANISM OF SEPSIS AND MULTIPLE ORGAN FAILURE

The observation of patients with sepsis and MOF at a point in time when the patients have a developing lactic acidemia has clearly brought attention to defective oxidative metabolism as being a major and fundamental physiologic abnormality of the septic state. The patients characteristically have an increase in cardiac output, which reflects the fact that the abnormality of tissue oxygen utilization is in the periphery and that the issue of oxygen delivery because of poor cardiac performance is not of critical significance until the later stages of the disease process. Interest in defective oxygen utilization has lead numerous investigators to pursue this fundamental cause of organ failure.

Considerable early attention focused on potential septic-associated injury to the mitochondria of parenchymal tissues. Experimental investigation into the effects of endotoxin on liver mitochondria resulted in considerable interest in injury to oxidative phosphorylation as the fundamental mechanism of defective oxygen utilization.[10,11] However, our investigations identified that bacterial infection actually resulted in an increase in the efficiency of oxidative phosphorylation rather than an injury state.[12,13] Furthermore, measurement of tissue oxygen tensions identified the paradox of poor tissue oxygen delivery at a

Table 11-1. Statistical Associations of Several Key Variables With the Emergence of Multiple Organ Failure in the Series of 553 Emergency Surgical Patients

Variable	No. of Patients	Number With MOF	P =
Hypovolemic shock	67	16	<0.05
Massive blood therapy	32	9	<0.05
Massive crystalloid therapy	35	10	<0.05
Chest injury	113	14	<0.05
Head injury	75	8	N.S.*
Long bone fractures	96	5	N.S.*
Septicemia	123	34	<0.01

From Fry DE, et al. Multiple system organ failure: The role of uncontrolled infection. Arch Surg 115:136, 1980. Copyright 1980, American Medical Association.

**N.S.*, Not significant; P >0.05

point in time when the experimental animals had normal arterial blood pressures and normal arterial blood gases.[12] The observations of tissue hypoxia led to early efforts with indocyanine green to measure liver blood flow in animal models of peritonitis.[14,15]

The development of galactose elimination kinetics as a method to estimate liver blood flow clearly identifies that effective perfusion of the liver progressively diminishes during the septic state while cardiac output is at a normal or supranormal level of performance.[16] Microscopic examination of liver tissue from animals in the septic state identifies the sequestration of neutrophils within the hepatic sinusoids.[17] Subsequent to neutrophil sequestration, one can identify focal areas of hepatic necrosis that appear to represent either ischemic injury or injury relating to local proinflammatory events.

The sequestration of neutrophils within the microcirculation led to investigations that would explain neutrophil–endothelial cell interaction that resulted in this sequestration phenomena. The activation of the complement cascade and the release of complement cleavage products serve as chemotactic signals for neutrophils. Because septic patients have been shown to have activation of complement through the alternative pathway,[18] we and others have explored activation of complement as a critical initiator of neutrophil sequestration and tissue level inflammation. Like humans, rats with peritonitis demonstrated activation of the complement cascade.[19] Experimentally, the activation of the complement cascade with zymosan results in the same hepatic microcirculatory injury that can be identified in animal models of actual bacterial infection.[20] These studies clearly identify that systemic activation of the complement cascade may be a potent activator of the septic response.

Another important activator of neutrophils has been tumor necrosis factor (TNF). TNF has generated considerable interest as a major proinflammatory signal that may have prominent mechanistic significance in the septic patient. In our investigations with TNF in experimental animals, TNF recreated many of the septic parameters in the experimental animal.[21] TNF resulted in an increase in cardiac output and a reduction in systemic vascular resistance and evoked a progressive decline in effective hepatic blood flow. Since TNF was principally identified as a product of activated macrophages, these data clearly implicated the macrophage as being a potentially pivotal cell in the evolution of the septic response.

Considerable information has emerged in recent years about the complex interactions between the neutrophil and the endothelial cell. This margination event truly begins the process of microcirculatory injury and the inflammatory lesions that are identified in the viscera of patients with organ failure. Margination was initially thought to be a neutrophil-mediated event with enhanced "stickiness" of the neutrophil. Recent data now implicate the endothelial cell with a critical role in neutrophil margination with the microcirculation.[22] Proinflammatory signals such as cytokines and chemotactic factors result in upregulation of P-selectin and E-selectin as adhesion receptors on the endothelial cell surface. The binding of the endothelial cell selectins to counterreceptors on the neutrophil and the similar binding of the constitutively expressed L-selectin of the neutrophil with its counterreceptor on the endothelial cell initiate the "rolling" phenomena of the neutrophil on the endothelial surface.[23] This rolling, in effect, slows the neutrophil migration through the microcirculation, and then a firm bond is established by the activated or transformed neutrophil with a similar constitutively expressed matching molecule on the endothelial cell. The tight bonding is mediated through neutrophil integrins (CD11-CD18 receptors) and the intercellular adhesion molecules (ICAMs) of the endothelial cell.[24] Thus a complex biologic process pathologically marginates neutrophils to the endothelial cells, and the activated neutrophils then release potent cellular products that mediate tissue injury.

Reactive oxygen intermediates and potent lysosomal enzymes released by the neutrophil then mediate the intravascular injury and the similarly identified perivascular inflammatory injury of the tissues. Lipid peroxidation products reflect these severe tissue-based injuries and the ultimate thrombosis of the microcirculation, which leads to ischemic vascular units. Activation of platelets may lead to the local release of thromboxane A_2 as a potent microcirculatory vasoconstrictor and aggregator of platelets, which further compromises the effective perfusion of the hepatic microcirculatory units.[25] The areas of ischemia create the well-recognized focal areas of necrosis. Focal necrosis then becomes itself an activator of the inflammatory cascade. Thus even when the primary infectious clinical event that initiated the septic process is eliminated, the patient may actually reach a point where the self-energizing local processes continue the progressive loss of microcirculation and the progressive loss of physiologic reserve of the organ. This becomes expressed clinically as failure of the organ cell affected.

UNIFYING CONCEPT OF INFLAMMATION, SEPSIS, AND MULTIPLE ORGAN FAILURE

Sepsis and MOF are the consequences of the normal and salutary local inflammatory processes that are unleashed at a systemic level of organization. All the pathophysiologic events of the human septic response can be identified in the soft tissue wound. If we understand the inflammatory events of the wound, we can understand the systemic events of human sepsis.

When a wound is created, blood vessels are disrupted, blood extravasates from the intravascular compartment, endothelial cells are damaged, and collagen is exposed. The magnitude of the tissue injury may be minimal (e.g., surgical incision) or may be great (jagged traumatic wound). In either case the critical elements of the human inflammatory response are activated.

First, the *coagulation cascade* is activated to initiate hemostasis. Activation of Hageman factor becomes significant for the intrinsic pathway of coagulation and leads to the transformation of prothrombin to thrombin and ultimately to the cleaving of fibrinogen to fibrin. The precipitation of fibrin at the wound surface becomes the natural protective biologic dressing to prevent bacteria from the external environment gaining access to deeper tissue spaces.

However, activation of Hageman factor becomes a foundation event in early inflammation. Activated Hageman factor activates mast cells, which then release a vast array of preformed inflammatory enzymes. Mast cell stimulation also upregulates the synthesis of other mediator compounds as well. The *mast cell* becomes an important component of acute inflammation in that its secreted products promote the relaxation of vascular smooth muscle and changes in the endothelial cell cytoskeleton. These mast cell–mediated events cause vasodilation and increased capillary permeability in the soft tissues about the perimeter of the injured tissue. The result is soft tissue edema from the extravasation of protein-rich plasma.

Activated Hageman factor initiates another series of protein reactions known collectively as the contact activating system. Activated Hageman factor mediates the cleavage of prekallikrein to kallikrein. In addition to its own physiologic properties, kallikrein leads to the generation of bradykinin. Bradykinin is bound to endothelial cell receptors, which upregulate the induced production of nitric oxide. Vasodilation is further mediated via this mechanism.

Injured tissue and exogenous contaminants of the wound activate yet another component of early inflammation. Complement proteins are sequentially activated by a stepwise series of reactions. Cleavage proteins particularly from the C3 and C5 components of the complement cascade have important functions and are collectively known as anaphylatoxins. They are potent activators of endothelial cell responses, opsonic proteins, and chemotactic agents.

Finally, exposed collagen, precipitated fibrin, and injured endothelial cells become biologic signals to activate platelets. Although the role of the platelet is generally appreciated in hemostasis, the platelet releases numerous vasoactive and proinflammatory signals as it degranulates with activation. Platelet activation begets more platelet activation so that vasoactive prostaglandin compounds cause vasoconstriction at areas of endothelial injury and collagen exposure. Vasoconstrictive and vasodilatory influences of these many areas of inflammation are regulated by separate components of the early inflammatory response. Vasoconstrictive influences predominate at the injured endothelium, whereas vasodilating influences predominate about the perimeter.

The net result of these early events in inflammation is to create a local environment with tissue edema that is rich with chemostatic signals. Diffusion of chemostatic signals from the epicenter of injury into the microcirculation become chemical beacons to upregulate adhesive molecules on circulating neutrophils. Neutrophil–endothelial cell interaction results in initial margination at the site, and diapedesis of the neutrophil is begun, with the chemotactic gradient providing chemical direction for movement. Neutrophil infiltration of the injured areas occurs within 12 hours. Contact of the neutrophil with foreign proteins (e.g., bacteria) initiates the process of phagocytosis. The edematous tissue planes now become aqueous channels to permit neutrophil entry. Recognition of unwanted macromolecules in need of phagocytosis is facilitated by nonspecific opsonins from plasma and from activated proteins (e.g., complement).

Monocytes are mobilized into the area of injury by the same chemotactic signals and probably by similar interaction with endothelial cells. The larger monocyte cells navigate into the injury site more slowly and are usually identified histologically at 24 hours. The monocyte orchestrates the severity and progression of the local inflammatory response. Large amounts of bacteria, fibrin debris, and effete self (e.g., dead tissue) elicits a diverse cytokine response. Foremost among these cytokine products is TNF. TNF has a host of biologic effects but upregulation of neutrophil phagocytic activity is of paramount significance at this juncture. Under the influence of TNF, neutrophils are driven to aggressive phagocytosis of offending particles. Extracellular release of lysosomal enzymes and reactive oxygen intermediates provide for digestion of the dead tissue matrix. Excessive phagocytosis with potent digestive enzymes results in death of many neutrophils. The resultant environment of inflammatory enzymes, liquefaction of tissue, foreign proteins, and dead neutrophils is known commonly as pus. The focus of liquefaction becomes a sustained stimulus to the further activation of all elements of inflammation.

Monocytes produce other cytokines that have endocrine functions. Interleukin-1, interleukin-6, and interleukin-8 have overlapping and redundant functions. The results are hypothalamic stimulation and fever, mobilization of neutrophils both from the bone marrow and from marginated reserves, and hepatic stimulation to produce acute phase reactants. The net effects of these acute phase responses are more neutrophils to the area of injury and more opsonic proteins.

Eradication of the offending stimulus within the area of the wound then initiates downregulatory processes. When the pus is drained, the dead tissue is gone, and the transgressing microbes are vanquished. An as yet poorly defined downregulatory series of events results in transformation from proinflammation to prowound healing.

With SIRS, the processes are the same as in the wound. However, the five initiator events (coagulation activation, mast cell activation, complement activation, contact-activating system activation, and platelet activation) are provoked systemically instead of locally. The plasma becomes a "sea" of chemotactic factors, which activates endothelium, neutrophils, and macrophages systemically. Systemic inflammation becomes the consequence. If the process is rapid and fulminant, profound vasodilation results in septic shock. When the process is more indolent and supportive care is more effective, the central circulation is supported, but tissue-level inflammation leads to ischemia and tissue destruction (Fig. 11-3).

Currently, the management of sepsis, septic shock, and MOF constitutes supportive care and attempts to treat infection. MOF and sepsis reach a critical biologic point where the disease is uncontrolled inflammation, and irradication of the original infectious event will still not likely reverse the process.

Attempts are now being made to control "run-a-way" inflammation. Antiendotoxin antibodies, anticytokine antibodies and receptor blockade, antiprostaglandin compounds, and antioxidants are but a few of the attempted strategies. All have failed because they compromise normal host responses. However, the wound holds the secrets for the treatment of sepsis and MOF in the same way that it illustrates the pathophysiology of the disease. The next generation of treatments for sepsis and MOF will hopefully focus on those natural mediator and effector systems that downregulate inflammation just as it is downregulated in the soft tissue wound.

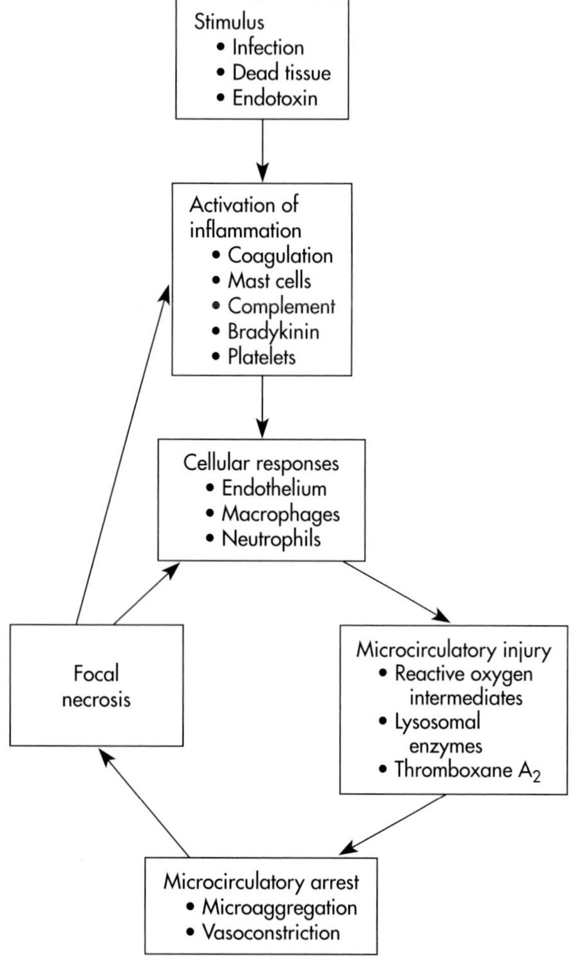

Fig. 11-3. Process of systemic inflammation, which leads to tissue injury. The critical point for emphasis is that tissue inflammation leads to tissue-level necrosis, which then becomes an inciting event to restimulate the entire process.

SUMMARY

MOF is a common cause of death in severely injured and critically ill patients. The emergence of this syndrome is strongly associated with the septic response, which is usually secondary to bacteria or bacterial cell products. This process may be activated from invasive infection or from dissemination of bacteria or bacterial cell products from areas normally contained from the host and host response, such as the gastrointestinal tract. The mechanism(s) underlying this systemic septic response remains uncertain, but activation of a variety of mediators and effectors that result in defective oxygen and substrate utilization in peripheral tissues appears to play a major role. Although much has been learned in the last decade regarding the pathogenesis of MOF and has positively impacted the management of the condition, identification of the specific mediators and effectors responsible for the defective utilization of oxygen and substrate will be important to lessen the lethality associated with this disorder.

REFERENCES

1. American College of Chest Physicians/Society of Critical Care Medicine Consensus Conference. Definition for sepsis and organ failure and guidelines for the use of innovative therapies in sepsis. Crit Care Med 20:864, 1992.
2. Siegel JH, et al. Physiologic and metabolic correlations in human sepsis. Surgery 86:163, 1979.
3. Cerra FB, et al. Septic autocannibalism: A failure of exogenous nutritional support. Ann Surg 192:570, 1980.
4. Skillman JJ, et al. Respiratory failure, hypotension, sepsis, and jaundice. Am J Surg 117:523, 1969.
5. Tilney NL, Bailey GL, Morgan AP. Sequential system failure after rupture of abdominal aortic aneurysms: An unsolved problem in postoperative care. Ann Surg 178:117, 1973.
6. Baue AE. Multiple, progressive, or sequential systems failure. Arch Surg 110:79, 1975.
7. Eiseman B, Beart R, Norton L. Multiple organ failure. Surg Gynecol Obstet 144:323, 1977.
8. Polk HC Jr, Shields CL. Remote organ failure: A valid sign of occult intraabdominal infection. Surgery 81:310, 1977.
9. Fry DE, et al. Multiple system organ failure: The role of uncontrolled infection. Arch Surg 115:136, 1980.
10. Schumer W, et al. Effect of endotoxemia on liver cell mitochondria in man. Ann Surg 171:875, 1970.
11. Mela L, Bacalzo LV, Miller LD. Defective oxidative metabolism of rat liver mitochondria in hemorrhage and endotoxin shock. Am J Physiol 220:571, 1971.
12. Fry DE, et al. Hepatic cellular hypoxia in murine peritonitis. Surgery 85:652, 1979.
13. Fry DE, et al. Alterations of oxygen metabolism in experimental bacteremia. Adv Shock Res 6:45, 1981.
14. Garrison RN, Ratcliffe DJ, Fry DE. Hepatocellular function and nutrient blood flow in experimental peritonitis. Surgery 92:713, 1982.
15. Asher EF, et al. Endotoxin, cellular function and nutrient blood flow. Arch Surg 118:441, 1983.
16. Schirmer WJ, et al. Galactose elimination kinetics in sepsis: Correlation of liver blood flow with function. Arch Surg 122:349, 1987.
17. Asher EF, et al. Experimental bacteremia and nutrient hepatic blood flow. Circ Shock 20:43, 1986.
18. Fearon DT, et al. Activation of the properdin pathway of complement in patients with gram-negative bacteremia. N Engl J Med 292:937, 1975.

19. Schirmer WJ, et al. Complement activation in peritonitis: Association with hepatic and renal perfusion abnormalities. Am Surg 53:683, 1987.
20. Schirmer WJ, et al. Systemic complement activation produces hemodynamic changes characteristic of sepsis. Arch Surg 123:316, 1988.
21. Schirmer WJ, Schirmer JM, Fry DE. Recombinant human tumor necrosis factor produces hemodynamic changes characteristic of sepsis and endotoxemia. Arch Surg 124:445, 1989.
22. Bevilacqua MP, Nelson RM. Selectins. J Clin Invest 91:379, 1993.
23. Lawrence MB, Springer TA. Leukocytes roll on a selectin at physiologic flow rates: Distinction from and prerequisite for adhesion through integrins. Cell 65:859, 1991.
24. Hynes RO. Integrins: Versatility, modulation, and signaling in cell adhesion. Cell 69:11, 1992.
25. Schirmer WJ, et al. Imidazole and indomethacin enhance hepatic perfusion in sepsis. Circ Shock 21:253, 1987.

12

Molecular Biology and Surgical Disease

Barbara Ann Zehnbauer and Timothy G. Buchman

The past decade has witnessed an explosion in knowledge concerning the molecular biology of the cell. Not only do we have a better understanding of how the cell behaves under normal physiologic conditions, but its response to perturbations within its environment are also more completely understood. Although our knowledge is just beginning to evolve, the impact of this knowledge on the care of patients with surgical disease is of special importance as strategies become available to alter intracellular processes. The purpose of this chapter is to organize and summarize advances in molecular biology as they impact on the care of patients by surgical specialists. The intent of this discussion is to provide a framework for interpreting new biologic knowledge in the context of clinical care. Accordingly, this chapter is organized into two parts. The first, labeled "Biologic Bases," reviews relevant fundamentals of molecular biology. The second, labeled "Application to Surgical Care," reviews an application that has proved to be of clinical significance and in so doing demonstrates how molecular biologic knowledge will increasingly become more and more relevant to surgical management of disease. Surgical care and molecular biology independently span broad areas of scientific knowledge and human endeavor. Thus the discussion of both the surgical aspects of care and of the molecular biology are superficial and incomplete, and the reader should be aware of this. It is hoped that this overview will stimulate additional interest and reference to more detailed discussion of molecular biologic issues.[1,2]

BIOLOGIC BASES

The fundamental unit of life is the cell. In contrast to unicellular organisms such as bacteria, complex eukaryotic organisms such as humans are multicellular and organized into specialized groups of cells that define tissues and organs. Such specialization requires sophisticated communications among cells, tissues, and organs. Neural, hormonal, and mechanical coupling are three familiar mechanisms that support the communications web. Communications signal cells to proliferate, to change their metabolic state, and even to die. In such complex organisms the survival of the cell is subordinate to the survival of the organism as a whole. The ordinary biology of such complex organisms necessarily includes deliberate destruction of constituent cells to support embryologic development, growth, and renewal. A schematic eukaryotic cell is illustrated in Fig. 12-1. The major structural divisions are the nucleus and the cytoplasm.

The Nucleus

The nucleus is the primary repository of information, which is encoded into DNA. Most DNA is in the nucleus; however, there is additional DNA in the mitochondria. (Some functional proteins require both mitochondrially coded and nuclearly coded subunits.) All eukaryotic DNA appears to consist of two polymeric strands, oriented in antiparallel fashion, each containing residues of the four nucleotides adenine, thymine, guanine, and cytosine (ATGC). The mitochondrial DNA is circular. The information is encoded into the particular sequence of these residues. The two strands contain different nucleotides but identical information content. Through the process of nucleotide residue ("base") pairing, the sequence of one strand is both necessary and sufficient to determine the sequence of the other. In this pairing process, an A on one strand predicts a T on the other, whereas a G on one strand determines a C on the other.

Operationally, the DNA is organized into genes, each of which is organized into regulatory and structural nucleotide sequences, the latter encoding the primary amino acid sequence of proteins. Genes are linearly arranged, interspersed with DNA of uncertain function, compacted by interaction with specialized proteins ("histones"), and organized into physically discrete units called chromo-

Supported in part by awards GM00581 and GM48095 from the National Institutes of Health.

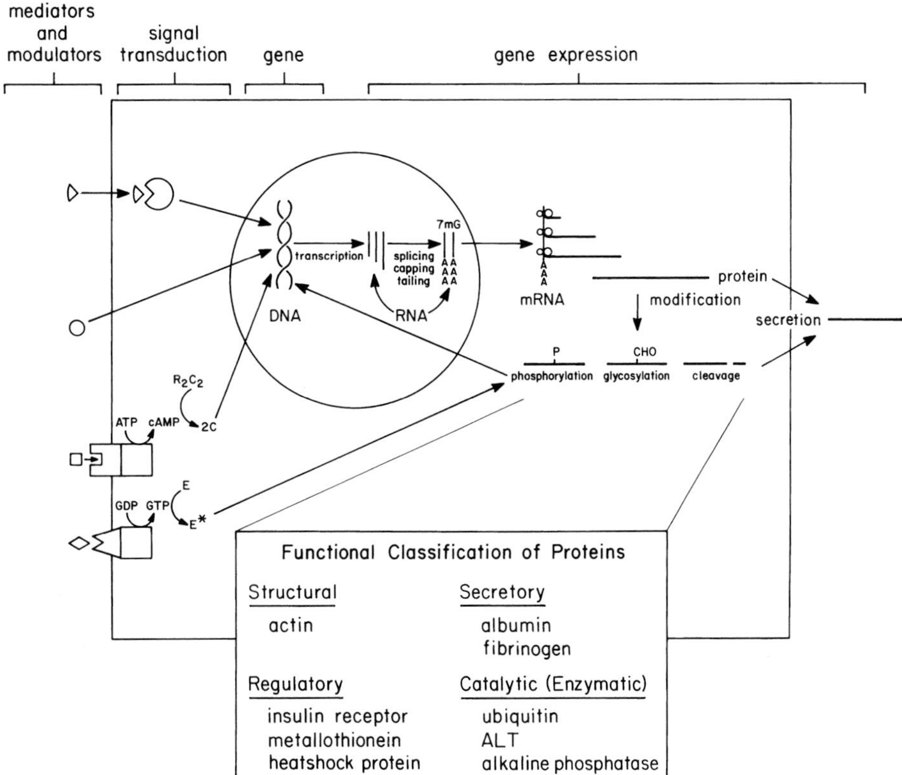

Fig. 12-1. Schematic diagram of regulation of eukaryotic gene expression. A hepatocyte is illustrated. At left are shown several mediators and modulators (i.e., cortisol *[wedge],* heat *[circle],* a β-agonist *[square],* and a cytokine *[diamond]).* The wedge transduces its signal by binding to a cytosolic receptor, which is transported to the nucleus, and the square exerts its effect via cAMP, which in turn releases regulatory subunits from catalytic subunits that travel to the nucleus. The diamond transduces by a typical protein kinase mechanism, phosphorylating a cytosolic protein that travels to the nucleus. Each of the factors can bind to regulatory DNA sequences and thereby regulate transcription of DNA into RNA. All subsequent steps are also susceptible to regulation. *ALT,* Alanine aminotransferase; *ATP,* adenosine triphosphate; *cAMP,* cyclic adenosine monophosphate; *GDP,* guanosine diphosphate; *GTP,* guanosine triphosphate; *mRNA,* messenger ribonucleic acid. (From Buchman TG. Regulation of gene expression: An overview for intensivists. Perspect Crit Care 3(2):64, 1990.)

somes. With the exception of germline cells, every normal human cell is thought to contain identical copies of DNA organized into 46 chromosomes, including 22 pairs of autosomes and 2 sex chromosomes. Each parent has contributed 22 autosomes and one sex chromosome. Paired autosomes (and in females the paired X chromosomes) contain similar genes. The homologous, information-containing regions of DNA of two chromosomes are called alleles. Where the alleles are identical, the human is said to be homozygous at that locus. Where the alleles are distinct, the human is said to be heterozygous at that locus. In males, sex chromosomes are unpaired so that the male is hemizygous for a particular locus on the X chromosome.

This encoded information must be replicated, and it must be expressed. The replication process precedes cell division (mitosis). The replication of DNA is semiconservative, meaning that each parent strand of DNA is used as a template to synthesize a daughter strand, and each parent-daughter couple reconstitutes the starting material. Key steps in this semiconservative replication are easily emulated in the laboratory. Since each replicate reconstitutes the parent, repetitive cycles of replication geometrically expand the number of copies (i.e., two become four, four become eight and so on). This geometric expansion is the basis of the polymerase chain reaction (PCR) (Fig. 12-2), which is now a standard investigational and diagnostic tool. Using PCR, a single molecule can be replicated a million-fold within a few hours.

To ensure fidelity, the cell contains extensive proofreading and repair mechanisms. (PCR replication in vitro is less precise, and errors occur commonly.) Despite the cell's checking mechanisms, errors can arise in both germline and nongermline cells. In general, the errors consist of deletion, insertion, substitution, and rearrangement of DNA sequences. These errors occur at basal rates, which are incremented by environmental factors including exposure to ionizing radiation, carcinogenic substances, and bi-

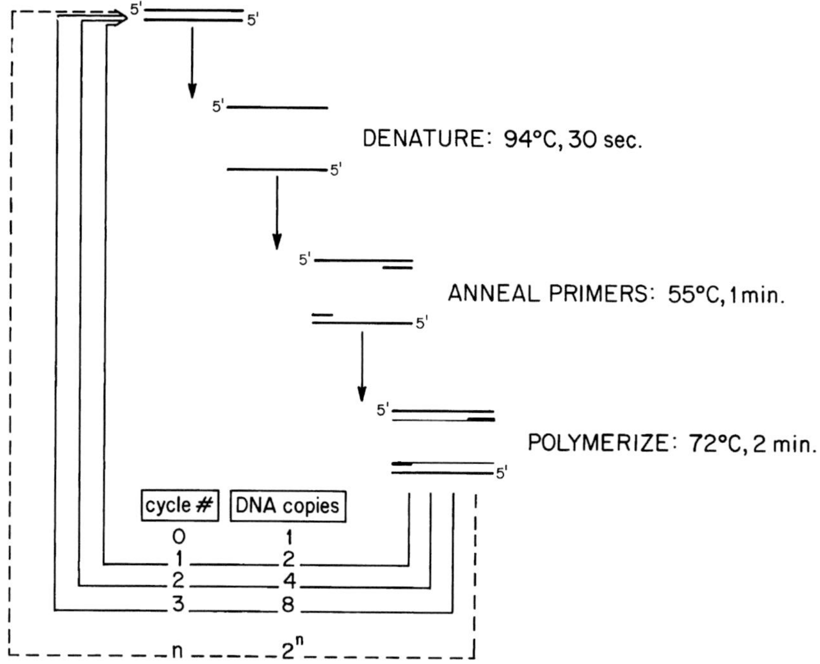

Fig. 12-2. Schematic diagram of the polymerase chain reaction (PCR). At the top of the diagram, a short (100 to 10,000 base pairs) region of double-stranded DNA is denatured by heating. Next, DNA primers, which are pieces of single-stranded DNA chemically synthesized to contain sequence complementary to the 3′ ends, are allowed to anneal by base pairing to their complements. The temperature is selected to allow only "correct" base pairing. Finally, a thermostable DNA polymerase extends or polymerizes from the primer. The result is two daughter molecules from each parent molecule. Since the primers, DNA polymerase, and free nucleotides are heat stable, the cycle can be completed merely by raising and lowering the temperature. The theoretical yield of this geometric "chain reaction" is 2^n, where *n* is the number of cycles. Although the process is in reality far less efficient, a few extra cycles are sufficient to compensate. Note that unlike DNA replication in the intact cell, this PCR process lacks ordinary editing functions and is therefore prone to errors.

ologic agents (certain viruses). One way to detect these errors is to determine the sequence of a DNA molecule; an outline of the process of sequencing is given in Fig. 12-3.

The expression of information, collectively called gene expression, can be both constitutive and regulated. Constitutive expression is relatively unaffected by intracellular or extracellular events. The nuclear component of gene expression is subject to complex regulation at the levels of transcription of DNA into an RNA copy; processing of that RNA into mRNA capable of being translated into protein; export of that mRNA from the nucleus into the cytoplasm; sequestration of RNA into a particular pool; and degradation of mRNA.

Gene Structure and Regulation of Gene Expression in the Nucleus

In general, each gene consists of three types of spatially discrete DNA sequences (see Fig. 12-4). The region of DNA that actually encodes the amino acid sequence of protein is called the coding region. This region includes coding sequences ("exons") and noncoding sequences ("introns"). These coding and noncoding sequences are transcribed as a whole, and subsequent processing ("splicing") excises the introns to create a piece of RNA in which the transcribed coding sequences are juxtaposed. Each gene also contains regulatory sequences, which typically flank the coding sequences. In some cases, however, relevant regulatory sequences have been found far distant from the coding sequences. Proximal regulatory sequences are typically organized into a "promoter" located near the DNA that codes for the amino terminus of the protein, at the site where transcription physically begins. Other regulatory sequences are located near the DNA that codes for the carboxyl terminus of the protein. These sequences typically encode information regarding stability and processing of the RNA transcript. It is important to note that the regulatory DNA sequences that affect the rate of transcription are not themselves transcribed, whereas regulatory sequences that affect RNA transcript processing are transcribed.

Surgeons commonly assay and manipulate transcriptional activity. Assays include tests for levels of estrogen

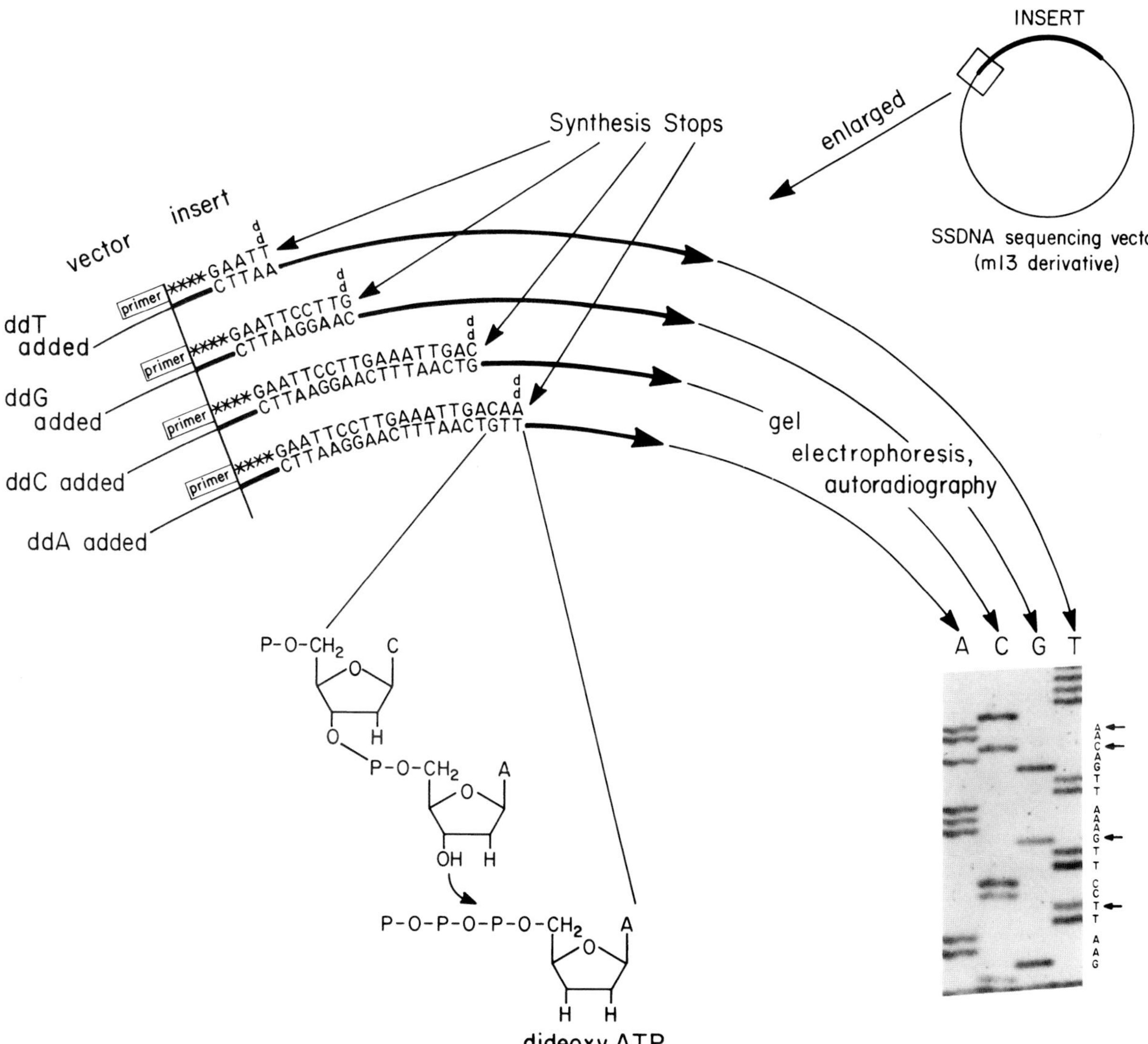

Fig. 12-3. Illustration of DNA sequencing using the classic dideoxy (Sanger) technique. As originally developed, DNA fragments to be sequenced were cloned into single-stranded bacteriophage. In this way a single primer based on phage (vector) sequence could be used to sequence any insert. (Today, many laboratories have benchtop primer synthesis machines that can custom synthesize any sequence.) After the primer was thermally annealed to its complementary sequence, the polymerization reaction was allowed to briefly proceed in the presence of radiolabeled nucleotide shown as **** and split into four reaction mixtures containing not only all four authentic nucleotide precursors (dATP, dCTP, dGTP, dTTP) but also a small amount of a dideoxynucleotide such as ddATP. As illustrated in the bottom portion of the figure, polymerization would proceed until a dideoxynucleotide was incorporated into the nascent chain. The absence of the 3′ hydroxyl group terminates the process ("synthesis stops"). Since all chains begin at the primer, knowing the particular dideoxynucleotide added and determining the length of the chain is sufficient to define the sequence. Each reaction mixture is separated by electrophoresis through a sieving gel, and autoradiography is performed to visualize the relative locations of the bands. The sequence is read "up" from bottom to top (i.e., from shortest to longest). The arrows to the right of the autoradiogram identify the specific bands illustrated in the four arcs of the figure. Although the bacteriophage target and autoradiography techniques are still employed, current use typically employs polymerase chain reaction (PCR) products as DNA targets and fluorescent tags read by a laser in an automated format in lieu of autoradiography. *ATP,* Adenosine triphosphate; *SSDNA,* single-stranded DNA.

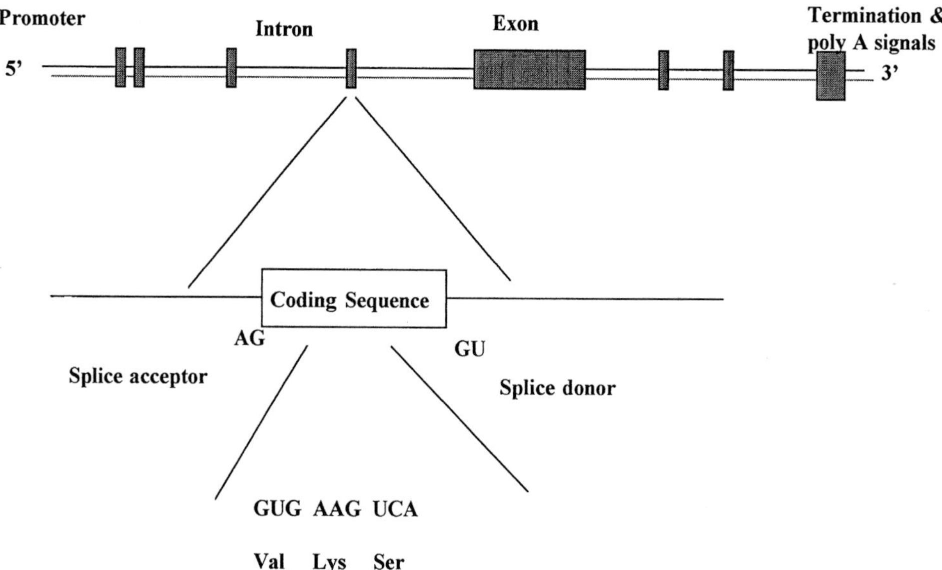

Fig. 12-4. Schematic diagram of gene structure and its relationship to expression. The top portion of the figure shows double-stranded DNA and illustrates the wide spacing between information-containing (stippled) regions. 5′ and 3′ labels indicate directionality of the top DNA strand; the bottom strand is antiparallel to the top. In the middle portion of the figure, the RNA relationship between an exon (coding sequence) and its flanking introns is shown. The sequences AG and GU (U is uracil, the ribonucleotide analog of T or thymidine) are common splice donor and splice acceptor sequences. In the bottom area the juxtaposed ribonucleotide triplets code for amino acids.

and progesterone receptor in breast cancer. These receptors are cellular proteins, which, on binding their ligand, translocate to the nucleus and activate transcription of specific genes. Similarly, the deliberate administration of glucocorticoids activates the soluble, cellular glucocorticoid receptor, which, on nuclear translocation, augments transcription of another class of genes. The administration of phosphodiesterase inhibitors such as the methylxanthines, aminophylline or theophylline, and amrinone increase the intracellular concentration of cyclic adenosine monophosphate (cAMP), which in turn activates a DNA-binding protein called CREB. Although it is important to understand that common interventions—diagnostic and therapeutic—may generally affect transcription of specific genes, the specific effects are beyond the scope of this discussion.

Common disease processes also have substantial effects on nuclear gene expression. Inflammatory cytokines (e.g., tumor necrosis factor-α and interleukin 1-β) alter the transcription rates of specific families of genes by their action on transcription factors such as NF-κB. These transcription factors are DNA-binding proteins, which bind to specific regulatory DNA sequences adjacent to coding regions of genes and thereby accelerate or attenuate transcription rates. Copies of a relevant regulatory sequence dispersed among many genes provide an important mechanism by which a single stimulus can affect transcription of many genes. Some regulatory DNA sequences confer cell specificity on gene expression: for example, both fibrinogen and albumin contain a regulatory sequence that is activated by transcription factors made exclusively by the liver. Other regulatory sequences confer responsiveness to external stimuli: during inflammation, activated factors accelerate transcription of fibrinogen but attenuate transcription of albumin.[3]

Although some stimuli may modulate transcription of relatively few genes, other stimuli that occur in the surgical patient have global effects. For example, resuscitation from deep shock triggers an intracellular stress response characterized by global suppression of all transcriptional activity except for transcription of a family of genes called heat shock genes. The products of these heat shock genes (so named because their transcription was first observed on heating cells) are intracellular proteins, which are crucial to cell survival during diverse forms of stress.[4] Other stresses that trigger transcription of gene families include inflammation (acute phase)[3] and oxidative stress.[5]

Processing of Transcripts Into mRNA

RNA has many roles in gene expression. It serves as a structural element in ribosomes (the site of protein translation), as the scaffold on which amino acids are transferred to nascent protein, and as the message encoding the amino acid sequence. The transformation of primary transcript into translatable message involves three canonical steps, each of which is subject to regulation.

The primary RNA transcript is a directional polymer of nucleotides. Each transcript has a free 5′ hydroxyl moiety in the ribose ring at one end of the molecule and a free 3′ hydroxyl moiety in the ribose ring at the other end of the molecule. We refer to these ends as the 5′ and 3′ ends of the molecule, respectively. The RNA molecule is "read" 5′→3′, and, in the case of mRNA, nucleotide residues near the 5′ end encode the amino terminus of the protein product.

The three steps required to transform a transcript into translatable message are (1) modification of the 5′ end to make it readable by the ribosome or "capping," (2) modification of the 3′ end to differentiate message from ribosomal or tRNA or "tailing," and (3) excision of nearly all the noncoding sequences (introns) from the raw transcript or "splicing." Some noncoding sequences are always left upstream of the 5′ end of the message and downstream of the 3′ end of the message. Not all modifications are required of all transcripts. For example, heat shock genes contain no introns and therefore do not require any splicing.

Capping involves transfer of one of a set of highly specialized nucleotides to the 5′ end of the RNA transcript. This nucleotide is typically modified—the most common modification is methylation—at an unusual position on the molecule. A common cap is 7′ methyl guanine. This cap is necessary to "tell" the ribosome that this particular piece of RNA is not a ribosome component but rather message to be translated.

Tailing involves transfer of ordinary adenosine residues (from adenosine triphosphate [ATP]) to the 3′ end of the molecule. Each RNA transcript destined to become message appears to contain a "tailing" signal sequence, typically ATAAA or a similar variant. The cell attaches up to 200 adenosine residues, and these residues are also necessary for the ribosome to differentiate mRNA from ribosomal or tRNA. This "poly A" tail shortens with time and appears to regulate the longevity of the RNA molecule in the cytoplasm.

Unlike capping and tailing, splicing involves rearrangement of the transcript, specifically excision of noncoding sequences and realignment of the coding sequences to make a translatable message (Fig. 12-4). This must be very precise. The splicing reactions are specified by distinct DNA sequences at both the 5′ and 3′ ends of the introns. The splice sites are unrelated to the reading frame of the mRNA. Mutations that alter splice sequences—deletions, insertion, or point mutations—may not change the reading frame but can produce a deleted or expanded, likely nonfunctional, protein.[6] The need for precision in the splicing reaction is dictated by the relationship between the four nucleotides and the 20 amino acids for which they must code. On purely combinatorial grounds, the four distinct nucleotides must be arranged into units no shorter than triplets coding for 20 amino acids, since $4^2 = 16$ and $4^3 = 64$. A one-nucleotide error in the splicing process may cause a "frame-shift," and the erroneously spliced product, its triplets out of phase, codes for meaningless polypeptide. This splicing is, at least in part, an intrinsic property of RNA; that is, at least some RNA molecules are capable of catalyzing their own splicing reactions.

The Cytoplasm

The cytoplasm is bounded by the cellular (cytoplasmic) and nuclear membranes. This space consists of a molecular cytoskeleton (microfilaments, intermediate filaments, and microtubules), organelles, and cytosol. Organelles, which include the endoplasmic reticulum (the largest organelle and the site of protein synthesis), the Golgi apparatus (the traffic police that sorts and directs proteins to their proper destination), and the lysosomes (which contain a battery of protein degradative enzymes), contain many essential information-processing functions. Organelles and the cytoskeleton rest in a supersaturated gel (cytosol). This cytosol contains proteins, molecules of intermediary metabolism, and water. Several cytosolic proteins (chaperons) function as molecular detergents, which maintain the solubility of the other components. Pathology in individual cytosolic components may be responsible for specific disease states. For example, Tay-Sachs disease is the result of the inability of lysosomes to degrade a specific ganglioside because of the absence of a specific acid hydrolase. However, the balance of this section focuses on general information processing.

RNA Stability and Accessibility

Synthesis and processing of RNA transcript in the nucleus are necessary but insufficient to describe and predict gene expression. Once transported to the cytoplasm, mRNAs are degraded at message-specific rates. For example, the mRNAs of many inflammatory cytokines are very prone to degradation because of the presence of a UA-rich sequence in the 3′ untranslated region of the message. Indeed, the upregulation of cytokine protein synthesis in response to an inflammatory challenge (such as bacterial endotoxin) begins with stabilization of that mRNA. Similarly, the expression of the major heat shock protein, hsp72, in response to weak stresses appears to be due to stabilization of the mRNA to the normal degradation pathways.[7] Such stabilization mechanisms provide for more-or-less instantaneous changes in translation rates of specific proteins independent of any (slower) change in transcription rates of their genes. It should be noted that the mere presence of mRNA in the cytoplasm may not be sufficient to guarantee access to ribosomes and translatability. Cells subjected to a heat shock stress selectively translate heat shock mRNA over other RNAs, which appear to be sequestered but can nevertheless be subsequently translated once the heat shock stress abates.

Translation of mRNA Into Protein

mRNA contains the (spliced) image of the coding portion of a specific gene. Translation of this message into a polypeptide chain involves not less than three discrete steps: initiation of the ribosome-mRNA complex; elongation of the nascent chain; and termination (release) of the completed polypeptide. Each of these steps is subject to regulation.

Initiation of the Ribosome-mRNA Complex

Ribosomes are bipartite structures, each consisting of specialized RNA and protein. In fact, the majority of intracellular RNA is ribosomal RNA. The two components of the ribosome are referred to as the small and large component. The initiation process involves the interaction of the small component of the ribosome, the mRNA, six (protein) initiation factors, guanosine triphosphate (GTP) as an energy source, and the initiator tRNA molecule. A key step in this process is read through the mRNA by the ribosome until it encounters the specific triplet of adenosine, uracil, and guanosine residues (AUG). Only after this initiation complex (known as the 40S complex because of its sedimentation characteristics) is formed does the large ribosomal component join to create a functional, translating ribosome (the 80S complex). Translation of RNA message begins with the insertion of the amino acid methionine at this AUG codon. Thus all known human proteins begin their syntheses with the amino acid methionine (coded by the triplet AUG) as the amino terminus (or N-terminus) of the nascent polypeptide. The initiator tRNA molecule therefore contains methionine. It is a special methionine residue because the N-terminus is "blocked" by a formyl acid residue. This N-terminus methionine is often modified or removed even before synthesis of the polypeptide is complete.

Elongation of the Nascent Chain

A series of peptide elongation factors facilitate the advancement of the ribosome along the mRNA molecule and the insertion of an appropriate tRNA molecule into the translation complex. Again, the energy source is GTP. tRNA molecules are small RNA molecules distinguished not only by their distinctive cloverleaf secondary structure but also by their covalent linkage to a single, specific amino acid. One leaf of the clover contains a highly exposed triplet anticodon capable of hydrogen bonding to the codons of mRNA. These tRNAs are the representation of the "second genetic code" that specifies the relationship between codons and amino acids. There are 61 codons, which use a similar number of discrete tRNA molecules to specify 20 amino acids, sometimes in a redundant fashion.

Termination of Protein Synthesis

The carboxy terminus (or C-terminus) of the nascent peptide chain is the site of elongation. The final amino acid residue added becomes the carboxy terminus of the protein. The signal that elongation must terminate is embedded in the mRNA molecule as a "stop" codon—UAA, UAG, or UGA—which does not direct the insertion of an amino acid by a tRNA molecule. When the ribosome encounters such a "stop" codon, the ribosome and completed protein release from the mRNA molecule. This final step also requires GTP hydrolysis, even though no new peptide bond is formed.

Polyribosomes

A single mRNA molecule can code for multiple copies of the protein molecule. There is no intrinsic reason that the translation mechanism must be linear (one copy completed before the next starts). Indeed, most actively translated messages exist as polyribosomal structures, with individual ribosomes marching down the mRNA strand, each reflecting a progressively longer peptide strand than the subsequent ribosome.

Posttranslational Processing of Polypeptides

Proteins have distinct conformations, intramolecular relationships, which, although they may be intrinsic to the sequence of peptide residues, do not typically form spontaneously. Rather, the nascent peptide is kept in a soluble state by the serial attachment of chaperon proteins ("chaperonins") until synthesis is complete. Detachment of these molecular detergents allows the protein to assume its preferred shape in the cytosol or in the membrane of an organelle. This change in conformation may juxtapose vicinal thiol groups of cysteine residues and thereby promote the formation of disulfide bridges within or between peptide strands. Chemical modification of the polypeptide may include addition of carbohydrates, cleavage of polypeptides into smaller polypeptide chains, and phosphorylation of the hydroxyl groups of amino acid residues such as tyrosine residues. Each of these modifications may be essential to the activity of the gene product or to the trafficking of the protein to the correct location for activity in the cell. Errors in these modifications, caused by either errors in the peptide sequence or in the machinery that executes the modifications (as occurs in the application discussed in the next section), can lead to altered or absent function. Moreover, when the gene product ordinarily serves a regulatory role, the abnormal gene product can have extraordinary effects on cell regulation and viability.

APPLICATION TO SURGICAL CARE

To illustrate the application of molecular biology to clinical surgical care, this section focuses on the recognition, localization, and clinical analysis of mutations in the *ret* proto-oncogene, which predispose to some forms of multiple endocrine neoplasia (MEN) including MEN2A,[8,9] familial medullary thyroid carcinoma (FMTC), and MEN2B.[9] Patients with MEN2A commonly develop medullary thyroid carcinoma and tumors of the parathyroid glands or adrenal glands (pheochromocytomas). It is therefore important to identify patients with mutations in the *ret* proto-oncogene not only because they are at risk for the tumors of MEN2[8-10] but also because the risk can be nearly eliminated by timely surgical intervention[11] and hormone replacement therapy.

As noted previously, errors in gene products can

markedly affect the phenotype of cells and in extreme cases can confer a malignant phenotype. Since human cells contain two allelic copies of most genes, the allelic error can be either dominant (a single copy of the error is sufficient for the malignant phenotype) or recessive (the normal allele overrides the abnormal allele, and expression of the malignant phenotype occurs only when a "second hit" occurs to inactivate the normal allele). Dominant allelic errors are characteristic of tumor genes or oncogenes, whereas recessive allelic errors occur in tumor suppressor genes. Familial MEN2 has a dominant inheritance pattern.

Identification of the Gene

The first step in the identification of the gene responsible for MEN2 syndromes was the performance of linkage analysis. This analysis is conducted on phenotypically normal cells—such as leukocytes—because every cell is expected to contain the pathologic gene. Such linkage analysis requires multiple generations of a large kindred because the investigator seeks to define a pattern of DNA markers that segregate according to the trait—in this case, MEN—under investigation (Fig. 12-5). Having identified the approximate location of the putative responsible gene by "the company it keeps," the next step is to identify a single affected individual in that kindred that keeps different company—implying that recombination has occurred between the putative gene and the marker. The process can be repeated with additional markers located progressively closer to the putative gene. The closer the marker is to the putative gene, the less likely it is that recombination will occur; therefore the resolution with which linkage analysis can define the site of a putative gene is related to the size of the kindred under study. Linkage analysis by several investigators studying different kindreds indicated that the gene(s) responsible for MEN2A, FMTC, and MEN2B localized to a region near the centromere of human chromosome 10.[12-15]

In unrelated studies, investigators comparing tumor tissue obtained from patients with sporadic thyroid cancers focused on a proto-oncogene variously called *trk* and *ret*. A proto-oncogene is a normal gene, which, when mutated, confers a malignant phenotype on cells. Mutated versions of this gene constitutively activate a tyrosine kinase product, that is, it leaves a particular protein(s) with a more or less permanently phosphorylated tyrosine residue. Mutated forms of this *ret* proto-oncogene (*ret* is the gene, and *ret* is the protein product), had first been defined as a dominant oncogene by classic DNA transformation assay[16] and overexpressed in both sporadic thyroid carcinomas and pheochromocytomas.[17] Importantly, *ret* also had been mapped to a region near the centromere of chromosome 10.[18] Thus *ret* was a candidate gene product as causation for one or more of the MEN2 syndromes.

When affected patients from MEN2 families were tested, neither germline nor phenotypically normal cells chromosomal rearrangements were observed. Moreover, there were neither rearrangements nor deletions detected in the particular neoplasias as had been observed in the sporadic papillary thyroid carcinomas. This suggested that if *ret* was not responsible for the cancer, perhaps a closely linked gene that segregated with *ret* could be the cause. It was necessary to clone a piece of DNA sufficient to span *ret* and two closely linked markers to resolve the ambiguity. Such a piece of DNA centered at chromosome

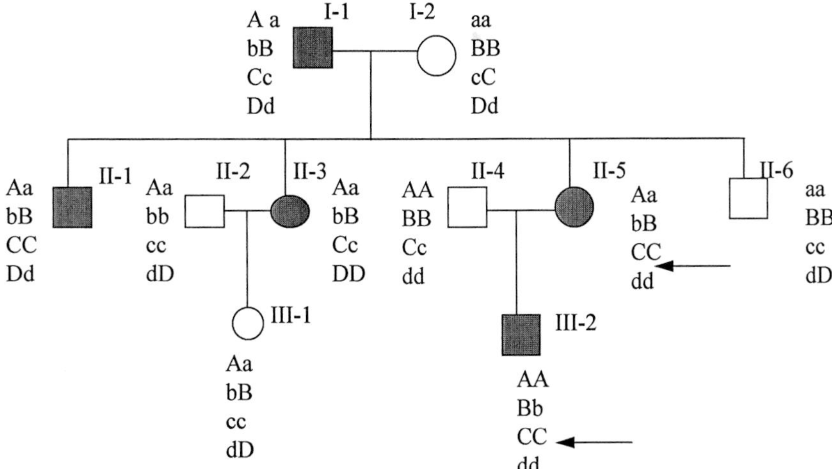

Fig. 12-5. Schematic diagram of data from linkage analysis showing segregation of autosomal dominant trait in this kindred. Individual I-1 has passed along the disease allele in linkage with the markers AbCD to his offspring II-1, II-3, and II-5. In daughter II-5 a recombinant event (noted by *arrow*) has occurred between markers C and D, but the disease allele has been retained. Moreover, her new disease-linked haplotype, AbCd has also been passed on to her son, III-2, who is affected. Individual II-6 did not inherit the disease allele from his unaffected father. Squares denote males, circles are females, filled symbols are affected with the disease, and open symbols represent the normal phenotype. Spouses II-2 and II-4 are unrelated to other members of the kindred.

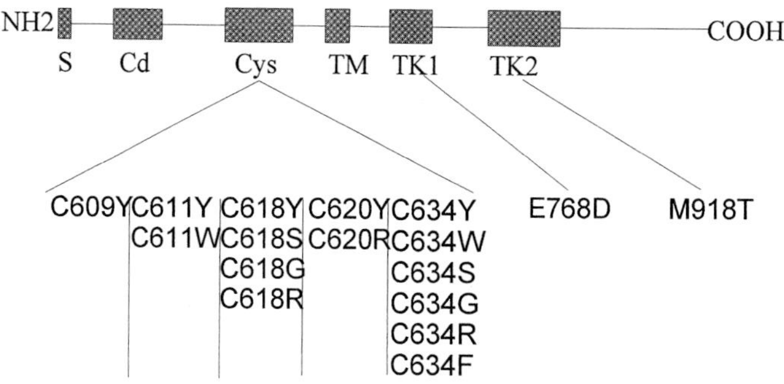

Fig. 12-6. Schematic diagram of the distribution of *ret* mutations. The *ret* protein is illustrated with amino (NH2) and carboxyl (COOH) termini; several discrete regions, including the cysteine-rich (Cys) region, are labeled. Within the cysteine-rich region, mutations in the germline DNA alter the cysteine residues normally located at positions 609, 611, 618, 620, and 634 to other amino acids. For example, C634F means that the cysteine at position 634 is changed to phenylalanine. The concentration of mutations at these cysteines could mean that this region is mutation prone, that mutations at other positions are silent, that mutations at other positions are lethal, or some combination thereof. (From Lips CJM, et al. Clinical screening as compared with DNA analysis in families with multiple endocrine neoplasia type 2A. N Engl J Med 331:828, 1994. Copyright © 1994 Massachusetts Medical Society. All rights reserved.)

10q11.2 (*q* is the long arm, and 11.2 defines a position very close to the centromere) was cloned with yeast artificial chromosomes (YACs).[19]

The YAC technique allows cloning of DNA fragments 100,000 to 500,000 base pairs in length, in contrast to conventional [plasmid and phage] techniques that can accommodate 100 to 10,000 base pairs. Contiguous, overlapping YACs—called contigs—can easily span millions of base pairs. The entire *Haemophilus influenzae* genome contains 1.8 million base pairs.[20]

Determination of the DNA sequence of these cloned fragments provided the nucleotide sequence information required to synthesize primers, which could then be used in PCR for more detailed study of each region of the gene(s). Of course, the sequence had been determined only for the DNA cloned into the YAC. It was necessary to discover the sites that set apart patients with MEN2 syndromes from their unaffected relatives.[21,22] The strategy used is called single-strand conformational variance (SSCV).[23] Such SSCV analysis of PCR-amplified areas allowed detection of single-base change variation(s). The method relies on the fact that single strands of DNA migrate differently through sieving gels than double-stranded DNA and moreover that even single-base changes ("mutations") can markedly alter the electrophorectic pattern.

Eventually, PCR amplification of regions spanning the entire *ret* gene followed by direct DNA sequencing confirmed point mutations in the germline DNA of patients with MEN2A, FMTC, and MEN2B. Remarkably, the mutations were localized to DNA coding for only five conserved cysteine codons in exons 10 and 11 (MEN2A and FMTC) or one methionine codon in MEN2B[24] (Fig. 12-6). These changes were not observed in DNA from unaffected relatives in these MEN families or other normal individuals. One specific point mutation was inherited in an autosomal dominant fashion by each affected family member within a given kindred. These observations cinched the cause-effect relationship between mutations in *ret* and familial MEN2 syndromes.

New MEN families—or, more precisely, affected and unaffected members of the kindred—undergo direct analysis of *ret* proto-oncogene to identify mutations. The techniques include direct DNA sequencing, SSCV analysis, and restriction fragment length polymorphism (RFLP) analysis. Each approach begins with the isolation of DNA from the peripheral blood lymphocytes of an affected family member. DNA sequences from exons 10, 11, and 16 (MEN2B only) are amplified by PCR because they are the "hot spots" for *ret* mutation. The PCR product may then be sequenced directly to identify the mutant codon or SSCV analysis. Certain mutations can create a palindromic sequence of nucleotides that serve as a recognition sequence for a sequence-specific endonuclease (restriction endonuclease). The latter enzymes, derived from bacteria, are thus important to clinical genetic analysis because they allow short DNA sequences (a physical attribute) to be analyzed as genetic markers without reference to functional characteristics of the gene product. Changes in the scission pattern give rise to RFLPs, which are readily detected by gel electrophoresis[25,26] (Fig. 12-7).

Each analytic approach has limitations. For example, the direct DNA sequencing strategy is the most costly method and may identify silent (nonfunctional) DNA substitutions. The SSCV technique does not identify which base pair has changed and may also identify benign DNA polymorphisms. The RFLP approach is limited because not all base changes produce a sequence that is recognized by a restriction endonuclease. A limitation common to all these strategies is that they address only a portion of the *ret* gene and therefore may miss *ret* gene mutations located in other coding regions or a flanking, regulatory sequence.

When a specific *ret* mutation has been identified for a MEN family, that mutation is sought in at-risk relatives or offspring. Detection of the distinct point mutation in

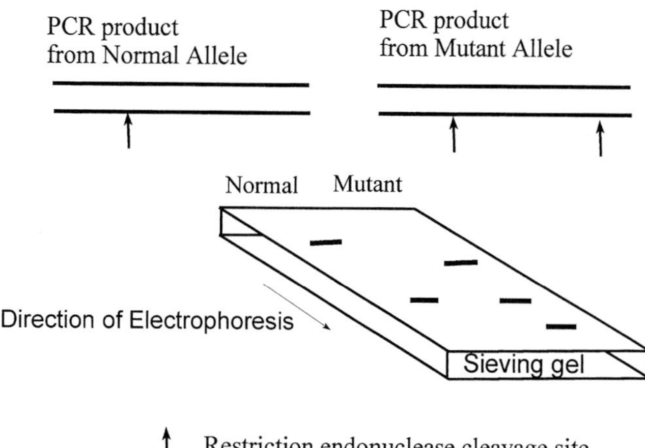

Fig. 12-7. Schematic illustration of restriction fragment length polymorphism (RFLP). The parallel lines represent double-stranded DNA amplified from a polymerase chain reaction (PCR). On the left is DNA amplified from a normal allele. On the right is DNA amplified from a mutant allele. The mutation, near the right terminus of the PCR product, creates a palindromic segment of DNA, which is recognized by a restriction endonuclease as a scission site. The cleavage product of the PCR material derived from the normal allele contains only two fragments, whereas the cleavage product from the mutant allele contains three fragments. These are separable by electrophoresis through a sieving gel and are readily visualized by staining with a fluorescent dye. Recall that unaffected individuals have two normal alleles so that cleavage of their PCR product should result in only two fragments. Affected individuals have a normal and a mutant allele; cleavage of their PCR product therefore contains four bands, a composite of the two patterns. This analysis is applicable only when the mutation creates a restriction endonuclease cleavage site.

some kindred members significantly refines the assessment of their risk for developing endocrine tumors and confirms that their offspring are at risk for inheriting both the gene and the syndromes: each offspring of an MEN patient has a 50% risk of inheriting the *ret* mutation. Ninety percent of individuals with *ret* mutations (in the regions defined above) develop medullary thyroid carcinoma by age 30. Thirty to fifty percent of those people develop pheochromocytomas, and another 30% develop parathyroid tumors. Kindred members who do not carry the *ret* mutation are at markedly less risk for these tumors, namely the risk associated with sporadic incidence observed in the general population. These genetically *ret* normal individuals, even though they are kindred members, may then be spared the routine physiologic monitoring by calcium-pentagastrin stimulation of calcitonin. The classic stimulation tests are uncomfortable, not without potential side effects, and difficult to administer to children, and variable levels may lead to inconclusive evaluations or failure to detect microscopic disease. Genetically positive relatives may choose surgical intervention such as thyroidectomy with hormone replacement to preempt the development of malignancy and metastasis and thereby improve the quality and duration of their lives.[11] Irrespective of the consultant's choice regarding preemptive surgery, the genetic predisposition to development of all manifestations of the MEN2 syndromes will influence decisions regarding the frequency and aggressiveness of clinical monitoring.

There are several risks that both surgeon and patient should acknowledge before undergoing genetic screening for *ret* mutations or any other germlike mutations. First, the significance of a laboratory error would be profound. It is therefore crucial that the laboratory performing the investigation adhere to stringent quality control procedures for clinical testing as opposed to the more lax procedures generally associated with a research laboratory. Second, any test result that reveals information about a person's genetic constitution must be maintained in strictest confidence by all medical staff including nurses, physicians, genetic counselors, and laboratory personnel. There is considerable potential for discrimination against the patient for insurance and employment when risk factors for disabling diseases, including malignancy, become known. It is recommended that consideration of these factors be discussed and documented during a genetic counseling session with the consultant as part of a formal consent process for genetic testing.

SUMMARY

The foregoing discussion highlights recent important advances in molecular biology and the potential impact they might have on the care of patients with surgical disease. A model of how such information can be applied in a particular patient care setting is reviewed and discussed. It is anticipated that such application will become more extensive in the years to come and that many diseases currently thought to be best treated with surgical extirpative processes will be managed successfully in the not-too-distant future with manipulation of fundamental molecular processes within cells. This being the case, it is incumbent on surgical specialists to be aware of this knowledge explosion and how advances in molecular biology will most assuredly impact on the treatment of surgical disease in future years.

REFERENCES

1. Buchman TG, Zehnbauer BA. Molecular biology in the intensive care unit: A framework for interpretation. New Horizons 3:139, 1995.
2. Daley MD, Siminovitch KA. Introduction to modern molecular biology: Fundamental concepts and techniques. New Horizons 3:146, 1995.
3. Pannen HJP, Robotham JL. The acute phase response. New Horizons 3:183, 1995.
4. DeMaio A. The heat shock response. New Horizons 3:198, 1995.
5. Camhi SL, Lee P, Choi AMK. The oxidative stress response. New Horizons 3:170, 1995.
6. Lorenzo MJ, et al. Multiple mRNA isoforms of the human RET proto-oncogene generated by alternate splicing. Oncogene 10:1377, 1995.
7. Pannen HJP, et al. Hepatic heat shock and acute phase gene expression are simultaneously induced but differently regulated after celiotomy in the anesthetized pig. Anesthesiology 83:850, 1995.
8. Asai N, et al. Mechanism of activation of the ret proto-oncogene by multiple endocrine neoplasia 2A mutations. Mol Cell Biol 15:1613, 1995.
9. Santoro M, et al. Activation of RET as a dominant transforming gene by germline mutations of MEN2A and MEN2B. Science 267:381, 1995.
10. Carson EB, et al. Ret gene silencing is associated with Raf-1-induced medullary thyroid carcinoma cell differentiation. Cancer Res 55:2048, 1995.
11. Wells SA, et al. Predictive DNA testing and prophylactic thyroidectomy in patients at risk for multiple endocrine neoplasia type 2A. Ann Surg 220:237, 1994.
12. Lairmore TC, et al. Familial medullary thyroid carcinoma and MEN 2B map to the same region of chromosome 10 as MEN 2A. Genomics 9:181, 1991.
13. Mathew CG, et al. A linked genetic marker for MEN2A on chromosome 10. Nature 328:527, 1987.
14. Mulligan LM, et al. Germ-line mutations of the ET proto-oncogene in MEN2A. Nature 363:458, 1993.
15. Simpson NE, et al. Assignment of MEN2A to chromosome 10 by linkage. Nature 328:528, 1987.
16. Takahashi M, Ritz S, Cooper GM. Activation of a novel human transforming gene, *ret,* by DNA rearrangement. Cell 42:581, 1985.
17. Santoro M, et al. The ret proto-oncogene is consistently expressed in human pheochromocytomas and medullary thyroid carcinomas. Oncogene 5:1595, 1990.
18. Donghi R, et al. The oncogene associated with human PTC is assigned to chromosome 10q11-10q12 in the same region as MEN 2A. Oncogene 4:521, 1989.
19. Lairmore TC, et al. A 1.5-megabase yeast artificial chromosome contig from human chromosome 10q11.2 connecting three genetic loci (RET, D10S94, and D10S102) closely linked to the MEN2A locus. Proc Nat Acad Sci U S A 90:492, 1993.
20. Fleischman RD, et al. Whole genome random sequencing and assembly of *Haemophilus influenzae.* Science 269:496, 1995.
21. Chi DD, et al. Predictive testing for multiple endocrine neoplasia type 2A (MEN 2A) based on the detection of mutations in the RET proto-oncogene. Surgery 116:124, 1994.
22. Donis-Keller H, et al. Mutations in the RET proto-oncogene are associated with MEN2A and FMTC. Hum Mol Genet 2:851, 1993.
23. Ceccherini I, et al. DNA polymorphisms and conditions for SSCP analysis of the 20 exons of the ret proto-oncogene. Oncogene 9:3025, 1994.
24. Lips CJM, et al. Clinical screening as compared with DNA analysis in families with multiple endocrine neoplasia type 2A. N Engl J Med 331:828, 1994.
25. Howe JR, et al. Improved predictive test for MEN2, using flanking dinucleotide repeats and RFLPs. Am J Hum Genet 51:1430, 1992.
26. Marsh DJ, et al. A rapid screening method for the detection of mutations in the RET proto-oncogene in multiple endocrine neoplasia type 2A and familial medullary thyroid carcinoma families. Genomics 23:477, 1994.

13

Physiologic Principles in Preparing Patients for Surgery

Henry J. Schiller, Kara C. Kort, and Lelan F. Sillin

Surgery can be considered "controlled trauma" that predictably alters the patient's normal physiology. These physiologic derangements may be more severe, and less well tolerated, in patients with concurrent illnesses, such as coronary artery disease or chronic obstructive pulmonary disease (COPD). The potential benefits of an operative procedure must be balanced against the potential risks of the procedure and the risks and benefits of management alternatives. It is imperative that the surgeon be able to recognize those features that may increase a patient's expected morbidity or mortality and to modify the perioperative management and operative plan accordingly. Just as "an ounce of prevention is better than a pound of cure," anticipating the patient's expected clinical course provides a better outcome than reacting to what may have been a preventable complication. An optimal outcome in surgery requires a thoughtful diagnostic workup, careful perioperative care, appropriate surgical procedure, and conscientious follow-up. Preoperative care remains an integral part of surgical care and is the ultimate responsibility of the surgeon. While preparing a patient for surgery may become routine, it is better to understand the physiologic principles involved rather than simply issuing "standard orders" by rote. A thoughtful evaluation based on a thorough knowledge of the natural history of the disease process involved, associated medical conditions, and the physiologic changes produced by them are essential for assessing the risk of treatment options and engaging in appropriate management of the patient's problems.

GENERAL ASPECTS OF PREOPERATIVE PREPARATION

A thorough history and physical examination should be performed along with a pertinent review of systems. All preoperative medications should be known, and allergies should be especially noted. Operative notes and pathology reports from prior surgical procedures frequently prove enlightening. One may obtain a general impression of the patient's physical condition by physical examination. Often a patient may pass or fail the "look test." Important features to note are the patient's apparent nutritional status and body habitus. Simple observations may give clues to clinically important conditions; for example, breathlessness, a barrel chest, clubbing, and cyanosis may indicate COPD. Patients in distress generally display an easily recognizable picture of vigilant anxiety. Assessment of a patient's functional status should also be assessed, as this may provide an important indication of underlying cardiac disease. Age greater than 70 has been implicated as a risk factor for postoperative cardiac complications.[1,2]

Ideally, patients should be kept NPO for 8 hours prior to an anesthetic to minimize the risk of aspiration. They should be well hydrated, and electrolytes should be within normal limits. Any active infection should be identified and treated preoperatively.

Surgical Consent

The surgeon must speak with the patient candidly about the proposed surgery. The patient should be given an explanation of the disease process, its expected course, and the indications for surgery. This should include a clear discussion of therapeutic alternatives. In discussing the specifics of the procedure, the patient should be informed of the expected rates of mortality and morbidity. Although it is unnecessary and counterproductive to intentionally frighten the patient, the surgeon has the medical, legal, and moral responsibility to inform the patient of potential complications or adverse outcomes. This is best done in the presence of a family member or another witness to prevent later misunderstandings. It is also desirable to obtain advance directives from the patient, in the event the patient is unable to participate in medical decision making later in the course of disease. Finally, the patient should be told what to expect postoperatively, including the tubes and lines one is likely to have in place, the amount of pain one is likely to experience despite analgesia, and regimens one is likely to undergo. Clear and honest communication increases the patient's confidence in the care he or she is receiving and will serve to strengthen the patient-physician relationship.

Nutrition

A patient's nutritional stores may be rapidly depleted by perioperative fasting and dietary restrictions. Moreover, the patient who is poorly nourished at the outset has fewer reserves and tolerates fasting poorly. Although fluid and electrolyte losses from recent emesis or diarrhea are easily documented, there is no specific laboratory measure for malnutrition. A serum albumin of less than 3.5 mg/dl may give a crude indication of malnutrition, but its long serum half-life (18 days) makes it relatively insensitive to acute perturbations in nutrition. Serum proteins with shorter circulating half-lives such as retinol-binding protein, prealbumin, and fibrinogen are also acute phase proteins and therefore may be artifactually elevated by recent infection or inflammation. Ultimately, history (weight loss, dietary habits), physical examination, and anthropometrics (e.g., triceps skinfold) should be used in concert with serum protein levels to determine a patient's nutritional reserve. In general, patients weighing 80% or less of ideal body weight or patients with recent, profound weight loss (greater than 10% ideal body weight) should be considered for preoperative hyperalimentation.[3,4] Enteral nutrition should be used in patients with a functioning gastrointestinal tract. Preoperative total parenteral nutrition should be given for at least 10 days preoperatively in malnourished patients. Consideration should be given for perioperative total parenteral nutrition even in well-nourished patients who will require bowel rest for more than 5 to 7 days.[4]

Obesity

Obesity, an all too common disorder in industrialized nations, provides additional physiologic stress including increased work of breathing and a requirement for a higher cardiac output. Comorbidities often seen in obese patients include respiratory insufficiency, coronary artery disease, hypertension, and diabetes mellitus.[5] Although the precise definitions of obesity and morbid obesity vary, in general a patient weighing more than 130% of his or her ideal body weight is at increased risk for perioperative complications, such as atelectasis, pneumonia, respiratory failure, deep venous thrombosis, or wound complications.[6]

There is usually little that can be done preoperatively to remedy obesity. Attention must therefore be directed toward the prevention of expected postoperative complications. Preoperative incentive spirometry, DVT prophylaxis, skin care, and early mobilization postoperatively may help decrease the risk of complications.

Integument

The integument is the largest organ of the body. The skins plays an invaluable role both as a barrier to conserve body heat and water and as a barrier to prevent infection from potential environmental pathogens. Trauma, or burns, that lead to major skin loss may predispose to hypovolemia from fluid loss and hypothermia from heat loss. Such patients must receive fluid resuscitation and must be kept warm. Percent skin loss may be determined by the "rule of nines"[7] so that an estimate of the patient's fluid requirements may be calculated by the Parkland formula.[8] Relatively minor skin trauma may predispose to infection by providing a portal of entry for resident skin flora.

Skin harbors a resident microbial flora and therefore represents not only a barrier to infection, which will be compromised by a surgical incision, but also a source of microbes with which to contaminate the surgical wound. For this reason, the skin ought to be scrubbed for surgery with povidone-iodine, hexachlorophene, or chlorhexidine.[9] This provide both mechanical cleansing to remove contaminants and debris and topical antiseptics to further decrease bacterial counts in the surgical field. Shaving the patient the night before surgery increases the incidence of wound infection compared to shaving just prior to the surgical incision.[9] This is doubtlessly due to compromise of the skin's microbial barrier function by microabrasions and nicks. Depilatory agents may be used in place of shaving, although risk of hypersensitivity reactions to these agents remains. Ideally, abrasions, rashes, eruptions, and furuncles are treated prior to operation, particularly in situations in which prosthetics are to be implanted. In the event this is not possible, incisions should be planned to avoid these areas. Preoperative antibiotics possessing gram positive coverage may be given for prophylaxis.

Antibiotic Prophylaxis

The incidence of postsurgical infection ranges from 2.8% to 7.6%, making it the second most common nosocomial infection, behind catheter-related urinary tract infection.[10] These range from simple skin infections to major sepsis, and they may have a profound impact on patient outcome and cost of care. Preexisting infections should be treated prior to elective operation to minimize the risk of postoperative infection. Prophylactic antibiotics administered perioperatively are clearly beneficial.[10,11] Conversely, prophylactic antibiotics administered after the skin incision is made do not achieve the desired effect and may be detrimental to both the patient and the institution by promoting the overgrowth of antibiotic-resistant bacteria.

Surgical procedures are classified as clean, clean contaminated, contaminated, or dirty. Clean cases involve no entry into the respiratory, gastrointestinal, or genitourinary tract and have no break in sterile technique. The incidence of postsurgical infection is only 2% to 5%, which decreases to 0.8% with perioperative antibiotic prophylaxis.[12] Since clean surgical cases comprise approximately 75% of all procedures, unless the patient has additional risk factors for infection (see accompanying box), antibiotics are withheld because of the low incidence of infection. The benefit of prophylactic antibiotics is difficult to demonstrate. Clean contaminated cases involve entry into the respiratory, gastrointestinal, or genitourinary tract without gross contamination of the surgical field. The incidence of postsurgical infection is 8% to 10%, which decreases to 1.3% with antibiotic prophylaxis. Contaminated wounds include open traumatic wounds, major breaks in sterile technique, or significant spillage from the gastrointestinal tract. In these wounds, the incidence of postsurgical infection is 20%, which decreases to 10.2% with antibiotic prophylaxis. Dirty cases involve fields with established infection and carry a 40% incidence of wound infection. Therapeutic, rather than prophylactic, antibiotic coverage is indicated for these cases.[12,13]

FACTORS INCREASING RISK OF POSTOPERATIVE INFECTION

- Duration of operation greater than 2 hours
- Emergency surgery
- Advanced age
- Placement of prosthetic material
- Medical conditions
  - Preexisting infection
  - Malignancy
  - Diabetes mellitus
  - Obesity
  - Malnutrition
  - Steroid usage
  - Immunoincompetence
  - Local vascular disease

Adapted from Neibart E. Preoperative preventive antimicrobial therapy. Mt Sinai J Med 58:19, 1991.

Prophylactic antibiotic coverage should be chosen according to the organisms most likely to cause infection. In general, first-generation cephalosporins (i.e., cefazolin) have been used because of their broad gram-positive and gram-negative coverage, their long half-life, low cost, and low toxicity. It is important to obtain adequate tissue levels prior to operation. Repeated doses should be administered during lengthy procedures.[14] Providing prophylactic antibiotic coverage beyond 24 to 48 hours is of no benefit and increases the risk of colonization or infection by antibiotic-resistant bacterial strains.[15]

Colonic surgery usually requires more significant preoperative regimens (Table 13-1). The colon contains the highest bacterial concentrations of any location in the body. The flora includes both aerobes and anaerobes. Although the latter predominate, some of the aerobes are particularly virulent (i.e., *Escherichia coli*). Consequently, postoperative infections are the major source of morbidity in colonic surgery. Although it is not possible to actually sterilize the colon, significant reduction in colonic flora can be achieved. A combination of mechanical colonic lavage preparation and oral nonabsorbable antibiotics prior to surgery is required to decrease infection rates.[16]

The standard prophylactic regimen still remains a combination of oral neomycin and oral erythromycin. Mechanical cleansing is achieved either with the traditional 3-day preparation using bisacodyl, magnesium citrate, and cleansing enemas or a 1-day preparation using a large vol-

Table 13-1. Bowel Preparation Regimen

Preoperative Day	Traditional Preparation	Polyethylene Glycol
3	Clear liquid diet Bisacodyl capsule orally at 6 PM	Regular diet as desired
2	Clear liquid diet Magnesium citrate 6% sodium, 296 ml orally at 10 AM, 2 PM, and 6 PM Cleansing enemas until clear rectal effluent	Regular diet as desired
1	Clear liquid diet Magnesium citrate 6% sodium, 296 ml orally at 10 AM and 2 PM Neomycin sulfate and erythromycin base, 1 g each orally at 1 PM, 2 PM, and 11 PM	Light breakfast as desired before 8 AM Polyethylene glycol 1 L hr orally × 5 hr or until clear rectal effluent Neomycin sulfate and erythromycin base, 1 g each orally at 1 PM, 2 PM, and 11 PM
0	NPO after midnight Rectal evacuation at 7 AM Cefoxitin or cefotetan, intravenous perioperative administration	NPO after midnight Rectal evacuation at 7 AM Cefoxitin or cefotetan, intravenous perioperative administration

Modified from Fleites RA, et al. The efficacy of polyethylene glycol–electrolyte solution versus traditional mechanical bowel preparation for elective colonic surgery: A randomized, prospective, blinded clinical trial. Surgery 98(4):708, 1985.

ume of orally administered polyethylene glycol–electrolyte lavage solution. One-day preparations have been found to be efficacious, safe, and relatively well tolerated preoperatively in addition to minimizing dietary alterations and reducing preoperative hospitalization.[17] Systemic intravenous antibiotics are often added to this regimen (i.e., cefoxitin or cefotetan); however, it remains controversial as to whether this provides any benefit over mechanical preparation with oral antibiotics.[10,16,18]

SPECIFIC ASPECTS OF PREOPERATIVE PREPARATION

Risks of Pulmonary Disease

Patients should be questioned regarding smoking history, chronic cough or sputum production, wheezing, or shortness of breath. Any history of chronic lung disease, pneumonia, chest injury, occupational exposures, or requirement for intubation should be obtained. Current exercise tolerance and medication use, particularly bronchodilators and corticosteroids, give an indication as to the severity of pulmonary disease. The physical examination should document body habitus, respiratory rate and effort, the presence and quality of breath sounds, the anteroposterior diameter of the chest, cyanosis, and clubbing. Patients over age 40 or patients with a history of cigarette smoking or pulmonary disease should receive a preoperative chest x-ray examination. Patients undergoing pulmonary resection should have formal pulmonary function testing, including spirometry, room air arterial blood gas determination, and split-lung perfusion testing. In abdominal and nonresective thoracic surgery, formal pulmonary function testing has not been shown to be superior to history and physical examination in predicting postoperative pulmonary complications.[19,20]

General anesthesia leads to depression of respiratory drive, particularly in response to hypercarbia and hypoxia. Tidal volume (TV), functional residual capacity (FRC), and thoracic volume decrease as the diaphragm loses tone and moves cephalad. The resulting atelectasis and preferential ventilation of the nondependent regions of the lungs leads to ventilation-perfusion mismatch, thereby increasing shunt fraction.[21]

High abdominal incisions, thoracotomy incisions, and median sternotomy predipose toward postoperative pulmonary complications. Pain and muscular splinting lead to inhibition of coughing and a decrease in TV. High abdominal incisions result in "diaphragmatic dysfunction" such that ventilation is more dependent on chest excursion.[22] Forced expiratory volume in one second (FEV_1) and vital capacity (VC) decrease from 25% to 50%, and the FRC decreases.[23] Cardiac surgery may result in dysfunction of the left hemidiaphragm, probably from left phrenic nerve injury incurred either during dissection of the left internal mammary artery at the thoracic inlet or by cold injury during slush cooling of the heart.[24] These predispose the patient to mucous plugging, atelectasis, and ultimately pneumonia. Although laparoscopic surgery largely avoids the muscle splinting seen with high abdominal incisions, absorption of carbon dioxide from the pneumoperitoneum occurs, predisposing to intraoperative hypercarbia and acidosis.[25] Smokers and patients with chronic lung disease are at increased risk for these postoperative pulmonary complications.

Smoking eventually leads to COPD, but even smokers with normal pulmonary function tests face an increased risk of pulmonary complication. Smoking both stimulates mucous secretion and impairs the mucociliary apparatus necessary to efficiently clear these secretions. Carbon monoxide found in cigarette smoke binds hemoglobin in preference to oxygen, thereby decreasing oxygen-carrying capacity. Moreover, cigarette smoking increases airway irritability, which may lead to perioperative bronchospasm and small airway dysfunction. Current smokers undergoing surgery can expect a 33% rate of pulmonary complications (mucus plugging, atelectasis, pneumonia, pleural effusion, or pneumothorax). Cessation of smoking for at least 2 months preoperatively decreases this rate to 14.5%, and cessation of smoking for more than 6 months decreases the rate of pulmonary complications to that of patients who have never smoked. Paradoxically, cessation of smoking for less than 2 months actually increases the rate of postoperative complications to 57%.[26]

Patients with chronic pulmonary disease either have a restrictive or an obstructive pattern. Restrictive diseases are generally characterized by a decreased forced vital capacity (FVC) and total lung capacity (TLC), whereas obstructive diseases are characterized by a decrease in the ratio of FEV_1/FVC. Patients with COPD, such as emphysema and chronic bronchitis, have an increased FRC and TLC but may have a decreased TV. Consequently, a greater respiratory rate is required to maintain an adequate minute ventilation. Carbon dioxide retention indicates severe disease. The presence of these chronic pulmonary diseases can be determined by history and physical examination. Subtle decrements in pulmonary function and the severity of overt pulmonary disease may be measured objectively by formal pulmonary function tests (PFTs), including clinical spirometry and arterial blood gas determination. In abdominal and nonresective thoracic surgery, PFTs are used to assess risk for postoperative pulmonary complications and to identify those patients likely to require specialized postoperative respiratory therapy or even postoperative mechanical ventilation. Unfortunately, this ideal has not been realized. Formal PFTs are not superior to a detailed history and physical examination for this purpose.[19,20] Conversely, clinical spirometry, split perfusion lung scanning, and preoperative arterial blood gas determinations do correlate with postoperative respiratory insufficiency and mortality in patients undergoing pulmonary resection. In general, the predicted FEV_1 postresection should exceed 800 ml.[27]

Patients preparing for general anesthesia should cease smoking at least 2 months beforehand. Moreover, they should be educated preoperatively regarding the importance of deep breathing and coughing. Those with preexisting pulmonary disease should receive preoperative bronchodilator therapy with either β-adrenergic agonists or ipratropium bromide (an atropine derivative).[23] Patients already receiving theophylline preparations should continue them. Aminophylline should not be administered prophylactically because the toxic-to-therapeutic index is small.[23] Patients with steroid-dependent COPD should receive stress-dose steroids perioperatively. Elective operation should be avoided in patients with active pulmonary infections, and prophylactic antibiotics with activity against *Haemophilus influenzae* and *Streptococcus pneumoniae* may be administered in those with chronic lung disease to suppress endogenous bronchial flora.[23] High-risk patients should additionally receive postural drainage and chest physiotherapy. Epidural analgesia may improve the diaphragmatic dysfunction seen with high abdominal incisions,[22] while pleural catheter analgesia may improve the respiratory mechanics after thoracotomy.[28]

Risks of Cardiovascular Disease

The cardiac history should detail exercise tolerance and symptoms of angina, dyspnea, orthopnea, paroxysmal nocturnal dyspnea, fatigue, palpitations, and syncope. Any history of myocardial infarction, congestive heart failure, valvular heart diease, or arrhythmia should be elicited. Examiners should listen for murmurs, clicks, extra heart sounds (S_3 and S_4), rales, and bruits. Blood pressure, heart rate, and pulses should be noted, as should the presence of jugulovenous distension, peripheral edema, and hepatomegaly. The results of previous cardiac testing should be reviewed.

During operation, the cardiovascular system is stressed both by anesthetic agents and by fluid shifts. The inhalation agents are generally myocardial depressants.[21] Loss of vascular tone during general, spinal, or epidural anesthesia may provoke hypotension, particularly in the hypovolemic patient. Postanesthetic recovery of vascular tone may result in fluid overload. Hypothermia results in vasoconstriction, and rewarming is associated with vasodilation and consequent hypotension. Longer procedures have greater evaporative fluid and heat losses, and more extensive procedures promote greater fluid loss into the "third space." The hypotension seen with induction of anesthesia can be minimized by adequate preoperative hydration. Patients requiring preoperative bowel preparation or those receiving chronic diuretic therapy may require additional fluids because of baseline volume contraction.

Hemodynamic Monitoring

Basic hemodynamic monitoring is performed noninvasively with pulse and blood pressure determinations. Urine output is followed as a crude indicator of visceral perfusion. Invasive monitoring is reserved for the hemodynamically unstable patient or those with underlying cardiac disease such as congestive heart failure, recent myocardial infarction, or significant coronary artery disease. It is also useful when urine output cannot be used as an indicator of visceral perfusion, such as patients with end-stage renal disease (ESRD) or with diabetes insipidus. The benefits derived from invasive monitoring must always be weighed against the complications, which generally include infection, thrombosis, and hemorrhage.

Percutaneous arterial catheters are used in patients requiring instantaneous, continuous blood pressure monitoring or for those requiring repeated arterial blood sampling. The catheters are usually placed in the radial artery after ensuring adequate ulnar artery collateral flow to the palmar arch by the modified Allen test.

Central venous catheters measure pressure in the superior vena cava. This equals right ventricular pressure at the end of diastole and therefore gives an approximation of right ventricular end-diastolic volume (right ventricular preload) in the normal, compliant heart. This is useful in patients with preserved myocardial function who may experience large fluid shifts during operation. Central venous catheters are generally inserted into either the internal jugular or the subclavian vein, although the femoral vein is also acceptable. Percutaneous insertion into the left internal jugular vein places the patient at risk for thoracic duct injury. Inadvertent arterial cannulation is risked at all insertion sites but is particularly worrisome in the subclavian position, where direct arterial compression for hemostasis is not generally possible. The subclavian approach also places the patient at risk for pneumothorax.

The Swan-Ganz, or pulmonary artery, catheter provides a better indication of left-sided cardiac function. The proximal port provides a central venous pressure. The distal port provides pulmonary artery pressures and the pulmonary capillary wedge pressure, which, in the absence of severe mitral stenosis, equals left ventricular end-diastolic pressure, giving an indication of left ventricular preload. Cardiac output may also be measured by thermodilution. These values, along with blood pressure, hemoglobin concentration, and saturation, may be used to calculate systemic vascular resistance, pulmonary vascular resistance, stroke work, oxygen delivery, and oxygen consumption. Complications of pulmonary artery catheter insertion are the same as those seen in central venous catheter insertion. In addition, the patient is at risk for ventricular arrhythmias, right bundle branch block, valvular injury, cardiac perforation, and pulmonary artery rupture. Moreover, catheter sepsis, endocarditis, venous thrombosis, and pulmonary infarction may develop over time. Therefore pulmonary artery catheterization should be performed only for specific indications.

Specific indications for preoperative pulmonary artery catheterization include the following.[29,30]

1. Myocardial infarction within the previous 3 months
2. Coronary artery bypass surgery within the previous 6 months
3. Refractory congestive heart failure
4. Symptomatic valvular heart disease
5. Unstable angina

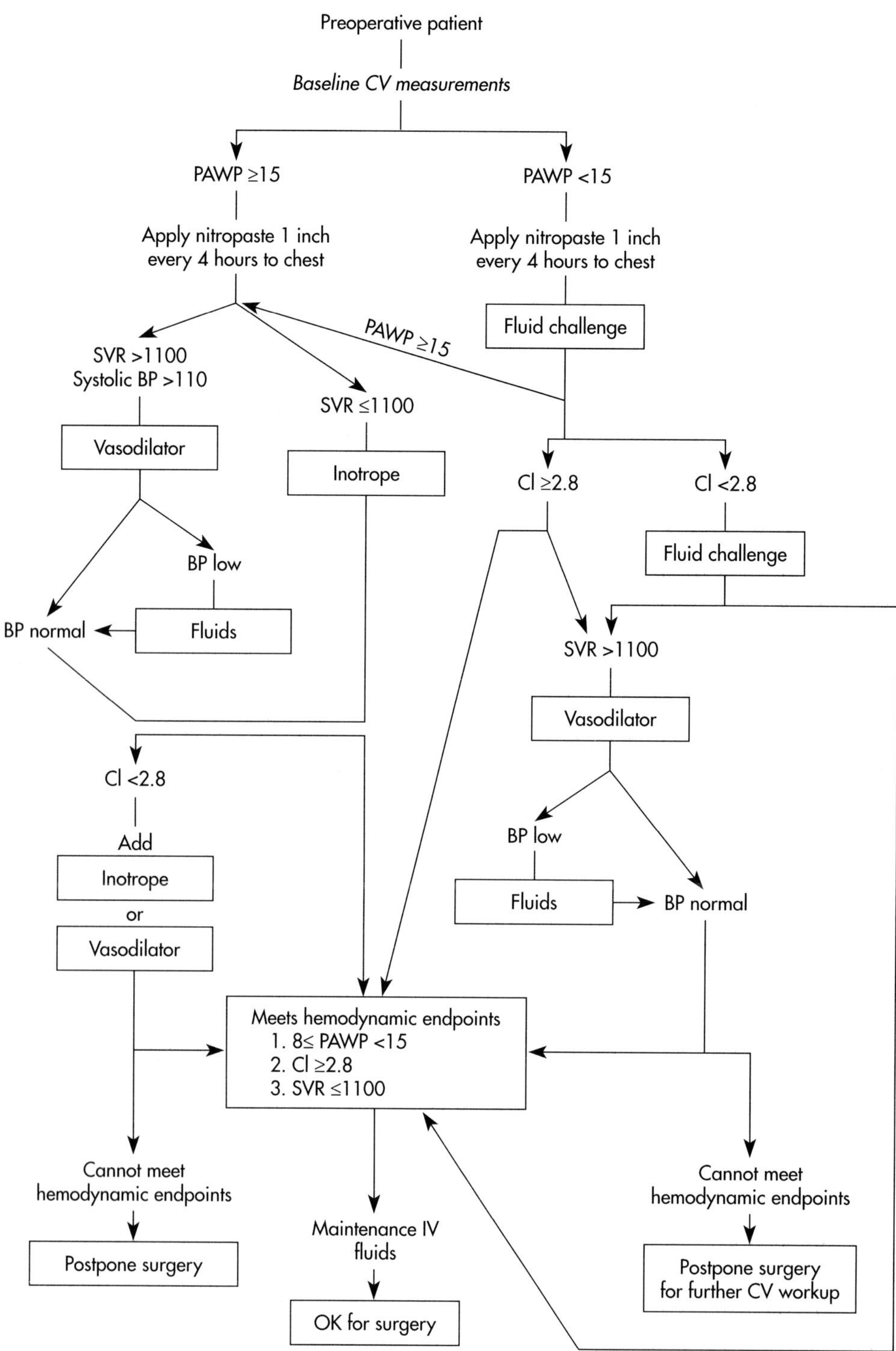

Fig. 13-1. Algorithm for preoperative cardiovascular tune-up. CV measurements were repeated after each intervention. Inotropes: dobutamine or dopamine. Vasodilators: nitroglycerin or nitroprusside. *CI,* Cardiac index; *CV,* cardiovascular; *PAWP,* pulmonary artery wedge pressure; *SVR,* systemic vascular resistance. Measurement units are mm Hg for pressure, dyne-sec cm^{-5} for resistance and $L/min/m^2$ for CI. (From Berlauk JF, et al. Preoperative optimization of cardiovascular hemodynamics improves outcome in peripheral vascular surgery: A prospective, randomized clinical trial. Ann Surg 214(3):289, 1991.)

A recent prospective randomized study by Berlauk et al.[30] exmained the utility of preoperative pulmonary artery catheterization in patients undergoing peripheral vascular surgery who lacked the above indications. Patients receiving pulmonary artery catheters were optimized to the following end points: pulmonary capillary wedge pressure ≥8 mm Hg, <15 mm Hg; cardiac index ≥2.8 L/min/m^2; and systemic vascular resistance ≤1100 dyne-sec cm^{-5} (Fig. 13-1). The death rate was decreased from 9.5% in the control group to 1.5% in the pulmonary artery catheter group, and the overall rate of complications (intraoperative arrhythmia, tachycardia or hypotension, postoperative cardiac morbidity, or early graft thrombosis) decreased from 42.9% to 16.2%. Pulmonary artery catheterization more than 12 hours preoperatively offered no advantage to that performed immediately preoperatively. Although these patients lacked specific indications for pulmonary artery catheter insertion, patients with peripheral vascular disease are known to be at high risk for cardiac complications.[31,32]

Coronary Artery Disease

The cardiovascular effects of anesthesia, along with fluid shifts, may stress those patients with coronary artery disease beyond their ability to respond appropriately. Perioperative myocardial infarction and/or death may result. Myocardial ischemia will, and infarction may, occur when the myocardial oxygen demand exceeds the myocardial oxygen supply. Patients with fixed coronary artery stenoses depend on maintaining coronary artery perfusion pressure above a critical level to prevent ischemia. In these patients, hypotension decreases coronary artery perfusion pressure. A reduction in mean arterial pressure of just 6% may provoke myocardial ischemia.[33] Coronary artery blood flow is dependent both on wall tension and diastolic filling time. In the failing ventricle, increasing preload (end-diastolic pressure) increases wall tension, thereby decreasing coronary perfusion. Tachycardia decreases diastolic filling time, also decreasing coronary perfusion.[34] In hypertensive patients, myocardial oxygen demand is increased, which may provoke ischemia and infarction.[34] Recent myocardial infarction increases the risk of reinfarction and death in the noncardiac surgery patient. In one study, a general anesthetic administered within 3 months of myocardial infarction resulted in a reinfarction rate of 37%. The rate decreased to 16% from 3 to 6 months after infarction to just 6% after 6 months, with an overall mortality of 50% in the

Table 13-2. Computation of the Cardiac Risk Index

Criteria	Multivariate Discriminant-Function Coefficient	"Points"
History		
Age >70 yr	0.191	5
MI in previous 6 mo	0.384	10
Physical Examination		
S_3 gallop or JVD	0.451	11
Important VAS	0.119	3
Electrocardiogram		
Rhythm other than sinus or PACs on last preoperative ECG	0.283	7
>5 PVCs/min documented at any time before operation	0.278	7
General Status		
Po_2 <60 or Pco_2 >50 mm Hg, K <3 or HCO_3^- <20 mEq/L, BUN >50 or Cr >3 mg/dl, abnormal SGOT, signs of chronic liver disease or patient bed ridden from noncardiac causes	0.132	3
Operation		
Intraperitoneal, intrathoracic or aortic operation	0.123	3
Emergency operation	0.167	4
TOTAL POSSIBLE		53 points

From Goldman L, et al. Multifactorial index of cardiac risk in noncardiac surgical procedures. N Engl J Med 297(16):845, 1977.
BUN, Blood urea nitrogen; *Cr,* creatinine; *ECG,* electrocardiogram; *HCO_3^-,* bicarbonate; *JVD,* jugular-vein distention; *K,* potassium; *MI,* myocardial infarction; *PACs,* premature atrial contractions; *Pco_2,* partial pressure of carbon dioxide; *Po_2,* partial pressure of oxygen; *PVCs,* premature ventricular contractions; *SGOT,* serum glutamic-oxalacetic transaminase; *VAS,* valvular aortic stenosis.

Table 13-3. Cardiac Risk Index

Class	Point Total	No or Only Minor Complication (N = 943)	Life-Threatening Complications* (N = 39)	Cardiac Deaths (N = 19)
I (N = 537)	0-5	532 (99)†	4 (0.7)	1 (0.2)
II (N = 316)	6-12	295 (93)	16 (5)	5 (2)
III (N = 130)	13-25	112 (86)	15 (11)	3 (2)
IV (N = 18)	>26	4 (22)	4 (22)	10 (56)

From Goldman L, et al. Multifactorial index of cardiac risk in noncardiac surgical procedures. N Engl J Med 297(16):845, 1977.
*Documented intraoperative or postoperative myocardial infarction, pulmonary edema, or ventricular tachycardia without progression to cardiac death.
†Figures in parentheses denote %.

Table 13-4. Modified Multifactorial Index

Variables	Points
Coronary artery disease	
Myocardial infarction within 6 mo	10
Myocardial infarction >6 mo	
Canadian Cardiovascular Society angina	5
Class 3	10
Class 4	20
Unstable angina within 3 mo	10
Alveolar pulmonary edema	
Within 1 wk	10
Ever	5
Valvular disease	
Suspected critical aortic stenosis	20
Arrhythmias	
Sinus plus atrial premature beats or rhythm other than sinus on last preoperative electrocardiogram	5
>5 ventricular premature beats at any time prior to surgery	5
Poor general medical status*	5
Age >70 yr	5
Emergency operation	10

From Detsky AS, et al. Cardiac assessment for patients undergoing noncardiac surgery: A multifactorial clinical risk index. Arch Intern Med 16:2131, 1986.
*Oxygen pressure <60 mm Hg; carbon dioxide pressure >50 mm Hg; serum potassium <3 mEq/L (<3 mmol/L); serum bicarbonate <20 mEq/L (<20 mmol/L); serum urea nitrogen >50 mg/dl (>18 mmol/L); serum creatinine >3 mg/dl (>260 mmol/L); aspartate aminotransferase, abnormal signs of chronic liver disease; and/or bedridden from noncardiac causes.

Table 13-5. Sensitivity, Specificity, and Confidence Interval (CI) (95%) for Seven Multivariate Predictors of Postoperative Ischemic Events

Predictors	Sensitivity	Specificity
	% (95% CI)	
Redistribution on thallium imaging	83 (65-94)	66 (59-75)
Q wave on ECG	47 (28-66)	85 (78-90)
Ischemic ECG changes after dipyridamole infusion	53 (32-72)	83 (77-88)
Age >70 yr	50 (30-69)	68 (61-75)
History of angina	53 (32-72)	75 (68-81)
History of ventricular ectopic activity	13 (1-28)	96 (86-100)
Diabetes	33 (18-53)	88 (75-100)

From Eagle KA, et al. Combining clinical and thallium data optimizes preoperative assessment of cardiac risk before major vascular surgery. Arch Intern Med 110:859, 1989.

reinfarcted patients.[35] Thus following myocardial infarction, elective procedures should be delayed 6 months. In the emergent setting, aggressive cardiac management with invasive hemodynamic monitoring can reduce the risk of reinfarction to approximately 6% in patients suffering myocardial infarction within the previous 6 months.[36]

Several investigators have proposed criteria to assess the risk of perioperative cardiac complications. Goldman et al.[1] identified nine risk factors that correlated with life-threatening and fatal cardiac complications in patients having noncardiac surgery (Table 13-2). These factors stratify patients into four risk categories (Table 13-3). Patients in Goldman class III (13 to 25 points) warrant preoperative cardiology consultation, whereas patients in Goldman class IV (26 points or more) should only undergo truly lifesaving procedures. Detsky et al.[2] modified the original Goldman criteria to account for both the type of operation and the presence of angina (Table 13-4). In patients undergoing vascular procedures both the Goldman and Detsky indexes appear to underestimate the risk of postoperative cardiac events.[31] Coronary artery disease may be found in up to 90% of patients undergoing major vascular surgery, and 60% of these patients may have a critical stenosis in at least one coronary artery.[32] Moreover, a significant proportion of patients with vascular disorders are unable to tolerate exercise stress testing because of claudication or other noncardiac problems. Eagle et al.[31] developed a cardiac risk assessment schema for these patients combining clinical criteria with preoperative dipyridamole-thallium testing. Clinical predictors for postoperative ischemic events are Q waves on electrocardiogram, age greater than 70 years, history of angina, history of ventricular ectopic activity, and diabetes. Variables on dipyridamole-thallium

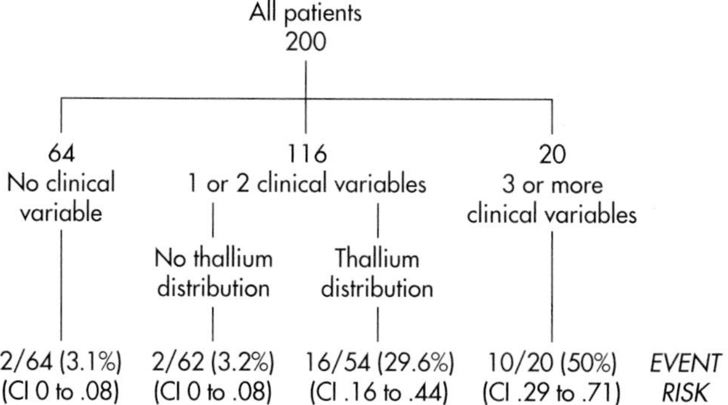

Fig. 13-2. Algorithm for using clinical variables and results of dipyridamole-thallium imaging to stratify cardiac risk as applied to this group of 200 patients. Event refers to postoperative cardiac ischemic events including unstable angina, ischemic pulmonary edema, myocardial infarction, or cardiac death. Clinical variables are Q wave on electrocardiogram, age greater than 70 years, history of angina, history of ventricular ectopic activity requiring treatment, and diabetes mellitus requiring treatment. *CI,* Cardiac index. (From Eagle KA, et al. Combining clinical and thallium data optimizes preoperative assessment of cardiac risk before major vascular surgery. Arch Intern Med 110:859, 1989.)

imaging that predict postoperative ischemia are ischemic electrocardiogram changes after dipyridamole infusion and redistribution on thallium imaging (Table 13-5). The algorithm Eagle et al.[31] applied to their study of 200 patients is presented in Fig. 13-2. Moderate-risk patients should undergo perioperative hemodynamic monitoring with pulmonary artery catheterization. High-risk patients should be referred for preoperative cardiac catheterization and possible coronary artery revascularization.

Congestive Heart Failure

Left ventricular dysfunction eventually leads to cardiac pump failure. Compensatory mechanisms include ventricular dilation and hypertrophy. As the ejection fraction decreases, end-systolic and end-diastolic volumes increase. This increases both end-diastolic and end-systolic ventricular pressures, resulting in increased wall stress, and increased myocardial oxygen consumption. As ventricular compliance decreases, cardiac output increasingly depends on diastolic filling time. Thus tachycardia is poorly tolerated.[37,38] The overall 5-year mortality in patients with congestive heart failure is 50%.[39] Predictors of mortality include poor functional capacity, high pulmonary capillary wedge pressure, low stroke work index, spontaneous ventricular arrhythmias, and elevated plasma levels of norepinephrine and renin.[38] Congestive heart failure is a risk factor for perioperative mortality.[1,2] Treatment consists of preload reduction with sodium restriction and diuretics. Digitalis improves myocardial contractility.[37] Afterload reduction with isosorbide dinitrate and hydralazine improves cardiac output and reduces long-term mortality.[40] Angiotensin-converting enzyme (ACE) inhibitors improve cardiac function, probably by both afterload reduction and interruption of the sodium and water retention characteristic of congestive heart failure.[41] ACE inhibitors also reduce long-term mortality.[41]

Hypertension

Chronic hypertension is associated with an increased risk for stroke (particularly lacunar infarcts),[42] renal failure,[43] and atherosclerotic diseases, including coronary artery disease, carotid artery disease, and peripheral vascular disease.[44,45] Hypertension is also an independent risk factor for myocardial infarction in otherwise healthy-appearing men.[46] Left ventricular hypertrophy and congestive heart failure are particularly ominous findings in these patients.[47,48] Effective long-term blood pressure control[49] can prevent these complications. Once established, blood pressure control does little to reverse end-organ damage.

Hypertension also has deleterious effects that can be minimized in the immediate perioperative period. Hypertension increases myocardial oxygen consumption by increasing myocardial wall tension.[34] Hypertensive patients with a preoperative diastolic blood pressure consistently ≥100 mm Hg have a 33% to 55% incidence of silent myocardial ischemia, whereas well-treated hypertensive patients have a 12% to 20% incidence.[50] Hypertension may be arrhythmogenic as well, particularly in patients with a history of ventricular ectopic beats.[51] Abrupt withdrawal of antihypertensive medications may result in rebound hypertension.

Hypertensive patients with the cardinal symptoms of headache, diaphoresis, and palpitations must have both plasma catecholamines and urinary metanephrines measured to exclude pheochromocytoma.[52] Patients with pheochromocytoma may develop hypertensive crisis during periods of stress or stimulation, such as induction of anesthesia or during intubation. Therefore α_1-adrenergic blocking agents, such as prazosin or phenoxybenzamine, should be administered preoperatively. These patients may be chronically volume depleted. Without preoperative fluid repletion, they may become hypotensive following extirpation of the tumor.[52]

Preoperatively, hypertensive patients should have the following:[22]

1. Antihypertensive medications maintained up to and following surgery
2. Systolic blood pressure not to exceed 160 mm Hg
3. Diastolic blood pressure not to exceed 110 mm Hg
4. Secondary causes of hypertension excluded

Valvular Heart Disease

In general, patients with asymptomatic valvular heart disease tolerate operation well. Bacterial endocarditis may develop in any patient with valvular abnormalities. Arrhythmias associated with valvular conditions may increase perioperative morbidity and mortality. Any history of rheumatic heart disease or cardiac murmurs, fevers, chills, dyspnea at rest or with exertion, and syncopal episodes should be sought, and exercise tolerance specifically documented. Valvular heart disease is usually diagnosed during the physical examination by the detection of cardiac murmurs. The examination should also seek to elicit evidence of rhythm disturbances, cardiomegaly, congestive heart failure (rales, jugulovenous distention, S_3 gallop, peripheral edema), or bacterial endocarditis (fever, petechiae, splinter hemorrhages, Janeway lesions).[53]

Mitral stenosis. Mitral stenosis results in impaired diastolic filling of the left ventricle, with elevation of left atrial and pulmonary venous pressures. In moderate mitral stenosis, symptoms of pulmonary venous hypertension develop with increased cardiac demand, such as with exercise or stress. With further reductions in mitral valve area, sustained pulmonary hypertension and right ventricular failure may ensue, leading to dyspnea even at rest. With left atrial enlargement, atrial fibrillation may occur. Fluid administration should be judicious. Indeed, the dyspneic patient with mitral stenosis often responds well to diuretics.[54] Maintenance of stroke volume and cardiac output is exquisitely dependent on left ventricular filling during diastole.[55] Heart rate must be well controlled to preserve adequate diastolic filling. Digitalis may be given preoperatively, both to prevent atrial fibrillation and to control the ventricular rate should atrial fibrillation occur.[56]

Mitral regurgitation. Mitral regurgitation results in volume overload of the left ventricle. With left ventricular contraction, a proportion of the stroke volume is regurgitated into the left atrium and the pulmonary veins. The left ventricle eventually dilates and hypertrophies to maintain forward cardiac output. Fatigue, dyspnea, and fluid retention may be seen. Pressure overload of the left atrium and pulmonary veins may occur but is generally less severe than that seen with mitral stenosis. Atrial fibrillation is common as the left atrium enlarges. Afterload reduction with vasodilators improves forward cardiac output. Inotropic agents decrease left ventricular volume, thereby decreasing the diameter of the mitral annulus and the degree of regurgitation. Digitalis is used to control the ventricular rate in atrial fibrillation.[54,56]

Aortic stenosis. The classic symptoms of aortic stenosis are angina pectoris, dyspnea, and syncope or dizziness with exertion.[57] Aortic stenosis results in an elevation of the left ventricular systolic pressure to maintain cardiac output. Concentric left ventricular hypertrophy develops, leading to increased ventricular wall tension and a greater myocardial oxygen demand. The pressure gradient across the aortic valve decreases systemic diastolic pressure, thereby limiting coronary artery blood flow. Because the myocardial oxygen supply is limited, angina becomes common. Exertional syncope results when the heart is no longer able to increase cardiac output to meet increased demand (fixed cardiac output). Ventricular arrhythmias are common with severe aortic stenosis and may be precipitated by exercise.[58] Left ventricular end-diastolic pressure and left ventricular end-systolic volume eventually increase to compensate for left ventricular outflow obstruction.[58] Patients with symptomatic aortic stenosis have a poor prognosis with a 30% expected mortality within 4 years.[59] Stroke volume depends on maintaining an adequate left ventricular diastolic pressure and preserving ventricular diastolic filling time. Therefore patients should be well hydrated, and the heart rate should be well controlled.[56]

Aortic regurgitation. Aortic regurgitation results in left ventricular dilation and hypertrophy. The left ventricle remains compliant so that end-diastolic pressure is only modestly elevated. As the severity of aortic regurgitation increases, left atrial and mitral valve dilation occurs. Symptoms seen with severe regurgitation are usually those of left ventricular failure with dyspnea, orthopnea, and paroxysmal noctural dypsnea. Patients respond to diuretics and digitalis. Hypertension should be well controlled. Vasodilators increase forward flow by decreasing ventricular afterload.[54,56]

Prosthetic heart valves. A properly functioning prosthetic heart valve in place should require no specific hemodynamic consideration. The patient is at increased risk, how-

CARDIAC CONDITIONS ASSOCIATED WITH ENDOCARDITIS

Endocarditis Prophylaxis Recommended
High-risk category

- Prosthetic cardiac valves, including bioprosthetic and homograft valves
- Previous bacterial endocarditis
- Complex cyanotic congenital heart disease (e.g., single ventricle states, transposition of the great arteries, tetralogy of Fallot)
- Surgically constructed systemic pulmonary shunts or conduits

Moderate-risk category

- Most other congenital cardiac malformations (other than above and below)
- Acquired valvar dysfunction (e.g., rheumatic heart disease)
- Hypertrophic cardiomyopathy
- Mitral valve prolapse with valvar regurgitation and/or thickened leaflets

Endocarditis Prophylaxis Not Recommended
Negligible-risk category (no greater risk than the general population)

- Isolated secundum atrial septal defect
- Surgical repair of atrial septal defect, ventricular septal defect, or patent ductus arteriosus (without residua beyond 6 mo)
- Previous coronary artery bypass graft surgery
- Mitral valve prolapse without valvar regurgitation
- Physiologic, functional, or innocent heart murmurs
- Previous Kawasaki disease without valvar dysfunction
- Previous rheumatic fever without valvar dysfunction
- Cardiac pacemakers (intravascular and epicardial) and implanted defibrillators

From Dajani AS, et al. Prevention of bacterial endocarditis: Recommendations by the American Heart Association. JAMA 277:1795, 1997.

ever, for endocarditis and thromboembolism. Patients with mechanical valves require long-term anticoagulation with warfarin, whereas those with tissue valves frequently require anticoagulation only for the first 3 to 6 months. If atrial fibrillation occurs, even patients with tissue valves should receive long-term anticoagulation.[60] Oral anticoagulation with warfarin should be halted 3 to 5 days prior to a planned surgical procedure to allow the prothrombin time (PT) to correct to less than 13 seconds. Therapeutic anticoagulation with intravenous heparin should be employed during this period. Heparin should be discontinued 6 to 12 hours prior to surgery and restarted within 6 hours postoperatively. Warfarin should be restarted as soon as the patient is tolerating oral liquids.[61] Reversing anticoagulation with vitamin K or fresh frozen plasma should be reserved for emergency situations because of the risk of thrombosis.[61]

DENTAL PROCEDURES AND ENDOCARDITIS PROPHYLAXIS

Endocarditis Prophylaxis Recommended*

Dental extractions
Periodontal procedures including surgery, scaling and root planing, probing, and recall maintenance
Dental implant placement and reimplantation of avulsed teeth
Endodontic (root canal) instrumentation or surgery only beyond the apex
Subgingival placement of antibiotic fibers or strips
Initial placement of orthodontic bands but not brackets
Intraligamentary local anesthetic injections
Prophylactic cleaning of teeth or implants where bleeding is anticipated

Endocarditis Prophylaxis Not Recommended

Restorative dentistry† (operative and prosthodontic) with or without retraction cord‡
Local anesthetic injections (nonintraligamentary)
Intracanal endodontic treatment; post placement and buildup
Placement of rubber dams
Postoperative suture removal
Placement of removable prosthodontic or orthodontic appliances
Taking of oral impressions
Fluoride treatments
Taking of oral radiographs
Orthodontic appliance adjustment
Shedding of primary teeth

From Dajani AS, et al. Prevention of bacterial endocarditis: Recommendations by the American Heart Association. JAMA 277:1797, 1997.
*Prophylaxis is recommended for patients with high- and moderate-risk cardiac conditions.
†This includes restoration of decayed teeth (filling cavities) and replacement of missing teeth.
‡Clinical judgment may indicate antibiotic use in selected circumstances that may create significant bleeding.

Endocarditis. Patients with significant valvular heart disease or prosthetic heart valves are at increased risk for the development of bacterial endocarditis. In patients at risk, prophylactic antibiotics should be started 1 hour prior to the procedure and continued for less than 24 hours. The boxes on pp. 302 and 303, and Tables 13-6 and 13-7 re-

OTHER PROCEDURES AND ENDOCARDITIS PROPHYLAXIS

Endocarditis Prophylaxis Recommended

Respiratory tract
- Tonsillectomy and/or adenoidectomy
- Surgical operations that involve respiratory mucosa
- Bronchoscopy with a rigid bronchoscope

Gastrointestinal tract*
- Sclerotherapy for esophageal varices
- Esophageal stricture dilation
- Endoscopic retrograde cholangiography with biliary obstruction
- Biliary tract surgery
- Surgical operations that involve intestinal mucosa

Genitourinary tract
- Prostatic surgery
- Cystoscopy
- Urethral dilation

Endocarditis Prophylaxis Not Recommended

Respiratory tract
- Endotracheal intubation
- Bronchoscopy with a flexible bronchoscope with or without biopsy†
- Tympanostomy tube insertion

Gastrointestinal tract
- Transesophageal echocardiography†
- Endoscopy with or without gastrointestinal biopsy†

Genitourinary tract
- Vaginal hysterectomy†
- Vaginal delivery†
- Cesarean section
- In uninfected tissue:
  - Urethral catheterization
  - Uterine dilatation and curettage
  - Therapeutic abortion
  - Sterilization procedures
  - Insertion or removal of intrauterine devices

Other
- Cardiac catheterization, including balloon angioplasty
- Implanted cardiac pacemakers, implanted defibrillators, and coronary stents
- Incision or biopsy of surgically scrubbed skin
- Circumcision

From Dajani AS, et al. Prevention of bacterial endocarditis: Recommendations by the American Heart Association. JAMA 277:1797, 1997.
*Prophylaxis is recommended for high-risk patients; optional for medium-risk patients.
†Prophylaxis is optional for high-risk patients.

Table 13-6. Prophylactic Regimens for Dental, Oral, Respiratory Tract, or Esophageal Procedures

Situation	Agent	Regimen*
Standard general prophylaxis	Amoxicillin	Adults: 2 g; children: 50 mg/kg orally 1 hr before procedure
Unable to take oral medications	Ampicillin	Adults: 2 g intramuscularly (IM) or intravenously (IV); children: 50 mg/kg IM or IV within 30 min before procedure
Allergic to penicillin	Clindamycin	Adults: 500 mg; children: 20 mg/kg orally 1 hr before procedure
	or	
	Cephalexin† or cefadroxil†	Adults: 2 g; children: 50 mg/kg orally 1 hr before procedure
	or	
	Azithromycin or clarithromycin	Adults: 500 mg; children: 15 mg/kg orally 1 hr before procedure
Allergic to penicillin and unable to take oral medications	Clindamycin	Adults: 600 mg/ children: 20 mg/kg IV within 30 min before procedure
	or	
	Cefazolin†	Adults: 1 g; children: 25 mg/kg IM or IV within 30 min before procedure

From Dajani AS, et al. Prevention of bacterial endocarditis: Recommendations by the American Heart Association. JAMA 277:1798, 1997.
*Total children's dose should not exceed adult dose.
†Cephalosporins should not be used in individuals with immediate-type hypersensitivity reaction (urticaria, angioedema, or anaphylaxis) to penicillins.

Table 13-7. Prophylactic Regimens for Genitourinary/Gastrointestinal (Excluding Esophageal) Procedures

Situation	Agents*	Regimen†
High-risk patients	Ampicillin plus gentamicin	Adults: Ampicillin 2 g intramuscularly (IM) or intravenously (IV) plus gentamicin 1.5 mg/kg (not to exceed 120 mg) within 30 min of starting procedure; 6 hr later, ampicillin 1 g IM/IV or amoxicillin 1 g orally Children: Ampicillin 50 mg/kg IM or IV (not to exceed 2 g) plus gentamicin 1.5 mg/kg within 30 min of starting procedure; 6 hr later, ampicillin 25 mg/kg IM/IV or amoxicillin 25 mg/kg orally
High-risk patients allergic to ampicillin/amoxicillin	Vancomycin plus gentamicin	Adults: Vancomycin 1 g IV over 1-2 hr plus gentamicin 1.5 mg/kg IV/IM (not to exceed 120 mg); complete injection/infusion within 30 min of starting procedure Children: Vancomycin 20 mg/kg IV over 1-2 hr plus gentamicin 1.5 mg/kg IV/IM; complete injection/infusion within 30 min of starting procedure
Moderate-risk patients	Amoxicillin or ampicillin	Adults: Amoxicillin 2 g orally 1 hr before procedure, or ampicillin 2 g IM/IV within 30 min of starting procedure Children: Amoxicillin 50 mg/kg orally 1 hr before procedure, or ampicillin 50 mg/kg IM/IV within 30 min of starting procedure
Moderate-risk patients allergic to ampicillin/amoxicillin	Vancomycin	Adults: Vancomycin 1.0 g IV over 1-2 hr; complete infusion within 30 min of starting procedure Children: Vancomycin 20 mg/kg IV over 1-2 hr; complete infusion within 30 min of starting procedure

From Dajani AS, et al. Prevention of bacterial endocarditis: Recommendations by the American Heart Association. JAMA 277:1799, 1997.
*Total children's dose should not exceed adult dose.
†No second dose of vancomycin.

view the indications for prophylaxis and the regimens recommended by the American Heart Association.[62]

Cerebrovascular Disease

Patients with carotid artery disease are at increased risk for stroke in the perioperative period. Patients with significant coronary disease or other stigmata of atherosclerosis should be questioned carefully for a history of transient ischemic attacks or amaurosis fugax. The carotid arteries should be evaluated for bruits and neurologic deficits. If any of these are present, duplex scanning provides a reliable, noninvasive screening test for carotid artery disease. All patients with symptomatic carotid artery disease or asymptomatic critical stenosis (>75%) should be evaluated for carotid endarterectomy prior to undergoing spinal or general anesthesia for an elective procedure.[63]

Risks of Liver Disease

Preoperative evaluation and management of the patient with liver disease is a challenging problem. The liver is involved in numerous metabolic and synthetic processes including amino acid, carbohydrate, and lipid metabolism, excretion of bilirubin and maintenance of glucose homeostasis. Predicting how a patient will respond not only to surgery but also to the effects of anesthesia can be extremely difficult. The evaluation of the patient with overt liver disease must include the cause of the disease (i.e., alcoholic cirrhosis, hepatitis), the chronicity of the disease, and the degree of hepatocellular injury based on both clinical findings and laboratory abnormalities. The magnitude of the surgery to be performed and the type of anesthesia to be administered must also be considered. Patients without overt liver disease but with abnormal liver function test results may require further workup.

Anesthesia

Anesthetic agents may exacerbate hepatic dysfunction. Although none of the currently used anesthetic agents are directly hepatotoxic, these agents, whether inhalational, spinal, or epidural, reduce hepatic blood flow by 30% to 50%.[64,65] Patients with completely normal liver function can develop asymptomatic elevations in transaminases. Those with known hepatic disease may develop clinically apparent impairment.[66] Moreover, impaired liver function may include impaired drug metabolism, thereby prolonging the action of anesthetic agents, sedatives, narcotic analgesics, or induction agents. These agents must be carefully administered with appropriate dosing. Sedative effects and hepatic encephalopathy must be closely monitored.[64]

Liver disease may lead to coagulopathy by several mechanisms. Hepatic disease can be associated with decreased synthesis and function of coagulation proteins, especially the vitamin K–dependent clotting factors.[67] Vitamin K deficiency is common particularly in patients with cholestatic disorders or those receiving antibiotics to suppress endogenous gut flora.[66] Liver disease may lead to qualitative or quantitative platelet abnormalities including the splenic sequestration seen with portal hypertension.

Coagulation factors must be checked preoperatively in any patient with known or suspected liver disease. Patients with obstructive jaundice should receive parenteral vitamin K preoperatively. Failure of vitamin K to correct a prolonged PT indicates severe hepatocellular function.[66] In this case, fresh frozen plasma must be used to achieve an adequate PT for surgery. Bleeding time should be obtained in all patients with less than 100,000 platelets/mm^3 and platelet transfusions considered in patients with elevated bleeding times and/or less than 50,000 platelets/mm^3.[66]

Obviously, purely elective surgery should be postponed in the patient with severe acute hepatic disease. Supportive care during the acute phase reduces operative risk. Operative considerations for specific hepatic disorders are discussed briefly in the following sections.

Acute Viral Hepatitis

Acute viral hepatitis increases operative morbidity and mortality.[68] Laboratory abnormalities seen in these patients include moderate-to-marked elevations in serum transaminase levels and mild elevations in alkaline phosphatase. Jaundice may or may not be present. The specific serologic diagnosis of the viral agent can usually be made.[64] If possible, laparotomy should be avoided in the setting of acute viral hepatitis. The increased availability of accurate serologic testing and radiologic and endoscopic diagnostic procedures usually establishes the diagnosis of hepatitis, thereby obviating the need for surgery.[64,66]

Alcoholic Liver Disease

Alcoholic liver disease can range from fatty liver (hepatic steatosis) to the more severe acute alcoholic hepatitis to cirrhosis. The patient with alcoholic fatty liver is not at increased risk for operative complications.[64,66] Mild elevations in transaminase and alkaline phosphatase may be seen and diagnosis confirmed by liver biopsy. Although elective surgery is not contraindicated, a period of abstinence may be beneficial by avoiding postoperative alcohol withdrawal.

Acute alcoholic hepatitis is more severe than acute viral hepatitis. Several studies have shown significantly increased morbidity and mortality of surgery in patients with alcoholic hepatitis.[69,70] Diagnosis should be made by percutaneous liver biopsy. Elective surgery is contraindicated in this group of patients and should be postponed until laboratory and clinical parameters are normal.

Chronic Hepatitis

Chronic hepatitis refers to a group of disorders characterized by chronic inflammation of the liver persisting for at least 3 to 6 months.[64] Chronic hepatitis is usually divided into chronic persistent form and chronic active form. Patients with chronic persistent hepatitis are usually asymptomatic with only mild laboratory abnormalities. This form is not considered a contraindication to elective surgery and these patients tolerate operation well.[64,71] Chronic active hepatitis is a more ominous disorder, which, unlike chronic persistent hepatitis, may progress to cirrhosis. Mild, asymptomatic anicteric patients with chronic active hepatitis tolerate elective surgery well,[71] whereas symptomatic patients with jaundice and significantly elevated serum liver function test levels have an increased perioperative mortality. Elective operation is contraindicated in these cases.[72]

Cirrhosis

The Child-Turcotte classification is a well-known system that attempts to correlate the severity of cirrhosis (and therefore the hepatic reserve) with expected operative mortality.[73] It grades the degree of ascites, encephalopathy, malnutrition, hyperbilirubinemia, and hypoalbuminemia in the cirrhotic patient. Although the classification was originally intended to evaluate patients undergoing portacaval shunting, it has since been generalized to nonshunt surgery. Patients are classified (A, B, and C) according to the severity of hepatic insufficiency. Mortality rates of 0% to 10%, 4% to 31%, and 19% to 76% are quoted for classes A, B, and C, respectively, for portacaval shunts and nonshunt operations.

In general, patients in Child class A tolerate surgery well, whereas patients in Child class C have a prohibitive operative mortality, thereby contraindicating elective surgery. Patients in Child class B must be assessed individually (see accompanying box).

The preoperative preparation of the cirrhotic patient should include evaluation of the metabolic alterations including hyponatremia, hypoalbuminemia, glucose intolerance, and possible oxygen desaturation.[64] Although these abnormalities may not be completely correctable preoperatively, they should be closely monitored both during and after operation. In addition, coagulation parameters must be evaluated and corrected preoperatively. Nutritional status should be optimized preoperatively when possible. Unfortunately, routine liver function biochemical tests (serum aminotransferase and alkaline phosphatase) tend to correlate poorly with the actual degree of hepatic impairment.[64]

With the availability and routine use of preoperative laboratory tests, the surgeon may encounter patients with unsuspected abnormal results from liver "function" tests while preparing for elective surgery. Although medical consultation may be obtained in these instances, the surgeon should be aware of the necessary further preoperative evaluation of these patients. History of recent drug use, past hepatitis or jaundice, blood transfusions, and general symptoms of liver disease such as malaise, fatigue, and arthralgia are important to elicit.[74] Physical examination should include potential evaluation for the signs of chronic liver disease such as cutaneous spider angiomata, parotid swelling, gynecomastia, palmar erythema, Dupuytren's contractures, organomegaly, ascites, encephalopathy, and poor nutritional status. A serum albumin level and a coagulation profile to assess the functional ability of the liver complement serum levels of bilirubin, alkaline phosphatase, serum glutamic-oxaloacetic transaminase (SGOT), serum glutamate pyruvate transaminase (SGPT), and lactate dehydrogenase (LDH) in assessing injury of the liver.[74]

Clearly patients with underlying liver disease are at increased surgical risk. Essential preoperative preparation of these patients must include correction of coagulopathy and electrolyte abnormalities (hypokalemia, hyponatremia), and control of ascites, hepatic encephalopathy, and infection.[74] Specifically, the PT should be corrected to within 3 seconds of control, preferably with vitamin K. Massive ascites may require paracentesis preoperatively.[75]

RELATIVE HEPATOLOGIC CONTRAINDICATIONS FOR ELECTIVE SURGERY

Active, acute viral hepatitis
Active, acute alcoholic hepatitis
Fulminant hepatitis
Icteric, symptomatic chronic active hepatitis
Contemplated ileostomy or colostomy in a cirrhotic
Contemplated abdominal surgery in OLT candidate
Prothrombin time greater than 3 seconds prolonged (despite vitamin K)
Child C cirrhotic

From Gholson CF, Provenza JM, Bacon BR. Hepatologic considerations in patients with parenchymal liver disease undergoing surgery. Am J Gastroenterol 85:487, 1990.
OLT, Orthotopic liver transplantation.

Risks of Kidney Disease

The kidney performs several important functions, including filtration and elimination of nitrogenous wastes and regulation of fluid volume, electrolyte concentrations, acid-base balance, and blood pressure, as well as performing certain endocrine functions. Moreover, urine output in the patient with normal renal function provides an important, albeit indirect, indication of visceral perfusion. Impairment of renal function generally increases both the risk of operation and the incidence of postoperative complications.[76-78]

Despite the kidney's many functions, renal insufficiency or failure in the surgical patient presents clinically as either oliguria or a rising serum creatinine. Patients with preexisting renal disease may have hypertension, hypoalbuminemia, lethargy, or anorexia.[79] Acute renal failure can be defined as a recent increase of serum creatinine of at least 0.5 mg/dl and reflects the inability of the kidneys to adequately eliminate nitrogenous wastes.[80] Renal creatinine clearance is used to estimate the glomerular filtration rate (GFR). The minimal obligatory urine volume output for an adult is 0.5 mg/kg/hr (1.0 mg/kg/hr in children), although nonoliguric renal failure may be present with seemingly adequate urine volumes. Chronic renal insufficiency predisposes the patient to further renal injury from either hypoperfusion or nephrotoxins.[81]

Acute renal failure is due to either prerenal, postrenal, or intrarenal lesions. Prerenal azotemia results from renal hypoperfusion; although this azotemia is reversible, it will progress to ischemic acute tubular necrosis (ATN) with continued hypoperfusion.[80] Homeostatic mechanisms maintain renal blood flow and GFR in the presence of hypovolemia or hypotension. The oliguria and azotemia seen in the prerenal state represents autoregulation with reabsorption of sodium and water to maintain or expand the effective circulating volume.[80] Causes of prerenal azotemia include hypovolemia, sepsis, neurogenic shock, congestive heart failure, and hepatorenal failure.[82] Whereas sodium and water reabsorption with circulating volume expansion is an appropriate response with a low effective circulating volume, it is an inappropriate response in congestive heart failure, which is characterized by an excessive circulating volume (fluid overload). Restoration of renal perfusion reverses prerenal azotemia. This requires volume administration in hypovolemia, and diuresis in congestive heart failure. Generally, the diagnosis of prerenal azotemia is supported by a high blood urea nitrogen/creatinine ratio (>20:1), a low urine sodium (U_{Na}<20), or a low fractional excretion of sodium (FE_{Na}<1%).[80,81]

Intrarenal acute renal failure may occur from a number of diseases, including the glomerulnephritides; but the most common form encountered in the surgical patient is ATN. ATN results from injury to the renal tubular epithelium, which is responsible for maintaining selective permeability to water and other solutes in ultrafiltrate, as well as for active transport of electrolytes, as is seen in the loop of Henle. Injury may result from hypoperfusion and ischemia or from any number of nephrotoxins. ATN may lead to either oliguric (<400 ml/day) renal failure or nonoliguric renal failure. The renal injury resulting in nonoliguric ATN is less severe than that resulting in the oliguric form.[80]

The causes of ischemic ATN are the same as those resulting in prerenal azotemia, although the insult is more severe. Hypovolemic shock, septic shock, neurogenic shock and congestive heart failure, or cardiogenic shock may result in ATN. Generally, ischemic ATN follows a recognizable period of profound hypotension.[80] The progression from prerenal azotemia to ATN represents a continuum; often restoration of renal perfusion restores some degree of renal function, representing the tubules of those nephons that have not yet succumbed to ischemia.[80] The diagnosis of ATN is supported by the presence of tubular casts on urinalysis, a high U_{Na} (>40) and a high FE_{Na} (>4%).[79,81]

Toxins leading to ATN include heme pigments (from myoglobin and hemoglobin), drugs (aminoglycoside antibiotics), and radiographic contrast agents. With rhabdomyolysis, myoglobin released into the circulation is filtered across the glomerulus. It precipitates in the lumen of the renale tubule; under acidic conditions, the heme moiety dissociates from the protein component and is taken up and metabolized by the tubular epithelium, to which it is ultimately toxic. Hemoglobinuria following massive hemolysis, as in transfusion reactions, causes ATN in an analogous fashion. ATN is prevented by maintaining high urine flow rates and alkalinizing the urine to prevent dissociation of the heme pigment from the globin. Aminoglycosides and radiographic contrast agents may both cause ATN in a dose-dependent fashion, possibly by direct toxicity to the tubular epithelium. These agents potentiate the injury incurred by ischemia or other nephrotoxins and are particularly toxic in the face of preexisting renal insufficiency.

Obstructive jaundice results in postoperative ATN in approximately 16% to 18% of patients. The mortality rate of renal failure in this setting correlates with serum bilirubin levels. Patients with serum bilirubin levels higher than 20 mg% had a mortality rate of 85%; those with levels lower than 10 mg% had a mortality rate of 33%.[75] Obstructive jaundice causes a decrease in total peripheral resistance, either because of peripheral vasodilation or an impairment of the vasoconstrictor response to pressor agents. This leads to a decrease in the effective plasma volume and explains the exaggerated hypotensive response seen with hemorrhage.[75,83] Moreover, obstructive jaundice also decreases renal blood flow.[75,83] The postoperative renal failure seen with obstructive jaundice may simply represent an ischemic ATN related to impaired hemodynamic responses and resultant hypotension, although endotoxin may also play a role. Bile salts bind and inactivate endotoxin, thereby preventing its absorption from the gut lumen.[83] The absence of bile salts in the gut lumen, as seen with obstructive jaundice, results in endotoxemia. This may explain the systemic and intrarenal hemodynamic effects seen with obstructive jaundice.[75,83] The use of oral bile salts appears to prevent endotoxemia.[83] Preoperative external biliary drainage has not been shown to be effective in decreasing the incidence of postoperative renal failure.[83] Current recommendations include preoperative hydration, avoidance of nephrotoxic agents, preoperative administration of mannitol (500 ml of 10% mannitol infused for a period of 1 to 2 hours prior to operation), and oral administration of bile salts preoperatively (sodium deoxycholate 500 mg every 8 hours for 48 hours).[83] The perioperative use of low-dose dopamine (3 μg/kg/min) appears not to be of benefit.[84]

Postrenal azotemia results from obstructive uropathy.[77,80] This commonly results from urethral obstruction, either caused by prostatic hypertrophy (in men) or Foley catheter blockage. Unilateral ureteric obstruction does not generally result in azotemia, as the contralateral kidney compensates by hyperfiltration.[82] If the obstruction is relieved early, postrenal azotemia is reversible. Persistent obstruction results in irreversible renal injury.[85] Foley catheterization usually excludes bladder outlet obstruction, although the Foley catheter itself may be occluded by blood clots or fibrinous exudate. Renal ultrasonography is useful to rule out ureteric obstruction.[86]

Chronic renal failure may result from any number of causes, including atherosclerosis, diabetes, hypertension, glomerulonephritis, ischemia, or exposure to nephrotoxins.[82] It must be recognized that these patients may lack the ability to concentrate or dilute their urine in response to fluid shifts or electrolyte disturbances.[87] Therefore fluid balance and electrolyte concentrations must be monitored meticulously. Excessive administration of potassium, magnesium, and phosphate should be avoided. Dosages of drugs that undergo renal excretion should be decreased according to the patient's estimated GFR. Exposure to nephrotoxins should be avoided. Chronic renal failure may also be associated with anemia which should be corrected preoperatively.[87,88]

Risk factors for the development of perioperative renal failure include preexisting renal insufficiency, diabetes mellitus, advanced age, jaundice, and aortic or cardiac surgery.[77,89] To preserve renal function, patients should be well hydrated prior to surgery and prior to the administration of potentially nephrotoxic agents. Fluid shifts and electrolyte loads should be minimized. Hypotension should be avoided. Invasive hemodynamic monitoring with pulmonary artery catheterization should be considered both in patients requiring cardiac optimization and in those undergoing surgery in which large fluid shifts can be anticipated. In the presence of oliguria, postrenal factors should be excluded, urine output should be carefully monitored, and prerenal factors (either hypovolemia or inadequate cardiac function) should be corrected.[87,88]

Patients with ESRD requiring dialysis have an increased risk for perioperative morbidity and mortality.[78,90] These patients have a high incidence of associated diseases, including diabetes mellitus, hypertension, and coronary artery disease. Complications include hyperkalemia, sepsis, hemorrhage, cardiac dysfunction, and hemodynamic instability.[78] Anemia is common because of decreased erythropoietin production. A hematocrit less than 25% should be corrected, either electively with recombinant human erythropoietin or emergently with blood transfusion.[87,91] The qualitative platelet dysfunction may be due to circulating guanidinosuccinic and hydroxyphenolic acids, which inhibit platelet factor 3 activity.[92] Dialysis improves platelet function, as will administration of cryoprecipitate, 1-deamino-8-D-arginine vasopression (DDAVP), or conjugated estrogens. Platelet transfusions are used for significant hemorrhage.[92] Ideally, the patient with ESRD should receive dialysis within 24 hours of operation.[88] Excessive hydration should be avoided. In patients with significant coronary artery disease, invasive hemodynamic monitoring should be considered.

Risks of Endocrine Disease

Diabetes Mellitus

Diabetes mellitus is a common disorder or carbohydrate metabolism with an estimated prevalence of between 2% and 5% in the United States.[93] The hyperglycemia associated with diabetes results from either a deficiency of insulin (type I) or a resistance to its action (type II). Complications from diabetes mellitus are common and include diabetic retinopathy, nephropathy, neuropathy, and an accelerated atherosclerosis. Diabetic sensory neuropathy usually has a "stocking and glove" distribution. Diabetic autonomic neuropathy may lead to postural hypotension, arrhythmias, gastroparesis, and urinary retention. Diabetes is the most common cause of blindness in the United States and is responsible for more than 25% of new cases of ESRD, and for more than 50% of all lower extremity amputations.[94]

As a result of the expected long-term sequelae of diabetes mellitus, approximately 50% of all diabetic patients eventually require surgery.[95] Because of the high incidence of coronary artery disease and renal dysfunction in this population, the expected perioperative morbidity and mortality in the diabetic patient are higher than that of the nondiabetic patient.[93] Furthermore, defects in wound healing and the immune system condemn the diabetic patient to a higher rate of wound complications.[96-98]

Although no prospective study demonstrates an improved surgical outcome in the euglycemic as opposed to the hyperglycemic patient,[99] hyperglycemia may lead to profound fluid and electrolyte depletion, altered immune function, and impaired wound healing.[96-98,100,101] Adequate insulin administration corrects the defects in granulocyte and fibroblast function seen with hyperglycemia.[101] Intuitively, it would seem that perioperative glycemic control should minimize surgical risk. Achieving glycemic control may be challenging because of the diabetogenic response elicited by the stress of surgery, anesthesia, and inflammation.[99] Part of the response to stress is an increased release of the counterregulatory hormones (epinephrine, glucagon, cortisol, growth factor) each of which either directly or indirectly stimulate glucose production.[99] In addition, these hormones are primarily catabolic, thereby promoting significant lipolysis and ketogenesis.[99]

Preoperative assessment. Prior to operation, the patient's type of diabetes should be determined and the patient's regimen for glycemic control should be clearly ascertained. The adequacy of recent glycemic control may be determined by reviewing blood glucose records and by obtaining a glycosylated hemoglobin level. Patients taking oral hypoglycemics should be screened for episodes of profound hypoglycemia, which is a common complication of these medications. Complications of diabetes should be identified preoperatively as well. Thus a thorough assessment of cardiovascular status and a determination of renal function (screening serum creatinine) are necessary, as is identification of any diabetic sensory or autonomic neuropathy.

Insulin and fluid administration. Plasma glucose levels should be tightly controlled perioperatively, avoiding hypoglycemia and hyperglycemia. The stress response to infection, inflammation, and surgery increases plasma glucose levels. Even moderate elevations in plasma glucose levels may result in glycosuria and therefore an osmotic diuresis. Although this may lead to volume depletion and electrolyte disturbances in non–insulin-dependent patients, it may progress to overt diabetic ketoacidosis in those who are insulin dependent.[99] If diabetic ketoacidosis is present, operation must be postponed until the patient's fluid volume is restored and the pH, electrolyte, and glucose levels are corrected.[93]

Preoperatively, the insulin dose must be adjusted for the fasting patient. All diabetic patients, both insulin and non–insulin dependent, should receive insulin therapy during surgery.[102] Indications for insulin therapy are summarized in the box on p. 309. A number of acceptable regimens for administration have been described, and no single regimen has been proved to be superior.[102] A common regimen used for insulin-dependent patients is to give fasting patients one half of their usual morning dose of intermediate-acting insulin subcutaneously on the morning of operation. The serum glucose is then checked every 2 to 4 hours and supplemental intermediate-acting insulin is ad-

INDICATIONS FOR INSULIN THERAPY DURING AN OPERATION

Always

All patients taking insulin—both insulin-dependent diabetes mellitus and non–insulin-dependent diabetes (NIDDM)

Patients with NIDDM treated with diet, oral hypoglycemic agents, or both but having chronic hyperglycemia (FBG >10 mmol/L and glycosylated Hb >0.1)

Variable

Patients with NIDDM treated with diet, oral hypoglycemic agents, or both, under good control
- Current FBG ≤10 mmol/L
- Glycosylated Hb 0.08 to 0.1
- Duration of operation less than 2 hours
- Use of glucose solutions not planned

From Gavin LA. Management of diabetes mellitus during surgery. West J Med 151:525, 1989. Reprinted by permission of The Western Journal of Medicine.
FBG, Fasting blood glucose; *Hb*, hemoglobin.

ministered according to a sliding scale dosage. This is continued until the patients can eat normally and resume their usual regimen.

Subcutaneous administration of insulin may result in erratic absorption and unpredictable serum levels, particularly with the hemodynamic changes seen perioperatively.[99,103,104,105] Intravenous administration of insulin offers the theoretic advantage of more predictable serum levels of insulin. Table 13-8 provides a guideline for perioperative intravenous insulin administration. Although fixed-rate insulin infusions offer no proven advantage over subcutaneous administration,[100,104] variable-rate infusions may be more useful to stabilize glucose levels.[106] Continuous intravenous insulin infusion is clearly superior to other methods when used intraoperatively,[107] although this unfortunately remains an underutilized technique.[108] If continuous intravenous insulin infusion is used, it generally is continued until the patient is eating.[99,109]

Preoperative intravenous fluids should provide dextrose to prevent hypoglycemia and the accumulation of ketones and free fatty acids. Five percent dextrose should be added to maintenance intravenous fluids, generally half normal saline, running at roughly 1 ml/kg/hr for adults. Since lactate is a gluconeogenic precursor, lactated Ringer's solution administered at a high infusion rate may produce hyperglycemia.[110] Thus additional fluid requirements should be met with dextrose-free solutions.

Table 13-8. Algorithm Guidelines for Perioperative Diabetes Management of Separate Insulin and Glucose Infusions

Insulin
- Regular, 25 U, in 250 ml normal saline (1 U/10 ml)

Infuse insulin intravenously from an infusion pump; flush 50 ml through line before connecting to patient; piggyback this line to the perioperative maintenance fluids infusion line

Monitor blood glucose levels hourly during operation and every 2-4 hr before and after operation once stable

Perioperative maintenance fluids must contain dextrose (5%)

Do the initial blood glucose measurement "stat" in the clinical laboratory

Blood Glucose		Insulin		
mmol/L	**(mg/dl)**	**U/hr**	**ml/hr**	**Fluids ml/hr**
≤4.4	(≤80)	0	0	125
4.5-5.5	(81-100)	0.5	5	125
5.6-7.8	(101-140)	1	10	125
7.9-10	(141-180)	1.5	15	125
10.1-12.2	(181-220)	2	20	125
12.3-14.4	(221-260)	2.5	25	100
14.5-16.6	(261-300)	3	30	100
16.7-18.9	(301-340)	4	40	100
>18.9	(>341)	5	50	100

Blood glucose ≤4.4 mmol/L, bolus with 50% dextrose in water (25 ml); once blood glucose >4.4 mmol/L, restart insulin infusion and recheck in 30 min

Decreased insulin needs
- Patients treated with diet, oral agents, or <50 U insulin per day

Increased insulin needs
- Sepsis, steroid therapy (renal transplantation), coronary artery bypass

If high-dose insulin is anticipated, a more concentrated insulin solution should be prepared to avoid excessive fluid intake

From Gavin LA. Management of diabetes mellitus during surgery. West J Med 151:525, 1989. Reprinted by permission of The Western Journal of Medicine.

Cortisol Metabolic Dysfunction

Cortisol is synthesized, stored, and secreted from cells of the adrenal cortex. Release is controlled primarily by the anterior pituitary hormone adrenocorticotropic hormone (ACTH). Cortisol influences the metabolism of glucose, amino acids, and fatty acids and potentiates the actions of glucagon and epinephrine in the liver.

Cortisol secretion, in response to increased ACTH production, is increased by acute stress including fever, pain, hemorrhage, and operative trauma. The glucocorticoid activity of cortisol maintains the responsiveness of small vessels to catecholamines, thereby maintaining vascular tone. Moreover, glucocorticoids influence the distribution of total body water to maintain intravascular volume.[111,112] Insufficient cortisol release in response to stress may be life threatening. It may result from primary adrenal gland insufficiency (addisonian crisis) or from suppression of the hypothalamic-pituitary-adrenal cortical axis, as is seen with chronic steroid therapy.

Signs and symptoms of chronic adrenal insufficiency are nonspecific and include weakness, nausea, fever, weight loss, lethargy, and even delirium. Hyponatremia and hyperkalemia result from mineralocorticoid (aldosterone) deficiency. Hypoglycemia may reflect glucocorticoid deficiency leading to diminished hepatic gluconeogenesis, even with elevated levels of glucagon and epinephrine. Hypercalcemia is also seen, and blood count differentials may reveal eosinophilia.[112] Acute adrenal insufficiency presents clinically as hypotension with a high cardiac output and a low systemic vascular resistance that is resistant to pressors but responds to glucocorticoid administration.[113]

Although circulatory collapse caused by adrenal insufficiency is a decidely uncommon complication of surgery (0.01% to 0.7% of cases),[114] patients at risk should be identified to receive perioperative stress doses of glucocorticoids. The functional status of the hypothalamic-pituitary-adrenal cortical axis should be assessed for receiving patients chronic glucocorticoid therapy, particularly if they show signs of Cushing's syndrome. While a plasma cortisol level of greater than 500 nmol/L is suggestive of adequate adrenal function, the 30-minute ACTH stimulation test provides an accurate screening test for adrenal dysfunction.[114]

Recommended stress doses of steroids typically consist of 50 to 100 mg of hydrocortisone given intravenously every 6 to 8 hours, followed by a steroid taper.[113] In a recent review, Salem et al.[114] recommended basing glucocorticoid dosing on the magnitude of surgical stress. They recommended the following dosing guidelines:

Minor surgical stress: 25 mg of hydrocortisone equivalent per day for 1 day

Moderate surgical stress: 50 to 75 mg of hydrocortisone equivalent per day for 1 to 2 days

Major surgical stress: 100 to 150 mg of hydrocortisone equivalent per day for 2 to 3 days

These doses may be continued for postoperative complications that extend the stress response. Patients already receiving baseline glucocorticoid therapy in excess of these recommended stress doses probably do not require additional perioperative coverage.

Pheochromocytoma

Pheochromocytomas are rare endocrine tumors of neural crest cells in the adrenal medulla or sympathetic ganglia that secrete catecholamines, often in dangerously high concentrations. While the majority are located within the adrenal glands, approximately 6% are ecoptic. Ten percent of pheochromocytomas may be bilateral,[115] and 8% to 10% are malignant.[116] These tumors account for hypertension in less than 0.1% of all patients, but they are estimated to cause the deaths of approximately 1000 Americans each year.[117]

Preoperative preparation of patients known to have this tumor is of major importance if the risks of excess catecholamine release such as malignant hypertension, stroke, myocardial infarction, or death are to be reduced. Suspicion of a pheochromocytoma should be heightened in a patient with unexplained episodic or sustained hypertension, headache, palpitations, and excessive sweating[118] precipitated by stimuli such as stress, exercise, or sexual activity. Other less common symptoms include, nervousness and anxiety, tremor, nausea with or without vomiting, weakness, and weight loss.

In those patients known to have a pheochromocytoma, preoperative localization is essential to safe, rapid surgical management. Occasionally, pheochromocytomas are found intraoperatively during an unrelated procedure or in females during pregnancy or parturition. In these situations, blood pressure and fluid management becomes critical. Determination of the 24-hour urinary catecholamine levels with or without epinephrine-norepinephrine fractionation[115] is used to confirm the diagnosis. Ninety-eight percent of patients with a pheochromocytoma have an elevated serum or urinary catecholamine level.[119] Plasma catecholamine levels greater than 2000 pg/ml are considered diagnostic of a pheochromocytoma. Epinephrine-norepinephrine fractionation has been successfully used in those patients with normal total catecholamine levels in whom pheochromocytoma is strongly suspected. An epinephrine fraction of greater than 20% correlates with a pheochromocytoma.

Pheochromocytomas 1 cm in size or greater are best localized by CT scan.[115,116] If CT scan fails to demonstrate the lesion, selective arteriography should be performed.[116] Ultrasound or MRI may be helpful in pregnant patients. Metaiodobenzylguanidine (MIBG) scintigraphy is most useful for extra-adrenal, recurrent, or metastatic disease.[119]

Surgical excision is the treatment for pheochromocytomas and should be performed before other elective procedures. Appropriate preoperative preparation reduces the morbidity and mortality associated with possible catecholamine release during induction of anesthesia or surgical manipulation of the tumor. Preoperative α-adrenergic blockade serves to reexpand plasma volume, control hypertension, and minimize blood pressure fluctuations intraoperatively. Phenoxybenzamine, 10 to 20 mg three to four times daily for 7 to 10 days before operation, blocks both postsynaptic (α_1-) and presynaptic (α_2-) adrenergic receptors.[116] More recently, prazosin, a selective α_1-blocker has been used (2 to 5 mg twice daily)[116] and provides acceptable α-adrenergic blockade with fewer side effects.[115]

Preoperative β-blockade is not routinely necessary in the absence of tachyarrhythmias. Should arrhythmias arise intraoperatively, intravenous propranolol can be administered.[115,116] β-Blockade should *never* be administered prior to α-blockade, as it may induce a pressor response, causing severe hypertension.

Thyroid Dysfunction

The normally functioning thyroid gland synthesizes, stores, and releases the thyroid hormones thyroxine (T_4) and triiodothyronine (T_3). These regulate many aspects of cellular metabolism including oxygen consumption and heat production, as well as potentiating the effects of the sympathetic nervous system. Release of these hormones into the circulation is mediated by thyroid-stimulating hormone (TSH) produced by the pituitary gland, which itself is regulated by a classic negative feedback system.

Thyroid hormone concentrations can be altered either as a result of primary thyroid dysfunction or the physiologic disturbances mediated by the body's stress response. Major operative trauma or injury impairs the normal peripheral conversion of T_4 to T_3, in part due to a rise in serum cortisol. Both circulating T_3 level and the total T_4 concentration are reduced but without the expected rise in TSH concentrations. Presumably total T_4 concentration is decreased with injury, whereas free T_4 levels remain normal.[120]

Hyperthyroidism, or thyrotoxicosis, results from excessive release of thyroid hormone and is associated with signs and symptoms of heat intolerance, sweating, palpitations, increased appetite, weight loss, and fatigue. More worrisome signs are tachycardia, atrial fibrillation, heart failure, and myopathy, which may develop in some patients. Thyrotoxicosis must be both recognized and treated prior to operation. Euthyroidism is the goal to avoid thyroid storm, which may be precipitated by the stress of anesthesia or surgery. Thyrotoxicosis is usually corrected preoperatively with a combination of antithyroid medication (methimazole or propylthiouracil) to inhibit thyroid hormone synthesis and exogenous thyroxine to counteract the trophic effects of TSH, thereby decreasing the vascularity of the gland.[121] β-Blockade is now standard therapy to control tachycardia and the hypertension perioperatively. Propranolol has been widely used, titrating the dose to maintain the pulse rate less than 80 to 100 beats/min. More recently, selective B_1-blocking agents such as metoprolol have been used to avoid bronchospasm in patients with reactive airway disease. The exclusive use of B_1-blockade to control thyrotoxicosis perioperatively has been advocated to avoid the low, but finite, incidence of agranulocytosis seen with the antithyroid agents. A prospective randomized trial compared the use of metoprolol to antithyroid agents for control of hyperthyroidism in patients undergoing thyroid surgery. There were no anesthetic or cardiovascular complications in either group; nor was any difference in consistency or vascularity of the gland noted.[122]

Hypothyroidism is relatively common, occurring in approximately 2% of the adult female population.[123] Signs and symptoms include cool dry skin, "puffy" features, cold intolerance, constipation, hoarseness, dry hair, brittle nails, nonpitting edema, slowed reflexes, and bradycardia. Hemodynamically, hypothyroidism is characterized by a low cardiac index, decreased stroke volume, decreased vascular volume, and an increased systemic vascular resistance.[124,125] Up to 30% of untreated patients may have pericardial effusions.[126] Hypothyroid-induced hypertension[127] and defects in lipid metabolism predispose these patients toward atherosclerosis. The diagnosis of primary hypothyroidism is confirmed by low serum T_4 levels and elevated TSH levels.

Surgical complications in patients with hypothyroidism include intraoperative hypotension and altered drug metabolism. Gastrointestinal and neuropsychiatric complications are more prevalent, but the risk of infection, operative bleeding, perioperative arrhythmias, hypothermia, and hyponatremia is not increased. Moreover, hypothyroidism predisposes toward heart failure during cardiac surgery.[128]

The hypothyroidism should be corrected toward euthyroidism prior to elective surgery, although this may be difficult in the patient with preexisting atherosclerotic coronary artery disease. The chronotropic and inotropic effects of thyroid hormone increase myocardial oxygen consumption, potentially leading to myocardial ischemia. Empiric recommendations exist for hormone replacement in patients with hypothyroidism and known or suspected ischemic heart disease. L-Thyroxine is started at a low dose of 25 μg/day and increased in 12.5 to 25 μg increments at 4- to 6-week intervals. Although the dose is usually reduced if worsening myocardial ischemia is evident, alternatively, β-blocking agents may be added.[123] Myocardial revascularization is indicated in patients unable to tolerate thyroid replacement.[123]

Risks of Hematologic Disease

Appropriate management of the surgical patient with a known hematologic disorder is extremely important to avoid potentially disastrous complications. More subtle, but no less important, is the workup of the patient in which a hematologic abnormality is discovered incidentally on routine preoperative testing.

Anemia

Preparation of the anemic patient involves consideration not only of the degree of anemia but also the cause of the anemia and how this may affect the patient's perioperative course.[129] The common assertion that the preoperative hemoglobin level should be at least 10 g/dl to avoid complications is not supported in the literature.[129] An otherwise healthy patient undergoing minor surgery should tolerate a hemoglobin level of 7 to 8 g/dl. A patient with significant COPD requiring general anesthesia should have a hemoglobin level of at least 10 g/dl even for minor surgery. In general, if significant blood loss is likely or if the general health status of the patient is questionable, the hemoglobin level should be kept around 10 g/dl.[130] Workup of the anemia should proceed prior to surgery, as this may uncover a condition (i.e., occult malignancy) that would alter the operative plan.[131]

Infection from blood transfusion involves a small, but finite, risk. With this in mind it becomes reasonable to determine a "safe" level of hemoglobin on an individual basis taking into consideration patient volume status, cause and chronicity of anemia, age, underlying cardiovascular disease, type of surgery, and anticipated blood loss.[129] Postoperatively, mild-to-moderate anemia has not been shown to have an adverse effect on wound healing.[132] History, physical examination, and a few routine laboratory tests can usually determine the cause of the anemia. Table 13-9 shows which tests are helpful in determining the various causes.

The surgical patients with sickle cell anemia may have

Table 13-9. Laboratory Tests to Determine the Cause of Anemia

Laboratory Value	Abnormality	Further Tests to Consider	Possible Diagnosis
Reticulocyte count	High		Hemolysis
	Low		Decreased red blood cell production
Mean corpuscular volume	High with low reticulocyte count	B_{12} and folate levels, liver function tests, thyroid function tests, bone marrow examination	Macrocytic anemia 2 degrees to vitamin B_{12} or folate deficiency, liver disease, hypothyroidism, or primary marrow disorders
Mean corpuscular volume	Low with low reticulocyte count	Serum iron, total iron-binding capacity, ferritin level, hemoglobin A_2	Iron deficiency, chronic malignant or inflammatory disease, thalassemia minor
Red blood cell	Low with normal mean corpuscular volume (normocytic anemia)	Renal function tests, Coombs' test, erythrocyte sedimentation rate, lactate dehydrogenase, bilirubin	Uremia, chronic disease, hemolysis, or bone marrow depression

Adapted from Fellin F, Murphy S. Hematologic problems in the preoperative patient. Med Clin North Am 71(3):477, 1987.

significant comorbidities in addition to anemia, including cardiomyopathy, congestive heart failure, chronic pulmonary disease, renal insufficiency, nephrotic syndrome, chronic liver disease, as well as other organ dysfunction. These patients usually have normal or increased blood volume and generally tolerate chronic hemoglobin levels of 6 to 9 g/dl without difficulty. Transfusions in these patients are not routinely necessary simply to increase oxygen carrying capacity, nor are they considered necessary for most surgical procedures.[129] For major surgery in which hypoxia, hypotension, or acidosis are likely to occur, exchange transfusions to reduce the hemoglobin S fraction to approximately 20% to 30% of total hemoglobin may be beneficial.[133]

The patient with an immunohemolytic anemia must be clearly identified to the blood bank far in advance of surgery, as finding compatible crossmatched blood may be extremely difficult, if not impossible, in the event of hemorrhage.[131]

Polycythemia

Polycythemia or erythrocytosis can be classified as relative or absolute. Relative erythrocytosis is the result of reduced plasma volume. Absolute erythrocytosis is further classified as either primary or secondary. Primary erythrocytosis or polycythemia vera is a neoplastic disorder characterized by increased red blood cell mass, splenomegaly, thrombosis, and leukocytosis. Secondary polycythemia can be physiologically appropriate in association with pulmonary disease, cardiac disease, or high altitudes. Polycythemia may be physiologically inappropriate as seen in patients with renal cysts or tumors of the kidney, liver, uterus, and posterior fossa.[129] Patients with polycythemia vera and its associated high hematocrit are known to have increased surgical morbidity and mortality likely caused by the increased risk of thromboembolic events.[134,135]

Once the cause of the erythrocytosis has been determined, phlebotomy is used to decrease the hematocrit to an acceptable level. Phlebotomy is usually performed removing 350 to 500 ml of blood every other day until the appropriate hematocrit is reached. Lesser amounts (200 to 300 ml) should be removed each time in the elderly or those patients with cardiac disease.[129] In primary polycythemia vera, the hematocrit should be decreased to less than 45% prior to surgery.[129] In patients with physiologically inappropriate erythrocytoses, the hematocrit should be reduced to at least 45% to 50% as well. In cases in which erythrocytosis is physiologically appropriate, one must weigh the risk of thromboembolic events against the risk of decreasing the oxygen-carrying capacity in a patient with cardiac or pulmonary compromise. For these patients, reducing the hematocrit to approximately 50% to 60% is suggested.[136]

Disorders of White Blood Cells

Abnormalities in white blood cell count, either leukopenia or leukocytosis, are usually associated with an underlying disease. As a result, the perioperative risks often are related to the underlying disorder. Leukocytosis may be seen with infections, neoplasms, or leukemia. Leukopenia may be seen with radiation, chemotherapy, or overwhelming infection.[129] An absolute neutrophil count of less than 1000/μL is associated with a higher incidence of bacterial infections.[131] Elective surgery should probably be postponed in the face of severe leukopenia. If urgent operation is required, the patient should be aggressively monitored for infection.[129,131]

Platelet Disorders

Platelet dysfunction must be characterized as either quantitative or qualitative. The patient with thrombocytopenia but without a qualitative platelet function defect has abnormal bleeding related to the platelet count. In general, excessive bleeding, even with severe trauma is rare with a platelet count greater than 100,000/μL. Platelet counts greater than 50,000/μL are considered adequate for most surgical procedures. Higher counts are usually preferable for most cardiac, neurologic, and some ophthalmologic surgery.[129,131] In addition, bleeding risk must be considered in any patient with fever, infection, sepsis, or anemia regardless of the platelet count.[129,131]

Evaluation of thrombocytopenia should identify the cause as related to either decreased production, sequestration, or increased destruction. Patients with primary production problems such as those secondary to neoplasms, aplastic anemia, or chemotherapeutic agents tend to show erythrocyte and leukocyte abnormalities as well.[129] Thrombocytopenia resulting from sequestration is seen with hypersplenism with or without splenomegaly. An accompanying anemia and leukopenia is seen with a normal marrow.[129] Thrombocytopenia secondary to increased platelet destruction can be seen with certain drugs, infection, idiopathic thrombocytopenia purpura, or disseminated intravascular coagulation (DIC).[129]

Drug-associated platelet dysfunction such as that seen with salicylates usually corrects within 1 week following discontinuation of the drug. Some drugs have a more prolonged effect and so repeated count and function should be obtained prior to proceeding with operation. Elective surgery should be postponed until the platelet defect is characterized and the underlying disorder is treated.[131,137] A low platelet count due to increased platelet destruction is unlikely to be improved by platelet transfusion. For nonelective surgery, if pathologic bleeding occurs, or if no therapy is available for the underlying disorder, platelet transfusion is appropriate.[131,137] In general, one unit of platelets will raise a platelet count by approximately 5,000 to 10,000/μL. For platelet consumption and bleeding due to DIC, the underlying cause must be treated and the patient should be transfused with platelet concentrates and fresh frozen plasma.[129] Although the normal lifespan of newly produced platelets is approximately 8 to 10 days, the expected lifespan of transfused platelets is between several hours and 3 days.[131] A posttransfusion platelet count is necessary before proceeding with surgery.[129,131]

Steroids are the initial therapy for idiopathic thrombocytopenia purpura (ITP). When a response is seen, splenectomy can be considered with the planned operative procedure. For patients not responding to steroids, splenectomy should be performed prior to elective surgery in an attempt to improve platelet counts. Preoperative intravenous gamma globulin should be given to patients unresponsive to steroid or splenectomy.[129]

PREOPERATIVE HEMOSTATIC EVALUATION

1. Have you ever bled for a long time or developed a swollen tongue or mouth after cutting or biting your tongue, cheek, or lip?
2. Do you develop bruises larger than a silver dollar without being able to remember when or how you injured yourself? If so, how big was the largest of these bruises?
3. How many times have you had teeth pulled, and what was the longest time that you bled after an extraction? Has bleeding ever started up again the day after an extraction?
4. What operations have you had, including minor surgery such as skin biopsies? Was bleeding after surgery ever hard to stop? Have you ever developed unusual bruising in the skin around an area of surgery or injury?
5. Have you had a medical problem within the past 5 years requiring a doctor's care? If so, what was its nature?
6. What medications, including aspirin or any other remedies for headaches, colds, menstrual cramps, or other pains, have you taken within the past 7 to 9 days?
7. Has any blood relative had a problem with unusual bruising or bleeding after surgery? Were blood transfusions required to control this bleeding?

From Rapaport SI. Preoperative hemostatic evaluation: Which tests if any? Blood 61:229, 1983.

Coagulation Defects

Adequate hemostasis is crucial to successful surgery. The history and physical examination are the most valuable screens for potential coagulation defects. However, as technology advances and more screening tests become available to the physician, one must consider which tests are appropriate. Several studies have looked at how useful and accurate some of these screening tests are and which ones, based on the history and surgery to be performed, should be obtained preoperatively.[137]

History should focus on any excessive bleeding with previous surgery, trauma or tooth extraction, drug use, renal or liver disease or any family history of bleeding disorders.[129] Physical examination should focus on petechiae, ecchymoses, jaundice, or hepatosplenomegaly.[129] Although history and physical examination are vital, laboratory screening tests are necessary for several reasons. They may protect against the failure to elicit an adequate history preoperatively. Some patients may not provide a reliable history. The patient may have a coagulation abnormality that causes bleeding only after surgery (e.g., factor XI deficiency), and the patient may never have had a surgical procedure. Moreover, a patient having undergone previous surgery may have only recently developed a coagulopathy.[137]

A preoperative screening questionnaire is recommended to identify the patient at risk (see accompanying box).

Patients undergoing minor surgery with no suspicious bleeding history require no further studies.[129,137] Patients having a major operation with no evidence of a bleeding history should have a PT, activated partial thromboplastin time (aPTT), and a platelet count.[138] A bleeding time should also be obtained in any patient with a suspicious or suggestive history who will be undergoing major surgery. This is particularly important in cardiac bypass surgery or prostate surgery where hemostasis could be further impaired or in any type of surgery in which excessive bleeding could be catastrophic (neurosurgery or ophthalmologic surgery).[129]

In general, the aPTT evaluates the intrinsic pathway of the coagulation cascade, whereas the PT evaluates the extrinsic and common pathway. Prolongation of the aPTT can be caused by a deficiency of factor XI, antibodies against a specific coagulation factor, by von Willebrand's disease (factor VIII R:WF deficiency), or in males a deficiency of factor VIII or IX (hemophilia A or B).[129] Lupus anticoagulant causes an artifactual prolongation of the aPTT but actually leads to a hypercoagulable state. Prolongation of the PT can be seen with factor VII deficiency, vitamin K deficiency, or liver disease. A prolongation of both the PT and aPTT is seen with liver disease, DIC, or vitamin K deficiency.[129,131]

Patients with known hemophilia A (factor VIII deficiency) can be treated specifically with factor VIII concentrate. Patients with severe hemophilia undergoing major surgery should receive 40 U/kg of factor VIII concentrate immediately before surgery.[129,131] Postoperatively, the dose is tapered according to the surgery performed, continuing longer for more major procedures. Patients with minor hemophilia undergoing major operative procedures can also be managed with cryoprecipitate that contains factor VIII. In addition, DDAVP can be used in mild hemophilia to raise factor VIII levels to the normal range.[129]

Patients with known hemophilia B (factor IX deficiency) can be treated similarly to those with hemophilia A. Factor IX concentrate is available; however, it contains activated clotting factors, and therefore the patient must be carefully monitored for thrombotic complications.

Preoperative preparation of the patient with von Willebrand's disease includes the use of DDAVP. A test dose is given preoperatively to evaluate response. Cryoprecipitate should be used for major surgical procedures.[129]

Liver disease can cause coagulation abnormalities by several mechanisms. The treatment and workup of coagulation problems associated with hepatic disease were discussed earlier in the chapter.

PROPHYLAXIS AGAINST THROMBOEMBOLISM

Surgical patients are at risk for developing venous thromboembolism on the basis of Virchow's triad (stasis, endothelial damage, and hypercoagulable state). The patient is at high risk of developing deep venous thrombosis while immobilized on the operating table. Effective prophylaxis regimens include the use of sequential compression devices on the lower extremities during surgery and the administration of subcutaneous heparin injections (5000 units every 8 to 12 hours) starting 2 hours prior to surgery. Recently, low-molecular-weight heparins have been shown to be efficacious for thromboembolism prophylaxis in both orthopedic and general surgical patients. The use of low-molecular-weight heparins has also been noted to cause fewer wound hematomas than unfractionated heparin does.[139]

HUMAN IMMUNODEFICIENCY VIRUS INFECTION AND THE ACQUIRED IMMUNODEFICIENCY SYNDROME

Patients infected with the human immunodeficiency virus (HIV), both those who have asymptomatic HIV and those who have progressed to the acquired immunodeficiency syndrome (AIDS), have a greater risk of morbidity and mortality, presumably because of their immunosuppression. The diagnosis of AIDS requires a positive HIV serology and the presence of either opportunistic infections, opportunistic tumors, neurologic complications resulting in encephalopathy, CD+4 T-lymphocyte percentage of less than 14%, or an absolute CD+4 count of less than 200/mm^3. Patients with end-stage AIDS can be expected to have a very poor outcome with surgical intervention, and so only conservative, palliative care should be offered to these patients. The difficulty remains, however, in identifying those HIV-positive and non–end-stage AIDS patients who may benefit from surgical intervention.

HIV infection, even in the absence of AIDS, appears to impair wound healing. Safavi et al.[140] presented a series of 48 HIV-positive patients undergoing anorectal surgery. Whereas essentially 100% of the wounds would be expected to heal in healthy patients, Safavi et al. found that only 69% of the wounds in HIV-positive patients healed. In patients with AIDS, only 26% of the wounds healed. CD+4 counts did not correlate with outcome.

Patients with AIDS undergoing emergent laparotomy, including appendectomy, have an expected perioperative mortality of 12% and an expected morbidity of 26%.[141,142] The presence of opportunistic infections, lack of ongoing prophylactic treatment for AIDS-related disease, and ongoing sepsis at laparotomy correlate with increased morbidity and mortality.[142] Binderow et al.[143] tried to predict outcome in 10 HIV-positive patients and 25 patients with AIDS undergoing major abdominal surgery, excluding appendectomy. The perioperative mortality for the group with AIDS was 33% compared to 10% for the HIV-positive group. Perioperative mortality correlated with serum albumin, which was significantly different in survivors (3.9 g/L) vs. nonsurvivors (2.8 g/L). Total and differential white blood cell counts do not seem to correlate with outcome.[141-143]

Based on the available studies[140-144] HIV-positive patients are more likely to benefit from surgery than patients with AIDS. Relatively minor procedures, such as for vascular access, or lymph node biopsy, are well tolerated without undue morbidity.[144] Ideally, HIV-positive patients and patients with AIDS undergoing elective surgery should be well nourished and free of opportunistic infection at the time of operation.

SUMMARY

The physiologic derangements accompanying surgery may, at times, exceed the patient's physiologic reserve, resulting in significant morbidity and mortality. It is the responsibility of the surgeon to balance the potential risks and benefits of an operative procedure with the available management alternatives to provide the patient with an optimal outcome. A thorough history and physical examination not only define the surgical disease process of interest but also identify associated comorbidities. Knowledge of the disease processes involved allows stratification of risk and the determination of the appropriate course of therapy. Ultimately, a thoughtful approach to the preoperative preparation of the surgical patient serves to minimize morbidity and mortality.

REFERENCES

1. Goldman L, et al. Multifactorial index of cardiac risk in noncardiac surgical procedures. N Engl J Med 297(16):845, 1977.
2. Detsky AS, et al. Cardiac assessment for patients undergoing noncardiac surgery; A multifactorial clinical risk index. Arch Intern Med 16:2131, 1986.
3. Smith LC, Mullen JL. Nutritional assessment and indications for nutritional support. Surg Clin North Am 71(3):449, 1991.
4. Ellis LM, Copeland EM, Souba WM. Perioperative nutritional support, Surg Clin North Am 71(3):493, 1991.
5. Reisin E, Frohlich ED. Obesity: Cardiovascular and respiratory pathophysiologic alterations. Arch Intern Med 141:431, 1981.
6. Mason ED, Renquist KE, Jiang D. Perioperative risks and safety of surgery for severe obesity. Am J Clin Nutr 55(Suppl):573S, 1992.
7. Lund CC, Browder NC. Estimation of areas of burns. Surg Gynecol Obstet 79:352, 1944.
8. Baxter CR. Crystalloid resuscitation of burn shock. In Polk HC, Stone HH, eds. Contemporary Burn Management. Boston: Little Brown, 1971.
9. Polk HC, et al. Guidelines for prevention of surgical wound infection. Arch Surg 118:1213, 1983.
10. Paluzzi RG. Antimicrobial prophylaxis for surgery. Med Clin North Am 77(2):427, 1993.
11. Kaiser AB. Overview of cephalosporin prophylaxis. Am J Surg 155(Suppl 5A):52, 1988.
12. Olson M, O'Connor M, Schwartz M. Surgical wound infections: A 5 year prospective study of 20,193 wounds at the Minneapolis VA Medical Center. Ann Surg 199:253, 1984.
13. Neibart E. Preoperative preventive antimicrobial therapy. Mt Sinai J Med 58(1):19, 1991.
14. Goldmann DA, Hopkins CC, Karchmer AW. Cephalothin prophylaxis in cardiac valve surgery: A prospective, double-blind comparison of two-day and six-day regimen. J Thorac Cardiovasc Surg 470, 1977.
15. Kaiser AM. Post-operative infections and antimicrobial prophylaxis. In Mandel G, Douglas G, Bettett J, eds. Principles and Practice of Infectious Disease, 3rd ed. New York: Churchill Livingstone, 1989.
16. Nichols RL, et al. Effect of preoperative neomycin-erythromycin intestinal preparation on the incidence of infectious complications following colon surgery. Ann Surg 178(4):453, 1973.
17. Fleites RA, et al. The efficacy of polyethylene glycol–electrolyte lavage solution versus traditional mechanical bowel preparation for elective colonic surgery: A randomized, prospective blinded clinical trial. Surgery 98(4):708, 1985.
18. Schoetz JD, et al. Addition of parenteral cefoxitin to regimen of oral antibiotics for elective colorectal operations: A randomized prospective study. Ann Surg 212(2):209, 1990.
19. Zibrak JD, O'Donnell CR, Marton K. Indications for pulmonary function testing. Ann Intern Med 112:763, 1990.
20. Williams-Russo P, et al. Predicting postoperative pulmonary complications: Is it a real problem? Arch Intern Med 152:1209, 1992.
21. Sykes LA, Bowe EA. Cardiorespiratory effects of anesthesia. Clin Chest Med 14(2):211, 1993.
22. Ford GT. Respiratory physiology in upper abdominal surgery. Clin Chest Med 14(2):237, 1993.
23. Hotchkiss RS. Perioperative management of patient with chronic obstructive pulmonary disease. Int Anesthesiol Clin 26(2):134, 1988.
24. Weiman DS, et al. Perioperative respiratory management in cardiac surgery. Clin Chest Med 14(2):283, 1983.
25. Wittgen CM, et al. Preoperative pulmonary function evaluation for laparoscopic cholecystectomy. Arch Surg 128:880, 1993.
26. Warner MA, et al. Role of preoperative cessation of smoking and other factors in postoperative pulmonary complications: A blinded prospective study of coronary artery bypass patients. Mayo Clin Proc 64:609, 1989.
27. Boysen PG. Perioperative management of the thoracotomy patient. Clin Chest Med 14(1):321, 1993.
28. Ferrante FM, et al. Intrapleural analgesia after thoracotomy. Anesth Analg 72:105, 1991.
29. Sola JE, Bender JS. Use of the pulmonary artery catheter to reduce operative complications. Surg Clin North Am 73(2):253, 1993.
30. Berlauk JF, et al. Preoperative optimization of cardiovascular hemodynamics improves outcome in peripheral vascular surgery: A prospective, randomized clinical trial. Ann Surg 214(3):289, 1991.
31. Eagle KA, et al. Combining clinical and thallium data optimizes preoperative assessment of cardiac risk before major vascular surgery. Arch Intern Med 110:859, 1989.
32. Hertzer NR, et al. Coronary artery disease in peripheral vascular patients. A classification of 1000 coronary angiograms and results of surgical management. Ann Surg 199:223, 1984.
33. Lieberman RW, et al. Hemodynamic predictors of myocardial ischemia during halothane anesthesia for coronary artery revascularization. Anesthesiology 59:36, 1983.
34. Leung JM. The role of hemodynamics in perioperative myocardial ischemia. Int Anesthesiol Clin 30(1):63, 1992.
35. Tarhan S, et al. Myocardial infarction after general anesthesia. JAMA 220:1451, 1972.
36. Rao TLK, Jacobs KH, El-Etr AA. Reinfarction following anesthesia in patients with myocardial infarction. Anesthesiology 59:499, 1983.
37. Just H, Drexler H, Hasenfuss G. Pathophysiology and treatment of congestive heart failure. Cardiology 84(Suppl 2):99, 1994.
38. Gradman AH, Deedwania PC. Predictors of mortality in patients with heart failure. Cardiol Clin 12(1):25, 1994.
39. McKee PA, et al. The natural history of congestive heart failure: The Framingham Study. N Engl J Med 285:1441, 1971.
40. Cohn JN, et al. Effect of vasodilator therapy on mortality in chronic congestive heart failure: Results of a Veterans Administration Cooperative Study. N Engl J Med 314:1547, 1986.
41. Greenberg B. Role of vasodilator therapy in congestive heart failure: Effects on mortality. Cardiol Clin 12(1):87, 1994.
42. Donnan GA, et al. Hypertension and stroke. J. Hypertens 12:865, 1994.
43. Epstein M. Hypertension as a risk factor for progression of chronic renal disease. Blood Press 1(Suppl):23, 1994.
44. Lip GY, Gammage MD, Beevers DG. Hypertension and the heart. Br Med Bull 50(2):299, 1994.
45. Lithell H. Pathogenesis and prevalence of atherosclerosis in hypertensive patients. Am J Hypertens 7(2):2S, 1994.
46. Shaper AG, Wannamethee G, Walker M. Physical activity, hypertension and risk of heart attack in men without evidence of ischaemic heart disease. J Hum Hypertens 8(1):3, 1994.
47. Devereux RB, et al. Left ventricular hypertrophy associated with hypertension and its relevance as a risk factor for complications. J Cardiovasc Pharmacol 21(Suppl 2):S38, 1993.
48. Schwartzkopff B, et al. Heart failure on the basis of hypertension. Circulation 87(Suppl 5):IV66, 1993.
49. Moser M. Effect of diuretics on morbidity and mortality in the treatment of hypertension. Cardiology 84(Suppl 2):27, 1994.
50. Allman KG, et al. Resistant hypertension and preoperative silent myocardial ischaemia in surgical patients. Br J Anaesth 73:574, 1994.

51. Sideris DA. High blood pressure and ventricular arrhythmias. Eur Heart J 14:1548, 1993.
52. Gifford RW, Manger WM, Bravo EL. Pheochromocytoma. Endocrinol Metab Clin North Am 23(2):387, 1994.
53. Rackley CE. Valvular heart disease. In Wyngaarden JB, Smith LH, eds. Cecil Textbook of Medicine, 17th ed. Philadelphia: WB Saunders, 1985.
54. Braunwauld E. Valvular heart disease. In Braunwauld E, ed. Heart Disease: A Textbook of Cardiovascular Medicine, 4th ed. Philadelphia: WB Saunders, 1992.
55. Leavitt JI, Coats MH, Falk RH. Effects of exercise on transmitral gradient and pulmonary artery pressure in patients with mitral stenosis or a prosthetic mitral valve: A Doppler echocardiographic study. J Am Coll Cardiol 17:1520, 1991.
56. Thomas SJ, Lowenstein E. Anesthetic management of the patient with valvular heart disease. Int Anesthesiol Clin 17(1):67, 1979.
57. Danielsen R, Nordrehaug JE, Vi-Mo H. Clinical and haemodynamic features in relation to severity of aortic stenosis in adults. Eur Heart J 12:791, 1991.
58. Driscoll DJ, et al. Cardiorespiratory responses to exercise of patients with aortic stenosis, pulmonary stenosis and ventricular septal defect. Circulation 87(Suppl I):I-102, 1993.
59. Kennedy KD, et al. Natural history of moderate aortic stenosis. J Am Coll Cardiol 17(2):313, 1991.
60. Turpie AGG. Preventing thromboembolism in patients with prosthetic heart valves. Cardiol Clin 12(3):487, 1994.
61. Madura JA, Rookstool M, Wease G. The management of patients on chronic coumadin therapy undergoing subsequent surgical procedures. Am Surg 60:542, 1994.
62. Dajani AS, et al. Prevention of bacterial endocarditis. JAMA 277:1794, 1997.
63. Callow AD, Trachtenberg JD. Diagnosis and surgical management of asymptomatic carotid stenosis. In Ernst CB, Stanley JC, eds. Current Therapy in Vascular Surgery, 3rd ed. St. Louis: Mosby, 1995.
64. Freidman LS, Maddrey WC. Surgery in the patient with liver disease. Med Clin North Am 72(3):453, 1987.
65. Ngai SH. Current concepts in anesthesiology. N Engl J Med 302:564, 1980.
66. Gholson CF, Provenza JM, Bacon BR. Hepatologic considerations in patients with parenchymal liver disease undergoing surgery. Am J Gastroenterol 85(5):487, 1990.
67. Kelly DA, Tuddenham EGD. Haemostatic problems in liver disease. Gut 27:339, 1986.
68. Harville DD, Summerskil WH. Surgery in acute hepatitis. JAMA 1984:257, 1963.
69. Greenwood SM, Leffler CT, Minkowitz S. The increased mortality rate of open liver biopsy in alcoholic hepatitis. Surg Gynecol Obstet 134:600, 1972.
70. Powell-Jackson P, Greenway B, Williams R. Adverse effects of laparotomy in patients with unsuspected liver disease. Br J Surg 69:449, 1982.
71. Runyan BA. Surgical procedures are tolerated well by patients with asymptomatic chronic hepatitis. J Clin Gastroenterol 8:542,1986.
72. Hargrove MD. Chronic active hepatitis: Possible adverse effects of exploratory laparotomy. Surgery 68:771, 1970.
73. Child CG, Turcotte JG. Surgery and portal hypertension. In Child CG, ed. The Liver and Portal Hypertension. Philadelphia: WB Saunders, 1964.
74. Conn M. Preoperative evaluation of the patient with liver disease. Mt Sinai J Med 58(1):75, 1991.
75. Coratelli P, Passavanti C. Pathophysiology of renal failure in obstructive jaundice. Miner Electrolyte Metab 16:61, 1990.
76. Schepens MA, et al. Risk assessment of acute renal failure after thoracoabdominal aortic aneurysm surgery. Ann Surg 219(4):400, 1994.
77. Novis BK, et al. Association of preoperative risk factors with postoperative acute renal failure. Anesth Analg 78:143, 1994.
78. Pinson CW, et al. Surgery in long-term dialysis patients: Experience with more than 300 cases. Am J Surg 151:567, 1986.
79. Rose BD. Diagnostic approach to the patient with renal disease. In Rose BD, ed. Pathophysiology of Renal Disease. New York: McGraw-Hill, 1987.
80. Rose BD. Acute renal failure—prerenal disease versus acute tubular necrosis. In Rose BD, ed. Pathophysiology of Renal Disease. New York: McGraw-Hill, 1987.
81. Kellen M, et al. Predictive and diagnostic tests of renal failure: A review. Anesth Analg 78:134, 1994.
82. Rose BD, Brenner BM. Mechanisms of progression of renal disease. In Rose BD, ed. Pathophysiology of Renal Disease. New York: McGraw-Hill, 1987.
83. Wait RB, Kahng KU. Renal failure complicating obstructive jaundice. Am J Surg 157:256, 1989.
84. Parks RW, et al. Prospective study of postoperative function in obstructive jaundice and the effect of perioperative dopamine. Br J Surg 81:437, 1994.
85. Turka LA. Urinary tract obstruction. In Rose BD, ed. Pathophysiology of Renal Disease. New York: McGraw-Hill, 1987.
86. Webb JA, et al. Can ultrasound and computed tomography replace high-dose urography in patients with impaired renal function? Q J Med 53:411, 1984.
87. Burke JF, Francos GC. Surgery in the patient with acute or chronic renal failure. Med Clin North Am 71(3):489, 1987.
88. Muller MC. Anesthesia for the patient with renal dysfunction. Int Anesthesiol Clin 22(1):169, 1984.
89. Kellerman PS. Perioperative care of the renal patient. Arch Intern Med 154:1674, 1994.
90. Solomonson MD, Johnson ME, Ilstrup D. Risk factors in patients having surgery to create an arteriovenous fistula. Anesth Analg 79:694, 1994.
91. Ziccardi VB, et al. Management of the oral and maxillofacial surgery patient with end-stage renal disease. J Oral Maxillofac Surg 50:1207, 1992.
92. Bick RL. Acquired platelet function defects. Hematol Oncol Clin North Am 6(6):1203, 1992.
93. Edelson GW, Fachnie JD, Whitehouse FW. Perioperative management of diabetes. Henry Ford Hosp Med J 38(4):262, 1990.
94. Feingold KR, et al. Diabetes mellitus. In Andreoli TE, et al. Cecil Essentials of Medicine, 2nd ed. Philadelphia: WB Saunders, 1990.
95. Root HF. Preoperative care of the diabetic patient. Postgrad Med 40:439, 1966.
96. Goodson WH III, Hunt TK. Wound healing and the diabetic patient. Surg Gynecol Obstet 149:600, 1979.
97. Goodson WH III, Hunt TK. Deficient collagen formation by obese mice in a standard wound model. Am J Surg 138:692, 1979.
98. Gottrup F, Adreassen TT. Healing of incisional wounds in stomach and duodenum: The influence of experimental diabetes. J Surg Res 313:61, 1981.
99. Hirsch IB, McGill JB. Role of insulin in management of surgical patients with diabetes mellitus. Diabetes Care 13:980, 1990.
100. Taitelman U, Reese EA, Bessman AN. Insulin in the management of the diabetic surgical patient. JAMA 237:658, 1977.
101. McMurry JF. Wound healing with diabetes mellitus better glucose control for better wound healing in diabetes. Surg Clin North Am 64(4):769, 1984.
102. Gavin LA. Management of diabetes mellitus during surgery. West J Med 151:525, 1989.
103. Galloway JA, et al. Factors influencing the absorption, serum insulin concentration, and blood glucose responses after injections of regular insulin and various insulin mixtures. Diabetes Care 4:366, 1981.
104. Hildebrand P, Sestoft L, Nielson SL. The absorption of subcutaneously injected short-acting soluble insulin: Influence of injection technique and concentration. Diabetes Care 6:459, 1983.

105. Goldberg NJ, et al. Insulin therapy in the diabetic surgical patient: Metabolic and hormone response to low-dose insulin infusion. Diabetes Care 4:279, 1981.
106. Watts NB, et al. Postoperative management of diabetes mellitus: Steady state glucose control with bedside algorithm for insulin adjustment. Diabetes Care 10:722, 1987.
107. Pezzarossa A, et al. Perioperative management of diabetic subjects: Subcutaneous versus intravenous insulin administration during glucose-potassium infusion. Diabetes Care 11:52, 1988.
108. Farkas-Hirsch R, Boyle PJ, Hirsch IB. Glycemic control in the surgical patient with IDDM [abstract]. Diabetes 38(Suppl 2):39A, 1989.
109. Alberti KGMM, Marshall SM. Diabetes and surgery. In Alberti KGMM, Krall LP, eds. The Diabetes Annual/4, New York: Elsevier, 1988, p 248.
110. Felig P, et al. Blood glucose and gluconeogenesis in fasting man. Arch Intern Med 123:293, 1969.
111. Fritz I, Levine R. Action of adrenal cortical steroids and norepinephrine on vascular responses of stress in adrenalectomized rats. Am J Physiol 165:456, 1951.
112. Knowlton AL. Adrenal insufficiency in the intensive care setting. J Intensive Care Med 4:35, 1989.
113. Claussen MS, Landercasper J, Cogbill TH. Acute adrenal insufficiency presenting as shock after trauma and surgery: Three cases and review of the literature. J Trauma 32(1):94, 1992.
114. Salem M, et al. Perioperative glucocorticoid coverage: A reassessment 42 years after emergence of a problem. Ann Surg 219(4): 416, 1994.
115. Havlik RJ, Cahow E, Kinder BK. Advances in the diagnosis and treatment of pheochromocytoma. Arch Surg 123:626, 1988.
116. Bravo EL, Gifford RW Jr. Pheochromocytoma: Diagnosis, location and management. N Engl J Med 311:1298, 1984.
117. Hauptman JB, Modlinger RS, Ertel NH. Pheochromocytoma resistant to alpha-adrenergic blockade. Arch Intern Med 143:2321, 1983.
118. Hull CJ. Pheochromocytoma diagnosis, preoperative preparation and anaesthetic management. Br J Anaesth 58:1453, 1986.
119. Malone MJ, et al. Preoperative and surgical management of pheochromocytoma. Urol Clin North Am 16(3):567, 1989.
120. Gann DS, Foster AH. Endocrine and metabolic responses to injury. In Schwartz SI, ed. Principles of Surgery, 6th ed. New York: McGraw-Hill, 1994.
121. Heimann P, Martinson J. Surgical treatment of thyrotoxicosis: Results of 272 operations with special reference to preoperative treatment with antithyroid drugs and L-thyroxine. Br J Surg 62:683, 1975.
122. Alderberth A, Stenstrom G, Hasselgren PO. The selective $beta_1$-blocking agent metoprolol compared with antithyroid drug and thyroxine as preoperative treatment of patients with hyperthyroidism. Results from a prospective, randomized study. Ann Surg 205(2):182, 1987.
123. Klein I. Thyroid hormone and the cardiovascular system. Am J Med 88:631, 1990.
124. Amidi M, et al. Effect of the thyroid state on myocardial contractility and ventricular ejection rate in man. Circulation 38:229, 1968.
125. Graettinger JS, et al. A correlation of clinical and hemodynamic studies in patients with hyperthyroidism with and without congestive heart failure. J Clin Invest 38:1316, 1959.
126. Kerber RE, Sherman B. Echocardiographic evaluation of pericardial effusion in myxedema. Circulation 52:823, 1975.
127. Streeten DH, et al. Effects of thyroid function on blood pressure. Recognition of hypothyroid hypertension. Hypertension 11:78, 1988.
128. Ladenson PW, et al. Complications of surgery in hypothyroid patients. Am J Med 77:261, 1984.
129. Fellin F, Murphy S. Hematologic problems in the preoperative patient. Med Clin North Am 71(3):477, 1987.
130. Rawstron RE. Anemia and surgery. A retrospective clinical study. Aust NZ J Surg 39:425, 1970.
131. Calandri C, Rand JH. Preoperative evaluation for hematologic status. Mt Sinai J Med 58(1):41, 1991
132. Heughan C, Grislis G, Hunt TK. The effect of anemia on wound healing. Ann Surg 179:163, 1974.
133. Dobson MB. Anesthesia for patients with hemoglobinopathies. Int Anesthesiol Clin 23:197, 1985.
134. Wasserman LR, Gilbert HS. Surgical bleeding in polycythemia vera. Ann NY Acad Sci 115:122, 1964.
135. Rigby PG, Leavell BS. Polycythemia vera: A review of fifty cases with emphasis on the risk of surgery. Arch Intern Med 5:622, 1960.
136. Golde DW, et al. Polycythemia: Mechanisms and management. Ann Intern Med 95:71, 1981.
137. Rapaport SI. Preoperative hemostatic evaluation: Which tests if any? Blood 61:229, 1983.
138. Eisenberg JM, Clarke JR, Sussman SA. Prothrombin and partial thromboplastin times as preoperative screening tests. Arch Surg 117:48, 1982.
139. Weitz JI. Low-molecular-weight heparins. N Engl J Med 337:688, 1997.
140. Safavi A, Gottesman L, Dailey TH. Anorectal surgery in the HIV+ patient: Update. Dis Colon Rectum 34(4):299, 1991.
141. Davidson T, et al. Emergency laparotomy in patients with AIDS. Br J Surg 78:924, 1991.
142. Whitney TM, et al. Emergent abdominal surgery in AIDS: Experience in San Francisco. Am J Surg 168:239, 1994.
143. Binderow SR, Cavallo RJ, Freed J. Laboratory parameters as predictors of operative outcome after major adominal surgery in AIDS- and HIV-infected patients. Am Surg 59:754, 1993.
144. Klatt EC. Surgery and human immunodeficiency virus infection: Indications, pathologic findings, risks and risk prevention. Int Surg 79:1, 1994.

PART TWO

THE ALIMENTARY TRACT
Esophagus and Stomach

14

Physiologic Dysfunction of the Esophagus

Peter F. Crookes and Tom R. DeMeester

Although the gastrointestinal tract is a continuous hollow tube, its various functions in the ingestion, digestion, and absorption of chemical energy and elimination of residue are performed separately in different compartments. Common to each compartment is the presence of a sphincter to separate it from adjacent compartments, a pumping mechanism to propel contents into the next most distal compartment, and the ability to maintain a distinct chemical and metabolic environment appropriate to its function (Fig. 14-1). The motor activity of each functional compartment generally has three components: a pump, a valve, and a receptacle (reservoir). Proximally, the pharynx functions as a pump, the upper esophageal sphincter (UES) and soft palate and epiglottis function as the valve, and the upper esophagus acts as the receptacle. The distal esophagus is characterized by higher amplitude contractility and pumps food through the valve (the lower esophageal sphincter [LES]) into the proximal stomach, which acts as a reservoir. The distal antrum behaves as a pump, propelling chyme through a valve (the pylorus) into the duodenum. Similarly, the small intestine pumps its contents through the ileocecal valve into a capacitance organ, the cecum. An important principle in this concept is that functional lesions in one part of the gastrointestinal tract tend to produce secondary effects proximally rather than distally. Thus problems originating in the stomach commonly cause gastroesophageal reflux disease (GERD) or symptoms referable to the cricopharyngeal area. This is important in elucidating the underlying pathophysiology of foregut symptoms.

Swallowing occurs in two phases. The chief function of the cervical phase is the transmission of lubricated food and liquid into the gastrointestinal tract while protecting the airway. The chief function of the second phase is propelling food into the stomach while protecting the esophageal mucosa from reflux of gastric juice. The commonest esophageal disease in Western society is GERD and its complications, followed by esophageal cancer, with esophageal motility disorders being less common still. All categories of esophageal disease are frequently referred to surgeons. Whereas in treating esophageal cancer, the primary goal of surgery is long-term survival, with quality of life being a secondary consideration, the situation in benign disease is quite different. The goal of surgery in benign esophageal disease is preservation of function. To accomplish this requires detailed understanding of the way in which diseases and their treatments can interfere with normal physiology.

ESOPHAGEAL PHYSIOLOGY
Pharyngoesophageal Segment

The tongue moves the bolus of chewed food into the posterior oropharynx and into the hypopharynx (Fig. 14-2, *A-D*). In concert with the posterior movement of the tongue, the soft palate is elevated (Fig. 14-2, *C-H*), thereby closing the passage between the oropharynx and nasopharynx. This partitioning prevents pressure generated in the oropharynx from being dissipated through the nose. During swallowing the hyoid bone moves upward and anteriorly, elevating the larynx and opening the retrolaryngeal space, bringing the epiglottis under the tongue (Fig. 14-2, *I-P*). The backward tilt of the epiglottis covers the opening of the larynx, helping to prevent aspiration.

The pressure in the hypopharynx rises abruptly during swallowing, creating a sizable pressure difference between the pharynx and the subatmospheric intrathoracic esophagus.[1] This pressure gradient produced by sequential pharyngeal contraction encourages the movement of food from the hypopharynx into the esophagus when the UES relaxes. The pharyngeal contraction passes through the UES as a postrelaxation contraction, the amplitude of which is higher than the peristaltic pressure in the upper esophagus, and this prevents retrograde escape of the bolus into the pharynx.

Esophageal Body

The pharyngeal activity in swallowing initiates the esophageal phase. The action of the body of the esopha-

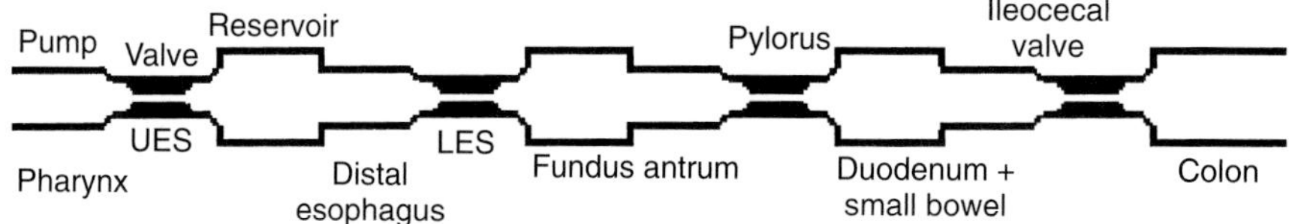

Fig. 14-1. Schematic representation of different functional components of the gastrointestinal tract. *LES,* Lower esophageal sphincter; *UES,* upper esophageal sphincter.

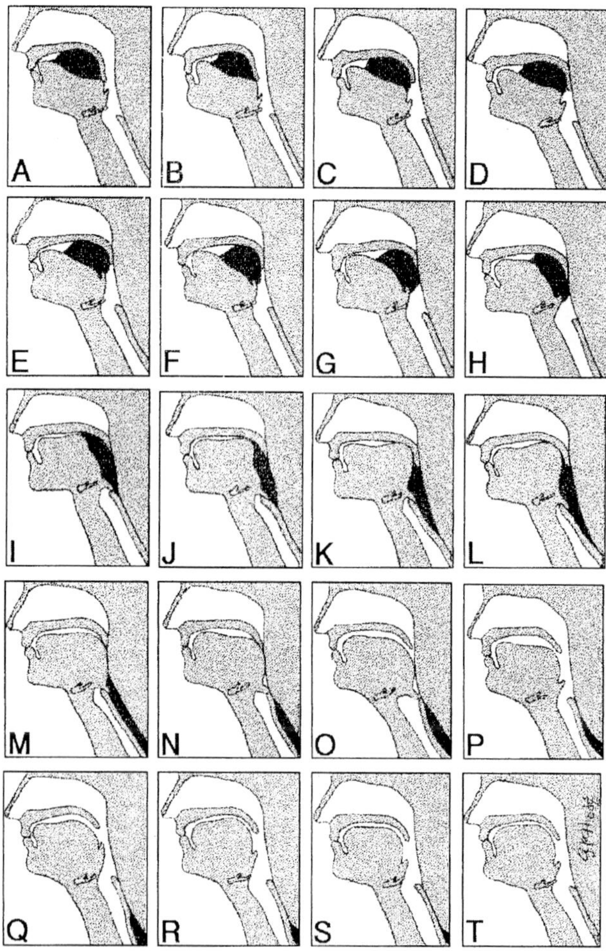

Fig. 14-2. Sequence of events during the pharyngeal phase of swallowing, showing the action of the tongue coordinated with the movement of the soft palate, larynx, and epiglottis during a swallow. (From Davenport HR. Physiology of the Digestive Tract, 5th ed. Chicago: Year Book Medical Publishers, 1982, p 37. As adapted from Rushmer RF, Hendron JA. J Appl Physiol 3:625, 1951. With permission.)

gus can be visualized as a worm-drive propulsive pump and is responsible for transmitting a bolus of food from the negative pressure environment of the distal esophagus into the positive pressure environment of the stomach. Effective and coordinated smooth muscle function in the lower third of the esophagus is therefore important in propelling food across this barrier. The peristaltic wave generates an occlusive pressure varying from 30 to 120 mm Hg. The peristaltic contraction initiated by a swallow (primary peristalsis) moves down the esophagus at 2 to 4 cm/sec and reaches the distal esophagus about 7 seconds after swallowing starts.[2] Esophageal peristalsis can also be produced without a swallow (secondary peristalsis) in response to esophageal distention. Secondary peristaltic waves tend to be of lower amplitude and less well organized than primary peristaltic waves. Orderly contraction of the muscular wall is impaired if the esophagus is not anchored at its distal end. Loss of this inferior anchor occurs with a large sliding hiatal hernia and can lead to inefficient propulsion.

Lower Esophageal Sphincter

The LES provides a pressure barrier between the esophagus and stomach and acts as the valve on the pump of the esophageal body. The sphincter normally remains actively closed except in two situations: (1) after a swallow, when it relaxes to allow passage of food into the stomach, and (2) when the fundus is distended with gas, it relaxes to allow venting of air. These non–swallow-induced relaxations are termed transient lower esophageal sphincter relaxations (TLESRs).[3] They are often associated with audible belching and are probably the mechanism of normal physiologic reflux.

The tonic resistance of the LES is a function not only of the LES *pressure* but of the *total length* over which the pressure is exerted. This length decreases as the stomach fills, rather like the neck of a balloon shortening as the balloon is inflated, and accounts for the tendency to reflux after a voluminous meal.[4] A third key feature of the LES is its position, in that a portion of that length *(abdominal length)* should be exposed to positive intra-abdominal pressure. During periods of increased intra-abdominal pressure, the resistance of the LES would be overcome if the abdominal pressure were not applied equally to the LES and stomach, causing the LES to collapse.[5] Think of sucking on a soft soda straw and picture how the hydrostatic pressure of the fluid causes the straw to collapse instead of allowing the liquid to flow up the straw in the direction of the negative pressure. If the abdominal length of the LES is inadequate, it cannot respond to an increase in the applied intra-abdominal pressure by collapsing and is thus more liable to result in reflux.

Stomach

The stomach has two main activities, secretory and motor. Secretion of acid by parietal cells is stimulated by vagal activity, histamine, and gastrin. Acid secretion may thus be reduced by vagotomy, the administration of H_2-blockers, or surgical removal of the source of gastrin (antrectomy). The output of the parietal cell into the gastric lumen requires the presence of a Na^+-H^+ pump, and this pump is blocked by proton pump inhibitors such as omeprazole.

The motor function of the stomach includes receptive relaxation of the fundus and the pumping and grinding function of the antropyloric region. As the stomach fills, the fundic muscle undergoes a vagally mediated receptive relaxation, thus keeping intragastric pressure in a steady state. By contrast, the motor activity of the gastric body and antrum are regulated by the gastric pacemaker, which is located on the upper part of the greater curvature. The pacemaker discharges with a regular rhythm of about three per minute and sweeps across the stomach from the greater curvature toward the pylorus. Food particles are swept toward the pylorus, which acts as a sizer: particles larger than 2 mm are returned to the proximal stomach for further milling. Gastric emptying is affected by the composition and consistency of the ingested meal. Liquids empty most rapidly, semisolids empty more slowly, and solids are the slowest to empty. The emptying of liquids and semisolids follows an exponential decline, whereas when solids are ingested, there is an initial plateau phase without any obvious emptying followed by a linear emptying of the foodstuff. Foods with a high protein content tend to empty most rapidly, whereas high fat and calorie composition in a meal tend to slow the rate of gastric emptying.

SYMPTOMS OF ESOPHAGEAL DISEASE

The cardinal symptom of esophageal disease is *dysphagia*. When the problem is in the pharyngoesophageal segment, there is difficulty in getting the food out of the mouth and into the esophagus. This is sometimes called "cervical" dysphagia, to be distinguished from "esophageal" dysphagia characteristic of lesions of the esophageal body or LES. *Aspiration,* manifested by coughing or choking during swallowing, is commonly worse with liquids than solids. A prominent cough on assuming the recumbent position suggests the presence of Zenker's diverticulum because retained food then flows back into the pharynx. Palatal paresis may cause nasal regurgitation because the pressure generated by the tongue is dissipated through the nose. Other symptoms commonly present reflect the concomitant involvement of other structures by the neural or muscular disease: the voice may be hoarse if there is paresis of a vocal cord, and it may sound "wet" because of uncleared secretions or nasal if there is palatal paresis. Similarly, the underlying condition may cause dysarthria.

In the esophageal body, dysphagia is often experienced as a sensation of food sticking or slowness in being transported to the stomach. It may be associated with burning pain (odynophagia) if there is mucosal ulceration. Esophageal dysphagia often develops slowly and causes patients unconsciously to modify their eating habits so that they deny or underestimate their difficulty. For this reason, it is important to take a detailed history enquiring about the extent to which the symptom has caused modification of their life-style: for example, if they need lots of liquids with their meals, if they cut food into small pieces, if they deliberately stay away from certain foods, if they are the last to finish a meal in company, or if they have given up eating in company. *Regurgitation* of food is sometimes described by the patient as vomiting. However, if the material tastes bland, it is clear that it has never entered the stomach; whereas regurgitated gastric contents taste sour or bitter. In the presence of a fixed mechanical obstruction, the patient may regurgitate saliva, which is described as "foam" or "phlegm."

The cardinal symptom of GERD is *heartburn* (i.e., a burning retrosternal discomfort) often beginning 1 hour or so after meals. In some patients, it is clearly precipitated by bending over or lying flat, a situation commonly associated with a profoundly defective sphincter. It may be relieved in the short term by antacids and for longer periods by consumption of H_2-blockers or omeprazole. It may be associated with acid regurgitation back into the throat or mouth, sometimes described as "acid belches."

Several categories of atypical symptoms resulting from esophageal dysfunction occur. *Pulmonary symptoms* include asthma (typically adult onset, steroid dependent, nonallergic) and episodic pneumonia. More proximal manifestations of esophageal disease, especially gastroesophageal reflux, are the development of "reflux laryngitis" characterized by erythema of the cords, and buccal erosion of dental enamel. Angina-like *chest pain* (sometimes called noncardiac chest pain) is often associated with esophageal motility disorders and increased esophageal acid exposure; it resembles angina pectoris in location and character but is not clearly related to exercise. *Epigastric pain and bloating* is primarily a gastric symptom but is often associated with gastroesophageal reflux disease.

These symptoms, although their pathogenesis can be readily understood, are not sufficiently specific to be the sole basis for planning therapy. Rather, their importance is to direct the physician to choose the correct sequence of confirmatory investigations.

INVESTIGATION OF ESOPHAGEAL DISEASE

Endoscopy

Endoscopy is generally the first investigation in patients with foregut symptoms, unless the chief complaint is dysphagia, when a "road map" should first be obtained by barium swallow. Endoscopy allows visualization of a wide range of disease processes and permits both biopsy and therapeutic measures. The chief risks are oversedation, aspiration, and instrumental perforation. Most patients have a spray of topical anesthesia and require intravenous sedation. Monitoring of heart rate and pulse oximetry must be carried out, and resuscitation equipment must be available. The endoscope is introduced through a mouth guard into the pharynx. The locations of esophageal landmarks are measured endoscopically from the incisor teeth (Fig. 14-3). The cricopharyngeus muscle is normally at 15 cm in the average adult. The tracheal bifurcation and indentation of the aortic arch is between 24 and 26 cm from the incisor teeth. This landmark is helpful in localizing intraluminal lesions. The position of the gastroesophageal junction is best identified during the initial introduction, before it is advanced into the stomach, to avoid reducing a sliding hiatal hernia. Once in the stomach, the scope is directed toward the pylorus and advanced into the second part of the duodenum, and the duodenum and stomach are systematically inspected as the scope is withdrawn. Turning the lens of the scope through 180 degrees (retroflexion) allows inspection of the fundus and cardia. Attention is paid to the "frenulum" of the gastroesophageal junction and to the closeness with which the cardia grips the scope. The instrument is then straightened and withdrawn through the cardia and esophagus. Three landmarks are measured in the region of the cardia: the level of the crura (observed as a slitlike narrowing that closes when the patient is asked to sniff), the level of the anatomic gastroesophageal junction (identified as the position where the stomach with vertically running rugal folds becomes the tubular esophagus with smooth mucosa), and the level of the squamocolumnar junction (Z-line). A hiatal hernia is present when the gastroesophageal junction is more than 2 cm above the crura. Barrett's esophagus is suggested when the squamocolumnar junction is more than 2 cm above the gastroesophageal junction. More recent evidence suggests that it may be diagnosed if any specialized epithelium (i.e., intestinal type, containing goblet cells) is identified within the region of the cardia. Esophagitis is recognized by the presence of redness, linear erosions, or ulceration of the mucosa and is generally classified on a graded scale of severity such as the Savary-Miller classification (see accompanying box). The most recent modification of this classification recognizes that Barrett's mucosa can coexist with any degree of esophagitis.[6]

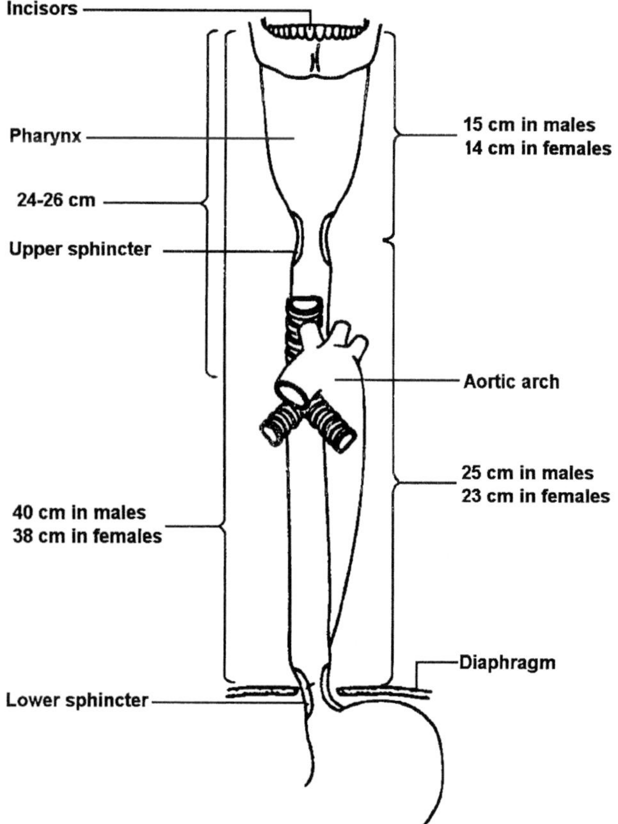

Fig. 14-3. Important clinical endoscopic measurements of the esophagus in adults.

Barium Upper Gastrointestinal Tract Studies

Barium upper gastrointestinal tract studies complement endoscopy in providing both structural and functional information, especially when the entire examination is recorded on videotape. Three areas of esophageal narrowing are noted on both barium esophagogram and endoscopy (Fig. 14-4). The first narrowing is at the site of the cricopharyngeus muscle, which often causes difficulty in introducing a rigid esophagoscope and is consequently the commonest site of endoscopic perforation. The left main bronchus and aortic arch cause narrowing of the middle third of the esophagus. The most distal narrowing of the esophagus is at the diaphragmatic hiatus and is caused by the LES mechanism. These normal points of narrowing tend to retard swallowed foreign objects. Also, corrosive liquid ingestion results in prominent mucosal injury at these sites since the liquid is slowed in passage.

The pharyngoesophageal region is evaluated while the patient is in the upright position. The hyoid bone, larynx, epiglottis, soft palate, and tongue are easily identified, and their relationship to the cricopharyngeal opening is determined. Aspiration, if observed, can be timed, and residual barium remaining after a swallow can be identified.

NEW SAVARY-MILLER FIVE-GRADE CLASSIFICATION OF REFLUX ESOPHAGITIS

Grade 1	Single or multiple erosions on a single fold; erosions may be erythematous or exudative
Grade 2	Multiple erosions affecting multiple folds; erosions may be confluent
Grade 3	Multiple circumferential erosions
Grade 4	Ulcer, stenosis, or esophageal shortening
Grade 5	Barrett's epithelium; columnar metaplasia in the form of noncircular (islands or tongues) or circular extensions

Esophageal body peristalsis is studied while the patient is in the supine position. A swallowed bolus normally generates a stripping wave, which clears the bolus completely. Residual material may stimulate a secondary peristaltic wave in the absence of a swallow. Motility disorders characterized by disorganized activity with simultaneous contractions give rise to "tertiary waves" often with a segmented appearance to the barium column, sometimes described as "rosary beading" or "corkscrew" appearance. A hiatal hernia, best seen with the patient in the horizontal position, may be found to be reducible when the patient is in the upright position. Barium studies are of little value in detecting reflux unless spontaneous reflux is observed while the patient is in the upright position.

Computed Tomography Scan

CT scanning of the esophagus is important in delineating the relationship of esophageal lesions to adjacent structures, especially the trachea, left main bronchus, and aorta. The esophagus normally appears as a flattened hollow structure with a thin wall. A more circular cross-sectional appearance with a fluid level is evidence of distal obstruction. The CT scan gives important information in staging esophageal tumors, as it can demonstrate involvement of adjacent structures (e.g., the trachea, involvement of lymph nodes, and distant metastases).

Endoscopy and barium studies are designed to give structural rather than functional information. Although they may confirm or refute the presence of tumors, strictures, ulcers, and diverticula, the functional information tends to be qualitative rather than quantitative. Measurement of function begins with two key investigations: esophageal manometry and 24-hour pH monitoring.

A

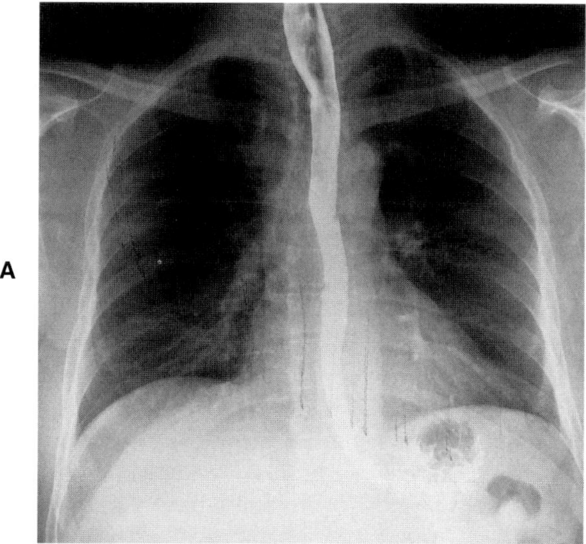

B

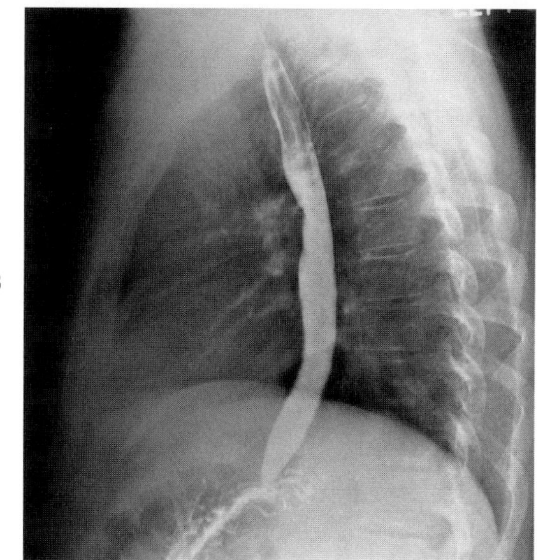

Fig. 14-4. Barium esophagogram **A,** Anteroposterior view. **B,** Lateral view.

Esophageal Manometry

Esophageal manometry is an investigative tool in which a catheter containing pressure sensors is inserted into the esophagus and used to measure pressures in the esophageal body and sphincters at rest and in response to swallowing. It is indicated in the following clinical situations:

1. *Nonobstructive dysphagia:* Patients with dysphagia in whom a structural (mechanical) cause has not been identified by endoscopy or esophagogram are likely to have a motility disorder, which can be detected only by manometry.
2. *Noncardiac chest pain:* Retrosternal chest pain in the absence of coronary artery disease is a frequent cause of morbidity and anxiety. Every year, it is estimated that 180,000 patients with central chest pain are found to have negative coronary angiography. Of these, 20% to 40% have a motility abnormality, of whom 50% are associated with increased esophageal acid exposure.[7]
3. *GERD:* The indications for manometry in patients with suspected GERD are chiefly to assess the status of the LES and to identify a motility disorder of the body. A defective sphincter is predictive of a poor long-term response to medical therapy but a good response to surgery. The presence of a named motility disorder or defective contractility in the esophageal body profoundly alters the operative strategy in patients with GERD and should always be sought by manometry prior to operative therapy.

Manometry is also known to be the most accurate way of locating the LES prior to placement of a pH electrode for 24-hour pH monitoring in patients suspected of having GERD. Finally, postoperative manometry objectively assesses if the goal of the operation has been attained and encourages the surgeon to modify his technique in light of the results.

The test is performed by passing the lubricated manometric catheter through the anesthetized nostril into the pharynx. The neck is then flexed, and the patient takes a swallow of water as the catheter is advanced through the relaxed cricopharyngeal sphincter into the esophagus. The catheter is further advanced until all recording ports are in the stomach. A manometric study consists of four components: assessment of the LES, LES relaxation, the esophageal body, and the UES.

Assessment of the Lower Esophageal Sphincter

As the catheter is slowly withdrawn in 1 cm increments, the high-pressure zone of the LES is reached by the uppermost transducer. The lower (distal) border of the LES is the point where the resting pressure rises above gastric baseline, and the upper border is the point where the resting pressure reaches esophageal baseline. Between these two points is the respiratory inversion point (RIP), where the positive deflections with inspiration change to negative deflections, the functional division between the abdomen and chest. Three components of the LES are measured. (1) The *resting pressure* is the pressure above gastric baseline measured in midrespiration at the RIP. The pressures in the high-pressure zone are a combination of the intrinsic pressure of the LES, the applied pressure of the intra-abdominal environment, and compression by the crura of the diaphragm. Generally, the applied intra-abdominal pressure is equal to the intragastric pressure and thus is usually disregarded. (2) The *overall length* of the sphincter is the distance from the distal border to the proximal border. (3) The *abdominal length* is the distance from the distal border of the LES to the RIP and represents the portion of the LES subject to fluctuations in intra-abdominal pressure. In hiatal herniation, the diaphragmatic and intrinsic components are sometimes separated rather than superimposed, resulting in a long high-pressure zone described as a "double hump." The effect of applied intra-abdominal pressure is negated if the abdominal length is too short.

These features are illustrated in the tracing in Fig. 14-5. The values for each of these components from each transducer are expressed as an average. The lower limits of normal (2.5th percentile) are a resting pressure less than 6 mm Hg, an overall length of less than 2 cm, or an abdominal length of less than 1 cm. If any one component is below normal, the sphincter is mechanically defective. A defect in one or even two components of the LES may be compensated by good esophageal body function, but when all three components are defective, excessive esophageal acid exposure is almost inevitable.[8]

All the pressures measured along the length of the sphincter and around its circumference during the pull-through may be treated as vectors having both magnitude and direction and hence integrated into a three-dimensional image, the volume (vector volume) of which is a measure of LES resistance (Fig. 14-6). A vector volume below the 5th percentile of normal is a more sensitive measure of mechanical deficiency of the LES than the parameters just described. The prevalence of a defective LES increases with increasing severity of GERD, being lowest in patients without evidence of endoscopic injury and highest in patients with stricture or Barrett's esophagus.[9]

Assessment of Lower Esophageal Sphincter Relaxation

The catheter is positioned with a transducer in the LES, and a series of swallows are obtained by giving boluses of 5 ml of water. The LES pressure normally drops to gastric baseline immediately after the swallow, before the oncoming peristaltic wave reaches the lower esophagus (Fig. 14-7).

Assessment of the Esophageal Body

After the LES study, the catheter is positioned so that the upper port is 1 cm below the UES: thus the transducers span the length of the esophageal body. The peristaltic response to 10 swallows of 5 ml of water is measured. Two key features are important to consider: contraction amplitude and wave progression. A typical pattern is shown in Fig. 14-8. Effective bolus transport depends on the presence of both features. Most commercially available manometric systems automatically measure these features and relate the results to those of normal subjects (Fig. 14-9).

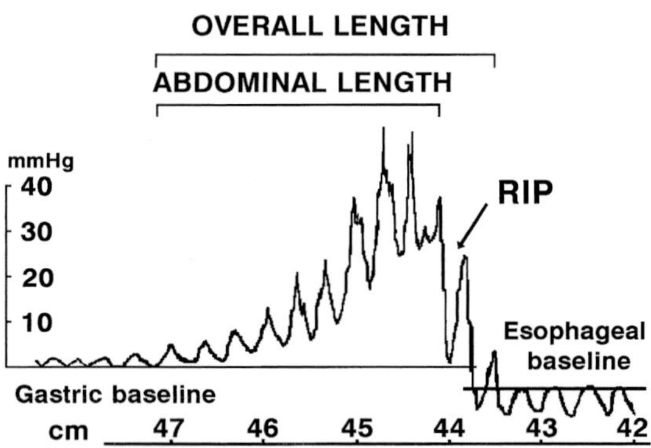

Fig. 14-5. Manometric tracing of a transducer being pulled through the lower esophageal sphincter showing the resting pressure, overall length, and abdominal length. *RIP,* Respiratory inversion point.

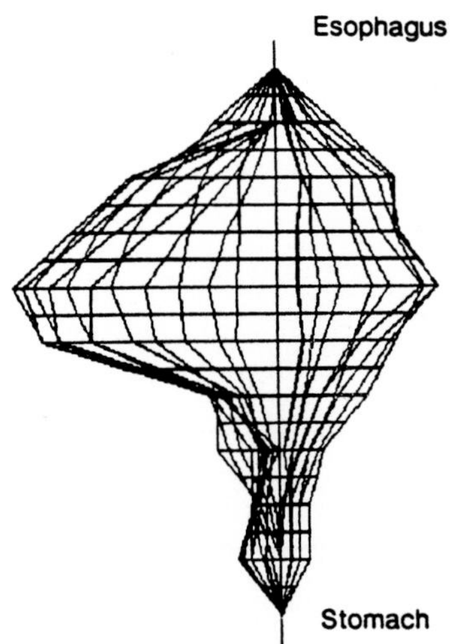

Fig. 14-6. Three-dimensional representation of the lower esophageal sphincter.

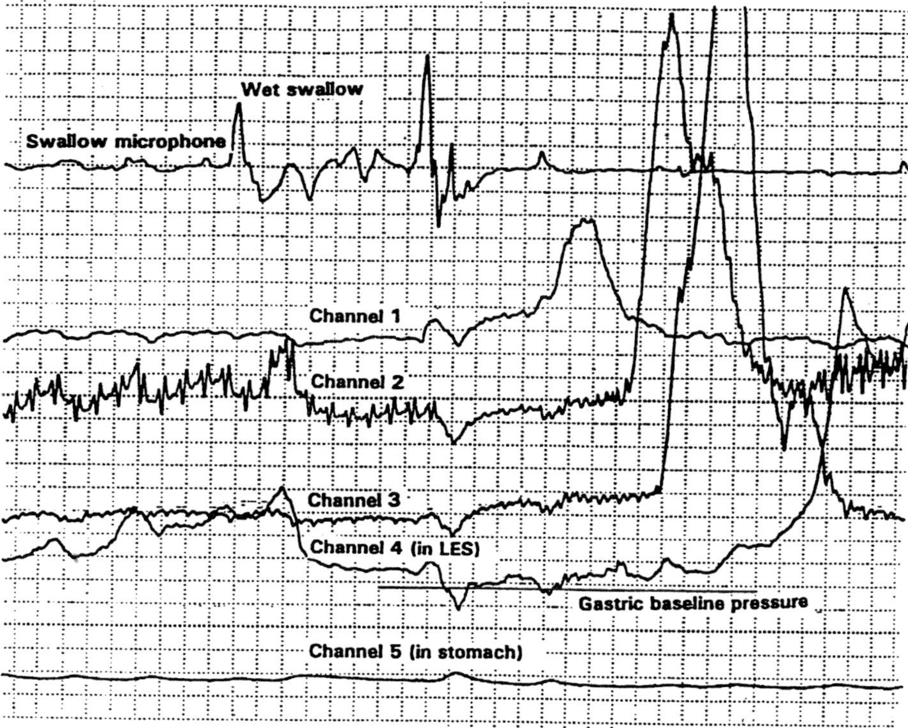

Fig. 14-7. Relaxation of the lower esophageal sphincter *(LES)* in response to a swallow.

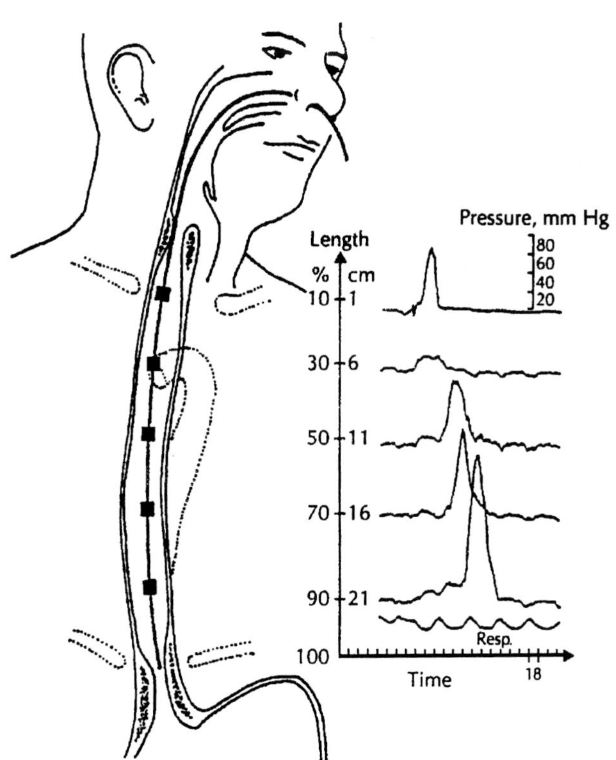

Fig. 14-8. Positioning of sensors in the esophageal body and typical peristaltic response to a swallow in a normal subject.

Assessment of the Upper Esophageal Sphincter

The position, length, and resting pressure of the UES and its relaxation with swallowing are assessed with a technique similar to that for the LES. The key features to be assessed are the adequacy of pharyngeal contraction and the timing and extent of UES relaxation. An indirect measure of UES "stiffness" or loss of compliance is the intrabolus pressure, which appears as a small separate prepharyngeal wave or a "shoulder" on the upstroke of the pharyngeal contraction wave.[10]

Measurement of Esophageal Acid Exposure

The development of 24-hour pH monitoring was a major advance in unraveling the pathophysiology of GERD. All previous tests had relied on the production of reflux by some kind of provocative maneuver, which often had little relevance to the patient's daily activities. The test made it possible to quantify the degree of reflux in normal individuals and to categorize different patterns of reflux in patients with GERD. Although 24-hour pH monitoring logically precedes manometry in the workup of suspected GERD, it is usually performed after the LES has been located by manometry. It is the principal method to make the diagnosis of GERD and has effectively replaced all other "dipstick" methods of measuring esophageal acid exposure. It is indicated in any patient with symptoms suggestive of GERD unless the symptoms are trivial or permanently abolished by a 12-week course of acid suppres-

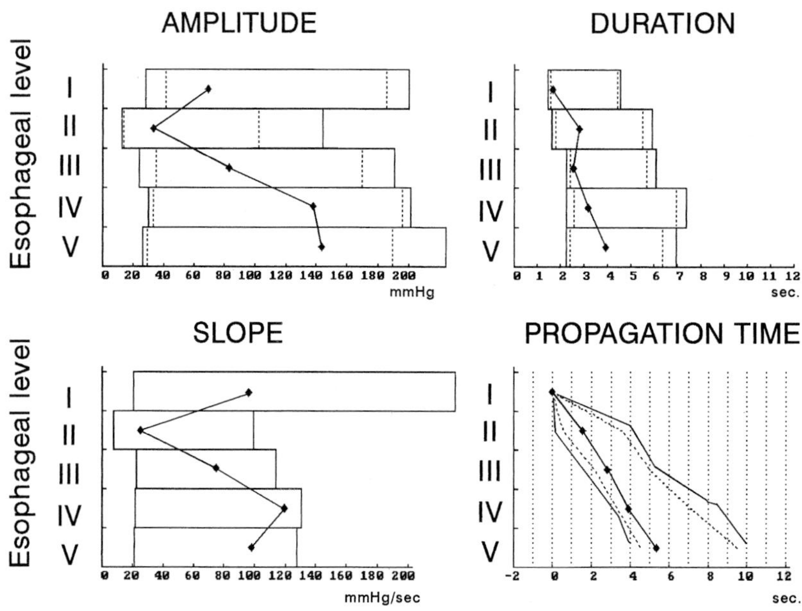

Fig. 14-9. Esophageal body motility characteristics in a patient, compared with normal values. The outer boxes represent the 5th and 95th percentile, and the inner the 10th and 90th percentile, of normal.

sion therapy. Symptoms may be typical (heartburn or regurgitation) or atypical (respiratory symptoms, chest pain, or pharyngeal manifestations). The need for continued acid suppression should stimulate objective study. This is especially important in patients who are being considered for antireflux repair.

It is important to realize that 24-hour esophageal pH monitoring is simply a measure of esophageal acid exposure, and an abnormal test result should not be equated with the presence of GERD. Rather, it should stimulate a search for the cause of the excessive acid exposure.

Conduct

Medications such as H_2-blockers and prokinetics should be discontinued for 48 hours prior to the procedure. Omeprazole may produce prolonged acid suppression, and it should be stopped for 2 weeks prior to pH monitoring. Glass pH electrodes are more accurate than antimony electrodes, especially for pH in the range 6 to 7. All pH probes should be calibrated before and after the test in buffer solutions at pH 1 and 7, and the drift in pH must be within of 0.2 U of the standard for accurate interpretation of the results. The pH probe is placed 5 cm above the manometrically determined upper border of the LES. The catheter is taped to the nostril and looped behind the ear to maintain a stable position with minimal patient discomfort. The pH values are recorded by a digital storage device strapped to the patient's side. The patient returns home and is instructed to carry out his or her normal daily activities but to avoid strenuous exertion. During the day the patient is asked to remain in the upright position and to eat items chosen from a diet sheet with a wide range of foods with a pH in the range of 5 to 7. Smoking and alcohol consumption are prohibited during the test. The patient is provided with a diary and asked to note the times of meals, retiring for sleep, and rising the following morning and to record the presence and duration of any symptoms.

Interpretation

Reflux episodes are defined as periods when the esophageal pH is less than pH 4. Normal (physiologic) reflux occurs in the form of short, rapidly cleared postprandial episodes. Abnormal esophageal acid exposure can be defined as that exceeding the 95th percentile of healthy normal subjects.[11] A typical tracing of a patient with excessive reflux is shown in Fig. 14-10. Some patients tend to experience reflux only while in the upright position, with reflux ceasing abruptly on lying down. Others experience reflux only when lying down. Patients who reflux both during day and night ("combined refluxers") tend to have the most profound loss of the LES and have more severe esophagitis.

A few episodes of long duration are more injurious than many brief episodes, even though the total acid exposure time may be similar. Thus a composite scoring system has been derived to integrate several different features of the pH record into a single measurement of esophageal acid exposure. The score is calculated from the six parameters shown in Table 14-1 and is produced by most commercially available computer software packages. When measured in the above way, esophageal acid exposure in normal subjects is independent of nationality or dietary

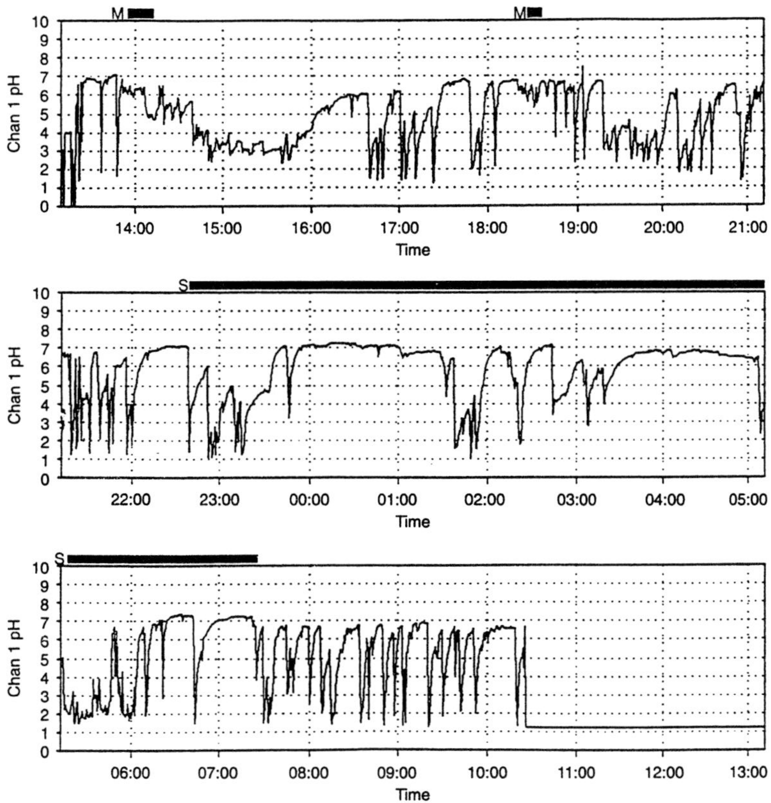

Fig. 14-10. A 24-hour pH record in a patient with both upright and supine reflux. Acid reflux is present when pH drops below pH 4. *M,* Meal period; *S,* supine period.

Table 14-1. Values of 24-Hour Esophageal pH Monitoring in 50 Healthy Volunteers for pH <4

	Mean	SD	Medium	Minimum	Maximum	95th Percentile
% Total time pH <4	1.5	1.4	1.2	0	6	4.5
% Upright time pH <4	2.2	2.3	1.6	0	9.3	8.4
% Supine time pH <4	0.6	1	0.1	0	4	3.5
Number of episodes	19	12.8	16	2	56	46.9
Number of episodes ≥5 min	0.8	1.2	0	0	5	3.5
Longest episode (minutes)	6.7	7.9	4	0	46	19.8
Composite score	6	4.4	5	0.4	18	14.7

habits; when the composite score is used, it is also independent of sex.[12] In addition to quantifying the actual time the esophageal mucosa is exposed to gastric acid, it gives a measure of the ability of the esophagus to clear refluxed acid and correlates esophageal acid exposure with the patient's symptoms.

In addition to the measurement of acid exposure, pH monitoring can also be used to detect excessive alkaline exposure (pH >7) in the esophagus. This is important clinically because it may be an indirect indication that the refluxing gastric juice is mixed with duodenal contents. A more direct measure of duodenogastric reflux (DGR) is now available using the bile probe (see the following). Evidence is emerging that components of bile and duodenal juice are important in the pathogenesis of Barrett's esophagus and its complications.[13]

Dual pH Probe Monitoring

Other esophageal function tests include *dual esophageal pH monitoring* for the investigation of patients who have respiratory symptoms such as nocturnal cough, wheeze, asthma, or recurrent pneumonia. Two pH electrodes are positioned in the esophagus, one 5 cm above the upper border of the LES and the other 1 cm below the lower border of the UES. A key feature of this test is the correlation between reflux episodes and subsequent respiratory symptoms experienced by the patient. If a clear relation can be established and there is no motility defect in the esophagus, abolition of reflux by surgery should be followed by good symptomatic relief.

Provocative Testing

In the standard acid reflux test (SART), the stomach is loaded with HCl; reflux in response to various straining maneuvers is detected by an esophageal pH probe. SART still has a place in patients with hypochlorhydria and a history suggestive of GERD.

The Bernstein test, in which hydrochloric acid is dripped into the esophagus via a nasogastric tube, is sometimes used to determine if a patient's symptoms are reproduced by acid exposure. The Bernstein test is basically a measure of esophageal mucosal sensitivity. It has been largely superseded by the use of 24-hour pH monitoring.

The edrophonium test is a stimulation test employing the anticholinesterase inhibitor edrophonium (Tensilon). It is occasionally performed for a patient with central chest pain in which an esophageal cause is suspected. Although edrophonium often causes marked increases in peristaltic amplitude, the end point of the test is reproduction of the patient's typical symptoms rather than the generation of a specific motility abnormality.

Ambulatory (24-Hour) Esophageal Manometry

Ambulatory esophageal manometry assesses esophageal body peristalsis during a 24-hour period. It is performed with a solid-state catheter having miniature transducers located at three levels in the esophageal body and a proximal sensor situated in the pharynx to flag swallows. The great advantage of ambulatory motility is the ability to record esophageal function during the patient's normal daily activities, especially during meals. It provides a much more comprehensive picture of esophageal function than is possible by stationary manometry. In health the esophagus becomes progressively more organized from the supine to the upright to the meal period, a feature which is reflected in the higher prevalence of effective peristaltic waves during meals.[14] Loss of this improved organization of esophageal activity during mealtimes is a subtle sign of motility disorder; when fewer than 50% of waves during the meal period are effective and peristaltic, there is a significant correlation with the presence of dysphagia.

Esophageal Bile Probe

Esophageal bile probe is a portable spectrophotometric device capable of continuously detecting the presence of bilirubin during a 24-hour period in the ambulatory setting. A fiber-optic cable is connected to a light source and a digital storage device and is worn on the patient's side (Bilitec 2000).[15] The light source emits light at the wavelength of maximal absorbance of bilirubin (453 nm). The light is transmitted across a 2 mm space to a white Teflon reflector, which reflects the light back to the probe. The absorbance of light at this wavelength is indicative of the presence of bilirubin, and the amount of light reflected back to the probe is proportionally reduced. A sentinel beam is also incorporated into the fiber-optic assembly to detect when loss of signal is due to a food particle blocking the reflectance of emitted light. The catheter bearing the bile probe is passed into the esophagus and positioned 5 cm above the upper border of the LES. One potential pitfall is that the yellow colorings in foodstuffs (e.g., butter) may give falsely high values, and the patient should not consume these foods while being monitored.

The function of the esophageal body and LES are affected by abnormalities in the stomach. The ability to study the stomach has lagged behind that of the esophagus because of the greater complexity of its functions.

Gastric Emptying

Gastric emptying is affected by the composition and consistency of the ingested meal. Protein empties faster than fats, and liquids faster than solids. Delayed gastric emptying may be an important etiologic factor in patients with GERD.

Gastric emptying is measured by radionuclide scanning of the stomach after a radiolabeled meal has been eaten. Anterior and posterior images of the area of interest are obtained by a gamma camera collimator for a period of 60 seconds every 15 minutes. Studies are best performed with patients in the upright position, but the patient must remain still during the entire study. Abnormalities in gastric emptying may be identified when the time taken to empty half the meal ($t_{1/2}$) is outside the normal range. More information may be obtained by plotting the patient's emptying curve against the normal values to see if and when the patient falls outside the normal range.

A recently developed technique to evaluate gastric emptying in an ambulatory setting is now available (Synectics, Irving, Texas). A portable Geiger counter is connected to a preamplifier and a digital storage device that can collect counts over a 24-hour period. The probe is passed transnasally and positioned in the proximal stomach 5 cm distal to the lower border of the LES. The patient then ingests up to three labeled meals over the ensuing 24 hours. This gives three measurements of gastric emptying and can be used to study the effect of posture, movement, and food composition. In addition, the gastric emptying probe can be combined with gastric pH monitoring or antroduodenal manometry.

Ambulatory (24-Hour) Gastric pH Monitoring

Gastric pH monitoring may be useful to identify DGR. Relative gastric alkalinization gives an indirect measure of DGR. The study is conducted similarly to that of esophageal pH monitoring, except that the pH probe is positioned in the fundus 5 cm below the lower border of the LES. Currently, more direct evaluation of DGR may be obtained by use of the gastric bile probe (see the following).

Gastric Acid Analysis

Gastric acid analysis is the traditional method for diagnosing gastric acid hypersecretion. The analysis is performed after an overnight fast in patients who have not ingested any antisecretory medications for 48 hours and omeprazole for 2 weeks. The stomach is intubated with a nasogastric tube, and basal acid output (BAO) is determined by collecting gastric secretions for four 15-minute periods. The maximal acid output (MAO) is determined by collecting 15-minute aliquots of gastric secretion during a 1-hour period following stimulation of the gastric secretory state with intravenous pentagastrin in doses of 6 μg/kg. The peak acid output (PAO) is determined by selecting the two consecutive highest stimulated periods. The values obtained are usually expressed as mEq/hr. Hypersecretion is present when BAO is greater than 5 mEq/hr, MAO is greater than 25 mEq/hr, or PAO is greater than 35 mEq/hr.

Gastric Bile Probe

The gastric bile probe (Bilitec 2000) can be used to detect bile in the stomach. The probe is positioned 5 cm below the lower border of the LES. It is a much more direct measure of DGR than monitoring of gastric pH. Early studies in our laboratory have indicated that gastric exposure to bilirubin (above the absorption threshold of >0.2) occurs up to 35% of the time in normal subjects maintaining a liquid diet. The technique is promising, and its role in the investigation of patients with suspected DGR is the subject of several ongoing studies.

Antroduodenal Motility

Antroduodenal motility is the technique used to study the motor function of the antrum and duodenum in response to a meal. Short-term studies (2 to 4 hours) may be performed with water-perfused catheters, but ambulatory studies with solid-state catheters are now possible. Computerized analysis is still being developed, and the method is likely to be valuable for investigation of gastroparesis and postoperative emptying disorders of the stomach.

Cholescintigraphy

Scintigraphic imaging of bile reflux into the stomach can be performed after intravenous injection of 5 μCi of Tc^{99m} iminodiacetic acid derivatives such as disofenin (DISIDA), followed by cholecystokinin stimulation of the gallbladder. Although the ability to quantitate gastric reflux by scintigraphy is an attractive concept, its specificity and sensitivity is low, and the test is likely to be replaced by more direct bile probe measurement in future.

ESOPHAGEAL MOTOR DISORDERS

Esophageal motor disorders primarily affect either the pharyngoesophageal segment or the esophageal body. Primary motor disorders of the esophageal body are muscular defects of unknown cause, whereas secondary motor disorders are the result of some systemic disease affecting the esophagus. In practice, the commonest secondary motor disorder is the impaired contractility associated with complicated GERD, but the term usually refers to a systemic connective tissue or neuromuscular disease such as scleroderma or polymyositis.

There are four identifiable categories of primary motor disorders, namely achalasia, diffuse esophageal spasm, nutcracker esophagus, and the hypertensive LES. A fifth "catch all" category termed nonspecific esophageal motor disorders includes those disorders where motor function is clearly abnormal, but the abnormalities do not fall into one of the four major categories mentioned. These categories are derived from the manometric features on stationary motility. The advent of ambulatory motility has shown that the disorders may not be as distinct as the classification implies. Intermediate forms exist. It is nevertheless convenient to use these categories until a broadly based consensus is reached.

Pharyngoesophageal Disorders

Disorders of the pharyngoesophageal phase of swallowing result from a discoordination of the neuromuscular events involved in chewing, initiation of swallowing, and propulsion of the material from the oropharynx to the cervical esophagus. The most common of pharyngoesophageal dysphagia are neuromuscular diseases.[16] The most important are cerebrovascular disease, myasthenia gravis, Parkinson's disease, motor neuron disease, multiple sclerosis, and muscular diseases such as myotonic dystrophy and polymyositis. Other important causes are structural lesions, and include tumors, Zenker's diverticulum, scarring of the tongue or pharynx from caustic injury, previous surgery, or radiation therapy. Rarely, pharyngoesophageal dysphagia may be caused by extrinsic compression from goiter or cervical spine osteophytes. All these diseases produce their effects by disrupting one or more of the components of the pharyngeal mechanism illustrated in Fig. 14-11.

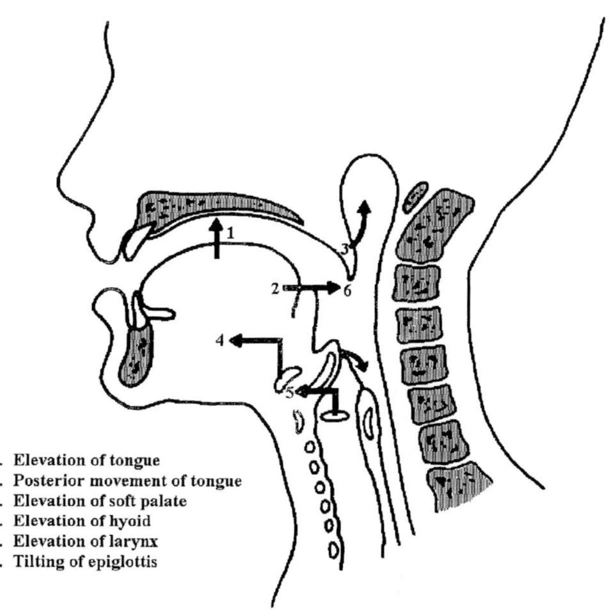

Fig. 14-11. Components of swallowing mechanism that may be disrupted by disease, resulting in dysphagia, aspiration, or nasal regurgitation.

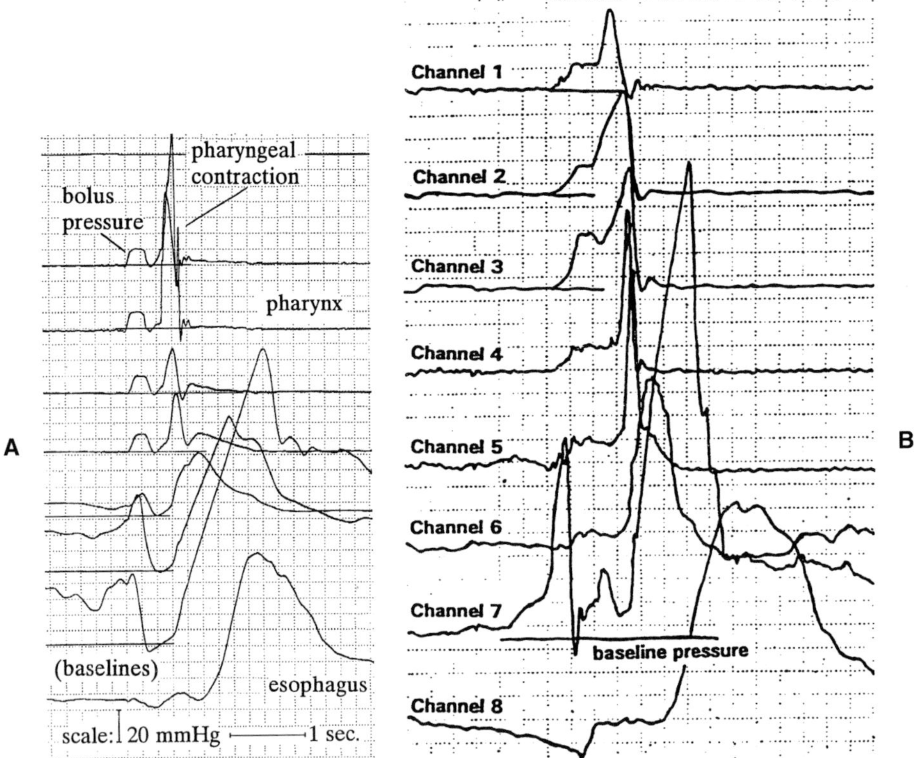

Fig. 14-12. Detailed manometric cricopharyngeal study of a normal subject **(A)** and a patient with elevated bolus pressure in channel 3 and incomplete upper esophageal sphincter relaxation in channel 7 **(B)**.

Weakness or immobility of the *tongue* produces difficulty in thrusting the bolus into the oropharynx, thus compromising oropharyngeal transfer. Paralysis of the *soft palate* prevents the oropharynx from being partitioned from the nasopharynx, thus preventing pressurization of the pharynx. This accounts for the frequent occurrence of nasal regurgitation and the nasal quality to the voice in such patients. If the *larynx* cannot be elevated, there is loss of airway protection, and patients are prone to aspiration. The *UES* may relax either incompletely, prematurely, or both. If pharyngeal pressure overcomes any residual pressure in the UES, swallowing may be normal, but incomplete UES relaxation in the face of inadequate pharyngeal pressure causes poor pharyngeal clearance of the bolus. Further, when the swallow is complete and the larynx and epiglottis have returned to their resting position, residual material in the hypopharynx is aspirated. Recent studies in which videoroentgenography and manometry were combined have demonstrated that in certain patients with pharyngeal swallowing disorders, notably Zenker's diverticulum or cricopharyngeal bar, the UES relaxes manometrically, but there is roentgenographic evidence of diminished opening and increased pressure in the bolus. This intrabolus pressure (Fig. 14-12) is recognized as a small wave just prior to the pharyngeal wave and is thought to reflect the compliance of the pharyngoesophageal segment. This pressure is elevated in the presence of muscle pathology, indicating reduced compliance.

Investigation

Videoroentgenography is crucial to evaluate oropharyngeal bolus transport, pharyngeal contraction, relaxation of the pharyngoesophageal segment, and the dynamics of airway protection during swallowing. It readily identifies a diverticulum (Fig. 14-13). Stasis of the contrast medium may occur in the valleculae or diverticulum, and in patients with a neurologic disorder a cricopharyngeal bar may be present, indicating a failure of the pharyngoesophageal segment to relax completely.

Carefully performed motility studies may demonstrate insufficient relaxation or premature contraction of the cricopharyngeus muscle, high sphincter pressure, inadequate pharyngeal pressurization, or an elevated intrabolus pressure. The latter suggests decreased compliance of the pharyngoesophageal segment.

Treatment

Therapeutic options in pharyngoesophageal disorders are limited by the nature of the pathology. In practice, nonsurgical treatment is limited to (1) drug treatment for a specific neurologic condition (e.g., myasthenia gravis or Parkinson's disease) and (2) therapy from a speech pathologist designed to train patients to maximize what function they possess. Patients with unilateral brain stem or cranial nerve lesions can to taught to swallow better by turning the head to the affected side. Aspiration can also be reduced by training patients to swallow against a closed glot-

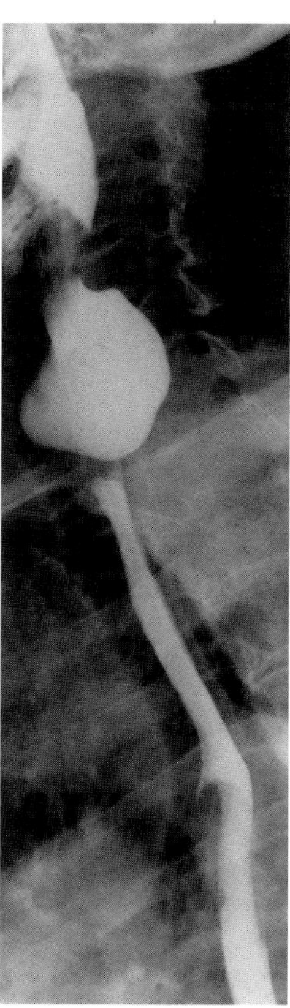

Fig. 14-13. Barium esophagogram in a patient with a Zenker's diverticulum.

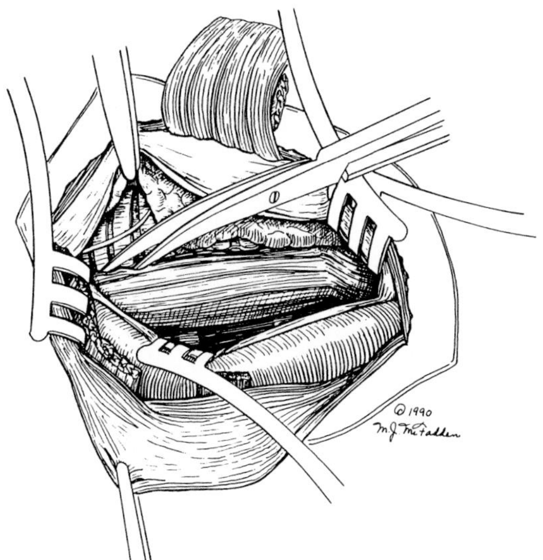

Fig. 14-14. Initial exposure for cricomyotomy via a left neck incision.

tis; if this is impossible because of vocal cord paresis, a Teflon injection into the affected vocal cord may allow improvement.

The surgeon's role is to reduce outflow resistance by performing cricomyotomy. Initially this was recommended only for patients with demonstrable failure of UES relaxation. More recently, a number of reports indicate that a wide variety of neuromuscular diseases may be improved by cricomyotomy. This is because a weak or uncoordinated pharyngeal contraction may be sufficient to permit improved swallowing if outflow resistance is reduced. The outcome of cricomyotomy is also affected by the presence of more distal esophageal disease: when gross GERD and an associated motility defect of the esophageal body coexist, the risk of aspiration of gastric juice is increased.

The surgical options in Zenker's diverticulum are either excision or suspension. Excision is sometimes recommended on the grounds that malignant change in the sac is prevented, but there is no evidence that excision carries any greater protective role than suspension, which effectively prevents stagnation of food material, thus removing the presumed cause of malignant change. Suspension also removes the risk of contamination of the operative site, the risk of subsequent breakdown of the closure site with fistula formation, and the risk of narrowing of the esophagus. Recurrence is likely if a concomitant cricomyotomy is not performed because the underlying defect that predisposed to the diverticulum persists. Histologic studies of esophageal muscle in Zenker's diverticulum show degenerative changes that correlate with decreased compliance noted manometrically. Thus all surgical procedures for this condition should include a myotomy of the cricopharyngeus muscle and proximal esophagus.

A longitudinal incision is performed along the anterior border of the left sternocleidomastoid muscle. The pharynx and cervical esophagus are exposed by retracting the sternocleidomastoid muscle and carotid sheath laterally and the trachea and larynx medially (Fig. 14-14). Care is taken not to injure the recurrent laryngeal nerve by avoiding the use of a metal retractor on the larynx. When a diverticulum is present, localization of the pharyngoesophageal segment is easy. The diverticulum is carefully freed from the overlying areolar tissue to expose clearly its neck and the underlying pharyngeal constrictor muscle. The fibers of the cricopharyngeal muscle, located inferior to the neck of the diverticulum, are divided down to the mucosa. The myotomy is extended cephalad to the diverticular neck by dividing 1 to 2 cm of inferior constrictor muscle of the pharynx and caudad by dividing the muscle fibers of the cervical esophagus for a length of 4 to 5 cm (Fig. 14-15). It can be difficult to identify the cricopharyngeus muscle in the absence of a diverticulum. When local anesthesia is used, the patient can be asked to swallow; this usually shows an area of persistent narrowing at the pharyngoesophageal junction. The myotomy is started in the easily identifiable cervical esophageal wall and extended cephalad 1 cm into the posterior pharyngeal muscle above the pharyngoesophageal junction. Critical in the performance of this operation is the maintenance of meticulous hemostasis. The venous pumping action of the lung can cause the development postoperatively of a large hematoma in the mediastinum, which at best delays the im-

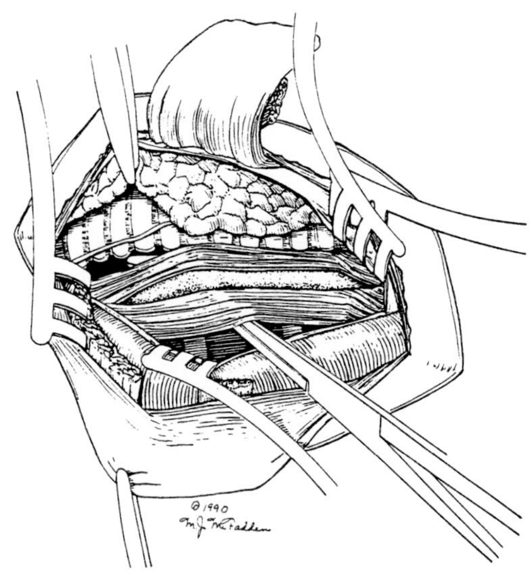

Fig. 14-15. Completed cricomyotomy.

provement in the patient's dysphagia and may result in laryngeal edema and the need for tracheostomy. The cervical wound is then closed without drainage, and oral alimentation is started the following day. The patient is usually discharged on the first or second postoperative day.

If the diverticulum is large enough to persist after myotomy, it may be suspended by suturing its apex to the prevertebral fascia using a nonabsorbable suture (i.e., diverticulopexy). If the diverticulum is excessively large so that it would be redundant if suspended, or its walls are thickened, a diverticulectomy should be performed. This may be achieved by a stapler applied in the transverse plane or a single layer of continuous or interrupted sutures. It is important to prevent narrowing during closure. Using a stapler to remove the diverticulum or suspending it has the advantage of preventing contamination of the wound. More recently, surgeons are exploring minimally invasive techniques to treat Zenker's diverticulum; the most popular involves the insertion of a modified endoscopic linear stapling device into the lumina of the esophagus and diverticulum and dividing the common wall between them. The cricopharyngeus muscle is necessarily divided in the process. Early results with this technique, which is restricted to large (>3 cm) diverticula, is encouraging in expert hands.

All operations on the cervical esophagus carry the risk of hematoma formation and recurrent nerve paralysis. If the diverticulum is opened rather than suspended, there is a significantly increased risk of salivary fistula and wound infection.

Finally, in patients who fail to benefit from reduction of outflow resistance and swallowing therapy, the only option is tube feeding. A percutaneous endoscopic gastrostomy (PEG) is inserted, and liquid feedings are given either through a continuous pump or by bolus injection. If aspiration of tube feedings from gastroesophageal reflux is a problem, a tube can be inserted through the PEG and fed into the distal duodenum under endoscopic control, but sometimes the upward angulation of the PEG causes the duodenal tube to flip back into the stomach. A formal jejunostomy is the most trouble-free solution but requires the patient be under general anesthetic.

Primary Motor Disorders of the Esophageal Body

Achalasia

Achalasia is the best known primary motility disorder of the esophagus. It is characterized by failure of esophageal body peristalsis and incomplete relaxation of the LES. It is generally thought to be caused by neuronal degeneration in the myenteric plexus, causing loss of activity of inhibitory neurons in the LES, leading to increased outflow resistance. The cause of the neuronal degeneration is obscure: there is some evidence that previous infection with varicella-zoster virus may be responsible.[17] Further, there is some experimental evidence that obstruction at the gastroesophageal junction may produce a condition with the radiologic and manometric features of achalasia. This corresponds to the clinical situation where features of achalasia develop in response to an infiltrating tumor of the cardia (pseudoachalasia) or after a tight Nissen fundoplication or Angelchik prosthesis. This evidence suggests that outflow resistance is a primary phenomenon and the degeneration of the esophageal body is a secondary phenomenon, a concept also supported by reports of return of peristalsis after relief of outflow obstruction.

All patients with achalasia have dysphagia, and most have regurgitation. Careful questioning is needed to distinguish regurgitation of esophageal contents from vomiting of gastric contents. Generally, it occurs during or at the end of a meal, and the material tastes bland rather than sour or bitter. Patients often have to leave the table to regurgitate and are usually slow eaters. Nighttime regurgitation causes staining of the pillow. Respiratory symptoms, caused by aspiration, are common and may precede the development of dysphagia. One further characteristic is the length of time, frequently several years, that the symptoms have persisted before the diagnosis is made. Patients are commonly told that their symptoms are due to "stress" and may be taking antidepressive or anxiolytic medication. Late in the disease, patients tend to lose weight and become socially isolated. Chest pain is common in achalasia, not always related to eating, and is sometimes due to trapped air causing distention. In some patients the occurrence of chest pain and the manometric finding of simultaneous contractions in the esophagus have led to the description of a subgroup termed vigorous achalasia. Recent evidence is casting doubt on this entity as a separate disease, and it is more likely that a continuous spectrum of clinical and manometric findings exists.

The roentgenographic appearance of achalasia depends on its stage. In the early stages it may be normal, and such patients may be falsely reassured. Later, esophageal dilation develops, and an air fluid level may be noted. Both of these indicate outflow obstruction. Barium is rarely seen to enter the stomach, and when a good view of the cardia is

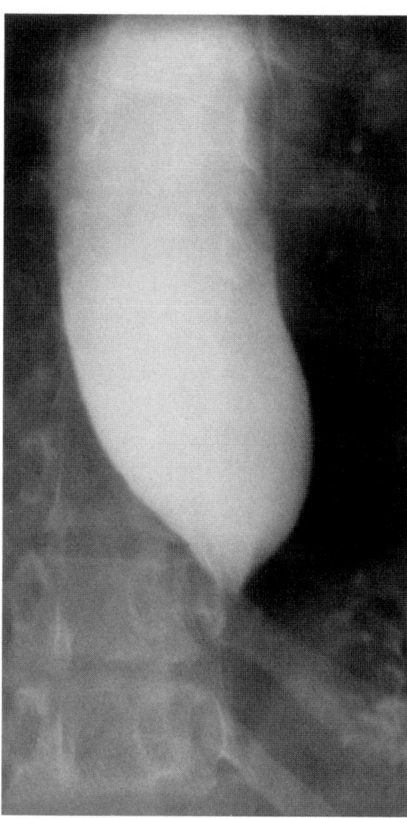

Fig. 14-16. Barium esophagogram demonstrating dilated esophagus and characteristic bird's beak deformity in achalasia.

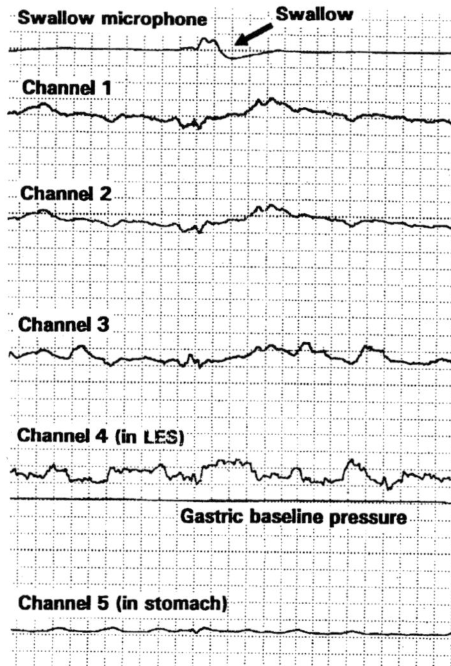

Fig. 14-17. Manometric tracing in achalasia, showing nonrelaxation of the lower esophageal sphincter *(LES)* and absent peristalsis.

obtained, it has a narrow tapering "bird's beak" appearance (Fig. 14-16). The late stage of achalasia is characterized by a tortuous, sigmoid esophagus, and an epiphrenic diverticulum may be present. Absence of the gastric air bubble may be noted and is due to the inability to propel swallowed air into the stomach.

Endoscopy frequently reveals residual liquid or food in the esophagus. Unlike a stricture the narrowing at the lower end permits the passage of the endoscope, usually with a characteristic "popping" sensation. In untreated cases mild esophagitis may be observed, sometimes attributed to fermentation or stagnation of esophageal contents. When the patient has had previous treatment for achalasia, such inflammation is likely to be caused by gastroesophageal reflux. In every patient with presumed achalasia, it is important to view the cardia from below with the endoscope retroflexed, as a small infiltrating gastroesophageal tumor may otherwise be missed.

Manometry is required to establish the diagnosis of achalasia. The classic features (Fig. 14-17) on stationary manometry are listed in the following:

1. Elevated LES pressure
2. Incomplete LES relaxation
3. Absence of esophageal body peristalsis
4. Positive intraesophageal body pressure

Not all patients have all four features. Sometimes the LES pressure is in the normal range, but it is never subnormal in untreated achalasia. Care is needed in interpreting LES relaxation. If the transducer is positioned in the lower part of the LES, upward movement of the LES during swallowing causes the transducer to be momentarily in the stomach, thus giving a spurious impression of relaxation. The transducer should be positioned in the proximal portion of the LES.

On swallowing, a low pressure wave is usually seen simultaneously in all levels in the esophagus. This is sometimes wrongly described as a simultaneous contraction, but it simply represents the pressure generated by the pharynx being transmitted to the esophageal body, which behaves as a fluid-filled cavity closed at its lower end. It is not unusual to find some peristaltic activity in the upper (skeletal muscle) esophagus. The intraesophageal pressure, which is subatmospheric in normal people, is typically positive in achalasia, reflecting resistance to outflow.

There are not many reports of 24-hour pH and motility studies in achalasia. In patients before dilation or operation, excessive acid exposure is rare. A characteristic pattern is the gradual fall in pH during a period of hours, often at night, probably as a result of fermentation of residual food material. When true reflux episodes do occur, they are prolonged because of the absence of peristalsis.

Treatment. Although some patients show a short-lived symptomatic and manometric response to calcium channel blocking agents, the mainstay of treatment in achalasia is either balloon dilation or surgery. The recent description of botulinum toxin injection has created much interest, but the reduction in LES pressure is small, and the follow-up very short. The role of botulinum toxin injection is therefore speculative at present.[18]

Balloon dilation has the advantages that it can be performed on an outpatient basis and has minimal recovery time. However, it is less likely to be effective than surgical treatment and frequently must be repeated. The risk of perforation of the lower esophagus is higher with this procedure than with any other form of esophageal instrumentation and varies from 2% to 10%. Some patients may be treated conservatively after perforation, but many require an emergency thoracotomy for closure. The risk of gastroesophageal reflux following dilation is not known, as large studies of 24-hour pH monitoring after dilation are lacking; but symptomatically the risk appears to be low.

All surgical procedures employ a variant of Heller's myotomy, in which the circular muscle of the lower esophagus is divided. In the United States most myotomies are carried out through the chest, but the abdominal route is favored in Europe. Regardless of the route chosen, four key principles are important, namely (1) adequate myotomy, (2) minimal hiatal disturbance, (3) antireflux protection without the creation of obstruction, and (4) prevention of rehealing. The advent of minimally invasive surgery has led to the development of thoracoscopic and laparoscopic myotomy, and these are now being extensively performed with early results comparable to open surgery. There is broad agreement that if the myotomy is performed through the abdomen, an antireflux procedure should be added and that a full Nissen wrap, however floppy, leads to long-term failure.[19,20] Either a posterior (Toupet) or anterior (Dor) hemifundoplication should be used. When approached through the chest, there is controversy about the need for an antireflux procedure, as it is claimed that less hiatal disturbance and more limited myotomy is possible by this route. Our preference is to add a partial fundoplication of the Dor type (covering the lower part of the myotomy) when performing open transthoracic myotomy but not when performing it thoracoscopically, since the enhanced view enables a more precise determination of the distal limit of the myotomy to be made.

Technique. Open Heller myotomy, a modified Heller myotomy, is usually performed through a left thoracotomy in the seventh intercostal space. The inferior pulmonary ligament is divided, and the left lung is retracted superiorly. The use of a double-lumen endotracheal tube with selective ventilation of the right lung greatly aids the exposure. An incision is made in the posterior mediastinal pleura over the esophagus, and the left lateral wall of the esophagus is exposed. Unless absolutely necessary, the esophagus is not circumferentially dissected. A nasogastric tube is passed to decompress the stomach. A 2 cm incision is made through the phrenoesophageal membrane into the abdomen along the left crus. This exposes the gastroesophageal junction and its associated fat pad. The latter is excised to expose the junction. A myotomy through all muscle layers is started on the esophageal body. The completed myotomy extends distally over the stomach to 1 to 2 cm below the junction and proximally on the esophagus for 4 to 5 cm (Fig. 14-18). Proximal extension of the myotomy can be performed if there is a vigorous component to the disease.

The muscle layer is dissected from the mucosa laterally for a distance of 1 cm. Care is taken to divide all minute muscle bands, particularly in the area of the junction. The persistence of small muscular fibers can cause a failure of the operation. The cardia is reconstructed by suturing the gastric fundic flap to the margins of the myotomy for a distance of 4 cm (Fig. 14-19) to prevent healing of the myotomy site and to provide reflux protection in the area of the divided sphincter. If an extensive dissection of the cardia has been done or if return of the cardia to the abdomen causes angulation, a more formal Belsey repair is

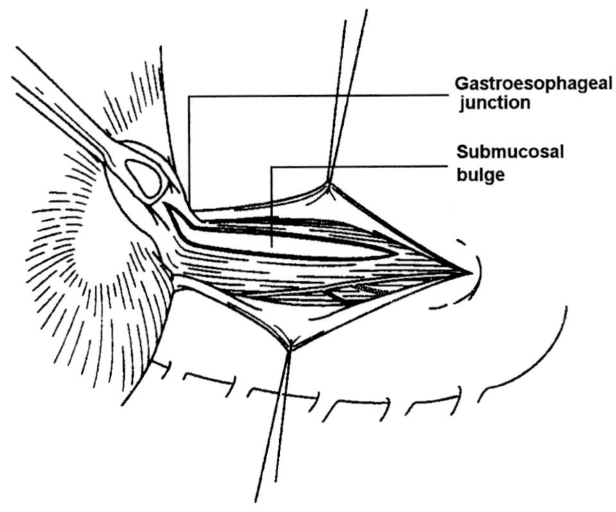

Fig. 14-18. Myotomy of the esophageal body and lower esophageal sphincter.

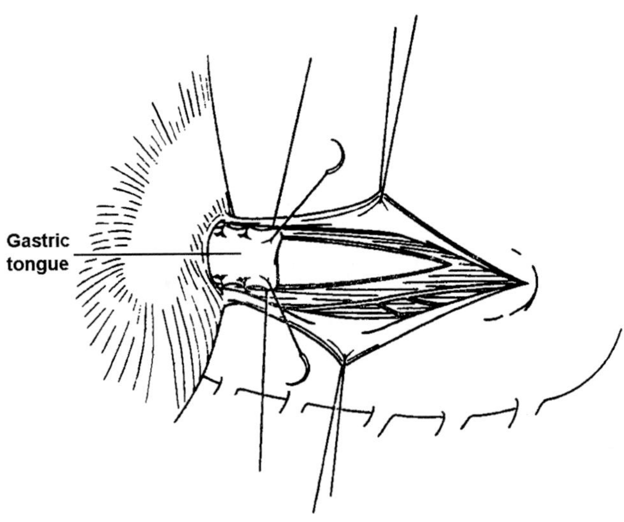

Fig. 14-19. Reconstruction of the cardia after myotomy. A tongue of gastric fundus is sutured to the distal 4 cm of the myotomy.

performed. The gastric fundic flap is allowed to retract into the abdomen and is maintained there by passing the tails of the tied apical sutures of the flap through the diaphragm (Fig. 14-20).

Before closure, the myotomy site is checked for perforation by insufflating air down the nasogastric tube with the myotomy site submerged in normal saline. If the mucosa is perforated at surgery, it should be carefully repaired using fine nonabsorbable sutures. The mucosa is usually covered by the tongue of gastric fundus brought up to perform the antireflux procedure. The same principles are followed exactly when performing the myotomy thoracoscopically, but the operator is aided by an assistant performing simultaneous endoscopy to visualize the gastroesophageal junction from within. This allows a precise delineation of the extent of myotomy.

Thoracoscopic myotomy is now becoming more popular and is performed via ports placed as shown in Fig. 14-21. The rigidity of the thoracic cavity obviates the need for gas insufflation. The principles of operation are the same except that the hiatal dissection is less. An L-shaped electrocautery hook is used to perform the myotomy and the lower limit of the incision is defined with the help of intraoperative flexible esophagoscopy to visualize the gastroesophageal junction. At the end of the procedure the cavity is filled with water, and air is insufflated via the endoscope to confirm mucosal integrity. No nasogastric tube is used after thoracoscopic myotomy.

Attention in the early postoperative period is directed to the chest. If used, the nasogastric tube is removed when the risk of gastric distention has passed, as judged by scanty aspirate, passage of flatus, and active bowel sounds. This is usually by the third or fourth day after open surgery. An esophagogram on the fifth to seventh postoperative day should demonstrate unimpaired passage of contrast into the stomach without extravasation. Wound infections should be rare, since the gastrointestinal tract is not opened. Mucosal perforations are usually easily seen and repaired at the time of surgery, but an unrecognized perforation is a serious complication and should be suspected in a patient with continuing fever or chest signs.

Late complications after either type of myotomy include persistent or recurrent dysphagia. Dysphagia returning in the first 3 months indicates either an incomplete myotomy, a healed myotomy, an improper antireflux repair, or the presence of megaesophagus. Dysphagia occurring 1 to 10 years postoperatively is more usually due to a reflux stricture or carcinoma. In general, the shorter the interval between primary surgery and recurrence of symptoms, the more likely the cause is a technical failure. In such patients, remyotomy or conversion of the fundoplication to a partial type has a good chance of success. When symptoms recur following an interval of several years, remyotomy is less likely to be successful, and esophageal replacement is required. In particular, the combination of a reflux stricture and an aperistaltic esophagus usually requires esophagectomy. Squamous carcinoma of the esophagus is said to be commoner in long-standing achalasia, but the magnitude of the risk is debated. There are several reports of adenocarcinoma developing in Barrett's esophagus after myotomy, presumably because of inadequate reflux protection.

Outcome. A single pneumatic dilation achieves adequate relief of dysphagia and pharyngeal regurgitation in about 60% of patients, although this figure falls to about 30% after 5 years. Close follow-up is required, and if dilation fails, myotomy is indicated. For those patients who have a dilated or tortuous esophagus, balloon dilation is dangerous, and surgery is the better option. Whether to treat newly diagnosed esophageal achalasia by forceful dilation or by operative cardiomyotomy remains controversial from the position of patient comfort, but the outcome

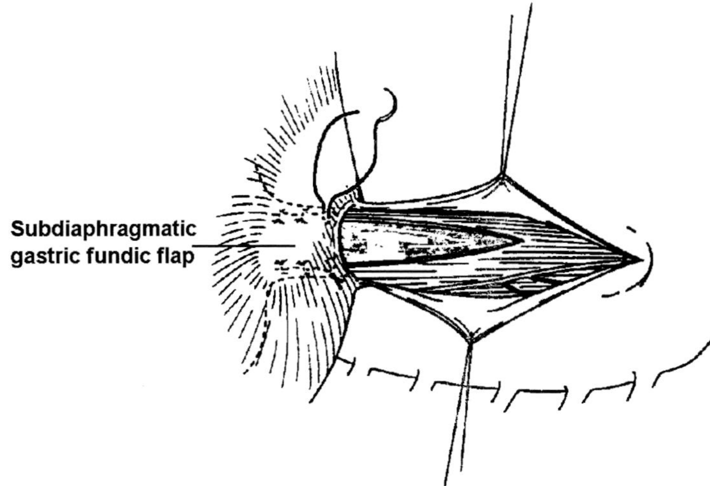

Fig. 14-20. Completed reconstruction of the cardia, illustrating the subdiaphragmatic portion of the gastric fundic flap. The tails of the tied apical sutures have been passed through the diaphragm and tied 2 cm apart at the margins of the myotomy.

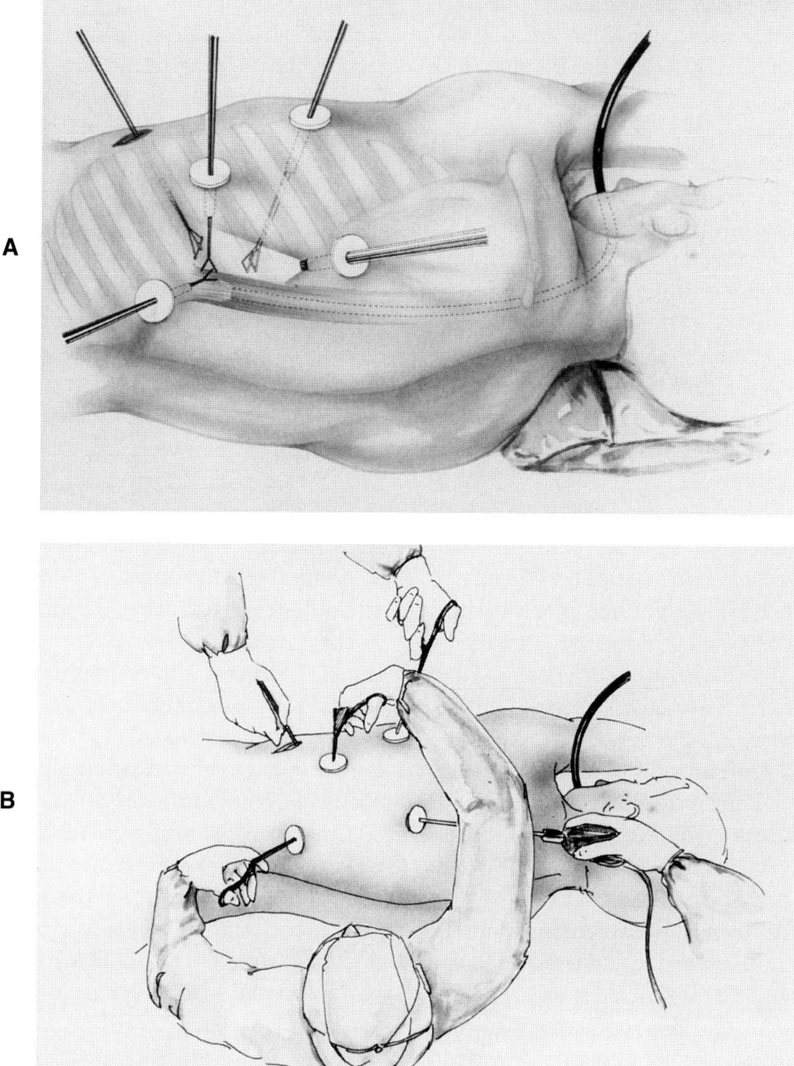

Fig. 14-21. A, Patient and surgeon positioning for thoracoscopic esophageal myotomy. **B,** Trocar ports. A single 2-inch incision and four thoracoports are used.

data support surgery. Only one controlled randomized study comparing the two modes of therapy has ever been performed. The results showed a clear advantage for surgery.[21] The study was criticized because the mode of dilation was thought to be inadequate, but the benefits persisted even when the dilation technique was changed. There are several large series that retrospectively describe the results obtained with the two modes of treatment, and their conclusions similarly support the superiority of surgical treatment over balloon dilation. Despite objections regarding variations in surgical and dilation techniques and the number of physicians performing the procedures, these collective data would appear to support operative myotomy as the initial treatment of choice. Although it has been reported that a myotomy after previous balloon dilation is more difficult, this has not been our experience unless the cardia has been ruptured. In this situation, operative intervention either immediately or after healing has occurred can be difficult.

Diffuse Esophageal Spasm

Diffuse esophageal spasm (DES) is an esophageal motor disorder characterized clinically by substernal chest pain and/or dysphagia. It differs from classic achalasia in that it represents a primary disease of the esophageal body, produces a lesser degree of dysphagia, causes more chest pain, and has less effect on the patient's general condition. True symptomatic DES is much more rare than achalasia. Roentgenographic abnormalities such as segmental spasm with compartmentalization of the esophagus or formation of a diverticulum are the anatomic correlates of the disordered motility function. The abnormal motility disorder usually occurs prior to the development of the roentgenographic findings. The development of a diverticulum may temporarily alleviate the symptom of initial dysphagia and replace it with postprandial symptoms of pain and regurgitation of undigested food, suggesting achalasia. In most patients with a diverticulum, simultaneous contractions of the esophageal body can be identified manometrically. If not, a traction etiologic factor for the diverticulum should be sought.

Manometric abnormalities in DES may be present over the total length of the smooth muscle portion of the esophageal body. In segmental esophageal spasm the manometric abnormalities are confined to a short segment of the esophagus. The classic manometric finding in these patients is the frequent occurrence of simultaneous and repetitive esophageal contractions, which may be of abnormally high amplitude or long duration. Key to the diagnosis of DES is that the esophagus retains a degree of peristaltic ability, in contrast to that of achalasia. A criterion of 20% or more simultaneous contractions in 10 wet swallows has been used to diagnose DES. This figure is arbitrary and often debated. More useful criteria may be developed based on ambulatory motility studies, especially during the meal period.

The LES in patients with DES usually shows normal resting pressure and relaxation on deglutition. A hypertensive sphincter with poor relaxation may also be present and may represent early achalasia. In patients with advanced disease the radiographic appearance of tertiary contractions appears helical and has been termed "corkscrew esophagus" or "pseudodiverticulosis."

DES is a benign disease in that it rarely causes nutritional problems and does not lead to life-threatening complications. For this reason, symptom control is the only significant goal of treatment. Medical treatment for DES is focused on abolishing strong simultaneous contractions and generally employs calcium channel blocking agents or long-acting nitrates. The surgical option is to perform myotomy of the esophageal body. Surgery for DES is not as strikingly successful as in achalasia and is considered only when medical treatment is ineffective. In general, the higher the incidence and extent of simultaneous contractions the more successful the myotomy will be. This is because the myotomy effectively abolishes the beneficial peristaltic contractions and the simultaneous contractions. Generally, if more than 70% of the esophageal contractions on ambulatory motility are simultaneous, the benefits of myotomy outweigh the loss of residual peristaltic waves.[22] Esophageal body myotomy should always be accompanied by myotomy of the LES (with partial fundoplication if performed by open surgery), as even a normal LES may impose an outflow resistance too great for the myotomized body to overcome.

Nutcracker Esophagus

The term *nutcracker esophagus* is used to describe a manometric abnormality in which by definition the amplitude of esophageal body peristalsis is greater than 2 standard deviations above normal. It came to light as increasing numbers of patients with noncardiac chest pain were investigated by esophageal manometry and is in fact the commonest primary motility disorder of the esophagus. However, ambulatory motility studies have shown that many of these patients are either normal or have features of diffuse spasm or a nonspecific esophageal motor disorder, and this disease may not be a genuine entity.

The dominant symptom of this condition is central crushing chest pain. It may have no relation to food ingestion but differs from angina in that it more frequently comes on at rest. Dysphagia or classic heartburn may be present but tends to be overshadowed by the chest pain.

These patients are usually referred from cardiologists with normal coronary angiograms and a request for esophageal motility testing. Barium radiography and endoscopy are not usually helpful. The pathognomic feature on manometry is the presence of prolonged high-amplitude waves, with a peak greater than 180 mm Hg. The cutoff point depends on the methodology of each laboratory. The waves are normally peristaltic. Many patients with noncardiac chest pain are found to have increased esophageal acid exposure; this subgroup is important to identify because they respond well to fundoplication.

Myotomy for isolated nutcracker esophagus with symptoms of chest pain has a low success rate, and the mainstay of treatment for these patients is muscle-relaxing drugs (e.g., nitrates and calcium channel blockers). If the diagnosis of DES is discovered by ambulatory manometry, myotomy is more likely to be successful.

Hypertensive Lower Esophageal Sphincter

The *hypertensive LES* is characterized by an elevated basal pressure of the LES (>95th percentile of normal). Typically, patients initially have chest pain and dysphagia. In about half of these patients with this manometric abnormality, the LES relaxation and esophageal body peristalsis are normal, but in the remainder there are associated motility disorders of the esophageal body, particularly hypertensive peristalsis and simultaneous contractions. Symptoms in these patients may be caused by a prolonged postrelaxation contraction of the LES. Myotomy of the LES may be indicated to reduce outflow resistance in patients not responding to medical therapy or dilations.

Nonspecific Esophageal Motor Disorders

Many patients complaining of dysphagia or chest pain of noncardiac origin demonstrate a variety of esophageal contraction patterns on esophageal manometry that are clearly out of the normal range but do not meet the criteria of a classic primary esophageal motility disorder. Esophageal manometry in these patients frequently shows an increased number of multipeaked or repetitive contractions, contractions of prolonged duration, nontransmitted contractions, an interruption of a peristaltic sequence at various levels of the esophagus, or contractions of low amplitude. These motility abnormalities have been termed nonspecific esophageal motility disorders. The significance of these abnormal contractions in the cause of chest pain or dysphagia is still unclear, and surgery plays no role in treatment of these disorders unless there is an associated diverticulum, in which case the diverticulum is suspended or resected and distal myotomy extending across the LES is performed. The finding of a nonspecific motor disorder may be important in a patient with proven GERD, as it may warn the surgeon of future trouble after a complete 360-degree Nissen fundoplication. The outcome of antireflux surgery in patients with nonspecific motor disorders depends on symptoms. A good result may be expected if the primary symptom is heartburn; but if the cough is the primary symptom, the outcome is less satisfactory.

It is important to realize that a clear distinction between the classic primary esophageal motility disorders and the nonspecific esophageal motility disorders is often not possible. Patients diagnosed as having a nutcracker esophagus often have only nonspecific esophageal motility abnormalities when studied repeatedly, and progression from a nonspecific esophageal motility disorder to classic DES during the course of the disease has been demonstrated. The finding of a nonspecific esophageal motility disorder therefore may represent only a manometric marker of an intermittent more severe esophageal motor abnormality. Combined ambulatory 24-hour esophageal pH and motility monitoring has shown that an increased esophageal exposure to gastric juice is common in patients diagnosed as having a nonspecific esophageal motility disorder. Furthermore, respiratory symptoms associated with GERD are increased in the presence of a nonspecific esophageal motility disorder. In some situations the motor abnormalities may be induced by the irritation of refluxed gastric juice; in other situations it may be a primary event unrelated to the presence of reflux. The distinction is important because correction of the reflux by total fundoplication cures the patient if the reflux is primary; but if the motility disorder is primary, total fundoplication may result in failure to improve the respiratory symptoms and in deterioration of the esophageal body.

Secondary Motor Disorders of the Esophagus

Many connective tissue and neuromuscular diseases affect the esophageal body, but the most significant is scleroderma, since most patients with this condition develop dysphagia. The loss of esophageal function is caused by replacement of the muscle of the lower esophagus and LES by fibrous tissue. The manometric hallmark of the condition is absence of LES pressure and severely impaired contraction amplitude in the smooth muscle portion of the esophagus. The grossly defective LES allows superimposed reflux-induced injury to occur, accelerating the loss of esophageal body function. Many patients develop a stricture. Antireflux surgery in this situation must involve a partial fundoplication, but some patients eventually require esophageal replacement. Sometimes the esophageal abnormality is combined with severe delay in gastric emptying. These patients are greatly improved by performing total gastrectomy and reconstruction via a Hunt-Lawrence jejunal pouch in a Roux-en-Y fashion.

Surgical treatment of motor disorders by myotomy cannot normally reverse the disease process but rather creates a defect to overcome an existing defect. In advanced disease when residual esophageal function has been destroyed, myotomy is ineffective. Further, the superimposition of an esophageal stricture on top of a primary motor disorder makes any procedure aimed at preserving the esophagus unlikely to succeed. In addition, if more than one myotomy has been attempted in the past, it is highly unlikely that any procedure short of esophagectomy will provide symptomatic relief. The indications and choice of esophageal substitute are considered in the section on esophageal replacement in benign disease (p. 352).

GASTROESOPHAGEAL REFLUX DISEASE

Gastroesophageal reflux is a normal phenomenon. Most normal people experience short episodes of reflux, usually after meals. GERD occurs when esophageal acid exposure exceeds that of a normal population. We define the disease quantitatively, that is by demonstrating increased esophageal acid exposure. Other definitions used in the past were either nonspecific (e.g., symptoms of heartburn or regurgitation) or indirect (e.g., the presence of a hiatal hernia) or detected the disease only when complications such as esophagitis were present. The ready availability of 24-hour esophageal pH monitoring allows us to quantitate the abnormality, objectively assess the response to treatment, and have a logical stepwise approach to therapy.

Symptoms attributed to GERD are very common in our community, as judged from sales of prescribed and over-the-counter antacids. It is estimated that 7% of Americans suffer daily heartburn and up to 30% use antacids at least once a month. Most people whose symptoms are controlled by such means do not consult a physician, and of those who do, few are referred to surgeons. The spectrum of such patients seen by a surgeon is thus variable and depends on local referral patterns.

Pathophysiology of Gastroesophageal Reflux Disease and Its Complications

Failure of the antireflux mechanism leading to increased esophageal acid exposure may be from a defect in the LES, the esophageal body, or the stomach, as discussed previously in the section on physiology. The most important cause is a mechanically defective LES. This accounts for about 50% to 60% of patients with increased esophageal acid exposure.[9] The presence of this mechanical defect helps explain why such patients respond poorly to long-term medical treatment. Other important causes of increased esophageal acid exposure are inefficient esophageal clearance of refluxed gastric juice and abnormalities of the gastric reservoir that augment physiologic reflux.

A complication is defined by the presence of tissue injury and includes esophagitis, stricture, and Barrett's esophagus. Studies of the natural history of GERD are few, and one of the most detailed comes from Lausanne, Switzerland,[6] where intensive endoscopic follow-up of a defined population for 30 years has shown that in about 45% of their patients the esophagitis develops as an isolated episode that does not return (Fig. 14-22). However, of the 55% who have recurrent disease, it progresses to a more severe degree in 42% (about 23% of the total). Why some patients develop complications and others do not is not known with certainty, but several factors are known to be associated with the development of complications as described in the following:

1. The status of the LES has emerged as a significant factor in several long-term studies.[23,24] For this reason, it predicts a poor response to medical treatment. Table 14-2 shows how the prevalence of a defective sphincter to is related to complications in 150 consecutive patients with proven gastroesophageal reflux. Note that Barrett's esophagus is almost always associated with a mechanically defective sphincter. Fig. 14-23 shows the relationship of LES resistance as measured by the vector volume technique to the degree of acid exposure for patients with and without injury. The fact that a clear inverse relationship between acid exposure and LES resistance is demonstrated even in patients without tissue injury is further evidence that LES failure is an early event in the pathogenesis of GERD but that patients with tissue injury have more profound impairment of LES function.
2. Any defect of esophageal clearance that prolongs the contact time between the gastric juice and the mucosa is likely to lead to increased esophageal injury. This may be due to failure of esophageal propulsion, as in primary motor disorders. More commonly the defect in

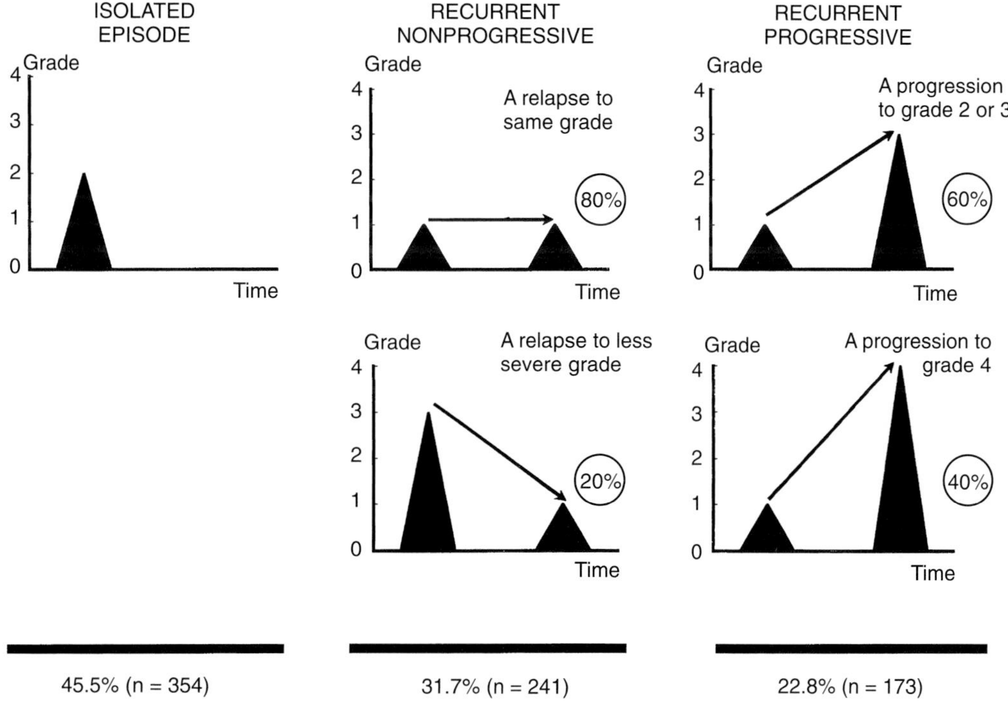

Fig. 14-22. Natural history of reflux esophagitis (Savary-Miller grades 1 through 3) in 759 patients receiving intermittent medical therapy. The recurrent nonprogressive form represents 32% of the entire group, and the recurrent progressive form accounts for 23% of the group. (From Monnier P, et al. Epidemiology and natural history of reflux esophagitis. Semin Laparosc Surg 2:2, 1995.)

Table 14-2. Complications of Gastroesophageal Reflux Disease in 150 Consecutive Patients

Complication	Number	Normal Lower Esophageal Sphincter (%)	Defective Lower Esophageal Sphincter (%)
None	59	58	42
Esophagitis	47	23*	77
Stricture	19	11	89
Barrett's esophagus	25	0	100

*Grade of esophagitis more severe with defective lower esophageal sphincter.

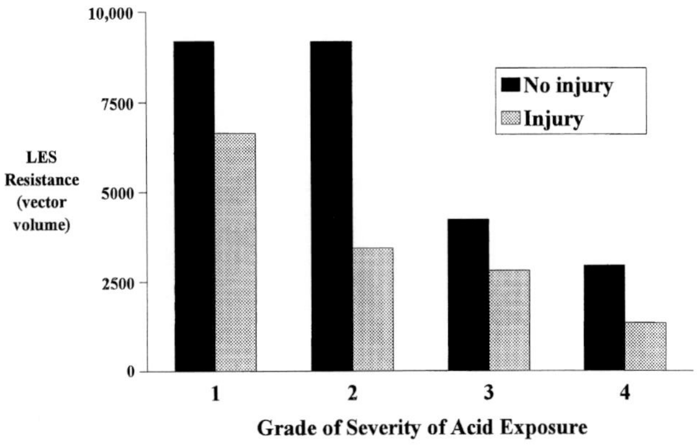

Fig. 14-23. Lower esophageal sphincter *(LES)* resistance (vector volume) in patients without injury (dark bars) and with mucosal injury (light bars). The pH severity score is based on the total time the esophagus is exposed to acid during 24-hour pH monitoring: Grade 1 = 0%-4%, grade 2 = 4%-8%, grade 3 = 8%-12%, grade 4 = >12%. There is a clear inverse relationship between acid exposure and lower esophageal sphincter resistance, even in the absence of tissue injury.

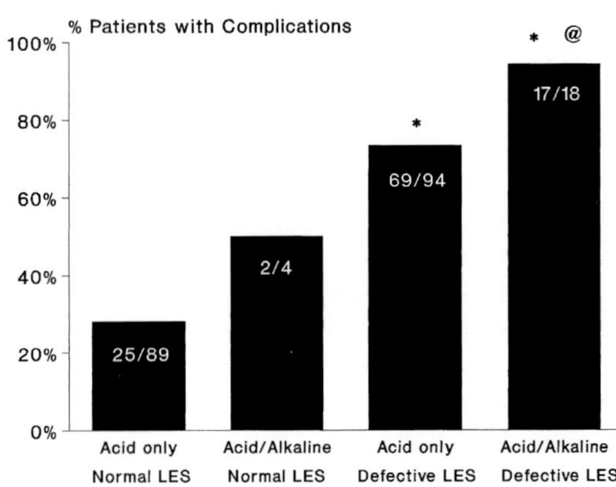

Fig. 14-24. The prevalence of complications in patients with gastroesophageal reflux disease related to the presence of a mechanically defective sphincter and the presence of acid vs. mixed (acid and alkaline) reflux. *LES,* Lower esophageal sphincter.

clearance is secondary to reflux-induced damage, creating a vicious cycle of increasing esophageal injury. Patients with strictures and Barrett's esophagus may thus have a profound defect in esophageal contractility. When the injury extends beyond the mucosa, the consequent interference with esophageal contractility may not revert to normal when the mucosa has healed. It is worth emphasizing that although the mucosa may heal by intensive acid suppression therapy, the abnormalities in the LES and esophageal body generally do not. This is because the mucosa is repeatedly being renewed, whereas muscle cells once damaged are unlikely to recover.

3. The presence of a hiatal hernia is also associated with more complications of GERD. The cause-and-effect relationship between hiatal herniation and GERD is controversial. Early workers used the terms hiatal hernia and reflux esophagitis as near synonyms, whereas later studies showed the feature that distinguished those with genuine reflux from those without reflux was not the presence of a hiatal hernia but rather the resistance to reflux imposed by the LES. More recently, as the diagnosis of hiatal herniation has become more standardized, it has become clear that the presence of a hiatal hernia interferes with the emptying of the distal esophagus and causes a defect in acid clearance.[25] Thus patients with GERD associated with a hiatal hernia have more complications of the disease than those without: conversely, the prevalence of hiatal herniation in patients with GERD increases as the complications become more severe. Most patients with Barrett's esophagus or stricture have a hiatal hernia.
4. The composition of the refluxed material also has an effect on the development of complications.[26] The injurious effect of refluxed juice depends on a number of interacting components. Acid alone in physiologic concentrations is not very damaging, but in high volume or in high concentration, as seen in patients with hypersecretion, the incidence of complications is increased. Pepsin-induced mucosal damage is likely only at a pH of 1 to 2.5; but in the presence of bile salts and a higher pH, trypsin may be more important. Not only is trypsin activated at a pH greater than 5, but the solubility of potentially injurious bile salts is greatest at neutral pH. In the clinical situation, complications of GERD are commoner when there is an alkaline component to the refluxate (Fig. 14-24). In Barrett's esophagus the development of complications such as stricture and ulceration is strongly associated with an increase in both acid and alkaline exposure. The presence of acid-alkaline reflux and the presence of a mechanically defective sphincter are independent determinants of mucosal damage; when these determinants are combined, the effects are additive. A patient with both features has a 95% incidence of complications.

Clinical Features

Symptoms may be classified as either typical (i.e., heartburn and regurgitation) or atypical (i.e., noncardiac chest pain, pulmonary problems such as asthma, recurrent pneumonia or progressive fibrosis, laryngeal symptoms such as hoarseness and aspiration, and loss of dental enamel).

Heartburn is easily the commonest symptom associated with GERD. Characteristically, it occurs 30 to 60 minutes after meals. Heartburn exacerbated by lying flat or bending over suggests a profound weakness of the LES. It may be associated with belching and regurgitation of acid up into the throat. If the regurgitated material comes from the esophagus, it tastes bland and suggests a motor disorder, and if it regurgitates from the stomach and tastes bitter, it suggests DGR.

If the regurgitation is associated with aspiration, a variety of respiratory symptoms may result. Sometimes the picture resembles asthma, and GERD should always be considered in managing this condition. A history of isolated episodes of pneumonia or frequent bouts of wheezing and coughing at night are also suggestive of GERD. Hoarseness may be present from laryngeal irritation.

Dysphagia resulting from GERD is usually insidious and results from a motility disorder secondary to esophagitis, loss of esophageal compliance from edema or fibrosis secondary to esophagitis, or from localized stricture formation. Patients usually localize dysphagia to the lower sternum, but we have found that cervical dysphagia was common in GERD. Patients' localization of the site of obstruction is not always reliable, but the general rule is that an obstructing lesion does not cause symptoms to be perceived distal to the lesion. It is common to find that heartburn ceases to be such a prominent symptom when a stricture has developed. By contrast, the sudden development or rapid progression of dysphagia suggests a tumor: in the absence of a history of heartburn a squamous cancer of the esophagus is likely, but if heartburn was prominent, the commonest cause is adenocarcinoma arising in Barrett's esophagus.

Angina-like chest pain, sometimes called noncardiac chest pain, is frequently caused by GERD. On questioning, patients with angina-like chest pain often admit to other classic symptoms of GERD but they tend to be mild and overshadowed by the chest pain. Of patients with chest pain and normal coronary angiograms, 50% have increased esophageal acid exposure, and 50% of the remainder can eventually be shown to have an esophageal cause. On the other hand, patients with angiographic lesions may have two causes for their chest pain, and some patients whose angina is poorly responsive to medical treatment may fall into this category.

Epigastric pain and nausea may be associated with symptoms of GERD and in these circumstances are usually due to pathologic DGR or delayed gastric emptying. It is important to recognize these entities before offering a patient antireflux surgery, since they may persist after operation, and the patient should be warned of their presence and the possibility of future medical or surgical therapy.

Bloating is mainly a gastric symptom suggesting gastric dilation secondary to aerophagia or delayed gastric emptying. It may be accompanied by adaptive relaxation of the abdominal muscles causing visible distention. Although sometimes thought to result from fundoplication, it is also a common complaint in medically treated disease.

Investigation

As outlined in the introduction, the initial investigations in most patients with foregut symptoms include a barium esophagogram and upper gastrointestinal tract endoscopy. In patients with GERD, these only uncover a pathologic lesion if either a complication of the disease such as esophagitis, stricture, or Barrett's esophagus or a potentially related condition such as hiatus hernia is present. The next step in investigation is physiologic testing of the esophagus and stomach (i.e., esophageal manometry and pH monitoring). Additional tests depend on the abnormalities uncovered by these basic assessments. Dual pH monitoring and chest roentgenography is helpful if there are respiratory symptoms, and gastric emptying tests, gastric acid analysis for hypersecretion, and esophageal and gastric bile probe monitoring may be required to elucidate gastric symptoms. Ambulatory esophageal motility may help define an esophageal motility disorder if stationary manometry is equivocal.

As a result of this process of investigation, a comprehensive understanding of the current status of the patient's esophageal function will be reached, enabling the physician to identify the etiologic factor responsible and predict the outcome of alternative treatments.

Complications of Gastroesophageal Reflux Disease

Esophagitis

Esophagitis is usually diagnosed by the presence of macroscopic erosions at endoscopy. Mere erythema of the mucosa is very subjective, especially on a video screen, and is consequently of little significance. Erosions first appear on the apex of distal mucosal folds and progress to affect multiple folds, eventually becoming confluent. Histologically, erosions are characterized by loss of surface epithelium and neutrophil infiltration. The histologic appearance of esophagitis when the epithelium is visually normal is more controversial. Reports of increased height of the basal cell layer of the squamous epithelium or increased depth of the papillae described in 1970 are now thought to be too nonspecific to be diagnostically useful. Rather, neutrophil infiltration is the hallmark of histologic esophagitis. Other markers include eosinophil infiltration or the presence of degenerate "balloon" cells in the epithelium. It is important to emphasize firstly that up to 50% of symptomatic patients with proven GERD have no evidence of esophagitis on endoscopy, and secondly that acid reflux is not the only cause of esophagitis: caustic ingestion is obvious from the history, and viral or fungal infection has specific histologic features, but pill-induced injury is an important nonreflux cause, which has no specific histologic appearance. This emphasizes the importance of documenting esophageal acid exposure before making the diagnosis.

Esophageal Ulceration

Historically, esophageal ulcers were the first clinical manifestation of GERD to be described. They resemble peptic ulcers in the stomach or duodenum, in that they have a tendency to penetrate deeply and lead to bleeding or perforation. They are found most commonly in association with Barrett's esophagus, often near the squamocolumnar junction, and when healed may lead to the high midesophageal stricture characteristic of that condition.

Esophageal Stricture

More severe esophagitis causes circumferential changes that may cause fibrosis in the deeper layers, leading to stricture and esophageal shortening. Strictures have an inflammatory component, as well as fibrous replacement of muscle, and improvement in the former is partly responsible for the improvement in dysphagia after corrective antireflux surgery or intensive medical treatment. Most reflux strictures occur at the distal end of the esophagus unless Barrett's esophagus is present, in which case the stricture is often higher. The development of a reflux stricture causes slowly progressive dysphagia for solids, usually following a long history of heartburn and regurgitation. Rapidly progressive dysphagia or severe weight loss are uncommon, and rather suggest malignancy.

Barrett's Esophagus

The condition whereby the tubular esophagus comes to be lined with columnar epithelium was first described by Norman Barrett in 1950, although he incorrectly believed it to be congenital in origin. It is now realized that it represents advanced GERD. In most practices it is found in 7% to 10% of patients with GERD. It is characterized endoscopically by the presence of velvety orange-red mucosa lining the tubular esophagus and histologically by the presence of columnar epithelium. The visual appearance at endoscopy can sometimes be confused with herniation of normal gastric mucosa above the crura, and in the past Barrett's esophagus was only diagnosed if the columnar mucosa extended 2 cm or more above the esophagogastric junction. The histologic hallmark of Barrett's esophagus is the presence of "specialized" columnar epithelium, which shows features of intestinal metaplasia, easily recognized by the presence of goblet cells. These features may be seen in biopsies specimens of segments less than 2 cm above the esophagogastric junction, sometimes called short-segment Barrett's esophagus.[27] Short segment Barrett's esophagus often appears as a small tongue of columnar epithelium extending above the Z-line into the lower esophagus. The presence of specialized epithelium is now regarded as the pathognomic feature of Barrett's esophagus regardless of how far it extends into the esophagus. Barrett's esophagus may exist on its own or may itself be complicated by ulceration, stricture, and malignant change.

Once Barrett's epithelium is present, medical therapy or antireflux surgery rarely causes it to regress. The most significant feature of Barrett's esophagus is its malignant potential. The metaplastic epithelium usually undergoes dysplastic change prior to becoming frankly neoplastic, but the changes may be focal and thus missed on biopsy examination. Most pathologists distinguish only two grades of dysplasia: low grade and high grade. High-grade dysplasia is synonymous with carcinoma in situ, and if the esophagus is removed for such a condition, foci of invasive carcinoma are found in 50% of the specimens. The exact magnitude of the risk of malignancy is debated and ranges from 1 per 50 to 1 per 150 patient-years. Even the most conservative estimates indicate a risk of 40 times that of the general population. Adenocarcinoma of the esophagus is rapidly increasing in most Westernized countries, and Barrett's esophagus is the only known risk factor. Whereas adenocarcinoma accounted for about 3% of esophageal cancers between about 1930 and 1970, since the mid-1970s its incidence has been rising at 10% per year, so that it now accounts for almost 50% of all esophageal cancers. The ratio of white/black patients is 7:1, and male/female is 5:1. At least some genetic factors must be involved to account for this predilection for white male patients. On the other hand, the sudden and alarming increase in incidence suggests an environmental cause, something which the large sales of acid suppressant medications, which are increasing at the same rate, are doing nothing to halt.

Physiologic dysfunction in Barrett's esophagus is characteristic of advanced reflux disease; a defective LES, poor distal esophageal body peristalsis, and fixed hiatal herniation are all common. Mucosal insensitivity is present and may explain why many patients seek medical help late in the course of the disease. Abnormal composition of gastric juice may be found: specifically the presence of duodenal juice. In the past this was inferred by the presence of so-called alkaline reflux (increased % time > pH 7) on esophageal pH monitoring, but recent reports using the Bilitec sensor for monitoring bilirubin confirm that Barrett's esophagus is frequently associated with excessive bile in the esophagus. Repetitive injury from noxious gastric juice can lead during the repair process to mutations in the p53 gene, a gene that controls programmed cell death. Adenocarcinoma arising in Barrett's esophagus has a significant incidence of p53 mutations.

Short Esophagus

The term *short esophagus* is used by surgeons to describe the situation in the operating room when the gastroesophageal junction cannot be brought down into the abdominal cavity without tension. Esophageal shortening begins to occur early in the development of GERD and has been demonstrated acutely in animals after perfusion of the esophagus with acid. Our own manometric studies demonstrated that shortening of the esophageal body increases as complications become more severe (Fig. 14-25). It is associated with shortening of the longitudinal muscle, hiatal herniation, and periesophageal inflammation. Radiologically it is associated with fixity of the hiatal hernia, that is, the hernia does not reduce in the upright position after a swallow. Any hernia greater than 5 cm in length is likely to be associated with esophageal shortening. Manometrically, the peristaltic amplitude in the distal esophagus is often subnormal. If this condition is detected only at the time of an abdominal fundoplication, the surgeon's options are severely limited: it is much better to detect it ahead of time and plan the operative strategy accordingly.

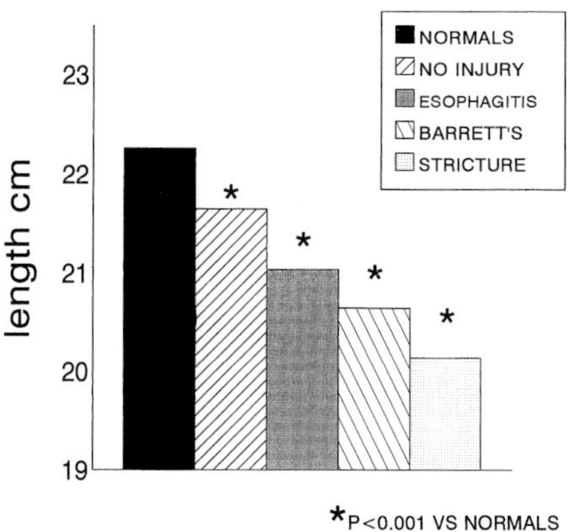

Fig. 14-25. Manometric esophageal length in normal subjects and patients with gastroesophageal reflux disease of increasing severity. Note that though it is maximal in advanced disease, it is detectable in mild disease.

Surgery in Gastroesophageal Reflux Disease

The aim of surgery is to restore the patient to a life free of symptoms, without the need to take regular medications and without undue social, dietary, or other life-style restrictions. The status of a patient whose reflux symptoms must be controlled by taking regular acid suppression therapy or prokinetic agents; avoiding late meals and rich or spicy food; eschewing tea, coffee, alcohol, tobacco, chocolate and peppermint; wearing only loose clothes; and sleeping propped up, perhaps in a double bed, cannot be considered ideal. The social and domestic disruption imposed by these restrictions is considerable and leads to noncompliance. Only two randomized trials have compared the relative merits of medical versus surgical treatment. Both showed a clear advantage for surgical treatment, but internists are reluctant to accept this conclusion, arguing that the medical treatment in both did not include omeprazole.[28] An ongoing trial comparing laparoscopic Nissen fundoplication with proton pump inhibitors may provide a conclusion more relevant to current practice. There is no doubt that proton pump inhibitors represent a great advance in the medical treatment of GERD, but until recently long-term use was discouraged by the FDA. Serum gastrin levels are usually raised in patients taking long-term omeprazole, and there are theoretical and experimental reasons to believe that the trophic effect of gastrin may predispose to neoplasia. In rats, gastric carcinoid tumors have been reported. Long-term use in patients with severe esophagitis generally heals the esophagitis if a big enough dose is given but is associated with atrophic gastritis. No reports of carcinoid tumors in humans have been attributed to omeprazole use. A limiting factor in the medical treatment of GERD is that treatment is focused only on acid suppression, ignoring the other potentially injurious components of the refluxate that continue to cause damage despite symptomatic relief.

The traditional reasons for an internist to refer a patient with GERD for surgery are an unsatisfactory response to medical treatment and the development of uncontrollable complications. These end points are very subjective and likely to be influenced by "gatekeeper" policies decided by insurance companies. We prefer an approach that aims to make the diagnosis and elucidate the pathophysiology at an early stage. This allows more accurate prognostic information to be given to the patient and the selection of rational and cost-effective therapy.

Who Benefits From Antireflux Surgery?

The first requirement for consideration of antireflux surgery is the objective demonstration of the presence of GERD by 24-hour pH monitoring. Second, the patient must have either symptoms or complications of the disease. Third, the disease should be caused by a defect appropriate to surgical therapy (i.e., a mechanically defective sphincter). Recent studies have indicated that a Nissen fundoplication has beneficial effects in addition to restoring the characteristics of the LES. It may accelerate gastric emptying and reduce the frequency of TLESRs. Consequently, even in patients without a defective sphincter, there are situations where a Nissen fundoplication corrects the underlying abnormality. The algorithm in Fig. 14-26 summarizes when patients should be studied in the course of their disease to determine when surgery is applicable.

Although it is usually straightforward to categorize patients in accordance with this recommended scheme, a number of anomalous pictures are worth bearing in mind:

1. If 24-hour esophageal pH monitoring is normal in a patient with unequivocal endoscopic esophagitis, the possibilities of alkaline, drug-induced, or retention esophagitis should be considered. If the patient also has a defective sphincter and a hiatal hernia, review the circumstances of the pH test. Sometimes patients have not stopped acid suppressant medication in time or have eaten so little during the test that it does not reflect normal daily life. Pure "alkaline" reflux occasionally occurs in the absence of acid reflux and may be detected by ambulatory bile probe monitoring.
2. If the sphincter is manometrically normal in a patient with increased esophageal exposure to gastric juice, the patient should be evaluated for an esophageal or gastric cause of increased acid exposure. In this situation the commonest abnormality is gastric hypersecretion.
3. Some patients with increased acid exposure and a mechanically defective sphincter who have no complication of the disease respond well to medical therapy, but they require long-term medication for continued relief. These patients should be given the option of surgery as a cost-effective alternative. At current prices, omeprazole 20 mg daily costs $140 per month, and many patients need double or even triple this dose.
4. Atypical symptoms of reflux such as respiratory manifestations often respond well to antireflux surgery. Pa-

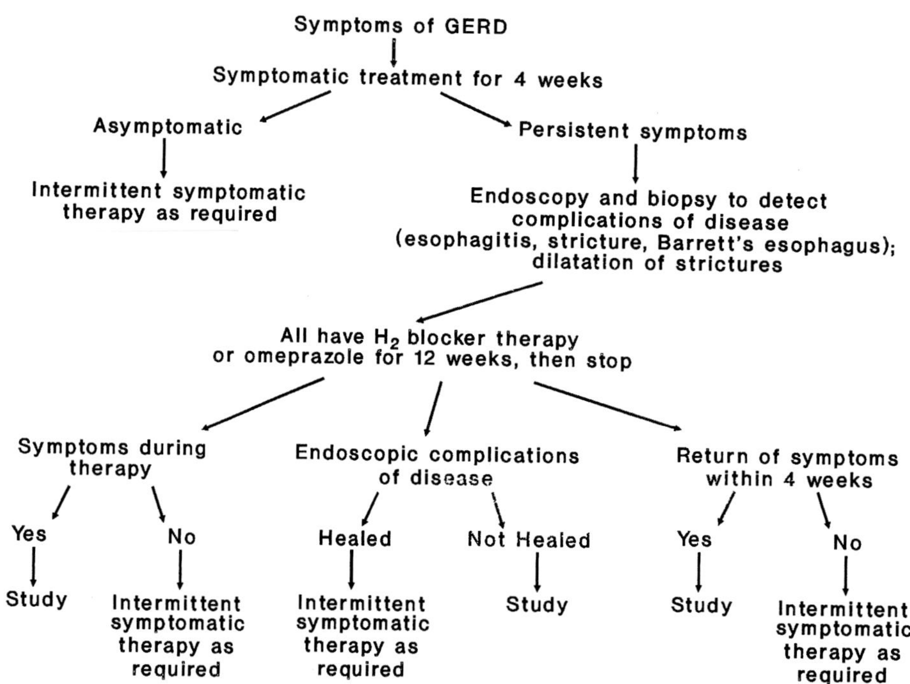

Fig. 14-26. Algorithm for selection of symptomatic patients for further study. *GERD,* Gastroesophageal reflux disease.

tients often record that omeprazole reduces heartburn but not regurgitation and coughing attacks. When respiratory symptoms are combined with typical symptoms such as heartburn and regurgitation, the results of antireflux surgery are generally good. When the respiratory symptoms are the only manifestation of GERD (i.e., in the absence of heartburn), the results of surgery are less beneficial. This is because many such patients have an associated motor disorder that encourages the retrograde transport of saliva even in the absence of gastroesophageal reflux or because the long-standing lung disease actually is primary and the reflux is secondary.

5. Complaints of epigastric pain, nausea, vomiting, and loss of appetite may be due to excessive DGR, which occurs in about 11% of patients with GERD. This problem is usually, but not invariably, confined to patients who have had previous upper gastrointestinal tract surgery. The coexistence of these gastric symptoms in a patient who also has typical symptoms of GERD should prompt a thorough evaluation of the stomach using the bile probe, 24-hour pH monitoring, or radionuclide scanning. In such patients the correction of only the incompetent cardia can result in a disgruntled individual who continues to complain of nausea and epigastric pain on eating. In rare cases surgery is necessary to control severe DGR by performing a bile diversion procedure as well. When the symptoms emerge after an antireflux repair, the administration of sucralfate (Carafate) can be helpful.

There are several important principles underlying antireflux surgery which, if ignored, risk failure of the mission of the operation and the production of unwanted postoperative symptoms. When faced with a number of potential operative solutions, adherence to underlying principles guides the surgeon to make a rational decision. Almost all antireflux operations work by plicating the lower esophagus with fundus. One notable exception is the Hill operation, but it requires intraoperative manometry in its performance and is not widely used outside Hill's own center. It may be valuable in a patient after previous gastric surgery. Other operations, such as those that use a ligamentum teres sling, are rarely used.

Only the fundus, and not the upper body of the stomach, should be used to construct the fundoplication. The fundus should be fully mobilized by dividing the short gastric arteries. The surgeon should take advantage of the ability of the fundus to relax in concert with the LES after a swallow. If the fundus is not adequately mobilized or is twisted around the lower esophagus under tension, the risk of postoperative dysphagia is high. The ideal position of the fundus is such that the anterior wall and the posterior wall envelop the lower esophagus, meeting approximately in the right lateral position, thus keeping the fundus of the stomach in its normal plane.

The fundus must be placed around the lower esophagus. In a patient with a hiatal hernia the gastroesophageal junction may not be obvious. An inexperienced operator may mobilize the lesser curve and create a fundoplication around the upper stomach, which may look tubular in this situation. This serious error causes both dysphagia and recurrent heartburn. It may be prevented when operating through the open abdomen by taking care to identify the gastroesophageal fat pad, keeping the dissection above the level of the hepatic branch of the anterior vagal nerve, and placing the fundoplication between the esophagus and the posterior vagus nerve. This is less of a concern in the laparoscopic approach, since the diaphragm is elevated and visualization of the cardia is improved. Preoperative recognition of esophageal shortening is the best preventive measure.

The fundoplication must lie comfortably in the abdomen without tension, requiring only closure of the crura to maintain it there. The whole fundoplication may ride up into the chest if the crura are not closed, if there is tension on the fundoplication because of undetected esophageal shortening, or both. This creates in effect an iatrogenic paraesophageal hernia. Although the fundoplication will function as an antireflux barrier even in the intrathoracic situation, the patient will experience postprandial chest pain as the intrathoracic portion of the stomach gets distended with air. Dragging the gastric mesentery through the hiatus into the chest increases the risks of ischemic ulceration and hemorrhage from the herniated pouch of stomach.

In creating an antireflux barrier the surgeon is to some extent playing off the risk of dysphagia against the risk of recurrent reflux. The Nissen fundoplication as originally described protected against reflux very effectively but at the expense of a substantial incidence of dysphagia and gas-bloat syndrome. The modern version of the Nissen operation, having a short 1 to 2 cm fundoplication constructed over a 60 FG bougie, using fully mobilized fundus to envelop the lower esophagus while keeping the fundus in its proper plane, has to a great extent overcome these early problems. Partial fundoplications, such as the Belsey operation, produce a lesser degree of resistance to outflow and are therefore appropriate for patients with poor esophageal body motility. However, the long-term recurrence rate is higher after the Belsey operation. More recently, there has been a resurgence of interest in partial fundoplications done through the abdomen because of the perceived risk of dysphagia and gas-bloat syndrome after the 360-degree Nissen fundoplication. These operations are variously named after their originators (e.g., Toupet, Dor, Watson, and Lind). Several randomized studies comparing partial and total fundoplications have found that partial fundoplications produce a lower incidence of early dysphagia and bloating, but the differences disappear with follow-up. Since the principles underlying the construction of these various partial fundoplications are similar to the Belsey operation, long-term failure may be a problem. Rather than adopt a blanket policy of performing partial fundoplications in all cases, it makes more sense to uncover the dominant physiologic abnormalities and tailor the operation accordingly.

Tailored Antireflux Operation

Patients with normal esophageal length and normal esophageal body motility are best served by a transabdominal Nissen fundoplication. This is now normally done via the laparoscopic route. Usually this situation is found in early disease before severe complications have developed. If the patient is obese or requires concomitant surgery on the lung or esophageal body, the transthoracic route is preferable.

The presence of a motility disorder alters the operative strategy. If the peristaltic amplitude is low (<20 mm Hg) in the distal third of the esophagus, a Nissen fundoplication would create too much resistance and lead to dysphagia. In this situation, the Belsey fundoplication is a better choice. Moreover, thoracic approach allows the surgeon to mobilize the esophagus to a much greater extent than is possible through the abdomen. Usually some degree of esophageal shortening is present when distal esophageal contractility is poor. In addition to extensive mobilization, a Collis gastroplasty can be created to produce an extra 5 cm of "neoesophagus" around which a Belsey procedure can be added. In the relatively rare situation where low distal peristaltic amplitude is associated with normal length, a transabdominal partial fundoplication is a reasonable option.

Generally, good relief of heartburn and regurgitation may be expected regardless of whether a nonspecific motor disorder is present or not. However, the relief of reflux-induced respiratory symptoms in the presence of a motility disorder is only one fourth as good as when the motility is normal. The presence of a motility disorder, even if it is due to reflux, is unlikely to change with surgery, suggesting that it is more a toxic effect than an irritating effect of the refluxate.

The combination of GERD and a named primary motor disorder such as achalasia and DES is rare unless myotomy or balloon dilation has been performed. In these circumstances the primary motor disorder should be treated by myotomy of the esophageal body and/or LES.

End-stage reflux disease (e.g., when there is an undilatable stricture, after multiple unsuccessful antireflux operations, or when Barrett's esophagus leads to high-grade dysplasia) is best served by esophageal replacement. The most durable substitute is the colon, and the functional results are especially good if the vagus nerves are intact. Fig. 14-27 summarizes the operative treatment of GERD depending on the stage of the disease.

Nissen Fundoplication

The steps in the performance of a transabdominal fundoplication are common to both the laparoscopic and open procedures and include the following:

1. Crural dissection, identification and preservation of both vagi and the anterior hepatic branch
2. Circumferential dissection of the esophagus
3. Crural closure
4. Fundic mobilization by division of short gastric vessels
5. Creation of a 1.5 to 2 cm loose fundoplication by enveloping the posterior esophagus with posterior fundic wall and the anterior esophagus with ante-

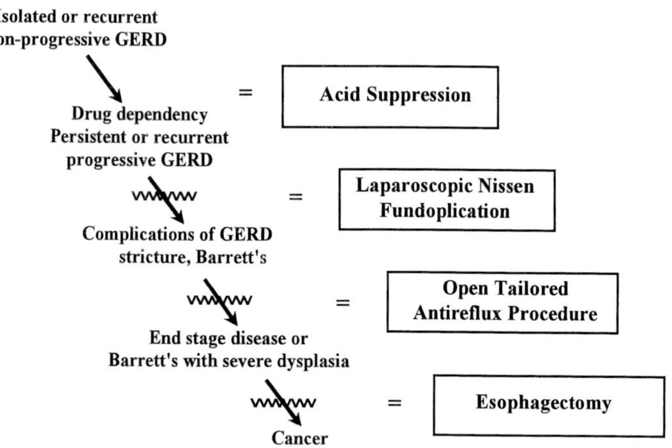

Fig. 14-27. Conceptual scheme for treatment of gastroesophageal reflux disease *(GERD)* depending on the stage of the disease.

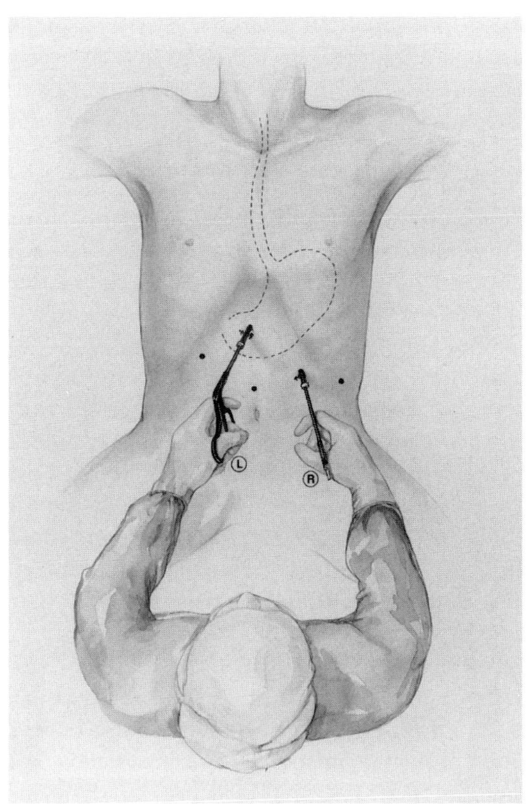

Fig. 14-28. Position of patient, surgeon, and trocars for laparoscopic antireflux surgery. The head of the table is elevated to 45 degrees, and the patient's hips and knees are slightly flexed.

rior fundic wall and approximating the fundic walls in the right lateral position to keep the fundus in the correct plane

Laparoscopic fundoplication has become commonplace and may soon replace traditional open Nissen fundoplication as the procedure of choice.[29] The patient should be placed in the supine position, in a modified lithotomy position, with the table elevated 30 to 45 degrees. The patient's knees should be only slightly flexed. If the patient's legs are sharply flexed at the knees, they interfere with the mobility of the instruments during the course of the procedure. Five 10 mm ports are used as indicated in Fig. 14-28. The camera is placed above the umbilicus, one third of the distance to the xiphoid process. The right-sided liver retractor is best placed immediately subcostal to the right of the xiphoid. This allows an acute angle toward the left lateral segment of the liver and thus the ability to push the instrument toward the operating table, lifting the liver. A second retraction port is placed laterally toward the left flank at the level of the umbilicus. The operating ports are placed in the right and left midclavicular lines, 2 inches below the costal margin. Placing the operating trocars on either side of the midline allows triangulation between the camera and the two instruments, avoiding the difficulty associated with the instruments being in direct line with the camera. The falciform ligament hangs low in many patients and provides a barrier around which the left-handed instrument must be manipulated. Most recently we have used a 12 mm universal port in the left midclavicular position to allow unhampered use of instruments of different diameters.

One of the most important elements of laparoscopic surgery is adequate retraction and safe exposure of the necessary structures. Laparoscopic fundoplication begins with exposure of the esophageal hiatus. A fan retractor is placed into the perixiphoid port to hold the left lateral segment of the liver toward the anterior abdominal wall. A Babcock clamp is placed into the left anterior axillary port, and the stomach is retracted caudad, exposing the esophageal hiatus. Commonly, a hiatal hernia must be reduced.

The key to the hiatal dissection is identification of the crura. In all except the most obese patients there is a very thin window in the gastrohepatic omentum overlying the caudate lobe of the liver. Dissection is begun by incision of this window above the hepatic branch of the anterior vagal nerve (Fig. 14-29). A large left hepatic artery arising from the left gastric artery is present in up to 25% of patients. It should be identified and avoided. Once opened, the outside of the right crus becomes evident. The peritoneum overlying the anterior aspect of the right crus is incised. The medial portion of the right crus leads into the mediastinum and is entered by blunt dissection with both instruments. At this juncture the esophagus usually becomes evident. The right crus is retracted laterally and the posterior or right vagal nerve is identified and kept with the esophagus. The anterior or left vagal nerve is left undisturbed.

The esophagus is lifted with a blunt-tipped grasper placed within the esophageal hiatus, and the dissection is carried inferiorly and laterally, exposing the medial and lateral aspects of the right crus. A large hiatal hernia often makes this portion of the procedure easier as it accentuates the diaphragmatic crura. On the other hand, dissection of a large mediastinal hernia sac can be difficult.

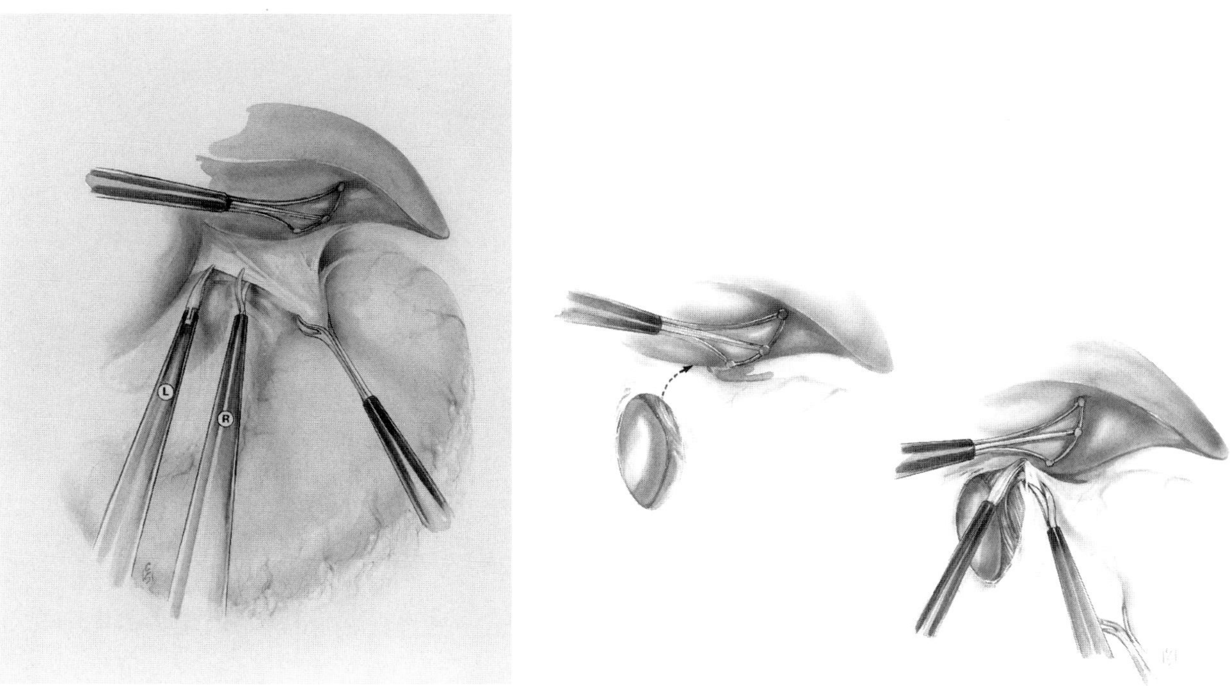

Fig. 14-29. Initial retraction for exposure of the esophageal hiatus. A fan retractor elevates the left lateral segment of the liver. A Babcock clamp retracts the esophageal fat pad.

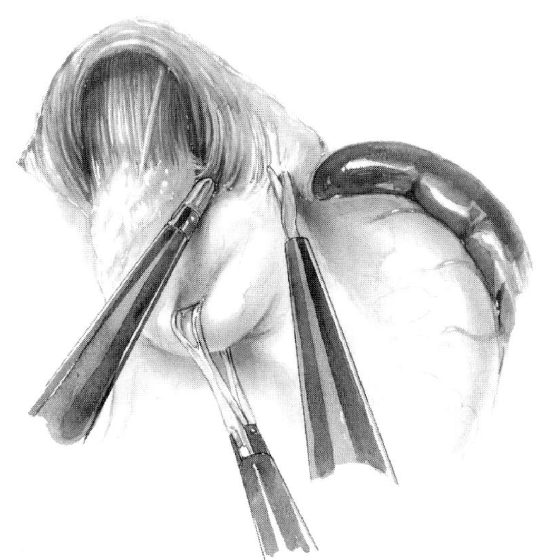

Fig. 14-30. Dissection of the left crus and the angle of His.

Following dissection of the right crus, attention is turned toward the angle of His, and a complete dissection of the lateral and inferior aspect of the left crus and the fundus of the stomach is performed (Fig. 14-30). This dissection is the key maneuver allowing circumferential mobilization of the esophagus. Failure to do so results in difficulty encircling the esophagus, particularly if approached from the right. Repositioning of the Babcock retractor toward the fundic side of the stomach facilitates retraction for this portion of the procedure.

The esophagus is mobilized by careful dissection of the anterior and posterior soft tissues within the hiatus. This can be difficult if the operating ports are placed too medially. In the presence of severe esophagitis and transmural inflammation with or without esophageal shortening, esophageal dissection may be particularly difficult. Following this dissection, a grasper is passed via the surgeon's left-handed port behind the esophagus and over the left crus. A Penrose drain is placed around the esophagus to facilitate further dissection and crural closure (Fig. 14-31).

The crura are dissected inferiorly to expose the V-shaped decussation. The esophagus is held anterior and to the left, and the crura are approximated with 3 to 4 interrupted 0 silk sutures, starting just above the aortic decussation and working anteriorly.

Complete fundic mobilization is necessary for construction of a tension-free fundoplication. The liver retractor is replaced with a second Babcock forceps to retract the upper stomach. The gastrosplenic omentum is suspended anteroposteriorly, in a clothesline fashion via both Babcock forceps, and the lesser sac is entered approximately one third the distance down the greater curvature of the stomach. The short gastric vessels are sequentially dissected (Fig. 14-32) and thrombosed with the harmonic scalpel. With caution and meticulous dissection the fundus can be completely mobilized in most patients.

The posterior wall of the mobilized fundus is gently brought behind the esophagus to the right side. The anterior wall of the fundus is brought anterior to the esophagus above the supporting Penrose drain (Fig. 14-33). Both

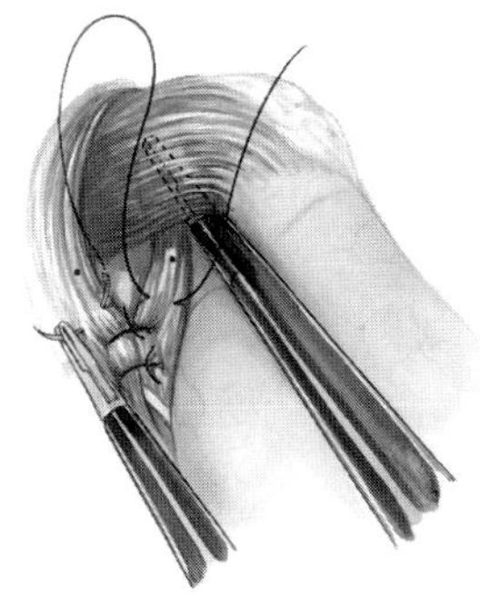

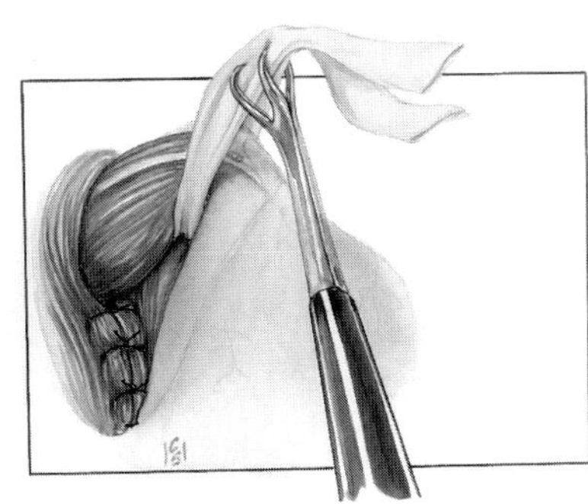

Fig. 14-31. *Left,* Closure of the crura with interrupted 2-0 silk. *Right,* Penrose drain around esophagus to facilitate exposure of the crura for closure.

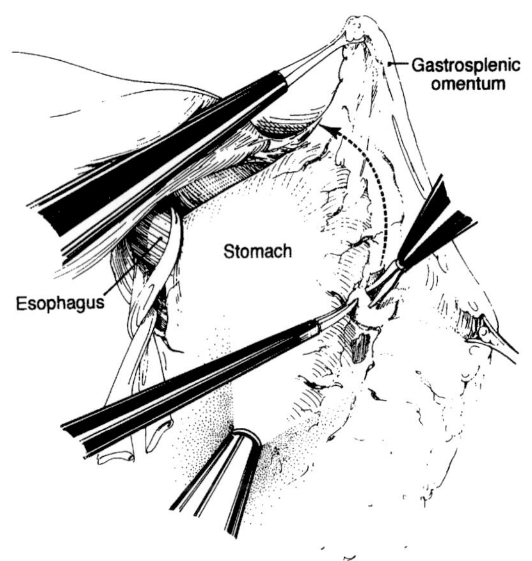

Fig. 14-32. Retraction of the gastrosplenic omentum in preparation for division of the short gastric vessels.

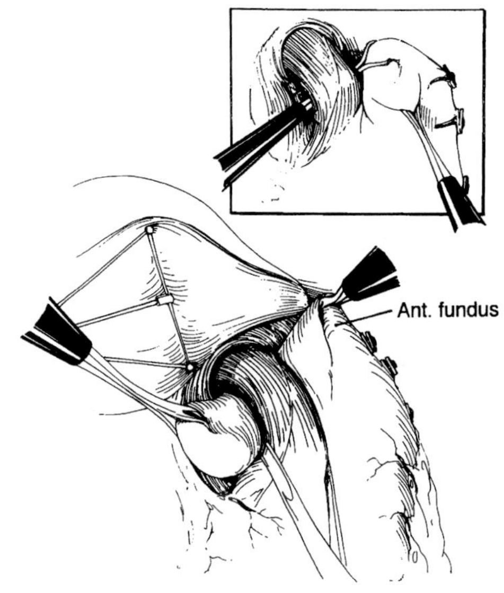

Fig. 14-33. Creation of the fundoplication. The posterior portion of the mobilized fundus is grasped by the Babcock forceps and pulled behind the esophagus.

posterior and anterior fundic lips are manipulated to allow the fundus to envelop the esophagus without twisting (Fig. 14-34). The laparoscopic visualization has a tendency to exaggerate the size of the posterior opening that has been dissected. If the right lip of the fundoplication has a bluish discoloration, the stomach should be returned to its original position and the posterior dissection enlarged. Once adequately placed, a 60 FG bougie is passed. The fundoplication is sutured with a single U-stitch of 2-0 Prolene buttressed with felt pledgets. The most common error is an attempt to grasp the anterior portion of the stomach to construct the fundoplication rather than the posterior fundus. The esophagus should comfortably lie in the untwisted fundus prior to suturing. Two anchoring sutures of 3-0 silk are placed above and below the U-stitch to complete the fundoplication. When finished, the suture line of the fundoplication should be facing in a right lateral direction. The bougie is replaced with a nasogastric tube, which should pass easily into the stomach. If it does not, intraoperative endoscopy should be performed.

Open Nissen fundoplication is less often performed today, but it is still easier when other complex procedures such as highly selective vagotomy or a bile diversion procedure are combined with the Nissen operation. Managing a patient with several previous upper abdominal operations may be more difficult. The principles of the open operation are identical to those described for the laparoscopic fundoplication. Exposure is aided by putting the patient in reverse Trendelenburg position and using a sternal retractor to elevate the liver and costal margin. For accurate positioning of the fundoplication around the esophagus and not stomach, its posterior lip is passed

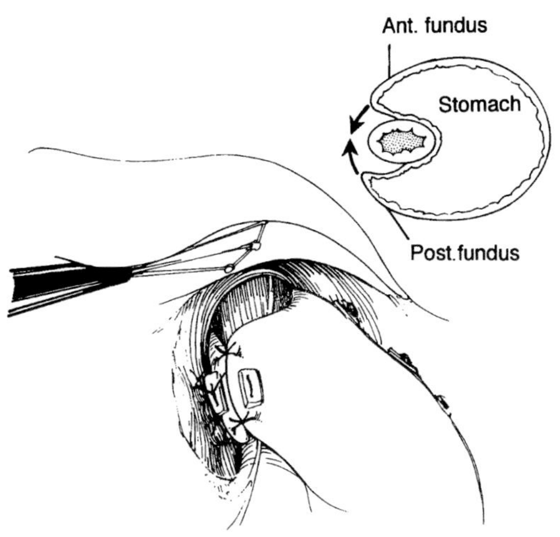

Fig. 14-34. Fixation of the fundoplication with a single horizontal mattress suture of 2-0 Prolene reinforced by Teflon pledgets. The 60 FG bougie passed just before the wrap is sutured ensures a floppy fundoplication. The inset shows the correct orientation of the wrap.

between the posterior vagus nerve and the esophageal wall.

For the transthoracic approach, a left posterolateral thoracotomy is made through the sixth intercostal space (i.e., above the seventh rib). Redo operations are easier through the seventh intercostal space (i.e., above the eighth rib). This allows better exposure of the abdomen through a peripheral diaphragmatic incision, in which the diaphragm is incised circumferentially 2 to 3 cm from the chest wall for a distance of approximately 10 to 15 cm. An adequate fringe of diaphragm must be preserved along the chest wall for reapproximation of the muscle. If further abdominal exposure is necessary, the thoracic incision can be extended diagonally across the rectus muscle to the abdominal midline, dividing the costal margin and the bridge of diaphragmatic muscle. Exposure is greatly facilitated by the use of a double-lumen endotracheal tube, allowing selective deflation of the left lung.

The principles of creating and securing the fundoplication are the same regardless of whether the approach is abdominal or thoracic, including fundic mobilization by division of the short gastric vessels and closure of the hiatus. Before creating the fundoplication, it is important to ensure that the gastroesophageal junction can be placed below the hiatus without tension. Several steps may be necessary to achieve this. The first is thorough mobilization of the esophagus up to the aortic arch. This involves ligation and division of the two bronchial arteries. Next, the branches of the left vagus nerve to the left pulmonary plexus can be divided in an effort to reduce the tension. If after this maneuver the tendency to ride up through the hiatus persists, a Collis gastroplasty is done (see the following). If a short fundoplication of 1 to 2 cm is used and the esophagus has been adequately mobilized, this step is rarely necessary in a patient in whom it was not planned from the outset.

At the completion of the procedure, a nasogastric tube should be able to be passed, without guidance from the surgeon, directly into the stomach to ensure that there has been no angulation of the distal esophagus. A chest tube for drainage of the pleural cavity is properly placed, and the chest incision is closed.

Belsey Mark IV Repair

The techniques of the Belsey Mark IV and the transthoracic Nissen operations are similar, differing only in the construction of the gastric fundoplication. The steps are illustrated in Figs. 14-35 to 14-37. To perform the Belsey Mark IV reconstruction, the esophagus and cardia are mobilized, and the fundus of the stomach is freed by dividing the short gastric vessels as it is brought up through the hiatus into the chest. The fundus is held in place by two rows of three horizontal mattress sutures placed equidistantly between the seromuscular layers of the stomach and the muscular layers of the esophagus. Each suture should obtain a firm grip of the esophageal wall. The first row of sutures is placed 1.5 cm above the external gastroesophageal junction and is tied only tightly enough to obtain tissue apposition without disrupting the muscle fibers of the esophagus. A second row of sutures is placed 1.5 to 2 cm above the first row, using the position of the previously placed sutures in the first row as a guide. Once again, the sutures in the second row are tied carefully to achieve tissue apposition without strangulation. The tails of these sutures are not cut, but are separately rethreaded on a large, thin Ferguson needle and passed 0.5 cm apart from each other through the diaphragm from the abdominal to the thoracic surface, 1 cm from the edge of the hiatus. These sutures must be carefully positioned so that the fundoplication is anterior and not lateral to the esophagus. Their placement is facilitated by the use of a spoon retractor to protect abdominal structures. The needle is guided along the inner surface of the spoon before passing it through the diaphragm. The fundoplication is gently replaced in the abdomen, and the diaphragmatic sutures are carefully tied.

Collis Gastroplasty

The Collis gastroplasty is best performed through the chest. A 4 to 5 cm gastric tube is created over a 48 Fr bougie placed along the lesser curvature of the stomach. This can be accomplished with a single application of a gastrointestinal linear (GIA) stapler/cutter placed along the fundic side of the bougie. To achieve a uniform diameter of the gastric tube throughout its length, gentle traction is exerted on the greater curvature prior to closure of the jaws of the stapler. The Belsey Mark IV fundoplication is then performed around the gastric tube as described above. Because of the absence of peristalsis in the gastric neoesophagus, we prefer the Belsey procedure to minimize outflow resistance.

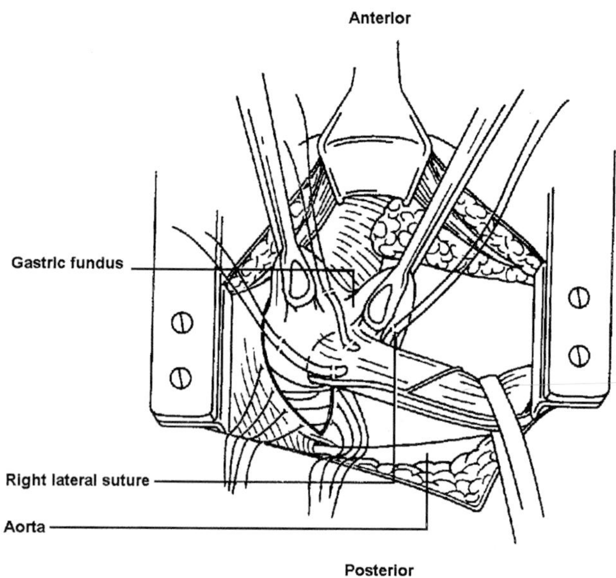

Fig. 14-35. Construction of the Belsey 240-degree fundic wrap showing placement of the first row of sutures 1.5 cm above the gastroesophageal junction.

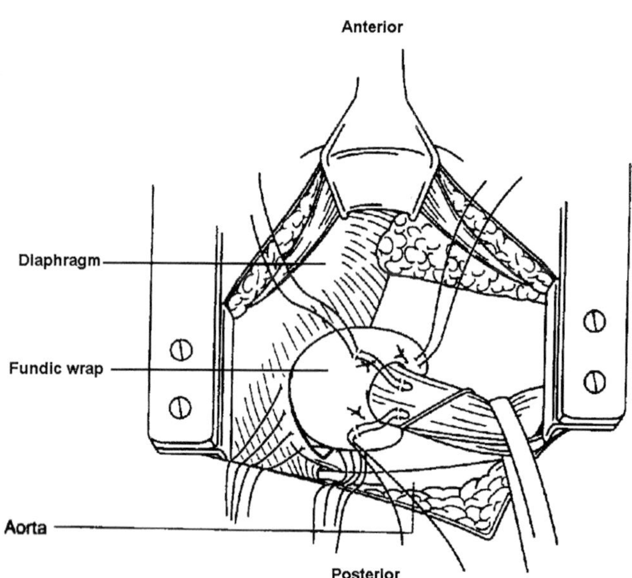

Fig. 14-36. Continued construction of the Belsey wrap showing placement of the second row of sutures 1.5 cm above the previously tied first row.

Other Partial Fundoplications

For reasons discussed above, partial fundoplications other than the Belsey procedure are rarely indicated. The most widely used is the transabdominal Toupet procedure, in which the anterior and posterior lips of the fundoplication are sutured, not to each other, but to the right and left crura and to the esophageal wall to produce a 270-degree fundoplication. The procedure can be performed without having to divide the short gastric arteries.

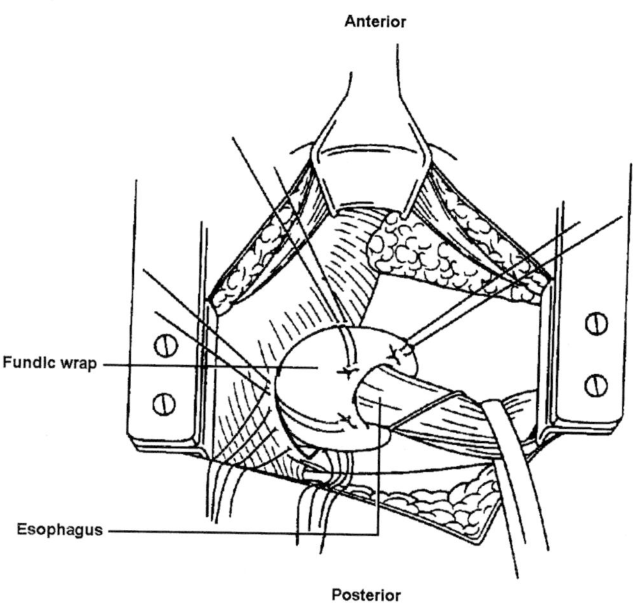

Fig. 14-37. Continued construction of the Belsey wrap showing how the tails of the second row of sutures are threaded through the diaphragm about 1.5 cm from the edge of the hiatus.

Intraoperative Complications

Splenic injury may occur from excessive traction on the greater curve of the stomach, and adhesions to the spleen must be carefully dissected in advance. Bleeding from minor or peripheral splenic injuries may be stopped by a combination of electrocautery and topical hemostatic agents and should not require splenectomy. The esophagus may be injured during the hiatal dissection or occasionally by the passage of the large bougie used to calibrate the fundoplication. The first may be avoided by careful dissection under direct vision. It is helpful if the surgeon conceives of the dissection as being a dissection of the crura rather than a dissection of the esophagus. This mindset helps establish the correct plane in the mediastinum. Bougie injury of the esophagus is more likely to occur in a patient with severe esophagitis or a stricture. A well-lubricated bougie should be passed with great gentleness by a knowledgeable anesthesiologist after the surgeon has relaxed the retraction on the Penrose drain to avoid angulation of the gastroesophageal junction. It is critical that the anesthesiologist pass the bougie with its pointed cone tip straight and not bent in the form of a J. In this position the bougie can rip the esophagus high in the thorax, and the situation can go undiscovered until fever and sepsis develop 48 to 72 hours after surgery.

Intraoperative hemorrhage creates great difficulties for laparoscopic fundoplication, since accumulated blood tends to pool in the hiatus and reduces overall illumination. The surgeon should avoid it by meticulous technique and avoid the use of irrigation where possible. Hemorrhage that endangers safe dissection by obscuring the surgeon's view is an indication for conversion to an open procedure.

Pneumothorax occasionally occurs if the mediastinal pleura is breached and the insufflated gas enters the pleural cavity. It is first manifested by an increase in peak inspiratory pressures. Ventilation may be improved by reducing the carbon dioxide insufflation pressure; but if this cannot be done without impairing exposure, the procedure should be converted to an open fundoplication.

If the surgeon has selected the patient correctly, he should not find himself in the unfortunate situation of performing an abdominal fundoplication but being unable to reduce the gastroesophageal junction into the abdomen. The options in this difficult predicament include conversion to a transthoracic approach or the transabdominal creation of a Collis gastroplasty tube by making a window with the EEA stapler and firing the gastrointestinal stapler between the window and the angle of His. Neither of these is ideal, and it is much better to anticipate the problem and plan the procedure accordingly.

Postoperative Management

After laparoscopic surgery, recovery is generally speedy. We remove the nasogastric tube the morning after surgery and commence liquids. If no dysphagia is experienced, soft foods are introduced later that day, and the patient goes home on the second postoperative day. As experience in laparoscopic fundoplication is gained, earlier discharge is becoming possible, and some surgeons have even performed it as an outpatient procedure. This is not yet standard practice. After open surgery, return of gastric and intestinal function is slower, and respiratory complications are more frequent because of the decreased ventilation caused by the pain of the long upper abdominal incision. Thus after either open abdominal or transthoracic repair, the patient is kept on nasogastric suction for approximately 5 days to prevent distention of the stomach during the healing period. Such distention can cause a breakdown of the repair. A barium swallow is obtained on the sixth to seventh postoperative day to demonstrate the unobstructed passage of barium into the stomach prior to starting a solid oral diet.

In the first 2 weeks, slight dysphagia may be experienced by the patient, but this disappears as the traumatic edema resolves. During this period, the patient should avoid swallowing large boluses of solid food, which might stress the repair. Dysphagia may occasionally persist for a longer period if an intramural hematoma at the site of the fundoplication developed. This usually is absorbed within 4 to 6 weeks, and the dysphagia subsides. Persistent dysphagia after this time in a patient with a previous stricture usually responds to a single dilation. Other important but preventable causes of persistent dysphagia after surgery are the presence of a motility defect and technical errors such as placing the fundoplication round the stomach or making it too long or too tight. One of the immediate benefits of an antireflux procedure is that from the time the patient recovers from anesthesia, the patient notes relief from heartburn and regurgitation. Before discharge, the patient should be counseled that until the habit of air swallowing is broken, he may experience increased flatus and mild gastric distention because of trapping of the air in the stomach. The patient also must be instructed that all medications should be taken in liquid or crushed form for at least 6 months to avoid a drug-induced esophageal injury.

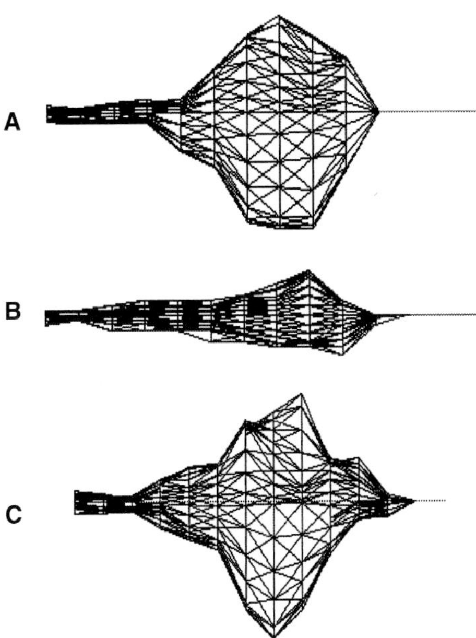

Fig. 14-38. Preoperative and postoperative three-dimensional representation of the lower esophageal sphincter in a patient with Barrett's esophagus. **A**, Normal. **B**, Preoperative. **C**, After Nissen fundoplication.

Results of Antireflux Surgery

When patients are correctly selected and the operation performed in conformity with the basic surgical principles outlined above, long-term relief of symptoms is achieved by more than 90% of patients.[30] Most patients experience some increase in flatulence and abdominal distention, but in the majority it quickly resolves. The open Nissen fundoplication has been most extensively studied both clinically and physiologically. Our own results show actuarial freedom from symptoms in 91% of patients at 10 years. The operation achieves this result by restoring the mechanical characteristics of the LES: that is, the overall length, intra-abdominal length, and the resting pressure. The effect of successful surgery can be visualized by three-dimensional representation of the LES (Fig. 14-38).

The outcome of complicated reflux disease is more variable and depends on residual esophageal function. Paradoxically, the outcome after a Collis-Belsey operation tends to be better than after a Belsey alone. This is probably because in patients suitable for the Belsey operation, that is, with normal esophageal length but poor contractility, the motility disorder is primary rather than secondary to reflux and does not improve after surgery. Most patients with strictures who have a good symptomatic response to dilation respond well to fundoplication. In Barrett's esophagus the ability of effective antireflux surgery to protect against the development of cancer is still not proven, but the clinical experience of most surgeons is that Barrett's cancers are exceedingly rare after fundoplication, whereas they most commonly occur in patients who have been treated medically for a long time. The American College of Gastroenterology keeps a registry of patients with Barrett's esophagus being followed after both medical and surgical treatment, and the incidence of dysplasia and cancer is significantly higher in the medically treated group. Thus the weight of evidence strongly urges that timely fundoplication is protective against cancer. Better still would be a policy of surgery in patients who are drug dependent before Barrett's esophagus develops.

Failed Antireflux Repairs

Patients with one or more previous unsuccessful antireflux operations constitute a particularly challenging group. In these patients it is especially important to obtain the fullest possible information about esophageal function. The reasons for a poor result may be either technical errors in performing the operation or inappropriate indications for operation. Several typical patterns are discernible:

1. The so-called slipped Nissen fundoplication may develop when the upper stomach rides up through the fundoplication and causes mainly dysphagia and some heartburn. It is more likely that the condition was created at the time of surgery because the surgeon did not mobilize the fundus or because unrecognized esophageal shortening led to inadequate mobilization of the gastroesophageal junction, causing the surgeon to wrap stomach around the upper stomach rather than lower esophagus. This problem usually necessitates a Collis-type gastroplasty to be combined with a Belsey repair, to ensure that the fundoplication sits below the diaphragm without tension.
2. When a fundoplication is created that is too tight, the patient develops dysphagia immediately postoperatively. Manometry shows a high-pressure nonrelaxing sphincter and may also show high-pressure simultaneous waves in the esophageal body, making it difficult to distinguish it from vigorous achalasia. Such patients highlight the importance of obtaining manometry on all patients before proceeding to antireflux surgery. In a patient with normal preoperative motility the cause is usually a fault in technique and can be corrected by constructing a looser fundoplication over a 60 FG bougie as described earlier. If manometry was not performed, the surgeon must assess clinically from a history of preoperative dysphagia the likelihood of an underlying motility disorder. The treatment of such a disorder must include a myotomy and partial fundoplication, as described in the motility disorders section.
3. Disruption of the fundoplication manifested clinically and physiologically by recurrent reflux has at least four predisposing causes:
   a. Inadequate suture technique includes taking inadequate bites of stomach or using flimsy or quickly absorbable material.
   b. Choice of operation: All partial fundoplications, such as the Toupet procedure are more prone to disruption than a Nissen operation. This is for three reasons: (1) the integrity of the repair depends on sutures to the esophageal wall, (2) the repair requires much more abdominal length of esophagus than a Nissen operation, and (3) placing the repair under tension.
   c. Unrecognized esophageal shortening leads to tension on the fundoplication, which may then become undone.
   d. Failure to mobilize the fundus properly by not dividing the short gastric vessels results in lateral tension on the repair.

Individual case reports of other complications after antireflux repairs include anatomic aberrations, such as the development of paraesophageal hernia, and fistulous complications from local penetrating sepsis. Examples of the latter are gastropleural and gastrobronchial fistulae.

Inappropriate patient selection also leads to dissatisfaction postoperatively. This most often occurs when the cause of the reflux is primarily a defect in the esophageal body or the gastric reservoir or when the operation has been performed for symptoms in the absence of objective documentation of the disease. Careful study of all patients prior to considering antireflux surgery minimizes the incidence of such problems.

The principles underlying treatment of these patients rely on the physiologic assessment of residual esophageal function. Generally, if a clear reason for the failure can be identified and the patient has only had one or two previous attempts at repair, a good result may be expected. Multiple previous operations or the presence of complex motility patterns should suggest the need for esophageal replacement, generally with colon.

Esophagectomy and esophageal replacement are occasionally indicated in the treatment of advanced GERD. To perform this operation safely and with good functional results requires the advantages of a specialist center where expertise in assessment, operative skill, and intensive care are readily available. In the absence of these facilities, the temptation to persist with ineffective medical treatment or attempt yet another antireflux operation is strong. The indications for esophagectomy are Barrett's esophagus with high-grade dysplasia and what is generally described as "burned-out esophagus" and includes failure of a third antireflux operation, a severe coexistent motility disorder, or the presence of an undilatable stricture. Either colon or stomach may be used to replace the esophagus. Colonic replacement is more difficult, requiring three anastomoses rather than one, but it has superior functional long-term results, particularly if it opens into a vagally innervated stomach. This is more likely to be the case in severe primary motility disorders, since after multiple operations at the gastroesophageal junction the vagal nerves are unlikely to be intact. In this eventuality the proximal stomach if left in situ would be a nonfunctioning atonic bag and contribute to upper abdominal discomfort. Therefore the proximal stomach is removed, and the colon graft is anastomosed to the antrum.[31]

ESOPHAGEAL CANCER

Esophageal carcinomas are of two types—squamous carcinoma and adenocarcinoma—which although differing profoundly in epidemiology, etiologic factors, relative incidence, and response to radiation therapy, present a similar clinical picture and are treated similarly from the surgeon's point of view. The surgeon's options depend more on the location and stage of the tumor than its histologic type.[32]

Etiology and Incidence

Squamous carcinoma accounts for the majority of esophageal carcinomas. Its incidence is highly variable, ranging from around 20 per 100,000 in the United States and Britain to 160 per 100,000 in certain parts of South Africa and the Hunan province of China, and even 540 per 100,000 in the Guriev district of Kazakhstan. The environmental factors responsible for these sharply localized high incidences have not been conclusively identified, although both additives from local foodstuffs (nitroso compounds in pickled vegetables and smoked meats) and deficiencies (zinc and molybdenum) have been suggested. In Western societies, smoking and alcohol consumption are strongly linked with squamous carcinoma. Other definite associations link squamous carcinoma with long-standing achalasia, lye strictures, tylosis (an autosomal dominant disorder characterized by hyperkeratosis of the palms and soles), and human papilloma virus.

Adenocarcinoma of the esophagus is now the fastest increasing cancer in the Western world, and the only significant risk factor is Barrett's esophagus. Longitudinal studies have variously estimated the risk from 1 per 50 patient-years of follow-up to 1 per 150 patient-years, as discussed in the section on gastroesophageal reflux. The increased incidence is of the same order of magnitude as the effect on lung cancer produced by smoking.

Clinical Features

Esophageal cancer is a disease affecting patients of advancing age, with dysphagia and weight loss being by far the most common symptoms at the time of diagnosis. In a few patients dysphagia does not occur, and symptoms arise from invasion of the primary tumor into adjacent structures or from metastases. Extension of the primary tumor into the tracheobronchial tree can cause stridor; if a tracheoesophageal fistula develops, coughing, choking, and aspiration pneumonia result. Severe bleeding from erosion into the aorta or pulmonary vessels occurs on rare occasions. Vocal cord paralysis may result from the invasion of either recurrent laryngeal nerve. Metastases are usually manifested by jaundice or bone pain. The situation is different in high incidence areas where screening is practiced. In these communities the most prominent early symptom is pain on swallowing rough or dry food.

Unfortunately, dysphagia usually presents late in the natural history of the disease because the lack of a serosal layer to the esophagus allows the smooth muscle to dilate with ease. As a result, the dysphagia becomes severe enough to motivate the patient to seek medical advice only when more than 60% of the esophageal circumference is infiltrated with cancer. Thus the disease is usually far advanced at the time of diagnosis. Tracheoesophageal fistula may be present in some patients on their first visit to the hospital, and greater than 40% have evidence of distant metastases. With tumors of the cardia, anorexia and weight loss usually precede the onset of dysphagia. The physical signs of esophageal tumors are those of distant metastases.

Investigations

Diagnosis

A large tumor causes no difficulty in interpretation on a barium esophagogram, since it produces an ulcerating, irregular lesion with upturned edges giving the so-called "apple core" appearance (Fig. 14-39). The ulcerating appearance of such advanced lesions on endoscopy is equally characteristic, and a biopsy specimen is easily obtained.

In early disease the diagnosis can be more difficult to make. The roentgenogram findings may be normal, and the only sign at endoscopy is a subtle color change in the

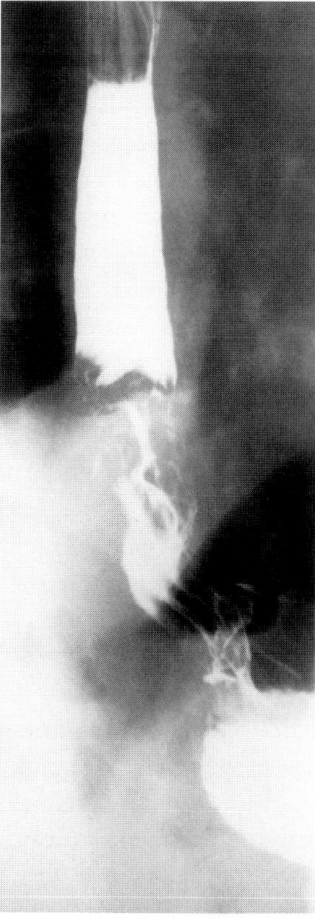

Fig. 14-39. Barium esophagogram in a patient with a large esophageal carcinoma demonstrating the "apple core" appearance.

mucosa, which may be enhanced by vital staining, or the presence of Barrett's metaplasia. Difficulties are known to occur in esophageal strictures, where biopsies are hard to obtain, and in presumed achalasia, where a small infiltrating tumor in the cardia may produce manometric and radiologic features indistinguishable from those of achalasia. The tumor may only be seen when the scope is retroflexed and the cardia is viewed from below. Early adenocarcinoma of the esophageal body may be found by biopsy of the edges of an ulcer or a small nodule within the Barrett's mucosa and on occasions serendipitously while confirming the presence of Barrett's metaplasia.

Detection of esophageal carcinoma by screening is worthwhile only in areas where the incidence of the disease is high. Mass screening based on cytologic specimens (obtained by swallowing a capsule or balloon with a net-like exterior and pulling it back through the cardia and esophagus) has been successfully used in China, but is not economically feasible in countries like the United States, where the prevalence is relatively low. Screening in this country is confined to high-risk groups, namely those with Barrett's esophagus.

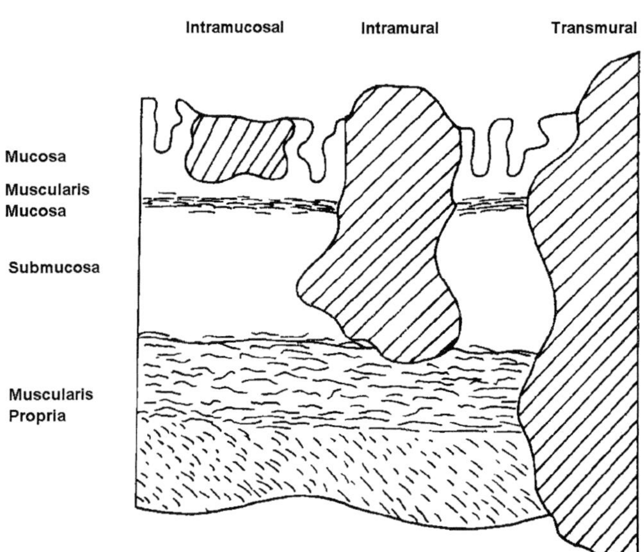

Fig. 14-40. Schematic representation of depth of penetration of tumors.

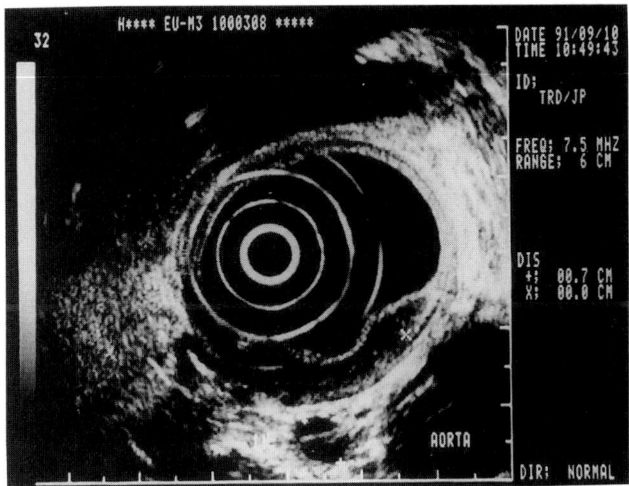

Fig. 14-41. Appearance of an early esophageal carcinoma on endoscopic ultrasonography. The normal layers of the esophagus are clearly visible.

Staging

The stage of the disease depends on the depth of penetration of the primary tumor and the presence of lymph node or distant metastases. Some idea of advanced spread may be obtained from clinical examination and features of the esophagogram (angulation of the barium column) or on endoscopy (tumors >8 cm in length). Such signs are only present in the most advanced tumors. Staging requires other imaging techniques to assess lesser degrees of spread. CT scanning is widely used but is not accurate in staging small tumors. MRI has not been shown to have any advantage over CT scanning in this regard. The results of endoscopic ultrasound are more promising in assessing the extent of small tumors within the esophagus itself and involvement of local lymph nodes. For these early lesions, classification of the former is conveniently done by defining the tumor as follows:

1. Intramucosal (limited by the muscularis mucosae)
2. Intramural (extending through the muscularis mucosae but not through all layers of the esophagus)
3. Transmural (extending through all layers of the esophageal wall)

This classification is graphically shown in Fig. 14-40. Our experience has shown that intramucosal tumors are usually identified by a positive biopsy result in the absence of an endoscopically visible mass, and intramural tumors are usually endoscopically visible masses that on endosonography do not penetrate the esophageal wall (Fig. 14-41). Transmural tumors are usually larger than 5 cm on endoscopic measurement and on endosonography extend through all layers of the esophageal wall.

Intramucosal tumors have a 5% incidence of involved lymph nodes, most of which are adjacent to the tumor. In contrast, once the tumor extends into the submucosa, the incidence of involved lymph nodes increases to 65% to 70%. The rich submucosal plexus of esophageal lymphatics presents little barrier to the spread of tumor (Fig. 14-42). In particular, adenocarcinoma commonly involves celiac axis and splenic artery nodes, just as in gastric cancer.

All these studies may need to be supplemented by information at the time of surgery (intraoperative staging), as unresectable tumor or distant metastases may be detected only during operation.

The most important goal in staging esophageal carcinoma is to determine if the end point of a surgical procedure is cure or palliation. A curative resection is one in which the tumor and all potentially involved lymph nodes

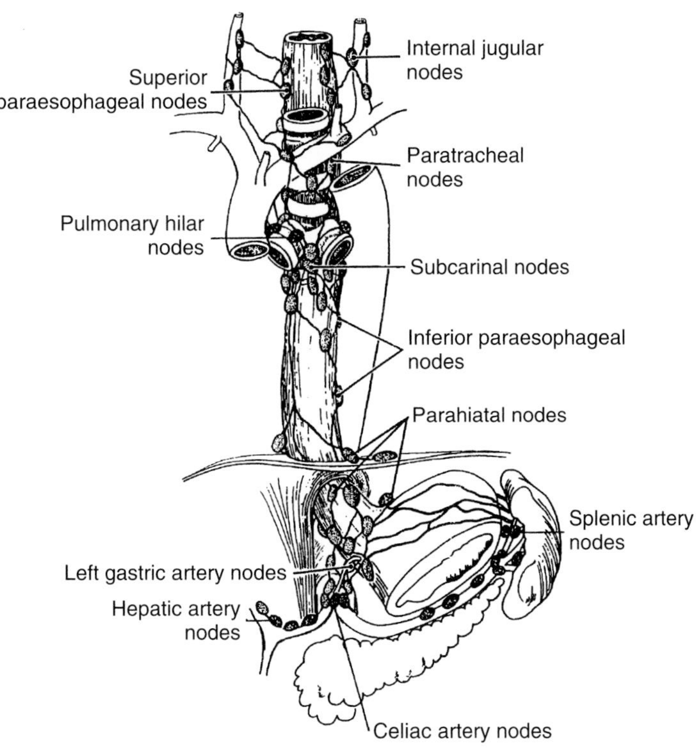

Fig. 14-42. Lymphatic drainage of the esophagus.

are removed en bloc, with the lesion being surrounded on all sides by normal tissue. Such a procedure is similar in principle to that carried out for head and neck tumors or for lung tumors. Making the distinction between curative and palliative procedures carries several benefits. It identifies the mission of the operation and emphasizes adequate surgery for cure and sufficient surgery for palliation. It does not conceal the curative benefits of surgery by diluting the results of survival with those of patients in which the procedure was done only for palliation. It also emphasizes the use of a more durable reconstruction of the gastrointestinal tract in patients operated for cure and identifies patients for multimodal therapy if surgical cure is not possible.

Treatment

The goal of treatment in esophageal carcinoma may be either curative or palliative. Until recently, the results of any form of treatment were so poor that many physicians regarded the disease as incurable from the time of presentation and advocated palliation as the only realistic aim. This pessimism is slowly being dispelled as the benefits of adequate surgery in appropriately selected patients become recognized. By contrast, nonsurgical therapies are entirely palliative. The factors that govern whether a curative or a palliative operation should be done are based on (1) the location of the tumor, (2) the age and fitness of the patient, and (3) the stage of the disease. Fig. 14-43 shows an algorithm of the clinical decisions important in the selection for curative or palliative therapy.

Tumor Location

Tumors in the cervical part of the esophagus, particularly those in the postcricoid area, constitute a well-defined pathologic entity in that the efferent lymphatics from the cervical esophagus drain directly into the paratracheal and deep cervical or internal jugular lymph nodes with minimal flow in a longitudinal direction. Almost all of them are squamous. For all practical purposes, tumors of the cervical esophagus are managed as though they were head and neck tumors. Lesions that are not fixed to the spine, do not invade the vessels, and do not have fixed cervical lymph node metastases should be resected. In most situations, preoperative chemotherapy and radiation are given. Often, the resection requires a laryngectomy with a pharyngogastrostomy and permanent tracheostomy. If lymph node metastases are present, the resection should be considered palliative and the larynx spared, since cure at this stage of disease is rare. Low cervical lesions that reach the level of the thoracic inlet are usually unresectable owing to early invasion of the great vessels and trachea. The length of the esophagus below the cricopharyngeus muscle is insufficient to allow palliative intubation or construction of a proximal anastomosis for a bypass procedure. Palliation of this tumor is very difficult, and patients with disease at this location have a very poor prognosis.

Tumors that arise within the middle or upper third of the thoracic esophagus lie too close to the trachea and aorta to allow an en bloc resection without removal of these vital structures. Consequently, in this location only

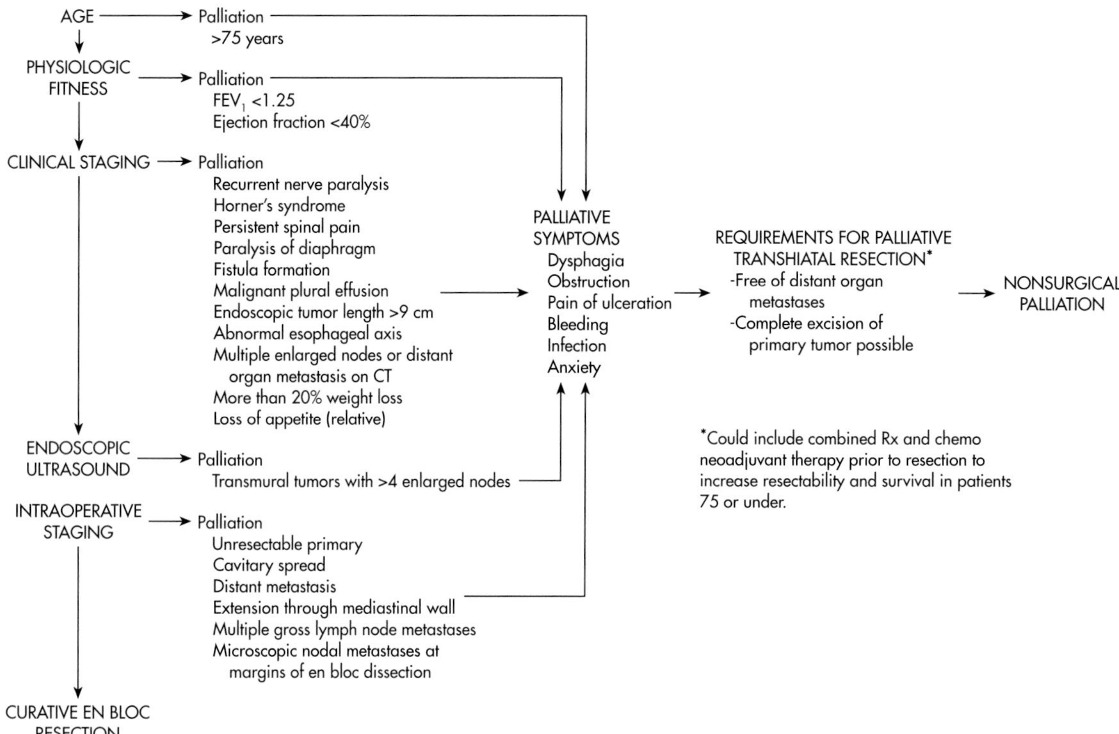

Fig. 14-43. Algorithm for overall management of esophageal cancer.

tumors that have not penetrated through the esophageal wall and have not metastasized to the regional lymph nodes are potentially curable. In essence, the resection for a tumor at this level is done similarly whether for palliation or cure, and long-term survival is a chance phenomenon. This does not mean that efforts to remove the adjacent lymph nodes when resecting such tumors should be abandoned. To do so may inadvertently leave metastatic disease behind and hamper the patient's overall survival. Preoperative chemotherapy and radiation therapy are most apt to be beneficial for tumors in this location, in that the reduction in size makes their removal easier and more complete.

Tumors of the cardia and lower esophagus are histologically different but clinically similar. Both tumors are amenable to en bloc resection. Unless preoperative and intraoperative staging clearly demonstrate an incurable lesion, an en bloc resection in continuity with a lymph node dissection according to the principles of surgical oncology should be performed.[33] If the resection is for palliation, a transhiatal esophagectomy is done.

Age

An en bloc resection for cure of carcinoma of the esophagus is unwise in patients older than 75 years because of the additional operative risk in face of a short life expectancy. Regardless of how favorable their pathology appears, a palliative resection is performed in these patients. This approach provides relief of symptoms with less surgery, and cure is still possible, though the chances are small.

Physiologic Status

It is important that patients undergoing esophageal resection have sufficient cardiopulmonary reserve to tolerate the operation. Consequently, the physiologic status of the patient affects the extent of surgery. The respiratory function is best assessed with the forced expiratory volume in 1 second (FEV_1), which ideally should be 2 L or more. Any patient with an FEV_1 of less than 1.25 L is a poor surgical candidate because that person carries a 40% risk of dying from his respiratory insufficiency within 4 years. In such a patient the chances of long-term survival, even if cured from the disease, do not justify an extensive en bloc resection. Cardiac reserve is best assessed noninvasively by using a gated radionuclide pool scan, which provides accurate information on wall motion and ejection fraction. A resting ejection fraction of less than 40% is an ominous sign. We prefer to perform a palliative resection in such a patient, regardless of how favorable the pathology appears.

Clinical Stage

Clinical factors that indicate an advanced stage of carcinoma and exclude cure by surgery are recurrent nerve paralysis, Horner's syndrome, persistent spinal pain, paralysis of the diaphragm, fistula formation, and malignant pleural effusion. Factors that make surgical cure unlikely include a tumor greater than 8 cm in length, abnormal axis of the esophagus on a barium roentgenogram, enlarged lymph nodes on CT scan, a weight loss of greater than 20% (of the patient's normal weight), and loss of appetite.

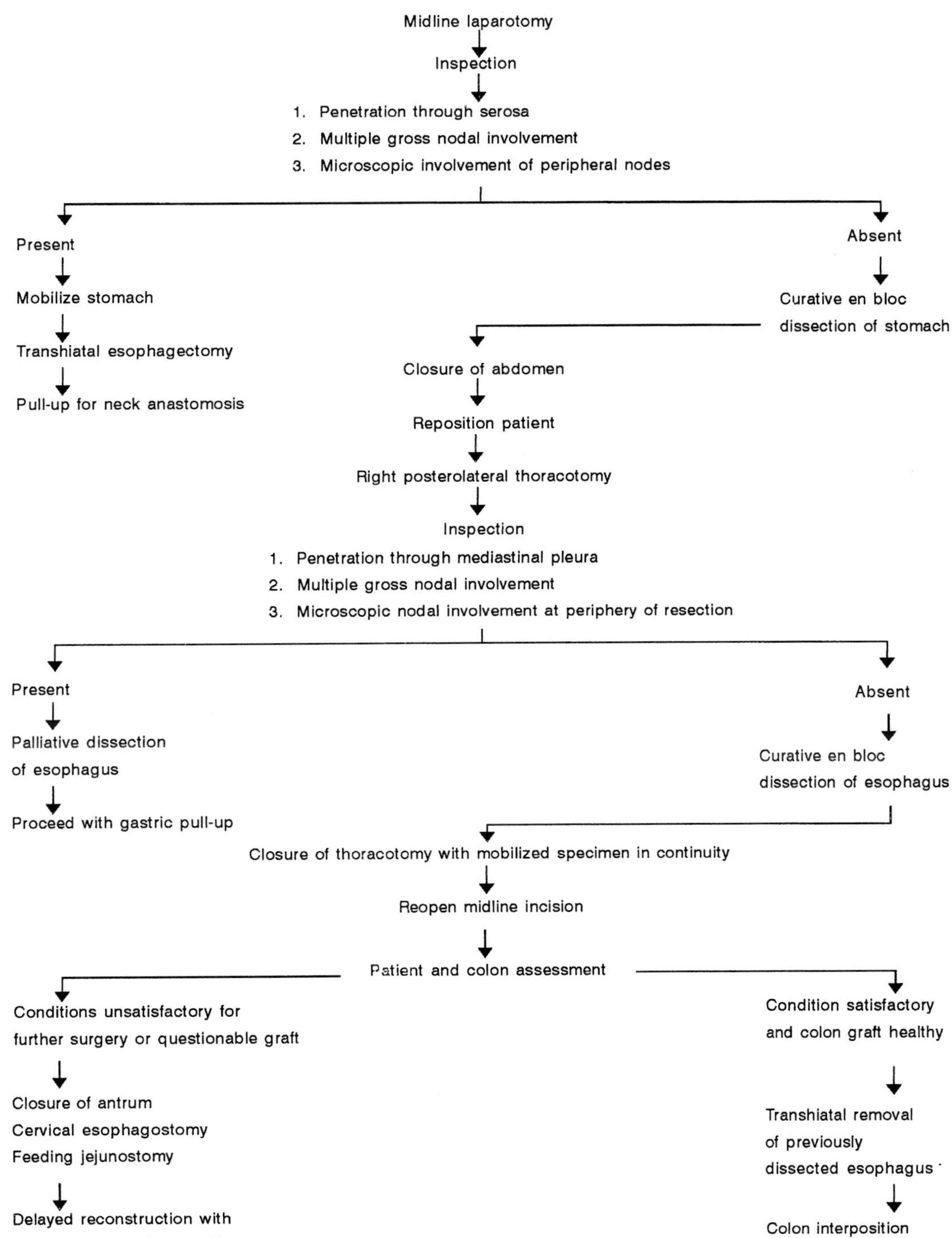

Fig. 14-44. Algorithm for intraoperative decision making for cancer of the lower esophagus.

Intraoperative Staging

Intraoperative staging is designed for intraoperative selection of favorable candidates for a curative en bloc resection. It is based on the observation that patients with a tumor that penetrates through the esophageal wall or has multiple or distant lymph node metastasis have a poor survival. It requires an operative approach that allows switching from a curative to a palliative resection. If during the course of an operation an incurable situation is identified, the surgeon should change to a palliative procedure. Fig. 14-44 shows an algorithm of intraoperative decision making. A curative en bloc dissection is abandoned if intraoperative staging reveals an unresectable primary tumor, cavitary spread of the tumor, distant organ metastasis, extension of the tumor through the mediastinal pleura, multiple gross lymph node metastases, or microscopic evidence of lymph node involvement at the margins of an en bloc resection (i.e., low paratracheal, portal triad, or subpancreatic periaortic lymph nodes). Our experience has shown that for cancers of the distal esophagus and cardia, patients with a favorable stage of disease can be identified by a combination of preoperative and intraoperative assessment with an 86% accuracy. Overall 5-year survival of patients after a curative en bloc resection was 40.6%. The benefits of en bloc esophagectomy are particularly seen in patients with fewer than four involved lymph nodes. These results support a clinical approach in which an en bloc resection of the esophagus and stomach and a durable reconstruction of the gastrointestinal tract is advocated for patients most apt to benefit.

Management of Patients Excluded From Curative Resection

If the patient's condition is considered incurable on preoperative or intraoperative evaluation, the severity of dysphagia or other incapacitating symptoms are assessed. We consider dysphagia for even semisolids an indication for a palliative resection. It is well documented that, if the patient is physiologically fit, a simple esophageal resection and reconstruction with esophagogastrostomy offers the best palliation. It allows the patient to eat without dysphagia and prevents the local complications of perforation, hemorrhage, fistula formation, and incapacitating pain. Occasionally, a patient is cured by a palliative resection, but this should not be used as justification for resection in the absence of dysphagia. The presence of a malignant pleural effusion, obvious mediastinal spread, or metastatic disease usually discourages a palliative resection.

Perioperative Management

The nutritional status of the patient is of paramount importance for the outcome of an esophageal resection. Low serum protein levels have a deleterious effect on the cardiovascular system, and a poor nutritional status affects the host resistance to infection and the rate of anastomotic and wound healing. A serum albumin level below 3.4 g/dl on admission indicates poor caloric intake and an increased risk of surgical complications, including anastomotic breakdown. In our experience a feeding jejunostomy tube provides the most reliable and safest method for nutritional support in patients who cannot consume an oral diet and have a functionally normal small bowel. In severely malnourished patients, the jejunostomy is performed as a separate procedure to allow for preoperative nutritional support. In these patients the abdomen is entered through a small supraumbilical midline incision. Otherwise, the jejunostomy tube is placed at the time of esophageal resection, and feeding is begun on the third postoperative day.

Conduct of Curative Resection

A curative procedure is conducted according to standard principles of surgical oncology, by performing an en bloc resection in continuity with the regional lymph nodes. It is attempted in a patient whose preresection physical condition and tumor characteristics have the potential for long-term survival.

Cervical Esophagus

In tumors of the cervical esophagus, the thoracic esophagus is removed by blunt dissection through a cervical and upper abdominal incision. A simultaneous en bloc bilateral neck dissection is performed, sparing the jugular veins at both sides. The larynx is often invaded with microscopic tumor, and a total laryngectomy in combination with an esophagectomy is necessary. It is our opinion that the larynx should be removed even if gross tumor cannot be visualized. The continuity of the gastrointestinal tract is reestablished by pulling the stomach up through the esophageal bed. A permanent tracheostomy stoma is constructed in the lower flap of the cervical incision. The 5-year survival rate ranges around 20%.

Upper and Middle Third

To remove tumors in the middle or upper third of the thoracic esophagus, we perform a standard esophagectomy. The procedure is performed through a right posterolateral or anterolateral thoracotomy, and the abdominal dissection is done through an upper midline incision. As many regional lymph nodes as possible are taken out with the specimen. Through a left neck incision the esophagus is divided, and the previously dissected thoracic esophagus is removed transhiatally. Gastrointestinal continuity is reestablished by pulling up the previously prepared stomach through the hiatus and anastomosing it to the esophagus in the neck. The operative mortality for this procedure is lower the more distal the tumor.

Lower Third

Tumors in the lower third of the thoracic esophagus and cardia are amenable either to an en bloc resection for cure or a limited palliative resection. En bloc resection implies removal of a tissue block surrounded on all sides by normal tissue (i.e., containing all possible extensions of the primary tumor) and requires a subtotal esophagectomy and a two-thirds gastrectomy in continuity with a block of tissue containing the following nodal groups: subcarinal, inferior paraesophageal, parahiatal, left gastric, celiac, hepatic, and splenic artery nodes (Fig. 14-45). The dissection is limited anteriorly by the pericardium; laterally by the left and right mediastinal pleura; and posteriorly by the intercostal arteries, aorta, and anterior vertebral ligaments. The proximal margin is the carina, the inferior margin is the celiac axis and common hepatic artery, and the lateral margins are the mediastinal pleura and a collar of diaphragmatic muscle around the esophageal hiatus. The resection is done through three incisions in the following order. First, exploration of the abdomen is performed through an upper midline incision, and the porta hepatis and subpancreatic nodes are examined by biopsy. If no metastases are identified, the incision is closed, and an en bloc dissection of the esophagus through a right posterolateral thoracotomy is performed with mobilization of the esophagus above the aortic arch. The thoracotomy is closed, the patient repositioned in the recumbent position, and the upper midline abdominal incision reopened to permit en

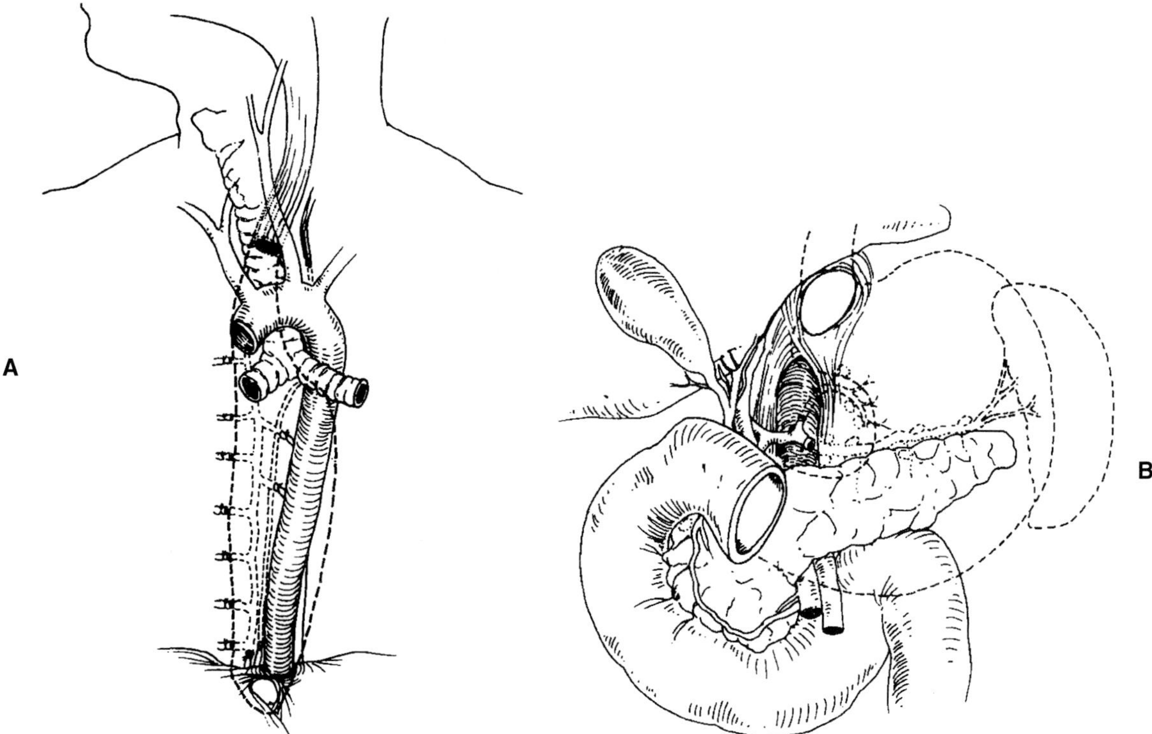

Fig. 14-45. Extent of resection in en bloc esophagectomy. **A,** Thoracic resection. **B,** Abdominal resection.

bloc dissection of the stomach and associated lymph nodes. The spleen and the splenic artery with its associated lymph nodes are removed by dissecting them off the superior border of the pancreas. A left neck incision is made to allow proximal division of the esophagus. The mobilized esophagus is removed transhiatally, and the stomach is divided at the angulus. Gastrointestinal continuity is reestablished with a left colon interposition. During the thoracic and abdominal dissection, intraoperative staging is done according to the algorithm. If during the course of the operation an incurable situation is identified, the en bloc resection is abandoned, and a palliative resection is performed in a manner similar to that described for tumors of the middle and upper thoracic esophagus. If preoperative staging has shown that the patient is a candidate for palliative resection, a transhiatal esophagectomy as described by Orringer is performed.

Operative mortality is 7% to 10% for en bloc esophagectomy, and overall 5-year survival is 41% in our experience. The benefits of en bloc resection are especially observed in those patients in whom four or fewer involved lymph nodes are observed[34] (Fig. 14-46). Overall 5-year survival after palliative esophagectomy is 14%.

Nonresectional Procedures

Resection is usually not possible if invasion of the trachea, bronchi, aorta, spine, or heart is found or when distal organ metastases are present. Further, the patient's general condition may be too poor to justify an extensive surgical procedure. In this situation relief of dysphagia requires reestablishing a conduit through which food may pass. The commonest methods are summarized below.

Intubation

Since the initial attempts at intubation by Leroy d'Etoilles in 1845 a number of tubes have been devised that are placed either by the pulsion or the traction technique. Most tubes are made of polyvinyl and have an internal diameter of 10 to 12 mm. The proximal end is funnel shaped to prevent caudal displacement and to direct food into it, whereas some also have a distal flange to prevent proximal dislodgment. Intubation is not applicable to tumors in the cervical or upper third of the thoracic esophagus because of the lack of room to seat the funnel below the cricopharyngeus muscle. Similarly, placement of the tube at the cardia may be difficult because of the angulation of the lumen of the esophagus. Most malignant strictures can be intubated using the flexible endoscope under sedation. The simplicity of the procedure belies the frequent occurrence of complications. These include perforation of the esophagus, reflux of gastric contents through the tube and aspiration, obstruction of the tube from distal tumor overgrowth, severe halitosis caused by decomposition of food adherent to the prosthesis, esophageal wall erosion, and obstruction of the tube by food. The use of self-expanding stents has reduced these somewhat. Despite these complications, intubation is a common method of palliation, and improvement occurs in nearly all patients,

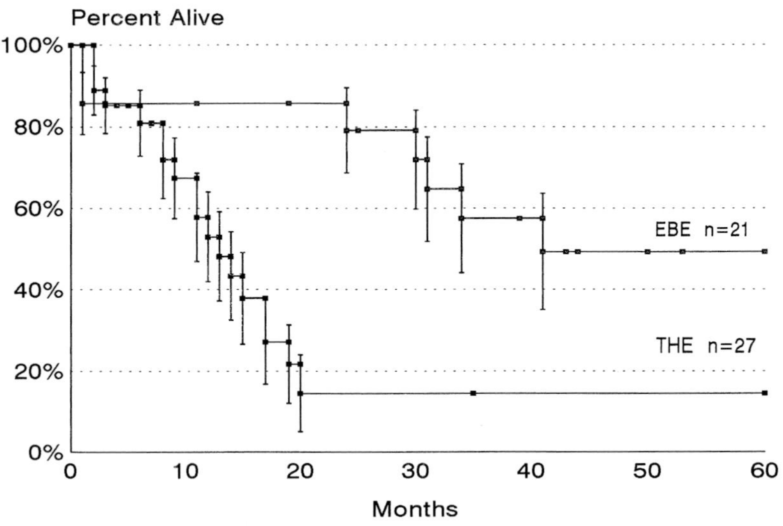

Fig. 14-46. Survival after en bloc esophagectomy (EBE) vs. transhiatal esophagectomy (THE) for cancer.

although only two thirds can manage a semisolid diet. Intubation usually signifies a last resort to palliate end-stage disease. The median survival after insertion of an esophageal tube for carcinoma is 2 to 4 months, but the benefit to the patient is well worth the risk, particularly in those who are unable to swallow their saliva.

Other methods of establishing a lumen in unresectable esophageal cancers are laser ablation or electrocoagulation. The former carries few complications but requires frequent repetition to maintain patency. The latter is useful only in circumferential tumors and requires fluoroscopy to position the heating electrode. In patients who have suffered multiple complications following attempted resection for cure or palliation and whose current health precludes future surgery, an extracorporeal tube connecting a cervical esophagostomy to a gastrostomy may provide beneficial relief of dysphagia.

Chemotherapy and Radiation Therapy

Nonsurgical modalities of treatment include chemotherapy and radiotherapy. Either modality may be given preoperatively, postoperatively, or instead of operation. Most published reports describe the outcome in uncontrolled series, and truly randomized comparisons are rare. The evidence may be summarized as follows.

Preoperative radiation given with the aim of improving resectability and reducing perioperative dissemination of tumor cells has not been found to increase resectability rates; rather, it may actually worsen the situation. A recent randomized trial combining preroperative dermatherapy and radiation and surgery for Barrett's adenocarcinoma found a slight advantage for the patient's treated with multimodal therapy compared to those having surgery alone.[36] Other similar trials are currently in progress and should be reported in the near future. Postoperative radiation may have an effect on reducing local recurrence, but any effect on survival is slight.

A wide variety of chemotherapeutic regimens have been used, although almost all include cisplatin combined with either bleomycin, 5-FU, or vindesine. A prolonged disease-free interval can be demonstrated in so-called responders, but overall survival is not. A combination of preoperative radiation and chemotherapy may produce an increase in the number of responders. Preoperative chemoradiation may be of value in cancer of the middle and upper thirds of the thoracic esophagus, a situation when curative surgery is rarely possible. However, there is a definite increase in surgical morbidity of esophagectomy after chemoradiation, especially of serious pulmonary problems consequent on the radiation-induced changes in the lungs.

Some studies have shown impressive results in patients with apparently unresectable tumors, treated by both radiotherapy and chemotherapy. However, the morbidity of these treatments can be considerable and includes not just unpleasant symptoms such as alopecia, nausea, vomiting, and diarrhea but also serious illness such as renal failure, pulmonary fibrosis, and septicemia. In consequence, the role of these treatments in the treatment and palliation of esophageal cancer is yet to be defined.[35]

SUMMARY

The most common esophageal disease in Western society is gastroesophageal reflux of gastric juice with its attendant complications, followed by esophageal cancer, with esophageal motility disorders being less common still.

Since all categories of esophageal disease are frequently referred to surgeons for management, it is mandatory that the underlying pathophysiologic perturbations be thoroughly understood if treatment measures are to prove successful. Whereas in treating esophageal cancer, the primary goal of surgery is long-term survival, with quality of life being a secondary consideration; the situation in benign disease is quite different. The goal of surgery in benign esophageal disease, such as reflux and motility disorders, is rather preservation of function.

REFERENCES

1. Kahrilas PJ, et al. Upper esophageal sphincter function during deglutition. Gastroenterology 95:52, 1988.
2. Kahrilas PJ, Dodds WJ, Hogan WJ. Effect of peristaltic dysfunction on esophageal volume clearance. Gastroenterology 94:73, 1988.
3. Mittal RK, et al. Transient lower esophageal sphincter relaxation. Gastroenterology 106:601, 1995.
4. DeMeester TR, et al. Clinical and in vitro analysis of determinants of gastroesophageal competence. Am J Surg 137:39, 1979.
5. Bonavina L, et al. Length of the distal esophageal sphincter and competency of the cardia. Am J Surg 151:25, 1986.
6. Monnier P, Ollyo J-B, Fontolliet C, Savary M. Epidemiology and natural history of reflux esophagitis. Semin Lap Surg 2:2, 1995.
7. DeMeester TR, et al. Esophageal function in patients with angina-type chest pain and normal coronary angiograms. Ann Surg 196:488, 1982.
8. Zaninotto G, et al. The lower esophageal sphincter in health and disease. Am J Surg 155:104, 1988.
9. Stein HJ, et al. Three-dimensional imaging of the lower esophageal sphincter in gastroesophageal reflux disease. Ann Surg 214:374, 1991.
10. Cook IJ, et al. Opening mechanisms of the human upper esophageal sphincter. Am J Physiol 257 (Gastrointest Liver Physiol 20):G748, 1989.
11. DeMeester TR, et al. Technique, indications and clinical use of 24-hour esophageal pH monitoring. J Thorac Cardiovasc Surg 79:656, 1980.
12. Jamieson JR, et al. Ambulatory 24-hour esophageal pH monitoring: Normal values, optimal thresholds, specificity, sensitivity, and reproducibility. Am J Gastroenterol 87:1102, 1992.
13. Attwood SEA, et al. Alkaline gastroesophageal reflux: Implications in the development of complications in Barrett's columnar-lined lower esophagus. Surgery 106:764, 1989.
14. Stein HJ, et al. Ambulatory 24-hour esophageal manometry in the evaluation of esophageal motor disorders and noncardiac chest pain. Surgery 110:753, 1991.
15. Bechi P, et al. Long-term ambulatory enterogastric reflux monitoring. Validation of a new fiber-optic technique. Dig Dis Sci 38:1297, 1993.
16. Duranceau A. Pharyngeal and cricopharyngeal disorders. In Pearson FG, ed. Esophageal Surgery. New York: Churchill Livingstone, 1995, p 389.
17. Robertson CS, Martin BAB, Atkinson MA. Varicella-zoster virus DNA in the oesophageal myenteric plexus in achalasia. Gut 34:299, 1993.
18. Pasricha PJ, et al. Intrasphincteric botulinum toxin for the treatment of achalasia. N Engl J Med 332:774, 1995.
19. Andreollo NA, Earlam RJ. Heller's myotomy for achalasia: Is an added antireflux procedure necessary? Br J Surg 74:765, 1987.
20. Topart P, et al. Long-term effect of total fundoplication on the myotomized esophagus. Ann Thorac Surg 54:1046, 1992.
21. Csendes A, et al. Late results of a prospective randomised study comparing forceful dilation and oesophagomyotomy in patients with achalasia. Gut 30:299, 1989.
22. Eypasch E, et al. Physiological assessment and surgical management of diffuse esophageal spasm. J Thorac Cardiovasc Surg 104:859, 1992.
23. Liebermann DA. Medical therapy for chronic reflux esophagitis; Long-term follow-up. Arch Intern Med 147:1717, 1987.
24. Kuster E, et al. Predictive factors of the long-term outcome in gastro-oesophageal reflux disease: Six year follow-up of 107 patients. Gut 35:8, 1994.
25. Sloan S, Rademaker AW, Kahrilas PJ. Determinants of gastroesophageal junction incompetence: Hiatal hernia, lower esophageal sphincter or both? Ann Intern Med 117:977, 1992.
26. Stein HJ, et al. Complications of gastroesophageal reflux disease: Role of the lower esophageal sphincter, esophageal acid and acid/alkaline exposure, and duodenogastric reflux. Ann Surg 216(1):35, 1992.
27. Schnell TH, Sontag SJ, Chejifec G. Adenocarcinoma arising in tongues or short segments of Barrett's esophagus. Dig Dis Sci 37:137, 1992.
28. Spechler SJ, Department of Veterans Affairs Gastroesophageal Reflux Disease Study Group #277. Comparison of medical and surgical therapy for complicated gastroesophageal reflux disease, in veterans. N Engl J Med 326(12):786, 1992.
29. Peters JH, et al. Clinical and physiologic comparison of laparoscopic and open Nissen fundoplication. J Am Coll Surg 180:385, 1995.
30. DeMeester TR, Bonavina L, Albertucci M. Nissen fundoplication for gastroesophageal reflux disease—Evaluation of primary repair in 100 consecutive patients. Ann Surg 204:9, 1986.
31. DeMeester TR, et al. Indications, surgical technique, and long-term function results of colon interposition or bypass. Ann Surg 208:460, 1988.
32. DeMeester TR, Barlow AP. Surgery and current management for cancer of the esophagus and cardia: Parts I and II. Curr Probl Surg 25(7-8):477, 1988.
33. DeMeester TR, Zaninotto G, Johansson K-E. Selective therapeutic approach to cancer of the lower esophagus and cardia. J Thorac Cardiovasc Surg 95:42, 1988.
34. Hagen JA, Peters JH, DeMeester TR. Superiority of extended en bloc esophagectomy for carcinoma of the lower esophagus and cardia. J Thorac Cardiovasc Surg 106:850, 1993.
35. Hilgenberg AD, et al. Preoperative chemotherapy, surgical resection, and selective postoperative therapy for squamous cell carcinoma of the esophagus. Ann Thorac Surg 45:357, 1988.
36. Walsh TN, et al. A comparison of multimodal therapy and surgery for esophageal adenocarcinoma. N Engl J Med 335:462, 1996.

15

Physiology of Gastric Secretion and Emptying

Kimberly S. Kirkwood and Haile T. Debas

Control of gastric secretion and emptying is brought about by complex interactions of nerves and humoral agents. The action of nerves at the effector cell (e.g., smooth muscle, oxyntic cell, gastric cell) requires the release of neurotransmitters, which, in addition to the classic cholinergic and adrenergic substances, include neuropeptides, amines (e.g., serotonin) and adenosine diphosphate (ADP). Some of the neuropeptides from nerve endings may be secreted into the interstitial fluid, through which they may be spread to adjacent cells: neurocrine transmission. The humoral agents arrive at their target cells not only by the classic endocrine (blood-borne) pathway, but also by diffusion through the interstitial fluid after their local secretion by endocrine cells within the wall of the stomach: paracrine transmission. Thus any response to a given stimulant or inhibitor is modulated by the ambient concentrations of paracrine and neurocrine agents in the local milieu of the target cells. The concept of local modulation therefore must be taken into consideration when interpreting gastric secretory or motor responses to exogenous stimulants. In general, much more is known about processes that stimulate secretion than those that inhibit it. Also mechanisms that control gastric secretion have been defined better than those that regulate motility. Thus any review of this subject must indicate not only the degree of knowledge achieved but also the state of ignorance that remains.

The aim of this chapter is to summarize the current knowledge of the physiology of gastric secretion and emptying in a manner relevant to the surgery of the stomach. Before discussion of gastric function, a brief review of the physiologic anatomy of the stomach is appropriate.

PHYSIOLOGIC ANATOMY

The traditional division of the stomach into three regions (the cardia, the body [corpus], and the antrum) is useful but only for describing gross pathology. In the past the body of the stomach has been regarded as the exocrine organ concerned with the secretion of acid and pepsin, the antrum as the endocrine organ for the release of gastrin, and the cardia as that buffer zone between the esophagus and the gastric corpus with no particular function. In truth, the entire stomach functions as both an endocrine and exocrine organ.

The esophagus enters the abdomen at the diaphragmatic hiatus, which is at the level of the T12 vertebra. The pyloroduodenal junction is at the level of the L1 vertebra. The stomach is fixed at these two points, from which it hangs in a J-shaped manner. The close proximity of the gastroesophageal junction and the pylorus should be appreciated.

Muscle Coat

The main muscle coat of the stomach consists of an outer longitudinal, middle circular, and inner oblique layer. The longitudinal muscle coat is concentrated along the lesser and greater curvatures of the stomach. The fibers of the middle circular layer are disposed at right angles to those of the longitudinal layer and completely encircle the stomach and become progressively thicker toward the pylorus. The inner oblique layer is concentrated largely over the anterior and posterior surfaces of the stomach and is deficient at the greater and lesser curvatures. At the pylorus there is an impressive thickening of the circular muscle layer, defining a distinct anatomic sphincter.

Mucosal Lining

The mucosal lining of the cardia of the stomach contains glands made up of simple columnar cells. No parietal or chief cells are present. The mucosa of the body of the stomach is characterized by the acid-secreting oxyntic (parietal) cells and the pepsin-secreting chief cells. On the surface the mucosa of the corpus contains gastric pits, each draining several gastric glands. The pits themselves are lined with mucous neck cells that maintain a thin layer of mucous gel over the surface of the entire mucosa (Fig. 15-1). The oxyntic cells are the most striking cells of the gastric glands of the proximal stomach. They contain large amounts of mitochondria in their cytoplasm, indicative of the high energy requirements of acid secretion. In terms of their mitochondrial content, the oxyntic cells are only second to the cells of the myocardium, another organ with high energy requirements. A most impressive morphologic transformation occurs in the oxyntic cell when it is stimulated. At rest the cell is filled with smooth membrane structures (tubulovesicles). On stimulation these structures decrease and become replaced by an expansion of the secretory canaliculus in the form of microvilli containing H^+,K^+-ATPase, the proton pump.[1]

The antrum is lined by pyloric gland mucosa containing principally mucus-secreting cells. A few scattered oxyntic cells are also found. In the human, unlike the dog, no pepsin is secreted in the antrum. In the midzone of the pyloric glands are scattered gastrin-secreting cells (G cells). The G cells are of the open type (i.e., they open into the lumen of the glands), and their apical surface is thrown into microvilli that come in contact with the contents of the gastric lumen. These microvilli are thought to represent chemical and pH sensors for the G cell.

Several other endocrine cells are scattered throughout the gastric mucosa from the cardia to the pylorus. In the proximal stomach of humans at least five endocrine cells have been identified (Table 15-1). D cells, which secrete somatostatin and some other unknown peptide; enterochromaffin (EC) cells, which secrete serotonin and various other peptides; enterochromaffin-like (ECL) cells, which have been shown recently to secrete histamine[2]; and P and X cells, whose function is unknown.[3] The human antral mucosa also contains D, EC, and P cells but no ECL or X cells. The somatostatin (D) cells in the antrum have long processes that end in fusiform swellings abutting on G cells (Fig. 15-2). Somatostatin is considered an important paracrine inhibitor of gastrin release.[4]

Neural Supply

The stomach receives both extrinsic and intrinsic nerve supply. The extrinsic pathway consists of both vagal and sympathetic nerve contributions. The intrinsic system, or enteric nervous system (ENS), is composed of interconnected neural plexuses within the bowel wall.

The extrinsic innervation of the stomach derives from the vagi and the sympathetic nervous system. It is no longer accurate to describe these nerves as purely cholinergic and adrenergic, respectively, because in truth both systems contain peptidergic and purinergic nerves. In addition, a certain number of adrenergic nerves are present in the vagi, and parasympathetic (cholinergic) nerves are present in the sympathetic fibers. Over 80% of the fibers in the vagi are afferent neurons carrying information back to the brain.

Table 15-1. Exocrine and Endocrine Cells of the Stomach and Their Secretory Products

Cells	Secretory Products	Primary Location
Exocrine		
Mucus	Mucus	Body, antrum
Oxyntic	Acid	Body
Chief	Pepsin	Body
Endocrine		
G	Gastrin	Antrum
D	Somatostatin	Diffuse
A*	Glucagon	
EC	Seratonin plus various peptides	Diffuse
ECL	Histamine	Body
P	Unknown	Diffuse
X	Unknown	Body

*In fetus or newborn; only exceptionally found in adults. *EC,* Enterochromaffin; *ECL,* enterochromaffin-like (cell).

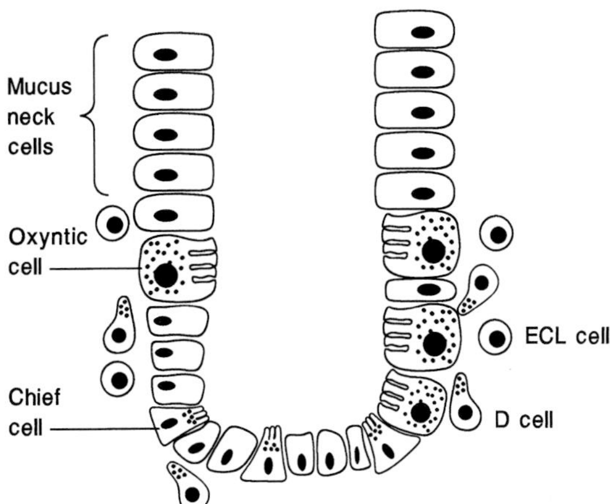

Fig. 15-1. Representation of a gastric gland demonstrating mucus cells and the close approximation of enterochromaffin-like cells *(ECL),* somatostatin-containing D cells, oxyntic cells, and chief cells.

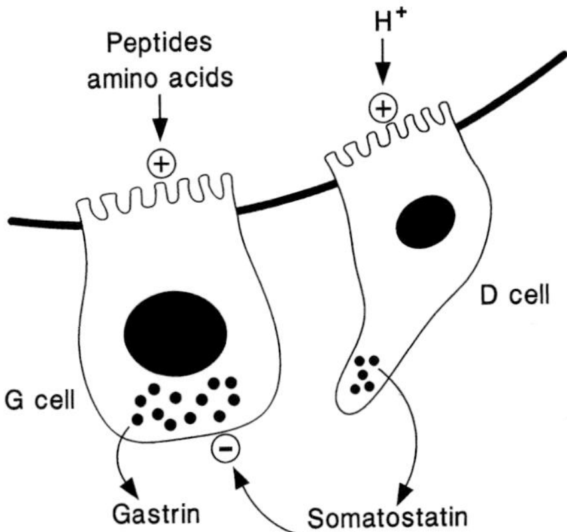

Fig. 15-2. Feedback loop regulating gastrin release from antral G cells. Luminal peptides and amino acids stimulate G cells to secrete gastrin leading to increased luminal acid. Acid, in turn, triggers somatostatin production from D cells, which inhibits gastrin release from G cells via a paracrine pathway.

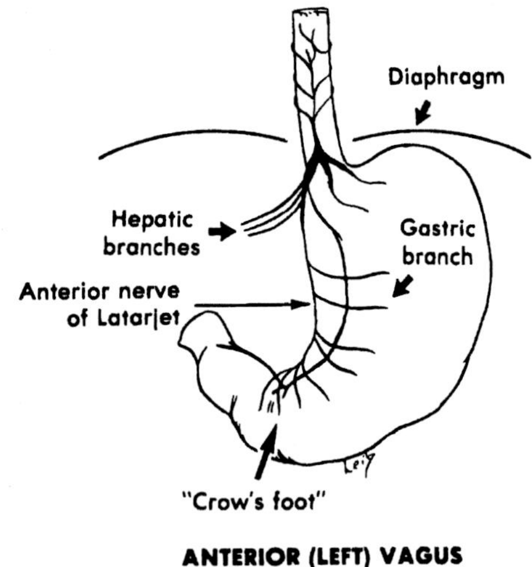

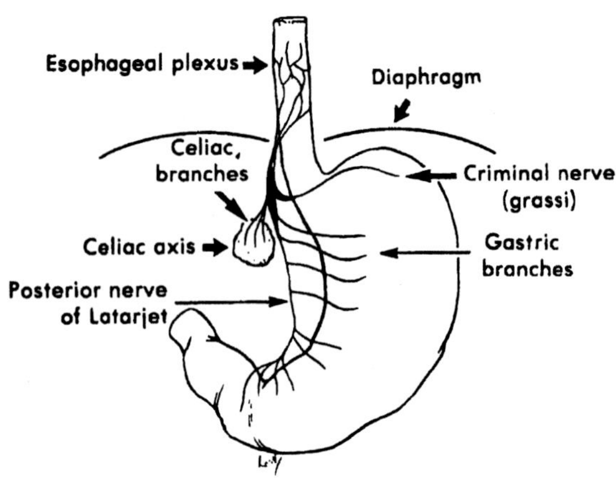

Fig. 15-3. Distribution of subdiaphragmatic vagi with their major branches.

The anterior (left) and posterior (right) vagus nerves enter the abdomen at the esophageal hiatus (Fig. 15-3). On the anterior surface of the abdominal esophagus, the anterior vagus nerve is present as a single trunk 60% of the time and as two or more trunks 40% of the time. By contrast, the posterior vagus nerves, often found to lie between the esophagus and the right diaphragmatic crus, form a single trunk in over 95% of cases. The extragastric vagal nerves come off the vagi proximal to or at the esophagogastric junction: the hepatic division from the anterior vagus nerve consisting toward the liver high in the lesser omentum, and the celiac division from the posterior vagus nerve running to the celial axis in proximity to the left gastric artery. These two branches are nearly always constant in their location and serve as useful guides to the identification of the main vagal trunks. Both vagi then give off gastric branches to the proximal stomach and continue on to the antrum as the nerves of Latarjet. An understanding of this anatomy is critical to the performance of a successful highly selective vagotomy for hyperacidity.

The sympathetic nerve distribution of the stomach, on the other hand, does not proceed along easily defined pathways. Sympathetic preganglionic neurons from the fifth to the tenth thoracic segments reach the celiac axis through the greater splanchnic nerve. Neurons with cell bodies in the celiac ganglion innervate the stomach. Sympathetic fibers are distributed to the stomach in the adventitia of the arterial supply and form a meshwork within the gastric wall. Adrenergic fibers innervate the three muscle layers (longitudinal, circular, and muscularis mucosae), but this innervation is sparse. Sympathetic innervation is more dense to the pyloric sphincter; in a number of species a rich network of substance P–staining fibers are found, raising the possibility that substance P neurons may mediate the relaxation of the pylorus (see discussion of substance P that follows). The major distribution of sympathetic fibers in the stomach is to the vasculature. Thus a proximal vagotomy also results in a partial sympathectomy resulting from devascularization of the lesser curvature of the stomach.

Much attention has been given recently to the ENS, which exhibits anatomic and physiologic independence from the CNS. In humans, the ENS of the entire gastrointestinal tract contains over 10^8 neurons compared to the number of efferent vagal fibers at the diaphragm of less than 2×10^3.[5] Therefore most enteric ganglion cells probably receive no vagal input. The ENS consists primarily of two main ganglionated plexuses (myenteric [Auerbach's] and Meissner's). The myenteric plexus lies between the circular and longitudinal muscle layers and forms more than one network of fibers connected to the ganglia. The myenteric neurons play an important role in the peristaltic reflex. Neurons located in the submucosa (Meissner's plexus) serve as vasomotor regulators and are largely responsible for control of secretory and absorptive function.[6] Several types of neurons have been identified in the ENS and are listed below:

1. Cholinergic (choline acetate transferase staining)
2. Serotonergic (containing or activated by serotonin)
3. Peptidergic
   a. Vasoactive intestinal polypeptide (VIP)
   b. Substance P
   c. Somatostatin
   d. Enkephalins
   e. Neurotensin
   f. Other peptides: Cholecystokinin (CCK), gastrin, pancreatic polypeptide

These peptidergic neurons are considered important in modulating the control of the microcirculation and of secretory and motor functions.

Blood Supply

The rich blood supply to the stomach is known to every surgeon and is derived from the celiac axis. The left gastric artery courses to the lesser curve near the gastroesophageal junction and curves downward to anastomose with the right gastric artery, the first branch of the hepatic artery. The greater curvature is supplied through the right and left gastroepiploic arteries. The right gastroepiploic artery is a branch of the gastroduodenal artery; the left gastroepiploic artery is a branch of the splenic artery. In addition, the splenic artery gives off the short gastric arteries that supply the fundus. Venous drainage is along the right and left gastric veins that join directly the portal vein and along the short gastric veins and the left gastroepiploic veins that join the splenic vein. The right gastroepiploic vein drains into the superior mesenteric vein. The rich blood supply to the stomach is what makes bleeding from gastric ulcers such a serious problem, requiring surgical intervention much more commonly than bleeding from duodenal ulcers.

NORMAL PHYSIOLOGY OF THE STOMACH

Motor Function

Electric Activity

The stomach, like the heart, has a natural pacemaker.[7] The gastric pacemaker is located high on the greater curvature of the body of the stomach and is composed of a group of specialized smooth muscle cells that generate cyclic changes in potential, called pacesetter potentials. These electric cycles appear regularly at a frequency of 3 cycles/min in humans and propagate distally from the pacemaker to the antrum. The pacesetter potential depolarizes smooth muscle cells as it spreads caudad and causes the cells to come close to their threshold for action potentials. Thus the pacesetter potential controls the frequency, rhythm, direction of propagation, and velocity of contraction. The action potential is associated with mechanical contractions and determines the strength of the contraction. The gastric electric activity is summarized in Fig. 15-4. If the proximal pacemaker is destroyed surgically, secondary pacemakers develop distally.

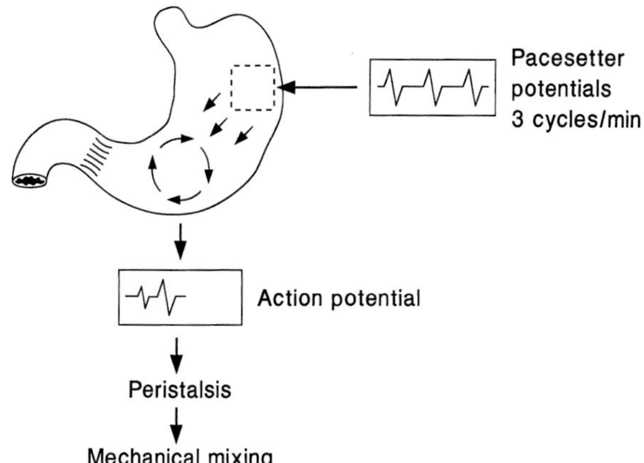

Fig. 15-4. Electric activity of the stomach and the motor activity of the distal stomach responsible for gastric emptying of solids. Peristaltic contractions triturate digestible solids to near liquefied form before they are emptied.

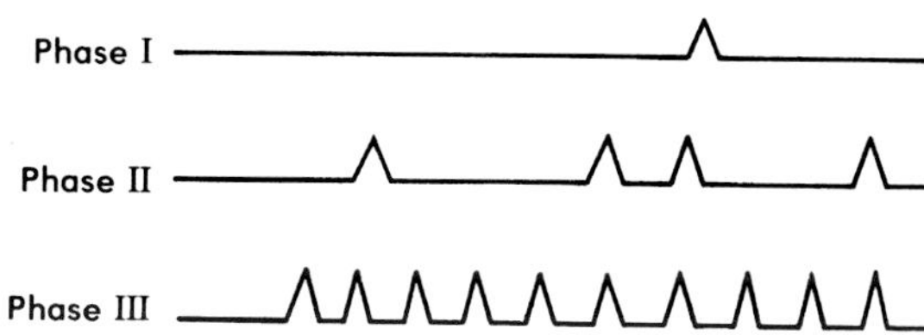

Fig. 15-5. The migrating myoelectric complex is initiated in the proximal stomach, and contractions during phase III sweep down to the pylorus, clearing the stomach of residue; hence the term *housekeeper potential* applied to it. Phase I is the quiescent phase, and contractions start to appear in phase II before they become numerous and repetitive in phase III.

During fasting, gastric motility demonstrates interdigestive motor cycles that occur every 1 to 2 hours.[8] Each interdigestive motor cycle consists of three phases. The quiescent period when there is no motor activity is phase I, followed by phase II in which irregular contractile activity is seen, followed by phase III when sweeping bursts of contractions occur (Fig. 15-5). The interdigestive motor complex has been called "the housekeeper potential" because the phase III contractions have the effect of clearing the stomach of its contents every 1 to 2 hours regularly.

Feeding disrupts the fasting cyclic motor activity, and the stomach responds to the neural, humoral, and mechanical stimulation imposed by the meal. The motor activities in the stomach are then directed toward delivering the gastric contents into the duodenum in appropriate volumes and particle sizes.

Mechanical Activity

The stomach is normally collapsed when empty. Feeding initiates "receptive relaxation" primarily of the fundus and upper body so that the meal is accepted without precipitous rise in intragastric pressure. Vagotomy interferes with this receptive relaxation so that the arrival of food to the stomach is associated with relatively higher increases in intragastric pressure. This phenomenon likely accounts for the feeling of "early satiety" described by some patients following vagotomy. Gastric emptying of liquids is thought to be primarily controlled by the proximal stomach. Low-amplitude tonic fundic contractions increase the intragastric pressure sufficiently to create a pressure gradient between the stomach and the duodenum. Liquids are thus squeezed out of the stomach much like wine is squeezed out of a Spanish bota bag. By contrast, the emptying of solid meals is under the control of the distal stomach and is associated with strong antral and antropyloric contractions. When solids are present in the stomach, ring contractions are stimulated to develop in the midbody, generating intraluminal pressures as high as 100 mm Hg.[9] These advance toward the pylorus, propelling the gastric contents caudad and pushing the food against a closed pylorus. The effect is propulsion and retropulsion of the food, ensuring good mixing with the liquid phase. The strong muscular contractions of the antropylorus region grind down solids into small particles. Only particles less than 1 mm in diameter are emptied into the duodenum. The ability of the stomach to discriminate between particle sizes is remarkable, and the phenomenon is not fully understood.

In summary, the ingestion of food is associated with disruption of the interdigestive motor complex and receptive relaxation of the proximal stomach. The classic view of gastric motility holds that emptying of liquids involves low-pressure tonic contractions and is controlled primarily by the proximal stomach; whereas the emptying of solids is a function of the distal stomach and is associated with contraction rings, high pressures, propulsion and retropulsion, and grinding down of food particles by the "antral pump." Recent studies suggest that the isolated distal stomach can produce transpyloric flow of liquids[10] and further that this region may play an important regulatory role in liquid emptying.[11]

Regulation of Gastric Emptying

The mechanisms that control and regulate gastric emptying involve both neural and humoral components. The receptive relaxation of the proximal stomach to feeding is mediated through vagal inhibitory reflexes, with the sensory receptors being located in the distal esophagus. The transmitters involved in receptive relaxation are unknown, but they are neither adrenergic nor cholingergic. Evidence has been produced that both dopamine and enkephalin may play a role. The main determinants of gastric emptying are (1) whether a meal is solid or liquid and (2) its nutrient content, acidity, and osmolality. Both osmoreceptors and pH-sensitive receptors are present in the upper small intestine. These factors are important in activating feedback inhibition of gastric emptying through neurohumoral pathways. Although a number of peptides, including gastric inhibitory polypeptide (GIP), glucagon, VIP, and neurotensin, have been proposed as mediators, only CCK has been shown to inhibit gastric emptying in physiologic doses.[12] CCK is released from the duodenum and upper jejunum by protein digests, fat, acid, and perhaps also by high osmolality and appears to act on the stomach via vagal afferent pathways.[13] Further evidence that brain centers are involved in the regulation of gastric emptying comes from experiments on mechanoreceptors in the stomach that respond to distention and on glucoreceptors in the first portion of the duodenum, both of which have been shown to influence the activity of neurons in the medulla (the nucleus tractus solitarii and the dorsal vagal nucleus).[14] The centers probably relay signals for both satiety and gastric emptying. In the duodenum, pH and osmoreceptors are present, and activation of these receptors delays gastric emptying. It is possible that CCK release may mediate in part the effect of low pH and high osmolality in slowing gastric emptying. A suggestion has also been made that the caloric content of the food passing into the duodenum may be important. It is possible that the receptors for all these mechanisms activate afferent vagal discharge.

The effects of vagotomy on gastric emptying that must be considered include both the direct effects of the operation on the stomach and the indirect effects resulting from the interruption of afferent vagal input from duodenal pH and osmoreceptors. Two important direct effects of truncal vagotomy on the stomach are the loss of receptive relaxation of the proximal stomach and loss of the relaxing effect on the pyloric sphincter. The later results in marked inhibition of emptying of both liquids and solids, and gastric distention and vomiting may occur. To prevent these sequelae the pyloris is often surgically bypassed or destroyed at the time of vagotomy. This results in acceleration of gastric emptying of liquids because of an increased luminal pressure between the stomach and the duodenum or jejunum with relatively normal emptying of solids. As expected, proximal gastric vagotomy that preserves the innervation of the antropyloric mechanism has little permanent effect on gastric emptying of either liquids or solids.

Measurement of Gastric Emptying[15]

Current methods for measuring gastric emptying have inherent problems, but progressive refinement has made available a number of useful techniques.[15] These techniques are of three types: intubative, radiologic, and radioisotopic. Intubative techniques are useful for providing a rough estimate of liquid emptying. In the most common one, "Hunt's test," a nasogastric tube is used to measure the residual volume 30 minutes after instillation of a solution containing a nonabsorbable marker (e.g., phenol red or polyethylene glycol). If gastric emptying is normal, the residual volume in the stomach should be less than one half the instilled volume. This procedure can also be used without the nonabsorbable markers as a bedside test. Fluoroscopic techniques, with both liquid barium and barium-impregnated solids, can be used to estimate emptying of liquids or solids.

Increased accuracy can now be obtained with radioisotopic imaging techniques. With the use of two different isotopes, one for liquid and the other for solid, emptying of liquids and solids can be studied simultaneously after the ingestion of a mixed meal. The commonly used markers are technetium 99m (^{99m}Tc) and indium-111.[15] The upper abdomen is scanned by a gamma camera and the data processed using a computer to determine the half-emptying times ($T_{1/2}$) for solid and liquid phases of gastric emptying. Recent advances include the ability to determine the effect of potential therapeutic pharmacologic interventions on gastric emptying in a given patient. Thus the relative efficacies of the various promotility agents can be determined for a patient with gastroparesis.[16]

Electrogastrography has recently been added to the armamentarium of the gastric physiologist interested in motility. It appears to offer great promise for measuring gastric myoelectric activity.[17] Studies are under way to assess the correlation of this technique with functional emptying characteristics of the stomach in health and disease.

Secretory Functions

Endocrine Stomach

As previously indicated, it is no longer valid to consider the distal stomach as an endocrine organ and the proximal stomach as an exocrine organ. Endocrine cells are found throughout the stomach. In addition, peptides and amines are found in neural elements within the wall of the stomach.[18] Peptides arrive at their target site, whether this be the oxyntic cell or a smooth muscle cell, in one of three ways.

Endocrine. Peptides are secreted through the basolateral membrane into the circulation. They circulate and arrive at the target cell through the blood stream. This appears to be the mechanism by which gastrin is delivered to the oxyntic cell. Clearly, peptides secreted by the endocrine cells of the intestine (e.g., CCK, secretin, GIP, and neurotensin) arrive at the oxyntic cell through the blood.

Paracrine. Some humoral agents are evanescent in the circulation, and they may reach their target cells by diffusion after being secreted into the interstitial fluid. Prime examples of paracrine agents are histamine and prostaglandins. In addition, a number of peptides may use this mode of delivery. The most important of these are somatostatin and VIP.

Neurocrine. Peptides are secreted from nerve endings and cross a small synaptic gap to the end plate or receptor to cause their actions. A prime example is bombesin or its mammalian counterpart, gastrin-releasing polypeptide (GRP). Another peptide that probably also acts as a neurotransmitter is substance P. A number of peptides (CCK, somatostatin, VIP, and substance P) are present in and secreted down the axons of the vagus nerves. What function these vagally transported peptides play is, as yet, undetermined.

Several peptides appear to exert their effects using multiple routes. Somatostatin secreted by the stomach acts via both endocrine and paracrine mechanisms on parietal and G cells.

In physiologic studies, peptides are usually administered into the blood stream to determine their action. Our inability to deliver them at the nerve terminal or interstitial fluid of the target organ represents a serious limitation in our ability to study any neurocrine or paracrine function they might have. From this discussion, it should be obvious that the target cells (e.g., the oxyntic cells) operate within a milieu in which a number of neural and humoral stimuli operate. Therefore in vivo responses represent reactions more to a perturbation of this chemical milieu than to that of a pure stimulus.

Gastric Peptides

The peptides found in measurable quantities in the stomach include gastrin, somatostatin, GRP, VIP, histamine, calcitonin gene–related peptide (CGRP), and substance P. In addition, a number of other peptides (e.g., neurotensin) are found in detectable quantities.

Gastrin. Gastrin is the most important hormone in the control of acid secretion. A second significant function relates to its trophic action on the oxyntic cell mucosa. In the Zollinger-Ellison syndrome (ZES) the marked hypertrophy of the rugae of the proximal stomach is caused by the trophic effect of high levels of circulating gastrin.

Biosynthesis and molecular heterogeneity of gastrin. Gastrin is synthesized as a prepropeptide that has the gastrin molecule sandwiched between extensions at both amino and carboxy terminals. Processing of this preprogastrin liberates glycine-extended progastrin, which then undergoes α-amidation to form the gastrin molecule with an amino terminal. Not one but a number of gastrin molecules are formed.[19] The important molecular forms of gastrin include (1) *big gastrin,* a 34-amino acid residue peptide (i.e., G-34) with a molecular weight of 3839 daltons; (2) *little gastrin,* with 17 amino acid residues (i.e., G-17) and a molecular weight of 2098; and (3) *minigastrin,* with 14 amino acids (i.e., G-14) and a molecular weight of 1833. All molecular forms of gastrin are found in both antral tissue and the circulation in both the sulfated and unsulfated forms. In the circulation, however, G-34 predominates, since its metabolic half-life (9 to 15 minutes) is approximately five times that of G-17.

Release of gastrin. The release of gastrin is regulated in a complex manner that is not completely understood[20] (Table 15-2). The most potent stimuli of antral gastrin release are luminal protein digests and amino acids.[21] Gastric distention and vagal stimulation are additional important stimulants of release. The mechanism by which protein digests release gastrin is thought to be by direct chemical action on the microvilli of the G cell. Release of gastrin by distention is largely mediated by acetylcholine and is blocked by atropine. By contrast, vagal modulation of gastrin release is complex involving both cholinergic and noncholinergic mechanisms. Calcium and prolonged alkalization (>8 hr) also release gastrin.

Inhibition of gastrin release is accomplished in several ways. The most important is by an acid negative feedback mechanism. When the pH in the antral lumen falls below 2.5, gastrin release is inhibited. Somatostatin, present in the antrum, is now thought to be an important modulator of gastrin release[4,22] (see Fig. 15-2). The release of somatostatin from antral tissue in vitro and antral veins in vivo has been shown to be reciprocal to that of gastrin. Somatostatin inhibits gastrin release, and in situ inactivation of somatostatin by somatostatin antiserum results in augmented release of gastrin.[23]

The vagus nerve mediates the cephalic phase of gastrin secretion. Vagal stimulation by sham feeding, insulin-induced hypoglycemia, or direct electric stimulation of the vagus nerve results in the release of gastrin. Interestingly, all forms of vagotomy also result in increased release of gastrin. Postvagotomy hypergastrinemia probably results not

Table 15-2. Major Determinants of Gastrin Release

Stimulate	Inhibit
Luminal peptides, amino acids	Luminal pH < 2.5
Gastric distention	Somatostatin
Vagal stimulation	
Vagotomy	
Prolonged alkalization	
Calcium	

only as a consequence of reduced acid secretion but also because of withdrawal of other vagal inhibitory influences.[24]

Actions of gastrin. The primary physiologic action of gastrin is stimulation of acid secretion, but indirect evidence also suggests that the trophic action of gastrin on the oxyntic cell is also physiologic. In pharmacologic doses gastrin has the following effects: increase in lower esophageal sphincter pressure, stimulation of pepsinogen and intrinsic factor secretion, stimulation of intestinal and gallbladder motility, and stimulation of pancreatic enzyme secretion.

Somatostatin. Somatostatin[25] is found both in the antrum and fundus of the stomach, where it is present both in endocrine cells and in nerve endings. It exists in two forms: somatostatin-14, (with 14 amino acid residues), the predominant gastric form,[26] and somatostatin-28, with an extra 14 amino acid extension of the amino terminal of the tetradecapeptide. D cells deliver somatostatin via cytoplasmic membrane processes to the vicinity of the target cell. Via paracrine secretion, D cells can thereby modulate acid secretion.[26,27] Somatostatin exerts its physiologic effect via both direct inhibition of oxyntic cell secretion and indirectly by inhibition of gastrin release[28] (see Fig. 15-2). Fundic somatostatin produces tonic inhibition of acid secretion. Antral somatostatin inhibits basal, postprandial, and vagal-stimulated gastrin release. Somatostatin also blocks the trophic effect of gastrin on the stomach. Varying pharmacologic effects on gastric emptying have been described, and these appear to be dose dependent.

Gastrin-releasing peptide. Erspamer et al.[29] first isolated a tetradecapeptide with potent acid and gastrin-stimulating action from the frog, *Bombina bombina.* Subsequently, bombesin-like immunoreactivity was shown in the mammalian brain and gut. McDonald et al.[30] isolated from intestinal extracts a mammalian peptide with structural similarity to bombesin. They called it gastrin-releasing peptide (GRP) because of its efficacy in stimulating gastrin release. Stimulation of acid secretion by bombesin and GRP is secondary to the release of gastrin.[31,32] The recent identification and cloning of an amphibian GRP distinct from bombesin suggests that a family of peptides with bombesin-like activity may regulate gastrin release.[33] In the mammalian stomach GRP is probably exclusively localized in nerves and not in endocrine cells[34] where it may be an important mediator of vagally induced gastrin release. GRP and bombesin are also potent inhibitors of gastric motor activity in the dog. When administered into the cisterna magna or the lateral ventricle of a number of animal species, bombesin causes inhibition of acid secretion, lowering of body temperature, and hyperglycemia.[35] Bombesin/GRP catabolism is mediated by neutral endopeptidase, a membrane-bound regulatory enzyme.[36]

Vasoactive intestinal polypeptide. VIP was initially isolated from hog intestinal extracts by Mutt and Said[37] and subsequently chemically characterized as a 27-n-amino acid peptide with strong homology to secretin, glucagon, and GIP. In the stomach, VIP is present mainly in the ENS, with VIP-containing fibers concentrated particularly at the gastroesophageal and pyloric sphincters and around the blood vessels of the lamina propria. Both vagal stimulation[38] and gastric distention[39] lead to VIP release. VIP is a predominantly inhibitory neurotransmitter that induces relaxation of the lower esophageal sphincter, inhibition of antral smooth muscle contraction, and relaxation of the proximal stomach. The effect of VIP on gastric acid secretion varies greatly among species, possibly related to mediation of VIP effects by local release of somatostatin.[27]

Histamine. Produced by both ECL cells[2] and mast cells in the gastric mucosa, accumulating evidence suggests that histamine may be a final common mediator of secretagog-induced acid secretion.[40] This notion is supported by both laboratory[41] and clinical studies demonstrating the high efficacy of H_2 receptor antagonists in blocking the acid secretory effect of both histamine and gastrin.[42]

Calcitonin gene–related peptide. CGRP, a 37 amino acid neuropeptide, is found in sensory afferent neurons in the gastric wall. Gastric CGRP appears to inhibit acid secretion via stimulation of somatostatin release.[43,44] Central CGRP, found in the dorsal vagal complex, increases gastric mucosal blood flow and prevents ulcer formation in animal models.[44]

Substance P. Substance P is an 11 amino acid peptide that is widely distributed throughout the gut and CNS. It is found in the vagus and spinal afferent nerves and in the intrinsic nerves of the stomach. Its precise role in the physiology of the stomach is unknown, but it probably functions as a neurotransmitter in control of blood flow, muscle contraction, and mediation of pain.

Exocrine Stomach

Control mechanisms of acid secretion

Basal acid secretion. The human stomach secretes small amounts of acid under conditions of no apparent stimulation. The normal subject secretes 1 to 5 mmol of HCl per hour under basal conditions (mean = 2.5 mmol/hr),[45] which represents 10% of maximal acid secretion. Both atropine and vagotomy reduce basal acid secretion by 75% to 90%, indicating the importance of tonic vagal-cholinergic control of basal secretion. The H_2 receptor antagonists, cimetidine and ranitidine, reduce basal acid secretion by greater than 90%, demonstrating an important role for histamine. Potentially important roles for the other neurocrine and paracrine substances discussed in the regulation of basal acid secretion have not yet been clearly defined. By contrast, there is no evidence that gastrin plays an important role in this control.

Stimulated acid secretion. The most important physiologic stimulus of acid secretion is food. Eating brings into play cephalic, gastric, and intestinal factors that stimulate acid secretion[46] (Table 15-3). The availability in recent years of gastrin monoclonal antibody has greatly facilitated animal research on the mechanisms that regulate acid release.

Table 15-3. Summary of Mechanisms Regulating Acid Secretion

Phase	Pathway	Mediator
Stimulation of Acid		
Cephalic	Vagus	Acetylcholine Gastrin Histamine
Gastric	Neural reflexes Hormonal	Acetylcholine Gastrin
Intestinal	Hormonal ?Neural	*Enteroxyntin** ?
Postabsorptive	Blood	Amino acids
Inhibition of Acid		
Cephalic	Vagus Central	? ?Neuropeptides
Gastric	Distention reflexes Paracrine	? Somatostatin
Intestinal	Hormonal	*Enterogastrone* Somatostatin, cholecystokinin Peptide YY, secretin
	Neural	?
Colonic	Hormonal	*"Cologastrone,"* Peptide YY

*Substances in italics have yet to be chemically characterized.

Cephalic phase. The thought, sight, smell, and taste of food stimulates several brain centers. The message is then transferred through the hypothalamus, mesencephalon, and brain stem to the vagal dorsal motor nucleus, whence efferent stimulation is sent to the oxyntic cell mucosa through the vagi. Vagal stimulation results in the direct activation of the oxyntic cell through the release of acetylcholine, resulting in acid release. Cephalic phase vagal stimulation activates both excitatory and inhibitory pathways of gastrin release, with the net effect being a mild elevation in circulating gastrin. The cephalic phase of acid secretion in humans can be estimated from studies that stimulate vagal centers either by modified sham feeding (chew-and-spit technique) or by insulin-hypoglycemia or 2-deoxyglucose. Modified sham feeding is by far the most physiologic test of the cephalic phase. The average response of healthy human individuals is about 50% of their maximal acid response to exogenous gastrin or histamine.

Gastric phase. Once food enters the stomach, both mechanical distention and the action of chemical constituents of the food result in the stimulation of acid secretion. Gastrin is the principal mediator of these effects. From studies in humans using glucose meals with intragastric titration, the distention factor has been estimated to account for 20% to 50% of the maximal acid response to a peptone meal. Distention activates both long vagovagal reflexes and short reflexes completed within the wall of the stomach.[47] In humans, gastrin release is sufficient to account for only a portion of the total acid released in response to gastric distention.[48] Species variability has impeded progress in delineating the factors important in this response. Dogs, for example, exhibit a pH-sensitive oxyntopyloric reflex inhibition of gastrin release that is not present in humans.[19]

Luminal nutrients provide the most potent stimulus of gastrin and acid release found in the gastric phase. Food in the stomach stimulates acid release by virtue of its chemical composition. Protein digests and amino acids (but not carbohydrates or fats) stimulate the G cell to secrete gastrin.

Intestinal phase. Once chyme enters the intestine, two additional phases of acid secretion are initiated: the intestinal phase and the postabsorption phase. These comprise a very small proportion of the total acid response to a meal. The intestinal phase is presumed to be caused by release of "entero-oxyntin," a stimulant of acid secretion originating from the intestine. Entero-oxyntin has not been fully isolated or chemically characterized[49,50]; however, in guinea pigs, its action on the oxyntic cell is mediated by both histaminergic and cholinergic pathways.[51] When liver extract is infused into the intestine of dogs with vagally denervated (Heidenhain) pouches of the proximal stomach, acid secretion from the pouches is stimulated only weakly. However, if intestinal perfusion of liver extract is combined with background stimulation with intravenous pentagastrin or histamine, there is marked potentiation with maximal acid production greater than the total of that obtained with liver extract alone and pentagastrin or histamine alone.[52] In humans, intraduodenal but not intrajejunal administration of amino acids stimulates gastric acid secretion. This mechanism is independent of serum gastrin or plasma amino acid levels,[53] thereby suggesting that local effects may be important in this response. The postabsorptive phase of acid secretion is caused by absorbed amino acids. Intravenous infusion of amino acids in humans is capable of stimulating acid secretory rates of 30% to 35% of maximum without increasing plasma gastrin concentrations.[54]

Inhibition of acid secretion. Much more is known about the mechanisms that stimulate acid secretion than those that inhibit it. Inhibitory signals may arise in the brain, the stomach, the small intestine, and the colon (see Table 15-3). The cephalic phase of inhibition is adduced from experiments in animals that show that sham feeding inhibits pentagastrin-stimulated acid secretion and that vagotomy increases Heidenhain pouch acid secretion.[55,56] Additionally, when some neuropeptides (bombesin, corticotropin-releasing factor, calcitonin, CGRP, neuropeptide) are injected into the CNS, inhibition of gastric acid secretion is observed. This effect is mediated by vagal afferents in the case of CGRP.[57] Whether these observations have physiologic relevance has yet to be established.

The best characterized inhibitory mechanism is the negative feedback inhibition of gastrin by acid in the lumen of the stomach.[58,59] When intragastric pH reaches 2, gastrin release by food is shut off. Aberrations in this negative feedback loop have been described in patients with duodenal ulcers.[59-61] In vitro studies using the isolated perfused stomach have elucidated several features of this feedback loop.[22,23,62] The emerging model suggests that somatostatin released in response to increasing luminal acid can act via a paracrine pathway to inhibit gastrin release and thereby lower gastric acid (see Fig. 15-2).

When chyme enters the small intestine, a number of inhibitory mechanisms, both neural and humoral, are activated. The most potent inhibitor of gastric acid secretion is fat in the upper intestine.[63] The mediator of fat-induced inhibition has been called "enterogastrone," but to date its chemical nature has not been defined. Using an intestinal transplant model in rats, Orloff et al.[64] have shown that neural and hormonal factors are important mediators of the enterogastric reflex. Specifically, somatostatin, and to a lesser extent CCK, seem to be important modulators of fat-induced inhibition of acid secretion.[64] Peptide YY (PYY) is another enterogastrone candidate whose physiologic role remains to be defined. Early work in this area was plagued with trouble associated with contaminated preparations[65] and difficulty differentiating physiologic from pharmacologic effects.[66]

The presence of acid and hyperosmolar solutions in the duodenum also inhibits acid secretion. Secretin seems to mediate intestinal acid-induced inhibition of gastric acid secretion.[67] Recent studies also implicate somatostatin in this reflex, as well as contribution by neural mechanisms.[68]

The colon has been identified as an endocrine organ. Both in dogs and humans, colonic perfusion with liver extract, peptone, or fats inhibits acid secretion.[69,70] Seal and Debas[69] have suggested the name "cologastrone" to designate this colon-derived inhibitor of the stomach. PYY, a peptide with strong structural homology to pancreatic polypeptide, has been found in abundance in the colon and terminal ileum.[71] Intravenous injection of PYY inhibits both acid and pancreatic secretion.[71] Colonic perfusion with fatty acid increases plasma PYY and concomitantly inhibits gastric acid secretion via a gastrin-independent mechanism.[72] It is not known if PYY is the only cologastrone.

Cellular and subcellular mechanisms of acid secretion.[58] Figure 15-6 illustrates the current working model of the cellular interactions critical to acid secretion. The ECL is now known to play a central role in the regulation of acid secretion. Histamine is the principal mediator of oxyntic cell acid release. In recent years, somatostatin has emerged as an important physiologic inhibitor of acid secretion, via effects on multiple target cells in this feedback loop.

The recent identification and cloning of several of the receptors important in acid secretion has greatly facilitated our understanding of cellular and postreceptor mechanisms in the oxyntic cell. Receptors are specific proteins that bind to specific ligands. They are synthesized by the cell and in many instances can be recycled. When the ligands bind to their specific receptors and form hormone-receptor complexes, intracellular mechanisms are activated that eventually result in the secretion of hydrogen ions into secretory canaliculi.

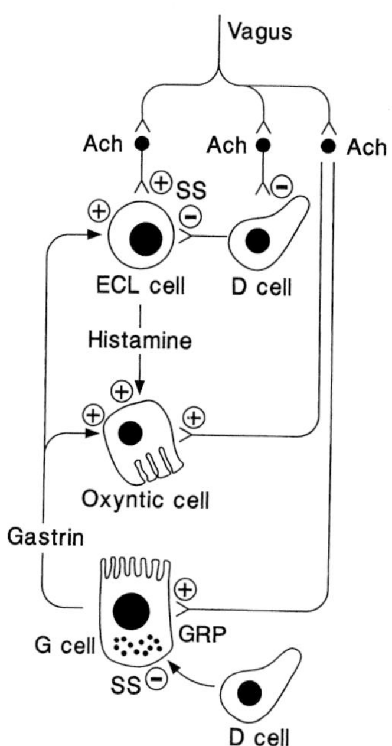

Fig. 15-6. Central role of the enterochromaffin-like cell *(ECL)* and of histamine in the regulation of acid secretion by the oxyntic cell. Note that both vagal discharge (*Ach* [acetylcholine]) and gastrin stimulate release of histamine from the enterochromaffin-like cell. Histamine diffuses through interstitial fluid in a paracrine manner to stimulate acid secretion. Note also that somatostatin *(SS)* secretion from the D cell exerts inhibitory modulation of the oxyntic cell in the parietal mucosa and of the G cell in the antrum. Vagal discharge inhibits somatostatin release from D cells. *GRP,* Gastrin-releasing peptide.

The oxyntic cell has three distinct receptors potentially important for stimulation of acid secretion on its surface (Fig. 15-7). These receptors are for acetylcholine, gastrin, and histamine. Recent evidence also supports the existence of somatostatin receptors on the oxyntic cell, which may mediate inhibitory effects on acid secretion.[73] The gastrin receptor, also known as the CCKB receptor, has been cloned and is a 7-transmembrane domain protein, which is a member of the G protein–coupled superfamily of receptors[74] (Fig. 15-8). Ligand binding activates phospholipase C-mediated calcium mobilization, resulting in stimulation of the proton pump. The importance of the gastrin receptor on the parietal cell in mediation of acid secretion has recently been questioned. Indeed, the evolving hypothesis is that gastrin acts primarily via its receptor on the ECL with histamine as the final mediator. The histamine receptor has also been cloned[75] and belongs to the same superfamily of receptors. Histamine binding leads to activation of the H^+,K^+-ATPase via an adenylate cyclase/cAMP-mediated pathway. The central importance of the histamine H_2 receptor is underscored by the high therapeutic efficacy of the H_2 receptor antagonist ranitidine

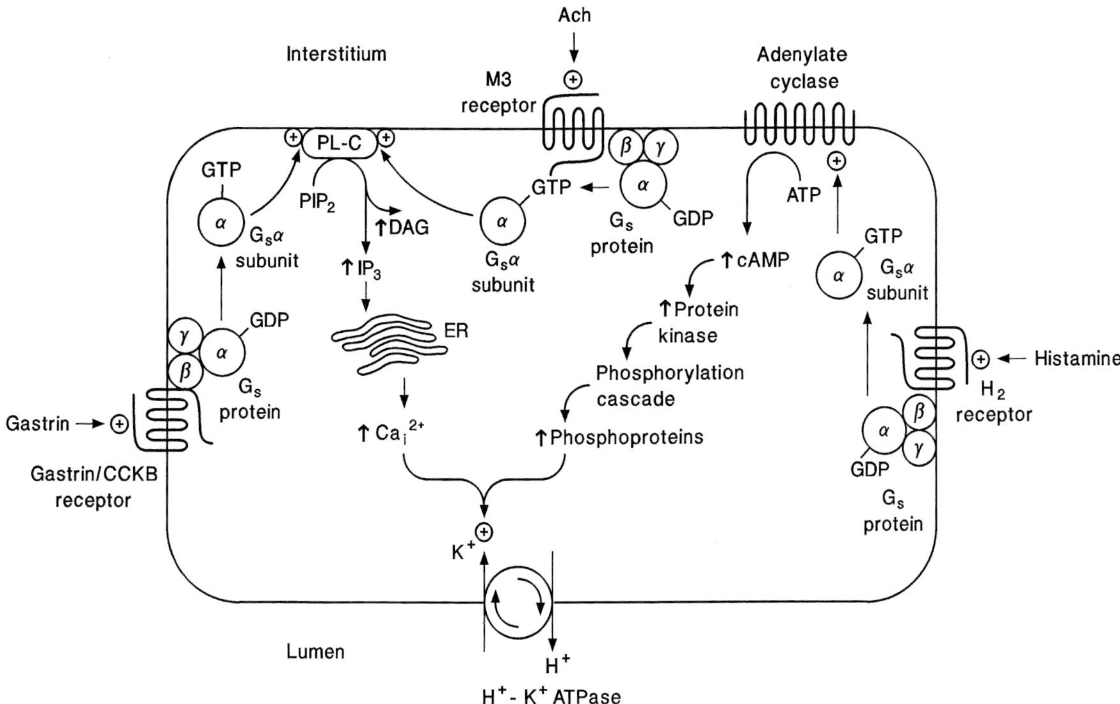

Fig. 15-7. Intracellular events following ligand binding in the oxyntic cell. Acetylcholine *(Ach)* and gastrin bind to receptor and activate guanine nucleotide-binding regulatory protein *(G protein)*, which stimulates phospholipase C *(PL-C)* to convert membrane-bound phospholipids to inositol triphosphate *(IP_3)*. IP_3, in turn, mobilizes calcium from intracellular stores leading to activation of the H^+,K^+-ATPase and H^+ extrusion into the gastric lumen. Histamine binding to H_2 receptors leads to activation of adenylate cyclase with resultant increases in cAMP and stimulation of kinase-mediated phosphorylation cascade, thereby activating the proton pump. *ATPase,* Adenosine triphosphatase; *cAMP,* cyclic adenosine monophosphate; *CCKB,* cholecystokinin; *DAG,* dianhydrogalactitol; *GDP,* guanosine diphosphate; *GTP,* guanosine triphosphate; *PIP2,* phosphatidylinositol 4,5 diphosphate.

in blocking acid secretion. Acetylcholine released from parasympathetic fibers of the autonomic nervous system binds to the muscarinic receptor (subtype M3) in the oxyntic cell[76] and activates acid release via increased intracellular calcium. Blockade of muscarinic receptors with pirenzepine leads to further reduction in gastric acid secretion in patients already taking H_2 receptor antagonists.[77] This additional effect is attributed to the different intracellular pathways affected by receptor binding by the two antagonists. Whatever cell surface receptor is activated and whichever intracellular pathway is used, the final event is the generation and activation of H^+,K^+-ATPase, which finds its way to the microvilli of the secretory vesicles. The H^+,K^+-ATPase is the proton pump that regulates the final step of secretion of H^+. Omeprazole, a proton pump antagonist, is an extremely effective inhibitor of gastric acid secretion because of its action on the final common pathway of acid secretion.

Function of gastric acid. The interposition of a highly acid medium between the environment and the intestinal tract serves to protect against colonization of the stomach and upper small intestine by bacteria. Bacterial colonization of the stomach and duodenum is known to occur in achlorhydric states, and achlorhydria is probably a factor in the cause of gastric malignancy, allowing the generation of nitrosamines. In addition, H^+ is necessary to convert pepsinogen into pepsin, which is required for the initial hydrolysis of protein into polypeptides. Acid is also required as a stimulus of secretin release from the duodenum so that a bicarbonate-rich watery pancreatic flow can occur.

Pepsin secretion. Pepsin is secreted by chief cells in the proenzyme form, pepsinogen, a protein with a molecular weight of 42,500. Three immunologically distinct aspartic proteinases can be found in human gastric mucosa: pepsinogen I (A), pepsinogen II (C), and a nonpepsinogen proteinase, slow-moving proteinase (SMP).[78,79] Group I pepsinogens (composed of five types, or isozymogens, of pepsinogen) are found only in the oxyntic mucosa in the peptic and mucous neck cells. Group II pepsinogens (two isozymogens) are found in the oxyntic, antral, and duodenal mucosa. Pepsinogen is converted to pepsin by acid, and thereafter pepsin autocatalyzes its generation. SMP has been localized to surface epithelial cells in both the fundic and pyloric glands.

Much less is known about the mechanisms that control pepsin secretion than those that control acid secretion. Va-

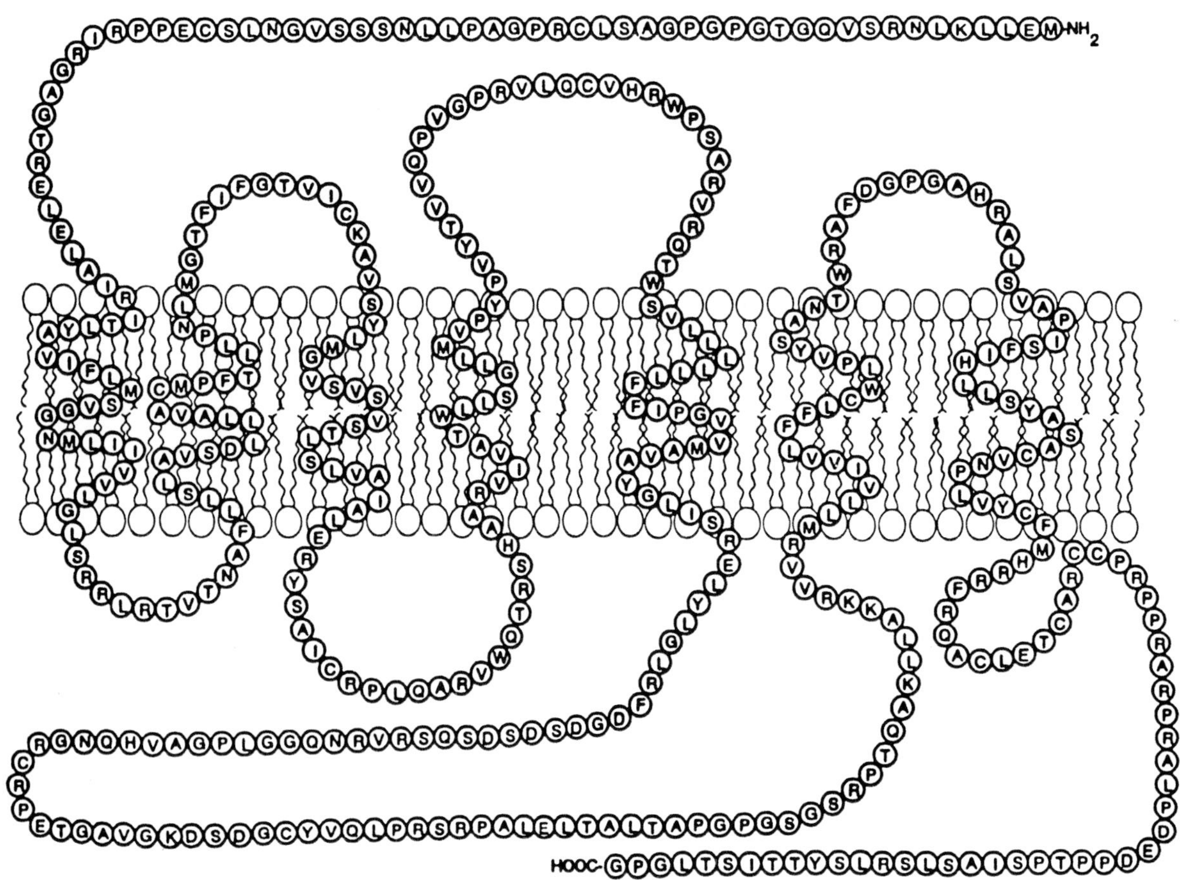

Fig. 15-8. Schematic representation of the molecular structure of the 7-transmembrane domain gastrin/CCKB receptor. (From Johnson LR, ed. Physiology of the Gastrointestinal Tract, 3rd ed. New York: Raven Press, 1994, p 1204.)

gal stimulation and cholinomimetic drugs are the most potent stimuli of pepsin secretion in humans. CCK is a potent stimulant of pepsin secretion in animals[80] via a mechanism involving mobilization of intracellular Ca^{2+} stores.[81] Atropine and vagotomy are potent inhibitors of pepsin secretion.[82]

Omeprazole inhibits pepsinogen synthesis and secretion.[83] Reduction in serum pepsinogen II levels has been correlated with the successful treatment of *Helicobacter pylori* gastritis using omeprazole in humans.[84]

Intrinsic factor secretion. Intrinsic factor[85] is secreted by the oxyntic cell in humans, and its secretion generally parallels that of acid. The intrinsic factor gene has been localized to human chromosome 11.[86] It is a 60,000 dalton mucoprotein that forms a complex with vitamin B_{12}, facilitating the absorption of the vitamin in the distal ileum. Intrinsic factor deficiency develops after total gastrectomy and in pernicious anemia. In the latter condition most patients have antibodies to intrinsic factor.

Secretion of gastric mucus and bicarbonate. Two additional exocrine secretory products of the stomach are mucus and bicarbonate. The stomach is lined by a mucous gel composed of protein, glycoproteins, and mucopolysaccharides.[87] The mucous gel is thought to protect the gastric mucosa from mechanical damage by food. Because of its ability to retain water, the mucous gel maintains a perpetual aqueous environment for the mucosal surface. It may also retain an alkaline atmosphere on the mucosal surface by trapping bicarbonate secreted by mucosal cells, the "mucobicarbonate barrier." Mucus is also thought to be important in maintaining the normal gastrointestinal flora while at the same time providing antibacterial and antiviral protection. The mucous gel is in a dynamic equilibrium, being continually solubilized by luminal pepsin on the one hand and secreted by mucosal cells on the other. The mechanisms that control mucus production are poorly understood.

Several recent studies emphasize the emerging clinical importance of gastric mucus. Reductions in mucin content leading to abnormal thinning of the gastric mucous gel layer have been found in experimental models of ethanol-induced gastric erosions.[88] Interestingly, proton pump inhibition prevented these alterations. *H. pylori,* a bacterium important in the pathogenesis of peptic ulcer disease, secretes proteases and lipases that break down mucin polymers, thereby reducing the integrity of the mucous coat.[89] These findings suggest that mucus may be an important barrier to the formation of ulcers.

Bicarbonate secretion by the gastric mucosa is a topic of recent great interest.[90] In vitro studies have shown that active bicarbonate secretion takes place in the oxyntic mucosa, whereas both active and passive secretion occur in the antrum. In vitro, calcium, carbachol, prostaglandins, glucagon, and dibutyryl-cGMP stimulate bicarbonate production. Secretin has been shown to stimulate gastric bicarbonate production in humans. In vitro inhibitors of bicarbonate secretion include acetylsalicylate, indomethacin, ethanol, α-adrenergic agents, glucagon, and parathormone. The magnitude of bicarbonate secretion relative to acid is small. The question then arises, what prevents uniform acidification of the mucous gel layer by secreted acid? The recent demonstration of a steep pH gradient across the mucous gel (luminal pH 2; epithelial pH 7) supports the notion of bulk transport of acid via channels away from the epithelial surface.[91] The epithelium may then remain protected by a bicarbonate-containing "cushion" deep in the gel layer. The importance of bicarbonate secretion is underscored by the recent finding that patients with a high relapse rate after treatment for duodenal ulcers have impaired gastric bicarbonate secretion.[92]

ABNORMAL PHYSIOLOGY

Abnormal motor and secretory function of the stomach develops as a result of either disease or surgical interventions of the stomach or of its innervation.

Motor Abnormalities

Transient Delay in Gastric Emptying

A transient delay in gastric emptying is seen most frequently in postoperative patients and in patients who have pancreatitis or peritonitis. The mechanism for this delay is unknown but is generally thought to involve neural reflexes or norepinephrine release. Usually gastric motor function returns with the resolution of the underlying disease, although protracted gastric atony lasting weeks to months is sometimes seen in acute pancreatitis. Transient delay in gastric emptying may also have metabolic causes, including hypokalemia, hypercalcemia and hypocalcemia, hypomagnesemia, hypothyroidism, uremia, hepatic coma, and hyperglycemia. Correction of the metabolic abnormality usually restores normal gastric emptying.

Chronic Impairment in Gastric Emptying

Diabetic gastroparesis. Diabetic gastroparesis, usually in individuals with insulin-dependent diabetes, may be present in symptomatic or asymptomatic form. Asymptomatic patients may become symptomatic following major abdominal surgery. Although it is attractive to attribute abnormal emptying to a form of "vagal neuropathy," this simplistic explanation is insufficient. Pathologic examination of excised vagal nerves from diabetic patients reveals degeneration and reduced fiber density; however, these findings occur irrespective of symptoms or objective evidence of abnormal emptying.[93] Surface electrogastrography indicates that diabetic patients in the hyperglycemic state exhibit abnormalities of gastric myoelectric activity.[94] Although delayed gastric emptying has been associated with hyperglycemic periods in diabetic patients,[95] correlation of these physiologic observations with specific abnormalities in myoelectric activity remains to be proved. It appears that while vagal neural degeneration is probably important, other factors such as dynamic gastric dysrhythmias also play a role in the pathophysiology of gastroparesis in diabetic patients.

Several prokinetic agents have achieved clinical usefulness in the treatment of diabetic gastroparesis. Metoclopramide has been shown to improve gastric emptying and reduce gastrointestinal tract symptomatology,[96] but its usefulness is limited by CNS side effects in some patients. Erythromycin, a macrolide antibiotic, likely increases gastric emptying via its activity as a motilin receptor agonist.[97] Cisapride, a recent addition to the pharmacologic armamentarium, improves gastric emptying, but its efficacy in reducing symptoms during long-term treatment requires further study.[98]

Postoperative delay in gastric emptying. Distressing problems in gastric emptying are occasionally seen after vagotomy and/or gastrectomy in the absence of gastric outlet obstruction.

Truncal vagotomy without drainage in dogs causes impairment of gastric emptying of both liquids and solids. When pyloroplasty is added, the emptying of liquids is accelerated, whereas the emptying of solids becomes normal. Similar changes are observed in humans when vagotomy was initially performed without a drainage procedure. About 30% to 40% of patients with vagotomy but without drainage develop significant impairment of gastric emptying. After vagotomy and drainage, about 5% of patients develop prolonged postoperative gastric stasis. Proximal gastric vagotomy in duodenal ulcer patients without drainage causes remarkably little impairment of gastric emptying. This is caused in part by the fact that the antropyloric mechanism is intact and in part perhaps by concomitant sympathectomy of the proximal stomach.

Accelerated Gastric Emptying

Procedures such as distal gastrectomy and vagotomy with drainage occasionally result in accelerated gastric emptying, leading to the dumping syndrome. The rapid entry of a hyperosmolar load into the jejunum or duodenum results in a rapid fluid shift from the intravascular space into the intestinal lumen and initiation of vasomotor symptoms that are in part caused by the release of bradykinin and serotonin. Avoiding rich carbohydrates in the diet, lying down for 20 minutes after eating, and avoiding drinking fluids with eating are elements in the conservative treatment of dumping. Refractory dumping has been successfully treated with the long-acting somatostatin analog, octreotide acetate.[99] Whether its efficacy results from a direct effect on intestinal motility[100] or via inhibition of peptide release remains unclear. In experimental animals, Becker et al.[101] have shown that electric pacing of the proximal small intestine through electrodes implanted on the serosa slows gastric emptying and ameliorates the dumping syndrome after vagotomy. This ingenious approach is yet to be tested in the clinical situation.

Tachygastria

An unusual cause of gastric atony develops when ectopic pacemakers appear in the stomach, leading to an irregular rhythm (slow wave frequency >4 cycles/min).[102] In this situation the stomach behaves much like the heart with ventricular fibrillation and is incapable of effective contractions that would lead to gastric emptying. The condition can occur de novo or may appear with diabetic gastroparesis, postoperative ileus, gastric carcinoma, and after vagotomy. Although in animal studies, electric pacing can abolish the tachygastria and restore normal gastric electric function,[103] results in humans have been less promising.[104] In contrast, erythromycin[104] and cisapride[105] appear to be effective both in normalizing electrogastrographic patterns and in improving symptoms.

Gastric Emptying Patterns in Peptic Ulcer Disease

Several investigators have reported delayed gastric emptying in gastric ulcer. The abnormality is more common in type II (prepyloric) ulcers and for the emptying of solids. Impaired gastric emptying, however, is by no means a universal finding in gastric ulcer. By contrast, accelerated gastric emptying is a common feature in duodenal ulcer and one that may be genetically transmitted.

Secretory Abnormalities

Secretory abnormalities can involve both the endocrine and exocrine stomach. Both hypersecretory and hyposecretory states may result.

Ulcerogenic Hypergastrinemic States

Conditions of hypergastrinemia associated with peptic ulceration include the ZES, G-cell hyperplasia or hyperfunction, the retained antrum, and the short gut syndromes. In ZES a gastrin-producing tumor is present usually in the pancreas and occasionally in the duodenum or elsewhere. In G-cell hyperplasia the number of gastrin-secreting cells in the antrum is increased. In G-cell hyperfunction the number of antral G cells is normal, but the cells hyperfunction. The latter two conditions are inherited as autosomal dominant diseases and are associated with hyperpepsinogenemia I.[106] In the retained antrum, G cells are excluded from the acid stream of the stomach and exposed to alkaline pancreatic and biliary secretion in the "duodenal stump." This condition occurs in patients undergoing Billroth II gastrectomy and results in hypersecretion of gastrin and recurrent peptic ulcer. These conditions can be distinguished from each other by performing the secretin and meal tests. In response to a bolus intravenous injection of secretin (2 U/kg), patients with ZES have a paradoxic rise in their serum gastrin (>125 pg/ml), whereas those with G-cell hyperplasia or hyperfunction and those with retained antrum have either no change or a decrease in their serum gastrin. By contrast, after the ingestion of a meal, patients with ZES have an increase in their serum gastrin by less than 10% of basal secretion, whereas those with G-cell hyperplasia or hyperfunction have exaggerated rises. Patients with retained antrum respond little or not at all to this meal.

Nonulcerogenic Hypergastrinemic States

Achlorhydric or hypochlorhydric conditions are associated with hypergastrinemia. The most important causes are pernicious anemia, previous proximal gastrectomy, and previous vagotomy (all types). Postvagotomy hypergastrinemia rarely results in elevation of serum gastrin beyond two or three times normal; but if a patient has a recurrent ulcer after vagotomy, ZES must be ruled out by the secretin test. Another cause of hypergastrinemia is renal failure when serum gastrin elevation is caused by failure of renal elimination of gastrin.

Prolonged therapy with the proton pump inhibitor omeprazole is emerging as the leading cause of hypergastrinemia. The near total ablation of acid secretion induced by omeprazole removes the normal feedback signal to the G cell leading to excess gastrin secretion.[107,108]

Ménétrier's Disease

Ménétrier's disease is characterized by enlarged gastric folds, cystic glandular dilation, hypoproteinemia, decreased acid secretion and increased gastric mucus production. Patients with this disease have increased levels of the peptide transforming growth factor-alpha (TGF-α) in gastric mucosa.[109] The recent demonstration of hypertrophic gastropathy, which resembles Ménétrier's disease in transgenic mice overexpressing TGF-α, suggests that this peptide may be important in the pathophysiology of Ménétrier's disease.[110]

SUMMARY

The aims of this chapter have been to (1) outline the normal anatomy of the stomach to indicate the complex neuroendocrine design of the gut, (2) describe the physiologic mechanisms that control the secretory and motor functions of the stomach, and (3) discuss abnormalities of secretion and motility. The transport of a number of peptides down the vagus nerve and the presence of peptides in vagal nerve terminals within the stomach wall have been described. The point has been made that peptides that control gastric function arrive at their target cell not only through the blood, as do classic endocrine substances, but also as neurocrine agents secreted in proximity to receptors on target cells and as paracrine agents diffusing to the target cells through the interstitial fluid after their secretion from neurons or endocrine cells.

In the control of the motor function of the stomach, the presence of the gastric pacemaker; the control of frequency, rhythm, and direction of propagation of electric activity and the ensuing velocity of contraction; and the role of the interdigestive motor complex that appears to sweep down the stomach regularly every 1 to 2 hours have been discussed. The mechanisms that regulate gastric emptying of liquids and solids and the methods for measuring gastric emptying have been outlined.

The complexity of the control of acid secretion has been addressed. It has been suggested that vagal stimulation causes acid secretion by direct cholinergic action on the oxyntic cell and by release of antral gastrin, which potentiates the direct cholinergic action. Gastrin is the most important hormone in the control of acid secretion; its molecular heterogeneity and the regulation of its release have been discussed. The mechanisms of inhibition of acid secretion have been discussed, and the cephalic (vagal), gastric, and intestinal components have been outlined. An evolving working model of the intercellular feedback mechanisms important in the regulation of acid secretion has been depicted. The subcellular mechanisms of acid secretion have been outlined, and the imperfection of our understanding of intracellular events has been emphasized. A number of motor and secretory abnormalities of the stomach have also been discussed to show the importance of understanding normal physiology to understand the abnormal. The advances that have been made in gastric physiology are impressive. But many serious gaps in our knowledge remain, and the reader must appraise the literature critically to see where major potential contributions can be made.

REFERENCES

1. Smolka A, Helander HF, Sachs G. Monoclonal antibodies against gastric H^+K^+-ATPase. Am J Physiol 245G:589, 1983.
2. Prinz C, et al. Histamine secretion from rat enterochromaffin-like cells. Gastroenterology 105:449, 1993.
3. Solcia E, et al. Human GEP endocrine-paracrine cells: Lausanne 1977 classification revisited. In Grossman MI, Brazier MA, Lechago J, eds. Cellular Basis of Chemical Messengers in the Digestive System. New York: Academic Press, 1981.
4. Schubert ML, et al. Paracrine regulation of gastric acid secretion by fundic somatostatin. (Part 1). Am J Physiol 252(4):G485, 1987.
5. Furness JB, Costa M. Types of nerves in the enteric nervous system. Neuroscience 5:1, 1980.
6. Surprenant A. Control of the gastrointestinal tract by enteric neurons. Ann Rev Physiol 56:117, 1994.
7. Weber J Jr, Kohatsu S. Pacemaker localization and electrical conduction patterns in the canine stomach. Gastroenterology 59:717, 1970.
8. Code CF, Marlett JA. The interdigestive myoelectric complex of the stomach and small bowel of dogs. J Physiol (Lond) 246:289, 1975.
9. Carlson HC, Code CF, Nelson RA. Motor action of the canine gastroduodenal function: A cineradiographic, pressure and electric study. Am J Dig Dis 11:155, 1966.
10. Malbert C-H, Mathis C. Antropyloric modulation of transpyloric flow of liquids in pigs. Gastroenterology 107:37, 1994.
11. Collins PJ, et al. Role of the proximal and distal stomach in mixed solid and liquid meal emptying. Gut 32:615, 1991.
12. Debas HT, Farooq O, Grossman MI. Inhibition of gastric emptying as a physiological action of cholecystokinin. Gastroenterology 68:1211, 1975.
13. Raybould HE. Capsaicin-sensitive vagal afferents and CCK in inhibition of gastric motor function induced by intestinal nutrients. Peptides 12:1279, 1991.
14. Ewart WR, Wingate D. Cholecystokinin octapeptide and gastric mechanoreceptor activity in rat brain. Am J Physiol 244G:613, 1983.
15. Minami H, McCallum RW. The physiology and pathophysiology of gastric emptying in humans. Gastroenterology 86:1592, 1984.
16. Datz FL, et al. Physiological and pharmacological interventions in radionuclide imaging of the tubular gastrointestinal tract. Semin Nucl Med 21:140, 1991.
17. Chen JD, McCallum RW. Clinical applications of electrogastrography. Am J Gastroenterol 88:1324, 1993.
18. Hokfelt T, et al. Peptidergic neurons. Nature 284:515, 1978.
19. Debas HT, et al. Proof of a pyloro-oxyntic reflex for stimulation of acid secretion. Gastroenterology 66:526, 1974.
20. Debas HT, et al. Release of antral gastrin. In Chey WY, Brooks FP, eds. Endocrinology of the Gut. Thorofare, N.J.: Charles B. Slack, 1974.
21. Lam SK, et al. Gastric acid secretion is abnormally sensitive to endogenous gastric released after peptone test meals in duodenal ulcer patients. J Clin Invest 65:555, 1980.
22. Schubert ML, Edwards NF, Makhlouf GM. Regulation of gastric somatostatin secretion in the mouse by luminal acidity: A local feedback mechanism. Gastroenterology 94:317, 1988.
23. Saffouri B, et al. Gastrin and somatostatin secretion by perfused rat stomach: Functional linkage of antral peptides. Am J Physiol 238:G495, 1980.
24. Hollinshead JW, et al. Hypergastrinemia develops within 24 hours of truncal vagotomy in dogs. Gastroenterology 88:35, 1985.
25. Konturek SJ. Somatostatin and the digestive system. Gastroenterol Clin Biol 1:849, 1977.
26. Lucey MR, Yamada T. Biochemistry and physiology of gastrointestinal somatostatin. Dig Dis Sci 34(Suppl 3):5S, 1989.
27. Schubert ML. The effect of vasoactive intestinal polypeptide on gastric acid secretion is predominantly mediated by somatostatin. Gastroenterology 100:1195, 1991.
28. Makhlouf GM, Schubert ML. Gastric somatostatin: A paracrine regulator of acid secretion. Metabolism 39(Suppl 2):138, 1990.
29. Erspamer V, et al. Occurrence of bombesin and alytesin in extracts of the skin of three European discoglossid frogs and pharmacological actions of bombesin on extravascular smooth muscle. Br J Pharmacol 45:333, 1972.
30. McDonald TJ, et al. A gastrin releasing peptide from the porcine nonantral gastric tissue. Gut 19:767, 1978.
31. Schubert ML, et al. Regulation of acid secretion by bombesin/GRP neurons of the gastric fundus. Am J Physiol 260:G156, 1991.
32. Schubert ML, Jong MJ, Makhlouf GM. Bombesin/GRP-stimulated somatostatin secretion is mediated by gastrin in the antrum and intrinsic neurons in the fundus. Am J Physiol 261:G885, 1991.
33. Nagalla SR, et al. Gastrin-releasing peptide (GRP) is not mammalian bombesin. Identification and molecular cloning of a true amphibian GRP distinct from amphibian bombesin in *Bombina orientalis*. J Biol Chem 267:6916, 1992.
34. Dockray GJ, Vaillant C, Walsh JH. The neuronal origin of bombesin-like immunoreactivity in the rat gastrointestinal tract. Neuroscience 4:1561, 1979.
35. Tache Y. Nature and biological actions of gastrointestinal peptides: Current status. Clin Biochem 17:77, 1984.
36. Bunnett NW, et al. Catabolism of gastrin releasing peptide and substance P by gastric membrane-bound peptidases. Peptides 6:277, 1985.
37. Mutt V, Said SI. Structure of porcine vasoactive intestinal octacosapeptide: The amino acid sequence: Use of kallikrein in its determination. Eur J Biochem 42:581, 1974.

38. Holst JJ, et al. Vagal control of the release of somatostatin, vasoactive intestinal polypeptide, gastrin-releasing peptide, and HCl from porcine non-antral stomach. Scand J Gastroenterol 27:677, 1992.
39. Schubert ML, Makhlouf GM. Gastrin secretion induced by distention is mediated by gastric cholinergic and vasoactive intestinal peptide neurons in rats. Gastroenterology 104:834, 1993.
40. Soll AH, et al. Modulation of histamine release from canine fundic mucosal mast cells. Am J Physiol 254:G40, 1988.
41. Lloyd KCK, et al. Role of gastrin, histamine, and acetylcholine in the gastric phase of acid secretion in anesthetized rats. Am J Physiol 262:G747, 1992.
42. Lloyd KCK, Debas HT. Peripheral regulation of gastric acid secretion. In Johnson LR, et al., eds. Physiology of the Gastrointestinal Tract, 3rd ed. New York: Raven Press, 1994, pp 1185-1226.
43. Wong HC, et al. Monoclonal antibody to rat alpha-CGRP: Production, characterization, and in vivo immunoneutralization activity. Hybridoma 12:93, 1993.
44. Tache Y, Raybould H, Wei JY. Central and peripheral actions of calcitonin gene-related peptide on gastric secretory and motor function. Adv Exp Med Biol 298:183, 1991.
45. Moore JG, Englert E. Circadian rhythm of gastric acid secretion in man. Nature 226:1261, 1970.
46. Richardson CT, et al. Studies in the mechanisms of food-stimulated gastric acid secretion in normal human subjects. J Clin Invest 58:623, 1976.
47. Grossman MI. Secretion of acid and pepsin in response to distension of vagally-innervated fundic gland area in dogs. Gastroenterology 41:718, 1962.
48. Soares EC, Zaterka S, Walsh JH. Acid secretion and serum gastrin at graded intragastric pressures in man. Gastroenterology 72:676, 1977.
49. Orloff MJ, Guillemin RCL, Nakaji NT. Isolation of the hormone responsible for the intestinal phase of gastric secretion. Gastroenterology 72:820, 1977.
50. Vagne M, Mutt V. Entero-oxyntin: A stimulant of gastric acid secretion extracted from porcine intestine. Scand J Gastroenterol 15:17, 1980.
51. Strodel WE, et al. Preliminary characterization of enterooxyntic activity on the guinea pig oxyntic cell. Endocrinology 117:376, 1985.
52. Debas HT, Slaff GF, Grossman MI. Intestinal phase of gastric acid secretion: Augmentation of maximal response of Heidenhain pouch to gastrin and histamine. Gastroenterology 68:691, 1975.
53. Lenz HJ, Hogan DL, Isenberg JI. Intestinal phase of gastric acid secretion in humans with and without portacaval shunt. Gastroenterology 89:791, 1985.
54. Isenberg JI, Maxwell V. Intravenous infusion of amino acids stimulates gastric acid secretion in man. N Engl J Med 298:27, 1978.
55. Preshaw RM. Inhibition of pentagastrin-simulated acid output by sham feeding. Fed Proc 32:410, 1973.
56. Sjodin L. Inhibition of gastrin-stimulated canine acid secretion by sham feeding. Scand J Gastroenterol 10:73, 1975.
57. Wei JY, Tache Y. Alterations of efferent discharges of the gastric branch of the vagus nerve by intracisternal injection of peptides influencing gastric function in rats. Gastroenterology 98:A531, 1990.
58. Sachs G, Berglindh T. Physiology of the oxyntic cell. In Johnson LR, et al., eds. Physiology of the Gastrointestinal Tract. New York: Raven Press, 1981.
59. Walsh JH, Richardson CT, Fordtran JS. pH dependence of acid secretion and gastrin release in normal and ulcer subjects. J Clin Invest 55:462, 1975.
60. Malagelada JR, et al. Gastric secretion and emptying after ordinary meals in duodenal ulcer. Gastroenterology 73:989, 1977.
61. Eysselein VE, et al. Regulation of gastric acid secretion by gastrin in duodenal ulcer patients and healthy subjects. Gastroenterology 102:1142, 1992.
62. Koop H, et al. Somatostatin-gastrin interactions in the rat stomach. Res Exp Med 188:115, 1988.
63. Kosaka T, Lim RKS. Demonstration of the humoral agent in fat inhibition of gastric secretion. Proc Soc Exp Biol Med 27:890, 1930.
64. Orloff SL, et al. Neural and hormonal mechanisms mediate the enterogastric reflex: A study in intestinal transplants in rats. Gastroenterology 101:734, 1991.
65. Maxwell V, et al. Effect of gastric inhibitory polypeptide on pentagastrin-stimulated acid secretion in man. Dig Dis Sci 25:113, 1980.
66. Yamagishi T, Debas HT. Gastric inhibitory peptide (GIP) is not the primary mediator of the enterogastrone action of fat in the dog. Gastroenterology 78:931, 1980.
67. Stollmaier W, Schwille PO. Endogenous secretin in the rat-evidence for a role as an enterogastrone but failure to influence serum calcium homeostasis. Exp Clin Endocrinol 99:169, 1992.
68. Orloff SL, et al. Intestinal acid inhibits gastric acid secretion by neural and hormonal mechanisms in rats. (Part 1). Am J Physiol 262(1):G165, 1992.
69. Seal AM, Debas HT. Colonic inhibition of gastric acid secretion in the dog. Gastroenterology 79:823, 1980.
70. Soon-Shiong P, Debas HT, Seal AM. Colonic inhibition of gastric acid secretion in man. Surg Forum 31:152, 1980.
71. Pappas TN, et al. Peptide YY inhibits meal-stimulated pancreatic and gastric secretion. Am J Physiol (in press).
72. Hashimoto T, et al. Intracolonic fat inhibits gastric acid secretion independent of gastrin release in the dog. Dig Dis Sci 36:888, 1991.
73. DelValle J, et al. Cellular mechanisms of somatostatin action in the gut. Metab Clin Exp 39(Suppl 2):134, 1990.
74. Wank SA, Pisegna JR, de Weerth A. Cholecystokinin receptor family. Molecular cloning, structure, and functional expression in rat, guinea pig, and human. Ann NY Acad Sci 713:49, 1994.
75. Gantz I, et al. Molecular cloning of the human histamine H_2 receptor. Biochem Biophys Res Commun 178:1386, 1991.
76. Pfeiffer A, et al. Human gastric mucosa expresses glandular M3 subtype of muscarinic receptors. Dig Dis Sci 35(12):1468, 1990.
77. Misawa T, et al. Effects of combined use of roxatidine and pirenzepine on gastric secretion in humans. Fukuoka Igaku Zasshi 81:242, 1990.
78. Samloff IM, et al. Slow moving proteinase. Isolation, characterization, and immunohistochemical localization in gastric mucosa. Gastroenterology 93:77, 1987.
79. Samloff IM. Pepsinogen, pepsins and pepsin inhibitors. Gastroenterology 60:586, 1971.
80. Tazi-Saad K, Chariot J, Roze C. Control of pepsin secretion by regulatory peptides in the rat stomach: Comparison with acid secretion. Peptides 13:233, 1992.
81. Miyamoto T, et al. Role of intracellular CA^{2+} and the calmodulin messenger system in pepsinogen secretion from isolated rabbit gastric mucosa. Gut 33:21, 1992.
82. Redfern JS, et al. Gastric acid and pepsin hypersecretion in conscious rabbits (Part 1). Am J Physiol 261(2):G295, 1991.
83. Tsukada S, et al. Effect of omeprazole on secretion, synthesis and the gene expression of pepsinogen in the guinea pig stomach mucosa. Cell Biochem Funct 12:113, 1994.
84. Hunter FM, et al. Serum pepsinogens as markers of response to therapy for *Helicobacter pylori* gastritis. Dig Dis Sci 38:2081, 1993.
85. Binder JJ, Donaldson RM. Effect of cimetidine on intrinsic factor and pepsin secretion in man. Gastroenterology 74:535, 1978.
86. Hewitt JE, et al. Human gastric intrinsic factor: Characterization of cDNA and genomic clones and localization to human chromosome 11. Genomics 10:432, 1991.
87. Allen A, Snarz D. The structure and function of gastric mucus. Gut 13:666, 1972.
88. Ishihara K, et al. Effect on gastric mucus of the proton pump inhibitor leminoprazole and its cytoprotective action against ethanol-induced gastric injury in rats. Arzneimittelforschung 44:827, 1994.

89. Slomiany BL, Slomiany A. Mechanism of *Helicobacter pylori* pathogenesis: Focus on mucus. J Clin Gastroenterol 14(Suppl 1):42S114, 1992.
90. Felmstrom G. Active alkalinization of amphibian gastric fundic mucosa in vitro. Am J Physiol 233(Suppl E):1, 1977.
91. Schade C, Flemstrom G, Holm L. Hydrogen ion concentration in the mucus layer on top of acid-stimulated and inhibited rat gastric mucosa. Gastroenterology 107:180, 1994.
92. Dal Santo P, et al. Gastric bicarbonate secretion in high-relapsing, smoking duodenal ulcer patients. Hepatogastroenterology 40:120, 1993.
93. Britland ST, et al. Vagus nerve morphology in diabetic gastropathy. Diabetic Med 7:780, 1990.
94. Jebbink RJ, et al. Hyperglycemia induces abnormalities of gastric myoelectrical activity in patients with type I diabetes mellitus. Gastroenterology 107:1390, 1994.
95. Horowitz M, Fraser R. Disordered gastric motor function in diabetes mellitus. Diabetologia 37:543, 1994.
96. Erbas T, et al. Comparison of metoclopramide and erythromycin in the treatment of diabetic gastroparesis. Diabetes Care 16:1511, 1993.
97. Peeters TL, et al. Effect of motilin on gastric emptying in patients with diabetic gastroparesis. Gastroenterology 102:97, 1992.
98. Richards RD, et al. Objective and subjective results of a randomized, double-blind, placebo-controlled trial using cisapride to treat gastroparesis. Dig Dis Sci 38:811, 1993.
99. Gray JL, Debas HT, Mulvihill SJ. Control of dumping symptoms by somatostatin analogue in patients after gastric surgery. Arch Surg 126:1231, 1991.
100. Richards WO, et al. Octreotide acetate induces fasting small bowel motility in patients with dumping syndrome. J Surg Res 49:483, 1990.
101. Becker JM, et al. Intestinal pacing for canine postgastrectomy dumping. Gastroenterology 84:383, 1983.
102. Hocking MP, Vogel SB, Sninsky CA. Human gastric myoelectric activity and gastric emptying following gastric surgery and with pacing. Gastroenterology 103:1811, 1992.
103. Telander RL, et al. Human gastric atony with tachygastria and gastric retention. Gastroenterology 75:497, 1978.
104. Hocking MP. Postoperative gastroparesis and tachygastria-response to electric stimulating and erythromycin. Surgery 114:538, 1993.
105. Rothstein RD, Alavi A, Reynolds JC. Electrogastrography in patients with gastroparesis and effect of long-term cisapride. Dig Dis Sci 38:1518, 1993.
106. Taylor IL, et al. Hypergastrinemic and hyperpepsinogenemic I duodenal ulcer disease. Ann Intern Med 95:421, 1981.
107. Shamburek RD, Schubert ML. Pharmacology of gastric acid inhibition. Baillieres Clin Gastroenterol 7:23, 1993.
108. Modlin IM, Nangia AK. The pathobiology of the human enterochromaffin-like cell. Yale J Biol Med 65:775, 1992.
109. Coffey RJ, et al. Roles for transforming growth factor-alpha in gastric physiology and pathophysiology. Yale J Biol Med 65(6):693, 1992.
110. Takagi H, et al. Hypertrophic gastropathy resembling Ménétrier's disease in transgenic mice overexpressing transforming growth factor alpha in the stomach. J Clin Invest 90:1161, 1992.

16

Gastritis and Peptic Ulceration

Stanley W. Ashley and Laurence Y. Cheung

Although there have been many recent major advances in our understanding of the pathophysiology of the stomach and duodenum, our knowledge is still far from complete. Despite the apparent complexity of normal gastric physiology, disorders appear primarily as some form of injury to the gastroduodenal mucosa. Two derangements of major importance are gastritis and peptic ulceration. These processes have traditionally been conceptualized as disturbances in the normal interplay between acid-pepsin secretion and gastroduodenal mucosal defense. Although the traditional concept of these disorders has recently been revolutionized by the recognition that infection with *Helicobacter pylori* plays a major role in chronic peptic ulcer, the theme of a balance between secretion and defense still provides a useful framework in which to organize the sometimes diverse clinical and laboratory data regarding pathogenesis and treatment.

Using this organization, the pathologic entities discussed in the following pages are characterized in terms of the disturbance in the normal balance between mucosal defense and acid-pepsin secretion. The spectrum extends from acute lesions, which predominantly stem from a defect in defense mechanisms, through gastric and duodenal ulcer, to the Zollinger-Ellison syndrome, which is the most obvious example of acid hypersecretion. Since the fairly similar medical and surgical therapies for these disorders primarily represent attempts to artificially restore this balance, they are approached first of all in terms of this concept and secondarily as they relate to the specific disease processes. Finally, recurrent ulceration after surgery is presented as an illustrative failure in these attempts to reestablish the normal interplay of secretion and defense.

PATHOPHYSIOLOGY OF GASTRITIS AND PEPTIC ULCERATION

The distinction between gastritis and ulceration is an important one. In general terms, gastritis represents inflammation confined to the mucosa of the stomach and can occur in both acute and chronic forms. Chronic gastritis is important primarily in its role in the pathogenesis of chronic peptic ulcer and is discussed in that context. Acute gastritis, on the other hand, is a commonly encountered problem for anyone involved in the care of the critically ill. It occurs typically after major physical or thermal trauma, shock, sepsis, head injury, and ingestion of a variety of chemical agents such as aspirin and alcohol. This lesion is generally classified under the generic term *stress erosion*. Stress ulcer has been used synonymously, although this designation actually represents a misnomer. True ulcers extend through the muscularis mucosae into the submucosa and muscularis (Fig. 16-1). Although this extension may occur occasionally in acute erosive gastritis, initiating massive hemorrhage from a large submucosal vessel, ulceration is usually chronic in nature. In fact, chronic gastric and duodenal ulcers are distinguished by the presence of an established inflammatory reaction.

Both acute and chronic ulcers have presented major obstacles to experimental study. A number of relevant animal models exist for acute lesions and have made possible the investigation of factors responsible for this type of disorder. Although no such model exists for chronic ulcer, this is by nature a chronic and recurrent disease, and this has permitted a variety of clinical studies. Investigators have made a very thorough examination of disturbances in acid secretion and its control in these patients. A major difficulty in these studies arises in the distinction between abnormalities of etiologic significance and those that merely represent a consequence of the ulcer diathesis itself. Although secretory abnormalities have been accessible through clinical studies, only recently have we begun to understand the role of mucosal defense mechanisms in chronic lesions.

Acute Gastritis

Although the precise mechanisms involved in the pathogenesis of acute gastric erosions are not known, current evidence suggests a multifactorial etiology.[1] Stress erosions are usually multiple, small, punctate lesions situated in the proximal acid-secreting portion of the stomach, although they may occasionally extend into the antrum and even

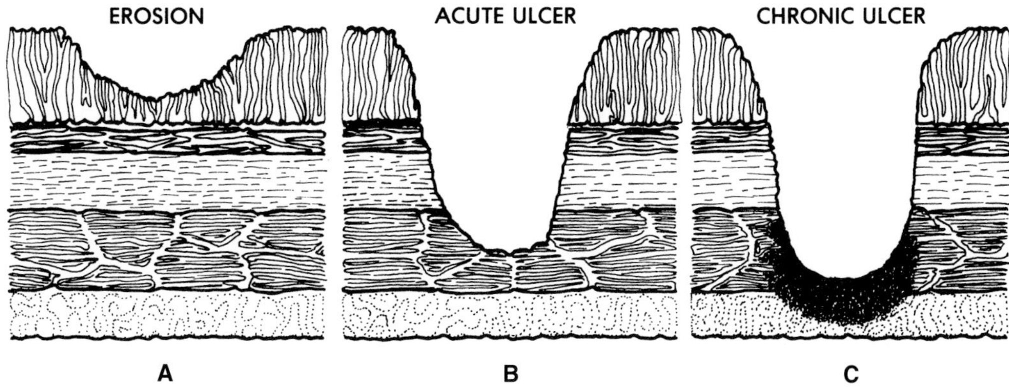

Fig. 16-1. Schematic representation of the distinction between acute erosion (**A**), acute ulcer (**B**), and chronic ulcer (**C**). Erosions are confined to the mucosa, whereas ulcerations extend through the muscularis mucosae to the submucosa and muscularis. Chronic ulceration is distinguished by the presence of established inflammatory reaction.

the duodenum. They occur in three main clinical settings, two of which are associated with a reduction in the ability of the gastric mucosa to protect itself against injury. First, virtually all patients with severe illness, trauma, burns, or sepsis develop these lesions, although the lesions achieve clinical significance only in a small percentage. When the lesions extend into larger submucosal vessels, life-threatening hemorrhage can result. In the setting of thermal injury, acute erosions have been distinguished as Curling's ulcers, although no real pathologic difference exists. Patients in this seriously ill group have multiple reasons for a depression of normal defense mechanisms, although, as is discussed later in the chapter, mucosal ischemia seems to be the predominant factor. The second setting for acute erosions is in the context of drug and chemical ingestion. Aspirin, a variety of other nonsteroidal anti-inflammatory drugs (NSAIDs), and alcohol may produce an acute erosive gastritis. These agents presumably directly alter gastric mucosal resistance, allowing back diffusion of acid and further damage. For the anti-inflammatory drugs, inhibition of the synthesis of prostaglandins, which appear to have multiple roles in the preservation of normal mucosal integrity, is probably the dominant mechanism. The third underlying condition associated with acute lesions (i.e., central nervous system trauma) is not so clearly related to a defect in mucosal defense. In fact, these patients have elevated levels of serum gastrin and, most likely, a secondary increase in acid secretion. This lesion, Cushing's ulcer, is characteristically deeper than other acute erosions and more frequently perforates.

Pathogenesis

Recent experimental observations have identified a number of factors that appear to contribute to acute erosive gastritis. Most reduce the ability of the stomach to protect itself against acute injury rather than increasing the amount of acid secretion. In fact, experimental evidence suggests that hemorrhagic shock and sepsis may actually result in a reduction in acid secretion. In general, however, Schwarz's "no acid, no ulcer" dictum remains valid, and complete neutralization of gastric acidity prevents the development of these lesions.[2]

Given that the presence of luminal acid is a necessary but not sufficient prerequisite for the development of stress lesions, it seems reasonable to postulate that some mechanisms may result in an increased back diffusion of hydrogen ion into the tissue. Davenport and Barr[3] noted that substances such as aspirin, bile salts, and alcohol reduced the normal barrier function of the gastric mucosa, allowing the backflux of hydrogen ions into the tissue. They postulated that this back diffusion might produce histamine release, vasodilation, and eventual bleeding (Fig. 16-2). This concept of a gastric mucosal barrier has been supported by a number of subsequent experimental studies with chemical-induced erosions. However, other models for stress lesions suggest that barrier disruption may not be an essential component of the pathologic process in all types of injury. For example, hemorrhagic shock and endotoxemia can produce lesions without overt evidence of a defect in the barrier.[4] Even in these instances, however, back diffusion of a smaller magnitude probably occurs. In severely traumatized or septic patients, endogenous bile salts may chemically disrupt the barrier. Clinical observations suggest that reflux of bile from duodenum to stomach is more common in critically ill patients, probably as a result of the adynamic ileus. Ritchie[5] has shown that the combination of acid, bile salts, and mucosal ischemia is remarkably ulcerogenic.

There is a general consensus among most investigators that mucosal ischemia is also a critical pathogenic factor. Many of these patients have experienced an episode of shock from hemorrhage, sepsis, or cardiac dysfunction, and decreased mucosal blood flow is a common denominator in many experimental models for stress erosion. It remains

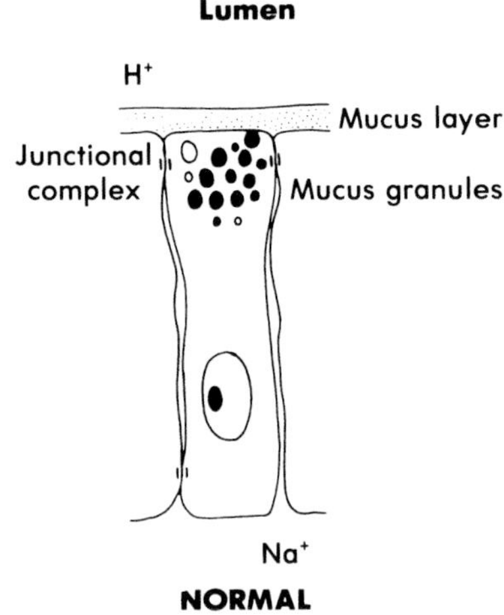

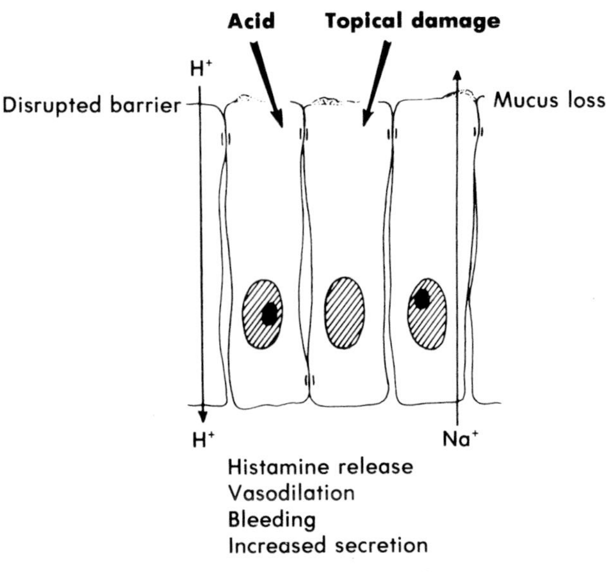

Fig. 16-2. Intact and disrupted gastric mucosal barrier. (From Sircus W, Smith AN, eds. Scientific Foundations of Gastroenterology. Philadelphia: WB Saunders, 1980.)

uncertain what the exact role of blood flow is in maintaining mucosal defense. The leading hypothesis is that it somehow functions to dispose of or buffer acid entering the tissue. Ischemia reduces this capacity, lowering intramucosal pH. Menguy[6] has also suggested that it may reduce mucosal resistance by secondarily producing a deficit of mucosal adenosine triphosphate and other high-energy phosphate intermediates. His animal experiments have demonstrated that this deficit is greater in the fundus than the antrum, possibly explaining the predisposition of this region to stress erosion.

Both systemic and gastric acid-base balance also appear to play important roles in gastric mucosal integrity. Acidosis has been shown to reduce the ability of the gastric mucosa to protect itself against injury in animal studies. The secretory status of the mucosa itself may be a critical factor. In concert with acid secretion, bicarbonate is released into the tissue, the so-called "alkaline tide." O'Brien and Silen[7] have demonstrated the importance of this release in mucosal protection. In animal studies the actively secreting stomach appears to be much more resistant to luminal acid than it is under conditions of secretory inhibition.

Mucus normally covers the gastric mucosa, and the possibility that this somehow has a protective role has stimulated considerable interest. It has been demonstrated that the mucus layer over surface epithelial cells may serve as an unstirred layer in which actively secreted bicarbonate neutralizes luminal acid before it can reach and damage the cells. However, the exact role of mucus and bicarbonate secretion in protecting the mucosa against acute lesions is as yet incompletely defined. The rate of epithelial renewal, or restitution, may also be a factor, presumably preventing the appearance of injury by replacing damaged mucosal cells. Gastrin and epidermal growth factor, a peptide found in salivary secretions, have both been shown to have trophic effects on the gastric epithelium. These agents inhibit the formation of erosions. Prostaglandins exert a protective effect in the gastric mucosa, and the inhibition of their production by aspirin and other NSAIDs may be a primary mechanism for gastric injury. Prostaglandins in high doses inhibit acid secretion, but even at lower concentrations they seem to exert what has been termed a "cytoprotective" effect. Experimental evidence suggests several possible mechanisms.[8] These agents increase mucosal blood flow and, in addition, have been shown to stimulate bicarbonate and mucus secretion, presumably enhancing a luminal buffer.

The recognition of these pathogenic mechanisms has provided a rationale for the prevention of stress erosions in critically ill patients. As a result, in recent years the incidence of clinically significant stress lesions has notably decreased. The prerequisite of acid secretion provides a basis for the regular use of antacid or H_2 receptor blockade, the efficacy of which has been demonstrated in a number of clinical trials. The correction of abnormalities in cardiac output and intravascular volume and the treatment of any septic focus may be critical in the prevention of mucosal ischemia. Adequate nutritional therapy is suggested by the concept of a mucosal energy deficit. Finally, the correction of systemic acid-base balance may also have a role. Ideally, as we continue to improve our management of at-risk patients, the incidence of these lesions will further decrease.

Clinical Manifestations and Diagnosis

The predominant clinical manifestation of erosive gastritis is gastrointestinal bleeding. Prodromal signs such as abdominal pain are infrequent. Although erosion formation can often be demonstrated within 24 hours after the acute insult, massive bleeding usually occurs after 7 to 10 days when the superficial erosion extends into larger submucosal vessels. Only rarely do erosions perforate.

If a high index of suspicion is maintained in conditions that predispose to this illness, diagnosis is usually fairly straightforward. Routine upper gastrointestinal series are of little value—the critical condition of these patients often precludes a good quality study; the erosions are usually too superficial to visualize; and should angiography become necessary, the contrast material may interfere. Upper endoscopy is the procedure of choice and is diagnostic in more than 90% of patients.[9] If the diagnosis remains in doubt, radionuclide scanning and visceral angiography may prove useful.

These patients are usually critically ill, and it is essential to stabilize and correct any predisposing conditions at the same time diagnostic maneuvers are being performed. Hypovolemia and coagulopathies should be identified and treated as early as possible. Large-bore nasogastric intubation, preferably with an Ewald tube, decompresses the stomach, eliminating the stimulating effects of distention and blood on acid secretion. In addition, it provides information about the rate of bleeding, clears the stomach for endoscopy, and allows saline lavage that alone controls the bleeding in greater than 80% of patients.[10] Although suggested by some, the efficacy of lavage, with iced solutions and levarterenol, for their vasoconstrictor effects, has not yet been demonstrated. Once the diagnosis is established, further steps in medical and, possibly, surgical management should be instituted.

Chronic Peptic Ulcer

The pathophysiologic mechanisms underlying chronic gastric and duodenal ulcer are different and are treated separately in the following discussion. However, despite attempts to make distinctions on the basis of such parameters as the type of pain, their clinical presentation and diagnosis are remarkably similar and are presented together.

Pathogenesis of Gastric Ulcer

Gastric ulcer is the next entity in this spectrum of gastroduodenal mucosal injury. Three forms are commonly recognized. Type I is the primary gastric ulcer, usually located in the proximal antrum and constituting the majority of gastric ulcers. Its pathogenesis has been generally associated with a disturbance in mucosal defense and hyposecretion of gastric acid. Type II gastric ulcer, which arises secondary to duodenal ulcer with pyloric stenosis, and type III, the prepyloric and channel ulcer, are often associated with acid hypersecretion, and both are assumed to be caused by duodenal ulcer. Only type I ulcerations are considered here.

As mentioned earlier, no really good experimental model exists for chronic peptic ulceration, and much of our current knowledge of its pathogenesis stems from epidemiologic and genetic studies.[11] In many instances the links between this body of information and the pathophysiology of chronic ulceration are speculative. For example, although the incidence of duodenal ulcer has declined in recent years, that of gastric ulcer, without apparent explanation, has remained relatively constant or even increased. Likewise, the role of dietary factors in the prevalence of gastric ulcer is unsubstantiated. The greater frequency of this lesion with advancing age may be related causally to an increased incidence of gastritis in the elderly and also to the greater consumption of NSAIDs. In addition, genetic factors seem to have a role. There is a definite familial aggregation of both gastric and duodenal ulcer.[12] However, unlike duodenal ulcer, as yet no genetic markers have been identified for this disease.

A number of risk factors have been recognized as important in the pathogenesis of this disorder. Probably the strongest association is with consumption of aspirin and NSAIDs.[13] In contrast with the effects of these agents in stress erosion where the injury is primarily topical, chronic ulcer seems to be most directly related to their systemic effects. Suppression of prostaglandin synthesis appears to be the common denominator. The prevalence of peptic ulcers in chronic NSAID users has been reported to range from 10% to 30%. Although most patients with gastric ulcer have an element of chronic gastritis in association with their ulcer, studies of gastrectomy specimens have revealed that habitual aspirin users may develop ulcers in otherwise normal mucosa.

Although the evidence to date is less convincing than that for duodenal ulcer as discussed below, *H. pylori* infection is also of significance in the pathogenesis of gastric ulcer.[14,15] The organism has been found in about two thirds of patients with gastric ulcer; in the third in whom this organism is not present, a history of chronic NSAID use can usually be obtained. Infection is associated with antral gastritis, and this may predispose to the development of chronic ulcer. However, 20% of patients who do not have ulcer are also colonized with *H. pylori*, and the factors explaining why only a minority of those infected develop ulceration remain poorly defined.

There also appears to be a correlation with cigarette smoking.[16] Nicotine reduces pyloric sphincter pressure and increases duodenogastric reflux. As will be discussed, this reflux may be an important factor in the development of gastric ulceration.

There are as yet no data to support the popular belief that irritants such as spices and curries may damage the gastric mucosa. One epidemiologic study has implicated coffee and soft drinks in ulcerogenesis, but did not distinguish between gastric and duodenal disease.[17] Although a relationship between psychologic factors and chronic ulceration has been suggested, patient studies have not been particularly revealing. No one personality pattern has been identified, and there are rather conflicting findings regarding the role of stressful life events.

Current theories suggest that there are two major but closely related physiologic abnormalities in gastric ulcer—duodenogastric reflux and damage to mucosal defenses.[18] In contrast to the hypersecretion noted in duodenal ulcer, gastric ulcer patients secrete in a range from normal to barely detectable. Although a few subjects have been reported with no detectable acid secretion or achlorhydria, in general it is believed that at least some acid-pepsin is required for ulceration. However, it is clear that the defect in these patients must include a significant disorder of defense.

It has been speculated that the most basic abnormality in gastric ulcer is a reflux of duodenal contents (i.e., biliary and pancreatic secretions) into the stomach, resulting in gastritis and eventual ulceration. Barium fluoroscopy and marker studies have in general demonstrated increased reflux in these patients, probably because of pyloric sphincter dysfunction.[19] Normally the pylorus has a low resting pressure that increases in response to acid, fat, amino acids, and cholecystokinin from the duodenum. In some gastric ulcer patients, low basal pressures have been documented, and in others pressure increases in response to duodenal infusion of acid or fat are significantly less than those of control subjects (Fig. 16-3). Pressure also rises less in response to exogenous cholecystokinin and secretin. It has been suggested that when these two hormones are released endogenously by acids or fat in the duodenum, the lack of response to them may be the primary mechanism for all these abnormalities. The pyloric malfunction presumably explains the increase in duodenogastric reflux.

The physiologic link between reflux and gastric ulceration has not been clearly established. Drainage of duodenal contents into the stomach in experimental animals produces a superficial gastritis that is worst in the antrum.[20] However, it has not been shown to result in chronic ulceration. Some patients with gastric ulcer do have an increase in bile acid conjugates in the stomach, both in the fasting state and after meals; and the severity of their gastritis seems to correlate with the concentration.[21] Bile acids (particularly deoxycholate and taurocholate), lysolecithin, and pancreatic secretions are the agents in duodenal contents speculated to have the most damaging consequences. It is believed that they damage the mucosa topically, disturbing the surface mucus layer and somehow producing a low-grade disruption of the gastric mucosal barrier.

Aspirin seems to have similar effects. Ion transport and metabolic processes such as adenosine triphosphate production may be altered. It has been suggested that patients with gastric ulcer are predisposed to this alteration by some inherent abnormality in mucus or bicarbonate secretion. Some data support a decrease in mucus secretion with atrophic gastritis, but it is very difficult to distinguish which disorder is the primary one.[22] No definite defect in the composition of gastric mucus has yet been demonstrated.

Chronic gastritis is the widely assumed intermediary step between the repeated injury to the gastric mucosal barrier by refluxing duodenal contents and the development of gastric ulceration. This concept of gastritis-producing ulceration is unproven, and chronic atrophic gas-

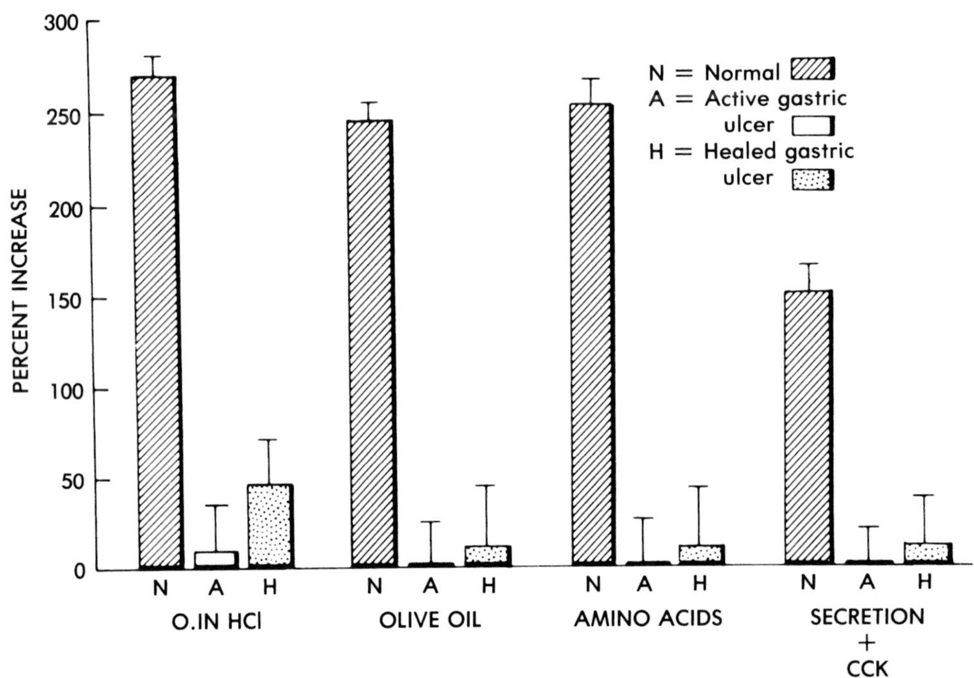

Fig. 16-3. Pyloric pressure responses to intraduodenal stimuli and exogenous hormonal administration in normal persons and patients with gastric ulcer before and after healing. Pyloric pressure is expressed as the percentage increase above basal pressure. In normal individuals, hydrochloric acid, olive oil, amino acids, and intravenous secretin increase pyloric pressure. In gastric ulcer these agents fail to produce a significant rise both before and after ulcer healing. *CCK,* Cholecystokinin. (From Fisher RS, Cohen S. Pyloric sphincter dysfunction in patients with gastric ulcer. N Engl J Med 288:273, 1973. Copyright © 1973 Massachusetts Medical Society. All rights reserved.)

tritis is very common in the elderly, found in approximately 40% of persons older than the age of 50.[23] Although chronic ulcer is usually associated with gastritis, the primary event has not been clearly established. Gastritis may be limited to only the area around the ulcer, but it usually persists after ulcer healing. The extension of the usual antral pattern of gastritis into the fundus helps to explain the generally low rates of acid secretion in patients with gastric ulcer. In addition, some increase in basal hydrogen ion back diffusion may also play a role. Gastrin cells are apparently spared the gastritis because, in response to the reduced acidity, fasting serum gastrin levels are usually slightly elevated and may double the normal increase after a meal.[24]

The pathologic anatomy of gastric ulceration has provided some insight into its pathogenesis. These ulcers usually occur along the lesser curvature at the incisura angularis, on the antral side of the junction between the corpus and antrum. Several possible explanations for this have been proposed.[25] Near the incisura angularis there are prominent muscle bundles underlying the mucosa that might somehow predispose to ulceration. With advancing age, the corpus-antral junction migrates cephalad; this occurs most rapidly along the lesser curvature. It has been suggested that ulcers develop when this junction overlies the muscle bundles. The bundles may somehow constrict the mucosal blood supply, increasing the susceptibility of the mucosa to acid-peptic injury. The concept that changes in mucosal blood flow may have a role in chronic ulceration is only conjecture. However, the blood supply is different on the lesser curvature. There mucosal capillaries and submucosal arteries are end vessels arising directly from the left gastric artery, whereas in the rest of the stomach they arise from an extensive submucosal plexus. Muscular contractions may constrict these end arteries and, without the usual system of anastomosing vessels, produce areas of focal mucosal ischemia.

In summary, gastric ulcer seems to result from a defect in gastric mucosal defense against digestion by acid-pepsin. Physiologic defects that may contribute to gastric ulcer are as follows:

1. Normosecretion or hyposecretion of acid
2. Duodenogastric reflux
   a. Pyloric sphincter dysfunction
3. Damaged gastric mucosal defenses
   a. Chronic gastritis
   b. Gastric mucosal barrier disruption
   c. Focal mucosal ischemia
   d. Defects in mucus or bicarbonate secretion

Hypersecretion cannot be incriminated in its pathogenesis. There is evolving evidence that pyloric dysfunction, acting through duodenogastric reflux, allows endogenous agents to exert injurious effects on the mucosa. These agents, in combination with acid-pepsin, produce ulceration in areas of reduced mucosal resistance. NSAIDs and *H. pylori* infection probably both can play a role in this reduction.

Pathogenesis of Duodenal Ulcer

More than gastric ulcer, duodenal ulcer has been linked to a disorder in acid-pepsin secretion, and more than 95% of duodenal ulcers occur in the first part of the duodenum, most within 3 cm of the junction between pyloric and duodenal mucosa.[26] This distribution suggests that gastric acid is crucial in the pathogenesis of duodenal ulcer. However, recent refinements in our knowledge have been made to complicate this theory.

Perhaps most dramatic has been the recognition of the association between duodenal ulcer and *H. pylori,* leading many experts to conclude that duodenal ulcer is in reality an infectious disease.[14,15] *H. pylori*–induced gastritis is found in more than 95% of duodenal ulcer patients. It causes a number of physiologic abnormalities, each of which may be related to ulcer formation. Meal-stimulated hypergastrinemia appears to be one consequence, perhaps leading to trophic effects on the parietal cell mass. *H. pylori* infection is also associated with a decrease in mucus hydrophobicity, the property presumed to be associated with acid impermeability. In addition, there is a strong link between infection and duodenitis, a common denominator in patients with duodenal ulcer. The best evidence for this role comes from data on the effects of treatment of *H. pylori* in patients with established ulcer; sustained eradication eliminates recurrence, as is discussed later in this chapter. However, a direct causal relationship does not exist; only a minority (10% over a lifetime) of individuals harboring *H. pylori* develop ulcers. Thus other factors must play a significant role.

As with gastric ulcer, much of our knowledge of the pathogenesis of duodenal ulcer stems from the indirect evidence of epidemiologic and genetic studies. There is considerable controversy regarding recent trends in the incidence of duodenal ulcer.[27] Several studies have reported major declines in the number of hospitalizations, complications, operations, and mortality figures for duodenal ulcer, perhaps implying some basic difference in the pathophysiology of the disease. However, others have disputed these suggested trends, implying that these changes may be more a reflection of other factors, such as differences in hospital disease classifications, an increase in patient self-medication with antacids, a greater willingness to treat ulcer on an outpatient basis, and an improved diagnostic approach with the advent of more widespread endoscopy.[12]

A number of risk factors have also been identified. As with gastric ulcer, there is a strong association with NSAIDs. Smoking is also associated with an increased incidence and also appears to impair the healing of duodenal ulcers. This appears to be a result of an associated decrease in prostaglandin synthesis, enhanced acid secretion, and reductions in duodenal and pancreatic bicarbonate secretion. Diet may play a role. For example, milk consumption was correlated with a decrease and coffee and soft drinks with an increase in the later development of ulcers.[17] Despite popular belief, however, there is no good evidence that a change in diet has a major effect on the disease.

There have been attempts to associate duodenal ulcer with a number of other chronic diseases, but as yet no common pathophysiologic mechanism has been identified. The increased incidence of duodenal ulcer in patients with chronic lung disease appears unrelated to the degree or treatment of the pulmonary disease, and, in fact, the ulcer often precedes the development of respiratory problems.[28] Cirrhosis seems to be associated with duodenal ulcer, and the finding that acid secretion is normal in these patients has led to the suggestion that a portal hypertension–induced alteration in mucosal blood flow may be involved.[29] Duodenal ulcers probably occur with increased frequency after renal transplantation, and this has fueled speculation regarding a relationship between steroids and ulcerogenesis.[30]

There is now very strong evidence that genetic factors play an important role in the pathogenesis of duodenal ulcer.[31] Until quite recently it was thought that peptic ulcer was a single disease, the result of complex interactions between many different genes and environmental factors. However, the recognition of several distinct, genetically determined subcategories of peptic ulcer has suggested instead that it is a heterogenous group of distinctly different diseases, in some instances the result of simple Mendelian genetics, all of which present as an ulcer of the gastroduodenum.[32] Initial evidence for a genetic basis came from familial aggregation and twin concordance studies, but this has been strengthened by the recognition of a number of rare genetic syndromes that all produce duodenal ulcer as a component of the phenotype. These include, among others, multiple endocrine neoplasia type I, which frequently presents as the Zollinger-Ellison syndrome; systemic mastocytosis; and an autosomal dominant disorder of tremor, nystagmus, narcolepsy, and ulcer.[23] In addition to this evidence, a number of discrete genetic subtypes of common duodenal ulcer have been identified by means of both biochemical and physiologic markers.[34] There is a group of patients with duodenal ulcer who have an elevation in serum pepsinogen I, the inactive precursor for pepsin, a characteristic that seems to be transmitted by an autosomal dominant pattern of inheritance. The risk of ulcer is increased only in hyperpepsinogenemic siblings. Other genetic subgroups have been identified by normopepsinogenemia, a pattern of rapid gastric emptying, and antral gastrin cell hyperplasia.

Empiric observations have repeatedly suggested that stressful life events and anxiety-producing situations affect the course of an individual patient's illnesses and may even be important in the initial pathogenesis.[35] A number of studies, particularly in patients with chronic gastric fistula, have demonstrated that emotions have an important effect on both gastric acid secretion and blood flow. Although animal studies with restraint and avoidance models implicate a role for stress in acute lesions, such a role has been nearly impossible to evaluate or clearly document in human studies. Attempts to identify an "ulcer personality" have not proven particularly fruitful.

In general, duodenal ulcer is associated with hypersecretion of acid. Patients with duodenal ulcer tend to secrete more both at rest and in response to stimulation than do normal control subjects[26] (Fig. 16-4). However, there is considerable overlap; in fact, there appears to be no direct relationship between the degree of acid hypersecretion and the severity of the ulcer diathesis. Multiple sources for this increase in acid secretion have been identified. Patients with duodenal ulcer have an average of 1.8 billion parietal cells as compared with 1 billion in control subjects.[36] Chief cell numbers increase in parallel, although the role of their secretory product, pepsin, in ulcerogenesis has not yet been clearly proven. Several explanations have been provided for this increase in secretory mass. In at least one subset of patients (i.e., those distinguished by hyperpepsinogenemia I), it probably occurs on a genetic basis. In others, it may be the acquired result of an increase in the release of trophic

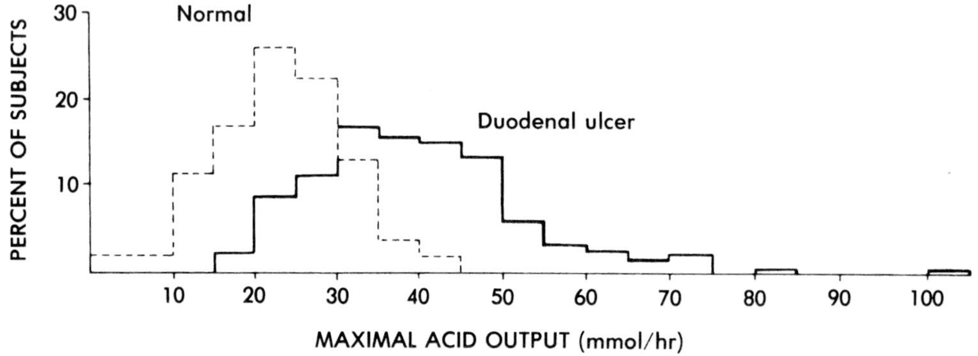

Fig. 16-4. Maximal acid response to intravenous infusion of histamine in normal men and men with duodenal ulcer. The median value is significantly greater in the patients with duodenal ulcer, although overlap is considerable, and approximately 70% of patients with duodenal ulcer fall within the normal range. (Data from Kirkpatrick, et al. From Grossman, MI, ed. Peptic Ulcer: A Guide for the Practicing Physician. Chicago: Year Book Medical Publishers, 1981.)

factors such as gastrin and histamine.[37] As mentioned, the hypergastrinemia associated with *H. pylori* infection may be significant in this regard. It may be that in some patients there is an increase not only in cell numbers but also in the capacity of the individual cell to secrete; this is a very difficult hypothesis to test. Secretory capacity tends to increase with longer duration of the disease, although it returns to control levels after ulcer healing.[38] The cause-and-effect relationship between this increase in secretory capacity and duodenal ulcer is by no means established.

There is also evidence that acid hypersecretion in some patients results from an increase in stimulation. There is an increase in basal secretion and in the ratio of basal secretion to total secretory capacity, suggesting that there is some increase in the background stimulus to acid secretion. Basal secretion probably results primarily from a combination of steady state vagal and histamine stimulation. Dragstedt[20] originally suggested that vagal hyperactivity might be the physiologic basis for duodenal ulcer. Studies demonstrating an increase in the acid secretory response to sham feeding and to insulin-induced hypoglycemia in patients with duodenal ulcer, both of which are believed to be mediated through the vagus nerve, provide some support for this hypothesis.[39] Because there is no satisfactory method for measuring gastric histamine release, it is very difficult to evaluate the suggestion that an increase in basal histamine stimulation is involved. One study did report a decrease in the histamine content and in the activity of histamine methyltransferase in the fundus of patients with duodenal ulcer, although this finding is very difficult to interpret.[40]

Patients with duodenal ulcer also secrete more acid in response to exogenous stimuli. With meals, some studies have demonstrated an increase in peak secretion, whereas others demonstrate a more prolonged response.[41] Although basal serum gastrin levels are usually not elevated and the actual gastrin content of the duodenal mucosa is normal, the increase in acid in response to meals seems to be greater. A decrease in gastrin degradation or a defect in inhibition rather than an increase in release could be occurring. Hyperacidity should inhibit antral gastrin secretion; thus gastrin levels in these patients may be inappropriately high in relation to their secretory capacity. Studies have variously shown defects in inhibition of both acid secretion and gastrin release in response to instilled acid or amino acids,[41] possibly reflecting defects in the intestinal phase of acid secretion. A host of disorders in secretory stimulation or inhibition by regulatory peptides, gut hormones, or absorbed food products may potentially be identified. There is also evidence for an increase in parietal cell sensitivity to secretogogs. For example, the dose of pentagastrin required to produce a half-maximal response is much reduced.[42] Explanations for this, such as an increase in parietal cell receptors or more efficient stimulation-secretory coupling, are merely speculative.

In addition to these disorders in acid secretion, some patients with duodenal ulcer have a motility abnormality. There is more rapid gastric emptying of meals, particularly liquids, and acid and food in the duodenum slow emptying to a lesser extent than in control subjects.[41] The etiologic basis for this rapid emptying is unclear. In some patients, as mentioned, there is evidence for a genetic pattern, whereas in others bulbar inflammation and ulceration may reduce the effectiveness of acid or food-sensitive mechanisms.

Thus both the tendency to secrete more acid and to empty it more rapidly contribute to an increase in the amount of acid delivered to the duodenum, lowering bulbar pH. However, despite the concept that duodenal ulcer, at least to a greater extent than gastric ulcer, represents a disorder in acid secretion, only about a third of patients secrete abnormally. In contrast, recent studies have clearly demonstrated a defect in duodenal acid disposal. Most patients with duodenal ulcer have a reduction in both basal and peak duodenal bicarbonate secretion[43] (Fig. 16-5). This is paralleled by a loss of mucosal buffering capacity. This appears to be the most prevalent physiologic abnormality in duodenal ulcer.

Defects in a variety of other duodenal defense mechanisms have been proposed. Impaired motility of the proximal duodenum, decreased production of prostaglandins, reduced bulbar mucosal blood flow, and defects in mucus

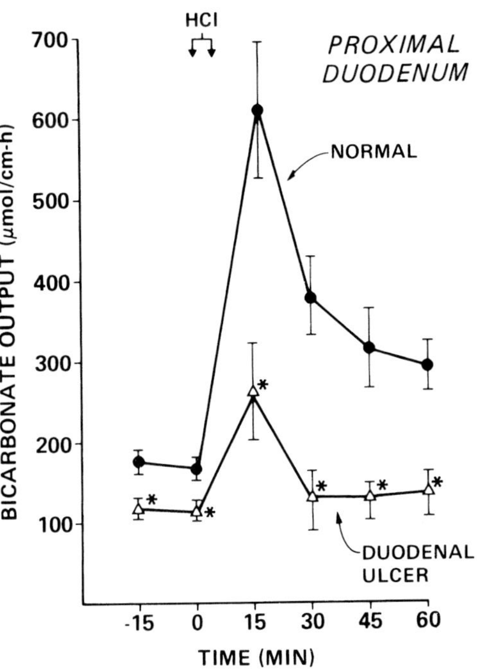

Fig. 16-5. Mean (±SE) values for proximal duodenal bicarbonate output in normal subjects and patients with duodenal ulcer. After basal output was measured for two 15-minute periods, the effect of a 5-minute infusion of 100 mM hydrochloric acid was measured. The asterisks denote $p < 0.01$. (From Isenberg JI, et al. Impaired proximal duodenal mucosal bicarbonate secretion in patients with duodenal ulcer. N Eng J Med 316:374, 1987. Copyright © 1987 Massachusetts Medical Society. All rights reserved.)

or bicarbonate secretion have been hypothesized but are difficult to demonstrate in humans. Chronic duodenitis, associated with *H. pylori,* may affect any of these parameters, setting the stage for ulceration.

In summary, consistent with current concepts of duodenal ulcer as a heterogenous group of disorders, a variety of abnormal physiologic patterns have been described:

1. Hypersecretion or normosecretion of acid
   a. Increase in parietal cell mass
   b. Increase in basal and stimulated secretion
   c. Decrease in secretory inhibition
2. Rapid gastric emptying
3. Defect in duodenal acid disposal or mucosal defense
   a. Impaired bicarbonate secretion

The common denominator in most patients appears to be *H. pylori* infection. In fact, recent evidence would suggest that, apart from NSAID-induced and some atypical ulcers, this disorder would not exist without *H. pylori.*

Clinical Presentation and Diagnosis of Peptic Ulcer

The physiologic manifestations and diagnostic possibilities in peptic ulcer disease are extensive and are discussed only briefly here. Gastric and duodenal ulcer often present in a very similar fashion. Classically, gastric ulcer has been associated with a gnawing or burning epigastric pain brought on by or closely following the secretory stimulus of eating. In contrast, duodenal ulcer pain is supposedly relieved by food or alkali and usually develops several hours after a meal when food has passed the duodenum and the crater is exposed to unbuffered gastric secretion. In fact, symptoms in these two processes are very nonspecific, and even the correlation of pain with the actual presence of peptic ulceration is a poor one.[38] Intractable pain has generally been considered an indication for surgery in peptic ulcer, but because of its nonspecific nature, such pain is very difficult to define. The actual physiology of ulcer pain is not known, although two explanations have been suggested. Acidic luminal contents may irritate afferent nerves within the ulcer crater itself or, alternatively, peristaltic waves passing through the ulcer might produce discomfort. The relative importance of these two possibilities has not been determined. Pain symptomatology in both gastric and duodenal ulcer tends to be chronic and recurrent. Usually these ulcers cannot be differentiated on the basis of clinical findings, although the mean age of patients with gastric ulcer is approximately 10 years greater than that of patients with duodenal lesions.[18] Gastric ulcers have a peak incidence from ages 50 to 65 years, whereas most duodenal ulcers develop in the fourth decade of life. Other common symptoms include nausea and weight loss, even in the absence of pyloric obstruction, and mild epigastric tenderness.

Diagnosis is usually fairly straightforward. Routine laboratory studies add little to the diagnostic workup. In the future, measurement of serum pepsinogen I by radioimmunoassay may prove useful in distinguishing familial ulcer disease.[34] Cultures for *H. pylori* should be obtained and salicylate levels may prove useful in identifying chronic users. Because of the overlap in rates between patients with ulcer and control subjects and because the rates have not been found to be useful in selecting therapy, secretory studies are not usually indicated. The two mainstays of diagnosis are upper gastrointestinal radiography and endoscopy. The decision of when to study a patient with dyspepsia is a complex issue requiring consideration of the character, severity, and duration of symptoms. The choice between radiography and endoscopy is not a simple one. However, at present, radiography is the more cost-effective procedure; with optimal double-contrast studies, greater than 90% of gastric and duodenal ulcer craters are detected, a sensitivity rate comparable to that achieved with endoscopy.[38] Endoscopy is indicated in the case of a poor-quality x-ray study. The question of malignancy in gastric ulcer complicates the decision; because 3% to 7% of gastric malignancies appear benign on x-ray studies, the use of endoscopy and biopsy in all cases has been recommended.[18] Other clinicians have suggested that endoscopy and biopsy are only necessary when gastric ulcers do not appear typically benign on standard x-ray studies, are large, or fail to heal with standard therapy.

Peptic ulcer may produce one of three main complications—hemorrhage, perforation, or obstruction. These can develop without any premonitory symptoms but typically appear as an abrupt change from preexisting dyspepsia. The pathophysiology of these complications is relatively simple; all basically result from the extension of ulceration and the accompanying inflammation deeper into the wall of the gastroduodenum.

When the crater extends into a major vessel, significant hemorrhage may result. About 15% to 20% of patients with peptic ulcer at some point develop gross bleeding, and occult blood loss is even more common.[18] Emergent bleeding requiring operation is most often the result of posterior erosion of a duodenal ulcer into the gastroduodenal artery. Bleeding gastric ulcers appear with hematemesis or melena in about equal frequency, whereas duodenal ulcers tend to produce melena alone.[38] Other symptoms stem from the resultant hypovolemia—transient ischemic attacks (TIAs) and other neurologic complaints, myocardial infarction, and intestinal ischemia. As with acute gastritis, it is important to stabilize the patient at the same time diagnostic maneuvers are performed. The diagnosis of upper gastrointestinal hemorrhage is confirmed by passage of a nasogastric tube. However, bleeding peptic ulcer accounts for only about a third of massive upper gastrointestinal bleeding; endoscopy is therefore indicated to identify the nature and site of the lesion.[44]

When the ulcer erodes through the full thickness of the gastroduodenum, it may produce a perforation or a penetration into surrounding structures. This occurs in 5% to 10% of patients with peptic ulcer.[44] With perforation, the spilled gastric juice incites both peritonitis and consequent catastrophic abdominal pain, marked tenderness, and ileus.

This peritoneal irritation also is responsible for the accompanying leukocytosis and hypovolemia from fluid sequestration. Pneumoperitoneum is present in 75% of patients.[45] Diagnosis is usually obvious. However, it may be more difficult if the perforation seals quickly—these patients occasionally seek medical attention only after a localized intra-abdominal abscess develops. If the perforation is diverted by the falciform ligament into the right colic gutter, it infrequently may be confused with appendicitis. Penetration into the biliary tract or colon can produce a fistula.

Gastric outlet obstruction develops, usually in the context of chronic ulcer disease, when secondary edema or scarring occludes the lumen. If edema is the result of a major lesion, the episode may be reversible either spontaneously or with a short course of intensive medical therapy, including nasogastric suction. However, if inflammatory scarring is the basis, improvement is unlikely. Obstruction develops in less than 5% of patients, usually with duodenal, but occasionally gastric, ulcer.[46] Onset is insidious, but patients usually have nausea, vomiting, and abdominal distention. Vomiting of hydrochloric acid may produce severe dehydration and a metabolic alkalosis. This is perpetuated by a paradoxic aciduria, as the kidney retains bicarbonate with sodium to maintain electroneutrality in the absence of the chloride lost in the vomitus. The diagnosis can be documented with barium x-ray examination, the saline load test consisting of a 400 ml residual one-half hour after gastric instillation of 750 ml of saline, or sequential scintiscanning with technetium-labeled liquids or solids. Endoscopy can differentiate atony from true obstruction when the diagnosis is in question.

Zollinger-Ellison Syndrome

Although uncommon, occurring in 0.1% to 1% of all patients with peptic ulcer, Zollinger-Ellison syndrome is the best understood form of gastroduodenal mucosal injury.[47] Physiologic abnormalities have been directly related to clinical manifestations and have provided the basis for refined diagnostic maneuvers.

Pathogenesis

This syndrome represents the extreme in the pathophysiologic spectrum, extending from disturbances in mucosal defense to those in acid secretion. Ulceration results from massive hypersecretion of acid, which is stimulated by ectopic gastrin production from a non-ß islet cell tumor, the gastrinoma. These tumors produce several forms of gastrin: the predominant form in the tumor is gastrin-17, whereas gastrin-34 with its longer half-life is the major circulating form. Gastrinomas may be located in the pancreas but have also been identified in the duodenum. Generally, they are assumed to represent ectopic lesions. The cells are histologically distinct from those in the antrum that normally produce gastrin, and gastrin cells have not been identified in the normal pancreas. Accompanying islet cell hyperplasia has been recognized, although its significance is not yet clear. In about 20% of patients there is an association with multiple endocrine neoplasia type I.[48] In this group the disease has a genetic basis. At least 20% of gastrinomas are multiple, and more than two thirds are malignant.[47] However, in general, they are very slow-growing, indolent tumors.

The parietal cell mass is expanded enormously, probably as a result of the trophic effects of gastrin. It has been estimated to be at least three to six times as large as that in normal individuals.[47] The physiologic effects of the resulting massive gastric secretion are most easily discussed in terms of the clinical features.

Clinical Manifestations and Diagnosis

More than 90% of patients with gastrinoma develop peptic ulcer during the course of their disease.[45] Symptoms tend to be more severe, unrelenting, and less responsive to therapy than those of usual ulcers. Most ulcers are located in the proximal duodenum. However, probably because of the greater acid secretion, gastric and more distal ulcerations also occur. Lesions are usually single and small, but multiple and giant ulcers have been described with greater frequency than in common duodenal ulcer.

Diarrhea is also a frequent symptom and may occur in the absence of gross ulceration. This is a consequence of the large quantities of hydrochloric acid.[37] There are frequently morphologic abnormalities throughout the small bowel, with stunted villi and mucosal inflammatory infiltrates. Brunner's glands, usually limited to the proximal duodenum, have been found as far distally as the ligament of Treitz. Steatorrhea is also a finding and probably results from two mechanisms. The low pH inactivates pancreatic lipase, impairing hydrolysis of dietary fats. In addition, bile salts are precipitated at low pH, reducing the formation of the micelles required for lipid absorption. Acidic conditions also appear to interfere with vitamin B_{12} absorption, although intrinsic factor secretion by the stomach is normal.

The diagnosis of gastrinoma has become increasingly refined. A search for this syndrome is warranted in patients with multiple, giant, or distal ulcers; ulcer disease refractory to the usual medical therapy; and recurrences after adequate surgery for peptic ulcer. Diagnostic techniques of some use include acid secretory studies and contrast radiography. These patients usually have elevated acid secretion, and basal acid output is usually greater than 60% of maximum.[49] However, there is considerable overlap with control subjects and common duodenal ulcer patients. Upper gastrointestinal x-ray films can reveal ulceration, prominent rugal folds indicating stimulated hypertrophy, dilated small intestine, and even the occasional tumor in the duodenum. Determination of basal serum gastrin levels by radioimmunoassay can be diagnostic; however, elevations may also be detected in several other pathologic conditions. In pernicious anemia, which is an atrophic and inflammatory gastric process that reduces the number of parietal cells but typically spares the antrum, hypergastrinemia results from both an increase in the number of gastrin cells and a loss of the normal acid feedback inhibition of secretion. Patients with renal insufficiency also develop elevated serum gastrins, although the mechanism has not yet been defined and gastrin clearance is normal even in anephric patients.[47] Antral gastrin-cell hyperplasia or hyperfunction occurs in a small proportion of patients with duodenal ulcer. These patients have hypergastrinemia and hypersecretion, although an actual increase in the number of gastrin cells has not been proved.

Three provocative tests have improved the specificity of biochemical diagnosis. For the secretin test, 2 U/kg of secretin is given intravenously over 30 seconds, and serum gastrin is measured 5 minutes before, immediately before, and at 5-minute intervals for one-half hour after injection. In normal patients and patients with duodenal ulcer, secretin has no significant effect, but in patients with Zollinger-Ellison syndrome there is a dramatic increase in serum gastrin levels. The mechanism for this is unknown, although it has been suggested that secretin may release gastrin by a direct local effect on blood flow to the tumor. For the calcium infusion test, calcium gluconate is given intravenously at a rate of 5 mg/kg for a 3-hour period, and serum gastrin levels are determined 30 minutes before and at half-hour intervals for 4 hours. In patients with Zollinger-Ellison syndrome there is usually more than a 400 pg/ml increase, possibly through release of peptide hormone through the calmodulin system, whereas much smaller increases occur in duodenal ulcer and other conditions. A combination test using both secretin and calcium appears to be even more sensitive. A third provocative test, the use of a standard meal, produces little change from basal levels in patients with gastrinoma when compared with the marked increase produced in control subjects or in patients with gastrin-cell hyperplasia. The secretion of the gastrinoma is independent of normal control mechanisms.

CT scanning and angiography are useful, not in the diagnosis of gastrinoma, but in preoperative tumor localization. In some cases, venous sampling has provided additional information for localization, although most surgeons perform exploration without invasive examinations.

PHYSIOLOGIC BASIS FOR TREATMENT IN GASTRITIS AND PEPTIC ULCER

Consistent with the general concept of a disturbance in the interplay between acid secretion and mucosal defense as the basis for these syndromes of gastroduodenal mucosal injury, the medical and surgical therapies of gastritis and peptic ulceration represent attempts to artificially restore this balance. Most treatments have approached this by methods designed to reduce acid secretion, although a few have been devised to improve mucosal resistance. These therapies are discussed first generally in terms of their physiologic mechanism of action and then briefly related to the specific disease entities.

Medical Therapy

In the past a variety of measures, generally unrelated to the pathophysiology of these lesions, were adapted empirically as part of the treatment regimen. Dietary therapy with frequent feeding of bland foods has not been shown to be particularly effective and has little if any effect on gastric acid secretion. Milk, another home remedy, is actually a strong secretory stimulus. Similarly, hospitalization for peptic ulcer was believed to improve healing, although recent evidence suggests that there is little, if any, added benefit.[18] On the other hand, several general measures probably are useful. Cigarette smoking has clearly been shown to retard ulcer healing and should be avoided.[38] Likewise, aspirin and NSAIDs have a detrimental effect on mucosal resistance and should not be prescribed. Coffee strongly stimulates acid secretion, and alcohol may damage the mucosa; at least moderation in their consumption should be suggested.

Pharmacologic therapy has been developed to restore the balance of secretion by three general mechanisms: neutralization of gastric secretion, inhibition of secretion, or protection of the gastric mucosa from further injury. Table 16-1 summarizes the classes of drugs available. A combination of drugs acting by different mechanisms may have more than an additive effect in improving ulcer healing.

Antacids are the oldest therapy. They reduce gastric acidity by reacting with hydrochloric acid to form a salt and water; inhibit peptic activity by the increase in pH; and bind bile acids, which may have a special role in the treatment of gastritis and gastric ulcer. Various antacids differ greatly in their buffering strength, absorption, taste, and side effects. Magnesium antacids tend to be the best buffers but cause significant diarrhea by a cathartic action. Aluminum antacids precipitate with phosphorus, resulting in occasional hypophosphatemia and, in addition, may produce significant constipation. Calcium compounds can cause a delayed acid secretory rebound, felt largely to result from the effect of absorbed calcium ion itself. For each equivalent of hydrochloric acid neutralized, bicarbonate is released in the tissue, and all these drugs may produce a systemic alkalosis. Normal renal function usually prevents this from becoming significant. Antacids are best taken an hour after meals because the food tends to prolong emptying. Many patients have found the large, frequent doses (30 ml of liquid antacid four to seven times daily) unacceptable.

The H_2 receptor antagonists are a group of agents that have revolutionized the treatment of peptic ulcer by directly reducing acid secretion. There are actually two types of gastric histamine receptors: (1) H_1, located on smooth muscle cells, and (2) H_2, located on the parietal cells. This class of drugs was devised to specifically block the histamine-H_2 receptor. Isolated cell studies indicate that there are three independent but mutually augmenting parietal cell receptors for histamine, acetylcholine, and gastrin.[50] Thus inhibition of the histamine receptor alone also re-

Table 16-1. Drugs for the Treatment of Gastritis and Peptic Ulcer

Class	Example	Mode of Action
Antacids	Aluminum hydroxide	Acid neutralization
H_2 receptor antagonists	Cimetidine	Secretory inhibition
Anticholinergics	Propantheline bromide	Secretory inhibition
Tricyclics	Pirezepine	Secretory inhibition
Substituted benzimidazoles	Omeprazole	H^+, K^+-ATPase inhibition
Prostaglandins	Misoprostol	Cytoprotection
Sulfated disaccharides	Sulcralfate	Protective coating
Licorice extracts	Carbenoxolone	Increase in mucus secretion
Colloidal bismuth	Bismuthate	Protective coating, eradicates *Helicobacter pylori*
Antibiotics	Nitroimidazole, tetracycline	Eradicates *H. pylori*

Modified from Stabile BE, Passaro E Jr. Duodenal ulcer: A disease in evolution. Curr Prob Surg 21:1, 1984.

duces the effects of acetylcholine and gastrin. These drugs consist of a five-member organic ring and a side chain similar to histamine itself. Cimetidine was the first employed clinically. Alteration of the ring and/or side chain has produced agents of increasing antagonistic potency and more specific gastric action. The physiologic effects include a decrease in both basal and stimulated acid secretion by what is believed to be competitive inhibition at the parietal cell level.[28] Pepsin output is also reduced. The decrease in antral acidity elevates serum gastrin levels. These agents also reduce gastric blood flow, a finding that may explain the observation that they may be less effective than antacids in preventing stress erosions. Cimetidine is the most widely used H_2 receptor antagonist. It is a potent inhibitor of acid secretion with a half-life of approximately 2 hours, requiring a dosage schedule of four tablets per day. Patient compliance is generally much improved over that with antacids. However, a number of significant side effects, including azospermia, gynecomastia, and a reversible central nervous system toxicity, have been described. This has led to the development of ranitidine and famotidine, longer acting agents that appear to be free of some of the side effects of cimetidine.

Anticholinergic agents act to inhibit the action of acetylcholine at muscarinic receptors. In the stomach they are believed to act directly at the parietal cell level. Atropine and propantheline (Pro-Banthine) are typical anticholinergic agents that, at equal doses, are even more potent than H_2 receptor antagonists.[28] However, side effects, including urinary retention, blurred vision, dry mouth, delayed gastric emptying, and mental disturbances, permit their use only at lower, less-effective doses. The tricyclic agents, including those with an antidepressant activity, are also thought to reduce acid secretion by an anticholinergic mechanism. Pirenzepine, which lacks antidepressant activity, appears to be as effective as cimetidine in the treatment of duodenal ulcer.[51]

An even more potent class of secretory inhibitors (i.e., the substituted benzimidazoles) has been developed. These agents selectively inhibit parietal cell H^+, K^+-ATPase, the enzyme responsible for acid secretion. Omeprazole, the member that was introduced first clinically, seems to be a highly potent agent that may be effective even in patients with refractory ulcers and gastrinoma. It is a weak base and accumulates selectively within the acidic environment of parietal cell. Long-term side effects may become evident, but at present the potential for this group of agents is enormous.

Four different agents seem to be effective by improving gastric mucosal resistance. The prostaglandins are naturally occurring fatty acids that prevent or heal mucosal injury by several mechanisms.[8] The methylated prostaglandin E_2 analogs are absorbed orally and significantly inhibit gastric acid secretion. However, at doses required for this effect, they also produce dramatic diarrhea. At lesser doses, they still exert a "cytoprotective" action, probably by increasing bicarbonate and mucus secretion and mucosal blood flow. Misoprostol, the most widely used analog, appears to be comparable to H_2 receptor antagonists in the healing of duodenal ulcers.

Sucralfate is related structurally to heparin, although it has no anticoagulant effects. Its unique mechanism of action is proving very effective in the treatment of established ulcer disease, and this drug is the only one of the agents presently in widespread clinical use that acts by enhancing resistance. It is an aluminum salt of sulfated sucrose that dissociates under the acidic conditions in the stomach. It has been proposed that the sucrose polymerizes and binds to proteins in the ulcer crater, producing a kind of protective coating that lasts up to 6 hours.[28] It inhibits peptic activity. Folkman et al.[52] have presented evidence that it may bind and concentrate endogenous basic fibroblast growth factor, stabilizing and concentrating this substance, which appears to be important in mucosal healing. The liberated aluminum hydroxide may have some slight additional antacid effect. Little of this is absorbed, so side effects are minimal.

Licorice extracts, the most frequently used of which is

carbenoxolone, a synthetic derivative, also act to enhance mucosal defense.[38] Glycyrrhetic acid appears to be the active moiety in these agents. They have no effect on acid secretion but actually enhance gastric mucus production and its thickness. This seems to reduce hydrogen ion back diffusion. Licorice extracts also appear to decrease pepsin secretion and inhibit peptic activity. Finally, they may increase epithelial cell half-lives. However, licorice extracts are absorbed systemically and have significant aldosterone-like effects, including sodium retention, hypertension, and hypokalemia, which have limited their use clinically.

Colloidal bismuth likewise coats exposed protein. It is the salt that chelates under acidic conditions and has been shown to protect against acute mucosal lesions in a variety of experimental models. An antipeptic activity has also been postulated to explain its effectiveness. In addition, it has activity against *H. pylori,* although complete eradication typically employs combined therapy with a nitroimidazole and either tetracycline or amoxicillin.

Surgical Therapy

The primary goal in the surgical treatment of gastritis or peptic ulcer is to eliminate the pathologic lesion while minimizing the consequent disruption of normal gastroduodenal physiology. Obviously, treatment must be individualized, depending on the specific type of lesion and its mode of presentation. However, the common theme behind all these procedures is to restore the normal balance between secretion and mucosal resistance. Surgically, it has been impossible to alter mechanisms of mucosal defense, and therefore all previous procedures have approached these diseases by attempting to reduce acid secretion as follows: (1) by decreasing the number of parietal cells, (2) by eliminating the hormonal stimulation from the antrum, or (3) by sectioning the vagus nerve. Basically four general operations have been devised to produce these results (Fig. 16-6). These are subtotal gastrectomy, vagotomy and drainage, vagotomy and antrectomy, and parietal cell vagotomy. A discussion of the physiologic rationale and consequences of these procedures would be impossible without at least briefly mentioning some of their undesirable side effects (i.e., the so-called postgastrectomy syndromes).

Subtotal gastrectomy, in the past a commonly performed procedure, is based on the reduction of acid and pepsin secretion by several mechanisms. It removes not only a major portion of the parietal and chief cells in the corpus but also the antral gastrin cells, eliminating the gastrin stimulus to secretion and also its trophic effects, resulting in atrophy of the remaining mucosa. This operation reduces basal and stimulated secretion by about 75% and 50%, respectively.[53] It also eliminates the antropyloric mixing mechanism or trituration by which food is reduced to chyme before entering the duodenum. In addition, emptying of both liquids and solids is more rapid. With removal of the pylorus, increased reflux of intestinal contents into the stomach may have major consequences in terms of the development of reflux gastritis. The choice between Billroth I reconstruction to the duodenal stump vs. Billroth II anastomosis to a more distal loop of jejunum has important physiologic consequences that should be considered in addition to their respective complications.

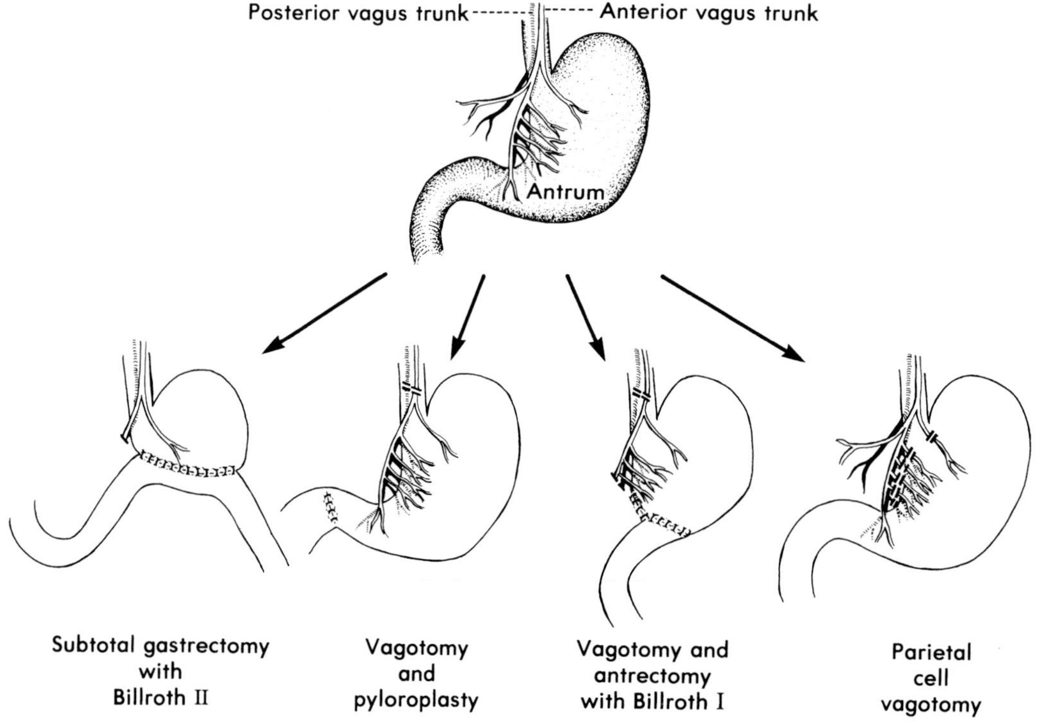

Fig. 16-6. Four most commonly used operative procedures for reduction of gastric acid secretion.

Billroth II eliminates the added stimulus to acid secretion from duodenal release of gastrin in response to passing chyme. However, it also prevents the meal from reaching pH and osmoreceptors in the proximal duodenum, which normally slow gastric emptying.

The rationale for truncal vagotomy is based on the elimination of direct cholinergic stimuli to acid-pepsin secretion. This withdrawal also makes parietal cells less responsive to histamine and gastrin and abolishes the vagal stimulus to release of antral gastrin. Basal and stimulated acid secretion are reduced by 80% and 50%, respectively.[31] Gastrin levels actually increase, probably as a result of a reduction in the normal acid inhibition of antral gastrin cells. Vagotomy also markedly alters gastric motility patterns. Both receptive relaxation and trituration are impaired. Gastric emptying of liquids is speeded, whereas solid evacuation may slow significantly, leading to overt gastric stasis in some patients. As a result, some form of emptying procedure (i.e., pyloroplasty or gastrojejunostomy) must be performed. These drainage operations also have important physiologic consequences. Pyloroplasty further speeds gastric emptying and, by reducing the period of contact between gastric contents and the antral mucosa, decreases acid secretion mediated through the direct gastric phase of stimulation. Gastroenterostomy may actually enhance secretion by producing antral gastrin release and eliminating the secretion of inhibitory factors normally generated by the passage of chyme through the duodenum. An increase in gastrin levels may result because of stasis in the partially excluded antrum and because the gastroenterostomy allows acid to empty and be neutralized before it can bathe the antrum. Both procedures eliminate the pyloric sphincter and produce duodenogastric reflux.

Vagotomy with antrectomy seems to combine some of the advantages of both these procedures. The simultaneous effects of vagotomy and antrectomy remove both the cholinergic and gastrin stimulus to acid secretion. Basal acid secretion is virtually abolished, whereas stimulated acid secretion is decreased by nearly 80%.[53] The rationale for this procedure was to preserve some of the reservoir function eliminated by a more subtotal gastrectomy. Dumping complications, the subject of another chapter, seem to be slightly less frequent than after more complete resection. Unlike reconstruction after a subtotal resection in which a Billroth II seems to be preferable both in terms of suture line tension and recurrence rates, experience has suggested that restoration of normal continuity with a Billroth I is more desirable after vagotomy and antrectomy.

The development of parietal cell vagotomy to treat ulcer disease is a prime example of the application of modern physiologic principles to the design of a practical surgical procedure. The rationale for this procedure is to eliminate vagal stimulation to the acid-secreting portion of the stomach without interrupting supply to the antrum or more distal gastrointestinal tract. Basically, the operation involves severing all the branches of the vagus along the lesser curvature that innervate the corpus and fundus. Basal and stimulated acid are reduced by greater than 75% and 50%, respectively.[31] In addition, the operation reduces the secretion of acid in response to gastric distention. Basal serum gastrin is increased, although the response to a meal is reduced. Receptive relaxation is again impaired, and emptying of liquids is more rapid than normal. However, antral peristalsis, trituration, and sphincter function are preserved. The emptying of solids is normal. The normal small bowel innervation preserves intestinal motility patterns and reduces the incidence of diarrhea and dumping. However, the lower complication rates are balanced by a somewhat higher incidence of recurrence.

The choice among surgical procedures is a very complex one. The most important single factor is the nature of the disease process itself, and this is considered in the following section. Although an elective procedure can be aimed directly at eliminating the pathophysiologic process, in an emergent situation attention must of necessity be directed to the complicated lesion. Other considerations in the choice among procedures include the respective operative mortalities and postoperative morbidities, the incidence of recurrent ulceration, the postgastrectomy side effects of the procedure, the long-term metabolic consequences of the operation (in terms of weight loss, bone disease, and anemia), and even the possible risk of gastric carcinoma. In addition, the familiarity of the operative surgeon himself with the techniques of various operative procedures is a crucial consideration.

Reliable data on the results of various operations have really only been generated over the last two decades. Published series in general have used different criteria for patient selection and have varied in how vigorously the incidence of side effects were pursued. Subtotal gastrectomy alone offers no advantage over the other procedures and is not as widely used today. Table 16-2 summarizes the data on the other three procedures. Briefly, mortality is lowest for highly selective vagotomy and greatest for vagotomy and antrectomy. The relative incidence of side effects is about the same for vagotomy with antrectomy or drainage and lower for the parietal cell operations. On the other hand, the incidence of recurrence is significantly lower

Table 16-2. Mortality, Side Effects, and Recurrence Rates for the Three Most Common Acid-Reducing Operations

Operation	Mortality (%)	Side Effects (%)	Recurrence (%)
Vagotomy and antrectomy	2	5	1
Vagotomy and drainage	1	5	10
Highly selective vagotomy	0.2	1	10

Modified from Grossman MI, ed. Peptic Ulcer: A Guide for the Practicing Physician. Chicago: Year Book Medical Publishers, 1981.

with vagotomy and antrectomy. Thus truncal vagotomy has both the high recurrence rate of parietal cell vagotomy and the unfavorable incidence of side effects of vagotomy and antrectomy. In general, vagotomy and drainage should have little place in the elective therapy of peptic ulcer. Even though this procedure is controversial, there is probably still a role for it in the emergent treatment of a patient for whom time is a critical factor; it can be performed considerably more quickly than a resection or the somewhat tedious parietal cell procedure.

Recently, laparoscopic approaches to operation for peptic ulcer have received increasing attention.[54] Although such techniques have not yet been refined enough to perform resections, vagotomy does appear to be feasible. Conventional highly selective vagotomy is demanding through the laparoscope, and most surgeons have employed a combination of posterior truncal vagotomy and either anterior seromyotomy or anterior highly selective vagotomy. As open operations, these techniques have results comparable to the highly selective procedure; the results with the laparoscope are too preliminary to adequately judge these procedures. So far most of these operations have been performed in the elective setting; as is discussed later in the chapter, with eradication of *H. pylori,* very few such procedures will be necessary in the future. Serious questions remain as to the applicability of laparoscopic techniques in the emergent setting. Neither hemorrhage or obstruction seem well suited to the laparoscope. It may be most applicable to the treatment of perforations, where patching and highly selective vagotomy seem most appropriate.

Treatment for Specific Entities

An exhaustive discussion of the specific treatment for each of these pathologic entities is beyond the scope of this chapter and has been provided elsewhere. What follows is a brief discussion of the basic principles of therapy in relation to the specific physiologic abnormalities of each disease. The various procedures are summarized in Table 16-3.

Table 16-3. Choice of Operative Procedure Based on Indication

Indication	Procedure
Acute gastritis	Vagotomy and pyloroplasty with oversewing of erosions or near-total gastrectomy
Gastric ulcer	Subtotal gastrectomy with ulcer excision
Duodenal ulcer	
Intractable pain	Parietal cell vagotomy
Perforation	Simple closure or closure and parietal cell vagotomy
Bleeding	Vagotomy and antrectomy with suture ligation of bleeding vessel or Vagotomy and pyloroplasty with suture ligation
Obstruction	Vagotomy and antrectomy
Zollinger-Ellison syndrome	Tumor resection or parietal cell vagotomy or total gastrectomy

Acute Gastritis

As mentioned previously, gastric evacuation and lavage halt bleeding in most patients with stress erosions. In addition, antacid administration is useful in preventing the development of further hemorrhage. The pH of gastric contents should be checked regularly, probably every hour; and magnesium or aluminum antacids that are insoluble and remain in the stomach for prolonged periods should be instilled to keep the pH above 5. One prospective randomized study comparing efficacies demonstrated antacid to be superior to cimetidine in the prevention of bleeding in critically ill patients.[28] Omeprazole appears to be equally as effective as antacids. Sucralfate may also be used. This latter drug has been associated with a decrease in pulmonary infections, presumably resulting from aspiration of gastric contents that become colonized when acid is neutralized with the antisecretory agents.

Intra-arterial infusion of vasopressin controls hemorrhage in approximately 80% of patients.[55] A variety of endoscopic techniques for controlling upper gastrointestinal hemorrhage have also been recently described, including the use of heater probe, bipolar electrocoagulation, and injection therapy with epinephrine. Although the initial experience with these techniques is encouraging, further validation in the setting of acute erosions is necessary. Transarterial embolization of bleeding vessels has been suggested, but as yet has not been adequately proven.

Surgery should be considered when the bleeding exceeds 6 to 8 U over 48 hours, but the underlying condition of the patient should enter into this decision. Mortality for surgery in this group of patients is in the range of 40%, and there is much controversy over the type of operation that offers the best chance of success.[9] No really good prospective trial has been performed, but some surgeons have advocated near-total gastrectomy in preference to the lesser procedures of vagotomy and pyloroplasty with oversewing of the bleeding erosions or partial gastrectomy with vagotomy. Generally, if the lesser procedures are successful, they are associated with a reduced morbidity and mortality but a greater incidence of rebleeding. Vagotomy is effective by reducing acid secretion and perhaps also by acutely decreasing mucosal blood flow. The oversewing of a few bleeding erosions is effective because, although there is most often a diffuse gastritis, only a few of these erosions have progressed into the deeper submucosal vessels, and it is these lesions that are responsible for the significant hemorrhage. Fairly satisfactory results have been obtained with the use of vagotomy and pyloroplasty with oversewing of bleeding erosions as the initial procedure, reserving total resection for those who rebleed.

Gastric Ulcer

Trials of medical therapy for chronic gastric ulcer have not been as distinctly successful as those for duodenal ulcer.

Several conclusive clinical studies have shown cimetidine to be significantly more effective than placebo in healing gastric ulcers, although prior investigators were unable to demonstrate this statistically.[18] Two considerations are important in evaluating the therapy for chronic ulcer—healing and pain relief. There is a trend to better pain relief with cimetidine or another H_2 receptor antagonist in most studies of gastric ulcer. On the other hand, antacids have not been shown to be effective; the physiologic reasons for this difference still are unclear. Likewise, the anticholinergic agents have not proved particularly useful in chronic gastric ulcer. Sucralfate appears to speed healing but at least in one study was less effective than cimetidine.[56] Omeprazole appears to be equally efficacious. Current recommendations suggest that these patients should receive cimetidine initially.[18] If *H. pylori* is involved, triple therapy is also instituted. After 2 weeks, if pain relief has not been achieved, a second medication should be added. At 8 weeks, follow-up x-ray films or endoscopy should be performed. If the ulcer is not completely healed, these studies should be repeated again at 12 and 15 weeks. Patients whose ulcers have not healed by this time should be offered surgery.

Gastric ulcer has generally been treated with surgery somewhat earlier than duodenal ulcer. There are several reasons for this approach. One is the fear of malignancy in benign-appearing ulcers. Improvements in the endoscopic diagnosis of cancer have reduced this risk, however. In addition, most data indicate that patients with gastric ulcer are more often hospitalized for their illness than patients with duodenal ulcer and gastric ulcer complications more often require operation, suggesting that gastric ulcer is a more virulent disease. Finally, the older patient with gastric ulcer has a distinctly higher mortality for a complication of the ulcer than the corresponding younger patient with a duodenal lesion.[31] Generally, surgery is recommended for the recurrent ulcer refractory to medical therapy, the ulcer that recurs during treatment with cimetidine, the ulcer that fails to heal within 12 to 15 weeks, or one of the complications of ulcer disease.

The elective surgical decisions in gastric ulcer are somewhat simpler than those in duodenal disease. As mentioned, prepyloric ulcers or those in association with duodenal ulcers share a common cause with duodenal lesions and should be treated as such. Parietal cell vagotomy for such lesions is associated with unacceptably high recurrence rates. For the usual type I gastric ulcer, gastric resection with or without vagotomy has proven effective. Usually it is unnecessary to remove a large amount of stomach for elective treatment of gastric lesions. The ulcer itself should be excised completely and submitted for pathology. Because gastric ulcer does not primarily result from a secretory disturbance, the use of vagotomy has been questioned. The specific operations for complications of gastric ulcer are similar in rationale to those performed for duodenal ulcer and are discussed in the following section.

Duodenal Ulcer

In many instances duodenal ulceration is an easily manageable disease entity, and some patients are able to self-medicate their disease with over-the-counter drugs, never seeking formal medical therapy. Of those who come to professional treatment, greater than 95% are controlled by pharmacologic therapy designed to reduce acid secretion.[38] Antacids are extremely effective, but their inconvenience has made cimetidine or another H_2 receptor blocker the drug of choice. Combination therapy is usually necessary only in refractory patients; antacids or cimetidine alone heal all but about 25% of duodenal ulcers within 4 weeks.[31] Sucralfate appears similar in efficacy to cimetidine, and there has been some conflicting evidence that it may reduce recurrence rates.[56] Colloidal bismuth, in a few clinical trials, also appears to equal the H_2 receptor antagonists. There is some question as to whether an actual ulcer crater need be documented by x-ray film or endoscopy before starting therapy; in fact, it has been suggested that the symptoms and potential complications should be the most important factors in determining treatment. Many ulcers heal, and most symptoms disappear with placebo.[57] However, even though pharmacologic treatment is more expensive, the more rapid response and greater probability of healing justify it.

None of these regimens affects the natural history of the disease process itself. With cessation of therapy, ulcers recur within 6 months in about 80% of patients.[38] Continuation of cimetidine at lower, perhaps only once daily, doses after healing has been shown to significantly reduce the risk of recurrence.[58] After healing, the relative merits of maintenance therapy vs. intermittent treatment for recurrences are still controversial and probably depend on the individual patient. The ultimate effect of routine medical therapy and maintenance treatment on the complication rate has not yet been determined and may not be with the advent of therapy for *H. pylori*. Recent studies, combining ulcer therapy with triple-drug therapy to eradicate this organism, have repeatedly demonstrated that this eliminates recurrence[4,15] (Fig. 16-7). This is undoubtedly the most significant development in this field in recent years.[59]

Classically the four indications for surgery include intractability and the complications of hemorrhage, perforation, and obstruction. Elective operation for intractability has become an increasingly rare occurrence because current medical therapy is so effective. The *H. pylori* data suggest that this may be an indication of the past, except in patients in whom this organism cannot be eradicated or who must continue to take NSAIDs. The decision entails weighing the relative risks and benefits of both medical and surgical therapy.

The choice of an operative procedure and its ultimate results depend critically on the indication for surgery and its specific pathophysiology. In the treatment of intractable pain, surgery is elective, the patient is adequately prepared for the procedure, time is not a crucial factor, and there is

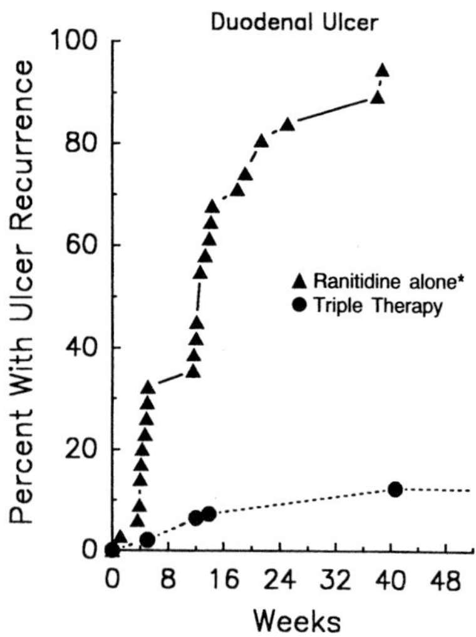

Fig. 16-7. Recurrence rates for duodenal ulcer after successful healing with ranitidine alone or ranitidine plus triple antibiotic therapy for *Helicobacter pylori*. The recurrence rate in patients healed with ranitidine alone was significantly greater ($P < 0.01$). (From Graham DY, et al. Effect of treatment of *Helicobacter pylori* infection on the long-term recurrence of gastric or duodenal ulcer: A randomized, controlled study. Ann Intern Med 116:705, 1992.)

little justification for exposing the patient to the potential for severe early or late postoperative complications. Under these circumstances, parietal cell vagotomy is probably the procedure of choice. The lumen of the gastrointestinal tract is not entered, reducing the risk of septic complications. In addition, because the normal functional anatomy of the stomach and pylorus are preserved and because distal vagal innervation is not interrupted, the potential for the serious long-term side effects of dumping and diarrhea is greatly reduced. Long-term data on these characteristics of treatment with the very recently developed laparoscopic approaches do not yet exist.

Hemorrhage is the principal cause of death from duodenal ulcer;[60] the current choice of operations remains difficult. These patients are critically ill and often have significant associated medical problems delaying the decision for surgery, although most studies indicate that early operation is the only way to reduce mortality and complications.[60] After preoperative stabilization, choice of procedure in these patients is usually limited to two possibilities. Initially the bleeding lesion itself should be addressed directly by control through suture ligation after pyloroduodenotomy. The choice between vagotomy and drainage vs. vagotomy and antrectomy is a controversial one. Vagotomy and pyloroplasty can be performed quickly and simply in the patient unable to tolerate any additional procedure. However, the addition of antrectomy, particularly with modern stapling techniques, does not add much in terms of time or morbidity and significantly reduces the risk of what may be a fatal recurrence. There is also accumulating evidence to suggest that oversewing the bleeding lesion, combined with highly selective vagotomy may be a reasonable option.

In the past, perforation was treated by simple closure, usually reinforced with omentum, the Graham patch. This is a rapid, often effective treatment and is still recommended for patients with preoperative shock, perforation exceeding 48 hours, and significant coexistent medical problems.[60] However, recent studies suggest that, of those treated with simple closure, 80% develop a recurrence, and one third require another operation.[61] Several recent studies have shown that, with proper patient selection, definitive treatment can be performed.[60] Both vagotomy and pyloroplasty and parietal cell vagotomy have been suggested. The latter seems to be receiving greater support.

Treatment for obstruction should both relieve this lesion and deal with the ulcer diathesis. Although there has been some hesitation in using vagotomy in the presence of already disturbed motility patterns, it should probably be included in the definitive operation. Vagotomy with antrectomy, resecting the scarred pylorus, is the procedure of choice, although vagotomy with gastroenterostomy has been applied by some surgeons.

Zollinger-Ellison Syndrome

Treatment of gastrinoma has taken some interesting turns in relation to our understanding of methods of control for this secondary disturbance in gastric physiology. In the past, the recognition that these tumors were frequently multicentric and metastatic (although slow growing) led to the use of the only operation believed to reliably and consistently reduce acid secretion: the total gastrectomy. Subsequently, with the advent of cimetidine, most clinicians adopted this pharmacologic therapy in preference to such a major procedure with its considerable accompanying morbidity and mortality. More recently there has been a trend back to surgery for several reasons. First, using a combination of intraoperative endoscopy to visualize duodenal lesions and thorough exploration of the head of the pancreas and hepatoduodenal ligament to localize others, much higher success rates have been reported for resection. Likewise, a number of trials have suggested that up to 25% of patients with gastrinoma who receive maintenance cimetidine therapy develop a complication of acid hypersecretion.[49] In addition, compliance problems and the recognition of long-term side effects with cimetidine have raised valid doubts about the desirability of continuing medical therapy. Recently, it has been proposed that, at least in those cases deemed unresectable, a parietal cell vagotomy may shift the dose-response curve of cimetidine, preventing breakthrough secretion.[49] Although there is accumulating evidence that ranitidine, famotidine, and omeprazole may be effective in treating those refractory to cimetidine without some of the adverse side effects, most patients with nonfamilial disease and no evidence of liver metastases should undergo exploration. Because of the generally low grade of this malignancy, if acid secretion is negated, long-term survival is possible. Little other effective treatment (e.g., radiotherapy or chemotherapy) is yet available.

RECURRENT ULCERATION AFTER SURGERY

Recurrent ulceration after surgery represents a failure of these attempts to restore the normal balance between acid secretion and mucosal defense and provides an interesting concluding perspective on the physiology of acid-peptic disease. Ulceration recurs in approximately 5% of patients who undergo surgery for peptic ulcer disease, although this incidence may be increasing as parietal cell vagotomy is applied with greater frequency in an attempt to reduce the general mortality and morbidity of ulcer surgery.[39] Ninety-five percent occur after surgery for duodenal ulcer; only a few ulcerations recur after gastric ulcer operations. In the past the vast majority were stomal ulcers, although, with increasing use of parietal cell vagotomy, duodenal ulcers are becoming more common.[46]

Pathogenesis

Multiple factors have been implicated in the pathophysiology of recurrent ulceration. However, an incomplete primary surgical procedure, which possibly results in an inadequate reduction in acid-pepsin secretion despite a technically sufficient operation, is by far the most frequent cause.[62] In these instances the wrong primary operation was chosen. On the other hand, the basis may be some failure in the original technique. Recurrences are more frequent when a new operation is used; specifically the experience of the surgeon seems to play an important role. The high incidence of incomplete vagotomy in some series has led to suggestions of intraoperative testing for completeness. After truncal vagotomy it is usually the right trunk that has been missed, whereas after a parietal cell operation fibers on the distal esophagus (i.e., the nerves of Grassi) are usually responsible. The high incidence of recurrence in some preliminary series with parietal cell vagotomy has been reduced as more experience with the operation is gained. In subtotal gastrectomy without vagotomy, insufficient resection of the acid-secreting region has been implicated. Retained antrum was a frequent cause for recurrence that has been eliminated by recognition and careful avoidance. This entity may still occur after antrectomy and Billroth II reconstruction when a portion of antrum is retained in the duodenal stump, sequestered from the inhibiting effects of gastric acid and thus still capable of stimulating acid secretion in the remaining stomach through release of the hormone gastrin.

Inadequate gastric drainage with stasis and distention-induced secretion has also been implicated as a cause of recurrent ulcer. Long afferent loops after Billroth II anastomoses that increase the distance between the stoma and the neutralizing effects of pancreatic and duodenal bicarbonate have been incriminated. Nonabsorbable sutures at the site of gastroenterostomy may also play a role.

Several etiologic sources for recurrent ulcer formation have been identified, unrelated to the original procedure. Two entities, gastrinoma and antral gastrin cell hyperplasia, can result in enough acid hypersecretion that ulceration results despite the adequacy of the initial operation. In addition, ingestion of aspirin, other anti-inflammatory agents, and even alcohol may damage the mucosa enough to allow ulcer recurrence. Malignancy may also appear as recurrent ulceration.

Clinical Manifestations and Diagnosis

Abdominal pain is the most common presentation.[62] In some instances it may be suggestive of ulcer; however, because of the disturbance in normal anatomy, it can be very atypical and difficult to distinguish from other postoperative symptoms. Approximately one half of patients may develop chronic or acute bleeding.[62] Others have weight loss, nausea and vomiting, gastric outlet obstruction, free perforation, and gastrojejunocolic fistula. Some degree of localized perforation is common.

Diagnosis is often difficult both in terms of the ulcer itself and its cause. Barium studies only detect 50% to 65% of recurrences—postoperative inflammatory changes can be very hard to distinguish from ulceration.[62] Endoscopy has been the procedure of choice for identification of the ulcer and can be diagnostic in the case of malignancy. Serum gastrin levels suggest the presence of gastrinoma or gastrin cell hyperplasia, which can be differentiated by secretin or calcium infusion tests. Acid secretory studies are not very helpful for two reasons. First, seldom have they been performed before surgery to know whether operation has altered the secretory capacity of the stomach, and, second, it has not been determined to what extent acid production must be decreased to indicate completeness of vagotomy. The Hollander insulin test has been shown to cause dangerous hypoglycemia, hypokalemia, and catecholamine release; in addition, it is frequently unreliable. Sham feeding–induced secretion, mediated through vagal pathways, appears to be a fairly good alternative test for completeness of vagotomy in the few published studies in which it has been used.

Treatment

Treatment for recurrence remains somewhat controversial. Before the availability of cimetidine, less than a third of recurrent ulcers healed with medical therapy, and about 40% of those recurred.[46] Cimetidine heals the majority of recurrences, however, and maintenance therapy may prevent redevelopment.[62] Surgery is indicated if the recurrent ulcer fails to heal or again recurs during medical therapy, if a complication develops, or if a compliance problem exists.

Two main approaches have been taken in the surgical therapy for recurrence. Sometimes the operative choice is made on the basis of the preliminary procedure. For example, if subtotal resection was performed, vagotomy may be added. Others specifically tailor the operation to the suspected cause. For suspected incomplete vagotomy, revagotomy is performed. Basically three options exist: vagotomy or revagotomy, resection or reresection, or the combination of vagotomy and antrectomy or gastrectomy. When no attempt is made to reduce acid secretion (e.g., after simple closure of a perforation) the recurrence rate is almost 50%.[62] Revagotomy alone has an approximate 15% recurrence rate, whereas the combination of revagotomy and resection has rates ranging from 1% to 12%.[63] The patient's general medical condition should play a role in decisions regarding therapy. For the poor-risk patient, transthoracic vagotomy may be the safest alternative. However, if the ulcer is large or some other lesion is suspected, laparotomy is mandatory. Gastric recurrence usually indicates that alkaline reflux gastritis plays a role, and surgery should include a Roux loop diversion. In a few instances, examination of the duodenal stump and resection of retained antrum may be all that is necessary.

SUMMARY

In the past three decades significant advances have been made in our understanding of basic gastric physiology and its disturbance in various disease states. A variety of experimental and clinical studies have helped to elucidate the factors responsible for acid secretion and for the capacity of the mucosa to withstand acid-pepsin digestion. Many of these principles have been successfully applied to our clinical management of the various syndromes of gastroduodenal mucosal injury. For example, the findings from a variety of experimental models for acute gastric injury have been used successfully in the preventive management of critically ill patients at risk for development of stress erosions. Likewise, in peptic ulcer the development of a host of therapeutic agents, especially H_2 receptor antagonists, was only possible after elucidation of the physiologic mechanisms of acid secretion and mucosal defense. Progress in the surgical management of acid-peptic disease is a prime example of the successful application of new physiologic principles to the development of more specific therapies. Thus the experimental definition of the importance of vagal pathways and antral gastrin in the control of gastric secretion has prompted the abandonment of the somewhat crudely oblative gastrectomy in favor of the more directed vagotomy and antrectomy. Quite recently, these principles in the control of acid secretion were combined with an understanding of the pathogenic importance of disruptions in vagal innervation and gastrointestinal continuity to the development of postoperative side effects known as the postgastrectomy syndromes. This led to the parietal cell vagotomy, probably the best example of the application of scientific principles to the development of new surgical procedures.

Very recent advances offer exciting possibilities for the future treatment of these disorders. The recognition of the role of *H. pylori* and the demonstration that treatment eliminates recurrence has revolutionized our thinking about acid-peptic disease. Elective operation, uncommon at present, will be increasingly rare. It has even been suggested that, as we learn more about this organism, colonization might be completely avoided, limiting the development of peptic ulcer to an increasingly small group of patients. It seems likely that operation for complications will continue, although in reduced numbers. It remains to be seen whether laparoscopic techniques can successfully be applied in this increasingly small group of patients. Thus there is every indication that this physiologic approach to gastritis and peptic ulceration will continue to enhance our clinical management.

REFERENCES

1. Cheung LY. Pathophysiology of stress-induced gastric mucosal erosions: An update. Surg Gastroenterol 1:235, 1982.
2. Schwarz K. Ueber penetrierende Magen-und Jejunalgeschwure. Beitr Klin Chir 67:96, 1910.
3. Davenport HW, Barr LL. Failure of ischemia to break the dog's gastric mucosal barrier. Gastroenterology 65:619, 1973.
4. Cheung LY, Reese RS, Moody FG. Direct effect of endotoxin on the gastric mucosal microcirculation and electrical gradient. Surgery 79:564, 1976.
5. Ritchie WP Jr. Acute gastric mucosal damage produced by bile salts, acid and ischemia. Gastroenterology 68:699, 1975.
6. Menguy R. Role of gastric mucosal energy metabolism in the etiology of stress ulceration. World J Surg 5:175, 1981.
7. O'Brien P, Silen W. Influence of acid secretory state on the gastric mucosal tolerance to back diffusion of H^+. Gastroenterology 71:760, 1976.
8. Miller TA, Jacobson ED. Gastrointestinal cytoprotection by prostaglandins. Gut 20:75, 1979.
9. Cheung LY. Treatment of established stress ulcer disease. World J Surg 5:235, 1981.
10. Lucas CE, Sugawa C, Riddle J. Natural history and surgical dilemma of "stress" gastric bleeding. Arch Surg 102:266, 1971.
11. Wormsley KG. The pathophysiology of duodenal ulceration. Gut 15:59, 1974.
12. Rotter JI. The genetics of peptic ulcer: more than one gene, more than one disease. Prog Med Genet 4:1, 1980.
13. Gillies MA, Skyring A. Gastric and duodenal ulcer, the association between aspirin ingestion, smoking, and family history of ulcer. Med J Aust 2:280, 1969.
14. Graham DY, Go MF. *Helicobacter pylori:* Current status. Gastroenterology 105:279, 1993.
15. Mertz HR, Walsh JH. Peptic ulcer pathophysiology. Med Clin North Am 75:799, 1991.
16. Wormsley KG. Smoking and duodenal ulcer [editorial]. Gastroenterology 75:139, 1978.
17. Paffenbarger RS Jr, Wing AL, Hyde RT. Chronic disease in former college students. XIII. Early precursors of peptic ulcer. Am J Epidemiol 100:307, 1974.
18. Richardson CT. Gastric ulcer. In Sleisenger MH, Fordtran JS, eds. Gastrointestinal Disease: Pathophysiology, Diagnosis, Management. Philadelphia: WB Saunders, 1983.
19. Fisher RS, Cohen S. Pyloric sphincter dysfunction in patients with gastric ulcer. N Engl J Med 288:273, 1976.
20. Dragstedt LR. The pathogenesis of duodenal and gastric ulcers. Am J Surg 136:286, 1978.
21. Du Plessis DJ. Pathogenesis of gastric ulceration. Lancet 1:974, 1965.
22. Baron JH. Current views on pathogenesis of peptic ulcer. Scand J Gastroenterol 170(Suppl 80):1, 1982.
23. Carter DC. Aetiology of peptic ulcer. In Sircus W, Smith AN, eds. Scientific Foundations of Gastroenterology. Philadelphia: WB Saunders, 1980.

24. Trudeau WL, McGuigan JE. Relations between serum gastrin levels and rates of gastric hydrochloric acid secretion. N Engl J Med 284:408, 1971.
25. Oi M, Oshida K, Sugimura S. The location of gastric ulcer. Gastroenterology 36:45, 1959.
26. Grossman MI, moderator. UCLA Conference: Peptic ulcer: New therapies, new diseases. Ann Intern Med 95:609, 1981.
27. Kurato JH, Honda GD, Frankl H. Hospitalization and mortality rates for peptic ulcers: A comparison of a large health maintenance organization and United States data. Gastroenterology 83:1008, 1982.
28. Peterson WL, Richardson CT. Pharmacology and side effects of drugs used to treat peptic ulcer. In Sleisenger MH, Fordtran JS, eds. Gastrointestinal Disease: Pathophysiology, Diagnosis, Management. Philadelphia: WB Saunders, 1983.
29. Kirk AP, Dooley JS, Hunt RH. Peptic ulceration in patients with chronic liver disease. Dig Dis Sci 25:756, 1980.
30. Owens ML, et al. Treatment of peptic ulcer disease in the renal transplant patient. Ann Surg 186:17, 1977.
31. Grossman MI, ed. Peptic Ulcer: A Guide for the Practicing Physician. Chicago: Year Book Medical Publishers, 1981.
32. McCarthy DM. Peptic ulcer heterogeneity and clinical implications [editorial]. Ann Intern Med 95:507, 1981.
33. Balard HS, Frame B, Hansock RJ. Familial multiple endocrine adenoma-peptic ulcer complex. Medicine 43:481, 1964.
34. Samloff IM. Pepsinogens and their relationship to peptic ulcer. In Rotter JL, Samloff IM, Rimoin DL, eds. The Genetics and Heterogeneity of Common Gastrointestinal Disorders. New York: Academic Press, 1980.
35. Wolf S. Peptic ulcer: Psychosomatic illness review: No. 3 in a series. Psychosomatics 23:1101, 1982.
36. Cox AJ. Stomach size and its relation to chronic peptic ulcer. Arch Pathol 54:403, 1952.
37. Johnson LR. The trophic action of gastrointestinal hormones. Gastroenterology 70:278, 1976.
38. Soll AH, Isenberg JI. Duodenal ulcer diseases. In Sleisenger MH, Fordtran JS, eds. Gastrointestinal Disease: Pathophysiology, Diagnosis, Management. Philadelphia: WB Saunders, 1983.
39. Feldman M, Richardson CT, Fordtran S. Effect of sham feeding on gastric acid secretion in healthy subjects and duodenal ulcer patients: Evidence for increased vagal tone in some ulcer patients. Gastroenterology 79:796, 1980.
40. Peden NR, et al. Gastric mucosal histamine and histamine methyltransferase in patients with duodenal ulcers. Gut 23:56, 1982.
41. Malagelada JR, et al. Gastric secretion and emptying after normal meals in duodenal ulcer. Gastroenterology 73:981, 1977.
42. Lam SK, et al. Gastric acid secretion is abnormally sensitive to exogenous gastrin released after peptone test meals in duodenal ulcer patients. J Clin Invest 65:555, 1980.
43. Isenberg JI, et al. Impaired proximal duodenal mucosal bicarbonate secretion in patients with duodenal ulcer. N Engl J Med 316:374, 1987.
44. Stabile BE, Passaro E Jr. Duodenal ulcer: A disease in evolution. Curr Probl Surg 21:1, 1984.
45. Walker C. Complications of peptic ulcer disease and indications for surgery. In Sleisenger MH, Fordtran JS, eds. Gastrointestinal Disease: Pathophysiology, Diagnosis, Management. Philadelphia: WB Saunders, 1983.
46. Stabile BE, Passaro E Jr. Recurrent peptic ulcer. Gastroenterology 70:124, 1976.
47. McGuigan JE. The Zollinger-Ellison syndrome. In Sleisenger MH, Fordtran JS, eds. Gastrointestinal Disease: Pathophysiology, Diagnosis, Management. Philadelphia: WB Saunders, 1983.
48. Priebe HJ, et al. Antacid versus cimetidine in preventing acute gastrointestinal bleeding: A randomized trial in 75 critically ill patients. N Engl J Med 302:426, 1980.
49. Modlin IM, Brennan MF. The diagnosis and management of gastrinoma. Surg Gynecol Obstet 158:97, 1984.
50. Soll AH, Grossman MI. The interaction of stimulants on the function of isolated canine parietal cells. Philos Trans R Soc Lond (Biol) 296:5, 1981.
51. Dal Monte PR, et al. Pirenzepine versus cimetidine in duodenal ulcer: A double-blind placebo-controlled short-term clinical trial. Hepatogastroenterology 27(Suppl):48, 1980.
52. Folkman J, et al. Duodenal ulcer: Discovery of a new mechanism and development of angiogenic therapy that accelerates healing. Ann Surg 214:414, 1991.
53. Kelly KA, Hinder RA. Evaluation of surgical procedures. In Sircus W, Smith AN, eds. Scientific Foundations of Gastroenterology. Philadelphia: WB Saunders, 1980.
54. Zucker KA, ed. Surgical Laparoscopy. St. Louis: Quality Medical Publishing, 1991.
55. Athanasoulis CA, et al. Control of acute gastric mucosal hemorrhage. Intraarterial infusion of posterior pituitary extract. N Engl J Med 290:597, 1974.
56. Marks IN, et al. Ulcer healing and relapse rates after initial treatment with cimetidine or sucralfate. J Clin Gastroenterol 3(Suppl 2):163, 1981.
57. Eshelman F, Sanzari N, DeFelice S. "Placebo" responsiveness of peptic ulcers [letter]. Gastroenterology 74:159, 1978.
58. Fitzpatrick WJF, Blackwood WS, Northfield TC. Bedtime cimetidine maintenance treatment: Optimum dose and effect on subsequent natural history of duodenal ulcer. Gut 23:239, 1982.
59. Al-Assi MT, Graham DY. Peptic ulcer disease, *Helicobacter pylori,* and the surgeon: Changing the guard. In Daly JM, ed. Current Opinion in General Surgery, 2nd ed. Philadelphia: Current Science, 1994, p. 120.
60. Jordan PH Jr. Peptic ulcer disease and early postoperative complications. In Sleisenger MH, Fordtran JS, eds. Gastrointestinal Disease: Pathophysiology, Diagnosis, Management. Philadelphia: WB Saunders, 1983.
61. Steiger E, Cooperman AM. Considerations in the management of perforated peptic ulcers. Surg Clin North Am 56:1395, 1976.
62. Feldman M. Postoperative recurrent ulcer. N Engl J Med 302:749, 1980.
63. Fromm D. Complications of Gastric Surgery. New York: John Wiley, 1977.

17

Derangements in Gastric Function Secondary to Previous Surgery

Thomas A. Miller and David W. Mercer

Although operative procedures on the stomach are less commonly performed today than they were a decade or two ago because of the decreasing incidence of gastric cancer and the ability to manage most forms of acid-peptic disease with various pharmacologic manipulations, gastric procedures are still performed with sufficient frequency that an understanding of those derangements that may be surgically induced is paramount to good surgical practice. Virtually any type of gastric operation is attended by some type of postoperative symptomatology; fortunately, the majority of these physiologic alterations can be managed with little patient inconvenience. Despite a surgeon's best efforts, however, a small percentage of patients subjected to gastric surgery develop untoward sequelae that can be devastating not only to a patient's sense of well-being but also to his ability to function in society and continue gainful employment. These physiologic aberrations can result from the loss of normal gastric reservoir function, transection of the vagus nerves, or interruption of normal pyloric sphincter function, or they may be directly related to the procedure performed to restore normal gastrointestinal continuity following treatment of the underlying disease. An understanding of the pathophysiology responsible for these various derangements is mandatory if successful management is to be effectively rendered.

DERANGEMENTS RELATED TO GASTRIC RESECTION OR INTERRUPTION OF NORMAL PYLORIC SPHINCTER FUNCTION

Dumping Syndrome

The dumping syndrome refers to the symptom complex that occurs following the ingestion of a meal when a portion of the stomach has previously been removed or the normal pyloric sphincter mechanism has been disrupted. Both an early and late form of this syndrome have been described, with the early form occurring considerably more frequently.

Early Dumping

The early form of the dumping syndrome usually occurs within 10 to 30 minutes following the ingestion of a meal and is associated with both gastrointestinal and cardiovascular symptomatology. The gastrointestinal symptoms include nausea and vomiting, a sense of epigastric fullness, eructations, crampy abdominal pain, and often explosive diarrhea. The cardiovascular symptoms include palpitations, tachycardia, diaphoresis, fainting, dizziness, flushing, and occasionally blurred vision. Characteristically these symptoms occur while the patient is seated at the table eating or shortly after arising. The symptom complex can develop after any operation on the stomach, but is especially common after partial gastrectomy with a Billroth II reconstruction in which as many as 50% to 60% of patients may be victims, especially if more than two thirds of the stomach has been removed. Less commonly it is observed after a Billroth I gastrectomy and in patients following vagotomy and drainage procedures, particularly if the type of drainage was a generous gastroenterostomy or a Finney-type pyloroplasty. Only rarely does this full-blown symptom complex supervene, and usually the gastrointestinal symptomatology is more frequently encountered than the vasomotor aberrations.

Although the exact sequence of events responsible for this syndrome remains to be defined, there is general agreement that it occurs because of the rapid passage of food of high osmolarity from the stomach into the small intestine.[1,2] This occurs because the previous gastric resection or interrupted pyloric sphincteric mechanism no longer allows the stomach to prepare its contents and deliver them to the proximal bowel in the form of small particles in isosmotic solution. Thus the resulting discharge of this hyperosmotic chyme into the small intestine induces a rapid shift of extracellular fluid into the intestinal lumen to achieve isotonicity. The luminal distention that follows and the autonomic responses induced by the resultant decrease in circulating plasma volume are thought to be responsible for many of the symptoms of this syndrome.

To what extent the contracted blood volume per se gives rise to the autonomic symptoms following dumping remains to be clarified, since several studies have failed to demonstrate a clear correlation between the severity of symptoms and the magnitude of blood volume derangements.[1] On the other hand, a number of studies have demonstrated that the release of several humoral agents is increased in patients with dumping and not in asymptomatic patients after gastrectomy, suggesting the agents are involved in the pathogenesis of this syndrome. Serotonin, for example, is released from the intestine in response to distention, and serotonin antagonists have been shown to benefit some patients with dumping symptoms.[3,4] Further evidence exists that plasma levels of a bradykinin-like substance are likewise elevated during dumping attacks and that bradykinin can reproduce many of the vasomotor components of the syndrome when administered exogenously.[5] Additionally, neurotensin[6] and vasoactive intestinal peptide[7] levels have been demonstrated to be increased in patients with the dumping syndrome. Finally, plasma enteroglucagon concentrations are increased after gastrectomy in symptomatic patients following a glucose challenge, in contrast to control subjects without the dumping syndrome.[8] In addition, this agent inhibits sodium and water absorption from the small intestine and through such a mechanism could account for the diarrhea that occurs in early dumping.

Generally, the symptoms associated with dumping are sufficiently obvious that the diagnosis can be made on this basis alone. It must be emphasized, however, that in any group of patients complaining of dumpinglike symptoms, a high proportion of individuals with social problems, various neuroses, and occasionally alcoholism may be present.[9] Thus if any doubt exists concerning the exact cause of the symptomatology, objective support for the diagnosis should be obtained, especially if a surgical procedure to correct the problem is potentially anticipated. This would include the demonstration of rapid gastric emptying on upper gastrointestinal barium study or by assessment with one of the currently available radionuclide techniques.[10] Another diagnostic approach is use of a provocation test in which a patient is given a meal of 200 ml of a 50% glucose solution in water.[11] In patients with the dumping syndrome, instillation of this liquid meal into the residual stomach has been shown to provoke the symptom complex concomitant with a fall in plasma volume.

It is of interest that the majority of patients subjected to gastric surgery complain of some dumpinglike symptoms in the early months following surgery. Most of these individuals, however, experience spontaneous relief and require no specific treatment.[12,13] Of those patients plagued with prolonged symptomatology, dietary measures alone can effect adequate management in most instances. Such measures should include avoiding foods containing large amounts of sugars, frequent feeding of small meals rich in protein and fat, and separating liquids from solids during a meal. If hot drinks elicit symptoms, as occurs in some patients, they should also be avoided. Lying down when symptoms do occur may likewise be beneficial, since gravity can aggravate dumping symptomatology. In some patients, carbohydrate gelling agents such as pectin have been ingested with the meal and shown to be of some success[14]; unfortunately, these agents are rather unpalatable and not readily tolerated for long periods of time.

Previously, serotonin antagonists were the only pharmacologic agents available that had potential benefit in the relief of dumping symptoms. Both methysergide maleate (Sansert) and cyproheptadine (Periactin) have been helpful in some individuals when given before meals.[3] Usually, however, large doses of such agents were required, which produced their own disagreeable side effects. Thus their use in any long-term fashion was limited.

Recently, the long-acting somatostatin analog, octreotide acetate (Sandostatin), has been shown to be highly effective in preventing the development of symptoms in the early dumping syndrome, both vasomotor and gastrointestinal.[15] Treatment with this synthetic analog of somatostatin was demonstrated to inhibit the hormonal responses associated with this syndrome and to completely ablate diarrhea.[15] In addition, intestinal motility is altered by octreotide acetate.[16] This peptide was demonstrated to not only inhibit gastric emptying, but was also demonstrated to induce a fasting or interdigestive small bowel motility pattern in patients with the dumping syndrome such that intestinal transit of an ingested meal was prolonged.[16] Thus Sandostatin appears to be a very promising agent in the nonoperative treatment of incapacitating early dumping syndrome by changing the hormonal response elicited by an ingested meal and by altering intestinal transit. Furthermore, the side effects associated with administration of this synthetic peptide are relatively innocuous,[15] consisting of occasional mild abdominal cramping immediately following its subcutaneous administration.

In the few patients (1% or less) who fail to respond to these treatment measures, operative intervention may become necessary. The physiologic rationale behind surgery should be to improve gastric reservoir function, decrease the rapid gastric emptying, or ideally accomplish both of these goals. Although a wide variety of surgical procedures have been used to manage dumping, the use of isoperistaltic or antiperistaltic jejunal segments has met with the greatest success in dealing with this problem in most centers (Fig. 17-1). With the former approach, a 10 to 20 cm loop of jejunum is interposed between the stomach and small intestine in an isoperistaltic fashion.[17,18] Over time this loop dilates and thereby promotes reservoir function. It also appears to delay gastric emptying, at least that of liquids. In the antiperistaltic approach a jejunal segment 10 cm in length is used, in which the jejunum is twisted on its mesentery so that its distal end is anastomosed to the stomach and its proximal end to the small intestine.[18,19] The resulting reversal in peristalsis permits the loop to act as a

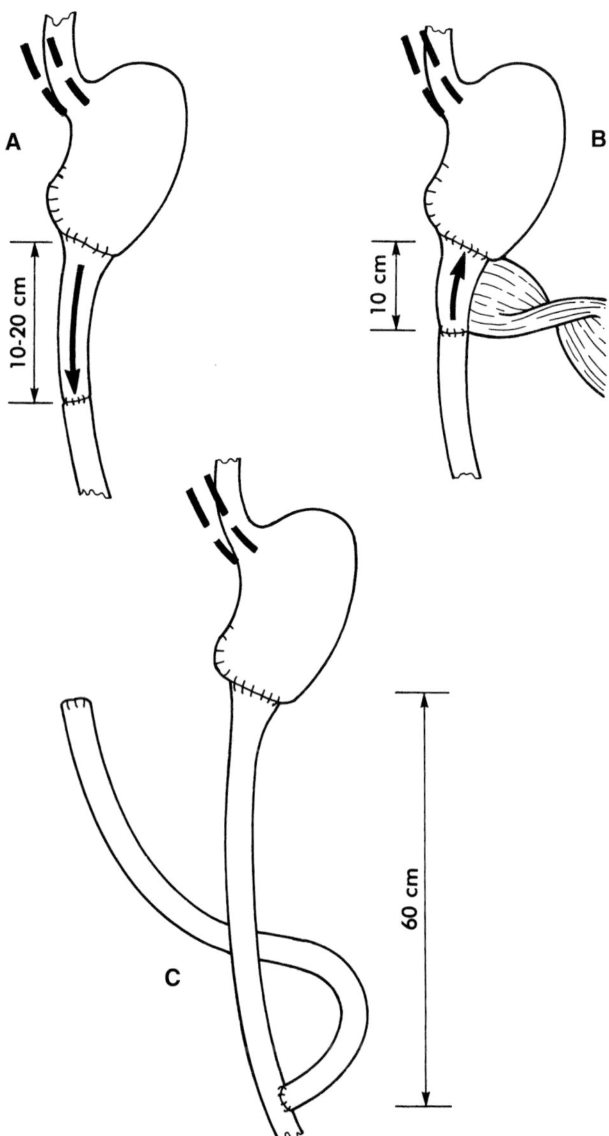

Fig. 17-1. Surgical approaches to treat the dumping syndrome. **A,** A 10 to 20 cm loop of jejunum is interposed between the stomach and the small intestine in an isoperistaltic fashion. **B,** A 10 cm loop of jejunum is twisted on its mesentery so that its distal end is anastomosed to the stomach, and its proximal end to the small intestine in an antiperistaltic fashion. **C,** A long-limb Roux-en-Y anastomosis where the jejunojejunostomy is fashioned approximately 60 cm from the gastrojejunostomy.

substitute pylorus, enabling it to slow the rate of gastric emptying and thereby allow more time for mixing and grinding of food before delivery into the small bowel. Published experience with this latter technique is now in excess of 10 years, demonstrating significant alleviation of symptoms in more than 90% of patients.[19] Another technique is the creation of a long-limb Roux-en-Y anastomosis to delay gastric emptying[20] (see Fig. 17-1). Whether this approach is superior to the use of isoperistaltic or antiperistaltic jejunal segments has yet to be determined.

Late Dumping

Late dumping occurs 2 to 3 hours after a meal and is considerably less common than its early counterpart. Like early dumping, the basic defect in this disorder is also rapid gastric emptying. In this situation, however, it is related specifically to carbohydrates and can be induced by meals containing large amounts of monosaccharides or disaccharides. When these sugars are delivered rapidly to the small intestine, they are quickly absorbed. The resulting hyperglycemia triggers the release of large amounts of insulin to control the rising blood sugar. In the attempt to normalize blood sugar, an actual "overshooting" occurs so that a profound hypoglycemia ensues. Catecholamine released by the adrenal gland is then activated, with the resulting symptoms of diaphoresis, tremulousness, light-headedness, tachycardia, and confusion. This symptom complex is indistinguishable from insulin shock.

As with early dumping, patients should be advised to ingest frequent small meals and markedly reduce their carbohydrate intake. Pectin has also been used in the treatment of this disorder, either alone or in combination with acarbose, an α-glucoside hydrolase inhibitor, a compound that delays carbohydrate absorption through impairment of intraluminal starch and sucrose digestion.[14,21] If these nonoperative approaches fail, the use of an antiperistaltic loop of jejunum between the residual gastric pouch and intestine has also been shown to effectively manage this problem (see Fig. 17-1). Not only does this loop delay gastric emptying, but it also results in a flattening of the glucose tolerance curve and an alleviation of the hypoglycemic symptomatology.[22]

Small Stomach Syndrome

If an excessive amount of the stomach has been removed, leaving only a small gastric pouch, some patients may develop the small stomach syndrome. This syndrome is characterized by extreme discomfort following the ingestion of even small amounts of food. Because of this unpleasant sensation and the fact that vomiting often occurs if any attempt is made to increase oral intake, patients with this disorder are frequently malnourished. The exact cause of this disorder is uncertain, but it probably develops because of the inability of the proximal stomach to dilate and receive a bolus of food without increasing intragastric pressure.[2] Normally the vagus nerve, which has been transsected in most of these patients, initiates distention of the stomach to allow accommodation of ingested food, a process known as receptive relaxation. If this vagally mediated action has been interrupted, such relaxation does not occur, and the intragastric pressure increases with distention on reception of food.

Unfortunately, treatment of this problem has remained extremely difficult. Although frequent small feedings and various liquid and enteral diets have been tried to alleviate symptoms, such nonoperative approaches have usually been unsuccessful. A number of operative approaches have

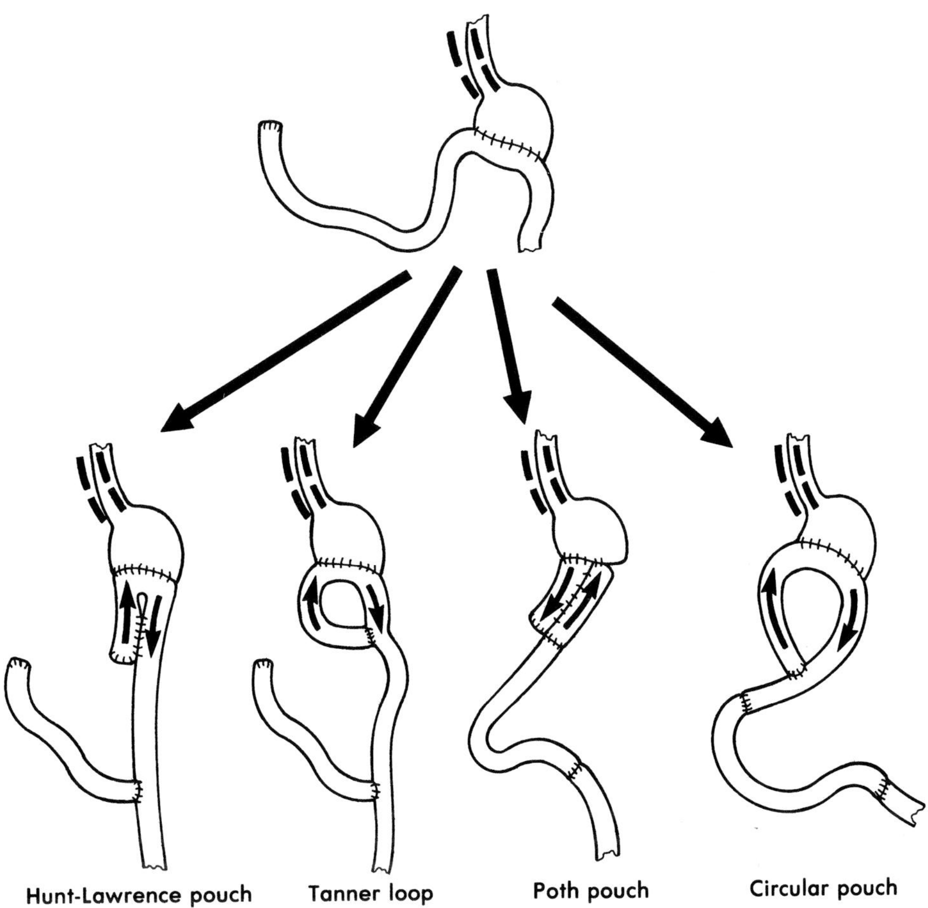

Fig. 17-2. Surgical management of the short stomach syndrome.

also been used with varying degrees of success. These have included procedures to enlarge the gastric reservoir through the creation of various pouches interposed between the stomach and intestine[23] (Fig. 17-2). Jejunal interposition with the use of an isoperistaltic limb has also been used to treat this disorder with reasonable success in alleviating symptoms and improving the underlying malnutrition problems.[24] In view of the difficulty in managing this disorder, the best approach is to prevent its development rather than to attempt to treat it when it occurs.

Metabolic Disturbances

Metabolic problems may develop following any type of gastric procedure, but they are more common and serious after partial gastrectomy than after vagotomy, and the incidence following gastrectomy is much greater if a Billroth II rather than a Billroth I approach has been used in reconstruction.[25] As with dumping, the severity of these disturbances is directly related to the extent of the gastric resection.

Anemia is clearly the most common metabolic derangement. Two major types have been identified: (1) that related to a deficiency of iron and (2) that related to an impairment in vitamin B_{12} metabolism. Of the two, iron deficiency is the more common, and more than 30% to 50% of patients carefully evaluated demonstrate this type of anemia following gastrectomy. The exact cause has remained elusive, but it appears to be related to a combination of (1) decreased iron uptake; (2) impaired iron absorption; and (3) chronic subliminal blood loss secondary to the hyperemic, friable gastric mucosa primarily involving the margins of the stoma where the stomach connects with the small intestine.[2,25] Generally, the addition of iron supplements to the patient's diet corrects this problem.

A megaloblastic anemia can also occur following subtotal gastrectomy (50% or greater) but only rarely develops after partial gastric resection (e.g., antrectomy). This problem is caused by a deficiency of vitamin B_{12} secondary to poor absorption of this substance because of the lack of intrinsic factor secretion in the gastric juice.[2,25] The more extensive the gastric resection, the more likely is this deficiency; it always occurs following total gastrectomy. If a patient develops a macrocytic anemia, a serum B_{12} level should be obtained. If this is abnormal, the patient should be treated by intramuscular injection of cyanocobalamin every 3 to 4 months indefinitely, since its administration orally is not a reliable route. The other cause of macrocytosis is a folate deficiency. This is a rare anemia following gastric resection, but it may coexist with an iron or vitamin B_{12} deficiency anemia. It is usually a consequence of inadequate oral intake and can generally be corrected by dietary supplementation.

Impaired absorption of fat is relatively common following any type of gastric operation, but the magnitude of fecal fat loss is usually small and of little importance clinically. Occasionally, steatorrhea is seen after a Billroth II gastrectomy and probably occurs as a result of inadequate mixing of bile salts and pancreatic lipase with ingested fat because of bypass of the duodenum. When this results, deficiencies in the uptake of fat-soluble vitamins may also be observed. For mild degrees of fat malabsorption, no treatment is indicated. If steatorrhea develops, pancreatic replacement enzymes are often effective in decreasing fat loss. Feeding with medium chain triglycerides is also of value, since these substances do not require bile and pancreatic lipase for absorption.

Occasionally, gastric resection is associated with the development of bone disease. Both osteoporosis and osteomalacia have been observed and appear to be caused by deficiencies in calcium absorption. If fat malabsorption is also present, the calcium problem is further aggravated, since free fatty acids bind calcium; further, fat malabsorption also inhibits the absorption of vitamin D, an important component in normal calcium balance.[2] The incidence of this problem clearly increases with the extent of gastric resection and is mainly an aberration associated with a Billroth II gastrectomy.[25,26] Usually the bone disease develops insidiously, and symptoms are generally not seen until 4 or 5 years after surgery. Occasionally, spontaneous fractures or unexplained aches and pains in the back or bones may be the only indication that a calcium deficiency exists. Treatment of this disorder is usually straightforward and includes the administration of calcium supplements (1 to 2 g/day) and vitamin D (500 to 5000 U daily). In patients developing postgastrectomy bone disease, serial serum calcium determinations are indicated, and adjustments in calcium supplementation and vitamin D administration are altered accordingly.

Weight loss is relatively common following surgical procedures on the stomach but is generally not a significant problem, except in those individuals who have had either all or substantial portions of their stomach removed, in which case considerable malnutrition may develop. The degree of weight loss correlates closely with such factors as the presence or absence of dumping, steatorrhea, diarrhea, abdominal discomfort during eating, and bilious vomiting.[27,28] Treatment of malnutrition is directed at improving nutritional balance by multiple small feedings, avoidance of factors that may precipitate the dumping syndrome, and dietary or pharmacologic management of diarrhea and/or steatorrhea. If such manipulations are not successful in treating this problem, some type of surgical procedure to delay gastric emptying and/or enhance the gastric reservoir effect, as outlined previously, may become necessary.

DERANGEMENTS RELATED TO GASTRIC RECONSTRUCTION

A number of disorders may develop following gastric resection that are directly related to the approach used to establish gastrointestinal continuity. All these problems are more commonly encountered in patients who have had a Billroth II gastrectomy, and the afferent loop and retained antrum syndromes occur exclusively in patients with this type of gastrectomy.

Afferent Loop Syndrome

The afferent loop syndrome is a mechanical problem produced by partial obstruction of the afferent loop resulting in its inability to empty its contents. Consequently, it can only occur following gastrectomy with a Billroth II type of reconstruction. A variety of causes can give rise to this obstruction, including angulation of the anastomosis with kinking, herniation of the afferent loop posterior to the efferent loop, stenosis of the gastrojejunostomy, volvulus, and adhesions (Fig. 17-3). This disorder is nearly always associated with the presence of a long (greater than 30 to 40 cm) afferent limb that has been anastomosed to the gastric remnant in an anticolic fashion. Both acute and chronic forms of this disorder have been recognized, but chronic afferent loop obstruction is clearly more common.[29,30]

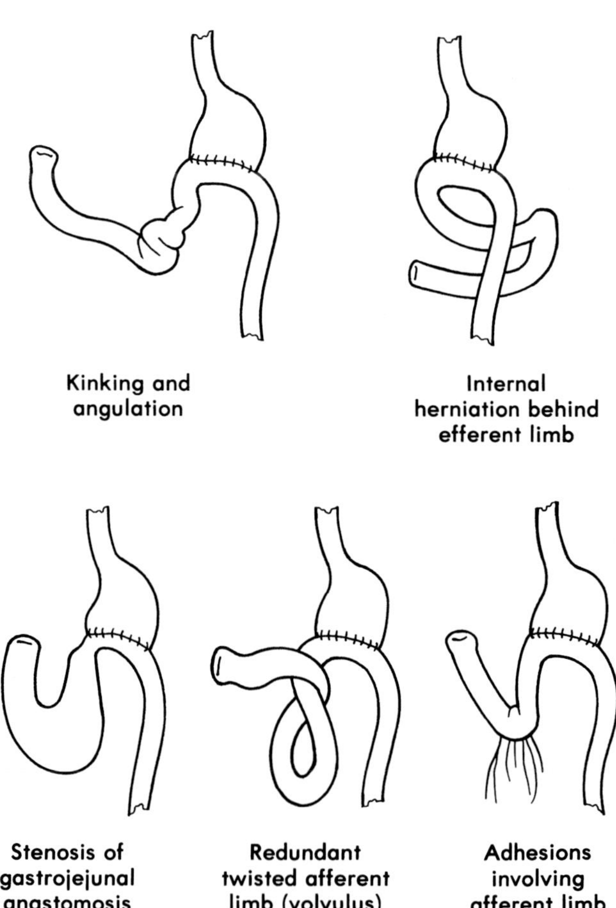

Fig. 17-3. Causes of the afferent loop syndrome.

From a pathophysiologic standpoint, the syndrome occurs because of an accumulation of pancreatic and hepatobiliary secretions within the obstructed loop, resulting in its distention. The stimulus for such secretion is the presence of food in the gastric remnant and efferent loop, which elicits the various neurohumoral mechanisms involved in normal digestion. Such distention results in epigastric discomfort and cramping. If the loop is only partially obstructed, the increasing intraluminal pressure is usually capable of overcoming it, following which the afferent loop empties its contents into the stomach, resulting in forceful (and sometimes projectile) vomiting of bilious material with immediate relief of symptoms. The vomitus lacks food, since any ingested meal has already passed into the efferent limb. If the obstruction is complete, necrosis and perforation of the loop can occur. This is a consequence of the surgical closure of the proximal duodenum that is performed during a Billroth II gastrectomy, resulting in a closed-loop type of obstruction. In this circumstance, constant abdominal pain is noted that can involve the entire upper abdomen, often more pronounced in the right upper quadrant, with radiation into the interscapular area. Unless this distention is surgically relieved, a lethal outcome may ensue from perforation and subsequent peritonitis.

In most patients suffering from the afferent loop syndrome, only partial obstruction of the afferent limb is present.[29,30] Symptoms may exist for months or sometimes even years. These symptoms are directly related to eating, at which time the hepatobiliary and pancreatic secretions distend the loop. Bile-stained material devoid of food is vomited after the meal has passed into the efferent limb, relieving symptoms; and the patient is relatively comfortable until the next meal. Obviously the degree of afferent loop obstruction influences the extent to which the patient is incapacitated by the symptoms and the need to seek medical treatment. If partial afferent loop obstruction has been present for a long period, it may be aggravated by the development of the blind loop syndrome. In this condition, bacterial overgrowth of enteric organisms proliferates in the static loop and binds with vitamin B_{12} and deconjugated bile acids.[2] This results in a systemic deficiency of vitamin B_{12} with the development of megaloblastic anemia and an inefficient micellization of fat that, if severe enough, can create steatorrhea.

The acute form of afferent loop obstruction may occur early after operation (within a few days) or may develop quite unexpectedly months to years following the Billroth II gastrectomy. In both circumstances it is caused by acute blockage of the afferent limb, as may occur with volvulus or herniation of the afferent loop posterior to the efferent loop. Because of the resulting closed-loop type of obstruction, acute afferent loop obstruction must be corrected by immediate operation. Although physical findings are usually nonspecific with the exception of the occurrence of a palpable abdominal mass in about one third of patients,[2] the associated pain and tenderness are usually severe enough to indicate the necessity of urgent operative intervention. Even if the diagnosis may not have been made before surgery, findings at surgery confirm the underlying cause.

In contrast to the diagnosis of the acute form, that of chronic afferent loop obstruction may be more difficult. Although symptoms are often suggestive of this abnormality, confirmation of the diagnosis may be difficult. Usually the dilated afferent limb is not demonstrable on plain films of the abdomen, and only occasionally do contrast barium studies of the stomach delineate the presence of an obstructed loop. Failure to visualize the afferent limb on upper endoscopy is suggestive evidence for the diagnosis. Hepatobiliary radionuclide imaging techniques have been used with some success in diagnosing the afferent loop syndrome.[2] With this technique the hepatic excretion of a previously administered radionuclide is followed after giving a patient a fatty meal or the hormone cholecystokinin. If the nuclide fails to pass into the stomach or distal bowel after being excreted into the afferent limb, the possibility of an afferent loop obstruction must be considered. Although this technique shows diagnostic promise, its clinical usefulness remains to be determined.

Because the afferent loop syndrome, whether acute or chronic, is a mechanical problem, operation is the only effective treatment. With few exceptions, a long afferent limb is usually the underlying problem. Thus treatment involves the elimination of this loop. A variety of procedures have been advocated to accomplish this feat, including the conversion of a Billroth II construction into a Billroth I anastomosis, enteroenterostomy below the stoma, and the use of a Roux-en-Y anastomosis[1] (Fig. 17-4). If the latter procedure is used, a concomitant vagotomy should also be performed to prevent marginal ulceration from the diversion of duodenal contents from the gastroenteric stoma.

Efferent Loop Obstruction

Compared to other derangements in gastric function following previous surgery, obstruction of the efferent limb of a gastrojejunostomy is relatively rare. Clearly the most common cause of such obstruction is herniation of the limb behind the anastomosis in a right-to-left direction.[31] This problem occurs because of the space that exists posterior to the anastomosis after construction of a gastrojejunostomy and has been described with both antecolic and retrocolic gastrojejunostomies. The preference for herniation in the right-to-left direction most likely results from the fact that the gastrojejunostomy lies to the left of the main mass of small intestine, thus making it mechanically easier for herniation to occur from right to left.[1] Although obstruction of the efferent loop is the usual circumstance with this type of herniation, it may also compress the mesentery of the afferent limb and thereby compromise its blood supply and/or obstruct the afferent limb as well.

Efferent limb obstruction following gastrojejunostomy from a retroanastomic hernia may occur at any time fol-

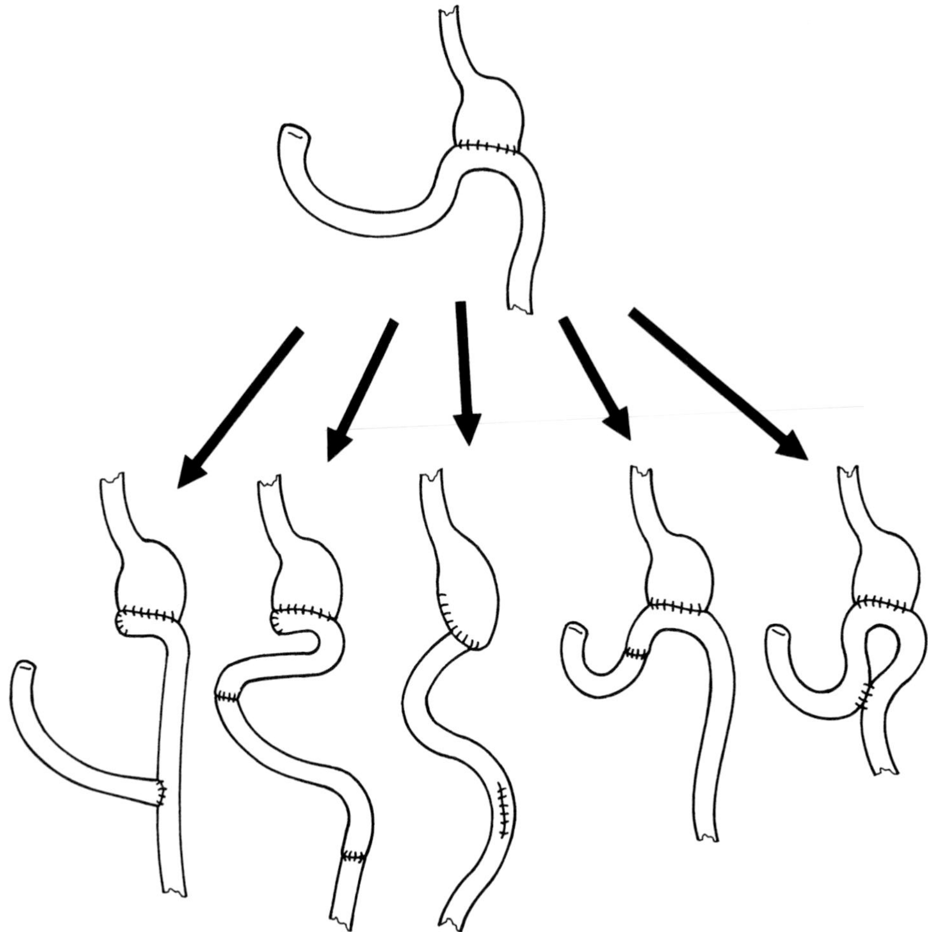

Fig. 17-4. Surgical management of the afferent loop syndrome.

lowing surgery, but more than half of the patients who develop this disorder do so within the first postoperative month. Diagnosis is frequently difficult. Initial complaints include colicky left upper quadrant pain; copious, bilious vomiting; and abdominal distention. Usually the most helpful diagnostic maneuver is a contrast barium study of the stomach in which barium fails to enter the efferent limb. Operative therapy is virtually always required and consists of reducing the retroanastomotic hernia and ensuring that the retroanastomotic space is securely closed to prevent recurrence of this condition.

Alkaline Reflux Gastritis

Reflux of bile into the stomach is relatively common following surgical procedures on this organ. In a small percentage of patients this reflux is associated with severe, continuous, unrelenting epigastric pain and bilious vomiting and weight loss.[2,32-36] Occasionally, this pain is substernal in nature, but despite its location, it is characteristically not relieved by food or antacids. The bilious vomiting may occur at any time during the day or night and not uncommonly awakens a patient from sleep. The diagnosis is made by taking a careful history along with a complete examination of the gastrointestinal tract including scintigraphic assessment of gastric emptying; gastroscopy in combination with multiple biopsy specimens taken away from the stoma; gastric analysis; gastric bile acid concentration content; and Tc-99m-labeled sulfur colloid to demonstrate reflux of bile into the gastric remnant. On endoscopic examination of the stomach, the mucosa is noted to be beefy red and friable and frequently demonstrates superficial erosions that may extend into the distal esophagus. Microscopically, both parietal and chief cells are greatly diminished, and superficial mucosal ulcerations are common with evidence of hemorrhage, atrophy, and intestinalization of the epithelial surface. It is not uncommon for achlorhydria to be present in many patients affected with this condition; and little, if any, response is elicited following stimulation with a secretagogue such as pentagastrin. Associated with these findings is the frequent demonstration of an iron deficiency anemia and weight loss. Since patients with this constellation of signs and symptoms are lacking in other explainable causes, the association of an alkaline gastric content, endoscopic gastritis in combination with bile reflux, and histologic confirmation of mucosal injury has been termed alkaline reflux gastritis.[2,35,36]

In most patients who develop alkaline reflux gastritis, gastric resection with restoration of gastrointestinal continuity with a Billroth II approach has been used.[2] The syndrome has also been reported after gastroduodenostomy or gastroenterostomy and in a few patients who have undergone vagotomy and drainage procedures.[33] Symptoms may develop any time following operation and have been observed as late as 20 years following surgery. Although bile reflux appears to be the inciting event, a number of problems remain unanswered with respect to the role of bile in its pathogenesis.[2,35,36] For example, both clinical and experimental reports indicate that enterogastric reflux is quite common following gastric surgery, although gastric mucosal injury is not an invariable consequence of this circumstance. In addition, asymptomatic patients frequently demonstrate histologic and endoscopic changes in the gastric epithelium not unlike those with symptoms of alkaline reflux gastritis. Finally, a clear correlation between the volume of bile and its composition (i.e., primary and secondary bile acid components) and the subsequent development of alkaline gastritis has never been proved. Thus although it appears that the syndrome does in fact exist, caution must be exercised to be sure that it is not overdiagnosed.

Although a variety of approaches have been used to manage the symptoms of alkaline reflux gastritis, medical treatment has usually failed in this condition. Antacids, H_2 = receptor antagonists (e.g., cimetidine), anticholinergics, and cholestyramine have been tried to relieve symptoms without consistently demonstrating efficacious results. Consequently, patients who have intractable problems with this disorder should undergo surgery. The principle underlying surgery is to divert the bile and pancreatic secretions away from the stomach. Although a large number of approaches have been used to accomplish this feat, the most effective operative procedure in terms of relieving symptoms, promoting weight gain, and reversing the findings seen in alkaline gastritis has been achieved with the use of a Roux-en-Y gastrojejunostomy in which the Roux limb has been 41 to 46 cm in length.[2,36,37]

Retained Antrum Syndrome

Occasionally, inadequate resection of the gastric antrum may occur during partial gastrectomy, even though the resection was carried beyond the pyloric sphincter. This happens because the antral mucosa may extend past the pyloric muscle for a distance of 0.5 cm.[38] The significance in remembering this is that a Billroth II anastomosis can result in the development of a retained antrum syndrome if residual antrum is included in the duodenal stump. This circumstance allows the retained antrum to be continually exposed to an alkaline pH from the duodenal, pancreatic, and biliary juices that may in turn stimulate the release of large amounts of gastrin with a corresponding continuous hypersecretion of hydrochloric acid in the gastric remnant. This highly ulcerogenic preparation is responsible for about 9% of recurrent ulcers following previous surgery for peptic ulcer disease and is associated with an incidence of recurrent ulceration as high as 80%.[39,40] This potential problem can virtually be eliminated if biopsy confirmation of duodenal mucosa is obtained during resection of the proximal duodenum at the time of a Billroth II gastrectomy.

If a patient develops a recurrent ulcer following previous gastrectomy for ulcer disease in which a Billroth II anastomosis was fashioned, the possibility of a retained antrum must be entertained. To exclude this possibility, a technetium scan may prove helpful.[41] In patients having a retained antrum, this scan demonstrates a hot spot that is adjacent to the area where normal uptake of technetium by the gastric mucosa of the remaining stomach occurs. Antral cuffs as small as 1 cm have been detected experimentally with this technique.[41] If a retained antrum is diagnosed, pharmacologic management with an H_2 receptor blocker may prove helpful in controlling the acid hypersecretion. If this is not effective, either conversion of the Billroth II anastomosis to a Billroth I reconstruction or excision of the retained antral tissue in the duodenal stump with reclosure should obviate the problem.

Jejunogastric Intussusception

Jejunogastric intussusception is a rare entity that results when the afferent or efferent limb intussuscepts into the stomach or residual gastric pouch. It may occur in any patient whose stomach has been anastomosed to the jejunum but has been most commonly seen following simple gastroenterostomy. Both acute and chronic variants have been described.[42] Although surgical intervention is the treatment of choice for both types of the disease, it is a surgical emergency in the acute variety to prevent strangulation of the intussuscepted bowel. Foster[43] has summarized the important features of diagnosis and has emphasized that any patient who has had gastric surgery (i.e., gastric resection or gastroenterostomy) and who subsequently develops the following should be suspected of having jejunogastric intussusception until proven otherwise:

1. Severe epigastric pain
2. Persistent vomiting (either bile-stained or bloody)
3. A palpable epigastric mass
4. Tenderness over the epigastrium
5. Any combination of these signs or symptoms

The more chronic form of the disease is less dramatic clinically and usually presents as recurrent episodes of vague upper abdominal pain that is exacerbated by meals. The pain ceases after eating because the intussuscepted limb reduces itself. Although jejunogastric intussusception may involve either the afferent or efferent limbs, the efferent limb is the more common intussuscipiens and is responsible for more than 80% of the reported cases.[42] Depending on findings at surgery, surgical approaches may include reduction of the intussuscepted intestine and/or its resection, takedown of the anastomosis, or its revision. Generally, the afferent and efferent limbs of jejunum are also fixed to adjacent tissue such as the mesocolon, colon, or stomach to prevent recurrence.

DERANGEMENTS RELATED TO VAGAL TRANSECTION

Postvagotomy Diarrhea

Diarrhea of varying degrees is relatively common following gastric surgery, and if carefully questioned, 30% or more of patients indicate some difficulty with this problem.[44] Fortunately, it is not severe in the majority of individuals and often disappears within the first 3 or 4 months following surgery. In many patients with diarrhea, it is part of the dumping syndrome. As the patient develops more discriminating eating habits, the dumping improves along with the diarrhea. Distinct from the diarrhea associated with an inadequate gastric reservoir, vagotomy itself is associated with alterations in stool frequency. As many as 30% to 70% of patients report an increased frequency in daily bowel movements following truncal vagotomy.[45-49] For a previously constipated patient, this is often viewed as beneficial. In some patients, actual diarrhea develops that may occur two to three times weekly or manifest itself once or twice a month, at which times it lasts 3 or 4 days. In others, it may be more explosive, resulting in the soiling of clothing. Between attacks, bowel movements may be entirely normal. Fortunately, most patients developing diarrhea following vagotomy find a dimunition in this problem with time.

The mechanisms responsible for postvagotomy diarrhea have remained elusive. That it indeed occurs is borne out by the Leeds/York trial, in which 7% of patients developed diarrhea following subtotal gastrectomy, compared to an impressive 23% who underwent resection of the same magnitude in combination with a truncal vagotomy.[46-48] Bacterial overgrowth in the upper gastrointestinal tract has been proposed as one possible mechanism on the basis of the observation that colonization of the jejunum with aerobic and anaerobic bacteria is relatively common following vagotomy. The problem with this hypothesis is that the degree of overgrowth does not appear to be different in patients developing postvagotomy diarrhea and those who are asymptomatic.[50] Denervation of the intestine in dogs following truncal vagotomy was shown to enhance the movement of small intestinal contents into the colon through a loss of the sphincteric mechanism of the ileal cecal valve.[51] Although a similar circumstance may occur in humans, data relative to that issue are unknown. However, other experimental observations have failed to uncover differences in small intestinal morphology, small intestinal fluxes of fluid and electrolytes, or the fecal output of fat in patients with and without vagotomy.[1] Some studies have suggested a more rapid gastric emptying in patients developing postvagotomy diarrhea compared with those without this problem, but consensus on this issue is far from uniform.[1] Although the incidence of postvagotomy diarrhea in patients who are subjected to selective vagotomy was initially reported as being less than a comparable group receiving truncal vagotomy, further follow-up with larger groups of patients has not borne out this contention.[1,52]

From a therapeutic standpoint, it is known that cholestyramine, an anionic exchange resin that absorbs bile salts and thereby renders them unabsorbable and inactive, can significantly decrease the severity of diarrhea in patients developing this problem following vagotomy.[53] The possible explanation for this relates to the finding of Allan et al.[51] who noted that although the total bile acid content in the stools of patients was not significantly greater in the presence or absence of diarrhea, those with postvagotomy diarrhea excreted more than twice the amount of chenodeoxycholic acid than vagotomy patients without diarrhea.

Because postvagotomy diarrhea is usually a self-limited disease, treatment should be symptomatic. In the 5% of patients in whom symptoms are severe and interfere drastically with life-style, cholestyramine is the treatment of choice. Ayulo[53] noted improvement within 1 to 4 weeks of treatment with this agent in almost all patients receiving the drug. Significant decreases in urgency, frequency, and severity of diarrhea were noted. Treatment consists of 4 g of cholestyramine with meals three times daily and adjusted to a maintenance dosage, allowing one to two well-formed bowel movements per day.[53]

Only in extremely rare instances is operative treatment justified for postvagotomy diarrhea. When diarrhea has remained incapacitating for at least 1 year following initial operation and fails to respond to cholestyramine therapy, remedial surgery is indicated. If patients are selected properly, this involves no more than 1% of all patients undergoing vagotomy. The operative procedure of choice is to interpose a 10 cm segment of reversed jejunum 70 to 100 cm from the ligament of Treitz[54] (Fig. 17-5). In patients subjected to this operation, sustained relief from diarrhea has resulted.

Postvagotomy Dysphagia

Although it is rare, occasionally after vagotomy a patient complains of dysphagia, which is usually noted within the first 2 weeks following operation. It is probably related to edema or an intramural hematoma of the esophagus resulting from injury to the esophageal wall at the time of vagal section and is more commonly noted after the transthoracic approach of performing a vagotomy than following a transabdominal procedure.[55,56] Radiologically the disorder resembles achalasia; but, unlike this disease, liquids pass easily, whereas solids usually evoke symptoms. Esophagoscopic and manometric findings are usually normal, indicating that both esophageal sphincter function and peristalsis are intact. Treatment is usually symptomatic

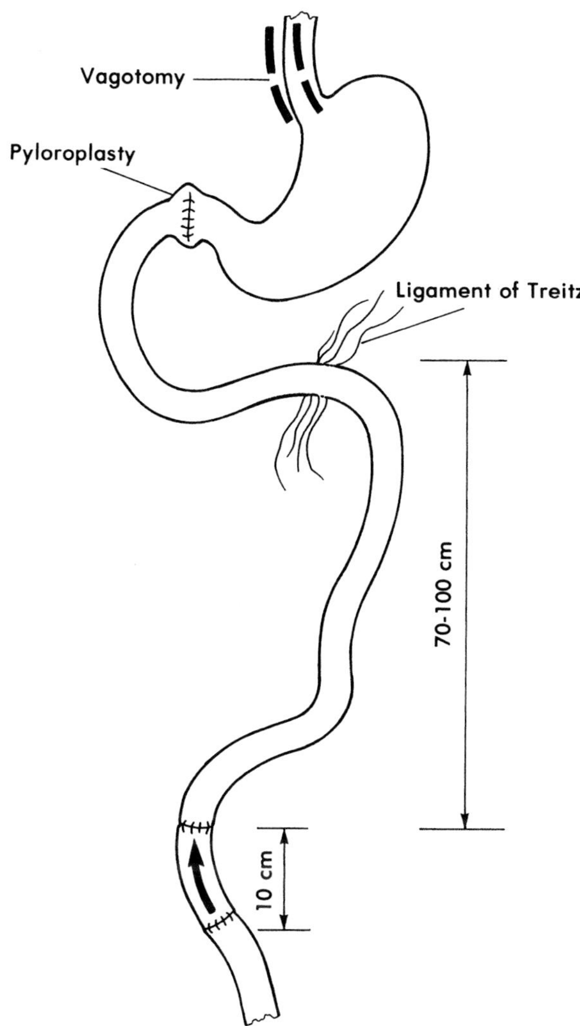

Fig. 17-5. Surgical management of postvagotomy diarrhea.

since the condition generally disappears spontaneously within 2 to 12 weeks of vagotomy. If dysphagia is particularly troublesome, esophageal dilation may be indicated with the use of a mercury-weighted bougie such as a Maloney dilator.

Postvagotomy Gastric Atony

Delayed gastric emptying is also a consequence of vagotomy, and it is for this reason that a drainage procedure must be performed when a truncal or selective vagotomy is performed. This relates to the normal function of the vagus nerve in adjusting gastric tone to the volume of the stomach so that peristalsis is initiated and coordinated properly. Since parietal cell vagotomy does not disrupt this function because of the maintenance of antral innervation, postvagotomy atony is not a problem with this procedure.

Sometimes after vagotomy (i.e., truncal or selective) and an apparently adequately performed drainage procedure, a patient may have persistent and bothersome gastric stasis that causes food to be retained in the stomach for several hours. Usually this is accompanied by no more than a feeling of fullness in the midepigastrium. At times this is associated with marked abdominal pain and rarer still with a functional gastric outlet obstruction.

The diagnosis of gastroparesis is confirmed on scintigraphic assessment of gastric emptying. However, to correctly establish the diagnosis of gastroparesis, other causes of delayed gastric emptying such as diabetes mellitus, electrolyte imbalance, drug toxicity, and neuromuscular diseases must be excluded. Further, mechanical causes of gastric hypomotility such as postoperative adhesions, afferent or efferent loop obstruction, and internal herniations must be ruled out. If endoscopic examination of the stomach reveals no evidence of a true anatomic obstruction and other causes of gastroparesis have been eliminated, watchful waiting is usually the treatment of choice. Occasionally, when observation fails, short-term treatment with various pharmacologic agents is indicated to improve gastric tone. Pharmacotherapy usually consists of using one of several gastrokinetic agents including metoclopramide,[57] cisapride,[58] and/or erythromycin.[59]

Metoclopramide exerts its gastrokinetic effects by acting as a dopamine antagonist and by cholinergic enhancing effects as a result of facilitation of acetylcholine release from enteric cholinergic neurons.[57] In contrast, cisapride, a newer gastrointestinal prokinetic agent without dopamine-antagonistic or cholinomimetic effects, exerts its actions by facilitation of acetylcholine release from the mesenteric plexus of the gut. Finally, erythromycin markedly accelerates gastric emptying by binding to motilin receptors on gastrointestinal smooth muscles, where it acts as a motilin agonist.[59,60] One of these three agents usually suffices to enhance gastric tone and improve gastric emptying.

Incomplete Vagal Transection

Since vagotomy is an important component of the surgical treatment of peptic ulcer disease, it is important that vagal transection of the acid-secreting portion of the stomach be complete. If this is not ensured, the patient is predisposed to the possibility of recurrent ulcer formation. The type of vagotomy influences the likelihood of this circumstance. In highly selective vagotomy (i.e., parietal cell) in which meticulous vagal denervation of the stomach is accomplished, an incomplete vagotomy is rarely a problem. In contrast, truncal vagotomy may be associated with a high incidence of incomplete transection because of the variability in size of the two vagal trunks, and their anatomic position. Although inadequate transection of either vagus nerve may occur during truncal vagotomy, the right vagus nerve is inadequately transected three times more frequently than the left vagus.[61,62] This relates to the fact that the right vagus nerve is frequently buried in the right periesophageal fibroareolar tissue—in contrast to the left vagus nerve, which usually hugs the anterior esophageal surface. The likelihood of incomplete vagotomy can be greatly lessened by confirming vagal transection histologically at the time of operation by frozen section examination of excised nerve tissue.

SUMMARY

Derangements in gastric function are common following operations on the stomach. These aberrations in normal physiology can result from a loss of gastric reservoir function when a portion of the stomach has been removed, from motility disturbances secondary to transection of the vagus nerves, or from interruption of the normal pyloric sphincter mechanism secondary to pyloroplasty; or they can be directly related to the type of reconstructive procedure that has been undertaken to restore normal gastrointestinal continuity. Although most patients experience some type of postoperative symptomatology following a gastric operation, many of these problems are short lived and abate with time. In a small percentage of patients, however, significant untoward sequelae result that may require substantial dietary manipulation and occasionally pharmacologic management to alleviate distressing signs and symptoms and enable a patient to function adequately in society. Occasionally, reoperation becomes necessary to correct the underlying physiologic dysfunction. Fortunately, patients in this latter category are less commonly seen today than they were a decade or so ago because of the decreasing incidence of gastric cancer and the development of new strategies to manage acid-peptic diseases of the stomach, both of which have resulted in fewer operative procedures involving the stomach.

REFERENCES

1. Fromm D. Complications of Gastric Surgery. New York: John Wiley, 1977.
2. Ritchie WP Jr, Perez AR. Postgastrectomy syndromes. In Moody FG, et al., eds. Surgical Treatment of Digestive Disease. Chicago: Year Book, 1986.
3. Johnson LP, et al. Serotonin antagonists in experimental and clinical "dumping." Ann Surg 156:537, 1962.
4. Reichle FA, et al. The effect of gastrectomy on serotonin metabolism in the human portal vein. Ann Surg 172:585, 1970.
5. Wang PY, et al. Kallikrein-kinin system in postgastrectomy dumping syndrome. Ann Intern Med 80:577, 1974.
6. Blackburn AM, et al. Elevation of plasma neurotensin in the dumping syndrome. Clin Sci 59:237, 1980.
7. Sagor GR, et al. Release of VIP in the dumping syndrome. Br Med J 282:507, 1981.
8. Bloom SR, Rorpton CMS, Thomson JPS. Enteroglucagon release in the dumping syndrome. Lancet 2:789,1972.
9. Eldkh J, et al. Long-term results of surgical treatment for dumping after partial gastrectomy. Br J Surg 61:90, 1974.
10. Donovan IA. The different components of gastric emptying after gastric surgery. Ann R Coll Surg Engl 58:368, 1976.
11. Lawson-Smith C, Thomson JPS. A dumping provocation test. Br J Surg 62:153, 1975.
12. Chaimoff CH, Dintsman M. The long-term fate of patients with dumping syndrome. Arch Surg 105:554, 1972.
13. Silver D, et al. The mechanism of the dumping syndrome. Surg Clin North Am 46:425, 1966.
14. Jenkins DJA, et al. Effect of dietary fiber on complications of gastric surgery: Prevention of post-prandial hypoglycemia by pectin. Gastroenterology 72:215, 1977.
15. Geer RJ, et al. Postgastric surgery syndromes: Octreotide in dumping syndrome—Efficacy of octreotide acetate in treatment of severe postgastrectomy dumping syndrome. Ann Surg 212:678, 1990.
16. Richards WO, et al. Octreotide acetate induces fasting small bowel motility in patients with dumping syndrome. J Surg Res 49:483, 1990.
17. Mackie CR, et al. The effect of isoperistaltic jejunal interposition upon gastric emptying. Surg Gynecol Obstet 153:813, 1981.
18. Remus NI, Williamson RCN, Johnston D. The use of jejunal interposition for intractable symptoms complicating peptic ulcer surgery. Br J Surg 69:265, 1982.
19. Sawyers JL, Herrington JL. Superiority of anti-peristaltic jejunal segments in management of severe dumping syndrome. Ann Surg 178:311, 1973.
20. Hocking MP, et al. Delayed gastric emptying of liquids and solids following Roux-en-Y biliary diversion. Ann Surg 194:494, 1981.
21. Speth PAJ, Jansen JBMJ, Lammers CBHW. Effect of acarbose, pectin, or a combination of acarbose with pectin, and placebo on postprandial reactive hypoglycemia after gastric surgery. Gut 24:798, 1983.
22. Fink WJ, et al. Treatment of postoperative reactive hypoglycemia by a reversed intestinal segment. Am J Surg 131:19, 1976.
23. Sawyers JL. Surgical management of post-gastrectomy syndrome. J Miss State Med Assoc 14:28, 1974.
24. Cuschieri A. Long-term evaluation of a reservoir jejunal interposition with an isoperistaltic conduit in the management of patients with small stomach syndrome. Br J Surg 69:386, 1982.
25. Alexander-Williams J, Donovan IA. Postgastrectomy and postvagotomy syndromes and their management. In Glass GBJ, Sherlock P, eds. Progress in Gastroenterology, vol 4. New York: Grune & Stratton, 1983.
26. Morgan DB, et al. Search for osteomalacia in 1228 patients after gastrectomy and other operations on the stomach. Lancet 2:1085, 1965.
27. Pryor JP, et al. The long-term metabolic consequences of partial gastrectomy. Am J Med 51:5, 1971.
28. Wheldon EJ, Venables CW, Johnson IDA. Late metabolic sequelae of vagotomy and gastroenterostomy. Lancet 1:437, 1970.
29. Jordon GL Jr. The afferent loop syndrome. Surgery 38:1027, 1955.
30. Mitty WE Jr, Grossi C, Nealon TF Jr. Chronic afferent loop syndrome. Ann Surg 172:996, 1970.
31. Rutledge RH. Retroanastomotic hernias after gastrojejunal anastomoses. Ann Surg 177:547, 1973.
32. Boren CH, Way LH. Alkaline reflux gastritis: A reevaluation. Am J Surg 140:40, 1980.
33. Bushkin FL, et al. Postoperative alkaline reflux gastritis. Surg Gynecol Obstet 138:933, 1974.
34. Davidson ED, Hersh T. The surgical treatment of bile reflux gastritis: A study of 59 patients. Ann Surg 192:175, 1980.
35. Ritchie WP Jr. Alkaline reflux gastritis: An objective assessment of its diagnosis and treatment. Ann Surg 192:288, 1980.
36. Ritchie WP Jr. Alkaline reflux gastritis: A diagnosis in search of a disease. J Clin Surg 1:414, 1982.
37. Fromm D. Ulceration of stomach and duodenum. In Fromm D, ed. Gastrointestinal Surgery. New York: Churchill Livingstone, 1985.
38. Ruding R, Hirdes WH. Extent of the gastric antrum and its significance. Surgery 53:743, 1963.
39. Allen WA, Welch CE. Gastric resection for duodenal ulcer. Ann Surg 115:530,1942.
40. Stabile BE, Passaro E. Recurrent peptic ulcer. Gastroenterology 70:124, 1976.
41. Chaudhuri TK, et al. Radioisotopic scan—A possible aid in differentiating retained antrum from Zollinger-Ellison syndrome in patients with recurrent peptic ulcer. Gastroenterology 65:697, 1973.
42. Wait JO, Beart RW Jr, Charboneau W. Jejunogastric intussusception. Arch Surg 115:1449, 1980.
43. Foster DG. Retrograde jejunogastric intussusception—Rare cause of hematemesis. Arch Surg 73:1009, 1956.

44. Goligher JC, et al. Several standard elective operations for duodenal ulcer. Ten to 16 year clinical results. Ann Surg 189:18, 1978.
45. Duthie HL, Kwong NK. Vagotomy or gastrectomy for gastric ulcer. Br Med J 4:79, 1973.
46. Goligher JC, et al. Five to eight year results of Leeds/York controlled trial of elective surgery for duodenal ulcer. Br Med J 2:781, 1968.
47. Goligher JC, et al. Clinical comparison of vagotomy and pyloroplasty with other forms of elective surgery for duodenal ulcer. Br Med J 2:787, 1968.
48. Goligher JC, et al. Five to eight year results of truncal vagotomy and pyloroplasty for duodenal ulcer. Br Med J 1:7, 1972.
49. Kronborg O. Clinical results 6 to 8 years after truncal vagotomy and drainage for duodenal ulcer in 500 patients. Acta Chir Scand 141:657, 1975.
50. Browning GC, Buchanan KA, MacKay C. Clinical and laboratory study of postvagotomy diarrhea. Gut 15:644, 1974.
51. Allan JC, Gerskovitch VP, Russell RI. The role of bile acids in the pathogenesis of postvagotomy diarrhea. Br J Surg 61:516, 1974.
52. Kennedy T. The vagus and the consequences of vagotomy. Med Clin North Am 58:1231, 1974.
53. Ayulo JA. Cholestyramine in postvagotomy syndrome. Am J Gastroenterol 57:207, 1972.
54. Herrington JL, et al. Treatment of severe postgastrectomy diarrhea by reversed jejunal segment. Ann Surg 168:522, 1968.
55. Edwards DA. Postvagotomy dysphagia. Lancet 2:90, 1970.
56. Suleiman SI, Maglad SA, Hobsley M. Dysphagia following selective vagotomy. Br J Surg 66:607, 1979.
57. McClelland RN, Horton JW. Relief of acute, persistent postvagotomy atony by metoclopramide. Ann Surg 188:439, 1978.
58. Camilleri M, et al. Gastric emptying problems. Effect of six weeks of treatment with cisapride in gastroparesis and intestinal pseudoobstruction. Gastroenterology 96:704, 1989.
59. Tack J, et al. Gastric emptying problems: Diabetic gastropathy—Effect of erythromycin on gastric motility in controls and in diabetic gastroparesis. Gastroenterology 103:72, 1992.
60. Peeters TL, et al. Gastric emptying problems: Motilin in diabetic gastroparesis—Effect of motilin on gastric emptying in patients with diabetic gastroparesis. Gastroenterology 102:97, 1992.
61. Fawcett AN, Johnston D, Duthie HL. Revagotomy for recurrent ulcer after vagotomy and drainage for duodenal ulcer. Br J Surg 56:111, 1969.
62. Venables CW. The value of a combined pentagastrin/insulin test in studies of stomal ulceration. Br J Surg 57:757, 1970.

Small and Large Intestine

18

Physiology of Digestion and Absorption

Gardiner Roddey and Joseph H. Sellin

The physiology of digestion and absorption involves the transformation of the vast array of foodstuffs eaten by humans into assimilable forms and then the transfer of these nutrients across an epithelial barrier. Simultaneously, this barrier must exclude bacteria, toxins, and an array of noxious compounds. Considering the complexity of the task, it is somewhat surprising, and comforting, that the gut usually accomplishes these functions without difficulties. However, derangements of this normally well-regulated system do occur and present significant clinical problems. Therapeutic intervention is based on an understanding of normal gut function.

This chapter describes the processes involved in the digestion and absorption of carbohydrate, protein, and fat; the mechanisms of intestinal fluid and electrolyte regulation; and the gastrointestinal tract's role in vitamin and mineral metabolism. Recent advances in our understanding of the physiology of digestion and absorption have centered on the molecular biology of specific transport proteins such as cystic fibrosis transmembrane conductance regulator (CFTR). Emphasis is placed on the clinical relevance of a knowledge of normal physiology. Rational approaches to the evaluation and management of malabsorption and diarrhea are also outlined.

PROTEIN ABSORPTION

Dietary proteins normally comprise 15% of total caloric intake. These complex substances are broken down in a stepwise manner into oligopeptides and amino acids, which are absorbed primarily in the upper small bowel (duodenum and jejunum). Specific transport pathways in small bowel enterocytes mediate active transport of these nutrients, which cross the enterocytes and then enter the portal circulation.

Protein digestion begins in the stomach. Pepsinogen, secreted by gastric chief cells, is converted to pepsin in the acidic environment of the gastric lumen and begins the process of protein digestion by breaking down dietary protein into polypeptide subunits. However, pepsin is not essential for normal protein digestion or absorption. Individuals who do not make pepsin (e.g., because of pernicious anemia or gastrectomy) still absorb protein efficiently.[1,2]

Polypeptides formed from digested protein within the intestinal lumen stimulate intestinal endocrine cells to release the hormone cholecystokinin-pancreozymin.* The pancreas responds to this hormonal stimulation by secreting peptidases, which serve to break protein down to oligopeptides and amino acids. The endopeptidases, trypsin, chymotrypsin, and elastase, cleave protein at specific interior sites. The exopeptidases, primarily carboxypeptidase, sequentially cleave off amino acids from a specific end of a polypeptide chain. The end result of this process of intraluminal digestion is a mixture of roughly equal amounts of amino acids and oligopeptides[3] (Fig.18-1). Because these compounds are polar and water soluble, they do not require bile salts or micelle formation in the absorptive process. However, because of their polar nature they cannot diffuse through cell membranes like lipids and require specific carriers to be transported across the mucosal membrane of the enterocyte.

Several distinct carrier proteins accomplish this task. Specific carrier systems appear to exist for neutral amino acids (e.g., leucine, phenylalanine, threonine) and for basic amino acids (e.g., arginine, lysine, cystine). These systems involve the coupling of amino acids with sodium to mediate movement across the apical membrane. Sodium (Na) movement into the cell is driven by a favorable electrochemical gradient (i.e., it is "downhill"). The coupling of amino acids with Na allows them to accumulate in the cell against a concentration gradient (Fig. 18-1). Once concentrated in the cell, diffusion across the basolateral membrane takes place.[2]

Several factors may affect this absorptive system. In a mixture of amino acids within the intestinal lumen, competition for binding to the carrier proteins is present. For

*Historically, cholecystokinin and pancreozymin were thought to be two separate hormones. Current evidence indicates that they are the same hormone. Many authors refer to cholecystokinin-pancreozymin as simply cholecystokinin (CCK).

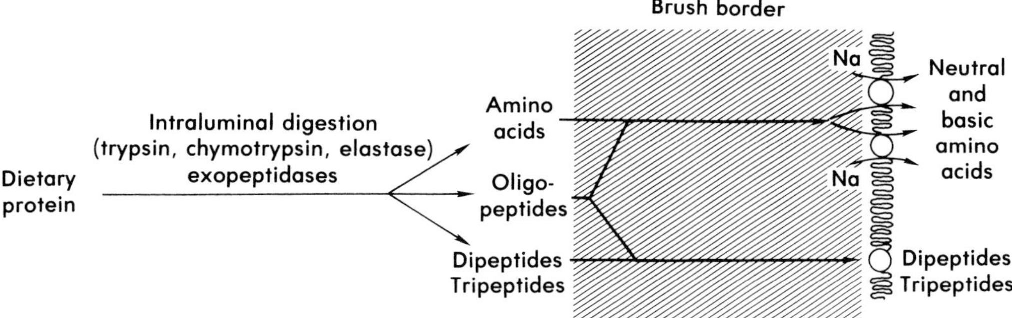

Fig. 18-1. Protein digestion and absorption. Intraluminal digestion of protein occurs primarily through the action of pancreatic enzymes *(left side of figure)*. Brush border enzymes play a relatively minor role and probably aid in the breakdown of residual oligopeptides *(crosshatched area)*. Amino acids, dipeptides, and tripeptides are then actively transported into the cell *(right side of figure)*.

example, amino acids with long side chains appear to have a higher affinity for the carriers and may inhibit the absorption of other amino acids with shorter side chains. Although Na is an absolute requirement for this carrier system, endogenous secretion of Na into the intestinal lumen is always sufficient for the system to be operative. Intraluminal pH affects this system only when extremely low (<2.5). Studies regarding the effects of dietary deprivation on protein absorption have been conflicting. It appears that diabetes is associated with increased transport activity of both the neutral and basic amino acids.[4] Intestinal and renal epithelial cells share similar transport systems, and in inherited metabolic disorders such as cystinuria and Hartnup disease, defects can be demonstrated in both organs.

Oligopeptides can be absorbed intact by the intestine without first being broken down into individual amino acids. Dipeptides and tripeptides are absorbed by a carrier system(s) different from those for amino acids. Tetrapeptides and larger protein digestive products are not absorbed intact. Although specific brush border dipeptidases and tripeptidases are on the small bowel mucosal membrane, the bulk of this enzyme activity is intracellular. Therefore it is likely that the majority of oligopeptides are absorbed and then subjected to intracellular hydrolysis[3,5] (see Fig. 18-1).

The presence of a specific transport system for oligopeptides has important physiological and clinical implications because this may be a major mechanism for absorption of dietary proteins. This system exhibits a higher rate of maximal uptake than the amino acid carriers and probably is not influenced as much by diabetes or diet. Recognition of oligopeptide absorption is necessary for the rational design of formulas for enteral nutrition.

CARBOHYDRATE ABSORPTION

Absorption of carbohydrates depends on a sequence of orderly steps involving intraluminal digestion, uptake across the luminal membrane of small bowel enterocytes by specific carriers, and subsequent entry into the mesenteric tributaries to portal blood in a manner analogous to protein absorption. However, unlike oligopeptides, oligosaccharides cannot be absorbed by enterocytes. Intraluminal digestion of carbohydrates is incomplete, and brush border enzymes are essential for the conversion of oligosaccharides into simple sugars that can be transported across the luminal membrane.

Carbohydrates are generally the chief source of calories. Starch, the major form of dietary carbohydrate, is a polymer of glucose with a molecular weight of 100,000 or greater; that is, one molecule of starch usually has more than 500 glucose subunits. The linkage between the glucose moieties determines the type of starch and its enzymatic degradation. Such types are classified by the spatial configuration of the glucosidic bond (α, β) and the carbon atoms involved in the linkage (1,4 or 1,6). Amylose is a straight chain of α-1,4 linked glucoses. The most common form of dietary starch is the branched starch amylopectin, which consists of α-1,4 chains and branch points created by α-1,6 linkages at every 20 to 25 residues (Fig. 18-2). Glycogen is a branched starch like amylopectin, but it has a greater frequency of α-1,6 linkages. Although only a minor dietary form of starch, glycogen is the major storage form of carbohydrate within the body.

Disaccharides comprise approximately one third of dietary carbohydrate. The two principal disaccharides are sucrose (glucose-fructose) and lactose (glucose-galactose). Several types of nondigestible carbohydrates are in the diet, chiefly the various forms of fiber (cellulose, hemicellulose, and pectin) and oligosaccharides found in legumes such as beans and lentils (raffinose, stachyose).

Digestion of starch begins in the mouth with salivary amylase but comes to a rapid halt in the acid environment of the stomach. Carbohydrate digestion is completed in the upper small bowel (primarily jejunum) and consists of two phases: intraluminal breakdown of starch and brush border hydrolysis of oligosaccharides (Fig. 18-3). Pancreatic α-amylase is primarily responsible for intraluminal digestion of starch. Because it is secreted in great excess, clinically significant amylase deficiency is extremely rare, even in cases of severe steatorrhea* associated with pancreatic insufficiency. α-Amylase is active only at the interior α-1,4 bonds of starch. It cannot hydrolyze 1,6 links, 1,4 links next to branch points, or the terminal glucose-glucose links. Therefore the final products of amylase digestion are the disaccharide maltose, the trisaccharide maltotriose, and α-limit dextrins (i.e., larger oligosaccharides of 5 to 10 glucose units containing the branch points) (see Figs. 18-2 and 18-3). Human amylase is inactive against β links; therefore cellulose, which is made up entirely of β-1,4 links, is not digested.

Next, maltose, maltotriose, and α-limit dextrins, along with dietary disaccharides, are broken down into simple sugars by specific brush border enzymes.[6] The end products of this process are glucose, galactose, and fructose (see Fig. 18-3). Glucose and galactose are transported across the luminal membrane of the cell by a carrier protein that couples the movement of sugar to sodium.[7] This transport mechanism is similar to Na-n-amino acid absorption. In the later stages of absorption, intraluminal concentrations of sugars may decrease; however, because of the Na coupling, active transport of sugars against a concentration gradient can occur. Fructose absorption occurs by facilitated diffusion (i.e., carrier-mediated, but not active, transport).

*Steatorrhea refers to excessive amounts of fat in the feces in excess of 7 g/day when a patient maintains a 100 g/day fat diet.

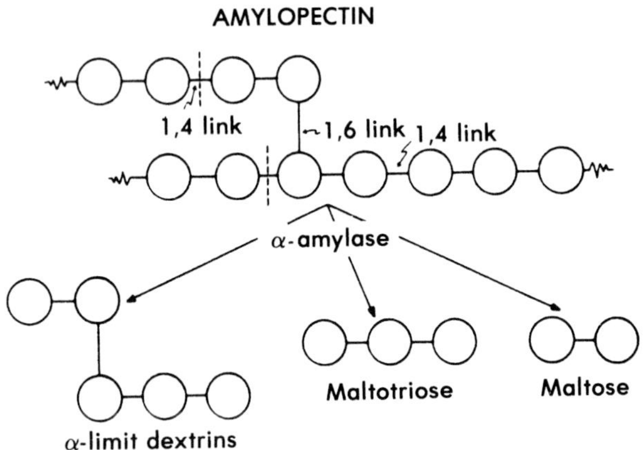

Fig. 18-2. α-Amylopectin and its final hydrolytic products are shown with glucose molecules *(circles)* joined by α-1,4 *(horizontal)* links or α-1,6 *(vertical)* links. (From Gray GM. Carbohydrate digestion and absorption. N Engl J Med 292:1225, 1975. Copyright © 1975 Massachusetts Medical Society. All rights reserved.)

Generally, transport into the cell is the rate-limiting step in this absorptive process. The hydrolytic capacity of the brush border enzymes provides an excess of monosaccharides for the transport carrier. The exception to this is lactose absorption, where the hydrolytic capacity of lactase is rate limiting. A complex regulatory mechanism appears to coordinate the activity of the brush border enzymes and the corresponding transport proteins.[8]

The overall design of carbohydrate absorption is to deliver maximal amounts of calories while introducing the least possible osmotic force into the duodenum and jejunum, where carbohydrates are primarily absorbed. A molecule of starch and a molecule of glucose have the same osmotic effect but vastly different caloric value. Intraluminal digestion of starch stops at the oligosaccharide stage, limiting the osmotic effect. The rapid absorption of monosaccharides into the intestine after action by brush border enzymes minimizes the potential for drawing fluid into the jejunum and duodenum. Under normal conditions this system is extremely effective; when disrupted, malabsorption may be compounded by osmotic diarrhea.

FAT ABSORPTION

The absorption of fat is complex and depends on the integrated function of the pancreas, biliary system, and intestinal mucosa. Much of this complexity is created by the problem of delivering a water-insoluble nutrient into an aqueous environment. Fat composes approximately one third of the typical American diet, although this percentage has been decreasing in recent years. The bulk of this

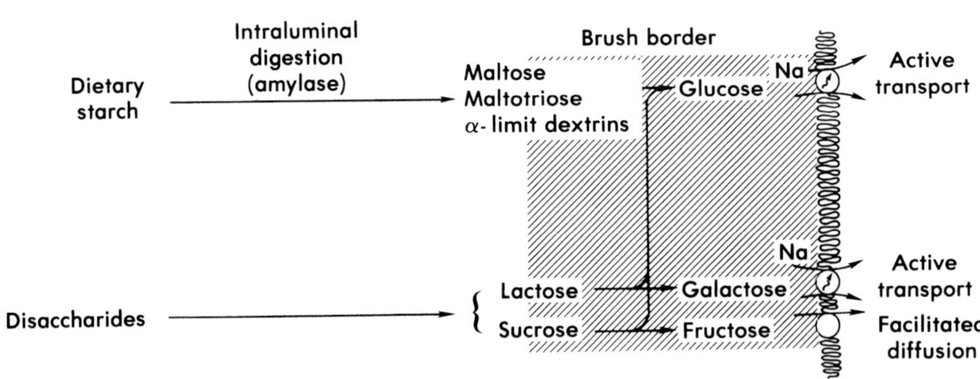

Fig. 18-3. Carbohydrate digestion and absorption. The principal intraluminal event is starch digestion by amylase *(left side of figure)*. The resulting maltose, maltotriose, and α-limit dextrins are broken down further by brush border enzymes, as are the disaccharides *(crosshatched area)*. Specific active transport systems, coupled to Na, exist for glucose and galactose. Fructose is absorbed by facilitated diffusion.

fat is the in the form of triglycerides (90%), phospholipids, cholesterol, fat-soluble vitamins, and other trace lipids.*

Dietary phospholipids are primarily derived from biologic membranes of foodstuffs. They are structurally similar to triglycerides, possessing a glycerol backbone and two ester links to fatty acids. In the third position, however, there is an ester link to phosphoric acid, which is then linked to a nitrogen-containing base (choline, serine, ethanolamine). Phospholipids are relatively resistant to lipase and are primarily degraded by phospholipase A_2, which requires calcium and bile salts as cofactors. An additional enzyme, nonspecific lipase, exhibits activity on cholesterol esters, monoglycerides, and trace fats.

One dietary source of fat comes replete with its own digestive enzyme. Human, but not cow, milk contains a nonspecific lipase that is acid resistant and therefore serves as an intestinal lipase for breast-fed infants. Considering the relatively low levels of lipase in the newborn, nature has provided an ingenious package to ensure that maximal nutritional benefit of human milk for the infant is achieved.

The intraluminal phase of digestion is crucial for fat absorption (Fig. 18-4). Dietary fat is mechanically broken down, emulsified into an oil phase, and finally solubilized within the upper small bowel lumen before being presented to the intestinal mucosa for transport through the enterocyte and into the lymph. The oil phase represents emulsified fat droplets of 2000 to 50,000 Å in size. Enzymatic digestion of the droplets by lipases forms calcium soaps (free fatty acids complexed with calcium) and a viscous isotropic phase of protonated fatty acids and monoglycerides. (A fat droplet remnant of undetermined composition generally remains after formation of the viscous isotropic phase.) The constituents of the viscous isotropic phase, fatty acids and monoglycerides, then interact with bile salts to form micelles.[9,10]

The primary enzymes responsible for fat digestion are lipase, phospholipase A_2, and nonspecific lipase (cholesterol esterase). Lipase has two sources: lingual and pancreatic. Lingual lipase is resistant to acid degradation in the stomach and prepares dietary fat for more efficient intestinal degradation. Pancreatic lipase is the major digestive enzyme for triglycerides. Extrapolations from in vitro activity suggest that a 1000-fold excess of lipase is secreted to handle the average daily fat intake. Lipase acts by hydrolyzing the two outside arms of triglyceride, yielding two fatty acids and a monoglyceride (see Fig. 18-4.)

In the setting of severe lipase deficiency there may still be a wide range in the magnitude of fat malabsorption. Recent studies on colipase serve to elucidate the variability of steatorrhea in these clinical states. Physiologic concentrations of bile salts in the upper gut inactivate pancreatic lipase by displacing it from its natural substrate, the triglyceride-containing fat droplet. Therefore without some additional factor, lipase could not digest triglycerides in its natural environment. That factor is colipase.[11]

Unlike lipase, colipase is not displaced from the surface of fat emulsions by bile salts. Colipase binds to the triglyceride substrate, then binds lipase, and serves as the necessary bridge to link the enzyme to its target. Thus colipase plays a crucial role in intraluminal fat digestion (see Fig. 18-4). Differences in colipase secretion in pancreatic insufficiency with severe lipase deficiency may account for some of the variability of fat malabsorption.[12]

The products of enzymatic digestion of dietary fat remain relatively water insoluble, primarily in the viscous isotropic phase (see Fig. 18-4). Bile salts provide the mechanism for bringing cholesterol, monoglycerides, fatty acids, and phospholipids into solution by forming micelles. Bile salts are detergents; like all detergents they are amphophiles, possessing both hydrophilic and hydrophobic

*These poorly characterized nonpolar lipids may represent industrial pollutants, residues from fossil fuels, degradation products from high-temperature cooking, natural products, and essential oils of plants; they account for the remainder of the fat in the diet.

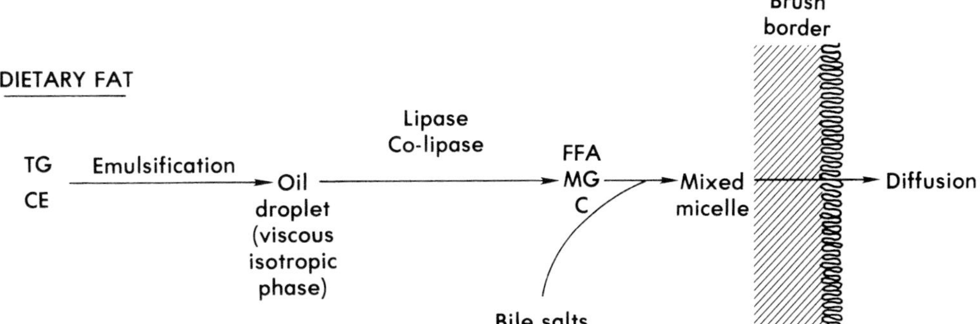

Fig. 18-4. Fat digestion and absorption. Dietary fats, triglycerides *(TG),* and cholesterol esters *(CE)* are emulsified to form fat droplets within the intestinal lumen. These droplets undergo a physiochemical transformation into a viscous isotrophic phase. At this stage the triglyceride is digested by pancreatic lipase. The resultant free fatty acids *(FFA)* and monoglyceride *(MG),* along with cholesterol *(C),* form mixed micelles with bile salts. The micelle then diffuses to the apical membrane. There are no brush border enzymes on specific membrane transport systems for fat absorption.

regions. Placed in an aqueous solution, bile salts spontaneously form into a particular three-dimensional arrangement called a micelle, in which the hydrophilic regions of the molecules are directed outward and the hydrophobic regions inward, thereby shielded from the aqueous environment. This formation occurs above a specific concentration of bile salts termed the critical micellar concentration (CMC). Depending on the types of bile salts involved, the CMC is generally in the range of 1 to 5 mM. Mixed micelles are formed with the products of lipase action shielded from the aqueous, polar environment of the intestinal lumen by the bile salts. Micelles are smaller (30 to 100 Å) than the fat emulsion and are truly in solution. Diglycerides and triglycerides are too bulky to be packaged in these micelles and must await lipase hydrolysis. Fat-soluble vitamins are solubilized by inclusion in mixed micelles.

Before absorption the mixed micelle and its constituent lipids must diffuse through two functional barriers: the apical membrane of the intestinal cell and the unstirred water layer (see p. 416), that portion of intestinal fluid immediately adjacent to the epithelium not subject to the bulk mixing that occurs normally within the lumen. The rate of diffusion is dependent on the thickness of the unstirred water layer, the concentration gradient across it, and the permeability coefficient of the micelle.[13,14] The micelle probably dissociates at the apical membrane. Fatty acids, cholesterol, and monoglycerides can then permeate through the lipid regions of the apical membrane into the cell interior. Unlike amino acids and sugars, they do not require a specific carrier protein. Whereas most dietary fat is absorbed in the duodenum and upper jejunum, bile salts generally remain in the intestinal lumen until they are reabsorbed in the terminal ileum.

Once inside the enterocyte, the digestive process is essentially reversed; monoglycerides and fatty acids are resynthesized into triglyceride. Through a series of enzymatic steps in the endoplasmic reticulum, triglycerides are reformed and then accumulate within the Golgi apparatus. However, before exiting across the basolateral membrane of the cell, the triglycerides must be suitably packaged for transport in lymph. This process is chylomicron formation.

Chylomicrons are large spheres (1000 to 5000 Å) with a core of hydrophobic lipids, primarily triglycerides, that also include cholesterol, cholesterol esters, fat-soluble vitamins, and trace fats. The surface is covered by phospholipids and specialized apolipoproteins. Although these apolipoproteins cover less than a quarter of the surface and account for about 1% of the mass, they are essential for chylomicron formation and transport. These proteins are made in the intestine; their rate of synthesis appears to be stimulated by fat absorption. Congenital absence of a certain apolipoprotein (abetalipoproteinemia) prevents the exit step of chylomicrons across the basolateral membrane of the cell.[9] Once in the subepithelial space, chylomicrons enter the central lacteal of the villus and the intestinal lymphatic system. Because of their size they cannot pass through the relatively tight junctions of the capillaries and are therefore excluded from the portal system.

One source of dietary fat is able to enter the portal system. Medium chain triglycerides (MCTs), with fatty acid chains of 6- to 10-carbon atoms, are metabolized somewhat differently than their long chain counterparts. About one third of an oral dose of MCT can be absorbed intact.[15] Pancreatic lipase acting at both the α and β positions can yield three medium chain fatty acids. These fatty acids may be absorbed directly into the portal blood independent of chylomicrons. The therapeutic implications of this distinct metabolism of MCTs is self-evident.

ENTEROHEPATIC CIRCULATION

Enterohepatic circulation is the process by which substances are recycled through biliary secretion, intestinal absorption, and hepatic uptake. Organic anions, drugs, and hormone metabolites undergo enterohepatic circulation, but the principal constituents are bile acids. Bile acids are a family of steroids synthesized by the liver from cholesterol. They are the physiologically most significant component of bile and serve several important functions: stimulation of hepatic bile flow, solubilization and excretion of cholesterol, micellarization of dietary lipid, and stimulation of intestinal fluid secretion.

Bile acids may be classified in several different ways: by the number of hydroxyl groups, by where they are synthesized, and by their conjugation. The number of hydroxyl groups determines, to a large extent, how water soluble the bile acid is; this, in turn, determines many of its functional characteristics. Cholic acid has three hydroxyl groups on its steroid nucleus: chenodeoxycholic and deoxycholic acids possess two hydroxyl groups, and lithocholic acid possesses a single hydroxyl group. Primary bile acids (cholic, chenodeoxycholic) are synthesized in the liver. The secondary bile acids (deoxycholic, lithocholic) have had a hydroxyl group removed by anaerobic bacteria in the intestine. All bile acids secreted into bile by the liver are conjugated; the two major conjugates are glycine and taurine.

The underlying biochemical mechanisms of conjugation are poorly understood. It appears that the system prefers taurine conjugation; however, because the relative supply of glycine is much greater, approximately two thirds of bile acids are glycine conjugates. No major functional difference is apparent between the two conjugates. Lithocholate may also be sulfated in addition to being conjugated with glycine and taurine. A small fraction of bile acids is glucuronidated. Conjugation has several important effects. It makes the bile acids more polar and therefore more water soluble. Additionally, conjugated bile acids are less likely to precipitate in an acid environment or to complex with calcium. Intestinal bacteria are capable of deconjugating bile acids. Because the small bowel is relatively sterile, deconjugation normally occurs in the colon. Therefore bacteria have two major effects on intestinal bile acid metabolism: (1) dehydroxylation (i.e., conversion of primary to secondary bile acids and (2) deconjugation.

There are two different mechanisms of intestinal absorption of bile acids: passive permeation, which occurs throughout the length of the gut, and active absorption, which is restricted to the terminal ileum. The difference in intestinal transport among the classes of bile acids is considerable, depending to a large extent on the physical characteristics of a particular bile acid. The more polar (conjugated) bile salts are well absorbed by the active transport mechanism in the ileum. This absorption is dependent on Na and is similar to other Na-coupled transport systems in the small bowel that link the intracellular accumulation of a solute to the downhill movement of Na across the apical membrane.

In contrast, passive absorption is greater for the less polar bile salts. The rate of passive absorption depends on two factors: (1) the concentration of the bile salt monomer within the intestinal lumen and (2) the passive permeability coefficient, which is inversely related to the polarity. Therefore bile acids that are unconjugated, or have fewer hydroxyl groups, are more easily absorbed passively.

Within this framework the passage of the different bile acids through the enterohepatic circulation can be traced. The primary bile acids, conjugated cholic and chenodeoxycholic acid, are poorly absorbed in the upper small bowel. Teleologically, this makes sense. Since a high concentration of bile salts is necessary for intraluminal fat digestion, it would be counterproductive to have bile acids absorbed in the jejunum. In the ileum, the active absorption of bile salts is efficient. The bile salts are transported across the ileal epithelium to the portal circulation and returned to the liver (Fig. 18-5). At this level of the gut, the bacterial metabolism of bile salts becomes significant. More than a quarter of ileal bile acid is either deconjugated or dehydroxylated (i.e., converted to secondary bile acids). These may then be absorbed passively and enter the enterohepatic circulation.

The fate of the two secondary bile acids is quite different. Deoxycholate, the dihydroxy bile acid formed from cholic acid, is well absorbed; once it is conjugated in the liver, deoxycholate is handled by the enterohepatic circulation in a manner quite similar to the primary dihydroxy bile acid, chenodeoxycholate. On returning to the liver, about two thirds of the lithocholate is conjugated with sulfate. The nonsulfated lithocholate is probably absorbed by the ileum, whereas the sulfated moieties pass into the colon. Here they may be deconjugated by bacteria; a fraction of this lithocholate is then passively reabsorbed and reenters the enterohepatic circulation (see Fig. 18-5).

Normally, the enterohepatic circulation is well regulated. A bile salt pool of approximately 2 g cycles itself through the enterohepatic circulation approximately six times daily, resulting in an intestinal bile acid secretion rate of 12 g/day. Approximately 0.5 g is lost in the stool daily; this is matched by an equivalent rate of bile acid synthesis by the liver. The turnover rate for the various bile acids varies. As one might expect, given its inefficient intestinal

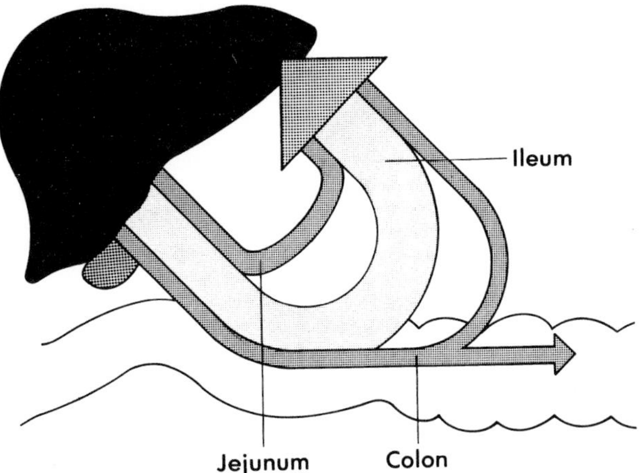

Fig. 18-5. Enterohepatic circulation. Bile acids secreted by the liver enter the intestine at the level of Vater's ampulla. In the jejunum, absorption occurs primarily by passive diffusion of conjugated bile acids. In the ileum, active transport of all bile acids occurs through an Na-dependent carrier. In the colon, passive diffusion of free bile acids occurs.

absorption, the pool of lithocholate (60 mg) is entirely turned over every 24 hours. Between 20% and 30% of the other major bile salts are excreted in the stool each day.

Disruption of the enterohepatic circulation may result in malabsorption and/or diarrhea. Ileal resection or dysfunction (e.g., Crohn's disease) blocks the reabsorption of bile acids. With small resections of the ileum (<100 cm), the passage of bile acids into the colon is increased. The dihydroxy bile acids are potent cathartics; they alter intestinal permeability and stimulate active electrolyte secretion.[16] Because there is considerable hepatic synthetic reserve, the increased fecal loss is compensated for by increased production. Therefore steatorrhea is mild, and the diarrhea that occurs is caused primarily by the effect of bile salts on the colon. With larger ileal resections (>100 cm), the liver can no longer produce enough bile acid to compensate for the fecal loss. Bile salt secretion drops significantly, and the steatorrhea becomes more severe (>20 g/day of fat) because of inadequate micelle formation in the small bowel. Diarrhea results in this setting from the increase in colonic long chain fatty acids, which like bile salts, stimulate secretion.

The enterohepatic circulation may be significantly altered by medications or in certain specific clinical settings. Cholestyramine, for example, functions as a binding resin and sequesters bile acids. Ursodeoxycholic acid, naturally occurring in bear bile and used in cholestatic diseases such as primary biliary cirrhosis, is itself a hydrophilic bile acid. Oral administration of ursodeoxycholic acid competitively inhibits the ileal absorption of endogenous hydrophobic bile acids, such as chenodeoxycholic and deoxycholic acid. Ursodeoxycholate becomes the major component of the bile salt pool. The consequences are diverse. Ursodeoxycholic acid increases the stability of biliary and hepatocyte membranes, increases transit and solubility of bile, and decreases expression of HLA class II antigens (the target of cytotoxin T cells). These effects may play a role in improving serum and tissue markers of cholestasis, which has been observed with ursodeoxycholic acid. Whether that will translate into improvement in end points such as mortality remains unclear.[17-19] Nevertheless, this may well explain the long-standing interest in Oriental folk medicine in bear gallbladder and bile.

In bacterial overgrowth, bile acid deconjugation in the small bowel is significant; therefore because unconjugated bile salts are less soluble, there may be a drop below the critical micellar concentration required for fat absorption. In cholestasis the block in enterohepatic circulation occurs either in the liver or in the biliary tree. In this setting the pattern of hepatic conjugation of primary bile acids is changed; more sulfates are formed, and subsequently renal excretion is greater.

FLUID AND ELECTROLYTE TRANSPORT

Physiologic Considerations

The average adult produces approximately 100 to 200 ml of stool water daily. Considering that the gut normally handles almost 10 L of fluid daily, this organ exhibits a highly efficient mechanism for conserving salt and water. Oral intake comprises only a small portion, approximately 1 L, of the total amount of gut fluid. The remainder consists of endogenous secretion from the salivary glands, stomach, pancreas, biliary tree, and the intestine itself. Even minor aberrations in this finely tuned system result in an increase in stool water and hence diarrhea.

The major factors involved in the gut's absorption of fluid are intestinal motility and epithelial transport. Traditionally, it was assumed that diarrhea was a consequence of hypermotility. Indeed, the term *diarrhea,* derived from the Greek, means "to run through." Over the last 20 years, the pendulum has swung in the opposite direction. With the recognition that cholera toxin causes the intestinal epithelium to actively secrete fluid and that sugar-containing solutions can counter this effect,[20,21] the major research emphasis has been on the mechanisms involved in epithelial transport, delineating the carriers, channels, and pumps involved in the movement of Na and chloride (Cl). Although motility clearly is important, its role in diarrhea is, as yet, unclear (i.e., is hypermotility [hyperthyroidism] or hypomotility [diabetic diarrhea] more important as a cause of diarrhea?). As a more thorough understanding of the intricacies of intestinal function are achieved, the pendulum is settling somewhere in the middle, with epithelia and muscle both playing a role. An intricate network, with input from nerves, endocrine and paracrine cells, and the immune system, forms a common regulatory system that modulates the roles of both salt and water transport and motility.[22]

Each section of the smoothly functioning intestine serves a special role in the epithelial transport of fluid, electrolytes, and nutrients. The jejunum absorbs fluid isosmotically secondary to Na-coupled nutrient absorption. The ileum absorbs Na-Cl and secretes bicarbonate (HCO_3), again isosmotically. Generally, the small bowel absorbs large volumes of fluid but does not concentrate the intestinal luminal contents. The colon, primarily the distal colon, is capable of absorbing Na against a concentration gradient and therefore is well adapted for its role of conserving salt and water.

Not only does electrolyte and nutrient absorption vary along the length of the gut, it also differs along the crypt-villus surface axis. In brief, intestinal epithelial cells originate from pluripotent stem cells located in the base of the crypts. As epithelial cells migrate upward from the crypt base toward the villus tip, they define the crypt-villus axis. During this upward migration, the epithelial cells begin to express additional transporters not found in the crypt cells. In addition, certain transporters expressed in crypt cells are lost as the cells migrate and mature. For example, in the jejunum, Na-coupled nutrient transporters are present primarily in the mature villus cells but absent in the crypt cells. Thus net absorption takes place in the villus cells, whereas net secretion occurs in the crypts. In contrast, Cl secretion occurs primarily in the crypt cells, not in the mature villus cells. Obviously, any pathologic process that primarily affects villus cells tilts the overall intestinal balance in favor of secretion, with diarrhea as the result.[22]

In crossing from lumen to blood, ions, solutes, and water face a series of barriers. The first barrier confronted is the unstirred layer of water and mucus coating the epithelium. The depth of this unstirred layer, which varies along the length of the gut, may play an important role in the rate at which certain ions and solutes are absorbed. In particular, the unstirred layer preferentially affects absorption of larger lipid-soluble molecules (e.g., long chain fatty acids) and solutes that are rapidly transported.[22] However, recent evidence suggests that this layer is much thinner, and hence more permeable, than previously appreciated.[23,24]

After penetrating the unstirred layer, ions and solutes face two possible routes of absorption. The first is between the cells through the tight junctions. Water, low molecular weight solutes, and ions move through this paracellular route passively in response to electrochemical and osmotic gradients. These gradients are established by active transport of ions and solutes through the cell (transcellular transport). Two-way traffic of ions occurs across the intestinal epithelia. Fluxes occur in a serosal-to-mucosal direction, as well as from mucosa to serosa. Net transport depends on the magnitude of the opposing fluxes. Alterations in one or both of the unidirectional fluxes may result in absorptive or secretory changes. Water movement occurs in response to osmotic gradients. Na is the principal ion driving absorptive flows, whereas active Cl secretion promotes movement of water into the intestinal lumen. Nutrients may have a crucial role in determining the rate of water transport. Carbohydrate malabsorption causes luminal retention of considerable osmotic force, resulting in either inhibition of water absorption or actual secretion. On the other hand, well-absorbed sugars and amino acids enhance water absorption.

All transport epithelia possess similar characteristics: a polarity of membranes with distinct apical (luminal) and basolateral (serosal) membranes; an Na pump (ouabain-inhibitable Na^+, K^+-ATPase) located on the basolateral membrane, exchanging intracellular Na for extracellular potassium (K); a characteristic electrochemical potential profile, in which the intracellular potential difference is negative and the intracellular Na concentration is low. Na entry into the cell is therefore "downhill" because of the favorable electric and chemical gradients, and the Na pump consumes energy (ATP) to extrude Na across the basolateral membrane. Intracellular Cl is generally above its electrochemical equilibrium; this means that Cl exit from the cell does not require energy. Given these common characteristics, what distinguishes one section of the intestine from another are the specific entry mechanisms for Na across the apical membrane and the response to a variety of hormonal, bacterial, neural, immunologic, and pharmacologic mediators of transport.

There are three basic mechanisms of Na entry across the apical membrane: (1) solute-coupled Na transport, (2) Cl-coupled Na transport, and (3) electrogenic Na absorption independent of other ions or solutes. In all cases Na absorbed across the apical membrane is extruded across the basolateral membrane by the Na pump[25] (Fig. 18-6).

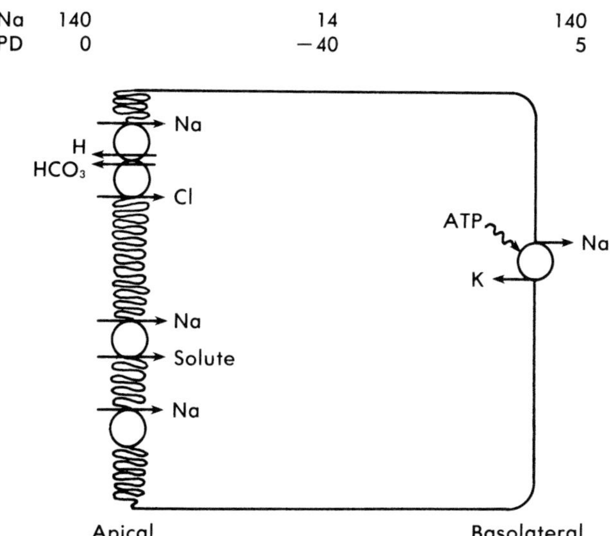

Fig. 18-6. Na absorptive pathways in the small bowel. A favorable electrochemical gradient exists for Na entry into the cell. The Na^+, K^+-ATPase on the basolateral border pumps Na out of the cell in exchange for K. Na enters the cell across the apical membrane through three different pathways: (1) coupled to Cl, in a system of Na-H, Cl-HCO_3 exchange; (2) coupled to solutes, such as glucose or amino acids; or (3) independently, in an electrogenic entry step. *Na,* Sodium; *H,* hydrogen; *HCO_3,* bicarbonate; *Cl,* Chloride; *K,* potassium; *PD,* potential difference. Numbers following Na and PD at top of figure refer to concentration of Na and PD in millivolts, respectively.

Solute-coupled Na absorption allows for accumulation of nutrients (mainly amino acids and glucose) in the enterocyte against a concentration gradient through linkage to downhill Na movement. Such Na-coupled transport mechanisms depend on the presence of both substances for the system (a carrier protein) to be operative. The transport may be either electrogenic or electroneutral depending on the charge of the cotransported solute. Finally, Na-glucose and Na–amino acid cotransporters are found throughout the small bowel but not in the colon. In contrast, specialized Na-coupled carrier proteins, such as those for bile acids, may be restricted to a limited region of the intestine.

One such carrier protein, an Na-glucose cotransporter named SGLT1, has recently been identified and cloned. Although multiple Na-glucose cotransporters operate elsewhere in the body, the evidence suggests that SGLT1 is the only Na-glucose cotransporter functioning at the brush border in small bowel epithelial cells.[26] Structurally, SGLT1 is a 664–amino acid protein that spans the apical membrane many times. It is distributed along the small bowel only, not the colon. Functionally, SGLT1 cotransports Na and glucose from lumen to enterocyte. Specifically, Na binds first to the protein's extracellular domain, thereby inducing a conformational change that allows glucose to bind alongside. In the absence of Na, glucose does not bind. A further conformational change induced by glucose binding flips the Na and glucose intracellularly. Na then dissociates along its concentration gradient. With Na now gone, SGLT1's affinity for glucose drops, and sugar is thereby released into the cytoplasm. From there, another glucose transporter (GLUT2) located at the basolateral membrane moves glucose into the extracellular milieu, with absorption into the blood coming still later.

Even before its identification, several interesting observations regarding the regulation of SGLT1 activity were made. First, because Na is absorbed down its electrochemical gradient, this process does not require energy. Hence, SGLT1's activity is, by definition, a type of facilitated diffusion. Second, the addition of one cotransported substance (glucose) to the lumen stimulates absorption of the other (Na). This latter observation forms the basis for oral rehydration therapy, in which patients with secretory diarrhea (from cholera, for example) are given glucose-rich oral therapy. In addition to the requisite electrolytes, this solution has a high concentration of glucose. The solution does not reverse or inhibit cholera toxin–mediated secretion; rather it stimulates the (Na-glucose) absorptive pathway. The absorptive movement of Na and glucose counters the effect of chloride secretion. This standoff between absorptive and secretory forces diminishes water flow into the intestinal lumen and hence diminishes diarrhea.

Finally, in animals, acute and chronic hyperglycemia appear to lead to paradoxical upregulation of SGLT1 activity and therefore to increased glucose absorption. Furthermore, this response seems to be both local and systemic. To whit, glucose infusion into the ileal lumen of anesthetized animals promotes glucose transport at the basolateral membrane of the same animal's jejunum. In addition, the response is rapid, occurring within hours. In contrast, acute hypoglycemia induced by insulin infusion, does not appear to affect sugar transport. Glucagon infusion, however, apparently does lead to increased SGLT1 activity (i.e., increased glucose absorption) at the brush border.[27] In sum, Na-glucose cotransport appears to be regulated at the luminal, paracrine, and systemic levels, and it is highly adaptable.

Na-Cl–coupled transport is found in a variety of epithelia. The nature of coupling is complex, and the existence of at least two different cotransport systems is probable. In the intestine Na-Cl absorption does not occur through a single transporter; instead, there are two coordinated, electrically neutral systems, one exchanging Na for H, the other Cl for HCO_3[28,29] (see Fig. 18-6). Since H + HCO_3 can combine to form water and carbon dioxide (CO_2), the net result is Na and Cl absorption. The two transporters are most likely synchronized by intracellular pH. Na-Cl-coupled transport is found in the jejunum, ileum, and colon. Molecular identification of several types of Na-H exchangers, with different kinetics and tissue distribution, has provided new insight into the complexities of absorption and secretion.

Na absorption that is not coupled to a solute or chloride is electrogenic because it involves net transfer of positive charge. Unlike the coupled transport systems that involve specialized protein carriers, this type of Na transport occurs through selective channels in the membrane that allow the passage of Na but exclude other cations and anions. This absorptive pathway is most readily apparent in the distal colon and can be blocked by the diuretic amiloride.

Cl, the principal ion governing secretion, accumulates within intestinal cells above its electrochemical equilibrium. The permeability (conductance) of the apical membrane for Cl determines the rate of the anion's movement across this membrane. The Cl conductance is controlled by several intracellular mediators—cyclic adenosine monophosphate (cAMP), cyclic guanosine monophosphate (cGMP), inositol triphosphate, and calcium. Stimuli (e.g., cholera toxin, which raises cAMP) that increase any of these three factors cause active Cl secretion and, secondarily, movement of water into the intestinal lumen.[30] In addition to increasing the Cl conductance of the apical membrane, these mediators also block the Na-Cl cotransport system. This antiabsorptive effect favors fluid accumulation within the intestinal lumen and an increase in diarrhea. However, these agents have no effect on Na absorption coupled to solutes such as sugars or amino acids. The therapeutic implications of this observation have led to oral rehydration therapy (described earlier), one of the more important medical developments in this century.

Another important medical development involving Cl secretion concerns cystic fibrosis (CF). The gene responsible for CF has recently been cloned, and its protein product identified. The protein, cystic fibrosis transmembrane conductance regulator (CFTR), is an apical transmembrane protein found in many tissues, notably respiratory and intestinal epithelia.[31] CFTR is activated by intracellular cAMP and protein kinase A to open and allow Cl to move down its concentration gradient into the intestinal lumen. Na and water follow. In CF, a missense mutation leads to defective Cl secretion and consequently dehydrated secretions. In humans, the primary organ affected is the lung.[32]

Structurally, CFTR belongs to a specific class of proteins, the ATP-binding cassette (ABC) superfamily. This superfamily consists of pumps, not channels.[32] CFTR structurally resembles these pumps, even possessing an ATP-binding site. However, this ATP-binding site does not appear to be an energy source supporting secretory activity. Contrary to expectations based on its structure, overexpression of CFTR is functionally associated with Cl channel activity. In general, channels do not require energy to function, and they allow fluxes, which are orders of magnitude higher than pumps. Because of this contradiction between structure and function, some have theorized that CFTR may function as both a channel and a pump. Accumulating evidence, however, supports the view that CFTR is the cAMP-activated Cl channel.

Although the specific gene product has been identified and studied intensively for several years, the precise defects underlying CF have not been fully elucidated. A major problem in CF may involve protein trafficking (i.e., the channel protein, although produced, never makes it to the proper place in the apical membrane.[33] Because CFTR is intimately associated with the Cl channel underlying most of intestinal secretion, the unfolding story of CF will provide new insights into intestinal secretory mechanisms.[34,35]

In sum, the intestinal epithelia has the capacity to either absorb or secrete. It is normally exposed to a vast array of absorbagogues and secretagogues, both from the luminal and serosal sides. These stimuli to absorption or secretion can be neural, hormonal, immunologic, or exogenous. They often act through second messengers as well (Table 18-1). Often, as is becoming increasingly clear for cholera toxin, a single agent exerts its effect through simultaneous actions at multiple levels: directly, at the enterocyte, and through neural, immune, and muscle targets. The transport function of the epithelium depends on the net sum of these stimuli. Knowledge of the pathways and their regulation aid in understanding the pathophysiology of diarrheal states and designing successful therapeutic strategies.

Clinical Implications

Acute diarrheas are frequent and generally self-limited. The diagnostic workup is straightforward: a stool search for blood, pus, and pathogens. Chronic diarrheas are less common and demand a logical clinical approach based on defining whether the diarrhea is secretory or osmotic in nature. This "paint can workup" requires serial 24-hour

Table 18-1. Intestinal Secretory Stimuli

Luminal	Serosal	Intracellular Mediator
Bacterial endotoxins (cholera, *Escherichia coli* heat labile toxins, *Shigella* organisms, *Staphylococcus aureus*)	Vasoactive intestinal peptide Prostaglandins	cAMP
Laxatives (castor oil, dioctyl sodium sulfosuccinate)		
Bile acids		
Dihydroxy fatty acids		?
Bacterial enterotoxins (*E. coli* heat-stable toxin)		cGMP
Detergents (bile acids?)	Acetylcholine Serotonin Substance P Neurotensin Bombesin	Calcium

cAMP, Cyclic adenosine monophosphate; *cgMP,* cyclic guanosine monophosphate.

stool collections for volume, electrolytes, osmolality, and fat. Frequently, stool volumes turn out to be normal, suggesting a functional cause and thereby shifting the emphasis of the workup. If stool volumes are increased (>500 ml/day), examination of the electrolytes and osmolality determines the type of diarrhea. In secretory diarrheas the osmolality can be accounted for by the ions in the stool water (calculated as the sum of Na and K, multiplied by 2). In osmotic diarrheas the osmolality is much greater than the concentration of measured ions.

Osmotic diarrheas may be caused by malabsorption of specific carbohydrates (lactose intolerance), ingestion of poorly absorbed solutes (laxatives containing magnesium), or unregulated entry of an osmotic load into the small bowel (postgastrectomy syndromes). Characteristically, in these conditions the diarrhea stops when nothing is taken by mouth. Secretory diarrheas may be caused by hormone-producing tumors. Vasoactive intestinal peptide, serotonin, calcitonin, gastrin, and prostaglandins have been implicated in the pathogenesis of tumor-related diarrheas. Bile salts, fatty acids, laxatives, and other drugs may produce a secretory diarrhea. Additionally, increased hydrostatic pressure or obstructed lymphatic drainage (Crohn's disease, lymphoma) may cause a similar clinical picture.

The clinical hallmark of a secretory diarrhea is continuation of the diarrhea while the patient is fasting. Hormone-induced diarrheas tend to be more voluminous than osmotic diarrheas, whereas those associated with lymphatic obstruction may have protein-losing enteropathy or lymphocytopenia. Once the presence of diarrhea and the broad category into which it falls have been established, attention can be focused on a more specific cause.

Cholera is the paradigm of a secretory diarrhea. An appreciation of the mechanisms underlying fluid loss and the rationale for oral rehydration therapy provide an understanding of the basic framework of intestinal transport. As a model of secretory diarrhea, cholera continues to provide new insights into intracellular trafficking, channel physiology, and the relations between epithelial transport and motility in the pathogenesis of diarrhea.

VITAMIN D AND MINERAL METABOLISM

The increasing recognition of the association between gastrointestinal dysfunction and metabolic bone disease emphasizes the importance of the gut and the liver in the regulation of mineral metabolism.[36] Vitamin D and calcium are the two critical factors in mineral homeostasis; their metabolism and actions are intertwined, and both are dependent on normal intestinal absorptive function. The role of the multiple metabolites of vitamin D, which may more properly be considered a prohormone, has been extensively studied during the last three decades. Significant questions remain over the physiologic role of some of the metabolites, the mechanisms of action of vitamin D, and the intestinal transport of calcium. It is now clear that vitamin D acts, at least in part, through the same mechanism as steroid hormones. Specifically, vitamin D binds an intracellular receptor, forming a complex. This complex then interacts with DNA in the cell nucleus, affecting transcription. In addition, vitamin D also acts through other, "nongenomic" mechanisms.[37] At the level of the enterocyte, vitamin D increases calcium absorption by inducing the cell to produce intracellular calcium-binding proteins.[38] Interestingly, the vitamin D intracellular receptor has been found in a variety of tumor cell lines. When vitamin D is added to these cell lines, their malignant potential appears to decrease. Thus in addition to its role in mineral metabolism, vitamin D may be important in tumorigenesis.[38]

Vitamin D has two major sources: (1) endogenous production, in which sterol precursors are converted to vitamin D by ultraviolet radiation, and (2) food that is either naturally rich in vitamin D (such as fatty fishes, eggs, and chicken liver) or has been fortified with vitamin D (such as milk). Vitamin D itself is biologically inactive. It is sequentially metabolized by the liver (25-hydroxylation) and kidney (1-hydroxylation) to produce 1,25 $(OH)_2$ vitamin D, the most potent of the vitamin D metabolites. The major regulatory step in this pathway is hydroxylation in the kidney. Both parathormone and low serum phosphate concentrations stimulate 1-hydroxylation. There is a feedback inhibition loop in which 1,25 $(OH)_2$ vitamin D leads to preferential hydroxylation at the 24- rather than the 1-position. The biologic role of 24,25 $(OH)_2$ vitamin D is unknown; it may simply represent a degradation pathway.[39] In addition, human placenta and human macrophages also possess 1-hydroxylase activity. These observations account, at least in part, for the bone loss associated with pregnancy and the hypercalcemia of granulomatous diseases.[38]

The major circulating vitamin D metabolite is the 25-OH form. Serum concentration generally reflects body stores.[40] In contrast, serum levels of 1,25 $(OH)_2$ vitamin D do not correspond well with the individual's vitamin status and may remain normal during deficiency.

Both vitamin D and 25-OH vitamin D have relatively long half-lives (weeks to months) and are stored primarily in fat and muscle. Interestingly, there is a seasonal variation in serum vitamin D levels, with higher values occurring during the summer when sun exposure peaks.[40] In addition, vitamin D and its metabolites circulate bound to plasma proteins, yet it is the unbound portion that accounts for the vitamin's activity. Consequently, agents that increase the production of these binding proteins increase measured levels of vitamin D without increasing activity.[38]

Because it is fat soluble, dietary vitamin D depends on intestinal bile salts and micelle formation for absorption. Vitamin D deficiency, likely caused by malabsorption resulting from insufficient bile, is seen in primary biliary cirrhosis. Although 25-hydroxylation is a necessary step in vitamin D metabolism, little correlation exists between the severity of hepatocellular disease and 25-hydroxylation. Drug-induced inductions of hepatic enzyme activity may increase the liver's metabolism of vitamin D and be associated with a deficiency. The most notable clinical example of this occurs with anticonvulsant therapy (e.g., phenytoin [Dilantin]). Although an enterohepatic circulation of vitamin D occurs, controversy exists regarding its significance.[41]

Calcium absorption depends on dietary intake, intraluminal factors, mucosal integrity, and hormonal status. The recommended minimal daily intake of calcium is 1000 mg; however, dietary intake in a substantial portion of the population (the lactase deficient, the elderly) and even "normals" may be inadequate. The principal food source for calcium is milk and milk products. Approximately one quarter of milk calcium is in the form of calcium citrate; the remainder appears to be in a colloidal calcium phosphate suspension. In other animal sources protein-bound calcium is present. In vegetables the predominant form is calcium salts (oxalates, phytates, or other organic anions).

Intraluminal factors, in addition to the source of the calcium, may determine the availability for absorption. To be absorbed, calcium must be ionized in the form of a soluble salt. Therefore when complexed with a fatty acid, oxalate, phytate, or cholestyramine, calcium is not absorbed. Recent studies have demonstrated that gastric acid secretion has a striking lack of effect on absorption of calcium salts,[42] thereby bringing into question the long-held role of the stomach in calcium absorption. Intraluminal factors can also increase calcium absorption. Most notably sugars, especially lactose,[43-45] have been shown to increase intestinal calcium absorption, presumably secondary to changes in fluid transport. Bile acids, amino acids, and certain antibiotics such as penicillin and chloramphenicol facilitate absorption by increasing calcium's solubility.

Calcium transport across the intestinal epithelium occurs by both active and passive mechanisms. At low intraluminal calcium concentrations, vitamin D–responsive active transport is dominant. This transport is most apparent in the duodenum. If intraluminal calcium concentration is increased sufficiently, passive diffusion can be demonstrated. Interestingly, the cecum and proximal colon may absorb calcium efficiently.[37] Although vitamin D clearly stimulates production of several specific transport proteins (calcium-binding protein, calcium-dependent alkaline phosphatases, calcium-ATPase), its stimulatory effect on calcium absorption may be related to changes in membrane structure and phospholipid metabolism.[46,47] Recent evidence suggests that calcium exits the cell across the basolateral membrane via an ATP-dependent calcium pump, an Na-Ca exchanger, and simple exocytosis.[48]

Intestinal transport, bone resorption, and renal excretion form a triad of regulatory sites for maintenance of serum calcium. Changes at one site generally stimulate a compensatory response at another. Parathormone and 1,25 $(OH)_2$ vitamin D act in concert to increase serum calcium. Parathormone has no direct action on the intestine but may alter calcium absorption indirectly by affecting vitamin D metabolism. Other factors may also play an important role: growth hormone, prolactin, estrogens, and granulomatous diseases such as sarcoidosis may increase calcium absorption. Glucocorticoids, thyroxine, thiazides, uremia, chronic acidosis, and aging decrease calcium absorption. These factors may act either directly on the intestine or alter vitamin D metabolism. Decreased calcium absorption is a common problem in gastrointestinal disease. Frequently, dietary intake is inadequate; lactose intolerance may compound this difficulty. Steatorrhea may result in intraluminal saponification with calcium binding to fatty acids. Additionally, steatorrhea is associated with vitamin D malabsorption. Loss of epithelial absorptive surface, either from resection or loss of mucosal integrity (e.g., in patients with sprue, inflammatory bowel disease, jejunoileal bypass), impairs calcium absorption. The principal liver disease associated with impaired calcium absorption is primary biliary cirrhosis, in which severe metabolic bone disease may be a crippling complication.

Magnesium deficiency is relatively uncommon because

obligatory fecal loss is minimal and the renal conservation mechanisms are extremely effective. However, magnesium deficiency can develop in a setting of renal disease, ketoacidosis, and malabsorption. Alcoholics appear particularly prone to develop magnesium deficiency. Because magnesium is necessary for parathormone's release from the parathyroid gland and its action on bone, magnesium deficiency should always be considered as a cause of hypocalcemia.

FOLIC ACID AND VITAMIN B_{12} METABOLISM

Folate and vitamin B_{12} are the two water-soluble vitamins that are essential for normal red blood cell production. Because isolated deficiencies of both these vitamins occur frequently, an understanding of their complex absorption pathways is important.

Folic Acid

Folate functions as a methyl donor in several vital reactions including purine synthesis, amino acid metabolism, and initiation of protein synthesis. Folate deficiency leads to megaloblastic changes in both the hematopoietic system and the intestinal epithelium.

Free folate consists of a pteroic acid moiety linked to L-glutamate. Most dietary folate is in a conjugated form, with a chain of several glutamates (polyglutamate folates). Absorption of folate depends on hydrolysis of the glutamic acid chain and subsequent transfer of the monoglutamyl product across the intestinal epithelium. The glutamic acid chain appears to be resistant to pancreatic digestive enzymes and is most likely broken down by brush border enzymes, which liberate free folic acid and amino acids. Polyglutamate folate, as such, is not absorbed.[49]

The rate-limiting step in folate absorption is entry across the apical membrane of the enterocyte. At low luminal concentrations of folate, a saturable, anion-exchange mechanism of facilitated diffusion exists. At high luminal concentrations, passive diffusion becomes evident. Alterations in pH affect the rate of intestinal uptake of folate; the optimum is pH 6.5. The epithelial cells reduce methylate folate, releasing methyltetrahydrofolate into the portal blood.

The body stores of folate are limited, in the range of 5 to 20 mg. The liver, which is the major storage site, contains primarily polyglutamate folate. Folate is excreted into the bile as the monoglutamate and undergoes an enterohepatic circulation with intestinal reabsorption. Folate deficiency may result from either inadequate intake or intestinal disease. Because the body stores of folate are small, individuals on a diet low in leafy green vegetables are particularly prone to folate deficiency; these include alcoholics, elderly people on tea and toast diet, and younger individuals eating primarily "junk food." Intestinal diseases such as gluten enteropathy and nontropical sprue are important causes of folate deficiency. Because megaloblastic changes of the intestinal epithelium can by themselves induce malabsorption, folate replacement is an essential first step in evaluating these patients.

States of increased folate demand can result in folate deficiency; the most notable example of this is pregnancy. Drugs may also contribute to folate deficiency. Anticonvulsants, most frequently phenytoin (Dilantin), have been implicated in folate deficiency. Sulfasalazine interferes with the intestinal absorption of folate; therefore individuals with inflammatory bowel disease who are taking this drug and may already have malabsorption or inadequate dietary intake are particularly prone to folate deficiency. Methotrexate blocks formation of the active form of folic acid (tetrahydrofolate) and therefore interferes with its biologic effects. Although diet is undoubtedly the major reason for folate deficiency in alcoholics, some evidence suggests that ethanol's toxic effect on the small bowel may impair folate absorption.[50] Because intestinal folate transport is inhibited by luminal alkalinization, patients with pancreatic insufficiency may exhibit supranormal folate absorption.

Vitamin B_{12}

Vitamin B_{12} (cobalamin) is an essential cofactor in the conversion of homocysteine to methionine. Cobalamin deficiency leads to a derangement in folic acid metabolism and subsequently DNA synthesis. This deficiency underlies the megaloblastic maturation pattern seen in hematopoietic and epithelial cells. Additionally, vitamin B_{12} is necessary for the conversion of methylmalonyl-CoA to succinyl-CoA. Disruption of this pathway causes accumulation of nonphysiologic fatty acids in neuronal lipids, the likely cause of the neurologic problems seen with vitamin B_{12} deficiency.

Because vitamin B_{12} is found only in animal products (meat and dairy foods), strict vegetarians are at risk for developing a deficiency. The body stores sufficient vitamin B_{12} to meet requirements for several years; therefore unlike folic acid deficiency, vitamin B_{12} deficiency does not develop acutely. As a corollary, individuals may malabsorb vitamin B_{12} for an extended period of time while their serum levels remain normal.

The absorption of cobalamin is complex and depends on gastric, pancreatic, and ileal function. Because vitamin B_{12} is relatively large (MW 1355) and possesses many polar groups, it cannot readily diffuse through membranes; therefore it depends on specific transport processes. A series of binding proteins is essential for vitamin B_{12} absorption: R proteins, intrinsic factor, and transcobalamin II. Considering the minute quantity of cobalamin in the diet ($\approx$ 10 μg/day), this system is highly efficient. The three binding proteins have a high affinity for cobalamin. Intrinsic factor is a glycoprotein produced by gastric parietal cells. R proteins, transcobalamin I, and transcobalamin III belong to a family of glycoproteins found in plasma, saliva, tears, bile, and gastric juice. Transcobalamin II is a circulating polypeptide that facilitates uptake of vitamin B_{12} into rapidly dividing cells. For the purpose of this discussion, the focus is only on the role of the gut in cobalamin absorption.

Cobalamin in food protein complexes is rapidly liberated in the acid environment of the stomach. Within this acid environment, cobalamin binds to salivary and gastric R proteins. In the duodenum the increased intraluminal pH decreases the affinity of R protein for intrinsic factor. More significantly, pancreatic proteases degrade R proteins, liberating the cobalamin to bind with intrinsic factor.[51] The intrinsic factor–cobalamin complex, which is resistant to proteolytic digestion, proceeds to the distal ileum. Specific receptors on the ileal brush border recognize and bind the complex, a process dependent on a neutral pH and calcium. The intrinsic factor–cobalamin complex then enters the ileal cell; the fate of intrinsic factor during this internalization has not been determined.[52] Cobalamin exits the ileal cell across the basolateral border into the portal circulation bound to transcobalamin II.

Although the role of R proteins in cobalamin absorption has been delineated, its significance is unknown. R proteins do not recognize the ileal cobalamin–intrinsic factor receptor, and therefore cannot mediate absorption. Individuals with R protein deficiency have been identified; no hematologic derangements are apparent in this condition. In pancreatic insufficiency, transfer of cobalamin from R proteins to intrinsic factor may be defective. This may cause an abnormal Schilling test (see later discussion), but it generally does not result in either a vitamin deficiency or megaloblastic changes. The most attractive hypothesis concerning their function centers on the possible protective role of R proteins.[53] In addition to vitamin B_{12}, bacteria produce many inactive cobalamin analogs. R proteins bind to these inactive analogs with a high affinity, whereas intrinsic factor is fairly specific for the bioactive cobalamins. Therefore R proteins may serve to bind and divert these unwanted cobalamin analogs.

Evaluation of cobalamin absorption is easily accomplished with a Schilling test. Radioisotopically labeled vitamin B_{12}, with and without intrinsic factor, can be administered orally and the relative rates of absorption can be calculated by measuring the 24-hour urinary excretion. Given the complexity of cobalamin absorption, several different pathologic entities may cause an abnormal Schilling test. Atrophic gastritis with achlorhydria may be associated with a failure of intrinsic factor production. Additionally, in atrophic gastritis, antibodies directed at either of the two intrinsic factor binding sites (for vitamin B_{12} or the ileal receptor) may be found. Gastric resection may remove the source of intrinsic factor production, and ileal resection may eliminate the site for intestinal absorption. Either pancreatic insufficiency or Zollinger-Ellison syndrome may lower duodenal and jejunal pH, thereby impeding the separation of R protein from cobalamin. Bacterial overgrowth may provide a competitive site for cobalamin uptake. Rare congenital deficiencies of either intrinsic factor, transcobalamin II, or the ileal receptor for the intrinsic factor–cobalamin complex, inhibit absorption. Finally, omeprazole has been shown to decrease cobalamin absorption, although the precise mechanism and the clinical significance of this information remain to be demonstrated.[5] Megaloblastic changes associated with folic acid deficiency may also affect the results. After appropriate clinical assessment, a modified Schilling test with either a course of antibiotics to treat overgrowth or pancreatic enzyme replacement may elucidate the cause of the cobalamin malabsorption.

WATER-SOLUBLE VITAMINS

Most water-soluble vitamins are relatively large, not freely diffusible in lipid because of their polar side chains, and found in the intestinal lumen in low concentrations. Therefore they are ideal candidates for carrier-mediated transport. Ascorbic acid, biotin, nicotinic acid, and thiamine possess Na-dependent active transport processes. Studies with riboflavin suggest a carrier-mediated absorption, whereas pyridoxine exhibits passive diffusion. Intestinal metabolism of pyridoxine, riboflavin, and thiamine appears to involve a phosphorylation step. Isolated malabsorption of these water-soluble vitamins is rare but in global malabsorption or dietary deprivation deficiencies may become clinically significant.

In addition to its role in intermediate metabolism, thiamine may have a specific role in nerve conduction. Clinical thiamine deficiency (beriberi) may appear as congestive heart failure or may have neurologic derangements such as peripheral neuropathy, Wernicke's encephalopathy, and the Korsakoff's syndrome. Wernicke's encephalopathy may present with horizontal nystagmus, lateral rectus muscle palsies, confusion, or coma. Korsakoff's syndrome involves recent memory loss with a compensatory, often colorful, confabulation. Clinically significant thiamine deficiency is found most frequently in alcoholics or globally malnourished individuals, including patients after gastric surgery.

Daily thiamine requirement may vary with the diet composition, increasing with more carbohydrates, decreasing with more fat. Therefore it is possible to precipitate overt signs of thiamine deficiency in a marginally compensated individual by administration of a large carbohydrate load. Routine administration of thiamine to alcoholics is aimed at preventing such an occurrence.

Deficiencies of other water-soluble vitamins, such as ascorbic acid, biotin, nicotinic acid, pyridoxine, and riboflavin, are sufficiently rare not to warrant detailed discussion. For a review of these vitamin deficiencies, the reader is referred to textbooks of nutrition.

IRON

Beyond the obvious relevance to hemoglobin production, recent work has suggested that the body's iron (Fe) status is important in coronary artery disease,[54] neoplastic cell growth,[55] viral hepatitis,[56] and immunocyte function.[57] Progress has also been made in fleshing out the still incomplete picture of iron metabolism.

The mechanisms of Fe excretion, through either bile, urine, or enterocyte sloughing, are extremely limited. Consequently, intestinal iron absorption is central to iron homeostasis. In men approximately 1 mg of Fe is absorbed daily, matching intestinal losses. In women absorption is somewhat higher, 1.5 mg/day. Rates of intestinal absorption clearly adapt to the body's overall needs; in states of Fe deficiency, the intestine increases its rates of absorption. the mechanisms for this autoregulation remain obscure.

Several factors affect Fe absorption even before Fe reaches its site of absorption. First, the type of Fe ingested is important. Dietary Fe may be plant Fe, heme, or inorganic salts (pharmacologic replacement). Heme Fe is more efficiently absorbed by mechanisms different from nonheme iron and is not affected by intraluminal events.[58] In contrast, nonheme iron absorption is influenced by intraluminal factors that either increase or decrease its solubility.[59] In addition, the chemical form of dietary iron is important. A ferrous (Fe^{2+}) compound is absorbed better than a ferric (Fe^{3+}) one. This may be related to the fact that $FeCl_2$ is much more soluble than $FeCl_3$ at neutral pH. Therefore factors that tend to reduce Fe, such as gastric acid, tend to increase its absorption. In pancreatic insufficiency, increased Fe absorption may be found; this is probably related to the high phosphate and bicarbonate concentrations found in normal pancreatic secretions, which alter the chemical form of Fe. Ascorbic acid also increases Fe absorption. In part, this results from its action as a reducing agent. Additionally, it may form a soluble complex with Fe, maintaining it in a more absorbable form. Other intraluminal factors, such as bile, amino acids, and succinic acid, further assist Fe absorption.

A variety of intraluminal binding agents may decrease Fe absorption. Phytate, phosphates, oxalate, and carbonate inhibit Fe absorption by forming insoluble complexes. Dietary fiber may also function as an intraluminal binder. There is evidence that other metallic cations such as cobalt and manganese (but not calcium or magnesium) may inhibit Fe absorption.

Two interactions within the stomach ready Fe for absorption when it reaches the proximal small bowel. First, the acid pH renders dietary Fe soluble. Next, gastric mucins bind Fe in a reaction that is again pH dependent. The mucin-Fe complex remains in solution as the pH rises with transit. This complex then reaches the chief site of Fe absorption, the proximal small intestine. Entry across the apical membrane of enterocytes is carrier-mediated, saturable, and energy dependent.[60] The identity of the carrier, however, remains obscure. Once within the cell, Fe is bound by a newly identified shuttle protein known as mobilferrin. If the body is Fe replete, mobilferrin delivers Fe to ferritin for storage. Alternately, in Fe deficiency, mobilferrin delivers the absorbed Fe to intracellular transferrin. This transferrin-Fe complex then enters the circulation across the basolateral membrane. Although the epithelium clearly adapts to the body's need for Fe, the specific mechanisms responsible for this adaptation have not been identified. Although ferritin, plasma transferrin saturation, and Fe content of mucosal cells have been proposed as possible regulatory mechanisms, they now seem unlikely candidates.[61] Finally, a small amount of Fe is absorbed by a simple diffusion via a paracellular route.[52]

Fe deficiency may occasionally result from an inadequate diet (almost exclusively observed in infants), achlorhydria, malabsorption syndromes such as nontropical sprue, duodenal bypass and/or resection, or increased metabolic demands (e.g., in pregnancy). As a practical matter, however, Fe deficiency must be assumed to be caused by blood loss until proven otherwise. Approximately half the body's Fe stores is found in red blood cells (2500 mg). One milliliter of packed red blood cells contains 1 mg of Fe. Since the rate of mobilization of Fe from nonheme stores is relatively slow, any compensation for acute blood loss is limited.

Fe overload syndromes may result from excessive Fe absorption. In hemochromatosis, Fe absorption may be as high as 4 mg/day. Because of the limited excretory mechanisms for this substance, total body Fe stores gradually and inexorably increase. Excessive Fe absorption is found in states of ineffective erythropoiesis or hemolysis. Increased dietary Fe can rarely cause overload. The classic example is Bantu siderosis, a form of Fe overload caused by ingestion of beer brewed in iron pots.

CLINICAL APPROACH TO MALABSORPTION

By combining clinical acumen with the rational use of diagnostic tests, physicians can establish a diagnosis of malabsorption, pinpoint a cause, and establish a rational therapeutic plan. Crucial to accomplishing this is an understanding of the pathophysiology of malabsorption and the principles underlying the diagnostic tests.[62] Individual patients may exhibit either global malabsorption or malabsorption of a specific nutrient; their initial clinical appearance varies accordingly. The cardinal symptom of global malabsorption is weight loss. Diarrhea is a common finding, but it is important to remember that not all diarrhea implies malabsorption; conversely, global malabsorption is not always accompanied by diarrhea. The development of bulky, floating, or oily stools suggests malabsorption. The presence of foul smelling stools is a less reliable indicator. Fatigue and lethargy are frequently present. The clinical appearance of malabsorption of a specific nutrient (e.g., vitamin B_{12}, lactose) may be more subtle and depends on the particular substance involved.

Generally, the first step is to confirm the presence of malabsorption by documenting the presence of steatorrhea. Fecal fat, rather than carbohydrate or protein, is used as the sensitive indicator of malabsorption for two fundamental reasons: successful fat absorption requires the pancreas, biliary system, and intestinal mucosa and therefore reflects the normal functioning of all three components. Additionally, and on a more pragmatic level, a reasonable correlation exists between unabsorbed dietary fat and fecal fat, whereas unabsorbed carbohydrate and protein are rapidly degraded by bacteria into ammonia, H, CO_2, and short chain fatty acids, disrupting the relationship between the actual unabsorbed and fecal components. Although it has generally been assumed that fatty acids are not attacked by bacteria,[63] recent studies suggest that there may be bacterial metabolism of fat.[9]

The gold standard for steatorrhea is a quantitative fecal fat collected during a period of 72 hours while the patient is ingesting a 100 g fat diet per day. A positive test result is defined as greater than 6 g per day of fecal fat excreted (>18 g/72 hr). A qualitative estimate of steatorrhea can be obtained with a Sudan stain of a stool sample.

Once the presence of steatorrhea is established, the next series of tests are designed to differentiate between mucosal and intraluminal defects. Intraluminal defects are associated with loss of pancreatic or biliary secretions or both or the failure of digestive enzymes to mix with food within the intestinal lumen. Mucosal defects imply a disruption of the normal epithelial function, either by loss of surface area or by disruption of the absorptive machinery of the epithelial cells. The classic tests for mucosal function include D-xylose absorption, small bowel x-ray examination, and small bowel biopsy. D-xylose is a poorly absorbed 5-carbon sugar. Because xylose does not require intraluminal digestion by pancreatic enzymes, it is generally regarded as an indicator of intestinal mucosal disease. Since the test is inexpensive, essentially risk free, and accurate, it is one of the primary tests in assessing malabsorption. After drinking a solution containing 25 g of D-xylose, urine is collected over a 5-hour period. Urinary excretion of 5 g or greater of D-xylose is normal. Severe bacterial overgrowth can sometimes lead to a falsely positive test result because intraluminal bacteria successfully compete with the mucosa for the sugar. After treatment for overgrowth, D-xylose absorption should return to normal.

Barium contrast studies of the small bowel are essential for diagnosing specific anatomic defects (e.g., strictures, jejunal diverticulum) and for assessing the mucosal pattern of the small bowel. The cardinal findings in intestinal disease include dilation of the intestinal lumen, thickening of mucosal folds, dilution of barium, and segmentation of the head of the barium column.[64] Thickening of folds generally indicates an infiltrative process (amyloidosis) or a response to hypoproteinemia. The new improved barium sulfate now used in contrast studies is "nondispersible"; therefore flocculation is no longer a reliable or common sign in malabsorption. Dilution of the barium is secondary to increased water within the intestinal lumen, a common finding in diarrhea associated with malabsorption. X-ray studies may indicate fairly specific abnormalities such as Crohn's disease that may elucidate the cause of a particular case of malabsorption. The small bowel series is an important diagnostic tool in a malabsorption workup; one proviso, however, is necessary: barium studies should be held in abeyance until all stool collections are complete.

The small bowel biopsy provides histologic confirmation of mucosal disease and frequently enables a specific diagnosis to be made.[65] Uncommon diseases such as abetalipoproteinemia, Whipple's disease, and immunodeficiency syndromes have diffuse lesions that are pathognomonic on small intestinal biopsy. Diagnostic small intestinal biopsies may also be obtained in diseases with patchy lesions (e.g., lymphoma, eosinophilic enteritis, amyloidosis, and Crohn's disease). The small bowel biopsy is probably most useful in the diagnosis of gluten enteropathy (nontropical sprue). In this disease the normal villous pattern is replaced by a "flat" mucosa in which the villi are absent, the crypts are hypertrophied, and the lamina propria contain increased numbers of inflammatory cells. Since sprue involves primarily the proximal small bowel, it is amenable to diagnosis by biopsy. However, subtotal villous atrophy occasionally can occur in tropical sprue and therefore, by itself, is not pathognomonic. Clinical and histologic improvement after withdrawal of dietary gluten can confirm the diagnosis. Partial villous atrophy is characterized by shortened, clubbed villi and increased numbers of inflammatory cells in the lamina propria and interepithelial spaces (Fig. 18-7). It is found in a number of intestinal diseases including tropical sprue, severe bacterial overgrowth, and radiation enteritis.

When a diagnosis that produces a patchy mucosal lesion is being considered, multiple biopsies are necessary. Normal results from a small bowel biopsy provide useful clinical information because they direct the malabsorption workup toward intraluminal defects caused by pancreatic insufficiency, bacterial overgrowth, and short bowel syndrome. Examples of the kinds of information that small bowel biopsy can provide are demonstrated in Fig. 18-7.

Accurate clinical assessment of pancreatic function is difficult and notoriously insensitive. The standard pancreatic secretion test assesses the increase in duodenal fluid and HCO_3 and pancreatic enzymes in response to secretion stimulated by secretin, CCK, or both. In severe chronic pancreatitis, both HCO_3 and volume are reduced. In carcinoma of the head of the pancreas, similar reductions may be found. In partial duct obstruction, HCO_3 secretion may be maintained while volume is decreased. Mild-to-moderate pancreatic insufficiency and carcinomas of the body and tail generally do not cause abnormalities in the pancreatic secretion tests.

Because of this insensitivity, attempts at developing tubeless pancreatic function tests have been numerous. Probably the most widely accepted of these newer tests is the bentiromide absorption test. Bentiromide absorption depends on peptide cleavage by chymotrypsin, which liberates *p*-aminobenzoic acid (PABA). PABA is subsequently absorbed and excreted into the urine, where it can be easily measured.[66] Bentiromide may not be available in the future.

The newer breath tests have simplified the diagnosis of malabsorption.[67] Although there is a wide array of breath tests, they are based on common principles: nutrients are absorbed in the small bowel, which is relatively sterile;

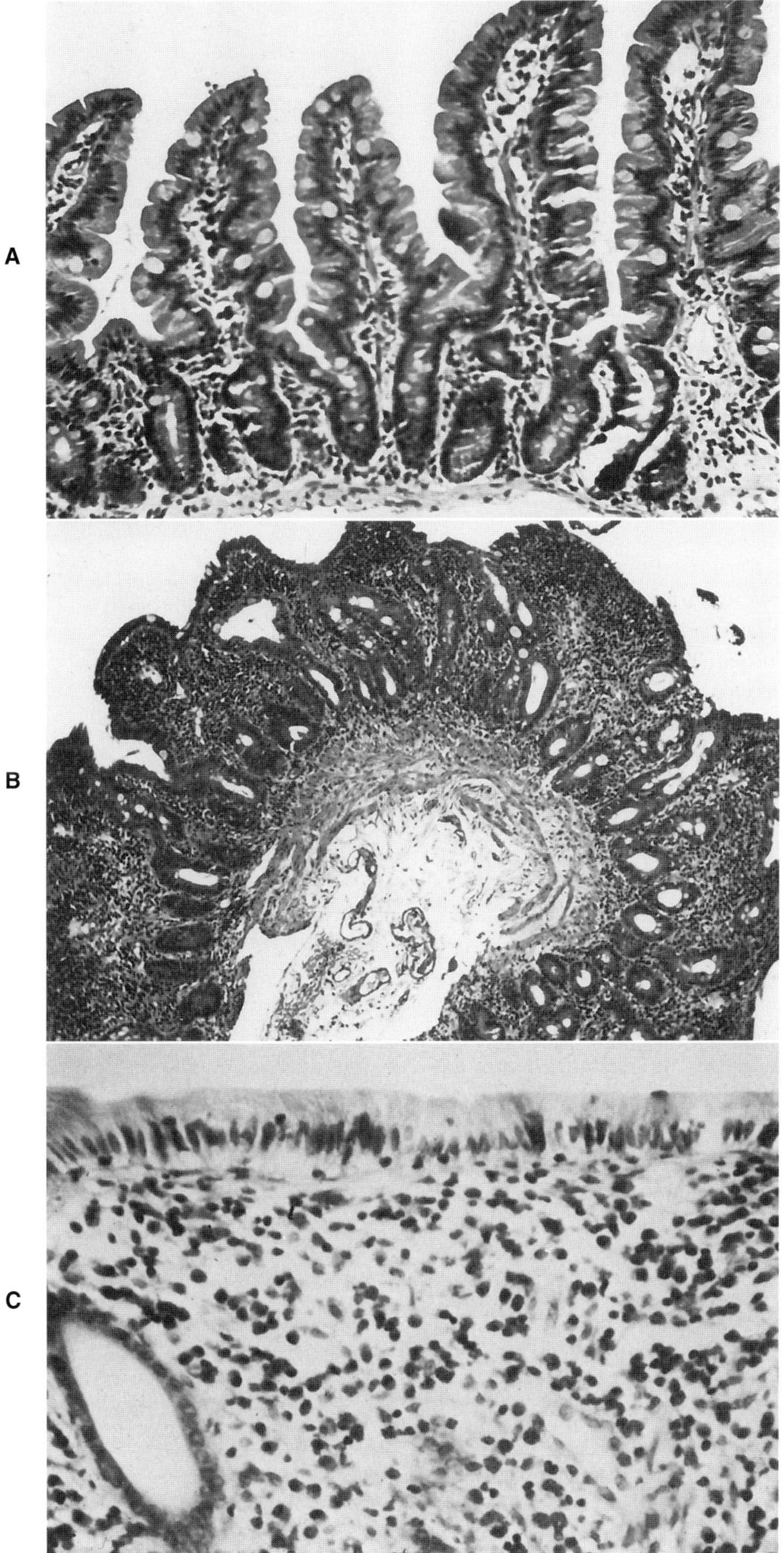

Fig. 18-7. Small bowel histology obtained by biopsy. **A,** Normal small bowel, with long slender villi, modest crypts, and a minimal number of inflammatory cells in the interstitium. **B,** Partial villous atrophy. The villi are clubbed and the crypts elongated. **C,** Subtotal villous atrophy. Villi are absent suggesting a "flat mucosa."

therefore they normally escape bacterial degradation. However, if unabsorbed, nutrients pass into the colon; or if there is significant bacterial contamination of the small bowel, intraluminal bacterial metabolism of the nutrients produces a gas (either carbon dioxide [CO_2] or hydrogen [H_2] that is freely diffusible across the gut wall into the systemic circulation. The gas is then excreted by the lungs.

Because H_2 is not normally expired, an increase in breath H_2 can be used as a sensitive signal for malabsorption. The situation is somewhat more complicated for CO_2. Because CO_2 is a normal constituent of expired air, a labeled form of carbon is necessary to detect CO_2 of gut origin. This can be accomplished by using either a radioactive isotope of carbon (^{14}C) that can be detected by standard scintillation counting techniques or a nonradioactive stable isotope (^{13}C). However, because the stable isotope is not as readily available and requires specialized mass spectroscopy for detection, this technology most likely is restricted to research centers.

The H_2 breath test has been used primarily to detect carbohydrate malabsorption. It has proven extremely useful in detecting lactase deficiency. In this situation an oral load of lactose is not absorbed because of a lack of the brush border disaccharidase enzyme. The sugar passes into the colon, where bacterial metabolism yields 2- and 3-carbon fragments, CO_2 and H_2. An increase in the amount of H_2 in expired air indicates malabsorption. Because the test is noninvasive, does not use radioisotopes, does not require blood drawing, and uses relatively simple equipment, it is ideal for assessing carbohydrate intolerance in children and pregnant women. This methodology can be easily applied to the study of other carbohydrates, including xylose, fructose, and glucose.

By radiolabeling one of the carbon atoms in the glycine conjugate of a bile acid, the enterohepatic circulation of bile salts can be assessed. Normally the terminal ileum efficiently absorbs the bile salts presented to it. However, if there is significant ileal dysfunction or small bowel bacterial overgrowth, the bile salt is deconjugated, the glycine is metabolized, and the $^{14}CO_2$ thus produced is excreted by the lungs. Therefore an abnormal ^{14}C-n-bile salt breath test can indicate ileal dysfunction or bacterial overgrowth. It cannot reliably distinguish between the two conditions.

The triolein breath test has been proposed as a substitute for a quantitative fecal fat collection. ^{14}C-Triolein is given with a standard oral fat load. Normal fat absorption results in a significant increase in expired $^{14}CO_2$, whereas steatorrhea is suggested by the lack of a $^{14}CO_2$ peak. This test differs from other breath tests in that the signal is found in normal results and does not depend on bacterial metabolism of the nutrient.[68]

Compared to recent technologic advances, the standard Schilling test may appear rather staid. Nevertheless, it can prove extremely useful in a general malabsorption workup in addition to its obvious application in detecting vitamin B_{12} malabsorption. It should be kept in mind that a Schilling test result may be abnormal in bacterial over-

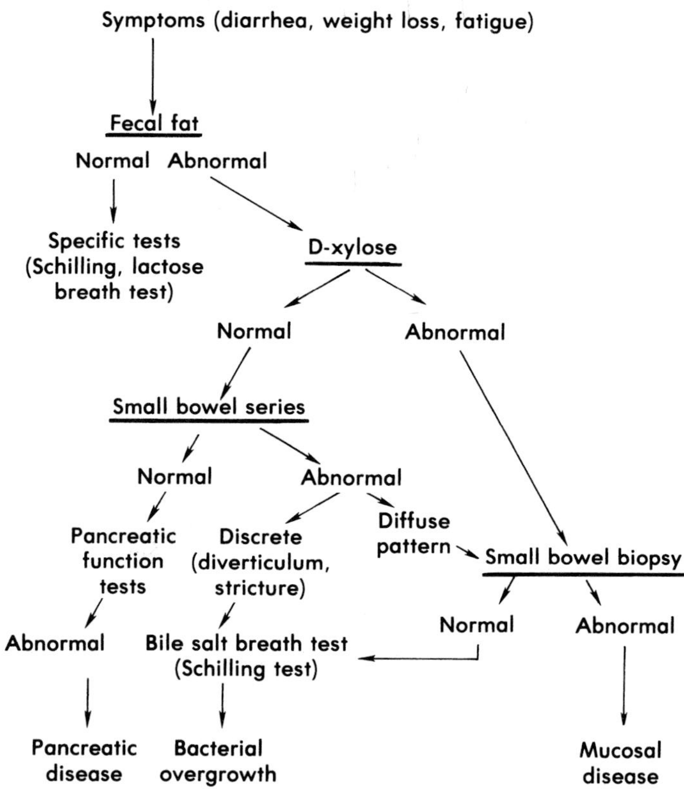

Fig. 18-8. Algorithm for a clinical approach to malabsorption.

growth (caused by bacterial metabolism of cobalamin), pancreatic insufficiency (secondary to lack of protease action on R protein), and ileal disease (with lack of the specific transporter). Because it is a sensitive indicator of malabsorption and readily available to every clinician, it remains a useful diagnostic tool.

A malabsorption workup can proceed in a rational fashion, applying diagnostic tests to answer a series of progressive questions:

Is global malabsorption (steatorrhea) present?
Is there any evidence of mucosal disease?
Is pancreatic function intact?
Is there malabsorption of a specific nutrient?

By following a standard algorithm, such as the one summarized in Fig. 18-8, the physician can proceed through a malabsorption workup quite efficiently.

MALABSORPTION IN SURGICAL PATIENTS

In surgical patients, syndromes causing malabsorption can occur as a consequence of operations on the intestinal tract. For example, overgrowth of bacteria in the small intestine occasionally occurs following a Billroth II gastrectomy. The accompanying diarrhea may limit the digestion and absorption of fats, protein, and carbohydrates. In addition, bacteria compete for vitamin B_{12}, potentially altering its absorption. Another example of surgically induced malabsorption results after extensive intestinal resection. Severe disturbances in the normal physiology of digestion and absorption may ensue, depending on the extent of resection. For a more detailed discussion of postsurgical malabsorption, please refer to the chapter on postsurgical derangements in intestinal function.

In addition to postsurgical syndromes, other conditions may alter intestinal function in surgical patients. Inflammatory bowel disease may severely alter the normal transport and absorptive mechanisms of the distal ileum, affecting both vitamin B_{12} absorption and enterohepatic circulation. More extensive involvement of the small intestine may cause abnormal calcium absorption. Deficiencies in vitamin K and iron may also be encountered. In inflammatory bowel disease a wide variety of effects on nutrient transport can be observed. These are directly related to the length of intestine.

Finally, surgeons routinely encounter cancer patients. Lymphomatous involvement of the intestinal wall may cause malabsorption. In addition, radiation can cause malabsorption because of the resulting fibrosis and endarteritis. Again, the length and segment of intestine involved determine the nature of the problem. Other diseases that can greatly alter digestion and absorption include celiac sprue, tropical sprue, and Whipple's disease. Because these disorders are only rarely seen by surgeons, the reader is referred to standard gastroenterology textbooks for a detailed discussion.

SUMMARY

Efficient absorption and digestion depend on integration of a series of complex events both within the intestinal lumen and at the epithelial border. Of the three major categories of food, only fats require emulsification and solubilization by micelles within the intestinal lumen before passive absorption across the epithelium. The products of carbohydrate and protein digestion use specific transport carriers at the apical border of the intestinal epithelium.

The movement of water is secondary to the active transport of ions. Specifically, Na is the major ion determining osmotic gradients favorable for water absorption, whereas Cl is the usual driving force for secretion. A host of hormones, peptides, drugs, immunologic factors, and bacterial toxins regulate the traffic of ions and water across the intestinal epithelium.

Diarrhea and malabsorption are the major clinical manifestations of dysfunction of the intestinal epithelium. An orderly clinical approach coupled with judicious use of basic diagnostic tests usually clarifies the cause of diarrhea (osmotic vs. secretory) or malabsorption (maldigestion vs. epithelial disease).

REFERENCES

1. Matthews DM, Adibi SA. Peptic absorption. Gastroenterology 71:151, 1976.
2. Sleisenger MH, Kim YS. Protein digestion and absorption. N Engl J Med 300:659, 1979.
3. Adibi SA, Kim YS. Peptide absorption and hydrolysis. In Johnson LR, et al., eds. Physiology of the Gastrointestinal Tract. New York: Raven Press, 1981.
4. Schedl HP, Wenger J. Adibi SA. Diglycine absorption in streptozoticin diabetic rats. Am J Physiol 235:E457, 1978.
5. Marcuard SP, et al. Omeprazole causes malabsorption of cyanocobalamin (vitamin B_{12}). Ann Intern Med 120(3):211, 1994.
6. Gray GM. Carbohydrate digestion and absorption. N Engl J Med 292:1225, 1975.
7. Kimmich GA, Randles J. Evidence for an intestinal Na^+: Sugar transport coupling stoichiometry of 2.0. Biochim Biophys Acta 596:439, 1980.
8. Rosensweig NS, Herman RH. Control of jejunal sucrase and maltase activity by dietary sucrose or fructose in man. J Clin Invest 46:186, 1967.
9. Patton JS. Gastrointestinal lipid digestion. In Johnson LR, et al., eds. Physiology of the Gastrointestinal Tract. New York: Raven Press, 1981.
10. Patton JS, Carey MC. Watching fat digestion. Science 204:145, 1979.
11. Gaskin KJ, et al. Colipase and maximally activated pancreatic lipase in normal subjects and patients with steatorrhea. J Clin Invest 69:427, 1982.
12. Gaskin KJ, et al. Colipase and lipase secretion in childhood-onset pancreatic insufficiency. Gastroenterology 86:1, 1984.
13. Wilson FA, Dietschy JM. Characterization of bile acid absorption across the unstirred water layer and brush border of the rat jejunum. J Clin Invest 51:3015, 1972.
14. Westergaard H, Dietschy JM. Delineation of the dimensions and permeability characteristics of the two major diffusion barriers to passive mucosal uptake in the rabbit intestine. J Clin Invest 54:718, 1974.
15. Riley JW, Glickman RM. Fat malabsorption—Advances in our understanding. Am J Med 67:980, 1979.
16. Heubi JE. Bile acid-induced diarrhea. In Lebenthal E, Duffey M, eds. A Textbook of Secretory Diarrhea. New York: Raven Press, 1990.
17. Cirillo NW, Zwas FR. Ursodeoxycholic acid in the treatment of chronic liver disease. Am J Gastroenterol 89(9):1447, 1994.
18. de Caestacker JS, et al. Ursodeoxycholic acid in chronic liver disease. Gut 32:1061, 1991.
19. Rubin RA, et al. Ursodiol for hepatobiliary orders. Ann Intern Med 121:207, 1994.
20. Kimberg DV, et al. Stimulation of intestinal mucosal adenylate cyclase by cholera enterotoxin and prostaglandins. J Clin Invest 50:1218, 1971.
21. Carpenter CC, et al. Site and characteristics of electrolyte loss and effect of intraluminal glucose in experimental canine cholera. J Clin Invest 47:1210, 1968.
22. Sellin J. Intestinal electrolyte absorption and secretion. In Sleisenger M, Fordtran JS, eds. Gastrointestinal Disease, 6th ed. Philadelphia: WB Saunders, 1993, p 1451.
23. Levitt H, et al. A reappraisal of the magnitude and implications of the intestinal unstirred layer. Gastroenterology 101(3):843, 1991.
24. Levitt I, et al. Human jejunal unstirred layer: Evidence for extremely efficient luminal stirring. (Part 1). Am J Physiol 262(3):G593, 1992.
25. Schultz SG. Cellular models of sodium and chloride absorption by mammalian small and large intestine. In Field M, Fordtran JS, Schultz SG, eds. Secretory Diarrhea. Bethesda, Md.: American Physiological Society, 1980.
26. Wright CEM. The intestinal Na+/glucose cotransporter. Annu Rev Physiol 55:575, 1993.
27. Debnam ES. Rapid adaptation of intestinal sugar transport. News Physiol Sci 9:84, 1994.
28. Fordtran JS, Rector FC, Carter NW. Mechanisms of sodium absorption in the human small intestine. J Clin Invest 47:884, 1968.
29. Liedtke CM, Hopfer U. Mechanism of Cl translocation across small intestinal brush border membrane. Am J Physiol 243:G263, 1982.
30. Frizzell RA, Heintze K, Stewart CP. Mechanisms of intestinal chloride secretion. In Field M, Fordtran JS, Schultz SG, eds. Secretory Diarrhea. Bethesda, Md.: American Physiological Society, 1980.

31. Anderson D, et al. Chloride channels in the apical membrane of normal and cystic fibrosis airway and intestinal epithelia. (Part 1). Am J Physiol 263(1):L1, 1992.
32. Fuller E, et al. CFTR! (Part 1). Am J Physiol 263(2):C267, 1992.
33. Morris AP, Frizzell RA. Vesicle targeting and ion secretion. In epithelial cells: Implications for cystic fibrosis. Annu Rev Physiol 56:371, 1994.
34. Gregory RJ, et al. Maturation and function of cystic fibrosis transmembrane conductance regulator variants bearing mutations in putative nucleotide binding domains 1 and 2. Mol Cell Biol 11:3886, 1991.
35. Higgins CF. Cystic fibrosis transmembrane conductance regulator (CFTR). Br Med Bull 48(4):759, 1992.
36. Kaplan MM. Metabolic bone disease associated with gastrointestinal diseases. Viewpoints Dig Dis 15:9, 1983.
37. Brasitus TA, Sitrin MD. Absorption and cellular actions of vitamin D. In Johnson LR, ed. Physiology of the Gastrointestinal Tract, 3rd ed. New York: Raven Press, 1994, p 1935.
38. Iqbal SJ. Vitamin D metabolism and the clinical aspects of measuring metabolites. (Part 2). Ann Clin Biochem 31:109, 1994.
39. Avioli LV, Haddad JG. The vitamin D family revisited. N Engl J Med 311:47, 1984.
40. van den Berg H. Vitamin D. Intern J Vit Nutr Res 63(4):257, 1993.
41. Clements MR, et al: Enterohepatic circulation of vitamin D: A reappraisal of the hypothesis. Lancet 1:1376, 1984.
42. Bo-Linn GW, et al. Evaluation of importance of gastric acid secretion in the absorption of dietary calcium. J Clin Invest 73:640, 1984.
43. Norman DA, Morawski SG, Fordtran JS. Influence of glucose, fructose, and water movement on calcium absorption in jejunum. Gastroenterology 78:22, 1980.
44. Kelly SE, et al. Effect of meal composition on calcium absorption: Enhancing effect of carbohydrate polymers. Gastroenterology 87:596, 1984.
45. Ziegler EE, Fomon ST. Lactose enhances mineral absorption in infancy. J Pediatr Gastroenterol Nutr 2:288, 1983.
46. Rasmussen H, et al. Role of changes in membrane lipid structure in the action of 1.25 dihydroxy-vitamin D_3. Fed Proc 41:72, 1982.
47. Wasserman RH, et al. Evidence for multiple effects of vitamin D_3 on calcium absorption. Proc Natl Acad Sci USA 79:7939, 1982.
48. Wasserman RH, et al. Intestinal calcium transport and calcium extrusion processes at the basolateral membrane. J Nutr 122(Suppl 3):662, 1992.
49. Rosenberg IH. Intestinal absorption of folate. In Johnson LR, et al., eds. Physiology of the Gastrointestinal Tract. New York: Raven Press, 1981.
50. Green PHR, Tall AR. Drugs, alcohol, and malabsorption. Am J Med 67:1066, 1979.
51. Allen RH, et al. Effect of proteolytic enzymes on the binding of cobalamin to R protein and intrinsic factor. J Clin Invest 61:47, 1978.
52. Turnberg LA, Riley SA. Digestion and absorption of nutrients and vitamins. In Sleisenger M, Fordtran JS, eds. Gastrointestinal Disease. Philadelphia: WB Saunders, 1993, p 999.
53. Kolhouse JF, Allen RH. Absorption, plasma transport and cellular transport of cobalamin analogues in the rabbit. J Clin Invest 60:1381, 1977.
54. Beard JL. Are we at risk for heart disease because of normal iron status? Nutr Rev 51(4):112, 1993.
55. Weinberg ED. Roles of iron in neoplasia. Promotion, prevention, therapy. Biol Trace Element Res 34(2):123, 1992.
56. Piperno A, et al. Relation between alpha-interferon therapy response and liver iron stores in chronic hepatitis C. Hepatology 18:90(A), 1993.
57. Kemp JD. The role of iron and iron binding proteins in lymphocyte physiology and pathology. J Clin Immunol 13(2):81, 1993.
58. Prasad AS, ed. Trace Elements and Fe Metabolism. New York: Plenum Publishing, 1978.
59. Schade SG, Cohen, RJ, Conrad HE. Effect of hydrochloric acid on iron absorption. N Engl J Med 279:672, 1968.
60. Manis J, Schacter D. Active transport of iron by intestine. Am J Physiol 203:73, 1962.
61. Conrad ME, Umbreit JN. A concise review: Iron absorption—The mucin-mobilferrin-integrin pathway. A competitive pathway for metal absorption. Am J Hematol 42:67, 1993.
62. Wilson FA, Dietschy JM. Differential diagnostic approach clinical problems of malabsorption. Gastroenterology 61:911, 1971.
63. Hoffman AF. Fat absorption and malabsorption. Viewpoints Dig Dis 9:13, 1977.
64. Kumar P, Bertram CI. Relevance of the barium follow through examination in the diagnosis of adult celiac disease. Gastrointest Radiol 4:285, 1979.
65. Trier JS. Diagnostic value of peroral biopsy at the small intestine. N Engl J Med 85:1470, 1971.
66. Lankisch PG. Tubeless pancreatic function tests. Hepatogastroenterology 28:333, 1981.
67. Hepner GW. Breath tests in gastroenterology. Adv Intern Med 18:25, 1978.
68. Newcomer AD, et al. Triolein breath test. Gastroenterology 76:6, 1979.

19

Normal Peristalsis and Abnormalities in Intestinal Motility

Erica A. Brotschi and James M. Becker

In 1899 Bayliss and Starling wrote, "In no subject in physiology do we meet with so many discrepancies of fact and opinion as in that of the physiology of the intestinal movements."[1] We know more about intestinal motility today than in 1899, but much uncertainty remains. The mechanisms that control intestinal movement are remarkably complex. Movement of food and secretions through the gastrointestinal (GI) tract depends on coordinated action of smooth muscle that makes up the gut wall. This chapter describes the mechanisms that control and organize contraction in GI smooth muscle. These control mechanisms are described in three categories: (1) myogenic mechanisms within the muscle tissue itself, (2) effects of local and long neural tracts, and (3) effects of GI hormones. This chapter also describes some important clinical problems associated with abnormal GI motor activity, or *motility.* Therapeutic approaches, especially drugs that influence GI motility, are discussed.

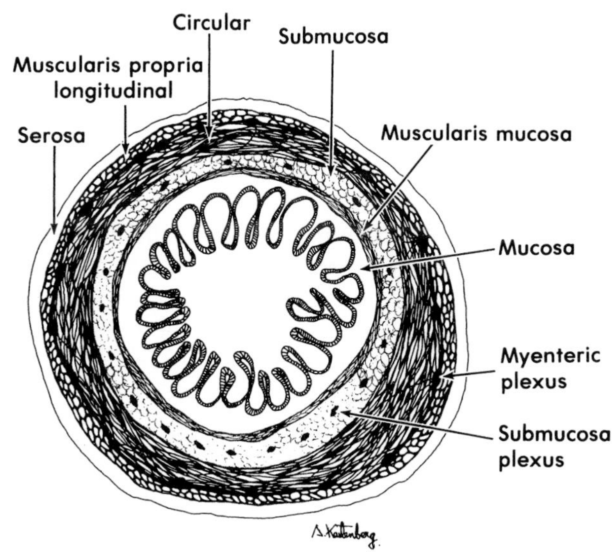

Fig. 19-1. Neuromuscular anatomy of the alimentary tract. Muscularis propria consists of both longitudinal and circular muscle groups.

GENERAL CONSIDERATIONS IN GASTROINTESTINAL MOTILITY

The primary role of the GI tract is to absorb water, electrolytes, and nutrients. Muscular activity of the wall of the GI tract generates several types of motion. *Propulsion* moves ingested food, secretions, and shed cells through the alimentary tract and directs them to sites of absorption. During this process, *mixing* occurs, which disperses food particles and increases their contact with the absorptive intestinal lining. Mixing also combines digestive secretions from the stomach, pancreas, and biliary tract with the intestinal contents. The GI tract also has a *reservoir* or storage function. This can involve active muscle relaxation. The colon stores unabsorbed contents from the small intestine while electrolytes are resorbed. Residual contents are then eliminated by defecation.

The anatomy of the alimentary tract is relatively consistent throughout its length (Fig. 19-1). Two anatomic features are particularly important for motility: the muscular wall of the gut and a complex network of intrinsic and extrinsic nerves that regulates every aspect of intestinal function, called the *enteric nervous system.*

From the midesophagus to the internal anal sphincter, the walls of the GI tract are composed of smooth muscle. In general, the smooth muscle of the alimentary canal is arranged in three layers. The inner layer is the muscularis mucosa. Around this is a circular layer of smooth muscle, which is surrounded by an outer longitudinal muscle layer. Between these muscle layers are the neural plexuses of the enteric nervous system. The submucosal (Meissner's) plexus is located between the muscularis mucosa and the circular muscle layer. The myenteric (Auerbach's) plexus is located between the longitudinal and circular muscle layers. The enteric nervous system receives input from local receptors and nerves in mucosa and smooth muscle. It is also regulated by input from the CNS through autonomic nerves including the vagus nerves, the pelvic parasympathetic nerves, and the sympathetic ganglia.

Motility of the GI tract is controlled by several mechanisms. *Myogenic control* arises from intrinsic rhythmic electric activity in the muscle tissue itself. This provides a pacemaker function analogous to the intrinsic rhythm of heart muscle. Myogenic control allows large numbers of muscle cells to contract in a coordinated pattern. Superimposed on myogenic control is input from the *enteric nervous system*. In general, enteric nerves determine whether contraction occurs, whereas myogenic control organizes the pattern of contraction. A further level of control results from secretion of the so-called *GI hormones.* These are a group of several dozen peptide neurotransmitters. These peptides are located within nerves of the enteric nervous system and often in the CNS as well. Some of the GI hormones are released into the gut lumen and into the blood during digestion. GI hormones may have both endocrine and paracrine effects that coordinate function of the gut, the pancreas, and the biliary tract.

Motility of the GI tract can be classified into three major patterns: tonic contractions, peristaltic waves, and segmenting contractions. *Tonic contractions* are sustained and generally produce low pressure (Fig. 19-2). Tonic contraction is observed in sphincter segments and is also involved in maintaining baseline tone in many smooth muscle types. The basic propulsive activity of the GI tract is *peristalsis,* which usually consists of rings of contraction moving in an aborad direction (Fig. 19-3, *A*) Cannon[2] proposed that intestinal distention is a major stimulus for peristaltic activity, and that distention leads to contraction above the site of distention and relaxation below it. This results in a directed contraction that propels luminal contents aborad (Fig. 19-4). *Segmenting contractions* are a pattern of motility that leads to mixing of intestinal content (Fig. 19-3, *B*).

MYOELECTRIC CONTROL OF INTESTINAL MOTILITY

Smooth muscle shows a rhythmic oscillation in membrane potential. This is probably related to rhythmic changes in ion flow across the membrane. Two important patterns of electric oscillation occur. Most types of smooth muscle show an intrinsic rhythmic fluctuation in membrane potential while at rest, called *slow waves.* In the GI tract, this slow wave rhythm has a major role in coordinating muscle contraction, just as the rhythmicity of cardiac muscle cells helps coordinate contraction of the heart. The slow waves, also called basic electric rhythm (BER) or electric control activity (ECA), are present both at rest and during contraction. Slow waves are often accompanied by slight rhythmic contractions or cyclic changes in resting muscle tension that can be measured in the laboratory. The second pattern of membrane electric activity consists of bursts of rapid fluctuation in potential. These bursts of larger electric fluctuations are called *spike potentials,* action potentials, or electric response activity (ERA). Spike potentials are superimposed on the slow waves. Spike potentials occur during rapid, complete depolarizations of smooth muscle cells. This is usually followed by obvious contractions.[3,4]

Slow Waves

Slow waves originate in the muscle cells themselves as an intrinsic fluctuation in membrane potential. The slow waves coordinate the pattern of membrane depolarization (Fig. 19-5). They establish the rhythm and polarity of intestinal contractions. In the small intestine the slow waves

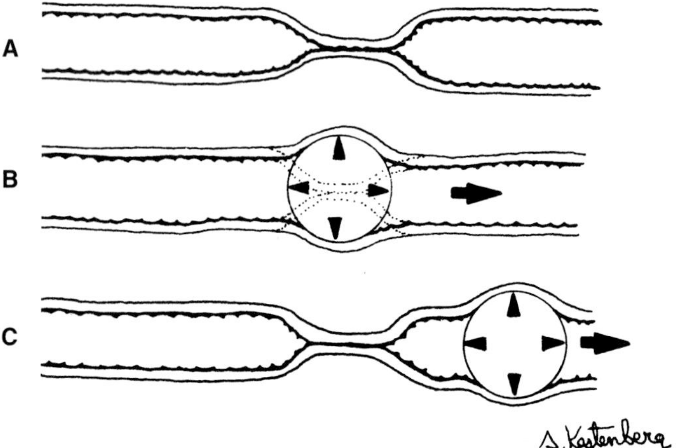

Fig. 19-2. Responses of gastrointestinal sphincters to intraluminal content. **A,** Tonic contraction of the sphincter at rest. **B,** Relaxation of the sphincter associated with passage of intraluminal content. **C,** Reestablishment of tonic contraction of the sphincter with aborad passage of the intraluminal bolus.

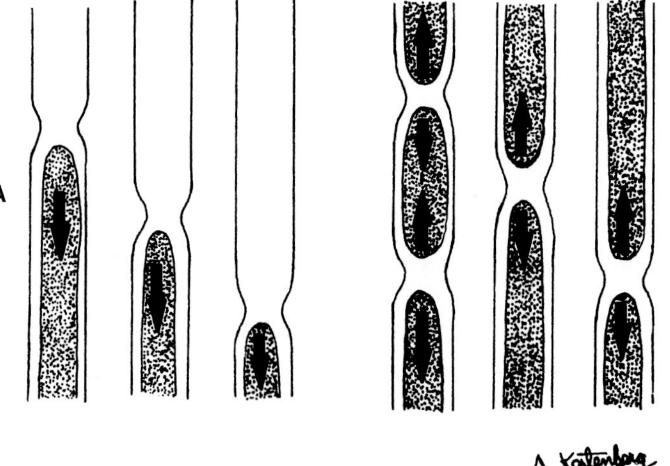

Fig. 19-3. A, Aborad movement of an intestinal peristaltic contraction. **B,** Segmental contraction of the bowel.

originate near the submucosa, either in circular muscle cells or in specialized submucosal cells.[5] The slow waves then spread to the longitudinal muscle layer. The frequency of the slow wave determines the maximum frequency of contraction in the bowel wall. This occurs because contractions are triggered by spike potentials, which occur only at one phase of the slow wave. Since only one contraction can occur during each slow wave, slow-wave frequency is also the maximum contractile frequency for a segment of bowel. Thus the slow wave serves as the pacemaker for a particular segment of bowel.

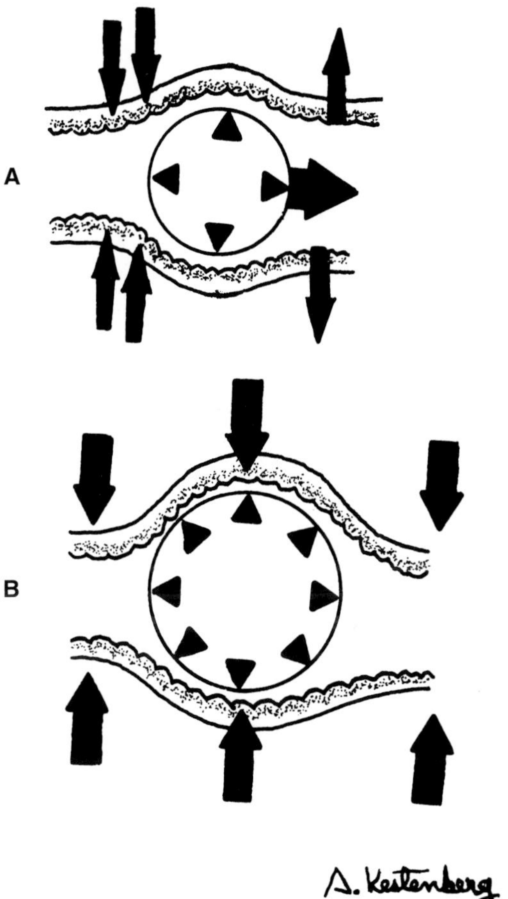

Fig. 19-4. **A,** According to Cannon's Law of the Intestine, physiologic distention of the bowel results in contraction orad to that point and relaxation aborad from that point with net aborad flow of intraluminal contents. **B,** Pathologic intraluminal distention of the bowel results in spasm and defective peristalsis with little or no aborad flow.

Each slow-wave oscillation lasts 2 to 3 seconds and results in a rhythmic change of membrane potential from about -70 to -25 or -30 mV. Segments of GI tract may be characterized on the basis of frequency of slow-wave oscillations.[6] In humans the slow-wave frequency of the stomach in vivo is 3 per minute, the duodenum 12 per minute, the jejunum 10 per minute, and the ileum 8 per minute. The slow-wave frequency declines progressively as more distal segments are measured.

Because of electric communication between smooth muscle cells, the more rapid slow-waves from a proximal segment of intestine "speed up" the slow-wave rate in adjacent distal segments. This tends to cause a slow wave that travels aborad along the bowel. This slow wave can serve as a pacesetter for organized peristaltic contraction. The effect of slow-wave electric activity in the intestine can be modeled using a relaxation oscillator. When two such oscillators are coupled, they influence one another. The one with lower intrinsic frequency increases in frequency so a pacemaker effect can be produced. By choosing appropriate intrinsic frequencies and coupling factors, a chain of oscillators can be modeled that gives slow-wave patterns like those recorded in the small intestine.

The cause of slow waves is a cyclic change in ion flux across the muscle cell membrane. The exact changes in ion flux are not completely understood. However, it is clear that depolarization or the "upstroke" phase of the slow wave corresponds to influx of calcium ions into the cells. The plateau phase of the slow wave reflects continuing calcium influx. Increased intracellular calcium is measurable within cells during the plateau of the slow wave. Repolarization may be due to efflux of potassium through calcium-activated potassium channels. The rise in intracellular calcium activates contraction in the cells and causes the small cyclic contractions that can be measured during slow waves.

Spike Potentials

Spike potentials, or action potentials, are rapid cycles of depolarization and repolarization that may occur superimposed on the slow wave (Fig. 19-5). Spike potentials oc-

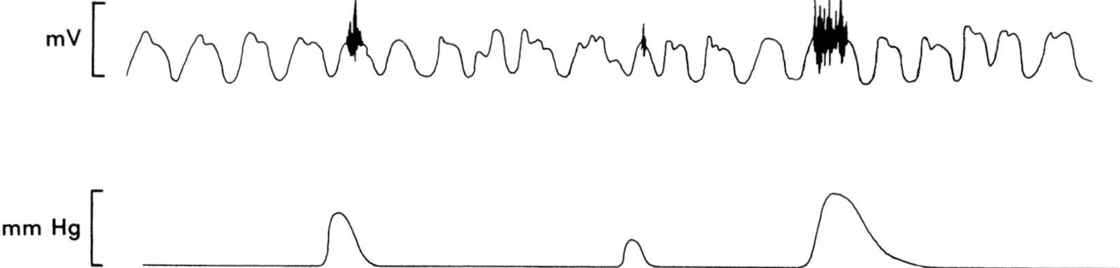

Fig. 19-5. Myoelectric slow waves with superimposed spike potentials *(upper tracing).* In general, slow waves determine the timing of spike potentials, which then initiate smooth muscle contractions *(lower tracing).* Recent evidence suggests that slow waves alone may induce contractions in certain regions of the gut.

cur only during the "peak" or depolarization phase of the slow wave. One slow wave may be associated with a series of spikes, or *burst*. This corresponds with a wave front of muscle contraction passing along the intestine. The basic slow wave acts as a pacesetter to organize smooth muscle contraction over long distances.

Whether spike potentials occur depends on the sum of excitatory and inhibitory stimuli acting on the muscle cell at the time of the slow wave. Most of these stimuli are neurotransmitters released by local nerves. Excitatory neurotransmitters stimulate the cell by binding to specific receptors. Receptor activation leads to depolarization (spike potentials) by causing rapid influx of calcium into the cells. This influx of calcium may occur either from the extracellular fluid or from calcium stored within the cell membrane.

Elevated intracellular calcium causes smooth muscle contraction. The mechanism by which calcium concentration regulates contraction is different in smooth muscle than in skeletal muscle. Increased intracellular calcium causes contraction in smooth muscle by a calmodulin-dependent mechanism. This may include activation of protein kinase C or other kinases. These kinases phosphorylate and activate myosin light chain kinase. Myosin light chain kinase in turn phosphorylates smooth muscle myosin, leading to increased cycling of cross-bridges between actin and myosin. This increased cross-bridge cycling leads to muscle contraction. The concentration of intracellular calcium appears to regulate contraction in most smooth muscle types.

Myoelectric Patterns in Various Parts of the Gastrointestinal Tract

In the duodenum, slow waves show a clear and consistent pattern. The frequency of the duodenal slow wave is 12 cycles per minute in humans and 18 cycles per minute in dogs. This frequency is driven by a pacemaker located in the wall of the first 5 to 6 cm of the duodenum. The pacemaker is the site of greatest intrinsic slow wave frequency. In the proximal jejunum a gradual decrease in the intrinsic frequency of the slow wave is found. The more rapid activity of the duodenal pacemaker ensures that the slow wave is propagated distally. This slow wave thus organizes peristaltic contraction along the duodenum. Abnormal function of the duodenal pacemaker may lead to disjointed duodenal contraction. This may occur due to duodenal trauma, inflammatory disease, resection of the first part of the duodenum, or vagotomy. Loss of the duodenal pacemaker may lead to abnormal gastric emptying.

Duodenal motility patterns appear to have a role in regulating motility of the distal common bile duct and the sphincter of Oddi. The sphincter area has a complex motility pattern that is regulated in part by a pacemaker in the biliary duct and in part by the electric and contractile activity of the duodenum.[7]

Characteristic motility patterns occur in the small intestine during fasting and after feeding (Fig. 19-6).[8] During fasting, activity follows a cyclic pattern called the *migrating motor complex* (MMC) or *interdigestive myoelectric complex* (IDMEC). As originally described by Szurszewski in 1969,[9] each cycle has four phases. Phase 1 has little or no contractile activity or electric spike activity. Phase II has intermittent spike activity and contractile activity. Phase III has maximum spike activity superimposed on every slow wave. This is associated with regular, strong contractile activity. Phase III is usually followed by a brief period of intermittent spike activity known as phase IV. The duration of an entire cycle is 90 to 120 minutes in humans. Each phase appears first in the distal esophagus, stomach, and duodenum and migrates down the small intestine. The migration takes about 2 hours. Eating abolishes the MMC cycle and induces intermittent contractile activity.

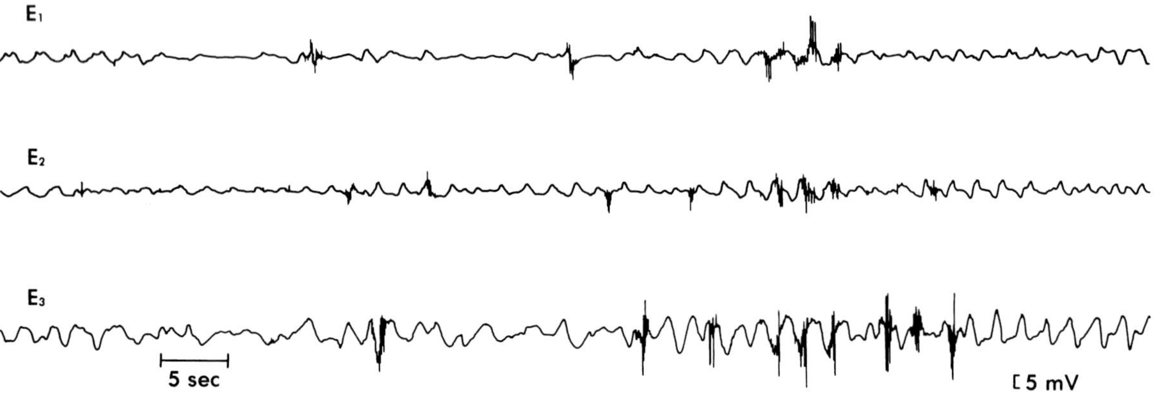

Fig. 19-6. Interdigestive myoelectric complex (IDMEC) recorded from sequential bipolar electrodes (i.e., E_1, E_2, and E_3) from the feline small intestine. Each cycle has four phases: phase I has little or no electric spike activity; phase II has intermittent spike activity; phase III has maximum spike activity, with spikes superimposed on every slow wave; and phase IV is again a period of only intermittent or absent spike activity.

The physiologic role of the MMC is unclear because the contractions are present only in the fasted state. In most species the MMC has no apparent role in mixing or propulsion of food. The MMC contractions may act as "housekeepers of the small intestine" by purging the small bowel of residual foods, secretions, and shed cells. The MMC may also limit the overgrowth of bacteria in the distal small bowel.[10] The factors that initiate and control the MMC are not well understood.[11] Neither vagotomy nor sympathectomy abolishes the MMC.[12] Although still controversial, motilin (a GI peptide found in high concentrations in the duodenal and jejunal epithelium) has been suggested to be the "interdigestive hormone" that regulates the initiation of cyclic motor activity in the small intestine.[13,14]

The control of motor activity in the colon is quite complex.[15] Most of the myoelectric activity in the colon is of low amplitude and apparently random. As descibed by Sarna[16,17] the colon shows four types of myoelectric activity: (1) electric control activity, (2) discrete ERA, (3) continuous ERA, and (4) the contractile electric complex (Fig. 19-7). The *ECA* is similar to the slow waves that were described in the proximal GI tract. The motor functions of the colon include mixing, temporary storage, and slow distal propulsion. These functions are apparently carried out by the random contractile activity recorded as *discrete and continuous ERA*.

In addition, high-amplitude propagated contractions occur occasionally in the colon, averaging six per 24-hour period in humans.[18] These powerful contractions are associated with myoelectric activity consisting of oscillations of potential called the *contractile electric complex*. These high-amplitude contractions correspond to radiologically identified "mass movements" of fecal content. They originate in the ascending colon and are propagated distally. They are often associated with defecation or an urge to defecate. Contractile activity in the entire colon increases on awakening from sleep. Colon contractile activity also increases almost immediately with food intake. The initial "cephalic" phase of increased colonic activity induced by food is neurally mediated.[19] Sham feeding or discussion of food increases colonic motility. Colon activity remains increased in the fed state, and colonic stimulation later in the fed period may be hormonally mediated.

Defecation is a complex motor phenomenon involving both voluntary and reflex activity. Normally the anal canal is closed by the *internal anal sphincter,* a thickening of rectal smooth muscle, and by the striated *external sphincter,* innervated by the pudendal nerve. When a mass movement distends the rectum with feces, the internal sphincter relaxes (the rectal inhibitory reflex) while the external sphincter constricts, producing the urge to defecate. If defecation is postponed, both muscles regain their normal tone. Defecation itself is controlled by a reflex center in the sacral cord, which is modulated by higher centers. Defecation is initiated when the internal sphincter relaxes reflexively and the external sphincter is relaxed voluntarily. Intra-abdominal pressure is increased by contraction of the abdominal muscles and by forced expiration against a closed glottis. The muscles of the pelvic floor are also relaxed, and this helps to straighten the rectal canal, permitting evacuation. In Hirschprung's disease, rectal distention fails to relax the internal anal sphincter, and therefore defecation cannot occur.

NEUROHUMORAL CONTROL OF INTESTINAL MOTILITY

Neurohumoral control of motor activity in the GI tract has historically been described at two levels. Stimuli from the CNS influence GI function through the *autonomic nervous system*. In addition, a much more complex level of neurohumoral control is exerted by the *enteric nervous system*. The enteric nervous system coordinates stimuli from the CNS with input from multiple types of receptors within the GI tract itself. The division between these two aspects of gut innervation is somewhat artificial.[20] The autonomic nervous system is actually just one of the mech-

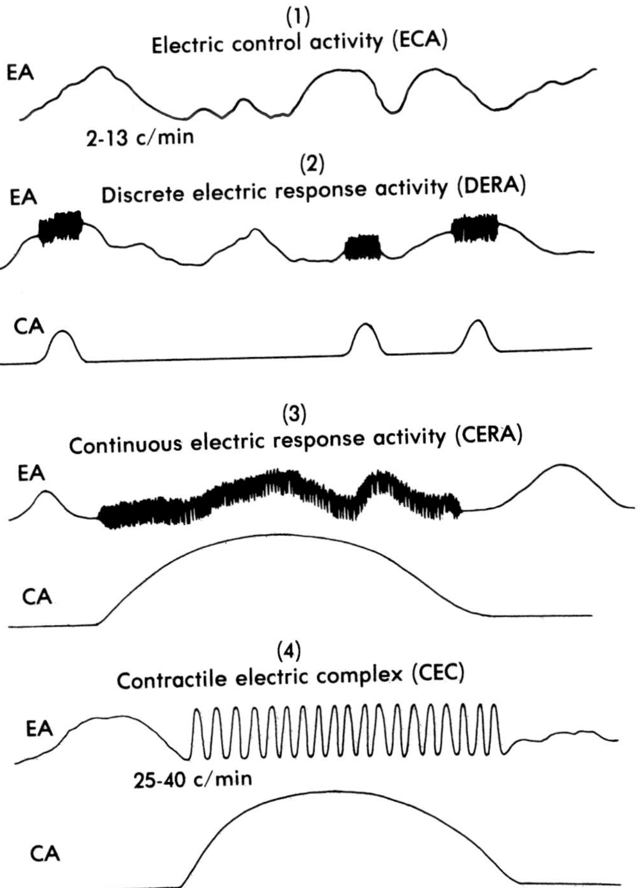

Fig. 19-7. Types of electric and contractile activity in the colon. *EA,* Electric activity; *CA,* contractile activity. (Modified from Sarna S. The control of colonic motility. In Chey WY, ed. Functional Disorders of the Digestive Tract. New York: Raven Press, 1983.)

anisms by which the brain influences the enteric nervous system. Characteristic neurotransmitters from both systems are found together in the vagus nerves: acetylcholine from the autonomic system and gastrin, cholecystokinin (CCK), and other peptides from the enteric nervous system.

Autonomic Nervous System

Autonomic neural pathways to the GI tract include the vagus nerves, the pelvic parasympathetic nerves, and the sympathetic ganglia. Branches of the vagus nerve supply parasympathetic input to the esophagus, stomach, and small intestine. The pelvic parasympathetic nerves supply the distal colon. The sympathetic nerve supply to the proximal GI tract comes through splanchnic nerves by way of the celiac ganglion. Sympathetic innervation to the colon comes through the hypogastric nerves from the superior and inferior mesenteric ganglia.

The major effect of the *parasympathetic nerves* is stimulatory to GI function and motility. The major parasympathetic neurotransmitter is acetylcholine. Acetylcholine is stimulatory to GI motility and many other digestive processes. GI muscle cells have muscarinic receptors for acetylcholine. Stimulation of acetylcholine receptors on muscle cells causes increased calcium influx into the cells. Elevated intracellular calcium then activates contraction. Many of the GI hormones that stimulate motility do so by releasing acetylcholine from intrinsic nerves. This can be demonstrated by showing that atropine, a muscarinic acetylcholine receptor antagonist, blocks the muscle contraction induced by the hormones.

The effect of *sympathetic nerves* on GI function is mainly inhibitory. Sympathetic nerves can be identified in the enteric nervous system, usually in close association with blood vessels.[21] Sympathetic nerves are also called *adrenergic* because they release norepinephrine or epinephrine, neurotransmitters that are also synthesized in the adrenal medulla. Adrenergic nerves are thought to presynaptically inhibit release of acetylcholine from cholinergic nerves.

Enteric Nervous System and Gastrointestinal Hormones

The enteric nervous system is a highly organized neural network that governs every aspect of GI function.[20] The enteric nerves are arranged in the submucosal and myenteric plexuses. The two plexuses are interconnected and also receive neural input from multiple types of receptors in the GI tract itself and from the CNS. The CNS input comes partly through autonomic nerves and partly through other nerves that release GI peptide hormones as neurotransmitters. The enteric nervous system regulates motility, as well as electrolyte secretion and absorption, vascular perfusion, and hormone secretion in the gut.

There are dozens of different neurotransmitters in the enteric nervous system. Many of the enteric neurotransmitters are also found in large amounts in the CNS, emphasizing the close relationship between the brain and the enteric nervous system.[22] Enteric neurotransmitters include nonpeptide molecules, which are important neurotransmitters in the CNS, such as adenosine triphosphate (ATP), acetylcholine, serotonin, and dopamine. Nitric oxide (NO) is an important GI neurotransmitter, causing smooth muscle relaxation.[23] In both vascular and GI tissues, NO is formed by an enzyme (NO synthetase) from the amino acid arginine and molecular oxygen. In GI smooth muscle, NO leads to hyperpolarization of the muscle, resulting in relaxation.

In addition to the autonomic neurotransmitters listed above, the enteric nervous system contains several dozen peptide neurotransmitters, the *GI hormones.* These peptide hormones are synthesized in nerves or in specialized neuroendocrine cells in the GI mucosa and pancreas. The list of these peptides has been increasing rapidly, with new ones discovered each year. Among the most widely studied of these peptides are CCK, gastrin, vasoactive intestinal peptide (VIP), somatostatin, and motilin. These peptides interact with specific receptors, either on nerves or on smooth muscle and other effector cells.

The smooth muscle receptors for these peptide hormones are G proteins, a class of guanosine triphosphate (GTP)–binding proteins.[24] The bound guanosine nucleotide is interconverted between GTP and guanosine diphosphate (GDP) as the receptor cycles between active and inactive forms. Hormonal binding to the G protein receptor activates muscle cell contraction by pathways involving phospholipid hydrolysis. Hydrolysis of phosphatidylinositol leads to generation of inositol phosphates, which release cellular calcium stores to raise intracellular calcium. Elevated intracellular calcium activates phosphorylation of the myosin light chain to cause contraction. Activation of G proteins may lead to hydrolysis of other membrane lipids such as phosphatidylcholine. Products of lipid hydrolysis also activate protein kinases, especially protein kinase C. Protein kinases may be involved in a second pathway leading to phosphorylation of the myosin light chain.[25]

The physiologic function of most peptide hormones is only partly understood. However, there is evidence that release of certain specific neurotransmitters regulates peristaltic activity in the intestine. By using specific inhibitors or measuring release of GI hormones into the vascular system, some candidate neurotransmitters for control of peristalsis have been identified. Neurotransmitters that probably mediate the contractile phase of peristalsis include acetylcholine and substance P.[22,26] The most likely neurotransmitters to mediate the relaxation phase of peristalsis include VIP, NO, somatostatin, and dynorphin, an endogenous opioid peptide. Increases in intraluminal pressure or stretching of the muscle wall of the gut causes release of these neurotransmitters. Motilin may be involved in generating the interdigestive contractile activity referred to as phase III of the MMC.[13,14]

The release of neurotransmitters to activate peristalsis is influenced by a variety of neural inputs.[27] These might include information from intestinal sensors of mechanical distention or luminal chemical stimuli. Input from the CNS through the autonomic and enteric neural tracts also influences the nerves that control peristalsis.

Endocrine Effects of Gastrointestinal Hormones

GI peptides are primarily neurotransmitters in the enteric nervous system. However, a few have an important role as endocrine hormones, controlling organ function distant from their site of synthesis and release. CCK is a classic GI endocrine hormone. CCK is synthesized by enteric nerves and also by neuroendocrine cells lining the duodenum and jejunum. Secretion of CCK is regulated by the CNS through cholinergic nerves, and occurs in response to sham feeding and ingested food. CCK is released or absorbed into the blood, where it circulates after a meal. Circulating CCK activates contraction of the gallbladder through a cholinergic mechanism.[28] It also acts directly on pancreatic acinar cells to stimulate pancreatic secretion. Two other peptide hormones with endocrine functions are gastrin and insulin. Both can have physiologic effects far from their site of release.

The GI peptides may also have paracrine effects: that is, effects on cells immediately adjacent to where the peptides are synthesized and released. GI peptides such as CCK and gastrin are synthesized in large amounts by neuroendocrine cells lining the GI tract. Large concentrations of these peptides are present in the gut lumen, but the paracrine effects of GI hormones are difficult to study, and little is known about them. In experimental preparations, luminal activity has been demonstrated for a few neurotransmitters. Serotonin has been shown to stimulate peristalsis when applied to the luminal surface of the gut. Luminal CCK stimulates peristalsis in the gut and contraction in the gallbladder. The paracrine effects of GI hormones may be important in vivo, but this has not been determined.

DISORDERS OF INTESTINAL MOTOR FUNCTION

Disorders of gut motility may involve any portion of the GI tract. The esophagus and stomach are responsible for a substantial proportion of GI motility problems, which are discussed elsewhere in this book (see Chapters 14 and 15). There are also a variety of causes for abnormal intestinal motility. These include systemic diseases, in which the motility disorder is part of a more generalized condition. Abnormal bowel motility may be associated with systemic diseases such as scleroderma and diabetes mellitus. A small group of patients have primary intestinal pseudo-obstruction. This is an uncommon, chronic illness related to abnormalities of gut neuromuscular function. The most common disorders of intestinal motility involve the colon and rectum. Patients often have subjective concerns about colonic function and elimination. Fortunately, colonic function is reasonably normal in most concerned patients. The problem can often be solved by simple changes of medication and diet. In patients who have true disorders of colon or rectal transit, various radiologic and manometric tests are useful in precisely defining the abnormality. The possibility of obstruction from cancer should always be considered and ruled out as a cause of change in bowel habit.

Abdominal surgery also affects GI motor activity.[29,30] A temporary loss of normal motility, called postoperative ileus, is generally of short duration. It is related to surgically entering the abdomen and manipulating the intra-abdominal contents, particularly the colon. More lasting effects on GI motility may follow surgical changes in anatomy such as vagotomy or resection of segments of intestine.[31] These anatomic changes can significantly alter intestinal motility or absorption and lead to long-term abnormalities of function.

Alterations in intestinal motility are often related to medications. These effects may occur from chronic use of medications, such as megacolon caused by anticholinergic drugs used in psychiatry. Short-term use of medications that alter intestinal contractility may also cause acute changes in bowel function. Since alterations in intestinal function caused by medications are very common, the effects of various drugs on GI motility are described.

Systemic Diseases Producing Intestinal Motor Dysfunction

A variety of systemic diseases may produce intestinal motor dysfunction, as shown in the box on p. 436.

In some cases the abnormal motility patterns these patients demonstrate clinically have been correlated with electrophysiologic abnormalities.[32] Patients with hypothyroidism or hyperthyroidism may show abnormal slow wave rhythm. Patients with abnormal or absent MMC activity may have associated bacterial overgrowth in the jejunum. For most clinical disorders of intestinal motility, however, the biochemical basis for abnormal motility and electrophysiologic abnormalities is not known.

Chronic Intestinal Pseudo-Obstruction

Chronic intestinal pseudo-obstruction (CIP) refers to a heterogeneous group of uncommon diseases of intestinal nerve and muscle. This condition presents with signs and symptoms of bowel obstruction, but no anatomic obstructing lesion is present. CIP may be called "idiopathic," but histologic abnormalities of enteric nerves or muscle have been shown to underlie the condition in many patients. One pathologic subtype, called *visceral neuropathy,* shows degeneration of enteric neurons. This condition may be familial or sporadic. A second pattern shows degeneration of intestinal smooth muscle cells, with vacuolization of smooth muscle and atrophy of mucle fibers. This subtype is called *hollow visceral myopathy* and appears to be genetically linked. These patients tend to be the most severely affected.

Patients with CIP show abnormal intestinal motility in both the fed and fasted state. Because of abnormal postprandial motility, food is not propelled through the intes-

DISEASES ASSOCIATED WITH SMALL INTESTINAL MOTOR DISORDERS

Chronic intestinal pseudo-obstruction syndromes
- Myopathies
- Visceral neuropathies

Paralytic ileus (acute intestinal pseudo-obstruction)
- Acute abdomen
- Abdominal surgery
- Electrolyte disturbances (especially potassium, calcium, magnesium, phosphorus, sodium)
- Drug effects

Mechanical obstruction

Autonomic neuropathies
- Diabetes mellitus
- Chagas' disease (trypanosomiasis)
- Cytomegalovirus infection

Collagen vascular diseases
- Progressive systemic sclerosis (scleroderma)

Myotonic dystrophy

Hyperthyroidism and hypothyroidism

Metabolic diseases
- Porphyria
- Amyloidosis

tine. During the fasted state, decreased MMCs lead to stasis and bacterial overgrowth in the small intestine. Patients with CIP present with abdominal pain and distention and other nonspecific alterations of bowel habit. In general, the patients have a long history of GI symptomatology. They may complain of both constipation and diarrhea, the diarrhea related to secondary bacterial overgrowth. They may be unable to eat without developing crampy abdominal pain, nausea, and vomiting. Abdominal x-ray films confirm dilation of the small bowel and often the colon. X-ray examination may not differentiate between pseudo-obstruction and mechanical bowel obstruction. Tests must be done to rule out systemic or mechanical causes for obstruction that may be treatable. Drug therapy has not been very successful in managing CIP. Nutritional support in the form of hyperalimentation has been of benefit. In general, surgery should be avoided in these patients, but limited success has been obtained with a combination of total parenteral nutrition and a venting gastrostomy or enterostomy.

Symptoms similar to those in CIP can be seen in the autonomic neuropathies of diabetes mellitus, Chagas' disease, amyloidosis, and scleroderma. As in CIP, these patients can be very difficult to treat, and surgery should be considered only as a last resort.

Severe Idiopathic Constipation

In a small proportion of patients with constipation, the condition is much more severe, persistant, and unresponsive to fiber and laxatives than normal.[33] These patients, usually women, often have stool frequencies of less than one per week despite the use of fiber and laxatives. Identifiable causes of constipation should be ruled out, including medications and endocrine or neurologic disorders. Colonoscopy is usually indicated to rule out an obstructing neoplasm. If the patient is indeed in good health except for constipation, further tests may identify specific abnormalities of colorectal function.

Idiopathic colonic dysmotility may lead to severe constipation, as demonstrated by extremely slow passage of radiologic markers through the colon. In severe cases, subtotal colectomy may be required.[34] Pathologic studies of the colons from these patients demonstrate abnormalities in the number and shape of neurons in the myenteric plexus, although it is unclear whether the neurologic abnormalities cause the abnormal contraction.[35]

Anorectal dysfunction occurs in a subgroup of patients with severe constipation who are unable to expel stool from the rectum.[36] As summarized by Sarna,[16,17] several abnormalities can cause abnormal rectal evacuation:

1. Inability of the rectum to sense distention and signal to the brain the need for evacuation
2. Loss of reflex internal sphincter relaxation in response to distention (a variant of Hirschsprung's disease)
3. Inability of the external sphincter to voluntarily relax
4. Inability of the puborectalis muscle sling to relax

The abnormalities in rectal emptying can be defined using anal manometry. The patient reports rectal sensation in response to distention of a balloon in the rectum. The pressure response (relaxation) of the internal sphincter to rectal distention is also measured. The length and strength of the internal (involuntary) and external (voluntary) anal sphincters is measured using a pull-through technique with a pressure catheter placed across the sphincters. Further information can be obtained using an x-ray test called cinedefecography. X-ray films of the patient during evacuation of rectal contrast material may confirm findings of rectal outlet obstruction.

Some investigators have found electrophysiologic studies to be useful in identifying and evaluating the status of the anal sphincter muscles after injury. This technique has also been used to confirm failure of the puborectalis muscle to relax in patients with outlet obstruction. Overall, electrophysiologic techniques have been of little value in the clinical evaluation of patients with idiopathic constipation.

If a clear diagnosis of Hirschsprung's disease can be made in an adult by anorectal manometry and perhaps by a full-thickness biopsy, a surgical approach is generally indicated.[37] The surgical management of adult Hirschsprung's disease, however, remains controversial. Although surgical opinions vary, it would appear that for short segment adult Hirschsprung's disease, anorectal myectomy is reasonable first-line surgical therapy. The best long-term results, however, are obtained with a Soave endorectal pull-through procedure, or a Duhamel retrorectal pull-through operation. Surgery has not been successful in the treatment of pelvic floor outlet obstruction. Use of puborectalis muscle incision or myectomy has produced variable results and may result in a patient who is incontinent of solid stool. Several recent reports have suggested that patients with dysfunction of the pelvic floor can be successfully treated with outpatient electromyographic biofeedback.[38]

For patients with severe chronic idiopathic constipation of colonic origin, definitive surgery is reserved only for patients truly refractory to medical management, which includes dietary manipulation and use of stool softeners, anticonstipation medications, and enemas. In patients with an unequivocal diagnosis of colonic inertia with normal anorectal function, several operative procedures have been advocated. While segmental colectomy seems appealing for patients with apparent segmental dilation of a portion of the colon, the results have been disappointing. Until better localization and documentation of segmental colonic motility is available, subtotal colectomy with ileorectal anastomosis appears to be the most effective operation for patients with colonic dysmotility and normal anorectal manometry findings.

Acute Pseudo-obstruction (Ogilvie's Syndrome) and Chronic Megacolon

Hospitalized patients may lose normal peristaltic activity in the colon, even though the colon is normal if examined pathologically. This loss of contractility may occur because of medications that affect motility or may follow medical illness, inactivity, or surgery. Colonic dilation occurs, which may lead to life-threatening volvulus or cecal perforation.

Patients without previous colonic disease can develop "acute pseudo-obstruction" while being treated for medical illness or recovering from surgery. This condition is characterized by massive colon dilation, often limited to the right colon and cecum. It was first described by Ogilvie in 1948.[39] The syndrome is characterized by progressive abdominal distention, usually with little pain. Vomiting, constipation, or diarrhea may occur. Peritoneal signs are absent unless perforation has occurred. Perforation of the cecum may occur if colon dilation is not treated promptly. The cecum is most likely to be damaged because it has the largest radius when the colon is distended. According to Laplace's law (tension = radius × pressure ÷ 2), wall tension is greatest in the segment of bowel with the largest radius.

Initial treatment for acute colon dilation consists of nasogastric suction, hydration, correction of electrolyte disturbances, and frequent position changes if possible. Colonoscopy should be performed to decompress the colon if the radiologic diameter of the cecum remains greater than 9 to 10 cm. More than one colonoscopy may be required to successfully decompress the colon. Colonoscopic decompression can avert surgery in many patients. If the colon cannot be decompressed colonoscopically, surgery is required to inspect and decompress the right colon, usually with a cecostomy or ileostomy. Right colectomy may be necessary if colonic distention has progressed to cecal infarction or perforation.

Patients who are chronically hospitalized may develop chronic constipation, accompanied by gradual enlargement and lengthening of the colon. This condition has been called "chronic megacolon" or "institutional colon." Constipation may result from lack of physical activity or from long-term use of drugs for psychiatric illness. Many drugs used for psychiatric disorders are anticholinergic and antidopaminergic and interfere with normal colonic motility. Patients with chronic megacolon are at risk for developing colonic volvulus. They may also develop acute episodes of pseudo-obstruction because of medication effects or electrolyte imbalance. If the megacolon leads to recurrent volvulus or to bouts of distention that seriously interfere with nutrition, colectomy should be considered.

Irritable Bowel Syndrome

Irritable bowel syndrome (IBS) is called a "functional" disorder of motility, since there is no apparent anatomic abnormality. IBS involves primarily the colon and sometimes more proximal parts of the GI tract. Common symptoms include abdominal pain and distention, often with alternating diarrhea and constipation. Colonic motility studies have recently identified clear abnormalities in patients with IBS. Manometric studies of the colon demonstrate that patients with IBS react aberrantly to distending stimuli, reporting pain at lower levels of colon distention than control subjects. Several investigators have also demonstrated alterations in slow wave frequency in colons of these patients. The symptoms of colitis may resemble those of IBS, and endoscopic evaluation to rule out colitis should be considered when making the diagnosis of IBS.

Diverticulosis

Diverticulosis may be due to high intraluminal pressures that cause herniation of the mucosa through the muscular wall of the colon. Studies of colon specimens from patients with diverticulosis demonstrate that colonic muscle in these patients is thickened and the luminal diameter is narrowed. Diverticuli occur between the mesenteric and antimesenteric tenia coli at sites where blood vessels transit the bowel wall. Manometric studies demonstrate higher pressures in the colon of patients with diverticulosis than in control subjects. Epidemiologic studies suggest that low fecal volume resulting from a refined Western diet is a major contributing factor in diverticulosis. Increasing the amount of fiber and bulk in the stool may be helpful.

Postoperative Motor Abnormalities

Paralytic ileus refers to the transient loss of intestinal peristalsis that occurs after operations involving the abdomen and retroperitoneum. Ileus also occurs as a response to peritonitis, abdominal trauma, and mechanical intestinal obstruction. Clinically, ileus is characterized by diminished bowel sounds and accumulation of gas and fluid within the bowel lumen. The pathophysiology of ileus is poorly understood. Factors around the time of surgery that may contribute to ileus include preoperative medication, anesthetic agents, analgesics, manipulation of bowel, mechanical or chemical irritation of the peritoneum, and electrolyte disturbances. Most of these variables can be controlled or altered without influencing the duration of ileus significantly. Incision of the abdominal wall and manipulation of the colon appear to be particularly important factors in inducing ileus.

The GI tract follows a predictable sequence in resuming motor function after postoperative ileus. Unless the small intestine is involved in the primary disease process, it resumes activity within 5 to 10 hours after abdominal surgery. When surgery is performed with spinal anesthesia, small intestinal peristalsis can be observed throughout the operative procedure. Gastric motility returns to normal within 24 hours. Colonic motility usually returns within 1 to 5 days. Studies have demonstrated that laparotomy does not affect small bowel slow wave frequency or its gradient along the small intestine. However, laparotomy does affect cycling of the small intestinal MMC, with disappearance of the MMC for 1 to 2 days after laparotomy.[40]

Postvagotomy syndromes refer to disorders of motility that occur after vagotomy. Since the vagus nerve is the main motor innervation to the stomach, vagotomy has a profound effect on gastric motor function.[31] Vagotomy also affects motility of the intestine, but clinical effects are variable. Diarrhea and hyperirritability of the small bowel may occur after vagotomy in animals and humans. Studies in humans do not show changes in the MMC after vagotomy. In all species, however, alterations in the myoelectric fed pattern or conversion to the fed pattern have been observed following vagotomy. These changes may explain decreases in jejunal and ileal transit time observed after vagotomy. The incidence of postoperative diarrhea following vagotomy ranges from 2% to 13% after proximal gastric vagotomy to 20% to 67% after truncal vagotomy and drainage. Selective vagotomy, in which the celiac and hepatic branches of the vagus nerves are identified and preserved, does not lead to a significant improvement over truncal vagotomy. There is evidence that postvagotomy diarrhea in humans may be due to rapid small bowel transit of bile acids, with incomplete absorption, subsequent colonic irritation, and diarrhea. Postvagotomy diarrhea is more common in patients who have undergone cholecystectomy. These patients have lost the storage function of the gallbladder and have continuous flow of bile into the intestine. Postvagotomy diarrhea often responds to treatment with cholestyramine, a resin that binds luminal bile salts.

Intestinal transection might be assumed to alter bowel motility by interrupting both myogenic and local neural pathways. However, in practice, evidence of altered motor activity after small bowel transection is surprisingly uncommon. A change in myoelectric pattern has been observed in humans after surgical transection and anastomosis, with MMC cycles occurring independently proximal and distal to the anastomosis. The MMC cycles become coupled across the anastomosis 30 to 100 days after surgery. However, these changes in myoelectric conduction do not usually interfere with intestinal function.

The duodenum is one region of the intestine where transection and reanastomosis may cause significant motor abnormalities. In the intact small intestine, there is a pacemaker in the proximal duodenum that determines the frequency of slow waves (or ECA) for the small intestine. After transection and reanastomosis, the intestine distal to the anastomosis is no longer entrained by the duodenal pacemaker. The frequency of the slow wave in the remaining small intestine slows to the basal frequency. Reverse propagation of the ECA may slow transit as well. Perhaps because of this, circumferential suture lines in the duodenum may cause delayed return of normal motility. This is seen commonly following pancreaticoduodenectomy, especially with the pylorus-preserving technique. One quarter to one half of patients receiving this operation develop delayed gastric emptying, attributed to loss of coordination between antrum, the pyloric area, and the proximal small intestine.

Sphincter of Oddi dysfunction refers to an uncommon syndrome of biliary type of pain that occurs in patients who have undergone cholecystectomy. Patients experience recurrent episodes of epigastric or right upper quadrant pain, sometimes accompanied by nausea and vomiting. Serum levels of amylase or liver enzymes may be elevated. The presence of retained common bile duct stones must be excluded before the diagnosis of sphincter of Oddi dysfunction can be considered.

A variety of tests have been proposed to diagnose sphincter of Oddi dysfunction, and the criteria for diagnosis have not been defined with certainty. Findings that suggest dysfunction may be present include slow emptying of contrast from the common duct during scintigraphic scanning or endoscopic retrograde cholangiopancreatography (ERCP). Further evidence includes elevated sphincter of Oddi pressure or an abnormally rapid contractile pattern measured during manometry of the sphincter at ERCP. Patients with this syndrome may also have prolonged dilation of the pancreatic or biliary duct following a fatty meal or an infusion of secretin. Patients in whom findings from one or more of these tests are abnormal may respond to biliary stenting, endoscopic sphincterotomy, or sphincteroplasty with relief of symptoms.[41,42]

Acute intestinal obstruction remains a frequently encountered and difficult-to-manage condition for the clinical surgeon. Intestinal obstruction is manifested by paroxysmal, crampy, abdominal pain and distention that is aggravated by eating and partially relieved by vomiting. It has been generally thought, based on clinical observations, intraluminal balloons, and direct observation of the gut, that motor activity is greatly increased proximal to the obstruction. Only recently has this been carefully assessed using manometric and electromyographic techniques.

Summers et al.[43] demonstrated experimentally that proximal to the site of obstruction spike burst frequency increased markedly, whereas distal to that obstruction spiking was depressed. When the obstruction was continued for more than 5 hours, the inhibition persisted distally, but proximal myoelectric spike activity and contractile activity gradually fell to control levels. After prolonged obstruction, the investigators observed clusters of regular intense spike bursts, preceded and followed by lengthening periods of absent motor activity. Further work from this group suggested that changes in luminal contents and nervous activity both contribute to the intestinal motility changes that accompany obstruction. Increased motor activity proximal to obstruction appeared to be mediated by cholinergic nerves. Some of the distal inhibition of spike bursts may be mediated by noncholinergic, nonadrenergic pathways, and some may result from diminished intraluminal contents.[44]

DRUGS THAT ALTER INTESTINAL MOTOR FUNCTION

Many common medications alter the motor activity of the intestine and may cause constipation or diarrhea in patients without intrinsic intestinal abnormalities. To assess and treat patients' complaints about bowel function, the physician must understand the effects common groups of drugs have on intestinal motility. Drugs can alter gut motor activity by several mechanisms:

1. Interactions with receptors in the brain or spinal cord to alter neural stimuli to the intestine
2. Interactions with receptors on intestinal muscle cells or intramural nerves
3. Changes in ion composition within smooth muscle cells, causing altered contractility of the muscle
4. Changes in fluid secretion or resorption in the intestinal lumen, with resulting changes in luminal volume

Drugs That Decrease Intestinal Motility

Opiates are classic inhibitors of intestinal propulsion and are used clinically to control diarrhea. The GI effects of morphine are mediated by receptors in the CNS and also by μ- and δ-opioid receptors in the intestine. Opiates decrease propulsive contractions in the intestine while causing a marked increase in muscle tone. This leads to slow intestinal transit, increased water absorption, and constipation. This mechanism underlies the effectiveness of narcotics for controlling diarrhea. Opiates that are of value in slowing intestinal transit include codeine, diphenoxylate (which is available only in combination with atropine, under the trade name Lomotil and others), and loperamide (trade name Imodium). These agents can produce physiologic dependence. They are best used for short-term control of diarrhea when the cause is known.

Anticholinergic drugs have been used for many years to control excessive motor activity of the GI and urinary tracts. The prototype for this group of drugs is atropine, a competitive antagonist for the muscarinic acetylcholine receptor. Acetylcholine is an important intestinal neurotransmitter that stimulates motor activity and secretion. Atropine has widespread GI effects including decreased GI secretion and peristalsis. Atropine is used along with diphenoxylate as an antidiarrheal agent, but its general usefulness is limited by side effects including dry mouth and visual changes. Other potent drugs with a similar mechanism of action include belladonna derivatives and oxybutynin, which is used for urinary bladder spasms. All these agents can cause decreased peristalsis and constipation. Constipation may be severe enough to require discontinuation of the drugs. Phenothiazines and related antipsychotic drugs are primarily antidopaminergic, but some have anticholinergic activity as well. Chlorpromazine has antimuscarinic activity and can cause constipation and decreased gastric emptying. Long-term effects of these drugs are often seen as chronic constipation and megacolon in patients with chronic psychiatric disorders.

Somatostatin analogs are a new group of drugs that mimic the potent peptide hormone somatostatin. Like somatostatin, these agents can act directly on smooth muscle cells. They block the effects of many other peptide hormones that stimulate GI secretion and motility. The commercially available agent in this class, octreotide, has its major surgical use in treating GI fistulas.

Calcium channel antagonists (nifedipine, verapamil, and diltiazem) are members of a class of drugs used widely to treat hypertension and ischemic heart disease. Smooth muscle and cardiac muscle both contain calcium channels that open in response to drugs, hormones, or changes in voltage across the cell membrane. These channels allow extracellular calcium to enter the cell to help activate contraction. Calcium channel antagonists affect the cardiovascular system by decreasing calcium stores and influx of calcium into muscle cells of the heart and blood vessels. Decreased calcium influx causes decreased cardiac contractility, decreased smooth muscle contraction, and vasodilation. These drugs have a similar effect on GI smooth muscle. In the intestine they decrease calcium influx into muscle cells and decrease contractility. The major GI effect of these drugs is constipation, which is very common. Nifedipine has been used to treat spastic disorders of the esophagus such as achalasia.

Drugs That Increase Intestinal Motility

Cholinergic drugs stimulate secretion and motility throughout the GI tract by interacting with receptors for acetylcholine. Drugs in this class such as bethanechol (Urecholine) may be used in surgical patients to treat urinary retention. Cholinergic drugs have also been given postoperatively to patients in an effort to shorten postoperative ileus, without significant improvement.

Antidopaminergic drugs are used in medical practice to promote gastric emptying and to decrease nausea and vomiting. Dopaminergic antagonists appear to suppress nausea and vomiting by a CNS effect, possibly on the chemoreceptor trigger zone. They also enhance gastric emptying by increasing antral contractility and decreasing receptive relaxation in the proximal stomach. Metoclopramide (Reglan) is the most widely used gastric prokinetic agent. It is a benzamide, structurally related to procainamide (Fig. 19-8). Metoclopramide appears to enhance gastric motility by releasing acetylcholine from local nerves, and its effect is blocked by atropine.[45] Metoclopramide also accelerates small intestinal transit time. Domperidone is another dopamine antagonist used as an antiemetic. It has effects on GI motility similar to metoclopramide, but its effects are not blocked by atropine.

Cisapride is another benzamide drug that stimulates GI motility. Its effects are blocked by atropine and are probably mediated by release of acetylcholine from enteric nerves. Cisapride differs from metoclopramide and domperidone, since it does not block the effect of dopamine. Cisapride increases motility of the colon and the small intestine and can cause diarrhea. It has been used to treat patients with severe chronic constipation. It is also used as an antireflux agent to enhance esophageal emptying in the treatment of esophagitis caused by gastroesophageal reflux.

Erythromycin is the best studied of a group of drugs that stimulate the receptor for motilin, an endogenous peptide neurotransmitter. Erythromycin enhances gastric emptying and may improve small bowel transit. It appears to improve symptoms in some patients with diabetic gastroparesis.

Prostaglandins are a group of biologically active lipids derived from arachidonic acid. Many prostaglandins and analogs have been chemically synthesized, and a few are approved for medical use. The prostaglandin E analog misoprostol is widely prescribed to suppress gastric acidity and diminish the ulcerogenic effect of nonsteroidal anti-inflammatory drugs. Prostaglandins may be endogenous regulators of GI motility. The effect of prostaglandins on GI smooth muscle has been studied. Prostaglandins can induce either contraction or relaxation of smooth muscle, depending on the type of prostaglandin and the source of the muscle. In the intestine, prostaglandins of the E class cause contraction of the longitudinal muscle layer but inhibit the circular muscle and decrease peristalsis. Despite the complex effects of prostaglandins on motility, they almost uniformly cause diarrhea. This is because prostaglandins stimulate adenylate cyclase activity in mucosal cells. The resulting rise in mucosal cAMP levels causes increased fluid and electrolyte secretion into the lumen of the intestine. The active secretion of fluid and electrolytes into the lumen causes diarrhea.

Laxatives cause increased defecation, either by adding bulk, altering fluid and electrolyte secretion into the lumen of the colon, or enhancing motility. With the exception of bulk-forming laxatives, most laxatives lead to decreased colonic function with long-term use. The treatment of constipation should be based on adequate dietary fiber and oral liquid and on avoiding medications associated with constipation when possible. Regular laxative use should be avoided if possible in patients without underlying colon abnormalities.

Many common laxatives contain salts or osmotic agents that are poorly absorbed. The osmotic effect causes increased fluid accumulation in the intestinal lumen, leading to defecation. Solutions containing magnesium salts, phosphate, or sulfate act by this mechanism. Other osmotic laxatives include the polyethylene glycol–electrolyte solutions (e.g., Colyte) that are used for bowel preparation for procedures, as well as lactulose and sorbitol. Bisacodyl (e.g., Dulcolax) and castor oil act both to reduce net absorption of luminal fluid and to stimulate motility.

INTESTINAL PACING

An exciting new approach to gut motility disorders is intestinal pacing. Experimental work has demonstrated that electric pacing can alter the frequency and direction of propagation of the enteric myoelectric pacesetter potential or slow wave, thereby affecting intestinal motility, transit, and absorption.[46] In experimental animals retrograde intestinal pacing has effectively ameliorated the postgastrectomy dumping syndrome[47] and the short bowel syndrome.[48] Antegrade pacing might be expected to enhance gastric emptying and further inhibit bile reflux in patients after Roux-en-Y conversion.[49] In addition, antegrade pacing might be expected to play some role in other disorders of intestinal atony or stasis.

Rapid improvement in technology and materials has made it possible to consider human implantation of an intestinal pacing unit in the near future in patients with GI

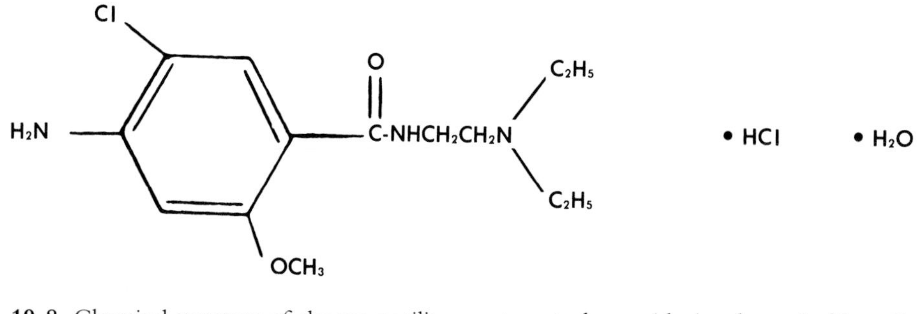

Cl
H_2N
O
C-NHCH$_2$CH$_2$N
C_2H_5
C_2H_5
OCH_3
• HCl • H_2O

Fig. 19-8. Chemical structure of the promotility agent, metoclopramide (methoxy-2-chloro-5-procainamide).

motility disorders. Further, if the units could be placed on the bowel nonsurgically, several conditions now refractory to currently available therapy might be readily treated by an intestinal pacing device.

SUMMARY

Motility of the GI tract depends on a highly integrated and coordinated response of the smooth muscle contained within the wall of the bowel. Small and large intestinal motility is controlled by three basic control mechanisms: myogenic, neural, and humoral. The organization of these control mechanisms is different in different anatomic sections of the GI tract. Understanding of these control mechanisms in both the physiologic and the pathologic state is incomplete, although this is improving rapidly with modern electrophysiologic, manometric, and histologic techniques. Motor disorders affect the entire GI tract. The disorders can be intrinsic to the alimentary canal, may reflect a generalized neural or myogenic dysfunction, or can result from surgical manipulation of the bowel or nervous system. These disorders are difficult to diagnose and treat.

Surgical therapy is seldom indicated for these disorders of motility; however, groups of patients are being identified with specific motor dysfunctions of the esophagus, stomach, and colon who may be amenable to surgical therapy. Several new promotility agents, including metoclopramide, domperidone, and cisapride, may be useful in the treatment of many hypomotility disorders. Opiates effectively delay GI transit and control diarrhea. Intestinal pacing is effective in experimental motility disorders and may ultimately be applicable to clinical disorders of intestinal motor function.

REFERENCES

1. Bayliss WM, Starling EH. The movements and innervation of the small intestine. J Physiol 24:110, 1899.
2. Cannon WB. The movements of the intestines studied by means of roentgen rays. Am J Physiol 6:251, 1906.
3. Becker JM, Duff WM, Moody FG. Myoelectric control of GI and biliary motility: A review. Surgery 89:466, 1981.
4. Bortoff A. Myogenic control of intestinal motility. Physiol Rev 56:418, 1976.
5. Post JM, Hume JR. Ionic basis for spontaneous depolarizations in isolated smooth muscle cells of canine colon. Am J Physiol 263:C691, 1992.
6. Christensen J, Schedl HP, Clifton JA. The small intestinal basic electric rhythm (slow wave) frequency gradient in normal men and in patients with a variety of diseases. Gastroenterology 50:309, 1966.
7. Becker JM, Moody FG. Sphincter of Oddi and biliary motility. In Condon RE, DeCosse JJ, eds. Surgical Care II. Philadelphia: Lea & Febiger, 1985.
8. Sarna S, Condon RE, Cowles VE. Enteric mechanisms of initiation of migrating myoelectric complexes in dogs. Gastroenterology 84:81, 1983.
9. Szurszewski JH. A migrating electric complex of the canine small intestine. Am J Physiol 217:1757, 1969.
10. Scott LD, Cahall DL. Influence of the interdigestive myoelectric complex on enteric flora in the rat. Gastroenterology 82:37, 1982.
11. Carlson GM, Bedi BS, Code CF. Mechanism of propagation of intestinal interdigestive myoelectric complex. Am J Physiol 222:1027, 1972.
12. Itoh Z, Aizawa I, Takeuchi S. Neural regulation of interdigestive motor activity in canine jejunum. Am J Physiol 240:G324, 1981.
13. Sarr MG, Kelly KA, Go VLW. Motilin regulation of canine interdigestive intestinal motility. Dig Dis Sci 28:249, 1983.
14. Bueno L, et al. Effects of motilin, somatostatin, pancreatic polypeptide on the migrating myoelectric complex in pig and dog. Gastroenterology 82:1395, 1982.
15. Misiewicz JJ. Human colonic motility. Scand J Gastroenterol 93(Suppl):43, 1984.
16. Sarna SK. Physiology and pathophysiology of colonic motor activity. Dig Dis Sci 36:998, 1991.
17. Sarna SK. Physiology and pathophysiology of colonic motor activity. Dig Dis Sci 36:827, 1991.
18. Bassotti G, Crowell MD, Whitehead WE. Contractile activity of the human colon: Lessons from 24 hour studies. Gut 34:129, 1993.
19. Rogers J, Raimundo AH, Misiewicz JJ. Cephalic phase of colonic pressure response to food. Gut 34:537, 1993.
20. Furness JB, Bornstein JC, Smith TK. The normal structure of GI innervation. J Gastroenterol Hepatol 1(Suppl):1, 1990.
21. Mawe GM, Gershon MD. Structure, afferent innervation, transmitter content of ganglia of the guinea pig gallbladder: Relationship to the enteric nervous system. J Compar Neurol 283:374, 1989.
22. Grider JR. Identification of neurotransmitters regulating intestinal peristaltic reflex in humans. Gastroenterology 97:1414, 1989.
23. Sneddon P, Graham A. Role of nitric oxide in the autonomic innervation of smooth muscle. J Auton Pharmacol 12:445, 1992.
24. Marston SB. The regulation of smooth muscle contractile proteins. Prog Biophys Mol Biol 41:1, 1982.
25. Washabau RJ, Wang MB, Ryan JP. Myosin light chain phosphorylation and contraction of guinea pig gallbladder smooth muscle. Am J Physiol 261:G952, 1991.
26. Donnerer J, Holzer P, Lembeck F. Release of dynorphin, somatostatin, substance P from the vascularly perfused small intestine of the guinea pig during peristalsis. Br J Pharmacol 83:919, 1984.
27. Mangel AW, Connor JA, Prosser CL. Effects of alterations in calcium levels on cat small intestinal slow waves. Am J Physiol 243:C7, 1982.
28. Brotschi EA, Pattavino J, Williams LF Jr. Intrinsic nerves affect gallbladder contraction in the guinea pig. Gastroenterology 99:826, 1990.
29. Condon RE, Sarna SK. Motility after abdominal surgery. Clin Gastroentrol 11:609, 1982.
30. Graber JN, et al. Relationship of duration of postoperative ileus to extent and site of operative dissection. Surgery 92:87, 1982.
31. Becker JM, Kelly KA. Implications of vagotomy. In Carter DC, ed. Clinical Surgery International: Peptic Ulcer, vol 7. Edinburgh: Churchill Livingstone, 1983.
32. Vantrappen GR, Janssens J. Intestinal motility disorders. Dig Dis Sci 29:458, 1984.
33. Read NW, et al, Impairment of defecation in young women with severe constipation. Gastroenterology 90:53, 1986.
34. Zenilman MD, et al, Successful surgical treatment of idiopathic colonic dysmotility. Arch Surg 124:947, 1989.
35. Krishnamurthy P, et al. Severe idiopathic constipation is associated with a distinctive abnormality of the colonic myenteric plexus. Gastroenterology 75:623, 1978.
36. Shouler P, Keighley MRB. Changes in colorectal function in severe idiopathic chronic constipation. Gastroenterology 90:414, 1986.
37. Wheatley MJ, et al. Hirschsprung's disease in adolescents and adults. Dig Dis Colon 33:622, 1990.
38. Fleshman JW, et al. Outpatient protocol for biofeedback therapy of pelvic floor outlet obstruction. Dis Colon Rectum 35:1, 1992.
39. Ogilvie H. Large-intestine colic due to sympathetic deprivation: A new clinical syndrome. Br Med J 2:671, 1948.
40. Waldhausen JHT, et al. Gastrointestinal myoelectric and clinical patterns of recovery after laparotomy. Ann Surg 211:777, 1990.
41. Parodi JE, Becker JM. Gallbladder and sphincter of Oddi motility. Curr Opin Gastroenterol 6:668, 1990.

42. Geenen JE, et al. The efficacy of endoscopic sphincterotomy after cholecystectomy in patients with sphincter of Oddi dysfunction. N Engl J Med 320:82, 1989.
43. Summers RW, Anuras S, Green J. Jejunal manometry patterns in health, partial intestinal obstruction, pseudo-obstruction. Gastroenterology 85:1290, 1983.
44. Prihoda M, Flatt A, Summers RW. Mechanisms of motility changes during acute intestinal obstruction in the dog. Am J Physiol 247: G37, 1984.
45. Albibi R, McCallum RW. Metoclopramide: Pharmacology and clinical application. Ann Intern Med 98:86, 1983.
46. Becker JM. Electrical pacing for post-surgical disorders of gastric motility. In Akkermans LMA, Johnson AG, Read NW, eds. Gastric and Gastroduodenal Motility. Surgical Science Series, vol 4. East Sussex, U.K.: Praeger Publishers, 1984.
47. Becker JM, et al. Intestinal pacing for canine post-gastrectomy dumping. Gastroenterology 84:383, 1983.
48. Gladden HE, Kelly KA. Electrical pacing for short bowel syndrome. Surg Gynecol Obstet 153:697, 1981.
49. Karlstrom L, et al. Ectopic jejunal pacemakers and enterogastric reflux after Roux gastrectomy: Effect of intestinal pacing. Surgery 106:486, 1989.

20

Intestinal Circulation and Vascular Disorders

David W. McFadden and Anthony J. Rongione

Intestinal homeostasis is entirely dependent on an adequate blood supply. Several factors, including the overall state of the general circulation, the extent of collateral blood flow, the response of the mesenteric circulation to autonomic regulation, circulating vasoactive substances, local humoral factors, and products of cellular metabolism before and after reperfusion, contribute to physiologic control of the intestine. Abnormalities in the intestinal blood supply at the macrocirculatory level may lead to a wide spectrum of disorders, ranging from mild postprandial abdominal pain (intestinal angina) to such profound abnormalities as intestinal gangrene.[1] Microcirculatory derangements can lead to impaired absorption, impaired motility, and poor anastomotic healing. This chapter discusses the normal anatomic and physiologic controls of intestinal blood flow and the current clinical methods of evaluating the integrity of the gastrointestinal circulation. The clinical manifestations of impaired gut circulation are also considered, along with current concepts in its management.

ANATOMY AND PHYSIOLOGY OF THE INTESTINAL CIRCULATION

The intestine is perfused by three main arterial systems that form an anastomotic system that provides a rich blood supply to the adjoining organs (Fig. 20-1). The celiac axis supplies the foregut structures primarily below the diaphragm. The superior mesenteric artery (SMA) is the main supplier of intestinal blood flow from the duodenojejunal junction to the midtransverse colon. The inferior mesenteric artery (IMA) supplies the hindgut from midtransverse colon to the rectum. In many areas, these systems overlap with an abundant blood supply; in other areas, there are weaknesses referred to as "watershed" areas. For instance, the collateral blood flow from the celiac artery to the SMA arises from the gastroduodenal artery, forming the pancreaticoduodenal arcades. Several arterial channels, including the marginal artery of Drummond, the central anastomotic artery, and the arch of Riolan, provide a generous collateralization between the SMA and IMA systems. Finally, the IMA has collateral pathways with

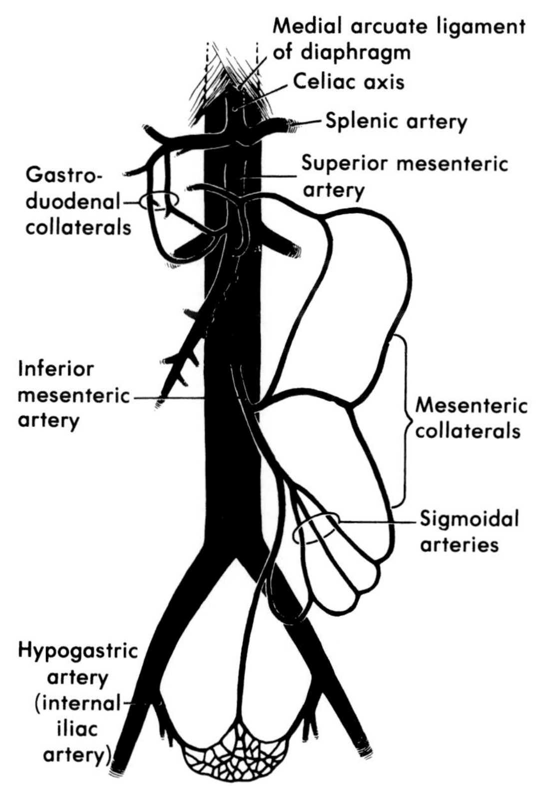

Fig. 20-1. Main arterial systems perfusing the gastrointestinal tract. (From Stoney RJ, Lusby RJ. In Haimovici H, ed. Vascular Surgery Principles and Techniques, 2nd ed. East Norwalk, Conn.: Appleton-Century-Crofts, 1984.)

the celiac axis through branches of the abdominal aorta, the femoral artery, the internal iliac branches, and aberrantly derived middle colic arteries. In total, more than 50 collateral pathways have been described for intestinal arterial blood flow, and asymptomatic occlusion of any one of the three main trunks is possible; occlusion of two or more vessels is frequently needed to produce symptomatic intestinal ischemia. Microscopically, extensive submucosal vascular plexi arise from the vasa recta and vasa brevia on the mesenteric border of the bowel. These serve a protective function through a central arteriole and provide a rich subepithelial capillary network within each villus at the cellular level. This plexus is much more extensive in the small bowel than in the colon, making the small intestine more resistant to ischemia.[2]

The fundamental arrangement of intestinal microvasculature is a circuit composed of a series of resistance arterioles, precapillary sphincters, capillaries, postcapillary sphincters, and the venous capacitance vessels. As a whole, the resistance arterioles are the primary determinants of vascular resistance and regulate blood flow to the splanchnic bed.

The venous drainage of the gastrointestinal tract is through tributaries of the superior and inferior mesenteric veins, which ultimately end in the portal vein. Small venules coalesce to form a system of venous arcades within the mesentary from which blood enters the main inferior and superior mesenteric veins. Each receives tributaries that correspond to the names and locations of paralleled arteries. The superior mesenteric vein drains the entire small intestine and the right half of the colon. The inferior mesenteric vein, a continuation of the superior hemorrhoidal veins, drains the left side of the large intestine from the upper rectum to the remainder of the transverse colon. The normal portal venous pressure is between 12 and 15 cm H_2O. Like the vena cava, the portal vein has no valves.

At rest, approximately 25% to 30% of total cardiac output is distributed to the intestines, equal to 30 to 70 ml/min/100 g tissue, or as much as one third of total blood volume.[3] Of this, 70% to 90% perfuses the mucosal-submucosal layers, with the remainder supplying the muscularis-serosal coats. Wide variances in reported blood flows are caused by the various measurement techniques (radioactive microspheres, inert gas washouts) and animal preparations (innervated, fasted, awake, or anesthetized). The physiology of intestinal circulation is still an evolving and often controversial science, but most published data[3,4] implicate three large groups of circulatory determinants: intrinsic (local metabolic vs myogenic), extrinsic or neural (sympathetic and parasympathetic nervous systems), and humoral (circulating or local vasoactive or neurohumoral agents).

The study of the intrinsic regulation of intestinal blood flow has long centered on the debate between metabolic and myogenic mechanisms. These interdependent mechanisms presumably control the immediate fluctuations in intestinal blood flow. Such well-documented physiologic phenomena as pressure-flow autoregulation, hypoxic vasodilation, and reactive hyperemia lend credence to the integral nature of intrinsic controls. The metabolic hypothesis of intrinsic regulation credits the accumulation of various tissue metabolites, such as H^+, K^+, hyperosmolarity of the blood, decreased local oxygen content, adenosine, the adenosine nucleotides, and a high concentration of carbon dioxide causing local acidosis, as the modifiers of local blood flow. Any situation creating an imbalance between tissue oxygen supply and demand would raise the local concentrations of these metabolites, with resultant vasodilation and hyperemia. The metabolic theory therefore states that it is oxygen delivery, rather than blood flow per se, that regulates the intestinal circulation.[3] The myogenic theory assumes that vascular resistance is proportional to arteriolar transmural pressure,[5] requiring the existence of arteriolar tension receptors. An acute decrease in perfusion pressure is compensated for by local regulatory mechanisms, so that flow reduction is proportionately less than the reduction in perfusion pressure.[6] The myogenic mechanism would therefore regulate and maintain constant intestinal capillary pressure and transcapillary fluid exchange.[7] Although more solid evidence exists in favor of the myogenic regulation of intestinal blood flow, the consensus is that both intrinsic mechanisms serve important functions.

The role that nitric oxide plays in the gastrointestinal tract has become increasingly important in the literature. Nitric oxide has been shown to regulate systemic blood pressure as well as local blood flow in the gastrointestinal vascular bed.[8] Mucosal blood flow, as stated, is dependent on the balance between the endothelial releases of substances that enhance and reduce flow. Evidence indicates that nitric oxide may be an important mediator of vascular tone in the gastrointestinal tract, in particular with gastric mucosal blood flow.[9-13] More recent data suggest that basal nitric oxide production is important in minimizing mucosal and microvascular barrier dysfunction associated with reperfusion of postischemic intestine.[14] The mechanism by which this occurs is still largely unknown; however, nitric oxide has been known to act as an antioxidant[15] and as an inhibitor of neutrophil adhesion to vascular endothelium and migration from blood vessels.[16] These results and others suggest that nitric oxide exerts a tonic relaxatory influence on the smooth muscle of intestinal vessels[17] and plays a protective role in intestinal mucosa.[18,19]

Blood flow autoregulation is a frequently used physiologic concept that describes the inherent ability of an organ to maintain a constant blood flow despite wide variations in arterial (perfusion) pressures. This response also serves to mediate autoregulatory escape, where initial hypoperfusion is rapidly ameliorated by arteriolar vasodilitation, restoring blood flow. Thus, it has been shown that this autoregulatory vasodilitation is responsible for the reactive hyperemia seen after occlusive states.[20] Intestinal autoregulation is neither as intense as in other organs (e.g., heart, kidney) nor as experimentally reproducible. However, it does appear to exist in "fed" animal preparations, as demonstrated by the constant blood flow that is maintained through a range of perfusion pressures between 40 and 125 mm Hg.[21] This physiologic action is related to vasodilation of the resistant vessels, largely in response to the release of the previously mentioned local metabolites.[6] An inherent sensitivity to oxygen concentration is in effect in fasted animal preparations, supporting a metabolic component as well.[7] Simple venous pressure increases appear to change blood flow by a myogenic mechanism, with increased vascular transmural pressure leading to raised arteriolar tone and vasoconstriction. In contrast, the metabolic theory would predict blood stagnation, increased interstitial metabolic products, and vasodilation.

The intrinsic autoregulatory system is also demonstrated in both the hypoxic and hypercapnic vasodilatory responses. An intestinal reactive hyperemia that is proportional to the length of time of arterial occlusion has been well described. This reactive hyperemia appears to affect the muscularis more prominently in experimental occlusions longer than 1 minute,[3,7] leading to increased motility after occlusion. Postprandial, or functional, hyperemia remains an unsettled phenomenon. In addition to metabolic and myogenic effects, the concomitant influence of locally produced hormones, neural reflexes, and changes in visceral smooth muscle tone have all been empirically implicated in this complex response.[3,7]

The extrinsic component of intestinal blood flow regulation comprises the generous sympathetic postganglionic vasoconstrictor fibers of the splanchnic intestinal nerves, which act primarily by activation of the α-adrenergic receptors. Stimulation of these fibers leads to release of norepinephrine, vasoconstriction of the precapillary resistance vessels, and decreased blood flow. However, as seen elsewhere in the body,[22,23] reduction of blood flow is associated with disproportionate vasoconstriction in the postcapillary venous beds that make up the capacitance vessels.[24] Within minutes of initial vasoconstriction, blood flow rises to nearly normal levels. The most reasonable explanation appears to be differential α- and β-adrenergic stimuli. A well-documented autoregulatory "escape" in experimental cases of prolonged electric splanchnic stimulation occurs within 1 to 2 minutes and may play a protective role in physiologic states of high sympathetic activity.[3] A reactive hyperemic response generally follows the cessation of sympathetic stimulation, concluding this triphasic response to splanchnic sympathetic activity.[3] Adrenergic stimuli also change intestinal motility, wall tension, and absorption and secretion, all of which have a profound effect on regional and local blood flow.[25] Therefore, it has not been possible to determine the net alteration in intestinal blood flow in the experimental model. At present, there is scant evidence to support other neurologic effects (vagal, cholinergic, sympathetic, or histaminergic) on intestinal blood flow, although motility is certainly affected.[3]

Numerous pharmacologic compounds affect intestinal blood flow when supplied intravascularly. The inherent difficulties in studying their effects and extrapolating them to possible physiologic roles is extremely complex and beyond the scope of this chapter. The accompanying box lists the more thoroughly investigated compounds according to their proposed vascular effects.

The naturally occurring catecholamines epinephrine and norepinephrine stimulate intense splanchnic vasoconstriction. Low circulating levels of epinephrine dilate the splanchnic vascular tree by selectively activating vascular β-receptors, whereas higher doses cause vasoconstriction. Similarly, dopamine in low doses (10^{-6} to 10^{-4} mol/L) causes mesenteric vasodilation because of its effect on specific splanchnic dopamine receptors. At higher doses, its crossover interaction with α-adrenergic receptors leads to vasoconstriction. Endogenously released dopamine is generally thought to be overwhelmed by concomitant epinephrine and norepinephrine release, so its circulating physiologic role is perhaps limited.[3] Dopamine's role in mesenteric circulation during exogenous infusion for myocardial disease is more important. The exogenous administration of catecholamines as vasopressors is the most common clinical condition seen, and their debilitating effects on intestinal perfusion are clinically well documented. Acetylcholine is generally believed to be a splanchnic vasodilator, but at higher doses this effect is counteracted by intestinal smooth muscle compression of the vascular bed.[26] Atropine in doses as high as 1 mg is able to block

PHARMACOLOGIC COMPOUNDS AFFECTING INTESTINAL BLOOD FLOW

Decrease	Increase
Norepinephrine	Epinephrine (β-effect)
Epinephrine (α-effect)	Dopamine
Methoxamine	Isoproterenol
Metaraminol	Dobutamine
Phenylephrine	Acetylcholine
Dopamine (α-effect)	Histamine
Vasopressin	Bradykinin
Angiotensin II	Sodium nitrate
Hexamethonium	Nitroprusside
Halothane	Aminophylline
Ouabain	Papaverine
Digoxin	Adenosine
Indomethacin	Caffeine
Aspirin	Diazepam
Meclofenamate	Gastrin
Prostaglandin E_1 (rat)	Pentagastrin
Prostaglandin E_2 (dog)	Secretin
Peptide YY	Glucagon
Neuropeptide Y	CCK
	Vasoactive intestinal polypeptide
	Substance P
	Prostaglandin E_1 (rabbit)
	Prostaglandin E_2 (pig)
	Prostaglandin I_2 (dog)
	Prostaglandin $F_{2\alpha}$ or $F_{2\beta}$
	Prostaglandin E_2
	Prostaglandin D_2
	Gastric inhibitory polypeptide
	Leukotrienes C4 and D4
	Thromboxane analogs
	Nitric oxide

the systemic effects of exogenously applied acetylcholine without demonstrable effects on intestinal vascular resistance.[26]

Histamine is an intestinal vasodilator that primarily mediates its effects by H_1 receptors, although the less numerous H_2 receptors in the small bowel may mediate a more sustained vasodilation. Vasopressin, as its name implies, is a potent constrictor of the mesenteric vasculature and may be physiologically important in the response to shock and gastrointestinal hemorrhage.[3] Vasopressin selectively affects the splanchnic resistance vasculature, and this response is disproportionately greater than that in the systemic circulation.[27] Another proposed physiologic vasoconstrictor is angiotensin. It appears to act by both its direct vascular effects and its potentiation of the catecholamine response to shock or blood loss after generation by renin release from the underperfused kidney during low-flow states.

The effect of circulating gastrointestinal hormones on the gastrointestinal circulation, as well as possible local effects by either localized agents (paracrine) or endoluminal secretion, remains an exciting new field of study. Difficulties in interpreting experimental data are generated by species' differences in response to individual gut hormones and the shortcomings of the various animal preparations in approximating a true physiologic condition. Gastrin, or pentagastrin, in addition to increasing gastric acid secretion, increases gastric mucosal blood flow and has a questionable effect on proximal small-intestinal blood flow. Secretin and cholecystokinin (CCK) vasodilate the small intestine in experimental animals, with selective mucosal hyperemia noted in cholecystokinin-infused animals. Glucagon is also a potent intestinal vasodilator in the cat, with vasodilating concentrations correlating well with those normally seen in the postprandial state. Serotonin, a potent stimulant of intestinal motility, does not appear to increase intestinal blood flow at normal circulating concentrations.[28] Substance P, vasoactive intestinal peptide, and gastric inhibitory polypeptide all tend to be vasodilators at pharmacologic doses but not physiologic levels. Somatostatin, however, appears to be a relatively selective vasoconstrictor of the upper gastrointestinal circulation at pharmacologic doses. This recent finding may have clinical significance in the treatment of upper gastrointestinal bleeding. Numerous substances are found in the intestinal lumen either basally or after vagal stimulation (serotonin, substance P, motilin, gastrin, peptide YY, somatostatin, vasoactive intestinal peptide, CCK), and the finding of a neurally independent mucosal hyperemia caused by endoluminal substance P has opened an entirely new field in the study of intraluminal, paracrine (or local) controls of mucosal blood flow.[29]

Prostaglandins are also released intraluminally into the small intestine, eliciting a wide range of responses in the gastrointestinal circulation. Variable intestinal responses, clear species differences, and rigorous assay techniques make this a difficult field of investigation, but one reviewer states that the splanchnic microcirculation quite likely will be shown to be controlled normally by locally released prostaglandins.[30]

The mesenteric circulation is affected by many systemic diseases and physiologic states that are beyond the scope of this chapter. The accompanying box illustrates some of these conditions.

REPERFUSION INJURY OF THE INTESTINE

After intestinal ischemia, reperfusion leads to a sequence of events that results in further tissue injury. Shorter periods of ischemia lead to alterations in microvascular permeability, whereas longer periods lead to disruption of the mucosal barrier, mediated primarily by reactive oxygen metabolites

DISEASES AFFECTING MESENTERIC CIRCULATION

Congenital	Metabolic	Inflammatory
Ehlers-Danlos syndrome	Hypertension	Polyarteritis nodosa
Pseudoxanthoma elasticum	Diabetes mellitus	Churg-Strauss syndrome
Marfan syndrome	Hypercoaguable states	Hepatitis B vasculitis
	Sickle-cell disease	Rheumatoid arthritis
	Pancreatitis	Systemic lupus erythematosus
	Neoplastic diseases	Sjögren's syndrome
	Sepsis	Scleroderma
		Dermatomyositis
		Hypersensitivity vasculitis
		Henoch-Schönlein purpura
		Behçet's disease
		Hemolytic-uremic syndrome
		Kawasaki syndrome
		Weber-Christian disease
		Takayasu's disease
		Cogan's syndrome

and polymorphonuclear leukocytes (PMNs). Several studies have demonstrated that most of the injury occurs on reperfusion.[31,32] Oxygen radical formation, specifically hydroxyl radical formation and its byproducts (dienes, lipid radicals, etc.) through the intestinal oxygen radical–producing enzyme xanthine oxidase, leads to extensive damage to tissues, including membrane lipids, nucleic acids, enzymes, and receptors.[33-37] Evidence supporting oxygen free radicals' involvement in reperfusion injury comes from several studies clearly documenting that antioxidants, xanthine oxidase inhibitors, and free-radical scavengers diminish tissue damage by detoxifying or limiting production of oxygen radicals.[38-40] Another source of reactive oxygen metabolites shown to be involved in reperfusion injury is the PMN, which contains a reduced nicotinamide adenine dinucleotide phosphate oxidase that reduces molecular oxygen to the superoxide anion and a myeloperoxidase that forms hypochlorous acid. It is postulated that xanthine oxidase–derived oxidants produced in epithelial and endothelial cells initiate the production and release of proinflammatory agents, subsequently attracting PMNs. The mechanism by which PMNs gain access to the tissue across the vascular wall is poorly understood, although PMN proteases have been implicated in both microvascular injury and disruption of the endothelial barrier.[41]

More recent literature suggests that activation of phospholipase A_2 during reperfusion seems to be instrumental in the development of hemorrhagic mucosal lesions after intestinal ischemia.[42] Phospholipase A_2 has been shown to increase the formation of cytotoxic lysophospholipids within the ischemic tissue, as well as to increase production of prostaglandins and leukotrienes.

CLINICAL EVALUATION OF INTESTINAL BLOOD FLOW

Although mesenteric vascular disease is a common entity in surgical practice, the diagnosis of acute mesenteric ischemia is frequently delayed. The search for effective preoperative and intraoperative indicators of intestinal blood flow and viability has been avid among general surgeons. The diagnosis of intestinal ischemia continues to be a challenge because the history and physical examination tend to be nonspecific. Many specialized laboratory and diagnostic tests have been used to aid in the diagnosis of intestinal ischemia. Previously, certain physical symptoms and signs (fever, constant rather than colicky pain, bloody stool, peritonitis) were used, generally unsuccessfully, to differentiate viability from nonviability.

Laboratory parameters were then used to assess this same differentiation. The use of creatinine kinase and its isoenzymes in the diagnosis of intestinal ischemia has not been proved. Although there have been isolated reports and limited studies of isoenzyme elevations in patients with intestinal ischemia,[43-46] these serum markers were found to be significantly elevated only in cases of advanced disease. Several other markers, including alkaline phosphatase, lactate dehydrogenase, and aspartate transferase, also showed elevations only in cases of advanced disease.[47] Other esoteric biochemical measurements (diamine oxidase, hexosaminidase, porcine ileal peptide, and venous and peritoneal phosphate) have been linked with intestinal ischemia,[48-53] but in limited and often contradictory studies. An elevated leukocyte count has been observed in numerous retrospective studies of mesenteric ischemia.[54,55] Because leukocyte count is elevated with most causes of surgical abdominal conditions, this is only a nonspecific indicator of intestinal ischemia. The finding of an acid-base disturbance implies a serious systemic illness, and no study has proved that either an acidosis or a base deficit is a reliable predictor of intestinal ischemia.[56] In summary, no single enzyme or combination thereof has been shown to be sensitive or specific enough to aid in the early diagnosis of intestinal ischemia.

Analysis of peritoneal fluid after lavage may assist in the accurate diagnosis of intestinal ischemia,[57] but this has not achieved widespread clinical acceptance. Tonometric pH measurement, a reflector of cellular metabolism and tissue oxygenation, has been found to be a sensitive and reproducible measurement of decreased intestinal blood flow,[58,59] and it may prove invaluable in the assessment of acute mesenteric ischemia. In this minimally invasive method, a tonometer attached to a silicone elastomer (Silastic) catheter is placed into the intestinal lumen. Saline solution is instilled into the balloon, allowed to equilibrate with intestinal pH, and then withdrawn for carbon dioxide determination. Intestinal pH measured in this fashion indirectly monitors cellular metabolism, assessing the adequacy of tissue oxygenation. In a recent prospective trial, gastric mucosal pH was the most reliable indicator of adequacy of tissue oxygenation, and it thus appears to be a simple and extremely effective way to monitor splanchnic blood flow.[60]

Abdominal radiographs are generally nondiagnostic, but a "gasless" abdomen and adynamic ileus have been described in association with mesenteric ischemia, thought to be caused by small-bowel spasm with subsequent distention and ileus. The most specific finding of intestinal ischemia is the presence of thumbprinting, caused by submucosal edema and hemorrhage. Gas in the bowel wall and portal venous gas are rare and considered terminal findings. Gas in the portal venous system is associated with necrotic bowel in more than two thirds of reported cases, with an associated mortality as great as 75%.[61] Barium examinations may help by revealing a thumbprinting pattern caused by submucosal hemorrhage and superficial mucosal ulcerations (Fig. 20-2). Transverse ridging and ulceration of the colonic wall have been reported in as many as 23% and 60% of patients, respectively.[62,63] Barium studies should not be done if gangrene, perforation, or peritonitis is suspected. Upper gastrointestinal tract series have been reported to be useful in patients with acute mesenteric ischemia, revealing such findings as thickened folds, ulcerations, stasis of barium in the affected bowel, and stenosis.[64] Although experience with computed tomography (CT) in intestinal ischemia is limited, there have been iso-

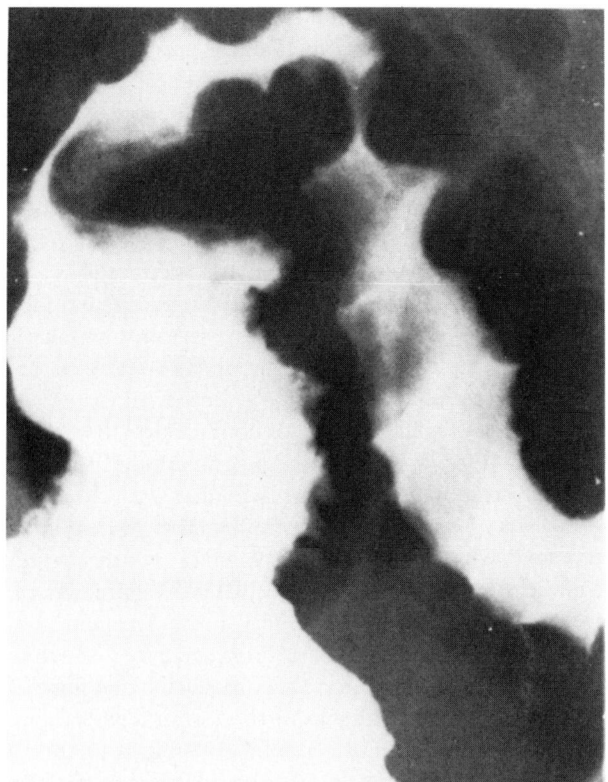

Fig. 20-2. Characteristic thumbprinting pattern seen in association with ischemic colitis. Spot-film taken during the filling phase of a barium enema. The smooth indentations (thumbprints) are the result of hemorrhage and/or edema in the submucosa. (From Wittenberg J. Radiology of the Colon. Baltimore: Williams & Wilkins, 1980.)

lated reports describing thickened bowel wall; dilated, fluid-filled loops of bowel; the target or double-halo sign; mesenteric edema; and thumbprinting[65] (see Fig. 20-2). Other specific findings, such as clot in the mesenteric vessels, pneumatosis, and portal venous gas, can be detected by CT. In a recent series, however, CT findings were nonspecific in 61% of patients.[66] Although CT may be nondiagnostic, it may be useful in excluding abdominal conditions other than ischemia. Ultrasonography is also commonly employed in the assessment of abdominal pain. Thickened bowel wall and portal venous gas can be seen clearly. Doppler ultrasonography is also being used to assess mesenteric blood flow in patients who may require angiography and intraoperative assessment of bowel viability. Magnetic resonance imaging (MRI) has shown promise in the diagnosis of intestinal ischemia. Both arterial and venous abnormalities can be identified, as well as bowel-wall thickening.[67] Again, large clinical trials that document the accuracy and reliability of one diagnostic test compared with another are lacking.

If the diagnosis of acute mesenteric ischemia is suspected, rapid early arteriography is considered the next step.[1,68-71] Arteriography has clearly been shown to improve survival before infarction and prior to laparotomy. It is extremely helpful in differentiating between occlusive and nonocclusive ischemia. The SMA origin is most commonly involved by atherosclerotic narrowing and subsequent thrombosis. Acute thromboses are always related to underlying atherosclerotic narrowing and usually involve the origins of any or all of the three main vessels. Embolic phenomena typically affect the SMA several centimeters distal to its origin, often at the orifice of the middle colic artery. The remainder of the emboli occlude at the origin of the right colic and ileocolic arteries, at points of anatomic narrowing. Emboli in the SMA appear as sharp, rounded filling defects with high-grade or subtotal obstruction of distal flow. Of note, almost half of all patients with an SMA embolus have an extramesenteric embolus, such as the loss of a femoral pulse.[68] Nonocclusive ischemic disease is characterized by segmental mesenteric arterial constriction, alternating areas of narrowing and dilitation of SMA branches, and spasm of the arcades. An associated proximal stenosis of the SMA is often seen. An important distinction must be made, however, from mesenteric venous thrombosis, which may be accompanied by arterial vasoconstriction. The treatment for these two disease entities may differ.[72] Both anteroposterior and anterolateral arteriographic views are necessary to adequately evaluate the arterial tree. The selective infusion of vasodilating agents (0.5 to 1.0 mg/min papaverine) has been advocated to maintain intestinal perfusion in both the occlusive and nonocclusive forms of acute mesenteric ischemia while other resuscitative measures are being undertaken and the surgical team is being assembled. Successful case reports of thrombolysis of acute arterial occlusions and angioplasty of high-grade SMA stenosis have been reported.[73-75] In summary, current arteriographic techniques do not allow quantitation of blood flow, but in the face of possible acute mesenteric ischemia, differentiation between occlusive and nonocclusive disease is necessary.[76]

Technetium 99m–labeled pyrophosphate, technetium 99m sulfur colloid–labeled leukocytes, technetium 99m–tagged albumin microspheres, technetium 99m–labeled methylene diphosphonate, and intraperitoneal xenon 133 are all radionuclides that have been used experimentally with some success; however, clinical trials are lacking. Numerous techniques involving radiolabeled particles have been investigated as preoperative indicators of intestinal ischemia. Intravascular injections of technetium 99m–labeled pyrophosphate, which binds to the extravasated extracellular calcium from ischemic cells, and technetium 99m sulphur colloid–labeled leukocytes, which migrate to areas of inflammation, have been used with moderate success in the laboratory, although clinical data remain unreported. The major shortcomings of these techniques are (1) their high background counts in other organs and (2) their need for advanced bowel ischemia (necrosis, transmural infarction) to obtain isotope uptake and the characteristic "hot spots" on isotope imaging.[77,78] An intraperitoneal injection technique with xenon 133, an inert gas, dissolved in normal saline solution has been reported to be successful in differentiating strangulated small-bowel obstructions from nonstrangulated small-bowel obstructions in laboratory animals, although this technique has never been tested clinically.[79] Its elucidation of acute mesenteric ischemia in laboratory animals has also been documented.[77] Intraperitoneally injected xenon 133 is quickly and equally absorbed by passive transperitoneal diffusion into ischemic and normal bowel.[77] It is promptly cleared by normally perfused bowel to the lungs. Poorly perfused intestine retains xenon 133, which is easily detectable externally by gamma-camera techniques. Diagnostic advantages include safety, rapidity of results (30 to 90 minutes), ability to detect early ischemia, and lack of interference by adhesions and moderate ascites.[80] More quantitative washout curve analysis may be needed, especially in critically ill, hypotensive patients who may have associated asymptomatic reduced splanchnic blood flow. In a recent series in anaesthetized pigs, the mucosal blood flow rate was determined by a local epimucosal application of xenon 133.[81] When compared with the microsphere entrapment technique, which measures blood flow in tissues and cannot be used in human studies, there were excellent correlations ($r = 0.89$ and $r = 0.996$, respectively) for blood flow rates in the small intestine and in the colon. Local washout of xenon 133 is an exciting new diagnostic tool, and appropriate clinical trials to test its efficacy are indicated. Other methods more commonly used in humans are laser Doppler velocimetry, hydrogen gas clearance, and iodoantipyrin clearance, all of which have been shown to have limitations.[82] For instance, the first technique is not quantitative. With a new technique that uses technetium 99m–labeled monoclonal antiplatelet antibodies, areas of ischemia have been detected experimentally as early as 90 minutes.[83] At present, clinical trials await.

Laparoscopy has been used extensively in surgery, and studies have shown that diagnostic laparoscopy can be performed and should be well tolerated in those with suspected intestinal ischemia.[84] Although there has been limited experience, fluorescein-assisted laparoscopy has proved as reliable as standard laparotomy.[85] Large series of data are lacking. It should be noted that despite a normal-appearing serosa on laparoscopy, negative laparoscopic findings do not indicate normal mucosa.

Although endoscopy has become an invaluable tool to the clinician, its role in determining intestinal viability is limited. Most cases of acute ischemia are out of the reach of the endoscope. It has, however, been shown to be a useful adjunct in those with suspected ischemic colitis.

Another method that holds clinical promise in assessing intestinal viability is reflectance spectrophotometry. This technique does not measure blood flow directly; however, it can measure oxygen saturation and hemoglobin concentrations in distinct patterns that correlate with different etiologies of acute ischemia.[86] Again, clinical trials are lacking.

The efficacy of any intraoperative method of assessing bowel circulation and viability quite naturally must be compared with experienced clinical judgment and must be a technique that involves no sophisticated equipment or risk to the patient. Most surgeons use normal bowel color, peritoneal sheen, mesenteric arterial pulsations, and the presence of spontaneous peristalsis as criteria. This assessment is based on experience and the obvious absence of these entities in infarcted bowel. The technique of applying warmed, moist packs to bowel of questionable viability for varying durations is almost universally accepted. The technique of second-look procedures, usually at 24 to 48 hours after the first laparotomy, is time honored, but it subjects the patient to additional anesthetic and metabolic stress. Simple transillumination of mesenteric vessels with a sterile light source has been suggested as an adjuvant naked-eye technique.[87] Reported attempts at clinical assessment of intestinal blood flow after ischemic insult have included various sophisticated but technically unwieldy methods, including electromyography, bowel-wall pH determinations, and radioactive microsphere injections. At present, most clinical debate focuses on two relatively simple and safe methods of mesenteric circulatory assessment: Doppler ultrasonography and intravenous injection of dyes.

The handheld, pencil-like, sterile Doppler ultrasonographic flow probe is used by applying it to the antimesenteric border of the bowel wall and to discrete mesenteric vessels. Most current probes penetrate tissue to a depth of 1 cm. The presence of a typical pulsatile arterial signal is claimed by proponents as an indication of adequate blood flow to that particular bowel segment.[88-90] Although this method has received enthusiastic support as a result of animal studies[91,92] and small clinical experiences,[93-95] its drawbacks include the impracticability of screening large areas of intestine and a lack of sensitivity,[96] especially for small, patchy areas of inadequate circulation along the bowel wall. In addition, it has been shown in a prospective clinical study to be of little or no value in cases of mesenteric venous occlusion.[97] Nevertheless, its quickness and facility of application have made it a generally useful tool that is popular among some surgeons.

Fluorescein dye is an organic compound that emits a gold-green fluorescence when exposed to UV light between 3600 and 4000 nm. It readily enters extracellular fluid after intravenous injections, whereupon its entrance into viable tissue occurs within minutes. A maximal intensity is reached within a few minutes of administration, with a gradual disappearance over 48 hours. It is nontoxic at normal dosage (10 to 15 mg/kg). There have been isolated reports of nausea and vomiting and rare anaphylactic reactions after injection.[98] Its success in detecting mesenteric arterial and venous occlusions is well documented,[99-101] with 96% sensitivity and 95% specificity reported, although a 17% false-positive rate has been reported for venous occlusions. In adults, two ampules of sodium fluorescein (1000 mg) are intravenously injected for 30 to 60 seconds. After the operating room lights have been dimmed, a Wood's lamp (3600 nm) is used to illu-

Table 20-1. Techniques to Assess Bowel Viability

Method	Reference	Mechanism	Advantages	Disadvantages
pH studies/tonometry	Myers et al.[108] Katz et al.[109]	Electromyography	Alkalotic serosal pH indicates irreversible ischemic damage	
Surface oximetry, pulse oximetry	Locke et al.[110] De Nobile et al.[111]	Transcutaneous oxygen monitoring (surface oxygen tension measurements)	Accurate intraoperative assessment of bowel perfusion; simple, accurate, and inexpensive	May miss segments of patchy ischemia
Photoplethysmography	Pearse et al.[92]	Monitors changes in tissue blood volume content by detecting alterations in reflected infrared light as a function of its absorption by hemoglobin	Highly sensitive to changes in blood flow	Impossible to quantitate waveforms; poorly specific
Myoelectric analysis	Khin and Daniel[112] Guisan et al.[113] Chou[114] Cabot and Kohatsu[115] Brolin et al.[116,117]	Predicts slow-wave activity in bowel wall serosal strain gauge	Simple and highly reliable	Artifact in baseline recordings allows much subjectivity

minate the operative field. Viable bowel shows a confluent yellow-green fluorescence, although a fine, granular pattern may be noted. Nonviable intestine demonstrates an absence of fluorescence, with only a perivascular fluorescent pattern or patches of nonfluorescence greater than 5 mm in diameter.[88] Because of sodium fluorescein's rapid transudation into the peritoneal cavity and its prolonged presence after injection, this test can really be performed only once within a 48-hour period, making it a one-shot examination.[88] To date, only four prospective trials have been published comparing the Doppler ultrasonographic flow probe analysis with sodium fluorescein injection in human mesenteric vascular disease[97,102,103]; all markedly support the fluorescein technique. The overall sensitivity and specificity of the sodium fluorescein technique were 100% and 100%, respectively, in the larger series,[102] whereas the figures were 50% and 58%, respectively, for Doppler ultrasonography. In fact, the clinical judgment of the senior operating surgeon in this study had better sensitivity and specificity than Doppler ultrasonography in identifying nonviable small intestine, 82% and 91%, respectively. Other dyes, including trypan blue, patent blue V dye, and bromophenol, have been also investigated, but without the success of fluorescein.[104-106] At present, the use of intravenous sodium fluorescein appears to be the investigation of choice in assessing mesenteric blood flow or adequacy of bowel perfusion in the intraoperative setting. In one recent if small series of patients (n = 16), however, the accuracies of clinical judgment, fluorescein, and Doppler ultrasonography were 50%, 56%, and 0% respectively, thereby recommending routine second-look explorations in patients with acute mesenteric ischemia.[107]

Table 20-1 compares various other techniques that are available to assess bowel viability.[108-117]

MESENTERIC VASCULAR DISEASE

Mesenteric occlusive vascular disease is classically divided into acute and chronic variants and arterial and venous origins. Many patients with acute manifestations, however, are demonstrating sudden deteriorations of chronic, often asymptomatic, visceral vascular disease. The arterial forms of acute mesenteric ischemia include SMA embolus, nonocclusive (obliterative) mesenteric ischemia, SMA thrombosis, and aneurysms of the splanchnic arteries.

Acute ischemic syndromes are the result of embolic occlusions of visceral branches of the abdominal aorta, thrombotic occlusions of a previously diseased branch of the mesenteric arterial system, mesenteric venous thrombosis, or nonocclusive mesenteric ischemia (low-flow syndrome).[1,88] The usual result of any of these conditions is intestinal infarction, with overall mortality rates ranging from 70% to 90%. Acute mesenteric ischemia is responsible for 0.1% of all hospital admissions in the United States, and because of the increase in the elderly proportion of the population, an aggressive approach to early diagnosis and intervention is warranted. Mortality from these conditions is directly related to the presence of frank bowel infarction and the frequent concomitant presence of significant cardiovascular disease. Attempts should be made to differentiate among the causes of acute mesenteric ischemia, because both treatment and prognoses differ. Currently, selective angiography is the gold standard for diagnosis and treatment of both occlusive and nonocclusive forms of acute intestinal ischemia.[71]

Nearly 70% of affected patients are older than 60 years, and more than 90% report the acute onset of abdominal pain, often crampy and central in location, as the most prominent symptom. Most patients describe the pain as severe or violent, and reported pain is generally disproportionate to the lack of physical findings. Abdominal pain followed by spontaneous bowel evacuation without significant physical findings is frequently seen in early occlusive mesenteric ischemia. Typically, patients with nonocclusive mesenteric ischemia initially have pain in the absence of defecatory urge.[1] Other clinical signs include vomiting, diarrhea, unexplained abdominal distention or tenderness, and melena. Bowel sounds range from hyperactivity in the early stages to absolute quiet as transmural necrosis proceeds. Occult blood is found 75% of the time in stool examination. A history of preexisting postprandial abdominal pain, "intestinal angina," is seen in about 10% of patients[118] and is an important diagnostic sign. Shock related to volume depletion or perforative sepsis is seen in one fourth of patients at initial examination. Hemoconcentration and leukocytosis greater than 20,000 cells/mm^3 are frequently seen, but no single test or combination of blood tests is diagnostic. Serum amylase level is elevated in one third of patients with mesenteric ischemia. It should be stressed that acute, severe abdominal pain in the absence of associated abdominal findings is usually the clearest sign of early mesenteric ischemia, especially in elderly patients, and at this stage most patients will not have intestinal infarction.[1] Furthermore, the development of abdominal or peritoneal signs implies infarction and significantly increases mortality risk. The use of plain and angiographic roentgenograms has already been mentioned as essential for diagnosis, and it is only noted here as a reminder for their rapid institution. Medical stabilization, metabolic correction, and invasive cardiovascular monitoring are integral efforts in these critically ill patients in the interim before surgery. Coexisting atherosclerotic heart disease, chronic airway disease, and diabetes mellitus are frequently encountered in these patients and require rapid attention.

Acute Mesenteric Arterial Embolism

Sixty percent of acute mesenteric arterial embolic events are amenable to surgery, making them the most important surgical cause of intestinal ischemia. They constitute 40% to 50% of all acute mesenteric vascular catastrophes. Bergan's triad of acute abdominal crisis, significant cardiac disease, and spontaneous gastrointestinal emptying is used descriptively for this disorder.[119] Affected patients are often younger, with no prior intestinal angina symptoms. An important historical or concomitant finding is the presence of arrhythmias in 70% of patients. Most of these arrhythmias are atrial tachyarrhythmias, although recent myocardial infarctions, previous arterial emboli, rheumatic heart disease, hypotension related to burns, pancreatitis, hemorrhage, and atherosclerotic heart disease are also known predisposing factors.[88,120] The oblique takeoff of the SMA favors embolization, with a total of 5% of all peripheral arterial emboli involving this vessel or a distal branch. Usually emboli lodge several centimeters distal to the SMA origin, occluding the middle colic artery (55%), right colic artery (16%), ileocolic artery (7%), or smaller peripheral branches (4%).[121] The usual source of emboli is left atrial or ventricular mural thrombi, but unusual emboli forms include those from bronchogenic carcinoma, atrial myxoma, aortic or mitral valvular prostheses, and the proximal aortic wall.[76]

Surgical management consists of (1) the identification and resuscitation of the patient at high risk; (2) plain films of the abdomen, arteriographic localization, and confirmation of the vascular abnormality; (3) preoperative papaverine infusion at 30 to 60 mg/hr with an infusion pump; (4) operative management; and (5) postoperative management that includes a possible second-look procedure. The patients are identified by observation of the previously mentioned signs, symptoms, and history. Resuscitation involves metabolic correction and monitored restoration of intravascular volume. Because of their constrictor effects on splanchnic blood flow, vasopressors and digitalis compounds should be avoided whenever possible. Antibiotic coverage is recommended when surgery is anticipated, and broad-spectrum coverage is the rule.[122]

After a brief but thorough resuscitative phase, early angiography is mandated. Lengthy delays before angiography not only allow further bowel ischemia but also obscure the radiologic diagnosis by allowing distal clot propagation. Femoral arterial access for angiographic evaluation is generally preferred, with biplanar selective injection of all three major splanchnic trunks. Some authorities recommend halving the usual dose of contrast medium because of these patients' tenuous fluid balance and to avoid renal failure.[120,123] Occlusion of the SMA or one of its branches with arterial spasm and a lack of collaterals (as seen with acute thrombosis) is the usual angiographic picture. The splanchnic vasoconstriction seen with SMA embolization is well documented,[124] and its persistence after embolectomy may be a reason for the frequent inability to restore adequate blood flow and for the frequent late reocclusions of distal vessels. Persistent precapillary arterial vasospasm has been seen experimentally after just 2 hours of partial SMA occlusion[125]; this possibly reflects myogenic control mechanisms. Because of this distal vasospasm, arterial vasodilators are selectively administered by most radiologists.[87,110] Tolazoline is used in an initial 25 mg bolus because of its rapid effect; further angiographic exposures are taken to ascertain this effect. If vasodilation is noted, a continuous intra-arterial infusion of papaverine is begun at 30 to 60 mg/hr. Glucagon at a rate of 1 μg/kg/min has also been shown to improve blood flow when administered parenterally. Tolazoline is neither as safe nor as efficacious as papaverine for continuous infusion. The clinical and angiographic responses to vasodilator therapy determine the duration of the papaverine infusion, which is usually continued for 12 to 24 hours.

Minor emboli are those limited to the branches of the SMA or to the SMA distal to the origin of the ileocolic artery. Patients with minor emboli and without peritoneal signs are managed conservatively with papaverine infusion and clinical observation. If peritoneal signs develop, papaverine infusion is continued and patients undergo prompt exploration. Patients with major emboli undergo prompt exploration unless peritoneal signs are lacking, perfusion distal to the embolus is adequate, or there are contraindications to surgery.

Operative management of this disorder is probably the least controversial aspect (Fig. 20-3). The SMA is dissected free through the base of the small-bowel mesentery, and linear arteriotomies are made, followed by embolectomy (and Fogarty catheterization to remove remaining clot) and vein patch graft closure of the arteriotomy. Because vein is preferred for patching, both legs should be prepared and draped within the operative field. The presence of palpable pulses distal to the arteriotomy must be documented before bowel evaluation and resection. If there is any question of the viability of the intestine, an attempt at arterial reconstruction is indicated. Although the dusky surface of the bowel wall may appear nonviable, this appearance can be deceiving. After revascularization, the entire gastrointestinal tract should be visualized for 15 to 30 minutes. Most patients require the resection of some intestine, followed by standard end-to-end anastamoses. As previously discussed, observational criteria, fluorescein injection, Doppler ultrasonography, or all three are used to select viable bowel for anastamosis and nonviable bowel for resection. Mortality risk is related to the amount of bowel resected, with resections of more than 50% approaching a 90% mortality.[120] The need for a second-look operation is decided on before closure; this decision is adhered to regardless of subsequent clinical improvement. Repeated angiography and postoperative continuation of intra-arterial papaverine are advocated by Boley et al.,[120] whose 55% survival figures are among the best reported.

The use of anticoagulants in SMA emboli is controversial.[119,120,126] The relative risks of significant intestinal bleeding versus the incidence of late postoperative thromboses leads most authorities to recommend some late (48 hours after the operation) anticoagulation. In patients awaiting a second-look procedure, low-molecular-weight dextran has been cited for both its plasma volume-expansion qualities and its antithrombotic properties. The duration of anticoagulation varies widely among patients. Thrombolytic therapy, as mentioned previously, remains highly experimental and controversial.

A variety of postoperative problems, both early and late, may arise. Sepsis, gastrointestinal bleeding, acute renal failure, pulmonary insufficiency, and myocardial dysfunction are all common and mandate admission of affected patients to an intensive care unit for several days. Unexplained acidosis, sepsis of unexplained origin, and refractory cardiovascular instability all suggest continuing bowel necrosis and may necessitate a second-look procedure.

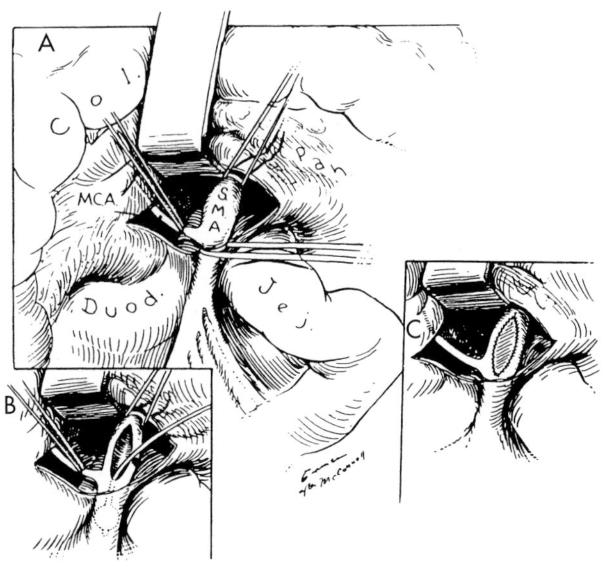

Fig. 20-3. Surgical management of embolism to the superior mesenteric artery. **A,** The artery has been isolated at the base of the transverse mesocolon and controlled with tapes. **B,** Longitudinal arteriotomy placed proximal to the origin of the middle colic artery. Fogarty catheter has been passed distally. **C,** Arteriotomy closure with a vein patch that may or may not be necessary. (From Boley SJ, et al. Surgery Annual. New York: Appleton-Century-Crofts, 1973.)

Acute Mesenteric Thrombosis

Acute thromboses of previously atherosclerotic SMA, celiac trunk, or IMA (in that order of frequency) are the most common cause of acute mesenteric ischemia. Various series report this entity to compose 44% to 82% of all mesenteric ischemic events.[1,118,121] The preoperative and postoperative management of affected patients are basically identical to that described in the earlier section, but several unique features of this condition merit further discussion.

Anatomically significant or complete atherosclerotic obstructions of any or all of the splanchnic major vessels are a frequent finding in many patients undergoing arteriography for other vascular disorders.[1,5,76,118] The presence of significant but usually hemodynamically incomplete collateral systems is also noted. These collateral systems may allow a longer "grace period" before infarction occurs, although survival statistics do not support this conjecture. They may also be responsible for the less dramatic clinical appearance of this disorder compared with embolic phenomenon. Both early clinical and early radiographic pictures often simulate a bowel obstruction. Abdominal pain, again out of proportion to clinical findings, associated with a history of cardiovascular disease is often the only early finding, although fever, shock, and melena eventually develop in many cases. Both abdominal symptoms and angiographic evidence of ischemic disease are necessary before laparotomy for this condition is performed.

Most of these patients have a significant gastrointestinal history. Between 50% and 70% have a significant history in the previous year of weight loss, diarrhea, abdominal pain, or the diagnosis of an abdominal bruit.[127] Many patients have undergone unsuccessful investigations in the preceding months for peptic ulcer or gallbladder disease, and many have diagnoses of psychiatric or functional abdominal pain. The exact percentage of patients with intestinal angina that progresses to frank bowel infarction is unknown. Overall mortality rate associated with acute thromboses averages 80%, with some series having almost two thirds of these patients undergoing either an "open and close" laparotomy or heroic massive bowel resections because of extensive intestinal necrosis.

Again, early arteriographic evaluation is necessary in these patients at high risk. Differentiation between arterial thrombus and embolus can be difficult, and these patients should be treated for SMA embolus. If possible, an angiographic catheter is placed into the vessels of concern, and papaverine infusion is begun. Glucagon therapy may also be instituted at this time. The simultaneous obstruction of both celiac and superior mesenteric vessels is usually ameliorated by restoring blood flow through just one of the involved vessels. Operatively, the SMA is more accessible and easier to manipulate than the celiac artery and is the preferred vessel for antegrade bypass. An autologous repair is recommended in a contaminated field resulting from intestinal infarction and necrosis.[128] All mesenteric vessels have a reputation for friability,[88] and handling them requires great care. The prompt relief of an obstructed SMA or celiac artery is the surgical goal. Although successful thromboendarterectomy has been reported,[129,130] most current authors favor venous graft or prosthetic bypass of the affected segment with the aorta or right iliac artery as the inflow vessel (Fig. 20-4). The preferred graft material is reversed autologous saphenous vein, although polyethylene terephthalate fabric (Dacron) is a suitable substitute. Reimplantation, if performed, is accomplished by transecting the artery distal to its disease and anastamosing directly to the aorta. Postoperative management is difficult because of the systemic nature of atherosclerosis.

Percutaneous balloon and laser angioplasties of the SMA have been performed.[131] Because of the reported complications of end-organ damage and rethrombosis, however, these procedures are not currently recommended.

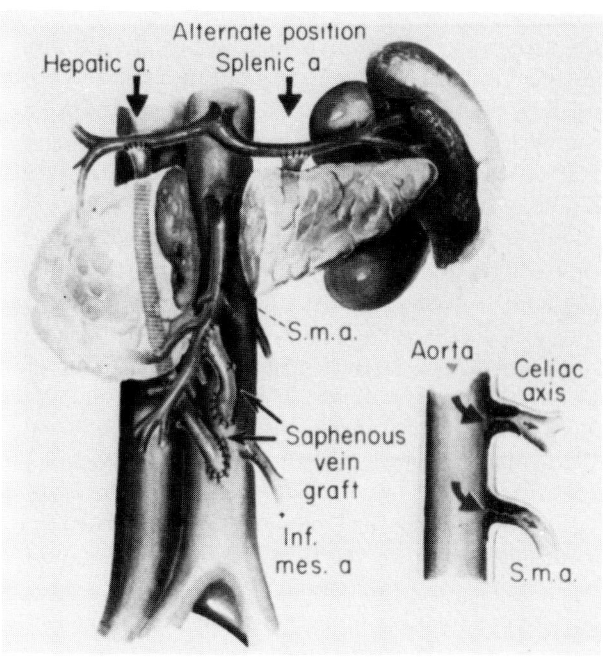

Fig. 20-4. Bypass of the atherosclerotic or thrombosed celiac artery or superior mesenteric artery (SMA). Artist's drawing showing saphenous bypass grafts to the celiac axis territory and SMA. The celiac axis graft passes behind the pancreas to connect with either the hepatic artery or the splenic artery. Atherosclerotic occlusions of the celiac axis and SMA are depicted in the lateral view of the aorta. (From Bergan JJ, Yao JST. In Rutherford RB, ed. Vascular Surgery, 2nd ed. Philadelphia: WB Saunders, 1984.)

Acute Mesenteric Ischemia After Aortic Surgery

Intestinal ischemia is an infrequent but serious complication of abdominal aortic surgery. Because of the significant association between aortic atherosclerotic disease and disease of the splanchnic arterial vessels, it is not uncommon for aortic revascularization procedures to create ischemic insults to the gut. Acute small or large intestinal ischemia, most commonly involving the left colon, may result from aortic surgery.[124] The reported incidence of significant colon ischemia varies between 0.2% and 10%, with mortality rates averaging 50% to 75%.[124,132,133] In a recent large clinical review of 2137 patients, the overall incidence of clinically significant ischemia was 1.1%. Small bowel ischemia occured in 0.2%, and 0.9% had colon ischemia.[134] Intestinal ischemia (primarily of the left colon) is seen five times more frequently after abdominal aortic aneurysm repair than after surgery for occlusive aortic disease.[135] In the latter situation, the IMA is already occluded, and the left colon receives its blood supply from collateral routes. In aneurysmal disease, inferior mesenteric flow is often intact, and the colon receives its major blood supply through this route.

Ischemia of the left colon may follow intraoperative ligation of the IMA if collateral circulation from above is compromised by coexistent SMA disease, by previous bowel resection, or by congenital interruption or absence of collateral routes. Congenital findings include aberrant takeoff of the middle colic artery (usually from the right colic artery) in 20% of cases and absence of the marginal artery of Drummond at the splenic flexure in 7%.[136] Other statistically significant implicated factors include prolonged crossclamp time; reoperative graft procedures;

ruptured aneurysm; the presence of hypoxemia, hypotension, or arrhythmias; operative colonic trauma; and digitalis toxicity.[134,136,137] Internal iliac artery flow compromised by occlusive or aneurysmal disease also limits bowel collateral flow. Embolization of thrombotic and atheromatous debris also occurs.[124] In the series by Brewster et al.,[134] the cause of small bowel ischemia was clearly related to postoperative thrombus or embolus. An aortoiliac steal syndrome has been described after simultaneous aortic reconstructions and lumbar sympathectomies, resulting in a 40% to 70% decrease in IMA flow.[138] In conclusion, patients at high risk for ischemic colitis after aortic surgery are those with an absence or occlusion of the marginal artery at the splenic flexure, absent middle colic artery, internal iliac arterial inflow disease, middle colic artery enlargement suggesting SMA occlusive disease, or aneurysms.[136]

Infarction of the small intestine is usually related to inopportune ligation of the IMA when it supplies most of the gastrointestinal tract through the meandering mesenteric artery. Careful examination of the preoperative arteriogram, especially lateral views, should alert the surgeon to this risk. If antegrade IMA flow is desired, this can be achieved by end-to-side aortic anastomosis. If end-to-end aortic anastomosis is preferred, IMA flow may be maintained by reimplantation into the graft. Because of the infrequent occurrence of colonic ischemia, routine reimplantation of the IMA is not advisable.[134]

Left-colon ischemia is prevented by ligation of the IMA immediately adjacent to the aorta to obviate interruption of its collateral channels. Careful vascular technique to avoid embolization is essential. Avoidance of hypotension and care to ensure patency of the hypogastric arteries are emphasized. Also, one must avoid trauma to collateral vessels by retractors. If the left colon appears ischemic on IMA clamping or division, if the IMA is patent but has little backflow, or if the IMA shows large ascending collateral vessels on preoperative angiographic examination,[124,139] an IMA reimplantation (Fig. 20-5) with Carrel button techniques or an aorta-IMA bypass should be performed, as previously mentioned.

If colonic ischemia occurs after surgery, symptoms are often late in appearing (48 to 72 hours). Lower left abdominal pain, watery guaiac-positive or bloody diarrhea, and systemic toxicity are the usual findings. Subclinical mucosal ischemia has been reported in 4% to 7% of patients,[124,139] but clinical ischemia reveals hemorrhagic ulcerations and mucosal edema with friability on sigmoidoscopy. If such findings occur, relaparotomy is necessary on an urgent basis. At the time of reoperation, all compromised bowel is resected and end-colostomy with distal Hartmann's procedure should be performed. Small bowel ischemia is treated similarly in an aggressive fashion, although sigmoidoscopic findings may only reveal melena. Again, if clinical doubt exists, early relaparotomy is performed. The primary focus, however, should be on identification of patients at high risk for bowel ischemia, so that appropriate preoperative studies may be obtained and the correct operative procedure can be performed.

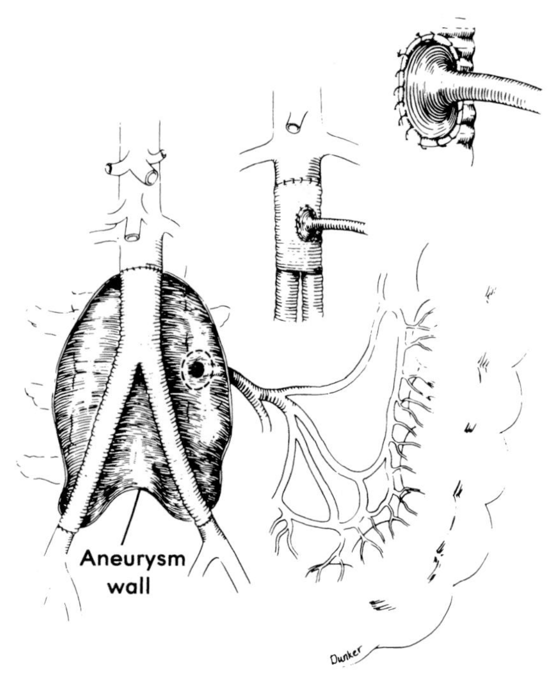

Fig. 20-5. Reimplantation of the inferior mesenteric artery (IMA) during abdominal aortic aneurysm surgery. Carrel path technique of IMA reconstruction. Excision of button of aneurysm wall surrounding IMA orifice facilitates repair. (From Ernst CB. Complications in Vascular Surgery, 2nd ed. Orlando, Fla.: Grune & Stratton, 1985.)

Mesenteric Venous Thrombosis

The syndrome of acute or subacute thrombosis of the mesenteric veins was first described more than 100 years ago by Elliot[140] and now constitutes fewer than 5% of all reported cases of mesenteric ischemia.[141] During the last 22 years, 71 cases of acute thromboses have been reported in the literature, with the largest series including seven patients.[142] Predisposing conditions include peritonitis or abdominal inflammation, abdominal trauma, portal hypertension, intra-abdominal tumors, adhesions, volvulus, decompression sickness, sickle-cell disease, polycythemia vera, coagulopathies (especially antithrombin III deficiencies and protein C and S deficiency), pregnancy, recent splenectomy, and the use of oral contraceptives.[1,76,88,143] More than 40% of patients have had previous deep vein thrombophlebitis of the lower extremity. The reported age range is from 11 months to 89 years, but most series report an average age of only 47 years.[144,145]

Presentations may be divided into two categories, subacute and acute.[146] The subacute category is far more common, often with a vague prodrome of crampy abdominal pain, distention, nausea, and lassitude lasting from a few days to several weeks without intestinal infarction.

Patients in this group are considered to have thrombi originating in small mesenteric veins or venules and then propagating proximally. Most often, the diagnosis is made during other radiologic examinations, and the symptoms typically subside spontaneously or after initiation of anticoagulant therapy. The more acute presentations are thought to represent primary thrombosis of large, often named, mesenteric veins.[93] Rarely are veins in the inferior mesenteric system involved. By the time of presentation, most patients have significant abdominal pain (>90%), tenderness, decreased bowel sounds, fecal occult blood, and distention. Laboratory investigations reveal leukocytosis, hemoconcentration, and copious, bloody peritoneal transudate. As venous pressure increases, myogenic mechanisms stimulate arteriolar vasoconstriction, which leads to capillary distention and leakage, with an abundant serosal transudation of bloody fluid. Additional anatomic findings include massive edema and cyanosis of the bowel wall as a result of interstitial edema, mesenteric arterial pulsations, compensatory mesenteric lymphatic engorgement, and mesenteric veins full of clot. Plain films of the abdomen, if abnormal, almost always reflect infarcted intestine. Classic, but frequently overlooked, radiographic findings include rigid, thick-walled segments of edematous bowel in which a small gas collection remains fixed in a straight or curved lumen on different radiographs.[144] Early selective angiography can be diagnostic, showing thrombus in the superior mesenteric vein, a delay in filling during the arterial phase, small artery spasm, poor emptying of arteries, failure of venous systems (including the portal vein) to opacify, reflux of contrast medium into the artery, and often opacification of thickened bowel wall as a result of transudation of contrast medium.[1,76,88,147]

Ultrasonography, CT, and MRI have all been used in the diagnosis of venous thrombosis.[148-150] A contrast-enhanced CT scan can establish a diagnosis in more than 90% of patients with mesenteric venous thrombosis. For this reason, there is no direct evidence supporting angiography instead of CT scan in establishing the diagnosis. MRI has the advantage of avoiding exposure of the patient to ionizing radiation. Treatment is similar to that discussed for other ischemic disorders of the splanchnic vasculature. In patients who do not yet have infarcted bowel identified by radiographic criteria, however, a trial of anticoagulant or thrombolytic therapy may be beneficial.[122,151] All other patients should undergo prompt exploration. An attempt at defining the extent of thrombosis, either by intraoperative ultrasonography or by direct injection of contrast into the venous system, has been shown to provide information valuable in defining surgical tactics.[142] Aggressive restoration of intravascular volume, preoperative heparin therapy, and antibiotics are administered before urgent laparotomy.[143] A small bowel resection is virtually always necessary. If palpable clot is present, a venous thrombectomy is performed through the superior mesenteric vein controlled inferior to the pancreas. A transverse venotomy is performed, and manual milking of the clot, as well as the use of Fogarty catheters, is employed to remove the thrombus. Most surgeons begin heparinization immediately, and warfarin compounds are continued for 3 to 6 months after surgery. If a predisposing coagulopathy exists, anticoagulation is continued indefinitely. Only nonviable bowel needs to be resected. In the earlier literature, a wide mesenteric resection was recommended to avoid leaving residual thrombotic veins behind that might later propagate clot. Recent data prove that with heparin therapy and second-look operations, this radical resection technique need no longer be used.[144-146,152] The mortality rate for this condition approaches 100% if untreated, but newer series report operative mortality rates averaging 20%, and falling below 15% with heparin therapy.[141,144-146,152] Rethrombosis is common, usually occuring early. It is seen in about one quarter of cases and carries a higher mortality rate of 60% to 80%.[144] Some surgeons routinely advocate second-look procedures because of this high rethrombosis rate.[144] In general, the prognosis is somewhat better than for mesenteric infarction caused by arterial occlusion, probably because of the shorter involved bowel segment. Certainly, a high index of suspicion and intensive care monitoring of the patient are warranted.

Nonocclusive Mesenteric Ischemia

The entity of nonocclusive mesenteric ischemia is a diverse series of interrelated events that accounts for 20% to 50% of all mesenteric infarctions in which autopsy data are included.[144-146,152] It involves the distribution of the SMA almost exclusively, and it is usually the consequence of both an anatomic defect (SMA stenosis in more than one third of patients) and some acute process that requires either an increase or a redistribution of cardiac output.[76] It has been shown in dogs that when the blood pressure falls below 15 mm Hg with a blood flow less than 10 ml/100 g tissue, irreversible ischemia develops. This results in a decrease in mesenteric perfusion pressure, with an accompanying splanchnic vasoconstriction initiated by myogenic mechanisms. This is clinically important because splanchnic hypersensitivity to angiotensin II, generated by the release of renin in the kidney, appears to be the fundamental mechanism underlying nonocclusive mesenteric ischemia.[153] As splanchnic vasoconstriction occurs, the critical closing pressures of small arteries are surpassed, leading to segmental microvascular collapse. This circumstance favors microthrombus formation, with a concomitant further reduction in blood flow.[1] If systemic hypotension also exists, increased endogenous catecholamines, exogenously administered catecholamines, or both may further constrict the splanchnic microcirculation, with eventual ischemia and necrosis. Local acidosis and thrombus formation lead to capillary sludging and hemoconcentration. Bowel distention is often present and further decreases blood flow by increasing mural pressure. This vicious physiologic circle continues until frank segmental bowel infarction occurs; untreated, this results in a mortality rate approaching 100%. A myriad of conditions have been associated with nonocclusive mesenteric ischemia. Most of patients with this disease have some underlying cardiac abnormality.

Digitalis compounds are potent in vitro contractors of arterial and venous smooth muscle in the gut that simultaneously decrease splanchnic blood flow and oxygen consumption. As many as 83% of patients with nonocclusive mesenteric ischemia are receiving digitalis compounds at diagnosis. Other conditions associated with this disorder include congestive heart failure; arrhythmias; cardiopulmonary bypass; cardiogenic or septic shock; administration of vasopressors, intravenous calcium, or both; major thermal injuries; and pancreatitis.

Patients are often already hospitalized for associated conditions when the disorder arises. Abdominal pain and evidence of a low-output state are the major diagnostic aids. Frequently, patients are examined for other acute abdominal processes, including cholecystitis, appendicitis, and bowel obstruction. The absence of abdominal pain in this condition is far more frequent than in occlusive mesenteric ischemia because of concomitant symptomatic conditions. Evidence of peripheral circulatory shutdown, acidosis, and hemoconcentration is often present. Plain abdominal roentograms often show only fluid-filled bowel loops. Arteriography is the single diagnostic tool that distinguishes this condition from occlusive mesenteric ischemia. In addition, careful angiography may reveal segmental spastic arterial constriction (chain of sausages),[88] and there may be a failure to visualize mesenteric vascular arcades or intramural vessels. The intra-arterial infusion of vasodilators (papaverine, glucagon, prostaglandins) while aggressive attempts to increase cardiac output and normalize intravascular volume are performed has been clinically reported with some success.[1,152,154] Repeated angiography is performed after vasodilator therapy has begun, to document improvement.

Unlike with other types of acute mesenteric ischemia, immediate surgery is not indicated for nonocclusive ischemia. Further, anesthesia and intraoperative manipulation decrease intestinal blood flow. Generally, 8- to 12-hour scrutiny of the patient while vasodilator therapy is administered and cardiac improvement is attempted is the initial treatment of choice. After this, or sooner if infarcted bowel is suspected, laparotomy should be performed in most of patients in clinically stable condition. Massive fluid replacement, cardiac support and a continuous epidural block to decrease splanchnic vasoconstriction have been recommended after operation.

Chronic Intestinal Ischemia

Chronic intestinal ischemia and its manifestation as intestinal angina were first described by Mikkelson in 1957.[155] The importance of this entity lies not only in its production of physical disability for the individual patient but also in its propensity for progression to life-threatening mesenteric infarction. After gradual occlusion of the main splanchnic arteries, three scenarios are possible: (1) intestinal infarction; (2) intestinal angina; and (3) established adequate collateral circulation. More than 50% of patients who die of SMA thrombosis previously had intestinal angina. These patients are classically in the sixth decade of life and are heavy smokers. Unlike with other types of peripheral vascular disease, female patients outnumber male patients by a ratio of 3:1. More than a third of these patients have associated atherosclerotic disease of the aorta or renal arteries. Atherosclerosis is the leading cause of the visceral artery stenoses that cause this syndrome, although extrinsic compression, neoplasms, and local inflammation have been implicated.[156] Less frequently, the stenosis results from compression of the celiac axis by a celiac ganglion or arcuate ligament of the diaphragm, compression from an expanding or dissecting aortic aneurysm, or thromboangiitis obliterans or periarteritis nodosa.

The classic triad of abdominal pain, weight loss, and diarrhea is seen in this condition.[124,157] Recurrent, crampy abdominal pain occurs 15 minutes to 1 hour postprandially; it is periumbilical and lasts from 1 to 3 hours. Because this pain commences soon after eating, it often causes a fear of eating, leading to significant weight loss that averages 20 to 25 pounds in most patients.[156,158] The severity depends on the amount of food ingested. Diarrhea, often containing occult blood, is seen in about one third of patients. Malabsorption is frequently seen, but specific diagnostic tests are not usually helpful. An abdominal bruit is heard in 50% of patients, but abdominal examination, even during attacks of pain, is frequently unremarkable. Because of the nature of the symptoms, patients are often investigated for the presence of an occult gastrointestinal neoplasm.[1,23,156,157,159]

Arteriography should be performed if malignancy investigation results are negative. Lateral views are mandatory in evaluating the celiac artery and SMA, whereas oblique views help demonstrate the IMA. Significant stenoses of both the celiac artery and the SMA are seen in 85% of patients,[156] and large collateral vessels are usually seen.

Treatment is reserved for patients with intestinal angina, weight loss that is documented, and angiographic evidence of advanced atherosclerosis. As noted in one study, treatment has evolved from simple thromboendarterectomy, or reimplantation of the SMA, to the current choices of transaortic endarterectomy or bypass grafting.[160] The same study shows that excellent long-term results can be obtained by complete revascularization in these patients. Proponents of transaortic endarterectomy cite the high incidence of concomitant aortic atherosclerosis found at operation and the ease of doing simultaneous one- or two-vessel endarterectomy. Many surgeons favor aortomesenteric retrograde bypass grafting because SMA atherosclerosis usually originates 5 to 15 mm from the main arterial ostium. Polyethylene terephthalate fabric (Dacron) grafts are preferred to saphenous vein grafts because of their resistance to kinking and better clinical results.[1,156,159,160] If gastrointestinal spillage or contamination occurs during surgery, vein grafting is preferred. Intraoperative pressure gradients greater than 35 mm Hg across the stenosed vessel are usually found, and although single-vessel bypass (usually of the SMA) generally leads to a good result, many surgeons recommend bifurcated grafts to both the celiac artery and the SMA because of substantial recurrence rates with a single bypass graft.[90] Pain relief is obtained for 90% of patients, and more than 75% regain lost weight and have improvement of malabsorption.

MISCELLANEOUS DISORDERS OF THE INTESTINAL VASCULATURE

Several rare, interesting, and controversial disorders of the mesenteric circulation are discussed briefly.

Celiac Artery Compression Syndrome

Celiac artery compression syndrome, also called *median arcuate ligament syndrome,* has been a controversial subject since its initial description in 1963 by Harjola.[161] It is briefly defined as compression of the celiac axis by either the median arcuate ligament of the diaphragm or fibrosed celiac ganglion tissue, leading to postprandial and often positional pain in the epigastrium, nausea, weight loss, and epigastric bruits. The histopathologic features suggest a chronic process of arterial compression, disordered and reduced blood flow, and significant intimal thickening in response to flow disturbances.[162] Women in younger age groups are more often affected than are men.[124] The variable anatomic positions of the celiac axis and median arcuate ligament may indeed lead to an anterior compression of the celiac axis, especially during expiration and various postural changes (Fig. 20-6). In median arcuate ligament syndrome, the lateral arteriogram shows eccentric compression of the celiac trunk along its superior border with caudal displacement, so that it lies adjacent to the SMA. In addition, 50% of patients with this problem have a celiac ganglion that interconnects around the axis with retroperitoneal fibrous and fatty tissue to form a thick and potentially compressing shield.[163] Both SMA and IMA systems normally provide excellent compensation for celiac arterial inflow decreases. In a series of 50 patients with symptoms undergoing arteriography, 24% were found to have at least a 50% stenosis of the celiac axis.[164] In addition, between 6% and 16% of healthy people have epigastric bruits indicating compromised flow through the celiac artery.[163] One large literature review of 330 patients with celiac artery compression syndrome documented postprandial abdominal pain and weight loss in only 30% and 50%, respectively.[163] In addition, alarming postoperative recurrence rates of 50% to 86%[124,165,166] have been reported after careful follow-up. The possibility of splanchnic nerve pain related to pulsatile compression of the celiac plexus by the celiac artery has been entertained as an explanation for this syndrome, with anecdotal reports of symptomatic relief after splanchnic ganglionectomy.[1,76]

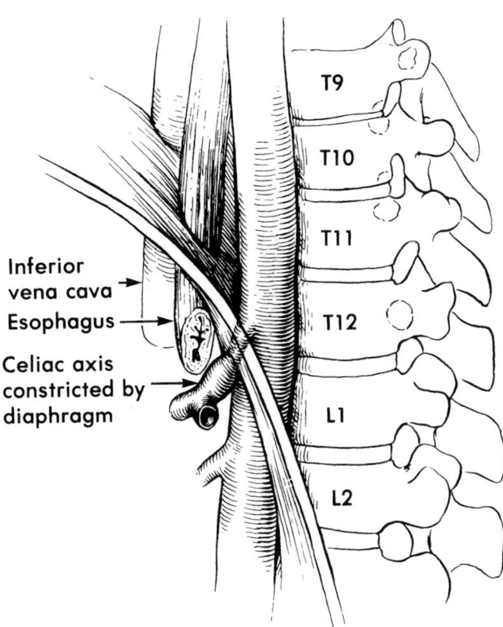

Fig. 20-6. Compression of celiac axis by median arcuate ligament of diaphragm. (From Stoney RJ, Lusby RJ. In Haimovici H, ed. Vascular Surgery Principles and Techniques, 2nd ed. East Norwalk, Conn.: Appleton-Century-Crofts, 1984.)

Despite debate concerning the origin of this entity and the significance of compromised flow through the celiac axis, median arcuate ligament and celiac plexus compression of the celiac artery do exist, and either or both may well be the cause of the syndrome in a few patients with otherwise negative results of evaluation.[118,167] Patients with postural, exercise, or respiratory components of their pain may do better after surgery. Surgical correction usually entails simple division of the constricting median arcuate ligament of the celiac ganglion. Bypass or vein patch angioplasty of the compressed segment is occasionally performed.[124,167] The documentation of this syndrome in monozygotic twins highlights the gross anatomic basis of the disorder and suggests a possible congenital mechanism.[162] It is clear that the debate regarding this entity's actual existence is far from over, and newer clinical studies of blood flow during attacks of pain may help resolve the problem and its clinical significance.

Vascular Compression of the Duodenum

Vascular compression of the duodenum is known by several names: *Wilkie's syndrome, SMA syndrome,* and *arteriomesenteric duodenal compression.* The procedure was well delineated by Wilkie[168] in a series of 75 patients in 1927. The symptoms of postprandial distention and vomiting with associated weight loss are caused by duodenal compression between the SMA or one of its branches and the aorta and vertebral bodies. Probably because of the attainment of an erect posture in humans, the SMA leaves the aorta at an acute angle through which pass the third and fourth portions of the duodenum[169] (Fig. 20-7).

Most affected patients are young (younger than 40 years), and 60% are female. Many claim that lying on the left side or in the knee-chest position alleviates the pain. Common associated conditions are prolonged bed rest, body cast, scoliosis, acute weight loss, and anorexia nervosa.[169-171] No affected patient has been described as obese. Diagnosis is based on classic symptomatology and cineradiography. Cineradiography reveals the classic to-and-fro churning of the duodenal contents proximal to the crossing of the SMA, with barium cascade over the incomplete obstruction.[169] Associated peptic ulcers are seen in 15% of patients.

Treatment is usually simple division of the ligament of Treitz. Occasionally, duodenojejunostomy is required in chronic cases. Weight gains have been reported to cure the condition in anorexic patients. Removal of body casts and mobilization, if feasible, should be attempted initially in appropriate patients before initiation of surgical intervention.

Visceral Artery Aneurysms

Aneurysms of the splanchnic arteries is a rare clinical entity. Most such aneurysms are asymptomatic and remain so until they rupture. Symptoms are related to clinical signs of acute blood loss. Features of rupture may include back or testicular pain when rupture is confined retroperitoneally. When in the peritoneal cavity, abdominal distention, spasm, and severe pain are typically present. Massive gastrointestinal bleeding may be present if there is rupture into the adjacent stomach or pancreatic duct. Among the visceral artery aneurysms, splenic arterial involvement is most common, accounting for 41% to 60%.[172] The overall incidence on autopsy is 0.78%, but these aneurysms are seen in 10% of geriatric patients and 7.1% of patients with portal hypertension. They are believed to evolve from arteriosclerosis, medial degeneration, or disorders of connective tissues, or by mycotic embolization.[173-175] Splenic artery aneurysm is the third most common intra-abdominal aneurysm, exceeded in incidence only by aneurysms of the infrarenal aorta and iliac vessels. Normally diagnosed in the sixth decade of life, these aneurysms are four times more common in women. Because pregnancy accentuates splenic blood flow, it is thought to be an etiologic factor. Hypertension is also believed to be of etiologic significance. Interestingly, 88% of female patients with this disease have had one or more pregnancies; 45% have had more than six.[124,172,176] Most patients are free of symptoms, and diagnosis is incidental by ultrasonography or the presence of curvilinear, ringlike (eggshell) calcifications in the left upper quadrant on plain abdominal radiographs. The development of referable symptoms implies impending rupture, with an associated mortality rate of 25%. Rupture during pregnancy, usually occurring in the third trimester, carries a mortality rate of 68%.[124] The ability of the lesser sac to contain splenic arterial rupture accounts for the better survival rate among nonpregnant patients.

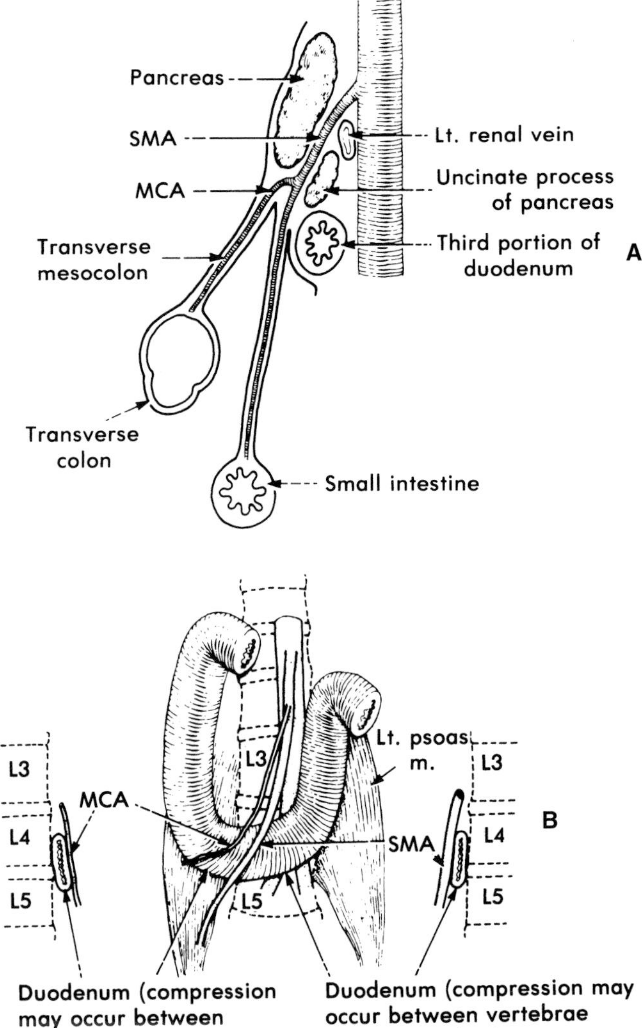

Fig. 20-7. Vascular compression of the duodenum by the superior mesenteric vessels. **A,** Diagrammatic sagittal section through the neck of the pancreas showing the relation of the third portion of the duodenum to the superior mesenteric artery *(SMA),* the middle colic artery *(MCA),* the aorta, and the mesentery. **B,** Anterior view of the duodenum, SMA, MCA, and the vertebral column. (From Akin JT, Gray SW, Skandalakis JE. Surgery 79:515, 1976.)

Most splenic artery aneurysms are atherosclerotic in origin, and associated vascular disease is common in these patients. Two thirds of splenic artery aneurysms are located in the main splenic artery before its arborization, and 40% are multiple.[172] Size ranges from 0.6 to 3 cm, although most are smaller than 2 cm.[172] The definitive study for the diagnosis of splanchnic artery aneurysms is selective mesenteric angiography, both before and after rupture if the clinical scenario allows. Elective surgery, usually entailing proximal and distal ligation of the aneurysm with obliteration of all feeding vessels to avoid splenectomy, is recommended for all patients with symptoms and for women of childbearing age without symptoms. Pregnant women should undergo elective excision, which has an operative mortality rate of less than 1%.[124,172] Asymptomatic aneurysms smaller than 2 to 3 cm in the elderly or high-risk patient should be watched. If rupture is detected, it usually necessitates a splenectomy to facilitate exposure for the ligation of the ruptured artery.

Hepatic artery aneurysms account for 16% to 20% of visceral artery aneurysms. Arteriosclerosis is the usual cause. Approximately three fourths are extrahepatic and 10% are mycotic.[172] The most common symptom is rupture, which occurs in 44% of patients[124,176]; right upper quadrant pain simulating cholelithiasis is also common. Complete visceral angiography is necessary to elucidate the intrahepatic aneurysm, which may require hepatic resection for cure. Rupture is usually equally divided between free intraperitoneal bleeding or intrabiliary hemorrhage, with resultant hemobilia and hematemesis. Because the risk for rupture is high, surgery is recommended for all hepatic artery aneurysms. Excision and bypass grafting, usually with autogenous vein graft, is the favored procedure. In the case of a ruptured hepatic artery aneurysm, an attempt should be made to reconstruct with autogenous vein graft, although most cases can be safely treated with ligation.

Celiac axis aneurysms account for only 3% of visceral artery aneurysms. Again, most are caused by arteriosclerosis, but a large number result from disorders of connective tissue and mycotic embolization. Most are asymptomatic, but because of their 80% rupture-associated mortality rate surgery is recommended if they are discovered.[124,176] Aneurysms of the celiac artery can usually be treated by excision without reconstruction. Rupture of a celiac artery aneurysm can be treated safely by ligation with or without bowel resection, depending on whether blood flow to the intestine has been compromised.

Pancreaticoduodenal artery aneurysms are rare, with only 34 cases reported in the literature.[177] Difficult exposure and identification at the time of surgery are the main problems in elective repair. Because 50% of these aneurysms ultimately rupture (generally into the peritoneal cavity) if left untreated, with an accompanying high mortality rate, surgical excision is the treatment of choice when they are diagnosed.

Intestinal Buerger's Disease

Fewer than a dozen verified cases of intestinal Buerger's disease, also known as *thromboangiitis obliterans,* have been reported since Buerger[178] first described this disorder of the peripheral vascular tree in 1908. Most cases involve the small intestine,[179] although the disease has been reported to occur in the sigmoid colon. A 40% mortality rate is reported. Peripheral ischemic problems are generally absent or minimal in these patients, implying a selective involvement of the mesenteric vessels. Buerger's disease more frequently involves smaller branches of the celiac and mesenteric arteries than the main stem branches.[180] Chronic or intermittent gastrointestinal problems, usually partial intestinal obstruction, are common in these patients and often are associated with weight loss. At the time of initial laparotomy, 40% of reported cases had an intestinal perforation without any typical clinical picture to indicate its likelihood. The need for careful observation of these patients, especially those with abdominal problems, and the realization that mesenteric disease acts independently of peripheral disease should be noted by the surgeon. Although it is suspected that cessation of smoking would alleviate the symptoms in these patients, clinical data supporting this assumption are lacking at present.

SUMMARY

The sophisticated array of intestinal functions relies on an intact vascular supply. In addition to the patency of a normal vascular tree, interdependent intrinsic and extrinsic regulatory mechanisms exist to effectively distribute 10% to 15% of total cardiac output to the gut. Intrinsic mechanisms include both myogenic and metabolic regulatory systems. Extrinsic controls include the generous but poorly understood parasympathetic and sympathetic nerve supply and numerous hormonal and neurohumoral influences.

Vascular disorders of the intestine are significant for the diagnostic challenge that they present, and for the substantial morbidity and mortality that they cause. For the operative clinician, a review of the clinical and experimental methods of determining intestinal viability supports intravenous fluorescein and experienced clinical judgment as the best intraoperative discriminators. Many vascular disorders feature similar symptoms, but careful attention to appropriate diagnosis leads to the best-directed therapy. When we better understand the pathophysiologic mechanisms that underly intestinal ischemia and its sequelae, new means of prevention and treatment will be developed in an attempt to reduce the high morbidity and mortality associated with each of these pathologic intestinal circulatory disorders.

REFERENCES

1. Siva WE. Intestinal vascular disease. In Cutler BS, et al., eds. Manual of Clinical Problems in Surgery. Boston: Little, Brown, 1984.
2. Spjut HJ, Margulis AR, McAlister WH. Microangiographic study of gastrointestinal lesions. Am J Roentgenol 92:1173, 1964.
3. Granger DN, et al. Intestinal blood flow. Gastroenterology 78:837, 1980.
4. Lanciault G, Jacobson ED. The gastrointestinal circulation. Gastroenterology 71:851, 1976.
5. Johnson PC. Myogenic nature of increase in intestinal vascular resistance with venous pressure elevation. Circ Res 6:992, 1959.
6. Folkow B. Regional adjustments of intestinal blood flow. Gastroenterology 52:423, 1967.
7. Granger DN, Kvietys PR. The splanchnic circulation: Intrinsic regulation. Annu Rev Physiol 43:409, 1981.

8. Iwata F, et al. Role of EDRF in splanchnic blood flow of normal and chronic portal hypertensive rats. Am J Physiol 260:H1299, 1991.
9. Pique JM, Whittle BJR, Esplugues JV. The vasodilator role of endogenous nitric oxide in the rat gastric microcirculation. Eur J Pharmacol 174:293, 1989.
10. Kitagawa H, Takeda F, Kohei H. Endothelium-dependent increases in rat gastric mucosal hemodynamics induced by acetylcholine and vagal stimulation. Eur J Pharmacol 133:57, 1987.
11. Thomas GR, et al. The effects of endothelium-dependent vasodilators on cadiac output and their distribution in the anaesthetized rate: A comparison with sodium nitroprusside. Br J Pharmacol 95:986, 1988.
12. Walder CE, Thiemermann C, Vane JR. Endothelium-derived relaxing factor participates in the increased blood flow in response to pentagastrin in the rat stomach mucosa. Proc Soc Lond (Biol) 241:195, 1990.
13. Pique JM, Esplugues JV, Whittle BJR. Endogenous nitric oxide as a mediator of gastric mucosal vasodilatation during acid secretion. Gastroenterology 102:168, 1992.
14. Kubes P. Ischemia-reperfusion in feline small intestine: A role for nitric oxide. Am J Physiol 264(1 Pt 1):G143, 1993.
15. Kanner J, Harel S, Granit R. Nitric oxide as an antioxidant. Arch Biochem Biophys 289:130, 1991.
16. Kubes P, Suzuki M, Granger DN. Nitric oxide: An endogenous modulator of leukocyte adhesion. Proc Natl Acad Sci USA 88:4651, 1991.
17. Pawlik WW, et al. Microcirculatory and motor effects of endogenous nitric oxide in the rat gut. J Physiol Pharmacol 44:139, 1993.
18. Stark ME, Szurszewski JH. Role of nitric oxide in gastrointestinal and hepatic function and disease. Gastroenterology 103:1928, 1992.
19. Guslandi M. Nitric oxide: An ubiquitous actor in the gastrointestinal tract. Dig Dis 1291:28, 1994.
20. Bulkley GB, Haglund UH, Morris JB. Mesenteric blood flow and the pathophysiology of mesenteric ischemia. In Bergan JJ, Yao ST, eds. Vascular Surgical Emergencies. Orlando, Fla.: Grune & Stratton, 1987, p 25.
21. Norris CP, et al. Autoregulation of superior mesenteric flow in fasted and fed dogs. Am J Physiol 237:H174, 1979.
22. Bailey RW, et al. Protection of the small intestine from nonocclusive mesenteric ischemic injury due to cardiogenic shock. Am J Surg 153:108, 1987.
23. Gershon MD, Erde SM. The nervous system of the gut. Gastroenterology 80:1571, 1980.
24. Rothe CF. Reflex control of veins and vascular capacitance. Physiol Rev 63:1281, 1983.
25. Jacob H, et al. Beta adrenergic blockade and the gastrointestinal system. Am J Med 74:1042, 1983.
26. Boatman DL, Brody MJ. Effects of acetylcholine on the intestinal vasculature of the dog. J Pharmacol Exp Ther 7:185, 1963.
27. Said SI. Vasoactive peptides: State of the art review. Hypertension 5(Suppl 1):17, 1983.
28. Zinner MJ, et al. The hemodynamic effects of intravenous infusions of serotonin in conscious dogs. J Surg Res 34:171, 1983.
29. Yeo CJ, Jaffe BM, Zinner MJ. Local regulation of blood flow in the feline jejunum. A possible role for edoluminally released substance P. J Clin Invest 70:1329, 1982.
30. Gallavan RH, Jacobson ED. Minireview: Prostaglandins and the splanchnic circulation. Proc Soc Exp Biol Med 20:391, 1982.
31. Parks DA, Granger DN. Contributions of ischemia and reperfusion to mucosal lesion formation. Am J Physiol 250:G749, 1986.
32. Perry MA, Wadhwa SS. Gradual reintroduction of oxygen reduces reperfusion injury in cat stomach. Am J Physiol 254:G366, 1988.
33. Schoenberg MH, et al. Studies on the oxygen radical mechanism involved in the small intestinal reperfusion damage. Acta Physiol Scand 124:581, 1985.
34. Younes M, et al. Inhibition of lipid peroxidation by superoxide dismutase following regional intestinal ischemia and reperfusion. Res Exp Med 187:9, 1987.
35. Granger DN. Role of xanthine oxidase and granulocytes in ischemia-reperfusion injury. Am J Physiol 255:H1269, 1988.
36. Parks DA, Granger DN. Ischemia-induced vascular changes: Role of xanthine oxidase and hydroxyl radicals. Am J Physiol 245:G285, 1983.
37. Granger DN, et al. Xanthine oxidase inhibitors attenuate ischemia-induced vascular permeability changes in the cat intestine. Gastroenterology 90:80, 1986.
38. Morris JB, et al. The direct, real-time demonstration of oxygen free radical generation of reperfusion following ischemia in rat small intestine. Gastroenterology 92:1541, 1987.
39. Zimmerman BJ, Grisham MB, Granger DN. Role of oxidants in ischemia/reperfusion-induced granulocyte infiltration. Am J Physiol 258:G185, 1990.
40. Achoenberg MH, et al. Posthypotensive generation of superoxide free radicals: Possible role in the pathogenesis of the intestinal mucosal damage. Acta Chir Scand 150:301, 1984.
41. Zimmerman BJ, Granger DN. Reperfusion-induced leukocyte infiltration: Role of elastase. Am J Physiol 259:H390, 1990.
42. Schoenberg MH, Beger HG. Reperfusion injury after intestinal ischemia. Crit Care Med 21:1376, 1993.
43. Lamar W, Woodward L, Statland B. Clinical implications of creatine kinase BB isoenzyme [letter]. N Engl J Med 299:234, 1978.
44. Graeber G, et al. Elevations of serum creatine phosphokinase in experimental mesenteric infarction. Surg Forum 31:148, 1980.
45. Graeber G, et al. Changes in serum total creatine phosphokinase (CPK) and its isoenzymes caused by experimental ligation of the superior mesenteric artery. Am J Surg 193:499, 1981.
46. Doran G. Appearance of creatinine kinase BB isoenzyme in the serum of a patient suffering from infarction of the colon. Clin Chim Acta 92:415, 1979.
47. DeToma G, et al. Enzymatic and metabolic changes in the peripheral serum after superior mesenteric artery ligation in dogs. Ital J Surg Sci 13:269, 1983.
48. Wollin A, Navert H, Bounous G. Effect of intestinal ischemia on diamine oxidase activity in rat intestinal tissue and blood. Gastroenterology 80:349, 1981.
49. Lobe T, et al. Hexosaminidase: A marker for intestinal gangrene in necrotizing enterocolitis. J Pediatr Surg 18:449, 1983.
50. Polson H, Mowat C, Himal H. Experimental and clinical studies of mesenteric infarction. Surg Gynecol Obstet 153:360, 1081.
51. Marks W, et al. Circulation concentrations of porcine ileal peptide but not hexosaminidase are elevated following 1 hour of mesenteric ischemia. J Surg Res 45:134, 1988.
52. Jamieson W, et al. The early diagnosis of massive acute intestinal ischemia. Br J Surg 69:S52, 1982.
53. May L, Berenson M. Value of serum inorganic phosphate in the diagnosis of ischemic bowel disease. Am J Surg 146:266, 1983.
54. Jenson C, Smith G. A clinical study of 51 cases of mesenteric infarction. Surgery 40:930, 1956.
55. Ottinger L, Austen G. A study of 136 patients with mesenteric infarction. Surg Gynecol Obstet 124:251, 1967.
56. Brooks D, Carey L. Base deficit in superior mesenteric artery occlusion: An aid to early diagnosis. Ann Surg 177:352, 1973.
57. Kosloske A, Goldthorn J. Paracentesis as an aid to the diagnosis of intestinal gangrene: Experience in 50 infants and children. Arch Surg 117:571, 1982.
58. Montgomery A, et al. Intramucosal pH measurement with tonometers for detecting gastrointestinal ischemia in porcine hemorrhagic shock. Circ Shock 29:319, 1989.
59. Poole J, Sammartano R, Boley S. The use of tonometry in the early diagnosis of mesenteric ischemia. Curr Surg 44:21, 1987.
60. Maynard N, et al. Assessment of splanchnic oxygenation by gastric tonometry in patients with acute circulatory failure. JAMA 270:1203, 1993.

61. Liebman PR, et al. Hepatic-portal venous gas in adults: Etiology, pathophysiology and clinical significance. Ann Surg 187:281, 1978.
62. Lida M, Matsui T, Fuchigami T. Ischemic colitis: Serial changes in double contrast barium enema examinations. Radiology 159:337, 1986.
63. Wittenberg J, et al. Ischemic colitis: Radiology and pathophysiology. AJR Am J Roentgenol 123:287, 1975.
64. Joffe N, Goldman H, Antonioli DA. Barium studies in small bowel infarction. Radiology 123:303, 1977.
65. Jones B, Fishman EK, Siegelman SS. Ischemic colitis demonstrated by computed tomography. J Comput Assist Tomogr 6:1120, 1982.
66. Smerud MJ, Johnson CD, Stephens DH. Diagnosis of bowel infarction: A comparison of plain films and CT scan in 23 cases. AJR Am J Roentgenol 154:99, 1990.
67. Hricak H, et al. Abdominal venous system: Assessment using MR. Radiology 156:415, 1985.
68. Boley SJ, Brandt LJ, Veith FJ. Ischemic disorders of the intestines. Curr Probl Surg 15:1, 1978.
69. Clark RA, Gallant TE. Acute mesenteric ischemia: Angiographic spectrum. AJR Am J Roentgenol 142:555, 1984.
70. Borden EB, Boley SJ. Early diagnosis of acute mesenteric ischemia. J Crit Illn 1:17, 1986.
71. Boley SJ, et al. Initial results from an aggressive roentgenological and surgical approach to acute mesenteric ischemia. Surgery 82:848, 1977.
72. Harward TRS, et al. Mesenteric venous thrombosis. J Vasc Surg 9:328, 1989.
73. Flickinger EG, et al. Local streptokinase infusion for superior mesenteric artery thromboembolism. Am J Radiol 140:771, 1983.
74. Pillari G, et al. Low-dose streptokinase in the treatment of celiac and superior mesenteric artery occlusion. Arch Surg 118:1340, 1983.
75. VanDeinse WH, Zawacki JK, Phillips D. Treatment of acute mesenteric ischemia by percutaneous transluminal angioplasty. Gastroenterology 91:475, 1986.
76. Williams LF. Vascular insufficiency of the intestines. Gastroenterology 61:757, 1971.
77. Gharagozloo F, et al. The use of intraperitoneal xenon for early diagnosis of acute mesenteric ischemia. Surgery 95:404, 1984.
78. Barth K, et al. Early imaging of experimental intestinal infarction with $_{99m}$Tc-pyrophosphate. Radiology 133:459, 1979.
79. Bulkley GB, et al. The use of intraperitoneal xenon 133 for imaging of intestinal strangulation in small bowel obstruction. Am J Surg 141:128, 1981.
80. Gharagozloo F, et al. Intraperitoneal xenon for the detection of early intestinal ischemia: Effects of ascites, adhesions, and misdirected injections. J Surg Res 34:581, 1983.
81. Mortensen PE, et al. Mucosal/submucosal blood flow in the gut wall determined by local washout of ^{133}xenon. Acta Physiol Scand 143(Suppl 603):75, 1991.
82. Granger DN, Kvietys PR. Recent advances in measurement of gastrointestinal blood flow. Gastroenterology 88:1073, 1985.
83. Oster Z, Som P, Zamora P. Mesenteric vascular occlusion: A new diagnostic method using a radiolabelled monoclonal antibody reactive with platelets. Radiology 171:653, 1989.
84. Kleinhaus S, Sammartano R, Boley S. Effects of laparoscopy on mesenteric blood flow. Arch Surg 113:867, 1978.
85. Kam DM, Scheeres DE. Fluorescein-assisted laparoscopy in the identification of arterial mesenteric ischemia. Surg Endosc 7:75, 1993.
86. Leung F, et al. Reflectance spectrophotometry for the assessment of astroduodenal mucosal perfusion. Am J Physiol 252:G797, 1987.
87. Ersek RA. Mesenteric transillumination for vascular 641- visualization. Surg Gynecol Obstet 152:339, 1981.
88. Perler BA, Zuidema GD. Mesenteric vascular occlusive disease. In Cameron JL, ed. Current Surgical Therapy 1984–1985. St. Louis: Mosby, 1984.
89. O'Donnell JA, Hobson RW. Operative confirmation of Doppler ultrasound in evaluation of intestinal viability. Surgery 83:705, 1978.
90. Wright GB, Hobson RW. Prediction of intestinal viability using Doppler ultrasound techniques. Am J Surg 129:642, 1975.
91. Shah SD, Andersen CA. Prediction of small bowel viability using Doppler ultrasound. Ann Surg 194:97, 1981.
92. Pearse WH, et al. The use of infrared photoplethysmography in identifying early intestinal ischaemia. Arch Surg 122:308, 1987.
93. O'Donnell JA, Hobson RW II. Operative confirmation of Doppler ultrasound in evaluation of mesenteric ischemia. Surgery 87:109, 1980.
94. Cooperman M, et al. Determination of viability of ischemic intestine by doppler ultrasound. Surgery 83:705, 1978.
95. Cooperman M, Martin EW, Carey LC. Evaluation of ischemic intestine by Doppler ultrasound. Am J Surg 139:73, 1980.
96. Ahn H, et al. Evaluation of laser Doppler flowmetry in the assessment of intestinal blood flow in the cat. Gastroenterology 88:951, 1985.
97. Mann A, Fazio VW, Lucas FV. A comparative study of the use of fluorescein and the Doppler device in the determination of intestinal viability. Surg Gynecol Obstet 154:53, 1982.
98. La Piana FG, Penner R. Anaphylactoid reaction to intravenously administered fluorescein. Arch Ophthalmol 79:161, 1968.
99. Marguggi RA, Greenspan M. Reliable intraoperative prediction of intestinal viability using a fluorescent indicator. Surg Gynecol Obstet 152:33, 1981.
100. Paes E, et al. Mesenteric infarct: New aspects of diagnosis and therapy. Chirurgie 59:828, 1988.
101. Gorey TF. Prediction of intestinal recovery after ischaemic injury due to arterial, venous and mixed arterial and venous occlusions. J R Soc Med 73:631, 1980.
102. Bulkley GB, et al. Intraoperative determination of small intestinal viability following ischemic injury. Ann Surg 193:628, 1981.
103. Mann A, Fazio VM, Lucas FV. A comparative study of the use of fluorescein and the Doppler device in the determination of intestinal viability. Surg Gynecol Obstet.
104. Dineen P, Goulian D, McSherry CK. A method of demonstrating intestinal viability. Am J Gastroenterol 45:335, 1966.
105. Myers MB, Cherry G. Use of vital dyes in the evaluation of the blood supply of the colon. Surg Gynecol Obstet 149:97, 1969.
106. Papachristou D, Fortner JF. Prediction of intestinal viability by intraarterial dye injection: A simple test. Am J Surg 132:572, 1976.
107. Ballard JL, et al. A critical analysis of adjuvant techniques used to assess bowel viability in acute mesenteric ischemia. Am Surg 59:309, 1993.
108. Myers MB, Cherry G, Gesser J. Relationship between surface pH and P_{CO_2} and the vascularity and viability of the intestine. Surg Gynecol Obstet 134:787, 1972.
109. Katz S, et al. New parameters of viability in ischemic bowel disease. Am J Surg 127:136, 1974.
110. Locke R, Hauser CJ, Shoemaker WC. The use of surface oximetry to assess bowel viability. Arch Surg 119:1252 1984.
111. De Nobile J, Guzzetta P, Patterson K. Pulse oximetry as a means of assessing bowel viability. J Surg Res 48:21, 1990.
112. Khin J, Daniel EE. The effects of ischemia on intestinal nerves and electrical slow waves. Am J Dig Dis 15:59, 1970.
113. Guisan YJ, Hreno A, Gurd FN. Effect of acute ischaemia on the motility of the small bowel in the awake dog. Eur Surg Res 7:32, 1975.
114. Chou CC. Relationship between intestinal blood flow and motility. Annu Rev Physiol 44:29, 1982.
115. Cabot RM, Kohatsu S. The effects of ischaemia on the electrical and contractile activities of the canine small intestine. Am J Surg 136:242, 1978.
116. Brolin RE, et al. Quantitative myoelectric determination of bowel viability. J Surg Res 41:557, 1986.

117. Brolin RE, et al. Comparison of five methods of assessment of intestinal viability. Surg Gynecol Obstet 168:6, 1989.
118. Hildebrand HD, Zierler RE. Mesenteric vascular disease. Am J Surg 139:188, 1980.
119. Bergan JJ, et al. Revascularization in treatment of mesenteric infarction. Ann Surg 187:430, 1975.
120. Boley SJ, Feinstein FR, Sammartano R. New concepts in the management of emboli of the superior mesenteric artery. Surg Gynecol Obstet 153:561, 1981.
121. Crawford ES, et al. Celiac axis, superior mesenteric artery, and inferior mesenteric arterial occlusion: Surgical considerations. Surgery 82:856, 1977.
122. Wells CL. Relationship between intestinal microecology and the translocation of bacteria. Antonie van Leeuwenhoek 58:87, 1990.
123. Kaufman SL, Harrington DP, Siegelman SS. Superior mesenteric artery embolization: An angiographic emergency. Radiology 124:625, 1979.
124. Rogers DM, et al. Mesenteric vascular problems: A 26 year experience. Ann Surg 195:554, 1982.
125. Boley SJ, et al. Persistent vasoconstriction: A major factor in nonocclusive mesenteric ischemia. Curr Top Surg Res 3:425, 1971.
126. Ottinger LW. The surgical management of acute occlusion of the superior mesenteric artery. Ann Surg 188:721, 1978.
127. Kwann JHM, Connolly JE. Prevention of intestinal infarction resulting from mesenteric arterial occlusive disease. Surg Gynecol Obstet 157:321, 1983.
128. Stoney RJ, Cunningham CG. Acute mesenteric ischemia. Surgery 114:489, 1993.
129. Rob C. Surgical diseases of the celiac and mesenteric arteries. Arch Surg 93:21, 1966.
130. Shaw RS, Rutledge RH. Superior mesenteric artery embolectomy in the treatment of massive mesenteric infarction. N Engl J Med 267:595, 1957.
131. Becker GH, Katzen BT, Dake MD. Noncoronary angioplasty. Radiology 170:921, 1989.
132. Johnson WC, Nasbeth DC. Visceral infarction following aortic surgery. Ann Surg 180:312, 1974.
133. Al Karawi MA, et al. Mesenteric vein thrombosis: Non-invasive diagnosis and follow-up (US + MRI) and non-invasive therapy by streptokinase and anticoagulants. Hepatogastroenterology 37:507, 1990.
134. Brewster DC, et al. Intestinal ischemia complicating abdominal aortic surgery. Surgery 109:447, 1991.
135. Redaelli CA, et al. Intestinal ischemia following replacement of the infrarenal aorta and aorto-iliac bifucation. Helv Chir Acta 58:589, 1992.
136. Siddharth P, Smith NL. An anatomic basis to prevent ischemia of the colon during operations upon the aorta. Surg Gynecol Obstet 153:71, 1981.
137. Kim MW, et al. Ischemic colitis after aortic aneurysmectomy. Am J Surg 145:392, 1983.
138. Kountz SL, Taub DR, Connolly JE. Aortoiliac steal syndrome. Arch Surg 92:490, 1966.
139. Ernst CB, et al. Inferior mesenteric artery stump pressure. Ann Surg 187:1, 1978.
140. Elliot JW. The operative relief of gangrene of the intestine due to occlusion of the mesenteric vessels. Ann Surg 21:9, 1895.
141. Kaleya RN, Boley SJ. Mesenteric venous thrombosis. In Najarian JS, Delaney JP, eds. Progress in Gastrointestinal Surgery. Chicago: Year Book Medical, 1989, p 417.
142. Gertsch P, et al. Acute thrombosis of the splanchnic veins. Arch Surg 128:341, 1993.
143. Abdu RA, Zakhour BJ, Dallis DJ. Mesenteric venous thrombosis—1911 to 1984. Surgery 101:383, 1987.
144. Khodadadi J, et al. Mesenteric venous thrombosis: the importance of a second look operation. Arch Surg 115:315, 1980.
145. Sack J, Aldret JS. Primary mesenteric venous thrombosis. Surg Gynecol Obstet 154:205, 1982.
146. Naitove A, Weissmann R. Primary mesenteric venous thrombosis. Ann Surg 161:516, 1965.
147. Clark AZ, Gallant TE. Acute mesenteric ischemia: Angiographic spectrum. AJR Am J Roentgenol 142:555, 1984.
148. Kidambi H, Herbert R, Kidami AV. Ultrasonic demonstration of superior mesenteric and splenoportal venous thrombosis. J Clin Ultrasound 14:199, 1986.
149. Matos C, et al. Mesenteric venous thrombosis: Early CT and ultrasound diagnosis and conservative management. Gastrointest Radiol 11:322, 1986.
150. Harward TRS, et al. Mesenteric venous thrombosis. J Vasc Surg 9:328, 1989.
151. Verbanck JJ, et al. Partial splenoportal and superior vative management. Gastroenterology 86:949, 1984.
152. Bynum TE, Jacobson ED. Non-occlusive intestinal ischemia. Arch Intern Med 139:281, 1979.
153. Bailey RW, et al. Protection of the small intestine from nonocclusive mesenteric ischemia injury due to cardiogenic shock. Am J Surg 153:108, 1987.
154. Russ JE, et al. Surgical therapy of non-occlusive mesenteric infarction. Am J Surg 134:638, 1977.
155. Mikkelson WP. Intestinal angina: Its surgical significance. Am J Surg 94:262, 1957.
156. Stoney RJ, Meacham PW. Chronic intestinal ischemia caused by visceral atherosclerosis. In Cameron JL, ed. Current Surgical Therapy, 1984—1985. St. Louis: Mosby, 1984.
157. Gluecklich B, et al. Chronic mesenteric ischemia masquerading as cancer. Surg Gynecol Obstet 148:49, 1979.
158. Zelenock GB, et al. Splanchnic arterio-sclerotic disease and intestinal angina. Arch Surg 115:497, 1980.
159. Connolly JE, Dwaan JH. Management of chronic visceral ischemia. Surg Clin North Am 62:345, 1982.
160. Calderon M, et al. Long-term results of the surgical management of symptomatic chronic intestinal ischemia. J Cardiovasc Surg 33(61):723, 1992.
161. Harjola PT. A rare obstruction of the celiac axis. Ann Chir Gynaecol Fenn 52:547 1963.
162. Bech F, et al. Median arcuate ligament compression syndrome in monozygotic twins. J Vasc Surg 19:934, 1994.
163. Brandt LJ, Boley SJ. Celiac axis compression syndrome: A critical review. Dig Dis 23:633, 1978.
164. Levin DC, Baltaxe, HA. High incidence of celiac axis narrowing in asymptomatic individuals. Am J Roentgenol 46:426, 1972.
165. Evans WE. Long-term evaluation of the celiac band syndrome. Surgery 76:867, 1974.
166. Plate G, Eklof B, Vang J. The celiac compression syndrome: Myth or reality? Acta Chir Scand 147:201, 1981.
167. Stanley JC, Fry WJ. Median arcuate ligament syndrome. Arch Surg 103:252, 1971.
168. Wilkie DPD. Chronic duodenal ileus. Am J Med Sci 173:643, 1927.
169. Akin JT, Gray SW, Skandalakis JE. Vascular compression of the duodenum: Presentations of ten cases and review of the literature. Surgery 79:515, 1976.
170. Pentlow BD, Dent RG. Acute vascular compression of the duodenum in anorexia nervosa. Br J Surg 68:665, 1981.
171. Price P, Clark CG. Wilkie's syndrome. J R Coll Surg Edinb 24:280, 1979.
172. Trastek VF, et al. Splenic artery aneurysms. Surgery 91:694, 1982.
173. Graham JM, McCollum CH, Debakey ME. Aneurysms of the splanchnic arteries. Am J Surg 140:797, 1980.
174. McNamara MF, Griska LB. Superior mesenteric artery branch aneurysms. Surgery 88:625, 1980.
175. Stanley JC, Thompson NW, Fry WJ. Splanchnic artery aneurysms. Arch Surg 101:689, 1970.
176. Busuttil RW, Brin BT. The diagnosis and management of visceral artery aneurysms. Surgery 88:619, 1980.

177. Chiou AC, Josephs LG, Mensoian JO. Inferior pancreaticoduodenal artery aneurism: Report of a case and review of the literature. J Vasc Surg 17:784, 1993.
178. Buerger L. Thromboangiitis obliterans: A story of the vascular lesions leading to presenile spontaneous gangrene. Am J Med Sci 136:567, 1908.
179. Deitch EA, Sikkema WW. Intestinal manifestations of Buerger's disease. Am J Surg 47:326, 1981.
180. Broide E, et al. Buerger's disease presenting as acute small bowel ischemia. Gastroenterology 104:1192, 1993.

21

Inflammatory Disorders of the Small Bowel and Colon

Carlos Alvarez, John Sayles, and Barbara Lee Bass

INFLAMMATORY BOWEL DISEASE

The intestinal tract is the target of a number of inflammatory disorders that vary considerably in underlying pathogenesis, pattern of presentation, and degree of seriousness in terms of morbidity and potential mortality. Appendicitis, for example, is usually an acute process, has a typical clinical presentation, and is cured by appendectomy. Inflammatory bowel disease (IBD), on the other hand, has a variable clinical presentation, is often characterized by relapses and remissions, and responds in a varying fashion to surgical intervention. This chapter summarizes the more important inflammatory processes involving the small bowel and colon, emphasizing the underlying physiologic dysfunction associated with each and the means by which physiologic function may be restored to normal or significantly improved through surgical intervention.

Crohn's disease (CD) and ulcerative colitis (UC) are the two broad clinical patterns of idiopathic intestinal inflammation grouped under the term *IBD*. The two diseases share a common origin in the medical literature; the first reported case of UC included small bowel involvement more consistent with CD.[1] Confusion between these entities persists today at times because of their variable, overlapping manifestations and clinical courses, as well as the difficulty in defining their etiologies. It is becoming increasingly evident that despite the shared histologic and clinical picture of uninhibited inflammation, these two entities probably represent the convergence of a number of heterogeneous initiating and propagating events. Despite exponential increases during the past 20 years in our understanding of intestinal inflammation and the intestinal immune system, the nature of these events remains uncertain.[2]

Epidemiology and Genetics

Incidence and prevalence of IBD vary widely, being generally higher in northern climates and industrialized countries.[3] Prevalence estimates for UC range from 5 to 100 cases/100,000 population, whereas for CD the range is from 10 to 90 cases/100,000 population. There has been a small but steady increase in CD incidence in the last 25 years, whereas the incidence of UC, after rising through the 1930s to the 1960s, now seems to be holding stable. Furthermore, it appears that the distribution of UC is changing, with an increasing proportion of disease limited to the distal large intestine and associated with a more favorable prognosis.[4] Both CD and UC show a bimodal age distribution, with peaks occurring during the third and seventh decades of life. Familial associations for both UC and CD have long been recognized, appearing stronger with CD. Twin studies corroborate this relationship, with monozygotic twins showing greater concordance rates than dizygotic pairs. Familial prevalence is not a strong independent risk factor, however; only 15% of patients have a relative with a confirmed diagnosis of IBD. The pattern of expression in families is consistent with multilocal inheritance, in which environmental factors may play an important role. Studies looking at race or ethnicity have shown higher rates prevalent among whites and Ashkenazic Jews. After immigration, however, the differences among races and ethnic groups in one region are seen to equilibrate at the prevalence level associated with that particular locale, further supporting the importance of environmental factors.

Pathogenesis

Infection

Because of the clinical and pathologic similarities to severe, chronic dysentery (see box on p. 465), infectious agents have been suspected in IBD from the early reports. There are striking similarities in histologic appearance between CD and tuberculosis enteritis, as noted initially by Crohn et al.[5] There is also a frequent temporal relationship between the onset of IBD and antecedent enteric infection. Current interest is centered around *Mycobacterium paratuberculosis,* the organism responsible for bovine granulomatous enteritis, which has been identified by DNA

PATHOLOGIC FEATURES OF IBD

Ulcerative Colitis	Crohn's Disease
Contiguous involvement proximal to rectum	Focal distribution ("skip lesions")
Crypt abscesses	Submucosal lymphoid aggregates
Goblet cell mucin depletion	Aphthous ulcers
Mucosal delimitation	Transmural (submucosal) inflammation
Mucosal polymorphonuclear leukocyte infiltrate	Transmural macrophage infiltrate
Lamina propia lymphocyte infiltrate	Noncaseating granulomas
Mucosal ulcerations	Deep linear ulceration
Pseudopolyps	Mucosal cobblestones
Friable mucosa	Wall fibrosis
Serosal sparing	Mesenteric fat "wrapping"
Small bowel spared	Rectum spared
	Fistula formation
	Perianal disease

polymerase chain-reaction analysis in the inflamed CD mucosa.[6] An alternative hypothesis, prompted by detection of viral RNA and antigens in granuloma adjacent to CD intestinal blood vessels, suggests that chronic measles (paramyxovirus) infection induces a chronic mesenteric vasculitis that causes mucosal ischemia and injury.[7] Epidemiologic studies by the same group support the possible involvement of the measles virus, or perhaps its vaccine. These findings await confirmation by other investigators. In the past, enthusiastic initial reports associating pathogenic microbes with IBD have been subsequently contradicted by follow-up studies. Consistent isolation of a specific microbe has not been possible, and there is substantial epidemiologic evidence against an infectious process. Clinical experience also argues against infection, because IBD does not respond to antibiotic therapy (except in certain settings), whereas it does improve with immunosuppressive medications.

Although microbial infection may not play a significant role, intestinal microflora may nevertheless be a factor in IBD by providing a persistent antigenic stimulus or providing stimulatory degradation products to a susceptible immune system. Certain bacterial components have received particular attention because of their ability to activate the immune system: formylmethionyl-leucyl-phenylalanine, a DNA-repair protein, and the cell wall components of endotoxin (lipopolysaccharide and peptidoglycan-polysaccharide).[8] All are found in the systemic circulation of patients with IBD at levels commensurate with disease activity, and all can induce variable degrees of enterocolitis in experimental animals. Because these molecules are excluded or neutralized by the barrier defenses of the normal intestine, their detection in the systemic circulation argues strongly for the presence of more fundamental defects in intestinal permeability, the immune response, or both.

Host Defenses

The human gastrointestinal tract has adjusted remarkably to an environment in which it is required to distinguish nutritional from harmful foreign material to carry out its normal function. How the intestine is able to make this distinction is currently unclear, but a derangement in this capability may be a basic defect in IBD. The normal gastrointestinal tract actively protects against pathogens and antigens by attacking, ignoring, neutralizing, or excluding them by means of a variety of host defenses. The nonimmune segment of these defenses is composed of salivary amylase; gastric acid; pancreatic, gastric, and intestinal digestive enzymes; the mechanical barrier formed by the epithelium; and the mucin secreted by the mucosa. The mechanical barrier, formed by enterocytes and their intercellular tight junctions, was once thought impermeable but is now understood to be selectively permeable. Permeability to small molecules is increased in active IBD, and perhaps in quiescent and preclinical disease states. However, increased permeability has not been shown conclusively to predate inflammation and may simply represent a nonspecific phenomenon paralleling disease severity and mucosal damage.[9]

A number of immunologic abnormalities have been detected in IBD[10] (see box on p. 466). The number of deranged factors identified, the multiple effects ascribed to each, and the counterregulatory relationships that exist among them make isolating a single element as the causative factor in IBD a daunting task. Indeed, the vast number of irregularities identified to date are not unique to IBD but are somewhat predictable in the presence of ongoing inflammation. Nevertheless, a number of factors suggest a central role for the mucosal immune system in IBD pathophysiology. IBD is manifested primarily and most severely in the intestine, although extraintestinal inflammation, particularly involving the skin, eye, joints, liver, and bile ducts, is associated with both UC and CD. Similarly, although systemic anti-inflammatory agents are often employed in therapy, locally active, poorly absorbed luminal preparations are often effective. The daily antigenic challenge from food and microbes provides the mucosal immune system (or one of its components) ample opportunity to malfunction.

Lymphocytes found in the epithelium, the lamina propia and in Peyer's patches, as well as immunglobulin (Ig) A-secreting plasma cells, epithelial M cells, and enterocytes, make up the immune component of the intestinal host defenses. The early lesion of CD, the apthous ulcer, invariably arises over Peyer's patches. The epithelial M cells normally lie in this location, functioning as antigen-presenting cells for the lymphocytes under them. The location of the apthous ulcer raises the possibility that dysfunction of either the M cells or Peyer's patch lymphocytes, or al-

IMMUNOLOGIC ABNORMALITIES IN IBD

Factors Increased	Factors Decreased
Serum IgA_1	Dimeric, secretory IgA
Mucosal IgG, IgG:IgA ratio	T-cell response to IL-2
pANCA (UC)	Mucosal IL-2, IL-4, interferon-γ
Major histocompatibility complex class II antigen expression by enterocytes	Monocyte IL-4 responsiveness
Mucosal IL-1, IL-6, IL-8	Mucosal mucin (UC)
Serum IL-2, IL-6, IL-10	Mucosal CD4+ (helper) T cells
Soluble IL-2 receptor	Mucosa vasoactive intestinal peptide (UC)
Mucosal CD8+ (cytotoxic) T cells	Mucosal substance P (CD)
Tumor necrosis factor–α	
CD14+ macrophages	
CD44v3 and v6 colonocyte surface antigen (UC)	
Mucosal substance P (UC)	
LP T-cell response to IL-2	
LP T cells (CD)	
Mucosal PGE_2 and LTB_4	
Serum intercellular adhesion molecule–1	
Tropomyosin	
Mucosal permeability (CD)	
IL-2 receptor	
Transferrin receptor	
4F2 antigen	

tered communication between them, may be of importance in the pathophysiologic process. Enterocytes may also be involved in the altered immune response because they can produce some of the inflammatory mediators seen in elevated levels in IBD. In UC, enterocytes have been shown to inappropriately express class II major histocompatibility antigens that regulate T-cell activity.

Auto-antibodies against enterocytes, as well as cytotoxic lymphocytes, have been detected in IBD, particularly in UC. Recent attention has been focused on antibodies against the P40 antigen of colon epithelial cells, which may be related to tropomyosin, a cytoskeletal protein.[11] Another set of auto-antibodies is targeted against an undetermined perinuclear cytoplasmic antigen in neutrophils (pANCAs). In some reports, as many as 70% of patients with UC express pANCAs, and as a group they are more likely to have sclerosing cholangitis and ileoanal pouch inflammation (pouchitis) after colectomy. Because few of these auto-antibodies have been consistently shown to be cytotoxic, the concept that IBD is innately an autoimmune process has fallen into disfavor.[12] The critics propose a paradigm that considers the intestinal cell an "innocent bystander," damaged by an altered inflammatory response that is unable either to eradicate the agent responsible for initiation of the response or to downregulate itself once that stimulus has been eliminated.[13] Auto-antibodies are seen as a reflection of the hyperactive immune reaction, rather than the cause. Although these auto-antibodies may have no pathogenic role, they may be helpful in identifying subsets of patients with IBD, as noted for pANCAs.

Both B and T cells in the mucosa are activated, as evidenced by high levels of expression of activation cell surface markers such as interleukin (IL)–2 receptor, transferrin receptor, and 4F2 antigen. Ratios of T-cell population are also altered, with a decrease in suppressor (CD4+) T cells with respect to cytotoxic (CD8+) T cells in the inflamed mucosa. Proliferation and activity of lymphocytes are under the control of cytokines. Levels of proinflammatory cytokines (IL-1, IL-2, IL-6, IL-8, and tumor necrosis factor–α) are elevated in active IBD. Levels of downregulating cytokines (IL-4, IL-10 and interferon–γ are depressed. There is an increased ratio of IgG to IgA produced by mucosal B cells. Because IgA acts primarily in the lumen to neutralize and exclude antigen, whereas antigen binding with IgG triggers the complement cascade and activates immunocytes, this change favors ongoing inflammation. Levels of arachidonic acid metabolites are markedly elevated in diseased tissue, although the increase is balanced between proinflammatory leukotrienes (LTs, such as LTB_4) and anti-inflammatory prostaglandins PGs, such as PGE_2).

Dietary and Environmental Factors

Diet has been implicated as a possible etiologic factor because of its importance in determining the local environment of the gastrointestinal tract. The "Western" diet (or its deficiencies) is also implicated, because of the higher prevalence of IBD seen in industrialized countries and the increased incidence observed as new immigrant groups assimilate Western habits. No specific food item (including caffeine, cow's milk, eggs, refined sugars, and wheat, among the many suspected) has been proved responsible. Psychologic factors have also been shown to have no relationship. Of the many other environmental factors also proposed to play a role, only tobacco use has been proved significant. UC is a disease of nonsmokers, and incidence is inversely related to smoking. A number of studies have shown a link between onset of UC or recurrence and cessation of smoking. Conversely, patients with CD smoke at twice the rate of the population in general.[14]

Clinical Presentation

UC can often be differentiated from CD on the basis of the history and physical examination. UC is characterized by the acute onset of abdominal pain, diarrhea, hematochezia, and tenesmus. The severity of symptoms corresponds to the extent of the disease. The manifestations of CD may be protean because of the potential for diffuse

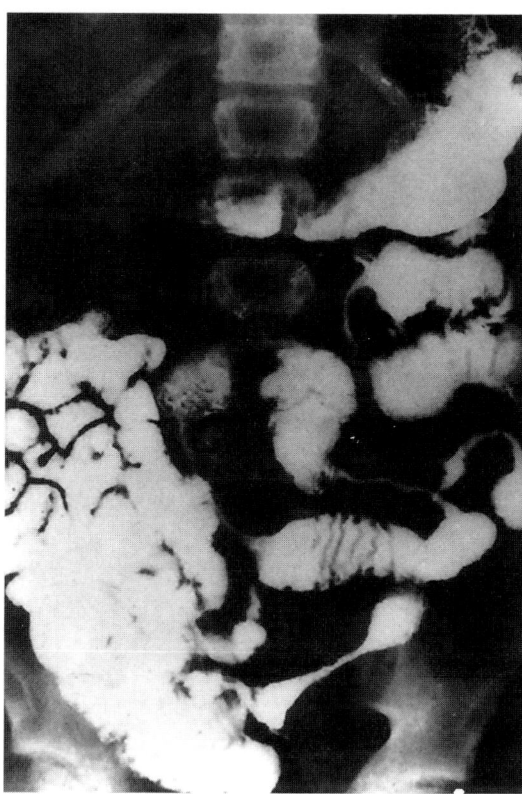

Fig. 21-1. Ulcerative colitis. Barium enema of a patient with panulcerative colitis revealing the cobblestone texture of the colonic mucosa and loss of haustral markings that give rise to the "lead pipe" appearance of the colon. (From Kirsner JB, Shorter RG. Inflammatory Bowel Disease, 4th ed. Baltimore: Williams & Wilkins, 1995.)

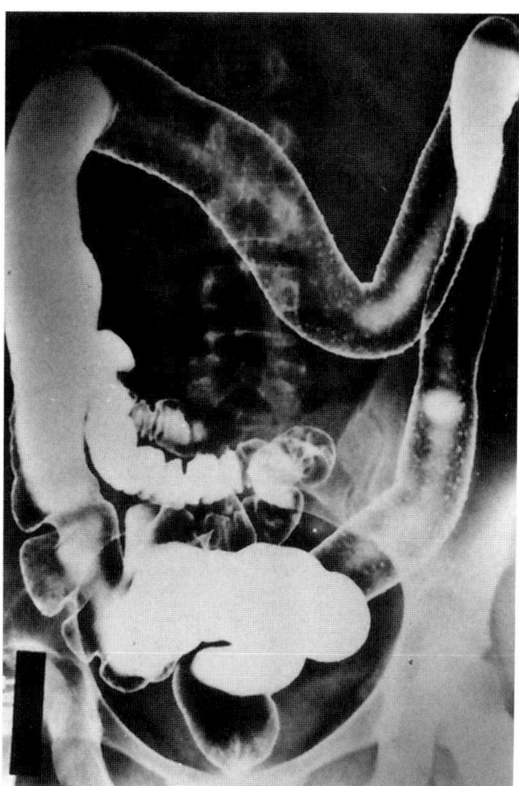

Fig. 21-2. Crohn's ileitis. Upper gastrointestinal and small bowel follow-through contrast study showing multiple long strictures distributed through many feet of small bowel, the characteristic pattern of skip lesions seen in this disease. Surgical management of skip lesions is dependent on their proximity and localization to a single region of the small bowel. Clusters of strictures are best managed by segmental resection, whereas diffuse skip-lesion strictures are optimally managed with stricturoplasty. (From Kirsner JB, Shorter RG. Inflammatory Bowel Disease, 4th ed. Baltimore: Williams & Wilkins, 1995.)

involvement of the entire gastrointestinal tract, and the disease typically presents in an insidious manner, often coming to medical attention only after a complication has developed. Chronic abdominal pain; nonbloody diarrhea; and such signs of systemic toxicity as fever, malaise, and cachexia are its cardinal features. As noted earlier, both types of IBD may be associated with extraintestinal manifestations, UC more commonly. The abdominal examination may be unremarkable in the patient with UC unless toxic megacolon is present. In CD, signs of obstruction or an inflammatory mass may be present in addition to perianal disease. Approximately 10% to 15% of patients, specifically those with severe colitis, have conditions that cannot be categorized at presentation as a specific form of IBD. Such "indeterminate" colitis eventually defines itself on long-term follow-up. Exclusion of infectious enteritis by a thorough travel and exposure history, as well as with stool and serologic studies, is of critical importance at initial diagnosis.

Other laboratory studies are not specific for IBD but may help identify correctable electrolyte or hematologic abnormalities. Acute-phase factors (C-reactive protein, sedimentation rate, etc.) are frequently monitored despite the lack of correlation with clinically or endoscopically determined disease severity. Monitoring of visceral protein levels (albumin, prealbumin, transferrin, etc.) in these chronically ill patients allows assessment of nutritional status. Colonoscopy can generally differentiate the two processes and rule out other causes of colitis, although examination and biopsy specimen interpretations are more accurate in the healing or quiescent stage. Once the diagnosis has been established, endoscopy should be employed cautiously, especially during flare-ups, when the risk of complication is high. Because the small bowel is less accessible to endoscopy, the diagnosis of CD there is dependent on small bowel radiographic contrast studies, which can best demonstrate mucosal lesions as well as delineate the number, location, and degree of stricturing and fistulization (Figs. 21-1 through 21-4). CT is reserved for cases in which abscess formation or advanced cancer is suspected.

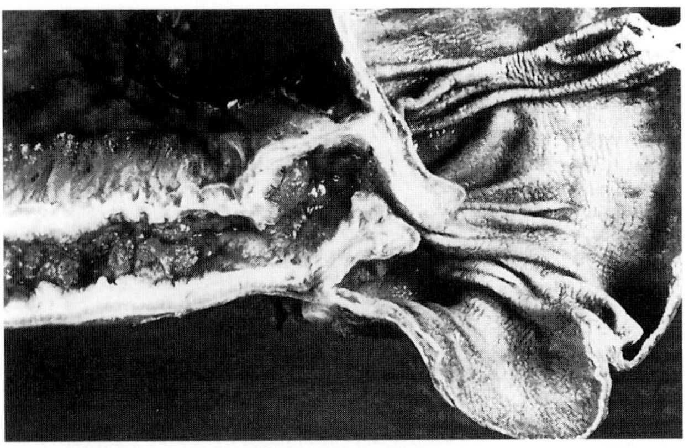

Fig. 21-3. Crohn's ileitis. Characteristic transmural inflammation of the terminal ileum with fibrosis of the intestinal wall. Note the abrupt cessation of the disease at the ileocecal valve and completely normal appearance of the cecal mucosa and wall. (From Corman ML. Colon and Rectal Surgery, 2nd ed. Philadelphia: JB Lippincott, 1989.)

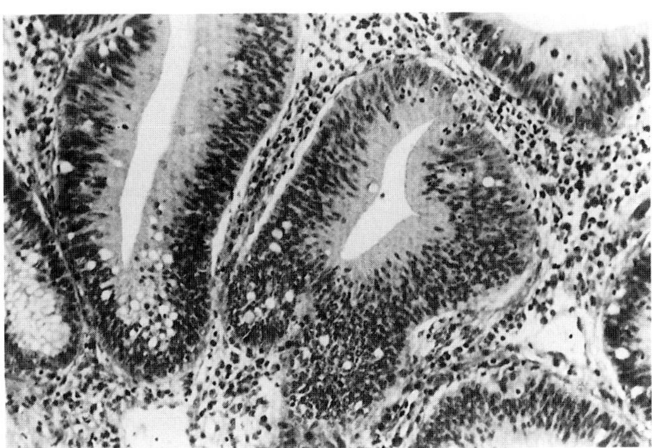

Fig. 21-4. Photomicrograph of biopsy specimen from a patient with ulcerative colitis. Moderate dysplasia with loss of polarity and proliferation of epithelial cells is noted. (Original magnification ×260. From Corman ML. Colon and Rectal Surgery, 3rd ed. Philadelphia: JB Lippincott, 1993.)

MEDICAL THERAPY FOR IBD

Crohn's Disease

Ileocolonic/Colonic Disease

Mild
- Sulfasalazine
- Metronidazole
- Mesalamine

Moderate to severe
- Prednisone

Severe
- Intravenous steroids

Small Bowel Disease

Mild
- Mesalamine
- Metronidazole

Moderate to severe
- Prednisone

Unresponsive to steroids
- Azathioprine/6-mercaptopurine

Fistula

Metronidazole
6-mercaptopurine/azathioprine/cyclosporine

Ulcerative Colitis

Colitis

Mild proctitis/left-sided colitis
- Oral sulfasalazine/mesalamine
- Topical mesalamine/steroids

Extensive mild to moderate colitis
- Oral sulfasalazine/mesalamine
- Topical agents for resistant proctitis

Moderate to severe colitis
- Prednisone

Severe colitis
- Intravenous steroids

Toxic Megacolon

Bowel rest
Frequent examinations
High-dose intravenous steroids
Intravenous broad-spectrum antibiotics

Maintenance Therapy

Oral sulfasalazine/mesalamine

Management

Medical Therapy

Anti-inflammatory therapy, beginning in the 1930s with sulfasalazine (SASP), has been the mainstay of medical management[15] (see accompanying box). The SASP molecule links 5-aminosalicyclic acid (5-ASA), responsible for the drug's therapeutic effects, with sulfapyridine, which was initially thought to act as an antibiotic but is now considered to serve essentially as a carrier. SASP's use is limited by allergic and dose-dependent side effects, attributed to the sulfa component, and by limited efficacy in severe UC and small intestinal CD. The exact mechanism of action is unknown, but the drug has been shown to inhibit a number of proinflammatory processes active in IBD, including release of IL-1 and other cytokines, mucosal antibody synthesis, arachidonic acid metabolism, and oxygen radical production. An intriguing recent report suggests that long-term SASP use may be protective against development of cancer.[16] Mesalamine, the unbound 5-ASA moiety, and olsalazine, a 5-ASA dimer, are newer, costlier formulations; they have fewer side effects than SASP but their efficacy is probably only equivalent.[17] Because patients are able to tolerate higher doses and bioavailability of 5-ASA is higher in the small bowel, mesalamine appears particularly well suited to management of small intestinal CD. Additionally, although there has been no demonstrated benefit of maintenance therapy with SASP after resection in CD, a number of recent trials have shown reduced recurrence with high-dose mesalamine.[18]

Moderate to severe exacerbations of IBD are treated with systemic glucocorticoids, which exert their therapeutic effects through nonspecific inhibition of inflammatory and immune function. Enema preparations can be used effectively as topical agents in distal UC. Until the advent of small intestine–active 5-ASA agents, symptomatic small bowel CD necessitated use of systemic steroids. There is no benefit to continued maintenance therapy with steroids after remission has been induced or after surgical resection. Steroid dependence warrants consideration of either alternative modes of therapy or surgical intervention because of the severe dose- and duration-related side effects associated with long-term steroid use.

The need for alternatives to glucocorticoids for severe disease has led to the use of immunosuppressant therapy for IBD, adapted from the organ transplantation experience. Two purine analogs, azathioprine and its metabolite 6-mercaptopurine, have been the most extensively and successfully used.[19] Their mechanism of action in IBD has not been determined, but it is likely that their specific inhibition of T cell and natural killer cell function and proliferation plays an important part. Their major benefit in IBD management has been their steroid-sparing effect and their ability to maintain remission. They have also been shown effective in the therapy of perianal and fistulous CD. One drawback is their delayed onset of activity, often requiring 3 to 6 months for improvement to become apparent. Neutropenia is the major dose-limiting side effect (or, some argue, the therapeutic goal). Close monitoring of the complete blood cell count is therefore essential. The increased incidence of malignancies, particularly lymphomas, associated with azathioprine use in the transplant population has not yet been noted in patients with IBD.

The folate inhibitor methotrexate has been used extensively in the treatment of rheumatoid diseases as an anti-inflammatory agent. The initial experience in IBD therapy with oral administration was disappointing, but controlled trials with parenteral dosing have since shown a steroid-sparing benefit. Toxic effects on the marrow, liver, and lungs need to be monitored for; these may limit the utility of methotrexate. Use of oral cyclosporine, a selective inhibitor of IL-2 synthesis used extensively in organ transplantation for its ability to suppress T-cell function, also failed initially to show efficacy. Recent trials have demonstrated a benefit in establishing remission in severe UC and complicated CD with intravenous cyclosporine. High rates of relapse after the drug is discontinued, together with the need to closely monitor serum levels and the high risk of nephrotoxicity with prolonged administration limit its current use to "salvage" therapy in cases of otherwise unresponsive disease.

There is little role for antibiotics in UC except in the perioperative period. On the other hand, patients with CD often require antibiotic treatment for perforating disease (phlegmons and abscesses). Metronidazole has specifically been shown to be efficacious in the management of perianal fistulous CD, and it may have a role in the management of moderately active CD, as well as in slowing the rate of recurrence after surgical resection.[19a,60] The negative relationship between smoking and UC has raised the possibility that nicotine might be of benefit. Indeed, adding transdermal nicotine to standard therapy improves symptoms in active UC, but in trials as single-agent maintenance therapy, no benefit has been noted.[20] The goal of therapy in IBD, particularly for CD, is symptomatic relief. As such, a number of medications with no presumable anti-inflammatory effect are used to aid the patient's comfort. These include antidiarrheal agents such as loperamide and atropine-diphenoxylate (Lomotil), bile-binding agents such as cholestyramine, and antidepressants. Narcotic use should be limited, because of the high risk of addiction related to the chronic nature of the underlying disorders. Avoidance of exacerbating factors, such as smoking for patients with CD, and nonsteroidal anti-inflammatory drugs is encouraged.

Patients with UC are at increased risk for development of adenocarcinoma. Although the same predisposing genetic alterations necessary for the progression from normal to adenomatous to malignant cell phenotype that has been shown to take place in sporadic colorectal cancer have been confirmed in UC; the cause of the increased risk and earlier development is unknown.[21,22] Cancer prophylaxis presupposes that colonoscopy can identify premalignant areas of dysplasia. Most protocols call for patients with long-standing (longer than 7 years) pancolitis to undergo colonoscopy every other year. Multiple biopsy samples are obtained to identify dysplastic mucosa. The benefit of such surveillance programs has been questioned from a cost-analysis viewpoint because a staggering number of colonoscopies and biopsies are required to identify the 12% of patients with UC who are likely to have cancer develop.[23] Others have criticized these programs for their shortcomings, noting that as many as 42% of patients are found to have invasive cancer when colectomy is carried out for dysplasia and as many as a third of these cancers are locally advanced or metastatic at the time of surgery.[24] Nevertheless, with the lack of alternatives, surveillance represents the best option for most patients.

Surgical Therapy

Surgical management of IBD is often viewed as a last resort. In UC, this tendency is largely the result of cultural aversion to ileostomy, which was at one time the only alternative to continued medical management. Delayed surgical intervention in CD is probably a reaction to the aggressive resectional approaches common in the past, which were based on the misguided notion that the disease could be eradicated and all too frequently created short bowel syndrome and parenteral nutrition dependency. The evolution of the ileoanal pouch procedure into an acceptable alternative to ileostomy for UC and the development of a more deliberate surgical approach to CD have radically altered current management and improved outcomes.

Surgical removal of the diseased colonic mucosa cures UC and eliminates the risk of carcinoma. Nevertheless, because the disease runs a variable course, surgery is reserved for the more aggressive patterns of UC. In order of frequency, the indications for surgery in UC are intractability, steroid dependence or intolerance, cancer prophylaxis (for patients with mucosal dysplasia) or treatment, fulminant presentation (toxic megacolon), perforation, and hemorrhage. An operation is required during the first year after diagnosis by as many as 30% of patients with severe colitis. The overall rates of colectomy vary widely, between 25% and 80%, at 25 years of follow-up.[4] The need for colectomy varies according to extent and severity of the disease. The likelihood of requiring surgery is six times greater for patients with pancolitis than for those with isolated proctitis, but approximately 15% to 20% of patients with initially limited distal disease have eventual progression to more extensive colitis. Early operation is usually necessary because of aggressive disease. Patients come to surgery later in the course of the disease either for intractable, recurrent disease or because of the risk for development or actual presence of cancer.

The choice of reconstructive method for UC is dictated by the clinical setting. Use of partial colon resection in any situation other than an emergency has been largely abandoned, on grounds that it leaves diseased tissue behind. When sepsis, hemorrhage, or toxic megacolon are present, or the possibility of advanced cancer exists, an abdominal colectomy and end-ileostomy with either a Hartmann pouch or a mucous fistula are performed. This strategy allows a restorative procedure at a later time. In the elective case, patient choice, moderated by consideration of age and body habitus, plays a large role. Many opt for restorative proctocolectomy, with removal of the distal rectal mucosa and the creation of an ileal reservoir with an ileoanal anastomosis. Because of the high risk of septic and anastomotic complications associated with steroid use, the pouch is usually rendered nonfunctional with the use of a temporary diverting ileostomy, which is taken down at a second operation after the pouch-anal anastomosis has healed. The morbidity of the pouch procedure (in its numerous configurations) compares favorably with that associated with proctocolectomy and ileostomy, although the requirement for multiple surgical procedures is clear. The one unexpected consequence of pouch formation has been the 20% to 40% incidence of idiopathic pouch inflammation, called *pouchitis*.[25] Pouchitis is unrelated to misdiagnosed Crohn's disease and is rarely observed in patients undergoing the pouch creation for familial polyposis. This is seen as further evidence of an underlying disorder in the regulatory mechanisms of inflammation in these patients. As noted earlier, many patients with pouchitis harbor pANCAs. In a small minority of patients, pouchitis is aggressive, necessitating long-term medical therapy. Most cases respond to short courses of metronidazole and nonsteroidal anti-inflammatory drugs.

Operation does not affect the natural history of CD; indeed, asymptomatic microscopic recurrence is found in 70% to 80% of patients at 1 year.[26] For this reason, surgical therapy is directed toward correcting complications, such as obstructing strictures, symptomatic internal fistulas, external fistulas, abscess formation from perforation, and persistent perianal disease. Surgical intervention should not be deferred indefinitely during multiple trials of ineffective medical therapy. This strategy risks worsening the nutritional condition of these patients and may lead to catastrophic complications from medical therapies. Of particular concern is the recent enthusiasm for use of immunosuppressants for fistulous disease, which increases the likelihood of septic morbidity. Surgery should be considered for chronic, unremitting symptoms when medical therapy has not affected prompt remission. Preoperative definition of the intestinal anatomy is essential to identify concurrent areas of disease, particularly with respect to strictures. Equally important is the radiographic definition of fistulous connections, which are generally but not exclusively found proximal to strictures. A major advance in the management of these patients has been the development of radiologically directed percutaneous drainage techniques. Used as temporizing measures to relieve the septic complications of abscess formation, these techniques allow nutritional optimization for these ill patients in preparation for definitive surgical intervention. Endoscopy may be necessary when enterocolonic fistulas are identified, to rule out colonic CD and the need for more extensive resection. Limiting resection to grossly normal margins at dominant stricture sites or at points of fistulization, rather than to microscopically normal margins, has been shown to be safe and preserves functional tissue.[27] As an extension of the concept that diseased tissue may be left in place, "strictureplasty" has been used to release stenotic regions when multiple areas of small bowel are involved.[28] Experience with strictureplasty in ileocolonic anastomotic strictures and colonic strictures is largely anecdotal and requires further evaluation. Resection remains the primary mode of treatment for colonic disease, and the benefits of proctectomy with ileostomy versus ileorectal anastomosis continue to be debated.

APPENDICITIS

Inflammation of the appendix is the most common acute surgical disease in North America. Long recognized as a potentially lethal entity, early reports of right lower quadrant disease refer to "perityphlitis," a process ascribed to acute pathology of the appendix in a classic article by Fitz in 1886.[29] Appendicitis may occur at any age but has a peak incidence in the 10- to 19-year-old age group, which corresponds to the increased lymphoid tissue found in the appendices of patients in this age group. During the last half century, the rate of appendicitis appears to be declining.[30]

The vermiform appendix is a wormlike appendage of the cecum found at the confluence of the three teniae coli. The appendicular artery, a branch of the ileocolic artery, provides the arterial blood supply to the appendix, which courses through its distinct mesentery. The narrow orifice of the appendix predisposes the lumen toward obstruction from either luminal or mural processes, both of which are causally linked to appendiceal inflammation. Although obstruction of the appendiceal lumen as the primary etiology of appendicitis has been debated, research starting with that of Wangensteen and Bowers[31] in the 1930s provides experimental and clinical support for this pathophysiologic mechanism. The most common cause of obstruction is a fecalith, a stone impacted at the orifice of the appendiceal lumen; this finding is noted in 30% of patients without symptoms, and as many as 90% of cases of gangrenous appendicitis are found to have an associated fecalith.[32] Less common causes of appendiceal obstruction include lymphoid hyperplasia, foreign bodies, intestinal worms, and neoplasms. The most common neoplasm of the appendix associated with appendicitis is the carcinoid tumor. Appendicitis associated with an adenocarcinoma or metastatic disease to the appendix has been reported rarely.

Although the precise mechanism by which luminal obstruction can result in appendiceal inflammation has not been determined, the following sequence is frequently described. Continued secretion of mucus and fluid by the appendiceal mucosa after luminal obstruction causes mural distention. The increased wall distention and tension elicit visceral afferent nerve stimulation, which is clinically manifested as vague, periumbilical abdominal pain. As the distention continues, lymphatic and capillary obstruction ensues and resident bacteria multiply, further worsening the hydrostatic pressure. As venous pressure is overcome, the mucosa becomes leaky and inflammation progresses to the serosa, initiating somatic nerve stimulation and parietal pain sensation localized to the right lower quadrant. Left untreated, venous thrombosis and arterial thrombosis follow, with consequent ischemia, eventually leading to gangrene and perforation.

Classic clinical presentation of appendicitis is unfortunately not always the rule. Typically, the pain begins with vague abdominal pain, which subsequently localizes to the right lower quadrant during the next 12 to 48 hours. Location, however, may vary in cases where the tip of the appendix is retrocecal, intrapelvic, or elevated by the uterus during pregnancy. Nausea, vomiting, and anorexia are frequently reported, and altered bowel habits may be noted. Low-grade fever and mild leukocytosis, along with a urinalysis showing a few leukocytes and erythrocytes, may be present. Physical examination typically reveals right lower quadrant tenderness with guarding, depending on the degree of inflammation present. If a mass is present, advanced disease associated with a large appendiceal phlegmon or abscess is likely.

Unfortunately, clinical findings and the course of the disease are often quite variable and subtle. Delay in diagnosis and treatment is common, particularly in infants, young children, and elderly persons. This variability in presentation in terms of both clinical course and physical findings and the potentially dire consequences of misdiagnosis have prompted efforts to develop a more definitive laboratory test or management algorithm. Multiple studies have investigated the value of leukocyte counts, C-reactive protein, phospholipase A_2, and sedimentation rate.[33] Clinical algorithms that selectively use abdominal radiography, ultrasonography, or CT scan with or without gastrointestinal contrast studies have also been investigated. Despite many such studies, no diagnostic algorithm has yet proved able to provide exceptional predictive value, and clinical assessment and judgment remain the diagnostic tools of choice.

Prompt recognition and appendectomy remain the mainstay in treating appendicitis and preventing complications. As described by McBurney,[34] a transverse right lower quadrant incision with delivery of the appendix and amputation at its base is the standard of care for acute appendicitis (Fig. 21-5). If perforation is noted, adequate ir-

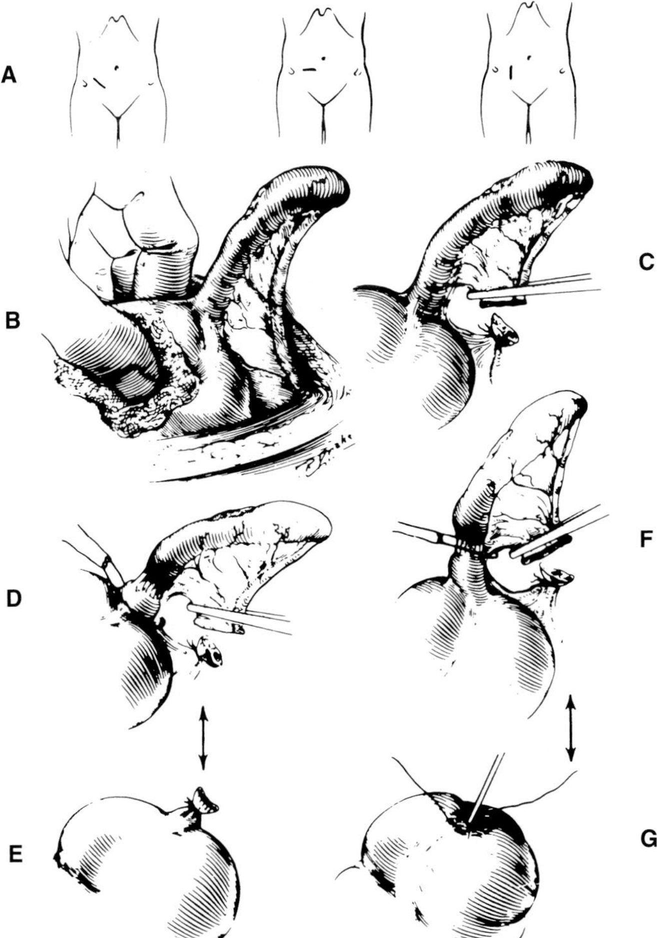

Fig. 21-5. Technique of appendectomy. **A,** Common incisions for the open appendectomy technique. **B,** Delivery of the appendix. **C,** Ligation and division of the mesoappendix. **D,** Ligation of the base of the appendix. **E,** Residual stump without inversion. **F,** Removal of the appendix with ligation. **G,** Inversion of ligated stump. (From Sabiston DC Jr, ed. Essentials of Surgery. Philadelphia: WB Saunders, 1987.)

rigation of the operative area and pelvis is added to the procedure and wound closure is delayed. Perioperative antibiotics can decrease the incidence of wound infection in acute appendicitis and are also indicated therapeutically in cases of right lower quadrant peritonitis with perforation. Infrequently, patients have "missed appendicitis," with the primary manifestation of a right lower quadrant abscess. Such abscesses can be managed with percutaneous drainage followed by interval appendectomy 2 to 3 months later.[35] Recently, laparoscopic appendectomy has also proved to be a satisfactory approach for patients with acute appendicitis. This modality may have particular value when diagnostic uncertainty is heightened. Several reports have noted less postoperative pain, shorter hospitalizations, and superior cosmetic results with this modality. Although laparoscopic appendectomy may be a safe procedure for uncomplicated appendicitis, its use in complicated appendicitis has not yet been established.[36]

MECKEL'S DIVERTICULUM

"Meckel's diverticulum is frequently suspected, often looked for and seldom found." So stated C. W. Mayo[37] regarding this congenital abnormality of the small intestine. A true diverticulum, a Meckel's diverticulum involves all layers of the small intestine and is the result of a remnant of the omphalomesenteric duct. In utero, this duct connects the primitive gut to the yolk sac and normally obliterates by 7 to 8 weeks of gestation. Failure of obliteration can result either in an ileoumbilical fistula, a cystic remnant along the duct, a fibrous band, or, most commonly, a Meckel's diverticulum. These diverticuli are usually found within 90 cm of the ileocecal valve; however, at least 180 cm of bowel proximal to the ileocecal valve should be evaluated prior to excluding a Meckel's diverticulum.[38] The blood supply to the diverticulum is from a remnant of the vitelline artery, which arises from the superior mesenteric artery and may or may not have its own mesentery. There is about a 2% (range 0.14% to 2.45%) incidence of this anomaly in the general population. Asymptomatic lesions are equally described in both sexes; however, symptomatic cases are described three times as frequently in men. There is an association between Meckel's diverticulum and certain congenital anomalies, including cleft palate, bicornuate uterus, and annular pancreas. There is also an increased incidence in Crohn's disease (6% to 18%), but the explanation for this is unknown.[39]

As many as 50% of Meckel's diverticuli contain ectopic gastrointestinal tissue. Gastric acid–secreting mucosa is most commonly present, but less frequently pancreatic tissue, Brunner's glands, colonic mucosa, or hepatobiliary tissue is identified. Inflammatory conditions may arise from acid secretion and ulceration of the adjacent ileal mucosa, which may lead to gastrointestinal hemorrhage. Obstruction of the orifice of the diverticulum by fecal matter, foreign bodies, or neoplastic tissue may elicit an inflammatory cycle similar to appendicitis. Carcinoids and adenocarcinomas have been found rarely in diverticuli.

In adults, the most common complication of Meckel's diverticulum is mechanical small bowel obstruction. Multiple patterns of obstruction have been described, including intussusception into the terminal ileum and right colon, volvulus of the attached small bowel around the fibrous mesenteric band, and internal herniation. Local inflammatory changes, with peptic ulceration and scarring, can also progress to lesions that cause obstruction. Incarceration in an abdominal hernia has been reported and is referred to as a *Littre's hernia.* Although first described for incarceration within a femoral hernia, this term is now generally applied to any hernia with an incarcerated Meckel's diverticulum. The complications associated with Meckel's diverticulum vary with the age of the patient. The pediatric population most commonly has painless hematochezia, whereas the adult population is more likely to show symptoms referable to diverticular inflammation or bowel obstruction. Because this anomaly is relatively rare, accurate diagnosis is often not established until laparotomy.

The presence of ectopic gastric mucosa in some Meckel's diverticuli has allowed the development of a noninvasive imaging procedure. Diverticuli containing functional gastric mucosa selectively take up ^{99m}(Tc)pertechnetate after intravenous injection. This gamma-emitting isotope can then be detected with external cameras. At least 1.8 cm^2 of ectopic gastric mucosa must be present to be detected with this scan. The accuracy of the scan in children approaches 90%; in the adult population, however, sensitivity is 62.5% and specificity is only 9%.[40]

Surgical management of symptomatic Meckel's diverticulum requires surgical segmental small bowel resection to remove all ectopic tissue and adjacent inflamed or ulcerated areas. The incidental finding of a Meckel's diverticulum presents less clear indications for excision. Lesions with a narrow orifice, an associated palpable mass, a fibrous band, or a vitelline vessel without a mesentery should be resected. The incidental Meckel's diverticulum that is free of signs of inflammation or scarring can be safely managed with simple excision from the antimesenteric surface of the small bowel, without segmental small bowel resection. This simplified approach is easily accomplished with a gastrointestinal stapling device. The risk of morbidity after elective, incidental excision has been reported to be 2%, compared with a 7% risk of morbidity after operation for symptomatic lesions. Excision of incidental Meckel's diverticuli thus appears warranted, provided there is no intraoperative finding to contraindicate this approach.[41]

JEJUNOILEAL DIVERTICULI

Diverticuli of the jejunum and ileum are rarely associated with clinical manifestations. Though such diverticuli are noted in 4.6% of the population at autopsy, they are described on only 0.5% to 2.3% of small bowel contrast studies.[42,43] These pseudodiverticuli are formed by herniation of the small bowel mucosa into the mesenteric fat at the sites where the vasa recta penetrate the bowel wall. The diverticuli, often multiple, are more frequently found in the proximal jejunum, probably because of the larger size of the vasa recta in this area of the small bowel, and are often not apparent on routine abdominal exploration because they are concealed within the mesenteric fat. They are thought to be acquired diverticuli, and increased intraluminal pressure, possibly associated with abnormal peristaltic action, may be responsible for their development.

Although these diverticuli are frequently clinically silent, clinical syndromes that may be associated with small bowel diverticuli include malabsorption, hemorrhage, inflammation, and obstruction. Extensive regions of small bowel diverticulosis may be associated with abnormal small bowel motility, with consequent stasis and bacterial overgrowth. A secondary malabsorption syndrome characterized by crampy abdominal pain, anemia, and diarrhea may ensue. Hemorrhage is rarely associated with these lesions, but they have been described as a cause of recurrent occult gastrointestinal hemorrhage. Obstruction of the orifice of the diverticulum with fecal material can result in acute inflammation, which may progress to peritonitis and perforation. Asymptomatic lesions, or those identified incidentally on upper gastrointestinal tract small bowel follow-through series, do not require surgical intervention. Lesions associated with acute inflammation or hemorrhage require emergency operation, with segmental small bowel resection.

COLONIC DIVERTICULAR DISEASE

Colonic diverticulosis is a common acquired structural disorder of the colon. Although it was first described in the eighteenth century, the pathologic significance of this disorder was not fully appreciated until the early twentieth century. This condition has increased in frequency during the last 80 years, with an autopsy prevalence rate of 5% in the early 1900s and one of 50% described more recently. Approximately 30% of all persons older than 45 years have diverticulosis, and as many as 70% of people older than 85 years have this condition. The condition is manifested equally among men and women.

The pathogenesis of colonic diverticuli remains unclear, although two factors seem to be operative in their development: weaknesses in the colonic wall and intraluminal pressure gradients. Intraluminal pressure recordings demonstrate a process termed *segmentation,* which allows small segments of the bowel to develop relatively high pressures. Patients with diverticulosis have similar resting pressures but generate markedly increased pressures with contraction. Diverticuli are most frequently identified in the sigmoid colon, the region where the highest pressures are generated (Fig. 21-6). The structural feature that predisposes toward diverticular development is the point where the vasa recta enter the bowel through the muscular wall. These perforating vessels cause weaknesses in the colon wall and are the sites where diverticuli form. The association of diverticular disease with increasing age may be explained by the decreased collagen synthesis and in-

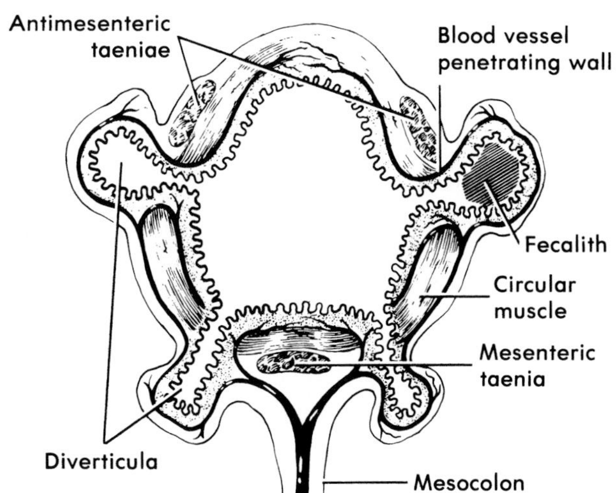

Fig. 21-6. Diverticulosis of the colon. Cross section of the colon depicting the sites where diverticuli form. Note that the antimesenteric portion is spared. Diverticuli originate at the site where the blood vessel penetrates the colonic wall. (From Way LW, ed. Current Surgical Diagnosis and Treatment, 7th ed. Los Altos, Calif.: Lange Medical Books, 1985.)

creased elastin content of the submucosa of the colon in elderly persons. Muscular thickening of the colonic wall, a condition termed *myochosis,* is present in younger people of the Western population at risk for this disease. This muscular abnormality constricts the lumen of the colon and leads to higher intraluminal pressures; it is thought to be the precursor of diverticulosis.[44] A low-residue diet typical of Western populations is associated with the risk of diverticulosis.[45] Diverticulosis is not present in African populations, where a high-residue diet is the norm. Population-shift studies have shown that Japanese immigrants, who have a low incidence of diverticulosis before immigration, acquire the same risk as the native U.S. population after adopting the low-residue regional diet of their new environment.

As many as 25% of patients with diverticulosis have a complication of this condition develop. Acute diverticulitis is the most common manifestation. Diverticulitis is caused by the obstruction of the orifice of the diverticulum by fecal material, with consequent bacterial overgrowth, inflammation, and eventual transmural inflammation and peritonitis. Advanced complications may be manifested by free or localized perforation, abscess formation, fistulization to adjacent viscera or the skin, and acute colonic obstruction. Bleeding is rarely associated with acute diverticulitis, although it is a well-described complication of diverticulosis. Acute diverticulitis is characterized by the gradual onset of crampy left lower quadrant pain. Altered bowel habits, including diarrhea or constipation, may be reported. More advanced disease is associated with fever, leukocytosis, and distinct left lower quadrant peritonitis. An abdominal CT scan to identify pericolonic inflammation and mesenteric streaking, with or without associated abscess, is the most sensitive radiographic study to identify acute diverticulitis. Contrast enemas are contraindicated, and plain abdominal films are of value only to rule out free perforation.

Mild cases of diverticulitis not associated with paralytic ileus can be treated with oral antibiotics on an outpatient basis. However, patients with fever, leukocytosis, or left lower quadrant peritonitis require hospitalization for intravenous antibiotic administration. Prompt evaluation with CT scan allows percutaneous drainage of localized abscess cavities preparatory to subsequent segmental colonic resection. Patients with diffuse peritonitis and those for whom initial nonoperative therapeutic measures fail should proceed to urgent laparotomy.

Surgical management is dictated by the operative findings.[46] If preoperative mechanical bowel preparation is possible, a one-stage procedure with resection and primary anastomosis is indicated. All involved bowel should be resected, particularly including the entire sigmoid colon. The distal margin of resection should be defined by the region in the upper rectum where the taeniae coli splay apart to become a confluent muscular layer. Patients with acute perforation, localized undrained abscess, or peritonitis should be treated with a two-stage procedure, with initial segmental resection of the inflamed bowel, descending colostomy, and a Hartman's rectal pouch. Rarely, the inflammatory process in the sigmoid colon is so severe as to warrant the older three-stage approach to this disease, in which a transverse colostomy to divert the fecal stream is performed at the initial setting, prior to subsequent sigmoid resection after the acute inflammatory process resolves and later closure of the colostomy. Elective surgical resection is generally recommended for patients younger than 40 years who have had one attack of diverticulitis severe enough to warrant hospitalization. Judgment regarding elective surgical management for older patients is based on medical comorbidities and suitability of the patient for elective colonic resection. Patients who have had a single attack of diverticulitis have a risk of recurrent disease exceeding 50%.

PSEUDOMEMBRANOUS COLITIS

With the advent of broad-spectrum antibiotics and their frequent use, the incidence of pseudomembranous colitis (PMC) caused by *Clostridium difficile* infection is increasing. PMC is characterized by diarrhea and colorectal mucosal inflammation. Original descriptions in the nineteenth century were of patients undergoing intestinal surgery for obstruction or ischemia, and occasional contemporary reports of PMC in immunocompromised patients attest to the possibility that PMC develops in the absence of antibiotic use. Nevertheless, the disease today is closely associated with antibiotic therapy.[47,48] Enteral medications appear to be slightly more likely to lead to disease than parenteral antibiotics, although greater frequency of use of parenteral agents in surgery makes them a common cause in this subset of patients. Agents most frequently implicated are cephalosporins, clindamycin, and lincomycin, but associations have been made with nearly all antibiotics except aminoglycosides, nitroimidazoles, and monobactams. Prolonged antibiotic treatment is most often involved, but a single dose of systemic therapy can lead to PMC.

C. difficile is most likely a minor component of the normal flora, although it is rarely cultured in individuals without symptoms. The organism can be transmitted from patient to patient by health care carriers and instruments, and nosocomial epidemics have been documented.[49] Once the organism is present, antibiotic-induced alterations in the normal colonic microflora may give *C. difficile* the proliferative advantage that leads to clinical disease. Of the various products that the bacterium secretes, two are toxins. Toxin A is weakly cytotoxic but elicits an inflammatory response characterized by vasodilatation and hemorrhage.[50] Toxin B is released from the cell membrane on lysis and is the basis for the commercially available cytotoxic assays. Both toxins are necessary for clinical disease.

A high index of suspicion is critical to allow a prompt therapeutic response. Watery diarrhea is the hallmark of the disease. Blood may be noted in the stool but is rare. Abdominal pain and low-grade fevers are characteristic but not specific in patients after abdominal operations. Mortality as great as 40% is documented for untreated patients; it drops to less than 10% with recognition and institution of appropriate measures. Stool cultures for the organism and stool assay for the *C. difficile* cytotoxin (toxin B) are diagnostic and readily available in most institutions. Whereas culture is the more sensitive test, cytotoxin assay is more specific.[51] The presence of leukocytes in the stool can be a more rapid, if less sensitive and specific, diagnostic aid. When the diagnosis is uncertain, endoscopy can be helpful. The rectum is involved in 75% of patients, with the right colon affected infrequently. Endoscopy reveals scattered patches of white plaque (the pseudomembranes) interspersed between normal appearing mucosa. Histologically, plaques are made up of fibrin, mucus, sloughed epithelial cells, and neutrophils. In the absence of pseudomembranes, the microscopic appearance can be difficult to differentiate from that of ischemic colitis.

Most patients show clinical improvement when the offending antibiotic is removed, although diarrhea may persist for more than a month. Relapses occur and carriers without symptoms pose a risk to the community. Therefore, even mild cases should be treated. Treatment consists of institution of *C. difficile*-specific therapy; the agents of choice are oral vancomycin and metronidazole. Although vancomycin may have a slight therapeutic advantage, its greater cost and the recent development of vancomycin-resistant *Enterococcus* species mandate that its use be reserved for severe cases or metronidazole-resistant PMC. Parenteral metronidazole can be used in patients unable to take oral medication; higher therapeutic doses are needed, however, and therapeutic failures are more common. Vancomycin enemas may also be effective. If continued antibiotic treatment is essential for treatment of concomitant disease, antibiotics not commonly linked to PMC, such as penicillin, ampicillin, aminoglycosides, erythromycin, or tetracycline, should be used if possible. Surgery is sometimes necessary in fulminant cases because of toxic megacolon or perforation. Despite the absence of gross right-sided disease in most cases, patients undergoing subtotal colectomy fare better than do those undergoing less extensive resections.[52]

RADIATION ENTERITIS

The beneficial effects of radiation on tumors became evident shortly after Roentgen invented his x-ray device 100 years ago. The harmful effects on normal tissue were reported soon thereafter, but it was not until the development of megavoltage external-beam radiation in the 1950s, which expanded the therapeutic role of irradiation, that intestinal damage began to be widely reported.[53] Despite efforts to limit injury by minimizing the radiation field and optimizing the dose administered, an increased incidence of gastrointestinal complications has been reported.[54] The increase is probably caused by the increased use of this modality for pelvic malignancies, as well as improved long-term patient survival. The synchronous administration of chemotherapy during radiation therapy to enhance radiosensitivity of the tumor may also lead to an increase in the incidence of radiation enteritis.

The acute effects of radiation are defined in experimental in vivo models.[55,56] Radiation energy induces its tumoricidal effects by denaturing DNA and forming oxygen free radicals. The sensitivity of normal tissues varies according to the proliferative rate of the cellular components. The alimentary tract, particularly the small bowel, is exquisitely sensitive to radiation because of the high rate of proliferation found throughout the intestinal epithelium. Mitotic activity in the crypts of the small intestine stops within hours after radiation exposure to single radiation doses of 500 to 1000 cGy (rads). Cell necrosis peaks at 6 to 8 hours. Conventional understanding proposed a proliferative burst during the next 24 hours by the remaining viable crypt cells. However, it is more likely that repair occurs by restitution, with flattening of the villi as residual cells spread out to cover the denuded areas of the epithelium. A leukocyte infiltrate is often present. The changes are associated clinically with nausea, vomiting, and diarrhea. The diarrhea results in part from malabsorption of nutrients and bile salts and can be ameliorated by cholestyramine.[57] Restitution from a single small-dose injury is complete by day 3, whereas after a course of treatment, histologic recovery requires 2 weeks. Symptomatic recovery may take as long as 6 months. With larger doses (>1500 cGy) and a proportionately larger cell kill, the re-epithelialization process is incomplete, the intestinal barrier function is lost, and septic death often results. Clinically, acute radiation enteritis is usually self-limited and responds to symptomatic therapy and conservative management.

Whereas acute injury is limited to the mucosa, chronic radiation enteritis involves the full thickness of the intestinal wall. It is seen 6 months to 12 years after exposure, generally correlates with the severity of the acute injury, and occurs through unknown mechanisms.[58] The most prominent and consistent histologic feature is obliterative sclerosis and intimal hyperplasia of the submucosal arterioles. This obstruction to blood flow likely results in ischemia and is responsible for the mucosal ulceration and atrophy typically associated with it. Inflammatory cells infiltrate the lamina propria, and the muscularis mucosa is hyperplastic and fibrotic. The normal appearance of the muscularis propria is preserved. Serositis, with infiltration by fibroblasts and inflammatory cells, is universally present. These changes are generally progressive.

Patients with chronic injury generally show acute signs of partial bowel obstruction superimposed on a history of chronic diarrhea and malabsorption. Because many have a prior history of abdominal surgery, cancer, or both, differentiating between radiation enteritis and tumor recurrence or adhesions may be difficult. Contrast upper and lower gastrointestinal tract series may be helpful, although findings must be differentiated clinically from other processes, primarily CD and ischemia. Such series also help define the location and extent of fistulous tracts and strictures, thereby guiding the operative approach. Most cases respond, at least initially, to conservative management with institution of bowel rest followed by a low-residue diet. As many as 40% of patients receiving radiation treatments have symptoms severe enough to require medical intervention at some point, and 2% to 5% require operative management. Fistula and stricture are the major indications for operation. Surgical intervention is hampered by the extensive serositis and dense vascular adhesions commonly encountered. Conservative measures, such as proximal enterostomy and enteroenteral bypasses, may be the most appropriate approach. Resection with reanastomosis can be safely carried out when the segment involved can be mobilized and the ends to be anastomosed are grossly normal in appearance.

Because of the progressive nature and difficult management once the disease is established, prevention is key. Focalization of the radiation field, optimization of the dose, and distention of the bladder during treatments minimize the risk of intestinal injury, although a recent report failed to demonstrate a relationship between amount of bowel exposed in the radiation field and surgical complications.[59] A number of intraoperative techniques have been suggested to prevent small bowel from dropping into the pelvis after such radical procedures as hysterectomy, exenteration, and abdominoperineal resection. These include reperitonealization of the pelvis, placement of omental and absorbable mesh slings across the pelvic brim, and insertion of saline- or silicone-filled pouches in the pelvic space. Numerous pharmacologic agents have been shown to ameliorate acute experimental radiation injury, including elemental diets, PGs, epidermal growth factor, glutamine, and sucralfate, but proof of clinical benefit is lacking for all but the last, and none have been shown to alter the course of chronic radiation enteritis.

SUMMARY

A large number of inflammatory disorders may adversely influence the normal physiology of the small bowel and colon. The inflammatory disorders of surgical significance include appendicitis, Meckel's diverticulitis, diverticular disease of the colon (and on occasion jejunum and ileum), CD, and UC. Other diseases that may require surgical intervention in selected situations include pseudomembranous colitis and radiation enteritis. The impacts that these disease processes have on intestinal function vary considerably in terms of disability and long-term sequelae. Appendectomy for appendicitis, for example, is usually associated with no long-term sequelae, in contrast to CD, in which a variety of mild to severe digestive disorders may plague the patient for most of his or her life, depending on the status of the disease, the frequency of relapses, the duration of remissions, and the type (or types) of surgical management rendered. An understanding of the physiologic derangements associated with each inflammatory disorder forms the basis for correction and for those surgical procedures that must be used to restore intestinal function to normal.

REFERENCES

1. Fielding JF. "Inflammatory" bowel disease. Br Med J 290:47, 1985.
2. Shanahan F. Pathogenesis of ulcerative colitis. Lancet 342:407, 1993.
3. Calkins BM, Mendeloff AI. The epidemiology of idiopathic inflammatory bowel disease. In Kirsner JB, Shorter RG, eds. Inflammatory Bowel Disease, 4th ed. Baltimore: Williams & Wilkins, 1995.
4. Farmer RG, Easley KA, Rankin GB. Clinical patterns, natural history, and progression of ulcerative colitis. A long-term follow-up of 1116 patients. Dig Dis Sci 38:1137, 1993.
5. Crohn BB, Ginzburg L, Oppenheimer GDL. Regional enteritis. JAMA 99:214, 1932.
6. Sanderson JD, et al. Mycobacterium paratuberculosis DNA in Crohn's disease tissue. Gut 33:890, 1992.
7. Wakefield AJ, et al. Crohn's disease: Pathogenesis and persistent measles virus infection. Gastroenterology 108:911, 1995.
8. Sartor RB, Bond TM, Schwab JH. Systemic uptake and intestinal inflammatory effects of luminal bacterial cell wall polymers in rats with acute colonic injury. Infect Immun 56:2101, 1988.
9. Howden CW, et al. Intestinal permeability in patients with Crohn's disease and their first-degree relatives. Am J Gastroenterol 89:1175, 1994.
10. Schreiber S, et al. The role of the mucosal immune system in inflammatory bowel disease. Gastroenterol Clin North Am 21:451, 1992.
11. Das KM, et al. Autoimmunity to cytoskeletal protein tropomyosin. A clue to the pathogenetic mechanism for ulcerative colitis. J Immunol 150:2487, 1993.
12. Shanahan F. The role of autoantibodies and autoimmunity in chronic inflammatory disorders of the gut. Curr Opin Gastroenterol 8:988, 1992.
13. Stenson WF. Interleukin-4 hyporesponsiveness in inflammatory bowel disease: Immune defect or physiological response? Gastroenterology 108:284, 1995.
14. Calkins BM. A meta-analysis of the role of smoking in inflammatory bowel disease. Dig Dis Sci 4:1841, 1989.
15. Hanauer SB, Baert F. Medical therapy of inflammatory bowel disease. Med Clin North Am 78:1413, 1994.
16. Pinczowski D, et al. Risk factors for colorectal cancer in patients with ulcerative colitis: A case-control study. Gastroenterology 107:117, 1994.
17. Sutherland LR, May GR, Shaffer EA. Sulfasalazine revisited: A meta-analysis of 5-aminosalicylic acid in the treatment of ulcerative colitis. Ann Intern Med 118:540, 1993.
18. McLeod RS, et al. Prophylactic mesalamine treatment decreases postoperative recurrence of Crohn's disease. Gastroenterology 109:404, 1995.
19. Pearson DC, et al. Azathioprine and 6-mercaptopurine in Crohn disease. A meta-analysis. Ann Intern Med 123:132, 1995.

19a. Rutgeerts P, et al. Controlled trial of metronidazole treatment for prevention of Crohn's recurrence after ileal resection. Gastroenterology 108:1617, 1995.

20. Thomas GA, et al. Transdermal nicotine as maintenance therapy for ulcerative colitis. N Engl J Med 332:988, 1995.
21. Fearon ER, Vogelstein B. A genetic model for colorectal tumorigenesis. Cell 61:759, 1990.
22. Kern SE, et al. Molecular genetic profiles of colitis-associated neoplasms. Gastroenterology 107:420, 1994.
23. Lynch DA, et al. Failure of colonoscopic surveillance in ulcerative colitis. Gut 34:1075, 1993.
24. Bernstein CN, Shanahan F, Weinstein WM. Are we telling patients the truth about surveillance colonoscopy in ulcerative colitis? Lancet 343:71, 1994.
25. Sandborn WJ. Pouchitis following ileal pouch-anal anastomosis: Definition, pathogenesis, and treatment. Gastroenterology 107:1856, 1994.
26. Rutgeerts P, et al. Predictability of the postoperative course of Crohn's disease. Gastroenterology 99:956, 1990.
27. Kotanagi H, et al. Do microscopic abnormalities at resection margins correlate with increased anastomotic recurrence in Crohn's disease? Retrospective analysis of 100 cases. Dis Colon Rectum 34:909, 1991.
28. Fazio VW, et al. Long-term follow-up of strictureplasty in Crohn's disease. Dis Colon Rectum 36:355, 1993.
29. Fitz RH. Perforating inflammation of the vermiform appendix: With special reference to its early diagnosis and treatment. Trans Assoc Am Physicians 1:107, 1886.
30. Addiss DG, et al. The epidemiology of appendicitis and appendectomy in the United States. Am J Epidemiol 132:910, 1990.
31. Wangensteen OH, Bowers WF. Significance of the obstructive factor in the genesis of acute appendicitis. Arch Surg 34:496, 1937.
32. Jones BA, et al. The prevalence of appendiceal fecaliths in patients with and without appendicitis. A comparative study from Canada and South Africa. Ann Surg 202:80, 1985.
33. Dueholm S, Bagi P, Bud M. Laboratory aid in the diagnosis of acute appendicitis. A blinded, prospective trial concerning diagnostic value of leukocyte count, neutrophil differential count, and C-reactive protein. Dis Colon Rectum 32:855, 1989.
34. McBurney C. Experience with early operative interference in the cases of disease of the veriform appendix. N Y Med J 50:676, 1889.
35. Vargas HI, Averbook A, Stamos MJ. Appendiceal mass: Conservative therapy followed by interval laparoscopic appendectomy. Am Surg 60:753, 1994.
36. Bonanni F, et al. Laparoscopic versus conventional appendectomy. J Am Coll Surg 179:273, 1994.
37. Mayo CW. Meckel's diverticulum. Mayo Clin Proc 8:230, 1933.
38. DiGiacomo JC, Cottone FJ. Surgical treatment of Meckel's diverticulum. South Med J 86:671, 1993.

39. Turgeon DK, Barnett JL. Meckel's diverticulum. Am J Gastroenterol 85:777, 1990.
40. Cooney DR, et al. The abdominal technetium scan (a decade of experience). J Pediatr Surg 17:611, 1982.
41. Cullen JJ, et al. Surgical management of Meckel's diverticulum. An epidemiologic, population-based study. Ann Surg 220:564, 1994.
42. Longo WE, Vernava AM III. Clinical implications of jejunoileal diverticular disease. Dis Colon Rectum 35:381, 1992.
43. Tsiotos GG, Farnell MB, Ilstrup DM. Non-Meckelian jejunal or ileal diverticulosis: An analysis of 112 cases. Surgery 116:726, 1994.
44. Watters DA, Smith AN. Strength of the colon wall in diverticular disease. Br J Surg 77:257, 1990.
45. Burkitt DP, Walker AR, Painter NS. Effect of dietary fibre on stools and the transit-times, and its role in the causation of disease. Lancet 2:1408, 1972.
46. Roberts PL, Veidenheimer MC. Current management of diverticulitis. Adv Surg 27:189, 1994.
47. Fekety R, Shah AB. Diagnosis and treatment of *Clostridium difficile* colitis. JAMA 269:71, 1993.
48. Kelly CP, Pothoulakis C, LaMont JT. *Clostridium difficile* colitis. N Engl J Med 330:257, 1994.
49. McFarland LV, et al. Nosocomial acquisition of *Clostridium difficile* infection, N Engl J Med 320:204, 1989.
50. Burakoff R, et al. Effects of purified *Clostridium difficile* toxin A on rabbit distal colon. Gastroenterology 109:348, 1995.
51. Gerding DN, Brazier JS. Optimal methods for identifying *Clostridium difficile* infections. Clin Infect Dis 16(Suppl 4):S439, 1993.
52. Lipsett PA, et al. Pseudomembranous colitis: A surgical disease? Surgery 116:491, 1994.
53. Walsh D. Deep tissue traumatism from Roentgen ray exposure. B M J 2:272, 1897.
54. Allen-Mersh TG, et al. Has the incidence of radiation-induced bowel damage following treatment of uterine carcinoma changed in the last 20 years? J R Soc Med 79:387, 1986.
55. Kinsella TJ, Bloomer WD. Tolerance of the intestine to radiation therapy. Surg Gynecol Obstet 151:273, 1980.
56. Yeoh EK, Horowitz M. Radiation enteritis. Surg Gynecol Obstet 165:373, 1987.
57. Yeoh E, et al. Effect of pelvic irradiation on gastrointestinal function: A prospective longitudinal study. Am J Med 95:397, 1993.
58. Coia LR, Myerson RJ, Tepper JE. Late effects of radiation therapy on the gastrointestinal tract. Int J Radiat Oncol Biol Phys 31:1213, 1995.
59. Letschert JG, et al. The volume effect in radiation-related late small bowel complications: Results of a clinical study of the EORTC Radiotherapy Cooperative Group. Radiother Oncol 32:116, 1994.

22

Intestinal Dysfunction Secondary to Previous Surgery

Mary E. Klingensmith and David I. Soybel

The principal function of the intestinal tract is absorption of food and water. Applied to the gastrointestinal (GI) tract, the terms *dysfunction* and *failure* thus imply the inability of the intestinal tract to absorb enough nutrients, minerals, or water to maintain weight and nutritional needs. However, these terms can also refer to alterations in GI motility, which can lead to visceral pain and diarrhea, or alterations in mucosal integrity, which can lead to chronic mucosal inflammation and bleeding. Such malabsorptive and mucosal inflammatory states are recognized complications of surgical procedures on the GI tract. In this chapter, we discuss four postoperative conditions of GI dysfunction: short bowel syndrome (SBS), blind-loop syndrome, ileal pouch inflammation, and diversion colitis. The pathogenesis and complications of each of these states are discussed, with an emphasis on alterations in enterocyte and colonocyte nutrition and function, luminal bacteriology, and neurohumoral milieu. Where possible, clinical correlations are used to detail symptoms, natural history, and therapeutic approaches to these disorders.

A BRIEF REVIEW OF DIGESTION AND MALABSORPTION

A combination of mechanical, enzymatic, and hormonal events are integrated in the digestive process that breaks down foodstuffs and permits absorption of fats, carbohydrates, and protein in the intestines. The capacity of the gut to absorb fluid and nutrients so efficiently is attributable to its massive surface area. Depending on the measurement technique used, the length of intestine has been estimated at 300 to 700 cm.[1] A dense arrangement of villi and microvilli accounts for the enormous surface area of the small bowel, which has been estimated to be 100 m^2.[1]

Both passive diffusion and active transport account for absorption of water, vitamins, and by-products of fat, carbohydrate, and protein catabolism. Of the 9 to 10 L fluid handled by the gut each day, about 2 L comes from oral intake. The remaining fluid consists of secretions, including gastric and pancreatic juices, bile, and succus entericus. The composition of these secretions varies with the site of origin. Gastric juice is composed of high concentrations of hydrochloric acid (about 100 mmol/L with sodium ion (Na^+) concentrations (20 mmol/L) much lower and potassium ion (K^+) concentrations (10 to 12 mmol/L) much higher than those found in plasma. In contrast, saliva, pancreatic secretions, and bile are high in bicarbonate ion (HCO_3^-). Ultimately, the secretions of the GI tract are efficiently absorbed, with the jejunum typically absorbing 3 to 5 L/day, the ileum absorbing 2 to 4 L/day, and the colon absorbing 1 to 2 L/day (Fig. 22-1).[2]

Different regions of the GI tract are responsible for absorption of different nutrients. The duodenum is the primary site of absorption for water, amino acids, simple sugars, and free fatty acids, whereas most carbohydrate absorption occurs in the jejunum. The ileum is unique in its role in bile salt, cholesterol, and vitamin B_{12} absorption (Fig. 22-2). Vitamins are adequately absorbed despite their extremely low concentrations in normal food (final luminal concentrations range from 10^{-6} to 10^{-8} mmol/L.)[3] Fat-soluble vitamins (A, D, E, and K) are absorbed by the same transport mechanism as fatty acids; they bind to the fatty acid–binding proteins found in the brush border of enterocytes. Active transport (often by sodium-dependent transport mechanisms) is required for absorption of water-soluble vitamins (vitamin C, niacin, and B vitamins).[3] Despite this regional specialization in transport functions, each region of the small intestine is capable of assuming the absorptive functions of the others to some extent.

An important contribution to normal gut function comes from its bacterial population. In patients with normal gastric acid secretion, the chyme entering the duodenum is sterile. The small numbers of bacteria that are found in stomach and proximal intestine are aerobic, gram-positive species found in the oropharynx. Distally, in the ileum and colon, gram-negative aerobes are present and anaerobic organisms predominate. Total bacterial counts

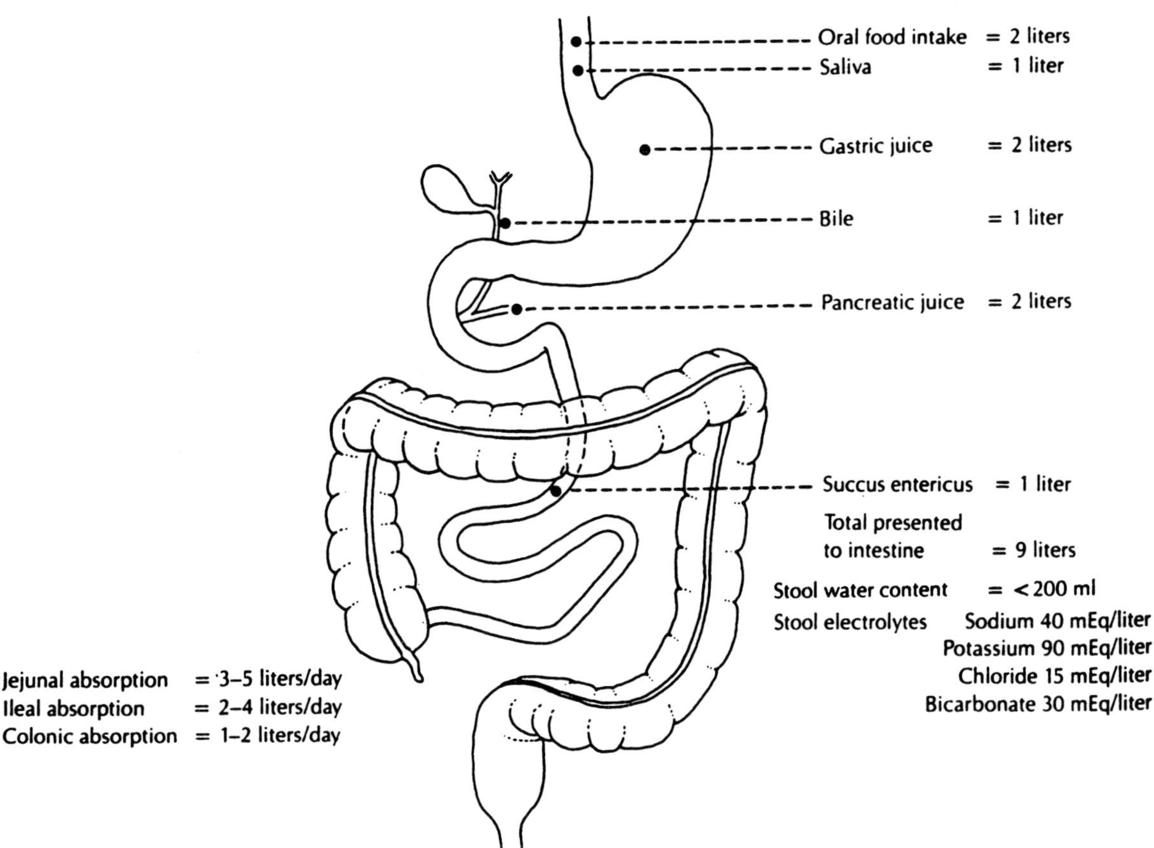

Fig. 22-1. Normal daily intestinal fluid balance. (From Chopra S, Trier JS. Diarrhea and malabsorption. In Chopra S, May RJ, eds. Pathophysiology of Gastrointestinal Disease. Boston: Little, Brown, 1989.)

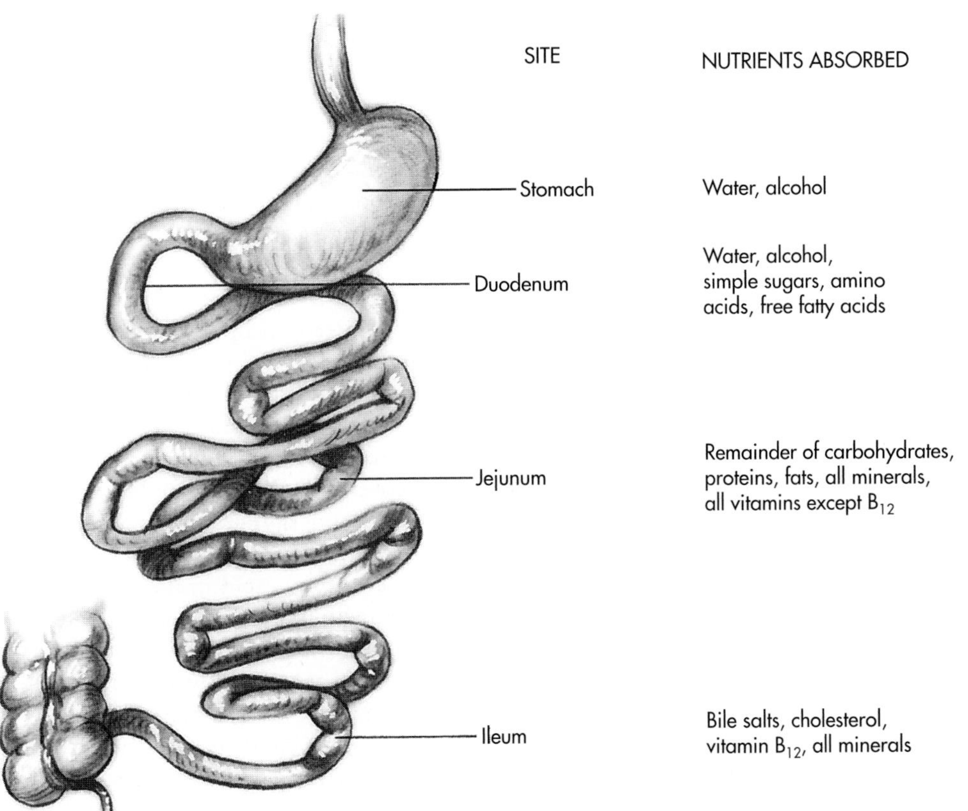

Fig. 22-2. Sites of nutrient absorption in the gastrointestinal tract. (From Davis JH, ed. Clinical Surgery. St. Louis: Mosby, 1987.)

Table 22-1. Signs and Symptoms of Malabsorption

Sign/Symptom	Cause
Diarrhea	Osmotic or secretory
Cramps, flatulence, distention	Bacterial degradation of carbohydrates
Weight loss	Nutrient malabsorption
Tetany, paresthesias, osteomalacia, pathologic fractures	Vitamin D, magnesium, calcium, phosphate deficiencies
Bruisability, ecchymoses	Vitamins K and C deficiency
Glossitis, cheilosis, stomatitis	Vitamins B complex, B_{12}, and C; folate; and iron deficiency
Amenorrhea, diminished libido	Protein deficiencies
Night blindness	Vitamin A deficiency
Acrodermatitis	Zinc and fatty-acid deficiency

in normal feces reach 10^{11} organisms (per gram). Control of the bacterial populations depends on intact motor activity of the intestines and the interactions of all species present. This ecology can be disturbed by antibiotic therapy or surgical reconstructions that result in stasis within intestinal segments. Intestinal bacteria serve several functions, including (1) metabolism of fecal sterols, releasing the short-chain fatty acids (SCFAs) that are an important food source for colonocytes; (2) metabolism of fecal bile acids, fat-soluble vitamins (e.g., vitamin K), and vitamin B_{12}; and (3) breakdown of complex carbohydrates and organic matter, leading to formation of carbon dioxide, hydrogen, and methane gases.[4] Only about 20% of intestinal gas is generated by bacterial metabolism. The other 80% represents swallowed air and is composed mainly of nitrogen. Considerable evidence suggests that the normal flora may contribute to baseline levels of intestinal secretion[4] and normal intestinal motility. Under baseline conditions, the small intestines in germ-free animals are frequently dilated, fluid filled, and without peristalsis.[4]

In discussing GI failure, it is important to distinguish between maldigestion and malabsorption. *Malabsorption* refers to the loss of absorption capacity for nutrients in the intestine itself. *Maldigestion* is the term used when pancreatic or biliary secretions fail to provide enzymes or bile necessary for carbohydrate, protein, or fat breakdown. Most commonly, this occurs in the setting of biliary obstruction or chronic pancreatitis. In extreme cases of SBS, hepatic synthesis of bile salts cannot keep pace with GI losses, and maldigestion may be superimposed on malabsorption.

Table 22-1 summarizes the clinical signs and symptoms of malabsorption and maldigestion. General and nonspecific symptoms such as diarrhea, cramps, flatulence, pain, and weight loss are common manifestations of maldigestion and malabsorption. Specific complications of vitamin and mineral deficiencies, such as pernicious anemia, osteomalacia, glossitis, and acrodermatitis are observed, but rarely in fulminant forms. A diagnosis of GI failure therefore relies on the demonstration of ongoing requirements for parenterally supplied nutrients, fluids, and electrolytes for the maintenance of body weight, nitrogen balance, and plasma protein and electrolyte composition. GI failure also often reflects imbalances between GI mucosa and the luminal milieu that lead to motility disorders, mucosal inflammation, and bleeding. SBS and blind-loop syndrome may be recognized by the former definition, whereas ileal loop pouchitis and diversion colitis are examples of the latter.

SHORT BOWEL SYNDROME

Etiology

The extensive surface area of the small bowel allows significant loss in length before nutritional compromise occurs. As much as 50% of the combined length of the jejunum and ileum can be resected safely. When more than 70% is resected (for remaining length less than 60 to 80 cm), life-threatening deficiencies occur unless total parenteral nutrition (TPN) is supplied.[1,5] SBS results from intestinal resection for disorders such as Crohn's disease, infarction (related to mechanical obstruction and strangulation or embolic events), radiation enteritis, volvulus, tumor, trauma, and fistulas. Intestinal bypass surgery, once used for treatment of morbid obesity, represented an intentional attempt to create SBS. In adults, the most common etiologic factors of SBS are Crohn's disease and mesenteric infarction.

Contributing Factors

Several factors have been identified as crucial in determining whether long-term SBS and dependence on TPN would result from a massive intestinal resection. Although it seems intuitively clear that the extent of resection would determine the likelihood of SBS, the crucial factor is the extent of small intestine *remaining*. The second most important factor is whether the colon and rectum have been preserved.

Table 22-2 summarizes data from a small series of patients reported on by Gouttebel et al.[6] They found that the presence of the colon and rectum considerably improved the prognosis for patients with less than 70 cm small intestine remaining after resection. In addition, the site of resection may contribute to the likelihood and rate of recovery of GI function. Normally, the jejunum does not contribute significantly to absorption of vitamin B_{12}, fat-soluble vitamins, or bile acids. In addition, transit time for food is more rapid in the jejunum than in the ileum. Thus, resection of the jejunum is better tolerated than resection of an equivalent length of ileum. An intact ileocecal valve, which allows normal intestinal emptying phases and less bacterial overgrowth of the ileum from reflux of colonic contents, also appears to improve the prognosis for recovery. Other important prognostic factors include the presence of disease in remaining segments and the age of the patient.[5]

Table 22-2. Relationship Between Length of Intestinal Remnant and Duration of Total Parenteral Nutrition

Group	N	Length of Small Bowel Remnant (cm)	Colon	Rectum	Duration of TPN (mo)
A	19	50-70	+	+	1-6
		80-150	+/−	+/−	
B	5	40-70	½	+	6-12
C	8	10-30	+/−	+/−	permanent
		<60	—	—	

From Gouttebel MC, et al. Total parenteral nutrition needs in different types of short bowel syndrome. Dig Dis Sci 31:718, 1986.
TPN, Total parenteral nutrition.

Clinical Manifestations and Natural History

The clinical characteristics of SBS result from maldigestion, malabsorption, dehydration, electrolyte abnormalities, and vitamin and nutrient deficiencies. Apart from these common clinical manifestations, massive enteral resection also disrupts the balance of circulating hormones and relationships between organs in the alimentary tract. At initial presentation, increased gastric acid secretion is common. This hypersecretion results from hypergastrinemia, which is presumably related to the loss of inhibitory hormones usually produced by the resected small-bowel segment.[5] This lower intraluminal pH causes impaired lipid degradation and can increase intestinal transit time. Gastric acid hypersecretion can be treated pharmacologically with H_2 blockers. The increased gastric acid secretion is temporary, typically resolving within 1 year.

Elevation of liver enzymes and serum bilirubin levels is also common in SBS, reflecting chronic liver disease and cirrhosis. The etiology of these liver abnormalities is not clear, and the body of literature on this topic is limited. It has been suggested that liver disease results from absorption of toxic by-products of bacterial metabolism.[5] In addition, cholesterol gallstones form in at least 30% of patients with SBS. Such stones appear to form because of the change in hepatic bile composition caused by interruption of the enterohepatic circulation, particularly in patients who have undergone ileal resection.[7] Patients requiring long-term TPN are also at risk for development of gallbladder sludge and acalculous cholecystitis.[7] The etiology of this latter complication reflects alterations in bile composition and gallbladder stasis.[7]

Other conditions encountered in the long term include renal calculi from increased colonic oxalate absorption and dehydration and osteomalacia from hypocalcemia and malabsorption of vitamin D. A rare but significant complication of SBS is D-lactic acidosis. This complication is observed when a patient with a short small bowel and an intact colon ingests large quantities of refined carbohydrates. The increased load of carbohydrate is not absorbed before reaching the colon and is metabolized by colonic bacteria to SCFAs and lactate. Acidification of luminal pH in the colon subsequently favors growth of anaerobic species (*Eubacterium, Bifidobacterium,* and *Lactobacillus* species) that produce D-lactate. This form of lactate is absorbed into the circulation and metabolized slowly, resulting in accumulation and systemic acidosis.[8] Neurologic manifestations include ophthalmoplegia, nystagmus, ataxia, and confusion. The patient seems intoxicated, but blood ethanol levels are normal. The diagnosis is made when serum D-lactate levels are found to be greater than 3 mmol/L (levels are normally undetectable).[8]

The natural history of patients with massive intestinal resection resulting in SBS has been simplified into three overlapping but clinically recognizable stages.[9] During stage I, patients have diarrhea, losing volumes of 2 to 3 L in eight to 10 bowel movements per day. Careful replacement of electrolytes, including calcium, magnesium, phosphate, and zinc, is imperative. Only TPN is tolerated at this stage, which typically lasts 1 to 3 months. Stage II, which lasts from a few months to longer than a year, requires prolonged parenteral and enteral nutritional adjustments. Oral intake is initiated and gradually increased. Parenteral support is tapered and then withdrawn when oral intake can exceed 2000 kcal/day without increase in diarrhea. Weight loss, anemia, and osteomalacia are common during this period. Finally, stage III occurs when maximal adaptation has been achieved. During this period, stable fluid and electrolyte losses and nutrient requirements are established. Some patients regain a relatively normal existence at this point; others must prepare to accommodate prolonged nutritional assistance with home TPN. The important lesson of this staging classification is that prognosis for recovery cannot always be assessed in the initial period after surgery. Recovery from massive enterectomy is slow and may continue as long as 2 years after operation.

Adaptation

Adaptation refers to recovery of digestive and absorptive functions that occurs in stage II after massive enteral resection. Clinical and experimental studies indicate that adaptation occurs in response to both luminal stimuli and alterations in the neurohumoral milieu. Recent work has focused on functional adaptation to such resections at the cellular and molecular levels. Lessons arising from studies performed at the bench are currently being applied in the management of these complex conditions.

Luminal Stimuli

The effects of luminal conditions on adaptation are well recognized.[10] After massive enteral resection, the remaining intestinal segments dilate and increase in length. Morphometric studies indicate that this increase in surface area is accompanied by hypertrophy of villous structures and proliferation of crypt cells.[1,5,11] Curiously, the former depends on exposure to pancreaticobiliary secretions stimulated by feeding, whereas the increase in crypt cell numbers seems to require the contents of gastroduodenal secretions, mediated through enterohormones such as epidermal growth factor (EGF).[1,5]

The composition of the chyme and luminal nutrients also contribute significantly to recovery of digestive and absorptive function. A group of French investigators demonstrated an early return to "enteral autonomy" when continuous enteral nutrition supplemented with tapioca was given within 2 weeks of bowel resection.[12] Tapioca increased the viscosity of the feeding, allowing increased intestinal transit time and thus increased time for absorption of nutrients. This study also suggested that elemental diets (predigested solutions that require no digestive effort from a short bowel) were associated with a slower intestinal adaptation than were polymeric diets supplemented with tapioca. It is unclear whether the inclusion of tapioca improves nutrient absorption on any basis other than simple slowing of intestinal transit. It is possible that a product of tapioca metabolism affects enterocyte activity, but as yet none has been identified. An additional supplement to enteral feeding that has been studied is pectin, a fermentable fiber. Pectin has been shown to delay gastric emptying and increase intestinal transit time, as well as to stimulate mucosal cell proliferation by itself and through its products of fermentation (SCFAs).[13]

Wilmore et al.,[14] in their extensive work in nutrition, demonstrated that supplemental enteral glutamine has hyperplastic effects in the mucosa of jejunum and ileum. This effect is also seen when glutamine is provided as a supplement to TPN. In studies in which enteral glutamine was implicated as responsible for the trophic effects, animals received either a glutamine-containing diet (glutamine as 25% of total amino acids) or an isocaloric and isonitrogenous diet lacking glutamine. These animals were studied after a 60% small intestine resection, and the glutamine-fed animals showed increased weight gain compared with the control animals. On light microscopic examination, the glutamine-fed animals had greater hyperplasia of the jejunum and ileum than did the control animals.[14]

Humoral Effects

Recent studies indicate that certain nutrients and biologically active substances are important in mucosal adaptation and regulation of GI functions after bowel resection. Many of these studies have led to advances in the therapeutic options available to clinicians and have allowed more complete provision of supplemental nutrition and pharmacologic assistance. One such substance is the amino acid glutamine. Initially, studies of the response to trauma and systemic stress identified marked increases in intestinal mucosal extraction of glutamine from the blood.[15] Further studies by Klimberg et al[16] demonstrated accelerated gut glutamine extraction after massive intestinal resection in rats. The importance of glutamine in the mucosal adaptive response was established when studies in rats demonstrated that administration of glutamine-enriched TPN was associated with trophic effects on intestinal mucosa, as compared with nonenriched but otherwise equivalent formulas.[17] TPN formulations enriched with glutamine also appear to attenuate the fluid retention and expansion of the extracellular compartment that accompany catabolic stress.[18] In addition, by virtue of its trophic effects on the mucosa, glutamine is thought to contribute to preservation of the integrity of the mucosal barrier of the GI tract, making bacterial translocation and sepsis less likely in patients under catabolic stress.[18]

In addition to the importance of amino acid composition of TPN formulas, it appears that the lipid composition can influence mucosal growth and adaptation after massive resection. Koruda et al.[19] demonstrated that the mucosal atrophy seen with TPN is reduced when SCFAs are added to TPN. This mucosal atrophy was studied in the rat intestine, assessing for mucosal weight, total protein, and DNA and RNA counts.

Recent work has also focused on circulating hormones or paracrine substances that regulate gastrointestinal mucosal function and motility and may influence recovery of these functions after massive intestinal resection. Secretion of circulating gastrin is increased in the initial period after such resections and is responsible for acid hypersecretion. Gastrin has well-recognized trophic effects on intestinal and colonic mucosa, and its role in early phases of adaptation after massive enterectomy is not known. Peptide YY (PYY) is a hormonal peptide released postprandially by endocrine L cells in the ileum and colon. Its well-recognized effects include inhibition of gastric acid secretion, delay of gastric emptying, slowing of intestinal transit time ("ileal brake"), and inhibition of pancreatic exocrine secretion.[8] A study by Bilchik et al.[20] examined the effects of PYY on water and electrolyte absorption in intact canine small bowel. They were able to demonstrate a dose-dependent increase in water and electrolyte absorption in both the ileum and jejunum in intact, unfed dogs when physiologic concentrations of PYY were administered intravenously. In further studies, they demonstrated that these increased absorptive effects were markedly augmented in fed dogs and postulated that PYY-agonists could have a therapeutic role in SBS, where intestinal absorption is reduced.[21] Finally, these investigators noted significant elevations of circulating PYY and expression of PYY messenger RNA in the intestinal mucosa in rats subjected to massive enterectomy.[22] These findings suggest that PYY could play an important role in mucosal adaptation after massive enterectomy, but further studies are needed to evaluate its trophic and proabsorptive effects in this setting.

Other potentially important circulating hormones in the adaptive response are neurotensin (NT) and enteroglucagon. NT has been studied extensively in this regard. This 13-residue peptide has been identified in discrete endocrine N cells distributed throughout the intestine, but with the highest concentration in the ileum.[23] Recent studies by Chung et al.[24] in animal models of massive intestinal resection demonstrated that exogenously administered NT accelerates intestinal regeneration. In addition, these investigators observed that NT affects mucosa growth and regeneration in more proximal intestinal segments (jejunum), but not in the ileum.[24]

More clinically oriented studies by Jacobs et al.[25] demonstrated a role for EGF as a therapeutic agent for patients with SBS. EGF, a substance produced by salivary gland tissue and by stem cells located in the intestinal crypts,[26] is a potent mitogen for intestinal mucosal cells. When given subcutaneously, EGF has trophic effects additive to those of glutamine on intestinal mucosa.[25]

Recently, anabolic hormone therapy has also been studied in clinical trials. Two recent studies suggest improved efficiency of TPN when recombinant growth hormone (GH) is given subcutaneously on a daily basis as a supplement to standard TPN.[27,28] In patients with gastrointestinal dysfunction receiving supplemental TPN, nutrient retention was improved when GH was given daily.[28] In addition, these investigators demonstrated a gain in lean body mass in patients treated with GH and TPN versus those receiving standard TPN alone. The patients studied gained more protein but less fat and had less expansion of their extracellular water compartment than did patients given standard TPN alone.[27] Such studies of exogenously administered EGF and GH do not necessarily implicate endogenous secretion of these hormones in the response to massive enterectomy. However, they do suggest the feasibility of identifying the neurohumoral responses to SBS and modulating their roles in mucosal growth and repair.

Enterocyte Adaptation

Although both luminal contents and circulating agents have been shown to have trophic effects on intestinal mucosa after bowel resection, the cellular and molecular responses of individual enterocytes to massive intestinal resection have also been a subject of increasing interest. Schulzke et al.[29] studied ileal remnants from rats after a 70% small intestinal resection. They observed a 250% increase in glucose-dependent electrogenic sodium absorption in ileal remnants. This increase was postulated to be due in part to increase in villus and microvillus surface area, but it may also have been influenced by increased ion transport rates of individual enterocytes.[29] Recent work by Hines et al.[30] focused on enterocyte adaptation on the molecular level. They demonstrated an upregulation of Na^+/glucose cotransporter messenger RNA in individual rat enterocytes from remaining ileum and jejunum after massive intestinal resection.[30] They also observed an upregulation of Na^+/K^+ adenosine triphosphatase in enterocytes from rats subjected to a 70% small-bowel resection.[31] With regard to amino acid transport, Menguy et al.[32] reported net increases in amino acid transport in rat enterocytes in SBS. However, in vesicles isolated from rabbit enterocytes, Sarac et al.[33] recently reported that such increases in enterocyte glucose and amino acid transport do not occur as quickly, despite histologic evidence of mucosal hypertrophy and hyperplasia. These authors noted that rats adapt quickly to SBS, whereas rabbits do not. Thus, experimental models are currently being developed to evaluate why adaptation occurs relatively quickly in some circumstances but not others. Further studies are needed to evaluate whether such differences reside at the cellular level or are caused by differences in neurohumoral milieu after massive enterectomy.

Management

The management of SBS is best conceptualized in the context of the three phases described previously. Initially, massive enterectomy is managed with the patient receiving no oral nutrition, fluid, or electrolytes. Intravenous fluid management must take into account maintenance as well as ongoing losses from fistulas, stomas, or early postoperative diarrhea. In many cases, management is complicated by ongoing intra-abdominal sepsis and by respiratory, hepatic, or renal failure. TPN is the mainstay of therapy in this early, acute phase. However, initiation of enteral feeding as early as is possible in the postresection period is advantageous.[34]

Enteral Feeding

Once a patient begins oral feeding, diet planning must include adequate oral fluid intake to account for losses. Several elecytrolyte-containing isotonic drinks are available, and these are useful for patients with SBS. As detailed previously, early institution of enteral feeding is beneficial, and additives, including glutamine, tapioca, and pectin, are of great benefit. Not only does early enteral feeding allow timely onset of the mucosal adaptive process, it also has been shown to be protective against postoperative sepsis. A meta-analysis by Moore et al.[35] demonstrated that surgical patients at high risk who were provided early postoperative enteral feeding had a lower incidence of postoperative septic complications than did those receiving standard TPN. Although most patients in this study were victims of trauma, and not affected by SBS, an extrapolation to the subgroup of patients recovering from a procedure resulting in SBS seems reasonable.

A prospective study by Messing et al.[36] revealed that patients adapt to enteral autonomy by consuming a hypercaloric, hyperprotein diet and use this as compensation for their increased fecal losses. They were also able to demonstrate a larger net absorption of carbohydrate compared with fat and protein. From their data, they were able to suggest that patients have a goal of net consumption of food equivalent to 2.5 times their basal energy expenditure. Woolf et al.[37] further characterized diet recommendations for patients with SBS. After studying patients who had been in clinically stable condition from a nutritional standpoint for at least a year, they proposed a diet that included an oral intake of 35 to 40 kcal/kg/day, with 80 to 100 g protein/day to counteract losses and maintain a positive nitrogen balance.

Dietary supervision is an important aspect of management. However, the clinician must constantly be aware of changes in nutritional needs as the patient adapts to SBS. The prolonged nature of this process was reviewed recently in the pediatric population, and a minimal period of 2 years was recommended before more radical intervention, such as intestinal transplantation, is entertained.[38] In addition, evidence that adaptation is still occurring at 2 years in the adult population was provided by Gouttebel et al.[39] in a recent study of calcium absorption in patients with SBS. They demonstrated continual increases in calcium absorption extending more than 2 years after major intestinal resection. Thus, both patient and clinician must be prepared for a prolonged period of dynamic nutritional needs after massive intestinal resection.

Pharmacologic Assistance

Pharmacologic interventions include antimotility agents, such as loperamide and codeine, to slow intestinal transit time; cholestyramine to bind bile salts and diminish diarrhea related to colonic irritation by bile salts; and H_2 blockers to inhibit increased gastric acid secretion.[1,5] Somatostatin, or its analog octreotide, has been used with success in diminishing small-bowel fistula output[40] and has been applied to patients with high intestinal output related to SBS to decrease sodium, potassium, and volume output.[41] Octreotide has proabsorptive effects on small-bowel mucosa through direct effects on intestinal ionic transport.[42] With a longer half-life than somatostatin, octreotide is highly bioavailable when given subcutaneously; recommended dosing 100 μg every 8 hours.[40] Human trials of exogenous PYY have not yet begun, but this too may prove beneficial in its proabsorptive effects. As discussed previously, exogenously administered EGF and GH may provide significant acceleration of the process of adaptation and hasten independence from TPN in a great many cases.

Surgical Treatment

Although surgical intervention is the culprit in causing SBS, in some cases return to the operating room can allow clinical improvement. Such interventions must be carefully considered, however, and less invasive measures are often warranted. The goal of surgical treatment of SBS is generally to increase either transit time or surface area.

Intestinal Lengthening

An isoperistaltic intestinal lengthening procedure was first described by Bianchi in 1980 and has since been applied successfully to limited numbers of patients in the pediatric population.[43] Reversed intestinal segments and colonic interposition have also been attempted for limited numbers of patients to slow peristalsis and increase absorption.[44]

Procedures to Increase Intestinal Absorption

Recirculating intestinal loops were conceived on the theory that enteral contents could recirculate several times prior to proceeding distally, thus enhancing absorption. In clinical practice, however, the results have not been encouraging, with high morbidity for little noted efficacy.[44] The presence of the ileocecal valve improves outcome in patients with SBS, leading to the development of surgical techniques for the construction of intestinal valves.[44] Others have suggested procedures to provide reversed electric intestinal pacing, theorized to initiate peristalsis in a retrograde direction.[44] Serosal patching is directed toward increasing mucosal surface area. Through patching of intestinal defects with colon serosa, abdominal wall, or prosthetic materials, an increase in absorptive surface area is gained through the growth of neomucosa on these surfaces.[45,46] The growth of neomucosa has been shown to be vigorous in experimental animals who have undergone massive enteric resection compared with those undergoing patching but not any resection.[45] The recommended timing of patching is at some point distinct from the initial resection. An increased risk of postoperative complications is possible, and patching has been shown to be successful in animals when performed 3 months after the initial resection.[46]

Tapering Enteroplasty

As one of the adaptive processes, bowel remaining after massive resection is known to dilate. Studies have shown that ineffective peristalsis occurs in these dilated segments as a result of failure of apposition of the bowel wall during contraction. The goal of tapering enteroplasty is to reduce the caliber of the bowel while preserving its length, thus enhancing peristaltic action.[44] This technique has seen more use and success among pediatric patients with SBS.

Small Bowel Transplantation

Perhaps the most promising operative intervention for the future is small bowel transplantation. Patients who are dependent on TPN but have problems with restricted venous access or catheter-related infections are the most likely candidates.[47] The harmful metabolic sequelae of long-term TPN, including liver impairment and metabolic bone disease, also make small bowel transplantation a liberating option. This is particularly true for children, whose long-term mortality with TPN (15%) is higher than that for adults.[48] Infection and malignancy are the only two absolute contraindications to bowel transplantation at this point.[49] The condition of the patient's liver must be assessed, and consideration of combined liver-bowel transplantation should be entertained. Multiple previous laparotomies complicate the procedure but are not considered a contraindication; indeed, many patients who have had failure of other operative procedures aimed at improving intestinal absorption often are candidates for transplantation. In the largest series reported to date, age of recipients ranged from 0.5 to 58 years, with the patients equally divided among adult and pediatric age groups. Among the 45 patients in that series, cumulative 1-year patient survival was 82%. Thirteen of the 45 patients in the series died, with postoperative deaths attributable to acute rejection and sepsis, lymphoproliferative disorders, pneumonia, or TPN catheter–related pulmonary embolus.[49] The process is accompanied by immunologic difficulties because the small bowel is rich in lymphoid tissue, increasing the incidence of graft-versus-host disease in recipients. Cyclosporine and the newer immunosuppressive agent FK 506 have allowed improved outcomes, both experimentally and clinically.[50] Paradoxically, the greatest challenge in the development of transplantation as an option in SBS management remains the identification of those patients who cannot achieve enteral "independence" by any other means.

THE BLIND-LOOP SYNDROME

Etiology

This syndrome can be precipitated by both postsurgical and nonsurgical states. Afferent loop stasis after Billroth II resection, presence of a continent ileostomy after colectomy, jejunoileal bypass, and loss of the ileocecal valve can all predispose toward blind-loop syndrome. Nonsurgical etiologies include strictures (as in Crohn's disease), fistulas, diverticuli, motility disorders (e.g., scleroderma, diabetes), and achlorhydria. Each of these etiologies has as a contributing factor either a state of allowing stasis or decreased acid production.

Pathophysiology

Blind-loop syndrome, synonymous with *bacterial overgrowth syndrome, stagnant loop syndrome,* and *contaminated small bowel syndrome,* is a state of malabsorption precipitated by stasis in the small bowel that allows increased replication and density of intestinal flora. There is a shift in the predominance of flora toward that more typical of the colonic environment, with increased gram-positive bacteria and facultative anaerobes. This results in hydrolysis and inactivation of bile salts and in competition for vitamins, especially B_{12}. A decrease in gastric acid secretion, with subsequent diminished bactericidal acid activity, can also facilitate creation of this overgrowth state. Malabsorption in blind-loop syndrome may be profound, yet the histologic examination of mucosa from affected segments is sometimes initially unimpressive. The brush borders and enterocytes appear unaffected according to light microscopy, yet higher-resolution examination shows the presence of swollen mitochondria and lipid deposits, suggesting altered intracellular processing.[51]

Presentation and Diagnosis

The clinical presentation varies according to the underlying etiology. Typically, patients have steatorrhea, weight loss, and fat-soluble vitamin deficiencies. A vitamin B_{12} deficiency syndrome is also common, resulting in a macrocytic anemia. Diagnosis begins with a high index of suspicion in the case of a patient with diarrhea, crampy abdominal pain, weight loss, and anemia who has a condition predisposing toward bacterial overgrowth. The tests useful in confirming a diagnosis of blind-loop syndrome vary, and generally the test that is least invasive and most readily available is used. Radiologic examination can confirm motility disorders or the presence of a blind intestinal loop. Barium studies, including enteroclysis, have proved particularly useful in these cases.[52,53]

Stool studies to demonstrate fat malabsorption or steatorrhea are helpful. A triolein breath test with carbon 14 that has been developed can eliminate the need in selected populations for traditional stool studies and determine, with sensitivity of 85% and specificity of 93%, the presence of fat malabsorption. The test shows decreased specificity in patients with concomitant obesity, diabetes, thyroid disease, or pulmonary disease, in whom the metabolism of absorbed [^{14}C]triolein or the excretion of breath [^{14}C]carbon dioxide may be impaired.[54]

Detection of inadequate absorption and excessive breakdown of bile acids can be achieved with a [^{14}C]cholylglycine-labeled bile acid breath test. This test can detect the increased bacterial deconjugation of bile salts in the colon, common in ileal resections, but cannot distinguish steatorrhea from choleric enteropathy (diarrhea from the irritative effects of deconjugated bile acids on colonic mucosa).[55]

A macrocytic anemia with a depressed serum vitamin B_{12} level suggests B_{12} deficiency. In bacterial overgrowth, this is caused by bacterial use of B_{12}, making less available for mucosal absorption. This can be distinguished from the B_{12} deficiency of pernicious anemia by means of a Schilling test. In this study, a small dose of radiolabeled vitamin B_{12} is given orally. Two hours later, a large "flushing" dose of unlabeled vitamin B_{12} is given intramuscularly, resulting in saturation of normal binding sites in plasma and renal excretion of that portion of radiolabeled B_{12} that had not been absorbed. A 24-hour urine collection is then analyzed for vitamin B_{12}, and malabsorption can be determined if less than 9% of the orally administered radioactive dose is recovered in the first 24-hour urine sample. Such a result in this stage of the test can be caused by pernicious anemia (lack of intrinsic factor), a paucity of ileal resorptive sites for vitamin B_{12}, or B_{12} malabsorption caused by bacterial overgrowth. To distinguish among these processes, a stage II test is performed in which intrinsic factor is given along with the dose of radioactive vitamin B_{12}. Normalization of the amount of B_{12} absorbed indicates pernicious anemia. Some laboratories advocate a stage III test to distinguish between bacterial overgrowth and lack of resorptive sites for B_{12} by administering antibiotics for 2 weeks to eradicate organisms causative in blind-loop syndrome prior to repetition of the stage I portion of the test.[56] (The following section on management gives recommended antibiotic coverage.) Table 22-3 summarizes the tests useful in diagnosing blind-loop syndrome.

Management

Clinical management of blind-loop syndrome includes replacement of nutritional deficits (vitamin B_{12} and fat-soluble vitamins) and antibiotic therapy. Aspiration of small-bowel contents for culture is not imperative but can help direct therapy; many institutions treat patients empirically with antibiotics directed toward *Bacteroides fragilis,* enterococci, *Escherichia coli,* and anaerobic lactobacilli bacilli because these are the organisms most commonly isolated in affected patients.[55] Antibiotic therapy is applied for 2 to 4 weeks; treatment can be reinstituted if relapse occurs. In particularly difficult cases, "pulse therapy" (1 week of antibiotic therapy every month) has been used with some success.[55] In selected patients with a chronically relapsing condition and clear surgically correctable lesion, such as stricture from Crohn's disease, operative intervention may be the best recourse.

POUCHITIS

Definition

Pouchitis, also called *acute reservoir ileitis,* occurs in patients with a continent ileal reservoir created by ileal pouch–anal anastamosis at the time of total colectomy (for ulcerative colitis, familial polyposis, etc.). It is a nonspecific idiopathic inflammation of the pouch mucosa that manifests by sudden increase in bowel movements (sometimes with blood), fecal incontinence, pelvic or low abdominal pain, and fever. Such inflammation occurs almost exclusively in patients undergoing surgery for ulcerative colitis and is extremely uncommon in patients undergoing surgery for familial polyposis. It has been recognized after construction of continent abdominal wall (Koch) pouches as well as anal pouches. Such inflammation and its attendant symptoms are not seen in patients where the pouch is used for urinary diversion.

Studies report an incidence of about 20%, ranging from 11% to 29%, with disparity possibly relating to length of follow-up and patient population studied.[57-59] Some investigators have suggested that the variable occurrence of pouchitis is related to the underlying disease process, with it being more common in patients who have undergone ileal pouch–anal anastamosis for ulcerative colitis as opposed to familial polyposis.[58] In addition, a male preponderance and concomitant presence of extraintestinal manifestations of the underlying disease have been noted.[60]

Contributing Factors and Pathophysiology

The rather high incidence of pouchitis among patients with chronic ulcerative colitis has led investigators to seek the factors that contribute to its development, in hopes of manipulating variables to decrease morbidity. Some clinicians have suggested that pouchitis may actually be a recurrence of the ulcerative colitis because histologic studies have shown colonic metaplasia in the pouches of affected individuals, particularly those with chronic pouchitis.[61] Further studies suggest that refractory pouchitis is an immunologic phenomenon because it frequently affects individuals with extraintestinal manifestations of ulcerative colitis, such as arthritis, and skin and eye changes.[60]

Studies of pouch size, stricture influencing outflow, and efficiency of pouch emptying have implicated stasis as a variable in the development of pouchitis. Careful surgical attention during pouch construction can help minimize stasis. Specifically, pouch sizes 150 cc in volume have been associated with a lower incidence of pouchitis than larger

Table 22-3. Tests Useful in Diagnosing Blind-Loop Syndrome

Test	Rationale
Radiologic study	Confirms presence of blind intestinal loop or motility disorder
Stool study	Demonstrates fat malabsorption by quantifying fecal fat
Triolein breath test	Detects fat malabsorption; test performed by injestion of [^{14}C]triolein with known quantity of fat; [^{14}C]carbon dioxide is detected in breath and expressed as percentage of the known dose of fat ingested
Bile acid breath test	Detects inadequate absorption and excessive breakdown of bile acids; uses [^{14}C]cholylglycine, which undergoes conversion to [^{14}C]carbon dioxide by bacterial deconjugation in the colon if ileal absorption sites are absent or diseased
Schilling test	Used to distinguish vitamin B_{12} deficiency caused by malabsorption from that caused by pernicious anemia
Aspiration of small bowel contents for culture	Suggestive of blind-loop syndrome if bacterial counts $>10^7$ microorganisms/μl; can be used to direct antibiotic therapy

(380 cc) pouches. The smaller size is believed to decrease stasis through more frequent and possibly more complete pouch emptying. In addition, outflow stricture is less likely if anastomoses are widely patent and exit sleeves are not excessively long.[57]

Analysis of stool from affected individuals has led to multiple hypotheses regarding pouchitis etiology. It has been suggested that bacterial overgrowth is responsible; others note no difference in bacterial density in affected versus control patients.[62] Further, a shift in the bacterial content toward aerobes has been noted, as well as a rise in the intraluminal pH of pouch contents, possibly influencing activity of pouch enzymes and resulting in a disruption of the protective mucous layer over the mucosal epithelium.[59] An analysis of SCFAs has revealed their decrease in stool of individuals with pouchitis, with the cause hypothesized to be a decreased concentration of the fermentable saccharides in affected pouches.[63]

Without definitive knowledge of the etiology of pouchitis, retrospective studies have been used in the attempt to implicate mechanisms. It is recognized that empirical therapy with metronidazole (Flagyl) improves symptoms in most patients. Paradoxically, it has not been possible to demonstrate a change in pouch bacterial density after treatment with metronidazole. In addition, although one study showed an improvement in histologic changes after treatment with metronidazole, another showed no efficacy greater than placebo effect.[62,64] The immunosuppressive actions of metronidazole have been suggested as key, yet similar symptomatic improvement has been noted with ciprofloxacin, which lacks these actions.[64]

Finally, the possibility of ischemia being related to pouchitis has been raised. The technical aspects of pouch creation, with movement of the intestinal pouch to a point low in the pelvis and potential for tension on both pouch-anal anastamosis and mesenteric blood supply, can predispose the pouch toward ischemia. Additionally, intermittent emptying of the pouch, with wall tension varying according to volume in the pouch, can result in intermittent episodes of wall ischemia. The possibilities that a reperfusion injury with creation of oxygen free radicals is involved led to a study of Levin et al.[65] in which allopurinol (an inhibitor of free-radical formation) was given enterally to patients with an acute episode of pouchitis. The treatment proved successful by symptomatic criteria, thus furthering the notion that free-radical formation arising from ischemia of the pouch wall may contribute to the pathophysiology of pouchitis.

Presentation and Diagnosis

Pouchitis is diagnosed on the basis of clinical, endoscopic, and histologic criteria; each of these can be suggestive of disease severity and used to track responses to therapeutic measures. However, there appears to be an inconsistent correlation between endoscopic and histologic findings and the clinical severity of the disease.

Endoscopically, swelling, erythema, and friability of the mucosa are noted; in moderate to severe cases, superficial ulceration that can progress to necrosis and copious mucopurulent exudate are noted.[58] Histologically, chronic inflammatory changes with villous atrophy are common, although some degree of inflammation has been noted in most pouches, regardless of whether the patient has clinical pouchitis. In cases where extensive inflammatory cell infiltration as well as crypt abscesses and ulcerations are seen histologically, there is a strong correlation with clinical symptomatology. Yet, because endoscopic and histologic findings do not always correlate with the clinical symptoms, many advocate relying on clinical presentation alone for diagnosis.[58]

Management

The management of pouchitis is thus based on both anecdotal and scientifically supported measures. A patient who has the symptoms of pouchitis can be treated empirically with either metronidazole or ciprofloxacin for a period of 1 to 2 weeks; some patients with relapsing episodes may require long-term low-dose "suppression" therapy with metronidazole. Additionally, steroids, allopurinol, cyclosporine enemas, and agents commonly used to control ulcerative colitis symptoms (salazopyrine or 5-aminosalicylic acid) have all been used, with some symptomatic relief.[58] Finally, in cases of chronic, unremitting symptoms of pouchitis, surgical correction of factors contributing to pouch stasis (size or anastomotic stricture) or even surgical removal of the pouch may be required.

DIVERSION COLITIS

Definition

A nonspecific inflammatory process can occur in segments of colon from which the fecal stream has been diverted. Termed *diversion colitis,* this entity was first recognized little more than a decade ago. Clinically, a patient may have crampy abdominal pain, mucous discharge, or rectal bleeding; the condition also may be totally asymptomatic.[66] Two prospective studies of patients undergoing colostomy closures, none of whom carried the diagnosis of inflammatory bowel disease, were done to investigate the incidence of diversion colitis. The patients studied had undergone colostomy creation for trauma, diverticulitis, cancer, protection of an anastamosis, or diversion of a fecal fistula. In one study, 70% of patients showed endoscopic evidence, histologic evidence, or both of diversion colitis; in the other study, this figure was 76%.[66,67] Importantly, none of these patients reported symptoms suggestive of diversion colitis. These authors concluded that diversion colitis is a common subclinical problem.

On gross examination, the affected colonic segment may show erythema, friability, edema, nodularity, and ulcerations. Histologically, nonspecific inflammation, crypt abscesses, mucin granulomas, and, as a hallmark, lymphoid hyperplasia are seen.[66] Because of the clinical, gross, and histologic findings, this process can be confused with inflammatory bowel disease, and clear distinction between the two is mandatory because the treatment modalities are radically different.

Pathophysiology and Colonocyte Nutrition

Diversion colitis raises important points about mucosal nutrition and the variables important in maintenance of colonocyte homeostasis. Colonic mucosa receives approximately 70% of its energy substrates from the lumen, most in the form of SCFAs produced by anaerobic fermentation of polysaccharides by bacteria.[68,69] The mechanism by which the colonic mucosa adapts to nutritional deprivation was investigated by Firmansyab et al.[69] In this study, rats were subjected to nutritional deprivation, and isolated colonocytes from these animals were compared with those from control animals. Colonocytes from malnourished animals showed a reduction in oxidative metabolism for all substrates except butyrate. The mechanism of this was unclear and perhaps related to a decreased cellular uptake of substrates or to alterations in catabolic enzyme activities. The functional significance of this altered energy metabolism was not proved in this study but was hypothesized to be sizable because the role of the colon in reabsorption of water and electrolytes requires energy.

The importance of butyrate, one of the SCFAs produced by fermentation of saccharides by bacteria, as a fuel source for colonocytes was investigated by Chapman et al.[68] They demonstrated that butyrate was a fuel source for colonocytes preferred to glutamine or glucose when provided in incubation to isolated colonocytes from healthy individuals. The use of the three substrates was followed through to CO_2 through a 2-hour period. They were able to demonstrate a significantly higher oxidation rate for butyrate, followed by glutamine and then glucose.

Luminal nutrients and bacteria to ferment those nutrients are necessary to maintain colonic mucosal integrity. Deprivation of butyrate for colonocytes to use as energy allows a nonspecific inflammatory process to affect colonic mucosa, resulting in friability and ulceration in the mucosal layer.[70] This process can be reversed by provision of SCFA irrigation over the affected mucosa, or simply by reconstitution of intestinal integrity to allow passage of the fecal stream over the affected segment. Fig. 22-3 is a pictorial summary of what colonocytes and enterocytes require for nutritional maintenance.

Management

For diversion colitis, all that is required to reverse the inflammatory process is reconstitution of the fecal stream. Clinical application of the knowledge that SCFAs, specifically butyrate, were important in colonocyte nutrition was performed by Harig et al.[70] In that study, patients with symptomatic diversion colitis were treated by irrigation of the affected colonic segments with a solution containing SCFAs. In the patients studied, the excluded colonic segments showed a notable absence of bacterial fermentation that would produce SCFAs. A twice-daily instillation of SCFAs for 4 to 6 weeks resulted in endoscopic and clinical improvement in the colitis, providing further evidence for the notion that colonocytes require SCFAs for maintenance of homeostatic mechanisms. For patients in whom reversal is not possible, instillation of SCFAs may produce symptomatic relief. Other aspects of medical management include corticosteroid enemas and oral steroids.[71] Results with steroids are mixed. Similarly, metronidazole has been beneficial to varying degrees.[71]

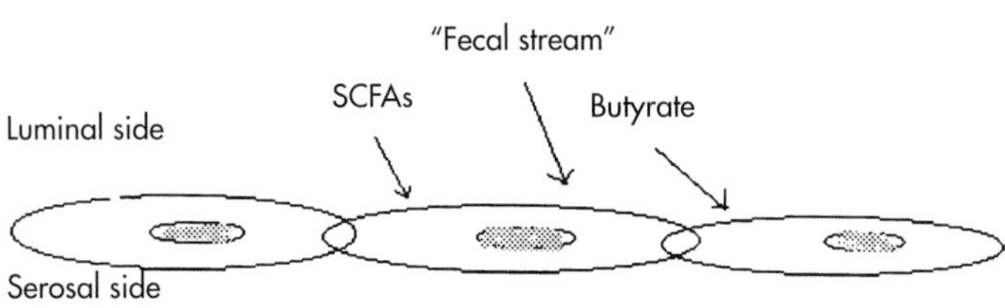

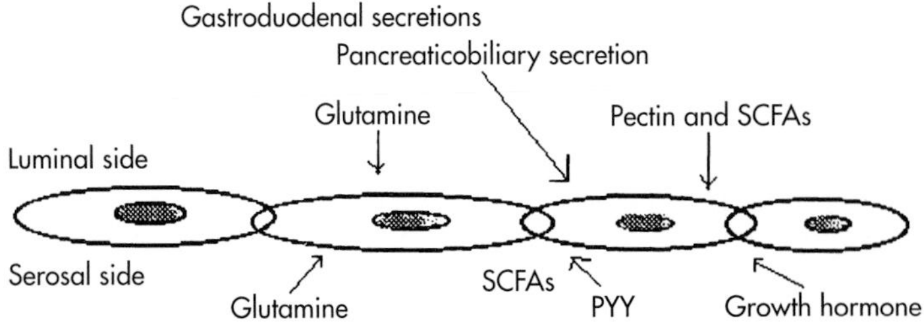

Fig. 22-3. Summary of substances involved in colonocyte and enterocyte nutrition. *PYY,* Peptide YY; SCFA, short-chain fatty acid.

CONCLUSION

The concept of GI dysfunction is evolving. Its components include alterations in secretory and absorptive functions, alterations in motility and peristalsis, and disturbances in luminal ecology and mucosal immune function. In this chapter, we reviewed syndromes that result from removal of large segments of small intestine, diversion of luminal contents from significant segments of small or large intestine, or creation of artificial organs for storage and emptying of feculent material. Management of SBS requires a detailed understanding of the extended natural history of the adaptation of remaining segments to loss of absorptive surface area and sudden alterations in the neurohumoral milieu that regulated gut function before the resection. Management of complications of procedures that create stasis or divert luminal contents requires an appreciation of mucosal-bacterial interactions and mechanisms that mediate the mucosal inflammatory response. We are just beginning to understand the nutritional needs of individual enterocytes and colonocytes, and the roles that bacteria play in normal enteric mucosal and motor functions. Further advances in these areas should improve our ability to manage the different syndromes that result in postoperative GI dysfunction.

REFERENCES

1. Obermayer-Pietsch BM, Krejs GJ. Short gut syndrome. In Bouchier IA, et al., eds. Gastroenterology: Clinical Science and Practice. London: WB Saunders, 1993.
2. Chopra S, Trier JS. Diarrhea and malabsorption. In Chopra S, May RJ, eds. Pathophysiology of Gastrointestinal Diseases. Boston: Little, Brown, 1989.
3. Spiller RC. Digestion and malabsorption of vitamins. In Bouchier IA, et al., eds. Gastroenterology: Clinical Science and Practice. London: WB Saunders, 1993.
4. Welch JP. Pathophysiology of bowel obstruction. In Bowel Obstruction: Differential Diagnosis and Clinical Management. Philadelphia: WB Saunders, 1990.
5. Rate AJ, Irving M. Short bowel syndrome. In Bayless TM, ed. Current Therapy in Gastroenterology and Liver Disease. St. Louis: Mosby, 1994.
6. Gouttebel MC, et al. Total parenteral nutrition needs in different types of short bowel syndrome. Dig Dis Sci 31:718, 1986.
7. Roslyn JJ, et al. Gallbladder disease in patients on long-term parenteral nutrition. Gastroenterology 84:148, 1983.
8. Westergaard H, Spady DK. Short bowel syndrome. In Sleisenger MH, Fordtran JS, eds. Gastrointestinal Disease. Philadelphia: WB Saunders, 1993.
9. Tilson MD. Pathophysiology and treatment of short bowel syndrome. Surg Clin North Am 60:1273, 1980.
10. Dowling RH. Intestinal adaptation. N Engl J Med 288:520, 1973.
11. Wilmore DW, et al. The role of nutrition in the adaptation of the small intestine after massive resection. Surg Gynecol Obstet 132:673, 1971.
12. Levy E, et al. Continuous enteral nutrition during the early adaptive stage of the short bowel syndrome. Br J Surg 75:549, 1988.
13. Allard JP, Jeejeebhoy KN. Nutritional support and therapy in the short bowel syndrome. Gastroenterol Clin North Am 18:589, 1989.
14. Wilmore DW, et al. The gut: A central organ after surgical stress. Surgery 104:917, 1988.
15. Souba WW, Wilmore DW. Postoperative alteration of arteriovenous exchange of amino acids across the gastrointestinal tract. Surgery 94:342, 1983.
16. Klimberg VS, et al. Intestinal glutamine metabolism after massive small bowel resection. Am J Surg 159:27, 1990.
17. O'Dwyer ST, et al. Maintenance of small bowel mucosa with glutamine-enriched parenteral nutrition. JPEN J Parenter Enter Nutr 13:579, 1989.
18. Scheltinga MR, et al. Glutamine-enriched intravenous feedings attenuate extracellular fluid expansion after a standard stress. Ann Surg 214:385, 1991.
19. Koruda MJ, et al. Effect of parenteral nutrition supplemented with short-chain fatty acids on adaptation to massive small bowel resection. Gastroenterology 95:715, 1988.
20. Bilchik AJ, et al. Peptide YY is a physiological regulator of water and electrolyte absorption in the canine small bowel in vivo. Gastroenterology 105:1441, 1993.
21. Bilchik AJ, et al. Peptide YY augments postprandial small intestinal absorption in the conscious dog. Am J Surg 167:570, 1994.
22. Bilchik AJ, et al. Peptide YY gene expression is an early adaptive response to massive small bowel resection. Surg Forum 44:126, 1993.
23. Izukura M, et al. Neurotensin augments intestinal regeneration after small bowel resection in rats. Ann Surg 215:520, 1992.
24. Chung D, et al. Differential trophic effects of neurotensin on small bowel mucosa. Surg Forum 42:128, 1991.
25. Jacobs DO, et al. Combined effects of glutamine and epidermal growth factor on the rat intestine. Surgery 104:358, 1988.
26. Wright NA, Pike C, Elia G. Induction of a novel epidermal growth factor-secreting cell lineage by mucosal ulceration in human gastrointestinal stem cells. Nature 343:82, 1990.
27. Byrne TA, et al. Anabolic therapy with growth hormone accelerates protein gain in surgical patients requiring nutritional rehabilitation. Ann Surg 218:400, 1993.
28. Ziegler TR, et al. Recombinant human growth hormone enhances the metabolic efficacy of parenteral nutrition: A double-blind, randomized controlled study. J Clin Endocrinol Metab 74:865, 1992.
29. Schulzke J, et al. Ion transport in the experimental short bowel syndrome of the rat. Gastroenterology 102:497, 1992.
30. Hines OJ, et al. Adaptation of Na+/glucose cotransporter following intestinal resection. J Surg Res 57:22, 1994.
31. Hines OJ, et al. Up-regulation of Na+, K+ adenosine triphosphatase after massive intestinal resection. Surgery 116:401, 1994.
32. Menguy R, Supulveda FV, Smith MW. Cellular adaptation of amino acid transport following intestinal resection in the rat. J Physiol 334:213, 1983.
33. Sarac TP, et al. Massive enterectomy alters brush-border amino acid and glucose transport. Surg Forum 45:184, 1994.
34. Bernard DKH, Shaw MJ. Principles of nutrition therapy for short bowel syndrome. Nutr Clin Pract 8:153, 1993.
35. Moore FA, et al. Early enteral feeding, compared with parenteral, reduces postoperative septic complications. Ann Surg 216:172, 1992.
36. Messing B, et al. Intestinal absorption of free oral hyperalimentation in the very short bowel syndrome. Gastroenterology 100:1502, 1991.
37. Woolf GM, et al. Nutritional absorption in short bowel syndrome. Dig Dis Sci 32:8, 1987.
38. Kurkchubasche AG, et al. Adaptation in short bowel syndrome: reassessing old limits. J Pediatr Surg 28:1069, 1993.
39. Gouttebel MC, et al. Intestinal adaptation in patients with short bowel syndrome. Dig Dis Sci 34:709, 1989.
40. Nubioloa-Calonge P, et al. Blind evaluation of the effect of octreotide (SMS 201-995), a somatostatin analogue, on small bowel fistula output. Lancet 2:672, 1987.
41. Nightingale JMD, et al. Short bowel syndrome. Digestion 45:77, 1990.
42. Anthone GJ, et al. Direct proabsorptive effect of octreotide on ionic transport in the small intestine. Surgery 108:1136, 1990.
43. Pokorny WJ, et al. Isoperistaltic intestinal lengthening for short bowel syndrome. Surg Gynecol Obstet 172:39, 1991.

44. Warner BW, Chaet MS. Nontransplant surgical options for management of the short bowel syndrome. J Pediatr Gastroenterol Nutr 17:1, 1993.
45. Bragg LE, Thompson JS. The influence of intestinal resection on the growth of intestinal neomucosa. J Surg Res 46:306, 1989.
46. Thompson JS. Growth of neomucosa after intestinal resection. Arch Surg 122:316, 1987.
47. Grant D. Intestinal transplantation: Current status. Transplant Proc 21:2869, 1989.
48. Schraut WH. Current status of small bowel transplantation. Gastroenterology 94:525, 1988.
49. Tzakis AG, et al. Intestinal transplantation. Annu Rev Med 45:79, 1994.
50. Starzl TE, et al. The many faces of multivisceral transplantation. Surg Gynecol Obstet 172:335, 1991.
51. Chadwick VS. Mechanisms of malabsorption and diarrhea. In Bouchier IA, et al., eds. Gastroenterology: Clinical Science and Practice. London: WB Saunders, 1993.
52. Herlinger H. Small bowel barium examination. In Gore RM, Levine MS, Laufer I, eds. Textbook of Gastrointestinal Radiology. Philadelphia: WB Saunders, 1994.
53. Schlegel DM, Maglinte DDT. The blind pouch syndrome. Surg Gynecol Obstet 155:541, 1982.
54. Turner JM, et al. [^{14}C]-Triolein absorption: A useful test in the diagnosis of malabsorption. Gut 28:694, 1987.
55. Carey WD. Malabsorption. In Achkar E, Farmer RG, Fleshler B, eds. Clinical Gastroenterology. Philadelphia: Lea & Febiger, 1992.
56. Nickoloff E. Schilling test: Physiologic basis for and use as a diagnostic test. Crit Rev Clin Lab Sci 26:263, 1988.
57. Fischer JE, et al. The pull-through procedure: Technical factors in influencing outcome, with emphasis on pouchitis. Surgery 114:828, 1993.
58. Fozard BJ, et al. Results of pouch surgery after ileo-anal anastomosis: The implications of pouchitis. World J Surg 16:880, 1992.
59. Ruseler-van Embden JGH, et al. Pouchitis: Result of microbial imbalance? Gut 35:658, 1994.
60. Subramani K, et al. Refractory pouchitis: Does it reflect underlying Crohn's disease? Gut 34:1539, 1993.
61. Luukkonen P, et al. Pouchitis—Recurrence of the inflammatory bowel disease? Gut 35:243, 1994.
62. Kmiot WA, et al. Mucosal morphology, cell proliferation and faecal bacteriology in acute pouchitis. Br J Surg 80:1445, 1993.
63. Clausen MR, et al. Short-chain fatty acids in pouch contents from patients with and without pouchitis after ileal pouch-anal anastamosis. Gastroenterology 103:1144, 1992.
64. Madden MV, et al. Double-blind crossover trial of metronidazole versus placebo in chronic unremitting pouchitis. Dig Dis Sci 39:1193, 1994.
65. Levin KE, et al. Role of oxygen free radicals in the etiology of pouchitis. Dis Colon Rectum 35:452, 1992.
66. Ferguson CM, Siegel RJ. A prospective evaluation of diversion colitis. Am Surg 57:46, 1991.
67. Orsay CP, et al. Diversion colitis in patients scheduled for colostomy closure. Dis Colon Rectum 36:366, 1993.
68. Chapman MAS, et al. New technique to measure mucosal metabolism and its use to map substrate utilization in the healthy human large bowel. Br J Surg 80:445, 1993.
69. Firmansyab A, et al. Isolated colonocyte metabolism of glucose, glutamine, *N*-butyrate, and beta-hydroxybutyrate in malnutrition. Gastroenterology 97:622, 1989.
70. Harig JM, et al. Treatment of diversion colitis with short-chain fatty acid irrigation. N Engl J Med 320:23, 1989.
71. Ernest DL, Schneiderman DJ. Other diseases of the colon and rectum. In Sleisenger MH, Fordtran JS, eds. Gastrointestinal Disease. Philadelphia: WB Saunders, 1989.

23

Hepatic Physiology

James H. Clark III and R. Patrick Wood

The liver has occupied an important place in history since the beginning of recorded time. As early as 2400 BC in ancient Babylon the liver from a sacrificed sheep was used in divination rituals. A particular question was asked and an answer gleaned from the topical anatomy of the liver.[1] This procedure of divine request was called hepatoscopy and was used to answer specific questions, usually regarding the royal family. According to Gray et al.,[2] hepatoscopy rested on two assumptions: (1) that the liver was the seat of life and of the soul and (2) that the god to whom the sacrifice was made entered the soul of the animal to be sacrificed. Therefore the soul of the animal reflected the soul of the god, and consequently the liver indicated the intentions of the god. Although ancient in its development, hepatoscopy remains in practice in some cultures today.[3] Even through the time of Galen (130-200 AD), the liver was still considered the seat of the soul. Knowledge of the anatomy and physiology of the liver developed slowly over the centuries, and even today researchers continue to try to unravel the mysteries still held by this unique organ. Mysteries such as how the mature liver retains its ability to regenerate, how this regeneration process is turned on and off, and how and why this process is affected by the vast array of liver diseases are but a few of the puzzles remaining to be solved. Although hepatoscopy is not practiced by medical professionals as it was in the ancient past, the reader is cautioned to remember that most modern hepatologists and liver surgeons continue to believe that the ancients were indeed correct about the central importance of the liver and the anatomic location of the soul.

PRACTICAL AND FUNCTIONAL ANATOMY OF THE LIVER

Surgeons must have an understanding of both the macroscopic and microscopic anatomy of the liver. Only then will they appreciate the role this anatomy plays in the pathophysiology of the liver and in the vast array of liver diseases, as well as the surgical and radiologic approaches to the liver.

Embryology

The liver is the largest organ in the body, weighing between 1200 and 1500 g in adults. In the newborn the liver accounts for 4% to 5% of total body weight because of its role in blood formation during the neonatal period.[4] The liver arises as the hepatic diverticulum from the endodermal lining of the foregut during the third to fourth week of gestation.[2] The hepatic diverticulum differentiates cranially into proliferating hepatic cords and caudally into the gallbladder and extrahepatic biliary system. These hepatic cords grow into the transverse septum, which also gives rise to the diaphragm. Mesenchymal cells derived from the transverse septum form the connective tissue elements of the hepatic stroma and the capsule of the liver. The "bare area" of the right lobe of the liver is a reminder of the joint embryologic origin of the liver and diaphragm.

During the fifth week of gestation, the hepatic cords are penetrated by a growing capillary network, which arises from the vitelline veins to form the primitive hepatic sinusoids. Once the portal vein begins branching within the forming hepatic parenchyma, the proximal portion of the primitive hepatic cords gives rise to the epithelium of the intrahepatic bile ducts. This primitive bile duct in the 8 mm embryo (5 to 6 weeks' gestation) is termed the ductal plate, which then undergoes remodeling to form the normal anastomosing system of bile ducts within the portal tracts. Bile canaliculi appear in the 10 mm embryo as intracellular spaces between immature hepatocytes. The liver rapidly enlarges during this stage. By day 32, most of the blood from the umbilical vein is trapped in the hepatic parenchyma that surrounds the venous channels.[2] During this time, the portal vein continues branching within the hepatic parenchyma. The right umbilical vein obliterates at the sixth week of gestation, leaving the left umbilical vein to carry placental blood to the fetus until birth. The ductus venosus is established in the 6-month embryo, permitting the direct flow of blood from the left umbilical vein to the inferior vena cava. The umbilical vein is often used in neonates as a site for intravenous access and this is one of the causes of portal vein thrombosis in these infants. Additionally, portal vein thrombosis in infants may be the result of an extension of the process that normally obliterates the umbilical vein and ductus venosus soon after birth. After the umbilical vein becomes obliterated, it remains as the round ligament within the falciform ligament. The umbilical vein may recanalize in patients who develop portal hypertension, resulting in the development of the caput medusae surrounding the umbilicus. When recanalization has occurred, this vein may be used by the vascular radiologist to gain access to the portal system.

As the liver continues to enlarge, it bulges out from the transverse septum and assumes a truly abdominal position in the ventral mesentery. The asymmetry between the right and left lobes of the liver also begins to become more pronounced during this period. By the third month of gestation, bile is produced and can be identified in the intestine by the fifth month. Stem cells from blood islands established from the mesoderm of the primitive yolk sac seed the liver and proliferate. Mature forms of erythrocytes, granulocytes, and platelets are produced in the liver between 9 and 24 weeks of gestation. Although blood production by the liver shuts down after seeding the bone marrow, the liver retains its ability for hemopoietic activity into adulthood and is a common site for extramedullary hematopoiesis in certain disease states.

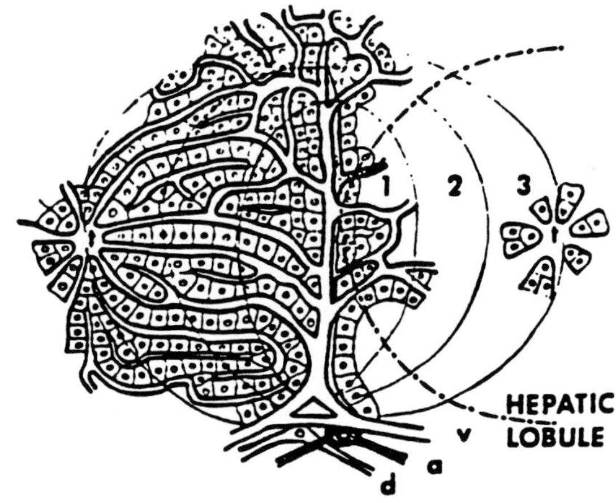

Fig. 23-1. Diagram comparing the hepatic acinus with zones 1, 2, and 3 to the hepatic lobule *(dotted line)*. Portal tract contains portal venule *(v)*, hepatic arteriole *(a)*, and hepatic duct *(d)*. *t*, Terminal hepatic venule. (From Thung SN, Gerber MA. Liver. In Sternberg SS, ed. Histology for Pathologists. New York: Raven Press, 1992, p 625.)

Histology

Parenchymal, interstitial, vascular, and ductal elements comprise the structural organization of the liver. The portal tracts contain the "portal triad" (bile duct, hepatic arterial branch, and portal vein branch), as well as lymphatic vessels and nerves, all of which are embedded in connective tissue. The condition of the arterioles, portal venules, bile ducts, central veins, as well as the amount, type, and location of any inflammatory cellular infiltrate, and the amount and location of fibrous tissue are used by the pathologist to help diagnose a variety of liver diseases. The hepatic sinusoids are formed of cords of hepatocytes lined by endothelial cells and reticuloendothelial cell elements known as Kupffer cells. Blood is not in direct contact with the hepatocytes but is separated from them by the endothelial lining cells of the sinusoids. Between the endothelial cells and the hepatocytes lies the space of Disse, the true business site of the liver. It is within this space that the exchange and flux of substance to and from the hepatocytes and the plasma take place. The large fenestrations between the endothelial lining cells of the sinusoids allow even relatively large macromolecules (albumin, globulins) to come in direct contact with the microvilli of the hepatocytes. Lymphatic fluid originates in the space of Disse, and this fluid flows in the same direction as bile. This anatomic arrangement is important in the cause of ascites in patients with liver disease.

Controversy remains regarding the correct anatomic description of the functional unit of the liver. Some authors believe it is represented by the *hepatic acinus* as described by Rappaport.[5,6] This unit (Fig. 23-1) is a regular, three-dimensional structure in which blood flows from a central access formed by the terminal portal venule and terminal hepatic arteriole in the portal tract into the sinusoids and empties into several terminal hepatic venules (central veins) at the periphery of the acinus. The *hepatic lobule* is believed by other authors to be the functional unit.[7,8] In the lobule (see Fig. 23-1) the efferent central vein has cords of hepatocytes radiating to several peripheral portal tracts. In a two-dimensional view the acinus occupies sections of several adjacent lobules. In the description of lesions of the liver the concept of the lobule is used to describe the location of an injury pattern as being centrilobular, midzonal, or peripheral (periportal). As shown in Fig. 23-1 the acinus is subdivided into zones 1, 2, and 3, with a decreasing oxygen gradient from zones 1 to 3. The hepatocytes in zone 1 are nearest the portal tract and correspond to the peripheral area of the lobule. Zone 2 corresponds roughly to the midzonal area of the lobule, and zone 3 corresponds to several centrilobular areas. The terminal branches of the hepatic arterial and portal venous system bring oxygen, nutrients, and substances to be metabolized or detoxified to the acinus. The terminal bile ducts provide egress for the secretory and excretory products of the acinus. The oxygen gradient, the metabolic heterogeneity, and the differential distribution of enzymes across the three zones of the acinus account for the zonal distribution of liver damage caused by ischemia or toxic substances, which is readily identifiable by light microscopy. When a patient with acute liver injury of unknown cause undergoes a liver biopsy, the pattern of injury on the biopsy specimen often provides the hepatic pathologist with clues as to the possible agent causing the injury. The pattern of injury is also essential in the histologic evaluation of biopsies from transplanted livers.

Functional Macroscopic Anatomy

Despite the long-standing teaching that the falciform ligament divides the right and left lobes of the liver, this concept has been demonstrated to be incorrect by a number of authors.[9,10] The right and left lobe of the liver is based on the arterial, portal venous, and biliary tract anatomy. The demarcation between the right and left lobes of the liver is a line that extends from the gallbladder fossa to the inferior vena cava. The right lobe is further subdivided into an anterior and posterior segment. The falciform ligament lies in the plane of the division of the left lobe into a medial and lateral segment. The quadrate lobe is a part of the medial segment of the left lobe and is not a true lobe. The caudate lobe, because of its unique vascular supply, is a distinct lobe adjacent to the vena cava on the medial segment of the left lobe. Because of its unique venous drainage directly into the vena cava, the caudate lobe may become massively enlarged when hepatic venous outflow is obstructed, as occurs in the Budd-Chiari syndrome.

Cousinaud[10] is most frequently credited with describing the segmental anatomy of the liver, as shown diagrammatically in Fig. 23-2. The liver is divided into eight segments based on the portal venous and hepatic arterial anatomy and the location of the hepatic veins. Using this classification system the classic left lobe of the liver includes segments 1 through 4, with the medial segment being segment 4, the left lateral segment being segments 2 and 3, and the caudate lobe being segment 1. The right lobe contains segments 5 through 8, with segments 5 and 8 being the equivalent of the anterior segment of the right lobe and segments 6 and 7 being the posterior segment of the right lobe.

Knowledge of segmental anatomy has allowed surgeons, in select patients, to perform segmental liver resection instead of resection of an entire lobe.[11,12] In addition, the techniques of reduced-size liver transplantation (transplantation of a lobe or part of a lobe rather than the entire liver),[13,14] split-liver transplantation (transplantation of two patients from a single donor liver),[15,16] and even living-related liver transplantation (taking a left lateral segment or the entire left lobe from a parent to transplant into a child)[17-20] were a direct outgrowth of the knowledge of the segmental anatomy of the liver.

The liver is unique in having a dual blood supply. The combined hepatic arterial and portal venous supply are necessitated by the unique location of the liver and its central role in maintaining metabolic homeostasis. There exists a reciprocal relationship between arterial and portal blood flow. This is regulated primarily by the arterioles within the liver; although a detailed review of hepatic hemodynamics is beyond the scope of this chapter, many of the physiologic processes and functions of the liver are intimately associated with this unique blood supply.[21-23]

The hepatic artery is one of the three branches of the celiac axis and, under normal circumstances, provides approximately 25% of the total blood flow and 50% to 75% of the oxygen to the liver, whereas the portal venous supply to the liver is the reciprocal of the arterial. Only 50%

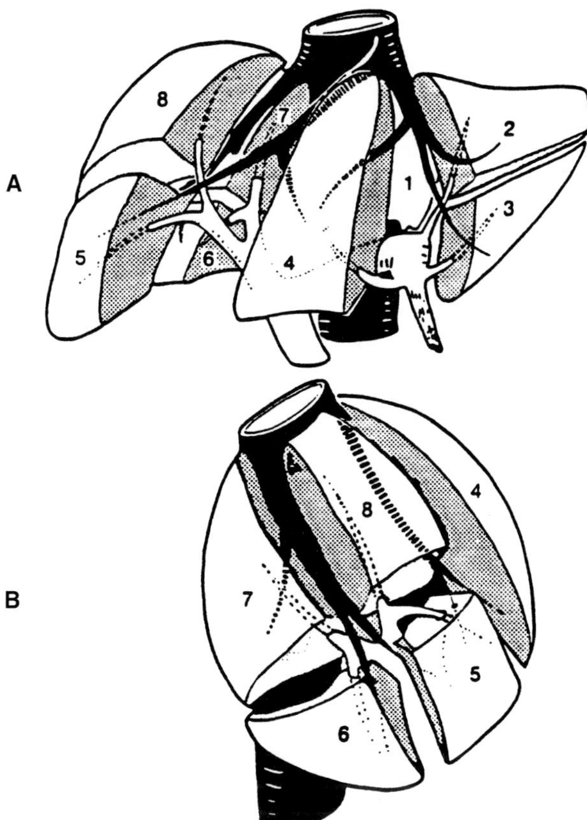

Fig. 23-2. The functional division of the liver and of the liver segments according to Couinaud's nomenclature: **A,** as seen in the patient; **B,** in the ex vivo position. (From Bismouth H, Aldridge MC, Kuntslinger F. Macroscopic anatomy of the liver. In McIntyre N, et al., eds. Oxford Textbook of Clinical Hepatology. Oxford: Oxford University Press, 1991, p 4. By permission of Oxford University Press.)

of people have a single hepatic artery in the "normal" location. Although the various arterial anomalies may have little impact on normal hepatic functions, the large number of anatomic variations are of vital concern for the hepatic surgeon and also the radiologist who performs hepatic arteriography or places catheters for intra-arterial chemotherapy.[24,25]

The hepatic portal system begins in the capillaries of the abdominal viscera and ends in the hepatic sinusoids. The veins of the portal system contain no valves, and obstruction of the outflow of this system at any site results in portal hypertension. Portal hypertension has traditionally been divided into three types: suprahepatic, intrahepatic, and subhepatic or prehepatic, based on the anatomic location of the obstruction to portal flow. Intrahepatic portal hypertension has been further subdivided into presinusoidal, sinusoidal, and postsinusoidal.[26,27] Presinusoidal portal hypertension, usually the result of thrombosis of the portal vein is associated with a normal wedged hepatic pressure. Sinusoidal and postsinusoidal portal hypertension are associated with an elevated wedged hepatic pressure. Except for identifying those diseases that are clearly associated with obstruction of the hepatic veins, there is little need to identify the precise location of the obstruction to portal vein flow in the most common forms of cirrhotic liver disease, as the therapeutic options to treat the portal hypertension are the same regardless of the anatomic location of the obstruction.

One complication with all forms of intrahepatic and suprahepatic portal hypertension is the association between elevated portal vein pressures and ascites formation. Increased pressure within the hepatic sinusoids results in a massive increase in hepatic lymph production, which when associated with a low serum oncotic pressure, results in the development of ascites.[28,29]

The hepatic veins have their origin in the microscopic central veins, which coalesce into progressively larger veins and terminate in the three main hepatic veins (right, middle, and left). The extraparenchymal portion of these veins is 1 to 1.5 cm and these veins join the anterior surface of the suprahepatic inferior vena cava just before it passes through the diaphragm to join with the right atrium. A detailed knowledge of the location of the main hepatic veins is crucial for decisions about resection of lobes and segments of the liver. As shown in Fig. 23-3, the major branches of the hepatic veins interdigitate with those of the portal vein. This anatomic arrangement has made possible direct access to the portal venous system from the hepatic veins through the hepatic parenchyma. This led to the development of the transjugular intrahepatic portosystemic shunt (TIPS) procedure. In this procedure the radiologist creates a false passage between a branch of the hepatic vein (usually the right) and a branch of the portal vein, creating an intrahepatic portosystemic shunt to relieve portal hypertension. Although it is too early to fully evaluate the results of this procedure, TIPS avoids the morbidity and mortality associated with major surgical procedures to relieve portal hypertension in patients with chronic liver disease.[30-33]

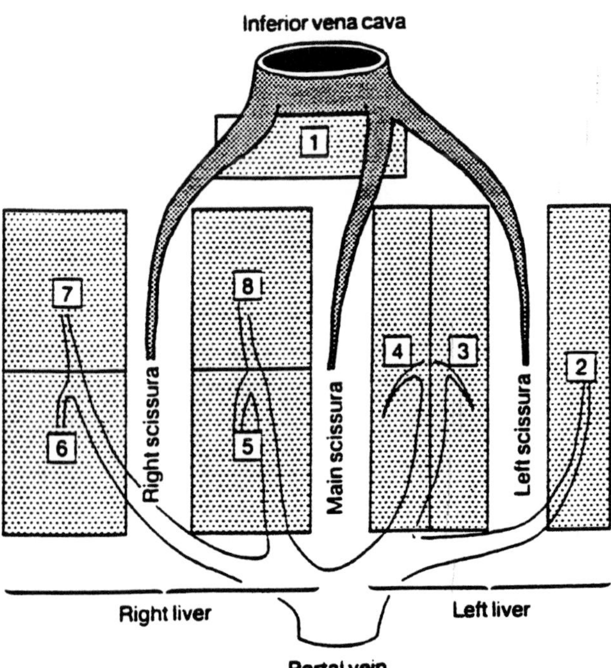

Fig. 23-3. Schematic representation of the functional anatomy of the liver. There are three main hepatic veins lying within the liver scissurae and dividing the liver into four sectors, each receiving a portal pedicle. The hepatic veins and portal pedicles are intertwined as are the fingers of two hands. (From Bismouth, H, Aldridge MC, Kuntslinger F. Macroscopic anatomy of the liver. In McIntyre N, et al., eds. Oxford Textbook of Clinical Hepatology. Oxford: Oxford University Press, 1991, p 5. By permission of Oxford University Press.)

Obstruction to outflow of the hepatic veins results in an immediate and sustained increase in pressure in the hepatic sinusoids. Outflow obstruction can be the result of heart failure,[34] congenital webs of the suprahepatic inferior vena cava,[35] thrombosis of the main hepatic veins,[36-39] or veno-occlusive disease of the smaller hepatic veins.[40-42] All these conditions result in the enlargement of the liver with development of portal hypertension and ascites. Because the increased resistance to venous outflow is reflected by a large rise in the pressure in the hepatic sinusoids, the influx of fluid into the space of Disse results in a marked increase in the amount of lymph produced. This can rapidly overload the capacity of the hepatic lymphatics, causing the development of massive ascites. The increased pressure in the sinusoid in acute portal hypertension results in reversal of flow in the portal vein, and the portal vein becomes the major site for venous outflow from the liver.

The caudate lobe, because of its unique location adjacent to the vena cava, has 3 to 50 small veins that drain directly into the vena cava. In patients with outflow obstruction the caudate lobe becomes enlarged, and these veins can dilate to provide another major site of venous outflow for the liver.

NORMAL HEPATIC FUNCTIONS

Overview

The liver occupies a unique location in the body. All blood collected from the digestive system must pass through the liver, and the liver receives up to 25% of the total cardiac output via the portal vein and hepatic artery. Only substrates directly absorbed in the mouth, upper esophagus, or the most distal rectum or substrates that pass directly into the lymphatics of the gut can enter the systemic circulation directly and avoid the first pass through the liver. A number of other factors also favor the central role of the liver in the maintenance of homeostasis. The liver represents approximately 3% of the total body weight, and the highly branching capillary system within the liver (hepatic sinusoids) provides a huge surface area in which the substances brought to the liver are exposed to the various types of liver cells. The liver both filters the incoming splanchnic blood to remove bacteria and other potentially toxic substances, as well as processing the huge variety of substrates absorbed from the gastrointestinal tract. The liver's unique dual blood supply allows simultaneous monitoring of the portal and systemic levels of hormones, available substrates, and the products of metabolism (glucose, lipids, and amino acids).

The maintenance of plasma level of metabolic substrates relies on the wide variety of synthetic and degradative pathways of the hepatocytes. The hepatocyte expresses phenotypically more of the human genome than any other cell in the body by using virtually every enzyme, receptor, and transport mechanism available in the genetic library.[43] The liver cannot be replaced by mechanical, physical, or biochemical supports that do not include the use of viable hepatocytes.[44-47] If a patient's liver fails, death follows within a short period of time. In humans the anhepatic state is not compatible with life for more than a few hours. The liver is unique among all solid organs in maintaining the ability to regenerate, even after massive subtotal resection or injury, if the appropriate conditions are present. The gradual loss of this regenerative capacity is central in the development of cirrhosis. Hepatic replacement therapy (liver transplantation) is presently the therapy of choice for most patients who develop acute fulminant hepatic failure (AFHF)[48,49] or complications related to chronic liver disease.[50,51] The hepatic functions important in the maintenance of normal homeostasis are outlined in the accompanying box, and these functions in normal and diseased states are discussed in the following sections.

HEPATIC FUNCTIONS

Filtration (Kupffer Cell of Reticuloendothelial System)

Capture and process incoming substrates and bacteria

Maintenance of Metabolic Homeostasis

Fundamental mechanisms

Capture
Intracellular metabolism
Storage
Release

Modulation of metabolic substrates

Carbohydrates: Glucose, fructose, galactose
Lipids: Fatty acids, glycerol, cholesterol
Amino acids: Protein synthesis and degradation

Specific Protein Synthesis

Secretory proteins: Albumin, acute phase reactants, carrier proteins
Coagulation proteins: Clotting proteins, anticoagulants, proteins, fibrinolytic proteins

Lipid Phase Metabolism

Drug metabolism
Bile formation

Filtration

Kupffer cells, derived from blood mononuclear cells, are fixed macrophages located within the sinusoids of the liver. These cells have a half-life of 3 to 16 weeks and represent between 70% to 90% of the body's functional reticuloendothelial system.[52,53] Kupffer cells have an incredible capacity to capture and process material entering the hepatic sinusoids. As much as 99% of bacteria found in the portal blood is filtered by the Kupffer cells. This enormous capacity to engulf material (phagocytosis) presented to the hepatic sinusoids depends, at least in part, on nonspecific opsonins, including fibronectin.[53] This process of phagocytosis is energy dependent and therefore can be profoundly affected by disease states. A decrease in the filtration function of the liver has been observed in patients with sepsis, alcohol abuse, trauma, hypoglycemia, hypothyroidism, and juvenile-onset diabetes. The depression of the reticuloendothelial system also occurs in cirrhotics as outlined in the accompanying box.

Metabolic Homeostasis

The capacity of the liver to regulate the body's metabolism may be divided into four broad categories: capture, intracellular metabolism, storage, and release. Capture represents the removal of a substrate from the blood across the hepatocyte or other liver cell. This may be accomplished by either active or passive transport processes and usually involves the generation of a gradient between the sinusoid and the internal milieu of the hepatocyte. Once inside the hepatocyte, substrates are either modified so that they are irreversibly lost to the plasma or changed to allow storage on a temporary or permanent basis. Many of these substances may be released when required for the maintenance of homeostasis. The liver's central role in the regulation of carbohydrates, lipids, and amino acids is described in the following. The variations in these metabolic responses in patients with liver disease are also examined.

MECHANISMS OF DEPRESSION OF THE RETICULOENDOTHELIAL SYSTEM

Intrahepatic shunting
Intrinsic defects in reticulendothelial system cells
Reduced serum opsonic activity
Circumstances worsening function of the reticuloendothelial system
- Alcohol intake
- Malnutrition
- Hypovolemia, shock
- Surgery
- Corticosteroid therapy

From Rimola A. In McIntyre N, et al., eds. Oxford Textbook of Clinical Hepatology. Oxford: Oxford University Press, 1991, p 1274. By permission of Oxford University Press.

Carbohydrate Metabolism

To sustain the function of the brain, adrenal medulla, and red and white blood cells, there is an obligatory requirement for glucose, which ranges between 160 and 180 g/day. With prolonged fasting a number of organs shift from glucose metabolism, and glucose requirements may be decreased to as little as 40 g/day after a prolonged fast.[54] Following an overnight fast, as in the patient awaiting a surgical procedure, 75% of the available glucose is produced from hepatic glycogenolysis and 25% from gluconeogenesis.[54] The total hepatic glycogen stores range from 60 to 80 g and are easily depleted by overnight fasting. Gluconeogenesis requires the presence of precursors including lactate, pyruvate, glycerol, or amino acids such as alanine, glutamine, and glycine. Of these, lactate is the most commonly used with increasing use of the products of protein breakdown and fatty acid oxidation with prolonged starvation.

In the fed state the factors that determine blood glucose concentration include the size of the glucose bolus, the rate of gastrointestinal absorption of glucose, the portion of the glucose load retained by the splanchnic tissues (especially the liver), the degree of associated suppression of hepatic glucose production, and the amount of glucose used by peripheral tissues.[54] Only 25% to 50% of an oral glucose load is removed in the first pass through the liver, with the majority of the absorbed glucose (up to 75%) being removed by the peripheral tissues, especially skeletal muscle, where it is converted to muscle glycogen.[54-56] The homeostatic responses to an oral glucose load are under hormonal control with insulin occupying the primary role in the regulation of plasma glucose levels in the fed state. Portal vein insulin levels are up to 10 times the systemic insulin levels, with 20% to 50% of the portal vein insulin extracted in the first pass through the liver.[54-57] The timing and magnitude of the insulin response is primarily responsible for blood glucose control. With an intact vagal system, stimulation of the release of insulin occurs prior to the rise in portal vein glucose concentration, and this results in an insulin-induced reduction in hepatic glucose production to 10% to 20% of normal values.[54] Insulin has little role in promoting glucose transport into hepatocytes, whereas in peripheral tissues (especially muscle), insulin causes a marked increase in the uptake of glucose by muscle cells. Elevated insulin levels also decrease lipolysis in adipose tissues, thereby reducing the amount of fatty acids and glycerol available to the liver. The reduction of these substrates results in decreased hepatic gluconeogenesis and glycogenolysis (Fig. 23-4). Insulin blocks hepatic glucose production at much lower serum levels than needed for maximal stimulation of glucose uptaking muscle. Therefore skeletal muscle is much more dependent on the magnitude of the insulin response, and the markedly elevated plasma insulin levels seen following oral glucose administration may be a consequence of the need for higher insulin levels for peripheral use of glucose. Because of the exquisite sensitivity of the liver to insulin, there is little difference in whether insulin is presented to the liver through the portal vein or systemic circulation. However, insulin administered peripherally does not undergo a first-pass extraction by the liver, and therefore higher serum insulin levels are obtained with peripherally administered insulin doses. This carries important implications in patients receiving total parenteral nutrition (TPN), especially when insulin is included in the TPN.

As noted earlier, insulin does not promote the hepatic uptake of glucose but rather blocks hepatic glucose production. Glucose entry into the hepatocytes is primarily dependent on the portal vein glucose concentration. Sinusoidal glucose levels must exceed the intracellular level for the flux of glucose to be into the hepatocyte. In addition, as yet poorly defined neural and intrahepatic factors may be important in increasing glucose use by the liver in the fed state.[54]

Starvation is a common and often iatrogenically induced condition in surgical patients. The regulation of carbohydrate metabolism in the face of starvation is dependent on a number of factors including the hormone milieu, the availability of gluconeogenic substrates, changes in the activity of key hepatic enzymes, and the autoregulation of hepatic glucose production.[54] Starvation results in a fall in serum glucose levels and a concomitant fall in serum and portal vein insulin levels. Glucagon, glucocorticoids, catecholamines, and growth hormone production are stimulated during starvation. A fall in insulin levels to baseline or below is responsible for the stimulation of gluconeogenesis and glycogenolysis within the hepatocytes. However, with brief periods of starvation, baseline insulin levels continue to exert an inhibitory effect on hepatic glucose production and block the unrestrained peripheral mobilization of fatty acids and gluconeogenic precursors to maintain the serum glucose at normal levels. As the serum glucose levels fall, glucagon levels rise and two thirds of the hepatic glucose production becomes secondary to glycogen breakdown, a process promoted by glucagon.[54] Sustained increases of growth hormone, cortisol, and catecholamines result in increased glucose production and help to maintain serum glucose levels within normal limits during prolonged fasting. Both the peripheral and hepatic actions of these hormones are important for the stimulation of hepatic glucose production during fasting. With fasting, less glucose is available for oxidation in the extrahepatic tissues. This changes the hormonal milieu and leads to muscle protein breakdown with the release of a lactate, pyruvate, and alanine and an increased rate of lipolysis in adipose tissues, resulting in increased free fatty acid and glycerol production. There is also an enhanced hepatic uptake of alanine and other gluconeogenic amino acids in response to glucagon and catecholamines. The increased use of these gluconeogenic substrates by the hepatocytes is not the result of hormonally mediated changes in the hepatocyte membrane transport system. Rather, it is the direct result of decreased intracellular concentration of these precursors as they are used for gluconeogenesis. This creates a gradient that allows transport of these substrates from the sinusoids into the hepatocytes. Fatty acid oxidation is also an important process that provides fatty acids to the hepatocytes, both as an energy source for gluconeogenesis and to increase mitochondrial acetyl-coenzyme A (acetyl-CoA).[58]

Hormonal regulation of key hepatic enzymes determines the rate and magnitude of both glycolysis and gluconeogenesis. The glycolytic or gluconeogenic flux depends on the activity of key hepatic enzymes that catalyze the nonequilibrium reactions in favor of either glycolysis or gluconeogenesis. The major regulatory sites of this process are shown in Fig. 23-4. The acute hormonal regulation of hepatic carbohydrate metabolism involves alterations in cytosolic cyclic adenosine monophosphate (cAMP) and calcium. This is true for virtually all the regulatory steps in carbohydrate metabolism.

The final factor that regulates carbohydrate metabolism is the level of blood glucose in the hepatic sinusoids. As noted above, the transport of glucose into the hepatocyte

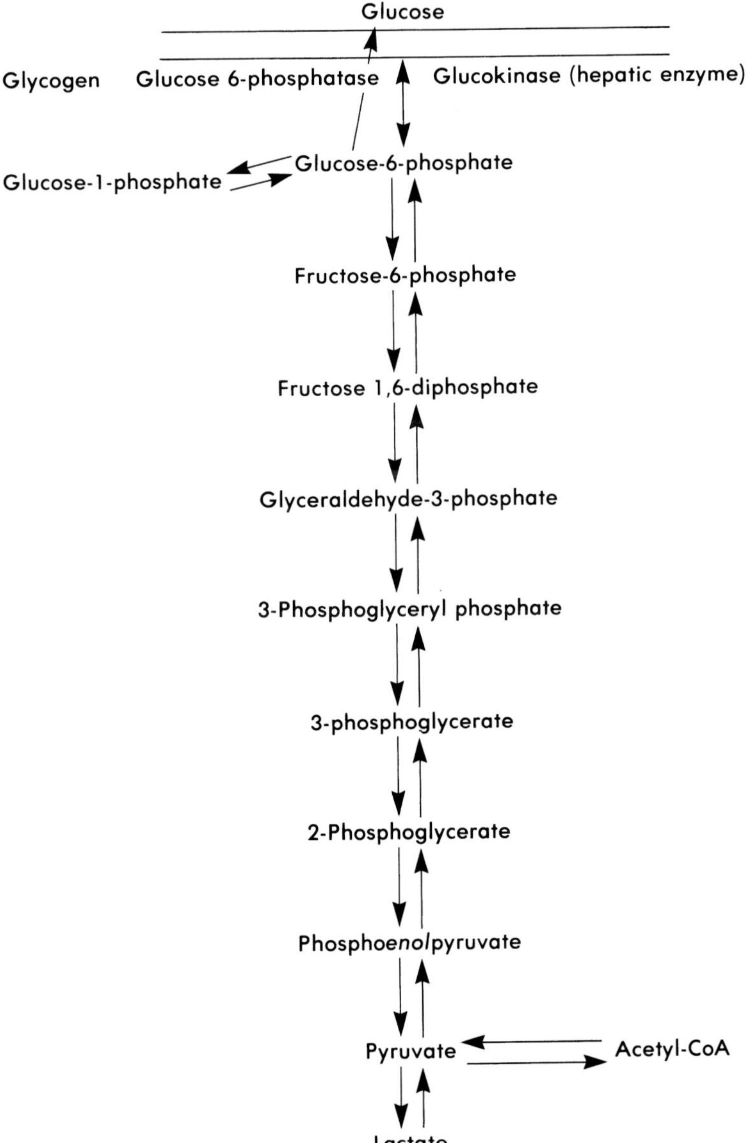

Fig. 23-4. Glycolysis-gluconeogenesis. These reactions are entirely cytoplasmic and, in response to mass action, readily reversible. Reversibility permits glycolysis and gluconeogenesis in the same cellular compartment. Mass action is determined by importation of substrate under the influence of insulin (glycolysis and glycogen synthesis), facilitated exit from the pathway (pyruvate entry into mitochondria for the Kreb's cycle), or the entry of products (lactate or amino acids) that promote gluconeogenesis, an event also regulated by glucagon. The location of the rate-limiting enzymatic pathways for both glycolysis and gluconeogenesis are identified. (Modified with permission from Merrell RC. Hepatic physiology. In Miller TA, ed. Physiologic Basis of Modern Surgical Care. St. Louis: CV Mosby, 1988, p 407.)

is not dependent on insulin and has a high capacity. Low portal vein glucose levels result in decreased glucose 6-phosphate production, which favors net glucose production. High intracellular glucose levels block the enzymes responsible for hepatic glucose production in favor of glycogen synthesis.

Carbohydrate metabolism in patients with chronic or acute liver disease is largely dependent on the severity of the patient's liver disease. End-stage liver disease is often associated with moderate-to-severe hypoglycemia. However, 80% of patients with moderate liver disease are actually glucose intolerant. There is a twofold to fourfold increase of incidence of diabetes in patients with chronic liver disease.[54-60] The mechanism of glucose intolerance in these patients is not completely understood. It is certainly multifactorial and results from the influence of nutritional factors, hepatic factors, insulin availability, tissue insensitivity to insulin, the presence of antimetabolic hormones, and portosystemic shunting.[54,61]

Patients with chronic liver disease suffer from varying degrees of malnutrition, and malnutrition itself has been associated with decreased insulin production. In most patients with cirrhosis, the glucose intolerance does not appear to be related to the diminished hepatic mass but rather to decreased exposure of the remaining hepatic mass to glucose and insulin, secondary to portosystemic shunting. The decreased exposure of the hepatocytes to glucose and insulin results in less stimulus for the cirrhotic liver to increase glycogen production. Many cirrhotic patients show a peripheral hyperinsulinemia, probably secondary to decreased hepatic extraction of insulin; in addition, they also demonstrate peripheral insulin resistance.[60,61] The role of the antimetabolic hormones such as glucagon, catecholamines, and growth hormone in carbohydrate metabolism in patients with liver disease has not been fully elucidated.

It is rare for stable cirrhotic patients to develop hypoglycemia with fasting. This may, in part, be due to the fact that only 20% of the functional hepatocyte mass is needed to maintain normal glucose homeostasis. Hypoglycemia is considered to be a poor prognostic sign both in patients with AFHF and in patients with chronic liver disease. Hypoglycemia should be managed, or better, prevented, by glucose infusion at a rate adequate to supply the tissues with the obligatory glucose requirement. This requires between 150 to 200 g of glucose every 24-hour period and may be provided as a 10% or 20% glucose solution as fluid requirements dictate. Supplemental glucose administration may also be required following extensive resection of the noncirrhotic liver, minor resections of the cirrhotic liver, or poor function of the liver following hepatic transplantation.

When cirrhotic patients fast, there is a more rapid transition to the pattern of hepatic metabolism described previously following starvation, and the decreased rate of delivery of gluconeogenic substrates and fatty acids may limit the liver's capacity for gluconeogenesis.[54] If gluconeogenesis cannot compensate for decreased glucose production from glycogenolysis, hepatic glucose production falls. Surgeons caring for or operating on patients with acute or chronic liver disease must be aware that adequate glucose must be supplied to these patients before, during, and after all surgical procedures. Impaired hepatic function may also change the use of the glucose supplied in TPN, and use of insulin in any patient with severe liver dysfunction must be carefully monitored.

Other important carbohydrates

Fructose. Sucrose is a disaccharide containing equimolar amounts of glucose and fructose and is a major component of the typical Western diet. Of the 300 g of carbohydrate normally ingested each day, 80 to 120 g is sucrose providing 40 to 60 g of fructose per day.[54] Sucrose is hydrolyzed by the brush border of the small intestine into glucose and fructose. Some of the fructose is used by the small intestine, and the remainder is passed into the portal venous blood. The liver is high in fructokinase, and most of the fructose is removed in the first pass through the liver. Much of the fructose is metabolized to glucose with 30% metabolized to pyruvate and lactate, making fructose a good precursor for glycogen production. The utilization of fructose is not dependent on insulin, and fructose administration leads to a rapid increase in the level of plasma triglycerides, which are carried on very-low-density lipoproteins (VLDLs). Patients with liver disease often experience an increase of serum fructose levels, which correlates with the severity of the liver disease and degree of portosystemic shunting.

Galactose. Lactose is a disaccharide with equimolar amounts of galactose and glucose. Galactose is an important dietary nutrient in infancy, and its clinical importance in later life depends on the quantity of milk and milk products consumed. Galactose is hydrolyzed in the small intestine epithelium into glucose and galactose, which are carried by the portal venous blood to the liver. Most of the galactose is removed in the first pass through the liver. The galactose is metabolized to glucose 1-phosphate, which can then be used for glycogen synthesis or can enter the glycolytic pathway.[54]

Lipids and Lipoprotein Metabolism

Dietary lipid is a major metabolic fuel for the body and a source of both fat-soluble vitamins and essential fatty acids. There are no specific recommendations for the total daily caloric intake of lipid or for the relative amounts of saturated or unsaturated fatty acids. However, 30% to 35% of the daily energy requirement would probably be provided in the form of fat.

Following ingestion of dietary fat, which is composed mainly of triglycerides of animal or plant origin, the fat is hydrolyzed by pancreatic lipases into fatty acids and monoglycerides. These are then associated with bile acids to form micelles that also incorporate cholesterol and fat-soluble vitamins into their core. These micelles are taken up by the intestinal mucosal cells, where the monoglycerides and fatty acids are reesterified into triglycerides. These triglycerides, together with cholesterol, cholesterol esters, phospholipids, apoproteins, and fat-soluble vitamins, are packaged into large particles called chylomicrons and leave the intestine via the intestinal lymph.[62] Unlike carbohydrates and amino acids, lipids are not carried directly to the liver in the portal vein but bypass the liver and enter the systemic circulation via the thoracic duct. Short-chain triglycerides do not require bile salts or pancreatic lipase for digestion and pass directly through the mucosal cells into the portal blood, where they are bound to albumin for transport to the liver in an unesterified form.

The major lipids in the plasma are (1) cholesterol, which is an important constituent of the plasma membrane of all cells and a precursor of bile acids and steroid hormones; (2) cholesterol esters, which store and transport cholesterol; (3) phospholipids, which are involved in many biochemical reactions and are important structural components of cell membranes; and (4) triglycerides, which are the major form in which fat is transported in plasma and the major storage form of energy in adipose tissue.[62] In plasma, lipids are associated with specific proteins. Although some unesterified fats and phospholipids are bound to albumin or other specific plasma proteins, the majority of plasma lipids are carried on complexes called lipoproteins. These large macromolecules are manufactured in the liver or intestine and contain cholesterol, phospholipids, specific polypeptides called apoproteins, and a small quantity of nonpolar lipids. Lipoproteins are classified on the basis of their physiochemical properties as chylomicrons, VLDLs, low-density lipoproteins (LDLs), and high-density lipoproteins (HDLs).[63-65] Triglycerides are mainly transported in chylomicrons and VLDLs, whereas LDLs are the lipoproteins that transport the majority of cholesterol.

Chylomicrons and VLDLs of intestinal origin are broken down by peripheral and hepatic lipases and lecithin-cholesterol acetyltransferases (LCATs).[66,67] Triglycerides from chylomicrons and VLDLs are hydrolyzed by lipoprotein lipases into free fatty acids, which are available for uptake in the periphery or by the liver. The liver is the major organ of traffic for lipid metabolism. Dietary lipids arriving from the gastrointestinal tract as chylomicrons or from the periphery as HDLs are bound to the hepatocytes by specific receptors and brought into the hepatocytes by the process of endocytosis. These intracellular vesicles are fused with liposomes to disassociate the receptor and the lipoprotein. The unbound lipid is available for several fates within the hepatocyte. It may be reprocessed into VLDLs and transported back into the sinusoids, or the triglycerides may be hydrolyzed to fatty acids and glycerol. Depending on the metabolic needs of the body, these substances can either be processed for energy or metabolized into other triglycerides or cholesterol.

Patients with acute or chronic liver disease of moderate severity experience a number of abnormalities in lipid and lipoprotein metabolism.[68-71] There is a decreased absorption of dietary lipids because of the reduced micelle formation that results from the decreased production of bile acids. This fat malabsorption causes mild-to-moderate steatorrhea, with a resultant loss of fat-soluble vitamins, especially vitamin K. The coagulopathy experienced by some patients with liver disease may be due to vitamin K deficiency secondary to fat malabsorption and may be corrected by parenteral administration of vitamin K. Patients with moderate liver disease or intrahepatic cholestasis often have markedly increased serum cholesterol levels.[71] This is primarily the result of decreased production of cholesterol esters because of the decreased synthesis of LCATs by the damaged liver, which results in a decrease in the conversion of cholesterol to cholesterol esters. Some groups have even used the serum level of LCATs as an indicator of the severity of liver disease.[72,73] The increased serum cholesterol can lead to the development of xanthomata. These lesions are the result of cholesterol deposition in the skin.[62] Patients with acute or chronic liver disease also experience a fall in VLDL production because of decreased hepatic synthesis of this lipoprotein. This may result in increased plasma levels of triglyceride-rich LDLs. The serum levels of nonesterified fatty acids (NEFAs) are also increased with moderate liver disease because of the increased release of NEFAs from the periphery and decreased removal of these substances by the diseased liver. Severe liver disease is also associated with abnormalities in platelet aggregation secondary to membrane changes caused by lipoprotein abnormalities.[74,75] Finally, severe liver disease may result in decreased synthesis of prostaglandin, as well as the production of other abnormal phospholipids.

Amino Acid Metabolism and Urea Production

Amino acid metabolism begins with dietary proteins being hydrolyzed within the intestinal lumen to amino acids and oligopeptides. The portal vein blood has high concentrations of amino acids, which unlike lipids are removed in a first pass through the liver. Some amino acids are used for protein synthesis and gluconeogenesis, while others are used for the synthesis of or conversion to nonessential amino acids.[76] There is a constant exchange of amino acids between the liver and the skeletal muscle. There is also a reamination of essential amino acids, and a release of amino acids for the rest of the body by the liver. The most important amino acids are glycine,[77] which is used in the conjugation of bile salts; alanine,[78] which is the major amino acid used for hepatic glucose production; and the branched-chain amino acids (BCAAs), leucine, valine, and isoleucine, which escape the first-pass uptake by the liver and are used primarily in skeletal muscle.[79] The fact that BCAAs are not metabolized in the liver has lead to their proposed use as a protein source in patients with liver disease.

The average protein turnover in a 70 kg man is between 250 and 300 g/day, which is much higher than the average daily protein intake of between 70 to 100 g.[80,81] There is an extensive turnover of endogenous proteins with release and reuse of amino acids, and this constant flux of amino acids accounts for a large portion of the basal energy expenditure, as shown in Fig. 23-5. Approximately 30 g of the endogenous pool of amino acids is fully metabolized each day, and approximately 32 g of dietary protein is needed to replace these amino acids.[82]

When amino acids are fully catabolized, the nitrogen may be removed by a number of mechanisms, but the major route is via urea synthesis and excretion. Unlike carbohydrates and fats, excess dietary amino acids must be broken down as they cannot be stored in the body. Hepatic protein synthesis accounts for about 15% of the total body protein turnover, with the splanchnic region as a whole responsible for up to 50%.[83,84] Skeletal muscle protein turnover is approximately twice that of the liver.

Following a protein-rich meal, the liver regulates the entry of amino acids into the systemic circulation; despite high portal vein concentrations, there is relatively little increase in the amino acid concentration in peripheral blood because of the first-pass extraction of amino acids by the liver. As noted previously, the BCAAs escape the first-pass extraction by the liver. A protein meal affects both the rate of hepatic protein synthesis and also the activity of key liver enzymes involved in amino acid catabolism.[76] Insulin release is stimulated by both protein and carbohydrate-rich meals. Insulin facilitates the uptake of amino acids into muscle and adipose tissue. The uptake of amino acids by skeletal muscle results in a fall in serum amino acid levels, especially levels of BCAAs.

Skeletal muscle and the liver play a major role in determining the plasma level of amino acids. Although muscle contains more than 50% of the total body pool of free amino acids, the urea cycle enzymes (Fig. 23-6) necessary for disposal of surplus nitrogen are almost exclusively located in the liver.[85] Both the liver and muscle participate in the interconversion of amino acids and their reentry into plasma. Glutamine and alanine are released from the muscle in amounts greater than that accounted for by protein synthesis, and the majority of these amino acids must come from the breakdown of BCAAs.[76]

Nonessential amino acids are readily oxidized in both the liver and muscle, whereas most essential amino acids are oxidized primarily in the liver.[86] Most of the gastrointestinal hormones seem to have reciprocal actions on muscle and the liver. When protein breakdown and release is stimulated in one organ, amino acid uptake tends to in-

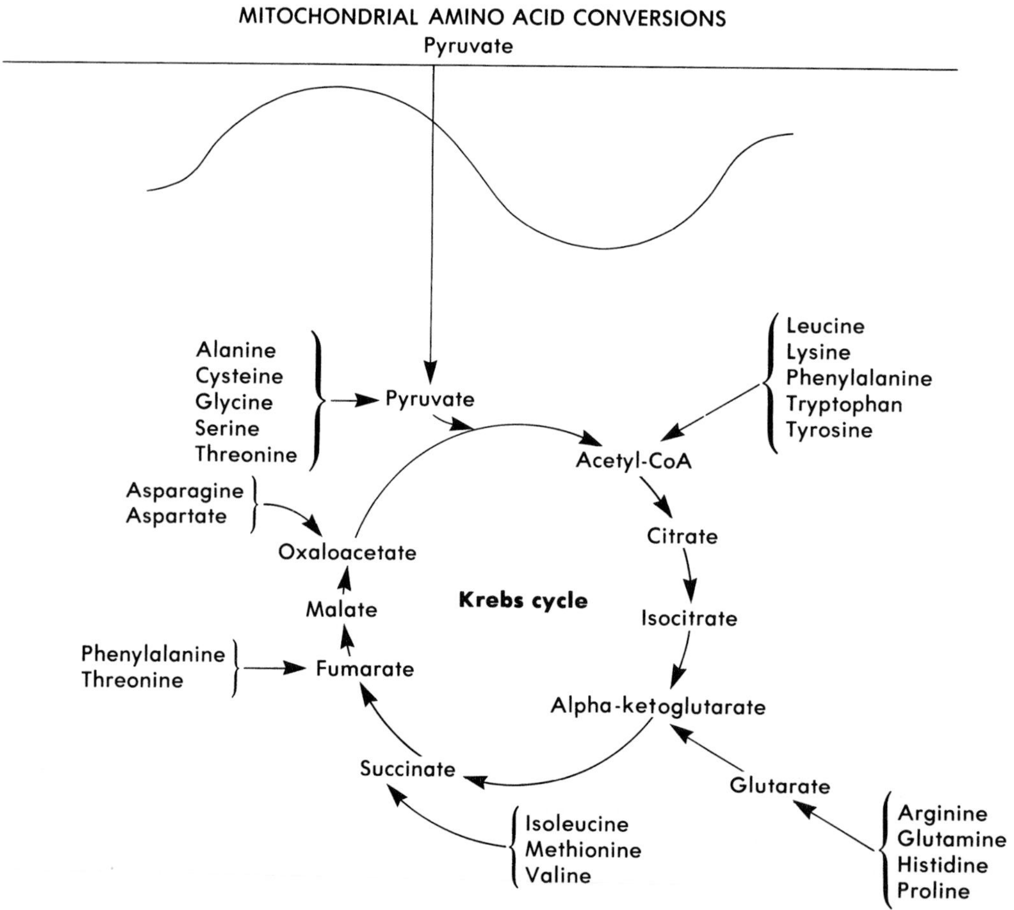

Fig. 23-5. Amino acid interconversion relies on cytoplasmic transamination, whereas metabolism of the carbon skeleton of the amino acid proceeds in the mitochondria. Most intermediates of the Krebs cycle can readily diffuse from the double convoluted membrane of the mitochondrion to participate in cytoplasmic intermediary metabolism. (From Merrell RC. Hepatic physiology. In Miller TA, ed. Physiologic Basis of Modern Surgical Care. St. Louis: CV Mosby, 1988, p 410.)

crease in the other. Insulin enhances amino acid uptake in the periphery and inhibits protein breakdown, resulting in a reduction in the plasma concentration of all amino acids except alanine. Glucocorticoids increase the level of free amino acids in muscle, plasma, and liver by stimulating protein breakdown and causing an increase in glutamine extraction and alanine production by the intestine.[76] Glucagon promotes the degradation of BCAA in muscle, increases alanine uptake by the liver, and stimulates both gluconeogenesis and ureagenesis.[87]

Plasma amino acid concentrations are often altered in patients with significant liver disease. In AFHF the plasma concentration of most amino acids is high, whereas plasma concentration of BCAA is low or normal.[88] This is due to the increased release and impaired uptake of amino acids by the damaged liver. As BCAAs undergo their metabolism predominantly in muscle, plasma levels are largely unaffected by liver disease. In patients with cirrhosis clearance of amino acids is reduced, and urea synthesis is also decreased. Increased peripheral protein breakdown may also contribute to the elevated plasma concentration of amino acids and may be stimulated by low insulin levels and higher levels of the catabolic hormones. Alterations in plasma levels of amino acids and alterations in ammonia metabolism and urea production have been incriminated in the genesis of hepatic encephalopathy. However, a direct correlation between plasma amino acid levels and the development of hepatic encephalopathy has not been established.[76] Hepatic encephalopathy is further discussed later in this chapter.

Ammonia and Urea Metabolism

Ammonia has a central role in nitrogen metabolism and is the major by-product of protein and nucleic acid catabolism as well as being a source of nitrogen for amino acids, nucleic acids, and other nitrogenous products.[76] Blood ammonia concentrations are normally very low, and elevated serum levels have been associated with the development of encephalopathy in patients with chronic and acute liver disease. The liver is the primary site of ammonia metabolism. The liver removes the ammonia presented to it and excretes it as the nontoxic product, urea (see Fig. 23-6).

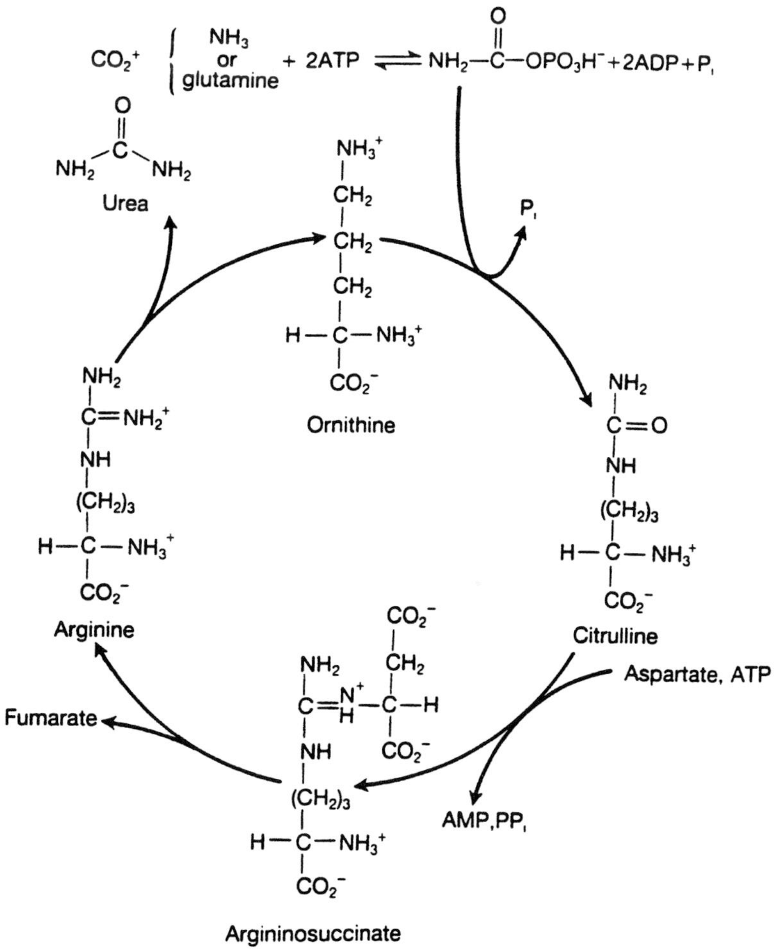

$$CO_2 + \left\{\begin{matrix} NH_3 \\ \text{or} \\ \text{glutamine} \end{matrix}\right. + 2ATP \rightleftharpoons NH_2{-}\overset{\overset{\displaystyle O}{\|}}{C}{-}OPO_3H^- + 2ADP + P_i$$

Urea: $NH_2{-}CO{-}NH_2$

Ornithine: $NH_3^+{-}CH_2{-}CH_2{-}CH_2{-}CH(NH_3^+){-}CO_2^-$

Citrulline: $NH_2{-}C(=O){-}NH{-}(CH_2)_3{-}CH(NH_3^+){-}CO_2^-$

Aspartate, ATP → AMP, PP_i

Argininosuccinate

Fumarate

Arginine: $NH_2{-}C(=NH_2^+){-}NH{-}(CH_2)_3{-}CH(NH_3^+){-}CO_2^-$

P_i

Fig. 23-6. The urea cycle. (From Herrmann R, McIntyre N. Amino-acid metabolism, urea production, and pH regulation. In McIntyre N, et al., eds. Oxford Textbook of Clinical Hepatology. Oxford: Oxford University Press, 1991, p 168. By permission of Oxford University Press.)

The liver also plays a central role in the metabolic regulation of the blood pH, since hydrogen ions released from ammonia during the synthesis of urea neutralize the excess bicarbonate produced by the breakdown of amino acids. Urea is an organic molecule that diffuses freely in the total body water, is not metabolized by human enzymes, and is ultimately excreted by the kidneys. Urea production takes place primarily within the liver, although much of the ammonia used for urea synthesis is derived from extrahepatic tissues. Only 25% of the ammonia used in urea synthesis reaches the liver from the portal vein, and the concentration of ammonia in the portal vein is 10 times higher than systemic blood levels.[76] Both amino acid and nucleic acid metabolism within the liver also produce ammonia.[89,90]

Ammonia appearing in the portal vein is the result of both bacterial action within the lumen of the gut and also production of ammonia by the small intestine through its metabolism of glutamine.[76,91] Most of the ammonia from the colon results from the bacterial degradation of urea and other nitrogenous substances.

Most of the surplus nitrogen (approximately 90%) in man enters the urea cycle for irreversible conversion to urea, which is excreted by the kidneys. The liver is quantitatively the major organ involved in urea synthesis, as the first two enzymes responsible for the production of urea are largely confined to the liver.[76] Regulation of these urea cycle enzymes is important, as ammonia is toxic and its production is variable. Short-term regulation of urea production appears to be achieved by alterations in the activity of the urea cycle enzymes, whereas long-term control seems to be affected by changes in enzyme concentrations. In addition, hepatic urea synthesis is subject to hormonal influences. Catabolic enzymes, including glucagon and glucocorticoids, are associated with increased levels of the urea cycle enzymes. Sepsis, surgery, and trauma are associated with increased levels of glucagon and glucocorticoids, which increase urea synthesis and contribute to the negative nitrogen balance observed in patients with these conditions.[92]

In patients with advanced liver disease, plasma urea levels tend to fall, and there is a reduction in the amount of urea excreted in the urine. Urea synthesis correlates with the severity of the liver disease. In well-compensated cirrhotic patients, baseline urea production is normal; but if these individuals are stressed, such as by major gastrointestinal bleeding, maximal urea production is significantly impaired. With advanced cirrhosis, there is a reduction in many of the urea cycle enzymes, and the decreased capacity for urea production is related to the loss of functional liver cell mass. In patients with liver disease, blood ammonia levels tend to rise as a result of portosystemic shunting, hepatocellular dysfunction, and an increase in ammonia production in the gastrointestinal tract.[76] This elevation in serum ammonia levels is associated with, but not solely responsible for, the development of hepatic encephalopathy, and therapeutic interventions are directed at reducing the ammonia production in the gut. This is accomplished by purging the gut with lactulose or reducing the bacterial flora with intraluminal antibiotics.

Because of reduced urea production and the use of diuretics, the liver's central role in the regulation of pH is also altered in patients with chronic liver disease. The liver has an additional role in the maintenance of acid-base balance because it is the major site of the metabolism of lactate. The liver removes 50% to 70% of the lactate produced each day, and the lactic acidosis experienced by patients with shock and inadequate tissue perfusion is due both to the increased production of lactate and the decreased hepatic metabolism.[76] In patients with acute or chronic liver disease the ability to metabolize lactate may be further compromised, potentially exacerbating any degree of the lactic acidosis.

Specific Protein Synthesis

Secretory Proteins

The hepatocyte is the principal site for synthesis and secretion of most of the plasma proteins, other than the immunoglobulins. With fasting, the synthesis of serum carrier proteins decreases.[93] With short-term fasting the reduced supply of available amino acids is compensated for by protein breakdown in the liver and extrahepatic sites, especially skeletal muscle. Although controversy exists, it appears that long-term alcohol ingestion inhibits protein secretion to a greater extent than protein synthesis.[94-96] Hormonal influences on hepatic production of carrier proteins varies depending on the clinical situation; in general, insulin, thyroid hormones, and growth hormones stimulate while glucagon reduces hepatic protein synthesis. The effects of glucocorticoids vary depending on which protein is studied.[97] The hepatocyte is the major site of synthesis and release of the acute phase proteins such as complement, ceruloplasmin, α_1-antitrypsin, fibrinogen, haptoglobin, and creative proteins.[98,99] The production of these proteins is stimulated by glucocorticoids and the inflammatory cytokines, interleukins-1 and -6, and tumor necrosis factor.

The effect of liver disease on production of hepatic secretory proteins is altered by a number of interdependent, but variable, factors, including the functional hepatocyte mass, nutritional status, availability of substrates, oncotic pressure, and hormone levels.[93]

The liver is the exclusive site of albumin biosynthesis, but albumin degradation takes place in almost all cells. Usually a steady state exists between albumin synthesis and degradation. The rate of albumin synthesis is regulated by a variety of factors including the availability of precursors and the extracellular oncotic pressure. The liver responds to decreasing oncotic pressure with an increased rate of albumin synthesis and secretion.[100] Albumin has two functions in the circulation. It is the most important regulator of plasma oncotic pressure and is the principal transport protein for many endogenous and exogenous substances. The serum concentration of albumin is the net result of three processes: synthesis, degradation, and distribution. Thus the serum albumin level does not necessarily correlate directly with the degree of hepatic dysfunction.[101]

As noted in the section on lipid metabolism, the liver is the primary site of the formation of lipoproteins, and these carrier proteins are vital for the transport of plasma lipids. Some of the other transport proteins synthesized in the liver include transferrin, the major transport protein for iron[102,103]; ceruloplasmin, the major transport protein for copper[104,105]; steroid-binding proteins[93]; thyroid hormone–binding proteins[106]; retinol-binding proteins[93]; and vitamin D–binding proteins.[107,108]

Clotting Proteins and Hemostasis

Normal hemostasis is a complicated interplay between several factors, including the blood vessel wall, platelets, and the normal plasma factors for both coagulation and fibrinolysis. A delicate balance exists between these complex systems, which prevents both bleeding and thrombosis, and the liver plays a central role in the regulation of this balance. In addition to being the major site of the synthesis of coagulation proteins, of naturally occurring anticoagulants, and of the proteins of the fibrinolytic system, the liver also plays a central role in clearing the blood of activated clotting factors and circulating activators of the plasminogen system.[109-111] The accompanying box shows the effects of liver disease on hemostasis.

EFFECT OF LIVER DISEASE ON HEMOSTASIS

Decreased Synthesis of Proteins

Coagulation: Factors XII, IX, VII, V, and II; fibrinogen, prekallikrein, kininogen
Anticoagulant: Proteins C and S, antithrombin III
Profibrinolytic: Plasminogen
Antifibrinolytic: 2-Antiplasmin, Cl-inhibitor, 2-macroglobulin, histidine-rich glycoprotein

Synthesis of Abnormal Proteins

Vitamin K–dependent factors
Factor VIII and von Willebrand's factor
Fibrinogen

Decreased Clearance Function

Activated coagulation factors
Plasminogen activators
Thrombin antithrombin III complexes

Abnormalities of Platelets

Disseminated intravascular coagulation
Lipoproteins

From Hoffman AL, et al. Hepatic regeneration: Current concepts and clinical implications. Semin Liver Dis 14(2):191, 1994. Reprinted with permission of Thieme Medical Publishers, Inc.

The liver is the major site for the production of all coagulation proteins except von Willebrand's factor. Vitamin K deficiency is associated with a fall in the plasma levels of actor IX (Christmas factor), factor X (Stuart factor), and factor VII. In addition, levels of prothrombin and the anticoagulant proteins, proteins C and S, are also diminished in patients with vitamin K deficiency. The coagulopathy experienced by patients with liver disease may be the result of vitamin K deficiency secondary to poor absorption of vitamin K from the gastrointestinal tract. Patients with more advanced liver disease may be unable to use the available vitamin K because of hepatocellular dysfunction. As shown in the box, patients with hepatocellular dysfunction also produce diminished amounts of the other proteins required for normal coagulation. Monitoring of the levels of coagulation factors, especially factor V, in patients with AFHF has been correlated with the likelihood for recovery from the acute liver injury.[112,113]

Patients with acute or chronic liver disease may also synthesize abnormal proteins. When insufficient vitamin K is present, the nonfunctional precursor forms of the coagulation proteins continue to be synthesized but are biologically inactive and cannot be converted to their active form without vitamin K. Patients with chronic liver disease may produce abnormal factor VIII and von Willebrand's factor and may synthesize fibrinogen, which is defective in its ability to polymerize.[111,114-116]

Fibrinolysis is a recognized complication of cirrhosis, liver surgery, and liver trauma. In addition to being the site for the synthesis of plasminogen, the liver is the main site for the synthesis of the major plasmin inhibitor, α_2-plasmin inhibitor. In patients with liver disease, there may also be an impaired clearance of plasminogen activators. The mechanism of increased fibrinolysis in patients with acute and chronic liver disease is therefore multifactorial.[117-119] The increased levels of circulating plasminogen activators are the direct result of decreased clearance and reduced inhibition of plasmin as the result of diminished synthesis of plasmin inhibitors. Disseminated intravascular coagulation (DIC) is also associated with acute and chronic liver disease. The pathogenesis of DIC is multifactorial and is dependent on the clinical condition of the patient.[120,121] In general, however, all patients seem to experience an increased activation of clotting factors secondary to the release of thromboplastic material in the presence of reduced concentrations of the main inhibitory proteins, antitrypsin III, protein C, and α_2-antiplasmin. In addition, this is coupled with an impaired removal of activated clotting factors and increased fibrinolytic activity as previously described.

Lipid Phase Metabolism

Drug Metabolism and Related Functions

Elimination of many drugs depends on their chemical modification, and the liver is the major site for this activity. Oxidation, acetylation, sulfation, methylation, hydroxylation, and addition of glucuronide or taurine residues are among the major reactions used in the liver to process these substances.[43] The diversity of substrate, which can be processed by the liver, seems incompatible with the exquisite specificity normally associated with enzymatic activity. Merrell states that "the fact that the capacity to detoxify twentieth-century drugs by enzymes evolved many millions of years ago is puzzling, unless one recalls that most drugs are derived from alkaloids that are plant products encountered in the diet. In fact, it was inevitable that consumption of plants would require the acquisition of enzyme pathways that could inactivate biologically active molecules absorbed from plant foods."[43] Substrate acceptance by the active sites of these enzymes may be dependent on induced modification of the active sites, once the cell has been exposed to the structure of a particular drug or substance. Although substrate induction of its specific metabolizing enzyme may be important, the broad induction of many enzymes can be brought about by a number of drugs, and it appears that these metabolizing enzymes can exist for many generations without being induced. This phenomenon may be responsible for the enormous variation in capacity to metabolize certain drugs seen between individuals. For most drugs a sixfold to tenfold variation in the metabolic rate of a substance among the populace is common.[122]

The chemical modification of drugs in the hepatocyte is localized to the smooth endoplasmic reticulum. The most prominent of the enzyme systems is the cytochrome P-450 system, and substrates must be rendered lipid soluble to gain access to these enzymes. This requirement compartmentalizes the drug-metabolizing activity from water-soluble metabolic intermediates that otherwise could serve as substrates for the enzymes. The products of endogenous metabolism that do participate in the reactions are appropriately lipid soluble and include bilirubin and cholesterol. Some of the by-products of the metabolism of these drugs by this fixed membrane system of the smooth endoplasmic reticulum are exported from the hepatocyte into bile, whereas other products leave the hepatocyte in a soluble form for renal excretion.[123]

The rate of hepatic metabolism of medications and other substances is variable in patients with acute or chronic liver disease. Because it is impossible to precisely establish the degree of hepatic dysfunction, there is an increased risk of toxicity following the administration of any drug metabolized by the liver, and extra thought must be used before prescribing any new medication to a patient with liver disease.

Bile Formation

A limited discussion of bilirubin, cholesterol, and bile acids is presented here, as these subjects are covered elsewhere in this book. Bilirubin is first solubilized by the addition of albumin to enable its transportation in blood.[9,124,125] Through a carrier-mediated membrane transport system, bilirubin enters the hepatocyte without albumin. A cytosolic protein ligand then binds to the bilirubin.[124-127] A smaller amount of bilirubin binds to the fatty acid–binding protein within the hepatocyte. Bilirubin is then solubilized by the conjugation of glucuronic acid to form bilirubin monoglucuronide and diglucuronide. This conjugation takes place in the endoplasmic reticulum of the hepatocyte.[124-127]

Cholesterol is oxidized in the endoplasmic reticulum of the hepatocyte to form cholic and deoxycholic acid.[128,129] In the bile, cholesterol is solubilized by the formation of micelles, with cholesterol occupying the hydrophobic center of the micelle.[128-130] The rate of formation of the bile salts is largely determined by the recirculation of the salts within the enterohepatic circulation. Bile salt or acid secretion is stimulated by the return of bile salts to the hepatocyte. In patients with a biliary fistula, the chronic loss of bile salts can increase bile salt synthesis 10-fold. Lecithin can be solubilized and incorporated into the bile acids to enable the micelle to solubilize increased amounts of cholesterol. Micelles are released into the bile, contributing to fat absorption within the gastrointestinal tract.[129,130]

Bile is released from the hepatocytes into the bile canaliculi. Bile canaliculi are channels lined by the plasma membrane of the hepatocytes. The fluid released into the canaliculi is isotonic.[131,132] Bile canaliculi converge to the bile ductules within the portal tracts. The composition of bile changes very little until bile enters the gallbladder, where it is concentrated. The liver produces 800 to 1000 ml of bile per day. However, the amount of bile released into the gastrointestinal tract may be much lower because of the reabsorption of fluid within the gallbladder.[131,132]

REGENERATION, REPAIR, AND CIRRHOSIS

The liver is unique among solid organs in having the capacity to respond to injury, which reduces the functioning hepatic mass by a dual process of hypertrophy and hyperplasia of the remaining hepatocytes.[133,134] This response is remarkable for a number of reasons. First, it occurs predictably and reproducibly in an organ in which mitotic activity is normally minimal in the adult. Second, new hepatocytes arise by proliferation of existing ones, despite the fact that these are cells with a wide range of specialized functions. Third, a similar response follows a second hepatectomy or repeated partial hepatectomies. Fourth, the proliferative response subsides when the original mass of the organ is restored. Fifth, the regeneration is not morphogenetic. Regeneration does not restore the lobe or the lobes that were removed but involves rather the enlargement of the part that remains. The factors controlling this response have been extensively investigated. The box on p. 505 lists all the known and suspected regulators of hepatic regeneration. When this response is initiated, hepatocytes both enlarge (hypertrophy) and increase in number (hyperplasia). The proliferation of hepatocytes may initially form two cell–thick hepatic plates, rosettes and pseudoducts, a configuration reminiscent of that seen in the fetal or neonatal liver. This response eventually remodels to assume the normal hepatic architecture, provided the agent

GROWTH REGULATORS OF HEPATIC REGENERATION

Growth-Stimulating Factors	Growth Inhibitory Factors
Hepatocyte growth factor	Transforming growth factor-β
Transforming growth factor-α	14 kDa protein
α-Fibroblast growth factor	Regenerating liver inhibitory factor-1
Epidermal growth factor	Rapamycin
Hepatocyte-stimulating substance	Interleukin-1
Insulin-like growth factor	Interleukin-6
Tumor necrosis factor	Interleukin-2
Hepatopoietins	

Hormones, Free Neurotransmitters, Nutrients, Immunosuppressive Drugs

Insulin	Glucagon
Catecholamines	Steroids (including sex hormones)
Calcium	Vitamin D
Parathyroid hormone	Triiodothyronine
Vasopressin	Angiotensin
Prolactin	Estradiol
Ions	Cyclosporine
FK506	Azathioprine (selected cases)
FKBP (receptor for FK506 and Rapamycin)	15-Deoxyspergualin
Prostaglandins	

From Lee CA, Kernoff PBA, Hutton RA. Haemostasis in liver disease. In McIntyre N, et al., eds. Oxford Textbook of Clinical Hepatology. Oxford: Oxford University Press, 1991, p 1236. By permission of Oxford University Press.)

responsible for the initial hepatic damage has been eliminated. Bile duct epithelium and mesenchymal elements, including Kupffer and epithelial cells, collagen, and reticulum, also take part in the regeneration response, although their proliferation lags behind that of the hepatocytes.

The extracellular matrix is a complex of collagen, proteoglycans, and noncollagenous glycoproteins that serves as the skeleton for the liver cells. In addition to the response of hepatocytes described above, cytokines released in response to liver injury also modulate the response of the other liver cells. A variety of cytokines have been shown to have either stimulatory or inhibitory effects on the regenerative process. Hoffman et al.[133] have noted that "regeneration can be viewed as an increase in cell mass without a concomitant increase in extracellular matrix with the net result initially being a decrease in extracellular matrix to cell mass ratio." When the cytokine-mediated balance is shifted by persistent injury, enhanced synthesis and assembly of matrix and decreased matrix degradation result in fibrosis and eventually cirrhosis.

In chronic or persistent injury the injured liver continues to attempt to repair and restore the functional hepatic mass. However, the regeneration takes place in the face of a proliferating extracellular matrix. This results in the vascular and reticulin architecture becoming disrupted with an associated loss of cell polarity, an uncoupling of hepatocytes, and the closure of gap junctions, all of which result in abnormal cell communication and function. Hepatic fibrosis appears to be simply an earlier stage of the cirrhotic process, distinguished by the fact that irreversible architectural disruption has not yet occurred. Therefore although cirrhosis is irreversible, fibrosis may be reversed with removal of the inciting agent.

DERANGED HEPATIC FUNCTION

Throughout this chapter, the normal functions of the liver and how these normal functions are altered by liver disease have been described. In assessing patients with chronic liver disease, the Child-Pugh classification (Table 23-1) continues to provide a reasonable correlation between the degree of hepatic dysfunction and the risk of a major surgical procedure. As this system was initially developed for patients undergoing portal decompressive procedures, the presence of a significant portal hypertension was inferred. Originally, the Child's classification included five straightforward, but somewhat subjective, parameters of hepatic function including the serum bilirubin and albumin levels, amount of ascites, the stage of encephalopathy, and the severity of malnutrition.[135] The Pugh modification dropped nutritional assessment in favor of the more measurable reflection of hepatic function, the prothrombin time.[136] The system categorizes the degree of hepatic dysfunction as A, B, or C and the surgical mortality rate correlates well with this clarification. The choice of the parameters examined was carefully calculated to reflect a variety of hepatic functions. Bilirubin metabolism requires

Table 23-1. Pugh's Modification of Child's Classification

Clinical and Biochemical Measurements	Points Scored for Increasing Abnormality		
	1	2	3
Encephalopathy*	None	1 and 2	3 and 4
Ascites	Absent	Slight	Moderate
Bilirubin (mg/100 ml)	1-2	2-3	>3
Albumin (g/L)	>35	28-35	<28
Prothrombin time (second prolonged)	1-4	4-6	>6
Child's A = 5-6 points (mortality = 3-10%)			
Child's B = 7-9 points (mortality = 10-30%)			
Child's C = 10-15 points (mortality = 50-80%)			

Adapted from McIntyre N. Symptoms and signs of liver disease. In McIntyre N, et al., eds. Oxford Textbook of Clinical Hepatology. Oxford: Oxford University Press, 1991, p 273. By permission of Oxford University Press.
*Grading of Trey, et al. N Engl J Med 274:473, 1966.

the conjugation and detoxification functions of the liver. In the stable cirrhotic patient a rise in bilirubin may indicate impairment of this system. Both albumin and prothrombin time reflect the synthetic capacity of the liver. Although serum albumin levels may be altered by factors other than hepatocellular dysfunction, low serum albumin levels, in general, reflect a significant impairment of normal hepatic function. The severity of the coagulopathy as measured by prolongation of the prothrombin time also reflects decreased hepatic protein synthesis. The presence of ascites not only reflects the derangement of the plasma oncotic pressure but also alteration of the portal venous pressure and the dynamics of lymph formation in the gastrointestinal tract and liver.

While the precise cause of hepatic encephalopathy remains unknown, the presence of encephalopathy reflects the diminished ability of the liver to capture and metabolize ammonia and other toxins from the gastrointestinal tract, either because of hepatic dysfunction or portosystemic shunting. Encephalopathy rarely occurs in patients who undergo total shunts for extrahepatic portal vein thrombosis associated with a normal liver. Nutritional deficiencies in patients with advanced liver disease are reflected most dramatically by muscle wasting. This results from the complex alterations of carbohydrate, lipid, and amino acid metabolism associated with advanced liver disease, which fails to provide an adequate pool of amino acids for continued production of structural proteins within the muscle.

Although chronic liver disease is most often associated with the gradual loss of hepatic function, AFHF is characterized by the rapid loss of virtually all vital hepatic functions, manifested by hypoglycemia, severe coagulopathy, hepatic coma, and multisystem organ failure. The mode of death of patients with chronic liver disease most often involves complications of bleeding or infection, whereas death of patients with AFHF usually follows the rapid deterioration of the patient to stage IV hepatic coma associated with the development of massive cerebral edema and eventual brain stem herniation.[137,138] Although patients with chronic liver disease may experience stage IV hepatic coma, they rarely develop cerebral edema. The reason that cerebral edema develops in patients with AFHF and not in patients with chronic liver disease is unknown.

For the surgeon facing an operative procedure on a patient with acute or chronic liver disease, many of the deranged hepatic functions significantly increase the patient's risk of morbidity and mortality.[139,140] In addition to the Child-Pugh classification for patients undergoing portal decompressive procedures, a number of other groups have developed prognostic scoring systems. However, none of these prognostic indexes are universally applicable to all patients with liver disease. This is understandable in view of the wide variation in the clinical course of patients with various liver diseases.[141-143] Newer surgical techniques, especially segmentectomies, have reduced the amount of liver mass removed while still providing an adequate resection of the hepatic malignancy. These procedures have allowed successful tumor resection in many patients who as a result of advanced liver disease would not have been able to tolerate a formal hepatic lobectomy.

EVALUATION OF THE LIVER

Liver function tests (LFTs) are used in the evaluation and management of patients with hepatic dysfunction. These tests often provide a sensitive, noninvasive method of screening for the presence of liver dysfunction. Patterns of abnormalities in the tests may provide a general impression of the type of liver disorder and give an indication of the severity of the liver dysfunction. Serial measurement of LFTs allow one to follow the course of the liver dysfunction and evaluate the response of the liver to therapeutic interventions. One of the limitations of LFTs is their lack of sensitivity; using these tests alone, it is often difficult to identify the precise cause of the liver disorder. Additionally, even a complete set of LFTs cannot fully assess the functional capacity of the liver because of the multitude of functions of this organ.

LFTs fall into four basic categories.[144] First are the tests that assess the liver's capacity to transport organic anions and metabolize drugs. These include the serum bilirubin level, the serum level of specific bile acids,[145-149] a variety of dye and breath tests,[150-153] and a number of clearance tests.[154-156] Each of these tests measures the liver's ability to clear endogenous or exogenous substances from the circulation. The second group of tests are those which detect injury to the liver cells. These are the enzyme tests including the aminotransferases and alkaline phosphatase. The third group are tests of the liver's biosynthetic capacity. These include measurements of serum albumin, ceruloplasmin, ferritin, lipoproteins, and blood-clotting factors, The final tests are those that detect chronic inflammation of the liver, faulty immunoregulation, or viral hepatitis. These include measurements of immunoglobulin levels, hepatitis serologies, and specific autoantibodies. Many of these tests are not truly LFTs because most of these substances are proteins made by the B lymphocytes and not the hepatocytes. However, many of these tests are quite specific for liver diseases.

Tests of Liver's Capacity to Transport Organic Anions and Metabolize Drugs

The total serum bilirubin level is a summation of two fractions of bilirubin: conjugated (direct) and unconjugated (indirect) bilirubin. The conjugated fraction represents the portion of bilirubin that has been solubilized in the liver by conjugation to glucuronic acid. This process forms bilirubin monoglucuronide and diglucuronide, both of which are referred to as the direct-reacting bilirubins. Unconjugated bilirubin is that fraction of the total bilirubin that has not been solubilized by the liver. Hyperbilirubinemia can be the result of several different mechanisms. Overproduction of bilirubin, hemolysis, damage to hepatocytes, and defects of conjugation or excretion are some of the causes of hyperbilirubinemia. The level of bilirubin elevation is not clinically specific to the degree of hepatocellular dysfunction. In the face of falling transaminase levels, a rise in serum bilirubin levels, coupled with a worsening prothrombin time, is usually associated with a poor prognosis. Dye tests[150,153] are rarely used in clinical practice and measurement of specific bile acids is usually of little use in routine clinical practice. The same may be said for the various breath tests[151,152] and the caffeine clearance test.[154] Galactose elimination capacity has been reported to be useful in the assessment of the hepatic reserve, but this test has not achieved widespread clinical application.[154-158]

Enzymes That Detect Hepatocellular Necrosis

Serum aminotransferases (formerly called transaminases) are the most sensitive indicators of liver cell injury. Alanine aminotranferase (ALT, also known as serum glutamate pyruvate transaminase [SGPT]) and aspartate aminotransferase (AST, also known as serum glutamic-oxaloacetic transaminase [SGOT]) are the most frequently measured enzymes. AST is found in a number of organs, making it a less-sensitive indicator of liver injury, whereas ALT is present in its highest concentrations in the liver. Unfortunately, the pattern of enzyme elevation for either of these transaminases is not indicative of the type of liver injury.

Enzymes That Detect Cholestasis

Alkaline phosphatase is a name given to a group of enzymes that catalyze the hydrolysis of a large number of organic phosphate esters. Because alkaline phosphatase is found in a number of tissues, especially bone, elevation of this enzyme is relatively nonspecific. The major value of the measurement of the serum alkaline phosphatase level is in the diagnosis of liver disorders associated with cholestasis. About 75% of patients with profound cholestasis have a fourfold increase in their serum alkaline phosphatase levels.[144] The enzyme 5′-nucleotidase catalyzes the hydrolysis of nucleotides such as adenosine 5′-phosphate. 5′-Nucleotidase is found in a variety of tissues including liver, intestine, brain, and endocrine pancreas. The major value of the measurement of 5′-nucleotidase is its specificity for hepatobiliary disease. A concomitant elevation of alkaline phosphatase and 5′-nucleotidase is highly suggestive that the elevated alkaline phosphatase is of hepatic origin. γ-Glutamyl transpeptidase (GGTP) is an enzyme found primarily in the bile ductular cells and like 5′-nucleotidase, an elevated GGTP confirms that the elevated alkaline phosphatase values are more likely of hepatic origin. The GGTP is also elevated in patients with alcoholic liver disease,[159] and following serial measurements of the GGTP along with the ALT is useful to monitor the transplanted liver for the presence of rejection.[160,161]

Tests of Liver's Biosynthetic Capacity

As discussed earlier in this chapter, most of the serum proteins (except immunoglobulins) are produced by the liver, and serial determination of these proteins has been used as an index of hepatic function. Serum albumin levels and the prothrombin time are the serum proteins most frequently monitored. Because abnormalities in the serum levels of both of these proteins may be due to a variety of factors, neither of these tests provide sensitive nor specific indications of the degree of hepatic dysfunction. However, normal serum albumin levels or prothrombin times do indicate that the liver's synthetic capacity is relatively intact.

Tests That Detect Inflammation or Altered Immunoregulation

Serum immunoglobulins are produced by B lymphocytes, and elevated serum levels do not directly indicate hepatic dysfunction. In a patient with chronic liver disease the immunoglobulin levels may be elevated because of the impaired extraction by the reticuloendothelial system in the hepatic sinusoids or the portosystemic shunting.[162] Elevated serum levels of a number of immunoglobulins may be helpful in the differentiation of the type of liver dysfunction. Very sensitive and specific serologic tests are available to detect hepatitis A, B, C, D, and E. The pattern of elevation of a number of nonspecific immunoglobulins such as antimitochondrial antibodies, antinuclear antibodies, and antismooth muscle antibodies may be useful in diagnosing specific liver disorders. Primary biliary cirrhosis, for example, is most commonly associated with marked elevation sin the serum levels of antimitochondrial antibodies and alkaline phosphatase.[163,164]

Additional Evaluation of the Liver

Radiology

It is beyond the scope of this chapter to provide a complete review of all the radiologic tests available to assess the liver, and comprehensive reviews have been published elsewhere.[165-174] At the present time, ultrasound provides the most useful noninvasive means to assess the liver. Ultrasound provides an accurate assessment of the hepatic parenchyma, detects the presence of lesions as small as 1 cm within the liver substance, identifies abnormalities within the biliary tree or gall bladder, and with the addition of Doppler accurately assesses the hepatic vasculature. Ultrasound is also useful to localize lesions for biopsy or drainage and is increasingly being used intraoperatively to assess for the presence of additional lesions when performing hepatic resection or cryosurgery.[168] The newer generation of CT scans and MRI, as well as new dynamic imaging techniques, provides an increasingly clear picture of the structure of the liver.[165,174] Radionuclear imaging techniques are also used to assess either the hepatic parenchyma or the biliary system, with the HIDA scan being the most commonly used.[170] Finally, invasive procedures such as percutaneous transhepatic cholangiography (PTC),[169] angiography,[166] placement of biliary stents,[167] TIPSS,[30-33] drainage of liver abscesses, or biopsy of hepatic lesions are part of the radiologist's armamentarium to assess and treat hepatic abnormalities.

SUMMARY

In ancient Greek mythology, Prometheus was punished by Zeus for giving fire to humans. He was condemned to have his liver consumed each day by a great bird, only to have it regenerate each night. As noted by Merrell,[43] this torture was certainly well considered in that no other organ is critical to life and yet is capable of remarkable healing and regeneration. Because of its central role in the anatomy and physiology of the body, the liver is subject to a huge variety of insults and injuries, as well as being primarily responsible for the maintenance of metabolic homeostasis. The liver remains unique among human organs in its ability to respond to injury by restoration of the functional hepatic mass. The loss of this regenerative capacity leads to the development of cirrhosis and eventual death from complications of liver failure. Perhaps the clearest indication of the importance of the liver is that it is highly unlikely that a mechanical device that does not include the use of living hepatocytes will ever be developed to replace the failing liver. It is perhaps unrealistic to imagine that any mechanical device will be able to duplicate the vast array of functions performed by the liver. Despite the tremendous advances that have been made in refining our understanding of hepatic anatomy and physiology, each year, more than 25,000 Americans die of cirrhosis, and more than 25 million are afflicted with diseases of the liver and biliary system.

REFERENCES

1. Sigerest HE. A History of Medicine: Primitive and Archaic Medicine, vol 1. New York: Oxford University Press, 1967.
2. Gray SW, et al. Surgical anatomy of the liver and associated extrahepatic structures. Contemp Surg 30:37, 1987.
3. Middleton J. Magic, Witchcraft and Curing. Garden City, N.Y.: Natural History Press, 1967.
4. Skandalakis JE. Surgical anatomy of the liver and associated extrahepatic structures. Contemp Surg 30:25, 1987.
5. Biolac-Sage P, LeBail B, Balabaud C. Liver and biliary tract history. In McIntyre N, et al., eds. Oxford Textbook of Clinical Hepatology, vol 1. Oxford: Oxford University Press, 1991.
6. Rappaport AM. Physioanatomic considerations. In Schiff L, Schiff ER, eds. Diseases of the Liver, 6th ed. Philadelphia: JB Lippincott, 1987.
7. Bismouth H, Aldridge MC, Kuntslinger F. Macroscopic anatomy of the liver. In McIntyre N, et al., eds. Oxford Textbook of Clinical Hepatology, vol 1. Oxford: Oxford University Press, 1991.
8. Thung SN, Gerber MA. Liver. In Sternberg SS, ed. Histology for Pathologists. New York: Raven Press, 1992.
9. Arias IM, et al., eds. The Liver: Biology and Pathobiology, 2nd ed. New York: Raven Press, 1988.
10. Couinaud C. LeFoie: Etudes anatomiques et chirurgicales. Paris: Masson, 1957.
11. Andrus CH, Kaminski DL. Segmented hepatic resection utilizing the ultrasonic dissection. Arch of Surg 121:515, 1986.
12. Scheele J, Stangl R. Segment orientated anatomical liver resections. In Blumgart LH, ed. Surgery of the Liver and Biliary Tract, 2nd ed., vol 2. New York: Churchill Livingstone, 1994.
13. Emond JC, et al. Reduced-size orthotopic liver transplantation: Use in the management of children with chronic liver disease. Hepatology 5:867, 1989.
14. Otte JB, et al. Size reduction of the donor liver is a safe way to alleviate the shortage of size-matched organs in pediatric liver transplantation. Ann Surg 211:146, 1990.
15. Emond JC, et al. Transplantation of two patients with one liver: Analysis of a preliminary experience with split liver graft. Ann Surg 212:14, 1990.
16. Rogiers X, et al. In situ splitting of the liver in the heart-beating cadaveric organ donor for transplantation in two recipients. Transplantation 59:1081, 1995.
17. Broelsch CE, et al. Liver transplantation in children from living-related donors. Ann Surg 214:428, 1991.
18. Emond JC. Living-related liver transplantation: Evaluation of donors and recipients. In The Liver Transplant Evaluation: Linking Risk Factors and Outcome, American Association for the Study of Liver Disease and International Liver Transplant Society, 1995, p 103.

19. Emond JC, et al. Improved results of living-related liver transplantation with routine application in a pediatric program. Transplantation 55(4):885, 1993.
20. Tanaka K, et al. Surgical techniques and innovations in living-related liver transplantation. Ann Surg 217(1):82, 1993.
21. Genecin P, Groszmann RJ. Hepatic blood flow, measurement, and physiological regulation. In McIntyre N, et al., eds. Oxford Textbook of Clinical Hepatology, vol 1. Oxford: Oxford University Press, 1991.
22. Mathie RT, Wheatley AM, Blumgart LH. Liver blood flow: Physiology, measurement and clinical relevance. In Blumgart LH, ed. Surgery of the Liver and Biliary Tract, 2nd ed., vol 1. New York: Churchill Livingstone, 1994.
23. Wynne HA, et al. The effect of age upon liver volume and apparent liver blood flow in healthy man. Hepatology 9:297, 1989.
24. Gibson RN, Hemingway AP. Radiological anatomy of the liver and biliary tract. In Blumgart LH, ed. Surgery of the Liver and Biliary Tract, 2nd ed., vol 1. New York: Churchill Livingstone, 1994.
25. Hiatt JR, Gabbay J, Busuttil RW. Surgical anatomy of the hepatic arteries in 1000 cases. Ann Surg 220(1):50, 1994.
26. Benoit JN, Granger DW. Splanchnic hemodynamics in chronic portal hypertension. Semin Liver Dis 6:287, 1986.
27. Ryley NG, McGee JO'D. Cirrhosis and portal hypertension: Pathological aspects. In Blumgart LH, ed. Surgery of the Liver and Biliary Tract, 2nd ed., vol 2. New York: Churchill Livingstone, 1994.
28. Arroyo V, et al. Ascites, renal failure, and electrolyte disorders in cirrhosis: Pathogenesis, diagnosis, and treatment. In McIntyre N, et al., eds. Oxford Textbook of Clinical Hepatology, vol 1. Oxford: Oxford University Press, 1991.
29. Witte MH, Witte CL, Dumont AE. Estimated net transcapillary water and protein flux in the liver and intestine of patients with portal hypertension from hepatic cirrhosis. Gastroenterology 80:265, 1981.
30. Conn HO. Transjugular intrahepatic portal-systemic shunts: The state of the art. Hepatology 17:148, 1993.
31. Roesslel M, et al. The transjugular intrahepatic portosystemic stent-shunt procedure for variceal bleeding. N Engl J Med 330:165, 1994.
32. Shiffman ML, et al. The role of transjugular intrahepatic portosystemic shunt for treatment of portal hypertension and its complications: A conference sponsored by the National Digestive Diseases Advisory Board. Hepatology 22(5):1591, 1995.
33. Wong F, Blendis L. Transjugular intrahepatic portosystemic shunt for refractory ascites: Tipping the sodium balance. Hepatology 22(1):358, 1995.
34. Collins P, McIntyre N. The liver in cardiovascular and pulmonary disease. In McIntyre N, et al., eds. Oxford Textbook of Clinical Hepatology, vol 2. Oxford: Oxford University Press, 1991.
35. Wang Z, et al. Recognition and management of Budd-Chiari syndrome: Report of one hundred cases. J Vasc Surg 10:149, 1989.
36. Becker C, Scheedegger J, Marincek B. Hepatic veins occlusion: Morphologic features on completed tomography and ultrasonography. Gastrointest Radiol 11:305, 1986.
37. Maddrey WD. Hepatic vein thrombosis (Budd-Chiari syndrome) possible association with the use of oral contraceptives. Semin Liver Dis 7:32, 1987.
38. Orloff MJ, Daily PO, Gerard B. Treatment of Budd-Chiari syndrome due to inferior vena cava occlusion by combined portal and vena caval decompression. Am J Surg 163:137, 1992.
39. Orloff MF, Orloff MS. Budd-Chiari syndrome and veno-occlusive disease. In Blumgart LH, ed. Surgery of the Liver and Biliary Tract, 2nd ed., vol 2. New York: Churchill Livingstone, 1994.
40. Ayash LJ, et al. Hepatic veno-occlusive disease in autologous bone marrow transplantation of solid tumors and lymphomas. J Clin Oncol 8:1699, 1990.
41. Bach N, Thung SN, Schaffner F. Comfrey herb tea induced hepatic veno-occlusive disease. Am J Med 87:97, 1989.
42. McDonald GB, et al. Veno-occlusive disease of the liver after bone marrow transplantation: Diagnosis, incidence and predisposing factors. Hepatology 4:116, 1984.
43. Merrell RC. Hepatic physiology. In Miller TA, ed. Physiologic Basis of Modern Surgical Care. St. Louis: CV Mosby, 1988.
44. Dixit V. Development of a bioartificial liver using isolated hepatocytes. Artif Organs 18:371, 1994.
45. Jauregui HO, Mullon CJ, Trenkler D, et al. In vivo evaluation of a hollow fiber liver assist device. Hepatology 21:460, 1995.
46. Nyberg L, et al. Evolution of the bioartificial liver: The need for randomized clinical trials. Am J Surg 166:512, 1993.
47. Sussman NL, Gislason GT, Kelly JH. Extracorporeal liver support: Application to fulminant hepatic failure. J Clin Gastroenterol 18:320, 1994.
48. Hoofnagle JH, et al. Fulminant hepatic failure: Summary of a workshop. Hepatology 21:240, 1995.
49. Lee WJ. Acute liver failure (review article). N Engl J Med 329(25):1862, 1993.
50. Fabry TL, Klion FM, eds. Guide to Liver Transplantation. New York: Igaku-Shoin Medical Publishers, 1992.
51. Maddrey WD, ed. Transplantation of the Liver. New York: Elsevier Publishing, 1988.
52. Fraser R, Day WA, Fernando NS. The liver sinusoidal cells: Their role in disorders of the liver, lipoprotein metabolism and atherogenesis. Pathology 18:5, 1986.
53. Nouri-Aria KT, Eddleston ALWF. Immunological functions of the liver. In McIntyre N, et al., eds. Oxford Textbook of Clinical Hepatology, vol 1, Oxford: Oxford University Press, 1991.
54. Kruszynska Y, McIntyre N. Carbohydrate metabolism. In McIntyre N, et al., eds. Oxford Textbook of Clinical Hepatology, vol 1, Oxford: Oxford University Press, 1991.
55. Ferrannini E, et al. The disposal of an oral glucose load in healthy subjects: A quantitative study. Diabetes 34:580, 1985.
56. Radziuk J, et al. Initial splanchnic extraction of ingested glucose in normal man. Metabolism 27:657, 1978.
57. Kruszynska YT, Home PD, Alberti KGMM. In vivo regulation of liver and skeletal muscle glycogen synthase activity by glucose and insulin. Diabetes 35:662, 1986.
58. Nosadini R, et al. Carbohydrate and lipid metabolism in cirrhosis: Evidence that hepatic uptake of gluconeogenic precursors and of free fatty acids depends on effective hepatic blood flow. J Clin Endocrinol Metab 58:1125, 1984.
59. Kelly D, et al. Skeletal muscle glycolysis, oxidation and storage of an oral glucose load. J Clin Invest 81:1563, 1988.
60. Taylor R, et al. Insulin action in hepatic cirrhosis: In vivo and in vitro studies. Hepatology 8:1615, 1988.
61. Creutzfeldt W, et al. Liver disease and glucose homeostasis. In Bianchi L, et al., eds. Liver in Metabolic Diseases. Lancaster: MTP Press, 1983.
62. Harry DS, McIntyre N. Plasma lipids and lipoproteins. In McIntyre N, et al., eds. Oxford Textbook of Clinical Hepatology, vol 1. Oxford: Oxford University Press, 1991.
63. Albero JJ, Segrest JP. Plasma lipoproteins—Part B: Characterization, cell biology and metabolism. In Colowick and Kaplan's Methods in Enzymology, vol 129. Orlando, Fla.: Academic Press, 1986.
64. McIntyre N, Harry DS. Lipids and lipoproteins. London: Wolfe Medical Publications, 1990.
65. Segrest JP, Albers JJ, eds. Plasma lipoproteins—Part A: Preparation, structure, and molecular biology. In Colowick and Kaplan's Methods in Enzymology, vol 128. Orlando, Fla.: Academic Press, 1986.

66. Glomset JA, Norum KR, Gjone E. Familial lecithin: Cholesterol acyltransferase deficiency. In Stanbury JB, et al., eds. The Metabolic Basis of Inherited Disease, 5th ed. New York: McGraw-Hill, 1988.
67. Quinn D, Shirai K, Jackson RL. Lipoprotein lipase: Mechanism of action and role in lipoprotein metabolism. Prog Lipid Res 22:5, 1983.
68. Avgerinos A, et al. Plasma lipid and lipoprotein response to carbohydrate feeding in cirrhotic patients. J Hepatol 6:315, 1988.
69. Avgerinos A, et al. Plasma lipid and lipoprotein responses to fat feeding in alcoholic liver disease. Hepatology 31:349, 1983.
70. Day RC, et al. Plasma lecithin-cholesterol acyltransferase and the lipoprotein abnormalities of parenchymal liver disease. Clin Sci 56:575, 1979.
71. Jahn CE, et al. Lipoprotein abnormalities in primary biliary cirrhosis. Gastroenterology 89:1266, 1985.
72. DeMartis M, et al. Pattern of lecithin-cholesterol-acyl-transferase (L-CAT) activity in the course of liver cirrhosis. J Int Med Res 11:232, 1983.
73. Simko V, Kelley RE, Dinscoy HP. Predicting severity of liver disease: Twelve laboratory tests evaluated by multiple regression. J Int Med Res 13(5):249, 1985.
74. Laffi G, et al. Altered platelet function in cirrhosis of the liver: Impairment of inositol lipid and arachidonic acid metabolism in response to agonists. Hepatology 8:1620, 1988.
75. Laffi G, et al. Altered renal and platelet arachidonic acid metabolism in cirrhosis. Gastroenterology 90(2):274, 1986.
76. Herrmann R, McIntyre N. Amino-acid metabolism, urea production, and pH regulation. In McIntyre N, et al., eds. Oxford Textbook of Clinical Hepatology, vol 1. Oxford: Oxford University Press, 1991.
77. Nyhan WL. Nonketotic hyperglycinemia. In Scriver CR, et al., eds. The Metabolic Basis of Inherited Disease, 6th ed. New York: McGraw-Hill, 1989.
78. Felig P. The glucose-alanine cycle. Metabolism 22:179, 1973.
79. Danner DJ, Elsas LJ. Disorders of branched chain amino acid and keto acid metabolism. In Scriver CR, et al., eds. The Metabolic Basis of Inherited Disease, 6th ed. New York: McGraw-Hill, 1989.
80. Hellerstein HK, Munro HN. Interaction of liver and muscle in the regulation of metabolism in response to nutritional and other factors. In Arias IM, et al., eds. The Liver: Biology and Pathobiology. New York: Raven Press, 1988.
81. Waterlow JC, Jackson AA. Nutrition and protein turnover in man. Br Med Bull 37:5, 1981.
82. Munro HN. Amino acid requirements and metabolism and their relevance to parenteral nutrition. In Wilkinson A, ed. Parenteral Nutrition. Edinburgh: Churchill Livingstone, 1972.
83. Gelfand RA, et al. Measurement of L-[1-14C] leucine kinetics in splanchnic and leg tissues in humans: Effect of amino acid infusion. Diabetes 37(10):1365, 1988.
84. Rothschild MA, Oratz M, Schreiber SS. Serum albumin. Hepatology 8(2):385, 1988.
85. Felig P. Amino acid metabolism in man. Annu Rev Biochem 44:933, 1975.
86. Elwyn D. The role of the liver in regulation of amino acid and protein metabolism. In Munro HN, ed. Mammalian Protein Metabolism. New York: Academic Press, 1970.
87. Felig P, et al. Amino acid metabolism during prolonged starvation. Eur J Clin Invest 48(3):584, 1969.
88. Record CO, et al. Plasma and brain amino acids in fulminant hepatic failure and their relationship to hepatic encephalopathy. Eur J Clin Invest 67:387, 1976.
89. Lowenstein JM. Ammonia production in muscle and other tissues: the purine nucleotide cycle. Physiol Rev 52:382, 1972.
90. Powers-Lee SG, Meister A. Urea synthesis and ammonia metabolism. In Arias IM, et al., eds. The Liver: Biology and Pathobiology. New York: Raven Press, 1988.
91. Weber FL Jr, Friedman DW, Fresard KM. Ammonia production from intraluminal amino acids in canine jejunum. Am J Physiol 254:264, 1988.
92. Hasselgran PO, et al. Current concepts of protein turnover and amino acid transport in liver and skeletal muscle during sepsis. Arch Surg 123:992, 1988.
93. Gerok W, Gross V. Secretory proteins: Synthesis, secretion and function. In McIntyre N, et al., eds. Oxford Textbook of Clinical Hepatology, vol 1. Oxford: Oxford University Press, 1991.
94. Baroana E, Lieber CS. Effect of alcohol on hepatic transport of proteins. Ann Rev Med 33:281, 1982.
95. Lieber CS. Alcohol, protein metabolism and liver injury. Gastroenterology 79:373, 1980.
96. Rothschild MA, Oratz M, Morland M. Effects of ethanol on protein synthesis and secretion. Pharmacol Biochem Behav 1(Suppl 13):31, 1980.
97. Tavill AS. Protein metabolism and the liver. In Wright R, et al., eds. Liver and Biliary Disease, 2nd ed. London: WB Saunders, 1985.
98. Gordon AH, Koj A. The acute phase response to injury and infection. In Research Monographs in Cell and Tissue Physiology. Amsterdam: Elsevier, 1985.
99. Kushner I. The phenomenon of the acute phase response. Ann N Y Acad Sci 389:39, 1982.
100. Rosenoer V, Oratz M, Rothschild M. Albumin: Structure, Function and Uses. Oxford: Pergamon Press, 1977.
101. Rothschild MA, Oratz M, Schreiber SS. Serum albumin in liver disease. In Bianchi L, et al., eds. Liver in Metabolic Diseases. Lancaster: MTP Press, 1983.
102. McKnight GS, et al. Transferrin gene expression: Effects of nutritional iron deficiency. J Biol Chem 255:144, 1980.
103. Morton AG, Tavill AS. The role of iron in the regulation of hepatic transferrin synthesis. Br J Haematol 36:383, 1977.
104. Sternlieb I. Copper and the liver. Gastroenterology 78:1615, 1980.
105. Sternlieb I. Copper and zinc. In Arias IM, et al., eds. The Liver: Biology and Pathobiology, 2nd ed. New York: Raven Press, 1988.
106. Cody V. Thyroid hormone interactions: Molecular conformation, protein binding and hormone action. Endocrinol Rev 1:140, 1980.
107. De Luca HF, Schoes HK. Vitamin D: Recent advances. Annu Rev Biochem 52:411, 1983.
108. Haddad JG. Transport of vitamin D metabolites. Clin Orthopaedics 142:249, 1979.
109. Carr JM. Hemostatic disorders in liver disease. In Schiff L, Schiff ER, eds. Diseases of the Liver, 7th ed. Philadelphia: JB Lippincott, 1993.
110. Kelly DA, Tuddenham EDG. Haemostatic problems in liver disease. Gut 27:339, 1986.
111. Lee CA, Kernoff PBA, Hutton RA. Effect of liver disease on other systems: Haemostasis in liver disease. In McIntyre N, et al., eds. Oxford Textbook of Clinical Hepatology, vol 2. Oxford: Oxford University Press, 1991.
112. O'Grady JG, et al. Early indications of prognosis in fulminant hepatic failure. Gastroenterology 97:349, 1989.
113. O'Grady JG, et al. Coagulopathy and fulminant hepatic failure. Semin Liver Dis 6:159, 1986.
114. Francis J, Armstrong DJ. Acquired dysfibrinogenemia in liver disease. J Clin Pathol 35:667, 1982.
115. Martinez J, Keane PM, Gilman PB. The abnormal carbohydrate composition of the dysfibrinogenemia associated with liver disease. Ann N Y Acad Sci 408:388, 1983.
116. Stein SF, Harker LA. Kinetic and functional studies of platelets, fibrinogen, plasminogen in patients with hepatic cirrhosis. J Lab Clin Med 99:217, 1982.
117. Boks A, Brommer EJP, Schalm SW. Hemostasis and fibrinolysis in severe liver failure and their relation to hemorrhage. Hepatology 6:79, 1980.

118. Francis RB Jr, Feinstein DI. Clinical significance of accelerated fibrinolysis in liver disease. Haemostasis 14:460, 1980.
119. Sprengers ED, Kluft C. Plasminogen activator inhibitors. Blood 69:381, 1987.
120. Carr JM. Disseminated intravascular coagulation in cirrhosis. Hepatology 10:103, 1989.
121. Verstraete M, Vermylen J, Collen D. Intravascular coagulation in liver disease. Annu Rev Med 25:447, 1974.
122. Kupfer A, Preisig R. Inherited defects of hepatic drug metabolism. Semin Liver Dis 3:341, 1983.
123. Griffeth LK, Rosen GM, Raukman EJ. Effects of model traumatic injury on hepatic drug metabolism in the rat. Drug Metab Dispos 13:398, 1985.
124. Hoffman AF. Overview of bile secretion. In Schultz SG, ed. Handbook of Physiology. Bethesda, Md.: American Physiological Society, 1989.
125. Vlahcevic ZR, Heuman DM, Hyleman PB. Regulation of bile acid synthesis. Hepatology 13:590, 1991.
126. Tiribelli C, Oxtrow JD. New concepts in bilirubin chemistry, transport and metabolism: Report of the international bilirubin workshop. Hepatology 11:303, 1990.
127. Tiribelli C, Oxtrow JD. new concepts in bilirubin chemistry, transport and metabolism: Report of the second international bilirubin workshop. Hepatology 17:715, 1993.
128. Bjorkhein I. Mechanism of bile acid biosynthesis in mammalian liver. In Danielsson H, Sjovall J, eds. Sterols and Bile Acids. Amsterdam: Elsevier Science, 1985.
129. Blitzer BL, Boyer JL. Cellular mechanisms of bile formation. Gastroenterology 82:346, 1982.
130. Carey MC, Small DM. Micelle formation by bile salts: Physical-chemical and thermodynamic considerations. Arch Intern Med 130:506, 1972.
131. Forker EL. Mechanisms of hepatic bile formation. Annu Rev Physiol 39:323, 1977.
132. Nathanson MH, Boyer FL. Mechanisms and regulation of bile secretion. Hepatology 14:551, 1991.
133. Hoffman AL, et al. Hepatic regeneration: Current concepts and clinical implications. Semin Liver Dis 14:190, 1994.
134. Weinbren K. Functions of the liver. In McIntyre N, et al., eds. Oxford Textbook of Clinical Hepatology, vol 1, Oxford: Oxford University Press, 1991.
135. Child CG, Turcotte JG. Surgery and portal hypertension. In Child CG, ed. The Liver and Portal Hypertension. Philadelphia: WB Saunders, 1964.
136. Pugh RNH, et al. Transsection of the oesophagus for bleeding oesophageal varices. Br J Surg 60:646, 1973.
137. Lidofsky SD, et al. Liver transplantation for fulminant hepatic failure: The role of intracranial pressure monitoring [abstract]. Gastroenterology 98:A604, 1990.
138. Moritz MJ, et al. Regeneration of the native liver after heterotopic liver transplantation for fulminant hepatic failure. Transplantation 55:952, 1993.
139. Garrison RN, et al. Clarification of risk factors for abdominal operations in patients with hepatic cirrhosis. Ann Surg 199:648, 1984.
140. Tinkoff G, et al. Cirrhosis in the trauma victim: Effect on mortality rates. Ann Surg 211:172, 1990.
141. Christensen E, et al. Updating prognosis and therapeutic effect evaluation in cirrhosis with Cox's multiple regression model for time-dependent variables. Scand J Gastroenterol 21:163, 1986.
142. D'Amico G, et al. Survival and prognostic indicators in compensated and decompensated cirrhosis. Dig Dis Sci 31:468, 1986.
143. Gines P, et al. Compensated cirrhosis: Natural history and prognostic factors. Hepatology 7:122, 1987.
144. Kaplan MM. Laboratory tests. In Schiff L, Schiff ER, eds. Diseases of the Liver, 7th ed. Philadelphia: JB Lippincott, 1993.
145. Ahlberg J, et al. Individual bile acids in portal venous and systemic blood serum in fasting man. Gastroenterology 73:1377, 1977.
146. Angelin B, et al. Hepatic uptake of bile acids in man: Fasting and postprandial concentrations of individual bile acids in portal venous and systemic blood venous. J Clin Invest 70:724, 1982.
147. Berry W. Reichen J. Bile acid metabolism: Its relation to clinical disease. Semin Liver Dis 3:330, 1983.
148. Jones MB, et al. Clinical values of serum bile acid levels in chronic hepatitis. Dig Dis Sci 26:978, 1981.
149. Milstein HJ, et al. Serum bile acids in alcoholic liver disease: Comparison with histological features of the disease. Am J Dig Dis 21:281, 1976.
150. Caesar J, et al. The use of indocyanine green in the measurement of hepatic blood flow and as a test of hepatic function. Clin Sci 21:43, 1961.
151. Hepner GW, Vesell ES. Assessment of aminopyrine metabolism in man by breath analysis after oral administration of ^{14}C aminopyrine: Effects of phenobarbital, disulfiram, and portal cirrhosis. N Engl J Med 291:1384, 1974.
152. Hoffman A. The aminopyrine demethylation breath test and the serum bile acid level: Nominated but not yet elected to join the common liver tests. Hepatology 4:152, 1982.
153. Shani M, et al. Sulfobromophthalein tolerance test in patients with Dubin-Johnson syndrome and their relatives. Gastroenterology 59:842, 1970.
154. Renner E, et al. Caffeine: A model compound for measuring liver function. Hepatology 4:38, 1984.
155. Shreeve WW, et al. Test for alcoholic cirrhosis by conversion of ^{14}C- or ^{13}C-galactose to expired CO_2. Gastroenterology 71:98, 1976.
156. Tygstrup N. Determination of the hepatic elimination capacity (Lm) of galactose by a single injection. Scand J Lab Clin Invest 18:118, 1966.
157. Henderson JM, Kutner MH, Bain RP. First order clearance of plasma galactose: The effect of liver disease. Gastroenterology 83:1090, 1988.
158. Henderson JM, et al. Distal splenorenal shunt with splenopancreatic disconnection: A 4-year assessment. Ann Surg 210:332, 1989.
159. Kaplan MM, et al. Biochemical basis for serum enzyme abnormalities in alcoholic liver disease. In Chang NC, Chan NM, eds. Early Identification of Alcohol Abuse. Research Monograph No 17, NIAAA, 1985.
160. Emond JC, et al. Rejection in liver allograft recipients: Clinical characterization and management. Clin Transplant 1:143, 1987.
161. Klintmalm GBG, et al. Rejection in liver transplantation. Hepatology 10:978, 1989.
162. Triger DR, Wright R. Hypergammaglobulinemia in liver disease. Lancet 1:1494, 1973.
163. Kaplan M. Primary biliary cirrhosis. In Schiff L, Schiff ER, eds. Diseases of the Liver, vol 1. Philadelphia: JB Lippincott, 1993.
164. Sherlock S. Primary biliary cirrhosis and vanishing bile ducts. In McIntyre N, et al., eds. Oxford Textbook of Clinical Hepatology, vol 2. Oxford: Oxford University Press, 1991.
165. Adam A, Roddie ME. Computed tomography of the liver and biliary tract. In Blumgart LH, ed. Surgery of the Liver and Biliary Tract, 2nd ed., vol 1. New York: Churchill Livingstone, 1994.
166. Allison ME. The kidney and the liver: Pre- and postoperative factors. In Blumgart LH, ed. Surgery of the Liver and Biliary Tract, 2nd ed., vol 1. New York: Churchill Livingstone, 1994.
167. Botet J. Interventional radiological techniques in the liver and biliary tract. In Blumgart LH, ed. Surgery of the Liver and Biliary Tract, 2nd ed., vol 1. New York: Churchill Livingstone, 1994.
168. Cosgrove DO. Ultrasound in surgery of the liver and biliary tract. In Blumgart LH, ed. Surgery of the Liver and Biliary Tract, 2nd ed., vol 1. New York: Churchill Livingstone, 1994.

169. Gibson RN. Percutaneous transhepatic cholangiography. In Blumgart LH, ed. Surgery of the Liver and Biliary Tract, 2nd ed., vol 1. New York: Churchill Livingstone, 1994.
170. Hoflin FG. Isotopic studies. In Blumgart LH, ed. Surgery of the Liver and Biliary Tract, 2nd ed., vol 1. New York: Churchill Livingstone, 1994.
171. Nissenbaum MA, vanSonnenberg E, D'Agostino HB. Interventional radiology in the liver, biliary tract, and gallbladder. In Schiff L, Schiff ER, eds. Diseases of the Liver, 7th ed., vol 1. Philadelphia: JB Lippincott, 1993.
172. Menu Y. Modern imaging of the liver and biliary tract. In McIntyre N, et al., eds. Oxford Textbook of Clinical Hepatology, vol 1. Oxford: Oxford University Press, 1991.
173. Taylor KJW, Kier R, Neuman R. Noninvasive imaging of the hepatobiliary system. In Schiff L, Schiff ER, eds. Diseases of the Liver, vol 1. Philadelphia: JB Lippincott, 1993.
174. Vock P. Magnetic resonance imaging. In Blumgart LH, ed. Surgery of the Liver and Biliary Tract, 2nd ed, vol 1. New York: Churchill Livingstone, 1994.

24

Portal Hypertension

James T. Mayes and J. Michael Henderson

Portal hypertension is caused by an increase in the resistance to portal venous flow as a result of many possible disease states. In almost all cases there is an associated alteration in splanchnic hemodynamics. As a direct result of the increased portal venous pressure, collateral flow is stimulated, and existing channels enlarge to form variceal channels connecting the portal and systemic circulation (Fig. 24-1). The most important site of variceal formation is in the distal esophagus and proximal stomach. Hemorrhage from these sites is one of the most significant complications of portal hypertension. Other clinical problems of portal hypertension are ascites formation, encephalopathy, and hypersplenism. Surgical therapy for portal hypertension requires a fundamental understanding of the severity of the underlying cause of the disorder, which is usually some form of liver disease. Liver transplantation has dramatically altered the treatment of advanced liver disease, so it is critical to remember that many of the operations to be discussed must be considered in this light.

ANATOMY

The liver has a dual blood supply from the hepatic artery and the portal vein. Arterial anatomy consists of right and left branches in 80% of cases arising from the proper hepatic artery, which arises from the common hepatic artery off the celiac axis. Important to note, however, is the 20% incidence of accessory or complete replacement of the right or left arteries with arterial branches arising from the left gastric artery or the superior mesenteric artery. Careful inspection of the lesser omentum in the region of the gastroesophageal junction reveals the accessory or replaced left arterial branches arising from the left gastric artery, and palpation along the right border of the hepatoduodenal ligament at the opening of Winslow's foramen identifies an accessory or replaced right hepatic arterial branch arising from the superior mesenteric artery. The hepatic artery, while contributing perhaps 25% to 30% of total flow to the liver, carries 60% to 70% of the oxygen supply and is the sole source of blood supply to the major bile ducts. The portal vein lies deep or dorsal to the hepatic artery and is formed at the junction of the superior mesenteric and splenic veins behind the neck of the pancreas. The portal vein then bifurcates at the liver hilus to feed the left and right hepatic lobes. Two other major veins contribute flow to the portal vein. The left gastric or coronary vein joins the portal or splenic vein close to their junction. This is the major vein leading to the gastroesophageal junction. The inferior mesenteric vein joins the splenic or superior mesenteric vein near their junction and is the collateral course to the hemorrhoidal plexus.

At a microscopic level (Fig. 24-2) a knowledge of the histologic anatomy and the circulation can help one understand pathophysiologic states. The fundamental unit of the liver is the lobule. Blood flows from portal venules and hepatic arterioles into sinuses in the lobule. At any one time 90% of the hepatic blood is found in these sinuses. The blood nourishes single plates of hepatocytes along a gradient of three zones as more and more nutrients are extracted on its path to the central vein in the lobule and back to the systemic circulation. The oxygen gradient of 200 to 400 torr from zone I to III can make "oxygen-poor" zone III the region most subject to hypoperfusion or hypoxic injury.[1] Toxic injuries tend to occur in zone I.

In summary, the liver circulation proceeds from major arteries and veins to the portal triads in the lobule. The blood percolates through the sinusoids and into the central vein. The central veins converge to form the major hepatic veins, which enter the inferior vena cava and return all blood to the systemic circulation.

PATHOPHYSIOLOGY

Normal hepatic blood flow constitutes 20% to 25% of the patient's cardiac output. Total flow is a combination of arterial and portal venous flow. What is unique is the ability of portal or arterial flow to compensate for deficits in each other. This is primarily achieved through the hepatic arterial buffer response whereby the arterial flow shows reciprocal responses to increases or decreases in portal venous flow. The current hypothesis for this is an adenosine washout, with a decrease in portal vein flow, allowing ac-

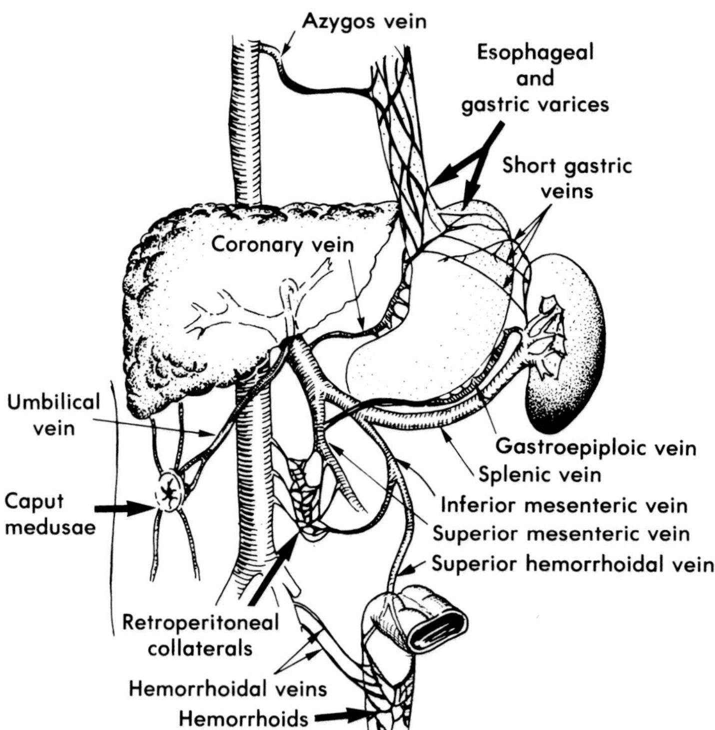

Fig. 24-1. Portosystemic collateral pathways develop where the portal venous and systemic venous systems are in close apposition *(large arrows)*.

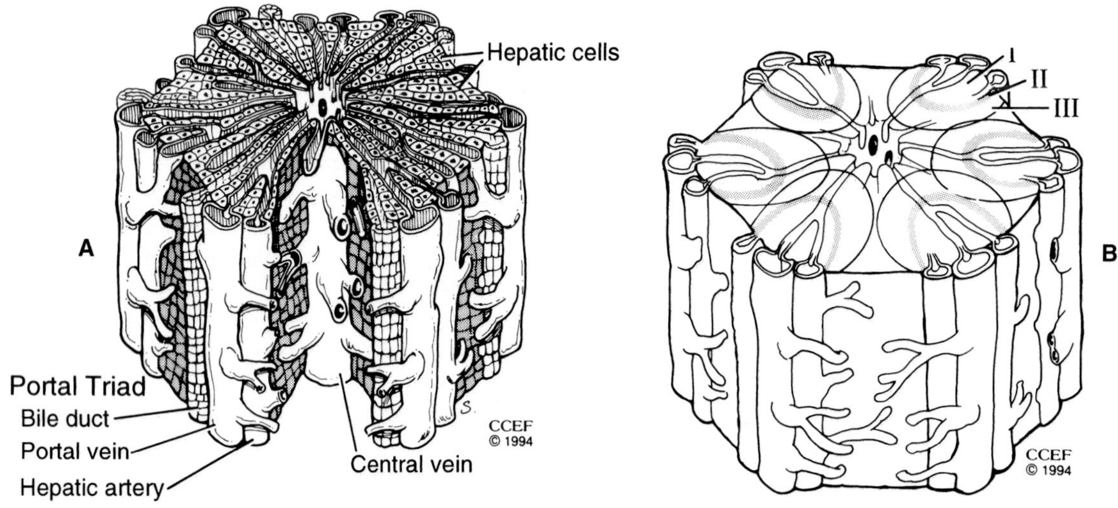

Fig. 24-2. A, Hepatic lobular anatomy. **B,** Hepatic zones of injury (Rappaport acinus zones).

cumulation of adenosine around terminal hepatic arterioles with resultant dilation.[2] This is a very potent response; although the hepatic arteriole is subject to all the usual vasoactive influences (e.g., catecholamines, neural influences), these are overridden by the intrinsic buffer response.

Portal hypertension exists when portal pressure generally exceeds 10 mm Hg. This can be determined by physical examination with evidence of caput medusae or splenomegaly with known liver disease. Another diagnostic modality is upper gastrointestinal endoscopy to demonstrate the presence of varices in the stomach and esophagus. A radiologic diagnosis can be made by measurement of the hepatic venous pressure gradient, which is the wedged hepatic vein pressure minus the free hepatic vein pressure. Gradients of greater than 10 mm Hg strongly suggest the diagnosis. This is analogous to measuring left

SOME CAUSES OF PORTAL HYPERTENSION

Presinusoidal

1. Portal/splenic vein thrombosis
2. Vascular malformations
3. Schistosomiasis
4. Biliary cirrhosis

Sinusoidal

1. Postnecrotic cirrhosis
   a. Virus, autoimmune, drugs
2. Alcoholic cirrhosis
3. Other cirrhosis

Postsinusoidal

1. Veno-occlusive disease
   a. Budd-Chiari syndrome
   b. Medication related

atrial pressures via a wedged pulmonary artery catheter. Another radiologic indication of portal hypertension is by either superior mesenteric artery or celiac artery injection with demonstration of varices or collateral flow in the venous phase.

With portal hypertension the hepatic component of portal flow is reduced and splanchnic venous pressure is increased. Both hepatic and mesenteric arterial flow increase, and splanchnic hyperemia develops. Collateral venous channels enlarge to allow venous outflow from the hyperemic gut. Cardiac output increases as the splanchnic arterial beds dilate and allow lower vascular resistance. A hyperdynamic circulation ensues, characterized by high cardiac output, low systemic vascular resistance, and splanchnic hyperemia.[3] The venous collaterals form in the distal esophagus and proximal stomach, the umbilical region through umbilical veins in the ligamentum teres, the retroperitoneal veins of Retzius, and the hemorrhoidal plexus. Rupture with resultant bleeding from these thin-walled, tortuous vessels most often occurs at the gastroesophageal junction, and at times it may be life threatening.[4]

Portal hypertension can be a result of many conditions (see accompanying box). *Presinusoidal portal hypertension* results from any venous occlusion or scarring of the terminal portal vein branches. Splenic vein thrombosis can result in segmental left-sided portal hypertension transmitted from the short gastric vessels thru esophageal and gastric varices. Portal venous obstruction for any reason can result in portal hypertension usually by thrombosis or external compression. Any other condition that increases portal flow, such as an arteriovenous malformation within the portal system, increases portal pressure. In addition to these vascular conditions, schistosomiasis and cholestatic forms of cirrhosis such as sclerosing cholangitis and primary biliary cirrhosis may result in presinusoidal portal hypertension. In these states the liver is injured in the portal triad or zone I levels first and the sinusoids are initially intact. Thus liver function is well preserved in most presinusoidal forms of portal hypertension until late in the course of the disease process.

Sinusoidal types of portal hypertension are the most common in the United States. This results from increased resistance to portal flow through the liver as a result of hepatocyte destruction and sinusoidal architectural disruption. The common theme is hepatocyte injury, cell death, lobular collapse, disorganized regeneration, collagen deposition and fibrosis. The major causes of this are toxins (alcohol), viruses (hepatitis and others), and autoimmune conditions. In sinusoidal types of portal hypertension, advanced liver disease usually presents concomitantly.[5]

Postsinusoidal portal hypertension can result when there is hepatic venous outflow obstruction. Classically, this condition is termed the Budd-Chiari syndrome when the large hepatic veins are occluded. Physiologically, small diffuse central venous disease has the same result. The pace at which the obstruction occurs frequently determines the degree of liver dysfunction. If the occlusion is relatively rapid, with little time for caudate lobe collaterals to form, near acute liver failure can result. In chronic forms, liver function can be preserved if compensatory outflow collaterals develop. Unfortunately, often an underlying myeloproliferative disorder or other malignancy has led to the thrombotic event.[6,7]

CLINICAL COMPLICATIONS OF PORTAL HYPERTENSION

Ascites

Ascites is a complication of portal hypertension for which the physiologists have two etiologic theories. The *overflow hypothesis* speculates that increased portal pressure leads to transudation and extravasation of fluid through capillaries and lymphatics into the abdominal space; this is aided by continued splanchnic hyperemia and further increases in portal pressure. On the other hand the *underfill hypothesis* states that the effective vascular volume is decreased and the resultant renal vasoconstriction and decreased fractional sodium excretion lead to fluid retention, through neural and aldosteronal mechanisms. Whatever the mechanism, the development of ascites is considered a sign of "decompensation" of cirrhosis.[8] Therapy is primarily medical, with bed rest, diuretics, and salt restriction. In most cases medical therapy is effective; however, in refractory cases, large-volume intermittent paracentesis can provide symptomatic relief. Surgical therapy may either reduce the portal hypertension with a large-diameter (>10 mm) side-to-side portosystemic shunt or shunt the ascites back into the systemic circulation via a peritoneal-venous shunt. In the latter method either a pressure activated Leveen-type or a manually pumped Denver-type shunt with a one-way valve mechanism can be used. Meticulous technique to minimize ascitic leak at the peritoneal insertion site and accurate placement of both the peritoneal and

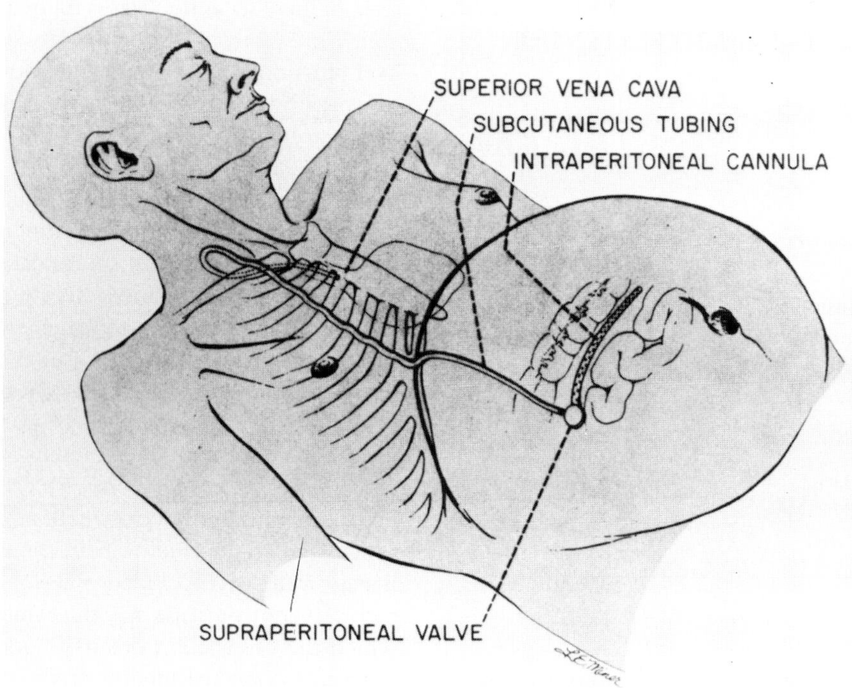

Fig. 24-3. Leveen peritoneovenous shunt transports ascites from the abdomen to the superior vena cava. (From Reinhardt GF, Stanley MM. Peritoneo-venous shunting for ascites. Surg Gynecol Obstet 145:420, 1977. By permission of Surgery, Gynecology, and Obstetrics.)

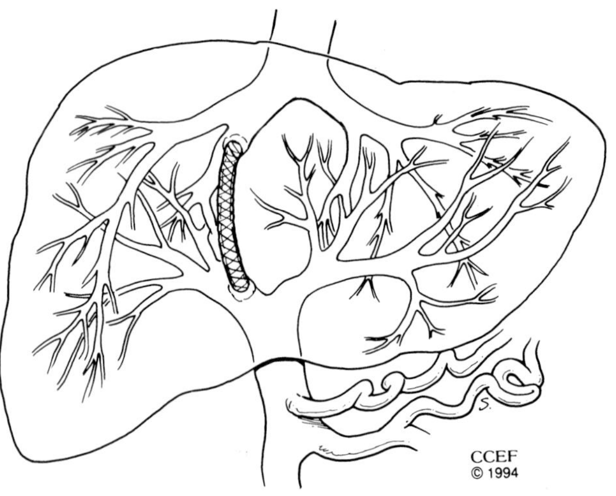

Fig. 24-4. Transjugular intrahepatic portosystemic shunt.

venous limbs are critical to success (Fig. 24-3). Antibiotic prophylaxis is required. However, controlled studies have not shown survival advantage of the surgically placed shunt over intermitten large-volume paracentesis.[9] Some authors have seen ascites controlled by using transjugular intrahepatic portosystemic shunt (TIPS) (Fig. 24-4). A low gradient needs to be achieved for success in ascites control.

Overall, however, it is to be remembered that survival in patients with medically intractable ascites is extremely poor.[10] These patients should be given every opportunity to seek hepatic transplantation.

Hepatic Encephalopathy

The liver provides many functions, but failure to detoxify is the functional derangement thought to cause hepatic encephalopathy. The two main etiologic factors in encephalopathy are hepatocellular failure and/or portosystemic shunting. The relative importance varies. Products from the diet, by-products of endogenous bacterial flora, material from gastrointestinal hemorrhage, absorbed medications, and breakdown products of normal metabolism flow through portal channels to the liver. It is hypothesized that some neurotoxic material is shunted around the liver via collaterals or simply overwhelms the poorly functioning liver's capacity and enters the brain. The main hypothesized materials include ammonia, γ-aminobutyric acid, and endogenous benzodiazepines.[11] These, plus other products, probably play a multifactorial role and give rise to the clinical condition termed hepatic encephalopathy. Encephalopathy covers a wide clinical spectrum. Low grades of encephalopathy may be subtle, characterized by sleep disturbances or episodes of mild disorientation or confusion. A simple number connection test (Trail test) can be used for diagnosis in these instances. In many cases, debilitating confusion or somnolence is the intermediate state. At the other end of the spectrum is deep coma. In acute liver failure, diffuse cerebral cellular swelling and brain herniation may result. Treatment is medical, aimed at removal

Table 24-1. Child Classification (Pugh-Turcotte Modified)

	Points		
	1	2	3
Bilirubin	<2 mg/dl	2-3	>3
Albumin	>3.5 g/L	3-3.5	<3
Ascites	None	Easily controlled	Poorly controlled
Encephalopathy	None	Mild	Disabling
Prothrombin time (seconds prolonged)	1-4	4-6	>6

Child class A = 5-7 points.
Child class B = 8-10 points.
Child class C = >10 points.

of precipitating factors and correction of metabolic abnormalities. This may be supplemented with lactulose, a disaccharide, which can stimulate bowel movements and provide an acidic enteric environment to minimize ammonia absorption. Metronidazole (Flagyl) or neomycin may be used to alter gut microflora. Protein restriction and avoidance of drugs metabolized in the liver also can minimize sedation. The degree of encephalopathy should be investigated by history or other tests in all patients with portal hypertension.

As with ascites, encephalopathy is an indication of advanced liver disease and is only effectively treated by transplantation.

Variceal Hemorrhage

Variceal hemorrhage develops in about 30% of patients with esophagogastric varices. These thin-walled vessels are located in a region where large differentials in intra-abdominal and intrathoracic esophageal luminal pressure are seen. The veins run submucosally for 2 to 3 cm at the gastroesophageal junction, whereas above and below this segment they are deep to the muscularis mucosae. In addition, this region is one of the narrower points of the gastrointestinal tract, and it is subject to some trauma with rough food boluses. Finally, acid reflux makes this area prone to erosions.[12] The initial bleeding is fatal in 20% to 50% of patients, and the risk of recurrence of the bleeding is 75% in the first year.[13] Therapy may be initiated prophylactically (i.e., before the first bleeding episode) or be therapeutic (i.e., to treat acute bleeding or prevent recurrent bleeding).

Prophylaxis

Many prospective randomized trials have studied surgical, endoscopic, and pharmacologic therapies to manage varices that have not bled.[14] Surgical prophylaxis is not indicated, because the morbidity of the operation usually exceeds the benefit.[16] Studies of sclerotherapy to prevent the initial bleed have had mixed results, but overall the morbidity exceeds the benefit and this is not currently recommended.[16] Trials of nonselective β-blockade have consistently shown a benefit of this treatment to lower the risk of initial bleeding.[17] Overall, this risk can be reduced from about 30% to 15% to 20% with propranolol or nadolol. The use of these agents is now recommended in most patients who have varices. Dosage should be sufficient to lower the resting heart rate 25% or bring the pulse to 60 beats/min.

Acute Variceal Bleeding

The initial assessment and management of the patient with upper gastrointestinal tract variceal hemorrhage should include standard resuscitative measures with airway protection and large-bore intravenous lines as the immediate priorities. The goal is to achieve hemodynamic stability and early endoscopy. Blood products, to include fresh frozen plasma and platelets, should be prepared immediately and a urinary catheter and nasogastric tube placed for monitoring. An ICU bed is usually needed. A rapid, thorough clinical and laboratory evaluation of the status of the patient, possible cause for variceal formation, and, in most cases, an assessment of the underlying liver reserve is needed. The type of liver disease, its duration, and the patient's baseline status as regarding ascites or encephalopathy must be determined. One should try to categorize the Child class (Table 24-1) of the patient, take a thorough history, perform a physical examination, and obtain laboratory data. From this early information the patient can be assessed for the likely need for liver transplantation. A patient receiving a Child "C" classification is likely to benefit from transplantation, whereas a Child "A" designation can usually be managed by other treatment strategies. If the patient is deemed a candidate, further therapeutic decisions can be made with this therapy in mind. An algorithm for the following discussion is shown in Fig. 24-5.

Diagnosis and initial therapy. Endoscopic gastroduodenoscopy (EGD) should be performed once stabilization occurs. Airway protection is paramount at this juncture, as sedation and encephalopathy can combine to allow aspiration. This immediate EGD is both diagnostic and therapeutic. Diagnosis depends on visualizing active bleeding, seeing stigmata of recent bleeding (a platelet

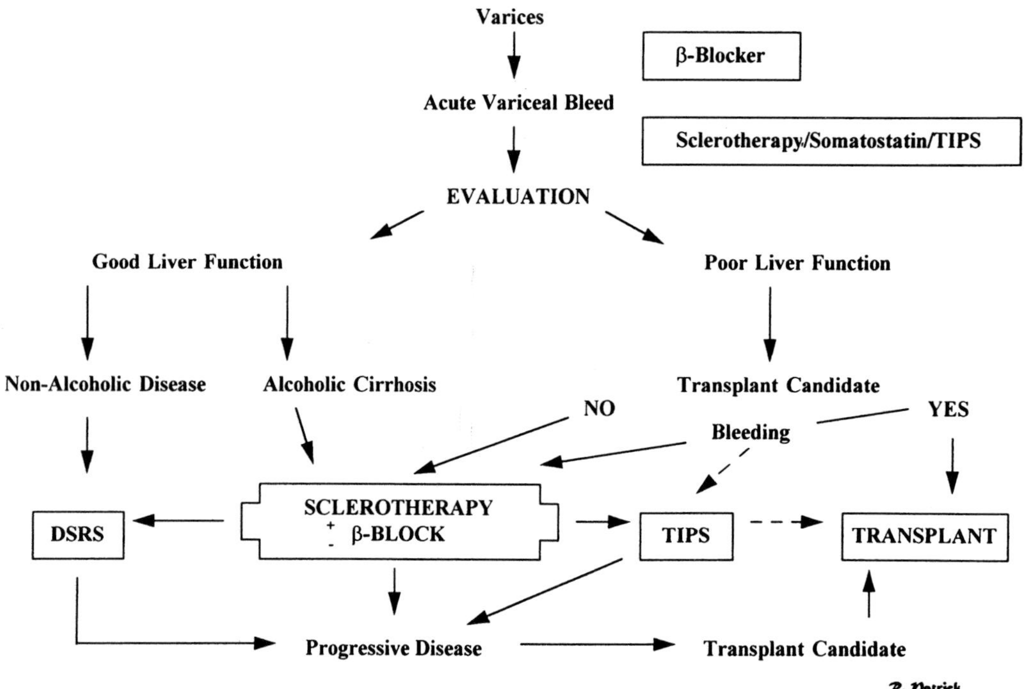

Fig. 24-5. Algorithm for portal hypertension and acute variceal bleeding management.

plug), or excluding other upper gastrointestinal tract sources of bleeding. Once the source of the bleeding is defined as variceal, an immediate sclerosis of the varix is successful in stopping hemorrhage in 90% of cases. In cases where initial sclerotherapy fails, other medical and radiologic options can be used before proceeding to surgical intervention.

Pharmacologic choices in acute variceal bleeding. Vasopressin may be used to lower portal pressure by constricting splanchnic arteriolar inflow to the portal system. Because of the general vasoconstriction in all arteriolar beds (e.g., myocardium), this agent must be used under close monitoring. The usual dose is 0.1 to 0.4 U/min by continuous infusion. Vasopressin is contraindicated in patients with known coronary artery disease and should be administered along with nitroglycerin to minimize coronary effects. The nitroglycerin dose is increased to maintain systolic blood pressure to ~100 mm Hg, usually beginning at 40 μg/min. This combination can successfully be used in 50% of patients and can be administered peripherally.

Somatostatin or its analog octreotide has been advocated. Several studies have shown the efficacy of this agent in stopping variceal hemorrhage is equal to vasopressin and to emergency sclerotherapy.[18] Its advantage over vasopressin is its selectivity for the splancnic bed, thus coronary and renal vasoconstriction do not occur. Indeed, this agent may replace vasopressin in the setting of acute variceal hemorrhage. Dosage of octreotide should be 25 to 50 μg/hr titrated for maximum efficacy and maintained for 3 to 4 days.

Other methods. Balloon tamponade with the Minnesota modification of the Sengstaken-Blakemore tube places direct pressure on the gastroesophageal plexus and is successful in 80% of cases. These tubes (Fig. 24-6) require ICU monitoring and airway protection with endotracheal intubation before use and should only be placed by those with experience in their maintenance. Esophageal perforation or necrosis can occur when pressure is too high for too long a period. The incidence of rebleeding is high when the balloon is deflated. Thus the balloon tamponade should be used only as a temporizing measure while more definitive therapy is planned.

The success of sclerotherapy and pharmacologic control of acute bleeding have markedly reduced the need for balloon tamponade.

The TIPS procedure (see Fig. 24-4) is the preferred method for decompression in the setting of acute refractory hemorrhage from esophagogastric varices. The radiologist inserts an expandable stent through the hepatic vein into the liver parenchyma and into a portal vein. The procedure has become widely available and by creating a nonselective portosystemic shunt (see the following) can successfully control variceal hemorrhage in many cases. The goal is to reduce the portal-to-hepatic vein gradient to 12 mm Hg or less, which can usually be achieved with stent expansion. This procedure can also be combined with selective variceal embolization.

Emergency surgical options for acute refractory bleeding are occasionally needed, but have largely been superceded by TIPS. Generally, the procedure with which the surgeon is most familiar should be used. (Further dis-

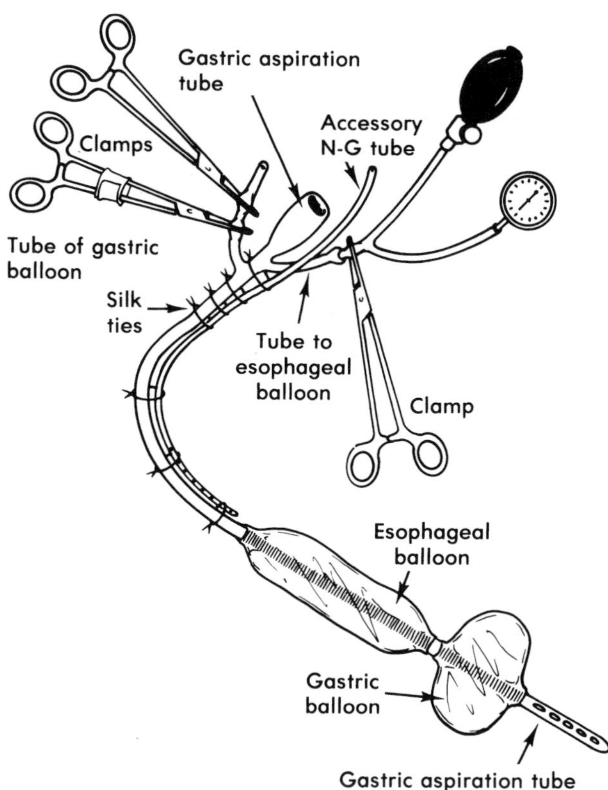

Fig. 24-6. The modified Sengstaken-Blakemore tube has an accessory nasogastric tube attached to prevent aspiration of secretions that accumulate above the esophageal balloon. (From Rikkers LF. Portal hypertension. In Goldsmith HS, ed. Practice of Surgery, vol 3. General Surgery. Hagerstown, Md.: Harper & Row, 1981.)

cussions of surgical options in the stabilized or chronic setting follow.) In unstable patients, mortality is quite high. Variceal decompression, either radiological or surgical, is required in only about 10% of patients in the acute setting.

Prevention of Rebleeding

Evaluation. The choice of an option for the long-term therapy of variceal hemorrhage depends on the cause of the patient's portal hypertension and on the severity and underlying cause of the liver disease. Laboratory data are helpful, and some sort of dynamic testing of liver function is becoming more common. Galactose elimination capacity[19] or lidocaine metabolite MEGX[20] assay can be useful in further documenting hepatic reserve.

The first decision is whether the patient needs a liver transplantation immediately or in the near future. In patients with Child class B and C disease (see Table 24-1) or in patients where a functional liver test shows poorly preserved hepatic function, a liver transplantation is probably the best option. Evaluation should then focus on ensuring that there are no contraindications for transplantation. In patients where liver transplantation is the goal, nonoperative therapy is preferred while the patient's name is on a transplantation waiting list. However, in many patients

Table 24-2. Some Pharmacologic Agents Lowering Portal Pressure

Category	Drug
β-Adrenergic antagonists nonselective	Propranolol Nadolol
Cardioselective	Atenolol Metoprolol
α/β	Labetalol
α-Antagonist	Prazosin Phenoxybenzamine
α_1- or α_2-Agonist	Clonidine Methoxamine
5-H Tryptamine antagonist	Ketanserin Ritanserin
Growth factor inhibitors	Somatostatin Octreotide
Vasoconstrictors	Vasopressin Triglycylvasopressin
Nitrodilators	Nitroglycerin Isosorbide dinitrate

with Child class A disease, other surgical therapy may be considered.

Nonoperative therapy

Pharmacologic therapy. Pharmacologic therapy to prevent variceal rebleeding has been extensively studied since the late 1980s. Many drugs such as β-blockers, calcium channel blockers, serotonin antagonists, nitrates, and α_2-agonists have been tried with varied outcomes (Table 24-2). Pathophysiologically, the goal has been to reduce the splanchnic hyperemia and/or the hyperdynamic systemic circulation. The most successful drug has been noncardioselective β-blockade, which reduces the risk of rebleeding from 75% to 40% to 50%. All medications have been limited to a degree by side affects, particularly lethargy and hypotension, and have a noncompliance rate of about 20%.[21]

Sclerosis. Chronic variceal sclerosis is an effective means of achieving long-term control of hemorrhage in some patients. Repeated sessions are necessary for the best results, with the goal of variceal obliteration. However, rebleeding occurs in 50% of patients by 4 to 5 years. This either occurs early because of failure to obliterate the varices or late with recurrence of gastric varices. Sclerosis can be used again if varices recur.

Overall, sclerosis fails in about 30% of patients.[22] Complications of sclerosis include esophageal stricture formation and dysphagia in about 10% of cases. Long-term survival and preservation of the existing liver function have been documented. Controlled trials of sclerotherapy have been subjected to meta-analysis. Sclerosis has been shown to be better than no therapy and shows no significant difference in survival compared to pharmacologic therapy or shunt surgery.[23,24] Individual studies can be found to support almost any position. The current trend is to advocate sclerotherapy for acute bleeding—implement an aggressive course for variceal obliteration—but recognize the need for other management in many patients.

TIPS. The TIPS procedure has been increasingly used in the acute setting to halt hemorrhage. Studies continue on its use for long-term therapy. If a greater than 10 mm diameter TIPS is used, all portal flow is diverted; but when reduced to 8 mm, a partial shunt occurs, preserving some portal flow to the liver.[25] The incidence of encephalopathy in patients with significant liver disease is 20% to 30% more than the incidence before the TIPS was placed. Also most studies show a 50% to 60% incidence of stenosis or occlusion of these bioartificial shunts by 1 year.[26] Repeated follow-up radiologic studies are crucial to the long-term success of TIPS, for rebleeding occurs if stenosis or occlusion go undetected and untreated. To date, follow-up is short (1 to 3 years), and rates of occlusion or stenosis (50%) and encephalopathy (20% to 30%) may relegate the procedure to a bridge therapy to transplantation. In that setting it appears promising.

Operative therapy. Operative therapy for the long-term treatment of variceal hemorrhage takes three forms: devascularization, nonselective shunts, and selective shunts. No one operation is applicable in every case. The choice depends on the hepatic hemodynamics, hepatic function, and the clinical circumstances. The surgeon undertaking these procedures is advised to perform mesenteric angiography in all cases to allow for the best decision making. When selective shunting is elected (discussion follows), left renal venography is necessary.

Devascularization. Devascularization operations range from the spectrum of simple splenectomy to extensive division and ligation of all periesophageal vessels up into the thorax combined with splenectomy—the Sugiura procedure. Many variations in between have been advocated. This group of operations has a role in instances of splanchnic thromboses where no shunt can be constructed. Splenectomy alone is curative for portal hypertension caused by isolated splenic vein thrombosis. The excellent results of the Sugiura procedure have been difficult to duplicate in the United States, although a recent series from Mexico has shown good results.[27] Esophageal transection and devascularization has been used with some success in patients with acute unstable conditions; however, rebleeding rates are high, and use of esophageal transection and devascularization cannot be recommended in otherwise "shuntable" patients. The advantage of these devascularization procedures is that liver perfusion and function are preserved (Fig. 24-7).

Nonselective shunts. The nonselective shunts totally divert portal flow to the systemic circulation, thereby decreasing portal pressure to normal. A side-to-side type of shunt is also effective in ascites control, as the portal vein serves as an outflow from the obstructed sinusoids. However, physiologic effects on the liver as a result of the total diversion can cause higher long-term rates of encephalopathy (approximately to 20% to 50%), particularly in those with poorer liver function. The exception to the overall reported experience is that of Orloff et al.,[28] who have obtained excellent results using portacaval shunt in an emergent setting in a primarily alcoholic population. The long-term patency is excellent when vein-to-vein anastomosis is used, but the risk of thrombosis with bioartificial material is 10% to 20% with long-term follow-up[29] (Fig. 24-8).

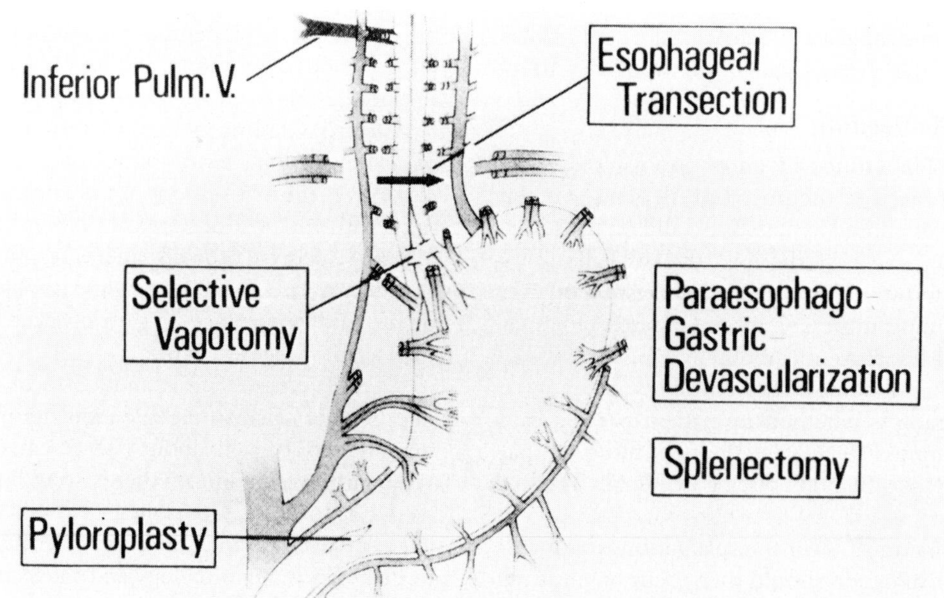

Fig. 24-7. Sugiura procedure. (From Sugiura M, Futagawa S. Further evaluation of the Sugiura procedure in the treatment of esophageal varies. Arch Surg 112:1318, 1977. Copyright 1977, American Medical Association.)

Selective shunts. Selective shunts provide decompression to the anatomic sites of variceal hemorrhage without reducing hepatic portal venous pressure. To date, two types of selective shunts have been described. Inokuchi and Sugimachi[30] have developed a left gastric vein–to–vena cava shunt. The published results are good but have been difficult to duplicate in the hands of others. The distal splenorenal shunt developed by Warren[31] is the selective shunt most used world wide. Results have been duplicated in several centers. In several randomized and nonrandomized studies the selective shunts provide equivalent control of bleeding and the advantage of a lower rate of encephalopathy (5% to 15%) compared to nonselective shunts. Presumably, this is because hepatic portal perfusion pressure is maintained. In patients with nonalcoholic cirrhosis, portal perfusion is maintained in 90% at long-term follow-up, but in alcoholic cirrhosis 50% of patients lose the selectivity through formation of new collateral veins to the shunt. Survival and encephalopathy risks do not change significantly in this group. Rates of rebleeding are not statistically different in the selective shunts vs. the nonselective shunts, but the risk of ascites formation is higher, since portal hypertension is maintained. However, in carefully selected, low-risk patients with preserved liver function, the selective shunt can provide good survival.[32] In addition, the shunt avoids dissection in the hepatic hilum, allowing for a technically easier liver transplantation should it be needed in the future. Finally, the vein-to-vein anastomosis provides good patency when compared to artificial materials (Fig. 24-9).

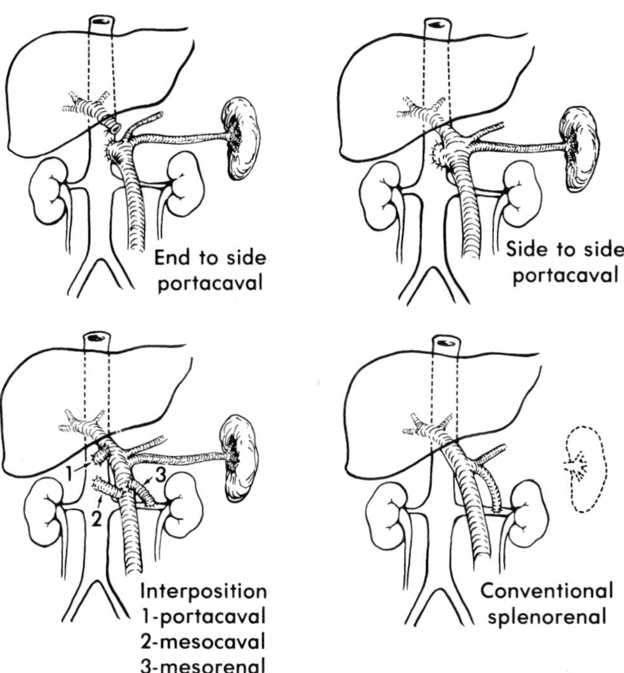

Fig. 24-8. Nonselective shunts decompress the entire portal venous system and divert all portal blood flow away from the liver.

SUMMARY

The surgeon's knowledge of the physiology of the liver and portal system is critical to the success of treating patients with portal hypertension. In most cases the complications of ascites and encephalopathy are managed medically. The surgeon's role in those cases that are refractory to medical management is almost exclusively in liver transplantation. For in such cases the fact that the disease is no longer medically responsive indicates extremely poor chances of long-term survival without transplantation. The surgeon needs the knowledge to make this decision.

When confronted with the complication of gastrointestinal hemorrhage from esophagogastric varices, the long-term success of surgical therapy hinges on the surgeon's knowledge and ability to properly select patients. The surgeon must be knowledgeable in all treatment options, in how to evaluate the patient, and in the indications for the available surgical options. In this selection process an un-

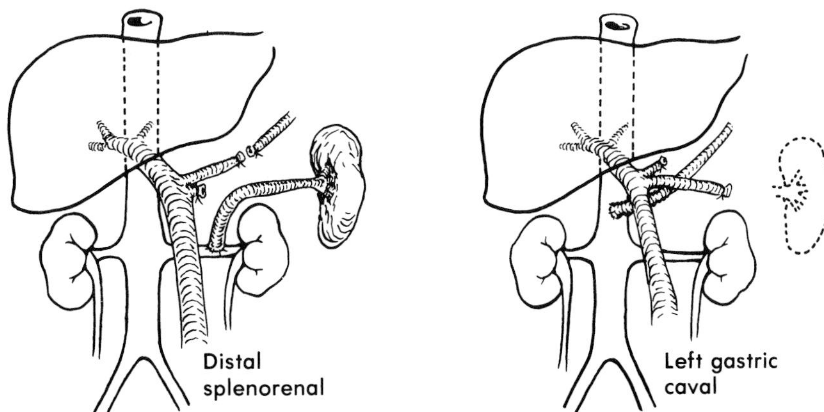

Fig. 24-9. Selective shunts decompress only the gastrosplenic component of the portal venous system and maintain portal hypertension and portal blood flow to the liver.

derstanding of liver physiology is paramount. In all but a few cases the choices are sclerotherapy/distal splenorenal shunt vs. sclerotherapy/transplantation waiting list.

REFERENCES

1. Sherlock S. Patterns of hepatocyte injuries in man. Lancet 1:782, 1982.
2. Lautt WW, Greenway CV. Conceptual view of the hepatic vascular bed. Hepatology 5:952, 1987.
3. Bomzon A, Blendis LM. The nitric oxide hypothesis and the hyperdynamic circulation in cirrhosis. Hepatology 20:1343, 1994.
4. Douglas BC, Baggenstoss A, Holinshead W. The anatomy of the portal vein and its tributaries. Surg Gynecol Obstet 91:562, 1950.
5. Groszman RJ, Atterbury CE. The pathophysiology of portal hypertension: A basis for classification. Semin Liver Dis 2:177, 1982.
6. Henderson JM, et al. Surgical options, hematologic evaluation and pathologic change in Budd-Chiari syndrome. Am J Surg 159:41, 1990.
7. Valla D, et al. Primary myeloproliferative disorders and hepatic vein thrombosis. A prospective study of erythyroid colony formation in vitro in 20 patients with Budd-Chiari syndrome. Ann Intern Med 103:329, 1985.
8. Llach J, et al. Prognostic view of arterial pressure, endogenous vasoactive systems and renal function in cirrhotic patients admitted to the hospital for the treatment of ascites. Gastroenterology 94:482, 1988.
9. Gines P, et al. Paracentesis with i.v. albumin infusion as compared to peritoneovenous shunting in cirrhosis with refractory ascites. N Engl J Med 325:829, 1991.
10. Gines P, et al. Compensated cirrhosis: Natural history and prognostic factors. Hepatology 7:122, 1987.
11. Record CO. Neurochemistry of hepatic encephalopathy. Gut 32:1261, 1991.
12. McCormack TT, et al. Perforating veins and blood flow in esophageal varices. Lancet 2:1442, 1983.
13. Graham DY, Smith JL. The course of patients after variceal hemorrhage. Gastroenterology 80:800, 1981.
14. Burroughs AK, D'Hyegere F, McIntyre N. Pitfalls in studies of prophylactic therapy for variceal bleeding in cirrhotics. Hepatology 6:1407, 1986.
15. Resnick RH, et al. A controlled study of the prophylactic portacaval shunt. A final report. Ann Intern Med 70:675, 1969.
16. The Veterans Affairs Cooperative Variceal Sclerotherapy Group. Prophylactic sclerotherapy for esophageal varices in men with alcoholic liver disease—A randomized, single blind, multi-center clinical trial. N Engl J Med 324:1779, 1991.
17. Groszmann RJ, et al. Hemodynamic events in a prospective randomized trial of propranolol versus placebo in the prevention of a first variceal hemorrhage. Gastroenterology 99:1401, 1990.
18. Silvain C, et al. Terlipressin plus transdermal nitroglycerin versus octreotide in the control of acute bleeding from esophageal varices: A multicenter randomized trial. Hepatology 18:61, 1993.
19. Henderson JM, Kutner MH, Bain RP. First-order clearance of plasma galactose: The effect of liver disease. Gastroenterology 83:1090, 1982.
20. Oellerich M, et al. Lidocaine metabolite formation as a measure of liver function in patients with cirrhosis. Ther Drug Monit 12:219, 1990.
21. Hayes PC, et al. Meta analysis of value of propranolol in prevention of variceal hemorrhage. Lancet 336:153, 1990.
22. Rikkers LF, et al. Shunt surgery versus endoscopic sclerotherapy for long-term treatment of variceal bleeding: Early results of a randomized trial. Ann Surg 206:261, 1987.
23. Henderson JM, et al. Endoscopic variceal sclerosis compared with distal splenorenal shunt to prevent recurrent variceal bleeding in cirrhosis. A prospective randomized trial. Ann Intern Med 112:262, 1990.
24. Fleig WE, et al. Prevention of recurrent bleeding in cirrhotics with recent variceal hemorrhage: Prospective, randomized comparison of propranolol and sclerotherapy. Hepatology 7:355, 1987.
25. Sarfeh IJ, Rypins EB, Mason GR. A systematic appraisal of portacaval H-graft diameters. Clinical and hemodynamic perspectives. Ann Surg 204:356, 1986.
26. Ring EJ, et al. Percutaneous intrahepatic portosystemic shunts to control variceal bleeding prior to liver transplantation. Ann Intern Med 116:304, 1992.
27. Orozco H, et al. Role of the distal splenorenal shunt in management of variceal bleeding in Latin America. Am J Surg 160:86, 1990.
28. Orloff MJ, et al. Long term results of emergency portacaval shunt for bleeding esophageal varices in unselected patients with alcoholic cirrhosis. Ann Surg 192:325, 1980.
29. Millikan WJ, et al. The Emory prospective randomized trial: Selective versus nonselective shunt to control variceal bleeding. Ten-year follow-up. Ann Surg 201:712, 1985.
30. Inokuchi K, Sugimachi K. The selective shunt for variceal bleeding: A personal perspective. Am J Surg 160:48, 1990.
31. Warren WD, et al. Selective transplenic decompression of gastroesophageal varices by distal splenorenal shunt. Ann Surg 166:437, 1967.
32. Henderson JM, et al. Selective shunt in the management of variceal bleeding in the era of liver transplantation. Ann Surg 216:248, 1992.

25

Calculous Disease of the Gallbladder and Common Bile Duct

Richard M. Sherry and Thomas R. Gadacz

Cholelithiasis and choledocholithiasis are common and costly digestive disorders. More than 10% of adult Americans have gallstones, and it is estimated that 600,000 patients undergo cholecystectomy annually.[1] This chapter is focused on the physiology and flow of bile, which is fundamental to understanding calculous disease of the gallbladder and common bile duct. The pathogenesis, natural history, and clinical aspects of gallstone disease are also considered.

BILE PHYSIOLOGY

Bile is a heterogenous fluid composed of bile salts, cholesterol, lecithin, pigments, inorganic ions, conjugated bilirubin, electrolytes, and water. Five hundred to 1500 ml of bile is secreted by the liver each day. Bile is essential for elimination of certain waste products and excretion of many drugs and toxins. Bile is necessary for the proper digestion and absorption of fats and is critical in cholesterol metabolism. Bile salts are the primary component of bile and together with cholesterol and lecithin account for 80% of its dry weight.[2,3] Familiarity with the metabolism of cholesterol, bile salts, and bilirubin is a prerequisite to understanding calculous disease of the gallbladder.

Cholesterol Metabolism

The word *cholesterol* is derived from the Greek words *chole* meaning bile and *stereos* meaning solid. Cholesterol is critical to cellular growth, differentiation, function, and regulation. Cholesterol is a key component of cell membranes and can be converted to steroid hormones, lipoproteins, bile salts, or excreted in bile. Cellular cholesterol content is affected by dietary intake and de novo hepatic synthesis. Lipoproteins in the serum serve as a source of cholesterol. This process is regulated by low-density lipoprotein (LDL) receptors located on the cell membrane that binds and internalizes lipoproteins. Lysosomal enzymes can metabolize these lipoproteins to free cholesterol.[4,5]

De novo synthesis in the liver accounts for the majority of cholesterol production (Fig. 25-1). Cholesterol is synthesized in a multistep fashion from acetate. The rate-controlling enzyme is hydroxy-methyl-gluteral coenzyme A (HMG-CoA) reductase that reduces 3-hydroxy-3-methylglutaryl CoA to melalonate. HMG-CoA activity is regulated by classic negative feedback control with cholesterol.[6] Melalonate is converted to intermediates that lead to cholesterol biosynthesis.

Free cholesterol can be stored in the form of cholesterol ester. This represents a metabolically inactive storage pool. Alternatively, free hepatic cholesterol is used for a variety of synthetic purposes including catabolism to form bile salts, or it can be eliminated by direct secretion into bile.

Bile Salt Metabolism

Bile salts are biologic detergents synthesized in the liver. They have multiple functions including the facilitation of cholesterol excretion in bile. Because bile salts are synthesized from cholesterol, they are also a major pathway for cholesterol elimination. Bile salts cycle between the intestine and liver in the enterohepatic circulation. The total amount of bile salts in the circuit is considered the bile salt pool. Bile, stored in the gallbladder during fasting, is released into the intestine following postprandial release of cholecystokinin (CCK). In the small bowel bile salts facilitate intraluminal solubilization and absorption of lipids. Ninety-five percent of circulating bile salts are absorbed in the distal ileum and returned to the liver, whereas approximately 500 mg/day are lost in the stool and are replaced by newly synthesized bile salts.[7] The bile salt pool circulates 8 to 10 times per day[8] (Fig. 25-2).

The synthesis of bile salts from cholesterol is controlled by the rate-limiting enzyme cholesterol 7α-hydroxylase. Ultimately chenodeoxycholate and cholate are produced. These primary bile salts are conjugated with taurine or

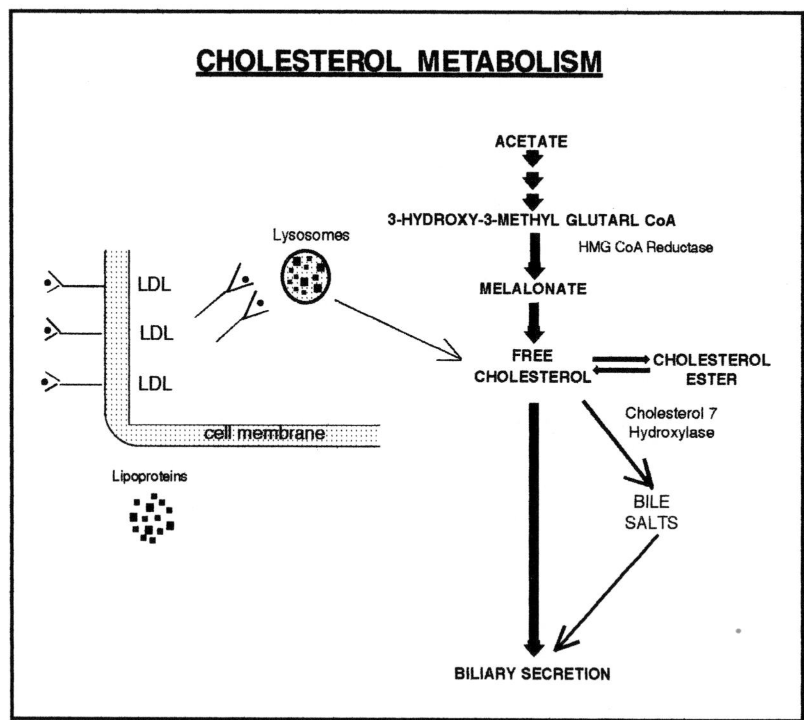

Fig. 25-1. Cholesterol is produced by de novo synthesis from acetate in a multistep process that is controlled by HMG-CoA reductase. Cholesterol is also produced from dietary lipoproteins. Free cholesterol is used for numerous synthetic processes including production of bile salts, or it can be excreted in bile. Bile salt synthesis from cholesterol is controlled by the rate-limiting enzyme cholesterol 7-α-hydroxylase. HMG-CoA reductase and cholesterol 7-α-hydroxylase are regulated in tandem under a host of clinical situations. *LDL,* Low-density lipoprotein. (From Sherry RM, Gadacz TR. Cholelithiasis and cholecystitis. In Zuidema GD, ed. Shackelford's Surgery of the Alimentary Tract. Philadelphia: WB Saunders, 1996.)

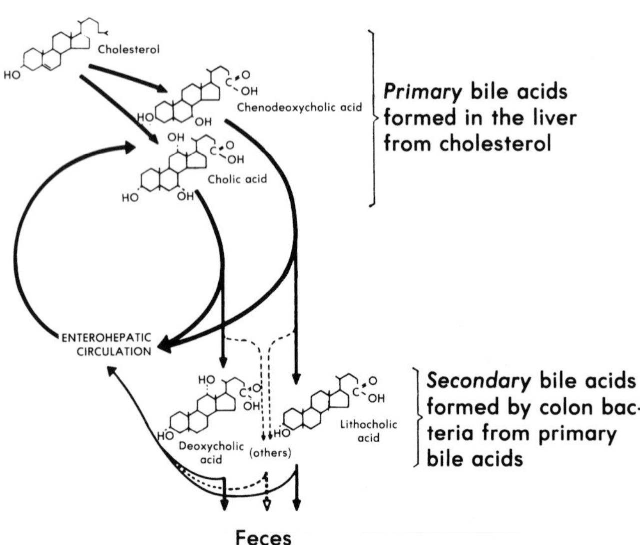

Fig. 25-2. Formation of primary and secondary bile acids from cholesterol and enterohepatic circulation of bile salts. (From Carey JB Jr. Bile salts and hepatobiliary disease. In Schiff L, ed. Disease of the Liver, 3rd ed. Philadelphia: JB Lippincott, 1969.)

glycine. Bacterial transformation in the intestine results in the formation of the secondary bile salts deoxycholate, ursodeoxycholate, and lithocholate.

Regulation of cholesterol 7α-hydroxylase is complex and incompletely understood. Hydrophobic bile salts (cholate, chenodeoxycholate, and deoxycholate) are potent inhibitors of bile salt synthesis. Hydrophilic bile salts have little effect on bile salt synthesis.[9,10] Thus bile salt synthesis is regulated in part by cycling hydrophobic bile salts that inhibit cholesterol 7α-hydroxylase. This serves to emphasize the importance of the enterohepatic circulation.

There appears to be a close relationship between cholesterol 7α-hydroxylase and HMG-CoA reductase because both enzymes are regulated in tandem under a variety of conditions. Bile fistula,[11] cholestryramine administration,[11] glucocorticoids,[12] and thyroid hormone[12] stimulate synthesis of both enzymes. Bile salt feeding inhibits both enzymes.[13] Ingestion of cholesterol[14] or melalonate[15] stimulates cholesterol 7α-hydroxylase but inhibits HMG-CoA activity. The parallel regulation of these two rate-limiting enzymes reflects the important interrelationship between bile salts and cholesterol.

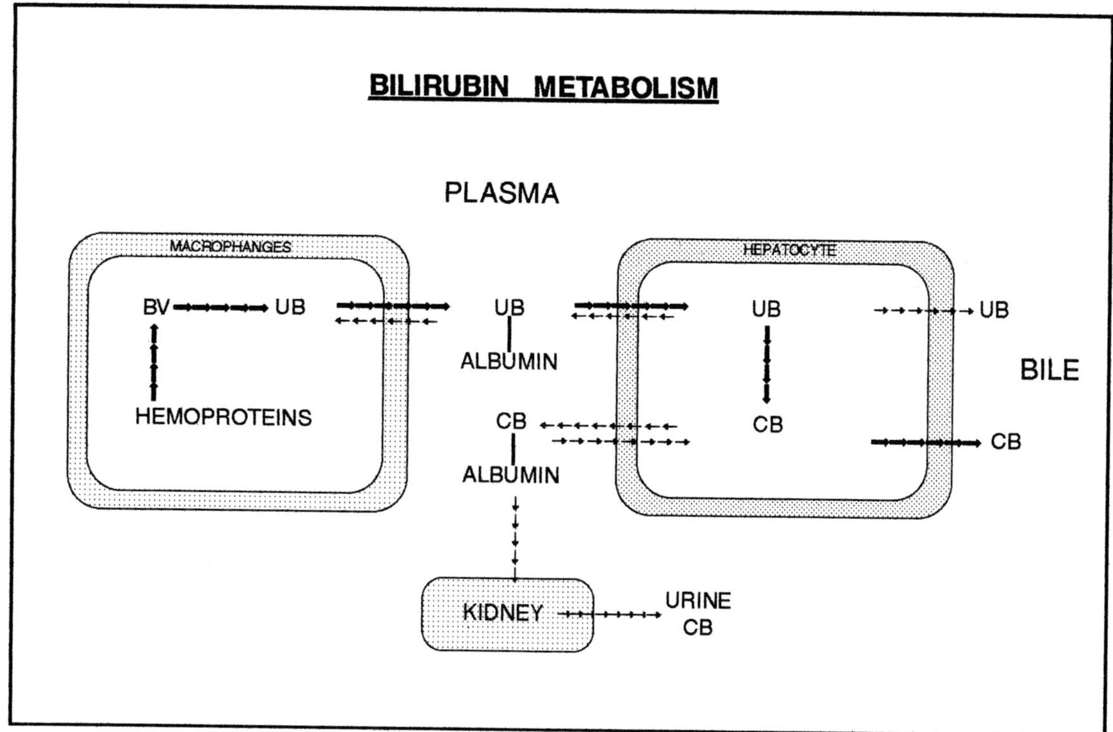

Fig. 25-3. Heme from hemoproteins including hemoglobin is converted to biliverdin *(BV)* by macrophages located in the bone marrow, spleen, and liver. Biliverdin is converted to unconjugated bilirubin *(UB)* and is found in plasma tightly bound to albumin. Unconjugated bilirubin is taken up by hepatocytes and is converted to conjugated bilirubin *(CB)*. Conjugated bilirubin (and to a lesser extent unconjugated bilirubin) is excreted in bile. Conjugated bilirubin, when present in plasma as a result of bile duct obstruction, can be excreted by the kidney. (Modified from Scharschmidt BF. Bilirubin metabolism, bile formation and gallbladder and bile duct function. In Sleisenger MH, Fordtran JS, eds. Gastrointestinal Disease. Philadelphia: WB Saunders, 1993.)

Bilirubin Metabolism

Bilirubin is a metabolic waste product generated as a result of the breakdown of senescent red blood cells or other nonhemoglobin hemoproteins. Macrophages in the bone marrow, liver, and spleen convert heme to biliverdin (Fig. 25-3). Biliverdin is rapidly converted to unconjugated (indirect) bilirubin, which circulates in plasma tightly bound to albumin because it is insoluble in water. Unconjugated bilirubin is taken up by hepatocytes, where it is conjugated to glucuronide making it water soluble. Conjugated (direct) bilirubin is then transported into the canaliculus and excreted into bile. Bilirubin is reduced by gut flora in the ileum and colon to urobilinogen and then oxidized to urobilin for excretion in feces. Normally only a trace amount of conjugated bilirubin passes back into plasma, and this is excreted by the kidney.

Daily bilirubin production in adults averages approximately 4 mg/kg.[16] The liver is usually efficient and can conjugate and excrete bilirubin so that the normal serum level is less than 1.5 mg/100 ml. With hemolysis there is a significant increase in the indirect fraction, and the total serum concentration is usually below 5 mg/100 ml. Both direct and indirect fractions are equally elevated with hepatocellular disease. With extrahepatic obstruction the direct fraction is elevated initially; if the obstruction is complete, the total bilirubin may reach 30 mg/100 ml.[17] Cholestasis follows a similar pattern and cannot be distinguished from extrahepatic obstruction on the basis of bilirubin values.

BILE FORMATION AND FLOW

Bile is formed in the liver by active transport of solutes by hepatocytes into the biliary canaliculus. This establishes an osmotic gradient and corresponding passive water flow.[18,19] Bile salts and inorganic electrolytes are the dominant osmotically active biliary solutes and consequently control canalicular bile formation (Fig. 25-4). Canalicular bile is considered to consist of two major components: a bile salt–dependent fraction and a bile salt–independent fraction. Each fraction generates approximately 50% of total canalicular bile flow.

Bile Salt–Dependent Fraction

Human studies have demonstrated a linear relationship between canalicular bile flow and bile salt output (Fig. 25-5). As noted before, most of the bile salts secreted into

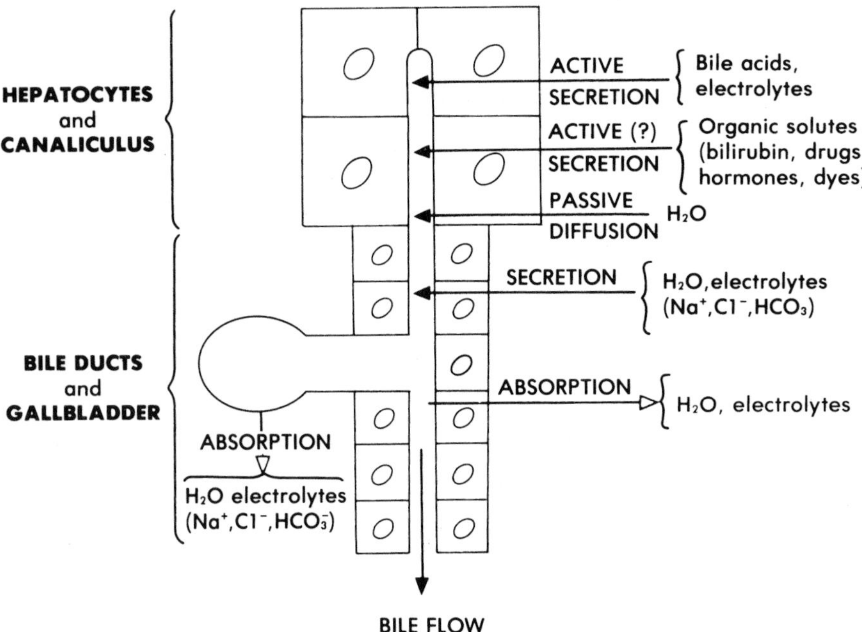

Fig. 25-4. Schematic representation of the formation of bile. Bile secretion begins in the canaliculus with active transport of bile salts (acids), inorganic electrolytes, and possibly other organic solutes. Secretion of these substances is followed passively by water flow into the canaliculus. Bile is concentrated in the gallbladder by the isotonic absorption of water and electrolytes. (From Scharschmidt BF. Bile formation and cholestasis, metabolism and enterohepatic circulation of bile acids, and gallstone formation. In Zakim D, Boyer TD, eds. Hepatology. Philadelphia: WB Saunders, 1982.)

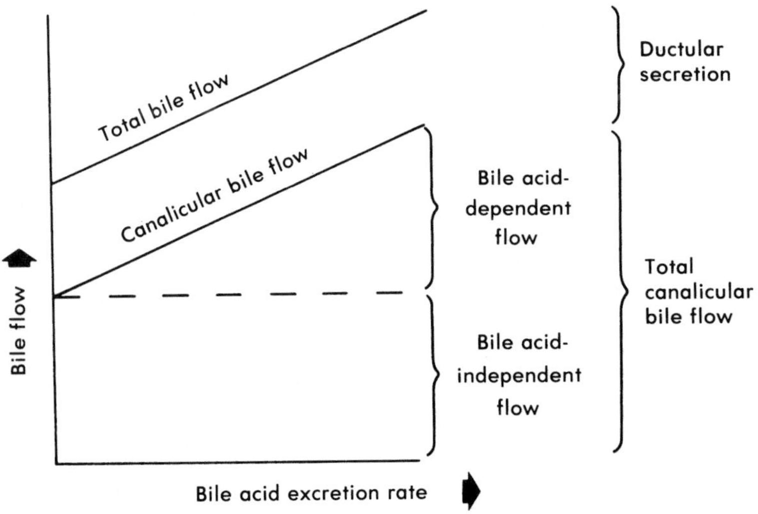

Fig. 25-5. Components of bile flow. Ductular secretion plus canalicular flow accounts for total bile flow. Canalicular flow has bile salt (acid)–dependent and bile salt (acid)–independent components. Bile-dependent canalicular flow varies directly with bile salt (acid) excretion rate. Although the other two components are shown as constant, there is some dependence on bile salt (acid) excretion rate. (Modified from Scharschmidt BF. Bile formation and cholestasis, metabolism and enterohepatic circulation of bile acids, and gallstone formation. In Zakim D, Boyer TD, eds. Hepatology. Philadelphia: WB Saunders, 1982.)

canalicular bile are the result of the extremely efficient extraction of bile salts from portal blood via the enterohepatic circulation. Only a small fraction is required to be produced by de novo hepatocyte synthesis. The uptake of bile salts by hepatocytes is largely by way of a sodium-dependent 49 kDa bile salt transport protein.[20,21] The mechanism of bile salt transport through the hepatocyte to the canaliculus involves both intracellular binding proteins and vesicular transport such as the endoplasmic reticulum.[22-24] Canalicular transport of bile salts is mediated by several mechanisms including two distinct adenosine triphosphate (ATP)–dependent glycoprotein transporters.[16]

The bile salt–dependent secretion of canalicular bile is a major determinant of phospholipid and cholesterol secretion into bile. Both phospholipid and cholesterol biliary output increase with bile salt–dependent bile flow but in a nonlinear fashion. Other factors effecting the biliary output of phospholipids and cholesterol include the noncontinuous nature of the enterohepatic circulation and the endogenous supply of phospholipids and cholesterol.[25] In summary, the primary and rate-limiting step in the bile salt–dependent fraction of canalicular bile flow is the bile salt uptake from the sinusoidal blood across the sinusoidal basal membrane of the hepatocyte. This process facilitates the concomitant secretion of phospholipid and cholesterol into canalicular bile.

Bile Salt–Independent Fraction

Theoretically, bile salt–independent canalicular bile secretion is the amount of bile secretion that occurs in the absence of bile salt output. The concentrations of sodium, potassium, chloride, and bicarbonate in hepatic bile are similar to those found in plasma, and it is these inorganic electrolytes that account for the majority of bile osmolality.[26] In fasting patients with a T-tube in the common bile duct, it has been estimated that the bile salt–independent bile secretion of electrolyte-rich solution is 50% of total canalicular bile production.[25,27] Recent evidence suggests that the active secretion of bicarbonate is the major controlling mechanism of bile salt–independent flow.[28-31] Interestingly, there is little evidence that other inorganic electrolytes, including sodium, chloride, or potassium are actively transported into the canaliculus or influence bile formation.[16] The major physiologic role of bile salt–independent bile formation may be to dilute the bile salt–dependent fraction of bile in the canaliculus.

Ductular Bile

Once bile leaves the canaliculus, it flows through and is modified by ductules and ducts, which secrete a hypertonic fluid composed primarily of water and electrolytes. In patients with an indwelling T-tube following cholecystectomy, ductular secretion is estimated to account for one third of total bile flow.[27] Bile ductular epithelium is capable of actively secreting fluid containing a high bicarbonate concentration.[32] The hormonal influence on bile secretion is at its greatest in the ductular system, where secretin, CCK, vasoactive intestinal peptide, and gastrin stimulate an increase in bile secretion through their effects on ductules and ducts. The duct system may adapt to a primarily absorptive function to help concentrate hepatic bile following cholecystectomy.[25]

Bile Flow

The direction and movement of bile flow within the biliary tract depends on multiple factors. Intrinsic and extrinsic factors play a part in this complex phenomenon of bile delivery to the gastrointestinal tract. In addition to the active transport of solutes such as bile salts and electrolytes, canalicular bile flow is facilitated by "peristalsis" of the canaliculi. Presumably contractile monofilaments are responsible for these contractions in the canaliculi. Support for these canalicular contractions is based on experimental work in which agents that inhibit microfilament function (i.e., cytochalasins and phalloidin) result in canalicular dilation and cholestasis in laboratory animals.[25,26]

The size of the bile salt pool is also an important determinant of bile flow. The smaller the bile salt load to the hepatocytes, the smaller the amount of bile salt–dependent canalicular bile flow, with a resultant increase in de novo synthesis of bile salts by the hepatocytes. Therefore derangements in the enterohepatic circulation by such diverse factors as terminal ileal disease, portal hypertension, or hepatocellular disease may decrease the amount or availability of bile salts to the hepatocytes and decrease bile flow. It is the bile salt load, not the capacity of the liver for bile salt secretion, that is the rate-limiting factor for bile salt–dependent bile secretion under normal conditions.[25]

Independent of their osmotic properties, bile salts may have direct secretory effects as well. The bile salts ursodeoxycholate and 7-ketolithocholate stimulate bile flow in the rat, perhaps by stimulation of canalicular bicarbonate secretion.[28] Increasing the bile salt load to the liver by the addition of exogenous bile salts to the diet increases the biliary secretion of phospholipids and cholesterol but in a nonlinear fashion, and this results in decreasing the saturation of bile with these substances. Sulfobromophthalein, iodipamide, and various anionic cholerectics (not bilirubin) also stimulate bile flow in human beings. Bile flow is at its lowest during fasting. Bile salts are then largely sequestered in the gallbladder, which minimizes their flux through the enterohepatic circulation and thereby significantly decreases bile salt–dependent canalicular bile formation.

Bile flow within the biliary tract also depends on regional differences in intraluminal pressures.[33] The maximal secretory pressure of the liver after manual occlusion of the common bile duct as measured in patients previously subjected to cholecystectomy ranged between 29 and 39 cm of water.[34] In the basal state the resistance of the sphincter of Oddi approximates 15 to 17 cm of water with a corresponding lower pressure in the common bile duct. The common bile duct pressure exceeds resistance to flow from the cystic duct with subsequent entrance of bile into the

Table 25-1. Neural, Hormonal, and Drug Influences on Bile Flow

	C*	D†	GB‡	CBD§	SO‖
Bile salts	↑¶				
Cholecystokinin		↑	↑		↑
Motilin			↑		
Insulin	↑				
Glucagon	↑				
Somatostatin	↓**		↓		
Secretin		↑	↑		↑
Vasoactive intestinal peptide		↑	↓		
Gastrin		↑	↑	↑	↑
Caerulein		↑	↑		↑
Pancreatic polypeptide			↓		
Progesterone			↓		
Estrogens	↓				
Thyroxine	↑				
Corticosteroids	↑				
Vagal input			↑	↑	↑
Sympathetic (alpha)			↑	↑	↑
Sympathetic (beta)			↓	↓	↓
Chlorpromazine	↓				
Phenobarbital	↑				
Iodipamide	↑				
Sulfobromphthalein	↑				
Ampicillin	↑	↑			

**C,* Canalicular bile flow.
†*D,* Ductular bile flow.
‡*GB,* Gallbladder contraction.
§*CBD,* Common bile duct.
‖*SO,* Sphincter of Oddi contraction.
¶↑, Increase flow or contraction.
**↓, Decrease flow or contraction.

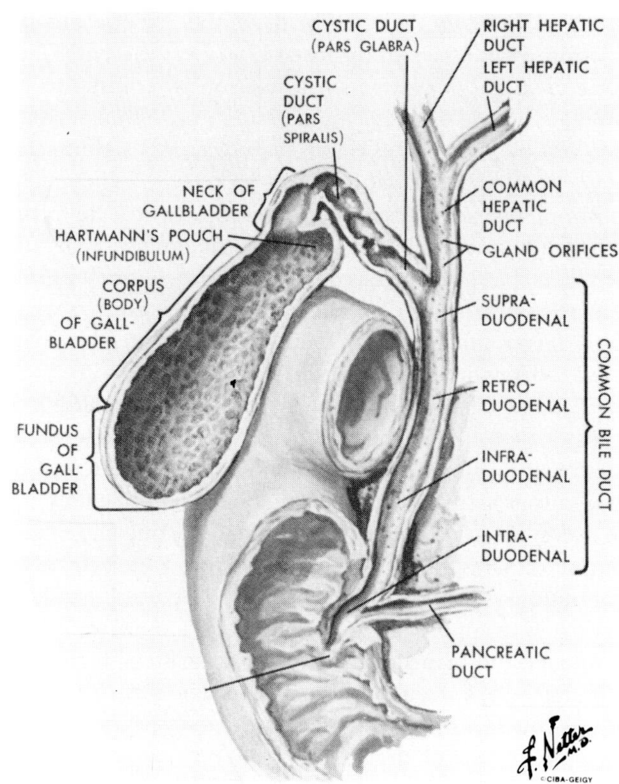

Fig. 25-6. Anatomy of gallbladder. (From Netter FH. CIBA Collection of Medical Illustrations, vol 3, part III. Indianapolis, Ind.: CIBA Pharmaceutical, Division of CIBA-GEIGY, 1964.)

gallbladder. The secretory rate of bile from the liver is minimal at this time. Once chyme enters the duodenum, hepatic bile secretion increases, and gallbladder contractions begin. Both of these events increase common bile duct pressure. Simultaneously, a decrease in pressure at the sphincter of Oddi occurs, allowing bile to flow into the duodenum. Although the significant effects of neurohumoral influences on the gallbladder, common bile duct, and sphincter of Oddi have been well described, their influence on the intrahepatic components of bile flow is less well delineated. Table 25-1 is a compilation of neurohumoral and drug influences on the biliary tract and bile flow.

GALLBLADDER

The gallbladder is a pear-shaped appendage of the common bile duct (Fig. 25-6). It is innervated by parasympathetic fibers from the hepatic branch of the anterior vagal trunk and numerous branches of the splanchnic tree. Histologically, it consists of an inner columnar mucosal layer similar to that seen in the intestine, a thin lamina propria, a thin layer of smooth muscle fibers, the perimuscular connective tissue, and a serosa[33] (Fig. 25-7). Its arterial supply is from the cystic artery, which is usually a branch of the right hepatic artery, and the venous drainage leads to both the liver and portal vein. Extensive lymphatics in the lamina propria ultimately drain into the cisterna chyli.

The gallbladder serves two functions. First, it concentrates bile by reabsorbing water and electrolytes from the relatively dilute hepatic bile. Second, during a meal the gallbladder contracts and delivers its contents into the small intestine. Both of these important functions are reviewed in the following.

Gallbladder Absorption

With its normal capacity of 20 to 40 ml, the gallbladder would be quickly filled with bile, which is secreted at volumes approximating 400 to 600 ml/day. However, the gallbladder has an enormous absorptive capacity. Within 4 hours up to 90% of the water present in hepatic bile can be removed and the gallbladder contents converted from an isotonic solution composed primarily of sodium chloride and sodium bicarbonate to a concentrated solution of impermeable bile salt anions.[18,35] The concentrations of sodium, calcium, and potassium increase, whereas chloride and bicarbonate anion concentrations decrease (Table 25-2). This absorptive process is largely the result of neutral sodium chloride transport.[36,37] The sodium gradient appears to be maintained by a Na^+, K^+-ATPase pump. In ad-

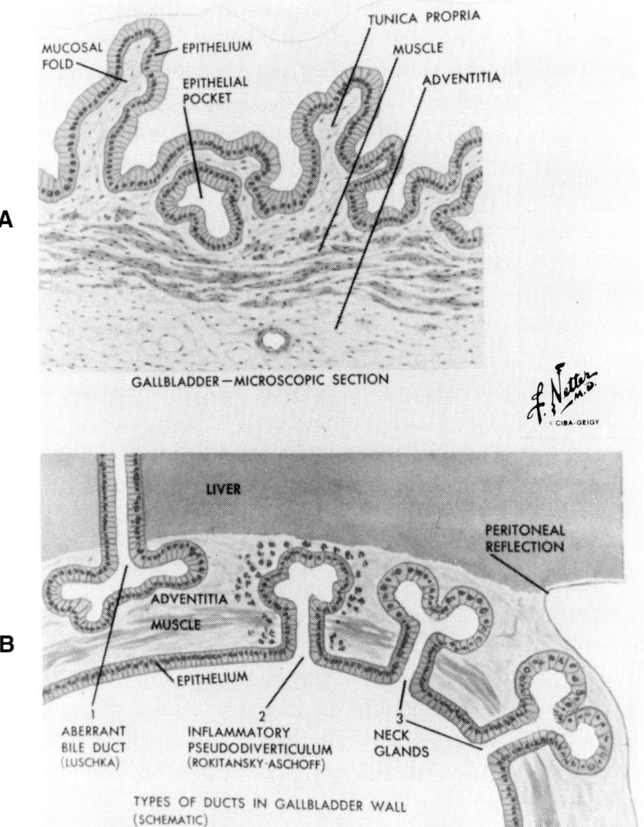

Fig. 25-7. A, Microscopic view of gallbladder. **B,** Microscopic view of types of ducts in gallbladder wall. (From Netter FH. CIBA Collection of Medical Illustrations, vol 3, part III. Indianapolis, Ind.: CIBA Pharmaceutical, Division of CIBA-GEIGY, 1964.)

dition to its potent absorptive function, animal models suggest that the gallbladder may exhibit net postprandial fluid secretion.[38] Normal human gallbladder mucosa is also capable of absorbing certain amino acids and sugars by specialized transport mechanisms as in the small intestine. A substantial concentration gradient exists for bile salts and bile pigments across the gallbladder wall, which is virtually impermeable to highly charged moieties such as taurocholate, sulfobromophthalein, and iodipamide (Cholografin). Weakly ionized substances such as unconjugated bilirubin and chenodeoxycholate are less well protected from diffusion. In the diseased gallbladder, permeability of highly ionized substances and water is increased. The cholecystographic nonvisualization of the gallbladder that is characteristic of inflammatory disease of this organ may be caused by the rapid absorption of iodipamide[37] and not just obstruction of the cystic duct.

Most gastrointestinal mucosa, the gallbladder epithelium included, is injured by direct exposure to high concentrations of bile salts. Under normal conditions, micellar stabilization of the bile salts helps to prevent injury to the gallbladder mucosa from these potentially damaging sub-

Table 25-2. Comparison of Hepatic and Gallbladder Bile

	Hepatic Bile	Gallbladder Bile
Percent solids	2-4%	10-12%
Na^+ (mEq/L)	140-150	200-300
Cl^- (mEq/L)	90-100	15-50
K^+ (mEq/L)	3.5-5	10-25
HCO_3^- (mEq/L)	25-40	10-20
Ca^+ (mEq/L)	25	10-20
Bilirubin (mg/100 ml)	20-60	200-300
Cholesterol (mg/100 ml)	130-230	400-700
Bile salts (mg/100 ml)	1000-2000	4000-9000

stances. The high concentration of bile salts in these micelles also decreases the lithogenic index of bile by enhancing cholesterol solubility, especially when the total lipid content is large.[39] Dilute bile (i.e., low concentrations of bile salts), on the other hand, has a decreased ability to solubilize cholesterol. In infected bile, bacterial deconjugation of bile salts occurs, resulting in enhanced absorption of these substances by the gallbladder epithelium. Such increased absorption of bile salts decreases the bile salt composition of bile (and thereby the solubility of cholesterol) and has direct injurious effects to the gallbladder mucosa, both of which may contribute to the formation of cholesterol gallstones.

Unconjugated bilirubin is also more rapidly absorbed from the gallbladder than conjugated bilirubin. Absorption appears to be linearly related to the luminal concentration of the pigment.[37,40] Calcium bilirubinate crystals are more likely to form in concentrated bile (i.e., bile in which the bile salt concentration is high) with its concurrent reduction in pH and increase in the ion product. Thus a high bile concentration is thought to be a contributory factor in the production of pigment stones rather than in the production of cholesterol stones, which are associated with dilute bile.[41]

Motor Function

Gallbladder filling is ensured by intraluminal common bile duct pressures high enough to permit free flow from the common hepatic duct into the cystic duct and gallbladder. The interdigestive storage of bile and the digestive release of bile are regulated by complex hormonal and neural systems.

The effect of several hormones on the gallbladder are listed in Table 25-1. CCK is a polypeptide containing 39 amino acids. It is released by the proximal small bowel (i.e., duodenum and proximal jejunum) endocrine and neuronal cells secondary to the presence of fat, peptones, essential amino acids, and magnesium sulfate. Vagal sectioning or the division of the thoracic sympathetics has no obvious effect on this release.[42] The mechanism of action of CCK on the gallbladder apparently involves acinar cell membrane binding leading to the release of membrane-bound Ca^{++} ions and a concomitant increase in intracellular cyclic guanosine monophosphate (cGMP), which then leads to gallbladder contraction and evacuation. The polypeptide, motilin, has also been suggested as an important physiologic modulator of gallbladder contraction.[26] Gastrin and caerulein (a CCK-like substance) also have demonstrable in vitro and in vivo CCK-like activity. Secretin seems to potentiate the action of CCK in vivo.[33] Pancreatic polypeptide and vasoactive intestinal peptide apparently inhibit gallbladder contraction by stimulation of adenyl cyclase activity in the gallbladder cells, which then promotes interdigestive relaxation. Somatostatin also promotes gallbladder relaxation, possibly by inhibiting CCK release from the proximal small bowel intestine.[25,42] The presence of bile salts in the proximal small intestine has been clearly shown to inhibit CCK release.[42]

Parasympathetic stimulation of the gallbladder musculature increases intracystic pressure but is not associated with gallbladder evacuation. Thus the physiologic significance of the vagal innervation of the gallbladder remains uncertain.[33] Vagotomy leads to dilation of the gallbladder with an increase in resting (fasting) volume up to 100%. However, following vagotomy the response of the gallbladder to CCK is unaffected, and emptying is unaltered.[26,41] A maintenance of tone may be the primary function of the parasympathetic innervation. In contrast, the adrenergic innervation of the gallbladder contains both excitatory and inhibitory fibers, with the overall tendency toward an inhibition of gallbladder motility. As with the parasympathetic system, the physiologic significance of this sympathetic innervation is uncertain.[33]

Under physiologic conditions, a meal produces strong gallbladder contractions, leading to bile flow into the duodenum within just a few minutes of its ingestion, presumably modulated by both neural and hormonal mechanisms as previously described. CCK has a major role in stimulating bile flow and gallbladder contraction and inducing relaxation of the sphincter of Oddi. As previously noted, sustained output of bile and bile salts into the duodenum depends on the bile salt return to the liver and reabsorption through the enterohepatic circulation.[43] Biliary secretion is associated with normal intestinal migratory motor complexes and involves both secretory and motor responses. The fasted (interdigestive phase) small intestine normally demonstrates a cyclic motor complex. Four separate phases have been identified. Phase I is characterized by the near-total absence of action potentials. In phase II there is persistent irregular action potential activity, with phase III demonstrating large action potentials on every pacesetter potential of that period. Phase IV shows a decline in incidence and intensity of action potentials.[41] The rise in bile secretion into the duodenum during phase II of the interdigestive motor cycle is predominantly caused by gallbladder contraction with simultaneous relaxation of the sphincter of Oddi. During phase I of the interdigestive motor cycle minimal amounts of bile enter the duodenum, with the majority entering the gallbladder because of the increased resting tone of the common bile duct and sphincter of Oddi. The cyclic delivery of bile into the small intestine is not completely determined by the gallbladder, as seen in patients following cholecystectomy who maintain some cyclic bile delivery, with the bile salt pool residing in the upper small bowel and biliary tree during the interdigestive phases.[43]

Investigation in both animal and human systems has revealed that gallbladder filling and emptying occurs in an alternating fashion during both the digestive and interdigestive phases. It appears the gallbladder acts like a "bellows" when contracting and that postprandial fluid secretion by the gallbladder mucosa may help to evacuate its content. These alternating episodes of filling and emptying may serve to mix concentrated gallbladder bile with fresh dilute bile during the interdigestive phase and thus prevent supersaturation of gallbladder bile.[44-46]

COMMON BILE DUCT

The common hepatic duct begins at the confluence of the major lobar bile ducts that drain each hepatic lobe. The common hepatic duct joins with the cystic duct to form the common bile duct. The common bile duct descends inferiorly and passes behind the first portion of the duodenum and through the substance of the head of the pancreas to enter into the duodenal lumen obliquely through the wall of its second part. In approximately 80% of cases, it forms a common channel with the main pancreatic duct called the ampulla of Vater.[25,33] During most of their passage through the duodenal wall these two structures are enclosed by a complex arrangement of intrinsic circular and longitudinal smooth muscle—the sphincter of Oddi (Fig. 25-8). Careful anatomic studies have demonstrated definitively that the sphincter of Oddi's musculature is anatomically and embryologically distinct from the duodenal musculature.[47] The motor activity of the sphincter of Oddi has a substantial role in bile delivery to the duodenal lumen.

Motility

In humans the common bile duct demonstrates a well-defined, spontaneous, rhythmic activity in vitro with three to five contractile waves per minute, each lasting 1 to 3 seconds.[33] The significance of these findings in vivo has not been delineated. The common bile duct musculature is oriented predominantly in the longitudinal direction and is probably more involved with maintaining tone than with intraluminal content propulsion.[48] True peristalsis, as seen in the intestine, is probably not present, nor is it necessary for efficient bile transport. Normally the pressure (11 to 13 cm of water) in the common bile duct is slightly less than the resting pressure or resistance of the sphincter of Oddi, which averages 15 to 17 cm of water. The pressure in the common bile duct exceeds any resistance to flow through the cystic duct so that normally bile enters the gallbladder rather than the duodenum. The efficient delivery of bile into the duodenum necessitates gallbladder

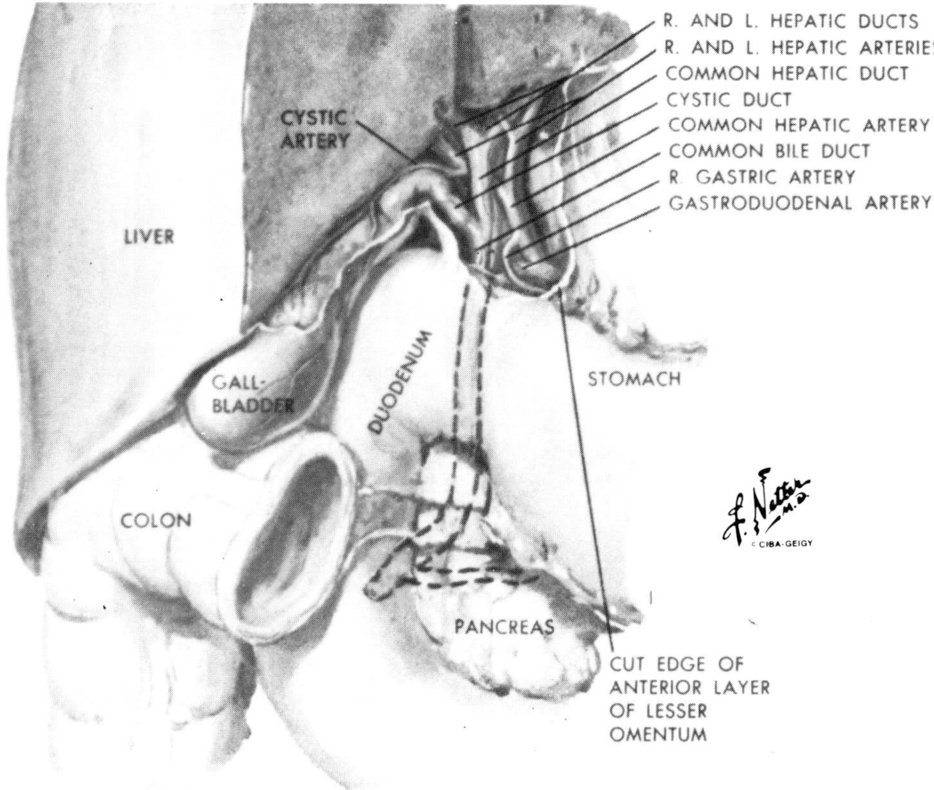

Fig. 25-8. Extrahepatic biliary tract system. (From Netter FH. CIBA Collection of Medical Illustrations, vol 3, part III. Indianapolis, Ind.: CIBA Pharmaceutical, Division of CIBA-GEIGY, 1964.)

contraction and relaxation of the choledochoduodenal junction.[33]

Sphincter of Oddi

Although changes in duodenal activity influence biliary duct pressures, the key factor appears to be the tone of the sphincter of Oddi. In vivo studies have documented the role of choledochoduodenal tone in the regulation of bile flow into the duodenum independent of duodenal motility.[49] Spontaneous rhythmic contraction of the sphincter of Oddi of myogenic origin has also been documented, which may represent a "milking" effect on bile delivery into the duodenum.[33] CCK acts directly on the musculature of the sphincter of Oddi as a relaxant and allows duodenal bile delivery.[25] As with the gallbladder, the neural influences on the common bile duct and the sphincter of Oddi are less quantitatively understood and are of questionable physiologic significance (see Table 25-1).

Resting common bile duct, main pancreatic duct, and sphincter of Oddi pressures do not appear to differ significantly between healthy patients and those with gallstones or common bile duct stones or those previously subjected to cholecystectomy, hepatic duct cancer, or chronic pancreatitis.[50] These observations diminish the likelihood of motility or pressure abnormalities as being of any major significance in the pathogenesis of biliary tract lithiasis.

PATHOGENESIS OF GALLSTONES

Cholesterol Stones

Seventy-five percent to 85% of the people in the United States who have gallstones have stones composed of 40% and usually greater than 60% cholesterol.[51] The three principal components of bile in gallstone formation are bile salts, lecithin, and cholesterol. Cholesterol is virtually insoluble in aqueous solution. Biliary solubilization and excretion of cholesterol are dependent on its interaction with lecithin and bile salts. Bile salts function as biologic detergents and form micelles with hydrophobic groups removed from contact with water and with hydrophilic groups exposed to water molecules (Fig. 25-9). Lecithin, which is also water insoluble, is the second most prominent solute in bile. It is incorporated into bile salt micelles and allows the micelles to swell and solubilize more cholesterol. Thus mixed lecithin–bile salt micelles are thought to solubilize cholesterol, providing a vehicle for its excretion.

Once cholesterol exceeds its maximal solubility in bile, it can crystallize to start a cascade that leads to gallstone formation. Admirand and Small[52] noted that the lipid composition of gallbladder bile in patients with cholesterol stones exceeded the limits of micellar cholesterol solubility. Healthy patients showed a lipid composition within the micelle only phase and showed no solid or liquid crystals. This relationship has been illustrated by a triangular

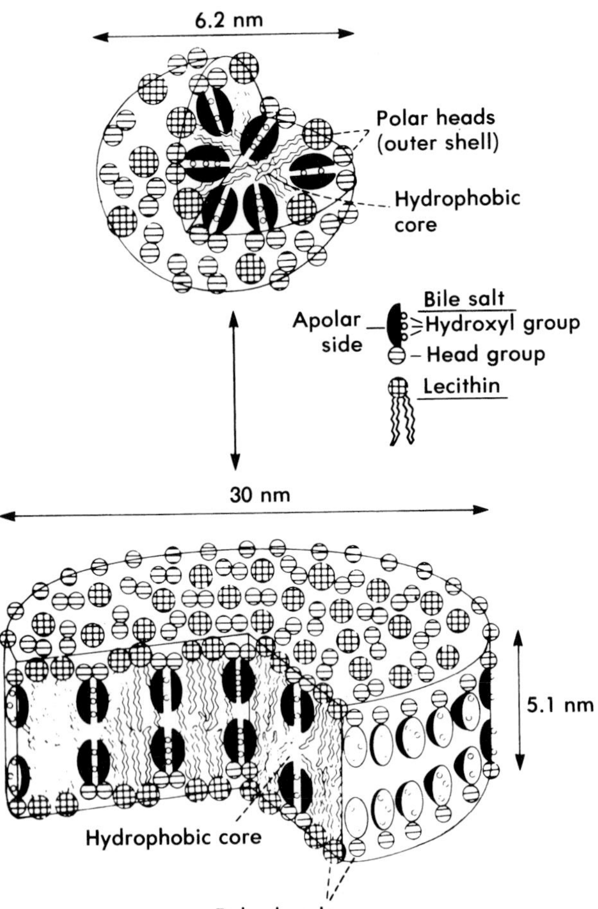

Fig. 25-9. Structure of a mixed micelle. If the solution is bile salt rich, the micelle is sphere shaped; whereas if it is lecithin rich, it is disk shaped. Lecithin-rich micelle is larger and capable of transporting a larger amount of cholesterol. Transition depends on the bile salt/lecithin molar ratio present in native bile. Bile salt molecules in both micellar forms are thought to form pairs (dimers) to avoid contact of the hydroxyl groups *(solid circles)* with the apolar environment of the micellar core. (Modified from Muller K. Structural dimorphism of bile salt/lecithin mixed micelles. A possible regulatory mechanism for cholesterol solubility in bile? X-ray structure analysis.Biochemistry 20:404, 1981. Reprinted with permission. Copyright © American Chemical Society.)

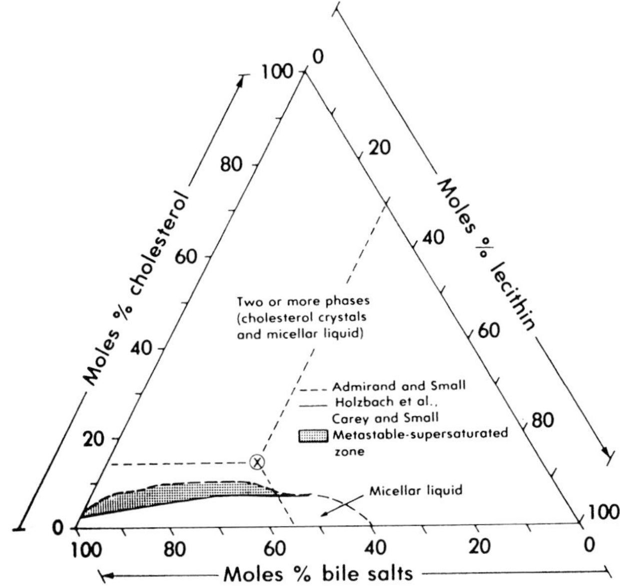

Fig. 25-10. Determination of cholesterol saturation index *(CSI)*. Tricoordinate phase diagram for representing by a single intersecting point *(x)* relative concentrations of cholesterol, lecithin, and bile salt in bile. In this scheme, relative concentration of each lipid is expressed as a percentage of the sum of the molar concentrations of all three. This manipulation permits representation of the relations between three constituents in two dimensions, the water content being invariant at, say, 90% (10% wt/vol solids). In this figure, for example, at point *(x)*, the relative concentration of bile salt from its coordinate is 55% (indicating 55% of the sum of all three lipids), whereas that for lecithin is 30%, and that for cholesterol is 15%. The range of concentrations found consistent with a clear aqueous micellar solution is limited to a small region at the lower left. A solution having the composition represented by point *x*, on the other hand, would initially be visually turbid and contain precipitated forms of cholesterol crystals in addition to bile salt mixed micelles. Last, a solution represented by a point falling in the shaded area below the dashed line would be unstable (i.e., metastable-supersaturated), meaning that by prediction it would be initially clear (micellar). Within a short time, however, various precipitated forms of cholesterol crystals would form, and such a solution would then be visually turbid, similar to all solutions above the dashed line. (From Holzbach RT. Pathogenesis and medical treatment of gallstones. In Sleisenger MH, Fordtran JS, eds. Gastrointestinal Disease: Pathophysiology, Diagnosis, Management, 3rd ed. Philadelphia: WB Saunders, 1983.)

coordinate plot that reflects bile salt, lecithin, and cholesterol equilibrium in aqueous solution (Fig. 25-10). An excess of cholesterol in relation to bile salts and lecithin results in either crystal formation or the lipid crystalline phase. Crystallization is probably a prerequisite for cholesterol gallstone formation, but marked saturation has been found in many patients without crystallization.[53] More recent data have challenged the mixed micelle concept of cholesterol solubilization and excretion. A large portion of biliary cholesterol exists in a vesicular form. It appears that the amphipathic molecules of bile salts and lecithin can form a lipid bilayer similar to that found in cell membranes. Cholesterol can be solubilized in the nonpolar portion of the bilayer.[54,55] In dilute bile or bile salt–poor solution the vesicular bilayers are stable and can solubilize greater quantities of cholesterol than can micelles. Concentration of bile in the gallbladder destabilizes the vesicles and leads to a transfer of cholesterol and lecithin to micelles. This has lead some authors to conclude that supersaturated bile becomes lithogenic only after it is concentrated in the gallbladder.[56]

Cholesterol saturated vesicles fuse and form crystals in a process known as nucleation. Cholesterol nucleation occurs by two general mechanisms. Homogenous nucleation is the random coalescence of cholesterol molecules that form a nidus for further cholesterol precipitation. This likely occurs in very highly saturated bile.[57,58] Heterogenous nucleation is a process in which precipitation occurs around an entity other than a crystal of pure cholesterol. Many different substances may act as nucleating agents to initiate precipitation of cholesterol from saturated bile. In fact, many cholesterol gallstones have a pigmented center, implicating some form of pigment nucleating agent. Nucleation occurs in the mucin gel that lines the gallbladder.[51] Mucin is a complex of glycoproteins secreted by gallbladder epithelial cells and is another key component of gallstones. Mucin glycoproteins accelerate cholesterol nucleation and serve as a matrix for stone growth.[59,60]

Normal gallbladder storage and motility may be disturbed under special circumstances and ultimately lead to gallstone formation. In pregnancy the residual volume of the gallbladder increases twofold over normal and is a presumed factor in the increased incidence of cholesterol gallstones in this population. Serum progesterone levels are elevated during the progesterone peak of the menstrual cycle and in women taking certain oral contraceptive pills. These conditions are associated with impaired gallbladder emptying or increased volume during fasting.[41,43,61,62] A sizable subgroup of cholesterol gallstone patients have been identified to have defective gallbladder emptying independent of clinical presentation, gallstone size, or gallstone number.[63] Defective gallbladder contractility has been shown to appear in the early stages of cholesterol gallstone formation in various animal models.[64] Multiple other factors may influence cholesterol gallstone formation, including calcium metabolism, pH, and neurohormonal factors.

Pigment Stones

Pigment stones are composed of a relatively high concentration of bilirubin and low concentration of cholesterol. The basic pathologic events resulting in pigment stones are similar to the development of cholesterol stones. A change in biliary composition occurs that results in an altered solubilization of unconjugated bilirubin, causing saturation and precipitation of calcium bilirubinate and insoluble salts. These stones are usually mulberry-like in appearance and are composed mainly of bilirubin and other pigment compounds. They account for about 15% to 25% of gallstones in the United States.

There are two types of pigment stones: brown and black. In the formation of both types, water-insoluble unconjugated bilirubin combines with calcium to form a calcium bilirubinate matrix that is the predominant component of pigmented stones.[3] Black pigment stones contain more inorganic components and mucin.[65] Black pigment stones are associated with hemolytic disorders, cirrhosis, long-term parenteral nutrition, ileal resections, and elderly patients. They are generally found only in the gallbladder. Brown pigment stones are associated with stasis and bacterial or parasitic infection. They occur predominantly in the Orient, although 50% of recurrent common bile duct stones in the United States are also of this variety.[66] Normally bile is sterile, but bacterial or parasitic infections of the biliary tract are not uncommon.[57] The critical role of infection in the formation of brown stones is supported by the finding that bacteria typically can be identified in the matrix of brown pigment stones but not from cholesterol or black pigment stones.[67] Improved public health conditions have resulted in a corresponding decrease in pigment stones and increase in cholesterol stones in the Orient.[66]

Risk Factors for Cholelithiasis

Heredity

The potential for genetic factors to cause cholesterol cholelithiasis has been documented in some Native Americans. Many Pima women have an inherited decrease in bile salt synthesis, which leads to a small pool of bile salts. Seventy-five percent of these women older than age 30 years have gallstones.[68] Marked racial differences are also known to exist as demonstrated by the fact that Mexican Americans have a higher prevalence of cholelithiasis than do whites or blacks.[69] It has also been shown that about twice as many patients with gallstones as matched controls without gallstones have first-degree relatives with gallstones.[70]

Obesity

Most overweight people have an overproduction of cholesterol; as a result, obese individuals have a prevalence of gallstones twice that of nonoverweight individuals.[71] About 25% of obese patients who lose weight rapidly develop cholesterol stones within 4 months. This occurs as a result of reduction in bile salt secretion in the presence of increased cholesterol mobilization from adipose tissue.[72] Although high cholesterol or polyunsaturated fatty acid diets can increase bile saturation, their role in cholesterol gallstone formation has not been confirmed.[73]

Hormones

The incidence of cholelithiasis in women is twice that of men. This most likely reflects the hormonal changes associated with pregnancy, birth control pills, and hormone replacement following menopause. Estrogen increases hepatic cholesterol secretion and probably decreases the bile salt pool, leading to increased bile saturation.[74] Cholesterol gallstones also occur frequently in men receiving estrogen for prostate cancer.[75]

Associated Medical Disorders

Patients with ileal disease or ileal resection are known to be at risk for cholesterol gallstones. This is due to a decreased absorption of bile salts (i.e., an interruption in the enterohepatic circulation) and a decrease in the bile salt pool. Similar alterations occurred in patients who had a jejunoileal bypass for morbid obesity. Fortunately, this operation is no longer performed for obesity. Patients receiving long-term total parenteral nutrition are at increased risk as a result of prolonged gallbladder stasis. In patients with diabetes, autonomic dysfunction leads to atony of the gallbladder, which may facilitate gallstone formation.[76] Patients with type IIb or type IV hyperlipoproteinemia also show an increased incidence of gallstone disease because of their associated metabolic disorder.[77] Drugs that reduce bile salt synthesis such as the hypolipidemic agent clofibrate can predispose a patient to cholelithiasis. Finally, vagotomy is frequently listed as a cause of gallstones; however, this has not been clearly established, since most patients regain normal motility function of the gallbladder following vagotomy.

CLINICAL SPECTRUM OF BILIARY DISEASE

Cholecystitis and Cholecystectomy

Biliary colic, chronic cholecystitis, and acute cholecystitis represent the spectrum of gallbladder disease. Biliary colic is right upper quadrant discomfort of short duration after a meal caused by obstruction of the cystic duct from a gallstone. It is usually an incomplete obstruction with little inflammatory response. Although called "biliary colic," the pain is not a true colic but a discomfort that gradually increases in severity, reaches a plateau, and then gradually decreases. It does not have the paroxysms of acute pain associated with intestinal obstruction (intestinal colic). Chronic cholecystitis is usually the result of multiple episodes of gallbladder inflammation, which eventually lead to a scarred gallbladder that has lost its functional ability to concentrate bile. As a result, functional studies of the gallbladder with radiocontrast materials show nonvisualization. Such patients usually have dull right upper quadrant discomfort following a meal that often is intermittent and that may last for several hours with little systemic response.

Acute cholecystitis refers to acute inflammation of the gallbladder and is caused by obstruction of the cystic duct by stones in at least 90% of cases. Infection of the gallbladder is probably also an important etiologic component, since bacteria of enteric origin may be cultured from gallbladder bile in two thirds or three fourths of patients with acute cholecystitis. In this disorder, a systemic response to the inflammation is common. This is characterized by right upper quadrant pain and tenderness, with a modest-to-moderate increase in temperature. In about 30% of patients a mass is palpable in the right upper quadrant. This mass usually represents omentum and bowel overlying the inflamed gallbladder. About 75% of patients with acute cholecystitis have had previous gallbladder symptoms. Laboratory studies may be abnormal, including a leukocytosis to 15,000 cells/mm and a slight increase in serum alkaline phosphatase, amylase, serum glutamic-oxaloacetic transaminase, and serum glutamate pyruvate transaminase. Occasionally, the bilirubin may be mildly elevated. A plain abdominal x-ray film is usually of little help in establishing the diagnosis and is more helpful in ruling out other diseases such as a perforated ulcer with free air and a urinary calculus. About 15% of patients have radiopaque gallstones demonstrable on this x-ray film. Air may occasionally be seen in the gallbladder wall or biliary tract if gas-forming organisms are present or if there is a fistula between the gallbladder and small intestine (cholecystoenteric fistula) from erosion of a gallstone into adjacent bowel that results from adherence of the bowel to the inflamed gallbladder.

The typical presentation of a patient with cholecystitis (acute or chronic) is the right upper quadrant abdominal pain occurring about 1 to 2 hours following a meal. The relationship to food is variable but consistent enough that it is probably caused by the emptying of fat from the stomach into the duodenum, which results in the release of CCK. CCK is a stimulant of gallbladder contraction, and with stones in the gallbladder the increased activity leads to a stone obstructing the cystic duct. The relationship between fat and CCK release and its effects on gallbladder contraction is probably the explanation for the common association of fatty and fried foods and the initiation of gallbladder pain in patients with cholelithiasis. Although acute cholecystitis is the result of cystic duct obstruction by an impacted stone or one attempting to pass from the gallbladder through the cystic duct and into the common duct, the majority of the time, it can occur without the presence of gallstones. Acalculous cholecystitis accounts for about 5% of all cases and is found in patients with sepsis, prolonged starvation, cystic artery occlusion, prolonged hyperalimentation, collagen vascular disease, and acquired immunodeficiency syndrome. The right upper quadrant pain and tenderness that occur with cholecystitis are attributed to distention and inflammation of the gallbladder. Gallbladder pain generally radiates around to the back and between the scapulae. The pain pattern may be short-lived if the stone dislodges itself from obstructing the cystic duct or persistent if the stone becomes impacted. The pain of gallbladder disease is contrasted with the pain associated with pancreatitis, which usually penetrates through to the back. On physical examination the tenderness that occurs in the right upper quadrant may be mild or severe and aggravated on inspiration, in which case it is referred to as Murphy's sign. This latter sign is usually elicited by the examiner by manually indenting the abdominal wall on the right side in the midclavicular line just below the costal margin and having the patient take a deep breath. With inspiration the diaphragm descends, pushing the liver down and anteriorly. With the indentation of the abdominal wall the gallbladder is struck, resulting in sharp pain. Murphy's sign refers to this particular maneuver of elicited pain on inspiration that is localized in the right upper quadrant and usually indicates an impacted stone in the cystic duct. Diffuse discomfort in the entire right upper quadrant is not considered a positive Murphy's sign and is usually more indicative of the resolution of cystic duct obstruction or the presence of liver disease. The position at which the localized tenderness of Murphy's sign is elicited may vary, especially if the patient has a large liver that may extend below the costal margin.

Specific diagnostic evaluation of cholecystitis can be placed in two general categories: patients with acute symptoms and those in whom symptoms have resolved. Those patients with acute symptoms should be evaluated promptly for biliary tract disease, since deterioration of the clinical course generally requires an emergency cholecystectomy. This is in contrast to patients with hepatitis and pancreatitis in whom medical support is the preferred treatment. Two studies are extremely helpful in diagnosing biliary tract disease under acute conditions: ultrasound and the radionuclide biliary scan. Both of these studies are noninvasive, rapid, and accurate and have low complication rates. Ultrasound provides information about the gallbladder anatomy, including thickening of the gallbladder wall and the presence or absence of pericystocolic fluid, and shows the presence of a stone or stones. Stones appear as an echogenic mass with acoustic shadowing. This has an accuracy approaching 90%. In a patient with typical symptoms of acute cholecystitis, confirmation of the presence of stones in the gallbladder with ultrasound usually provides sufficient information to justify proceeding with a cholecystectomy. In contrast to ultrasound, technetium-99 radionuclide scanning is a functional test of the gallbladder. This test is performed by injecting technetium intravenously, coupled with various iminodiacetic acid (IDA) derivatives (e.g., 2,6-dimethyl acetanilid [HIDA], paraisopropyl iminodiacetic acid [PIPIDA], 2,6-diisopropyl acetanilid [DISIDA]). The injected radioisotope is excreted by the hepatocytes into bile and concentrated in the gallbladder. Within 5 to 10 minutes of injection the liver is imaged, and shortly afterward the bile ducts and gallbladder are visualized. The visualization of the liver and bile ducts without visualization of the gallbladder is considered an abnormal test result. Since ingestion of fat before this test results in gallbladder contraction and its emptying, it is important that the patient is fasted before the test is begun to prevent a falsely abnormal outcome. Assuming that the test has been performed properly, it is necessary to rely on clinical symptoms for interpretation of nonvisualization of the gallbladder. A symptomatic patient with nonvisualization has acute cholecystitis. Chronic cholecystitis is suggested when symptoms have abated and the gallbladder does not visualize. The various iminodiacetic radionuclide compounds that image the biliary tract are related to the bilirubin level. The technetium HIDA scan images the biliary tree when the bilirubin is under 6 mg/100 ml. The other compounds visualize the biliary tree at higher bilirubin levels. In the patient with hyperbilirubinemia it is important to select the appropriate radionuclide material to ensure adequate imaging of the biliary tract. If this is not done, poor visualization of the liver and bile duct occurs and could be misinterpreted. In this circumstance, poor imaging does not indicate complete biliary obstruction but rather parenchymal liver disease.

The selection of ultrasonography, radionuclide scanning, or oral cholecystography depends on the clinical presentation of the patient and the resources available to the clinician. Most clinicians prefer a radionuclide scan in acute conditions and an ultrasound in asymptomatic patients. The combination of sonography and radionuclide scanning under acute conditions combines anatomy and function; therefore the tests complement one another.

Patients with acute cholecystitis should be admitted to a general surgical service, resuscitated with intravenous fluids, have concomitant medical problems stabilized, and undergo cholecystectomy at the earliest convenient time once the diagnosis is confirmed with ultrasound or radionuclide study. Additional therapy such as parasympathetic drugs, nasogastric suction, and H_2 receptor antagonists have not been shown to affect the course of the disease. Unless the patient is febrile and has evidence of bacterial infection or is at risk from endocarditis, antibiotics are used only in the periods immediately before, during, and after surgery. Antibiotics that have good tissue penetration for gram-negative organisms are preferred. The main purpose of antibiotics in these patients is to decrease the incidence of a wound infection, since cholecystectomy is considered a clean contaminated case. Observing the patient until symptoms subside or performing cholecystectomy in 6 to 8 weeks during another hospitalization should rarely be necessary. The clinical condition of the patient should be the factor that determines the timing of the operation. The golden period of 72 hours has not been substantiated despite anecdotal reports. Data exist that refute the practice of delayed operation (i.e., 6 to 8 weeks) if the patient cannot undergo a cholecystectomy within 72 hours of the onset of acute cholecystitis.[78]

In contrast to symptomatic patients who do not fair well when followed, multiple epidemiologic studies have confirmed that asymptomatic patients with gallstones generally have an indolent course.[79,80] Two percent of asymptomatic patients with gallstones initially present with serious symptoms or a complication. The validity of this approach is reinforced by reports that almost all patients experience symptoms prior to the development of complications, and less than 2% present initially with a serious complication.[79] It should also be noted that the utilization of laparoscopic cholecystectomy should not alter the management of patients with silent gallstones. In highly selected patients the presence of gallstones, even when asymptomatic, can be an indication for cholecystectomy.

The indications for cholecystectomy in patients with asymptomatic gallstones include the following conditions. Children with gallstones almost always develop symptoms and should be considered for cholecystectomy. Patients with sickle cell disease and gallstones may present a difficult diagnostic problem during sickle cell crisis, and consequently most experts recommend an elective operation. Since a nonfunctioning gallbladder indicates advanced disease and 25% of these individuals develop symptoms, elective cholecystectomy is recommended. A calcified gallbladder wall is an indication for cholecystectomy because approximately half these patients have an associated gallbladder cancer. Large stones (>2.5 cm in diameter) are more frequently associated with acute cholecystitis, and cholecystectomy may be warranted. The natural history of asymptomatic gallstones in diabetic patients is not well defined. Prophylactic cholecystectomy for diabetic patients is not recommended.[1] Although diabetic individuals have an increased mortality with emergency cholecystectomy, these patients also have increased operative risk with elective surgery. The increased risk associated with these patients appears to be related to a high incidence of coexisting medical problems rather than as a direct result of the diabetes.

Choledocholithiasis

Common bile duct stones (i.e., choledocholithiasis) can be divided into primary and secondary types. About 15% of patients with gallbladder stones have simultaneous stones in the common bile duct. These stones are virtually always the same chemically as those in the gallbladder. Primary choledocholithiasis is more difficult to prove and is the subject of much clinical controversy. Generally, a 2-year asymptomatic interval after previous cholecystectomy is required before stones found in the common duct can be considered to be primary. The incidence of primary choledocholithiasis varies from 4% to 90%, depending on the criteria used for its identification.[81]

More than 50% of primary common bile duct stones are pigment stones. These are light, soft, crushable yellow or brown stones, often found in association with sludge or debris in other parts of the biliary tree but routinely absent in the gallbladder if this organ has not been previously removed. Primary stones are usually associated with common bile duct dilation, biliary tract infection, advanced patient age, a long history of biliary tract disease, and multiple previous surgical interventions on the biliary tree. Secondary stones in the common duct found in association with primary gallbladder disease and gallstones are rarely associated with biliary tract infection or pathologic changes in biliary tree histology.[81,82] Although controversial, stasis is thought to be a leading factor in primary choledocholithogenesis. Previous operations on the biliary tract or trauma to the sphincter of Oddi may contribute to stasis in the bile ducts, since the bile duct dilates following these circumstances. Stasis also occurs with age and seems to correlate with duct dilation and stone formation. The relationship between a motility disorder, stasis, and stone formation is not well defined, but there seem to be several correlations. The stones found in dilated bile ducts are usually pigmented and more frequently occur in elderly patients. Congenital diseases associated with ductular dilation such as Caroli's disease are also associated with primary stone formation.[83]

The role of biliary infection in the genesis of pigment stone formation has been discussed previously. An interrelationship between infection and stasis is thought to promote mucosal inflammatory changes that lead to dilation and extrusion of calcium and abnormal mucus that may act as nidi for stone formation.[84] Periampullary duodenal diverticula are also associated with a high incidence of common bile duct calculous disease,[85] probably because of incompetent choledochoduodenal sphincter function and bacterial contamination.

Another method of classifying common duct stones is according to the chemical composition of the stone. This has major therapeutic implications, since cholesterol stones are amenable to dissolution and pigment stones cannot be safely dissolved. Following cholecystectomy and comon duct exploration, the stones should be saved and incubated in monoctanoin. If the stones dissolve within 5 days, the cholesterol content is sufficiently high (>60%) that any retained common duct stones can be dissolved. Currently, monoctanoin is the preferred compound to dissolve retained cholesterol common duct stones. Monoctanoin is a medium chain diglyceride and is described in more detail in the following section.

Of the approximately 15% of patients who have choledocholithiasis in combination with cholelithiasis, as many as 50% of them demonstrate no clinical evidence of common duct disease. Most of the others experience jaundice, biliary colic, cholangitis (see the following), or pancreatitis as a result of obstruction from the stones. Because of the fluctuating nature of the obstruction, serum bilirubin levels are usually less than those seen with malignant disease and rarely exceed 15 mg/100 ml. At initial surgery for cholelithiasis, historical suspicions (jaundice, cholangitis, pancreatitis) or physical manifestations (palpable stone, dilated common bile duct, filling defects seen on cholangiography before and during surgery) may lead the surgeon to perform a common bile duct exploration with stone removal by means of irrigation, forceps, balloon catheter, or sphincterotomy. It is now common to remove common duct stones laparoscopically using a host of techniques. In addition, the use of preoperative endoscopic retrograde cholangiopancreatography (ERCP) for removal of a common duct stone can be considered. The surgically opened common bile duct is usually closed over a soft T-tube to stent the traumatized duct to lessen postoperative edema, protect the suture line, and allow postoperative radiologic evaluation and treatment, if necessary, for retained stones.

Cholangitis

Cholangitis usually signifies bacterial infection of an obstructed common bile duct, generally resulting from stones within the duct (i.e., choledocholithiasis), a stricture occluding the diameter of the duct lumen (often resulting from surgical injury), or a neoplasm occluding the duct. Charcot's triad (right upper quadrant pain, jaundice, fever, and chills) is seen in approximately two thirds of these patients. Most of these patients respond to intravenous broad-spectrum antibiotics unless the duct is virtually totally occluded. In this latter circumstance, the cholangitis becomes suppurative and usually presents with shock and mental status changes in addition to Charcot's triad, warranting urgent resuscitation, antibiotic coverage, and surgical drainage of the duct by means of laparotomy (i.e., choledochotomy). In selected cases, percutaneous or endoscopic drainage of the duct has been successful. If either of these methods is used and the patient does not respond, adequate drainage must be obtained with a large T-tube placed during operation.

Nonsurgical Therapy for Gallstone Disease

Insights into the pathophysiology of gallstone formation have generated investigation of alternatives to cholecystectomy for treating gallstone disease. These alternatives have become less attractive as a result of laparoscopic cholecystectomy. A nonsurgical approach to cholelithiasis may be useful for patients deemed to be poor surgical risks or for prophylactic treatment in special circumstances. In general, these methods should not be considered standard approaches to cholelithiasis and cholecystitis.

Oral and Contact Dissolution Therapy

Chenodeoxycholate and ursodeoxycholate are bile salts approved for use as litholytic agents for gallstone disease. Chenodeoxycholate expands the bile salt pool and reduces cholesterol by suppression of the key enzyme for cholesterol synthesis HMG-CoA reductase.[86] Ursodeoxycholate expands the bile salt pool and reduces intestinal absorption of cholesterol.[87] The use of these medications is limited to symptomatic patients with cholesterol stones and functioning gallbladders who have minimal disease. If the stones are radiopaque, show evidence of calcification, or can be seen on CT scan, bile salt therapy is not likely to be successful. If the gallbladder does not function, bile salts do not reach the stones. It must be emphasized that bile salts dissolve only cholesterol gallstones. The gallstone dissolution rate with bile salts varies depending on patient selection and bile salt dosage. In the National Cooperative Gallstone Study, 14% of the patients had complete dissolution of stones within 2 years.[88] With chenodeoxycholate, 41% of the patients had significant diarrhea, and 3% had significant hepatotoxicity. European trials using higher doses of chenodeoxycholate coupled with a low cholesterol diet found that 75% of patients showed complete dissolution following 12 months of therapy.[89,90] Treatment with ursodeoxycholate seems to have a higher success rate and lower complication rate compared to treatment with chenodeoxycholate. Approximately 50% of patients develop recurrence of gallstones following cessation of therapy.

Gallbladder stones can be dissolved also by instilling potent organic solvents directly into the gallbladder through a percutaneous catheter. Monoctanoin and methyl tert-butyl ether are the best-studied agents. Niether agent is suitable for oral ingestion. Patients with stones likely to respond to contact dissolution are very similar to those who respond to bile salt therapy because only noncalcified cholesterol stones can be dissolved by these solvents. Unlike bile salt therapy, large stones may be effectively treated with contact dissolution.

Gallstone dissolution with monoctanoin is safe and in highly selected patients has been reported to be over 90% successful.[91] This infusion may require 4 to 21 days of continuous therapy. Complete dissolution with methyl tert-butyl ether generally occurs in less than 12 hours.[92] There are significant side effects, and it is important that it not leak from the gallbladder. Methyl tert-butyl ether cannot be infused into the common duct, and its general use is still considered to be investigational.

Fragmentation

Fragmentation of gallstones can be accomplished using extracorporeal shock wave lithotripsy (ESWL). Studies to date document that ESWL is safe and has few serious complications. It appears to be most effective in patients with a single gallstone 20 mm in diameter or smaller. It has been reported to render up to 90% of highly selected patients (single small stones) stone free.[93] Patients with 20 to 30 mm gallstones and those with up to three stones have stone clearance rate of about 60%. Recurrence rates are approximately 10% during the first year.[94] It has been demonstrated that adjuvant bile salt therapy is essential. The disadvantages to ESWL include a high incidence of treatment related biliary colic, the need for prolonged bile salt therapy, the possibility of recurrence, and a lack of long-term post ESWL follow-up. The use of ESWL for treatment of gallstones is considered to be investigational.

Malignancy and Calculous Disease

Biliary cancer is a rare disease in the United States. The development of biliary cancer appears to be related to chronic inflammation of the biliary system. Cholelithiasis has been implicated as an etiologic factor because as many as 70% to 90% of patients have gallstones and the risk of malignant degeneration appears to correlate with the length of time gallstones have been present. As noted earlier as many as 60% of patients with porcelain gallbladders from chronic cholecystitis develop carcinoma of the gallbladder. Cholangiocarcinoma is associated with ulcerative colitis, Crohn's disease, biliary atresia, sclerosing cholangitis, Caroli's disease, and hepatolithiasis.

Gallbladder cancer is a disease of the elderly; 75% of patients are older than 65 years at the time of diagnosis. Most patients are women, and histologically most primary tumors are adenocarcinoma. Like gallbladder cancer, most patients with bile duct malignancies are in the older age group, although they may appear in patients as young as 20 years old.

The signs and symptoms associated with cancer of the gallbladder are similar to those occurring in other types of biliary tract disease. Pain in the right upper quadrant in association with nausea, vomiting, and occasionally weight loss are relatively frequent. At some point in the disease process, jaundice may be encountered in as many as 50% of patients, and the gallbladder is palpable in as many as 25% of patients. Such findings are usually attributed to benign gallbladder disease. It is for this reason that the diagnosis is rarely made before operation. Many of the symptoms associated with gallbladder cancer are also found in patients with bile duct malignancies. Because of the obstructive nature of biliary tract malignancy, jaundice is more commonly encountered and is often associated with clay-colored stools, diarrhea, and a dark "tea-colored" urine. Because these findings are common to all patients with obstructive jaundice, the diagnosis of bile duct carcinoma is also usually confirmed only at the time of operation. The treatment of carcinoma of the gallbladder has generally been dismal because of early metastases and extension of the tumor beyond the gallbladder by the time of diagnosis. Even when cholecystectomy in combination with resection of all or part of the right lobe of the liver is attempted as a curative procedure, the overall 5-year survival rate averages no more than 2% to 3%. Adjuvant postoperative radiation therapy is controversial although several small series suggest a small benefit. Obviously, earlier diagnosis and resection when the tumor has been confined to the gallbladder is the only hope of effecting a cure in patients with this devastating tumor.

The outcome in patients with bile duct carcinoma is just as discouraging. The overall 5-year survival rate in patients with this disease approaches 10% to 15%. Like gallbladder cancer, the treatment is operative (i.e., resection of the affected bile duct). For distal bile duct lesions, this usually involves a pancreaticoduodenectomy (Whipple procedure). For middle common duct or low hepatic duct tumors, bile flow is reestablished with a Roux-en-Y choledochojejunostomy approach in which the proximal duct is anastomosed to a jejunal loop following resection of the common hepatic and common bile duct. Tumors at the hilum of the liver, if resectable, provide a more formidable problem in terms of reestablishing bile flow. The tumor is resected with some hepatic parenchyma, and reconstruction consists of a Roux-en-Y hepaticojejunostomy, in which the anastomosis is fashioned between the hilum of the liver and the bowel rather than between individual bile ducts and the intestine.

Most reports of chemotherapy for cancers of the gallbladder, bile ducts, and intrahepatic cholangiocarcinomas suggest a similar response rate of about 20% with hepatic artery infusion being somewhat higher. Many series suggest radiation therapy improves survival of patients with biliary duct cancers who have not had a complete surgical resection. The role of radiation therapy after complete resection is more controversial.

SUMMARY

A knowledge of the physiology of bile composition, secretion, and flow and their relationships to biliary pathology is crucial to understanding the pathogenesis of calculous disease of the gallbladder and biliary tree. The complex fluid called bile is produced and modified in the hepatic bile canaliculi in both bile salt–dependent and bile salt–independent fractions and later supplemented by the addition of ductular bile. Bile flow depends on multiple factors, including active transport, peristalsis, and the size of the bile salt pool. The unique interaction between bile salts, phospholipids, and cholesterol into micelles facilitates lipid absorption from the gut. Disproportionate changes in the amounts of any of these substances may lead to saturated bile with lithogenic tendencies. The gallbladder and common bile duct are often the site of gallstone formation. Symptomatic patients with gallstones should have a cholecystectomy.

REFERENCES

1. Kalser SC. National Institutes of Health Consensus Development Conference Statement on Gallstones and Laparoscopic Cholecystectomy. Am J Surg 165:390, 1993.
2. Donovan JM, Carey MC. Physical-chemical basis of gallstone formation. Gastroenterol Clin North Am 20:47, 1991.
3. Saunders KD, Cates JA, Roslyn JL. Pathogenesis of gallstones. Surg Clin North Am 70:1197, 1990.
4. Cooper AD. Metabolic basis of cholesterol gallstone disease. Gastroenterol Clin North Am 20:21, 1991.
5. Goldstein JL, et al. Receptor-mediated endocytosis: Concepts emerging from the LDL receptor system. Annu Rev Cell Biol 1:1, 1985.
6. Cooper AD. Hepatic lipoprotein and cholesterol metabolism. In Zakim D, Boyer TD, eds. Hepatology a Textbook of Liver Disease. Philadelphia: WB Saunders, 1990.
7. Vlahcevic ZR, Heuman DM, Hyleman PB. Physiology and pathophysiology of enterohepatic circulation of bile acids. In Zakim D, Boyer TD, eds. Hepatology a Textbook of Liver Disease. Philadelphia: WB Saunders, 1990.
8. Brunner H, et al. Gastric emptying and secretions of bile acids, cholesterol, and pancreatic enzymes during digestion: Duodenal perfusion studies in healthy subjects. Mayo Clin Proc 49:851, 1974.
9. Heuman DM, et al. Regulation of bile acid synthesis: I. Effects of conjugated urso deoxycholate and cholate on bile acid synthesis in chronic in chronic bile fistula in the rat. Hepatology 8:358, 1988.
10. Heuman DM, et al. Regulation of bile acid synthesis: II. Effect of bile acid feeding on enzymes regulating hepatic cholesterol and bile acid synthesis in the rat. Hepatology 8:892, 1988.
11. Danielsson H, Einarsson K, Johansson G. Effects of biliary drainage on individual reactions in the conversion of cholesterol to taurocholic acid. Eur J Biochem 2:44, 1967.
12. Balasubramaniam S, Mitropoulos KA, Myant NB. Hormonal control of the activities of cholesterol 7α-hydroxylase and hydroxymethyl-gluteryl-CoA-reductase in rats. In Matern S, Hackanschmidt J, Back P, eds. Advances in Bile Acid Research III. Bile Acid Meeting. Stuttgart: Verlag, 1974.
13. Shefer S, et al. Regulatory effects of sterols and bile acids on hepatic 3-hydroxy-3-methyl glutaryl CoA-reductase and cholesterol 7-α-hydroxylase in the rat. J Lipid Res 14:573, 1973.
14. Raicht RF, et al. Sterol balance studies in the rat. Effects of dietary cholesterol and B-sitosterol on sterol balance and rate limiting enzymes of sterol metabolism. Biochim Biophys Acta 388:374, 1975.
15. Mok HgL, von Bergmamm K, Grundy SM. Kinetics of enterohepatic circulation during fasting: Biliary lipid secretion and gallbladder storage. Gastroenterology 78:1023, 1980.
16. Scharschmidt BF. Bilirubin metabolism, bile formation and gallbladder and bile duct function. In Scharschmidt BF, Feldman M, eds. Gastrointestinal Disease. Philadelphia: WB Saunders, 1993.
17. Zimmerman HJ. The differential diagnosis of jaundice. Med Clin North Am 52:1417, 1968.
18. Scharschmidt BF. Bile formation and cholestasis. In Zakim D, Boyer T, eds. Hepatology. Philadelphia: WB Saunders, 1989.

19. Van Dyke RW, Lake JR, Scharschmidt FF. Cellular mechanisms of hepatic fluid and electrolyte transport. In Forte JP, ed. Volume on Salivary, Pancreatic, Gastric and Hepatobiliary Secretion. Handbook of Physiology. Bethesda, Md.: American Physiological Society, 1986.
20. Ananthanarayanan M, von Dippe P, Levy D. Identification of the hepatocyte Na-dependent bile acid transport protein using monoclonal antibodies. J Biol Chem 263:8338, 1988.
21. Wieland T, et al. Identity of hepatic membrane transport systems for bile salts, phalloidin, and antamanide by photoaffinity labeling. Proc Natl Acad Sci USA 81:5232, 1984.
22. Goldsmith MA, Huling S, Jones AL. Hepatic handling of bile salts and protein during intrahepatic cholestasis. Gastroenterology 84:978, 1983.
23. Lamri Y, et al. Immunoperoxidase localization of bile salts in rat liver cells: Evidence for a role of the Golgi apparatus in bile salt transport. J Clin Invest 82:1173, 1988.
24. Suchy FJ, et al. Intracellular bile acid transport in rat liver as visualized by electron microscope autoradiography using a bile acid analogue. Am J Physiol 245:G681, 1983.
25. Paumgartner G, Sauerbruch T. Secretion, composition and flow of bile. Clin Gastroenterol 12:3, 1983.
26. Scharschmidt BF. Bile formation and gallbladder and bile function. In Sleisenger MH, Fordtran JS, eds. Gastrointestinal Disease: Pathophysiology, Diagnosis, Management, 3rd ed. Philadelphia: WB Saunders, 1983.
27. Boyer JL, Bloomer JR. Canalicular bile secretion in man: Studies utilizing the biliary clearance of [^{14}C] mannitol. J Clin Invest 54:773, 1974.
28. Dumont M, Erlinger S, Uchman S. Hypercholesterosis induced by ursodeoxycholic acid and 7-ketolithocholic acid in the rat: Possible role of bicarbonate transport. Gastroenterology 79:82, 1980.
29. Lake J, Van Dyke RW, Scharschmidt BF. Effects of Na replacement and amiloride on ursodeoxycholic acid–stimulated choleresis and biliary bicarbonate secretion. Am J Physiol 252:G163, 1987.
30. Lake JR, et al. Bile acid induced bile flow and bile acid biotransformation. Inhibition of ursodeoxycholate stimulated hypercholeresis in the rat by sodium substitution, amiloride or amiloride analogues is associated with replacement of biliary unconjugated ursodeoxycholate by its glucuronide. Gastroenterology 95:454, 1988.
31. Renner EL, et al. Ursodeoxycholic acid choleresis: Relationship to biliary bicarbonate secretion and study of the effects of amiloride analogues. Am J Physiol 254:G232, 1988.
32. Hardison WG, Norman JC. Electrolyte composition of the secretin fraction of bile from the perfused pig liver. Am J Physiol 214:758, 1968.
33. Ryan JP. Motility of the gallbladder and biliary tree. In Johnson LR, ed. Physiology of the Gastrointestinal Tract. New York: Raven Press, 1981.
34. Kjellgren K. Persistence of symptoms following biliary surgery. Ann Surg 152:1026, 1960.
35. Soloway RD, Balistreth WF, Trotman BW. The gallbladder and biliary tract. In Bouchier IAD, ed. Recent Advances in Gastroenterology 5. Edinburgh: Churchill Livingstone, 1984.
36. Frizzell RA, Dugas M, Schultz SG. Intracellular chloride activities in rabbit gallbladder: Direct evidence for a coupled NaCl-influenced process. J Gen Physiol 65:769, 1975.
37. Rose RC. Absorptive functions of the gallbladder. In Johnson LR, ed. Physiology of the Gastrointestinal Tract. New York: Raven Press, 1981.
38. Svanik J, et al. Variations in concentrating function of the gallbladder in conscious monkey. Gastroenterology 86:919, 1984.
39. Carey MC, Small DM. The physical chemistry of cholesterol solubility in bile: Relationship to gallstone formation and dissolution in man. J Clin Invest 61:998, 1978.
40. Ostrow J. Absorption by the gallbladder of bile salts, sulfomophthalein and iodipamide. J Lab Clin Med 74:482, 1969.
41. Bouchier IAD. Biochemistry of gallstone formation. Clin Gastroenterol 12:25, 1983.
42. Rehfield JF. Cholecystokinin. Clin Gastroenterol 9:593,1980.
43. Malagelada JR. Gastric, pancreatic, and biliary responses to a meal. In Johnson LR, ed. Physiology of the Gastrointestinal Tract. New York: Raven Press, 1981.
44. Abiru H, Sarna SK, Condon RE. Contractile mechanisms of gallbladder filling and emptying in dogs. Gastroenterology 106:1652, 1994.
45. Howard PJ, Murphy GM, Dowling RH. Gallbladder emptying patterns in response to a normal meal in healthy subjects and patients with gallstones: Ultrasound study. Gut 32:1406, 1991.
46. Radberg G, et al. Contraction and evacuation of the gallbladder studied simultaneously by ultrasonography and ^{99m}Tc-labeled diethyl-iminodiacetic acid scintigraphy. Scand J Gastroenterol 28:709, 1993.
47. Boyden EA. The anatomy of the choledochoduodenal junction in man. Surg Gynecol Obstet 104:641, 1957.
48. Ludwick JR. Observations on the smooth muscle and contractile activity of the common bile duct. Ann Surg 164:1041, 1966.
49. Ono K, et al. Bile flow mechanisms in man. Arch Surg 96:869, 1968.
50. Csenoes A, et al. Pressure measurements in the biliary and pancreatic duct systems in controls and in patients with gallstones, previous cholecystectomy, or common bile duct stones. Gastroenterology 77:1203, 1979.
51. Sharp KW, Gadacz TR. Selection of patients for dissolution of retained common duct stones with monoctanoin. Ann Surg 196:137, 1982.
52. Admirand WH, Small DM. The physicochemical basis of cholesterol gallstone formation in man. J Clin Invest 47:1043, 1968.
53. Sedaghat A, Grundy SM. Cholesterol crystals and the formation of cholesterol gallstones. N Engl J Med 302:1274, 1980.
54. Somjen GJ, Gilat T. A non-micellar mode of cholesterol transport in human bile. FEBS Lett 156:265, 1983.
55. Somjen GJ, Gilat T. Contribution of vesicular and micellar carriers to cholesterol transport in human bile. J Lipid Res 26:299, 1983.
56. Carey MC, Cahalane MJ. The enterohepatic circulation. In Arias I, et al., eds. The Liver: Biology and Pathobiology. New York: Raven Press, 1988, p 573.
57. Bennion LJ et al. Development of lithogenic bile during puberty in Pima Indians. N Engl J Med 300:873, 1979.
58. Evans DM, Wessler EL. Physiochemical considerations in gallstone pathogenesis. Hosp Pract 9:133, 1974.
59. Gallinger S, et al. Effect of mucus glycoprotein on nucleation time of human bile. Gastroenterology 89:648, 1985.
60. Heuman DM, Moore EW, Vlahcevic ZR. Pathogenesis and dissolution of gallstones. In Zakin D, Boyer TD, eds. Hepatology: A Textbook of Liver Disease. Philadelphia: WB Saunders, 1990, p 1480.
61. Braverman DZ, Johnson ML, Kern F, Jr. Effects of pregnancy and contraceptive steroids on gallbladder function. N Engl J Med 302:362, 1980.
62. Honore LH. Cholesterol cholelithiasis in adolescent females. Arch Surg 115:62, 1980.
63. Pomereranz IS, Shaffer EA. Abnormal gallbladder emptying in a subgroup of patients with gallstones. Gastroenterology 88:787, 1985.
64. Fridhandler TM, Davison JS, Shaffer EA. Defective gallbladder contractility in the ground squirrel and prairie dog during the early stages of cholesterol gallstone formation. Gastroenterology 85:830, 1983.
65. Trotman BW, Soloway RD. Pigment gallstone disease: Summary of the National Institute of Health International Workshop. Hepatology 2:879, 1982.
66. Horbach RT. Pathogenesis and medical treatment of gallstones. In Sleisenger MH, Fordtran JS, eds. Gastrointestinal Disease: Pathophysiology, Diagnosis, Management, 3rd ed. Philadelphia: WB Saunders, 1983.
67. Kaufman HS, et al. The role of bacteria in gallbladder and common duct stone formation. Ann Surg 209:584, 1989.

68. Grundy SM, et al. Mechanism of lithogenic bile formation in American Indian women with cholesterol gallstones. J Clin Invest 51:3026, 1972.
69. Diehl AK, et al. Clinical gallbladder disease in Mexican-American, Anglo, and Black women. South J Med 73:438, 1980.
70. Gilat T, et al. An increased familial frequency of gallstones. Gastroenterology 84:242, 1983.
71. Maclure KM, et al. Weight, diet, and the risk of symptomatic gallstones in middle-aged women. N Engl J Med 321:563, 1989.
72. Broomfield PH, et al. Formation and prevention of lithogenic bile and gallstones during loss of weight. N Engl J Med 519:1567, 1988.
73. Letkof IR, et al. Diet in the formation and treatment of cholesterol gallstones. In Cohen S, Soloway RD, eds. Contemporary Issues in Gastroenterology: Gallstones. New York: Churchill Livingstone, 1985, p 113.
74. Marks JW, Schoenfield LJ. Formation and treatment of gallstones. In Schiff L, Schiff ER, eds. Diseases of the Liver, 7th ed. Philadelphia: JP Lippincott, 1993.
75. Henriksson P, et al. Estrogen-induced gallstone formation in males: Relation to changes in serum and biliary lipids during hormonal treatment of prostate cancer. J Clin Invest 84:811, 1989.
76. Haber GB, Heaton KW. Lipid composition of bile in diabetics and obesity-matched controls. Gut 20:518, 1979.
77. Ahlberg J, et al. Prevalence of gallbladder disease in hyperlipoproteins. Am J Dig Dis 24:459, 1979.
78. McArthur P, et al. Controlled clinical trial comparing early with interval cholecystectomy for acute cholecystitis. Br J Surg 62:850, 1975.
79. Friedman GD, Raviola CA, Fireman B. Prognosis of gallstones with mild or no symptoms: 25 years of follow up in a health maintenance organization. J Clin Epidemiol 42:127, 1989.
80. McSherry CK, et al. The natural history of diagnosed gallstone disease in symptomatic and asymptomatic patients. Ann Surg 202:59, 1985.
81. Lygidcikis NJ. Incidence and significance of primary stones of the common bile duct in choledocholithiasis. Surg Gynecol Obstet 157:434, 1983.
82. Madden JL. Primary common duct stones. In Cameron J, ed. Current Surgical Therapy. Philadelphia: BC Decker, 1984.
83. Witlin LT, et al. Transhepatic decompression of biliary tree in Caroli's disease. Surgery 91:205, 1982.
84. Saharia PC, Zuidema GD, Cameron JL. Primary common duct stones. Ann Surg 185:598, 1977.
85. Lotveit T, Osnes M, Larsen S. Recurrent biliary calculi: Duodenal diverticula as a predisposing factor. Ann Surg 196:30, 1982.
86. Salem G, Nicolau G, Shefer S. Chenodeoxycholic acid inhibits elevated hepatic HMG-CoA reductase activity in subjects with gallstones. Clin Res 21:523, 1973.
87. Hardison WG, Grundy SM. Effect of ursodeoxycholate and its taurine conjugate on bile acid synthesis and cholesterol absorption. Gastroenterology 87:130, 1984.
88. Schoenfield LJ, Lachin JM, Chenodiol (chenodeoxycholic acid) for dissolution of gallstones. The National Cooperative Gallstone Study. A controlled trial of efficacy and safety. Ann Intern Med 95:257, 1981.
89. Maudgal DP, Kupfer RM, Northfield TC. Factors affecting gallstone dissolution rate during chenic acid therapy. Gut 24:7, 1983.
90. Maudgal DP, et al. Low cholesterol diet: Enhancement of effect of CDCA in patients with gallstones. Br Med J 2:851, 1978.
91. Gadacz TR. The effect of monoctanoin on retained duct stones. Surgery 89:527, 1981.
92. Thistle JL, Nelson PE, May GR. Dissolution of cholesterol gallbladder stones using methyl tert-butyl ether. Gastroenterology 90:1775, 1986.
93. Sackmann M, et al. The Munich gallbladder lithotripsy study. Results of the first five years with 711 patients. Ann Intern Med 114:290, 1991.
94. Nahrwold DL. Gallstone lithotripsy. Am J Surg 165:431, 1993.

26

Pancreatic Exocrine Function

Gordon L. Kauffman, Jr., and Robert L. Conter

Pancreatic exocrine function consists of protein synthesis, which occurs in the acinar cell, and bicarbonate production, which occurs in the centroacinar and ductular cells. Although control mechanisms for protein and bicarbonate secretion are quite different, pancreatic disease usually results in a similar reduction in both products.

Much information regarding the processes of pancreatic protein synthesis and bicarbonate production has been derived from experiments conducted in various animal preparations. With respect to information on pancreatic exocrine function, this chapter mentions the experimental model and identifies differences in species. When it is available, information derived from human studies is presented.

HISTORIC CONSIDERATIONS

In the midnineteenth century Claude Bernard observed that pancreatic secretion plays a significant role in the digestion and absorption of fats. He noted that fats were emulsified in the lumen of the duodenum only in the portion distal to the entrance of the pancreatic duct. In the late nineteenth century Ivan Pavlov observed that pancreatic secretion was partly controlled by both the vagus nerve and duodenal mucosal acidification. It was also noted that these two stimuli caused the pancreas to secrete fluid of different composition. Vagal nerve stimulation caused the release of a thick, viscous, enzyme-rich fluid, whereas duodenal acidification was associated with high-volume fluid output of very low enzyme concentration. When it was clear that duodenal acidification caused pancreatic stimulation, even in the vagally and sympathetically denervated gland, most investigators believed that reflex neural connections between the duodenum were not involved.

Further experimentation on the acidification of isolated and denervated jejunal segments showed similar pancreatic secretory stimulation. In 1902 at the Physiological Laboratory of University College in London, Bayliss and Starling injected extracts of jejunal mucosal scrapings into the blood stream, which resulted in the production of a pancreatic secretion. The substance responsible for this observation was named secretin; 3 years later the term *hormone* was suggested for the chemical messengers produced in one organ and released into the blood, affecting a different target organ. More recently Palade and coworkers were awarded the Nobel Prize in Medicine for their studies on the cellular and subcellular events associated with pancreatic acinar cellular protein synthesis and secretion.

ANATOMIC CONSIDERATIONS

Embryology

Formation of the ventral and dorsal endodermal outgrowths, which ultimately form the pancreas, arises from the abdominal foregut in the fourth week of human gestation.[1] The ventral pancreatic bud is initially bilobed and arises from the lateral aspects of the hepatic duct at its entry into the gut tube. The larger dorsal pancreatic bud is a single outgrowth arising from the dorsal aspect of the gut tube, rostral to the hepatic duct. During the fifth week the left lobe of the ventral pancreas disappears, and in the sixth week both dorsal and persisting ventral pancreatic buds have ductal systems that open into the gut tube. The dorsal duct opens directly into the gut lumen, whereas the ventral duct usually opens with the hepatic duct. In the region of the future stomach the gut tube dilates and rotates. This rotation is caused by unequal growth of the original dorsal and ventral borders of the gut tube.

Rotation of the stomach and liver causes the duodenum to be pulled across to the right from its original midline position. As this occurs, the dorsal mesentery of the duodenum, which contains the dorsal pancreas, approaches the dorsal body wall, and the ventral body wall comes into contact with the dorsal pancreas to the right of the midline. During the seventh week of gestation the dorsal and ventral elements of the pancreas fuse in their retroperitoneal position to form a single organ. The duct of the larger dorsal bud is Santorini's duct, which directly enters the lumen in the descending portion of the duodenum. The duct of the ventral bud is Wirsung's duct, which opens into the origin of the hepatic duct, later becoming

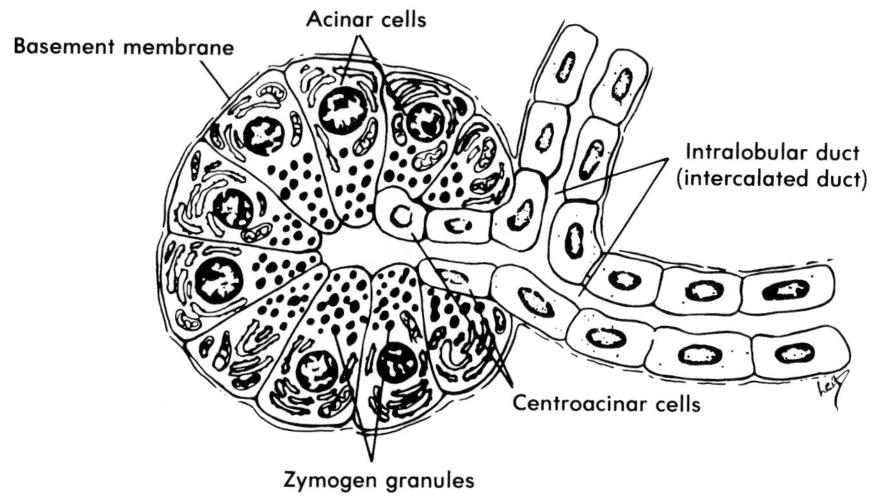

Fig. 26-1. Exocrine acinus of the pancreas.

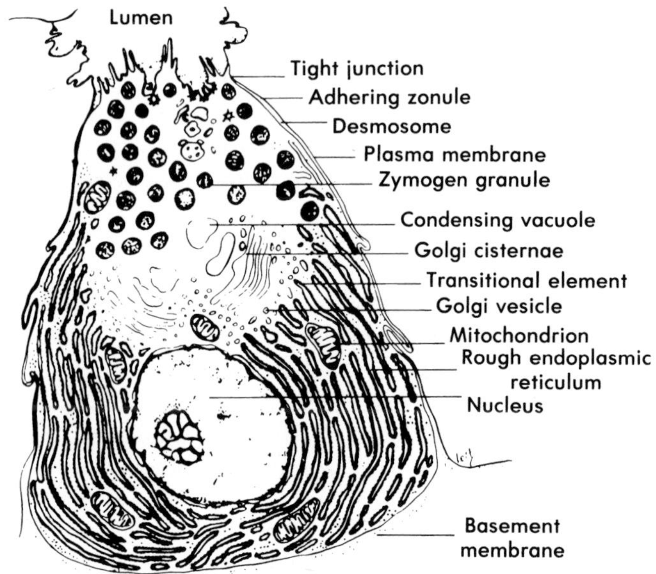

Fig. 26-2. Diagram of pancreatic acinar cell.

the common bile duct. In humans Wirsung's duct is usually the larger and more constant of the two, but Santorini's duct is patent in about 70% of persons.

The pancreas grows rapidly by elongation of the primitive ducts and overgrowth of numerous side branches that arise in groups and assume a lobular arrangement.[2] The columnar epithelium of the main duct takes on a cuboidal configuration in the smaller branches. Acini, the secreting units of the exocrine pancreas, consist of pyramidal cells whose apexes are directed toward the lumen of the duct; they begin to appear along the lateral wall and distal ducts in the third month of development (Fig. 26-1). The ducts from which the acini arise are lined by centroacinar cells. Proximal to the centroacinar cells the ducts elongate and form intercalated ducts, which connect to form intralobular ducts lined by columnar epithelium. During the fourth month the lobules enlarge and connective tissue diminishes, resulting in coalescence and lobe formation. Small granules also appear in the cytoplasm of the acinar cells in the fourth month. These zymogen granules increase in number and accumulate in the apical cytoplasm (Fig. 26-2). Morphologically these acinar cells appear capable of secretion, but no evidence suggests secretory activity during prenatal life.

Gross Anatomy

The pancreas is a solid glandular organ, weighing 70 to 110 g and lying in the retroperitoneum below the left hepatic lobe and posterior to the stomach. It is bordered on the right by the duodenum and on the left by the spleen. The pancreatic head, including the uncinate process, lies within the curvature of and is intimately apposed to the duodenum. The neck, body, and tail of the pancreas extend to the left, crossing the midline, with the tail reaching the root of the splenorenal ligament. The common bile duct and the main pancreatic duct either join (90%) or open separately (10%) into the medial aspect of the second position of the duodenum.[3]

Blood Supply

The major arteries supplying the pancreas are the celiac trunk, situated above the neck of the pancreas, and the superior mesenteric artery, located below the pancreatic neck. Two pancreaticoduodenal arcades, the anterior and posterior, are derived from the union of the anterior and posterior branches of the superior and inferior pancreaticoduodenal arteries and supply the head region. Superior pancreaticoduodenal arteries are branches of the gastroduodenal artery, whereas the inferior pancreaticoduodenal arteries originate from the superior mesenteric artery. The neck and body of the pancreas derive their blood supply from the dorsal pancreatic artery, which may arise from the proximal splenic artery, the celiac trunk, or the superior mesenteric artery; from branches of the dorsal pancreatic artery that enter the posterior surface of the pancreas and pass in the direction of the tail; and from branches of the splenic artery. The tail of the pancreas is supplied primarily by branches of the splenic artery.

A rich vascular anastomotic complex is present in the pancreatic tissue. From the vessels at the exterior of the gland, branches pass internally to form an interlobular plexus, from which a single intralobular artery supplies individual islets of Langerhans as a vascular tuft. From these tufts, blood then passes to the acini. Such a vascular arrangement, with hormone-rich blood from the islets of Langerhans supplying the acini, is considered a portal system.[4] This anatomic configuration is consistent with the hypothesis that islet hormones may affect pancreatic exocrine function. Although comprising less than 2% of pancreatic mass, the islets receive 15% to 25% of total pancreatic blood flow.[5]

The functional relationship between pancreatic secretory activity and pancreatic blood flow is poorly understood. No data exist on the effect of a meal on pancreatic blood flow. Several studies suggest that stimulated pancreatic secretory exocrine activity occurs before any measured change in blood flow. Small amounts of intraintestinal hydrochloric acid stimulate bicarbonate secretion, whereas significantly larger amounts of hydrochloric acid are required to increase blood flow.[6] Physiologic *systemic concentrations* of secretin or cholecystokinin (CCK) that stimulate pancreatic secretion seem to have almost no effect on pancreatic blood flow.[7,8] These observations suggest that under physiologic conditions pancreatic blood flow is not a limiting factor for exocrine function. Pancreatic blood flow is autoregulated, perhaps by both neural and humoral mechanisms, to provide maintenance of blood flow to the pancreas under conditions of mean arterial pressure reduction.[9]

Venous blood from the pancreas directly or indirectly enters the portal vein. Blood from the pancreatic head drains either into the gastroepiploic venous system or directly into the portal vein and drains from the neck, body, and tail into the inferior mesenteric vein or into the splenic vein, which joins with the superior mesenteric vein to form the portal vein.

Neural Input

The extrinsic autonomic innervation of the pancreas occurs through both sympathetic and parasympathetic pathways. Afferent *parasympathetic* fibers pass from the pancreas to the inferior ganglion of the vagus nerve, from which fibers travel in the vagus nerve to terminate in the dorsal nucleus of the vagus nerve in the brain.[10] Efferent parasympathetic fibers originate in the dorsal vagal nucleus and are contained in the posterior trunk, which contains fibers from both the anterior and the posterior trunks. These fibers pass through the celiac axis ganglia but do not synapse there. The efferent parasympathetic fibers synapse with cell bodies within the interlobular septa of the pancreas.

Sympathetic innervation of the pancreas originates from the thoracolumbar region.[11] Cell bodies for efferent sympathetic innervation are found in the lateral columns of dorsal segments 5 through 10. The fibers reach the ganglionated dorsal and lumbar sympathetic trunks; they then travel to the prevertebral abdominal sympathetic plexuses (the celiac and superior mesenteric). From these plexuses the sympathetic efferent fibers reach the pancreas along with the arterial supply. Afferent sympathetic fibers originate in the pancreas and reach the dorsal nerve roots by many of the lumbar and greater splanchnic nerves.

Peptidergic neural activity, in which the neurotransmitter is a peptide stored in nerve terminals and released on stimulation to act on a specific local receptor, has been described in the pancreas. Peptidergic neurons are identified by immunofluorescent techniques, using specific antipeptide antibody, and their function is determined by the effect of exogenous administration of the substance on that organ. Vasoactive intestinal polypeptide (VIP) immunoreactivity has been identified in nerves supplying the pancreas.[12] In pigs vagal activity stimulates both pancreatic enzyme and fluid and electrolyte secretion, as well as increased VIP concentration in the pancreatic venous blood. In humans VIP has a weak secretin-like action, whereas the high doses required to stimulate pancreatic secretion are accompanied by significant side effects.[13] These data suggest that vagally stimulated pancreatic secretion may be mediated in part through VIP-ergic nerves. Nerves containing enkephalin and substance P have also been identified in the pancreas.[12] Exogenous enkephalin administration suppresses pancreatic secretion. The interactions between peptidergic neural activity and other modulating peptides appear to be complex and are not yet fully understood.

Acinus

The functional unit of the exocrine pancreas is the acinus[14] (see Fig. 26-1).Grossly the lobular structure of the pancreas is visible, with the lobules separated by fine connective tissue continuous with that surrounding duct epithelium. Subunits of the lobule are the acini, composed of spheric or short tubular masses of cells. Most cells in the acinus are acinar cells, which form these spherically arranged cellular masses. The smaller centroacinar cells mark the beginning of the ductular system. The lumen draining the acinus is an intercalated duct that communicates with intralobular and interlobular ducts and finally with the main pancreatic duct. The intercalated ducts are lined by centroacinar cells that are smaller than acinar cells. Intralobular and interlobular ducts are striated and lined with low columnar epithelial cells very similar in appearance to centroacinar cells. The synthesis and release of enzymes and bicarbonate, the two major functions of the exocrine pancreas, occur in the acinar cell and duct cells, respectively.

The supporting matrix of the pancreas consists of type IV and V collagen, laminin, and heparin sulfate proteoglycans.[15] The extracellular spaces contain types I and II collagen and fibronectin. The former are produced by the epithelial cells, whereas the latter are a product of fibroblasts. There is a suggestion that aberrations in synthesis, deposition, and turnover of the basal lamina are associated with neoplastic transformation.

PHYSIOLOGIC CONSIDERATIONS

Acinar Cell

Histology

By weight, acinar cells account for more than 80% of the pancreas (see Fig. 26-2). The pyramid-shaped cells are oriented with their apexes, which contain the secretory granules, facing the lumen of the acinus (see Fig. 26-1). The density of these apical zymogen granules may vary as a function of secretory state. The midportion of the acinar cell contains the Golgi complex (apparatus). The basal region, with intense basophilic staining, contains the endoplasmic reticulum. The acinar cell nuclei are located in the basal region. A plasma membrane, which is rather straight basally and laterally but forms microvilli apically, envelops the acinar cell. This cell is designed for the synthesis, packaging, and release of enzymes.

Junctional complexes, a major barrier between duct lumen and pancreatic interstitial space, firmly attach acinar cells to each other and to centroacinar cells. They occur at the apical portion of the lateral plasma membrane and consist of three morphologically defined structures: (1) tight junctions, found near the duct lumen; (2) adhering zonules, where the lateral plasma membranes of two cells are within 200 angstrom units (Å) of each other but are not fused; and (3) the zonula adherens, containing desmosomes. These functional complexes are impermeable to macromolecules and secretory proteins (molecular weight, 16,000 to 95,000). Integrity of junctional complexes appears to depend on calcium.

Acinar cells communicate with each other by specialized areas in the lateral plasma membrane called *gap junctions.* At these points the plasma membranes of the adjacent acinar cells are within 20 Å of each other. Freeze-fracture techniques have identified pores between cells with an inner diameter of 200 to 1000 daltons, which permits the movement of small molecules between adjacent acinar cells. The integrity of the gap junction depends on both calcium and intracellular pH.[14,16]

Ultrastructure

The subcellular structure of the acinar cell is highly organized for enzyme synthesis, packaging, and secretion. The plasmalemma is divided into two domains, apical and basolateral, which are structurally and functionally distinct.[17,18] The former possesses microvilli with an outer glycocalyx layer. Filament bundles within each microvillus allow for enhancement of the number and length of the microvilli. The basolateral plasmalemma possesses smooth surfaced small vesicula invaginations that may be important for fibrinolytic activity. The concentration of basolateral lectin-binding sites is lower than in the apical plasmalemma; however, the receptor for CCK is found exclusively on this portion of the membrane.[19] The most striking feature is the extensive rough endoplasmic reticulum (RER) and the accumulation of zymogen granules in the apical cytoplasm. RER, consisting of parallel membranous cisternae and interconnecting tubules, that have numerous ribosomes attached to their cytoplasmic surface, primarily is found in the basal cytoplasm. RER also stores calcium in vesicles termed calcisomes. Calcium is held in this compartment by calcium-binding proteins, calsequestrin, and calrecticalin.[20,21] The appearance of the basal cytoplasm is related to the density of the ribonucleoprotein in the basal region. Mitochondria, with cristae and intramitochondrial granules, are situated between the cisternae of the RER. The nucleus, also found in the basal region of the cell, contains peripherally accumulated chromatin. The Golgi complex consists of stacks of flattened cisternae and smooth-surfaced vesicles. These vesicles are located between the stacks and the ER, interconnected by tubular elements referred to as the cis-Golgi network. This represents the intermediate compartment and plays a role in ER–Golgi membrane transport. Condensing vacuoles are formed by exocytosis of the trans–Golgi cisternae in the lumen of the trans–Golgi cisternae.[22]

Transport between various compartments of the Golgi complex involves the budding of vesicles from one compartment with fusion into another, a process that requires adenosine triphosphate (ATP) and low-M_r guanosine triphosphate (GTP) binding. Vectorial movement is from cis- to trans-stacks within the Golgi complex.[23]

Protein sorting is thought to occur in the trans–Golgi network or immediately after exit from the Golgi complex. Zymogen granules are generated by the fusion of similarly sized molecules. Granule-to-granule fusion may, in fact, occur as restraints to fusion are removed.

The condensing vacuole is pinched off the membrane that is then recycled to the Golgi complex for reuse. The presence of highly charged, glycosylated residues within the granules of the condensing vacuole make it electron dense.

The majority of intracellular protein degradation occurs in lysosomes that are organelles containing a large number of hydrolytic enzymes. The pH within the various compartments is critical to the function of each: Golgi stacks, 7; condensing vacuole, 5.6; zymogen granules, 6.5; and lysozomes, 5.3. The mechanisms of regulating intracellular pH are not known.[24]

At intervals around the periphery of the nucleus, the outer and inner nuclear membranes fuse, producing nuclear "pores" approximately 60 nm in diameter. One or more large dense nucleoli may be found within the acinar cell nucleus cells.[14,16]

Cellular Mechanisms of Acinar Cell Protein Synthesis, Packaging, and Release

The process by which the acinar cell synthesizes and releases proteins is orderly, proceeding from the basal to the apical region of the cell. The basic steps involve synthesis and segregation in the RER, chemical and structural modification in the RER and Golgi complex, followed by storage in secretory granules and exocytosis. The cytosol is the component of the cytoplasm in which protein synthesis begins. The functionally interconnected membrane-bound cistanae are the components defining exocytic and endocytic activities.[25] Proteins destined for export are synthesized in the RER and subsequently processed and sorted to the correct destinations along the pathway of secretion.

The processes by which the acinar cell synthesizes, packages, and releases protein products have been defined by combined autoradiographic and cell fractionation techniques.[26] In addition, pulse-chase experiments, in which small pieces of pancreas are incubated in labeled amino acid medium, then in cold amino acid medium, have clearly demonstrated a narrow band of labeled amino acids that move through the secretory machinery of the cell. Radioactivity is highest in the granular endoplasmic reticulum immediately after labeling, in the Golgi apparatus at 10 minutes, in the condensing vacuoles at 40 minutes, and in the zymogen granules at 2 hours (Fig. 26-3).[14,27]

Amino acids required for protein synthesis enter the acinar cell by active transport linked to sodium ion (Na^+) movement down an electrochemical gradient.[28] An amino acid destined to be immediately incorporated into a protein is picked up by an appropriate transfer ribonucleic acid (tRNA) molecule once it enters the cell. Excess nonactivated amino acids enter an ultracellular pool where they can exchange with other amino acids by the same carrier mechanism.[29]

Proteins for export from the acinar cell are synthesized in ribosomes attached to the cytosolic portion of the RER.[30] This signal hypothesis has been developed as an explanation for the mechanisms by which a given messenger RNA (mRNA) molecule is translated on a bound or free ribosome. The process of protein synthesis begins with transcription of mRNA in the nucleus with subsequent movement into the cytosol in association with cytosolic ribosomes at the 5′ portion of the mRNA. As translation proceeds, amino acid sequence numbering 16 to 25 serves as the targeting signal sequence that determines whether the protein completes translation. This amino acid sequence associates with a signal recognition protein (SRP) that halts translation, preventing deleterious proteins from being released into the cytosol.[31] Next the mRNA-SRP-signal sequence complex associates with the specific SRP receptor on the RER, following which the SRP moiety dissociates from the complex and translation proceeds. The SRP, free in the cytosol, is able to participate in further protein synthesis. As the nascent peptide grows, it assumes a linear configuration through the RER membrane into a channel. When the termination sequence of the mRNA is reached, the polypeptide becomes free in the cisternae of the RER. Proteins destined to become an integral part of the protein membrane possess a hydrophobic sequence that arrests the protein in a transmembrane configuration and subsequent cotranslational or posttranslational modification.[25]

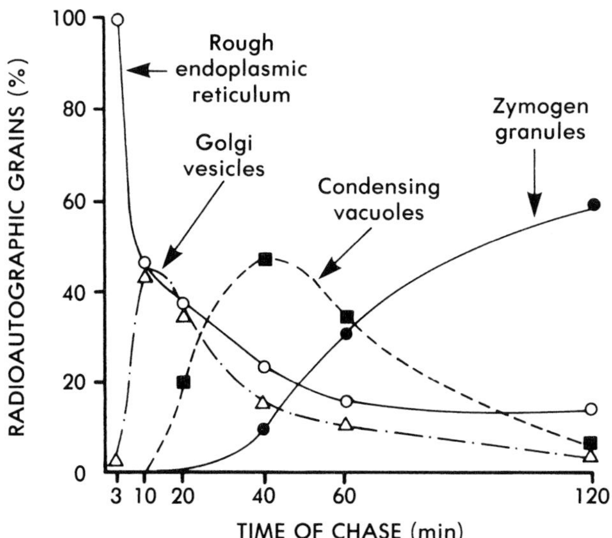

Fig. 26-3. Vectorial movement of secretory proteins in the pancreatic acinar cell derived from pulse-chase experiments using radiolabeled amino acids. (Redrawn from Gorelick FS, Jamieson JD. Structure-function relationships of the pancreas. In Johnson LR, ed. Physiology of the Gastrointestinal Tract. New York: Raven Press, 1981.)

Several modifications of the protein occur during movement from the ribosome to the cisternae of the endoplasmic reticulum. These include both biochemical and tertiary structural changes, which may account for the irreversible segregation of proteins within the RER. A signal peptidase cleaves the signal peptide from proteins with an amino terminal signal peptide extension. Cell surface–targeted proteins are anchored to the internal side of the RER by a glycosylphosphatidal inositol group. Others have a mannose-rich core oligosaccharide added.

Further modification within the RER lumen ensures correct folding necessary for entry into the secretory pathway. Some of these "chaperon" enzymes are protein disulfide isomerases, BiP and GRP78. Once correctly folded, many proteins undergo higher order association or oligomerization related to disulfide bonding. Thus the RER plays a crucial role in producing only proteins designed to benefit the cells, the organ, and the organism. Abnormalities in folding prevent the release of the protein from the RER as occurs with the cystic fibrosis transmembrane regulator that functions as the chloride channel.[32,33]

Once in the cisternae, the proteins remain membrane bound within the acinar cell. Secretory proteins move from the cisternae to the Golgi complex within 20 to 30 minutes. This transfer mechanism is highly specific for the RER portion of the pathway and appears to require cyclic coating and uncoating of vesicular carriers. The intermediate compartment between the RER and Golgi complex is the site in which the targeting and recycling of transport vesicles between the two compartments occurs. It also contains brefeldin A, which blocks the anterograde but not the retrograde movement of vesicles from the RER to the Golgi complex.[34] Transport of vesicles from the RER to the Golgi complex is regulated by low-M_r GTP-binding proteins related to the ras family of oncogenes.[35] They function as molecular "switches" that allow membrane fusion to proceed in the GTP-bound form, events which are dependent on the rate and extent of GTP association and dissociation. Entry of proteins, either membrane or secretory, appears to be a passive process. Once properly folded and processed, the protein enters a transport vesicle that shuttles it to the translational side of the Golgi complex, at which point fusion of the membranes allows the protein to be delivered to the Golgi cisternae.

The primary functions of the Golgi complex are to concentrate the proteins into condensing vacuoles and to provide for posttranslational modification. Concentration may occur by interaction of the predominantly basic secretory proteins with polyanionic substances on the translational side of the Golgi complex or by condensation sorting, in which proteins aggregate in the secretory granuli by their selective removal from the bulk flow pathway. Posttranslational modification in the Golgi complex involves terminal sulfation of proteoglycans and proteolytic cleavage of the propeptides to the final secretory product.

Protein sorting also occurs within the Golgi complex in addition to routing constitutive proteins to their organelles or membrane destinations. The sorting signal is not known.

Mature secretory granules then move from the Golgi complex to the apical portion of the acinar cell cytoplasm. Stimulus-secretion coupling is spacially and temporally separated in the acinar cell. Considering that a humoral stimulant binds to the basal membrane and the secretory response is at the apical membrane, it has been suggested that the cytosolic message results from either membrane phosphatidyl inositol hydrolysis or activation of adenylate cyclase. Microtubules or microfilaments of the actin-myosin system play an important role in the movement of secretory granules to the site of exocytosis. With appropriate acinar cell stimulation, the contents of these mature vacuoles are released into the lumen by exocytosis. For this process to occur, the zymogen granule membrane must recognize the appropriate fusion position within the plasma membrane of the acinar cell. Following this recognition, fusion of the zymogen granule membrane with the plasmalemma occurs at the site of exocytosis.[36] After discharge of the contents of the zymogen granule, the membrane is thought to be recycled.[37]

It has been shown that the rate of zymogen content biosynthesis is an order of magnitude greater than that of the granular membrane proteins and that there is direct morphologic confirmation of secretory granule reutilization. A cycle of membrane association with zymogen granule membranes of a novel rab 3–like protein and its relocation to the trans side of the Golgi complex accompanying exocytosis has been described.[38]

Composition of Pancreatic Enzyme Secretion

The major categories of pancreatic enzyme secretion include (1) proteolytic (chymotrypsinogen, trypsinogen, proelastase, procarboxypeptidase A and B), which accounts for nearly 70% of the pancreatic digestive mass[39]; (2) amylolytic (α-amylase); (3) lipolytic (lipase, esterase, phospholipase A, cholesterol esterase); and (4) nucleolytic (ribonuclease, deoxyribonuclease) enzymes. Additional secreted enzymes include colipase, trypsin inhibitor, sulfated polyanionic peptidoglycans, and soluble acid lipoproteins.

Under most physiologic conditions the relative concentrations of these enzymes remain constant in the pancreatic juice of each species.[40] Analysis of the enzyme profile in subcellular fractions of pancreatic acinar cells has identified the same ratios of one enzyme to another, as in secreted juice.[41] These observations have supported the theory of "parallel" pancreatic enzyme secretion, however, other studies have shown that one enzyme may be secreted into pancreatic juice preferentially at a higher rate than others, suggesting that in some situations enzyme secretion may not occur in a parallel fashion.[42,43] Thus the composition of proteins in the zymogen granules possibly can be changed by certain stimuli, either through equilibration with specific cytosolic enzymes or from subpopulations of acinar cells that have differing profiles of enzymes within their zymogen granules.

Long-term pancreatic secretory adaptation to change in diet has been rather conclusively proved in the rat.[44] Prolonged feeding of a high-carbohydrate diet produces a significant increase in pancreatic amylase content.[45] Diets high in protein and fat given over a prolonged period cause an elevation of pancreatic trypsinogen and lipase content, respectively.[46,47] It is unknown whether a similar adaptation to diet occurs in humans.

Centroacinar and Duct Cells

Histology

Centroacinar cells are irregular in shape and are wedged between acinar cells within the acinus (see Fig. 26-1). In histologic sections these cells are distinguished by their pale staining, which is related to the low-density cytoplasm. Cells lining the small ductules, although more regular in shape, are structurally similar to the centroacinar cell. As the ductular system enlarges from the acinus to the main pancreatic duct, the duct cells assume a more columnar appearance.

Ultrastructure

Centroacinar and duct cells, in contrast to acinar cells, have a poorly developed granular endoplasmic reticulum and Golgi complex, no zymogen granules, and few mitochondria.[48] A unique feature of the centroacinar and duct cells is the large nucleus with indentations. The nucleus occupies a large portion of the cell, leaving only a rim of cytoplasm between nucleus and plasma membrane. Infolding of the lateral plasma membrane is more extensive than occurs in the acinar cell. The centroacinar cell possesses a single cilium, which is in contact with the fluid in the acinar lumen. These cells have apical microvilli. Supporting the contention that they are responsible for fluid and electrolyte secretion is the localization of carbonic anhydrase to these cells and the presence of a nonchloride anion, which most likely is bicarbonate. Connections between duct cells and acinar cells or other duct cells are through terminal bars, as described for acinar–acinar cell interaction.

Cellular Mechanisms of Water and Electrolyte Secretion

The ductular elements and centroacinar cells appear to be the primary site of electrolyte secretion, with a contribution from the acinar cell. The following observations support this hypothesis:

1. Alloxan treatment reduces electrolyte secretion with concomitant destruction of ductular elements but not of acinar cells.[49]
2. A copper-free diet with penicillamine supplement[50] or ethionine feeding[51] causes almost total acinar cell atrophy but only partly reduces the maximum electrolyte secretory response to secretin.
3. Carbonic anhydrase, the enzyme necessary for rapid production of bicarbonate (HCO_3^-), has been shown to be present in the centroacinar and ductular cells but not in the acinar cell.[52]
4. Micropuncture experiments demonstrate that HCO_3^- concentration of pancreatic juice increases in the ducts, particularly in the extralobular ducts.[53,54]

Specific ion requirements for pancreatic electrolyte secretion have been identified. Reduction in extracellular Na^+ to a value of ≤80 mM results in a significant reduction in pancreatic secretory rate.[55] Replacement of Na^+ by lithium ion (Li^+) also causes a significant inhibition of pancreatic secretion.[56] Similarly, removal of potassium ion (K^+) from the nutrient solution reduces pancreatic secretion more than 50%, whereas substitution of rubidium for K^+ restores the secretory response to secretin. Chloride (Cl^-) is also required for full pancreatic secretory response to secretin but can be substituted by bromide (Br^-) or iodine (I^-) with little effect on pancreatic secretory function.[57] Finally, HCO_3^- is required for full secretory response to secretin stimulation.[58]

Under conditions of maximum stimulation, HCO_3^- concentration in secreted fluid is fivefold to sixfold greater than in plasma.[54] The electric potential across the duct epithelium is lumen negative relative to the interstitial fluid.[59] Based on these two findings, it has been postulated that the transport of HCO_3^- against an electrochemical gradient is an active process. In contrast, Na^+, K^+, and Cl^- appear to be passively distributed across the duct epithelium. The source of secreted HCO_3^- is thought to be primarily plasma, although metabolically generated CO_2 may also make a minor contribution. Two facts support this hypothesis: (1) the rate of pancreatic secretion is directly related to perfusate (plasma) HCO_3^- concentration, and (2) when carbon-14 (^{14}C)-labeled HCO_3^- is added to perfusate, it appears rapidly in pancreatic juice.[60] It has been estimated that more than 95% of secreted HCO_3^- is derived from plasma.

The initial step in HCO_3^- secretion from the centroacinar and duct cells is the diffusion of CO_2 into the cytosol and its hydration to H_2CO_3, a reaction that is catalyzed by carbonic anhydrase. After the dissociation of H_2CO_3 into H^+ and HCO_3^-, the free proton is translocated across the basolateral membrane either by an electrogenic H^+-ATPase or a Na^+/H^+ exchanger, resulting in accumulation of HCO_3^- in the cytosol. It is thought that HCO_3^- ions cross the apical membrane in exchange for Cl^-. The rate at which this Cl^-/HCO_3^- exchanger recycles is dependent on luminal concentration [Cl^-], which itself is dependent on opening of an apical Cl^- channel. Secretin-activation of the duct cell is thought to open this apical Cl^- channel serving as a control of the secretory mechanism. As HCO_3^- exits the cytosol at the apical membrane, a current is generated that equals the current across the basolateral membrane during secretion. A portion of this current is accounted for by K^+ flux through K^+ channels and cycling of the H^+-ATPase and Na^+, K^+-ATPase[61] (Fig. 26-4).

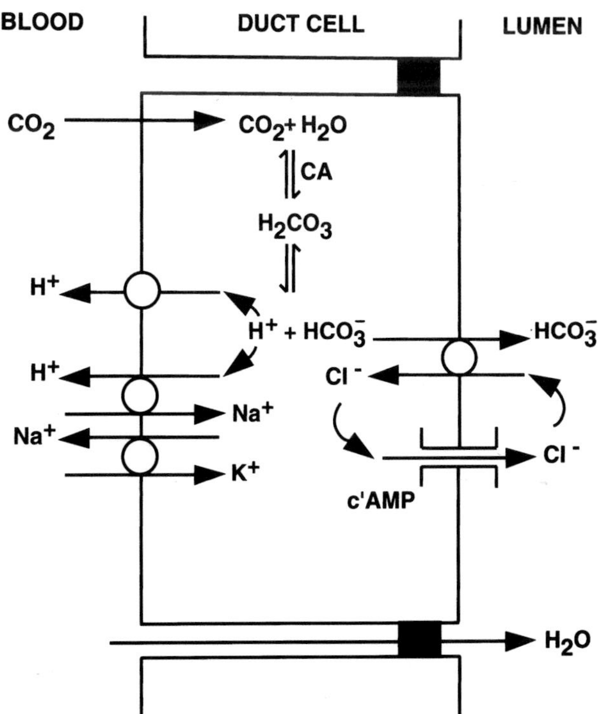

Fig. 26-4. Proposed mechanism of pancreatic duct cell HCO_3^- secretion. Carbon dioxide *(CO_2)* diffuses from the blood into the duct cell, where it is hydrated to carbonic acid by carbonic anhydrase *(CA)*. The dissociation of carbonic acid to $H^+ + HCO_3^-$ provides a source of bicarbonate secretion, as the proton is translocated across the basolateral membrane. Bicarbonate exits the cytosol at the apical membrane in exchange for chloride. (Redrawn from Argent BE, Case RM. Cellular mechanism and control of bicarbonate secretion. In Johnson LR, ed. Physiology of the Gastrointestinal Tract, 3rd ed. New York: Raven Press, 1994.)

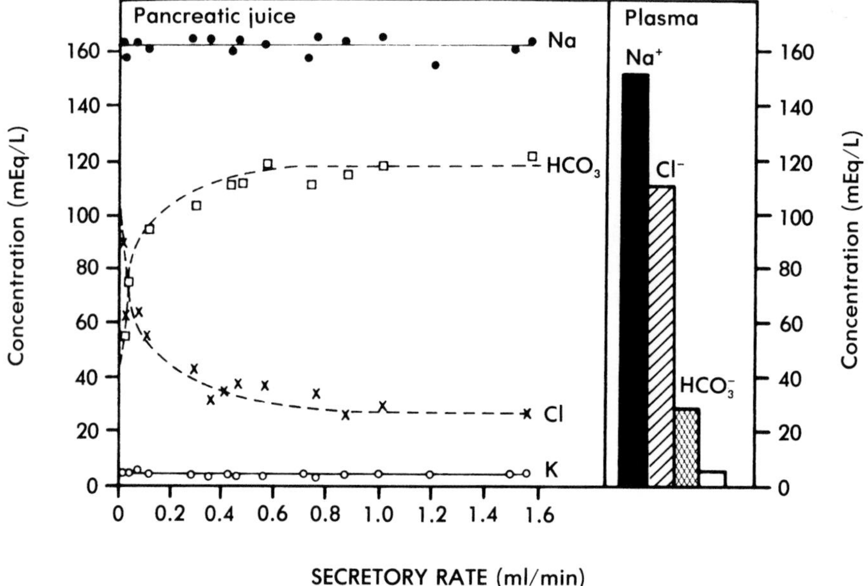

Fig. 26-5. The change in sodium *(Na^+)*, potassium *(K^+)*, chloride *(Cl^-)*, and bicarbonate *(HCO_3^-)* as a function of secretory rate in the dog. (Redrawn from Bro-Rasmussen F, Killmann SA, Thaysen JH. The composition of pancreatic juice as compared to sweat, parotid saliva, and tears. Acta Physiol Scand 37:97, 1956.)

Movement of water is passive due to concentration gradients. Pancreatic secretion is isosmotic with plasma at all rates of secretion.

Composition of Pancreatic Water and Electrolyte Secretion

The principal anions in pancreatic juice are HCO_3^- and Cl^-; the cations are Na^+ and K^+. Other ionic constituents include Ca^{++}, Mg^{++}, Zn^{++}, HPO_4^- and SO_4^-. The two major anions vary reciprocally during secretory stimulation and total 150 mM. The concentration of Na^+, the major cation is nearly 160 mM. At low secretory flow rates, the Cl^- concentration is high, and the HCO_3^- low. During stimulation, HCO_3^- concentration exponentially increases, whereas Cl^- exponentially decreases. The rate of secretion has no influence on Na^+ concentration[62,63] (Fig. 26-5).

Three theories have been proposed to explain this pattern of anion secretion. The unicellular theory postulates that all cells secrete both HCO_3^- and Cl^- but that the secretory rate of each is a function of degree of stimulation. The exchange diffusion hypothesis suggests that the major anion secreted is HCO_3^- but that along the ductal system HCO_3^- is exchanged for Cl^-; thus a low flow rate would allow more time for HCO_3^- and Cl^- exchange, resulting in a high Cl^- concentration. This hypothesis would also explain the higher HCO_3^- concentration observed at higher flow rates.

The third theory, which has some experimental support, has been termed the two-component hypothesis. This suggests that the acinar cell secretes Cl^-, whereas the centroacinar and duct cells secrete HCO_3^-. The anion content of the pancreatic juice is an admixture of the secretion from different types of cells, with $HCO3_3^-$ added to a Cl^--rich acinar cell secretion. Micropuncture studies indicate that at high flow rates higher Cl^- concentrations are present in the interlobar ducts, with a progressive decline in Cl^- and rise in HCO_3^- concentrations in samples obtained from sequentially larger ducts (Fig. 26-6). The following observation also supports this hypothesis: rats in which the acinar cells have been destroyed by chronic penicillamine treatment are still able to increase HCO_3^- concentration in secretory fluid during stimulation.

Stimulants and Inhibitors of Pancreatic Secretion

Signal Transduction Pathways

One of two functionally distinct sequences of intracellular biochemical change is initiated by individual stimulants of pancreatic secretion. Certain secretagogs, acetylcholine (Ach), CCK, gastrin, substance P, and bombesin, interact with a specific plasma membrane receptor and cause a rise in cytosolic calcium concentration.[64,65] Changes in the transmembrane potential and conductance associated with these receptor-agonist interactions are mediated by a rise in cytosolic Ca^{++} concentration as a result of opening of Ca^{++}-sensitive cation channels. This occurs due to cleavage of polyphosphoinositides and production of inositol triphosphate (IP_3) and diacylglycerol (DAG). The pathway involves the activation of GTP-binding proteins or G proteins that are a family of proteins with specific and unique α-subunit and shared β- and γ-subunits. After the recep-

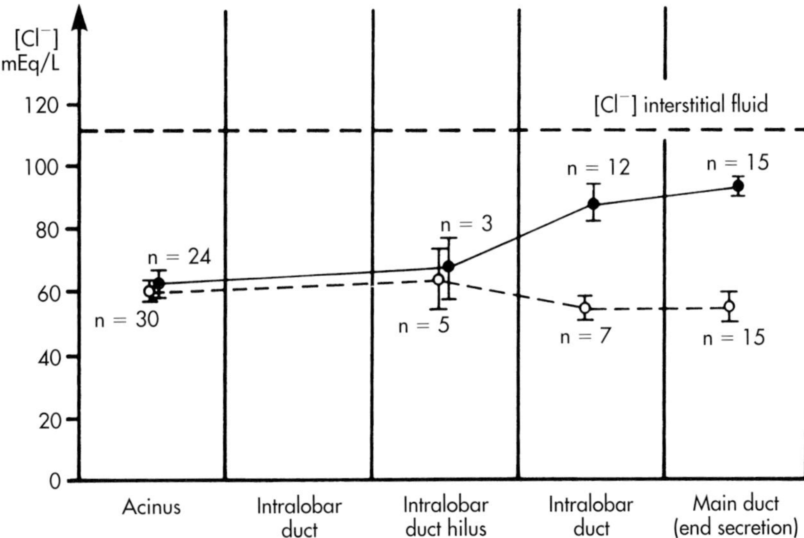

Fig. 26-6. Free flow chloride *(Cl^-)* concentrations in samples from micropuncture experiments under basal (○) and secretin-stimulated (●) conditions. (Redrawn from Schulz F. Electrolyte ⊕ fluid secretion in the exocrine pancreas. In Johnson LR, ed. Physiology of the Gastrointestinal Tract. New York: Raven Press, 1981.)

tor binds to its ligand, it interacts with the G protein to catalyze the phosphorylation of GDP_1 bound to the α-subunit, to GTP. The α-subunit then dissociates from the β- and γ-complex and activates the effector, phospholipase C. Stimulation of phospholipase C activity causes the hydrolysis of PI(4,5)P_2 and the formation of 1,4,5-IP_3 and DAG. Both molecules appear to be primary intercellular messengers. Subsequently, 1,4,5-IP_3 induces the release of Ca^{++} from the endoplasmic reticulum or specialized organelles referred to calcisomes[66] (Fig. 26-7).

Following receptor interaction, other secretagogs, including secretin and VIP, produce a rise in cytosolic cyclic adenosine monophosphate (cAMP) by activation of adenylate cyclase and cAMP-dependent protein kinase.[67] Cytologic calmodulin is an ubiquitous acidic protein that binds 4 mol Ca^{+2}/mol protein. Calmodulin is responsible for activating several enzymes including multiple protein kinases, protein phosphates, and cyclic nucleotide phosodiesterases, resulting in the secretory response. G proteins regulating adenylate cyclase are either stimulatory (G_S) or inhibitory (G_I) based on the presence of distinct α-subunits, which can be distinguished on their sensitivity to cholera and pertussis toxins, respectively.[68,69] Potentiated responses to combinations of secretory stimulants occurring independent of the second messenger associated with each suggest a cytosolic interaction of these signal transduction pathways.[70]

Neural Stimulants of Pancreatic Secretion

In all species studied, vagal stimulation produces an increase in both pancreatic bicarbonate and enzyme secretion.[71-73] Exogenous secretin potentiates this neural response.[74] Cholinergic agents produce rates of bicarbonate and enzyme secretion similar to those obtained during vagal stimulation. Atropine blocks vagally and cholinergically stimulated pancreatic secretion, but significant species selectivity exists for volume, bicarbonate, and enzyme secretory inhibition.[71-73] In humans vagal stimulation induced by hypoglycemia augments secretin-stimulated pancreatic protein output. Truncal vagotomy, although reducing bicarbonate response to exogenous stimulants by approximately 25%, does not affect maximum enzyme secretion but does reduce sensitivity to submaximum stimulation.[75]

VIP has been suggested as a possible local neurotransmitter for vagal stimulation of pancreatic bicarbonate secretion.[76] VIP neurons appear to encircle the cell bodies of intrapancreatic ganglia and directly innervate pancreatic ducts. In addition, vagally induced bicarbonate secretion was decreased by a specific VIP antibody. Although these findings are strongly supportive for regulation of pancreatic bicarbonate secretion by VIP, the importance of VIP in vagally mediated pancreatic secretory response to a meal is unknown.

Splanchnic nerve stimulation is usually associated with inhibition of pancreatic exocrine secretion. The mechanism is thought to be related to intense vasoconstriction and blood flow inhibition; however, splanchnic nerve stimulation has been shown to inhibit pancreatic secretion even when the vasoconstriction has been abolished pharmacologically.[64] Exogenous administration of adrenergic agonists or antagonists, however, may also produce changes in heart rate, cause discharge of hormones, and alter neural activity by their effects at central or other peripheral sites. To date, no clear-cut pattern has emerged on adrenergic regulation of basally or meal-stimulated pancreatic exocrine secretion.

Local neural pathways, probably cholinergically medi-

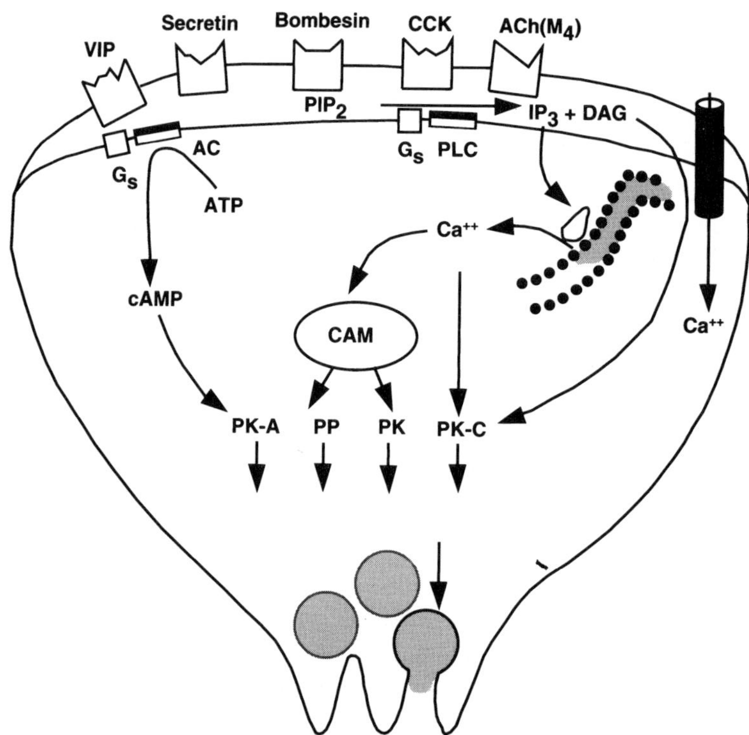

Fig. 26-7. Proposed mechanism of stimulus-secretion coupling of pancreatic acinar cell protein secretion. The binding of peptide and neurotransmitter liquids to their specific receptors results in G protein–coupled activation of cytosolic second messengers. Activation by cholecystokinin, acetylcholine, and bombesin, through a stimulatory GTP-binding protein *(Gs)* leads to the release of Ca^{++} from intracellular stores and Ca^{++} influx. Diacylglycerol *(DAG)* is subsequently formed from phosphatidylinositol 4,5 bisphosphate, by phospholipase C and activates protein kinase C *(PKC)*. Activation by secretion or vasoactive intestinal polypeptide, also acting through a stimulatory GTP-binding protein, causes the formation of adenylate cyclase, cyclic AMP *(cAMP)* and activation of protein kinase A *(PKA)*. Phosphorylation of structural and regulatory proteins results in release of cellular products found in the cytosolic vacuoles.

ated, also appear to play a significant role in pancreatic secretion. The rapidity with which intraduodenal and intrajejunal stimulants produce an increase in pancreatic secretory response has led to the hypothesis that duodenojejunopancreatic neural connections produce a physiologic reflex that significantly facilitates at least the rapid pancreatic response to intraluminal stimulants.[77]

Receptors and Agonists on Pancreatic Acinar Cells

Receptors for humoral stimulants, neurotransmitters, and growth factors have been described in the pancreatic acinar cell. Certain peptides, such as CCK-related peptides are potent secretagogs and have marked trophic effects that are associated with increased DNA and RNA content, perhaps because of activation of early c-*myc*, c-*fos*, and c-*jun* gene expression. Receptor binding results in either activation of phospholipase C and activation of C (PKC) or the activation of adenylate cyclase and activation of A protein kinase (PKA), resulting in enzyme secretion.

Cholecystokinin. CCK is a polypeptide of 33 amino acids. CCK_A receptors are localized to the basolateral membrane of the acinar cell.[78,79] The CCK_A receptor has a high affinity for CCK and its analogs sulfated in the seventh position from the carboxy terminus. This receptor has a low affinity for gastrin, which is sulfated in the sixth position from the carboxy terminus. A second class of CCK receptors is the CCK_B/gastrin receptor, which has equal affinity for gastrin and CCK; however, it is not a biologically active receptor in the pancreatic acinar cell.

CCK is a product of the I cells in the duodenum and proximal jejunum. Preprocholecystokinin is a 115 amino acid that undergoes specific enzymatic cleavage to form the biologically active peptide. The peptide sequence for biologic activity is Trp-Met-Asp-Phe-NH_2, and for full biologic activity the tyrosine of the seventh position must be sulfated.[80] The largest biologically active circulating form is the CCK-58. In humans, CCK-33 is a major circulating form. The half-life of CCK is 2 to 7 minutes.

Primary stimulants of CCK release are intraluminal fats, proteins, and amino acids. Two naturally occurring, trypsin-sensitive peptides act within the human to stimulate CCK release. Monitor peptide, a 61-amino acid protein, is produced by the pancreas and secreted into the pancreatic juice, stimulating CCK release. CCK-releasing peptide is a product of the intestine and may be important in basal secretion of CCK.[81,82]

Secretin. Secretin is a polypeptide of 27 amino acids that derives its name from the stimulatory effects it produces on pancreatic bicarbonate secretion. Interestingly, as noted earlier, Bayliss and Starling identified this humoral stimulant of pancreatic secretion in 1902, which not only caused the scientific community to rethink Pavlov's emphasis on an exclusively neural reflex mechanism of pancreatic exocrine secretion but also ushered in the systematic study of humoral agents and the endocrine system.

Secretin is a strong stimulant of pancreatic bicarbonate and volume output and a relatively weak stimulant of protein output.[83] The whole secretin molecule is required for full biologic activity. The half-life of secretin is about 3 minutes. The intracellular second messenger of secretin-induced pancreatic bicarbonate output is cAMP.[75]

There appears to be only one type of secretin receptor. Secretin has marked structural similarities to VIP and growth hormone–releasing factor (GRF). Of all the secretin-VIP–related peptides, secretin has a 900-fold higher affinity for its receptor than VIP or the others.

Secretin is a basic 27–amino acid peptide of which the carboxy terminus valine is amidated. The cells of origin of secretin, S cells, have been characterized in the proximal small bowel on the basis of secretin production and morphology. The S cells are localized to the villi in the duodenum and proximal jejunum with a frequency of 6 cells/100 mucosal epithelial cells. Release of secretin occurs during mucosal exposure to endogenous hydrochloric acid, the threshold being an intraluminal pH of ≤4.5. Other intraluminal substances causing secretin release are bile salts, fatty acids, sodium oleate, and herbal extracts. Somatostatin inhibits secretin release.

Release of secretin from S cells is mediated by a secretin-releasing factor, a peptide that is sensitive to proteolytic digestion.[84] This forms a negative feedback loop by which secretin release is inhibited because of the activity of pancreatic proteases on this peptide, resulting in attenuation of secretin release.

Secretin occupation of the secretin receptor causes an 80-fold increase in cytosolic cAMP, and activation of protein kinase A. Rather than affecting protein secretion, secretin is thought to regulate the Na^+, K^+-ATPase that modulates electrolyte secretion.

Other receptors. Other receptors have been shown to exist on the acinar cell. Muscarinic cholinergic receptors, M_1-M_5 belong to the family of G protein–coupled receptors. The human M_4 receptor is larger than the other muscarinic receptors and may represent the primary physiologic muscarinic cholinergic receptor on the acinar cell. Through the PKC signal transduction pathway, muscarinic receptor activation results in enzyme secretion. A high-affinity receptor for VIP has been shown to stimulate adenylate cyclase with activation of PKA, resulting in enzyme secretion.

Pancreatic Response to a Meal

The total pancreatic secretory response to a meal is a complex interaction between neural and humoral events. This response has been divided into cephalic, gastric, and intestinal phases. Technical experimental constraints and species differences in response to diversion of chyme and pancreatic and biliary secretions make it difficult to provide definitive statements about specific mechanisms regulating pancreatic responses to a meal. Many existing deductions are based on in vivo and in vitro experimental data in animals.

In dogs and human beings, pancreatic enzyme secretion in response to a meal represents only 70% to 80% of its maximum secretory capacity. It is presently unknown (1) whether a meal simply does not evoke physiologic mechanisms at a magnitude compatible with maximum pancreatic secretion or (2) whether some neural or humoral mechanism evoked by a meal exerts an inhibitory effect on pancreatic secretory activity.

Cephalic phase. Visual and olfactory stimuli increase more pancreatic protein than bicarbonate secretion.[85,86] In the dog the cephalic phase of pancreatic enzyme secretion is approximately 25%, and bicarbonate secretion is 10% to 15% of maximum secretory capacity. The cephalic phase of pancreatic secretion appears to be mediated by the vagus nerves, with efferent fibers acting either directly or indirectly on the pancreas to elicit acinar cell secretion of enzymes.[87-89] Atropine greatly reduces or abolishes the pancreatic response to sham feeding, whereas truncal vagotomy completely inhibits the response. A major site of action of sham feeding–induced cholinergic efferent activity is probably directly on the pancreas, since vagal stimulation of the extracorporeally perfused in situ dog pancreas induces pancreatic secretion. Sham feeding does not result in CCK release, and CCK antagonists do not alter the pancreatic response to sham feeding. Sham feeding is a strong stimulant of gastric acid secretion, and it has been suggested that gastric acid augmentation of the cephalic pancreatic response is due to the release of secretin. With background secretin infusion, sham feeding has been shown to increase pancreatic secretion to 50% of CCK-stimulated maximum response in humans.[90] Gastric antral acidification, which inhibits the cephalic phase of gastrin release, abolishes the cephalic phase of pancreatic secretion, suggesting that in the dog the cephalic phase of pancreatic secretion may be largely caused by gastrin release.[91] In human beings gastrin is also a stimulant of pancreatic enzyme secretion[92]; however, the rapidity with which the pancreas responds to visual and olfactory stimulation, 2 to 4 minutes, suggests that a direct neural component also exists.[93]

The potential central mechanisms that mediate the cephalic effects of pancreatic secretion have only recently been investigated. In anesthetized dogs the central stimulatory areas for pancreatic secretion included the dorsal and ventral middle hypothalamus, the mamillary body, and parts of the ventromedial and dorsomedial nuclei.[94] The pathway for electric and chemical stimulation of these areas appears to be through the dorsal motor nucleus and the nucleus of the solitary tract because both atropine and vagotomy block the pancreatic secretory effects of central stimulation. Electric stimulation of the medial amygdaloid nucleus in rats significantly increases water secretion and bicarbonate secretion. These augmented pancreatic secretory responses, however, are abolished by bilateral truncal vagotomy.

Many of the peptides found in the gastrointestinal tract have also been isolated within the CNS and may play a regulatory role in pancreatic secretion. Vasoactive intestinal peptide, a structural homolog to secretin, has been isolated in numerous sites within the CNS and stimulates the secretion of enzymes, water, and bicarbonate from the pancreas. Secretin has been found in the CNS of rats and pigs. In the rat the highest concentrations occur in the pineal and pituitary glands followed by the thalamus and hypothalamus. Central injection of secretin into the left lateral ventricle of rats induces significant increases in pancreatic volume and bicarbonate output. This centrally induced pancreatic secretory response appears to be mediated by a cholinergic mechanism.[95]

Gastric phase. Several studies have made precise observations leading to the conclusion that the control over pancreatic secretion exerted by the stomach is substantial. It is now clear that gastrin is not a significant contributor to the gastric phase of pancreatic secretion. The most compelling evidence for this is that the plasma levels of gastrin required for stimulation of pancreatic secretion are higher than those measured after ingestion of food. Currently, it appears that the gastric phase of pancreatic secretion is mediated by one or more "gastropancreatic reflexes." Distention of either the gastric body or the gastric antrum results in an increase in pancreatic protein output with a lesser effect on bicarbonate secretion.[96,97] The latter antropancreatic reflex is abolished by anticholinergics and vagotomy but not by antral acidification, suggesting that gastrin release is not the mediator of this reflex but rather a true neural cholinergic reflex. Gastric proteolysis releases oligopeptides, which may stimulate the pancreas after they enter the small intestine. The stomach also tightly controls the rate of entry of chyme into the intestine, as well as the size of solid food particles, which in turn determines the rate of release of digestive products.[98] In these various ways the stomach controls the intestinal phase of pancreatic secretion, which is perhaps the most important phase.

Two studies have evaluated meal-stimulated pancreatic secretory activity following an 80% gastrectomy. Meal-stimulated pancreatic secretion was only minimally affected by this surgical procedure, which removes the gastrin-producing cells while greatly disturbing gastric emptying.[99,100] Another study on the effect of gastrin release in relation to the gastric phase of acid secretion demonstrated that distention of innervated canine antral pouches with an alkaline solution increased both pancreatic enzyme secretion and gastrin release, although distention with an acidic solution produced a similar pancreatic secretory response while blocking gastrin release.[101]

Intestinal phase. Neural interactions and enteropancreatic reflexes probably account for the earliest pancreatic responses following a meal. Although the denervated pancreas does respond to intestinal stimuli when experimentally transplanted, the magnitude of the protein secretory response following a meal is reduced approximately 50% when compared to the innervated pancreas.[102] Denervation does not interfere with the gland's capacity to secrete protein, water, or bicarbonate. Both truncal vagotomy and atropine reduce the pancreatic response to intraluminal oleate and tryptophan by nearly 50%. These observations suggest that innervation is required for full secretory response to intestinal stimulants.

In an attempt to evaluate the relative contribution of the neural and humoral components of this rapid enteropancreatic response, a comparison of the latency of protein secretory response was made between instillation of intraluminal stimulants and intraportal administration of CCK. Amylase output was shown to occur within 0.30 to 0.33 minute of intestinal oleate or tryptophan perfusion, whereas 0.59 minute was required for the response to intraportal CCK administration.[77] Atropine or truncal vagotomy increased the latency to intraluminal stimulants by a factor of nearly 10, whereas no effect on the latency to intraportal CCK administration was observed. These observations suggest that the earliest pancreatic response to intestinal perfusion with oleate or tryptophan is neurally mediated. Similar experiments recently have found that the latency of pancreatic bicarbonate output in response to intraduodenal tryptophan was 62 seconds; to oleate, 64 seconds; to intraportal CCK, 28 seconds; and to secretin, 45 seconds.[103] These data suggest that differences may exist in the neural component between stimulated pancreatic enzyme and bicarbonate output. The dependent and interdependent interactions of neural and humoral components on enteropancreatic reflexes are complex and controversial and require further investigation. Recently, it has been suggested that enteropancreatic reflexes mediate potentiation of acid-induced pancreatic bicarbonate output by amino acids but not by fatty acids.

The role of gut hormones in the negative feedback regulation of pancreatic exocrine secretion has been well established in rats. This feedback is mediated via CCK and secretin through trypsin-sensitive releasing peptides. In dogs, however, the postprandial pancreatic secretion appears to be mediated through the release of secretin rather than CCK. In humans humoral feedback regulation of pancreatic exocrine secretion in the intestinal phase appears to be mediated by the release of CCK. A negative feedback regulation of pancreatic secretion of bicarbonate and enzyme in human volunteers has been demonstrated to be mediated via both CCK and secretin.[104,105]

Acidification. In addition to the neural component of postprandial pancreatic secretion, intraduodenal acid, fat, and amino acids stimulate pancreatic secretion by humoral mechanisms. When the duodenum is acidified to a pH of 4.5, acid load rather than concentration appears to be an important determinant of pancreatic volume and bicarbonate output[106,107] (Fig. 26-8). For equal and titratable acid loads, pancreatic bicarbonate secretion is greater for strong than for weak acids. Pancreatic bicarbonate response to intestinal acidification is also partly a function of the length of intestine acidified.[108] Neutralizing duodenal contents reduces postprandial pancreatic bicarbonate output by about 50%.[109] The threshold pH, above which pancreatic bicarbonate secretion does not occur, is 4.5 in dogs[110] but may be slightly lower in humans.[111]

These observations suggest that acid entering the duodenum after a meal is a potent stimulus for pancreatic bicarbonate and volume secretion. Following a mixed meal, chyme entering the duodenum may have a pH of 2 to 2.5,[112] which indicates that under physiologic conditions duodenal acidification does contribute to pancreatic bicarbonate and volume secretory response. Pancreatic bicarbonate output following duodenal acidification by a permeable acid (lactic acid) or an impermeable acid (acidified albumin) is not significantly different, suggesting that pancreatic response to intestinal acidification is a function of acid-receptor activation at the intestinal lumen.[113]

One can reasonably conclude that duodenal acidification causes a release of endogenous secretin, which then acts on the pancreas, since primarily bicarbonate and volume output rather than protein output are stimulated.

Secretin potentiation. The concentration of secretin in the gastrointestinal mucosa is greatest in the duodenum.[114] Lower concentrations are found distal to the duodenum.

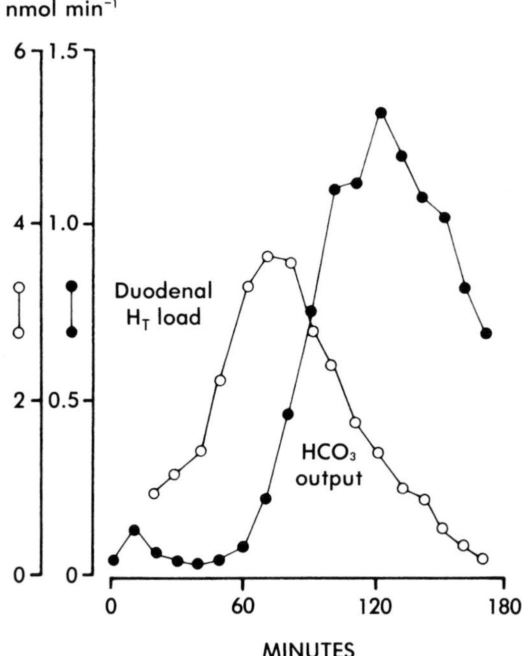

Fig. 26-8. Duodenal acid *(H_t)* load and pancreatic bicarbonate *(HCO_3^-)* response to a meal in dogs. (Redrawn from Moore EW, Verine HJ, Grossman MI. Pancreatic bicarbonate response to a meal. Acta Hepato-Gastroenterol 26:30, 1979.)

Secretin-like immunoreactivity has been found in S cells, which are present between the crypts and villi. Although plasma concentration of secretin, as measured by radioimmunoassay, has been shown to increase during duodenal acidification,[115] the data on plasma secretin concentrations following a meal have been inconsistent. Some investigators have been unable to detect a rise in plasma secretin concentration, whereas others observing a rise have also found it to be smaller than would be expected for the magnitude of pancreatic bicarbonate response[116,117] (Fig. 26-9). Several explanations may exist for this apparent discrepancy.

First, the magnitude of pancreatic bicarbonate response to a meal is much less than the maximum secretin-stimulated bicarbonate response. Second, during a meal hydrochloric acid secreted by the parietal cells is buffered by weak meal proteins, so the gastric effluent into the duodenum has a pH range of 2 to 4. Thus the secretin response

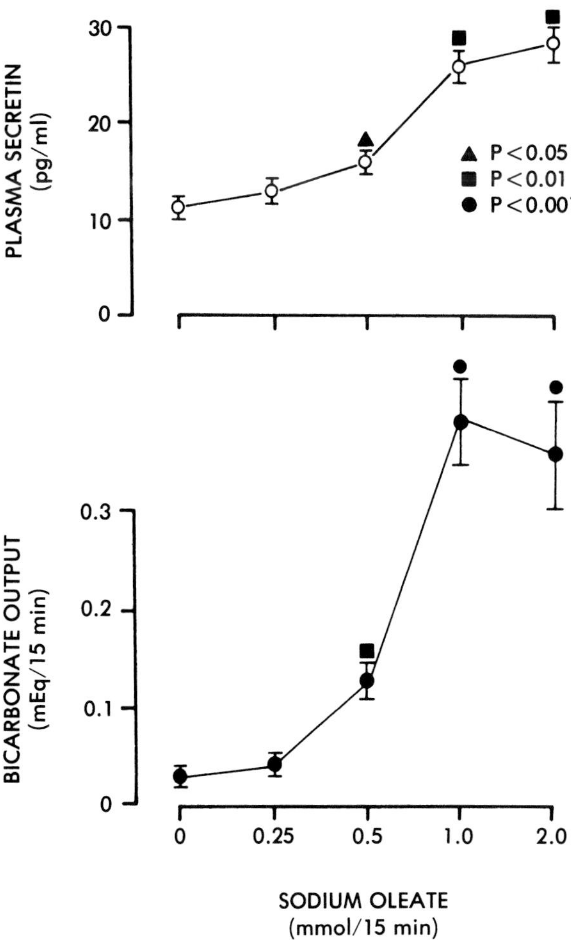

Fig. 26-9. Effect of increasing concentrations of intraduodenal oleate on plasma immunoreactive secretin concentration and pancreatic bicarbonate output in dogs. (Redrawn from Faichney A, et al. Effect of sodium oleate on plasma secretin concentration and pancreatic secretion in dogs. Gastroenterology 81:458, 1981. Copyright 1981 by The American Gastroenterological Association.)

to a meal would not be expected to be as great as the response to duodenal acidification with hydrochloric acid, a strong acid.

Finally, small increases in plasma secretin concentration following a meal, with a relatively greater pancreatic bicarbonate response than would be expected for that increase, may be explained by the physiologic responses to the administration of more than one stimulatory peptide producing secretory responses that are greater than the sum of the individual responses. This effect has been termed potentiation. Potentiation of pancreatic bicarbonate secretion has been shown with CCK and secretin, gastrin and secretin, caerulein and secretin, secretin and L-phenylalanine but not with secretin and bethanechol.[118]

Additional evidence supports the role of secretin in postprandial pancreatic bicarbonate response. One study found that treatment with antisecretin antiserum reduced bicarbonate output by 80% following a meal in dogs.[119]

These correlations among duodenal acidification, pancreatic bicarbonate secretion, and small changes in plasma secretin concentration suggest that the pancreatic bicarbonate response to a meal is partly mediated by secretin release from the duodenum and proximal small intestine.

Fatty acids. Intraduodenal and intraintestinal products of fat digestion stimulate pancreatic bicarbonate and protein secretion. Intraluminal triglycerides and diglycerides are not stimulants until hydrolyzed.[120] Fatty acids of less than nine carbons do not stimulate pancreatic secretion; those with more than nine carbons, as well as monoglycerides, do stimulate secretion[121,122] (Fig. 26-10). Responses to these stimulatory fatty acids are dose related, being directly related to the length of intestine to which they are exposed and inversely related to the individual rate of absorption from the intestine.[120]

The pancreatic bicarbonate and protein response to intraluminal fatty acids varies and therefore gives few clues as to the mediators. Medium chain fatty acids stimulate more bicarbonate than protein than do amino acids.[123] Relative secretory rates vary with the intraluminal concentration of an individual fatty acid, as indicated by the observation that pancreatic bicarbonate relative to protein output rises with increasing oleate concentrations. Intraluminal fatty acids possibly stimulate the release of either CCK or secretin, a function of concentration, or the primary mechanism may be CCK release in a milieu that provides for potentiation of interactions with endogenous humoral agents such as secretin. Studies have shown that intrajejunal perfusion with oleate and decanoate augments the pancreatic bicarbonate response to duodenal acidification and potentiates submaximum secretin-stimulated bicarbonate secretion.[123,124] The stimulation of gallbladder contraction by fatty acids suggests that significant amounts of CCK are released under these conditions. Basal plasma CCK concentrations in humans are low.[125,126] Postprandial plasma CCK concentrations increase significantly, and high concentrations are measured even following instillation of intraduodenal fat.[127]

One study demonstrated that intraduodenal oleate produced a concomitant increase in immunoreactive plasma CCK, pancreatic protein output, and gallbladder pressure

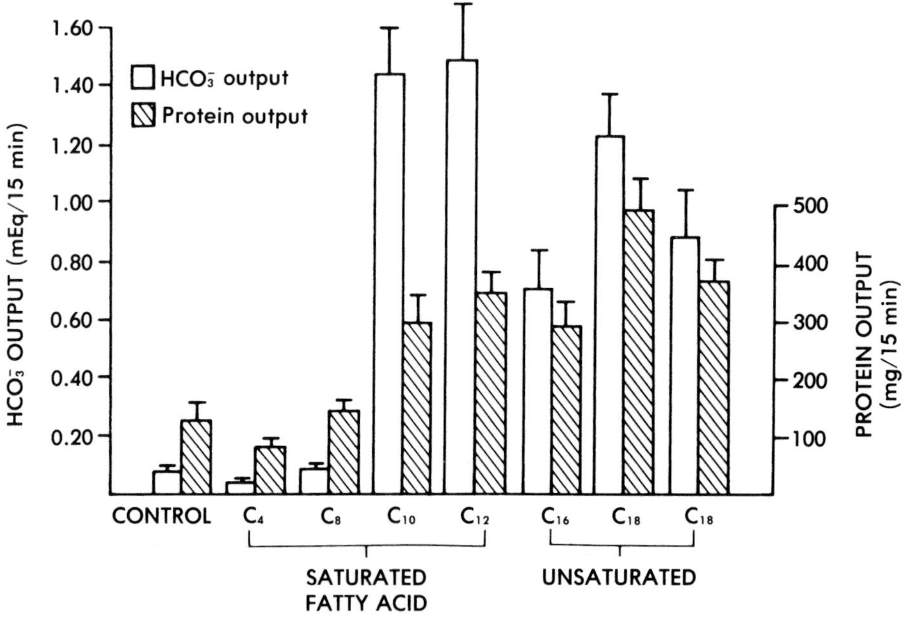

Fig. 26-10. Pancreatic bicarbonate *(HCO_3^-)* and protein outputs in response to different fatty acids, 80 mM, administered intraduodenally in dogs. (Redrawn from Meyer JH. Release of secretin and cholecystokinin. In Thompson JC, ed. Gastrointestinal Hormones. Austin, Tex.: University of Texas Press, 1975.)

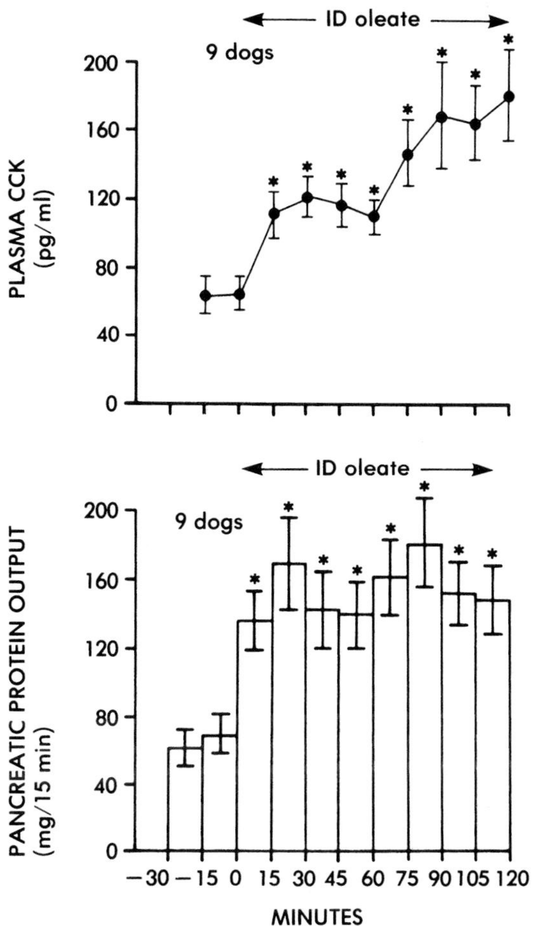

Fig. 26-11. Change in plasma CCK concentration and pancreatic protein output in response to intraduodenal oleate perfusion in dogs. (Redrawn from Fried GM, et al. Release of cholecystokinin in conscious dogs. Gastroenterology 85:1113, 1983. Copyright 1983 by The American Gastroenterological Association.)

in the dog (Fig. 26-11).[128] Truncal vagotomy caused a 45% reduction in pancreatic protein output and completely abolished the gallbladder response but had no effect on the change in immunoreactive plasma CCK. In dogs intraduodenal oleate greatly increases pancreatic volume and bicarbonate secretion and is accompanied by a small but significant increase in plasma secretin concentration.[129] Intravenous lipid administration to dogs does not appear to stimulate the pancreas to secrete bicarbonate or protein (Fig. 26-12).[130] These observations suggest that intraintestinal fats stimulate the release of both secretin and CCK, which in turn produce responses in pancreatic bicarbonate and protein output.

Amino acids and peptides. Intraduodenal and intrajejunal perfusion with products of protein digestion cause the pancreas to secrete fluid that has a high protein concentration of low volume, a response similar to that produced by neural stimulation or exogenous CCK administration.[92,131,132] In the dog the two most potent amino acids that provoke this response are phenylalanine and tryptophan, whereas in humans they are methionine, valine, and phenylalanine. Protein output is stimulated in the canine pancreas to the same degree by polypeptides, oligopeptides, and individual L-amino acids[133,134] (Fig. 26-13). In humans trypsin, amylase, and lipase are secreted when neutral amino acids bathe the lumen of the proximal jejunum.[131] In rats diversion of intestinal contents stimulates pancreatic secretion; in this species the presence of trypsin in the lumen apparently inhibits pancreatic secretion, a negative feedback mechanism.[135] This is not the case in dogs,[136] and in humans it is not clear whether such a negative feedback mechanism exists.[137] Large quantities of pancreatic proteases delivered to the duodenum have been shown to suppress pancreatic exocrine output in healthy control subjects and patients with chronic pancreatitis.[138]

CCK is found primarily in the jejunal mucosae of dogs, with the duodenal and ileal mucosas having somewhat lower concentrations.[114] In humans the predominant

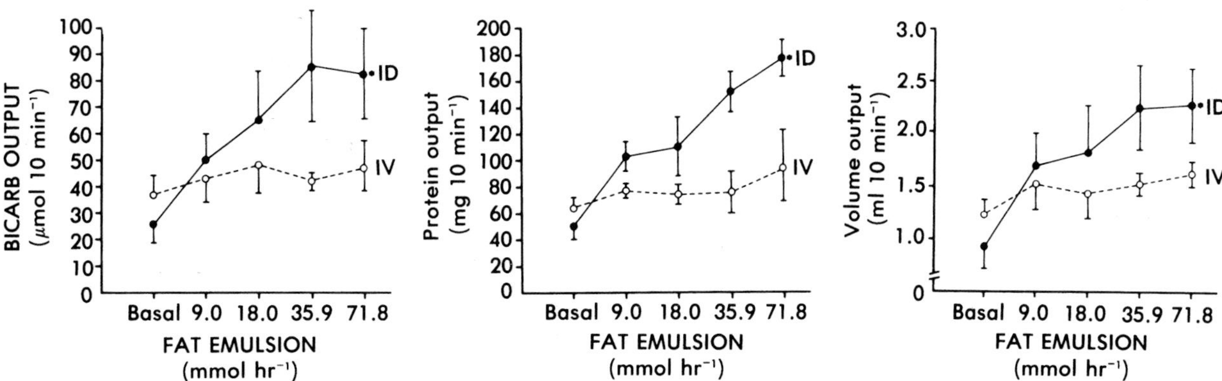

Fig. 26-12. Pancreatic volume, protein, and bicarbonate responses to graded doses of fat emulsion administered intraduodenally *(ID)* or intravenously *(IV)* in dogs. (From Stabile BE, et al. Intravenous mixed amino acids and fats do not stimulate exocrine pancreatic secretion. Am J Physiol 246:G274, 1984.)

plasma form of CCK is the octapeptide, which has been shown to increase from 0.5 to 6 fomol/ml^{-1} following a mixed meal.[126] Intraduodenal infusion of L-tryptophan and L-phenylalanine is associated with a doubling of plasma CCK-like immunoreactivity. As with secretin, these low concentrations and relatively small increases observed following a meal suggest that the pancreatic enzyme secretory response to a meal depends on potentiated interactions between peptides. This has recently been demonstrated in the dog, with intraduodenal perfusion of protein digestive materials potentiating acid-induced bicarbonate but not protein output.[139] As with fats, parenteral administration of amino acid–containing solutions probably does not stimulate pancreatic bicarbonate or protein output in the dog (Fig. 26-14).[130]

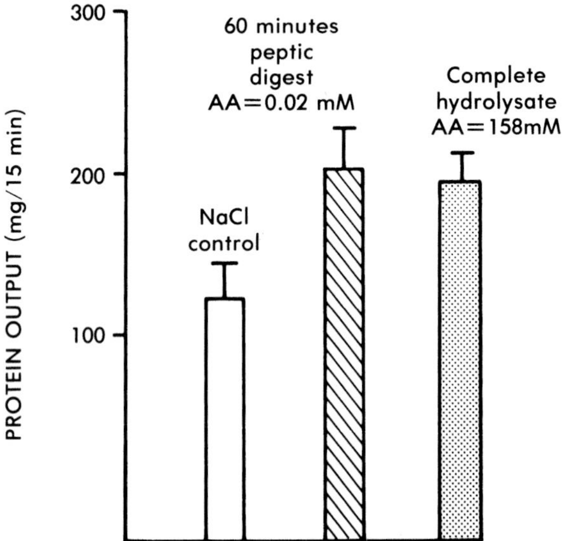

Fig. 26-13. Pancreatic protein responses in dogs to perfused peptic digestive material of 1.75% bovine serum albumin and to an amino acid mixture with a composition similar to a theoretically complete hydrolysate of bovine serum albumin. (Redrawn from Meyer JH. Release of secretin and cholecystokinin. In Thompson JC, ed. Gastrointestinal Hormones. Austin, Tex.: University of Texas Press, 1975.)

Summary of intestinal phase. A variety of neural and humoral mechanisms contribute to the intestinal phase of pancreatic exocrine secretion. The early response appears to be primarily neural and cholinergic. Intact vagal-vagal innervation is a prerequisite for full activity. Intraintestinal acid stimulates pancreatic bicarbonate and volume secretion, which is probably mediated in part by secretin release. Intraintestinal fats stimulate both pancreatic bicarbonate and protein secretion, which is most likely mediated partly by secretin and CCK release. Intraintestinal peptides and amino acids stimulate pancreatic protein secretion, which is probably mediated in part by CCK release. Radioimmunoassay studies suggest that the change in plasma concentration of these two peptides is small, implicating potentiated interactions between peptides for realization of full pancreatic secretory activity.

PANCREATIC FUNCTION TESTS

Serum Concentrations of Pancreatic Enzymes

The most frequently measured pancreatic enzyme in the blood is amylase. Pancreatic ductal obstruction causes a rise in serum amylase concentration. Amylase may also be derived from the salivary glands, intestine, fallopian tube, breast, and liver. Specific isozymes of amylase provide information regarding the source of serum enzyme elevation. Measurement of the activity of total serum amylase either in the basal state or after stimulation of pancreatic exocrine secretion is of little value in the detection of chronic pancreatitis. In acute pancreatitis serum amylase may rise rapidly fivefold to ten-fold and return to normal

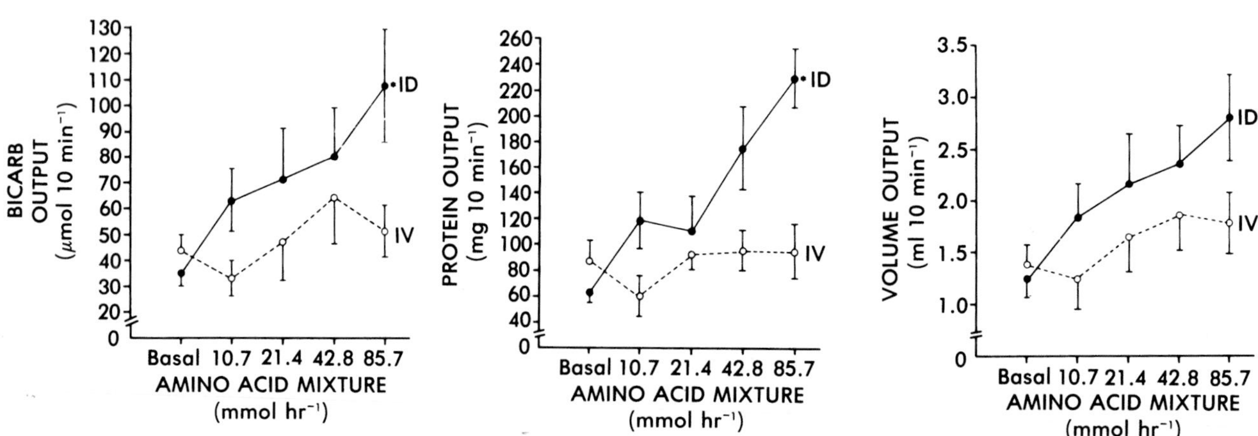

Fig. 26-14. Pancreatic volume, protein, and bicarbonate responses to graded doses of mixed amino acids administered intraduodenally *(ID)* or intravenously *(IV)* in dogs. (From Stabile BE, et al. Intravenous mixed amino acids and fats do not stimulate exocrine pancreatic secretion. Am J Physiol 246:G274, 1984.)

within a few days. Unfortunately, in conditions such as chronic pancreatitis, serum amylase concentration may be normal or subnormal. Other conditions that may cause hyperamylasemia include perforated duodenal ulcer, intestinal obstruction, acute mesenteric infarction, and acute cholecystitis. The elevation of the pancreatic isozyme of amylase in a patient with abdominal pain is a very useful indicator of acute pancreatitis. Serum concentrations of this isozyme rise with increasing age, and increased concentrations are found in healthy individuals and in patients with chronic liver disease, chronic renal failure, or acute pancreatitis. Less than one half of patients with pancreatic exocrine insufficiency, however, demonstrate a low pancreatic isoamylase concentration.[104]

Urine Concentrations of Pancreatic Enzymes

In acute pancreatitis urinary amylase may be elevated for a longer period than serum amylase and therefore represents a more sensitive test than serum amylase. Urinary clearance of amylase increases in acute pancreatitis. In healthy persons the ratio of amylase clearance to creatinine clearance is less than 5%, whereas in patients with acute pancreatitis it is often significantly higher. Unfortunately, the lack of specificity of this test limits its clinical usefulness.

Stool Concentrations of Pancreatic Enzymes

Although trypsin and chymotrypsin are detectable in feces, only chymotrypsin is resistant enough to enteric degradation to warrant its measurement to assess exocrine function. Fecal chymotrypsin concentrations directly correlate with exocrine pancreatic secretion in response to the secretogogs CCK and secretin. Clinically, however, fecal chymotrypsin measurement appears to have merit only in those patients with severe exocrine function impairment.[105]

Pancreatic Secretory Tests

Fecal Fat

Fat malabsorption and steatorrhea resulting from pancreatic insufficiency occurs when stimulated lipase output decreases to less than 10% of normal. Fat in the stool is measured for 72 hours during the ingestion of a diet containing 70 to 100 g of fat each day. Values greater than 7% of ingested fat appearing in the stool are considered abnormal. A less labor-intensive test involves the microscopic examination of a single stool sample for oil, which is felt to be equally as sensitive as the quantitative 72-hour measurement.[140]

Exogenous Secretin and Cholecystokinin Duodenal Drainage

Measurement of ductular and acinar cell function can be evaluated simultaneously by means of duodenal intubation and collection of exogenously stimulated pancreatic exocrine secretions. The secretagogs should be administered at a constant rate of intravenous infusion at doses that produce a near maximum response. When properly performed, the sensitivity and specificity approach 85% to 95%. The results of secretin and CCK stimulation of pancreatic secretion correlate with the degree of histologic abnormalities observed in surgical specimens (Table 26-1).

Accurate sampling can be a difficult problem. Some pancreatic juice may not be sampled, and that sampled may have varying amounts of bilious contamination. Even with this potential for minor error, patients with malabsorption secondary to pancreatic disease usually have less than 80 mEq/L of bicarbonate in duodenal drainage following secretin administration. The secretin test results may be normal or abnormal in patients with acute pancreatitis.[141]

Endogenous Stimulation of Pancreatic Secretion (Lundh Test)

To conduct the Lundh test, a tube is placed in the very proximal jejunum, and the patient drinks 300 ml of a test meal consisting of corn oil, milk, and dextrose.[142] After the meal, at specific intervals, jejunal aspirates are analyzed for trypsin and perhaps for fats, fatty acids, and bile salts. In healthy persons trypsin output increases two to three times over basal values, and trypsin concentration remains relatively constant. Trypsin concentration that is reduced by more than 90% compared to normal values suggests rather severe pancreatic insufficiency.[142] The Lundh test, however, provides no direst information on pancreatic bicarbonate secretion.

Clinical Usefulness of Exogenous Secretagog and Lundh Tests

Clinically, the secretin/CCK and Lundh tests are infrequently used. Unless properly performed, the results of both tests may be affected by dilution of pancreatic secretions with meal contents or intestinal juices, autodegradation of secreted enzymes, or partial neutralization or absorption of secreted bicarbonate. Consequently, standard deviation of the mean in "normal" subjects may vary from 25% to 60%, even using dye dilution indicators to correct for volume and direct pancreatic duct cannulation. Pancreatic exocrine secretory tests in 33% to 50% of patients with chronic pancreatitis or carcinoma of the pancreas are within the "normal" range. Despite their limitations, exogenous secretagog stimulation with duodenal sampling is

Table 26-1. Response to Secretin Test

Patient	Mean Volume (ml/kg^{-1})	Mean Maximum Bicarbonate Output (mEq/L^{-1})
Normal	3.2	108
Acute pancreatitis	2.4	93
Chronic pancreatitis	2.7	57
Carcinoma of pancreas	1.3	83

Modified from Dreiling D. Pancreatic secretory testing in 1974. Gut 16:653, 1977.

thought to be more sensitive than the Lundh test in early chronic pancreatitis.

Other Tests

Bentiromide and pancreolauryl tests. If duodenal intubation cannot be accomplished, evaluation of pancreatic exocrine function can be performed by the oral ingestion and digestion of test substrates. For the bentiromide test, N-benzoyl-*l*-tyrosyl-*p*-aminobenzoic acid (NBT-PABA) is a peptide substrate for chymotrypsin. The Pancreolauryl test requires the ingestion of fluorescein dilaurate (FDL) as a substrate for cholesterol ester hydrolase. The metabolites of each substrate are measured in the urine. Since the substrates rely on enteric absorption and liver conjugation and excretion, any preexisting pathobiology in these organ systems may interfere with these measurements. In general, results of these oral tests of pancreatic exocrine function are reliably abnormal only in the presence of severe exocrine insufficiency.[143]

Breath tests. Several variations of breath tests using labeled carbon in either a triglyceride, to measure fat digestion by pancreatic lipase, or cornstarch, to measure carbohydrate hydrolysis, have been used clinically. The triglyceride, cholesterol-octanoate, and H_2/CO_2 breath tests are diagnostic only in patients with severe pancreatic insufficiency.

Therefore in the evaluation of the patient with abdominal pain, other tests such as ultrasound, computed tomography, and perhaps endoscopic retrograde cholangiopancreatography are more cost and time effective than those tests requiring duodenal intubation and/or ingestion of a test substrate. Similarly, in patients with pancreatic insufficiency, the condition is usually clinically obvious, and the diagnosis does not depend on performing these tests. More than 85% of pancreatic exocrine function must be lost before malabsorption becomes clinically apparent. By that time test results are almost universally positive. Pancreatic supplements may be prescribed, assuming that the clinical response is indicative of pancreatic insufficiency.

Pancreatic function tests are sufficiently insensitive to establish the diagnosis of chronic pancreatitis or pancreatic cancer in the absence of malabsorption, although they do effectively diagnose pancreatic exocrine insufficiency. In the occasional patient with malabsorption secondary to pancreatic insufficiency, these tests effectively establish the diagnosis; however, in most cases of pancreatic insufficiency, pancreatic disease is clinically obvious.

Exocrine pancreatic inhibition. Although the vast majority of investigative efforts have focused on stimulatory factors of pancreatic secretion, substantial evidence suggests that inhibition of basal and meal-induced pancreatic exocrine secretion may be an equally complex process. The contributions of cholinergic, adrenergic, and peptidergic neural input to pancreatic exocrine inhibition have been alluded to earlier in this chapter. A variety of hormones have been proposed as putative inhibitors of exocrine pancreatic secretion. It remains unclear how each peptide is involved in the component phases of meal-induced secretion, yet it seems obvious that meal-induced release occurs.

Hormones that inhibit exocrine function include somatostatin, which inhibits pancreatic bicarbonate and enzyme secretion in response to food, as well as exogenous secretin and CCK; pancreatic polypeptide, which at physiologic doses inhibits meal-induced and exogenously stimulated secretion; pancreatic glucagon, which inhibits secretin- and CCK-induced output in dogs and humans; and galanin, which inhibits meal-induced exocrine secretion. Other potential inhibitors include peptide YY, neuropeptide Y, calcitonin, and calcitonin gene–related peptide.[144]

SUMMARY

Normal pancreatic exocrine secretion consists of a protein component that includes proteolytic, amylolytic, lipolytic, and nucleolytic enzymes important in the normal digestion of carbohydrates, protein, and fats. A watery, bicarbonate component also is important for the neutralization of acidic chyme that is emptied into the duodenum from the stomach. This secretion is under complex control and includes various neural and humoral mechanisms.

The pancreatic secretory response to a meal has been divided into cephalic (vagal), gastric (through the hormone gastrin), and intestinal phases. The earliest response to a meal appears to be primarily mediated through neural and cholinergic mechanisms and requires an intact vagus nerve for full activity. Antral gastrin release modulates this secretory response through stimulation of pancreatic enzyme output. Following delivery of acidic chyme into the proximal duodenum, pancreatic bicarbonate and volume secretion is elicited and probably is partly mediated by release of the hormone secretin from the duodenal mucosa. Intraintestinal fats stimulate both pancreatic bicarbonate and protein secretion, which is most likely mediated by a combination of secretin and CCK release from the duodenum. Intraintestinal peptides and amino acids stimulate pancreatic protein secretion, probably primarily through CCK release. Since plasma concentrations of secretin and CCK are small in response to a meal, potentiated interactions between these two hormones are implicated in full pancreatic secretory activity. Conversely, the role of inhibitors in basal and meal-induced pancreatic exocrine secretion requires additional study.

REFERENCES

1. McLean JM. Embryology of the pancreas. In Howat HT, Sarles H, eds. The Exocrine Pancreas. London: WB Saunders, 1979.
2. Conklin JL. Cytogenesis of the human fetal pancreas. Am J Anat 111:181, 1962.
3. Berman LG, et al. A study of the pancreatic duct system in man by the use of vinyl acetate casts of postmortem preparations. Surg Gynecol Obstet 110:403, 1960.
4. Henderson JR, Daniel PM. A comparative study of the portal vessels connecting the endocrine and exocrine pancreas, with a discussion of some functional implications. Q J Exp Physiol 64:267, 1979.

5. Lifson N, et al. Blood flow to the rabbit pancreas with special reference to the islets of Langerhans. Gastroenterology 7:466, 1980.
6. Chung RS, Safaie-Shirazi S. The effect of secretin on pancreatic blood flow in the awake and anesthetized dog. Proc Soc Exp Biol Med 173:620, 1983.
7. Aune S, Semb LS. The effect of secretin and pancreozymin on pancreatic blood flow in the conscious and anesthetized dog. Acta Physiol 76:406, 1969.
8. Conter RL, Washington L, Kauffman GL Jr. Stimulated pancreatic exocrine secretion does not require pancreatic hyperemia in rats: Potential cholinergic role. Dig Dis Sci 38:1270, 1993.
9. Kvietys PS, et al. Pancreatic Circulation: Intrinsic regulation. Am J Physiol 242(Gastrointest Liver Physiol 5):G596, 1982.
10. Govaerts JP, Kiekens R. Role of vagal innervation on pancreatic secretion. Surgery 62:942, 1968.
11. Harris PF. Anatomy. In Howat HT, Sarles H, eds. The Exocrine Pancreas. London: WB Saunders, 1979.
12. Larsson LI. Innervation of the pancreas by substance P, enkephalin, vasoactive intestinal polypeptide and gastrin/CCK immunoreactive nerves. J Histochem Cytochem 27:1283, 1979.
13. Domschke S, et al. Vasoactive intestinal peptide: A secretin-like partial agonist for pancreatic secretion in man. Gastroenterology 73:478, 1977.
14. Gorelick FS, Jamieson JD. Structure-function relationships of the pancreas. In Johnson LR, ed. Physiology of the Gastrointestinal Tract. New York: Raven Press, 1981.
15. Ingbert DE, Madri JA, Jamieson JD. Neoplastic disorganization of-pancreatic epithelial cells-cell relations. Role of basement membrane. Am J Pathol 121:248, 1985.
16. Dixon JS. Histology: Ultrastructure. In Howat HT, Sarles H, eds. The Exocrine Pancreas. London: WB Saunders, 1979.
17. Ekholm R, Zelander T, Edlund Y. The ultra-structural organization of the rat exocrine pancreas. J Ultrastruct Res 7:61, 1962.
18. Maylie-Pfenninger MF, Jamieson JD. Distribution of cell surface saccharides on pancreatic cells. J Cell Biol 90:77, 1979.
19. Rosenzwig SA, Miller LJ, Jamieson JD. Identification and localization of cholecystokinin binding sites on rat pancreatic plasma membranes and acinar cells: A biochemical and autoradiographical study. J Cell Biol 96:1288, 1983.
20. Opas M, et al. Regulation of expression and intercellular distribution of calreticulin, a major calcium binding protein of non-muscle cells. J Cell Physiol 149:160, 1991.
21. Michalak M, et al. Calreticulin. Biochem J 285:681, 1992.
22. Saraste J, Kuismanen E. Pathways of protein sorting and membrane traffic between the rough endoplasmic reticulum and the Golgi complex. Semin Cell Biol 3:343, 1992.
23. Kreis TE. Regulation of the vesicular and tubular membrane traffic of the Golgi complex by proteins. Curr Opin Cell Biol 4:609, 1992.
24. Orci L, Ravalzzola M, Anderson R. The condensing vacuole of the exocrine cells in more acidic than the mature secretory vesicle. Nature 326:77, 1987.
25. Rapoport TA. Transport of proteins across the endoplasmic reticulum membrane. Science 258:931, 1992.
26. Palade G. Intracellular aspects of the process of protein secretion. Science 189:347, 1975.
27. Jamieson JD, Palade GE. Intracellular transport of secretory proteins int he pancreatic exocrine cell. II. Transport to condensing vacuoles and zymogen granules. J Cell Biol 34:597, 1967.
28. Begin N, Scholefield PG. The uptake of amino acids by mouse pancreas in vitro. 1. General characteristics. Biochem Biophys Acta 90:82, 1964.
29. van Venrooij WJ, et al. Relationship between extracellular amino acids and protein synthesis in vitro in the rat. Eur J Biochem 30:426, 1972.
30. Redman CM, Siekevitz P, Palade GE. Synthesis and transfer of amylase in pigeon pancreatic microsomes. J Biol Chem 241:1150, 1966.
31. Rapiejko PJ, Gillmore R. Protein translocation across the ER requires a functional GTP-binding site in the alpha subunit of the signal recognition particular receptor. J Cell Biol 117:493, 1992.
32. Lingappa VR. Control of protein topology at the endoplasmic reticulum. Cell Biophys 19:1, 1991.
33. Bonifacino JS, Lippincott-Schwartz J. Degradation of proteins within the endoplasmic reticulum. Curr Opin Cell Biol 3:592, 1991.
34. Saraste J, Palada GE, Farquhar MG. Temperature-sensitive steps in the transport of secretory proteins throughout the Golgi complex and in exocrine pancreatic cells. Proc Natl Acad Sci U S A 83:6425, 1986.
35. Rothman JE, Orci L. Molecular dissection of the secretory pathway. Nature 355:409, 1992.
36. Creutz CE, Pazoles CJ, Pollard HB. Self association of synexin in the presence of calcium. J Biol Chem 254:553, 1979.
37. Meldosi J. Membranes and membrane surfaces: Dynamics of cytoplasmic membranes in pancreatic acinar cells. Philos Trans R Soc Lond (Biol) 268:39, 1974.
38. vander Sluijs P, et al. The small GTP-binding protein rab4 controls an early sorting event in the endocystic pathway. Cell 70:729, 1992.
39. Scheele G, Bartelt D, Bieger W. Characterization of human exocrine pancreatic proteins by two-dimensional isoelectric focusing/sodium dodecyl sulfate gel electrophoresis. Gastroenterology 80:461, 1981.
40. Scheele GA, Palade GE. Studies on the guinea pig pancreas: Parallel discharge of exocrine enzyme activities. J Biol Chem 250:2660, 1975.
41. Kraehenbuhl JP, Rocine L, Jamieson JD. Immunocytochemical localization of secretory proteins in bovine pancreatic exocrine cells. J Cell Biol 72:406, 1977.
42. Dagorn JC, Sohel J, Sarles H. Now parallel secretion of enzymes in human duodenal juice and pure pancreatic juice collected by endoscopic retrograde catheterization of the papilla. Gastroenterology 73:42, 1977.
43. Rothman SS. Trypsin and chymotrypsin secretion from the rabbit pancreas in vitro. Am J Physiol 211:777, 1966.
44. Grossman MI, Greengard H, Ivy AC. The effect of dietary composition on pancreatic enzymes. Am J Physiol 138:676, 1943.
45. Desmuelle P, Reboud JP, Ben Abdeljlil A. Influence of the composition of the diet on the enzyme content of the rat pancreas. In de Reuck AUS, Cameron MP, eds. Ciba Foundation Symposium on the Exocrine Pancreas. Boston: Little, Brown, 1962.
46. Morisset J, Dunnigan J. Effects of glucose, amino acids and insulin on adaptation of the exocrine pancreas to diet. Proc Soc Exp Biol Med 140:1308, 1971.
47. Robberecht P, et al. Rat pancreatic hydrolases from birth to weaning and dietary adaptation after weaning. Am J Physiol 221:376, 1971.
48. Schulz F. Electrolyte and fluid secretion in the exocrine pancreas. In Johnson LR, ed. Physiology of the Gastrointestinal Tract. New York: Raven Press, 1981.
49. Grossman MI, Ivy AC. Effect of alloxan upon external secretion of the pancreas. Proc Soc Exp Biol Med 63:62, 1946.
50. Folsch UR, Creutzfeldt W. Pancreatic duct cells in rats: Secretory studies in response to secretin, cholecystokinin-pancreozymin, and gastrin in vivo. Gastroenterology 73:1053, 1977.
51. Almeida AL, Grossman MI. Experimental production of pancreatitis with ethionine. Gastroenterology 20:554, 1952.
52. Carter MJ. Carbonic anhydrase: Isoenzymes, properties, distribution and functional significance. Biol Rev 47:465, 1972.
53. Lightwood R, Reber HA. Micropuncture study of pancreatic secretion in the cat. Gastroenterology 72:61, 1977.
54. Schulz I, Yamagata A, Weske M. Micropuncture studies on the pancreas of the rabbit. Pflugers Arch 308:277, 1969.

55. Rothman SS, Brooks FP. Pancreatic secretion in vitro in "Cl^--free," "Co_2-free" and low Na^+ environment. Am J Physiol 209:790, 1965.
56. Case RM, Scratchard T. The secretion of alkali metal ions by the perfused cat pancreas as influenced by the composition and osmolality of the external environment and by inhibitors of metabolism and Na^+,K^+-ATPase activity. J Physiol 242:415, 1974.
57. Case RM, Harper AA, Scratchard T. Ionic requirements for pancreatic secretion. Proc Int Anion Physiol Sci XXIV Washington Abstr 230, 1968.
58. Schultz I. Influence of bicarbonate, $CO_2$1 and glycodiazine buffer on the secretion of the isolated cat pancreas. Pflugers Arch 329:283, 1971.
59. Swanson CH, Solomon AK. Micropuncture analysis of the cellular mechanisms of electrolyte secretion by the in vitro rabbit pancreas. J Gen Physiol 65:22, 1975.
60. Case RM, Scratchard T, Wynne RD. The origin and secretion of pancreatic juice bicarbonate. J Physiol (Lond) 210:1, 1970.
61. Argent BE, et al. The pancreatic duct cell: Report on a conference. Pancreas 7:403, 1992.
62. Bro-Rasmussen F, Killmann SA, Thaysen JH. The composition of pancreatic juice as compared to sweat, parotid saliva, and tears. Acta Physiol Scand 37:97, 1956.
63. Case RM, Harper AA, Scratchard T. The secretion of electrolytes and enzymes by the pancreas of the anesthetized cat. J Physiol 201:335, 1969.
64. Case RM, Clausen T. The relationship between calcium exchange and enzyme secretion in the isolated rat pancreas. J Physiol 235:75, 1973.
65. Williams JA, Chandler D. Ca^{++} and pancreatic amylase release. Am J Physiol 228:1729, 1975.
66. Volpe P, et al. "Calcisome," a cytoplasmic organelle, the inositol, 1,4,5-triophosphate-sensitive Ca^{2+} store of non-muscle cells? Proc Natl Acad Sci U S A 85:1091, 1988.
67. Peikin SR, et al. Kinetics of amylase release by dispersed acini prepared from guinea pig pancreas. Am J Physiol 235:E743, 1978.
68. Burnham DB, Williams JA. Activation of protein kinase activity in pancreatic acini by calcium and cAMP. Am J Physiol 246:G500, 1984.
69. Edervenn AGH, et al. Phosphorylation of low molecular mass cytosolic proteins by protein kinase C and protein kinase A in the rabbit exocrine pancreas. Eur J Biochem 185:461, 1989.
70. Gardner JD, Jensen RT. Regulation of pancreatic enzyme secretion in vitro. In Johnson LR, ed. Physiology of the Gastrointestinal Tract. New York: Raven Press, 1981.
71. Hickson JD. The secretion of pancreatic juice in response to stimulation of the vagus nerves in the pig. J Physiol (Lond) 206:275, 1970.
72. Holst JJ, Schaffalitzky de Muckadell OB, Fahrenkrug J. Nervous control of pancreatic exocrine secretion in pig. Acta Physiol Scand 105:33, 1979.
73. Magee DF, White TT. Influence of vagal stimulation on secretion of pancreatic juice in pigs. Ann Surg 161:605, 1965.
74. Hickson JD. The secretory and vascular response to nervous and hormonal stimulation in the pancreas of the pigs. J Physiol (Lond) 206:299, 1970.
75. Wormsley KG. Pancreatic secretion: Physiological control. In Duthie HL, Wormsley KG, eds. Scientific Basis of Gastroenterology. Edinburgh: Churchill Livingstone, 1979.
76. Lee KY, et al. A hormonal mechanism for the inter-digestive pancreatic secretion in dogs. Am J Physiol 251:G759, 1986.
77. Singer MV, et al. Latency of pancreatic enzyme response to intraduodenal stimulants. Am J Physiol 238(Gastrointest Liver Physiol 1):G23, 1980.
78. Williams JA, et al. Quantitative electron microscopy autoradiographs of [^{125}I]-cholecystokinin in pancreatic asini. Am J Physiol 243:G291, 1982.
79. Rosenzwig SA, Miller LJ, Jamieson JD. Identification and localization of cholecystokinin-binding sites on the rat pancreatic plasma membranes and acinar cells: A biochemical and autoradiographic study. J Cell Biol 96:1288, 1983.
80. Stening GF, Grossman MI. Gastrin related peptides as stimulants of pancreatic and gastric secretion. Am J Physiol 217:262, 1969.
81. Iwai K, et al. Purification and sequencing of a trypsin-sensitive cholecystokinin-releasing peptide from rat pancreatic juice. J Biochem 262:8956, 1987.
82. Lu L, Louie D, Owyang C. A cholecystokinin releasing peptide mediates feedback regulation of pancreatic secretion. Am J Physiol 256:G430, 1989.
83. Debas HT, Grossman MI. Pure cholecystokinin: Pancreatic protein and bicarbonate response. Digestion 9:464, 1973.
84. Li P, et al. Mechanism of acid-induced releasing secretin in rats: Presence of a secretin releasing factor. J Clin Invest 86:1474, 1990.
85. Novis BH, Bank S, Markes IM. The cephalic phase of pancreatic secretion in man. Scand J Gastroenterol 6:417, 1971.
86. Sarles H, et al. Cephalic phase of pancreatic secretion in man. Gut 9:214, 1968.
87. Defillip C, Solomon TE, Valenzela JE. Pancreatic secretory response to sham feeding in humans. Digestion 23:217, 1982.
88. Katschinski M, et al. Cephalic stimulation of gastrointestinal secretory and motor responses in humans. Gastroenterology 103:383, 1992.
89. Bergman RN, Miller RE. Direct enhancement of insulin secretion by vagal stimulation of the isolated pancreas. Am J Physiol 226:481, 1973.
90. DeFillipi C, Solomon TE, Valenzuela JE. Pancreatic secretory response to sham feeding in humans. Digestion 23:217, 1982.
91. Preshaw RM, Cooke AR, Grossman MI. Sham feeding and pancreatic secretion in the dog. Gastroenterology 50:171, 1966.
92. Valenzuela JE, Walsh JH, Isenberg JI. Effect of gastrin on pancreatic enzyme secretion and gallbladder emptying in man. Gastroenterology 71:409, 1976.
93. Pavlov IP. The Work of the Digestive Gland, Lecture VII. London: Griffin, 1992.
94. Furukawa N, Okada H. Effects of stimulation of the hypothalamic area on pancreatic exocrine secretion in dogs. Gastroenterology 97:1534, 1989.
95. Conter RL, Hughes MT, Kauffman GL Jr. Intracerebroventricular secretin enhances pancreatic volume and bicarbonate response in rats. Surgery (in press).
96. White TT, Lundh G, Magee DF. Evidence of existence of a gastro-pancreatic reflex. Am J Physiol 198:725, 1960.
97. White TT, McAlexander RA, Magee DF. The effect of gastric distension on duodenal aspirates in man. Gastroenterology 44:48, 1965.
98. Meyer JH, et al. Sieving of solid food by the canine stomach and sieving after gastric surgery. Gastroenterology 76:804, 1979.
99. MacGregor I, Parent J, Meyer JH. Gastric emptying of liquid meals and pancreatic and biliary secretion after subtotal gastrectomy or truncal vagotomy and pyloroplasty in man. Gastroenterology 72:195, 1977.
100. Thomas JW, Mason FE. The effects of gastric exclusion operations on pancreatic exocrine secretion. Surgery 75:461, 1974.
101. Debas HT, Yamagishi T. Evidence for pyloropancreatic reflex for pancreatic exocrine secretion. Am J Physiol 234:E468, 1978.
102. Wang CC, Grossman MI. Physiological determination of release of secretin and pancreozymin from intestine of dogs with transplanted pancreas. Am J Physiol 164:527, 1951.
103. Singer MV. Latency of pancreatic fluid secretory response to intestinal stimulants in the dog. J Physiol 339:75, 1983.
104. Kelleher J, Lowsowsky MS, Ruddell WSJ. Assessment of rapid pancreatic isoenzyme assay as a screening test for pancreatic disease. Br Med J 18:791, 1983.
105. Dürr HK, et al. Faecal chymotrypsin: A study on its diagnostic value by comparison with the secretin-cholecystokinin test. Digestion 17:404, 1978.

106. Meyer JH, Way LW, Grossman MI. Pancreatic bicarbonate response to various acids in duodenum of the dog. Am J Physiol 219:964, 1970.
107. Moore EW, Verine HJ, Grossman MI. Pancreatic bicarbonate response to a meal. Acta Hepato-Gastroenterol 26:30, 1979.
108. Meyer JH, Way LW, Grossman MI. Pancreatic response to acidification of various lengths of proximal intestine in the dog. Am J Physiol 219:971, 1970.
109. Annis D, Hallenbeck GA. Effect of excluding pancreatic juice from duodenum on secretory response of pancreas to a meal. Proc Soc Exp Biol Med 77:383, 1951.
110. Grossman MI, Konturek SJ. Gastric acid does drive pancreatic bicarbonate secretion. Scand J Gastroenterol 9:299, 1974.
111. Fahrenkrug J, et al. pH threshold for release of secretin in normal subjects and in patients with duodenal ulcer and patients with chronic pancreatitis. Scand J Gastroenterol 13:177, 1978.
112. Malagelada JR, Go VLW, Summerskill WJH. Different gastric, pancreatic, and biliary responses to solid-liquid or homogenized meals. Dig Dis Sci 24:101, 1979.
113. Solomon TE, Grossman MI, Meyer JH. Pancreatic response to intestinal perfusion with lactic acid or acidified albumin. Am J Physiol 235:E560, 1978.
114. Rayford PL, Miller TA, Thompson JC. Secretin, cholecystokinin and newer gastrointestinal hormones. N Engl J Med 294:1093, 1976.
115. Lee KY, Tai HH, Chey WY. Plasma secretin and gastrin responses to a meat meal and duodenal acidification in dogs. Am J Physiol 230:784, 1976.
116. Miller TA, et al. The effect of fat on secretin release. Ann Surg 187:303, 1978.
117. Schaffalitzky de Muckadell OB, Fahrenkrug J. Secretion pattern of secretin in man: Regulation by gastric acid. Gut 19:812, 1978.
118. Beglinger C, Grossman MI, Solomon TE. Interaction between stimulants of exocrine pancreatic secretion in dogs. Am J Physiol 246:G173, 1984.
119. Chey WY, et al. Effect of rabbit antisecretin serum on postprandial pancreatic secretion in dogs. Gastroenterology 77:1268, 1979.
120. Malagelada JR, et al. Regulation of pancreatic and gallbladder functions by intraluminal fatty acids and bile acids in man. J Clin Invest 58:493, 1976.
121. Meyer JH. Release of secretin and cholecystokinin. In Thompson JC, ed. Gastrointestinal Hormones. Austin: University of Texas Press, 1975.
122. Meyer JH, Jones RS. Canine pancreatic responses to intestinally perfused fat and products of fat digestion. Am J Physiol 226:1178, 1974.
123. Fink AS, Luxenburg M, Meyer JH. Regionally perfused fatty acids augment acid-induced canine pancreatic secretion. Am J Physiol 245(Gastrointest Liver Physiol 8):G78, 1983.
124. Fink AS, Meyer JH. Intraduodenal emulsions of oleic acid augment acid-induced canine pancreatic secretion. Am J Physiol 245(Gastrointest Liver Physiol 8):G85, 1983.
125. Byrnes DJ, et al. Radioimmunoassay of cholecystokinin in human plasma. Clin Chim Acta 111:81, 1981.
126. Walsh JH, Lamers CB, Valenzuela JE. Cholecystokinin-octapeptidelike immunoreactivity in human plasma. Gastroenterology 82:438, 1982.
127. Jansen JBMJ, Lamers CBHW. Radioimmunoassay of cholecystokinin in human tissue and plasma. Clin Chim Acta 131:305, 1983.
128. Fried GM, et al. Release of cholecystokinin in conscious dogs: Correlation with simultaneous measurements of gallbladder pressure and pancreatic protein secretion. Gastroenterology 85:1113, 1983.
129. Faichney A, et al. Effect of sodium oleate on plasma secretin concentration and pancreatic secretion in dog. Gastroenterology 81:458, 1981.
130. Stabile BE, et al. Intravenous mixed amino acids and fats do not stimulate exocrine pancreatic secretion. Am J Physiol 246:G274, 1984.
131. Go VLW, Hoffman AF, Summerskill WHJ. Pancreozymin bioassay in man based on pancreatic enzyme secretion: Potency of specific amino acids and other digestive products. J Clin Invest 49:1558, 1970.
132. Meyer JH, et al. Canine gut receptors mediating pancreatic responses to luminal L-amino acids. Am J Physiol 231:669, 1976.
133. Meyer JH, Kelley GA. Canine pancreatic responses to intestinally perfused proteins and protein digests. Am J Physiol 231:682, 1976.
134. Meyer JH, Kelly GA, Jones RS. Canine pancreatic response to intestinally perfused oligopeptides. Am J Physiol 231:678, 1976.
135. Schneeman BO, Lyman RL. Factors involved in the intestinal feedback regulation of pancreatic enzyme secretion in the rat. Proc Soc Exp Biol Med 148:897, 1975.
136. Sale JK, et al. Chronic and acute studies indicating absence of exocrine pancreatic feedback inhibition in dogs. Digestion 15:540, 1977.
137. Krawisz BR, et al. In the absence of nutrients pancreatic-biliary secretions in the jejunum do not exert feedback control of human pancreatic or gastric function. J Lab Clin Med 95:13, 1980.
138. Slaff J, et al. Protease-specific suppression of pancreatic exocrine secretion. Gastroenterology 87:44, 1984.
139. Fink AS, et al. Digests of protein augment acid-induced canine pancreatic secretion. Am J Physiol 242(Gastrointestin Liver Physiol 4):G634, 1982.
140. Lankisch PG. Progress report: Exocrine pancreatic function tests. Gut 23:777, 1982.
141. Gullo L, Sarles H, Mott C. Functional investigation of the exocrine pancreas following acute pancreatitis. Rendic Gastroenterol 4:18, 1972.
142. Lundh G. Pancreatic exocrine function in neoplastic and inflammatory disease: A simple and reliable new test. Gastroenterology 42:275, 1962.
143. Boyd EJS, Wormsley KG. The assessment of chronic pancreatitis. In Burns GP, Banks S, eds. Disorders of the Pancreas: Current Issues in Diagnosis and Management. New York: McGraw-Hill, 1992, p 283.
144. Mannon P, Taylor FL. The pancreatic polypeptide family. In Walsh JH, Dockray GJ, eds. Gut Peptides. New York: Raven Press, 1994, p 341.

27

Acute and Chronic Pancreatitis

Mark T. Toyama, Stanley W. Ashley, and Howard A. Reber

Pancreatitis is an inflammatory process involving the pancreas that can manifest in acute and chronic forms.[1] Acute pancreatitis is usually associated with full recovery of exocrine and endocrine function when the underlying inflammation has resolved. Under most circumstances, chronic pancreatitis is associated with permanent impairment of both exocrine and endocrine function. The development of chronic pancreatitis may be insidious or may involve repeated episodes of acute inflammation indistinguishable clinically from acute pancreatitis. Despite the overlap that may exist between the acute and chronic forms of pancreatitis, they are distinct clinical entities and are discussed as such in this chapter.

ACUTE PANCREATITIS

Pathology

In mild forms of acute pancreatitis, pancreatic edema is the most prominent feature.[2] Grossly, the pancreas appears boggy and indurated. Microscopically, the pancreatic lobules are separated by edematous fluid without evidence of hemorrhage. There is a variable amount of interlobular infiltration by inflammatory cells. The acinar cells show no evidence of necrosis, and blood flow appears to be maintained in the small capillaries and venules. In severe cases, the edema and accompanying inflammation may extend throughout the retroperitoneum and to surrounding organs. Acute fluid collections often develop. Fat necrosis is common in acute pancreatitis and appears as raised, whitish-gray areas in the retroperitoneum, omentum, or mesentery.

If the initial inflammatory process progresses, pancreatic necrosis can occur. Grossly, the pancreas appears first hemorrhagic and then frankly necrotic. The surface of the pancreas may appear dark and devitalized, although it can look normal if the dead tissue is located deep within the gland. The acinar cells undergo nuclear and cytoplasmic degeneration, in association with thrombosis of the nutrient vessels that supply the individual lobules. Necrotic areas are found adjacent to healthy lobules, along with an intense inflammatory reaction and cellular infiltration. Interstitial hemorrhage can also occur.

Early in the disease, the acinar cell organelles responsible for protein synthesis appear abnormal. However, zymogen granules remain intact until late in the process of acinar cell necrosis. It is then that pancreatic enzymes may be released as the terminal event of acinar cell death.

Pathogenesis

Acute pancreatitis may result from a variety of causes (see accompanying box). It is generally believed that these inciting factors initiate a common chain of events leading to autodigestion of the pancreas. In all forms of acute pancreatitis, it has been proposed that pancreatic enzymes, normally inactive and confined to acinar cells or ducts, pass instead into the interstitium of the gland, where they are activated and digest the gland itself.[3] The mechanisms of this final common pathway are poorly defined, although recent findings suggest that enzyme activation may actually occur within the acinar cells themselves. In the normal

ETIOLOGIES OF ACUTE PANCREATITIS

Biliary tract disease (e.g., cholelithiasis)
Alcohol
Drugs
Trauma
Hyperparathyroidism (elevated calcium)
Malnutrition (protein/calorie deficit)
Hyperlipidemia
Pancreatic duct obstruction
Duodenal obstruction
Infection
Ischemia
Familial
Scorpion venom
Idiopathic

pancreas, inactive enzymes are packaged in zymogen granules that fuse with the cell membrane and release their contents into the ductal lumen when secretion occurs. In several animal models of acute pancreatitis, Steer et al.[4] showed that the zymogen granules fail to fuse with the membrane and instead join with lysosomes (colocalization) (Fig. 27-1). The lysosomes contain the enzyme cathepsin B, which may convert trypsinogen to trypsin within the living cell. Steer proposed that this could be the event initiating autodigestion and inflammation, but this hypothesis remains controversial.

In any case, activated enzymes and inflammatory mediators are then released into the interstitium, retroperitoneum, and peritoneal cavity. Absorption of these potential toxins is believed to account for some of the systemic effects of the disease. However, the severity of the systemic illness and the progression of changes within the gland may be related to factors other than the direct effects of pancreatic enzymes.[5,6] Some pancreatic enzymes can activate humoral systems throughout the body. For example, trypsin generates bradykinin from kallikrein in experimental acute pancreatitis. Complement factors (C3a and C5a) have also been recovered from the serum in significant quantities during acute pancreatitis in both experimental animals and humans; trypsin can also activate many of these factors. Such secondary humoral systems are undoubtedly important in the development and perpetuation of the cardiovascular, pulmonary, and renal complications seen in acute pancreatitis, but their exact roles remain to be determined.

Mechanisms

Acute pancreatitis in humans is most commonly associated with the passage of gallstones through the bile ducts into the duodenum, but a number of other causes have been identified. Although the mechanisms responsible for the initiation of pancreatitis in these situations are unknown, several hypotheses have been proposed on the basis of clinical and experimental evidence: (1) pancreatic duct obstruction, (2) common-channel phenomenon, (3) reflux of activated enzymes into the pancreatic duct, and (4) alterations in pancreatic duct permeability.

Pancreatic Duct Obstruction

This hypothesis applies most directly to gallstone-associated disease. Even when gallstones are not found obstruct-

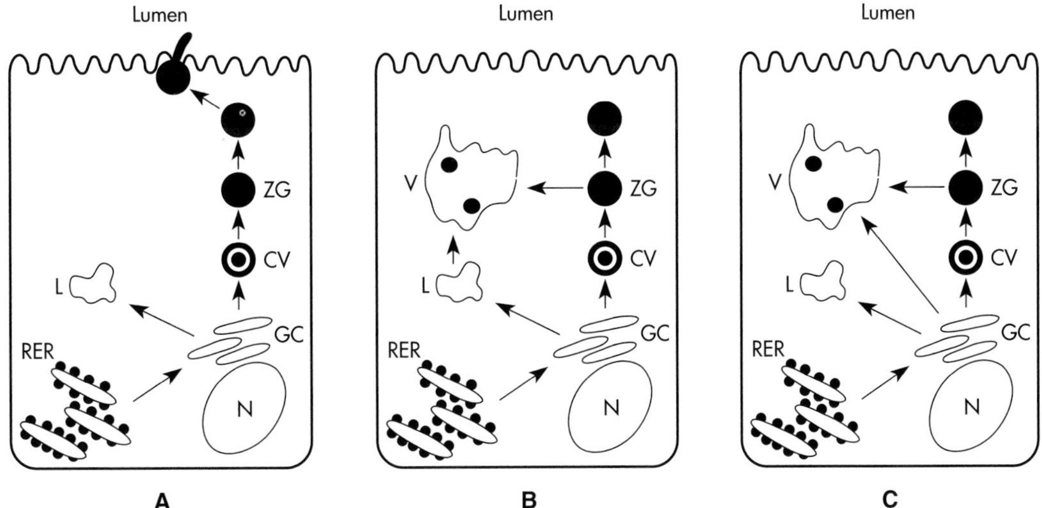

Fig. 27-1. Intracellular transport of digestive enzymes and lysosomal hydrolases. Digestive enzymes and lysosomal hydrolases are synthesized in the rough endoplasmic reticulum *(RER)*. Newly synthesized enzymes are transported to the Golgi complex *(GC)* adjacent to the nucleus *(N)*. **A,** Normal separation of lysosomal hydrolases, which are transported to lysosomes *(L)* and digestive enzymes. Digestive enzymes are then concentrated in condensing vacuoles *(CV)* and zymogen granules *(ZG)* that fuse with the luminal plasma membrane and release their contents into the luminal space by exocytosis. **B,** Changes induced in mice fed the choline-deficient, ethionine-supplemented diet, which blocks exocytosis and causes digestive enzymes and zymogen granules to accumulate. The zymogen granules fuse with lysosomes (crinophagy), causing the formation of large vacuoles *(V)* that contain both lysosomal hydrolases and digestive zymogens. **C,** In rats given infusions of supramaximal doses of cerulein, transport to the Golgi complex is unaffected. Impaired separation of lysosomal hydrolases and digestive zymogens results in the formation of large vacuoles that contain both types of enzymes. Mature zymogen granules also fuse with these vacuoles by a process analogous to crinophagy. Exocytosis at the luminal plasma membrane is blocked. (From Steer ML, Medolesi J. The cell biology of experimental pancreatitis. N Engl J Med 316:149, 1987. Copyright 1987 Massachusetts Medical Society.)

ing the ampulla, they can be recovered in the stool of 85% to 90% of patients with gallstone-associated pancreatitis.[7] Although the exact mechanisms remain controversial, passage of gallstones through the common duct and ampulla could initiate pancreatitis in a variety of ways. Direct obstruction of the pancreatic duct could occur through impaction of a gallstone at the ampulla. Alternatively, the passage of a stone could cause inflammation with spasm of the sphincter of Oddi and common duct obstruction at the point where it enters the duodenum. Interestingly, sphincter spasm has been shown to occur in experimental animals after ingestion of alcohol, so this hypothesis may also be relevant in alcohol-induced disease.

The relationship between pancreatic duct obstruction and pancreatitis has not been clearly defined, although it is known that secretion of pancreatic juice into the obstructed duct leads to intraductal pressure.[8] This pressure could rupture the ducts, and pancreatic enzymes could then leak into the interstitium. Although this scenario makes conceptual sense, the experimental evidence is contradictory. For example, in most animal models, complete obstruction of the duct produces pancreatic atrophy rather than acute pancreatitis. In contrast, prolonged secretory stimulation against a totally obstructed duct leads to hemorrhagic pancreatitis in dogs.[9] Such total obstruction is probably not common clinically, but partial obstruction during secretion does occur and may cause pancreatic edema.[10] Most experiments that have examined the effects of increased pressure in the pancreatic duct have used forceful retrograde injection at pressures as great as 300 mm Hg. Histologic examination shows that ducts rupture at these pressures. However, the maximum pressure that is generated by active secretion in an obstructed pancreatic duct is only about 40 mm Hg, and this pressure alone is not associated with pancreatitis.[11] Although ductal obstruction is probably important, it is likely that other factors must be operative. The various hypotheses are not mutually exclusive, and it may be that elements of each are important in different settings.

Common-Channel Hypothesis

The common bile and pancreatic ducts usually join for a variable distance, before they open into the ampulla of Vater and the duodenum. If this "common channel" is long enough (e.g., >1 cm), it could become obstructed by a gallstone. In such a circumstance, the common channel may have particular significance in the pathogenesis of acute pancreatitis. If the channel itself is obstructed, bile could reflux under pressure into the pancreatic duct and damage it. Pancreatic and biliary manometry during secretory stimulation have shown that the pressure in the pancreatic duct is generally greater than that in the bile duct. Thus, if there is reflux of bile into the pancreatic duct, it probably would occur passively and at low pressure. Even at low pressures, however, bile can be injurious. For example, experimental exposure of the ducts to deconjugated bile salts during low-pressure perfusion damages the ducts. The resultant increase in pancreatic duct permeability permits leakage of large molecules (e.g.. pancreatic enzymes) out of the ductal lumen.[12] Because deconjugation of bile salts frequently results from bacterial infection of the bile, reflux of these substances into the pancreatic duct could be an inciting mechanism in some cases of pancreatitis. Reflux of contrast material into the pancreatic duct has been demonstrated by cholangiography in patients with gallstone pancreatitis. Reflux has also been shown, however, in patients with gallstone disease but without pancreatitis. Thus, the exact role of biliary-pancreatic duct reflux in the initiation of acute pancreatitis remains incompletely defined.

It may be that some other factor is necessary, in addition to ductal obstruction and an increase in duct permeability. For example, recent studies suggest that duct obstruction results in an increased release of duodenal cholecystokinin (CCK) and an elevated plasma CCK level. This could stimulate pancreatic secretion and might also play a role in the pathogenesis of pancreatitis. There is experimental evidence that the severity of pancreatitis is greater when CCK levels are high.[13]

Reflux of Activated Pancreatic Enzymes

Enzymes secreted into the pancreatic ducts are inactive, and they remain so until activation in the duodenum, where they are exposed to enterokinase. Pancreatitis could result from reflux of activated enzymes from the duodenum back into the pancreatic duct. Normally, the sphincter of Oddi effectively prevents reflux, but stone passage may at least temporarily inhibit the efficacy of this sphincter mechanism. Destruction of the ampulla, which allows free communication between the duodenum and the pancreatic duct, has produced hemorrhagic pancreatitis in experimental animals. However, patients who have undergone sphincteroplasty do not have an increased incidence of pancreatitis. Reflux of duodenal contents into the pancreatic duct has not been demonstrated in humans. Thus, there are no clinical analogies to suggest that this mechanism is important in human disease. In addition, experimental perfusion of normal pancreatic ducts with activated enzymes at normal pressures does not induce acute pancreatitis.[14]

Duct Permeability

During pancreatic secretion, the pancreatic duct normally contains inactive pancreatic enzymes. Because most of these enzymes are large molecules (e.g., 25 to 50 kd), they remain within the duct lumen. As discussed previously, however, experimental exposure of the ducts to bile salts, ethanol, or elevated ductal pressures increases the permeability of the ducts. It is in this setting that pancreatic enzymes can leak into the interstitium. If the enzymes are activated, acute pancreatitis occurs. Thus, duct permeability may be important in human disease.[1]

Other Mechanisms

Alcohol. Like bile, ethanol is known to induce pancreatitis. Several theories have been proposed to explain ethanol's effects on the pancreas.[15] For example, the toxic-metabolic hypothesis suggests that ethanol (or its metabolic by-product acetaldehyde) has a direct cytotoxic effect on the pancreas, and that this initiates the pancreatitis. The ductal plug theory postulates that ethanol alters pancreatic secretion so that it contains an abnormally high protein concentration. As a result, precipitation of protein occurs in the small pancreatic ducts, obstructing them. This ductal obstruction leads to the characteristic pancreatic inflammation. There is some evidence to support each of these hypotheses, and both may be important. The role of ethanol in the development of pancreatitis is discussed more fully in the section on chronic pancreatitis.

Hyperparathyroidism. Early studies found that the incidence of pancreatitis among patients with hyperparathyroidism was as high as 20%, but more recent reports indicate a lower figure of 1% to 2%.[16] These differences may reflect the fact that hyperparathyroidism is recognized earlier today in most patients because of the wide use of modern automated laboratory analyses. Thus, the disease usually is diagnosed before pancreatitis develops. The cause of acute pancreatitis in patients with hyperparathyroidism is unknown. Elevated serum concentrations of parathyroid hormone (PTH) and hypercalcemia both have been implicated, but elevation of PTH in experimental animals does not produce pancreatitis.[17,18] On the other hand, hypercalcemia does increase pancreatic duct permeability and allows the development of pancreatitis in animals. Acute pancreatitis has been reported in patients with hypercalcemia from a number of causes other than hyperparathyroidism. In every case, the pancreatitis resolved after removal of the abnormal parathyroid tissue or reduction of the serum calcium concentration.[16] In evaluating such patients, it is important to exclude other causes of pancreatitis before concluding that the pancreatitis will resolve with treatment of the endocrine abnormality.

Hyperlipidemia. Hyperlipidemia is an occasional cause of abdominal pain and pancreatitis.[19] It may be primary, caused by one of the familial forms of lipid disorders, most commonly type V (Fredrickson and Lees classification). It also may be secondary caused by the ingestion of certain drugs (e.g., estrogen contraceptives). In patients with hyperlipidemia the course of the pancreatitis generally parallels the elevation of the serum triglycerides. Thus, as the concentrations of lipid decreases, the abdominal pain and pancreatitis subside. The mechanism of the pancreatitis in hyperlipidemia is not known. Experiments in dogs have shown that high concentrations of free fatty acids in the pancreatic microcirculation damage the pancreas.[20] These fatty acids are thought to injure the capillary endothelium or the acinar cell membranes directly. The generation of free-radical oxygen metabolites may be important and has recently received increasing attention in this and other forms of the disease.

Drugs. Pancreatitis caused by specific drugs is uncommon. Anticholinesterases, azathioprine, 2,3-dideoxyinosine, L-asparaginase, salicylates, thiazide diuretics, valproic acid, *Vinca* alkaloids, and estrogen have been most firmly established as possible causative or contributory agents. Pancreatitis may subside in a patient after withdrawal of any of these drugs and recur when the drug is reinstituted. Weaker associations have been observed with biguanides, cisplatin, antituberculous agents, cyclosporine A, H_2-blocking agents, loop diuretics, 6-mercaptopurine, metronidazole, pentamidine, steroids, sulfonamides, sulindac, and tetracycline.[21-23] The pathogenesis of the pancreatitis associated with these drugs is unknown, but they may act as a trigger or cofactor in the induction of the inflammation.

Infection. Pancreatitis has been associated with viral, bacterial, and parasitic disorders.[24-27] Among the viral agents, mumps and coxsackie virus are most common. Pancreatitis is also more common in patients with AIDS; this is probably the result of associated cytomegalovirus infection. The precise mechanisms are unknown

Ischemia. Acute pancreatitis has been described in after aortic aneurysm rupture, in other shocklike states, and after cardiopulmonary bypass.[28] In these patients, ultrastructural studies of the pancreas showed alteration in the cellular synthetic organelles, but the zymogen granules were released only after cell necrosis. These morphologic findings are similar to the changes that occurred in the other experimental models discussed previously.

In hypotensive patients, the onset of pancreatitis parallels the damage to the other organs sensitive to poor perfusion. Commonly, renal failure is also present in patients with ischemia-related acute pancreatitis. Although there is strong evidence that impaired perfusion of the pancreas during shock can cause pancreatitis, the role of ischemia in nonshock conditions remains to be determined. Evidence is accumulating to suggest that microvascular stasis is important in the evolution of other forms of the disease, and this is under active study.[29,30]

Multifactorial Origin of Pancreatitis

The pathogenesis of pancreatitis is probably multifactorial. For example, a common channel may predispose some patients toward pancreatitis through duct obstruction or reflux of bile. Increased duct permeability could follow either event. Physical and biochemical changes in acinar cells from a toxin such as ethanol or from ischemia may affect the synthesis, storage, activation, and discharge of pancreatic digestive enzymes, causing pancreatitis in other cells.

The sequential development of pathologic changes after the initiation of acute pancreatitis requires further study. Although the pancreas may continue to secrete enzymes that could cause progressive gland necrosis, this seems unlikely because the zymogen granules appear to remain in the cells until late in the disease. Secretory studies during acute pancreatitis in humans indicate that the response to stimulation is impaired. This impairment may continue for several weeks, even in the patient without symptoms. Experimental studies in animals corroborate these findings. Thus, the role of secretion in the initiation and progression of pancreatitis (as well as that of inhibition of secretion in its treatment) remains unclear.

Ischemia may play a role in the conversion of edematous pancreatitis into the necrotizing form because ischemia itself is known to produce pancreatitis. Moreover, the necrosis of pancreatic tissue in edematous pancreatitis is associated with small-vessel thrombosis. Animal studies have shown that large-vessel occlusion can convert edematous pancreatitis to a form of pancreatitis characterized by hemorrhage and necrosis. In our current state of knowledge, it is uncertain whether vascular thrombosis is the cause or effect of the necrosis.

Pathophysiologic Effects of Pancreatitis

Fluid Sequestration

In response to inflammation, patients with acute pancreatitis may sequester 2 L or more of fluid in the abdominal cavity and retroperitoneum. The most frequent site of fluid accumulation is the lesser sac; other sites are the spaces posterior to the pancreas and anterior to the kidneys. In most patients with uncomplicated edematous pancreatitis, ascitic fluid is straw-colored and without necrotic debris. It becomes blood-tinged, or "prune juice–colored," in more severe forms. The color of the fluid obtained from paracentesis at hospital admission has been used to predict the severity of disease.

Fat Necrosis

Fat necrosis is the result of local or systemic pancreatic enzyme activation in patients with acute pancreatitis.[31] Locally, it is found within the intralobular septa of the gland, in the retroperitoneum, and in the abdominal cavity. Although the fluid sequestered in the abdominal cavity contains a variety of enzymes, only lipase in combination with colipase causes necrosis of fat. These necrotic areas are sharply demarcated from the healthy fat in omentum or mesentery and appear as whitish-gray, firm plaques. Chemical analysis of the plaques reveals high concentrations of lipase, calcium, and free fatty acids. It is thought that calcium binds with the free fatty acids in the process of saponification. Although this may contribute to the reduction in serum calcium seen in some patients with severe pancreatitis, there are probably multiple causes for the hypocalcemia.

Fat necrosis is also occasionally found outside the abdominal cavity, in the subcutaneous tissue of the extremities and in the bone marrow. The subcutaneous lesions, which are similar morphologically to the abdominal ones, appear during an episode of acute pancreatitis. Histologically, these areas of fat necrosis are similar to those noted in the abdomen. Serum amylase concentrations are usually elevated, even though serum lipase concentrations may be normal, perhaps as a result of the consumption of lipase in the process of lipolysis. The extent of fat necrosis throughout the body correlates with the severity of the disease. Patients with multiple sites of involvement are less likely to survive. The lesions frequently disappear with resolution of the disease or after pancreatectomy.

Peripheral fat necrosis also may occur in the joints, where a significant synovitis can develop. Arthrocentesis reveals a cloudy or creamy fluid with elevated concentrations of lipase.

Cardiovascular Effects

Hypovolemia resulting from the fluid sequestration and systemic capillary leak that result from the release of inflammatory mediators may account for oliguria, decreased cardiac output, and hypotension seen during acute pancreatitis. However, hypovolemia alone cannot account for all the systemic manifestations of the disease.

The usual response to fluid sequestration in uncomplicated acute pancreatitis is a compensatory increase in cardiac output. Pulse rate and cardiac contractility normally increase in response to mild hypovolemia. In severe pancreatitis, however, this myocardial response may be impaired. In this situation, the pulse rate may increase but the cardiac output does not. Even when intravascular volume is restored by intravenous fluid administration, there may be a variety of abnormalities in cardiovascular function (see accompanying box). These include a progressive depression of left ventricular stroke work, accompanied by an increasing pulmonary capillary wedge pressure.[32] Not only is cardiac output decreased, but tissue perfusion also falls.[33] Interestingly, no histologic changes have been noted in the myocardium of patients who died of acute pancreatitis, and such noninvasive tests of the heart as echocardiography have not demonstrated structural abnormalities.[2]

Humoral factors released from the pancreas may be important in the development of cardiovascular complications. For example, bradykinin and other members of the kallikrein system are increased both in patients and in experimental animals with acute pancreatitis. These substances are known to alter cardiac and vascular function in ways that could explain the changes seen. The effects of pancreatic enzymes on cardiac function have not been studied.

A myocardial depressant factor (MDF) has been isolated from the serum of experimental animals with acute pancreatitis and those with hypovolemic shock.[33] The production of MDF in experimental pancreatitis is temporally related to the release of lysosomal enzymes from pancreatic acinar cells. A substance thought to be MDF has been isolated from the serum of patients with hypovolemic shock, but it has not been isolated from patients with pancreatitis. Thus, the role of MDF in mediating the

CHANGES IN CARDIOVASCULAR FUNCTION IN ACUTE PANCREATITIS

Depressed contractility
Decreased left ventricular stroke work
Decreased systemic vascular resistance
Decreased tissue perfusion
Electrocardiographic abnormalities
ST-segment and T-wave changes

cardiovascular alterations associated with pancreatitis remains to be determined.

Renal Alterations

Oliguria is common in patients with acute pancreatitis and fluid sequestration. In uncomplicated disease, the urinary output increases when intravascular volume is overfilled. In more severe cases, acute renal failure may ensue, and oliguria may persist for 3 days or longer. In most patients with uncomplicated disease, the blood urea nitrogen (BUN) rises to approximately 40 mg/dl and the creatinine rises to approximately 6 mg/dl. These levels promptly return to normal with adequate fluid replacement.[34]

In some patients with acute pancreatitis, renal function may be impaired without any history of hypotension. In such cases, there is often microscopic evidence of a membranous glomerulopathy and acute tubular necrosis. Other studies have demonstrated fat emboli in the small renal arterioles. These observations have not been investigated experimentally. In fact, some investigators have noted hypertension during the first 72 hours of acute disease.[35] The cause is unknown, but in these patients, the systemic and renal vascular resistances are both elevated and the renal plasma flow and glomerular filtration rate are both decreased. The significance of these observations and the mechanisms responsible are unknown.

Respiratory Alterations

From 50% to 60% of patients with acute pancreatitis exhibit arterial hypoxemia, with a partial pressure of oxygen (Po_2) of less than 70 mm Hg while breathing room air.[2,36] Most have rapid improvement as the disease resolves, but some patients show a progressive impairment of oxygenation. There may be a significant lag between the appearance of hypoxemia and radiographic evidence of pulmonary disease. Sterile pleural effusions are common in patients with pancreatitis, and analysis of this fluid often reveals a high concentration of amylase. The volume of the pleural effusion, however, is not usually sufficient to account for the ventilatory abnormalities. Ventilation, gas exchange, and the pulmonary circulation all may be affected during acute pancreatitis (see accompanying box).

CHANGES IN RESPIRATORY FUNCTION IN ACUTE PANCREATITIS

Decreased ventilation

Vital capacity
Forced expiratory capacity in 1 second/forced vital capacity

Decreased efficiency of gas exchange

Carbon monoxide–diffusing capacity

Decreased oxygen-carrying capacity of hemoglobin

Ventilation-perfusion mismatch results from the reduction in both pulmonary capillary blood flow and alveolar ventilation. The decrease in capillary blood flow does not appear to be cardiogenic. A transient increase in pulmonary vascular resistance has been noted on occasion,[37,38] but this finding does not account for the decreased capillary flow in most patients.

Most patients with acute pancreatitis have ventilatory abnormalities. The vital capacity is decreased approximately 25%, and the ratio of the forced expiratory volume in 1 second to forced vital capacity is reduced by 20% to 35%. The efficiency of pulmonary gas exchange, measured by the carbon monoxide diffusion capacity, is also reduced by approximately 25% in most patients. The oxygen-carrying capacity of hemoglobin is also impaired, but this does not appear to be related to decreased 2,3-diphosphoglycerate levels or to hemoglobin concentration. Despite these ventilatory abnormalities, most patients do not require assisted ventilation.

The mechanisms of pulmonary injury in acute pancreatitis are unknown.[5] Sepsis may account for respiratory failure in patients with infection, but many patients in whom pulmonary dysfunction develops have only uncomplicated, sterile disease. High concentrations of pancreatic enzymes in the circulation at the time of acute pancreatitis may also contribute to respiratory failure. Intravenous infusion of trypsin in sheep increases pulmonary lymph flow and pulmonary transvascular protein clearance. Advance treatment of these animals with a trypsin inhibitor (e.g., aprotinin [Trasylol]) prevents the increased pulmonary vascular permeability.[39] Pulmonary leukostasis with capillary sludging also results from trypsin infusion and is inhibited by aprotinin pretreatment.

Free fatty acids in the circulation can cause respiratory failure, and they may be released as the result of fat digestion by lipase. Serum triglyceride levels are elevated in some patients, particularly those with a history of chronic alcoholism or disorders of lipid metabolism. Experiments performed with isolated dog lungs have confirmed the injurious effects of free fatty acids.[40] Furthermore, histologic studies of diseased lungs in pancreatitis patients have demonstrated the presence of fat emboli.[41]

Phospholipase A_2 (PLA_2) has also been recovered from the serum of patients with acute pancreatitis in whom failure developed respiratory. The magnitude of pulmonary derangement appears to correlate closely with the degree of PLA_2 elevation. The proposed mechanism of action of PLA_2 is through the dissolution of pulmonary surfactant. In patients with the highest levels of PLA_2, neither peritoneal lavage nor pancreatectomy alters the course of the respiratory failure.

Endocrine Alterations

Significant abnormalities also occur in the metabolism of glucose and calcium (Table 27-1). Elevated blood glucose concentrations (130 to 200 mg/dl) occur in 50% to 75% of patients with acute pancreatitis. However, glucosuria

Table 27-1. Endocrine Abnormalities in Acute Pancreatitis

Abnormality	Proposed Mechanism
Hyperglycemia (130-200 mg/dl) (returns to normal 18 to 21 days after resolution of pancreatitis)	Serum glucagon concentrations greater than serum insulin concentrations in basal and stimulated states Elevation of growth hormone
Hypocalcemia (true or ionized fraction)	Hyperglucagonemia Hypercalcitonemia Hypoalbuminemia Hypomagnesemia Defect in parathyroid metabolism

occurs in only approximately one third of patients with hyperglycemia. Although blood sugar levels greater than 200 mg/dL are associated with increased mortality rates,[42] this is only a reflection of the severity of the pancreatitis. Death rarely occurs as the result of the hyperglycemia itself; most deaths are from other complications.

A number of factors contribute to hyperglycemia.[2] In general, serum concentrations of both glucagon and insulin are elevated in patients with any form of stress. However, serum insulin concentrations are not high enough to prevent hyperglycemia. In patients with acute pancreatitis, the serum glucagon concentrations are much higher, and the insulin concentrations are lower than in patients with stress from other causes. Serum concentrations of growth hormone and cortisol, both of which also produce hyperglycemia, are also elevated in patients with acute pancreatitis.

Intravenous infusion of arginine or alanine stimulates moderate secretion of both glucagon and insulin in healthy individuals. In patients with acute pancreatitis, these secretagogues produce an increase in serum glucagon that is nine to 10 times normal and 50% greater than that seen in patients with other forms of stress. Likewise, serum insulin concentrations after secretagogue infusion are two to six times that seen in the normal response to stress.

The fasting hyperglycemia, hyperglucagonemia, and abnormal response to alanine and arginine infusion all resolve as the pancreatitis improves. During the first 48 to 72 hours after the onset of disease, there is significant fasting hyperglycemia along with hyperglucagonemia and hypoinsulinemia. The elevated concentrations of glucagon and glucose usually return to normal within 18 to 21 days after resolution of pancreatitis, but the hyperglucagonemia resolves spontaneously and unpredictably. Administration of large amounts of insulin to these patients to correct the elevated blood glucose may produce dangerous hypoglycemia, and mild hyperglycemia should be tolerated.

Mild hypocalcemia is frequent in patients with pancreatitis, and a number of factors may contribute to this. Some of the serum calcium is normally bound to albumin, and hypoalbuminemia is common because vascular permeability is increased and albumin is lost from the intravascular space. In this situation, the serum ionized calcium level is often normal, despite a low total serum calcium. Fat necrosis, with saponification of calcium, may also account for the loss of as much as 1 to 2 g calcium.

PTH production, release, and peripheral activity in response to hypocalcemia are all normal in this setting. Patients with true ionized hypocalcemia have appropriately elevated serum PTH concentrations,[43] which decrease as serum ionized calcium returns to normal. Hypocalciuria and decreased tubular reabsorption of phosphate indicate normal action of PTH in the kidney. Infusion of PTH into patients with acute pancreatitis and hypocalcemia results in increased serum calcium and urinary cyclic adenine monophosphate, indicating unimpaired action of the hormone.

Serum concentrations of calcitonin are elevated to as much as six times normal in hypocalcemic patients with pancreatitis. There is evidence that the increase in serum calcitonin precedes the hypocalcemia.[44] Infusion of glucagon in healthy individuals increases serum calcitonin concentrations. Thus, hyperglucagonemia may account for the hypercalcitoninemia. On the other hand, infusion of glucagon in patients with acute pancreatitis does not increase serum calcitonin levels, nor does it reduce ionized calcium concentrations further.[2]

Hypomagnesemia may also be present in patients with acute pancreatitis. This is important because hypocalcemia may be impossible to correct without also treating the hypomagnesemia.

Physiologic Basis of Diagnosis

The diagnosis of acute pancreatitis is based on the patient's history, physical findings, laboratory study results (Table 27-2), and observation of the clinical course after institution of treatment.[45]

Clinical Appearance

Clinically, the patient with acute pancreatitis usually is seen with midepigastric or right upper quadrant pain that radiates to the back. The onset of pain may be related to eating a large meal or consuming alcohol. The severity of the pain is variable, although in most cases it is significant enough to cause the patient to seek medical treatment. The pain is often unrelenting and associated with nausea and vomiting. Low-grade fever is common. In severe cases, tachycardia and orthostatic hypotension may reflect hypo-

Table 27-2. Laboratory Diagnosis of Acute Pancreatitis

Enzyme Elevation	Principle*
Serum amylase concentration	Release of enzyme into circulation
Urinary amylase excretion (amylase/creatinine clearance ratio)	Increase renal clearance of amylase in acute pancreatitis
Isoamylases	Increased *P*-amylase specific to pancreas in acute pancreatitis
Serum lipase	Release from acinar cells or ducts into circulation, no renal clearance

*There may be a failure in the elevation of serum enzymes and amylase/creatinine clearance ratio in patients with acute pancreatitis that is superimposed on chronic pancreatitis.

CONDITIONS ASSOCIATED WITH HYPERAMYLASEMIA

Intra-abdominal

Pancreatic disorders

Acute pancreatitis
Chronic pancreatitis
Trauma
Pseudocysts
Carcinoma
Abscess
Pancreatic ascites
Early cystic fibrosis

Extrapancreatic disorders

Biliary tract disease
Intestinal obstruction
Mesenteric infarction
Perforated ulcer
Peritonitis
Appendicitis
Ruptured ectopic pregnancy
Ruptured aortic aneurysm
Salpingitis
Afferent loop syndrome

Extra-abdominal

Salivary gland disorders

Parotitis
Trauma
Mumps
Postirradiation inflammation

Decreased amylase excretion

Renal failure
Macroamylasemia

Liver disorders

Hepatitis
Cirrhosis

Miscellaneous

Pneumonia
Pancreatic pleural effusion
Mediastinal pseudocyst
Head trauma
Burns
Diabetic ketoacidosis
Pregnancy
Drugs
Bisalbuminemia
Anorexia nervosa and bulimia
Alcoholism

volemia resulting from significant fluid sequestration.

Physical examination typically reveals abdominal tenderness and guarding in the upper abdomen, although the entire abdomen may be diffusely tender. The tenderness is a result of the peritoneal irritation by intraperitoneal fluid, which may contain pancreatic enzymes and other noxious substances. Bowel sounds are decreased or absent. There may be splinting of respirations and decreased breath sounds over the lung bases. In patients with hemorrhagic pancreatitis, blood may dissect throughout the retroperitoneum, resulting in a bluish discoloration in the flanks (Turner's sign) or in the periumbilical area (Cullen's sign).

Most patients with acute pancreatitis have an elevated serum amylase concentration.[46] However, other intra-abdominal conditions may also be associated with moderate elevations in serum amylase level (see accompanying box), and some of these (e.g., acute cholecystitis, small-bowel infarction, and duodenal perforation) can mimic acute pancreatitis. Thus, an elevated serum amylase concentration alone does not always distinguish pancreatitis from another disorder requiring operation.

Amylase is produced in different forms, or isozymes, designated as salivary (S) and pancreatic (P). The S-isoamylase is the predominant form in normal serum, constituting approximately 60% of the total. The pancreas is the only source of *P*-isoamylase, whereas *S*-isoamylase is found in the salivary glands, lungs, and prostate gland. In acute pancreatitis, the elevated serum amylase is predominantly the P-isoamylase. Thus, measurement of the specific pancreatic fraction in patients with suspected acute pancreatitis may increase the specificity of the test. However, isoenzyme measurements in patients with acute illness are usually not necessary, are impractical, and have not found wide clinical application.

During acute pancreatitis, the renal clearance of amylase increases compared with that of creatinine (amylase/creatinine clearance ratio [ACCR], normally 0.01 to 0.03) and large amounts of P-isoamylase are found in the urine.[47] The renal clearance of amylase usually does not change when the serum amylase level is increased for other reasons. Thus, the ACCR may help to differentiate acute pancreatitis from elevated amylase levels from other intra-abdominal processes. Because the ACCR may be abnormally elevated in other conditions, such as diabetic ketoacidosis and thermal burns, its specificity is limited.

Determination of the serum lipase concentration may be more valuable.[46,48] The major source of lipase is the pancreas, and there are no known isoenzymes of this substance. The serum lipase concentration increases at approximately the same time as does serum amylase in patients with acute pancreatitis and provides the same sort of information. Lipase is not excreted in the urine, and its clearance cannot be measured. The assay originally was difficult, but it is now easier and more standardized. As a result, it has become more valuable in identifying patients with acute pancreatitis.

Other pancreatic enzymes (trypsin, elastase, PLA_2, carboxylic ester hydrolase, and ribonuclease) and proteins (pancreas-specific protein and pancreatic stone protein [PSP]) have been measured in the serum and body fluids of patients with acute pancreatitis. Although these tests may provide some additional specificity for pancreatitis when the diagnosis is equivocal, they are not widely available, nor are they used in most institutions.

Prediction of Severity

Most patients with acute pancreatitis have mild disease that resolves spontaneously without complications. For these patients, medical therapy is largely supportive. In contrast, intensive medical monitoring and care are critical for the survival of patients with more severe disease. These patients should be identified early in the course of their disease. Thus, estimation of the severity of an attack of acute pancreatitis is important to assess potential morbidity and mortality and to plan therapy. In individuals who have more than one attack, there is no correlation in severity among the individual episodes, and each must be evaluated alone. Ranson[49,50] demonstrated that a number of factors predict the severity of pancreatitis and the likelihood of death (see accompanying box). The mortality rate correlated closely with the number of these criteria that were met. Patients with more than four of Ranson's signs were more likely to have necrotizing pancreatitis, to have significant complications, and to die. Even though patients with fewer than four signs were likely to have milder disease, however, many still had serious complications, some of which necessitated surgery. Ranson's system is cumbersome to use, requires 48 hours for full definition, and has only been validated for the beginning of an attack of pancreatitis. A variety of other systems have therefore evolved. For example, Satiani and Stone[51] identified a variety of clinical parameters that can be evaluated at admission (see

PARAMETERS FOR PREDICTING SEVERITY OF ACUTE PANCREATITIS ON THE BASIS OF LOCAL AND SYSTEMIC CRITERIA

Ranson's Criteria

Initial

Age >55 years
WBC >16,000
Blood glucose >200 mg/dl
Serum LDH >350 IU/L
Serum AST >250 Sigma Frankel U/dl

During initial 48 hours

Hematocrit fall >10%
BUN rise >5 mg/100 ml
Serum calcium concentration <8 mg/dl
HCO_3^- deficit >4 mEq/L
Arterial Po_2 <60 mm Hg
Fluid sequestration >6 L

Satiani and Stone

Oral temperature >39° C
Respiratory distress (arterial Po_2 <60 mm Hg)
Shock necessitating extensive resuscitation
WBC >15000
Serum calcium <7 mg/dl

AST, Aspartate transaminase; *HCO_3^-,* bicarbonate ion; *LDH,* lactate dehydrogenase; *WBC,* white blood cell count.

box on p. 570). The Acute Physiologic and Chronic Health Evaluation II system also accurately predicts the severity of the disease, and it has the advantage that it can be applied at any time during the illness.[52] Paracentesis has also been used to estimate the severity of the pancreatitis.[42] Hemorrhagic pancreatitis is more likely to be associated with larger volumes of fluid during the initial aspiration (>10 ml free fluid) and with free fluid that is brown, purple, or dark straw-colored. Because this is an invasive study, it is not widely used. Grading of the magnitude of the abnormality detected on abdominal computerized tomographic (CT) scanning also may be of predictive value.[53,54] With contrast enhancement, the diagnosis of necrosis can be established by CT scan. Typically, the necrotic area fails to enhance as does the normal pancreas (Fig. 27-2).

The degree of elevation of the serum enzyme levels bears no relationship to the severity of the disease.[55] Evaluation of concentrations of inflammatory markers,[56,57] such as C-reactive protein, complement factors, protease inhibitors, and leukocyte enzymes, may be more helpful in predicting severity, but further evaluation is needed.

The combination of clinical assessment and measurement of biochemical abnormalities gives the best initial index of the severity of pancreatitis. Derangements in other organ systems generally indicate severe disease and the need for aggressive management to minimize the risk of morbidity and mortality. The patient with severe disease is typically somewhat anxious and tachycardic. The mucous membranes appear dry, and the urine output may be low. Often, the patient is tachypneic and the PO_2 is reduced. The hematocrit, creatinine level, and BUN may all be elevated. Significant hypocalcemia (<8 mg/dl) is also predictive of a poor prognosis. All these indicators suggest the need for careful monitoring, usually in the intensive care unit.

A

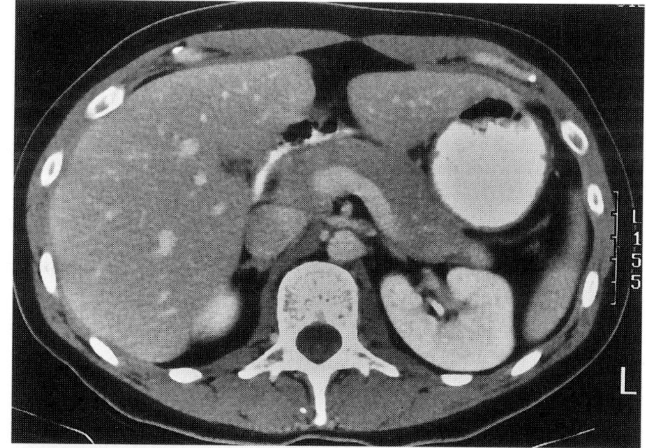

B

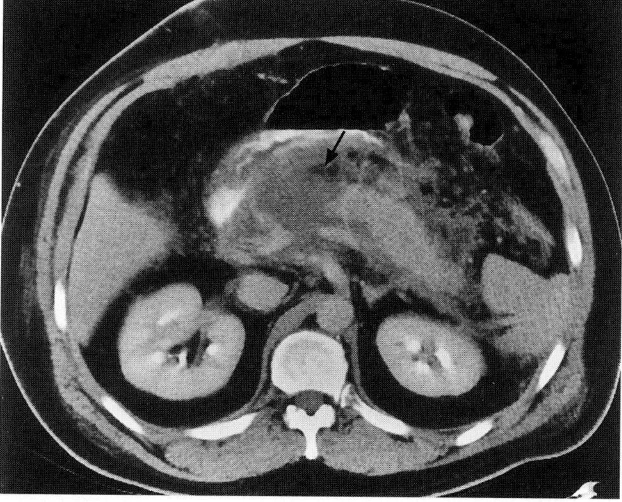

Fig. 27-2. A, Contrast-enhanced CT scan of healthy pancreas, demonstrating relatively uniform enhancement of the pancreatic parenchyma. **B,** Contrast-enhanced CT scan of pancreatic necrosis. A relatively large area of the pancreas *(arrow)* fails to enhance with contrast injection.

Treatment of Acute Pancreatitis

Medical Treatment

The primary mode of therapy for acute pancreatitis is medical; surgery is reserved for complications of the disease. Medical treatment has taken two different approaches. The first attempts to limit the progression of the pancreatitis. The second is directed toward the restoration of fluid and electrolyte losses, the treatment of other associated physiologic derangements, and the relief of pain. The stimulation of pancreatic secretion is avoided. Nasogastric suction has been employed to decrease the amount of gastric acid entering the duodenum, reducing the release of secretin that would stimulate pancreatic water and bicarbonate secretion. The production of gastric acid can be further limited by the administration of atropine, cimetidine, or omeprazole. Food is withheld because dietary fat and protein are the primary stimuli for CCK release, which stimulates pancreatic enzyme secretion. Although controlled trials have failed to demonstrate that any of these modalities are of benefit, usually oral intake is interdicted and nasogastric suction is initiated because of the ileus and vomiting that often accompany acute pancreatitis. Glucagon and somatostatin have also been used to inhibit pancreatic secretion. Clinical trials with glucagon did not show any improvement in mortality or morbidity rates.[58] The use of somatostatin analogs continues to be debated, but there is still no convincing evidence of their value for these patients.[59-61] The ineffectiveness of efforts to treat the pancreatitis by suppressing secretory activity has been frustrating. On the other hand, there is evidence that the acutely inflamed gland is normally unresponsive to secretory stimuli, and these efforts may therefore be superfluous. It also may be that the damage has already been done by the time the patient seeks treatment, and that such therapy at that stage is too late.

As previously noted, proteolytic enzyme activity may be important in the development of the systemic complications of acute pancreatitis. Efforts have therefore been made to limit the action of pancreatic enzymes released during pancreatitis. Trypsin is normally produced when trypsinogen is activated by enterokinase in the duodenum. Trypsin can then activate all the other pancreatic enzymes. Although trypsin is normally inactivated by antiproteases in serum and tissue, these may be rapidly consumed during acute disease. The degree of antiprotease saturation is probably important, because the amount of free (active) trypsin in the circulation correlates with disease progression. The trypsin inhibitor aprotinin has been used to inactivate free trypsin in response to this rationale. Unfortunately, clinical trials have not shown any beneficial effect. The reasons for this failure are not clear, but it could be that other enzymes are activated independently and contribute to the systemic complications. Alternatively, proteases may not be of primary importance in the disease and its complications, or aprotinin may not be a sufficiently potent trypsin inhibitor. On the other hand, some studies have demonstrated a limitation of the severity of respiratory failure in animals given aprotinin before the induction of pancreatitis.[39] As with the other therapies, the problem may be that they have to be administered *before* the pancreatitis has been initiated to be effective.

Prophylactic antibiotics are of no benefit as a routine treatment in mild to moderately severe acute pancreatitis.[32,62-64] In the setting of severe pancreatic or peripancreatic necrosis, however, broad-spectrum antibiotics (e.g., imipenem) should be used. These were shown in a multicenter, controlled trial to decrease the incidence of infection.[34,65]

The conservative management of acute pancreatitis demands close follow-up, with frequent reexamination of the patient. Temperatures of 101° to 102° F are common during the early course of the disease and rarely signals that an infection is present at this early stage. The presence of an infection may be heralded later, however, by the return of fever and leukocytosis.

Most patients tolerate uncomplicated episodes of pancreatitis well. Severe cases may necessitate prolonged supportive treatment, and significant morbidity can result from associated malnutrition. Parenteral nutrition is useful in this clinical setting,[66] but studies indicate that this form of nutrition by itself does not influence the course of the disease.[67] The same is true for enteral nutrition with elemental diets. Recent evidence of the beneficial effects of enteral feeding in a variety of clinical settings suggest that this might also be desirable in pancreatitis if appropriate access can be achieved.[68]

Peritoneal Lavage

Peritoneal lavage has been used to prevent the absorption of toxins and activated enzymes from ascitic fluid, which may be responsible for the systemic manifestations of the disease. A percutaneous lavage catheter is inserted into the abdomen and 1 L fluid is infused into the peritoneal cavity, where it remains for 30 to 60 minutes before drainage. This process is repeated multiple times during the subsequent 24 to 36 hours. Although randomized trials have failed to show a decrease in mortality,[69] there has been a reluctance to give up this form of treatment, and it continues to be evaluated in various subsets of patients.[50]

Endoscopic Retrograde Cholangiopancreatography

As already discussed, gallstone pancreatitis often is associated with the passage of a stone through the ampulla.[70] Although most stones pass easily, some may be too large and become impacted in the ampullary orifice, where the continued obstruction produces severe and persistent pancreatitis. When this happens, endoscopic retrograde cholangiopancreatography (ERCP) with sphincterotomy and stone extraction or surgical sphincteroplasty and stone removal are indicated.[71] In some studies,[72] the endoscopic approach has been shown to be effective. Because it avoids the morbidity of open operation, it is preferred.

Surgical Treatment

Uncomplicated acute pancreatitis should be managed medically. If the clinical course is complicated by pancreatic or peripancreatic necrosis with infection, or if the patient's condition fails to improve with maximal medical therapy, surgery may be indicated.[73,74] The details of these operations, when indicated, are discussed with the specific complications.

Complications of Acute Pancreatitis

Pancreatic Infection

Infection should be suspected in a patient with pancreatitis when symptoms persist despite medical treatment, or when they return after temporary recovery. At that time, a contrast-enhanced CT scan should be done. Poor enhancement of the pancreatic tissue indicates pancreatic necrosis, which may be infected in as many as 70% of cases. If gas bubbles are seen in the region of the pancreas on the CT scan, infection is presumed to be present. Otherwise, local fluid or necrotic tissue should be aspirated percutaneously, Gram stained, and cultured. Aspiration is safe, and the chance of missing an infection as a result of sampling error is low. If infection is proved, operation is indicated. Percutaneous drainage is inadequate because the small tubes quickly become plugged by the thick, particulate material. If the clinician is unable to prove infection, the CT scan and aspiration are repeated at weekly intervals. Deterioration in the patient's condition, however, may necessitate earlier aspiration or even operation.[75,76]

At operation, the lesser sac is entered, the fluid is drained, and the necrotic pancreas is debrided. Large sump drains are then placed for postoperative lavage and drainage, which may be required for many weeks. A feeding jejunostomy tube is also placed in most of these critically ill patients. Even if all the patient's caloric needs cannot be supplied this way, it is important to maintain the integrity of the gut mucosa by providing luminal nutrients. There is evidence from patients with other critical illnesses that this decreases the incidence of bacterial translocation and may prevent the "sepsis syndrome." Reoperation to drain recurrent infection may be necessary in as many as 20% of patients.

Pseudocysts

Peripancreatic fluid collections occur in many patients with pancreatitis, but they resolve spontaneously in most cases. In about 2% of patients with acute pancreatitis, the fluid persists and a mature pseudocyst develops. Pseudocysts should be suspected when recovery from the acute episode is prolonged or complicated in any way; an ultrasonographic or CT examination confirms their presence. Pseudocysts result from local exudation of fluid during acute inflammation of the pancreas. There may be direct communication with a pancreatic duct. The enzyme content of the fluid is usually high (amylase >1000 IU/L). The inflammatory reaction in the adjacent organs and tissues produces a fibrous capsule that matures during a 4- to 6-week period. Complications of pseudocysts include rupture, infection, hemorrhage, and gastrointestinal or biliary obstruction.

Cysts larger than 5 to 6 cm and those accompanied by symptoms should be drained once they have developed a mature capsule. Although percutaneous drains have been used, drainage is usually accomplished surgically by draining the cyst into the adjacent stomach (cystogastrostomy) or to a Roux-en-Y loop of jejunum. The cysts typically disappear quickly after such drainage is established. Infected cysts are usually drained externally.

Pancreatic Ascites

This disorder is caused by the chronic leakage of fluid into the peritoneal cavity from a pseudocyst or from a disrupted pancreatic duct. The clinical syndrome is characterized by ascites and malnutrition and is frequently seen in patients with alcoholism and chronic pancreatitis. Thus, the patient may be thought to have decompensated cirrhosis, and the pancreatic disease may be overlooked. The diagnosis is confirmed if the amylase and protein concentrations in the ascitic fluid are high (often >1000 IU/L and >2.9 g/dl, respectively). An ERCP should be obtained to demonstrate the site of leakage. In some cases, the leak may seal spontaneously during a period of medical management with parenteral nutrition and somatostatin inhibition of pancreatic secretion. If it does not, surgery is required. Usually, this necessitates internal drainage at the point of the leak into a Roux-en-Y jejunal limb.

CHRONIC PANCREATITIS

Chronic pancreatitis is characterized by permanent destruction of exocrine pancreatic tissue, with eventual pancreatic insufficiency. Ninety percent of cases of chronic pancreatitis are the result of alcohol ingestion. The remainder are a consequence of a variety of conditions, including hyperparathyroidism, protein malnutrition, and pancreatic duct obstruction. Usually patients with alcoholic chronic pancreatitis have consumed alcohol heavily (100 to 200 g/day) for 5 to 10 years before symptoms occur. Acute pancreatitis caused by gallstones rarely leads to chronic pancreatitis, although acute attacks recur until the offending stones have been removed. Patients with chronic pancreatitis may also have repeated episodes of acute pancreatic inflammation; these are indistinguishable from the acute pancreatitis that occurs in a patient with a previously normal pancreas. Although severe abdominal pain is the most common complaint in patients with chronic pancreatitis, sometimes pain is absent. The initial symptoms are then usually those of steatorrhea from fat malabsorption, caused by acinar cell destruction and exocrine insufficiency. Diabetes may occur as well because islet cell function is also compromised. Even though some subjects with chronic alcoholism never show evidence of pancreatic disease during life, as many 50% have morphologic abnormalities of the pancreas evident at autopsy.

Pathology

Grossly, the pancreas in chronic pancreatitis is firm, fibrotic, smaller than normal, and with rounded edges. Its anteroposterior diameter may be increased. If the main pancreatic duct is dilated, it may be palpable as a longitudinal ridge on the anterior surface of the gland. In some cases, the inflammatory process extends to surrounding organs, with duodenal, biliary, and colonic fibrous strictures that can produce mechanical obstruction. Pseudocysts are also common.

Histologically, intralobular and extralobular fibrosis is distributed randomly throughout the gland. Proteinaceous precipitates, some of which may be calcified, are found in the small ducts. As the disease progresses, the small pancreatic ducts as well as the main duct may dilate. As the fibrosis progresses, the amount of exocrine and endocrine tissue decreases.

Intrapancreatic inflammation of nerves is common in advanced cases and may be a cause of the pain that many patients have. Recent studies also demonstrated that the perineural nerve sheath is disrupted so that it may no longer provide a barrier between the surrounding connective tissue and the internal neural components.[77] These changes could make the nerves more susceptible to noxious stimuli within the pancreas.

Pathogenesis of Chronic Pancreatitis

Alcohol

Chronic alcohol consumption alters secretory physiology in ways that may influence the development of chronic pancreatitis.[78] The protein concentration of the pancreatic juice increases, which may promote the precipitation of obstructing protein plugs within the small ducts. The concentration within the juice of citrate, normally secreted in parallel with protein, decreases. Because citrate dissolves pancreatic stones and decreases calcite crystal formation, lower concentrations favor the formation of stones.

Citrate is not the only stabilizer of calcium in pancreatic juice. PSP, a nonenzymatic protein with a molecular weight of 13 kd, is synthesized in the acinar cells and may also be important.[79] This PSP is able to prevent the precipitation of calcium carbonate in a supersaturated solution of calcium that mimics the ionic composition of pancreatic juice. In at least two thirds of patients with chronic calcifying pancreatitis from a variety of causes (alcoholic, hereditary, and idiopathic), PSP concentration in pancreatic juice is lower than normal. Low PSP levels may also play a role in the pathogenesis of chronic pancreatitis by predisposing toward intraductal calculus formation.

Recent evidence suggests that the pancreas, like the liver, is able to metabolize ethanol.[80] The acetaldehyde that is produced may form toxic oxygen free radicals that could damage the pancreas.[81] Chronically high levels of acetaldehyde could also lower the level of a proteinase inhibitor.[82] This might make the pancreas more susceptible to damage from pancreatic enzymes. The possibility that patients with alcoholic pancreatitis may metabolize ethanol differently also continues to be investigated.[83]

Pancreatic Duct Obstruction

The role of pancreatic duct obstruction in chronic pancreatitis has not been completely defined. Partial and complete main pancreatic duct obstruction in experimental animals and humans causes pancreatic duct dilation and progressive acinar tissue atrophy, with replacement of lobules by fibrous tissue. The fibrosis is distributed uniformly throughout the gland, unlike in the alcoholic variety, where the changes are randomly distributed. This is probably because of the random nature of small-duct obstruction caused by protein plugs in alcoholic chronic pancreatitis. However, it suggests that ductal obstruction is an important feature that leads to similar tissue destruction in these patients as well.

The degree of obstruction is important in the development of both functional and histologic changes. In cats, obstruction of the main pancreatic duct by more than 75% of the luminal diameter for 12 weeks impaired bicarbonate, water, and protein secretion.[84] Lesser degrees of obstruction also decreased enzyme secretion, but the ability to produce high concentrations of bicarbonate was retained. The histologic changes correlated well with the secretory changes. Periductal fibrosis and duct dilation were most impressive in cats with greater degrees of obstruction, but some perilobular fibrosis and acinar atrophy were found in all animals. Unrelieved obstruction resulted in progressive secretory impairment and replacement of the gland with fibrous tissue.

Pancreatic duct obstruction may cause pancreatitis in patients with a ductal stricture. Pancreatitis also may develop in patients with pancreas divisum, where the etiology is thought to be an obstructing accessory papilla. In this anatomic variant, the minor papilla is the sole opening through which most of the pancreatic secretions must drain. Only the secretions from the uncinate process empty through the major papilla. If the obstruction is relieved before irreversible parenchymal changes occur, chronic pancreatitis may be averted.

Malnutrition

In certain tropical countries, malnutrition may cause atrophy of the pancreatic parenchyma, pancreatic calcifications, and diabetes mellitus.[85,86] The pancreas actively synthesizes enzyme protein, and alterations in diet may change the nature of the enzymes produced. Thus, chronic malnutrition may alter the composition of the pancreatic secretions and injure the pancreas. Others have suggested that the ingestion of a specific food (e.g., cassava) in large quantities may be responsible for the chronic pancreatitis.[85,86] Patients with nutritional pancreatitis have recurrent episodes of severe abdominal pain during adolescence. The pain subsides after a few years, and relatively long pain-free periods may follow. During the patient's late teens or early twenties, diabetes becomes clinically manifest and the patient again seeks medical care. Characteristic signs and symptoms of diabetes are found, including microangiopathy. At this stage of the disease, abdominal radiographs reveal pancreatic calcifications in many cases.

Pancreatic Blood Flow

Recent studies have suggested that reduction in pancreatic blood flow may play a role in the pathophysiology of chronic pancreatitis.[9] Pancreatic blood flow is low in cats with chronic pancreatitis from partial duct obstruction, and it falls further with secretory stimulation. Normally, pancreatic blood flow increases with stimulation. This reduction is associated with decreases in tissue oxygen content and parenchymal acidosis, suggesting that the pancreas may be ischemic.[87,88] Similar reductions in pH were noted in patients undergoing operations for painful chronic pancreatitis. Pancreatic ischemia could explain both the progressive parenchymal destruction and the pain that these patients suffer. Surgical decompression of the duct, which reduces the elevated interstitial pressures, also returns pancreatic blood flow toward normal. This suggests that the pathophysiology of chronic pancreatitis is similar to that of compartment syndrome, in which the elevated pressures in the fibrotic, noncompliant gland compromise arterial inflow and the ability of the pancreas to respond to physiologic stimuli.

Diagnosis

The diagnosis of chronic pancreatitis is usually straightforward, especially in patients with alcoholism, diabetes, upper abdominal pain, and radiographically determined pancreatic calcifications. In some patients, the diagnosis is less obvious. A CT scan or ultrasonography may demonstrate the shrunken, constricted, and calcified pancreas characteristic of the disease. ERCP also may demonstrate ductal abnormalities, such as multiple constrictions and areas of intervening dilatation, the "chain of lakes" appearance (Fig. 27-3).

Because the pancreas possesses a large functional reserve, steatorrhea does not occur until about 85% of its function has been lost.[89] Then, diarrhea and loose, bulky stools result from the malabsorption of fat. Tests of pancreatic secretory function can detect milder functional ab-

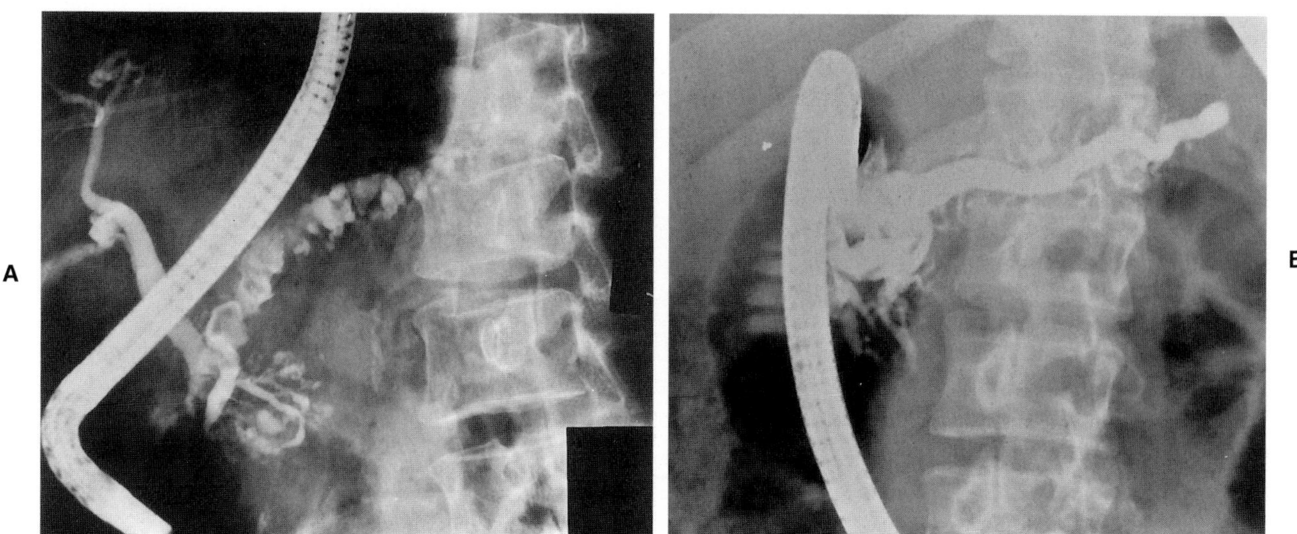

Fig. 27-3. A, ERCP from a patient with chronic pancreatitis. The pancreatogram demonstrates the "chain of lakes" pattern of multiple ductal dilatations separated by areas of obstructing stricture. **B,** Pancreatogram demonstrating a uniformly dilated pancreatic duct.

Table 27-3. Characteristics of Pancreatic Juice in Healthy Patients and Those With Chronic Pancreatitis

	Volume (ml/kg/hr)	$[HCO_3^-]$ (mEq/L)	HCO_3^- output (mEq/hr)*	Lipase output (KU/hr)*	Trypsin output (KU/hr)*
Healthy patients	3-5	100-135	15-35 mEq/hr	150	35
Patients with chronic pancreatitis	2	90	10 mEq/hr	25	10

*Output (the total number of kallikrein units or millequivalents) is a reflection of volume *and* concentration.

normalities. The most sensitive test requires intubation of the duodenum with a gastroduodenal tube for collection of pancreatic juice. Pancreatic secretion is stimulated by CCK or secretin given intravenously or with a standard meal. Duodenal juice is collected and analyzed for enzyme and bicarbonate content. In chronic pancreatitis, the volume of secretion is low and the concentrations of enzymes and bicarbonate are reduced (Table 27-3). The hormonal stimulation method is preferred, because it is easier to standardize and the results are simpler to interpret. Both tests are somewhat cumbersome to perform, however, so they are not used widely. An alternative test that is simpler but less sensitive is more popular. Bentiromide, a synthetic peptide linked to para-aminobenzoic acid (PABA), is fed to the patient with a standard meal. Chymotrypsin in the pancreatic juice selectively cleaves the bentiromide molecule to liberate PABA. PABA is absorbed and excreted in the urine, where it is assayed. Patients with pancreatic insufficiency excrete less PABA than do healthy patients. Unfortunately, even the most sensitive techniques probably detect only moderately advanced pancreatic insufficiency; that is, more than 50% loss of function. Other biochemical tests have been proposed but have not shown routine clinical efficacy.[90] The major value of secretory testing is to differentiate pancreatic insufficiency from other causes of malabsorption, such as celiac disease. Serial testing may be useful in an individual patient to study progressive deterioration.

ERCP is more sensitive than are function tests in the diagnosis of chronic pancreatitis, but it also has limitations. In one study, the sensitivity of ERCP was evaluated in a group of 200 patients known to have the disease.[72] Disappointingly, 15% of the patients without pancreatic calcifications (a group among whom the diagnosis would depend heavily on the ability to show ductal abnormalities) had normal ERCP findings. In 7.5% of the patients, the study could not be performed for technical reasons.

Medical Treatment

Treatment is directed primarily toward the relief of pain and the management of malabsorption and diabetes.[91]

Pain

Early in the disease, abdominal pain may occur only in association with recurrent episodes of inflammation. With progression, the pain becomes more frequent and each episode lasts longer, so that patients may experience discomfort daily or even continuously. Frequently, patients consume alcohol in an attempt to relieve the discomfort, and many also become addicted to narcotics. This complicates efforts to evaluate the efficacy of various interventions because reports of pain may be an effort to obtain narcotics. Every effort should be made to eliminate the use of alcohol. Pain and the frequency of acute episodes of inflammation may decrease, but there is no evidence that the rate of pancreatic destruction is slowed. Abstinence is more likely to benefit those with early disease, who still have residual pancreatic function. With advanced disease, in which most exocrine function has been lost, the relationship between continued drinking and the persistence of pain is less clear. On the other hand, these patients are more likely to have spontaneous pain relief as the disease progresses and secretory function is lost.

The observation that the pain is related to secretory function has provided a rationale for several therapeutic strategies. Somatostatin has been used to inhibit pancreatic secretion, and it may relieve pain in some patients. Prospective trials are ongoing to evaluate the efficacy of this approach. Oral pancreatic enzymes have also been used to relieve pain. The theory is based on the observation that in animals low levels of intraduodenal proteases, which are typical of chronic pancreatitis, cause CCK release and elevated plasma CCK concentrations. This stimulates pancreatic secretion and is thought to provoke pain. Exogenous enzymes restore the physiologic inhibition of CCK release, which lowers circulating levels of the hormone, avoids secretory stimulation, and relieves pain. Although this approach may be effective in some patients (e.g., middle-aged women with mild idiopathic chronic pancreatitis), no improvement is seen in most.[92,93] The validity of the concept itself is controversial.

Malabsorption

Many of these patients lose weight because eating provokes pain and they voluntarily reduce their food intake. However, malabsorption can also be an important cause of weight loss and malnutrition. Malabsorption occurs when more than 90% of pancreatic enzymes fail to enter the duodenal lumen. Carbohydrates continue to be well absorbed, but proteins and fats are lost in the stool in excessive amounts. Although the creatorrhea generally does not produce symptoms, the steatorrhea may produce bulky, foul-smelling stools and diarrhea. These symptoms should be treated. Generally, patients should be given diets with liberal amounts of carbohydrate (400 g or more) and protein (100 to 150 g), with as much fat as can be tolerated without the production of diarrhea. Pancreatic enzymes should be provided in an amount that supplies about 30,000 U lipase with each meal. If symptoms continue, gastric acid antisecretory drugs should be prescribed to raise the gastric pH. In some patients who secrete large amounts of hydrochloric acid, the low gastric pH destroys the lipase before it even mixes with the chyme. An alternative is to change the enzyme preparation to one that is enterically coated, which protects the enzymes while they are in the acidic environment of the stomach. In the duodenum or proximal small bowel, where the pH rises above 5, the protective coating is dissolved and the enzymes are released. Even when an optimal treatment regimen has been established, fat malabsorption cannot be corrected completely.[91,94]

Diabetes

Insulin-dependent diabetes mellitus occurs in about 40% of patients with chronic pancreatitis. Such diabetic complications as retinopathy and peripheral vascular disease may be less common than among patients with adult-onset diabetes mellitus, but they still occur. Complications related to insulin therapy are more common, because many patients with chronic pancreatitis are unreliable, with a history of alcoholism and narcotic addiction. Patients with chronic pancreatitis have low basal serum insulin concentrations that do not rise adequately after eating. In contrast, insulin concentrations are characteristically high in patients with adult-onset diabetes and increase as much as twofold with eating. Although the islets are relatively well preserved in chronic pancreatitis, the surrounding tissue is fibrotic. This fibrotic tissue may prevent the hormones insulin and glucagon from entering the lymphatics and capillaries that drain the islets. Because hypoglycemic insulin reactions are common, mild hyperglycemia and glucosuria should be tolerated. An insulin dose of 20 to 40 U/day usually suffices.

Surgical Management

The most common indication for surgery is refractory pain. Two surgical approaches have been used, (1) drainage operations to relieve ductal obstruction and (2) resection operations to remove diseased pancreatic tissue. Patients with a dilated duct (>7 mm) are usually candidates for the former; if the duct is narrow, resection is preferred. Information about ductal anatomy and other associated abnormalities (e.g., pseudocysts) is obtained with an abdominal CT scan and ERCP, which should be done in most patients. Patients with a history of alcoholism who have stopped drinking but still have pain are usually the best surgical candidates.

Drainage Procedure

The lateral (longitudinal) pancreaticojejunostomy (Puestow procedure) is the standard operation (Fig. 27-4). A longitudinal incision is made in the pancreas that extends through the anterior wall of the main pancreatic duct for its entire length. Stones and debris are removed, and a Roux-en-Y limb of jejunum is sutured to the opened pancreas along its length so that the pancreatic juice drains directly into the small intestine.

Although 85% of patients have immediate relief of pain, it recurs in 30% to 50% within 5 years. The mechanism by which the operation relieves pain is unclear. The Puestow procedure reduces the elevated interstitial pressures in these patients, and the degree of pain relief cor-

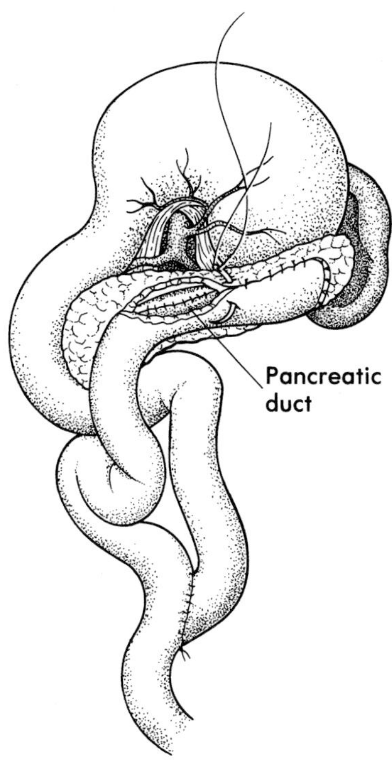

Fig. 27-4. Lateral (longitudinal) pancreaticojejunostomy (Puestow procedure) is the most frequently used drainage procedure for chronic pancreatitis. A Roux-en-Y limb of jejunum is sutured to the opened pancreatic duct along its length. (From Way L. Current Surgical Diagnosis and Treatment. Los Altos, Calif.: Lange Medical Books, 1985. Used with permission.)

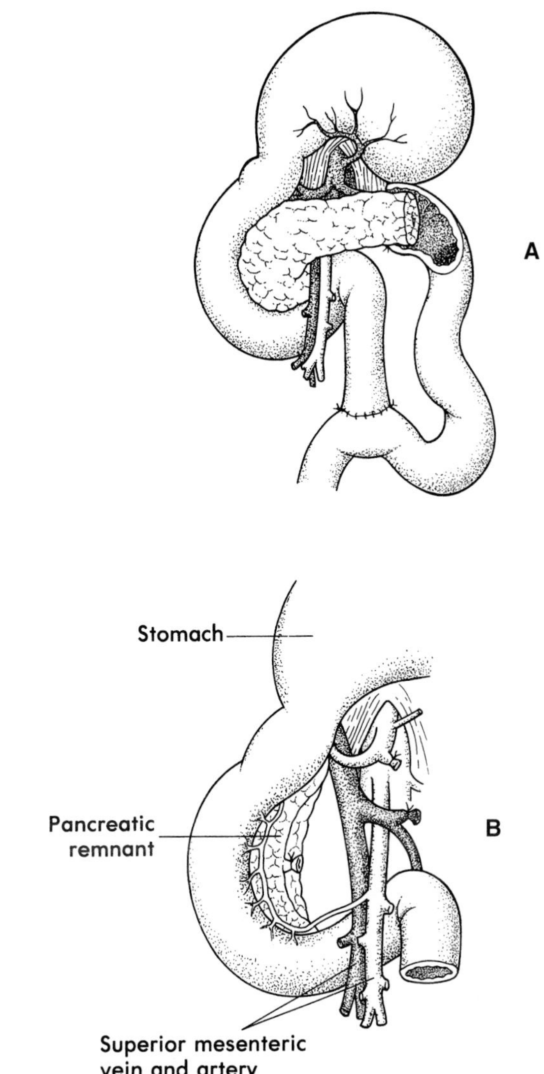

Fig. 27-5. Surgical resection for chronic pancreatitis. **A,** Distal resection of the pancreas with pancreaticojejunostomy. **B,** Subtotal pancreatectomy. (From Way L. Current Surgical Diagnosis and Treatment. Los Altos, Calif.: Lange Medical Books, 1985. Used with permission.)

relates with the magnitude of reduction.[95] In an animal model, ductal decompression was also associated with a return of pancreatic blood flow toward normal.[14] This suggests that the pain may be ischemic in nature and that restoration of blood flow is important for pain relief.

Ductal drainage operations also might be expected to improve exocrine insufficiency because pancreatic enzymes can empty more easily into the gut. Because the pancreatic juice is diverted away from the duodenum, however, poor mixing of the gastric chyme with the pancreatic juices might be expected. In practice, these procedures almost never have a clinically significant impact on the degree of malabsorption. Whether drainage operations slow the destruction of pancreatic tissue, or even promote the regeneration of functional parenchyma, is controversial.[94] One recent study suggested that the progressive losses of both exocrine and endocrine pancreatic function were delayed by drainage.[96] At this time, however, surgery should not be performed either to slow the progress of the disease or to promote improvement in pancreatic function.

Resection

After resection, pain is relieved in about 85% of cases, which is similar to the rate for drainage operations. However, the relief is more likely to be permanent than after a Puestow procedure. Operative mortality and morbidity rates are only marginally higher than with the drainage operations. Diabetes, which requires insulin for its management, is, however, likely to occur after major pancreatic resections. This can be a life-threatening problem in irresponsible patients with a history of alcoholism or addiction to narcotics.

Resections of the tail of the pancreas of 40% or less (Fig. 27-5) usually do not worsen pancreatic insufficiency. Resections of 50% to 80% of the distal pancreas produce significant steatorrhea in at least 20% of the patients. Diabetes mellitus also worsens in as many as 30%. In patients undergoing 80% to 95% distal resections, 50% have worsening of both steatorrhea and diabetes.

Distal resections do not alter gastric emptying and the mixing of food with pancreatic juice. Pancreaticoduo-

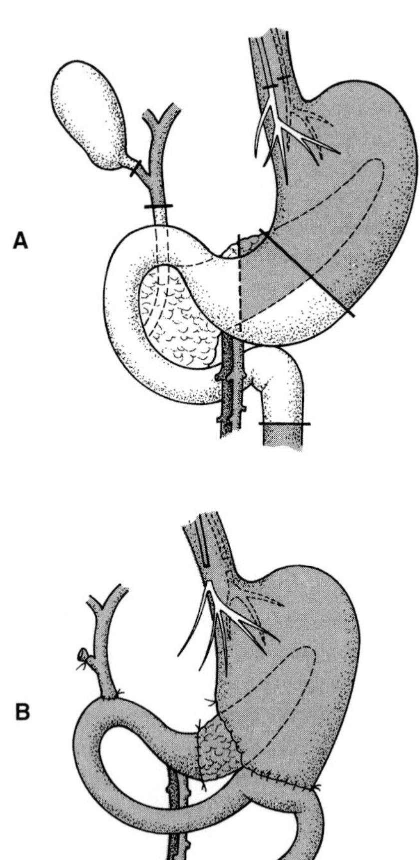

Fig. 27-6. Pancreaticoduodenectomy (Whipple procedure). **A,** Preoperative anatomic relationships. **B,** Postoperative reconstruction showing pancreatic, biliary, and gastric anastomoses. A cholecystectomy (if gallstones are present) and bilateral truncal vagotomy are also part of the procedure. In many cases, the distal stomach and pylorus can be preserved, and vagotomy is then unnecessary. (From Way L. Current Surgical Diagnosis and Treatment. Los Altos, Calif.: Lange Medical Books, 1985. Used with permission.)

denectomy (Fig. 27-6) alters both. At least half of all patients have troublesome steatorrhea after this operation, which involves distal gastrectomy and gastrojejunostomy as well as pancreatic resection. Because at least 50% of the pancreas remains after this procedure, the changes incident to the gastric surgery are probably responsible for some of the malabsorption.

After pancreaticoduodenectomy, diabetes worsens in about 10% of patients. When total pancreatectomy is performed, all patients require insulin and pancreatic enzyme replacement. Hypoglycemic episodes are more common in this group, probably because of the absence of pancreatic glucagon.

SUMMARY

Although we have learned a great deal about the pathophysiology of pancreatitis, many of the basic mechanisms remain obscure. In the case of acute pancreatitis, a number of inciting factors have been identified, but the final common pathway leading to autodigestion and its systemic manifestations has not yet been elucidated. Uncomplicated acute pancreatitis usually resolves without altered digestive function or permanent damage to other organ systems affected during the acute disease. It is still not clear why only pancreatic edema develops in one patient and the disease progresses to hemorrhagic necrosis in another. We are now able to reliably assess the severity of the disease and use this information to tailor treatment and predict complications and survival for individual patients. Recovery is generally complete, and acute pancreatitis generally does not recur if the cause (e.g., gallstones) is removed.

Chronic pancreatitis is associated with permanent damage to the gland. Digestive and endocrine functions are altered according to the degree of glandular damage. Although the cause of the pancreatitis may be removed, there is usually no improvement in either endocrine or exocrine function. In many cases, these changes are progressive. Systemic manifestations of chronic pancreatitis are related to the degree of digestive impairment (e.g., malabsorption), the degree of endocrine impairment (e.g., diabetes mellitus), and the inciting cause (e.g., alcoholism). Patients with chronic pancreatitis may also have recurrent episodes of acute pancreatitis.

REFERENCES

1. Gyr KD, Singer MV, Sarles H, eds. Pancreatitis: Concepts and Classification. Amsterdam: Excerpta Medica, 1984.
2. Austin J, Reber HA. The pathologic features of acute pancreatitis. In Howard J, Jordan G, Reber HA, eds. Surgical Diseases of the Pancreas. Philadelphia: Lea & Febiger, 1986.
3. Wedgewood K, Reber HA. Acute pancreatitis: The concepts of pathogenesis. In Howard J, Jordan G, Reber HA, eds. Surgical Diseases of the Pancreas. Philadelphia: Lea & Febiger, 1986.
4. Steer ML. How and where does acute pancreatitis begin? Arch Surg 127:1350, 1992.
5. Malik AB. Pulmonary edema after pancreatitis: Role of humoral factors. Circ Shock 10:71, 1983.
6. Popieruitis AS, Thompson AG. The site of bradykinin release in acute experimental pancreatitis. Arch Surg 98:73, 1969.
7. Acosta JM, Ledesma CL. Gallstone migration as a cause of acute pancreatitis. N Engl J Med 290:484, 1974.
8. Austin JL, et al. Effect of partial duct obstruction and drainage on pancreatic function. J Surg Res 28:426, 1980.
9. Herman RE, Davis JH. The role of incomplete pancreatic duct obstruction in the etiology of pancreatitis. Surgery 48:318, 1960.
10. McMahon MJ, Playforth MJ, Pickford IR. A comparative study of methods for the prediction of severity of attacks of acute pancreatitis. Br J Surg 67:22, 1980.
11. Hallenbeck GA. Biliary and pancreatic intraductal pressures. In Code CF, ed. Handbook of Physiology. Baltimore: Williams & Wilkins, 1967.
12. Mosely J, Reber HA. The effect of bile salts on the pancreatic duct mucosa. Br J Surg 67:59, 1980.
13. Toriumi Y, et al. Octreotide and cholecystokinin antagonist reduce edema in obstruction-induced acute pancreatitis. J Lab Clin Med 122:450, 1993.
14. Wedgewood KR, Farmer RC, Reber HA. A model of hemorrhagic pancreatitis in cats—Role of 16,16-dimethyl prostaglandin E2. Gastroenterology 90:32, 1986.

15. Nordback IH, et al. The role of acetaldehyde in the pathogenesis of acute alcoholic pancreatitis. Ann Surg 214:671, 1991.
16. Bess MA, Edis AJ, VanHeerden JA. Hyperparathyroidism and pancreatitis. JAMA 243:246, 1980.
17. Elliott DW. Pancreatitis associated with hyperparathyroidism. In Howard JM, Jordan GJ, Reber HA, eds. Surgical Diseases of the Pancreas. Philadelphia: Lea & Febiger, 1986.
18. Kelly TR. Relationship of hyperparathyroidism to pancreatitis. Arch Surg 97:267, 1968.
19. Sanfey H, Cameron JL. Pancreatitis associated with hyperlipemia. In Howard JM, Jordan GJ, Reber HA, eds. Surgical Disease of the Pancreas. Philadelphia: Lea & Febiger, 1986.
20. Saharia P. Acute pancreatitis with hyperlipemia: Studies with an isolated perfused canine pancreas. Surgery 82:60, 1972.
21. Mallory A, Kern F. Drug-induced pancreatitis: A critical review. Gastroenterology 78:813, 1980.
22. Satake K, Nakashima Y. Drug-induced pancreatitis. In Howard JM, Jordan GJ, Reber HA, eds. Surgical Diseases of the Pancreas. Philadelphia, Lea & Febiger, 1986.
23. Underwood TW, Frye CB. Drug-induced pancreatitis. Clin Pharm 12:440, 1993.
24. Adler JB, Mazzotta SA, Barkin JS. Pancreatitis caused by measles, mumps, and rubella vaccine. Pancreas 6:489, 1991.
25. Aloia T, et al. Candida in pancreatic infection: A clinical experience. Am Surg 60:793, 1994.
26. Ozsvar Z, Deak J, Pap A. Possible role of coxsackie-B virus infection in pancreatitis. Int J Pancreatol 11:105, 1992.
27. Khuroo MS, et al. Worm extraction and biliary drainage in hepatobiliary and pancreatic asariasis. Gastrointest Endosc 39:680, 1993.
28. Warshaw AL, O'Hara PJ. Susceptibility of the pancreas to ischemic injury in shock. Am J Surg 188:197, 1978.
29. Bockman DE. Microvasculature of the pancreas: Relation to pancreatitis. Int J Pancreatol 12:11, 1992.
30. Lefer AM. Vascular mediators in ischemia and shock. In Cowley RA, Trump BF, eds. Pathophysiology of Shock, Anoxia, and Ischemia. Baltimore: Williams & Wilkins, 1982.
31. Lee PC, Howard JM. Fat necrosis. Surg Gynecol Obstet 148:785, 1979.
32. Bradley EL, et al. Hemodynamic consequences of severe pancreatitis. Ann Surg 198:130, 1983.
33. DiCarlo V, et al. Hemodynamic and metabolic impairment in acute pancreatitis. World J Surg 5:329, 1981.
34. Goldstein DA, Llach F, Massry SG. Acute renal failure in patients with acute pancreatitis. Arch Intern Med 136:1363, 1976.
35. Sankaran S, Lucas CE, Walt AJ. Transient hypertension with acute pancreatitis, Surg Gynecol Obstet 138:225, 1974.
36. Nath BJ, Warshaw AL. Pulmonary insufficiency. In Bradley EL, ed. Complications of Pancreatitis. Philadelphia: WB Saunders, 1982.
37. Halmagyi DF, et al. Pulmonary hypertension in acute hemorrhagic pancreatitis. Surgery 76:637, 1974.
38. Miyashiro A, Grosberg SJ, Wapnick S. Reversible pulmonary hypertension and cardiac failure with recurrent pancreatitis. Chest 71:669, 1977.
39. Tahamont MV, et al. Increased lung vascular permeability after pancreatitis and trypsin infusion. Am J Pathol 109:15, 1982.
40. Kimura T, et al. Respiratory failure in acute pancreatitis. Ann Surg 189:509, 1979.
41. Lankisch PG, Rahlf G, Koop H. Pulmonary complications in fatal acute hemorrhagic pancreatitis. Dig Dis Sci 28:111, 1983.
42. Ranson JHC, Spencer F. The role of peritoneal lavage in severe acute pancreatitis. Ann Surg 187:565, 1978.
43. Imrie CW, et al. Parathyroid hormone and calcium homeostasis in acute pancreatitis. Br J Surg 65:717, 1978.
44. Canale DD, Donabedian RK. Hypercalcitoninemia in acute pancreatitis. J Clin Endocrinol Metab 49:738, 1975.
45. Moosa AR. Diagnostic tests and procedures in acute pancreatitis. N Engl J Med 311:639, 1984.
46. Warshaw AL, O'Hara PJ. Laboratory diagnosis of acute pancreatitis. In Howard JM, Jordan GJ, Reber HA, eds. Surgical Diseases of the Pancreas. Philadelphia: Lea & Febiger, 1986.
47. Johnson SG, Ellis CJ, Levitt MD. Mechanisms of increased renal clearance of amylase/creatinine in acute pancreatitis. N Engl J Med 295:1214, 1976.
48. Pezzilli R, et al. Serum amylase and lipase concentrations and lipase/amylase ratio in assessment of etiology and severity of acute pancreatitis. Dig Dis Sci 38:1265, 1993.
49. Ranson JH. The role of surgery in the management of acute pancreatitis. Ann Surg 211:382, 1990.
50. Ranson JH, et al. Prognostic signs and the role of operative management in acute pancreatitis. Surg Gynecol Obstet 139:69, 1974.
51. Satiani B, Stone HH. Predictability of present outcome and future recurrence in acute pancreatitis. Arch Surg 114:711, 1979.
52. Wilson C, Heath DI, Imrie CW. Prediction of outcome in acute pancreatitis: A comparative study of APACHE II, clinical assessment and multiple factor scoring systems. Br J Surg 77:1260, 1990.
53. Freeny PC. Angio-CT: Diagnosis and detection of complications of acute pancreatitis. Hepatogastroenterology 38:109, 1991.
54. London NJM, et al. Rapid-bolus contrast-enhanced dynamic computed tomography in acute pancreatitis: A prospective study. Br J Surg 78:1452, 1991.
55. Lebenthal E, Rolston DD, Holsclaw DS. Enzyme therapy for pancreatic insufficiency: Present status and future needs. Pancreas 9:1, 1994.
56. Dominguez-Munoz JE, et al. Monitoring of serum proteinase-antiproteinase balance and systemic inflammatory response in prognostic evaluation of acute pancreatitis. Results of a prospective multicenter trial. Dig Dis Sci 38:507, 1993.
57. Heath DI, et al. Role of interleukin-6 in mediating the acute phase protein response and potential as an early means of severity assessment in acute pancreatitis, Gut 34:41, 1993.
58. Olazabal A, Fuller R. Failure of glucagon in the treatment of alcoholic pancreatitis. Gastroenterology 74:489, 1978.
59. Buchler MW, Binder M, Friess H. Role of somatostatin and its analogues in the treatment of acute and chronic pancreatitis. Gut 35:S15, 1994.
60. Gjorup I, et al. A double-blinded multicenter trial of somatostatin in the treatment of acute pancreatitis. Surg Gynecol Obstet 175:397, 1992.
61. Ladas SD, Raptis SA. Conservative treatment of acute pancreatitis: The use of somatostatin. Hepatogastroenterology 39:466, 1992.
62. Finch WT, Sawyers JL, Schenker S. A prospective study to determine the efficacy of antibiotics in acute pancreatitis. Ann Surg 183:667, 1976.
63. Howes R, Zuidema GD, Cameron JL. Evaluation of prophylactic antibiotics in acute pancreatitis. J Surg Res 18:197, 1975.
64. Bradley EL. Antibiotics in acute pancreatitis: Current status and future directions. Am J Surg 158:472, 1989.
65. Pederzoli P, et al. A randomized multicenter clinical trial of antibiotic prophylaxis of septic complications in acute necrotizing pancreatitis with imipenem, Surg Gynecol Obstet 176:480, 1993.
66. Pisters PW, Ranson JH. Nutritional support for acute pancreatitis. Surg Gynecol Obstet 175:275, 1992.
67. Sax HC, et al. Early total parenteral nutrition in acute pancreatitis: Lack of beneficial effects. Am J Surg 153:117, 1987.
68. Parekh D, Lawson HH, Segal I. The role of total enteral nutrition in pancreatic disease. S Afr J Surg 31:57, 1993.
69. Schroder T, et al. Pancreatic resection versus peritoneal lavage in acute necrotizing pancreatitis. A prospective randomized trial. Ann Surg 214:663, 1991.
70. Patti MG, Pellegrini CA. Gallstone pancreatitis. Surg Clin 70:1277, 1990.
71. de-Vergilio C, et al. Gallstone pancreatitis: The role of preoperative endoscopic retrograde cholangiopancreatography. Arch Surg 129:909, 1994.

72. Sahel J. The usefulness of endoscopic retrograde pancreatography for the classification of chronic pancreatitis. In Gyr KF, Singer MV, Sarles H, eds. Pancreatitis: Concepts and Classification. New York: Elsevier North-Holland, 1984.
73. Reber HA, Smale B. Planned operation for acute pancreatitis: The American experience. In Howard JM, Jordan GJ, Reber HA, eds. Surgical Diseases of the Pancreas. Philadelphia: Lea & Febiger, 1986.
74. Reber HA, McFadden DW. Indications for surgery in severe pancreatitis—State of the art. Int J Pancreatol 15:83, 1994.
75. Hill MC, et al. The role of percutaneous aspiration in the diagnosis of pancreatic abscess. Am J Radiol 141:1035, 1983.
76. Schurawitzki H, et al. CT-guided percutaneous drainage and fluid aspiration in intensive care patients. Acta Radiol 33:131, 1992.
77. Bockman DE, et al. Analysis of nerves in chronic pancreatitis. Gastroenterology 94:1459, 1988.
78. Sarles H, Devaux MA, Noel-Jorund MC. Action of ethanol on the pancreas. In Gyr KF, Singer MV, Sarles H, eds. Pancreatitis: Concepts and Classification. New York: Elsevier North-Holland, 1984.
79. Malagalada J-R. The pathophysiology of alcoholic pancreatitis. Pancreas 1:270, 1986.
80. Clemente F, et al. Biochemical events in rat pancreatic cells in acute and chronic alcohol intoxications. In Gyr KE, Singer MV, Sarles H, eds. Pancreatitis: Concepts and Classification. New York: Elsevier North-Holland, 1984.
81. Day CP, et al. Investigation of the role of polymorphisms at the alcohol and aldehyde dehydrogenase loci in genetic predisposition to alcohol-related end-organ damage. Hepatology 14:798, 1991.
82. Brecher AS, Pavlock JL. Acetaldehyde decreases the antitryptic activity of alpha 1 proteinase inhibitor. Alcohol 9:181, 1992.
83. Sing M, Simcek H. Ethanol and the pancreas: Current status. Gastroenterology 98:1051, 1990.
84. Reber HA, et al. Pancreatic blood flow in cats with chronic pancreatitis. Gastroenterology 103:652, 1992.
85. Balasegaram M. Pancreatitis in the tropics. In Howard JM, Jordan GJ, Reber HA, eds. Surgical Diseases of the Pancreas. Philadelphia: Lea & Febiger, 1986.
86. Pitchumoni CS. "Tropical" or "nutritional pancreatitis"—An update. In Gyr KF, Singer MV, Sarles H, eds. Pancreatitis: Concepts and Classifications. New York: Elsevier North-Holland, 1984.
87. Karanjia ND, et al. Pancreatic ductal and interstitial pressures in cats with chronic pancreatitis. Dig Dis Sci 37:268, 1992.
88. Toyama MT, et al. Pancreatic tissue oxygenation in chronic pancreatitis. Pancreas 9:805, 1994.
89. DiMagno EP, Go VLW, Summerskill WHJ. Relations between pancreatic enzyme outputs and malabsorption in severe pancreatic insufficiency. N Engl J Med 288:813, 1973.
90. Goldberg DM, Durie PR. Biochemical tests in the diagnosis of chronic pancreatitis and in the evaluation of pancreatic insufficiency. Clin Biochem 26:253, 1993.
91. Austin JL, Reber HA. Chronic pancreatitis. In Rakel RE, ed. Conn's Current Therapy. Philadelphia: WB Saunders, 1985.
92. Mossner J. Is there a place for pancreatic enzymes in the treatment of pain in chronic pancreatitis? Digestion 54(Suppl 2):35, 1993.
93. Ihse I, Permerth J. Enzyme therapy and pancreatic pain. Acta Chir Scand 156:281, 1990.
94. Patel AG, et al. Changes in pancreatic interstitial pH during the evolution of chronic pancreatitis [abstract]. Gastroenterology 106:A313, 1994.
95. Ebbehoj N, et al. Pancreatic tissue fluid pressure during drainage operations for chronic pancreatitis. Scand J Gastroenterol 25:1041, 1990.
96. Nealon WH, Thompson JC. Progressive loss of pancreatic function in chronic pancreatitis is delayed by main pancreatic duct decompression. A longitudinal prospective analysis of the modified Puestow procedure. Ann Surg 217:466, 1993.

28

The Jaundiced Patient

Attila Nakeeb and Henry A. Pitt

The term *jaundice,* or *icterus,* refers to a yellow staining of the skin, mucous membranes, and body fluids by bilirubin. Serum bilirubin concentration is normally between 0.5 and 1.3 mg/dl. Jaundice usually becomes clinically apparent when the serum bilirubin concentration exceeds 2.0 mg/dl. Because bilirubin preferentially concentrates in elastic tissue, the yellowish discoloration of jaundice may first become apparent in the sclera of the eye.

During the past 50 years, significant advances have been made in our understanding of the pathophysiology, diagnosis, and management of jaundice. Biochemists have elucidated normal bilirubin metabolism and have described specific defects that result in different clinical syndromes. Such imaging techniques as ultrasonography (US), computed tomography (CT), percutaneous transhepatic cholangiography (PTC), and endoscopic retrograde cholangiography (ERC) have dramatically changed the diagnostic approach to the patient with jaundice.

Many of these techniques have led to newer therapeutic options, such as percutaneous transhepatic drainage (PTD), endoscopic sphincterotomy (ES), percutaneous or endoscopic balloon dilatation, and the placement of endoprostheses to relieve biliary obstruction. Similarly, advances in perioperative and operative management have resulted in improved operative survival among patients with jaundice. Before a discussion of the various diagnostic and therapeutic modalities available for the management of jaundice, normal and abnormal bilirubin metabolism are reviewed, a classification system of jaundice is presented, and the multiple pathophysiologic effects of jaundice are explained.

BILIRUBIN METABOLISM

In adults, between 250 to 350 mg bilirubin is produced each day. Approximately 80% to 85% of this bilirubin is derived from the destruction of senescent red blood cells by the reticuloendothelial system. The remaining 15% to 20% comes from the breakdown of nonhemoglobin proteins, such as myoglobin and the cytochromes. The metabolism of bilirubin is reviewed in Fig. 28-1. In reticuloendothelial cells, the microsomal enzyme heme oxygenase cleaves heme into biliverdin. Biliverdin is then reduced to bilirubin by the cytosolic enzyme biliverdin reductase before being released into the circulation. In this unconjugated form, bilirubin is water insoluble and is transported to the liver tightly bound to albumin.

The liver removes unconjugated bilirubin and other organic anions bound to albumin from plasma. Once the bilirubin-albumin complex enters the sinusoidal circulation of the liver, three distinct metabolic phases are recognized: (1) hepatocyte uptake, (2) conjugation, and (3) excretion into bile. Unconjugated bilirubin is transported across the sinusoidal membrane of the hepatocyte into the cytoplasm. Although the exact mechanism is unknown, a series of carrier proteins is thought to be responsible for this process. Once inside the hepatocyte, unconjugated bilirubin is again bound by a cytoplasmic protein, in this case a glutathione S-transferase. The microsomal enzyme uridine diphosphate-glucuronyl transferase then conjugates the insoluble unconjugated bilirubin with glucuronic acid to form the water-soluble conjugated forms bilirubin monoglucuronide (15%) and bilirubin diglucuronide (85%). Conjugated bilirubin is then excreted from the hepatocyte into the bile canaliculus by an active-transport mechanism.

Excretion into bile is the rate-limiting step in bilirubin metabolism. After excretion, bile flows through the biliary ductal collecting system, may be stored in the gallbladder, and enters the duodenum. In the terminal ileum and colon, bilirubin is converted by bacterial enzymes into the colorless urobilinogen. From 10% to 20% of the urobilinogen is then reabsorbed from the intestine into the portal circulation, creating an enterohepatic circulation. This recycled urobilinogen may be reexcreted either into the bile by the liver or into urine by the kidney. The remaining urobilinogen in the intestine is converted to fecobilinogen, which gives stool its characteristic brown color.

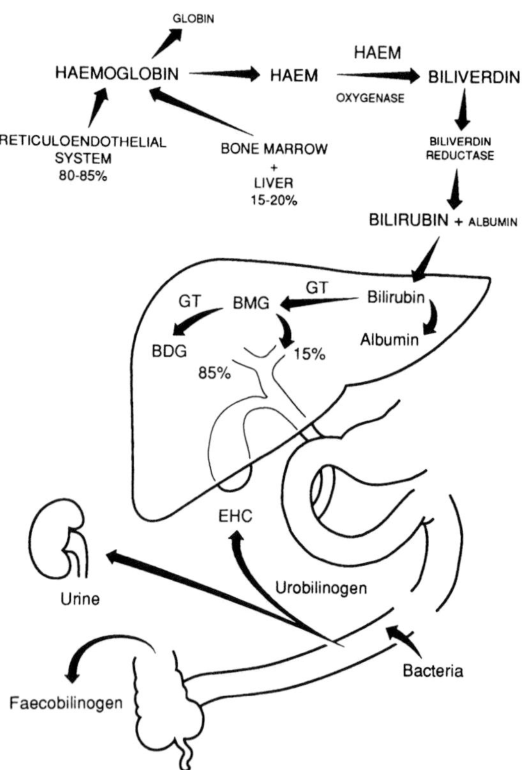

Fig. 28-1. Schematic representation of normal bilirubin metabolism. *BMG,* Bilirubin monoglucouronide; *EHC,* enterohepatic circulation; *GT,* glucuronyl transferase; *HAEM,* heme. (From Lippset PA, Pitt HA. Jaundice: Mechanisms and differential diagnosis. In Toouli J, ed. Surgery of the Biliary Tract. Edinburgh: Churchill Livingstone, 1993, p 49.)

Normal bilirubin metabolism can be summarized as a series of steps: (1) production, (2) uptake by the hepatocyte, (3) conjugation, (4) excretion into bile ducts, and (5) delivery to the intestine. Jaundice can result from defects in any of these steps of bilirubin metabolism.

CLASSIFICATION OF JAUNDICE

Numerous systems for the classification of jaundice have been proposed, with factors such as pathogenic mechanisms, disease processes, and treatment regimens. However, the most widely accepted classification system is one that relates jaundice to an alteration in normal bilirubin metabolism. In this system, jaundice may result from (1) increased production of bilirubin, (2) impaired uptake of bilirubin, (3) impaired conjugation of bilirubin, (4) impaired transport or excretion of bilirubin into the bile canaliculus, or (5) obstruction of the intrahepatic or extrahepatic biliary tree (Table 28-1). Overproduction, impaired uptake, and impaired conjugation of bilirubin all lead to a predominately unconjugated hyperbilirubinemia. Impaired transport and excretion and biliary ductal obstruction result in hyperbilirubinemia that is primarily conjugated. Some patients have multiple defects in normal metabolism. For example, a patient with biliary obstruction from tumor may acquire secondary hepatocellular dysfunction. Therefore, these classification systems may be simplifications of more complex disease processes.

Increased Production

Overproduction of bilirubin can result from either congenital or acquired hemolysis. Hereditary causes include spherocytosis, thalassemia, and sickle-cell disease. Acquired causes of hemolysis include sepsis, burns, infections, drugs, transfusion reactions, and acquired autoimmune diseases. When the capacity of the liver to remove bilirubin from the circulation is exceeded, unconjugated hyperbilirubinemia occurs. The total bilirubin level in hemolysis rarely exceeds 4 to 5 mg/dl. If underlying hepatocellular dysfunction is also present, however, much higher bilirubin levels may occur.

Impaired Uptake and Conjugation

Impaired uptake of unconjugated bilirubin by hepatocytes can be caused by drugs, prolonged fasting, sepsis, and viral hepatitis. Gilbert syndrome, the most common cause of unconjugated nonhemolytic hyperbilirubinemia, affects between 2.5% and 7% of the population. Gilbert syndrome is a congenital defect that results in unconjugated hyperbilirubinemia because of reduced bilirubin glucuronyl transferase levels within hepatocytes. The bilirubin level fluctuates according to the clinical state but rarely exceeds 3.0 mg/dl.

Neonatal jaundice results from an immaturity of the hepatic conjugating and transport system. This problem occurs between the second and fifth days of life, and it usually disappears by 2 weeks, as the enzyme systems mature. In the Crigler-Najjar syndromes, there is either complete absence of glucuronyl transferase activity (type I) or a marked decrease in glucuronyl transferase activity (type II). Type I disease is usually fatal within the first year of life.

Impaired Transport or Excretion

Impairment of bilirubin transport or excretion into the bile canaliculus results in intrahepatic cholestasis, which is also referred to as *medical jaundice.* Impaired bilirubin transport and excretion into the bile canaliculus after conjugation result in increased serum levels of conjugated bilirubin. Hepatitis, either viral, alcoholic, or drug-induced, is the most common cause of intrahepatic cholestasis. Cirrhosis, a diffuse fibrotic process in the liver, usually caused by chronic alcohol consumption, may result in hepatocellular failure. Drugs such as estrogens, oral contraceptives, and anabolic steroids also may cause a defect in the excretion of bilirubin.

Genetic defects in the hepatic excretion of bilirubin and other organic anions across the hepatocyte membrane exist in both Dubin-Johnson and Rotor's syndromes. In Dubin-Johnson syndrome, pigments accumulate within hepatocytes, causing the liver to turn black. Rotor's syndrome has a similar defect in hepatic storage of bilirubin,

Table 28-1. Classification of Jaundice

Defect in Bilirubin Metabolism	Predominant Hyperbilirubinemia	Examples
Increased production	Unconjugated	Congenital hemoglobinopathies, hemolysis, multiple transfusions
Impaired hepatocyte uptake	Unconjugated	Gilbert's syndrome, drug induced
Reduced conjugation	Unconjugated	Neonatal jaundice, Crigler-Najjar syndrome
Impaired transport and excretion	Conjugated	Hepatitis, cirrhosis, Dubin-Johnson syndrome, Rotor's syndrome
Biliary obstruction	Conjugated	Choledocholithiasis, benign strictures, peri-ampullary cancer, cholangiocarcinoma

except that no pigment accumulates within the liver parenchyma.

Biliary Obstruction

Jaundice caused by biliary obstruction is often referred to as *surgical jaundice.* With biliary obstruction, hyperbilirubinemia, is primarily conjugated, but unconjugated bilirubin is often also moderately elevated. Common causes of surgical jaundice, depicted in Table 28-1, are the primary focus of the remainder of this chapter.

PATHOPHYSIOLOGY OF JAUNDICE

Biliary obstruction produces local effects on the bile ducts that lead to derangements of hepatic function and, ultimately, widespread systemic effects. Patients with jaundice are at increased risk for development of hepatic dysfunction, renal failure, cardiovascular impairments, bleeding problems, infections, and wound complications, and for death after surgery. Several authors have reported a direct correlation between operative mortality rate and the degree of jaundice. In one such analysis of 155 patients undergoing operations on the bile duct, Pitt et al.[1] reported that mortality rate was significantly increased among patients with bilirubin greater than 10 mg/dl (Table 28-2). In this analysis, mortality rates were 3% for 101 patients with bilirubin less than 5 mg/dl, 9% for 23 patients with bilirubin between 5 and 10 mg/dl, and 23% for 31 patients with bilirubin greater than 10 mg/dl.

In addition to bilirubin levels, (1) underlying malignancy, (2) advanced age, (3) low hematocrit or albumin level, and (4) high white blood cell count, alkaline phosphatase activity, or creatinine level have all been identified as risk factors for death in patients with obstructive jaundice. Among these factors, subsequent studies have suggested that albumin and creatinine are the best predictors.

Hepatobiliary Association

The biliary system normally has a low pressure. In the setting of complete or partial biliary obstruction, biliary pressure can approach 30 cm H_2O. This increase in biliary pressure has been correlated with increased counts of bacteria in the bloodstream.[2] Ultimately, the increase in biliary pressure leads to the dilatation of the extrahepatic and intrahepatic biliary tree. With long-standing obstruction, intrahepatic bile ductule proliferation occurs and results in biliary cirrhosis.

Table 28-2. Correlation of Serum Bilirubin With Postoperative Mortality

Bilirubin (mg/dl)	Patients (N)	Mortality (%)
<1.5	61	3.3
1.5-5	40	2.5
5-10	23	8.7
10-20	22	18.2*
>20	9	33.3*

Modified from Pitt HA, et al. Factors affecting mortality in biliary tract surgery. Am J Surg 141:68, 1981.
*p <0.01 versus patients with bilirubin <5 mg/dl.

The secretory, metabolic, and synthetic functions of hepatocytes are altered by biliary obstruction.[3] When biliary pressure is greater than 20 cm H_2O, hepatic bile secretion is diminished. Similarly, patients with jaundice have a decreased capacity to excrete drugs, such as antibiotics, that are normally secreted into bile. The increased concentration of bile acids associated with obstructive jaundice results in inhibition of the hepatic cytochrome P_{450} enzymes and therefore a decrease in the rate of oxidative metabolism in the liver. The synthetic function of the hepatocyte is also decreased with obstructive jaundice, as evidenced by decreased plasma levels of albumin, clotting factors, and secretory immunoglobulins.

Kupffer's cell, a tissue macrophage, is the predominant cell type of the hepatic reticuloendothelial system. Normally, infectious agents, damaged blood cells, cellular debris, fibrin degradation products, and endotoxin that are absorbed or formed in the portal circulation are effectively filtered by Kupffer's cells and removed from the systemic circulation. Obstructive jaundice has been shown to have a profound effect on the ability of Kupffer's cells to clear bacteria, colloid, and endotoxin.[4,5]

Renal Association

The association between jaundice and postoperative renal failure has been known for many years. The reported incidence of postoperative acute renal failure is approximately 10%. Moreover, the mortality rate among patients with jaundice in whom renal failure develops has been reported to be as high as 75%.[6] Several theories have been proposed to explain this renal failure in patients with jaundice. Among these theories are the possibilities that (1) bile pigments damage renal tubules, (2) renal perfusion is decreased, (3) renal tubules are more sensitive to anoxia and hypotension, and (4) endotoxins cause renal damage. Although multiple factors may be involved, this last theory is currently the most widely accepted.

Endotoxin has been found in the peripheral blood of approximately 50% of patients with obstructive jaundice.[7,8] This phenomenon may be the result of a lack of bile salts in the gut lumen that normally prevent absorption of endotoxins and inhibit anaerobic bacterial growth, as well as of the decreased hepatic clearance of endotoxin by Kupffer's cells. Endotoxin also causes renal vasoconstriction with redistribution of renal blood flow away from the cortex and disturbances in coagulation, including the activation of complement, macrophages, leukocytes, and platelets.[7] As a result, glomerular fibrin and peritubular fibrin are deposited. This deposition, in combination with reduced renal cortical blood flow, results in the tubular and cortical necrosis observed in patients with jaundice and renal failure.

Certain bile salts have been shown to be efficacious in preventing the development of postoperative renal dysfunction. In a study by Evans et al.,[9] two of nine patients with jaundice not receiving oral sodium taurocholate before surgery had acute renal failure. Creatinine clearance in these patients decreased from a mean of 85 to 55 ml/min. In contrast, none of nine patients with jaundice treated before surgery with oral bile salts had renal failure, and mean creatinine clearance increased from 79 to 99 ml/min. In a study by Cahill,[8] 54% of 24 patients with jaundice not given oral bile salts before surgery were found to have systemic endotoxemia, which was associated with renal impairment in two thirds of all cases. In comparison, none of eight patients with jaundice given 500 mg sodium deoxycholate every 8 hours for 48 hours before surgery had portal or systemic endotoxemia. Moreover, none of these eight patients showed evidence of renal impairment.

Cardiovascular Association

In addition to the hepatic dysfunction and increased propensity toward development of renal failure, obstructive jaundice is known to cause severe hemodynamic disturbances. Experimental animals with obstructive jaundice tend to be hypotensive and exhibit an exaggerated hypotensive response to hemorrhage. Studies in experimental animals have demonstrated that bile duct–ligated animals have (1) decreased cardiac contractility, (2) reduced left ventricular pressures, and (3) impaired response to β-agonist drugs such as isoproterenol and norepinephrine.[10,11] In a study of nine patients with obstructive or cholestatic jaundice, Lumlertgul et al.[12] showed a significantly blunted response in left ventricular ejection fraction compared with that of healthy volunteers after the infusion of the positive inotrope dobutamine. The effect of obstructive jaundice on the peripheral vasculature is to cause a decrease in total peripheral resistance.

In addition to the direct effects of jaundice on the heart and peripheral vasculature, jaundice results in hypovolemia. The increased serum levels of bile acids associated with obstructive jaundice have both diuretic and natriuretic effects on the kidney. In dogs, the infusion of bile into the renal artery results in increased urinary flow, natriuresis, and kaliuresis. This diuretic effect may be mediated by increased prostaglandin E_2 production by the kidney.[13] The combination of hypovolemia, depressed cardiac function, and decreased total peripheral resistance most likely makes the patient with jaundice more susceptible to the development of postoperative shock than are those without jaundice.

Coagulation

Disturbances of blood coagulation are also commonly present in patients with jaundice. The most frequently observed clotting defect in patients with biliary obstruction is prolongation of the prothrombin time (PT). This problem results from impaired vitamin K absorption from the gut, related to a lack of intestinal bile. This coagulopathy is usually reversible by the parenteral administration of vitamin K. Decreased bile levels in the small intestine may also result in diminished absorption of other fat-soluble vitamins and fats, causing weight loss and loss of calcium. This latter factor, as well as the previously mentioned increase in circulating endotoxin, may further contribute to clotting abnormalities.

In experimental animals, endotoxin affects factors XI and XII and causes platelet and direct endothelial damage.[7] Moreover, endotoxin release in patients with jaundice results in a low-grade disseminated intravascular coagulation (DIC), with increased fibrin degradation products. Hunt et al.[14] have shown that patients with jaundice who have circulating endotoxin or increased fibrin-degradation product levels before surgery are at increased risk for hemorrhagic complications. In addition to problems with endotoxemia, patients with cirrhosis may have even more complicated clotting abnormalities, such as problems with thrombocytopenia from hypersplenism and fibrinolysis.

Immune System

Surgery in the patient with jaundice is associated with a significant rate of postoperative septic complications. Patients with jaundice have a number of defects in cellular immunity that make them more susceptible to infection. Cainzos et al.[15] demonstrated an association between jaundice and altered delayed-type hypersensitivity. Only 16% of 118 patients with jaundice, compared with 76% of 59 healthy subjects, were found to be immunocompetent when tested with a battery of seven skin antigens. Several authors have shown impaired T-cell proliferation,[16] decreased neutrophil chemotaxis,[17] and defective bacterial phagocytosis[18] after bile duct ligation in rats. As mentioned earlier, the ability of the reticuloendothelial system, specifically liver Kupffer's cells, to clear bacteria and endotoxin from the circulation is also reduced in obstructive jaundice.

The absence of bile from the intestinal tract also plays a role in the infectious complications seen in patients with obstructive jaundice. Bacterial translocation from the gut has been shown to be increased in the setting of bile duct obstruction.[19] Obstruction causes a disruption of the enterohepatic circulation and results in the loss of the emulsifying antiendotoxin effect of bile acids. Therefore, a larger pool of endotoxin is available within the intestine for absorption into the portal circulation. The combination of a lack of bile in the intestine and the impairment of cellular immunity and reticuloendothelial cell function most likely results in the observed increase in septic and infectious complications seen among patients with jaundice.

Wound Healing

Delayed wound healing and a high incidence of wound dehiscence and incisional hernias have been observed among patients undergoing surgery for the relief of obstructive jaundice. Patients with obstructive jaundice have decreased activity of the enzyme propylhydroxylase in their skin. Propylhydroxylase is necessary for the incorporation of proline amino acid residues into collagen, and its activity has been used as a measure of collagen synthesis. Grande et al.[20] measured skin propylhydroxylase activity in 95 patients with extrahepatic bile duct obstruction and 123 control patients without jaundice undergoing cholecystectomy. The patients with jaundice had only 11% of the skin propylhydroxylase activity shown by the control patients. In the subgroup of patients who had jaundice related to malignancy, the propylhydroxylase activity was less than 7% of control value. With relief of obstruction, the activity increased to 22% of control values. Interestingly, in patients with jaundice related to benign obstruction, the activity increased to 100% of control values.

Other Factors

Other problems that face patients with jaundice are anorexia, weight loss, and resultant malnutrition. Appetite is adversely influenced by the lack of bile salts in the intestinal tract. In addition, patients with pancreatic or periampullary malignant lesions may have partial duodenal obstruction or abnormal gastric emptying, perhaps related to tumor infiltration of the celiac nerve plexus. Patients with pancreatic or ampullary tumors may also have pancreatic endocrine and exocrine insufficiency. This latter problem may further compound other nutritional defects, which in turn may multiply the immune deficits of the patient with jaundice.

In recent years, it has become clear that the many physiologic derangements that occur with obstructive jaundice take a long time to reverse. For example, Koyama et al.[3] showed that hepatic mitochondrial function does not return to normal even 7 weeks after relief of obstruction. This same prolonged effect of obstructive jaundice has been noted with lymphocyte, polymorphonuclear leukocyte, and Kupffer's cell function. Therefore, even patients who have had temporary relief of biliary obstruction by means of percutaneous or endoscopic stents are likely to remain at risk for the development of significant complications after surgery.

DIAGNOSTIC APPROACH

When confronted with a patient with jaundice, the objective of the physician is to identify any potentially treatable causes of the condition. The most important distinction is whether the jaundice has been caused by intrahepatic cholestasis or extrahepatic obstruction. Fortunately, the distinction between medical and surgical jaundice can be made relatively easily with a careful history, physical examination, review of serum chemistries, and radiologic evaluation. An algorithm for the evaluation of the patient with jaundice is shown in Fig. 28-2. The following discussion presents an approach to the patient with jaundice that allows accurate diagnosis without subjecting the patient to needless risk, discomfort, or expense.

Clinical Evaluation

The first and most important step in the workup of the patient with jaundice is to obtain a careful history. Important historical points to consider include occupational exposures, travel history, recent exposures to hepatitis, and contacts with jaundiced persons. Similarly, any exposure to transfusions, blood tests, tattoos, or body fluids should be noted. The patient should be questioned about drug ingestion, with special attention to alcohol and other hepatotoxins. A family history regarding hemolytic anemias or congenital hyperbilirubinemias also may be helpful. A history of previous surgery, especially biliary operation, raises the suspicion of a benign biliary stricture or retained common duct stones. Hepatitis after transfusion or halothane toxicity may also appear after a surgical procedure.

The time of onset and course of jaundice should be determined; these can often give a clue to the diagnosis. Viral hepatitis may be suspected if the jaundice is of rapid onset and is associated with nausea and anorexia. A history of biliary colic points toward choledocholithiasis. Pancreatic cancer, on the other hand, is more likely to be associated with progressive, painless jaundice and weight loss. The presence of fever, chills, and upper abdominal pain in addition to jaundice (Charcot's triad) is suggestive of cholangitis, which occurs more often in patients with choledocholithiasis than in those with malignant obstruction. The presence of pruritus suggests cholestasis and mandates the exclusion of extrahepatic bile duct obstruction.

On physical examination, the abdomen should be carefully palpated. A small liver may be discovered in cases of severe cirrhosis or hepatitis. A tender liver edge may be found in cases of hepatitis, congestive heart failure, or alcoholic hepatitis. A palpable, nontender gallbladder may be noted in cases of pancreatic or ampullary carcinoma

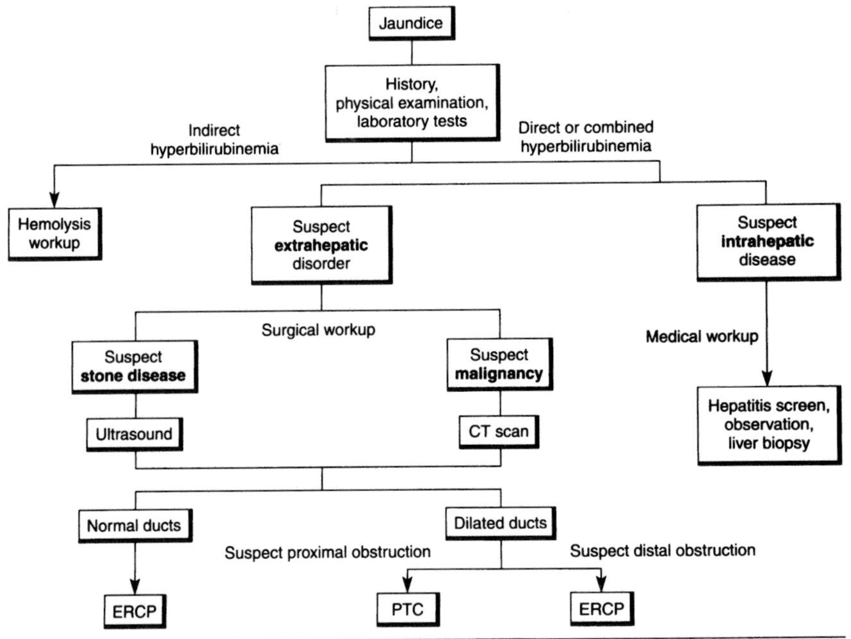

Fig. 28-2. Algorithm for the evaluation of jaundice. *ERCP,* Endoscopic retrograde cholangiopancreatography; *PTC,* percutaneous transhepatic cholangiography.

(Courvoisier's sign). A tender gallbladder, on the other hand, may be palpated in a patient who has choledocholithiasis with associated cholecystitis. Any signs of cirrhosis (ascites, spider angioma, or periumbilical venous enlargement) should also be noted.

The color of the patient's urine and stool should be carefully noted. Total obstruction of the biliary tract results in acholic, pale stools, increased bilirubin in the urine, and absence of urine urobilinogen. If excess urinary bilirubin is detected, then serum conjugated bilirubin levels are usually elevated. Stools that are black or silver suggest the presence of blood, which may indicate an ampullary lesion that is both bleeding and obstructing the distal bile duct.

Biochemical Evaluation

Along with the history and physical examination, biochemical evaluation is an integral part of the initial workup of the patient with jaundice. Hyperbilirubinemia is the sine qua non of jaundice, and the level of bilirubin indicates the severity of the disease process. Moreover, bilirubin levels can be used to follow disease progression. The routine laboratory tests that should be performed on all patients with jaundice include determinations of direct (conjugated) and indirect (unconjugated) bilirubin levels, alkaline phosphatase activity, serum transaminase activities, and amylase activity. The urine should also be tested for bilirubin and urobilinogen.

Patients with hemolysis have an increase in the indirect (unconjugated) fraction of bilirubin, whereas the direct (conjugated) bilirubin level remains normal. As stated previously, the total bilirubin concentration in hemolysis rarely exceeds 4 to 5 mg/dl. Bilirubin is absent in the urine of patients with hemolysis, because indirect bilirubin is not excreted by the kidney. If hemolysis is suspected, further laboratory tests should include complete blood cell count, blood smear, reticulocyte count, erythrocyte fragility test, and Coombs' test.

The amino acid transaminases aspartate aminotransferase (AST; formerly SGOT) and alanine aminotransferase (ALT; formerly SGPT) are serum markers for hepatocyte damage. AST is found in liver, heart, kidney, skeletal muscle, and brain tissue. ALT is found predominantly within hepatocytes, making ALT more specific for identifying liver injury.

In cases of hepatic parenchymal disease, broad derangements in liver function tests are seen. The concentrations of both conjugated and unconjugated fractions of bilirubin are increased. With the increased level of conjugated bilirubin in the serum, bilirubinuria develops. In patients with acute hepatitis, serum ALT and AST are markedly elevated. In contrast, alkaline phosphatase and bilirubin levels may be only slightly elevated in these patients, and the serum amylase activity is usually normal. As in hepatitis, the serum transaminases are elevated in alcoholic liver disease, with serum AST levels usually greater than twice serum ALT levels. In the patient with cirrhosis, serum bilirubin levels increase in proportion to the degree of parenchymal damage. Albumin, and factors V, VII, IX, and X, prothrombin, and fibrinogen are all synthesized in the liver. Therefore, the measurement of serum albumin levels and PT may be helpful in assessing the degree of parenchymal liver injury.

In extrahepatic obstruction, the fraction of direct bilirubin is increased, along with a moderate increase in indirect bilirubin. The highest elevations of bilirubin are usually found in patients with malignant extrahepatic obstruction, in whom bilirubin levels may exceed 20 mg/dl. With malignant obstruction, the alkaline phosphatase activity is elevated to the same degree. Results of other liver function tests are usually normal or only slightly elevated, and the amylase concentration is usually normal. Common bile duct stones, on the other hand, rarely cause an increased bilirubin level greater than 10 to 12 mg/dl. With choledocholithiasis, alkaline phosphatase activity is usually also elevated to a moderate degree. As a gallstone passes through and momentarily obstructs the ampulla of Vater, serum transaminase levels may rise transiently. In this setting, hyperamylasemia may also develop. If long-standing extrahepatic obstruction is present, liver damage and fibrosis can occur, resulting in a combined intrahepatic and extrahepatic biochemical profile.

Serum alkaline phosphatase activity, often a more sensitive indicator of obstruction, may be elevated when the bilirubin level is normal. This circumstance occurs most commonly with incomplete or partial obstruction. However, increased alkaline phosphatase activity may also result from bone disease. If this possibility is suspected, serum 5′-nucleotidase or serum γ-glutamyltransferase levels should be measured, because both parallel changes in alkaline phosphatase activity from a hepatobiliary source and are not found in bone.

By obtaining a careful history, performing a physical examination, and interpreting laboratory tests, an experienced clinician can usually accurately differentiate intrahepatic diseases from extrahepatic obstruction. O'Connor et al.[21] reported that the respective accuracies in diagnosing extrahepatic obstruction by clinical evaluation, CT, US, and biliary scintigraphy were 84%, 81%, 78%, and 68%, respectively. This analysis suggests that clinical evaluation is comparable to noninvasive radiologic tests for the detection of extrahepatic biliary obstruction. Although the sensitivity of clinical examination in this study was 95%, however, the specificity was only 76%. Thus, nearly one fourth of patients with diagnoses of extrahepatic obstructive disease actually have hepatocellular disease. Therefore, although the history and physical examination are vital in evaluating the patient with jaundice, further tests are usually essential to diagnose the specific cause of jaundice.

Radiologic Evaluation

The goals of the radiologic evaluation of the patient with jaundice include (1) the confirmation of clinically suspected extrahepatic biliary obstruction by the demonstration of a dilated biliary tree, (2) the identification of the cause and site of extrahepatic biliary obstruction, and (3) the selection of patients for whom surgical or interventional radiologic or endoscopic treatment is indicated.

Abdominal Plain Films

The likelihood of a plain abdominal radiograph's providing diagnostic information in the patient with jaundice is low. Abdominal radiography may reveal gallstones, a calcified gallbladder wall, or the outline of a distended gallbladder. Approximately 15% to 20% of gallstones are radiopaque and can be visualized by radiography. However, cholangiography is still necessary to determine whether common duct stones are present and to rule out other causes of jaundice, such as hepatic parenchymal disease or an obstructing tumor. Plain radiographs may also be diagnostic of a spontaneous biliary fistula when air is present in the biliary tree or of emphysematous cholecystitis when air is noted in the gallbladder lumen or wall.

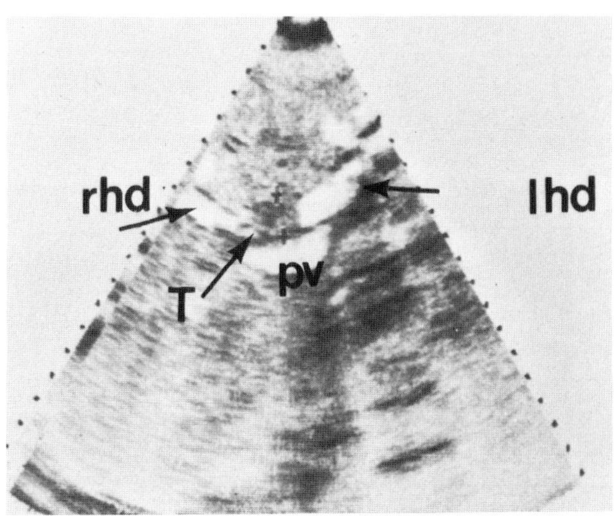

Fig. 28-3. Ultrasonic demonstration of Klatskin's tumor *(T)* anterior to portal vein *(pv)* and at the bifurcation of the right *(rhd)* and left *(lhd)* hepatic ducts. (From Pitt HA, Roslyn JJ, Tompkins RK. Surgical resection of bile duct cancer. In Wanebo HJ, ed. Hepatic and Biliary Cancer. New York: Marcel Dekker, 1986.)

Ultrasonography

US is commonly performed as the initial screening procedure in the patient with jaundice. US is noninvasive, inexpensive, and widely available. Dilated intrahepatic bile ducts are a reliable sign of extrahepatic biliary obstruction, and most series report that US can detect dilatation of the intrahepatic or proximal extrahepatic bile ducts with an accuracy rate of at least 80%.[22,23] The normal extrahepatic bile duct diameter is less than 10 mm, and normal intrahepatic duct diameter is less than 4 mm. Dilated ducts are easily detectable by US and often can be identified before the onset of clinical jaundice (Fig. 28-3).

Failure of US to detect dilated ducts usually indicates an intrahepatic source of jaundice. In this setting, continued observation, screening tests for hepatitis, or liver biopsy may be indicated. However, the absence of ductal dilatation does not entirely rule out extrahepatic obstruction. In intermittent or partial obstruction, the intrahepatic biliary tree may not be dilated. Likewise, in long-standing obstruction, especially if secondary biliary fibrosis or cirrhosis is present, dilated ducts may not be seen. In those cases where extrahepatic obstruction is suspected despite negative results of US, direct cholangiography by either the transhepatic or endoscopic route may be necessary.

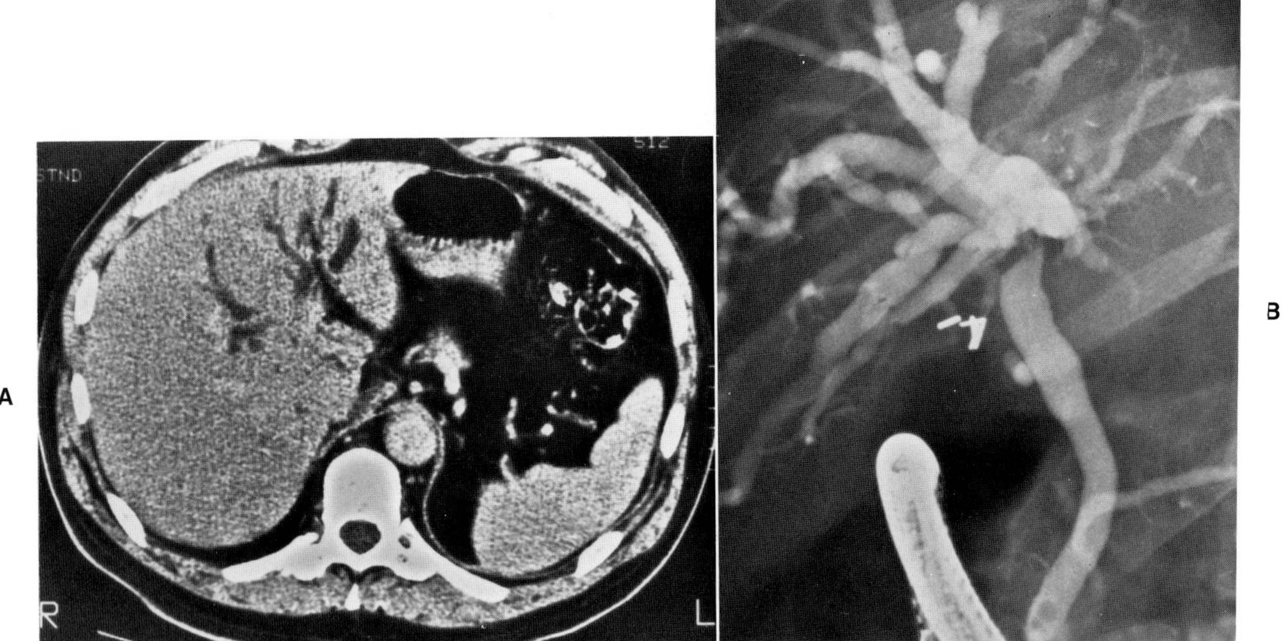

Fig. 28-4. A, CT of a patient demonstrating dilation primarily on the left, but also of the right hepatic duct. **B,** Endoscopic retrograde cholangiography in same patient showing a defect in the proximal common hepatic duct related to a cholangiocarcinoma.

US can differentiate between extrahepatic obstruction and hepatocellular causes of jaundice in as many as 96% of cases.[24] Unfortunately, US is limited in its ability to identify the cause and exact location of an obstructing lesion. The anatomic level of the obstruction can be estimated in as many as half of the patients. The cause of the obstruction is evident in a far lower proportion. This low yield in determining the cause of obstruction is caused by a failure to visualize the entire common bile duct, especially the distal third, and an inconsistency in the ability of US to detect common duct stones. The distal end of the bile duct is frequently obscured by duodenal or colonic gas. Studies indicate that US successfully identifies the presence of common bile duct stones in at most 70% of patients. Therefore, although US is a valuable initial step in the evaluation of the jaundiced patient, further diagnostic studies such as computed tomography or direct cholangiography are usually necessary to identify the cause and exact location of the obstruction.

Computed Tomography

CT can also be used to differentiate intrahepatic disease with nondilated ducts from extrahepatic obstruction. CT is more than 90% accurate in detecting the presence of ductal dilation. This success rate is slightly higher than that of US because CT provides better definition of anatomic structures and can use contrast media to enhance delineations (Fig. 28-4).

The accuracy of CT in determining the site and cause of obstruction is controversial, with rates ranging between 30% and 96%.[23,25] This wide range in reported accuracy of CT for diagnosing the cause and anatomic location of an obstructing lesion results primarily from differences in the reported ability of CT to detect obstructing common bile duct stones. CT shows the common bile duct in cross section instead of longitudinally, and small stones in the common bile duct may not be identified. As Table 28-3 indicates, CT is more likely to identify the cause and location of extrahepatic biliary obstruction than is US. In a study of 103 patients, Baron et al.[22] showed that CT was slightly more accurate than US in identifying the presence of biliary obstruction (96% vs 87%). Moreover, the precise level of obstruction was shown by CT in 88% of patients compared with 60% for US. The cause of obstruction was predicted accurately by CT in 70% of cases and by US in only 38%. In addition, CT scanning, especially with newer spiral techniques, can also provide highly accurate information regarding retroperitoneal extension, vascular invasion, and spread to the liver in malignant causes of biliary obstruction.

In summary, CT and US have similar value in the diagnosis of biliary ductal dilation. CT may be the preferred initial screening procedure for obese patients or patients with suspected malignancy. Most authorities agree that CT is slightly more accurate than US in detecting the nature and anatomic level of obstruction. CT also has the advantage of being able to routinely visualize the pancreas; it therefore is probably the screening procedure of choice if

Table 28-3. Comparison Between Ultrasonography and Computed Tomography in the Diagnosis of Jaundice

Criterion	US	CT
Identification of ductal dilatation	80% to 85%	>90%
Identification of cause of obstruction	35% to 40%	40% to 80%
Patient selection	Thin patients, pregnancy, suspected choledocholithiasis	Obese patients, bowel gas, suspected malignancy
Other factors	Less expensive, no radiation	More expensive, radiation

a periampullary tumor is suspected. On the other hand, US is less expensive, more widely available, and does not expose the patient to radiation. Therefore, US should be performed initially if stone disease is suspected.

Magnetic Resonance Imaging

The use of magnetic resonance imaging (MRI) in the evaluation of the patient with jaundice is relatively new and still undergoing evaluation. MRI is capable of detecting intrahepatic and extrahepatic biliary dilatation. However, the sensitivity of MRI has not yet been compared with that of either US or CT to determine its clinical usefulness. T2-weighted images in the coronal and sagittal planes may also be used to obtain a magnetic resonance cholangiogram and pancreatogram (MRCP). Wallner et al.[26] described the identification of a dilated biliary tree in 11 of 13 patients with obstructive jaundice, with the cause of obstruction determined in eight of these patients. A more prominent role for MRI may lie in its ability to define venous anatomy and identify potential portal vein involvement by pancreatic and periampullary tumors.

Biliary Scintigraphy

Technetium 99m–labeled iminodiacetic acid (IDA) derivatives (H-IDA, DIS-IDA, PIP-IDA) are injected intravenously, rapidly extracted from the blood, and excreted into the bile. These radionuclide scans provide functional information about the liver's ability to excrete radiolabeled substances into a nonobstructed biliary tree. Biliary scintigraphy is useful in the workup of neonatal jaundice, the detection of bile leaks, and the diagnosis of acute cholecystitis. Cholescintigraphy also provides a method of noninvasively evaluating the patency and function of biliary-enteric anastomoses and of studying the kinetics of bile flow in patients with suspected disorders of biliary motility.

Biliary scintigraphy plays only a limited role in the evaluation of a patient with jaundice. The technique has been shown to be useful in the diagnosis of complete common bile duct obstruction. Any appearance of the nucleotide in the gastrointestinal tract indicates patency of bile flow into the duodenum. However, other available noninvasive tests, such as US and CT, have generally been shown to be more accurate and are therefore preferred.

Percutaneous Transhepatic Cholangiography

Direct cholangiography is indicated if dilated bile ducts are visualized on US or CT, or if the clinical suspicion of extrahepatic biliary obstruction remains high despite negative results of US or CT scan. Cholangiography may be performed percutaneously or endoscopically. PTC involves the cannulation of intrahepatic bile ducts with a thin, flexible Chiba needle under radiographic control, followed by the injection of contrast material to outline the bile ducts. PTC is successful in differentiating intrahepatic from extrahepatic obstruction in as many as 96% of cases.[27]

PTC is highly accurate in defining the site and cause of extrahepatic obstruction (Fig. 28-5); it can define the site of an obstructing lesion in approximately 95% of patients and the cause of the obstruction in nearly 90% of cases.[28] Diagnostic cholangiography can also be combined with a series of therapeutic maneuvers, such as the insertion of biliary stents or endoprostheses, percutaneous stone extraction, biliary dilation, and cholangioscopy. In addition, cholangiography provides an anatomic road map of the biliary tree that is useful during surgical procedures.

The success rate of entering a bile duct during PTC increases with the experience of the radiologist. In patients with dilated intrahepatic ducts, PTC is nearly 100% successful. In patients with nondilated bile ducts, the success rate is approximately 70%. Although PTC is an invasive procedure, it has an acceptably low complication rate.[29] The major complication rate of PTC at most centers is less than 5%. The most commonly reported complications include hemorrhage (2.5%), sepsis (2.5%), bile peritonitis (1.8%), and pneumothorax or empyema (1.8%). The procedure-related mortality rate is approximately 0.5%. Even with more frequent passes of the needle (as many as 15 attempts), no increase in the complication rate has been reported. Thus, in the management of the patient with jaundice, the advantages of PTC are the ability to (1) establish a diagnosis, (2) determine the site and cause of obstruction, and (3) provide specific anatomic detail.

Endoscopic Retrograde Cholangiography

ERC is the other option for direct visualization of the biliary system (Fig. 28-6). The technique of ERC requires a skilled endoscopist who is capable of cannulating the sphincter of Oddi with a side-viewing duodenoscope and then filling the biliary tree with contrast material in a retrograde fashion. The success rate of ERC is approximately 85% to 90% and improves with the experience of the endoscopist. ERC is able to define the site and cause of extrahepatic obstructive jaundice in 75% to 90% of patients.[23,30] As with PTC, the complication and mortality

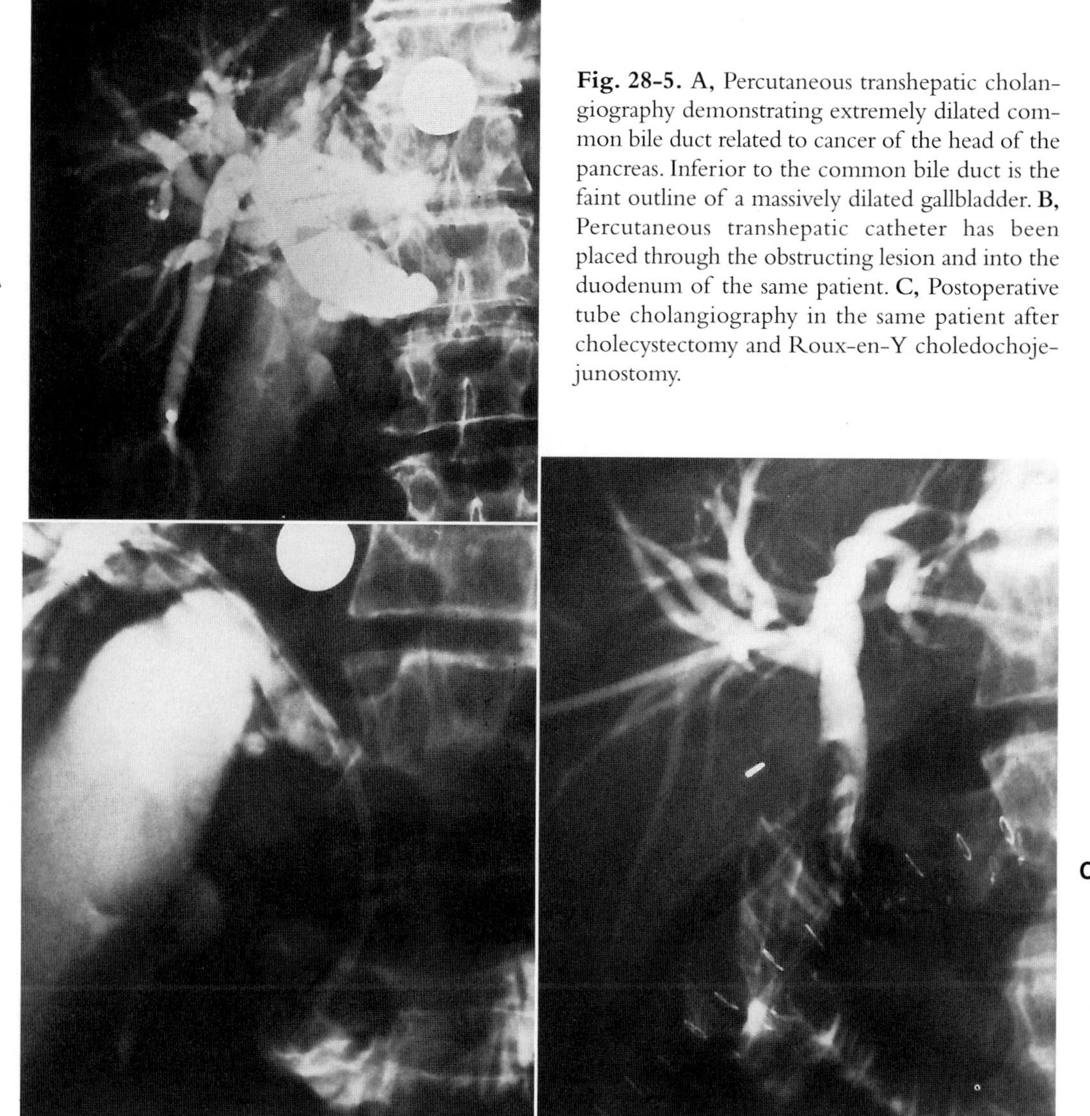

Fig. 28-5. A, Percutaneous transhepatic cholangiography demonstrating extremely dilated common bile duct related to cancer of the head of the pancreas. Inferior to the common bile duct is the faint outline of a massively dilated gallbladder. **B,** Percutaneous transhepatic catheter has been placed through the obstructing lesion and into the duodenum of the same patient. **C,** Postoperative tube cholangiography in the same patient after cholecystectomy and Roux-en-Y choledochojejunostomy.

rates associated with ERC are acceptably low. In a review of 10,000 ERCs, Bilbao et al.[31] reported a complication rate of less than 3% and a mortality rate of less than 0.1%. The two major complications of the procedure are sepsis and acute pancreatitis. Prophylactic antibiotics should be administered before the procedure if biliary obstruction is suspected.

In the patient with jaundice who is found to have dilated ducts on US or CT, direct cholangiography by either PTC or ERC is the next procedure to be used (Table 28-4). PTC is less expensive, is more widely available, requires less expertise, and has a higher success rate if dilated ducts are present than ERC. In patients with total biliary obstruction, PTC provides the surgeon with information about the proximal biliary tree, whereas ERC frequently only delineates the anatomy of the distal bile duct. PTC is the preferred procedure if therapeutic manipulations such as biliary drainage, balloon dilation, or endoprosthesis placement are necessary for hilar bile duct lesions. ERC may be difficult or impossible to perform in patients with ampullary stenosis or altered gastrointestinal anatomy related to previous surgery.

In several instances, however, ERC is preferable to PTC. PTC is contraindicated in patients with an uncorrectable coagulopathy or with significant ascites. ERC allows endoscopic visualization of the upper gastrointestinal tract and ampullary region. Therefore, lesions can be sampled and varices can be identified during the course of ERC. Moreover, cannulation and injection of the pancreatic duct with contrast medium is often helpful in patients with suspected pancreatic cancer. In patients with postcholecystectomy symptoms or sphincter of Oddi dyskinesia, ERC enables visualization and cannulation of the ampulla and manometric pressure recordings. As with

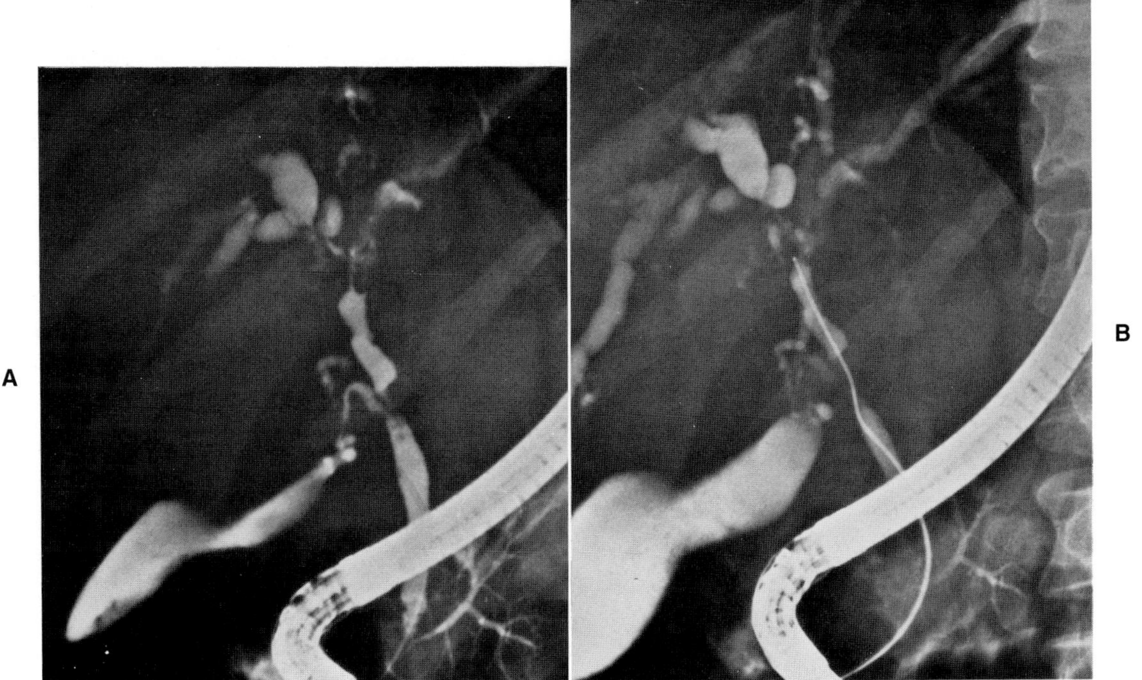

Fig. 28-6. A, Endoscopic retrograde cholangiography demonstrating an extensive cholangiocarcinoma involving the hilum of the liver and the common hepatic-cystic duct junction. **B,** Attempt to establish nasobiliary drainage in the same patient was unsuccessful because of the difficulty of draining the most proximal hilar lesion.

Table 28-4. Comparison of Percutaneous Transhepatic Cholangiography (PTC) and Endoscopic Retrograde Cholangiography (ERC)

Criterion	PTC	ERC
Success rate	>90% with dilated ducts, 70% with nondilated ducts	80% to 90% with either dilated or nondilated ducts
Identification of cause of obstruction	90% to 100%	75% to 90%
Complications	5% (range 3% to 10%)	5% (range 2% to 7%)
Mortality rate	0.2% to 0.9%	0.1% to 0.2%
Expense	Less	More
Skill required	Less	More
Patient selection	Proximal lesions, altered gastroduodenal anatomy, failed ERC	Distal lesions, pancreatic pathology, coagulopathy, ascites, failed PTC

PTC, therapeutic manipulations such as ES and stenting may be carried out in conjunction with ERC.

In summary, the method of direct cholangiography, either PTC or ERC, is individually chosen in each case. In certain situations, such as totally obstructing proximal lesions, PTC may be the procedure of choice. On the other hand, when noninvasive studies suggest periampullary or pancreatic pathology, ERC provides additional useful information. The choice between these two procedûres may ultimately be decided by the expertise of the radiologists and endoscopists at an individual institution.

Angiography

Celiac and superior mesenteric angiography is not a routine investigative procedure in the patient with jaundice. Angiography is performed in patients with cirrhosis and bleeding esophageal varices prior to portosystemic or transhepatic shunts, or for therapeutic infusion of intraarterial vasopressin. In patients with jaundice and active gastrointestinal bleeding, hemobilia can be diagnosed and treated with selective embolization by skilled invasive radiologists.

Angiography may also be of benefit in predicting resectability of pancreatic and periampullary neoplasms. Dooley et al.[32] evaluated visceral angiography in 90 patients with periampullary neoplasms undergoing resection at Johns Hopkins Hospital. Among 62 patients with normal angiograms, 48 (77%) neoplasms were resectable. In 17 patients with angiograms suggesting vascular encasement, the resectability rate was 35%. None of the remaining 11 patients with vessel occlusion had resectable disease. This group therefore concluded that major-vessel occlusion rules out resection, and that major-vessel encasement makes resection less likely. However, angiography increases hospital cost, and exposes the patient with jaundice, who is already at an increased risk for renal failure, to an additional contrast dye load. Angiography should therefore be used selectively, only when resection is seriously contemplated.

Endoscopic Ultrasonography

Endoscopic US (endosonography) is a relatively new modality that may be of some benefit in the evaluation of the patient with jaundice. A potential use is in the assessment of patients with malignant jaundice. Grimm et al.[33] reported that endoscopic US was able to accurately predict resectability in 88% of 26 patients with pancreatic cancer. A limitation of this technique, however, is that endoscopic US may have difficulty differentiating tumor infiltration of a vessel from simple compression. The addition of a pulsed Doppler component may aid in this differentiation.

Advocates of endoscopic US also claim that this technique can differentiate normal lymph nodes from those containing metastatic tumor. Normal lymph nodes are hyperechoic, with indistinct margins, whereas lymph nodes containing cancer are hypoechoic, with well-defined margins. In one analysis of 25 patients,[33] endosonography was 72% accurate in diagnosing lymph node metastasis. In this study, the sensitivity was 82%, but the specificity was only 50%. Preoperative study of patients with pancreatic cancer suggested that endoscopic US was superior to conventional US, CT, and angiography in predicting resectability.[34] Although it is promising, the ultimate role of endoscopic US in the evaluation of malignant jaundice awaits further analysis.

Laparoscopy

Laparoscopy has recently been proposed as a useful technique for the staging of suspected pancreatic or ampullary malignancy. Liver and peritoneal metastases not detected by CT or US can be identified by direct examination of the peritoneal cavity. The application of laparoscopic US provides the ability to assess mesenteric or portal vessel involvement, as well as deeper liver lesions. In a study from Edinburgh, laparoscopy was shown to be 65% accurate in predicting resectability (sensitivity 100%, specificity 50%) in 40 patients with a periampullary malignancy without distant metastases.[35] The addition of laparoscopic US increased the accuracy of predicting resectability to 89% (sensitivity 92%, specificity 88%). Thus, the authors suggest that the combination of laparoscopy and laparoscopic US is a valuable technique in staging suspected periampullary malignancies. Whether this new technology is as effective as the combination of CT and angiography or as spiral CT in successfully predicting resectability remains to be determined.

Liver Biopsy

The developments in the past decade in US and CT have made percutaneous liver biopsy unnecessary in most cases of jaundice caused by extrahepatic obstruction. However, numerous indications for liver biopsy remain. If clinical and laboratory data indicate intrahepatic cholestasis, and if dilated bile ducts are not present on US or CT scans, a liver biopsy is usually the next test. Liver biopsy may be useful if results of diagnostic studies are negative or equivocal, or if parenchymal disease is suspected along with extrahepatic obstruction.

A liver biopsy can aid in the diagnosis of intrahepatic cholestasis, storage diseases, unexplained hepatomegaly, and liver infections. Among the cholestatic causes of jaundice in which a liver biopsy may be helpful are hepatitis, cirrhosis, drug-induced cholestasis, primary biliary cirrhosis, and sclerosing cholangitis. Other indications for percutaneous liver biopsy are diseases such as amyloidosis, glycogen-storage disease, and liver infections such as tuberculosis, histoplasmosis, and coccidiomycosis.

Liver biopsy is a relatively safe procedure. In reviews of large series of liver biopsy procedures, mortality rates of 0.01% to 0.02% and serious complication rates of 0.2% to 0.4% have been reported. The most frequent complications of liver biopsy are hemorrhage and bacteremia. This latter problem occurs most frequently in patients with chronic bile duct infections. Percutaneous liver biopsy is contraindicated if the patient is uncooperative, or if an uncorrectable coagulation defect is present. If the patient has a prolonged PT or partial thromboplastin time (PTT) or a diminished platelet count, attempts should be made to correct these abnormalities with vitamin K, fresh-frozen plasma, or specific component therapy. If the coagulopathy persists and liver biopsy is essential, laparoscopic or open liver biopsy must be considered.

MANAGEMENT

Once it has been determined that extrahepatic biliary obstruction is the cause of jaundice, a surgeon should become intimately involved in the management of the patient. Extrahepatic biliary obstruction, or surgical jaundice, may be the result of either benign or malignant disease processes. Jaundice from benign lesions can be caused by congenital defects, complications of gallstone disease, and inflammatory or traumatic strictures of the bile duct. Malignant causes of extrahepatic biliary obstruction include cholangiocarcinomas, gallbladder cancers, and cancers of the head of the pancreas, ampulla, or duodenum. Prior to a discussion of the management of common causes of "surgical" jaundice, important issues in the general management of the jaundiced patient are described.

Assessment of Risk

In the past, the only option for the relief of obstructive jaundice was operative. However, with the development of therapeutic techniques such as percutaneous and endoscopic stenting, balloon dilatation, and ES, many nonoperative options for the relief of obstructive jaundice are now available. The surgeon must determine the safest and most efficacious form of therapy for each individual patient, as well as adequately prepare the patient for surgery or nonoperative therapeutic interventions.

In an effort to determine which patients undergoing biliary surgery were at greatest risk, Pitt et al.[1] analyzed 15 clinical and laboratory parameters in 155 consecutive patients. These authors found eight factors (advanced age, malignant obstruction, anemia, leukocytosis, hyperbilirubinemia, increased alkaline phosphatase activity, increased creatinine level, and hypoalbuminemia) to be associated with an increased risk of death after surgery. Subsequent analyses by Hunt,[14] Blamey et al.,[36] and Dixon et al.[37] confirmed these findings. In these analyses, the most consistent predictors of outcome were shown to be the presence of malignancy, elevated serum bilirubin level, hypoalbuminemia, and increased serum creatinine level. In a 1987 report, Little[38] defined a mortality index that employs albumin level, creatinine level, and a cholangitis score (see accompanying box) to predict which patients with jaundice are at increased risk. In a prospective study of 40 patients, Little's mortality index was 100% accurate in predicting outcome. Thus, the assessment of nutritional status, renal function, and sepsis may be the most important factors to consider when attempting to determine who should be an operative candidate.

LITTLE'S MORTALITY INDEX

Mortality Index* =

$0.0016 \times$ serum creatinine (μmol/L)
$-0.0227 \times$ albumin (g/L)
$+ 0.0641 \times$ cholangitis score
$+ 0.6935$

Cholangitis score

0 If afebrile
1 If temperature <37.5° C
2 If temperature >37.5° C without rigors
3 If temperature >37.5° C with rigors, right upper quadrant pain
4 If fever with shock and/or mental changes (obtundation)

*An index of 0.4 or greater is associated with a high risk of death.

Management Issues

Patients with obstructive jaundice and those with hepatocellular disease severe enough to cause jaundice are likely to have many secondary problems. Patients with jaundice are at increased risk for the development of renal failure, gastrointestinal bleeding, infections, and wound complications (see the section on the pathophysiology of jaundice). Cardiac, pulmonary, and renal function must be considered in every patient undergoing major abdominal surgery. In addition, special attention must be focused on nutritional status, coaguability, immune function, and presence or absence of biliary sepsis. Patients with chronic liver disease and cirrhosis may also have ascites and encephalopathy, which may require specific treatment.

Cardiopulmonary

In assessing cardiopulmonary status, the patient's age, history of recent myocardial infarction, presence of congestive heart failure, significant valvular aortic stenosis, and disturbance of normal cardiac rhythm have all been correlated with increased operative risk.[39] In addition, patients with severe pulmonary disease may not be candidates for extensive abdominal surgery.

Renal

Patients with jaundice, especially those with cirrhosis and cholangitis, are at increased risk for development of renal insufficiency. The maintenance of adequate blood volume is extremely important if renal complications are to be avoided. However, fluid management can be quite complex in patients with jaundice. These patients often benefit from invasive hemodynamic monitoring with central venous catheters, and in some cases pulmonary artery catheters, to assist in assessing intravascular volume. In 1967, Dawson[40] suggested that the liberal use of preoperative mannitol, resulting in an osmotic diuresis, and intravenous fluids could achieve the goal of maintaining an adequate blood volume while protecting the kidneys. As mentioned in the section on pathophysiology, preoperative treatment with oral bile salts may also be effective in preventing postoperative renal problems.

Nutrition

Malnutrition is a significant risk factor for surgery in the setting of obstructive jaundice. Halliday et al.[41] noted that patients who died in the postoperative period after surgery for obstructive jaundice had a significant reduction in body weight, midarm circumference, total body potassium level, and reactivity to skin-test antigens. In a study from Italy, enteral hyperalimentation was found to significantly decrease operative morbidity and mortality in a group of patients treated with 20 days of preoperative percutaneous biliary drainage.[42] Although most patients with benign biliary problems are adequately nourished, various degrees of malnutrition are frequently present in patients with malignant obstruction. Therefore, patients with malignant obstructive jaundice should be evaluated for evidence of malnutrition, and nutritional support should be instituted if necessary.

Coagulation

Patients with obstructive jaundice, cholangitis, or cirrhosis are all susceptible to excessive intraoperative bleeding. The most common clotting defect in patients with obstructive jaundice is prolongation of the PT, which is usually reversible by the administration of parenteral vitamin K. Patients with severe jaundice or cholangitis may also have DIC, which may necessitate infusion of platelets and fresh-frozen plasma. Reversal of DIC also requires control of the underlying sepsis, which usually includes biliary drainage and systemic antibiotics.

In patients with cirrhosis, clotting abnormalities may be more complicated and include (1) thrombocytopenia related to hypersplenism, (2) prolongation of PT and thromboplastin time PTT, and (3) fibrinolysis. Vitamin K should be administered if the PT is prolonged. If no effect is seen, or the PTT is also prolonged, fresh-frozen plasma should be given. Thrombocytopenia can usually be managed by intraoperative platelet infusions. If the patient has a shortened clot lysis time and hypofibrinogenemia, ϵ-aminocaproic acid may be indicated.

Pruritus

Pruritus is often a distressing problem in the patient with jaundice. The exact cause of pruritus remains obscure, but increased bile salts, histamines, and central nervous system opiate receptors have been implicated.[43] For some patients, relief from itching can be obtained by bile salt–binding agents such as cholestyramine. Various sedatives and antihistamines can also provide relief from itching for patients with jaundice. However, relief of biliary obstruction remains the most effective method of managing this problem.

Cholangitis

Biliary sepsis has also been identified as a major risk factor in the patient with jaundice. Cholangitis occurs when there is either partial or complete obstruction of the bile duct, resulting in increased intraluminal pressure, and infected bile is present behind the obstruction. Patients with cholangitis have right upper quadrant abdominal pain, fever, and jaundice (Charcot's triad). Patients with "toxic" cholangitis, Charcot's triad plus shock and mental confusion (Reynold's pentad), face significant mortality risk with appropriate antibiotic therapy alone, and therefore require emergency biliary decompression.

Gigot et al.[44] identified seven prognostic factors that are indications for urgent biliary decompression. These factors include (1) acute renal failure, (2) liver abscesses, (3) cirrhosis, (4) high malignant stricture, (5) prior PTC, (6) female gender, and (7) advanced age. However, emergency surgical treatment is associated with significant morbidity and mortality. Therefore, both percutaneous and endoscopic biliary drainage have been proposed as effective therapy for the 5% to 10% of patients with cholangitis unresponsive to conservative therapy. Lai et al.[45] showed in a series of 82 patients with severe acute cholangitis that endoscopic drainage is associated with lower morbidity (34% vs 66%) and mortality (10% vs 32%) rates than is operative drainage.

Antibiotic Coverage

Because of the depressed immune system that accompanies jaundice, adequate antibiotic coverage needs to be provided for the treatment of cholangitis and prior to any manipulation of the biliary tree. Under normal conditions, bile, the biliary tree, and the liver are sterile. However, biliary stasis, obstruction, biliary-enteric anastomoses, and foreign bodies predispose the biliary system toward infection. The organisms most commonly isolated from the biliary tree include *Escherichia coli, Klebsiella pneumonia, Enterococcus* species, and, with increasing frequency, the anaerobe *Bacteroides fragilis.* Approximately two thirds of patients with bactibilia have gram-negative aerobes in the bile, and 25% to 30% have enterococci. Anaerobes are found in the bile of older patients, those with cholangitis, and those with complex biliary problems and indwelling tubes.[46]

Four factors must be considered when choosing antibiotics for the patient with jaundice. These properties include (1) the antibacterial spectrum of the antibiotic, (2) serum and liver concentrations, (3) biliary excretion, and (4) toxicity. For many years, the combination of a penicillin and an aminoglycoside has been recommended to cover the gram-negative aerobes and enterococci. However, concern about the nephrotoxicity of aminoglycosides, especially in patients with jaundice has led to a search for less toxic agents. Options include ureidopenicillins, third-generation cephalosporins, and monobactams. The ureidopenicillins piperacillin and mezlocillin have been shown to be effective in patients with cholangitis. Mezlocillin was able to cure cholangitis in 84% of patients (20/24), compared with only 41% (9/22) treated with a combination of ampicillin and gentamicin.[47] In a prospective study of 96 patients from Johns Hopkins, University of California–Los Angeles, and Olive View Medical Center, piperacillin was shown to be as effective as the combination of tobramycin and ampicillin.[16]

In patients with biliary obstruction and cholangitis, serum levels of antibiotics are more important than are biliary excretion levels. The biliary excretion of antibiotics is significantly reduced in the setting of biliary obstruction, making it difficult to achieve high bile levels of antibiotics in the situations where they are most needed. Therefore, antibacterial specificity and toxicity are the most important factors considered in the selection of antibiotic therapy.

Prophylactic antibiotics should be administered to all patients undergoing operative or nonoperative manipulations of the biliary tree, including cholangiography and sphincterotomy. Meijer et al.[48] published a meta-analysis of 42 controlled clinical trials of antibiotic prophylaxis in biliary tract surgery. They demonstrated that patients undergoing prophylactic antibiotic therapy had a 9% lower incidence of infection. The authors also concluded that second- and third-generation cephalosporins were no more effective in preventing infection than were first-generation cephalosporins. Therefore, in uncomplicated cases, a broad-spectrum first-generation cephalosporin usually provides adequate coverage for prophylaxis.

Preoperative Drainage

During the 1970s, surgical relief of biliary obstruction in patients with severe jaundice was associated with postoperative morbidity in 40% to 60% and with mortality in 15% to 20% of patients. During this same period, numerous authors reported that PTD could be performed with little morbidity. For this reason, preoperative PTD was recommended and supported by retrospective and nonrandomized studies. However, prospective, randomized studies failed to demonstrate any advantage of preoperative biliary drainage. In a study by Pitt et al.,[49] hospital mortality rate was 8% among patients undergoing preoperative PTD and 5% among patients who underwent surgery without preoperative PTD.

Lai et al.[50] recently documented similar results when endoscopic drainage was used to decompress the biliary tree before the operation. Several other studies confirmed these findings (Table 28-5).[49-52] Moreover, preoperative biliary tract drainage has been shown to significantly lengthen the hospital stay for these patients. Thus, although retrospective analyses suggested that preoperative drainage might be beneficial, prospective, randomized studies have not supported this finding.

A criticism of these prospective studies is that the duration of preoperative drainage (10 to 18 days) may not have been long enough to reverse the multiple metabolic and immunologic abnormalities associated with severe obstructive jaundice. Both animal and human studies demonstrate that recoveries of various metabolic and immune functions require at least 6 weeks after the relief of biliary obstruction.[5,53-55] Similarly, animal studies strongly suggest that return of bile to the intestinal tract has significant advantages over external biliary drainage.[56]

Although the data suggest that preoperative biliary drainage may not be of any benefit in routine cases, this maneuver may have some value in selected patients with advanced malnutrition, biliary sepsis, and hilar malignancies necessitating liver resection. Preoperatively placed catheters are also of value in the operating room during difficult biliary dissections, as well as in aiding in the placement of long-term transhepatic stents.

Benign Disease

Choledocholithiasis

The most common benign cause of obstructive jaundice is choledocholithiasis. The incidence of stones in the bile ducts of patients undergoing cholecystectomy is approximately 10% to 15%, and the incidence of retained bile duct stones after cholecystectomy and common bile duct exploration has been 5% to 10%. The most common symptoms of choledocholithiasis are pain, jaundice, and fever. Biliary colic results from intermittent obstruction of the cystic or common duct. With choledocholithiasis, serum bilirubin levels usually range from 2 to 8 mg/dl, with a mean of approximately 5 mg/dl. Fever and chills result from the cholangitis that often accompanies choledocholithiasis. Positive bile cultures are found in almost 90% of patients with primary bile duct stones. Patients with common duct stones require treatment to prevent the complications of choledocholithiasis. These complications include cholangitis, liver abscesses, secondary biliary cirrhosis, and pancreatitis.

Prior to the development of endoscopic and laparoscopic techniques, open cholecystectomy with common bile duct exploration was the treatment of choice for choledocholithiasis. In the era of laparoscopic cholecystectomy and ES, however, the management of choledocholithiasis has become more controversial. The options for treatment now include (1) preoperative endoscopic retrograde cholangiopancreatography (ERCP) and sphincterotomy for patients with suspected choledocholithiasis, (2) conversion to open common bile duct exploration, (3) laparoscopic common bile duct exploration, or (4) postoperative ERCP and ES.

ES is accepted as a valuable technique in the management of choledocholithiasis in patients who have previously undergone cholecystectomy. ES is a relatively safe and effective procedure for the removal of common duct stones that can achieve a clearance rate of almost 90%.[57] In recent series, procedure-related death occurs in fewer than 1% of patients, with major postprocedure morbidity averaging 8% (Table 28-6). The long-term complication

Table 28-5. Results of Randomized Trials Comparing Preoperative Biliary Drainage

Authors	No. of Patients	Type of Drainage	No Drainage	Preoperative Drainage
Hatfield et al.[51]	55	Transhepatic	15	14
McPherson et al.[52]	65	Transhepatic	19	32
Pitt et al.[49]	75	Transhepatic	5	8
Lai et al.[50]	85	Endoscopic	14	15

Table 28-6. Mortality, Morbidity, and Late Complications of Endoscopic Sphincterotomy

Complications	Mean (%)	Range (%)
Mortality	1.1	0.4-1.7
Major morbidity	8.2	4.4-8.7
Hemorrhage	2.8	1.8-5
Pancreatitis	2.7	0.6-3.3
Cholangitis/impaction	1.8	0.8-2.3
Duodenal perforation	1	0.2-1.5
Emergency surgery	1.5	0.4-2.4
Unsuccessful procedure	9.8	3.4-14
Late complications		
Gallbladder problems	14.9	14.7-15.2
Recurrent stones	5.9	2.8-20.5
Sphincter stenosis	3	0.8-3.7

rate is 13% and includes sphincter stenosis and recurrent stones.[58]

In the late 1980s and early 1990s, it was shown that preoperative ERCP was of no value in decreasing morbidity and mortality associated with open surgical management of choledocholithiasis.[59,60] With the widespread use of laparoscopic cholecystectomy, preoperative ERCP has been suggested for patients at high risk for common duct stones. With this approach in 400 patients undergoing laparoscopic cholecystectomy, Lillemoe et al.[61] demonstrated that ERCP and ES were required in 11% and 3.5%, respectively. Moreover, postoperative ERCP and ES were required in only 1.5% and 0.8% of patients.

Until recently, the options for the management of choledocholithiasis discovered during operation were either postoperative ERCP or open bile duct exploration. With the development of new equipment and techniques for laparoscopic common duct exploration, open surgery and sphincterotomy may be avoidable. Laparoscopic duct exploration can be accomplished by intubating the cystic duct or by creating a choledochotomy. In the transcystic duct approach, the cystic duct is dilated and common duct stones can be retrieved with a basket under fluoroscopic guidance or direct vision by means of a flexible choledochoscope.

In a review of three series with a total of 272 patients, the success rate was 93%, with a morbidity rate of 5% and a mortality rate of 0.7%.[62] Laparoscopic choledochotomy is technically challenging, but it has the advantage of being able to extract larger impacted stones and perform intrahepatic choledochoscopy. Results with this technique have also been good. Franklin et al.[63] reported a series of 80 patients with only two retained calculi, whereas Berci and Cuschieri[64] reported one retained stone among 43 patients. The morbidity rates were 5% and 7% and the mortality rates were 1% and 2%, respectively. As surgeons gain more experience with laparoscopic techniques and appropriate equipment becomes available, more patients may be able to undergo laparoscopic bile duct exploration for the management of choledocholithiasis.

Bile Duct Strictures

Causes of benign bile duct strictures include operative injury, inflammatory disorders such as pancreatitis and sclerosing cholangitis, and infectious agents. Because the vast majority of benign bile duct strictures occur after iatrogenic injuries to the bile duct, this discussion focuses on the management of such strictures.

The exact incidence of bile duct injury during open cholecystectomy has been estimated at 0.1% to 0.2%. With the advent of laparoscopic cholecystectomy, this rate has increased to approximately 0.3 to 0.5%. Factors such as acute inflammation, anatomic variants, excessive bleeding, obesity, lack of adequate assistance, and the surgeon's experience have been associated with bile duct injuries during laparoscopic cholecystectomy. Bile duct strictures can also occur at sites of previous biliary-enteric anastomoses. Ischemia of the anastomosis from excessive dissection of the duct prior to anastomosis is a likely cause of such strictures.

The clinical presentation of postoperative strictures is variable, with nearly 80% being identified within 1 year of the initial operation. Patients in whom strictures develop early after cholecystectomy usually have either progressive elevations in serum bilirubin and alkaline phosphatase activity or bile leaks, whereas patients seen months or years after surgery often have cholangitis. Excessive pain in the early postoperative period may also be an indication that bile is leaking.

Prior to the definitive management of benign bile duct strictures, adequate control of biliary sepsis by either endoscopic or transhepatic biliary drainage and optimal nutritional status are important. Once these goals have been accomplished, three options for the management of the stricture include (1) surgical excision with reconstruction, (2) percutaneous balloon dilatation, and (3) endoscopic dilatation and stenting.

The goals of surgical therapy are to reestablish the flow of bile from the liver to the proximal intestine and to prevent the formation of a recurrent stricture. These goals are best achieved by the creation of a Roux-en-Y biliary-enteric anastomosis. Principles to be observed in the surgical repair of bile duct strictures include complete resection of the stricture, trimming back of the proximal bile duct to expose healthy biliary mucosa, and the creation of a tension free mucosa-to-mucosa anastomosis to a 40 to 60 cm Roux-en-Y jejunal limb.[65] The need for transanastomotic stenting remains controversial. However, long-term Silastic stents can be useful to decompress the biliary tree in the postoperative period, provide access for the removal of retained intrahepatic stones, and ensure a patent biliary anastomosis during the period of healing and scar contracture.

The success rate for surgical management of benign bile duct strictures varies between 80% and 90%, with a mortality rate less than 5% and a morbidity rate of 20%

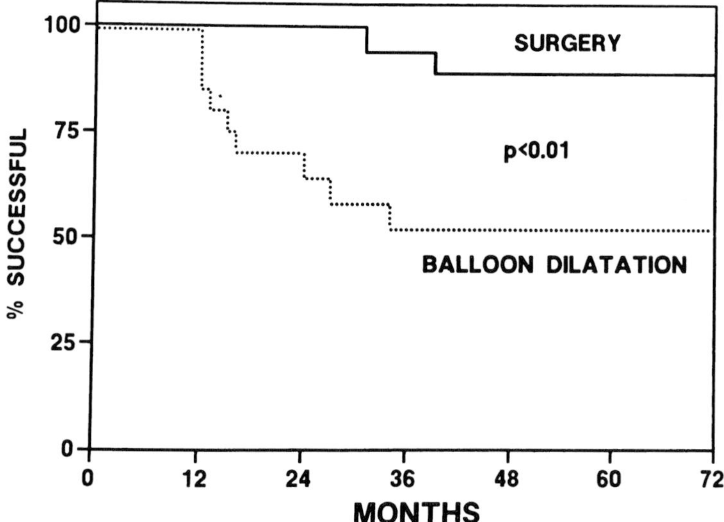

Fig. 28-7. Actuarial success rates after 72 months for surgery (89%) and balloon dilatation (52%). The difference is statistically significant (p <0.01). (From Pitt HA, et al. Benign postoperative biliary strictures. Operate or dilate? Ann Surg 210:417, 1989.)

to 30%.[66] Pitt et al.[67] examined the factors influencing outcome after surgical repair of bile duct strictures and determined that better results are achieved in younger patients (<30 years), patients undergoing primary stricture repairs, repairs with a Roux-en-Y jejunal loop, and stenting of the anastomosis for longer than 1 month.

Nonoperative options for the management of a benign bile duct strictures are percutaneous or endoscopic balloon dilatation and stenting. Both techniques involve intubating the biliary system (from above in the case of percutaneous dilatation and from below with endoscopic dilatation), crossing the stricture with a guide wire under fluoroscopic guidance, inflating an angioplasty-type balloon to dilate the stricture, and then stenting the lesion. With both techniques, patients often require multiple stricture dilatations. Results for both procedures are similar, with success rates ranging between 55% to 87% for percutaneous dilatation and 53% to 96% for endoscopic dilatation.[68] The complication rate for transhepatic dilatation ranges between 20% and 30%, including cholangitis, bleeding, and bile leaks. The mortality rate is 1%. The complications associated with endoscopic balloon dilatation are similar to those reported for ES, with cholangitis, pancreatitis, bleeding, and perforation of the duodenum occurring in 8% to 10% of patients.

When analyzing data on the efficacy of nonoperative stricture management, the length of follow-up is important. Surgical experience has demonstrated that strictures may recur many years after treatment. In a report from Johns Hopkins Hospital, Pitt et al.[18] compared the results of operative stricture repair with Roux-en-Y hepaticojejunostomy and long-term stenting in 25 patients with percutaneous balloon dilatation in 20 patients (Fig. 28-7). Eighty-eight percent of patients in whom the condition was managed surgically had a successful outcome at 57 months, whereas only 55% of patients treated with dilatation had a good outcome at 59 months. Therefore, these authors recommended that surgical therapy should be offered to young, healthy patients and that nonoperative therapy should be reserved for patients with a prohibitive operative risk or a short life expectancy.

Choledochal Cysts

Choledochal cysts are congenital dilatations of the biliary tree. The cystic dilatation may either involve the extrahepatic biliary tree alone or have associated intrahepatic dilatation. Recent evidence suggests that an anomalous junction of the pancreaticobiliary ducts may be responsible for the formation of choledochal cysts. ERCP has demonstrated that in most patients with choledochal cysts, the bile duct and pancreatic duct join more than 15 mm from the ampulla of Vater, resulting in a long common channel that allows pancreatic juice to reflux into the biliary tree and alter the bile duct wall.

Clinical manifestations of choledochal cysts are quite variable. Epigastric pain, jaundice, and an abdominal mass are the most common symptoms at presentation. Management of choledochal cysts is primarily surgical. In the past the standard surgical therapy was internal drainage of the cyst by creating a cystoduodenostomy, a cystogastrostomy, or a cystojejunostomy. However, patients with choledochal cysts have 20 times greater than normal risk for development of a biliary malignancy. Therefore standard therapy should be complete surgical excision of the dilated bile duct and reconstruction with a Roux-en-Y loop of jejunum.

Malignant Disease

Periampullary Carcinoma

Periampullary cancers are a group of malignant neoplasms that arise near or at the ampulla of Vater. Adenocarcinoma

Table 28-7. Results of Operative Versus Nonoperative Palliation of Malignant Obstructive Jaundice

			Relief of Jaundice (%)		Mortality (%)		Complications (%)		Recurrent Jaundice (%)		Late Duodenal Obstruction (%)	
Reference	**N**	**Stent**	**Surgery**	**Stent**	**Surgery**	**Stent**	**Surgery**	**Stent**	**Surgery**	**Stent**	**Surgery**	**Stent**
Bornman et al.[70]	50	Transhepatic	76	84	20	8*	32	28	16	38	0	14
Shepard et al.[71]	48	Endoscopic	92	82	20	9*	56	30	0	30*	4	9
Anderson et al.[69]	50	Endoscopic	88	96	24	20	20	36	—	—	0	0
Smith et al.[72]	201	Endoscopic	91	92	14	3*	29	11*	2	36*	7	17*

*p <0.05 versus surgical palliation.

of the head of the pancreas accounts for 40% to 60% of periampullary cancers, whereas ampullary (20% to 40%), distal bile duct (10%), and duodenal (10%) locations account for the rest. Because of the location of these tumors, they are usually associated with obstructive jaundice. Noninvasive imaging demonstrates dilated intrahepatic and extrahepatic bile ducts and a dilated gallbladder. Once extrahepatic biliary obstruction has been determined, the patient should undergo direct cholangiography by either PTC or ERCP. ERCP offers the advantage of the ability to sample duodenal or ampullary lesions for biopsy and also provides the ability to obtain a pancreatogram.

Liver metastases and peritoneal implants are the most common site of distant spread in periampullary carcinomas. Contrast-enhanced dynamic CT scanning can usually detect liver metastases that are larger than 1 cm. Unfortunately, almost 15% of liver metastases are smaller than 1 cm and may not be seen on CT. Similarly, peritoneal implants are usually 1 to 2 mm in diameter and can only be seen by direct vision. Once distant metastases have been identified, survival is limited, and a conservative approach is indicated.

In patients with malignant obstruction of the biliary tract, endoscopic and percutaneous placement of biliary stents have been proposed as alternatives to surgical palliation. Four prospective, randomized trials comparing nonoperative biliary stenting with surgical biliary bypass for malignant obstructive jaundice have been published.[69-72] As Table 28-7 demonstrates, operative and nonoperative techniques are equally effective in relieving jaundice. Nonoperative therapy, however, was associated with a lower complication rate and shorter initial hospital stays. Advocates of surgical palliation criticize these studies on two counts. First, the 30-day in-hospital mortality rate for the surgical arms of these studies was high, ranging from 14% to 24%. In a recent analysis by Lillemoe et al.[73] of 118 consecutive patients undergoing palliative surgical therapy for periampullary carcinoma at Johns Hopkins Hospital, the hospital mortality rate was only 2.5%. The second reason that surgical palliation is favored by some authors is that nonoperative palliation is frequently associated with the late complications of recurrent jaundice and gastric outlet obstruction.

Surgery offers the only chance for the simultaneous palliation of the three major complications of periampullary carcinoma: biliary obstruction, gastric outlet obstruction, and pain. Surgical palliation should consist of either a choledochojejunostomy or hepaticojejunostomy for the relief of jaundice, a retrocolic gastrojejunostomy for the prevention of duodenal obstruction, and intraoperative chemical splanchinectomy for the control of pain. In a prospective, randomized trial, Lillemoe et al.[74] demonstrated that the intraoperative injection of 50% alcohol into the celiac plexus at the time of surgery significantly reduces and prevents the development of pain in patients with unresectable cancer.

If a chance for surgical cure exists, the Whipple procedure (pancreatoduodenectomy) is the procedure of choice. Several recent reports have documented perioperative mortality rates of 2% to 3% after pancreatoduodenectomy. Trede,[75] from Mannheim, Germany, recently reported an operative mortality rate of 2.5% in 118 pancreatoduodenectomies performed for cancer and 81 performed for chronic pancreatitis. The Johns Hopkins group recently reported a series of 145 consecutive pancreatoduodenectomies without any deaths.[76] With these acceptable mortality rates, and because the differentiation among periampullary cancers cannot always be made at the time of surgery, we continue to advocate pancreatoduodenectomy for periampullary tumors causing jaundice.

Cholangiocarcinoma

Cholangiocarcinoma can occur in any portion of the biliary tree. A clinically useful classification system of cholangiocarcinoma divides them into intrahepatic, perihilar, distal, and diffuse types. The intrahepatic tumors are managed similarly to primary liver tumors, and the distal cholangiocarcinomas are managed with pancreatoduodenectomy. The perihilar tumors, or Klatskin's tumors, comprise two thirds of all cholangiocarcinomas and are the most difficult to manage.

More than 90% of cholangiocarcinomas are associated with jaundice. In cases of malignant jaundice, serum bilirubin can be markedly elevated, attaining levels between 20 and 30 mg/dl. US and CT examinations in patients with perihilar tumors usually reveal dilated intrahepatic ducts, collapsed gallbladder and extrahepatic biliary tree, and a normal pancreas. A primary tumor mass

Table 28-8. Mortality and Survival of Hilar Versus Liver Resection for Perihilar Cholangiocarcinoma

				Actuarial Survival (%)		
Resection	**Patients**	**Operative Mortality (%)**	**Mean Survival (mo)**	**1 yr**	**3 yr**	**5 yr**
Hilar	201	8	21	76	21	7
Liver	188	15	24	61	28	17

From Boerma EJ. Research into the results of resection of hilar bile duct cancer. Surgery 107:597, 1990. Used with permission.

can be identified in only 21% of patients by US and in only 40% by CT scanning.[16] Direct cholangiography can be performed by either ERC or PTC. PTC may be preferable for perihilar tumors because it provides delineation of the proximal extent of the tumor. Transhepatic stents also provide access to the biliary system for intrahepatic cholangioscopy and can be useful technical aids in performing hilar dissections and in placing large-bore transhepatic Silastic catheters.

Palliative therapy in patients with cholangiocarcinoma includes both nonoperative and operative procedures. Criteria that exclude patients from surgery include poor general medical condition, distant metastasis, tumor extension into secondary biliary radicles of both hepatic lobes, and portal vein or main hepatic artery encasement. In patients with liver or peritoneal metastases who have had percutaneous transhepatic stents placed before operation, operative palliation may only involve cholecystectomy and tumor biopsy. In patients with locally advanced but unresectable tumors, the options for palliation include Roux-en-Y choledochojejunostomy with intraoperative placement of large-bore Silastic stents and segment III bypass to the left intrahepatic ducts. Nonoperative palliation consists of the percutaneous transhepatic placement of Silastic stents or endoscopic placement of endoprostheses. A recent study comparing percutaneous and operative palliation for unresectable hilar cholangiocarcinoma demonstrated that the in-hospital mortality rate was lower (7% vs 14%) and the mean survival was significantly longer (8 vs 5 months) for the surgically treated group.[77]

Patients with resectable perihilar cholangiocarcinoma are typically treated with resection of the extrahepatic biliary tree and reconstruction with a Roux-en-Y loop of jejunum with or without transhepatic stents. Recently, the trend around the world has been to perform more extensive surgery by adding partial hepatectomy to resection of the extrahepatic biliary tree to achieve a higher cure rate for perihilar cholangiocarcinoma.

In 1990 Boerma[78] reported a collective review of 389 patients with hilar cholangiocarcinoma resected since 1980 (Table 28-8). The data show an increase in both operative mortality rate and 5-year survival, with median survival unchanged, when partial hepatectomy is combined with resection of the extrahepatic biliary tree. Thus, if operative morbidity and mortality could be reduced, both median and 5-year survivals should increase. Nimura et al.[79] have achieved this goal. This group places multiple transhepatic catheters before operation to relieve jaundice and performs extensive flexible choledochoscopy to map out the full extent of tumor before major liver resection. Most patients undergo resection with an operative mortality rate of less than 5% and a 5-year survival of approximately 30%. Thus, if partial hepatectomy can be performed safely in patients with perihilar cholangiocarcinoma, this aggressive approach should give the patient the greatest opportunity for cure.

SUMMARY

During the past few decades, tremendous strides have been made in our ability to care for the patient with jaundice. Clinicians now have a better understanding of normal bilirubin metabolism and can classify the diseases that cause jaundice as defects in normal metabolism. Similarly, scientists are beginning to elucidate the multiple pathophysiologic effects of jaundice, and thus explain why patients with jaundice are at risk for increased morbidity and mortality during surgery. Our ability to accurately diagnose the cause of jaundice has increased with the development of noninvasive and invasive imaging techniques such as US, CT scanning, PTC, and ERC. In comparison, the roles of endoscopic and laparoscopic US and MRI are still being defined. These advances in diagnostic imaging have led to new and effective nonoperative therapeutic options for the relief of jaundice. ES, balloon dilatation, and the placement of endoprostheses for obstructive jaundice can all be performed in the patient with jaundice as primary therapy or as an adjunct to surgical therapy. However, the surgeon must decide which options will be the most efficacious, safe, and cost-effective in the diagnosis and treatment of each patient with jaundice.

REFERENCES

1. Pitt HA, et al. Factors affecting mortality in biliary tract surgery. Am J Surg 141:66, 1981.
2. Stewart L, Pellegrini CA, Way LW. Cholangiovenous reflux pathways as defined by corrosion casting and scanning electron microscopy. Am J Surg 155:23, 1988.
3. Koyama K, et al. Experimental and clinical studies on the effect of biliary drainage in obstructive jaundice. Am J Surg 142:293, 1981.
4. Holman JM, Rikkers LF. Biliary obstruction and host defense failure. J Surg Res 32:208, 1982.
5. Clements WD, et al. Effects of extrahepatic obstructive jaundice on Kuppfer cell clearance capacity. Arch Surg 128:200, 1993.
6. Wait RB, Kahng KU. Renal failure complicating obstructive jaundice. Am J Surg 157:256, 1989.
7. Hunt DR, et al. Endotoxemia, disturbance of coagulation, and obstructive jaundice. Am J Surg 144:325, 1982.

8. Cahill CJ. Prevention of postoperative renal failure in patients with obstructive jaundice—The role of bile salts. Br J Surg 70:590, 1983.
9. Evans HJR, et al. The effect of preoperative bile salt administration on postoperative renal function in patients with obstructive jaundice. Br J Surg 69:706, 1982.
10. Jacob G, et al. Cardiac function and responsiveness to β-adrenoceptor agonists in rats with obstructive jaundice. Am J Physiol 265:G314, 1993.
11. Melzer E, Krepel Z, Bar-Meir S. Recovery of pressor response to norepinephrine following relief of the obstructed common bile duct in the rat. Res Exp Med 193:163, 1993.
12. Lumlertgul D, et al. The jaundiced heart: Evidence of a blunted response to positive inotropic stimulation. Ren Fail 13:15, 1991.
13. Green J, Better OS. Circulatory disturbance and renal dysfunction in liver disease and in obstructive jaundice. Isr J Med Sci 30:48, 1994.
14. Hunt DR. The identification of risk factors and their application to the management of obstructive jaundice. Aust N Z J Surg 50:476, 1980.
15. Cainzos M, et al. Hyperbilirubinemia, jaundice and anergy. Hepatogastroenterology 39:330, 1992.
16. Thompson JE, et al. Broad spectrum penicillin as adequate therapy for acute cholangitis. Surg Gynecol Obstet 171:275, 1990.
17. Andy OJ, et al. Peritoneal neutrophil chemotaxis is impaired in biliary obstruction. Am Surg 58:28, 1992.
18. Pitt HA, et al. Benign postoperative biliary strictures. Operate or dilate? Ann Surg 210:417, 1989.
19. Deitch EA, et al. Obstructive jaundice promotes bacterial translocation from the gut. Am J Surg 159:79, 1990.
20. Grande L, et al. Obstructive jaundice and wound healing. Br J Surg 77:440, 1990.
21. O'Connor KW, et al. A blinded prospective study comparing four current noninvasive approaches in the differential diagnosis of medical vs. surgical jaundice. Gastroenterology 84:1498, 1983.
22. Baron RL, et al. A prospective comparison of the evaluation of biliary obstruction using computed tomography and ultrasonography. Radiology 145:91, 1982.
23. Thomas MJ, Pellegrini CA, Way LW. Usefulness of diagnostic tests for biliary obstruction. Am J Surg 144:102, 1982.
24. Taylor KJW, Rosenfield AT, Spiro HM. Diagnostic accuracy of gray-scale ultrasonography for the jaundiced patient: A report of 275 cases. Arch Intern Med 139:60, 1979.
25. Pedrosa CS, Casanova R, Rodriquez R. Computed tomography in obstructive jaundice. I. The level of obstruction. Radiology 139:627, 1981.
26. Wallner BK, et al. Dilated biliary tract: Evaluation with MR cholangiography with T2-weighted contrast-enhanced fast sequence. Radiology 181:805, 1991.
27. Gold RP, et al. Transhepatic cholangiography: The radiological method of choice in suspected obstructive jaundice. Radiology 133:39, 1979.
28. Gibbons CP, Griffiths GJ, Cormack A. The role of percutaneous transhepatic cholangiography and grey-scale ultrasound in the investigation and treatment of bile duct obstruction. Br J Surg 70:494, 1983.
29. D'Agostino HB, et al. Imaging and radiologic intervention of the biliary tree. In Braasch JW, Tompkins RK, eds. Surgical Diseases of the Biliary Tract and Pancreas. St. Louis: Mosby, 1994, p 68.
30. Pasanen PA, et al. Diagnostic accuracy of ultrasound, computed tomography, and endoscopic retrograde cholangiopancreatography in the detection of obstructive jaundice. Scand J Gastroenterol 28:185, 1991.
31. Bilbao MK, et al. Complications of endoscopic retrograde cholangiopancreatography (ERCP): A study of 10,000 cases. Gastroenterology 70:314, 1976.
32. Dooley WC, et al. Is preoperative angiography useful in patients with periampullary tumors? Ann Surg 211:649, 1990.
33. Grimm H, et al. Endoluminal ultrasound for the diagnosis and staging of pancreatic cancer. Baillieres Clin Gastroenterol 4:869, 1990.
34. Rosch T, et al. Staging of pancreatic and ampullary carcinoma by endoscopic ultrasonography: Comparison with conventional sonography, computed tomography, and angiography. Gastroenterology 102:188, 1992.
35. John TG, et al. Carcinoma of the head of pancreatic head and periampullary region: Tumor staging with laparoscopy and laparoscopic ultrasonography. Ann Surg 221:156, 1995.
36. Blamey SL, et al. Prediction of risk in biliary surgery. Br J Surg 70:535, 1983.
37. Dixon JM, et al. Factors affecting morbidity and mortality after surgery for obstructive jaundice: A review of 373 patients. Gut 24:845, 1983.
38. Little JM. A prospective evaluation of computerized estimates of risk in the management of obstructive jaundice. Surgery 102:473, 1987.
39. Goldman L, et al. Multifactorial index of cardiac risk in noncardiac surgical procedures. N Engl J Med 297:845, 1977.
40. Dawson JL. The incidence of postoperative renal failure in obstructive jaundice. Br J Surg 52:663, 1967.
41. Halliday AW, Benjamin IS, Blumgart LN. Nutritional risk factors in major hepatobiliary surgery. J Parenter Enter Nutr 12:43, 1988.
42. Foshi D, et al. Hyperalimentation of jaundiced patients on percutaneous transhepatic biliary drainage. Br J Surg 73:716, 1986.
43. Gillespie DA, Vickers CR. Pruritus and cholestasis: therapeutic options. J Gastroenterol Hepatol 8:168, 1993.
44. Gigot JF, et al. Acute cholangitis: Multivariate analysis of risk factors. Ann Surg 209:435, 1989.
45. Lai ECS, et al. Endoscopic biliary drainage for severe acute cholangitis. N Engl J Med 326:1582, 1992.
46. Lippset PA, Pitt HA. Biliary infection: Prophylaxis and treatment. In Toouli J, ed. Surgery of the Biliary Tract. Edinburgh: Churchill Livingstone, 1993, p 59.
47. Gerecht WB, et al. Prospective randomized comparison of mezlocillin therapy alone with combined ampicillin and gentamicin therapy for patients with cholangitis. Arch Intern Med 149:1279, 1989.
48. Meijer WS, Schmitz PIM, Jeekel J. Meta-analysis of randomized, controlled clinical trials of antibiotic prophylaxis in biliary tract surgery. Surgery 70:283, 1990.
49. Pitt HA, et al. Does preoperative percutaneous biliary drainage reduce operative risk or increase hospital cost? Ann Surg 201:545, 1985.
50. Lai ECS, et al. Preoperative endoscopic drainage for malignant obstructive jaundice. Br J Surg 81:1195, 1994.
51. Hatfield ARW, et al. Preoperative external biliary drainage in obstructive jaundice. Lancet 2:896, 1982.
52. McPherson GAD, et al. Preoperative percutaneous transhepatic biliary drainage: The results of a controlled trial. Br J Surg 71:371, 1984.
53. Greve JW, et al. Suppression of cellular immunity of obstructive jaundice is caused by endotoxins: A study with germ-free rats. Gastroenterology 98:478, 1990.
54. Kennedy JA, et al. Modulation of immune function and weight loss by L-arginine in obstructive jaundice in the rat. Br J Surg 81:1199, 1994.
55. Thompson RLE, et al. Development and reversibility of T lymphocyte dysfunction in experimental obstructive jaundice. Br J Surg 77:1229, 1990.
56. Rughneen PT, et al. Impaired specific cell-mediated immunity in experimental biliary obstruction and its reversibility by internal biliary drainage. J Surg Res 41:113, 1986.
57. Cotton PB, Vallon AG. British experience with duodenoscopic sphincterotomy for removal of bile duct stones. Br J Surg 68:373, 1981.
58. Hawes R, Cotton PB, Vallon AG. Follow-up 6 to 11 years after duodenoscopic sphincterotomy for stones in patients with prior cholecystectomy. Gastroenterology 98:1008, 1990.

59. Neoptolemos JP, et al. Precholecystectomy endoscopic cholangiography and stone removal is not superior to cholecystectomy, cholangiography, and common duct exploration. Am J Surg 163:227, 1992.
60. von Stiegmann G, et al. Endoscopic cholangiography and stone removal prior to cholecystectomy. Arch Surg 124:787, 1989.
61. Lillemoe KD, et al. Selective cholangiography: Current role in laparoscopic cholecystectomy. Ann Surg 215:669, 1992.
62. Phillips EH. Controversies in the management of common duct calculi. Surg Clin North Am 74:931, 1994.
63. Franklin ME, Pharand D, Rosenthal D. Laparoscopic common bile duct exploration. Surg Laparosc Endosc 4:119, 1994.
64. Berci G, Cuschieri A. Practical Laparoscopy. London: Bailliere Tindall, 1986.
65. Lillemoe KD, Pitt HA, Cameron JL. Current management of benign bile duct strictures. Adv Surg 25:119, 1992.
66. Langer JC, et al. Carcinoma of the extrahepatic bile ducts: Results of an aggressive surgical approach. Surgery 98:752, 1985.
67. Pitt HA, et al. Factors influencing outcome in patients with postoperative biliary strictures. Am J Surg 144:14, 1982.
68. Moote DJ, Malone DE. Non-operative management of benign bile duct strictures. In Toouli J, ed. Surgery of the Biliary Tract. Edinburgh: Churchill Livingstone, 1993, p 327.
69. Anderson JR, et al. Randomized trial of endoscopic endoprosthesis versus operative bypass in malignant obstructive jaundice. Gut 30:1132, 1989.
70. Bornman PC, et al. Prospective controlled trial of transhepatic biliary endoprosthesis versus bypass surgery for incurable carcinoma of head of pancreas. Lancet 1:69, 1986.
71. Shepard HA, et al. Endoscopic biliary prosthesis in the palliation of malignant obstruction of the distal common bile duct: A randomized trial. Br J Surg 75:1166, 1988.
72. Smith AC, et al. Randomised trial of endoscopic stenting versus surgical bypass in malignant low bile duct obstruction. Lancet 344:1655, 1994.
73. Lillemoe KD, et al. Current status of surgical palliation of periampullary carcinoma. Surg Gynecol Obstet 176:1, 1993.
74. Lillemoe KD, et al. Chemical splanchnicectomy in patients with unresectable pancreatic cancer. Ann Surg 217:447, 1993.
75. Trede M. The surgical treatment of pancreatic carcinoma. Surgery 97:28, 1985.
76. Cameron JC, et al. One hundred and forty-five consecutive pancreaticoduodenectomies without mortality. Ann Surg 217:430, 1993.
77. Nordback IH, et al. Unresectable hilar cholangiocarcinoma: percutaneous versus operative palliation. Surgery 115:597, 1994.
78. Boerma EJ. Research into the results of resection of hilar bile duct cancer. Surgery 107:597, 1990.
79. Nimura Y, et al. Combined portal vein and liver resection for carcinoma of the biliary tract. Br J Surg 78:727, 1991.

29

Splenic Physiology and Dysfunction

Steven A. Blau and Barry A. Levine

Nearly 2000 years ago, Galen declared the spleen an organ of mystery, and despite our sophisticated modern technology, some of that mystery persists. Our ignorance of some of the more important aspects of splenic physiology led as recently as 25 years ago to the rather casual extirpation of the organ for trivial injuries, and even today splenectomy is performed as a diagnostic technique in establishing the extent of neoplastic disease. Moreover, many of our assumptions of splenic function in humans come from animal studies, and their extrapolation to our patients may not be justified. For the surgeon today the major operation performed on the spleen is still its complete removal. The goal of this chapter is to define for the reader the indications for that procedure, the physiologic and pathophysiologic processes that underlie it, and the alternatives and alternate therapies that may be considered.

ANATOMY

The spleen is a solid, purplish-red organ, which in "normal" adults weighs 50 to 250 g and is located in the posterior left upper quadrant at the level of the 8th to 11th ribs. All factors being equal, the weight of the spleen is greater in whites than in blacks and is greater in males than in females. Further, the weight of the spleen decreases with age. In size, it averages about 12 × 7 × 4 cm in young adults and tends to involute with age. Its shape, sometimes described as a coffee bean, is consequent in part to the organs that it abuts, principally the diaphragm, stomach, and left kidney, and its surface may evidence persistent "fetal lobulations." It is attached to the underside of the left hemidiaphragm by the splenophrenic ligament, laterally to the visceral peritoneum by a condensation of the peritoneal tissue, by the lienorenal ligament to the left kidney, by the splenocolic ligament to the splenic flexure of the colon, and to the stomach by the gastrosplenic ligaments. With the exception of the last, these "ligaments" are largely avascular except in patients with advanced portal hypertension. The gastrosplenic ligament, though, is always vascular, containing as it does the vasa brevia or short gastric vessels.

The principal arterial supply of the spleen is the splenic artery, which arises from the celiac trunk and courses along the superior margin of the pancreas before entering the splenic hilum. Flow through the short gastric vessels also contributes to the splenic inflow. At the hilum, the splenic artery divides into six or eight segmental branches that are true end arteries; it is this arrangement that allows segmental splenectomy. Venous drainage of the spleen is via the splenic vein, which courses behind the head of the pancreas, joining the inferior mesenteric vein and subsequently the portal vein. Small gastric veins also contribute to the venous drainage of the spleen.

The spleen is covered by a 1 to 2 mm thick fibrous capsule, which contains major afferent and efferent blood vessels, nerves, and lymphatic vessels. In dogs and cats the capsule is more a fibroelastic layer with numerous bands extending into the splenic pulp. In response to circulating catecholamines the organ can actually contract, allowing "autotransfusion" of blood within the spleen. In humans the paucity of smooth muscle makes this response to hypotension unlikely. The capsule of the spleen is thicker in the young, than in the adult, and may become fibrotic and scarred in the elderly, especially in those with a previous history of injury or infarction. The capsule is covered with a thin layer of peritoneal mesothelium.

Beneath the capsule the spleen is divided into three components: the red pulp, the white pulp, and the marginal zone between them (Figs. 29-1 and 29-2). The white pulp can be visualized grossly as uniformly distributed 1 to 2 mm white nodules, and the white pulp is intimately associated with the arterial circulation of the spleen. The splenic artery divides into trabecular arteries, which leave the trabeculae and enter the white pulp as large central arteries. These are ensheathed with dense accumulations of lymphocytes (predominantly T cells), plasmacytes, and macrophages. This cylindric cuff is termed the periarterial lymphoid sheath (PALS). The PALS becomes more attenuated as the arteries branch into arterioles, but this cuffing can still be seen around the penicilliary arterioles. Lymphoid follicles (which contain

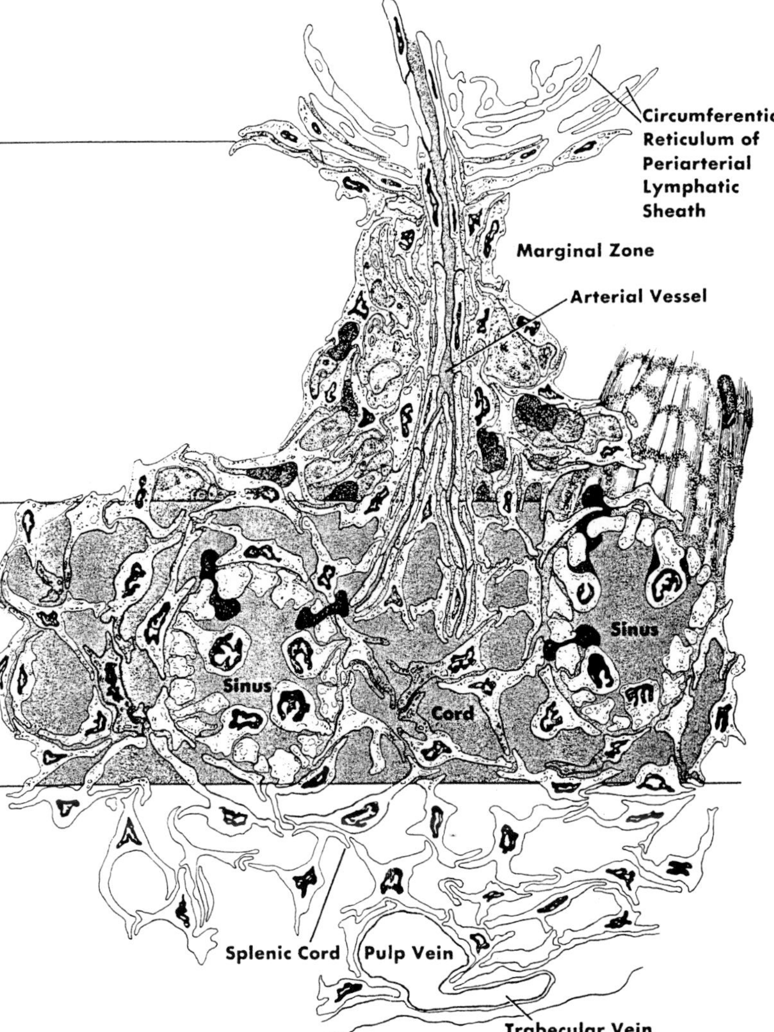

Fig. 29-1. Diagram illustrating the circulation of the red pulp and demonstrating both closed *(left)* and open *(right)* phases of venous circulation. (From Weiss L. The Cells and Tissues of the Immune System: Structure, Function, Interactions. Englewood Cliffs, N.J.: Prentice-Hall, copyright © 1972, p 60. Reprinted with permission.)

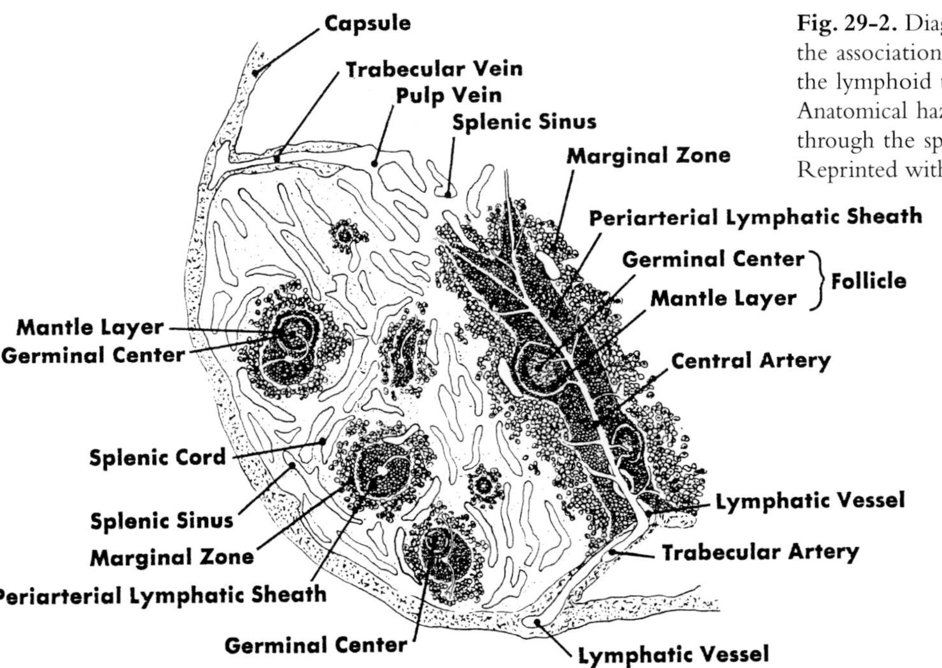

Fig. 29-2. Diagram of splenic white pulp showing the association between the arterial network and the lymphoid tissue. (From Weiss L, Tavassoli M. Anatomical hazards to the passage of erythrocytes through the spleen. Semin Hematol 7:372, 1970. Reprinted with permission.)

B lymphocytes) occur periodically as outgrowths of the PALS, usually at arterial branch points. The scaffolding of the white pulp is composed of a meshwork of cells with long dendritic cytoplasmic processes and silver-staining reticulin fibers.

Like the spleen itself, the morphology of the white pulp varies with the age of the patient and his or her immunologic status. The white pulp is fully developed at birth, reaches a peak at puberty, and then gradually involutes at a variable rate. The white pulp appears inactive or hypoplastic in both infants and in the elderly. In immunologically unstimulated adults, no germinal centers are seen, whereas in the spleens of children or young adults, secondary germinal centers are usually observed. In these immunologically active states, distinct zones corresponding to the lymphoid subpopulations may be observed. The germinal center or follicle is surrounded by a mantle zone composed of small B lymphocytes. This is then encased by a marginal zone that marks the division between the red and white pulp. This marginal zone is an extension of the PALS and thus contains many T lymphocytes. A zone of perifollicular venous sinuses surrounds this marginal zone.

The course of the arteries within the white pulp exhibits a number of variations. Some tributaries end with the PALS and others within the marginal zone. Some go to the periphery of the PALS, curve around and follow the perimeter of the marginal zones, and form the marginal sinuses between the red and white pulp. Still others leave the white pulp entirely and enter the red pulp as penicilliary arteries. Some of these terminal vessels are surrounded by lymphocytes from the attenuated PALS, and others are surrounded by a sheath of phagocytic cells. This anatomy is important to the immunologic functions of the spleen. It is thought that the marginal zone of the white pulp represents the site of the initial localization, trapping, and processing of antigens.

The red pulp is much simpler and is composed of vascular sinuses, the cords of Billroth, and the terminal arterial branches, where much of blood filtration occurs. The splenic sinuses are unique structures, lined by spindle-shaped endothelial cells with long cytoplasmic projections aligned along the longitudinal axis of the sinus. There are no desmosomes or tight junctions along this wall, but neither are there true spaces between the cells. Erythrocytes, granulocytes, and platelets squeezing through these potential "apertures" may be observed by electron microscopy. The basement membrane, which encircles the sinus, is discontinuous and fenestrated and is composed of a grid of transversely oriented reticular "ring fibers," which are attached to cordal macrophages. Conspicuously absent from the sinus is collagen. Structurally, the sinus resembles a barrel, with ring fibers being analogous to the hoops and endothelial cells the staves.[1] The adventitial surface of the sinus wall is covered by processes of the reticular cells of the cords of Billroth, fixed cells of the monocyte/macrophage series.

Controversy continues as to whether the red pulp circulation is "closed," that is, endothelially lined throughout, or whether it is "open" with the blood circulating within the mesh before entering the sinuses themselves. There is support for both theories depending on the species studied, the pathology involved, and environmental factors.[2] That both states exist is supported by experiment rather than political compromise. The bulk of the evidence suggests that the majority of blood flows through the "closed" system. This corresponds to a functionally rapid component with the blood flowing rapidly between arteriole and venous sinus. The open system corresponds to a functionally slower component with cells forced to percolate within a meshwork composed of cordal macrophages before they enter the venous sinuses. Stagnation in the pulp is probably the site of removal of abnormal, defective, or senescent erythrocytes. The environment within these cords is acidotic and hypoxic and contains limited quantities of available energy substrate.

EMBRYOLOGY

The spleen arises from the mesoderm and is unique embryologically in neither being a midline structure nor the remnant of what arose as a bilaterally symmetric structure. At about the fifth week of gestation, the spleen arises as a condensation of mesenchymal cells between the layers of the left dorsal mesogastrium, the mesentery suspending the stomach from the dorsal wall of the peritoneal cavity. Thin-walled blood vessels appear in the splenic tissue by the eighth or ninth week of development; as the vessels proliferate, reticular cells and fibers form sheaths around them.

Lymphocytes appear during the fourth month of gestation. Although both B and T lymphocytes are seen, B cells predominate during gestation. By the 19th week, surface markers for all immunoglobulin types are found within the developing spleen. The red and white pulp are distinguishable by the sixth month, although no germinal centers are seen in the fetal spleen. Secondary germinal centers are not seen generally until about 3 weeks prior to birth. Despite this, IgM and some IgG antibodies are synthesized during the third trimester. IgA and IgE are not synthesized during fetal life but make their appearance during the first year of neonatal life. Phagocytic function by cordal macrophages begins early in fetal life, and phagocytosis has been seen as early as the 12th week of gestation.

Histologically, the fetal spleen has been considered a hematopoietic organ, largely because of the recovery of precursor cells as early as the second trimester. These cells decrease in number during the fifth month as other sites subsume the responsibility for hematopoiesis. At birth, only occasional hematopoietic precursors are seen. This picture may be erroneous, based largely on conventional histology (finding the cells within the fetal spleen) or by inference from studies of nonhuman mammals. The precursor cells recovered are not part of the dividing pool, and other more primitive cells are not seen. Moreover, these same cells can be seen circulating in the fetal blood.

The consensus today[1] is that these cells within the spleen have been filtered out of the circulation and that the human spleen plays a minimal, if any, role in fetal hematopoiesis.

PHYSIOLOGY AND FUNCTION OF THE SPLEEN

The primary function of the spleen (see accompanying box) is probably filtration of the peripheral blood. Three processes of filtration can be seen in the handling of erythrocytes, namely, "culling" or destruction of erythrocytes, "pitting" or removal of particulate material or inclusions from the erythrocyte with return of viable cells to the circulation, and "erythroclasis" or destruction of the red blood cell by fragmentation. Each erythrocyte passes through the spleen nearly 1000 times a day.

Culling eliminates normal but aging erythrocytes and abnormal red blood cells.[3] Hereditary spherocytosis is an example of the latter. An abnormal spleen can also cull perfectly normal erythrocytes and other formed blood cells with consequent cytopenias. Culling can also be used to describe the removal of other circulating cells such as immature granulocytes, antibody-coated platelets, and particulate material such as bacteria or colloidal carbon in experimental models.[1]

SPLENIC FUNCTIONS

Filtration

1. Culling: Erythrocyte (or other blood cell) destruction
   a. Physiologic (as the red blood cells age)
   b. Pathologic
      (1) Associated with blood cell abnormalities
      (2) Associated with primary splenic changes
2. Pitting ("face-lifting" of erythrocytes)
   a. Removal of cytoplasmic inclusions
   b. Remodeling of cell membranes
3. Erythroclasis: Destruction of abnormal red blood cells with liberation into circulation of erythrocyte fragments
4. Removal of other particulate material (e.g., bacteria, colloidal particles)

Reservoir

1. Storage of normal sequestration of platelets, erythrocytes, granulocytes, iron

Hematopoietic

1. Erythropoiesis, granulopoiesis, megakaryopoiesis
2. Lymphocytic and macrophage production

Immunologic

1. Trapping and processing of antigen
2. "Homing" of lymphocytes
3. Lymphocyte transformation and proliferation
4. Antibody and lymphokine production
5. Macrophage activation

From Wolf BC, Neiman RS. Disorders of the spleen. In Wolf BC, Neiman RS, eds. Major Problems in Pathology, vol 20. Philadelphia: WB Saunders, 1989.

Pitting removes particulate material or inclusions from red blood cells with return of viable cells to the circulation. The recovery of cells with these inclusions is diagnostic of splenectomy or asplenia. These cells include those with Howell-Jolly bodies (which are remnants of nuclear material), Heinz bodies (denatured hemoglobin), Pappenheimer bodies (siderotic granules), and malarial parasites.

Erythroclasis involves the destruction of erythrocytes by fragmentation; as opposed to the situation with culling, the fragments are returned to the peripheral blood and are removed in subsequent passages through the spleen.[1] This phenomenon occurs in autoimmune hemolytic anemia, thalassemia, and the hemoglobinopathies, especially hemoglobin C disease and hemoglobin S disease.

The barriers to the passage of the red blood cell are only partially anatomic. The cells must pass around various cytoplasmic processes just to get near the sinuses, and then they must enter through the fenestrated basement membrane of the sinus. The principal barrier, though, seems to lie in the plasticity of the red cell membrane, since these passages are much smaller than the diameter of the erythrocytes. The cords of Billroth also produce a hostile environment. Plasma is skimmed off, and the blood in the pulp cords has a higher hematocrit and is more viscous.[4] Stagnation of erythrocytes decreases the available oxygen and increases lactic acidosis, producing an acidotic, hypoxic environment.[5] The mature erythrocyte, lacking mitochondria, is dependent on glycolysis for its energy needs, and even with abundant substrate the cell produces energy less effectively in a hypoxic environment. With inadequate substrate the cell cannot maintain its membrane-dependent ion pumps. The reticulocyte, on the other hand, although a larger cell, is more likely to withstand its passage than an aging erythrocyte. The reticulocyte is still capable of oxidative phosphorylation because of the few remaining cytoplasmic mitochondria that can metabolize glucose efficiently and maintain cell membrane integrity. The cords contain macrophages that are rich in lysosomal acid hydrolytic enzymes, which may be released into the cords if the cells are disrupted.[6] Moreover, the available data suggest that the erythrocyte membrane becomes progressively thinner and more fragile with aging.[7]

The spleen may also play a role in the maturation of the reticulocyte to a mature erythrocyte, by eliminating a high molecular weight membrane–protein complex.[8] This decreases the surface area of the cell and changes the cell membrane surface. Temporary sequestration in the spleen alters the surface charge of the reticulocyte, making it more negative, as is the case with the mature erythrocyte.[1] This may be consequent to a change in the orientation of membrane fatty acids.

In humans the spleen is a very poor red blood cell

reservoir, containing at most 40 ml of blood.[9] This is in contradistinction to the dog, whose spleen pools a significant volume of blood during sleep and contracts to return the blood when the animal awakens.[1] This difference in function can be intimated from the structure of the capsule of the human spleen, which contains little or no smooth muscle and is therefore incapable of contraction. In experimental models of shock in dogs the spleen is frequently removed prior to the experiment so as to eliminate this autonomic "autotransfusion." The human spleen, though, may be an effective reservoir for platelets. As much as one third of the body platelet mass is held in the red pulp.[10] Large numbers of mature granulocytes are also stored within the normal spleen. Blood pools within the spleen in conditions of splenomegaly regardless of the cause.[11] The spleen plays an important role in iron metabolism because of its role in erythrocyte destruction,[3] and the iron recovered from erythrocyte hemoglobin is transferred to the plasma and returned to the bone marrow. In some hemolytic conditions, though, the splenic macrophages may become engorged with iron, overwhelming their ability to return iron to the bone marrow.[3]

The human fetal spleen is considered by many to be a hematopoietic organ, a conclusion based on microscopic evidence of normoblasts and megakaryocytes in fetal specimens.[1] Immunohistologic and cytochemical techniques have demonstrated very few primitive precursor cells within the human fetal spleen,[12] and the discovery of normoblasts may represent filtration of circulating cells rather than in situ hematopoiesis.[1] The human fetal liver, however, is a hematopoietic organ. With regard to hematopoiesis, some investigators have suggested that the normal adult spleen exerts a mild inhibitory effect on the bone marrow through a circulating hormone termed "splenin" by Dameshek.[13] There is little current evidence, though, to support this idea.[1] Although it does not play a role in the formation of erythrocytes, the spleen certainly plays a role in the production of lymphocytes and macrophages.

The white pulp of the spleen is the body's largest lymphoid organ[1] and, as such, is capable of trapping and processing antigens with the resultant production of lymphokines and antibodies and the activation of the complement cascade system. The spleen responds not to local antigenic stimulation, of course, but to disseminated blood-borne antigens such as circulating bacteria. The white pulp of the spleen is compartmentalized into B- and T-cell zones with some overlap between them. The PALSs and marginal zones are composed predominantly of T lymphocytes.[14,15] T-helper cells predominate by a 3:1 or 4:1 ratio in these areas. There are some T cells found in the red pulp, but these are mainly suppressor/cytotoxic cells.[16] The majority of the B lymphocytes are found in the germinal centers and in the mantle zones,[14] although B cells may also be found in the marginal zone.[16] Rare B lymphocytes are found in the PALS.[1]

The distribution of immunoglobulin-containing B cells follows the pattern seen in reactive lymph nodes with immunoglobulin-bearing B cells being abundant in the marginal and mantle zones and absent in the majority of the germinal centers.[15] IgM staining is seen in these mantle and marginal zone B cells, but IgG is absent. IgG expression is limited to scattered cells within the red pulp. IgD is expressed predominantly in the mantle zones, whereas only rare IgA staining is found at the periphery of the follicles.

Macrophage cells are rarely found in the white pulp, but numerous such cells can be seen in the red pulp. Natural killer (NK) cells are scattered throughout the red pulp but appear only in the germinal centers of the white pulp. The red pulp, however, contains a far greater number of lymphocytes and macrophages than it does NK cells.[1]

The lymphocytes in the splenic white pulp represent a dynamic rather than a static population, as circulating lymphocytes enter the spleen and selectively "hone" into the white pulp. If antigen is present, the lymphocytes undergo activation and proliferation with resulting germinal center formation and production of both antibodies and lymphokines. If no antigen is present, the lymphocytes return to the circulation.

The marginal zone appears to play a key role in the initial trapping and processing of antigens.[17] Labeled particulate antigens appear first in the red pulp and then concentrate in the marginal zone.[18] Recent experiments suggest that the marginal zone lymphocytes may be of a unique immunologic phenotype and that they may be of central importance in the immune response to carbohydrate antigens.[19] Following initial localization within the marginal zones, antigens then penetrate the germinal center. The primary follicles enlarge and develop germinal centers within 3 or 4 days following exposure to a given antigen. The germinal centers diminish in size approximately 10 days after removal of the antigenic stimulation and return to the inactive state after about 4 weeks. Of course, the second set of phenomena is operant within the spleen, and the morphologic sequence occurs more rapidly on re-presentation of a specific antigen.

The immunologic function of the spleen is of prime importance in the debate over splenic salvage (see discussion of postsplenectomy sepsis and its prevention). Some investigators continue to believe that adults are not more susceptible to infection after splenectomy, although children and those adults with underlying hematologic or neoplastic disorders definitely are.

The spleen appears to play a key role in the body's defense against encapsulated bacteria and in the removal of other circulating particulate antigens. More specifically, the spleen is most important in the rapid antibody production following challenge with previously unencountered antigens.[20] The liver, although it can subsume some responsibility for clearing particulate matter, is less effective than the spleen, especially when the level of specific antibody is low or absent as it would be in the early stages of bacteremia.[20] In the spleen, antigens have a prolonged exposure to antigen-processing cells in the marginal zone and to the cordal macrophages. In the liver, not only are there far fewer macrophages, but the circulation time is shorter. Some investigators have reported efficient production of antibody in splenectomized animals when particulate antigen is injected subcutaneously or intraperitoneally.[21] The spleen is necessary, however, for the production of these early-appearing antibodies when the particulate antigen appears by intravenous challenge.

But why the particular sensitivity of splenectomized humans to encapsulated microorganisms? The polysaccharide coat of the bacteria provides a protective antiphagocytic property,[22] and the impaired clearance of these bacteria implies an inefficient production of opsonizing antibody and the absence of splenic phagocytosis. In the asplenic patient the liver is called on to clear circulating antigen, but it can only do so in the presence of high titers of specific antibody. It is inefficient in clearing these antigens with lower or no antibody, and it cannot produce the opsonizing proteins.

Which antibody class is deficient in the asplenic patient continues to be a subject of controversy as well. Although most investigators describe impaired production of IgM (which is usually the first antibody produced in response to antigen challenge), others have also described a deficiency in mounting an IgG response in splenectomized individuals.[23]

The complement system is also involved in the opsonization of particulate organisms. The C3b fragment binds to bacteria and antigen-antibody complexes, and both neutrophils and macrophages contain C3b receptors. This system seems to survive splenectomy intact.[24] The spleen also manufactures a tetrapeptide (threonine-lysine-proline-arginine) "tuftsin," which is believed to be an integral part of the circulating γ-globulin "leucokinin." Tuftsin plays a role in phagocytosis by coating circulating polymorphonuclear leukocytes and in some poorly understood manner facilitates phagocytosis.[25] A deficiency in tuftsin could thus enhance susceptibility to infection. Tuftsin deficiency is described after splenectomy,[25] but the data do not necessarily implicate this deficiency in the clinical problems following splenectomy.

SPLENOMEGALY AND HYPERSPLENISM

The terms *splenomegaly* and *hypersplenism,* although used interchangeably by some authors, are different phenomena. Splenomegaly, strictly speaking is the enlargement of the spleen, usually sufficient to make the spleen palpable on physical examination. In some instances the spleen can be enlarged but still not be palpable because it is enlarged from a smaller-than-normal starting point. Hypersplenism, as defined by Dameshek,[13] includes evidence of cytopenia of one or more peripheral blood lines, bone marrow hyperplasia commensurate with the cytopenia, splenomegaly, and correction of the cytopenia following splenectomy. This classic definition is not always accepted, and many authors believe that splenic dysfunction can occur in the absence of splenomegaly and, moreover, that the absence of a response to splenectomy does not mean the original condition was not a manifestation of hypersplenism. Another common definition is that of Crosby,[26] who defined hypersplenism as a detrimental increase in splenic activity "when a person is hematologically better off without his spleen."

Primary hypersplenism is applied to clinical situations where the spleen is histologically normal and there is no acceptable explanation for the splenomegaly or the cytopenia. This definition remains controversial, and the disease is rarely, if ever, encountered. Usually secondary hypersplenism occurs consequent to the sequestration of abnormal blood cells in an intrinsically normal spleen or when the sequestration is of normal cells and is consequent to splenic disease. Hypersplenism secondary to portal hypertension, for instance, falls into the second group in the above classification.

Before one proceeds to specific diseases of the spleen, note must be made of the diagnostic tests available in the evaluation of splenic size and function. The widespread use of CT scanning has, of course, added another means of evaluating splenic size to clinical examination. Splenic function is best evaluated by liver-spleen scanning with sulfur methionine, but this evaluates only one aspect of splenic function, namely the ability of the organ to take up the sulfur colloid. This test does not demonstrate immunologic function of the spleen, a situation addressed in greater detail when autotransplantation of splenic fragments is discussed (p. 622). Examination of the peripheral blood smear is a very important means of evaluating splenic function. The appearance of Howell-Jolly bodies, Pappenheimer bodies, and Heinz bodies is strongly suggestive of asplenia or postsplenectomy states. Finally, ^{51}Cr-tagged erythrocyte scanning is a useful technique for localizing red blood cells and determining the amount of sequestration localized to the spleen, liver, or the other components of the reticuloendothelial system.

DISEASES INVOLVING THE SPLEEN

Diseases of Red Blood Cells

Diseases of red blood cells include disease of erythrocyte membranes, diseases of erythrocyte metabolism, and diseases of hemoglobin.

Diseases of Erythrocyte Membranes

Diseases of erythrocyte membranes can be divided into hereditary spherocytosis (HS), hereditary elliptocytosis (HE), and hereditary pyropoikilocytosis (HPP).

Hereditary spherocytosis. HS is the most common hereditary anemia among people of northern European descent, occurring at a frequency of 1 in 5000. The disorder is seen in other populations less frequently.[27] Although once considered a single disease with a hereditary pattern of autosomal dominance, today variations in the severity of the disease are recognized, and in some cases an autosomal recessive pattern of inheritance is described.[27] The classic description is, of course, of the most severe form of the disease, and the patients have anemia, jaundice, and splenomegaly of varying degrees. Although the condition may be severe enough to warrant transfusion during the neonatal period,[28] many patients have a disorder that may remain clinically silent.[29] The anemia here is characteristically mild, but sudden exacerbations may occur. These are commonly due to hemolysis in conditions of stress or infection[30] and are usually self-limited; the patients do not require transfusion. However, aplastic crises, which may be associated with viral infections, can be severe, with anemia leading to cardiac decompensation and even death.[30] Hemolytic crises are commonly associated with increases in unconjugated bilirubin and splenomegaly.

Jaundice is most common during the neonatal period, and 30% to 50% of clinically stable adults with HS report neonatal jaundice.[28] After the neonatal period, icterus is mild and intermittent.[30] Palpable splenomegaly occurs in 75% to 82% of patients, but as implied earlier, there is no association between splenomegaly and the severity of the disease.[27] The liver is normal in both size and function, but cholelithiasis is a significant problem. Gallstones have been seen in children as young as 5 years and in 43% to 85% of adults.[27] Unusual and otherwise unexplainable complications of HS include chronic leg ulceration and a slowly progressive demyelinating process of the spinal cord that has been described in a small number of patients with HS.[27] The symptoms of the disease are affected by its severity, the frequency of transfusions, and the complications of therapy. In patients with severe HS who require multiple transfusions, there are skeletal changes and growth retardation similar to those seen with thalassemia and hemosiderosis, and multiple endocrine disorders resulting from iron overload have been seen in patients not being managed with iron chelation therapy.

The peripheral blood of these patients demonstrates microspherocytes, spherocytes, and normal-appearing cells. Before splenectomy the mean hemoglobin averages 11.3 to 14.6 g/dl and the reticulocytosis ranges 5% to 20%.[29] Automated indexes of red blood cell morphology may be normal consequent to the heterogenous population. The mean corpuscular hemoglobin concentration of the spherocytes may actually be increased because of the relative dehydration of the spherocyte in comparison to the normal discoid erythrocyte. Bone marrow examination reveals erythroid hyperplasia and normoblasts may account for 25% to 60% of nucleated cells.[27]

The single best test for determining the degree of spherocytosis is the determination of osmotic fragility because of the spherocyte's lower membrane surface area:volume ratio. Erythrocytes are placed in saline solutions of decreasing osmolarity, with osmotic fragility defined either as the saline concentration that produces any hemolysis, complete hemolysis, or hemolysis of 50% of the cells. Occasionally, it is necessary to preincubate the erythrocytes for 24 hours to allow depletion of intracellular energy stores before increased osmotic fragility can be demonstrated. Another technique is osmotic gradient ektacytometry in which the erythrocyte is subjected to a laminar shear stress field in a viscometer with the changes in shape monitored by laser diffractometry.[31] This single measurement can detect alterations in red blood cell surface or volume.

The pathophysiologic defect in the HS erythrocyte has been the subject of much study, and many putative mechanisms have been discarded. Earlier proposed defects included alterations in intracellular metabolism, protein phosphorylation, and ion permeability, but these have been inconsistent and may be secondary to the primary lesion that lies in the erythrocyte membrane.[30] Spectrin (which is actually two different but homologous subunits) is the largest protein associated with the erythrocyte membrane and appears to be responsible for both its strength and deformability. Spectrin accounts for 25% to 30% of total membrane protein. Spectrin deficiency to a variable degree was found in all patients with HS in whom the assay was performed,[32] and the magnitude of the deficiency correlated with the severity of the disease.[32] The cause for the spectrin deficiency is presently unknown, and the condition is complicated by additional reports of spectrin dysfunction in patients with HS.[27] Finally, sporadic reports implicate other, less common membrane proteins.

The mechanisms by which the spleen contributes to the anemia of this condition have already been discussed. First, the morphologic structure of splenic cords requires the deformability of the erythrocyte to successfully course through them, and the HS erythrocyte is clearly less deformable. Second, hypoxia and acidosis within the spleen contribute to "splenic conditioning," a process by which erythrocyte lipid loss occurs, leading to decreased membrane surface area, increased spheroidicity, and increased osmotic fragility. Finally, splenic macrophages may play a role either by direct erythrophagocytosis or by oxidant damage.

Therapy for patients with HS consists of splenectomy, and after this procedure the hematocrit generally rises to normal levels and the reticulocytosis falls. Hemolytic and aplastic crises are prevented, and the risk of traumatic rupture of the very enlarged spleen is eliminated. Although the risk of cholelithiasis increases the longer the spleen is left in situ, the recognition of the risks of overwhelming postsplenectomy sepsis has encouraged most clinicians to withhold this option until late childhood or early adolescence.

Hereditary elliptocytosis and hereditary pyropoikilocytosis.[27] Mild HE is most frequently found in blacks and Europeans. At least two genetically different forms are seen, both of which are inherited in an autosomal dominant manner. In the heterozygous state the patient usually exhibits no ill effects. The reticulocytosis is mild and sufficient to prevent anemia, and the abnormal morphology is readily apparent on the peripheral smear. The patient with a sporadic hemolysis variant also suffers from a mild disease except during the periods of splenic sequestration. Homozygous HE is rare and is characterized by severe hemolysis necessitating transfusion. The patients commonly exhibit pallor, jaundice, and splenomegaly. The reticulocytosis in these patients is as high as 20%, and death during infancy has been reported.

Mild HE with poikilocytosis or pyknocytosis produces a moderately severe anemia during the neonatal period, and patients may require transfusion; however, the disease seems to improve during the first few years of life, coming to resemble mild HE. Jaundice has been described, but splenomegaly is not usually present during the early neonatal period. This condition is more common in blacks, but has been reported in whites as well.

HPP is a rare disease that has been found only in blacks in which the erythrocyte's response to in vitro heating is abnormal. These erythrocytes undergo budding and fragmentation at several degrees below that at which normal erythrocytes fragment. The clinical picture associated with this condition becomes manifest during infancy and early childhood and includes moderate-to-severe anemia, pallor, jaundice, splenomegaly, and occasionally hepatomegaly. The peripheral smear exhibits elliptocytes, spherocytes, fragments, and cells with budlike projections. These shrunken and fragmented cells exhibit a profoundly decreased mean corpuscular volume when evaluated with a Coulter counter.

Stomatocytic elliptocytosis occurs with a frequency of up to 15% among the indigenous coastal population of New Guinea. Although the cells are abnormal on peripheral smear, the disease is generally mild, with anemia being uncommon. HE with spherocytosis is an autosomal dominant disorder that is usually mild and found in patients of European origin. Severe hemolytic anemia has been described, however, and fatal cases have been reported. The disease in the laboratory is similar to HS except that osmotic fragility is variably increased.

Each of these diseases has been associated with specific defects in the structure of the erythrocyte membrane, most of which are defects in one or the other subcomponent of spectrin. As with HS, splenectomy is effective therapy, eliminating the need for transfusion to control the anemia; but since not all patients actually have an anemia, the surgical option should be considered individually. Moreover, in some of these conditions the disease essentially "burns itself out"; for patients with HPP, for instance, splenectomy is routinely withheld until the age of 2 years and only after the patient has demonstrated that the disease is not of the transient variety.

Diseases of Erythrocyte Metabolism

The mature circulating erythrocyte is incapable of oxidative phosphorylation consequent to the loss of mitochondria and is therefore totally dependent on anaerobic glycolysis to meet its energy requirements. Intracellular energy (adenosine triphosphate [ATP]) is necessary for cation transport, glutathione synthesis (to prevent oxidative injury), methemoglobin reduction, adenine nucleotide salvage, and maintenance of its discoid shape. The generation of high levels of 2,3-diphosphoglycerate (2,3-DPG) in the Embden-Meyerhof glycolytic pathway modulates oxygen-hemoglobin affinity and may affect membrane stability. The rate of glycolysis in erythrocytes is slower than that of many other tissues, but their metabolic needs are obviously less. With aging, intracellular enzyme levels decrease, and without a nucleus or ribosomes, these cannot be replaced. Eight glycolytic pathway enzyme deficiencies have been identified as being associated with congenital nonspherocytotic hemolytic anemia. Because of the exceptionally stressful environment with the spleen, splenic destruction of these abnormal red blood cells may be a factor in the pathophysiology of these diseases, and splenectomy may play a role in their therapy. These enzyme defects usually demonstrate an autosomal recessive mode of inheritance, and they are rare.

Pyruvate kinase (PK) deficiency is the second most common enzymopathy associated with congenital nonspherocytic hemolytic anemia after glucose-6-phosphate dehydrogenase deficiency. Approximately 300 cases have been described in all ethnic groups, but the disease is most common in north Europeans. Its presentation is variable with about a third of the patients presenting with neonatal jaundice. About a third of these patients require transfusion, and some patients die during the neonatal period. In some infants the anemia improves with maturation. In more mild cases the anemia is less severe, and the diagnosis may not be established until later in childhood or even during adult life. As with other hemolytic anemias, episodes of severe anemia may occur as a result of transient bone marrow suppression associated with infection. Hemolytic crises are exceedingly uncommon; however, sufficient hemolysis occurs for choleithiasis to be a problem, and at least 10% of adults have this condition. Chronic leg ulceration has been reported in association with this enzymopathy.

The specific enzyme defect affects the conversion of phosphoenolpyruvate to pyruvate and the generation of ATP from adenosine diphosphate (ADP). Individuals who are heterozygous for the disease have about 50% of the PK enzyme in their red blood cells and are clinically healthy. A number of different kinetic patterns of PK mutations have been described.

The injury to the red blood cell in this condition is consequent to the failure to generate energy with resulting cell swelling and destruction. The gradual decrease in the glycolytic enzymes under normal conditions might lead one to believe that the PK-deficient red blood cells that are destroyed would be the oldest. Unfortunately, there is evidence of increased energy requirement in young erythrocytes. Moreover, reticulocytes may suffer, although they are able to generate energy by oxidative phosphorylation because in the spleen hypoxia forces an increased reliance on anaerobic glycolysis. The enzyme defect also leads to a rigidification of the cell membrane consequent to the loss of water and potassium. Finally, the accumulation of 2,3-DPG that occurs proximal to the enzyme deficiencies actually may be of benefit by decreasing oxygen affinity. This latter finding may explain the increased exercise tolerance of patients with PK deficiency, which exceeds that expected on the basis of the patients' anemia.

Splenectomy is of considerable benefit in patients with anemia but is not necessarily curative. It should result in a decrease in the need for autologous blood transfusion, and a gain of several grams in baseline hemoglobin usually results. Reticulocytosis can rise after splenectomy consequent to the decreased clearance of these cells once the spleen has been removed. Alternative therapies that focus on the enzyme deficiency have included the provision of alternate substrate for energy production, but clinical studies have been inconclusive.

Splenectomy has been applied in only a limited fashion to patients suffering from the other glycolytic enzymatic deficiencies. It has decreased transfusion needs but not eliminated the anemia in patients with hexokinase deficiency (converting glucose to glucose-6-phosphate) and phosphoglycerate kinase deficiency (the enzyme that converts 1,3-DPG to 3-phosphoglycerate). Splenectomy has been beneficial in severe cases of glucose phosphate isomerase deficiency (the enzyme that converts glucose 6-phosphate to fructose 6-phosphate). Experience with splenectomy has been limited in cases of phosphofructokinase deficiency (the enzyme that converts fructose 6-phosphate to fructose 1,6-diphosphate). There was no benefit of splenectomy in the single patient with triose phosphate isomerase deficiency (the enzyme that converts dihydroxyacetone phosphate to glyceraldehyde-3-phosphate and back again). Splenectomy has not been advised in patients with diphosphoglycerate mutase (the enzyme that converts 1,3-DPG to 2,3-DPG) because the anemia has not been severe enough to warrant it. Finally, no patient has undergone splenectomy for aldolase deficiency (the enzyme that converts fructose 1,6-diphosphatase to dihydroxyacetone phosphate and glyceraldehyde-3-phosphate).

Glucose 6-phosphate deficiency is the most common erythrocyte enzyme abnormality associated with hemolytic anemia. This X-linked disorder affects millions of people around the world but occurs with the highest frequency among individuals of Mediterranean descent. It affects approximately 15% of African-Americans. Hemolysis is most common in men but can occur in women as well, since heterozygous women have the enzyme defect in some of their red blood cells. In most cases the hemolysis is in response to specific agents that produce an oxidative stress with depletion of intracellular glutathione. The hemoglobin is oxidized, resulting in sulfhemoglobin and Heinz bodies. Although splenic destruction of these abnormal cells occurs, therapy is generally directed at avoiding known drugs with splenectomy being performed only in the most severe cases associated with chronic nonspherocytic hemolytic anemia to reduce the rate of erythrocyte destruction.

Diseases of Hemoglobin

Diseases of hemoglobin include hemoglobinopathies, thalassemias, and acquired "autoimmune" hemolytic anemia.

Hemoglobinopathies. A large number of unstable hemoglobins have been identified in humans, although most reports describe only a single individual or family. These share a common instability and denature within the red blood cell, either spontaneously or following oxidative stress. The inheritance pattern of unstable hemoglobin disease is autosomal dominant, and all affected patients are heterozygous for the affected gene, as homozygous disease would almost certainly be lethal. The clinical picture associated with these defects is variable and includes severe, moderate, or mild hemolytic anemia. On the other hand, some patients may be completely asymptomatic. Hemolysis is consequent to the precipitation of the unstable hemoglobin as Heinz bodies and the removal of these in the spleen along with attached portions of the cell membrane. These cells, now with a decreased cell surface area, are less deformable. Patients with mild disease require little or no therapy other than the avoidance of oxidant drugs if these have been implicated in hemolysis for the specific hemoglobinopathy. Splenectomy has been advocated in patients with moderate disease and has generally been effective in reducing the severity of the disease. In patients with severe disease, splenectomy has been less successful, probably because other reticuloendothelial organs such as the liver or lymph nodes can subsume the spleen's function in destroying these cells. Splenectomy is, of course, not indicated in mild disease, although it may prevent hemolytic crises and decrease the incidence of cholelithiasis. When advocated, splenectomy is deferred until after age 6 years for the now-recognized postsplenectomy infectious risks.

Whereas unstable hemoglobins are rare causes of congenital hemolytic anemia, sickling syndromes in which the hemoglobin polymerizes when deoxygenated are common. The long fibers produced distort the membrane resulting in the classic sickle shape. Sickling results in poorly deformable cells and increased adherence to cells of the reticuloendothelial system and to vascular endothelium. This leads to both hemolysis and vaso-occlusive episodes.

Hemoglobin S is probably the most common hemoglobinopathy seen in clinical practice. The gene is widespread throughout equatorial Africa; in some tribes, half the population carries the gene. Among American blacks, the incidence of the gene is about 87%. The gene, moreover, is not restricted to blacks, as it appears in parts of Turkey, Saudi Arabia, southern India, Sicily, Cyprus, and Greece. It is suggested that heterozygous individuals have an increased resistance to malaria, and the geographic pattern of the gene resembles the geographic distribution of malaria.

Symptoms of sickle cell anemia (the homozygous state with 76% to 100% of the circulating hemoglobin being hemoglobin S) first appear during the neonatal period as hemoglobin F production is replaced by adult hemoglobin production (hemoglobin S rather than hemoglobin A). As affected individuals enter adolescence, new problems arise such as growth retardation, and vaso-occlusive crises increase in frequency. Hemorrhagic strokes, cardiac failure, and chronic renal disease are seen in adults. Aplastic crises in which the bone marrow response is inadequate to maintain the hematocrit are commonly associated with viral infections. Acute anemia can also occur secondary to acute splenic sequestration. Despite the prominence of the spleen in this condition, there is no indication for splenectomy in these patients. Instead, the spleen infarcts over time consequent to occlusion of blood within it. Scarred fibrotic splenic remnants are all that are usually found in adults; in prospective studies, asplenia can be seen as early as 4 months of age and was present in most children by 12 months of age. The asplenia of sickle cell anemia is the paradigm for asplenia in patients about to undergo splenectomy for other conditions. These patients are at increased risk of infections from encapsulated organisms, especially *Streptococcus pneumoniae.* The risk for sepsis or meningitis is 20 to 600 times that of age-matched controls, and the mortality approaches 35%. Therapy includes polyvalent pneumococcal vaccines, which have decreased the incidence of infection and mortality but are not always effective, as many patients continue to suffer infection with this microorganism. Prophylactic penicillin, both long- and short-acting, has been reported to decrease the incidence of pneumococcal disease in children. There is a danger to extrapolating the experience in these patients to the splenectomized patient because other immunologic defects have been demonstrated in the patient with sickle cell anemia such as defective C3b fixation to the bacterial surface and inactivation of the complement system consequent to high circulating free hemoglobin levels. These additional immunologic defects have not been reported in the asplenic patient following splenectomy. The patient with hemoglobin SS disease is more likely to require cholecystectomy and splenectomy.

The more common sickle cell trait is rarely associated with morbidity. Sickling can occur in these patients (whose hemoglobin S content ranges from 20% to 45% of circulating hemoglobin) under hypoxic conditions or during prolonged periods of strenuous exercise. Splenic infarction has been reported in individuals with sickle cell trait during flights in unpressurized aircraft and during vigorous exercise at high altitudes. Because splenic sequestration is rare, splenectomy is not indicated. Moreover, splenic function seems to be normal in afflicted individuals.

Additional hemoglobinopathies have been reported. The combination of hemoglobin C with hemoglobin S results in patients whose disease can be as severe as those with hemoglobin SS disease. These patients may manifest splenomegaly, suffer from acute attacks of splenic sequestration, and develop splenic infarction. Splenomegaly, but not acute sequestration, is seen in patients with sickle cell trait and thalassemia.

Thalassemias. Thalassemia (Mediterranean anemia) is a constellation of syndromes reflecting specific mutations that decrease the rate of synthesis of the globulin chains that make up the hemoglobin tetramer. The disease may be divided into α-, β-, and γ-types according to the chain involved and into major or minor depending on whether the patient is heterozygous or homozygous for the mutation. Combinations of mutations have also been reported. The disease is relatively common in the Mediterranean basin and in the United States in people of southern European ancestry. The pathophysiology of the disease lies not so much in the failure to produce hemoglobin tetramers, but in the relative overproduction of the non-thalassemic globulin chains and abnormal hemoglobins. These can precipitate, damage the red blood cell membranes, and shorten red blood cell survival.

α-Thalassemia can occur from the deletion of one or more α-globulin genes. Single deletions are asymptomatic. Deletion of two of the genes produces the α-thalassemia trait, which is associated with a mild anemia. Loss of three copies of the gene produces a moderately severe hemolytic anemia associated with splenomegaly and hypersplenism in some individuals. Finally, deletion of all four genes produces an individual incapable of producing fetal hemoglobin and manifests as severe intrauterine hemolytic anemia. Furthermore, the consequent defect in oxygen transport usually results in stillbirth. There is no indication therefore for splenectomy in any of the α-thalassemia variants.

The genetics of β-thalassemia are simpler because there is only a single pair of β-globulin alleles. The disease that develops, however, is affected by the amount of β-globulin produced and the compensatory production of γ-globulin. The single gene defect results, then, in either a silent carrier state or β-thalassemia trait, a disease characterized by microcytosis, hypochromasia, and mild anemia with pregnant women being the individuals most likely to require transfusion therapy. Thalassemia intermedia occurs with the inheritance of two defective genes, but the disease is less severe than thalassemia major or Cooley's anemia where there is no production of β-globulin at all. Individuals with thalassemia intermedia have a moderately severe anemia (hemoglobin levels average 6 to 9 g/dl). These patients may need transfusions occasionally, but they are not transfusion dependent. Splenomegaly, hypersplenism, and often hepatomegaly are common symptoms of thalassemia intermedia, and these patients may require cholecystectomy for their bilirubin stones.

β-Thalassemia major may not be obvious at birth because circulating hemoglobin composed of α- and γ-globulins is synthesized in adequate amounts. The relatively greater solubility of the hemoglobin H produced and its delayed precipitation within the erythrocyte lead to peripheral hemolysis. The erythrocytes of patients with this disease have a decreased survival when compared to normal red blood cells. By ^{51}Cr survival studies, their half-life ranges from 7 to 22 days (with normal half-life being

25 days). During the first year of life, however, the decrease in γ-globulin synthesis produces the disease. Patients who do not receive transfusion during the first decade of life usually die. They manifest a severe anemia with massive hepatosplenomegaly. The spleen enlarges probably because of two phenomena, splenic sequestration of erythrocytes and erythroid hematopoiesis. The bone marrow hypertrophy weakens the skeleton and predisposes these patients to pathologic fractures. In patients who survive into the second decade of life, the complications of iron overload consequent to both transfusion and to hemolysis become a part of the pathophysiology of the disease. Growth and development are impaired. Hepatic hemosiderosis usually leads to abnormalities of liver function and may produce cirrhosis. Diabetes may result from iron overload in the pancreas, and cardiac conduction defects from hemosiderosis are common. Iron chelation therapy is mandatory if the patient is to survive the second decade of life. Splenic erythropoiesis can be suppressed with maintenance of hemoglobin levels above 12 g/dl, and these patients should be regularly transfused with leukocyte-poor packed red blood cells every 3 to 4 weeks. These patients should also receive desferrioxamine to decrease iron toxicity. Splenectomy is indicated when the annual blood requirement exceeds 200 to 250 ml of packed cells per kilogram body weight.[33] This criterion is usually met when the patients reach 6 or 8 years of age. Splenectomy does not eliminate the need for maintenance transfusion therapy, it merely decreases the frequency of transfusions. The septic mortality of patients with thalassemia after splenectomy is among the highest of any group coming to splenectomy, and these patients make the best case for overwhelming postsplenectomy sepsis and the need to be vigilant for it. The mortality of this disease has decreased recently, perhaps as a result of improved prophylaxis (both pneumococcal vaccine and prophylactic penicillin therapy) against infection. The increasingly apparent immunosuppression associated with blood transfusion may also play a role in the septic complications of these patients seen after splenectomy.

Finally, defects in the genes for γ- and β-globulin synthesis and for γ-, δ-, and β-genes have been reported in small numbers of patients. These aberrations are generally managed in a fashion similar to that of patients with β-thalassemia.

Acquired "autoimmune" hemolytic anemia. Hemolytic anemia may occur consequent to antibodies that are directed against antigens on the erythrocyte cell membrane. This may result in intravascular hemolysis or extravascular hemolysis in the liver or spleen. In addition to the site of red blood cell destruction or fatal injury, autoimmune hemolytic anemia may be classified by its cause or by the type of antibodies present. For most patients with this condition, the cause is idiopathic. Defined causes include drug reactions, associated collagen vascular diseases, infections (especially viral and mycoplasmal), and lymphoid malignancy. Alternatively, these are termed primary and secondary autoimmune hemolytic anemia.

The distinguishing feature of this disease is a positive direct Coombs' test in which hemolysis of red blood cells is identified in vitro. The attached antibodies are described as warm reactive if they bind to red blood cells most avidly at 37° C or cold reactive in that they have increased affinity as the temperature approaches 4° C. Warm-reactive antibodies are usually IgG class but less commonly are IgM or IgA class. Macrophages within the spleen (and, to a lesser extent, the liver) have receptors for the Fc portion of the IgG attached to these red blood cells. This leads to recognition, binding, and removal of the antibody with a portion of the cell membrane causing a change in the cell's surface. This increasingly spherical cell is more vulnerable to injury coursing through the splenic sinusoids and is eventually removed from the circulation. This destruction is not complement mediated. Red blood cells coated with both IgG and complement are destroyed by the reticuloendothelial system and not just the spleen.

Warm-reactive drug-related hemolytic anemia can be caused by a number of different medications. There are two types of antibodies: those directed against the red blood cell antigens and those directed against the drug (hapten type) in which the red blood cell is an "innocent bystander." Methyldopa, for instance, produces the former picture.

Cold-reactive antibodies are usually of the IgM class (rarely IgA or IgG) and bind to red blood cells in the peripheral circulation such as exposed portions of the fingertips, the nose, or the ears where the temperature is lower, rather than in the central circulation. Cold-reactive antibodies produce intravascular hemolysis by complement-mediated red blood cell lysis or, less often, by sequestration in the liver (secondary to receptors directed against the C3b portion of complement) with subsequent destruction. These patients have an underlying chronic hemolysis that is aggravated by exposure to cold. Furthermore, Raynaud's phenomenon or acrocyanosis can occur consequent to intracapillary red blood cell agglutination.

Patients with secondary autoimmune hemolytic anemias usually seek medical attention for the underlying disease. Splenomegaly is found in 50% of these patients. Examination of the peripheral smear demonstrates spherocytosis and a secondary reticulocytosis. Bone marrow aspirates demonstrate increased erythroid activity. In severe cases of hemolysis, urine sample results are positive for myoglobinuria. The definitive test for this disease is ^{51}Cr-tagged red blood cell sequestration studies, and this test also allows a rational decision regarding the role of splenectomy.

The therapy for autoimmune hemolytic anemia secondary to mycoplasmal pneumonia and viral diseases is observation, as the disease is usually acute and self-limited. More often, however, the disease is chronic with a waxing and waning severity over months or years. The initial therapy for the chronic condition is corticosteroids. The majority of patients demonstrate a clinical response to high-dose steroids (60 to 100 mg prednisone per day) in a median of 7 days. Failure to improve by 3 weeks is considered a signal of steroid failure. Following a successful response to corticosteroids, the dose is tapered for a period of 3 to 6 months with close follow-up for signs of recrudescence. In about two thirds of patients a complete remission is seen. Patients who fail to respond to steroids or who relapse with tapering are candidates for splenectomy. If splenic sequestration was demonstrated, response rates of 80% or better are reported, especially for patients with primary, warm-reactive antibodies. Failure of splenic sequestration does not constitute a reason to avoid splenectomy, as many of these patients achieve at least a partial response. This may be explained by the spleen's role in the *production* of IgG. Finally, in patients who fail both steroids and splenectomy, immunosuppressive drugs such as cyclophosphamide or azathioprine have been successful.

Diseases of Platelets

Idiopathic Thrombocytopenic Purpura

Idiopathic thrombocytopenic purpura (ITP) is a relatively common disease wherein antibody-coated platelets are sequestered and destroyed in the spleen. This was demonstrated first and effectively managed by William Harrington, then a hematology trainee, who in 1951 was voluntarily transfused with plasma obtained from a patient with ITP and promptly developed a severe thrombocytopenia.[34] ITP may occur spontaneously or be associated with such other disorders as chronic lymphocytic leukemia or systemic lupus erythematosus. In Evans's syndrome, ITP occurs concomitantly with an autoimmune hemolytic anemia. The disease may be acute, as it often is seen in children, or chronic. In acute disease the precipitating event is usually a viral infection, and the disease is usually self-limited. When acute disease occurs in adults, it is usually a result of a drug sensitivity reaction. Chronic ITP is most often seen in women (in one series[35] the average age was 36 and the average platelet count was 33,000 cells/mm^3), and it is here that definite IgG platelet antibodies are found. The incidence of chronic ITP seems to be increasing. Not only is the spleen the site of sequestration and destruction of these platelets, but the spleen is also the major site of production of these antibodies. Destruction of platelets proceeds with complement fixation or with phagocytosis facilitated by antiplatelet IgG.

The patient's clinical presentation includes spontaneous bleeding, petechiae, purpura, mucosal bleeding, and epistaxis. Menorrhagia is common. Spontaneous bleeding is unlikely until the platelet count falls below 50,000 and is usually severe with platelet counts of 20,000 or less. Children with the acute form of ITP have a 1% or 2% incidence of intracranial hemorrhage, a complication that is rare in adults. Some investigators have suggested that the presentation should determine the aggressiveness of the management with "dry purpura" with petechiae and ecchymosis being considered a less severe disease than "wet purpura" with active bleeding from mucosal surfaces.[36]

The diagnosis of ITP requires normal counts of erythrocytes and leukocytes and the demonstration of thrombocytopenia. Bone marrow aspirates should demonstrate increased platelet production, commonly four or five times normal. Splenic sequestration of platelets can be demonstrated by nuclide studies. The older studies used ^{51}Cr-labeled homologous platelets,[37] but recently ^{111}In-labeled autologous platelets have been reported.[38] The older chromium technique was criticized because of the disadvantages of poor labeling in severe cases of thrombocytopenia and of poor yield of external counting methods.[37] The newer technique may more accurately assess splenic sequestration (which is not the sole problem in all patients) and increase the yield of therapeutic splenectomy.[38] Splenomegaly occurs rarely in this disease.

The therapy for the acute form of the disease is entirely conservative, and these patients usually recover spontaneously. Patients with the chronic form of ITP are usually treated with steroids (prednisone 1 mg/kg/day), and the majority respond at least transiently with an increased platelet count within 3 to 7 days. Complete remission with steroids is rare, however, and thrombocytopenia recurs with tapering of the steroid dose. Splenectomy is eventually required in about two thirds of adults.[39] Patients who fail to respond to steroids usually have a favorable and permanent response to splenectomy, but patients who have responded to steroids usually have an even greater chance of benefiting from splenectomy. Should splenectomy, then, be the first treatment of choice? Perhaps. Although steroid treatment increases preoperative platelet counts, infectious complications are increased in patients who have received steroids for prolonged periods of time. This argues for very brief courses of steroid therapy. Both splenectomy and steroids are associated with a decrease in antiplatelet IgG. Since antineoplastic agents such as cyclophosphamide and vincristine can also produce this fall in IgG, some have advocated their use in refractory patients with ITP, but the clinical response rate is poor.

Preoperative management of the patient scheduled for splenectomy frequently includes adjunctive measures to increase platelet count. In addition to steroids, plasmapheresis to reduce antiplatelet antibody levels and high-dose intravenous γ-globulin to saturate macrophage Fc receptor have been employed. Preoperative administration of platelets is usually unnecessary and would probably be futile prior to clamping the splenic artery. Prompt increases in platelet count have encouraged many surgeons to avoid platelet transfusion altogether, but many administer transfusions after clamping the splenic pedicle to decrease the risk of wound hematoma and intra-abdominal bleeding. Pneumococcal vaccine is recommended to prevent the specific infectious complications of these encapsulated bacteria after splenectomy. The vaccine should be administered prior to splenectomy in order to maximize the antibody titers. The vaccine is even more important in the few children whose ITP becomes chronic and who require splenectomy. After splenectomy, 80% of patients should have normal platelet counts within 6 weeks; another 15% have subnormal levels but do not require platelet transfusion therapy. In addition to previous response to steroids, age less than 60 years, a short duration of thrombocytopenia, and a prompt thrombosis after splenectomy are associated with long-term splenectomy success.

Today, splenectomy remains the second course of therapy, although few studies have documented an increased life expectancy with splenectomy as opposed to no additional therapy. This is because only a small number of patients are at risk of fatal bleeding with low platelet counts. Splenectomy is a palatable choice of therapy, moreover, because the age of the patients who suffer from the disease makes the perioperative morbidity and risks of the operation less problematic. Because splenectomy in elderly patients is felt to be associated with significant risks, alternative therapies for patients who fail steroid therapy have been considered. These include the vinca alkaloids, colchicine, danazol, alkylating agents, and cyclosporine. Higher dose pulse steroids have recently been reported to be of value,[40] a technique that is appealing financially as well as physiologically. Nonpharmacologic techniques for steroid failures include radiotherapy.[41]

Examination of the resected spleen may be of value in predicting the patient's response to splenectomy. The characteristic finding of prominent secondary follicles and the presence of foamy macrophages are not found universally. In a recent series, secondary follicles were found in 28% of a series of 83 patients, and this finding was associated with age (the patients were younger), sex (they were more likely to be female), a higher rate of antibody production, and a greater response to splenectomy in terms of subsequent platelet counts. In contrast, the eight patients with neither prominent secondary follicles nor foamy macrophages did significantly poorer.[42]

Despite a dramatic initial response to splenectomy, some patients develop recurrent disease. In many cases this may represent disease consequent to accessory spleens missed at the initial operation or "caused" by the splenectomy itself. In one series 65% of 43 patients benefited from accessory splenectomy with maintenance (at least early on) of platelet counts in excess of 100,000 cells/mm^3.[43] The presence of accessory spleens, however, may not be sufficient to justify a return to the operating room. In a series of 216 patients, Coon[44] found accessory spleens at autopsy in patients without recurrent disease and an absence of splenic tissue in most of the patients who did relapse.

The future of splenectomy for this disease should be based on accurate localization studies that confirm the spleen as an active participant in platelet sequestration.

Thrombotic Thrombocytopenic Purpura

Thrombotic thrombocytopenic purpura was initially described in 1924[45] and is primarily a disease of the microvasculature with deposition of "hyaline" material composed of aggregated platelet and fibrin in subendothelial and intraluminal sites. This leads to arteriolar occlusion. The platelet count is reduced, possibly consequent to platelet deposition and thrombosis. A microangiopathic anemia develops probably consequent to the passage of erythrocytes through damaged arterioles. The remaining clinical signs include purpura, fever, renal failure, and neurologic manifestations of seizures, coma, or aphasia. The disease is more common in females than males, and its usual age of onset is between 10 and 40 years. Hepatosplenomegaly occurs in about a third of patients. Peripheral smears confirm the anemia, the thrombocytopenia, and the fragments of red blood cells consistent with the microangiopathy. The bone marrow aspirate reveals the compensatory increase in erythroid precursors with normal or increased megakaryocyte activity.

The cause of this disease remains unclear and this impacts adversely on its management. Allergic reaction, autoimmunity, infection, and unspecified toxins have been considered etiologic agents. Antiplatelet drugs such as aspirin and dipyridamole have been used and have increased survival, as has plasmapheresis. When plasmapheresis has been employed, it has been combined in some centers with exchange transfusion. Steroids as antiimmune agents have also been employed. The majority of survivors of this disease, though, have had splenectomy, and many of these patients are also receiving concomitant steroid therapy. Whether this is a valid indication for splenectomy is controversial, however, since no direct link to the spleen has been established in the pathophysiology of this disease. Histologic evaluation of spleen specimens has not been effective in elucidating the controversy. Although germinal centers have been found in a high proportion of spleens removed, they are not a universal finding.[46] The splenic pathology is clearly different from that of the ITP spleen, however, with prominent periarteriolar deposits, hemophagocytosis, and hemosiderosis.[46] Splenectomy as a salvage procedure is supported, at the very least, by the fact that this is an almost fatal disease in the absence of remission.[47]

HIV-Related Thrombocytopenia

Autoimmune thrombocytopenic purpura was first reported[48] in 1982, and it is estimated that 5% to 15% of HIV-infected individuals suffer from thrombocytopenia. This finding is independent of the cause of the infection or the clinical and immunologic status of the patient.[49] Splenectomy has been advocated for this disease based on the experience with other forms of autoimmune ITP. As with that disease, pharmacologic treatment is sometimes effective, but the duration of the platelet response is limited. Pharmacologic agents in this condition include zidovudine (AZT), steroids, and danazol. These patients generally tolerate the operation well with minimal morbidity despite their immunosuppressed states, and more than half in one large series with a mean follow-up of 42 months had a persistent complete response.[50] Outright failures are uncommon. Splenectomy is warranted in these patients because of the increasing life expectancy of the HIV-positive population. Concerns that splenectomy might be a factor in converting asymptomatic HIV to AIDS have not been confirmed.

Diseases of White Blood Cells

Splenic Neutropenia

Splenic neutropenia is a relatively rare condition characterized by severe neutropenia that is uncommonly associated with thrombocytopenia or hemolytic anemia. Although it is associated with splenomegaly, the hypothesis that the neutrophils are destroyed because of the decreased transit time and exposure of the neutrophils to a hostile environment in the spleen is not convincing. Neutrophils, unlike erythrocytes, are capable of oxidative glycolysis and would be more capable of surviving the relative hypoxia and acidosis of the pulp because of the increased efficiency of oxidative phosphorylation in the generation of ATP. Splenic-derived immunoglobulins directly against the neutrophil cell surface would be a better theory for this disease. These patients usually have recurrent infections, and one could hypothesize that the infection was the cause of the neutropenia by eliciting a response within the spleen. On the other hand, with as many as 40% of patients having neutrophil counts of less than 1000 cells/mm^3, one could argue that the infections are simply the result of the neutropenia.

Steroids have been advocated at least transiently in the management of patients with this disease, but the majority of patients require splenectomy. Splenectomy is curative in 95% of patients who undergo the operation.

Malignant Diseases of the Spleen

Lymphoma and Lymphocytic Leukemia

The spleen as a lymphoid organ is often involved in chronic lymphocytic leukemia and in lymphoma, and these patients sometimes suffer a pancytopenia secondary to infiltration of the spleen. The hypersplenism observed in some of these patients, along with the severe splenomegaly has sometimes been considered an indication for splenectomy. Removal of a grossly enlarged organ would decrease the risk of spontaneous rupture, but this procedure exposes the patient to the risk of postsplenectomy infectious complications, and this may especially be a problem in the patient who is receiving chemotherapy. Alternatively, splenectomy might actually be of benefit to the patient by allowing increased doses of chemotherapy, since the baseline leukocyte and platelet counts are increased after the operation.

Compromise would dictate that the decision to perform splenectomy be based on the results of chromium-labeled erythrocyte studies. The patients with splenic sequestration, especially in the absence of significant liver uptake, would be good candidates for splenectomy. When splenectomy is performed in these patients, there is generally a benefit achieved by splenectomy. Although some patients without documented splenic sequestration benefit from the operation in terms of improvement in anemia and platelet count, this indication for splenectomy seems weak. Splenectomy as part of a staging laparotomy remains a valid indication as discussed further in the following section.

Hodgkin's Disease

Hodgkins's disease is a unique lymphoid malignancy that is highly treatable with radiotherapy and/or chemotherapy with the therapy dictated by the stage of the disease. Disease is staged according to the Ann Arbor system developed at the University of Michigan, and chemotherapy is recommended for patients with stage III-B disease and stage IV disease. Stage III disease implies disease on both sides of the diaphragm, and stage IV disease implies extralymphoid metastases, especially spread to the bone marrow. A and B refer to a constellation of systemic complaints including fever and weight loss, with B being the expression of disease in which these complaints are present. Radiotherapy is reserved for less advanced disease.

The key to management of the patient with Hodgkin's disease is accurate staging; despite the advances of ultrasonography, liver-spleen scanning, and CT scans, accurate staging requires staging laparotomy and splenectomy. Clinical examination is of little value in deducing splenic involvement. Splenomegaly is generally uncommon. Splenic weights of involved spleens are greater than those of uninvolved spleens, but this distinction is of mean weight; there is considerable overlap. The principles of staging laparotomy were established decades ago, and the operation still includes, in addition to the splenectomy, biopsies of both lobes of the liver, complete abdominal exploration, and lymph node biopsies of nodes in mesenteric, splenic, caval, iliac, portal, and celiac areas. Iliac crest bone marrow biopsies are also performed. Since many patients survive the disease, many centers move the ovaries on their pedicle to a position behind the uterus, thereby decreasing the incidence of radiation injury.

Removing an involved or uninvolved spleen allows the radiation ports to be designed smaller. It also allows increased doses of chemotherapy because of the increase in baseline platelet and leukocyte count. Splenectomy does not affect the overall survival from the disease. The price of splenectomy here, as elsewhere, is an increased susceptibility to infection, and this risk is increased in patients who received both total nodal radiotherapy and combined chemotherapy. Children are at the highest risk for sepsis. Patients who receive less aggressive therapy (i.e., radiation alone or chemotherapy alone) have a decreased risk for sepsis. The organisms of which the patient is at risk are the usual ones seen in the asplenic state, namely *S. pneumoniae* and *Haemophilus influenzae.*

In addition to the immunologic effects of splenectomy, patients with Hodgkin's disease have a selective impairment of cell-mediated immunity. Several studies have suggested that this is related to a serum factor produced by the spleen or by a focus of Hodgkin's disease within the spleen. The splenectomized patient is relieved of this immunologic burden.

Consideration of the infection risks of splenectomy has prompted some groups to perform partial splenectomy as part of the staging laparotomy, rather than a complete splenectomy. Their review of the pathology suggests that the incomplete specimen is adequate for staging the disease. This management has not become the standard in the oncology literature, and partial splenectomy may be a less appropriate technique than total splenectomy and autotransplantation.

Myeloid Metaplasia

In patients with myeloid metaplasia, the normal hematopoietic centers in the bone marrow cease to function as the marrow is replaced by fibrous tissue. The liver, which was a hematopoietic organ in fetal life, and the spleen, which in humans probably was not, become the site of extramedullary hematopoiesis. In this disease, nearly all patients exhibit hepatosplenomegaly on physical examination. These patients are usually anemic consequent to inadequate hematopoiesis, and mild thrombocytopenia is seen in a third of the patients. Late in the disease the splenomegaly may be associated with secondary hypersplenism; the patient gets more harm from the spleen than benefit from it as a site of hematopoiesis, in which case splenectomy may prove beneficial. The decision to remove the spleen should be based on chromium-tagged red blood cell sequestration studies. When the spleen is the site of red blood cell destruction, splenectomy usually decreases the frequency of transfusions to maintain the hematocrit. The increase in platelet count may be sufficient to decrease the incidence and severity of associated bleeding complications.

Infiltrative and Rheumatoid Diseases

Felty's Syndrome

Felty's syndrome is a rheumatoid disease characterized by leukopenia, splenomegaly, and chronic rheumatoid arthritis. Associated findings include anemia, hepatomegaly, chronic weight loss, and increased susceptibility to infection. Although the neutropenia would suggest an antibody directed against some leukocyte surface antigen, the removed spleen is characterized most often by simple passive congestion. The average neutrophil count in these patients is below 2000 cells/mm^3. The weight of the resected spleen ranges from 500 to 1400 g, not surprising considering the incidence of splenomegaly. Splenectomy has been effective in 70% to 80% of these patients,[51] and relapses after splenectomy are rare. Attempts to avoid splenectomy have included steroids, but the benefits of corticosteroids are both inconsistent and short-lived.

Sarcoidosis

Anemia and thrombocytopenia have been reported in patients with sarcoidosis. Splenomegaly is present in about a quarter of patients with this disease, but only about 20% of the patients with splenomegaly demonstrate hypersplenism. Hypersplenism, moreover, can occur in the absence of clinically apparent splenomegaly, presumably consequent to infiltration by noncaseating granulomata. Finally, hypersplenism can occur even in the absence of obvious sarcoid infiltration. The anemia and thrombocytopenia here are presumably consequent to entrapment and sequestration, but splenic phagocytosis has also been considered part of the pathophysiology. An immune etiologic factor for the hemolysis has been proposed but is not supported by the fact that most patients are direct Coombs' negative.

Most of the patients who have anemia and thrombocytopenia have already manifested other signs of sarcoidosis. The hemoglobin in these patients is commonly below 8 g/dl and the platelet count below 100,000 cells/mm^3. Compensatory reticulocytosis is usually seen, and results from bone marrow aspirates reveal generalized hyperplasia. ^{51}Cr-tagged erythrocyte scanning has been useful in selecting the patients for splenectomy.[52] Corticosteroids have not been demonstrated to be effective in this condition.

Gaucher's Disease

Gaucher's disease is an autosomal recessive disease that results in a deficiency in lysosomal glucocerebrosidase and a consequent accumulation of glycolipid cerebrosides throughout the body. Three types have been described, each with a different degree of enzyme deficiency. More than 99% of patients suffer from type I disease, the form seen in adults; type II is the most serious and occurs in infancy. The incidence in the general population is less than 1 in 40,000, but the incidence in Ashkenazi Jews is estimated at 1 in 450 to 1 in 640. Both the onset of disease and the rate of progression are variable, with some patients manifesting the disease at birth and others only in old age. Moreover, because of variable severity of the symptoms, some patients are never diagnosed as having the disease. Pathophysiologically, the disease begins with the accumulation of glucocerebroside within the lysosomes of reticuloendothelial cells. The characteristic lipid-laden Gaucher cells are particularly abundant within the red pulp of the spleen, sinusoids of the liver, lymph nodes, bone marrow, and alveolar capillaries. Splenomegaly is usually the earliest sign of Gaucher's disease because the spleen is the predominant reservoir of excess glucocerebroside. The splenomegaly is usually painless, and the splenic enlargement demonstrates the progression of the disease. The splenic weight averages about 2700 g, and splenic infarction can occur. There is an association between splenic size and disease duration and the risk of splenic infarction.[53]

Although liver function test results are frequently abnormal and fibrotic changes in the liver are common, cirrhosis is seen only in severe cases, and frank hepatic failure is rare. Bone manifestations of Gaucher's disease range from skeletal changes characterized by a failure of remodeling of the distal femur, proximal tibia, and other bones to growth retardation and spontaneous fractures. Acute, recurrent episodes of aseptic osteomyelitis can occur. Neurologic manifestations are limited to patients with type II and III disease. Malignancy has been seen in some series of patients, and splenectomy has been implicated in the pathogenesis of this condition. A review of multiple series, however, demonstrated a 7.3% incidence of cancer in patients requiring splenectomy and a 9.4% incidence in those who did not undergo splenectomy.[53] Although Gaucher cells are found in the bone marrow, most of the hematologic manifestations of the disease are consequent to hypersplenism. Over time, blood transit time is reduced, and this accelerates the removal of platelets, erythrocytes, and neutrophils. The thrombocytopenia is frequently severe enough to cause significant hemorrhage, but usually averages less than 100,000 cells/mm^3. A mild, normochromic, normocytic anemia with hematocrits below 30% is observed in 80% of patients with Gaucher's disease. In one series the white blood cell count averaged 4150 cells/mm^3.[53]

Patients with severe hypersplenism and thrombocytopenia benefit from splenectomy. Splenectomy, however, increases the risk for overwhelming sepsis and the rate of progression of both hepatic and osseous disease; partial splenectomy has therefore been advocated in Gaucher's disease. The decision to perform partial splenectomy in a quarter of the patients in one large series[53] was associated with both a reduction in subsequent bone disease and decreased effectiveness in recovery of platelet and white blood cell counts. Relapses of hematologic disease after splenectomy are rare and are attributable to bone marrow failure, sequestration by the other elements of the reticuloendothelial system, accessory spleens, and (in the patients managed by partial splenectomy) hypersplenism in the splenic remnant.

Corticosteroids are not indicated in Gaucher's disease because the hematologic manifestations are not consequent to an immunologic disorder. Medical therapy with alglucerase, a mannose-terminated form of human placental glucocerebrosidase, may, however, eliminate the manifestations of this disease altogether. Hepatosplenomegaly is reduced in most patients within months of administration of this drug.[54] In one series, liver and spleen volumes decreased in 6 months from 7% to 64% and 8% to 84% by 12 months, respectively.[55] Hemoglobin increases have been seen in all patients within 4 months of treatment, although the response was more rapid in patients who had undergone previous splenectomy. The picture with thrombocytopenia was similar. The response of the platelet count is slower than that of the erythrocyte count, and this response too is more rapid in the splenectomized patient. Long-term effects of alglucerase therapy are unknown; patients develop antienzyme antibodies, which so far have not affected the response to the drug. These data suggest a decreasing role for splenectomy in the future with the surgical option being a consideration only in cases of splenic infarction.

Other Diseases of the Spleen

Splenic Artery Aneurysm

Splenic artery aneurysms are rare and occur most frequently in women, usually as a manifestation of medial dysplasia of the arterial wall. In men, atherosclerosis is the most common cause for these aneurysms, which can also be associated with pancreatitis, trauma, or arteritis secondary to septic emboli. When asymptomatic, the aneurysms can be found on plain abdominal radiographs as egg-shell calcifications in the left upper quadrant. The symptoms are usually vague when they occur, and the signs and symptoms of rupture are those of an acute hemoperitoneum. Resection is advised in both symptomatic and asymptomatic patients, especially women of childbearing age who are at increased risk for rupture during pregnancy.

Splenic Cysts

Splenic cysts may be parasitic or nonparasitic, with the former being almost exclusively caused by echinococcal disease. In areas of the world where hydatid disease is endemic, such as South America, Australia, and Greece, two thirds of splenic cysts are echinococcal. In the United States, where parasitic disease is rare, nonparasitic cysts are encountered with greater frequency. These cysts can be "true" cysts, in that they are lined with epithelium, or pseudocysts. These latter are more common and are thought to represent liquefaction of old hematomas or areas of inflammation and infarction. True cysts of the spleen are rare and include epidermoid and dermoid cysts, cystic hemangiomas, and cystic lymphangiomas.

The symptoms of splenic cysts are vague and usually include left upper quadrant fullness. Symptoms can also be secondary to diaphragmatic irritation and compression of adjacent viscera when they are large. Nonparasitic cysts may be candidates for aspiration. Large cysts and those of uncertain origin should be approached operatively. Splenectomy remains a valid operation, but partial splenectomy may be possible and may avoid the infectious complications of splenectomy. Marsupialization and external drainage have fallen into disrepute because of infection, bleeding, and recurrence of the cyst.

Splenic Vein Thrombosis

Splenic vein thrombosis is an uncommon cause of acute upper gastrointestinal variceal hemorrhage, which secondarily leads to the development of collateral venous channels via the short gastric veins when the spleen's primary venous outflow is blocked. More than half the cases of splenic vein thrombosis are consequent to acute pancreatitis. Other associated conditions include pancreatic carcinoma, pseudocyst, retroperitoneal fibrosis, and myeloproliferative disorders. The diagnosis can be confirmed by celiac angiography, and the therapy is splenectomy. Alternative therapies include splenic artery embolization. In the asymptomatic patient, elective splenectomy or splenic artery embolization should be considered, since the risk of severe hemorrhage is always present.

Portal Hypertension and Secondary Hypersplenism

Hypersplenism may result from portal hypertension, regardless of its cause. Although portal hypertension is most often seen consequent to Laënnec's cirrhosis, postnecrotic cirrhosis, primary biliary cirrhosis, schistosomiasis, and hepatic vein thrombosis (Budd-Chiari syndrome) can cause this syndrome. Acute splenic vein thrombosis or portal vein thrombosis can produce massive splenomegaly and hypersplenism. The pathophysiology in this condition is straightforward and simple: there is a rise in splenic venous pressure and a consequent increase in splenic volume. Within the spleen, the trabeculae become thickened and sclerosed, and a greater percentage of central arterioles end within the reticular substance of the splenic cord. Normal blood flow becomes more circuitous, and the cellular elements of the blood spend an increased time within the spleen.

Although 80% of patients with portal hypertension may have splenomegaly and hypersplenism is common, the major manifestations of portal hypertension occur outside the spleen. Moreover, the major hematologic complication of portal hypertension is exsanguinating hemorrhage from esophageal varices and not anemia or thrombocytopenia caused by hypersplenism. The therapy for the patient with this disease is usually directed at the underlying portal hypertension; the various shunt procedures that decrease portal pressures usually result in a resolution of both the splenomegaly and the hypersplenism. Persistence of these conditions suggests that the spleen has been damaged by chronic pressure elevation with consequent fibrosis of the splenic capsule and trabeculae. These patients should be considered candidates for splenectomy if chromium-tagged red cell sequestration studies document splenic sequestration. Splenectomy should not be considered in patients with hypersplenism associated with portal hypertension as a substitute for a shunting procedure.

Infectious Diseases of the Spleen

Splenic Abscess

Splenic abscesses are relatively rare complications in the modern era of antibiotics. They are usually consequent to distant bacteremias or secondary infections in a spleen damaged by infarction (from sickle cell disease or iatrogenic splenic artery embolization or splenic artery ligation or interruption), trauma, or parasitic infection. The enteric organisms, *Escherichia coli* and *Klebsiella,* are frequent offenders. When splenic abscess is consequent to endocarditis, staphylococcal and streptococcal species are causative organisms. Finally, in the immunosuppressed patient, opportunistic organisms such as *Nocardia* and *Candida* are reported.

The patient commonly presents with fever, and left upper quadrant tenderness is frequently noted. Although physical examination may suggest the diagnosis, CT scans have become the definitive diagnostic technique. Liver-spleen scans are useful but probably unnecessary. Management is surgical with coverage with the appropriate parenteral antibiotics. The abscess, which frequently extends beyond the splenic capsule, is drained and the spleen removed. Splenic salvage, although possible in some cases, has not been performed usually because of the fear of spreading the infection consequent to abscess disruption during manipulation out of the left upper quadrant. The mortality of splenic abscess is high and is usually consequent to the underlying disease that led to the abscess. Percutaneous drainage has been advocated by some aggressive interventional radiologists, but this modality should be considered (if at all) only in patients with a single abscess and in those in whom there are major contraindications to splenectomy.

Infectious Mononucleosis

Infectious mononucleosis typically affects young adults and is characterized by fever, sore throat, lymphadenopathy, and hepatosplenomegaly. The peripheral smear usually demonstrates atypical lymphocytes, which are believed to be T lymphocytes reacting to B lymphocytes infected with the Epstein-Barr virus. The diagnosis is confirmed by finding serum heterophil antibodies on a "mono" spot test. In this disease the spleen is palpable in more than 50% of patients, and spontaneous rupture of an enlarged spleen may occur. A palpable spleen is not an indication for elective splenectomy or any therapy directed against the spleen because in the overwhelming majority of these patients the disease spontaneously resolves without splenic rupture.

HYPOSPLENISM

The most common cause of hyposplenism is, of course, splenectomy. Acquired atrophy of the spleen can be caused by a number of diseases, but sickle cell disease is the most common. In this disease the splenic microvasculature becomes clogged with sickled cells, and in advanced stages the spleen becomes fibrotic and autoinfarcted. Functional hyposplenia, though, precedes the atrophy and can be seen in the splenomegalic phases of this disease in infants.[56] Splenic atrophy may also occur consequent to infarction from stagnation of platelets in essential thrombocytosis. Functional asplenia can occur with infiltration of the spleen in patients with leukemia and lymphoma. Partial or complete atrophy of the spleen without infarction is an uncommon complication of some malabsorption syndromes including tropical sprue and ulcerative colitis.

Therapeutic irradiation may result in splenic atrophy as well, a modality considered for some patients with ITP. Congenital asplenia is rare and is usually associated with cardiovascular abnormalities and occasionally pulmonary malformations and situs inversus viscerum.[57] Congenital hypoplasia is somewhat less rare.

The peripheral smear provides a ready diagnostic test for hyposplenism. Erythrocyte inclusion bodies, which are usually cleared by the spleen, are found in the peripheral blood in its absence, whether that absence is anatomic or functional. The most characteristic finding is of Howell-Jolly bodies, which represent cytoplasmic fragments of nuclear material; this finding persists for the life of the individual.[58] Heinz bodies, which represent denatured hemoglobin, can be found in the blood after splenectomy but usually as a consequence of exposure to oxidative drugs. They persist for several weeks after the drug exposure but disappear even in the absence of the spleen.[59] Pappenheimer bodies, which are iron granules, can be seen as well.

Erythrocytes with "pits" or "pocks" that represent inclusions or excess cell membranes can be found with phase contrast microscopy after splenectomy. Although some of these cells are seen in eusplenic individuals, their numbers increase with asplenia.[60] Normally, the cell membrane of reticulocytes is modified by the cell's transit through the spleen. Target cells are found after splenectomy.[61] These cells are thinner-than-normal erythrocytes and have a greater area-to-volume ratio. Since their hemoglobin cannot fill the entire cell, it appears to be deposited along the periphery as a central rim surrounded by a lucent halo. These cells have decreased osmotic fragility. They increase in number during the weeks following splenectomy, suggesting that they are produced after splenectomy and not formed from preexisting erythrocytes. Acanthocytes, characterized by multiple irregular surface projections, can also be seen in the peripheral smear. Nucleated red blood cells are rarely seen after splenectomy, suggesting that other components of the reticuloendothelial system are capable of assuming this role after the spleen has been removed. The life span of erythrocytes that are cleared by the spleen is not changed after splenectomy, again suggesting that the reticuloendothelial system has subsumed this role.

Leukocytosis can be seen after splenectomy, but it is usually short lived, and the white blood cell count returns to normal in the weeks after splenectomy in 75% of patients. About 60% of patients develop a relative or absolute lymphocytosis, though, and 30% a relative or absolute monocytosis.[62] Thrombocytosis is a common finding after splenectomy, increasing almost immediately. The platelet count usually normalizes within 1 month.[63] Dangerously high levels of platelets can occur in patients who undergo splenectomy for myeloproliferative disorders such as polycythemia vera and essential thrombocythemia.[64] Anticoagulant therapy may be necessary in such patients to prevent thromboses.

SPLENIC TRAUMA

The spleen is one of the most commonly injured abdominal organs in both blunt and penetrating trauma and is frequently injured during operations in the upper abdomen, the victim of injudicious placement of retractors or excessive traction on the stomach with avulsion of the vasa brevia. As recently as the early 1970s, the management of even trivial injuries was simple (i.e., the spleen was removed). Repair was felt to carry a prohibitive risk of rebleeding and the organ was not necessary to normal life anyway. This approach was considered appropriate despite the publication by King and Schumacker[65] in 1952 in which overwhelming postsplenectomy sepsis was described. The ensuing years have demonstrated that the infectious risks for splenectomy are real and can be life threatening.[66] Although these risks are more likely in the patients with underlying hematologic diseases or neoplasms where a staging laparotomy with splenectomy was performed, there is still a risk for infection posed by splenectomy in even normal individuals. Avoiding splenectomy in noniatrogenic trauma has evolved along a number of lines: (1) avoiding operation entirely, (2) using the techniques of interventional radiology, and (3) trying to preserve at least a portion of spleen by various techniques of splenic repair and splenorrhaphy.

Pediatric trauma victims are uncommonly managed by diagnostic peritoneal lavage because of the fear that a positive tap will lead to laparotomy. This management technique is justified by the small amount of free peritoneal blood necessary to produce a "positive" tap (a red blood cell count of greater than 100,000 cells/mm^3) and the ability of even a trivial liver or spleen injury to produce that amount of blood. Many of these patients have "indicated" but not "therapeutic" laparotomies on the basis of the peritoneal lavage. More importantly, many patients with splenic injuries are subjected to splenectomy. The ability of the child's spleen to bleed and then heal supports avoiding laparotomy. In the absence of other injuries, close observation and transfusion may avoid the need for operation.

The problem with this management technique is, of course, the need to be sure that injuries to colon or small bowel are not present, since these will not heal spontaneously. The liver-spleen scans have been replaced by CT scanning, but even these are not definitive diagnostic tools with regard to other injuries. Fever, increasing abdominal pain, and signs of peritonitis are indications that suggest a reconsideration of the initial management plan. The CT scan is important in establishing the degree of splenic injury and in evaluating the amount of free intraperitoneal blood. Many studies now support the nonoperative management of these patients even in the presence of free blood within the peritoneal cavity.

These patients are commonly hospitalized in the intensive care unit to allow frequent and competent observation. Blood transfusions are administered, in some cases, up to a full replacement of intravascular volume. Patients are kept at strict bed rest for 48 to 72 hours and then followed in the hospital for at least a week and sometimes longer. After discharge they are advised to avoid strenuous physical activity, including contact sports.

Although it is clear that this technique can avoid splenectomy, the burden of blood transfusion is again becoming a questionable therapeutic technique. These patients may require more transfusions avoiding operation than they would require if they had undergone exploratory laparotomy and splenic salvage. The known risk of blood-borne pathogens, including HIV, may have decreased with the increasing sophistication of blood banking, which now detects a good portion of non-A, non-B hepatitis in blood bank blood, but we are ignorant of the next pathogen to be discovered. Moreover, there is increasing evidence that blood is an immunosuppressive agent, and these patients may be exposed to a significant risk of infection during their hospital stay. These infectious risks are, of course, less than the risks of splenectomy in this pediatric population.

The success of this management plan in children has been extended to adults in a few centers. Again these patients are carefully monitored after they have undergone CT scans that demonstrate only splenic or splenic and hepatic injuries. The tolerance of adult trauma surgeons to blood loss and transfusion is somewhat less than that of the pediatric surgeons. Nevertheless, some patients can avoid operation even with significant splenic injuries.

In some centers with aggressive interventional radiologists, splenic artery embolization has been used to avoid operation, but this technique is not without complications. Moreover, this represents a degree of sophistication beyond that of most trauma centers, let alone most hospitals.

The usual management of the patient with a splenic injury is laparotomy. For severe injuries of the spleen, those where bleeding is severe and the injury extends into the hilum, splenectomy remains the operation of choice. In the elderly or unstable patient the choice of the surgeon is the most expeditious technique to control blood loss, and that remains splenectomy. For most trauma surgeons the number of associated injuries or the presence of an associated colon injury is not a factor in choosing to preserve the spleen.

The anatomy of the spleen and of its blood supply makes salvage actually rather simple. Compression of the splenic artery between the index and forefinger as the vessel courses in the tail of the pancreas or at the hilum effectively reduces blood loss sufficiently to assess the situation. Mobilization of the spleen out of the posterior left upper quadrant by division of its attachments to the diaphragm, colon, and kidney not only allows a complete assessment of the organ but makes compression of the splenic artery easier. These "ligaments" are generally not vascular. The 1 to 2 mm thick fibrous capsule can readily hold stitches. The capsule is thicker and more reliable in the young patient, but most surgeons can place these sutures successfully in even the elderly patient. Finally, the division of the splenic artery into segmental arteries makes segmental splenectomy possible.

Lacerations of the spleen that do not progress to the hilum can be repaired with suture. Injuries of the tip can be amputated with oversewing of the raw edge with suture and sometimes a pedicle of omentum. Abraded surfaces are amenable to topical hemostatic agents such as microcrystalline collagen, Surgicel, or topical thrombin–soaked sponges. Small areas of persistent bleeding may afterward be amenable to suture splenorrhaphy. At our trauma center, about half the techniques involve the use of a biodegradable polyglycolic acid (PGA) mesh, which is applied around the spleen and effectively tamponades the injury. The majority of spleens with penetrating injuries are thus saved at our institution, as are more than a third of the injuries consequent to blunt trauma. Most of the spleens where splenorrhaphy is attempted are, in fact, salvaged. Few patients require splenectomy for a failed splenorrhaphy during the initial laparotomy, and recurrent bleeding is rare in our institution, as it is in the literature.

Our experimental studies have suggested that PGA mesh does not function as a cofactor in infection when the animal is challenged with stool or stool mixed with blood. These patients are at risk for developing fluid collections around the mesh, which, when they require aspiration, usually fail to grow bacteria. The chemical changes associated with the hydrolysis of the PGA mesh, however, have been associated with an increase in the incidence of left pleural effusion and left-sided atelectasis when compared to the alternative techniques of splenic salvage. The amount of spleen that must be preserved to assure immunologic capacity is not known.

When the splenic injury is too severe to allow for repair or the patient too unstable to allow it, splenectomy becomes the indicated procedure. Care is taken, of course, to avoid injury to the contiguous structures, especially the colon. The vasa brevia are securely ligated, and the pancreatic tail is left uninjured. When the pancreatic tail is injured or when there is a suspicion of injury, pancreatic drainage by a closed suction catheter is recommended. The use of octreotide (Sandostatin) to decrease pancreatic secretion in cases of suspected injury is supported by the data that demonstrated a decreased rate of pancreatic leak in elective pancreatic resections.

The complications of splenectomy include the discovery on peripheral smear of target cells and cells with Howell-Jolly bodies and other inclusions. These are not associated with clinical sequelae. Despite the absence of a spleen to remove senescent erythrocytes, red blood cells continue to maintain normal life expectancies. Thrombocytosis occurs after splenectomy, but the platelet counts usually decrease (although they remain higher than those of healthy age-matched patients) and do not pose a threat of thrombosis. Platelet counts over a million are generally considered indications for antiplatelet agents, but counts that high are rare in victims of trauma, being more compatible with patients whose splenectomy was indicated for their myeloproliferative disorders.

POSTSPLENECTOMY SEPSIS AND ITS PREVENTION

The major long-term complication of splenectomy is overwhelming infection, a picture similar to that of patients who become asplenic because of diseases such as sickle cell anemia. The earliest suggestion of this problem was published in 1919 in a paper[67] that cautioned against the indiscriminate removal of the spleen because of an increased susceptibility to infection. The seminal paper by King and Shumacker[65] in 1952 described five cases of infection in children younger than 1 year of age who had undergone splenectomy for HS and focused attention on the problem. Singer's review[66] in 1973 described 2795 patients and focused on the diseases associated with the splenectomy performed. This study demonstrated that the highest risk was for patients undergoing splenectomy for hematologic diseases such as thalassemia, acquired hemolytic anemias, and HS but that patients undergoing splenectomy for trauma or even incidental splenectomy were at an increased incidence both for sepsis and for death caused by sepsis. Subsequent studies have concluded that the risk is highest for thalassemia and such reticuloendothelial system diseases as Hodgkin's disease, histiocytosis X, and the Wiskott-Aldrich syndrome.[18,68] The overall incidence of sepsis was 4.2%, and the overall mortality was 2.5%. The risk of infection was highest in children younger than 4 years. The risk for overwhelming sepsis is greatest in the 2 years following splenectomy,[18] but fatalities have occurred decades after splenectomy,[69,70] well into adult life. Although a series of 740 adults undergoing splenectomy during World War II had an increased mortality, which included death caused by pneumonia and ischemic heart disease, it is unclear whether this really represents death caused by infection rather than as a consequence of congestive heart failure. These studies have been retrospective. The only large prospective paper demonstrated a 2% risk of infection in children undergoing splenectomy.[71]

The clinical picture of fulminant sepsis has led to the term *overwhelming postsplenectomy sepsis.* The classic picture is of a previously healthy individual who develops a mild upper respiratory infection that rapidly progresses to nausea, vomiting, headache, confusion, shock, coma, and death. Laboratory tests reveal hypoglycemia commonly, and there is evidence of disseminated intravascular coagulopathy. Blood cultures sometimes demonstrate as many as 10^6 organisms/mm^3. Bacteria can be seen on peripheral smears in some cases. Multiorgan hemorrhage and the Waterhouse-Friderichsen syndrome are sometimes seen at autopsy. *S. pneumoniae* is reported in more than half the cases.[68] The other bacteria commonly noted include *Neisseria meningitidis, E. coli,* and *H. influenzae.* Staphylococcal and other streptococcal varieties have been associated with the syndrome as well. Patients with pneumococcal sepsis frequently have no obvious site of primary infection. Less common infections in splenectomized patients leading to overwhelming sepsis and death include malaria and babesiosis,[1] a malaria-like organism whose disease is usually self-limited in healthy people. There is no evidence for an increased risk for viral infections in splenectomized individuals. Overall mortality still averages 50%, and mortalities as high as 80% have been described in pneumococcal infections. The lack of good follow-up on trauma patients, many of whom have decreased life expectancies because of associated disease (e.g., HIV infection) and life-styles (urban trauma), makes it difficult to establish incidence figures for splenectomies performed for this condition.

The cause of postsplenectomy sepsis can be inferred from the immunologic consequences of splenectomy, namely decreased serum tuftsin and properidin levels, decreased serum IgM, impairment of the alternate pathway of complement activation, and reduced response to particulate antigens. In addition to recognizing the syndrome at the patient's initial examination, the options for prevention of overwhelming sepsis include avoiding splenectomy, preserving splenic tissue when able, autotransplantation of splenic tissue to avoid asplenia, prophylactic antibiotics, and polyvalent pneumococcal vaccine and vaccines directed against *H. influenzae.*

The focus is on *S. pneumoniae* because this is the bacterium most often associated with fatal sepsis. The splenectomized patient seems to be at risk not for an immunologic "forgetting" of the previous experience with the specific antigen but at risk for a new exposure to antigens not previously seen. Support for this idea comes from the finding that many of the subtypes found in fatal cases are unusual ones.[72] Polyvalent pneumococcal vaccines containing the largest number of antigens would probably be the best choice for the splenectomized individual. Controversy exists, however, over whether this management is truly successful in controlling sepsis in adults. The risk of sepsis is less in adults and the longevity of the antigenic stimulation is limited. The manufacturer of Pneumovax recommends against repeated administration of the vaccine to asplenic individuals. Finally, the question of timing of administration has not been completely elucidated. The best time to expose the patient to these new antigens is before splenectomy. When this is impossible—as in emergency splenectomy—some surgeons advocate withholding the vaccine until the acute stress response has lessened.

Antibiotic prophylaxis against streptococcal species has its appeal and has been shown to decrease infections in patients who underwent splenectomy as part of their staging for Hodgkin's disease.[68] But what are the indications for this prophylactic administration? Surely, the patient with an acute febrile upper respiratory tract illness would be a candidate for penicillin. Whether penicillin should be administered for surgical procedures such as dental extractions as it is in patients at risk for endocarditis is less easily defended.

Avoiding splenectomy has been discussed under the

specific diseases for which splenectomy is considered, and the surgeon and the referring physician should be cognizant of the potential immunologic consequences of splenectomy. In general, of course, the benefits of splenectomy outweigh this risk. Some surgeons, however, have suggested limiting the amount of splenic tissue removed, as in staging laparotomy, suggesting hemisplenectomy.

For patients who must undergo splenectomy for trauma, consideration should be given to autotransplantation of the splenic tissue. Extrapolating from animal studies wherein splenic autotransplantation reversed some of the immunologic sequelae of splenectomy, many investigators have used this technique in their patients. In general, thin slices or homogenates of the spleen are implanted into omental pouches. In one series, the splenic sections were placed in a preperitoneal, subfascial pouch.[73] The autograft is usually marked with radiopaque clips. Complications of this technique have been rare and have included two cases of intestinal obstruction consequent to adhesions.[74,75] Focal abscess formation has also been reported.[50,76,77] This incidence of infection has prompted some investigators to avoid autotransplantation in the presence of bowel injuries, although others have not demonstrated an increased rate of infection in patients with hollow viscus injuries.

Animals studies, usually performed in rats and mice, have suggested the superiority of the omental site when compared to subcutaneous placement of the grafts, both in terms of the histologic appearance of the tissue and its reticuloendothelial function. In these models, splenic implants decreased the mortality in splenectomized animals challenged with pneumococci by aerosol inhalation or intratracheal injection. One study also demonstrated a marked decrease in mortality in animals challenged intranasally with *H. influenzae.* Increased clearance of pneumococci has been demonstrated, but only one group demonstrated a completely normal clearance after splenic transplantation.

In man the benefits of transplantation are more difficult to evaluate, and extrapolating from rodent studies is fraught with risks. The benefits observed are consequent to the assays used, since it is not possible to deliberately challenge these patients with virulent bacteria. Most authors report a gradual reduction in postsplenectomy thrombocytosis and a gradual increase in IgM levels back to normal. Peripheral blood smears demonstrate the gradual loss of the postsplenectomy features of Howell-Jolly bodies and target cells on the peripheral smear. Radionuclide scans have demonstrated functional splenic tissue, which takes up the radionuclide. Despite splenic transplantation, there are numerous case reports of fatal postsplenectomy infection. The available data, which are largely retrospective, demonstrate that transplantation is simple and carries minimal risk of its own, but that its benefit to the patient is unclear. The best conclusion is that prospective studies are warranted.

SUMMARY

The spleen continues to be an organ of mystery, participating as its does as a hematologic, a reticuloendothelial, and an immunologic structure. Management of the diseases affecting the spleen requires a thorough knowledge of the underlying physiology and especially the immunology; armed with this, the surgeon can be an active participant in the management of the patient and not merely a technician. Recognition must be made of the new advances in the nonsurgical management of these diseases and in our own developing surgical armamentarium.

REFERENCES

1. Wolf BC, Neiman RS. Disorders of the spleen. In Wolf BC, Neiman RS, eds. Major Problems in Pathology, vol 20. Philadelphia: WB Saunders, 1989.
2. Witte CL, Witte MH. Circulatory dynamics of the spleen. Lymphology 16:60, 1983.
3. Crosby WH. Normal functions of the spleen relative to red blood cells. A review. Blood 14:399, 1959.
4. Weiss L, Tavassoli M. Anatomic hazards to the passage of erythrocytes through the spleen. Semin Hematol 7:372, 1970.
5. Crowell JW, Ford RG, Lewis VM. Oxygen transport in hemorrhagic shock as a function of the hematocrit ratio. Am J Physiol 196:1033, 1959.
6. Sutton JS, Weiss L. Transformation of monocytes in tissue culture into macrophages, epithelioid cells, and multinucleated giant cells. An electron microscopic study. J Cell Biol 28:303, 1966.
7. Stewart WB, et al. Age as affecting the osmotic and mechanical fragility of dog erythrocytes tagged with radioactive iron. J Exp Med 91:147, 1950.
8. Lux SE, John KM. Isolation and partial characterization of a high molecular weight red cell membrane protein complex which is normally removed by the spleen. Blood 7:261, 1952.
9. Ebert RV, Stead EA. Demonstration that in normal man no reserves of blood are mobilized. Am J Med Sci 201:655, 1941.
10. Amorosi EL. Hypersplenism. Semin Hematol 2:249, 1965.
11. Jandl JH, Aster RH. Increased splenic pooling and the pathogenesis of hypersplenism. Am J Med Sci 253:383, 1967.
12. Wolf BC, Luevano E, Neiman RS. Evidence to suggest that the human fetal spleen is not a hematopoietic organ. Am J Clin Pathol 80:140, 1983.
13. Dameshek W. Hypersplenism. Bull NY Acad Med 31:113, 1955.
14. Grogan TM, Jolly CS, Rangel CS. Immunoarchitecture of the human spleen. Lymphology 16:72, 1983.
15. Grogan TM, et al. Further delineation of the immunoarchitecture of the human spleen. Lymphology 17:61, 1984.
16. Hsu SM, Cossman J, Jaffe ES. Lymphocyte subsets in normal human lymphoid tissue. Am J Clin Pathol 80:21, 1983.
17. Weisman IL, et al. The lymphoid system, its normal architecture and the potential for understanding the system through the study of lymphoproliferative diseases. Hum Pathol 9:25, 1978.
18. Eicher ER. Splenic function: Normal, too much and too little. Am J Med 66:311, 1979.
19. MacLennan ICM, et al. The lymphocytes of splenic marginal zones. A distinct B-cell lineage. Immunol Today 3:305, 1982.
20. Kitchens CS. The syndrome of post-splenectomy fulminant sepsis. Case report and review of the literature. Am J Med Sci 274:303, 1977.
21. Sullivan JL, et al. Immune response after splenectomy. Lancet 1:178, 1978.
22. Knecht JC, Schiffman G, Austrian R. Some biological properties of the pneumococcus type 37 and the chemistry to its capsular polysaccharide. J Exp Med 132:475, 1970.

23. Hosea S, et al. Impaired immune response of splenectomized patients to polyvalent pneumococcal vaccine. Lancet 1:804, 1981.
24. Hosea SW. The role of the spleen in pneumococcal infection. Lymphology 16:115, 1983.
25. Constantopoulos A, et al. Defective phagocytosis due to tuftsin deficiency in splenectomized subjects. Am J Dis Child 125:663, 1973.
26. Crosby WH. Hypersplenism. Annu Rev Med 13:217, 1962.
27. Mentzer WC, Wagner GM, eds. The Hereditary Hemolytic Anemias. New York: Churchill Livingstone, 1989.
28. Trucco JI, Brown AK. Neonatal manifestations of hereditary spherocytosis. Am J Dis Child 113:263, 1967.
29. Schilling RF. Hereditary spherocytosis: A study of splenectomized persons. Semin Haematol 13(Suppl 3):169, 1976.
30. Becker PS, Lux SE. Hereditary spherocytosis and related disorders. Clin Haematol 14:15, 1985.
31. Mohandas N, Chasis JA, Shohet SB. The influence of membrane skeleton on red cell deformability, membrane material properties, and shape. Semin Hematol 20:225, 1983.
32. Agre P, Orringer EP, Bennett V. Deficient red-cell spectrin in severe recessively inherited spherocytosis. Med Intell 306(Suppl 19):1155, 1982.
33. Cohen AR, Markenson AI, Schwartz E. Transfusion requirements and splenectomy in thalessemia major. J Pediatr 9:100, 1980.
34. Schwartz RS. Treating chronic idiopathic thrombocytopenia—A new application of an old treatment [editorial]. N Engl J Med 330:1609, 1991.
35. Schwartz SI, Hoepp LM, Sachs S. Splenectomy for thrombocytopenia. Surgery 88:497, 1980.
36. McMillan R. Chronic idiopathic thrombocytopenia purpura. N Engl J Med 304:1135, 1981.
37. Aas K, Gardner F. Survival of blood platelets labelled with chromium 51. J Clinical Invest 37:1257, 1958.
38. Najean V, et al. The site of platelet destruction in thrombocytopenic purpura as a predictive index of the efficacy of splenectomy. Br J Haematol 79:271, 1991.
39. Bussel J. Autoimmune thrombocytopenic purpura. Hematol Oncol Clin North Am 4:179, 1990.
40. Anderson JC. Response of resistant idiopathic thrombocytopenia purpura to pulsed high-dose dexamethasone therapy. N Engl J Med 339:1560, 1994.
41. Calverley DC, Jones GW, Kelton JG. Splenic radiation for corticosteroid-resistant immune thrombocytopenia. Ann Intern Med 116:977, 1992.
42. Chang C-S, Li C-Y, Cha SS. Chronic idiopathic thrombocytopenia purpura. Splenic pathologic features and their clinical correlation. Arch Pathol Lab Med 117:981, 1993.
43. Montefusco PP, Geiss AC. Accessory splenectomy in management of idiopathic thrombocytopenic purpura. Contemp Surg 32:73, 1988.
44. Coon WW. Splenectomy for idiopathic thrombocytopenic purpura. Surg Gynecol Obstet 164:225, 1987.
45. Moschcowitz E. Hyaline thrombosis of the terminal arterioles and capillaries: A hitherto undescribed disease. Proc NY Pathol Soc 24:21, 1924.
46. Saracco SM, Farhi DC. Splenic pathology in thrombocytopenic purpura. Am J Surg Pathol 14:223, 1990.
47. Wells AD, et al. Role of splenectomy as a salvage procedure in thrombocytopenic purpura. Br J Surg 78:1389, 1991.
48. Morris L, et al. Autoimmune thrombocytopenic purpura in homosexual men. Ann Intern Med 96:714, 1982.
49. Polk BF, et al. Predictors of the acquired immunodeficiency syndrome developing in a cohort of seropositive homosexual men. N Engl J Med 316:61, 1987.
50. Alonso M, et al. Splenectomy in human immunodeficiency virus–related thrombocytopenia. Br J Surg 80:330, 1993.
51. O'Neal J Jr, et al. The role of splenectomy in Felty's syndrome. Ann Surg 167:81, 1978.
52. Bertino J, Myerson RM. The role of splenectomy in sarcoidosis. Arch Intern Med 106:213, 1960.
53. Fleshner PR, et al. A 27-year experience with splenectomy for Gaucher's disease. Am J Surgery 161:69, 1991.
54. Whittington R, Goa KL. Alglucerase: A review of its therapeutic use in Gaucher's disease. Drugs 44:72, 1992.
55. Pastores GM, Sibille AR, Grabowski GA. Enzyme therapy in Gaucher disease type 1: Dosage efficacy and adverse effects in 33 patients treated for 6 to 24 months. Blood 82:408, 1993.
56. Pearson HA, Spencer RP, Cornelius EA. Functional asplenia in sickle-cell anemia. N Engl J Med 281:923, 1969.
57. Putschar WGJ, Manion WC. Congenital absence of the spleen and associated anomalies. Am J Clin Pathol 26:429, 1959.
58. Pepper OHP, Austin JH. A twenty-eight year follow-up on a splenectomy for hemolytic anemia. Persistence of Howell-Jolly bodies. J Am Med Assoc 122:870, 1943.
59. Selwyn JG. Heinz bodies in red cells after splenectomy and after phenacetin administration. Br J Haematol 1:173, 1955.
60. Corrigan JJ Jr, VanWyck DB, Crosby WH. Clinical disorders of splenic function: The spectrum from asplenism to hypersplenism. Lymphology 16:101, 1983.
61. Singer K, Miller EB, Dameshek W. Hematologic changes following splenectomy in man with particular reference to target cells. Am J Med Sci 202:171, 1941.
62. McBride JA, Dacie JV, Shapley R. The effect of splenectomy on the leukocyte count. Br J Haematol 14:225, 1968.
63. Hirsh J, Dacie JV. Persistent post-splenectomy thrombocytosis and thromboembolism. Br J Haematol 12:44, 1966.
64. Gordon DH, et al. Post-splenectomy thrombocytosis: Its association with mesenteric, portal, and/or renal vein thrombosis in patients with myeloproliferative disorders. Arch Surg 113:713, 1978.
65. King H, Schumacker HN. Splenic studies. I. Susceptibility to infection after splenectomy performed in infancy. Ann Surg 136:239, 1952.
66. Singer R. Postsplenectomy sepsis. Perspect Pediatr Pathol 1:285, 1973.
67. Morris DH, Bullock FD. The importance of the spleen in resistance to infection. Ann Surg 70:513, 1919.
68. Leonard AS, et al. The overwhelming postsplenectomy sepsis problem. World J Surg 4:423, 1980.
69. Evans D. Postsplenectomy sepsis 10 years or more after operation. J Clin Pathol 38:309, 1985.
70. Grinblat J, Bilboa Y. Overwhelming pneumococcal sepsis 25 years after splenectomy. Am J Med Sci 270:523, 1975.
71. Walker W. Splenectomy in childhood: A review of cases in England and Wales 1960–4. Br J Surg 63:36, 1976.
72. Gopal V, Bisno AL. Fulminant pneumococcal infections in "normal" asplenic hosts. Arch Intern Med 173:1526, 1977.
73. Traub A, et al. Splenic reticuloendothelial function after splenectomy, spleen repair, and spleen autotransplantation. N Engl J Med 298:1389, 1978.
74. Bem C, Echun D. Regeneration of the spleen and splenic autotransplantation [letter]. Br J Surg 78:1276, 1991.
75. Buyukunal C, Danismend N, Yeker D. Spleen-saving procedures in paediatric splenic trauma. Br J Surg 74:350, 1987.
76. Moore FA, et al. Risk of splenic salvage after trauma. Analysis of 200 adults. Am J Surg 148:800, 1984.
77. Nielsen JL, et al. Demonstration of splenic functions following splenectomy and autologous spleen implantation. Acta Chir Scand 150:469, 1984.

30

Gastrointestinal Hemorrhage

Joseph E. Miller and Kenneth R. Sirinek

Acute hemorrhage from the gastrointestinal (GI) tract has been recognized by clinicians for over 5000 years.[1] Initial descriptions of sanguineous discharges appear both in ancient Chinese manuscripts and Egyptian papyri. The Ebers papyrus, with its extensive description of symptoms, findings, and complications, recorded hemorrhage as a possible sequela of peptic ulceration. Hippocrates also recognized bleeding from peptic ulceration but unfortunately recommended phlebotomy as appropriate treatment. Further understanding of the clinical significance of GI tract hemorrhage came from the early writings of both Galen and Avicenna. Later significant, but not always correct, contributions included those of Littre, Morgagni, and Ewald. In fact, as late as 1891, Ewald included application of leeches to the abdomen as therapy.

The modern era of understanding and therapy for GI tract hemorrhage followed developments in several disparate medicine-related fields.[1] Discovery of the ABO blood group system by Landsteiner, coupled with techniques to preserve blood and infuse fluids parenterally, made blood transfusion, and thus, successful resuscitation from hemorrhage, a reality. Forty years after Röntgen's discovery of x-rays, Hampton's use of barium contrast studies of the GI tract to detect the source of GI tract bleeding revolutionized diagnosis. An even greater delay ensued between the inception of general anesthesia and the first reported series of patients undergoing successful operation to control GI tract bleeding sites. The most significant recent contribution was the refinement of the endoscope, since its clinical introduction over a century ago, into a useful, and clinically applicable, diagnostic and therapeutic instrument.

GI tract hemorrhage is a common clinical problem crossing national and socioeconomic boundaries. A report in 1981 indicated that 25,100 patients per year required hospitalization in England and Wales for GI tract hemorrhage.[1] In the United States such bleeding accounted for 1% to 2% of all medical and surgical hospital admissions during a similar time period.[2] In the 1960s and 1970s, annual rates of GI tract bleeding were reported at 48 to 144 episodes per 100,000 population, which translated into an estimated 150 hospitalized patients per 100,000 population in the United States.[3] At the lesser end of the scale is an admission rate of only 47 per 100,000 for a defined population from the Oxford region of England.[4] Despite this threefold difference in reported geographic incidences, there appears to be no difference in rate of GI tract hemorrhage when rural and urban areas are compared.[5] High-risk rates for GI tract bleeding have been correlated with specific aspects of peptic ulcer disease.[5] High-risk categories include patients with blood group O, widows and single persons, persons in stress-producing occupations, and the seasons of fall and spring. Advancing age seems to be a specific risk factor for all patients with GI tract bleeding, which is independent of the cause. Recent studies indicate that almost 50% of such patients are older than 60 years of age.[1]

Mortality rates have remained essentially stable at 5% to 12% during the past 50 years.[6] This continued high rate of mortality is due to the offsetting nature of an aging patient base vs. medical advances such as the introduction of blood transfusion, intensive care units, sophisticated monitoring equipment, and new therapeutic modalities. Risk factors for mortality and morbidity include older age, associated illness, coagulopathy, immunosuppression, magnitude of hemorrhage (measured by transfusion requirement), inaccurate diagnosis, bleeding during hospitalization, rebleeding, and endoscopic features (e.g., arterial spurting, a visible vessel, variceal bleeding).[7,8] Eighty percent of episodes of GI tract hemorrhage are self-limited. The remaining 20% of patients have a 30% to 40% mortality.[7]

It would appear that the negative medical aspects of an aging population have offset the beneficial effects of evolving medical technology related to the patient with GI tract hemorrhage. If further strides at reducing the morbidity and mortality associated with GI tract bleeding are to be made, every clinician must be familiar with the pathophysiologic response to hemorrhage, the various GI tract abnormalities likely to give rise to bleeding, the principles and strategies underlying diagnosis, and the therapeutic approaches based on cause. These components are important in the management of the patient with GI tract hemorrhage and form the basis of this chapter.

ETIOLOGY OF GASTROINTESTINAL TRACT HEMORRHAGE

Hemorrhage from the GI tract can stem from many sites and have many diverse causes. Generally, hemorrhage occurs from an abnormality with the GI tract, although a disease process in an adjacent organ with secondary involvement of the GI tract may be the inciting cause. Occasionally, a systemic disorder such as a coagulation problem may be the major underlying factor. Eight major disease categories leading to hematemesis, melena, and hematochezia (frank and/or occult) are shown in the accompanying box. No attempt has been made to make this list all inclusive; rather, representative causes have been listed for each major category. When all causes of GI tract bleeding are considered as a whole, 50% of the episodes of GI tract bleeding occur during hospitalization, and upper GI tract bleeding is much more commonly encountered than that arising from lesions distal to the ligament of Treitz.[8]

Upper Gastrointestinal Tract Bleeding

The national American Society of Gastroenterological Endoscopy survey on upper gastrointestinal bleeding involved 2225 patients and reported that 75% of upper GI tract bleeding was due to acid-peptic disease with equal numbers of patients with gastritis, gastric ulcer, and duodenal ulcer. Another 5% to 15% of upper GI tract hemorrhages occurred in patients with varices, esophagitis, duodenitis, and Mallory-Weiss tears.[9] The local incidence in a defined geographic setting varies from institution to institution, depending on the population of patients served by a given hospital. The majority of upper GI tract bleeding encountered in metropolitan hospitals serving patients with minimal or no health insurance is due to gastritis and gastroesophageal varices, whereas private community hospitals see a higher incidence of hemorrhage in patients with peptic ulcer disease.

Peptic Ulcer Disease

If one combines the incidence of bleeding from both duodenal and gastric ulcers, peptic ulcer disease is responsible for hemorrhage in almost 50% of patients. It has been estimated that 25% of hospitalized ulcer patients have GI tract bleeding if followed for a 10-year period.[9] The frequency of bleeding is directly related to the duration of the disease; however, there appears to be a slightly greater tendency for hemorrhage to occur during the first year of disease than in subsequent years of follow-up. GI tract bleeding from an ulcer usually presents as hematemesis or melena, but occasionally hematochezia may be the only sign of bleeding from the upper GI tract. Melena without hematemesis occurs most often in the presence of a competent pyloric sphincter and usually indicates that the ulcer is in the duodenum rather than the stomach. Gender does not appear to be a risk factor for hemorrhage. Seventy percent of patients with an ulcer and hemorrhage are men, reflecting the fact that men have a higher incidence of ulcer disease. Onset of ulcer disease late in life is associated with a higher incidence of bleeding, with the highest incidence of hemorrhage occurring during the fifth decade of life.[10] However, age per se does not appear to be the most important factor. There is an increased incidence of bleeding in patients with duodenal ulcer and blood group O.

Hemorrhage is also more common in patients with postbulbar ulcers, especially when they occur in the older age group. GI tract hemorrhage is the first sign of peptic ulcer disease in approximately 10% of patients. Melena or hematemesis occurs in about 50% of patients with a gastrinoma (Zollinger-Ellison syndrome). Hematemesis and melena may also occur from recurrent ulceration following any operation originally performed to manage peptic ulcer disease. Bleeding has been found to be the presenting symptom in 40% of patients with recurrent ulcers following a Billroth II gastrectomy.[9] Ulceration is always located on the afferent jejunal limb of the anastomosis because of the relative inability of small intestinal mucosa to withstand acid-peptic digestion. Barium contrast study is a poor diagnostic test for this entity, which can readily be visualized by upper GI tract endoscopy.

MAJOR SOURCES OF GASTROINTESTINAL TRACT HEMORRHAGE

Inflammatory
- Esophagitis
- Gastritis
- Stress ulcer
- Gastric ulcer
- Duodenal ulcer
- Stomal ulcer
- Regional enteritis
- Ulcerative colitis
- Diverticulitis

Neoplasms
- Adenocarcinoma
- Polyps
- Leiomyoma

Vascular
- Esophageal varices
- Hemangioma
- Angiodysplasia
- Aortointestinal fistula
- Hemorrhoids

Mechanical
- Hiatus hernia
- Mallory-Weiss syndrome
- Diverticulosis

Anomalies
- Duplications
- Meckel's diverticulum

Systemic Disease
- Uremia
- Collagen diseases

Blood Dyscrasias
- Hemophilia
- von Willebrand's disease

Other
- Epistaxis
- Hemoptysis
- Bleeding from oropharyngeal cavity
- Malingering

Acute Gastritis

Acute hemorrhagic gastritis, accounting for ~25% of patients with upper GI tract hemorrhage, is composed of a variety of acute erosive diseases of the stomach. Histologically, these lesions (usually multiple and diffuse) are erosions rather than ulcers, since they generally do not penetrate to the level of the muscularis mucosae as is typical of a true ulcer. They may, however, coexist with true peptic ulcers. These lesions may be secondary to various drugs or arise as a result of stress. Drug-induced gastritis generally occurs in patients taking nonsteroidal anti-inflammatory drugs (NSAIDs) such as aspirin, indomethacin, and naproxen. Individuals receiving long-term steroid management may also have such erosive lesions. Excessive alcohol consumption is likewise associated with erosive gastritis.

Bleeding from drug-induced erosive gastritis may be minimal or massive. In either case, it can generally be managed with aggressive nonoperative therapy by discontinuing the inciting drug and ensuring that the gastric acid production is adequately diminished (as with H_2 receptor blockers or omeprazole) or neutralized (as with antacids). A gastric mucosal barrier protector (sucralfate) or prostaglandin E_2 replacement (misoprostol) is also effective. Although these medications do not stop hemorrhage, they promote healing to lessen the chance of rebleeding. Only rarely is a surgical procedure necessary to control such bleeding.

Acute stress gastritis (also called stress ulceration) of the stomach and/or duodenum is a source of GI tract hemorrhage in the acutely ill patient under a variety of clinical circumstances. It must not be confused with acute hemorrhage from chronic peptic ulcer disease that may be exacerbated by the stress of an acute illness.[11] The causes and circumstances that result in stress ulcerations are diverse. Although some overlap exists, there appear to be a number of separate clinical situations in which stress ulcers develop, including the following:

1. The patient sustaining trauma secondary to an operation, accident, or violent act is at risk for stress ulcer formation in the immediate posttrauma period.
2. A critically ill patient with sepsis, jaundice, renal failure, or pulmonary failure—usually found in the intensive care unit—can start bleeding from the gastric mucosa at various stages of organ failure.
3. Patients suffering from major thermal injury develop a Curling's ulcer.
4. Patients with intracranial trauma or disease, both preoperatively and postoperatively develop lesions known as Cushing's ulcers.
5. There is absence of an underlying disorder in 25% of patients.

The onset of the multiple lesions that make up stress ulceration is insidious, and their development is usually painless. It is thought by some to be an imbalance between offensive and defensive mucosal factors. Considered offensive to the gastric mucosa are acid, pepsin, bile, and external irritants (e.g., ethanol, NSAIDs). Considered defensive are mucosal blood flow, mucus, bicarbonate, endogenous prostaglandins, and new epithelial cells. In the patient without a nasogastric tube, the bleeding remains undetected until the individual vomits blood or passes a melanic stool. Hemorrhage from acute stress gastritis may occur within the first 24 hours after injury, but the usual onset of bleeding develops at 5 to 10 days after the initial insult. In patients at risk for the development of stress gastritis, prophylactic therapy as noted above has dramatically lessened the incidence of bleeding from this entity.

Esophagogastric Varices

Bleeding from varices is a manifestation of portal hypertension and accounts for 14% of the patients with upper GI tract hemorrhage.[12] The bleeding point is usually a tear in the esophageal mucosa secondary to rupture of a varix within 2 cm proximal or distal to the esophagogastric junction. This lesion must be differentiated from a Mallory-Weiss tear in which no varix lies below the mucosal disruption. It must be remembered that patients with varices secondary to portal hypertension frequently may bleed from other upper GI tract sources. Merigan et al.[13] found that varices were responsible for the bleeding in only 53% of patients with cirrhosis. Outstanding features of variceal bleeding include the magnitude of blood loss that can occur and the high mortality rate associated with such lesions. The elevated venous pressure and massive distention of the varices are factors responsible for the large amount of acute blood loss.

Esophagitis and Mallory-Weiss Tears

Esophagitis and Mallory-Weiss tears are the cause of upper GI tract hemorrhage in 10% of patients.[12] Bleeding from esophagitis usually occurs in association with a hiatal hernia and gastroesophageal reflux. Typically, such bleeding is slow and usually presents as chronic blood loss. Patients with this problem can usually be managed without an operation. If the mucosa in the distal esophagus is particularly friable, suture control of the bleeding may become necessary at the same time that an antireflux procedure is performed.

The Mallory-Weiss syndrome represents a tear in the gastric mucosa near the esophagogastric junction. This tear, 3 to 20 mm long and 2 to 3 mm wide, extends in a longitudinal direction. It often follows an episode of forceful retching and/or vomiting. The mucosal disruption extends through the mucosa and submucosa, usually sparing the muscularis mucosae. It presents as hematemesis in 85% of cases with a 4:1 predominance in males. Usually there is a history of alcohol abuse. There is spontaneous cessation of bleeding in 90% of cases.[14,15] Occasionally, surgical intervention becomes necessary, in which case oversewing of the bleeding mucosal edges through a high gastrotomy is performed. Most of these lesions are confined to the stomach just below the esophagogastric junction. Occasionally, the lesion may straddle the esophagogastric junction, and only rarely does it involve the distal esophagus alone. More than two thirds of patients with this entity have an associated hiatal hernia.

Other Sources of Bleeding

The entities described above are responsible for approximately 85% of all episodes of acute blood loss from the upper GI tract. The remaining 15% arise from a variety of miscellaneous causes. These include various vascular abnormalities such as a Dieulafoy malformation (lesion) or vascular ectasias, blood dyscrasias, and tumors (e.g., leiomyomas or leiomyosarcomas) that grow in the gastric submucosa and erode into the plexus of veins and arteries supplying the stomach. Occasionally, a gastric carcinoma may erode into an underlying vessel. Usually bleeding from these neoplastic causes is mild. Other sources of upper GI tract hemorrhage include hemobilia, erosion of a pancreatic pseudocyst into the stomach, an aortoduodenal fistula, and invasion of a pancreatic cancer into the duodenum.

Lower Gastrointestinal Tract Bleeding

Bleeding from the small intestine and colon is much less frequent than that arising proximal to the ligament of Treitz. Nonetheless, it can be severe and may arise from any site from the ligament of Treitz to the anus.[16] The hemorrhage may be occult or massive with melena or hematochezia. Three to 5% of all GI tract hemorrhages arise from sites between the second portion of the duodenum and the ileocecal valve and are from a vascular ectasia in a majority of patients.[17,18] Causes of brisk bleeding include angiodysplasia, neoplasms, jejunal diverticula, Crohn's disease, an aortoenteric fistula, Meckel's diverticulum, duplication cyst, and hemangioma. Neoplasms may be benign tumors (e.g., leiomyomas), polyps (usually malignant), or frank cancers such as carcinoma, sarcoma, lymphoma, and occasionally a leukemic implant. Occult hemorrhage is most likely from angiodysplasia, adenocarcinoma, lymphoma, carcinoid tumor, Crohn's disease, gastrinoma, vasculitis, medications, and infectious causes. Bleeding is common in patients with inflammatory bowel disease involving the jejunum and ileum but is usually intermittent and frequently occult. Massive hemorrhage from such a source is distinctly uncommon.

Intussusception can be seen in all age groups but is particularly common in childhood and generally occurs before the age of 2 years. Its presentation as lower GI tract bleeding is manifest by the passage of dark clots and occasionally stool that has the consistency and appearance of "currant jelly."[16] A Meckel's diverticulum may also bleed and occasionally is an initial cause of small bowel bleeding in children and young adults. This bleeding occurs because there is ectopic gastric mucosa in the diverticulum, which causes peptic ulceration of nearby ileal mucosa.[19] When such a circumstance arises, an ulcerlike pain in the periumbilical region of the abdomen often precedes bleeding.

Bleeding from colonic sources comprises the vast majority of causes of lower GI tract hemorrhage.[20] Although massive hemorrhage is much less common than that observed from lesions proximal to the ligament of Treitz, substantial bleeding can occur from a number of lesions distal to the ileocecal valve. These include diverticular disease of the colon, vascular malformations, and ischemic colitis.[21] Both benign and malignant tumors may also cause bleeding, but this is much more likely to be occult and intermittent.

Literature from the 1980s commonly reported that vascular ectasias are an equal or more frequent source of lower GI tract bleeding than diverticulosis in people older than the age of 60.[22,23] Although diverticula may occur anywhere throughout the large intestine, diverticular bleeding is usually from the right colon even though the majority of colonic diverticula are found in the sigmoid colon. Fortunately, it stops spontaneously in most patients, even though recurrent episodes are frequent. It must be emphasized that the existence of documented diverticula does not necessarily ensure that bleeding is coming from this source. In fact, other sources of hemorrhage have been identified in as many as 50% of patients with diverticular disease. Vascular abnormalities of the colon were thought to be infrequent causes of lower GI tract bleeding a decade or two ago, but now they are recognized as being relatively common.[16,23] In fact, arteriovenous malformations of the right colon are the major cause of lower GI tract hemorrhage of obscure origin. Most patients with angiodysplastic disorders of the colon are older than 60 years of age, and many have associated cardiac disease. For unexplained reasons, an association with aortic stenosis commonly exists.

Another important cause of colonic bleeding that also generally occurs in older patients is ischemic colitis.[21] The left colon is most often involved. This entity represents a syndrome of hypoperfusion resulting from decreased intestinal blood flow. The mucosal ischemia leads to necrosis and then hemorrhage. Generally, the disease is self-limiting, and because the full thickness of the intestinal wall is not involved, surgical intervention is usually not indicated. An exception to this is ischemic colitis caused by ligation of the inferior mesenteric artery during repair of an abdominal aortic aneurysm. On barium enema a characteristic "thumbprinting" sign is noted that represents a combination of muscle spasm, submucosal edema, and minute mucosal ulcerations. Mucosal blebs are commonly seen in the affected colonic segment on colonoscopic examination.

Initially with ulcerative colitis there may be massive bleeding from the lower GI tract, but usually the hemorrhage is more modest. Patients with this disorder are critically ill and have a history of recurrent diarrhea and abdominal pain consistent with the diagnosis. When the friable colonic mucosa is seen on endoscopic evaluation, the explanation for bleeding in this disorder becomes apparent. Generally, the marked malnutrition and chronic anemia associated with the colitis requires colonic resection to effect adequate treatment.

Finally, bleeding from the lower GI tract may arise from various neoplastic lesions and disorders of the anus and rectum.[24] Usually such bleeding is modest and self-limiting. If blood is not mixed with stool or appears on the toilet paper, it usually indicates a source in the anorectal region such as a hemorrhoid, an anal fissure or ulcer, or proctitis. If blood is mixed with stool, the possibility of a colonic polyp or malignancy becomes more likely. In either case a careful rectal examination and colonoscopy should be carried out to determine the specific diagnosis.

PATHOPHYSIOLOGIC ALTERATIONS IN GASTROINTESTINAL TRACT HEMORRHAGE

Acute GI tract hemorrhage has usually been described by clinical terms that estimate both the rate of bleeding and volume of blood lost. These descriptors range from minor or trivial, through moderate, and finally to severe or torrential. The magnitude of the physiologic response needed to maintain homeostasis parallels the degree of acute blood loss. Blood loss beyond an individual's compensatory mechanisms results in hypovolemic shock and, if untreated, eventually leads to death. Thus the term "shock," in its most basic definition, connotes a state in which the circulation fails to meet the nutritional and metabolic needs of the cell because of inadequate tissue perfusion.

The clinical manifestations of acute GI tract bleeding depend on the rate and total amount of blood loss and yield signs and symptoms that correlate with the severity of shock.[25] A progression of organ involvement beginning with skin and progressing to kidney, then heart, then brain, is usually seen. Associated disease such as hypertension or congestive heart failure, as well as the use of various medications (i.e., antihypertensives, calcium channel blockers) by a given patient may alter the timing and magnitude of this normal physiologic response.

Mild hemorrhagic shock manifested by orthostatic hypotension occurs with loss of less than 20% of the circulating blood volume. Adrenergic vasoconstriction of blood vessels to the skin and skeletal muscles results in extremities that are pale and cool to palpation. The patient may complain of feeling cold, weak, lethargic, or thirsty. Moderate shock represents loss of 20% to 40% of the blood volume. A low urine output signals this stage and is the most sensitive indicator of hypovolemia. In contrast, tachycardia and hypotension may not occur until late and are relatively poor indicators of a compromised vascular compartment. The patient in severe shock has lost more than 40% of blood volume. A rapid, thready pulse and hypotension occur in conjunction with either oliguria or anuria. Signs of myocardial ischemia may be apparent on an electrocardiogram. Ischemia to the central nervous system in its earliest stages is usually manifested as agitation and restlessness. In a more severe form the patient may be obtunded or unconscious.

DIAGNOSIS OF GASTROINTESTINAL TRACT HEMORRHAGE

Initial investigation to determine the source (see box, p. 625) and the cause of GI tract hemorrhage should begin shortly after the patient has been stabilized. Thus the patient's history, physical examination, and laboratory tests should be an integral part of medical care that is rendered simultaneously with early resuscitation and the placement of monitoring equipment. A sense of urgency should be applied to this workup phase to either identify or eliminate possible serious sequela. The major diagnostic goal during this early stage is to determine whether the bleeding originates from the upper or lower GI tract with the ligament of Treitz serving as the established boundary between these two segments. The prognostic significance of this determination is that bleeding from the lower GI tract is usually intermittent, of smaller volume, and therefore not as acutely life threatening as that arising from the esophagus, stomach, or duodenum.

History and Physical Examination

Salient features of the patient's illness should be elicited. In this regard a family member may provide important additional information. A history of hematemesis localizes the hemorrhage to a site proximal to the ligament of Treitz, often proximal to the pylorus. Hematemesis refers to the vomiting of blood that may be either bright red or brown and precipitated, in which case it resembles coffee grounds. Melena and hematochezia are less reliable indicators of the bleeding site. Melena is defined as the passage of black, tarry stools. It most often occurs from a bleeding site proximal to the jejunum but may accompany more distal lesions. The tarry color is usually attributable to the action of gastric acid on hemoglobin, resulting in the production of hematin. However, melena can accompany other bleeding lesions throughout the GI tract (usually proximal to the ileocecal valve) and is secondary to the effects of bacteria and various digestive enzymes on the intraluminal blood. Hematochezia is defined as the passage of red blood from the rectum, and it usually heralds bleeding from the lower GI tract, particularly the colon or rectum. However, it is occasionally observed in patients with a massive upper GI tract hemorrhage.

A history of peptic ulcer disease, abuse of alcohol, or the use of NSAIDs suggests an upper GI tract bleeding source. Dysphagia may indicate an esophageal lesion. Weight loss and anorexia are suggestive of a malignancy. A history of inflammatory bowel disease in a patient with hematochezia should point to the lower GI tract as the site of hemorrhage. If the patient has had a previous bleeding episode, the possibility that the bleeding is from the same lesion is greatly increased.

Physical findings often indicate the extent of vascular volume depletion. Thus careful evaluation of pulse and blood pressure (both upright and supine), skin color, and presence or absence of diaphoresis gives an indication of the magnitude of hemorrhage. The stigmata of certain diseases may also be noted on physical examination and direct one's attention to the possible site of bleeding. For example, the findings of spider angiomas, abdominal venous distention, palmar erythema, jaundice, testicular atrophy, and muscle wasting are often found in patients with cirrhosis and portal hypertension. The presence of melanin spots on the oral mucosa, lips, and digits suggests Peutz-Jeghers syndrome and that the hemorrhage may be caused by the presence of polyps in the small intestine. In any patient with petechiae and ecchymoses, the possibility of a hemorrhagic diathesis must be considered and excluded. Finally, a careful examination of the oropharynx and nose should be done because hematemesis may actually arise from swallowed blood secondary to nasopharyngeal bleeding.

Laboratory Tests

An important early step in the evaluation of a patient with GI tract hemorrhage is determination of the hematocrit. This provides a baseline against which subsequent determinations can be compared. The initial hematocrit may be normal or decreased, depending on the rate of blood loss and the degree of extracellular fluid shift that has occurred to maintain circulating blood volume. Repeat hematocrit readings during initial resuscitation and at 2- to 4-hour intervals are mandatory to determine the adequacy of blood replacement. A low hematocrit in the face of what was thought to be adequate transfusion therapy or a falling hematocrit after initial resuscitation indicates continued bleeding.

Other laboratory tests of importance include coagulation studies, a liver function profile, serum electrolytes, and a determination of blood urea nitrogen (BUN). Coagulation studies, including platelet counts, provide an assessment of the adequacy of clotting factors. Derangements in blood clotting commonly occur following multiple blood transfusions (dilutional coagulopathy) and can actively aggravate the hemorrhage that one is attempting to control. Demonstration of hepatocellular dysfunction may not only aid in diagnosis (e.g., varices in a patient with cirrhosis) but may also indicate the need for replacement therapy (e.g., vitamin K, fibrinogen) to treat a coagulation problem. In an otherwise normal patient, BUN elevation suggests the presence of bleeding proximal to the ligament of Treitz. The metabolic breakdown products of digested blood that are absorbed in the proximal gut are then reflected in the BUN level. It is important to remember that patients with renal failure demonstrate platelet dysfunction, and replacement/supplementation may be necessary.

Techniques to Localize the Site and Cause of Bleeding

If a patient has hematemesis, a bleeding site proximal to the ligament of Treitz is virtually assured. In contrast, hematochezia can result from a lesion in the colon or from rapid passage of blood secondary to a bleeding site in the upper GI tract. Similarly, melanic stools may result from bleeding lesions from the nasopharynx all the way to the proximal colon. Aspiration of bloody gastric contents with a soft nasogastric tube in a patient with melena or hematochezia confirms bleeding proximal to the ligament of Treitz. However, absence of blood in a gastric aspirate by no means rules out an upper GI tract source. The bleeding either may have stopped before placement of the tube or may have originated from a site distal to a competent pyloric sphincter. Because of these limitations, special diagnostic procedures are generally needed to delineate the site and cause of GI tract hemorrhage.[9]

These procedures may either localize or exclude various sites as sources of hemorrhage. In addition, they may demonstrate an associated pathologic lesion that could be a potential, but not the actual cause of bleeding. These special procedures include endoscopy, barium contrast radiography, radionuclide imaging, arteriography, and exploratory celiotomy.

Use of any of these special techniques depends on its availability and assessed accuracy rate at each individual institution. Use of a particular procedure varies with the clinical presentation of the patient. Endoscopy provides the best help in patients with suspected upper GI tract bleeding, whereas radionuclide scanning and arteriography are commonly used in those patients with presumed distal bleeding sites. The order of use and the timing of these special procedures vary considerably among physicians and surgeons. Some clinicians believe that the routine use of special diagnostic procedures in suspected upper GI tract bleeding is seldom indicated, since 80% to 90% of patients with upper GI tract hemorrhage stop bleeding spontaneously.[26] They contend that the small advantage gained in terms of localizing the bleeding site is offset by the associated complication rate of these procedures. Others contend that controlled trials have failed to show any reduction in mortality rates associated with early diagnosis provided by special diagnostic techniques.[27,28] Steer and Silen[26] have cautioned that the lack of merit of these diagnostic maneuvers has not been proven; rather, therapeutic improvements or the willingness to use them have lagged behind diagnostic innovations.

In contrast, others advocate a vigorous diagnostic approach to all patients with GI tract hemorrhage, particularly those with upper GI tract bleeding.[29] Clinicians holding this viewpoint argue that the bleeding site should be expeditiously identified because hemorrhage may recur or persist in 25% of patients, and early surgical intervention may be required in 10% to 25%.[9] Further, patients requiring an early operation (e.g., a vessel in the base of an ulcer, spurting bleeder) can be confidently identified. With this approach, Palmer[29] was able to demonstrate the bleeding lesion in 93% of his patients with upper GI tract bleeding. Further justifying early diagnostic intervention, he noted that 40% of his patients who had had a prior hemorrhagic episode were bleeding from a different site. Most clinicians stand somewhere between these extremes in management and individualize the need for special diagnostic approaches for a given patient.

Endoscopy

Esophagogastroduodenoscopy (EGD) performed with a flexible fiber-optic instrument should be the first diagnostic maneuver in the majority of patients with suspected or proven (i.e., hematemesis or bloody gastric aspirate) upper GI tract hemorrhage. Generally, the diagnostic accuracy using this technique approaches 90%.[30,31] An overall complication rate of 0.9% has been recorded for a large series of patients undergoing EGD, with about half the complications classified as major (e.g., perforation, aspiration, or bleeding).[32]

The timing of endoscopy remains controversial. Proponents of early endoscopy want to identify those patients who will need immediate surgical intervention.[26] Endoscopy during the active bleeding phase has the advantage of correctly identifying the source in the patient with a possibility of more than one lesion (e.g., gastritis vs. esophageal varices, as may occur in the cirrhotic patient with portal hypertension). Such a vigorous diagnostic approach has led to a greater appreciation of the frequency with which acute mucosal lesions cause massive bleeding.[9] However, Peterson et al.[28] in 1981 showed that endoscopy within 4 hours of onset of hemorrhage did not reduce known morbidity and mortality rates. The benefits of early diagnosis must be weighed against the small but increased risk of complications secondary to endoscopy that may occur when it is performed during the acute bleeding phase. Fifty percent of the morbidity and mortality caused by endoscopy is cardiopulmonary related. Endoscopy is contraindicated in patients experiencing acute myocardial infarction or ventricular arrhythmias or those with an acute abdomen. Although they recognize the risks, the majority of experienced surgical endoscopists still prefer early endoscopy to plan possible short-term and long-term therapy.

In most patients with lower GI tract bleeding, anoscopy and colonoscopy should be performed following a careful digital rectal examination. Absence of blood above the rectum in the acutely bleeding patient implicates the anorectal region as the bleeding site. If bleeding is present above the rectum, careful inspection of the colonic mucosa on colonoscopy may demonstrate an inflammatory, ischemic, or neoplastic lesion that could be responsible for the hemorrhage. If active bleeding is present or the colon is filled with a considerable amount of fecal material, colonoscopy may not be helpful because of the obstructed view that exists in such an unprepared bowel.

Barium Contrast Radiography

The accuracy of barium contrast radiography in the diagnosis of acute upper GI tract hemorrhage has been reported at only 20% to 50%.[30,31] Cello and Thoeni[33] contend that barium examinations have no role in the evaluation of acute GI tract bleeding. Additional limitations of barium studies in the diagnosis of upper GI tract causes of hemorrhage include the inability to examine a patient in the upright position when actively bleeding, the presence of blood clots in the stomach, and blurred films secondary to movement in an acutely distressed individual.[9] Further, the use of contrast radiography in diagnosing a colonic source of bleeding in lower GI tract hemorrhage has proven to be no better.[26] The identification of colonic diverticula on barium enema, a lesion commonly found in elderly patients, may lead one to believe falsely that this is the source of hemorrhage, when in fact another cause is present. In addition, the use of barium in both upper and lower GI tract examinations may preclude the subsequent use of angiography. Thus rarely, if ever, are barium studies of value during initial evaluation of a patient with GI tract hemorrhage. Instead, such studies should be reserved to evaluate the patient who has clearly stopped bleeding.

Radionuclide Imaging

Radionuclide imaging with either technetium 99m (^{99m}Tc) sulfur colloid or ^{99m} Tc pertechnetate–labeled red blood cells is an effective noninvasive technique that can identify bleeding when the rate is as low as 0.1 ml/min[34,35] (Fig. 30-1). With ^{99m}Tc-sulfur colloid imaging, scans of the abdomen are obtained shortly after intravenous injection of this nuclide to look for its extravasation from the vascular system.[34] Labeling red blood cells with ^{99m}Tc pertechnetate is generally a more sensitive method because the labeled erythrocytes are retained in the vascular compartment for a longer period of time than with ^{99m}Tc sulfur colloid, and thus repeated scanning is permitted for periods as long as 24 to 36 hours after the intravenous injection. Use of this nuclide permits detection of slow or intermittent bleeding.[35] The accuracy with both techniques has been quite impressive,

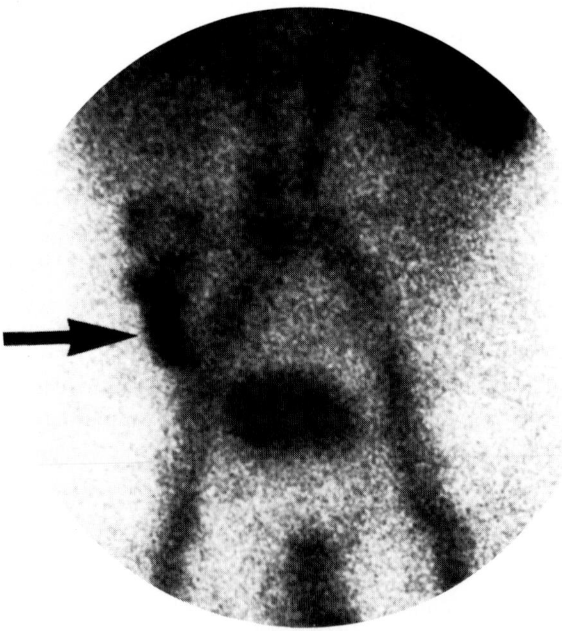

Fig. 30-1. Radionuclide scan using ^{99m}Tc pertechnetate–labeled red blood cells. Arrow indicates bleeding site in right colon.

and the absence of any associated side effects from either of these nuclides has been an especially attractive feature. In anatomic regions of the GI tract where endoscopic evaluation is not possible (i.e., small intestine and occasionally large intestine when adequate preparation for colonoscopic examination cannot be obtained), information derived from radionuclide imaging may be of considerable value. In addition, in patients with intermittent bleeding, use of this methodology as a screening test for active bleeding should reduce the incidence of negative results from angiographic studies. The major deficit of radionuclide scanning is that the procedure usually identifies only a general abdominal region where bleeding exists rather than a specific anatomic site. The one exception is a ^{99m}Tc-pertechnetate scan, which may demonstrate ectopic gastric mucosa present in a Meckel's diverticulum (a Meckel's scan) or an enteric duplication cyst.

Angiography

For less pronounced bleeding or hemorrhage that appears intermittent, radionuclide scanning should generally precede angiography. If endoscopic examination of the upper GI tract or colon fails to reveal a site of bleeding or if the mucosa cannot be adequately evaluated (e.g., bleeding too rapid, visualization of colonic mucosa obscured by feces and/or blood), selective visceral angiography should be performed. This is especially true if evidence of massive bleeding exists (e.g., continued hypotension and/or dropping hematocrit in spite of "adequate" blood transfusions). Angiography involves catheterization of the celiac and/or mesenteric arterial systems through a percutaneous femoral arterial approach. This technique can demonstrate a bleeding site if the rate of hemorrhage at the time of examination is in excess of 0.5 ml/min.[10,36] If a bleeding site is present, contrast medium escapes from the vasculature into the lumen of the involved segment, which is easily recognized on x-ray films. Arteriography may also be helpful in the demonstration of nonbleeding lesions when abnormal vasculature is present. Examples of such lesions include the vascular blush of a tumor, a vessel displaced by a tumor, an arteriovenous fistula, a visceral aneurysm, or vascular ectasia. Angiography should provide an accurate diagnosis of the cause of bleeding in approximately 75% of patients in whom it is performed.[36] This diagnostic accuracy occurs with a background complication rate of less than 2%.[37] Selective angiography has been particularly valuable in identifying bleeding sites in the small bowel and colon, which are areas that are notoriously difficult to identify with other diagnostic procedures. Once a site of bleeding is diagnosed, various techniques can be used through the angiographic catheter to stop the hemorrhage. These approaches are described in more detail later in this chapter (see discussion of interventional angiography).

Exploratory Celiotomy

On rare occasions the procedures just discussed fail to identify a site of continuing hemorrhage. As a last resort diagnostic and therapeutic maneuver, an abdominal exploration may be undertaken. When this becomes necessary, careful evaluation of the entire GI tract is mandatory. This requires careful inspection of the serosal surface in the search for an identifiable bleeding lesion. Particular efforts should be used to identify a primary vascular abnormality such as a vascular malformation, fistula, or ectasia, since these lesions are usually the responsible culprits. Several ancillary maneuvers have been recommended, including perioperative endoscopy, Doppler probes, injections of various dyes such as methylene blue to detect increased areas of blood flow, and transillumination of the bowel. Their success rates in defining the source of bleeding, however, have been low.[26] Occasionally, intraluminal blood appears to be localized to a specific segment of the intestinal tract, suggesting that the hemorrhage may be originating from that site. Unfortunately, when celiotomy becomes a diagnostic maneuver, its success in identifying the bleeding site has been only modest. More often than not, the operation proves to be of little benefit. Another hemorrhagic episode, along with the increase in morbidity and mortality attendant to rebleeding, must occur before the procedures described above are successful in establishing its cause. This is in addition to the risks of exposing a critically ill patient to a major operation.

INITIAL TREATMENT

Initial treatment of the patient with acute GI tract bleeding involves two major components: (1) resuscitation, and (2) placement of appropriate monitoring devices. As in most emergency situations, the ABCs apply, and maintenance of an airway and breathing should be assured. Treatment may range from applying nasal cannula oxygen to intubation and mechanical ventilation. Two large-bore intravenous catheters should be placed into available peripheral veins to secure adequate means to infuse crystalloid solutions and blood components. A cutdown on a peripheral vein may be indicated in some patients. Placement of a pulmonary artery catheter may be indicated in certain clinical situations (i.e., an elderly patient, associated heart and/or lung disease). In the majority of patients this is not necessary, but this should not deter rapid treatment.

Blood should be obtained for hematologic indexes, coagulation profile, serum chemistries, hepatic and renal function studies, and for type and crossmatch for 4 to 6 U of packed red blood cells and fresh frozen plasma. Insertion of a Foley catheter is mandatory to monitor urine output. If the patient is hypotensive, the patient's legs may be elevated or the patient may be placed in the Trendelenburg position. A nasogastric tube should be placed for decompression of the stomach to prevent vomiting and possible aspiration of gastric contents. If facilities are available, the patient should be admitted to an intensive care unit.

Initial intravenous fluid resuscitation should be carried out with either normal saline or lactated Ringer's solution. The rate of fluid infusion depends on the specific patient's condition and response to therapy. The patient in shock should be given a rapid infusion of at least 1 L or more of fluid. Further therapy is dictated by the response to this initial therapy as monitored by blood pressure, heart rate, and urine output. In spite of these measures the patient in shock may require volume expansion with fresh frozen plasma or albumin.

When packed red blood cells (PRBCs) are available, transfusion depends on response to the initial fluid bolus, rate and amount of blood loss, hematocrit changes, and continued or recurrent bleeding. Hemodilution is not an immediate response, and equilibration of the hematocrit may take 6 hours or more. Therefore an admission hematocrit of less than 30% may indicate a significant acute blood loss requiring early transfusion. With continued or recurrent bleeding, the blood bank should be notified to keep ahead of blood use by at least 6 U. One unit of fresh frozen plasma should be given for every 4 U of PRBCs to lessen the effects of a dilutional coagulopathy.

During the initial phase of resuscitation vital signs should be obtained frequently (every 15 minutes). This should include urine output, since it is the most sensitive indicator of adequacy of intravascular volume. Pulmonary wedge pressure and cardiac output are additional hemodynamic parameters that are available in patients with pulmonary artery catheters. There may be a role for an arterial catheter to monitor blood pressure changes closely in the unstable patient. Once the patient has responded to emergency therapy, vital signs may be obtained on an hourly basis. A portable chest x-ray film and electrocardiogram should be obtained once the patient has been stabilized.

Hemodynamic monitoring, nasogastric tube aspiration, and serial hematocrits should continue to detect recurrent bleeding. Certain diagnostic efforts to ascertain the site and source of hemorrhage may be initiated at this time, beginning even in the transiently stable patient with an examination of the upper GI tract by means of flexible fiber-optic endoscopy. If bleeding recurs, an emergency operation may be indicated. Special diagnostic and therapeutic measures may be indicated in certain disease states (i.e., placement of a Sengstaken-Blakemore tube in a patient with portal hypertension and bleeding esophageal varices). These considerations are discussed in subsequent sections of this chapter.

MANAGEMENT OF GASTROINTESTINAL TRACT HEMORRHAGE

In the management of the patient with GI tract hemorrhage, three priorities are paramount. These include resuscitation, identification of the bleeding site, and the use of measures to arrest the bleeding. Principles underlying resuscitation have already been briefly reviewed. Similarly, diagnostic maneuvers to localize the site of bleeding have been discussed. This section describes the various nonoperative and operative strategies currently used to bring about cessation of bleeding.

Nonoperative Therapy

Gastric Lavage

The placement of a nasogastric tube is both a diagnostic and a therapeutic maneuver. Detection of blood in the gastric aspirate confirms a bleeding site proximal to the ligament of Treitz. The nasogastric tube can also be used to gauge the magnitude, persistence, and/or recurrence of bleeding from the upper GI tract. When blood is detected, every effort should be made to aspirate it and remove any clots that may be present in the gastric lumen. The purpose of such aspiration is to lessen gastric distention. This enhances contraction of the gastric musculature, which often assists in the arrest of a gastric bleeding site. It also eliminates the stimulus to secrete gastric acid through gastrin release, which may further irritate the bleeding site. An additional purpose for aspiration is to reduce fibrinolysis at the bleeding site, which can be aggravated by blood remaining in the stomach. Effective aspiration is generally best accomplished with a large-bore nasogastric or orogastric tube (No. 30 French or larger) or ideally an Ewald tube.

Although no controlled trials are available for comparison with room temperature lavage solutions, traditionally gastric lavage has been performed with ice-cold solutions of saline or water. It remains to be determined, however, whether the temperature is truly that important. Generally, the stomach is lavaged with 60 ml aliquots of solution at a time. This volume allows adequate fragmentation of clots and aids in the successful evacuation of any blood that may remain in the stomach while producing minimal distention. With this approach, many clinicians have found that active bleeding from upper GI tract sources has often stopped. Palmer[2] reported that bleeding stopped for at least a few hours in two thirds of his patients when lavage was properly performed. Opponents of lavage contend that it may precipitate recurrent bleeding by washing off clots, it increases the risk of aspiration of gastric contents, and it is probably of little value since bleeding stops spontaneously in 80% to 90% of patients, regardless of the therapy used.[26]

Whether gastric lavage is truly a necessary exercise will probably never be a settled issue, but there is no question that it does provide a means of gauging the rate of bleeding and determining whether other therapeutic endeavors (e.g., arteriography) are necessary. In addition, most clinicians agree that it is an appropriate procedure to perform in preparation for emergency endoscopy when continued hemorrhage is present.

Balloon Tamponade

Balloon tamponade was first introduced by Sengstaken and Blakemore in 1950 for the control of bleeding from gastroesophageal varices.[9] The present modification is a triple-lumen tube with gastric and esophageal balloons. Endotracheal intubation is a mandatory prerequisite to prevent aspiration. The position of the tube must be verified by x-ray film before gastric balloon inflation to prevent inadvertent inflation in the distal esophagus. Once correct positioning has been assured, the gastric balloon should be inflated with 150 to 200 ml of normal saline, and gentle traction should be applied to maintain compression at the esophagogastric junction. If bleeding persists, the esophageal balloon may be inflated with air to 40 to 60 mm Hg pressure. Balloons must be deflated at 24 hours to prevent esophageal necrosis. If bleeding recurs, the balloons may be reinflated for another 12 to 24 hours while plans are being made for some additional therapeutic maneuver. Initial success occurs in about 90% of patients so treated. However, two thirds of these patients rebleed when the balloons are deflated. This treatment modality should be viewed as a temporizing procedure to prevent exsanguination from gastroesophageal varices. Major complications, including aspiration and esophageal rupture, have been reported.

Intravenous Vasopressin

Vasopressin, a cyclic octapeptide, also called antidiuretic hormone, is synthesized in the hypothalamus and stored in the posterior pituitary gland. Its endogenous release is a physiologic response during shock to preserve the integrity of the intravascular compartment following hemorrhage or severe dehydration. Vasopressin is a potent vasoconstrictor acting at the level of the arterioles and precapillary sphincters. It is this latter property that has prompted the use of exogenously administered vasopressin as a therapeutic drug to arrest hemorrhage from the GI tract.

Since its introduction by Kehne et al.[38] in 1956 in patients with bleeding gastroesophageal varices, vasopressin has become an accepted clinical modality for the control of GI tract hemorrhage. In initial reports vasopressin was given as an intravenous bolus of 20 U during a 20-minute period. This method of administration resulted in a myriad of side effects that included hypertension, bradycardia, coronary vasoconstriction, cardiac arrhythmias, water retention, and extremity gangrene.[39] In an attempt to avoid these adverse effects, Nusbaum et al.[40,41] recommended selective intra-arterial infusion of vasopressin at a decreased dosage for control of both variceal and nonvariceal upper GI tract bleeding. More recent studies have shown that a continuous intravenous infusion of vasopressin is as effective as an intra-arterial infusion.[42-44] Additional benefits (i.e., ease of administration, universal availability without the need for special equipment and personnel, and avoidance of treatment delay) have made the intravenous route of vasopressin administration the treatment of choice under most circumstances.[44] The most efficacious uses of vasopressin have been recognized in control of bleeding from gastric mucosa, gastroesophageal varices, and colonic lesions.

Although vasopressin has been shown to control upper GI tract hemorrhage, its efficacy in terms of decreasing morbidity and mortality rates has been questioned. In a placebo-controlled trial Fogel et al.[45] noted that a continuous intravenous infusion of vasopressin (40 U/hr) neither controlled bleeding nor altered the outcome in a group of 60 patients with GI tract hemorrhage. Lack of efficacy occurred in patients with bleeding from both variceal and nonvariceal sites. In contrast, other studies have shown a reduction in mortality rates, transfusion requirements, and operating time when this agent is used to control bleeding before and during surgery.[46,47] The therapeutic efficacy of these studies vs. that of Fogel's group may be secondary to the higher dosage (60 vs. 40 U/hr) of vasopressin used in the latter studies. Experimental evidence exists that such increased vasopressin dosages result in significant reductions in splanchnic arterial blood flow without compromising either cardiac output or coronary blood flow below those mild reductions seen with extremely small vasopressin dosages.[48] Present clinical recommendations for vasopressin therapy include administration in the emergency center, the intensive care unit, and the operating room. Once the diagnosis of GI tract bleeding has been made, the patient may be given an initial loading bolus of vasopressin (20 U for 20 minutes) before infusion of large amounts of blood or crystalloid. This keeps the splanchnic circulation vasoconstricted during restoration of the intravascular volume and thereby prevents continued or recurrent hemorrhage from the GI tract. This should be followed by a continuous intravenous infusion of vasopressin at 60 U/hr. An initial lower dose is indicated in the older patient with a history of myocardial dysfunction. In contrast, vasopressin should not be given to the patient with angina or the individual with a documented history of myocardial infarction. In patients deemed suitable for vasopressin therapy, treatment is usually continued for at least 24 hours after bleeding has ceased. Vasopressin dosage should then be tapered off to prevent hypotension secondary to an expanded intravascular compartment with ensuing vasodilation. If GI tract bleeding recurs, therapy may be restarted, but success is less likely, and other measures most likely must be used. Similar dosages of vasopressin have been used intraoperatively without any adverse effects.[47] Reductions in cardiac output may be offset with isoproterenol. Dopamine is contraindicated because of its splanchnic vasodilatory action.[49,50]

Intravenous Somatostatin

More recently, somatostatin and its longer acting analog octreotide have been used to stop upper GI tract hemorrhage. Somatostatin occurs naturally in plasma as a 14–amino acid cyclic peptide or in a 28–amino acid version. Its plasma half-life is 2 to 6 minutes, whereas octreotide has a serum half-life of 113 minutes after subcutaneous injection. The action of octreotide in controlling upper GI tract hemorrhage is thought to result from splanchnic vasoconstriction, prompting a decrease in splanchnic arterial inflow and a decrease in portal venous pressure.[51]

Treating hemorrhage from esophageal erosions, gastroesophageal varices, portal hypertensive gastropathy, and gastric and duodenal ulcers has been reported. However, its efficacy in treating acutely bleeding esophageal varices, either alone or in combination with injection sclerotherapy, is the most investigated use in the literature currently. In a randomized, double-blind trial from Denmark in 1995, 86 patients were studied comparing intravenous somatostatin vs. placebo.[52] There was no difference between the two study groups for the number of units of blood transfused or the need for gastroesophageal balloon tamponade. Further, the authors of this study reported a meta-analysis of three similar trials involving 290 patients that showed no improvement in survival.

These results are in contrast to findings from Liverpool by Baxter and Jenkins,[53] who reported that the initial control of acute variceal bleeding and the incidence of recurrent bleeding in the first 5 days after initiation of therapy are similar in patients treated with either somatostatin or sclerotherapy. Another study by Sung et al.[54] from Hong Kong showed an improvement in the incidence of rebleeding (9% vs. 38%) after endoscopic variceal ligation in combination with octreotide infusion over endoscopic ligation alone. It is not yet clear from the literature what role octreotide will have in the treatment of the patient with acutely bleeding gastroesophageal varices.

Transendoscopic Therapy

For the past decade there has been marked enthusiasm for the development of safe and effective endoscopic techniques for the treatment of upper GI tract hemorrhage. Purported advantages of these techniques include treatment under direct vision as the diagnosis is made and prevention of an emergency operation with its attendant morbidity and mortality. These techniques include injection of a bleeding vessel with a sclerosant or polymer, injection of the vessel and surrounding tissue with epinephrine, topical application of hemostatic agents, thermocoagulation, electrocoagulation, and laser photocoagulation.[55]

Cyanoacrylate tissue adhesives, as well as fibrinogen and thrombin, have been applied as an aerosol to a bleeding surface by means of an endoscopic catheter.[56] In addition, an electrically heated thermal probe can be passed through an endoscope and pressed against a bleeding lesion. Radiofrequency electric current has been used for coagulation for the past 60 years. Electrocoagulation is performed by intermittent bursts of energy with resultant tissue desiccation.[56] The bipolar technique is purported to have the theoretic advantage of less deep tissue injury. In contrast, the monopolar electrode has the advantage of superficial deposition of energy during tissue desiccation by spark jumping/arcing. This fulguration can coagulate large caliber vessels better than the methods in which the electrodes are in contact with the tissue. In addition, surrounding tissue edema from the heat injury helps keep the vessel closed. Use of this technique has been associated with a success rate of 95% without significant complications.[56]

The word *laser* is an acronym for light amplification by stimulated emission of radiation. The laser is a device that produces an intense beam of radiation of precise wavelength in the optical region of the spectrum. Laser photocoagulation has been accomplished with both argon and Nd:YAG lasers. The Nd:YAG laser has been more effective because of its greater tissue penetration. However, the risk of tissue damage is also increased. Reports to date have shown that both lasers have a 60% to 90% success rate in arresting acute upper GI tract hemorrhage.[56]

A variety of sclerosing agents have been used to halt bleeding from esophagogastric varices including a 1:100,000 solution of epinephrine, 98% ethanol, or 5% morrhuate sodium. Success has varied from 75% to more than 90%.[57-59] Through an endoscope the sclerosing agent is usually injected directly into a bleeding vessel or adjacent to it. Also endoscopically placed rubber band ligation of esophageal varices can be used during an episode of acute hemorrhage with good results.[60]

Interventional Angiography

Localization of GI tract bleeding sites and the control of bleeding with intra-arterial vasopressin or transcatheter embolization are therapeutic applications of selective visceral angiography. In most circumstances endoscopy should precede angiography, since endoscopic localization of the bleeding site should facilitate the angiographic procedure (i.e., celiac axis vs. superior mesenteric artery vs. inferior mesenteric artery.) Arteriography is routinely performed using the femoral route and standard Seldinger technique. For lower esophageal and gastric lesions the left gastric artery is selectively catheterized. Duodenal bleeding requires a celiac arteriogram followed by selective studies of the gastroduodenal and pancreaticoduodenal arteries. Superior mesenteric arteriography is obtained for small bowel lesions and suspected right colon sites. Superior and inferior mesenteric arteriograms are obtained for a suspected colonic bleeding site. Once the site of bleeding has been demonstrated by extravasation of contrast media into the gastric or intestinal lumen, treatment may be instituted with either intra-arterial vasopressin or by transcatheter vessel occlusion.[61]

Vasopressin should be infused at a rate of 0.2 U/min for 20 minutes followed by a second arteriogram.[62] If bleeding persists, the dosage of vasopressin is increased to 0.4 U/min for 20 minutes and once again is followed by a second angiogram. If bleeding still persists, vasopressin infusion should be abandoned as a method of therapy, and transcatheter occlusion should be considered. For those in whom bleeding is controlled, vasopressin is usually infused at the dosage at which cessation of bleeding occurred for an additional 12 to 24 hours. The dosage is then halved over two subsequent 12-hour treatment periods. The catheter is kept patent with a saline infusion for another 24-hour period. If bleeding recurs, transcatheter occlusion is considered; if not, the catheter is removed.[62]

Transcatheter occlusion of a bleeding vessel has been accomplished using combinations of autologous blood clot or Gelfoam. Isobutyl with cyanoacrylate has also been used to create permanent occlusion. More commonly, detachable small balloons and coils attached to angiographic catheters have been used for the control of hemorrhage. The embolization procedure is performed through the arteriography catheter. Repeat angiograms are obtained to document successful vessel thrombosis and control of the bleeding site (Fig. 30-2).[62]

Hemorrhage from the distal esophagus can be demonstrated by selective left gastric arteriography and successfully controlled by selective intra-arterial vasopressin administration in the majority of patients.[62] Therapeutic success includes control of bleeding from esophagitis, Mallory-Weiss tears, tumors, and endoscopic trauma. Mucosal hemorrhage secondary to gastritis or superficial erosions can be controlled in 84% of patients, whereas bleeding from a gastric ulcer can be stopped with infusion of vasopressin into the left gastric artery in about two thirds of patients.[62] In contrast, hemorrhage from a duodenal ulcer can be controlled with vasopressin infusion in only 50% of patients. The dual blood supply of the duodenum (celiac axis and superior mesenteric artery) is probably responsible for this failure rate. The other half require transcatheter embolization of the superior (via the gastroduodenal artery) and inferior (via the superior mesenteric artery) pancreaticoduodenal arteries. Infusion of vasopressin into the superior mesenteric artery decreases portal venous pressure 25% to 35% and stops variceal bleeding in slightly over half of patients. Percutaneous transhepatic portal vein catheterization followed by transcatheter occlusion of the coronary vein is another successful treatment modality but has a significantly higher complication rate.[62]

A

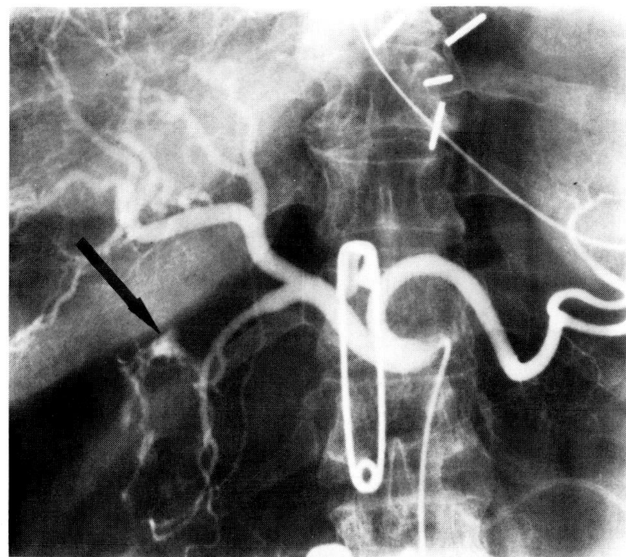

B

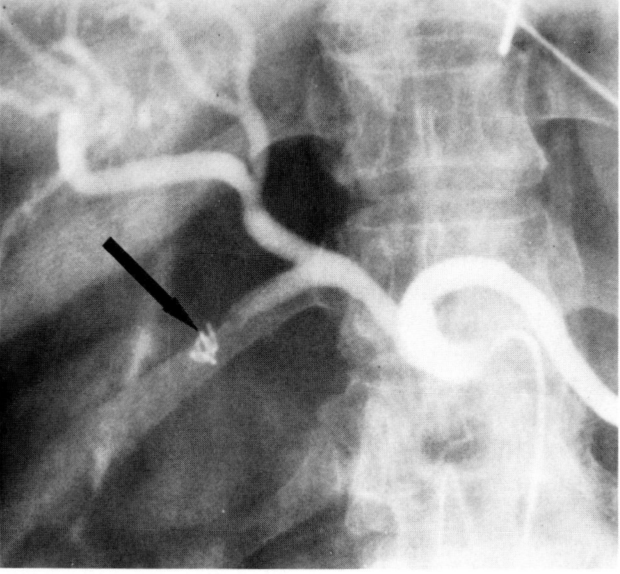

Fig. 30-2. Selective celiac arteriogram showing extravasation *(arrow)* from posterosuperior pancreatoduodenal artery **(A)** and control of bleeding site by transcatheter embolization of coil *(arrow)* in gastroduodenal artery **(B)**.

Infusion of vasopressin into the superior mesenteric artery can also successfully control hemorrhage from small bowel tumors, vascular malformations, diverticula, and angiodysplasia of the right colon. Intra-arterial vasopressin successfully controls acute colorectal bleeding in as many as 90% of patients.[62] Recurrent bleeding occurs in about 25% of these patients within 24 hours. Lower GI tract bleeding requires cannulation of the inferior mesenteric artery, if it is patent. Left colon lesions are less responsive to this mode of therapy and may require earlier surgical intervention.

In the early 1980s, experimentation was initiated to develop an interventional angiographic procedure for portal decompression. What emerged was the transjugular intrahepatic portosystemic shunt (TIPS). Under fluoroscopy, a catheter is passed through the superior vena cava and inferior vena cava into a hepatic vein. The catheter is then forced out of the vein and through the hepatic parenchyma until a portal vein branch is reached. The resulting channel is balloon dilated, and an expandable stent is left in place to maintain patency.

In a review by Kerlan et al.[63] in 1995, the TIPS procedure was successfully accomplished in 95% to 100% of patients in whom it was attempted. Residual portosystemic pressure gradient was 9 to 15 mm Hg. Short-term control of variceal hemorrhage was obtained in 81% to 94% of patients. Procedure mortality was 1.3%, whereas 30-day mortality was 3% to 15%. Uncontrolled encephalopathy occurred in 5% of patients. Recurrent GI tract bleeding occurred in 18% to 31% of patients. Of these, recurrent gastroesophageal variceal bleeding was usually due to stenosis or occlusion.[63]

The major problem with the TIPS procedure has been long-term patency. One-year patency rates range from 25% to 66%. Pseudointimal hyperplasia in the stent appears to be the cause of stenosis and/or occlusion. Balloon dilation of the stenosis in patients with either recurrent variceal hemorrhage, Duplex scanning abnormalities, or worsening ascites resulted in an 83% to 85% 1-year patency rate and a 79% to 90% 2-year patency rate.[63]

Operative Therapy

To optimize the clinical management of patients with GI tract hemorrhage, consultation between medical and surgical gastroenterologists should occur soon after admission. This combined initial approach should identify those patients needing only medical therapy. In addition, such cooperation minimizes the chances of unnecessary delays, with the attendant increased risks, for patients requiring emergency surgical treatment. Accepted guidelines for triage of this latter group remain controversial, therefore a working classification should be established for each institution.

Classic indications for emergency surgical intervention routinely include persistent hypotension or shock in spite of adequate resuscitative measures and significant recurrent bleeding during maximal medical therapy. Additional criteria are the requirements for more than 6 U of blood during the first 24 hours of treatment or for 3 U/24 hr to maintain stable hemodynamic indexes. The source of bleeding, age of patient, associated critical illness, and availability of blood products are additional mitigating circumstances that may modify the therapeutic approach.

In 1991 Branicki et al.[64] reported that emergency surgery was required in 15% to 30% of patients with GI tract bleeding, including 10% to 15% of patients with a bleeding peptic ulcer. This variability is most likely secondary to differing patient populations and also to reported incidences of specific causes from a particular institution. The national American Society of Gastroenterological Endoscopy survey on upper gastrointestinal bleeding, which contains data from 277 physicians across the nation, reflects an unbiased sampling. From this database Silverstein et al.[65] reported in 1981 that there was an overall series mortality rate of 11%. There was an 8.5% mortality rate for those receiving only medical therapy. Those patients who underwent an operation (15.6%) had an overall surgical mortality rate of 26%. Of the operations, 85% were emergency procedures with a 30% mortality vs. 10% mortality for elective operations. Mortality rates also varied widely for major diagnostic categories.

Prior to operation the patient should be brought to the best possible hemodynamic state. A secure intravenous route for continued blood and fluid replacement must be in place. A urinary catheter should be inserted to monitor the adequacy of hydration. In many patients, particularly the elderly, a pulmonary artery catheter may also be of value. Four to six units of crossmatched PRBCs and a sufficient amount of fresh frozen plasma and platelets should be on hand, with more available on demand. A nasogastric tube should be placed to decompress the stomach before induction of general anesthesia. At operation all the contents of the abdomen must be carefully explored in a systematic fashion.

Upper Gastrointestinal Tract

Hematemesis and/or blood in the nasogastric aspirate implicates a site proximal to the ligament of Treitz, even though the specific source of upper GI tract bleeding may not have been localized before surgery. With the extensive use of endoscopy and arteriography, the bleeding site, if possible, should be documented before surgery to allow for the planning of an appropriate surgical approach. Absence of signs of portal hypertension should direct attention to the stomach and duodenum as the most common sites of bleeding. Some lesions (i.e., gastric cancer, leiomyoma) are readily apparent. Others (i.e., duodenal ulcer) may be identified only after careful palpation.

Superficial lesions of the stomach or duodenum may be missed and require direct inspection of the gastroduodenal mucosa. A generous (~6 cm) longitudinal anterior antropyloroduodenotomy is made for exploration. All gastric contents including clotted and nonclotted blood should be evacuated. Sponges should be placed distally in the duodenum to prevent reflux of previously shed blood and bile. If a bleeding ulcer is found in the duodenal bulb, it can usually be controlled by suture ligation followed by closure of the incision in a transverse fashion (Heineke-Mikulicz pyloroplasty). To ensure continued control of hemorrhage after operation, suture ligation of the gastroduodenal artery both superior and inferior to the duodenal bulb is often added. Finally, a bilateral truncal vagotomy is accomplished. If a bleeding site is not found, a separate vertical gastrotomy is then made and extended to within a few centimeters of the gastroesophageal junction. Division of the short gastric vessels may be necessary to facilitate thorough examination of the proximal stomach.

When all these procedures fail to demonstrate the origin of bleeding, attention should be directed to the duodenum for evidence of a postbulbar ulcer, diverticulum, or neoplasm. A gastrectomy or ulcer operation is contraindicated if the bleeding has stopped without identification of a specific lesion. The pyloroduodenotomy and gastrotomy should be closed longitudinally and the patient observed for recurrent hemorrhage. The latter group, in which no lesion or source of bleeding is identified, should comprise a very small minority of patients.

Esophageal lesions. Nonvariceal esophageal bleeding is rarely a cause for an emergency operation. Blood loss is usually on a chronic basis and can be treated either medically or by an elective operation once the site and cause have been established. If an emergency operation is required, it is often associated with a high mortality rate, primarily because of the occurrence of such lesions in an older age group of patients. Only 10% of patients with the Mallory-Weiss syndrome require surgical intervention for persistent or recurrent bleeding. The surgical procedure includes proximal gastrotomy with suture closure of the submucosal bleeding site. Postoperative rebleeding has been reported in 10% of such treated patients, with surgical mortality as high as 10%.[66]

Variceal hemorrhage. Treatment of the patient with acute variceal hemorrhage remains a therapeutic dilemma. A recent study of 85 consecutive patients with endoscopically proven, clinically significant, variceal hemorrhage reported a 42% 6-week mortality for those treated medically.[67] One third of the patients experienced rebleeding within 6 weeks. It was therefore concluded that any substantial improvement in long-term survival must result from a decrease in early mortality. Intravenous infusion of vasopressin with adjunctive use of balloon tamponade, transhepatic embolization, and sclerotherapy should control the acute episode of variceal bleeding in 75% to 90% of patients.[46] Oversewing of the bleeding varix, although "quick and easy," has an unacceptably high failure rate.

Another approach to stopping gastroesophageal variceal hemorrhage or preventing recurrent hemorrhages is to decompress the portal circulation. Various operations have been used with this in mind. Total portal blood flow diversion is achieved with end-to-side portacaval shunting. This approach controls the bleeding; however, accelerated liver failure and the occurrence of hepatic encephalopathy have limited its use. Partial portal flow diversion is achieved with side-to-side shunts, portacaval H-graft shunts, or "Warren" distal splenorenal shunts.[68,69] Emergency portosystemic shunts for persistent bleeding have reported surgical mortality rates as high as 50%.[67] More recently emergency, side-to-side portacaval shunts have been performed with a 30-day mortality of 24%.[70] This is in contrast to a 3.5% mortality when the same operation is performed on an elective basis. Hemodynamic instability and lack of a complete workup in the acutely bleeding patient (determination of cause of portal hypertension, evaluation of the rebleeding risk and functional capacity of the remaining liver, and angiographic delineation of arterial supply and venous drainage of the visceral organs) are the prime reasons for the increased mortality.

Successful liver transplantation alleviates the portal hypertension and essentially "cures" the patient. In data from the UCLA Tissue Typing Laboratory covering 11,980 patients from 1987 to 1993, 1- and 5-year survival rates of patients with liver transplantations performed for alcoholic liver disease are 81% and 65%, respectively.[71] This compares to survival rates of 78% and 65%, respectively, for liver transplantation for all indications. The best outcome occurred in patients with cholestatic jaundice.[71] Frequently, sclerotherapy and/or the TIPSS procedure are used to control variceal hemorrhage in transplantation candidates until a suitable donor liver becomes available.

Gastric ulcer. Operative therapy for the bleeding gastric ulcer, as with other operations, must first control the hemorrhage. Biopsies of the ulcer should be taken to exclude malignancy. Herrington and Davidson[72] have categorized gastric ulcers based on location and recommended an operation to match. Briefly, an antral or prepyloric ulcer is managed with a 60% distal gastrectomy with Billroth I anastomosis and a truncal vagotomy. A lesser curve ulcer at the incisura is treated with a 60% distal gastrectomy extended to excise the ulcer, and a Billroth I anastomosis is performed.

If the patient is unstable, an anterior gastrotomy and ulcer oversewing is performed immediately. This is followed at a later date with an elective Billroth I gastrectomy and truncal vagotomy. For the frail patient with multiple comorbid conditions, gastrotomy, biopsy, oversewing of the bleeding site, truncal vagotomy, and drainage is the most expeditious management, even though the risk of rebleeding is higher. There have been limited studies to support the use of parietal cell vagotomy and ulcer oversewing to treat acute hemorrhage from a gastric ulcer. Most studies select good-risk patients for this procedure, and parietal cell vagotomy has not been widely embraced by the surgical community as a treatment option.[73-76]

Duodenal ulcer. Hemorrhage from a duodenal ulcer remains the most frequent cause of massive upper GI tract bleeding.[65] Although there is no consensus among surgeons regarding the best operation for such lesions, the choice should be tailored to the physiologic reserve of the patient. High-risk patients should undergo a procedure that is both effective in controlling the bleeding and can be performed expeditiously. Oversewing of the bleeding point, combined with truncal vagotomy and pyloroplasty, is an appropriate therapeutic choice in this setting.[72] More latitude for choice of surgery exists in the low-risk patient. In this latter group the mortality for a truncal vagotomy and gastric resection is similar to that for a truncal vagotomy and pyloroplasty.[66]

Overall surgical mortality rates, inclusive of both emergency and elective patients, range between 5% and 10% and show a direct correlation with age of the patient and the volume of blood transfused. Recurrent hemorrhage has been found to be less in patients undergoing truncal vagotomy and partial gastrectomy (5%) than in patients undergoing truncal vagotomy and pyloroplasty (10%).[66] Multiple-organ failure is responsible for two thirds of the deaths for both groups of patients.[65]

Hemorrhage from a late recurring ulcer after a prior drainage procedure is usually not massive. The site is most often at the stoma. In a series of 117 patients only 4% required an emergency operation.[66] For high-risk patients, oversewing the bleeding point with revagotomy is the procedure of choice. Revagotomy (usually by means of a transthoracic route) and resection are optimal treatments for most healthy surgical candidates under nonemergent conditions.

Stress ulceration. The therapy of choice for stress ulceration is prevention. Once bleeding has started, an emergency operation is required in about 7% to 10% of these patients.[66,77] A variety of surgical strategies have been recommended, including truncal vagotomy and pyloroplasty, gastrectomy, total gastrectomy, and gastric devascularization.[66] The surgical mortality for these procedures has been similar, ranging from 30% to 50%.

Lower Gastrointestinal Tract

The need for surgical management of a continuing source of bleeding distal to the ligament of Treitz depends on the underlying cause and whether nonsurgical approaches such as angiography have been successful in bringing about its cessation. If an underlying malignancy is a possible cause, exploratory celiotomy should be performed and resection of the involved intestine and lymph node drainage routes carried out. Even if hemorrhage is successfully arrested with nonsurgical maneuvers, demonstration of a small intestinal source would generally require an operation (usually elective), since the exact cause cannot be discerned in most instances. Even though 70% to 80% of small bowel hemorrhages (excluding duodenum) are caused by vascular ectasias, the possibility of a small bowel neoplasm must always be entertained.[18] Again, a local resection including lymphatic drainage routes is appropriate. If other sources of small bowel bleeding such as a Meckel's diverticulum, various duplications, and congenital arteriovenous malformations are likely sources and bleeding can be arrested without an operation, observation is usually indicated. Surgical therapy should be reserved for those patients who may develop recurrent hemorrhage.

If a colonic polyp is the responsible bleeding source, it generally should be removed, since the likelihood of recurrent bleeding is high and the possibility of an underlying malignancy is always present. Under most circumstances such polyps can be removed during colonoscopy. Bleeding is not uncommonly observed in patients with inflammatory bowel disease, but it is usually modest and can be managed with conservative therapy. In the event that severe bleeding occurs from ulcerative colitis, subtotal or total colectomy is almost always indicated. In contrast, bleeding from Crohn's disease of a recurrent nature is best controlled by limited intestinal resection, if possible.

Management of colonic bleeding from either diverticulosis or an arteriovenous malformation has been the subject of considerable controversy.[20,23] Most surgeons recommend a conservative approach if nonsurgical maneuvers can control such bleeding and reserve surgery for those individuals in whom recurrent hemorrhage becomes a problem. Generally, segmental resection of the bleeding site is adequate treatment in this group of patients.

Recently, a more aggressive stance has been taken with respect to angiodysplastic abnormalities because the natural history of this disorder is one of recurrent bleeding. Thus, Boley et al.[20] recommended that the demonstration of a vascular malformation on angiography, with or without evidence of active bleeding, warrants colonic resection. This is generally accomplished as an elective procedure if active bleeding can be controlled. Since virtually all these abnormalities are limited to the right colon, resection of that portion of the intestine is carried out. As mentioned earlier, the large majority of colonic diverticular hemorrhages also originate in the right colon.

Occasionally, massive hemorrhage from the colon occurs in which all attempts at diagnostic localization prove unrewarding. In this circumstance total abdominal colectomy becomes necessary as a lifesaving maneuver.

OCCULT HEMORRHAGE

Occult GI tract bleeding encompasses a spectrum of clinical definitions. To the majority of clinicians occult bleeding means intermittent, chronic, slow blood loss from the GI tract. To others the term means anemia coupled with a positive test result for blood in the stool. Finally, occult bleeding has been defined in terms of continued blood loss from an undetermined site in spite of exhaustion of available diagnostic modalities.

Small physiologic amounts of blood are shed normally into the digestive tract (0.5-1 ml/day).[78,79] Chronic blood loss of a larger volume may occur without producing specific symptomatology. The patient may have a history of melena or intermittent episodes of a small amount of bright red blood per rectum. Additional vague symptoms of weakness and chronic fatigue may be the only reason for seeking medical advice. Demonstration of a microcytic, hypochromic anemia without known blood loss from another source in these patients warrants a thorough examination of the GI tract. Although the barium contrast upper GI tract series may detect a potentially responsible lesion, there is no proof that that particular entity is the cause of bleeding. In Palmer's series[2] of 1400 patients, 59% had another nonbleeding lesion found during the course of evaluation. Therefore EGD should be performed in all patients with occult bleeding. The source of bleeding is found in as many as 40% of patients who undergo upper endoscopy for workup of iron deficiency anemia and/or melena. Anoscopy and colonoscopy should be obtained to identify potential colorectal sources of bleeding. In contrast to its general lack of usefulness for acute GI tract bleeding, colonoscopy has found the source of bleeding in 30% to 40% of patients with chronic blood loss.[80] The majority of lesions found have included polyps, vascular malformations, and superficial ulcerations.

Selective visceral angiography has been quite useful in patients with occult bleeding. The bleeding site has been identified in approximately 50% of patients; in another 25% to 30% of these patients the angiograms have demonstrated a highly suspicious lesion.[80] As already noted, radionuclide imaging with labeled red blood cells is a noninvasive technique that may prove helpful in identifying the source of hemorrhage but is less specific in demonstrating the actual anatomic site. Furthermore, it is hampered by the minimal limits on rates of hemorrhage. The use of exploratory celiotomy to diagnose the site of occult GI tract bleeding has been generally unsuccessful. In one series the use of intraoperative endoscopy at the time of celiotomy increased the diagnostic yield to 80% in a group of patients subjected to this diagnostic maneuver, although this has not been a uniform experience.[26,80]

In the face of these diagnostic modalities, a group of patients will continue to carry the diagnosis of occult GI tract bleeding. Care must be taken to ensure proper follow-up for these individuals. Serial hematocrits should be obtained to assess the degree of anemia and to indicate any episodes of acute bleeding superimposed on the chronic anemia. The patient and/or family must be instructed to look for recurrent symptoms, the presence of melena, and to routinely test the stool for occult blood. The most important factor is to ensure continuity of care to prevent the patient from being lost to follow-up.

SUMMARY

Hemorrhage from the GI tract is responsible for approximately 1% to 2% of all hospital admissions, and 50% of episodes occur during hospitalization. Overall mortality ranges from 5% to 12%. Hemorrhage originating from a source proximal to the ligament of Treitz (accounting for ~80% of occurrences) is referred to as upper GI tract hemorrhage, whereas hemorrhage distal to this anatomic boundary is termed lower GI tract hemorrhage. Common causes of upper GI tract hemorrhage include duodenal ulcer, acute gastritis, gastric ulcer, gastroesophageal varices, esophagitis, and Mallory-Weiss mucosal tears. Common causes of lower GI tract hemorrhage include diverticulosis, angiodysplasia/vascular extasias, ischemic colitis, and various neoplastic, infectious, and inflammatory lesions of the small and large intestine.

In the management of any patient with GI tract hemorrhage, three priorities are paramount. These include resuscitation, identification of the underlying bleeding site, and the use of appropriate measures to stop the bleeding. Hematemesis virtually always implicates a source of bleeding proximal to the ligament of Treitz, whereas melena and hematochezia are less reliable indicators of the underlying bleeding site. Endoscopy provides the best help in locating the site of bleeding in patients with suspected upper GI tract hemorrhage, whereas radionuclide scanning and arteriography are commonly used when a distal bleeding site is presumed. With the availability of various endoscopic and angiographic techniques to control bleeding, the vast majority of patients with GI tract hemorrhage can be managed without an operation. In those patients requiring surgical management, the type of procedure is determined by the underlying cause. For a bleeding peptic ulcer, for example, surgical management may require truncal vagotomy and partial gastrectomy, whereas an angiodysplastic lesion of the colon usually necessitates a right colectomy. In a small percentage of patients, the source of GI tract bleeding remains occult in spite of a vigorous diagnostic investigation. In this group of patients, careful follow-up is mandatory. Continued surveillance of the GI tract with various endoscopic maneuvers, barium contrast studies, and on occasion radionuclide scanning and/or angiography to search for sources of unexplained anemia identifies the underlying cause in a majority of these individuals.

REFERENCES

1. Allan RN. History, epidemiology, mortality. In Dykes PW, Keighley MRB, eds. Gastrointestinal Haemorrhage. Boston: Wright PSG, 1981.
2. Palmer ED. Upper gastrointestinal hemorrhage. JAMA 231:853, 1975.
3. Cytler JA, Mendeloff AI. Upper gastrointestinal bleeding: Nature and magnitude of the problem in the U.S. Dig Dis Sci 26(Suppl):90, 1981.
4. Schiller KFR, Truelove AC, William DG. Haematemesis and melena with special reference to factors influencing the outcome. Br Med J 2:7, 1970.
5. Johnston SJ, et al. Epidemiology and course of gastrointestinal haemorrhage in north-east Scotland. Br Med J 3:655, 1973.
6. Gilbert DA. Epidemiology of upper gastrointestinal bleeding. Gastrointest Endosc 36(Suppl 5):S8, 1990.
7. Fleischer D. Etiology and prevalence of severe persistent upper gastrointestinal bleeding. Gastroenterology 84:538, 1983.
8. Gostout DJ, et al. Acute gastrointestinal bleeding: Experience of a specialized management team. J Clin Gastroenterol 14:260, 1992.
9. Bogoch A. Hematemesis and melena. I. Etiology and medical aspects. In Bockus HL, ed. Gastroenterology, vol I. Philadelphia: WB Saunders, 1974.
10. Baum S, et al. The operative radiographic demonstration of intraabdominal bleeding from undetermined sites by percutaneous selective celiac and superior mesenteric arteriography. Surgery 58:797, 1965.
11. Skillman JJ, Silen W. Stress ulceration in the acutely ill. Ann Rev Med 27:9, 1976.
12. Gardner B, Richardson JD. Gastrointestinal bleeding. In Polk HC, Stone HH, Gardner B, eds. Basic Surgery. Norwalk, Conn.: Appleton-Century-Crofts, 1983.
13. Merigan TC, et al. Gastrointestinal bleeding with cirrhosis: A study of 172 episodes in 158 patients. N Engl J Med 263:579, 1980.
14. Graham DY, Schwartz JT. The spectrum of the Mallory-Weiss tear. Medicine 57:307, 1978.
15. Sugawa C, Benishek D, Walt AJ. Mallory-Weiss syndrome. Am J Surg 145:30, 1983.
16. Boley SJ, Sammartano R, Adams A. The nature and etiology of vascular ectasis of the colon. Gastroenterology 72:650, 1977.
17. Netterville R, Hardy J, Martin R. Small bowel hemorrhage. Ann Surg 167:949, 1968.
18. Harford W. Gastrointestinal angiodysplasia: Clinical features. Endoscopy 20:144, 1988.
19. Rutherford RB, Akers DR. Meckel's diverticulum: A review of 148 patients with special reference to the pattern of bleeding and to mesodiverticular vascular bands. Surgery 59:618, 1966.
20. Boley SJ, Brant LJ, Frank MS. Severe lower intestinal bleeding: Diagnosis and treatment. In Torsoli A, ed. Gastrointestinal Emergencies, Clinics in Gastroenterology. Philadelphia: WB Saunders, 1981.
21. Bray SJ, et al. Lower intestinal bleeding in the elderly. Am J Surg 137:57, 1979.
22. Baum S, et al. Angiodysplasia of the right colon: A cause of gastrointestinal bleeding. AJR Am J Roentgenol 129:789, 1977.
23. Boley SJ, et al. Lower intestinal bleeding in the elderly. Am J Surg 137:57, 1979.
24. Moody FG. Rectal bleeding. N Engl J Med 290:839, 1974.
25. Gann DS, Amaral JF. Pathophysiology of trauma and shock. In Zuidema GD, Rutherford RD, Ballinger WF, eds. The Management of Trauma. Philadelphia: WB Saunders, 1985.
26. Steer ML, Silen W. Diagnostic procedures in gastrointestinal hemorrhage. N Engl J Med 309:646, 1983.
27. Dronffield MW, et al. A prospective randomised trial of endoscopy and radiology in acute upper-gastrointestinal-tract bleeding. Lancet 1:1167, 1977.
28. Peterson WL, et al. Routine early endoscopy in upper-gastrointestinal-tract bleeding: A randomized controlled trial. N Engl J Med 304:925, 1981.
29. Palmer ED. Upper Gastrointestinal Hemorrhage. Springfield, Ill.: Charles C Thomas, 1970.
30. Hoare AM. Comparative study between endoscopy and radiology in acute upper gastrointestinal hemorrhage. Br Med J 1:27, 1975.
31. McGinn FP, et al. A prospective comparative trial between early endoscopy and radiology in acute upper gastrointestinal haemorrhage. Gut 16:707, 1975.
32. Gilbert DA, Silverstein FE, Tedesco FJ. National ASGE survey on upper gastrointestinal bleeding: Complications of endoscopy. Dig Dis Sci 26(Suppl):55, 1981.
33. Cello JP, Thoeni RF. Gastrointestinal hemorrhage: Comparative values of double contrast upper gastrointestinal radiology and endoscopy. JAMA 243:685, 1980.

34. Alavi A. Detection of gastrointestinal bleeding with ^{99m}Tc-sulfur colloid. Semin Nucl Med 12:126, 1982.
35. Winzelberg GG, et al. Detection of gastrointestinal bleeding with ^{99m}Tc-labelled red blood cells. Semin Nucl Med 12:139, 1982.
36. Baum S. Angiography and the gastrointestinal bleeder. Radiology 143:569, 1982.
37. Hessel SJ, Adams DF, Abrams HL. Complications of angiography. Radiology 138:273, 1981.
38. Kehne JH, Hughes FA, Gompertz ML. The use of surgical Pituitrin in the control of esophageal varix bleeding. Surgery 39:917, 1956.
39. Swan KG, Hobson RW, Kerr JC. Experimental observations and clinical recommendations on vasopressin for control of gastrointestinal hemorrhage. Am Surg 43:545, 1977.
40. Nusbaum M, et al. Pharmacologic control of portal hypertension. Surgery 62:299, 1967.
41. Nusbaum M, et al. Clinical experience with selective intra-arterial infusion of vasopressin in the control of gastrointestinal bleeding from arterial sources. Am J Surg 123:165, 1972.
42. Chojkier M, et al. A controlled comparison of continuous intraarterial and intravenous infusion of vasopressin in hemorrhage from esophageal varices. Gastroenterology 77:540, 1979.
43. Johnson WC, et al. Control of bleeding varices by vasopressin: A prospective randomized study. Ann Surg 186:369, 1977.
44. Thomford NR, Sirinek KR. Intravenous vasopressin in patients with portal hypertension. J Surg Res 18:113, 1975.
45. Fogel MR, et al. Continuous intravenous vasopressin in active upper gastrointestinal bleeding: A placebo-controlled trial. Ann Intern Med 96:565, 1982.
46. Levine BA, Gaskill HV, Sirinek KR. Portosystemic shunting remains procedure of choice for control of variceal hemorrhage. Arch Surg 120:296, 1985.
47. Sirinek KR, Martin EW, Thomford NR. Peripheral vasopressin provides safe and adequate control of portal hypertension during shunt operations. Am J Surg 131:103, 1976.
48. Gaskill HV, Sirinek KR, Levine BA. Hemodynamic effects of vasopressin: Can larger doses be safely given? Arch Surg 118:434, 1983.
49. Sirinek KR, Thomford NR. Isoproterenol in offsetting adverse effects of vasopressin in cirrhotic patients. Am J Surg 129:130, 1975.
50. Teterick CE, et al. The portal hypertensive effect of dopamine. J Surg Res 22:671, 1977.
51. Hanisch E, Doertenbach J, Usadel KH. Somatostatin in acute bleeding oesophageal varices. Drugs 44(Suppl 2):24, 1992.
52. Gtøzsche PC, et al. Somatostatin versus placebo in bleeding oesophageal varices: Randomised trial and meta-analysis. Br Med J 310:1495, 1995.
53. Baxter JN, Jenkins SA. Somatostatin: An alternative to sclerotherapy? Scand J Gastroenterol 29(Suppl 207):17, 1994.
54. Sung JJY, et al. Prospective randomised study of effect of octreotide on rebleeding from oesophageal varices after endoscopic ligation. Lancet 346:1666, 1995.
55. Pitcher JL. Therapeutic endoscopy and bleeding ulcers: Historical overview. Gastrointest Endosc 36(Suppl 5):S3, 1990.
56. Silverstein FE, Gilbert DA, Auth DC. Endoscopy hemostasis using laser photocoagulation and electrocoagulation. Dig Dis Sci 26(Suppl):31, 1981.
57. Hennessey TPJ, et al. Acute and chronic management of varices by injection sclerotherapy. Surg Gynecol Obstet 154:375, 1982.
58. Johnston GW, Rodgers HW. A review of 15 years experience in the use of sclerotherapy in the control of acute haemorrhage for oesophageal varices. Br J Surg 60:797, 1973.
59. Terblanche J, et al. Acute bleeding varices: A five-year prospective evaluation of tamponade and sclerotherapy. Ann Surg 194:521, 1981.
60. Stiegmann GV, et al. Endoscopic elastic band ligation for active variceal hemorrhage. Am Surg 55:124, 1989.
61. Rahn NH, et al. Diagnostic and interventional angiography in acute gastrointestinal hemorrhage. Radiology 143:361, 1982.
62. Kadir S, Athanasoulis CA. Angiographic management of gastrointestinal bleeding. Ann Rev Med 30:41, 1979.
63. Kerlan RK Jr, et al. Transjugular intrahepatic portosystemic shunts: Current status. AJR Am J Roentgenol 164:1059, 1995.
64. Branicki FJ, et al. Emergency surgical treatment for nonvariceal bleeding of the upper part of the gastrointestinal tract. Surg Gynecol Obstet 172:113, 1991.
65. Silverstein FE, et al. The national ASGE survey on upper gastrointestinal bleeding. I. Study design and baseline data. Gastrointest Endosc 27:73, 1981.
66. Larson DE, Farnell MB. Upper gastrointestinal hemorrhage. Mayo Clin Proc 58:371, 1983.
67. Graham DY, Smith JL. The course of patients after variceal hemorrhage. Gastroenterology 80:800, 1981.
68. Henderson JM. The distal splenorenal shunt. Surg Clin North Am 70(2):405, 1990.
69. Rypins EB, Sarfeh IJ. Small-diameter portacaval H-graft for variceal hemorrhage. Surg Clin North Am 70(2):395, 1990.
70. Levine BA, Sirinek KR. Direct portacaval anastomosis—Safe and effective in patients with previous abdominal operations. Am J Surg 152:721, 1986.
71. Dawson S III, et al. Dumont-UCLA liver transplantation: Analysis of the first 1000 patients. Clin Transplants 189:95, 1994.
72. Herrington JL, Davidson J. Bleeding gastroduodenal ulcers: Choice of operations. World J Surg 11:304, 1987.
73. Hoffman J, et al. Parietal cell vagotomy as an emergency procedure for bleeding peptic ulcer. Ann Surg 206:583, 1987.
74. Johnston D. Division and repair of the sphincteric mechanism of the gastric outlet in emergency operations for bleeding peptic ulcer. Ann Surg 186:723, 1977.
75. Jordan PJ Jr. Surgery for peptic ulcer disease. Curr Probl Surg 28:265, 1991.
76. Miedema BW, et al. Proximal gastric vagotomy in the emergency treatment of bleeding duodenal ulcer. Am J Surg 161:64, 1991.
77. Borch K, et al. Hemorrhagic gastritis. Acta Chir Scand 154:211, 1987.
78. Ahlquist DA, McGill DB, Schwartz S. Fecal blood levels in health and disease—A study using Hemoquant. N Engl J Med 312:422, 1985.
79. Herzog P, et al. Cecal blood loss in patients with colonic polyps: A comparison of measurements with ^{51}Chromium-labelled erythrocytes and with the hemoccult test. Gastroenterology 83:957, 1982.
80. Bowden TA, et al. Occult gastrointestinal bleeding: Locating the cause. Am Surg 46:80, 1980.

31

Acute Abdominal Pain: Physiology of the Acute Abdomen

Stuart I. Myers and Thomas A. Miller

The term *acute abdomen* refers to the sudden unexpected onset of acute abdominal pain, usually accompanied by other symptoms such as nausea, vomiting, anorexia, and abdominal distention. Such pain may be secondary to many etiologic possibilities, all of which can present clinically in a variety of ways, depending on the underlying anatomic focus of disease, the duration of the pathophysiologic process, and the specific pathology involved. Accurate diagnosis of the cause of an acute abdomen depends on the physician's understanding of the embryology, anatomy, neurophysiology, and natural history of each potential specific etiologic factor. The goal of this chapter is to examine the physiologic derangements responsible for the development of the acute abdomen and how such knowledge aids in its diagnosis and treatment.

EMBRYOLOGY OF ABDOMINAL VISCERA

Acute abdominal pain can originate from virtually any intra-abdominal structure, and at times even from extra-abdominal sources. Thus diagnosis of the underlying disease process responsible for the development of an acute abdomen requires accurate knowledge of the embryology of these abdominal structures and extra-abdominal organs such as the heart, lungs, and esophagus.

Development of the Heart, Lungs, and Diaphragm

The vascular system of the human embryo starts to develop between 3 and 4 weeks of gestation. The original cardiogenic plexus that will form the heart is located anterior to the prochordal and the neural plates. As the central nervous system grows rapidly in the cephalic direction, it extends over the central cardiogenic area. The heart tubes come to lie in a new area ventral to the foregut as it descends into the pericardial cavity. At the beginning of the fourth week, the partitioning into chambers and the ingrowth to the heart of the autonomic nerves begin[1-3] (Fig. 31-1). The central tendon of the diaphragm (as well

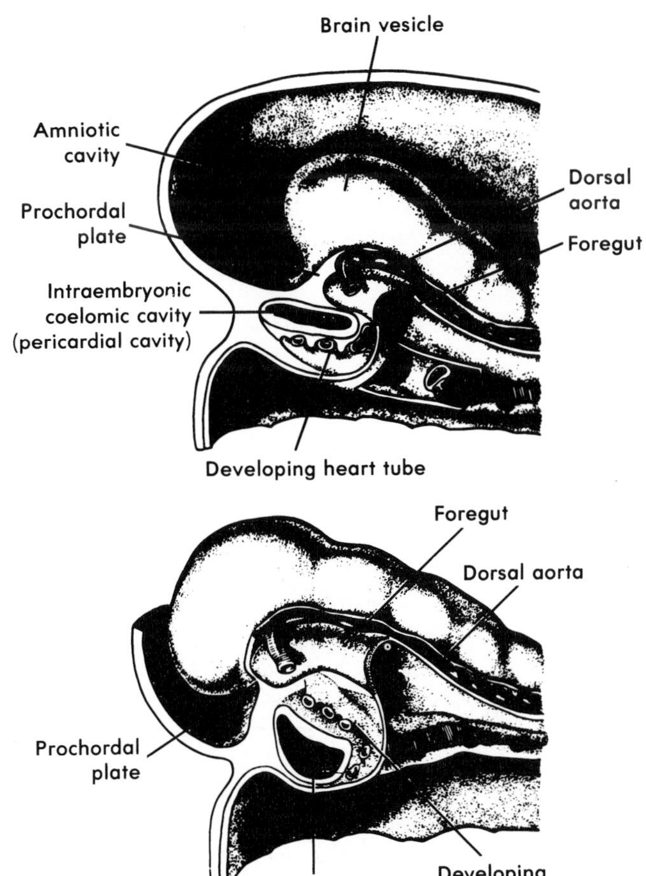

Fig. 31-1. Results of the rapid growth of the brain vesicles on the position of the pericardial cavity and the developing heart tube. Initially the angiogenetic cell clusters and the pericardial cavity are located in front of the prechordal plate. As a result of the rotation along a transverse axis through the prechordal plate, the cardiogenic plexus finally comes to lie dorsal to the pericardial cavity. (From Langman J. Medical Embryology, 2nd ed. Baltimore: Williams & Wilkins, 1969.)

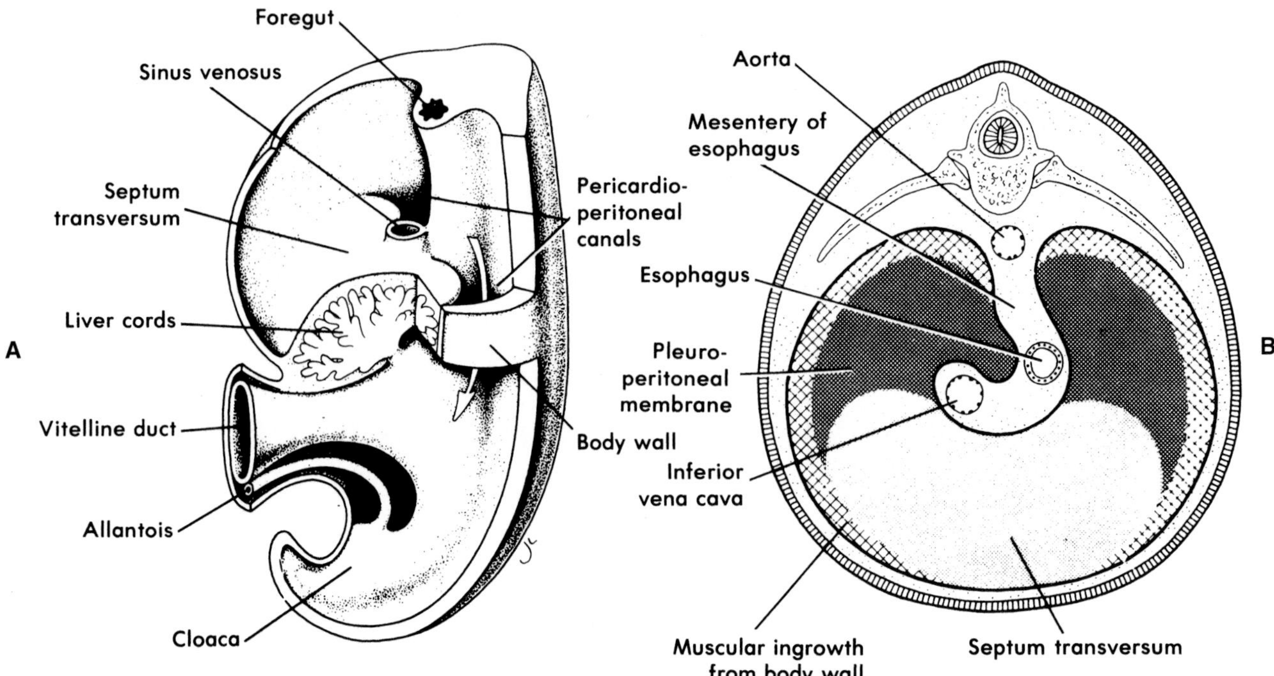

Fig. 31-2. **A,** Model of a portion of an embryo of approximately 5 weeks. Parts of the body wall and the septum transversum have been removed to show the pericardioperitoneal canals. Note the size and thickness of the septum transversum and the liver cords penetrating the mesenchyme. **B,** Schematic representation of the definitive diaphragm, indicating the origin of the various components. (From Langman J. Medical Embryology, 2nd ed. Baltimore: Williams & Wilkins, 1969.)

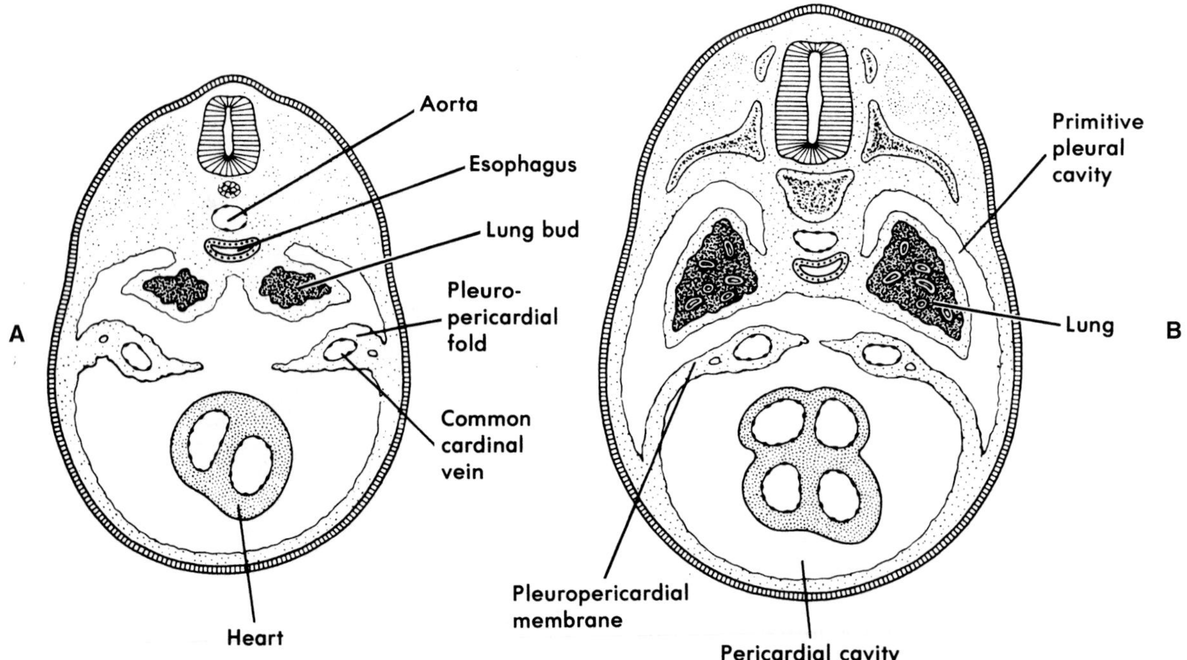

Fig. 31-3. Schematic drawings at two successive stages of development showing the transformation of the pericardioperitoneal canals into the primitive pleural cavities and the formation of the pleuropericardial membranes. **A,** Note the relationship of the common cardinal vein to the pleuropericardial ridge. **B,** As a result of the expansion of the pericardioperitoneal canals, the mesenchyme of the body wall is split into the pleuropericardial membranes and the definitive body wall. (From Langman J. Medical Embryology, 2nd ed. Baltimore: Williams & Wilkins, 1969.)

as part of the liver) originates from the septum transversum. However, this does not separate the pericardial cavity from the abdominal contents because the lateral aspects of the pericardioperitoneal canals remain open and connect the cavities. These canals are vitally important to the growing lung buds and eventually contain most of the lung growth and become the primitive pleural cavities. The caudal expansion of the pericardioperitoneal canals is limited by the pleuroperitoneal fold that originates from the cranial ligament of the original mesonephros. This fold expands in an anterior and medial direction and by the seventh week fuses with the mesentery of the esophagus and the septum transversum to form the diaphragm. Invading myoblasts from the body wall contribute to the development of the muscle of the diaphragm. These myoblasts are derived from the third through the fifth cervical segments, and their innervation (i.e., phrenic nerve) remains as the central diaphragm descends from the original position in the neck to its adult position. The peripheral portion of the diaphragm, formed from the body wall, retains its innervation by the lower seven intercostal nerves that supply the adjacent body wall[1-3] (Figs. 31-2 and 31-3).

Development of the Gut

The gut begins to develop during the fourth week of gestation. The primitive gut is derived from both the endoderm (which gives rise to most of the epithelium and glands) and the mesoderm (which gives rise to muscular and fibrous parts surrounding the endodermal lining). The epithelium of the primitive mouth and anus is derived from surface ectoderm and develops separately from the primitive gut tube. Because of this circumstance, the ectodermal and endodermal elements of these two regions develop separate blood supplies, lymphatic drainage systems, and neural innervations. The gut tube is comprised of a foregut, midgut, and hindgut. Each of these regions has its own blood supply and nervous innervation and retains these distinctions throughout development and into adulthood.

Foregut

The foregut extends from the pharynx to the duodenum at the level of entrance of the common bile duct. Caudal to the primitive pharynx and respiratory tract is the narrow esophagus, which widens to form the stomach and duodenum. During formation, the stomach rotates around its longitudinal axis in a 90-degree clockwise fashion that results in its left side facing anteriorly and its right side facing posteriorly. The left vagus nerve thus becomes anterior, and the right vagus nerve becomes posterior in its location. The posterior portion of the stomach also grows more than the anterior portion during this rotation, which gives rise to the greater and lesser curvatures. Of further note, the duodenum takes on its U-shaped loop configuration during this rotation and rotates to the right to assume its retroperitoneal location. The liver bud develops as a ventral outgrowth of endoderm and grows into the septum transversum to form the liver and the various components of the biliary tract. The pancreas develops as separate ventral and dorsal buds that arise from endoderm distal to the liver bud. The ventral pancreatic bud develops into the major portion of the pancreatic head, whereas the dorsal bud develops into the dorsal pancreas, which consists of the superior pancreatic head, the uncinate process, and the pancreatic body and tail. Although not actually part of the foregut, the spleen develops from mesenchymal cells derived from the stomach mesentery and obtains a similar blood supply to the foregut, that is, the celiac artery[1-3] (Figs. 31-4 to 31-6).

Midgut

The midgut can be separated into cranial and caudal portions. The cranial portion includes the duodenum distal to the entrance of the common bile duct, all the jejunum, and the proximal part of the ileum. The caudal portion includes the distal ileum, appendix, ascending colon, and

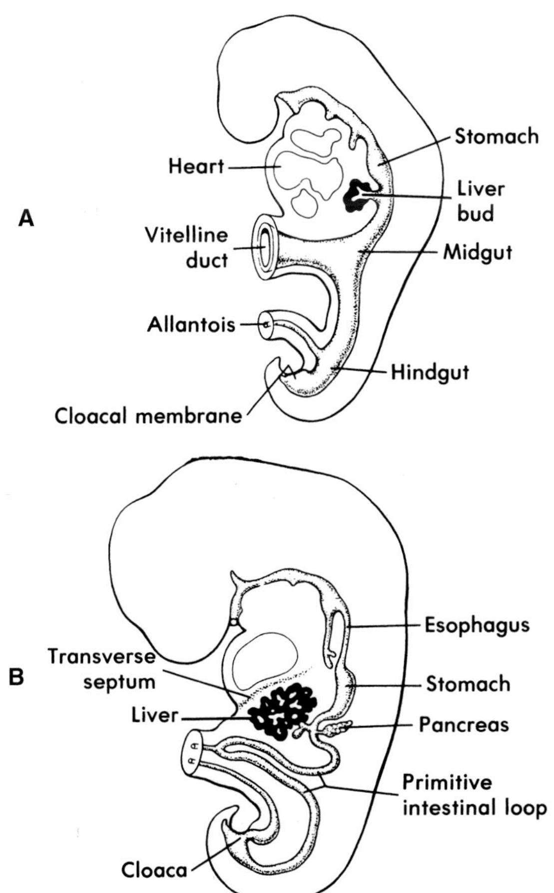

Fig. 31-4. A, Drawing of a 3 mm embryo (approximately 25 days) to show the primitive gastrointestinal tract. Note the formation of the hepatic diverticulum. The hepatic diverticulum is formed by the entodermal epithelial lining of the terminal part of the foregut. **B,** Drawing of a 5 mm embryo (approximately 32 days). The epithelial liver cords penetrate the mesenchyme of the transverse septum. Note the primary intestinal loop. (From Langman J. Medical Embryology, 2nd ed. Baltimore: Williams & Wilkins, 1969.)

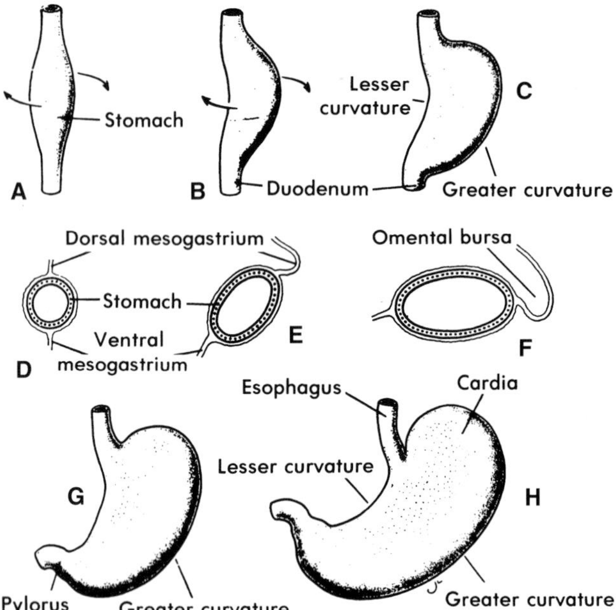

Fig. 31-5. Schematic representation of the positional changes of the stomach. **A, B,** and **C,** Rotation of the stomach along its longitudinal axis as seen from anterior; **D, E,** and **F,** in transverse section the effect of rotation on the peritoneal attachments; **G** and **H,** rotation of the stomach around the anteroposterior axis (seen from anterior). (From Langman J. Medical Embryology, 2nd ed. Baltimore: Williams & Wilkins, 1969.)

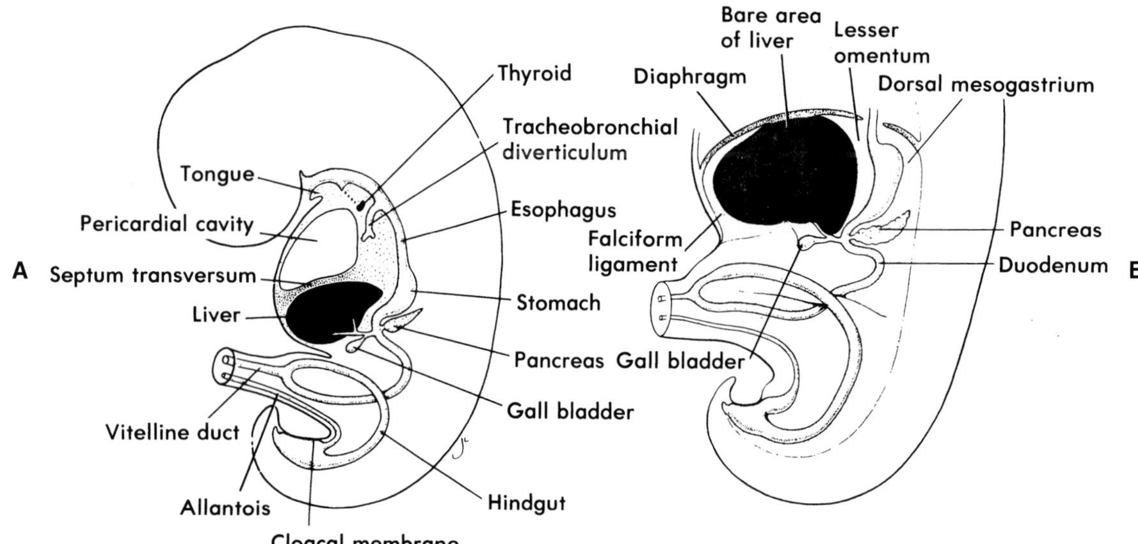

Fig. 31-6. A, Drawing of a 9 mm embryo (approximately 36 days). The liver expands caudally into the abdominal cavity. Note condensation of mesenchyme in the area between the liver and the pericardial cavity, foreshadowing the formation of the diaphragm. **B,** Drawing of a slightly older embryo. Note falciform ligament extending between liver and anterior abdominal wall, lesser omentum between liver and anterior abdominal wall, and lesser omentum between liver and foregut (stomach and duodenum). The liver is entirely surrounded by peritoneum, except in its contact area with the diaphragm. This area is known as the bare area of the liver. (From Langman J. Medical Embryology, 2nd ed. Baltimore: Williams & Wilkins, 1969.)

the proximal two thirds of the transverse colon. The apex of the midgut is represented by the vitelline or omphalomesenteric duct. This duct, when patent in the adult, persists of a Meckel's diverticulum. The midgut greatly elongates during its development, forming the primary intestinal loop. The cranial portion elongates much more than the caudal portion. This elongation causes a physiologic herniation during the sixth week of gestation as the abdominal cavity temporarily becomes too small to adequately contain the primary intestinal loop. At this stage of development, the primary intestinal loop also rotates 270 degrees in a counterclockwise direction around the axis of the superior mesenteric artery from which it derives its blood supply. After the third month the greatly elongated small intestinal loops and colon begin to return to the abdominal cavity, which by now has also developed to an adequate size to accommodate these structures. The jejunum returns first and lies normally on the left side, whereas the cecum enters last, lying in the right upper quadrant at first and then descending into its permanent position in the right lower quadrant[1-3] (Fig. 31-7).

Hindgut

The hindgut extends from the origin of the distal one third of the transverse colon to the cloacal swelling. The cloacal membrane represents the contact area between the surface ectoderm and endoderm of the cloaca. The hindgut is at first connected to the cloaca as is the allantois. As further development occurs, a urorectal septum forms in the angle between the allantois and the hindgut, dividing the cloaca into its two portions: an anterior urogenital sinus and a posterior anorectal canal. Thus the cloacal membrane also divides into two distinct areas, an anal membrane and a urogenital membrane separated by the

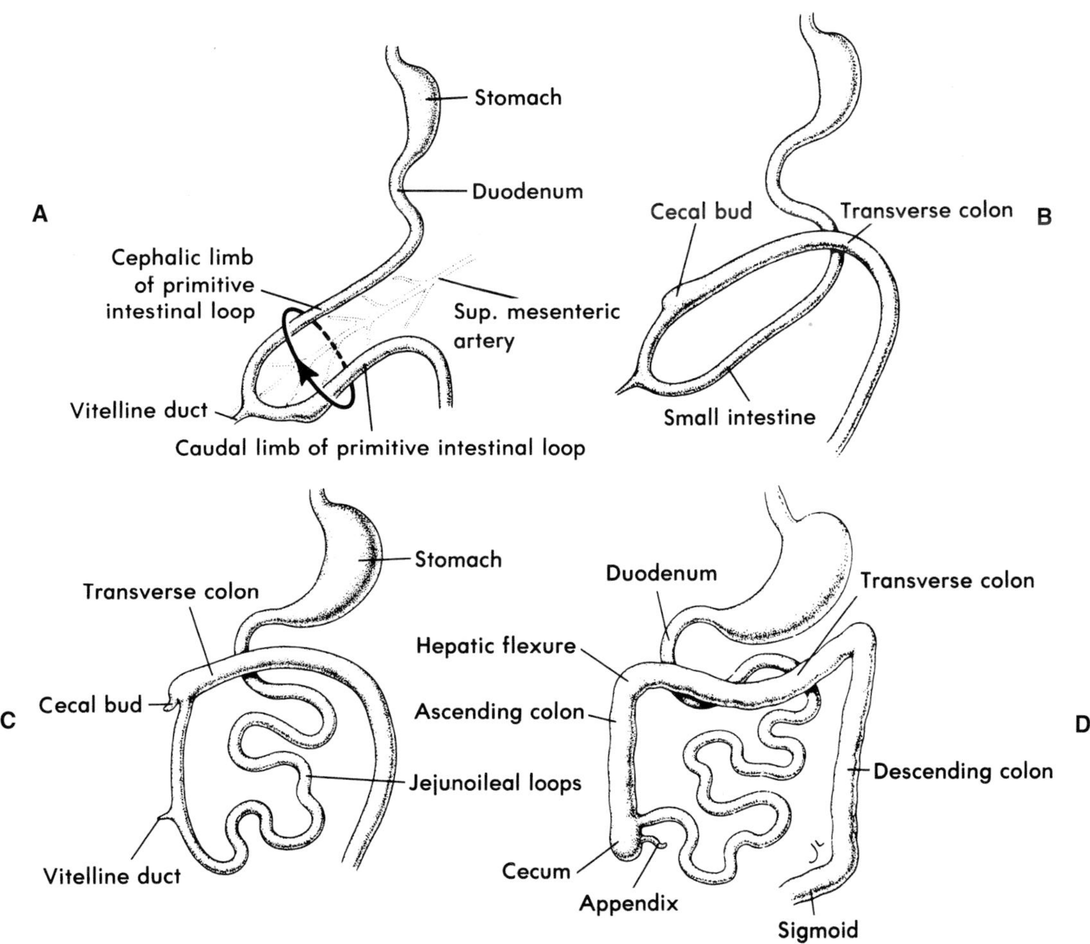

Fig. 31-7. A, Schematic drawing of the primitive intestinal loop before rotation (lateral view). The superior mesenteric artery forms the axis of the loop. Arrow indicates the direction of the anticlockwise rotation. **B,** Similar view as in **A,** showing the primitive intestinal loop after 180-degree anticlockwise rotation. The transverse colon passes in front of the duodenum. **C,** Anterior view of the intestinal loops after 270-degree anticlockwise rotation. Note the coiling of the small intestinal loops and the position of the cecal bud in the right upper quadrant of the abdomen. **D,** Similar view as in **C,** with the intestinal loops in the final position. Cecum and appendix are located in the right lower quadrant of the abdomen. (From Langman J. Medical Embryology, 2nd ed. Baltimore: Williams & Wilkins, 1969.)

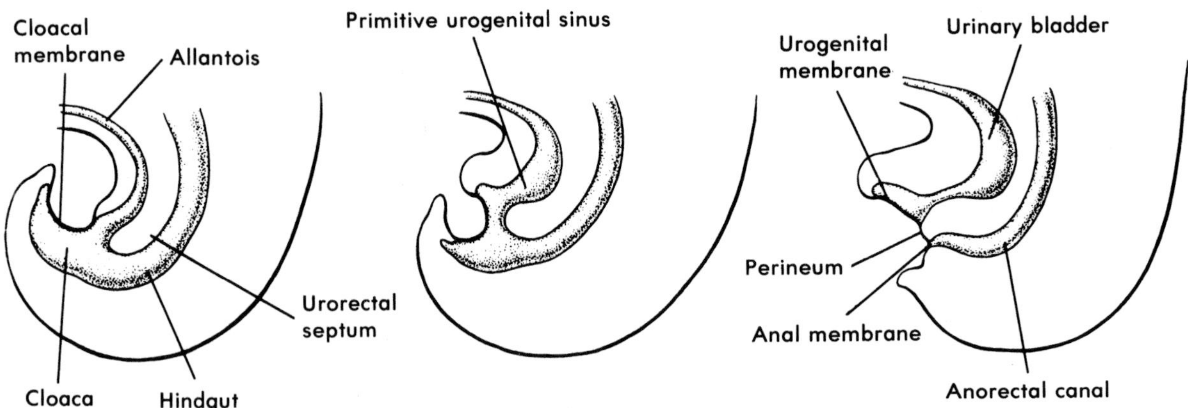

Fig. 31-8. Drawings of the cloacal region in embryos at successive stages of development. Note route of descent followed by the urorectal septum (from figure on left to figure on right) and the formation of the anorectal canal and the perineum. (From Langman J. Medical Embryology, 2nd ed. Baltimore: Williams & Wilkins, 1969.)

perineum. The anal membrane forms on the bottom of the proctoderm and becomes surrounded by mesenchymal swellings that develop into the anal glands. By the ninth week, the anal membrane ruptures, forming an open communication between the hindgut and the outside of the body. The upper part of the anorectal canal develops from the hindgut and its endoderm and is supplied by the artery of the hindgut, the inferior mesenteric artery. The lower portion of the anorectal canal forms from the surface ectoderm and is supplied by its vascular supply, the internal iliac artery[1-3] (Fig. 31-8).

Development of Mesenteries

Initially during development, the foregut, midgut, and hindgut are in contact with the posterior abdominal wall. At the 8 mm embryo stage this mesenchymal bridge becomes membranous, forming the dorsal mesentery. The divisions of this mesentery derive their names from the organs to which they are attached. These divisions are the dorsal mesogastrium in the area of the stomach, the mesoduodenum in the area of the duodenum, and the dorsal mesocolon in the area of the colon. The dorsal mesentery of the primary intestinal loop is termed the mesentery proper. Throughout development the mesentery serves as the conduit through which traverses the arterial blood supply, venous and lymphatic drainage routes, and neural pathways that supply the gut. In spite of rotational changes that take place in the gut and the ultimate fixation of the duodenum and ascending and descending portions of the colon to the retroperitoneum, the neural pathways and the vascular supply and drainage routes remain within the dorsal mesentery, originating as midline structures.

The permanent retroperitoneal position of the duodenum results from the rotational changes in the stomach and duodenum already described, as well as pressure effects attendant to the enlarging pancreas. The duodenum and pancreas become pressed against the dorsal body wall. The mesoduodenum fuses with the adjacent somatic peritoneum; and both structures disappear, as most of the duodenum becomes fixed in the retroperitoneum, except the proximal duodenum, which remains intraperitoneal and attached to a dorsal mesoduodenum. In similar fashion the ascending and descending colons assume their adult positions in the peritoneal cavity, with their mesenteries becoming adherent to the adjacent somatic peritoneum with subsequent fusion and fixation of these structures to the retroperitoneum. The cecum and appendix do not fix and are free intraperitoneal structures. The transverse colon retains its mesentery and covers the duodenum with an additional peritoneal layer that later fuses with the greater omentum.

The peritoneum is composed of continuous visceral and parietal layers. Although both layers are derived from mesoderm, each develops separately. The visceral layer is derived from splanchnic mesoderm originating from the gut tube, and its blood supply is through visceral vessels. In contrast, the parietal layer is derived from somatic mesoderm originating from the lining on the inside of the body cavity, and its blood supply is through blood vessels of the body wall. Similarly, the nerve supply to each layer differs. The visceral layer is supplied by autonomic nerves (i.e., sympathetic and parasympathetic), and the parietal layer is supplied by somatic innervation (i.e., spinal nerves). The pathways involving the sensation of pain differ from each layer and differ in quality as well. Visceral pain is dull, crampy, and aching; whereas parietal pain is sharp, often severe, and persistent[1-3] (Figs. 31-9 and 31-10).

Development of the Urogenital Tract

Development of the urogenital tract is equally complex and begins as a growth of intermediate mesoderm parallel to the dorsal mesentery that forms the rudimentary pronephric glomeruli and pronephric ducts. These glomeruli evolve in the thorax and are replaced by devel-

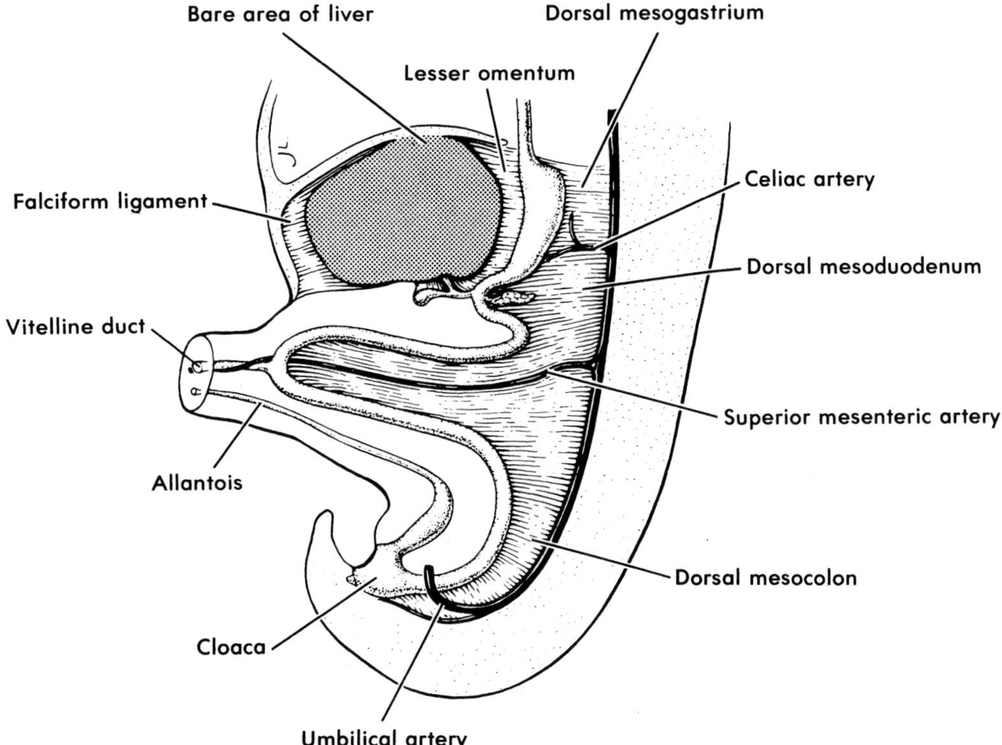

Fig. 31-9. Schematic drawing showing the primitive dorsal and ventral mesenteries. Note how the liver is connected to the ventral abdominal wall and to the stomach by the falciform ligament and lesser omentum, respectively. The superior mesenteric artery runs through the mesentery proper and continues toward the yolk sac as the vitelline artery. (From Langman J. Medical Embryology, 2nd ed. Baltimore: Williams & Wilkins, 1969.)

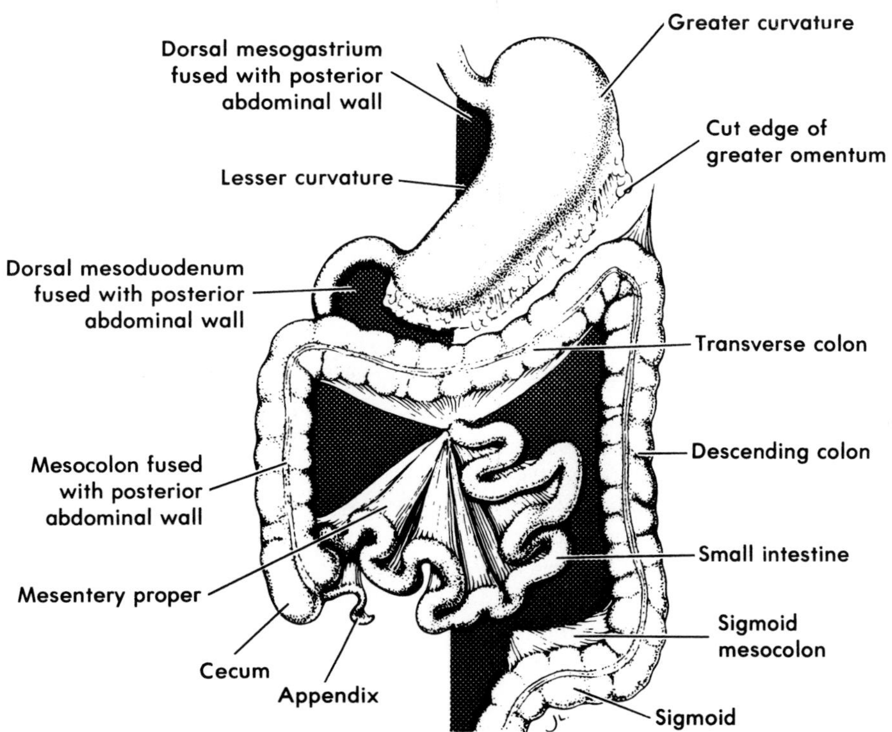

Fig. 31-10. Frontal view of the intestinal loops after removal of the greater omentum. The cross-hatched areas indicate the parts of the dorsal mesentery that fuse with the posterior abdominal wall. Note the line of attachment of the mesentery proper. (From Langman J. Medical Embryology, 2nd ed. Baltimore: Williams & Wilkins, 1969.)

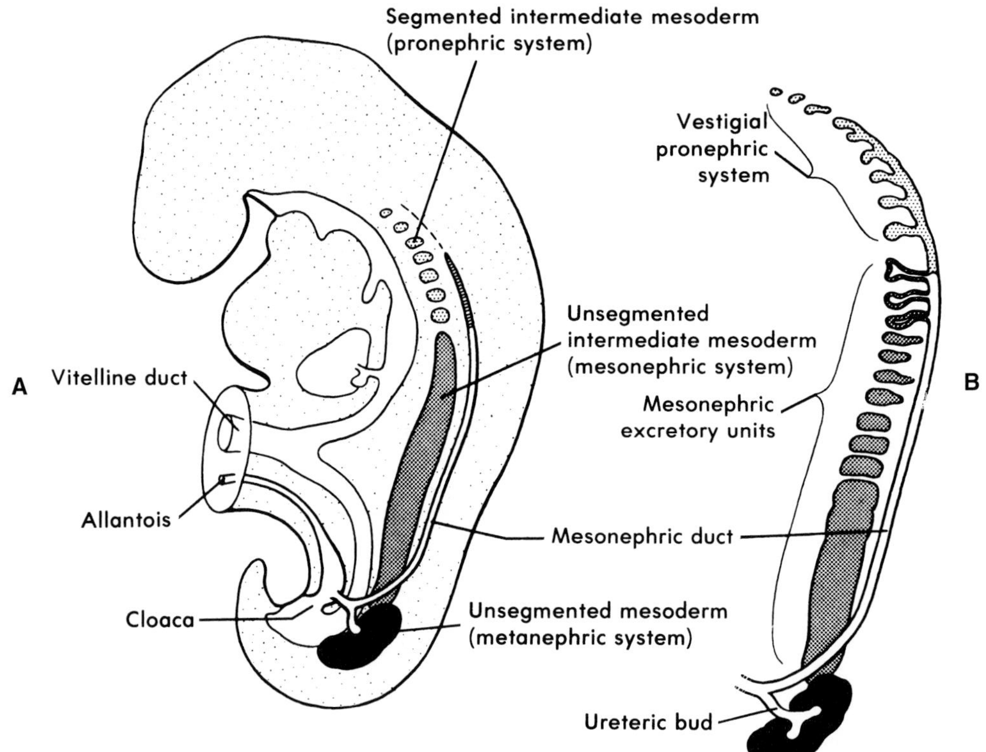

Fig. 31-11. **A,** Schematic diagram showing the relation of the intermediate mesoderm of the pronephric, mesonephric, and metanephric systems. In the cervical and upper thoracic regions the intermediate mesoderm is segmented; in the lower thoracic, lumbar, and sacral regions it forms a solid, unsegmented mass of tissue, the nephrogenic cord. Note the longitudinal collecting duct, initially formed by the pronephros but later taken over by the mesonephros. **B,** Schematic representation of the excretory tubules of the pronephric and mesonephric systems in a 5-week-old embryo. The ureteric bud penetrates the metanephric tissue. Note the remnant of the pronephric excretory tubules and longitudinal collecting duct. (From Langman J. Medical Embryology, 2nd ed. Baltimore: Williams & Wilkins, 1969.)

opment of mesonephric glomeruli that lie between T8 and L4 vertebrae. The degeneration of the pronephric glomeruli is accompanied by a degeneration of the proximal pronephric duct. The remaining pronephric duct is called the mesonephric duct. The mesonephros itself only functions for months 2 and 3 of gestation and is replaced by the metanephros. The ureteric bud arises from the caudal end of the mesonephric duct and grows into the intermediate mesoderm, which begins to develop the metanephric cap. The metanephric cap develops the glomerular capsule, the convoluted tubules, and the loop of Henle. The ureteric cap develops the major and minor calyces, collecting tubules, renal pelvis, and ureters. The forming kidneys initially develop in the pelvis but later ascend to take their adult positions. When the ascent is complete, they are then innervated by autonomic nerves[1-3] (Figs. 31-11 through 31-15).

The genital ridges appear in the fourth week and lie between the mesonephros and dorsal mesentery along the midline. These ridges are the earliest gonads and are formed from coelomic epithelium and mesenchyma. The

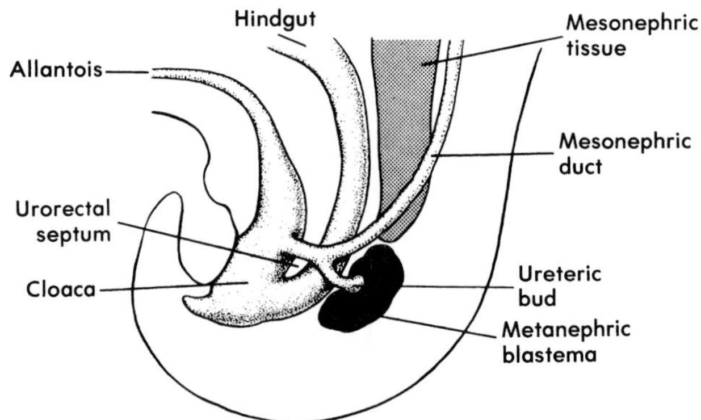

Fig. 31-12. Schematic drawing to show the relationship of the hindgut and cloaca at the end of the fifth week. The ureteric bud begins to penetrate the metanephric blastema. Note the urorectal septum, which will grow in caudal direction to divide the cloaca into the urogenital sinus and anorectal canal. (From Langman J. Medical Embryology, 2nd ed. Baltimore: Williams & Wilkins, 1969.)

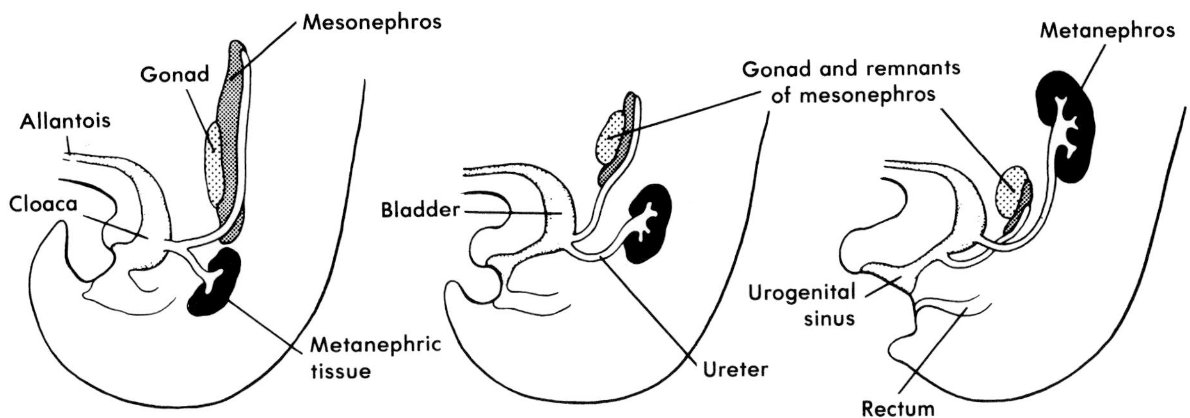

Fig. 31-13. Ascent of the kidney. Note the change in position between the metanephros and mesonephric system. The mesonephric system degenerates almost entirely, and only a few remnants persist in close contact with the gonad. In both the male and female embryo the gonad descends from its original level to a much lower position. (From Langman J. Medical Embryology, 2nd ed. Baltimore: Williams & Wilkins, 1969.)

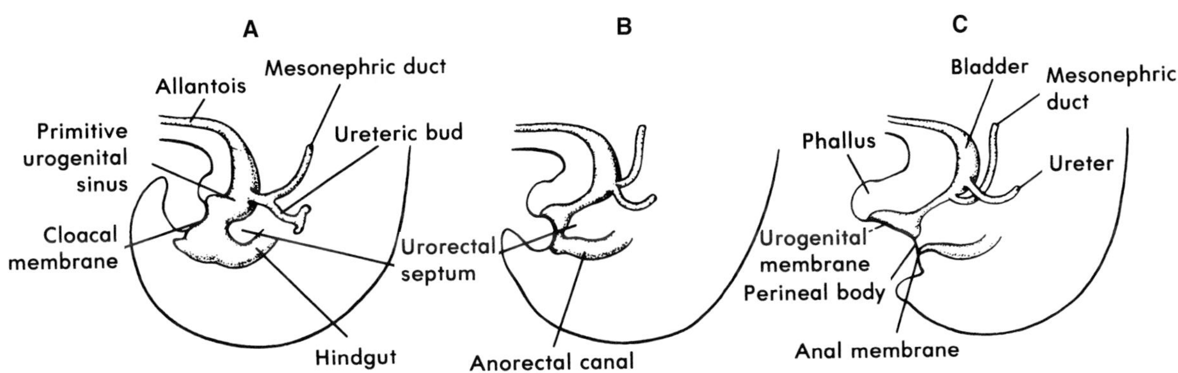

Fig. 31-14. Diagrams showing the division of the cloaca into the urogenital sinus and anorectal canal. Note that the mesonephric duct is gradually absorbed into the wall of the urogenital sinus and that the ureters enter separately. **A,** End of fifth week. **B,** 7 weeks. **C,** 8 weeks. (From Langman J. Medical Embryology, 2nd ed. Baltimore: Williams & Wilkins, 1969.)

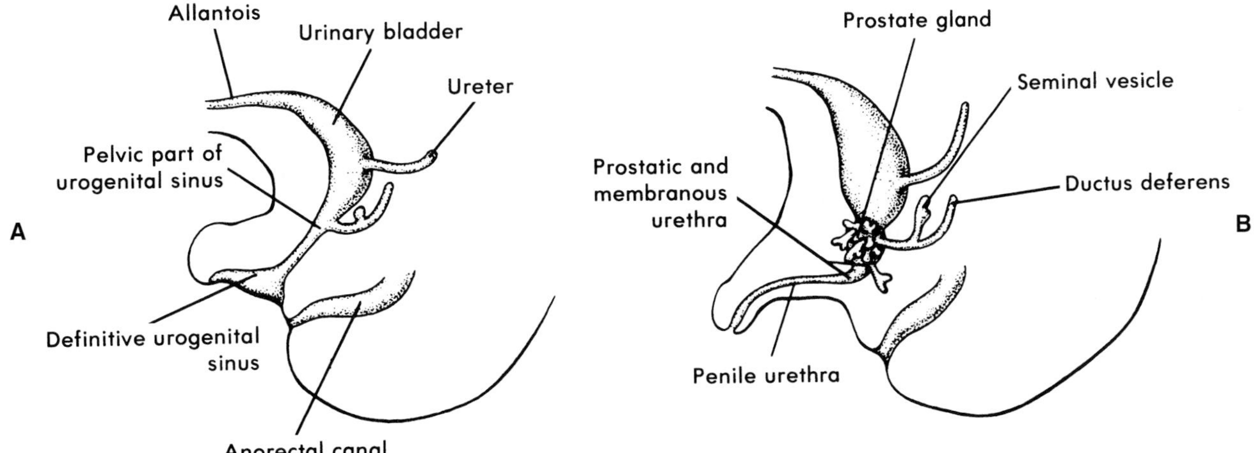

Fig. 31-15. A, Development of the urogenital sinus into the urinary bladder, the pelvic part of the urogenital sinus, and the definitive urogenital sinus. **B,** In the male the urogenital sinus develops into the prostatic, membranous, and penile portions of the urethra. The prostate gland is formed by outbuddings of the urethra, whereas the seminal vesicles are formed by an outbudding of the ductus deferens. (From Langman J. Medical Embryology, 2nd ed. Baltimore: Williams & Wilkins, 1969.)

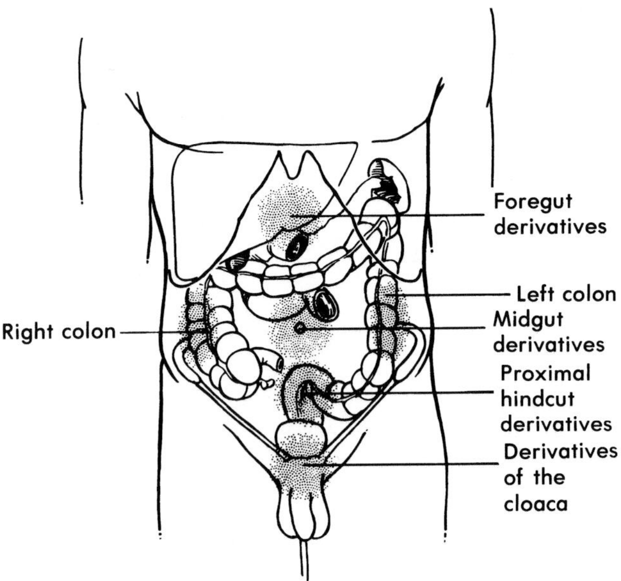

Fig. 31-16. Visceral pain from most parts of the gastrointestinal tract is felt in the midline at four levels that are related to the four embryologic divisions of the tract. The exception is visceral pain from the right or left side of the colon that may be felt in the right or left flank, respectively. (From Currie DJ. Abdominal Pain. New York: Hemisphere Publishing, 1979.)

germ cells appear in the yolk sac at the sixth week of development and migrate to the genital ridges. The germ cells either form the male testis or the female ovary. The testis comes to lie 10 segments below its level of origin in the second month as the body elongates and is thus a shift in position in relation to the body wall. The testis remains in close proximity to the inguinal canal until the seventh month, when it descends through the inguinal ring into the scrotum. The testis retains its original blood supply from the aorta. The female ovary descends less than the testis, but it still descends to a level below the pelvic rim.

The male and female embryos develop two pairs of genital ducts during the sixth week of development, the wolffian ducts and the müllerian ducts. The müllerian ducts arise from the coelomic epithelium from the urogenital ridge and cranially open in the coelomic cavity with a funnellike structure that forms the abdominal ostia of the fallopian tube and the remainder of the fallopian tube. Caudally the müllerian duct runs lateral to the mesonephric duct and crosses the midline to fuse with the müllerian duct from the opposite side and forms a septum that fuses and forms the uterovaginal canal. The caudal portion of the fused müllerian ducts continues to grow caudally to the wall of the urogenital sinus. The wolffian ducts open on either side of the ureterovaginal canal into the urogenital sinus. In the male the wolffian duct forms the ductus deferens, and the müllerian duct disappears. In the female the müllerian ducts continue development to form the oviducts, uterus, and part of the vagina.

Embryologic Basis of Abdominal Pain

Knowledge of the embryologic development of structures within the abdomen can add greatly in the anatomic localization of abdominal pain. Since the normal embryologic development of abdominal viscera proceeds with bilateral midline sensory innervation, pain arising from such viscera is usually described as being in the abdominal midline. The position of pain in the midline is determined by the embryologic origin of the viscera involved. An epigastric location of abdominal pain is typical of a foregut origin. Umbilical midline pain is more typical of pain arising from the midgut. Hypogastric (i.e., lower abdominal) midline pain is more indicative of an origin from hindgut structures. Finally, pain arising in the pelvis is more typical of disease originating from structures derived from the cloaca (Fig. 31-16).

PHYSIOLOGY OF PAIN MEDIATION[4-8]

Anatomic Pathways

For the sensation of abdominal pain to occur, receptors for pain known as nociceptors must be activated by some damaging stimulus. When this occurs, such nociceptive input is transmitted from the site of origin to the central nervous system through small, thinly myelinated or unmyelinated fibers termed the A-delta and C-neuronal fibers, respectively. The A-delta fibers are rapidly transmitting and give the sensation of a sharp, pricking, well-localized type of pain. These fibers, measuring 3 to 4 μm in diameter, are distributed principally to muscle and skin and are primarily involved with the transmission of somatic pain through spinal nerves. In contrast, the C-fibers are more slowly transmitting and give rise to the sensation of a dull, sickening, poorly localized type of pain that is more gradual in its onset and of longer duration. These fibers are located in the walls of hollow viscera and in the capsule of solid organs; they are also found in muscle, periosteum, and parietal peritoneum. These fibers are primarily involved in the transmission of visceral pain through the autonomic nervous system. Much of the gastrointestinal tract is also innervated by branches of the vagus nerve. Despite the fact that 90% of these fibers are sensory, they do not appear to be involved with the mediation of pain, since the ability to feel pain arising from abdominal viscera is unaltered following vagotomy. Most of the afferent input from the vagus nerves appears to be concerned with modulation and regulation of gastrointestinal motility and secretion.

The neural pathways responsible for pain mediation differ, depending on whether the pain is derived from the abdominal wall or originates in the intra-abdominal viscera. The anterior and lateral abdominal walls are supplied by nerves arising from spinal segments T7 through L1; the posterior abdominal wall by L2 through L5. Pain arising from the abdominal wall is transmitted to the spinal cord through the spinal nerves (Fig. 31-17). Because such pain fibers enter the spinal cord on the same side from which the focus of pain arises, it is perceived as originating on

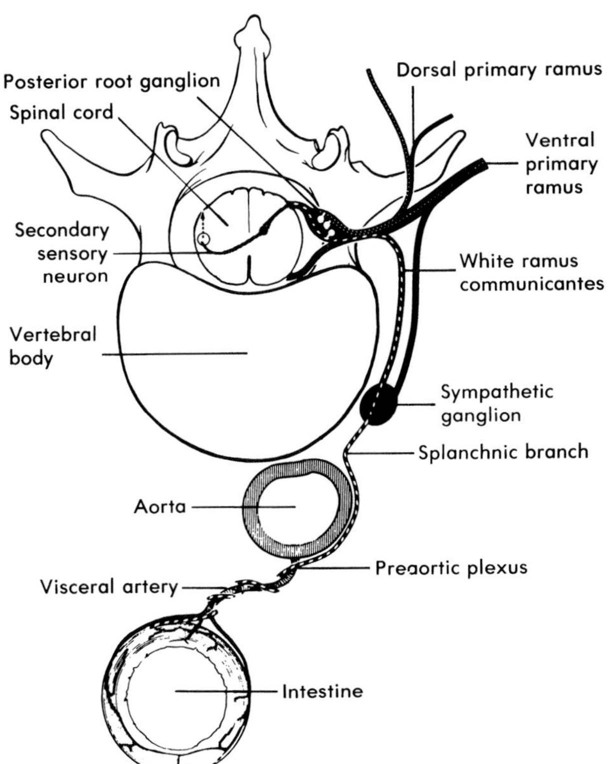

Fig. 31-17. Pathways of the peripheral processes of the cells of a typical posterior root ganglion. Some pass through the spinal nerve to the skin or other somatic structures with the dorsal or ventral primary rami. Others supply the viscera through the white rami communicantes, sympathetic ganglia and trunk, and preaortic plexus to reach a viscus such as the intestine by traveling with its artery. (From Currie DJ. Abdominal Pain. New York: Hemisphere Publishing, 1979.)

that side (i.e., right or left). Further, such pain is additionally localized to the area of the abdomen from which it originates (e.g., right upper abdomen vs. right lower abdomen). In contrast, pain arising from intra-abdominal viscera is generally felt in the midline because sensory input from such viscera generally enters the spinal cord on both sides. As previously noted, the embryologic derivation of these viscera determines whether this pain is perceived in the epigastrium, the periumbilical region, the hypogastrium, or the pelvis. The innervation of the gut depends on its embryologic origin. In general, the initial position of each structure (e.g., diaphragm, foregut) determines its segmental afferent innervation that remains with that structure even though its anatomic location may change during later development in utero. Afferent nerves innervate viscera as part of the plexus that is located around the arterial supply to that viscus. Thus foregut structures (including the spleen) derive their arterial supply from the celiac artery. Sensory innervation is derived from nerves originating from the celiac plexus. Pain sensation is mediated by the greater splanchnic nerves (T5 to T9 spinal cord level). The arterial supply to the midgut is the superior mesenteric artery and its branches. Afferent sensory input is from the lesser and least splanchnic nerves (T8 to L1 spinal levels). The pancreas is interesting, since it develops at the border of the foregut and midgut and derives arterial and afferent innervation from both the celiac and superior mesenteric arteries and plexuses. The hindgut receives separate arterial and afferent supply proximally and distally. The proximal hindgut is supplied by the inferior mesenteric artery and the nerve fibers from the interior mesenteric plexus (T12 to L1 spinal cord levels). The distal hindgut receives its blood supply from the paired internal iliac arteries and its nerve branches, the lowest splanchnic nerve (T11 to L1 spinal segments), and the hypogastric plexus (S3 to S5 spinal segments). These nerve branches form the pelvic plexus, which arborizes distally with branches of the internal iliac artery (Fig. 31-18).

Sensory innervation of the genitourinary structures is also important to a proper understanding of the presentation of acute abdominal pain. The kidneys, ureter, vault of bladder, and gonads are supplied by visceral afferent nerves entering the spinal cord at T10 to L2. The sensory supply of the kidney, ureter, and gonads is from T10 to L1. The vault of the bladder derives its afferent nerve supply from T11 to L2 through the hypogastric plexus. The base of the bladder, ovary, uterine cervix, and upper vagina are cloacal structures and receive their blood supply from the internal iliac arteries and their afferent nerve supply from the hypogastric and pelvic plexuses. The rest of the uterus is supplied solely by the hypogastric plexus (T12 to L1) (see Fig. 31-18). The absolute number of nociceptive visceral afferent nerve fibers in any individual splanchnic nerve is quite small. The majority of sensory neurons and nerve fibers within these nerves are part of the enteric nervous system. These nerves are mostly involved with physiologic regulation of intestinal motility and secretion.[1-8]

Whether pain fibers are derived from visceral structures or the abdominal wall, they enter the spinal cord through the posterior nerve root (see Fig. 31-17). They then bifurcate and ascend or descend a distance of one to three spinal segments, forming part of what is termed the tract of Lissauer. The ganglion cells of these neurons have been separated histologically by Rexed[9] (on the basis of longitudinal arrangement of the neurons into columns and their underlying cytoarchitecture) into 10 lamina designated by I to X. Rexed laminae I, II, and III represent those neurons that terminate in the marginal zone and substantia gelatinosa; laminae IV, V, and VI in the nucleus proprius; and laminae VII and VIII in the intermediolateral nucleus. The proximal extension from the cell body located in the dorsal root ganglion of the first-order neuron passes into the spinal cord, ultimately synapsing in the dorsal horn, primarily in laminae I, V, and X.[5,10] Somatic nerves or nociceptors primarily synapse in laminae II to IV.[5,10,11] These second-order neurons are either relay cells that project axons that ultimately decussate in the anterolateral fasciculus to the brain stem and thalamus or interneurons that transmit pain information to other neu-

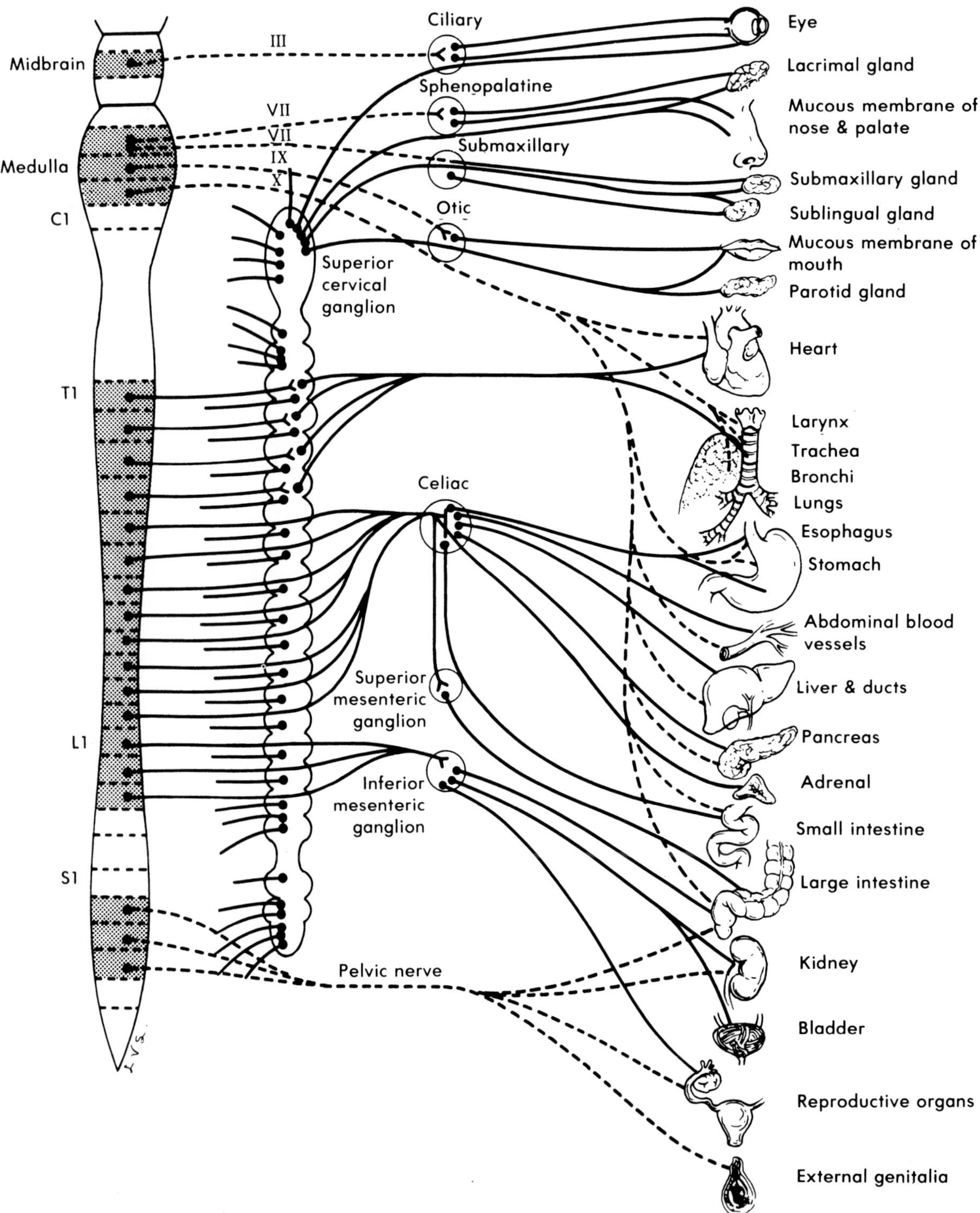

Fig. 31-18. Schematic representation of the transmission of visceral and somatic pain from its site of origin to the brain. (From Way LW. Abdominal pain and the acute abdomen. In Sleisenger MH, Fordtran JS, eds. Gastrointestinal Disease: Pathophysiology, Diagnosis, Management, 3rd ed. Philadelphia: WB Saunders, 1983.)

rons or relay cells. The second-order neuron then begins at the level of synapse in the dorsal horn, crosses the midline to the contralateral ventral region of the spinal cord, and ascends to the level of the thalamic nuclei, pons, and medulla, traveling primarily in the spinothalamic tract and the spinoreticular tract. Third-order neurons are then distributed from these basilar areas to higher levels of cortical perception, primarily to the somatosensory cortex, where ultimate pain perception is appreciated, and additionally to the limbic and frontal cortex, where the associated phenomenon of nausea, vomiting, and other physiologic responses are precipitated (Fig. 31-19).

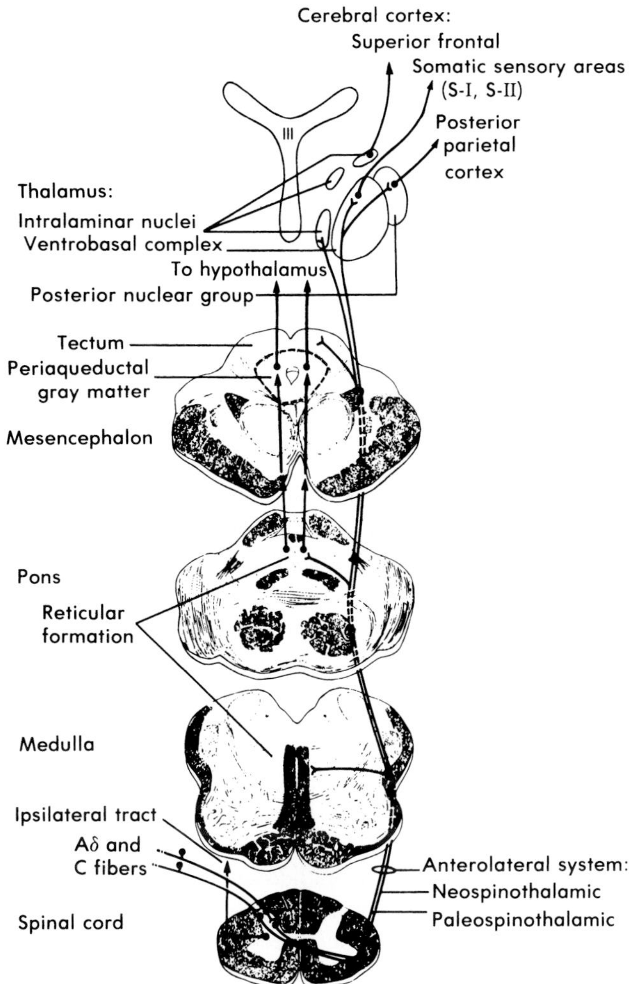

Fig. 31-19. Diagram of the autonomic nervous system. The visceral afferent fibers mediating pain travel with the sympathetic nerves, except for those from the pelvic organs, which follow the parasympathetics of the pelvic nerve. Sympathetics are represented here by solid lines; parasympathetics by dashed lines. (From Kandel ER, Schwartz JH, eds. Principles of Neuronal Science, 2nd ed. New York: Elsevier, 1985. Copyright 1985 by Elsevier Science Publishing Co.)

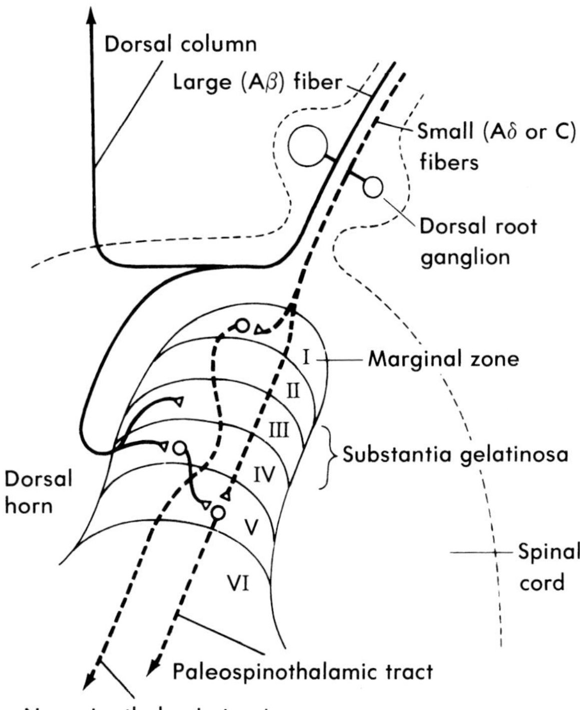

Fig. 31-20. Schematic drawing of dorsal horn of the spinal cord illustrating that nociceptive neurons, the axons of which form the ascending anterolateral system, are found in laminas I and V of the dorsal horn. Neurons in the marginal layer (lamina I) receive input primarily from small A and C fibers, but there is greater convergence of large- and small-fiber input on nociceptive neurons in lamina V. This difference is reflected in the electrophysiology of these cells. Many nociceptive neurons in the marginal layer do not respond to nonpainful touch stimuli, whereas those in the deeper layers display a wider dynamic range. (From Kandel ER, Schwartz JH, eds. Principles of Neuronal Science, 2nd ed. New York: Elsevier, 1985. Copyright 1985 by Elsevier Science Publishing Co.)

The dorsal horns of each spinal segment also contain inhibitory neurons for pain, which can affect the overall perception of pain. Inhibitory neurons begin initially in the periaqueductal gray area of the midbrain, traversing to structures in the medulla and reticular formation. Neuronal elements then descend to the level of substantia gelatinosa and release endogenous opioids and enkephalins. These substances activate inhibitory interneurons to decrease the ascending nociceptive pain information emanating from the various organs[12-14] (Fig. 31-20).

To further expand on the complexity of interactions regulating nociceptors, the cell bodies in Rexed laminae V of the dorsal horn receive information from both somatic and visceral pain fibers. This complex input of nociceptors contributes to the phenomenon of referred pain.[5,10]

The complex interactions of the afferent fibers just described can lead to the transmission of pain impulses or occasionally the inhibition of this transmission. Melzack and Wall[15] suggested a gate-control theory to explain this interaction. This theory proposed that the thick fibers within the substantia gelatinosa may actually exert a negative feedback effect (inhibitory) on the transmission of the thin fibers. Thus when excited, the thin fibers that ordinarily cause stimulation on the first transmission or "T" cells and the transmission of pain impulses could at times have their effects overridden by the thick fibers as if these latter fibers were acting as a gate. Complicating this potential interaction is the additional influence of the higher centers of the brain, which also can exert their influence by changing the threshold to pain impulse transmission through a positive or negative feedback effect.[4,8,15] The gate-control theory was proposed before the current understanding of the presence of many neuroactive sub-

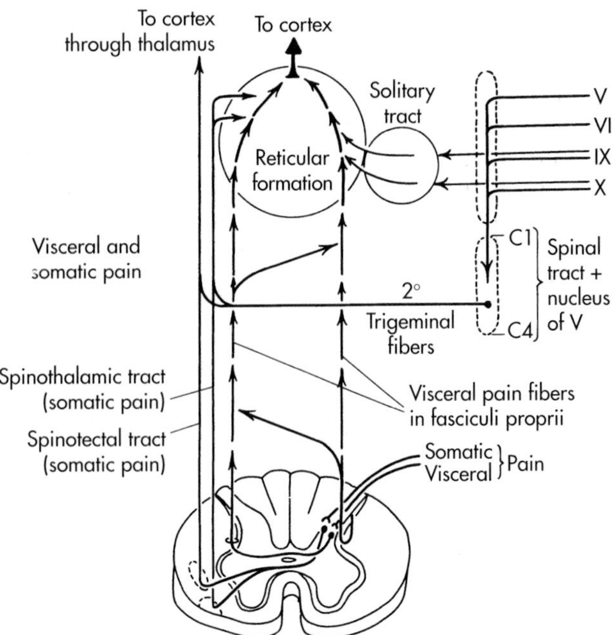

Fig. 31-21. The anterolateral system of spinothalamic, spinoreticular, and spinotectal fibers conveys information about pain to several regions of the brain stem and diencephalon. (From Kandel ER, Schwartz JH, eds. Principles of Neuronal Science, 2nd ed. New York: Elsevier, 1985. Copyright 1985 by Elsevier Science Publishing Co.)

stances described below was known and is presently being debated as an acceptable explanation for the mediation of pain. Whether such a gate does in fact exist remains to be established (Fig. 31-21).

Role of Neuroactive Agents in Mediating Pain

The classic pain pathways of nociception have been further complicated in complexity by the discovery of many neurogenic substances within the peripheral nervous system, spinal cord, and supraspinal nervous system that are now known to interact with neural impulses to both augment and inhibit transmission. Over the past 10 years, an increasing number of these substances have been identified in various animal species. A comprehensive discussion of these agents and the experimental evidence implicating their role in nociception are beyond the scope of this chapter. Only those agents thought to be important in the mediation of abdominal pain are discussed. These include the endogenous opioid system, substance P, and the monoamines.

Three major families of endogenous opioids have been described, each being derived from a different precursor molecule that contains the classic enkephalin sequence (Tyr-Gly-Gly-Phe), which indicates that it is indeed an opioid peptide.[4,8,16] The first family is the β-endorphin/corticotropin family, which has propiomelanocortin as its precursor. This precursor contains one opioid peptide sequence from which the β-endorphins, corticotropins, and melanotropins are derived. The β-endorphins are located primarily in the hypothalamus, have a limited axonal distribution, and are thought not to have activity in endogenous nociception. The second family is the enkephalin group, which is derived from the precursor molecule proenkephalin. Proenkephalin contains seven copies of the opioid sequence, six having a metenkephalin core and the other a leuenkephalin core (from which enkephalin is derived). The enkephalins are found in the spinal cord, amygdala, caudate, periductal gray, locus caeruleus, nucleus magnus raphae, and the thalamic periventricular nuclei of the brain. The third family is the dynorphin/neoendorphin family, derived from the precursor, prodynorphin. Prodynorphin has three opioid sequences that have a leuenkephalin core that gives rise to the dynorphins and neoendorphins. These substances are distributed within the spinal cord, amygdala, caudate, periaqueductal gray, locus caeruleus, and the magnocellular neurosecretory nuclei of the hypothalamus.[17,18]

Experimental studies have found a variety of subtypes of the enkephalins and dynorphins. These subtypes possess differences in amino acid structure and sequence. In addition, they have been shown pharmacologically to have different states of enzymatic degradation. Thus within each opioid family, different subtypes could be located in different areas of the nervous system that could conceivably modify neural transmission by speed and duration of action.

The complexity of the opioid system is further demonstrated by the discovery of at least five subtypes of the opioid receptors themselves. Such receptors have been classified as μ-, κ-, δ-, σ-, and the most recent ϵ-. The endogenous opioids and exogenous opiates (morphine, fentanyl, sufentanil) exert their effects by a complex interaction of agonism/antagonism on these receptors. The μ-receptors predominate in the brain stem and subcortical regions of the brain but are infrequently seen within the spinal cord. These receptors are highly selective to morphine and are responsible for most opiate and opioid analgesic properties. The β-receptors are the primary effectors of supraspinal analgesia, and the two major side effects associated with opiates are respiratory depression and decreased gastrointestinal motility.

Two separate subclasses of μ-receptors (μ_1 and μ_2) have been identified and discovered to have differing pharmacologic properties. Almost all the analgesic properties of opiates are derived from the μ_1-subclass. Additionally, the major side effects associated with opiates are not observed with selective stimulation of μ_1-receptors.

It appears that μ_2-receptor activation results in most of the side effects of opiates. This receptor is also known as the classic morphine selective receptor.

The κ-receptors are found predominantly in cortical and spinal locations and are the preferred site of the endogenous dynorphins. The classic drug that has been associated with this receptor (as well as the σ-receptor) is pentazocine. Although the analgesia is classified as both spinal and supraspinal, the effects on spinal pain transmission predominate. The κ-receptors exert their effects fully in a μ-tolerant individual, demonstrating that its actions are separate and independent of μ-stimulation.

The δ receptors make up the third group of opioid receptors responsible for analgesia. These receptors mediate spinal analgesia, primarily acting as antinociception for thermal stimuli. Thermal injury is not mediated by the κ-receptor class. Both enkephalins and β-dynorphins bind to these receptors; the enkephalins are the more selective of the two. The receptors have also been located diffusely in the cortical regions of the brain and may act either synergistically with or may modulate the activity of μ-receptors. The side effect most commonly associated with δ receptors is respiratory depression due to a decrease in the respiratory rate.

The σ-receptor appears to be unrelated to analgesia. It is probably responsible for some of the more addicting side effects of opiates, as with opium and heroin. Pentazocine is one of the classic compounds, along with heroin, that is an agonist for this receptor.

The last receptor class is the ϵ-receptor. It is highly selective for the β-endorphins, lacks affinity for the enkephalins, and does not appear to be related to analgesia. Little is known about ϵ-receptor function, and its role remains unclear.[19]

Substance P comprises the next major group of neuroactive substances. Substance P has been shown to increase both vascular permeability and bronchial smooth muscle contraction and has been found in primary afferent nerves involved in nociception in animal studies.[20] Patients with familial dysautonomia, a disease in which severe diminished pain and temperature threshold sensitivity exists, have depleted levels of substance P in the substantia gelatinosa.[21] Further, the effects of substance P seem to be blocked by exogenous morphine.[22] Taken together, these findings suggest that substance P is involved in nociception. Calcitonin gene–related peptide is another neuropeptide that exists in the neurons of the dorsal root ganglion (B1, B1-6). Substance P and calcitonin gene–related peptide are the two primary neurochemicals that coexist in the primary afferent neurons located in the dorsal root ganglion. Substance P and calcitonin gene–related peptide are transported and released centrally in the spinal cord and released at the level of the dorsal root ganglion.[7,23]

The third major family of neuroactive substances is the monoamines. The monoamines exert their effects both in the spinal cord and supraspinally. The action of the level of the dorsal horns of the spinal cord seems to be inhibition of those neurons excited by the nociceptive pathway. This antinociceptive effect appears to be initiated supraspinally and mediated through descending pathways to the level of the dorsal root nuclei. Serotonin is one of these monoamine substances.[24] It is located in serotoninergic cell bodies in the nucleus magnus raphae that give rise to pathways that descend in the dorsolateral white matter to the dorsal root, where they terminate in the Rexed laminae and exert their inhibitory effects on those neurons responsible for nociception. Norepinephrine has been found to modify nociception at the level of the dorsal root nuclei.[25] The other effect of the monoamines has been suggested by studies that have shown an inhibition of morphine analgesia by monoamine depletion through reserpine pretreatment, destruction of the nucleus magnus raphae, and interruption of the descending dorsolateral columns of the spinal cord. Thus the monoamines could influence nociception through several mechanisms.

The foregoing discussion emphasizes that the sensation of pain (abdominal or otherwise) is the expression of complex interactions between the anatomic divisions of the nervous system and the biologic interaction of various neurogenic agents at all levels of the spinal and supraspinal nervous system.

TYPES OF ABDOMINAL PAIN[1,26-30]

Visceral Pain

A previously noted, sensory receptors within the wall of the abdominal viscus and its derivatives are responsible for the type of pain referred to as visceral pain (see Figs. 31-17 and 31-18). The major forces that give rise to this type of pain are related to changes in geometry such as stretching or sudden distention as may occur in the wall of the gut, resulting in increased tension on the wall of the particular viscus affected. For those viscera that are hollow, these pain fibers are located within the muscular wall; in organs such as the liver, spleen, and kidneys, which are solid in consistency, the nerve endings of these pain fibers are located in their respective capsules and result in pain from stretching of the capsule as may occur from parenchymal swelling in a condition such as hepatitis.

Those factors thought to be directly responsible for the development of visceral pain include inflammation and ischemia. Inflammation, either chemically or bacterially induced, is thought to lower the pain threshold for a given stimulus and thereby sensitizes the nerve endings of pain fibers. The exact mechanism responsible for this remains unknown but may be related to the release of various vasoactive substances such as bradykinin, histamine, serotonin, and eicosanoids. Ischemia also causes visceral pain. Again the mechanism is not clear, but possible routes of mediation include the accumulation of acidic metabolic end products, the release of various vasoactive substances, and the lowering of the pain threshold to various other stimuli. Both spasm and overdistention of a hollow viscus presumably cause pain from the resultant decrease in normal blood flow to the muscle of the viscus wall. The ischemia then sets into motion the stimulation of nerve endings of pain fibers through the proposed mechanisms already noted. An example of spasm of a hollow viscus would be the ureter during attempted passage of a ureteral calculus. An example of overdistention of a hollow viscus is that which occurs during intestinal obstruction.

The mediation of visceral pain is transported from visceral structures through the autonomic nervous system. The major route is through sympathetic nerves, except for those of the middle and upper esophagus and pelvic organs, which follow parasympathetic pathways. The cell bodies for these afferent nerves are located in the dorsal routes of the spinal cord and the homologous cranial nerve ganglia. Further transmission of pain then occurs through the various pathways of the spinal cord already described, being ultimately received in the cerebral cortex. Such pain is perceived as being dull, aching, or cramping. Depending on the region of the gastrointestinal tract from which it arises, it is perceived in the abdominal midline in the epigastrium (foregut structures); periumbilical region (midgut structures); lower abdomen (hindgut structures), the latter also being referred to as the hypogastrium; or the pelvis (cloacal structures).

Visceral pain always indicates the earliest manifestation of intra-abdominal disease but does not necessarily indicate that surgical intervention will be required for treatment. A patient often has visceral pain from the disordered motility secondary to food poisoning or a viral gastroenteritis, but usually the diagnosis is sufficiently obvious that any surgical considerations are clearly unwarranted. It is when visceral pain becomes supplanted by somatic pain, as is caused by other disease processes, that surgical intervention becomes a likely possibility.

Somatic Pain

Somatic pain (also referred to as parietal pain) is the type of pain that arises from irritation of the parietal peritoneum (see Fig. 13-17). It is mediated mainly by spinal nerve fibers that innervate the abdominal wall. Like those pain fibers mediating visceral pain through sympathetic pathways, these fibers also enter the spinal cord through the dorsal route ganglia and travel to the cerebral cortex for interpretation through the previously described pathways in the spinal cord. In contrast to visceral pain, which is perceived in one of three regions of the abdomen (i.e., epigastric, periumbilical, hypogastric), somatic pain is more localized and is perceived as arising from one of four quadrants of the abdominal wall (i.e., the right upper quadrant, right lower quadrant, left upper quadrant, or left lower quadrant).

Therefore, in a determination of the source of the pain, one must be familiar with those organs that normally reside in each of these quadrants. For example, the right lower quadrant includes the appendix, the cecum, the ascending colon, the distal ileum, and in the case of a female the right fallopian tube and ovary. In contrast to visceral pain, in which a change in geometry is responsible for the stimulation of nerve endings, somatic pain arises in response to acute changes in pH or temperature, as may occur in bacterial or chemical inflammation. In addition, somatic pain may arise in response to a sudden increase in pressure as may occur in an incision. Somatic pain is perceived as being sharp and pricking and is often constant.

Referred Pain

Referred pain is the phenomenon that occurs when pain is perceived in an area of the body other than the site of its origin. The pain usually arises in a deep structure; is superficial in its distant presenting location; and is often intense, sharp, and localized in the distant site. It occurs because of the existence of shared central pathways for afferent neurons arising from different sites. For example, visceral pain fibers synapsing in the spinal cord with pain fibers from the skin may give rise to a painful sensation in the skin itself as though it originated there even though the source of the pain was actually from some visceral structure. An example of this would be a ruptured spleen that results in irritation of the left hemidiaphragm (supplied by cervical nerves 3, 4, and 5) being perceived as arising in the left shoulder, also supplied by the same nerve roots. Other common areas of referred pain that may present on the surface of the body are shown in Figs. 31-22 and 31-23. Being aware of such referred pain patterns can often assist in the diagnosis of intra-abdominal pathology when other evidence of disease is lacking.

In summary, abdominal pain may consist of visceral pain, somatic pain, referred pain, or components of all three types of pain. Visceral pain is commonly associated with autonomic responses of sweating, nausea, pallor resulting from the central ramification of the nociceptive fibers through thalamic areas to the limbic system and the frontal cortex.

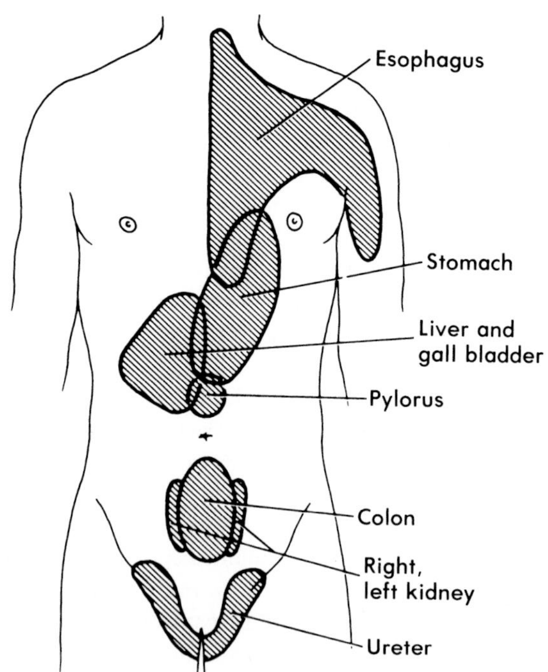

Fig. 31-22. Anterior areas of visceral referred pain. (From Cheung LY, Ballinger WF. Manifestations and diagnosis of gastrointestinal disease. In Hardy JD, ed. Hardy's Textbook of Surgery. Philadelphia: JB Lippincott, 1983.)

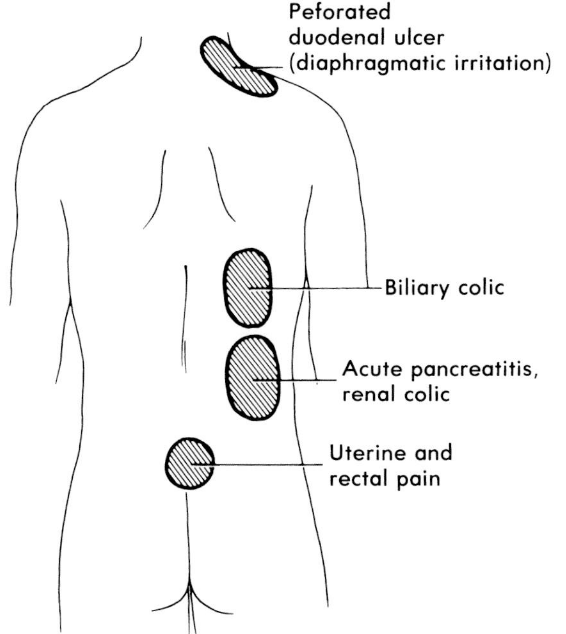

Fig. 31-23. Posterior areas of visceral referred pain. (From Cheung LY, Ballinger WF. Manifestations and diagnosis of gastrointestinal diseases. In Hardy JD, ed. Hardy's Textbook of Surgery. Philadelphia: JB Lippincott, 1983.)

EVALUATION OF THE PATIENT WITH ABDOMINAL PAIN[1,26-29]

In any patient who presents with the acute onset of abdominal pain, an orderly and systematic approach to diagnosis must be undertaken to determine whether surgical intervention is required. The more intense and severe the pain is, the more likely surgery is indicated (see accompanying box). Usually a thoughtfully conducted history and physical examination in combination with appropriate laboratory studies provide the necessary information relevant to diagnosis and the assurance as to whether surgery is indicated. The types of disease processes that may be responsible for the onset of acute abdominal pain are summarized below.

History

A careful history is absolutely mandatory in determining the characteristics of the pain and the likelihood of a given diagnosis. The *character* and *onset* of the pain are particularly important in this regard. Colicky pain usually indicates some type of obstructive process and represents disordered motility. This type of pain is associated with intestinal obstruction, the passage of a ureteral calculus, and acute cholecystitis. It signifies hyperperistalsis of smooth

---

CLASSIFICATION OF CAUSES OF ABDOMINAL PAIN ACCORDING TO RATE OF DEVELOPMENT OF THE PAIN

Sudden Onset (Instantaneous)

Perforated ulcer
Rupture of abscess or hematoma
Rupture of esophagus
Ruptured ectopic pregnancy
Infarct of abdominal organ, heart, or lung
Spontaneous pneumothorax
Ruptured or dissecting aortic aneurysm

Rapid Onset (Minutes)

Perforated viscus
Strangulated viscus (strangulated obstruction, torsion)
High small intestinal obstruction
Pancreatitis
Acute cholecystitis; biliary colic
Mesenteric infarction
Ureteral or renal colic
Ectopic pregnancy
Pneumonitis
Peptic ulcer
Diverticulitis
Appendicitis (less commonly than gradual onset)

Gradual Onset (Hours)

Appendicitis
Strangulated hernia
Low mechanical small bowel obstruction
Cholecystitis
Pancreatitis
Duodenal ulcer
Gastritis
Gastric ulcer
Mesenteric lymphadenitis
Terminal ileitis (regional enteritis; Crohn's disease)
Meckel's diverticulum
Sigmoid diverticulitis
Ulcerative colitis
Perforated tumor (usually of the colon or stomach)
Intraabdominal abscess
Ectopic pregnancy before rupture
Threatening abortion
Ureteral colic
Cystitis or pyelitis
Salpingitis (pelvic inflammatory disease)
Prostatitis
Urinary retention
Mesenteric cyst
Small bowel tumor or infarct

From Way LW. Abdominal pain and the acute abdomen. In Sleisenger MH, Fordtran JS, eds. Gastrointestinal Disease: Pathophysiology, Diagnosis, Management, 3rd ed. Philadelphia: WB Saunders, 1983.

muscle in its attempt to push fluid past the obstruction. Between such colicky episodes the pain greatly lessens or subsides entirely. The more intense the pain, the more noxious the stimulus of pain usually is. Thus when a viscus has perforated or a major arterial vessel has become occluded, the pain may be excruciating in nature. Such pain is usually persistent and unrelenting. Similarly, pain associated with some infectious process (e.g., appendicitis, intra-abdominal abscess) is also usually sustained and may even become more severe with time. Clues to the underlying cause of pain may also be indicated by the type of onset. Pancreatitis is often gradual and not uncommonly follows an alcoholic binge. In contrast, a perforated hollow viscus such as occurs with a peptic ulcer or a ruptured abdominal aortic aneurysm produces the sudden onset of pain that frequently is associated with the sensation of impending doom.

The *location* of pain is also helpful in establishing the underlying diagnosis. This is particularly true with somatic pain that is produced by irritation of the parietal peritoneum. An understanding of referred pain and the patterns by which a given intra-abdominal disease process may express itself is frequently of great help in pinpointing the underlying cause. Thus unexplained back pain may actually represent disease in the pancreas or biliary tract. Of equal importance is the *duration* of pain. The longer the duration, the more likely a surgical problem exists. This is particularly true if the pain has existed for longer than 5 or 6 hours.

In addition to pain, associated factors that may give clues to its underlying cause include a history of previous intra-abdominal disease. Thus the development of acute pain in the patient who has been taking H_2 receptor blockers for control of peptic ulcer disease suggests that it may be related to an aggravation of that process. Similarly, a previous diagnosis of gallstones by ultrasonography or cholecystography indicates the possibility that the present pain problem may be associated with acute cholecystitis. Although vomiting suggests some obstructive process, it is also commonly encountered with other intra-abdominal processes, making it a less specific diagnostic aid.

Physical Examination

The overall appearance of the patient often gives valuable clues concerning the severity of the intra-abdominal process. The magnitude of the pain is often reflected in the facial expression and in the body habitus. A relative immobility or unwillingness to change postural positions suggests an underlying peritonitis. Similarly, flexion of the hips with the knees drawn up to maintain comfort suggests tension on the abdominal wall and the presence of peritoneal irritation. Finally, any restriction of diaphragmatic excursion with respiration also suggests peritoneal irritation.

Actual examination of the abdomen gives more specific information. Any localized or generalized distention should be noted, since this may indicate peritonitis or the presence of intestinal obstruction. Similarly, sites where hernias are likely to occur should be examined, since incarceration may be the cause of the pain. Particularly important in evaluating the abdomen is auscultation and careful palpation. In the presence of peritonitis, bowel sounds are routinely diminished and often absent. In contrast, hyperperistalsis with high-pitched bowel sounds suggests some type of intestinal obstruction. Palpation is especially helpful and not only reveals areas of tenderness but also the extent, if present, of muscle rigidity. Tenderness usually suggests peritoneal irritation, and the area where this is most maximal suggests the anatomic point of underlying disease. In eliciting the presence or absence of tenderness, it is important to emphasize that palpation should be gently performed and that the palpation should begin at that portion of the abdomen most removed from the point of suspected disease. Rigidity (also called guarding) represents a protective mechanism on the part of the abdominal musculature to limit peritoneal irritation from the underlying intra-abdominal disease process. Its presence generally indicates underlying peritoneal irritation even though its absence does not exclude that possibility. In patients with a perforated abdominal viscus, rigidity is often diffuse, giving rise to what is known as a "boardlike" abdomen. In this circumstance not only is the abdomen rigid in palpation throughout but diffuse tenderness is also observed that is usually quite severe.

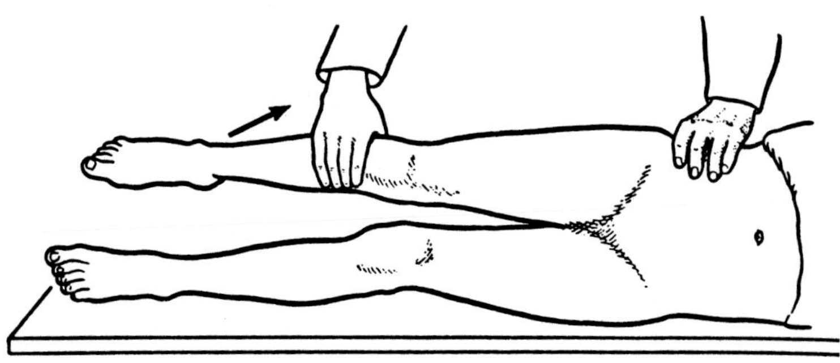

Fig. 31-24. Method of performing the iliopsoas (sometimes called psoas) test. (From Silen W. Cope's Early Diagnosis of the Acute Abdomen, 15th ed. New York: Oxford University Press, 1979.)

Rebound tenderness is another manifestation of peritoneal irritation and generally parallels the extent of tenderness. It is usually elicited by deeply palpating the tender area and then quickly releasing the examining hand. On release, sudden, immediate pain results. More gentle ways of demonstrating rebound tenderness include light percussion over the area in question and jarring the abdomen by either shaking the patient's bed or asking him to cough. With both of these latter maneuvers, the inflammatory focus within the abdomen irritates the adjacent parietal peritoneum and causes localized pain, thereby stimulating the rebound phenomenon.

In any patient who comes to the physician with acute abdominal pain, several other maneuvers are also appropriate to complete the examination. These include a rectal examination and also a pelvic examination in the case of a female patient. The pliability of the rectal walls allows careful examination of the entire lower pelvis through gentle palpation to determine the presence or absence of pain, masses, or unusual swellings that could represent a pelvic appendicitis. Similarly, a pelvic examination in the woman not only further aids in obtaining such information but is also helpful in determining the presence or absence of ovarian, fallopian tube, or uterine disease as a possible explanation for the abdominal pain.

Two special maneuvers that may prove helpful diagnostically are the *psoas sign* and the *obturator sign*. The psoas sign is elicited by stretching the peritoneum over the psoas muscle by extension of the thigh at the hip (Fig. 31-24). If an infection involving the psoas sheath exists, as may occur with a psoas abscess or a pelvic or retrocecal appendix, pain is elicited in this maneuver. The obturator sign is performed by internally rotating the thigh and thereby stretching the obturator fascia, (Fig. 31-25). Again, if inflammation is present involving the obturator fascia, as may occur with appendicitis, pain is elicited by this maneuver.

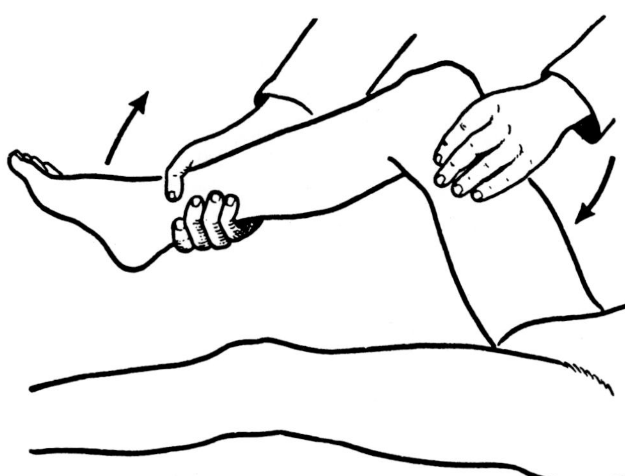

Fig. 31-25. Method of performing the obturator test. (From Silen W. Cope's Early Diagnosis of the Acute Abdomen, 15th ed. New York: Oxford University Press, 1979.)

Occasionally, the skin may be exquisitely sensitive to gentle touch in the dermatome corresponding to that innervated by the same nerve roots supplying an area of parietal peritoneum that is being irritated by an intra-abdominal inflammatory process. Such hypersensitivity is termed hyperesthesia. Although not commonly present, *hyperesthesia* is also a clue to the underlying source of abdominal disease.

Laboratory Tests

In any patient developing acute abdominal pain, adequate evaluation should include a number of laboratory tests. A complete white blood cell count with differential is often helpful in determining whether a bacterial or viral infection is responsible for the underlying abdominal disease. The hematocrit is less helpful but may indicate evidence of anemia or hemoconcentration from accompanying dehydration. Urinalysis may demonstrate pyuria or hematuria, in which case a renal cause of abdominal pain is suggested. Occasionally, an inflamed appendix overlying the ureter reveals similar abnormalities. Liver function studies and amylase determinations in the serum often assist in determining whether the underlying source of disease resides in the pancreas, liver, or biliary tree.

Radiologic studies may also be of help in defining the underlying diagnosis. An upright film of the abdomen, for example, may demonstrate free air under the diaphragm, indicating a perforated viscus or air/fluid levels suggestive of intestinal obstruction. Since pneumonia may masquerade as a cause of upper abdominal pain, the chest x-ray film is also helpful in excluding an underlying pneumonic process. In patients in whom the history and physical examination are suggestive of biliary tract or pancreatic disease, abdominal ultrasound is often of value. This may reveal the presence of acute cholecystitis (with or without gallstones), pancreatitis, a pseudocyst of the pancreas, or some other unsuspected inflammatory process. Similarly, ultrasound may demonstrate an unsuspected abdominal aortic aneurysm. Although barium contrast studies are usually not indicated in the workup of patients with acute abdominal pain, occasionally such information is helpful, particularly if intestinal obstruction is present, in excluding a large bowel obstruction or defining more accurately the source of small bowel obstruction. Obviously, each patient must be individualized and careful judgment rendered in the choice of tests ordered.

APPENDICITIS: PROTOTYPE OF ABDOMINAL PAIN[1,26,29,31]

Among the various intra-abdominal pathologic processes that may be responsible for the acute development of abdominal pain, appendicitis is clearly the most common. For this reason, a discussion of its clinical presentation is appropriate and highlights in practical terms the pain patterns that occur when a particular intra-abdominal organ is diseased and the accompanying physical findings that may be expected.

Appendicitis is basically an obstructive process in which the appendiceal lumen, usually at its opening into the cecum, is obstructed by a fecalith, mucus plug, tumor, or some foreign body. Because the epithelial surface distal to this obstruction continues to maintain its normal secretory processes, the accumulated intraluminal fluid that would ordinarily be discharged into the cecal lumen now results in appendiceal distention. The resultant stretch in the appendiceal wall triggers pain receptors that are carried by visceral afferent nerves to the spinal cord. Such painful information is then transported through the spinothalamic tracts of the spinal cord to the patient's cerebral cortex for interpretation. Because the appendix is a midgut structure, this visceral stimulation presents itself as a periumbilical pain, which is usually colicky in nature, coincident with attempts of the appendiceal musculature to overcome the obstructive process. Accompanying this development of periumbilical pain is a reflex ileus that is nearly always manifested by the feeling of anorexia and often is associated with nausea and vomiting. As the pathologic process within the appendiceal wall persists, invasion by microorganisms with secondary inflammation eventually results, with a gradual onset of a low-grade fever and an accompanying leukocytosis. At this point in the pathologic process, the obstruction may still be reversible, particularly if caused by a mucous plug or a small fecalith, which may be dislodged by the continuing muscular contractions of the appendix. If this circumstance does not supervene, however, the inflammation progresses further, resulting in edema of the appendiceal wall to involve the whole organ distal to the site of obstruction. When this occurs, the neighboring parietal peritoneum becomes irritated, and its stimulation leads to a change in the character of the pain, which now moves from the periumbilical region to become localized in the right lower quadrant. Accompanying this localization, the pain becomes much more pronounced and constant.

In addition to this sequence of events, important physical findings now become evident that are generally not present when only the visceral expression of pain is manifested. Thus the patient now has tenderness on palpation of the right lower quadrant with evidence of abdominal rigidity (guarding) and rebound tenderness, all manifestations of peritoneal irritation. In some patients, hyperesthesia may also be present. The point of maximal tenderness in appendicitis is usually at an anatomic location known as McBurney's point, a site two thirds of the distance from the umbilicus to the right anterior superior iliac spine. Usually by this point in the disease, nausea is much more pronounced, vomiting is frequently present, and clear evidence of fever and leukocytosis can generally be demonstrated. Bowel sounds are also diminished and may be absent entirely. Thus the derivation of the appendix as a midgut structure and its anatomic location in the right lower abdomen make the clinical presentation of this disease entirely consistent with what one would expect.

Although the clinical presentation described above is typical of the majority of cases of appendicitis, it cannot be emphasized too strongly that no evaluation of abdominal pain is complete without a rectal examination (and if the patient is a female, a pelvic examination). Not only do these examinations help to rule out another cause for the abdominal pain that may simulate appendicitis such as a tubo-ovarian abscess from pelvic inflammatory disease, but occasionally the appendix, which is normally anteriorly displaced, resides in a retrocecal location or is located more posteriorly along the pelvic brim (Fig. 31-26). In either of these situations the physical manifestations of disease in the right lower quadrant may be less pronounced or not present at all, thus suggesting another cause for the abdominal pain. A rectal and pelvic examination may be especially helpful in this setting by revealing tenderness on palpation of the right rectal or vaginal walls. Other diagnostic maneuvers that may further secure the diagnosis include the demonstration of a positive psoas sign and/or obturator sign (see Figs. 31-24 and 31-25). Another complicating factor in the presentation of appendicitis is its occurrence during pregnancy. As the uterus increases in size from the developing fetus, the cecum and appendix move superiorly to the right upper quadrant. Thus the diagnosis of appendicitis must be entertained when a pregnant patient complains of right upper quadrant pain.[1]

The ultimate outcome of appendicitis, if left untreated, is perforation. This may take the form of a generalized

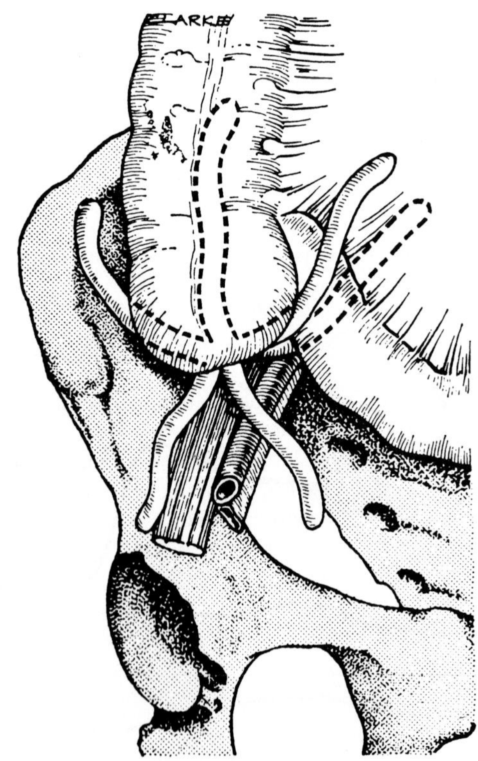

Fig. 31-26. Various possible positions of the appendix. (From Silen W. Cope's Early Diagnosis of the Acute Abdomen, 15th ed. New York: Oxford University Press, 1979.)

peritonitis if the inflammation involving the appendix has not been contained by the surrounding omentum. If protection by the omentum has occurred, the peritonitis is usually greatly modified and may remain localized to the right lower quadrant or ultimately develop into an appendiceal abscess. The cause of the perforation is probably multifactorial in origin and includes the local pressure effects from the increasing intraluminal pressure, local tissue ischemia from the obstructing lesion (particularly if induced by a fecalith), and the buildup of acid metabolites from the resultant anaerobic metabolism and cellular death that results when the obstructed appendix impedes the venous and lymphatic drainage that ultimately supervenes from the increased intraluminal pressure. Under most circumstances perforation can be expected to occur within 36 to 48 hours following the onset of appendicitis. For this reason surgical intervention with appendectomy should be undertaken once the diagnosis has been made.

PAIN PATTERNS ARISING FROM INTRA-ABDOMINAL VISCERA[1,26,29,31,32]

This section describes the common types of pain arising from intra-abdominal disease and the pathways responsible for this pain. Tables 31-1 and 31-2 summarize the descriptions of pain and the sequential innervation for the various viscera involved.

Esophagus

Although the esophagus is primarily an intrathoracic organ, its distal portion resides within the abdomen; therefore an understanding of pain patterns arising from this organ is mandatory if the cause of acute abdominal pain is to be correctly diagnosed. Sensory afferent pain fibers from the esophagus are derived from the upper six thoracic segments of the spinal cord. Visceral pain is mostly a result of distention of the esophagus and is felt anteriorly from the suprasternal notch to the epigastrium. Somatic pain is usually caused by inflammation or neoplastic infiltration of the esophagus and radiates to the back. If the pain stimulus is severe, reflex spinal arcs are excited, leading to regional muscle contraction that can then result in restriction of inspiration, severe chest pain (resembling angina), tachypnea, and shortness of breath. Additional pain can be felt in the distribution of the cervical sympathetics (e.g., face, jaw, neck, arms). The usual esophageal pain is a deep thoracic pain at the level of the pathologic lesion. Thus a disease process developing in the upper esophagus generally produces pain in the neck, whereas disease in the lower esophagus is commonly felt in the region of the lower sternum or xiphoid process but may also occur in the epigastrium.

Common presentations of esophageal pain are seen with pyrosis, spasm, stricture, and spontaneous rupture. *Pyrosis* is a common disorder most frequently caused by regurgitated gastric contents. Acid with bile is a stronger stimulus for this pain than acid alone. Lower esophageal sphincter tone that normally prevents pyrosis is decreased by large meals, air swallowing, and physical exertion. Pyrosis is increased by bending forward, stooping, tight clothing, and in the obese. Dysphagia associated with pyrosis implies a concomitant stricture. Esophageal *spasm* is a motility disorder that has symptoms of intermittent pain and dysphagia. This pain is increased by cold liquids, gastroesophageal reflux, and stress. The motility of the lower half of the esophagus has been shown to have increased tertiary contractions with abnormal (decreased) peristal-

Table 31-1. Sensory Innervation of the Viscera

	Viscera	Artery	Nerve Plexus	Primary Pain	Referred Pain
Heart	Heart	Coronaries	Cardiac	Central chest	Shoulder, arm, neck
Esophagus	Esophagus	From aorta	Esophageal	Central chest	Midline back
Foregut	Stomach, pancreas, liver, gallbladder, proximal duodenum	Celiac	Celiac	Midepigastrium	—
Midgut	Distal duodenum, jejunum, ileum, ascending and transverse colon	Superior mesenteric	Superior mesenteric	Umbilicus	—
Proximal hindgut	Descending and sigmoid colon	Inferior mesenteric	Inferior mesenteric	Hypogastrium	—
Gonads	Testis, ovary	Gonadal	Renal	Gonad	Umbilicus
Proximal urinary	Kidney, ureter	Renal	Renal	Costomuscular, loin	Groin, scrotum, labia
Bladder, body of uterus	Bladder, body of uterus	Internal iliacs	Hypogastric	Hypogastrium	Groins
Cloaca	Rectum, upper anus, cervix, upper vagina, base of bladder, prostate	Internal iliacs	Pelvic	Midpelvis	Midsacrum

From Currie DJ. Abdominal Pain. New York: Hemisphere Publishing, 1979.

Table 31-2. Segmental Innervation of Walls of Body Cavities and Predominant Sensory Innervation of Viscera

	Cervical 2 3 4 5 6 7 8	Thoracic 1 2 3 4 5 6 7 8 9 10 11 12	Lumbar 1 2 3 4 5	Sacral 1 2 3 4 5
Parietes				
Central diaphragm	3—5			
Thoracic walls		1 — 12		
Anterior and lateral abdominal walls		5 —	— 1	
Posterior abdominal wall			1 — 4	
Pelvic walls				1 — 5
Viscera				
Heart		1 — 6		
Esophagus		1 — 6		
Thoracic aorta		3 — 12		
Derivatives of foregut		5 — 9		
Testis, ovary		10–11		
Derivatives of midgut		10 —	— 1	
Kidney, ureter		10 —	— 1	
Vault of bladder		11 —	— 2	
Derivatives of proximal hindgut		12 —	— 1	
Body of uterus		12 —	— 1	
Abdominal aorta			1 — 4	
Derivatives of cloaca				3–4

From Currie DJ. Abdominal Pain. New York: Hemisphere Publishing, 1979.

sis. Severe pain is accompanied by diffuse muscle spasm and the distribution of pain described above. *Stricture* of the esophagus can be benign or malignant. The presentation and evolution of symptoms range from pain with swallowing to steady and severe thoracic and back pain. The several presentations depend on the underlying disease process. Spontaneous *rupture* usually follows vomiting after a large meal or alcoholic binge. The patient has sudden severe thoracic pain, usually in the region of the xiphosternum (since most ruptures occur in the lower esophagus), and shock.

Occasionally, the diagnosis of retrosternal pain, often indicative of esophageal disease, can be confused with myocardial ischemia (i.e., angina). Reflux esophagitis and hiatal hernia can both mimic the pain of myocardial ischemia. In distinguishing between these possibilities and a true cardiac origin of the pain, it should be remembered that reflux-induced pain from the esophagus is usually relieved by antacids and food, whereas myocardial pain is not.

Stomach and Duodenum

The afferent nerves to the stomach and duodenum that mediate pain arise from spinal cord segments T5 through T9 and travel through the greater splanchnic nerves and the celiac plexus. Visceral pain is felt in the midepigastrium, and this is by far the most common presentation. Somatic pain is also felt in the midepigastrium; but if it arises from the stomach, it may also be experienced in the left upper quadrant. Somatic pain is usually secondary to spread of the inflammatory or neoplastic infiltrate process outside the serosa of the stomach or duodenum. Referred pain is quite rare.

The vagus nerves also are involved with sensory innervation to the stomach. However, any decrease in the pain of acid-peptic disease following vagotomy is not caused by an interruption of direct pain pathways but rather by a diminution in gastric acid secretion. Under normal conditions the gastric sensory afferents are not usually responsive to acid and bile, and pinching the normal gastric mucosa does not lead to pain. However, congestion and inflammation in the mucosa, as seen in ulcer disease or gastritis, can decrease the threshold to these noxious stimuli.

The most common conditions leading to gastric and duodenal pain are acid-peptic disease and its complications, gastritis, postgastrectomy syndromes, neoplasia, gastric volvulus, and a strangulated paraesohageal hiatal hernia. The peptic ulcer pain can arise from the stomach, duodenum, and lower esophagus or at the site of the previously fashioned gastrojejunostomy. This pain can be decreased by neutralizing gastric acid secretion. Severe disease also involves pain arising from smooth muscle contraction of the surrounding viscus. Duodenal ulcers can cause burning or gnawing superficial pain. This pain characteristically has times of severity associated with increasing levels of acid bathing the ulcer. The pain increases 2 to 3 hours after meals and at bedtime. It is decreased by food and antacids fairly promptly. The symptoms also seem to be worse in the fall and spring, for reasons not entirely defined. The pain of a penetrating duodenal ulcer is secondary to the posterior penetration of the ulcer and its surrounding inflammation. It presents as a constant, deep, dull aching back pain that may or may not occur with the more typical epigastric pain usually seen in duodenal ulcer disease.

Perforation of an ulcer (usually duodenal) presents with sudden, severe diffuse abdominal pain caused by the spread of chemical irritants throughout the peritoneal cavity. This pain is associated with guarding, often diffuse (giving rise to a boardlike abdomen), and rebound tenderness, both findings associated with peritonitis. In contrast, pain is not a hallmark of hemorrhage as the blood tends to buffer the ulcer. Gastritis can present with pain similar to peptic ulcer disease but is usually decreased less easily by antacids and is more steady in character. The pain of postgastrectomy syndromes is associated with the size of the gastric pouch, the presence of an afferent loop syndrome, dumping, alkaline reflux, gastritis, and obstruction. The mechanisms of pain are similar to those described above.

Liver

The liver capsule is sensitive to stretch and inflammation, in contrast to the parenchyma of the liver itself, which is not sensitive to pain. The surrounding peritoneum can also respond to inflammation or growth of the liver. Pain arising from the right lobe of the liver and surrounding peritoneum travels by way of afferent nerves involving the sixth through twelfth thoracic segments, whereas pain syndromes involving the left lobe are mediated through nerves reaching the sixth and seventh thoracic segments, in both cases reaching the spinal cord through the greater splanchnic nerves and the celiac ganglia. Afferent pain fibers from the surrounding peritoneum also travel by way of the phrenic nerves. Pain from an expanding liver capsule can often be felt as right upper quadrant pain that may be increased with breathing. Common disorders with these symptoms are hepatitis, congestive hepatomegaly, and expanding hematoma.

Spleen

The parenchyma of the spleen, like the liver, is insensitive to pain. The splenic capsule, however, is sensitive to stretching, and the surrounding parietal peritoneum is sensitive to inflammation and blood. When present, visceral pain of the spleen is felt as a dull vague epigastric pain, but this is generally not common. Somatic pain of the surrounding peritoneum is common and is usually stimulated by blood from rupture of an injured spleen. The pain is commonly referred to the top of the left shoulder. Sudden sharp left upper quadrant pain can be caused by splenic rupture or splenic infarction. Splenic infarcts are not common but have two broad causes. The first is emboli, which can emanate from the heart during myocardial infarction or atrial fibrillation, endocarditis, or aneurysm formation. The second broad category is hematologic. Etiologic factors in this group result in splenic arterial thromboses and are most commonly represented by sickle cell disease, leukemia, and polycythemia vera. Massive splenomegaly can cause a dull aching left upper quadrant pain by traction on the peritoneal attachments of the spleen.

Gallbladder and Bile Ducts

The spectrum of gallstone disease can produce all the types of pain previously described for the stomach, duodenum, liver, or spleen. The gallbladder and bile ducts arise from the foregut, and pain is transmitted to the spinal cord through the greater splanchnic nerves (T5-T9) and the celiac plexus. The pain sensation mediated by the paired splanchnic nerves is interpreted by the brain as arising in the abdominal midline (epigastric region) and is called biliary colic. Uncomplicated biliary colic is not really a "colic" but a steady, dull, deep visceral pain arising in the upper epigastrium. This visceral presentation can be caused by distention of the gallbladder with stones, cystic duct obstruction, or distal obstruction of the common bile duct. Severe biliary colic can be associated with pain radiating to the back and pain on contraction of the lower intercostal muscles. The pain caused by intercostal contraction is felt as a tightness or constricting sensation and can mimic the pain originating from myocardial ischemia.

Acute inflammation of the gallbladder changes the midline deep visceral pain of biliary colic to a more severe somatic pain involving the right upper quadrant. If the inflammation spreads to the serosa and involves the peritoneum, the parietal peritoneal irritation can cause pain referred to the inferior angle of the scapula; diaphragmatic irritation can cause pain referred to the right shoulder. In as many as 10% of patients with acute cholecystitis, both a right upper and left upper quadrant pain may be present. One patient out of 25 with acute inflammation has left upper quadrant pain only. As the inflammation progresses, the pain generally becomes localized to the right upper quadrant, and its severity relates to both somatic and visceral components. As the inflammation becomes further advanced, the upper abdominal and lower thoracic muscles become rigid and tender. This acute progressive inflammation can further progress to gangrene and perforation of the gallbladder, leading to the formation of a paracholecystic abscess or diffuse peritonitis.

Pancreas

Sensory innervation of the pancreas is similar to that of the gallbladder, with sensory afferent pain fibers arising from the greater splanchnic nerves (T5 to T9) and the celiac plexus. Visceral pain and somatic pain are present in the midepigastrium. Referred pain is present in the back at the level of the first lumber vertebra.

Visceral pancreatic pain is not common but can be classically demonstrated during pancreatic duct injection during retrograde endoscopic examination. This pain is constant, midline, and midepigastric. Abdominal pain is not present early in the course of the pancreatic cancer. Unfortunately, visceral pain tends to be mild to moderate, resulting in delayed diagnosis. Later in the disease process, visceral pain can evolve and is caused by pancreatic duct obstruction. The local spread of tumor can infiltrate surrounding perineural tissue, and the pain can spread.

Somatic pain is much more common with diseases of the pancreas and is produced in states of inflammation (e.g., acute pancreatitis). The sensory afferent fibers for somatic pain are carried in the first lumbar nerve. This nerve does not have good localization to the anterior abdominal wall; for this reason the pain of acute pancreatitis commonly presents as back pain without signs of anterior wall peritoneal irritation (anterior abdominal wall muscle rigidity or tenderness). The back pain is referred and originates from stimulation of the posterior parietal peritoneum.

Small Intestine

The sensory innervation of the small intestine is that of the midgut and consists of visceral afferent fibers from T10 to L1 splanchnic nerves through the superior mesenteric ganglion. Visceral pain commonly emanates from mechanical obstruction and is located in the midline at the level of the umbilicus. Midgut somatic pain involves local parietal peritoneal stimulation. The pain is felt locally at the site of stimulation and is associated with surrounding muscle contraction or guarding. Common causes for midgut somatic pain are ischemia, inflammation, tumor infiltration, and traction on the mesentery. Referred pain from the midgut is quite rare.

Mechanical small bowel obstruction presents as crampy periumbilical pain with obstipation, abdominal distention, and nausea and vomiting. Distention of the bowel causes this visceral presentation of abdominal pain. The lower the level of obstruction, the greater is the distention. The higher the level of obstruction, the earlier nausea and vomiting are seen. If the obstruction evolves into ischemic, gangrenous, or inflamed bowel, the components described for somatic small bowel pain come into play.

Intestinal ischemia can be acute or chronic. Acute intestinal ischemia can be caused by an arterial embolus or in situ thrombosis distal to a narrowed visceral artery. The pain produced is a sharp steady pain and is thought to be caused by acid-metabolite accumulation or anoxia in the ischemic tissue. Progression of the ischemia leads to edema and hemorrhage into the bowel wall that can become transmural, resulting in watery or bloody diarrhea. The presentation of sudden vascular occlusion of the small bowel is acute abdominal pain followed by watery or bloody diarrhea and shock. This syndrome is most commonly seen with occlusion of the superior mesenteric artery and only rarely with the celiac artery. Intestinal ischemia can occur as a result of mechanical small bowel obstruction and can have signs and symptoms of both processes.

Large Bowel and Rectum

Like the appendix, which has already been discussed, the proximal large bowel (including the cecum, ascending colon, and most of the transverse colon) is derived embryologically from the midgut and has a vascular and sensory supply similar to the other midgut structures. Visceral pain presents as periumbilical pain that can include the right side of the abdomen when distention of the cecum is such that traction on the mesentery occurs. Similar to the small bowel, somatic pain presents over sites of inflammation, obstruction, tumor infiltration, or ischemia; referred pain is rare.

The distal large bowel, from the splenic flexure (to include the distal transverse colon) to the distal sigmoid, develops from the hindgut. The vascular supply is from the inferior mesenteric artery, and the neural innervation is from nerve segments T12 to L1 and the inferior mesenteric plexus. Visceral pain is felt in the suprapubic area in the midline. Left-sided pain can be caused by traction of the mesentery by distention of the left colon, either lower left-sided pain from distention in the descending colon or in the upper left quadrant from distention of the splenic flexure. The sigmoid colon is attached to peritoneum proximally and distally, so distention is felt in the midline as visceral pain above the pubis.

The pathologic entities most commonly affecting the distal colon are carcinoma, diverticular disease, colitis, and ischemia. These disease entities can present with simple visceral pain or complex variations of visceral and somatic pain. Carcinoma is usually and unfortunately insidious in its growth and becomes symptomatic only when it causes partial or complete obstruction. Symptoms can range from obstipation, diarrhea, or complete colonic obstruction. Diverticulosis is associated with a variety of complications, including bleeding, obstruction, and inflammation that may result in perforation or abscess formation. Mild obstruction is perceived as visceral pain; in contrast, hemorrhage is painless unless it causes diarrhea and cramping. Inflammation and infection localizes somatic pain to the anatomic area involved, which is most commonly the left lower quadrant. Ischemia causes symptoms as mentioned in the above section. Colitis and/or an irritable colon present generally with two regions of pain: the left lower quadrant and the hypogastric area. The pain is crampy in nature and associated with diarrhea.

The rectum develops from the cloaca and is thus quite different in its sensory and vascular supply from that of hindgut structures. The arterial supply is the internal iliac arteries, and the afferent sensory nerve supply is from the pelvic splanchnic nerves (S3 and S4) and the pelvic plexuses. Visceral and somatic rectal pain is appreciated centrally in the pelvis and can be referred to the midsacral region in the midline.

Abdominal Aorta and Iliac Arteries

Pain from these retroperitoneal structures is unusual. The sensory afferent visceral nerves that mediate pain arise from the lumbar nerves (L1 to L4), and somatic pain is perceived in the back at this level. Referred pain is unusual. Pathologic processes of the aorta and iliac arteries that cause painful symptoms are acute occlusion of these vessels and aneurysmal dilation and rupture. Acute occlusion presents with pain from the level of the occlusion distally that can be accompanied by pallor, pain, pulselessness, paresthesias, and paralysis of the extremities. Acute occlusion also presents with abdominal or back pain at the level of occlusion. Aneurysmal dilation can cause compression and erosion of the surrounding viscera, which would present as visceral or somatic pain of these structures. Erosion of the aneurysm into a viscus can lead to hemorrhage as well.

Female Pelvic Viscera

The sensory innervation of the uterus and the fallopian tubes originates between segments T12 and L1 of the spinal cord. These spinal roots send fibers to the lumbar sympathetic ganglia and periaortic plexus and inferiorly to the hypogastric plexus and the bilateral pelvic plexuses. The afferent nerves branch with the hypogastric artery to send branches to the fallopian tubes and uterus. Visceral pain localizes in the midline of the suprapubic area. Severe visceral pain from the uterus can radiate to the groins (L1) or, as in pregnancy, the inner thighs (L2). Somatic pain is felt in the localized anatomic area experiencing the peritoneal irritation. Ectopic pregnancy, salpingitis, and spontaneous incomplete abortions can cause severe somatic pelvic pain.

The sensory innervation of the cervix is from pelvic splanchnic nerves (i.e., spinal segments S3 and S4) and the pelvic plexus. Visceral pain is felt centrally in the pelvis, as is somatic pain. Severe pain can radiate to the midsacral region in the midline. The sensory innervation of the ovaries is from the T10 and T11 spinal segments because of their embryologic development high in the posterior abdominal cavity. Visceral pain may be periumbilical, whereas direct somatic pain is felt locally at the area of pathology. Ovulation and its bleeding can cause severe abdominal pain, which is usually short lived, and not lasting more than 24 hours. Torsion of the ovary and functional or neoplastic cysts of this organ can present with acute abdominal pain.

Genitourinary System

The genitourinary system is made up of the kidneys, bladder, ureter, urethra, and in the male the prostate and testes. Each anatomic division is described separately.

The urinary bladder receives sensory afferent nerves from the thoracic and lumbar nerves (T11 to L2 to the vault), the hypogastric plexus (to the base), and the pudendal nerves. The urinary bladder develops from the cloaca and is supplied by the hypogastric artery. Visceral pain is felt in the hypogastrium and somatic pain in the suprapubic area. Referred pain is felt in the groins. Pain from the bladder is commonly from distention. Pain from such distention can emanate from several sources: the bladder itself, through its visceral and somatic afferent nerves, and through traction on the parietal peritoneum. Bladder pain is most commonly sensed in the suprapubic area, but also is felt in the back and the upper lumbar regions. Inflammatory processes involving the urinary bladder are common causes of abdominal pain.

The base of the bladder, prostate, and urethra receive sensory innervation from the pelvic splanchnic nerves (S3 and S4) and the pelvic plexuses. Visceral pain is felt in the central pelvis as is somatic pain. Referred pain is felt in the midsacral region of the back and the distal end of the urethra. Inflammation of the base of the bladder or urethra is a common cause of pain that is felt at the tip of the urethra on urination. Common associated findings with this pain are urgency, frequency, and dysuria.

The testes have a similar sensory innervation to that of the ovary, since both structures develop medial to the kidney and are supplied by thoracic splanchnic nerves T10 and T11 and the renal plexus. Visceral pain is felt in the groin and lower abdomen, and when severe, is associated with nausea, vomiting, and weakness. Somatic pain is also felt over the gonads, and referred pain is felt in the umbilical region.

The kidney, renal pelvis, and upper ureter are innervated by the thoracic, least splanchnic and lumbar splanchnic nerves, and the renal plexus. Visceral pain is felt in the costomuscular region (angle between the 12th rib and the lateral border of the erector spinae muscles). Somatic pain localizes over the site of irritation; referred pain is rare for these structures. The lower ureter receives the same sensory innervation as the aforementioned structures. Visceral pain caused by obstruction of the lower ureter can also be felt in the costomuscular region but is commonly perceived in the scrotum as well. Somatic pain is localized in the lower abdominal quadrant ipsilateral to the irritation. Pain may be referred to the groin, scrotum, or in the female the labia.

The most common pathologic causes of acute pain are urinary calculi, infections, or neoplasia. Slow, insidious obstruction may not cause discomfort, but rapid obstruction causes severe renal colic. Renal colic is thought to be from distention of the ureter and renal pelvis and not from muscular contraction. This pain can last for considerable periods of time, often up to 6 hours. The pain is constant and subsides only with relief of the obstruction or following administration of some analgesic. When ureteral obstruction presents on the right side, the associated pain can be easily confused with acute cholecystitis or appendicitis.

SOURCES OF ABDOMINAL PAIN NOT ARISING FROM INTRA-ABDOMINAL PATHOLOGY

Although intra-abdominal lesions are responsible for the development of the acute abdomen in most cases, the acute onset of abdominal pain may also arise from other sources. Any pneumonic process involving the pleura can present at times as abdominal pain. Usually this pain presents in the upper abdomen and is more commonly encountered when the lower lobes of the lung or lower thoracic cage is the site of pathology.[1] Diseases that may present in this fashion include pneumonia, pulmonary emboli, and pneumothoraces. Similarly, various cardiac disorders occasionally present as abdominal pain, particularly in the region of the upper epigastrium or left upper quadrant. Examples include both acute and chronic pericarditis and myocardial ischemia, especially if the left ventricle is involved.

Although most intra-abdominal lesions ultimately present physical findings affecting various portions of the abdominal wall, it must not be forgotten that pathology within the abdominal wall itself may be responsible for the onset of acute abdominal pain. In this regard the most common abdominal wall lesions found are hernias. Such hernias are generally painful and are usually easily demonstrable because of their associated mass effect and the fact that pain arises where hernias are usually located. Further, the pain of reducible hernias tends to be relieved when they are reduced, but incarcerated (nonreducible) and strangulated (incarcerated hernias in which the blood supply to the hernial contents is compromised) hernias produce constant symptoms. Because the contents of incarcerated and strangulated hernias involve intraperitoneal structures, they not infrequently present with symptoms referable to both the abdominal wall and intra-abdominal pathology. Inguinal hernias cause symptoms in the groins, whereas epigastric hernias cause symptoms (often vague) of the upper midline. Periumbilical hernias cause symptoms around the umbilicus and spigelian hernias at the lateral border of the junction of the middle and lower thirds of the rectus muscle. The rectus muscle itself can also present with acute pain caused by intramuscular hemorrhage induced by anticoagulation or strenuous muscle effort. This condition often produces a painful mass in the lower left or right quadrants, depending on the size of the resulting hematoma.

An important part of the differential diagnosis of acute abdominal pain is any infection that involves the posterior root ganglia and nerves. The most common infections responsible for this are herpes zoster (reactivation of chicken pox virus) and syphilis. Herpes zoster can be caused by malnutrition, trauma, leukemia, neoplasia, and immunosuppression. The pain arises in the dermatomes (area of skin supplied with afferent nerve fibers by a single posterior spinal root) infected with the virus and often is excruciating. Tabes dorsalis denotes a condition in which there is degeneration of the posterior root ganglia and/or axons in the posterior columns of the spinal cord following infection with syphilis, usually 5 to 20 years earlier. This disease, although presently rare, can present with shooting abdominal pains at any level of the abdomen, usually associated with other neurologic deficits.

Although the aforementioned conditions are the more common nonintra-abdominal sources responsible for abdominal pain, a wide variety of other lesions can also present as an acute abdomen, even though rare. Thus the astute physician must bear in mind the possibility of these lesions in the workup of any patient who develops the acute onset of abdominal pain. Among these various disorders are diabetic ketoacidosis, hyperparathyroidism, lead intoxication, hemochromatosis, acute porphyria, epilepsy, essential hyperlipemia, drug addiction, primary peritonitis, and any number of wide assortment of psychiatric disorders.

ACUTE ABDOMINAL PATHOLOGY AND CHEST PAIN

In addition to the abdominal pain presentations just enumerated, it must be emphasized that intra-abdominal disease may on occasion present primarily as chest pain suggestive of a cardiac cause. This is particularly true of biliary colic, which can present with upper epigastric midline or chest pain. Associated pain in the right upper quadrant or referred pain to the right inferior angle of the scapula that occurs with gallbladder disease but not with ischemic heart disease helps differentiate these diagnoses. When biliary pain is limited to the chest or upper epigastrium, a careful evaluation must be made of the patient's cardiovascular system. Abscess formation or inflammation in the subphrenic spaces can also present with chest pain, although the pain in these situations (usually perceived in the right or left lateral chest) is more atypical than the usual pain presentation with cardiac ischemia.

Studies have shown that one in four patients admitted to the hospital with chest pain has a problem referable to the gastrointestinal tract. Also one patient in five evaluated for biliary tract disease has myocardial pathology as the cause. Thus one must carefully consider the possible roots of sensory innervation to distinguish among those structures that could serve as the source for abdominal pain.

SUMMARY

The term *acute abdomen* is the designation used to denote the clinical condition characterized by the acute onset of abdominal pain, usually in association with other findings such as nausea and vomiting, anorexia, and abdominal distention. A wide variety of intra-abdominal and extra-abdominal pathologic lesions may be responsible for this condition, many of which have the potential of being life-threatening conditions. For this reason the underlying diagnosis must be promptly made and appropriate treatment measures instituted. To accomplish this in the most judicious fashion, the treating physician must obtain an accurate database and be able to extrapolate these data within a fund of knowledge encompassing the anatomy, the embryology, the neurophysiology, and the natural history of each potential cause. This database derives from the initial history and physical examination, supported by various laboratory tests and radiologic studies. The differential diagnosis of the acute abdomen can be challenging, even to the most astute physician, but is ultimately successful when approached from this frame of reference.

REFERENCES

1. Currie DJ. Abdominal Pain. New York: Hemisphere Publishing, 1979.
2. Langman J. Medical Embryology, 2nd ed. Baltimore: Williams & Wilkins, 1969.
3. Patten BM. Human Embryology, 2nd ed. New York: McGraw-Hill, 1959.
4. Adams RD, Victor M. Principles of Neurology. New York: McGraw-Hill, 1985.
5. Antonson DL. Abdominal pain. Pediatr Endosc 4:1, 1994.
6. Budd K. Pain. London: Update Publication, 1982.
7. Hamilton AB, Zeltzer LK. Visceral pain in infants. J Pediatr 125:S95, 1994.
8. Kandel ER, Schwartz JH. Principles of Neuroscience, 2nd ed. New York: Elsevier Science Publishing, 1985.
9. Rexed B. A cytotectonic atlas of the spinal cord in the cat. L Comp Neurol 100:297, 1954.
10. Ness TJ, Gebhart GF. Visceral pain: A review of experimental studies. Pain 41:167, 1990.
11. Klein KB, Mellinkoff SB. Approach to the patient with abdominal pain. In Tadataka Y, Alpers DH, eds. Textbook of Gastroenterology. Philadelphia: JB Lippincott, 1991, p 660.
12. Beal JM, Raffensperger JG. Diagnosis of Acute Abdominal Disease. Philadelphia: Lea & Febiger, 1979.
13. Harrington-Kiff JG. Pain. London: Update Publication, 1982.
14. Ruch TC. The pathophysiology of pain. In Ruch TC, Patton HD, eds. Physiology and Biophysics: The Brain and Neural Function. Philadelphia: WB Saunders, 1979.
15. Melzack R, Wall PD. Pain mechanisms. Science 150:971, 1965.
16. Rossier J. Opioid peptides have found their roots. Nature 298:221, 1982.
17. Ninkovic M, et al. The distribution of multiple opiate receptors in bovine brain. Brain Res 214:163, 1981.
18. Rance MJ. Multiple opiate receptors—Their occurrence and significance. In Bullingham RES, ed. Opiate Analgesia—Anesthesiology, vol I. London: WB Saunders, 1983.
19. Poole JC, Jahr JS. Opiate receptors: A review of analgesic properties and pharmacological side effects. J La State Med Soc 144:106, 1992.
20. Jessell TM. Fifty years of substance P. Nature 295:551, 1982.
21. Pearson J, Brandeis L, Cuello AC. Depletion of substance P–containing axons in substantia gelatinosa of patients with diminished pain sensitivity. Nature 295:61, 1982.
22. Husobuchi Y. Elevated CSF level of substance P in arachnoiditis is reduced by systemic administration of morphine. Pain 1(Suppl):S257, 1981.
23. Fitzgerald M. Development of pain pathways and mechanisms. In Arnand KJS, McGrath PJ, eds. Pain in Neonates. New York: Elsevier Science Publishing, 1993.
24. Reddy SVR, Yatish TC. Spinal noradrenergic terminal system mediates antinociception. Brain Res 189:391, 1980.
25. Svelt WH. Neuropeptides and monoaminergic neurotransmitters: Their relation to pain. J R Soc Med 73:482, 1980.
26. de Domball FT. Diagnosis of Acute Abdominal Pain. New York: Churchill Livingstone, 1981.
27. MacBride CM. Signs and Symptoms, 5th ed. Philadelphia: JB Lippincott, 1970.
28. Mackenzie J. Symptoms and Their Interpretation. London: Shaw & Sons, 1909.
29. Silen W. Cope's Early Diagnosis of the Acute Abdomen, 15th ed. New York: Oxford University Press, 1979.
30. Sinclair DC, Weddell G, Feindel WH. Referred pain and associated phenomena. Brain 71:184, 1948.
31. Kirkpatrick JR. The Acute Abdomen—Diagnosis and Management. Baltimore: Williams & Wilkins, 1984.
32. Capps JA, Coleman GH. An Experimental and Clinical Study of Pain in the Pleura, Pericardium, and Peritoneum. New York: MacMillan, 1932.

32

Neoplastic Disorders of the Gastrointestinal Tract

Michael W. Mulholland, Walter E. Longo, and Anthony M. Vernava III

Neoplasia of the gastrointestinal tract is commonly encountered in the practice of surgery. Although tumors can arise in virtually any region of the gut, the incidence of neoplasia in the colon and rectum far exceeds other anatomic sites. This chapter summarizes the types of tumors likely to occur in the alimentary tract, again emphasizing the underlying physiologic dysfunction associated with each of them and the means by which normal physiology is restored when surgery becomes necessary.

Neoplastic Disease of the Stomach, Small Bowel, and Colorectum

Michael W. Mulholland

GASTRIC NEOPLASMS

Gastric cancer is a lethal disease that remains among the top 10 causes of cancer-related deaths in the United States.[1] Since gastric neoplasms are frequently recognized only at an advanced stage, they cannot be controlled by operation alone; as a consequence, surgical cure rates remain unacceptably low.

In the first eight decades of this century, the incidence of gastric cancer declined in the United States. In 1980 the incidence of gastric cancer in males (10 cases per 100,000 of population) was one fourth the incidence observed in 1930. Approximately 23,000 new cases were reported in 1990.[1] The causes of gastric cancer are unknown, and the factors contributing to its continued prevalence have not been identified.

Benign Lesions

Benign tumors of the stomach comprise between 5% and 10% of all gastric neoplasms and arise primarily in the epithelium or underlying submucosa. Those tumors of epithelial origin present clinically as polypoid lesions and may either be sessile or pedunculated. Unless they are located in the distal stomach where they may alter normal gastric emptying, they are usually asymptomatic and often discovered as incidental findings on upper gastrointestinal endoscopy or barium study. Their major importance surgically is that they may harbor an underlying malignancy (see the following discussion).

Benign tumors arising from the submucosa are commonly found within the gastric wall and almost invariably represent smooth muscle tumors known as leiomyomas. These lesions are generally of little clinical significance unless they compromise the blood supply to the overlying epithelium secondary to excessive growth. When this occurs, a central ulceration of the epithelium and underlying leiomyoma develops that has been known to culminate in a massive upper gastrointestinal hemorrhage. Distinguishing lesions of this nature from their malignant counterparts may be very difficult.

Other benign tumors of the stomach may also occur. Generally, they are asymptomatic and discovered as incidental findings at autopsy, on endoscopy, or during radiologic studies of the stomach. Examples include neurofibromas, lipomas, carcinoid tumors, and occasionally a remnant of a pancreatic rest (i.e., ectopic pancreas).

Premalignant Lesions

Gastric Polyps

The presence of gastric polyps increases the risk of developing gastric carcinoma.[2] The increase in risk relates to polyp histology, size, and number. In terms of malignant potential, benign gastric neoplasms may be categorized in two broad groups: hyperplastic and adenomatous polyps. Hyperplastic gastric polyps are considered to have negligible neoplastic potential, and most affected individuals are asymptomatic. Microscopically, the polyp contains histologically normal gastric mucosa without atypia. Complications are unusual, with occult gastrointestinal bleeding occurring in less than 20% of cases. Endoscopic removal is sufficient treatment.

In contrast to hyperplastic polyps, adenomatous polyps have an increased risk for malignant degeneration. Mitotic figures and atypia are more common than in hyperplastic polyps, and both markers of malignant potential increase with increasing polyp size. The incidence of carcinoma is greatest for polyps more than 2 cm in diameter. The risk of gastric cancer is increased when multiple adenomatous polyps are present.

Endoscopic polypectomy is indicated for pedunculated adenomatous polyps; endoscopic treatment is sufficient treatment if the polyp can be removed completely and shows no evidence of invasion on microscopic examination. For sessile lesions or those larger than 2 cm, operative excision is appropriate. After treatment of an adenomatous polyp, endoscopic surveillance of the gastric mucosa is indicated. The presence of an adenomatous polyp indicates that the entire gastric mucosa is at an increased risk for the development of cancer.

Gastritis

Strong, but circumstantial, evidence supports a role for chronic gastritis in the development of gastric carcinoma.[3] Both atrophic gastritis and gastric cancer occur with increased frequency in elderly populations. Gastritis is often observed in mucosa adjacent to gastric cancer. Mucosal dysplasia and intestinal metaplasia, the presence of intestinal glands within the gastric mucosa, are observed in association with chronic gastritis. Intestinal metaplasia is also commonly noted in association with gastric cancer.

A potential role for *Helicobacter pylori* in gastric carcinogenesis has received considerable attention recently but must still be considered conjectural.[4,5] In industrialized nations the frequency of *H. pylori* infection in patients with gastric adenocarcinoma is similar to the incidence in age-matched control subjects. In contrast, an increased prevalence of *H. pylori* infestation has been reported in regions of the world with high gastric cancer rates. Serologic evidence for prior infection, as reflected by anti–*H. pylori* antibodies, has also been reported in patients with gastric cancer. The decreased incidence of gastric cancer in developed countries observed during the early decades of this century has been postulated to be due to reduction in *H. pylori* infestation secondary to improved nutrition and hygiene.

A relationship between gastric malignancy and chronic gastritis associated with pernicious anemia has been recognized for some time. Atrophic gastritis is characterized by fundic mucosal atrophy, with loss of parietal and chief cells, hypochlorhydria, and hypergastrinemia. Atrophic gastritis confined to the fundic mucosa occurs in 3% of people older than 60 years. For individuals affected by pernicious anemia for more than 5 years, the risk of gastric cancer is doubled relative to age-matched control subjects. This increased risk dictates prompt investigation of new digestive symptoms in patients with long-standing pernicious anemia. In contrast to fundic gastritis, antral gastritis, which is observed in patients with peptic ulceration, has no demonstrated malignant potential.

Previous Gastric Surgery

Gastric cancer is more likely to develop in individuals who have undergone prior gastric resection, but the relative risk for developing gastric malignancy is low.[6,7] Prospective studies with long-term follow-up indicate that the risk of gastric carcinoma begins to increase at 15 years after gastric resection, with a tripling of the relative risk noted after 25 years. This level of risk is not sufficient to justify regular endoscopic surveillance in asymptomatic postgastrectomy patients but does suggest that new symptoms should be aggressively investigated.

Adenocarcinoma

Clinical Presentation

The symptoms produced by gastric cancer are not specific and must be distinguished from a number of unrelated gastroduodenal diseases.[8] Epigastric pain resembling symptoms produced by peptic ulceration is present in 70% of patients with early gastric carcinoma. In some patients the pain may be relieved, at least temporarily, by antacids, leading to diagnostic delay. Anorexia, nausea, and weight loss become increasingly common with disease progression. Proximal gastric lesions produce dysphagia in approximately 20% of patients. Antral lesions may cause symptoms of gastric outlet obstruction. Occult gastrointestinal blood loss and anemia are common; melena is noted in 20% and acute gastrointestinal hemorrhage in 10%. Perforation is rare in gastric carcinoma.

Physical examination is normal in patients with early gastric cancer. Stool testing reveals guaiac-positivity in one third. Abnormal physical findings such as abdominal mass, hepatomegaly, and supraclavicular adenopathy usually reflect advanced disease. Cachexia is prominent, even in the absence of luminal obstruction. There are no laboratory tests specific for gastric neoplasms. Serum tumor markers are neither sensitive nor specific enough to be diagnostically useful.

Diagnosis and Screening

Fiber-optic endoscopy is the most appropriate diagnostic method when gastric neoplasm is suspected. Early gastric carcinomas may appear polypoid or as flat indurated lesions. Advanced carcinomas are usually ulcerated, with an irregular, beaded border and a base that is necrotic and shaggy. The ulcer may relate to an underlying mass. Differentiation of benign and malignant gastric ulcers requires endoscopic biopsy. Diagnostic accuracy exceeds 95% if multiple biopsies are obtained. Accuracy is enhanced by the addition of direct brush cytology.

Single-contrast barium examinations have a diagnostic accuracy approximating 80%. When double-contrast (air and barium) techniques are used, diagnostic yield increases to 90%. Typical x-ray findings indicating gastric carcinoma include ulceration, gastric mass, disruption of mucosal detail, and distortion of the gastric contour. Because biopsy is necessary to definitively distinguish benign and malignant gastric ulceration, endoscopy has largely supplanted barium contrast studies for diagnostic purposes.

CT scans may be used as a primary diagnostic test and to evaluate extragastric spread.[9] CT scans performed with intraluminal contrast readily demonstrate infiltration of the gastric wall by tumor, gastric ulceration, and hepatic metastasis (Figs. 32-1 and 32-2). CT scans are less reliable with regard to the presence of lymphatic metastases or malignant invasion of adjacent organs (Fig. 32-3). Because of these limitations, CT scans cannot replace histologic staging and do not eliminate the necessity for laparotomy in most cases.

Endoscopic ultrasonography uses an endoscopically directed probe with transducer frequencies between 7.5 and 12 MHz. The gastric wall, acoustically coupled to the transducer by instillation of water, is visualized as a five-layered structure with alternating echogenic and low-echo layers. Endoscopic ultrasound is useful for evaluating gastric submucosal lesions and in distinguishing them from invasive gastric neoplasms or gastric compression by adjacent organs or disease processes. Benign leiomyomas appear as round, smooth, hypoechoic masses contiguous with muscularis propria.[10–12]

Gastric adenocarcinomas have several features that may be detected by endoscopic ultrasound. Malignancy is suggested by size (>3 cm), destruction of normal wall layers, irregular margins, and hypoechoic foci caused by necrosis. The depth of intramural invasion caused by gastric cancer can be determined in four fifths of cases. Early gastric cancer, defined as a lesion confined to the mucosa and submucosa, can be differentiated from invasive cancer by endoscopic ultrasound in 90% of cases. Gastric adenocarcinoma can usually be distinguished from gastric lymphoma based on ultrasonographic characteristics. Using current techniques endoscopic ultrasound is unacceptable for nodal staging of gastric cancer, with an accuracy of 50% to 80%. Evaluation for hepatic and distant metastasis requires CT scanning.

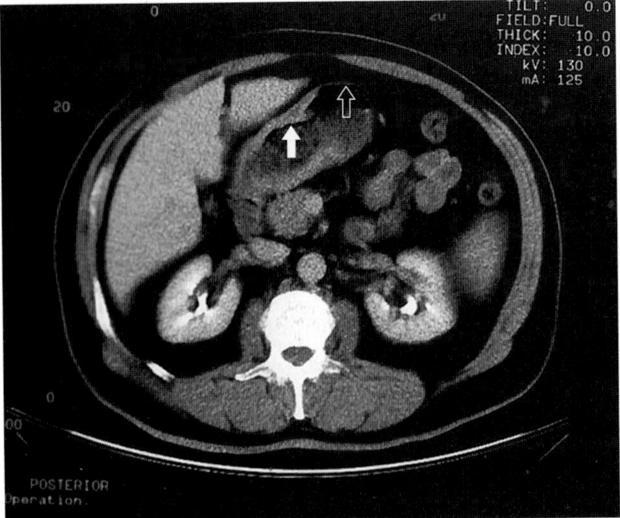

Fig. 32-1. CT scan of antral carcinoma. Note differences in gastric wall thickness for involved *(closed arrow)* and uninvolved areas of the stomach *(open arrow)*.

Pathology

In the United States, gastric adenocarcinomas are distributed with approximately equal frequency in the proximal and distal regions of the stomach.[13,14] Forty percent of cases involve the proximal stomach, which is defined as the esophagogastric junction, fundus, or body, and an equal proportion arise in the antrum. In 15% of cases the stomach is diffusely involved at the time of diagnosis; widespread infiltration is also known as linitis plastica. Proximal

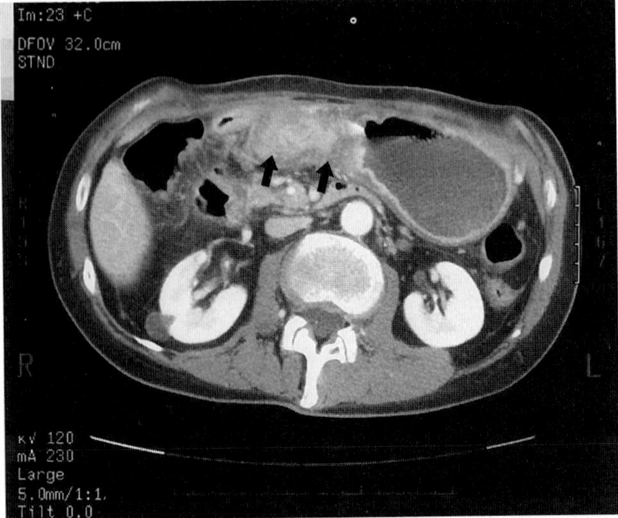

Fig. 32-2. CT scan of large antral adenocarcinoma *(arrows)* causing gastric outlet obstruction. Note air-fluid level in the stomach.

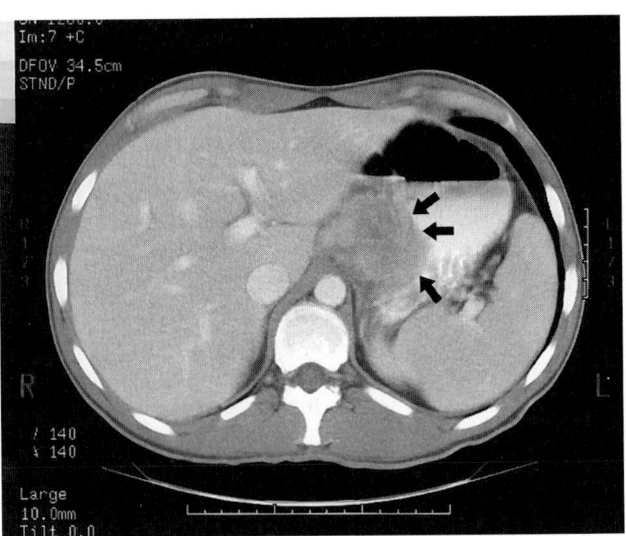

Fig. 32-3. Large gastric adenocarcinoma with involvement of perigastric lymph nodes, causing displacement of the lesser curvature of the stomach *(arrows)*.

gastric involvement is more frequent in elderly patients.

Gastric adenocarcinoma occurs in intestinal and diffuse histologic subtypes. In the intestinal form, malignant gastric cells form glands. The intestinal form of gastric cancer is associated with chronic gastritis, mucosal atrophy, and intestinal metaplasia and dysplasia. The intestinal subtype of gastric cancer is more common in geographic areas of high cancer prevalence and occurs with increased frequency in older patients. The intestinal subtype more frequently demonstrates blood-borne metastases.

The diffuse type of gastric adenocarcinoma infiltrates the gastric wall as a sheet of loosely adherent cells. Lymphatic invasion is common, and intraperitoneal metastases are frequent (Fig. 32-4). The diffuse subtype of gastric adenocarcinoma is observed more commonly in geographic areas of low cancer incidence (e.g., United States) and occurs more frequently in younger patients. The prognosis is worsened for patients with diffuse subtype histology.

Although the size, location, and degree of tumor differentiation (the less differentiated, the less favorable) directly influence the prognosis in gastric cancer, the two major factors influencing survival in potentially resectable tumors are the extent of spread through the gastric wall and the presence or absence of regional *lymph node involvement.* The TNM system of classifying gastric carcinoma emphasizes these two prognostic factors and is currently the major system of staging this disease in the United States (see accompanying box). With this staging scheme the extent of disease is defined in terms of the degree of penetration of the primary tumor through the gastric wall, designated by the letter T; the extent of regional lymph node involvement, designated by the letter N; and the presence or absence of distant metastases, designated by the letter M.

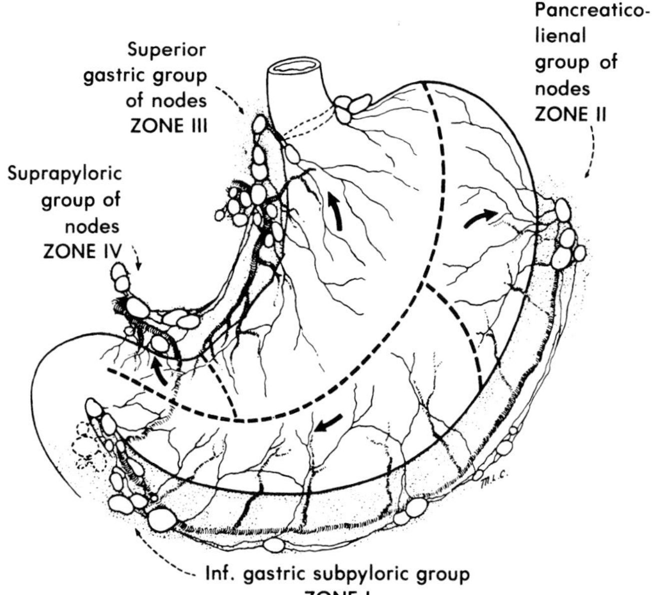

Fig. 32-4. Routes of lymphatic spread for carcinoma of stomach. (From Coller FA, Kay EB, McIntyre RS. Regional lymphatic metastases of carcinoma of the stomach. Arch Surg 43:748. Copyright 1941, American Medical Association.)

Surgical Treatment

While surgical resection offers the only chance for cure of gastric cancer, most patients have an advanced stage of disease at the time of diagnosis. The operative treatment of gastric adenocarcinoma has focused on the extent of gastric resection needed for potentially curable lesions, the role of perigastric lymphadenectomy, the need for disease-free proximal and distal resection margins, the role of splenectomy, and the treatment of involved adjacent organs.

For early gastric cancer involving the antrum, distal subtotal gastrectomy including 80% of the stomach provides adequate 5-year survival without increasing operative morbidity (Fig. 32-5). Proximal gastric lesions may require total gastrectomy or esophagogastrectomy to remove the tumor. Regardless of the extent of gastric resection, patients with advanced tumors have poor long-term survival because of the effects of transmural invasion with lymphatic and hematogenous spread.[15-17]

Gastric cancer frequently demonstrates intramural

TNM CLASSIFICATION

Primary Tumor (T)

- T1 Limitation of the tumor to mucosa and submucosa, regardless of its extent or location
- T2 Tumor involvement of the mucosa and submucosa (including the muscularis propria), with extension to or into the serosa but not penetration through the serosa
- T3 Tumor penetration through the serosa without invasion of contiguous structures
- T4 Tumor penetration through the serosa and invasion of contiguous structures

Nodal Involvement (N)

- N0 Absence of regional lymph node metastases
- N1 Perigastric lymph node involvement within 3 cm of the primary tumor along the lesser or greater curvature
- N2 Regional lymph node involvement more than 3 cm from the primary tumor, which can be removed at surgery, including those nodes located along the left gastric, splenic, celiac, and common hepatic arteries
- N3 Other intra-abdominal lymph node involvement that cannot be adequately removed at surgery such as the para-aortic, hepatoduodenal, retropancreatic, and mesenteric nodes

Distant Metastasis (M)

- M0 No known evidence of distant metastases
- M1 Distant metastases present

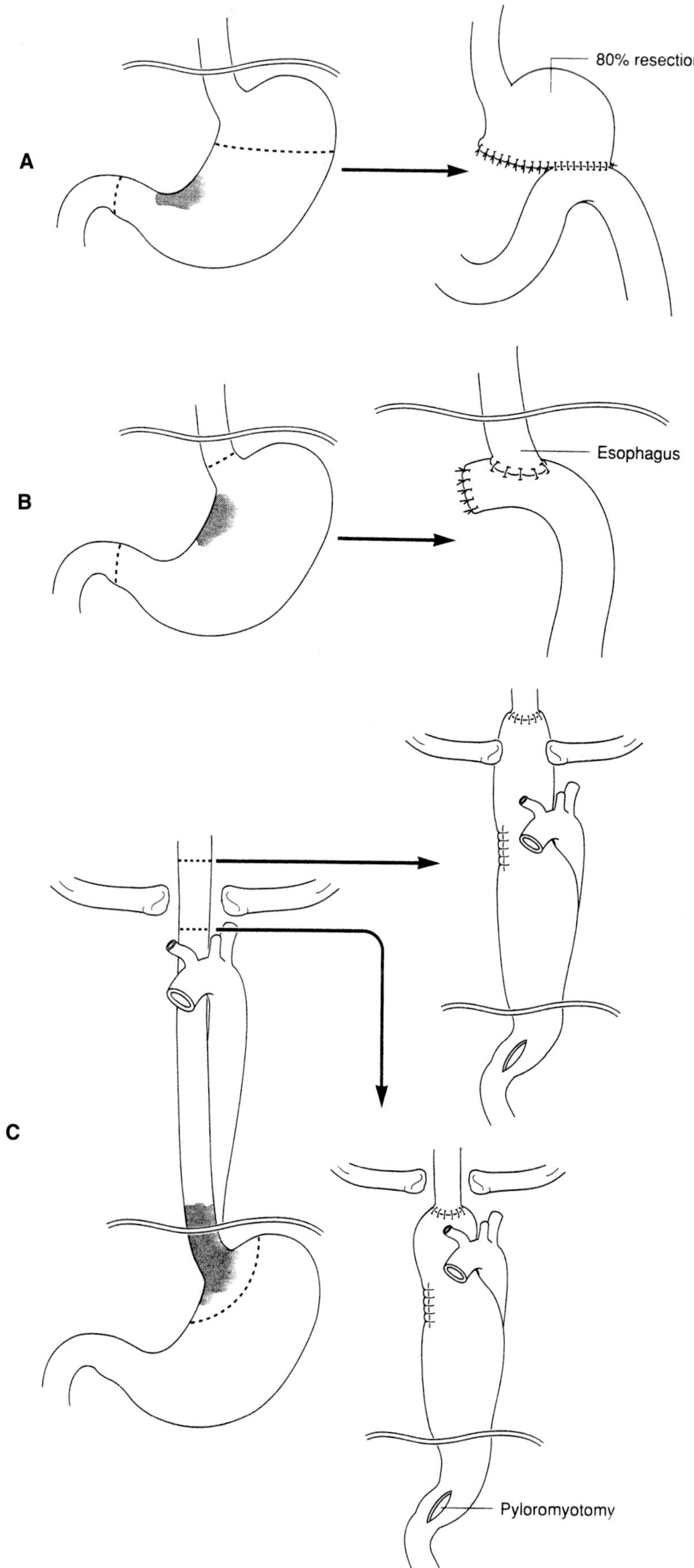

Fig. 32-5. Surgical options for treatment of gastric adenocarcinoma. **A,** Subtotal gastrectomy with gastrojejunal reconstruction. **B,** Total gastrectomy followed by esophagojejunostomy. **C,** Esophagogastrectomy with intrathoracic or cervical reconstruction. (From Mulholland MW. Gastric neoplasms. In Greenfield LJ, et al., eds. Surgery: Scientific Principles and Practice. Philadelphia: JB Lippincott, 1993, p 714.)

spread, related to the extensive anastomosing lymphatic network within the wall of the stomach. The extent of gastric resection is determined by the need to obtain a margin of resection free of microscopic disease.[18] Microscopic tumor involvement of the resection margin is associated with a high risk for anastomotic recurrence. Retrospective studies suggest that a resection margin 6 cm from the tumor mass is necessary to minimize anastomotic recurrence.

The role of radical lymphadenectomy in the treatment of gastric adenocarcinoma is controversial. The largest favorable experience has been reported by Japanese surgeons.[19-22] In Japan an improvement of approximately 10%, stage for stage, has been reported for patients with advanced disease treated with extended lymphadenectomy. These results have not been confirmed in other Asian series or in western countries.[23,24] In one retrospective trial, extended lymphadenectomy increased morbidity caused by intra-abdominal sepsis but did not improve cancer cure rates.[23] Histologically involved lymph nodes are frequently present in the splenic hilum and along the splenic artery, but routine splenectomy has not been demonstrated to improve outcome. If resection of adjacent organs is required for local control of direct invasion, operative morbidity is increased, and long-term survival is unusual.

Chemotherapy and Radiation Therapy

Single-agent chemotherapy, used as an adjuvant after potentially curative surgery, has not been proved to be beneficial. No definitive studies exist to show that multiple-agent combinations based on 5-fluorouracil are more effective than single agents when used as adjuvants.[25] Likewise, with disseminated disease, chemotherapy does not have proven efficacy in treatment of patients with disseminated gastric cancer.[26] Single-agent chemotherapy protocols have partial response rates of 25% to 30%, but complete responses have not been reported. Because of the lack of complete response, single-drug regimens have not had impact on long-term survival. Increases in mean survival have been proven with multiple-agent chemotherapy. The use of radiation therapy has modest benefit.

Gastric Lymphoma

Clinical Features

Non-Hodgkin's lymphomas represent 5% of malignant gastric tumors, with the stomach as the most common organ involved in extranodal lymphoma. Patients are considered to have primary gastric lymphoma if the stomach is exclusively or predominantly involved with the tumor. Gastric lymphoma has peak incidence in the sixth and seventh decades, and is distinctly unusual in children and young adults. Symptoms include epigastric pain, weight loss, anorexia, nausea, and vomiting; initial symptoms are indistinguishable from those caused by gastric adenocarcinoma. Occult gastrointestinal hemorrhage and anemia are observed in the majority of patients, but acute bleeding is rare.

Diagnosis

Upper gastrointestinal endoscopy is the diagnostic method of choice. Endoscopic biopsy, combined with brush cytology, provides the correct diagnosis in 90% of cases. Submucosal extension without ulceration of the overlying mucosa may occasionally render endoscopic biopsy nondiagnostic. In this circumstance, endoscopic ultrasonography is quite sensitive in detecting submucosal lymphomatous infiltration. Contrast x-ray findings are similar to those noted for adenocarcinoma. When gastric lymphoma is diagnosed, evidence of systemic involvement should be sought. CT scans of the chest and abdomen, bone marrow biopsy, and biopsy of enlarged peripheral lymph nodes should be performed.

Treatment

A multimodality treatment program, with gastrectomy as the first step, is currently the most common approach for primary gastric lymphoma.[27-30] However, the role of gastrectomy for gastric lymphoma is unsettled; substantial numbers of patients have been treated with chemoradiation therapy alone. In arguing for gastrectomy before chemoradiation therapy, the risk of therapy-induced hemorrhage or perforation has frequently been cited.[31] This risk has probably been overstated; perforation in primary gastric lymphomas treated with cytolytic agents instead of resection approximates 5%. In this regard, endoscopic ultrasonography to detect full-thickness involvement of the gastric wall may be useful in selection of patients for primary chemoradiation therapy.

If gastrectomy is elected, extended resection is not indicated. In contrast to adenocarcinoma, microscopically positive resection margins do not lead to anastomotic recurrence when radiotherapy is administered postoperatively. In patients with stage I disease, surgery may be curative, and no further therapy is required. Patients with stage II primary gastric lymphoma should be considered to have systemic disease and require systemic therapy in addition to surgery and/or radiotherapy. Postoperative radiation to the gastrectomy site improves local and regional control, with local recurrence observed in less than 15% of treated patients.

Gastric Carcinoid

Gastric carcinoids are rare tumors, accounting for 3% to 5% of all gastrointestinal carcinoids and only 0.3% of gastric neoplasms. The incidence of gastric carcinoids may have been underestimated in older reports because of misclassification as gastric carcinoma. Patients with pernicious anemia have increased risk for development of gastric carcinoids, in addition to increased risk for gastric adenocarcinoma. According to one hypothesis, gastric carcinoids develop as a result of chronic trophic stimulation of enterochromaffin-like cells by hypergastrinemia associated with pernicious anemia.[32,33] Typically, carcinoid tumors developing in association with pernicious anemia are located in the gastric body or fundus. The antrum is not involved.

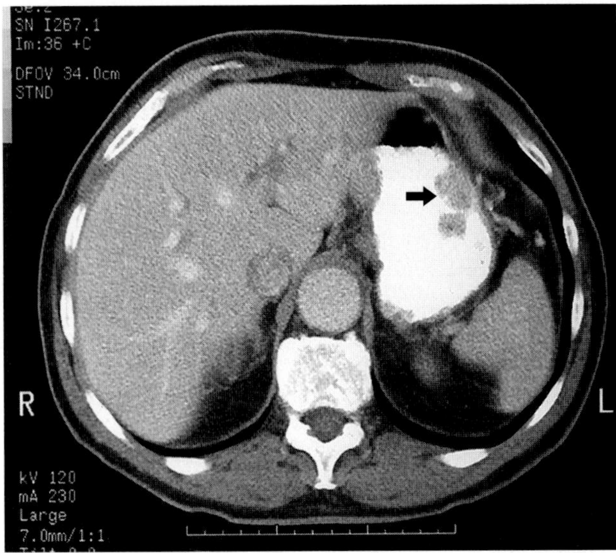

Fig. 32-6. CT scan of patient with polypoid gastric carcinoid *(arrow)* arising from the anterior wall of the fundus. The size of the lesion predicts malignant behavior.

The tumors are composed of monotonous hyperchromatic cells originating in the submucosa or within the basal area of gastric glands. Malignant potential is closely related to tumor size. Invasion is uncommon in tumors less than 2 cm in diameter but is noted with increasing frequency in larger tumors.

Most patients are asymptomatic, and the tumors are discovered incidentally during endoscopy performed for some other problem. Small carcinoids are pink to yellow submucosal nodules in the proximal stomach. Multiple tumors are frequent. When larger tumors cause ulceration of the overlying mucosa, symptoms are similar to those of gastric ulcer or gastric adenocarcinoma (Fig. 32-6). Endoscopic biopsy, performed deeply enough to sample the submucosa, is usually diagnostic. Gastric resection is indicated in almost all cases because of the potential for malignant degeneration. Unlike midgut carcinoids, metastatic gastric carcinoids are not associated with the carcinoid syndrome.

Gastric Sarcomas

Gastric sarcomas, derived from the mesenchymal components of the gastric wall, constitute approximately 3% of gastric malignancies. Leiomyosarcomas are most common, whereas angiosarcomas and fibrosarcomas are rare. Sarcomas occur most frequently in the sixth and seventh decades of life. Because the tumors are located extraluminally, they may achieve large size before causing symptoms. Ischemic ulceration of the overlying mucosa may cause gastrointestinal hemorrhage, epigastric pain, or weight loss. In this circumstance, symptoms are similar to those produced by adenocarcinoma. Because sarcomas frequently reach large size by the time of diagnosis, an epigastric mass may be detected on physical examination.

Grossly, the tumors are firm and grayish white. Compressed fibrous tissue separating tumor from normal smooth muscle may be present. Eventually, large tumors outgrow their blood supply, and central necrosis is common. Leiomyosarcomas are graded histologically, with the frequency of mitotic figures an important indicator of malignant potential. Greater than 5 to 10 mitoses per 10 high-power fields denotes increased metastatic potential. With benign leiomyomas, mitoses are absent or rare.

Metastasis occurs by the hematogenous route, and hepatic dissemination is common. Intraperitoneal spread is frequent, as is local intraperitoneal recurrence after resection. Lymphatic metastasis is observed in less than 10% of patients. En bloc resection of the tumor and involved structures is the treatment of choice.[34] Radical lymphadenectomy is not indicated because of the low frequency of lymphatic metastasis, but uninvolved resection margins must be ensured histologically. Leiomyosarcomas are not radiosensitive, and chemotherapy has not been shown to improve survival. Overall survival approximates 50%.

SMALL BOWEL NEOPLASMS

Benign Tumors

Small intestinal tumors are infrequent relative to neoplasms of the esophagus, stomach, or colon. Benign neoplasms of the small intestine may be derived from the epithelial layer, lymphoid tissue, or mesenchymal tissues. Epithelially derived adenomas are most frequent. Small intestinal adenomas are similar to those derived from the colon in that both tubular and villous features may be present. For reasons that are not clear, the periampullary region of the duodenum is the most common location for villous tumors in the duodenum. Approximately 90% of sporadic and familial polyposis villous tumors are discovered in the second portion of the duodenum.[35] Leiomyomas are the most common benign mesenchymal tumor; these neoplasms are derived from smooth muscle cells of the muscularis propria or blood vessel wall.

Clinical Presentation

The majority of benign tumors produce symptoms by the sixth decade of life. Partial small bowel obstruction is the most common problem, manifested as pain or emesis. Bowel obstruction may be produced by circumferential tumor growth, but more commonly is due to intussusception of the tumor mass. Although occult blood loss is frequent, weight loss, gross hemorrhage, and melena are unusual. The latter symptoms increase the likelihood of a malignant process.

Therapy

Benign duodenal adenomas are amenable to endoscopic resection if they are not sessile. Tubular and tubulovillous adenomas have a low malignant potential; if single-stage endoscopic removal is not feasible, piecemeal resection is an option. Villous adenomas have a malignant potential similar to villous tumors of the colon. Thirty percent of villous tumors of the duodenum have foci of invasive cancer. This increased risk mandates total excision. Sessile lesions involving the ampulla of Vater should be treated with operative excision to preserve biliary and pancreatic ductal patency.

Malignant Tumors

Clinical Presentation

Abdominal pain secondary to partial small bowel obstruction is the most common symptom in patients with malignant small bowel tumors. Symptoms caused by complete obstruction, perforation, or bleeding are less frequent. Nonspecific symptoms such as anorexia and malaise are common but not helpful. In the absence of overt small intestinal obstruction, physical examination is usually normal; in patients with lymphoma or sarcoma, abdominal masses may be palpable.

Partial or complete obstruction occurs in half of patients with malignant small intestinal neoplasms. In contrast to most benign tumors, malignant neoplasms cause annular constriction of the small bowel lumen. A malignant tumor may occasionally act as an intussuscipiens. Carcinoid tumors may generate an intense desmoplastic reaction involving the mesentery, with fixation and angulation of the bowel contributing to obstruction. Occult gastrointestinal hemorrhage is frequent. Gross bleeding may be caused by erosion of tumor into an artery within the mesentery or by tumor necrosis. Bowel perforation is very uncommon with adenocarcinomas but occasionally is reported with lymphomas or leiomyosarcomas caused by ischemic necrosis of a transmurally invasive tumor. Duodenal tumors involving the periampullary area may cause obstructive jaundice. Metastatic carcinoid neoplasms may be biochemically active and cause the carcinoid syndrome.

Diagnostic Studies

Radiologic contrast studies are the usual diagnostic tests for patients suspected of harboring small bowel tumors. Barium swallow used to evaluate the stomach and duodenum is followed by small bowel examination. Fluoroscopy is performed to monitor the passage of contrast to the cecum. Diagnostic yield is increased by a double-contrast technique in which an effervescent solution is ingested with the contrast. Enteroclysis is another form of small bowel contrast study in which a tube is passed fluoroscopically through the stomach and into the duodenum. Methylcellulose is mixed with the barium to improve mucosal detail. In addition to information on small intestinal mucosa, enteroclysis can be used to determine distensibility of the small intestine. Enteroclysis is most useful in cases of intermittent or partial obstruction.

CT scanning is useful in determining tumor resectability, demonstrating invasion of adjacent organs or distant metastasis. Newer CT techniques are sensitive for detection of major vascular involvement, exophytic masses, or tumor necrosis. Major vascular encasement, invasion of contiguous organs, distant lymphadenopathy, and hepatic metastases may indicate the lack of potential for curative resection.[36,37]

Enteroscopy, endoscopic examination of the small intestine, has an important role in the diagnosis of small intestinal tumors. Enteroscopy is performed using a long endoscope, 160 to 170 cm in length, passed orally. With persistence, satisfactory evaluation of the mucosa is accomplished in 50% to 70% of patients.[38-40] The bowel wall may also be examined using specially designed ultrasound probes passed endoscopically. In the small bowel, endoscopic ultrasound is limited to the duodenum and periampullary area. Modern probes can visualize the duodenal wall, ampulla, distal common bile duct, pancreas, proximal portal vein, and regional lymph nodes. An accurate assessment of mural penetration by tumor and the status of proximate lymph nodes is possible in most cases. Accuracy rates approximating 80% for staging of periampullary and common bile duct carcinomas have been reported.[41]

Adenocarcinoma

Total excision is the only definitive therapy for duodenal and periampullary tumors. Periampullary local excision is appropriate only for tumors without evidence of invasion. Because of the high incidence of local recurrence if tumors with an invasive component are treated by local resection, it is imperative to prove that a locally excised tumor is benign. Endoscopic biopsy alone is not adequate, as endoscopic biopsy fails to include malignant tissue in 50% of cases.[42] With local excision, reimplantation of the common duct is necessary, using a technique derived from transduodenal sphincteroplasty.[43]

Pancreaticoduodenectomy is the standard procedure for curative resection of periampullary adenocarcinoma and is frequently necessary for larger nonmalignant neoplasms involving the ampulla of Vater or the second or third portions of the duodenum. Referral centers with surgical expertise have reported operative mortality rates less than 5% and significant procedure-related morbidity less than 20%.[44] Adenocarcinoma of the jejunum or ileum should be treated by segmental small intestinal resection with mesenteric resection to include draining lymphatics.

For small bowel adenocarcinomas, there are no effective chemotherapy agents for use as adjuvants to surgical resection. 5-Fluorouracil and the nitrosoureas have been reported to have partial response rates of 10% to 20% but have not been demonstrated to increase disease-free survival. Small intestinal adenocarcinomas are radioresistant.

Prognosis

Five-year survival rates for patients with small intestinal adenocarcinoma approximate 5% to 30%.[45] Survival is severely impacted by the presence of lymph node metastases. In one recent report, patients without lymph node metastases had 5-year survival of 70%; survival was 13% in node positive patients. Overall survival rate was 24% in another recent report.[46]

Carcinoid Tumors

Pathogenesis

Carcinoid tumors are categorized according to the embryologic segment in which they develop: foregut, midgut, or hindgut.[47] Grossly, the typical carcinoid tumor is bright yellow, and associated with a dense desmoplastic infiltration of collagen. Carcinoid tumors demonstrate a histochemical affinity for silver stains (argentophillic staining). Results from immunocytochemical staining using antibodies to a variety of gastrointestinal peptides or neuronal markers such as neuron-specific enolase are typically positive. Many carcinoid tumors produce and secrete humorally active compounds. Tumor products identified in blood, urine or tumor tissue include 5-hydroxytryptamine (serotonin), 5-hydroxytryptophan, histamine, substance P, prostaglandins, catecholamines, kallilkrein, gastrin, somatostatin, adrenocorticotropic hormone (ACTH), and insulin.[48] Hormonal products secreted into the mesenteric venous effluent by carcinoid tumors are metabolized by the liver, and for this reason, most carcinoid tumors are biochemically silent until extraintestinal metastases develop.

Histologically, carcinoids are composed of uniform population of cells with monotonous nuclei and cytoplasm. Few mitotic figures are noted, although all carcinoids are potentially malignant. Carcinoids may appear similar to undifferentiated adenocarcinomas or other anaplastic tumors. In such cases, immunocytochemical staining with antibodies directed against a variety of peptide hormones, silver staining, and electron microscopy to demonstrate secretory granules may be needed to confirm the diagnosis.

Clinical Presentation

Small nonmetastatic carcinoids are asymptomatic and are usually discovered incidentally at laparotomy performed for an unrelated reason. Larger lesions usually become symptomatic with bowel obstruction resulting from luminal obstruction by tumor mass or mesenteric desmoplastic reaction.

The appendix is the most common site of origin of carcinoid tumors, with a small intestinal location ranking second. When they occur in the small bowel, they are usually found within 2 or 3 feet of the ileocecal valve as hard, white nodules arising in the deep aspect of the mucosa. In contrast to appendiceal carcinoids, in which metastases are uncommon, as many as 35% to 40% of ileal carcinoids have spread to regional nodes when first identified at surgery. The likelihood of metastases is related to their size, with tumors larger than 2 cm in diameter having metastasized in 80% to 90% of cases.[47,48]

Since carcinoid tumors arise from enterochromaffin cells throughout the gut, they are members of the amine precursor uptake and decarboxylase (APUD) family. Thus it is not surprising that they are associated with neoplasms involving other enterochromaffin tissues, including medullary carcinoma of the thyroid and pheochromocytoma. This coexistence of a second neoplasm has been noted in as many as 30% to 53% of patients with carcinoid tumors.[47,48]

Carcinoids that have metastasized to the liver may develop systemic symptoms that are collectively known as the *carcinoid syndrome.* Intermittent flushing and diarrhea are the most disabling symptoms. The flushing may last from seconds to minutes and can be precipitated by foods, alcohol, physical stress, and anesthetic induction. Flushing may be accompanied by bronchospasm, cutaneous suffusion, and development of telangiectasia. Right-sided heart failure has been associated with the carcinoid syndrome due to endocardial and valvular fibrosis of the right side of the heart. The peculiar cardiac lesions are thought to be caused by high levels of vasoactive amines in venous blood entering the heart.

The exact biochemical events responsible for this syndrome remain to be fully clarified, but an abnormality in serotonin metabolism has been clearly implicated.[47,48] Under normal conditions, approximately 1% of dietary tryptophan, the immediate precursor of serotonin, is metabolized to produce this substance. In contrast, as much as 50% to 60% of tryptophan may be diverted into the serotonin pathway with the presence of a functioning carcinoid tumor. Usually, any excess in serotonin production is broken down in the liver to 5-hydroxyindoleacetic acid (5-HIAA), which is then excreted in the urine. However, in patients with metastatic carcinoid tumor implants, this breakdown is impaired, with the subsequent release of serotonin into the systemic circulation. It is this enhanced release of serotonin and perhaps other unidentified substances that gives rise to the carcinoid syndrome. Since available liver parenchyma, even in the presence of metastatic implants, attempts to catalyze as much serotonin as possible, even though this event is not completely successful, levels of 5-HIAA in the urine are greatly increased. This urinary measurement provides the chemical basis for the diagnosis of a functioning carcinoid tumor.

Diagnosis

Diagnostic studies for small intestinal carcinoid tumors presenting with intestinal obstruction are similar to those used for other small intestinal tumors. When the carcinoid syndrome is suspected, biochemical testing is directed at detecting serotonin overproduction. An elevation in urinary 5-HIAA is the most consistent finding. Urine collection must be rigorously controlled, as a number of foods (tomatoes, pineapples, bananas) and medications (phenothiazines) can cause false positive test results. Urinary 5-HIAA levels in excess of 10 mg/dl are highly suggestive of the carcinoid syndrome.

Treatment

Surgery is the only curative treatment available for carcinoid tumors of the small intestine. Even when curative operation is not possible, surgery is usually important in the palliation of patients with metastatic disease.[49] In planning an operation, it is important to realize that anesthetic induction can precipitate the development of carcinoid crisis. Carcinoid crisis refers to a life-threatening syndrome of persistent generalized flushing culminating in cardiovascular collapse. Cardiovascular derangements include tachycardia, arrhythmia, and shock. For patients with known metastatic carcinoid tumor, the long-acting somatostatin analog octreotide should be immediately available during laparotomy. Intravenous administration of octreotide to a patient with carcinoid crisis suppresses the release and action of a number of vasoactive compounds from the tumor and may be lifesaving.[50] Preoperative prophylaxis with octreotide has been advocated.[51]

There is a clear correlation between the ability of a carcinoid tumor to metastasize and its size. Metastatic risk is relatively low for tumors less than 1 cm.[48] Segmental resection should include en bloc wedge resection of mesentery. Multicentric disease exists in 20% to 30% of patients.

For patients with single hepatic metastases, hepatic resection is appropriate if tumor-free margins can be achieved. Unfortunately, hepatic metastases are usually diffuse and not amenable to resection. If surgery is not possible, octreotide is the most effective agent for palliation of flushing and diarrhea. Octreotide suppresses release of vasoactive compounds elaborated in hepatic metastases. The drug is administered by subcutaneous injection; clinical effects persist 6 to 8 hours. Tachyphylaxis is unusual, and a significant proportion of patients (25% to 30%) experience relief for up to 2 years. Radiotherapy has no proven benefit for metastatic carcinoid tumors and chemotherapy achieves partial response rates of only 30% to 40%. Chemotherapy-induced partial responses have not been associated with increased survival.

Prognosis

Overall 5-year survival in one large series was 75% in patients who underwent complete resection for cure and 19% in patients with distant metastases.[52] Development of the carcinoid syndrome has a significant negative impact on survival. Patients with nonmetastatic disease who undergo curative resection have survival rates that are not significantly different from the general population. Even the presence of nodal metastases, if completely resected, is associated with survival times of 10 to 15 years.

Lymphoma

Predisposing Factors

Non-Hodgkin's lymphoma of the small intestine comprises 20% of all gastrointestinal lymphomas. The ileum is involved more frequently than the jejunum. The risk of small intestinal lymphoma is increased in patients with solid organ transplantation, celiac sprue, idiopathic steatorrhea, Crohn's disease, and AIDS.

The frequency of lymphoma in transplantantation recipients has been estimated to be 40 to 400-fold higher than that of the normal population. Transplantation-associated lymphomas are often extranodal and occur in the gastrointestinal tract and the central nervous system at increased rate. The disease is often systemic by the time of diagnosis, but isolated intestinal disease has been reported. Lymphomas developing in the setting of organ transplantation are almost always of B-cell type. Serologic evidence of Epstein-Barr virus infection suggests a causative role for the virus.[53,54]

Approximately 5% of patients with sprue develop lymphoma; the incidence increases with age.[55] Intestinal lymphoma as a complication of celiac sprue typically presents as an exacerbation of chronic symptoms or abrupt clinical deterioration after a stable, relatively mild course. Sprue-associated tumors are T-cell lymphomas. Other malabsorptive states associated with an increased risk of intestinal lymphoma include idiopathic steatorrhea and dermatitis herpetiformis. Lymphomas most frequently occur in children or after age 50.

Pathology

Although celiac disease–associated lymphomas are predominantly T cell in origin, most intestinal lymphomas are of B-cell origin. Although the majority of small bowel lymphomas are non-Hodgkin's in type, the incidence of primary Hodgkin's disease has risen recently, especially in patients with AIDS. In the United States primary small intestinal lymphomas usually are localized to a segment of small bowel.

Clinical Presentation

Symptoms associated with small intestinal lymphoma are nonspecific and include abdominal pain, weight loss, and intestinal obstruction. Palpable masses, present in 50% of patients, are noted more frequently than in patients with adenocarcinoma. In contrast to small intestinal adenocarcinoma, perforation in association with lymphoma is not rare. Perforation is common in patients with AIDS and is associated with worsened prognosis.[56,57] Contrast studies demonstrate partial small bowel obstruction, mucosal infiltration, and mass effect. CT scanning is helpful in demonstrating segmental wall thickness, the relationship of the tumor to adjacent structures, abdominal lymphadenopathy, and splenic and hepatic involvement.[58]

Treatment

Localized disease is best treated by surgical resection. When curative resection is not possible, peritonitis from perforation or luminal obstruction may still mandate surgical exploration. Staging laparotomy including splenectomy is not appropriate for non-Hodgkin's lymphoma of the small bowel. Splenic involvement can usually be identified noninvasively by CT or MRI. Liver biopsy and para-aortic node sampling are recommended at laparotomy, as these procedures have little morbidity and alter staging and management in 30% of patients.

Multidrug chemotherapy is usually recommended when resected lesions involve mesenteric lymph nodes. For advanced disease with or without partial surgical debulking, combination chemotherapy and radiation therapy may provide palliation.

The prognosis for intestinal lymphomas is dependent primarily on the stage of the tumor at the time of diagnosis. For stage I or II disease, 5-year survival rates approximate 80%; with advanced disease, survival beyond 1 year is unusual. Variables associated with improved prognosis include younger age, lower stage, and surgical resection.[59] Multicentricity is common, and as a result malabsorption and malnutrition are problematic.

Sarcoma

Pathology

Sarcomas account for 10% to 20% of malignant tumors of the small intestine. Peak incidence occurs in the fourth and sixth decades of life. Leiomyosarcomas are the most frequent histologic type; fibrosarcomas and liposarcomas occur with lower frequency. Kaposi's sarcoma, recently noted with increased frequency, is common in patients with AIDS. Kaposi's sarcoma is usually diffuse and rarely confined to the small intestine. Small intestinal sarcomas may grow extraluminally to very large size before causing symptoms. Small intestinal sarcomas are usually hypervascular; even so, central tumor necrosis is often seen as tumors outgrow blood supply. When the central necrosis communicates with the intestinal lumen, hemorrhage is manifest as melena. Lymph node metastasis is rare. Small intestinal sarcomas metastasize hematogenously, usually to the liver.

Tumor size and the number of mitotic figures per high-power microscopic field predict malignant biologic behavior. Tumors greater than 1 cm in diameter have a high risk for metastasis, regardless of histologic features.[60] Cellular atypia is associated with increased mitotic rate and poor prognosis. Symptomatic tumors are more likely to be malignant than benign.

Clinical Presentation

In concert with other small intestinal tumors, sarcomas present with vague symptoms of abdominal pain or bloating. In contrast to adenocarcinomas, abdominal mass on physical examination is frequently observed with sarcomas. The tumors often develop extraluminally. Bowel obstruction may be due to extrinsic luminal compression in addition to circumferential growth. With contrast radiography, a cavity communicating with the bowel lumen indicates central tumor necrosis and strongly suggests sarcoma. CT scanning with oral contrast can also be used to document an extrinsic mass with central tumor necrosis suggestive of sarcoma. CT scanning may also be used to demonstrate hepatic, intraperitoneal, or pulmonary metastases, which are noted in 30% of cases.

Treatment

The only curative therapy for small intestinal sarcomas is surgical resection with en bloc removal of the mesentery and associated lymph nodes. Failure is usually due to local or regional intraperitoneal recurrence. Extended lymph node dissection is not appropriate. Duodenal sarcomas require pancreaticoduodenectomy. Adjuvant chemotherapy and radiotherapy have no documented survival benefit.

Long-term survival depends on histologic grade of the tumor, size of the tumor, and number of mitoses per high-power field. For incompletely resected tumors of low grade, 5-year survival approximates 50% to 80%.[61,62] Patients with high-grade sarcomas have survival rates of 5% to 20%.[61,62] The development of recurrent intra-abdominal disease is associated with a median survival of 8 months.[60]

COLORECTAL NEOPLASMS

Carcinoma of the colon and rectum is diagnosed in 155,000 cases annually in the United States, making it the second most common malignancy.[1] Although curable when discovered at an early stage, carcinomas of the colon and rectum also represent the second leading cause of cancer-related deaths.

Risk Factors

Polyps

Colorectal polyps are the strongest risk factor for the development of colon cancer. Nonneoplastic polyps have no risk for malignant degeneration; this category includes juvenile polyps, inflammatory polyps, and hyperplastic polyps. In contrast, neoplastic polyps have the potential to develop into malignant tumors, with the degree of risk related to histologic type and size. Neoplastic polyps can be categorized as tubular, tubulovillous, or villous adenomas. Tubular adenomas are the most common and have the lowest risk of malignant transformation. Tubulovillous adenomas comprise 15% of neoplastic polyps. Villous adenomas, which have the highest risk for developing invasive cancer, represent an additional 10%. Most adenomas demonstrate some degree of cellular atypia or dysplasia. In modern grading systems, high-grade dysplasia denotes carcinoma in situ. Carcinoma in situ is distinguished from invasive cancer by lack of penetration of the muscularis mucosae. Invasive cancers are associated with adenomatous polyps in 5% of cases, with 22% of tubulovillous adenomas and with 40% of villous lesions.[63]

Inherited Syndromes

Familial polyposis coli is a rare inherited syndrome characterized by the development of large numbers of colonic polyps and colon cancer in early adulthood. Familial polyposis coli is transmitted as an autosomal dominant trait; affected individuals begin to develop adenomatous polyps in the teenage years. Eventually, hundreds of polyps line the colon. Unless prophylactic proctocolectomy is performed, development of colon cancer is uniform by age 50.

The Lynch syndromes represent two forms of familial colon cancer that are not associated with polyposis. The syndromes are more properly termed hereditary nonpolyposis colorectal carcinoma (HNPCC).[64,65] HNPCC type I, is an autosomal dominant syndrome associated with colon cancers that typically develop between 30 and 50 years of age. Unlike sporadic colon cancer or that associated with familial polyposis coli, tumors have a predilection for the right colon, with 60% to 90% of tumors developing in the proximal large bowel. The second Lynch syndrome, also called cancer family syndrome, includes the features of the first Lynch syndrome but is associated with premature onset cancers of the uterus, ovaries, and stomach. Familial forms of colon cancer have been estimated to account for 5% to 10% of all cases of colon malignancy.

Inflammatory Bowel Disease

A definitive association for development of colon cancer exists for patients with ulcerative colitis. The risk of colon cancer is related to the extent of colonic involvement, severity of disease, and duration of illness. Approximately 3% of patients with symptomatic ulcerative colitis develop colon cancer during the first decade after the onset of disease. With greater chronicity, risk increases appreciably, rising to a 20% incidence in the succeeding 10 years.[66] Patients with ulcerative colitis who develop cancer have tumors with pathologic staging and cure rates comparable to noncolitic patients.[67] The presence of Crohn's disease is also associated with an increased risk for colon cancer, although to a lesser degree than ulcerative colitis.

Diagnosis

Unless an individual is enrolled in a screening program, the diagnosis of colorectal cancer is usually made on the basis of symptoms. Most cancers become symptomatic because of gastrointestinal blood loss or malignant bowel obstruction. When bleeding is slow and occult, initial symptoms are often those of iron deficiency anemia with easy fatigue and dyspnea. A more rapid hemorrhage may cause melena, especially for right-sided colon cancers, or red or maroon stools in left-sided or rectal cancers.

Malignant colonic obstruction is most commonly associated with cancers of the descending or sigmoid segments of the colon. Colon cancer involving the ileocecal valve may be associated with small intestinal obstruction. Colonic obstruction causes abdominal distention, lower abdominal pain, nausea, and vomiting. If obstruction is complete, colonic perforation may occur in the proximal bowel or at the site of the tumor. Rectal obstruction is heralded by a change in bowel habits and the passage of stools of decreasing caliber. Symptoms of tenesmus, perineal pain, and urgency usually indicate penetration of the rectal wall by the tumor.

Diagnostic evaluation begins with abdominal and rectal examinations. Stool should be obtained for testing for occult bleeding. Flexible fiber-optic sigmoidoscopy has largely supplanted rigid proctosigmoidoscopy as instruments measuring 65 cm have become available. The bowel is examined after cleansing enemas. An examination of the rectum, sigmoid colon, and descending colon segments can be performed in most patients without sedation. Physician training with this technique is straightforward; patient acceptance is high.

Colonoscopy using a 180 cm fiber-optic instrument is the most important diagnostic method for evaluation of the colon. Colonoscopy is preferred because of the ability to obtain mucosal biopsy samples, to distinguish other lesions that may mimic colon cancer, and to perform therapeutic maneuvers such as polypectomy. Colonoscopy is associated with a definite incidence of complications, including perforation or hemorrhage; these complications require surgical intervention in an estimated 0.1% of examinations.

Barium contrast enema may also be used for the diagnosis of colonic neoplasms. A double-contrast technique in which air and barium are insufflated provides superior mucosal detail relative to single-contrast examination. Colon cancers produce a disruption of the smooth mucosal contour. Circumferential lesions have an apple core appearance. Barium enema consistently visualizes the right colon, which is not reached in 5% of colonoscopic examinations. Proctoscopy should always be performed in conjunction with barium enema because the anal canal and distal rectum are not well visualized by this technique.

Pathology

The risk of developing metastatic disease is predicted by the level of tumor invasion of the bowel wall and by tumor involvement of pericolic lymph nodes. Initially, intramural expansion of an adenocarcinoma is characterized by growth of the tumor into the bowel lumen. Continued growth usually extends transversely rather than longitudinally. Transverse growth leads to circumferential compromise of the bowel lumen. The incidence of lymphatic metastasis increases as the tumor penetrates successive histologic layers of the bowel wall.

The prognosis in colorectal cancer is directly related to the extent of spread at the time of diagnosis. Although a number of staging procedures have been proposed over the last several decades, the original Dukes' classification continues to have considerable merit.[68] This classification is summarized in the accompanying box and is based on the extent of disease and its confinement to the bowel wall or pericolic tissues and the absence or presence of involved nodes. Involvement of regional nodes decreases the likelihood of survival by approximately 50% when patients

DUKES' CLASSIFICATION OF COLORECTAL CANCER

Stage A	Limited to bowel wall
Stage B	Extension of cancer through the bowel wall into pericolic tissues, but without lymph node involvement
Stage C	Cancer involving not only the bowel wall, but also extending into regional nodes

Table 32-1. Other Modifications of Dukes' Classification of Colorectal Cancer*

Stage	Astler, Coller—1954	Gunderson, Sosin—1974
A	Tumor limited to mucosa	Tumor limited to mucosa
B1	Tumor extension into muscularis propria, but not through it	Tumor textention through mucosa, but still within bowel wall
B2	Tumor extension through muscularis propria, but without nodal involvement	Tumor extension through entire bowel wall, but without nodal involvement
B3	—	Tumor adherent to or invading adjacent organs, but without nodal involvement
C1	Tumor limited to bowel wall, but nodes nevertheless positive	Tumor limited to bowel wall, but nodes nevertheless positive
C2	Tumor extension through entire bowel wall, nodes also positive	Tumor extension through entire bowel wall, nodes also positive
C3	—	Tumor adherent to or invading adjacent organs, nodes also positive

Adapted from Astler VB, Coller FA. The prognostic significance of direct extension of carcinoma of the colon and rectum. Ann Surg 139:846, 1954; and Gunderson LL, Sosin H. Areas of failure at reoperation (second or symptomatic look) following "curative surgery" for adenocarcinoma of the rectum. Cancer 34:1278, 1974.

*None of these classifications includes stage D. Convention, however, assigns patients to stage D if the patients have distant metastases or locally unresectable tumor.

are evaluated 5 years after diagnosis. Distant spread beyond regional nodes generally represents incurability, and very few patients are alive beyond 1 year following diagnosis. Other modifications of the Dukes' classification are shown in Table 32-1. Many oncologists currently use the TNM staging system. Its relationship to the Dukes' staging system is shown in the box on p. 681.

The liver is the most common site of hematogenous metastases from colorectal cancers. Overall, approximately 50% of patients develop hepatic involvement.[69] The reason that hepatic metastasis is so common is incompletely understood. Undoubtedly, anatomy plays an important role. The portal system is the venous drainage of the colon and upper rectum, and the liver is the first capillary bed that tumor emboli encounter. The lung is the next most common site of metastasis for colorectal tumors. Rectal tumors occasionally metastasize to pelvic and vertebral bones. Colon cancers may metastasize directly to peritoneal surfaces if full-thickness invasion has occurred. The occurrence of widespread intraperitoneal metastasis, termed carcinomatosis, is not associated with long-term survival.

Treatment

Neoplastic Polyps

For adenomatous polyps without a malignant component, endoscopic polypectomy is the preferred treatment. Pedunculated polyps can be removed endoscopically using a cautery-equipped snare. Small to medium-sized sessile polyps can also be removed endoscopically, although this may require more than one endoscopic session. When an endoscopically resected polyp contains a microscopic focus of cancer, one must decide whether further therapy is required. A polyp is considered to contain an in situ malignancy if the tumor cells do not penetrate the muscularis mucosae of the polyp. In situ cancers in polyps do not have the potential for metastasis and do not require further therapy. For endoscopic polypectomy to be considered adequate therapy, the polyp resection margin should be tumor free and the tumor should be well differentiated and without evidence of lymphatic or vascular invasion.[70-72] If these criteria do not apply, endoscopic resection of the cancer-containing polyp should be followed by segmental colectomy. Occasionally, larger villous tumors of the colon cannot be resected endoscopically; segmental colectomy is appropriate in this instance.

Colorectal Cancer

For colon and rectal cancers, preoperative evaluation for synchronous cancers and metastatic disease is important. Physical examination may reveal ascites, hepatomegaly, or inguinal or supraclavicular adenopathy. Laboratory investigation should include a complete blood count, liver function studies, and determination of carcinoembryonic antigen (CEA). An elevation in alkaline phosphatase is a sensitive indicator of hepatic metastasis. Preoperative measurement of CEA is important for postoperative follow-up. A complete colonoscopy or barium enema is necessary to detect coexisting synchronous colon neoplasms. CT scanning is a sensitive method for detecting hepatic metastases, involvement of adjacent structures or malignant ascites. For rectal neoplasms, CT scanning should be performed routinely to assess factors that influence resectability (extension of tumor to pelvic side wall, involvement of ureters or bladder, encasement of major vascular structures).

Operative therapy for colorectal cancers commences with a careful appraisal of peritoneal surfaces and intraperitoneal organs, particularly the liver. The presence of intraperitoneal metastasis may occasionally mandate pal-

STAGING CLASSIFICATION OF COLORECTAL CANCER*

TNM System

Primary tumor

Tx	Primary tumor cannot be assessed
T0	No evidence of tumor in resected specimen (prior polypectomy or fulguration)
Tis	Carcinoma in situ
T1	Invades into submucosa
T2	Invades into muscularis propria
T3/T4	Depends on whether serosa is present

Serosa present

T3	Invades through muscularis propria into subserosa Invades serosa (but not through) Invades pericolic fat within the leaves of the mesentery
T4	Invades through serosa into free peritoneal cavity, or through serosa into a continguous organ

No serosa (distal two thirds of rectum, posterior left or right colon)

T3	Invades through muscularis propria
T4	Invades other organs (vagina, prostate, ureter, kidney)

Regional lymph node involvement

NX	Nodes cannot be assessed (e.g., local excision only)
N0	No regional node metastases
N1	1-3 positive nodes
N2	4 or more positive nodes
N3	Central nodes positive

Distant metastasis

MX	Presence of distant metastases cannot be assessed
M0	No distant metastases
M1	Distant metastases present

Dukes' Staging System Correlated With TNM

Dukes A	T1, N0, M0 (stage I) T2, N0, Mo (stage I)
Dukes B	T3, N0, M0 (stage II) T4, N0, M0 (stage II)
Dukes C	T (any), N1, M0; T (any), N2, M0 (stage III)
Dukes D	T (any), N (any), M1 (stage IV)

Modified Astler-Coller (MAC) System Correlated With TNM

MAC A	T1, N0, M0 (stage I)
MAC B1	T2, N0, M0 (stage I)
MAC B2	T3, N0, M0 (stage II)
MAC B3	T4, N0, M0 (stage II)
MAC C1	T2, N1, M0; T2, N2, M0 (stage III)
MAC C2	T3, N1, M0; T3, N2, M0 (stage III) T4, N1, M0; T4, N2, M0 (stage III)
MAC C3	T4, N1, M0; T4, N2, M0 (stage III)

From Greenfield LJ, et al., eds. Surgery: Scientific Principles and Practice, 2nd ed. Philadelphia: Lippincott Raven, 1997.

*In all pathologic staging systems, particularly those applied to rectal cancer, the abbreviations *m* and *g* may be used; *m* denotes microscopic transmural penetration; *g* or *m* + g denotes transmural penetration visible on gross inspection and confirmed microscopically.

liative treatment only. The goals of surgical resection of colorectal cancer are threefold: (1) to perform en bloc resection with margins of normal colon proximal and distal to the tumor; (2) to obtain tumor-free margins laterally if a transmurally invasive tumor has involved adjacent structures; and (3) to resect pericolic lymph nodes. Microscopically, colon cancer rarely extends intramurally more than 2 cm beyond the point of gross involvement. Margins of greater than 2 cm are not difficult to achieve for the intraperitoneal colon. However, for cancers involving the mid rectum, margins greater than 2 cm may be difficult if sphincteric function is to be preserved. Immediately paracolic and mesenteric lymph nodes are removed during curative colon resection. Extensive bowel resections in efforts to perform a more radical lymphadenectomy or resection of central or retroperitoneal lymph nodes are not appropriate; operative morbidity is substantially increased without concomitant improvements in survival. Occasionally, resection of adjacent organs is necessary if they are involved by direct tumor extension.[73]

Cancers of the cecum and ascending colon require right hemicolectomy (Fig. 32-7). The ileocolic, right colic, and branches of the middle colic arteries are divided and the encompassed mesentery is resected. If the tumor involves the hepatic flexure, the middle colic artery is divided at its origin and the bowel resection is carried further to the left side. Mobilization of the colon for performance of a right hemicolectomy exposes the right ureter, right gonadal vessels, inferior vena cava, superior mesenteric vein, and duodenum; these structures must be carefully protected.

Cancers arising in the transverse colon should be treated by a transverse colectomy. This procedure requires ligation of the middle colic artery. Colon cancers involving the splenic flexure should be resected via segmental resection of the splenic flexure and descending colon such that the transverse colon is anastomosed to the descending colon. A left hemicolectomy, which removes the mid transverse colon to the distal sigmoid colon, is appropriate for tumors arising from the descending colon. In this procedure the inferior mesenteric artery is divided. When the sigmoid cancer involves the sigmoid colon, segmental sigmoid colectomy is required with ligation of the sigmoid artery. Mobilization of the left colon exposes the left ureter, gonadal vessels, and inferior mesenteric vein.

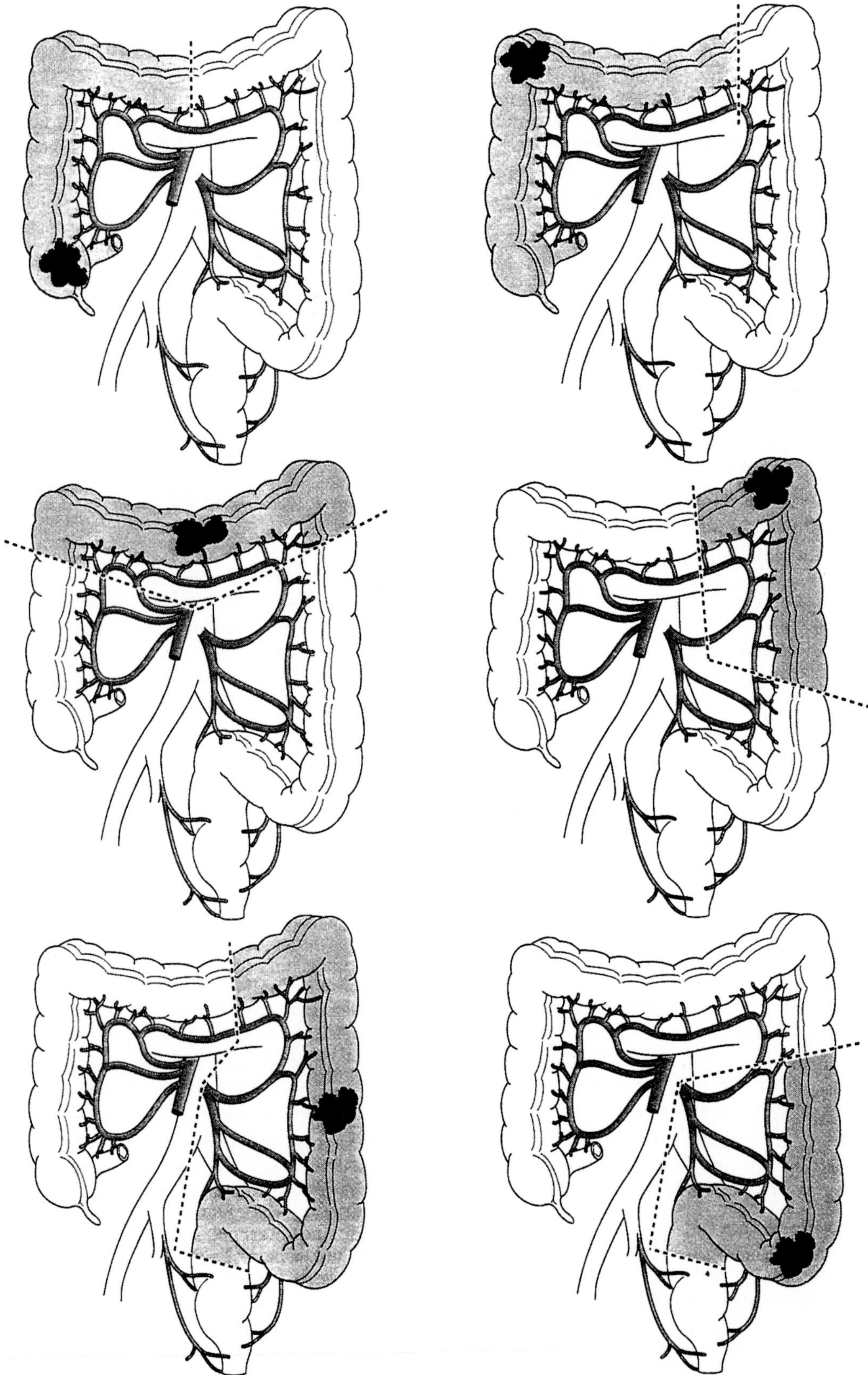

Fig. 32-7. Operative procedures used for resection of colon adenocarcinoma based on location of the lesion. (From Chang A. Colorectal cancer. In Greenfield LJ, et al., eds. Surgery: Scientific Principles and Practice. Philadelphia: JB Lippincott, 1993, p 1024.)

Operative treatment of rectal cancer is based on the position of the tumor within the rectum. The upper third of the rectum is defined as that portion from the rectosigmoid junction to a point 12 cm from the anal verge. The upper portion of the rectum is partially covered with peritoneum. The middle third of the rectum extends to a point 6 to 8 cm from the anal verge; the middle portion of the rectum is entirely below the peritoneal reflection. The lower third of the rectum extends caudally to the anal verge.

Cancers involving the upper third of the rectum are removed via anterior resection. The peritoneal reflections of the rectum are divided and the rectum is mobilized from the presacral space. The mesenteric vessels are divided at the level of the sigmoidal artery. Branches of the superior rectal artery are also divided. The mesorectum corresponding to this distribution is removed along with the colorectal segment. Anastomosis is performed using sutures or a stapling device passed via the anus.

Cancers of the middle third of the rectum, in the area between 6 and 12 cm from the anal verge, are usually managed by techniques that attempt to preserve sphincteric function.[74] The pelvic dissection includes division of the rectal peritoneal reflections, mobilization of the rectum to the level of the pelvic floor, and ligation of sigmoidal and superior rectal arteries. Division of the bowel wall should be performed so that a grossly normal margin is obtained distally while still leaving sufficient rectum above the sphincteric complex to permit anastomosis. The development of transanal end-to-end (EEA) staplers has been vital in this regard. When attempting sphincter-saving procedures for mid rectal tumors, the length of distal mucosal margin is crucial. Less than 5% of patients have microscopic intramural spread of tumor cells more than 2 cm from the palpable tumor, and there is no improvement in local recurrence rates when distal margins are greater than 2 cm. If possible, a surgical margin of 2 to 3 cm should be achieved. If this margin cannot be obtained and still permit a safe anastomosis, abdominoperineal resection should be performed. The length of the rectum between the tumor and pelvic floor can usually be increased as the rectum is mobilized from its pelvic attachments.

Cancers located in the lower third of the rectum, less than 6 cm from the anal verge, usually require abdominoperineal resection. This procedure includes wide excision of the rectum, including lateral pelvic attachments and mesorectum. A permanent colostomy is required. The superior rectal vessels are ligated at their origin from the left colic artery . The pelvic floor muscles are excised en bloc with the anus. The perineum is closed primarily.

Adjuvant Therapy

Radiation therapy, used as an adjuvant to surgical resection, has been demonstrated to reduce the incidence of local tumor recurrence in rectal cancer.[75-78] For stage II rectal cancers the incidence of local recurrence (approximately 30%) is reduced to 5% with adjuvant radiation therapy. For stage III rectal cancers, adjuvant radiation therapy reduces pelvic recurrence from approximately 50% to 10%. However, improved local control has not translated into prolonged survival; distant metastases still occur. Adjuvant radiation therapy for cancers of the intraperitoneal colon has not been proven to be beneficial but may be considered in specific circumstances such as tumor perforation or adherence to adjacent structures. Radiation of the intraperitoneal colon has increased toxicity because of inclusion of small bowel in the treatment field.

Adjuvant chemotherapy has established benefit for patients with stage III colon cancer. In one study, patients with stage III disease were shown to have improved disease-free survival when treated with 5-fluorouracil and levamisole.[79] The benefit in patients with stage II tumors was equivocal. The National Surgical Adjuvant Breast and Bowel Project has reported improved survival in stage II and III patients using 5-fluorouracil, semustine, and vincristine.[80] The National Institutes of Health recommend that patients with stage III colon cancer be offered adjuvant postoperative chemotherapy as standard treatment.[81]

The combination of adjuvant chemotherapy with radiation has proved effective in improving both local control and survival in patients with rectal cancer. In a randomized, prospective trial, patients with stage II or III rectal cancer who received chemotherapy had improved local tumor control and increased overall survival.[82] The National Institutes of Health have recommended that patients with stage II or III rectal cancers should undergo postoperative chemotherapy and radiation as a standard part of their care.[81]

Neoplasms of the Anal Canal and Anal Margin

Walter E. Longo and Anthony M. Vernava III

Anal and perianal malignancies of the gastrointestinal tract are rare, representing approximately 1% to 5% of all anorectal tumors. A number of risk factors have been identified, such as prior sexually transmitted diseases, anoreceptive intercourse, and chronic benign anal conditions such as pruritus ani.[83] Recently human papillomavirus (HPV) infection has been shown to confer an increased risk of anal cancer. Evidence supporting this observation includes the fact that many patients have simultaneous anal neoplasia and genital viral infections and that both these entities are associated with HPV genotypes 16 and 18.[84] Other factors, such as carcinogenic compounds (e.g., tobacco), simultaneous infection with other viruses, the immunocompromised state, and genetic mutations, may act in concert with HPV to transform epithelial abnormalities, including dysplastic lesions, into cancer. Although these lesions may occur at any age, the median age is 50 to 60 years. Males more commonly develop anal *mar-*

gin lesions, whereas anal *canal* tumors are nearly equally distributed between males and females.

Anal neoplasms are divided into those arising within the anal canal and those found at the anal margin. Secondary invasion from an adenocarcinoma of the rectum that descends into the anal canal may also occur. Lesions in the perianal skin act similarly to other cutaneous lesions found elsewhere. Neoplasms of the anal canal and anal margin may be either invasive or in situ. Nevertheless, these anal and perianal lesions present much confusion as to anatomic location and staging. One area of confusion relates to the anatomic location of the anal canal. Most surgeons agree that the proximal end of the anal canal corresponds to the anorectal ring. However, much disagreement exists about its distal limit. This limit has been chosen as the dentate line, the mucocutaneous junction, or the anal verge. Depending on the definition used, the anal margin would correspond to that region caudal to the distal limit of the anal canal. Until a uniform description is agreed on, it is important for authors to state clearly which definitions they are using to report results of treatment. A second area of confusion involves staging. A number of staging techniques have been proposed. Dukes' stages cannot be applied because the tumor spreads to inguinal and iliac nodes, which are not routinely removed. Popular staging methods include TNM (tumor, node, metastasis) classification and the International Union Against Cancer (UICC). Once the diagnosis is confirmed, examination of both groins, colonoscopy, chest x-ray examination, and CT scan of the abdomen and pelvis should be performed to determine the tumor's confinement to the site of origin or its distant spread.

Neoplasms of the *anal margin* are generally slow growing and late to metastasize. Nevertheless, despite their surface location, they are frequently detected late, often years after the onset of symptoms. This circumstance is frequently due to neglect, either by the patient or the physician, and to the fact that both benign disease and neoplasia may coexist concomitantly, with the latter being missed. Squamous cell carcinoma of the anal margin often resembles lesions found elsewhere in the skin. The lesions commonly have rolled everted edges with central ulceration. Treatment is wide local excision; occasionally a split-thickness skin graft may be required to cover the defect. Recurrent disease is often treated by reexcision. Abdominoperineal resection is reserved for lesions that have destroyed the sphincteric mechanism, rendering the patient incontinent. The 5-year survival rate varies from 40% to 100% for most lesions.[85] Advanced disease results in a poorer prognosis. Basal cell carcinoma is an extremely rare lesion. Grossly this lesion is similar to a cutaneous basal cell carcinoma found elsewhere in the body; it is superficial, mobile, and rarely metastasizes. This lesion must be distinguished from basaloid carcinoma, which has an entirely different origin and behavior. Treatment of this lesion is local excision. Although local recurrence is common, it can be treated by reexcision. This tumor is almost uniformly curable.[86]

There are two cancerous lesions at the anal margin that generally involve in situ histopathology, specifically Bowen's disease and Paget's disease. Bowen's disease is an intraepithelial squamous cell carcinoma. Patients commonly present with nonspecific complaints of anal itching, burning, or bleeding. Examination of the perineum in symptomatic patients usually reveals raised, irregular scaly lesions with eczematoid features. Diagnosis is confirmed by biopsy, which reveals characteristic bowenoid cells, which are multinucleated giant cells giving a "halo effect." In the absence of invasive malignancy, wide local excision is the treatment of choice. Mapping of the perianal and the anal canal with four-quadrant random biopsies is recommended because Bowen's cells may extend beyond the gross margin of the lesion.[87] Although Bowen's disease was once felt to represent a cutaneous manifestation of a predisposition to the development of malignant tumors elsewhere, recent evidence has failed to support the view that this condition is a marker for internal malignancy.[88] Paget's disease of the anus is an intraepithelial adenocarcinoma. Most patients complain of intense pruritus and a perianal rash. Microscopically, perianal Paget's disease is characterized by Paget's cells (PAS positive) located immediately above the basal layer. Wide excision and mapping is the treatment of choice for this disease. Recurrent lesions are reexcised. In the absence of invasive malignancy, the patient is cured.[89] Unlike Bowen's disease, the incidence of associated malignancies with Paget's disease approaches 50%. In both lesions long-term follow-up is necessary to identify recurrence of the disease or progression to invasive malignancy.

There are other rare anal margin tumors. The Buschke-Löwenstein tumor, or giant condyloma acuminatum, represents a verrucous carcinoma. It is a well-differentiated squamous cell carcinoma that can be distinguished from large condylomata only by invasion into local tissues. It may also originate from within the anal canal. Wide local excision with clear margins is the treatment of choice. Abdominoperineal resection is reserved for lesions that involve the anal sphincter.[90] Kaposi's sarcoma is a malignancy whose incidence and aggressiveness increases with immunosuppression. Treatment is palliative; it is reserved for symptomatic lesions and may involve excision, ablation, radiation, or chemotherapy. The prognosis is poor and is usually related to the severity of coexisting opportunistic infections. Leukemia cutis is an extremely painful lesion that involves infiltration of the perianal area by leukemic cells. It may first appear as a fistula, an abscess, or a tender erythematous area with marked cellulitis. These signs usually indicate advanced disease and carry a poor prognosis. Treatment is aimed at aggressive management of septic perianal complications of the leukemia. Mycosis fungoides is a fatal cutaneous malignancy of the lymphoreticular system. Treatment is aimed at managing the systemic disease.

The majority of epithelial tumors in the *anal canal* are squamous cell cancers or their histologic variants, such as the cloacogenic (transitional) tumors and the mucoepidermoid lesions. When treatment and outcome are discussed, all three histologic lesions are considered interchangeably. Anal canal carcinomas spread along the superior rectal, internal iliac, or inguinal lymphatic channels. It is estimated that in up to 20% of patients inguinal lymph node metastases are present at the time of diagnosis and that in up to 30% pelvic lymph node involvement is noted.[91] It is for this reason that these lesions must be treated with multimodality therapy. The patients often come to the attention of the physician with a painless lump in the anus, or they may have rectal bleeding, tenesmus, anal pain, fecal incontinence, or inguinal adenopathy; some patients are entirely asymptomatic. Biopsy demonstrates epidermoid carcinoma originating from the stratified squamous epithelium. Treatment of this lesion has changed from radical surgery to multimodality therapy. Local excision alone gives a high local recurrence rate and poor survival. Some advocate this treatment when the tumor involves only the submucosa. Abdominoperineal resection results in poor local control, a permanent colostomy, and, at best, a 50% survival at 5 years. Originally chemotherapy and radiation were used to enhance local control of disease in patients who subsequently underwent abdominoperineal resection. Among Nigro's first six patients treated in this fashion, no cancer was found in the operative specimen in five.[92] This finding led to chemoradiation with local excision as the treatment of choice for epidermoid cancer of the anal canal.[93] Although there have been several modifications to Nigro's original protocol, external beam radiotherapy (3000-5000 cGy) with administration of 5-fluorouracil and mitomycin C remains the treatment of choice. One can expect local control in 90% of patients and 5-year survival rates between 70% and 80%. If metastatic tumor is suspected in the groin, or if it subsequently develops, inguinal lymphadenopathy should be performed. In the absence of palpable nodes, lymphadenectomy should not be performed. Radical radiotherapy produces survival rates that approach those of chemoradiation; however, it carries a high rate of anal complications necessitating fecal diversion.

Once the patient has been successfully treated, follow-up initially involves proctoscopic examination and biopsy of the scar performed 4 weeks after treatment. This approach allows for desquamanation of nonviable tumor cells. The patient is followed up with a yearly proctoscopic examination with biopsy of the scar and, if necessary, intrarectal ultrasound, including imaging of the anal canal and anal margin. Patterns of failure are manifest by either local recurrence, regional spread, or distant metastasis. Local failure is characterized by either persistent disease or recurrent disease. Persistent disease is defined as either partial response or no response to treatment, which implies that the original therapy failed to eradicate disease. Recurrent disease is defined as tumor that returns after an initial period of complete clinical response. Local failure is best managed by abdominoperineal resection.[94] Such treatment, however, does not ensure survival for most individuals. There are currently some promising reports on the use of additional chemotherapy and radiation in the management of locally advanced disease. Regional failure involving spread to the inguinal lymph nodes is best treated by groin dissection followed by chemotherapy and radiation therapy. Distant visceral metastases have a poor prognosis, rarely allowing for one to be free of disease, and relapse is often anticipated.

Carcinoma in a hemorrhoidectomy specimen poses a challenge. If the pathologist reports a focus of carcinoma in a hemorrhoidectomy specimen, the patient should be reexamined in 4 weeks under anesthesia with performance of reexcision and mapping of the pedicle from which the hemorrhoid was removed. If biopsies are negative, follow-up at 3-month intervals is done for 1 year. If no adverse development occurs by 1 year, the patient is considered cured. If either persistent tumor after reexcision of the hemorrhoid specimen or recurrent is identified, chemoradiation is performed.[95]

The remainder of tumors seen in the anal canal are rare. Anal canal melanoma is suspected when a deeply pigmented lesion is noted in or surrounding the anorectum. However, a number of these lesions may be amelanotic. Up to 40% of lesions will have metastasized at the time of the diagnosis. The virulence and resistance of melanoma to treatment is accounted for by its obscure location and by the fact that it is usually not diagnosed until the tumor has grown to considerable size. This lesion is radioresistant and does not consistently respond to chemotherapy and immunotherapy. The surgical approach to this neoplasm is controversial. The majority of patients with melanoma succumb from distant metastasis. Wide local excision can provide local control, and most patients retain fecal continence. Abdominoperineal resection provides improved local control. Long-term survival has occurred only in patients with tumor <3 mm in depth (15% 5-year survival) following abdominoperineal resection.[96]

Anal canal adenocarcinomas are rare tumors arising from anal glands or chronic fistulas. They are slow growing and invasive. An accurate diagnosis requires a deep biopsy. Because of the rarity of this lesion, no comparative studies allow for rigorous analysis of treatment options. Wide local excision can be performed for small superficial and well-differentiated lesions. Otherwise, abdominoperineal resection is indicated. Postoperative adjuvant therapy may be of some benefit.[97] Prognosis depends on the stage of disease and the depth of invasion. Anal sarcomas are extremely rare and may be intraluminal or extraluminal. A variety of histologic types resembling any mesodermal tissue can occur. Abdominoperineal resection is the favored treatment, with 5-year survival between 20% and 30%.[98]

SUMMARY

The foregoing discussion emphasizes the plethora of tumors that can occur in the alimentary tract. Despite recent advances in our understanding of the pathogenesis of these various lesions, surgery still plays an essential role in management. For example, the treatment of choice for gastric cancer continues to be surgical resection of the neoplasm to include en bloc removal of lymph node drainage routes. Under most circumstances a subtotal gastrectomy should be performed, not only because the morbidity and mortality associated with this procedure is less than that with total gastrectomy, but also because survival rates have been at least as good, if not better, than those with more extensive procedures. Since most gastric malignancies occur in the mid body or distal portions of the stomach, subtotal resection can generally be performed without undue technical difficulty. Similarly, with neoplastic disorders of the small bowel, colorectum, and anus, altered physiology can usually be restored to normal or near-normal following surgical resection of the underlying tumor, unless widespread metastases have taken place. In this circumstance, life span is short; in addition to the primary disease, other organ systems are also adversely affected, allowing only supportive care rather than permanent reversal of the underlying pathophysiologic processes. Major advances are being made, however, in understanding the various causes of these lesions, and some progress has been made in using other types of treatment, such as radiation and/or chemotherapy either as an adjunct to surgical management or in place of it where surgical resection would not be prudent. Until such time as the etiologic factors responsible for the development of different types of gastrointestinal neoplasia are precisely defined and preventive measures can be appropriately instituted, surgery will continue to play an important role in care.

REFERENCES

1. Silverberg E, Boring CC, Squires TS. Cancer statistics, 1990. CA 40:9, 1990.
2. Harju E. Gastric polyposis and malignancy. Br J Surg 73:532, 1986.
3. Wyatt JI. Gastritis and its relation to gastric carcinogenesis. Semin Diagn Pathol 8:137, 1991.
4. Veldhuyzen van Zanten, Sherman PM. *Helicobacter pylori* infection as a cause of gastritis, duodenal ulcer, gastric cancer and nonulcer dyspepsia: A systematic overview. Can Med Assoc J 150:177, 1994.
5. Parsonnet J, et al. *Helicobacter pylori* infection and the risk of gastric carcinoma. N Engl J Med 325:1127, 1991.
6. Lundegardh G, et al. Stomach cancer after partial gastrectomy for benign ulcer disease. N Engl J Med 319:195, 1988.
7. Toftgaard C. Gastric cancer after peptic ulcer surgery: A historic prospective cohort investigation. Ann Surg 210:159, 1989.
8. Meyers WC, et al. Adenocarcinoma of the stomach: Changing patterns over the past 4 decades. Ann Surg 205:1, 1987.
9. Andaker L, et al. Evaluation of preoperative computed tomography in gastric malignancy. Surgery 109:132, 1991.
10. Nicholson DA, Shorvon PJ. Review article: Endoscopic ultrasound of the stomach. Br J Surg 66:487, 1993.
11. Greenberg J, et al. Computed tomography or endoscopic ultrasonography in preoperative staging of gastric and esophageal tumors. Surgery 116:696, 1994.
12. Caletti G, et al. Accuracy of endoscopic ultrasonography in the diagnosis and staging of gastric cancer and lymphoma. Surgery 113:14, 1993.
13. Waneba HJ, et al. Cancer of the stomach: A patient care study by the American College of Surgeons. Ann Surg 218:583, 1993.
14. Boddie AW, McBride CM, Balch CM. Gastric cancer. Am J Surg 157:595, 1989.
15. Heberer G, et al. Results of gastric resection for carcinoma of the stomach: The European experience. World J Surg 12:374, 1988.
16. Moreaux J, Bougaran J. Early gastric cancer: A 25 year surgical experience. Ann Surg 217:347, 1993.
17. Nakane Y, et al. Prognostic differences of adenocarcinoma arising from the cardia and the upper third of the stomach. Ann Surg 7:423, 1993.
18. Shiu MH, et al. Influence of the extent of resection on survival after curative treatment of gastric cancer: A retrospective multivariate analysis. Arch Surg 122:1347, 1987.
19. Maruyama K, Okabayashi K, Kinoshita T. Progress in gastric cancer in Japan and its limit of radicality. World J Surg 11:418, 1987.
20. Noguchi Y, et al. Radical surgery for gastric cancer: A review of the Japanese experience. Cancer 64:2053, 1989.
21. Korenaga D, et al. Long-term survival in Japanese patients with far advanced carcinoma of the stomach. World J Surg 12:236, 1988.
22. Adachi Y, et al. Role of lymph node dissection and splenectomy in node-positive gastric carcinoma. Surgery 116:837, 1994.
23. Robertson CS, et al. A prospective randomized trial comparing R1 subtotal gastrectomy with R3 gastrectomy for antral cancer. Ann Surg 220:176, 1994.
24. Dent DM, Madden MV, Price SK. Randomized comparison of R1 and R2 gastrectomy for gastric carcinoma. Br J Surg 75:110, 1988.
25. Gastrointestinal Tumor Study Group. A combination chemotherapy and combined modality therapy for locally advanced gastric carcinoma. Cancer 49:1771, 1982.
26. Findlay M, Cunningham D. Chemotherapy of carcinoma of the stomach. Cancer Treat Rev 19:29, 1993.
27. Rao A, et al. Management of gastrointestinal lymphoma. Am J Oncol 7:213, 1984.
28. Shiu MH, et al. Recent results of multimodal therapy of gastric lymphoma. Cancer 58:1389, 1986.
29. Mittal B, Wasserman TH, Griffith RC. Non-Hodgkin's lymphoma of the stomach. Am J Gastroenterol 78:780, 1983.
30. Gobbi PG, et al. The role of surgery in the multimodal treatment of primary gastric non-Hodgkin's lymphoma: A report of 76 cases and review of the literature. Cancer 65:2528, 1990.
31. Bozzetti F, et al. Role of surgery in patients with primary non-Hodgkin's lymphoma of the stomach: An old problem revisited. Br J Surg 80:1101, 1993.
32. Creutzfeldt W. The achlorhydria—carcinoid sequence: Role of gastrin. Digestion 39:61, 1988.
33. Borch K, Renvall H, Liedberg G. Endocrine cell proliferation and carcinoid development: A review of new aspects of hypergastrinaemic atrophic gastritis. Digestion 35(Suppl 1):106, 1986.
34. Shiu M, Farr G, Papachristou D. Myosarcomas of the stomach: Natural history, prognostic factors and management. Cancer 48:177, 1982.
35. Galandiuk S, et al. Villous tumors of the duodenum. Ann Surg 207:234, 1988.
36. Kazerooni EA, Quint LE, Francis IR. Duodenal neoplasms: Predictive value of CT for determining malignancy and tumor resectability. AJR Am J Roentgenol 159:303, 1992.
37. Dudiak KM, Johnson D, Stephens DH. Primary tumors of the small intestine: CT evaluation. AJR Am J Roentgenol 152:995, 1989
38. Allison DJ, Hemingway AP, Cunningham DA. Angiography in gastrointestinal bleeding. Lancet 2:30, 1982.
39. Lewis BS, Waye JD. Total small bowel enteroscopy. Gastrointest Endosc 33:435, 1987.
40. Bowden TA. Endoscopy of the small intestine. Surg Endosc 69:1237, 1989.
41. Mukai H, et al. Evaluation of endoscopic ultrasonography in the pre-operative staging of carcinoma of the ampulla of Vater and common bile duct. Gastrointest Endosc 39:676, 1992.
42. Ryan DP, Shapiro RH, Warshaw AL. Villous tumors of the duodenum. Arch Surg 203:301, 1986.
43. Ross RK, et al. Epidemiology of carcinomas of the small intestine:Is bile a small bowel carcinogen? Br J Cancer 63:143, 1991.

44. Lowell JA, et al. Primary adenocarcinoma of the third and fourth portions of the duodenum. Arch Surg 127:557, 1992.
45. Ouriel K, Adams JT. Adenocarcinoma of the small intestine. Am J Surg 197:66, 1984.
46. Desa LA, et al. Primary jejunoileal tumors: A review of 45 cases. World J Surg 15:81, 1991.
47. Feldman JM. Carcinoid tumors and the carcinoid syndrome. Curr Prob Surg 26:831, 1989.
48. Thompson GB, et al. Carcinoid tumors of the gastrointestinal tract: Presentation, management and prognosis. Surgery 98:1054, 1985.
49. Strodel WE, et al. Surgical therapy for small-bowel carcinoid tumors. Arch Surg 118:391, 1983.
50. Kvols LK, et al. Treatment of malignant carcinoid syndrome: Evaluation of a long-acting somatostatin analog. N Engl J Med 319:663, 1986.
51. Basson MD, et al. Biology and management of the midgut carcinoid. Am J Surg 165:288, 1993.
52. Godwin DJ. Carcinoid tumors: An analysis of 2,837 cases. Cancer 36:560, 1975.
53. Haber DA, Mayer RJ. Primary gastrointestinal lymphoma. Semin Oncol 15:154, 1988.
54. Cohen JI. Epstein-Barr virus lymphoproliferative disease associated with acquired immunodeficiency. Medicine 70:137, 1991.
55. Cooper BT, et al. Celiac disease and malignancy. Medicine 59:249, 1980.
56. Davidson T, et al. Emergency laparotomy in patients with AIDS. Br J Surg 78:924, 1991.
57. Domizio P, et al. Primary lymphoma of the small intestine. A clinicopathological study of 119 cases. Am J Surg Pathol 17:429, 1993.
58. Dodd GD. Lymphoma of the hollow abdominal viscera. Radiol Clin North Am 28:771, 1990.
59. Rackner VL, Thirlby RC, Ryan JA. Role of surgery in multimodality therapy for gastrointestinal lymphoma. Am J Surg 161:570, 1991.
60. Licht JD, Weissmann LB, Antman K. Gastrointestinal sarcomas. Semin Oncol 15:181, 1988.
61. Akwari OE, et al. Leiomyosarcoma of the small and large bowel. Cancer 42:1375, 1978.
62. Chiotasso PJP, Fazio VW. Prognostic factors of 28 leiomyosarcomas of the small intestine. Surg Gynecol Obstet 155:197, 1984.
63. Cannon-Albright LA, et al. Common inheritance of susceptibility to colonic adenomatous polyps and associated colorectal cancers. N Engl J Med 319:533, 1988.
64. Lynch HT, et al. Management of hereditary site-specific colon cancer. Arch Surg 112:170, 1970.
65. Boland CR, Troncale FJ. Familial colonic cancer without antecedent polyposis. Ann Intern Med 100:700, 1984.
66. Devroede GJ, et al. Cancer risk and life expectancy of children with ulcerative colitis. N Engl J Med 285:17, 1979.
67. Gyde SN, et al. Survival of patients with colorectal cancer complicating ulcerative colitis. Gut 25:228, 1984.
68. Dukes CE. Cancer of the rectum. J Pathol Bacteriol 35:323, 1932.
69. August DA, Ottow RT, Sugarbaker PH. Clinical perspective of human colorectal cancer metastasis. Cancer Metastasis Rev 3:303, 1984.
70. Haggitt RC, et al. Prognostic factors in colorectal carcinomas arising in adenomas: Implications for lesions removed by endoscopic polypectomy. Gastroenterology 89:328, 1985.
71. Wilcox GM, Anderson PB, Colacchio TA. Early invasive cancer in colonic polyps. Cancer 57:160, 1986.
72. Stein BL, Coller JA. Management of malignant colorectal polyps. Surg Clin North Am 73:47, 1993.
73. Curley SA, Evans DB. Resection for cure of carcinoma of the colon directly invading the duodenum or pancreatic head. J Am Coll Surg 179:587, 1994.
74. Yeatman TJ, Bland KI. Sphincter-saving procedures for distal carcinoma of the rectum. Ann Surg 209:1, 1989.
75. Mohiuddin M, Marks G. Adjuvant radiation therapy for colon and rectal cancer. Semin Oncol 18:411, 1991.
76. Fisher B, et al. Postoperative adjuvant chemotherapy or radiation therapy for rectal cancer: Results from NSABP protocol R-01. J Natl Cancer Inst 80:21, 1988.
77. Gastrointestinal Tumor Study Group. Survival after postoperative combination treatment for rectal cancer. N Engl J Med 315:1294, 1986.
78. Tepper JE, et al. Postoperative radiation therapy for rectal cancer. Int J Radiat Oncol Biol Phys 13:5, 1987.
79. Moertel CG, et al. Levamisole and fluorouracil for adjuvant therapy of resected colon carcinoma. N Engl J Med 322:352, 1990.
80. Wolmark N, et al. Postoperative adjuvant chemotherapy or BCG for colon cancer: Results from NSABP protocol C-01. J Natl Cancer Inst 80:30, 1988.
81. Steele GD Jr, et al. National Institutes of Health Consensus Development Conference statement-adjuvant therapy for patients with colon and rectal cancer. JAMA 264:1444, 1990.
82. Krook JE, et al. Effective surgical adjuvant therapy for high-risk rectal carcinoma. N Engl J Med 324:709, 1991.
83. Wexner SD, Milsom JW, Dailey TH. The demographics of anal cancers are changing: Identification of a high-risk population. Dis Colon Rectum 30:942, 1987.
84. Noffsinger A, Witte D, Fenoglio-Presier CM. The relationship of human papillomaviruses to anorectal neoplasia. Cancer 70:1276, 1992.
85. Greenall MJ, et al. Epidermoid cancer of the anal margin. Pathologic features, treatment, and clinical results. Am J Surg 149:95, 1985.
86. Nielsen OV, Jensen SL. Basal cell carcinoma of the anus. A clinical study of 34 cases. Br J Surg 68:856, 1981.
87. Beck DE, et al. Perianal Bowen's disease. Dis Colon Rectum 31:419, 1988.
88. Reymann F, et al. Bowen's disease and internal malignancy. Arch Dermatol 124:677, 1988.
89. Beck DE, Fazio VW. Perianal Paget's disease. Dis Colon Rectum 30:263, 1987.
90. Chu QD, et al. Giant condyloma acuminatum (Buschke-Lowenstein tumor) of the anorectal and perianal regions. Dis Colon Rectum 37:950, 1994.
91. Cummings BJ. Treatment of primary epidermoid carcinoma of the anal canal. Int J Colorectal Dis 2:107, 1987.
92. Nigro ND, Vaitkevicius VK, Considine B. Combined therapy for cancer of the anal canal. Dis Colon Rectum 17:354, 1974.
93. Nigro ND, et al. Combined preoperative radiation and chemotherapy for squamous cell carcinoma of the anal canal. Cancer 51:1826, 1983.
94. Longo WE, et al. Recurrent squamous cell carcinoma of the anal canal. Ann Surg 200:40, 1994.
95. Corman ML. Malignant tumors of the anal canal. In Corman ML, ed. Principles of Colon and Rectal Surgery. Philadelphia: JB Lippincott, 1993.
96. Ross M, Pezzi C, Pezzi T. Patterns of failure in anorectal melanoma. A guide to surgical therapy. Arch Surg 125:313, 1990.
97. Jensen SL, et al. Adenocarcinoma of the anal ducts: A series of 21 cases. Dis Colon Rectum 31:268, 1988.
98. Beck DE, Wexner SW. Anal neoplasms. In Beck DE, Wexner SD, eds. Fundamentals of Anorectal Surgery. New York: McGraw-Hill, 1992.

33

Mechanical Disorders of the Stomach, Duodenum, and Intestine

Stacey L. Mazzacco and Daniel T. Dempsey

Under normal circumstances, the primary function of the stomach and intestine is to provide the body with adequate hydration and nutrition. This function, accomplished through various absorptive mechanisms throughout the gastrointestinal (GI) tract, occurs optimally only in the setting of proper peristaltic activity to move food through the alimentary system and may be pathologically altered by two basic mechanisms. The first is a narrowing of the bowel lumen by either intrinsic or extrinsic means. This narrowing, or partial obstruction, can progress to total obstruction of the lumen, resulting in a complete bowel obstruction. The second mechanism is one of ineffective peristalsis, a state referred to as *adynamic ileus* or *pseudo-obstruction,* depending on the clinical scenario. In both instances, normal GI physiology is altered. Discussion of this alteration forms the basis of this chapter.

MECHANICAL DISORDERS OF THE STOMACH AND DUODENUM

Gastric Outlet Obstruction

Etiology and Pathophysiology

Gastric outlet obstruction in the adult is usually caused by peptic ulcer disease or cancer. In *acute* ulcer disease, the pyloric channel may be obstructed by edema. Alternatively, normal antropyloric function may be disrupted by the inflammatory process. Contained perforation of the ulcer with extrinsic compression by mass effect is less common. *Chronic* peptic ulcer disease produces obstructive scarring of the pyloric channel. Adenocarcinomas of the distal stomach and pancreas are the most common malignancies associated with gastric outlet obstruction. Other less common etiologies include idiopathic (hypertrophic) pyloric stenosis, proximal duodenal webs, posttraumatic (including postoperative) stricture, and a variety of primary or secondary gastric motor disorders[1] (see accompanying box).

Volume and electrolyte depletion from vomiting may be severe in patients with gastric outlet obstruction. The characteristic finding is hypokalemic, hypochloremic metabolic alkalosis with extracellular fluid volume depletion.[2] Because of the sodium and potassium depletion, sodium is avidly absorbed and exchanged for hydrogen in the distal renal tubule. This results in paradoxic aciduria (an acidic urinary pH in the setting of alkalemia).

The effects of gastric outlet obstruction on gastric motor function are poorly understood. Acute gastric outlet obstruction presumably results in overdistention and loss of motor tone. Chronic obstruction causes hypertrophy of the muscularis propria and may result in gastric enlargement. More sophisticated techniques of assessing myoelectric activity and motor function of the obstructed stomach may guide diagnosis and treatment in the future.[3]

CAUSES OF CHRONIC GASTRIC RETENTION WITHOUT MECHANICAL OBSTRUCTION

Drugs
Diabetes
Gastric surgery
Pain, trauma
Peritonitis
Contiguous inflammation (e.g., pancreatitis)
Neuromuscular diseases
Central nervous system disease
Pseudo-obstruction
Collagen vascular disease
Idiopathic cause

Modified from Graham DY. Ulcer complications and their nonoperative treatment. In Sleisinger MH, Fordtran JS, eds. Gastrointestinal Disease, 5th ed. Philadelphia: WB Saunders, 1993, p 698.

Historically, the saline load test was often used as an index of the degree of obstruction. If 400 ml or greater remained in the stomach 30 minutes after gastric instillation of 750 ml saline solution, the result was positive. Because liquids may empty by gravity, whereas solids require intact gastric motor function, the saline load test should be abandoned in favor of more quantitative assessments, such as nuclear scintigraphy.

Significant nutritional defects may be present, especially in the patient who has had symptoms for weeks or months. Clinically significant protein or calorie deficits are indicated by ≥15% weight loss (measured after return to euvolemic status), serum albumin ≤3 g/dl, assessment of dietary history, and functional evaluation (e.g., muscle fatigability). Deficiencies in micronutrients (calcium, iron, magnesium, trace elements, and vitamins) may also be evident.

Diagnosis and Treatment

The clinical presentation of gastric outlet obstruction may be acute or chronic. The most common symptoms are nausea, nonbilious vomiting, epigastric pain, and bloating. The last two symptoms usually occur postprandially. Patients with nonmalignant obstruction do feel hunger and do not report early satiety, perhaps because the capacitance function of the proximal stomach is not affected and autonomic innervation is not disturbed by the disease process.

Epigastric fullness and tympany may be evident on physical examination and a "succussion splash" may be elicited in some patients. This last finding is the audible sound of fluid heard in the left upper quadrant on auscultation of the abdomen during its gentle movement. A palpable mass usually indicates malignancy. Tachycardia and orthostatic hypotension reflect volume depletion. Cardiac irritability and muscle weakness may reflect electrolyte abnormalities, particularly those associated with potassium losses from vomiting.

The history and physical examination suggest the diagnosis. Vital signs, urinary output, and measurements of serum electrolytes should guide the repletion of fluid and electrolyte deficits with isotonic saline and potassium chloride solutions (the latter should be given only after reassurance regarding adequate renal function). Repletion of magnesium, as well as of calcium and iron (both of which are absorbed in the stomach and duodenum), may be necessary. Diagnosis is confirmed and etiology is sought by endoscopy, scintigraphy, and upper GI tract radiologic evaluation.

Total parenteral nutrition should be initiated if the patient is severely malnourished or will receive nothing by mouth for at least 7 days. Whether preoperative gastric decompression, often practiced for 5 to 7 days, hastens postoperative return of gastric function is unknown. Because postoperative return of normal gastric emptying is not always prompt, temporary Stamm gastrostomy and feeding jejunostomy may be useful adjunct procedures.

Definitive treatment of mechanical gastric outlet obstruction depends on the underlying cause. All patients with peptic ulcer disease should be treated with intravenous antisecretory drugs and evaluated for *Helicobacter pylori* infection. Although as many as 46% of these patients (presumably those with "acute" ulcer) show improvement after a few days of nasogastric suction and intravenous therapy, the risk of recurrent obstruction in the "pre-*Helicobacter* era" was greater than 50%.[4,5] Most patients admitted to the hospital with gastric outlet obstruction caused by peptic ulcer disease should therefore be considered for definitive operation (vagotomy and gastrojejunostomy or vagotomy and antrectomy with Billroth-II reconstruction). Lesser procedures (parietal cell vagotomy with dilation; endoscopic balloon dilation) have been tried, with variable results.[6-8] Whether aggressive treatment of *H. pylori* in patients infected with this bacterium will alleviate obstruction and obviate surgery remains to be seen.

Patients with outlet obstruction caused by malignant disease should undergo resection or palliative gastrojejunostomy (a vagotomy should be considered if survival longer than 6 months is anticipated). Laparoscopic vagotomy and gastrojejunostomy offer a useful option in some patients with benign or malignant obstruction.[9] Webs and hypertrophic pyloric stenosis may be treated with endoscopic dilatation or operative stricturoplasty.

Duodenal Obstruction

Etiology and Pathophysiology

Duodenal obstruction in the adult may cause symptoms similar to gastric outlet obstruction. However the vomitus may be bilious, and the alkalosis tends to be less pronounced because alkaline duodenal contents are vomited along with gastric acid. Postprandial pain may be significant, presumably because of postcibal secretion into an obstructed duodenal loop, which may be intermittently closed at the upper end by the pylorus, creating a closed loop. Pyloric relaxation and retrograde discharge of contents from the distended duodenal loop relieve the pain (and often result in bilious vomiting with food).

The most common causes of duodenal obstruction in the adult are cancer (pancreatic, duodenal, and recurrent colon cancers), duodenal ulcer disease (gastrinoma should be considered in the case of a duodenal ulcer distal to the bulb), pancreatitis, and congenital problems (webs, intraluminal diverticula [windsock deformity]). In the patient with trauma or receiving anticoagulation, duodenal hematoma should be considered. Rare causes of duodenal obstruction include the "SMA syndrome" (obstruction of the duodenum proximal to the site where the superior mesenteric artery [SMA] traverses the distal duodenum), radiation fibrosis, idiopathic retroperitoneal fibrosis, gallstones (Bouveret's syndrome) and paraduodenal hernia. Duodenal atresia, annular pancreas, and Ladd's bands (associated with malrotation of the midgut) are important causes in the pediatric patient (see Chapter 66). Although they are unusual in the adult, Ladd's bands should always be considered, because midgut volvulus and infarction remain a possibility even in the adult patient.[10]

Diagnosis and Treatment

The diagnosis of duodenal obstruction is suggested by the history and confirmed by endoscopic gastroduodenoscopy and radiologic evaluation of the upper GI tract with small bowel follow-through. Ladd's bands with malrotation may be ruled out if the latter evaluation shows the cecum in its normal right lower quadrant location. Computed tomographic scan should be done if malignancy is suspected, and enteroscopy may be indicated in certain cases. Angiography is necessary to assess the frontal and lateral SMA-aortic angle in the rare case of suspected SMA syndrome.[11]

The treatment of duodenal obstruction is dictated by the cause but should be guided by duodenal physiology. Whereas gastric outlet obstruction entails one functional problem (emptying of the stomach), duodenal obstruction presents at least two, emptying of the stomach *and* emptying of duodenal contents. Duodenal distention causes pain and nausea but also causes gastric hypomotility. In these patients, physiologic stimuli (e.g., eating) deliver normal volumes of bile and pancreatic juice to the duodenum; these, along with duodenal secretions, cause duodenal distention in the setting of normal pyloric function.

Gastrojejunostomy for duodenal obstruction relies on retrograde transpyloric decompression of the duodenum into what may be a poorly functioning stomach and yields poor results. It should be avoided in the patient with benign disease. Duodenojejunostomy, duodenoduodenostomy, and stricturoplasty are much more physiologically sound and yield better results. They are easily applied to most patients with benign duodenal obstruction (webs, distal ulcers, SMA syndrome, annular pancreas). Furthermore, they are not ulcerogenic, so vagotomy or long-term acid suppression is not required unless the cause of obstruction is peptic ulcer disease. Loop gastrojejunostomy may be appropriate, however, for the patient with duodenal obstruction from pancreatic carcinoma where the bile has been diverted above the duodenum and the pancreatic duct is obstructed by the tumor. These patients admittedly have limited survival and should be maintained on acid-suppressive therapy. Malrotation in the adult with symptoms should be treated promptly with operative division of Ladd's bands and cecal fixation in the right lower quadrant.

Gastric Volvulus

Etiology and Pathophysiology

Most clinically significant cases of gastric volvulus are associated with paraesophageal hiatal hernia or some other diaphragmatic defect and are referred to as *supradiaphragmatic* or *secondary volvulus*.[12] Less commonly, the twist is not associated with a diaphragmatic defect (*subdiaphragmatic* or *primary volvulus*) and is thought to be caused by unusually lax gastric attachments or a high left hemidiaphragm (e.g., occurring after left pulmonary resection or left phrenic nerve injury). Usually, the stomach rotates on this long axis (organoaxially), giving rise to the term *upside-down stomach*. This is the volvulus usually seen with paraesophageal hiatal hernia. Volvulus along the shorter transverse axis (mesenteroaxial) or a combination of these two rotations may also be seen (Fig. 33-1).

The important pathophysiologic features of gastric volvulus are vascular compromise, poor gastric emptying,

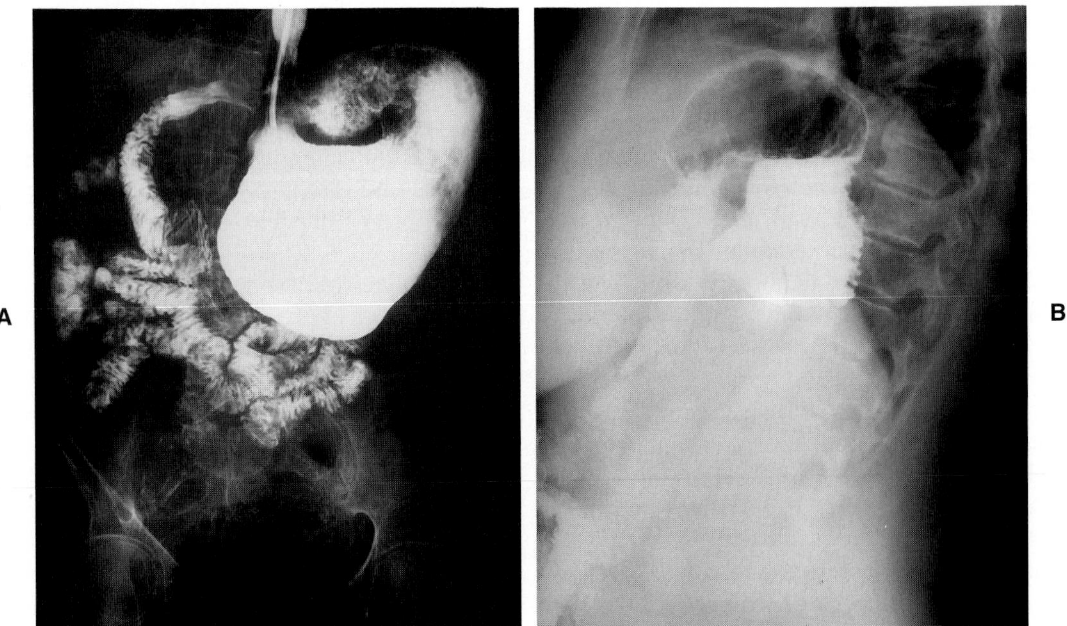

Fig. 33-1. Barium studies characteristic of mesenteroaxial **(A)** and organoaxial gastric volvulus **(B)**.

and compression of adjacent viscera. The twist may obstruct the distal stomach, so that ingestion of food and air causes prolonged gastric distention. This often compresses adjacent organs (e.g., esophagus, heart, lung), causing postprandial symptoms (e.g., dysphagia, arrhythmia, dyspnea). The volvulus, closed-loop distention, and (in supradiaphragmatic cases) narrow-neck hernia sac result in ischemia and gastric infarction in some patients.

Diagnosis and Treatment

Although some patients with acute gastric volvulus have severe epigastric and chest pain, retching, diaphoresis, and tachycardia, most have chronic, intermittent symptoms.[13] Usually, these symptoms are related to eating and include pain, dysphagia, bloating, palpitations, and the sensation that belching or vomiting would give relief but without the ability to do so. Plain radiographs of the chest and abdomen usually appear abnormal. Meglumine diatrizoate (Gastrografin) swallow is diagnostic and should be done before the passage of a nasogastric tube because acute gastric volvulus may appear much like spontaneous esophageal rupture (Boerhaave's syndrome).

Treatment depends on the clinical scenario. If gastric ischemia or infarction is suspected, emergency operation is indicated. If symptoms settle with gastric decompression, or if they are chronic and severe, prompt elective operation is planned. Repair of the diaphragmatic defect is essential. Ideally, the sac is removed, but if this cannot be accomplished safely, the stomach must be completely disconnected from the peritoneum of the hernia sac. Gastropexy or gastrostomy should be added.

Disorders of Gastric Motility

Etiology and Pathophysiology

Although the pathophysiology of most GI motility disorders is poorly understood,[14] it is important to consider gastroduodenal motor dysfunction in the differential diagnosis of many of the more common disorders discussed previously. GI motility disorders are generally classified as idiopathic, neuropathic, myopathic, metabolic, or iatrogenic (e.g., medication related).[15] Some syndromes are thought to have a heterogeneous pathogenesis. A simpler but less organized classification divides disorders into primary and secondary.[16] In practice, secondary gastropareses are more common than primary.

Chronic idiopathic gastroparesis causes a measurable delay in gastric emptying of solids, and to a lesser extent liquids, on scintiscan. Electrogastrography may demonstrate abnormal myoelectric activity, and pressure measurements demonstrate decreased antral contractile activity. Dyscoordinated antropyloric function may also be present. Diabetic gastroparesis is thought to be neuropathic, resulting from diabetes-induced damage to the extrinsic autonomic gastric innervation. Postprandial antral hypomotility and pylorospasm are characteristic findings on gastric manometry.[17] Amyloidosis and systemic sclerosis may produce gastrointestinal dysmotility by damaging both intrinsic nerves and muscularis propria. Postoperative gastroparesis is iatrogenic, and its etiology is multifactorial. In many patients, a preexisting motility problem may not be identified, and an operation such as truncal vagotomy and drainage, truncal vagotomy and antrectomy, or gastric resection makes the problem worse. If gastrointestinal continuity is reestablished with a Roux-en-Y procedure in which the anastomosed segment has measurable motility and myoelectric abnormalities, gastric emptying may be worsened even further.[18] This is especially true if a large vagotomized gastric remnant remains. Duodenogastric reflux is a poorly understood phenomenon that may be pathologic in a small number of patients.[19] Measurements show increased gastric reflux of duodenal bile on scintigraphy and abnormal antral alkalinization. Gastric emptying is usually normal.

Diagnosis and Treatment

Primary or secondary gastroparesis or pathologic duodenogastric reflux should be considered in patients with symptoms of gastric or duodenal obstruction in whom no lesion is found. It should be noted, however, that these motor disorders may be associated with lesions more commonly associated with obstruction, namely ulcers and previous operation. The single most useful test in evaluating these gastric motility disorders is scintigraphy.[20] By means of simple, noninvasive techniques, gastric emptying of solids and liquids, as well as duodenogastric reflux and gastroesophageal reflux, may be quantitated. The treatment of these disorders is largely medical (promotility agents, dietary counseling, bile salt–binding resins), and surgery is palliative. Irreversible operations should therefore be avoided. An ill-conceived operation or reoperation often makes the problem worse.

MECHANICAL DISORDERS OF THE SMALL BOWEL

Small Bowel Obstruction

There are three broad categories of small bowel obstruction according to the origin of the lesion: (1) intrinsic (the lesion arises from within the bowel wall), (2) extrinsic (the lesion is extraintestinal and compresses the bowel wall), and (3) obturation (the lumen is obstructed by material such as feces, bezoars, parasites, or gallstones). Extrinsic lesions are by far the most common cause, with adhesions and hernias accounting for approximately 70% to 75% of all cases of small bowel obstruction.[21,22] Intrinsic obstruction by tumor constitutes the third most common cause of small bowel obstruction but is the most common cause of large bowel obstruction.

Intrinsic lesions causing small bowel obstruction are either congenital, inflammatory, or neoplastic. An inflamed Meckel's diverticulum may cause obstruction or act as a lead point for intussusception. Volvulus may occur if congenital malrotation exists, or the intestine may twist around a fibrotic remnant of the yolk stock. Acute inflammatory conditions of the bowel such as Crohn's disease and diverticulitis may also cause obstruction through local edema and stricture formation. In addition, complicated cases of Crohn's disease or diverticulitis resulting in perforation, abscess formation, and fistulization can extrinsically obstruct the bowel lumen through a mass effect. Stricture may occur from chronic ischemia, Crohn's disease, or radiation.

Obstructions may also result from small bowel neoplasms. Among malignant small bowel neoplasms causing obstruction, adenocarcinoma is the most common, although epidemiologic reports suggest that carcinoid is the most common tumor of the small bowel.[23] Carcinoids are more frequently found in the distal small bowel, whereas adenocarcinoma tends to occur in the more proximal small bowel.

Another infrequent cause of intrinsic small bowel obstruction is intramural hematoma occurring in the patient with trauma or, rarely, spontaneously in persons receiving anticoagulation. Even if not initially obstructing, these lesions may eventually produce symptoms related to stricture formation.

Extrinsic lesions are the most common cause of small bowel obstruction. Congenital lesions, such as annular pancreas and Ladd's band related to congenital malrotation, are rare in the adult. Postoperative or inflammatory adhesions remain the most common cause of small intestinal obstruction, followed by hernias. External compression of the small bowel from various neoplastic conditions, including diffuse carcinomatosis and extraintestinal neoplasms, may result in obstruction. Other miscellaneous etiologies include volvulus and SMA syndrome.

The final, and least common, type of obstruction is related to obliteration of the small bowel lumen by foreign bodies, including gallstones ("gallstone ileus"), bezoars, parasites, and balloons of intraluminal tubes.

Etiology

Adhesions. Intraperitoneal adhesions are the most common cause of intestinal obstruction in Western society, and they are the most likely cause in the patient who has previously undergone abdominal surgery. The physiologic mechanisms of adhesion formation have not been completely elucidated. However, it is evident that intraperitoneal irritation by surgery or previous intraabdominal infection, such as pelvic inflammatory disease, may initiate the process.[24] In addition, ischemic peritoneum is particularly susceptible to adhesion formation. Dense fibrous bands form between loops of bowel or between bowel and parietal peritoneum. These bands may result in progressive decrease in luminal diameter by external compression, may create a fixed defect through which the bowel can herniate, or may provide an axis around which loops of bowel could volvulize. The last two situations in particular may compromise blood supply, creating a closed loop of bowel that is susceptible to strangulation. This represents a surgical emergency that necessitates immediate operative intervention.

Hernia. Hernia comprises the second most common cause of bowel obstruction in the Western world. Hernias can be classified as external, in which there is an abnormal protrusion of intraabdominal tissue through a defect in the abdominal wall, or, less commonly, internal, in which the intra-abdominal tissue protrudes through abnormal openings in mesentery or the peritoneum. In either case, the defect may be acquired or congenital. The most frequently encountered hernias are inguinal and umbilical. A hernia is defined as *reducible* if its contents are returned freely to the abdominal cavity, *incarcerated* if the contents are unable to be reduced, and *strangulated* if the incarcerated contents become ischemic with compromised blood supply. The less frequently encountered hernias are those with a higher incidence of strangulation (femoral, obturator, paraduodenal).

Intussusception/volvulus. *Intussusception* is defined as a telescoping of one segment of bowel into another (Fig. 33-2). It occurs mostly in infants, with 80% of cases being observed in the first 2 years of life.[25] It has been hypothesized that inflamed lymphoid tissue in the terminal ileum may act as a lead point by causing focal wall motion abnormalities, with subsequent kinking of bowel and invagination of this segment into the more distal bowel by a peristaltic wave. Although lead points are found in only 5% of pediatric cases,[26] as many as 80% of adult cases have a discrete lead point, usually a neoplasm.[27] Thus, intussusception in the adult is an indication for operation and resection, whereas careful hydrostatic reduction with barium enema is often used in children.

Volvulus, by contrast, is commonly seen in adults. It results when the intestine twists on its mesentery. Vascular

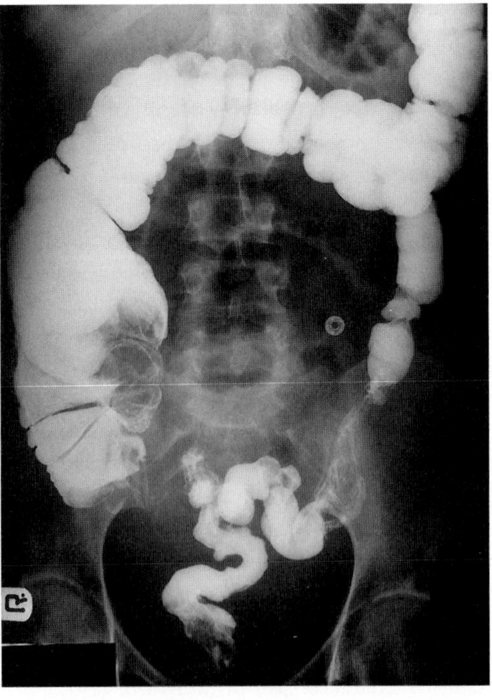

Fig. 33-2. Barium enema study demonstrating ileocolic intussuception. The terminal ileum is seen as a filling defect within the proximal colon.

compromise may result through direct occlusion of mesenteric vessels or creation of a closed-loop obstruction, with resultant increases in wall tension, venous obstruction, and eventual arterial insufficiency. Volvulus may occur in either the small or large bowel; however, the pathogeneses are different. Volvulus of the small bowel in the adult is usually caused by a fixed adhesive band around which the usually mobile loops of small bowel may twist. The adhesive band may be inflammatory (e.g., postoperative adhesion), congenital (e.g., omphalomesenteric duct), or iatrogenic (e.g., jejunostomy tube). Volvulus related to malrotation is rare but can occur in adults. In contrast, the colon is usually fixed in the retroperitoneum, and is susceptible to torsion only in an area that may be freely mobile, namely the cecum or more commonly the sigmoid.

Pathophysiology

Absorption/secretion. The GI tract accumulates 6 to 8 L of salivary, gastric, pancreatic, and intestinal secretions per day,[28] with most of this fluid reabsorbed along the intestine tract. The normal secretory and absorptive capacities of the bowel are markedly altered in bowel obstruction. Classic studies on small bowel obstruction revealed a net decrease in the absorptive capacity and a net increase in secretory activity. In early intestinal obstruction, there is a decrease in absorption with little change in secretion. With progressive dilatation, secretion is augmented and absorption remains decreased,[29,30] resulting in marked intraluminal fluid accumulation and distention, a process further exacerbated by luminal gas and swallowed air. These effects are potentiated in the closed-loop type of obstruction. Distention causes increasing secretion and initiates a positive-feedback loop that induces high intraluminal pressures, with risk of ischemia and perforation.

Fluid accumulates not only intraluminally but also within the wall of the distended gut (edema) and eventually in the peritoneum.[31] These various sources of fluid loss can be quite substantial (6 L), resulting in profound hypovolemia, electrolyte disturbance, and shock. Volume replacement is an essential aspect of preoperative management of the patient with obstruction, and it can usually be accomplished with a balanced salt solution such as lactated Ringer's solution or normal saline, with the addition of 20 to 30 mEq/L potassium chloride (if urine output is present). Depending on the magnitude of dehydration, several liters of fluid may be required to restore fluid and electrolyte balance. Response of resuscitation may be measured by heart rate, blood pressure, central venous pressures, and maintenance of urinary output greater than 30 ml/hr. In elderly patients or those with underlying renal or cardiac disease, pulmonary artery catheters may be useful for monitoring resuscitation.

Intestinal blood flow. Intestinal blood flow is directly related to intraluminal pressures.[32-37] Clinically, the longer a mechanical obstruction exists, the greater the degree of distention, with a concomitant increase in intraluminal pressures. Multiple classic experiments have demonstrated decreases in mucosal blood flow with progressive increases in intraluminal pressures. However, these experimentally induced pressures are often much greater than those encountered in the setting of a simple mechanical small bowel obstruction. Sustained intraintestinal pressures of 5 to 15 mm Hg, representing only a mild elevation beyond normal intraluminal pressure, have been reported in experimental models of simple small bowel obstruction. In contrast, pressures greater than 15 to 30 mm Hg are required to impair capillary flow. The ability of the gut to distend as well as decompress proximally prevents tremendous pressure increases. When this ability is lost, as in the closed-loop obstruction, intraluminal pressures as high as 43 mm Hg have been reported.[38] Thus, it is reasonable to conclude that simple obstruction will usually not compromise bowel viability, whereas closed-loop obstruction may result in the loss of regional blood flow, with subsequent ischemic changes and tissue death.

Direct compression of vascular elements, whether by volvulus, intussusception, hernia, or adhesive bands, is an obvious source of ischemia. Most of these strangulations are essentially venous in character, and classic experiments demonstrated that death is more rapid from simple venous occlusion than from arterial and venous ligation simultaneously.[39] In the setting of venous occlusion, the patient may have a large amount of blood lost into the bowel, resulting in profound shock that necessitates both blood and fluid resuscitation. At the time of surgery, all nonviable intestine must be resected, with viable margins assessed by Doppler signals or the use of fluorescein dye. The choice of primary closure versus ostomy depends on the clinical situation and the judgment of the surgeon.

Bacterial overgrowth, translocation, and antibiotic prophylaxis. In the healthy human, the proximal GI tract is relatively bacteria-free, with a resident bowel flora of streptococci, lactobacilli, diphtheroids, and fungus in only small quantities, less than 10^4 organisms/ml.[40] In the terminal ileum, coliform and bacteroides may be isolated, but again in low concentrations (10^5 to 10^8 organisms/ml) compared with the normal colonic flora concentration of 10^9 to 10^{12} organisms/g stool.

Peristalsis continually clears bacteria from the bowel lumen. In the setting of obstruction, this mechanism fails and bacterial stasis and overgrowth occur, with the accumulation of primarily coliform and anaerobic bacteria.[41-43] Alterations in the mucosal layer of the intestinal tract may also play a role in bacterial adherence and overgrowth in obstructed intestine.[44] It has been postulated that these changes, especially in the setting of vascular compromise, may promote bacterial translocation across the intestinal wall, leading to systemic infection and possibly sepsis.[45] The role of antibiotics in bowel obstruction remains controversial.[21,46] Generally, the longer the obstruction has been present, allowing distention of the bowel wall and the overgrowth of intestinal flora, the more likely that antibiotic prophylaxis will be of value. As the likelihood of ischemia increases, as determined by history, physical examination, and laboratory values, the threshold for using prophylactic antibiotics decreases, especially if resection is anticipated. Generally, if bowel distention has been present for longer than 24 hours, broad-spectrum antibiotics should be administered before surgery and continued for 2 to 3 days after the operation.

Motility alterations. Clinically, small bowel obstruction is heralded by the onset of crampy abdominal pain interrupted by periods of quiescence. This correlates with the results of several studies that reveal an increase in motor activity in bowel proximal to the obstruction.[47,48] This is postulated to result from a reflex response of the myenteric receptor to distention, creating increased cholinergic stimulated myoelectric activity. This hypermotility begins initially in the segment just proximal to the obstruction, progresses cephalad with time, and is characterized by irregular spike burst activity accompanied by a loss of the normal migrating motor complex (MMC) observed in the GI tract during the fasting state.[49-51] In unobstructed bowel, the MMC ("housekeeper potential") originates cyclically in the stomach and progresses to the terminal ileum, propelling any retained foodstuffs through the gut between meals.

Distal to the site of obstruction, there are also alterations in motility manifested by a loss of the MMC, with an accompanied increase in irregular spike bursts. This distal activity is less vigorous than the myoelectric bursts seen proximally, perhaps related to postulated long neural inhibitory reflexes or modulation of intramural mechanoreceptors by the lack of GI contents passing through the distal segment.[52] It seems as though peristaltic activity remains both proximal and distal to the obstruction but is grossly abnormal.

In the setting of partial small bowel obstruction, the normal MMC is also lost and replaced by periods of intense spike burst activity, with however, longer periods of quiescence. This activity remains confined to the area of obstruction and does not progress orally as in the setting of complete small bowel obstruction. Normal MMC patterns are reestablished 2 to 3 days after release of the partial obstruction.

These changes occur in the acute period. Prolonged obstruction leads to progressively decreased motor activity and eventually paralysis.

Diagnosis and Treatment

The principal signs and symptoms of intestinal obstruction are colicky abdominal pain, distention, vomiting, lack of flatus or defecation, and, with prolonged symptoms, dehydration with decreasing urinary output and eventual shock. The severity of these complaints depends on the degree of the obstruction and the region of intestine involved. More proximal sites of obstruction result in the early onset of vomiting as a result of the rapid accumulation of salivary, gastric, biliary, and pancreatic secretions. In addition, distention is less prominent because the secretions may be almost completely expelled with emesis. In lower intestinal obstructions, vomiting is less pronounced and may initially be absent. With prolonged distal obstruction, as normal peristalsis and clearance of resident bowel flora are abolished and bacterial overgrowth occurs, the vomitus may take on a characteristic feculent odor and consistency. Distention becomes more pronounced, especially with complete obstruction, as swallowed air and gastrointestinal secretions accumulate proximal to the obstruction. The normal GI tract secretes approximately 6 to 7 L fluid per day, making it easy to appreciate the massive dilatation that can occur during a short period in the absence of normal clearance mechanisms.

Pain is also a characteristic symptom of intestinal obstruction and is usually crampy and intermittent in nature, corresponding to the vigorous contractions of the peristaltic bowel as it attempts to push fluid and gas beyond the point of obstruction. This activity translates into the hyperactive, high-pitched sounds observed on auscultation. A metallic tinkling of bowel sounds results from the large air-fluid interface present in obstructed bowel. Between periods of peristalsis, the abdomen is quiet and the pain is less pronounced. The onset of continuous abdominal pain with subsequent peritoneal signs is more ominous, indicating the possibility of strangulation and ischemia.

Most patients with bowel obstruction report some change in bowel habits preceding the onset of other symptomatology. These changes may be subtle, such as changes in frequency of defecation, or dramatic, such as complete cessation of fecal passage and flatus as seen with complete obstruction. In addition, patients with colorectal carcinoma may report progressive narrowing of stool caliber, as well as change in color indicative of passage of blood.

From a laboratory standpoint, any patient with suspected intestinal obstruction should have a complete blood cell count, electrolyte profile, blood urea nitrogen, and creatinine determination performed. Other useful studies are arterial blood gas, serum lactate, and amylase determinations. The patient with obstruction usually has profound dehydration and may exhibit any combination of electrolyte and acid-base imbalances. Hemoconcentration as a result of dehydration usually increases hemoglobin and hematocrit. Patients with high obstruction usually have a hypochloremic, hypokalemic metabolic alkalosis as a result of hydrogen, sodium, and chloride losses with emesis. Volume contraction is a contributing factor to the alkalosis that may be present to a variable extent. Metabolic acidosis may be seen as a result of combined presence of dehydration and ketosis of starvation. A profound acidosis indicated by decreased bicarbonate, low pH, and increased lactate levels heralds the presence of a strangulated segment of bowel. Although modest elevation in white blood cell count may be seen with intestinal obstruction, marked leukocytosis with an accompanying leftward shift suggests ischemia. The serum amylase activity may be elevated in intestinal obstruction as a result of leakage of amylase and lipase into the peritoneal space, usually from a compromised intestinal wall. Urinanalysis shows a high specific gravity and ketonuria.

In the large majority of cases with compromised small bowel, the obstruction is complete. Thus important aids in the diagnosis of intestinal obstruction are plain radiographs and limited contrast studies. An obstruction series should include upright and supine abdominal films. In a patient too debilitated to sit upright or stand, lateral decubitus films suffice. Of course, pneumoperitoneum or pneumatosis indicates the need for operation. The presence of air-fluid levels in the bowel, often in a stepladder configuration, is the hallmark of small intestinal obstruction (Fig. 33-3). Because peristalsis remains functional beyond the obstruction, gas is expelled from that point distally. Thus, proximal distention and gasless distal bowel suggest complete small bowel obstruction, mandating early operation. Small bowel and colonic distention suggests paralytic ileus or distal colon obstruction with incompetent ileocecal valve. The pattern of air-fluid levels suggests the level of obstruction. High duodenal obstruction may yield a double-bubble sign, indicating gas in both the stomach and proximal duodenum. Valvulae conniventes are pronounced in jejunal rather than ileal obstruction, and haustra are present in colonic obstruction. Haustra may be distinguished from valvulae because they do not traverse the entire bowel lumen on plain radiography. Location of the air-fluid levels may also provide a clue to their origin, with the small bowel usually remaining more central on radiography, and the colon being confined to the peripheral region of the abdomen.

It may be difficult to differentiate mechanical small bowel obstruction from paralytic ileus or to distinguish complete from partial obstruction. In this setting, small bowel follow-through with thin barium will rule out or confirm the presence of an obstructing lesion (either partial or complete) and allow estimation of transit times of small bowel contents. Transit times are greatly increased in paralytic ileus. Antegrade barium studies should be avoided if imminent operation is deemed necessary. The hyperactive bowel sounds and intense colicky abdominal pain characteristic of small bowel obstruction are absent in the patient with paralytic ileus unless the source of ileus is related to peritoneal irritation caused by pancreatitis, cholecystitis, pneumonitis, or trauma. Differentiating these two entities is important, because an ileus is managed nonoperatively and bowel obstruction usually requires operative intervention.

In addition to demonstrating air-fluid levels and possibly confirming the site of obstruction, plain radiographs may be helpful in other respects. For example, foreign bodies, as well as renal or biliary calculi or fecaliths, may be visualized radiographically, which helps to sort out underlying pathology in less clear cases. Gallstones seen radiographically may themselves be the obstructing lesions in

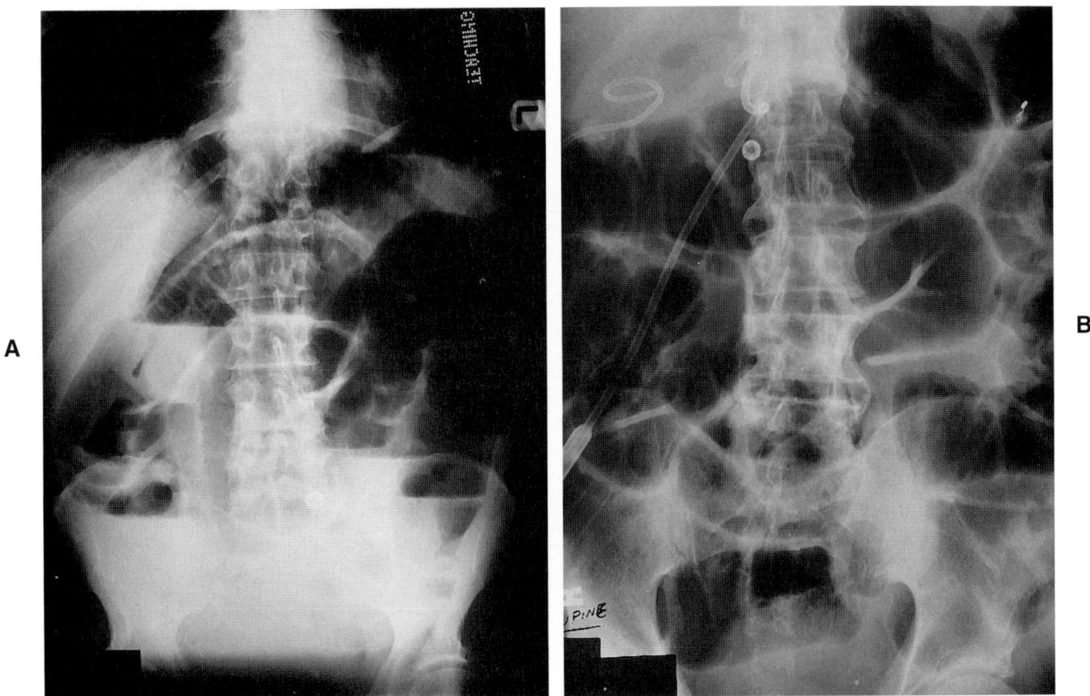

Fig. 33-3. Characteristic upright abdominal radiograph of small bowel obstruction revealing distended small bowel, multiple air-fluid levels, and paucity of air within the colon **(A)**. Bowel gas patterns in paralytic ileus are similar, except air is seen throughout both small and large bowel **(B)**.

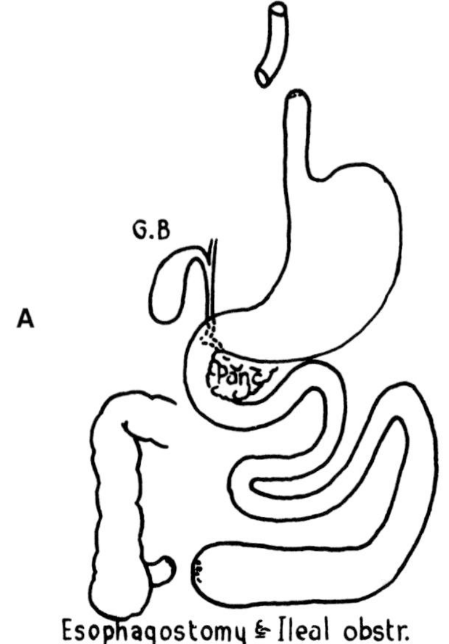

Fig. 33-4. Classic experiments designed to prevent bowel distention by diverting esophagostomy **(A)** demonstrated increased survival in the canine model of complete ileal obstruction. Survival among control animals (surgical creation of complete ileal obstruction) averaged 7 days, whereas survival in the experimental group averaged 35 days **(B)**. (From Wangensteen OH, Rea J. The distention factor in simple intestinal obstruction. Surgery 5:327, 1939.)

B

ESOPHAGOSTOMY AND ILEAL OBSTRUCTION (WANGENSTEEN & REA, SURGERY 5:327, 1939)

Operation	*Dog No.*	*Initial Weight (kg.)*	*Saline Solution (cc.)*	*Survival in Days*	*Gas (cc.)*	*Fluid (cc.)*	*Weight at Death (kg.)*	*Remarks*
Esophagostomy+feeding for 1 month; then closure of the distal esophageal opening and terminal ileal obstruction+saline solution	1	24.0	1,500	19	100	150	16.5	Dogs 1-7 showed no distension of the gut except for segment 15 to 20 cm. proximal to ileal obstruction
	2	20.0	1,500	20	150	50	16.0	
	3	17.5	1,500	32	0*	100	12.0	
	4	26.0	1,500	40	50	50	15.2	Dog 4 received 2 transfusions of citrated blood, 300 cc. each. Total plasma protein just before death, 4.5 gm. %
	5	15.9	1,500	29	0*	350	12.5	
	6	17.0	1,500	45	50	60	11.5	
	7	18.5	1,500	34	0*	90	10.0	
	8	18.0	1,500	33	175	150	13.5	Slight distention
	9	15.0	1,500	33	600	800	9.5	Died with a volvulus; gut markedly distended
	10	20.0	1,500	45	1,000	350	14.5	Stomach and jejunum are contracted; received 4 transfusions of citrated blood, 300 cc. each, after ileal obstruction
	11	18.3	1,500	57	100	125	12.5	Ileum was distended and contained 500 gm. of semisolid fecal material; this dog received a total of 5 transfusions of citrated blood, 300 cc. each, after the ileal obstruction; just before the animal was sacrificed, plasma protein 4.4 gm. %, plasma chlorides 676 mg. %, and non-protein nitrogen 60.6 mg. %
Average survival				35.2				

* Too small to be measured accurately.

gallstone ileus. Because the gallstone enters the bowel through a cholecystoenteric (usually duodenal) fistula and usually obstructs the narrowest part of the small bowel (terminal ileum), pneumobilia and multiple loops of distended small bowel are pathognomonic of gallstone ileus.

Decompression of the intestine has classically been shown to increase survival[53] (Fig. 33-4). The early management of suspected partial or complete bowel obstruction includes the passage of intestinal tubes. Shorter tubes, such as nasogastric and nasoduodenal tubes, function by aspirating swallowed air and upper GI tract secretions, thereby minimizing further intestinal distention. In most cases nasogastric tubes are as effective as nasointestinal tubes.[54] Longer enteric tubes may be placed fluoroscopically to decompress distal intestinal contents, facilitating the relief of intestinal obstruction. The preferred method of decompressing a complete obstruction is operative because of the higher risks of strangulation with complete obstruction. These longer tubes may be used in more prolonged fashion in individuals with terminal illnesses, for example, those with extensive intraabdominal malignancies.[55]

The following principles guide the management of small-bowel obstruction:

1. Clinical judgment (even that of experienced surgeons) is notoriously *bad* at predicting which patients with small bowel obstruction will be found to have compromised bowel.
2. The great majority of cases of compromised bowel in small bowel obstruction occur in the setting of complete obstruction.
3. The patient with *clear* evidence of partial small bowel obstruction (and neither fever, tachycardia,

leukocytosis, tenderness, nor unremitting pain) does not have compromised bowel.

For years, general surgeons have trained with the adage, "Never let the sun rise or set on an intestinal obstruction." This was born out of the tremendous morbidity and mortality associated with the delay in diagnosis and definitive therapy of a strangulated obstruction, and it is still a reliable dictum. With the advent of nasogastric decompression and aggressive resuscitation, it has become increasingly acceptable to manage incomplete obstruction, and in a few rare instances complete obstruction, nonoperatively. For instance, few surgeons are anxious to operate on an anastomotic obstruction in a patient in stable condition during the postoperative period. Bowel compromise is unusual in this setting, and most cases of postoperative small bowel obstruction (many of which may be persistent ileus) resolve uneventfully with nonoperative treatment. However, the clinician must ever be alert for the conversion of a simple obstruction to a strangulating obstruction, heralded by an increase in abdominal pain and associated peritoneal signs, increasing white blood cell count, fever, and acidosis.

The surgeon must also bear in mind that most obstructions (complete and partial) have etiologies that are readily corrected by operation—adhesions, hernias, neoplasms, and volvulus. Two obvious and common exceptions are intussusception in an infant treated with barium enema and sigmoid volvulus in an elderly person treated initially with sigmoidoscopic decompression. The important principles of operative management of small-bowel obstruction are simply stated: (1) relieve the obstruction; (2) remove compromised (ischemic, perforated) bowel; and (3) avoid spillage of GI contents.

Motility Disorders of the Small Intestine

Etiology and Pathophysiology

Paralytic ileus is the most common acute motor disorder of the small intestine. It is usually associated with an acute intraperitoneal or retroperitoneal pathologic process or operation. The pathophysiology of acute paralytic ileus is unclear, but perturbations in the enteric nervous system, the endocrine system, and GI muscle are almost certainly involved.

Chronic intestinal pseudo-obstruction is a rare condition with multiple possible causes.[56] It should be considered in patients with symptoms of recurrent small bowel obstruction, especially if these remain unexplained at operation. Marked chronic enlargement anywhere along the GI tract (megaduodenum, megajejunum, megacolon) may occur. Mechanical obstruction must be ruled out, even in patients with known pseudo-obstruction, because vascular compromise and perforation may ensue if a mechanical obstruction is missed.

Diagnosis and Treatment

The clinical presentation of small bowel motility disorders may be remarkably similar to that of patients with mechanical small bowel obstruction. Signs and symptoms include distention, pain, obstipation, vomiting, and dehydration. Plain radiographs may show small bowel distention with air-fluid levels. Colonic distention is common. Upper GI tract series and small bowel follow-through with thin barium are useful to rule out mechanical obstruction. Results of esophageal manometry are usually abnormal in patients with chronic intestinal pseudo-obstruction, as are those of scintigraphic transit scans. The ingestion of nonabsorbable radiopaque markers may be helpful in identifying the site of functional obstruction along the alimentary tract.

Treatment of acute paralytic ileus consists of nasogastric decompression (long intestinal tubes do not pass without peristalsis), intravenous fluids, nutritional support, mobilization (ambulation if possible), and therapy for any associated causative diseases (e.g., pancreatitis). Operation is rarely indicated unless perforation is likely.

Treatment of chronic intestinal pseudo-obstruction is largely medical and includes promotility agents; dietary, nutritional, and psychologic counseling; intermittent antibiotics for bacterial overgrowth; and treatment of diarrhea or constipation. Long-term parenteral alimentation may be necessary. Acute exacerbations are treated with intravenous hydration, tube decompression, and antibiotics as needed. Operation is palliative and is indicated if mechanical obstruction is expected, to place decompressive gastrostomy and jejunostomy tubes, and to manage complications (e.g., stercoral perforation).[57]

MECHANICAL DISORDERS OF THE COLON

Colonic Obstruction

Etiology and Pathophysiology

Most mechanical colon obstructions are caused by cancer, volvulus, or diverticulitis, in decreasing order of frequency. In contrast to small bowel obstruction, most large bowel obstructions (60% to 65%) are a result of intrinsic neoplasms, usually in the left side of the colon.[58] Postulated reasons for this phenomenon include the steadily decreasing caliber of the intra-abdominal colon as it progresses from right to left, combined with the more solid character of stool in the left colon. In addition, there is a higher frequency of circumferential tumor within the left colon. Inflammatory processes, most commonly diverticulitis, account for approximately 10% of all large bowel obstructions. Uncommon intrinsic etiologies of obstruction include inflammatory bowel disease, ischemic stricture, postradiation stricture, and intussusception.

The most common external cause (and second most common cause overall) of large bowel obstruction is volvulus, accounting for approximately 10% to 15% of large bowel obstructions. Volvulus usually affects the sigmoid (75%) or cecum (20%) (Fig. 33-5). Transverse colon volvulus is rare (5%). Sigmoid volvulus results when the colon is elongated and distended by such factors as chronic constipation or high fiber intake, making the bowel more likely to volvulize on itself.[58]

Finally, obturating lesions, such as rectal foreign bodies and stool impaction, can cause large bowel obstruction.

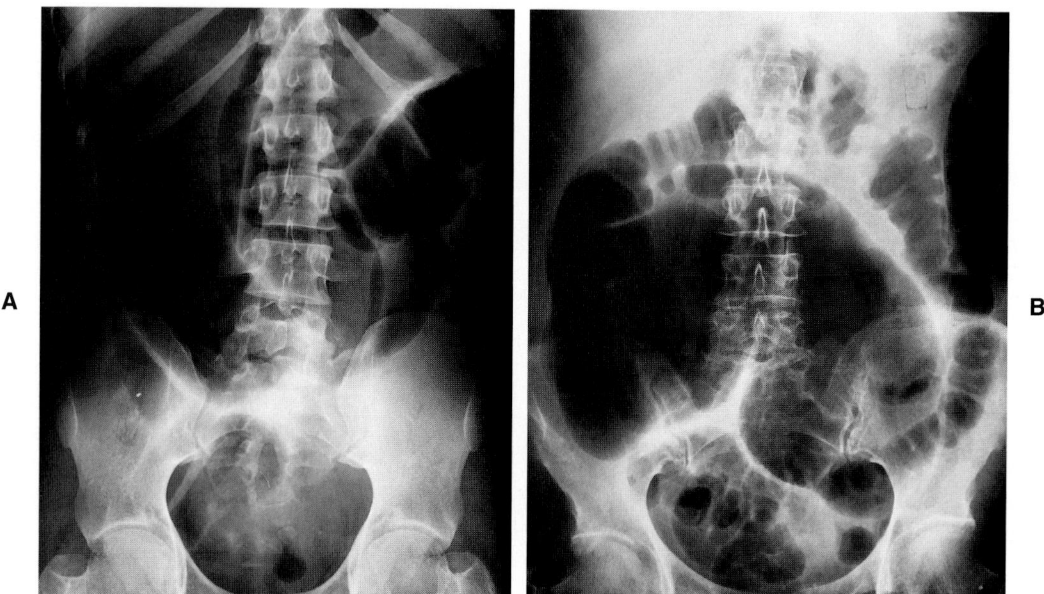

Fig. 33-5. The "bent inner tube" sign of sigmoid volvulus. The distended loop of sigmoid colon is directed to the right upper quadrant, with its base located in the left lower quadrant **(A)**. In contrast, the "coffee bean deformity" of cecal volvulus is directed toward the left upper quadrant, with its base in the right lower quadrant **(B)**.

Less common extrinsic etiologies of colonic obstruction include hernias, carcinomatosis, extraintestinal tumor, and pelvic recurrence of rectal carcinoma.

Diagnosis and Treatment

Patients with an obstructing colon cancer or colon volvulus have progressive distention and obstipation. Nausea and vomiting are variable, depending on the competence of the ileocecal valve. Peritoneal signs suggest compromised bowel or perforation. Acute colon obstruction not uncommonly complicates acute diverticulitis. Although resolution of the colon blockage usually heralds the resolution of the acute attack, progressive colonic distention may be an indication for operation in acute diverticulitis. Alternatively, chronic partial obstruction of the sigmoid from chronic diverticular disease is associated with cramps, distention, and difficult defecation. Operation for obstruction is more often indicated in chronic diverticulitis.

The diagnostic workup of colon obstruction consists of plain radiography (obstruction series), sigmoidoscopy, and limited barium enema. Plain films suggest the diagnosis. Operation is indicated if cecal diameter is 12 cm or greater.

Sigmoidoscopy rules out rectal pathology and may be diagnostic of obstructing rectosigmoid cancer or diverticulitis. Air insufflation should be negligible. Careful barium enema documents obstruction and should be terminated when complete obstruction or extravasation is seen. Sigmoidoscopy is successful in reducing the sigmoid volvulus in approximately 85% of cases, with emergency laparotomy and sigmoid resection with end-colostomy reserved if endoscopy is unsuccessful or colonic ischemia is suspected. Because of the high rate of recurrence, elective sigmoid resection, usually with primary anastomosis, should be scheduled after successful reduction. Unlike sigmoid volvulus, which is seen as a large bowel obstruction, cecal volvulus is seen as a small bowel obstruction. Colonoscopic detorsion is ineffective in this instance, and laparotomy should be undertaken to reduce the volvulus and prevent recurrence through a definitive procedure such as cecal resection, cecostomy, or cecopexy. Resection with primary anastomosis is acceptable if irreversible cecal damage has occurred. Obstructing colon cancer may be managed initially with loop colostomy, resection, and Hartman operation or rarely with resection and primary anastomosis following on-table mechanical cleansing of the obstructing colon. Intractable acute obstruction from acute diverticulitis is managed with Hartmann's operation, whereas chronic obstruction from chronic diverticular disease is treated with resection and primary anastomosis.

Colonic Dysmotility
Etiology and Pathophysiology

Colonic dysmotility may mimic mechanical obstruction from tumor, diverticulosis, stool, or volvulus. Presentation may be acute (e.g., Ogilvie's syndrome or toxic megacolon) or chronic (e.g., colonic inertia or idiopathic megacolon). Most deaths from colonic dysmotility occur in the acute group from perforation or fulminant colitis. The pathophysiology of acute colonic ileus is unclear, but motor function is often abnormal in the setting of fulminant mucosal inflammation. Medications (e.g., narcotics) or op-

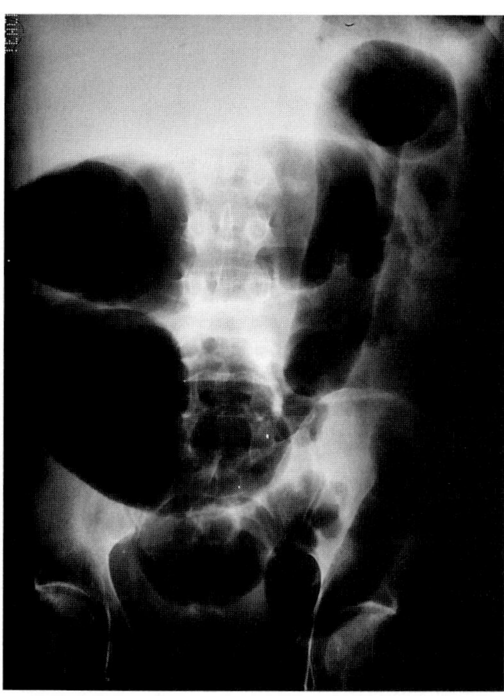

Fig. 33-6. The massive colonic dilatation associated with Ogilvie's syndrome.

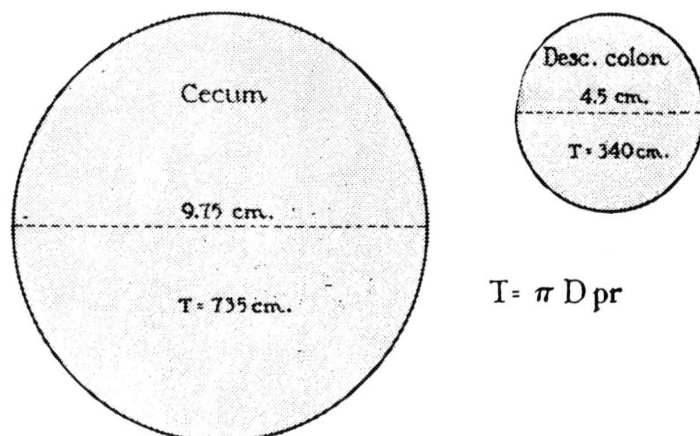

Fig. 33-7. As the colon dilates in cases of obstruction or ileus, wall tension is greatest in the region of largest diameter, as dictated by Laplace's law. The risk of perforation increases with increasing wall tension. (From Wangensteen OH. Intestinal Obstruction. Springfield, Ill.: Charles C Thomas, 1937, p 51.)

erations (e.g., hip replacement) may precipitate colonic ileus. Chronic colon dysfunction may be congenital (e.g., adult Hirschsprung's disease) or acquired (e.g., laxative abuse). In practice, most cases of acute and chronic colonic dysfunction are idiopathic.

Experimental evidence has revealed bowel distention, not sustained increases in intraluminal pressures, to be the hallmark of simple obstruction.[37] This carries important implications in colonic obstruction or acute colonic ileus, especially in patients with competent ileocecal valves and with the massive dilatation that frequently accompanies Ogilvie's syndrome (Fig. 33-6). Laplace's law dictates that wall tension is the product of radius times internal pressure. The cecum is the widest portion of the GI tract, with the largest radius. When the cecum distends and pressure increases in this setting, wall tension increases and the risk of perforation becomes substantial[22,59] (Fig. 33-7). Cecal diameters greater than 12 cm on abdominal radiographs are of great concern and necessitate operative decompression with either a transverse colostomy or a cecostomy. Colonoscopy may be used for decompression in individuals with Ogilvie's syndrome.

Diagnosis and Treatment

Diagnostic evaluation in the patient with colonic dilatation is focused on answering three questions: (1) Is there distal obstruction? (2) Is this a manifestation of colonic dysmotility, and if so, was the hypomotility caused by mucosal disease? (3) Is the viability of the colon compromised? This evaluation is done by physical examination, plain abdominal radiography, proctosigmoidoscopy, and limited retrograde barium study. Complete distal obstruction requires urgent operative decompression. If distal obstruction is ruled out, acute distention may be caused by mucosal disease (e.g., "megacolon" from inflammatory bowel disease, or *Clostridium difficile* colitis), ischemia, or some other poorly understood cause (for example, opioids, stroke, and reflex dysmotility after major orthopedic surgery). In the setting of clinical toxicity, megacolon associated with mucosal disease should be treated by subtotal colectomy and ileostomy. Segmental ischemia may be treated with partial colectomy. In either case, margin viability cannot be assessed by gross inspection, and frozen-section confirmation is important. Diagnostic evaluation in the adult patient with chronic colonic dysfunction is designed to rule out colonic obstruction, global motility disorder, and adult short-segment Hirschsprung's disease, and to confirm colonic dysfunction.

On plain radiographs, patients with colonic obstruction or dysfunction and a competent ileocecal valve show colonic dilatation and little small bowel and rectal gas. In contrast, those with incompetent valves may have radiographic evidence of small bowel and colonic distention. Paralytic ileus results in air-fluid levels evenly distributed throughout the gastrointestinal tract, and at times it may be extremely difficult to differentiate from colonic obstruction in the setting of an incompetent ileocecal valve. Barium enema is often useful in these circumstances to exclude the colon as a site of obstruction. Colonoscopy may also be used in this setting; it has the advantage of facilitating cecal decompression. Other important tests include anorectal manometry, ingestion of radiopaque markers, scintigraphy, and defecography. In colonic inertia or idiopathic megacolon, anorectal manometry shows normal relaxation of the internal sphincter in response to rectal distention (provided that normal sensory threshold exists). This feature is absent in adult short-segment Hirschsprung's disease. A deep mucosal biopsy sample of the distal rectum in the latter disease may show a paucity of ganglion cells, but this may also be seen in healthy subjects. Total abdominal colectomy and ileoproctostomy are indicated if colonic hypomotility is confirmed in the patient with severe symptoms and relatively normal gastric emptying and small bowel transit. Adult Hirschsprung's disease may respond to internal sphincterotomy or distal proctectomy with coloanal anastomosis. Frozen-section confirmation of proximal resection margins is necessary to confirm ganglion cells.

SUMMARY

Mechanical disorders of the GI tract result when the normal digestive and absorptive functions of the stomach, duodenum, or intestine are altered by either an obstructive process or a derangement in motility. Depending on the site of obstruction, these patients have a fairly predictable history and physical examination. An understanding of the underlying pathophysiologic changes common to these disorders allows early correction of underlying metabolic derangements and paves the way for ultimate surgical intervention designed to restore normal GI function.

REFERENCES

1. Graham DY. Ulcer complications and their nonoperative treatment. In Sleisinger MH, Fordtran JS, eds. Gastrointestinal Disease, 5th ed. Philadelphia: WB Saunders, 1993, p 698.
2. Adrogue HJ, Madias NE. Management of life-threatening acid-base disorders. N Engl J Med 338:107, 1998.
3. Parkman HP, et al. Electrogastrography and gastric emptying scintigraphy are complementary for assessment of dyspepsia. J Clin Gastroenterol 24:214, 1997.
4. Jaffin BW, Kaye MD. The prognosis of gastric outlet obstruction. Ann Surg 201:176, 1985.
5. Matthews JB, Silen W. Operations for peptic ulcer disease and early postoperative complications. In Sleisinger MH, Fordtran JS, eds. Gastrointestinal Disease, 5th ed. Philadelphia: WB Saunders, 1993, p 713.
6. Mentes AS. Parietal cell vagotomy and dilatation for peptic duodenal stricture. Ann Surg 212:597, 1990.
7. Lindor KD, Ott BJ, Hughes RW, Jr. Balloon dilatation of upper digestive tract strictures. Gastroenterology 89:545, 1985.
8. Kuwada SK, Alexander GL. Long-term outcome of endoscopic dilation of nonmalignant pyloric stenosis. Gastrointest Endosc 41:15, 1995.
9. Brune IB, et al. Laparoscopic gastrojejunostomy and endoscopic biliary stent placement for palliation of incurable gastric outlet obstruction with cholestasis. Surg Endosc 11:834, 1997.
10. Fukuya T, Brown BP, Lu CC. Midgut volvulus as a complication of intestinal malrotation in adults. Dig Dis Sci 38:438, 1993.
11. Raissi B, Taylor BM, Taves DH. Recurrent superior mesenteric artery (Wilkie's) syndrome. Can J Surg 39:410, 1996.
12. Wasselle JA, Norman J. Acute gastric volvulus: pathogenesis, diagnosis, and treatment [review]. Am J Gastroenterol 88:1780, 1993.
13. Harriss DR, et al. Paraesophageal hiatal hernia: When to operate. J R Coll Surg Edin 37:97, 1992.
14. Kusano M, et al. Further classification of dysmotility-like dyspepsia by interdigestive gastroduodenal manometry and plasma motilin level. Am J Gastroenterol 92:481, 1997.
15. Schuffler MD, Sinahan MN. Intestinal obstruction and pseudo-obstruction. In Sleisinger MH, Fordtran JS, eds. Gastrointestinal Disease, 5th ed. Philadelphia: WB Saunders, 1993, p 898.
16. Malagelada J-R, Azpiroz F, Mearin F. Gastroduodenal motor function in health and disease. In Sleisinger MH, Fordtran JS, eds. Gastrointestinal Disease, 5th ed. Philadelphia: WB Saunders, 1993, p 486.
17. Mearin F, Camilleri M, Malagelada JR. Pyloric dysfunction in diabetes with recurrent nausea and vomiting. Gastroenterology 90:1919, 1986.
18. Schirmer BD. Gastric atony and the Roux syndrome. Gastroenterol Clin North Am 23:327, 1994.
19. Wilson P, et al. Pathologic duodenogastric reflux associated with persistence of symptoms after cholecystectomy. Surgery 117:421, 1995.
20. Parkman HP, Miller MA, Fisher RS. Role of nuclear medicine in evaluating patients with suspected gastrointestinal motility disorders. Semin Nucl Med 25:289, 1995.
21. Levine BA, Aust JB. Surgical disorders of the small intestine. In Sabiston DC Jr, ed. Essentials of Surgery. Philadelphia: WB Saunders, 1987.
22. Wangensteen OH. Historical aspects of the management of acute intestinal obstructions. Surgery 65:363, 1969.
23. DiSario JA, et al. Small bowel carcinoma: epidemiological and clinical characteristics from a population based registry. Am J Gastroenterol 89:699, 1994.
24. Tanphiphat C, Chittmittrapat S, Prosopsunti K. Adhesive small bowel obstruction. Am J Surg 154:283, 1987.
25. Stevenson RJ. Non-neonatal intestinal obstruction in children. Surg Clin North Am 65:1217, 1985.
26. Ziegler MM. Gastrointestinal problems after the first month of life. In Hardy JD, ed. Hardy's Textbook of Surgery. Philadelphia: JB Lippincott, 1988.
27. Nagorney DM, Starr MG, McIlrath DC. Surgical management of intussusception in the adult. Ann Surg 193:230, 1981.
28. Guyton AC. Textbook of Medical Physiology. Philadelphia: WB Saunders, 1986.
29. Shields R. The absorption and secretion of fluid and electrolytes by the obstructed bowel. Br J Surg 25:774, 1965.
30. Wright HK, O'Brien JJ, Tilson MD. Water absorption in experimental closed segment obstruction of the ileum in man. Am J Surg 121:96, 1971.
31. Chappuis CW, Cohn I Jr. In Fielding LP, Welch JP, Moore FD, eds. Intestinal Obstruction. Clinical Surgery International, vol 13. Edinburgh: Churchill Livingstone, 1987, p 32.
32. Enochsson L, Nylander G, Ohman U. Effects of intraluminal pressure on regional blood flow in obstructed and unobstructed small intestine in the rat. Am J Surg 144:558, 1982.
33. Ruf W, Suehiro GT, Pressler U. Intestinal blood flow at various intraluminal pressures in the piglet with closed abdomen. Ann Surg 19:157, 1980.
34. Gatch WD, Trusler HM, Ayers KD. Effects of gaseous distention on bowel obstruction: Incarceration of intestine by gas traps. Arch Surg 14:1215, 1927.
35. Oppenheimer MJ, Mann FC. Intestinal capillary circulation during distention. Surgery 13:548, 1943.
36. Shikata J, Shida T, Amino K. Experimental studies on the hemodynamics of the small intestine following increased intraluminal pressure. Surg Gynecol Obstet 156:155, 1983.
37. Ohman U. Studies on small intestinal obstruction. I. Intraluminal pressure in low small bowel obstruction in the cat. Acta Chir Scand 141:413, 1975.
38. Burgett GE, Martzliff K, Suckon G. The closed intestinal loop: Relation of intra loop (jejunum) pressure to the clinical condition of the animal. Arch Surg 21:289, 1936.
39. Wangensteen OH. The early diagnosis of acute intestinal obstruction with comments on pathology and treatment. Dis Colon Rectum 25:65, 1982.

40. Gurbach SL. Intestinal microflora. Gastroenterology 60:1110, 1971.
41. Sykes PA, Boulter KH, Schofield PF. The microflora of the obstructed bowel. Br J Surg 63:721, 1976.
42. Gupta S, Reddy KRRM, Samyal SC. Bacterial flora in acute small bowel obstruction. Chemotherapy 26:446, 1980.
43. Bishop RF, Allcock EA. Bacterial flora of the small bowel in acute intestinal obstruction. Br Med J 1:766, 1960.
44. Banwill JC, et al. Intestinal microflora after feeding phytohemagglutinins *(Phaseolus vulgaris)* to the rat. Appl Environ Microbiol 50:68, 1983.
45. Deitch EA, et al. Obstructed Intestine as a Reservoir for Systemic Infection. Am J Surg 159:394, 1990.
46. Brolin RE. Partial small bowel obstruction. Surgery 95:145, 1984.
47. Antoncic RF, Lawson H. The muscular activity of the small intestine in the dog during acute obstruction. Ann Surg 114:415, 1941.
48. Summers RW, et al. Acute intestinal obstruction: An electromyographic study in dogs. Gastroenterology 85:1301, 1983.
49. Prihoda M, Glatt A, Summers RW. Mechanisms of motility changes during acute intestinal obstruction in the dog. Am J Physiol 247:G37, 1984.
50. Enochsson L, et al. Myoelectric motility patterns during mechanical obstruction and paralysis of the small intestine in the rat. Scand J Gastroenterol 1987:22, 969.
51. Coelho JHC, et al. Gastrointestinal motility following small bowel obstruction in the opossum. J Surg Res 41:274, 1986.
52. Carlson RS, Wangensteen OH. Motor activity of the distal small bowel in intestinal obstruction. Proc Soc Exp Biol Med 27:676, 1930.
53. Wangensteen OH, Rea J. The distention factor in simple intestinal obstruction. Surgery 5:327, 1939.
54. Fleshner PR, et al. A prospective randomized trial of short versus long tubes in adhesive small bowel obstruction. Am J Surg 170:366, 1995.
55. Wolfson PJ, et al. Use of the long tube in the management of patients with small intestinal obstruction due to adhesions. Arch Surg 120:1001, 1985.
56. Patel R, Christensen J. Chronic intestinal pseudo-obstruction: Diagnosis and treatment. Gastroenterologist 3:345, 1995.
57. Murr MM, Sarr MG, Camilleri M. The surgeon's role in the treatment of chronic intestinal pseudoobstruction. Am J Gastroenterol 90:2147, 1995.
58. Stanislov GU, Fabrisio M. Obstruction of the large bowel. In Cameron JL, ed. Current Surgical Therapy. St. Louis: Mosby, 1992.
59. Miller LD, Mackie JA, Rhoads JE. The pathophysiology and management of intestinal obstruction. Surg Clin North Am 42:1285, 1962.

34

Physiologic Derangements of the Rectum and Anus

D.C.N.K. Nyam, Francis Antony Frizelle, and John H. Pemberton

The *anorectum* is the terminal part of the gastrointestinal tract. Its anatomy and several unique physiologic parameters combine to facilitate fecal continence and defecation. An understanding of the normal anorectal and pelvic floor anatomy and physiology is important in the appreciation of the role that abnormal physiology plays in the etiology of several common anorectal disorders.

RECTUM

General Anatomy

About 15 to 18 cm long, the rectum extends from the sigmoid colon to the anorectal ring. Anatomically, the rectum begins at the level of the third sacral vertebra. Surgically, however, it is typically described as starting at the level of the sacral promontory.[1] The rectum is divided into three parts, depending on its relationship to the peritoneum. The cranial third is covered with peritoneum on the anterior and lateral sides, almost encircling it save for a short mesorectum. The middle third is covered only anteriorly by peritoneum, whereas the caudal third is devoid of peritoneal covering.

The level of the anterior peritoneal reflection varies. It is usually 5 to 7.5 cm above the anal verge in women and 7 to 9 cm in men.[2] The peritoneum is reflected from the rectum onto the pelvic side walls to form the perirectal fossa. In women, the anterior peritoneum reflects onto the vagina and uterus, whereas in men it reflects onto the seminal vesicles and bladder.

At the junction between the rectum and sigmoid colon, the taeniae coli disappear as the longitudinal muscle spreads out to encircle the rectum as a continuous muscle layer (Fig. 34-1). Intraluminally, the sigmoid becomes rectum when it gives way to the smoother rectal mucosa.[3] In addition, the rectum has no appendices epiploicae, haustra, or mesentery.[4]

The rectum descends caudally along the curve of the sacrum, initially downward and then forward to end at the anorectal ring. The anorectal ring is formed by the pelvic floor muscles, along with the external and the internal anal sphincters. The anal canal continues below the anorectal ring by turning abruptly downward and backward, terminating at the anal verge.

The rectum has three curves, the upper and lower convex to the right and the middle convex to the left. The infoldings of these curves form the valves of Houston on the luminal aspect. These valves incorporate all layers of the rectal wall except the longitudinal muscle layer. The middle, most consistent valve usually marks the lever of the peritoneal reflection.[2] When the rectum is completely mobilized, it can usually be elongated by as much as 5 cm.

Fascial Attachments

The rectum and mesorectum are enveloped by a thin layer of pelvic fascia, the fascia propria. Below the anterior peritoneal reflection, condensations of this fascia on either side form the lateral ligaments that lie between the rectum to the pelvic side walls. They act as supports for the rectum and must be divided to ensure full mobilization of the rectum. Accessory branches of the middle rectal artery sometimes traverse the ligaments. Generally, the main middle rectal artery travels toward the rectum on the top of the levator muscles.

Below S4, the retrorectal fascia (Waldeyer's fascia) forms a thick layer that must be incised sharply for complete posterior rectal mobilization. Condensation of areolar tissue anteriorly in the extraperitoneal rectum (Denonvillers' fascia) extends down to the pelvic floor, separating the rectum from the prostate gland and seminal vesicles in men and from the vagina in women.

Anal Canal

The anal canal extends from the hairy skin of the anal verge to the anorectal ring. At rest, the lateral walls form an anterioposterior slit.[5] The anal canal is closely related to both internal and external sphincters. The coccyx is posterior, and the ischiorectal fossa is lateral. Anteriorly, it is related to the urethra in men and the lower vagina in women.

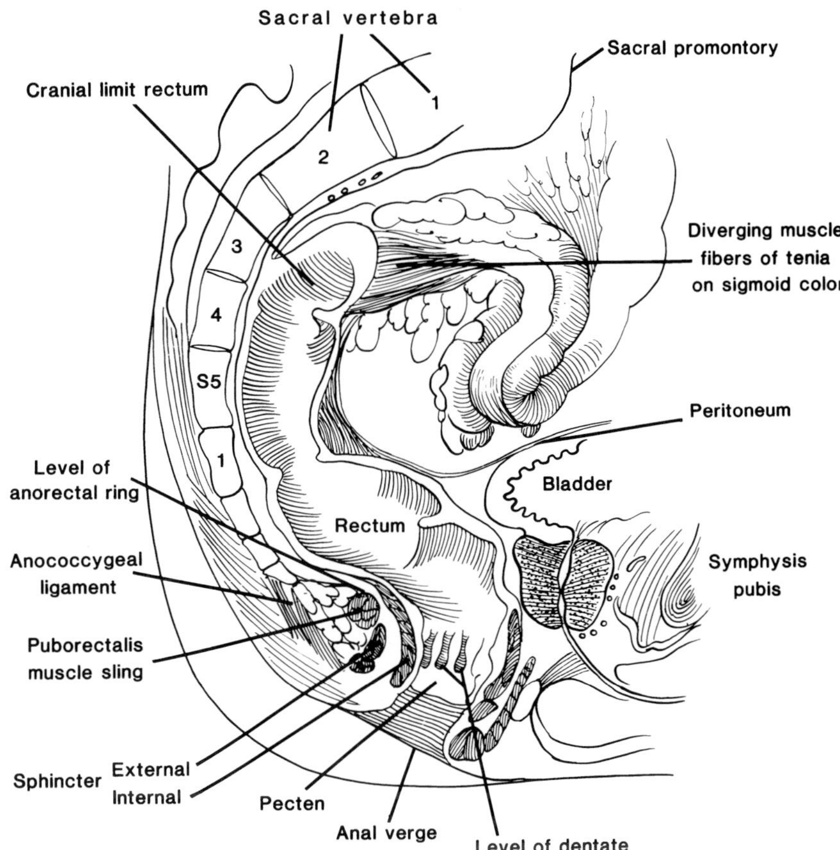

Fig. 34-1. Diagram of the rectum as it courses through the pelvis. The rectum descends downward from S3 to the level of the coccyx, then downward and forward to end at the anorectal ring. The tenia diverge at the level of S2 to S3, providing a visual landmark distinguishing sigmoid from rectum. (From Pemberton JH. Anatomy and physiology of the anus and rectum. In Condon RE, ed. Shackelford's Surgery of the Alimentary Tract, vol 4. Philadelphia: WB Saunders, 1991, p 242. Used with permission.)

Anal Canal Epithelium

The epithelium of the anal canal starts as a continuation of the rectal mucosa cranially and ends as squamous epithelium of skin. Approximately 2 cm cranial to the anal verge is the pectinate or dentate line. This line joins the anal valves and is located at the junction of the middle and distal thirds of the internal anal sphincter. Above each valve is an anal crypt, which is connected to anal glands. These vary in number from four to 10 and traverse the mucosa to end in either the submucosa, internal anal sphincter, or the intersphincteric plane. It is from these glands that perianal abscesses and fistulas arise.

Above the anal valves are 12 to 14 columns of Morgagni. The mucosa in this region consists of several layers of cuboidal cells, which blend at variable distances from the anal verge to a single layer of columnar cells characteristic of rectal mucosa.[1] This area above the dentate line is called the *anal transition zone.*

Caudal to the dentate line, the anal canal is lined by modified squamous epithelium devoid of hair and glands. Grossly, this appears smooth, thin, and stretched.[1] It changes to typical squamous epithelium with hairs and glands at the anal verge. It is important to realize that none of the mucosal boundaries described are the same all the way around the anal canal.[6]

Musculature of the Anal Canal

Smooth muscle. The circular muscle of the rectum continues as the internal anal sphincter and ends as bulb 1 to 1.5 cm caudal to the dentate line (Fig. 34-2). This is palpable as a distinct rounded edge slightly cranial to the termination of the external anal sphincter complex. The internal anal sphincter is about 2.5 to 4 cm in length and about 0.5 cm thick. Some fibers of the longitudinal muscle and puborectalis pass between the internal and external sphincters and are attached to the perianal dermis. These are called *corrugator cutis ani.*

Striated muscle. The external sphincter complex envelops the whole length of the internal anal sphincter. It consists of three parts, deep, superficial, and subcutaneous. This elliptical muscle is continuous with the puborectalis superiorly. Inferiorly, the subcutaneous part extends distal

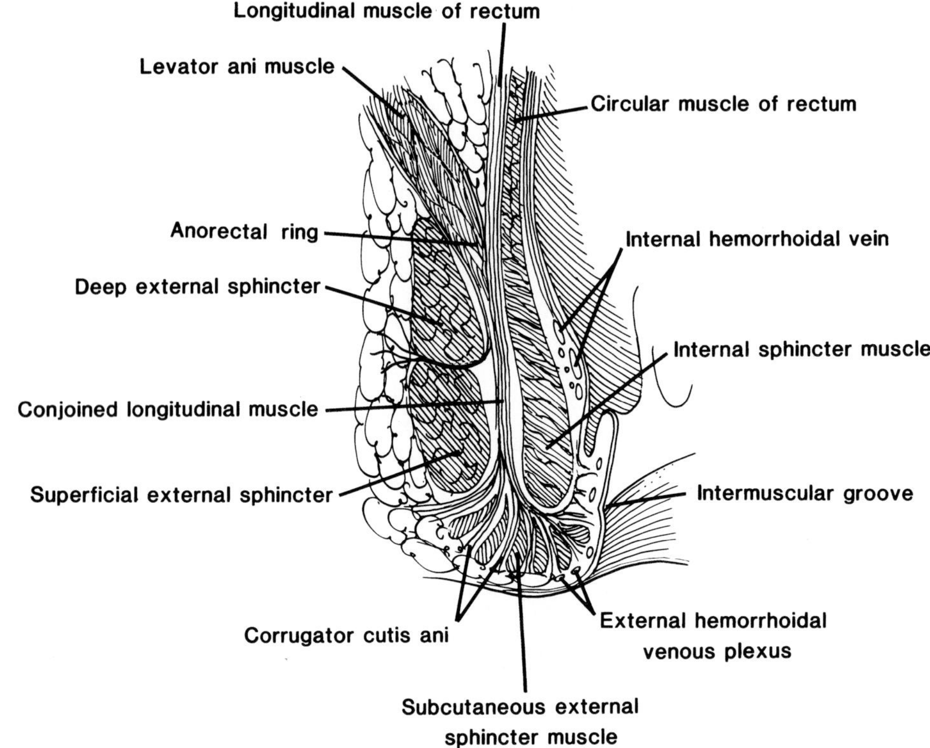

Fig. 34-2. The voluntary and involuntary muscles of the anorectum and their relationships to the topography of the anal canal. (From Pemberton JH. Anatomy and physiology of the anus and rectum. In Condon RE, ed. Shackelford's Surgery of the Alimentary Tract, vol 4. Philadelphia: WB Saunders, 1991, p 242. Used with permission.)

to the internal anal sphincter. The muscle is attached posteriorly in a continuous fashion with the puborectalis, sacrococcygeal raphae, coccyx, and skin. Anteriorly, it is similarly attached to the puborectalis, transverse perineal muscle, and skin.[7]

Pelvic Floor

The pelvic diaphragm provides a firm surface for fixation of the pelvic viscera and through which the gastrointestinal and genital tracts traverse. The levator ani consists of three muscles that form the posterior portion of the diaphragm (Fig. 34-3). The iliococcygeus originates from the ischial spine and obturator fascia to insert on S4, S5, and the anococcygeal raphae. The pubococcygeus originates from the obturator fascia and pubis and passes posteriorly, caudally, and medially, where fibers from both sides decussate. The puborectalis arises next to the pubococcygeus from the pubis and proceeds posteriorly alongside the anorectal junction. Fibers from either side merge to form a sling behind the rectum at the anorectal junction. The anorectal ring that results is important because division almost inevitably results in fecal incontinence.

The rectococcygeus that is present bilaterally and attaches the rectum to the coccyx is involuntary. The coccygeus muscles, in contrast, are voluntary and arise from S5 and the coccyx. The superficial and deep transverse perineal muscles arise from the pubis and ischium, respectively. They insert into the perineal body and serve to fix this central tendon. In men, these muscles merge with the external urinary sphincter and allow voluntary control of voiding.[7]

Para-anal Spaces

These potential spaces are important as sites of perianal infections (Fig. 34-4). The ischiorectal fossa is bounded inferiorly by the perineal skin, anteriorly by the transversus perinei muscles, posteriorly by the sacrotuberous ligament and the gluteus maximus muscle, medially by the external sphincter and levator ani, and laterally by the external obturator muscle. Alcock's canal, containing the pudendal vessels and nerves, passes in the lateral wall. The contents of this space include fat, the inferior hemorrhoidal vessels and nerves, and the scrotal or labial vessels.

The perianal space surrounds the anal verge and is continuous with the ischiorectal fat laterally. It also extends upward into the intersphincteric space. It contains the most caudal part of the external sphincter, the inferior hemorrhoidal vessels, and the external hemorrhoidal plexus. This space is tightly bound down by the corrugator cutis.

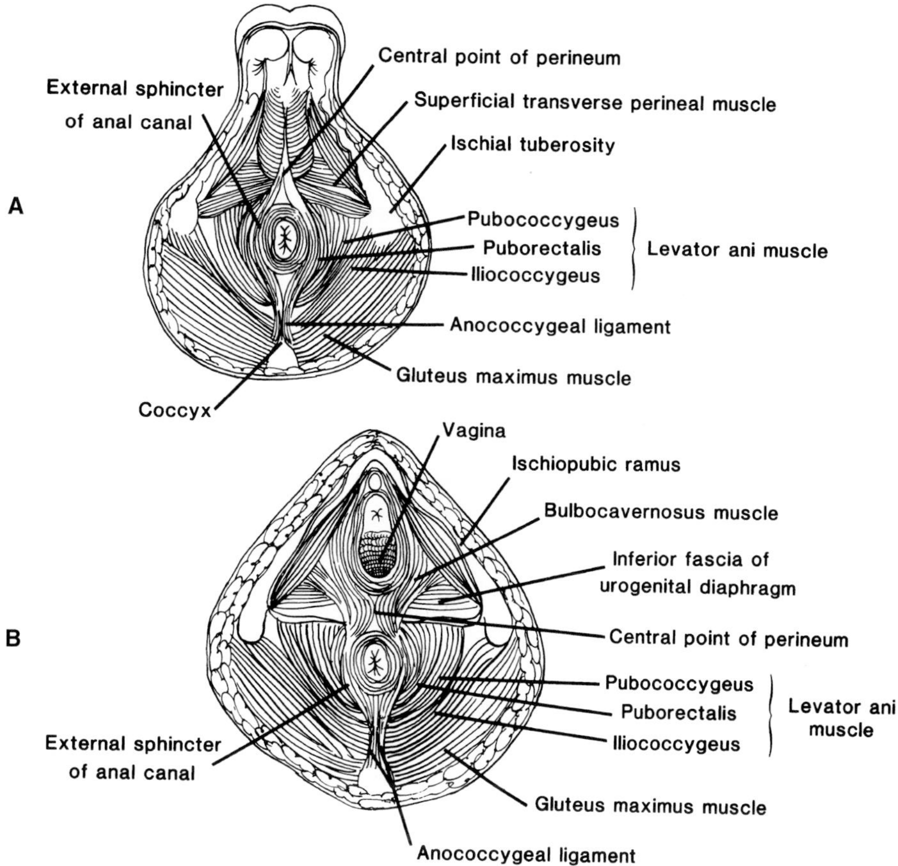

Fig. 34-3. The levator ani muscles in men **(A)** and in women **(B)**. (From Pemberton JH. Anatomy and physiology of the anus and rectum. In Condon RE, ed. Shackelford's Surgery of the Alimentary Tract, vol 4. Philadelphia: WB Saunders, 1991, p 242. Used with permission.)

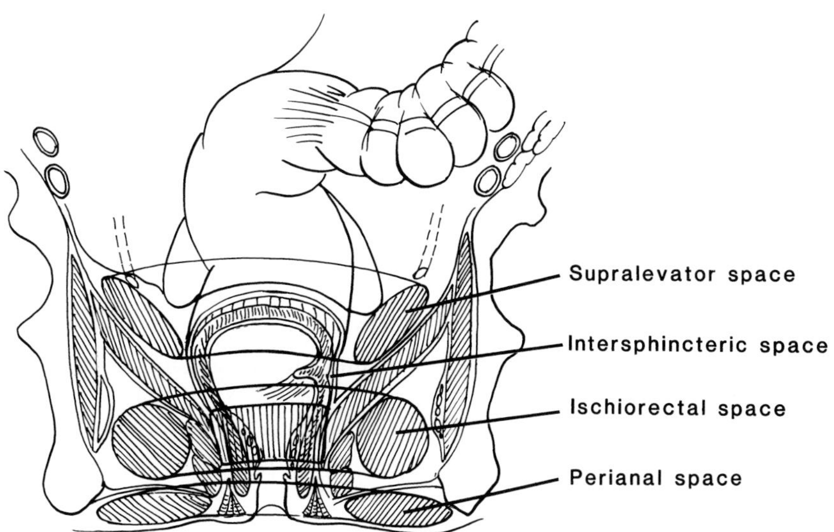

Fig. 34-4. The para-anal and pararectal spaces (coronal view). (From Pemberton JH. Anatomy and physiology of the anus and rectum. In Condon RE, ed. Shackelford's Surgery of the Alimentary Tract, vol 4. Philadelphia: WB Saunders, 1991, p 242. Used with permission.)

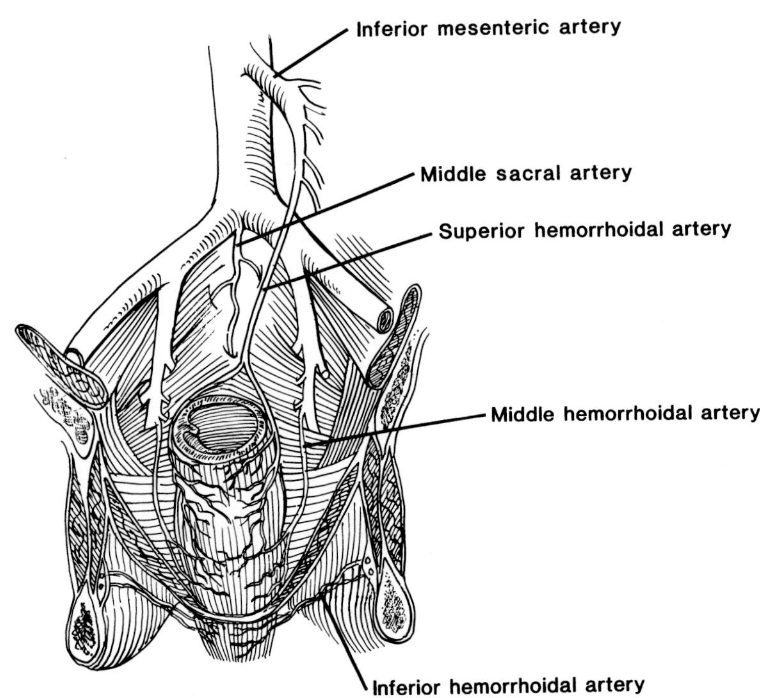

Fig. 34-5. The vasculature of the rectal and anal canal. Note that the middle hemorrhoidal artery, if present, is small and lies immediately on top of the levator ani musculature, *not* in the lateral rectal stalks. (From Pemberton JH. Anatomy and physiology of the anus and rectum. In Condon RE, ed. Shackelford's Surgery of the Alimentary Tract, vol 4. Philadelphia: WB Saunders, 1991, p 242. Used with permission.)

Blood Supply

The blood supply of the rectum and anal canal is predominantly from the superior and inferior rectal arteries. The middle rectal artery has a variable supply (Fig. 34-5).

The superior rectal artery directly continues the inferior mesenteric artery. It descends to S3, at which point it divides into left and right branches. These in turn divide into anterior and posterior branches that enter the rectal wall and descend in the submucosa. Three main branches reach the anal canal—the right posterior, right anterior, and left lateral. There are little extramural midline arterial anastomoses along the entire length of the rectum.

The inferior rectal artery branches from the pudendal artery, itself a branch of the internal iliac artery. It passes through the external anal sphincter and ascends in the submucosa.

The middle rectal artery branches from the internal iliac artery. It passes above the levator ani, not through the lateral ligaments. Small branches of this vessel may, however, pass through the ligaments. In contrast to the extramural arterial system, there is a rich intramural anastomotic network.

The venous drainage generally follows the arterial supply. The superior rectal veins drain into the portal system through the inferior mesenteric vein. The middle and inferior rectal veins drain into the systemic system. There are abundant anastomoses existing between the two systems.

Lymphatics follow the vascular system (Fig. 34-6). The upper two thirds of the rectum drains to the inferior mesenteric nodes. The lower third, however, drains into both the inferior mesenteric and internal iliac nodes. Below the dentate line, the drainage is usually to the inguinal lymph nodes, but it can also drain to the inferior mesenteric or along the inferior rectal artery. Retrograde lymphatic spread below the level of a rectal cancer has been described when there is extensive cancerous involvement of the proximal draining lymphatics.[8]

Nerve Supply

The rectum and upper anal canal are supplied by both components of the autonomic nervous system (Fig. 34-7). The sympathetic system causes inhibition of smooth muscle contraction of the rectum and contraction of the internal sphincter, thus promoting continence. The parasympathetic response is that of rectal wall contraction and relaxation of anal sphincter, promoting defecation.

The sympathetic supply arises from L1 to L3. These lumbar sympathetics run along the inferior mesenteric artery and form the inferior mesenteric plexus. The postganglionic fibers then follow the arterial supply to terminate in the upper rectum. The lower rectum is innervated by the presacral nerves, which arise from the terminal

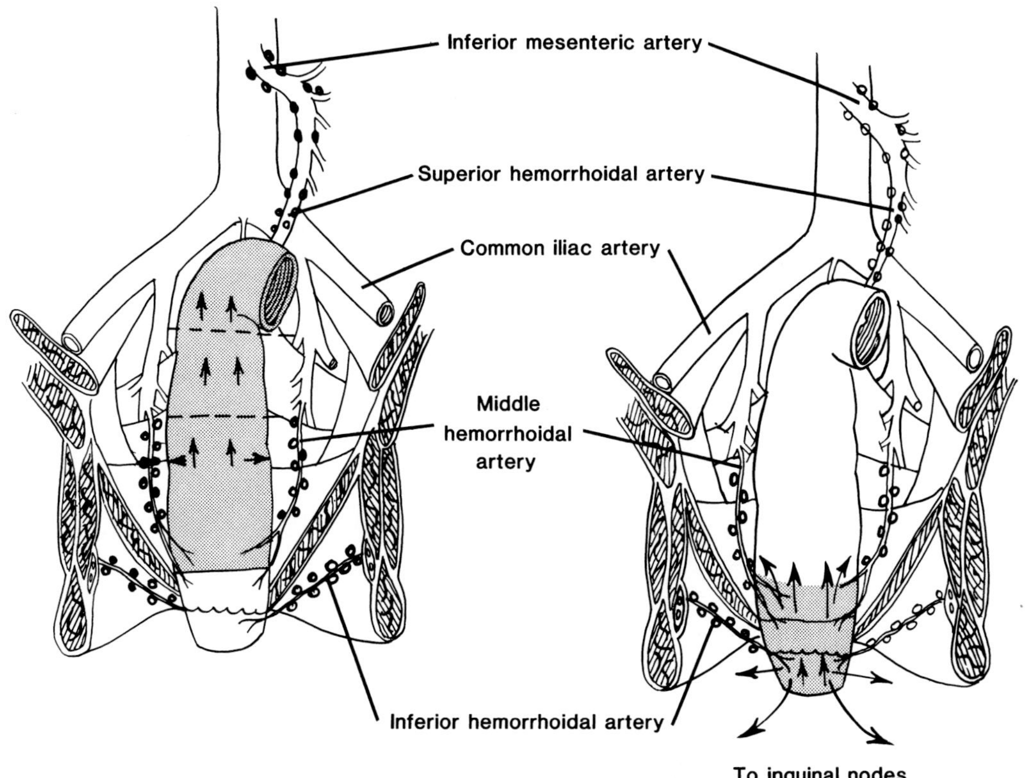

Fig. 34-6. The lymphatic drainage of the rectum and anal canal. The "watershed" area is the dentate line; tumors below the dentate metastasize to the inguinal lymph node chain, whereas tumors above metastasize to the internal iliac and inferior mesenteric nodes. (From Pemberton JH. Anatomy and physiology of the anus and rectum. In Condon RE, ed. Shackelford's Surgery of the Alimentary Tract, vol 4. Philadelphia: WB Saunders, 1991, p 242. Used with permission.)

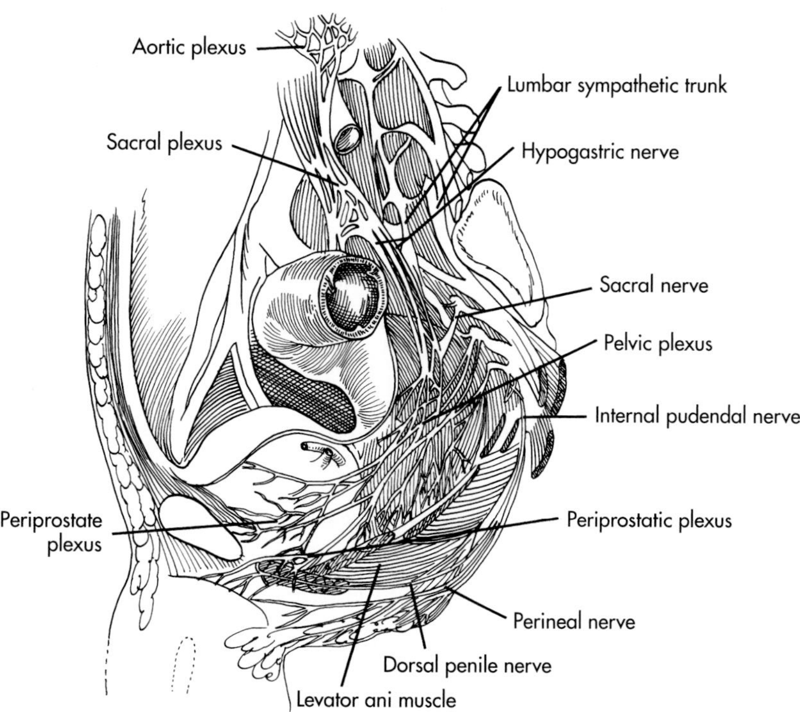

Fig. 34-7. Complex diagram of the innervation of the rectum, anal canal, and anterior structures. (From Pemberton JH. Anatomy and physiology of the anus and rectum. In Condon RE, ed. Shackelford's Surgery of the Alimentary Tract, vol 4. Philadelphia: WB Saunders, 1991, p 242. Used with permission.)

branches of the aortic plexus and lumbar splanchnics. These divide below the sacral promontory to form the right and left hypogastric nerves, which in turn pass to the right and left hypogastric plexuses situated lateral to the lower third of the lateral ligaments. Branches from these plexuses supply the lower rectum, upper anal canal, bladder, and genital organs.

Parasympathetic innervation of the rectum originates from S2, S3, and S4. The nervi erigentes are formed from S3 and S4 and join the sympathetic nerves in the pelvic plexus to be distributed to the inferior mesenteric plexus (supplying the upper rectum), pelvic plexus (supplying the bladder, genital organs, and internal sphincter) and periprostatic plexus (supplying the prostate, seminal vesicles, corpora cavernous, vas deferens, ejaculatory ducts, and bulbourethral glands).[9] These nerves lie outside the fascia enclosing the mesorectum and can be preserved during surgery by careful dissection in this plane.

Erection is controlled by parasympathetic input. Emission is controlled by sympathetic inflow. Ejaculation is controlled by parasympathetic activity.

Somatic pelvic nerves arise from S3, S4, and S5. They cross under the levator ani fascia, supplying the muscle and anal canal. The pudendal nerve arising from S2, S3, and S4 enters the perineum through Alcock's canal, giving out the inferior hemorrhoidal, perianal, and dorsal penile or clitoral nerves.

Sensation

Although there are many nonmyelinated nerve fibers in the rectum, organized endings are generally lacking. Receptors for distention are probably outside the rectal wall. These sensations are carried by parasympathetic nerves to S2, S3, and S4.

From about 1 to 1.5 cm above the anal valves to the anal verge, free nerve endings are present. These include Meissner's corpuscles (touch), Krause's bulbs (cold), Golgi-Mazzoni corpuscles (pressure), and genital corpuscles (friction). Sensation is carried through the inferior hemorrhoidal branch of the pudendal nerve.

NORMAL PHYSIOLOGY OF THE ANUS AND RECTUM

The two main functions of the rectum and anus are the maintenance of fecal continence and defecation. The two processes are complex and interrelated.

Fecal Continence

The mechanisms facilitating fecal continence include (1) the anal high-pressure zone (the internal and external anal sphincters); (2) the anorectal angle and the coordinated activity of the pelvic floor musculature; (3) anorectal sensory and reflex mechanisms; (4) compliance, tone, and capacity of the rectum; (5) rectal filling and emptying; (6) motility and evacuability of the rectum; (7) motility of the anal canal; and (8) stool volume and consistency.

Anal High-Pressure Zone

The mean length of the anal canal is 4.2 cm. Women have shorter anal canals than do men (4.0 vs 4.4 cm).[10]

Resting anal pressure. The internal and external sphincters contribute to maintaining the resting anal pressure (Fig. 34-8). The internal anal sphincter contributes about 85% of the resting tone, with the remainder provided by the external sphincter.[11] The pressure increases distally, with the highest pressure 1 to 2 cm proximal to the anal verge. The length of the high-pressure anal zone is 2.0 to 4.0 cm in women and 2.5 to 4.0 cm in men. This zone is the main resistance to the passage of stools. The mean resting anal pressure in men is 90 cm H_2O.[12] It is lower in women[13] and also decreases with age.[14]

Resting pressures exhibit longitudinal and radial varia-

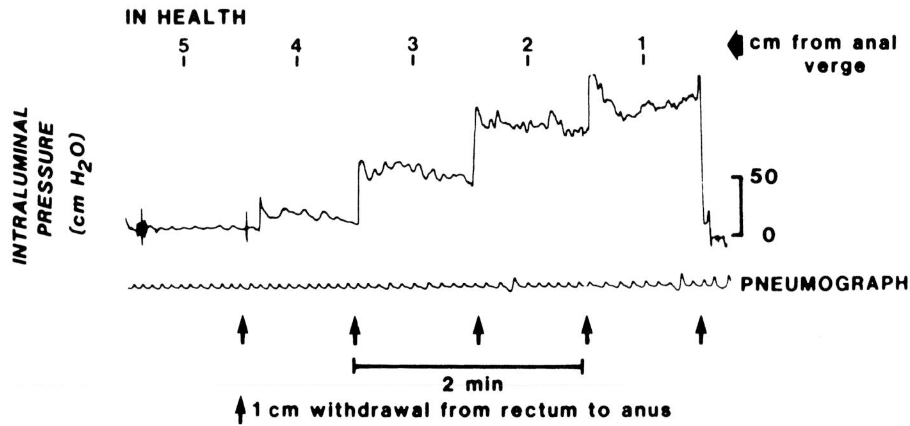

Fig. 34-8. Single-channel recording of anal sphincter resting pressures from the anal canal. Superimposed on the resting pressure are small oscillations of pressure that occur at a frequency of 15 cycles/min with an amplitude of about 10 mm Hg. (From Pemberton JH. Anatomy and physiology of the anus and rectum. In Condon RE, ed. Shackelford's Surgery of the Alimentary Tract, vol 4. Philadelphia: WB Saunders, 1991, p 242. Used with permission.)

tion. This is partly explained by the anatomic arrangements of the anal sphincters and puborectalis. Therefore, proximally the resting pressure is higher posteriorly and lowers posteriorly near the anal verge, whereas in the midanal canal, the pressure is more equally distributed (Fig. 34-9). In women, the anterior resting pressures are highest distally, whereas they are highest proximally in men.[13] The pressures increase with increased intra-abdominal pressure and erect posture.

The internal sphincter is smooth muscle and thus has a constant tone. The external sphincter and levator complex also maintain a constant tone, mediated by a low sacral reflex. This reflex is inhibited during straining to defecate.

Squeeze pressure. Intra-anal canal pressure can increase to more than twice resting levels during maximal squeeze effort generated by the external anal sphincter and puborectalis. It exhibits longitudinal and radial variations similar to resting pressures. Maximal squeeze pressure elevation lasts less than 1 minute because the sphincter fatigues rapidly (Fig. 34-10). This mechanism is therefore likely to be effective only in preventing leakage on presentation of the content to the proximal canal at inopportune times. The squeeze pressure is unlikely to maintain fecal continence from hour to hour. Continence is more likely a result of the differential pressure between the rectum (6 cm H_2O) and the anal canal (90 cm H_2O).[15]

Anorectal Angle

This angle is formed by the anterior pull of the puborectalis muscle as it envelops the anorectal junction (Fig. 34-11). The angle measures 102 ± 18 degrees[16] and helps maintain hour-to-hour fecal continence of solid content. Increases in squeeze pressure and Valsalva's maneuver decrease the angle to 81 ± 19 and 87 ± 23 degrees, respectively, augmenting anorectal continence. The puborectalis maintains continuous activity, even during sleep.

This mechanism of continence is augmented by a flutter-valve effect in situations where the intrarectal pressure

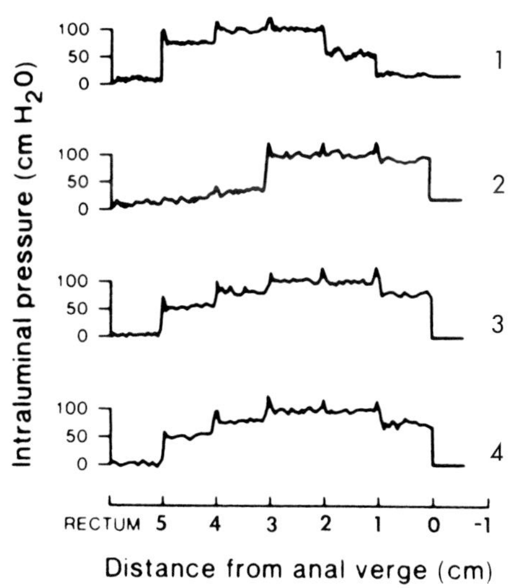

Fig. 34-9. Perfused four-channel recordings of resting anal canal pressure (*1,* posterior; *2,* anterior, *3,* right lateral, *4,* left lateral). A stepped pull-through technique was used. Note that on pulling the probe into the anal canal, pressures are recorded posteriorly first and anteriorly last. This is caused by the presence of puborectal muscle high in the anal canal and its absence low in the canal. (From Pemberton JH. Anatomy and physiology of the anus and rectum. In Condon RE, ed. Shackelford's Surgery of the Alimentary Tract, vol 4. Philadelphia: WB Saunders, 1991, p 242. Used with permission.)

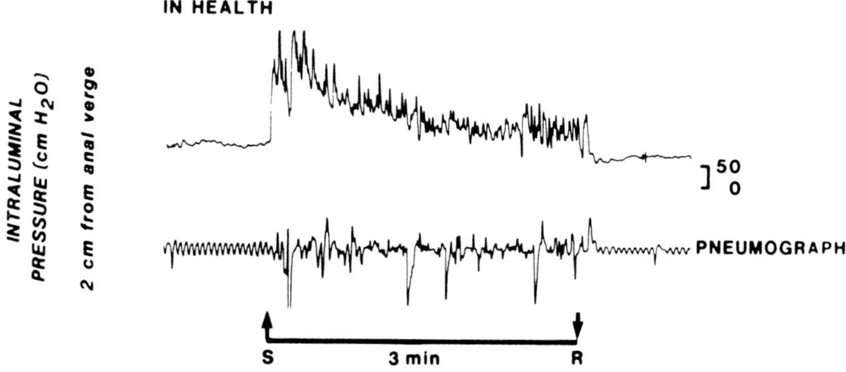

Fig. 34-10. Anal canal squeeze pressure recorded by a perfused probe positioned about 2 cm proximal to the anal verge. This is a single-channel recording. The overall duration of elevated pressure was 3 minutes, but the duration of maximal pressure was less than 1 minute. (From Pemberton JH. Anatomy and physiology of the anus and rectum. In Condon RE, ed. Shackelford's Surgery of the Alimentary Tract, vol 4. Philadelphia: WB Saunders, 1991, p 242. Used with permission.)

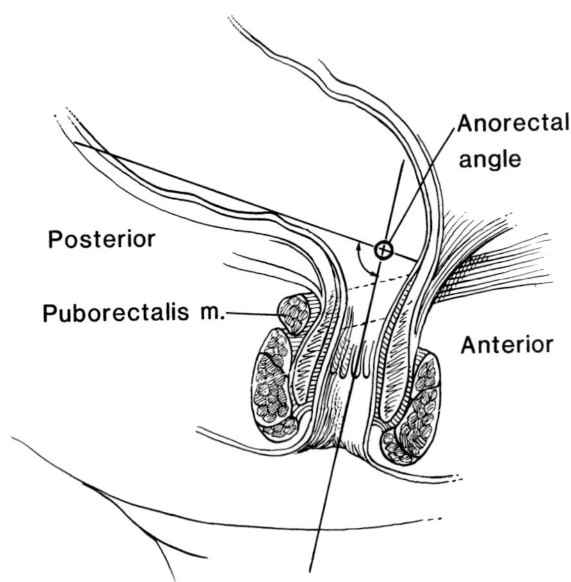

Fig. 34-11. Diagram of the angulation between the rectum and anal canal. This angle is formed by the pull of the puborectalis muscle, which is directly anteriorly. (From Pemberton JH. Anatomy and physiology of the anus and rectum. In Condon RE, ed. Shackelford's Surgery of the Alimentary Tract, vol 4. Philadelphia: WB Saunders, 1991, p 242. Used with permission.)

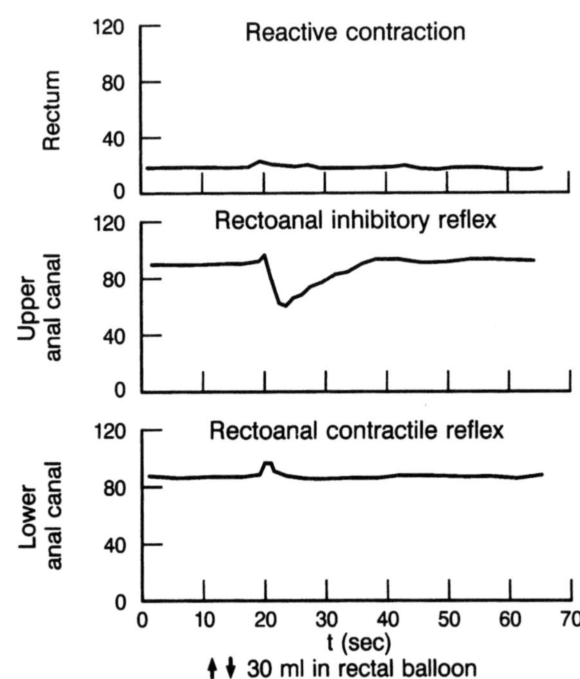

Fig. 34-12. The rectoanal sphincter inhibitory response is composed of three parts: (1) reactive rectal contraction, (2) decreased anal canal pressure proximally, and (3) increased anal canal pressure distally. The decrease in resting pressure lasts approximately 20 seconds and is thought to be caused by relaxation of the internal anal sphincter. The brief increase in pressure distally may be caused by reactive contraction of the external anal sphincter. (From Pemberton JH. Anatomy and physiology of the anus and rectum. In Condon RE, ed. Shackelford's Surgery of the Alimentary Tract, vol 4. Philadelphia: WB Saunders, 1991, p 242. Used with permission.)

surpasses the resting anal canal pressure. Such situations include Valsalva's maneuver, lifting, and coughing.

During defecation, the anorectal angle must be overcome to evacuate solid contents. Flexing the hips 90 degrees while sitting increases the anorectal angle beyond 100 degrees. This straightening process is further enhanced during defecation when the puborectalis and external anal sphincter become electrically silent. This, however, does not occur at every act.

Passage of flatus results from a decrease in the anorectal angle and an increase in anal sphincter and intrarectal pressure. Fluids, on the other hand, are passed when the anorectal angle increases, anal sphincter pressure decreases, and intrarectal pressure increases. These differences may explain how flatus is passed and liquid continence is maintained.

Anorectal Sensation

Sensory mechanisms allow discrimination of contents (liquid, semisolid, and solid) and detection of urgency. Sensory receptors are thought to reside in either the rectal muscles or the pelvic floor musculature. Preservation of sensation after coloanal anastomoses and restorative proctocolectomy supports the presence of receptors in the pelvic floor.

Flatus generates a lower intrarectal pressure than do solids.[12] The ability to differentiate intrarectal pressures may be important in discriminating rectal contents. Sensory perception has also been found in the proximal anal canal mucosa.[17]

When the upper anal canal distends, the rectal wall contracts slightly. At the same time, the external anal sphincter causes a transient rise in resting pressure in the distal anal canal (rectoanal contractile reflex). This is followed almost immediately by a transient relaxation of the internal sphincter in the proximal anal canal, resulting in a decrease in resting pressure. This is the rectoanal sphincter inhibition response (Fig. 34-12). The amplitude and duration of relaxation vary directly with rectal distention. They are mediated by nonadrenergic, noncholinergic nerves in the myenteric plexus of the internal sphincter. This intramural reflex is modulated by sacral spinal cord.

Rapid intermittent distention of the rectum causes prolonged relaxation of the internal sphincter, whereas continuous distention causes an initial relaxation followed by a return to resting pressure.[18] The latter is probably an exponential adaptation of the rectum to distention. Transient relaxation of the internal anal sphincter is thought to allow recognition by the proximal anal canal mucosa (sampling reflex). With continued rectal distention, the external sphincter is inhibited. This results in urgency. The sampling reflex has been shown to occur between 4 to 10 times an hour in healthy ambulatory individuals.[19] This

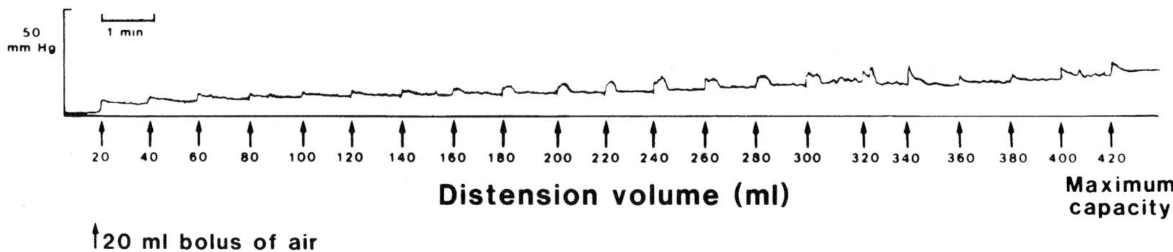

Fig. 34-13. Effect of distention of an intrarectal balloon on rectal pressure. Rectal accommodation ensures little rise in intraluminal pressure, even at 420 ml inflation. (From Pemberton JH. Anatomy and physiology of the anus and rectum. In Condon RE, ed. Shackelford's Surgery of the Alimentary Tract, vol 4. Philadelphia: WB Saunders, 1991, p 242. Used with permission.)

supports the finding of internal sphincter relaxation and external sphincter and puborectalis muscle contraction after passage of contents into the rectum.[20] It does not, however, explain the maintenance of continence after ileoanal anastomosis, because the response is then absent. Continence is also unaffected when local anesthetics are applied to the anal canal mucosa.

Compliance, Tone, and Capacity of the Rectum

Receptive relaxation is the term for the ability of the rectum to accommodate passively to distention. This causes the intrarectal pressure to increase transiently and then gradually return to preinflation levels, thereby maintaining a lower intrarectal pressure relative to the anal canal pressure.

Urgency normally develops after distention with 200 ml saline solution. The maximal tolerable volume is in the region of 400 ml. The intraluminal pressure remains low, even with this volume (Fig. 34-13).

Rectal compliance is decreased in active ulcerative colitis, radiation proctitis, and ischemic proctitis. Patients with these conditions often have frequency, urgency, and tenesmus, with episodes of incontinence. In Hirschsprung's disease, the compliance is increased by a functional megarectum.

Rectal Filling and Emptying

The rectum usually remains empty, protected as it is from the sigmoid contents by the natural angle between the rectum and sigmoid, the valves of Houston, and its resting contractile activity, which is greater than that in the sigmoid. Instillation of saline solution or artificial stool into the rectum results in progressive accommodation to increasing volumes. About half of this instilled volume promptly refluxes into the sigmoid and remains there. At the time of evacuation, the sigmoid colon empties into the rectum first. This is followed by evacuation of the rectal volume[21] (Fig. 34-14). These findings suggest that the sigmoid colon plays an active role in maintaining overall enteric continence. Only when the sigmoid colon is sufficiently filled does it empty partially into the rectum.

Duodenal-cecal transit time is increased by distention of the rectum with a balloon. This occurs during fasting as well as after feeding.[22] Gastric emptying is also delayed by rectal distention.[23] These decreases may help slow down the enteric transit until the rectum can be emptied at a socially convenient time.

Motility of the Rectum

The resting rectal pressure is about 6 cm H_2O. Three types of rectal contractile activity have been described: (1) simple contractions, which occur at 5 to 10 cycles/min; (2) slower contractions, which occur at about 3 cycles/min with amplitudes as great as 100 cm H_2O; and (3) slow, propagated contractions, which occur infrequently with high amplitude.[24]

Ambulatory manometric studies have demonstrated three types of motor activity: (1) isolated prolonged contractions of 10 to 20 seconds' duration occurring mainly during waking hours, (2) clusters of contractions of relatively low amplitude occurring at a frequency of 5 to 6 cycles/min and lasting 1 to 2 minutes with a periodicity of 20 to 30 minutes, predominantly in the postprandial period, and (3) runs of powerful phasic contraction greater than 50 mm Hg amplitude occurring at 2 to 3 cycles/min and lasting 3 to 10 seconds.

These last happen periodically about every 92 minutes in the day and 56 minutes at night.[25] These complexes of regular sustained contractions are termed *rectal motor complexes* (RMCs). They occur more regularly and frequently during sleep (Fig. 34-15). Although they resemble interdigestive migrating motor complexes of the small bowel, there does not appear to be synchrony between these two complexes.[15,25] RMCs are disrupted after meals for about 150 to 180 minutes. The function of RMCs is unknown, but it may be to keep the rectum empty. It has also been shown that the rectal tone varies little during fasting and increases significantly after a meal.[26]

Motility of the Anal Canal

The anal canal has a unique motility pattern. Slow waves with small oscillations occur at frequencies of 10 to 20 cycles/min, with an amplitude of 5 to 25 cm H_2O superimposed on the resting tone. There is also a slow-wave gradient in the anal canal, with the frequency being high-

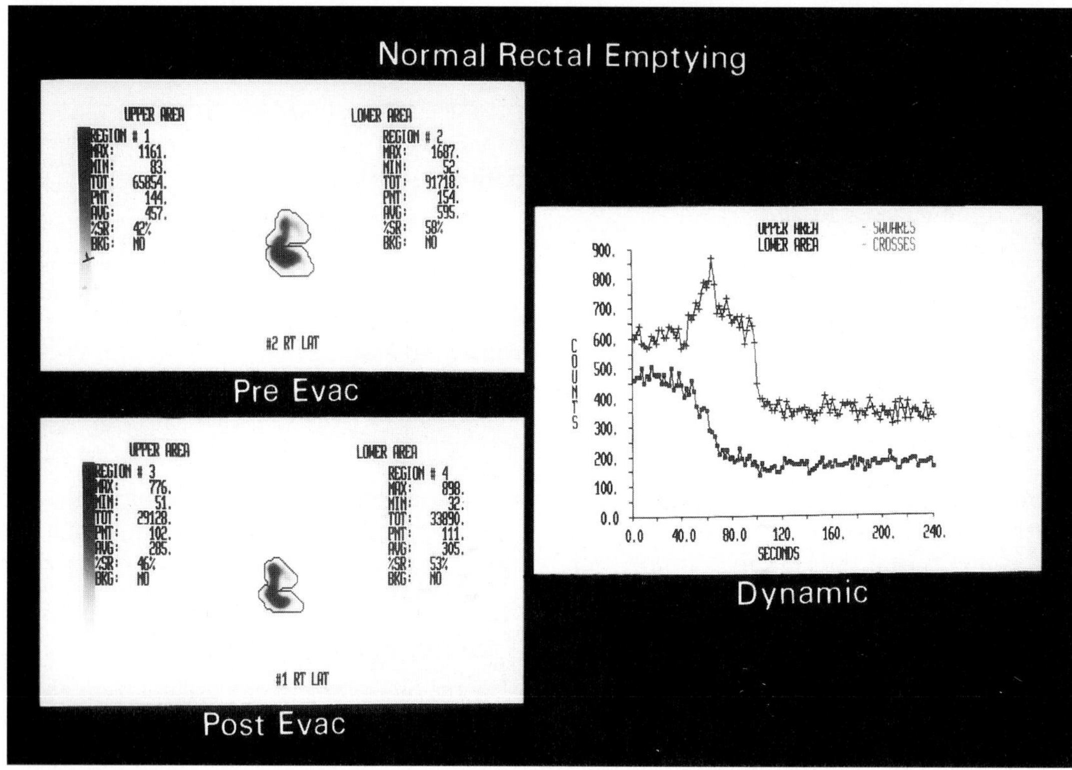

Fig. 34-14. Patterns of rectal filling and emptying recorded from a healthy volunteer. Evacuation dynamics are observed by gamma camera imaging of ^{99m}Tc-labeled artificial stool. *Upper left:* The infused artificial stool distributes into the sigmoid colon and rectum. *Below left:* A postevacuation scan. *Right:* A dynamic record of evacuation from the sigmoid colon *(boxes)* and rectum *(triangles)*. Note that the sigmoid colon empties into the rectum first (counts decrease in the sigmoid and rise in the rectum), and then both evacuate together. The mean percentage evacuation among healthy volunteers is approximately 75% to 85%. (From Pemberton JH. Anatomy and physiology of the anus and rectum. In Condon RE, ed. Shackelford's Surgery of the Alimentary Tract, vol 4. Philadelphia: WB Saunders, 1991, p 242. Used with permission.)

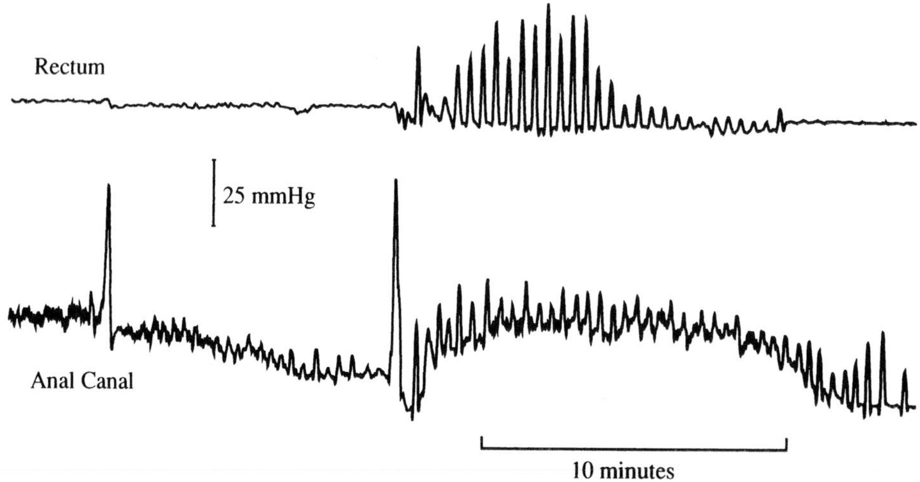

Fig. 34-15. Recording from one rectal *(top)* and one anal *(bottom)* canal transducer in a control subject. The rectal transducer recorded a typical rectal motor complex (RMC). Note that the anal canal began to contract *before* the start of the RMC. Throughout the RMC, the anal canal maintained an increased basal pressure, and contractile activity was likewise increased. As the RMC disappeared, contractile activity in the anal canal decreased, as did the baseline pressure. (From Pemberton JH. Anatomy and physiology of the anus and rectum. In Wexner SD, Beck DE, eds. Textbook of Anorectal Surgery. New York: McGraw-Hill, 1992, p 22. Used with permission.)

est distally.[27] This may tend to propel contents back into the rectum, keeping the anal canal clean and thus ensuring continence.

Ultraslow waves can be found in 40% of normal subjects. These have an amplitude of 30 to 100 cm H_2O with a duration of about 33 seconds and a frequency of 3 cycles/min.[28] They are associated with high resting anal pressures. Electromyographic studies have shown that both slow and ultraslow waves represent regular fluctuations of the internal sphincter activity.[10]

Coordination of Anorectal Motility

Prolonged ambulatory manometric studies have demonstrated that RMCs are always accompanied by a rise in mean anal canal pressure and contractile activity. This maintains a greater pressure in the anal canal relative to rectal pressure,[15] a gradient that helps to preserve fecal continence (Fig. 34-16).

Stool Volume and Consistency

Most of the water from the 1500 ml small bowel content that enters the cecum is absorbed, producing about 150 ml of stool each day.[29] This is normally passed at a frequency that varies from 3 stools/day to 3 stools/week.

If the consistency (which is usually firm) or volume of stools changes suddenly, the mechanisms of continence are stressed. If small pellets of hard stool are introduced slowly into the rectum, rectal distention and perception of rectal contents may not occur. This may account for the finding that volunteers passed large, deformable stools more readily and with less straining than they did small, hard pellets.[30] Others have found that semisolid stools are more

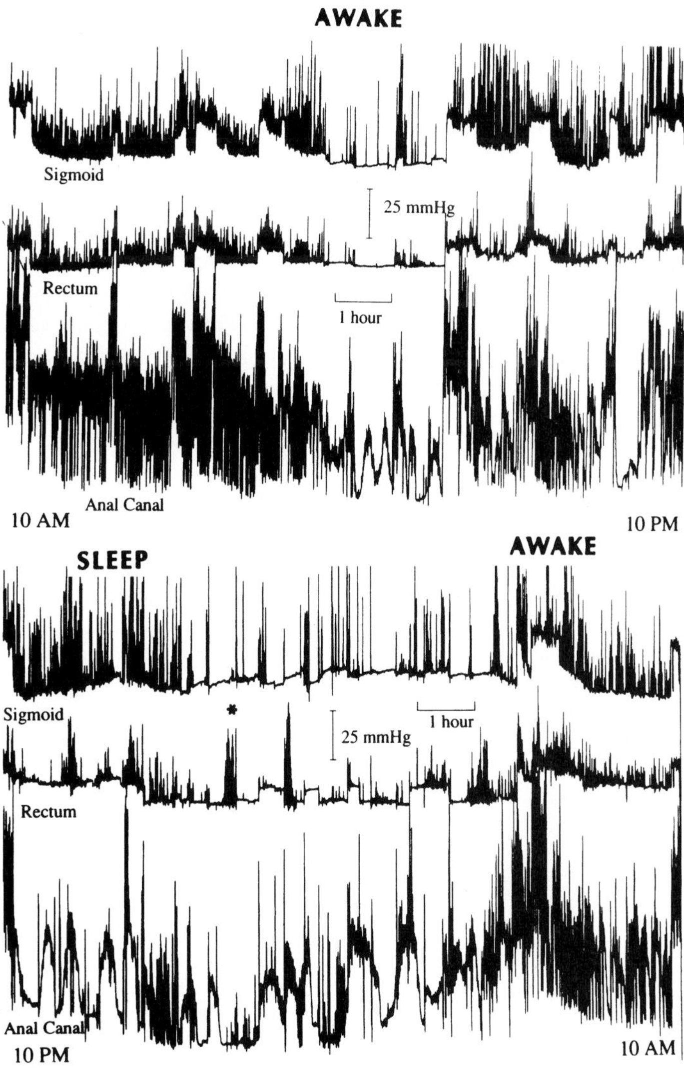

Fig. 34-16. Nocturnal variations in rectal and anal canal mean pressures in a healthy subject. Cyclic decreases in pressure in the anal canal occurred several times, with the lowest pressure approximating 15 to 20 mm Hg. However, a rectal anal canal pressure differential was always present. (From Pemberton JH. Anatomy and physiology of the anus and rectum. In Wexner SD, Beck DE, eds. Textbook of Anorectal Surgery. New York: McGraw-Hill, 1992, p 19. Used with permission.)

completely evacuated than are either solid or liquid stools.[31] On the other hand, liquid stools presented suddenly to the rectum in large volumes will quickly overcome the continence mechanism, even in healthy individuals.

The influence of stool volume and consistency can be used to restore continence in some patients. It is useful predominantly in patients with low resting and squeeze pressures or those with an obtuse anorectal angle.

Defecation

The physiology of defecation has not been well studied. A likely sequence of events is described here (Fig. 34-17).

When the volume of sigmoid colon contents is sufficiently large to trigger contractions, the contents are emptied into the rectum. Rectal distention is sensed by stretch receptors there. Intermittent, progressive rectal distention initiates the rectoanal inhibitory response, resulting in internal anal sphincter relaxation. Concurrently, the external sphincter contracts, preventing leakage. The nature of the contents is thus perceived by the sensory nerve–rich proximal anal canal. If the decision is made to evacuate, the sitting position is assumed, rendering the anorectal angle less acute. Intraabdominal and intrarectal pressures rise with straining. These increased pressures result in coordinated reflex relaxation of the internal and external sphincters, as well as the puborectalis.

Some healthy subjects pass without further straining, whereas others need to strain to initiate rectal emptying. With straining, the puborectalis muscle relaxes further and the pelvic floor descends to form a funnel with the outlet at the top of the anal canal. The intra-abdominal pressure is thus transmitted directly to the fecal bolus, expelling it.

Once initiated, defecation proceeds either continuously or as passage in bits preceded by periodic straining. The pattern depends on stool consistency and individual habit.

When emptying is complete, a closing reflex occurs. Here, the external sphincter and puborectalis muscles transiently contract, restoring the anorectal angle.[32] This promotes recovery of the internal sphincter tone, closing the anal canal.

Defecation can be deferred by voluntary contraction of the external sphincter and puborectalis, causing the contents in the upper anal canal to be returned to the rectum. Passive accommodation allows the rectal pressure to remain low and the urge to defecate to be suppressed by cortical pathways.

Tests of Colonic and Anorectal Function

Manometry, electromyography, and nerve stimulation measure motor complex function. Defecating proctography, scintigraphic balloon topography, scintigraphic evacuation, and colonic transit studies evaluate the complex, coordinated activity of continence and defecation.

Anorectal Manometry

Manometry typically measures resting and squeeze pressures of the anal canal high-pressure zone, defines the maximum capacity and distensibility of the rectal ampulla, and measures the presence of the rectoanal inhibitory response. Different techniques give widely different results. It is therefore important to have controls for a particular technique. No method has been shown to be superior to another.

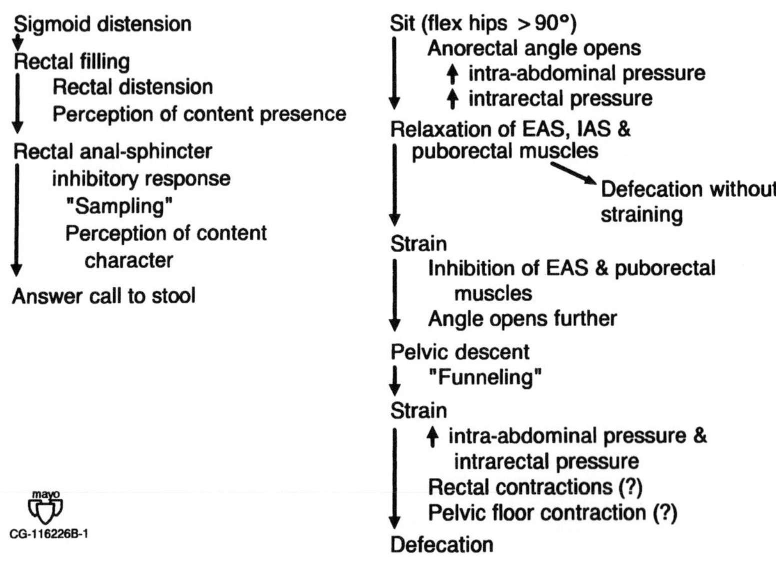

Fig. 34-17. A hypothesis proposed for the sequence of normal defecation. (From Pemberton JH. Anatomy and physiology of the anus and rectum. In Condon RE, ed. Shackelford's Surgery of the Alimentary Tract, vol 4. Philadelphia: WB Saunders, 1991, p 242. Used with permission.)

The appliance with a perfused four-channel methylmethacrylate probe with four 0.14 cm channels oriented 90 degrees apart is shown in Fig. 34-18. These channels are perfused with normal saline solution at a rate of 0.3 ml/min through a low-compliance pneumohydraulic perfusion system.

This technique provides a sequential pull-through resting pressure profile in four quadrants. Maximum squeeze pressures are measured in the same way, with the subject consciously squeezing the anal canal. The probe is used to measure the pressures sequentially at the proximal, middle, and distal anal canal.

The probe is then repositioned in the proximal anal canal. A balloon traverses the middle of the probe to allow measurement of rectal capacity and inhibitory reflex. This is inflated and immediately deflated in 5 ml increments to elicit proximal anal relaxation—the rectoanal sphincter inhibitory response. The maximum tolerable volume measures the rectal capacity.

Electromyography

A standard concentric needle is used for electromyographic assessment. The external anal sphincter and puborectalis are studied at rest, during sphincter squeezing and Valsalva's maneuver in which defecation is actively prevented, and during straining stimulating attempted defecation. Single-fiber techniques are useful for calculation of fiber densities.

Nerve Stimulation

Spinal and terminal motor latencies are determined by stimulating either over L1 or L4 (supplying the external anal sphincter and puborectalis) or at the exit of the pudendal nerve from the pudendal canal (pudendal nerve terminal motor latency) and recording the arrival of the stimulus at the puborectalis muscle or the external anal sphincter.

Mucosal Sensation

Electrosensitivity and temperature sensation measurements in the anal canal are novel techniques designed to attempt to quantify the subjective parameter of anal canal sensation. Electrosensitivity sensory thresholds are found to be elevated in patients with incontinence and hemorrhoids and reduced in cases of anal fissure.[33] The more complex technique of measuring temperature sensation also shows impairment of sensation in patients with incontinence.[19]

Defecating Proctogram

This documents the act of defecation with x-rays (Fig. 34-19). Recently, the use of videoproctography has gained popularity. It provides a real-time assessment of defecation. Rectal intussusception is among the most useful findings. Another, albeit uncommon, finding is a sigmoidocele. In addition, the resting and straining anorectal angles can be calculated. The main difficulty is that positive findings are often misinterpreted. For example, rectal intussusception also occurs in half of healthy volunteers.[34] The results therefore need to be interpreted in the light of a good history and physical examination.

Scintigraphic Balloon Topography

This demonstrates the movement of the anorectal angle and pelvic floor through low radiation exposure with scintigraphic techniques. In healthy subjects, maneuvers such as sphincter squeeze and Valsalva's maneuver narrow the angle and lower the junction.[16] In patients with disorders of continence, the normal movements of the anorectal angle and junction may be disturbed.[35]

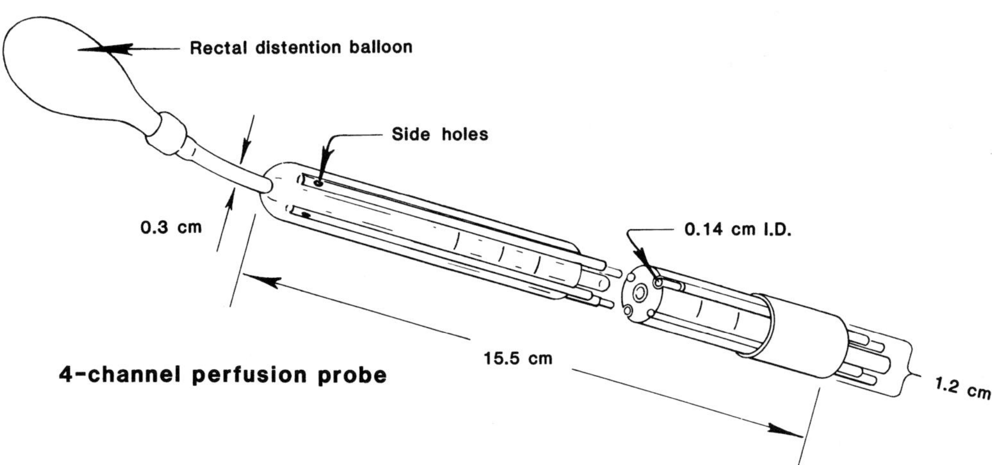

Fig. 34-18. Four-channel probe with 0.14 cm probes orientated 90 degrees apart used for anal manometry. (From Pemberton JH. Anatomy and physiology of the anus and rectum. In Condon RE, ed. Shackelford's Surgery of the Alimentary Tract, vol 4. Philadelphia: WB Saunders, 1991, p 242. Used with permission.)

A

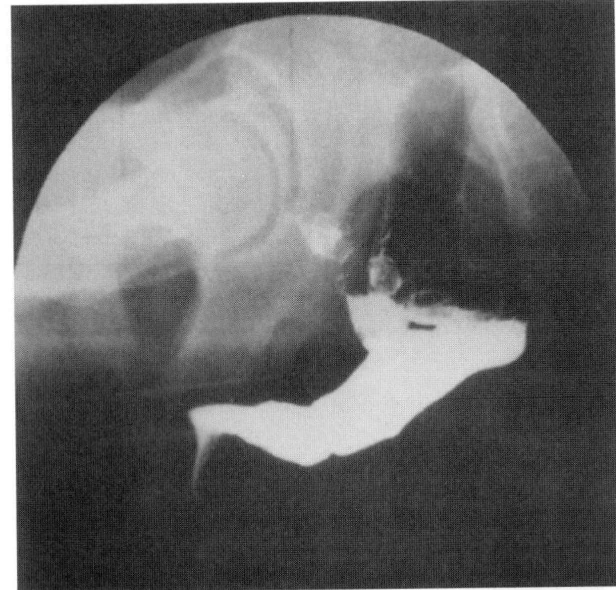

B

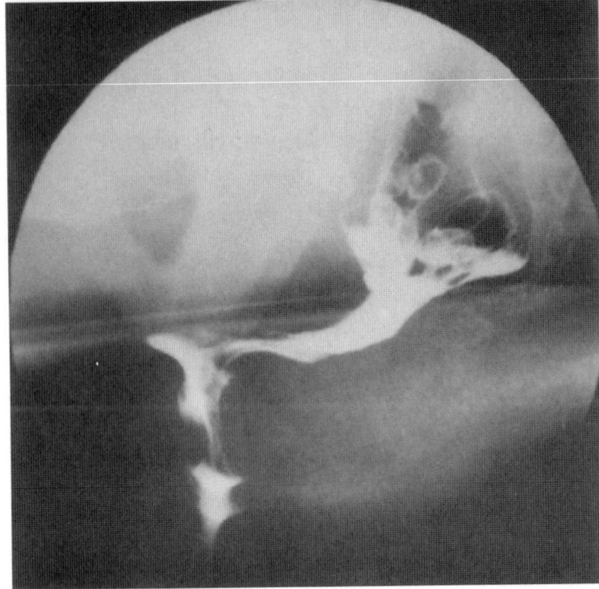

Fig. 34-19. Normal defecating proctogram, before **(A)** and after **(B)** defecation. (From Pemberton JH. Anatomy and physiology of the anus and rectum. In Condon RE, ed. Shackelford's Surgery of the Alimentary Tract, vol 4. Philadelphia: WB Saunders, 1991, p 242. Used with permission.)

Scintigraphic Evacuation

This test uses radiolabeled artificial stools to quantify the efficiency and pattern of evacuation.[21] The artificial stool is introduced into the rectum at a preestablished maximal rectal capacity. As the subject defecates, gamma cameras record the pattern and calculate the efficiency of evacuation. Abnormal emptying efficiency and patterns have been shown in patients with continence disorders.[35]

Colonic Transit

Small, radiopaque markers ingested orally can be used to quantify transit time. Twenty markers are ingested on each of 3 days, and a plain abdominal radiograph is taken on days 4 and 7. Studies with serial radiography were used to calculate transit times in healthy subjects. Total colonic transit was 35.0 ± 2.1 hours; segmental transits were 11.3 ± 1.1 hours for the right colon, 11.4 ± 1.4 hours for the left colon, and 12.4 ± 1.1 hours for the rectosigmoid. Men have been found to have significantly shorter whole-colon transit times than do women (33 ± 4 vs 47 ± 4 hours). This difference was apparent to some extent in the right and left colon but not in the rectosigmoid. Age, however, has not been shown to have any effect on colonic transit.[36]

Findings of transit markers in any segment of the colon indicate slow transit. If the markers are found in the rectum, additional tests may be indicated to exclude outlet obstruction as the cause of the holdup.

Disordered Anorectal Physiology

Hemorrhoids

Anal cushions are part of the normal anatomy of the anal canal. These discrete masses have a thick submucosa containing blood vessels, smooth muscle, and connective tissue. Hemorrhoids should therefore be considered to occur only when these cushions are abnormal (Fig. 34-20). This happens when the vascular cushions slide down, prolapse, become congested, enlarge, bleed, or thrombose.[7] The vascular cushions are found consistently in the left lateral, right anterolateral, and right posterolateral positions. Smaller, secondary cushions may be present between the main cushions. External hemorrhoids by definition arise below the dentate line. They are covered by squamous epithelium and are well innervated. Internal hemorrhoids arise above the dentate line and are lined with nonsensitive rectal mucosa.

The precise etiology of hemorrhoids is unknown. One hypothesis is that the anal cushion prolapses outward on repeated straining with time.[37] Hard stools and diarrheic stools promote straining, and irregular bowel habits are commonly found in patients with hemorrhoids. Straining may cause engorgement of the cushions, making them more susceptible to prolapse.

Internal sphincter dysfunction has also been proposed as a cause of hemorrhoids. This may produce submucosal venous stasis and impair emptying of the internal hemorrhoidal plexus, resulting in enlarged internal hemorrhoids.[38]

Some anorectal physiologic derangements are found in patients with hemorrhoids. Ultraslow pressure waves have been recorded in the anal canal in 50% of patients with hemorrhoids, compared with 5% of healthy individuals. The frequency gradient of intraluminal contractile activity was found to be absent.[39] Higher resting sphincter pressures have also been recorded in patients with hemorrhoids than in healthy subjects. This finding, however, is not universal.[40] Furthermore, the abnormally high pressures may be a result, rather than the cause, of hemorrhoids. Patients with hemorrhoids have also been documented as having an increased sensory threshold compared with control subjects.[32]

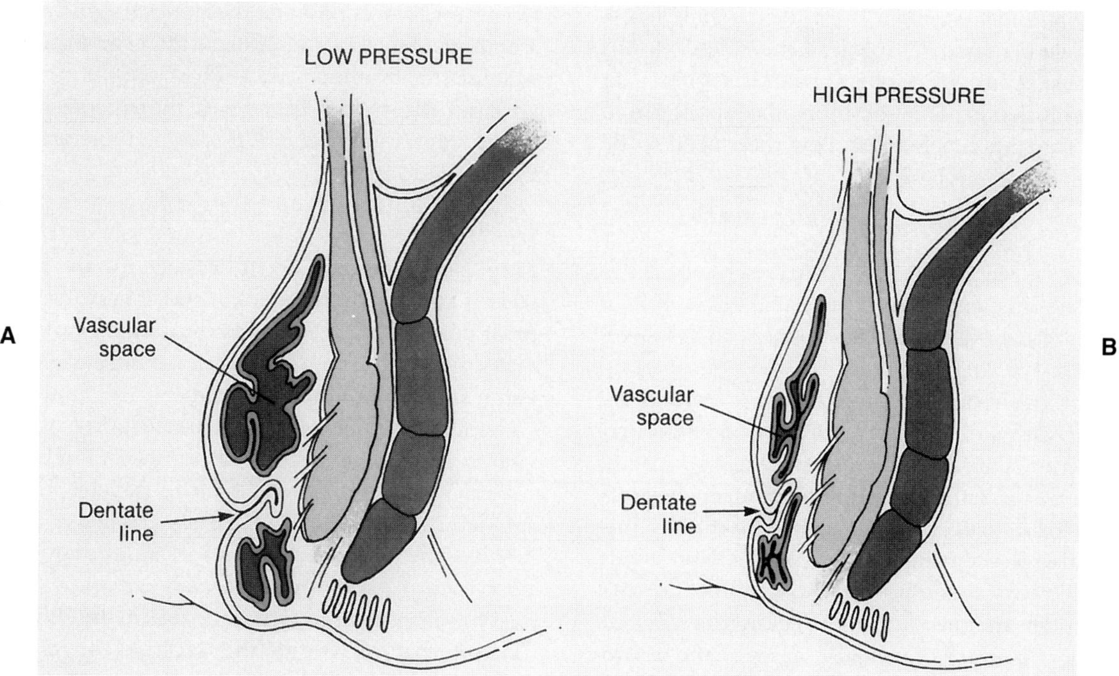

Fig. 34-20. Diagrammatic representation of normal vascular channels **(B)**, which become significant hemorrhoids with dilatation of the vascular space **(A)**. (Adapted from Gordon PH, Nivatvongs S, eds. Principles and Practice of Surgery for the Colon, Rectum, and Anus. St. Louis: Quality Medical Publishing, 1992.)

Bleeding is the most common presenting symptom. This may be in the form of staining on the toilet paper, dripping, or squirting into the toilet bowl. Larger hemorrhoids may prolapse. When the prolapse becomes chronic, mucous discharge and fecal leakage may result, causing pruritus and perianal excoriation. Pain is not a common symptom of uncomplicated internal hemorrhoids. It is usually a result of thrombosis and strangulation and indicative of the presence of a concomitant fissure or abscess.

The importance of a good history and physical examination, including a digital examination and proctoscopy, is not only to confirm the diagnosis but also to exclude the presence of other perianal and rectal disorders. On this basis, all patients should undergo proctoscopy or flexible sigmoidoscopy. More detailed bowel imaging should be considered in older patients reporting first-time bleeding or in anyone with an atypical history.

External hemorrhoids become surgically significant when they thrombose. This is seen as an excruciatingly painful bluish subcutaneous nodule beneath the perianal skin. Sensory nerve fibers and a tight compartment account for the pain when thrombosis and congestion occurs. If patients are seen early in the course of pain, excision of the overlying skin and evacuation of the clot results in almost instantaneous relief. Acute pain subsides after a few days, however, facilitating conservative, nonoperative management.

Internal hemorrhoids have been graded according to severity. First-degree internal hemorrhoids generally do not protrude below the dentate line on straining. Second-degree hemorrhoids are larger and, because the submucosal tissue cannot fully support them, prolapse into the anal canal on defecation. They reduce spontaneously on cessation of straining. Third-degree hemorrhoidal prolapse requires manual reduction. Fourth-degree hemorrhoids have redundant rectal mucosa and overstretched submucosa that cannot retain them in the normal position. They are permanently prolapsed.

The aim in the management of hemorrhoids is symptomatic relief. Most first-degree hemorrhoids that bleed are managed by local measures, such as sitz baths and suppositories. Education in bowel habits, implementation of appropriate dietary changes, such as bulk-forming agents (e.g., psyllium hydrophilic mucilloid [Metamucil, Konsyl]), and sufficient liquids are important. Surgery is rarely indicated. Injection sclerotherapy, coagulation diathermy, and infrared photocoagulation have been used in an attempt to cause fixation of the hemorrhoids and prevent prolapse, but they are probably no more efficacious than bulking agents.

Second-degree hemorrhoids, which prolapse into the anal canal, are more troublesome and are treated with banding. A ligator is passed through an anoscope to grasp the redundant tissue well above the hemorrhoidal mass, and a rubber band is fired to its base. This procedure is done in the outpatient setting. The ligated tissue sloughs on day 3 to 5, resulting in scarring and fixation of any residual hemorrhoids. Persistent third-degree and almost all fourth-degree hemorrhoids require hemorrhoidectomy, which involves excision of the hemorrhoidal tissue.

Hemorrhoids that become thrombosed or strangulated can progress to gangrene. Surgery may then need to be carried out on an urgent basis.

Fissure In Ano

Anal fissures, or ulcers in the anal canal, usually occur below the dentate line, extending to the anal verge. Pain is the main presenting complaint, associated with sphincter spasm (increased resting anal pressure) and constipation. This results in a vicious cycle of difficulty in defecation, pain, and aggravation of the fissure. Bright-red blood may line the stools or stain the toilet paper. Other symptoms include pruritus ani, difficulty in micturition, or dyspareunia. Digital examination and anoscopy are usually impossible because of the pain. The diagnosis is often made with a careful history and inspection. An examination with the patient under anesthesia may be required to exclude other perianal conditions or primary causes of the fissure.

The most frequent cause is the passage of dry, hard, large stools. Most fissures occur posteriorly at the 6 o'clock position. This may be related to the poorer blood supply in the posterior midline.[41] Fissures in other anatomic positions should raise the suspicion of associated disease processes. These include severe diarrhea, Crohn's disease, and carcinoma of the anal canal.

Chronic anal fissures are associated with a swelling or skin tag on the anal verge. This is the sentinel pile. Internally, a hypertrophic anal papilla is often found at the dentate line. High resting anal pressures, predominantly contributed by the internal anal sphincter, have been associated with anal fissures.[42] The normal internal sphincter relaxation response is followed by an overshoot.[43] It is still unclear whether the high resting pressures are a cause or an effect. In addition, ultraslow waves can be recorded in as many as 80% of patients with anal fissures.[38] These ultraslow waves are associated with high anal canal resting pressures and disappear when the high pressures are reduced by lateral internal sphincterotomy to a level found in control subjects without ultraslow waves. Ultraslow waves may therefore be a manifestation of increased internal anal sphincter activity.[44]

Anal fissures have been thought to be ischemic ulcers. Anodermal blood flow at the posterior midline is less than in other segments of the anal canal. The perfusion of the anoderm at the posterior commissure is strongly inversely related to anal canal pressure.[45]

Most fissures respond to conservative management with stool bulkers, dietary advice, and sitz baths. Chronic anal fissures usually necessitate a lateral sphincterotomy. The aim is to alleviate internal anal sphincter spasm by releasing a portion of the underlying internal anal sphincter that is in spasm, disrupting the vicious cycle. Anal dilatation should be relegated to the archives, because it produces an uncontrolled disruption of the sphincters and may result in a high incidence of incontinence. Occasionally, low-pressure anal fissures are found. These should not be treated with sphincterotomy because of the potential for incontinence. An advancement flap may be more appropriate in these situations.[46]

Fistula In Ano

Fistulas in ano usually occur between the area infected, abscessed anal gland, and the skin and are usually the result of prior perianal sepsis. The classification of Parks et al.[47] divides them into intersphincteric, transphincteric, supralevator, and extrasphincteric fistulas.

Patients are seen with recurrent perianal sepsis, discharge and soiling, a perianal lump, or, rarely, blood per rectum. Extrasphincteric fistulas traverse the external sphincter into the ischiorectal fossa, whereas supralevator fistulas arise above the muscles of anal continence. These two types of fistula are fortunately rare.

The surgical treatment of fistula in ano is fistulotomy. The internal opening of the tract and the relationship of the tract to the puborectalis must be defined before surgery, because the commonest problems after fistula surgery are recurrence and incontinence.

Goodsall's rule helps in finding the internal opening (Fig. 34-21). A transverse line drawn across the anus in the coronal plane divides anterior from posterior fistulas. Anterior fistulas have a direct radial tract, with the internal opening at the nearest crypt. Posterior fistulas almost always open in the posterior midline and then track dorsally around the anus for a variable distance. External openings greater than 3 cm from the anal verge usually arise in the posterior crypts and suggest the presence of Crohn's disease. An accurate definition of the track allows complete fistulotomy, which in turn decreases recurrence rate (Fig. 34-22).

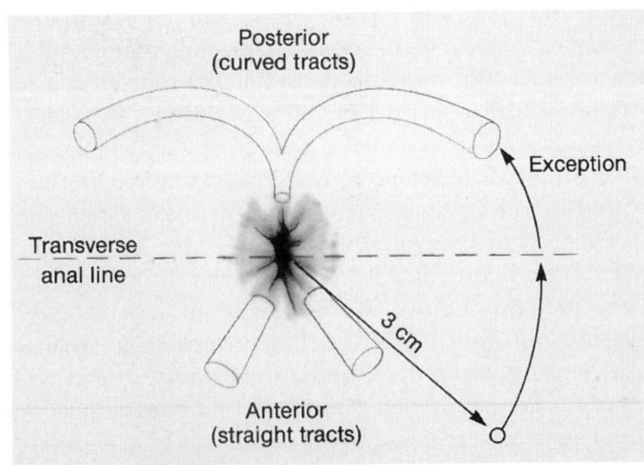

Fig. 34-21. Goodsall's rule. (From Gordon PH, Nivatvongs S, eds. Principles and Practice of Surgery for the Colon, Rectum, and Anus. St. Louis: Quality Medical Publishing, 1992.)

The relationship of the track to the sphincters and puborectalis provide an estimate of the amount of muscle that needs to be incised during fistulotomy. If there is concern about the amount of sphincter damage, the fistula track may be partially cut or not cut at all and a seton may be inserted. The seton cuts through the sphincters slowly, allowing scar formation proximal to the migrating seton. The sphincters therefore do not spring apart as they would at fistulotomy. The track can be laid open when there is sufficient fibrosis or when it has migrated down to a level where this can be done without jeopardizing continence. In addition, a seton also allows drainage of the fistula, thus clearing sepsis.

Perianal and Perirectal Abscesses

These usually arise from infections in the anal glands, sometimes as a result of obstruction of the anal gland duct related to feces or trauma. Abscesses are also associated with Crohn's disease, ulcerative colitis, carcinoma, pelvic infections, and previous surgery.

These abscesses are classified anatomically as perianal, ischiorectal, intersphincteric, and supralevator. Infection spreads downward in the intersphincteric plane towards the anal verge. Pain and localized swelling are the usual complaints. Less commonly, an abscess tracks supralevatorly or outside the external sphincters into the ischiorectal fossa. In these situations, there usually is exquisite pain and tenderness but no palpable induration externally. Patients may be toxic, with fever and leukocytosis. As well as tracking upward, the abscess may spread circumferentially around the anus, forming a horseshoe abscess. In addition to these symptoms, the patient may have bleeding and purulent discharge per rectum and also may have diarrhea.

Treatment of these abscesses involves surgical drainage. Antibiotics are required only in the presence of extensive cellulitis or immunosuppression. After the operation, patients must have sitz baths and dietary education to ensure good bowel habits.

Approximately one third of patients with perianal abscess eventually have a fistula in ano. There is some controversy regarding whether a fistula should be sought and fistulotomy should be performed at the initial surgery. The search for a fistula may in fact cause a false track and result in unnecessary sphincter damage. Furthermore, it is not known whether fistulas present at the index surgery persist after drainage of the abscesses. We have performed fistulotomies in patients with abscesses when they are clearly present. Patients who subsequently have a fistula can then have it laid open as a second procedure.

Rectal Prolapse

When the full thickness of the rectum intussuscepts through the anus, rectal prolapse occurs. Herniation of the pouch of Douglas is an associated feature, but not the cause. Rectal prolapse was classified by Theuerkauf et al.[48] into (1) incomplete (mucosal prolapse) and (2) complete (full-thickness wall prolapse), with the latter classified as (a) first-degree (high or early concealed), (b) second-degree (externally visible on straining), or (c) third-degree (externally visible).

Rectal prolapse affects women six times more often than it does men.[49] It is not related to parity.[50] Patients report a perianal lump or its effect on continence. Initially, it protrudes only after defecation, but with time it occurs with minor increases in intra-abdominal pressure, such as coughing and sneezing. Some degree of fecal incontinence is almost always present. Difficulty in moving the bowels may be described as constipation or obstructed defecation.

Examination may reveal a pathognomonic large, mucosa-covered mass with a sulcus between the rectal wall

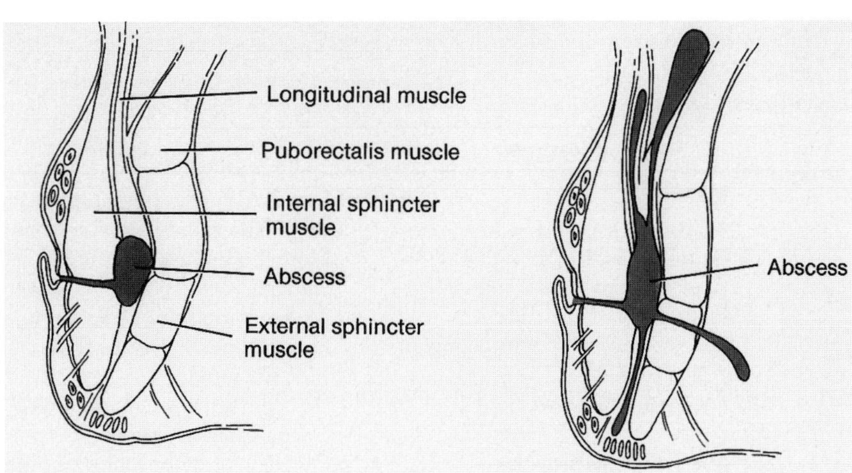

Fig. 34-22. Avenues of extension for an anal fistula. *EMG,* Electromyogram. (From Gordon PH, Nivatvongs S, eds. Principles and Practice of Surgery for the Colon, Rectum, and Anus. St. Louis: Quality Medical Publishing, 1992.)

and anal canal. The overlying mucosa may show traumatic ulceration and nonspecific inflammation. It is important to exclude the possibility that the mass is merely prolapsing hemorrhoids or mucosal. Poor anal tone is often evident on rectal examination, as is a component of perineal descent. More occult forms of rectal prolapse (type 2a) can often be diagnosed only with a defecating proctogram.

Although the exact etiology of intussusception is unknown, several abnormalities are associated with rectal prolapse. These include a defect in the pelvic floor with separation of the levator ani and a weakened endopelvic fascia, an abnormally deep pouch of Douglas, a patulous weak anal sphincter, and a loss of the normal horizontal position of the rectum caused by its loose attachment to the sacrum and pelvic walls.

Electromyographic studies in patients have shown complete inhibition of the puborectalis muscles on straining, which may predispose them toward prolapse. Some patients with rectal prolapse also have abnormal perineal descent and fecal incontinence, suggesting that prolonged staining may progressively cause pudendal neuropathy from stretch. This results in a lax puborectalis and external sphincter, allowing progression of the prolapse. These pelvic floor abnormalities cannot be directly responsible for the rectal intussusception because it begins 6 to 8 cm above the puborectalis muscle.

It is postulated that patients with difficulty in expelling bowel contents may strain at stool for prolonged periods. This is sometimes the result of a failure of the puborectalis muscle to relax. The prolonged increased intra-abdominal pressure may cause the lax rectum to intussuscept. With continued straining, the pudendal nerve and pelvic nerves are repeatedly stretched, thus partially denervating the pelvic floor and external sphincter muscles. Some degree of incontinence results. As the rectum descends, the sensation of fullness causes further straining at stool. This sequence of events is not present in every patient with rectal prolapse; some have no abnormality of the puborectalis or external sphincter denervation, nor is every patient incontinent.

Treatment of the prolapse is difficult, as evidenced by the abundant number of operations and approaches that have been devised. These include resection of redundant and prolapsing bowel (from above or transanally), reconstruction of the pelvic floor, suspension or fixation of the prolapsed bowel (with or without foreign materials), and reduction in size of the subcutaneous passage with a silicone elastomer (Silastic), synthetic, or steel suture wire (which aims at tightening the anus, thereby preventing further prolapse). The high failure rate is probably the result of treating only the prolapse, not the cause, which unfortunately is still unclear.

Fecal Incontinence

Complete fecal incontinence is defined as the uncontrolled passage of solid feces, whereas *partial incontinence* is defined as the uncontrolled passage of liquid or flatus. Incontinence must be distinguished from urgency, which is frequently accompanied by the passage of liquid stool.

A frequently identifiable cause of incontinence is some form of sphincter injury. This is often the result of anorectal surgery (internal sphincterotomy, fistula surgery, hemorrhoidectomy, anal dilatation, coloanal anastomosis, and low anterior resection) or childbirth. Obstetric injuries occur more commonly after obstructed labor, use of forceps,[51] and a third-degree tear or episiotomy. Rectal trauma, irradiation, and rectal prolapse are also associated with incontinence. A large number of patients have no identifiable specific cause (idiopathic fecal incontinence).

Idiopathic fecal incontinence has been shown to be associated with several physiologic abnormalities (Table 34-1). Most patients have low resting and squeeze pressures and abnormal external anal electromyograms suggestive of a neuropathy.[52] Abnormally elevated rectal pressures have also

Table 34-1. Tests of Fecal Incontinence

Test	Measures	Indication
Anal manometry	RAP	Low RAP with internal sphincter damage
	MSP	Low MSP with external sphincter damage
	Rectoanal inhibitory reflex	More pronounced in pruritus ani
Directional anal manometry	Anal sphincter pressure vector	Sphincter defects
Single fiber EMG	Fiber density	Deinnervation-reinnervation injury
Pudendal nerve motor terminal latency	Speed of travel of signal along pudendal nerve	Pudendal nerve damage from childbirth or straining
Defecating proctogram	Movement of pelvic floor	Descending perineum syndrome Occult intussusception
Endoanal ultrasonography	Maps sphincter defects	Obstetric or other sphincter injuries
Electrosensitivity	Sensitivity of anal mucosa electrical stimulation	Probably no clinical value

From Sagar PM, Pemberton JH. Anorectal and pelvic floor function: Relevance to continence, incontinence and constipation. Gastroenterol Clin North Am 25:171, 1996. Used with permission.
RAP, Resting anal pressure; *MSP,* maximum squeeze pressure; *EMG,* electromyogram.

been recorded in some patients. These pressures intermittently exceed anal canal pressures, causing leakage.[53]

Many patients with idiopathic fecal incontinence also have an obtuse anorectal angle. By itself, the obtuse angle does not result in incontinence. If it occurs concomitantly with inadequate resting and squeeze anal pressures, however, then incontinence is inevitable.[31] On the other hand, a normal angle (competent puborectalis) with inadequate anal sphincters can usually maintain continence to solid stools.[54]

The most likely cause of idiopathic fecal incontinence is progressive neuropathic damage to the striated muscles of the pelvic floor and external anal sphincter, as well as weakness of the internal anal sphincter.[55] This is supported by electromyographic findings of decreased activity and motor unit potentials that have larger amplitude and longer duration in the puborectalis and external anal sphincter. The single-fiber density of the external sphincter is increased, which is consistent with a denervation-renervation pattern. The pudendal nerve latencies are also found to be significantly increased in these patients.[53] Most patients with idiopathic fecal incontinence have only a distal conduction delay.[56] This can be differentiated from a cauda equina syndrome by transcutaneous electrical stimulation of the spinal cord to measure the spinal nerve motor latency.

There is a reduced sensitivity of the internal anal sphincter to noradrenaline in incontinence. This is caused by the absence of an α-adrenergic excitatory component of the intramural nerves.[57]

The assessment of fecal incontinence starts with a thorough history to define the presence and severity of incontinence, as well as any likely cause. Careful examination of the anus and rectum and proctoscopy are essential. Specific examinations are then used as indicated (Fig. 34-23). Anorectal manometry determines the presence or absence of the anorectal inhibitory reflex. The presence of the reflex eliminates the suspicion of Hirschsprung's disease. Basal resting and squeeze pressures do not correlate with the severity of incontinence; nor do they predict postoperative results. Defecography assesses the anorectal angle. Electromyography is useful after trauma to locate the severed ends of the external sphincter. Pudendal nerve terminal motor latency is useful in assessing neuropathy,[58] the presence of which usually implies a lower probability of successful sphincter repair. Rectal compliance may be found to be low after radiotherapy. Endoanal ultrasonography is an excellent means of delineating the sphincter anatomy and can define specific anatomic sphincter defects[59] (Fig. 34-24).

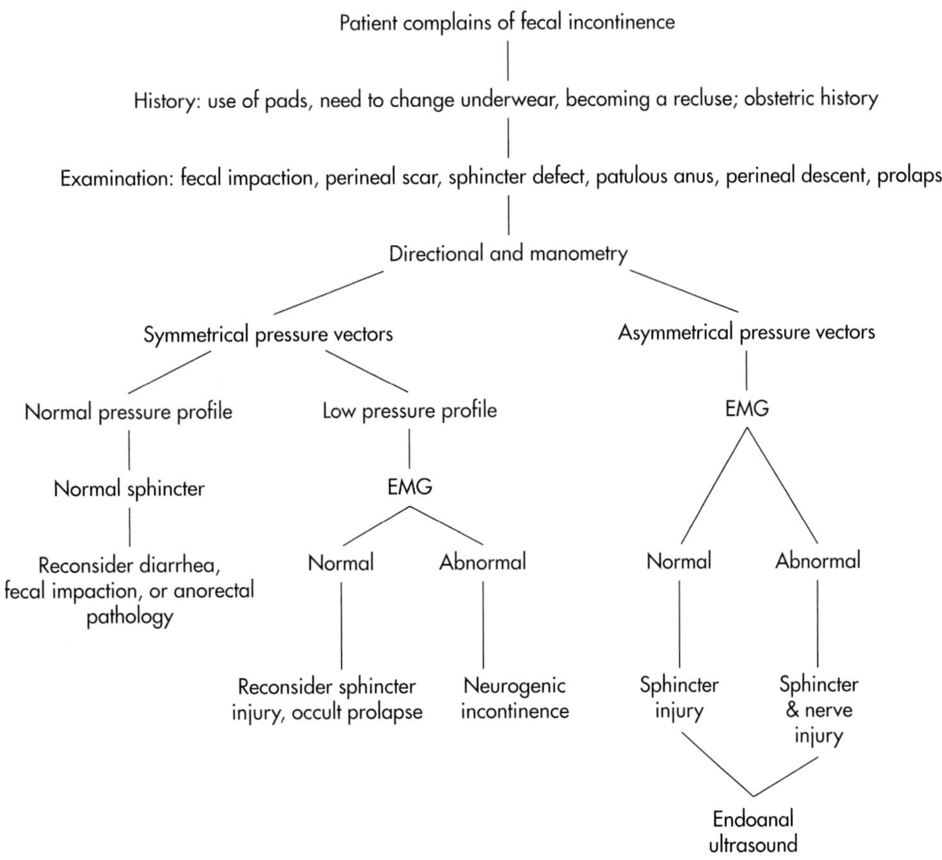

Fig. 34-23. Investigation of fecal incontinence. *EMG,* Electromyogram. (From Sagar PM, Pemberton JH. Anorectal and pelvic floor function: Relevance to continence, incontinence and constipation. Gastroenterol Clin North Am 25:176, 1996. Used with permission.)

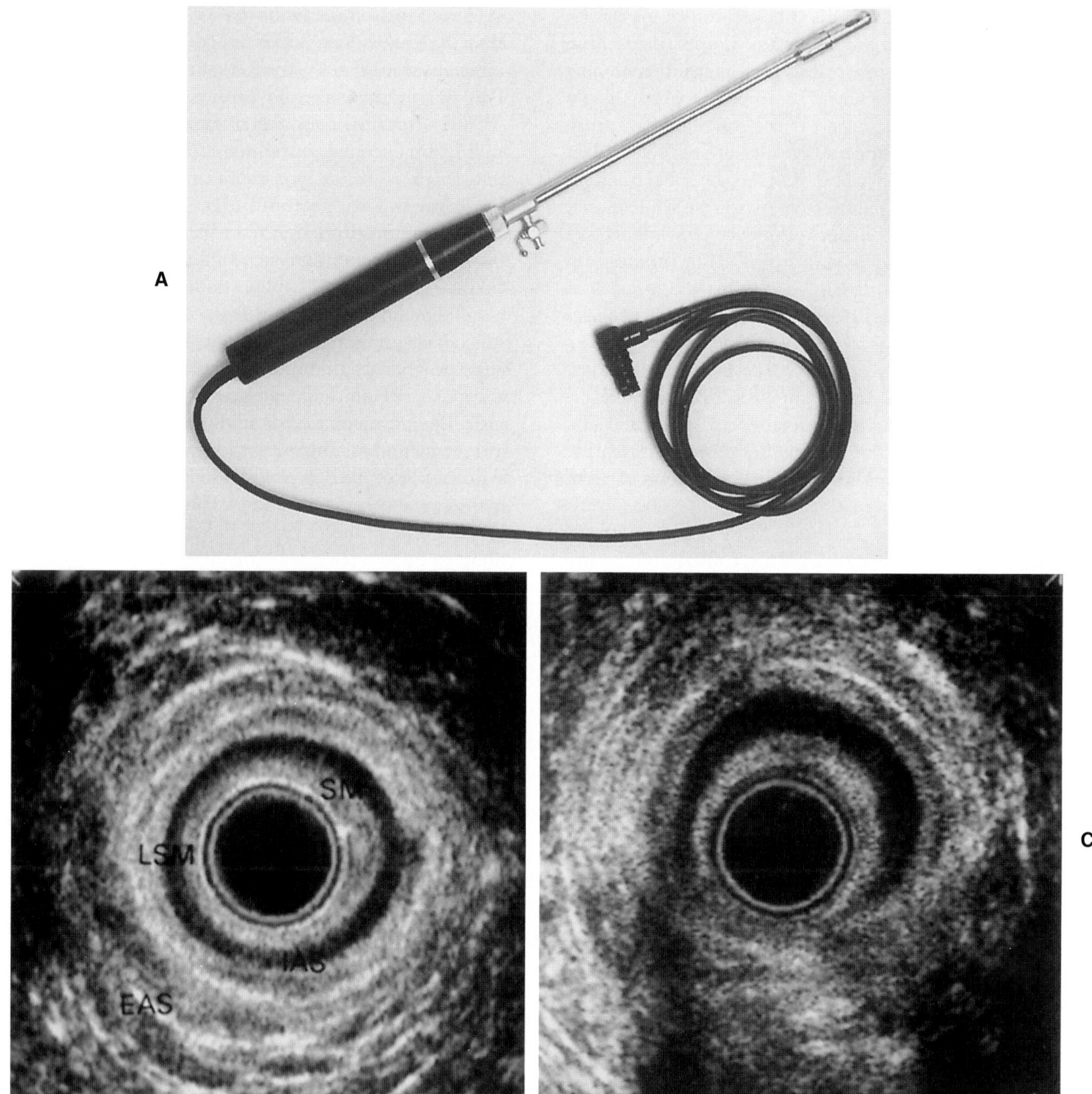

Fig. 34-24. Anal ultrasonography. **A,** Ultrasonographic apparatus, the assembled probe; **B,** normal appearance with a hyperechoic ring of submucosa *(SM),* hypoechoic internal anal sphincter *(IAS),* hyperechoic longitudinal smooth muscle *(LSM),* and the outer speckled external anal sphincter *(EAS);* **C,** anterior defect of the internal sphincter caused by a traumatic forceps delivery. These ultrasonographic views are oriented with the posterior plane in the 9 o'clock position. (From Bartram CL, Brunett SJO. Atlas of Anal Endosonography. London: Butterworth-Heinemann, 1991. Used with permission.)

If the etiology of incontinence is secondary, treatment is directed toward the primary cause. Symptomatic diarrhea may, however, be improved with dietary changes and perineal exercises. Biofeedback training has been found to be useful for most patients without a specific sphincter defect. This involves placing a balloon in the rectum with pressure transducers attached to a visual display. The patient is then taught to respond to rectal sensation, initially with the help of visual display and eventually without it.

Specific sphincter defects should be repaired. The most common repair is an overlapping repair. Although it is extremely controversial, if there is no anatomically definable disruption, a postanal repair has been advocated. Why this operation works at all is unknown.

Muscle transpositions to encircle the anal sphincters in the hope of augmenting its function have been tried, with mixed results. These have used the gluteus and gracilis muscles. Lately, the stimulated gracilis muscle has gained

EXTRACOLONIC CAUSES OF CHRONIC CONSTIPATION

Faulty Diet and Habits

Inadequate bulk (fiber)
Excessive ingestion of foods that harden stools (e.g., cheese)
Lack of exercise
Ignoring the call to stool

Pharmacologic

Analgesics
Antacids
Anticholinergics
Anticonvulsants
Antidepressants
Antiparkinsonian
Diuretics
Ganglionic blockers
Hypotensives (monoamine oxidase inhibitors)
Iron
Laxative abuse
Metallic intoxication (arsenic, lead, mercury, phosphorus)
Opiates (especially codeine)
Psychotropics (especially phenothiazines)

Metabolic and Endocrine

Diabetes mellitus
Uremia
Hypothyroidism
Hypercalcemia
Hypokalemia
Hyperparathyroidism
Amyloidosis
Hypopituitarism
Phaeochromocytoma
Pregnancy
Porphyria

Psychiatric

Depression
Psychoses
Anorexia nervosa

Neurologic

Iatrogenic

Resection of nervi erigentes
Immobilization

Spinal

Neoplasm
Lumbosacral cord trauma
Paraplegia
Multiple sclerosis
Tabes dorsalis
Shy-Drager syndrome
Meningocele

Cerebral

Neoplasm
Stroke
Parkinson's disease

Peripheral

Autonomic neuropathy
Ganglioneuromatosis (von Recklinghausen's disease)

From Pemberton JH. Management of constipation. In Swash M, Henry MM, eds. Coloproctology. Oxford: Butterworth-Heinemann, 1992. Used with permission.

popularity.[60,61] The gracilis, which has been transposed around the anal canal, is hooked to a pacemaker that continuously stimulates the muscle. The muscle undergoes changes when stimulated continuously to behave like a smooth muscle with tonic response. Defecation is initiated by use of a magnet mechanism to switch off the pacemaker, thus relaxing the neosphincter. Patient selection and motivation are vital in the outcome of these procedures.

The artificial anal sphincter was developed through an extension of the artificial urinary sphincter. Long-term results of these devices should be available in the near future. Occasionally, a permanent colostomy may give patients the only relief possible from the constant soilage and embarrassment of severe fecal incontinence.

Constipation

This ill-defined term as been taken to mean stools that are too small, too hard, or difficult to expel; to mean prolonged, repeated attempts at defecation, or to mean the need for manual assistance. The variety of symptoms makes it imperative that the patient be asked what specifically is meant by *constipation*. Because the parameters are difficult to assess objectively, stool frequency remains the clinical guide. This depends on diet, sex, and the presence of disease. By definition, constipation is said to exist when a patient has no more than 2 bowel movements per week.

There are many causes of constipation, including endocrine and metabolic disorders, side effects of drugs, psychologic imbalance, faulty diet, congenital problems such as megacolon or megarectum, rectal tumors, and sigmoid volvulus (see accompanying box). However, the most common causes of functional severe chronic constipation is colonic dysmotility, disordered defecation, or a combination of the two (Fig. 34-25).

Colonic dysmotility. Slow-transit constipation is an idiopathic disorder of colonic motility characterized by a radiologically normal-appearing colon but prolonged transit time. It occurs primarily in women. The stool interval increases gradually until stools occur 1 or 2 weeks apart. Fiber supplements paradoxically worsen the constipation. Laxatives are usually taken in increasingly large amounts, until spontaneous passage of stool becomes impossible.[62] The cause of slow-transit constipation has been attributed to an abnormality in the myenteric plexus,[63] deficient rectal sensation (no call to stool), disordered defecation, laxative abuse, psychologic problems, and reduced stool volume.

The other main disorder of colonic motility is the constipation-predominant variant of the irritable bowel syndrome (IBS) also known as *normal-transit constipation*. The likely pathophysiology of IBS is an enhanced motor re-

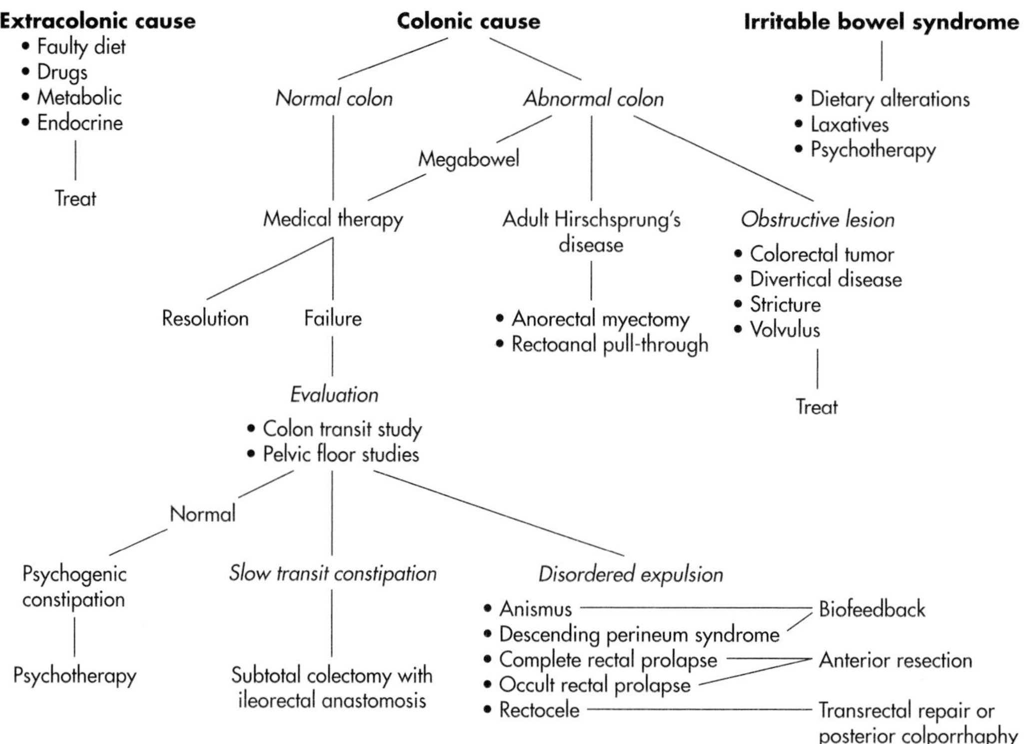

Fig. 34-25. Causes of chronic severe constipation in adults. (From Pemberton JH. Management of constipation. In Swash M, Henry MM, eds. Coloprotology. Oxford: Butterworth-Heinemann, 1992, p 417. Used with permission.)

Table 34-2. Tests of Anorectal Function for the Patient With Constipation

Test	Measures	Indication
Anal manometry	Increased RAP	Fissure in ano
	Increased MSP	Puborectalis spasm
	Absent rectoanal inhibitory reflex	Hirchsprung's disease
Radiopaque marker, studies	Intestinal transit	Colonic inertia
Scintigraphic studies	Colonic transit	Colonic inertia
Defecating proctography	Dynamic movements of pelvic floor	Occult intussusception
Balloon expulsion	Ability to evacuate rectum	Obstructed defecation
% Evacuation of stool	Efficiency of evacuation	Obstructed defecation

From Sagar PM, Pemberton JH. Anorectal and pelvic floor function: Relevance to continence, incontinence and constipation. Gastroenterol Clin North Am 25:175, 1996. Used with permission.
RAP, Resting anal pressure; *MSP,* maximum squeeze pressure.

sponse of the colon to meals, stress, and luminal distention.[64,65] Patients with constipation-predominant IBS, unlike those with slow-transit constipation, have episodes of diarrhea and normal colonic transit time; they show an appropriate response to stool bulking.

A challenge lies in differentiating these two conditions, because the results of surgery for IBS are nearly always unsatisfactory (Table 34-2). Appropriate dietary habit and psychologic management strategies are often valuable.

Abnormal defecation. Abnormal defecation results from failure of the striated muscles of the pelvic floor to relax on straining (anismus), failure of the internal sphincter to relax on rectal distension (Hirschsprung's disease), rectal intussusception (occult rectal prolapse), anterior rectal herniation (rectocele), posterior rectal herniation, and deficient or ignored rectal distention.

Of these only Hirschsprung's disease is well characterized pathophysiologically. The role of surgery is clearly defined; the aganglionic segment of the rectum is removed, and a normal defecation pattern is restored.

Anismus, or *puborectalis paradox,* is a condition in which the pelvic floor fails to relax on straining.[66] If the puborectalis does not relax, the anorectal angle does not straighten, thus causing an obstructive type of defecation. Some patients are found to have not only failure of relaxation but contraction of the puborectalis. This finding is not diagnostic, because puborectalis paradox can be a normal finding in healthy individuals who are not constipated.[67] The clinical presentation should be taken as an important indicator in the assessment of a patient with anismus. These may include an inability to initiate defecation, incomplete evacuation, a history of manual evacuation, assuming contorted postures for defecation, laxative and enema abuse, leakage, and rectal pain.

A rectocele fills with stool preferentially, instead of allowing evacuation.[68] Some women place a finger in the vagina to prevent filling of the rectocele while straining to pass. Others manually evacuate the rectocele, and some push up on the perineum. Surgical repair when defecation problems are present often gives good results. The mere presence of an asymptomatic rectocele, however, does not warrant surgical intervention.

Herniation of the posterior rectal wall backward and downward through the levator plane has also been described. The causes of these posterior hernias are not clear. They are probably caused by a relaxed puborectalis on straining, which allows the rectum to balloon posteriorly and caudally, making defecation difficult.

When the presence of stool in the rectum is not perceived, the rectoinhibitory response is often blunted or absent. Stools then accumulate in the rectum, resulting in a megarectum. Whether this is primary (congenital) or secondary (acquired) is not known. Occasionally, patients ignore the sensation of stool in the rectum. It becomes a habit, and large volumes of stools that become difficult and painful to pass accumulate. This condition is often associated with behavioral problems. One study found that 30% of women did not experience the desire to defecate.[69]

In addition to a full history and physical examination, specific questions on the history of constipation, laxative use, and diet often give valuable clues to the underlying cause. Examination should include a digital examination and careful inspection of the anal region for fissures, hemorrhoids, fistulas, and abscesses. Proctosigmoidoscopy with a barium enema or colonoscopy should be undertaken in anyone at risk for colorectal cancer. Transit-time studies are helpful to differentiate colonic from pelvic floor causes of constipation. The different tests outlined to assess the different components of the pelvic floor can be done as indicated. In particular, manometry can rule out or confirm Hirschsprung's disease, and electromyography is useful in puborectalis paradox.

Careful assessment followed by simple guidance and dietary advice may help a significant number of patients who do not have a specific cause for their constipation. They should be advised to answer the call to stool, undertake regular exercise, and consume adequate fiber and fluids (Fig. 34-26).

Colonic causes of constipation with normal pelvic floor function are probably best treated with a total colectomy and ileorectostomy if the symptoms warrant surgery.[70,71] Abnormal pelvic floor function responds to

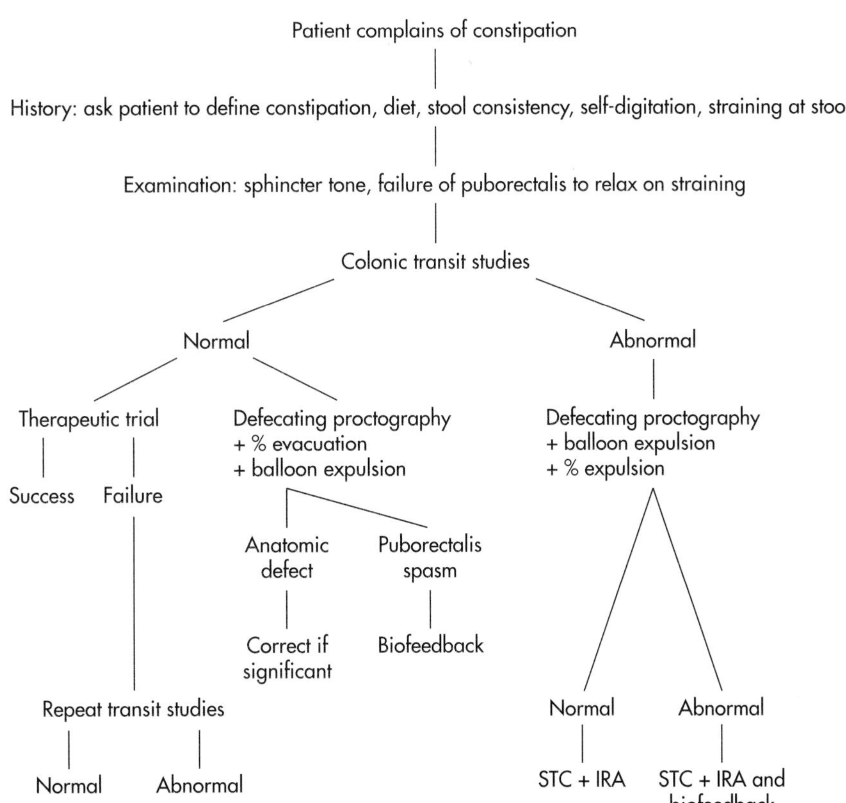

Fig. 34-26. Management of constipation in adults. *IRA,* Ileorectal anastomosis; *STC,* slow-transit constipation. (From Sagar PM, Pemberton JH. Anorectal and pelvic floor function: Relevance to continence, incontinence and constipation. Gastroenterol Clin North Am 25:417, 1996. Used with permission.)

pelvic floor retraining.[72] Anatomic problems such as rectoceles, rectal prolapses, and aganglionosis, on the other hand are best managed surgically.

SUMMARY

Tests of anorectal function need to be tailored to individual patients. The tests enumerated in this chapter are most useful when they identify an anatomic or physiologic abnormality for which there are successful medical or surgical treatments. For instance, for patients with fecal incontinence, anal manometry and intra-anal ultrasound are the most useful tests. Sphincter injuries identified by such maneuvers should be repaired, whereas neurogenic fecal incontinence documented by normal anatomy and inability to squeeze the pelvic floor (documented by manometry) is best treated with biofeedback initially. The tests most useful for patients with constipation are colonic transit time, determination of descent of pelvic floor on straining, and ability to defecate a balloon. Patients who are proven to have colonic inertia respond best to total colectomy and ileorectal anastomosis, whereas those with pelvic floor dysfunction respond best to pelvic floor retraining (biofeedback). Patients who are identified by these tests as having no quantifiable physiologic abnormalities are best referred to their physicians for the management of presumed irritable bowel syndrome. A complete understanding of the anatomic and physiologic interactions between the rectum and the anus in maintaining fecal incontinence and promoting normal defecation is becoming increasingly important in the management of patients who present with difficult functional abnormalities of the colon, rectum, and anus.

REFERENCES

1. Goligher JC. Surgery of the Anus, Rectum and Colon, 5th ed. London: Balliere, 1984.
2. Goldberg SM, Gordon PH, Nivatvongs S. Essentials of Anorectal Surgery. Philadelphia: JB Lippincott, 1980.
3. Wood BA, Kelly AJ. Anatomy of the anal sphincters and pelvic floor. In Henry MM, Swash M, eds. Coloproctology and the Pelvic Floor, 2nd ed. London: Butterworth-Heinemann, 1992.
4. Symington J. The rectum and anus. J Anat 23:106, 1989.
5. Phillips SF, Edwards DAW. Some aspects of anal incontinence and defecation. Gut 6:396, 1965.
6. Walls EW. Observations of the microscopic anatomy of the human anal canal. Br J Surg 45:504, 1958.
7. Gordon PH, Nivatvongs S. Surgical anatomy. In Gordon PH, Nivatvongs S, eds. Principles and Practice of Surgery for the Colon, Rectum, and Anus, St. Louis: Quality Medical Publishing, 1992.
8. Quer EA, Daklin DC, Mayo CW. Retrograde intramural spread of carcinoma of the rectum and rectosigmoid: A microscopic study. Surg Gynecol Obstet 96:24, 1953.
9. Lane RHS, Parks AG. Function of the anal sphincter following colo-anal anastomosis. Br J Surg 64:596, 1977.
10. Bouvier M, Gonella J. Nervous control of the internal sphincter in the cat. J Physiol 310:457, 1981.
11. Frenckner B, Euler CV. Influence of the pudendal block on the function of the anal sphincters. Gut 16:482, 1975.
12. Goligher JR, Hughes ESR. Sensitivity of the rectum and colon; Its role in the mechanism of anal continence. Lancet 1:543, 1951.
13. Mc Hugh SM, Diamant NE. Anal canal pressure profile; A reappraisal as determined by rapid pull thru technique. Gut 28:1234, 1987.
14. Pemberton JH, Phillips SF. Colonic absorption. Perspect Colon Rectal Surg 1:89, 1988.
15. Ferrara A, Pemberton JH, Hansen RB. Relationship between anal canal tone and rectal motor activity. Dis Colon Rectum 34:4, 1993.
16. Barkel DC, et al. Scintigraphic assessment of the anorectal angle in health and after ileal pouch-anal anastomois. Ann Surg 208:42, 1988.
17. Parks AG. Anorectal incontinence. Proc Soc Med 68:681, 1975.
18. Block IR, Enquist IF. Studies pertaining to local spread of carcinoma of the rectum in females. Surg Gynecol Obstet 112:41, 1961.
19. Miller R, et al. Anorectal temperature sensation; A comparison of normal and incontinent patients. Br J Surg 74:511, 1987.
20. Ihre T. Studies on anal function in continent and incontinent patients. Scand J Gasteroenterol 9(Suppl 25):1, 1974.
21. O'Connell PR, Kelly KA, Brown ML. Scintigraphic assessment of neorectal motor function. J Nucl Med 27:460, 1986.
22. Kellow JE, Gill RC, Wingate DL. Modulation of human upper gastrointestinal motility by rectal distension. Gut 28:864, 1987.
23. Youle MS, Read NW. Effect of painless rectal distension on gastrointestinal transit of solid meal. Dig Dis Sci 29:902, 1984.
24. Scharli AF, Kiesewetter WB. Defecation and continence; Some new concepts. Dis Colon Rectum 13:81, 1970.
25. Kumar D, et al. Prolonged anorectal manometry and external anal sphincter electromyography in ambulant human subjects. Dig Dis Sci 35:641, 1990.
26. Bell AM, et al. Variations in muscle tone of the human rectum; recordings with an electromechanical barostat. Am J Physiol 260:917, 1991.
27. Hancock D. Measurement of anal pressure and motility. Gut 17:645, 1976.
28. Kerremans R. Morphological and Physiological Aspects of Anal Continence and Defecation. Brussels: ED Arscia, 1969.
29. Phillips SF, Giller J. The contribution of the colon to electrolyte and water conservation in man. J Lab Clin Med 81:733, 1973.
30. Bannister JJ, et al. Effect of the stool size and consistency on defecation. Gut 28:1246, 1987.
31. Ambroze WL, et al. The effect of stool consistency on rectal and neorectal emptying. Dis Colon Rectum 34:1, 1993.
32. Bartolo DCC, et al. Differences in anal sphincter function and clinical presentation in patients with pelvic floor descent. Gastroenterology 85:68, 1983.
33. Roe AM, Bartolo DCC, Mortensen NJ. New method for assessment of anal sensation in various anorectal disorders. Br J Surg 73:310, 1986.
34. Shorran PJ, et al. Defecographic findings in young healthy volunteers. Gut 29:A1361, 1987.
35. Pezim M, Pemberton JH, Phillips SF. The immobile perineum; pathophysiologic implications in severe constipation [abstract]. Dig Dis Sci 32:924, 1984.
36. Metcalf AM, et al. Simplified assessment of segmental colonic transit. Gasteroenterology 92:40, 1987.
37. Thompson WHF. The nature of hemorrhoids. Br J Surg 62:542, 1975.
38. Hancock BD. The internal sphincter and anal fissure. Br J Surg 64:92, 1977.
39. Waldron DJ, et al. Prolonged ambulant assessment of anorectal function in patients with prolapsed hemorrhoids. Dis Colon Rectum 32:968, 1989.
40. Lin JK. Anal manometric studies in hemorrhoids and anal fissures. Dis Colon Rectum 32:839, 1989.
41. Klosterhalfen B, Vogel P, Rixen H. Topography of the inferior rectal artery; A possible cause of chronic primary anal fissure. Dis Colon Rectum 29:248, 1986.
42. Cerdan FJ, de Leon AR, Azpiroz F. Anal sphincter measures in fissure in ano before and after lateral sphincterotomy. Dis Colon Rectum 25:198, 1982.

43. Nothman BJ, Schuster MM. Internal anal sphincter derangement with anal fissures. Gasteroenterology 67:216, 1974.
44. Schouten WR, Blankensteijn JD. Ultra slow wave pressure variations in the anal canal before and after lateral internal sphincterotomy. Int J Colorectal Dis 7:115, 1992.
45. Schouten WR, Briel JW, Auwerda JJ. Relationship between anal pressure and anodermal blood flow. The vascular pathogenesis of anal fissures. Dis Colon Rectum 37:664, 1994.
46. Nyam DCNK, et al. Island advancement flaps in the management of anal fissures. Br J Surg 82:326, 1995.
47. Parks AG, Porter NH, Hardcastle J. The syndrome of the descending perineum. Proc Soc Med 59:477, 1966.
48. Theuerkaulf FJ Jr, Beahrs OH, Hill JR. Rectal prolapse: Conservation and surgical treatment. Ann Surg 171:819, 1970.
49. Kupfer CA, Goligher JC. One hundred consecutive cases of complete prolapse of the rectum treated by operation. Br J Surg 17:21, 1974.
50. Boutsis C, Ellis H. The Ivalon sponge wrap operation for rectal prolapse. An experience with 26 patients. Dis Colon Rectum 17:21, 1974.
51. Sultan AH, et al. Anal sphincter trauma during instrumental deliver. Int J Gynaecol Obstet 43:263, 1993.
52. Read NW, et al. A clinical study of patients with fecal incontinence and diarrhea. Gasteroenterology 76:747, 1979.
53. Read NW, et al. Use of anorectal manometry during rectal infusion of saline to investigate sphincter function in incontinent patients. Gasteroenterology 85:105, 1983.
54. Varma KK, Stephens D. Neuromuscular reflexes of rectal continence. Aust N Z J Surg 41:263, 1972.
55. Wormack DJ, et al. The role of pelvic floor denervation in the etiology of idiopathic fecal incontinence. Br J Surg 73:404, 1986.
56. Kiff ES, Swash M. Slowed conduction in the pudendal nerves in idiopathic (neurogenic) fecal incontinence. Br J Surg 71:614, 1984.
57. Speakman CT, et al. Abnormalities of innervation of internal anal sphincter in fecal incontinence. Dig Dis Sci 38:1961, 1993.
58. Snooks SJ, Swash M, Henry MM. Abnormalities in central and peripheral nerve conduction in patients with anorectal incontinence. J R Soc Med 78:294, 1985.
59. Sultan AH, et al. Anal endosonography for identifying external sphincter defects confirmed histologically. Br J Surg 81:463, 1994.
60. Williams NS, et al. Development of an electrically stimulated neosphincter. Lancet 338:1166, 1991.
61. Baeten CGM, et al. Dynamic gracilloplasty for treatment of fecal incontinence. Lancet 338:1163, 1991.
62. Christensen J. Motility of the colon. In Johnson LR, ed. Physiology of the Gastrointestinal Tract. New York: Raven Press, 1987, p 665.
63. Krishnamurthy S, et al. Severe idiopathic constipation is associated with a distinctive abnormality of the colonic myenteric plexus. Gastroenterology 88:26, 1985.
64. Connell AM, Jones FA, Rowlands EN. Motility of the pelvic colon. IV. Abdominal pain associated with colonic hypermotility after meals. Gut 6:165, 1965.
65. Rogers J, Henry MM, Misiewicz JJ. Increased segmental activity and intraluminal pressures in sigmoid colon of patients with irritable bowel syndrome. Gut 30:634, 1989.
66. Preston DM, Leonard-Jones JE. Anismus in chronic constipation. Dig Dis Sci 30:413, 1985.
67. Jones PN, et al. Is paradoxical contraction of puborectalis muscle of functional importance? Dis Colon Rectum 30:667, 1987.
68. Ihre T, Selingson U. Intussusception of the rectum internal procidentia; Treatment and results in 90 patients. Dis Colon Rectum 18:391, 1975.
69. Read NW, et al. Impairment of defecation in young women with severe constipation. Gasteroenterology 90:53, 1986.
70. Pemberton JH, Rath DM, Illstrup DM. Evaluation and surgical treatment of severe chronic constipation. Ann Surg 214:403, 1991.
71. Wexner S, Daniel N, Jagelman DG. Colectomy for constipation: Physiologic investigation is the key to success. Dis Colon Rectum 34:851, 1991.
72. Chan CW, et al. Long term results of pelvic floor training in patients with pelvic floor dysfunction [abstract]. Dis Colon Rect 38:18, 1995.

35

Physiology of Respiration

Courtney Crim

The human species, like other mammals, requires a consistent and continuous supply of oxygen and elimination of metabolically derived carbon dioxide for optimal function of peripheral tissues and cells. Although both the heart and lungs participate in these processes in a coordinated fashion, the lungs are unique in accomplishing these goals because they are the means by which oxygen is delivered to the body and carbon dioxide is eliminated, both through a series of passageways commonly called the *tracheobronchial tree* and across diffusion barriers known as the *alveolar-capillary membrane.* This chapter reviews the physiologic constructs of ventilation and diffusion in the lungs and the mechanics of how this breathing apparatus accomplishes these goals.

CELLULAR RESPIRATION

At the cellular level, aerobic energy metabolism involves a complex process that has been defined as *respiration*. This process requires not only the delivery of adequate substrates, such as carbohydrates and fats, but also sufficient amounts of oxygen and blood flow to remove the produced carbon dioxide. The lungs play a critical role in this process, which is coupled with the cardiovascular system to ensure adequate gas transport from the external environment to and from the tissues.

This interplay of the cardiovascular and respiratory systems can be illustrated by examining the metabolic changes that occur in exercising muscle. Muscle contraction is dependent on an adequate supply of adenosine triphosphate (ATP), which in turn is principally generated from mitochondrial oxidation of stored carbohydrates (glycogen) and fats (triglycerides). Although ATP acts as the coupling agent for transfer of energy from substrates to actual cell function (e.g., muscle contraction), creatine phosphate serves as the "storage depot" for the high-energy phosphate bonds. Creatine phosphate replenishes ATP during its use and is itself resynthesized during oxidative phosphorylation. The *respiratory quotient* (RQ) is defined as the molar ratio of carbon dioxide produced to oxygen used. The consumption of carbohydrates as the sole energy source would result in an RQ of 1, whereas the use of released free fatty acids would result in an RQ of 0.7. During normal cellular respiration, there is approximately equal use of fats and carbohydrates as substrates and thus an RQ of approximately 0.85.

At the onset of muscle activity, there is an initial delay before a constant oxygen delivery is reached. This initial oxygen deficit results in increased lactate production and creatine phosphate depletion. Although this initial rise in lactate is usually transient, with increasing muscle work an "anaerobic threshold" is reached at which plasma lactate level rises progressively. Protons released with the formation of lactic acid react with bicarbonate, leading to excess carbon dioxide production. The molar ratio of carbon dioxide exhaled to oxygen intake in the lungs is referred to as the *respiratory exchange ratio* to distinguish it from the RQ. It is therefore conceivable that the respiratory exchange ratio may differ from RQ above the anaerobic threshold. At the end of exercise, there is a delay before oxygen intake returns to resting levels. This "oxygen debt" is related to the aerobic metabolism of lactate, resynthesis of muscle energy reserves, and replenishment of tissue oxygen stores.

Several mechanisms come into play to meet these increased metabolic demands. Local vasodilatation occurs immediately, presumably as a result of regional changes in the concentrations of lactate, ATP, and potassium, as well as tissue hypoxia. Cardiac output increases to facilitate tissue carbon dioxide removal and augment oxygen delivery. An increased oxygen extraction may be evidenced by a widened arteriovenous oxygen difference. In the lungs, this increase in cardiac output results in the distention of the capillary bed, as well as recruitment of previously closed vessels. Alveolar ventilation ($\dot{V}_A$) increases in concert with the carbon dioxide output, and the fraction of dead space ventilation ($\dot{V}_{DS}$) declines. The net effect is to improve pulmonary gas exchange, leading to enhanced oxygen uptake and carbon dioxide elimination.

It is therefore obvious that in patients with concomitant disease of the cardiovascular or respiratory systems, the ability to meet increased organ system metabolic demands may be seriously compromised. Oxygen delivery to peripheral tissues is jeopardized in patients with low–cardiac output states from valvular heart disease or myocardial dysfunction. This problem is further exacerbated if peripheral vascular disease coexists. Hypovolemia, in either the presence or absence of anemia, compromises the adaptation to metabolic stress. Increases in hemoglobin concentration to levels greater than normal have been shown to improve maximum oxygen consumption and performance in healthy subjects.[1] It is plausible that a similar response may occur in certain disease states. Furthermore, with hypovolemia, the ability to recruit and distend the pulmonary capillary bed is limited, which in turn may impair the ability to optimize gas exchange in the lungs. Similarly, individuals with underlying pulmonary parenchymal, airway, or vascular disease may exhibit defects in gas transfer at the alveolar-capillary interface and maldistribution of ventilation or perfusion with ventilation-perfusion mismatch. With pulmonary vascular disease, the ability to recruit the pulmonary circulation as cardiac output increases (for example, to compensate for hypovolemia or other increases in metabolic demands) is impaired. The cumulative effect is an inability to augment oxygen uptake during periods of increased metabolic stress.

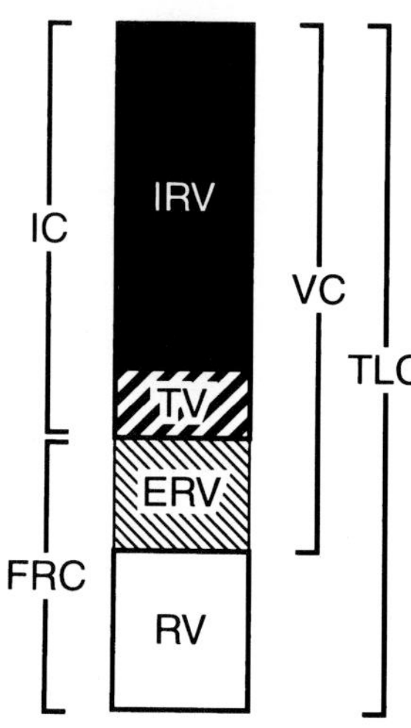

Fig. 35-1. The subdivisions of lung volumes and the determination of the various lung capacities: tidal volume *(TV),* inspiratory reserve volume *(IRV),* expiratory reserve volume *(ERV),* residual volume *(RV),* inspiratory capacity *(IC),* functional residual capacity *(FRC),* vital capacity *(VC),* and total lung capacity *(TLC).*

VENTILATION

The primary function of the tracheobronchial tree is to conduct air to the alveolar surface, where gas exchange occurs. As such, the airway system can be viewed as being divided into three zones. The conductive zone is concerned with bulk flow of air to the gas exchanging regions and includes the trachea and bronchi down to the level of the terminal bronchioles. This constitutes the anatomic dead space. The transitory zone carries out both conductive and respiratory functions and includes the region of the respiratory bronchioles to the alveolar sacs. The respiratory zone consists of the alveoli, across which gas exchange occurs. Diffusion is the predominant mechanism of gas transport in this region. The region of the lung distal to the terminal bronchiole, the acinus, is taken to represent the basic functional unit of the lung. It is also the smallest anatomic lung unit that can be visualized roentgenographically, ranging from 6 to 10 mm in diameter.[2,3]

Lung Volumes and Ventilation

The maximum amount of air that can be contained within the lungs is called the *total lung capacity* (TLC). Because capacities represent the sum of two or more volumes, the TLC can be divided into the residual volume (RV), which represents the volume of air remaining after a maximal expiration, and the vital capacity (VC), which equals the maximum amount of air that can be expired after a maximal inspiration (Fig. 35-1). Although the size of the subdivisions vary with age, sex, weight, and height, VC is normally about 75% of the TLC and the RV constitutes the remaining 25%. The tidal volume (V_T), the volume of gas inspired or expired during each respiratory cycle, averages between 400 and 600 ml. The volume of air in the lungs after a quiet expiration (the resting end-expiratory position) is the functional residual capacity (FRC). The position of the FRC represents the balance of forces from the elastic recoil between the lungs and chest wall. It is approximately 40% of the TLC and acts as a buffer against extreme changes in alveolar oxygen tension (PO_2) with each breath. Lung volumes and capacities that do not include the RV can be measured directly with a spirometer. Techniques used to measure compartments that do contain the RV include helium dilution, nitrogen washout, and whole-body plethysmography. The last technique is considered the gold standard, because both helium dilution and nitrogen washout may underestimate lung volumes in the presence of significant obstructive airway disease.

Early studies conducted with inhaled radioactive tracer gases demonstrated regional differences in the ventilation of the lung. For example, in an upright subject, ventilation is greater at the bases than at the apices. If the individual assumes a supine position, ventilation is now greater in the posterior lung. This regional difference in ventilation occurs because the gravitational forces on the lung result in a greater (less negative) intrapleural pressure in the dependent lung regions. At FRC, the nondependent lung units are more distended than are those in the dependent regions and thus expand less during the inspiratory phase. At lung volumes approaching RV, the intrapleural pressure exceeds intraluminal airway pressure, which results in closure of the peripheral airways. Thus, the initial portion of a breath taken from RV enters the alveoli in the lung apices (in the upright position). As FRC is approached, the distribution of ventilation shifts to the dependent lung zones.

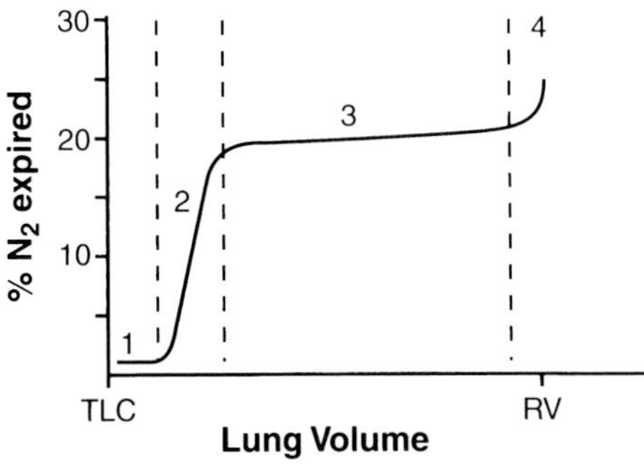

Fig. 35-2. Single-breath nitrogen washout for determination of closing volume. A single breath of 100% oxygen is inspired from RV to TLC, and the concentration of nitrogen during the subsequent expiration is measured. *Phase 1* represents oxygen-containing dead-space gas; *phase 2,* mixture of dead-space and alveolar gas; *phase 3,* alveolar gas from both dependent and nondependent lung zones; *phase 4,* alveolar gas from the nondependent lung zone containing a relatively high concentration of nitrogen. The inflection point at the beginning of phase 4 indicates the CV.

The distribution of ventilation and the volume at which airways in the dependent lung regions close can be assessed by the single-breath nitrogen washout test. The subject inspires a single breath of 100% oxygen from residual volume to TLC and the concentration of nitrogen is measured during the subsequent exhalation (Fig. 35-2). Phase 1 represents the expiration of dead-space oxygen. Phase 2 occurs as nitrogen-containing alveolar gas mixes with dead-space gas and rises to a plateau (phase 3). Phase 3 represents the washout of alveolar gas. At low lung volumes (approaching RV), the airways at the lung bases (oxygen containing) close, and only the alveoli at the apices continue to contribute to the expired volume. Because the concentration of nitrogen is higher in these apical lung units (from the nitrogen-containing dead-space gas during the single-breath maneuver), an abrupt increase in the nitrogen concentration is observed. The volume of air expired from this point represents the closing volume (CV). In normal young people, the CV is about 10% of the VC, but it may be undetectable in some individuals. In adults, the CV increases with age, and in individuals older than 60 years and in supine subjects older than 45 years, it may occur at a lung volume that exceeds the FRC. This occurrence is likely because the FRC decreases 0.5 to 1.0 L on assumtion a supine position.[4,5] The reduction in FRC appears to be multifactorial and includes an elevation of the diaphragm, a decrease in the cross-sectional chest area, and a shift in central blood volume from the thorax to the abdomen.[4] If the CV encroaches on the FRC, dependent lung units may close during a portion of the respiratory cycle,[6] which in turn results in atelectasis and arterial hypoxemia. This may become a significant problem for some bedridden postoperative patients.

Although a restrictive ventilatory defect is defined by a reduced TLC, measurement of the VC by spirometry is the best bedside marker. Conditions that reduce VC include diseases of the chest cage (e.g., kyphoscoliosis, ankylosing spondylitis), pleural disease (e.g., effusions), neuromuscular disease, interstitial lung disease, and severe airways obstruction (TLC, however, is normal or increased with this condition). Other potentially useful information that can be obtained from the spirogram includes the forced expiratory volume in 1 second (FEV_1) and the ratio of the FEV_1 to the forced expired VC ($FEV_{1\%}$). The usefulness of these parameters in predicting postoperative complications is controversial,[7] but it most likely depends on the type of surgery (e.g., thoracic vs abdominal) and underlying cardiopulmonary risk factors.

The main function of the respiratory system is to maintain optimal alveolar and arterial levels of oxygen and carbon dioxide. This is accomplished through ventilation. However, although the ventilatory process supplies just enough oxygen to meet the metabolic demands, determination of the minute ventilation ($\dot{V}_E$), and specifically the $\dot{V}_A$, gives useful information about carbon dioxide balance. If an individual is in a steady-state, it can be shown that

$$863 \times \dot{V}CO_2 = \dot{V}_A \, PCO_2$$

or

$$863 \times \dot{V}CO_2 = (\dot{V}_E - \dot{V}_D)PCO_2$$

where $\dot{V}CO_2$ is carbon dioxide production and PCO_2 is carbon dioxide tension. From the first equation, it is obvious that for constant carbon dioxide production, arterial PCO_2 is inversely related to $\dot{V}_A$. From the second relationship, two other principles are obvious. First, for a resting 70 kg subject with normal $\dot{V}_{DS}$ and $\dot{V}CO_2$, a $\dot{V}_E$ of approximately 80 to 100 ml/kg/minute would result in an arterial PCO_2 in the range of 35 to 45 mm Hg. This serves as one rationale for initiating mechanical ventilation for patients with respiratory failure with tidal volumes in the range of 8 to 10 ml/kg. Ventilation with large tidal volumes has been associated with lung injury as a result of alveolar and capillary injury and surfactant inactivation.[8-10] Moreover, if the $\dot{V}_D$ is small and relatively constant compared with $\dot{V}_E$, then arterial PCO_2 is inversely related to $\dot{V}_E$. For example, an arterial PCO_2 of 70 mm Hg in a patient who is receiving a $\dot{V}_E$ of 8 L/min can be corrected to 40 mm Hg by increasing the $\dot{V}_E$ to 14 L/per min. Failure of this relationship to hold would imply a dynamic rather than steady state of either carbon dioxide production, $\dot{V}_{DS}$ or both, the cause of which should be investigated rigorously.

DIFFUSION

As mentioned previously, the conducting zone of the respiratory system moves fresh gas to the respiratory zone by bulk flow. The uptake of oxygen from the inspired air into the circulation depends on several factors. Some of these factors are intrinsic to the gas molecule of interest; for example, its tissue solubility. Carbon dioxide is more tissue soluble than is oxygen and therefore diffuses at a faster rate. Other factors include the distance across which diffusion must occur (the alveolar-capillary interface), the alveolar surface area, and the driving pressure gradient of the gas between the alveolus and the capillary blood. In addition, the measured diffusing capacity is influenced by the rate at which marker gas combines with hemoglobin, the amount of hemoglobin, and the rate at which hemoglobin is delivered to the pulmonary circulation (the effects of cardiac output on the size of the pulmonary capillary bed).

Although from a clinical standpoint the diffusion of oxygen is of interest, it is technically difficult to measure directly. The test is therefore routinely performed with a single-breath inhalation of a low concentration of carbon monoxide. Carbon monoxide has size and molecular weight similar to those of oxygen. Moreover, because of its higher affinity for hemoglobin than that of oxygen, the partial pressure of dissolved carbon monoxide is low in the red blood cell. For this reason, the pressure gradient for carbon monoxide diffusion remains constant. The diffusing capacity measures the conductance of the lung as a "whole" to carbon monoxide, and by extrapolation to oxygen. Principally, it is altered by any condition that results in a maldistribution of ventilation to perfusion. Likewise, a decrease in the lung volume from surgical resection results in a lower diffusing capacity by decreasing the total surface area for diffusion. Anemia and low–cardiac output states can also give a low diffusing capacity. The carbon monoxide diffusing capacity averages around 35 ml/min/mm Hg and is considered abnormal when it is reduced by 20% to 25%.

PULMONARY BLOOD FLOW AND VENTILATION-PERFUSION MATCHING

Optimal gas exchange occurs when there is perfect matching of alveolar ventilation to perfusion. Just as the distribution of ventilation increases in the dependent portions of the lung, so does pulmonary blood flow. This progressive increase in blood flow, described by West et al.,[11] is a function of the relationships among alveolar, arterial, and venous pressures.[11] Regional lung perfusion is greater in zone 3, where both arterial and venous pressures exceed alveolar pressure. However, perfusion is minimized in zone 1, where alveolar pressure is greater than both arterial and venous pressures. Failure to appreciate this difference can have important ramifications during pulmonary artery catheterization. For example, attempts to estimate left ventricular filling pressure with the tip of the catheter in a zone 1 position may actually reflect alveolar pressure, giving erroneous information.

Normally, each liter of blood flow through the lungs is matched with 0.8 L alveolar ventilation. With the multiple inert gas elimination technique, however, there is a narrow distribution of ventilation/perfusion ($\dot{V}/\dot{Q}$) ratios centered around a value of 1.0 for both ventilation and blood flow.[12] Both dead space ($\dot{V}/\dot{Q} \approx \infty$) and true shunt ($\dot{V}/\dot{Q} = 0$) can also be quantified with this technique. At present, this procedure is relegated to the research setting and is not clinically available. To assess altered arterial blood gases as a result of impaired gas exchange, measurement of the alveolar-arterial oxygen gradient ($PAO_2 - PaO_2$) while breathing room air has been the traditional method. An increase in the $PAO_2 - PaO_2$ (normally 2.5 + 0.21 × age with the SD ≈ 6[13]) implies $\dot{V}/\dot{Q}$ mismatch ($\dot{V}/\dot{Q} \neq 1$) or true shunt. Calculation of this gradient is of limited use for patients requiring supplemental oxygen because the "normal" gradient increases with increasing inspired oxygen concentration (FIO_2). Recently, it has been demonstrated that measurement of the arterial to alveolar oxygen ratio (a/APO_2) is more stable than is the $PAO_2 - PaO_2$ with changing FIO_2[14] because its computation normalizes for any given FIO_2. Therefore, the determination of the a/APO_2 (lower normal limit = 0.75) is probably a better parameter to use when assessing abnormal gas exchange.

Detection of a gas exchange abnormality by the demonstration of a reduced a/APO_2 would suggest either an increase in $\dot{V}DS$ or venous admixture (including true shunt). Measurement of physiologic dead space (the sum of anatomic dead space and wasted ventilation from lung units with high $\dot{V}/\dot{Q}$ ratios) can be performed by using a modification of the Bohr equation

$$VDS/VT = (PaCO_2 - PECO_2)/PaCO_2$$

where *VDS* is dead space volume, $PaCO_2$ is arterial PCO_2, and $PECO_2$ is mixed expired PCO_2. Normally, VD/VT is no greater than 0.3. Calculation of this ratio is not routinely performed clinically. However, elevation in $\dot{V}DS$ may be suspected in circumstances where the overall $\dot{V}E$ is increased relative to the "normal" $PaCO_2$.

Determination of true shunts and the degree of venous admixture (true shunts plus lung regions of low $\dot{V}/\dot{Q}$ ratios) can be quantified by the shunt equation

$$\dot{Q}S/\dot{Q}T = (CcO_2 - CaO_2)/(CcO_2 - C\bar{v}O_2)$$

where $\dot{Q}S$ is the shunted (true shunt or admixed venous blood) flow, $\dot{Q}T$ is the cardiac output, CcO_2 is the pulmonary end-capillary blood content, CaO_2 is the arterial oxygen content, and $C\bar{v}O_2$ is the mixed venous oxygen content. The true shunt can be determined by having the subject breathe 100% oxygen, thereby eliminating the contribution of lung units with low $\dot{V}/\dot{Q}$ ratios. Normally, true anatomic shunt is about 2% of the cardiac output whereas the venous admixture should be less than 10%.

GAS TRANSPORT TO THE PERIPHERY

The delivery of oxygen to the tissues is in one of two forms, (1) that dissolved in plasma and (2) that which is combined with hemoglobin. The dissolution of oxygen in plasma obeys Henry's law with a solubility coefficient of 0.0031 ml O_2/mm Hg/dl blood. On the other hand, 1 g hemoglobin is capable of combining with 1.39 ml oxygen. Thus, 100 ml arterial blood with 15 g fully saturated hemoglobin and a PaO_2 of 100 mm Hg would carry approximately 21 ml oxygen. Because of the cooperative binding of oxygen by hemoglobin (as described by the sigmoid shape of the oxyhemoglobin dissociation curve) the oxygen saturation of hemoglobin only begins to decline significantly at a Po_2 less than 60 mm Hg. Because the tissue Po_2 is on the order of 5 mm Hg, with mitochondria requiring a Po_2 of only 0.5 to 1.0 mm Hg,[15,16] there exists a large gradient for diffusion of oxygen from the blood. Other factors that effect oxygen release from hemoglobin (a rightward shift in the dissociation curve) include increases in temperature, hydrogen ion concentration, carbon dioxide, and 2,3-diphosphoglycerate. The release of oxygen at the tissue level is coupled with the uptake of carbon dioxide (the Bohr and Haldane effects). Carbon dioxide produced from cell metabolism is carried back to the lungs as dissolved carbon dioxide (solubility coefficient of 0.67 ml CO_2 /mm Hg/dl blood) and carbamino compounds (from protein binding), but principally as bicarbonate. Most of the bicarbonate carried in the plasma is formed in the erythrocyte by carbonic anhydrase. Its diffusion from the red cell is counterbalanced by a shift of chloride ions in accordance with the Gibbs-Donnan equilibrium. On return of the venous blood to the lung, the higher Po_2 leads to a reversal of these processes, thereby facilitating the release of carbon dioxide and uptake of oxygen.

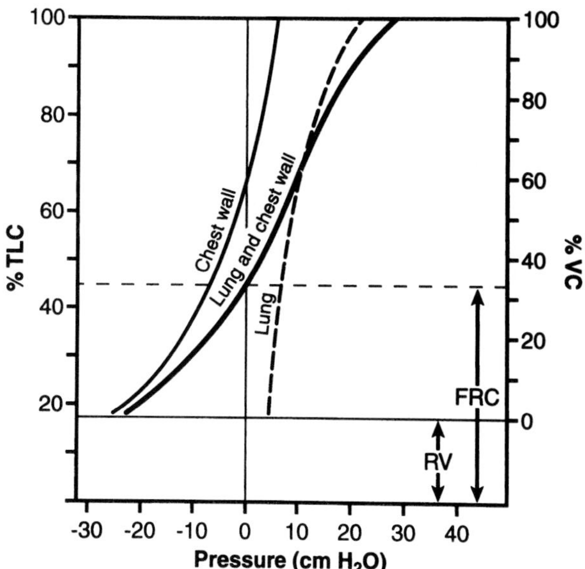

Fig. 35-3. Pressure-volume (compliance) curves of the lung, chest wall, and algebraic sum. The compliance, the slope at any point along the curve, decreases at both large and small lung volumes. *FRC,* Functional residual capacity; *RV,* residual volume; *TLC,* total lung capacity; *VC,* vital capacity.

LUNG MECHANICS

The process of gas exchange requires the flow of gas and blood to the alveoli and alveolar capillaries, respectively. At end-expiration (at FRC), the intrathoracic pressure is normally subatmospheric (because the elastic lung tends to recoil inward and away from the thoracic cage). Active contraction of the inspiratory muscles of respiration further lowers intrathoracic pressure and enlarges the thorax. This active contraction of the inspiratory muscles provides (1) the force necessary to overcome the elastic recoil of the lungs and thorax (compliance), (2) the force required to overcome frictional resistance from the movement of the tissues of the lung and thorax (tissue resistance—rarely significant, even in disease states), and (3) the force necessary to overcome frictional resistance to airflow through the airways (resistance). At end-inspiration, the potential energy created by contraction of the inspiratory muscles is stored in the elastic tissues of the lungs and thorax. If airway resistance is negligible, the elastic recoil causes the lungs and thorax to passively return rapidly to FRC. If the expiratory resistance opposing elastic recoil is abnormally great (e.g., bronchospasm, chronic obstructive pulmonary disease), active contraction of the expiratory muscles of respiration may be needed (unless the time for expiration is lengthened).

Thus, the mechanical properties of compliance and resistance of the lung are the principal determinants of the work that must be performed by the respiratory muscles during respiration. Pressure-volume curves can be generated from which the compliance of both the lungs and the chest cage may be examined (Fig. 35-3). Because inspiration of the V_T occurs as a result of changes in intrathoracic pressure (changes induced by contraction of the respiratory muscles), compliance (C) is defined as a volume change (ΔV) produced by a unit pressure change (ΔP):

$$C = \Delta V/\Delta P$$

Resistance (R) is the ΔP required for a unit of airflow (F; i.e., airway pressure gradient required to flow a volume of air into the lungs):

$$R = \Delta P/F$$

Therefore, a patient with poorly compliant lungs (e.g., adult respiratory syndrome, pulmonary edema, fibrosis) or significant elevation in airways resistance (e.g., acute asthma, chronic obstructive pulmonary disease) would have to significantly increase the degree of contraction of the respiratory muscles to generate a normal V_T.

In the physical sense, work is a force acting over a distance, or in the case of either compression or expansion of a gas, is the pressure-volume product. Consequently, if the volume of air (inspired or expired) is plotted as a function of pressure, then the area lying between the curve and the volume axis represents the work performed (Fig. 35-4). Because the direct measurement of lung compliance requires the placement of a balloon catheter in the esophagus, this determination is not routinely performed clinically. Similarly, airway resistance is not directly measured in an intensive care unit setting. In mechanically ventilated patients, however, the total respiratory compliance can be quantified and the total resistance can be qualitatively assessed. These parameters can be determined by observing the ventilator-delivered pressure wave during an unassisted breath

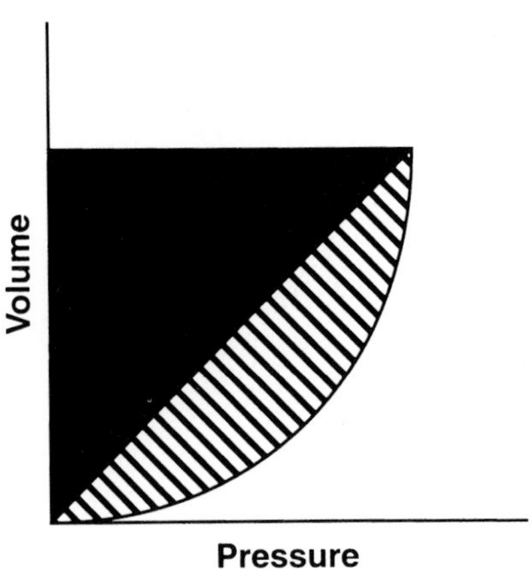

Fig. 35-4. The mechanical work required to overcome the compliance of the respiratory system *(triangular area)* and the airway resistance *(curved loop)* during lung inspiration. The total work is the sum of the two.

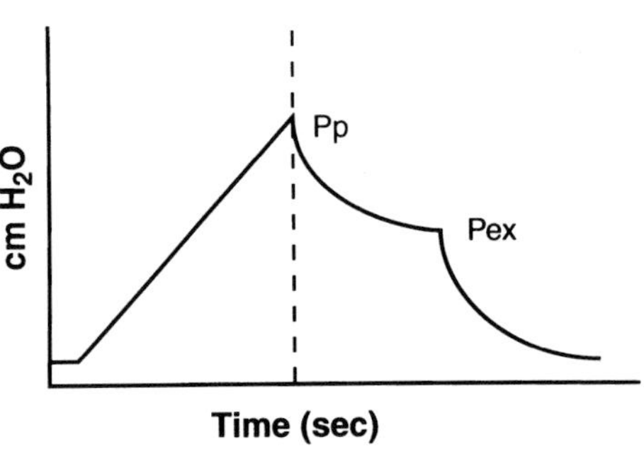

Fig. 35-5. Pressure tracing from a volume-cycled ventilator with constant (square-wave) flow delivery. An end-inspiratory hold is applied at the vertical dashed line. The peak *(Pp)* and static *(P_{EX})* pressures are as indicated. The Pp − P_{EX} difference represents the pressure gradient required to overcome flow resistive work. The P_{EX} − baseline pressure difference is that necessary for compliance work.

while applying an occlusion on the expiratory limb of the ventilator circuit (Fig. 35-5). The difference between the "plateau" or end-inspiratory pressure and the baseline pressure (e.g., positive end-expiratory pressure) represents the distending pressure required to keep the lungs and chest cage inflated with the delivered VT, thus the total compliance. The difference between the peak airway and end-inspiratory pressure reflects the pressure that is required to overcome the flow-resistive properties of the system. The total compliance measured as described is normally 60 to 100 ml/cm H_2O. In most clinical scenarios it can be assumed that the compliance of the chest cage is invariant. Therefore, any observed changes in the measured compliance usually indicates a change in the lung component.

Decreases in lung compliance, as in pulmonary edema and atelectasis, or increases in the total resistance, with conditions such as bronchospasm and chronic obstructive pulmonary disease, result in an increased work of breathing. Such increases in respiratory work may significantly increase the oxygen cost of breathing and impede weaning from mechanical ventilation.[17] It has been for this type of problem that pressure-support ventilation has been advocated as a mode to decrease work of breathing.[18,19] The technology is now becoming available whereby work of breathing can be measured directly at the bedside and therapeutic interventions applied.[20]

CONTROL OF BREATHING

The primary function of the respiratory system is to maintain homeostatic levels of alveolar and arterial oxygen and carbon dioxide so that cellular respiration can proceed without hindrance. To maintain this fine balance requires the integration of the entire respiratory apparatus with the cardiovascular system. The respiratory system needs to respond to inputs from various organs regarding their metabolic needs, thereby optimizing gas exchange for subsequent delivery. Although mathematic models[21-23] have been employed in an attempt to explain the intricacies of respiratory control, these techniques have not yet been able to accurately mimic the complexity of the control system in humans. The respiratory apparatus can be arbitrarily divided into (1) sensors for afferent inputs, (2) the central controller (the central nervous system respiratory center), and (3) the effectors (the lungs and respiratory musculature).

Sensors

Peripheral and central chemoreceptors respond to changes in arterial PO_2, PCO_2, and pH.[24] Whereas the carotid bodies respond to all three stimuli, the aortic bodies appear not to be stimulated with alterations in hydrogen ion concentration, and may in fact be depressed.[25] Despite a high metabolic rate, the carotid body receives a large blood flow (2000 ml/min/100 g tissue) and has an arteriovenous oxygen difference of 0.15 volume%. The glomus cell, the key chemosensor in the carotid body, has well-defined afferent synapses with the carotid sinus branch of the glossopharyngeal nerve. The glomus cell has cytosolic vesicles that are rich in catecholamines, principally dopamine. However, other putative transmitters, such as acetylcholine, norepinephrine, and neuropeptides, are also present in the glomus cell and may also play a role in the response of the carotid body to hypoxia.[26] Recently, several investigations have examined the cellular and molecular mechanisms underlying the chemotransduction pathways. Although the mechanisms remain unclear, recent experiments demonstrate the presence of oxygen-sensitive K^+ and Ca^{+2} channels[27] that influence dopamine release, which in turn is paralleled by an increase in the frequency of carotid sinus nerve action potentials. It appears that the signal transduction process can also be mediated in part by intracellular calcium,[28] G proteins,[29] and phosphatidylinositol.[30] Furthermore, neurons within the carotid body, as well as branches of the carotid sinus and glossopharyngeal nerves, have been shown to have the capacity to synthesize nitric oxide; inhibition of its synthesis results in an augmented chemoreceptor response to hypoxia.[31] The carotid body also receives both sympathetic and parasympathetic efferent input that regulates carotid body blood flow. In summary, the stimulus-response mechanisms of the carotid body, although multifaceted, appear to be well coordinated to transduce sensory inputs to the central controller.

The central chemoreceptors have been localized to three areas on the ventrolateral surface of the medulla and are sensitive to extracellular hydrogen ion concentration. The blood-brain barrier is not freely permeable to either hydrogen ions or bicarbonate, but it is permeable to carbon dioxide. Thus, hypercapnic respiratory acidosis would be a greater stimulus than a comparable degree of metabolic acidosis. A low pH caused by metabolic acidosis stimulates the peripheral chemosensors, resulting in increased ventilation. This lowers arterial P_{CO_2} and consequently elevates cerebrospinal fluid (CSF) pH, producing an attenuation of the ventilatory response to the acidosis. Similarly, the acute ventilatory response to hypoxia through stimulation of the peripheral chemoreceptors would be partially offset by the consequent hypocapnic alkalosis. Understanding this difference in ventilatory drives can be crucial in weaning patients with chronic hypercapnia from mechanical ventilation. A patient with chronic hypercapnia would be expected to have CSF elevations in both carbon dioxide and bicarbonate. Hyperventilation of the patient to a normal P_{CO_2} would in time decrease the CSF P_{CO_2} and bicarbonate concentration. Subsequent attempts to wean the patient would result in an acute rise in both arterial and CSF P_{CO_2}, with a fall in pH. Because the patient's altered lung mechanics would preclude an increase in minute ventilation, acute respiratory failure would ensue.

The central controller also receives inputs from receptors located in the respiratory tract and lungs. The nose, epipharynx, and larynx contain afferent nerve fibers that respond to chemical and mechanical stimulation. The trachea also contains irritant receptors, stimulation of which results in coughing and bronchoconstriction. Within the lung are three major classes of receptors: irritant receptors in the airways, pulmonary stretch receptors that lie in the airway smooth muscle; and the juxtapulmonary capillary receptors, or J-receptors. The pulmonary stretch receptors are also thought to be involved in the Hering-Breuer inspiratory inhibition reflex, whereas the J-receptors are believed to be stimulated by increases in pulmonary interstitial fluid volume. Stimulation of these latter receptors may explain the dyspnea observed in pulmonary edema and interstitial lung diseases. From the muscles of respiration come afferents from Golgi tendon organs in the diaphragm and muscle spindles in both the internal and external intercostals.

Central Controller

The central respiratory controller is located within the central nervous system and composed of the voluntary cortical centers and the automatic centers in the brain stem.[32] Located in the rostral pons are the pneumotaxic center, the apneustic center (in the pontine reticular formation near the pontomedullary border), and the medullary center. The medullary center is grouped into two distinct areas of respiratory neurons, the dorsal respiratory group (DRG) and ventral respiratory group (VRG). The DRG contains primarily inspiratory cells, whereas the VRG consists of both inspiratory and expiratory cells. All the sensory input from the respiratory tract, as well as the peripheral chemoreceptors, is believed to project near or onto the DRG. It is hypothesized that the primary site of respiratory rhythm generation originates from the DRG, which in turn drives the VRG. One potential mechanism to explain the medullary respiratory rhythm invokes rhythmic inhibition of the tonically active expiratory cells by the inspiratory cells of the VRG. Axons from both the DRG and VRG descend in the contralateral spinal cord to synapse with and influence the phrenic nerve and spinal respiratory motor neurons. The pneumotaxic center does not appear to be important in the generation of rhythmic respirations. Its role is believed to be in modulating both phasically and tonically the inspiratory cut-off mechanism during lung inflation. The apneustic center, believed to be the site of the normal inspiratory cutoff switch, receives inputs from the pneumotaxic center. Apneusis, the cessation of rhythmic respiration as a result of prolonged inspiration, arises from damage to this center.

Effectors

The net effect of the sensory input to the respiratory center is to modulate the magnitude of the neuronal discharges to the respiratory apparatus. Quantification of this neuronal output is not easily performed, and surrogate markers have been used, all with some limitations. For example, diaphragmatic electromyograms represent the output to only one of the respiratory muscles and also a process one step removed from the actual neural output. Although phrenic nerve electrical activity is measurable, this is rarely performed in the clinical setting. Measurement of the ventilatory response to either hypoxia[33] or carbon dioxide[34] has been commonly performed as an index of the respiratory drive. The hypoxic response curve has a hyperbolic shape with the $\dot{V}_E$ only beginning to rise when the Pa_{O_2} falls to 50 to 60 mm Hg. On the other hand, the carbon dioxide–response curve is linear, with the chemosensitivity quantified as the slope $\Delta\dot{V}_E/\Delta P_{CO_2}$. However, because ventilation is the output variable, these tests are also influenced by altered lung mechanics. Consequently, they may not accurately reflect respiratory center output. One easily performed clinical measurement that is not influenced by poor airway resistance or lung compliance in the inspiratory mouth pressure that is generated in the first 100 msec (0.1 sec) after the occlusion of the airway (P_{100} or $P_{0.1}$).[35] The subjects must be unaware of the airway occlusion, because their response to the occlusion becomes influential after 0.15 seconds. As an index of the respiratory center output, the P_{100} depends only on the neural output and the effectiveness of the respiratory musculature (the neuromuscular component of the respiratory center output).

PERIOPERATIVE PULMONARY ASSESSMENT

Identification of patients at risk for postoperative respiratory complications remains a challenge for the clinician and surgeon. Although many clinical investigations have focused on patients undergoing lung resectional surgery, studies conducted in patients undergoing nonthoracic surgery have been recently reviewed.[7,36] Many of the earlier reports suffered from the lack of a consensus regarding what constitutes a pulmonary complication. For example, end points such as dyspnea, atelectasis, and sputum production may not be as reliable or important indicators as respiratory failure resulting in prolonged mechanical ventilation, prolonged hospital stay, or death. With these caveats, thoracic and upper-abdominal operations appear to be associated with more postoperative pulmonary complications than procedures performed distant from the thorax. Likewise, the types of intraoperative and postoperative anesthesia and analgesia, as well as their routes of administrations, can affect the development of complications. However, newer surgical techniques, such as laparoscopic cholecystectomy and video-assisted thoracoscopic surgery, appear to be associated with fewer serious respiratory complications.[37,38]

Patients undergoing lung resection are viewed as being at particular risk for respiratory complications. Frequently, patients with bronchogenic carcinoma have underlying lung disease from a prior smoking history. To illustrate this point, a recent multicenter study demonstrated an in-hospital mortality rate of 3.8% after wedge resection, 4.2% after lobectomy, and 11.6% after pneumonectomy.[39] Preoperative pulmonary function testing has been advocated in an attempt to detect individuals at particular risk for postoperative complications. However, routine spirometry is probably not warranted for every patient scheduled for a "low-risk" surgical procedure. With the exception of an arterial P_{CO_2} greater than 45 mm Hg, routine arterial blood gas values do not accurately predict the likelihood of postoperative complications.[40,41] For patients undergoing lung resection surgery, spirometry with diffusing capacity should be performed. Patients with borderline lung function should also be considered for quantitative lung scanning to predict postoperative lung function. In a recent study of 47 patients undergoing either lobectomy or pneumonectomy, there were no deaths among patients with a predicted postoperative FEV_1 of 40% or more than the predicted value, whereas a value less than 40% was associated with a 50% mortality rate.[42] In addition, both the predicted postoperative FEV_1 and diffusing capacity were predictive of serious respiratory complications.[42] Certain patients who do not meet these criteria may still be considered candidates for surgical resection. Several groups have shown that in patients with borderline lung function, performance of an incremental exercise test with measurement of maximal oxygen consumption may be predictive of respiratory complications.[43,44] In a recent study by Morice et al.,[44] patients with lung lesions and either FEV_1 less than 40% predicted, a projected postoperative FEV_1 33% or less than predicted, or an arterial P_{CO_2} greater than 45 mm Hg underwent a graded exercise test. There were no deaths among the patients who achieved a maximal oxygen consumption of 15 ml/kg/minute, and 75% of those patients had uncomplicated postoperative courses.[44]

Other factors have been demonstrated to affect respiratory function after surgery. In one study of 200 patients undergoing elective coronary artery bypass grafting, patients who had stopped smoking for 2 months or less prior to surgery had a fourfold greater pulmonary complication rate than did patients who had stopped for more than 2 months.[45] The complication rate among patients who had ceased smoking for more than 6 months was equal to that among individuals who had never smoked.[45] Postoperative pain control with intercostal nerve block or patient-controlled analgesia results in fewer respiratory complications. Chest physiotherapy, with or without bronchodilators, can also prevent or reverse the hypoxemia from postoperative atelectasis.

SUMMARY

The lungs play a critical role in the supply of oxygen to meet tissue needs. This function is exquisitely controlled by optimally matching lung ventilation to pulmonary perfusion. Although several clinical parameters can be used to assess overall gas exchange and tissue oxygen use, none are sensitive or specific enough in the clinical arena to evaluate the metabolic processes at the organ or tissue level. Abnormal lung mechanics can interfere with gas exchange and significantly increase the work of breathing. These altered lung mechanics may also hinder the weaning of patients from ventilatory support, so the recognition of this potential problem is crucial. Measurement of lung function may allow the clinician to determine which patients are at risk for postoperative respiratory complications. However, these studies might not be warranted in some patients undergoing nonthoracic procedures. Smoking cessation, adequate pain relief, early ambulation, and chest physical therapy are other modalities that can minimize postoperative pulmonary morbidity.

REFERENCES

1. Woodson RD. Hemoglobin concentration and exercise capacity. Am Rev Respir Dis 129(Suppl):72, 1974.
2. Gamsu G, et al. Roentgenographic appearance of the human pulmonary acinus. Invest Radiol 6:171, 1971.
3. Lui YM, Taylor JR, Zylak CJ. Roentgen-anatomical correlation in the individual human pulmonary acinus. Radiology 109:1, 1973.
4. Hedenstierna G, et al. Functional residual capacity, thoracoabdominal dimensions, and central blood volume during general anesthesia with muscle paralysis and mechanical ventilation. Anesthesiology 62:247, 1985.

5. Linderholm H. Lung mechanics in sitting and horizontal postures studied by body plethysmographic methods. Am J Physiol 204:85, 1963.
6. Hedenstierna G, et al. Airway closure in each lung of anesthetized human subjects. J Appl Physiol 50:55, 1981.
7. Zibrak JD, O'Donnell CR. Indications for preoperative pulmonary function testing. Clin Chest Med 14(2):227, 1993.
8. American College of Chest Physicians Consensus Conference. Mechanical ventilation. Chest 104:1833, 1993.
9. Parker JC, Hernandez LA, Peevy KJ. Mechanisms of ventilator-induced lung injury. Crit Care Med 21:131, 1993.
10. Wyszogrodski I, et al. Surfactant inactivation by hyperventilation: Conservation by end-expiratory pressure. J Appl Physiol 38:461, 1975.
11. West JB, Dollery CT, Naimark A. Distribution of blood flow in isolated lung: Relation to vascular and alveolar pressures. J Appl Physiol 19:713, 1964.
12. Wagner PD, et al. Continuous distributions of ventilation-perfusion ratios in normal subjects breathing air and 100% O_2. J Clin Invest 54:54, 1974.
13. Mellemgaard K. The alveolar-arterial oxygen difference: Its size and components in normal man. Acta Physiol Scand 67:10, 1966.
14. Gilbert R, Keighley JF. The arterial/alveolar oxygen tension ratio. An index of gas exchange applicable to varying inspired oxygen concentrations. Am Rev Respir Dis 109:142, 1974.
15. Katz IR, Wittenberg JB, Wittenberg BA. Monamine oxidase: An intracellular probe of oxygen pressure in isolated cardiac myocytes. J Biol Chem 259:7504, 1984.
16. Wittenberg BA, Wittenberg JB. Oxygen pressure gradients in isolated cardiac myocytes. J Biol Chem 260:6548, 1985.
17. Henning RJ, Shubin H, Weil MH. The clinical measurement of the work of breathing for the clinical assessment of ventilator dependence. Crit Care Med 5:264, 1977.
18. MacIntyre NR. Respiratory function during pressure support ventilation. Chest 89:677, 1986.
19. MacIntyre NR. Pressure support ventilation: effects on ventilatory reflexes and ventilatory-muscle workloads. Respir Care 32:447, 1987.
20. Banner MJ, et al. Partially and totally unloading respiratory muscles based on real-time measurements of work of breathing. Chest 106:1835, 1994.
21. Bennett FM. Limitations of the open loop gain concept in studies of respiratory control. Ann Biomed Eng 18:533, 1990.
22. Noshiro M, et al. Nonlinear identification of the P_{CO_2} control system in man. Comput Methods Programs Biomed 40:189, 1993.
23. Saidel GM, Chang YA. CO_2 control of breathing: Parameter estimation and stability evaluation. Med Eng Phys 16:135, 1994.
24. Berger AJ, Mitchell RA, Severinghaus JW. Regulation of respiration. N Engl J Med 297:92, 1977.
25. Sampson SR, Hainsworth R. Responses of aortic body chemoreceptors of the cat to physiological stimuli. Am J Physiol 222:953, 1972.
26. Gonzalez C, et al. Carotid body chemoreceptors: From natural stimuli to sensory discharges. Physiol Rev 74:829, 1994.
27. Montoro RJ, et al. Oxygen sensing by ion channels and chemotransduction in single glomus cells. J Gen Physiol 107:133, 1996.
28. Buckler KJ, Vaughan-Jones RD. Effects of hypoxia on membrane potential and intracellular calcium in rat neonatal carotid body type I cells. J Physiol 476:423, 1994.
29. Cachero TG, et al. Effects of fluoride and cholera and pertussis toxins on sensory transduction in the carotid body. Am J Physiol 269:C1271, 1995.
30. Strosznajder RP. Acute hypoxia modulates arachidonic acid metabolism in cat carotid bodies. Role of dopamine. Acta Neurobiol Exp 56:535, 1996.
31. Wang ZZ, et al. Localization and actions of nitric oxide in the cat carotid body. Neuroscience 60:275, 1994.
32. Berger AJ, Mitchell RA, Severinghaus JW. Regulation of respiration. N Engl J Med 297:138, 1977.
33. Weil JV, et al. Hypoxic ventilatory drive in normal man. J Clin Invest 49:1061, 1970.
34. Read DJC. A clinical method for assessing the ventilatory response to carbon dioxide. Aust Ann Med 16:20, 1967.
35. Whitelaw WA, Derenne JP, Milic-Emili J. Occlusion pressure as a measure of respiratory center output in conscious man. Respir Physiol 23:181, 1975.
36. Wait J. Southwestern Internal Medicine Conference: Preoperative pulmonary evaluation. Am J Med Sci. 310:118, 1995.
37. Meyers MC. Southern Surgeons Club. A prospective analysis of 1518 laparoscopic cholecystectomies. N Engl J Med 324:1073, 1991.
38. Daniel TM, et al. Thoracoscopic surgery for diseases of the lung and pleura. Ann Surg 217:566, 1993.
39. Romano PS, Mark DH. Patient and hospital characteristics related to in-hospital mortality after lung cancer resection. Chest 101:1332, 1992.
40. Olsen GN, et al. Pulmonary function evaluation of the lung resection candidate: A prospective study. Am Rev Respir Dis 111:379, 1975.
41. Tisi GM. Preoperative evaluation of pulmonary function, validity, indications and benefits. Am Rev Respir Dis 119:293, 1979.
42. Markos J, et al. Preoperative assessment as a predictor of mortality and morbidity after lung resection. Am Rev Respir Dis 139:902, 1989.
43. Smith TP, et al. Exercise capacity as a predictor of post-thoracotomy morbidity. Am Rev Respir Dis 129:730, 1984.
44. Morice RC, et al. Exercise testing in the evaluation of patients at high risk for complications from lung resection. Chest 101:356, 1992.
45. Warner MA, et al. Role of preoperative cessation of smoking and other factors in postoperative pulmonary complications: A blinded prospective study of coronary artery bypass patients. Mayo Clin Proc 64:609, 1989.

36

Common Pulmonary Derangements, Respiratory Failure, and Adult Respiratory Distress Syndrome

J. David Richardson

The understanding of pulmonary derangements is of critical importance for the surgeon involved in the care of seriously ill patients of any type. Discussion of pulmonary dysfunction in the surgical patient must be limited in scope because of the myriad abnormalities that affect the lung. This chapter focuses on the functional anatomy and physiology of the lung, respiratory failure (particularly adult respiratory distress syndrome [ARDS]), and other topics of pulmonary physiology commonly encountered by surgeons.

FUNCTIONAL ANATOMY OF THE LUNG

The trachea and major airways act as conduits for the passage of air into the lungs where gas exchange actually occurs. However, the trachea and major bronchi are not merely passive conduits through which air passes. They perform an important function in the protection of the lungs from inhaled particles. The mucociliary action of the major airways is one of the first barriers in the lung's defense mechanism. The trachea branches into the main stem bronchi, and subsequently the airways undergo 22 to 25 subdivisions with the last 8 to 10 sequential divisions occurring within the lung parenchyma. The terminal bronchioles are present at about the sixteenth division and are the most distal airways to have continuous mucosal lining. Respiratory bronchioles with partial mucosal lining alternating with alveoli are distal to the terminal bronchioles. The alveolar ducts are next in succession and eventually terminate in the alveolar sacs. These successive branchings of the airways provide a huge surface area for potential gas exchange. There are approximately 300 million alveoli with a surface area of 7 m^2 in the adult lung.[1]

The mucosa consists of an epithelial lining, basement membrane, and lamina propria. Pseudostratified columnar epithelium lines the large airways and consists of ciliated cells and goblet cells. The goblet cells secrete mucus, and the ciliated cells actively propel particulate matter proximally toward the trachea. Each ciliated cell contains approximately 200 cilia that are capable of 1000 beats/min. It is estimated that the mucus produced by the goblet cells is propelled along with entrapped particles toward the mouth at a rate of 10 to 20 mm/min. This provides the first barrier in the lungs' defense system for particles that have reached the tracheobronchial tree. Other goblet cells are present in the respiratory mucosa and produce immunologically active substances such as IgA. There are numerous speculations about the potential role of this immunoglobulin in lung defense, but the exact function is not known.

The next line of host defense in the lung consists of the alveolar macrophage. The origin of the pulmonary macrophage is from both the interstitial tissue of the alveolar wall and from within the alveolus itself. The pulmonary macrophage apparently arises from a pluripotential cell such as a circulating monocyte and differentiates into a mature macrophage or remains dormant until needed for macrophage differentiation. Pulmonary macrophages actively engulf bacteria and inert particles. They are endowed with an elaborate enzyme system that allows them to engulf and to complete intracellular killing of engulfed microorganisms. In experimental systems the alveolar macrophages are capable of engulfing and killing 95% of aerosolized bacteria within 4 hours of exposure to the organism.[2]

In addition to macrophages there are four other major cellular components of the alveolar wall: two types of epithelial cells, fibroblasts, and endothelial cells. The two types of epithelial cells lining the alveoli are referred to as type I and type II pneumocytes. The type I cells are thin in shape and cover most of the alveolar surface. Electron microscopic studies demonstrate few intracellular organelles, and type I cells appear to be relatively inert. The thin layer and low metabolic activity suggest that these cells have adapted to yield maximum oxygen exchange with a minimum of caloric expenditure.[3]

Type II pneumocytes are cuboidal in shape, are fewer

in number and cover less surface area than type I epithelium, have an abundance of intracellular organelles, and are metabolically active. The type II cell has at least two critical functions. The first is production of a surfactant that is a lipoprotein containing large amounts of saturated lecithins. Lipoprotein is a surface-active compound that stabilizes the surface tension existing between the air-tissue interface in the lung. The surfactant has an extremely short half-life and thus must be constantly produced by the type II cells. These cells apparently are able to store surfactant in organelles and release this substance as needed, providing the cell is not injured by a process such as ARDS. The second function of type II pneumocytes is a replicative one, since they alone have the ability to regenerate after a lung injury such as ARDS. In the pathologic condition of ARDS, necrosis of type I cells rapidly occurs, and only type II cells are seen until the reparative process is well under way (see discussion of adult respiratory distress syndrome). Type II cells appear to have the potential of regenerating new type I cells.

Fibroblasts are the fourth cellular element located within the alveolar wall. They are thought to produce the connective tissue stroma that provides the architectural framework for the lung. These cells are relatively inert during periods of normal lung function, but they may be activated by a number of stimuli, resulting in severe fibrosis in cases of idiopathic pulmonary fibrosis and ARDS.

The fifth cellular component is the endothelial cell, which lines the extensive alveolocapillary membrane. These cells are water permeable but do not readily permit passage of macromolecules under ordinary circumstances. The metabolic role of the endothelial cells is continuing to be elucidated, but it is known that these cells secrete prostaglandins and have the potential to deactivate many bioactive compounds such as histamine and serotonin.

NORMAL FUNCTION OF THE LUNG

Ventilation

The force that moves air into or out of the lung is the pressure relationship between the alveoli and the atmosphere. Changes in alveolar pressure are primarily dictated by inspiratory and expiratory muscle activity. When alveolar pressure is greater than atmospheric pressure, the air is expelled and the lungs deflated. Conversely, a fall in alveolar pressure below that of atmospheric pressure assures a movement of air into the alveoli, and the lungs expand. Thus the pressure relationships dictate flow, although flow can be modified by resistance changes within the airway system. Muscular activity by the intercostal muscles and diaphragm cause enlargement of the thoracic cage and a decrease in intrapleural pressure. The rapidity and degree of inspiratory effort largely determines the rate of flow and volume of air delivered to the alveoli. During normal quiet ventilation, expiration occurs passively—until the static recoil pressure of the lung that is imparted by the active inspiratory phase of ventilation is negated by the outward recoil pressure of the chest wall. At this point the intra-alveolar pressure should equal atmospheric pressure, and expiration ceases until voluntary contraction of expiratory muscles occurs, resulting in an increased intrapleural and hence increased intra-alveolar pressure, which results in an active expiratory effort.

Tests of Ventilation

There are myriad tests of ventilation, and a discussion of many of them is beyond the scope of this chapter. I only consider some of the more common and clinically useful tests of lung function. The simplest and most informative test of ventilation relies on forced expiration. The forced expiratory volume (FEV) is that volume of gas that can be exhaled over a unit of time (usually 1 second: FEV_1). The forced vital capacity (FVC) represents the total volume of gas that can be exhaled after a full inspiration. The relationship between the FEV_1 and the FVC can be useful in determining normal lung dynamics or an obstructive or restrictive pattern (Table 36-1). The values shown in Table 36-1 indicate that a normal 70 kg person exhales about 80% of a roughly 5 L FVC in 1 second. Patients with either obstructive or restrictive pulmonary diseases have a decreased FVC, but the relationship of the FEV_1 to the FVC varies greatly. In obstructive lung disease the percent of exhaled gas in 1 second is relatively low; in a restrictive pattern the percent exhaled within 1 second is relatively high.

Disease processes that increase airway resistance have a dramatic effect on the FEV. Causes of increased airway resistance include asthma, chemical irritants, cigarette smoke, chronic bronchitis with structural changes in the airway, and airway obstruction secondary to a foreign body or retained bronchial secretions. Patients with chronic obstructive lung disease secondary to chronic bronchitis or emphysema have several factors that affect pulmonary function and the delayed FEV_1/FVC. The mucosal lining of the airways may be thickened, and that, combined with excessive secretions, leads to increased pulmonary resistance to air flow. Actual destruction of lung tissue may occur with a decrease in the number of small airways of the terminal bronchioles and secondary increased resistance. Additionally, even though the lung volume may be greatly increased with emphysema, there is a loss of normal elastic recoil of the lung. As alveolar walls lose structural integrity, there is a tendency for collapse of the smaller airways because of a loss of support from the lung paren-

Table 36-1. Relationship of Forced Expiration Patterns to Pulmonary Disease

	FEV_1 (L)	FVC (L)	Percent
Normal	4	5	80
Obstructive	1.4	3.3	39
Restrictive	3	3.3	90

FEV_1, Forced expiratory volume; *FVC*, forced vital capacity.

chyma. All these factors tend to increase airway resistance and thus act as an obstruction to normal gas flow within the airway.

Restrictive lung disease usually occurs because of interstitial fibrosis. The total volume of the lung is reduced, but the elastic recoil pressure of the lung is high; therefore the FEV_1/FVC is high. In the clinical situation there is a great deal of overlap between obstructive and restrictive disorders, and mixed patterns of lung disease are extremely common. Thus these illustrations represent an oversimplification of the disease process involved.

Compliance of the lung is represented by an expression that defines a change in volume for a given change in pressure. This change in volume is greatly affected by changes in small airways that produce increased resistance. This concept of decreased compliance or stiff lungs is discussed extensively in the section on ARDS.

Certain terms are necessary to understand the concept of ventilation. The first of these terms is *total ventilation.* Total ventilation represents the additive effects of *alveolar ventilation* and *total dead space ventilation.* It must be remembered that when gas is taken into the lungs, only a portion goes to the alveoli to participate in gas exchange at the alveolocapillary membrane. The volume of gas that goes to the alveoli is called *alveolar ventilation.* A certain amount of gas fills the conducting airways and is designated *anatomic dead space ventilation.* There may also be a portion of gas that goes to alveoli that are not perfused and therefore cannot participate in gas exchange; such alveolar gas is referred to as *physiologic dead space.* The elimination of carbon dioxide is directly related to alveolar ventilation but may not be directly related to total ventilation, since an increase in dead space must cause an increase in total ventilation if the alveolar ventilation is to remain constant. Therefore simple determination of minute ventilation does not necessarily provide accurate information about the adequacy of alveolar ventilation. However, the effectiveness of alveolar ventilation can be simply determined by measurement of arterial partial pressure of carbon dioxide (PCO_2) and increases or decreases in PCO_2 reflect hypoventilation or hyperventilation, respectively, at the alveolar level.

The body has an elaborate system for the maintenance of PCO_2 within a narrow normal range by alterations as needed in the alveolar ventilation. An increase in PCO_2 causes an increased diffusion of carbon dioxide into the cerebrospinal fluid (CSF), resulting in a decrease in CSF pH. This decrease in CSF pH stimulates ventilation through central chemoreceptor neurons located in the medulla. Conversely, a decrease in PCO_2 increases the pH and depresses respiration by the same mechanism. Diaphragmatic excursion accounts for muscular activity necessary for adequate ventilation during quiet resting ventilation. As the minute ventilation increases, accessory muscles of respiration, including abdominal and intercostal musculature, must be used.

Exchange of Oxygen and Carbon Dioxide

The exchange of oxygen and carbon dioxide is the principal function of the lungs and requires a coordinated effort of the individual components of the respiratory cycle to proceed smoothly. Respiratory muscle function, nondiseased airways, alveoli, and normal pulmonary vasculature must be present if the gases and blood are to reach the critical point of gas exchange at the alveolocapillary level. Figure 36-1 illustrates the pressure relationships between the alveolar and blood interface that allow gas exchange. The oxygen tissue tension is approximately 40 mm Hg,

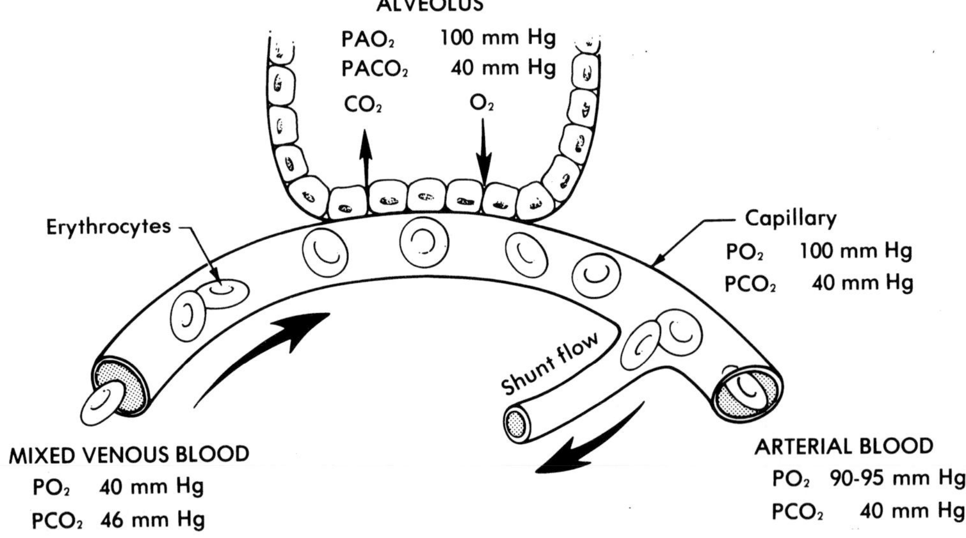

Fig. 36-1. Relationship between driving pressures for oxygen *(O_2)* and carbon dioxide *(CO_2)* exchange at alveolocapillary membranes. *$PaCO_2$,* Partial pressure of arterial carbon dioxide; *PaO_2,* partial pressure of arterial oxygen; *PCO_2,* partial pressure of carbon dioxide; *PO_2,* partial pressure of oxygen.

and that of the alveoli is 100 mm Hg, allowing a 60 mm Hg gradient for adequate gas exchange. Carbon dioxide is approximately 25 times more soluble than oxygen. Thus the gradient difference between arterial carbon dioxide (40 mm Hg) and venous carbon dioxide (46 mm Hg) permits adequate carbon dioxide uptake by tissues and exchange at the alveolus.

The oxygen requirements for resting human adults is approximately 150 to 250 ml/min. The volume of oxygen carried in the blood is dependent on the concentration of hemoglobin, and the partial pressure of oxygen (Po_2) with 1 g of hemoglobin binding is about 1.34 ml of oxygen. About 98% of oxygen is transported as oxyhemoglobin, and only a small amount of oxygen or carbon dioxide is carried in a simple solution. The oxygen-carrying capacity is therefore markedly affected in cases of severe anemia in which the hemoglobin concentration is greatly reduced. Therefore 15 g of hemoglobin that is 97% saturated transports 20 volumes percent of oxygen, whereas 7.5 g of hemoglobin of equal saturation carries only 10 volumes percent of oxygen. The transport of oxygen is also affected by the oxyhemoglobin desaturation curve (see Chapter 35 for more detailed discussion). The Po_2, for example, at 50% saturation (P_{50}) at a temperature of 37.5° C and a plasma pH of 7.4 is 26.5 mm Hg. Increasing the percent saturation from approximately 50% to 90% results in a marked increase in Po_2 (i.e., the steep portion of the oxyhemoglobin saturation curve). However, once the saturation reaches about 90%, there is a relatively small incremental change in Po_2 because of the flatness of the curve at this point. Increases in temperature and decreases in plasma pH result in a shift of this curve to the right with a greater degree of oxygen in solution. The chemical intermediary that is present within the red blood cell and is responsible for oxygen transport appears to be 2,3-diphosphoglyceric acid (2,3-DPG). Oxygen forms a bond with this substance, allowing much more oxygen to be transported by erythrocytes than would be carried dissolved in a simple solution. This bond between oxygen and 2,3-DPG is not stable, and the oxygen can be released or "off-loaded" from the molecule under conditions such as decreased pH. The storage of blood results in a marked decrease in the concentration of 2,3- DPG and a decrease in the P_{50}.

Hypoxemia

Hypoxemia is rarely caused by abnormalities in oxygen-diffusing ability, although such an abnormality may be a cofactor with other mechanisms. The common causes of hypoxemia are alveolar hypoventilation, ventilation-perfusion ($\dot{V}A/\dot{Q}$) mismatching, or an increase in the intrapulmonary shunts.

The alveoloarterial gradient ($A\text{-}aDo_2$) may be useful in determining the oxygen exchange across the lung. Ordinarily, the $A\text{-}aDo_2$ is less than 20 mm Hg, with this difference resulting from the 5% of cardiac output that normally shunts across the lung without being oxygenated. The $A\text{-}aDo_2$ may be calculated after breathing 100% oxygen for 20 minutes and is useful in determining the cause of hypoxemia.

The causes of alveolar hypoventilation are indicated in the accompanying box. In alveolar hypoventilation that results in hypoxemia, the hypoxemia is caused by a direct decrease in the Po_2 in the alveoli and therefore must be reflected in a decreased Po_2 at the arterial level. Thus there is no abnormality of oxygen exchange across the lung, and the $A\text{-}aDo_2$ is normal in alveolar hypoventilation (Table 36-2). In ventilation-perfusion mismatching, the capillary blood is directed to alveoli that are being ventilated where the ventilation-perfusion ratio is less than 1. Thus the blood from low ventilation areas has a Po_2 that is less than normal. As the amount of ventilation-perfusion inequality increases, there is a greater likelihood that hypoxemia will result. In this situation increasing the inspired oxygen content (Fio_2) increases the Po_2, since the alveoli are being ventilated. In fact, raising the Fio_2 to higher levels results in an $A\text{-}aDo_2$ that is nearly normal.

Shunting of blood represents a different situation, since blood perfuses the capillaries of alveoli that are not ventilated. Therefore there is no potential for oxygen transport in this situation, and increases in Fio_2 do not produce concomitant increases in Po_2. In fact, if the shunt fraction increases to greater than 30%, the rise in Fio_2 to 1 has virtu-

CAUSES OF ALVEOLAR HYPOVENTILATION

Thoracic Wall and Neuromuscular Abnormalities

Trauma
Kyphoscoliosis
Obesity
Guillain-Barré syndrome
Myasthenia gravis
Neuromuscular blockade (such as curare)
Poliomyelitis (anterior horn cell disease)
Bilateral diaphragmatic paralysis
Severe malnutrition (muscular atrophy)
Myxedema
Pleural restrictive disease
Upper airway obstruction

Central Respiratory Depression

Idiopathic hypoventilation
Sleep apnea syndrome
Pickwickian syndrome
Central nervous system–altering drugs (opiates, sedatives, anesthetics)
Central nervous system trauma } Medulla abnormality
Central nervous system infections } Medulla abnormality
Stroke

Table 36-2. Evaluation of Hypoxemia

Causes of Hypoxemia	Pathologic Process	PCO_2 Level	Response of PO_2 to Increased FIO_2	A-aDO_2
Alveolar hypoventilation	Decreased PaO_2 and subsequent PO_2	Elevated	Rises	Normal (<20 mm Hg; PAO_2 >500 mm Hg FIO_2 = 1)
Ventilation-perfusion mismatching	Higher percentage of pulmonary blood flow perfusing portions of lung with ventilation-perfusion ratio <1 Lower percentage of fully oxygenated blood and resultant hypoxemia	Normal or decreased	Rises	Near normal with high FIO_2 (PAO_2 >500 mm Hg if FIO_2 = 1)
Shunting	Blood perfusing capillary bed of unventilated alveoli	Normal or decreased	No change	Marked difference that increases as percentage of blood increases

A-aDO₂, Alveoloarterial gradient; *FIO₂*, fraction of inspired oxygen; *PaO₂*, partial pressure of arterial oxygen; *PCO₂*, partial pressure of carbon dioxide; *PO₂*, partial pressure of oxygen.

ally no effect. The shunt fraction can be calculated by the formula:

$$\frac{Qs}{Qt} = \frac{O_2\text{ Content capillary} - \text{Arterial } O_2 \text{ content}}{O_2 \text{ Content capillary} - \text{Mixed venous } O_2 \text{ content}}$$

where Qs is the shunt flow, and QT is the total flow.

The arterial oxygen content and mixed venous oxygen content can be calculated from measurements of the partial pressure and percent saturation of the arterial and mixed venous blood obtained from a pulmonary artery catheter. The capillary oxygen content is more difficult to ascertain accurately, since its measurement is based on the assumption that either the arteriovenous difference for oxygen is fixed or that the partial pressure of oxygen at the arterial and capillary level is 100% saturated. Neither of these assumptions is likely to be true with respiratory failure, and thus formulas used to calculate shunt fraction may introduce error. Therefore if the patient has a major shunt, there is relatively little effect from increasing the FIO_2. Likewise, both ventilation-perfusion abnormalities and shunts may be present in the same patient, and the relative contribution of each is difficult to determine without very sophisticated techniques that are not clinically practical.

CLINICAL DISORDERS OF THE LUNG

Acute Respiratory Failure

There is no uniform definition of respiratory failure that would be applicable to all patients, since age, presence of chronic pulmonary disease, and inspired oxygen concentration greatly affect the patient's blood gas status. For this discussion I define acute respiratory failure as acute dyspnea, PO_2 of less than 50 mm Hg while breathing room air, PO_2 greater than 50 mm Hg, and a decreased arterial pH (<7.35). Not all patients have all these findings; however, two are usually present, and hypoxemia is the most important of these.[4]

Respiratory failure has been divided into types I and II. Patients with type I respiratory failure have hypoxemia with a normal or low PCO_2. This type of failure is more common in patients with ARDS and usually is accompanied by poor lung compliance. Patients with type II respiratory failure have both hypoxemia and hypercapnia. These conditions usually result from chronic obstructive lung disease or central nervous system defects resulting in alveolar hypoventilation.

The causes of acute respiratory failure may range from defects in the brain or spinal cord to the level of the alveolus. The myriad causes of acute respiratory failure are shown in the box on p. 743. The type I pattern of respiratory failure is of greater clinical importance to surgeons than type II, and the problem of ARDS is discussed in detail in the following section.

Adult Respiratory Distress Syndrome

ARDS was described in 1967 by Ashbaugh et al.[5] in 12 adult patients with the clinical features of dyspnea, hypoxemia, decreased pulmonary compliance, and diffuse alveolar infiltrates that resembled pulmonary edema even though there was no prior history of lung disease or congestive heart failure. The term *ARDS* was derived because Ashbaugh et al. believed that a defect in surfactant metabolism in adults similar to that seen in premature infants might be responsible for the abnormalities observed. Although decreased surfactant levels have been measured in bronchopulmonary lavage fluid from patients with ARDS, it is believed that these changes are secondary rather than primary factors in its cause. Moore et al.[6] described the clinical behavior of pulmonary insufficiency following shock and trauma and began to identify many factors that were thought to be contributory, including fluid overload, massive blood transfusion, thromboembolism, fat embolism, and aspiration.

CAUSES OF ACUTE RESPIRATORY FAILURE

Brain

Stroke
Bulbar poliomyelitis
Drug overdose (such as narcotics)
Central alveolar hypoventilation
Anesthetic depression
Cerebral edema
Myxedema

Spinal Cord

Guillain-Barré syndrome
Spinal cord trauma
Poliomyelitis
Amyotrophic lateral sclerosis

Neuromuscular System

Myasthenia gravis
Tetanus
Curare-like agents
Neuromuscular blocking antibiotics
Botulism
Organophosphate insecticides
Peripheral neuritis
Multiple sclerosis
Severe depletion—K^+, Mg^+, PO_4

Thorax and Pleura

Muscular dystrophy
Massive obesity
Kyphoscoliosis
Flail chest
Rheumatoid spondylitis
Pneumothorax
Pleural effusion

Upper Airway

Sleep apnea (obstruction)
Tonsillar hypertrophy
Vocal cord paralysis
Tracheal obstruction
Epiglottitis
Laryngeal edema

Cardiovascular

Cardiogenic pulmonary edema
Pulmonary embolism
Uremia

Lower Airway and Alveoli

Aspiration
Smoke inhalation
Severe asthma
Chronic obstructive lung disease
Adult respiratory distress syndrome
Pulmonary fibrosis
Cystic fibrosis
Bilateral pneumonia
Atelectasis
Pulmonary contusion
Fat embolism syndrome
Near drowning
Radiation injury
Pancreatitis
Microembolization

The critical role of sepsis in the cause of ARDS was defined by Fulton and Jones[7] in an evaluation of injured patients at the University of Louisville. In a study of 399 high-risk trauma patients, ARDS developed in 44 patients. Sepsis was present in 40 of the 44 patients and appeared to be the primary causative factor along with a history of shock, direct chest injury, and several of the factors previously noted. The important role of sepsis, which is often occult at the time pulmonary insufficiency develops, was confirmed by Walker and Eiseman.[8] Thus a hallmark of prevention or control of ARDS is prevention and/or treatment of sepsis, even though this has been an elusive goal.

It appears that ARDS represents a final common pathway to a variety of noxious stimuli or injuries to the lung.[9,10] Potential causes of ARDS include the following:

Air embolism
Aspiration
Burns
Cardiopulmonary bypass
Drug overdose
Disseminated intravascular coagulation
Eclampsia
Fat embolism syndrome
Near-drowning
Oxygen toxicity
Pancreatitis
Pulmonary contusion
Sepsis
Smoke inhalation
Trauma

Some common features of ARDS are frequently used to describe symptoms in a variety of syndromes that in part may be related to ARDS, including shock lung, wet lung, Da Nang lung, noncardiogenic pulmonary edema, capillary leak syndrome, pulmonary contusion, congestive atelectasis, and adult hyaline membrane disease. ARDS is a clinical syndrome, and thus clinical criteria must be used for diagnosis, since there is no single laboratory test that can be equated with the condition. Diagnostic criteria may vary slightly from one clinical series to another but generally include the following[11,12]:

1. History of an event resulting in respiratory failure
2. Exclusion of pulmonary or cardiac disease as the primary cause of the respiratory failure
3. Respiratory distress as manifested by dyspnea, hypoxemia, and tachypnea
4. Diffuse pulmonary infiltrates on chest radiograph
5. PO_2 less than 50 mm Hg with FIO_2 concentration greater than 0.6, reduced pulmonary compliance, increased shunt fraction, and increased dead space ventilation

Several studies have refined the risk factors thought to contribute to ARDS. Fowler et al.[13] prospectively followed 936 patients with a variety of conditions thought to predispose to ARDS, including sepsis, cardiopulmonary bypass, multiple transfusions, pulmonary contusion, pelvic fracture, severe pneumonia, disseminated intravascular coagulation, and aspiration of gastric contents. The incidence of ARDS for those with a single risk factor was 5.8%, but the addition of multiple factors increased the risk of ARDS to 24.6%. The lowest risk factor was cardiopulmonary bypass, whereas sepsis was the highest. A study by Pepe et al.[11] in Seattle confirmed the additive effect of multiple risk factors on the likelihood of the development of ARDS.

One of the difficulties of dealing with clinical trials regarding ARDS has been the clinical variability in using the above described definition for this disorder. Similarly, the above definition does not provide an index of the severity of the disorder. With this in mind, Murray et al.[14] expanded the definition of ARDS and offered a scoring system that would allow for better staging of the disease. The scoring system uses a score of "0 to 4," which evaluates chest x-ray consolidation, the hypoxemia ratio, the amount of positive end-expiratory pressure (PEEP) required, and the respiratory compliance when measured (Table 36-3). The use of such a scoring system better allows comparisons between those with a moderate illness and those with severe life-threatening ARDS. The use of such scoring may explain some of the reported discrepancies in the incidence of this disorder as well.

Pathology

One of the reasons commonly given for inclusion of a variety of insults in the definition of ARDS is that the lung seems to respond to diverse injuries in a remarkably constant pathologic nature.[15] However, the simplistic approach that ARDS merely represents noncardiac pulmonary edema or capillary leak is probably not realistic in light of the complex pathologic process that occurs.[16] The pathologic phases of ARDS are listed below and illustrated in Figs. 36-2 to 36-6:

1. Phase 1 (early reversible)
   a. Interstitial edema
   b. Fibrin deposition in pulmonary microvasculature
   c. ±Alveolar edema
   d. Grossly heavy, edematous, ±hemorrhagic
2. Phase 2 (early progressive)
   a. Perialveolar hyaline membranes
   b. Capillary congestion
   c. Interstitial edema

Table 36-3. Scoring of Adult Respiratory Distress Syndrome

Score	No. of Quadrants With Alveolar Consolidation on Chest X-Ray Examination	Ratio Pa_{O_2}/F_{IO_2} (torr)	PEEP Score (cm H_2O)	Respiratory Compliance (ml/cm H_2O)
0	0	>300	≤5	≤80
1	1	225-299	6-8	60-79
2	2	175-224	9-11	40-59
3	3	100-174	12-14	20-39
4	4	<100	≥15	≤19

Adapted from Murray JF, Matthay MA, Luce JM. An expanded definition of the adult respiratory distress syndrome. Am Rev Respir Dis 138:720, 1988. Official journal of the American Thoracic Society. Copyright © American Lung Association.
F_{IO_2}, Fraction of inspired oxygen; *Pa_{O_2}*, partial pressure of arterial oxygen; *PEEP*, positive end-expiratory pressure.

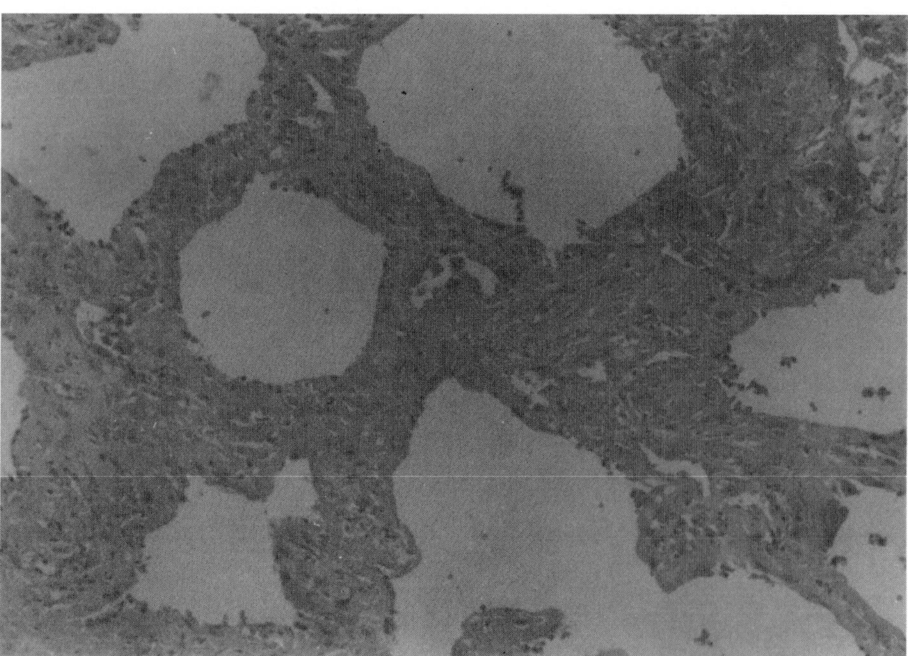

Fig. 36-2. Low-power view of resolving adult respiratory distress syndrome with marked thickening of airways but resolution of hyaline membranes.

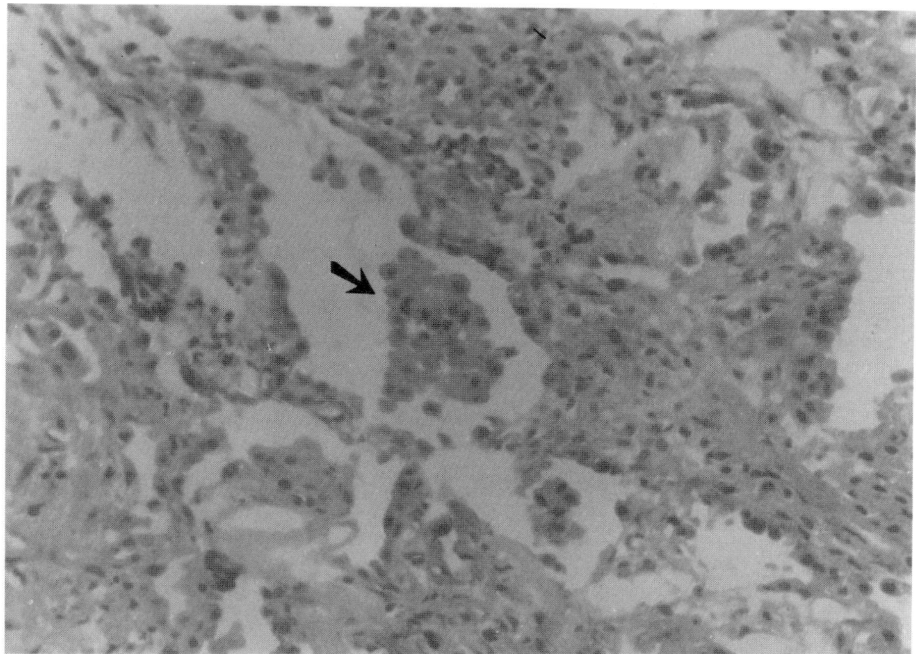

Fig. 36-3. Early phase of adult respiratory distress syndrome characterized by thickened alveoli and sloughing of pneumocytes into alveolus *(arrow)*.

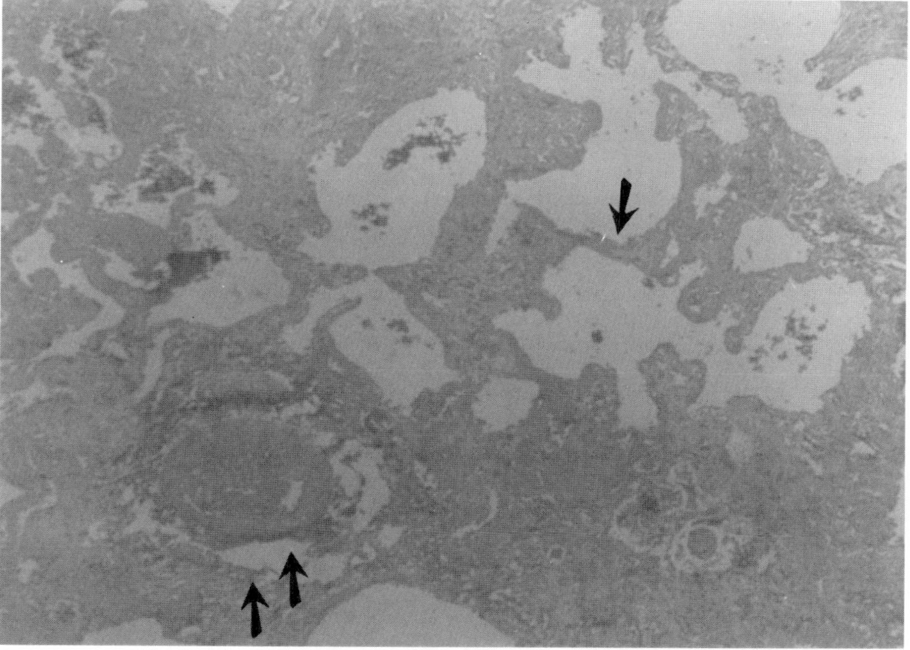

Fig. 36-4. Hyaline membranes *(single arrow)* noted around alveoli, but alveoli are still distinguishable histologically. Vessel thrombosis *(double arrow)* contributes to increased pulmonary artery pressure.

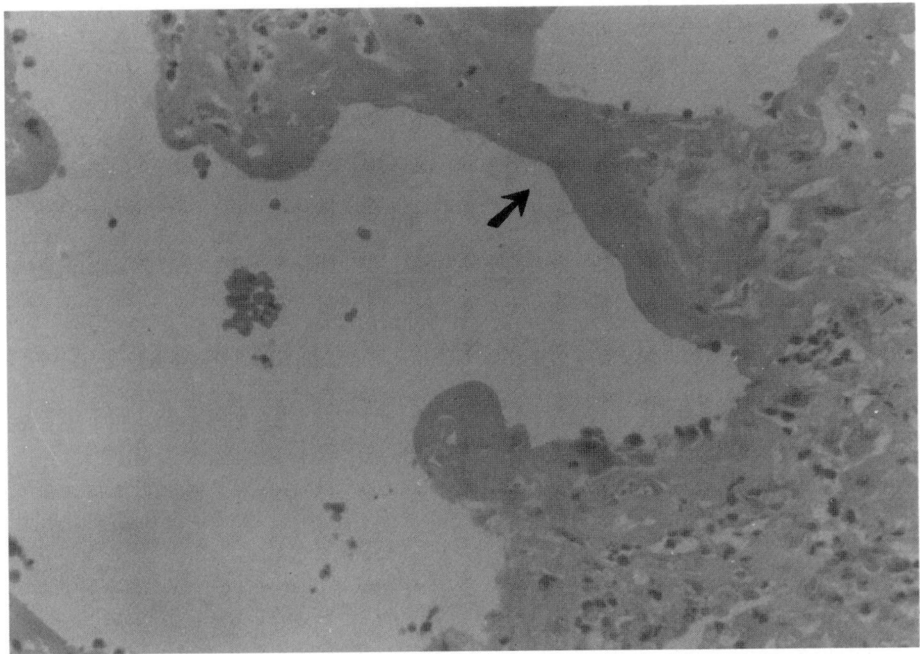

Fig. 36-5. A close view of changes in hyaline membrane *(arrow)* around alveolar wall.

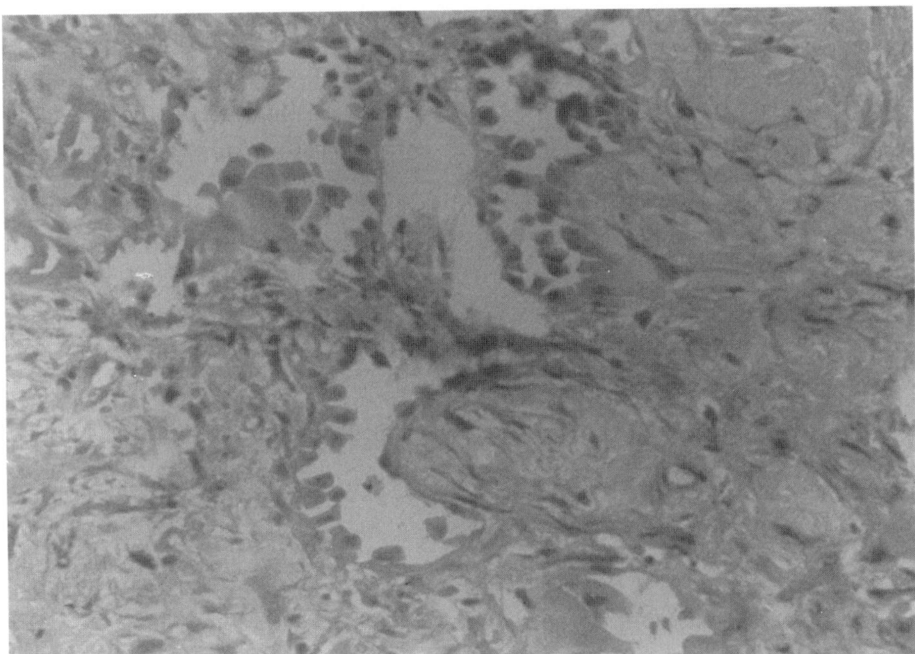

Fig. 36-6. Later stages of adult respiratory distress syndrome reveal alveolar wall nearly destroyed, walls markedly thickened, and loss of capillaries.

3. Phase 3 (late progressive)
   a. Decreased congestion and edema
   b. Perialveolar interstitial fibrosis
   c. Increased type II pneumocytes
   d. Decreased number of capillaries
4. Phase 4 (resolving)
   a. Gradually improving architecture
   b. Decreased fibrosis

The type I alveolar-lining cell is more prone to injury than the type II cuboidal cell, and the type I cells rapidly undergo necrosis. In the earliest phase of ARDS, alveolar edema and interstitial edema are present. There is active deposition of fibrin, platelets, and leukocytes. The second phase is characterized by hyaline membranes rich in eosinophilic-staining material, which surrounds the alveolar ducts. This phase usually occurs 4 to 5 days after the inciting event that produced ARDS. The late progressive phase is characterized by increased interstitial fibrosis and an increase in type II pneumocytes. These type II cells proliferate, resulting in a thickened alveolar septum. Superinfection with bacteria or fungi may also occur, further complicating the pathologic condition. The final phase leads either to further fibrosis and eventual death or to gradual resolution of the process, presumably resulting from the action of scavenger alveolar macrophages. Interstitial fibrosis and intra-alveolar fibrosis centered primarily around the alveolar ducts appear to be the major long-term consequence of ARDS. These changes occur rapidly, and increased collagen contact was noted in the lungs of all patients who survived more than 12 days.

Parallels have been drawn between idiopathic pulmonary fibrosis and ARDS. Each is characterized by acute alveolar injury manifested by interstitial inflammation, hemorrhage, and edema, followed by a proliferative phase with an increase in type II pneumocytes, culminating in the eventual loss of the alveolar structure and subsequent fibrosis. A variety of mechanisms have been implicated as potential mediators of the fibrotic response even though the exact cause is uncertain. It is known that alveolar macrophages are capable of stimulating fibroblast proliferation and may act to increase pulmonary fibrosis. Whether they initiate the fibrosis in ARDS remains to be defined.

Pathophysiology

The initial inciting event in the production of ARDS is believed to occur from a capillary leak presumably resulting from damage to the pulmonary capillary endothelium[17,18] as previously discussed. Potential causes of the capillary endothelial injury are the following:

1. Direct injury
    a. Toxins (gases, inhalants)
    b. Acid aspiration
    c. Oxygen toxicity
2. Granulocyte injury
    a. Oxygen-free radicals (complement mediated)
    b. Proteolytic enzymes
    c. Platelet activating factor
    d. Arachidonic acid metabolites
3. Arachidonic acid pathway
    a. Leukotriene
    b. Thromboxane
    c. Prostaglandin
4. By-product of coagulation
    a. Fibrin
    b. Fibrin degradation products

Protein-rich fluid leaks into the interstitium and Starling forces result in accumulation of edematous fluid. Eventually, alveolar edema occurs as the tension in the alveolar wall is overcome. Surfactant abnormalities then develop, and widespread alveolar collapse occurs with a resultant noncompliant or stiff lung. Profound hypoxemia then develops as a result of shunting and ventilation-perfusion mismatch. Presumably the shunt occurs because of blood flow through areas of severe alveolar edema and collapse. Noncompliant lungs are clinically reflected by the high-peak pressures required to deliver an adequate tidal volume. The combination of interstitial and alveolar edema along with the active bronchoconstriction induced by arachidonic acid metabolites is the most likely cause for the loss of lung compliance.

Pathogenesis of interstitial edema formation. It is important to recognize what appear to be two separate reactions responsible for the formation of interstitial edema that may occur in patients who undergo shock, trauma, infection, or a variety of other noxious insults. An initial reaction occurs within seconds and results from functional alterations that may be entirely reversible. On the other hand, a *delayed reaction,* which may occur after several hours, is associated with specific changes within the wall of the capillary endothelial interface that may result in more permanent and long-lasting changes. The vasoconstriction that occurs after early leukocyte adherence results primarily in veno-constriction with elevation of capillary filtration pressures.[19] Thromboxane and other mediators cause a rapid increase in capillary filtration by producing a functional loosening or increasing in pore size of the interendothelial junctions. This, in combination with increased filtration pressures, causes a rapid increase in capillary filtration and an increase in pulmonary lymph production, which is noted with experimental injury.

The ongoing production of proteinases from the granulocytes and macrophages, however, begins to destroy the vessel wall and leads to a low-pressure edema and capillary leak, which is an ongoing process. This later capillary vascular leakage is caused by structural changes within the vessel wall itself in contrast to the functional changes that occur early after stimulation of the inflammatory pathways.

Lung volumes are also decreased with ARDS.[20] The mechanisms responsible for decreased lung volume might include fluid-filled alveoli, atelectasis, compression of alveoli by interstitial edema, and surfactant abnormalities with resultant increased surface tension.

Although the specific causes of ARDS are unknown, intense investigation has yielded much information about the potential physiologic mechanisms responsible for this disorder (or as the case may be, this group of disorders). One of the observations that led to a current theory on the pathogenesis of ARDS was made in the late 1960s regarding dialysis patients.[21] It was noted that patients developed severe leukopenia while undergoing hemodialysis. It was initially supposed that the leukocytes were trapped on the cellophane membrane of the dialyzer; however, it was later observed that many of these patients had a marked decrease in Po_2 at the time the leukocyte count decreased. A search for the mechanism of this sequence of events prompted a series of laboratory experiments in which sheep plasma exposed to a hemodialyzer was reinfused into the animals. These animals developed both sudden profound leukopenia and pulmonary dysfunction. Examination of fresh lung specimens from these sheep disclosed that the pulmonary vasculature was filled with leukocytes, particularly granulocytes and monocytes, such as were depleted from the blood.[22,23]

The use of the sheep lymph fistula model[24] produced much of the physiologic framework for the current theories on the pathogenesis of ARDS. It was observed in such experimental preparations that the infusion of activated complement components resulted in pulmonary artery hypertension, profound neutropenia, arterial hypoxemia, and increased pulmonary lymph flow, suggesting a capillary leak. Furthermore, if the animals were rendered granulocytopenic before the infusion of activated complement, its effects could be obviated.

Virtually all clinicians and investigators involved in ARDS research now agree that a triggering of a diffuse inflammatory reaction in the lungs' microvasculature seems to be one of the key factors in the development of this disorder. It is now well recognized that a series of humoral alterations may occur as a result of shock, multiple trauma, infection, endotoxin, or lipopolysaccharide administration, etc.

Much work has been focused on the isolation of a particular mediator for the initiation of these events, often ignoring the interaction of other important pathways that are responsible for inflammatory reactions within the lung. It now seems clear that no one mediator is responsible in and of itself for the initiation of ARDS. Rather a variety of mediators and various cascade systems, which have the potential for persisting for a long period of time, seem to be responsible for the mechanisms involved in disturbing the vascular tone not only in the lungs but in other organs as well (see accompanying box).

Organization of mediator systems. Neuhof[25] has stressed that a "hierarchy" of mediator systems have developed, each of which is interrelated with the other (Fig. 36-7). The *cascade systems,* including complement, kallikrein-kinin, and coagulation-fibrinolytic system, are found at the highest levels of the hierarchy of the humoral systems. The humoral systems may be stimulated by a wide variety of endogenous and exogenous substances. The functional linkage of these systems inevitably leads to an activation of all of them to a varying degree. Thus activation rarely produces response in a single cascade but rather in multiple systems in an integrated fashion. Likewise, products of these systems induce a synthesis of arachidonic acid, metabolites, and lung tissue and secondarily stimulate granulocytes, platelets, mast cells, and fibroblasts in the development, enhancement, and eventual liberation of mediators that may alter vascular permeability. Thus attempts at blocking one arm of the inflammatory response generally have proven futile because other arms of the system induce processes that tend to bypass the area, which has been pharmacologically blocked.

At the next level, responding to these higher organized cascades, are cells that may form and release various mediators. These include cellular elements such as granulocytes, platelets, mast cells, smooth muscles, and endothelial cells.

At the lowest level in this chain of responses are the end organ or final mediators, which become effector instruments on various organs. These would include various proteases, eicosanoids, and various target-activated oxygen molecules.

FACTORS INVOLVED IN THE INFLAMMATORY RESPONSE IN ADULT RESPIRATORY DISTRESS SYNDROME

Cellular Components	Noncellular Components
Granulocytes	Cascade systems including complement, coagulation, and fibrinolytic systems
Monocytes	Proteolytic and antiproteolytic systems
Macrophages	Arachidonic acid metabolites
Erythrocytes	Platelet activating factor
Platelets	Vasoactive substance (e.g., kinins)
Endothelial cells	Cytokines (tumor necrosis factor, interleukin-1)
Epithelial cells (e.g., respiratory)	
Connective tissue cells (e.g., mast cells, fibroblasts)	

Each of the humoral cascade systems plays some role in the pathogenesis of ARDS. The activation of the complement system following a noxious stimulus appears to be the primer that activates the rapid generation and release of mediators. The initial adverse hemodynamic reactions are induced mainly by direct or indirect effects of factors of activated complement, which includes C3a and C5a. These factors induce histamine release from mast cells and granulocytes, which may act as chemoattractants and may also stimulate granulocytes and monocytes. The preterminal and terminal complement complexes C5b-8 C5b-9 may stimulate arachidonic acid metabolites or the eicosanoids. These eicosanoids, produced as a result of activation through a variety of the cascade systems (particularly complement), may cause a multiplicity of deleterious effects including thromboxane production and direct effects on the alveolocapillary interface. Such effects may result in specific physical injury with formation of pores facilitating capillary leak.

Granulocytes and macrophages as sources of mediators and producers of injury

Granulocytes. Granulocytes are found extremely early within the injured lung following virtually any experimental preparation that renders an ARDS-like picture. Lipopolysaccharide stimulation causes intensive granulocyte stimulation via the complement activation system, which begins very early. The potential for direct bacterial toxins to cause direct "pore forming" also occurs. Specific pore-forming bacterial toxins include staphylococcal α-toxin, *Escherichia coli* hemolysin, and *Pseudomonas aeruginosa* cytotoxin. Once these pores are formed, activated polymorphonuclear cells adhere to the endothelium and eventually to structures of the basement membrane.

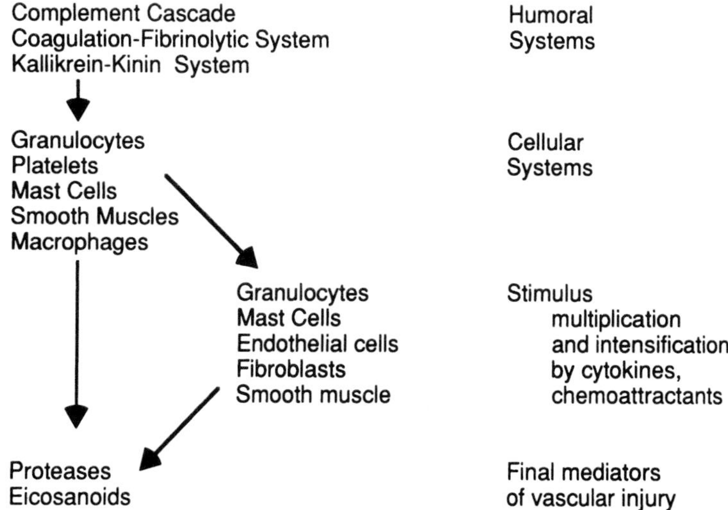

Fig. 36-7. Hierarchy of mediator systems. (Adapted from Neuhof A. Actions and interactions of mediator systems and mediators in the pathogenesis of ARDS and multi-organ failure. Acta Anaesthesiol Scand 35[Suppl 95]:7, 1991.)

There are a variety of other mechanisms through which neutrophilic injury to the lung may occur.[22,26-28]

1. Oxygen-free radicals, which are toxic metabolites derived from molecular oxygen and include superoxide anions, hydrogen peroxide, singlet oxygen ion, and the hydroxy radical, are believed to be injurious to the lung. Furthermore, all these oxygen by-products are capable of being produced by enzyme systems present in neutrophils. Studies of cultured lung endothelial cells exposed to granulocytes and activated complement show direct cellular injury. Accumulating evidence suggests that "free radical scavengers" such as superoxide dismutase and catalase may ameliorate some of these effects.
2. Proteases released by neutrophils may activate complement, Hageman factor, and plasminogen in the blood, producing both direct pulmonary injury and activating other deleterious pathways that produce pulmonary endothelial damage.
3. Neutrophils release various metabolites of arachidonic acid including prostaglandins, thromboxanes, and leukotrienes. These substances may promote vasoconstriction, alter capillary permeability, and act as chemoattractants for other neutrophils.
4. Neutrophils also release platelet-activating factor, which promotes platelet and neutrophil agglutination and increased vascular permeability. Furthermore, normal lung defense mechanisms such as α_1-antitrypsin, are permanently deactivated by the superoxide radical and high concentrations of oxygen.

Macrophages. Macrophages, which are strongly stimulated by endotoxins through a mechanism of specific binding sites, may themselves be toxic by releasing a variety of proteases. These include elaboration and release of elastase, cathepsin B, and various collagenases. In addition, the macrophages synthesize complement factors and various cytokines such as interleukin-1 (IL-1) and tumor necrosis factor (TNF).[29]

The interrelationship between the macrophage and other cellular elements is illustrated in Fig. 36-8. Macrophages through the elucidation of IL-1 and TNF stimulate granulocytes that may have already been stimulated by complement and other cascade pathways. Additionally, IL-1 and TNF act as mitogens on fibroblasts, and this activity along with other stimuli appears to be responsible for much of the fibrosis of lung tissue seen in the pathologic sections taken from patients with ARDS.

Additionally, IL-1 and TNF stimulate endothelial cells directly, which induces a change in the shape of the cell and leads to adherence of leukocytes. There also appears to be an upregulation of the adherence molecules such as endothelial leukocyte adhesion molecule-1 and intracellular adhesion molecule 1 (ICAM-1), which lead to further sticking of leukocytes.

Thus the macrophage acts in two ways as both a direct and indirect contributor to potential lung and other organ injury in ARDS. First, as a producer of direct toxins such as various proteinases, which may lead to destruction of the endothelial and alveolar wall, and secondly through the production of various cytokines such as TNF and IL-1.

Timing of inflammatory activation (Fig. 36-9). The granulocyte reaction that occurs via the classic cascade stimulation, such as the complement pathway, is known to begin in minutes but appears to be a relatively short-lived process. On the other hand, macrophage stimulation may induce a prolonged response with continued generation of inflammatory mediators that may act as the ongoing motor for the development of ARDS and multiple-organ failure. The timing of the inflammatory activation occurring in different pathways varies greatly, with complement activation beginning almost immediately through its stimulation of granulocytes. On the other

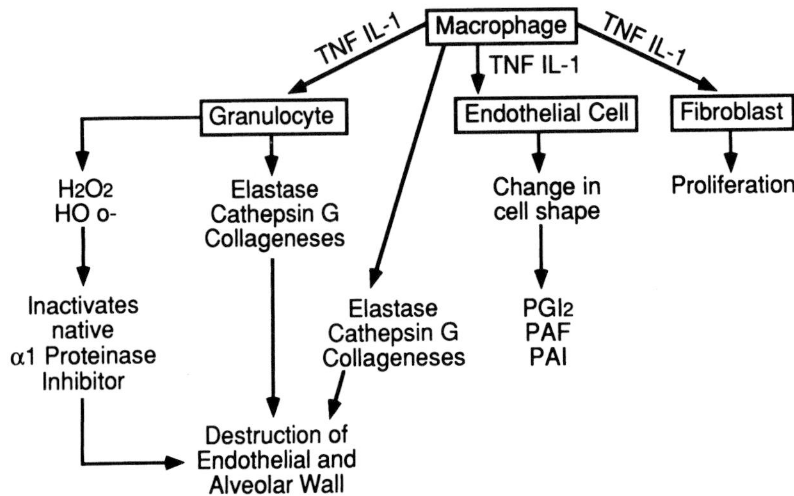

Fig. 36-8. Interrelationship between macrophage and other cellular elements. *H_2O_2*, Hydrogen peroxide; *HO_0-*, hydroxy radical; *IL-1*, interleukin-1; *PAF*, platelet-activating factor; *PAI*, plasminogen activator inhibitor; *PGI_2*, prostaglandin I_2; *TNF*, tumor necrosis factor.

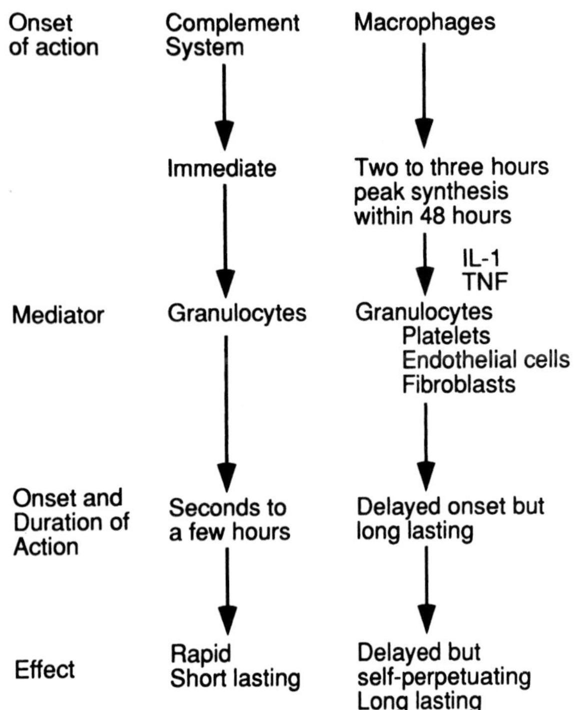

Fig. 36-9. Timing of inflammatory activation. *IL-1*, Interleukin-1; *TNF*, tumor necrosis factor.

hand, macrophage activity usually requires 2 to 3 hours before its cytokine production kicks into gear. Generally, the point of peak synthesis is within 48 hours. The elaboration and release of IL-1 and TNF then act as ongoing stimuli to granulocytes and various cellular effectors. Under most conditions, the duration of the complement system of activation persists for a few hours, and that of the macrophages, while more delayed, may be very long lasting and self-perpetuating.

Coagulation fibrinolytic system. It seems clear that the coagulation system is also involved in ARDS, although it is not well understood whether this is a primary or secondary event.[30] The activation of the cascade system, the kallikrein-kinin system, and the coagulation-fibrinolytic system tend to stimulate granulocytes and other target cells. The formation of various fibrin products within the alveoli impair surfactant production, which directly leads to the formation of microatelectasis.

It has been known for a number of years that patients with ARDS have a high incidence of pulmonary vascular occlusion as measured angiographically. Furthermore, both an increased platelet consumption and sequestration in the lung are noted in patients with ARDS. A variety of experiments conducted primarily by Malik et al.[31] indicated that complement neutrophils, fibrin and fibrin degradation products are essential components for the development of ARDS following microembolization. The observation that heparin and fibrinogen depletion did not block the development of ARDS in experimental animals shows that not every portion of the coagulation system is equally important in inciting the chain of events that may lead to ARDS. Additionally, certain coagulation products may induce lung injury directly. The infusion of thrombin antigen D (one of the fibrin degradation products) causes an increased capillary permeability with hypoxemia.[32]

In the normal animal the reticuloendothelial system (RES) plays a major role in the clearance of both aggregates and products of fibrin degradation (FDPs). Saba et al.[33] elucidated the role of fibronectin as an important component of this critical RES function. Fibronectin is a protein of 450,000 molecular weight that is located on platelet membranes throughout the RES. Fibronectin appears to function as an opsonin in removal of aggregates and FDPs. It has been observed that patients with ARDS may have a depletion of fibronectin. Since fibronectin can

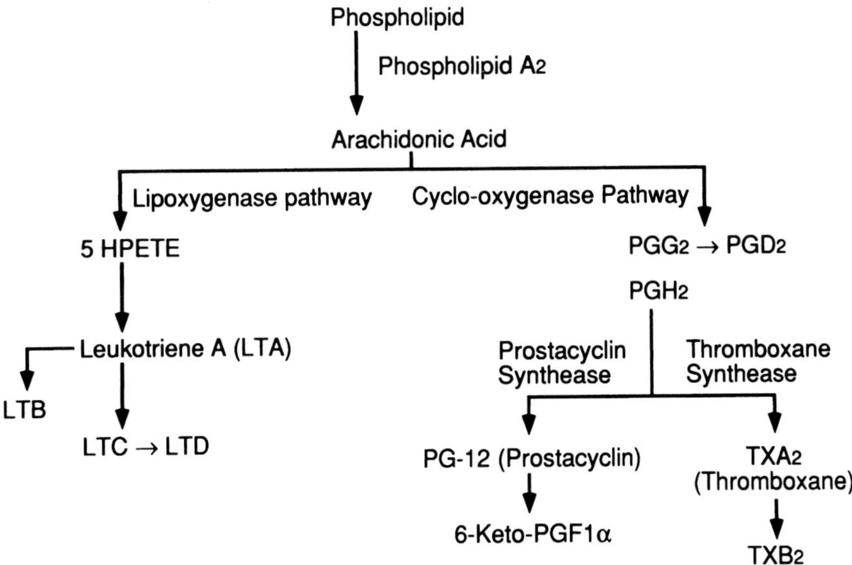

Fig. 36-10. The role arachidonic acid metabolites play in adult respiratory distress syndrome. *LTB, LTC,* and *LTD,* leukotrines B, C, and D; *PGG_2, PGD_2,* and *PGH_2,* prostaglandins G_2, D_2, and H_2.

be infused in cryoprecipitate, it was hoped that this substance might be beneficial in the treatment of ARDS. Although there was an initial wave of enthusiasm for the therapeutic effects of fibronectin, clinical confirmation of its effectiveness has not been forthcoming. Undoubtedly, like many other attempts at single-agent therapy, fibronectin is only one piece of the puzzle.

Role of arachidonic acid metabolites. Arachidonic acid is found in endothelial cells throughout the body and acts as a precursor to a number of pathways of potential importance in ARDS.[34] Arachidonic acid may be converted through the cyclooxygenase pathway to prostaglandins or thromboxanes or through the lipoxygenase pathway to the leukotrienes.

Arachidonic acid metabolites may be released by neutrophils, platelets, and pulmonary endothelium. Thromboxanes appear to be potent pulmonary vasoconstrictors and bronchoconstrictors and lead to increased pulmonary vascular permeability, all of which are seen in ARDS. Increased pulmonary vascular resistance is observed in patients with ARDS and most laboratory models under experimental conditions that simulate this syndrome. Vasoconstriction is produced by several arachidonic acid metabolites, including prostaglandins E_2, F_2, H_2, and by thromboxane A_2. There is a two-phase response to infuse endotoxin in experimental animals. In the first phase an acute rise in pulmonary vascular resistance begins approximately 1 hour following infusion and can be blocked by thromboxane synthetase inhibitors; this suggests that the first phase is mediated by arachidonic acid metabolites. The second phase begins within 3 to 5 hours following endotoxin challenge and does not respond to arachidonic acid inhibitors, which suggests that this effect is not related to thromboxane.

A key to the understanding of all prostaglandin function is that for each action mediated by a prostaglandin there apparently is an opposite or antagonistic function mediated by another prostaglandin.[35] The lung is no exception, and prostaglandin E_1 and I_2 (prostacyclin) have favorable properties that counteract the deleterious effects of thromboxane. Prostacyclin has powerful vasodilating properties and acts as an antagonist to platelet and neutrophil aggregation. The search for possible clinical applications of prostacyclin or for agents such as thromboxane that alter deleterious prostaglandins continues. Although a number of interesting observations have been made in the laboratory, none have yet had any widespread clinical use in the treatment of ARDS.

There has been increased interest in the role of arachidonic acid metabolites in ARDS, especially the leukotrienes (Fig. 36-10). Much of the work on the leukotrienes has been done by Samuelsson[36] of the Karolinska Institute in Stockholm, who shared the 1982 Nobel Prize for Physiology and Medicine. Work with pure leukotrienes has shown a variety of biologic effects, some of which are summarized as follows[34,35]:

1. Pulmonary effects (leukotrienes C_4, D_4, E_4)
   a. Potent bronchoconstrictors
   b. Direct action on peripheral airways
2. Microvascular effects (leukotrienes C_4, D_4)
   a. Arteriolar vasoconstrictor
   b. Leakage of macromolecules
   c. Direct action on vessel wall (does not require histamine, prostaglandin, or granulocytes)
3. Effects on leukocytes (leukotriene B_4)
   a. Increased leukocyte adhesion to small vessel endothelium
   b. Increased interstitial leukocytes (? potential me-

diator of migration of leukocytes from blood to areas of inflammation)

c. Activated neutrophils causing aggregation, degranulation, and superoxide production

Leukotrienes C_4, D_4, and E_4 (all containing cysteine) appear to act directly on the postcapillary venule wall to increase pulmonary vascular permeability. They are potent bronchoconstrictors in humans. Additionally, leukotriene B_4 appears to have direct stimulating effects on leukocytes that produce agglutination, degranulation, and release of free oxygen radicals, which have been implicated with lung injury as previously discussed.

It is difficult to say with certainty to what extent the leukotrienes are involved in the clinical production of lung injury in ARDS. However, there is clear involvement in a variety of experimental conditions that could lead to ARDS. Such information leads one to speculate that these substances are in fact important copromoters of injury in patients with ARDS.

Potential Therapeutic Interventions

If the progenitor of ARDS is the triggering of an inflammatory response, it is only logical that experimental efforts would have been made to study the effects of various anti-inflammatory agents in the treatment of ARDS. An excellent review of these efforts has been published by Metz and Sibbald.[37] Attempts to alter endothelial injury have focused on two primary fields of investigation: the use of high-dose corticosteroid therapy and the use of agents to alter arachidonic acid metabolism.[38] The theoretic advantages of corticosteroids include inhibition of phospholipase, which is the initial step in arachidonic acid metabolism. Although the empiric use of high-dose steroids for the treatment of ARDS is practiced in many centers, there are no data to justify this practice. There is an assumption that such steroid treatment has few side effects, but experimental laboratory studies demonstrated that a single dose of methylprednisolone markedly depressed the ability of both healthy and injured animals to clear aerolized bacteria from their lungs.[2] Given the propensity for patients with ARDS to develop nosocomial pneumonia, the empiric use of steroids is probably not justified.

A randomized trial from Dallas included 81 acutely ill patients requiring mechanical ventilation and judged to be at high risk for the development of ARDS.[39] Sodium methylprednisolone succinate (30 mg/hr) was used in about half the patients and placebo in the remainder. There was no difference in the number of patients who developed ARDS; however, there was a higher incidence of infectious complications in the steroid-treated group. Ashbaugh and Maier[40] believe that sodium methylprednisolone succinate is useful in preventing the pulmonary fibrosis that can occur with ARDS. In 10 consecutive patients who were not responding to conventional treatment, lung biopsies were performed and pulmonary fibrosis documented. High-dose methylprednisolone (125 mg every 6 hours) therapy was initiated and continued until oxygenation began to improve. Eight of these patients survived. These two studies illustrate the difficulty in defining the proper role of steroid therapy because the studies compared different patient groups and used greatly different doses of methylprednisolone. Further studies are needed to properly define the role steroids play in the treatment of ARDS.

The arachidonic acid pathway has several key steps in which various antiinflammatory agents might be efficacious (see Fig. 36-10). Methylprednisolone has been used to inhibit the synthesis of products of the arachidonic acid cascade by a specific blockade of phospholipase A_2. There are two concerns with the use of methylprednisolone. First, there is a concern as to whether any type of posttreatment model would be effective. Second, there is concern about the possible increase in infectious complications in these steroid-treated patients. Postinsult treatment with methylprednisolone has been used in two experimental studies of a porcine model of acute lung injury with conflicting data. There have also been several clinical trials on the use of methylprednisolone in the therapy of ARDS. Methylprednisolone was used as prophylaxis[41] against ARDS and in high-risk traumatized patients, and in one study there was the suggestion that treated patients developed a lower incidence of lung injury than control patients with similar trauma scores. In another study, however, ARDS developed more commonly in methylprednisolone-treated patients. Additionally, three randomized double-blind placebo-controlled trials have been done and have likewise yielded conflicting results. The overall summation of these reports tends to offer no compelling evidence on the utility of methylprednisolone.

There has been considerable interest in the inhibition of various eicosanoids in the treatment of ARDS. Ibuprofen, indomethacin, and meclofenamate have the theoretic benefit of blocking the cyclooxygenase pathway, leading to decreased thromboxane synthesis. Experimentally, several of these agents have been shown to be effective in a variety of experimental models in ameliorating certain problems such as decrease in capillary leak and decreasing pulmonary hypertension. These agents appear to be more effective when given as pretreatment, but their efficacy has not been determined in widespread clinical trials.

Clinical Management

Although there is no direct and specific "magic bullet" for the treatment of ARDS, there are certain goals of therapy that must be strongly considered[42] (see box on p. 753). The strategies for the treatment of ARDS include the maintenance of adequate oxygen delivery through increasing PaO_2 by whatever means necessary and increasing cardiac index as appropriate to ensure adequate oxygen delivery. The use of PEEP for recruitment of alveoli has been one of the constant strategies employed by most physicians caring for patients with inadequate oxygen delivery. Newer ventilator strategies such as inverse-ratio ventilation, high-frequency jet ventilation, and permissive hy-

STRATEGIES FOR TREATMENT OF ADULT RESPIRATORY DISTRESS SYNDROME

Increase Oxygen Delivery

Increase arterial PO_2

Continuous positive airway pressure
Positive end-expiratory pressure
Pressure support
Newer ventilatory strategies (e.g., inverse-ratio ventilation, high-frequency jet ventilation, permissive hypercapnia)
Extracorporeal membrane oxygenation

Increase cardiac index

Fluids
Inotropes
Vasodilators/vasoconstrictors

Modulation of Fluid Balance

Invasive
Cardiac monitoring
Diuretics
Low left atrial filling pressure
Ultrafiltration

Prevent and Treat Underlying Cause of Sepsis

Antibiotics
Debride devitalized tissue, drain abscesses
Selective gut decontamination

Pharmacologic Manipulations

Anti-inflammatory agents (methylprednisolone, nonsteroidal anti-inflammatory drugs)
Oxygen radical scavengers
Pentoxifylline

Nutritional Support

Enteral when possible
Parenteral

percapnia have their proponents and are currently being studied at this time. The use of extracorporeal membrane oxygenation is of benefit in various forms of respiratory failure in neonates and children, but its role is less well understood and defined in adults with ARDS.

Fluid balance should be modulated with an attempt, as much as possible, to avoid overhydration.[43] The use of ultrafiltration in grossly overhydrated patients is occasionally a very useful technique.

The treatment of infection is paramount for the surgeon. Devitalized tissue must be debrided and any abscesses or nidus of infection must be thoroughly investigated and treated whenever possible. The use of techniques such as selective gut decontamination have received a mixed review in the numerous studies on its efficacy. To date, there is no compelling evidence that selective whole gut decontamination prevents ongoing multiple-organ failure.

Table 36-4. Effects of Cardiac Output and Partial Pressure of Oxygen (PO_2) on Oxygen Availability

Cardiac Output (L/min)	PO_2	Available Oxygen (ml/min)
5	60	900
5	40	750
4	60	720
4	40	600

Peters[44] has described the following potentially lifesaving steps to assist the surgeon caring for a patient with ARDS:

1. Determine the adequacy of alveolar ventilation. If the patient has a PCO_2 that is elevated or even normal, ventilatory support is needed. A normal PCO_2 in the face of hypoxemia indicates inappropriate alveolar ventilation.
2. Establish maintenance of cardiac output as a first priority of therapy. Factors controlling cardiac output are (a) preload filling pressure, (b) afterload vascular resistance, and (c) contractility of the myocardium. The most common cause of decreased cardiac output in surgical patients is inadequate preload as a result of hypovolemia. Additionally, maintaining an adequate cardiac output has a direct effect on the oxygen available for tissue demands. Table 36-4 shows the effect of variations in cardiac output and PO_2 on available oxygen. The importance of maintaining an adequate cardiac output in the face of low PO_2 is well demonstrated.
3. Limit FIO_2 to as low a level as possible to prevent further oxygen toxicity (below 0.4 to 0.5, if possible).
4. Institute PEEP or continuous positive airway pressure (CPAP) if the shunt fraction is above 20%.
5. Suspect pneumothorax if peak inspiratory pressures suddenly increase, and institute rapid treatment.
6. Mobilize the patient.

By increasing functional residual capacity (FRC), the use of PEEP tends to improve oxygenation greatly in patients with ARDS, permitting a lower FIO_2 to accomplish the same acceptable level of tissue oxygenation. This increase in FRC is apparently the result of prevention of airway closure and recruitment of unventilated alveoli. The ventilation of previously collapsed but perfused alveoli decreases shunting and improves hypoxemia. This increase in FRC may increase static lung compliance as well. There are many controversies about the use of PEEP that are beyond the scope of this chapter but have been excellently reviewed.[45,46] Although it is clear that PEEP improves oxygenation, its effect on the clinical course of ARDS is less certain. In fact, it has not been uniformly accepted that PEEP actually improves survival.[47] Pepe et al.[48] have reported a randomized trial of prophylactic PEEP in patients at high risk for the development of ARDS. Unfortunately, this study did not confirm the efficacy of "early PEEP" in the amelioration or prevention of ARDS.

Prichard[49] suggested several possible mechanisms to decrease lung extravascular fluid volume: (1) decrease of transvascular hydrostatic gradient; (2) increase of colloid oncotic pressure; (3) reversal of endothelial injury; and (4) increase of pulmonary lymphatic clearance. Careful attention to fluid balance with monitoring of the left ventricular filling pressure of the heart may decrease the net fluid flux into the lung. Thus the goal is to assure adequate filling of the left ventricle without elevating the pulmonary capillary wedge pressure (PCWP). If the PCWP is elevated, judicious administration of diuretics may ameliorate some of the fluid flux into the lung. Low-dose dopamine (4 to 10 mg/kg) may aid in promoting a diuretic response without deterioration of cardiac dynamics. There has been a great deal of interest in the use of colloid to raise colloid osmotic pressure and circumvent the pulmonary edema seen in patients with ARDS. However, the ability to maintain normal colloid osmotic pressure during the capillary leakage phase is virtually impossible, since there is a rapid movement of macromolecules from the pulmonary vascular spaces to interstitial spaces. The value of blood or colloid-containing fluids is that better filling pressures can be maintained with less volume requirements than if crystalloid solutions alone are infused.

Smoke Inhalation and Pulmonary Dysfunction Following Burns

Abnormalities in the airways and lungs are common problems following burn injury. The abnormalities may include smoke inhalation (with or without any surface burn), direct thermal injury to the airway, and alterations in pulmonary function as a result of the burn wound.

A critical element of smoke inhalation is the nature of the chemical injury induced by the substance under combustion. Many models of experimental smoke inhalation using wood or charcoal as the source of smoke failed to produce the lethal inhalational injury often observed in patients.[50] It is now clear that much of the lethality of smoke inhalation results from combustion of plastic and synthetic materials that release aldehydes and organic acids, which are direct toxins to the upper and lower airways. Chlorine, ammonia, and sulfur compounds may also be by-products of combustion and result in the formation of potent acids and bases, causing further airway injury. Direct injury to the major airways and a marked increase in bronchial blood flow may lead to formation of severe edema,[51] which is manifested in increased airway resistance. Bronchoconstriction may occur as a direct result of toxins on the airways or through a mediator such as the leukotrienes. Clinically, this phase is marked by wheezing that may be severe. An increase in dead space ventilation is also observed. Ventilation-perfusion abnormalities occur as a result of alveolar collapse from bronchospasm and peribronchiolar edema. Many patients with severe burn injury have frothy edematous fluid evident in their major airways and alveoli. The source of this edematous fluid may be direct alveolar injury with an increase in lung water or may be caused by retrograde flow of the severe mucosal edema of the bronchi. Studies in humans have tended to confirm the latter as the cause of the severe edema that is observed clinically.

Some authors have included smoke inhalation as a cause of ARDS.[48] It is clear that there is a prompt migration of neutrophils into the bronchial mucosa following such inhalation. This process is probably related to complement activation that triggers the cascade of physiologic consequences described in the previous section on ARDS.

Direct pulmonary or upper airway burns are probably a lesser cause of airway and/or lung injury than is commonly believed. Burns occurring in a closed space, particularly if associated with facial burns and burns of the nasal hairs, must be suspected of producing direct thermal injury. Direct thermal burns are usually confined to the upper airway, since the oropharynx and the nasopharynx quickly dissipate heat. Thus direct upper airway injury with edema and the potential for airway obstruction are of major concern after such thermal injuries. Furthermore, the patient must be closely observed for progressive swelling that continues throughout the first 24 to 36 hours after injury. The need for high-volume fluid resuscitation to treat a major cutaneous burn undoubtedly worsens the edema and increases the potential for obstruction. Although the presence of carbonaceous sputum or the observation of soot in the airways leads to a high index of suspicion for direct thermal injury to the airway, these findings correlate poorly with the need for intubation.

Determinations of carbon monoxide levels should be obtained in such burn patients. Direct observation of the color of the arterial blood is necessary because a bright red color may be an early indicator of high carbon monoxide levels in the blood. Carbon monoxide preferentially binds with the hemoglobin molecule (CO-Hgb) instead of oxygen and interferes with the ability of hemoglobin to off-load oxygen at the cellular level. When levels of CO-Hgb are in the 20% to 40% range, the symptoms may be difficult to recognize but usually include nonspecific central nervous system manifestations. Coma and even death (from severe cerebral hypoxia) are likely to occur with CO-Hgb levels in the range of 40% to 50% and greater than 60%, respectively.[52]

Demling[52] noted a number of pulmonary effects that may result from the burn wound. Particularly, thromboxane A_2 is released from burn tissue and, as discussed in the section on ARDS, has a number of potentially deleterious consequences, including bronchoconstriction with increased airway resistance and decreased compliance and vasoconstriction with resultant pulmonary artery hypertension.

There is no specific therapy for smoke inhalation at this time. Usually, ventilatory support is promptly required in severe cases. The ventilatory therapy should be aimed at providing appropriate levels of oxygenation with the least possible FIO_2 and PEEP to avoid oxygen toxicity and barotrauma. Unfortunately, many patients with smoke inhalation injury require high levels of inspired oxygen and PEEP. Nosocomial pneumonias are common, and aseptic technique should be practiced when providing ventilatory therapy.

Pulmonary Contusion

Pulmonary contusion represents a direct injury to the lung, causing localized alveolar flooding with erythrocytes. Pulmonary contusion has been acknowledged as an entity since World War II when "traumatic wet lung" was recognized as a clinical syndrome. Clinicians have always believed that fluid administration had an adverse effect on pulmonary contusion. In the decade between 1965 to 1975, enormous strides were made in the recognition of pulmonary contusion as a distinct entity, and the ability to produce effective laboratory models contributed greatly to the understanding of this problem. Although pulmonary contusion is often included among the causes of ARDS, it appears to have a different pathologic mechanism than the neutrophil-induced capillary leak phenomenon now thought to be the hallmark of ARDS.

A number of studies by Fulton and Peter[53-55] provide much of the understanding of the physiology of pulmonary contusion. Fulton and Peter developed a model of experimental contusion and found that the PO_2 was a progressive change that worsened over the first 24 hours after injury. Histologic studies of the lung taken immediately after injury showed only interstitial hemorrhage with little or no edema present. Two hours after injury there was significant edema present with a marked thickening of alveolar walls but no appreciable cellular infiltration. By 24 hours there was loss of normal alveolar architecture and profuse round cell infiltration.

Physiologic studies using a model of severe lung injury showed decreased blood flow and increased pulmonary vascular resistance in the injured lung. Consequently, there was a marked increase in blood flow in the noncontused lung. These changes were also progressive. Furthermore, it was noted that surfactant was decreased between 24 and 48 hours with a decreased compliance and worsening of lung mechanics.[56] The infusion of saline with or without blood produced a further fall in PO_2. When saline was rapidly infused, a marked rise in pulmonary artery pressure occurred with a shift of blood flow to the opposite lung and a subsequent increase in edema of the noncontused lung. Increased lung water was noted in both the contused and noncontused lungs.

Richardson et al.[57] and Trinkle et al.[58] developed a less severe injury model that produced an isolated contusion to study the effects of various manipulations on more limited injury. They noted that the administration of fluid caused an increase in the zone of edema surrounding the central area of contusion. The greater the volume of fluid given and the more rapid its rate of administration, the more severe was the injury produced. In studies of combined pulmonary contusion and shock, colloid did not prevent lung edema but did provide a more efficient resuscitation in terms of restoring hemodynamic parameters with less lung water produced in the area of contusion. Methylprednisolone was the only agent studied that decreased the extent of the pulmonary contusion.

These studies led to a series of clinical recommendations that seem valuable in the care of patients with pulmonary contusions and flail chest[59]: (1) judicious use of crystalloid solutions, avoiding unnecessary administration of sodium-containing solutions and the raising of pulmonary vascular pressure above physiologic limits; (2) liberal use of blood for resuscitation—this is done not to increase colloid osmotic pressure but to limit the amount of crystalloid required for resuscitation; (3) use of intravenous diuretics (usually 20 mg furosemide) for patients who receive excessive crystalloid resuscitation; and (4) avoidance of use of corticosteroids in this clinical setting because, although methylprednisolone limits the size of the contusion experimentally, there is concern about its effect on lung defenses.

One of the most controversial areas in surgical physiology concerns the debate of the appropriate use of crystalloid vs. colloid solutions for the resuscitation of injured patients. A brief attempt to summarize the pros and cons of this discussion is in order for the neophyte in surgical physiology. To understand the issues concerning crystalloid and colloid, it is important to understand some basic precepts of capillary physiology. In 1896, Starling reported his observations on the absorption of fluids from connective tissue spaces into small vessels. Starling hypothesized that fluid flux was predicated by the equation:

$$\text{Net fluid flux} = K\ (\Delta P - \Delta\pi)$$

where K is the permeability of the membrane of the vessel wall; ΔP is the hydrostatic pressure gradient; and $\Delta\pi$ is the protein osmotic gradient across the wall.

If at least a portion of the deleterious effects of many noxious insults on lung (e.g., ARDS resulting from sepsis, pulmonary contusion, smoke inhalation, or aspiration injury) was caused by the net movement of fluid into the lung, attempts were made to modify factors shown in the Starling equation. The three factors that could be altered were wall permeability, hydrostatic pressure gradient, and osmotic pressure gradient. There are few, if any, known methods to correct wall permeability abnormalities in the clinical setting, so attempts focused on means to affect hydrostatic and osmotic pressure gradients. One potential method to alter osmotic pressure in a way that would limit fluid movement into the lung was to infuse albumin solution in an attempt to raise the colloid osmotic pressure within the vascular system. Proponents of this approach believed that the lung was better protected from edema formation with a colloid resuscitation and that hydrostatic pressure was less likely to be elevated.[60,61]

Unfortunately, in many situations that are deleterious to the lung (e.g., ARDS and smoke inhalation), there is an alveolocapillary leak; and if the pores in the capillary are large enough to allow protein and solute to cross the vessel wall, the osmotic pressure gradient, $\Delta\pi$, disappears. If this occurs, then

$$\text{Net fluid flux} = K\ \Delta P$$

where K is membrane permeability and ΔP is pressure gradient. Since this is a common occurrence in many of the important problems affecting the lung, it obviates most of the potential value of colloid infusion. In fact, since colloid may be sequestered in the connective tissue pores, it may actually promote a net fluid accumulation outside the vessel. This fact plus the high cost of colloid-containing solutions makes their use in conditions that result in alveolocapillary leak undesirable.

Clinical trials have shown that when overinfusion is avoided (and thus alter the ΔP), even large volumes of balanced salt solutions (crystalloids) are well tolerated.[62]

Pulmonary Embolism

The etiologic factors and clinical findings associated with pulmonary embolism are generally well recognized.[63] The physiologic consequences of pulmonary embolism are manifested through several mechanisms. The occlusion of pulmonary arteries by clots leads to alveoli that are ventilated but not perfused, resulting in wasted ventilation or increased dead space ventilation. Initially, there is a reflex airway constriction that tends to limit ventilation to unperfused areas, but within 24 hours this reflex appears relatively unimportant in limiting ventilation-perfusion imbalance. The redistribution of blood flow from unperfused areas leads to a relative overperfusion of other alveoli, further increasing the ventilation-perfusion mismatch. Surfactant production is impaired after 24 hours, leading to local atelectasis and edema that may result in congestive atelectasis that grossly resembles pulmonary infarction. Pulmonary infarction is actually an unusual event, probably occurring in less than 10% of cases of pulmonary embolism caused by the lungs' dual blood supply.

It also appears that pulmonary embolism initiates a humoral reflex mechanism that causes generalized pulmonary vasoconstriction. The cause of this vasoconstrictive mechanism is not precisely understood and a variety of medications have been implicated. Serotonin, bradykinin, and prostaglandins have been incriminated as the substances that cause generalized pulmonary vasoconstriction and that further heighten ventilation-perfusion imbalance. Hypoxemia without carbon dioxide retention is commonly seen following pulmonary embolus. There is an increase in the physiologic shunt and dead space ventilation. Experimental embolism studies suggest that most cases of hypoxemia are the result of ventilation-perfusion inequity. Thus the addition of supplemental oxygen generally results in rapid improvement in hypoxemia (as opposed to a large shunt where addition of oxygen fails to improve hypoxemia).

The pulmonary vascular bed has a large capacitance with a number of vascular beds that are unused under normal circumstances. These vascular beds may be "recruited" under conditions of vascular occlusion by pulmonary embolus. Thus about 50% of the vasculature of the lung must be occluded before pulmonary hypertension occurs. The development of a major embolus may lead to an increase in pulmonary artery pressure. If this pressure is high and sustained, right ventricular failure may result, although this event is certainly not the usual case.

Studies involving patients with pulmonary emboli have documented the consequences of these physiologic events.[36] Abnormalities noted in patients with pulmonary emboli include the following:

1. *Hyperventilation:* Eighty-three percent of patients had a minute ventilation of greater than 8 L.
2. *Pulmonary restriction:* More than 80% of patients had a decreased vital capacity. Possible mechanisms might include chest splinting because of pleural pain or decreased lung compliance on the basis of surfactant loss and congestive atelectasis.
3. *Bronchoconstriction:* A decrease in the FEV_1 and in maximum midexpiratory flow rate may occur as a reflex mechanism or through the release of substances such as those discussed in the section on ARDS.
4. *Hypoxemia:* Hypoxemia appears to be secondary to ventilation-perfusion inequality.
5. *Pulmonary hypertension:* Pulmonary hypertension occurs to a variable degree depending on the extent of the pulmonary embolism.

Atelectasis

Atelectasis is derived from a Greek term meaning "airless" and refers to a loss of volume of the lung (either lobar, segmental, or subsegmental). The term may be confusing because a number of mechanisms of atelectasis have been proposed[64] and are outlined as follows:

1. Absorption atelectasis occurs following obstruction of a major bronchus or multiple secondary bronchi with subsequent resorption of the air in the distal lung. This type of atelectasis is of major concern to the surgeon because the obstructing agent may be a mucous plug, foreign body, or tumor.
2. Passive atelectasis refers to a condition resulting from a space-occupying condition in the thorax such as a pneumothorax or hydrothorax.
3. Compression atelectasis follows a space-occupying lesion within the lung parenchyma such as might result from a tumor or emphysematous bulla. In both the passive and compression types of atelectasis, the lung being compressed may be completely normal initially.
4. Adhesive atelectasis occurs in the presence of patent bronchi and presumably is secondary to surfactant abnormalities. It is seen in association with pneumonia and other inflammatory conditions of the lung.
5. Cicatrization atelectasis refers to an airless condition of the lung associated with pulmonary fibrosis.

Atelectasis secondary to bronchial obstruction by tumor or foreign body may be associated with a variety of symptoms such as secondary pneumonia or wheezing, depending on the location and degree of obstruction involved. In some patients significant bronchial obstruction does not cause atelectasis because the lobe may continue to be ventilated by the passage of air from nonobstructed segments into the obstructed portion through interlobar communications. This phenomenon is referred to as *collateral ventilation* and explains why atelectasis may not be apparent even when a tumor or foreign body results in near total bronchial obstruction. Therefore the absence of atelectasis on a chest radiograph does not rule out the possibility of a central obstructing lesion in the bronchus.

The pathophysiology of atelectasis may be related to three major factors, each of which contributes to bronchial obstruction in the postoperative patient: (1) a decrease in the cough or expulsion mechanism from the bronchus; (2) changes in bronchial secretions leading to tenacious adherent sputum; and (3) a reduction of bronchial caliber, which may occur as a result of direct airway trauma caused by conditions such as intubation, edema, or inflammation. Many classic studies on the incidence of atelectasis were published in the 1940s and 1950s and may no longer be applicable to patients because today greater emphasis is placed on pulmonary care. Atelectasis occurred in 10% of thoracic and upper abdominal procedures reported by Moersch in 1943[65] but in only 4% of nonabdominal operations. Kurzweg[66] studied the incidence of postoperative pulmonary complications and found on the average they occur in 2.5% to 3% of all operations. However, complications were much higher in abdominal operations, particularly upper abdominal procedures, occurring in 10% to 20% and 20% to 30%, respectively. Atelectasis involving smaller airways ("microatelectasis"), which may not be diagnosed by chest radiography, is presumably present even more frequently.

The clinical examination should be adequate for early diagnosis of atelectasis in most patients. Bronchial breathing or moist rales occurring most commonly at the lung bases are the hallmark of the clinical condition. A chest radiograph need not be routinely obtained in the typical patient with postoperative atelectasis. Atelectasis may be manifested by tachypnea, fever, and tachycardia, but these are late signs. The cause of the fever is presumably infection secondary to bacterial proliferation in the atelectatic area of the lung. Shields[67] demonstrated in 1949 that intravenously administered bacteria tend to localize at the site of atelectasis. Collapse of the lung also interferes with the lung's host defenses and does not permit adequate macrophage function in engulfing bacteria.

Successful treatment of atelectasis depends on prompt mobilization of bronchial secretions by deep breathing, coughing, and nasotracheal suctioning if necessary. In patients with major areas of collapse that involve an entire segment or lobe of the lung or in patients in which effective nasotracheal suctioning cannot be performed, therapeutic bronchoscopy is indicated to remove secretions and mucous plugs. Increased mobilization of the patient is helpful when possible. Pain medication should be judiciously used to help avoid splinting to alleviate postoperative pain without producing harmful respiratory depression. Through the years mechanical means of pushing air into the lungs, such as intermittent positive pressure breathing, have fallen into disrepute because of their ineffectiveness, their cost, and the risk of nosocomial infection.

Pneumonia

Pneumonia is one of the most common pulmonary derangements affecting surgical patients. Postoperative pneumonia may be initiated by atelectasis or acquired as a nosocomial infection in patients treated by endotracheal intubation or tracheostomy and mechanical ventilation. In a patient hospitalized for community-acquired pneumonia, the typical signs of infection—productive cough, purulent sputum, fever, and rales—are usually present. Leukocytosis is the rule, and an infiltrate is generally present on the chest radiograph. The diagnosis of pneumonia in a postoperative patient is occasionally somewhat more difficult because the classic signs may be absent or altered by other conditions occurring in the postoperative state. A report from the University of Louisville School of Medicine has used the following criteria for the diagnosis of postoperative pneumonia[68]:

1. New postoperative infiltrate seen on chest x-ray film
2. A temperature of at least 38° C for at least 24 hours
3. Purulent sputum production and/or cultured pathogens
4. Antibiotic therapy deemed to be needed to treat the pulmonary process

Although these specific criteria may be challenged, it is important to define the clinical parameters necessary to make a diagnosis before effective study of this condition can be undertaken. With the criteria outlined above, which my associates and I hoped would eliminate those patients with atelectasis, the incidence of pneumonia was 1.3% of all operated cases over a 7-year period. This rate compares with an incidence of 0.75% of all surgical patients reported by the National Nosocomial Infection Study[69] but is much lower than the 17% reported by Garibaldi et al.[70] However, the latter study did not require culture evidence of pneumonia and undoubtedly included many patients with atelectasis.

The mortality rate for patients with postoperative pneumonia is high (from 15% to 50%), with the specific rate dependent on the diagnostic criteria. Certain risk factors are predictors of a poor outcome including (1) gram negative pneumonitis, particularly *Pseudomonas;* (2) signs of remote organ failure; (3) bilateral pneumonia; (4) emergency operation preceding pneumonia; (5) positive results from blood culture; (6) postoperative peritonitis; and (7) pneumonia acquired while receiving mechanical ventilation. It is postulated that several of these risk factors, including positive results from blood culture, the development of bilateral pneumonia, and the occurrence of multiple-organ failure, represent a breakdown of host defense mechanisms and thus ensure a high mortality.

Further analysis of patients with postoperative pneumonia indicate that the following three etiologic mechanisms are involved: (1) following atelectasis (as discussed in the previous section); (2) following aspirations; and (3) following the introduction of mechanical ventilation for hypoxemia.

Aspiration is a major risk factor for the development of pneumonia in surgical patients. The following list indicates various conditions that predispose to aspiration:

1. Alteration of consciousness
   a. Head injury
   b. Stroke, seizure, coma
   c. Alcohol intoxication
   d. Drug overdose
   e. Cardiac arrest
   f. General anesthesia, oversedation
2. Derangements of swallowing mechanism and esophageal function
   a. Tracheostomy
   b. Laryngeal lesions (e.g., carcinoma, ulcers)
   c. Pseudobulbar palsy
   d. Esophageal obstruction (e.g., cancer, benign stricture)
   e. Incompetent lower esophageal sphincter (with or without hiatal hernia)
   f. Achalasia
   g. Zenker's or epiphrenic diverticulum
   h. Tracheoesophageal fistula
   i. Nasogastric intubation
3. Defective cough reflex
   a. Following local anesthesia of larynx and trachea
   b. Neuromuscular disorders

Drugs that alter the state of consciousness such as general anesthesia and postoperative pain medications are particularly important to surgeons. Likewise, alcohol intoxication, substance abuse, and head injuries are frequently encountered in patients who suffer traumatic injuries. A variety of disorders of swallowing and esophageal function are commonly seen by surgeons and may predispose the patients to aspiration. The treatment of pneumonia depends in large part on which of the three etiologic mechanisms mentioned previously is responsible for the pulmonary infection. If the pneumonia occurs as a consequence of atelectasis, vigorous pulmonary toilet with nasotracheal suction and/or therapeutic bronchoscopy as indicated usually results in a prompt resolution of the process. Antibiotics specific to the pathogen cultured should be instituted, but mechanical treatment to eliminate the source of bronchial obstruction seems the most important part of the treatment regimen.

The treatment of aspiration pneumonia is more conventional. A variety of specific treatment recommendations for pneumonia following aspiration includes the following:

1. Bronchopulmonary lavage to remove acid and/or particulate matter from the airways
2. Corticosteroids to obviate the inflammatory response produced by the low pH in the tracheobronchial tree
3. Empiric use of antibiotics (to cover a broad spectrum or narrow spectrum such as oral cavity flora)
4. Selective use of antibiotics (based on organisms seen on Gram's stain of aspirated material or on culture results)

No one protocol for the treatment of aspiration has been proven with randomized trials to be more effective than other treatment modalities. At the University of Louisville School of Medicine, I use the following guidelines in the management of aspiration:

1. Heavy emphasis is placed on preventing aspiration.
2. If aspiration has been observed or is thought to have occurred, liberal use is made of therapeutic bronchoscopy.
3. Corticosteroids are not used for the treatment of aspiration.
4. Cultures are obtained, but antibiotics are not used, until clinical and radiologic evidence of pneumonitis exists.

Bronchoscopy has little, if any, role in the removal of acid from the tracheobronchial tree, since acid absorption through mucosa is almost instantaneous; however, bronchoscopy is useful in the removal of particulate matter that may be a nidus for the development of infection. My associates and I have avoided corticosteroids because of their deleterious effects on pulmonary host defenses as noted previously in this chapter.

One final type of pneumonia that is seen with increasing frequency in surgical patients is that occurring in the immunocompromised patient. The causative agents for pneumonia in immunosuppressed patients are rarely encountered in community-acquired pneumonia. Etiologic agents are bacterial (either gram-negative or gram-positive organisms or *Mycobacterium*), fungal (including *Aspergillus, Cryptococcus, Candida,* or *Nocardia*), protozoan *(Pneumocystis),* or viral (e.g., cytomegalovirus or herpes). When the patient with alterations in immune status develops pneumonia, vigorous diagnostic techniques must often be used to obtain adequate specimens for special staining, culture, and light microscopy and even electron microscopy to aid in establishing a diagnosis. Reliance on simple sputum cytology is often not adequate in this clinical setting, and a biopsy of involved lung parenchyma may be mandatory despite the critical nature of the patient's illness. The means of obtaining a biopsy of affected lung depend in large measure on the skill and experience of the physician obtaining the specimen. Acceptable techniques include percutaneous needle biopsy, transbronchial biopsy, and open lung biopsy. Empiric treatment often is necessary in these desperately ill patients and initially must be based on the likelihood of the patient's having a specific diagnosis.[71] Patients with AIDS tend to have a high incidence of infection caused by *Pneumocystis, Legionella,* and *Mycoplasma.* Patients with defects in cellular immunity not related to AIDS have the additional risks for gram-negative or gram-positive bacterial pneumonias and eventually may need empiric coverage. The neutropenic patient has a higher risk of *Pseudomonas* infection in addition to those previously mentioned and may require empiric treatment with carbenicillin or piperacillin.

Pneumothorax

Pneumothorax occurs when air escapes from the pulmonary parenchyma and causes the lung to collapse away from the chest wall. In simple or closed pneumothorax, this condition is not progressive, the mediastinal structures are not shifted, and the opposite lung is not compressed. In contrast, a tension pneumothorax is caused by the progressive accumulation of air within the thoracic cavity, leading to a shift in the cardiomediastinal structures with possible compression of the contralateral lung.

Tension pneumothorax results from a one-way valve phenomenon in which air enters the thoracic cavity from an opening in the pulmonary parenchyma or the chest wall. Air enters the pleural space during inspiration but cannot escape during expiration. The increased pleural pressure decreases venous return to the heart by kinking or distorting the low pressure vena cava and/or by direct pressure on the cava. Hypotension and complete circulatory collapse may occur within minutes if the condition is not promptly treated.

Pneumothorax may occur with a variety of conditions:

1. Trauma
   a. Blunt
   b. Penetrating
2. Iatrogenic
   a. Nerve blocks
   b. Subclavian catheters
3. Barotrauma
   a. Mechanical ventilation
   b. PEEP
4. Rupture of abnormal pulmonary parenchyma
   a. Congenital bleb
   b. Pneumatocele
   c. Emphysematous bulla
   d. Catamenial (?)
5. Idiopathic

Both penetrating and blunt trauma commonly result in a pneumothorax. Blunt trauma may be associated with a pneumothorax caused by laceration of the lung from a rib fracture. However, a pneumothorax may also occur in the absence of rib fractures because of the sudden compression of the chest wall against a closed glottis. This rapid increase in the intrathoracic pressure leads to a disruption of the alveoli and to a subsequent pneumothorax. A pneumothorax may also result from barotrauma in which the increased pressure on the airway (usually from positive pressure mechanical ventilation and PEEP) results in a "blow-out" type of alveolar injury with secondary air leak.

Pneumothorax may occur because of disease or abnormality in the underlying lung tissue. Spontaneous pneumothorax often results from apical blebs that appear to be congenital in nature. Likewise, acquired conditions such as bulbous emphysema or pneumatocele following staphylococcal pneumonia result in a thinning of the pulmonary parenchyma that may leak air and result in a pneumothorax.

The type of physiologic defect produced in the lung by a simple pneumothorax is a restrictive one. The degree of restriction and secondary respiratory compromise is determined by the degree of pneumothorax. In relatively mild cases (<30% pneumothorax), the degree of physiologic insult may be mild. However, an increase in the degree of pneumothorax or bilateral pneumothoraces may result in more serious respiratory compromise.

It is important in estimating the degree of pneumothorax to remember that the lung is a three-dimensional cylinder rather than a two-dimensional structure as seen on chest radiograph. If only the loss in diameter on the chest radiograph is considered, the decrease from 20 cm to 16 cm is considered to be a 20% pneumothorax. If, however, the lung is regarded as a sphere, the volume loss with such a change in diameter is much greater. The volume may be determined by $V = \pi r^3$; thus the diameter reduction from 20 to 16 cm causes a radius change from 10 to 8 cm. This decrease results in a net volume loss of 50% rather than the 20% calculated by simple measurement of diameter loss.

Treatment of a pneumothorax varies depending on its cause, the degree of clinical embarrassment produced, and associated factors. A small simple pneumothorax resulting from blunt trauma or arising spontaneously may be safely observed and may resolve without treatment. Large degrees of collapse should be treated. Aspiration is occasionally successful if a continuing air leak is not present. If the patient is moderately symptomatic, has bilateral pneumothoraces, or will require positive pressure ventilation (for surgery or mechanical ventilation), a thoracostomy tube should be inserted and connected to an underwater seal to produce a negative pressure and aid in lung reexpansion.

Flail Chest

Flail chest is defined as the paradoxic motion of a segment of chest wall such that the flail area is depressed with inspiration (and its negative intrathoracic pressure) and is moved outward during expiration (Fig. 36-11). A flail chest occurs when a group of ribs are fractured in more than one area or when there is a costochondral separation and a lateral rib fracture. The physiologic abnormalities resulting from flail chest have been controversial. It was once believed that the lung functioned as a bellows and that the loss of chest wall rigidity because of a flail chest caused a "to-and-fro" movement of air from one hemithorax to another rather than the normal effective exchange of air. The concept of to-and-fro motion was termed *pendelluft.* The concept was demonstrated invalid in a series of stud-

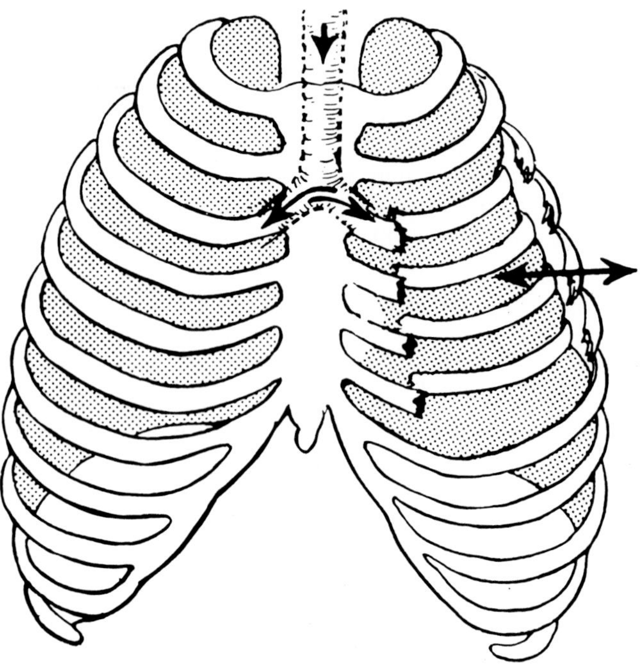

Fig. 36-11. Fracture of chest wall in two locations is necessary for development of flail chest. Classic concept of altered mechanics causing "to-and-fro" movement of air between major bronchi *(double arrow)* has largely been dispelled.

ies by Maloney et al.[72] The hypoxemia associated with flail chest probably has two origins: (1) there is associated damage to the underlying lung in the form of pulmonary contusion (see Pulmonary Contusion); and (2) the loss of mechanical stability and flail motion may lead to a loss of lung volume. Considerable clinical experience suggests that pulmonary contusion is the primary mode that renders the patient hypoxemic.

Treatment of flail chest has gone through several historic phases. Initial attempts to treat flail chest relied on external mechanical stabilization through a traction device or by tapes or belts. The introduction of the piston-driven ventilator led to the development of internal pneumatic stabilization[73] in which the patient's respiratory drive was eliminated by rendering the patient alkalotic and allowing the ventilator to "stabilize" the flail segment. The patient was generally maintained on mechanical ventilation until the flail segment stabilized. Unfortunately, this method of treatment was associated with continued high mortality secondary to complications of therapy such as nosocomial pneumonia, tracheostomy and endotracheal tube complications, and electrolyte disorders.

There has been a trend toward selective management of flail chest[59,74] depending on the degree of hypoxemia produced and the extent of the flail segment. The basic tenets of this treatment include (1) avoidance of overresuscitation with crystalloid infusion, which may worsen a pulmonary contusion; (2) vigorous pulmonary toilet to control secretions and prevent atelectasis; and (3) selective use of endotracheal intubation and early extubation and weaning from mechanical ventilation based on physiologic parameters rather than chest wall instability. Large series involving many patients have shown that this is a safe and effective method of treating patients with flail chest.

PULMONARY AND MEDIASTINAL NEOPLASIA

Tumors of the Lung

A variety of neoplastic disorders may affect the lung. Clinically, they may manifest themselves with symptomatology similar to other pulmonary disorders, including wheezing, coughing, hemoptysis, pain, or at times an unexplained pneumonia caused by a pneumonitis distal to the site of the tumor. Occasionally, a patient may be totally symptom free; and an unexplained solitary pulmonary nodule, called a coin lesion, is identified on a chest x-ray film that has been obtained for an entirely different reason. Such nodules are sharply circumscribed, are localized in the peripheral lungs, are 5 cm or less in diameter, and may or may not demonstrate calcification. At least half these lesions turn out to be malignant; and the larger their size, the more likely a malignancy is present. For this reason all solitary pulmonary nodules must be considered malignant until proven otherwise.[75] Unfortunately, routine studies such as bronchoscopy, sputum sample analysis, and even transthoracic biopsy are usually nondiagnostic. Consequently, the majority of patients who have such lesions initially must undergo exploratory thoracotomy to confirm the diagnosis. If the lesion is benign, a wedge resection of the lung is generally adequate management. In contrast, malignant lesions should be treated with a formal lobectomy or pneumonectomy to enhance the chances of cure. In fact, compared with other presentations of pulmonary cancer, an undiagnosed pulmonary nodule is usually the only stage of bronchogenic cancer in which a good-to-excellent chance for cure can be expected.

Of the various kinds of benign neoplasms that may affect the bronchopulmonary tree, hamartomas (mixed tumors) are the most common.[76] Other types include fibrous mesotheliomas, various xanthomatous and inflammatory pseudotumors, and other rare lesions such as lipomas and myoblastomas. Benign tumors are generally slow growing and often first present with bronchial obstruction, pneumonitis, or hemoptysis. Such tumors account for only 1% to 2% of all pulmonary neoplasms and surgical excision consisting of enucleation or wedge resection offers an excellent prognosis.

Malignancies are the most frequently encountered neoplasms of the lung; and, of the various types encountered, bronchogenic carcinoma is responsible for as many as 93% of them.[77] Presently, this is the most common malignancy in men (and is becoming a frequently diagnosed tumor in women) and is clearly associated with cigarette smoking and probably atmospheric pollution as well. Most carcinomas arise from the bronchial epithelium and typically involve the upper lobes of the lung (63%). The various cell

Table 36-5. Cell Types and Characteristics of Carcinoma of Lung

Type of Carcinoma	Percent	Sex	Growth Characteristics
Epidermoid	50	75% in men	Occurs in major bronchi, causing distal atelectasis, tends to spread by lymphatics
Undifferentiated large cell	20	38% in women	Located more peripheral from hilus of lung, spreads by lymphatics and blood stream
Small cell (oat cell)	9	80% in men	Very cellular and largely extrabronchial, causing little or no atelectasis, early lymphatic and hematogenous spread
Adenocarcinoma	20	30% in women	Majority occur in periphery of lung, metastasize by blood stream
Bronchiolar or alveolar cell	1	—	Occurs as a diffuse, patchy pneumonia and as a slow-growing, well-circumscribed local lesion

From Richardson JD. Hemoptysis, cough, and other symptoms of pulmonary lesions. In Polk HC Jr, Gardner B, Stone HH, eds. Basic Surgery, 4th ed. St. Louis: Quality Medical Publishing, 1993, p 310.

types with their growth characteristics and frequency of occurrence are shown in Table 36-5.

Most patients who develop carcinoma of the lung have a long history of sustained cigarette smoking. Typical symptoms associated with carcinoma include cough, wheezing, hemoptysis, and occasionally fever, all caused by pneumonitis distal to the site of the tumor. Pain is a relatively late symptom and generally indicates chest wall extension. Weight loss is usually not seen until the cancer is quite advanced. If the tumor involves the thoracic or superior pulmonary sulcus at the root of the neck, a *Pancoast's syndrome* may result. This includes involvement of the brachial plexus, the sympathetic ganglia at the base of the neck, Horner's syndrome (ptosis, miosis, enophthalmos, and decreased sweating on the involved side), and frequently destruction of ribs and vertebrae and loss of strength in the upper arm of the affected side.

As many as 20% of patients initially have symptoms remote from the lung, indicating metastatic disease. Typical sites of metastasis include the liver and brain. Other extrapulmonary manifestations are related to various humoral agents that may be secreted by the tumor. An adrenocorticotropic hormone (ACTH)–like substance elaborated by oat cell carcinoma may closely mimic Cushing's syndrome. In addition, a parathormone-like substance produced by some squamous cell carcinomas simulates clinical findings typical of primary hyperparathyroidism. A syndrome of inappropriate antidiuretic hormone may also occur, manifested by water retention and symptoms of hyponatremia. Although the exact mechanism responsible for this condition remains to be determined, pulmonary osteoarthropathy is frequently associated with carcinoma of the lung. This condition is different from arthritis because the bones rather than the joints are tender, and x-ray films of the fingers demonstrate a fine linear deposition of calcium along the periosteum. Clubbing of the fingers also occurs in patients developing carcinoma of the lung, the mechanism again remaining yet undefined.

Because of the relatively poor prognosis that exists in patients who develop carcinoma of the lung, care must be taken to ensure the tumor's resectability and to prevent an unnecessary thoracotomy. The absolute and relative signs of inoperability are summarized in Table 36-6. In determining such information, CT scanning is often helpful in assessing mediastinal nodes. If mediastinal adenopathy is present, mediastinoscopy should be performed to determine the presence of metastases. This technique involves an incision above the suprasternal notch through which a fiber-optic mediastinoscope is introduced into the superior mediastinum, enabling identification of lymph nodes and the ability to biopsy them. This technique is especially useful in diagnosing central lesions, in which tissue samples for malignancy prove positive in about 65% of cases. The technique is, however, less suitable for more peripheral lesions.

When first diagnosed, more than 50% of patients have inoperable carcinoma of the lung. Another 25%, when explored, are discovered to have nonresectable lesions because of neoplastic extension into the mediastinum or carina. Of those patients actually amenable to surgical excision, only about 8% (or two of the initial 100 patients) live for 5 years. The type of surgical procedure performed relates to the nature and extent of the tumor and may range from a segmental resection to a total pneumonectomy.

Of those tumors found to be surgically resectable, a malignant solitary pulmonary nodule without lymph node involvement is generally associated with a 50% 5-year survival rate. Squamous cell carcinoma without node metastases treated by lobectomy or pneumonectomy yield 30% to 35% 5-year survival rates. If nodal involvement is present in either of these circumstances, the 5-year survival rate drops to 10% or less. For those tumors that are histologically adenocarcinomas or undifferentiated large cell cancers, the survival rate is even more dismal.

A particular circumstance that continues to remain controversial with respect to treatment involves that patient who is believed to be surgically resectable in other respects but has positive mediastinal lymph nodes.[78] Although some investigators recommend surgical treatment combined with radiography for squamous cell carcinoma,[79] the

Table 36-6. Signs of Inoperability in Lung Cancer

Absolute Signs	Relative Signs
Lymphatic spread to cervical axillary, or remote mediastinal nodes	Mediastinal nodes (may be removed at operation)
Distant spread to other organs (brain, bone, kidneys, adrenals, etc.)	Phrenic nerve paralysis
Small cell cancer (some controversy)	Pericardial extension
Superior vena cava syndrome	May be excised but usually will be unresectable at operation
Malignant pleural effusion	Chest wall extension; chest wall can often be excised
Widened carina (with biopsy-proven cancer)	Superior sulcus (pancoast tumor) may be resected after a course of radiation therapy
Paralyzed vocal cord (invasion of recurrent laryngeal nerve)	

From Richardson JD. Hemoptysis, cough, and other symptoms of pulmonary lesions. In Polk HC Jr, Gardner B, Stone HH, eds. Basic Surgery, 4th ed. St. Louis: Quality Medical Publishing, 1993, p 311.

generally dismal outcome in the experience of most surgeons has suggested that radiotherapy alone is the treatment of choice for this stage of the disease.[80] Radiation therapy may also be of value in the prevention of hemoptysis or bronchial obstruction by reducing the tumor mass in patients who have unresectable lesions.

The role of multiple-drug chemotherapy in the management of bronchogenic carcinoma remains to be clearly defined. Recent experience in the treatment of oat cell carcinoma has been extremely encouraging, resulting in an objective response rate (i.e., measurable decrease in tumor size) in as many as one third of patients so treated.[81] With such therapy, patients who normally would have succumbed from their disease in less than 6 months are now surviving as long as 2 years or more. Whether similar success rates will be demonstrated with other types of carcinomas must await further study.

Although the preceding has centered around bronchogenic carcinoma, other malignancies, collectively known as the bronchial adenomas, may also affect the lungs. The two most common types are carcinoid (85%) and cylindromas (12%), also called the adenoid cystic type. These tumors are generally located in the walls of the major bronchi. When examined bronchoscopically, usually only a small amount of the tumor is visible, with a much larger portion of it extending outside of the bronchus, a situation known as the *iceberg effect*. Of these two types, the cylindromas are usually more aggressive and tend to invade adjacent tissues and metastasize to nodes more frequently. Treatment of both types depends on their size and location. Accordingly, procedures used in their treatment range from sleeve resection of the bronchus for very small lesions to lobectomy or pneumonectomy for larger lesions. As many as 90% of patients with these tumors are cured after surgical resection, with the carcinoid type of lesion being more favorable in this regard.

Tumors of the Mediastinum

In addition to tumors directly involving the pulmonary parenchyma, a number of neoplastic conditions may also arise in the mediastinum.[82] These tumors are generally asymptomatic, except when they grow large enough to cause compression of an adjacent structure. They usually first come to the attention of a physician when noted on a routine chest film. The particular source of the tumor in a given patient depends on the particular mediastinal compartment in which the tumor arises. As an example, the anterior mediastinum contains the thyroid gland, the thymus, and the pericardium; accordingly, tumors arising in this location develop from these structures. A summary of the types of tumors arising in various portions of the mediastinum is detailed in the accompanying box.

COMMON MEDIASTINAL TUMORS

Anterior Mediastinal Compartment

Parathyroid adenomas
Thyroid tumors, goiters, and cysts
Thymic tumors and cysts
Teratomas
Pericardial cysts

Superior Mediastinal Compartment

Thyroid tumors
Parathyroid adenomas
Bronchogenic cysts
Lymphomas

Middle Mediastinal Compartment

Lymphatic tumors
Lymphomas
Bronchogenic cysts

Posterior Mediastinal Compartment

Neurogenic tumors
Neurilemomas
Ganglioneuromas
Gastroenteric cysts

Because a malignant process must always be considered when a mediastinal tumor is diagnosed, surgical excision is the treatment of choice. For virtually all benign lesions and for most malignant processes, complete cure can be expected with such surgical approach.

SUMMARY

This chapter has dealt with some basic physiologic mechanisms involved in the pulmonary derangements commonly encountered in surgical patients. The lung seems to have a limited number of ways of reacting to injury, and thus a variety of noxious stimuli tend to produce abnormalities of the lung that behave similarly. Many of these abnormalities have been included in a discussion on the ARDS. It seems clear that for surgical patients sepsis is the most common provocation of ARDS.

The physiology and basic principles of treatment of a number of other commonly encountered disorders such as smoke inhalation, pulmonary contusion, atelectasis, pneumonia, pneumothorax, flail chest, and pulmonary neoplasms are also discussed. A thorough understanding of the basic physiologic mechanisms underlying these common problems is crucial for any surgeon who deals with critically ill patients.

REFERENCES

1. West JB. Pulmonary Pathophysiology. Baltimore: Williams & Wilkins, 1982.
2. Richardson JD, et al. Lung bacterial clearance following pulmonary contusion. Surgery 86:730, 1979.
3. Whitcomb ME. The lung—Normal and diseased. St. Louis: Mosby, 1982.
4. Balk R, Bone RC. Classification of acute respiratory failure. Med Clin North Am 67:551, 1983.
5. Ashbaugh DG, et al. Acute respiratory distress in adults. Lancet 2:319, 1967.
6. Moore FD, et al. Posttraumatic Pulmonary Insufficiency. Philadelphia: WB Saunders, 1969.
7. Fulton RL, Jones CE. The cause of posttraumatic pulmonary insufficiency in man. Surg Gynecol Obstet 140:179, 1975.
8. Walker L, Eiseman B. The changing patterns of posttraumatic respiratory distress syndrome. Ann Surg 181:693, 1975.
9. Bone RC, et al. Adult respiratory distress syndrome—Sequence and importance of development of multiple organ failure. Chest 101:320, 1992.
10. Cunningham AJ. Acute respiratory distress syndrome—Two decades later. Yale J Biol Med 64:387, 1991.
11. Pepe PE, et al. Clinical predictors of the adult respiratory distress syndrome. Am J Surg 144:924, 1982.
12. Petty TL, Fowler AA. Another look at ARDS. Chest 82:98, 1982.
13. Fowler AA, et al. Adult respiratory distress syndrome: Risk with common predispositions. Ann Intern Med 98:593, 1983.
14. Murray JF, Matthay MA, Luce JM. An expanded definition of the adult respiratory distress syndrome. Am Rev Respir Dis 138:720, 1988.
15. Blaisdell FW. Pathophysiology of the respiratory distress syndrome. Arch Surg 108:44, 1974.
16. Jones JG, Minty BD, Royston D. The physiology of leaky lungs. Br J Anaesth 54:705, 1982.
17. Anderson RR, et al. Documentation of pulmonary capillary permeability in the adult respiratory distress syndrome accompanying human sepsis. Am Rev Respir Dis 119:869, 1979.
18. Stevens JH, Raffin TA. Adult respiratory distress syndrome—Etiology and mechanisms. Postgrad Med J 60:505, 1984.
19. Gadek JE. Adverse effects of neutrophils on the lung. Am J Med 92:6A, 1992.
20. Gattinoni L, et al. CT scan in ARDS—Clinical and pathological insights. Acta Anaesthesiol Scand 35(Suppl 95):87, 1991.
21. Kaplow LS, Goffinet JA. Profound neutropenia during the early phase of hemodialysis. JAMA 203:1135, 1968.
22. Fantone JC, Kunkel SL, Ward PA. Chemotactic mediators in neutrophil-dependent lung injury. Annu Rev Physiol 44:283, 1983.
23. Jacob HS. Complement-mediated leucoagglutination—A mechanism of tissue damage during extracorporeal perfusions, myocardial infarction, and in shock. Q J Med 207:289, 1983.
24. Staub NC, et al. Preparation of chronic lung lymph fistulas in sheep. J Surg Res 19:351, 1975.
25. Neuhof A. Actions and interactions of mediator systems and mediators in the pathogenesis of ARDS and multi-organ failure. Acta Anaesthesiol Scand 35(Suppl 95):7, 1991.
26. Hosea J, et al. Role of complement activation in a model of adult respiratory distress syndrome. J Clin Invest 66:375, 1980.
27. Sacks T, et al. Oxygen radicals mediate endothelial cell damage by complement-stimulated granulocytes. J Clin Invest 61:1161, 1978.
28. Wong C, Flynn J, Demling RH. Role of oxygen radicals in endotoxin-induced lung injury. Arch Surg 119:77, 1984.
29. Nathan CF. Secretory products of macrophages. J Clin Invest 71:319, 1985.
30. Bone RC, Francis PB, Pierce AK. Intravascular coagulation associated with adult respiratory distress syndrome. Am J Med 61:585, 1976.
31. Malik AB, et al. Role of blood components in mediating lung vascular injury after pulmonary vascular thrombosis. Chest 83:215, 1983.
32. Manwaring O, Thorning D, Curreri PW. Mechanism of acute pulmonary dysfunction produced by fibrinogen degradation products. Surgery 84:85, 1978.
33. Saba TM, et al. Cryoprecipitate reversal of opsonic surface binding glycoprotein deficiency in septic surgical and trauma patients. Science 201:622, 1978.
34. Seale JP. Prostaglandins, slow-reacting substances (leukotrienes) and the lung. Aust N Z J Med 11:550, 1981.
35. Miller TA. Protective effects of prostaglandins against gastric mucosal damage: Current knowledge and proposed mechanisms. Am J Physiol 245:G601, 1983.
36. Samuelsson B. Leukotrienes: Mediators of immediate hypersensitivity reactions and inflammation. Science 220:568, 1983.
37. Metz C, Sibbald WJ. Anti-inflammatory therapy for acute lung injury: A review of animals and clinical studies. Chest 100:110, 1991.
38. Kopolovic R, et al. Effects of ibuprofen on a porcine model of acute respiratory failure. J Surg Res 36:300, 1984.
39. Weigelt JA, et al. Early steroid therapy for respiratory failure. Arch Surg 120:536, 1985.
40. Ashbaugh DG, Maier RV. Idiopathic pulmonary fibrosis in adult respiratory distress syndrome. Arch Surg 120:530, 1985.
41. Petty TL, et al. Contemporary clinical trials in acute respiratory distress syndrome. Chest 101:550, 1992.
42. MacNaughton PD, Evans TW. Management of adult respiratory distress syndrome. Lancet 339:469, 1992.
43. Mitchell JP, et al. Improved outcome based on fluid management in critically ill requiring pulmonary artery catheterization. Am Rev Respir Dis 145:990, 1992.
44. Peters RM. Lifesaving measures in acute respiratory distress syndrome. Arch Surg 138:368, 1979.
45. Kuckelt W, et al. Effect of PEEP on gas exchange, pulmonary mechanics, and hemodynamics in adult respiratory distress syndrome (ARDS). Intensive Care Med 7:177, 1981.
46. Weisman IM, Rinaldo JE, Rogers RM. Positive end-expiratory pressure in adult respiratory failure. N Engl J Med 307:1381, 1982.

47. Springer RR, Stevens PM. The influence of PEEP on survival of patients in respiratory failure: A retrospective analysis. Am J Med 66:196, 1979.
48. Pepe PE, Hudson LD, Carrico JC. Early application of positive end-expiratory pressure in patients at risk for adult respiratory distress syndrome. N Engl J Med 311:281, 1984.
49. Prichard JS. Edema of the Lung. Springfield, Ill.: Charles C Thomas, 1982.
50. Stephenson SF, et al. The pathophysiology of smoke inhalation injury. Ann Surg 182:652, 1975.
51. Moylan JA, Alexander LG. Diagnosis and treatment of inhalation injury. World J Surg 2:185, 1978.
52. Demling RH. Early pulmonary abnormalities from smoke inhalation. JAMA 251:771, 1984.
53. Fulton RL, Peter ET. The progressive nature of pulmonary contusion. Surgery 67:499, 1970.
54. Fulton RL, Peter ET. Physiologic effect of fluid therapy after pulmonary contusion. Am J Surg 126:773, 1973.
55. Fulton RL, Peter ET. Compositional and histologic effects of fluid therapy following pulmonary contusion. J Trauma 14:783, 1974.
56. Nichols RT, Pearce HJ, Greenfield LJ. Effects of experimental pulmonary contusion on respiratory exchange and lung mechanics. Arch Surg 96:723, 1968.
57. Richardson JD, et al. Pulmonary contusion and hemolyse—Crystalloid versus colloid replacement. J Surg Res 16:330, 1974.
58. Trinkle JK, et al. Pulmonary contusion, pathogenesis and effect of various resuscitative measures. Ann Thorac Surg 16:569, 1973.
59. Richardson JD, Adams A, Flint LM. Selective management of flail chest and pulmonary contusion. Ann Surg 196:103, 1982.
60. Lutz PL, et al. Pulmonary edema related to changes in colloid oncotic and pulmonary artery wedge pressure in patients after acute myocardial infarction. Circulation 51:350, 1975.
61. Skillman JJ, Restall DS, Salzman EW. Randomized trial of albumin versus electrolyte solutions during abdominal aortic operations. Surgery 78:291, 1975.
62. Virgilio RW, et al. Crystalloid versus colloid resuscitation: Is one better? Surgery 85:129, 1979.
63. Sasahara AA, et al. Clinical and physiologic studies in pulmonary thromboembolism. Am J Cardiol 20:10, 1967.
64. Fraser RG, Pare JAP. Diagnosis and Diseases of the Chest. Philadelphia: WB Saunders, 1978.
65. Moersch HJ. Bronchoscopy in treatment of postoperative atelectasis. Surg Gynecol Obstet 77:435, 1943.
66. Kurzweg FT. Pulmonary complications following upper abdominal surgery. Am Surg 19:967, 1953.
67. Shields RT. Pathogenesis of postoperative pulmonary atelectasis. Arch Surg 58:489, 1949.
68. Martin LF, et al. Postoperative pneumonia. Arch Surg 119:379, 1984.
69. Centers for Disease Control. National Nosocomial Infection Study Report, 1976, Annual Summary. Atlanta: Centers for Disease Control, 1978.
70. Garibaldi RA, et al. Risk factors for postoperative pneumonia. Am J Med 70:677, 1981.
71. Masur H, Shelhamer J, Parillo JE. The management of pneumonia in immunocompromised patients. JAMA 253:1769, 1985.
72. Maloney JV, Schmutzer KJ, Raschke E. Paradoxical respiration and 'pendelluft.' J Thorac Cardiovasc Surg 41:291, 1961.
73. Avery EE, Morch ET, Benson DW. Critically crushed chests: A new method of treatment with continuous mechanical hypoventilation to produce alkalotic apnea and internal pneumatic stabilization. J Thorac Surg 32:301, 1956.
74. Trinkle JK, et al. Management of flail chest without mechanical ventilation. Ann Thorac Surg 19:355, 1975.
75. Dedrick CG. The solitary pulmonary nodule and staging of lung cancer. Clin Chest Med 5:345, 1984.
76. Oldham HN Jr. Benign tumors of the lung and bronchus. Surg Clin North Am 60:825, 1980.
77. Chung CK, et al. Carcinoma of the llung: Evaluation of histological grade and factors influencing prognosis. Ann Thorac Surg 33:599, 1982.
78. Pearson FG, et al. Significance of positive superior mediastinal nodes identified at mediastinoscopy in patients with resectable cancer of the lng. J Thorac Cardiovasc Surg 83:1, 1982.
79. Kirsh MD, Rotman H, Argenta L. Carcinoma of the lung—Results of treatment over 10 years. Ann Thorac Surg 21:371, 1976.
80. Byfield JE. Radiation therapy, local tumor control, and prognosis in bronchogenic carcinoma: Current status and future prospects. Am J Surg 143:675, 1982.
81. Ihde DC. Current status of therapy for small cell carcinoma of the lung. Cancer 54:2722, 1984.
82. Silverman NA, Sabiston DC Jr. Mediastinal masses. Surg Clin North Am 60:757, 1980.

37

Normal Cardiac Function

Andrew C. Fiore and Andrew S. Wechsler

As a component of the cardiovascular system, the heart is responsible for maintaining adequate blood flow to meet the metabolic needs of the body. This is accomplished by the integration of neural, metabolic, anatomic, and physiologic subsystems that combine to form the intact, functioning human heart. An understanding of cardiac function must consider each of these factors, since a knowledge of only one, or even several, without an appreciation of the others gives an incomplete picture of the physiologic mechanisms responsible for this function. In discussing cardiac physiology, it is appropriate to begin with the molecular events underlying contraction and relaxation, to provide the basis for understanding the performance of the intact organ.

MOLECULAR MECHANISMS IN CONTRACTION AND RELAXATION

The basis of cardiac function is the relationship between the contractile proteins actin and myosin. The nature of this relationship determines to a large extent the characteristics of activation and relaxation in individual muscle cells and in the intact heart. As in skeletal muscle, the functional unit of cardiac muscle is the sarcomere. The sarcomere is composed principally of four proteins.[1] These are the previously mentioned contractile proteins actin and myosin and the regulatory complex consisting of tropomyosin and troponin. In electron micrographs the sarcomere appears as an arrangement of thick and thin filaments. This arrangement is shown schematically in Fig. 37-1. The thick filament exists as an aggregate of myosin molecules. Myosin consists of a pair of heavy, coiled polypeptide chains, each of which is attached to a globular head region.

These head regions project from the axial core of the myosin aggregate and form cross-bridges to the thin filament (Fig. 37-2). The thin filament is made up of actin in association with troponin and tropomyosin. Actin is a globular molecule that polymerizes to form a double-stranded α-helical filament. Actin filaments attach to the Z line of the sarcomere and project inward as the thin filament. Here they interact to various degrees with the thick filament. This interaction is regulated by troponin and tropomyosin.

Tropomyosin spans the length of the thin filament, and the tropinin complex is normally located at every seventh actin site.[2] Troponin consists of several subgroups that are responsible for binding calcium ions and for regulating the formation of attachments between actin and the myosin by way of the cross-bridges.[3] In the resting state, tropomyosin blocks binding sites on actin so that cross-bridge interaction is prevented. The presence of calcium bound to the troponin complex leads to a conformational change in tropomyosin, such that the actin-myosin association is no longer blocked.

The head region of myosin is the enzymatically active portion of the molecule.[1] Adenosine triphosphate (ATP) binds here and is hydrolyzed to adenosine diphosphate (ADP) and phosphorus (P). In this form the affinity of myosin for actin is enhanced, such that if calcium is present, an actin-myosin complex is formed. As the hydrolysis products are released from the complex, the myosin head undergoes a conformational change that displaces the actin filament relative to the myosin. In this manner, force generation and shortening are accomplished. The addition of ATP to the actin-myosin complex results in dissociation of the filaments. The ATP is once again hydrolyzed, and the process repeats.[4-8]

Force generation during activation depends to a large extent on the number of cross-bridge attachments that are formed.[9] This number is a function of the degree of filament overlap and the level of calcium present. The rate of shortening is a measure of the ATPase activity of myosin.[10] It has been established that myosin exists in several forms that are distinguished by the composition of their heavy chains.[11] These various forms differ in their ATPase kinetics and thus in their rate of fiber shortening.[12] The composition of the myosin subunits is genetically determined; however, it has been shown to change in response to such hormones as thyroxin and to chronic elevations in mechanical loading of the muscle.[13,14]

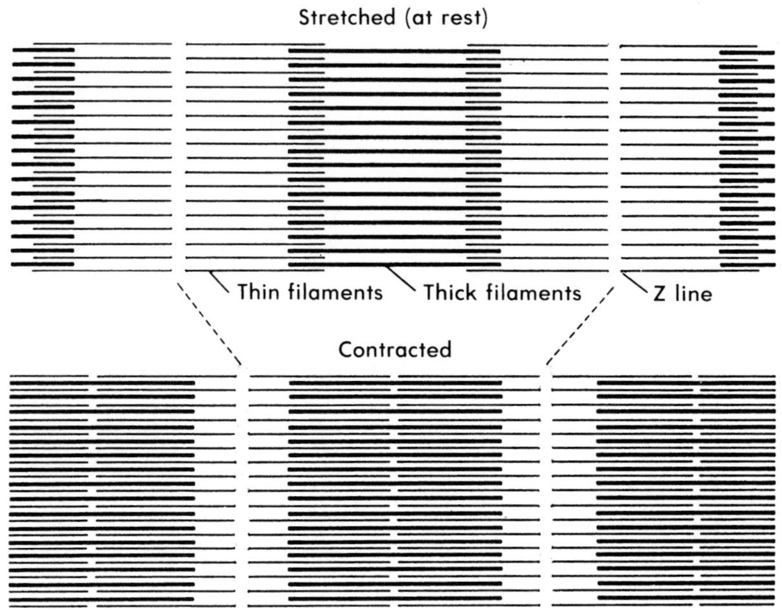

Fig. 37-1. Schematic diagram showing the pattern of thick and thin filaments of one sarcomere. Degree of filament overlap varies with the phase of contraction. (From Murray J, Weber A. The cooperative action of muscle proteins. Sci Am 230[2]:58, 1974.)

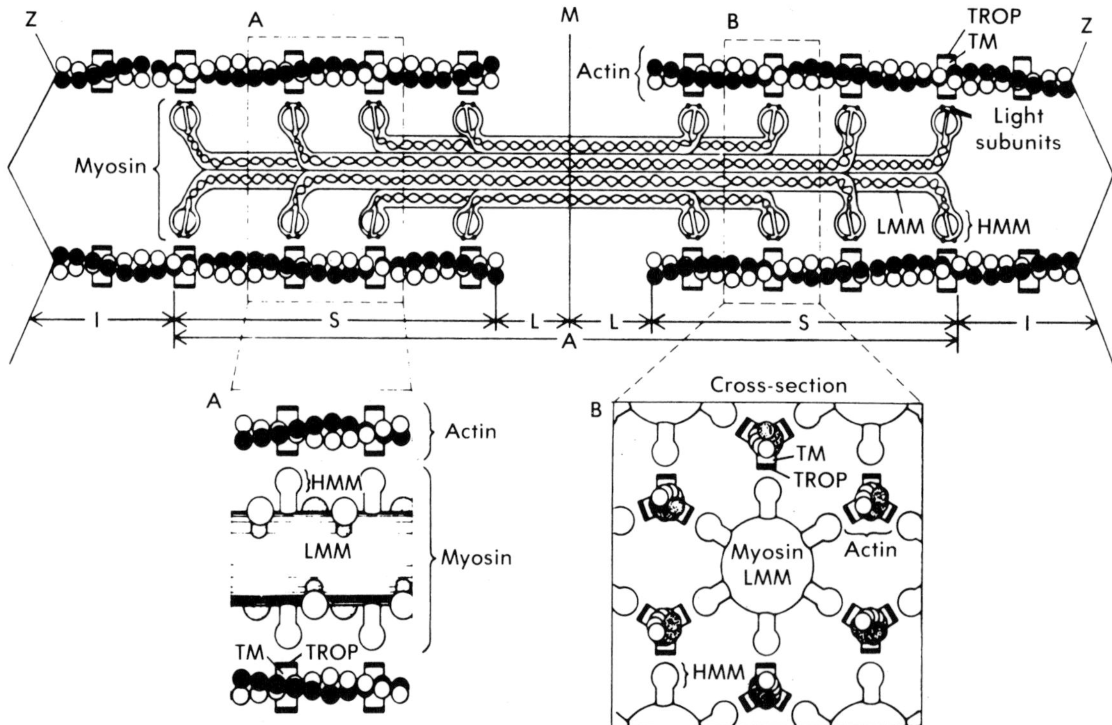

Fig. 37-2. Detailed representation of filament structure. Helical tails of the myosin molecules form a rigid, rodlike structure. Globular heads project from this toward the actin filament. **A-B,** Three-dimensional relationships. Each myosin is seen to interact with six actin filaments *(B).* Note steric hindrance provided by troponin *(TROP)* and tropomyosin *(TM). HMM,* Heavy meromyosin; *LMM,* light meromyosin. (From Mason DT, et al. Mechanisms of cardiac contraction. In Sodeman WA Jr, Sodeman TM, eds. Sodeman's Pathologic Physiology, 6th ed. Philadelphia: WB Saunders, 1979.)

Excitation-Contraction Coupling

Myocardial contraction is initiated following a rise in cytosolic calcium. During the plateau phase of the cardiac action potential, a small number of calcium ions enter the muscle cell through slow channels. These ions do not significantly alter myoplasmic calcium (Ca^{++}), but they do cause release of calcium stores from the sarcoplasmic reticulum.[15] This release significantly elevates myoplasmic Ca^{++}. Calcium is now available to bind to troponin, and muscle activation occurs. This process, in which calcium entry triggers intracellular calcium release and muscle activation, is called excitation-contraction coupling (Fig. 37-3).

It is interesting to note the amplification of the effects of calcium in this process. The small number of ions entering the cell through the slow channel causes the release of intracellular stores that raises the myoplasmic Ca^{++} from a resting value of 10^{-7} M to 10^{-5} M.[4] In turn, each calcium ion that binds to troponin activates seven actin-binding sites. This two-step amplification illustrates the exquisite sensitivity of the muscle cell to calcium.[16]

Muscle relaxation depends on the presence of adequate levels of ATP, which act to dissociate the actin-myosin complexes and provide energy for the restoration of myoplasmic Ca^{++} to resting levels. The latter is accomplished primarily by a calcium-activated ATPase in the membrane of the sarcoplasmic reticulum. In addition, smaller amounts of calcium are extruded from the cell through an Na^+/Ca^{++} exchange mechanism that operates secondary to the Na^+, K^+-ATPase of the sarcolemma and is not voltage dependent, as are the slow channels.[9,17,18]

MECHANICS OF ISOLATED MUSCLE

Much of what is known about the nature of cardiac function has been learned from studies of isolated muscle. Under these conditions, it is possible to finely control the loading of the muscle while making accurate measurements of force development and shortening characteristics. From these studies, three factors have arisen that determine the behavior of isolated muscle. They are muscle preload, afterload, and contractile state.[19,20]

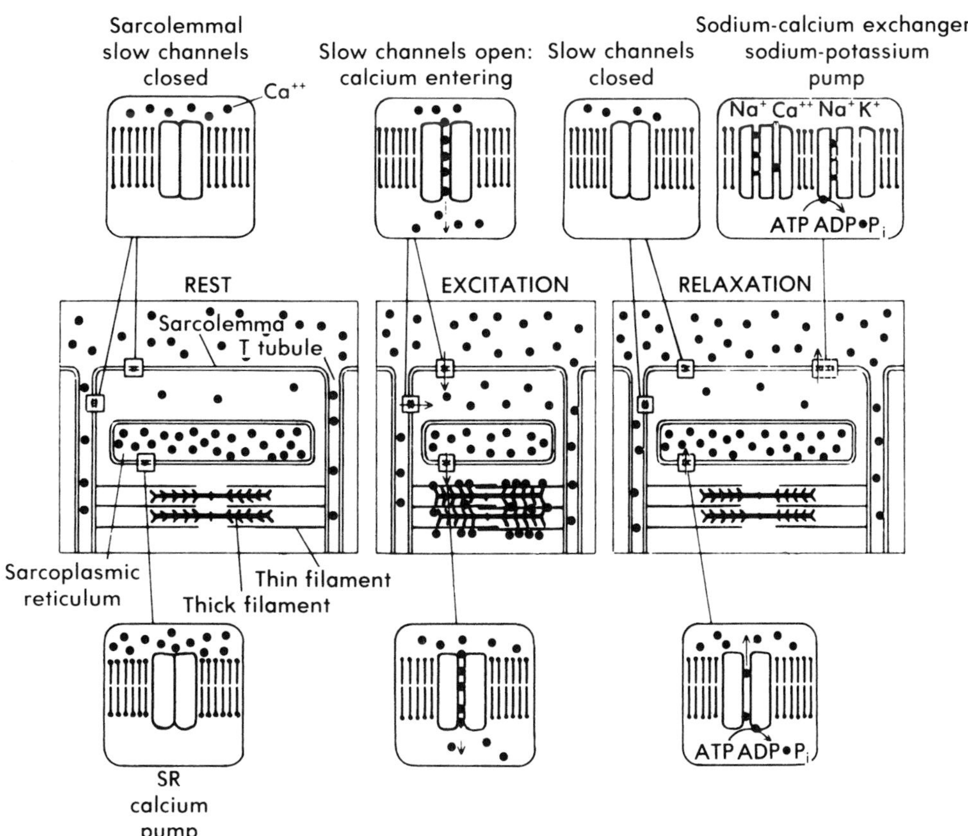

Fig. 37-3. Representation of the transmembrane calcium movements during a contraction cycle. At rest, calcium concentration in the sarcoplasm is low compared with the extracellular space and the interior of the sarcoplasmic reticulum. Slow channel is closed, and Ca^{++} pumps are inactive. During excitation, the slow channel opens, allowing a small number of extracellular Ca^{++} ions to enter the cell. This entry triggers a release of Ca^{++} from the sarcoplasmic reticulum (SR), and contraction proceeds. Relaxation is accomplished by the active restoration of resting gradients. *ADP,* Adenosine diphosphate; *ATP,* adenosine triphosphate; P_i, inorganic phosphate. (From Katz AM, Smith VE. Relaxation abnormalities. I. Mechanisms. Hosp Pract 19[1]:69, 1984.)

Preload is defined as the distending force, or load, that is placed on a muscle before contraction. The preload and the distensibility of the muscle are the determinants of the initial length of the muscle before contraction. The load encountered by the muscle after activation is defined as the afterload. The magnitude of the afterload determines the nature of the subsequent contraction. If the muscle is able to generate a force equivalent to the afterload, shortening occurs. Such a contraction is termed isotonic, since the force developed by the muscle is equal to the load and therefore remains constant during shortening. If the muscle is unable to generate force equal to the load, no external shortening occurs and the contraction is said to be isometric. Contractility refers to the intrinsic ability of the muscle to contract independently of loading conditions. This meaning will become clearer as the characteristics of muscle activation are explained.

Isotonic contractions are useful for studying the shortening characteristics of isolated muscle. From these studies, several fundamental principles of cardiac muscle mechanics have been developed. The first of these defines the relationship between afterload and shortening. As the afterload is increased, the extent of muscle shortening and the velocity of shortening decrease.[19] This effect is shown in isolated cat papillary muscle in Fig. 37-4.

Cardiac muscle exhibits length-dependent properties: the length of the muscle before contraction affects the nature of the contraction. As initial muscle length is increased, there is an increase in both the extent and the velocity of shortening (Fig. 37-5). A third property of cardiac muscle involves the response of the muscle to inotropic agents. Positive inotropes enhance the contractility of the muscle, as defined by an increase in the rate and extent of shortening generated from a given preload. Fig. 37-6 shows the effects of a positive inotrope on the velocity and extent of shortening. A unique feature of the force-velocity relationship is that it allows an estimation of the contractile state of the muscle. Theoretically, the velocity of muscle shortening at zero load should be determined only by the kinetics of the actin-myosin association. Since any muscle contraction is necessarily loaded to some extent by the preload, the velocity of shortening at zero load (V_{max}) can be obtained only by extrapolation of the force-velocity curve to zero load. For the relationship shown in Fig. 37-6, the addition of norepinephrine resulted in an increase in the extrapolated value of V_{max}. In contrast, Fig. 37-5 demonstrates the required load independence of contractility as suggested by the stable estimates of V_{max}.[19]

Isometric contractions provide a convenient means to study force development in isolated muscle. When a muscle is stimulated to contract isometrically, the amount of force (tension) developed depends only on the length before contraction and the inotropic state of the muscle. Variations in afterload are not a factor, since by definition the magnitude of the afterload always exceeds the force-generating capability of the muscle. Increasing the initial length of the muscle at a given contractile state results in an increase in the level of resting tension borne by the muscle (Fig. 37-7). As the length of the muscle increases, the peak force generated from any given length also increases (see Fig. 37-7), as does the rate of force development (*dF/dt*). The addition of Ca^{++} has the effect of a positive inotrope on the isometric preparation. Specifically, resting tension is unaffected, but the peak force, time to peak force, and *dF/dt* are enhanced.

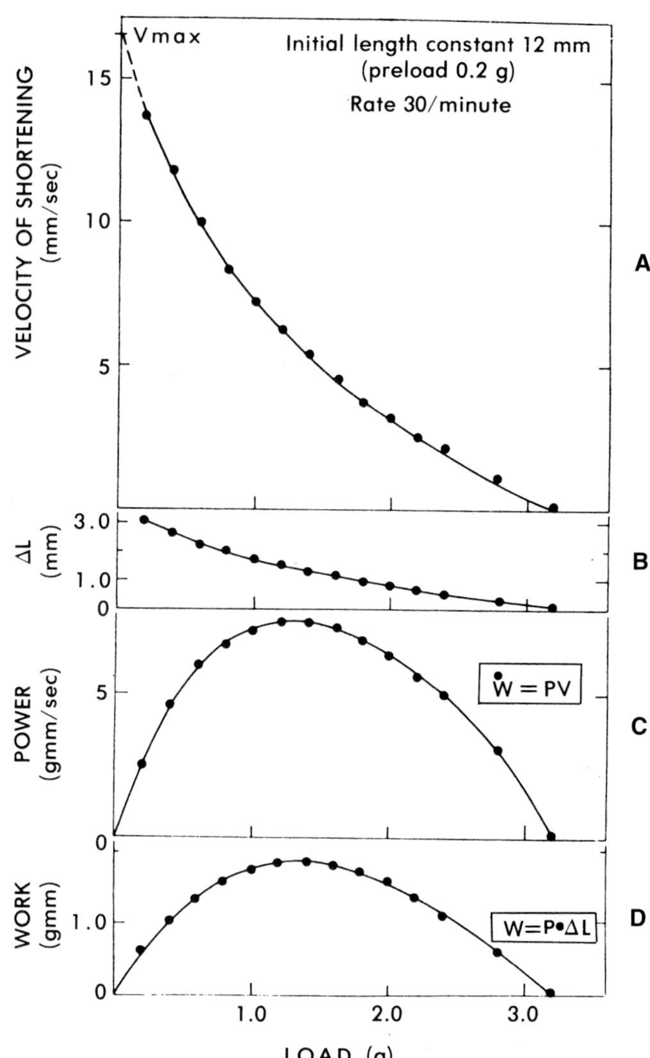

Fig. 37-4. Force-velocity relations for isolated cat papillary muscle. **A,** Velocity of the isotonic contraction is seen to be a decreasing function of load. Extrapolation of the velocity at 0 load *(dashed line)* provides an estimate of maximum velocity *(V_{max})*. **B,** Extent of shortening (Δ*L*) also decreases with increasing load. **C-D,** Concomitant effects of increasing load *(P)* on power and work *(W)*. *PV*, Load × velocity of muscle shortening. (From Sonnenblick EH. Implications of muscle mechanics in the heart. Fed Proc 21[Suppl 12]:975, 1962.)

When a muscle fiber is distended, a point is reached at which force development is maximum. The length at this point is termed L_{max}. Further increases in muscle length beyond L_{max} result in a reduction in the amount of developed

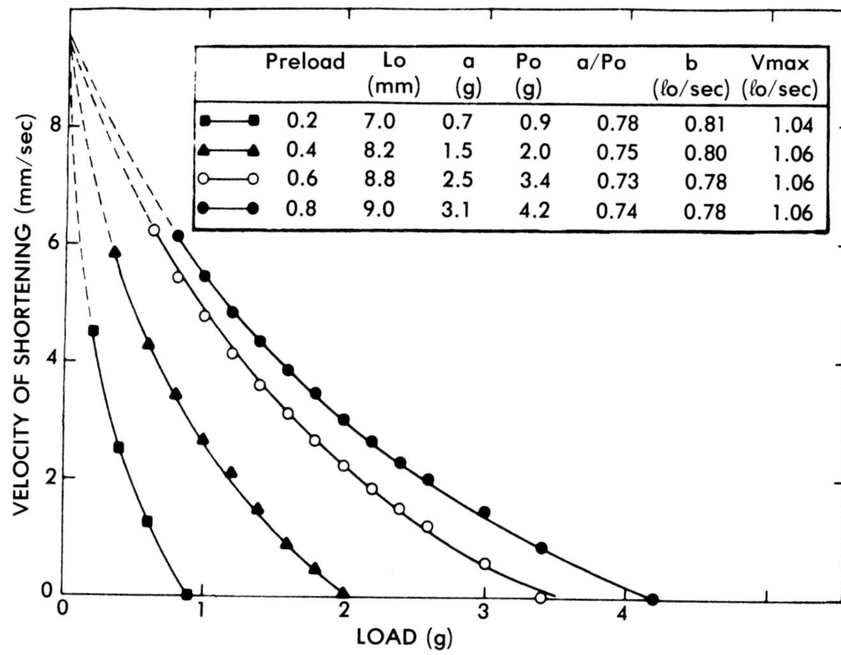

Fig. 37-5. Effects of varied preload on the force-velocity relations of cat papillary muscle. As the preload is increased, the velocity of shortening increases. However, the maximum velocity (V_{max}) does not change. (From Sonnenblick EH. Implications of muscle mechanics in the heart. Fed Proc 21[Suppl 12]:975, 1962.)

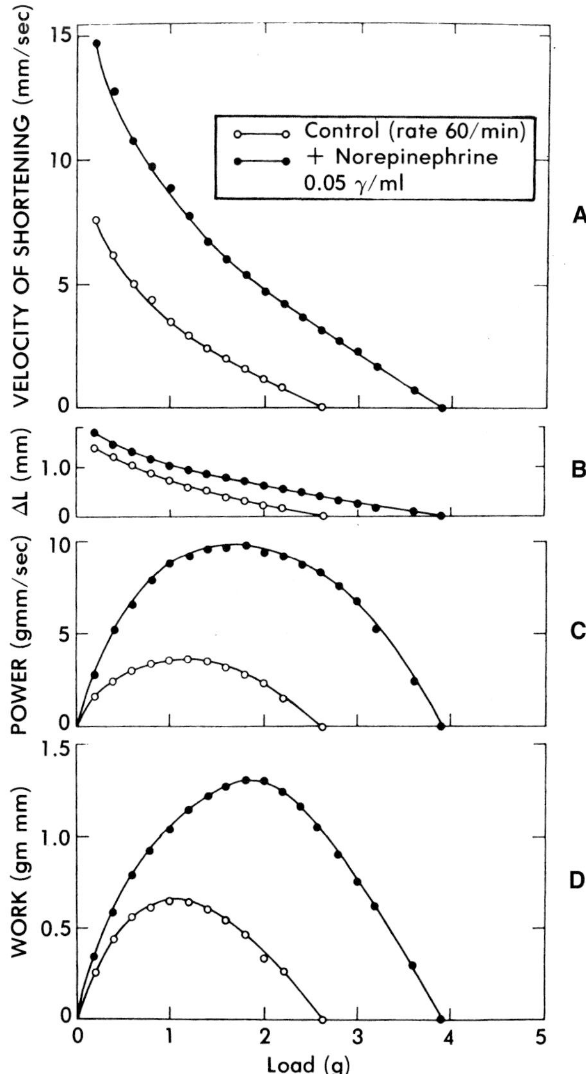

Fig. 37-6. A, Application of norepinephrine causes an increase in the velocity of shortening and maximum velocity. **B,** Amount of muscle shortening is also increased at any shortening load. C and **D** show concomitant effects of load on power and work. (From Sonnenblick EH. Implications of muscle mechanics in the heart. Fed Proc 21[Suppl 12]:975, 1962.)

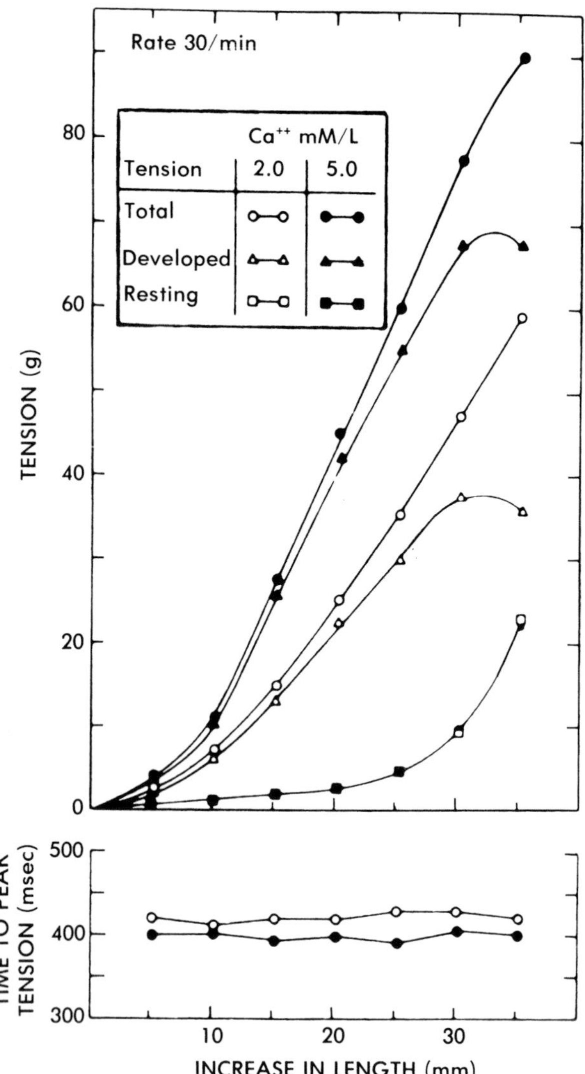

Fig. 37-7. When a muscle contracts isometrically, the amount of tension that is developed depends on the length and inotropic state of the muscle. In this figure the upward exponential curve *(squares)* represents the resting tension existing in the muscle as it is stretched to increasing lengths. Developed tension *(open triangles)* generated during isometric contraction from each length increases as the muscle is stretched. Addition of calcium does not affect the resting length tension curve but does cause an upward displacement of developed tension. (From Braunwald E, ed. Heart Disease, 2nd ed. Philadelphia: WB Saunders, 1984.)

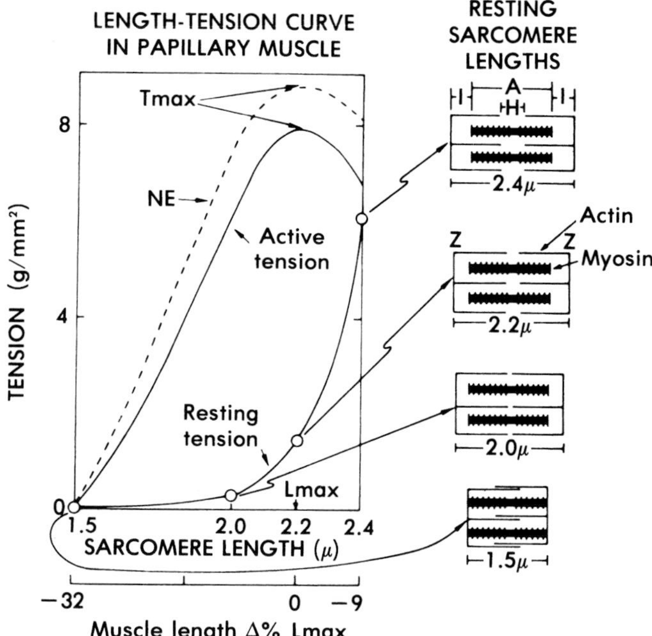

Fig. 37-8. Representation of the relationship between active tension, resting tension, and filament overlap in the feline right ventricle. These relationships form the basis of the Frank-Starling principle as seen in the intact heart. Note that the degree of active tension that is developed depends on the extent of filament overlap. Maximum active tension *(T_{max})* is developed at a sarcomere length of 2.2 μm *(L_{max})*, which also corresponds to the optimum length for filament interaction. *NE,* Norepinephrine. (From Mason DT, et al. Mechanisms of cardiac contraction. In Sodeman WA Jr, Sodeman TM, eds. Sodeman's Pathologic Physiology, 6th ed. Philadelphia: WB Saunders, 1979.)

tension.[4] This and other length-dependent properties of the muscle can be explained in part by relating the various muscle lengths to the degree of overlap in the thick and thin filaments of the sarcomere (Fig. 37-8). At rest, sarcomere length, defined as the distance between adjacent Z lines, averages 1.8 μm. As the muscle is lengthened, sarcomere length increases. More importantly, there is an increase in the degree of overlap between the chemically active portions of the thick and thin filaments. Since the potential for the formation of force-generating cross-bridges is increasing, there is a concomitant increase in the amount of force developed. The length of the sarcomere at L_{max} averages 2.2 μm.[4] At this distance the thick and thin filaments are arranged such that all myosin heads lie adjacent to actin filaments. In this state the probability of interaction between the filaments is greatest; hence force generation is greatest. With the application of large forces, cardiac muscle can be distended beyond L_{max}. Little change occurs in the amount of filament overlap, even though active tension declines sharply. This decline has been attributed to damage of the myocyte as a result of the large deformations produced by this loading force.[21] This relationship explains why overdistention of the heart (excessive filling) results in deterioration of cardiac function.

Examination of the resting force–length relationship reveals a nonlinear relationship between applied force and deformation.[22] This behavior is illustrated in the resting length–tension curves of Figs. 37-7 and 37-8. At the lower ranges of preload a given increment in applied force results in a relatively large degree of fiber deformation. In the upper range the same increment in applied force results in a smaller deformation. This behavior is a manifestation of the mechanical properties of the tissue. The significance of this property will become evident when filling of the intact heart is discussed.

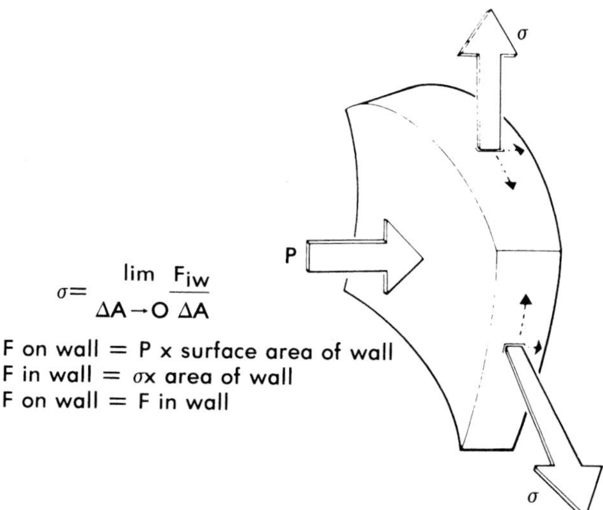

Fig. 37-9. Section removed from the wall of the left ventricle is acted on by a force *(F)* equal to the product of the chamber pressure *(P)* multiplied by the area over which it acts. For this element to be in equilibrium, opposing forces exist in the wall, which precisely balance this load. These forces are called wall stresses. This figure shows the loading pressure and the two principal resultant forces. (From Sandler H, Ghista DN. Mechanical and dynamic implications of dimensional measurements of the left ventricle. Fed Proc 28[4]:1344, 1969.)

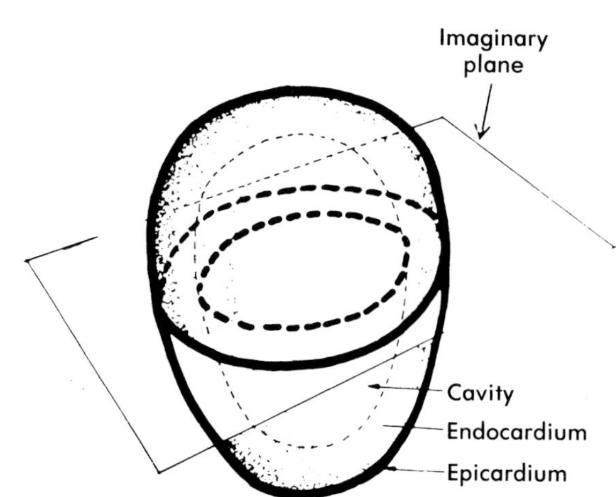

Fig. 37-10. Net wall force concept considers that the ventricle is divided by an imaginary plane located at the level of interest. Net wall force is simply the force necessary to hold the ventricle together at the given level. It is equal to the ventricular pressure multiplied by the area of the chamber involved in the plane. (From Hefner LL, et al. Relation between mural force and pressure in the left ventricle of the dog. Circ Res 11:654, 1962. By permission of the American Heart Association.)

FUNCTION OF THE INTACT HEART

The heart is composed of a complex array of muscle fibers that are arranged to form the various cardiac chambers. Each of these fibers operates under the same basic principles as those that have been established for isolated muscle, namely a dependence on preload, afterload, and contractility. Heart rate is a fourth determinant of the heart's performance per unit of time. Each of these factors finds its analog at the organ level, and together they determine the ability of the intact heart to establish and maintain the circulation of blood in the body.

Wall Forces

The force relationships that govern the function of muscle fibers in the intact heart are determined by chamber pressures and geometries. At any point in the cardiac cycle the pressure within a given chamber exerts a load on the wall of the chamber. This load (in dynes) is equivalent to the product of the pressure (dynes/cm^2) and the area over which the pressure acts (cm^2). In accordance with Newton's law of motion, this load must be precisely balanced by opposing forces in the wall. These forces, normalized to the areas over which they act, are known as wall stresses.[23] Fig. 37-9 shows the chamber pressure acting on a section of the wall of the left ventricle and the two principal resultant forces. Assuming an ellipsoidal representation for the left ventricle, application of the Laplace relationship results in the following expression for the meridional (σ_1) and equatorial (σ_2) components of stress:

$$\frac{\sigma_1}{R_1} + \frac{\sigma_2}{R_2} = \frac{P}{h}$$

where R_1 and R_2 represent the principal radii of curvature for the ellipsoid; P is the ventricular pressure; and h is the wall thickness. A number of expressions are available for independent solutions of σ_1 and σ_2 based on ventricular dimensions and pressure. These expressions and their limitations have been reviewed.[24]

An alternative method of conceptualizing force considers only the net force existing in the wall rather than the normalized force.[25] The net wall force at any level may be calculated by imagining that the ventricle has been transected by a plane (Fig. 37-10). The force necessary to hold the ventricle intact, then, is the net force acting in the wall at that level. This force is equal to the product of the ventricular pressure and the area of the chamber included in the plane. For a sphere this force is constant at any level. For an ellipsoid the net force depends on the plane of the section. If the section is made normal to the long axis of the ventricle, the pressure x area product is equivalent to the net force in the meridional direction. The magnitude of this force decreases as the plane of section is moved toward the poles of the ellipse, since chamber area is decreasing.[26] Wall thickness also decreases toward the poles[27]; therefore stresses and deformation tend to remain uniform. If the plane of section is considered in the long axis, the pressure x area product approximates the equatorial component of wall force. Fig. 37-11 shows pressure, equatorial wall stress, and net wall force for the left ventricle during one cardiac cycle.

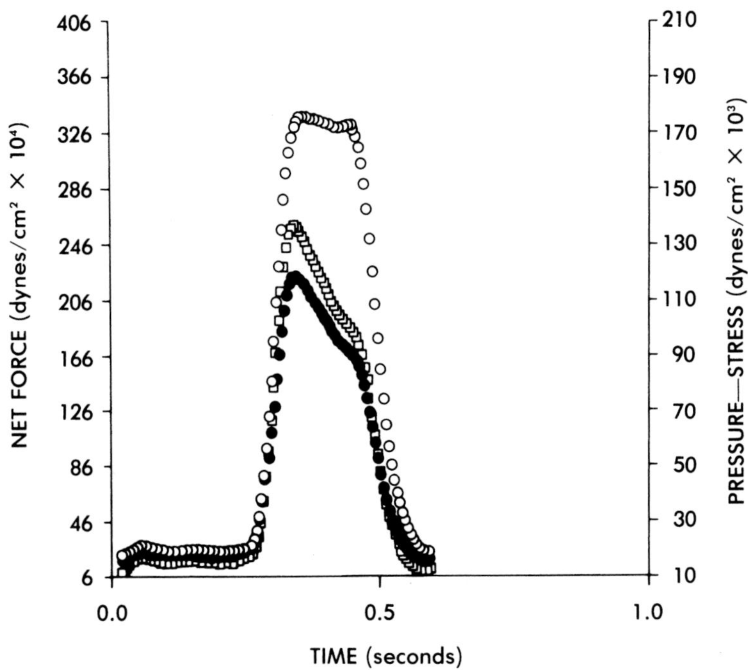

Fig. 37-11. Left ventricular *(LV)* pressure and wall forces for one cardiac cycle in the canine heart. Shown here are pressure *(open circles),* equatorial wall stress *(open squares),* and net wall force *(closed circles).* Note the fall in stress and wall force as the ventricle unloads itself during ejection.

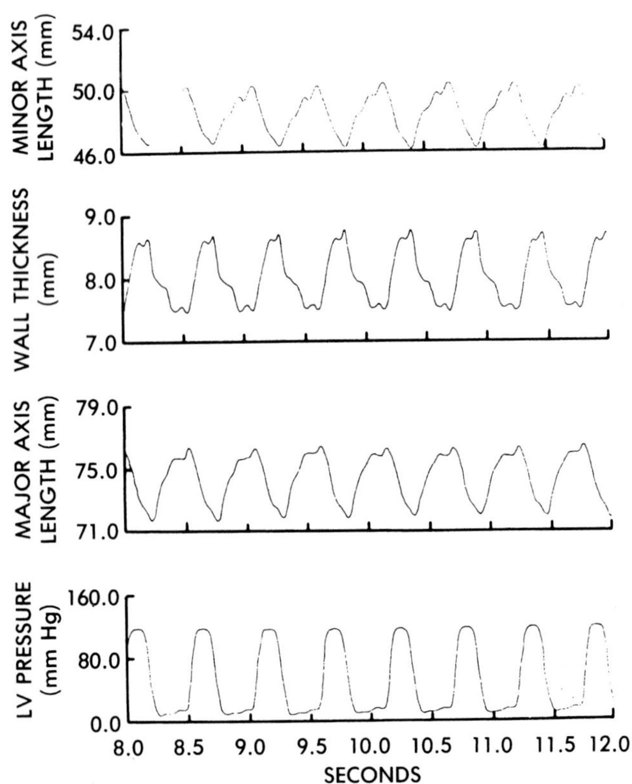

Fig. 37-12. Left ventricular *(LV)* chamber dimensions and pressure in the conscious dog.

Ventricular Geometry and the Cardiac Cycle

Efforts to quantify ventricular function often begin with the adoption of simplified geometric models. The normal left ventricle has been represented as an ellipsoidal shell, a sphere, or a cylinder, with various degrees of success. Even during the dynamic events of filling and ejection, accurate determinations of ventricular dimensions can be obtained with the appropriate use of these models. The elliptical model of left ventricular geometry is often used because it accurately represents the configuration of the left ventricle throughout the cardiac cycle.[23,27] In this model the left ventricle is considered as a general ellipse axisymmetric about its major axis, having a finite but varying wall thickness. The base-to-apex (major) axis is consistently greater than the transverse (minor) axis. The thickness of the ventricular wall is maximum in the equatorial minor axis plane and tapers to a minimum value at the poles of the ellipse.[27] During the cardiac cycle, muscle shortening produces variations in ventricular dimensions, with the resultant generation of pressures and volume displacements. Figure 37-12 illustrates left ventricular chamber dimensions and pressure for several beats. The complex anatomy, configuration, and contraction pattern of the right ventricle have precluded efforts to model this chamber accurately with simple geometric reference figures. Accordingly, the remainder of this section describes the pattern of hemodynamic events in both chambers, with the inclusion of dimensional information for the left ventricle.

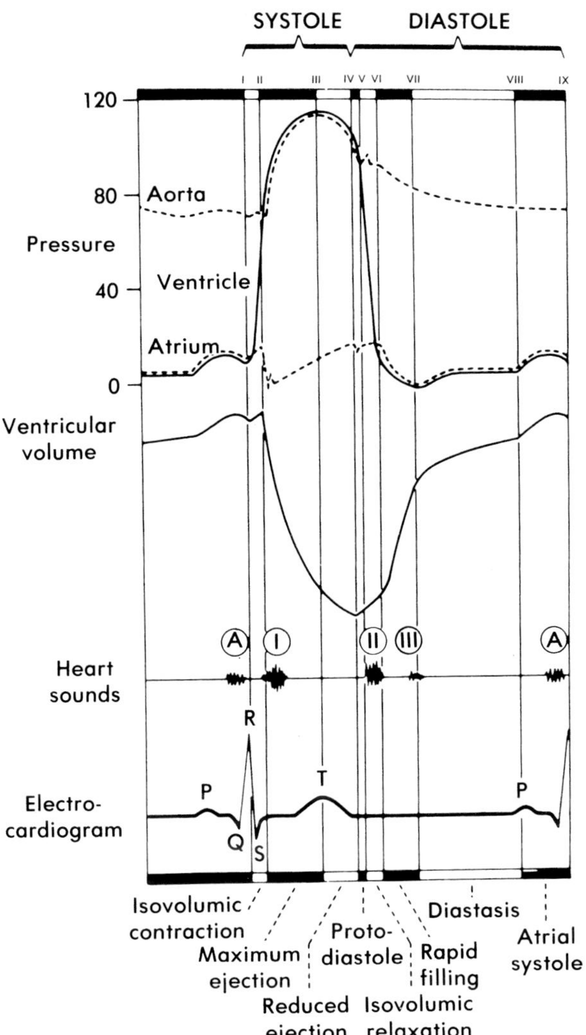

Fig. 37-13. Phases of the cardiac cycle. Shown are left ventricular pressure and volume and the correlation of these measurements to left atrial and aortic pressures, heart sounds, and the electrocardiogram. *A,* Atrial sound; *I,* first heart sound; *II,* Second heart sound; *III,* third heart sound. (From Katz AM. Physiology of the Heart. New York: Raven Press, 1977.)

The cardiac cycle can be thought of as beginning with atrial contraction, as indicated by the P wave of the electrocardiogram (Fig. 37-13). Atrial contraction provides a final, active increment in ventricular filling before systole.[28] With the onset of the QRS complex, the period of isovolumic ventricular contraction begins. This marks the beginning of ventricular systole. As ventricular pressures rise above atrial pressures, the atrioventricular valves close. The vibrations generated by the abrupt closure of these valves are responsible for the first heart sound. In the left ventricle the minor axis dimension shortens, the major axis lengthens, and the thickness of the ventricular wall increases,[27] resulting in an ellipsization of the chamber. During this period there is a rapid rise in the rate of pressure generation *(dP/dt).* This parameter reaches a maximum value at the onset of the ejection phase. Ejection begins when pressure within each of the ventricles rises above the pressures in their respective outflow tracts. The higher ventricular pressures result in an opening of the semilunar valves, and the phase of rapid ejection ensues. Rapid ejection is followed by reduced ejection as pressures in the ventricles and great arteries fall.

In left ventricular ejection the minor and major axes shorten, and the wall becomes thicker, resulting in a decrease in internal chamber volume. In the canine heart the major axis, minor axis, and wall thickness changes account, respectively, for 9%, 47%, and 44% of volume output during systolic ejection.[27] In the right ventricle, contraction occurs in a peristaltic wave moving from the sinus region toward the conus.[29] As ventricular and arterial pressures fall, flows in the great vessels reverse. This point marks the end of systole and the beginning of the first phase of diastole, known as protodiastole. Protodiastole ends with the closure of the semilunar valves, which produces the second heart sound. Such closure is also marked by the incisura of the arterial pressure tracing. Protodiastole is followed by the period of isovolumic relaxation. During this period the geometric patterns observed during isovolumic contraction generally are reversed, and the peak fall in *dP/dt* occurs. Ventricular pressures fall until they are less than pressures in the atria. The atrioventricular valves open, and diastolic filling begins.

Diastolic filling is composed of several phases. The first of these is the rapid filling phase, during which rapid volume expansion occurs. This phase is sometimes associated with an audible third heart sound. As the ventricles become full, the rate of filling slows, and the period of diastasis is approached. During diastole the left ventricle becomes more spherical as the minor axis dimension increases with respect to the major axis, and the wall becomes thinner.[27] The end of diastole is marked by atrial systole and the generation of the fourth heart sound.

At slow heart rates the atrial contribution to ventricular filling is minimal. At more rapid heart rates or with stenosis of the atrioventricular valves, the contribution of atrial systole to ventricular filling becomes more important. In the failing heart the contribution by atrial systole can result in a 20% to 30% increase in cardiac output.

Diastolic Behavior

Relaxation

Diastole represents the period of relaxation and filling in the cardiac cycle. During relaxation the ion fluxes that occurred during the process of excitation-contraction coupling are reversed, and the contractile proteins assume their resting configurations.

In the filling phases of diastole the relaxed sarcomeres lengthen as the ventricles distend with blood and the initial muscle length for the next beat is determined. Relaxation is often thought of as a passive event, since pressures and flows are rapidly falling; however, it is a period of considerable metabolic activity, requiring the presence of ATP initially to dissociate the actin-myosin complexes and later to provide the energy for the active transport, which restores the resting ion gradients. For relaxation to occur, sarcoplasmic Ca^{++} must be reduced to a level such that Ca^{++} dissociates from the troponin complex. This activity is accomplished by pumps in the membrane of the sarcoplasmic reticulum and to a lesser extent by transport mechanisms in the sarcolemma.[9]

The common feature of these transport processes is the requirement for ATP. In light of this, abnormalities of relaxation have been explained in part on the basis of reduced ATP availability in the injured or diseased heart.[30] An additional role has been suggested for ATP in the relaxation process. Adding ATP to a cell that has normal levels of ATP results in an enhancement of the uptake of Ca^{++} by the sarcoplasmic reticulum. Thus ATP may act in a regulatory manner in controlling Ca^{++} transport. Slight reductions in cellular levels as a result of moderate degrees of energy deprivation could result in impaired relaxation, even though sufficient levels are available to saturate the primary transport mechanisms.[9]

Filling

The importance of the filling events of diastole as determinants of cardiac function was first noted by Frank in the late nineteenth century. Frank observed a direct relationship between end-diastolic volume and the force of contraction in the isolated frog heart.[31] Later, Starling made similar observations in the mammalian heart. This work culminated in the concept of the Frank-Starling relationship, which was simply stated as "the energy of contraction, however measured, is a function of the length of the muscle fiber."[32]

In the intact heart, diastolic filling determines the length of the muscle fibers before contraction and therefore influences the force of contraction. The nature and extent of this filling, in turn, are influenced by a number of factors; among these are the level of filling pressure, the material properties of the myocardium, the geometry of the chamber, and such external forces as pericardial and pleural pressures.[30]

Within any of the cardiac chambers the filling pressure produces distending forces within the wall of the chamber. These forces are a function of the magnitude of the pressure and the size and shape of the chamber. The resulting distention produced by a given increment of force is governed by the material properties of the myocardium. Because these forces act to determine the length of the muscle fibers before contraction, they may be considered analogs to the preload previously described for isolated muscle.

The "material properties" of the myocardium refer specifically to the elastic and viscous characteristics of the muscle. An elastic material deforms when acted on by an external force and recovers from the deformation when the force is removed. For a substance with linear elastic properties, deformation (e) is related to the force (f) as:

$$f = E\,(e)$$

where E, the slope of the relationship, is known as the coefficient of elasticity or Young's modulus.[33] An increase in E reflects an increase in the stiffness of the material. In a viscoelastic material, force is a function of both deformation and the rate of deformation. Heart muscle is known to possess both elastic and viscous properties.[34] The analysis of these properties and their influence on diastolic filling is complicated by the fact that the elastic properties, and possibly the viscous properties, are nonlinear entities.[34]

When a force is applied along the long axis of an isolated papillary muscle, the deformation of the muscle

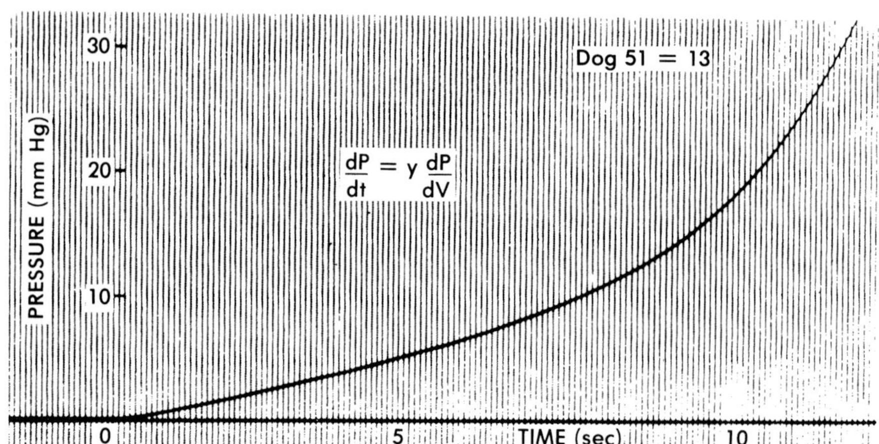

Fig. 37-14. Relationship between pressure *(dP)* and volume *(dV)* (expressed as time *(dt)* of infusion of volume at a constant rate) in the isolated, arrested canine heart. The relationship is approximately linear in the lower pressure ranges and becomes exponential in the upper range. The increasing instantaneous slope of the pressure-volume curve reflects the increase in chamber stiffness that occurs as the ventricle is filled. (From Diamond G, et al. Diastolic pressure-volume relationship in the canine left ventricle. Circ Res 29:267, 1971. By permission of the American Heart Association.)

obeys the following relationship, assuming that the rate of deformation is small so that viscous effects are not important[22]:

$$F = \alpha \left[e^{\beta(x-x^*)} - 1\right]$$

where x is the muscle length, x* is the resting muscle length, and α and β are elastic constants analogous to the coefficient of elasticity of Equation 2. F is the fiber stress. Stress is an expression of normalized force, here equal to the applied force divided by the cross-sectional area of the muscle specimen. This nonlinear elasticity of heart muscle is the principal factor affecting the relationship between diastolic pressure and volume in the intact left ventricle.[35] Fig. 37-14 shows the pressure-volume curve obtained by slowly filling a canine heart with saline. Several important points are apparent from this illustration. First, even though the ventricle is composed of muscle that displays exponential elastic behavior, the relationship between pressure and volume is not truly exponential. It is approximately linear in the lower pressure ranges and approaches exponentiality in the upper pressure ranges. Second, the elastic nature of the myocardium resist deformation above a filling pressure of about 20 mm Hg. The significance of the second factor is that the increasing stiffness of the cardiac muscle prevents overextension of the individual sarcomeres, permitting the heart to function on the ascending limb of the Frank-Starling relationship, where increased volume results in increased output.

Systolic Function

The peak force that can be generated at a given contractile state and end-diastolic volume is attained in the isovolumically contracting heart.[36] As the end-diastolic volume is raised, the peak developed force increases in a linear fashion (Fig. 37-15). This behavior demonstrates the operation of the Frank-Starling relationship in the intact ventricle, where force generation is an increasing function of fiber length, expressed here as end-diastolic volume. The line that results from relating peak force to initial volume defines the limit of force generation for the ventricle. When the ventricle is permitted to eject, this line also defines the limit of systolic shortening.[36]

Figure 37-16 depicts the pressure-volume relationships for an ejecting ventricle under changing conditions of preload and afterload. Contraction 1, originating from end-diastolic volume A, contracts isovolumically to point *B*. At point *B* the ventricular pressure just exceeds aortic pressure, and ejection begins. During ejection (points *B* to *C*), the force sustained by the muscle fibers in the wall of the ventricle represents the afterload. Ejection continues until a point is reached at which muscle force is maximum for a given volume (point *C*). This point contracts the isovolumic pressure-volume line and represents the end of systolic shortening. When preload is altered as in contraction 3, there is a change in stroke volume, but the extent of fiber shortening does not change. Contraction 3 still proceeds to point *C*. Increasing the afterload by augmenting

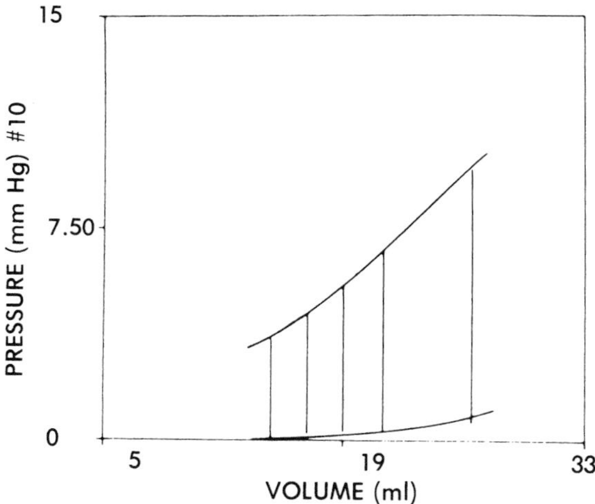

Fig. 37-15. Development of pressure in the isovolumically contracting canine left ventricle. As resting volume is increased, the peak generated pressure increases. Line connecting the peak pressures defines the limit of force generation for the contracting ventricle. (From Strauer BE, ed. The Heart in Hypertension. Heidelberg: Springer-Verlag, 1981.)

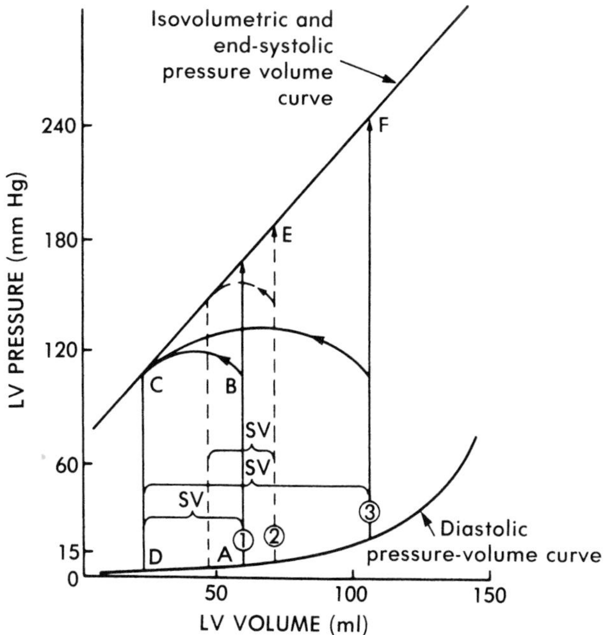

Fig. 37-16. Schematic diagram of the pressure-volume loops for several beats under various loading conditions. Contraction 1 is considered control, contraction 3 shows the effects of increased preload, and contraction 2 shows the effects of increased afterload on stroke volume *(SV)* and pressure generation. Points *E* and *F* represent the peak pressures that could be generated if the ventricle were to contract isovolumically from preloads at points 2 and 3, respectively. Note that points *E* and *F* define the limit for shortening in the ejecting heart. See text for further details. *LV,* Left ventricular. (From Braunwalk E, ed. Heart Disease, 2nd ed. Philadelphia: WB Saunders, 1984.)

aortic pressure (contraction 2) results in both decreased stroke volume and a change in the extent of fiber shortening. Thus the degree of fiber shortening in the ejecting heart is determined by the instantaneous load borne by the muscle, not by alterations in loading before contraction.[36] The ability of the ventricle to generate force is influenced by the contractile state of the muscle. A change in contractility is represented by a change in the peak force.

Electrical Activity

Electrically excitable tissues communicate within themselves and with other structures through the generation of action potentials. Within the heart there are certain cells that generate spontaneous action potentials, which propagate and serve as a stimulus to initiate contraction. This property is referred to as automaticity. A second property, intrinsic to the electrical activity of the heart, is conductivity. Conductivity describes the low-resistance intercellular connections that permit any depolarization to be spread throughout the mass of the heart.

Under normal circumstances, contraction of the heart is initiated by action potentials generated in the sinoatrial node.[37] This structure, located at the junction of the right atrium and the superior vena cava, has the highest rate of intrinsic pacemaker activity found in the heart. Actin potentials generated here spread slowly over the right and left atria, with resultant atrial contractions. Excitation moves to the cardiac ventricles through the atrioventricular node. In contrast to the atria, impulse conduction through this structure is extremely slow. This delay permits the completion of atrial contraction before ventricular activation. Having passed through the AV node, the wave of excitation enters the bundle of His, a structure located in the subendocardium of the right surface of the interventricular septum. The bundle of His then divides into right- and left-sided branches, which ramify in the fibers of the Purkinje system. The Purkinje system extends over the subendocardial surfaces of both ventricles. Its electric activity is characterized by a high conduction velocity, which permits near-simultaneous activation of the ventricles.

Many factors affect the nature of pacemaker activity and excitation in the heart. These include neural, hormonal, physiochemical, and pathologic influences. These influences often exert their effects by alterations of events occurring at the cellular level, specifically by inducing changes in the transmembrane electric potential and ion movement.[38] Transmembrane electric potential (V_m) in cardiac cells comes about as a result of an unequal distribution of ions across the cell membrane. In cardiac cells, as in most other cells of the body, the internal potassium concentration is high and the internal sodium concentration is low. The contribution of each of these ions to the net charge on the membrane can be estimated from the Nernst equation.[39] For an unspecified ion X:

$$E = \frac{58}{Z} \log \frac{[X\ out]}{[X\ in]}$$

where E is the equilibrium potential resulting solely from ion X, and Z is the charge number of the ion. If the membrane is permeable only to X, V_m equals E. When more than one ion is involved, V_m becomes a weighted average of the equilibrium potential of each ion. The weighting factors depend on the relative conductance of each ion. Conductance (g) is the reciprocal of resistance and is an expression of the ease with which an ion can cross the cell membrane. Thus in general terms, for a cell permeable to ions A, B, and C, V_m could be approximated from the equation:

$$V_m = \frac{gA}{gA + gB + gC} E_A + \frac{gB}{gA + gB + gC} E_B + \frac{gC}{gA + gB + gC} E_C$$

where in the case of cardiac tissue, the major ions involved in transmembrane flux are Na^+, K^+, and Ca^{++}, such that:

$$V_m = \frac{gNa}{gNa + gK + gCa} E_{Na} + \frac{gK}{gNa + gK + gCa} E_K + \frac{gCa}{gNa + gK + gCa} E_{Ca}$$

In the quiescent cardiac cell, K^+ permeability greatly exceeds Na^+ and Ca^{++} permeability—or in terms of conductances, gK greatly exceeds gCa and gNa. Given this fact, Equation 6 then reduces to the Nernst equation for K^+, and the resting V_m equals or approaches E_K.

Action potentials in cardiac tissue result from changes in the relative conductances of the principal ions Na^+, K^+, and Ca^{++}. Ion concentrations across the membrane actually change very little. The arrival of an action potential causes a rise in the resting V_m toward threshold value for the particular cell. Once threshold is achieved, a complex pattern of conductance changes ensues. Cardiac muscle cells and cells of the Purkinje system have a high relative gK at rest. Membrane potential is -80 to -90 mV, and threshold is approximately -60 mV. When cardiac muscle cells are stimulated, gNa becomes markedly elevated in what is known as phase 0 of the action potential (Figs. 37-17 and 37-18). Sodium ions are now better able to cross the membrane. Note that this movement is favored by both chemical and electric gradients, so it occurs quite rapidly. The net inward movement of positive charge causes depolarization of the cell; V_m moves toward and then past 0 mV. As the cell depolarizes, gNa falls, completing phase 0. Phase 1 is characterized by a rapid fall in V_m thought to be the result of a transient increase in membrane permeability to chloride (Cl^-). Phase 2 is the plateau phase of the action potential. This is brought about by a slow inward Ca^{++} and Na^+ current balanced by an outward K^+ current. Repolarization occurs in phase 3 and is a result of a further increase in gK combined with an inactivation of the slow inward current of phase 2.

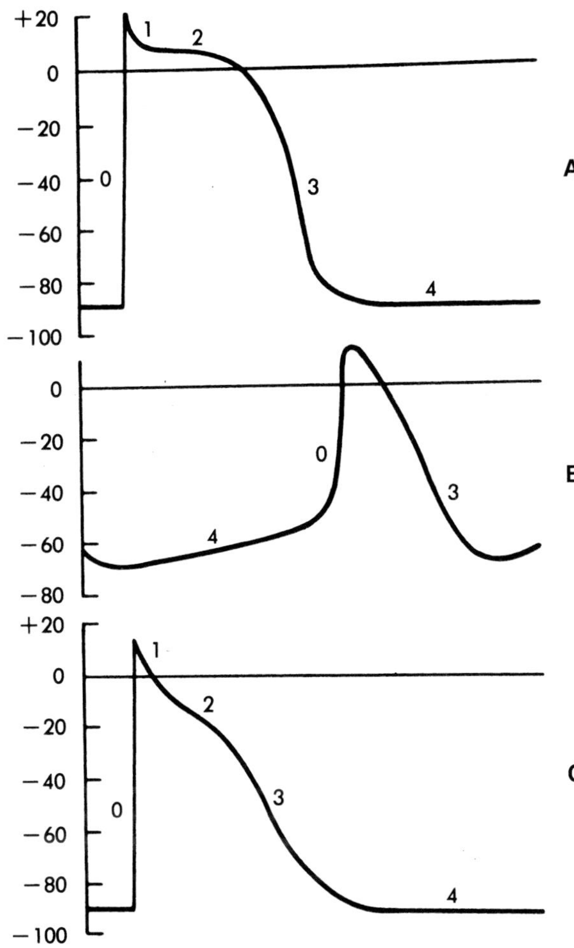

Fig. 37-17. Action potentials seen in various cardiac tissues. **A**, Ventricular muscle cell. **B**, Sinoatrial node. **C**, Atrial muscle. Time base for **B** is half that of **A** and **C**. (From Berne RM, Levy MN, eds. Physiology. St. Louis: Mosby, 1983.)

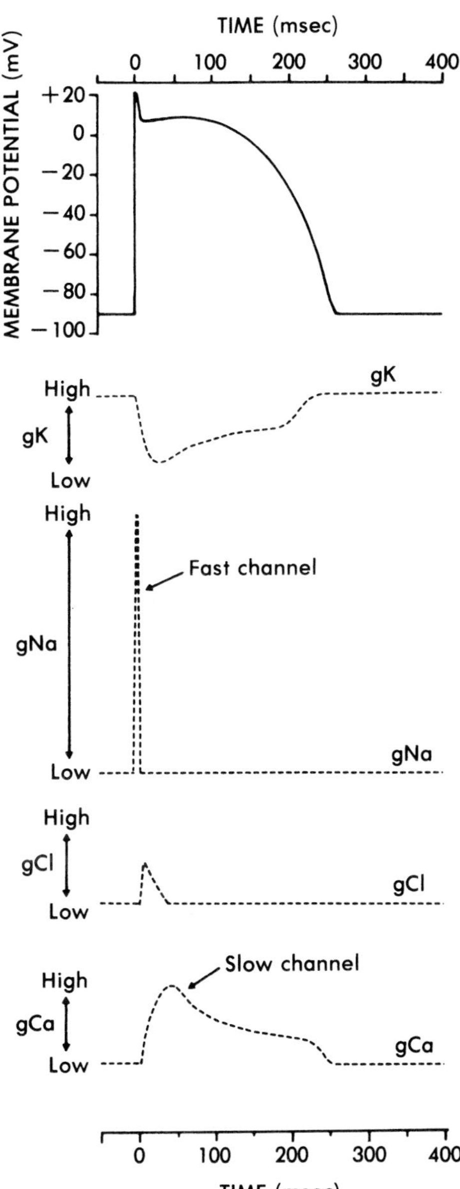

Fig. 37-18. Conductance changes seen within a Purkinje fiber. Typical action potential is shown at the top, with the accompanying changes in conductance for potassium *(gK)*, sodium *(gNa)*, chloride *(gCl)*, and calcium *(gCa)*. (From Katz AM. Physiology of the Heart. New York: Raven Press, 1977.)

There are striking differences between action potentials seen in the nodal structures and those just described (see Fig. 37-17). Recordings from cells of the SA node reveal a less negative resting potential, a decreased rate of phase 0 depolarization, no plateau, and a reduced rate of phase 3 depolarization. Perhaps most significant is the behavior that nodal tissue displays in phase 4. During this phase V_m is not constant but moves steadily toward threshold. The basis for this behavior is believed to be a time-dependent decrease in the outward K^+ movement in the presence of a small, steady, inward movement of Ca^{++}. The loss of the K^+ current disrupts the balance of charge and results in membrane depolarization. When the membrane potential reaches threshold, an action potential is generated. In this manner, nodal tissue serves as a pace generator for the heart. The rate of pacemaker activity depends on the minimum phase 4 V_m, the rate of depolarization, and the threshold potential.[40] These factors are under neural and hormonal controls that act to vary the heart rate[13] (Fig. 37-19). For example, increased vagal activity results in the release of acetylcholine at the SA node. This has the effect of increasing gK, which hyperpolarizes the membrane and slows the heart rate. Conversely, catecholamines can increase the inward phase 4 Ca^{++} current, which would increase both the rate of depolarization and the heart rate (see next section on neural control).[18,38,40,41]

Neural Control

The sympathetic and parasympathetic divisions of the autonomic nervous system act in concert to regulate cardiac function. Sympathetic effects are excitatory and are medi-

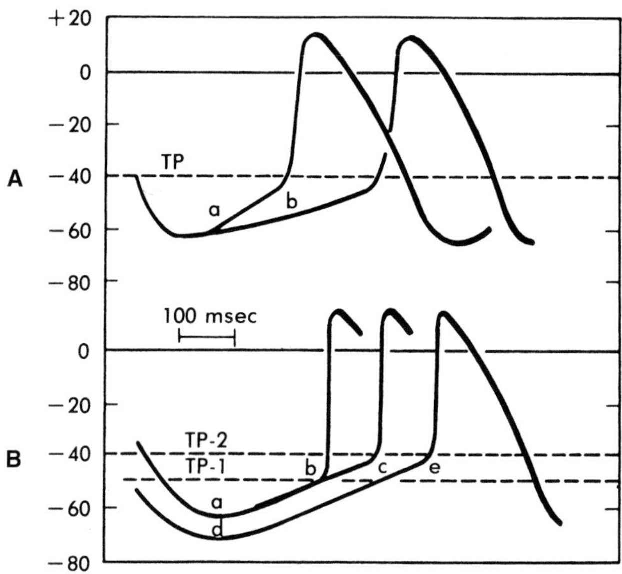

Fig. 37-19. Altering rate of pacemaker activity. **A,** Rate of firing is slowed by a decrease in the rate of phase 4 depolarization. Threshold potential *(TP)* is not changed. **B,** Changing threshold at a given rate of phase 4 depolarization can alter heart rate by changing the time required to reach TP (tracings a-b and a-c). Hyperpolarization can also influence rate (tracings a-e). (From Berne RM, Levy MN, eds. Physiology. St. Louis: Mosby, 1983.)

ated through nerve fibers distributed to the atria, ventricles, and nodal tissue. Parasympathetic influences are generally inhibitory and act predominantly on atrial and nodal tissues.

The terminal regions of the sympathetic fibers synthesize and store norepinephrine, which is released as a result of nerve stimulation. Norepinephrine acts on β-adrenergic receptors imbedded in the membrane of the cardiac cell. β-receptors in the myocardium are of two types, β_1 and β_2. β_1-receptors are distributed exclusively to the ventricles, and their activation results in an increase in ventricular contractility.[42,43]

The mechanism of action is thought to involve increases in the level of cyclic adenosine monophosphate (cAMP), which in turn promotes the phosphorylation and activation of calcium channels in the membrane.[44,45] The net effect of β_1-stimulation is an increase in calcium influx, which causes an increase in the contractile state of the muscle.[12] β_2-receptors are found in the atria. The activation of these receptors results in an increased heart rate through their positive chronotropic effects.[8] The stimulus for activation of β_2-receptors differs from that of β_1 types in that β_2-receptors are sensitive to epinephrine and norepinephrine.

Parasympathetic effects are mediated by fibers of the vagus nerve that are distributed to the atria, and, to a lesser extent, to the ventricles. Activation of these fibers results in a release of acetylcholine, which causes a depression of cardiac function characterized by a reduction in heart rate and atrial contractility. Ventricular contractility is affected to a lesser extent.[46] The diminution in ventricular function seen during vagal stimulation can be explained in part by reduced ventricular filling, which occurs secondarily to the fall in atrial contractility.[4] Acetylcholine produces its negative chronotropic effects by hyperpolarizing the nodal tissue. Hyperpolarization is a consequence of the increase in potassium permeability caused by the application of acetylcholine. Acetylcholine also binds to muscarinic receptors on the sympathetic nerve fibers. Activation of the muscarinic receptors results in reduced catecholamine release during sympathetic stimulation. Thus the inhibitory influences of parasympathetic activity are more pronounced when sympathetic activity is high.[46]

In recent years an increasing emphasis on neural control of heart function has been evolving. Trauma, anesthesia, and anxiety evoke major alternations in cardiovascular function and may be the precipitants of arrhythmias or cardiac dysfunction.

Coronary Flow and Myocardial Oxygen Consumption

The energy imparted by the heart to the blood during the process of ejection is linearly related to three factors: heart rate, stroke volume, and developed aortic pressure. A rise in any of these three variables leads to an increase in myocardial oxygen consumption. Minute work of the heart is defined as the product of these three parameters. Changes in stroke volume are associated with the greatest efficiency and the lowest energy cost to the heart, whereas increases in heart rate and blood pressure are costly and require the greatest increase in myocardial oxygen delivery.

Because heart rate and blood pressure figure so much more prominently in the determination of myocardial oxygen consumption than stroke volume, two clinical indexes based on heart rate and aortic pressure have been developed for estimation of myocardial oxygen consumption. These are the *double product* (heart rate multiplied by the blood pressure) and the *tension time index* (the average ejection pressure of the left ventricle multiplied by the duration of ejection). Both of these indexes correlate well with cardiac oxygen consumption, but neither takes into account the effect of ventricular dilation or altered contractility. It is obvious from this discussion that myocardial oxygen consumption can be decreased and the efficiency of the heart improved by a reduction in heart rate and a decrease in mean arterial blood pressure (vasodilation).

The flow of oxygenated blood into the myocardium is controlled by the coronary circulation. Blood flow is regulated to ensure an environment of aerobic metabolism to support cardiac work. To accomplish this goal, the coronary circulation possesses two unique features:

1. Under basal conditions, there is a high degree of oxygen extraction (coronary sinus oxygen saturation is 20% to 30%) so that the heart can adjust to changing oxygen needs by only a small increment in oxygen extraction.
2. Accordingly, increasing oxygen requirements must be met by proportionate increases in coronary flow.

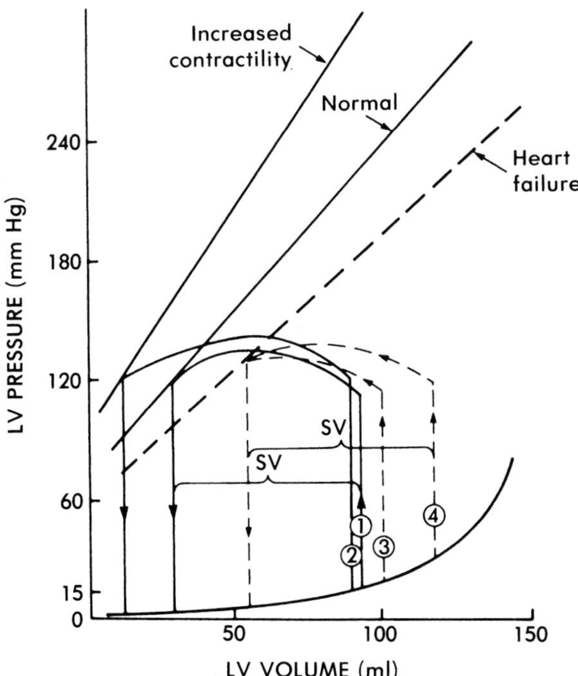

Fig. 37-20. Conceptual pressure-volume loops for hearts at three contractile states. Note the effect of the contractile state on the stroke volume *(SV)* generated from similar preloads at points *1, 2,* and *3.* During heart failure, SV may be decreased despite a slightly larger end-diastolic volume at a comparable level of aortic pressure (see contraction 3). If end-diastolic volume is further increased, SV may be restored (see contraction 4). *LV,* Left ventricular. (From Braunwald E, ed. Heart Disease. 2nd ed. Philadelphia: WB Saunders, 1984.)

HEART FAILURE

Contraction 3 in Fig. 37-20 represents a decreased contractile state, as might be seen in conditions of heart failure.[28,47,48] Failure occurs when the heart can no longer pump blood commensurate with the needs of the body. This condition can occur as a result of depression in the intrinsic contractility of the muscle or as a result of the imposition of increased loading conditions on ventricular ejection.[49] The heart can compensate in several ways. Contractile state can increase with endogenous catecholamine release. Also muscle preload can be augmented by the increased filling pressure that often accompanies the reduced pumping ability of the failing ventricle. Hypertrophy and/or chamber dilation also can occur.

Associated with these compensatory mechanisms are certain detrimental factors that may contribute to the eventual failure of the heart. Increased preload results in an increased level of wall stress throughout diastole. Wall stress has been shown to be related to myocardial oxygen consumption[50]; therefore incorporation of this mechanism necessarily increases the flow requirements of the myocardium. As chamber enlargement occurs, several aspects of active force relations are affected. From the net wall force concept developed earlier, it is simple to see how an increase in chamber size results in a decrease in the efficiency of the ventricular contraction. Recall that wall force (F) is equal to the product of chamber pressure (P) and area (A). Rearranged, this gives $P = F/A$. The generation of a given pressure within the large ventricle (larger A) then requires the existence of a greater wall force. A second aspect of chamber enlargement concerns the unloading of the ventricle during systole. In a normal heart the muscle load (stress) peaks soon after the onset of ejection and then declines through the remainder of systole (see Fig. 37-11). This occurs because the chamber size decreases more than the pressure increases, resulting in a partial unloading of the ventricle. To generate a given stroke volume, the enlarged heart undergoes a smaller degree of systolic shortening. It therefore unloads itself less than would a smaller heart ejecting the same volume. Worsened ejection resulting from prolonged high wall tension creates an afterload mismatch in the coupling of the heart of the periphery. Vasodilator therapy normalizes this loading of the heart and thereby facilitates ejection. At the same time, smaller volumes and wall tension decrease myocardial oxygen consumption.

SUMMARY

For many years the complexity of the cardiovascular system prevented the systematic study of its properties. Although that complexity remains, several basic principles by which the heart functions have been determined. These principles include the dependence of myocardial performance on preload, afterload, and contractility. Preload is defined as the distending force, or load, that is placed on cardiac muscle before contraction. The preload and the distensibility of the muscle are the determinants of the initial length of the muscle before contraction. The load encountered by cardiac muscle after activation is defined as the afterload. The magnitude of the afterload determines the nature of the subsequent contraction. Contractility refers to the intrinsic ability of cardiac muscle to contract, independent of loading conditions. Heart failure occurs when the heart can no longer pump blood commensurate with the needs of the body. This condition can occur as a result of depression in the intrinsic contractility of cardiac muscle or as a result of the imposition of increased loading conditions on ventricular ejection. Understanding the interplay among these various parameters and how their imbalance can be corrected or lessened, both medically and surgically, underlies the rationale for treatment in patients with cardiac dysfunction.

REFERENCES

1. Morkin E. Contractile proteins of the heart. Hosp Pract 18(6):97, 1983.
2. Bremel RD, Weber AM. Cooperation with actin filament in vertebrate skeletal muscle. Nature (New Biol) 238:97, 1972.
3. Weber A, Murray JM. Molecular control mechanisms in muscle contraction. Physiol Rev 53:612, 1973.
4. Braunwald E, Sonnenblick EH, Ross J. Contraction of the normal heart. In Braunwalk E, ed. Heart Disease. Philadelphia: WB Saunders, 1984.

5. Spudich JA. How molecular motors work. Nature 372:515, 1994.
6. Ebashi S. Excitation-contraction coupling and the mechanism of muscle contraction. Annu Rev Physiol 53:1, 1991.
7. Elliott GF, Worthington CR. How muscle may contract. Biochim Biophys Acta 1200:109, 1994.
8. Honerjager P. Pharmacology of bipyridine phosphodiesterase III inhibitors. Am Heart J 121:1939, 1991.
9. Katz AM, Smith VE. Relaxation abnormalities. I. Mechanisms. Hosp Pract 19(1):69, 1984.
10. Schwartz K, et al. Myosin isoenzymic distribution correlates with speed of myocardial contraction. J Mol Cell Cardiol 13:1071, 1981.
11. Samuel JL, et al. Distribution of myosin isozymes with single cardiac cells: An immunohistochemical study. Circ Res 52:200, 1983.
12. van Breeman C, Aaronson P, Loutzenhiser R. Na-Ca interactions in mammalian smooth muscle. Pharmacol Rev 30:167, 1979.
13. Hoh JFY, McGrath PA, Hale PT. Electrophoretic analysis of multiple forms of rat cardiac myosin: Effects of hypophysectomy and thyroid replacement. J Mol Cell Cardiol 10:1053, 1978.
14. Rupp H. The adaptive changes in the isoenzyme pattern of myosin from hypertrophied rat myocardium as a result of pressure overload and physical training. Basic Res Cardiol 76:79, 1981.
15. Fabiato A, Fabiato F. Calcium and cardiac excitation-contraction coupling. Annu Rev Physiol 41:473, 1979.
16. Barry WH, Bridge JHB. Intracellular calcium homeostasis. Circulation 87:1806, 1993.
17. Katz AM. Physiology of the Heart. New York: Raven Press, 1992.
18. Swynghedauw B, Coraboeuf E. Cardiac hypertrophy and failure. In Willerson JT, Cohn JN, eds. Cardiovascular Medicine. New York: Churchill-Livingstone, 1995, p 771.
19. Sonnenblick EH. Implications of muscle mechanics in the heart. Fed Proc 21:975, 1962.
20. Katz AM. Regulation of cardiac contraction and relaxation. In Willerson JT, Cohn JN, eds. Cardiovascular Medicine. New York: Churchill-Livingstone, 1995, p 790.
21. Sonnenblick EH, et al. Redefinition of the ultrastructural basis of the cardiac length-tension relations. Circulation 48(Suppl 4):65, 1973.
22. Glantz SA, Kernoff RS. Muscle stiffness determined from canine left ventricular pressure-volume curves. Circ Res 37:787, 1975.
23. Sandler H, Ghista DN. Mechanical and dynamic implications of dimensional measurements of the left ventricle. Fed Proc 28(4):1344, 1969.
24. Yin FCP. Ventricular wall stress. Circ Res 49(4):829, 1981.
25. Hefner LL, et al. Relation between mural force and pressure in the left ventricle of the dog. Circ Res 11:654, 1962.
26. Weber KT, et al. Contractile mechanics and the interaction of the right and left ventricles. Am J Cardiol 47:686, 1981.
27. Rankin JS, et al. The three-dimensional dynamic geometry of the left ventricle in the conscious dog. Circ Res 39(3):304, 1976.
28. Foex P, Leone BJ. Pressure-volume loops: A dynamic approach to the assessment of ventricular function. J Cardiothorac Vasc Anesth 8:84, 1994.
29. Meier GD, et al. Contractile function in canine right ventricle. Am J Physiol 239(8):H794, 1980.
30. Grossman W, Barry WH. Diastolic pressure-volume relations in the diseased heart. Fed Proc 39:148, 1980.
31. Frank O. On the dynamics of cardiac muscle. Am Heart J 58(2):282, 1959.
32. Starling EH. The Linacre lecture on the law of the heart. London: Longmans Green, 1918.
33. Mirsky I, Pasipoularides A. Elastic properties of normal and hypertrophied cardiac muscle. Fed Proc 39:156, 1980.
34. Pouleur H, et al. Diastolic viscous properties of the intact canine left ventricle. Circ Res 45:410, 1979.
35. Glantz SA. Computing indices of diastolic stiffness has been counterproductive. Fed Proc 39:162, 1980.
36. Weber KT, Janicki JS. The heart as a muscle-pump system and the concept of heart failure. Am Heart J 98(3):371, 1979.
37. DiFrancesco D. Pacemaker mechanisms in cardiac tissue. Annu Rev Physiol 55:455, 1993.
38. Naccarelli GV, Willerson JT, Blomqvist CG. Recognition and physiologic treatment of cardiac arrhythmias and conduction disturbances. In Willerson JT, Cohn JN, eds. Cardiovascular Medicine. New York: Churchill-Livingstone, 1995, p 1282.
39. DeVoe RD, Maloney PC. Principles of cell homeostasis. In Mountcastle VB, ed. Medical Physiology, 14th ed. St. Louis: Mosby, 1980.
40. Campbell DL, Rasmusson RL, Strauss HC. Ionic current mechanisms generating vertebrate primary cardiac pacemaker activity at the single cell level: An integrative view. Annu Rev Physiol 54:279, 1992.
41. Coraboeuf E, Nargeot J. Electrophysiology of human cardiac cells. Cardiovasc Res 27:1713, 1993.
42. Hedberg A, Minneman KP, Molinoff PB. Differential distribution of beta-1 and beta-2 adrenergic receptors in cat and guinea-pig heart. J Pharmacol Exp Ther 213:503, 1980.
43. Homcy CJ, Vatner ST, Vatner DE. Beta-adrenergic receptor regulation in the heart in pathophysiologic states: Abnormal adrenergic responsiveness in cardiac disease. Annu Rev Physiol 53:137, 1991.
44. Feldman AM. Classification of positive inotropic agents. J Am Coll Cardiol 22:1223, 1993.
45. Leier CV. Current status of non-digitalis positive inotropic drugs. Am J Cardiol 69:120G, 1992.
46. Levy MN, Martin PJ. Neural control of the heart. In Berne RM, ed. Handbook of Physiology, Section 2, The Cardiovascular System, vol 1. The Heart. Bethesda, Md.: American Physiological Society, 1979.
47. Folkow B, Svanborg B. Physiology of cardiovascular aging. Physiol Rev 73:725, 1993.
48. Klug D, Robert V, Swynghedauw B. Role of mechanical and hormonal factors in cardiac remodeling and the biologic limits of myocardial adaptation. Am J Cardiol 71:46A, 1993.
49. Braunwald E. Pathophysiology of heart failure. In Braunwald E, ed. Heart Disease. Philadelphia: WB Saunders, 1984.
50. McDonald RH Jr, Taylor RR, Gingolani HE. Measurement of myocardial-developed tension and its relation to oxygen consumption. Am J Physiol 211:667, 1966.

38

Heart Failure and Resuscitation

Reynolds M. Delgado III, Camelia A. Davtyan, and Heinrich Taegtmeyer

When the patient thinks there is something amiss with his heart, he fears it may fail. It is therefore necessary that the doctor should understand what heart failure is and the signs by which it is made manifest.—Sir John Mackenzie, 1916[1]

Heart failure is a systemic disease caused by an impairment of efficient energy transfer in heart muscle. Clinically, heart failure exists when the heart fails in one or both of its primary functions: during diastole to receive blood into the ventricles under low pressure, during systole to propel blood into the systemic circulation under high pressure.[2] Since the heart is both a consumer and provider of energy, a restriction in energy consumption (e.g., as it occurs in ischemic heart disease) results in impaired energy delivery to the rest of the body.[3] Impaired energy delivery, in turn, causes adaptive and ultimately maladaptive responses of the organism as a whole.

This chapter focuses on aspects of heart failure most commonly encountered in the practice of surgery. The first part of the chapter reviews the etiology, pathophysiology, clinical manifestations, therapy, and prognosis of acute and chronic heart failure. A discussion of chronic heart failure is important, as it is often a comorbid condition in surgical patients and may significantly alter the care and prognosis of the patient. The second part of the chapter discusses the principles of cardiopulmonary resuscitation, since cardiopulmonary arrest (also termed "sudden death") is the extreme form of acute heart failure. The discussion includes the pathophysiology and etiology of cardiopulmonary arrest and techniques of resuscitation.

Heart Failure

FEATURES OF HEART FAILURE

Irrespective of the causes of heart failure, it is useful to distinguish its clinical features, which can occur either alone or in combination with one another. These features include acute and chronic, high-output and low-output, right ventricular and left ventricular, backward and forward, as well as systolic and diastolic heart failure.[4]

The rapidity with which symptoms of heart failure develop depends on the underlying pathophysiology and on the time allowed for compensatory mechanisms to develop. Acute heart failure occurs within minutes or hours and may be caused by loss of cardiac muscle from acute myocardial infarction, volume overload, or arrhythmias. Chronic heart failure develops over months or years, and may be due to a slow loss of functional myocardium (e.g., as in hypertensive cardiomyopathy). In addition, a patient with chronic heart failure may achieve a well-compensated state, only to experience a superimposed acute exacerbation of heart failure; for example, caused by arrhythmias, volume overload, systemic infection, or noncompliance with medications.

In the hospitalized patient with symptoms and signs of pulmonary edema, it is often difficult to distinguish an acute exacerbation of chronic heart failure (i.e., acute on top of chronic heart failure) from a new presentation of acute heart failure. This is especially difficult in patients in the perioperative period, in patients with renal failure, and in those receiving blood products or intravenous fluids. Thus it is important to understand the etiology and pathophysiology of the various forms of acute and chronic heart failure so that effective diagnostic and therapeutic decisions may be made.

ETIOLOGY AND NATURAL HISTORY OF HEART FAILURE

Heart failure can occur as the result of three general derangements. First, mechanical or anatomic abnormalities may be present within the heart, in the coronary circulation, or in the pulmonary or systemic vascular bed and may result in inefficient pump function. Second, functional myocardial abnormalities may occur as a result of long-standing pressure or volume overload, primary myocardial disease, or myocarditis. Third, rhythm disturbances may bring the rhythmic function of the heart out of order and lead to

CARDIAC AND SYSTEMIC ABNORMALITIES RESULTING IN HEART FAILURE

Structural Myocardial Abnormalities

Cardiomyopathies (hypertrophic, dilated, restrictive)
Inadequate myocardial mass (myocardial infarction, hypoplasia)
Presbycardia (senile cardiomyopathy)
Dysdynamic (ventricular aneurysm)

Metabolic

Endocrine (thyroid dysfunction, acromegaly, pheochromocytoma, hypoparathyroidism, diabetes mellitus)
Thiamine deficiency (beri-beri)
Ischemia
Acidosis

Infections

Viral, bacterial, rickettsial, parasitic, fungal

Inflammatory

Connective tissue disease
Rheumatic fever

Toxic

Drugs (doxorubicin [Adriamycin], disopyramide, antituberculosis therapy, sulfonamides, heroin, cocaine, amphetamines, alcohol)
Cobalt, iron, lead
Radiation

Infiltrative

Amyloidosis
Glycogen storage disease
Mucopolysaccharidosis
Leukemia
Wegener's granulomatosis
Uremia

Cor Pulmonale

Acute (pulmonary embolus)
Chronic (emphysema)

Arrhythmias

inefficient pump action. In each situation the development of heart failure may be acute or chronic. In addition, certain causes of cardiac dysfunction may lead to reversible disease, whereas others, especially those that are chronic and cause intrinsic myocardial changes, may lead to progressive, irreversible derangements. A list of the different causes of heart failure is shown in the accompanying box.

Mechanical or Anatomic Abnormalities Causing Heart Failure

A hallmark of chronic heart failure is an initial phase of adaptation to environmental changes, which is followed by deadaptation of the heart muscle.[5] Adaptation is characterized by hypertrophy, which is brought about either by pressure overload or by volume overload of the heart. When presented with a patient whose main problem is heart failure, an important early step for the physician is to establish the cause of the compensatory hypertrophy. An increased pressure load on one or both of the ventricles may be due to systemic or pulmonary hypertension, aortic or pulmonary valve stenosis, pulmonary embolus, or coarctation of the aorta. An increased volume load may be caused by a valvular regurgitant lesion, an increased filling pressure, or a shunt between the systemic and pulmonary circulation such as an arteriovenous fistula, an atrial septal defect, or a patent ductus arteriosus. Obstruction to ventricular filling leads to a volume overload upstream from the stenotic lesion. Examples are mitral or tricuspid valve stenosis or rare congenital abnormalities such as cor triatriatum. Pericardial constriction and tamponade cause an extrinsic mechanical force that may lead to a restrictive pattern of heart failure. Other mechanical causes of heart failure include endocardial or myocardial restrictive disease, ventricular aneurysm, and ventricular asynergy.

Intrinsic Myocardial Abnormalities Causing Heart Failure

Intrinsic myocardial abnormalities may cause heart failure either because of primary myocardial diseases, such as hypertrophic cardiomyopathy, or because of secondary influences such as viral infection. Although there are many primary and secondary causes of heart failure, the clinical presentation and treatment are very similar. Identification of the cause is crucial because treatment of the underlying disease may afford partial or complete reversal of the heart failure.

Rhythm and Conduction Disturbances Causing Heart Failure

Rhythm and conduction system abnormalities may lead to symptoms and signs of heart failure. Extreme tachycardia such as seen in sinus tachycardia greater than 150 beats/min, ventricular tachycardia, atrial fibrillation or flutter, paroxysmal supraventricular tachycardia (atrioventricular nodal reentrant tachycardia), or multifocal atrial tachycardia, may cause symptoms and signs of cardiac failure, often with a normal blood pressure. Electric asynchrony and conduction disturbances, as in atrial dysrhythmias and bundle branch blocks, cause a decrease in cardiac output and can lead to heart failure, especially in patients with underlying impaired ventricular function.

The most common underlying abnormalities that result in heart failure include systemic hypertension and coronary artery disease. When the different causes of heart failure were evaluated in a long-term follow-up of 9405 subjects in the Framingham study, it was found that nearly 90% of patients with heart failure have a history of hypertension, coronary artery disease, or both.[6] Other causes, including the different forms of cardiomyopathies, make up the remaining 10%. These findings are shown in Fig. 38-1.

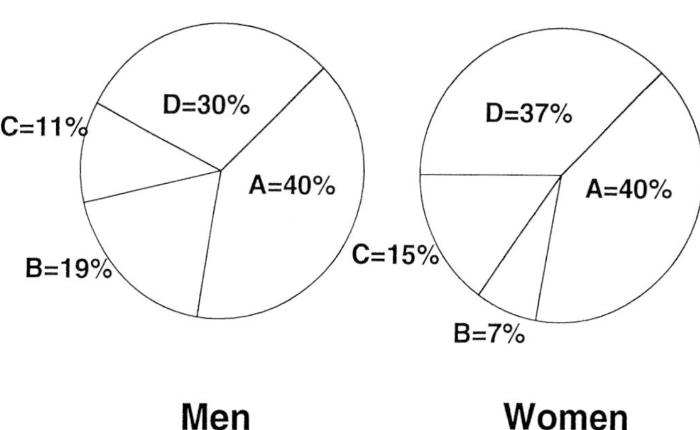

Fig. 38-1. The prevalence of coronary artery disease and hypertension among 9405 male and female Framingham study subjects with congestive heart failure. *A* = Coronary artery disease plus hypertension; *B* = coronary artery disease alone; *C* = neither hypertension nor coronary artery disease; *D* = hypertension alone. (Adapted from Ho KK, et al. The epidemiology of heart failure, the Framingham study. J Am Coll Cardiol 22(Suppl A):6A, 1993.)

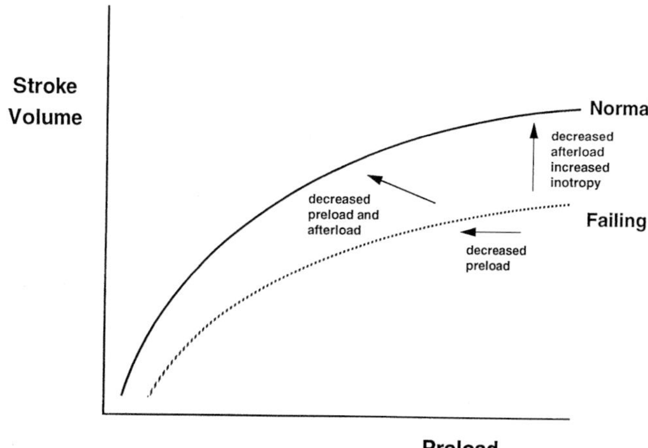

Fig. 38-2. Frank-Starling curves in the normal heart and in heart failure. An improvement in inotropy or reduction in afterload improves the ventricular performance. Reducing the preload alone does not improve performance, since there is no physiologically relevant "descending limb" of the curve. Combining preload reduction with either a reduction in afterload or a direct inotropic stimulus provides better systolic function and a reduction in ventricular filling pressure.

PATHOPHYSIOLOGY OF HEART FAILURE

As stated earlier, heart failure is a systemic disease that begins and ends with the heart. Just as the causes of heart failure may be varied, there are different pathophysiologic mechanisms leading to the clinical entity of heart failure. Cellular biochemical mechanisms may be at work either as the precipitators of acute heart failure or as mediators of chronic heart failure. Pressure overload, volume overload, or both may be initiating factors. Heart failure may be due to loss of contractility from loss of heart muscle, abnormal muscle proteins, or impaired energy metabolism. Lastly, heart failure may also arise from extrinsic influences such as increased pericardial or pleural pressures.

Biochemical Derangements

The heart consumes energy locked in the chemical bonds of fuel molecules through their controlled combustion and converts chemical energy into physical energy (predominantly mechanical pump work).[3] When this ability is impaired, it results in functional and metabolic abnormalities in the rest of the body, commonly referred to as "heart failure." This may occur, for example, because of lack of supply of oxygen, as in coronary artery disease, or in inappropriate use of fuels, as in a cardiomyopathy. Ultimately, the increased energy demands and impaired energy production lead to a state of energy starvation with subsequent further cardiac deterioration (decreased capillary density, decreased number of mitochondria, increased connective tissue). Other organs deteriorate because the heart no longer effectively provides energy in the form of substrates and oxygen to the rest of the body.

Mechanical Derangements

Left ventricular function is dependent on the filling pressure of the ventricle (preload) and contractility (Fig. 38-2), as well as the resistance of blood flow out of the ventricle (afterload) (Fig. 38-3). The impedance is the sum of resistance in small arteries and arterioles (resistance vessels) and compliance in larger arteries (conductance vessels). The normal left ventricle is able to adjust to changes in resistance through an increase in contractility. This increase is caused by an increase in ventricular filling pressure (Frank-Starling mechanism). After the ventricle has faced increased loading conditions for some time, the Frank-Starling curve becomes depressed, such that a higher loading condition no longer elicits a comparable increase in contractility. Thus the now dysfunctional ventricle does not respond as well to changes in loading conditions or increases in resistance.[7]

Abnormal Cardiac Contractility

The mechanism by which cardiac contractility becomes impaired is unclear and may vary significantly depending on the cause. Loss of cardiac muscle may occur because of loss of myofibrillar protein, as seen in acute myocardial infarction. In chronic heart failure, muscular contraction may be compromised because of decreased activity of myofibrillar actinomyosin, or myosin adenosinetriphosphatase (ATPase) proteins.[8,9] Additional abnormalities may occur because of decreased release or reuptake of calcium by the sarcoplasmic reticulum,[10] decreased sodium/potassium exchange, or decreased cyclic adenosine monophosphate (cAMP) caused by decreased β-receptor activity[11] or decreased coupling with adenylate cyclase across the sarcolemma.[7]

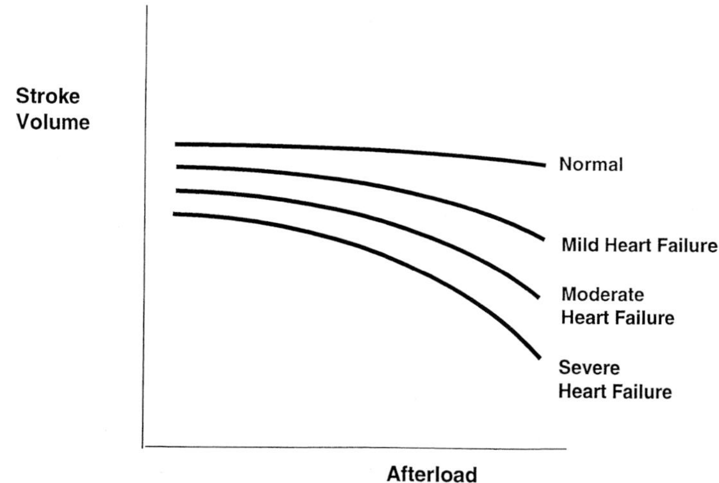

Fig. 38-3. The relationship between ventricular function and afterload in the normal heart and in heart failure. Small increases in afterload may lead to a significant decline in ventricular function. Conversely, decreasing afterload improves the systolic performance of the failing heart.

We have observed that heart failure can also be caused by impaired substrate flux through metabolic pathways. An example is the acute decrease in contractile function of the working rat heart perfused with ketone bodies as the only substrate, which is completely reversible on addition of glucose. This substrate-induced contractile dysfunction occurs because of inhibition of the Krebs citric acid cycle at the level of the enzyme α-ketoglutarate dehydrogenase and is reversed through replenishment of citric acid cycle intermediates by pyruvate carboxylation.[3]

Extrinsic Mechanisms

In addition to abnormal loading conditions, other extracardiac factors influence cardiac performance. For example, pericardial disease may produce an extrinsic mechanical stress that may impair myocardial relaxation, leading to a restrictive pattern of heart failure. In a similar way, increased pleural pressures may affect contractility, as seen in tension pneumothorax or mechanically ventilated patients with positive end-expiratory pressure. All these factors may decrease cardiac output, leading to high filling pressures and poor forward flow, thus causing the clinical syndrome of heart failure.

COMPENSATORY MECHANISMS

In both the heart and the body, the responses to altered pathophysiology are initially adaptive and later maladaptive. As we discuss the adaptive compensatory mechanisms in both systems, we recognize that the maladaptive responses in the body lead to the clinical presentation of heart failure.

Myocardial Compensatory Mechanisms

It is well recognized that in heart failure there are alterations of myocardial structure, changes in the contractile function of myocytes, and changes in blood flow to the heart. The myocardial response to volume, as well as to pressure overload, results in an increase of contractile units (hypertrophy) and thus a change in myocardial composition. This change leads to accelerated cell death with increased loading of the remaining normal cells.[12]

The mediators of ventricular remodeling and hypertrophy are local (autocrine) and systemic (neuroendocrine). The autocrine mediators are angiotensin, endothelin, endothelin-derived relaxing factor, prostaglandin I_2, and prostaglandin E_2. The systemic mediators include the renin-angiotensin system,[9] sympathetic stimulation,[13] vasopressin, and atrial natriuretic peptide (ANP). Some of these mediators are vasoconstrictors, others are dilators, and it is the imbalance between these mediators that leads to decompensation and clinical manifestations in heart failure.

Overload on the ventricles causes changes in gene expression, altered synthesis of myocardial proteins, and abnormal membrane assembly, resulting in preferential synthesis of fetal isoforms of several proteins, which have a shortened life span. In addition, there is evidence of overexpression of cellular proto-oncogenes c-fos, c-myc, and c-jun in response to myocardial overload, leading to altered protein synthesis and thus an abnormal myocardial structure.[12]

Pressure or volume overload on the ventricles results in an increase in length of the sarcomeres and an increase in the total muscle mass. This mechanism allows maintenance of an elevated ventricular systolic pressure (in the case of volume overload) without depressed contractility. As heart failure advances, the alterations in contractility make this compensatory mechanism less and less efficient, ultimately resulting in depressed ventricular function.[8]

Following the sustained increase in stroke volume, there is cardiac dilation and an increased rate of relaxation. The

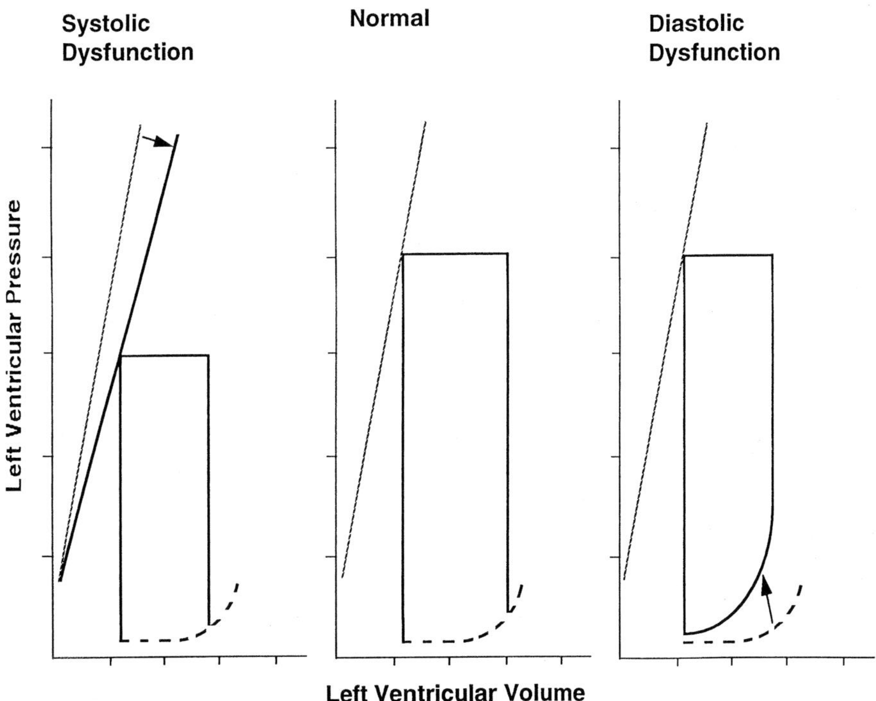

Fig. 38-4. Pressure volume loops comparing normal left ventricular function with impaired systolic and diastolic function. In systolic dysfunction, contractility is depressed and there is diminished capacity to eject blood into a high pressure aorta. In diastolic dysfunction, there is diminished capacity to fill at low diastolic pressure. The left ventricular ejection fraction is low in systolic dysfunction and normal in diastolic dysfunction.

combination of the above leads to an adequate cardiac performance until a phase of "exhaustion" is reached, which is characterized by lysis of myofibrils, interstitial fibrosis, a decreased capillary density in relation to myocytes, impaired coronary flow reserve, and ultimately deterioration of cardiac performance.

Ventricular relaxation during diastole is also altered in the failing, hypertrophied heart.[14] In this "diastolic dysfunction" the delay in relaxation with pressure overload interferes with diastolic filling and leads to elevated left ventricular filling pressures (Fig. 38-4). Sometimes this mechanism alone can be severe enough to cause clinically advanced heart failure.

Systemic Compensatory Mechanisms

Depressed systolic function of the heart leads to an inadequate effective arterial volume, which in turn triggers a series of humoral responses. Adrenergic stimulation, renin release, aldosterone secretion, and excessive release of vasopressin act to ensure adequate perfusion to vital organs.

The adrenergic system in heart failure is characterized by increased levels of circulating norepinephrine.[13] These levels correlate inversely to the severity of ventricular dysfunction and to prognosis. For example, in acute heart failure following myocardial infarction, the compensatory increase in norepinephrine in the early stages later becomes deleterious because of increased afterload and arrhythmogenicity. In chronic heart failure the prolonged increase of circulating norepinephrine leads to a downregulation of cardiac β-adrenergic receptors with a decrease in their density and subsequent reduction in contractility. Reversal of this downregulation may be achieved with β_1-antagonists, which have been shown in some studies to be beneficial in low doses in the treatment of heart failure, possibly by restoring the responsiveness to adrenergic inotropic stimulation.[15]

Aldosterone secretion is stimulated by decreased renal blood flow and increased sympathetic activity.[13] The release of renin leads to increased production of angiotensin II, which causes increased afterload and stimulates myocardial hypertrophy. The increased production of aldosterone increases retention of sodium and water with a further increase in preload. This chain of events leads to the so-called "vicious cycle of heart failure" (Fig. 38-5). Reversal of these effects by angiotensin converting enzyme inhibitors has been shown to decrease mortality in heart failure of different etiologies.[16-18]

Other systemic changes that occur in heart failure include changes in the levels of vasopressin, ANP, and peripheral oxygen delivery. The circulating levels of vasopressin are elevated in heart failure because of an abnormal response to serum osmolality. This causes systemic vasocon-

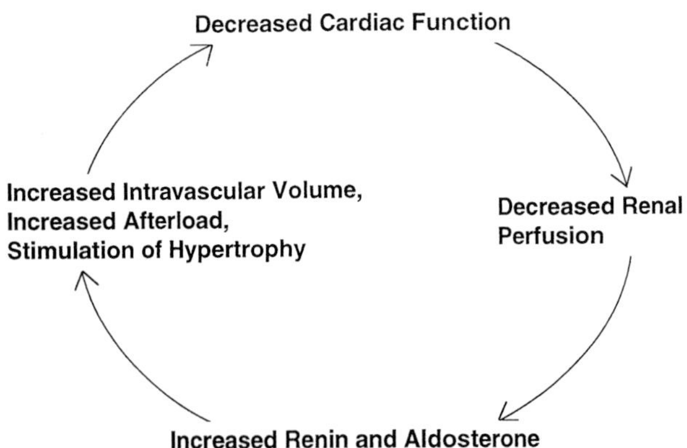

Fig. 38-5. This "vicious cycle of heart failure" begins with an impaired cardiac function, leading to a low cardiac output and thus decreased renal perfusion. The subsequent release of renin and aldosterone causes an increased intravascular volume, increased afterload, and stimulation of left ventricular hypertrophy, all of which exacerbate cardiac dysfunction.

striction and perhaps contributes to hyponatremia in the later stages of the disease. ANP is a counterregulatory hormone opposing vasoconstriction and sodium and water retention, thus protecting the heart from volume overload. In acute heart failure, ANP inhibits the synthesis of renin, opposes the effects of angiotensin II, and stimulates renal excretion of sodium and water, thus, decreasing preload. Finally, there is a change in peripheral oxygen delivery in heart failure caused by the redistribution of cardiac output toward vital organs, an altered oxyhemoglobin dissociation curve, and an increased oxygen extraction by tissues.

The compensatory mechanisms in heart failure are a "double-edged sword," as they support myocardial performance in the early stages of heart failure but later cause undesirable effects leading to accelerated deterioration of the failing heart. Thus the goal in treatment of heart failure is to modify these compensatory mechanisms using pharmacologic agents to break the cycle of maladaptive changes.

CLINICAL MANIFESTATIONS OF HEART FAILURE: A SERIES OF OPPOSING ADJECTIVES

Heart failure is characterized by a number of factors: sodium and water retention, dyspnea or fatigue (limitation of exercise tolerance), neurohormonal activation, decreased peripheral blood flow with subsequent lowering of end-organ metabolism, impaired systolic function, ventricular arrhythmias, and ultimately decreased survival.[7]

In describing the clinical features of heart failure it is useful to consider a series of opposing adjectives (see accompanying box). These descriptions are useful particularly early in the course of the disease, but they do not necessarily signify fundamentally different disease states. Late in the course of the disease, the differences between these forms often become less distinct.[5]

CLINICAL ADJECTIVES USED IN DESCRIBING HEART FAILURE

Acute vs. chronic
Right vs. left sided
High vs. low output
Forward vs. backward
Systolic vs. diastolic
Primary vs. secondary
Latent vs. overt
Reversible vs. irreversible
Compensated vs. refractory (intractable)
Stable vs. unstable

Right vs Left Ventricular Failure

The distinction between right and left ventricular failure was first proposed by Harrison et al.[19] in 1932. Pure right ventricular failure is most commonly caused by cor pulmonale from chronic lung disease and increased pulmonary vascular resistance. The symptoms include edema, congestive hepatomegaly, systemic venous distention, weakness, fatigue, and central nervous system symptoms. The signs include an elevated central venous pressure, hepatojugular reflux, ascites, pleural/pericardial effusion, bowel edema (causing anorexia, nausea, vomiting, and malabsorption), and cachexia. Left heart failure is characterized by poor cardiac output, an increased left ventricular filling pressure, and pulmonary congestion. The symptoms include dyspnea, orthopnea, paroxysmal nocturnal dyspnea, cough, nocturia, and hemoptysis. The signs are tachycardia, auscultatory gallop, inspiratory rales, expiratory wheezes, and pulsus alternans. Many patients with advanced left ventricular failure develop right ventricular failure, and a combination of both left and right ventricular failure is a common clinical presentation. This is especially true for patients with mitral stenosis and patients with a dilated cardiomyopathy.

High-Output vs Low-Output Heart Failure

The description, high output/low output, relates the cause to the typical clinical features. High-output heart failure is characterized by decreased peripheral resistance often in the absence of sodium and water retention. Etiologies known to cause high-output heart failure include hyperthyroidism, anaemia, arteriovenous fistula, beriberi, Paget's disease of the bone, Albright's syndrome, multiple myeloma, hypernephroma with bone metastases, cirrhosis, and acute glomerulonephritis. Low-output heart failure is characterized by retention of sodium and water and often an elevated peripheral vascular resistance and is caused by anything that decreases the cardiac output, including left ventricular dysfunction, and restrictive influences on the heart.

Forward vs Backward Heart Failure

The concepts of forward and backward heart failure date back to 1913 and 1832, respectively[20,21]; although they are old concepts, they retain clinical utility today. Forward heart failure involves inadequate discharge of blood into the arterial system, which leads to decreased renal perfusion, activating the renin-aldosterone axis and causing sodium and water retention, mental obtundation, and hypotension. In backward heart failure the ventricle fails to discharge its contents normally, and the end-diastolic volume and the pressure in the atria and ventricles are elevated, leading to pulmonary and venous congestion and sodium and water retention. The manifestations are hepatomegaly, ascites, and peripheral edema.

Systolic vs Diastolic Dysfunction

Systolic dysfunction leads to increased filling pressures and pulmonary congestion, decreased cardiac output, redistribution of flow toward vital organs, decreased stroke volume, and increased left ventricular end-diastolic volume with dilation of the ventricle.[22] There is a growing recognition of diastolic dysfunction (heart failure with normal heart size and ejection fraction) as a cause for impaired pump function of the heart.[23] As seen in Fig. 38-3, this diastolic dysfunction or "input failure" is characterized by the inability of the ventricle to relax and fill normally, leading to an increased filling pressure, increased ventricular end-diastolic pressure, and a decreased stroke volume because of decreased myofibrillar stretch and impaired diastolic filling. It is important to recognize that traditional therapy aimed at stimulation of systolic ejection may be ineffective or even deleterious in pure diastolic dysfunction.[14,23]

Other Adjectives Used to Describe Heart Failure

There are other adjectives of value in describing heart failure, which may relate to cause, treatment, and prognosis. In *reversible heart failure* the manifestations disappear if the underlying cause is removed early in the course of the disease. Examples include ischemia, valvular lesions, constrictive pericarditis, infectious endocarditis, hypertension, and most of the causes of high-output heart failure. *Irreversible heart failure* occurs when the manifestations do not disappear after precipitating factors are eliminated; in fact, they are often progressive. The classic example is myocardial infarction with extensive myocardial necrosis. Other factors leading to irreversibility include isolated myocardial cell loss and interstitial fibrosis with plastic transformation of the adjacent myocardium.

The commonly used term *congestive heart failure* refers to abnormal circulatory congestion caused by impaired heart function but also caused by peripheral circulatory and sympathetic renal compensatory mechanisms. A *congested state* is an expanded intravascular volume with preserved ventricular function, for example, caused by vigorous volume infusions, anemia, beriberi, etc. It is often difficult to distinguish congestive heart failure from a congested state, especially in the postoperative patient and in patients in renal failure. It often becomes necessary to use invasive monitoring with determination of cardiac output and pulmonary capillary wedge pressure to make the distinction. If the precipitating factors persist, the congested state may become congestive heart failure (ventricular function becomes impaired).

Primary heart failure refers to diseases arising from the myocardium such as congenital heart diseases, neuromuscular diseases, myocarditis, and presbycardia (senile heart). *Secondary heart failure* occurs because of other factors such as ischemic disease, systemic disorders, and metabolic and inflammatory diseases. *Unstable heart failure* means a severe circulatory derangement, which is life threatening if not aggressively treated, and includes acute pulmonary edema and cardiogenic shock. *Transient heart failure* ("flash pulmonary edema") is often seen in patients with diastolic dysfunction resulting from hypertension and following cardiopulmonary bypass.

Special Considerations

Often a patient with chronic, well-compensated heart failure is hospitalized for a surgical procedure or other reasons and experiences an exacerbation of heart failure, leading to worsening of symptoms or signs of heart failure. There are many factors that may underly the exacerbation, and most often it can be corrected by simply removing the offending cause; however, sometimes the cause leads to a direct worsening of ventricular function, which is irreversible and leads to unstable heart failure or a new level of compensation at a worsened functional class (see accompanying box).

EVENTS PRECIPITATING OR EXACERBATING HEART FAILURE IN PATIENTS WITH COMPENSATED DISEASE

Changes in environment or diet
Noncompliance with medical therapy
Arrhythmias
Myocardial ischemia
Anemia
Drugs: Nonsteroidal anti-inflammatory drugs, corticosteroids, calcium channel blockers, β-blockers
Thyroid dysfunction
Metabolic deficiencies
Infections
Worsening renal function
Pulmonary embolism
Pregnancy
Emotional factors
Myocarditis
Endocarditis
Systemic hypertension
Myocardial infarction

THE NEW YORK HEART ASSOCIATION CLASSIFICATION OF HEART FAILURE

Functional Capacity

Class I: Patients with cardiac disease, but without resulting limitation of physical activity. Ordinary physical activity does not cause undue fatigue, palpitation, dyspnea, or anginal pain.

Class II: Patients with cardiac disease resulting in slight limitation of physical activity. They are comfortable at rest. Ordinary physical activity results in fatigue, palpitation, dyspnea, or anginal pain.

Class III: Patients with marked limitation of physical activity. They are comfortable at rest. Less than ordinary activity causes fatigue, palpitation, dyspnea, or anginal pain.

Class IV: Patients with cardiac disease resulting in inability to carry on any physical activity without discomfort. Symptoms of heart failure or of the anginal syndrome may be present even at rest. If any physical activity is undertaken, discomfort is increased.

Objective Assessment*

A. No objective evidence of cardiovascular disease
B. Objective evidence of minimal cardiovascular disease
C. Objective evidence of moderately severe cardiovascular disease
D. Objective evidence of severe cardiovascular disease

*For example, physical examination, electrocardiogram, chest x-ray examination, cardiac catheterization, echocardiography, radiologic imaging, stress testing.

The New York Heart Association classification of heart failure (see accompanying box) has gained broad acceptance as the standard clinicians use to communicate with one another regarding the severity of heart failure. It is based on subjective and objective findings, with the objective assessment being based not only on physical examination but also on noninvasive and invasive tests to evaluate cardiac status. It is accepted that the severity of symptoms may not necessarily be matched by equivalent degrees of impaired structure and function of the heart.[24]

THERAPY

Broad Objective: Correct the Deranged Physiology

The goal in treatment of heart failure is to correct the deranged physiology while establishing and treating the underlying cause. Despite this, prevention of heart failure exerts far more salutary effect on public health than treatment. Prevention of the most common causes involves early and vigorous treatment of hypertension, hyperlipidemia, diabetes, and the promotion of life-style changes to lower the risk of coronary artery disease. In addition, the early use of thrombolytic therapy in acute myocardial infarction decreases the risk of development of heart failure. Finally, the identification and management of the specific causes and precipitating factors in heart failure are important (see accompanying box).

Once the diagnosis of heart failure is made, the therapeutic challenge is to alleviate symptoms and prolong life by correcting the abnormal physiology. The normal cardiac physiology involves both metabolic and mechanical derangements.[25] The correction of mechanical derangements involves the increase in supply of energy substrates and blood flow to meet the increased energy demands. For example, coronary revascularization may improve ventricular performance in patients with coronary artery disease and depressed ventricular function. The treatment of the normal mechanical properties of the heart may include the reversal of maladaptive hypertrophy with angiotensin converting enzyme (ACE) inhibitors or an increase in contractility with digoxin. The correction of systemic derangements involves lowering preload with salt restriction, diuretics, and venous vasodilators and lowering afterload with arterial vasodilators. The control of heart rate and rhythm is also important, and this can be achieved with β-blockers, antiarrhythmics, and pacemakers if needed. Lastly, in suitable patients with refractory heart failure, the treatment of choice may be cardiac transplantation; however, this option is limited by a supply of donor organs that is only a fraction of the demand.

Treatment of Acute Heart Failure

General Principles

The therapy of acute heart failure and cardiogenic shock involves treatment modalities that are both similar and dissimilar to those used in chronic heart failure. The most prominent features include a clinical assessment of the intravascular volume status, invasive hemodynamic monitoring, inotropic pharmacologic therapy, and mechanical assist devices. The goal in treating hemodynamically unstable patients is to optimize oxygen delivery to vital organs by increasing cardiac output and decreasing pulmonary venous congestion. In the critical care setting, this therapy is assisted by a peripheral arterial catheter (for assessment of arterial pressure) and a balloon-tipped, flow-directed pulmonary artery catheter (for assessment of left ventricular filling pressure and cardiac output).[26,27]

Before considering invasive or complicated techniques to treat acute heart failure, it is important to remember there are frequently simple derangements contributing to pump failure that may be easily corrected. For example, acid-base imbalances, electrolyte abnormalities, and hypoxia may directly contribute to myocardial depression and should be aggressively corrected. In addition, arrhythmias, such as sinus bradycardia or atrioventricular block or dissociation may contribute to a low cardiac output. Finally, mechanical complications of acute myocardial infarction, such as mitral regurgitation caused by papillary muscle infarction, ventricular septal rupture, and ventricular free wall rupture may be the culprit in acute heart failure and require immediate surgical intervention.

Specific Measures

In the patient with acute heart failure the inadequate cardiac output may be increased by the following means. First, by increasing the end-diastolic volume or preload through volume expansion, one augments cardiac output by utilizing the Frank-Starling mechanism. Inotropic agents such as dopamine, dobutamine, norepinephrine, and digitalis increase cardiac output by directly increasing contractility. Lowering afterload with agents such as nitroprusside and ACE inhibitors improves cardiac output by decreasing resistance to ventricular ejection. Decreasing the degree of ischemia in patients with coronary artery disease may influence cardiac output by improving ventricular wall motion. When the stroke volume is fixed, cardiac output can be augmented by increasing the heart rate with a pacemaker or a positive chronotropic agent. When these measures are undertaken, it is important to weigh the possible negative effects on the myocardium caused by an increase in oxygen demand with the need to improve the cardiac output.[28]

An increase in pulmonary venous pressure is corrected by decreasing total circulating blood or fluid volume with diuretics or phlebotomy or by facilitating peripheral venous pooling with vasodilators or rotating tourniquets. In addition to decreasing the intravascular volume, diuretics also facilitate venous pooling.[29]

Mechanical Assist Devices

In the setting of acute myocardial infarction, mechanical circulatory assistance devices such as the *intra-aortic balloon pump* (IABP) increase arterial pressure during diastole (diastolic augmentation) to maintain or enhance coronary arterial perfusion pressure and lower preejection and ejection pressures (systolic unloading) to reduce myocardial work and oxygen demand.[28,30] In addition, the IABP improves the hemodynamic status and has been shown to reverse the shock syndrome. Despite these acute hemodynamic effects, the ultimate prognosis in patients using the IABP is not significantly improved. Indications for circulatory assistance using the IABP are cardiogenic shock secondary to myocardial infarction or myocardial depression following cardiac surgery, acute heart failure refractory to medical therapy, and recurrent life-threatening ventricular arrhythmias unresponsive to medication and/or pacing. In addition to these indications the IABP is commonly used in the stabilization of patients who are hemodynamically compromised immediately after myocardial infarction while waiting for catheterization or cardiac surgery. Placement of an IABP is contraindicated in patients with irreversible brain damage, chronic end-stage heart disease, severe associated disease, or an incompetent aortic valve.[26]

The *left ventricular assist device* (LVAD) is an extracorporeal or intracorporeal pump that provides the power to shunt oxygenated blood from the left ventricle to the ascending aorta, while reducing the workload of the ventricle. It is used most commonly in patients with end-stage heart failure as a bridge to cardiac transplantation and in patients with stunned myocardium, when cardiac function is slow to recover.

Metabolic Support

Recently, the concept of providing metabolic support for the ischemic myocardium with glucose, insulin, and potassium has stimulated new interest in the treatment of acute heart failure refractory to conventional therapy.[31] The administration of a solution of high doses of glucose, insulin, and potassium (the latter to prevent hypokalemia) has demonstrated utility in improving ventricular function in patients with acute heart failure, especially after elective hypothermic ischemic arrest.[31,32] Although it has been thought that the accumulation of glycolytic products worsens the functional effects of ischemia, the provision of glucose and insulin improves contractile function in myocardial infarction in the acutely ischemic, reperfused myocardium.[33] It is thought that the glucose, insulin, and potassium solution preserves cell integrity (e.g., through preserving glycogen stores, activating ATP-sensitive potassium channels, and maintaining sodium and potassium ATPase activity).

Treatment of Chronic Heart Failure

The basic principles in the treatment of chronic heart failure are to first eliminate precipitating factors, second to determine if systolic dysfunction or diastolic dysfunction prevails and treat accordingly, and finally to identify and correct any other underlying cause. Patients may have purely systolic or diastolic dysfunction, but frequently they have some combination of the two.[5,34] As stated earlier, the ultimate goal in treatment of chronic heart failure is the reduction of morbidity and mortality.

Approach to Asymptomatic Heart Failure

Irrespective of its cause, systolic dysfunction has an asymptomatic, a symptomatic, and a refractory stage. In the asymptomatic patient the treatment consists of modification of risk factors for coronary artery disease such as smoking, hypertension, hyperlipidemia, and obesity. Whereas strenuous physical activity may overtax the circulation of the patient with compensated heart failure, regular aerobic exercise can enhance the efficiency of the cardiovascular system, with a resultant increase in exercise tolerance.[35] ACE inhibitors inhibit the maladaptive myocardial hypertrophy and may prevent progression to the symptomatic stage and are thus very important in the treatment of the asymptomatic patient. There is mounting evidence that ACE inhibitors influence intracellular signaling cascades, which have effects on growth and thus may inhibit growth of overloaded myocardial cells.[36]

Approach to Symptomatic Heart Failure: Importance of Triple Therapy

In the symptomatic patient the goals of therapy are to relieve symptoms and to prolong life. Specifically, the hallmarks of treatment involve lowering the heart's workload, increasing contractility, controlling sodium and water retention, and controlling associated arrhythmias. The workload may be lowered by physical and emotional rest, treatment of obesity, and the use of preload and afterload reducing agents. ACE inhibitors have been shown to be of greatest benefit; however, the combination of nitrates and hydralazine have also shown benefit.[16,37,38] In addition, ACE inhibitors have been shown to affect favorably long-term outcome in patients who have heart failure as a result of myocardial infarction by decreasing adverse left ventricular remodeling.[17] Digoxin continues to be the only positive inotropic agent available for oral administration. Long-term administration of digoxin has been shown to reduce morbidity and mortality when combined with afterload reduction and diuretics.[16] Sodium and water retention can be modulated by the use of a low-sodium diet and diuretics. Precautions must be taken when using diuretics to avoid electrolyte imbalances. The combination of afterload reduction, digitalis, and diuretics forms the cornerstone of the management of chronic symptomatic heart failure. Finally, it is important to preserve or restore normal sinus rhythm.[39]

Special Considerations

There are a number of special considerations in the treatment of heart failure, some of which have already been mentioned but are summarized once more here in context. First, the identification of diastolic dysfunction and pure right ventricular failure is important, as the treatment of these unique physiologic derangements is different from that of systolic left ventricular dysfunction.[40] Second, in severe heart failure the prevention of and treatment of thombotic complications and arrhythmias is important. Lastly, the pharmacokinetics of many drugs may be altered in heart failure, even in the absence of renal impairment.

Diastolic Dysfunction

In contrast to the fundamental defect in systolic dysfunction, patients with isolated diastolic dysfunction have normal or often enhanced contractile function of the left ventricle (as measured by the ejection fraction). However, these patients also have dyspnea and fatigue and develop pulmonary edema in the same way as patients with systolic dysfunction. The key problem in this syndrome is that increased ventricular stiffness (or reduced compliance) leads to limitations on the use of preload reserve because of rapid increases in cardiac filling pressures at normal or slightly increased cardiac volume.[14] Since the left ventricle contracts normally, there is no need to attempt to conserve or improve left ventricular function with inotropic agents. Similarly, there is no benefit from preload reduction, which may even worsen the situation. Treatment is instead directed at improving relaxation characteristics, mitigating the effects of an abnormal compliance, and prolonging diastole to allow for improved ventricular filling. Calcium channel blocking agents and β-blocking agents have offered the best utility in this effort. ACE inhibitors cause regression of left ventricular hypertrophy and may have direct myocardial effects that improve diastolic function. Lowering of blood pressure into the normal range is of paramount importance and should be done with one of these three agents.

Arrhythmias

As ventricular performance deteriorates in chronic heart failure and the cardiac muscle is remodeling in response to overload, electrophysiologic abnormalities develop. The majority of patients with severe chronic heart failure have ventricular arrhythmias often manifested by ventricular tachycardia and ventricular fibrillation. It would be expected that patients with the most frequent or serious arrhythmias would be at greatest risk of sudden death, but this does not seem to be the case. Complex ventricular arrhythmias are more a reflection of the severity of the patient's hemodynamic and functional status rather than a specific pathophysiologic event. Nonsustained ventricular tachycardia occurs in 40% to 60% of patients with the New York Heart Association class III-IV heart failure, and sudden death may occur in 40% of patients in class III-IV. Antiarrhythmic therapy may suppress ventricular arrhythmias but does not prolong life in these patients.[7] Furthermore, antiarrhythmic drugs appear to be most proarrhythmic in these myopathic ventricles. Some of these drugs were actually shown to increase mortality in certain circumstances (such as class IC agents following myocardial infarction).[41,42] Thus the jury is still out on the utility of antiarrhythmic therapy in patients with advanced heart failure.

Anticoagulation

Dilated atria and/or ventricular chambers can be the site of thrombi; however, because of its inherent morbidity, routine anticoagulation for prevention of thromboembolic events is not uniformly recommended. Patients with echocardiographic evidence for mural thrombi, presenting with a history of systemic or pulmonary embolism, or patients with a history of atrial fibrillation should be anticoagulated. Otherwise, the risks of complications from chronic anticoagulation, including intracranial or gastrointestinal hemorrhage, do not warrant the expected benefits.[43]

Altered Pharmacokinetics

In heart failure, decreased gastric emptying delays absorption and decreases the peak plasma concentration of digoxin, furosemide, and bumetanide. Decreased first-pass metabolism in the liver increases the concentration of nitrates, morphine, and hydralazine. Decreased biotransformation to active forms causes diminished activity of ACE inhibitors. Thus the use of various medications necessitates frequent monitoring of blood levels, electrolytes, and clinical effects of the medication.

Right Ventricular Infarction

Right ventricular infarction, which occurs in less than 7% of patients with acute myocardial infarction, may lead to right ventricular failure. The hemodynamic picture in these patients is characterized by markedly elevated right atrial and right ventricular end-diastolic pressures with a normal or reduced right ventricular systolic pressure, normal or reduced pulmonary artery systolic pressure, and a normal or slightly elevated pulmonary capillary wedge pressure. Because of a markedly reduced right ventricular output, the left ventricle filling pressure becomes inadequate, and left ventricular output therefore decreases. Volume expansion to maintain right ventricular filling pressure and output has been the mainstay of treatment in the acute phase. Vasodilators may improve right ventricular output and therefore left ventricular filling pressure and output in the long term.[26,27,42]

Therapy of Refractory Heart Failure: Cardiac Transplantation

Refractory heart failure does not respond to conventional therapy, and thus more aggressive therapies must be used, usually in an inpatient setting. Inotropic support with parenteral inotropes such as dobutamine, dopamine, and the phosphodiesterase inhibitors amrinone and milrinone has been used widely to alleviate the symptoms and signs of heart failure temporarily. Removal of excess fluid by paracentesis, thoracentesis, or dialysis may be necessary. Mechanically assisted circulation with the IABP or the left or right ventricular assist device may become the last resort but usually only as a bridge to transplantation. Cardiac transplantation has a greater than 60% 5-year survival; however, the greatest hurdle is the timely procurement of donor organs, which limits this option to relatively few patients.[44]

Future of Treatment Strategies for Chronic Heart Failure

The future of treatment of chronic heart failure will involve the development of new high-technology devices to augment or supplant the pumping function of the heart and also the elucidation of the genetic basis of heart failure and attempts to alter this genetic destiny. In addition, as more knowledge becomes available about the complex neurohormonal interactions involved in heart failure, new therapies such as the use of low-dose β-adrenergic blocking agents may come into use.[21,45] Both modalities merit a brief mention.

Total Artificial Heart

A new emphasis in the concept of the total artificial heart (TAH) has emerged, and prototypes are being developed at institutions in the United States and Japan. The new generation of TAH will be totally implantable with no transcutaneous implements. Power will be supplied by transmission of energy through intact skin to a subcutaneous receiver from battery packs worn by the patient. The development teams believe that new technology in microminiaturization and computer-aided design will enable the new TAH to overcome the pitfalls of the existing Jarvic TAH such as thrombosis and infection. It is hoped that this technology will supplant cardiac transplantation and become a therapeutic option for both chronic and acute heart failure. The current estimate is that a safe and effective device will be available for clinical human testing by the year 2000.[46]

Gene Therapy

Gene therapy is aimed at correction of abnormal cardiac gene expression, and it is believed that the gene response to overload may lead to cell death. The target gene(s) has(have) not been identified; however, the genes responsible for some specific cardiac disease states have been found, and research is underway to develop treatments based on them.[47] For example, it has been shown that a mutation on a specific site on chromosome 14 encoding myosin heavy chain is associated with familial hypertrophic cardiomyopathy, and thus theoretically the reversal of this mutation could prevent the development of this disease.[48]

Resuscitation

Cardiopulmonary arrest is the extreme form of acute heart failure. During cardiopulmonary arrest there is the cessation of systemic blood circulation and effective ventilation. Basic life support, or cardiopulmonary resuscitation (CPR), provides artificial ventilation and circulation until advanced cardiac life support (ACLS) can be initiated. Modern CPR has revolutionized the treatment of sudden death and began with the observation of Kouwenhoven et al.[49] in 1960 that rhythmic depression of the sternum in animals produced pulsations in arterial pressure and permitted successful closed-chest electric defibrillation after prolonged ventricular fibrillation. Since the introduction of this technique, many modifications have been proposed, but none have consistently been proven superior to the basic idea that to be successful the pump function of the heart must be maintained and/or restored. Because of the poor long-term survival rates of patients receiving CPR, it has been difficult to quantitate the survival benefit of traditional CPR or any newer techniques.[50] The clinical scenarios in patients most likely to be successfully resuscitated using traditional CPR are outlined in the box on p. 792.

PATHOPHYSIOLOGY OF CARDIOPULMONARY RESUSCITATION

Blood flow during CPR is maintained by a generalized increase in intrathoracic pressure, causing blood to move from the vascular structures of the thorax to the peripheral circulation. When the chest compression is released, blood flows back from the peripheral structures to the thorax. The flow is maintained in the antegrade direction by the valves in the heart and the veins and can reach 1.7 L/min.[51] Some investigators have proposed that the increase in pleural pressures rather than compression of the heart results in blood flow to the periphery.[52] It has been shown that mechanical ventilation alone increases intrathoracic pressures. Translocation of blood from the pul-

CLINICAL SCENARIOS OF PATIENTS MOST LIKELY TO BE SUCCESSFULLY RESUSCITATED WITH TRADITIONAL CARDIOPULMONARY RESUSCITATION

1. Witnessed sudden arrest caused by ventricular fibrillation outside the hospital, when electric countershock can be performed within approximately 7 to 8 minutes
2. Hospitalized patients with primary ventricular fibrillation and ischemic heart disease
3. Cardiac arrest in the absence of life-threatening coexisting conditions
4. Primary respiratory arrest
5. Arrest caused by hypothermia, drug overdose, or airway obstruction

monary into the systemic bed with forward flow can be achieved with the left heart chamber as a conduit.[53] Forceful, rhythmic cough can also generate systolic pressures equivalent to normal cardiac activity and sustain cardiac output during asystole, maintaining cerebral blood flow and peripheral flow.[54] Paradoxically, the compression of the heart and the increase in intrathoracic pressure with CPR can lead to pulmonary edema in one third to one half of patients, representing a major cause of hypoxemia during resuscitation. Some investigators have found that pulmonary artery mean pressure and pulmonary capillary wedge pressures increase within 5 to 10 minutes of CPR and return to baseline within 5 minutes of effective spontaneous circulation.[55]

The experimental strategies to increase the effectiveness of CPR are aimed at making pleural pressures more positive during cardiac emptying and more negative during filling. The former can be achieved by inflation of the lungs during chest compressions and the use of a pneumatic vest. The latter is accomplished with chest cuirass, stimulation of the inspiratory muscles, negative airway pressure during the filling phase, and increasing the abdominal pressure during filling.[56]

Cerebral Blood Flow During Cardiopulmonary Resuscitation

Irreversible brain damage occurs within 4 to 6 minutes of anoxia. Although isolated neurons show complete recovery after 20 to 60 minutes of anoxia, the postischemic damage is due to hypoperfusion secondary to vasospasm and the release of oxygen-derived free radicals from injured tissues and neuronal calcium overload. Experimental techniques used to preserve cerebral function during CPR include calcium channel blockers, free radical scavaging agents, transient postresuscitation hypertension, retrograde arterial perfusion with low-viscosity solutions, anticoagulation, hypothermia, barbiturate coma, and hyperosmotic solutions.[57] None of these have been shown to be consistently effective in clinical trials. Excessive volume loading is actually detrimental to cerebral perfusion because of cerebral edema or shunting of blood through extracerebral vessels.[58]

Coronary Blood Flow During Cardiopulmonary Resuscitation

The basal myocardial oxygen consumption is 30% to 40% of normal during ventricular fibrillation; thus if coronary perfusion cannot meet this demand, the likelihood of successful defibrillation is low. Coronary blood flow decreases from 30% to 5% of normal within the first 20 minutes of CPR. This decrease in flow may be due to epinephrine, direct heart compression, abdominal compression, or negative pleural pressure during the filling phase.

Other methods employed to increase the effectiveness of CPR include vigorous volume infusion and the use of glucose-containing fluids. These methods are controversial because they may increase cerebral damage during ischemia or after reperfusion or may cause pulmonary edema.[53] High doses of epinephrine may increase aortic pressure and coronary flow, and the α-receptor stimulation may restore a spontaneous heartbeat; however, the β-receptor activity increases oxygen consumption and may be detrimental.[59] Calcium channel blockers theoretically would decrease intracellular damage and postischemic cerebral and coronary vasospasm, but their negative inotropic and chronotropic action precludes their use. Sodium bicarbonate corrects systemic acidosis, which may compromise cardiac function, suppresses spontaneous cardiac activity, decreases the threshold for ventricular fibrillation, and impairs cardiac and peripheral response to catecholamines. Despite these beneficial effects, bicarbonate may also exacerbate central nervous system acidosis, produce a paradoxic intracellular acidosis, change the oxygen dissociation curve so as to decrease oxygen delivery, increase osmolality, and cause hypernatremia. Studies have failed to show an improved outcome with its use in CPR.

Ventilation during CPR should be achieved with endotracheal intubation if at all possible. This method is the best at achieving oxygenation during arrest. Other less-effective methods are mouth-to-mouth ventilation, mouth-to-mask ventilation, esophageal obturator, or multiluminal airway device.[60]

ADVANCED CARDIAC LIFE SUPPORT

The initial objective of ACLS has been the treatment of life-threatening arrhythmias. The prototypical arrhythmias causing cardiopulmonary arrest are ventricular tachycardia and ventricular fibrillation, which are treated with a series of electric countershocks to achieve defibrillation to normal rhythm. This has been shown to be very successful especially in patients in the intensive care unit setting when defibrillation can be accomplished early. If another rhythm is the cause of the arrest or if ventricular tachycardia or fibrillation persists after countershock, endotracheal intubation, chest compressions, intravenous access, and delivery of medications should take precedence over other measures.[60]

When ventricular fibrillation is successfully electrically cardioverted, 70% to 80% of patients convert to a rhythm that is capable of supporting adequate perfusion if cardioversion is done within 3 minutes of onset.[60] If ventricular fibrillation persists after the initial countershocks, epinephrine should be given prior to further attempts. The use of antiarrhythmic agents is encouraged, although whether there are true benefits is controversial.

Asystole is frequently the initial rhythm identified in patients with cardiac arrest found outside the hospital and in critically ill inpatients. This rhythm carries the worst prognosis with less than 2% of patients surviving hospitalization. In addition to epinephrine and atropine, the use of transcutaneous and transvenous pacing should be encouraged if they can be instituted in a short period of time.

Pulseless electric activity, formerly also termed electromechanical dissociation, can be due to metabolic and mechanical derangements. This is a disturbance frequently encountered in the traumatized or burned patient where hypovolemia, cardiac tamponade, tension pneumothorax, acidosis, and hypoxia are prevalent. Other causes may include pulmonary embolus and a large myocardial infarction. After ACLS has been initiated, each of the possible causes should be investigated and treated immediately.

CARDIOPULMONARY ARREST FOLLOWING TRAUMA

The approach to the patient with cardiopulmonary arrest as a result of trauma is different than the patient with arrest as a result of a primary cardiac or pulmonary event. The causes of arrest associated with trauma may include exsanguination with hypovolemia and diminished oxygen delivery, diminished cardiac output resulting from tension pneumothorax or pericardial tamponade from penetrating trauma, or direct trauma to the heart or great vessels. In addition, there may be causes that may not be as readily apparent as the purely mechanical causes, such as cardiovascular collapse or primary respiratory arrest resulting from a neurogenic response to severe central neurologic injury and trauma associated with a primary arrest, such as in the patient who suffers ventricular arrhythmias while driving a car.

The management of patients who suffer arrest associated with trauma begins with immediate evaluation of the airway and electrocardiographic rhythm. Ventilation should be accomplished as first priority, since the tolerance of pulselessness may be extended in patients who have achieved adequate oxygenation. While establishing an adequate airway, in-line stabilization of the neck should be performed, and lateral neck supports, strapping, and backboards should be used to prevent worsening of a possible neck injury. If after airway control and defibrillation of dysrhythmias there is no pulse or blood pressure, chest compressions may have to be initiated. In penetrating injury to the chest the thorax should be vented if there is asymmetry of breath sounds or an increase in airway resistance. A thorough survey of the body should be made for penetrating injury that may cause pneumothorax or tension pneumothorax. Once identified, a penetrating injury should be sealed, and immediate monitoring for (and relief of) tension pneumothorax should be performed. Emergency thoracotomy permits direct massage of the heart and allows relief of tamponade, control of thoracic and extrathoracic hemorrhage, and aortic cross-clamping.[60] Open cardiac massage increases cardiac output and aortic pressures more than standard CPR; however, it has been shown that there is no benefit of this procedure if initiated after 30 minutes of standard CPR.[53]

When a patient becomes pulseless as a result of intravascular volume loss, functional long-term survival is unlikely unless single-organ hemorrhage can be rapidly terminated, along with aggressive volume resuscitation, blood transfusions, and circulatory support. Patients with prehospital arrest caused by multiple-organ hemorrhage, as is commonly seen with blunt trauma, rarely survive neurologically intact, despite rapid prehospital and trauma center response. Those who survive prehospital arrest associated with trauma are generally young, have penetrating injuries, have received early endotracheal intubation, and undergo rapid transport by highly skilled paramedics to a definitive care facility.[60]

MONITORING THE EFFECTIVENESS OF CARDIOPULMONARY RESUSCITATION

Cardiopulmonary resuscitation is most effective when the mean and diastolic aortic pressures are maintained continually at an adequate level. These are the critical pressures that define perfusion of oxygenated blood to the coronary arteries and systemic circulation. In addition, adequate aortic pressures are needed to promote effective circulation of emergency medications such as catecholamines and antiarrhythmics. However, if the left atrial pressure is as high as the aortic pressures, there may not be forward flow even with adequate aortic pressures, and the result may be reverse flow and pulmonary edema. This situation may be encountered, for example, in patients with mitral or aortic valvular dysfunction.

Arterial pH and PO_2 do not correlate well with outcome in CPR except in the extreme. With a very high pH, for example, there may be failure of defibrillation. A very low pH portends a poor outcome. Arterial lactate levels are an indicator of perfusion with oxygenated blood and have an inverse correlation with outcome. Mixed venous or coronary venous pH and PCO_2 do not correlate with outcome; however, failure to eliminate carbon dioxide as measured by an increased mixed venous carbon dioxide and a low end-tidal carbon dioxide tension is associated with the onset of ventricular fibrillation.[61]

MORBIDITY, MORTALITY, AND PROGNOSIS

With in-hospital cardiopulmonary arrest, there is a 55% rate of successful resuscitation; however, only 15% of the patients survive the hospitalization.[62] The extent of prearrest morbidity plays an important role in the outcome of CPR. Approximately one out of five survivors suffer serious permanent brain damage, and this complication is most correlated to the amount of time in cardiopulmonary arrest prior to beginning CPR and ACLS.

The most important prognostic factors are a prolonged delay in onset of CPR, a prolonged duration of CPR, age less than 40 or greater than 70, the presence of hypotension and lactic acidosis after arrest, severe hypoxia before arrest, azotemia, hyperglycemia, and comorbid conditions such as sepsis, renal failure, and malignancy.[60]

SUMMARY

As the general population ages, acute and chronic heart failure is an increasingly important cause of morbidity and mortality in the adult surgical patient. While there are a large number of causes and exacerbating factors for heart failure, management issues may be similar. With this in mind, it is important to understand the pathophysiology of heart failure, as the treatment is aimed directly at influencing and hopefully reversing the maladaptive physiologic mechanisms both within the heart and systemically. Although there is a great promise in the future for metabolic, molecular biologic, and sophisticated mechanical treatments for acute and chronic heart failure, early diagnosis and aggressive treatment while excluding reversible causes is and will remain the hallmark of treatment of heart failure.

After more than 30 years of use, CPR remains a desperate effort to treat cardiopulmonary arrest, and unfortunately the benefits are limited to only a small number of patients. It is interesting that despite many efforts at change, the original technique of CPR has changed little throughout the years. Perhaps the greatest impact in the future will be the development of improved measures at prediction and prevention of arrest and improvement in postresuscitation measures.

REFERENCES

1. Mackenzie J. Principles of Diagnosis and Treatment in Heart Affections. London: Oxford University Press, 1916, p 38.
2. Grossman W. Personal communication, 1995.
3. Taegtmeyer H. Energy metabolism of the heart, from basic concepts to clinical applications. Curr Probl Cardiol 11:64, 1994.
4. Isselbacher K, ed. Harrison's Principles of Internal Medicine. New York: McGraw Hill, 1994, p 989.
5. Braunwald E, ed. Heart Disease: A Textbook of Cardiovascular Medicine, 4th ed. Philadelphia: WB Saunders, 1992, p 393.
6. Ho KK, et al. The epidemiology of heart failure, the Framingham study. J Am Coll Cardiol 22(Supple A):6A, 1993.
7. Willerson JT, ed. Treatment of Heart Diseases, London: Gower Medical Publishing, 1992, p 2.3.
8. Gerdes AM, et al. Structural remodeling of cardiac myocytes in patients with ischemic cardiomyopathy. Circulation 86:426, 1992.
9. Weber KT, Brilla CC. Pathological hypertrophy and cardiac interstitium: Fibrosis and renin-aldosterone system. Circulation 86:426, 1991.
10. Langer GA. Calcium and the heart: Exchange at the tissue, cell and organelle levels. FASEB J 6:893, 1992.
11. Ungerer M, et al. Altered expression of beta-1 adrenergic receptors in the failing human heart. Circulation 87:454, 1993.
12. Schwartz K, et al. Switches in cardiac muscle gene expression as a result of pressure and volume overload. Am J Physiol 262:364, 1992.
13. Goldsmith SR, Hasking GJ, Miller E. Angiotensin II and sympathetic activity in patients with CHF. J Am Coll Cardiol 21:1107, 1993.
14. Goldsmith SR, Dick C. Differentiating systolic from diastolic heart failure: Pathophysiologic and therapeutic considerations. Am J Med 95:645, 1993.
15. Bristow MR. Pathophysiologic and pharmacologic rationales for clinical management of chronic heart failure with beta blocking agents. Am J Cardiol 71:12C, 1993.
16. The CONSENSUS Trial Study Group. Effects of enalapril on mortality in severe congestive heart failure. N Engl J Med 316:1429, 1987.
17. Pfeffer MA, et al. The effect of captopril on mortality and morbidity in patients with left ventricular dysfunction following myocardial infarction: Results of the survival and ventricular enlargement (SAVE) trial. N Engl J Med 327:669, 1992.
18. The SOLVD Investigators. Effect of enalapril on mortality and the development of heart failure in asymptomatic patients with reduced LV ejection fraction. N Engl J Med 327:685, 1992.
19. Harrison TR, et al. Congestive heart failure. The mechanism of dyspnea on exertion. Arch Int Med 50:690, 1932.
20. Hope JA. Treatise on the Diseases of the Heart and Great Vessels. London: Williams-Kid, 1832.
21. Mackenzie J. Diseases of the Heart, 3rd ed. London: Oxford University Press, 1913.
22. Carabello B. Clinical assessment of systolic dysfunction. ACC Curr J Rev 23:25, 1994.
23. Bonow RO, Udelson JE. Left ventricular diastolic dysfunction as a cause of congestive heart failure: Mechanisms and management. Ann Intern Med 117:502, 1992.
24. Dolgin M, ed. Nomenclature and Criteria for Diagnosis of Disease of the Heart and Great Vessels, 9th ed. New York: Little Brown, 1994, p 253.
25. Scheuer J. Metabolic factors in myocardial failure. Circulation 87(Suppl 7):VII54, 1993.
26. Chatterjee K. Acute Heart Failure, Critical Care Management. Boston: Little Brown, 1975, p 203.
27. Passmore J Jr, et al. Hemodynamic Support of the Critically Ill Patient in Cardiopulmonary Critical Care. Orlando, Fla.: Grune & Stratton, 1986, p 359.
28. Braunwald E, et al. Effects of drugs and of counterpulsation on myocardial oxygen consumption. Circulation 40(Suppl 4):220, 1969.
29. Dikshit K, et al. Renal and extrarenal hemodynamic effects of furosemide in congestive heart failure after acute myocardial infarction. N Engl J Med 288:1087, 1973.
30. Kantrowitz A, et al: Initial clinical experience with intra aorta balloon pumping in cardiogenic shock. JAMA 203:135, 1968.
31. Taegtmeyer H. The use of hypertonic glucose, insulin and potassium (GIK) in myocardial preservation. J Appl Cardiol 6:255, 1991.
32. Grandinak S, et al. Improved cardiac function with glucose-insulin-potassium after coronary bypass surgery. Ann Thorac Surg 48:484, 1981.
33. McElroy DD, Walker WE, Taegtmeyer H. Effects of glycogen on function and energy metabolism of the isolated rabbit heart after hypothermic ischemic arrest. J Appl Cardiol 4:455, 1989.
34. Hurst JW, ed. Current Therapy in Cardiovascular Diseases. Chicago: Mosby–Year Book, 1993.
35. Uren NG, Lipkin DP. Exercise training as therapy for chronic heart failure. Br Heart J 67:430, 1992.
36. Katz AM. Treating heart failure: Yesterday, today and tomorrow. Adv Cardiovasc Med 1:1, 1994.

37. Cohn JN, et al. Effects of vasodilator therapy on mortality in chronic congestive heart failure: Results of a Veterans Administration Cooperative Study (V-HeFT). N Engl J Med 314:1547, 1986.
38. Goldman S, et al. Mechanisms of death in heart failure: The vasodilator-HF trials. Circulation 3(87)(Suppl 6):VI-24, 1993.
39. Hochleitner M, et al. Usefulness of physiologic dual-chamber pacing in drug resistant idiopathic dilated cardiomyopathy. Am J Cardiol 66:198, 1990.
40. Gaash WH. Diagnosis and treatment of heart failure based on LV systolic or diastolic dysfunction. JAMA 271:1276, 1994.
41. Armstrong PW, Moe GW. Medical advances in the treatment of congestive heart failure. Circulation 88:2941, 1993.
42. Parrillo JE. Current Therapy in Critical Care Medicine, 2nd ed. Philadelphia: BC Decker, 1991.
43. Clinical Practice Guideline #11. Rockville, Md.: Agency for Health Care Policy and Research, 1994, p 11.
44. DEFIBRILAT Study Group. Actuarial risk of sudden death while awaiting cardiac transplantation in patients with atherosclerotic heart disease. Am J Cardiol 68:545, 1991.
45. Sonnenblick EH, LeJemtel TH. Heart failure: Its progression and its therapy. Hosp Pract Sept:75, 1993.
46. Lenfant C. Report of the task force on research in heart failure. Circulation 90:1118, 1994.
47. Watkins H, et al. Characteristics and prognostic implications of myosin missense mutation in familial hypertrophic cardiomyopathy. N Engl J Med 326:1108, 1992.
48. Hejtmancik JF, et al. Localization of the gene for familial hypertrophic cardiomyopathy to chromosome 14q1 in a diverse US population. Circulation 83:1592, 1991.
49. Kouwenhoven WB, Jude JR, Knickerbocker GG. Closed-chest cardiac massage. JAMA 173:1064, 1960.
50. Tucker KJ, et al. Cardiopulmonary resuscitation: Historical perspectives, physiology, and future directions. Arch Intern Med 154:2141, 1994.
51. Rudikoff MT, et al. Mechanisms of blood flow during cardiopulmonary arrest. Circulation 61:345, 1980.
52. Chandra N, et al. Contrasts between intrathoracic pressures during external clot compression and cardiac massage. Crit Care Med 9:789, 1981.
53. Schleien CL, et al. Controversial issues in cardiopulmonary resuscitation. Anesthesiol 71:133, 1989.
54. Criley YM, et al. Modification of cardiopulmonary resuscitation based on cough. Circulation 74(Suppl 4):42, 1986.
55. Ornato YP, et al. Rapid changes in pulmonary vascular hemodynamics with pulmonary edema during CPR. Am J Emerg Med 3:237, 1985.
56. Einagle V, et al. Interposed abdominal compress and carotid blood flow during CPR. Chest 93:1206, 1988.
57. Safar P, Bricher NG. Cardiopulmonary Cerebral Recirculation, 3rd ed. Philadelphia: WB Saunders, 1988, p 229.
58. Lumpkin JR, Safar P. Brain resuscitation after cardiac arrest. In Harwood AL, ed. CPR. Baltimore: Williams & Wilkins, 1982, p 55.
59. Stiell IG, et al. High-dose epinephrine in adult cardiac arrest. N Engl J Med 327:1045, 1992.
60. Lundberg GD, ed. Guidelines for cardiopulmonary resuscitation and emergency cardiac care. JAMA 268:2214, 1992.
61. Gudipati CV, et al. Expired carbon dioxide: A noninvasive monitor of CPR. Circulation 77:234, 1988.
62. Burns R, et al. Prediction of in-hospital cardiopulmonary arrest outcome. Arch Intern Med 149:1318, 1989.

39

Assisted Circulation

Michael P. Macris, Steven M. Parnis, and O. Howard Frazier

Low cardiac output is an altered physiologic state that results from many diseases of the myocardium and that may necessitate mechanical circulatory assistance. Whatever its origin, low cardiac output is usually accompanied by varying degrees of dysfunction of the kidneys, brain, or lungs or by failure of these vital organs. Such failure manifests clinically as oliguria or anuria; as paresis, paralysis, or sensorial changes caused by decreased cerebral blood flow; or as hypoventilation, ventilation-perfusion imbalances, or alveolocapillary blocks in pulmonary gas exchange. Other failure states (i.e., hepatic or hematologic shortcomings) may coexist and may affect any of the 5000 enzyme systems and metabolic pathways of the liver, the quantity and quality of circulating hemoglobin, and the integrity of the coagulation factors. These failure states may also cause generalized mitochondrial dysplasia and disrupt critical oxidative phosphorylation and cytochrome function in all organ systems.[1]

Low cardiac output may be produced by a wide variety of etiologic factors, all of which adversely affect myocardial function, resulting in depressed cardiac performance and inadequate oxygen delivery to tissues. The triggering mechanisms may vary, however, and include blood loss resulting from a vascular injury, third-space sequestration related to pancreatitis, or endotoxemia resulting from an intra-abdominal abscess. These mechanisms may lead to diverse consequences such as myocardial depression caused by hypoxia, acidosis, or calcium shifts; arrhythmias; inadequate filling pressures; inadequate preload; changes in afterload; systemic and pulmonary vasoconstriction or vasodilation; and variations in capillary permeability.

As these variables have become better appreciated and their effects on cardiac function more fully understood, support of the failing circulation has left the realm of fantasy and become a realistic option for numerous critically ill patients. Many who would previously have died of a low cardiac output state are now surviving as our knowledge broadens with respect to the optimal timing and duration of mechanical assistance, as well as the potential for recovery and rehabilitation. Because of our exponential success in supporting patients with end-stage cardiac disease and subsequently returning them to meaningful, productive lives, the implant duration for some devices has been extended to longer than a year, after which successful heart transplantation has been performed.

HISTORICALAL PERSPECTIVE

Although it is one of the simplest organs in the body, the heart is absolutely essential to survival because it pumps blood and other substances to and from the tissues. Despite the attempts of LeGallois[2] to replace the heart in 1812, most surgeons considered this organ untouchable until the midtwentieth century. The development of a clinical system of extracorporeal circulation in the early 1950s provided the basis for surgical procedures on the open heart.[3] With the introduction of safer, more reliable oxygenators, extracorporeal oxygenation and support of the circulation became an established modality. Progress was furthered in 1956 when Kolff[4] designed a coil-type membrane oxygenator for clinical use and in 1962 when Cooley et al.[5] introduced an economical, disposable bubble oxygenator.

Because of these developments and the growing importance of heart disease as a cause of death in the United States, scientists became interested in creating a total artificial heart (TAH) that would serve as a functional substitute for the natural heart. In 1958 Kusserow[6] described an intra-abdominal pump for partially replacing the right side of the heart. Later, he and Clapp[7] developed a pump that could be attached to the back of a dog to assist the left side of the heart. As early as 1958 Akutsu and Kolff[8] reported that they had replaced a dog's heart with an air-driven reciprocating pump that supported the animal for 5½ hours. Kolff described this pump as "a mechanical prosthetic heart that completely substitutes for the natural heart, anatomically and physiologically."[8]

Because of this early success, researchers believed that mechanical support of the heart was a straightforward problem and that the TAH would soon see clinical use. They did not fully realize the limitations of the biomaterials, pump designs, and driving and power systems available at that time. Nevertheless, steady improvements in the various types of pumps led to increased survival of experimental animals.[9,10] In 1969 the feasibility of short-term clinical support with a pneumatically driven TAH was demonstrated by Cooley et al.,[11] who supported a patient for 64 hours with a heart made of Dacron reticular fabric. The patient's own heart had been refractory to weaning from cardiopulmonary bypass.

While attempts were in progress to develop a TAH, various cardiac assist devices were also being tested. These systems were generally less complex than the TAH, as was the surgery necessary to implant them. In 1971 Bernhard et al.[12] reported they had achieved right and left ventricular bypass for 85 and 170 days, respectively, in calves; moreover, 16 calves had survived for 7 to 42 days with simultaneous biventricular bypass. In that same year Takagi et al.[13] reported the 2-month survival of a calf with a left ventricular assist device (LVAD).

Because these devices required a pneumatic power source and because materials failure, hemolysis, and thrombosis remained serious problems, little progress was made clinically during this period. DeBakey[14] reported two cases in which LVADs were used clinically for 4 to 10 days. Similarly, Kantrowitz et al.[15] used an LVAD to support the failing circulation after cardiac surgery. Clinical application by other investigators was almost nonexistent.

As the 1970s unfolded, the clinical use of assist devices increased, particularly in the case of the intra-aortic balloon pump (IABP), which is still an important modality in the treatment of low cardiac output. Developed in 1961 by Moulopoulos et al.,[16] the IABP is based on the principle of counterpulsation. Kantrowitz et al.[17] first demonstrated its potential clinical usefulness in 1967. Clinical application of the IABP, as well as other approaches to the failing circulation, was championed by other investigators including Dennis (1961), DeBakey (1963), Norman[18] and Cooley (1975), Bernhard et al. (1976),[19] Thoma et al. (1977),[20] Pierce et al. (1977),[21] and Turina et al. (1977).[22] By the end of the 1970s ventricular assistance had become an established clinical reality.

During the 1980s TAHs were implanted in a handful of patients with the goal of permanent cardiac replacement. Despite initially successful results, these patients invariably died of infection or thromboembolism. Therefore the United States government placed a moratorium on permanent TAH implantation. Like ventricular assist devices (VADs), however, TAHs have proved valuable as short-term bridges to cardiac transplantation.

In the 1990s the emergence of tether-free temporary VADs has enabled patients to leave the hospital and enjoy near-normal lives, thereby fulfilling the vision of the original pioneers of these devices.

CARDIOPULMONARY BYPASS

The prototype of assisted circulation is the extracorporeal heart-lung machine, or cardiopulmonary bypass (CPB) circuit. Its clinical introduction more than 40 years ago made modern cardiac surgery possible and paved the way for the development of other assist devices to support the failing circulation. Thus a discussion of assisted circulation would not be complete without a brief consideration of CPB and an understanding of how it works physiologically.

Because open heart surgery requires a quiet, blood-free operative field, the function of the patient's heart and lungs must be assumed by a CPB circuit during surgery. The physiologic goal of CPB is to maintain an adequate blood flow and mean arterial pressure, thereby allowing optimal end-organ perfusion during elective cardiac arrest. A blood flow of 40 to 60 ml/kg body weight/min can provide a cardiac index of approximately 2.5 L/min/m^2, which is adequate for an anesthetized adult.

All CPB circuits have a venous reservoir, a gas exchange device (oxygenator), a blood pump, a heat exchanger, blood filters, and an arterial line filter (Fig. 39-1). Venous blood is drained into the oxygenator by means of passive flow, which depends on the central venous pressure and on the oxygenator's being positioned lower than the operating table. Once the blood has passed through the pump and traversed the oxygenator, it is returned to the patient's body. An arterial heat exchanger, which controls the temperature of the blood, is usually incorporated into the oxygenator. Before returning to the body, the blood passes through an arterial line filter, which ensures that no air is accidentally injected into the patient.

Suction devices are necessary to remove excess blood from the operative field and to decompress the heart. Most procedures involve the use of two suction pumps, each connected to an individual pump head. Suctioned blood goes to a cardiotomy reservoir, where it is filtered to remove platelet-leukocyte aggregates and fibrin before entering the oxygenator.

Oxygenator

By providing contact between a broad film of blood and a suitable gas mixture, the oxygenator serves as an artificial lung, which oxygenates the venous blood and removes carbon dioxide. The two main types of oxygenators are bubble and membrane. *Bubble oxygenators* create a large blood-gas surface, injecting oxygen directly into the blood. This process creates a foaming action, in which gas bubbles are forced to the surface as a result of the hydrostatic pressure exerted by the blood. The bubbles are removed by an antifoaming agent before the blood is returned to the patient. *Membrane oxygenators* interpose a gas-permeable membrane between the oxygenating gas and the blood. Gas transfer depends on the particular membrane's permeability to the individual gases and on the gases' pressure gradient across the membrane.

Of these two types of oxygenators, the membrane variety is more widely used today because it minimizes trauma to platelets and erythrocytes[23-27] and provides a better hemodynamic response.[28] For open heart operations in which the pump time is expected to be prolonged, the

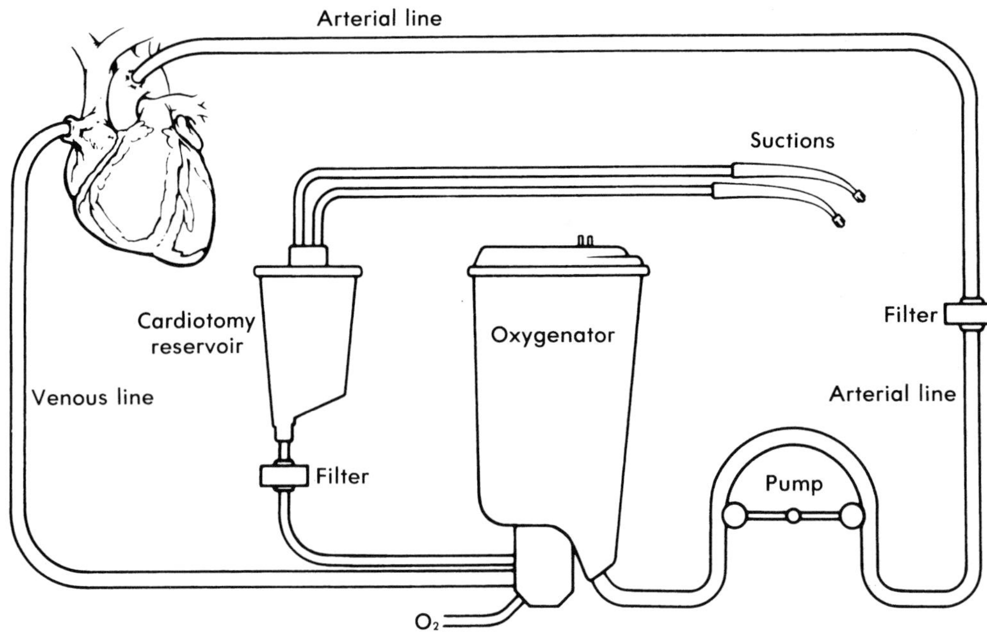

Fig. 39-1. The cardiopulmonary bypass circuit.

membrane oxygenator is especially the more appropriate choice.

Blood Pump

The pump component of the CPB circuit provides for blood flow through the unit and maintains artificial systemic circulation and end-organ perfusion during cardiac arrest. Blood pumps used for CPB systems are of either the positive-displacement type (roller pump) or the centrifugal type. The *roller pump* produces flow by compressing the wall of a collapsible tube between the roller and the backing plate of the roller head, propelling the blood column ahead of the roller and out of the pump. No direct contact occurs between the blood and the roller itself, and no valves are necessary. In contrast, *centrifugal pumps,* such as the Medtronic BioMedicus BP 50 and 80 models, use the principle of a constrained vortex to propel blood. In this arrangement, the spinning of a series of rotator cones imparts a circular motion to the blood, generating a centrifugal force that gives rise to pressure and flow.

In contrast to the body's own physiologic system, both types of pumps provide nonpulsatile perfusion. Various techniques have been used to create pulsatile flow during CPB. Although the merits of pulsatile and nonpulsatile flow have been debated,[29-31] most cardiac procedures today use nonpulsatile flow, with acceptable results.

Surgical Considerations

Cannulation Techniques

Venous return is diverted into the CPB circuit through cannulas in the vena cava, right atrium, or femoral vein, depending on the type of cardiac procedure. Double-caval cannulas provide the best decompression of the venous system but fail to remove blood that enters the right atrium from the coronary sinus and the thebesian veins.[32] Systemic venous return can also be diverted to the circuit by a single large-caliber cannula, which is introduced into the right atrium and the inferior vena cava through the right atrial appendage. The choice of cannula depends on the type of surgical procedure.

Femoral vein cannulation for femorofemoral bypass is indicated when the patient has had one or more previous open heart procedures resulting in extensive adhesions. Surgery on the ascending aorta and aortic arch also requires cannulation of the femoral vessels.

Arterial cannulation for delivery of oxygenated blood is done through a major artery, usually the ascending aorta. The femoral artery may be cannulated if the operation involves the ascending aorta and the aortic arch or if the patient has had previous open heart surgery, as already mentioned.

Prevention of Cardiac Distention

Decompression of the heart, particularly of the left ventricle, is accomplished by placing a sump in the left atrium through the right superior pulmonary vein or the apex of the left ventricle. Excess blood in the pericardium or in the operative field is removed with additional suction devices and is returned to the circuit, thus minimizing blood loss. These additional suction devices are responsible for most of the blood trauma previously attributed to the oxygenator.[33]

Prevention of Air Embolization

To prevent systemic or coronary air embolization, intracardiac air must be removed before CPB is terminated. Air can be present in the pulmonary veins, left atrium, or left ventricle. During restoration of left ventricular function, air is aspirated from the ascending aorta by a suction needle connected to a roller pump. The patient is placed in Trendelenburg's position, and a 19-gauge needle is inserted repeatedly into the left ventricular cavity to remove air that may be trapped within the multiple recesses of the endocardial surface. Manual inflation of the lungs by the anesthesiologist forces blood from the pulmonary veins into the left atrium and helps evacuate air from the pulmonary vasculature.

Systemic Responses

Cardiopulmonary bypass results in several hemodynamic changes that directly affect patient management. An initial decrease in blood pressure is attributed to hemodilution,[34] hypothermia, or relative hypovolemia. This initial hypotension is followed by an increase in systemic vascular resistance, which is attributed to the release of endogenous catecholamines and activation of the renin-angiotensin system.[34,35] Because this increased vascular resistance may render the patient hypertensive, intraoperative vasodilator therapy may be necessary to reduce the left ventricular afterload before CPB is discontinued. Reported hypotension after rapid reinfusion of bronchial venous drainage is attributed to the release of vasodilator prostaglandins, which are produced by the lungs during the period of minimal pulmonary perfusion.[36] Cerebral blood flow, based on flow velocity through the middle cerebral artery, is increased during CPB; this increase is attributed to hemodilution rather than cerebral autoregulatory mechanisms.[37]

Fluid shifts during and after CPB have been adequately described but are still not well understood. An increase in extracellular water is accompanied by a decrease in the red blood cell mass, which persists during the early postoperative period, mainly in patients who received crystalloid priming solution.[38] A decrease in sodium excretion is accompanied by a marked increase in potassium excretion, which accounts for the extensive potassium replacement required by these patients.[38,39] The glomerular filtration rate is enhanced, probably because of the increase in extracellular volume that occurs during the first 2 postoperative days.

During CPB the lungs are neither ventilated nor perfused. Pulmonary changes include loss of surfactant, alveolar septal edema, and leukocytic sequestration.[40,41]

Alterations in host-defense mechanisms and in the complement system during CPB are a major concern in the prevention of postoperative infections. A reduction in the opsonic capacity of the host-defense system is attributed to decreased levels of the third component of complement (C3) and of the hemolytic activity of complement. This reduction in opsonic capacity is believed to result from hemodilution and complement consumption.[42] Other studies have shown a decrease in the proliferative responses of lymphocytes.[43] Hypothermia has been found to inhibit mobilization of leukocytes from the bone marrow; this inhibition is thought to be the source of the neutrophilia seen during CPB.[44]

Overall, CPB can maintain the body in a nearly normal hemodynamic state and acid-base balance, permitting cardiac surgeons to perform complex procedures in a motionless, bloodless field.

INTRA-AORTIC BALLOON PUMP

The IABP is widely used for the circulatory support of patients with postoperative left ventricular failure, cardiogenic shock after acute myocardial infarction, unstable angina refractory to medical treatment, or recurrent myocardial ischemia after acute myocardial infarction.[45-48] The IABP is an intravascular volume-displacement device that augments the patient's existing circulation. Balloon inflation and deflation is precisely synchronized with the cardiac cycle. Inflation is initiated during diastole after the aortic valve closes, and deflation is synchronized with systole. The balloon and driveline, which are constructed of nonthrombogenic, biocompatible materials, are commonly inserted percutaneously via the right or left femoral artery. The driveline is attached to a portable pneumatic drive console.

Hemodynamic Effects

Balloon actuation leads to a reduction of left ventricular outflow impedance during systole, phase shifting of the peak arterial pressure contour into diastole, and augmentation of the stroke volume and cardiac output (by 500 to 800 ml/min).[49] Balloon pumping also causes a marked increase in coronary perfusion pressures during diastole, a reduction in left ventricular volumes and filling pressures, and a decrease in left ventricular chamber radii, wall tensions, and oxygen consumption.[50-52] The myocardial oxygen supply/demand ratio is increased.[53,54] Moreover, right-sided cardiac performance is improved because of a balloon-induced decrease in left-sided cardiac filling pressures.[55]

From a physiologic standpoint, IABP actuation produces alternating hemodynamic effects that cannot be replicated by pharmacologic agents. The first effect, diastolic augmentation, depends on rapid displacement of the aortic blood volume at end systole. This volume displacement, which results from inflation of the balloon in the descending thoracic aorta, increases diastolic perfusion pressures in the coronary arteries and peripheral circulation. Because balloon inflation is timed to begin after closure of the aortic valve, myocardial and tissue perfusion are enhanced without an increase in myocardial work or ejection impedance.

The second effect, a reduction in left ventricular ejection impedance or "unloading," is caused by rapid deflation of the balloon at end diastole. The ensuing reduction in aortic blood volume produces a marked decrease in intra-aortic pressure. As systole begins, aortic pressure and impedance are lowered. The reduction in left ventricular ejection impedance increases the ejection fraction and re-

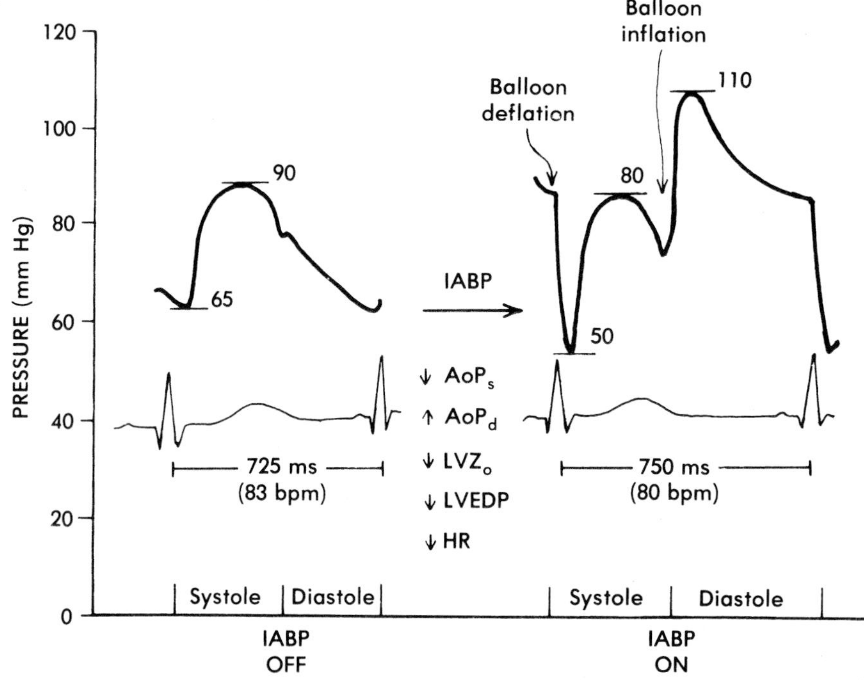

Fig. 39-2. Arterial blood pressure tracing and electrocardiogram with and without intra-aortic balloon pump *(IABP)* support. Balloon actuation decreases the heart rate *(HR)* and systolic aortic pressure *(AoP_s)* while it increases the diastolic aortic pressure *(AoP_d)*. *bpm,* Beats per minute; *LVEDP,* left ventricular end-diastolic pressure; *LVZ_o,* left ventricular impedance; *ms,* milliseconds; *pressure,* arterial blood pressure (mm Hg).

duces the developed wall tension, thereby augmenting the stroke volume and cardiac output (Fig. 39-2).

Balloon actuation also accomplishes the following goals:

1. Decreases the heart rate and systolic aortic pressure (afterload), thus decreasing myocardial oxygen consumption
2. Increases the diastolic aortic pressure (by augmenting the diastolic gradient for coronary and systemic perfusion), stroke volume index, and cardiac index
3. Lowers the mean pulmonary capillary wedge pressure, which can be equated with the left atrial and left ventricular end-diastolic pressures (preload)
4. Decreases the total pulmonary vascular resistance

The latter decrease affects the right side of the heart by lowering the systolic pulmonary artery pressure (afterload) and the mean right atrial pressure, which can be equated with the right ventricular end-diastolic pressure (preload). The indexes for left and right ventricular systolic work per minute are essentially unchanged. These effects reduce the myocardial oxygen demand, improve all the indexes of myocardial oxygen supply, and enhance cardiac performance.

The foregoing benefits are more pronounced in the presence of reduced coronary blood flow. In such cases, counterpulsation may actually increase myocardial oxygen consumption, presumably by improving the oxygen supply to previously underperfused areas of myocardium. This effect is particularly important in attempting to limit a myocardial infarction. Other possible benefits include a reflex reduction in systemic vascular resistance, which may contribute to the decrease in left ventricular afterload, and the opening of potential collateral coronary channels.

Indications for Use

The main indications for IABP counterpulsation are precardiotomy, intraoperative, or postcardiotomy low cardiac output states; the need for a bridge to cardiac transplantation; and postinfarction cardiogenic shock unresponsive to intensive medical management. Except in the bridge-to-transplant population, the IABP can reverse the hemodynamic abnormalities in a substantial number of patients, depending on the severity of the deficits. Balloon counterpulsation also helps stabilize the condition of many critically ill patients so that emergency coronary arteriography and left ventricular angiography can be performed with reasonable safety. Determination of the need for emergency revascularization, infarctectomy, mitral valve replacement, or repair of ruptured interventricular septa during continued IABP support is extremely helpful. The striking reversal of preinfarction anginal pain and ST segment abnormalities with balloon counterpulsation provides clinical and electrocardiographic confirmation of the IABP's instantaneous effects. The balloon's value in stabilizing patients with refractory, life-threatening ventricular dysrhythmias and in resuscitating patients from cardiac arrest is well recognized.

Insertion Techniques
Percutaneous Femoral Approach

Percutaneous access can be rapidly obtained in the catheterization laboratory with fluoroscopic guidance or in the operating room or at the bedside without fluoroscopy. After the femoral artery has been percutaneously entered with a 16-gauge needle, a guide wire is advanced into the vessel. An introducer sheath/dilator catheter is inserted, and the balloon is advanced into the descending thoracic aorta so that it lies distal to the origin of the left subclavian artery and above the origins of the renal arteries. Correct positioning is checked by means of portable chest radiography; the balloon is then repositioned, if necessary, or is sutured in place.

Datascope Corporation introduced a sheathless balloon insertion technique designed to reduce the incidence of limb ischemia. This technique's only disadvantage is the need for fluoroscopy during insertion, because the balloon cannot be later repositioned.

Direct Femoral Approach

Under selected circumstances the balloon may be inserted through a short segment of prosthetic vascular graft anastomosed to the femoral artery, thereby allowing temporary vascular access. This technique is useful in the operating room when percutaneous insertion is unsuccessful. In addition, the low cardiac output encountered in the operating room frequently obscures the femoral artery pulse, which must be located precisely if the percutaneous route is used.

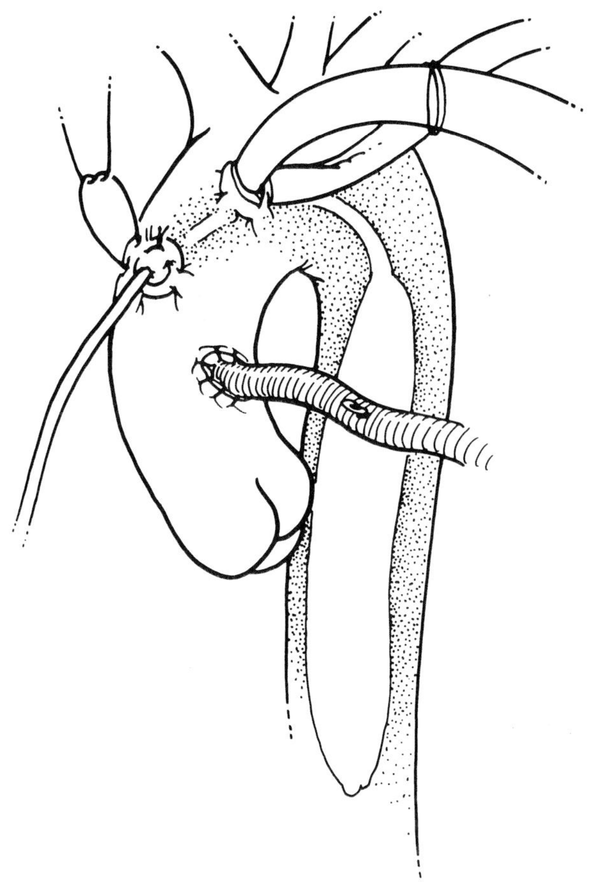

Fig. 39-3. Technique of transthoracic insertion of an intra-aortic balloon pump (IABP). In this diagram the heart has been deleted to better show the IABP insertion site in the ascending aorta of a patient undergoing aortocoronary bypass grafting.

Transthoracic Approach

In some patients, neither femoral artery is suitable for balloon insertion because of extensive atherosclerotic aortoiliac disease, tortuosity, or small size. Under these circumstances, the transthoracic approach is used.[56,57] To obviate the need for general anesthesia and a repeat sternotomy for balloon removal after use of the transthoracic route, some investigators advocate sewing a woven graft to the aorta and introducing the balloon through this graft, much as in the transfemoral approach. Removal is then accomplished with the use of local anesthesia by simply exposing the graft, withdrawing the balloon, and ligating the graft.[58-61] Despite its advantages, this approach increases the risk of graft infection, thromboembolism, and graft-aorta disruption.[62]

In the transthoracic approach, a purse-string suture is placed on the right lateral aspect of the ascending aorta to facilitate balloon insertion. A stab incision is made in the center of the purse-string suture, and the device is advanced to the appropriate position in the descending thoracic aorta (Fig. 39-3). Pumping is initiated in the same manner as for transfemoral insertion. Hemostasis is achieved at the aortotomy site by tightening the purse-string suture around the catheter. The catheter is secured with the ends of the suture and is brought out through the inferior portion of the incision. In postoperative patients who require transthoracic insertion, the sternum is left open and only the skin is closed; the sternum is later closed in delayed fashion.[63] This technique reduces compression of an acutely dilated heart and decreases the amount of surgical manipulation required at the time of balloon removal. After being weaned from the balloon, the patient is returned to the operating room, the sternotomy is reopened, and the mediastinum is explored. Thrombus is removed, and surgical hemostasis is carefully obtained.

Postoperative Care and Complications

To assess the immediate postoperative progress of IABP recipients, Norman et al.[64] developed a system of scoring in which systemic vascular resistance is plotted against the cardiac index (Fig. 39-4). This system has proved to be a simple, yet accurate, method of evaluating a patient's cardiovascular status. Patients who remain in class A during the first 8 hours after balloon implantation usually survive. Those who remain in class C for the first 8 hours invari-

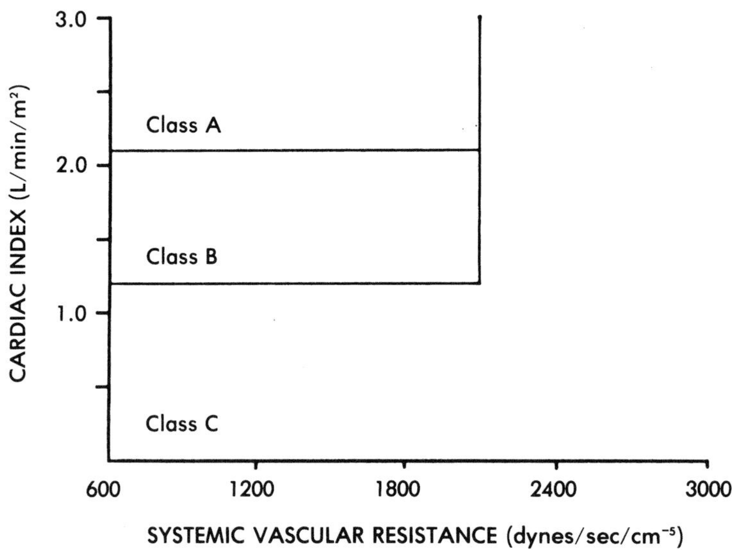

Fig. 39-4. The Texas Heart Institute's scheme for classifying patients who require an intra-aortic balloon pump. Cardiac index is plotted against systemic vascular resistance. Class A: CI (L/min/m^2) >2.1 and SVR (dynes/sec/cm^{-5}) <2100; Class B: CI = 2.1 to 1.2 and SVR <2100; Class C: CI <1.2 and SVR >2100.

ably fail to survive. Pharmacologic manipulation can be used to reduce systemic vascular resistance as appropriate and to elevate the cardiac output with inotropic agents or digitalis if required.

Few complications of IABP have been reported.[65] Lower limb ischemia can occur, however, and aortic dissection has been observed.[65] If ischemia occurs, the balloon should be removed as quickly as possible, and a Fogarty catheter thrombectomy should be performed, along with angioplasty. If the balloon cannot be removed, a femorofemoral crossover graft may be used to supply the involved artery distal to the site of balloon insertion.

In our experience the IABP has been a safe and reliable method of mechanical cardiac support. Insertion is generally easy and rapid, and the device increases the oxygen supply and decreases the oxygen demand of the myocardium while concomitantly improving the cardiac output. When used to support the failing heart, this technique consistently yields survival rates of 55% to 60%.[66,67]

VENTRICULAR ASSIST DEVICES

VADs are a more effective form of cardiac assistance than the IABP. Since the early 1980s a full range of VADs has become available for right ventricular, left ventricular, and biventricular support. These systems are constructed of biocompatible materials and yield either pulsatile or nonpulsatile flow. They offer three degrees of implantability, depending on the location of the pump and energy source (external to the patient's body, partially implantable, or fully implantable).

Unlike volume-displacement devices, which augment the existing circulation, VADs are volume-capturing pumps that augment or supplant native cardiac function, thereby providing an advanced form of mechanical support. Device filling and ejection are not generally synchronized with the cardiac cycle as in IABP use. Depending on the specific model, VADs may be implanted through an open chest approach or via a femoral artery cut-down. Moreover, they can provide short-term support (<2 weeks), intermediate-term support (2 weeks to 30 months), or long-term support (>6 months).

Because LVADs are the most widely used VADs and the only ones suitable for long-term implantation, this section focuses on devices for supporting the left ventricle.

Hemodynamic Effects

Use of an LVAD, with capture of most of the ventricular volume, results in the following changes:

1. A profound reduction in left ventricular outflow resistance during systole (or diastole), to such an extent that the aortic valve may not open and the LVAD captures all available cardiac output
2. A decrease in left ventricular pressure
3. Augmentation of the stroke volume and cardiac output (through the pump) up to 10 L/min[68,69]

The LVAD also produces a proportionate major increase in coronary perfusion pressures during diastole; a marked reduction in left ventricular volumes and filling pressures; and a profound decrease in left ventricular radius, wall tension, and oxygen consumption. As with the IABP but to a far greater extent, the myocardial oxygen supply is increased, but demand is reduced, and right-sided cardiac performance is proportionately improved because of LVAD-induced decreases in left-sided cardiac filling pressures.[70,71]

A clear understanding of the LVAD's clinical effectiveness is best gained by viewing the biologic and prosthetic left ventricles as two pumps that are connected in parallel during asynchronous LVAD actuation. Each pump has its own pressure-volume relationship, stroke volume, output, and stroke work. The net effect of LVAD actuation can be predicted as the result of an integrated biologic-prosthetic in-parallel pump system.

The pump system can be further understood if left-sided heart failure is viewed as a reduction in contractility, accompanied by decreased forward blood flow. This failure to generate pressure and displace volume can extend over a wide spectrum of states, ranging from compensated to decompensated. Biologic left ventricular performance can be assessed on the basis of the ejection fraction (the ratio of stroke volume to end-diastolic volume). Within limits, the stroke volume can be enhanced by augmenting the filling volume (Frank-Starling response) or by augmenting myocardial contractility with catecholamines or digitalis.[71] Reductions in ejection impedance produce elevated ejection fractions and stroke volumes, whereas increases in ejection impedance have the opposite effect.[72]

Biologic left ventricular function is greatly influenced by asynchronous LVAD actuation, and complete capture of the cardiac output can be achieved without opening of the biologic aortic valve. During periods of ventricular fibrillation or standstill, the systemic, pulmonary, and coronary circulations can be completely supported by the LVAD if pulmonary vascular resistance is low.

Myocardial oxygen consumption is principally determined by four hemodynamic variables: (1) peak developed wall tension, which is governed by systolic pressure and cardiac size; (2) contractile state; (3) heart rate; and (4) external stroke work.[73] When the LVAD's low impedance during biologic systole is substituted for left ventricular outflow (aortic) impedance, the peak systolic left ventricular pressure is greatly reduced, and myocardial oxygen consumption is correspondingly decreased. Left ventricular chamber size, stroke work, and heart rate are also reduced. Moreover, during biologic diastole, LVAD ejection produces an increase in both systemic and coronary blood flow.[51]

The LVAD's effectiveness primarily results from its ability to reduce left ventricular ejection impedance during biologic systole and to eject blood during biologic diastole. LVAD actuation can be compared with vasodilator (nitroprusside) therapy and IABP actuation, both of which cause lesser reductions in left ventricular impedance. Vasodilator therapy, IABP use, and LVAD actuation are escalating methods of achieving moderate-to-profound afterload reductions.

Indications for Use

The decision to use an LVAD is primarily based on (1) the inability to wean a patient from CPB despite optimal pharmacologic support and IABP use or (2) the need for a bridge to cardiac transplantation.

These devices are particularly useful in keeping transplantation candidates alive until a suitable donor heart can be located. When evaluated for cardiac transplantation, adults with terminal cardiomyopathies generally show reversible pulmonary vascular changes. Most patients have right ventricular hypertrophy, which is probably related to pumping against the elevated resistance that results from chronic left ventricular failure. Accordingly, simple unloading of the left ventricle usually provides adequate temporary support. With the newer LVADs, patients can even leave the hospital and undergo rehabilitation, so that they are in optimal condition at the time of transplantation.[74] Experience with these systems is yielding valuable insights that will hasten the day when long-term ventricular assistance can be used as an alternative to heart transplantation.[75-79]

Implantation Techniques

Except for the Hemopump, which is inserted via a femoral artery cut-down, LVADs must be implanted through a median sternotomy and an extended midline abdominal incision. The pump is placed in the left upper quadrant of the abdomen. Its inlet tube is passed through the diaphragm and positioned in the left ventricular apex. The outlet conduit is anastomosed to the ascending aorta. The driveline is connected percutaneously, through a separate incision, and is coupled to the external console.[80]

Postoperative Care and Complications

Immediate postoperative management is aimed at preventing right ventricular failure and controlling hemorrhage, which may be related either to the coagulopathy induced by prolonged CPB or to the underlying disease state and incipient organ failure.

TOTAL ARTIFICIAL HEART

In the race to produce a safe, effective TAH for long-term use, researchers have been slowed by their inability to develop a system as effective as the natural heart. A TAH must be able to maintain the circulation during normal patient activity, yet be flexible enough to augment cardiac output during increased activity. Moreover, the device must be acceptably safe and complication free. Although numerous problems must be overcome before permanent implantation is feasible, many experts believe that a safe, effective TAH for permanent use will become available within the next decade. The patients most likely to benefit from such a device will be those with end-stage cardiac disease and increased pulmonary vascular resistance or with acute global cardiac failure.

Meanwhile, pneumatically actuated TAHs are available for short-term use in bridge-to-transplant cases, and electrically actuated TAHs are undergoing experimental trials in animals.

Pneumatic Total Artificial Heart

A pneumatic TAH consists of two separate blood pumps that have smooth, seam-free blood-contacting surfaces.

The inflow and outflow ports each contain a prosthetic valve that ensures unidirectional flow. During implantation the pump's inflow cuffs and outflow Dacron grafts are attached to the remnant atria and great vessels. (Anatomically, the TAH is more restricted than the LVAD because of the need for alignment with these structures.) Each ventricle is independently actuated by a percutaneous driveline that connects with an air-driven power source. Energy from the power source collapses the bladders within the pumping chambers, causing blood to eject into the outlet conduit and thoracic aorta.

Pneumatic systems have two major disadvantages: (1) the large percutaneous drivelines that exit through the patient's skin pose a constant risk of infection and (2) the bulky power units that drive the system do not allow the patient much mobility. Therefore they are used only for patients who need short-term support while awaiting cardiac transplantation.

Electric Total Artificial Heart

The electric TAH incorporates a small electric motor and is therefore totally implantable, with no need for large external drivelines and drive units. Power is transmitted across the patient's intact skin, and small internal and external batteries allow unlimited patient mobility. Although not yet ready for clinical use, these pumps offer the best potential for long-term, and eventually permanent, implantation.[81,82]

SUMMARY

The prototype of assisted circulation is the extracorporeal heart-lung machine, or CPB circuit. Its development more than four decades ago made modern cardiac surgery possible and paved the way for other devices designed to support the failing circulation. Among the mechanical assist devices currently used in the clinical setting, the most successful short-term device is the IABP, which is generally the first choice for initial support in cases of cardiac failure. The IABP instantaneously benefits the circulatory system by decreasing the systolic arterial pressure (afterload) and heart rate, while increasing the diastolic perfusion pressure and cardiac output but not the mean arterial pressure.

LVADs are more hemodynamically effective than IABPs during profound left ventricular failure because LVADs can capture the total cardiac output and augment systemic and coronary perfusion; moreover, these devices can function in the absence of an intact electrocardiographic signal and during ventricular fibrillation or standstill. If support can be maintained, ventricular recovery can occur, even if the myocardium is severely depressed.

Presently being evaluated clinically, electrically actuated devices offer increasingly longer durability and reliability and are expected to be useful in several settings. Possible candidates include patients with advanced ischemic or idiopathic cardiomyopathy refractory to surgical or medical management, as well as those refractory to (or dependent on) pharmacologic, IABP, or short-term LVAD support. Long-term cardiac assistance also appears feasible as a primary method of treating intraoperative or postinfarction myocardial failure or as a bridge to cardiac transplantation. Whereas the TAH can maintain the entire circulation satisfactorily, its major current benefit lies in its ability to support the failing circulation until cardiac transplantation can be performed.

Mechanical cardiac assist devices have proved effective in both augmenting and capturing the cardiac output in patients who require short-term circulatory support. The need for a reliable long-term support system has not yet been met. Experimental studies are promising, however, and should eventually produce devices capable of providing partial or total long-term support.

REFERENCES

1. Gibbon JH Jr. Artificial maintenance of circulation during experimental occlusion of the pulmonary artery. Arch Surg 34:1105, 1937.
2. LeGallois JJC. Experiences sur le principe de la vie, Paris, 1812. (Nancrede JG, Nancrede NC, translators. Philadelphia, 1813).
3. Gibbon JH Jr. Application of a mechanical heart and lung apparatus to cardiac surgery. Minn Med 37:171, 1954.
4. Kolff WJ. Disposable membrane oxygenator (heart-lung machine) and its use in experimental surgery. Cleve Clin Q 23:69, 1956.
5. Cooley DA, Beall AC Jr, Grondin P. Open heart surgery using disposable oxygenators. Scientific exhibit at the American College of Surgeons Forty-Eighth Annual Clinical Congress. Atlantic City, N.J.: 1962.
6. Kusserow BK. A permanently indwelling intracorporeal blood pump to substitute for cardiac function. Trans Am Soc Artif Intern Organs 4:227, 1958.
7. Kusserow BK, Clapp JF III. Partial substitution of ventricular function over extended periods by a mechanical pump. Trans Am Soc Artif Intern Organs 7:332, 1961.
8. Akutsu T, Kolff WJ. Permanent substitutes for valves and hearts. Trans Am Soc Artif Intern Organs 4:230, 1958.
9. Akutsu T, et al. A sac type of artificial heart inside the chest of dogs. J Thorac Cardiovasc Surg 47:512, 1964.
10. Nosé Y, et al. Elimination of some problems encountered in total replacement of the heart with an intrathoracic mechanical pump: Venous return. Trans Am Soc Artif Intern Organs 12:301, 1966.
11. Cooley DA, et al. First human implantation of cardiac prosthesis for staged total replacement of the heart. Trans Am Soc Artif Intern Organs 15:252, 1969.
12. Bernhard WF, et al. Biventricular bypass: Physiologic studies during induced ventricular failure and fibrillation. J Thorac Cardiovasc Surg 62:859, 1971.
13. Takagi H, et al. Pathophysiologic studies on prolonged continuous pumping of series-type left heart assist device in calves. Trans Am Soc Artif Intern Organs 17:189, 1971.
14. DeBakey ME. Left ventricular bypass pump for cardiac assistance: Clinical experience. Am J Cardiol 27:3, 1971.
15. Kantrowitz A, Krakauer J, Sherman JL. A permanent mechanical auxiliary ventricle. J Cardiovasc Surg 9:1, 1968.
16. Moulopoulos SD, Topaz S, Kolff WJ. Extracorporeal assistance to the circulation and intraaortic balloon pumping. Trans Am Soc Artif Intern Organs 8:85, 1962.
17. Kantrowitz A, et al. Initial clinical experience with intraaortic balloon pumping in cardiogenic shock. JAMA 203(2):135, 1968.
18. Norman JC. An intracorporeal (abdominal) left ventricular assist device (ALVAD). XXX. Clinical readiness and initial trials in man. Cardiovasc Dis Bull Tex Heart Inst 3(3):249, 1976.

19. Bernhard WF, et al. A left ventricular aortic blood pump for circulatory support in postoperative patients with acute left ventricular failure. In Unger F, ed. Assisted Circulation. Berlin: Springer-Verlag, 1979.
20. Thoma M, et al. Drive technology of mechanical circulation support systems—Consequences from clinical experience. Med-Markt Acta Medicotech 5:150, 1978.
21. Pierce WS, et al. Prolonged mechanical support of the left ventricle. Circulation 58(Suppl 1):133, 1978.
22. Turina M, Bosio R, Senning A. Clinical applications of paracorporeal, uni and biventricular artificial heart. Trans Am Soc Artif Intern Organs 25:625, 1978.
23. Boers M, et al. Two membrane oxygenators and a bubbler: A clinical comparison. Ann Thorac Surg 35(4):455, 1983.
24. Hessel EA, et al. Membrane vs. bubble oxygenator for cardiac operations: A prospective randomized study. J Thorac Cardiovasc Surg 80(1):111, 1980.
25. Siderys H, et al. A comparison of membrane and bubble oxygenation as used in cardiopulmonary bypass patients. J Thorac Cardiovasc Surg 68(5):708, 1975.
26. Van Den Dungen JJAM, et al. Clinical study of blood trauma during perfusion with membrane and bubble oxygenators. J Thorac Cardiovasc Surg 83(1):108, 1982.
27. Wright JS, et al. Some advantages of the membrane oxygenator for open-heart surgery. J Thorac Cardiovasc Surg 69(6):884, 1975.
28. Liddicoat JE, et al. Membrane vs. bubble oxygenator: A clinical comparison. Ann Surg 181(5):747, 1975.
29. Hickey PR, Buckley MJ, Philbin DM. Pulsatile and nonpulsatile cardiopulmonary bypass: Review of a counterproductive controversy. Ann Thorac Surg 36(6):720, 1983.
30. Wesolowski SA, Fisher JH, Welch CS. Perfusion of pulmonary circulation by non-pulsatile flow. Surgery 33:370, 1953.
31. Wesolowski SA, Sauvage LR, Pinc RD. Extracorporeal circulation: The role of the pulse in maintenance of the systemic circulation during heart lung bypass. Surgery 37:663, 1955.
32. Bennet EV, et al. Comparison of flow differences among venous cannulas. Ann Thorac Surg 36(1):59, 1983.
33. Solis RT. Blood filtration during cardiopulmonary bypass. J Extra-Corporeal Tech 6:64, 1974.
34. Putman EA, Manners JM. Vascular resistance during cardiopulmonary bypass; Its effect on vascular performance in the immediate post bypass period. Anesthesia 38(7):635, 1983.
35. Cooper TJ, et al. Factors relating to the development of hypertension after cardiopulmonary bypass. Br Heart J 54(1):91, 1985.
36. Lajos TZ, Venditti J, Vennuto R. Hemodynamic consequences of bronchial flow during cardiopulmonary bypass. J Thorac Cardiovasc Surg 89(6):934, 1985.
37. Lundar T, et al. Cerebral perfusion during nonpulsatile cardiopulmonary bypass. Ann Thorac Surg 40(2):144, 1985.
38. Cohn LH, Angell WW, Shumway NE. Body fluid shifts after cardiopulmonary bypass. I. Effects of congestive heart and hemodilution. J Thorac Cardiovasc Surg 62(3):423, 1971.
39. Pacifico AD, Digerness S, Kirklin JW. Acute alterations of bodily composition after open cardiac operations. Circulation 41:331, 1970.
40. Royston D, et al. The effect of surgery with cardiopulmonary bypass on alveolar-capillary barrier function in human beings. Ann Thorac Surg 40(2):139, 1985.
41. Svennevig JL, et al. Should the lungs be ventilated during cardiopulmonary bypass? Clinical, hemodynamic, and metabolic changes in patients undergoing elective coronary artery surgery. Ann Thorac Surg 37(4):295, 1984.
42. Van Velzen-Blad H, et al. Cardiopulmonary bypass and host defense functions in human beings. I. Serum levels and role of immunoglobulins and complement of phagocytosis. Ann Thorac Surg 39(3):207, 1985.
43. Van Velzen-Blad H, et al. Cardiopulmonary bypass and host defense functions in human beings. II. Lymphocyte function. Ann Thorac Surg 39(3):212, 1985.
44. Quiroga MM, et al. The effect of body temperature on leukocyte kinetics during cardiopulmonary bypass. J Thorac Cardiovasc Surg 90(1):91, 1985.
45. Buckley MJ, et al. Hemodynamic evaluation of IABP in man. Circulation 41(Suppl II):11, 1970.
46. Dunkman WB, et al. Clinical and hemodynamic results of IABP and surgery for cardiogenic shock. Circulation 46:465, 1972.
47. Kramer JS, et al. Clinical management ancillary to phase-shift balloon pumping in cardiogenic shock: Preliminary comments. Am J Cardiol 27:123, 1979.
48. Scheidt S, et al. Intraaortic balloon counterpulsation in cardiogenic shock: Report of a cooperative clinical trial. N Engl J Med 288(19):979, 1973.
49. Igo SR, et al. Intraaortic balloon pumping: Theory and practice—Experience with 325 patients. Artif Organs 2(3):249, 1978.
50. Schelbert HR, Covell JW, Burns JW. Observations on factors affecting local forces in the left ventricular wall during acute myocardial ischemia. Circ Res 29:306, 1971.
51. Spotnitz HM, Covell JW, Ross J. Left ventricular mechanics and oxygen consumption during arterial counter-pulsation. Am J Physiol 217:1352, 1969.
52. Weber KT, Janicki JS. Intraaortic balloon counter-pulsation: A review of physiological principles, clinical results and device safety. Ann Thorac Surg 17:602, 1974.
53. Igo SR, et al. Determinants of induced subendocardial ischemia as reflected by DPTI/TTI ratios, in occluded and nonoccluded zones of bovine left ventricle. Physiologist 17:253, 1974.
54. Philips PA, Miyamoto AM. Application of the supply-demand ratio for the early detection of subendocardial ischemia. In Norman JC, ed. Coronary Artery Medicine and Surgery: Concepts and Controversies. New York: Appleton-Century-Crofts, 1975.
55. Holub DA, et al. Changes in right ventricular function associated with intraaortic balloon pumping (IABP) in the cardiogenic shock patient. Clin Res 25:553A, 1977.
56. Gueldner TL, Lawrence GH. Intraaortic balloon assist through cannulation of the ascending aorta. Ann Thorac Surg 19(1):88, 1975.
57. Ugorji CC, et al. Transascending aortic intraaortic balloon insertion with delayed sternal closure: A retrospective analysis. Cardiovasc Dis Bull Tex Heart Inst 7(3):307, 1980.
58. Krause AH, Bigelow JC, Page US. Transthoracic intraaortic balloon cannulation to avoid repeat sternotomy for removal. Ann Thorac Surg 21:562, 1976.
59. McCabe JC, et al. Complications of intraaortic balloon insertion and counter-pulsation. Circulation 57(4):769, 1978.
60. Roe BB, Chatterjee K. Transthoracic cannulation for balloon pumping: Report of a patient undergoing closed chest decannulation. Ann Thorac Surg 21:568, 1976.
61. Tchervendov CI, Salerno TA. Preliminary experience with a new technique of insertion and removal of the intraaortic balloon pump into the ascending aorta [letter to the editor]. J Thorac Cardiovasc Surg 87:475, 1984.
62. Nunez L, et al. Transthoracic cannulation for balloon pumping in a "crowded aorta." Ann Thorac Surg 30:400, 1980.
63. Frazier OH, et al. Morbidity in balloon counterpulsation: Transfemoral versus transthoracic insertion. Trans Am Soc Artif Intern Organs 30:108, 1984.
64. Norman JC, et al. Prognostic indices for survival during postcardiotomy intraaortic balloon pumping: Methods of scoring and classification, with implications for left ventricular assist device utilization. J Thorac Cardiovasc Surg 74(5):709, 1977.
65. Isner JM, et al. Complications of the intraaortic balloon counterpulsation device: Clinical and morphologic observations in 45 necropsy patients. Am J Cardiol 45:250, 1980.
66. Bedderman C, et al. Intraaortic balloon pumping in women: Effects of balloon size on survival. Thorac Cardiovasc Surg 28:428, 1980.

67. McGee MG, et al. Retrospective analyses of the need for mechanical circulatory support (intraaortic balloon pump/abdominal left ventricular assist device or partial artificial heart) after cardiopulmonary bypass: A 44-month study of 14,168 patients. Am J Cardiol 46:135, 1980.
68. Berger RL, et al. Successful use of a paracorporeal left ventricular assist device in man. JAMA 243(1):46, 1980.
69. Norman JC. Partial artificial hearts: Mechanical closing of the ventricle. Artif Organs 2(3):235, 1978.
70. Daly BDT, et al. Right ventricular effects of left ventricular unloading with an abdominal left ventricular assist device in the calf. Physiologist 17(3):205, 1974.
71. Patterson S, Starling EH. On the mechanical factors which determine the output of the ventricles. J Physiol 48:357, 1914.
72. Sarnoff SJ. Myocardial contractility as described by ventricular function curves; Observations on Starling's law of the heart. Phys Rev 35:107, 1955.
73. Sonnenblick EH, Ross J Jr, Braunwald E. Oxygen consumption of the heart: Newer concepts of its multifactorial determination. Am J Cardiol 22:328, 1968.
74. Frazier OH, et al. Improved mortality and rehabilitation of transplant candidates treated with a long-term implantable left ventricular assist system. Ann Surg 222:327, 1995.
75. Frazier OH. The development of an implantable, portable, electrically powered left ventricular assist device. Semin Thorac Cardiovasc Surg 6:181, 1994.
76. Wampler RK, Baker BA, Wright WM. Circulatory support of cardiac interventional procedures with the Hemopump cardiac assist system. Cardiology 84:194, 1994.
77. Myers TJ, Macris MP. Clinical experience with the HeartMate left ventricular assist device. Heart Failure Dec 1994/Jan 1995:247, 1994/1995.
78. Wasler A, et al. A comparison between intraperitoneal and extraperitoneal left ventricular assist system placement. ASAIO J 42:M573, 1996.
79. Macris MP, et al. Development of an implantable ventricular assist system. Ann Thorac Surg 63:367, 1977.
80. Radovancevic B, Frazier OH, Duncan JM. Implantation technique for the HeartMate left ventricular assist device. J Cardiac Surg 7:203, 1992.
81. Parnis SM, et al. Chronic in vivo evaluation of an electrohydraulic total artificial heart. ASAIO J 40:M489, 1994.
82. Kung RT, et al. Progress in the development of the ABIOMED total artificial heart. ASAIO J 41:M245, 1995.

40

Congenital Heart Lesions

Ralph S. Mosca and Edward L. Bove

The surgical treatment of congenital heart defects has progressed at a rapid rate since its beginning more than half a century ago. Numerous technical achievements have been made possible by advances in many fields. Precise knowledge of anatomy and physiology, detailed noninvasive diagnostic capabilities, better perfusion and myocardial preservation techniques, and improved neonatal intensive care have all played major roles in allowing the management of congenital heart disease to progress to this extent. Nearly all congenital heart defects are now amenable to surgical repair. This chapter discusses the pathophysiology underlying some of the cardiac defects more commonly encountered by the pediatric cardiac surgeon and covers the physiologic rationales behind their treatment.

ADJUSTMENTS IN THE CIRCULATION AFTER BIRTH

Although it is beyond the scope of this chapter to discuss in detail the physiology of the intrauterine circulation and its adaptation to extrauterine life, a brief description is included to aid in the understanding of the topics to follow.

Oxygen-enriched placental blood returns to the fetus through the umbilical vein and then passes through the liver. There it joins the inferior vena caval return and enters the right atrium. Much of this blood passes across the patent foramen ovale by preferential streaming into the left atrium, left ventricle, and ascending aorta, where it is distributed to the brain and coronary circulations (Fig. 40-1). Superior vena caval return is directed across the right atrium, tricuspid valve, and right ventricle to be ejected into the pulmonary artery. Nearly all this blood passes across the patent ductus arteriosus (PDA) into the descending aorta. Because the ductus is nonrestrictive, both ventricles essentially function as a unit and eject blood against the same overall resistance. However, systemic vascular resistance is low because of the placental circulation, and pulmonary vascular resistance (PVR) is high in the nonaerated fetal lung, resulting in less than 10% of the fetal cardiac output going to the lungs.

At birth, the placenta is eliminated from the circulation, resulting in an abrupt rise in systemic vascular resistance. Expansion of the lungs leads to a fall in PVR. As arterial and alveolar partial pressure of oxygen (PO_2) increase, PVR falls further and pulmonary blood flow rises, resulting in an increase in left atrial pressure and functional closure of the flap valve of the foramen ovale. The increase in arterial PO_2 also causes constriction of the smooth muscle in the wall of the ductus arteriosus, closing the duct and completing the separation of the two circulations. PVR falls to adult normal levels within 2 to 4 weeks in the term infant.

CONGESTIVE HEART FAILURE

Simply defined, congestive heart failure is the failure of myocardial oxygen supply to meet oxygen demand. The classic findings of congestive heart failure in infants include tachypnea, tachycardia, diaphoresis, and hepatomegaly. Peripheral edema and rales are not typically noted in infants. The neonatal myocardium is already functioning at maximal stroke volume and can only increase cardiac output by increasing heart rate. Further, the neonatal myocardium has a reduced density of contractile elements. For these reasons, the already stressed neonate with limited cardiac reserve is easily susceptible to congestive heart failure. Congenital heart disease typically results in congestive heart failure in either of two ways, volume overload or pressure overload.

Volume overload occurs with either a large communication between the systemic and pulmonary circulations or valvular regurgitant lesions (Fig. 40-2). When a left-to-right shunt occurs, the volume of shunted blood depends on the relative resistances of the two vascular beds. As the PVR falls during the first few weeks of life, pulmonary blood flow may increase dramatically, producing a large volume overload of the left ventricle. Because this shunt depends on a falling PVR, congestive failure from volume overload is not usually seen until 2 or 3 weeks of age.

Pressure overload results from an obstruction to ventricular emptying. This obstruction is usually located at the level of the semilunar (pulmonary or aortic) valve, but it

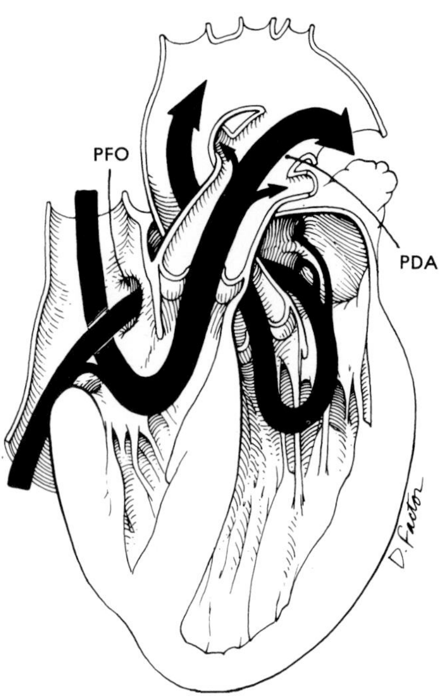

Fig. 40-1. Course of the intracardiac circulation before birth. Most inferior vena caval blood passes across the patent foramen ovale *(PFO)* to the left atrium. The superior vena caval return is directed predominantly across the patent ductus arteriosus *(PDA)*.

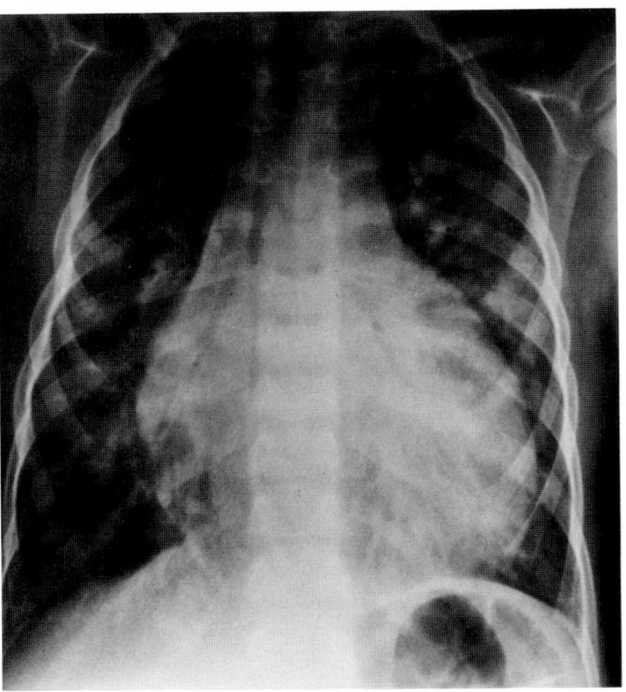

Fig. 40-2. Chest radiograph of a patient with atrial septal defect. There is cardiomegaly and an increase in pulmonary vascular markings as a result of the large left-to-right shunt.

may be seen with subvalvular or supravalvular blockage. When the ventricle can no longer eject an adequate blood volume through the obstruction, pulmonary and systemic venous congestion with congestive heart failure result.

Cyanosis

Cyanosis is a blue discoloration of the skin and mucous membranes caused by the presence of at least 5 g/dl unsaturated circulating hemoglobin. When it is noted in infancy, the administration of 100% oxygen is a reliable test to establish the presence of intracardiac shunting related to congenital heart disease. If the Po_2 in the right radial artery rises above 250 mm Hg, cyanotic heart disease is virtually eliminated. Although values less than 250 mm Hg are not certain indicators of cardiac disease, a Po_2 less than 100 mm Hg generally indicates a cardiac problem.

Cyanosis resulting from congenital heart disease may be caused by decreased pulmonary blood flow with intracardiac right-to-left shunting or by abnormalities of intracardiac mixing. When cyanosis is caused by decreased pulmonary blood flow, two conditions are necessary, obstruction to flow into the lungs and an intracardiac communication between the two circulations proximal to the obstruction. The obstruction may be located anywhere between the systemic venous atrium (tricuspid atresia) and the branch pulmonary arteries (tetralogy of Fallot). Resistance to flow through the obstruction is at least that through the communication, allowing desaturated blood to enter the systemic circulation directly.

Cyanosis may also occur as a result of inadequate mixing of the blood between the systemic and pulmonary circulations. This situation is classically seen in transposition-type physiology. Although total systemic and pulmonary blood flow may be normal or increased, the effective flow is reduced. That is, the amount of desaturated blood actually reaching the lungs and the amount of fully saturated blood reaching the body are decreased. This condition is discussed more fully later in this chapter.

Finally, common mixing occurs when desaturated and saturated blood freely mix, allowing some desaturated blood to reach the body. This can occur at atrial (common atrium), ventricular (common or single ventricle), or great vessel level (truncus arteriosus).

OBSTRUCTIVE LESIONS

Coarctation of the Aorta

Coarctation is a narrowing in the thoracic aorta most commonly located just distal to the left subclavian artery, opposite the insertion of the ductus arteriosus or ligamentum arteriosum (Fig. 40-3, *A*). Obstruction to left ventricular emptying results in a pressure overload of the ventricle, which may lead to congestive heart failure. In infancy, associated defects often dictate the hemodynamic condition. When the ductus arteriosus is patent, blood may flow from the pulmonary artery across the duct into the descending aorta (Fig. 40-3, *B*). In this situation, differential cyanosis is present, with desaturated blood perfusing the lower extremities and saturated blood perfusing the upper body.

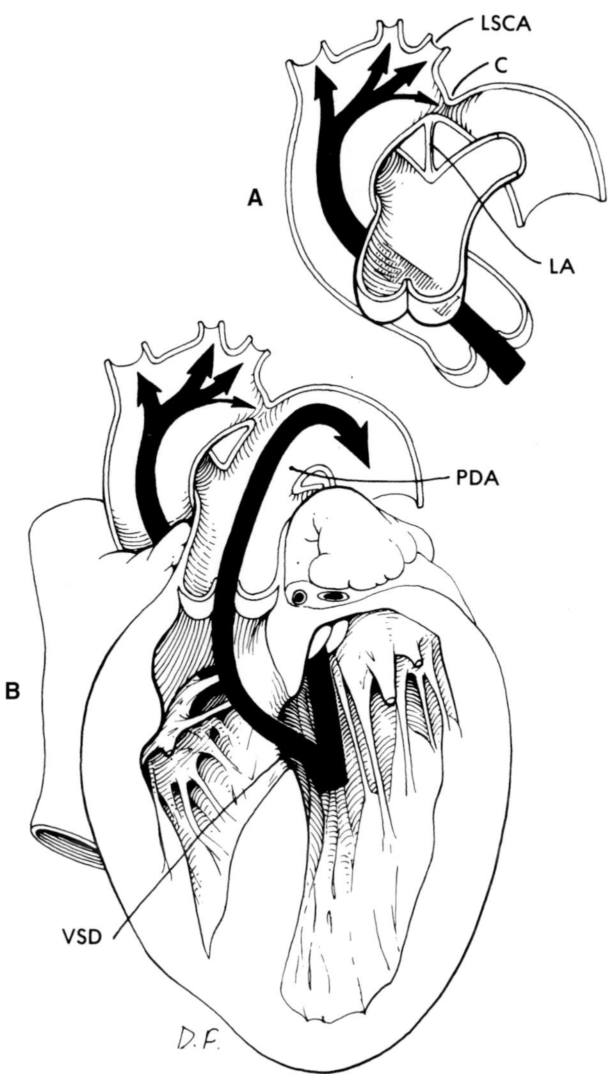

Fig. 40-3. Hemodynamic abnormalities in coarctation *(C)* of the aorta. **A,** Pathophysiology in the older child or adult. **B,** In infancy, patent ductus arteriosus *(PDA)* allows blood flow to the descending aorta from the right ventricle. *LA,* Ligamentum arteriosum; *LSCA,* left subclavian artery; *VSD,* ventricular septal defect.

Approximately 20% of patients have an associated ventricular septal defect (VSD). The impedance to left ventricular emptying imposed by the coarctation increases the left-to-right shunt and results in severe congestive heart failure from combined pressure and volume overload. Other obstructive lesions in the left side of the heart may also be seen with coarctation; most common is aortic stenosis related to a bicuspid aortic valve.

When coarctation results in congestive heart failure in infancy, nonoperative treatment carries a high mortality rate. Most patients with coarctation, however, do not have symptoms, and the defect is not found until after infancy. The discovery of upper-extremity hypertension with diminished or absent femoral pulses typically leads to the diagnosis. Flow murmurs over the back and palpable pulsations in the subscapular area from prominent collaterals may be present. All extremity pulses must be carefully palpated. A decrease in the left arm pulse may indicate involvement of the origin of the left subclavian artery in the coarctation. Plain chest radiographs may show dilation of the aorta proximally and distally to the narrowed segment (3 sign) and notching of the ribs related to enlarged intercostal arteries. In the past, aortography was generally recommended to accurately define the anatomy of the coarctation before surgical repair. Today, noninvasive techniques, including Doppler echocardiography and magnetic resonance imaging, are generally adequate to delineate the anatomy. In rare cases, the coarctation may be in an unusual location.

The exact cause of hypertension in coarctation remains obscure. The etiology in older patients is apparently more than obstruction alone, because relief of coarctation in adulthood does not result in the restoration of normal blood pressure in every case. It seems certain that in these cases a renal mechanism is in part responsible. In a classic experiment performed by Scott and Bahnson,[1] coarctation was surgically created in dogs. The resultant hypertension was relieved by removal of one kidney and transplantation of the other above the level of the coarctation. When abnormal plasma renin activity is unmasked by volume depletion, abnormally high renin-angiotensin activity has been found in patients with coarctation.[2]

Virtually all patients with hemodynamically significant coarctation of the aorta should undergo operative repair. The ideal age for repair in the child without symptoms is not well defined, but it has been moved earlier and earlier in recent years. Repair is probably best accomplished between the ages of 1 and 3 years. Earlier operation may increase the risk of recoarctation with growth of the aorta, whereas delaying repair beyond childhood increases the chance of persistent hypertension.[3] The presence of congestive heart failure in infancy dictates operative intervention, regardless of age or size.

The classic surgical technique remains resection of the narrowed segment with end-to-end anastomosis. The benefits of this technique include removal of all the ductal tissue, thus decreasing the risk of recoarctation. The potential disadvantages include the need for greater dissection, increased technical difficulty, and the possibility of tension at the repair site. Concerns about growth of the aorta in the face of a circumferential suture line have been minimized by the use of absorbable suture material and further alleviated by good results with other similar neonatal repairs, such as the arterial switch procedure.

We prefer the resection and end-to-end anastomosis in virtually all cases. However, the subclavian angioplasty procedure, first reported by Waldhausen and Norwald in 1966[4] (Fig. 40-4), is preferred by some groups. Although this technique does not remove all the ductal tissue and is not suitable for augmentation of more proximal aortic narrowing, it is technically easier and avoids suture line

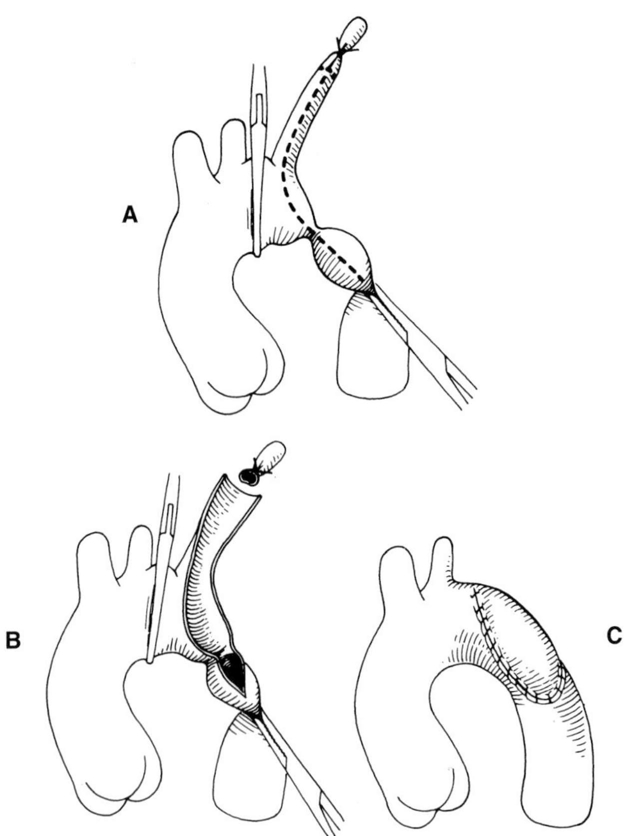

Fig. 40-4. Repair of coarctation with the subclavian angioplasty technique. **A,** Left subclavian artery is mobilized and divided distally. **B,** Longitudinal incision through the artery and adjacent aorta is made. This incision must extend distally beyond the coarctation until normal aorta is reached. **C,** Completed repair.

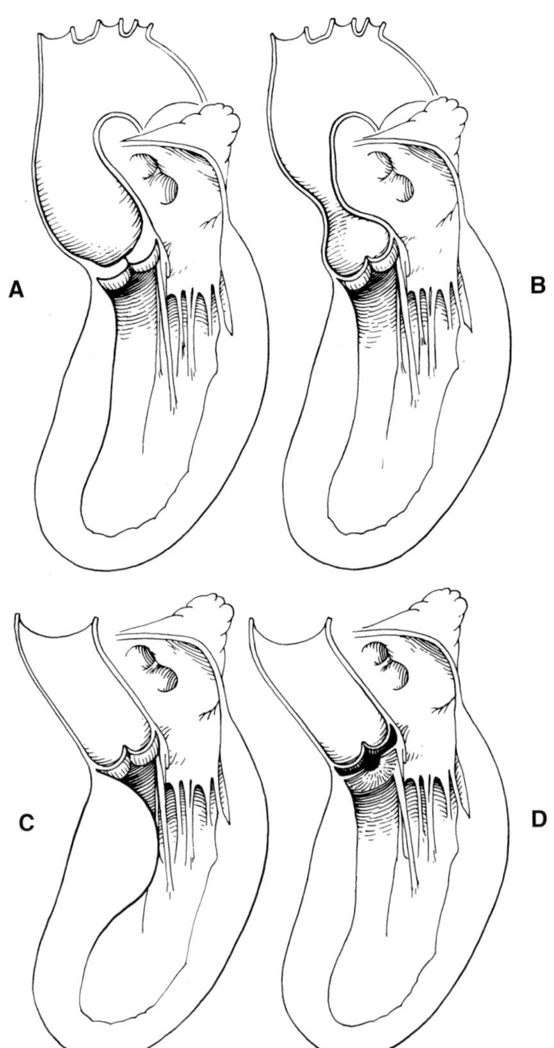

Fig. 40-5. Anatomic types of left ventricular outflow tract obstruction. **A,** Valvular stenosis related to a bicuspid aortic valve. Note the poststenotic dilation of the ascending aorta. **B,** Hourglass narrowing of the ascending aorta, resulting in supravalvular stenosis. **C,** Subvalvular stenosis resulting from diffuse hypertrophy of the ventricular septum. **D,** Subvalvular stenosis resulting from a discrete subaortic membrane.

tension. Division of the subclavian artery can, on occasion, lead to disparate upper extremity growth.

Synthetic patch aortoplasty retains abnormal ductal tissue and may lead to aneurysm formation on the aortic wall opposite the patch (also reported with subclavian flap technique). This technique should be used only in cases of discrete recoarctations in which mobilization for end-to-end repair is not feasible.

Coarctation associated with a large VSD is best treated by a single-stage complete repair through a median sternotomy. During a period of circulatory arrest, the coarctation is resected and repaired with the mobilized distal aortic segment used to augment the transverse aortic arch if necessary. The VSD is then closed from a transatrial approach.

Aortic Stenosis

The most common cause of obstruction to left ventricular ejection is aortic stenosis. The obstruction is typically located at the level of the valve, but it may be subvalvular or supravalvular (Fig. 40-5). Valvular aortic stenosis is usually caused by a bicuspid aortic valve with varying degrees of fusion of the commissures, although fused tricuspid valves may also be found. A dome-shaped unicusp valve may result in significant obstruction in infancy. Subvalvular aortic stenosis may be discrete or diffuse. In the discrete form, a fibrous membrane is found just below the aortic valve leaflets. The diffuse form is seen in obstructive cardiomyopathies, such as idiopathic hypertrophic subaortic stenosis or muscular tunnel–type subvalvular hypoplasia. In supravalvular stenosis, the obstruction is most commonly caused by an hourglass deformity of the ascending aorta just above the valve.

Valvular aortic stenosis may be seen at any age. In infancy, severe stenosis may cause congestive heart failure.[5] In most children, however, an asymptomatic heart murmur is detected on physical examination beyond the neonatal period. When symptoms are present in childhood, exertional dyspnea, syncope, and angina pectoris are the usual manifestations. Syncope is caused by the inability of the left ventricle to maintain adequate cerebral blood flow through a narrow, fixed orifice valve during exercise. Angina pectoris, although rare in childhood, may be seen when pressure overload results in significant left ventricular hypertrophy and myocardial blood flow does not adequately perfuse the thickened, hypertensive ventricular muscle.

Indications for operation in patients with valvular aortic stenosis include syncope, congestive heart failure, or angina with a significant left ventricular outflow tract gradient. A significant gradient is usually considered to be at least 50 mm Hg, unless cardiac output is greatly diminished. The timing of operative intervention in the child without symptoms who has moderate or severe obstruction is less well defined. Electrocardiographic changes indicating left ventricular strain or ischemia, either at rest or induced during exercise, are considered definite indications. Severe gradients, greater than 70 mm Hg, are best treated promptly, even in the absence of symptoms or electrocardiographic changes.

Options for relief of critical aortic stenosis in the neonate include open valvotomy, transventricular dilatation, and transcatheter therapy. The standard approach has been open valvotomy with cardiopulmonary bypass. Relief of valvular aortic stenosis is accomplished by direct incision of fused commissures. The incision is stopped 1 to 2 mm from the annulus to avoid detaching all leaflet support and creating significant aortic regurgitation. In a true bicuspid valve, rudimentary commissures must not be incised, or a flail leaflet will result. Although satisfactory reduction of the gradient can usually be accomplished, it may be difficult to provide complete relief of obstruction in all cases.[6] Certain bicuspid valves may not lend themselves to valvotomy and may remain obstructive despite lack of commissural fusion. Although a few studies have reported good results with open aortic valvotomy,[7,8] the mortality rates have remained high in most series. This may be in part because congenital aortic stenosis is a heterogeneous, complex disorder in which the aortic valvular and annular substrates may not be conducive to direct operative intervention.

Transventricular dilatation, first described by Trinkle et al.[9] in 1975, provides a simple and effective technique of closed aortic valvotomy in infants. Through an apical left ventricular approach, progressive dilatation of the valve is accomplished with or without cardiopulmonary bypass. Transventricular dilatation provides effective relief of the obstruction without creating significant aortic insufficiency, and it avoids the myocardial ischemia inherent in open techniques.[10]

Transcatheter therapy through the femoral, umbilical, or carotid arteries is also quite effective in the neonatal population. The risks of balloon aortic valvotomy continue to include inadvertent aortic cusp perforation, with resultant severe aortic insufficiency as well as arterial injury.

The goal of treatment of neonates and infants with critical aortic stenosis is to establish an effective aortic orifice, thereby relieving the left ventricular pressure overload without inducing hemodynamically significant aortic insufficiency. Few of these patients are cured by their initial procedure. Because of the complexity of the disease (valvular stenosis, annular hypoplasia, varying degrees of subaortic stenosis, and the turbulent flow as a result of these), most patients require further operative intervention. Replacement of the aortic valve with a pulmonary autograft (Ross procedure) can be performed at any age, even in the neonate, and is the optimal procedure when more conservative treatment fails.

Operation for subvalvular stenosis is recommended for the same indications as in valvular obstruction. The required gradient may be somewhat less for discrete subvalvular stenosis, however, because resection of the membrane is more often curative.[11] Many patients with untreated discrete subvalvular stenosis later have progressive aortic regurgitation related to turbulence beneath the valve. Early resection of the membrane, often combined with a septal myectomy, may prevent this complication. Diffuse, muscular left ventricular outflow tract obstruction is more difficult to relieve. Transaortic resection of hypertrophied septal muscle, an aortoventriculoplasty, or bypass of the obstruction by insertion of a valved conduit from the left ventricular apex to the aorta is often needed.[12,13]

Supravalvular aortic stenosis is the least common site of left ventricular outflow tract obstruction. Isolated supravalvular aortic stenosis is rare in infants and may occur as part of the Williams syndrome in older children. This lesion is also highly variable, ranging from a membranous ringlike constriction, the classic hourglass deformity, to a diffuse form involving much of the aorta and brachiocephalic vessels. The coronary arteries are exposed to high pressure, and degenerative changes may be seen early in life. Indications for operation include a gradient greater than 50 mm Hg and evidence of coronary obstruction. Repair involves a longitudinal incision in the ascending aorta, extended proximally into both the noncoronary and right coronary cusps in an inverted Y configuration. The patch is then extended as far distally as necessary to relieve the obstruction.

LEFT-TO-RIGHT SHUNTS

Atrial Septal Defect

Atrial septal defect (ASD) accounts for approximately 10% of all congenital cardiac lesions. The defect in the septum allows blood to flow from the left to the right atrium, producing a volume overload of the right ventricle and pulmonary circulation. The shunt is directed from left to right because of the greater diastolic compliance and lower diastolic pressure in the right-sided chambers. Moderate-sized defects result in pulmonary blood flow from one and one half to three times the systemic flow, whereas in large defects the pulmonary to systemic flow ratio exceeds 3 to 1. In most cases, pulmonary artery pressure and systemic blood flow remain normal.

ASDs often occur as isolated lesions and tend to remain asymptomatic until early adult life.[14] When present, symptoms are often nonspecific and consist of fatigue or mild dyspnea on exertion. In the presence of a large left-to-right shunt, overt congestive heart failure can occur at any age. Most commonly, however, nearly normal activity is maintained until the third or fourth decade of life, when symptoms of congestive heart failure become manifest.

Any chronic left-to-right shunt may eventually produce changes of pulmonary vascular occlusive disease. Although these changes occur more frequently and earlier in life with defects that cause an increase in both pulmonary blood flow and pressure, uncomplicated ASDs may result in irreversible pulmonary occlusive changes. This problem is discussed more fully in the following section concerning VSDs.

Most ASDs occur in the center of the atrial septum and are referred to as *ostium secundum ASDs* (Fig. 40-6). In approximately 5% to 10% of patients, the defect is located high in the atrial wall, where the superior vena cava joins the right atrium. These defects, known as *sinus venosus ASDs,* are almost always associated with drainage of the right upper lobe pulmonary veins to the right atrium or superior vena cava. About 5% of patients have another variety of defect, called *ostium primum ASDs.* These defects, which are located low in the septum, are part of a more complex anomaly referred to as *endocardial cushion defect.*

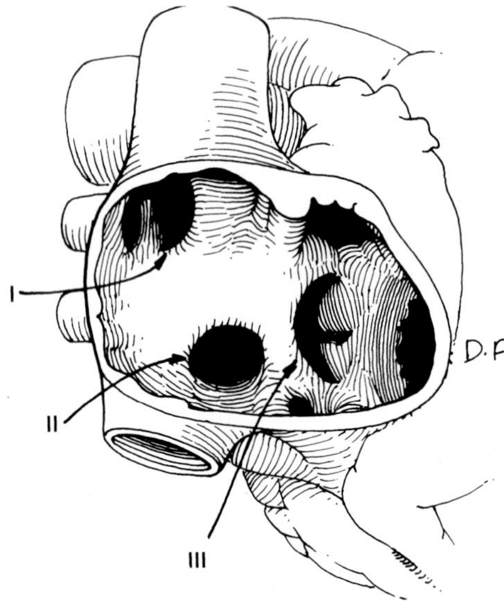

Fig. 40-6. Locations of the three common types of atrial septal defect. The sinus venous defect is shown with anomalous drainage of the right upper lobe pulmonary vein *(I).* The ostium secundum defect is in the midportion of the septum *(II).* The ostium primum defect is located in the base of the septum, with its inferior edge formed by the continuity of the tricuspid and mitral valves *(III).* Note the cleftlike anomaly in the anterior leaflet of the mitral valve visible through the defect.

In its simplest form, the ostium primum ASD is associated with a cleft in the anterior leaflet of the mitral valve. Mitral regurgitation may be present and can be severe.

Any ASD in which the ratio of pulmonary to systemic blood flow (Q_p/Q_s) is at least 1.5:1 should be closed. Operative correction prevents the long-term complications of congestive heart failure and pulmonary vascular occlusive disease. Studies on patients who did not undergo surgery indicated that life expectancy is significantly reduced, to the fourth or fifth decade of life. To prevent these complications, elective repair before school age is advised.

The technique of repair involves suture closure during cardiopulmonary bypass in most patients. Through an incision in the right atrium, the anatomy is easily exposed. In large defects, a patch of pericardium or polytetrafluoroethylene (Gore-Tex) may be necessary to avoid tension on the edges of the repair. In sinus venosus defects with partial anomalous pulmonary venous return, closure is achieved by modifying the patch to redirect the pulmonary veins to the left atrium. Ostium primum ASDs must also be repaired with a patch, because no lower rim of atrial septum is present. The lower edge of this defect is the junction of mitral and tricuspid valves on the crest of the ventricular septum. If significant mitral regurgitation is present before the operation, the valve should be studied carefully at operation and a valvuloplasty should be performed.[15]

Ventricular Septal Defect

Excluding bicuspid aortic valve, ventricular septal defect (VSD) is the most common congenital structural cardiac anomaly. It accounts for 20% to 25% of all cardiac lesions and is estimated to occur in two of 1000 live-born infants. The hemodynamics, symptoms, and treatment depend on the size of the VSD and on the magnitude of the shunt. With a small VSD, right ventricular pressure remains normal, Q_p/Q_s is less than 1.5:1, and symptoms are usually absent. Moderate-sized defects have right ventricular pressure as great as half of systemic levels and a Q_p/Q_s as great as 2.5:1 or 3:1. Some degree of congestive heart failure is often present, but growth is usually normal. A large VSD is present when the Q_p/Q_s exceeds 3:1. Right ventricular pressure usually exceeds half that of the left ventricle, but it may be normal when PVR is low. Severe congestive heart failure and poor growth are often found.

Approximately 50% of VSDs discovered in infancy undergo spontaneous reduction in size or complete closure. Thus all defects are initially managed medically, with early surgical intervention reserved for those with refractory congestive heart failure. Small VSDs usually do not require treatment, and nearly all eventually close. Spontaneous closure is less likely with larger defects but may still occur.

In response to the increasing pulmonary blood flow seen with moderate and large VSDs, pulmonary arteriolar resistance rises, and pulmonary artery pressure may also become elevated. Sustained increases in pulmonary artery flow and pressure can lead to early development of pulmonary vascular occlusive disease. Irreversible changes in resistance may become apparent by 2 years with an isolated large VSD or by 6 months in patients with associated trisomy 21. These changes have been classified by Heath and Edwards[16] on a histologic level. The early changes in the small pulmonary arteries and arterioles of medial hypertrophy (grade I) and intimal proliferation (grade II) are considered reversible. More advanced changes, consisting of intimal fibrosis (grade III) and progressive dilation lesions with eventual arterial necrosis (grades IV through VI), are irreversible.

Cardiac catheterization documents the magnitude of the shunt, right ventricular and pulmonary artery pressures, and PVR. Left ventricular cineangiography and two-dimensional echocardiography delineate the locations and number of VSDs. Associated defects, including coarctation, aortic stenosis, PDA, and pulmonary stenosis, are common and must be identified.

VSDs may be single or multiple. Most VSDs are single and located high in the membranous portion of the ventricular septum, just beneath the aortic valve. These defects are classified by their relationship to structures in the right ventricle.[17,18] The typical high VSD, referred to as an *infundibular* VSD, can be found beneath the anteroseptal commissure of the tricuspid valve (Fig. 40-7). Inlet VSDs are located more inferiorly, beneath the septal leaflet of the tricuspid valve, and subarterial VSDs occur high in the septum immediately below the pulmonary valve. When a VSD extends to the annulus of the tricuspid valve, it is referred to as *perimembranous;* otherwise, it is a muscular defect. Muscular defects occurring in the heavily trabeculated portion of the septum are more likely to be multiple.

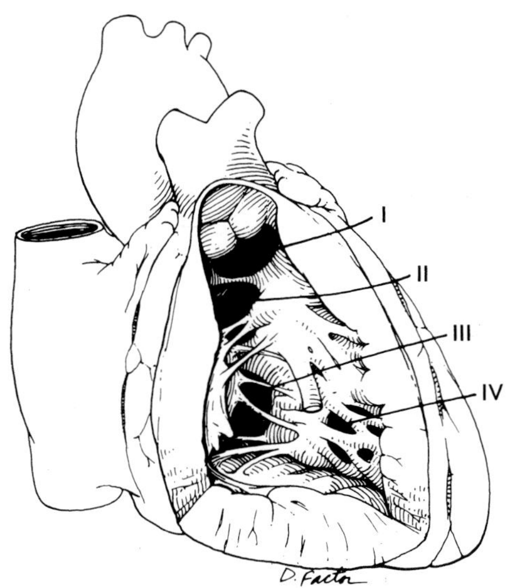

Fig. 40-7. Locations of the common types of ventricular septal defect. Subarterial defects *(I)* are located in the infundibular portion of the septum, beneath the pulmonary valve. In the most common type, perimembranous infundibular *(II),* part of the defect edge is formed by the tricuspid valve. Inlet defects *(III)* are found more inferiorly, beneath the septal leaflet of the tricuspid valve. Muscular defects *(IV)* are remote from the valve annulus.

The indications for surgery depend on the hemodynamic situation and presence of symptoms. With moderate and large VSDs, persistent severe congestive heart failure (often with failure to thrive) despite medical management is an operative indication. When heart failure is well controlled medically, the primary factors influencing the decision to operate are the pulmonary arterial pressure and PVR. These should be assessed by 12 months of age. If the pulmonary arterial pressure is greater than half of systemic levels by this age, surgical intervention should be carried out to prevent progressive changes in PVR. Moderate defects with minimal symptoms and normal pulmonary artery pressure and PVR may continue to be observed, because late spontaneous closure could still occur. If VSDs do not close by 3 to 5 years of age, operative therapy is indicated.

If the PVR is severely elevated, above two thirds of systemic resistance, VSD closure may be contraindicated. When PVR reaches this level, it will often progress further and eventually exceed that of the systemic circulation. Reversal of flow through the defect then occurs (Eisenmenger's syndrome), and cyanosis results. Closure of the VSD in this situation would result in right-sided heart failure and shortened life expectancy.

The optimal surgical treatment of VSDs consists of patch closure. In infants, deep hypothermia with reduced flow on cardiopulmonary bypass is used to facilitate exposure and reduce operative risk. The operative approach for most defects is through the right atrium and tricuspid valve. A patch of polytetrafluoroethylene (Gore-Tex) is sutured to the right ventricular side of the defect edge; care is taken not to injure the conduction tissue, which must be precisely located for each VSD.[19] In complex lesions, the atrioventricular node and bundle of His may be identified with endocardial mapping. Subpulmonary defects are best closed through the right atrium or pulmonary artery. Anterior muscular VSDs can often be quite difficult to close because they are obscured by the heavy trabeculations of the right ventricle. Apical muscular defects may require a small apical left ventriculotomy for proper exposure. In each case, initial exposure and evaluation through the tricuspid valve allow the surgeon to plan the best approach.

Complete repair in infancy may not be advisable in all cases. When multiple defects are found, for example, palliation with pulmonary artery banding may be indicated. With constriction of the main pulmonary artery, the resistance to flow into the lungs is markedly increased, reducing the magnitude of the left-to-right shunt and controlling congestive heart failure. Further, the pulmonary vascular bed is protected against the development of pulmonary vascular occlusive disease, allowing complete repair to be done at less risk when the patient is older. Because of the good results of complete repair of most congenital heart defects in infants, multiple complicated VSDs may be one of the few remaining indications for pulmonary artery banding in infants.

Patent Ductus Arteriosus

Patent ductus arteriosus (PDA) is the most common cause of left-to-right shunting at the great artery level. Because aortic pressure is greater than pulmonary artery pressure throughout all phases of the cardiac cycle, shunting occurs in both systole and diastole. This gives rise to the typical continuous or machinery-like murmur. Additionally, the diastolic runoff into the low-resistance pulmonary circulation results in a wide pulse pressure and bounding arterial pulses. A large PDA may allow substantial left-to-right shunting and significant heart failure. Pulmonary artery pressure and PVR may be elevated as described in the previous section, resulting in eventual pulmonary vascular occlusive disease.

The anatomy of the duct is quite constant. Its aortic end originates just distal to the left subclavian artery, and it enters the pulmonary artery bifurcation or proximal left pulmonary artery.

Any duct that remains patent beyond infancy should be closed. Elective closure is usually recommended in early childhood. A large PDA in a patient with heart failure and pulmonary hypertension should be closed immediately. Small PDAs may be complicated by bacterial endarteritis, aneurysm formation, or calcification. Closure prevents these complications.

The operative approach is through a left thoracotomy. Exposure of the duct is easily accomplished after opening the mediastinal pleura. Care must be taken to avoid injury to the recurrent laryngeal nerve. Closure of the duct may be done by simple ligation, usually over a length of duct, by division and suture or by hemoclip occlusion in premature infants. Recently, new forms of therapy have been introduced, including transluminal placement of coils, umbrellas or clamshell devices[20-22] and clipping of the PDA by means of video-assisted thoracoscopy.[23]

RIGHT-TO-LEFT SHUNTS

Tricuspid Atresia

Tricuspid atresia is an uncommon defect in which the tricuspid valve is completely absent. The ASD that is invariably present shunts all vena caval blood directly to the left atrium. The degree of cyanosis depends on the amount of pulmonary blood flow. When no communication between left and right ventricles is present, the ductus arteriosus is the sole source of flow to the lungs (Fig. 40-8, *A*). These patients are deeply cyanotic in early infancy, and emergency prostaglandin infusion may be necessary.[24] Prostaglandins of the E type relax the smooth muscle in the wall of the duct and are used to maintain ductal patency before palliative surgery.

In some cases a VSD allows blood to flow from the left ventricle directly to the hypoplastic right ventricle and then to the pulmonary circuit (Fig. 40-8, *B*). Depending on the size of this communication, cyanosis may be mild. However, these VSDs often undergo spontaneous reduction in size, thus decreasing pulmonary blood flow as the child grows. Less commonly, the aorta and pulmonary artery are transposed, and the pulmonary artery receives the direct output of the left ventricle, resulting in an increase in pulmonary blood flow and pressure.

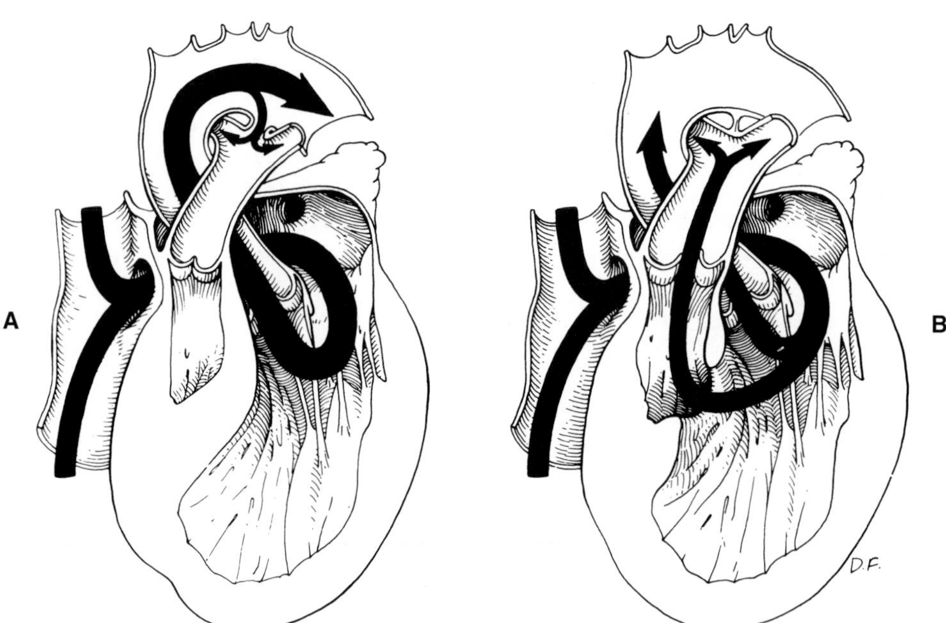

Fig. 40-8. **A,** Tricuspid atresia with normally related great vessels and without a ventricular septal defect. Pulmonary blood flow is duct dependent. **B,** When a septal defect is present, forward flow across the pulmonary valve can occur.

The initial surgical treatment of tricuspid atresia with decreased pulmonary blood flow is aimed at increasing this flow by a systemic artery–to–pulmonary artery shunt.[25,26] The modified Blalock-Taussig procedure, in which an interposition graft of polytetrafluoroethylene (Gore-Tex) is placed between the sides of the subclavian and pulmonary arteries, is the most commonly used operation[27] (Fig. 40-9). This procedure provides a source of pulmonary blood flow with minimum risk of increasing PVR or causing congestive heart failure. A relatively large graft (4 or 5 mm) is used, even in infants, because flow is limited by the smaller-sized native vessels. With growth of the subclavian and pulmonary arteries, flow can potentially increase and maintain effective palliation. Other shunt procedures are used much less commonly today. These include the Waterston (ascending aorta–to–right pulmonary artery), Potts (descending aorta–to–left pulmonary artery), and Glenn (superior vena cava–to–right pulmonary artery) anastomoses.

The shunt procedure is then followed in many circumstances by a bidirectional Glenn or hemi-Fontan procedure. This second stage removes the volume load imposed by the aortopulmonary shunt, improves the effective pulmonary blood flow, and may allow ventricular remodeling prior to the Fontan procedure.

The third stage, and the most satisfactory form of treatment for tricuspid atresia, was first reported in 1971 by Fontan and Baudet.[28] Originally done by direct connection of the right atrium to the pulmonary artery or hypoplastic right ventricle, this procedure is now most commonly performed with the lateral tunnel technique.[29] A tube of appropriately sized polytetrafluoroethylene (Gore-Tex) is opened longitudinally and sewn within the atrium to incorporate the orifices of the superior and inferior venae cavae without obstructing the pulmonary venous return (Fig. 40-10). Many centers now routinely incorporate a fenestration of the lateral baffle to allow a small degree of mixing of saturated and desaturated blood. This serves as a "pop-off" mechanism, limiting systemic venous pressures to an extent and preserving cardiac output, albeit with desaturated blood. Later, the fenestration is closed by means of a snare device or by transcutaneous umbrella occlusion, restoring normal systemic oxygenation and eliminating left ventricular volume overload. Although the early results with this procedure have been most gratifying, long-term follow-up is lacking and a late rise in the hazard function for survival has been noted.[30-32] Specifically, the late effects of chronic venous hypertension and lack of pulsatile pulmonary blood flow are unknown.

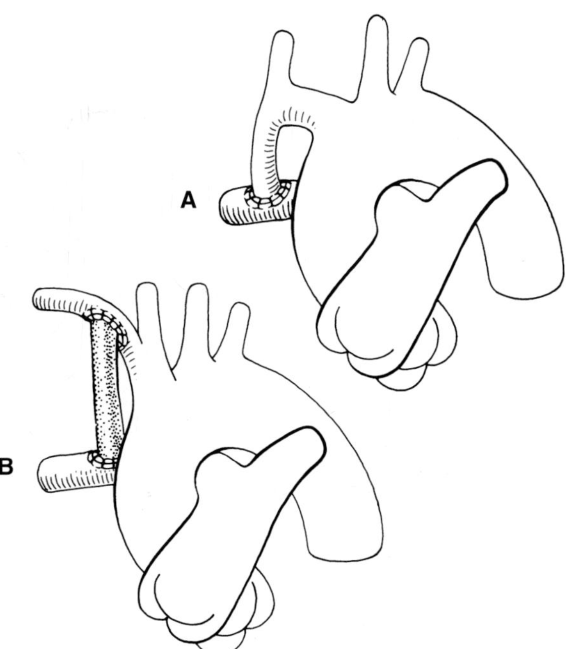

Fig. 40-9. A, Standard Blalock-Taussig anastomosis between the right subclavian and pulmonary arteries. **B,** Modification of the procedure with an interposition polytetrafluoroethylene graft.

Tetralogy of Fallot

The most common congenital heart defect resulting in cyanosis is tetralogy of Fallot. In this abnormality, obstruction to pulmonary blood flow occurs at the level of the right ventricular outflow tract, usually as the result of a combination of infundibular and pulmonary valvular stenoses (Fig. 40-11). The basic anatomic defect is anterior and superior displacement of the infundibular (outlet) portion of the ventricular septum. This obstructs right ventricular outflow and results in a large malalignment VSD (Fig. 40-12). Overriding of the aorta above the VSD and right ventricular hypertrophy (related to obstruction) complete the tetrad.

The clinical status of patients with tetralogy of Fallot depends on the severity of the right ventricular outflow tract obstruction. In its severest form, pulmonary atresia may be present with duct-dependent pulmonary blood flow. More commonly, infundibular obstruction coexists with varying degrees of pulmonary valve hypoplasia, resulting in moderate cyanosis. Patients with tetralogy of Fallot may have hypercyanotic "tet" spells. These occur when the dynamic portion of the obstruction is transiently worsened as a result of increased contractility of the muscle in the right ventricular outflow tract, often in combination with a decrease in systemic vascular resistance. Pulmonary blood flow is dramatically reduced, with an increase in the right-to-left shunt across the VSD.

Complete repair is now possible with good results in the infant and neonate.[33] It is believed that by early repair the consequences of severe right ventricular hypertrophy (ventricular systolic and diastolic dysfunction), can be reduced or eliminated. In addition, early re-establishment of normal pulsatile pulmonary arterial blood flow may improve the development of alveoli and intraparenchymal pulmonary arteries.[34] Contraindications to repair in infancy may include significant hypoplasia of the pulmonary

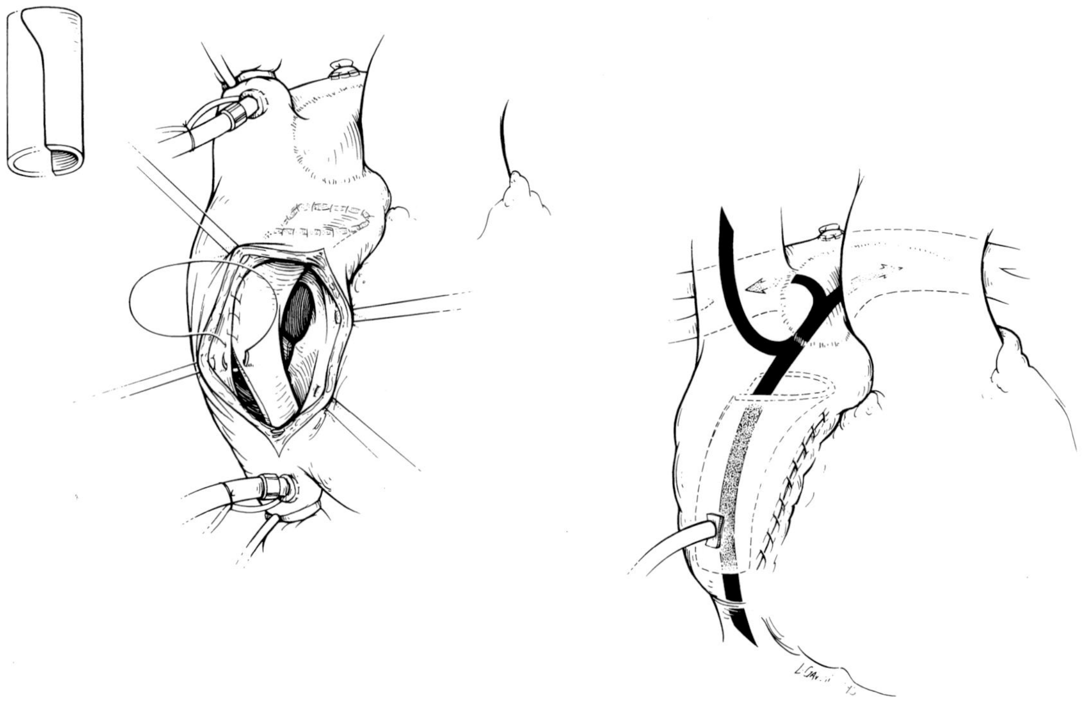

Fig. 40-10. Fontan procedure (lateral tunnel technique). Following a hemi-Fontan reconstruction, the inferior vena caval blood is tunneled within the atrium to the confluent pulmonary arteries.

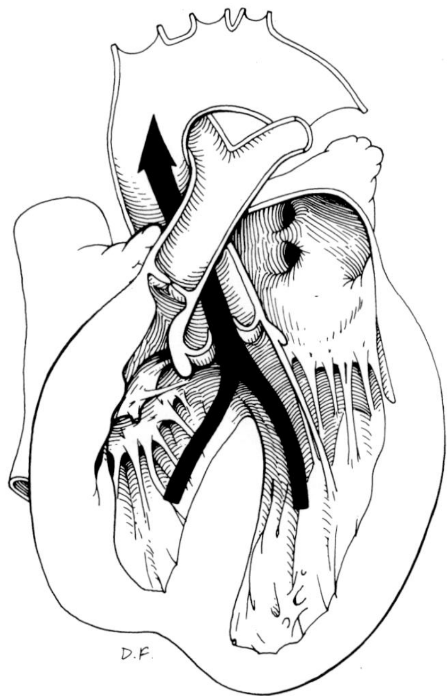

Fig. 40-11. Typical anatomy in tetralogy of Fallot. The large ventricular septal defect with overriding of the aorta is shown. The right ventricular outflow tract obstruction results in desaturated blood crossing the ventricular septal defect directly into the aorta.

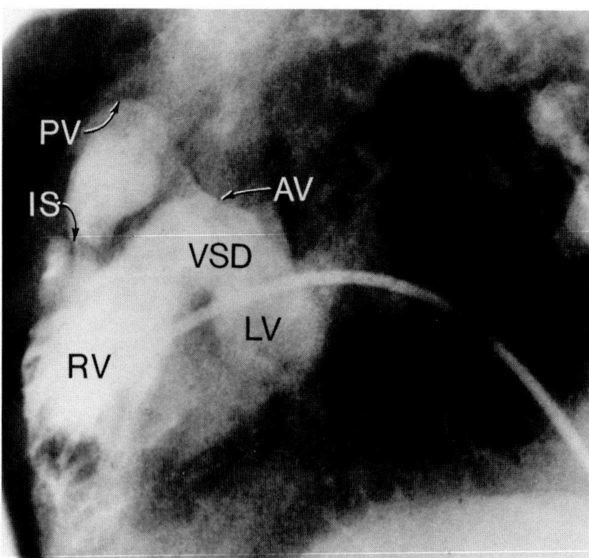

Fig. 40-12. Cineangiogram from a patient with tetralogy of Fallot. *AV,* Aortic valve; *IS,* infundibular stenosis; *LV,* left ventricle; *PV,* pulmonary valve; *RV,* right ventricle.

arteries and the origin of the anterior descending coronary artery from the right coronary artery. Because relief of the obstruction in the latter situation may require the insertion of a valve-bearing conduit or allograft, repair may best be postponed until the patient reaches an age at which a larger conduit may be inserted.

Complete repair includes relief of right ventricular outflow tract obstruction and closure of the VSD. Relief of the obstruction is governed by the individual anatomy. Whenever possible, pulmonary valve function should be preserved and resection of right ventricular muscle should be minimized.[35] In the past, the standard repair involved a right ventriculotomy to close the VSD and divide or resect the obstructing muscle bundles. Obstruction at the level of the pulmonary valve or annulus was dealt with by a commissurotomy or transannular patch as necessary. In the vast majority of patients, this can be performed through a transatrial approach across the tricuspid valve. In neonates and infants, obstructing muscle bundles need only be divided, not resected. If pulmonary valvular stenosis is present, a comissurotomy is performed. Pulmonary valvular hypoplasia is treated with a limited (<10 mm) transannular patch. Only in cases of true infundibular hypoplasia are a formal ventriculotomy and large outflow tract patch needed.

The operative mortality rate for repair of tetralogy of Fallot is 5% or less. Transatrial repair in the neonatal and infant period may improve the development of the pulmonary vascular bed and help to avoid the late sequelae of a right ventriculotomy (right ventricular dysfunction and ventricular dysrhythmias).

INADEQUATE MIXING

Transposition of the Great Arteries

In transposition of the great arteries (TGA), two separate and parallel circulations—systemic and pulmonary—are present. In the simplest form of TGA, the aorta arises from the right ventricle and receives the desaturated systemic venous return and the pulmonary artery arises from the left ventricle and receives oxygenated pulmonary venous blood (Fig. 40-13). Some exchange of blood between the two circulations (mixing) must be present to sustain life. This most commonly occurs by means of an interatrial communication allowing saturated blood to pass from the left to the right atrium and then to the right ventricle and aorta. An equal amount of desaturated blood must pass from right to left atrium to reach the pulmonary circulation. The adequacy of this mixing determines the amount of saturated venous blood reaching the aorta (effective systemic blood flow) and desaturated venous blood reaching the pulmonary artery (effective pulmonary blood flow), and thus the clinical status of the infant.

Even with adequate intracardiac mixing, the neonate with TGA has noticeable cyanosis. Quite often, the interatrial defect is restrictive, and profound cyanosis is detected within hours of birth. Arterial P_{O_2} may be less than 25 to 30 mm Hg, and progressive acidosis during the first days of life can occur. The clinical presentation is also influenced by the presence of associated lesions. In approximately 10% of cases, a large VSD or hemodynamically significant pulmonary stenosis is present. When only a VSD is present, cyanosis is lessened because mixing occurs at both the atrial and ventricular levels. Because total pulmonary blood flow is elevated further, however, severe congestive heart failure usually results. If pulmonary stenosis is also present, volume overload is reduced, tending to lessen the effect of the VSD. When pulmonary stenosis is particularly severe, with or without a VSD, total pulmonary blood flow may be reduced to a level below normal, and cyanosis may be worsened. Finally, communication between the two circulations may also occur from a PDA. Similar to the situation with a large VSD, both effective and total pulmonary blood flows are increased, improving oxygenation but resulting in congestive heart failure.

The initial treatment of an infant with TGA is aimed at improving the intracardiac mixing by enlarging the ASD. This is performed in the cardiac catheterization laboratory after the diagnosis has been established. The procedure, known as *balloon atrial septostomy* and originated by William Rashkind in 1966, involves passage of a balloon-tipped catheter from the right to the left atrium across the foramen ovale. The procedure can be performed in the catheterization laboratory or in the intensive care unit, with echocardiographic guidance used for accurate catheter placement. Once the catheter tip has been posi-

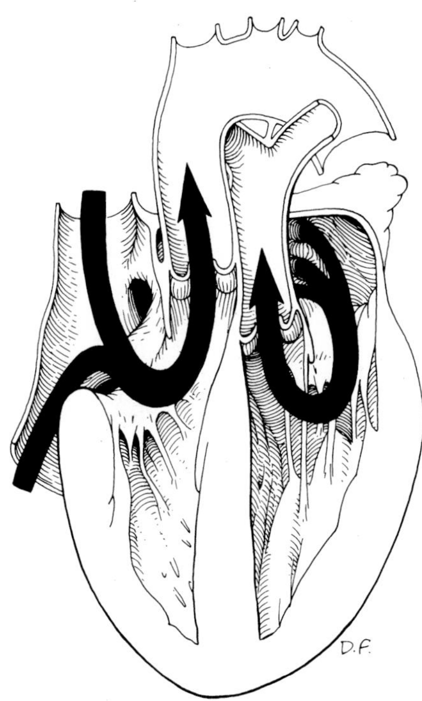

Fig. 40-13. Anatomy of transposition of the great arteries. The aorta arises from the right ventricle, and the pulmonary artery arises from the left ventricle.

tioned in the left atrium, the balloon is inflated and the catheter is forcibly withdrawn to tear a portion of the atrial septum. This procedure is repeated two or three times to ensure a wide patency in the septum. Improvement in arterial oxygenation is usually noted immediately after the septostomy.

A few neonates may continue to have unsatisfactory oxygenation even with a large ASD.[36] The poor mixing in these cases may be caused by failure of the PVR to fall to its normally low level after birth. The diastolic compliances of the two ventricles remain about equal, and no mixing of blood between the two sides occurs. When this is coupled with closure of the ductus arteriosus, effective pulmonary blood flow may be poor. This situation may be treated temporarily by the administration of a prostaglandin infusion, maintaining ductal patency and allowing mixing at the great vessel level.[37,38] This restores satisfactory oxygenation for a few days until PVR falls.

When TGA is associated with a large VSD, significant congestive heart failure and pulmonary hypertension may be apparent very early in life. Prior to the arterial switch repair, banding of the main pulmonary artery to reduce pulmonary blood flow and pressure was indicated. This procedure, however, invariably results in a drop in arterial PO_2 because pulmonary blood flow is reduced by the band. An adequate interatrial communication is mandatory. If severe pulmonary stenosis is present and pulmonary blood flow and pressure are below normal, a systemic artery–to–pulmonary artery (Blalock-Taussig) shunt may be performed.

Correction of TGA may be performed at the atrial, ventricular, or great vessel level, depending on the exact anatomy and associated defects. Prior to the 1980s, physiologic correction was achieved at the atrial level by redirecting venous inflow. This technique was first successfully performed by Senning in 1959 and revised by Mustard in 1964. Mustard's procedure involves complete removal of the atrial septum, followed by the placement of a "baffle" (usually pericardium) to repartition the atria (Fig. 40-14). Vena caval blood drains behind the baffle to the mitral valve, left ventricle, and pulmonary artery, and the pulmonary veins drain to the tricuspid valve and then to the systemic circulation through the right ventricle. In the Senning procedure, little prosthetic material is used because redirection of venous inflow is done with the patient's own atrial tissue. Although it is more difficult to perform, Senning's operation may allow better growth and function of the atrial chambers. The operative mortality rates for both procedures are low (<5%), even in infancy, and long-term results are good. Significant technical complications, such as obstruction to caval (usually superior vena caval) or pulmonary venous flow and troublesome atrial arrhythmias, continue to be a problem.

The major long-term difficulty with both the Mustard and the Senning procedures is the possible failure of the right ventricle to perform at systemic workloads for long periods.[39] Late congestive heart failure, often with tricuspid insufficiency, has been recognized in a small percentage of children. Careful studies of right ventricular function late after repairs have shown impaired performance even in patients without symptoms. The exact cause remains unclear. Most children, however, have excellent long-term results after Mustard or Senning operations.

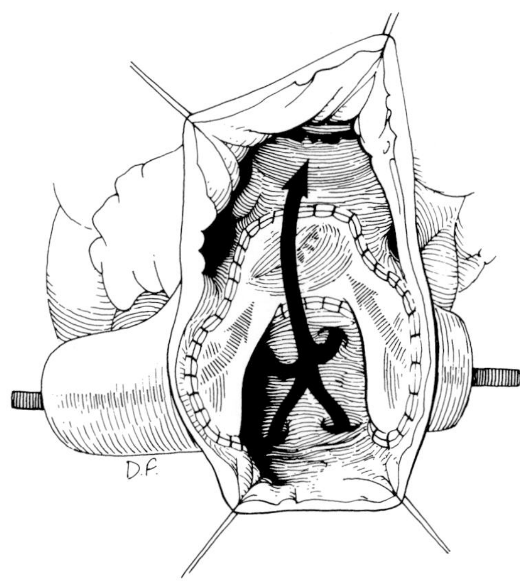

Fig. 40-14. Appearance of the atrial baffle in the Mustard procedure. Superior and inferior vena caval blood passes behind the patch to the mitral valve. The pulmonary venous blood passes over the patch to the tricuspid valve.

During the last decade, the arterial switch has emerged as the procedure of choice in patients with TGA (Fig. 40-15). The arterial repair of TGA has the benefit of restoring the left ventricle as the systemic pump.[40] Although early operative mortality rates were quite high, current techniques have reduced the risk to acceptable levels. These technical improvements include the refinement of coronary transfer, repair of the pulmonary artery with a pantaloon pericardial patch, and superior myocardial protection. Successful performance of this procedure seems to require that the left ventricle be prepared to pump against systemic resistance. Patients with TGA and a large VSD retain high pressure in the left ventricle and are ideal candidates for arterial repair. Banding of the pulmonary artery to raise left ventricular pressure in some patients with TGA and intact ventricular septum has been advocated to prepare the left ventricle for an arterial switch procedure.[41] When arterial repair is done within the first month of life, however, preliminary banding is unnecessary.

In patients with TGA, large VSD, and left ventricular outflow tract obstruction (pulmonary stenosis), repair can be carried out at both the ventricular and great vessel levels. The VSD is closed in a way that diverts left ventricular blood through the defect into the aorta (Fig. 40-16). The main pulmonary artery is ligated and the right ven-

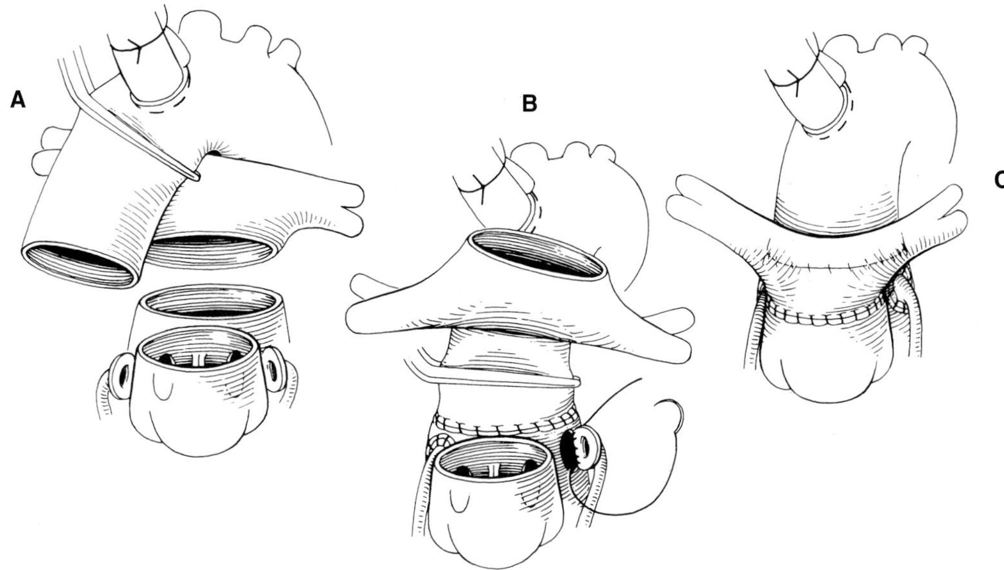

Fig. 40-15. Steps in the performance of the arterial switch procedure. **A,** The pulmonary artery is transected just proximal to its bifurcation. The aorta is transected at the same level. The coronary arteries are removed with wide buttons of adjacent aorta. **B,** The distal aorta is brought behind the pulmonary artery confluence and anastomosed to the proximal pulmonary artery. The coronary arteries are then relocated to the new aorta. **C,** The right ventricular outflow tract is reconstructed by anastomosing the distal pulmonary artery confluence to the proximal aorta.

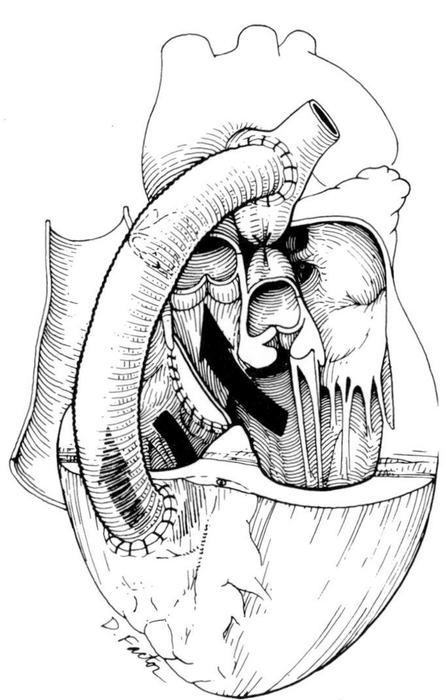

Fig. 40-16. Repair of transposition of the great arteries with ventricular septal defect and pulmonary stenosis. The defect is patched to place both great vessels in continuity with the left ventricle. The pulmonary artery is ligated proximally. The right ventricle is then connected to the distal pulmonary artery with a valved conduit.

tricle is connected to the pulmonary artery bifurcation with a valved extracardiac conduit. The left ventricle is restored as the systemic pump, and the coronary arteries do not require relocation.[42]

HYPOPLASTIC LEFT HEART SYNDROME

Hypoplastic left heart syndrome (HLHS) is a collective term referring to a spectrum of congenital heart defects with varying degrees of hypoplasia of left-sided cardiac structures. The vast majority of patients with HLHS (84%) have aortic and mitral atresia, hypoplasia, or stenosis (classic HLHS), whereas 16% have a malaligned atrioventricular canal defect.[43] A coarctation is present in more than 80% of patients.

Patients with HLHS have complex cardiopulmonary physiology. The pulmonary arteries, ductus arteriosus, and descending aorta are arranged in parallel circulations. Q_p/Q_s depends on the balance between PVR and systemic vascular resistance.

Because of its hypoplasia and obstructed outflow, the left ventricle is essentially a nonfunctional structure. Pulmonary venous return is directed across an ASD and mixes with the systemic venous return. The right ventricle provides both the pulmonary and systemic output. Coronary and systemic perfusion is maintained through the ductus arteriosus. In most cases, the PVR declines after birth, leading to excessive pulmonary blood flow. Although this produces good arterial oxygen saturations, the systemic perfusion may be poor, resulting in metabolic acidosis. Without intervention, HLHS is almost uniformally fatal in the first weeks of life. Initial therapy is directed at maintaining an adequate PDA with prostaglandin E. This allows the child's overall condition to stabilize.

Surgical options for the treatment of HLHS consist of neonatal cardiac transplantation or staged reconstruction. In the best of situations, neonatal cardiac transplantation is associated with a 1-year survival of 80% to 90%.[44] However, because of the limited supply of organ donors, approximately 15% to 25% of patients die while awaiting organ transplantation. In addition, the patient faces the need for lifelong immunosuppression, with its attendant risks.

For these reasons, many centers have opted to pursue palliative repair in this group of patients. The repair of HLHS involves three separate procedures; the Norwood, bidirectional Glenn, and Fontan procedures. The Norwood operation connects the right ventricle and pulmonary valve to the augmented ascending, transverse, and descending aorta and provides a limited amount of pulmonary blood flow through a modified Blalock-Taussig shunt. Performed at 6 months, the bidirectional Glenn procedure consists of division of the aortopulmonary shunt and connection of the superior vena cava to the cephalad portion of the right pulmonary artery. This decreases the volume load on the right ventricle and improves the effective pulmonary blood flow. A fenestrated Fontan procedure is then planned at 18 months to channel the desaturated inferior vena caval blood to the undersurface of the right pulmonary artery. First-stage reconstruction is now associated with an 85% to 90% in-hospital survival, and the actuarial survival for the three stages together is approximately 75% at 2 years.[45]

Overall, the outlook for patients born with HLHS has improved dramatically during the past few years. Cardiac transplantation offers good intermediate results but is plagued by donor shortages and the need for immunosuppression. Results of palliative procedures have improved greatly but three operative procedures are required, and the right ventricle is retained as the systemic ventricle. Further study is needed to better categorize which patients benefit most from these treatment modalities.

SUMMARY

Successful surgical treatment of most forms of congenital heart disease is now possible. However, the surgeon must be knowledgeable about more than just cardiac anatomy to achieve this success. In particular, a thorough understanding of cardiac physiology in infants and children is essential, so that a well-conceived treatment plan can be devised for even the most complex of anomalies. In some cases, one or more palliative procedures may be necessary, either because no definitive repair is ultimately possible or because it is best postponed until the patient is older. These procedures must provide satisfactory immediate palliation and, in addition, must ensure that ultimate repair can be performed with the lowest possible risk to the patient.

Early corrective surgery, now routinely performed for many defects, is expected to significantly reduce the associated complications of congenital heart disease. The elimination of pulmonary vascular disease, chronic cyanosis, and long-standing congestive heart failure are only a few examples of the advantages of early correction. However, examining the benefits of surgical repair in light of the late results is increasingly important. The development of ventricular dysfunction and electrophysiologic abnormalities are examples of potentially serious consequences that may detract from an apparent early success. In some cases, a number of late studies have led to alterations in surgical technique designed to maintain excellent long-term functional results. These evaluations serve as a stimulus for cardiac surgeons to continue to strive for improvement in the treatment of congenital heart disease.

REFERENCES

1. Scott HW Jr, et al. Study of the renal pressure system in experimental coarctation of the abdominal aorta. Am Surg 43:771, 1977.
2. Parker FB, et al. Preoperative and postoperative renin levels in coarctation of the aorta. Circulation 66:513, 1982.
3. Simsolo R, et al. Long-term systemic hypertension in children after successful repair of coarctation of the aorta. Am Heart J 115:1268, 1988.
4. Waldhausen J. Repair of coarctation of the aorta with a subclavian flap. J Thorac Cardiovasc Surg 51:532, 1966.
5. Sandor CGS, et al. Long-term follow-up of patients after valvotomy for congenital valvular aortic stenosis in children. J Thorac Cardiovasc Surg 80:171, 1980.
6. Ankeney JL, Tzeng TS, Liebman J. Surgical therapy for congenital aortic valvular stenosis. J Thorac Cardiovasc Surg 85:41, 1983.
7. Buich M, et al. Open valvotomy for critical aortic stenosis in infancy. Br Heart J 63:37, 1990.
8. Messina LM, et al. Successful aortic valvotomy for severe congenital valvular aortic stenosis in the newborn infant. J Thorac Cardiovasc Surg 88:92, 1984.
9. Trinkle JK, et al. Closed aortic valvotomy and simultaneous correction of associated anomalies in infants. J Thorac Cardiovasc Surg 69:758, 1975.
10. Mosca RS, et al. Critical aortic stenosis in the neonate: A comparison of balloon valvuloplasty and transventricular dilatation. J Thorac Cardiovasc Surg (in press).
11. Shem-Tov A, et al. Clinical presentation and natural history of mild discrete subaortic stenosis. Circulation 66:509, 1982.
12. Bjornstad PG, et al. Aortoventriculoplasty for tunnel subaortic stenosis and other obstructions of the left ventricular outflow tract. Circulation 60:59, 1979.
13. Sweeney MS, et al. Apioaortic conduits for complex left ventricular outflow obstruction: 10-year experience. Ann Thorac Surg 42:609, 1986.
14. Craig RJ, Selzer A. Natural history and prognosis of atrial septal defect. Circulation 37:805, 1968.
15. Losay J, et al. Repair of atrial septal defect primum. J Thorac Cardiovasc Surg 75:248, 1978.
16. Heath D, Edwards JE. The pathology of hypertensive pulmonary vascular disease: A description of six grades of structural changes in the pulmonary arteries with special reference to congenital cardiac septal defects. Circulation 18:533, 1958.
17. Becker AE, Anderson RH. Classification of ventricular septal defects—A matter of precision. Heart Vessels 1:120, 1985.
18. Lincoln C, et al. Transatrial repair of ventricular septal defects with reference to their anatomic classification. J Thorac Cardiovasc Surg 74:183, 1977.

19. Milo S, et al. Surgical anatomy and atrioventricular conduction tissues of hearts with isolated ventricular septal defects. J Thorac Cardiovasc Surg 79:244, 1980.
20. Rashkind WJ, Cuaso CC. Transcatheter closure at patent ductus arteriosus. Pediatr Cardiol 1:3, 1979.
21. Sato K, et al. Transfemoral plug closure of patent ductus arteriosus: Experience in 61 consecutive cases treated without thoracotomy. Circulation 51:337, 1975.
22. Rothenberg SS. Transcatheter versus surgical closure of patent ductus arteriosus. N Engl J Med 330:1014, 1994.
23. Laborde F, et al. A new video-assisted thoracoscopic surgical technique for interruption of patent ductus arteriosus in infants and children. J Thorac Cardiovasc Surg 105:278, 1993.
24. Freed MD, et al. Prostaglandin E_1 in infants with ductus arteriosus–dependent congenital heart disease. Circulation 64:899, 1981.
25. de Brux JL, et al. Tricuspid atresia. J Thorac Cardiovasc Surg 48:378, 1978.
26. Dick M, Fyler DC, Nadas AS. Tricuspid atresia: Clinical course in 101 patients. Am J Cardiol 36:327, 1975.
27. Blalock A, Taussig HB. The surgical treatment of malformations of the heart. JAMA 128:189, 1945.
28. Fontan F, Baudet S. Surgical repair of tricuspid atresia. Thorax 26:240, 1971.
29. Jonas RA, Castaneda AR. Modified Fontan procedure: Atrial baffle and systemic venous to pulmonary artery anatomic techniques. J Cardiac Surg 3:91, 1988.
30. Fontan F, et al. Repair of tricuspid atresia in 100 patients. J Thorac Cardiovasc Surg 85:647, 1983.
31. Fontan F, et al. Outcome after a "perfect" Fontan operation. Circulation 81:1520, 1990.
32. Sanders SP, et al. Clinical and hemodynamic results of the Fontan operation for tricuspid atresia. Am J Cardiol 49:1733, 1982.
33. Touati G, et al. Primary repair of tetralogy of Fallot in infancy. J Thorac Cardiovasc Surg 99:396, 1990.
34. Rabinovitch M, et al. Growth and development of pulmonary vascular bed in patients with tetralogy of Fallot with or without pulmonary atresia. Circulation 64:1234, 1981.
35. Bove EL, et al. The influence of pulmonary insufficiency on ventricular function following repair of tetralogy of Fallot. J Thorac Cardiovasc Surg 85:691, 1983.
36. Mair DD, Ritter DF. Factors influencing systemic arterial oxygen saturation in complete transposition of the great arteries. Am J Cardiol 31:742, 1973.
37. Benson LN, et al. Role of prostaglandin E_1 infusion in the management of transposition of the great arteries. Am J Cardiol 44:691, 1979.
38. Lang P, et al. Use of prostaglandin E_1 in infants with D-transposition of the great arteries and intact ventricular septum. Am J Cardiol 44:76, 1979.
39. Benson LN, et al. Assessment of right ventricular function during supine bicycle exercise after Mustard's operation. Circulation 65:1052, 1981.
40. Jatene AD, et al. Anatomic correction of transposition of the great vessels. J Thorac Cardiovasc Surg 72:364, 1976.
41. Yacoub M, et al. Clinical and hemodynamic results of the two-stage anatomic correction of simple transposition of the great arteries. Circulation 62(suppl 1):1190, 1980.
42. Marcelletti C, et al. The Rastelli operation for transposition of the great arteries. J Thorac Cardiovasc Surg 72:427, 1976.
43. Bharati S, Lev M. The surgical anatomy of hypoplasia of aortic tract complex. J Thorac Cardiovasc Surg 88:97, 1984.
44. Bailey L, et al. Pediatric heart transplantation: Issues relating to outcome and results. The Loma Linda Pediatric Heart Transplant Group. J Heart Lung Transplant 11:5267, 1992.
45. Iannettoni MD, Bove EL, Mosca RS. Improving results with first-stage palliation for hypoplastic left heart syndrome. J Thorac Cardiovasc Surg 107:934, 1994.

SUGGESTED READINGS

Bave AE, et al., eds. Glenn's Thoracic and Cardiovascular Surgery, 6th ed. Norwalk, Conn.: Appleton & Lange, 1996.

Castaneda AR, et al. Cardiac Surgery of the Neonate and Infant. Philadelphia: WB Saunders, 1994.

Garson A Jr, Bricker JT, McNonara DG, eds. The Science and Practice of Pediatric Cardiology. Philadelphia: Lea & Febiger, 1990.

41

Acquired Cardiac Disorders

Glenn J.R. Whitman, David A. Fullerton, and Andrew C. Fiore

In contrast to congenital heart disease, in which surgical intervention is usually required to restore the underlying pathophysiology to normalcy, acquired cardiac disorders are often amenable to medical management. Notwithstanding this circumstance, several diseases are still best treated surgically and will probably remain so for many years to come. Acquired heart disease in which surgical management plays a prominent role forms the basis for this chapter. The first section focuses on ischemic heart disease and abnormalities of the cardiac valvular system, and on the role that surgery plays in correcting disordered physiology in these conditions. The second section concentrates on diseases that require surgical attention less commonly, but in which the cardiac surgeon still renders important help in the delivery of optimal care. These disorders include cardiac dysrhythmias, pericardial disease, and cardiac tumors.

Ischemic and Valvular Heart Disease

Glenn J.R. Whitman and David A. Fullerton

ISCHEMIC HEART DISEASE

The Coronary Circulation

Coronary Arteries (Fig. 41-1)

The right coronary artery (RCA) and left coronary artery originate from the aorta just above the aortic valve cusps. In fact, the positions of these two arteries within the sinuses of Valsalva designate the right and left coronary cusps. The third cusp is referred to as the *noncoronary cusp* because it does not have an associated coronary os. The left main coronary artery, which travels posterolaterally to the left behind the pulmonary artery, divides into two main branches, the left anterior descending coronary artery (LAD) and the left circumflex coronary artery. The LAD emerges from behind the pulmonary artery to course anteriorly within the interventricular groove. The initial tributary of the LAD is usually the first diagonal, which runs over the anterolateral surface of the left ventricle, followed by the first septal perforator, which emerges at a right angle from the LAD and penetrates into the interventricular septum. The LAD may then give off more diagonal and septal branches. The left circumflex coronary artery descends posteriorly from the left main coronary artery. In 80% to 85% of cases, it terminates with branches to the posterolateral wall of the left ventricle. In the remainder, it extends to the crux of the heart and then gives off the posterior descending coronary artery (PDA), which runs in the posterior interventricular groove. The branches of the circumflex artery are referred to as *obtuse marginals* and cover the lateral and posterolateral portion of the left ventricle.

The RCA runs in the right atrioventricular groove, where in 80% to 85% of cases it gives off the PDA, continuing with terminal branches to the posterior left ventricular wall. The RCA feeds the anterior surface of the right ventricle with acute marginal branches.

Coronary Veins

Three venous systems drain the coronary circulation. (1) The coronary sinus located in the posterior atrioventricular groove receives blood from the great, middle, and small cardiac veins. The great cardiac vein ascends along the LAD and then follows the circumflex artery to empty into the coronary sinus. The middle cardiac vein follows the PDA, again emptying into the coronary sinus. The small cardiac vein follows the RCA in the atrioventricular groove before it, too, joins the coronary sinus. (2) The thebesian veins are tiny venous orifices that drain directly into any of the four chambers of the heart. (3) The anterior cardiac veins drain the right ventricular coronary system, traversing the right ventricular free wall and crossing the atrioventricular groove to empty directly into the right atrium.

Coronary Blood Flow

The heart extracts a greater percentage of delivered oxygen than any other organ in the body. In fact, the heart

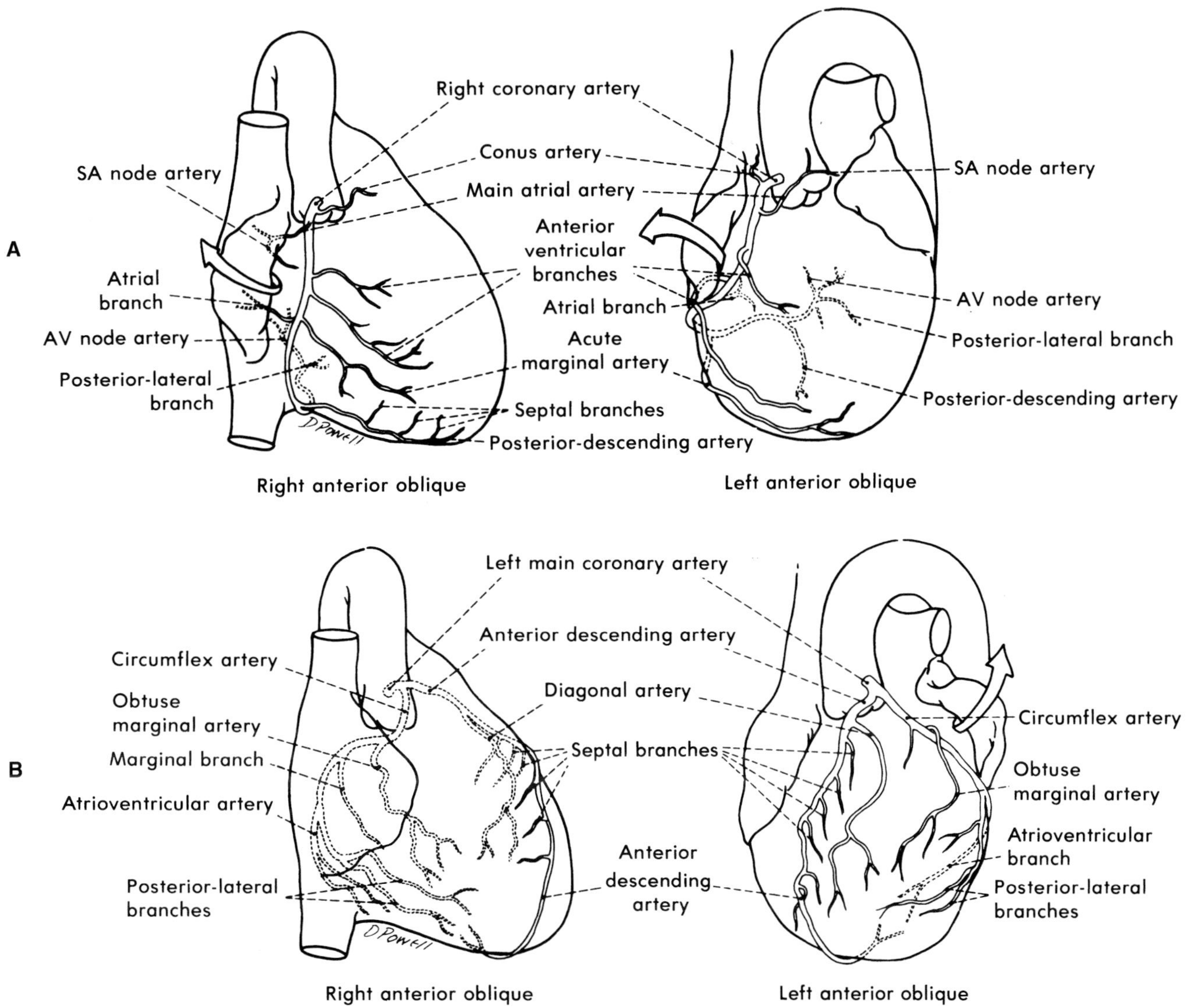

Fig. 41-1. A, Diagram of the RCA circulation in the right anterior oblique and left anterior oblique projections. **B,** Diagram of the left coronary arterial circulation in the right anterior oblique and left anterior oblique projections. (From Peter RH. Coronary arteriography. In Sabiston DC Jr, Spencer FC, eds. Gibbon's Surgery of the Chest, 4th ed. Philadelphia: WB Saunders, 1983.)

uses 60% to 70% of the oxygen supplied, as opposed to only 25% for the body as a whole. Coronary sinus oxygen content is only 4 to 6 ml oxygen/dl blood, which corresponds to an oxygen tension of approximately 24 mm Hg and a hemoglobin oxygen saturation of only 20% to 30%. Therefore, even at rest, the heart is extracting oxygen maximally, and, unlike in other organs, increased oxygen demand can only be met by increased delivery, rather than increased oxygen extraction.

The most important factor that regulates coronary blood flow is perfusion pressure. Myocardial blood flow occurs almost entirely during diastole, because during systole, cavitary left ventricular pressure equal to that of aortic pressure prevents coronary flow. Coronary flow also depends on coronary luminal diameter. In general, obstruction is considered clinically significant when luminal diameter decreases to two thirds of baseline. Myocardial blood flow thus depends on diastolic pressure as well as coronary arterial patency. Tachycardia can therefore lead to ischemia not only by increasing oxygen demand, but also by limiting diastolic perfusion time.

A variety of metabolic factors regulate coronary circulation as well. In fact, these autoregulatory capabilities increase blood supply to the heart in response to increased myocardial oxygen requirements. The most important metabolic regulator of this phenomenon is the potent vasodilator adenosine.[1] Increased oxygen demand increases adenosine triphosphatase (ATP) use, with a resultant in-

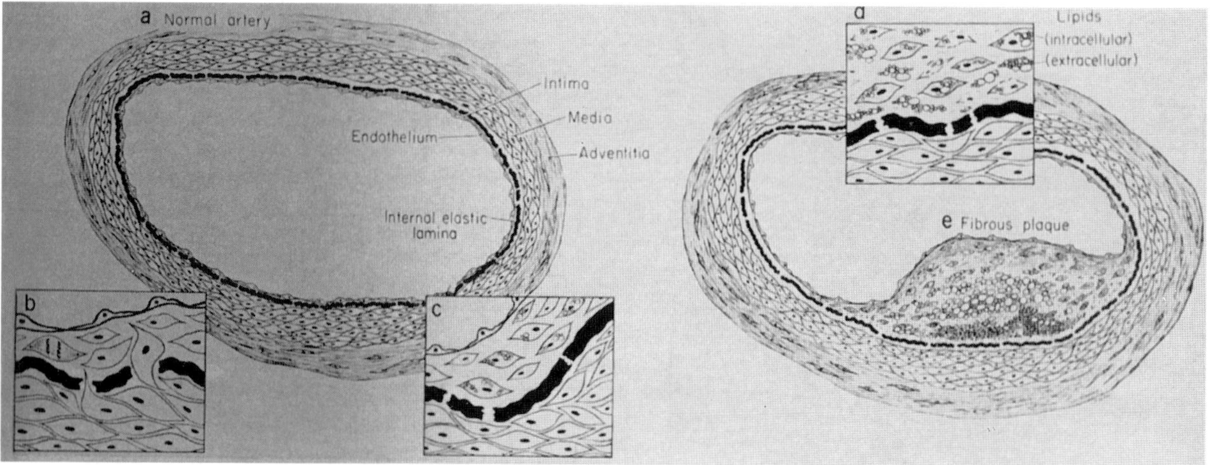

Fig. 41-2. Developmental stages of the lesions of atherosclerosis. **A,** The normal muscular artery consists of an internal intima with endothelium and internal elastic lamina. The smooth muscle of the vessel wall is in the media, and the thin adventitial layer contains connective tissue and vasovasorum. With age, the thin, sparsely muscled intima increases in thickness and smooth muscle cell content. **B,** In the first phase of an atherosclerotic lesion, there is focal thickening of the intima with smooth muscle cells and extracellular matrix. There is also initial accumulation of intercellular lipid deposits. **C,** Extracellular lipid may also develop. **D,** When both intracellular and extracellular lipids are present in the earliest phase, this is referred to as a *fatty streak.* **E,** Fibrous plaque results from continued accumulation of fibroblasts covering proliferating smooth muscle cells laden with lipids and cell debris. The lesion becomes more complex as continuing cell degeneration leads to ingress of blood constituents and calcification. (Modified from Glomset JA, Ross R. Atherosclerosis and the arterial smooth muscle cell. Science 180:1332, 1973. Copyright 1973 by the American Association for the Advancement of Science. Reproduced with permission from the publishers and authors.)

crease in adenosine concentration because it is a direct breakdown product of ATP. This results in coronary vasodilation and increased oxygen delivery. Conversely, thromboxane A_2 is thought to play a crucial role in coronary vasoconstriction. Interestingly, it is released by platelets, particularly in the setting of platelet clumping, a situation that occurs almost universally in the setting of angina with myocardial infarction (MI).[2]

Coronary Atherosclerosis

The lesion (Fig. 41-2). Atherosclerotic lesions all have in common a mixture of proliferating smooth muscle with a tissue matrix consisting of collagen, elastin, and proteoglycans formed by these cells, as well as the accumulation of intracellular and extracellular lipid. The lesions characteristically occur within the intima and progress from benign, fatty streaks to complicated, occlusive plaques. It is known that fatty streaks may occur as early as the first decade of life. With time, particularly in populations at risk, the fatty streaks develop into a fibrous plaque, a protruding lesion that may become obstructive. The subintimal smooth muscle cell proliferation that goes along with this fibrous plaque is the factor most responsible for this protrusion. With time, the fibrous plaque may enlarge, become calcified, and degenerate on its intimal surface, resulting in ulcerations that are thrombogenic. Organization of clot with platelet clumping on this surface not only causes increased obstruction to flow but, as stated previously, may release thromboxane A_2, further exacerbating the compromised delivery of blood and therefore oxygen to the myocardium.

Risk factors. A number of established risk factors predispose patients toward atherosclerosis.[3] These include advanced age, male sex, genetic predisposition, hypertension, diabetes mellitus, hyperlipidemia, and cigarette smoking. Aging has a complex association with the development of atherosclerosis, because many other risk factors are associated with aging as well. Genetic factors appear to have a direct effect on endothelial cell biology and predisposition toward the development of atherosclerosis. It is well documented that men are three times more likely than women to acquire coronary disease, and, in fact, the development of ischemic syndromes occurs on the average 10 years earlier in affected men than in affected women. The risk of coronary artery disease increases with increasing blood pressure; among patients with blood pressure >160/95 mm Hg, the incidence of coronary disease is five times greater than among those who are normotensive. Of most importance is the fact that control of hypertension decreases this risk. Diabetes mellitus is clearly associated with coronary artery disease. The risk of coronary disease is increased at least twofold in patients with diabetes, with the risk even higher among those with juvenile-onset diabetes. Unfortunately, it is not certain that rigorous control of hyperglycemia decreases coronary mortality rate in this population. The Lipid Research Clinics Trial[4] demonstrated an unequivocal association between cholesterol level and morbidity and mortality from coronary artery disease. Furthermore, as with hypertension, decreasing the levels of hyperlipidemia decreases the risk of coronary disease. Interestingly, high-density lipoproteins (HDLs), which contain approximately 20% of total plasma cholesterol, protect one from coronary disease. HDL level is known to be raised by exercise and estrogens and decreased by cigarette smoking. Cigarette smoking is one of the most important risk factors for the development of coronary artery disease, not simply because it is so clearly related to its development but because its cessation so clearly decreases the risk. In patients who smoke only one pack of cigarettes per day, the death rate from coronary artery disease is 70% higher than in nonsmokers. Furthermore, cigarette smoking appears to potentiate other risk factors.

Because of our recognition that atherosclerosis may begin as early as the first or second decade of life, primary prevention of this disease must begin early. The importance of understanding the risk factors for coronary disease and eliminating or modifying those over which we have control cannot be overemphasized.

Clinical Presentation of Ischemic Heart Disease

The clinical presentation of ischemic heart disease can take many forms. As many as 25% of patients with positive stress test results because of coronary occlusive disease may have no symptoms. Similarly, some acute MIs may occur silently. In fact, in some patients sudden cardiac death is the first and only manifestation of this disease process. Another subset of patient without typical symptoms may have progressive heart failure. This in general is caused by a slow, diffuse loss of ventricular function associated with increasing coronary obstructions. This entity is often referred to as *ischemic cardiomyopathy.* Most commonly, however, when significant coronary obstructive disease is present, angina pectoris results.

The typical description of angina is as a pressure or heaviness felt in the middle of the chest, radiating to the left shoulder and down the left arm. Abdominal pain, nausea, belching, jaw pain, and hand heaviness or numbness are less typical manifestations of cardiac ischemia. In almost all cases, however, stable angina pectoris is brought on by reproducible increases in myocardial demand for a pathologically limited oxygen supply. Emotional excitement or stress, exposure to cold, eating, and exercise are typical historical events that trigger demand-induced angina. In unstable angina, however, the symptom of chest pain may occur at rest, or even when the patient is sleeping. These patients are exhibiting a phenomenon of myocardial ischemia without demonstrable changes in myocardial oxygen demand. This reflects a situation in which the supply of blood to the myocardium is so marginal that spontaneous coronary vasoreactivity alone may lead to symptoms. Prinzmetal's or variant angina is a less typical form of angina that also may occur spontaneously without increasing myocardial oxygen demand. It is thought to result from spontaneous coronary arterial spasm, but it is almost always associated with underlying fixed atherosclerotic lesions. Patients may have ST-segment elevation, as opposed to the more typical ST-segment depressions associated with classical angina. Angina may be graded according to the Canadian Heart Classification scheme. Class I patients have no symptoms, class II patients have angina on significant exertion, class III patients have angina on mild exertion, and class IV patients have symptoms at rest.

On physical examination, there is usually no detectable sign of coronary artery disease. There may be evidence of associated peripheral vascular disease, however, with loss of pulses or presence of bruits in the carotid arteries, abdominal aorta, or femoral arteries. Xanthomas or hypertensive retinal changes provide evidence of the presence of risk factors for coronary disease.

Laboratory studies are useful only in detecting risk factors such as diabetes, hyperlipidemia, or hyperthyroidism. Anemia, of course, can exacerbate underlying coronary insufficiency. Results of electrocardiographic (ECG) examination are frequently normal, but some patients have evidence of old MIs, clearly indicating the presence of coronary disease. Stress testing is an ideal physiologic examination for assessing the functional significance of coronary disease. In this study, the patient undergoes graded exercise on a treadmill with continuous ECG monitoring. If the patient shows signs or symptoms of angina pectoris associated with typical ischemic. ECG changes, this is considered a positive test result. Specificity of the test is improved dramatically if it is combined with the administration of thallium. Thallium is a radioactive isotope that is distributed intracellularly, like potassium. When thallium is injected during exercise, if a patient has coronary ischemia, the involved area of myocardium fails to pick up thallium and a defect is present on the scan. As the patient recovers from exercise and ischemia resolves, the myocardial defect fills in, suggesting the reversible nature of the problem. A defect on a thallium scan that never fills in is a sign of irreversibly scarred, nonviable myocardium.

Despite the specific and sensitive nature of thallium stress testing, coronary arteriography although invasive, is the only way to make a definitive anatomic diagnosis of coronary artery disease. It is indicated in patients with atypical presentations in whom it is important to rule out a definitive diagnosis of coronary disease. Otherwise, patients with classic anginal symptoms and ECG changes in whom the diagnosis is not in question should undergo coronary arteriography if the condition is refractory to medical therapy, they are candidates for revascularization, or both. If patients have suspected severe coronary disease, such as left main or severe proximal three-vessel disease, regardless of symptoms, coronary arteriography should be performed to document this condition in preparation for revascularization. Well-known survival benefits accrue to patients who undergo surgery after such documentation. Diagnostic coronary arteriography should also be performed in patients with other cardiac diseases, such as valvular heart disease, in whom valve surgery is planned but in whom there is a risk of concomitant coronary disease.

The medical management of coronary disease includes the identification and reduction of controllable risk factors. Once the disease presents itself in the form of clinically significant ischemia, however, the focus for the clinician is on decreasing myocardial oxygen uptake and increasing myocardial oxygen supply. It therefore follows that patients with hyperthyroidism or anemia, one of which affects oxygen demand and the other supply, should have these underlying conditions corrected.

In general, though, there are three classes of drugs in the armamentarium of the physician that are useful for treating ischemic heart disease. Nitrates are the most commonly used agents. They primarily dilate venous capacitance blood vessels, with resultant decreases in preload, wall tension, and oxygen uptake. Although nitrates do not appear to increase coronary blood flow in the normal heart, improvement in coronary collateral blood flow does occur in patients with ischemic heart disease. β-Adrenergic blocking agents also reduce myocardial oxygen demand by decreasing both cardiac contractility and heart rate. These agents may also reduce blood pressure and systemic vascular resistance, further reducing the work of the heart. Finally, calcium-channel blocking agents, such as nifedipine and diltiazem, decrease myocardial oxygen uptake by decreasing ventricular contractility. By causing arterial dilation, they diminish systemic vascular resistance as well, and they are particularly effective in patients with a component of coronary vasospastic disease.

Acute Myocardial Infarction

MI is one of the most common diagnoses of hospitalized patients in the United States. Approximately 1.5 million MIs occur each year, with an early mortality rate of approximately 25%. More than half of these deaths occur before the patient even reaches the hospital.

Acute MI is the direct result of interruption of blood supply to the myocardium. It almost always occurs as the result of coronary arterial thrombosis at the site of a significant stenosis over a complicated plaque. Although the acute event associated with acute MI is thrombosis, cardiac catheterization studies show that within days 20% to 30% of culprit coronary arteries are patent. This is more common in nontransmural MI than in transmural MI.

A major determinant of prognosis after an acute MI is the amount of ventricular myocardium that undergoes necrosis. In patients who have ejection fractions >50% after MI, 3-year survival is close to 90%, but when ejection fraction after MI falls to <37%, 3-year survival is only 50%. Loss of 25% of ventricular myocardium leads to symptomatic cardiac dysfunction, whereas the loss of more than 40% is frequently associated with cardiogenic shock and death. Therefore, efforts to treat patients who are having an acute MI should be focused on decreasing myocardial loss by improving flow to the area at risk as soon as possible. Interestingly, although well-developed collaterals may not prevent demand-induced angina, they may significantly diminish the loss of myocardium after an acute MI.

Presentation

Pain is the most common presenting complaint in patients with MI. It is by no means universally present, however; 20% to 25% of patients have no symptoms. Interestingly, acute MIs associated with the LAD distribution frequently result in sympathetic hyperactivity, with tachycardia and hypertension, whereas inferior MIs involving the RCA frequently have parasympathetic activity with bradycardia and hypotension. The classic ECG picture of an acute MI is the development of Q waves and elevated coved ST segments in leads reflecting the affected areas (Fig. 41-3). In fact, the type of MI can frequently be characterized by the associated ECG changes. Transmural infarctions usually cause Q waves, whereas subendocardial or nontransmural MIs are usually characterized by transient ST-segment changes with inverted T waves, without the development of Q waves. The most sensitive method available to us for diagnosing MI lies in the evaluation of specific cardiac isoenzymes released by necrotic myocytes in large enough quantities to be detected in the blood. In particular, serum levels of creatine kinase (CK), a cardiac enzyme involved with high-energy phosphate metabolism, are increased after MI, rising within 8 to 24 hours and returning to normal within 1 to 2 days. CK is found in brain (CK-BB) and muscle (CK-MM), and it can rise significantly after a variety of clinical scenarios, such as stroke, surgery, cardiac catheterization, or simple intramuscular injection. It is therefore crucial to measure the cardiac-specific isoenzyme, CK-MB, when ruling out an MI.

Medical Treatment

During the early phase of MI, oxygen should be administered, heart rhythm should be monitored, and lidocaine should be given to prevent ventricular fibrillation in case of warning arrhythmias. Within 4 to 6 hours of the onset of continued chest pain, a significant amount of myocardium may still be salvageable. Initial treatment should be to control pain, usually with intravenous morphine. Decreasing pain has a significant therapeutic benefit because it decreases myocardial oxygen demand, helping to limit infarct size. Intravenous nitroglycerin should be initiated, because it may diminish infarct size, decrease the risk of sudden cardiac death, and lower the incidence of congestive heart failure.[5] β-Blockers have also been shown to limit infarct size and decrease early mortality rates.

In the mid 1970s it was hypothesized that the administration of thrombolytic agents could lead to the dissolution of coronary thromboses, reversing the process precipitating the MI. A consequent European trial of strep-

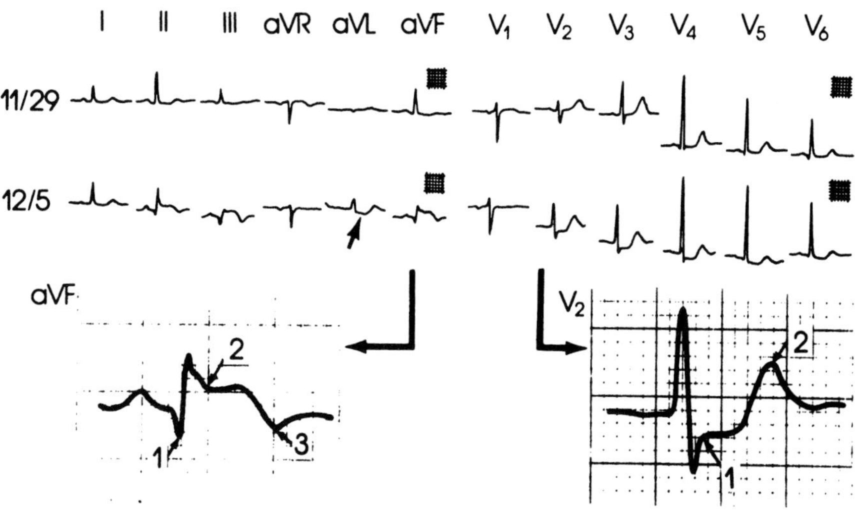

Fig. 41-3. Acute inferior wall MI. The ECG of 11/29 shows minor nonspecific ST-segment and T-wave changes. On 12/5, an acute MI occurred. There are pathologic Q waves *(1)*, ST-segment elevation *(2)*, and terminal T-wave inversion *(3)* in leads II, III, and aVF, indicating the location of the infarct on the inferior wall (see text). Reciprocal changes are seen in aVL *(small arrow)*. Increasing R-wave voltage with ST depression and increased voltage of the T wave in V_2 is characteristic of true posterior wall extension of the inferior infarction. (From Wilson JD, et al. Harrison's Principles of Internal Medicine. New York: McGraw-Hill, 1990, p 957. Used with permission.)

tokinase (SK) revealed a significant benefit when the drug was given within 12 hours of acute MI.[6] Since then, thrombolytic trials have established without doubt the benefits of this approach, showing that thrombolysis reopens acutely occluded coronary arteries in most cases, restoring flow and reducing mortality rate.[7] Three intravenous thrombolytic agents are currently approved by the Food and Drug Administration: SK, recombinant tissue-type plasminogen activator (rtPA), and anisoylated plasminogen SK activator complex (APSAC). The most widely used is SK, which has been effective in several very large trials and is inexpensive. APSAC was developed to enable treating physicians to give one intravenous bolus dose in a few minutes, with maintenance of the effect for several hours because of its long half-life. However, APSAC has not been significantly better than SK, and its prolonged half-life has become a drawback rather than a benefit. rtPA, produced by recombinant DNA techniques, is more effective than SK. It also yields higher patency rates and generates less of a systemic fibrinolytic effect. However, rtPA is several times more expensive than SK, and it thus may not be cost-effective.

What is clear is that the earlier the thrombolytic treatment, the greater the impact on post-MI morbidity and mortality, with the greatest benefit accruing to those patients treated within 1 to 2 hours of the onset of symptoms. Heparin and antiplatelet drugs should be added to thrombolytic therapy, particularly to rtPA, which has a short half-life and exerts little antithrombin effect because it does not generate excessive fibrin-degradation products. Hemorrhage is the major problem with all thrombolytic agents, occurring commonly at the site of vascular access. Strokes occur in fewer than 1% of patients but may be catastrophic because of their hemorrhagic nature.[8]

Mechanical Intervention in Acute Myocardial Infarction

After thrombolytic therapy with early recanalization, the issue remains whether anything more need be done in the acute setting. Despite early reperfusion, significant residual stenoses remain in the culprit coronary arteries. The TIMI-II trial[9] compared immediate cardiac catheterization with percutaneous transluminal coronary angioplasty (PTCA) with elective cardiac catheterization and PTCA only if ischemia developed during the hospital course. The more invasive approach failed to provide any increased benefit with respect to early or late mortality rates. As a result of this and other studies, cardiac catheterization and mechanical intervention should be withheld in most patients after acute MI unless patients exhibit ischemia during their hospital stay or have poor results of a predischarge low-level exercise stress test.

Indications for Surgery After Acute Myocardial Infarction

Postinfarction angina. Recurrent chest pain occurs in 10% to 15% of patients after acute MI, an incidence increased to 30% to 35% among patients who receive thrombolytic therapy. It is well recognized that after MI the mortality rate may increase several fold if infarct extension occurs.[10] Infarct extension is a powerful predictor of post-MI mortality risk, as seen by an increase in the average 1-year mortality rate from approximately 18% to 65% if infarct extension occurs. Thus, postinfarction angina is an indicator of continued myocardial ischemia and a harbinger of infarct extension. It should be regarded as an indication for cardiac catheterization with mechanical intervention, either PTCA or coronary bypass surgery.

Cardiogenic shock. Cardiogenic shock after MI is uncommon, only occurring in approximately 7% of patient with acute MI. Shock after acute MI is associated with a 65% mortality rate, compared with a mortality rate of only 4% if shock is not present. The risk factors for development of cardiogenic shock after acute MI are age >65 years, ejection fraction <35% on admission, a large MI as evaluated by peak CK-MB serum concentration, a history of diabetes mellitus, and a history of previous MI. Because shock develops after hospitalization in more than 50% of patients, identifying patients with these risk factors is important because it might possibly allow early intervention to prevent development of shock.

Animal studies have shown that in cases of prolonged regional MI, intervention with emergency revascularization may decrease the amount of damage sustained by the myocardium. By focusing on ways to decrease myocardial energy expenditure during early reperfusion, as well as decreasing cell swelling and oxidant injury and improving intermediary cellular metabolism, a significant decrease in myocardial injury can be achieved. This has led to a prospective study evaluating the effect of coronary bypass surgery on patients in cardiogenic shock after MI.[11] If surgery occurred within 18 hours of the onset of shock, mortality rate was reduced from 65% to 7%, whereas if surgery occurred within 18 hours, mortality rate was 31%, still a definite improvement from medical therapy. At centers capable of performing surgery of this kind, this may be an ideal approach to patients in shock after MI. However, these results have not been duplicated by other institutions. Until they are, they must be viewed as preliminary.

Ventricular septal defect. A ventricular septal defect occurs in approximately 2% of patients after MI. This complication, which occurs when the myocardium is at its weakest, approximately 3 to 5 days after an MI, has an associated medical mortality rate of more than 90%. It is seen most frequently in elderly hypertensive female patients with anterior transmural infarcts. The initial medical therapy involves decreasing afterload as much as possible, invariably with the use of the intraaortic balloon pump as well as vasodilator therapy. Preload is optimized and surgery is performed immediately. Early operation, before the complications of shock occur, appears to carry a much better survival rate.[12]

Acute mitral regurgitation. As with ventricular septal defect, acute papillary muscle rupture with mitral regurgitation occurs in only 2% of patients after acute MI. Posteroinferior MIs lead to this complication more frequently than do anterior MIs, almost certainly because the circumflex artery and PDA distributions are the most crucial blood supplies to the papillary muscles. This complication presents similarly to a ventricular septal defect. As opposed to the pattern in patients with an acute VSD, however, the pulmonary capillary wedge pressure shows prominent V waves and there is no right ventricular hemoglobin oxygen saturation step up. Medical therapy involves maximizing afterload reduction through use of an intraaortic balloon pump. Early surgery, although it carries a high risk, decreases mortality rate from 90% to less than 50%. If the mitral valve apparatus can be preserved, mortality risk can be decreased even further.

Free wall rupture. Like the previous two complications, ventricular free wall rupture occurs at a time when the myocardium is at its weakest, 3 to five days after acute MI. The medical mortality rate is exceedingly high (>90%) because the patients die acutely in tamponade. Surgical case reports cite dramatic rescues of these patients, but in general, for successful treatment, free wall rupture must be small and contained, allowing time for diagnosis and operative intervention. Most commonly, free wall rupture leads to pericardial tamponade, cardiogenic shock, and death.

Revascularization

Angioplasty

In the mid 1970s, Gruentzig and Hoff designed a balloon dilatation catheter for use in the coronary arteries and initiated the important treatment option for patients with ischemic heart disease currently known as percutaneous transluminal coronary angioplasty (PTCA). Under fluoroscopic guidance, a catheter is directed into the coronary artery. A guide wire is then placed across the obstructing lesion, and a balloon catheter is then passed over the guide wire and positioned in the midportion of the lesion. Under fluoroscopic control, the balloon is inflated to 4 to 10 atm pressure for 20 to 60 seconds in an effort to reduce the degree of coronary obstruction. The indications for PTCA are the same as those for coronary artery bypass surgery, which is the main alternative revascularization technique. Patients with intractable symptoms and those with proximal coronary stenoses that place a large amount of myocardium at risk are potential candidates for angioplasty. The ideal lesion is a symmetric, focal stenosis in a proximal epicardial vessel. PTCA is contraindicated if there is significant disease in the left main coronary artery, if the target coronary artery is <2 mm in diameter, if there are multiple significant obstructive lesions in the same artery, or if there are complex obstructive lesions involving arterial bifurcations. The primary risk of angioplasty is dissection of the coronary artery with acute closure, which occurs in approximately 3% of cases and usually requires emergency coronary bypass surgery. Otherwise, the risks are similar to those of coronary arteriography and include cerebral vascular accidents and local arterial trauma. Under development are atherectomy catheters that incorporate tiny rotating blades for lysis of atheromatous plaque, as well as laser-tipped catheters that vaporize intraluminal obstructions. Coronary stents are also becoming popular. These small, implantable cylindric devices are designed to maintain patency of diseased arteries when more conventional balloon angioplasty is ineffective. Successful dilation of favorable coronary arterial obstructive lesions occurs in more than 90% of PTCA attempts, with an immediate complication rate of only 3%. The most significant long-term problem with PTCA is the high incidence of restenosis, which occurs in between 20% to 40% of patients within the first 4 to 6 months after the initial PTCA.[13] Although redilatation of recurrent stenotic lesions may be carried out successfully, many of these patients ultimately require coronary bypass surgery.

Coronary Artery Bypass Surgery

Coronary bypass surgery is among the most commonly performed operations in the United States today, with more than 250,000 procedures performed yearly. The goal, as with PTCA, is to treat ischemic heart disease by relieving the imbalance between myocardial oxygen supply and demand.

Indications (see accompanying box). In general, data from clinical trials and retrospective studies show that as the number of diseased major coronary arterial segments increases, the greater the survival benefit from coronary bypass surgery. Three major prospective, randomized coronary bypass surgery studies, the CASS,[14] the Veterans Affairs Cooperative Study,[15] and the European Cooperative Study,[16] are in large part responsible for how we treat patients with ischemic heart disease. Patients with intractable symptoms were not involved in these studies; those patients, in general, should undergo bypass surgery because it is the most successful way to relieve angina. These three studies have provided us with the anatomic indications for bypass surgery, which include left main stenosis and double- and triple-vessel disease involving the proximal LAD.

INDICATIONS FOR CORONARY BYPASS SURGERY

Anatomy

1. Left main disease
2. Triple-vessel disease involving the proximal LAD, with normal or diminished ejection fraction
3. Double-vessel disease involving the proximal LAD, with normal or diminished ejection fraction

Symptoms

1. Unstable (crescendo) angina
2. Post-MI angina
3. Acute coronary occlusion after PTCA
4. Symptoms unsuccessfully controlled with medical therapy
5. Controlled symptoms, but with unacceptable lifestyle

As stated previously, the most common indication for bypass surgery continues to be angina refractory to medical therapy. Bypass surgery can be expected to eliminate angina in more than 90% of patients at 1 year, with benefit continuing for 60% of patients at 5 years.

Patients being medically treated for unstable angina require aggressive therapy, including nitrates, β-blockers, and calcium-channel blockers. Often, heparin anticoagulation is necessary. If the patient continues to have angina while receiving maximal medical therapy, urgent revascularization is indicated. Finally, as noted before, emergency coronary bypass surgery is necessary in approximately 3% of patients who have coronary occlusive complications after PTCA. Most of these occlusions result from coronary dissections proximal or distal to the site of dilatation. Most patients in the midst of an evolving MI have some attenuation of the ischemic injury by placement of an intra-aortic balloon counterpulsation device before transport to the operating room. If hemodynamic instability continues despite balloon pump support, portable cardiopulmonary bypass perfusion with femoral arterial and femoral venous cannulation may allow sufficient time to stabilize the patient's condition for an operation.

Surgical technique. In coronary artery bypass surgery, the diseased portion of the coronary artery is bypassed by creation of an alternative conduit for delivery of blood beyond the stenosis. Grafts are constructed by making an end-to-side anastomosis to the coronary artery distal to the obstruction. The proximal end of the vein graft is usually sutured end to side to the ascending aorta. Use of arterial grafts has increased in recent years. The most commonly used arterial graft is the left internal thoracic artery, which is used as a pedicle retaining its origin at the subclavian artery with a distal end-to-side anastomosis to the diseased coronary artery. Most commonly, this is the LAD. The right internal thoracic artery may be used as either a pedicle graft or a free graft as well when more than one arterial graft is desired. In a much more limited fashion, the gastroepiploic artery, the radial artery, and the inferior epigastric artery have been used as conduits. The main benefit of these grafts is improved long-term patency; the 10-year patency of the internal thoracic artery is between 90% and 95%, whereas saphenous vein grafts have only a 50% 10-year patency.

To maintain a quiet, bloodless field, cardiopulmonary bypass must be employed for coronary bypass surgery (Fig. 41-4). With the patient on bypass and the heart empty, the distal ascending aorta is cross-clamped and potassium cardioplegic solution injected into the aortic root, causing nearly instantaneous cardiac arrest. The cardioplegic solution is usually between 4° and 10° C, to induce rapid myocardial cooling. In addition, topical iced saline solution may be employed to provide surface cooling of the heart. The most important protective effects of cardioplegia are hypothermia and potassium, which causes arrest of the heart in diastole. Decreasing myocardial temperature to 10° to 15° C decreases the metabolic rate by as much as 80%, with mechanical arrest lowering the metabolic rate to as little as 5% of the normothermic, working heart.

A great deal of investigative effort has gone into determining the best type of cardioplegic solution. Again, though, the most important aspects of arresting the ischemic heart are maintaining hypothermia as well as mechanical arrest. Newer techniques employ initial warm induction of arrest followed by cold cardioplegia. Furthermore, on completion of the operation, administration of a warm dose of cardioplegic solution before removal of the cross-clamp has also been advocated. Both of these techniques are used in an attempt to allow the metabolic machinery to perform reparative processes before asking the heart to perform any mechanical work. In fact, some surgeons prefer to do the entire operation with the patient and the heart warm, while cardioplegic solution is being administered continuously.[17] During the past several years, retrograde cardioplegic administration has come into vogue. Delivery of cardioplegic solution through the coronary sinus and the coronary veins may yield enhanced myocardial protection because significant coronary stenoses can prevent the homogeneous antegrade delivery of cardioplegic solution. Retrograde cardioplegia is also useful in the presence of significant aortic insufficiency, because effective delivery of cardioplegic solution in an antegrade fashion is severely hindered by an incompetent aortic valve.

The distal anastomoses are generally performed with the aid of optical magnification. In addition to individual vein or thoracic artery graft anastomoses, two or more distal anastomoses can be constructed from a single vein or thoracic artery. These sequential grafts are favored when multiple distal sites are planned for anastomoses, or when there is a shortage of suitable conduit material. Sequential

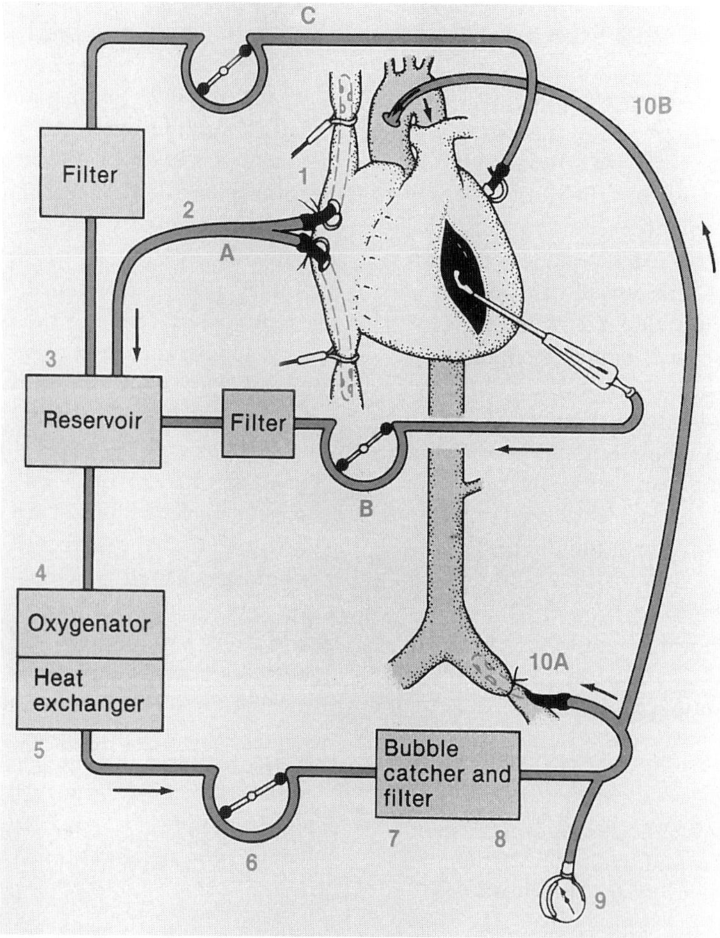

Fig. 41-4. Schematic diagram of a typical cardiopulmonary bypass circuit. Blood is drained by gravity from the venae cavae *(1)* through venous cannula *(2)* into a venous reservoir *(3)*. Blood from surgical field suction and from a ventricular vent (if used during operation) is pumped *(B, C)* into a cardiotomy reservoir (not shown) and then drained into a venous reservoir *(3)*. Venous blood is oxygenated *(4)*, temperature adjusted *(5)*, raised to arterial pressure *(6)*, filtered *(7-8)*, and returned to the patient by way of a cannula in either the aorta *(10B)* or femoral artery *(10A)*. Arterial line pressure is monitored *(9)*. (Modified from Nose Y. The Oxygenator, vol 2. St. Louis: Mosby, 1973. Used with permission.)

grafting is achieved by performing side-to-side anastomoses between the conduit and recipient artery and ending the graft with an end-to-side anastomosis to the most distal coronary artery. After completion of the distal anastomoses and initiation of reperfusion, a partially occluding side-biting clamp is placed on the ascending aorta and the proximal anastomoses are constructed.

Rarely, if the recipient coronary artery is diffusely diseased with no available site for the distal anastomoses, the surgeon may be required to perform an endarterectomy to allow a reliable graft-to-artery anastomosis. Coronary endarterectomy sites are more vulnerable to early thrombosis and reocclusion, and this should be performed only if there is no alternative. Because patients with such diffuse disease are already likely to have poor outcomes, it has been difficult to demonstrate a beneficial effect from coronary endarterectomy.

Postoperative management. After the operation, cardiac surgical patients are monitored in an intensive care unit with careful hemodynamic evaluation. Arterial blood pressure, central venous pressure, pulmonary artery pressures, cardiac output, mixed venous oxygen saturation, and urinary output all provide valuable information regarding the adequacy of tissue perfusion and organ function. Mediastinal and chest tube drainage should be monitored hourly and, in fact, can be transfused to minimize the use of banked blood products. All patients have a capillary leakage syndrome after cardiopulmonary bypass and fluid accumulation, with a marked increase in total body sodium such that patients typically gain between 5 and 10 kg. Most patients are able to be extubated within 4 to 12 hours of surgery and thereafter can be transferred to a step-down unit, where continuous monitoring for arrhythmias, gentle diuresis to attain preoperative weight, and early ambulation are achieved.

Compared with other populations, the patient after cardiac surgery provides an opportunity for sophisticated management and optimization of cardiac output (CO). In the early postoperative period, hypovolemia, increased systemic vascular resistance, hypothermia, and arrhythmias (both bradycardic and tachycardic) may all contribute to low CO. Management of these patients is both challenging and rewarding, because the cause of low CO is almost always reversible.

Low cardiac output *(see box).* When the calculated cardiac index is less than 2 L/min/m^2, despite optimization of heart rhythm, preload, and afterload, an inotropic agent is invariably indicated. If a patient remains in cardiogenic shock despite significant inotropic support, consideration should be given to placement of an intra-aortic balloon pump. The balloon, which may be inserted percutaneously through the femoral artery, is positioned just beyond the subclavian artery takeoff of the aorta. Balloon inflation and deflation are timed so that intra-aortic balloon counterpulsation increases coronary artery perfusion pressure during diastole and, as a result of active deflation, maximally decreases afterload during systole. Rarely, if shock persists, a left ventricular–assist device should be considered. However, the cause of persistent low CO in the early postoperative period should be pursued aggressively, with any reversible cause identified. Left ventricular–assist device support is extremely labor intensive and costly, and it should only be considered if myocardial failure is considered to be reversible, or if the patient needs a bridge to transplantation.

Postoperative complications. The major complications after open-heart surgery include bleeding, tamponade, infection, and stroke. Platelet function and blood clotting factors are severely altered after bypass and may not return to normal for as long as 36 hours. Average postoperative blood loss is between 400 and 800 ml and, as stated previously, may be reinfused to decrease the need for homologous blood transfusions. When bleeding exceeds a rate of 200 ml/hr for 4 hours or longer, return to the operating room for correction of any surgical cause of the bleeding should be considered. Before then, all medical causes of coagulopathy should be corrected aggressively. It is simple and safe to give additional protamine to reverse the residual heparin used during bypass, but transfusions of platelets, fresh-frozen plasma, or cryoprecipitate should be considered only if indicated by coagulation studies.

Cardiac tamponade is a potentially lethal cause of low CO early after operation. Clinically, one sees a decreased CO increasing filling pressures, and a narrowed pulse pressure. Pulsus paradoxus and a widened mediastinal silhouette are frequently seen. Transesophageal echocardiography has made this diagnosis more easily established and should be used without hesitation when faced with this possible diagnosis.

The major wound complication facing surgeons after coronary bypass is sternal infection with mediastinitis, dehiscence, or both. This complication occurs in as many as 2% to 4% of patients, with the incidence increased when bilateral thoracic arteries are used, particularly in elderly patients and those with diabetes. Staphylococci are the most common organisms, and because of the devastating nature of this complication, most patients receive antistaphylococcal prophylaxis in the perioperative period.

CAUSES OF LOW CARDIAC OUTPUT AFTER CORONARY BYPASS

1. Inadequate preload
2. Excessive afterload
3. Poor ventricular contractility
   a. Perioperative ischemia
   b. Poor myocardial preservation
4. Arrhythmia
5. Severe acidosis
6. Tension pneumothorax
7. Tamponade

Cerebral vascular accidents may be the most tragic of postoperative complications. Stroke is usually caused by atherosclerotic emboli that probably originate from the aorta, loosened by cannulation, cross-clamping, or the construction of the proximal anastomoses. Underlying cerebral vascular disease combined with hypotension during bypass contributes to this problem. Strokes occur in 1% to 2% of patients at low risk but may occur in as many as 10% of octogenarians. No data suggest that the investigation of asymptomatic carotid bruits prior to open-heart surgery with subsequent combined coronary bypass and carotid endarterectomy would reduce the incidence of stroke after surgery. In patients who have both symptomatic carotid and coronary disease with significant stenosis of the carotid, however, a combined procedure is usually carried out.

Risk factors for operative death (Table 41-1). The assessment of the patient's mortality risk after bypass surgery is an important component of the preoperative evaluation in coronary artery disease. Furthermore, as issues regarding quality assurance and the delivery of efficient, cost-effective health care loom ever larger in our society, scrutiny of the benefits and risks associated with this most expensive of medical procedures has come increasingly in vogue. Clearly, patients with concurrent medical problems, such as cerebral vascular disease, pulmonary or renal insufficiency, diabetes, and morbid obesity, are at higher risk for development of postoperative complications. Poor ventricular function is among the most important factors increasing the mortality rate after bypass surgery.[18] Operative risk is also increased when patients require additional operative intervention, such as valve repair or replacement. It is well documented that increasing age itself increases mortality rate. In the CASS study,[14] the mortality rate among patients older than 70 years was nearly 8%, compared with an overall mortality rate of 3%. It has also been stated that women have a higher mortality rate after bypass surgery than do men. The explanation for this is not exactly clear, but may be related to the fact that women undergoing coronary bypass surgery are on average 10 years older than men and have a higher incidence of unstable angina, preoperative congestive heart failure, hypertension, and diabetes. It is more than conceivable that the higher risk for women is related to these increased risk factors.[19]

Table 41-1. Prediction of the Risk for Operative Death

	Low	Medium	High
Age (yr)	60	75	75
Sex	Male	Female	Female
Diabetes	No	Yes	Yes
Unstable angina	Yes	No	Yes
Ejection fraction (%)	65	35	25
Three-vessel disease	Yes	Yes	Yes
Operative incidence	First	First	Redo
Predicted mortality rate (%)	0.8	3.4	12

Based on The Society of Thoracic Surgery National Cardiac Database Risk Stratification Algorithm. Minneapolis: Summit Medical Systems.

Reoperative coronary bypass surgery has become increasingly frequent during the past several years, accounting for close to 10% of the patients undergoing bypass surgery in 1992. Reoperative surgery has a higher mortality rate than does primary bypass surgery because of its technical difficulty resulting from pericardial adhesions and scar formation, as well as the fact that patients undergoing reoperation are older and have more advanced coronary disease.[20]

Long-term results. Most series show elimination of angina in 90% of patients at 1 year, with approximately 70% of patients remaining free of any cardiac event at 3 years. Although relief from symptoms is unquestioned, controversy exists regarding the long-term functional benefit of bypass surgery. However, functional improvement in left ventricular ejection fraction has been documented after bypass surgery and can be attributed to improved contractility in the myocardial regions in which there had been demonstrable ischemia prior to surgery.

Clinical improvement obviously depends at least in part on short- and long-term graft patency. The overall occlusion rate for saphenous vein bypass grafts is 5% to 20% during the first operative year and 2% to 4% annually thereafter, for an occlusion rate of approximately 30% at 5 years and 50% at 10 years. Use of the internal thoracic graft has become increasingly favored because of its 95% 1-year and 90% 10-year patency rates. Excellent late internal thoracic artery graft patency clearly correlates with increased patient survival, reduced symptoms, and fewer reoperations. In a study at the Cleveland Clinic, where internal thoracic artery grafts have been used extensively, the 10-year survival rate among patients with saphenous vein grafts for triple-vessel disease was 71%, compared with 83% in a comparable group of patients who had an internal thoracic artery graft to the LAD. Approximately 80% of all patients undergoing primary coronary bypass surgery survive for 10 years, and use of the internal thoracic artery graft improves 10-year survival to close to 90%. Furthermore, about one in seven patients who have had only vein grafts require reoperation at 15 years, twice the reoperation rate for those patients who received at least one thoracic artery bypass.

Patients who undergo reoperation have approximately twice the primary operative mortality rate, because the operation is technically more difficult and because the patients are older, with more severe atherosclerotic disease. In addition, total revascularization is more difficult for technical reasons, and symptomatic relief is therefore usually of shorter duration as well.

Transplantation vs High-Risk Coronary Surgery

In deciding whether to recommend transplantation or bypass surgery to a patient at high risk as a result of severely depressed left ventricular function, it is important to assess whether the myocardium is viable. In patients with ischemic but viable myocardium, ventricular function may improve after bypass surgery once adequate blood flow is restored. The term *hibernating myocardium* has been used to describe ventricular dysfunction caused by inadequate coronary flow.[21] This should be distinguished from an ischemic cardiomyopathy, which implies irreversible myocardial dysfunction. Anginal symptoms suggestive of reversible ischemia are often a useful measure of myocardial viability.

Patients whose only symptom is heart failure should be approached with caution. Currently, myocardial viability may best be assessed by thallium scanning, either with exercise or at rest. Myocardium that takes up thallium either early or late is presumed to be viable. In this way, one may be able to estimate the possibly dramatic potential for improved ventricular function with revascularization in the patient who has severely depressed ventricular function but viable myocardium. In a patient with these findings, especially if angina is present, surgery rather than transplantation is indicated if there is operable coronary disease. In patients with congestive heart failure and no evidence of viable myocardium, however, bypass surgery clearly carries high risk and little benefit, and transplantation should be considered.

VALVULAR HEART DISEASE

Aortic Valve Disease

Aortic Valvular Stenosis

The normal aortic valve consists of three equal-size leaflets attached to the aortic wall, forming the three aortic sinuses. As mentioned in the section on coronary artery disease, the coronary arteries arise from two of these sinuses, thereby defining the left, right, and noncoronary cusps.

Pathologic anatomy. The most common cause of left ventricular outflow tract obstruction is aortic valvular stenosis. Supravalvular and subvalvular obstructions occur much less commonly. Aortic stenosis is the most common isolated valvular abnormality found in humans. Although congenital valvular stenosis may cause symptoms immediately, a congenital bicuspid valve is usually asymptomatic at birth and becomes symptomatic in the sixth to eighth decade of life. The turbulent flow across the bileaflet valve leads to fibrosis and calcification, so that stenosis develops with time. Rheumatic aortic stenosis, initially an inflammatory lesion, leads to fusion of the leaflet commissures, with thickening and calcification of the cusps themselves. Retraction of the leaflet borders, which occurs commonly, leads to regurgitation as well. In rheumatic aortic valvular disease, mitral involvement is invariably also present. In degenerative or senile aortic stenosis, normal leaflet stress leads to calcification and cusp immobility. This calcification can extend either inferiorly onto the anterior mitral leaflet or upward along the aorta, occasionally causing coronary osteal stenosis (see Fig. 41-1).

Pathophysiology. Narrowing of the left ventricular outflow tract becomes important when it obstructs flow, causing a transvalvular pressure gradient. In the presence of a normal CO, a transvalvular gradient of 60 mm Hg or a calculated valve area of less than 0.7 cm^2 is considered severe aortic stenosis. The normal response to aortic stenosis, a process that in itself can take years, is the development of left ventricular hypertrophy. This hypertrophy initially leads to a decrease in compliance, with an elevation in the left ventricular end-diastolic pressure. With progressive hypertrophy and loss of ventricular compliance, atrial contraction plays an increasingly important role in left ventricular filling, so loss of a normal sinus mechanism (such as atrial fibrillation) can cause acute decompensation in these patients. Furthermore, with severe aortic stenosis, prolongation of the systolic ejection time and a concomitant elevation in left ventricular end-diastolic pressure act to decrease diastolic coronary blood flow, with a resultant oxygen debt. The subendocardium may become chronically ischemic, with cell death and fibrosis. In this situation, the left ventricle begins to fail as stroke volume decreases and cardiac output falls. Paradoxically, follow-up of a patient with aortic stenosis may reveal a low or a decreasing aortic gradient during a period of years, which should not be confused with resolving or stable aortic valvular disease but rather indicates a failing left ventricle with a decreased stroke volume and therefore a decreased transvalvular gradient.

The clinical course of aortic stenosis may be divided into two phases. The initial phase involves hypertrophy of the left ventricle as it compensates for increasing afterload. Angina, the hallmark of this stage of aortic stenosis, results from the imbalance of myocardial oxygen demand and myocardial oxygen delivery. The second stage involves the onset of left ventricular dysfunction, which is the result of a progressively stiffening ventricle that requires increasing preload for adequate filling, with resultant pulmonary hypertension, shortness of breath, and dyspnea on exertion.

Diagnosis. Although auscultation of the patient with aortic stenosis reveals a systolic murmur best heard at the base of the heart at the left sternal border radiating up into the neck, this murmur can also be associated simply with normal systolic ejection. However, a slow, prolonged rise in the arterial pulse, as opposed to a sharp upbeat, is a palpable indicator that significant ventricular outflow tract obstruction is present. Doppler echocardiography has become an invaluable tool in the noninvasive detection of aortic stenosis. The peak aortic valvular gradient can be calculated by the following formula[22]:

$$\Delta = 4 \cdot V^2$$

where Δ is the peak gradient and V is the maximal measured blood velocity (in meters per second) across the valve. The most accurate measure of left ventricular outflow tract obstruction is determined invasively by cardiac catheterization, where a simultaneous aortic and ventricular pressure measurement can determine the exact aortic gradient (in the case of atrial fibrillation, this is the only acceptable means of determining this number). The aortic valve area (AVA, in square centimeters) may then be determined by the Gorlin formula[23]:

$$AVA = \frac{AVF}{44.5\ (\text{Gradient})^{1/2}}$$

where *AVF* is aortic valve flow, which equals CO in milliliters per minute divided by the systolic ejection period (in seconds per minute), and 44.5 is the empiric orifice constant (obtained by comparing calculated with measured AVA at operation or post mortem). For quick calculations, this simplifies to:

$$AVA = \frac{CO}{(\text{Gradient})^{1/2}}$$

Patients frequently have symptoms when the AVA is <1 cm^2, whereas they invariably have symptoms when the area is <0.7 cm^2.[24] Angina is usually the earliest symptom in patients with aortic stenosis. The mean survival after its onset is 4.7 years. However, when a patient has syncope, survival is typically decreased to less than 3 years, whereas when a patient has dyspnea and congestive heart failure, survival is on the order of 1 to 2 years[25] (Fig. 41-5).

Treatment. The only effective therapy for symptomatic aortic stenosis is operative. Symptoms alone are an indication for aortic valve replacement. Occasionally, a patient with aortic stenosis may have no symptoms. The appropriate timing of surgery in such patients is not clear. Timely surgery provides the opportunity for resolution of left ventricular hypertrophy, whereas allowing the condition to persist may lead to irreversible myocardial fibrosis with dysfunction. In general, patients without symptoms with progressive left ventricular hypertrophy should be offered surgical therapy because survival is superior to that with medical therapy.[26] An unwritten dictum is that all patients with aortic stenosis should be given the opportunity for surgical therapy because it is so effective in leading to reversal of symptoms. With progressive fibrosis and irreversible myocardial dysfunction, however, an occasional patient may have a decrease in ejection fraction out of proportion to the increase in wall stress caused by the aortic stenosis. With this "end-stage aortic stenosis" (in which contractility has decreased out of proportion to the increase in wall stress), patients derive little benefit from surgical therapy.[27,28]

In patients with good ventricular function, aortic valve replacement has an associated mortality rate of 2% to 8%. Perioperative risk factors include age, left ventricular function, preoperative New York Heart Association functional classification, and pulmonary function. The projected 5-year survival for patients after aortic valve replacement is 80% to 85%. Although symptoms are generally relieved in all patients, improvement in ejection fraction with resolution of left ventricular hypertrophy may require months to occur.[29,30] In patients with aortic stenosis as well as coronary artery disease, valve replacement and myocardial revascularization should be performed concurrently.[31]

Percutaneous aortic balloon valvuloplasty is a "noninvasive" alternative to surgical therapy for aortic stenosis. In this procedure, either one or two balloon catheters are placed retrogradely through the aortic orifice and inflated in an effort to crack the calcium that is retarding valvular motion. The immediate results show an increase in the AVA of 50%, with a 3% to 10% mortality rate and a sim-

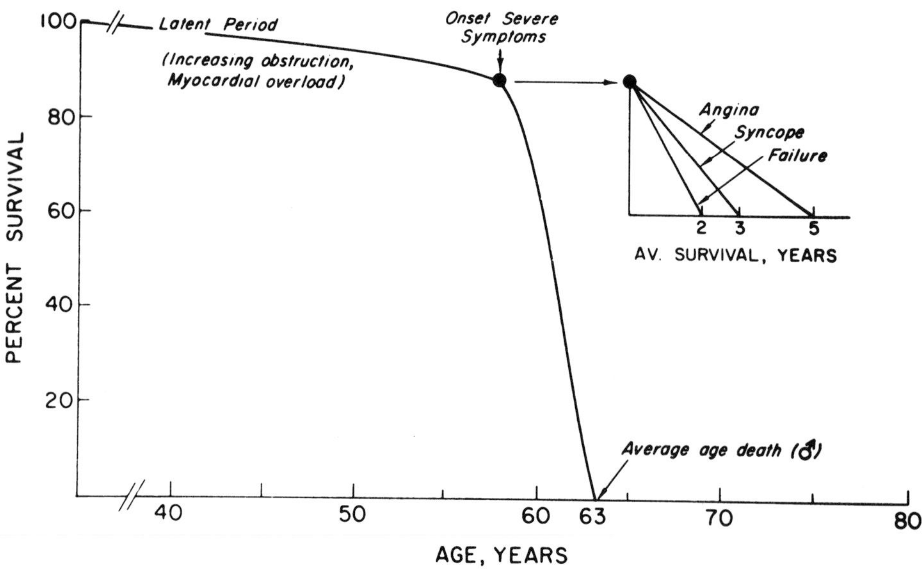

Fig. 41-5. Average course of medically treated valvular aortic stenosis in adults (postmortem data). Although one can understand the difficulty in operating on the patient without symptoms, the severe slope of the curve mandates that patients be seriously considered for surgery at the onset of symptoms. (From Ross J, Braunwald E. Aortic stenosis. Circulation 38 (Suppl 5):v61, 1968. Reproduced with permission. Copyright 1968, American Heart Association.)

ilar stroke rate.[32] Long-term results are abysmal, with a 1-year mortality rate of 25% and a 30% to 35% symptomatic recurrence rate during that period. With recurrence of symptoms, death, hemodynamic evidence of restenosis, or a combination of these occurring in more than 50% of patients at 6 months, percutaneous aortic balloon valvuloplasty cannot compete with surgical valve replacement. If it has a role at all, it should be limited to the aged and frail patient whose long-term prognosis is also abysmal.

Aortic Insufficiency

Pathologic anatomy. Incompetence of the aortic valve may be the result of either primary valvular or aortic root disease.[33] Rheumatic fever is a major cause of aortic insufficiency. As discussed with aortic stenosis, it causes retraction of the cusps, which prevents adequate apposition and leads to a central leak. Congenital bicuspid valves with time become calcified and generally lead to aortic stenosis. Occasionally, however, bicuspid valves have a redundant leaflet that leads to regurgitation. Myxoid degeneration of the aortic valve, as seen in Marfan syndrome, Ehlers-Danlos syndrome, and cystic medial necrosis, may lead to redundancy, prolapse, and regurgitation. Infective endocarditis with bacterial destruction of the leaflets may also lead to valvular insufficiency. Ascending aortic dissection as a result of either trauma or hypertensive atherosclerotic disease often leads to loss of commissural suspension, with resultant leaflet prolapse. Furthermore, severe aortic dilatation causes annular stretching (as seen in annuloaortic ectasia, syphilis, and ankylosing spondylitis), which leads to annular dilatation and central vascular incompetence.

Pathophysiology. With aortic regurgitation, there is a significant increase in preload, where end-diastolic volume is the result of both normal left ventricular filling through the mitral valve as well as left ventricular filling through the incompetent aortic valve. At the expense of an increase in left ventricular wall stress, ejection fraction remains normal as stroke volume and end-diastolic volume increase. Left ventricular dilatation increases wall tension, which increases myocardial oxygen demand. To counteract this, left ventricular wall thickness increases to maintain a wall thickness to cavity radius ratio that preserves myocardial efficiency. With time, however, left ventricular volume may become enormous. Increasing wall thickness does not keep pace with this increasing left ventricular dilation. Sharply increased wall tension develops, with resulting systolic dysfunction. At this point, an elevation in left ventricular end-diastolic pressure occurs and patients have symptoms (Fig. 41-6). Acute aortic regurgitation, on the other hand, such as occurs with dissections or endocarditis, leads to extremely high left ventricular end-diastolic pressures as a result of the acute increase in end-diastolic volume in the unconditioned ventricle. In these patients, symptoms develop immediately.

Diagnosis. Patients with aortic insufficiency have a characteristic pattern on physical examination that results from the wide pulse pressure associated with this disease.

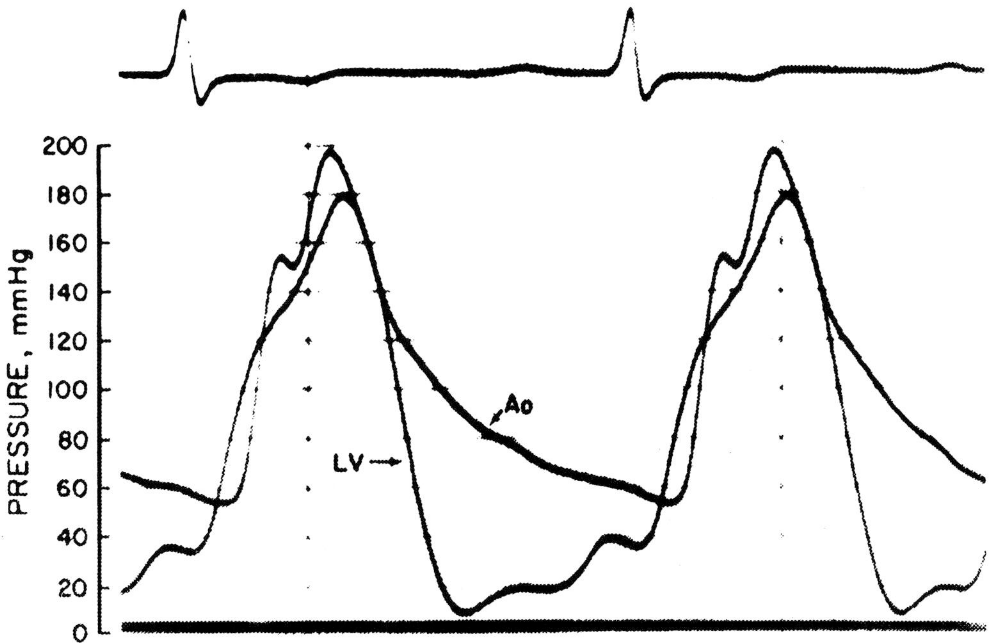

Fig. 41-6. Simultaneous left ventricular and aortic pressure-time curves in a patient with severe aortic insufficiency. Note that in this patient with extremely severe aortic insufficiency, the left ventricle has become less and less compliant, and at end-diastole the aortic pressure and left ventricular end-diastolic pressure have nearly equalized. (From Grossman W. Cardiac Catheterization, Angiography, and Intervention. Philadelphia: Lea & Febiger, 1991. Used with permission.)

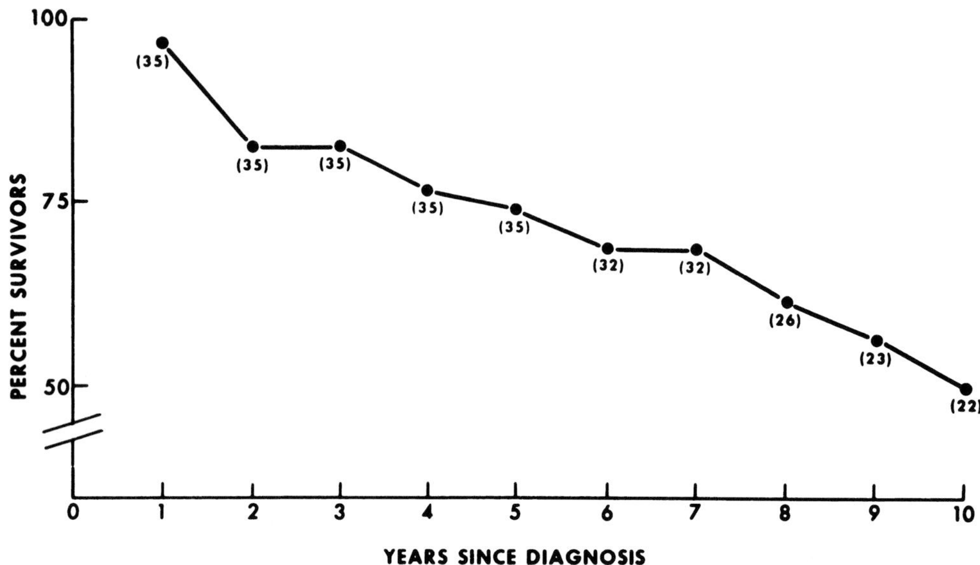

Fig. 41-7. Survival of patients with of medically treated aortic insufficiency. Unlike with aortic stenosis, cardiac failure from aortic insufficiency occurs much more gradually. Consequently, it is much more difficult to discern where one should intervene, particularly in the patient without symptoms. (From Rapaport E. Natural history of aortic and mitral valve disease. Am J Cardiol 35:221, 1975. Used with permission.)

The peripheral pulses rise and fall abruptly (Corrigan's or water-hammer pulse), the head may bob with each systolic stroke (Musset's sign), and the capillaries visibly pulsate (Quincke's sign). Auscultation reveals a soft S_2 with a high-frequency, diastolic, regurgitant murmur best heard at the left sternal border. A mid to late diastolic rumble can be heard (Austin Flint murmur); this represents rapid diastolic flow across the mitral valve that is becoming narrowed as a result of rapid ventricular filling caused by the aortic insufficiency.

Clinical course. In chronic aortic regurgitation, symptoms occur late after left ventricular dilatation and myocardial dysfunction.[34] Symptoms occur as a result of elevation in left ventricular end-diastolic pressure, again a situation that occurs later in the course of the disease, because early on, left ventricular volumes increase to maintain compliance. Interestingly, nocturnal angina can occur as the result of a slow heart rate, so that diastolic pressure in the coronary arteries is low and left ventricular end-diastolic pressure is high, compromising blood flow and oxygen delivery to the endocardium. Acute aortic regurgitation, however, is poorly tolerated, and patients have symptoms almost immediately. This is the result of extremely poor compliance of the ventricle and an excessively high diastolic volume.

Management. Patients with symptomatic aortic insufficiency require surgical therapy, because survival with medical therapy is only a few years from the onset of symptoms. The patient with no symptoms or mild symptoms but with moderate to severe aortic insufficiency presents a dilemma. Frequently, diuretics and afterload reduction may be able to maintain these patients for a considerable period before they have symptoms. Without surgery, 75% of patients survive 5 years from the time of diagnosis, and 50% of patients survive 10 years[35] (Fig. 41-7). Despite the lack of symptoms, however, irreversible myocardial dysfunction occurs. The goal of the clinician should be to intervene before this happens. When end-systolic volume is less than 30 ml/m^2, prognosis after surgical therapy is still excellent. With progressive systolic dysfunction, however, end-systolic volumes may rise above 90 ml/m^2, a situation that frequently portends permanent postoperative disability. End-systolic volumes between 30 and 90 ml/m^2 have intermediate short- and long-term results.[36] Indications for surgical therapy in the patient without symptoms thus should rest on serial echocardiography or radionuclide ventriculography to discern systolic dysfunction or decreasing ejection fraction. Despite good exercise tolerance, when systolic dysfunction occurs, surgery should be recommended.

The mortality rate associated with aortic valve replacement for aortic insufficiency is approximately 4% to 6%, somewhat higher than that seen in aortic stenosis.[37-39] As discussed, long-term survival depends on preoperative left ventricular function.

Mitral Valve Disease

Surgical Anatomy

The mitral valve apparatus is composed of the left ventricular papillary muscles, the mitral valve chordae tendineae, the mitral valve leaflets, and the mitral valve annulus. By means of the chordae tendineae, the mitral leaflets are connected to the apical region of the left ventricle. Normal function of the valve depends on the coordinated interaction of these components. The mitral valve has two leaflets joined at two commissures. The anterior leaflet (also called the *aortic leaflet*) is broad and relatively square in shape. It is attached to the anterior one-third circumference of the mitral valve annulus and is in fibrous continuity with the aortic valve annulus. The posterior leaflet (also called the *mural leaflet*) is narrower and relatively rectangular. It is attached to the posterior two-thirds circumference of the mitral annulus. Each leaflet is attached by chordae to each of two papillary muscles arising from the luminal surface of the left ventricle, the anterior-lateral and the posterior-medial papillary muscles. The blood supply of the anterior-lateral papillary muscle is from the diagonal branches of LAD or by obtuse marginal branches of the circumflex coronary artery. The posterior-medial papillary muscle is supplied by the PDA coronary artery, which is usually the terminal branch of the RCA.

The mitral valve functions to permit antegrade blood flow from the left atrium into the left ventricle during diastole and to prevent reflux of blood from left ventricle into the left atrium during systole. Blood flows antegrade through the mitral valve when the left atrial pressure exceeds left ventricular pressure. As the ventricle contracts during systole, closure of the valve is effected by several mechanisms. Once the left ventricular pressure exceeds left atrial pressure, leaflet closure is initiated, and the rate of blood flow from the atrium into the ventricle is decelerated. At the same time, contraction of the left ventricular muscle at the base of the heart serves to narrow the mitral annulus; echocardiographic data suggest that the annular area decreases by approximately one third from end-diastole to midsystole.[40] This reduction in annular area helps achieve leaflet approximation. During systolic contraction, papillary muscle contraction pulls the chordae taut, preventing prolapse of the leaflets. Any disease process that interferes with the normal function of any portion of the mitral valve apparatus may result in mitral stenosis or regurgitation.

Mitral Stenosis

Rheumatic fever is the primary cause of mitral stenosis.[41] Other etiologies of mitral stenosis are rare and include congenital mitral stenosis and stenosis resulting from collagen vascular diseases such as systemic lupus erythematosus and rheumatoid arthritis. Two thirds of patients with rheumatoid mitral stenosis are female. After resolution of acute rheumatic fever, most patients remain free of symptoms for at least two decades before development of symptoms of mitral valve disease. Thereafter, patients have progressively more and worse symptoms.[42]

The normal mitral valve orifice measures 4 to 6 cm^2 in cross-sectional area. A mitral valve area (MVA) of 2 cm^2 is considered moderate mitral stenosis. At this degree of narrowing, flow across the mitral valve may be accomplished only by generation of an abnormally high pressure gradient across the valve. An MVA of 1 cm^2 is considered critical mitral stenosis, because flow across the valve (CO) is relatively fixed; even extremely high pressure gradients across the valve are unable to increase flow (Fig. 41-8). As with the aortic valve, the MVA may be calculated according to the Gorlin formula (for the mitral valve, the constant is 38 rather than the 44.5 used for the aortic valve):

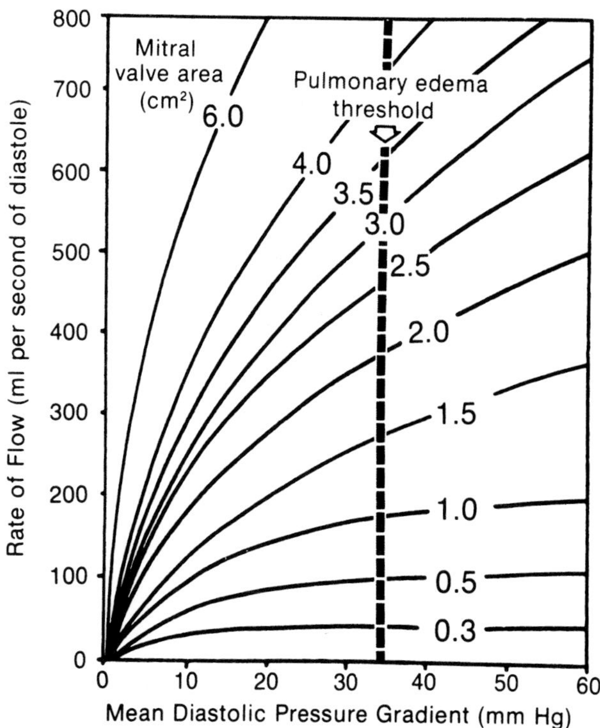

Fig. 41-8. The relationship between mean diastolic gradient across the mitral valve and the rate of flow across the mitral valve per second of diastole. When the valve area is ≤1.0 cm^2, little additional flow can be achieved despite an increased pressure gradient. (From Wallace AG. Pathophysiology of cardiovascular disease. In Smith LH Jr, Thier SO, eds. Pathophysiology: The Biological Principles of Disease. The International Textbook of Medicine, vol 1. Philadelphia: WB Saunders, 1981, p 1192.)

$$\text{MVA} = \frac{\text{Flow rate across valve}/38}{(\text{Mean gradient across valve})^{1/2}}$$

For any given MVA, the magnitude of the transvalvular gradient is proportional to the square of the transvalvular flow rate; doubling the CO quadruples the transvalvular pressure gradient. Increased left atrial pressure results in increased pulmonary venous pressure, and in turn increased pulmonary capillary pressure. Should the transvalvular gradient culminate in a left atrial pressure greater than 25 mm Hg, pulmonary edema may result. For this reason, exertional dyspnea is commonly the first symptom of mitral stenosis.

Patients frequently first have symptoms with the onset of atrial fibrillation. Chronically elevated left atrial pressure produces left atrial distention, ultimately producing atrial fibrillation. With the onset of atrial fibrillation, diastolic time is shortened; the same volume of blood must flow from left atrium to ventricle in less time, which further increases left atrial pressure. The atrial kick contributes approximately 30% to the presystolic transvalvular gradient in patients with mitral stenosis. Its loss with the onset of atrial fibrillation eliminates this mechanical advantage, and left atrial pressure rises and CO declines.[43]

The contractile function of the left ventricle is typically well preserved in mitral stenosis. The hemodynamic features of mitral stenosis are notable for a reduced CO at rest (because of the mechanical obstruction of the stenotic valve), which rises subnormally with exercise along with pulmonary hypertension. The pulmonary hypertension is derived from retrograde transmission of elevated left atrial pressure, pulmonary arterial vasoconstriction, and obliterative structural changes in the pulmonary circulation produced by chronic left atrial hypertension. Pulmonary hypertension may become severe, resulting in impaired right ventricular function and tricuspid regurgitation.

Diagnosis. Patients with mitral stenosis typically are seen with easy fatigue, dyspnea on exertion, and orthopnea. As noted previously symptoms may develop with the onset of atrial fibrillation. A history of rheumatic fever is noted in approximately one half of cases. If the left atrial enlargement is sufficient to compress surrounding structures, patients may report dysphagia or hoarseness.

On cardiac auscultation, an opening snap of the mitral valve is common as a result of sudden tensing of the valve leaflets by the chordae as the valve leaflets achieve their opening excursion. The opening snap may be heard within the first 100 msec after the second heart sound. Mitral stenosis produces a low-pitched, rumbling diastolic murmur best heard at the apex. The murmur is often difficult to appreciate but may be provoked by maneuvers that increase CO. Pulmonary hypertension is suggested by a loud pulmonary component of the second heart sound. With pulmonary hypertension, an enlarged right ventricle may shift the left ventricle posteriorly, making the murmur extremely difficult to hear (silent mitral stenosis).

The chest roentgenogram is significant for left atrial enlargement. There may be elevation of the left main stem bronchus and posterior displacement of the esophagus on the lateral radiographic view. Pulmonary venous hypertension typically results in cephalization of pulmonary blood flow.

Two-dimensional echocardiographic evaluation of mitral stenosis reveals thickened mitral valve leaflets and restricted leaflet motion as the valve opens. The left atrium is typically enlarged, and the left ventricular cavity is usually reduced in size. Mitral annular calcification and left atrial thrombus are identifiable on echocardiography. Doppler echocardiography provides a functional estimate of the severity of mitral stenosis. The peak velocity of blood flow across the valve is increased, allowing an estimate of the transvalvular gradient (see the section on the aortic valve).

Medical treatment. Medical treatment of mitral stenosis is of limited efficacy. The focus of medical treatment is to minimize pulmonary edema with diuretics and to control the ventricular rate with digoxin. Because left atrial thrombus may form, patients in atrial fibrillation should have anticoagulation with warfarin.

Surgical treatment. Because of the efficacy of surgical treatment, the natural history of mitral stenosis is now unclear. However, after acute rheumatic fever, most patients remain free of symptoms for 20 to 25 years. Once these patients have symptoms, at least 5 years is required for the progression of symptoms from mild to severe. According to the study of Olesen[44] of patients in the presurgical era, 40% of symptom-free patients with mitral stenosis had significantly worsened condition or were dead within 10 years. Among patients with mild symptoms, the number was 80%. Munoz et al.[45] reported a 45% 5-year survival rate for medically treated patients with mitral stenosis and mitral regurgitation. In a comparable population undergoing mitral commissurotomy, 5-year survival rate was 80%.

The first report of successful surgical correction of mitral stenosis appeared in 1923; Cutler and Levine[46] reported successful relief of mitral stenosis by incision of the valve with a knife introduced through an apical left ventriculotomy. In 1925, Souttar[47] performed the first successful closed mitral commissurotomy through the left atrial appendage. After the reports of Harken et al.[48] in 1948 and Bailey[49] in 1949, closed mitral commissurotomy became widely used for mitral stenosis. Despite excellent long-term results after closed mitral commissurotomy,[50] by the mid 1970s, this technique was supplanted by open mitral commissurotomy. Closed mitral commissurotomy is now of historical interest only.

Although closed mitral commissurotomy offered good palliation of mitral stenosis, open mitral commissurotomy offers several advantages.[51] First, the valvuloplasty may be performed under direct vision. The primary reason for failure of closed mitral commissurotomy was residual stenosis, not restenosis.[52,53] In as many as 75% of patients, the subvalvular apparatus of the mitral valve contributes significantly to the stenosis.[54] The open technique allows precise and maximal division of fused commissures, as well as of fused chordae.[55] In addition, calcium may be sharply debrided from the valve, and any residual mitral insufficiency may be corrected at the time of operation. Finally, the closed technique offers the disadvantages of potentially dislodging left atrial thrombus, resulting in intraoperative embolization and stroke.

The results of open mitral commissurotomy are excellent. Operative mortality rate is usually reported as 0.2% to 2%, and in most series, the need for reoperation is reported to be 2% per year.[55]

Balloon mitral valvuloplasty. Inoue et al.[56] reported the first successful percutaneous balloon mitral valvuloplasty in 1984. The valvular pathology of mitral stenosis makes the valve unsuitable for balloon dilation. Nonetheless, this procedure is now an alternative to surgical relief of mitral stenosis in a small, select group of patients. After creation of a hole in the interatrial septum, a balloon catheter is introduced through the mitral valve and inflated within its orifice. The procedure is based on the idea that the inflated balloon will split fused commissures. As noted previously, however, the subvalvular apparatus contributes significantly to the stenosis, and this region is not addressed by balloon dilation. Immediate hemodynamic improvement is noted in most patients, with a significant reduction in transvalvular gradient, improved CO, and reduction in pulmonary arterial pressure.[18] However, these hemodynamic benefits are not long-standing, and the complication rate is significant. Reported mortality rates range from 0% to 4%,[57] comparable to that of open mitral commissurotomy. Approximately 30% of patients are left with a significant atrial septal defect.[58] Stroke is reported as a complication of the procedure in 3% to 4%.[59] Recurrence of mitral stenosis is noted in as many as 30% to 40% of patients within 1 year.[60] The small subset of patients with the best results from balloon mitral valvuloplasty are those with soft, pliable leaflets without calcification and without stenosis of the subvalvular apparatus. Such patients are, of course, rare. Thus, although balloon mitral valvuloplasty attempts to spare the patient a more invasive procedure, the patient is actually exposed to greater risk of complication and death. At the same time, the results are inferior to open mitral commissurotomy, which must be considered the procedure of choice.

Mitral Regurgitation

Structural abnormalities of any component of the mitral valve apparatus (mitral leaflets, chordae tendineae, and papillary muscles) may result in mitral regurgitation. Rheumatic fever remains the most common cause of mitral regurgitation; it results in deformity and retraction of the leaflets and shortening of the chordae. Other causes include perforation by trauma and infective endocarditis. Calcification of the mitral annulus may result in annular rigidity, preventing valve closure, and mitral annular dilation resulting from left ventricular dilation may likewise preclude leaflet apposition during systole. Chordal rupture may result from trauma, endocarditis, rheumatic fever, or diseases of collagen formation. Chordae to the posterior leaflet rupture more frequently than do those to the anterior. Coronary arterial disease may produce infarction of the papillary muscle, resulting in mitral regurgitation. Infarction in distribution of the anterior descending coronary artery may necrose the anterior-lateral papillary muscle, whereas the posterior-medial muscle may infarct if blood flow through the PDA artery is interrupted. Mitral regurgitation caused by MI typically is seen as a new murmur several days after infarction.

Pathophysiology. The regurgitant mitral valve offers an alternative route by which blood may exit from the left ventricle. During both isovolumetric contraction and systole, blood is preferentially ejected into the low-pressure left atrium. The volume of the regurgitant flow (regurgitant fraction) depends on the size of the regurgitant orifice and the afterload against which the left ventricle must work to pump blood through the aortic valve. The regurgitant fraction is increased with increased left ventricular preload and increased afterload, both of which dilate the left ventricle, thereby enlarging the mitral annulus and regurgitant orifice. Because the valve leaks during systole, the volume of regurgitant flow also increases as heart rate (number of systoles per minute) increases. To maintain an adequate systemic blood flow (CO), the left ventricle becomes volume overloaded; it must pump the combined volume of systemic and regurgitant flows. Because the left ventricle is able to beat against the reduced resistance of the left atrium, parameters of systolic function (ejection fraction) are *increased* in mitral regurgitation. However, as with aortic insufficiency, the left ventricle ultimately fails, with chronic volume overload. In fact, *normal* values of systolic function indicate significant contractile dysfunction of the left ventricle. An ejection fraction of 40% to 50% in the setting of mitral regurgitation indicates severe left ventricular contractile dysfunction.[41]

As in mitral stenosis, left atrial hypertension results from mitral regurgitation. This pressure is transmitted retrogradely into the pulmonary circulation; if high enough it produces pulmonary hypertension. The magnitude of the left atrial pressure is a function of the compliance of the left atrium (Fig. 41-9). A normal or low compliance of the left atrium, such as may occur in acute mitral regurgitation, results in a relatively rapid rise in left atrial pressure. On the other hand chronic, slowly developing left atrial volume overload may create significant enlargement of a compliant left atrium, with relatively low left atrial pressure.

Diagnosis. Symptoms result from the degree of mitral regurgitation, the rate of its progression, the degree of pulmonary hypertension, and the magnitude of left ventricular contractile dysfunction. Symptoms in patients with chronic mitral regurgitation typically do not occur until the left ventricle begins to fail. Patients with mild mitral regurgitation may remain free of symptoms for most of their lives.[61] The onset of atrial fibrillation does impair the patient's functional status, but not to the same degree as with mitral stenosis. With moderate to severe chronic mitral regurgitation, patients may be free of symptoms for long periods. However, this lack of symptoms may be deceptive, because the contractile function of the left ventricle may be slowly deteriorating. Once symptoms occur, left ventricular contractile dysfunction may be irreversible.

The natural history of mitral regurgitation is obscure, because surgical intervention has effectively altered this history. In the presurgical era, however, approximately 80% of patients with severe mitral regurgitation survived 5 years and 60% survived 10 years.[35]

On cardiac auscultation, a holosystolic murmur is best heard at the apex and radiates to the axilla and left scapular region. The ECG is notable for left atrial enlargement and, frequently, atrial fibrillation. The chest roentgenogram

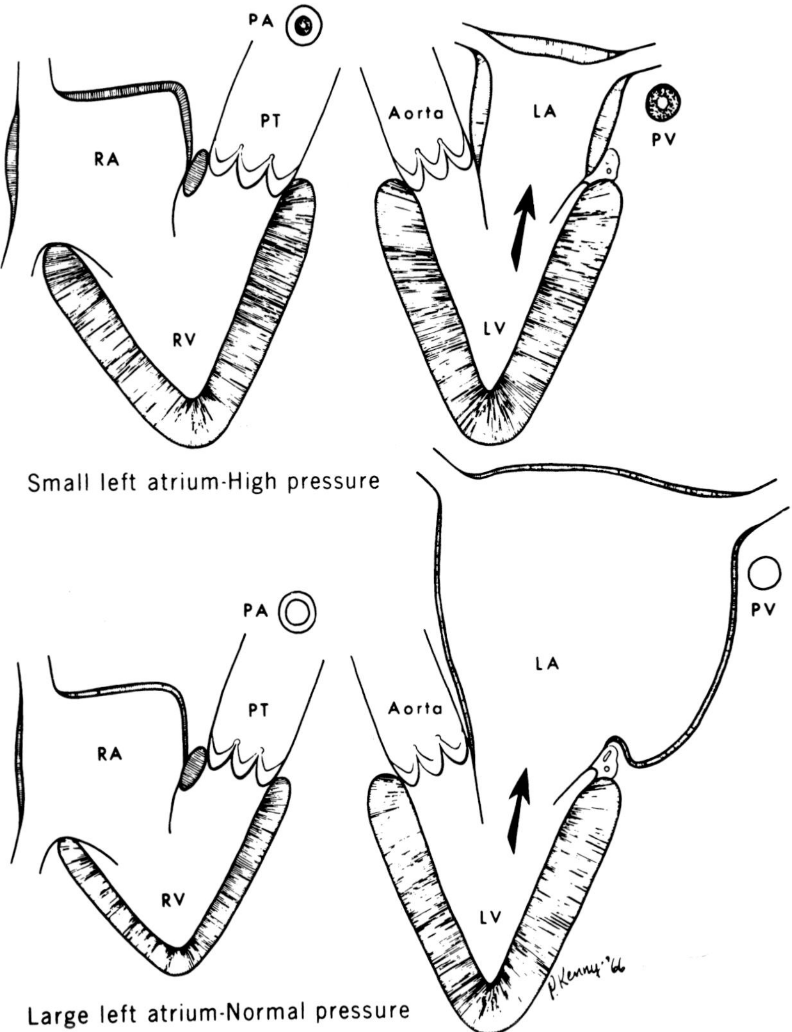

Fig. 41-9. Syndrome of mitral regurgitation. When mitral regurgitation occurs abruptly in patients with previously normal hearts, left atrial compliance is normal. This results in a rapid increase in left atrial pressure. On the other hand, the insidious development of mitral regurgitation allows the left atrial compliance to increase along with its size, attenuating the rise in left atrial pressure. *LA,* Left atrium; *LV,* left ventricle; *PA,* pulmonary artery; *PT,* pulmonary trunk; *PV,* pulmonary vein; *RA,* right atrium; *RV,* right ventricle. (From Roberts WC, et al. Nonrheumatic valvular cardiac disease. A clinicopathologic survey of 27 different conditions causing valvular dysfunction. Cardiovasc Clin 5:403, 1973. Used with permission from FA Davis, Company, Philadelphia.)

is significant for cardiomegaly and left atrial enlargement. Pulmonary venous hypertension may be manifested by cephalization of pulmonary blood flow and pulmonary edema.

Echocardiography is extremely valuable in confirming the diagnosis and severity of mitral regurgitation. Transesophageal echocardiography is particularly effective in providing an anatomic explanation for the regurgitation, such as perforated leaflets, poor leaflet coaptation, or ruptured chordae. Doppler echocardiography reveals a high-velocity jet of regurgitant blood flow into the left atrium during systole. The severity of the valve regurgitation is a function of the distance from the mitral annulus that the jet can be visualized (into the pulmonary veins) and the size of the left atrium. Contrast ventriculography performed at cardiac catheterization likewise demonstrates regurgitation during systole.

Management. The cornerstone of medical management is diuresis and afterload reduction with angiotensin-converting enzyme inhibitors.[41] The importance of afterload reduction cannot be overemphasized. Because blood leaving the left ventricle travels the path of least resistance, lowering systemic vascular resistance increases systemic CO.

The indications for surgical intervention are (1) symptoms despite medical management or (2) evidence of deteriorating left ventricular contractile funcation, as determined by echocardiography or contract ventriculography. Surgical correction of mitral regurgitation should be undertaken before left ventricular contractile dysfunction becomes irreversible; the operative mortality rate increases substantially as the ventricle fails.

The two surgical options are repair and replacement of the valve. The final decision regarding which of these options to employ is made during the operation after inspection of the valve. There are several advantages to mitral valve repair rather than replacement. First, with mitral valve replacement, there is loss of the mitral valve apparatus connecting the mitral annulus to the apex of the left ventricle by means of the chordae and papillary muscles. In the long term, this may lead to left ventricular dysfunction.[40] Mitral valve repair preserves this apparatus. Second, the risks associated with a prosthetic valve, such as prosthetic valve endocarditis and thromboembolic complications, are avoided. Third, the operative mortality rate associated with mitral valve repair is 0% to 4%, which is lower than the 2% to 8% reported for mitral valve replacement.[54]

Cardiac Dysrhythmias, Pericardial Disease, and Cardiac Tumors

Andrew C. Fiore

CARDIAC DYSRHYTHMIAS

Cardiac function can be adversely influenced by changes in both cardiac rhythm and cardiac rate, but in actuality, perturbations in cardiac output (CO) are more commonly rate related. Healthy individuals in sinus rhythm have a frequency of cardiac contraction that can vary considerably. In optimally physically conditioned individuals, resting heart rates may be as low as 40 to 50 beats/min, although most healthy persons range from 60 to 90 beats/min. Cardiac rate can vary across a wide range (40 to150 beats/min) without eliciting symptoms. With the induction of exercise, however, symptoms generally occur at each end of this spectrum, and especially in individuals with underlying cardiovascular pathology. Although dysrhythmias can generally be managed medically, certain situations may necessitate surgical intervention.

Bradycardias

In patients with symptomatic bradycardia, implantation of a pacemaker may be indicated to increase the heart rate. The common types of symptomatic bradycardia include (1) congenital heart block, (2) acquired heart block, (3) iatrogenic heart block, (4) sick sinus syndrome, (5) atrial fibrillation, and (6) bradycardia-tachycardia syndrome.

Patients with congenital heart blocks are frequently free of symptoms because the heart is in other respects structurally and functionally normal. As the child enters adolescence and early adulthood, maintenance of adequate exercise tolerance may require pacemaker implantation. In elderly patients, in whom acquired heart block usually occurs, ischemic heart disease is commonly the underlying etiology. Symptoms may be evoked with minimal exercise and occasionally arise even under resting conditions. Acquired heart block is a common cause of syncope (Stokes-Adams attacks). Sudden cardiac death may occur in this situation as the rhythm degenerates into asystole as a result of the development of ventricular escape beats from the block and the resultant ventricular tachycardia and fibrillation.

Because the arterial supply to the atrioventricular node is derived from a branch of the right coronary artery, acute MI resulting from occlusion of this artery may give rise to heart block. This occurs because the resultant ischemia from the coronary occlusion alters the normal function of the atrioventricular node. Although the heart block associated with acute MI usually resolves, these patients are candidates for prophylactic, temporary pacemakers. Occasionally, permanent pacemaking is required.

In patients undergoing repair of damaged valves or septal defects, or complex intra-atrial repairs associated with congenital heart disease, postoperative heart block may occur. Not uncommonly, such blockade does not manifest immediately after operation. Because cardiac surgeons have encountered this situation with sufficient frequency, temporary pacing wires are routinely placed in these patients at the time of surgery, so that external pacing can be administered rapidly should circumstances necessitate this approach.

Chronic sinus bradycardia is typically referred to as the *sick sinus syndrome*. In this condition, heart rates in the range of 30 to 40 beats/min are characteristic. Although sudden cardiac death is much less likely than with complete heart block, the symptoms are essentially the same. The bradycardia is usually regular but can on occasion be irregular, and it typically occurs in older patients, many of whom have ischemic heart disease, although this is not a requirement for the syndrome to occur. Permanent pacemaking is usually required in patients with this condition.

Although chronic atrial fibrillation is effectively managed medically in most patients, significant bradycardia can at times occur, necessitating pacemaker placement. It must be determined, however, that the bradycardia is not related to digitalis toxicity before a pacemaker is placed. This can be determined by stopping the digoxin therapy to see whether the bradycardia is resolved.

In patients with the bradycardia-tachycardia syndrome, profound episodes of supraventricular tachycardia requiring digoxin prophylaxis produce profound symptomatic bradycardia related to the digoxin therapy necessary to manage tachycardia. The explanation for this effect is not clear, but the treatment of this syndrome requires the placement of a pacemaker to enable the administration of sufficient doses of digoxin to manage the tachycardia.

Pacemaker Placement

When pacemakers were first introduced approximately 40 years ago to manage cardiac dysrhythmias, they were placed in the left side of the chest through a formal thoracotomy. The pacemakers were large and heavy, and the pacing leads were sutured to the ventricular myocardium. Furthermore, the batteries needed to operate these pacemakers were generally short-lived and required replacement at least every 2 years, often more frequently. In addition, the lead systems were undependable. Much progress has been made in the development of pacemakers during the last several decades, so that current pacemakers approach the size and weight of a silver dollar, use lithium batteries that have life spans of 10 or more years, and possess lead systems that are remarkably dependable.

Current pacemaker management makes use of both epicardial and endocardial methodologies. The epicardial approach employs a subxiphoid access to the pericardium in which the lead is screwed into the undersurface of the right ventricle and the battery box itself is implanted subcutaneously, usually in the left upper abdominal quadrant. This technique requires general anesthesia for the lead placement, but the battery box can easily be replaced with local anesthesia. The endocardial approach employs a catheter system that uses the cephalic, subclavian, or jugular vein, through which the catheter tip is advanced and impacted into the apex of the right ventricle. In this circumstance, the battery box is implanted in a subcutaneous pocket inferior to the clavicle. Compared with the epicardial approach, this strategy of pacemaker management is less dependable, requires more time to position the pacemaker, and is associated with a small but real hazard of perforating the right ventricle. Its major advantage with respect to the epicardial approach is that it can be carried out entirely with local anesthesia. These two approaches are schematically represented in Fig. 41-10.

A wide variety of pacemakers are presently available. Despite their current level of sophistication compared with older models, they all fire on "demand" when they do not sense a QRS complex. They all have the capability to be programmed for such modalities as rate, size of electrical impulse, and sensing level after implantation. In recent years, there has been a trend toward dual-chamber pacemakers that pace the atria and ventricles sequentially as well as pacemakers that sense changes in the native sinus rate (in response to a stimulus such as exercise) and thereby change the rate of ventricular firing. These newer systems, although expensive, have been demonstrated to be extremely beneficial in the vast majority of pacemaker candidates, particularly for patients with exercise intolerance or chronic congestive heart failure.

Not all patients with dysrhythmias require cardiac pacemaker implantation. Guidelines for the use of pacemakers are summarized in the box on p. 843.

Evaluation of Pacemakers Before Attempting Surgery

In patients about to undergo general anesthesia and surgery, it is mandatory that the surgical and anesthesia teams determine that the pacemaker is sensing and functioning normally. After the pacemaker has been properly identified, the currently active program can be retrieved by interrogation with the manufacturer's programmer. The first issue is to identify whether the patient is pacemaker dependent. If the pacemaker fails, does it have a dependable and adequate intrinsic rhythm? If the answer to this question is no or cannot be determined because the pacemaker is not programmable, a backup method of main-

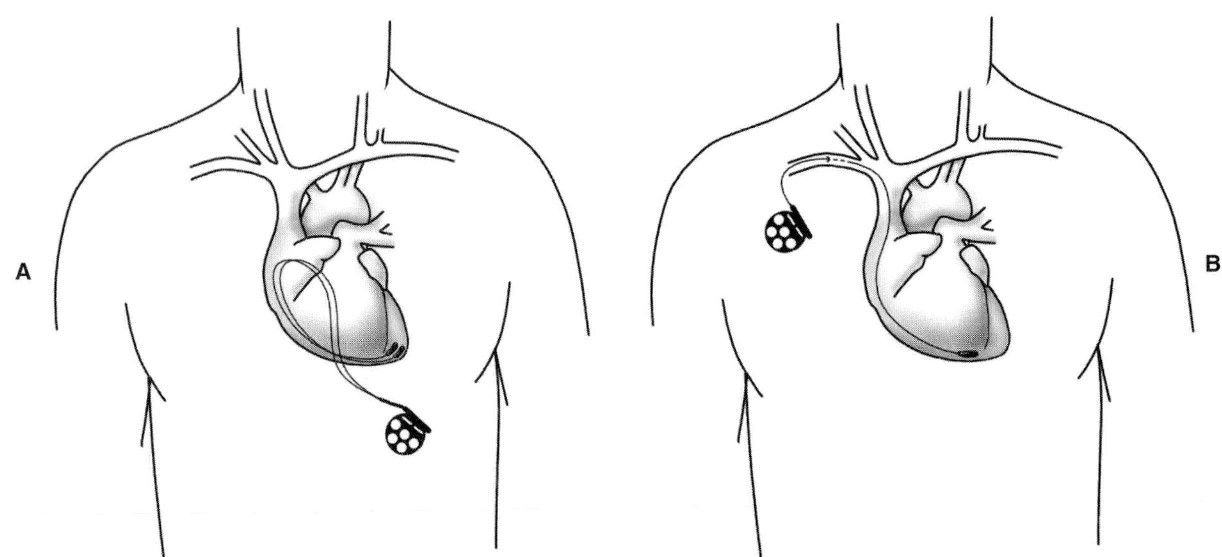

Fig. 41-10. Schematic representation of the two approaches currently used for pacemaker placement. **A,** *Epicardial approach* employs subxiphoid access in which pacemaker lead is secured to undersurface of right ventricle and battery box is implanted subcutaneously in left upper abdominal quadrant. **B,** *Endocardial approach* uses subclavian (or cephalic or jugular) vein for access in which pacemaker tip is impacted into apex of right ventricle and battery box is implanted subcutaneously inferior to clavicle.

taining a heart rate must be defined. This is particularly important because electrocautery can induce pacemaker failure. Most pacemaker manufacturers recommend against use of electrocautery in any patient without an adequate intrinsic rhythm. Unipolar cautery is far more hazardous than bipolar cautery. Electrocautery can, by its noise level, be misinterpreted by the pacemaker and cause inhibition of the pacemaker that is reversible when the cautery is turned off. Thus, frequently, electrocautery can cause the pacemaker to revert to a backup mode. This usually is a ventricular demand mode. The most severe problem the electrocautery may cause is complete and permanent loss of pacing. The best way to manage a pacemaker during the use of electrocautery is to program the generator to ventricular demand mode at a rate sufficient to minimize competition with the intrinsic heart rate. The simplest way to achieve this is to place a permanent magnet over the pacemaker. This prevents inhibition by electrocautery.

If a permanent loss of pacemaker function occurs in the operating room, with no intrinsic heart rate, the quickest and most efficient method of inducing an intrinsic rate is to begin intravenous infusion of a β-stimulant, such as isoproterenol. After this maneuver, a temporary transvenous pacemaker should be inserted.

GUIDELINES FOR CARDIAC PACEMAKER IMPLANTATION

Accepted

In patients with symptoms and chronic conditions

Atrioventricular block
- Complete (third-degree)
- Incomplete (second-degree)
  - Mobitz type I (rare indication)
  - Mobitz type II
- Incomplete with 2:1 or 3:1 block

Sinus node dysfunction (symptomatic)
- Sinus bradycardia
- Sinoatrial block, sinus arrest
- Bradycardia-tachycardia syndrome

Controversial

In patients with symptoms

Bifascicular/trifascicular intraventricular block
Hypersensitive carotid sinus syndrome

In patients without symptoms

Third-degree block
Second-degree atrioventricular block Mobitz type II
Transient complete or Mobitz type II atrioventricular block with bundle-branch block in selected situations (e.g., acute myocardial infarction)
Congenital atrioventricular block
Sinus bradycardia with heart rates <45 beats/min, with long-term drug therapy necessary
Overdrive pacing for ventricular tachycardia

Not Warranted

Syncope of undetermined cause
Sinus bradycardia, sinoatrial block, or sinus arrest without symptoms
Bundle-branch blocks
Mobitz type I block (asymptomatic)

Modified from AMA Council on Scientific Affairs. The use of cardiac pacemakers in medical practice. JAMA 254:1952, 1985.

Tachycardias

In addition to problems with bradycardia, tachycardias can also pose difficulties that may require surgical intervention if medical management is not efficacious.

Supraventricular Tachycardias

Supraventricular arrhythmias, the most common rhythm disturbances encountered in surgical practice, usually occur in the postoperative period. Typical arrhythmias of this variety include atrial flutter, paroxysmal atrial tachycardia, and atrial fibrillation. The diagnosis of these dysrhythmias is made with ECG testing. Most of these disturbances can be managed medically with drugs such as verapamil, digoxin, and diltiazem, or with combinations of these agents. On rare occasions, such medical management does not prove efficacious, and because of the rapid ventricular rate emanating from these dysrhythmias, emergency cardioversion is required.

A more worrisome supraventricular tachycardia that does not respond as well to medical management is the Wolff-Parkinson-White (WPW) syndrome. This disorder is caused by reentry of cardiac excitation impulses through an anomalous muscle bundle, known as the bundle of Kent, that connects the atrial and ventricular myocardia, which are normally electrically separate (Fig. 41-11). This bundle has been demonstrated in a variety of positions in the atrioventricular groove or junction of the atrial and ventricular septa, having been previously mapped experimentally. The seriousness of this condition is that the Kent bundle can conduct as many as 400 beats/min with degeneration into ventricular responses characterized by tachycardia or fibrillation, with the potential for cardiac arrest. On ECG, patients with the WPW syndrome demonstrate a short PR interval (less than 0.12 seconds) and small delta waves at the beginning of the QRS complex. Although a wide variety of antiarrhythmic drugs have been used to manage this syndrome (including procaine, quinidine, propranolol, verapamil, and amiodarone), such therapy has not proved especially successful. Fortunately a means of ablating the Kent bundle surgically is now available. First introduced at Duke University in 1968, this modality has proved efficacious, and many patients treated with interruption of the Kent bundle have had successful outcomes and have gone on to live normal lives. Recent experience with catheter-delivered radiofrequency ablation of the Kent bundle has also proved effective and has supplanted the surgical approach.

The success encountered with treating the WPW syndrome surgically has been extended to other mechanisms of tachycardia, such as concealed accessory connections,

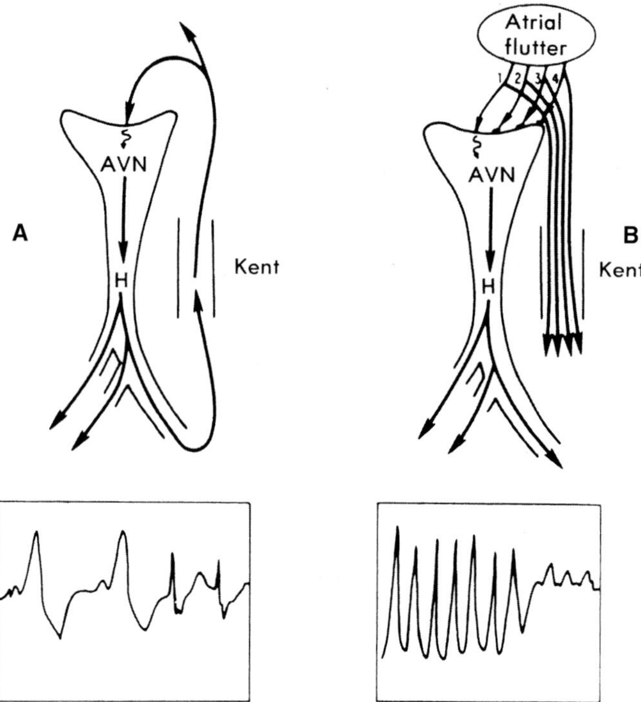

Fig. 41-11. Two tachycardias found in patients with WPW syndrome are shown. **A,** Reentry type. The wide QRS of preexcitation changes to a narrow QRS during the reentry tachycardia *(box).* **B,** Fast ventricular response during atrial flutter. The rhythm strip shows the rapid ventricular response progressing to ventricular fibrillation *(box).* (From Sealy WC, Selle JG. Surgical treatment of supraventricular arrhythmias. In Roberts AJ, Conti CR, eds. Current Surgery of the Heart. Philadelphia: JB Lippincott, 1987. Used with permission.)

nodal and atrial tachycardia, and even refractory atrial fibrillation. Treatment of this last arrhythmia, the maze procedure, consists of a series of atrial incisions to prevent atrial reentry and allow sinus node impulses to activate the entire atrial myocardium. In so doing, this procedure restores atrioventricular synchrony.

Ventricular Tachycardia

Ventricular dysrhythmias are much more serious than supraventricular tachycardias because of the rate-induced depression of CO that can degenerate into life-threatening ventricular fibrillation. Most patients with sustained ventricular tachycardias have significant ischemic heart disease and have had one or more MIs, resulting in varying degrees of both reversible and nonreversible ischemic damage. Among patients surviving MI, significant ventricular tachycardias may occur in as many as 5%. Despite the recent development of new antiarrhythmic drugs, approximately one third of patients with ventricular tachycardia do not have adequate control with them.

In this subset of patients, "mapping" the various areas of the epicardium and endocardium that induce ventricular tachycardias electrically and then resecting this area has proved efficacious in controlling the ventricular dysrhythmias. The mapped areas usually comprise subendocardial scar tissue that, from a surgical standpoint, are relatively easy to resect unless vital structures such as the mitral apparatus, membranous septum, and aortic annulus are involved in the scarred area. In such cases, local cryoblation has been substituted and proved useful.

Although the risk associated with this type of surgery is substantial, it is directly related to the degree of left ventricular function. The less dysfunction, the better is the outcome. As many as 70% to 80% of patients surviving this type of surgery have relief of their tachycardia without the need for further drug therapy or have substantial reduction in the drug requirements to manage their ventricular dysrhythmias.

Implantable cardioverter-defibrillator. Patients who have had a documented cardiac arrest (sudden cardiac death syndrome) in the absence of a documented MI within the preceding 48 hours and who are not candidates for antiarrhythmic drug therapy, as documented by electrophysiologic study, should have an implantable cardioverter-defibrillator (ICD) implanted. This device, which is similar in size to a pacemaker, is implanted to sustain any cardioversions for several years.

Candidates for ICD placement usually have severe coronary artery disease and prior MI. The infarction zone provides the scarring and slow conduction needed for the reentrant arrhythmias (ventricular tachycardia or ventricular fibrillation). As expected, this patient population is in extremely debilitated condition, with low ejection fractions and chronic congestive heart failure. Consequently, these patients are good candidates for ICD insertion, rather than long-term antiarrhythmic drug therapy, which is associated with negative inotropic effects.

This type of therapy is extremely expensive ($12,000 to $20,000 per generator; $2000 to $8000 per lead system). It is, however, worthwhile for selected individuals at high risk.

PERICARDIAL DISEASE

The *pericardium* is a fibrous sac that surrounds and envelops the heart. Its purpose is to fix the heart anatomically within the mediastinum, act as a barrier to the spread of infection from surrounding structures such as the lungs, and reduce friction between the enclosed heart and surrounding organs. In the nondiseased state, the pericardium has little or no effect on cardiac hemodynamics. Two specific pericardial disorders, however, may necessitate surgical intervention. These include pericardial effusion with tamponade and chronic constrictive pericarditis.

Pericardial Effusion With Tamponade

Pericardial effusion by itself is not uncommon. It can occur in response to acute viral pericarditis, MI, congestive heart failure, and various immune disorders, such as rheumatoid arthritis and lupus erythematosus. In these conditions, the effusion is usually moderate and self-limited, and it abates with treatment of the underlying condition. In patients with chronic uremic pericarditis or malignant involvement of the pericardium, such as may occur from neoplastic spread of bronchogenic carcinoma, excessive amounts of effusion may collect in the pericardial sac so that adverse stresses are placed on the contracting heart and cardiac dynamics are severely impaired. This state of pericardial tamponade can significantly compress the heart, not only by compressing the great veins and atria with substantial reduction of venous return to the ventricles but also by impeding the optimal filling of the ventricles during diastole, so that CO is severely depressed despite normal systolic function.

The fluid accumulating in the pericardial sac that gives rise to tamponade may be serous or sanguineous, depending on the underlying cause. Inflammatory disorders, such as viral infections or immune diseases, usually result in a serous fluid. Liquid or clotted blood within the pericardium is commonly associated with uremic pericarditis, as well as with malignant pericardial involvement. Occasionally, the pericardial sac fills with blood after cardiac surgery but this is rare with modern cardiovascular procedures if proper postoperative drainage techniques are employed. Cardiac trauma from penetrating injury, and rarely from blunt trauma, may also produce pericardial tamponade. In these settings, the pericardium is normal and a relatively small volume of blood (as little as 150 to 200 ml) may produce the tamponade, in contrast to those sustaining tamponade from more chronic pericardial disease, in which the volume may approach 1 L or more of fluid before symptoms develop. Although uncommon, trauma from within the heart as a result of a perforating transvenous pacemaker lead or the placement of a central venous pressure or Swan-Ganz catheter can produce unsuspected tamponade. Thus, any patient who becomes hypotensive for unknown reasons in the presence of one of these devices may have a cardiac perforation.

The clinical presentation of pericardial tamponade is usually characterized by a triad of physical signs, including arterial hypotension, increased jugular venous pressure, and distant (or muffled) heard sounds. Facial cyanosis may also be present, as well as a paradoxic pulse. This latter sign is a drop in arterial blood pressure of 10 mm Hg or more with inspiration. It is usually an exaggeration of the normal response to ventilation and is distinctly more prominent in individuals subjected to positive-pressure ventilation.

In patients with suspected pericardial tamponade, management depends on "how tight" the effusion is. This tightness is reflected in the degree of hypotension and elevation of venous pressure from the tamponade. In individuals with only moderate tamponade, a Valsalva maneuver is helpful in determining its seriousness. If palpable radial pulses are not lost with a Valsalva maneuver, the situation is not critical. Another useful approach to determine the seriousness of the tamponade is to test a patient's blood pressure response to a rapid infusion of intravenous fluid. If the tamponade is only moderate, a significant rise in arterial blood pressure should occur from this fluid bolus; in contrast, more serious degrees of tamponade blunt this response. The presence of an unexplained supraventricular dysrhythmia is a sign of significant tamponade and of the potential for incipient circulatory failure, especially if intermittent sinus arrest exists.

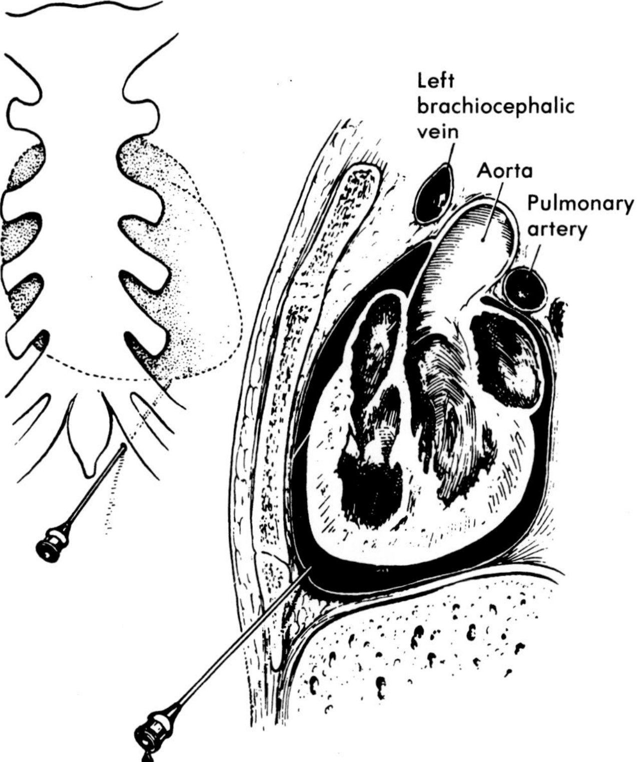

Fig. 41-12. For pericardiocentesis, a 16-gauge plastic-sheathed needle is introduced beneath the costal margin and passed through the properitoneal fat and into the pericardial cavity through the tendinous part of the diaphragm. (From Edwards EA, Malone PD, Collins JJ Jr. Operative Management of the Thorax. Philadelphia: Lea & Febiger, 1972. Used with permission.)

It is essential in the analysis of suspected pericardial effusion that an echocardiogram be obtained. This modality is extremely useful in patients with pericardial effusions and potential pericardial tamponade. An echocardiogram can determine the location and characteristics of the fluid (loculated or free floating) and also ascertain to a reasonable extent whether the pericardial tamponade is of physiologic significance. In addition, it can be used to guide the insertion of a needle into the pericardial space to aspirate fluid, especially if this is deemed to be the appropriate treatment.

Once significant tamponade has been deemed to exist, fluid drainage may be accomplished percutaneously by pericardiocentesis with either a needle or catheter placement (Fig. 41-12). Alternatively, surgical intervention through a subxiphoid pericardial window can be performed. Situations in which traumatic hemopericardium exists require a sternotomy or thoracotomy for optimal management. It needs to be emphasized that if the tamponade is considered to be of only modest proportions and is not life-threatening, great care should be taken to determine the benefit of the pericardiocentesis. This technique, although useful in urgent tamponade, can result in cardiac puncture and actually worsen the situation.

An important principle in managing a patient with tamponade is that endotracheal intubation should be avoided. The reason for this is that positive-pressure ventilation frequently causes cardiac arrest in individuals with significant tamponade. Consequently, preparation and draping in the operating room should be carried out prior to induction of anesthesia and intubation, so that rapid decompression may be achieved in the event that it becomes necessary.

A generous subxiphoid window, instead of formal pericardiectomy, is usually adequate to decompress the pericardial sac in patients with uremic or malignant pericardial tamponade. After removal of the subxiphoid bone, the pericardium is opened between two silk stitches and the window is created. The fluid is aspirated and sent for appropriate cultures while the pericardium is formally sampled for biopsy. An angled chest tube is placed within the pericardial cavity along the diaphragmatic surface and exits through a separate stab-wound incision in the skin. This tube is removed when the drainage ceases. Although pericardial effusions can recur after subxiphoid window, this is distinctly uncommon.

Chronic Constrictive Pericarditis

Chronic constrictive pericarditis is the other condition of surgical significance involving the pericardium. This form of pericarditis is produced in response to chronic infectious tuberculosis and histoplasmosis, various collagen-vascular diseases, and, less commonly, after what appears to be uncomplicated cardiac surgery or MI, with the development of Dressler's syndrome (characterized by fever, pericardial friction rub and pain, and often pericardial effusion). The pericardial-epicardial scarring can be severe, with obliteration of the pericardial space, thickening of the pericardium (sometimes as much as 1 inch or more), and severe fibrosis and calcifications in which calcific deposits may actually grow in the myocardium. Pathophysiologically, this massive pericardial thickening induces several aberrations, including obstruction of venous return with severe diastolic cardiac dysfunction. Physical signs attendant on this condition are similar to those of severe congestive heart failure with elevated venous pressure, edema, hepatomegaly, and ascites. If calcification is not apparent on chest radiography, the diagnosis may not be evident. Cardiac catheterization is usually diagnostic. This latter modality usually shows small ventricular cavities, diastolic pressures within 5 mm Hg of each other, jugular venous distention with measured mean arterial pressures above 10 mm Hg, and the typical "dip and plateau" pattern of diastolic right ventricular pressure (the square-root sign).

Because surgical management of chronic constrictive pericarditis can be difficult and dangerous, and it may tax the skill of the most accomplished cardiac surgeon, a median sternotomy incision should be used with cardiopulmonary bypass. The absence of an epicardial-pericardial plane can make this procedure bloody. Therefore, a cell saver and aprotinin should be employed. Careful attention must be paid to freeing the atria and venae cavae, as well as the ventricles, with recognition of the fact that the visceral pericardial layer may be as important as the parietal layer. This visceral pericardiectomy is complicated by the occasional "invasion" of the ventricular myocardium itself by calcific deposits. The pericardium should be removed from the phrenic nerve anteriorly, but it also should be removed posterior to the phrenic nerve. Complete removal of the constricting pericardium restores the left ventricular pressure volume loop to normal or nearly normal. Operative mortality rate for this procedure ranges between 10% and 20% and is adversely influenced by the severity of heart failure, elevation of right atrial pressure, and comorbid disease. Long-term results are poorest in patients with radiation pericarditis, and in all cases results vary primarily in proportion to the preoperative severity of heart failure.

CARDIAC TUMORS

The most common tumor of the heart is a metastatic neoplasm. Approximately 10% to 20% of patients who die of disseminated cancer have cardiac metastases. The most common tumors to metastasize to the heart are from leukemia (50% of these patients have cardiac metastases), breast cancer, lung cancer, lymphoma, and melanoma. Metastatic disease to the heart usually does not warrant surgical intervention, except if it is associated with pericardial effusion and tamponade. Pericardial drainage is best accomplished in these terminally ill patients through subxiphoid pericardiotomy. This operation is performed with local anesthesia and provides reliable relief of symptoms, a recurrence rate of 3%, and minimal morbidity.

Primary tumors of the heart are rare. The incidence ranges between 0.002% to 0.19%. Approximately 75% of primary cardiac tumors are benign, and 15% of these are myxomas. Although myxomas can arise in any cardiac chamber, 90% occur in the atria; 75% are observed in the left atrium and 15% to 20% are found in the right atrium. Myxomas are distinctly rare in children. The peak incidence is the third to fourth decade of life, they are more common in women than in men, and 94% are solitary. About 5% of myxomas are familial, with an autosomal dominant inheritance. Familial patients tend to be younger, are equally likely to be male or female, and frequently have multicentric tumors. Most important, familial myxomas have the highest recurrence rate (20% to 60%).

Atrial myxomas arise from the interatrial septum near the oval fossa. Right atrial myxomas are most common in women and are broad based. Left atrial tumors are round, lobulated, gelatinous, and frequently pedunculated with a stalk. Consequently, they are quite mobile. Their color is usually white or yellow-brown, and they frequently are covered with thrombus. The average size is 5 cm. Myxomas arise from endocardium, not from a thrombotic origin as was formerly speculated. Myxomas have developed after cardiac trauma, especially atrial septal defect closure.

Constitutional symptoms include weight loss, fever, and lethargy. This clinical presentation is associated with leukocytosis, elevated sedimentation rate, thrombocytopenia, and elevated C-reactive protein. Immunoglobulin G levels and interleukin-6 are also elevated.

Clinical presentation is related most commonly to obstruction to blood flow within the heart. Left atrial myxomas mimic mitral stenosis or, less commonly, mitral regurgitation. Right atrial myxomas produce features of right heart failure, including venous distention, ascites, hepatomegaly, and peripheral edema.

Systemic embolization, the second most common mode of presentation, occurs in 30% to 40% of patients. Most commonly the tumor embolus goes into an intracranial vessel, producing a transient ischemic attack or complete stroke. Less commonly, embolization to the lower extremity occurs. Histologic examination of surgically removed peripheral emboli can establish a diagnosis of an otherwise unsuspected tumor.

The most useful diagnostic test is echocardiography, which establishes a diagnosis in nearly every case. Transesophageal echocardiography is particularly sensitive to detect small tumors, and it can be useful in the operating room to make certain that the entire mass has been removed.

Surgical resection employs cardiopulmonary bypass and bicaval cannulation, with care taken to avoid manipulation of the heart because myxomas are friable and can embolize. After aortic cross-clamping and cardioplegic arrest, the left atrium is opened widely, and the location of the myxoma is determined. In most cases, it is attached with a stalk to the interatrial septum. A second incision in the right atrium allows excision of the stalk with the atrial septum, followed by gentle removal of the mass through the left atrium. The surgically created atrial septal defect is closed with autologous pericardium. The operative mortality rate is 1% to 3%, and the recurrence rate in nonfamilial cases is 1% to 5%.

SUMMARY

Aberrations in normal cardiac function can occur when disease adversely affects cardiac rate and rhythm, the efficiency of cardiac pumping, and the optimization of cardiac loading. Acting either alone or in various combinations, derangements in each of these activities can seriously affect circulatory dynamics throughout the body and thereby jeopardize adequate delivery of oxygen and nutrients to ensure cellular health and function. Although most acquired cardiac defects lend themselves to nonsurgical management strategies, the cardiac surgeon still plays a key role in restoring disturbed physiology to a normal or nearly normal condition. As reviewed in this discussion, both ischemic heart disease and valvular heart disease are commonly best managed with modern surgical techniques to reroute blood to ischemic myocardium and improve the pumping capability of the four cardiac chambers by either repairing diseased valves or replacing them with suitable substitutes, respectively. Less commonly, surgical expertise may also prove useful in managing various dysrhythmias, pericardial problems, or cardiac tumors. Despite the need for surgical intervention, and the conditions in which it may prove useful, the goal of the surgeon is the same as that of the medical counterpart, namely to restore the function of the heart to as nearly normal as possible when its intrinsic performance has failed to meet this expectation.

REFERENCES

1. Berne RM. The role of adenosine in the regulation of coronary blood flow. Circ Res 47:807, 1980.
2. Robertson RM, et al. Thromboxane A_2 in vasotonic angina pectoris. N Engl J Med 304:998, 1981.
3. McGill H. Risk factors for atherosclerosis. Adv Exp Med Biol 104:273, 1977.
4. The Lipid Research Clinics Program. The Lipid Research Clinics coronary primary prevention trial results: II. The relationship of reduction in incidence of coronary heart disease to cholesterol lowering. JAMA 251:365, 1984.
5. Flaherty JT, et al. A randomized prospective trial of intravenous nitroglycerin in patients with acute myocardial infarction. Circulation 54:766, 1976.
6. European Cooperative Study Group for Streptokinase Treatment in Acute Myocardial Infarction. Streptokinase in acute myocardial infarction. N Engl J Med 301:797, 1979.
7. Fry ETA, Sobel BE. Coronary thrombosis. Prog Cardiol 2:199, 1990.
8. Tiefenbrunn AJ, Sobel BE. The impact of coronary thrombolysis on myocardial infarction. Fibrinolysis 3:1, 1989.
9. TIMI Study Group. Results of thrombolysis in myocardial infarction (TIMI) phase II trial. N Engl J Med 320:618, 1989.
10. Maisel AS, et al. Prognosis after extension of myocardial infarct: The role of W wave on non-Q wave infarction. Circulation 71:211, 1985.
11. Allen BS, et al. Studies on prolonged acute regional ischemia IV. Myocardial infarction with left ventricular failure. J Thorac Cardiovasc Surg 98:691, 1989.
12. Daggett WM, et al. Improved results of surgical management of postinfarction ventricular septal rupture. Ann Surg 196:269, 1982.
13. King SB III, Talley JD. Coronary arteriography and percutaneous transluminal coronary angioplasty: Changing patterns of use and results. Circulation 79(Suppl 1):19, 1989.
14. Myers WO, et al. Medical versus early surgical therapy in patients with triple-vessel disease and mild angina pectoris: A CASS registry study of survival. Ann Thorac Surg 44:471, 1987.
15. Detre KM, et al. Long-term mortality and morbidity results of the Veterans Administration randomized trial of coronary artery bypass surgery. Circulation 72(Suppl 5):84, 1985.
16. Varnauskas E, The European Coronary Surgery Study Group. Twelve-year follow-up of survival in the randomized European coronary surgery study. N Engl J Med 319:332, 1988.
17. Gundry SR, et al. Retrograde continuous warm blood cardioplegia: Maintenance of myocardial homeostasis in humans. Ann Thorac Surg 55:358, 1993.
18. Grove FL, et al. Factors predictive of operative mortality among coronary artery bypass subsets. Ann Thorac Surg 56:1296, 1993.
19. Barbir M, et al. Coronary artery surgery in women compared with men: Analysis of coronary risk factors and in-hospital mortality in a single centre. Br Heart J 71:408, 1994.
20. Lytle BW, et al. The effect of coronary reoperation on the survival of patients with stenoses in saphenous vein bypass grafts to coronary arteries. J Thorac Cardiovasc Surg 105:605, 1993.

21. Braunwald E, Rutherford JD. Reversible ischemic left ventricular dysfunction: Evidence for the hibernating myocardium. J Am Coll Cardiol 8:1467, 1986.
22. Yeager M. Comparison of Doppler derived pressure gradient to that determined at cardiac catheterizatin in adults with aortic valve stenosis: Implications for management. In Weyman AE, ed. Principles and Practice of Electrocardiography. Philadelphia: Lea & Febiger, 1994, p 525.
23. Gorlin R, Gorlin SG. Hydraulic formula for calculation of area of stenotic mitral valve, other cardiac valves, and central circulatory shunts. Am Heart J 41:1, 1951.
24. Lombard JT, Selzer A. Valvular aortic stenosis. Clinical and hemodynamic profile of patients. Ann Intern Med 106:292, 1987.
25. Olesen KH, Warburg E. Isolated aortic stenosis—The late prognosis. Acta Med Scand 160:437, 1957.
26. Copeland JB, et al. Long-term follow-up after isolated aortic valve replacement. J Thorac Cardiovasc Surg 74:875, 1977.
27. Carabello BA, et al. Hemodynamic determinants of prognosis or aortic valve replacement in critical aortic stenosis and advanced congestive heart failure. Circulation 62:42, 1980.
28. Fifer MA, et al. Myocardial contractile function in the aortic stenosis as determined from the rate of stress development during isovolumic systole. Am J Cardiol 44:1318, 1979.
29. Kennedy JW, Doces J, Stewart DK. Left ventricular function before and following aortic valve replacement. Circulation 56:944, 1977.
30. Pantely G, Morton M, Rahimtoola SH. Effects of successful, uncomplicated valve replacement on ventricular hypertrophy, volume and performance in aortic stenosis and in aortic incompetence. J Thorac Cardiovasc Surg 75:383, 1978.
31. Miller DS, et al. Surgical implications and results of combined aortic valve replacement and myocardial revascularization. Am J Cardiol 43:494, 1979.
32. Safian RD, et al. Balloon aortic valvuloplasty in 170 consecutive patients. N Engl J Med 319:169, 1988.
33. Olson LJ, Subramanian R, Edwards WD. Surgical pathology of pure aortic insufficiency: A study of 225 cases. Mayo Clin Proc 59:835, 1984.
34. Alpert JS. Chronic aortic regurgitation. In Dalen JE, Alpert JS, eds. Valvular Heart Disease, 2nd ed. Boston: Little, Brown, 1987, p 283.
35. Rapaport E. Natural history of aortic and mitral valve disease. Am J Cardiol 35:221, 1975.
36. Borow K, et al. End-systolic volume overload from valvular regurgitation. Am J Med 68:655, 1980.
37. Bonow RO, et al. Survival and function results after valve replacement for aortic regurgitation from 1976 to 1983: Impact of preoperative left ventricular function. Circulation 72:1244, 1985.
38. Greves J, et al. Peroperative criteria predictive of late survival following valve replacement for severe aortic regurgitation. Am Heart J 101:300, 1981.
39. Lytle BW, et al. Replacement of aortic valve combined with myocardial revascularization: Determinants of early and late risk for 500 patients. 1967–1981. Circulation 68:1149, 1983.
40. Rankin JS. Mitral and tricuspid valve disease. In Sabiston DC Jr, ed. Textbook of Surgery: The Biological Basis of Modern Surgical Practice, 13th ed. Philadelphia: WB Saunders, 1992, p 2026.
41. Braunwald E. Valvular heart disease. In Braunwald E, ed. Heart Disease. A Textbook of Cardiovascular Medicine. Philadelphia: WB Saunders, 1992, p 1007.
42. Bowe JC, et al. Course of mitral stenosis without surgery: 10 and 20 year perspectives. Ann Intern Med 52:741, 1960.
43. Thompson ME, Shaver JA, Leon DT. Effect of tachycardia on atrial transport in mitral stenosis. Am Heart J 94:297,1977.
44. Olesen KH. The natural history of 271 patients with mitral stenosis under medical treatment. Br Heart J 24:349, 1962.
45. Munoz S, et al. Influence of surgery on the natural history of rheumatic mitral and aortic valve disease. Am J Cardiol 35:234, 1975.
46. Cutler EC, Levine SA. Cardiotomy and valvulotomy for mitral stenosis: Experimental observations and clinical notes concerning an operated case with recovery. Boston Med Surg J 188:603, 1923.
47. Souttar HS. The surgical treatment of mitral stenosis. Br Med J 2:603, 1925.
48. Harken DE, et al. The surgical treatment of mitral stenosis. N Engl J Med 239:801, 1948.
49. Baily CP. The surgical treatment of mitral stenosis (mitral commissurotomy). Dis Chest 15:377, 1949.
50. Ellis LB, Harken DE. Closed valvuloplasty for mitral stenosis. A twelve-year follow-up of 1571 patients. N Engl J Med 270:643, 1964.
51. Montoya A, et al. The advantages of open mitral commissurotomy for mitral stenosis. Chest 75:131, 1979.
52. Higgs LA, et al. Mitral restenosis: An uncommon cause of recurrent symptoms following mitral commissurotomy. Am J Cardiol 26:34, 1970.
53. Harken DE, et al. Reoperation for mitral stenosis. A discussion of postoperative deterioration and methods of improving mitral and secondary operation. Circulation 23:7, 1961.
54. Kirklin JW, Barrett-Boyes BG. Mitral valve disease without tricuspid valve disease. In Cardiac Surgery, 2nd ed. New York: Churchill Livingstone, 1993, p 425.
55. Smith WM, et al. Open mitral valvotomy: Effect of preoperative factors on result. J Thorac Cardiovasc Surg 82:738, 1981.
56. Inoue K, et al. Clinical application of transvenous mitral commissurotomy by a new balloon catheter. J Thorac Cardiovasc Surg 87:394, 1984.
57. Nishimura RA, Holmes DR Jr, Reeder GS. Percutaneous balloon valvuloplasty. Mayo Clinic Proc 65:198, 1990.
58. Tuzcu EM, Block PC, Palacios IF. Comparison of early versus late experience with percutaneous mitral balloon valvuloplasty. J Am Coll Cardiol 17:1121, 1991.
59. Block PC. Early results of mitral balloon valvuloplasty (MBV) for mitral stenosis: Reports from the NHLBI Registry. Circulation 78(Suppl 2):II489, 1978.
60. Nobuyoshi M, et al. Indications, complications and short-term clinical outcomes of percutaneous transvenous mitral commissurotomy. Circulation 80:782, 1989.
61. Stapleton JF. Natural history of chronic valvular disease. In Frankl WS, Brest AN, eds. Cardiovascular Clinics. Valvular Heart Disease: Comprehensive Evaluation and Management. Philadelphia: FA Davis, 1986, p 105.

SUGGESTED READINGS

Surgery for Cardiac Dysrhythmias

Belott PH, Reynolds DW. Permanent pacemaker implantation. In Ellenbogen KA, Kay GN, Wilkoff BL, eds. Clinical Cardiac Pacing. Philadelphia: WB Saunders, 1995, p 447.

Bocker D, et al. Do patients with an implantable defibrillator live longer? J Am Coll Cardiol 21:1638, 1993.

Bonnet CA, Fogoros RN. Clinical experience with antiachycardia pacing. In Ellenbogen KA, Kay GN, Wilkoff BL, eds. Clinical Cardiac Pacing. Philadelphia: WB Saunders, 1995, p 744.

Ellenbogen KA, Kay GN, Wilkoff BL, eds. Clinical Cardiac Pacing. Philadelphia: WB Saunders, 1995.

Furman S, Schwedel JB. An intracardiac pacemaker for Stokes-Adams seizures. N Engl J Med 261:948, 1959.

Guiraudon GM, et al. Encircling endocardial ventriculotomy: A new treatment for life-threatening ventricular tachycardia. Ann Thorac Surg 26:438, 1977.

Harken AH, Josephson ME, Horowitz LN. Surgical endocardial resection for the treatment of malignant ventricular tachycardia. Ann Surg 190:456, 1979.

Kim SG, et al. Long-term outcomes and modes of death of patients related with nonthoracotomy implantable defibrillators. Am J Cardiol 75:1229, 1995.

Levine PA, et al. Electrocautery and pacemakers: Management of the paced patient subject to electrocautery. Ann Thorac Surg 41:313, 1996.

Lowe JL, Sabiston DC. The surgical management of cardiac arrhythmias. J Cardiovasc Surg 1:1, 1986.

May CD, et al. The impact of implantable cardioverter defibrillator on quality of life. PACE Pacing Clin Electrophysiol 18:1411, 1995.

Mirowski R, et al. Termination of malignant ventricular arrhythmias with an implantable automatic defibrillatory in human beings. N Engl J Med 303:322, 1980.

Morse DP, et al. A Guide to Cardiac Pacemakers, Defibrillators and Related Products. Durham, N.C.: Droege Computing Services, 1991.

Phibbs B, et al. Indications for pacing in the treatment of bradycardia. JAMA 252:1307, 1984.

Sealy WC, Anderson RW, Gallagher JJ. Surgical treatment of supraventricular tachyarrhythmias. J Thorac Cardiovasc Surg 73:511, 1977.

Strathmore NF. Interference in cardiac pacemakers. In Ellenbogen KA, Kay GN, Wilkoff BL, eds. Clinical Cardiac Pacing. Philadelphia: WB Saunders, 1995, p 539.

Weirich WL, Gott VL, Lillihei CV. Treatment of complete heart block by the combined use of myocardial electrode and an artificial pacemaker. Surg Forum 8:360, 1958.

Zipes DP, Roberts D. Results of the international study of the implantable pacemaker cardioverter-defibrillator. A comparison of epicardial and endocardial lead systems. Circulation 92:59, 1995.

Pericardial Disease

Blalock A, Burwell CS. Chronic pericardial disease. Surg Gynecol Obstet 73:433, 1941.

Caccavale RJ, et al. Pericardial disease. In Kaiser LR, Daniel TM, eds. Thoracoscopic Surgery. Boston: Little, Brown, 1993, p 177.

Dressler W. The post-myocardial infarction syndrome. Arch Intern Med 103:28, 1959.

Guberman B, et al. Cardiac tamponade in medical patients. Circulation 64:40, 1981.

Hancock EW. Diseases of the pericardium, cardiac tumors, and cardiac trauma. Sci Am Med 13:1, 1997.

Seifer FC, et al. Surgical treatment of constrictive pericarditis: Analysis of outcome and diagnostic error. Circulation 72 (Suppl 2):II264, 1985.

Shabetai R. The pericardium. New York: Grune & Stratton, 1981.

Cardiac Tumors

Bortolotti U, et al. Surgical excision of intracardiac myxomas: A 20-year follow-up. Ann Thorac Surg 49:449, 1990.

Burke AP, Virmani R. Cardiac myxoma: A clinicopathologic study. Am J Clin Pathol 100:671, 1993.

Castells E, et al. Cardiac myxomas: Surgical treatment, long-term results and recurrence. J Cardiovasc Surg 34:49, 1993.

Ensberding R, et al. Diagnosis of heart tumors by transesophageal echocardiography. Eur Heart J 14:1223, 1993.

Farrah MG. Familial cardiac myxoma: Study of patients with myxoma. Chest 105:65, 1994.

Harvey WP. Clinical aspects of cardiac tumors. Am J Cardiol 21:328, 1968.

Heath D. Pathology of cardiac tumors. Am J Cardiol 21:315, 1968.

Miralles A, et al. Cardiac tumors: clinical experience and surgical results in 74 patients. Ann Thorac Surg 52:886, 1991.

Murphy MC, et al. Surgical treatment of cardiac tumors: A 25 year experience. Ann Thorac Surg 49:612, 1990.

Reynen K. Cardiac myxomas. N Engl J Med 333:1610, 1995.

Silverman NA. Primary cardiac tumors. Ann Surg 191:127, 1980.

Thomas CR, et al. Primary malignant cardiac tumors: Update 1992. Med Pediatr Oncol 20:519, 1992.

PART FOUR

THE URINARY SYSTEM

42

Physiology of Urine Formation

Alan S. Tonnesen

The kidney serves three major functions. First, it maintains fluid and electrolyte homeostasis, which is considered briefly in this chapter and discussed more fully in Chapter 2. Second, the kidney functions as an endocrine organ; it produces the active metabolite of vitamin D and erythropoietin and also serves as both a target organ and an organ of catabolism for various peptide hormones. Third, the kidney is an organ of excretion for certain intermediate and end products of metabolism, and for several drugs. Because of the central role of the kidney in metabolic processes, it is not surprising that renal failure is characterized by protean clinical manifestations.

OVERVIEW OF FLUID AND ELECTROLYTE HOMEOSTASIS

In healthy individuals, remarkable constancy exists in the total amount of fluid, electrolytes, and solutes in the body as a whole, as well as in the individual compartments within the body. This constant internal environment is maintained by rapid adjustments in the rates of excretion of solutes and waste material in response to wide variations in the rates of intake and body metabolism. The amount and composition of the fluid in the cells differ from those of the extracellular fluid. The ionic composition and volume of the cells are maintained by specific ion pumps and channels in the cellular membranes. Although critical to survival of the organism, these transport processes are not considered further in this chapter, except as they pertain to vectorial transport of fluids and solutes by the kidney.

The kidney in healthy persons is the major organ of regulation for control of fluid and electrolyte balance. Its ability to accomplish this is manifested by the fact that variations in intake of several orders of magnitude result in no change in the amount of fluid or electrolytes in the body and no alteration in the composition of either the fluid or cellular compartments of the body. This concept is illustrated schematically in Fig. 42-1.[1-3] In an individual ingesting or receiving 100 mEq sodium daily, the 24-hour urinary excretion is also 100 mEq. When such an individual decreases the intake of sodium to 10 mEq or increases it to ≥200 mEq daily, a rapid adjustment in excretion occurs so that input and output are matched. The transient net gains or losses of sodium in healthy individuals are clinically insignificant. Unlike sodium, water is lost and gained from the body by nonrenal routes. Nonetheless, the major adjustments to altered intake of water are mediated by alterations in the rate of urinary excretion. The same general schema holds for other electrolytes. General, as well as specific, mechanisms modulate the renal response to alterations in intake and permit maintenance of overall balance.

The operation of such feedback systems involves sensor and effector mechanisms. Many processes exist for detecting changes in the amount or composition of fluid compartments of the body. Sensors for alterations in the extracellular fluid volume, for example, are located within the heart, great blood vessels, and central nervous system; they have also been found experimentally in the liver, gastrointestinal tract, and the kidney itself. Perturbations in volume or composition of the extracellular fluid result in changes in the levels of systemic and locally produced hormones and nerve traffic to the kidney, which affect the renal transport of fluid and electrolytes. As discussed later, the renal response is modulated in specific subsegments of the nephron that are responsive to these stimuli. Renal mechanisms regulate the rates of absorption and secretion of specific solutes and water. Mechanisms that affect the rates of transport of several electrolytes, nonelectrolytes, and water simultaneously have also been identified.

RENAL PHYSIOLOGY

Renal Blood Flow

The kidneys account for 0.5% of the total body mass but receive 20% to 25% of the total cardiac output. This high rate of blood flow in relation to renal mass is necessary to support glomerular filtration but far exceeds the normal metabolic needs of the kidney. The distribution of blood

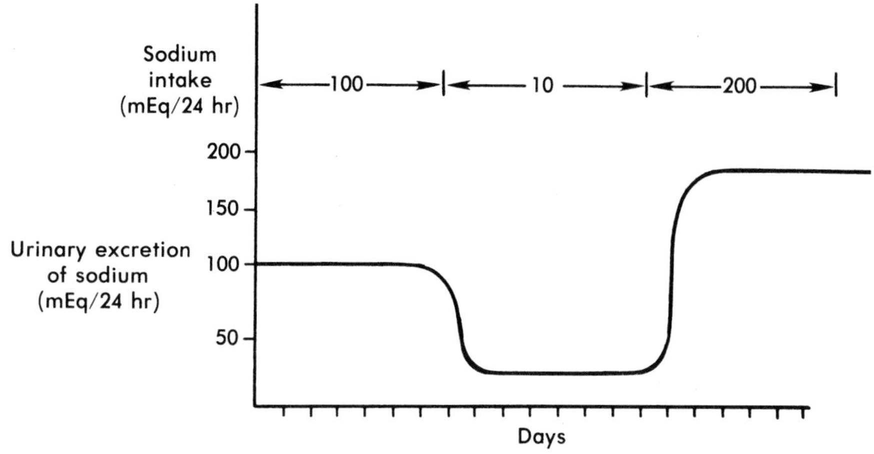

Fig. 42-1. Influence of sodium intake on urinary excretion of sodium.

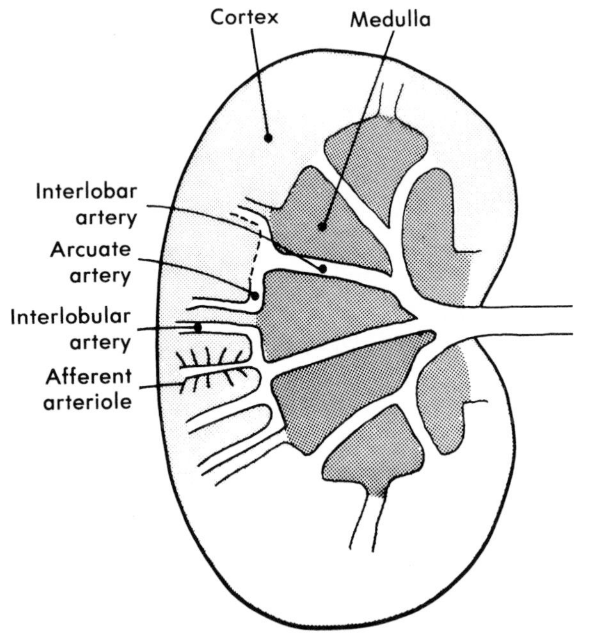

Fig. 42-2. Schematic representation of the major arterial renal vasculature.

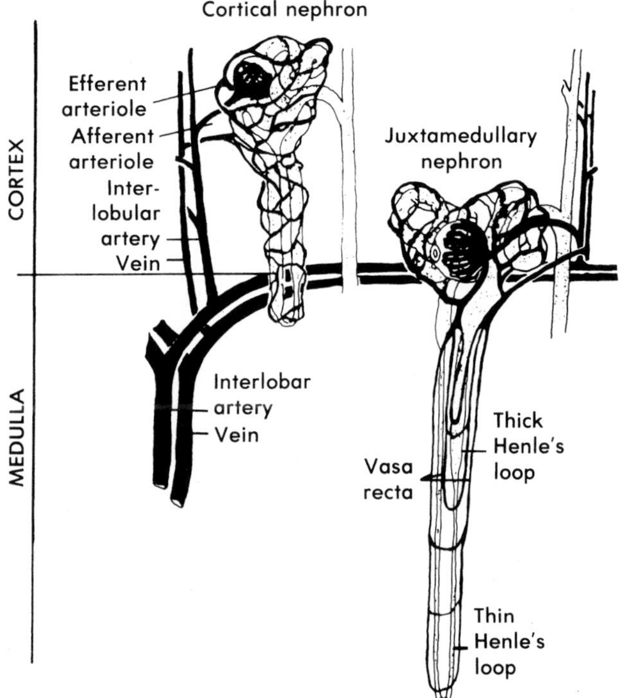

Fig. 42-3. Schematic comparison of the postglomerular vasculature of the superficial and juxtamedullary nephrons. Note the vasa recta arising from the juxtamedullary efferent arteriole. The density of the vasculature becomes progressively less as it descends into the medulla. (Modified from Pitts RF. Physiology of the Kidney and Body Fluids. Chicago: Year Book, 1974.)

flow within the kidney roughly parallels the distribution of glomerular filtration: highest in the superficial cortex and diminishing progressively toward the medulla.[4]

Anatomy

The renal artery (or arteries) enters the kidney at the hilum (Fig. 42-2). The main renal artery divides into branches, forming interlobar arteries. At the level of the corticomedullary junction, the interlobar arteries divide to form the arcuate arteries, which travel parallel to the renal surface. The interlobular arteries arise from the arcuate arteries and subsequently divide into the afferent arterioles. The afferent arteriolar smooth muscle cells form circumferential rings. These arterioles break up into the glomerular capillary tufts, reunite to form the efferent arteriole, and, as they surround the renal tubules, become the peritubular capillaries (Fig. 42-3). In superficial nephrons, peritubular capillary surrounds the proximal tubule of the nephron of origin. The peritubular capillaries of the deeper nephrons do not necessarily arise from the glomerulus of the same nephron. The proximal tubules of juxtamedullary nephrons are perfused by efferent vessels of midcortical nephrons. Efferent vessels of juxtamedullary nephrons form endothelial or sphincter types.[5] Those of the endothelial type have thin walls and perfuse the loops of Henle and collecting tubules of the outer medulla. Those of the sphincter type have long, muscular efferents and extend deeper into the medulla. The smooth muscle cells are irregular and form incomplete layers. Juxtamedullary efferent arterioles divide into vasa recta. The vasa recta descend in parallel with Henle's loops and form an anastomosing system that becomes progressively less dense from the outer to the inner medulla. The peritubular capillaries and vasa recta empty into the interlobular veins. These drain to the arcuate veins, which finally join to form the renal veins.[4]

Medullary flow originates from the efferent arterioles of the juxtamedullary nephrons.[6] The medulla is divided into an outer and an inner zone. The outer zone is subdivided into an outer (adjacent to the cortex) and an inner stripe. The descending vasa recta are formed near the junction of the outer and inner stripe of the outer medulla.[6] The descending vasa recta coalesce into a vascular bundle. The capillary network surrounding the tubules in the outer stripe of the outer medulla is supplied primarily by branches from the efferent arteriole[6] and is relatively sparse. The inner stripe is occupied mainly by the thick ascending limbs and is supplied only by the vasa recta.[6] Capillaries in the inner stripe form ascending vasa recta, which do not join the vascular bundles and thus do not form a countercurrent circuit.[6] The inner medulla is supplied by the descending vasa recta. Thus, the blood reaching the inner medulla has not perfused tubules.[6] The proximal descending vasa recta are surrounded by smooth muscle cells, a prominent basement membrane, and a thick continuous endothelium.[5] The endothelium of the ascending vasa recta is thinner, similar to that of most other capillaries.[5] Capillaries of the inner medulla form ascending vasa recta, which enter the vascular bundles before passing through the outer medulla. The flow through the ascending vasa recta exceeds descending vasa recta flow by the amount of fluid reabsorbed, and ascending vasa recta outnumber descending vasa recta by more than 2:1. Ascending flow may exceed descending flow by 30% to 300% depending on the state of antidiuresis.[5] This exposes blood from the inner medulla to a countercurrent relationship with blood from the inner stripe.[5] Although this is useful for maintaining the corticomedullary solute concentration gradient, it also reduces oxygenation of the blood entering the inner medulla.[6] The oxygen tension of the medulla is only about 10 mm Hg, and it is associated with a reduced redox state of the medullary cells.[6] These capillary-like vasa recta are susceptible to compression by cellular swelling. Accordingly, these relationships contribute to the severe ischemic damage to the third segment of the proximal tubule and the thick ascending limb cells that are located

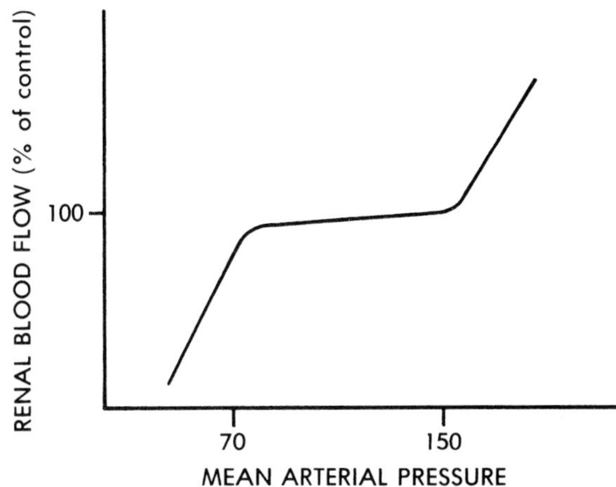

Fig. 42-4. Autoregulation of renal blood flow. As the mean systemic arterial pressure varies over wide ranges, the renal blood flow remains relatively constant.

predominantly in the outer and inner stripe of the outer medulla. Distribution of resistance along the renal vascular bed is believed to be approximately 25% prior to the afferent arteriole, 50% along the afferent arteriole, and 30% along the efferent arteriole.[7]

Regulation of Blood Flow

Renal blood flow (RBF) manifests the property of *autoregulation* (Fig. 42-4), a term that describes the constancy of RBF in the face of changes in mean arterial pressure ranging from 70 to 180 mm Hg. The mechanism of autoregulation has not been totally clarified. The myogenic theory postulates that in response to an increase in pressure, the afferent arteriole vasoconstricts. Thus, the resistance in the afferent arteriole increases and RBF is held constant. Others have suggested that the tubuloglomerular feedback (TGF) mechanism and renal nerves also are necessary for complete and efficient autoregulation.

Plasma flow to the cortex averages 2.0 ml/g tissue/min and accounts for approximately 90% of the total renal plasma flow. The outer medulla receives about 1.0 ml/g tissue/min and accounts for about 9% of the total renal plasma flow. Blood flow to the inner medulla accounts for only about 1% of total renal plasma flow.[8-10] The relative distribution of RBF between the cortex and medulla is under metabolic control and may vary under different conditions. During water diuresis, RBF increases, but a relatively greater increase in flow occurs to the outer medulla than to the cortex. Increased sodium intake tends to elevate outer cortical blood flow, with less influence on inner cortical flow. The mechanisms controlling the intrarenal distribution of blood flow are not completely clarified, but they may include the sympathetic nervous system, the renin-angiotensin system, prostaglandins, and antidiuretic hormone (ADH).

Autoregulation is an intrinsic myogenic property of the preglomerular vessels, especially the afferent arteriole, and appears to control as much as 40% of the preglomerular resistance.[7,11,12] The myogenic theory of autoregulation postulates that the afferent arteriole constricts from an inherent stretch mediated response if pressure increases. It has been proposed that flow-induced vasodilation plays a role in response to falling perfusion pressure.[6] As pressure falls, the decreasing rate of fluid delivery to the distal nephrone will invoke TGF-mediated vasodilation (see later discussion). The resulting increased shear stress may induce further vasodilation by an endothelium-dependent action. The vasoconstrictive responses of the interlobular and arcuate vessels depend on the presence of blood, as demonstrated experimentally by the absence of vasoconstriction when perfused in vivo with blood-free solution. This latter response is dependent on an intact endothelium, leading to speculation that the endothelium itself functions as the stretch transducer. Others have suggested that renal nerves are necessary for complete and efficient autoregulation. Autoregulation is impaired in hypertensive patients and animals,[6] and after renal ischemia. The clinical consequence is that such patients require a higher than normal blood pressure to sustain normal renal blood flow.

TGF is the phenomenon of reduced glomerular plasma flow and GFR induced by an increased rate of delivery of sodium chloride to the macula densa cells of the distal tubule. It appears to be responsible for about 25% of renal vascular tone.[12] TGF and autoregulation interact. When the TGF mechanism is overwhelmed by rapid tubular flow (e.g., fluid loading, diuresis), autoregulation is intact. When TGF is inactivated by absence of tubular flow, however, renal plasma flow falls passively as perfusion pressure falls.[12] The clinical analogies of this situation are urinary tract obstruction and intratubular obstruction after tubular necrosis. If the set point of the TGF mechanism changes, the position of the autoregulatory myogenic curve also changes. Both dopamine and adenosine are found in distal tubular fluid and influence TGF reactivity from the luminal side. Dopamine-1 agonists inhibit and adenosine-1 receptor stimulation increases TGF reactivity. High dietary salt intake stimulates secretion of dopamine and inhibits adenosine secretion by the proximal tubule. Both effects depend on an adrenal product.[12] TGF is blunted when intravascular volume is acutely or chronically expanded, and it is enhanced when depleted. Pharmacologic doses of atrial natriuretic peptide also attenuate TGF-mediated decreases in RBF induced by either hypertonic saline solution infusion or adenosine infusion.[13] The overall response to increased volume status is to inhibit TGF-mediated decreases in RBF and GFR. This probably facilitates excretion of a volume load.

Renal sympathetic nerve activity (RSNA) or norepinephrine causes α_1-mediated vasoconstriction, with some preference for the afferent arteriole. α_2-Agonists cause intracellular cyclic adenosine monophosphate (cAMP) levels to increase, which may blunt the vasoconstriction.[14] Although RSNA seems to decrease cortical flow more than medullary flow, renal denervation causes a marked increase in inner medullary flow, suggesting basal adrenergic-mediated vasoconstriction. RSNA provides a mechanism for rapid response to changes in cardiovascular performance. RSNA suppression should theoretically protect the vulnerable medullary circulation during ischemic or hypoxic periods. RSNA may be suppressed by subarachnoid or subdural local anesthetics, and to a lesser extent by volatile inhalational anesthetics and acute spinal cord injury.

Various chemical mediators also influence RBF. Angiotensin II (AII) increases efferent tone more than afferent tone and medullary more than cortical tone. The renal vasoconstrictor response occurs at levels of AII lower than required to elicit systemic vasoconstriction.[15] The effects are direct and may also relate to increased norepinephrine release and potentiation of adenosine-induced vasoconstriction.[7] The effects of AII are blunted by prostaglandins. The renal vasoconstriction induced by salt restriction is related to AII. AII reduces inner medullary flow in doses that do not change total RBF. In addition, the juxtaglomerular nephrons appear to be more sensitive to AII than are superficial nephrons. This may be related to the release of prostacyclin I_2 (PGI_2) in the superficial nephrons. Medullary vessels may be constricted in the basal state by AII, as indicated by an increase in medullary flow during angiotensin-converting enzyme inhibition or AII-receptor blockade.[5]

Vasopressin contracts the vasa recta by a V1-receptor–mediated mechanism. Stimulation of V2 receptors may also contribute indirectly to constriction.[5,7] Despite this action, superficial cortical flow tends to fall more than medullary flow. This should facilitate the formation of a concentrated urine by increasing the proportion of the GFR derived from juxtamedullary nephrons.

Adenosine has complex effects on renal vascular resistance (RVR). Acute administration decreases RBF, but chronic infusion causes vasodilation. In isoflurane-anesthetized rats, adenosine induced systemic hypotension but did not change RVR.[16] When adenosine was used to treat post–coronary bypass hypertension, RBF fell by 44% because of a mean blood pressure reduced to 80 mm Hg but vasodilation failed to occur; that is, RVR remained constant. The ratio of preglomerular to postglomerular RVR increased as indicated by a reduction of filtration fraction.[17] GFR and filtration fraction fall regardless of effects of RBF, indicating an increase in the ratio of afferent to efferent arteriolar tone.[7] Adenosine appears to potentiate the vasoconstrictive effect of AII on the afferent arteriole.[7] The effects of adenosine can be blocked by theophylline.[7] Adenosine receptors present in the inner medulla appear to cause vasodilation independent of effects elsewhere in the kidney.[5] Renal ischemic insults leading to adenosine generation have the potential to cause a positive-feedback cycle of increasing ischemia. Indeed, animal experiments suggest a protective role for 8-phenyltheophylline in ischemic acute renal failure.

Prostaglandins do not control resting RBF, but they blunt the vasoconstrictive effects of most or all renal vasoconstrictors. This is associated with an increase in intracellular cAMP.[14,15] PGI_2 (prostacyclin) has a half-life of about 3.5 minutes. Bradykinin, substance P, arachidonate, thrombin, interleukin-1, platelet-derived growth factor, and adenine nucleotides stimulate PGI_2 synthesis and release.[18] When prostaglandin synthesis is blocked, total RBF does not fall under normal circumstances. In contrast, the papillary circulation may be under the influence of prostaglandins in the basal state.[5] Patients treated with nonsteroidal anti-inflammatory drugs have lost an important protective mechanism and may be more susceptible to renal ischemia.

Acetylcholine causes vasodilation, especially of the medullary circulation, and increases RBF. Muscarinic receptor stimulation releases endothelial derived-relaxing factor (EDRF).[18,19] Cholinergic fibers accompany the interlobar, arcuate, interlobular arteries, afferent arterioles, and vasa recta.[5] The effects on medullary flow may be mediated by prostaglandin release, because cyclo-oxygenase inhibitors abolish the vasodilation. The physiologic role is uncertain.

Bradykinin is a potent renal vasodilator with a predominant effect on the efferent arteriole and in the papillary circulation.[5] Kallikrein, the enzyme responsible for production of bradykinin, is found in the kidney and is stimulated by aldosterone, AII, and prostaglandins.[7] Despite this, no definite physiologic role for bradykinin has been defined.

Atrial natriuretic peptide (ANP) has the capacity to dilate the afferent and constrict the efferent arteriole, although the net effect on RBF is variable. When the afferent arteriole has been preconstricted, especially by AII, ANP causes vasodilation. The medullary circulation vasodilates in response to ANP.[5] The net effect is to decrease the ratio of afferent to efferent resistance, which leads to an increase in filtration fraction.

Endothelin (ET)[17-20] is a potent vasoconstrictor.[7] It increases renal vascular resistance and decreases GFR and decreases sodium excretion. ET-1 (found in vascular tissue), ET-2 (a more potent vasoconstrictor than ET-1), and ET-3 (possibly neural) species exist. ET receptors are found in vascular smooth muscle, adrenal glomerulosa, glomeruli, and the medullary vasculature. Receptor density is greater in the vasa recta than in the cortex, suggesting a predominant effect on medullary circulation. There are at least two receptor types on vascular smooth muscle. One type, ETA, binds ET-1 and ET-2 but shows only limited binding of ET-3, whereas the other, ETB, binds all three agonists. ET-1 generates inositol triphosphate and diacylglycerol, which increase intracellular calcium concentration. This leads to intense and long lasting vasoconstriction of the efferent (more than the afferent) arterioles and glomerular mesangial cell constriction.[21,22] Thrombin, shear stress, AII, interleukin-1, arginine vasopressin, and epinephrine stimulate ET production. ET also stimulates EDRF and PGI_2 production, causing a counterregulatory loop. ANP, prostaglandin E_2 (PGE_2), PGI_2 and calcium-channel blockade reduce the renal effects of ET. The vasoconstriction of small (but not large) arteries is inhibited by calcium-channel blockade. ET stimulates ANP production and aldosterone and renin release. Injured endothelium generates ET, thromboxane A_2, and AII, which lead to prolonged vasoconstriction. The combination of renal vasoconstriction and glomerular contraction lead to decreased GFR.

EDRF[19,20,23] is nitric oxide (NO) or a closely related substance. Its actions are produced by the enzyme guanylate cyclase. This enzyme also is activated by the nitrovasodilators nitroprusside, nitroglycerin, and nitrates. Some vasodilator agents (acetylcholine, histamine-1 receptor agonists, thrombin, adenosine triphosphate [ATP], bradykinin, AII, α_2-receptor agonists, arachidonic acid) act only in the presence of intact endothelium; that is, they are endothelium dependent. Acetylcholine-induced vasodilation of the efferent arteriole is mediated by NO, whereas afferent dilation is not. Endotoxin and interleukin-1 induce NO production and release. Activation of these receptors increase calcium concentration, which activates type II NO synthase. Similarly, ANP stimulates accumulation of intracellular cyclic guanosine monophosphate independently of the endothelium by activating the particulate form of guanylate cyclase. EDRF has a half-life of only a few seconds; it is destroyed by superoxide anions. EDRF causes vasodilation, inhibits platelet aggregation and adhesion, and potentiates these effects caused by PGI_2. EDRF reduces renin release in vitro and inhibits release of ANP from the cardiac atria. EDRF probably is important in regulating basal RBF, because inhibitors of NO generation reduce RBF.[18] After ischemic renal injury, EDRF-mediated vasodilation is impaired, whereas the vasoconstrictor response to renal nerve stimulation is enhanced, suggesting loss of EDRF production. Inhibition of NO action by hemoglobin and myoglobin may contribute to heme pigment–induced renal failure through the resultant inhibitory effects on vasorelaxation.

Physiologic Significance of Blood Flow Alterations and Distribution

Alterations in RBF may play a role in overall fluid and electrolyte metabolism by the kidney.[9] The glomerular filtration rate (GFR) depends on plasma flow. Alterations in the ratio between the GFR and the renal plasma flow (the filtration fraction) may affect the rates of water and solute absorption in the proximal convoluted tubule. Alterations in RBF may be a contributing factor in the concentration-dilution function of the kidney. At least under experimental circumstances, however, changes in RBF can be dissociated from alterations in renal function.

Alterations in the distribution of RBF between the outer and inner zones of the kidney have also been postulated as factors in the renal excretion of electrolytes. Some have suggested that the long-looped juxtamedullary nephrons are "sodium-retaining" nephrons, whereas those on the cortex absorb less sodium. Thus, sodium excretion in the urine could be affected by the distribution of RBF through greater or lesser perfusion of salt-retaining or salt-wasting nephrons. Despite some support for this hypothesis, considerable evidence also suggests that alterations in the distribution of RBF are not the sole or even major mechanism in maintaining sodium and water balance.

Glomerular Filtration

The initial process of urine formation is the generation of an ultrafiltrate of plasma across the glomerular capillaries.

Anatomy

Blood enters the glomerular capillaries from the afferent arteriole. The glomerular capillary endothelial cell is the initial barrier encountered by plasma. These endothelial cells are extremely thin, and a large proportion of the surface area is occupied by diaphragmed and unusually large fenestrae (50 to 100 nm),[20] indicating that this potential route of diffusion or convection could sieve only formed elements of blood, not dissolved proteins or electrolytes. Functionally, endothelial fenestrae appear to permit passage of molecules at least as large as 6.1 nm in radius. The glomerular capillary basement membrane lies adjacent to the endothelial cells. This membrane, which is produced by the mesangial cells of the glomerulus, is composed of glycoproteins with fixed negative charges. This charge serves to retard the passage of proteins, which are negatively charged. In addition, the glomerular capillary membrane behaves as if pierced with pores of fixed molecular dimensions. The estimated size of these pores is of such magnitude as to exclude large proteins but not small solutes, and it represents the anatomic correlate of the reflection coefficient (see later discussion).

Thus, the basement membrane excludes macromolecules on the basis of both charge and size. The glomerular capillary basement membrane abuts the processes of the visceral epithelial cells, the podocytes. The physical space between the podocytes is large. The podocytes, however, are also lined by negative charges and thus serve to retard the passage of negatively charged proteins into the proximal tubule.

Filtration Barrier

Because of the anatomic features just outlined, the glomerular capillary filtration apparatus acts as a highly efficient semipermeable membrane system that effectively excludes passage of molecules with a radius greater than 38 to 44 Å but allows ready passage of molecules less than 20 Å.[24] Functionally, endothelial fenestrae appear to permit passage of molecules at least as large as 6.1 nm in radius. The basement membrane excludes molecules larger than 6.1 nm, partially retards passage of those with a radius of 5.2 nm, and is freely permeable to molecules with a radius of 3.0 nm. The foot processes block passage of molecules with radii as small as 3.0 nm. It is important to note that these dimensions do not correspond to clearly identifiable structural pores; rather, they reflect the functional characteristics of the filtration barrier.

Glomerular Dynamics

An understanding of the process of glomerular filtration can be appreciated by considering the components of the modified Starling equation:

$$SNGFR = K_f\,[(HP_{gc} - HP_t) - (OC_{gc} - OC_t)]$$

where *SNGFR* is the single-nephron GFR, *Kf* is the permeability (ultrafiltration) coefficient, which is equivalent to the product of the hydraulic conductivity of the glomerular capillary membranes and the surface area available for filtration, *HPgc* is the hydrostatic pressure in the glomerular capillary bed, *HPt* is the hydrostatic pressure in the most proximal regions of the proximal tubule (Bowman's space), *r* is the reflection coefficient, *OCgc* is the oncotic pressure in plasma perfusing the glomerular capillary apparatus, and OC_t is the oncotic pressure of the tubular filtrate. Normally, OC_{gc} is equal to 22 to 25 mm Hg at the arteriolar end of the glomerular capillary bed, and OC_t is essentially zero. The reflection coefficient *r,* ranges from 0 for molecules that cross the membrane as easily as water to 1.0 for molecules larger than about 50. The ultrafiltration coefficient (K_f) is directly proportional to surface area and hydraulic conductivity. In rats, it is 2 to 5 nl/min/mm Hg, although the variability of this estimate is quite high.[25] The glomerular capillary endothelial cell, the basement membrane, and podocytes of the visceral epithelial cells form a semipermeable membrane.

Contractile mesangial cells are connected to the basement membrane.[14] These cells can contract and decrease the K_f in response to ET-1,[5,7,20] arginine vasopressin, AII, sympathetic nerve stimulation, norepinephrine, and thromboxane.[26] This response is associated with a rise in cytosolic calcium. Dopamine, α_2-agonists, EDRF,[20] and PGE_2 increase intracellular cAMP and relax mesangial cells.[14]

The net ultrafiltration pressure gradient is equal to the mean hydrostatic pressure gradient minus the mean oncotic pressure gradient as the plasma traverses the glomerular capillary from the afferent to the efferent arteriole[27] (Fig. 42-5). The hydrostatic pressure in the proximal tubule remains relatively constant. The glomerular capillary pressure drops by only a few millimeters of mercury as it traverses the capillary bed. As a result, the hydrostatic gradient from capillary to Bowman's space is relatively constant from the afferent to the efferent end of the arteriole. By contrast, however, the oncotic pressure (from protein concentration) in the glomerular capillary rises as water is removed from the capillary space. The concentration of protein, and thus the oncotic pressure, is higher in the efferent than in the afferent arteriole. The oncotic pressure in the tubular fluid is zero.

The net ultrafiltration pressure gradient at any point along the glomerular capillary is equal to the difference between the hydrostatic pressure gradient and the oncotic pressure gradient (see Fig. 42-5). The net ultrafiltration pressure is greatest at the afferent arteriolar end of the glomerulus where the oncotic pressure is lowest, and becomes progressively lower as the oncotic pressure rises. Fil-

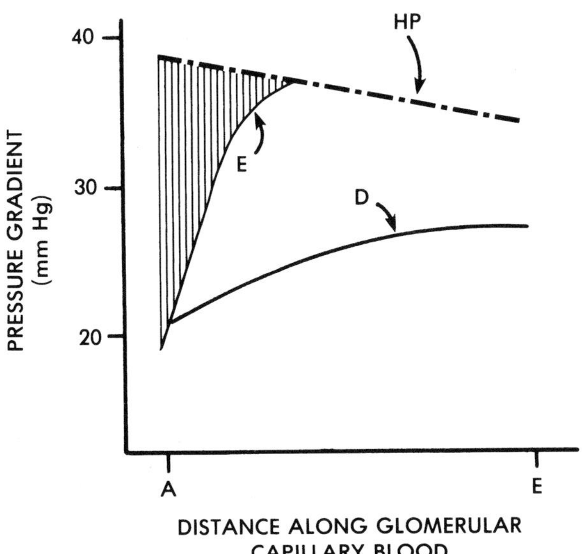

Fig. 42-5. Effect of glomerular plasma flow on the mean ultrafiltration pressure gradient. *A* represents the afferent arteriolar end of the glomerular capillary bed, whereas *E* represents the efferent arteriolar end. The *HP* line is the hydrostatic pressure gradient; that is, the difference between glomerular hydrostatic pressure and the pressure in the early proximal tubule. Curves *E* and *D* on the graph represent the rise in colloid osmotic pressure as plasma passes from *A* to *E*. The vertically shaded area limited by curve *E* and *HP* on the graph is proportional to the mean ultrafiltration gradient during states of low flow, when filtration equilibrium exists. The area limited by curves *D* and *HP*, which is obviously much larger, represents the gradient during high glomerular plasma flow, when filtration disequilibrium exists. Thus, high glomerular plasma flow maintains a higher mean ultrafiltration pressure gradient, supporting a higher GFR. (Modified from Maddox DA, Brenner BM. Glomerular filtration of fluid and macromolecules: The renal response to injury. Annu Rev Med 28:91, 1977. Reprinted with permission from the Annual Review of Medicine, © 1977 by Annual Reviews, Inc.)

tration can proceed until the oncotic pressure in the glomerular capillary becomes equal to the hydrostatic pressure gradient. The net pressure for ultrafiltration across the entire glomerulus is thus determined by the geometric mean of the difference between the hydrostatic pressure gradient curve and the oncotic pressure gradient curve (see Fig. 42-5).

Glomerular plasma flow does not at first appear to be represented in the Starling equation. Glomerular plasma flow is a critical determinant of the GFR, however, and determines both the hydrostatic and the oncotic pressure gradients. A consideration of the effects of extreme examples gives an indication of the importance of glomerular plasma flow in determining the rate of filtration.

As illustrated in curve *E* of Fig. 42-5, the efferent arteriole may be considered as nearly closed. In this circumstance, a net pressure gradient for ultrafiltration exists at the afferent arteriolar end of the capillary, and filtration proceeds. Initially, the net gradient for ultrafiltration is high, but as the macromolecules in the glomerular capillary plasma are rapidly concentrated by loss of filtered water, the oncotic pressure rises to a level that ultimately equals the hydrostatic pressure gradient. Filtration equilibrium is thus attained, and the entire potential surface area for filtration is not used. If the efferent arteriole is now released momentarily, and a fresh bolus of plasma is allowed to enter, ultrafiltration occurs. It continues until the ultrafiltration pressure gradient is again reduced to zero.

By extrapolating to normal conditions, one can thus appreciate that the total rate of filtration (the GFR) depends heavily on plasma flow rate. This dependency derives from progressive displacement of the equilibrium pressure point toward the efferent end of the capillaries. In other words, with no change in hydraulic conductivity, increases in the rate of glomerular capillary blood flow recruit greater areas of the capillary for filtration.

In contrast to the previous circumstance, an alternative situation exists in which glomerular plasma flow is high, as shown by curve *D* in Fig. 42-5. If the rate of plasma flow is high enough that filtration equilibrium is not obtained by the efferent end of the glomerulus, the entire filtering surface area is used for ultrafiltration, and the rate of filtration depends less on glomerular plasma flow. As Fig. 42-5 indicates, the areas between the hydrostatic pressure gradient curve and the oncotic pressure gradient curve are greatly different in states of low and high plasma flow. The shaded areas between the two curves represent the total ultrafiltration pressure gradient acting to cause filtration across the glomerular capillary bed. Thus, the higher is the glomerular capillary plasma flow, the lower is the oncotic pressure gradient resisting filtration, the higher is the hydrostatic pressure gradient favoring filtration, and the larger the surface area exposed to pressures that favor filtration.

Regulation of Glomerular Filtration Rate

Although the determinants of the GFR are well described, the factors regulating the rates of filtration are still incompletely understood. The two major factors are the glomerular plasma flow and the hydraulic permeability of the filtration barrier. Each of these variables may be affected independently by disease conditions, hormones, and drugs. The GFR filtration exhibits two interesting phenomena, autoregulation and TGF regulation. Autoregulation of the GFR is similar to that observed for RBF. As blood pressure changes across wide ranges, the GFR remains constant. The precise mechanisms responsible have not been as extensively clarified as those involved in autoregulation of RBF. To some extent, autoregulation of RBF helps regulate GFR.

The phenomenon of TGF regulation of GFR is manifested by decreases in the rate of glomerular filtration associated with increases in the rate of flow of tubular fluid through Henle's loop.[28,29] A reduction in the glomerular capillary blood flow and a decrease in hydraulic conductivity account for the reduction in filtration. TGF appears to decrease GFR by vasoconstriction and a reduction in hydraulic conductivity when distal fluid delivery increases,[28,29] such as after furosemide administration.[30] The juxtaglomerular apparatus is the functional link between distal fluid delivery and preglomerular vasoconstriction.[31] The transport of chloride or sodium, or the osmolality of the tubular fluid at a distal nephron site, may be the triggering stimulus. At high distal delivery rates, GFR may be depressed by 50%.[31] TGF leads to a reduction in GFR on infusion of hypertonic saline solution, which increases intravascular volume, and by infusion of adenosine, a proposed stimulatory agent. Conversely, pharmacologic doses of ANP suppress TGF-mediated reductions in GFR.[14] Changes in volume status reset the TGF system; dehydration sensitizes, and volume expansion blunts the response.[14,31] TGF is suppressed in early and hyperactive in later phases of chronic hypertension.[30] Hyperglycemia suppresses TGF sensitivity, leading to increased GFR. The TGF loop operates more efficiently to reduce glomerular filtration when tubular fluid flow increases than to increases filtration in response to reductions in tubular flow. The exact signal initiating the response is still controversial. It has also been proposed that this triggering step is transduced through the renin-angiotensin system to cause alterations in the rate of renal plasma flow. This occurs by presumably altering the tone of the afferent arteriole or by altering the surface area for filtration through a direct effect on the mesangial cells of the glomerulus.

AII and prostaglandins also interact to control GFR. AII leads to a reduction in GFR by reducing RBF and Kf. This is associated with increased PGE_2 production. PGE_2 leads to vasodilation, which may further lower GFR, but it also stimulates release of renin from the afferent arteriole. This causes generation of AII, which then causes efferent arteriolar constriction. This raises HP_{gc}, and thus GFR. Increased protein ingestion also raises RBF and GFR by depressing TGF. Low protein intake potentiates the reduction in GFR induced by high distal flow rates; that is, it potentiates TGF.[31] Glucocorticoids support normal GFR, and pharmacologic doses increase GFR above normal.[32] The effect is caused by increased glomerular plasma flow related to nearly equal reductions in afferent and efferent resistances, at least in rats, but it may cause a decrease in the ratio of afferent to efferent resistance in humans.[32] This may be related to accelerated ANP release or to increased plasma amino acid levels. Steroids also blunt AII-induced constriction.[32] Calcitonin gene–related peptide, but not calcitonin itself, raises GFR and inhibits AII-induced glomerular mesangial cell contraction when infused systemically. Calcitonin gene–related peptide normally is released locally by nerve terminals. Thus, its precise physiologic effect is not known.[33]

Age also affects GFRs. Premature infants have low GFR because of incomplete nephrogenesis and high renin-induced renal vasoconstriction.[34] Nephrogenesis is complete at 34 weeks after conception, with no further nephron addition. GFR declines by approximately 1% per year after the age of 30 years. Explanations include vascular injury, high protein intake, accumulation of subclinical acute injuries, and immune damage. This is not reflected in the serum creatinine because of a parallel reduction in muscle mass.

Drug-induced effects on GFR vary considerably. Calcium-channel antagonists augment GFR in circumstances involving renal vasoconstriction, especially vasoconstriction caused by norepinephrine or AII.[26,30] This occurs because the afferent arteriole dilates more than the efferent arteriole, leading to increased HP_{gc}. Thus, when calcium-channel antagonists are administered, GFR increases to a greater degree than does RBF. GFR usually does not change in normotensive individuals, but it usually increases in hypertensive patients.[30] α_1-Antagonists generally do not change GFR. α_1-Agonists, which cause central sympatholysis, have no consistent effect on GFR. β-Adrenergic antagonists generally cause a reduction of GFR. Angiotensin-converting enzyme inhibitors usually cause GFR to increase.[30] However, if GFR is being supported by AII-induced efferent constriction and blood pressure falls significantly or there is arterial inflow obstruction, GFR may fall despite an increase in RBF.[35] The reduction in GFR is caused by a fall in glomerular capillary pressure related to a disproportionate decrease in efferent arteriolar resistance, despite increased RBF. Nonspecific vasodilators usually cause no change in GFR.[30] In contrast, adenosine generally reduces GFR and urinary flow rate. When adenosine was used to treat hypertension after operations, the GFR fell 52% and urinary flow rate fell by 76%. When used in normotensive patients, RBF (−50%), GFR (−60%) and urinary flow (−78%) all fell. Filtration fraction fell in each group, most likely because of preglomerular vasoconstriction.[17] Nonsteroidal anti-inflammatory agents block the production of prostaglandins. If the renin-angiotensin system has been activated, there may be unopposed vasoconstriction and glomerular constriction, with a marked fall in GFR.[36]

Glomerular Ultrafiltrate

The process of filtration results in the formation of an ultrafiltrate of plasma. This is a solution containing no formed elements and with a greatly reduced protein content. The electrolyte composition of the ultrafiltrate, however, is not identical to that of plasma. Because of the differences in protein content in the glomerular capillary blood as compared with that in Bowman's space, a separation of charge occurs. Anions and cations distribute asymmetrically across this membrane to achieve electrochemical equilibrium. Thus, the concentrations of anions such as chloride are higher and the concentrations of cations such as sodium are lower in the fluid of Bowman's space than in the capillary blood.

Tubular Function

The kidney filters approximately 144 L of fluid daily. The renal tubules reabsorb back into the bloodstream vast quantities of this filtrate (98% to 99.5%) to match the rate of urinary excretion with the rate of fluid intake into the body. In addition, the kidney directly adds certain substances and drugs into the tubular fluid for ultimate excretion. The composition and volume of the glomerular filtrate are progressively altered as it is transported down the length of the nephron.

Physiology of Renal Transport Mechanisms

Renal tubular cells are polar cells with one side facing the tubular fluid (the luminal or apical membrane) and one side facing the interstitium of the kidney and the peritubular capillaries (the basolateral membrane; Fig. 42-6). Vectorial transport in either the absorptive or secretory direction involves the operation of specific transport proteins and ion channels in the given membranes and the permeability properties of the tubule itself. The specialized nature of each nephron segment derives from differences in the types of proteins in the membranes and differences in permeability.

Despite these regional differences, it is worth considering some general factors that account for vectorial transport.[37] First, some transport processes are capable of displacing substances across membranes against an electrochemical gradient, a process known as *active transport.* These processes require the expenditure of metabolic energy. If the transport process directly requires hydrolysis of high-energy compounds, it is termed *primary active transport.* The best example of such a transport process is the sodium-potassium ATPase Na^+-K^+ ATPase enzyme pump located in almost all cells of the body, including the basolateral membrane of renal tubule cells. The activity of this pump accounts for most of the oxygen consumption of the kidney beyond that required for cellular maintenance. This protein serves both an enzymatic role (hydrolysis of ATP) and a transport function. Na^+-K^+ ATPase translocates three sodium molecules out of the cell in exchange for two potassium molecules into the cell. Thus, the pump is electrogenic and results in displacement of charge. Because of the action of Na^+-K^+ ATPase, the concentration of potassium inside the cell is considerably higher than that of plasma. Conversely, the concentration of sodium is lower. The basolateral membrane of renal tubular cells is more permeable to potassium than to sodium. Intracellular potassium diffuses out of the cell down its electrochemical gradient and renders the inside of the cell electronegative.

The electrochemical gradients generated across the membranes of the cells can also be harnessed for the transport of other solutes. This process ultimately requires metabolic energy, but by itself the process does not result in hydrolysis of high-energy compounds. Such a process, if it involves a specific transport protein (mediated transport), is designated as *secondary active transport.* The operation of this type of mechanism can be illustrated by the reabsorption of glucose and the secretion of protons in the proximal convoluted tubule. The luminal membrane of the proximal convoluted tubule contains a transport protein with affinity for sodium and glucose. Both sodium and glucose must be on the carrier protein for the transporter to be active. The energy for the translocation of sodium and glucose from the lumen into the renal cell derives from the electrochemical gradient for sodium across the luminal membrane. Thus, glucose transport, which can be described as a sodium-dependent cotransport system, is a secondary active transport process. The sodium entering the cell through this mechanism is removed across the

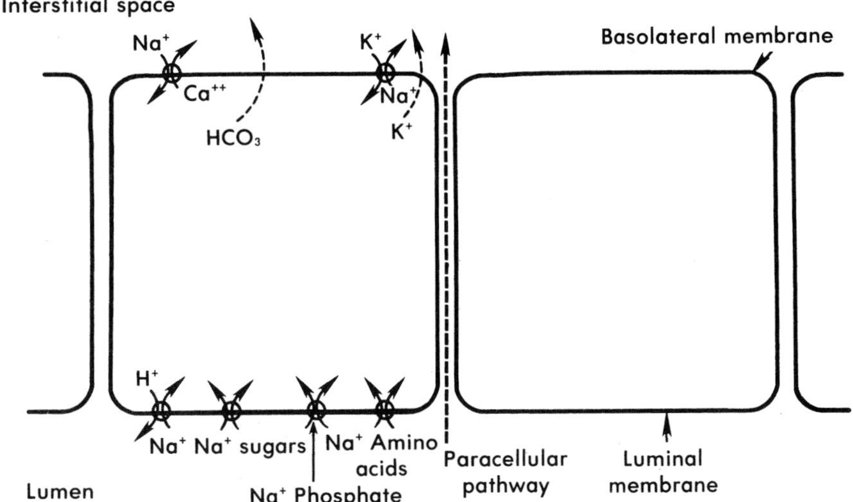

Fig. 42-6. Schematic representation of renal tubular cells. Not all mediated and passive transport pathways are illustrated. Sodium-dependent cotransport systems for sugars, phosphate, and amino acids and the countertransport system for sodium and hydrogen ions in the luminal membrane are shown. Na^+-K^+ATPase and sodium-calcium exchange are illustrated in the basolateral membrane. The *interrupted line* shows passive diffusion pathways for bicarbonate and potassium across the basolateral membrane and for water and some solutes between the cells (the paracellular pathway).

basolateral membrane by the Na^+-K^+ ATPase pump. The glucose is metabolized or exits across the basolateral membrane into the blood. Several other cotransport systems analogous to that of glucose but involving different transport proteins have been described in the brush border membrane of the proximal tubule.[37] Examples include the sodium-dependent phosphate and amino acid transporters that mediate the reabsorption of these solutes from the lumen.

Glucose is normally completely reabsorbed by the proximal tubule by a saturable sodium-glucose cotransporter mechanism. Glucosuria results when glucose delivery to the proximal tubule exceeds the maximal rate of transport (approximately 300 mg/min). The rate of delivery of glucose to the proximal tubule is determined by the plasma level of glucose and the GFR (GFR $\times$ $P_{glucose}$). Certain critically ill patients, such as those with burns and trauma, have markedly elevated GFR and moderately elevated blood glucose, resulting in glycosuria. In the early stages of diabetic nephropathy, glomerular hyperfiltration also leads to a lowered plasma glucose concentration threshold for glycosuria. Amino acids are essentially completely absorbed by the proximal tubule by the organic acid cotransport system. Tubular damage increases the quantity of amino acid lost in the urine, contributing to negative nitrogen balance.

The electrochemical gradient for sodium can also be used for sodium-dependent counter-transport systems. Counter transporters (antiporters) require the presence of both sodium and another molecule, but as sodium moves into the cell, down its concentration gradient, the other molecule is removed from the cell. In the proximal tubule, hydrogen ion generated by the cell exchanges for sodium in the lumen. This sodium-proton counterexchanger is also a secondary active transport process. Another well-described countertransport system is the sodium-calcium countertransporter. This transport protein is probably located in the basolateral membrane of the cell.

In addition to cation transport systems, anion-exchange transport systems have been identified in various segments of the nephron and appear to be located in the brush border and basolateral membranes. These transport systems are important in the renal excretion of organic metabolites such as urate and oxalate. An organic base transport system has also been identified. In distal nephron segments, a hydrogen ion ATPase has been located that is important in the renal excretion of acid. Finally, membranes of renal tubule cells also have finite passive permeabilities to electrolytes and nonelectrolytes. The movement of electrolytes and nonelectrolytes by diffusion is governed by electrochemical driving forces and the permeability of the membrane to the solute.

The presence of and the factors controlling the activity of specific transport proteins, whether primary pumps, cotransporters, countertransporters, or ion channels in specific nephron segments, are areas of great investigational interest and research. The location of specific transport proteins is segregated in specific nephron segments, a finding that permits specialization of function along the length of the nephron. In addition, the amount and activity of these transport proteins are under metabolic control.

Thus, in the final analysis, input to the kidney from peripheral sensors or drugs alters the rates of transport within cells of the renal tubules directly by changing the activity or amount of the transporters or indirectly by altering critical electrochemical gradients across the cell membranes. It is important to note, however, that in certain nephron segments, particularly the proximal tubule, fluid and electrolytes can "back-leak" from the interstitium into the lumen through a paracellular pathway between the cells. In such "leaky" epithelia, the rates of back-leak may have important effects on the net rates of transport.

Absorptive and Secretory Functions of Renal Tubules

Several organizational levels of renal tubules exist. The nephron can be subdivided into subsegments, each of which differs in morphology, function, and response to drugs, hormones, and other stimuli. This is termed *axial heterogeneity.* Differences also may exist in the function of anatomically similar segments in superficial nephrons compared with juxtamedullary nephrons; this has been termed *internephronal heterogeneity.* Although internephronal heterogeneity may be of some physiologic importance, it is useful to view the kidney as a single nephron, as illustrated in Fig. 42-7. As glomerular filtrate courses along the nephron, its composition and volume are progressively altered by the presence of the transport processes in the cells of the subsegment, the relative concentration gradients across the membranes of the cells, and the paracellular pathways. Each nephron segment receives tubular fluid different in composition from that in the preceding segment.[38]

Proximal convoluted tubule. The proximal convoluted tubule reabsorbs approximately 60% of filtered sodium and water. The osmolality of the fluid in the proximal tubule is nearly isotonic with plasma. Sodium is reabsorbed by the sodium-dependent cotransport and countertransport processes described earlier and by the diffusion of sodium into the cell. The sodium entering the cell ultimately is removed from the cell by the Na^+-K^+ ATPase pump in the basolateral membrane. Some of the sodium pumped into the interstitium leaks back into the lumen through the paracellular pathway. In the process of flow along the proximal tubule, the bulk of the filtered glucose, amino acids, and bicarbonate is reabsorbed. A significant amount of phosphate is also reabsorbed. Thus, the glomerular filtrate is rendered free of glucose, amino acid, and bicarbonate by the end of the proximal tubule. As bicarbonate is removed, the chloride concentration rises to 20 to 40 mEq/L above plasma, creating conditions for chloride to diffuse out of the lumen through the paracellular pathway. The permeability to organic solutes is low, preventing their backward diffusion.

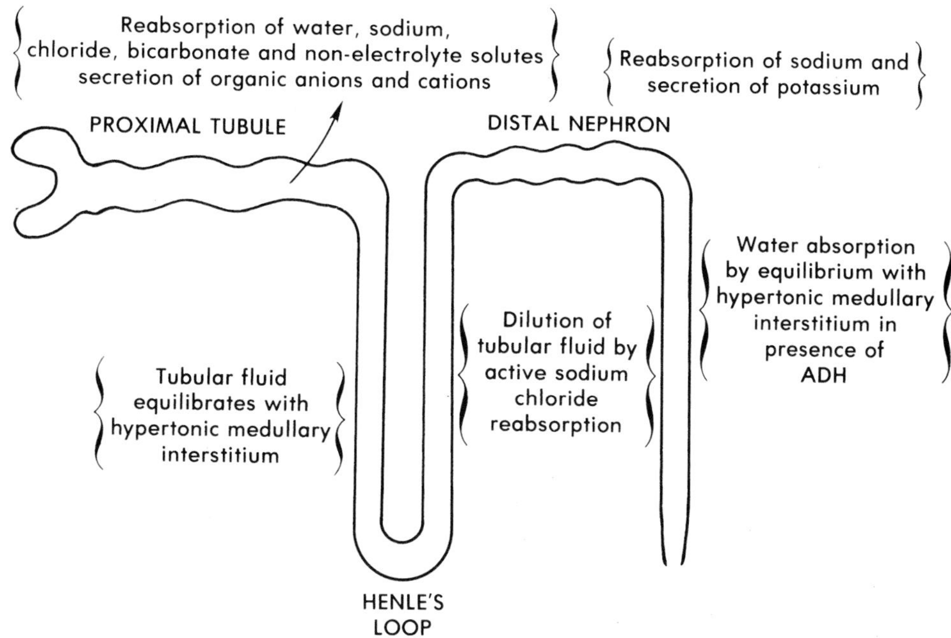

Fig. 42-7. Stylized nephron illustrating the major anatomic divisions and the major fluid and electrolyte transport functions of each division.

The proximal convoluted tubule is a water-permeable segment. As sodium and solutes are removed by transport systems, the luminal fluid becomes hypotonic relative to that of the interstitial space. It is also believed that the effective osmolality of the ions in the interstitial space exceeds that of the tubular fluid. Water therefore rapidly equilibrates across the proximal tubule by moving through the paracellular pathway. Because of the high permeability to water in the proximal tubule, the luminal fluid is maintained nearly iso-osmolar.

The proximal convoluted tubule also adds substances to the tubular fluid. Organic anions and bases are removed from blood and translocated into the cells by specific transport proteins in the basolateral membrane. Once inside the cell, these anions and cations can gain access to the tubule fluid by passive or mediated mechanisms across the luminal membrane. Proximal tubule cells also produce ammonia, which can diffuse into the lumen, undergo protonation to NH_4^+, and thereby become "trapped" in the tubular fluid.

Thin limbs of Henle's loop. In contrast to the proximal tubule, the thin limbs perform little in the way of mediated transport. The descending limb segment of Henle's loop is highly water permeable but impermeable to electrolytes and solutes. The osmolality of the interstitium is progressively higher from the cortex to the tip of the papilla. With the lack of transport systems, the low permeability to solutes, and the high permeability to water in the descending limb, the tubular fluid is progressively concentrated as it equilibrates with the hypertonic interstitium. Thus, at the bend of the Henle's loop, the tubular fluid volume is considerably reduced and its concentration of solutes is increased as water is abstracted. In humans, osmolality at the tip of Henle's loop can be as high as 1200 mOsm/kg of water. The water permeability of the ascending limb, unlike that of the descending limb, is low, whereas the permeabilities to urea and sodium are higher. As a result, sodium diffuses down its concentration gradient from the lumen into the interstitium, whereas urea enters the tubular fluid. The net result is a progressive dilution of fluid in the thin ascending limb.[39] The Na^+-$2Cl^-$-K^+ co-transporter in the luminal membranes moves one sodium, two chloride, and one potassium ions from the tubular lumen into the cell. Loop diuretics block this transporter. Chloride moves down its electrochemical gradient through a basolateral chloride channel and by means of a basolateral K^+-Cl^- co-transporter. Potassium passes down its concentration gradient from the cytosol into the lumen through potassium channels and into the interstitium by means of the K^+-Cl^- co-transporter. The net result is a small electrical gradient across the cell, with the lumen positive with respect to the interstitium. This causes sodium to move through a paracellular pathway from lumen to interstitium.[40] The medullary thick ascending limb has a higher capacity for sodium absorption and higher concentrations of Na^+-K^+ ATPase and mitochondria than does the cortical thick ascending limb. Thus, the absorption from the medullary portion is greater than from the cortical. Mineralocorticoids increase luminal sodium uptake by means of the Na^+-H^+ antiporter. As fluid moves up this nephron segment, the tubular fluid is progressively diluted as sodium is removed by this secondary active transport process. Fluid exiting the thick ascending limb is reduced in osmolality to less than that of plasma (100 to

150 mOsm/kg water). This fluid is hypotonic regardless of the osmolality of the excreted urine. The absorbed sodium chloride is partly retained in the interstitium of the medulla and is critically important in the renal handling of water. The thick ascending limb also reabsorbs calcium and magnesium.

Distal nephron segments. Several anatomic and functional subsegments are included in the term *distal nephron*. Considered as a whole, however, this segment finely regulates the composition and volume of the excreted urine. The proximal tubule subserves bulk reabsorption, whereas the distal nephron is responsible for regulation of urinary volume and composition. The distal nephron continues to reabsorb sodium from the filtrate. In addition, the distal nephron (specifically the cortical collecting tubule) secretes potassium. Almost all the potassium that appears in the urine derives from secretion in the distal tubule. The absorption of sodium and the secretion of potassium are influenced by aldosterone. The distal nephron also reabsorbs calcium and, in the absence of parathyroid hormone, phosphate. Hydrogen ions are secreted in the distal portion of the nephron, probably by a hydrogen ion ATPase located in the luminal membrane. Water permeability remains extremely low in the distal convoluted tubule, and the tubular fluid remains hypotonic. The osmolality of the distal tubular fluid is largely caused by urea. The cortical collecting duct epithelium is relatively impermeable to urea and, in the absence of ADH, to water. The presence of ADH renders the cortical collecting duct permeable to water. ADH also increases the water permeability of the medullary collecting duct. Urea permeability in the medullary collecting duct is greater than that of the cortical portion and increases in response to ADH.

These considerations are important in understanding the mechanisms involved in the concentration and dilution of urine.

Renal Modulation of Fluid and Electrolyte Homeostasis

Water. In healthy humans excreting maximally concentrated urine, approximately 500 ml/day is required to excrete obligatory solutes. The normal kidney is also able to generate approximately 20 L solute-free water. In other words, a healthy individual could ingest or receive as much as 20 L water daily, excrete all of it, and not alter the volume or composition of any water compartment in the body. The development of maximum urinary dilution and concentration depends on precise interactions between almost every nephron segment. This integrated system is disrupted by several renal diseases and drugs, resulting in an early loss of maximum concentrating and diluting ability. Under such conditions, the range of fluid intake that can be accommodated may be severely restricted, and the intake of water may have to be adjusted to conform to the regulatory range of the kidney.

Concentration of the urine depends critically on the presence of ADH. Arginine vasopressin is the mammalian ADH. ADH is produced in the supraoptic nucleus of the hypothalamus and translocated to the posterior pituitary gland for storage and release. The regulation of ADH release is normally under control of the osmolality of the immediate extracellular fluid environment near the osmole receptors in the supraoptic and paraventricular nuclei of the hypothalamus.[41] The range of regulation is narrow, and the gain of the system is high (Fig. 42-8). ADH secretion is almost completely suppressed when plasma os-

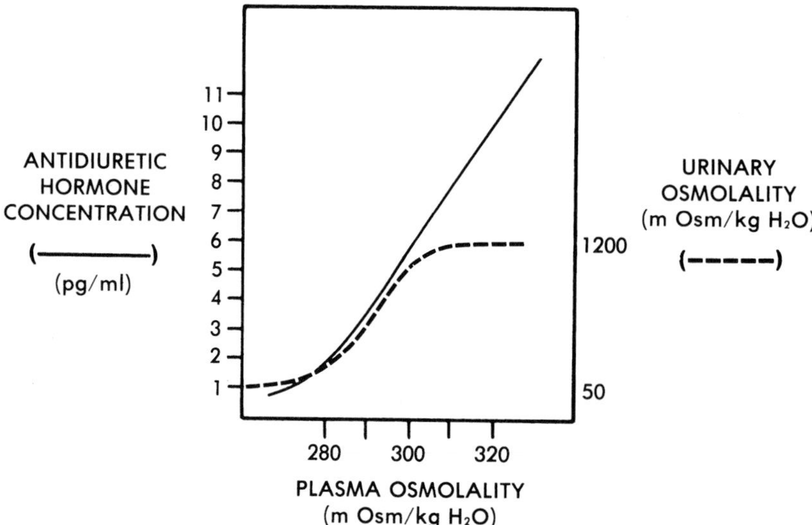

Fig. 42-8. Relationship between extracellular fluid osmolality (represented by plasma osmolality) and ADH concentration and urine osmolality. As plasma osmolality rises, ADH levels rise. As the ADH level rises, the urine osmolality increases to its maximum value of about 1200 mOsm/kg water. Despite further elevations of ADH concentration, urine osmolality dose not rise higher.

molality is less than 280 mOsm/kg water and becomes greatest when osmolality exceeds 290 mOsm/kg water.

Although the osmolality of the plasma is the major determinant of ADH release, it is important to note that ADH release can occur in response to nonosmolar stimuli. Both depletion of the intravascular volume and hypotension can result directly in release of ADH and in a resetting of the relationship between osmolality and plasma ADH concentration so that ADH is released at lower osmolalities. Depletion of intravascular volume by 8% to 15% is sufficient to stimulate ADH release, despite normal plasma osmolality. Similarly, hypotension causes ADH release despite a normal osmolality of the plasma and a normal intravascular volume. Finally, a variety of other stimuli, loosely called "stressful," (pain, nausea, and vomiting) cause ADH release in the presence of normal plasma osmolality, volume status, and blood pressure. Although several drugs, including narcotics, have been implicated in stimulating ADH release, it appears that this is not a primary pharmacologic effect. If a drug causes hypotension, nausea, or anxiety, ADH is released. If these side effects are avoided, no change in plasma ADH level occurs. On the other hand, ethanol inhibits ADH release because of inhibition of calcium channels in the pituitary. The reduction in ADH levels contributes to the diuretic effect seen during acute intoxication.

ADH binds to specific receptors on the basolateral membrane of the collecting duct cells. Adenylate cyclase is then activated, and cAMP is produced. cAMP activates protein phosphatases, which through additional metabolic steps cause a change in the water permeability of the cells of the collecting duct. The increase in the water permeability of the collecting duct allows the fluid within the lumen to come into osmotic equilibrium with the hypertonic medullary interstitium. ADH also alters the urea permeability of the medullary collecting ducts. In addition to its effects on water permeability, ADH increases the rate of sodium chloride transport in the thick ascending limb of Henle's loop and may also decrease plasma flow to the medulla of the kidney. These actions tend to increase the tonicity of and limit the removal of solute from the interstitium and also to enhance the formation of a concentrated urine when distal tubule fluid equilibrates with interstitial fluid. The maximum tonicity of the urine that can be achieved thus depends on a normal response by distal tubule cells to ADH and the tonicity of the medullary interstitial fluid. The tonicity of the interstitial fluid depends in turn on the delivery of filtrate to the thick ascending limb of Henle's loop, the reabsorption of sodium chloride in the thick ascending limb, and the diffusion to urea out of the collecting ducts.

Water and electrolyte balance are also under the control of the renin-angiotensin-aldosterone system. Renin, an enzyme produced by the kidney, is the rate-limiting step in this system. Its release is stimulated by an intrarenal baroreceptor mechanism, by β-adrenergic stimulation, and by changes in the delivery of sodium or chloride to the distal nephron. Prostaglandins and calcium also appear to be important in the mechanism underlying its release. Once released, renin causes the conversion of angiotensinogen, a precursor protein produced in the liver, to angiotensin I (AI). A second enzyme, angiotensin-converting enzyme, which is found in all vascular beds (with particularly high levels in the lung), then catalyzes the conversion of AI to angiotensin AII, the most active product of the system. AII causes vasoconstriction, elicits the production of aldosterone by the adrenal cortex, stimulates water ingestion (thirst), and has important interactions with the sympathetic nervous system, as well as inhibiting further renin release.

Aldosterone production and release by the adrenal cortex are also enhanced by hyperkalemia and negative sodium balance. Further, adrenocorticotropic hormone may play a permissive role in its production. The predominant action of aldosterone is to stimulate the reabsorption of sodium and secretion of potassium by the distal nephron; it thus minimizes the amount of sodium that is excreted in the urine.

As a whole, the renin-angiotensin-aldosterone system is activated by states of inadequate circulating plasma volume or extracellular fluid volume and abnormalities in their composition. It responds by enhancing electrolyte reabsorption and fluid intake and by causing vasoconstriction.[42] (For additional discussion of this system, see Chapters 2 and 46.)

Sodium. Approximately 20,000 mEq sodium is filtered by the kidneys each day. The kidney is the sole organ of excretion of sodium in normal individuals, and the urinary excretion of sodium matches the dietary intake. In an average healthy person, sodium ingestion ranges from 50 to 250 mEq/day. Thus, the urinary excretion of sodium is less than 1% of the filtered load. Sixty percent of filtered sodium is reabsorbed in the proximal convoluted tubule. Sodium is also reabsorbed in the thick ascending limb of Henle's loop and the distal nephron. In the distal nephron, aldosterone enhances the rate of sodium reabsorption. Various organs sense the intake of sodium. The rates of absorption at multiple sites within the kidney can be altered by many mechanisms. In addition to stimuli generated outside the kidney, the kidney is capable of directly altering its own rates of reabsorption when the intake of sodium varies.

In an individual with normal renal function, the urine can be rendered almost free of sodium. In conditions of excess intake of sodium, the kidney is capable of excreting all this cation, at least as much as intakes of several hundred milliequivalents per day. These renal adjustments in the rates of reabsorption of sodium occur in many nephron segments. In the proximal convoluted tubule, the rate of sodium reabsorption is increased in states of depletion of the extracellular fluid volume and decreased in states of expansion. These altered rates of transport are mediated by changes in the concentrations of circulating factors, local factors generated by the kidney, renal nerve traffic, and renal hemodynamic factors. Collectively, these stimuli affect the rate of sodium and water transport out of the lumen of the proximal tubule and the rate of back-leak through the paracellular pathway.

It has been demonstrated, however, that changes in the rates of reabsorption in the proximal tubule alone do not necessarily result in changes in the urinary excretion of sodium. This is because of the capacity of downstream nephron segments to compensate and independently adjust their rates of sodium reabsorption. Thus, the response to a change in the extracellular fluid volume must also involve a change in the rates of sodium reabsorption in Henle's loop and in distal nephron segments. In response to a volume challenge or an increase in sodium intake, for example, the rate of aldosterone secretion is reduced; this factor decreases the rates of sodium reabsorption in the distal nephron. Similarly, sodium depletion results in increased rates of reabsorption in Henle's loop and in the distal nephron segments. The response to alterations in sodium intake are thus integrated across a range of sodium intakes by many mechanisms acting on several subsegments of the nephron. Drugs, disease states of the kidney, and clinical conditions engendering the development of substances that directly or indirectly affect the tubular reabsorption of sodium may limit the kidney's ability to regulate the rates of sodium excretion.[43]

Potassium. Unlike sodium, the urine cannot be rendered free of potassium. Despite this, the range of potassium intakes that can be tolerated is quite large. The renal responses to rapid alterations in potassium intake are slower than those for sodium. In humans, rates of potassium ingestion and excretion can be increased progressively without change in the plasma or tissue concentration of potassium as long as such step increases in intake occur during several days. Sudden and large increases in potassium intake can overwhelm both the capacity of the kidney to excrete the load and the ability of other tissues to sequester potassium.

Filtered potassium is reabsorbed in the proximal convoluted tubule. The major regulatory site for potassium excretion is the distal nephron. In this segment, potassium is taken up across the basolateral membrane into the cell by the operation of the Na^+-K^+ ATPase pump. The potassium content of the cells of the distal tubule is above electrochemical equilibrium. A finite permeability of the luminal membrane to potassium permits potassium to diffuse out of the cell into the lumen. The process across the luminal membrane is passive and governed by the prevailing electrochemical gradients from cell to lumen.

The major determinant for potassium secretion appears to be the concentration of potassium in the luminal fluid. When luminal flow is high, the secreted potassium is rapidly diluted, and the gradient for potassium secretion is maintained. In states of low flow, the cell-to-lumen potassium concentration gradient is rapidly decreased, and the absolute rate of secretion is diminished. Thus, flow rate past the distal tubule is a major factor influencing the urinary secretion and excretion of potassium. Another factor is the electric potential difference from the cell to the lumen of the distal tubule. The lumen's negative potential difference is generated by the tubular reabsorption of sodium. The greater the rate of sodium reabsorption, the more negative the voltage in the lumen. The link between sodium and potassium transport therefore derives not from the presence of a countertransport process but rather from electrochemical coupling.

Aldosterone increases the rate of potassium secretion by several mechanisms.[44] It increases the permeability of the luminal membrane to potassium; enhances the rate of sodium reabsorption, rendering the tubule lumen more electronegative; and increases the activity of the Na^+-K^+ ATPase pump. The rate of aldosterone secretion is influenced by the renin-angiotensin system and by the plasma concentration of potassium. Sodium depletion can stimulate the renal production of renin, which ultimately results in stimulation of aldosterone secretion. The generated aldosterone thus serves a role in sodium conservation. Increases in dietary intake of potassium can directly increase the secretion of aldosterone. The aldosterone serves to increase urinary excretion of potassium.

It is important to note that aldosterone is not the only factor affecting potassium metabolism. In addition to urinary excretion, potassium is taken up and released by other tissues of the body. Although those nonrenal mechanisms can help modulate the plasma concentrations of potassium, they do not serve to eliminate potassium from the body. The renal excretion of potassium may be affected by kidney diseases, various hormones, and therapeutic drugs.[45-47]

Increased ammonium excretion, but not production, decreases potassium excretion by an effect on the collecting duct.[48] Acidosis impairs and alkalosis stimulates potassium secretion by the distal nephron.[48] Calcitonin increases fractional potassium excretion.[33] As the GFR falls, fractional excretion of potassium rises. Thus, hyperkalemia is not seen until the end stages of kidney failure. Any drug or condition that increases the delivery of sodium to the distal nephron (proximal or loop diuretics, osmotic diuresis) or that causes increased distal sodium absorption, leads to potassium wasting.

Bicarbonate. The metabolism of food results in the generation of hydrogen ion at approximately 1 mEq/kg body weight/day of nonvolatile acid. This acid must be excreted by the kidney. The kidney filters approximately 3500 mEq bicarbonate, which must be reabsorbed. Although the overall body production of acid is only 70 mEq/day in a 70 kg individual, the kidney must secrete 3500 + 70 mEq/day to reabsorb filtered bicarbonate and dispose of metabolic acid. The bulk of filtered bicarbonate is absorbed in the proximal tubule by a process linked with the secretion of protons in the lumen. Sodium ions and protons undergo counterexchange in this nephron segment. The secreted protons combine with filtered bicarbonate and, under the influence of carbonic anhydrase, are converted to carbon dioxide and water. The carbon dioxide readily crosses the luminal membrane into the cell. Within the cell, carbon dioxide is hydrated to carbonic acid (catalyzed by carbonic anhydrase), which dissociates into a hydrogen ion and a bicarbonate ion. This bicarbonate exits through the basolateral membrane and is returned to the blood. The hydrogen ion is then secreted into the luminal fluid.

The rate of reabsorption of bicarbonate in the proximal tubule is influenced by several factors. In general, when the rates of sodium reabsorption are enhanced or inhibited in the proximal tubule, parallel changes occur in the capacity for bicarbonate reabsorption. Systemic acid-base conditions and potassium balance also affect the rates of bicarbonate reabsorption. Bicarbonate that escapes reabsorption in the proximal tubule can be reabsorbed in more distal nephron sites by a proton pump that requires ATP. The capacity of the distal nephron for bicarbonate reabsorption, however, is limited. The net result of these processes is to reclaim filtered bicarbonate but not to dispose of metabolic acid.[49]

Nonvolatile acids. Nonvolatile acids are excreted by two processes. First, hydrogen ions that are secreted into the lumen are buffered by the conversion of dibasic sodium phosphate to monobasic sodium phosphate, a process known as the *formation of titratable acid.* Approximately 30 mEq (~40%) acid is eliminated by this mechanism each day, and the amount is relatively fixed. Second, nonvolatile acid excretion occurs through the renal production of ammonia, from the metabolism of glutamine. Ammonia is a gas that diffuses into both the lumen and the peritubular capillary blood. In the lumen, ammonia is protonated to ammonium ion, and in this state it is trapped in the lumen because of the lower permeability of the ionized species. The collecting duct secretes most of the ammonium ion that appears in the urine. The ammonia accumulated in the medullary interstitium provides a gradient to move into the collecting duct lumen, where it can combine with secreted hydrogen.[52] The concentration of ammonia in the interstitium is 100 to 1000 times higher than in arterial plasma because of a countercurrent multiplication.[50] The more acid in the luminal fluid, the more ammonia is converted to ammonium ion and the lower is the luminal ammonia concentration. This circumstance supports the continued movement of ammonia from interstitium to lumen. This process is known as *nonionic diffusion trapping.* In response to acidosis, an increase in the rate of renal ammonia production is the major mechanism for eliminating fixed acid from the body. Bones and other tissues can act as temporary buffers, but, ultimately, excretion by the kidney is required.[51,52]

Calcium and magnesium. Calcium is reabsorbed in the proximal tubule, Henle's loop, and certain subsegments of the distal nephron. Magnesium, on the other hand, is reabsorbed predominantly in Henle's loop. Acutely and chronically, the reabsorption of calcium and probably that of magnesium are affected by parathyroid hormone (PTH). The absolute rates of excretion of these substances, however, depend on the balance between delivery to the kidney and the renal transport mechanisms. In states of PTH excess, for example, the absolute rates of calcium absorption by the kidney are increased, despite the absolute rates of excretion also being increased. Kidney diseases and drugs such as diuretics can influence the renal excretion of calcium.[53-55]

Phosphate. Filtered phosphate is reabsorbed by a sodium-dependent mechanism in the proximal tubule. In the presence of permissive amounts of PTH, phosphate rejected from the proximal tubule cannot be reabsorbed in more distal nephron segments. The rate of phosphate reabsorption in the proximal tubule is influenced by PTH and vitamin D. PTH, through specific receptors in the proximal tubule and the generation of cAMP, inhibits the tubular reabsorption of phosphate and is a major regulating factor. Increases in the ingestion of phosphate transiently reduce the plasma concentration of ionized calcium and result in the release of PTH. PTH causes a phosphaturia and a normalization of the serum concentrations of phosphate and ionized calcium. Other hormones, including corticosteroids, glucagon, and insulin, can affect handling of phosphate by the kidney. In addition, abnormalities in phosphate metabolism are intimately involved in the genesis of the multifactorial systemic manifestations of advanced renal disease. Hypophosphatemia also affects renal function and can result in a decreased rate of reabsorption of bicarbonate and calcium.[53,55]

Other metabolites. The kidneys also excrete a variety of metabolic waste products and drugs. Well-described organic acid and organic base secretory systems are present in the kidney. In general, organic compounds are taken up at the antiluminal border of the cell and secreted into the lumen. Some of these substances, such as urate, are also reabsorbed by the kidney. Thus, urate undergoes bidirectional tubular transport. The excretion of organic compounds is complex and influenced by kidney disease, drugs, and hormones.

Tubular Function in Renal Disease

The ability of the kidney to regulate rates of excretion and contribute to overall body homeostasis may be affected by several factors. Drugs and disease conditions may selectively alter one or another specific transport process. Diffuse parenchymal disease is often characterized by many abnormalities. Compensating mechanisms may provide a margin of reserve, which blunts the clinical expression of the abnormality. For example, even when as much as 90% of renal function is destroyed, the serum concentrations of calcium, phosphate, and potassium may be normal. With additional damage, abnormalities in plasma concentrations of these substances become evident. In such circumstances, intake must be matched to output to maintain homeostasis. One characteristic of renal disease is the loss of the kidney's ability to regulate water and sodium balance, resulting in the excretion of relatively fixed amounts of solutes. Intake that exceeds the kidney's ability to excrete results in increases in body water and solutes, whereas limitations in intake may result in states of depletion.[56]

CLINICAL ASSESSMENT OF RENAL FUNCTION

Urinalysis

Urinalysis has long been used as a screening test for renal or systemic disease.[57] Typical tests that are components of the urinalysis include measurement of urinary glucose, protein, pH, and specific gravity, as well as microscopic examination. The use of urinalysis in the diagnosis of specific disease conditions is a critical part of the preoperative evaluation of patients and in follow-up of patients in the postsurgical period.[58]

Urine Osmolality and Specific Gravity

The term *specific gravity* refers to the weight of a fixed volume of solution expressed as a multiple of the weight of the same volume of pure water. The addition of physiologic solutes to water generally increases density and thus specific gravity. Unfortunately, the relationship between the concentration of solute in the solution (osmolality) and the specific gravity depends heavily on the nature of the solute. For example, a small amount of protein greatly increases specific gravity but changes osmolality little. Osmolality is thus a far more useful measure of urinary concentration than is specific gravity. The potential differences in a given patient between urinary osmolality and urinary specific gravity are important to remember, because specific gravity measurements are often used in clinical medicine as an index of the kidney's concentrating ability. The specific gravity of a voided urine specimen, for example, may indicate a value representative of normal renal concentrating ability (e.g., 1.018), when in fact the urinary osmolality is the same as in plasma. (See the prior discussion on water regulation and the following section on urine osmolality and urinary flow rate.)

Urinary pH

Urinary pH varies greatly, from 4.4 to 8.0, and reflects the need of the body to excrete acid or base to maintain plasma pH at 7.4. A persistently alkaline urine (pH >7) is seen in metabolic alkalosis and may indicate urinary tract infection with a urea-splitting organism. A relatively alkaline urine is found in patients with renal tubular acidosis, a condition caused by incomplete reabsorption of bicarbonate or insufficient secretion of hydrogen ion. A discussion of these complex disorders is beyond the scope of this chapter.

Proteinuria

By definition, proteinuria refers to excretion of more than 100 mg protein in 24 hours. A small amount of protein, especially of low molecular weight, is filtered by the glomerulus, but the bulk of it is reabsorbed in the proximal tubule. When found in the urine, protein usually reflects glomerular disease but may also indicate renal tubular defects, polycystic kidneys, infection, hypertension, or renal vein thrombosis. The molecular weight of the protein is often helpful in distinguishing its etiology. Urinary protein of large molecular weight (>55 kd) generally indicates glomerular basement membrane injury (glomerulonephritis), whereas low–molecular-weight urinary protein indicates renal tubular injury (acute tubular necrosis, infection). In many glomerular diseases, the excretion of larger proteins increases dramatically. When protein excretion exceeds 3.5 g/24 hr, the diagnosis of nephrotic syndrome is made. Many etiologies of nephrotic syndrome exist and are considered in detail in Chapter 43.

Glycosuria

Glycosuria occurs when the amount of glucose filtered exceeds the capacity of the proximal tubular reabsorption mechanism. Thus, glycosuria occurs in the presence of elevated glucose level (e.g., >180 mg/100 ml), elevated GFR, or reduction in tubular transport function related to disease or drugs. Glycosuria in the absence of high exogenous carbohydrate loads and stress usually means that a patient has diabetes mellitus. The two common tests for urine glucose are copper reduction, which detects many substances other than glucose, and glucose oxidase, which is much more specific. False-positive glucose oxidase results may be seen if the specimen is contaminated with hydrogen peroxide or hypochlorites, and false-negative results may occur in the presence of L-dopa or aspirin.

Urinary Sediment

Microscopic examination of the urinary sediment can give important information regarding the level within the urinary tract at which disease is active. The presence of casts containing cellular elements implies parenchymal renal disease, whereas free red blood cells can arise at any level. Likewise, white blood cell casts indicate inflammatory renal disease, and casts composed of epithelial cells are associated with tubular damage.

Various types of urinary crystals may also be important aids to diagnosis of disease. Crystals of calcium oxalate or calcium phosphate may mean that the patient has hypercalcemia or calcium-containing renal calculi. Uric acid crystals reflect hyperuricosuria and uric acid stone formation and may indicate that the patient has gout or other diseases associated with hyperuricemia. Similarly, cystine crystals indicate that the patient probably has cystinuria, because such crystals are almost never found in the urine under normal conditions. Finally, triple-phosphate crystals indicate the presence of urinary tract stones produced by infection with urea-splitting organisms. For greatest clinical value, such determinations should be obtained before administration of diuretics.

Renal Function Tests

Tests of renal function can be classified as those predominantly related to (1) RBF, (2) GFR, and (3) tubular transport function.[58]

Renal Blood Flow

Clinical measurement of RBF is indirect, and methodologic problems hamper the interpretation of data. The most frequently used method is the clearance measurement of substances that are actively secreted into the urine and whose clearance is limited primarily by renal plasma flow. *p*-Aminohippuric acid (PAH) is one such substance. Approximately 85% to 95% of PAH is cleared from plasma in one passage through the kidney under normal circumstances. Renal plasma flow is equal to the clearance of any substance divided by its extraction ratio. The calculation of the extraction ratio requires the measurement of the concentration of the substance in the renal venous plasma. Clearance of a substance such as PAH is not higher than the renal plasma flow. It must be emphasized, however, that a reduction in PAH clearance may be caused by a decrease in tubular secretory function, which results in a lowered extraction ratio, as well as by a reduction in renal plasma flow. Because of the nonspecificity of such clearance techniques, they are not widely used today in the clinical setting.

RBF flow can also be estimated by various radiologic methods, including angiography and scans of the kidney with radioisotopes.[59] Although useful in experimental studies, determination of the rates of RBF with these techniques is not usually employed clinically. Rather, the clinical use of measuring RBF by nuclear scanning or angiography is to determine (1) the patency of the vascular tree in suspected cases of renovascular catastrophies and renal transplants and (2) the relative as opposed to the absolute differences in blood flow between the kidneys.

Glomerular Filtration Rate

The serum creatinine concentration (SCr) is typically used clinically to evaluate renal filtration function. The rationale for this measurement is based on the observation that 95% to 98% of creatinine is derived from muscle, its turnover is relatively constant (<2% per day), and nearly all creatinine is excreted in the urine. SCr indicates the balance between creatinine excretion by the kidney and creatinine production by muscle. The total excretion of creatinine is proportional to the muscle mass of the body, and derangements in muscle mass must be considered in interpreting the SCr. Although SCr of 1.2 or 1.4 mg/dl may be consistent with a normal GFR in a muscular young man, a similar plasma value in an elderly, inactive woman could indicate a 50% to 75% reduction in GFR. Further, muscle injury can elevate the SCr even though GFR is normal. The use of SCr is also limited by the requirement for a steady state. If the GFR is unstable, changes in SCr will lag behind by 1 to 2 days.

Because of the difficulties inherent in assessing renal filtration function with static measurements of SCr, the GFR is often estimated by measuring the creatinine clearance (CCr). *Clearance* is defined as the volume of plasma (or blood) from which all of a given substance (e.g., creatinine) is removed per time unit, which would explain the resulting rate of disappearance from the plasma. It is a two-compartment model in which it assumed that all of the substance is removed from some proportion of the plasma flow, whereas none is removed from another portion. Urinary clearance is the classic method for estimating GFR. An ideal marker of GFR should be eliminated only by glomerular filtration. The marker should not be produced, metabolized, secreted, or reabsorbed by the kidney. Further, the marker molecule should be of a size to allow unimpeded permeability, lack significant electrical charge, be minimally protein bound, and be nontoxic. The formula of Cockcroft predicts CCr most accurately in patients with normal function.[60] The Cockroft formula performs well in estimating GFR provided that the patient's renal function is stable. Ideal body weights should be used in the obese and those who have muscle wasting. Obviously, calculated clearances cannot be used to assess acute changes.[61] The formula employed for men is

$$CCr = [(140 - Age) \times Wt]/(SCr \times 72)$$

where CCr is in milliliters per minute, age is in years, *Wt* is weight in kilograms, and SCr is milligrams per deciliter. The result is multiplied by 0.85 for women.

Unfortunately, CCr is not a perfect measure of GFR because it is the result of both filtration and secretion, which results in an overestimate of the true GFR by as much as 30%. The overestimation increases as GFR falls and SCr rises. Thus, CCr represents the maximum likely GFR. Despite these shortcomings and the difficulties in obtaining quantitative collections of urine, the safety and simplicity of measuring CCr warrant its use in estimating GFR. For more accurate estimation of the GFR, measurement of inulin clearance can be employed. Inulin is a carbohydrate that is filtered but not metabolized, secreted, or reabsorbed. Its clearance rate is considered to be the best measurement of true GFR. Because of methodologic problems, it is not commonly used, however.

Urea clearance has also been used to measure GFR, but it is less accurate than CCr. Blood urea nitrogen (BUN) reflects the balance between protein and amino acid catabolism and excretion. Urea is freely filtered, but its excretion is proportional to urine flow rate as a result of recycling in the medulla. This dependence on urinary flow rate leads to a characteristic finding in prerenal azotemia as a result of dehydration, hypovolemia, and heart failure. Urea clearance is diminished more than is CCr. Thus, BUN rises proportionately more than does SCr, increasing the BUN:creatinine ratio above the usual 10:1 to more than 20:1.

Tubular Transport Function

Fractional rates of solute excretion. Tests of tubular function include determinations of the fractional rates of excretion of a solute, the concentration of the solute in the urine, and the urinary osmolality. The term *fractional excretion (FE)* is defined as the ratio of the amount of a substance filtered at the glomerulus that is excreted in the urine; this is expressed as a percentage. The FE rate can be calculated as the clearance of a substance divided by the clearance of a glomerular filtration marker. Thus, the FE of solute *s* is calculated from the following expression:

$$FE_s(\%) = \frac{C_s}{C_{cr}} \times 100 = \frac{(U_s \times \dot{V}) \div P_s}{(U_{cr} \times \dot{V}) \div P_{cr}} \times 100 = \frac{U_s/P_s}{U_{cr}/P_{cr}} \times 100$$

where C is the clearance; U_s and P_s are the urinary and ultrafiltrable plasma concentrations of the solute; U_{cr} and P_{cr} are the urinary and plasma concentrations of the glomerular filtration marker creatinine; and $\dot{V}$ is the urinary flow rate. Normal FE rates for the major solutes of plasma have been determined. For example, in healthy humans, the FE of urate is approximately 7% to 10% of the filtered load. In patients with tubular defects in the absorption of urate or in individuals receiving a drug that inhibits the absorption of urate, the FE of urate rises. The FE of any solute can be determined to evaluate tubular function. Because urate and phosphate are handled predominantly in the proximal convoluted tubule, calculation of the FE of these two substances can be used to reflect transport activity in this nephron segment.

A frequently used clinical test is the determination of the FE rate of sodium.[62,63] In healthy individuals, the FE of sodium is less than 1%. The FE of sodium increases when sodium is ingested, when diuretics are administered, or when renal tubular disease is present. In a patient with signs of fluid overload, a low FE rate of sodium is inappropriate. In a patient with normal hydration or in a patient who is volume depleted, an FE of sodium greater than 1% is inappropriate and may indicate renal tubular disease or administration of diuretics.

The measurement of urinary sodium concentration alone is of less value than the determination of the FE rate. The urinary sodium concentration is determined not only by the degree of sodium reabsorption but also by the degree of urinary dilution. Thus, the excretion of 100 mEq sodium in 1 L of urine results in a sodium concentration of 100 mEq/L. The excretion of the same 100 mEq in 3000 ml of urine results in a concentration of only 33 mEq/L. In the presence of the same absolute and fractional rates of excretions of sodium, the sodium concentration can vary threefold.

Urine osmolality and urinary flow rate. The measurement of the osmolality of urine is useful when interpreted together with the clinical condition of the patient because urinary concentration depends on the integrated function of multiple nephron segments, determination of the urine osmolality is a relatively sensitive test of tubular function. When urine osmolality should be elevated, such as in hyperosmolality of the plasma, hypovolemia, or hypotension, the findings of an iso-osmolar urine suggests that the kidney is incapable of producing a concentrated urine. The finding of a high urine osmolality conversely suggests that integration of nephron function is relatively intact.

The measurement of urinary output is probably the most frequently performed renal function test. As a single measure of renal function, however, the urinary flow rate is not specific. Patients with severe renal failure may have normal urinary flow rates. The urinary flow rate depends on the intake or administration of water, the concentration of ADH, the tonicity of the medullary interstitium, the response of the kidney to ADH, the GFR, and the tubular reabsorption of sodium. Because so many factors can influence the measured urinary flow rate, this determination is not usually of clinical value as a measure of tubular function. However, quantitative measurement of the urinary output is of value in specific clinical situations.

CLINICAL CORRELATIONS
Effects of Anesthesia and Surgery on Renal Function

Physicians have recognized since the beginning of this century that anesthetics can influence renal function. Most studies involving currently used anesthetics have been performed on humans, but exact mechanisms by which the observed changes are produced have not been clarified. Despite this lack of information, total RBF, as measured by PAH clearance, falls by 20% to 40% during anesthesia with potent inhalational anesthetics or during balanced anesthesia with nitrous oxide, narcotics, and muscle relaxants. These changes occur in the absence of major changes in blood pressure. The same anesthetics generally cause a somewhat lesser reduction (20% to 30%) in GFR. The effects of anesthesia on RBF and GFR are increased as the depth of anesthesia is increased. Vigorous hydration before the induction of anesthesia blunts but does not totally prevent the changes in RBF and GFR. With deeper levels of anesthesia, hydration has no effect on the decrease in blood flow and filtration rate. Subarachnoid and epidural anesthesia have few direct effects on renal plasma flow and GFR.

In response to anesthesia, the urinary flow rate decreases even more than does either the GFR or the rate of renal plasma flow. The decrease in urinary flow rate is usually accompanied by a modest increase in urine osmolality, although urine osmolalities greater than 700 to 800 mOsm/kg water are unusual. The effects of inhalational anesthesia and regional anesthesia on the urine flow rate appear to be similar.

The mechanisms responsible for the changes in renal function after induction of anesthesia are unclear. It has been demonstrated that well-conducted general anesthesia is not associated with significant elevations in plasma renin activity, nor in the plasma concentration of vasopressin. Almost all modern general anesthetics and regional blocks tend to cause a reduction in renal sympathetic nerve activity (RSNA) and in catecholamine concentrations.

Methoxyflurane has been reported to be an indirect renal toxin that results in renal injury.[64] The toxicity of this agent is caused by the generation of inorganic fluoride from the metabolism of methoxyflurane; the typical patient has polyuria that is resistant to therapy with vasopressin. The only other anesthetic that releases significant amounts of fluoride is enflurane. Only extremely prolonged and deep anesthesia with this agent, however, has resulted in fluoride levels associated with changes in renal function.[65] Aside from these two agents, no general anesthetics are associated with direct renal toxicity. The observed changes in renal function after anesthesia are not usually associated with morphologic changes. These functional changes are rapidly reversed when the anesthetic state is discontinued.

When surgery is performed during the anesthetic state, several additional changes in renal function occur. Renal plasma flow and GFR may decrease further, and ADH release is greatly stimulated. ADH concentrations often increase to levels that are supramaximum for urinary concentration. The effect of surgery on ADH concentrations may be blunted somewhat by increasing the depth of anesthesia. In addition, after the surgical stimulus, stimulation of RSNA and of renin release may occur. When surgery is performed, the changes in renal plasma flow and GFR persist into the immediate postoperative period. The degree and the duration of renal function depression increases roughly in proportion to the magnitude of the surgical procedure performed. The factors responsible for this persistent suppression of renal function have not been well clarified.

Alterations in Renal Function in Response to Systemic Diseases

In addition to primary diseases of the kidney, renal function may be altered by systemic diseases. The renal response to depletion of the extracellular fluid volume, regardless of etiology, in patients with normal renal function is a decrease in the urinary excretion of sodium and water. This response reflects the influence of normal homeostatic mechanisms that attempt to maintain the fluid volume of the body. Diseases characterized by external losses of fluid and electrolytes or blood, as well as clinical conditions characterized by no external loss but rather by a sequestration of fluids within the body (as in patients with pancreatitis, in whom fluid is lost from the vascular to the interstitial space), may initiate this response. In patients with diseases such as cirrhosis or heart failure, in whom total body fluid may be increased although the "effective" circulating volume is decreased, this response is also triggered.

In all these conditions, body sensors detect a state of volume depletion and initiate a series of stimuli that result in sodium and water avidity by the kidney. This response is adaptive in the cases of sequestration and internal shifts but may be maladaptive in a patient with congestive heart failure. The characteristics of conditions in which a decreased effective circulating volume occurs are

1. A decrease in the GFR and a rise in BUN and SCr
2. A rise in the BUN/SCr ratio
3. A low urinary concentration of sodium, usually less than 20 mEq/L, on a spot sample of urine
4. A rise in urine osmolality to greater than 800 mOsm/kg water
5. Fractional excretion of sodium less than 1%

The administration of diuretics; the presence of high rates of excretion of nonelectrolyte osmoles such as glucose, mannitol, or urea; and renal disease may render these urine indices of volume depletion nondiagnostic. In the absence of these confounding variables, the urinary indices reflect the intact nature of the renal response to loss of effective circulating volume. If a patient, who by other criteria is volume depleted, manifests inappropriately high rates of excretion of sodium (>40 mEq/L on a spot sample of urine or an FE of sodium >1%) in the absence of a diuretic or high osmolar loads, the possibility of acute or chronic renal injury must be considered. As a clinical rule, urinary excretion of sodium or preferably the FE of sodium and the urine osmolality, should be obtained immediately when assessment of fluid balance is required. For maximum clinical value, such determinations should be obtained before administration of diuretics.

In a patient who by other criteria appears to have expansion of the extracellular fluid volume but whose urinary excretion of sodium is low and urinary osmolality is high, the physician must consider that the kidney may be sensing effective circulating volume as inadequate. In such a patient, central hemodynamic monitoring may indicate that the central volume is appropriate or overexpanded and that the renal response reflects hormonal or nervous override of normal volume regulatory mechanisms. Hemodynamic monitoring may also indicate that the central volume is depleted, despite the apparent presence of fluid excess by other criteria. Under such circumstances, the renal response is appropriate.

Liver Disease and the Kidney

Patients with advanced liver failure, and especially those with hepatic cirrhosis, acquire a characteristic type of renal dysfunction termed *hepatorenal syndrome (HRS)*. This syndrome consists of renal dysfunction characterized by a reduction in GFR, severe sodium retention (urinary sodium usually <10 mEq/L), and severe oliguria. Hepatic coma, ascites, relative hypotension, and jaundice are frequently present. Further, the severity of these abnormalities does not correlate well with the degree of renal dysfunction. Small amounts of protein are found in the urine, and hyaline and granular cases are typical in patients with HRS. Impaired renal concentrating ability usually occurs, although the urine osmolality is often modestly elevated. The most characteristic abnormality is the extremely low concentrations of sodium found in the urine. This has been attributed primarily to a reduction in distal delivery of sodium to the tubules because of reduced filtration and enhanced proximal reabsorption.

One of the most prominent and consistent findings in patients with HRS is an alteration in RBF. In patients with cirrhosis and HRS, angiography reveals severe attenuation of interlobar arteries, with loss of visualization of arcuate and interlobular arteries.[59] The constriction may be segmental, giving a beaded appearance. The nephrogram is diminished, with a loss of the normal distinction between cortex and medulla. The arterial washout phase is prolonged, and the renal vein is rarely visualized. Xenon scans reflect a labile diminution in flow, which affects the superficial cortex to a greater degree than the juxtamedullary region. This renal vasoconstriction is not reversed by α-adrenergic blockade. Autopsy reveals no evidence of this vasoconstriction. Of further interest, kidneys from patients with HRS have been successfully transplanted, with no vasoconstrictive problems after transplantation.

The GFR is severely reduced in HRS. Consequently, SCr is usually in the range of 4 to 6 mg/dl. The reduction in GFR appears to be functional and is probably related to the severe abnormalities in renal blood flow and its distribution, because most investigators do not report any characteristic pathologic abnormality of kidneys at autopsy or after biopsy in patients with HRS. Although glomerular sclerosis has been found in some patients, it does not correlate with the degree of renal dysfunction.

Although ADH, PTH, the kallikrein-kinin system, natriuretic hormone, vasoactive intestinal peptide, and prostaglandins have all been proposed as possibly playing a role in the pathogenesis of this syndrome, the renin-angiotensin-aldosterone system has received the most attention in studies of HRS. Patients with cirrhosis but not HRS have elevated plasma renin activity and aldosterone concentrations. Whereas renin levels correlate inversely with sodium excretion, aldosterone levels do not.[66] It seems unlikely that elevated aldosterone levels are primarily responsible for the profound sodium retention found in patients with HRS, because sodium excretion can be dissociated from plasma aldosterone levels by various experimental manipulations in these patients.[67-70]

Much debate has surrounded the role of disturbances in extracellular and plasma fluid volumes and the distribution of cardiac output in patients with HRS. The concept of "effective circulating blood volume" has been invoked to explain the apparent paradox of an increased extracellular fluid volume seen in these patients associated with renal responses usually found in states of volume depletion. Volume expansion by intravenous infusion of fluid, by body immersion in water, or by reinfusion of ascitic fluid usually causes an increase in GFR and sodium excretion. Unfortunately, in the case of administration of intravenous fluids, the net sodium and water balance are positive. The relative hypovolemia has been explained by splanchnic pooling, a reduction in colloid osmotic pressure related to hypoalbuminemia, and an increase in vascular capacitance related to systemic vasodilation. Because some patients do not respond to these factors, this proposed concept to account for the findings in HRS cannot entirely explain the observed abnormalities. An alternate proposal suggests that sodium and water retention are the primary events that cause the expanded extracellular fluid volume and vasodilation. This hypothesis, however, fails to explain why some patients *do* respond to augmentation of their intravascular volume with diuresis. Thus, no adequate explanation exists at present for the abnormalities.

Bilirubin per se does not cause the renal functional abnormalities seen in HRS, but bile salts do induce vasodilation, hypotension, and sodium retention when administered long term. In contrast, acute bile duct ligation in dogs, which induces bile stasis within the liver, has been reported to cause an increase in GFR and sodium excretion.[71]

A final hypothesis to explain HRS speculates that the deranged liver performance in patients with cirrhosis permits the passage of endotoxin produced in the gut into the systemic circulation. The endotoxin then produces the characteristic hemodynamic and renal functional changes.[72] It has been further postulated that patients with jaundice but without cirrhosis may be at risk for increased endotoxin absorption because of a deficiency of bile acids in the lumen of the gut. Currently available data are only suggestive, and no studies have shown that low levels of endotoxin can produce the entire spectrum of observed clinical abnormalities.

The treatment of HRS has been unsuccessful unless hepatic function improves. It is critical to maintain intravascular volume throughout any illness in patients with preexisting liver disease. Because systemic hemodynamics are often abnormal in patients with cirrhosis, invasive monitoring is frequently required. The choice of fluid for maintenance of intravascular volume remains controversial. In some patients, establishment of a peritoneovenous shunt restores intravascular volume, diminishes the volume of ascites, and improves renal function. Crystalloid infusion alone rarely causes more than a transient improvement and uniformly results in accumulation of massive amounts of edema and ascitic fluid. Protein-containing solutions produce a more lasting response, but no data show that these improve survival. The use of vasodilators and vasopressors in these patients is also controversial. When hypotension is clearly present, some patients have improvement in urinary output when dopamine is used to restore normotension. As with fluid resuscitation, however, little evidence suggests that survival is improved. Although dialysis supports life in patients with HRS, it is often difficult to remove significant amounts of fluid without producing severe hypotension. Thus, unless the liver itself improves, treatment of the associated renal dysfunction in patients with HRS is rarely effectual.[73]

Abnormalities in Urinary Volume

Oliguria

Oliguria may be defined as a urinary flow rate that is reduced below the level capable of excreting obligatory solutes. Osmolar excretion is calculated by multiplying the urine flow rate by the urine osmolality. The daily osmolar load averages 12 mOsm/kg body weight/day, which is equivalent to an osmolar excretion rate of 0.5 mOsm/kg/hr. Because each milliliter of urine is capable of excreting

1 mOsm (maximum urinary concentration, approximately 1000 mOsm/L water), it is unlikely that osmolar excretion is adequate if the urinary output is less than 0.5 ml/kg/hr. In the setting of acute renal failure, oliguria is often stated to be 400 ml/day.

Oliguria or a low osmolar excretion suggests that GFR is reduced. However, the presence of a "normal" urinary output is no guarantee that the GFR is normal. In healthy persons, the kidney normally reabsorbs 98% to 99% of the glomerular filtrate. Any reduction in the efficiency of the concentrating mechanism results in excretion of a larger fraction of the glomerular filtrate. For example, if the fractional excretion of filtrate were to rise to 10%, a GFR of 10 ml/minute (10% of normal) would result in a urinary output of 1 ml/min, or 60 ml/hr. Thus, although the presence of oliguria indicates that renal function is impaired, the absence of oliguria provides no assurance that function is not impaired. Because the excretion of catabolic products depends primarily on glomerular filtration, most chemical and clinical abnormalities of oliguric renal failure can be observed in patients despite the presence of a "normal" urinary output.

Polyuria

Polyuria is defined literally as a large volume of urine.[74] Generally, this implies that the urinary output exceeds the flow rate required to maintain a balance of fluid within body compartments; if allowed to persist, it will result in a depletion of extracellular fluid volume. The clinical recognition of an excessive urinary output, or polyuric state, is occasionally difficult. A urinary output greater than 300 ml/hr suggests the diagnosis of polyuria. One must recognize, however, that it is appropriate for the body to excrete fluid administered in excess of body needs.

"True" polyuria results from two primary mechanisms, each of which evolves from the known physiology of the kidney. The first is an osmotic diuresis. This form of diuresis results when the proximal tubule fails to reabsorb the bulk of the filtered solute. This may be caused by tubular epithelial disease, an overload or saturation of reabsorptive mechanisms, or nonabsorbable, osmotically active substances. Osmotic diuretics increase medullary blood flow, which reduces the solute concentration in the medullary interstitium. Whereas approximately 50% of the volume entering the descending limb is normally reabsorbed, less than 10% may be reabsorbed during an osmotic diuresis. In the distal nephron segments, the absolute amount of sodium chloride that is reabsorbed probably increases, but the ability to compensate for proximal defects is limited. In the collecting duct, water reabsorption is limited by the lack of a hypertonic medullary interstitium. The presence or absence of ADH becomes less important in these circumstances. During osmotic diuresis, the urine approaches iso-osmolality.

An osmotic diuresis is frequently encountered in surgical patients. Hyperglycemia saturates the reabsorptive capacity of the proximal tubule when the blood sugar approaches 180 to 300 mg/100 ml. The administration of mannitol or urea represents therapeutic attempts at attaining an osmotic diuresis. Fluid and electrolyte resuscitation after injury and in the perioperative period results in positive water and electrolyte balance. During recovery, the hormonal mechanisms mediating this retention abate, and the excess is excreted. Radiocontrast agents employed in various radiologic procedures typically have osmolalities higher than 1000 mOsm/kg water and routinely produce an osmotic diuresis. With damage to the proximal tubule, sodium reabsorption is depressed, and an osmotic diuresis may ensue.

The second example of a "true" polyuria is seen in the patient undergoing water diuresis. In contrast to an osmotic diuresis, in which the urinary osmolality is relatively isotonic, water diuresis results in production of an extremely dilute urine (urinary osmolality of 50 to 100 mOsm/kg water). A water diuresis may result from either a lack of ADH or an inability of the collecting duct to respond normally to ADH. Low ADH concentrations are normally seen in the presence of hypoosmolality of the extracellular fluid. A pathologic lack of ADH (diabetes insipidus) may be seen in patients with hypothalamic and pituitary lesions and after surgery on the pituitary gland and hypothalamus.[75] In the normal kidney with a GFR of 100 ml/min, 60 to 70 ml/min is reabsorbed by the proximal tubule. Half of the remaining fluid, or 15 to 20 ml/minute, is reabsorbed in Henle's loop. If no further reabsorption occurs, as in the case of diabetes insipidus, as much as 15 ml/min (or 900 ml/hr) could be excreted as urine. Urinary flow rates of this magnitude are not usually observed, however, because diabetes insipidus rapidly results in hypovolemia, a reduction in GFR, and an increase in the percentage of electrolytes and fluid reabsorbed in the proximal tubule.

Thus, a urinary output in excess of 900 ml/hr suggests that mechanisms other than or in addition to diabetes insipidus are present. These considerations are especially important in the management of patients after head trauma and pituitary or brain surgery.[76]

Use of Diuretics

Diuretic agents generally inhibit sodium absorption in one or more nephron segments. This action may cause secondary effects that reduce urinary concentration potential. Thus, most diuretics increase both sodium and water excretion. Agents that inhibit sodium absorption before the distal tubule increase potassium excretion by mechanisms already outlined. Diuretic action leads to secondary effects by changing intravascular and extracellular volume and the concentration of sodium and potassium ions. For example, volume depletion lead to activation of the sympathetic and renin-angiotensin-aldosterone system.

General indications for diuretic administration include hypertension, extracellular fluid volume expansion, intravascular hypervolemia, therapeutic hypovolemia, and diagnostic purposes. Extracellular fluid volume overexpansion occurs in several diseases, including heart, kidney, and liver failure. Edema impairs brain, heart, lung, liver, and gut function. Diuresis may improve function in edematous conditions, but it is critical not to introduce intravascular hypovolemia during the perioperative period. When the intravascular volume exceeds that required for optimizing cardiac function, diuresis may improve overall cardiovascular condition. Hypertensive patients often have subnormal intravascular volume. About one third of patients with essential hypertensive have exacerbation of blood pressure when sodium chloride is administered, and their pressure is more easily controlled by mild sodium depletion. In recent years, the use of diuretics as primary therapy has been decreasing. Of particular interest, it is not advisable to control hypertension before or after operations with diuretics, because of the consequent hypovolemia. Dehydration therapy may reduce tissue edema, leading to a desire to induce diuresis. The evidence that dehydration improves outcome after brain or lung injury is minimal. The goal in dehydration is to reduce tissue fluid volume without inducing hypovolemia. This is difficult to maintain for prolonged periods, because the source of the diuresed fluid is necessarily from the intravascular space. Diagnostic uses of diuretics to differentiate between prerenal and intrinsic renal failure have largely been discredited. Patients with intrinsic acute renal failure may have a diuretic response, whereas those with prerenal azotemia may not.

The major diuretics in use in the in-hospital situation are the osmotic diuretics and the high-ceiling loop diuretics. Osmotic diuretics, such as mannitol, are filtered by the glomeruli and act as a nonreabsorbable solute in the proximal tubule.[77] In the proximal tubule, they sustain osmolality, which prevents water absorption, because the proximal tubule cannot produce large osmotic gradients because of its high water permeability. This dilutes the remaining intratubular sodium. Because the sodium pump in this segment cannot generate large concentration gradients, sodium and water reabsorption are diminished. The thick ascending limb can generate high concentration gradients, but the massively increased sodium load exceeds the absorptive capacity of the distal nephron. Normally, high collecting duct permeability leads to water reabsorption if the medullary interstitium is concentrated. However, the increase in fluid flow into the loop of Henle dilutes the concentration of the interstitium. The net result is an increase in sodium and water excretion, with urine osmolality tending to become iso-osmotic. It needs to be emphasized, however, that because an agent such as mannitol obligates water relative to sodium, vigorous administration may result in hypernatremia. It is also important to remember that the kidney is the sole route of excretion of mannitol. Systemic administration of mannitol to a patient whose GFR is reduced may result in a failure to obtain diuresis and, more importantly, the retention of unwanted osmoles in the plasma.

The major clinical uses of agents such as mannitol may be (1) the purposeful reduction of the extracellular fluid volume in patients with cerebral edema, (2) the initiation of an increase in the urinary flow rate in patients with specific types of drug overdoses, and (3) the preparation of some patients for procedures that may be associated with renal injury. The third use derives from experimental observations that high urinary flow rates may protect the kidney from some types of acute renal injury.[78,79] The translation of these animal observations to the clinical domain, however, must be made with great caution.

The loop-acting diuretics operate from the luminal side of the tubule and appear to inhibit a sodium chloride cotransport system in the luminal membrane of Henle's loop. Examples of this group of diuretics include furosemide, bumetanide, and metolazone (Zaroxolyn). They gain access to tubular fluid by the organic anion secretory system and, depending on the degree of binding to plasma proteins, by filtration. The diuretic response depends on the delivery of sodium chloride to the thick ascending limb of Henle's loop. Failure to observe a diuretic response thus may derive from failure of the drug to be secreted, such as in patients with renal disease, in patients with retention of organic anions that compete for the secretory site, or in circumstances when a greatly enhanced rate of sodium reabsorption in the proximal convoluted tubule and reduced delivery of filtrate to the thick ascending limb occur. The dose-response relationship of the loop-acting diuretics is such that relative degrees of impaired rates of secretion (and thus the diuretic response) may be overcome by administration of higher doses of the drug.

The major indication for potent loop-acting diuretics is to reduce the extracellular fluid volume.[80,81] If administered in excess or inappropriately, the loop-acting diuretics can cause depletion of the extracellular fluid volume, hypokalemia, and alkalosis. The attendant depletion of the extracellular fluid volume results in increases rates of fluid and electrolyte transport in the proximal tubule, a decrease in delivery of filtrate to the Henle's loop, and thus a partial internal brake on the unmodified effect of diuretics to deplete the extracellular fluid volume. Such protection, however, is only relative, is often incomplete, and depends on the operation of normal homeostatic mechanisms. In the clinical use of these drugs, such defense mechanisms cannot always be documented as being present, and the drugs must be used with caution. Frequent monitoring of the state of hydration of the patient is required. If, in addition to the diuretic, sodium and fluids are administered to match the urinary output, or if the patient has internal sources of fluids that can be mobilized (edema, effusions), the extracellular fluid volume tends to be sustained, and the delivery of filtrate to the site of diuretic action and the distal nephron tends to be maintained. This may result in high rates of potassium excretion and hypokalemia.

A less commonly used group of diuretics is the thiazide group. These agents act on the distal convoluted tubule to inhibit sodium reabsorption. They also induce vasodilation when administered long term. This action may partially counteract their volume-depleting effects. Thiazides are used primarily to manage blood pressure in patients with hypertension.

It has been suggested that diuretics may be of value in maintaining renal function in conditions where acute renal injury is likely to occur.[78,79] As with mannitol, experimental data indicate that pretreatment with loop diuretics may be of value.[79] In clinical circumstances, however, the injurious event or toxin usually occurs before diuretics are administered. Perhaps the most widely disputed issue pertaining to the surgical patient is the use of diuretics in the oliguric patient with suspected acute renal failure. Before diuretics are used, the etiology of the oliguria must be evaluated. If such an evaluation results in the diagnosis of acute renal injury (vasomotor nephropathy or acute tubular necrosis), controversial recommendations exist regarding the use of diuretics. Most studies suggest that neither the degree nor the duration of acute renal failure is altered by the use of loop-acting diuretics.[82,83] Some studies indicate a worsening degree of renal injury. Nonetheless, a finite number of oliguric patients with acute renal injury respond to diuretic administration by converting from an oliguric to a nonoliguric form of acute renal failure. Although diuretics do not alter the course or outcome, it is easier to manage patients with polyuric acute renal failure than those with oliguria.

To date, no clinical or laboratory signs are available to indicate which patients would be responsive to diuretics. As a practical and pragmatic approach, it is recommended that patients with oliguria be thoroughly evaluated. If acute renal failure is the most probable diagnosis and the patient is normally hydrated, 200 to 400 mg furosemide can be administered as a single intravenous bolus. If no response is obtained, further diuretic administration should be halted. In a patient who is severely overloaded with fluid and unresponsive to diuretics, dialysis or continuous ultrafiltration may be required to remove the excess fluid.[81,84]

SUMMARY

The kidney is responsible for maintenance of fluid and electrolyte balance; participates in several endocrinologic systems, including regulation of vitamin D homeostasis, the renin-angiotensin system, erythropoietin production, and catabolism of peptide hormones; and serves as the excretory route for endogenously produced and exogenously administered substances. In maintaining fluid and electrolyte balance, the kidney responds to several hormones, including aldosterone, parathyroid hormone, and antidiuretic hormone, to alter excretion in a way designed to adjust output to match intake.

Fluids and electrolytes are regulated by the production of a large volume of plasma ultrafiltrate through glomerular filtration, from which varying components are reabsorbed by the renal tubular system before excretion. In addition, several specific secretory transport processes accelerate excretion of a variety of substances. The proximal renal tubule reabsorbs about 60% of the filtered sodium and water in isotonic ratios and removes almost all the bicarbonate, glucose, and amino acids. It also adds several organic acids and bases to the tubular fluid. Henle's loop and its associated vascular bundles set the stage for the production of concentrated and diluted urine. The descending limb performs little active transport, whereas the thick ascending limb is extremely active in reabsorbing sodium from the filtrate before its entry into the distal nephron. The distal nephron segments finely regulate the composition of the excreted urine in terms of sodium, potassium, hydrogen ions, and water concentration.

The clinical assessment of renal function is closely related to an understanding of renal physiology and consists of examination of the formed elements in the urine as well as of the chemical composition of the urine. Specific tests of RBF, GFR, and tubular transport can also be evaluated. Many systemic diseases, as well as anesthesia, drugs, surgery, and various bodily insults, can greatly alter renal function, with the potential for permanent renal damage. Only by clearly appreciating the dynamics of normal kidney physiology can the physician appropriately recognize derangements in renal function and thus initiate judicious treatment before irreversible injury ensues.

REFERENCES

1. Bonventre JV, Leaf A. Sodium homeostasis: Steady states without a set point. Kidney Int 21:880, 1982.
2. Seely J, Levy M. Control of extracellular fluid volume. In Brenner BM, Rector FC, eds. The Kidney, 2nd ed. Philadelphia: WB Saunders, 1981.
3. Skorecki KL, Brenner BM. Body fluid homeostasis in man: A contemporary overview. Am J Med 70:77, 1981.
4. Thurau K, Levine DZ. The renal circulation. In Rouiller C, Muller AF, eds. The Kidney: Morphology, Biochemistry, Physiology. New York: Academic Press, 1971.
5. Chou SY, Porush JG, Faubert PF. Renal medullary circulation: Hormonal control. Kidney Int 37:1, 1990.
6. Hays SR. Ischemic acute renal failure. Am J Med Sci 304:93, 1992.
7. Stein JH. Regulation of the renal circulation. Kidney Int 38:571, 90.
8. Ladefoged J, Munch O. Distribution of blood flow in the kidney. In Fisher JW, ed. Kidney Hormones. London: Academic Press, 1971.
9. Maher JF. Pathophysiology of renal hemodynamics. Nephron 27:215, 1981.
10. Navar LG, et al. Intrinsic control of renal hemodynamics. Fed Proc 41:3022, 1982.
11. Carmines PK, et al. Determinants of renal microvascular autoregulation behavior in normal and hypertension rats. Kidney Int 39(Suppl 132):S89, 1991.
12. Haberle DA, et al. Renal blood flow control by tubuloglomerular feedback (TGF) in normal and spontaneously hypertensive rats—A role for dopamine and adenosine. Klin Wochenschr 69:587, 1991.
13. Loftus JP, Redfield MM, Burnett Jr JC. Atrial natriuretic factor inhibits saline-mediated decreases in renal hemodynamics. Kidney Int 38:227, 1990.
14. Kon V. Neural control of renal circulation. Miner Electrolyte Metab 15:33, 1989.
15. Hollenberg NK. Renal perfusion and function. The implications of converting enzyme inhibition. Am J Med 84(Suppl 4A):9, 1988.
16. Sperry RJ, et al. The influence of hemorrhage on organ perfusion during deliberate hypotension in rats. Anesthesiology 77:1171, 1992.

17. Zall S, Milocco I, Ricksten S-E. Effects of adenosine on renal function and central hemodynamics after coronary artey bypass surgery. Anesth Analg 76:493, 1993.
18. Henrick WL. Southwestern Internal Medicine Conference: The endothelium—A key regulator of vascular tone. Am J Med Sci 302:319, 1991.
19. King AJ, Brenner BM. Endothelium-derived vasoactive factors and the renal vasculature. Am J Physiol 260:R653, 1991.
20. Luscher TJ, et al. Endothelium-derived relaxing and contracting factors. Kidney Int 39:575, 1991.
21. Ballermann B, Marsden P. EDRF and endothelin-I release by glomerular endothelial cells. Clin Invest Med 14:508, 1991.
22. Gandhi CR, Berkowitz DE, Watkins WD. Endothelins—Biochemistry and pathophysiologic actions. Anesthesiology 80:892, 1994.
23. Luscher TF, Bock HA. The endothelial L-arginine/nitric oxide pathway and the renal circulation. Klin Wochenschr 69:603, 1991.
24. Brenner BM, Hostetter TH. Mechanisms of glomerular barrier function. Contrib Nephrol 26:9, 1981.
25. Oken DE. Does the ultrafiltration coefficient play a key role in regulating glomerular filtration in the rat? Am J Physiol 256:F505, 1989.
26. Loutzenhiser RD, Epstein M. Renal hemodynamic effects of calcium antagonists. J Cardiovasc Pharmacol 12(Suppl 6):S48, 1988.
27. Maddox DA, Brenner BM. Glomerular filtration of fluid and macromolecules: the renal response to injury. Annu Rev Med 28:91, 1977.
28. Haberle DA, von Baeyer H. Characteristics of glomerulo-tubular balance. Am J Physiol 244:F355, 1983.
29. Kiil F. Mechanisms of glomerul-tubular balance: The whole kidney approach. Renal Physiol 5:209, 1982.
30. Frei U, Schindler R, Koch KM. Influence of antihypertensive therapy on renal function. Clin Invest 70:S120, 1992.
31. Wright FS, Okusa MD. Functional role of tubuloglomerular feedback control of glomerular filtration. Adv Nephrol 19:119, 1990.
32. Baylis C, Handa RK, Sorkin M. Glucocorticoids and control of glomerular filtration rate. Semin Nephrol 10:320, 1990.
33. Kurtz A, Muff R, Fischer JA. Calcitonin gene products and the kidney. Klin Wochenschr 67:870, 1989.
34. Shaffer SG, Weismann DN. Fluid requirements in the preterm infant. Clin Perinatol 19:233, 1992.
35. Suki WN. Renal hemodynamic consequences of angiotensin-converting enzyme inhibition in congestive heart failure. Arch Intern Med 149:669, 1989.
36. Straer JD, Rondeau E, Lacave R. Role of the renin-angiotensin system in the regulation of glomerular filtration. J Cardiovasc Pharmacol 14(Suppl 4):S21, 1989.
37. Warnock DG, Eveloff J. NaCl entry mechanisms in the luminal membrane of the renal tubule. Am J Physiol 242:F561, 1982.
38. Knepper M, Burg M. Organization of nephron function. Am J Physiol 244:F579, 1983.
39. Kokko JP. Transport characteristics in the thin limbs of Henle. Kidney Int 22:449, 1982.
40. Greger R, Velazqyez H. The critical thick ascending limb and early distal convoluted tubule in the urinary concentrating mechanism. Kidney Int 31:590, 1987.
41. Schrier RW, Berl T, Anderson RJ. Osmotic and nonosmotic control of vasopressin release. Am J Physiol 236:F321, 1979.
42. Berliner RW. Mechanisms of urine concentration. Kidney Int 22:201, 1982.
43. Knox FG, et al. Role of hydrostatic and oncotic pressures in renal sodium reabsorption. Circ Res 52:491, 1983.
44. Young DB, Paulsen AW. Interrelated effects of aldosterone and plasma potassium on potassium excretion. Am J Physiol 244:F28, 1983.
45. Giebisch G. Newer aspects of renal tubular potassium transport. Contrib Nephrol 21:106, 1980.
46. Jamison RL, Work J, Schafer JA. New pathways for potassium transport in the kidney. Am J Physiol 242:F297, 1982.
47. Wright FS. Potassium transport by successive segments of the mammalian nephron. Fed Proc 40:2398, 1981.
48. Tannen RL. Effect of potassium on renal acidification and acid-base homeostasis. Semin Nephrol 7:263, 1987.
49. Chan YL, Biagi B, Giebisch G. Control mechanisms of bicarbonate transport across the rat proximal convoluted tubule. Am J Physiol 242:F532, 1982.
50. DuBose TD, Good DW. Effects of diuretics on renal acid-base transport. Semin Nephrol 8:282, 1988.
51. Masora EJ. An overview of hydrogen ion regulation. Arch Intern Med 142:1019, 1982.
52. Warnock D, Rector FC. Renal acidification mechanisms. In Brenner BM, Rector FC, eds. The Kidney, 2nd ed. Philadelphia: WB Saunders, 1981.
53. Dennis VW, Stead WW, Myers JL. Renal handling of phosphate and calcium. Annu Rev Physiol 41:257, 1979.
54. Dirks JH. The kidney and magnesium regulation. Kidney Int 23:771, 1983.
55. Lang F. Renal handling of calcium and phosphate. Klin Wochenschr 58:985, 1980.
56. Bricker NS, Fine LG. The renal response to progressive nephron loss. In Brenner BM, Rector FC, eds. The Kidney, 2nd ed. Philadelphia: WB Saunders, 1981.
57. Graff SL. A Handbook of Routine Urinalysis. Philadelphia: JB Lippincott, 1982.
58. Haycock GB. Old and new tests of renal function. J Clin Pathol 34:1276, 1981.
59. Adams DR, Hollenberg NK, Abrams HL. Angiography of renal failure. In Griffith JH, ed. Radiology of Renal Failure. Philadelphia: WB Saunders, 1976.
60. Rhodes PJ, et al. Evaluation of eight methods for estimating creatinine clearance in men. Clin Pharm 6:399, 1987.
61. Gault MH, et al. Predicting glomerular function from adjusted serum creatinine. Nephron 62:249, 1992.
62. Harrington JT, Cohen JJ. Measurement of urinary electrolytes—Indications and limitations. N Engl J Med 293:1241, 1975.
63. Pru C, Kjellstrand CM. The clinical usefulness of the FeNa test in acute renal failure: A critical analysis. Proc Dial Transplant Forum 10:240, 1980.
64. Mazze RI, Trudell JR, Cousins MJ. Methoxyflurane metabolism and renal dysfunction: Clinical correlation in man. Anesthesiology 35:247, 1971.
65. Cousins MJ, et al. Metabolism and renal effects of enflurane in man. Anesthesiology 44:44, 1976.
66. Rosoff L Jr, et al. Renal hemodynamics and the renin-angiotensin system in cirrhosis: Relationship to sodium retention. Dig Dis Sci 24:25, 1979.
67. Better OS, Schrier RW. Disturbed volume homeostasis in patients with cirrhosis of the liver. Kidney Int 23:303,1983.
68. Epstein M. Deranged sodium homeostasis in cirrhosis. Gastroenterology 76:622, 1979.
69. Epstein M. Determinants of abnormal renal sodium handling in cirrhosis: A reappraisal. Scand J Clin Lab Invest 40:689, 1980.
70. Skorecki KL, Brenner BM. Body fluid homeostasis in congestive heart failure and cirrhosis with ascites. Am J Med 72:323, 1982.
71. Bailey ME. Endotoxin, bile salts and renal function in obstructive jaundice. Br J Surg 63:774, 1976.
72. Richman AV, Gerber LI, Balis JU. Peritubular capillaries: A major target site of endotoxin-induced vascular injury in the primate kidney. Lab Invest 43:327, 1980.
73. Papper S. Hepatorenal syndrome. Contrib Nephrol 23:55, 1980.
74. Baylis PH, Gaskill MB, Robertson GL. Vasopressin secretion in primary polydipsia and cranial diabetes insipidus. Q J Med 50:345, 1981.
75. Notman DD, Mortek MA, Moses AM. Permanent diabetes insipidus following head trauma: Observations in ten patients and an approach to diagnosis. J Trauma 20:599, 1980.

76. Schrier RW, Szatalowicz VL. Disorders of water metabolism. Contrib Nephrol 21:48, 1980.
77. Warren SE, Blantz RC. Mannitol. Arch Intern Med 141:493, 1981.
78. de Torrente A, et al. Effects of furosemide and acetylcholine in nonepinephrine-induced acute renal failure. Am J Physiol 4:131, 1978.
79. Levinsky NG, Bernard DB, Johnson PA. Enhancement of recovery of acute renal failure. In Brenner BM, Stern JM, eds. Acute Renal Failure: Contemporary Issues in Nephrology, vol 6. New York: Churchill Livingstone, 1988.
80. Brater DC. Determinants of response to loop diuretics. Fed Proc 42:1694, 1983.
81. Heidenreich O, Greven J, Weintze K. Diuretic agents: Actions on a molecular level. Clin Exp Hypertens 5:177, 1983.
82. Brown CB, Ogg CS, Cameron JS. High dose furosemide in acute renal failure: A controlled trial. Clin Nephrol 15:90, 1981.
83. Kleinknecht D, Ganeval D, Gonzales-Duque LA. Furosemide in acute oliguric renal failure: A controlled trial. Nephron 17:51, 1976.
84. Lant AF. Modern diuretics and the kidney. J Clin Pathol 34:1267, 1981.

43

Obstruction of the Urinary Tract

Marko R. Gudziak and Joseph N. Corriere, Jr.

Obstructive diseases of the urinary tract can be congenital or acquired, can occur at any level in the organ system, and can be found at all ages and in both sexes. Most patients eventually develop signs or symptoms related to the disease process causing the obstruction, the obstructed urinary tract organs per se, or renal failure symptoms secondary to progressive loss of functioning renal tissue. With the more liberal use of noninvasive diagnostic imaging modalities such as ultrasound, as well as the routine use of laboratory studies, more and more totally asymptomatic patients with obstructive uropathy are being discovered, even in the prenatal period. Fortunately, most obstructive problems are reversible if discovered at an early stage, so a high index of suspicion of their presence can help prevent needless morbidity and mortality. In the following discussion an emphasis is placed on the physiologic derangements in renal function and in the function of the renal collecting system that occur during both the urinary obstruction and the reparative process after the obstruction has been relieved.

INCIDENCE OF OBSTRUCTIVE DISORDERS

Because of the variety of lesions that can cause obstructive uropathy, it is difficult to give a true overall incidence of this disease process. One must go back to the pioneering work of Campbell[1] cataloging pediatric urologic disorders to get a sense of the problem in children, where it is the most common renal collecting system disorder that requires surgical correction. In an autopsy study of 15,919 patients 15 years old or younger, he found 316 to have hydronephrosis, an incidence of 1.99%. The majority of the patients, 256 (81%), were younger than 1 year old, and 148 (57.8%) of these infants were boys. Only 14 (4.4%) were between the ages of 3 and 10 years, and 11 (3.5%) were between 11 and 15 years of age. Campbell found over half the hydronephroses to be bilateral and more than 80% of the lesions to have their origin above the level of the bladder.

A concomitant series of 512 children whose diseases were recognized clinically rather than at autopsy had a less skewed age distribution. Only 114 (22.3%) were younger than 1 year of age, 124 (24.2%) were between 1 and 2 years of age, and 234 (45.7%) were between the ages of 3 and 10 years. Forty children (7.8%) were between the ages of 11 and 15 years. However, as with the autopsy series, more than 80% of the lesions were secondary to supravesical disorders. The screening of patients with both prenatal and postnatal ultrasound is changing these figures because asymptomatic hydronephrotic kidneys are being found more and more frequently. Prenatal ultrasound detects hydronephrosis in as many as 1.4% of fetuses, with it persisting postnatally in half of that percent.[2]

During middle age, pelvic disease in women and ureteral calculus disease in both sexes account for most cases of obstructed ureters. Indeed, the prevalence of calculi causing renal colic or hematuria and acute or chronic hydroureteronephrosis is about 5% in women and 10% in men in the United States.[3] Later in life, bladder outlet obstruction, specifically benign prostatic hyperplasia (BPH), causes voiding symptoms in approximately 50% of men older than 60, and about 10% of men older than 40 eventually need a prostatectomy.[4] The number of men having prostatectomies has dropped during the last decade with the advent of new noninvasive treatments for BPH.

NORMAL FUNCTION

Renal Pelvic and Ureteral Function

The collecting system of the upper urinary tract, the renal pelvis and ureter, is a tubular extension of the renal collecting tubules. Physiologically, it is a continuous structure with only anatomic distinctions. The function of this unit is to convey urine from the kidney to the bladder. The smooth muscle of the ureter can be divided into inner longitudinally coursing bundles and an outer layer of circular and oblique muscle. Urine does not flow passively but is actively propelled by ureteral peristalsis. A bolus of urine entering the renal calyces and pelvis stimulates a pelvic contraction that is propagated along the ureter by cell-to-cell propagation of action potentials. Neurotransmission is thought to occur by diffusion rather than any direct transmission.[5] Resection of any segment of the collecting system does not seem to disturb function of the unit.

The ureter receives sympathetic input from T10 though L2 spinal segments. Parasympathetic input is from S2 to S4. The role of this autonomic input is unclear. Normal ureteral peristalsis does not require autonomic input. Propagation originates in pacemaker sites in the intrinsic smooth muscle of the minor calyces.[6] Autonomic input may affect urine transport by affecting the peristaltic frequency and bolus volume.[7] As a urine bolus enters the ureter, the ureteral walls must coapt behind the bolus to move it forward efficiently. Baseline or resting pressure in the ureter is 0 to 5 cm H_2O (approximately 6.5 mm Hg) with peristaltic contractions of 20 to 80 cm H_2O occurring two to six times per minute.[8,9] During acute obstruction, as from a ureteral calculus, ureteral pressure will rise to 50 to 70 mm Hg. During chronic obstruction the mean intrapelvic pressures are about 21 mm Hg.[8] During a brisk diuresis the ureter can generate pressures as high as 110 mm Hg.[10] Renal pelvic pressures decrease in time after acute obstruction. The ureter enters the bladder at an oblique angle and then travels in a submucosal tunnel before opening into the bladder proper. This configuration produces a flap valve effect, which prevents urine in the bladder from refluxing back into the ureter.

Bladder Function

The main functions of the urinary bladder are to store urine produced by the kidney at low pressure and to act as an efficient voiding mechanism. The urinary bladder or detrusor muscle is composed of a meshwork of smooth muscle fibers without any hierarchic organization, unlike the ureter. The spherical geometry and viscoelastic properties allow the bladder to maintain low tension during increases in urine volume. In other words, in the normal bladder, intravesical pressure does not rise or rises very little as the bladder fills within a physiologic range. This is termed compliance. A normal bladder is highly compliant. The syncytial arrangement of the detrusor muscle facilitates efficient evacuation. Because of its unique ureterovesical junction, the bladder protects the upper urinary tract and renal parenchyma from high pressures of voiding and prevents bacteria from ascending to the kidney.

The bladder and its outlet are innervated by the parasympathetic, sympathetic, and somatic nervous systems. The parasympathetic motor nerves from spinal cord segments S2 to S4 are carried to the bladder and posterior urethra by the pelvic nerves. The sympathetic nerves from spinal cord segments T10 to L2 are carried to this same area by the hypogastric nerves. The somatic sensory and motor nerves from spinal cord segments S2 to S4 are carried to the striated muscles of the pelvic floor by the internal pudendal nerves. Also, afferent sensory nerves from the bladder and urethra carry proprioception, pain, and temperature in the pelvic nerves and to some extent in the hypogastric nerves.[11]

As the bladder fills with urine, the muscle fibers lengthen and increase their intramural tension. This increased tension is sensed by afferent mechanoreceptors, which travel through the pelvic nerve to higher centers, resulting in the sensation of fullness. Central control of micturition and storage appears to be centered in the rostral pons in the pontine micturition center (PMC). The PMC seems to regulate bladder capacity and coordinate the activity of the bladder and external urethral sphincter.[12] The sensation of distention can normally be suppressed by the cerebral cortex until volitional voiding is desired.

Immediately before voiding or active bladder contraction, the striated muscles of the pelvic floor and external urethral sphincter relax. The detrusor muscle then contracts with stimulation from sacral parasympathetics, resulting in release of urine when detrusor pressure exceeds urethral resistance. During the voiding cycle typical bladder pressure ranges from 40 to 60 cm H_2O in men and are somewhat lower in women because the shorter female urethra provides less resistance to outflow.

The role of sympathetic input to the bladder is less clear. It appears to be more important in urine storage and continence than in the act of micturition.[11] Sympathetic input to the lower urinary tract is tonic during bladder filling. It appears to inhibit the detrusor smooth muscle, thus allowing accommodation of larger volumes of urine and increasing urethral resistance. It also inhibits transmission in vesical parasympathetic ganglia.[13]

TYPES OF LESIONS

Obstructing lesions of the urinary tract are best divided into intrinsic diseases of the organ system and extrinsic diseases that secondarily cause urinary tract obstruction (Fig. 43-1). Obviously, the bulk of the congenital disorders are found in children, commonly in the neonatal period or infancy, whereas renal and ureteral calculi are the most common causes of obstructive uropathy in young and middle-aged adults. BPH and urethral strictures are seen in males in later life, which is also the time when genitourinary tract tumors occur and can cause urinary tract obstruction. Bladder outlet obstruction rarely occurs in neurologically intact women; when it occurs, it is usually a result of overzealous urethral suspension. Ureteral strictures are usually caused by surgical trauma but may be associated with ureteral calculi or tuberculosis. Virtually any retroperitoneal or pelvic neoplastic or inflammatory process can secondarily involve and obstruct the ureters. The more common problems encountered are shown in the box on p. 879.

CLINICAL PRESENTATION

Obstruction of the upper urinary tract is usually accompanied by flank pain. This discomfort is caused by distention of the collecting system and renal capsule and quickly dissipates when the obstruction is relieved. The pain is usually caused by acute obstructions, not chronic problems. If the obstruction occurs in the upper portion of the ureter, the pain may radiate into the ipsilateral testicle in the male. If low in the ureter, near the bladder, the pain

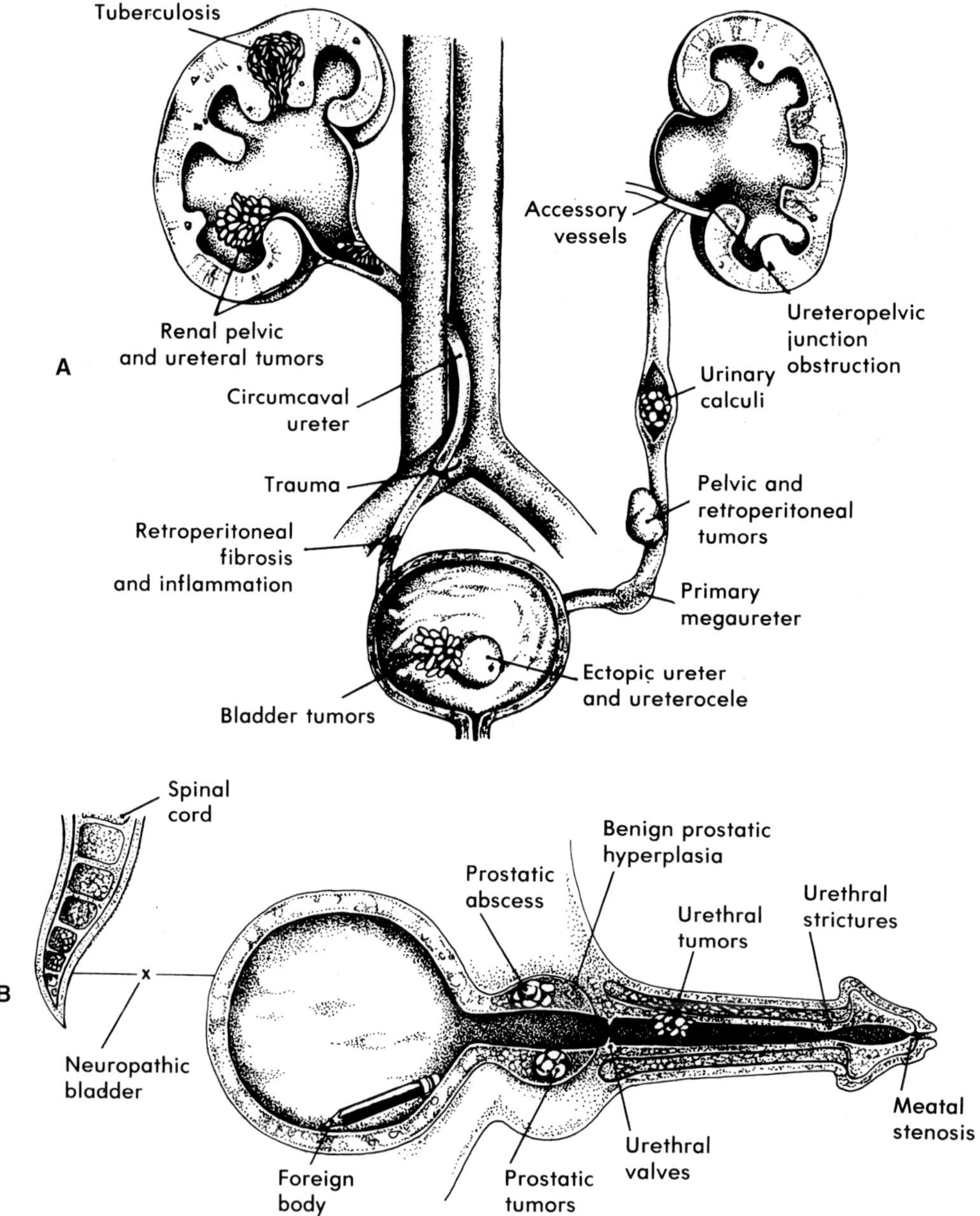

Fig. 43-1. A, Causes of upper urinary tract obstruction. **B,** Causes of lower urinary tract obstruction.

may be felt in the ipsilateral scrotum, labia, or inner aspect of the thigh. This is known as referred pain and is related to the common nerve supply shared by the urinary and genital systems.

Afferent nerve terminals exist in the renal capsule and parenchyma and the epithelium and smooth muscle of the renal pelvis and ureter. The sympathetic nerve supply is mainly from the celiac ganglia and aortic plexus. Preganglionic fibers are received through the lesser and least splanchnic nerves from the T6 through L1 Ganglia. The hypogastric plexus receives impulses from the bladder (S2 through S4), whereas the pudendal nerve supplies the urethra.

Visceral pain travels to the lateral spinothalamic tract up the cord to the premotor cortex of the frontal lobes. The T10 through T12 and L1 segments are the visceral afferents for the kidney and ureter but also serve the margin of the diaphragm, large bowel, ovary, fallopian tube and uterus, appendix, duodenum, small bowel, gallbladder, pancreas, testes, spleen, and abdominal aorta. The afferent somatic nerves of these segments are also represented in this area.

This common segment innervation is present because of normal intrauterine organ migration. During development the kidney arises in the lower lumbar and sacral regions and ascends to its final flank position, whereas the gonads and genital ducts develop high in the abdomen and

COMMON CAUSES OF URINARY OBSTRUCTION

Intrinsic Diseases of the Urinary Tract

Congenital disorders

Ureteropelvic junction lesions
Primary megaureter
Ectopic ureter
Ectopic ureterocele
Neuropathic bladder disease
Urethral valves
Detrusor sphincter dyssynergia
Ureteral dysplasia (prune-belly syndrome)

Metabolic and inflammatory disorders

Urinary calculi
Blood clots
Fungus balls
Sloughed papillae (papillary necrosis)
Renal, ureteral, or vesical tuberculosis
Urethral strictures
Prostatic inflammatory diseases
Meatal stenosis
Foreign body

Neoplastic disorders

Benign prostatic hyperplasia
Renal pelvic and ureteral tumors
Bladder tumors
Prostatic tumors
Urethral tumors

Traumatic disorders

Ureteral stricture (postsurgical)
Urethral stricture

Extrinsic Obstruction of the Ureter

Vascular lesions

Accessory vessels
Aortic, iliac aneurysms
Ovarian vein syndrome
Circumcaval (retrocaval) ureter

Pelvic and retroperitoneal masses

Pregnancy
Enlarged uterus—benign, malignant disorders
Hydrometrocolpos
Ovarian lesions
Embryologic remnants (cysts of Gartner's duct)
Pelvic and retroperitoneal tumors, primary and metastatic
Pelvic lipomatosis
Lymphocele
Uterine prolapse

Inflammatory diseases

Retroperitoneal fibrosis
Retroperitoneal abscess
Retroperitoneal hemorrhage
Tubo-ovarian abscess; pelvic inflammatory disease
Appendiceal or diverticular abscess
Endometriosis
Granulomatous (Crohn's) disease of the bowel

descend approximately 10 segments below this level of origin to eventually descend into the scrotum.

Referred pain is through a viscerosomatic reflex arc. The afferent fiber enters the cord to form a synapse with a cell in the lateral horn of the gray matter. This cell's preganglionic fiber connects with a sympathetic ganglion whose postganglionic fiber connects to a peripheral spinal nerve. This connection to peripheral nerves accounts for the hyperesthesia or pain referred from visceral pathologic conditions to dermatomes innervated by somatic nerves originating at the same cord levels. The genitofemoral and ilioinguinal nerves are the usual pathways for referred pain to the groin and upper inner thighs.

Although classically described as colicky pain caused by contraction and relaxation of the ureter, the discomfort may be constant in nature. The patient is restless and cannot get into a comfortable position. Frequency and urgency may be seen if the obstructing lesion is near the bladder and irritating that organ. Commonly, reflex nausea and vomiting may be present; if the obstructed renal unit is infected, bacteremia, fever, and chills may develop. Usually urine volume is not noticeably changed when only one kidney is totally obstructed. Anuria occurs with bilateral obstruction or in the patient who has a solitary obstructed kidney.

When acute ureteral obstruction occurs, hematuria may be seen and is usually secondary to damage of the transitional epithelium of the upper urinary tract by the offending lesion, usually a calculus. When chronic obstruction is present, it is common for veins in the submucosa of the renal pelvis to become quite large and thin walled. Minimal trauma to these chronically distended renal units may cause these veins to rupture, and blood is present in the urine. This is a particularly common first sign of a dilated collecting system structure in children.

Chronic obstruction of the upper urinary tract is usually virtually asymptomatic. Vague abdominal complaints may be elicited, especially after a large fluid intake. If obstruction is of a long-standing bilateral nature, symptoms of chronic renal failure, namely, polyuria and polydipsia, as well as fatigue, may be present.

Patients with infravesical obstruction usually have all the symptoms of prostatism—frequency, urgency, hesitancy, nocturia, a slow intermittent urinary stream, and perhaps (overflow) urinary incontinence. Some patients have complete urinary retention. Hematuria may be present because of rupture of distended mucosal veins in the bladder, urethra, or prostate; if the patient has an infected lower urinary tract, dysuria is a common complaint. Patients with neuropathic bladder disease usually mimic the patient with bladder neck obstruction but also have complaints relative to their primary neurologic problem.

EXAMINATION AND DIAGNOSTIC STUDIES

Physical Examination

Patients who have obstructed renal units may have tenderness in the costovertebral angle or in the abdomen at the level of the obstructing lesion. Infected, septic patients may be febrile. A tender mass in the flank may indicate a long-standing obstructing kidney, and a midline suprapubic mass may indicate a distended bladder. Children with the prune-belly syndrome do not have the anterior abdominal muscles but have bilateral undescended testicles and chronic hydronephrosis.

A large, smooth prostate on rectal examination in an elderly man suggests benign prostatic hyperplasia. The size of the prostate, however, does not correlate with the degree of obstruction that it causes. A nodular prostate at any age suggests a neoplasm of that organ. Bowel or pelvic organ lesions may be palpated on rectal or vaginal examination, as may masses extrinsic to these organ systems. The external sphincter tone, bulbocavernosus reflex, perineal sensation, and lower extremity function should be noted in patients suspected of having neurologic disorders. One should check for periurethral masses and palpate the length of the urethra. Finally, inspection of the urethral meatus for stenosis should not be overlooked.

Laboratory Evaluation

A urinalysis is helpful in the diagnosis of bilateral obstructive uropathy, for concentrating ability is lost in the course of this disease process. White blood cells and bacteria may be found if infection is present. Urinary tract infections should be confirmed by a urine culture. Hematuria may be seen.

Serum chemistries, especially a blood urea nitrogen and creatinine, are necessary to monitor renal function. Serum electrolytes should be measured, especially in the azotemic patient. A creatinine clearance may be necessary to help plan and follow therapeutic measures that will be instituted. If a carcinoma of the prostate is suspected, a prostate-specific antigen (PSA) level should be determined. In patients with suspected urothelial tumors, a cytologic evaluation of urine may be helpful. Stone chemistries eventually may be needed if the patient is found to have a urinary tract calculus.

Imaging Studies

Radiographic studies with contrast agents are the most useful tests to determine the level of urinary tract obstruction and to obtain diagnostic information about the cause of the obstruction. In the patient with normal or near-normal renal function, the first procedure ordered should be an intravenous urogram (IVU). Most of the time, this study is sufficient to diagnose upper tract lesions, but retrograde or antegrade pyelograms may be needed if the kidney is poorly functioning. In the child a voiding cystourethrogram, in conjunction with a renal ultrasound, is usually all that is required.

Although good quality urograms are possible even in the face of moderate azotemia,[14] the diabetic patient with severely compromised renal function may develop a further reduction in function with iodinated contrast materials.[15] In these situations, as well as in the neonate, who has poor renal function because of age, and in pregnant women, ultrasound evaluation may be a better first-choice study; at least it should be used to corroborate the diagnosis.

The nuclear renal scan is also used in children, but it does not give the fine anatomic detail of an IVU. Its use in conjunction with a diuretic can evaluate the physiologic function of a dilated upper urinary tract by determining emptying time of the renal pelvis.[16] Computed tomography may also be useful, especially in complicated cases of intrinsic or extrinsic upper urinary tract disease. Finally, if a urethral stricture is suspected, a retrograde urethrogram is the appropriate study to perform to delineate the problem. If a bowel lesion is under consideration, barium studies of the gastrointestinal tract should also be obtained.

Diseases of the bladder and urethra in the adult are best diagnosed by cystoscopy and panendoscopy. Up to 40% of the time the cystogram phase of an IVU demonstrates supposed abnormalities that are not actually present or are interpreted as normal even though a lesion is present in the bladder. Biopsies of bladder lesions and the sampling of individual kidney urine for cytologic analysis are also easily accomplished through a cystoscope.

Urodynamic Studies

Urodynamic studies (UDS) can be performed on both the upper and lower urinary tract and are probably the most reliable indicators of urinary obstruction. A renal isotope drainage study in conjunction with a diuretic can give a good indication of the presence of obstruction.[16] With a large capacious renal pelvis and ureter, however, diagnosing obstruction may be difficult using intravenous urography or nuclear renography. The Whitaker test is superior in assessing and quantifying obstruction in the hydronephrotic kidney.[17] This involves percutaneously placing a catheter into the renal pelvis and measuring pressure in the pelvis while a constant flow of saline is infused. Elevated pressure develops in an obstructed system but not in an nonobstructed system.[18] The Whitaker test, if done with contrast material under fluoroscopy, also provides anatomic detail and shows the level of the obstruction.

As in the upper urinary tract, UDS are the most reliable

method of determining whether obstruction is present and the only way of physiologically quantifying the degree of bladder outlet obstruction. In addition, UDS can assess the contractility of the bladder, compliance, and neurologic lesions affecting the bladder. Measuring the rate and volume of urine flow, one can calculate a voiding flow rate. This is not, however, a good indicator of obstruction by itself. By measuring both bladder pressure and urine flow simultaneously one can obtain and truly make a diagnosis of obstruction.[19]

A cystometrogram (CMG) involves filling the bladder through a urethral catheter and measuring bladder sensation, intravesical pressures at various volumes, checking for uninhibited bladder contraction, and then seeing if the detrusor muscle contracts. This provides a reasonable indication of bladder function. When this is performed using intravesical contrast through a small urethral catheter with pressure-sensing ports or microtransducers and observed fluoroscopically, the presence of obstruction can be diagnosed and the level of obstruction accurately determined.[20]

CONSEQUENCES OF OBSTRUCTION ON RENAL FUNCTION

To gain an understanding of the effects of obstructive uropathy on the urinary tract, it is best to consider the organ system as a closed space with an opening for fluid to enter at one end and a relief valve at the other end. Despite obstruction occurring in the system, fluid continues to enter the space. Because of this, the collecting system must dilate to accept the increased volume. Although leaks may develop to relieve the inevitable increase in pressure, the final outcome, because the kidneys are enclosed by a fairly indistensible capsule, is compression and destruction of the renal parenchyma, a phenomenon called hydronephrosis (Fig. 43-2).

Three major mechanisms lead to renal parenchymal damage in urinary tract obstruction: (1) the pressure effect on the kidney, (2) ischemia, and (3) concomitant pyelonephritis. As the hydronephrosis progresses, the parenchyma is compressed. The renal papillae take the brunt of the pressure, but eventually the cortex is obliterated as well. The total renal blood flow decreases in time, and the transmission of increased intratubular pressure to the surrounding vasculature decreases postglomerular blood flow. Pressure is also exerted on the vasa recta and eventually on the preglomerular vessels, especially the interlobar, arcuate, and interlobular arteries. Secondary renal infection is promoted by obstruction and is so common that obstructive uropathy should always be looked for in the patient with an unexplained urinary tract infection, especially if fever, chills, and flank pain are prominent complaints.

The sequence of renal dysfunction that results from obstruction follows[21]:

1. Loss of concentrating ability
2. Reduced ability to excrete acid
3. Decreased glomerular filtration
4. Decreased renal blood flow after initial increase
5. Decreased sodium and water reabsorption

Since the first damage occurs in the medulla of the kidney, it follows that tubular function would be affected initially. In all ages the first defect seen is an inability of the organ to concentrate urine. Exogenous vasopressin does not correct the lesion, which is caused by a decrease in the corticopapillary interstitial osmotic gradient. The reduced ability to excrete acid and the subsequent inability to reduce the urinary pH are probably caused by damage to the collecting ducts. Some investigators believe this pH effect is only seen when glomerular filtration decreases, whereas others believe it is secondary to a decrease in the total number of nephrons.

The reduction in glomerular filtration rate (GFR) is dependent on the degree and duration of obstruction and whether the obstruction is unilateral or bilateral.[22] The increases in peritubular capillary pressure and interstitial pressure that occur with obstruction reduce GFR within 20 minutes of unilateral obstruction, and the permeability of the tubular walls increases. This leaky fluid is removed through the renal lymphatics.[23]

In contrast to these findings, renal blood flow (RBF) increases to about 50% of normal within the first 1 to 2 hours after obstruction. This is most likely caused by release of a vasodilating prostaglandin.[24] This increase in flow seems limited to the renal cortex and falls within 6 hours of the occlusion to approximately 30% of normal

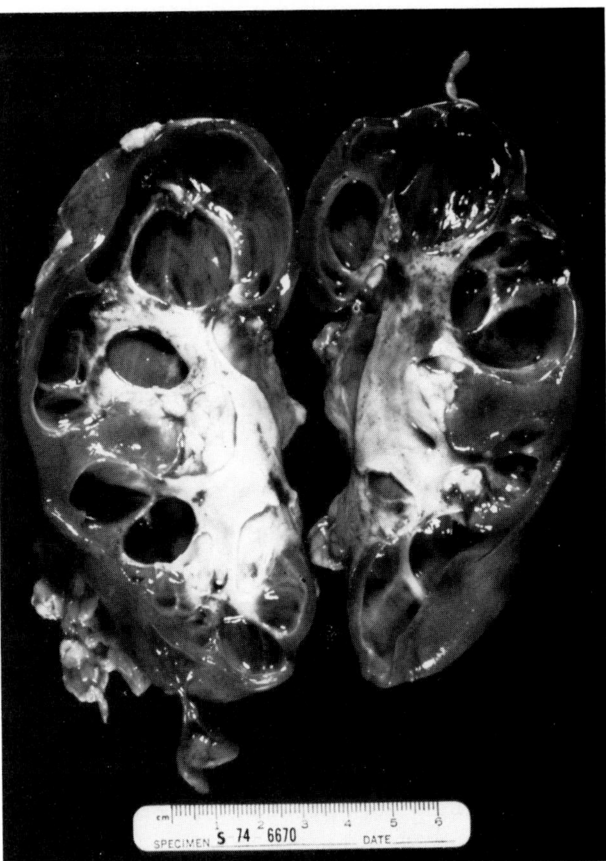

Fig. 43-2. Hydronephrosis with renal parenchymal thinning.

because of a progressive increase in the resistance of the afferent arterioles. Although initially the decrease in GFR allows for a more complete absorption of sodium, with prolonged obstruction, urinary sodium concentration is increased, urinary osmolality is decreased, and a dilute urine is excreted. This is caused by impaired salt and water reabsorption rather than by hyperfiltration by undamaged nephrons.[25]

The effects of bilateral renal obstruction are surprisingly less severe than those of unilateral renal obstruction. Intratubular pressure rises higher in bilateral obstruction but declines in a few hours. Similarly, glomerular capillary pressure increases more rapidly with bilateral occlusion but falls to normal, not below normal as with unilateral obstruction. It appears that afferent arteriolar resistance does not increase as much in this situation. The reason for these differences is unclear. A possible explanation is that when both kidneys are blocked, the composition of the circulating blood—increased amounts of plasma potassium, phosphate, creatinine, urea, and total solutes, as well as other normally eliminated substances—may relax vascular smooth muscle.[26] It should be noted that serum sodium does not change in serum concentration during bilateral renal obstruction.

Postobstructive Diuresis

In some patients with azotemia, an osmotic diuresis of a varying intensity may ensue after relief of obstruction. It is more marked after an acute, complete blockage or an acute blockage superimposed on a chronic, partial obstruction. The mechanism of this diuresis is the sudden increase in GFR, which allows a rapid large delivery of sodium to the tubules with decreased reabsorption in the proximal tubules and probably the distal tubules.[27] The exact mechanism of postobstructive diuresis is unknown, but studies have shown buildup of a natriuretic factor in the plasma of animals with bilateral ureteral obstruction.[28]

It should be stressed that this phenomenon does not happen in the presence of a normal kidney, and most patients who have their obstructive uropathy relieved either have no significant natriuresis or have a physiologic diuresis that results in release of pathologically retained sodium and a reduction of total body sodium to normal. Most of the time this diuresis is gone within 72 hours.[29]

Renal Recovery After Relief of the Obstruction

After removal of a unilateral obstruction, GFR rapidly returns to normal. Glomerular capillary pressure rises and then falls a few hours after relief of the obstruction.[30] Renal blood flow remains low after the relief. Both of these effects are attributed to a persistent elevation in afferent arteriolar resistance. Because of these effects, urine osmolality and the reabsorption of sodium and water remain impaired. The speed and amount of return to normal function depend on the magnitude of permanent damage sustained by the nephron units.

Release of bilateral renal obstruction produces similar effects except in patients who develop postobstructive diuresis. In these patients the sodium balance is usually restored in 3 days, but the concentrating defect may persist for a longer period.

Therapeutic Considerations

In the unilateral obstructed kidney, tube drainage and repair or removal of the obstructing lesion are all that is necessary to obtain maximum recovery because total renal function in the patient is at a level sufficient for normal body function. However, azotemic patients with bilateral obstruction or obstruction of a solitary kidney are at risk for severe postobstructive diuresis after relief of the obstruction. These patients must be observed closely to prevent vascular collapse from a massive diuresis. After the urine is removed from the distended collecting system or bladder, cultured, and measured, careful hourly monitoring of urine output is initiated. If urine output exceeds 200 ml/hr the physician is notified. An alert and conscious patient is able to restore lost volume through the normal thirst mechanism. The natriuresis can be very brisk. Electrolytes should be monitored and vital signs checked frequently to assess for hypovolemia. If the patient has a severe pathologic loss of sodium or is unconscious or unable to keep up with urine loss by oral intake, sodium replacement is needed. An intravenous solution of 0.5 normal saline or lactated Ringer's solution replacing 50% of urine output is started. The diuresis should resolve in 72 hours. If urine output is still copious, the patient may be overhydrated. The diuresis can be perpetuated by overzealous hydration. If the azotemia persists, prolonged tube drainage or temporary diversion may be necessary to return the renal function to a level sufficient to allow surgical repair of the obstructing lesion. In most cases bilateral renal obstruction is due to bladder outlet obstruction. If patients require prolonged bladder drainage, they should be taught self-intermittent catheterization (SIC). This is done using clean, not sterile technique and is associated with fewer complications and morbidities than indwelling urethral or suprapubic catheters.

CONSEQUENCES OF OBSTRUCTION ON THE UPPER URINARY TRACT

When obstruction of the ureter occurs, action potentials and contractions increase. The baseline pressure rises to approximately 70 mm Hg in a few hours, and the ureter eventually becomes an open fluid-filled space. The walls are unable to coapt even though action potentials still occur.[31] Eventually, however, they cease, and the hydraulic pressure falls to normal as the ureter dilates, sometimes to gigantic proportions, to accommodate its increased fluid load. Ureteral pressures continue to decline for 6 to 8 weeks to approximately 15 mm Hg.[32]

Postobstructive Recovery

The ureter that is still dilated after the obstruction has been removed has a decreased ability to develop intraluminal pressures required for urine transport. Despite muscle hypertrophy and increased contractility, the increase in ureteral diameter changes the thickness/radius ratio in the Laplace relationship. Removal of the obstructing lesion and prolonged drainage many times are all that is needed to return the ureter to normal function. However, if the side walls cannot coapt, ureteral motility may not be sufficient to propel a bolus of urine from the kidney to the bladder. Tapering the ureter by folding, plication, or surgical removal of a strip of muscle to decrease its circumference often improves its performance.[33] The tapered ureter can then coapt its walls more easily and generate higher intraluminal pressures.[34]

CONSEQUENCES OF OBSTRUCTION ON BLADDER FUNCTION

The detrusor muscle of the urinary bladder supplies a finite amount of contractile energy during voiding. It is essentially myogenic, and the amount of energy increases with bladder filling, reaching a maximum at 250 to 450 ml. The muscle fibers of the detrusor muscle probably follow Starling's law and are more efficient when lengthened up to a point where they then begin to decompensate.[35]

During infravesical outlet obstruction, bladder outlet resistance increases, which decreases the voiding flow rate but does not affect the power or total energy of the detrusor muscle. A higher voiding pressure develops by passive adaptation. Voiding pressures of more than 100 cm H_2O can develop. As obstruction progresses, more energy is needed for one void. Because available energy is limited, the voided volumes decrease, and residual urine develops when the need exceeds the energy supply.

The detrusor muscle develops large endoscopically visible muscle bundles known as trabeculae. The smooth muscle cells do not really hypertrophy or develop hyperplasia; instead, a massive connective tissue buildup occurs between the muscle bundles.[36] The bladder becomes stiffer and less compliant, tending to reduce detrusor muscle strength. Eventually, the bladder may fail to contract at all, and the patient develops urinary retention.

The effects of obstruction on the upper urinary tract, as discussed earlier, obviously may develop with infravesical obstruction. It has been shown that patients with chronically elevated intravesical pressures (>40 cm H_2O) develop upper urinary tract deterioration (i.e., hydronephrosis and vesicoureteral reflux).[37] At times, the vesicoureteral junction becomes distorted by pathologic conditions within the bladder (mainly pressure), and vesicoureteral reflux develops. When this occurs, the high intravesical pressure of voiding may be transmitted to the kidneys and ureters, accelerating the destructive process to these organs. Vesicoureteral reflux also allows bacteria in the bladder to infect the kidneys.

Postobstructive Recovery of the Bladder

The tissue changes in the bladder wall with partial urethral obstruction, namely, thickening of the musculature and the increase in intracellular connective tissue, seem to be reversible if the duration of obstruction does not exceed 8 weeks.[38] In severe or prolonged obstruction, permanent morphologic and functional damage occurs. At times, the bladder is so damaged it is unable to contract at all. Most of the time, however, even if bladder recovery is not complete, adequate detrusor muscle contractions are possible to empty the bladder in an efficient manner if the obstruction has been adequately removed.

Therapeutic Considerations

Acute postoperative urinary retention is not unusual, particularly after a spinal anesthetic or inguinal or perianal surgery such as for hemorrhoids, and it can occur even in younger patients. If the bladder is allowed to become overdistended, it can suffer a myogenic injury from being overstretched. These patients should be managed with clean intermittent catheterization (CIC). The patient should initially be started on a catheterization schedule of every 4 to 5 hours. The catheterization interval is then adjusted depending on urine output. The goal should be to prevent bladder distention and keep total bladder volume (voided volume plus postvoid residual) less than 400 ml, which is a normal bladder capacity. CIC should be continued until the patient is able to void spontaneously and the postvoid residual is consistently less than 75 ml.

In the patient who has had chronic bladder outlet obstruction, recovery of detrusor muscle function may take weeks or even months. Prolonged drainage with an indwelling urethral catheter or suprapubic tube should be avoided. Indwelling catheters are associated with an increased incidence of infection, calculi, urethral strictures and fistulae, alteration in compliance, hydronephrosis and vesicoureteral reflux, and renal failure.[39] Patients should be treated with CIC. Although the drug bethanechol increases bladder muscle contractility, it is ineffective in this clinical setting.[40] α-Blockers are somewhat effective in treating bladder outlet obstruction secondary to BPH.[41] α-Blockers have also been used to prevent postoperative urinary retention.[42]

SUMMARY

Urinary tract obstruction is a fairly common problem seen at all ages and in both sexes. Mild obstructions may have minimum or no effects on renal function or urine transport and storage and need little or no therapy. Indeed, anatomic dilation of the collecting system does not of itself mean pathologic physiology—all that dilates is not obstructed. On the other hand, sudden total blockage or silent chronic occlusion may lead to acute or chronic renal failure and be life threatening.

Imaging and physiologic studies are now quite refined and, for the most part, exacting in determining the site of obstruction and its significance. Unfortunately, other than improving drainage and awaiting self-repair, there is little to offer in terms of treatment to the urinary tract that has been damaged by the process. We are able, however, to understand what damage has been done and how to support the organism in lieu of normal renal and collecting system function while awaiting recovery.

REFERENCES

1. Campbell M. Urinary obstruction. In Campbell M, ed. Clinical Pediatric Urology. Philadelphia: WB Saunders, 1951.
2. Livera LN, et al. Antenatal ultrasonography to detect fetal renal abnormalities: A prospective screening programme. Br Med J 298:1421, 1989.
3. Johnson CM, et al. Renal stone epidemiology: A 25 year study in Rochester, Minnesota. Kidney In. 16:624, 1979.
4. Lytton B, Emery JM, Harvard BM. The incidence of benign prostatic obstruction. J Urol 99:639, 1968.
5. Weiss RM. Ureteral function. Urology 12:114, 1978.
6. Morita T, Ishizuka G, Tsuchida S. Initiation and propagation of stimulus from the renal pelvic pacemaker in pig kidney. Invest Urol 19:157, 1981.
7. Morita T, et al. Ureteral urine transport: changes in bolus volume, peristaltic frequency, intraluminal pressure and volume of flow resulting from autonomic drugs. J Urol 137:132, 1987.
8. Michaelson G. Percutaneous puncture of the renal pelvis intrapelvic pressure and the concentrating capacity of the kidney in hydronephrosis. Acta Med Scand 559(Suppl):1, 1974.
9. Ross JA, Edmond P, Kirkland IS. Behavior of the Human Ureter in Health and Disease. Edinburgh: Churchill Livingstone, 1972.
10. Swenson O, Fischer JH, Smyth BT. Studies of normal and abnormal peristalsis. Med J Aust 146:805, 1959.
11. Raezer DM, et al. Autonomic innervation of canine urinary bladder. Cholinergic and adrenergic contributions and interaction of sympathetic and parasympathetic nervous systems in bladder function. Urology 2:211, 1973.
12. de Groat WC. Anatomy and physiology of the lower urinary tract. Urol Clin North Am 20:383, 1993.
13. de Groat WC, Booth AM, Yashimua N. Neurophysiology of micturition and its modification in animal models of human disease. In Maggi CA, ed. The Autonomic Nervous System: Nervous Control of the Urogenital System, vol 3. London: Harwood Academic Publishers, 1993, p 227.
14. Talner LB. Urographic contrast media in uremia. Radiol Clin North Am 10:421, 1972.
15. Van Zee BE, et al. Renal injury associated with intravenous pyelography in non-diabetic and diabetic patients. Ann Intern Med 89:51, 1978.
16. Koff SA. Ureteropelvic junction obstruction: Role of newer diagnostic methods. J Urol 127:898, 1982.
17. Wolk FN, Whitaker RH. Late followup of dynamic evaluation of upper urinary tract obstruction. J Urol 128:346, 1982.
18. Whitaker RH. The Whitaker test. Urol Clin North Am 6:529, 1979.
19. Schäfer W. Principles and clinical application of advanced urodynamic analysis of voiding function. Urol Clin North Am 17:553, 1990.
20. McGuire EJ. Urodynamic studies in prostatic obstruction. In Fitzpatrick JM, Krane RJ, eds. The Prostate. New York: Churchill Livingstone, 1989, p 103.
21. Gillenwater JY, et al. Renal function one week after release of chronic unilateral hydronephrosis in man. Kidney Int 7:179, 1975.
22. Suki W, et al. Patterns of nephron perfusion in acute and chronic hydronephrosis. J Clin Invest 45:122, 1966.
23. Heney NM, O'Morchoe PJ, O'Morchoe CCC. The renal lymphatic system during obstructed urine flow. J Urol 106:455, 1971.
24. Gaudio KM, et al. Renal perfusion and intratubular pressure during ureteral occlusion in the rat. Am J Physiol 238:F205, 1980.
25. Wilson DR. Micropuncture study of chronic obstructive nephropathy before and after release of obstruction. Kidney Int 2:119, 1972.
26. Jaenike JR. The renal functional defect of postobstructive nephropathy. The effects of bilateral ureteral obstruction in the rat. J Clin Invest 51:2999, 1972.
27. Howards SS. Post-obstructive diuresis: A misunderstood phenomenon. J Urol 110:537, 1973.
28. Wilson DR, Honrath U. Cross circulation study of natriuretic factors in post obstructive diuresis. J Clin Invest 57:380, 1976.
29. McDougal WS, Wright FS. Defect in proximal and distal sodium transport in postobstructive diuresis. Kidney Int 2:304, 1972.
30. Dal Canton A, et al. Effects of 24 hour unilateral ureteral obstruction on glomerular hemodynamics in rat kidney. Kidney Int 15:457, 1979.
31. Backlund L. Experimental studies on pressure and contractility in the ureter. Acta Physiol Scand 59(Suppl 212):1, 1963.
32. Vaugh ED Jr, Sorenson EJ, Gillenwater JY. The renal hemodynamic response to chronic unilateral complete ureteral occlusion. Invest Urol 8:78, 1970.
33. Keating MA, Retik AB. Management of the dilated obstructed ureter. Urol Clin North Am 17:291, 1990.
34. Weiss RM. Clinical correlations of ureteral physiology. Am J Kidney Dis 2:409, 1983.
35. Schäfer W. Detrusor as the energy source of micturition. In Hinman F Jr, ed. Benign Prostatic Hypertrophy. New York: Springer-Verlag, 1983.
36. Barnard RJ, Dixon JS, Gosling JA. A clinical and morphological evaluation of the trabeculated urinary bladder. Prog Clin Biol Res 78:285, 1981.
37. McGuire EJ, et al. Prognostic value of urodynamic testing in myelodysplastic patients. J Urol 126:205, 1981.
38. Magasi P, Csontai A, Ruszinko B. Beitrage zur blasenwamtre-generation. Z Urol Nephrol 62:209, 1969.
39. Selzman AA, Hampel N. Urologic complications of spinal cord injury. Urol Clin North Am 20:453, 1993.
40. Wein AJ, et al. The effect of oral bethanechol chloride on the cystometrogram of the normal male adult. J Urol 120:330, 1978.
41. Caine M, Pfau A, Perlberg S. The use of alpha adrenergic blockers in benign prostatic obstruction. Br J Urol 48:225, 1976.
42. Goldman G, et al. Alpha-adrenergic blocker for posthernioplasty urinary retention. Arch Surg 123:35, 1988.

44

Renal Failure

Marc I. Lorber

Although the advent of maintenance dialysis and transplantation has dramatically altered management strategies, renal failure continues to present an extremely challenging constellation of problems in clinical surgery. Prior to the early 1960s, progressive uremia was managed symptomatically with severe protein and salt restriction. Unless spontaneous recovery of renal function occurred, the inexorable downhill course, ultimately resulting in coma and death, was well characterized. During the German occupation of the Netherlands in World War II, Willem Kolff developed the forerunner of the modern hemodialysis machine.[1] By 1960 long-term maintenance of patients using hemodialysis became realistic, and previously fatal problems were transformed into a new group of chronic illnesses.[2] Just as maintenance hemodialysis became more commonplace, the ultimate goal of renal replacement therapy by transplantation enjoyed parallel success with the introduction of effective prophylactic immunosuppression.[3] Although maintenance hemodialysis, and renal transplantation have altered the outlook for patients with chronic renal failure (CRF), the advent of these technologies has impacted little on the overall mortality associated with the development of acute renal failure (ARF) requiring dialysis. This chapter details the pathophysiology and management of patients with ARF and CRF.

NORMAL RENAL FUNCTION

The physiology of urine formation and excretion has been detailed in Chapter 42, but the salient features as they relate to renal failure merit reemphasis. Each human kidney contains approximately 1 million nephrons that collectively respond to the metabolic alterations and fluid and electrolyte changes in the body to achieve internal homeostasis (Fig. 44-1). Extracellular fluid volume regulation is initiated as blood passing through the afferent renal arteriole is subjected to glomerular filtration. A fraction of the water and accompanying dissolved solute is separated from the formed cellular elements and macromolecules in the blood. The glomerular filtrate generally excludes substances with molecular weights greater than 70,000 daltons, whereas small-molecular-weight substances (less than 15,000 daltons) are uniformly included. Middle-range molecules are filtered in a more selective fashion.

The glomerular filtration mechanism maintains a relatively high hydrostatic pressure because of the unique anatomy of the glomerulus placing the glomerular capillary bed between two arteriolar structures. Renal blood flow is regulated primarily at the arteriolar level, and the glomerular filtration rate (GFR) relates directly to renal blood flow. The fraction of renal blood flow represented by GFR has been termed the *filtration fraction*. Renal blood flow normally approximates 25% of cardiac output. Therefore if the normal renal blood flow is 600 ml/min

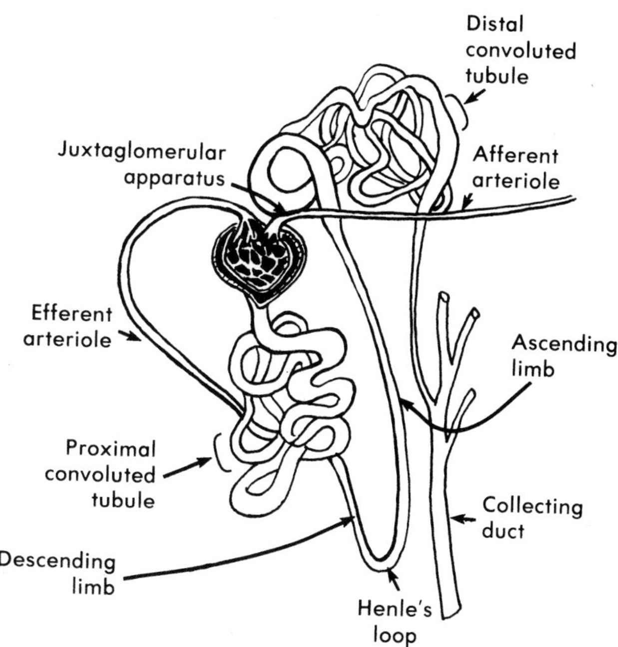

Fig. 44-1. Anatomy of an isolated nephron. Each nephron functions as an independent filtration unit in production of the final urinary product, reflecting excesses of water, electrolytes, metabolic by-products, as well as various other toxins. The human kidney normally contains 1 million nephrons.

per kidney and GFR is approximately 120 ml/min, the normal filtration fraction is 0.2.

The GFR can be measured directly using micropuncture techniques; however, its estimation using the concept of solute clearance is employed more often in the clinical setting, as shown by the relationship:

$$\text{Clearance} = \frac{\text{Urine concentration} \times \text{Urine volume}}{\text{Plasma concentration}}$$

Clearance of a particular substance can be used to predict GFR accurately only if the substance is neither secreted nor reabsorbed by the renal tubular system. Inulin represents such a substance, and inulin clearance has become the standard for estimation of GFR. The clinical setting would be more conveniently served if an endogenously produced substance could be used. Clearance of creatinine, a by-product of skeletal muscle metabolism, closely parallels the value obtained using inulin clearance. Thus for most clinical purposes, creatinine clearance (CrCl) is measured to estimate GFR.

Approximately 80% of available solids and water present in the glomerular filtrate are reabsorbed in the proximal renal tubule. The proximal tubular filtrate maintains an isosmotic relationship with the blood; however, the process of reabsorption may also require energy expenditure (active transport). Although some substances such as glucose are absorbed very efficiently by the proximal tubule, other substances are reabsorbed partially (e.g., sodium) or not at all (e.g., creatinine). The process is further complicated by the active and passive secretion of certain substances. The countercurrent exchange mechanism found within the renal medulla enhances the reabsorption of solute and water as the filtrate traverses Henle's loop. The ascending limb of Henle's loop represents an additional site of active electrolyte and thereby passive water reabsorption. The energy-dependent processes whereby chloride and sodium reabsorption occur are crucial for maintenance of normal tubular function.

By the time the distal convoluted tubule is encountered, approximately 90% of the glomerular filtrate has been reabsorbed. The final reabsorption processes are controlled hormonally by aldosterone and antidiuretic hormone (ADH). Aldosterone mediates sodium reabsorption and potassium and hydrogen ion excretion. ADH regulates additional water reabsorption by its modulating effects on collecting duct and distal tubular permeability. Thus the final urinary product reflects excesses of water, electrolytes, and metabolic by-products, as well as products of drug metabolism and other potentially toxic substances.

RENAL DYSFUNCTION

Abnormal renal function impacts on surgical practice in several different settings, including (1) ARF among injured or critically ill patients recovering from major surgery, (2) chronic renal dysfunction in patients with various surgical disorders unrelated to their renal disease, (3) angioaccess for hemodialysis, and (4) surgical care of patients with CRF by renal transplantation. Therefore the surgeon caring for patients with renal dysfunction should be well versed in the consequences of altered renal physiology and the resultant effects on homeostasis.

Renal disease can involve alterations in glomerular function alone, tubular function alone, or both in combination. Glomerular dysfunction can result in two basic pathophysiologic abnormalities: (1) diminished glomerular filtration and (2) increased glomerular capillary permeability. Thus patients with renal insufficiency can manifest diminished filtration by reduced clearance of metabolic by-products and reduced urinary volume. When such a pure glomerular lesion results in reduction of glomerular blood flow as might occur, for example, in acute glomerulonephritis, the kidney remains able to concentrate the urinary filtrate, but dilute urinary excretion may not be possible. Further, increased permeability of the glomerular capillaries results in a diminution of the normal barrier to macromolecules. Frequently, large amounts of protein losses occur, whereas glomerular filtration and blood flow, as measured by clearance, might remain unaffected. Persistent proteinuria with hypoproteinemia and negative nitrogen balance, as observed in the nephrotic syndrome, leads to a cascade of events, including reduction of relative blood volume, activation of the renin-angiotensin-aldosterone system, and stimulation of ADH secretion with resultant sodium and water retention and peripheral edema. When glomerular injury is severe, permanent loss of function with the associated irreversible morphologic changes of glomerular sclerosis or necrosis is observed.

Acute renal tubular injury, as has been associated with aminoglycoside nephrotoxicity, can be localized to particular anatomic regions. The site of injury can often be determined by the results of specific clinical measurements. Proximal tubular injury, for example, can affect renal regulation of substances that are normally reabsorbed at that level of the nephron. Therefore since essentially all the glucose and protein present in the glomerular filtrate are normally reabsorbed in the proximal renal tubule, urinary excretion of those substances in the absence of other demonstrable pathology suggests a proximal tubular injury. Similarly, injury to transport mechanisms located in the ascending limb of Henle's loop results in abnormal handling of monovalent anions and cations, including chloride, sodium, potassium, and hydrogen. Perhaps more importantly, damage to these energy-dependent ion exchange mechanisms causes altered renal medullary osmolarity with impairment of the concentrating ability of the kidney.

Finally, alterations in responsiveness to the sodium-conserving influence of aldosterone and to the effects of ADH on water reabsorption in the distal tubule result in an inability to excrete an adequately concentrated urinary product. In this latter circumstance, however, one must remember that insufficient hormonal stimulation (i.e., ADH in diabetes insipidus) or end-organ insensitivity to appropriate hormone levels may also adversely affect the ability of the kidney to concentrate urine.

Although isolated renal tubular damage to a specific anatomic region is possible, it is more common to observe a clinical condition that results from a combination of insults causing global tubular damage. Further, because renal tubular cells are metabolically very active and cellular turnover is high, these cells are capable of regeneration following injury. Thus renal failure resulting from tubular damage can be completely reversible. This is in direct contrast to glomerular pathology, which frequently progresses and leads to irreversible renal failure.

Acute Renal Failure (Table 44-1)

Despite improved technology allowing effective substitution of lost renal function in critically ill patients through dialysis, ARF continues to be associated with mortality rates in excess of 70%.[4-6] Naturally, those figures reflect more directly the complexity and severity of clinical conditions treated in intensive care units; however, it seems clear that uremic problems accompanying ARF require special attention, particularly when complications such as infection, poor nutrition, and multiorgan dysfunction occur.

Classification of Acute Renal Dysfunction

Acute renal dysfunction has characteristically been classified as prerenal, renal, or postrenal according to the etiologic nature of the precipitating event. It is important to recognize that prerenal azotemia and renal failure due to acute tubular necrosis (ATN) comprise the overwhelming majority of ARF cases observed among hospitalized patients.

Prerenal azotemia. Prerenal azotemia or failure (elevated blood urea nitrogen [BUN] and serum creatinine concentrations) indicates a condition resulting in diminished renal blood flow, usually because of decreased effective circulatory volume, and thereby altered renal function. Among the many potential etiologic factors, acute hemorrhage, dehydration, "third-space" gastrointestinal losses, sepsis and resultant peripheral vasodilation, peritonitis, cardiac failure, renal artery injury or embolization, and pancreatitis represent some of the more common considerations.

The underlying mechanism in each of these situations is renal hypoperfusion and/or ischemia. Reduction of arterial volume or pressure results in afferent arteriolar dilation with concomitant increases in vasomotor tone at the efferent renal arteriole.[7] This vasomotor process of renal autoregulation allows maintenance of GFR at the expense of blood delivery to the peritubular regions. Mean arterial pressures below 80 to 90 mm Hg precipitate, through hormonal and autonomic responses, a progressive fall in renal blood flow. When the precipitating event can be identified and corrected early, actual renal pathology does not ensue, thus the term *prerenal azotemia.* However, sustained reduction in renal blood flow causes intense global renal vasoconstriction as the attempt to maintain GFR becomes less successful. The resultant cellular hypoxia, often termed *vasomotor nephropathy,* represents the final common pathway leading to true ARF.[7,8] Ischemic injury creates the cycle resulting in tubular damage, filtrate back-leak, intraluminal obstruction from cellular swelling, further vasoconstriction, and alterations in glomerular permeability, ultimately resulting in persistent ARF. Histologically, the injury appears as a tubular cell insult, thus the term *acute tubular necrosis (ATN),* which has become a frequently used clinical designation.

Postrenal azotemia. Renal dysfunction resulting from urinary obstruction is known as postrenal azotemia. Obstruction can occur at any level of the urinary collecting system. Renal calculi, blood clots, tumors, and papillary necrosis represent a few of the more common intrinsic upper urinary tract findings leading to this condition. External retroperitoneal abnormalities, including retroperitoneal fibrosis, neoplasia, massive retroperitoneal hemorrhage, or rarely massive intraperitoneal hemorrhage or ascites leading to elevated intra-abdominal pressure, can also result in postrenal azotemia by obstructing normal urinary flow through the ureters. Accidental surgical ligation of a ureter may also be a cause. Lower urinary tract abnormalities that can result in postrenal azotemia include bladder calculi, blood clots, prostatic hypertrophy, and carcinoma. Finally, retroperitoneal urinary extravasation, as may occur from an injury to the urinary tract such as a gunshot wound, can mimic postrenal azotemia because the urinary product becomes reabsorbed rather than excreted. As with prerenal azotemia, the postrenal form need not be associated with actual renal pathology unless the cause of obstruction is sustained and not relieved.

Renal azotemia. Specific abnormalities of the kidneys that develop acutely can also result in overt ARF. The most frequently observed abnormalities encountered by the surgeon include ATN, pigment nephropathy from free myoglobin or hemoglobin, direct nephrotoxicity from drugs or radiographic contrast materials, and acute interstitial nephritis also usually from drugs.

ATN represents the end stage of ischemic insult, as discussed earlier; again, it constitutes approximately 75% of ARF cases observed among hospitalized patients. ATN is usually considered a reversible injury; however, when ischemia is severe and prolonged, acute cortical necrosis and irreversible renal failure result.

Extensive trauma or mismatched blood transfusion can cause hemolysis and/or muscle destruction. The resultant hemoglobinuric or myoglobinuric renal failure occurs because of accumulation of pigment casts in the proximal tubular lumen and accumulation of breakdown products in the tubular cells.[9] This causes intense vasoconstriction, as well as proximal tubular obstruction that prevents effective glomerular filtration. Similarly, radiographic contrast agents are directly toxic to renal tubular cells and also induce intense renal vasoconstriction.[10,11] It is important to realize that the propensity toward contrast-induced renal failure is markedly increased among patients with diabetes and/or underlying renal dysfunction.

Table 44-1. Common Causes of Acute Renal Dysfunction

Diagnosis	Clinical Manifestations	Primary Level of Injury	Preventive or Therapeutic Measures
Prerenal			
Hypovolemia True volume loss Intravascular volume redistribution	Volume contraction with or without oliguria	Reduced GFR; 2 degrees decreased blood flow	Volume repletion
Cardiac failure	Oliguria, peripheral edema, pulmonary edema	Pump failure	Improve cardiac performance
Hepatorenal syndrome	Hepatic dysfunction; ascites, oliguria; peripheral edema	Reduced GFR 2 degrees to altered hemodynamics	Diuresis; peritoneovenous shunt; liver transplantation
Intrarenal			
Acute tubular necrosis	Oliguria, anuria, polyuria, isosthenuria, uremia	Pantubular	Volume repletion, avoid hypotension
Radiographic contrast	Usually oliguric ARF	Pantubular	Minimize contrast volume; hydrate; avoid other nephrotoxins
Aminoglycosides	Usually nonoliguric ARF	Proximal tubule; 2-degree immune response	Hydration; drug levels; avoid nephrotoxins
Other antimicrobials	Usually nonoliguric ARF	Tubular, secondary immune response	Adequate hydration; avoid nephrotoxins
Cyclosporine/tacrolimus	Oliguric or nonoliguric uremia	Afferent arteriole	Drug level mitoring; avoid excessive dose
Acute heme pigment load	Hemoglobinuria/myoglobinuria	Proximal tubule	Urinary alkalinization hydration; diuresis
Organic solvents/heavy metals	Oliguric or nonoliguric ARF	Pantubular/glomerular	Hydration; diuresis; chelating agents
Acute glomerulonephritis	Hypertension; proteinuria; hematuria; active sediment	Glomerular	Treat infection; supportive care
Acute interstitial nephritis Allergic/infectious	Fever; rash; eosinophilia; oliguria	Pantubular; interstitial	Discontinue offending agent; corticosteroids
Intratubular crystal formation Acute uric acid nephropathy	Oliguria; renal calculi	Pantubular	Control uric acid; hydration; urinary alkalinization
Hypercalcemia	Reduced concentrating ability; nephrocalcinosis	Distal tubule	Hydration; forced diuresis; mithramycin
Hyperoxaluria	Reduced concentrating ability	Pantubular	Hydration; oxalate-binding agents; discontinue oxalate-rich foods
Vascular Vasculitis Malignant hypertension Hemolytic uremic syndrome Thrombotic thrombocytopenic purpura Post partum	Renal insufficiency in a setting consistent with underlying systemic disease; active urinary sediment; characteristic renal biopsy findings	Vascular; glomerular	Appropriate therapy for underlying disease; control hypertension; corticosteroids/immunosuppressants; supportive care
Postrenal			
Ureteral obstruction Intrinsic Extrinsic	Oliguria; collecting system dilation	Ureter; extrinsic compression	Correct underlying abnormality
Bladder outlet obstruction	Oliguria; collecting system dilation	Prostate; urethra	Correct underlying abnormality

ARF, Acute renal failure; *GFR,* glomerular filtration rate.

The mechanisms underlying drug toxicity to the kidney vary depending on the particular drug. The aminoglycoside antibiotics represent a typical group of drugs that exert toxicity through renal vasoconstriction, alterations in glomerular capillary permeability, and direct tubular cell disruption.[12,13]

Finally, acute interstitial nephritis or glomerular nephritis can result following induction of immune responses in the kidney to various drugs or microorganisms.[14]

Diagnosis

Critically ill patients are extremely vulnerable to alterations in intravascular volume and renal perfusion that can result in acute renal injury. The most direct clinical determinations that allow assessment of renal perfusion include measurements of urinary volume, urinary specific gravity, electrolyte excretion, examination of the urinary sediment, and serum determinations of creatinine and BUN (Table 44-2). Adjunctive information regarding the status of cardiac and respiratory function, as well as direct central hemodynamic measurements, have become indispensable tools in the management of complicated illnesses.

The measurement of urinary output over time provides an important direct determination of the adequacy of renal perfusion. The minimum hourly urinary excretion should approximate 0.5 ml/kg of body weight. In the absence of urinary obstruction and cardiac pump failure, assuming the kidney is otherwise intact, urine production below that rate implies inadequate circulating blood volume. Although a decrease in urine output is frequently seen in renal disease, it is important to remember that oliguria does not necessarily accompany significant renal injury. Direct nephrotoxic injury from various sources results in nonoliguric renal failure (1000 to 1500 ml urine daily) in 25% to 50% of patients.[15]

The intact nephron is capable of concentrating the urine to approximately 1300 mOsm/L (specific gravity, 1.040). This is slightly more than a fourfold increase over the normal plasma osmolarity, which is approximately 300 mOsm/L (specific gravity, 1.010). Oliguria from prerenal azotemia can usually be differentiated from azotemia induced by renal tubular injury (ATN) by measuring the urine specific gravity. In prerenal azotemia, the urine is highly concentrated, usually with a sodium level <10 and high specific gravity (approaching 1.040). In contrast, when ATN occurs, tubular function is disrupted, usually resulting in isotonic urine (sodium, >20) and iso-osmolar specific gravity (1.010). As a cautionary note, the urinary osmolarity and specific gravity may be misleading in critically ill patients. These measurements can be altered by significant proteinuria, glycosuria, and the use of radiographic contrast materials, mannitol, furosemide, or other osmotically active drugs or metabolites.

Among alternate methods developed to assist in differentiating ARF from prerenal azotemia, the calculation of fractional sodium excretion (FENa) has in the past been considered discriminating by some investigators.[16] FENa represents the percentage of sodium in the initial glomerular filtrate that is excreted in the urine. The calculation requires simultaneous determinations of plasma sodium (PNa) and CrCl with similar urinary determinations. FENa is calculated by dividing the product of urinary sodium (UNa) and total urinary volume (V) by the total sodium filtered as follows:

$$\text{FENa (\%)} = \frac{(\text{UNa})\ (\text{V})}{(\text{PNa})\ (\text{CrCl})}$$

Normally the FENa represents less than 1% of the filtered sodium load, whereas patients with ARF tend to excrete larger quantities of sodium despite oliguria, and patients with prerenal azotemia conserve urinary sodium. However, limitations in practical application among patients with intrinsic renal insufficiency and nonoliguric ARF have diminished the clinical value of this calculation.

Examination of the urine and urinary sediment frequently yields additional important information. Hemoglobin from hemolysis and myoglobin from rhabdomyolysis can be readily identified. Proteinuria can be screened using urinary dipstick evaluation. Prerenal azotemia is frequently associated with small amounts (1+, 2+), whereas heavier proteinuria suggests intrinsic renal injury. The urinary sediment can assist in the differentiation of infection

Table 44-2. Diagnostic Indexes in Acute Renal Failure

Index	Normal Value	Prerenal Azotemia	Acute Tubular Necrosis	Obstruction
Urinary volume	≥0.5 ml/kg	≤0.5 ml/kg	Variable	Variably diminished
Urinary specific gravity	1.003-1.025	≥1.020	1.010	Variable
Urinary sodium	Variable	<20 mEq/L	>40 mEq/L	>40 mEq/L
Urinary fractional sodium excretion	<1%	<1%	>3%	>3%
Creatinine clearance	100-120 ml/min	Normal-to-mild reduction	Progressive reduction	Variable
Serum creatinine	0.6-1.3 mg/dl	Mild elevation	Progressive elevation	Variable elevation
Blood urea nitrogen (BUN)	10-20 mg/dl	Elevation	Progressive elevation	Variable
BUN/creatinine ratio	10:1	>20:1	Variable	Variable

and primary renal disorders. Prerenal azotemia is associated with occasional fine granular and hyaline casts, whereas ATN is characterized by large numbers of tubular epithelial cells, epithelial cell casts, and coarse granular casts. Red blood cells and red blood cell casts frequently suggest acute glomerulonephritis.

Creatinine, a normal end product of creatine phosphate metabolism in muscle, is a substance that is primarily filtered but not reabsorbed by the nephron. Its clearance has already been discussed as an estimate of GFR. If one assumes that muscle mass remains constant, daily creatinine production also remains constant, averaging 10 to 20 mg/kg/day. The normal serum creatinine is 0.6 to 1.3 mg/100 ml in the patient with normal renal function. Patients with abnormal renal function therefore sustain elevation in serum creatinine as urinary clearance diminishes. Total renal failure is associated with a serum creatinine rise at an average rate of 1 to 2 mg/100 ml/day.

Similarly, BUN directly reflects adequacy of renal function. The incremental daily rise in BUN approximates 20 to 25 mg/day in the complete absence of glomerular filtration. However, since urea production is less constant than creatinine, BUN determination is much less discriminating in distinguishing prerenal from renal azotemia. The BUN/creatinine ratio is much more useful in this regard. A ratio in excess of 20:1 frequently signifies prerenal azotemia, whereas a ratio of 10:1 or less might indicate intrinsic renal disease.

Prevention

The kidneys are relatively well protected from ischemic insult because of their normally high blood flow. The metabolic, hormonal, and hemodynamic alterations associated with critical illness, however, greatly increase their vulnerability to various forms of injury. The high mortality that frequently accompanies ARF should serve as appropriate warning that the emphasis should be on prevention. Thus important aspects of prevention should be initiated during the period of preoperative evaluation and preparation.

Radiographic studies employing hyperosmotic contrast agents, vigorous bowel preparation, and restricted fluid intake can result in significant dehydration and increased susceptibility to ARF. Similarly, endogenous intravascular fluid losses associated with the third-space phenomenon in patients with pancreatitis, bowel obstruction, peritonitis, and so on may result in severe intravascular dehydration, as can fever, fistulous drainage, vomiting, and diarrhea. All these states of severe volume loss and dehydration make the kidneys vulnerable to the development of ARF.

The history and physical examination therefore can provide indispensable data to the clinician in determining patients at risk. Preexisting illnesses that can increase the incidence of ARF include hypertension, diabetes mellitus, and renal insufficiency. Symptoms or signs suggesting urinary obstruction, such as decreased urinary stream, incomplete bladder emptying, and urinary urgency or frequency, should be fully evaluated before elective surgery. Abnormal laboratory studies indicating renal problems or dehydration demand complete investigation. Except in life-threatening situations, no patient should undergo major surgical intervention without having electrolyte disturbances and associated dehydration corrected first.

Often the accepted approach is to begin intravenous fluid therapy the evening before surgery. This is particularly important when the patient has been subjected to an extensive preoperative evaluation, has been receiving short-term or long-term diuretic therapy, or may otherwise be suspected of having mild dehydration. Selected patients, including the elderly, those with preexisting cardiac disease, and those determined to be at increased risk, should undergo preoperative preparation to optimize volume status. This is generally best accomplished with central venous cannulation or ideally with right-sided heart catheterization with a Swan-Ganz catheter, 12 to 24 hours before planned surgery. Cardiac filling pressures and output can thereby be maximized and renal perfusion optimized.

The intraoperative management of patients undergoing major procedures demands communication and cooperation between the anesthesiologist and surgeon. Hypovolemia or the peripheral vasodilation of anesthesia with resultant renal vasoconstriction should be minimized. The catecholamine discharge associated with operative trauma alone can have deleterious effects on renal blood flow. Diminished renal perfusion can result from anesthetic-related myocardial depression, myocardial ischemia, or cardiac arrhythmia. Hemorrhage, or spasm from reperfusion following major vascular occlusion, can result in renal hypoperfusion and acute renal injury.

Direct renal injury can result from the use of nephrotoxic medications. The nephrotoxicity associated with the aminoglycoside antibiotics is well known. Penicillins, cephalosporins, and sulfonamides can precipitate acute interstitial nephritis. Inhibitors of prostaglandin biosynthesis, such as aspirin and nonsteroidal anti-inflammatory agents,[17] affect glomerular autoregulation and can prevent intrarenal vasodilation and resultant hypoperfusion injury. Narcotics, such as morphine and meperidine, diminish GFR, and various anesthetic agents stimulate ADH release, thereby diminishing urinary output. Vasoactive amines with α-adrenergic activity mediate renal vasoconstriction and can precipitate renal ischemia. The nonpulsatile flow during cardiopulmonary bypass can also contribute to ARF. Thus a good understanding and judicious use of necessary but toxic drugs and appropriate use of technology required during complex surgical procedures must be supplemented with good surgical technique to minimize the incidence of serious renal insult.

Management

Despite preventive measures, the surgeon frequently faces situations likely to result in ARF. Available evidence suggests that nonoliguric renal failure is prognostically preferable to the oliguric form of ARF.[18] Because fluid overload and serious electrolyte abnormalities are less often encountered in nonoliguric renal failure, dialysis can often be avoided. Further, avoiding the need for fluid restriction permits more effective supportive care, including correction of severe nutritional deficits. These considerations have suggested that efforts to convert oliguric to nonoliguric ARF might be desirable. Although controversy continues, experimental and clinical evidence suggests that the conversion of oliguric ARF to nonoliguric ARF is sometimes possible.[14,19] In practical terms this controversy has provided a rational clinical approach to the patient who develops acute oliguria. Depending on the clinical situation, a *single* test challenge with fluids and/or high-dose intravenous diuretics (12.5 to 25 g mannitol; 200 to 400 mg furosemide) can influence and perhaps modify the degree of renal injury. Furosemide should be administered at rates no greater than 15 mg/min, and repeated high doses should be avoided to reduce the risk of ototoxicity. A favorable response would suggest less severe injury, at least some preservation of function, and the necessity for continued volume repletion. A poor response alternately indicates the need to change the management approach to prevent the additional sequelae of ARF.

Although the clinical relevance remains somewhat controversial, administration of agents such as essential amino acids,[20] ATP-$MgCl_2$,[21] thyroxine,[22] and atrial natriuretic peptide (hANP)[23] have each been demonstrated to ameliorate the incidence and severity of experimentally induced ATN. More extensive clinical trials are presently ongoing; however, promising preliminary results have been reported following trials using ATP, thyroxine, and hANP.

Fluid and electrolytes. Measures to prevent acute volume overload should accompany the diagnosis of oliguric ARF. Total daily fluid intake is restricted to the sum of urinary output and approximate insensible loss. The sodium chloride load should be estimated for each patient, with insensible loss replaced with 5% dextrose solution and urinary output with 0.45% saline. Without the usual compensatory capacity of the kidneys, it is essential to monitor fluid status closely because hyponatremia (sodium, 120 mEq/L) from too much free water or hypernatremia from too little free water can result in neurologic abnormalities (see Chapter 2).

Oliguric ARF requires careful monitoring of serum potassium. Acute hyperkalemia is particularly troublesome in the critically ill, catabolic patient. Serum potassium levels approaching 6 mEq/L require urgent therapy, especially when associated with muscle weakness, electrocardiographic changes, or a rapid rate of rise. Immediate temporizing maneuvers should include intravenous administration of sodium bicarbonate (45 mEq) if the patient is acidemic or glucose and insulin (start with 25 g, 50% glucose solution plus 10 to 15 U regular insulin) to redistribute potassium into cells. A glucose/insulin infusion may also be of value for short-term therapy. This must include close glucose monitoring (every 2 to 3 hours) with avoidance of hypoglycemia. Following these acute maneuvers, aggressive attempts to remove potassium from the body must also occur. Ion exchange resins such as sodium polystyrene sulfonate (Kayexalate, 30 to 50 g per dose) have been particularly effective. Kayexalate administered into the intestinal tract exerts its hypokalemic influence through cationic exchange. However, Kayexalate is constipating, and it is advisable to concomitantly administer sorbitol to promote catharsis. Although Kayexalate can be administered orally or by enema, it is more effective and complications are fewer following oral administration. Importantly, Kayexalate should not be administered by enema during the early postoperative period because acute colonic perforation can result.

Largely because of the loss of renal acid-base regulatory capacity, acidosis and less frequently alkalosis become major management considerations in renal failure. The setting of ARF is often associated with requirements for parenteral nutrition, a catabolic state, intestinal bicarbonate losses, and lactic acidosis or ketoacidosis. Although sodium bicarbonate administration can alleviate the metabolic acidosis, volume is frequently rate limiting, and dialysis support may become necessary. The restriction of protein can slow the rate of metabolic acid accumulation; however, this maneuver may not be advisable for the critically ill patient who is already severely protein depleted.

Hypocalcemia, hypermagnesemia, and hyperphosphatemia also complicate management in patients with ARF. Because seriously ill patients are often hypoalbuminemic, ionized calcium can be normal even when total serum calcium levels are greatly reduced. This effect can be measured directly or estimated using the knowledge that total calcium is reduced approximately 0.8 mg/dl for every 1 mg/dl reduction in serum albumin. Phosphate binders (usually calcium carbonate or aluminum hydroxide) are generally employed to control hyperphosphatemia. Calcium and phosphate abnormalities should be corrected simultaneously to avoid exceeding a calcium phosphate product of 70, the level above which injury to the cardiac conducting system, central nervous system, vascular endothelium, and kidneys has been described.[24,25]

Uremia. The symptomatic manifestation of renal failure is called *uremia*. The toxic complications associated with uremia are outlined in Table 44-3. Although actual uremic symptoms have been etiologically linked to middle-molecular-weight nitrogenous metabolites (500 to 10,000 daltons), the BUN remains the best clinical gauge of impending uremic symptomatology. When renal function deteriorates below 10% of normal or BUN exceeds 100 mg/dl, uremic symptoms generally become apparent. However, among diabetic patients symptoms can occur when BUN values are much lower than 100 mg/dl. Common complaints such as leg muscle or abdominal cramping, nausea, vomiting, and diarrhea can be largely ascribed to alterations in autonomic tone resulting from progressive metabolic acidosis. Acidosis also can precipitate development of Kussmaul respiration, depression in cardiac contractility, glucose intolerance, central nervous system

Table 44-3. Toxic Complications of Uremia

Toxicity	Pathophysiology	Systemic Manifestations
Cardiac	Metabolic acidosis, calcium oxalate deposition ? Circulating toxins Aseptic inflammation	Decreased myocardial contractility, myocardial calcifications, heart failure, pericarditis
Central nervous system	? Circulating toxins Metabolic acidosis	Lethargy, headaches, tremor, seizures, coma
Coagulation	Platelet dysfunction	Hemorrhagic diathesis
Dermatologic	? Tissue deposition of toxins ? Melanin deposition	Pruritus, hyperpigmentation
Endocrine	Generalized reduction in hormone levels, end-organ hyporesponsiveness, abnormal hormonal metabolism	Glucose intolerance, sexual dysfunction, hypothyroidism
Gastrointestinal	Enhanced vagal tone, metabolic acidosis	Nausea, vomiting, diarrhea, anorexia
Peripheral nervous system	?Circulating neurotoxins ?Guanidines	Peripheral neuropathy
Pulmonary	Hypervolemia, metabolic acidosis, capillary leak	Pulmonary edema, cardiac failure, Kussmaul respiration

depression, and encephalopathy. The cause of uremic pericarditis remains controversial; however, aseptic inflammation describes the characteristic histopathology. Deposition of uncleared metabolites, calcium, and phosphate into tissues can produce severe pruritus. Also, as discussed later in this chapter, platelet function abnormalities of uremia result in development of a hemorrhagic diathesis. The potential risks of therapy (dialysis) must be weighed against the consequences of delay when initiation of dialysis is considered. Usually, early institution of therapy for critically ill patients is sensible because fluid and electrolyte balance are frequently labile, and the nutritional requirements for these individuals can be more effectively addressed.

Dialysis. The widespread availability of dialysis support has dramatically altered therapeutic options for patients with ARF. The important initial decisions regarding institution of dialysis are those of timing and methodology. Acute renal dysfunction with severe fluid overload, acidosis, and hyperkalemia with associated multiorgan system dysfunction can present formidable management dilemmas. Additional indications for emergency dialysis include acute toxin loads that are dialyzable (e.g., methanol, ethylene glycol, and salicylates). Similarly, uremic complications such as encephalopathy, pericarditis, and bleeding caused by platelet dysfunction are at least partly reversible with dialysis. Aggressive initiation of dialysis is frequently advisable to facilitate nutritional support and obviate metabolic complications in severely ill, catabolic patients. The relative advantages and disadvantages of various dialysis strategies are discussed in the following and summarized in Table 44-4.

Hemodialysis. Hemodialysis remains the mainstay in therapy for ARF. The principles of osmotic diffusion are put into practice as toxic solutes are removed. Concentration gradient, molecular size, and degree of protein binding represent primary considerations. Clearance is generally greater for small-molecular-weight molecules that are not protein bound and lower for larger molecules, as well as those with high degrees of protein binding. Ten to 15 hours of dialysis per week is usually required to achieve the equivalent clearance of toxic materials that would result if 10% renal function was present. However, recent years have seen the advent of more efficient, "high-flux" dialyzers, which arguably may reduce the time required to effect adequate therapy. Fluid removal can also be accomplished with dialysis because of the hydrostatic pressure gradient across the membrane interface between the blood and dialysate. The quantity of fluid removal can be manipulated by altering the magnitude of the pressure gradient across the membrane in relation to the fixed ultrafiltration coefficient of the particular dialyzer being used.

Because hemodialysis is accomplished extracorporeally and flow must exceed 200 ml/min (adults), specialized vascular access is necessary. Until recent years, acute hemodialysis required high-flow, arteriovenous (AV) shunts. Refinement in technology allowing *single-needle dialysis* altered the approach to vascular access for ARF. Hemodialysis in the setting of ARF is usually accomplished through central venous catheterization using one of several specially designed double-lumen catheters. This approach has been reasonably safe and effective. Acute complications are limited to those associated with subclavian vein catheterization primarily including hemothorax, pneumothorax, and the later risk of catheter sepsis.

Unfortunately, the evolving experience with prolonged use of these large-bore, relatively stiff catheters has been associated with a dramatic rise in the incidence of central

Table 44-4. Interventional Therapy for Acute Renal Failure

Method	Advantages	Disadvantages
Hemodialysis	Rapid, efficient and widely available; treatment is intermittent	Requires high-flow vascular access; requires sophisticated equipment and personnel; large fluid and electrolyte shifts; hemodynamic instability; requires anticoagulation
Peritoneal dialysis	Slow, gradual dialysis; no anticoagulation required; minimal equipment and technical support	Less predictable fluid removal; less efficient; risk for peritonitis; requires suitable peritoneal membrane
Continuous hemofiltration	Continuous dialysis; very efficient fluid removal; effective even in setting of hemodynamic instability; amenable to maintenance of nutritional support	Requires anticoagulation; requires sophisticated personnel; with venovenous approach, requires sophisticated equipment

venous thrombosis, a potentially catastrophic complication.[26] Some have suggested that the incidence might be minimized by preferentially using the right internal jugular approach and softer Silastic catheters, but unambiguous data to support that claim have not been forthcoming. Regardless, most would agree that whenever feasible, central venous dialysis should serve only as a temporary measure with more durable, surgically created AV fistulae and prosthetic shunts providing for long-term hemodialysis needs.

Additionally, single-needle dialysis technique can also be accomplished by femoral vein cannulation. However, many clinicians consider this latter approach less desirable because of requirements for frequent insertion and removal of catheters, the higher incidence of hemorrhagic and thrombotic complications, and the increased risk for infection associated with groin cannulation.

Peritoneal dialysis. The peritoneum as a dialysis membrane was initially suggested in 1926 by Rosenak and Siwon.[27] Although effective, early techniques were associated with unacceptably high morbidity and mortality. Peritoneal dialysis has waxed and waned in popularity oven the years, but it remains an effective and in many ways advantageous technique for renal substitution. The installation of sterile dialysate into the peritoneal cavity is straightforward, and well-designed catheters that maximize efficiency and minimize morbidity are readily available. Solutes are removed by the concentration gradient between the dialysate and those present in the interfacing capillary bed, depending on molecular charge and size. Fluid is removed by creating as osmotic gradient, usually by the addition of hypertonic glucose to the dialysate. This results in water movement into the peritoneal cavity, which can then be drained externally through the catheter.

Urea clearances of 10 to 15 ml/min can be achieved using peritoneal dialysis, and uremic symptomatology can be prevented. Peritoneal dialysis is considerably less stressful hemodynamically, accomplishes dialysis in a slower and more continuous fashion with less dramatic electrolyte flux, and requires less specialized personnel and equipment when compared to hemodialysis. It is frequently too inefficient for application to highly catabolic patients with acute electrolyte abnormalities or fluid overload, and peritonitis is a significant risk. It can, however, maintain metabolic status once acute emergency situations are overcome.

Continuous hemofiltration. An important advance in management of ARF in the intensive care setting came with development of the hemofilter, an extracorporeal device using semipermeable capillary tubes to allow continuous selective filtration of fluid and solutes from blood.[28-31] The pore size of hemofilter capillary tubes allows passage of molecules less than approximately 10,000 daltons with a high ultrafiltration coefficient, permitting large volumes of ultrafiltration. The initial technique, called continuous arteriovenous hemofiltration (CAVH), required high-flow arterial and venous access with filtration pressure supplied by the pulse pressure gradient. Solutes were removed more slowly than by standard hemodialysis; however, the rate was adequate to maintain metabolically stable individuals. Importantly, ultrafiltrate volumes in excess of 500 ml/hr with solute clearances approximating 20 to 25 ml/min have been maintained at normal arterial pressure. Unfortunately, critically ill patients are often highly catabolic, and intermittant hemodialysis was necessary to maintain adequate metabolic control. Additionally, the required indwelling arterial and venous catheters were an important source of morbidity. Finally, patients experiencing periods of relative hypotension were unable to maintain adequate filtration pressure using the CAVH technique.

However, the potential benefits of continuous hemofiltration were quickly recognized, and strategies were designed to address the shortcomings of CAVH. Continuous arteriovenous hemodiafiltration (CAVHD) uses diffusive rather than convective solute clearance. Dialysate infused to bathe the outside of the capillary tubes was used to provide countercurrent flow and improved solute clearance. This approach has been shown to provide adequate metabolic clearance, even for highly catabolic individuals.

An important advance in continuous hemofiltration technology was provided when a blood pump was used to supply filtration pressure through a single dual lumen ve-

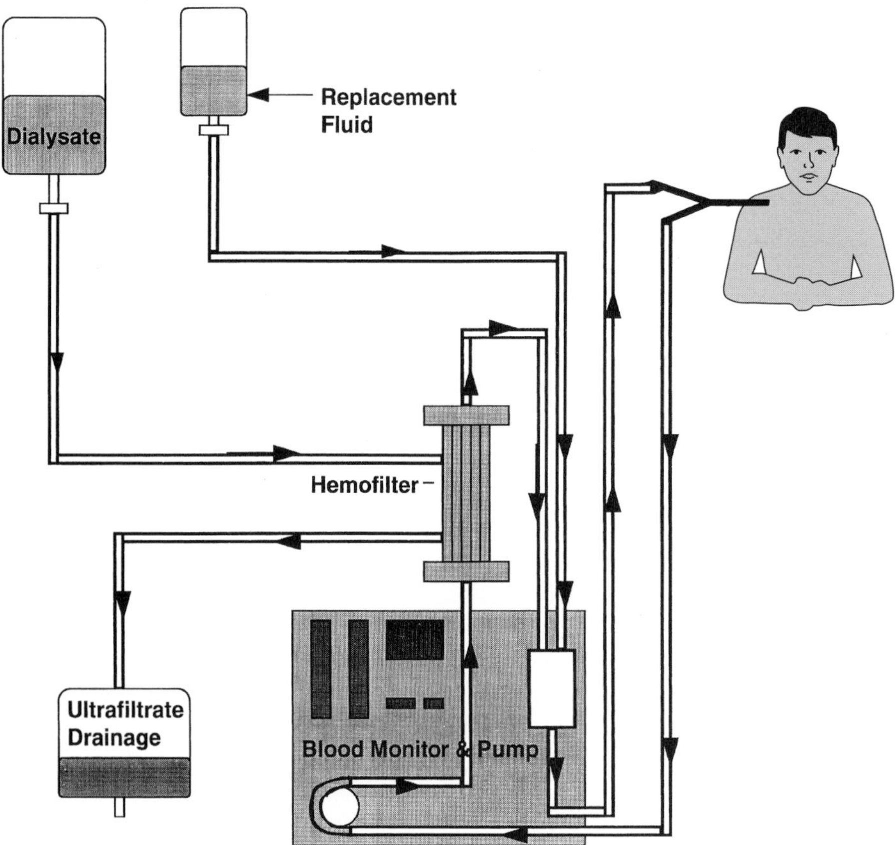

Fig. 44-2. Continuous venovenous hemofiltration (CVVH) provides for large-volume ultrafiltration using a dual-lumen, single-needle technique. Filtration pressure is applied using a blood pump, and the large volume of ultrafiltrate can be replaced using an individualized, patient-specific formula. Replacement fluids generally consist of appropriate electrolytes, glucose, amino acids, etc., to maintain homeostasis and to meet nutritional needs. Continuous venovenous hemodiafiltration (CVVHD) is used when improved solute clearance is required (e.g., critically ill, highly catabolic patients).

nous catheter (Fig. 44-2). As continuous venovenous hemofiltration (CVVH) and continuous venovenous hemodiafiltration (CVVHD) techniques have been refined, many of the earlier difficulties with CAVH were solved.[28,32,33] Although CVVH and CVVHD require sophisticated equipment and nursing personnel, several studies have documented their effectiveness in controlling azotemia, even among hypotensive, highly catabolic patients in the intensive care unit. Importantly, the morbidity associated with large-bore arterial cannulation has also been eliminated.

As with CAVH, CVVH replacement fluid is composed of needed electrolytes such as sodium, chloride, bicarbonate, calcium, magnesium, and so on. Additionally, glucose and amino acid solutions of appropriate composition are included to support nutritional requirements. Volume is determined by the patient's hemodynamic status and regulated according to hourly needs. Critically ill patients with associated ARF typically require a minimum of 40 kcal/kg energy and 1 g/kg protein to achieve adequate nutritional support.[34,35] These nutritional requirements are easily administered using continuous hemofiltration. As described, when greater solute clearance is desired, dialysate can be infused through the hemofilter (CVVHD) to more than double the efficiency of small molecule clearance in shorter times than required for conventional hemodialysis.[28] CVVH and CVVHD have demonstrated their value, particularly when renal support for patients requiring parenteral nutrition in the intensive care unit are considered. The reduced hemodynamic stress, coupled with the ability to more effectively achieve homeostasis through appropriate volume/nutritional replacement, commend CVVH and CVVHD as potentially superior renal replacement therapy for such critically ill, highly catabolic patients.

Chronic Renal Failure

ARF, diagnosed early and treated aggressively, is usually reversible and results in no permanent impairment of kidney function. In contrast, CRF represents a substantial and permanent loss of nephron function that, depending on its magnitude, can severely alter the body's ability to maintain homeostasis. Although ischemic injury leading to ATN accounts for most cases of ARF, it uncommonly progresses to CRF. Diabetes mellitus, hypertension, various forms of glomerulonephritis, congenital abnormalities of the genitourinary tract, metabolic derangements, and infection compose a list of the more common causes of CRF in approximately descending order.

As the population of patients with CRF has increased in size, it has become apparent that certain unique problems must be addressed when surgical diseases are considered. Procedures for hemodialysis and peritoneal dialysis access are common; however, CRF is also associated with several surgical diseases that may require operative intervention. Although the anemia of CRF has in large part been eliminated since the advent of recombinant erythropoietin therapy, poor nutrition, coagulopathy, fluid and electrolyte disturbances, endocrinologic derangements, cardiovascular diseases, and alterations in host defense remain important confounding problems associated with care of patients with CRF. Cooperation and teamwork among the surgery, nephrology, and anesthesiology teams have fostered the development of effective strategies that provide optimum management, including surgical intervention, with acceptably low morbidity and mortality for this high-risk patient population.

Vascular Access for Hemodialysis

Maintenance hemodialysis is usually accomplished using a surgically created internal AV fistula or a subcutaneous AV shunt of prosthetic material. The versatility of the radiocephalic AV fistula first described in 1966 by Brescia et al.[36] has been well documented. Long-term patency rates have been good, infection rates low, and overall satisfaction acceptably high.[37-39] Other sites where endogenous AV fistulas can be surgically created to provide effective dialysis access include the median cubital vein and brachial artery at the elbow and the cephalic vein and brachial artery in the mid-upper arm (Fig. 44-3). The major disadvantages of the surgically created AV fistula is that several weeks of maturation are necessary before sufficient venous dilation occurs to allow adequate flow for dialysis, and increasingly patients have inadequate superficial venous outflow to support fistula maturation. However, when anatomically feasible, the endogenous AV fistula remains the hemodialysis access of choice for most situations.

Frequently, endogenous AV fistula creation is not feasible. Experience with various methods for creation of external AV shunts has been unrewarding, therefore the subcutaneous AV shunt has become the most common operative strategy. Most surgeons currently favor the subcutaneous AV shunt using expanded polytetrafluoroethylene (PTFE). The requirements for placement include an artery and vein that are in proximity and amenable to vascular anastomosis. Comparison of patency rates indicate that PTFE shunts are less durable than primary AV fistulas; however, 60% to 80% figures at 2 years postoperatively have been frequently reported.[40,41]

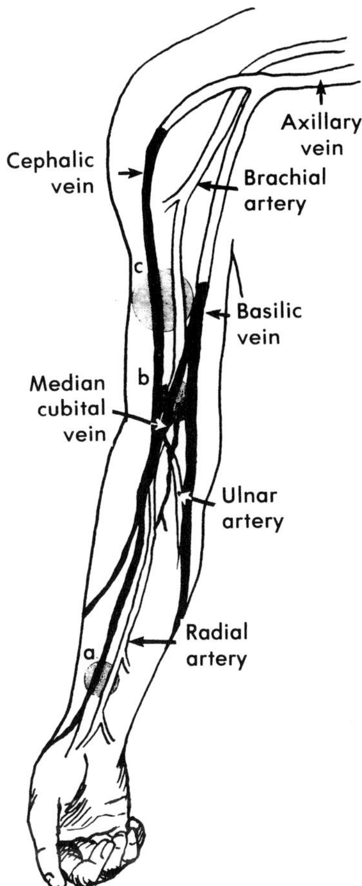

Fig. 44-3. Potential sites for creation of endogenous arteriovenous fistula for hemodialysis. The most frequently used arteriovenous fistula is created by joining the radial artery and cephalic vein at the wrist *(a)*. Other potentially suitable anastomoses include the brachial artery and medial cubital vein at the elbow *(b)* and the brachial artery and cephalic vein at the mid-upper arm *(c)*.

As nephrologists have focused efforts toward assuring adequacy of dialysis, an additional consideration has become more widely recognized, that of inadequate solute clearance. When difficulties with solute clearance are identified, evaluation should focus on potential anatomic abnormalities despite grossly adequate AV shunt function. Distal venous stenosis or occlusion, frequently in the area of the subclavian vein, innominate vein, or superior vena cava, is the most frequent cause. When suspected, this clinically important problem should be considered and thoroughly evaluated. Venous Doppler ultrasound examination provides a good screening approach; however, significant clinical suspicion should be evaluated angiographically. The most common cause of chronic AV shunt failure has been venous stenosis resulting from pseudointimal hyperplasia at the PTFE-venous anastomosis. Angiographic dilation has been attempted, but long-term maintenance of patency frequently requires operative revision. Assuming the remaining venous outflow is unaffected, excellent results have been enjoyed using PTFE angioplasty across the stenotic segment. Alternatively, central venous stenoses and occlusions have proved difficult management dilemmas. Percutaneous angioplasty with or without intravascular stenting has been attempted with mixed results. Frequently, this problem requires creation of new AV access using an alternative site away from the area of central venous abnormality.

Secondary Hyperparathyroidism

The abnormalities of calcium and phosphorus metabolism that result in abnormal parathyroid hormone production and chief cell hyperplasia represent an additional surgical disease peculiar to the CRF patient population (see Chapter 55). Depending on the criteria used, sequelae from secondary hyperparathyroidism have been estimated in 10% to 45% of patients undergoing long-term hemodialysis. Fortunately, severe problems including bone pain, pathologic fractures, metastatic calcifications, intractable pruritus, marked fatigue, and muscle weakness, occur in only a minority of patients; however, dramatic improvement has been documented following parathyroidectomy.[42]

Other Surgical Diseases

Patients with CRF are certainly not protected from developing surgical illness unrelated to their renal dysfunction. Although they develop and require care for the entire spectrum of disease entities, patients with CRF develop some diseases at rates above those of the age-matched population without renal failure. Pericardial abnormalities, including pericarditis and tamponade, represent complications of uremia that can be minimized by effective dialysis. Such complications can be life threatening, and severe cases may require pericardiectomy.

Similarly, the incidence and progression of atherosclerotic vascular disease is accelerated among individuals suffering CRF. Beyond the usual concerns related to cardiac disease, lower extremity vascular disease, and stroke, the possibility of mesenteric ischemia should always be considered during evaluation of abdominal pain in patients with CRF. Finally, although a high risk, major cardiac and atherosclerotic disease can be effectively treated in this population with acceptable operative results.

Uremic gastrointestinal disturbances have been well documented; again, most are effectively controlled with adequate dialysis. Peptic ulcer disease has been reported to occur more often among dialysis and transplantation recipients, possibly related to the gastric damaging effects of urea and steroids, the latter being a common component of the immunosuppression regimen in transplantation. Nonetheless, the association between corticosteroids and gastric ulceration remains controversial.

Perioperative Care

A recurrent theme characterizing the requirements for successful management and therapy of surgical disease cannot be overemphasized when considering care of CRF patients: *attention to detail.* The lack of normal renal autoregulatory mechanisms greatly diminishes the margin for error, and seemingly minor indiscretions in management can become life-threatening clinical dilemmas. Initial evaluation of these patients must ensure that respiratory and cardiovascular function is acceptable; previously undetected abnormalities that could adversely affect outcome must also be identified and corrected. Other preoperative measures, such as bowel preparation, should proceed as for the patient without renal failure. Ensuring that the patient is adequately dialyzed during the preoperative period is especially important. Optimization of cardiovascular and pulmonary function requires appropriate fluid balance. Adequate removal of uremic "toxins," normalization of electrolyte balance, and correction of severe anemia are crucial. Finally, in the elective setting, a period of vigorous nutritional supplementation can be extremely beneficial.

Another important aspect of the preoperative management program is timing and frequency of dialysis. When possible, it is advisable to avoid dialysis during the early postoperative period. Dialysis should therefore be planned for the day immediately preceding proposed surgery. Usual guidelines dictate a 4- to 5-hour hemodialysis or a 12-hour peritoneal dialysis session. Alternatively, patients maintained by chronic ambulatory peritoneal dialysis (CAPD) generally continue to receive dialysis until called to the operating room, at which time the peritoneal cavity is simply drained. Because electrolyte fluxes, particularly potassium, can be a major difficulty during anesthesia, surgery should not be performed before confirming preoperative optimization of serum levels. Most patients well tolerate transient postdialysis hypokalemia; thus potassium supplements are usually not administered unless hypokalemic symptomatology, such as a cardiac arrhythmia, develops. The efficacy of preoperative dialysis using a low-potassium dialysis bath becomes problematic, however, when a patient requires digitalis therapy. In that situation, care must be taken to avoid hypokalemia because of the increased incidence of digitalis toxicity associated with potassium depletion.

The hemorrhagic diathesis of renal failure was first recognized in the eighteenth century. Attempts to understand the nature of uremic bleeding were initiated in the mid-1950s, and recent advances allowing improved understanding of platelet biochemistry and physiology have begun to define underlying mechanisms.[43] Abnormal availability of platelet-membrane phospholipid ("platelet factor 3") has been extensively documented in renal failure. Similarly, decreased platelet adhesiveness and defective platelet-platelet interaction have been consistently observed among patients with uremic coagulopathy.[44-46] Bleeding time was improved by dialysis, and several dialyzable agents, including urea, guanidine succinate, and phenols, have been hypothesized as etiologic agents.[45,47] However, as experience mounted, it became clear that dialysis alone was insufficient to reverse uremic coagulopathy, and attention was redirected to abnormalities in platelet-membrane phospholipid.

Abnormalities in arachidonic acid metabolism and abnormalities in the factor VIII-von Willebrand's complex have been shown to be important in the pathogenesis of the hemostatic defect in renal failure.[48,49] Transfusion with cryoprecipitate, or the synthetic ADH analog, 1-deamino-8-D-arginine vasopressin (DDAVP), which causes the release of von Willebrand's factor multimers from endothelial cells, effectively normalizes bleeding time in uremic patients.[48,50] This has been an important observation for surgeons because the ability to control abnormal uremic bleeding reduces the risk associated with operative intervention.

Again, adequate dialysis remains the optimum therapy for the uremic hemorrhagic diathesis, and well-dialyzed patients have significantly reduced incidence of perioperative and postoperative bleeding complications. The surgeon must remain extremely cautious, and ensure complete intraoperative hemostasis. When problems arise despite control of "surgical" bleeding, cryoprecipitate (10 U) or DDAVP (0.3 μg/kg) should be administered. Although cryoprecipitate can be repeatedly administered with reasonable expectation that uremic hemorrhage will be controlled, repeated administration of DDAVP has been associated with tachyphylaxis.

Although in the past anemia was a near-universal finding among patients with CRF, this situation has changed dramatically during recent years. Earlier studies extensively documented that chronically anemic patients tolerate induction of anesthesia and subsequent surgical procedures. However, the widespread introduction of recombinant erythropoietin therapy has reduced the importance of anemia in surgical management of patients with end-stage renal disease (ESRD).[51] Most patients with ESRD are effectively managed with regular intravenous recombinant erythropoietin in dose ranges of 25 to 50 U/kg, usually three times weekly. This approach has maintained relatively normal hematocrit, and several investigations have documented the beneficial effects on quality of life.

Evidence has documented compromised host defenses in CRF.[5] The increased incidence of septic complications may be diminished by a good dialysis program; however, prophylactic perioperative antibiotics seem appropriate. The usual approach has been to administer broad-spectrum antibiotics with antistaphylococcal activity beginning preoperatively and continuing for 24 to 48 hours following surgery. Additional measures include meticulous aseptic technique and frequent examination of operative wounds with early and aggressive drainage when infection occurs.

The safe conduct of anesthesia and anesthetic management in the patient with renal failure require the same careful thought and attention to detail as is appropriate for any patient. Again, it should be emphasized that the margin for error is greatly diminished when considering patients with CRF. Volume status, electrolyte management, and hemodynamic considerations demand careful attention and precise regulation. Although transfusion is usually not a prerequisite to induction of anesthesia, red blood cell replacement must be ensured. Many drugs are metabolized abnormally by the patient with renal failure, and agents must be chosen carefully. Dosage schedules also require appropriate alterations. Finally, anesthetic agents, particularly those used for neuromuscular blockade, present unique management challenges in patients with CRF. Pancuronium and D-tubocurarine have been particularly problematic because of their effects on intracellular electrolyte balance, most importantly the tendency toward release of intracellular potassium and resulting hyperkalemia. Fortunately, newer agent used for neuromuscular blockade are safer and less problematic when considering anesthesia for CRF.

Following surgery, patients with CRF require strict attention to fluid and electrolyte replacement. Parameters other than urinary output must be employed to estimate volume replacement. Operative blood loss can be combined with the physical examination to estimate replacement therapy. It is also necessary to estimate third-space volume losses and losses from drains and fistulas when considering postoperative fluid management. Frequently, when major surgery is performed, monitoring of central venous pressure or preferably pulmonary artery pressures becomes indispensable in the postoperative care of patients with CRF.

Electrolyte disturbances in patients with CRF can occur rapidly during the postoperative period. Surgical trauma with resultant tissue damage, transfusion of banked blood, and the tendency toward acidosis favor release of intracellular potassium stores and hyperkalemia. Patients with CRF therefore require close and frequent monitoring to determine the need for early dialysis. The timing of postoperative dialysis is critical, since one must frequently choose an appropriate compromise between volume and electrolyte status and the increased risk of bleeding from requisite anticoagulation during dialysis. When one also considers the possibility of uremic coagulopathy further complicating this decision, the necessity for careful attention to detail during the entire perioperative period becomes obvious.

SELECTION OF CANDIDATES FOR RENAL TRANSPLANTATION

The safety and success of renal transplantation is well documented and now widely accepted worldwide. Kidney transplantation, when applied to appropriate patients with ESRD, offers the greatest opportunity for full rehabilitation and return to productive life. Improved immunosuppression and management strategies after the widespread introduction of cyclosporine during the 1980s resulted in a dramatically better outlook. Similarly, newer agents such as tacrolimus, mycophenolate mofetil, rapamycin, brequinar, deoxyspergualin, and leuflonimide promise greater things to come. Additionally, rapid progress using experimental strategies designed to effect specific immunologic manipulation should see clinical application in the relatively near future.

Who among the ESRD population are appropriate candidates for renal transplantation? Although most individuals with ESRD are possible transplantation candidates, several important issues must be considered. Medical and psychosocial factors have a major impact on an individual's ability to achieve successful transplantation and rehabilitation from ESRD. The pretransplantation evaluation must therefore be designed to identify those factors that could ultimately prove detrimental to a successful outcome (see accompanying box).

Prior to the widespread use of cyclosporine-based immunosuppression, consensus dictated that transplantation should be reserved for younger patients with ESRD. Renal transplantation was contraindicated for patients older than 50 to 55 years. However, little detrimental effect has been documented among older renal transplantation recipients receiving cyclosporine-based immunosuppression protocols. Deaths in this age group were usually unrelated to immunosuppression or complications of immunosuppressive therapy. Those observations resulted in a widespread belief that age alone should not be considered absolute, and renal transplantation can be considered for older patients with acceptable expectation for success.

Although recurrence of the original renal disease after transplantation has been uncommon, this possibility should be considered in some settings. Among various forms of glomerulonephritis, membranoproliferative and focal sclerosing variants have been reported to recur more often after renal transplantation.[52] Reports suggesting recurrent glomerulonephritis also have rarely implicated immunoglobulin A nephritis, glomerulonephritis associated with systemic diseases such as Henoch-Schönlein purpura, and membranous glomerulonephritis. Among other systemic diseases associated with renal failure, including systemic lupus erythematosus, scleroderma, sickle-cell disease, amyloidosis, Fabry's disease, and cystinosis, the general experience indicates that transplantation can be successfully performed.[53] However, it remains important to stress that associated problems manifest by these patients place them at higher-than-average risk. Primary oxalosis, a rare autosomal recessive disorder of glyoxalate metabolism, has been associated with a high incidence of recurrent renal failure because of oxalate deposition in the transplanted organ.[54] Some of these patients have been successfully treated with combined liver and renal transplantation.

Diabetes mellitus is the most common systemic disorder for which kidney transplantation has been performed. When considering the type I population of diabetic patients, nephropathy has been estimated to occur in 15 patients per 1 million population per year in the United States.[30] This group has represented a challenging patient population with many serious associated medical problems. Although diabetic patients represent a group at increased risk, primarily because of associated vascular and microvascular complications, successful transplantation is frequently performed. Studies have now followed diabetic patients for extended time periods after renal transplantation. Three-year actuarial graft survival under cyclosporine immunosuppression has been reported at 80%.[55] Biopsy data have substantiated that changes consistent with diabetic glomerulopathy occur in almost all diabetic renal transplantation recipients[56]; however, deterioration in renal function has not been well documented. The diabetic patient therefore has benefited from renal transplantation, but associated risks primarily caused by complications of vascular and microvascular disease result in increased morbidity and mortality.

Absolute contraindications to renal transplantation are few but include irreversible central nervous system disease, severe liver insufficiency when combined hepatic and renal transplantation is not appropriate, active infection, ma-

PRETRANSPLANTATION EVALUATION

General

History and physical examination
Nutritional assessment
Detailed psychosocial evaluation
Complete hematologic evaluation
Chest roentgenogram

Gastrointestinal Evaluation

Upper gastrointestinal contrast study (selected patients)
Upper gastrointestinal endoscopy (selected patients)
Lower gastrointestinal contrast study (selected patients)
Lower gastrointestinal endoscopy (selected patients)

Biliary Evaluation

Ultrasound examination

Cardiovascular Evaluation

Electrocardiogram
Noninvasive cardiac stress testing with radionuclide imaging
- All diabetic patients
- When clinically indicated

Coronary arteriography (when imaging results are positive)

Urologic Evaluation

Urinalysis with culture
Voiding cystourethrogram (when clinically indicated)
Cystoscopy (when clinically indicated)

Immunologic Evaluation

Histocompatibility testing
Immunologic profile
Transfusion history
Hepatitis serologic screening
Cytomegalovirus testing
HIV testing/Western blot if results are positive
Epstein-Barr virus testing

lignancy, or advanced systemic disease. As previously discussed, several contributing factors can collectively render renal transplantation inappropriate. Therefore, in practice, patients are selected for transplantation after detailed evaluation of individual medical and psychosocial considerations in an attempt to optimize ultimate rehabilitation.

A complete medical profile of potential renal transplantation recipients is critical to the pretransplantation evaluation (see box on p. 898). The history, physical examination, laboratory results, specific organ system, and immunologic examinations provide important prognostic data. A clinical psychologist or social worker provides information ensuring that potential financial and social difficulties may be anticipated and addressed. The pretransplantation evaluation frequently identifies abnormalities better handled before initiation of immunosuppressive therapy. Any necessary dental work should be completed before transplantation. Surgical procedures, including cholecystectomy for gallstones, have increased in importance with the widespread use of cyclosporine because of the agent's hepatotoxic side effects and its recent association with development of biliary calculous disease.[57] Also procedures such as splenectomy for hypersplenism and parathyroidectomy for symptomatic secondary hyperparathyroidism should be performed when indicated. Similarly, infectious diseases should be treated and their resolution assured before transplantation and initiation of immunosuppression. Careful attention to these pretransplantation details can pay tremendous dividends in the form of reduced posttransplantation morbidity and mortality.

Results following renal transplantation in management of ESRD have been gratifying. Patients can now be offered this therapeutic option with confidence, and widespread analysis has documented 5-year allograft and patient survival under cyclosporine therapy exceeding 70% and 90%, respectively, for recipients of primary cadaveric allografts. Similarly, recipients of haploidentical grafts from living related donors enjoy 90% graft and 98% patient survival at 5 years. Importantly, these improved results have been underscored by the important observation that 89% of patients successfully transplanted were considered vocationally rehabilitated.

SUMMARY

The widespread application of maintenance dialysis and renal transplantation has dramatically improved the outlook for patients suffering from renal failure. This also has impacted substantially on surgical diseases because patients can now be effectively managed in the presence of severely compromised or absent renal function. Abnormal renal function and physicians' ability to manage its sequelae affect surgical practice in various settings: ARF complicating the clinical course of injured or critically ill patients postoperatively, CRF in patients requiring surgery for operative disorders unrelated to their renal disease, angioaccess for hemodialysis, and renal transplantation.

ARF has been classified according to the cause of the precipitating events into prerenal azotemia and failure, intrinsic renal failure, and postrenal or obstructive forms. Largely because of associated complications, including infection, poor nutrition, and multiorgan dysfunction, ARF continues to result in high mortality rates exceeding 70%. Clinical indexes such as measurements of urinary volume, urinary specific gravity, electrolyte excretion, examination of the urinary sediment, and serum determinations of BUN and creatinine allow the clinician to assess renal function accurately. The high mortality associated with development of ARF emphasizes the necessity for preventive measures, including adequate hydration, optimum cardiac performance, identification of structural genitourinary abnormalities, and judicious use of potentially nephrotoxic medications.

When faced with a situation likely to result in ARF, the surgeon must be prepared to provide effective management strategies to minimize adverse sequelae. Fluid and electrolyte balance, acid-base regulation, and avoidance of uremic complications are essential. The methodology used and the timing in initiating interventive support for the ARF patient are extremely important. Hemodialysis remains the mainstay in support of patients with severe ARF; however, peritoneal dialysis and the more recently developed technique of continuous hemofiltration have specialized applications.

Patients with CRF continue to increase in numbers, primarily as the result of improved long-term management using dialysis and transplantation. Surgery for hemodialysis and peritoneal dialysis access, parathyroidectomy for secondary hyperparathyroidism, pericardiectomy for uremic pericarditis, gastrointestinal disorders, and the general spectrum of surgical diseases require strict attention to detail. The ability of the surgery, anesthesiology, and nephrology teams to cooperate closely during the preoperative, operative, and postoperative periods is essential to the successful outcome for this complex patient population.

Finally, renal transplantation has become widely accepted as the therapy of choice for patients with ESRD. Advances in immunosuppressive regimens have improved the posttransplantation prognosis such that patients can be offered this modality with confidence not only for a high degree of technical success but also for an excellent probability of vocational rehabilitation.

ACKNOWLEDGMENT

The author would like to express sincere appreciation to Dr. Margaret J. Bia for critical review and helpful suggestions in completing this manuscript.

REFERENCES

1. Billingham RE. Dedication: Proceedings of the Sixth International Congress of the Transplantation Society. Transplant Proc 9:37, 1977.

2. Graham WB. Historical aspects of hemodialysis. Transplant Proc 9:49, 1977.
3. Starzl TE. Experience in Renal Transplantation. Philadelphia: WB Saunders, 1964.
4. Abl AM, Buckley MI, Austen WG. Etiology, incidence, and prognosis of renal failure following cardiac operations. J Thorac Cardiovasc Surg 71:323, 1976.
5. Kasishe BL, Kjellstrand CM. Perioperative management of patients with chronic renal failure and postoperative renal failure. Urol Clin North Am 10:35, 1983.
6. Wilkins RG, Faraghen EB. Acute renal failure in an intensive care unit: Incidence, prediction, and outcome. Anesthesia 38:628, 1983.
7. Brezis M, Rosen S, Epstein FH. Acute renal failure. In Brenner BM, Rector FC, eds. The Kidney. Philadelphia: WB Saunders, 1986.
8. Flamenbaum W. Pathophysiology of acute renal failure. In Solez K, Whelton A, eds. Acute Renal Failure. New York: Marcel Dekker, 1984.
9. Flemenbaum W, et al. Acute renal failure associated with myoglobinuria and hemoglobinuria. In Brenner BM, Lazarus JM, eds. Acute Renal Failure. Philadelphia: WB Saunders, 1983.
10. Byrd L, Sherman RL. Radiocontrast-induced acute renal failure: A clinical and pathophysiologic review. Medicine (Baltimore) 58:270, 1979.
11. Mudge GH. Nephrotoxicity of urographic radiocontrast drugs. Kidney Int 18:540, 1980.
12. Bennett WM, Luft F, Porter GA. Pathogenesis of renal failure due to amino glycoside and contrast media. Am J Med 69:767, 1980.
13. Kaloyanides GJ, Pastoriza-Munoz E. Aminoglycoside nephrotoxicity. Kidney Int 18:571, 1980.
14. Anderson RJ, Linus SL, Bernz AS. Nonoliguric renal failure. N Engl J Med 296:1134, 1977.
15. Swartz RD. Interventive support for acute renal failure in the critically ill patient. In Bartlett RH, Whitehosue WM, Turcotte JG, eds. Life Support Systems in Intensive Care. Chicago: Year Book Medical Publishers, 1984.
16. Miller TR, et al. Urinary diagnostic indices in acute renal failure. Ann Intern Med 89:47, 1978.
17. Brezin JH, et al. Reversible renal failure and nephrotic syndrome associated with nonsteroidal anti-inflammatory drugs. N Engl J Med 301:1271, 1979.
18. Rasmussen HH, Ibels LS. Acute renal failure: Multivariant analysis of causes and risk factors. Am J Med 73:211, 1982.
19. Schrier RW. Acute renal failure. Kidney Int 15:205, 1979.
20. Abel RM, et al. Improved survival from acute renal failure after treatment with intravenous essential L-amino acids and glucose. N Engl J Med 288:695, 1973.
21. Siegel NH, Gaudio KM, Kashgarian M. Adenine nucleotides in prevention of acute renal failure. In Robinson RR, ed. Nephrology. New York: Springer-Verlag, 1984, p 800.
22. Siegel NJ, Gaudio KM, Katz LA. Beneficial effect of thyroxin on recovery from toxic acute renal failure. Kidney Int 25:906, 1984.
23. Mann JFE, et al. Atrial natriuretic factor in patients with renal insufficiency: A placebo controlled, randomized study. Nephrol Dial Transplant 4:776, 1989.
24. Hanley DA, Sherwood LM. Secondary hyperparathyroidism in renal failure. Med Clin North Am 62:1319, 1978.
25. Sutton RAL, Dirks JH. Calcium and magnesium: Renal handling and disorders of metabolism. In Brenner BM, Rector FC, eds. The Kidney. Philadelphia: WB Saunders, 1986.
26. Welchel JD. Central venous hemodialysis access catheters: A review of technical considerations and complications. In Vascular Access for Hemodialysis II. Chicago: Precept Press, 1991, p 123.
27. Rosenak S, Siwon P. Experimentelle untersuchungen ueber die peritoneale assucheidung harnpflichtigen substanzen aus dem blute. Mitt a d Gronzgeb D Med U Chir 39:391, 1926.
28. Clark WR, et al. A comparison of metabolic control by continuous and intermittent therapies in acute renal failure. J Am Soc Nephrol 4:1413, 1994.
29. Kramer P, et al. Intensive care potential of continuous arteriovenous hemofiltration. Trans Am Soc Artif Intern Organs 28:28, 1982.
30. Kramer P, et al. Management of anuric intensive care patients with arteriovenous hemofiltration. Int J Artif Organs 3:225, 1980.
31. Kramer P, et al. Continuous arteriovenous haemofiltration: A new kidney replacement therapy. Proc Eur Dial Transplant Assoc 18:743, 1981.
32. Macias WL, et al. Continuous venovenous hemofiltration: An alternative to continuous arterio-venous hemofiltration and hemodiafiltration in acute renal failure. Am J Kidney Dis 18:451, 1991.
33. Storek M, et al. Comparison of pump driven and spontaneous continuous hemofiltration in postoperative acute renal failure. Lancet 337:452, 1991.
34. Abel RM. Nutritional support in the patient with acute renal failure. J Am Coll Nutr 2:33, 1983.
35. Mault JR, et al. Starvation: A major contributor to mortality in acute renal failure. Trans Am Soc Artif Intern Organs 29:390, 1983.
36. Brescia MJ, et al. Chronic hemodialysis using venipuncture and a surgically created arteriovenous fistula. N Engl J Med 275:1089, 1966.
37. Ehrenfeld WK. Surgical techniques for hemodialysis access. In Barker WF, ed. Peripheral Arterial Disease. Philadelphia: WB Saunders, 1975.
38. Ishihara AM. The current state of the art for vascular access in hemodialysis. Contemp Cont Dial Sept:29, 1980.
39. Rohn MS, et al. Arteriovenous fistulas for long-term dialysis. Arch Surg 113:153, 1978.
40. Jenkins AM, Buist TAS, Glover SD. Medium term follow-up of 40 autogenous vein and forty polytetrafluoroethylene grafts for vascular access. Surgery 88:667, 1980.
41. Tellis VA, et al. Expanded polytetrafluoroethylene graft fistula for chronic hemodialysis. Ann Surg 189:101, 1979.
42. Campbell DA, Dafoe DC, Swartz RD. Medical and surgical management of secondary hyperparathyroidism. In Thompson NW, Vinik AI, eds. Endocrine Surgery Update. New York: Grune & Stratton, 1983.
43. Deykin D. Uremic bleeding. Kidney Int 24:698, 1972.
44. Castaldi PA, Rozenberg MC, Stewart JH. The bleeding disorder of uremia: A qualitative platelet defect. Lancet 2:66, 1966.
45. Rabiner SF, Hrodek O. Platelet factor 3 in normal subjects and patients with renal failure. J Clin Invest 47:901, 1968.
46. Salzman EW, Neri LL. Adhesiveness of blood platelets in uremia. Thromb Diath Haemorh 15:84, 1966.
47. Eknoyan G, et al. Platelet function in renal failure. N Engl J Med 280:677, 1969.
48. Mannucci PM, et al. D-amino-8-D-arginine vasopressin shortens the bleeding time in uremia. N Engl J Med 308:8, 1983.
49. Ruggeri ZM, et al. Multivein composition of factor VIII/von Willebrand factor following administration of DDAVP: Implications for pathophysiology and therapy of von Willebrand's disease subtypes. Blood 59:1272, 1982.
50. Janson PA, et al. Treatment of the bleeding tendency in uremia with cryoprecipitate. N Engl J Med 303:1318, 1980.
51. Erslev AJ. Erythropoietin. N Engl J Med 324:1339, 1991.
52. Kreis H. Transplanted kidney: Natural history. In Hamburger J, et al. eds. Renal Transplantation. Baltimore: Williams & Wilkins, 1981.
53. Sreepada TK. Hemodialysis and transplantation in systemic diseases. In Friedman E, ed. Renal Failure. New York: John Wiley, 1978.
54. Scheinman JI, Najarian JS, Mauer SM. Successful strategies for renal transplantation in primary oxalosis. Kidney Int 25:804, 1984.

55. Najarian JS, et al. A single institution, randomized, prospective trial of cyclosporine versus azothioprine, antilymphocyte globulin for immunosuppression in renal allograft recipients. Ann Surg 201:142, 1985.
56. Mauer SM, et al. Development of diabetic vascular lesions in normal kidneys transplanted into patients with diabetes mellitus. N Engl J Med 295:916, 1976.
57. Lorber MI, et al. Hepatobiliary and pancreatic complications of cyclosporine therapy in 466 renal transplant recipients. Transplantation 43:35, 1987.

45

Neurogenic Bladder and Urinary Diversion

George S. Benson

Urinary continence and micturition are processes that are controlled by complex neurologic mechanisms. When normal neurologic control is lost, a variety of lower urinary tract syndromes, which are collectively known as *neurogenic bladder disease,* may be produced. Because these syndromes are commonly encountered in the practice of surgery, a familiarity with their pathophysiology is mandatory if urinary tract complications are to be prevented. This chapter summarizes the anatomy and physiology of normal urinary continence and micturition and provides a classification of neurogenic bladder disease to aid in diagnosis and management. In addition, several important aspects of normal lower urinary tract function are poorly understood and controversial. These controversies, particularly as they relate to the clinical management of neurogenic bladder disease, are also discussed.

ANATOMY AND PHYSIOLOGY OF CONTINENCE AND MICTURITION

Anatomy of the Bladder and Its Outlet

Embryologically and anatomically the urinary bladder can be divided into the detrusor and trigone. Contrary to classic thinking, the detrusor musculature is not composed of outer and inner longitudinal and middle circular muscle layers, but rather is composed of a meshwork of smooth muscle fibers, many of which run at right angles to each other.[1] In the region of the bladder neck, muscle bundles arch toward and away from the bladder outlet in such a manner that, with contraction of the detrusor musculature, the bladder neck is pulled up and open. The ureters enter the bladder posteriorly near the superior portion of the trigone and course through submucosal "tunnels" to the level of the ureteral orifices. The length of the submucosal "tunnel" is an important factor in the prevention of vesicoureteral reflux during bladder contraction.

Functionally, the bladder is better divided into body and base than into detrusor and trigone.[2] The base is defined as that part of the bladder circumferentially distal to the level of the ureteral orifices and the body as that part proximal to the ureteral orifices. Neuroanatomically and neuropharmacologically, all portions of the bladder base differ from the bladder body; these differences are discussed in the following paragraphs.

A solid body of clinical data convincingly demonstrates that a continence mechanism exists in the area of the bladder neck and proximal urethra in both the male and the female.[3] The existence of an anatomic sphincter composed of annular fibers in the area of the bladder neck was denied by Clark in 1883,[4] and over the past century, most investigators have reiterated Clark's observation. However, many anatomic studies done by careful investigators present remarkably conflicting results concerning the anatomy of the bladder neck and proximal urethra.

Those advocates of the "no anatomic sphincter" position differ among themselves on the muscular anatomy of the bladder neck. Woodburne[1] concluded that the "muscle in this region does not constitute a sphincter of annular fibers." The "arching muscle fascicles which arch toward and then away from the urethral opening and do not encircle it" were viewed by him as "an opening mechanism rather than a sphincter."[1] The closure properties of this region were postulated to be secondary to its high concentration of elastic tissue. Common to most of the "no anatomic sphincter" descriptions is the belief that at least part of the urethral musculature is a direct continuation of the detrusor. Thus Woodburne[1] states that in the human "its (bladder) internal longitudinal fascicles are traceable directly downward into the submucosal layer of the urethra." According to Tanagho and Smith,[5] "the proximal urethra of the male and the whole urethra in the female consist of two muscular layers, (1) an inner longitudinal coat (a direct continuation of the inner longitudinal coat of the bladder); and (2) an outer circular coat of oblique fibers that are the direct continuation of the outer longitudinal coat of the bladder." The sphincter mechanism, according to these investigators, "is achieved by the oblique and circular fibers around the urethra. Because of their special arrangement, these muscle fibers are occlusive in the passive relaxed state and they do not hinder the active opening of the bladder neck during voiding."[5]

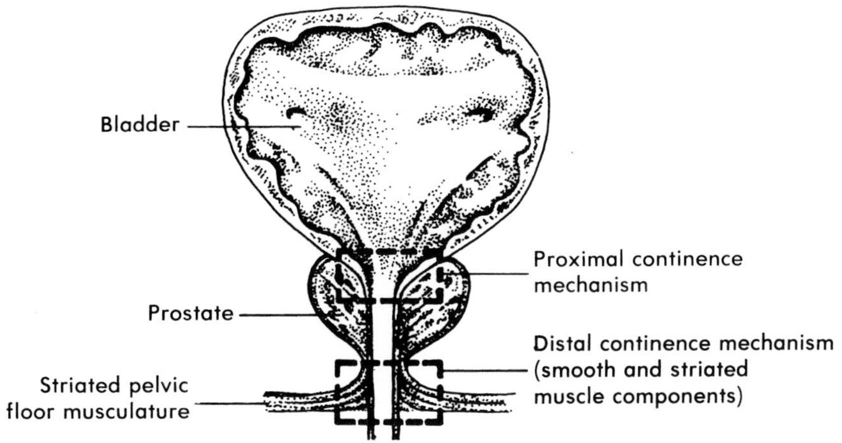

Fig. 45-1. Proximal and distal continence mechanisms in the male.

Another viewpoint concerning the muscular anatomy of the bladder neck is that a definite sphincteric muscle completely encircling the bladder neck does exist. Gosling[6] has reported that, at least in the male, the "bladder neck smooth muscle is histologically and histochemically different from that which comprises the detrusor" and that "a complete circular collar" is present, which also surrounds the preprostatic portion of the urethra.

In the male, but not in the female, a second continence mechanism is present in the area of the membranous urethra (that part of the urethra traversing the striated musculature of the pelvic floor)[3] (Fig. 45-1). The membranous urethra contains not only smooth muscle but also elastic tissue. In addition, periurethral striated muscle extending from the bladder neck to the level of the membranous urethra has been recognized for years. The issue of whether this periurethral striated muscle forms part of the complex musculature of the perineum or whether this intrinsic striated musculature is anatomically separate from the external striated musculature of the pelvic floor has not been resolved.[7]

Innervation of the Bladder and Its Outlet

The bladder and its outlet are innervated by the two divisions of the autonomic nervous system (parasympathetic and sympathetic) and by the somatic nervous system.[8] The terms *parasympathetic* and *sympathetic* should not be confused with the terms *adrenergic* and *cholinergic*. Parasympathetic and sympathetic are anatomic terms that signify the location of the cell bodies of autonomic nerves. Parasympathetic nerves originate in the craniosacral portions and sympathetic nerves in the thoracolumbar portion of the spinal cord. Cholinergic and adrenergic are physiologic terms that indicate the type of neurotransmitter released at nerve terminals. The neurotransmitter released by cholinergic nerves is by definition acetylcholine, whereas the adrenergic neurotransmitter is a catecholamine. Cholinergic nerves include somatic motor neurons, preganglionic autonomic fibers, and postganglionic parasympathetic fibers. Postganglionic sympathetic fibers are, in general, adrenergic in nature, and the catecholamine responsible for neurotransmission in the lower urinary tract is norepinephrine.

The primary motor nerve supply to the bladder is carried through the pelvic nerve, a parasympathetic nerve derived from sacral segments S2 to S4. Classically, micturition has been viewed as a relatively simple spinal reflex. Bladder distention stimulates afferent fibers that are also carried in the pelvic nerve. These sensory fibers enter the cord through the posterior sacral roots and synapse with the pelvic nerve nuclei in the intermediolateral portion of the cord. Preganglionic efferent fibers then exit the cord in the ventral nerve roots and are carried to peripheral ganglia in the pelvic nerve. In the ganglia these preganglionic fibers then synapse with postganglionic cholinergic fibers, which innervate the bladder and urethra. The view that normal micturition is controlled by a sacral spinal reflex is no longer thought to be true. Relatively recent experimental evidence has demonstrated that voiding is controlled not by a spinal reflex but rather by a pontine micturition center.[9,10] Sensory afferent fibers carried in the pelvic nerve do not synapse with efferent nerve cell bodies in the spinal cord but are carried directly to the pons. These afferent fibers synapse with nerve fibers that descend in the spinal cord and then synapse with pelvic nerve cell bodies in the sacral spinal cord (Fig. 45-2). Thus the peripheral parasympathetic pathways controlling bladder function are the same in both the sacral reflex arc and the pontine micturition schemes, and both viewpoints incorporate cerebral control of micturition. The spinal cord organization of the micturition reflex is, however, significantly different. DeGroat and Steers[11] have clearly demonstrated that normal voiding is governed by the pontine micturition center. Following spinal cord injury, however, voiding can occur via the more primitive sacral spinal reflex.

Acetylcholinesterase positive (presumptive cholinergic) nerves have been identified by light microscopy in all ar-

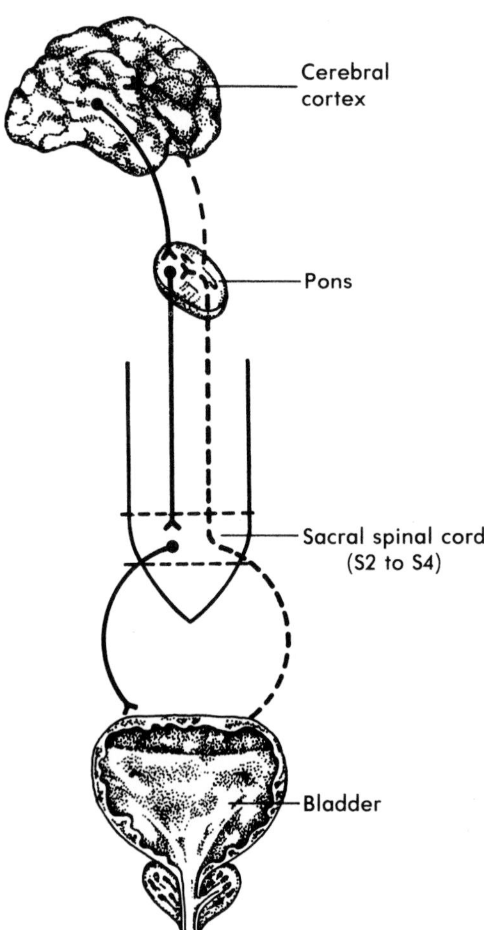

Fig. 45-2. Bladder innervation. Bladder distention results in increased afferent activity in the pelvic nerve. These sensory fibers ascend in the spinal cord to finally synapse with nerves in the pons. Stimuli are then carried in nerve tracts from the pons to again synapse with parasympathetic nerves in the sacral spinal cord.

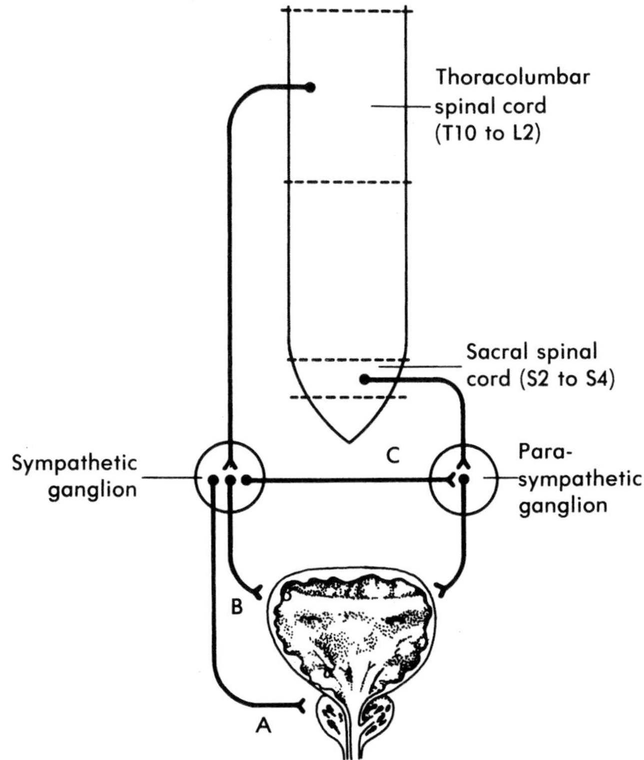

Fig. 45-3. Sympathetic innervation of the lower urinary tract. *A,* α-Adrenergic receptor stimulation of the bladder base and urethra; *B,* β-adrenergic receptor stimulation of the bladder body; *C,* α-adrenergic receptor–mediated inhibition of parasympathetic ganglionic transmission.

eas of the bladder. In vitro bladder muscle strips respond by contracting when stimulated with acetylcholine; this contraction with acetylcholine stimulation is blocked by pretreating the muscle strips with cholinergic muscarinic receptor-blocking agents (atropine, propantheline).[12] This evidence supports the contention that the parasympathetic neurotransmitter responsible for bladder contraction is acetylcholine and that voiding is therefore a cholinergically mediated event. In vivo stimulation of the pelvic nerve also causes bladder contraction. Unlike the in vitro situation, however, the bladder contraction cannot be completely abolished with pretreating the experimental animal with atropine. This relative atropine resistance of the urinary bladder has led to the hypothesis that at least part of the parasympathetic bladder innervation is noncholinergic.[8] Several putative neurotransmitters, including vasoactive intestinal polypeptide (VIP), enkephalin, adenosine triphosphate, and others, are currently being investigated.

The bladder and its outlet are also innervated by the sympathetic division of the autonomic nervous system. Preganglionic sympathetic nerves arise from the thoracolumbar portion of the spinal cord (T10 to L2). These preganglionic fibers synapse in ganglia located near the spinal cord (paravertebral ganglia), between the paravertebral ganglia and end organ (preganglia), or near or within the end organ (peripheral ganglia). Postganglionic sympathetic fibers then innervate the end organ itself. In addition, sympathetic neurons synapse with parasympathetic ganglia, and adrenergic stimulation has been demonstrated to slow neurotransmission through parasympathetic ganglia[13] (Fig. 45-3).

Morphologically, the various regions of the bladder and its outlet vary remarkably with respect to their adrenergic innervation. The bladder base and urethra are densely innervated by adrenergic fibers, whereas adrenergic fibers in the bladder body are sparse. In addition, muscle bath and radioligand-binding studies have demonstrated that the bladder base and urethra have a high concentration of α-adrenergic receptors and a low concentration of β-adrenergic receptors. Conversely, the bladder body contains more β-adrenergic receptors than α-adrenergic receptors.[14] In the lower urinary tract, stimulation of α-adrenergic receptors causes smooth muscle contraction, whereas stimulation of β-adrenergic receptors causes relaxation.[2] With sympathetic nerve stimulation, the bladder base and urethra contract (through α-adrenergic receptors), and the bladder body relaxes (through β-adrenergic receptors). These actions are viewed as promoting urine storage.

As previously discussed, the anatomy of the striated musculature in the area of the membranous urethra is not well understood. The innervation of the musculature in this region is equally controversial. The nerve supply to the entire perineal striated musculature is generally thought to be somatic in nature. These fibers originate in the sacral cord (S2 to S4) and are carried in the pudendal nerve. Several researchers believe that the portion of the pelvic floor striated musculature that is located periurethrally (intrinsic striated musculature) is anatomically separate from the extrinsic striated musculature of the perineum. Furthermore, evidence has been presented that this intrinsic striated musculature, or urethral striated sphincter, is not innervated by the pudendal nerve but rather by autonomic nerves coming from the pelvic plexus.[15]

Micturition and Continence (A Simplified Scheme)

Although our understanding of normal lower urinary tract anatomy and physiology is far from complete, a relatively simple approach to patient care, integrating consistent basic science findings and clinical observations, enables the physician to rationally treat most patients with neurogenic bladder disease.

The lower urinary tract has two primary functions: urine emptying (micturition) and urine storage (continence). Micturition is primarily a parasympathetically mediated event. Afferent impulses signaling bladder distention synapse with efferent fibers that exit from the sacral spinal cord. Conscious cerebral control over the micturition reflex occurs through pathways that facilitate or inhibit the pontine micturition reflex. Efferent stimuli (primarily cholinergic) cause the bladder to contract. With bladder contraction, the bladder base is pulled up and open; when intravesical pressure exceeds the intraurethral pressure, micturition occurs.

Under normal circumstances, continence requires the absence of uninhibited bladder contractions. In females the only continence mechanism, or "continence zone," is located in the area of the bladder neck and proximal urethra. The bladder neck and proximal urethra are thought to remain closed by two mechanisms: (1) the inherent elasticity of the tissue and (2) contraction of the smooth muscle in this area (mediated through α-adrenergic receptors). In the male two "continence zones" are present. The proximal continence area is composed of the bladder neck and proximal urethra. The second or distal continence mechanism is located near the area of the membranous urethra. This distal continence mechanism is also thought to be dependent on the inherent elasticity and α-adrenergic receptor–mediated contraction of the smooth muscle of the urethra. The importance of the striated musculature of the pelvic floor in helping to maintain passive continence is controversial. In normal micturition, however, the pelvic floor musculature reflexly relaxes just before detrusor contraction. In some pathologic states, contraction of the pelvic floor striated musculature with detrusor contraction can cause functional obstruction of urine flow in the area of the membranous urethra.[16]

DIAGNOSIS AND CLASSIFICATION OF NEUROGENIC BLADDER DISEASE

Diagnosis

Symptoms

Patients afflicted with neurogenic bladder disease may have a variety of symptoms. In fact, many patients with neurogenic bladder disease are incorrectly diagnosed because their initial symptoms so closely mimic other types of urologic disease. For instance, hesitancy, straining to void, decrease in the force and caliber of the urinary stream, and urinary retention are symptoms not only of bladder outlet obstruction (secondary to urethral stricture, benign prostatic hyperplasia, or prostatic carcinoma) but also of some types of neurogenic bladder disease. Dysuria and fever are symptoms not only of uncomplicated infections in otherwise healthy patients but also of infection complicated by lower urinary tract dysfunction. In general, patients with neurogenic bladder disease are more prone to infection than the general population. Urinary urgency can occur secondary to bladder outlet obstruction, but it also can be seen when normal cortical function is lost and uninhibited contractions occur. Severe urgency can lead to urgency incontinence, which should be differentiated from stress incontinence and from overflow incontinence secondary to urinary retention.

History

In patients who have any of these symptoms, a diagnosis of neurogenic bladder disease should at least be entertained. Does the patient have a history of cerebrovascular disease, disk disease, diabetes mellitus, multiple sclerosis, or back or pelvic trauma or surgery? Does the patient have any neurologic symptoms, weakness, paresthesias, blurred vision, or tremor? Since sacral segments S2 to S4 innervate the rectum and penis as well as the bladder, a history of constipation, fecal incontinence, or impotence should be ascertained. A careful history of medications taken by the patient should also be obtained. Many drugs, including antihistamines, antidepressants, and over-the-counter cold remedies, have anticholinergic or sympathomimetic side effects and can significantly alter lower urinary tract function.

Physical Examination

A complete physical examination should be performed with special attention directed to the urologic and neurologic systems. Palpation of the abdomen may reveal masses (hydronephrotic kidneys or a distended bladder). A rectal examination in males to evaluate the prostate gland and rectal sphincter tone is mandatory. Females should undergo a pelvic examination to exclude pelvic masses, cystocele, or a urethral diverticulum.

A neurologic examination should include an evaluation of sensation of the perineal or saddle area, which is supplied by sacral segments S2 to S4. The bulbocavernosus reflex is often helpful in determining the status of the afferent and efferent limbs of the sacral reflex. This reflex is elicited by squeezing the glans penis or clitoris and determining the presence of an immediate contraction of the external anal sphincter, which can be felt with an examining finger in the rectum. Although this reflex cannot be elicited in all neurologically intact individuals and it does not directly test bladder innervation, the presence of a bulbocavernosus reflex is indicative that at least some reflex activity through the sacral spinal cord is intact.

Laboratory, Radiologic, and Urodynamic Evaluation

Any patient with suspected neurogenic bladder disease must have a urinalysis and urine culture to rule out infection and a serum creatinine to estimate renal function. Determination of the blood glucose to screen for diabetes and a serologic screening test for syphilis may be required. An excretory urogram is usually necessary to evaluate any ureteral or renal changes secondary to bladder dysfunction or vesicoureteral reflux. Specifically, hydronephrosis, urinary tract stones, and renal scarring secondary to pyelonephritis can be evaluated with this study. A renal ultrasound can be performed instead of an excretory urogram and is the screening study of choice for children. A voiding cystourethrogram is often required to rule out vesicoureteral reflux, particularly in children with congenital neurologic defects such as myelodysplasia. In addition, various neurologic studies may be necessary to exclude specific neurologic lesions. Head or spine computed tomographic scans, magnetic resonance imaging scans, myelograms, and electromyograms are often indicated in these patients to confirm or exclude suspected neurologic disease.

The diagnosis and management of most patients with neurogenic bladder disease is usually dictated by the results of urodynamic studies. Objective measurements of lower urinary tract function are extremely helpful; the extent of the urodynamic evaluation necessary to adequately manage patients with neurogenic bladder disease is, however, controversial.[17,18]

The cystometrogram is the most useful study in objectively assessing lower urinary tract dysfunction. For this study the patient is asked to empty the bladder; then a catheter is inserted, and residual urine volume measured. Water or carbon dioxide is then instilled into the patient's bladder at a given rate, and the intravesical pressure is recorded as the bladder is filled (Fig. 45-4).

Bladders in healthy individuals demonstrate accommodation; that is, intravesical pressure increases little with relatively large increments in volume. In addition to residual urine volume, the bladder capacity can be estimated. Although bladder capacity varies greatly from patient to patient, the bladder capacity of most individuals falls in the 300 to 500 ml range. The presence or absence of bladder sensation and the presence of uninhibited bladder contractions and normal detrusor contractions can be ascertained. Although a variety of classifications for neurogenic bladder disease exist, most of them depend heavily on the findings of the cystometrogram to categorize types of bladder dysfunction.

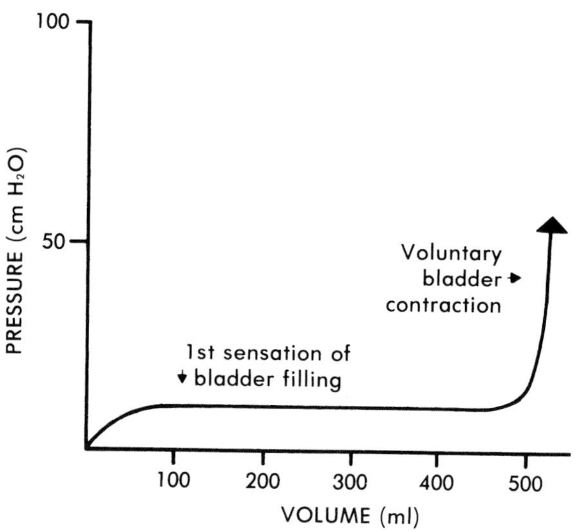

Fig. 45-4. Normal cystometrogram.

The cystometrogram can be performed simultaneously with other studies to yield additional information. Normally, pelvic floor striated muscle electromyographic activity diminishes just before the onset of a bladder contraction. When functional obstruction at the level of the membranous urethra is suspected (detrusor–striated sphincter dyssynergia), a combined cystometrogram and pelvic floor electromyogram can be performed. An increase in electromyographic activity during bladder contraction is characteristic of this lesion (Fig. 45-5).

Determination of the voiding flow rate is helpful to rule out obstruction. Maximum voiding flow rates are related to the voided volume; nomograms exist for the interpretation of results into normal or obstructed patterns.[19] The voiding flow rate can be performed simultaneously with other parameters of lower urinary tract function. For example, the recording of urine flow rate, intravesical pressure, and pelvic floor electromyographic activity can be obtained simultaneously with a fluoroscopically monitored voiding cystourethrogram. Combined studies such as these may give additional diagnostic information in difficult clinical situations.

The bethanechol supersensitivity test is occasionally helpful in determining the integrity of bladder innervation. This test is based on the principle that denervated smooth muscle becomes supersensitive to neurotransmitters.[20] The cystometrogram is performed and the intravesical pressure at 100 ml of volume recorded. Bethanechol

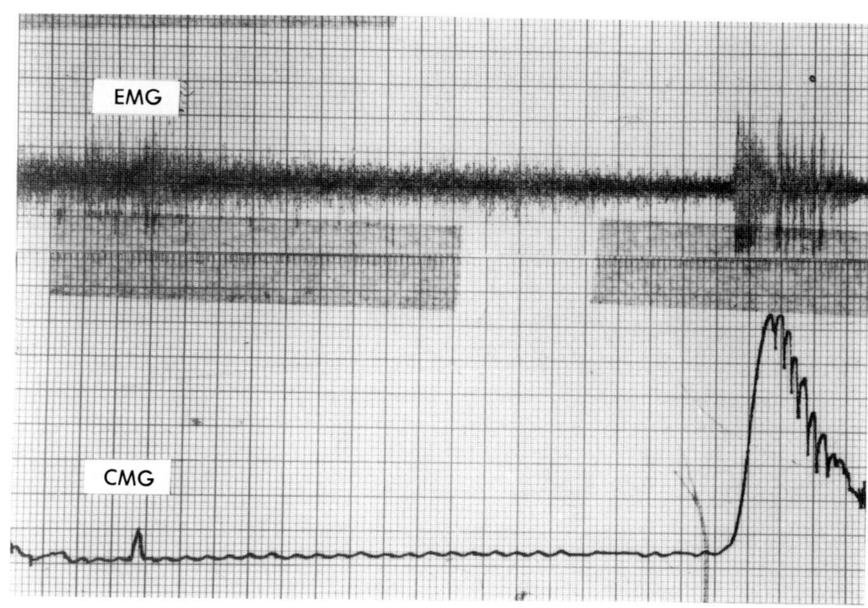

Fig. 45-5. Combined cystometrogram and pelvic floor striated muscle electromyogram in patient with detrusor–striated sphincter dyssynergia. (Note increase in electromyographic activity at time of bladder contraction.)

chloride (0.35 mg/kg), a muscarinic cholinergic receptor agonist, is then injected subcutaneously. Cystometrograms are done at 15 minutes, 30 minutes, and 45 minutes following the injection of bethanechol. The intravesical pressure during these subsequent cystometrograms at 100 ml volume is again recorded. An increase of 15 cm of water over the preinjection value is considered positive. Although this test is used primarily to determine the intactness of the motor innervation to the bladder, the bethanechol supersensitivity test has also been reported to be positive in cases of patients with only sensory neuropathy.[21] Several clinical entities that cause false-positive results (notably cystitis) limit the usefulness of this study.[22] Other diagnostic studies have been developed in an attempt to measure the integrity of bladder innervation. Sacral latency times can be measured by a stimulating electrode placed on the penis and a recording electrode placed on the external anal spincter. This study measures the conduction time of nerve impulses carried through the afferent pudendal nerve, sacral cord, and motor pudendal nerve. Like the clinically useful bulbocavernosus reflex, it does not directly test bladder innervation but does give some information concerning the integrity of the sacral spinal cord.

Classification of Neurogenic Bladder Disease

Numerous schemes exist for the classification of neurogenic bladder disease.[23] The classification of Lapides[24] is one of the oldest and simplest and the one familiar to most physicians. Although many patients do not fit exactly into one of the categories of the Lapides classification, this scheme nevertheless provides a framework for understanding many of the principles of neurogenic bladder disease.

The Lapides classification is based primarily on the cystometrogram. This scheme categorizes patients as having neurologic disease that affects (1) sensory nerves to the bladder, (2) motor nerves to the bladder, (3) both motor and sensory nerves to the bladder, (4) descending and ascending spinal cord tracts, or (5) the cerebral cortex.

Sensory Neurogenic Bladder (Fig. 45-6)

If only the peripheral sensory nerves from the bladder or the sensory components of the ascending spinal cord tracts are interrupted, the patient is not aware of bladder filling and may initially have painless urinary retention and overflow incontinence. One might anticipate that the cystometrogram results would be normal except for the absence of bladder sensation. This is usually not the case, however. Typically, the patient with sensory neurogenic bladder disease voids infrequently and with time develops a large bladder capacity. With overdistention, the bladder loses its ability to effectively contract and empty. The cystometrogram commonly demonstrates a large residual urine volume, a large bladder capacity, absent or reduced sensation, and no uninhibited bladder contractions; frequently, no detrusor activity can be demonstrated. By far the most common cause of sensory neurogenic bladder disease is diabetes mellitus. Any diabetic patient with voiding symptoms or recurrent urinary tract infections should be evaluated for sensory neurogenic bladder disease. This is particularly important in older diabetic men with signs and symptoms of outlet obstruction from benign prostatic hy-

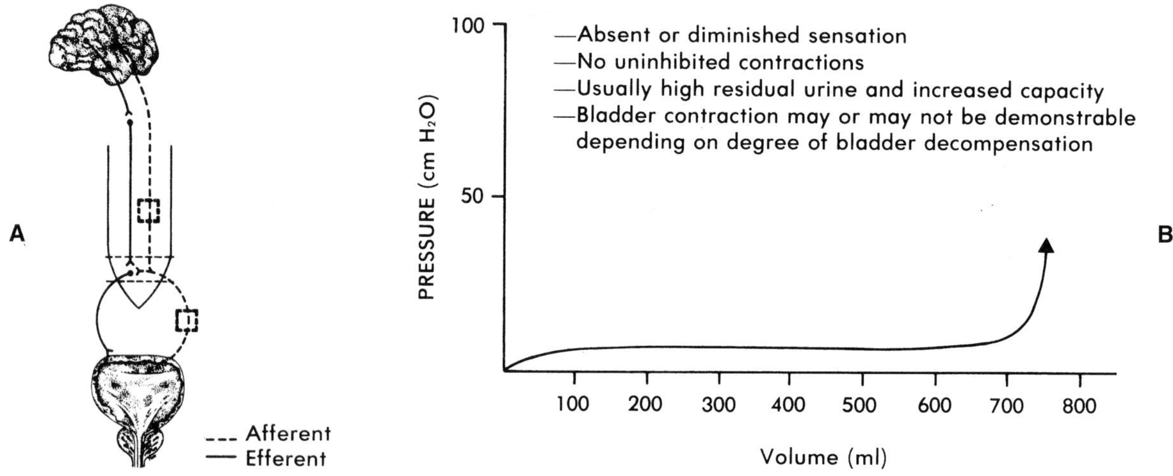

Fig. 45-6. Sensory neurogenic bladder. **A,** Site of lesion indicated by box. **B,** Cystometrogram.

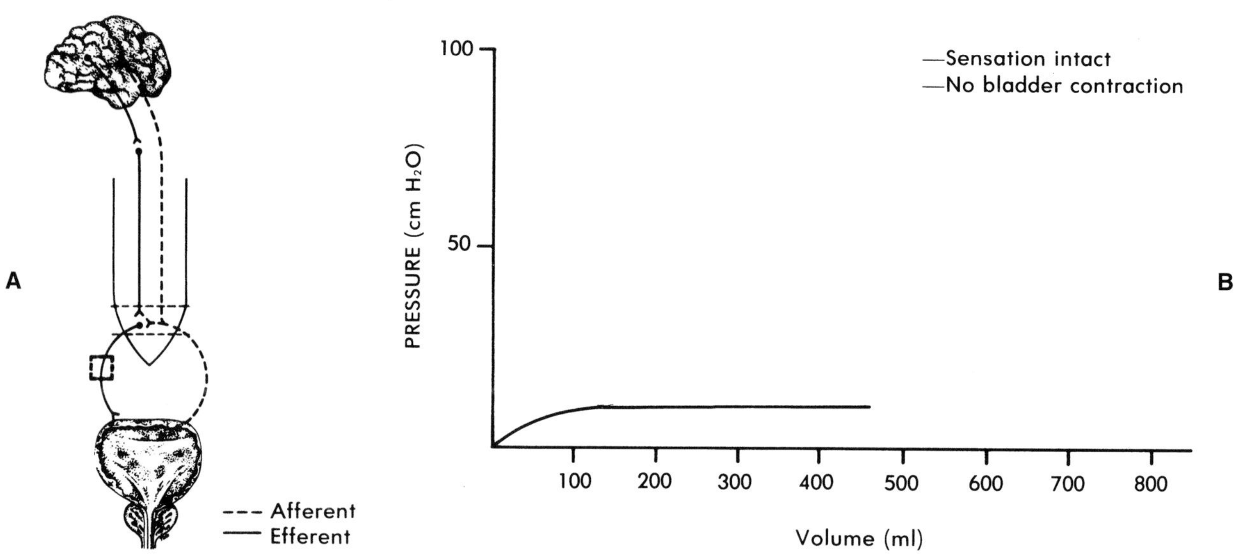

Fig. 45-7. Motor neurogenic bladder. **A,** Site of lesion indicated by box. **B,** Cystometrogram.

perplasia. Other diseases (multiple sclerosis, pernicious anemia, and central nervous system syphilis) can selectively damage the sensory innervation of the bladder and may also occur with sensory neurogenic bladder disease.

Motor Neurogenic Bladder (Fig. 45-7)

This uncommon lesion occurs with diseases that damage only the parasympathetic motor supply to the bladder. As both the motor and sensory nerves to the bladder are carried in the pelvic nerve, injury to the pelvic nerves by surgery or trauma usually does not result in a pure motor neurogenic bladder. Patients with motor neurogenic bladder disease typically have acute painful urinary retention. After the bladder is emptied, cystometrogram results are usually normal except for the inability of the patient to initiate a detrusor contraction. Sensation is intact, and uninhibited detrusor contractions are absent.

Motor neurogenic bladder disease is occasionally seen with a herniated lumbar disk and may be associated with viral illnesses such as herpes zoster, mononucleosis, and infection with cytomegalovirus.[25] Another cause of acute painful urinary retention, particularly in young women, is psychogenic urinary retention.[26] This entity can be very difficult to differentiate from motor neurogenic bladder disease. Usually, extensive neurologic and urodynamic studies, including bethanechol supersensitivity testing, are necessary to rule out significant underlying pathologic conditions. Psychogenic urinary retention should be a diagnosis of exclusion made only after the viral diseases noted earlier and multiple sclerosis are excluded.

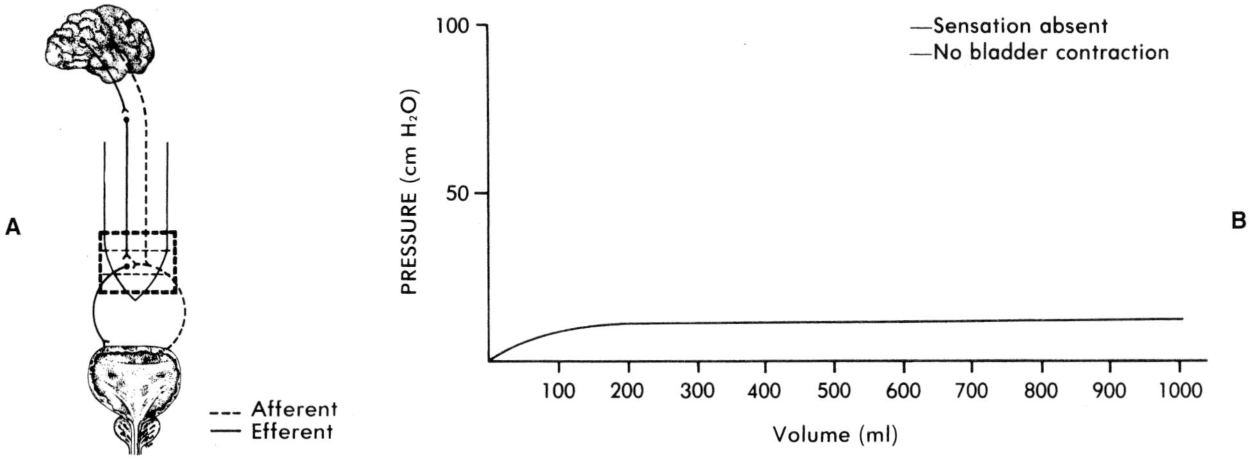

Fig. 45-8. Autonomous neurogenic bladder. **A,** Site of lesion indicated by box. **B,** Cystometrogram.

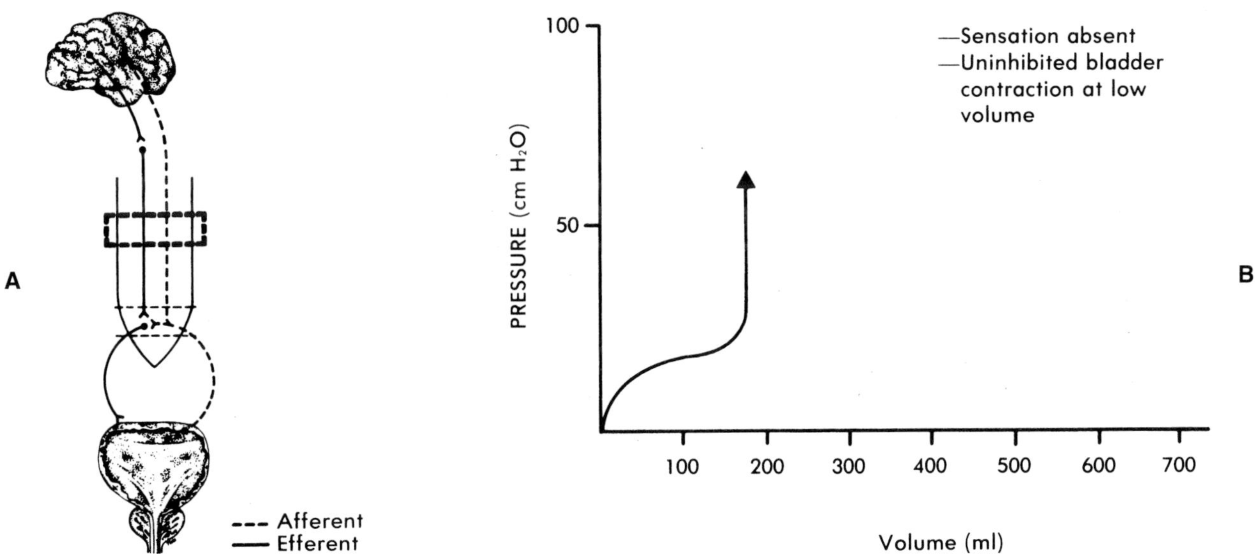

Fig. 45-9. Reflex neurogenic bladder. **A,** Site of lesion indicated by box. **B,** Cystometrogram.

Autonomous Neurogenic Bladder (*Fig. 45-8*)

If both the motor and sensory components of the parasympathetic bladder innervation are disrupted, the bladder is effectively denervated. Patients usually have urinary retention, and overflow incontinence may occur. The patient may void to some extent by abdominal straining, but effective bladder emptying is rarely achieved. The cystometrogram typically demonstrates a high residual urine volume, large bladder capacity, a lack of sensation, and no uninhibited or voluntary detrusor contractions. Voiding flow rates in patients with autonomous neurogenic bladders usually demonstrate a low maximum sustained flow rate and an intermittent stream.

Any lesion affecting the sacral spinal cord, cauda equina, or pelvic nerves may produce this lesion. Trauma to the sacral portion of the spinal cord or cauda equina and congenital lesions such as myelomeningocele result in autonomous neurogenic bladders. In addition, patients who have undergone extensive pelvic surgery such as abdominoperineal resection for colon cancer are at significant risk to develop this lesion.

Reflex Neurogenic Bladder (*Fig. 45-9*)

According to the Lapides classification, which is based on the concept of a spinal reflex arc, reflex neurogenic bladder disease is seen in patients who have complete spinal cord lesions above the level of S2. When the ascending and descending spinal cord tracts are interrupted, the patient exhibits uncontrolled and uninhibited reflex-mediated bladder contractions secondary to bladder filling.

Since reflex voiding cannot be inhibited by higher centers, patients with reflex neurogenic bladder disease usually have incontinence. A cystometrogram demonstrates a complete lack of sensation and uninhibited bladder contractions (usually at low bladder volumes).

As previously discussed, voiding is normally controlled by a pontine (not spinal cord) micturition center reflex. Following suprasacral spinal cord injury, reflex bladder contractions usually develop. The neural mechanisms responsible for bladder contractions following suprasacral spinal cord transection have been investigated by DeGroat and Steers.[11] Kittens reflexly void through a sacral spinal reflex. With maturation of the animal, however, voiding occurs through the pontine micturition center rather than through a simple sacral spinal reflex. With interruption of the ascending and descending spinal cord tracts, it is hypothesized that the infantile or sacral reflex again becomes operational. Presumably, similar events occur in man.

Patients with reflex neurogenic bladder disease usually empty their bladders unless detrusor–striated sphincter dyssynergia is present. As previously discussed, patients with this syndrome exhibit contraction instead of relaxation of the striated pelvic floor musculature at the time of detrusor contraction. Functional obstruction to urine flow in the area of the membranous urethra may occur. This diagnosis should be considered in all patients with reflex neurogenic bladder disease who carry high residual urine volumes. A combined cystometrogram-striated muscle electromyogram shows a dyssynergic pattern, and a voiding cystourethrogram shows the level of obstruction to be in the area of the membranous urethra.

The majority of patients with reflex neurogenic bladder disease are traumatic paraplegics. Transverse myelitis, multiple sclerosis, spinal cord vascular disorders, abscesses, and tumors are also responsible for this disorder.

Uninhibited Neurogenic Bladder (*Fig. 45-10*)

When a lesion develops in the cortical regulatory pathways, the ability to suppress reflex bladder contractions is lost. During bladder filling, all is normal until the point of first sensation. At this point, a sudden desire to void occurs; the patient is unable to inhibit this desire, and normal coordinated micturition occurs. The bladder empties completely, and the stream is uninterrupted. Patients with cortical lesions and uninhibited neurogenic bladder disease do not exhibit detrusor–striated sphincter dyssynergia.[9]

Patients with this type of neurogenic bladder disease usually have urgency and urgency incontinence. A cystometrogram reveals a small residual urine volume, intact sensation, and uninhibited bladder contractions. The cystometrogram findings are very similar to those seen with reflex neurogenic bladder disease. Bladder sensation, however, is absent in the presence of a reflex bladder and present in patients with an uninhibited neurogenic bladder.

Uninhibited neurogenic bladder disease is common in elderly patients. Cerebrovascular disease and Parkinson's disease are common causes. Multiple sclerosis may occur with any type of neurogenic bladder disease, and the patient with an uninhibited neurogenic bladder is no exception.

MANAGEMENT OF NEUROGENIC BLADDER DISEASE

A working knowledge of a classification scheme for neurogenic bladder disease, such as the Lapides classification previously discussed, is essential to an understanding of the pathophysiology involved. A simpler scheme, however, has been devised to assist in the therapy for these patients and is based on the premise that the urinary bladder has two functions: urine emptying and urine storage.[23] Despite the varied neurologic lesions that can lead to bladder dysfunc-

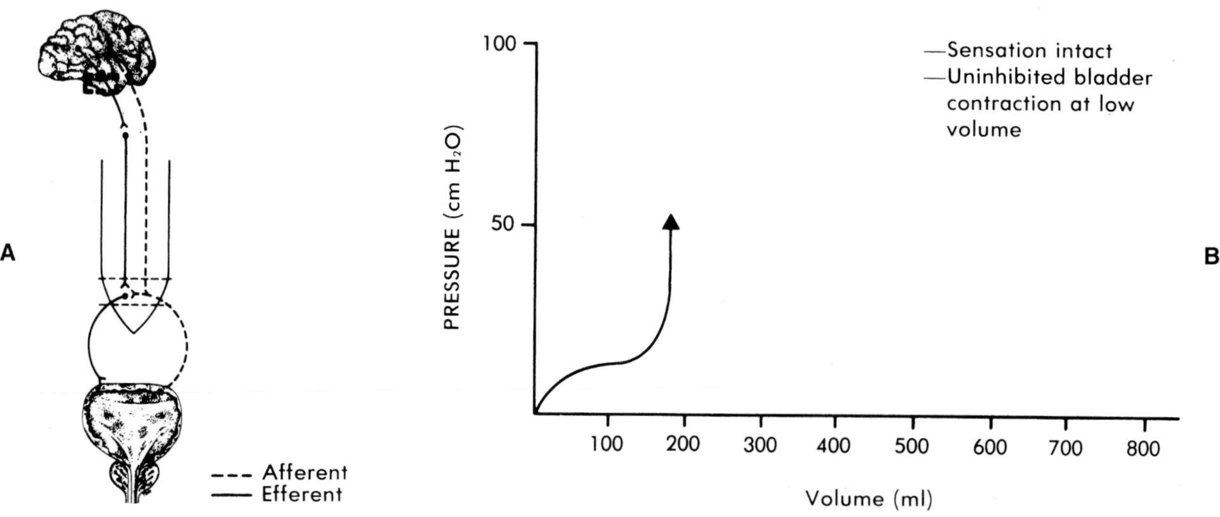

Fig. 45-10. Uninhibited neurogenic bladder. **A,** Site of lesion indicated by box. **B,** Cystometrogram.

tion, patients with neurogenic bladder disease have either failure of urine emptying or failure of urine storage. If the patient's symptoms are the only factor taken into consideration, clinical mistakes regarding management are often made. For example, without a careful examination, which many times requires urodynamic assessment, the patient with overflow incontinence secondary to urinary retention may be viewed as having a failure of bladder storage rather than as having primarily a problem in bladder emptying.

In addition to control of the patient's bladder symptoms, the status of the patient's upper urinary tracts should always be kept in mind. Bladder dysfunction commonly results in renal deterioration because of hydronephrosis, vesicoureteral reflux, infection, or stone disease. The most common long-term cause of death in traumatic paraplegics, for example, is renal disease.[27]

Failure to Empty

Various methods are presently used to achieve bladder emptying; the method of choice varies depending on the status and compliance of each individual patient.

Catheter Drainage

Although efficacious for short-term use, catheter drainage (either urethral or suprapubic) is usually not the best treatment for the long-term problem of bladder emptying. In males complication rates (urethral strictures and fistulas, infection, bladder stones) are particularly high with urethral catheter drainage. Long-term catheter drainage should be used only when other therapeutic options are not effective.

Clean Intermittent Self-Catheterization

Clean intermittent self-catheterization (CIC) is the therapy of choice in most patients with failure of bladder emptying secondary to neurogenic bladder disease. During the last decade, this form of therapy has gained widespread popularity because of patient acceptance and relatively low complication rates.[28] Many patients who formerly would have been treated with more radical therapeutic alternatives (urinary diversion) are presently being managed successfully with CIC (Fig. 45-11).

Patients are taught to catheterize themselves at approximately 4-hour intervals using a clean (not sterile) technique. Some degree of manual dexterity is required; the patient's neurologic disease cannot greatly limit use of the upper extremities. The use of CIC is applicable to children and adults and is particularly useful in those children with neurogenic bladder disease secondary to myelodysplasia.

Urinary tract infection is the most common complication in patients treated with CIC. These infections are usually easily treated, and the infection rate with CIC is far lower than that seen in patients with permanent indwelling catheters. Patients using CIC need periodic assessment of the upper urinary tracts by excretory urography or ultrasonography because renal deterioration has been reported in these patients.

Pharmacologic Therapy

Theoretically, any drug that causes the bladder to contract or causes the bladder outlet to relax should promote bladder emptying. Bethanechol chloride, a muscarinic cholinergic agonist, has been used for more than 30 years for this

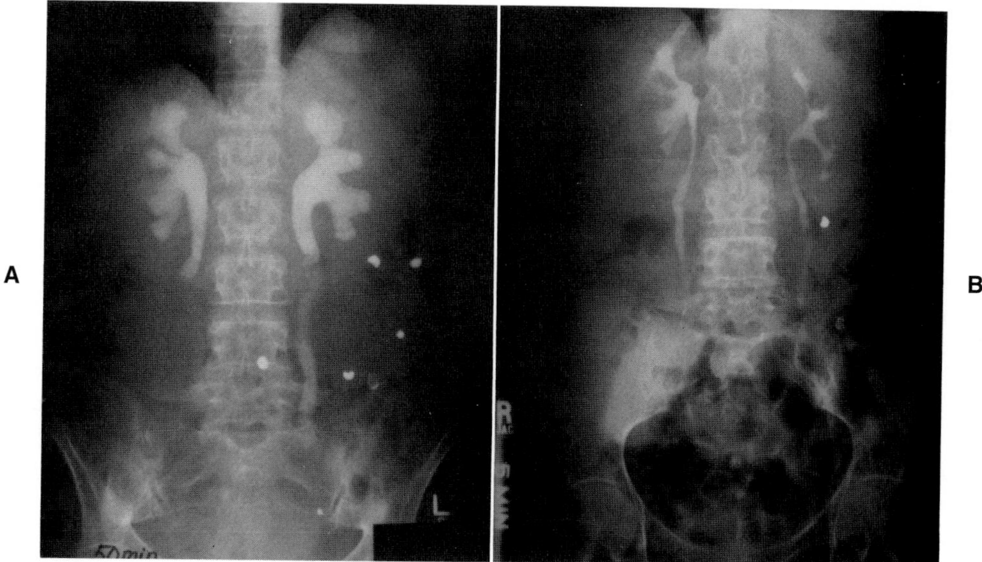

Fig. 45-11. Patient with sensory neurogenic bladder secondary to diabetes mellitus. Patient had 1000 ml of residual urine. **A,** Excretory urogram at time of diagnosis demonstrating bilateral hydroureteronephrosis. **B,** Excretory urogram after 6 months' treatment with clean intermittent self-catheterization demonstrating resolution of the hydroureteronephrosis.

purpose. This acetylcholinesterase-resistant drug is pharmacologically active and does cause bladder contraction. Recent studies, however, have questioned the clinical usefulness of this compound.[29] Specifically, patients treated with bethanechol have shown no improvement in objective measurements such as residual urine volumes or voiding flow rates. These results are not surprising when one considers that a coordinated bladder contraction is probably not produced by bethanechol and that stimulation of muscarinic receptors also results in urethral smooth muscle contraction, thereby increasing outlet resistance. Although the use of bethanechol to promote bladder emptying remains controversial, evidence favors the position that its use in most clinical situations is not efficacious.

An attempt has also been made to use drugs to promote bladder emptying by decreasing outlet resistance. As previously discussed, stimulation of α-adrenergic receptors in the bladder base and urethra causes contraction of smooth muscle in this area and thereby increases outlet resistance. α-Adrenergic blocking agents do decrease outlet resistance and have been used clinically.[30] However, the responses seen with such agents as phenoxybenzamine and prazosin are often not clinically significant, and troublesome side effects, notably postural hypotension, do occur.

External Sphincterotomy

Patients with spinal cord lesions above the sacral spinal cord may not achieve bladder emptying because of detrusor–striated sphincter dyssynergia. Patients with demyelinating diseases and occasionally neurologically intact children also manifest this syndrome. Many patients, particularly paraplegics with detrusor–striated sphincter dyssynergia, can be successfully managed with CIC. When CIC is not a viable therapeutic option (e.g., in patients with neurologic disease who have limited or no use of their upper extremities) or when persistent infections or upper urinary tract deterioration occur while CIC is being perfomed, a surgical procedure designed to decrease urethral resistance in the area of the membranous urethra is usually warranted.

Although pudendal neurectomy has been used successfully in some patients, external sphincterotomy is the surgical treatment of choice at the present time. External sphincterotomy is performed endoscopically by resecting a portion of the urethra and periurethral striated musculature in the area of the membranous urethra with a resectoscope. Tissue is preferably removed from the 12 o'clock position. Incisions in the 3 o'clock and 9 o'clock positions have been reported to result in a high incidence of postsphincterotomy impotence.[31] Damage to the paired penile cavernosal nerves that course near the membranous urethra may be the cause of the impotence.

Cutaneous Vesicostomy

Cutaneous vesicostomy is an excellent method of treating young children with neurogenic bladder disease with failure to empty. In children the dome of the bladder can be easily mobilized and brought to the skin; the bladder wall is sutured to the anterior rectus fascia, and a stoma flush with the skin is created in the midline of the lower abdominal wall. This simplified Blocksom technique results in few complications (primarily stomal stenosis and bladder herniation) and is now preferred over previously used types of vesicostomy in which skin flaps were mobilized and brought down to the bladder wall.[32]

Urine exiting the stoma can be collected in diapers. When the child reaches an age when other therapy such as CIC can be instituted, the vesicostomy can be closed. This form of urinary diversion is generally not suitable for adults, primarily because of problems with collecting devices.

Failure to Store

In general, patients whose primary problem is one of urine storage (incontinence) are more difficult to treat than those whose primary problem is failure to empty. Patients with neurogenic bladder disease who fail to store urine and are therefore incontinent have either uninhibited bladder contractions or decreased bladder neck and urethral resistance.

Pharmacologic Therapy

Although evidence does exist that demonstrates that the urinary bladder in in vivo models is relatively atropine resistant, uninhibited bladder contractions associated with reflex or uninhibited-type neurogenic bladder disease can be treated with anticholinergic agents. Many patients, particularly those with uninhibited-type neurogenic bladders, obtain significant relief from their symptoms of urgency and urgency incontinence when so treated. A variety of drugs with anticholinergic activity, including propantheline, methantheline, and oxybutynin, have been used.

Drugs are also occasionally effective in increasing bladder outlet resistance. α-Adrenergic receptor agonists (phenylpropanolamine, ephedrine, and pseudoephedrine) have been used with some success. Imipramine, a tricyclic antidepressant, is a clinically efficacious drug that promotes urine storage. The mechanism by which this drug acts on the lower urinary tract is not entirely understood. Imipramine does possess anticholinergic and direct smooth muscle depressant activity. In the central nervous system, imipramine has been demonstrated to have a cocainelike effect in that it blocks the reuptake of norepinephrine into nerve terminals. The net effect of this action is to enhance adrenergic activity. Peripherally, this sympathomimetic effect would increase outlet resistance (α-adrenergic receptor stimulation) and relax the bladder body (β-adrenergic receptor stimulation) and thus, at least theoretically, promote continence.[12]

In some clinical situations, drugs are intentionally used to convert a bladder that fails to store into a bladder that does not empty. For example, a patient with a spinal cord injury and incontinence secondary to uninhibited bladder contractions can be treated with anticholinergic agents

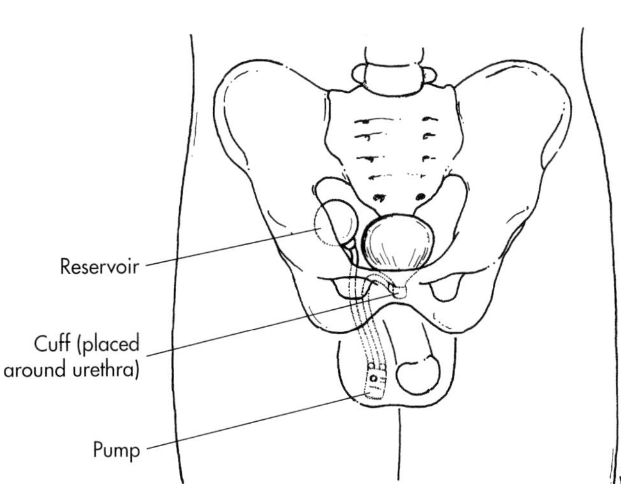

Fig. 45-12. Artificial urinary sphincter.

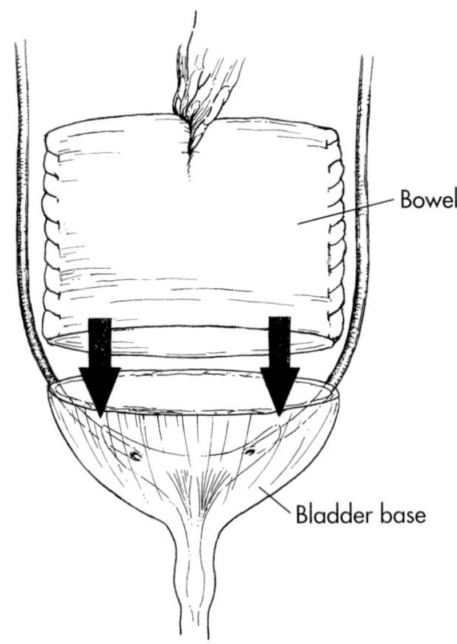

Fig. 45-13. Augmentation cystoplasty. An isolated segment of bowel is opened along its antimesenteric border and used as a "patch" to reconstruct the bladder.

with the hope of causing urinary retention. The urinary retention then can be managed by CIC.

Clean Intermittent Self-Catheterization

Occasionally, patients with incontinence secondary to uninhibited bladder contractions can be treated by CIC alone. Patients who are successfully treated with this technique usually not only have uninhibited bladder contractions but also carry high postvoiding residual volumes. If the bladder can be periodically drained and never reaches a volume high enough to initiate a reflex detrusor contraction, continence may be achieved.

Long-Term Catheter Drainage

For previously discussed reasons, long-term catheter drainage is not the preferred method to achieve continence in most patients. However, in some patients, particularly elderly women, catheter drainage may be a reasonable choice of therapy.

Artificial Urinary Sphincter

In the past, numerous mechanical devices have been used in an attempt to achieve continence secondary to low outlet resistance. Many of the initial devices were implanted perineally, compressed the urethra, and increased urethral resistance essentially by creating an artificial stricture. The artificial sphincter, the most widely used device at present, consists of an inflatable cuff inserted around either the bladder neck or the bulbous urethra.[33] Patients can deflate the cuff to void and inflate the cuff to achieve continence by transferring fluid to and from a reservoir by a pump mechanism implanted into the scrotum or labia (Fig. 45-12).

Augmentation Cystoplasty

Patients with neurogenic bladder disease who develop noncompliant bladders with high intravesical pressure are at risk for developing vesicoureteral reflux, hydronephrosis, and deterioration of renal function.[34] Children with myelodysplasia frequently have this complication. The goal of therapy is to reduce intravesical pressure. If anticholinergic medication is not effective, the therapy of choice is an augmentation cystoplasty. This surgical procedure consists of resecting most of the bladder, leaving intact only the trigone, ureteral orifices, and bladder neck. An isolated segment of ileum (ileocystoplasty) or colon (colocystoplasty) is then used as a "patch" to reconstruct that part of the bladder that has been removed (Fig. 45-13). Particularly in children, the use of stomach (gastrocystoplasty) has recently gained popularity. The goal of all these procedures is to produce a "bladder" that functions as a low pressure reservoir. Emptying is achieved by CIC.

SUPRAVESICAL URINARY DIVERSON

When all other forms of therapy fail in patients with either failure to empty or failure to store, a supravesical urinary diversion can be performed as a last resort. Tube diversions (i.e., nephrostomy) are generally not suited for long-term urinary diversion for multiple reasons (infection, stone formation, and the necessity for frequent tube changes). In most patients, supravesical urinary diversion is best achieved by either an ileal or colon conduit or, in rare situations, by a ureterosigmoidostomy. Before the development of many of the treatment modalities already discussed (particularly CIC, drug therapy, and the artificial urinary sphincter), many patients, particularly children with neurogenic bladder disease, underwent supravesical

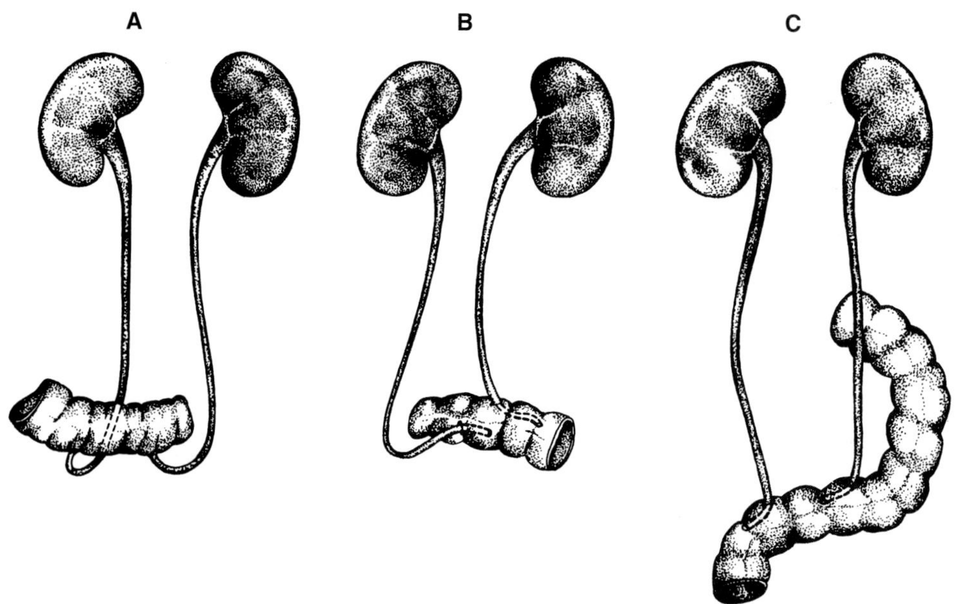

Fig. 45-14. Types of supravesical urinary diversion. **A**, Ileal conduit. **B**, Colon conduit. **C**, Ureterosigmoidostomy.

urinary diversion. Because of the success of other forms of treatment, many of these patients have undergone "undiversion."[35]

Ureters brought directly to the skin usually undergo stomal stenosis. For this reason, most operations designed to divert urine supravesically have either (1) used a segment of bowel, which is interposed between the ureters and skin (ileal or colon conduit), or (2) anastomosed the ureters directly into the intact bowel (ureterosigmoidostomy) (Fig. 45-14). Most patients with neurogenic bladder disease have undergone urinary diversion with either an ileal or colon conduit. An absolute contraindication to ureterosigmoidostomy is an incompetent anal sphincter, and many patients with neurogenic bladder disease also have significant problems with fecal, as well as urinary, control.

Although descriptions of surgical technique vary greatly, the performance of each of these procedures uses several basic principles. The ureters are divided well into the pelvis to ensure adequate ureteral length. One ureter is tunneled behind the colon mesentery to reach the opposite side. In performing an ileal or colon conduit, an appropriate length of bowel is isolated for use as the conduit, and then a bowel anastomosis is performed to reestablish bowel continuity. One end of the conduit is closed. Both ureters are attached to the ileum or colon by using a ureteral mucosa–to–bowel mucosa anastomosis. The open end of the conduit is then anastomosed to the skin. Some surgeons prefer colon conduits over ileal conduits because the thicker colon wall allows the ureters to be "tunneled," thereby creating an antirefluxing anastomosis. In a ureterosigmoidostomy the colon is left in continuity and the ureters are usually anastomosed to the sigmoid by means of a "tunneled" antirefluxing technique.[36]

Early surgical complications seen with ileal and colon conduits include ureteral leak at the site of anastomosis, intestinal obstruction or fistula, ureteral obstruction, and rarely necrosis of the conduit. Late surgical complications include pyocystis (secondary to the bladder being defunctionalized), stomal stenosis, intestinal obstruction, ureteral obstruction, calculi, and parastomal hernia. Long-term follow-up of patients (particularly children) who have undergone ureteroileal diversion has shown a high rate of upper urinary tract deterioration (increasing hydroureteronephrosis, calculi, and pyelonephritis).[37] This realization has led to increasing reluctance to perform urinary diversion into ileal conduits on children with neurogenic bladder disease.

Surgical complications from ureterosigmoidostomy include pyelonephritis, ureterocolonic anastomosis stricture, and calculi. In addition, a late complication of ureterosigmoidostomy is adenocarcinoma of the colon, which usually occurs at the site of the ureteral anastomosis.[38] The incidence of colon cancer associated with ureterosigmoidostomy has been calculated to be 500 times greater than the incidence in the normal population. Studies in rats have indicated that the presence of a fecal stream is necessary for the development of carcinoma. Whether carcinogenic factors are present in urine or feces or both is unclear. Only one case report exists of a carcinoma in a colon conduit urinary diversion where the fecal and urinary streams had been divided.[39] Most surgeons agree that patients with ureterosigmoidostomy should be followed up with stool examinations for blood and routine sigmoidoscopy or colonoscopy.

Table 45-1. Electrolyte Changes With Ureteral Diversion

	Ureterosigmoidostomy	Ileal or Colon Conduit	Jejunal Conduit
Serum chloride	↑↑	↑	↓
Serum sodium	Normal	Normal	↓
Serum potassium	Normal to reduced	Normal	↑
Acidosis	Present (50–80%)	Present (2–15%)	Present (35%)

In addition to local surgical complications, systemic effects relating primarily to fluid and electrolyte disorders occur in patients whose urine has been diverted into bowel segments. In 1950 Ferris and Odel[40] reported that 80% of patients who had undergone a ureterosigmoidostomy had an elevated serum chloride level and 77% had at least some degree of metabolic acidosis. The primary event leading to this syndrome appears to be colonic absorption of chloride.[41] Hyperchloremia and acidosis may also occur in patients with ileal and colon conduits. The incidence and severity of this syndrome in conduits, however, is much less than with ureterosigmoidostomy. This difference is most likely related to both the amount of time urine is in contact with the bowel mucosa and the smaller mucosal surface area of conduits. In addition, patients with ureterosigmoidostomies tend to have slightly decreased serum potassium levels but markedly reduced total body potassium. The mechanism for potassium loss is probably potassium secretion by the colon. Patients with ileal or colon conduits uncommonly demonstrate clinical manifestations of electrolyte imbalance and rarely need treatment. Patients with ureterosigmoidostomies, however, commonly need therapy to correct their acidosis and hypokalemia.

Patients undergoing ureteral diversion into a jejunal conduit develop a syndrome that differs from that described for other types of diversions.[42] Specifically, these patients exhibit hypochloremia, hyponatremia, hyperkalemia, and acidosis (Table 45-1). Sodium and chloride are lost and potassium is absorbed from the conduit. Hypovolemia and hyponatremia decrease the glomerular filtration rate, which further aggravates the acidosis and hyperkalemia. Treatment of these patients is the administration of salt.

Diversion of urine into the bowel is occasionally complicated by encephalopathy associated with hyperammonemia.[43] This syndrome is usually seen when coexistent hepatic disease interferes with urea synthesis. Increased blood ammonia levels are thought to be secondary to absorption of urinary ammonia by the bowel coupled with the action of bacterial urease, which increases urinary ammonia levels.

CONTINENT URINARY DIVERSION

The fact that patients with standard ileal or colonic conduit urinary diversions are required to wear bags to collect urine from the conduit has led to interest in more socially acceptable forms of supravesical urinary diversion. A large number of continent urinary diversion procedures have been described; all these operations have several features in common. All the procedures are designed to create a low-pressure reservoir for urine storage. They possess an antireflux mechanism and a urinary continence mechanism. Patients periodically empty the reservoir by catheterizing the continent stoma, and the need for a urine collecting bag is therefore obviated.

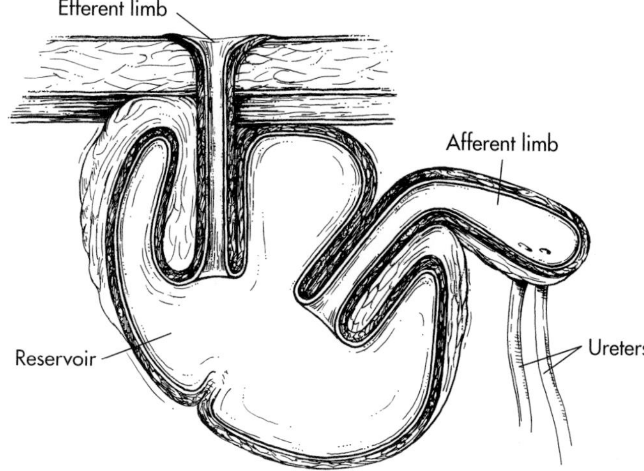

Fig. 45-15. Continent urinary diversion. A low-pressure reservoir is created and is emptied by intermittent catheterization of the efferent limb.

The proliferation of newly described continent diversions underscores the fact that the creation of the perfect continent diversion remains to be described. Low-pressure reservoirs have been created by opening the bowel along the antimesenteric border and then folding it into a sphere. This technique reduces the pressure in the reservoir by eliminating unidirectional peristaltic waves. The catheterizable Kock pouch relies on the nipple valve, a form of compression continence mechanism in both the afferent limb, to prevent reflux, and in the efferent limb, to achieve urinary continence (Fig. 45-15). In contrast to the Kock pouch, which is constructed of ileum, the Indiana pouch is a reconfigured ileocolonic reservoir. The Indiana pouch uses double imbrication over a catheter to reduce the lumen of the ileocecal valve and distal ileum to create a compression continence mechanism. The creation of continent urinary diversions is a technically demanding procedure with high complication and reoperation rates.[44] Long segments of bowel are used, and patients must be monitored for the development of pernicious anemia. Like patients with ureterosigmoidostomies, the development of hyperchloremic acidosis is a potential problem, particularly when the reservoir is constructed from colon.[45] Long-term follow-up of patients with continent diversions is necessary before this new form of diversion can be adequately compared with standard conduit urinary diversion.

SUMMARY

Although knowledge of the anatomy, neurophysiology, and neuropharmacology of the lower urinary tract is far from complete, clinically useful classification systems exist that allow accurate diagnosis and effective therapy for most patients with neurogenic bladder disease. In addition, the widespread use of increasingly sophisticated urodynamic studies has made possible more accurate diagnoses and objective means to evaluate therapeutic modalities. Relatively new forms of therapy (including pharmacologic manipulation, self-intermittent catheterization, and the artificial sphincter) have obviated the need for supravesical urinary diversion in most patients.

REFERENCES

1. Woodburne RT. Anatomy of the bladder and bladder outlet. J Urol 100:474, 1968.
2. Raezer DM, et al. Autonomic innervation of canine urinary bladder: Cholinergic and adrenergic contributions and interaction of sympathetic and parasympathetic systems in bladder function. Urology 2:211, 1973.
3. Turner-Warwick R, et al. A urodynamic view of prostatic obstruction and the results of prostatectomy. Br J Urol 45:631, 1973.
4. Clark SL. Some remarks on the anatomy and physiology of the urinary bladder and sphincter of the rectum. J Anat Physiol 17:442, 1883.
5. Tanagho EA, Smith DR. The anatomy and function of the bladder neck. Br J Urol 38:54, 1966.
6. Gosling JA. The structure of the bladder and urethra in relation to function. Urol Clin North Am 6:31, 1979.
7. Gosling JA, et al. A comparative study of the human external sphincter and periurethral levator ani muscles. Br J Urol 53:35, 1981.
8. Wein AJ, Raezer DM. Physiology of micturition. In Krane RJ, Siroky MD, eds. Clinical Neuro-urology. Boston: Little, Brown, 1979.
9. Blaivas JG. The neurophysiology of micturition: A clinical study of 550 patients. J Urol 127:958, 1982.
10. Bradley WE, Timm GW, Scott FB. Innervation of the detrusor muscle and urethra. Urol Clin North Am 1:3, 1974.
11. DeGroat WC, Steers WD. Autonomic regulation of the urinary bladder and sexual organs. In Loewy AD, Spyer KM, eds. Central Regulation of the Autonomic Functions. Oxford: Oxford University Press, 1990, p 318.
12. Benson GS, et al. Adrenergic and cholinergic stimulation and blockade of the human bladder base. J Urol 116:174, 1976.
13. DeGroat WC, Saum WR. Adrenergic inhibition in mammalian parasympathetic ganglia. Nature 321:188, 1971.
14. Levin RM, Wein AJ. Quantitative analysis of alpha and beta adrenergic receptor densities in the lower urinary tract of the dog and rabbit. Invest Urol 17:75, 1979.
15. Donker PJ, Droes JTPM, Van Ulden BM. Anatomy of the musculature and innervation of the bladder and urethra. In Williams DI, Chisholm GD, eds. Scientific Foundations of Urology, vol 2. Chicago: Year Book Medical Publishers, 1976.
16. Blaivas JG, et al. Detrusor–external sphincter dyssynergia. J Urol 125:542, 1981.
17. Hinman F, Jr. Urodynamic testing: Alternatives to electronics. J Urol 121:643, 1979.
18. McGuire EJ, Woodside JR. Diagnostic advantages of fluoroscopic monitoring during urodynamic evaluation. J Urol 125:830, 1981.
19. Siroky MB, Olsson CA, Krane RJ. The flow rate nomogram. II. Clinical correlation. J Urol 123:208, 1980.
20. Lapides J, et al. Denervation supersensitivity as a test for neurogenic bladder. Surg Gynecol Obstet 114:241, 1962.
21. Harris JD, Benson GS. Positive bethanechol chloride supersensitivity test in hereditary sensory neuropathy. J Urol 124:923, 1980.
22. Merrill DC, Rotta J. A clinical evaluation of detrusor denervation supersensitivity using air cytometry. J Urol 111:27, 1974.
23. Wein AJ. Classification of neurogenic voiding dysfunction. J Urol 125:605, 1981.
24. Lapides J. Cystometry. JAMA 201:618, 1967.
25. Michaelson RG, Benson GS, Friedman HM. Urinary retention as the presenting symptom of acquired cytomegalovirus infection. Am J Med 74:526, 1983.
26. Barrett DM. Evaluation of psychogenic urinary retention. J Urol 120:191, 1978.
27. Hackler RH. A 25-year prospective mortality study in the spinal cord injured patient: Comparison with the long-term living paraplegic. J Urol 117:486, 1977.
28. Lapides J, et al. Further observations on self-catheterization. J Urol 116:169, 1976.
29. Wein AJ, et al. The effects of bethanechol chloride on urodynamic parameters in normal women and in women with significant residual urine volumes. J Urol 124:397, 1980.
30. Caine M, Perlberg S, Meretyk S. A placebo-controlled double-blind study of the effect of phenoxybenzamine in benign prostatic obstruction. Br J Urol 50:551, 1978.
31. Hackler RH. Surgical treatment of the adult neurogenic bladder dysfunction. In Krane RJ, Siroky MB, eds. Clinical Neuro-urology. Boston: Little, Brown, 1979.
32. Duckett JW, Jr. Cutaneous vesicostomy in childhood: The Blocksom technique. Urol Clin North Am 1:485, 1974.
33. Scott FB. The artificial sphincter in the management of incontinence in the male. Urol Clin North Am 5:375, 1978.
34. McGuire EJ, et al. Prognostic value of urodynamic testing in myelodysplastic patients. J Urol 126:205, 1981.
35. Allen TD. Undiverting the ileal conduit. J Urol 124:519, 1980.
36. Goodwin WR, Scardino PT. Ureterosigmoidostomy. J Urol 118:169, 1977.
37. Shapiro SR, Lebowitz R, Colodny AH. Fate of 90 children with ileal conduit urinary diversion a decade later: Analysis of complications, pyelography, renal function, and bacteriology. J Urol 114:289, 1975.
38. Parsons CD, Thomas MH, Garrett RA. Colonic adenocarcinoma: A delayed complication of ureterosigmoidostomy. J Urol 118:31, 1977.
39. Chiang MS, et al. Carcinoma in a colon conduit urinary diversion. J Urol 127:1185, 1982.
40. Ferris DO, Odel HM. Electrolyte pattern of the blood after bilateral ureterosigmoidostomy. JAMA 142:634, 1950.
41. Stamey TA. The pathogenesis and implications of the electrolyte imbalance in ureterosigmoidostomy. Surg Gynecol Obstet 103:736, 1956.

42. Golimbu M, Morales P. Electrolyte disturbances in jejunal urinary diversion. Urology 1:432, 1973.
43. McDermott WV. Diversion of urine to the intestines as a factor in ammoniagenic coma. N Engl J Med 256:460, 1957.
44. Skinner DG, Lieskovsky G, Boyd S. Continent urinary diversion. J Urol 141:1323, 1989.
45. Davidsson T, et al. Absorption of sodium and chloride in continent reservoirs for urine: Comparison of ileal and colonic reservoirs. J Urol 151:335, 1994.

46

Renovascular Hypertension

James C. Stanley and Linda M. Graham

Renovascular hypertension secondary to renal artery occlusive disease is the most common form of surgically correctable hypertension. High blood pressure in patients with this disease follows critical reductions in renal perfusion with activation of the renin-angiotensin system. This physiologic response results in restoration of renal blood flow toward normal, but it does so at the expense of producing systemic hypertension. Considerable knowledge exists regarding the physiologic basis for increased blood pressure associated with renal artery stenoses, the histologic and morphologic character of the most common renal artery diseases, the clinical manifestations and means of diagnosing renovascular hypertension, and the therapeutic options in treating this disease.

PHYSIOLOGIC BASIS OF RENOVASCULAR HYPERTENSION

The renin-angiotensin system is of paramount importance in renovascular hypertension. Its role in cardiovascular homeostasis was first proposed by Tigerstedt and Bergman,[1] who in 1898 demonstrated that intravenous injection of saline extracts of rabbit kidney caused immediate elevations in blood pressure of up to 20 minutes' duration. They introduced the term *renin* as the substance responsible for this phenomenon. The humoral basis of renovascular hypertension was advanced further when it was noted that renal venous blood in hypertensive animals exhibited greater vasoconstrictor activity than that from normotensive dogs.[2] Braun-Menendez et al.[3] called the vasopressor substance responsible for this activity "hypertensin," whereas Page[4] and Page and Helmer[5] named this nonrenin vasoactive substance "angiotonin." These two groups subsequently agreed to call this substance "angiotensin." Skeggs et al.[6] later documented that angiotensin existed in two forms, known as angiotensins I and II.

Extensive studies have defined the most important elements in the renin-angiotensin system that contribute to blood pressure control. These include (1) renin, produced in the kidney; (2) angiotensinogen, produced in the liver; (3) angiotensin converting enzyme, which is most active in the endothelium of the lung; (4) angiotensin II, produced from angiotensin I by angiotensin converting enzyme; and (5) aldosterone, produced in the adrenal gland (Fig. 46-1).

Renin is produced by the juxtaglomerular apparatus of the kidney (Fig. 46-2). Major components of this anatomic region include (1) myoepithelioid cells or granular cells, located on the wall of the afferent arterioles; (2) the macula densa, which is a specialized region of tubular epithelial cells, located in the glomerular hilus at the transition of Henle's loop to the distal convoluted tubule; and (3) lacis cells, located in the region of the efferent glomerular arteriole and the macula densa. The lacis cells are intimately associated with the glomerulus and are anatomically similar to mesangial cells. An interrelationship clearly exists between these structures, with the function of the juxtaglomerular apparatus being translation of various signals into altered glomerular filtration and secretion of renin.

Mechanisms controlling renin production and its release from the kidney are very complex.[1,7-9] Renal baroreceptors appear responsible for release of renin from juxtaglomerular cells, with these cells specifically acting as stretch receptors. The cellular basis for activation of these receptors seems to involve the calcium ion, with experimental evidence documenting an inverse relationship between renin release and intracellular calcium levels. Stimuli for renin release also include pressure changes at the afferent renal arteriole level, renal interstitial volume and pressure changes. The importance of the tubular fluid milieu and the macula densa has been well established, with changes in sodium and chloride content of tubular fluid altering renin release. However, the relative importance of macula densa receptors in activation of the renin-angiotensin system in renovascular hypertension is uncertain. Stimulation of postganglionic sympathetic neurons to renal arterioles, many of which end in the region of the juxtaglomerular apparatus, also causes increased renin release. This may be due to afferent arteriolar constriction with decreased stretch of intrarenal vascular receptors and

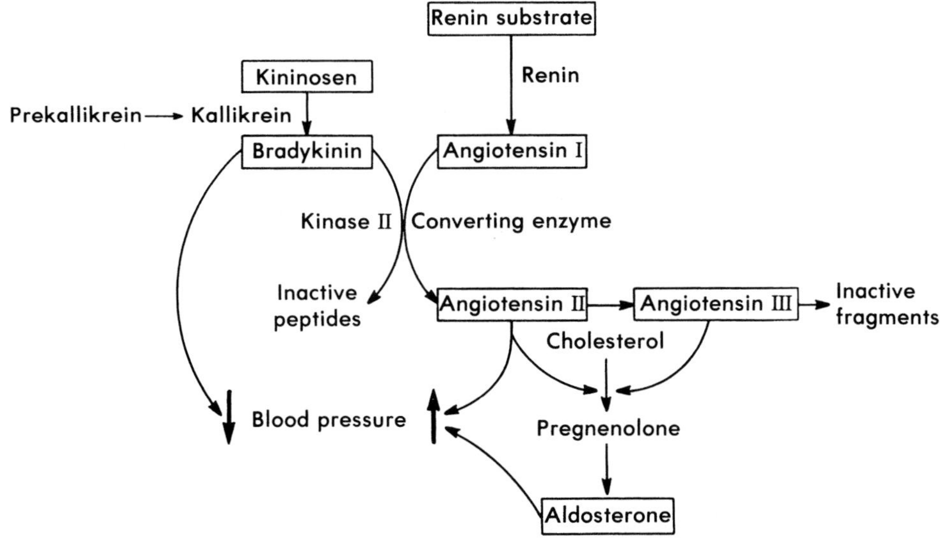

Fig. 46-1. Renin-angiotensin system interrelation with aldosterone and bradykinin in regulation of blood pressure.

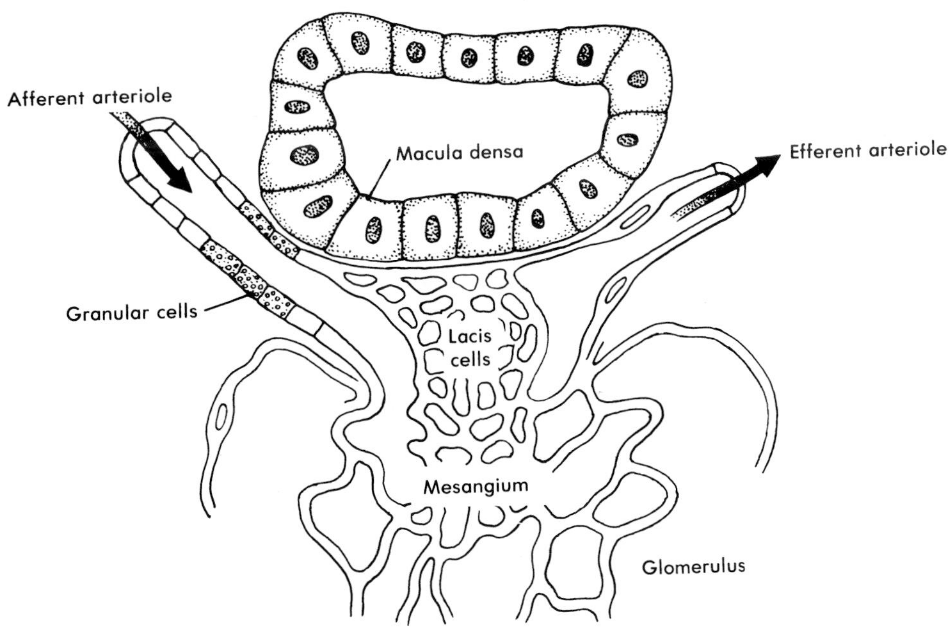

Fig. 46-2. Anatomic components of the juxtaglomerular apparatus.

decreased sodium load to the macula densa, but it is more likely a direct result of catecholamine action on β-adrenergic receptors of the juxtaglomerular cells. Clearly, the factors initiating renin synthesis in the kidney are complicated, and only recently has the molecular basis of the renin-angiotensin system become better understood.[10-14,]

Renin, a proteolytic enzyme, is active at a neutral pH on its only known substrate, angiotensinogen. The renin gene in humans is located on chromosome 1[15] (Figs. 46-3 and 46-4). It consists of nine exons and an additional miniexon, interrupted by eight introns.[16] The renin gene is transcribed into renin mRNA and translated into a preprorenin molecule with a molecular weight of 45,000.[17] Following cleavage and glycosylation in the rough endoplasmic reticulum, prorenin is produced with a molecular weight of 47,000. It is transferred into the Golgi complex, where it is rapidly secreted and processed to active renin, a single-chain polypeptide with a molecular weight of approximately 38,000.[18] Extrarenal renin or reninlike enzymes (isorenins) have been found in the submaxillary salivary gland, uterus, placenta, and brain. No documentation exists that these latter substances are functionally important in elevating blood pressure.

Renin, once synthesized, is stored as granules within

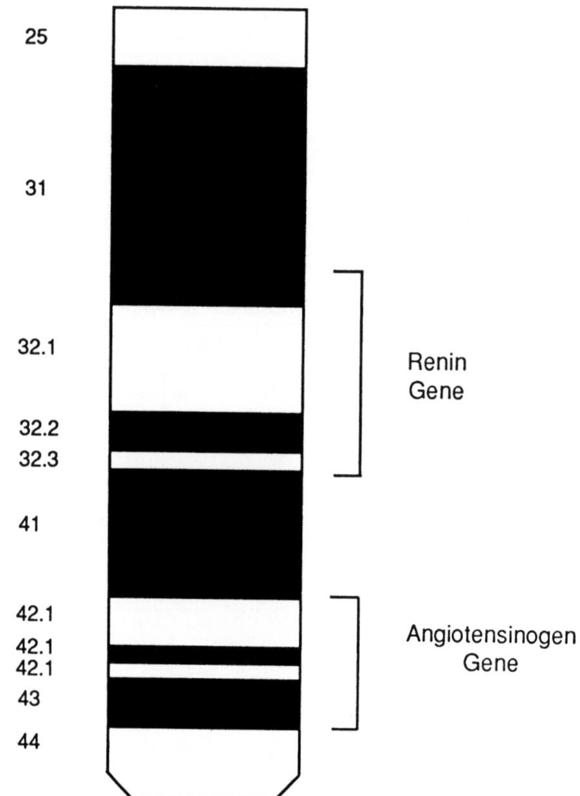

Fig. 46-3. Chromosome 1 contains both the human renin and angiotensinogen genes.

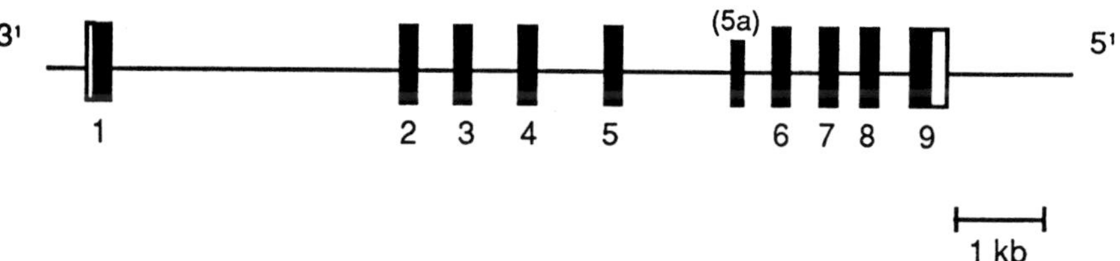

Fig. 46-4. Human renin gene, consisting of nine exons and eight introns, with a 9bp miniexon (5a) of unknown function located between exon five and six. This gene is approximately 12.18 kb in length. The coding sequence *(black boxes)* is contained in the second to eighth exons and portions of the first and ninth exons.

the juxtaglomerular cells, and in some instances as granules within the arteriolar wall. The release of both prorenin and renin into the extracellular space occurs by exocytosis. Renin has a half-life of approximately 20 to 30 minutes. Peripheral levels of circulating renin appear to be in a steady state, the sum of renin activity from both renal veins being approximately 48% greater than that in the infrarenal vena cava or arterial circulation.[19] The major site for removal and clearance of renin is the liver.[20]

Biochemical events related to the renin-angiotensin system have been relatively well defined (Fig. 46-5). The primary and perhaps only function of renin is the hydrolysis of the circulating renin substrate, *angiotensinogen,* to form angiotensin I. Angiotensinogen is an α_2-globulin with a molecular weight of 60,000, produced in the liver. The human gene for angiotensinogen is located on chromosome 1[21] (Figs. 46-3 and 46-6). It is composed of five exons interrupted by four introns.[22] The nucleotides encoding for the angiotensin I peptide are located within the second exon. Gene expression is subject to a variety of physiologic and pathophysiologic stimuli, including steroid hormones, angiotensin II, salt loading, and various drugs. Angiotensinogen itself is not vasoactive.

Angiotensin I, the decapeptide produced by the renin substrate–renin reaction, is relatively inactive. It does exert some effect on the adrenal medulla, the sympathetic and central nervous systems, and the renal arterioles. Quantita-

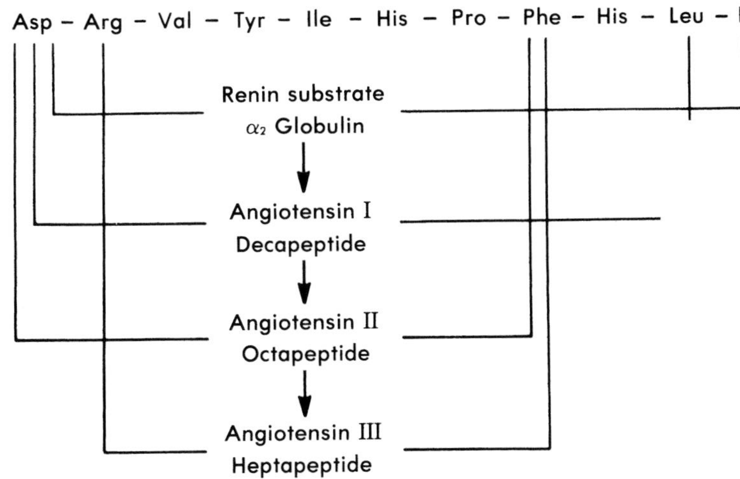

Fig. 46-5. Biochemical composition of renin substrate and the angiotensins.

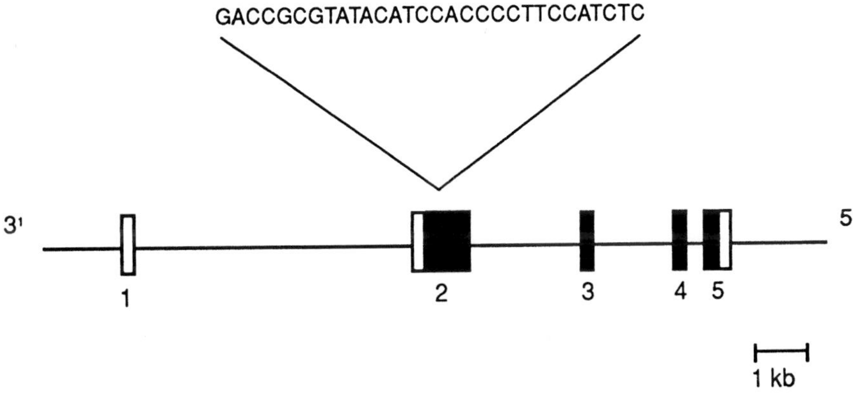

Fig. 46-6. Human angiotensinogen gene, consisting of five exons and four introns. This gene is approximately 14.55 kb in length. The coding sequence *(black boxes)* for angiotensinogen is contained in the second to fifth exon. The second exon contains the coding sequence for angiotensin I.

tion of this intermediary is the basis for many radioimmunoassays of renin activity.

Angiotensin II is produced when two C-terminal peptides are cleaved from angiotensin I by a carboxypeptidase known as angiotensin converting enzyme. The resulting octapeptide is the major contributor to the vasoactive element of renovascular hypertension. Angiotensin II stimulates liver production of angiotensinogen, but in normal individuals it provides a continuous negative feedback on the renal release of renin. Angiotensin II has a half-life of approximately 4 minutes.

Angiotensin III, which is a heptapeptide, is derived by aminopeptidase cleavage of angiotensin II to l-desaspartyl-angiotensin II. Angiotensin III has biologic activity, although its levels are so low that its physiologic importance is questioned. Angiotensin III inhibits angiotensin II. Perhaps its most relevant effect is stimulation of aldosterone synthesis.

Aldosterone, a mineralocorticoid, is secreted from the zona glomerulosa of the adrenal cortex. The biosynthesis of this substance initially involves cleavage of the side of cholesterol to form pregnenolone. This step is facilitated by both angiotensin II and III. Aldosterone increases renal conservation of sodium and water, with a resultant expansion of the extracellular fluid volume and an eventual increase in blood pressure.

Angiotensin converting enzyme is a zinc metallopeptidase responsible for the generation of angiotensin II from angiotensin I by removing C-terminal peptides. The enzyme has a molecular weight of 150,000 to 180,000. Its gene has been mapped to chromosome 17q23 in humans.[23,24] Angiotensin converting enzyme has its highest concentration in the lung on the surface of endothelial cells. It also can be found at lower levels in the blood and kidney, as well as in other vascular beds. Conversion of angiotensin I to angiotensin II, at physiologic concentrations, has been shown to occur in a single passage through the lungs.

Angiotensin converting enzyme also plays an important role in the metabolism of the vasodepressor *bradykinin.* At least two enzymes appear responsible for the inactivation of bradykinin. The first is kinase I, which cleaves the carboxyl terminal arginine of bradykinin. The second enzyme, kinase II, cleaves the carboxyl terminal dipeptide group, Phe-Arg. Kinase II and angiotensin converting enzyme are considered the same, in that they have nearly identical substrate specificities, cofactor requirements, and antigenic specificities.

The most common technique for determination of plasma renin activity involves measurement of angiotensin I generation using a radioimmunoassay. Plasma renin activity is expressed as the hourly rate of angiotensin I generation per unit of volume assayed. The assay involves two phases: (1) incubation of plasma to generate angiotensin I and (2) measurement of generated angiotensin I by the radioimmunoassay. Actual renin secretion is calculated as the renal arteriovenous difference in renin activity multiplied by renal plasma flow, and it is usually expressed as nanograms/millimeter/hour. Assay methods may vary among laboratories, often making interlaboratory comparisons difficult.

Angiotensins have actions on the cardiovascular system, central nervous system, adrenal gland, and kidneys (Fig. 46-7). The effects on cardiac activity, vascular smooth muscle reactivity, and salt and water metabolism are profound, and all contribute to increased arterial pressure. The most important consequence of renal artery occlusive disease is the production of angiotensin II, which by weight is one of the most potent pressor substances known. Angiotensin II acts directly on the arteriolar smooth muscle of nearly all vascular beds. The splanchnic, renal, and cutaneous circulations are most sensitive to its effects. Despite an acceptance of the central importance of angiotensin in the generation of renovascular hypertension, the relevance of absolute plasma levels remains unknown. The end-organ sensitivity to these vasoactive substances is often impossible to predict because it is different in various physiologic and pathologic settings. In addition, the exact role in renovascular hypertension of locally secreted renin and locally generated angiotensin remains poorly defined.

Hemodynamic responses to activation of the renin-angiotensin system depend on the rate at which renal blood flow is decreased, as well as whether one or both kidneys are at risk. Acute reductions in renal blood flow result in prompt blood pressure increases and increased plasma renin levels. Experimental animal models of renovascular hypertension are defined as two kidney–one clip (2K-1C), two kidney–two clip (2K-2C), or one kidney–one clip (1K-1C), depending on whether one or both renal arteries are constricted.

In instances of 2K-1C renovascular hypertension, where the total renal mass is not affected, the hypertension is characterized by renin hypersecretion from the affected kidney and contralateral suppression of kidney renin production.[25,26] Sodium avidity within the affected kidney is counterbalanced by continuous sodium excretion from the contralateral kidney, resulting in relative intravascular volume depletion. This form of hypertension is angiotensin II dependent and responds to angiotensin antagonists and converting enzyme inhibitors.

When the entire renal mass is at risk with 2K-2C or 1K-1C renovascular hypertension, pathophysiologic alterations are quite different and undoubtedly relate to changes other than vasoconstriction. Angiotensin II is known to be involved with sodium retention, decreases in glomerular filtration, stimulation of aldosterone produc-

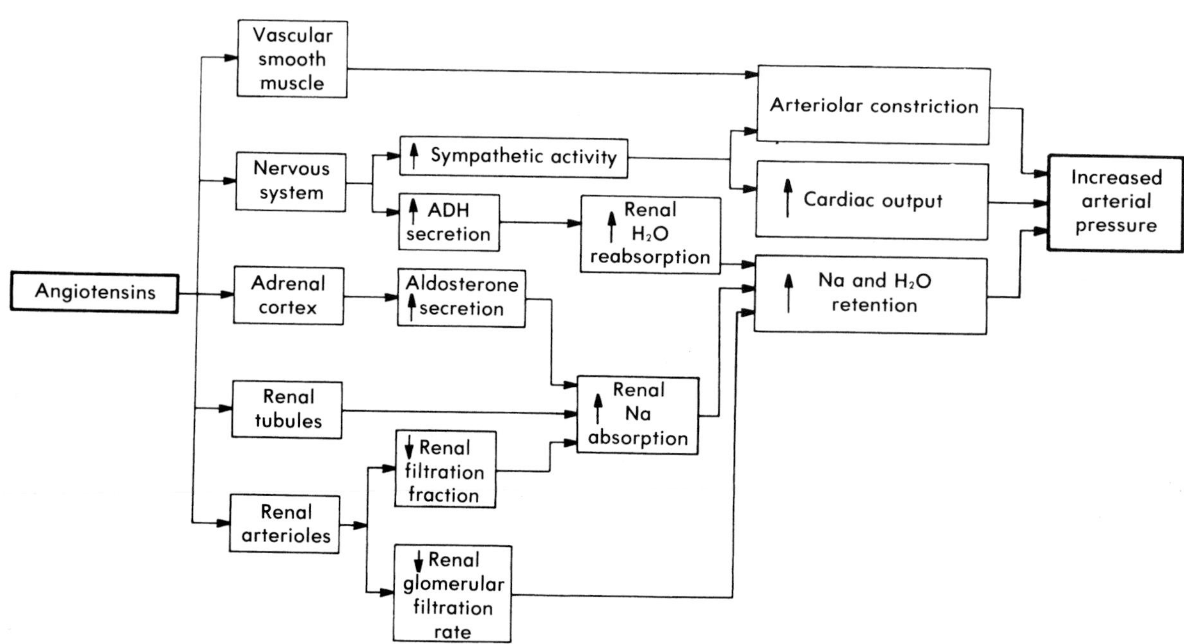

Fig. 46-7. Effects of angiotensins contributing to increased arterial pressure.

tion, and stimulation of norepinephrine release from the adrenergic nervous system. These effects may occur acutely, but in chronic 2K-2C or 1K-1C renovascular hypertension it appears that sodium retention accounts for late reductions in renin secretion, although the absolute renin activity may be abnormal in relation to the existing state of sodium balance. Studies have been unable to demonstrate that blood pressure elevations depend on the renin-angiotensin system in sodium-replete chronic renovascular hypertension. In fact, angiotensin receptor antagonists or converting enzyme inhibitors are effective in reducing elevated blood pressures only when the subjects are depleted of sodium.

PATHOLOGY OF RENAL ARTERY STENOTIC AND OCCLUSIVE DISEASE

The importance of renal artery narrowings to renovascular hypertension was firmly established by the classic canine experiments of Goldblatt et al.[27] first published in 1934. Sustained hypertension was produced in these and subsequent studies by gradual reductions in renal artery blood flow using an intricate vascular clamp (Fig. 46-8). Although Goldblatt's investigations suggested that renovascular hypertension was simply a consequence of renal ischemia, subsequent studies have disproven the importance of simple ischemia per se. Certain hemodynamic signals appear more essential in the control of renin release, the most obvious being decreased mean perfusion pressure. In this regard critical stenoses causing at least a 70% to 80% reduction in the renal artery's cross-sectional area are necessary to induce a pressure gradient. These critical lesions are a cause of renin release from the kidney and are the focus for understanding the importance of renal artery stenotic disease.

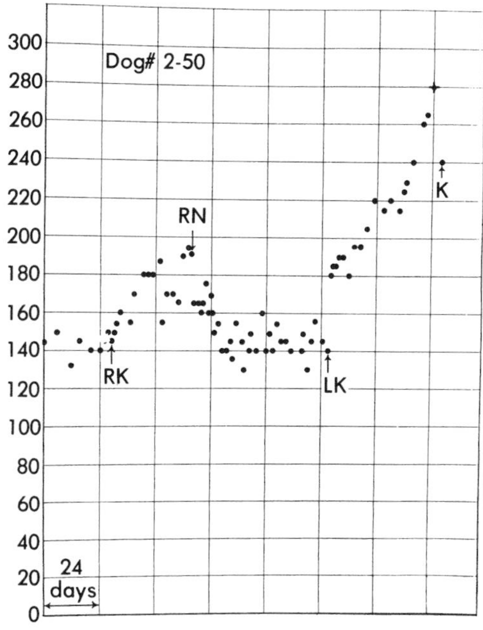

Fig. 46-8. Graph of a dog's mean blood pressure in Goldblatt's experiment. *RK,* Right main renal artery moderately constructed; *RN,* right nephrectomy; *LK,* severe construction of left main renal artery; *K,* animal sacrificed. (From Goldblatt H. The pathogenesis of experimental hypertension due to renal ischemia. Ann Intern Med 11:69, 1937.)

Various types of occlusive disease affect the renal arterial circulation, ranging from common macrovascular diseases to unusual microvascular arteriopathies associated with connective tissue diseases. Although relatively uncommon, renal artery emboli, spontaneous dissections, and traumatic occlusions are occasionally associated with acute forms of renin-mediated hypertension. The most often encountered causes of hypertension secondary to renal artery occlusive disease are those associated with atherosclerosis, arterial fibrodysplasia, and developmental renal artery stenoses.[28-31]

Atherosclerosis

Atherosclerosis is the most common renal artery occlusive disease, accounting for approximately 95% of reported cases of renovascular hypertension. Atherosclerotic renovascular lesions are usually recognized in the sixth decade of life. Men are twice as likely as women to exhibit this disease. It is important to note that some degree of atherosclerotic renal artery stenotic disease affects nearly half the elderly population and that this is not always associated with elevated blood pressures.

Atherosclerotic renal artery occlusive disease typically involves the proximal third of the vessel with eccentric or concentric stenoses. In nearly 80% of patients these lesions represent a "spill-over" stenosis associated with aortic atherosclerosis (Fig. 46-9). Such lesions are bilateral in three quarters of patients. When unilateral, the lesions seemingly affect the right and left sides with equal frequency, although the left renal artery often appears more severely diseased. Subendothelial and medial accumulation of cholesterol-laden foam cells and fibrosis are present in these lesions. Necrosis, hemorrhage, deposition of cholesterol crystals, calcification, and luminal thrombus formation are characteristic of complicated atherosclerotic plaques associated with advanced disease.

Arterial Fibrodysplasia

Arterial fibrodysplasia is the second most common type of renal artery disease, affecting nearly 5% of patients with renovascular hypertension. Renal artery stenoses caused by dysplastic disease are a heterogeneous group of lesions classified by the specific pathologic process and region of the vessel wall most affected. These lesions include intimal fibroplasia, medial fibrodysplasia, and perimedial dysplasia.[31] The latter two entities appear to be a continuum of the same disease process. Each category has certain characteristic features that deserve mention.

Intimal Fibroplasia

Intimal fibroplasia accounts for approximately 5% of all dysplastic renal artery lesions. It affects infants and young adults more often than the elderly, and occurs with equal

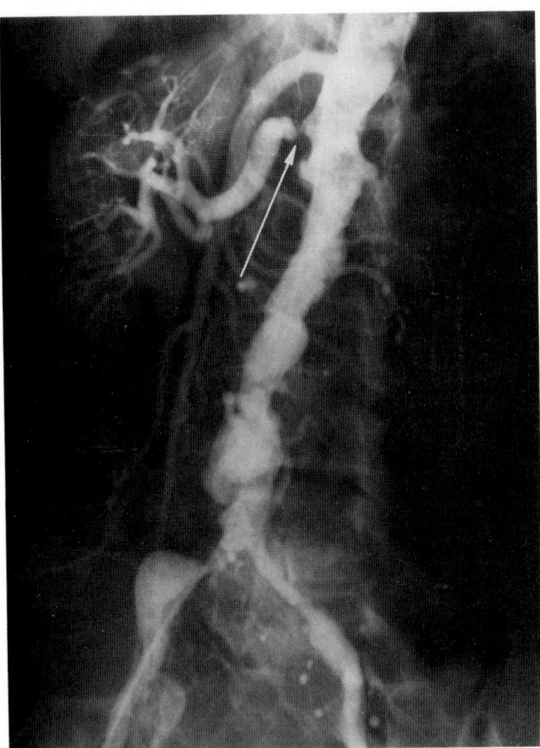

Fig. 46-9. Characteristic proximal disease in atherosclerotic renal artery stenosis.

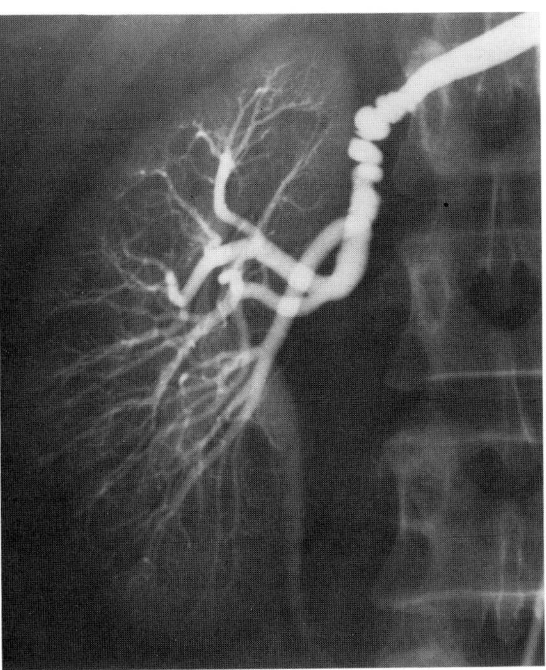

Fig. 46-10. Arterial fibrodysplasia. Serial stenoses and intervening macroaneurysmal outpouchings are characteristic of medial fibrodysplasia.

frequency in female and male patients. The cause of primary intimal fibroplasia is unknown, although some of these lesions may represent persistent myointimal cushions, originally occurring during fetal development. Secondary intimal fibroplasia has been attributed to trauma and the sequela of an earlier arteritis. Progression of intimal fibroplasia may cause an accelerated proliferation of fibrous tissue and rapid compromise of the arterial lumen.

Intimal fibroplasia usually appears as long, tubular stenoses of the main renal artery or weblike segmental renal artery lesions in young patients and as smooth, focal stenoses in adults. Proximal intimal stenoses are most often secondary lesions associated with aortic hypoplasia or coarctations, frequently in patients with neurofibromatosis.[32,33] Subendothelial accumulations of irregularly arranged mesenchymal cells surrounded by loose fibrous connective tissue are typical of these intimal lesions that protrude as hillocks of tissue into the vessel lumen. The internal elastic lamina is usually intact, but partial fragmentation may occur.

Medial Fibrodysplasia

Medial fibrodysplasia is the most common dysplastic renal artery disease, accounting for 85% of such stenoses. It invariably affects women. Clinical presentation occurs most often during the fourth decade of life. This disease in its classic form has not been encountered before menarche. Medial fibrodysplasia appears to be a systemic arteriopathy in certain patients, with the internal carotid, superior mesenteric, and external iliac arteries being the extrarenal vessels most often affected. The cause of medial fibrodysplasia remains poorly defined but appears associated with estrogenic effects on smooth muscle in women during their reproductive years, unusual stretch forces on affected vessels, and mural ischemia resulting from a paucity of vasa vasorum blood flow.[31]

Morphologic changes of medial fibrodysplasia range from solitary stenoses in the middle and distal main renal artery to multiple constrictions with intervening mural dilations. The latter produce this lesion's classic string-of-beads appearance (Fig. 46-10). Actual macrovascular aneurysms, usually occurring at branchings, affect nearly 13% of patients with arterial fibrodysplasia[34] but are rarely a cause of hypertension.[35] Extension of medial fibrodysplasia into segmental branches occurs in approximately 25% of cases. Bilateral disease affects nearly 60% of patients and is usually most severe in the right renal artery. Unilateral lesions more commonly involve the right renal artery, with isolated disease of the right and left renal arteries existing in 30% and 10% of patients, respectively. Progression has been recognized in approximately 20% of patients, occurring more frequently in premenopausal women.

Diffuse medial fibrodysplasia is typified by severe disorganization of smooth muscle and the predominance of myofibroblasts, that appear responsible for excessive accumulations of ground substance encroaching on the vessel lumen.[31,36] These stenoses occur adjacent to areas of atrophic smooth muscle and medial thinning, which are responsible for the mural dilations. Peripheral medial fibrodysplasia is a second form of this disease. It is characterized by fibroproliferative changes and loss of normal smooth muscle limited to the outer portion of the media. The latter findings are usually associated with less severe stenoses than occur with diffuse disease. Both the diffuse and peripheral forms of this disease may be observed in the same vessel.

Perimedial Dysplasia

Perimedial dysplasia accounts for nearly 10% of dysplastic renal artery disease. It invariably affects women, with its recognition usually occurring during the fifth decade of life. This particular dysplastic lesion appears to be more progressive than medial fibrodysplasia. Only 20% of patients have bilateral disease. Perimedial disease appears as solitary or multiple constrictions without intervening mural dilations. These stenoses involve distal portions of the main renal artery, usually without branch involvement. Excessive accumulation of elastic tissue in inner adventitial regions is characteristic of perimedial dysplasia. Abnormal increases in medial ground substances may also accompany this type of renal artery dysplasia. Certain histologic and ultrastructural features are common to both perimedial dysplasia and medial fibrodysplasia. Although perimedial dysplasia is classified as a separate pathologic entity, this may not be an appropriate distinction.

Developmental Renal Artery Stenoses

Developmental renal artery stenoses represent a third category of renal artery occlusive disease. Most are ostial in location, and many are associated with abdominal aortic narrowings. There is no gender predilection, and most are encountered in late childhood.[28,32,33] Nearly 80% of patients with these stenoses have multiple renal arteries. It is believed that most of these lesions evolve because of faulty union of the metanephric vessels to the aorta during fetal development; at the same time the two embryonic aortas fuse to become a single vessel. Other developmental stenoses are seen in association with neurofibromatosis, in which case a growth disturbance of mesenchymal tissue is likely to underlie the hypoplastic character of these renal arteries. Fragmentation of the internal elastic lamina, incomplete formation of the media, and excesses of perimedial elastic tissue typify the stenoses of these diminutive vessels.

CLINICAL MANIFESTATIONS

The exact prevalence of renovascular hypertension among all patients with elevated diastolic blood pressures is unknown but is probably close to 1%. It clearly occurs much more often in individuals having moderate or severe diastolic blood pressure elevations, with as many as 5% of such patients exhibiting underlying renovascular hypertension.

Clinical findings suggestive of renovascular hypertension include (1) systolic-diastolic upper abdominal bruits, (2) initial diastolic blood pressures greater than 115 mm Hg or sudden worsening of mild preexisting essential hypertension, (3) development of hypertension during childhood, or (4) sudden development of high blood pressure after age 50. Drug-resistant hypertension and malignant hypertension are also more likely to be associated with renovascular hypertension. Patients whose renal function deteriorates while receiving multiple antihypertensive drugs, especially angiotensin converting enzyme inhibitors, must also be tested for renal artery stenotic disease and renovascular hypertension. Clinical screening of patients is important before undertaking diagnostic studies for suspected renovascular hypertension. Otherwise, the costs of indiscriminate evaluations for this type of hypertension would be prohibitive.[37]

DIAGNOSIS OF RENAL ARTERY STENOSIS AND SECONDARY HYPERTENSION

Many diagnostic and prognostic tests for renovascular hypertension represent methods of defining the anatomic presence of renal artery disease or pathophysiologic derangements of renal function due to the stenotic disease.

Contrast Arteriography

In the past, conventional contrast arteriography has been a standard study for the evaluation of all patients with suspected renovascular hypertension. Oblique aortography and multiple-plane selective renal arteriography can precisely define the morphologic character and extent of a stenotic lesion. Collateral vessels circumventing a stenosis are evidence of a lesion's hemodynamic and functional importance. Pressure gradients of approximately 10 mm Hg are necessary for development of collateral circulation, and the same degree of pressure change is associated with activation of the renin system. Accordingly, collateral vessels circumventing a renal artery stenosis are invariably associated with increased renin release. Thus the importance of an otherwise benign-appearing stenosis may be established when collateral vessels are present (Fig. 46-11) or when dilution defects representing noncontrast-containing blood from collateral vessels entering the poststenotic portion of the vessel are identified with selective renal arteriography. Pharmacoangiographic vasodilatory and vasoconstrictive manipulations have been advocated as a means to demonstrate nonparenchymal renal artery collateral vessels circumventing a critical stenosis.[38] Digital subtraction arteriography following intra-arterial contrast injection has become commonplace. This technique allows the use of smaller amounts of contrast agents as compared to conventional arteriography, lessening potential nephrotoxicity. This is especially relevant in patients with preexisting impairment of renal function.

Arteriographic evidence of arterial nephrosclerosis should not be considered an indication that renal revascularization or angioplasty will not have a beneficial effect on blood pressure. This is in keeping with previous reports

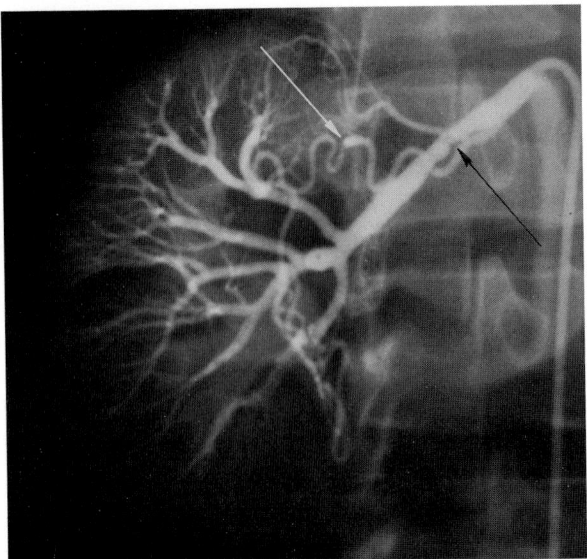

Fig. 46-11. Arteriogram of a benign-appearing stenosis *(black arrow)* associated with a large collateral vessel *(white arrow)* circumventing the lesion, defining hemodynamic significance of the stenosis and implicating its functional importance. (From Stanley JC, Graham LM, Whitehouse WM Jr. Renovascular hypertension: Limitations and errors of diagnostic and prognostic investigations. In Bernhard VM, Towne JM, eds. Complications in Vascular Surgery. Orlando, Fla.: Grune & Stratton, 1985.)

that biopsy evidence of nephrosclerosis is of limited prognostic value.[39]

Magnetic Resonance Angiography

Application of magnetic resonance technology to vascular imaging, especially with gadolinium enhancement, has evolved to a sufficient extent that it often provides high-resolution images of the renal arteries.[40] Magnetic resonance angiography is not available at all institutions, and recent advances require further evaluation before it becomes widely used in assessing patients suspected of renovascular disease. Nevertheless, its noninvasiveness and lack of nephrotoxicity make it an attractive diagnostic test.

Deep Abdominal Renal Artery Ultrasonography

Hemodynamically significant renal artery narrowings, and in many instances functionally important narrowings, may often be identified by imaging the renal arteries and characterizing flow velocity patterns through these vessels with abdominal duplex ultrasonography.[41-43] Such studies have been advocated in screening for renovascular disease and are useful in establishing the existence of a stenosis when peak systolic velocities are in the range of 180 to 200 cms/sec and the ratio of these velocities to those in the aorta approaches 3.5. Unfortunately, this technology does not provide discrimination of renal artery lesions exceeding 60% cross-sectional narrowing. Failure to identify a main renal artery in cases where no parenchymal flow signal exists suggests existence of a main renal artery occlusion. However, occluded accessory or segmental renal arteries may go unrecognized and thus contribute to false negative assessments.

Renin Activity of Peripheral and Renal Venous Blood

Renin activity in peripheral and renal venous blood provides information about the functional importance of renal artery disease. To reduce interpretive errors evolving from minor fluctuations in basal renin activity, the renin-angiotensin system should be stimulated before sampling blood for renin assays. Blood samples for renin assays in the peripheral and renal circulations should be obtained simultaneously, or nearly simultaneously, with the patient tilted to a semiupright position. Sodium intake should be limited to 20 mEq/day and a diuretic administered for 3 days before testing. Renin-suppressing drugs are discontinued when possible. Blood pressure elevations in such circumstances should be controlled with renin-stimulating agents such as hydralazine. The effect of converting enzyme inhibitors in stimulating renin release and thus improving renin assay results has not been achieved in general practice.

Renal Vein Renin Ratios

Renal vein renin ratios (RVRRs) are calculated by dividing the renin activity in venous blood from the affected kidney by that from the contralateral kidney. An RVRR greater than 1.48 indicates functionally important renovascular disease.[25,26] Because this test compares one kidney to another, it is not helpful in the presence of bilateral disease when both kidneys exhibit equal elevations of renin secretion. In fact, approximately 15% of patients benefiting from surgery have an RVRR less than 1.48 (Fig. 46-12).

Renal:Systemic Renin Index

Renal:systemic renin index (RSRI) is an expression of a single kidney's renin secretion. It is calculated by subtracting systemic renin activity from an individual kidney's venous renin activity and dividing the remainder by the systemic renin activity.[25] In nonrenovascular hypertension, renal venous activity from each kidney is usually 24% higher than systemic activity.[19] Thus the total of both kidneys' activity is usually 48% higher than systemic levels, balancing hepatic degradation and establishing a steady state.

In renovascular hypertension the RSRI of the affected kidney becomes greater than 0.24. This is normally accompanied by suppression of contralateral kidney renin production with a drop in its RSRI below 0.24. In the case of bilateral renal artery disease this servomechanism may be lost, and autonomous release of renin from both kidneys may cause the sum of the individual RSRIs to be greater than 0.48. Renin production then exceeds normal hepatic degradation, and a hyperreninemic state evolves.

RSRI documentation of renin hypersecretion and suppression allows differentiation of patients most likely to be cured or improved following treatment (Fig. 46-13). The

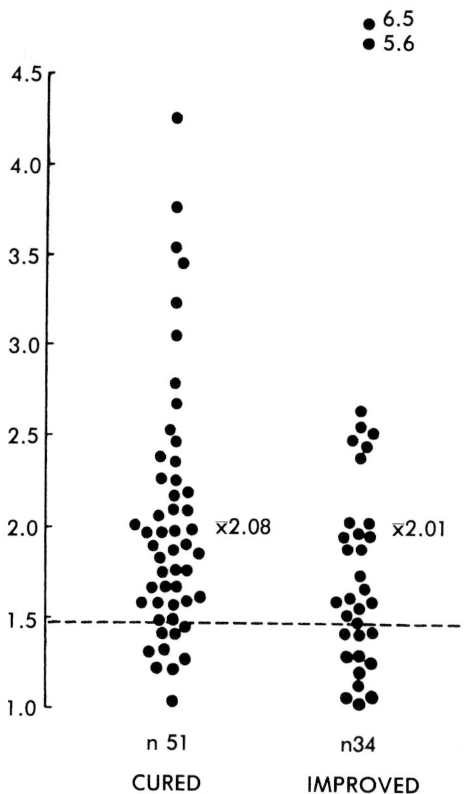

Fig. 46-12. Renal vein renin ratios, reflecting their limited diagnostic and prognostic value. (Modified from Stanley JC, Gewertz BL, Fry WJ. Renal:systemic renin indices and renal vein renin ratios as prognostic indicators in remedial renovascular hypertension. J Surg Res 20:149, 1976.)

validity of ischemic renin hypersecretion (RSRI > 0.48) from the kidney being revascularized and contralateral renin suppression (RSRI < 0.24, approaching 0) in identifying patients who will be cured has been well documented.[25,26,44] However, the prognostic accuracy of RSRI may be limited in that approximately 8% of patients who are cured do not exhibit contralateral renin suppression.[44]

Angiotensin-Converting Enzyme Inhibitor Hypotensive Response

Angiotensin-converting enzyme inhibitors may reveal the existence of renovascular hypertension by inhibiting angiotensin II generation and producing obvious reductions in blood pressure. Use of converting enzyme inhibitors offers a more sensitive means than administration of competitive antagonists to angiotensin receptors for detecting angiotensin II–dependent blood pressure elevations. However, the specificity of such studies is very low, perhaps because converting enzyme is the same as kinase II, and its inhibition causes accumulations of bradykinin with its subsequent blood pressure lowering effect in nonrenin-mediated forms of hypertension.

Hypertensive Urography

Hypertensive urography is a poor diagnostic test for renovascular hypertension because of its limited sensitivity.[45] Bilateral or segmental disease often precludes recognition of gross differences in contrast excretion between the two kidneys. In a large series of patients with proven renovascular hypertension, urograms were abnormal in only 27% of pediatric patients, 48% of patients with arterial fibrodysplastic disease, and approximately 72% of patients

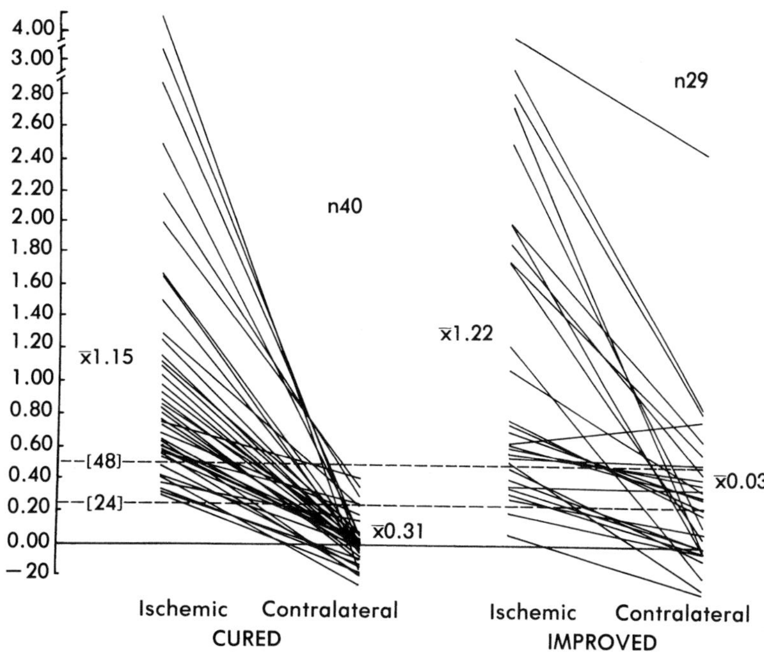

Fig. 46-13. Renal:systemic renin indexes, depicting their prognostic usefulness. (From Stanley JC, Fry WJ. Surgical treatment of renovascular hypertension. Arch Surg 112:1291, 1977. Copyright 1977, American Medical Association.)

with atherosclerotic lesions.[46] Nevertheless, rapid-sequence urography may contribute to the diagnosis of renovascular hypertension when (1) at least a 1-minute delay in contrast appearance occurs within the collecting system of the affected kidney compared to that of the contralateral kidney; (2) a length discrepancy is found, with the right kidney being 2 cm shorter than the left or the left 1.5 cm shorter than the right; and (3) hyperconcentration of contrast in the collecting system of the affected kidney is observed on late urograms. Ureteral or pelvic irregularities caused by large collateral vessels may also accompany these urographic features.

Isotopic Renography

Isotopic renography has been used with both imaging and analysis of the washout curve of several tracers, the most common being ^{99m}Tc-DTPA (diethylenetriamine pentaacetic acid), ^{123}I or ^{131}I orthoiodohippurate, ^{99m}Tc-MAG$_3$ (mercaptoacetylglycyl glycylglycine), ^{99m}Tc-DMSA (dimercaptosuccinic acid), and ^{99m}glucoheptonate. These compounds provide an assessment of both renal blood flow and excretory function. Unfortunately, different states of hydration and intrarenal vascular resistance often result in flow abnormalities with false positive studies in nonrenovascular hypertensive patients. The specificity and sensitivity of current studies are both approximately 75%. However, the sensitivity may be improved by administration of an angiotensin converting enzyme inhibitor to block the compensatory change in glomerular filtration, causing it to fall on the side of a stenosis. The sensitivity of the renogram increases to more than 80%, and the specificity of such a modified study approaches 85%. Renal perfusion-excretion ratios and more sophisticated computer programs offer a potential means of increasing the predictive value of radionuclide screening for renovascular hypertension, but they are not yet in widespread use.

Split Renal Function Studies

Split renal function studies of altered individual renal function were among the first tests used for suspected renovascular hypertension.[47] These studies involve ureteral catheterization to sample urine from each kidney. Two specific tests have been used most widely: (1) the Howard test, designed to document reduced urine volume, as well as increased sodium and creatinine concentration from the affected kidney, and (2) the Stamey test, performed after a urea-induced osmotic diuresis and an infusion of *p*-aminohippuric acid (PAH), with the affected kidney usually producing a smaller volume of urine and greater concentration of PAH than the normal kidney. Using standard criteria, few patients with essential hypertension had abnormal results from studies, but only half those with proven renovascular hypertension had positive results from diagnostic tests. Investigators from Vanderbilt University proposed liberalizing the diagnostic criteria for split renal function studies, with a positive test result defined as constant lateralization to the affected kidney having 25% less urine volume and a 15% increase in creatinine concentration.[47] Greater sensitivity was obtained using such criteria, but appreciable numbers of results from studies in patients without renovascular hypertension became positive.

TREATMENT

Therapeutic results in renovascular hypertension relate to an accurate diagnosis and proper execution of an appropriate intervention, whether the intervention is arterial reconstructive surgery, ablative surgery, transcatheter renal infarction, percutaneous transluminal angioplasty, or institution of drug therapy. The specific type of renovascular disease being treated is also relevant to the expected therapeutic outcome.

Data from an earlier prospective Mayo Clinic series suggest increased patient survival among individuals with both fibrodysplastic and atherosclerotic renovascular disease treated surgically compared to those treated medically.[48] A prospective *randomized* study comparing medical and surgical therapy has yet to be published. Nevertheless, long-term drug therapy has not been favored by most physicians responsible for the care of these patients.

Drug Therapy

Antihypertensive drugs developed during the past two decades have resulted in major improvements in the medical management of patients with renovascular hypertension.[49,50] Vasoconstriction assumes greatest importance with a unilateral stenosis in patients having a normal contralateral kidney (2K-1C). Excessive sodium retention and hypervolemia become important factors in patients with bilateral renal artery stenoses (2K-2C), in those with unilateral stenoses affecting a solitary kidney (1K-1C), or in patients with contralateral parenchymal disease. Blood pressure elevations in most, if not all, patients with renovascular hypertension may be reduced by appropriate drug interventions. However, side effects, compliance, and effects on renal function must be considered before pursuing drug treatment.

β-Blocking agents are usually the first drugs administered in known cases of renovascular hypertension, with subsequent reductions in renin release causing a lowering of the blood pressure.[51] Propranolol and atenolol are most frequently used, although other β-blockers are also effective in treating renovascular hypertension. High doses of these drugs may be required to control the blood pressure, although in most cases suppression of renin release may be accomplished with very small doses. In instances of more refractory hypertension, especially that caused by bilateral renal artery stenoses or unilateral lesions with contralateral parenchymal disease, addition of a standard diuretic such as a thiazide, a hydrogenated thiazide, or substituted compound is recommended. In cases of impaired renal function secondary to decreased blood flow, a loop diuretic such as furosemide provides a more effective diuretic action.

Angiotensin converting enzyme inhibitors, such as captopril and enalapril, are used for treating hypertension in general. Antihypertensive effects other than decreased angiotensin II generation, such as those involving bradykinin, probably occur with the use of these agents. Angiotensin converting enzyme inhibitors may be supplemented with β-blockers or diuretics in resistant hypertension. In more severe hypertension, vasodilators such as minoxidil may be required. It is important to recognize the deleterious effects of converting enzyme inhibitors on renal function. This becomes especially evident in patients with bilateral renal artery stenoses, in cases of unilateral stenosis together with contralateral parenchymal disease, or when stenosis occurs in a solitary kidney.[52] In these instances severe deterioration of glomerular filtration may occur, and use of these agents is contraindicated.

Percutaneous Transluminal Renal Angioplasty

In 1978 Gruntzig et al.[53] were the first to report the use of percutaneous transluminal angioplasty in the management of renovascular hypertension. This method of treatment has important patient safety and cost benefits. However, certain issues must be considered, including (1) differences in treating various types of renal artery disease, (2) the frequency of being unable to catheterize or dilate a given type of stenosis, (3) the long-term effects of angioplasty on the vessel wall, (4) the incidence of renal and extrarenal complications, and (5) the durability of a successfully performed dilation.

Intimal fibroplastic and medial fibrodysplastic stenoses and isolated arteriosclerotic stenoses appear most amenable to percutaneous angioplasty (Fig. 46-14). Ostial lesions associated with developmental aortic anomalies represent diminutive vessels with considerable elasticity that are less likely to be successfully dilated.[54] Medial fibrodysplasia with multiple stenoses in series can often be easily dilated; but difficulties may occur initially in traversing extensive disease with the guide wire, and extension into segmental vessels increases the hazards of dilation. Percutaneous transluminal angioplasty of atherosclerotic stenoses may be limited by an inability to dilate "spill-over plaque" from extensive aortic disease. These aortic-associated lesions appear most responsible for the high recurrence rate when treating atherosclerotic occlusive stenoses.[55] Stenting after balloon angioplasty may be useful in these patients, but studies to support the routine use of stents do not exist. Nevertheless, the potential benefits following successful percutaneous transluminal angioplasty in carefully selected patients with renovascular hypertension approach 90%.[56,57]

Complications following dilation of both atherosclerotic and dysplastic lesions are uncommon, with renal complications probably not occurring in more than a few percent of cases. Extrarenal complications most often relate to hemorrhage at the site of arterial catheterization, which rarely threatens the patient's limb or life. Percutaneous transluminal renal angioplasty must be considered as an alternative to other therapies for renovascular hypertension in appropriately selected patients.[58-60]

Surgical Options

Many operative interventions for the treatment of renovascular hypertension have evolved over the past few decades. The most common operations are bypass procedures, ex vivo reconstructions, and endarterectomy.

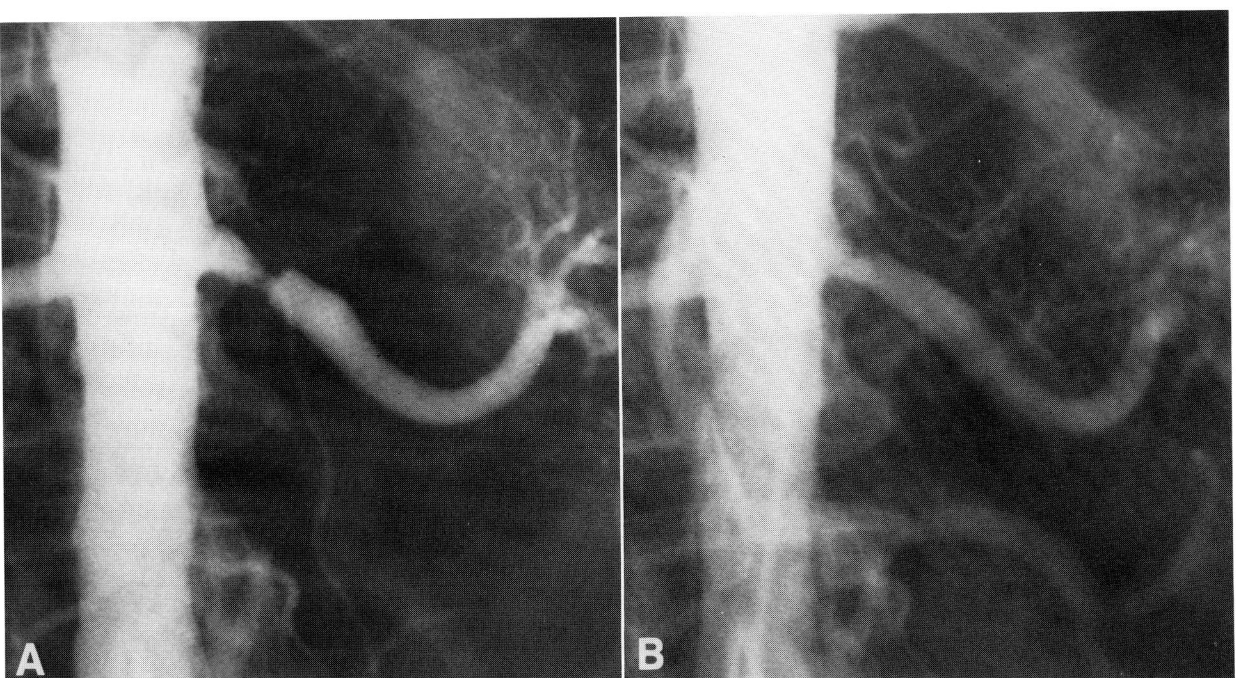

Fig. 46-14. Percutaneous transluminal angioplasty. Renal artery stenosis. **A,** Before dilation. **B,** After dilation.

Bypass Procedures

Bypass procedures are the most frequently used means of renal revascularization for both atherosclerotic and fibrodysplastic stenoses (Fig. 46-15). Autogenous saphenous vein is the graft employed most often. Autogenous internal iliac arteries are the preferred graft when undertaking bypasses in pediatric patients,[33,61] in that vein grafts placed in younger patients often are associated with late aneurysmal changes.[62,63] Prosthetic grafts of knitted Dacron or expanded Teflon are used when autogenous conduits are not available. Limitations of prosthetic grafts relate to their potential for infection and technical difficulties in anastomosing them to small arteries. Although most bypass procedures are fashioned as aortorenal reconstructions, the aorta may be an inappropriate site for the graft to originate. In these latter circumstances, nonanatomic reconstructions with grafts originating from the hepatic or splenic arteries may be best for the patient.[64,65] In some patients with ostial disease, especially in the pediatric-aged group,[33] aortic reimplantation of the normal renal artery beyond its stenosis may be better than a conventional bypass.

Ex Vivo Renal Artery Reconstruction

Ex vivo renal artery reconstruction is an alternative to in situ repair for treating select cases of complex renovascular hypertension.[66-68] This technique allows temporary removal of the kidney for precise microsurgical repair of the diseased vessel. Disruption of preexisting collateral channels, the need to cool the kidney, and the longer duration of such procedures are disadvantages of ex vivo reconstructions. This form of reconstruction is most applicable when treating multiple stenoses and aneurysms of segmental vessels.

Endarterectomy

Endarterectomy has been advocated in the treatment of most atherosclerotic renal artery stenoses.[69-71] A transaortic approach with an aortotomy extending along the lateral aorta from the level of the superior mesenteric artery to below the renal orifices anteriorly is usually preferable to a direct longitudinal renal arteriotomy and local endarterectomy (Fig. 46-16). Endarterectomy through the transected infrarenal aorta during aortic reconstructive procedures has gained favor over bypass reconstructions in certain patients.[72]

Results of Surgical Therapy

The benefits of surgical therapy for renovascular hypertension have been documented from many centers. Loss of life during renovascular surgery occurs infrequently today, with overall operative mortality in most large series usually being less than 0.5%. Renal preservation and maintenance of renal function is clearly very important in assessing clinical experiences. Cumulative primary and secondary nephrectomy rates should not exceed 10%. Nephrectomy may provide good early results but obviously leaves the patient at considerable risk if contralateral disease evolves later. The incidence of nephrectomy during second surgery for failed primary procedures approaches 43% and emphasizes the importance of an appropriately performed primary revascularization.[73]

Contemporary surgical treatment of renovascular hypertension has resulted in excellent outcomes. Differences among the various series usually reflect the most prevalent renal artery disease entity causing the secondary hypertension (Tables 46-1 to 46-3).[74] Pediatric patients with renovascular hypertension are most likely to be cured after

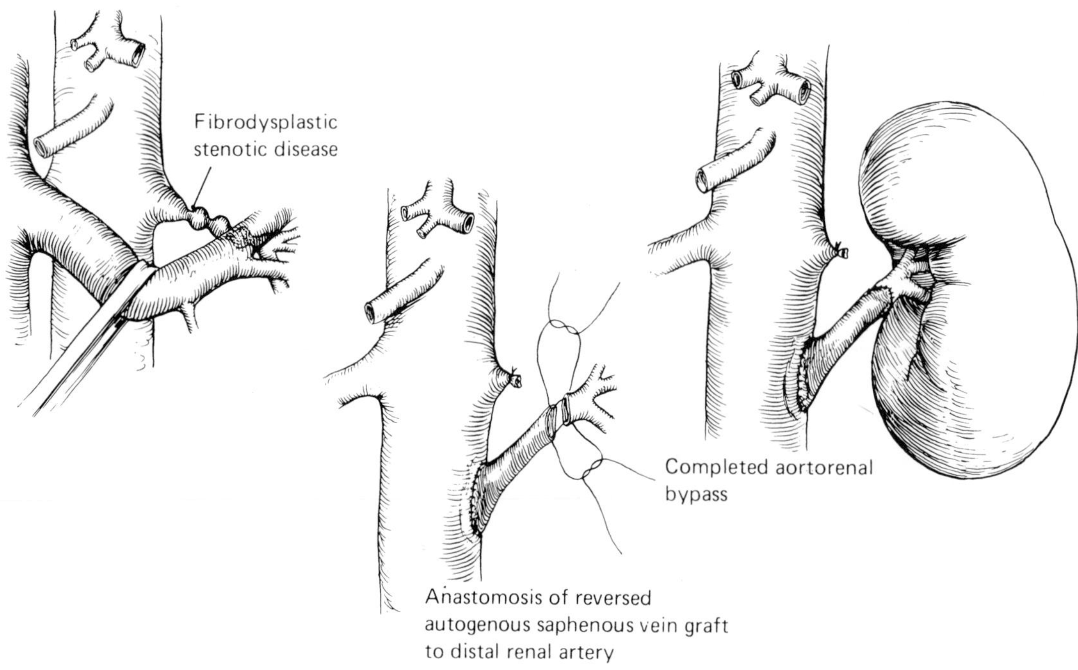

Fig. 46-15. Renal revascularization. Bypass procedure with autogenous saphenous vein.

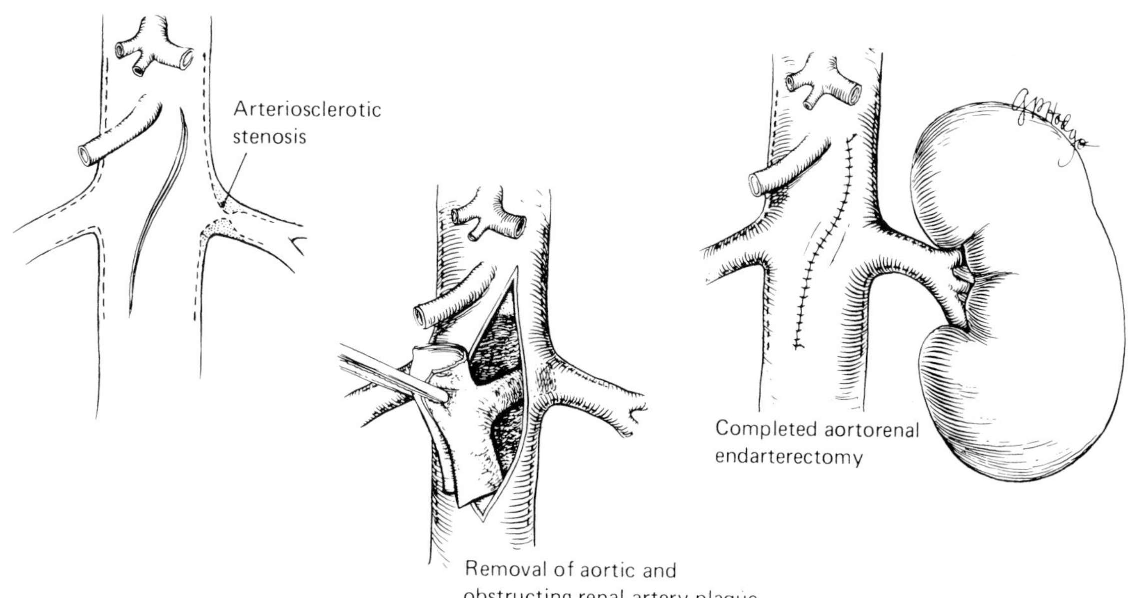

Fig. 46-16. Renal revascularization by performance of an endarterectomy.

Table 46-1. Pediatric Renovascular Hypertension

Institution	No. of Patients	Operative Outcome (%)			Surgical Mortality (%)
		Cured	Improved	Failed	
University of Michigan	55	83.5	14.5	2	0
Cleveland Clinic	27	59	18.5	18.5	4
University of California Los Angeles	26	84.5	7.5	4	4
Vanderbilt University	21	68	24	8	0
University of Pennsylvania	17	76.5	23.5	0	0
Argentinian Institute Buenos Aires, Argentina	15	53	13	27	7
University of California San Francisco	14	86	7	0	7

From Stanley JC. The evolution of surgery for renovascular occlusive disease. Cardiovasc Surg 2:195, 1994.

Table 46-2. Fibrodysplastic Renovascular Hypertension, Adults

Institution	No. of Patients	Operative Outcome (%)			Surgical Mortality (%)
		Cured	Improved	Failed	
University of Michigan	144	55	39	6	0
Baylor College of Medicine	113	43	24	33	0
Cleveland Clinic	92	58	31	11	Unstated
University of California San Francisco	77	66	32	1.3	0
Mayo Clinic	63	66	24	10	Unstated
University Hospital Leiden Leiden, The Netherlands	53	53	34	13	2
Vanderbilt University	44	72	24	4	2.3
Columbia University	42	76	14	10	Unstated
University of Lund Malmo, Sweden	40	66	24	10	0

From Stanley JC. The evolution of surgery for renovascular occlusive disease. Cardiovasc Surg 2:195, 1994.

Table 46-3. Arteriosclerotic Renovascular Hypertension, Adults

Institution	No. of Patients	Operative Outcome (%) Cured	Improved	Failed	Surgical Mortality (%)
Baylor College of Medicine	360	34	31	35	2.5
Bowman Gray	152	15	75	10	1.3
University of Michigan	135	29	52	19	4.4
University of California San Francisco	84	39	23	38	2.4
Cleveland Clinic	78	40	51	9	2
Columbia University	67	58	21	21	Unstated
University of Lund Malmo, Sweden	66	49	24	27	0.9
Hospital Aiguelongue Montpellier, France	65	45	40	15	1.1
Vanderbilt University	63	50	45	5	9
Indiana University	52	31	61	8	5.8

From Stanley JC. The evolution of surgery for renovascular occlusive disease. Cardiovasc Surg 2:195, 1994.

Table 46-4. Results of Surgical Treatment of Renovascular Hypertension in Specific Patient Subgroups, University of Michigan Experience

Subgroup	No. of Patients	Postoperative Status (%)*† Cure	Improvement	Failure	Operative Mortality (%)
Pediatric disease	34	85	12	3	0
Arterial fibrodysplasia	144	55	39	6	0
Arteriosclerosis					0
Focal renal artery disease	64	33	58	9	8.5
Overt extrarenal disease	71	25	47	28	

From Stanley JC. The evolution of surgery for renovascular occlusive disease. Cardiovasc Surg 2:195, 1994.
*Represents outcome of 415 operations (346 primary, 59 secondary), including initial nephrectomy in 17 patients.
†Cure: Blood pressures were 150/90 mm Hg or less for a minimum of 6 months postoperatively during which no antihypertensive medications were administered. *Improvement,* Normotensive while receiving drug therapy or if diastolic blood pressures ranged between 90 and 100 mm Hg but were at least 15% lower than preoperative levels. *Failures,* Diastolic blood pressures greater than 90 mm Hg but less than 15% lower than preoperative levels or greater than 110 mm Hg. Lower pressure standards were used in evaluating pediatric patients.

restoration of renal blood flow, with a beneficial response expected in approximately 95% of such cases. Adults with arterial fibrodysplasia benefit from surgery more often than those with atherosclerotic disease, which probably reflects the fact that coexisting essential hypertension and nephrosclerosis is quite uncommon in younger patients with arterial fibrodysplasia compared to those with atherosclerosis.

Atherosclerotic renovascular hypertension has often been considered a homogenous disease entity. However, at least two clinical subgroups of patients with atherosclerotic lesions exist: (1) those having focal renal artery disease, whose only clinical manifestation of their atherosclerosis is secondary renovascular hypertension, and (2) those with clinically overt extrarenal atherosclerosis. The severity and duration of hypertension, age, and sex distribution in these two subgroups are often similar, but the surgical outcomes are very different. Improved renal function following revascularization is a well-recognized event, occurring most often among patients with profound preoperative impairment in renal function.[75-78]

Surgical treatment of renovascular hypertension may be best portrayed by reviewing results within four specific subgroups treated in an early University of Michigan series (Table 46-4). Patients were categorized as (1) pediatric patients up to 17 years in age, (2) adults with fibrodysplastic disease, or (3) adults having atherosclerotic renal artery lesions *without* overt extrarenal atherosclerotic cardiovascular disease, or (4) adults who have atherosclerotic renal artery lesions *with* overt extrarenal atherosclerotic cardiovascular disease.[46] Patients in the fourth subgroup included those with extracranial cerebrovascular disease (cerebrovascular accident or transient ischemic attacks), coronary artery disease (angina pectoris or myocardial infarction), aneurysmal disease of the abdominal aorta or its branches, and symptomatic peripheral arterial occlusive disease. All patients undergoing surgical intervention in this early University of Michigan experience were failures of previous medical management. However, none was receiving angiotensin converting enzyme inhibitors, which clearly might have rendered some of them normotensive. Surgical therapy was most beneficial in the pediatric and adult fibrodysplastic categories, where 97% and 94% of patients, respectively, were cured or improved. Outcomes were also satisfactory in adults with focal atherosclerotic disease, with 91% being cured or improved. Adults exhibiting clinically overt generalized atherosclerosis had a 72% beneficial response to surgery, but only 25% were cured. It was among this subgroup of patients with widespread atherosclerosis that this series' only surgical mortality existed. Operative deaths did not occur in the other three subgroups.

SUMMARY

Renovascular hypertension, the most common cause of surgically correctable high blood pressure, results from altered renal circulatory hemodynamics causing the release of renin. Renin is produced in the juxtaglomerular apparatus of the kidney and released into the systemic circulation. Renin acts on angiotensinogen, an α_2-globulin produced in the liver, to form the decapeptide, angiotensin I. This latter substance is cleaved of two amino acids by angiotensin converting enzyme to produce angiotensin II. Angiotensin II, an octapeptide, is a potent vasopressor responsible for contraction of vascular smooth muscle, representing the vasoconstrictive component of renovascular hypertension. Indirectly, angiotensin II acts to increase production of aldosterone with subsequent retention of sodium, the latter representing the volume component of renovascular hypertension. This renin-mediated form of hypertension can be altered by several drug interventions, including those diminishing release of renin, blocking the conversion of angiotensin I to angiotensin II, or causing direct relaxation of vascular smooth muscle. However, derangements of renovascular hypertension are best reversed by correction of the altered renal hemodynamics that usually result from renal artery stenosis. Surgical intervention with renal revascularization and percutaneous transluminal angioplasty are presently the most appropriate means to this end.

REFERENCES

1. Tigerstedt R, Bergman PG. Niere und kreislauf. Scand Arch Physiol 8:223, 1898.
2. Fasciolo JC, Houssay BA, Taquini AC. Blood-pressure raising secretion of the ischemic kidney. J Physiol (Lond) 94:281, 1938.
3. Braun-Menendez E, et al. La substancia hipertensora de la sangre del rinon isquemiado. Rev Soc Argent Biol 15:420, 1939.
4. Page IH. On the nature of the pressor action of renin. J Exp Med 70:521, 1939.
5. Page IH, Helmer OM. A crystalline pressor substance (angiotonin) resulting from the reaction between renin and renin-activator. J Exp Med 71:29, 1940.
6. Skeggs LT Jr, et al. Existence of 2 forms of hypertension. J Exp Med 99:275, 1954.
7. Davis JO, Freeman RH. Mechanisms regulating renin release. Physiol Rev 56:1, 1976.
8. Keeton TK, Campbell WB. The pharmacologic alteration of renin release. Pharmacol Rev 31:81, 1981.
9. Peach MJ. Renin-angiotensin system: Biochemistry and mechanisms of action. Physiol Rev 57:313, 1977.
10. Hackentahl E, et al. Morphology, physiology, and molecular biology of renin secretion. Physiol Rev 70:1067, 1990.
11. Krieger JE, Dzau VJ. Molecular biology of hypertension. Hypertens 18(Suppl I):13, 1991.
12. Lynch KR, Peach MJ. Molecular biology of angiotensinogen. Hypertens 17:263, 1991.
13. Morris BJ. Molecular biology of renin. I. Gene and protein structure, synthesis and processing. J Hypertens 10:209, 1992.
14. Morris BJ. Molecular biology of renin. II. Gene control by messenger RNA, transection and transgenic studies. J Hypertens 10:337, 1992.
15. Gifffiths LR, et al. The β subunit of coagulation factor VIII is linked to renin and the Duffy blood group to α-spectrin on human chromosome 1. Hum Hered 39:107, 1989.
16. Hobart PM, et al. Human renin gene: Structure and sequence analysis. Proc Natl Acad Sci USA 81:5026, 1984.
17. Pratt RE, Ouellette AJ, Dzau VJ. Biosynthesis of renin: Multiplicity of active and intermediate forms. Proc Natl Acad Sci USA 80:6809, 1983.
18. Pratt RE, et al. Human renin biosynthesis and secretion in normal and ischemic kidneys. Proc Natl Acad Sci USA 84:7837, 1987.
19. Sealey JE, et al. The physiology of renin secretion in essential hypertension: Estimation of renin secretion rate and renal plasma flow from peripheral and renal vein renin levels. Am J Med 55:391, 1973.
20. Schneider EG, et al. The hepatic metabolism of renin and aldosterone: A review with new observations on the hepatic clearance of renin. Circ Res 26-27(Suppl I):175, 1970.
21. Gaillard-Sanchez I, et al. Assignment by *in situ* hybridization of the angiotensinogen gene to chromosome band 1qr, the same region as the human renin gene. Hum Genet 84:341, 1990.
22. Fukamizu A, et al. Structure and expression of the human angiotensinogen gene. J Biol Chem 265:7576, 1990.
23. Hubert C, et al. Structure of the angiotensin I–converting enzyme gene. J Biol Chem 266:377, 1991.
24. Mattei M-G, et al. Angiotensin-I converting enzyme gene is on chromosome 17. Cytogenet Cell Genet 51:1041, 1989.
25. Stanley JC, Gewertz BL, Fry WJ. Renal:systemic renin indices and renal vein renin ratios as prognostic indicators in remedial renovascular hypertension. J Surg Res 20:149, 1976.
26. Vaughan ED Jr, et al. Renovascular hypertension: Renin measurements to indicate hypersecretion and contralateral suppression, estimate renal plasma flow, and score for surgical curability. Am J Med 55:402, 1973.
27. Goldblatt H, et al. Studies on experimental hypertension. I. The production of persistent elevation of systolic blood pressure by means of renal ischemia. J Exp Med 59:347, 1934.
28. Graham LM, et al. Abdominal aortic coarctation and segmental hypoplasia. Surgery 86:519, 1979.
29. Stanley JC. Morphologic, histologic and clinical characteristics of renovascular fibrodysplasia and arteriosclerosis. In Bergan JJ, Yao JST, eds. Surgery of the Aorta and Its Body Branches. New York: Grune & Stratton, 1979.
30. Stanley JC. Pathologic basis of macrovascular renal artery disease. In Stanley JC, Ernst CB, Fry WJ, eds. Renovascular Hypertension. Philadelphia: WB Saunders, 1984.
31. Stanley JC, et al. Arterial fibrodysplasia: Histopathologic character and current etiologic concepts. Arch Surg 110:551, 1975.
32. Stanley JC, et al. Developmental occlusive disease of the abdominal aorta and the splanchnic and renal arteries. Am J Surg 142:190, 1981.
33. Stanley JC, et al. Pediatric renovascular hypertension: A thirty-year experience of operative treatment. J Vasc Surg 21:212, 1995.
34. Stanley JC, Fry WJ. Renovascular hypertension secondary to arterial fibrodysplasia in adults. Arch Surg 110:992, 1975.

35. Stanley JC, et al. Renal artery aneurysms: Significance of macroaneurysms exclusive of dissections and fibrodysplastic mural dilations. Arch Surg 110:1327, 1975.
36. Sottiurai V, Fry WJ, Stanley JC. Ultrastructure of smooth muscle, myofibroblasts and fibroblasts in human arterial dysplasia. Arch Surg 113:1280, 1978.
37. McNeil BJ, et al. Measures of clinical efficacy: Cost-effectiveness calculations in the diagnosis and treatment of hypertensive renovascular disease. N Engl J Med 293:216, 1975.
38. Bookstein JJ, et al. Pharmacoangiographic manipulation of renal collateral blood flow. Circulation 54:328, 1976.
39. Vidt DG, et al. Surgical treatment of unilateral renal vascular disease: prognostic role of vascular changes in bilateral renal biopsies. Am J Cardiol 30:827, 1972.
40. Prince M, et al. Breath-hold 3D Gadolinium enhanced MR angiography of the abdominal aorta and its major branches. Radiology 197:785, 1995.
41. Hansen KJ, et al. Renal duplex sonography: Evaluation of clinical utility. J Vasc Surg 12:227, 1990.
42. Hoffman U, et al. Role of duplex scanning for the detection of atherosclerotic renal artery disease. Kidney Int 39:1231, 1991.
43. Kohler TR, et al. Noninvasive diagnosis of renal artery stenosis by ultrasonic duplex scanning. J Vasc Surg 4:450, 1968.
44. Stanley JC, Fry WJ. Surgical treatment of renovascular hypertension. Arch Surg 112:1291, 1977.
45. Thornbury JR, Stanley JC, Fryback DG. Hypertensive urogram: A nondiscriminatory test for renovascular hypertension. Am J Roentgenol 138:43, 1982.
46. Stanley JC, et al. Operative therapy of renovascular hypertension. Br J Surg 63(Suppl):S63, 1982.
47. Dean RH, Rhamy RK. Split renal function studies in renovascular hypertension. In Stanley JC, Ernst CB, Fry WJ, eds. Renovascular Hypertension. Philadelphia: WB Saunders, 1984.
48. Hunt JC, Strong CG. Renovascular hypertension: Mechanisms, natural history and treatment. In Laragh JH, ed. Hypertension Manual. New York: Dun-Donnelly, 1975.
49. Vidt DG. Advances in the medical management of renovascular hypertension. Urol Clin North Am 11:417, 1984.
50. Zweifler AJ, Julius S. Medical treatment of renovascular hypertension. In Stanley JC, Ernst CB, Fry WJ, eds. Renovascular Hypertension. Philadelphia: WB Saunders, 1984.
51. Buhler FR, et al. Propranolol inhibition of renin secretion. N Engl J Med 287:1209, 1972.
52. Hricik DE, et al. Captopril-induced renal insufficiency in patients with bilateral renal-artery stenosis or renal-artery stenosis in a solitary kidney. N Engl J Med 308:373, 1983.
53. Gruntzig A, et al. Treatment of renovascular hypertension with percutaneous transluminal dilatation of a renal-artery stenosis. Lancet 1:801, 1978.
54. Martin EC, Diamond NG, Casarella WJ. Percutaneous transluminal angioplasty in nonatherosclerotic disease. Radiology 135:27, 1980.
55. Grim CE, et al. Percutaneous transluminal dilatation in the treatment of renovascular hypertension. Ann Intern Med 95:439, 1981.
56. Sos TA, et al. Percutaneous transluminal renal angioplasty in renovascular hypertension due to atheroma or fibromuscular dysplasia. N Engl J Med 309:274, 1983.
57. Tegtmeyer CJ, Kellum CD, Ayers C. Percutaneous transluminal angioplasty of the renal artery: Results and long-term follow-up. Radiology 153:77, 1984.
58. Canzanello VJ, et al. Percutaneous transluminal renal angioplasty in the management of atherosclerotic renovascular hypertension: Results in 100 patients. Hypertens 13:163, 1989.
59. Klinge J, et al. Percutaneous transluminal renal angioplasty: Initial and long-term results. Radiology 171:S01, 1989.
60. Weibull H, et al. Percutaneous transluminal renal angioplasty versus surgical reconstruction of atherosclerotic renal artery stenosis: A prospective randomized study. J Vasc Surg 18:841, 1993.
61. Stoney RJ, et al. Aortorenal arterial autografts: Long-term assessment. Arch Surg 116:1416, 1981.
62. Stanley JC, Fry WJ. Pediatric renal artery occlusive disease and renovascular hypertension: Etiology, diagnosis, and operative treatment. Arch Surg 116:669, 1981.
63. Stanley JC, Ernst CB, Fry WJ. Fate of 100 aortorenal vein grafts: Characteristics of late graft expansion, aneurysmal dilatation, and stenosis. Surgery 74:931, 1973.
64. Khauli RB, Novick AC, Ziegelbaum M. Splenorenal bypass in the treatment of renal artery stenosis: Experience with sixty-nine cases. J Vasc Surg 2:547, 1985.
65. Moncure AC, et al. Use of the splenic and hepatic arteries for renal revascularization. J Vasc Surg 3:196, 1986.
66. Belzer FO, Raczkowski A. Ex vivo renal artery reconstruction with autotransplantation. Surgery 92:642, 1982.
67. Brekke IB, et al. Fibro-muscular renal artery disease treated by extracorporeal vascular reconstruction and renal autotransplantation: Short- and long-term results. Eur J Vasc Surg 6:471, 1992.
68. Terpstra JL, van Schilfgaarde R, Zwartendijk J. Extracorporeal renal surgery. Neth J Surg 33:165, 1981.
69. Clair DG, et al. Safety and efficacy of transaortic renal endarterectomy as an adjunct to aortic surgery. J Vasc Surg 21:926, 1995.
70. Hansen KJ, et al. Contemporary surgical management of renovascular disease. J Vasc Surg 16:319, 1992.
71. Stoney RJ. Transaortic renal endarterectomy. In Rutherford RB, ed. Vascular Surgery. Philadelphia: WB Saunders, 1984.
72. Stoney RJ, et al. Renal endarterectomy through the transected aorta: A new technique for combined aortorenal atherosclerosis. A preliminary report. J Vasc Surg 9:224, 1983.
73. Stanley JC, et al. Reoperation for complications of renal artery reconstructive surgery undertaken for treatment of renovascular hypertension. J Vasc Surg 2:133, 1985.
74. Stanley JC. The evolution of surgery for renovascular occlusive disease. Cardiovasc Surg 2:195, 1994.
75. Dean RH, Lawson JD, Hollifield JW. Revascularization of the poorly functioning kidney. Surgery 85:44, 1979.
76. Dean RH, et al. The effect of renal vascularization on kidney function. J Surg Res 22:443, 1977.
77. Jamieson GG, et al. Reconstructive renal vascular surgery for chronic renal failure. Br J Surg 71:338, 1984.
78. Whitehouse WM, Jr, et al. Chronic total renal artery occlusions: Effects of treatment on secondary hypertension and renal function. Surgery 89:753, 1981.

PART FIVE

THE CENTRAL AND PERIPHERAL NERVOUS SYSTEMS

47

Altered States of Consciousness

Gage Van Horn and Alan H. Lockwood

The relationships between mind and body have generated intense thought by philosophers and scientists throughout history. In early medical manuscripts, clinical descriptions of unconsciousness following head injuries supported Platonic notions of consciousness and its localization to the head. Descartes attributed consciousness to the pineal gland, but operated from a philosophic rather than an observational base. Franz Joseph Gall's concept that specific mental faculties were attributable to specific brain centers set the stage for the modern era of neurologic investigation that relates structure and function through careful experimentation and observation. Brodmann, who identified and mapped anatomically distinct regions of the cerebral cortex linked subsequently with specific neural functions, and Cajal, who developed the neuronal theory of cerebral function, facilitated this relationship between structure and function.

Surgeons frequently provide care for patients with impaired consciousness. Major surgical procedures require the administration of general anesthesia. Drugs useful in alleviating postoperative pain and potentiating anesthetic agents also affect consciousness and may prolong postoperative lethargy. Surgeons are often the first physicians called on to evaluate unconscious patients, particularly in emergency rooms. Some must serve as the only treating physician for a comatose patient. Successful approaches to the diagnosis and management of patients with altered consciousness necessitate an understanding of the pathophysiologic principles that relate neural structure and function. This chapter deals with those principles.

ANATOMIC AND PHYSIOLOGIC BASIS OF NORMAL CONSCIOUSNESS

In 1949 Moruzzi and Magoun[1] reported that stimuli applied to the reticular formation in the brain stem and the lower diencephalon interrupted high-voltage, slow synchronous EEG activity and replaced it with low-voltage, fast activity. This activation was the same type observed after environmental stimuli such as eye opening and provided evidence for a reticular origin of EEG and behavioral activation. Additional studies led to the conclusion that the neural pathways involved in activation were multisynaptic and depended on the integrity of thalamic projection areas (Fig. 47-1). French and Magoun[2] placed lesions in the reticular formation of monkeys and induced coma that persisted until the animal died or was killed, confirming the importance of the reticular formation in the mediation of consciousness. Clinical and neuropathologic findings from five patients with persistent coma were reported by French[3] in 1952. Three patients had extensive destructive lesions in the reticular formation, a fourth had lesions in the rostral projections of the reticular formation, and the fifth had nearly complete cortical ablation due to presumed tertiary syphilis. French concluded that destruction of the ascending reticular activating system, its rostrally projecting fibers, or the entire cerebral cortex would produce coma. These notions have withstood careful scrutiny by Plum and Posner[4] who reported similar conclusions.

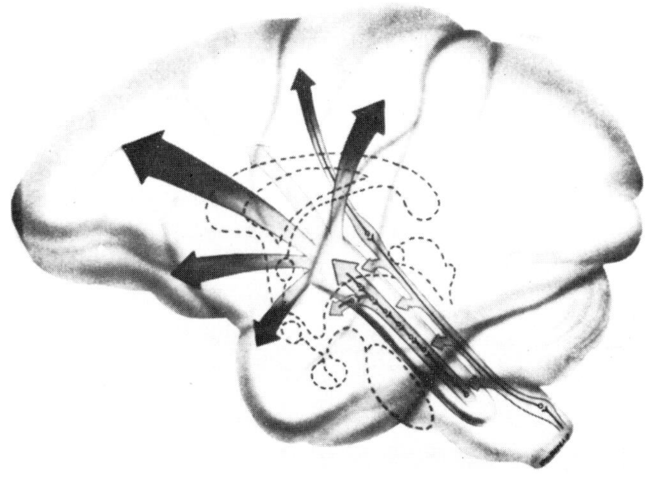

Fig. 47-1. Multisynaptic neural pathway activation *(arrows)* originating in the reticular formation. (From Magoun HW. Brain Mechanisms in Consciousness. Oxford: Blackwell Scientific Publications, 1954.)

Although the reticular formation appears grossly homogeneous, even early microscopic studies by Cajal indicated that the region was anatomically heterogeneous. More recently, combined anatomic and physiologic studies have shown that the reticular formation is the site of origin of neurons that have very large projections and complex neurophysiologic interrelationships.

Neuropharmacologic studies of the reticular formation show additional heterogeneity. Neurons containing norepinephrine, serotonin, dopamine, and enkephalins have been identified by using specific fluorescent techniques, autoradiographic ligand-binding studies, or immunohistochemical stains. Among the catecholaminergic nuclei in the reticular formation, the locus ceruleus has been the most completely described because of its characteristic appearance under the light microscope and because of the large amount of norepinephrine in the neurons. Lesions of the locus ceruleus increase the length of time that animals spend in a quiet but wakeful state.[5] This nuclear group appears to be important in coordinating neural inputs from the environment and viscera and relating them to the rest of the brain.[6]

Although no single homogeneous neuronal group has been identified in the reticular formation as the site of neural activity that determines wakefulness, the notion that this region of the brain stem does in fact control vigilance retains clinical usefulness. The complexities within the reticular formation, demonstrated by the types of studies mentioned previously, make it likely that the region identified by Moruzzi and Magoun[1] is the site where neural interactions determining consciousness have their highest density, either at a synaptic level or because of the physical proximity of neuronal elements. This region is the site where minimum lesions have maximum effects on consciousness.

In humans, both a quantitative and qualitative element of consciousness are recognized. The quantitative aspect, or level of consciousness, can be rated on a continuum between complete alertness through lethargy and stupor to coma and is mediated by the reticular formation. Qualitative consciousness, which includes cognition, memory, language, and special sensory processing, is mediated by regions of the cerebral cortex and their interaction with subcortical, often thalamic, centers. In a clinical setting, an examiner describes the quantitative, on-off aspect of the level of consciousness on the basis of responses to alerting stimuli (such as a spoken word or shout) or in more extreme cases to noxious stimuli. Qualitative aspects of consciousness can be evaluated only in individuals with a quantitative aspect of consciousness that is sufficient to permit interpersonal communication. The mental status examination—tests designed to measure orientation, memory, and cognition—evaluates this qualitative aspect of consciousness and the integrity of cerebral regions mediating the activity.

Although it is usually easy to determine whether or not patients are conscious, there are occasional patients in whom this determination is difficult. Certain patients with severe lower brain stem destructive lesions may be conscious but unable to interact with the environment because of quadriplegia and the inability to move the oral and pharyngeal muscles required for speech. Plum and Posner[4] described these patients as being "locked in" by their neurologic lesions. Akinetic mutism or, more properly, the persistent vegetative state[7] is an increasingly common condition in which the patient gives the appearance of consciousness, possibly by visual tracking, but exhibits no evidence of cognition. This condition may be seen after head injury, cardiopulmonary arrest, or less frequently other causes of nontraumatic coma.

MECHANISMS FOR ALTERED CONSCIOUSNESS

Lesions that affect consciousness do so by destroying, damaging, or interfering with the normal function of the reticular formation or the cerebral cortex. The mechanisms for altered consciousness can be broadly divided into structural vs. metabolic categories. In nearly 400 cases of coma of unknown origin, supratentorial or infratentorial destructive lesions accounted for a little more than 30%, whereas nearly 70% of the patients had metabolic abnormalities such as drug intoxication, infections, or anoxia.[4] Surgeons occasionally attend patients with multiple causes for their coma. Trauma, a common cause of reduced consciousness in a surgical practice, may coexist with a metabolic encephalopathy. The intoxicated alcoholic may have a subdural hematoma, or a metabolic abnormality may cause a driver to lose control of a car, resulting in an injury that may divert attention from an underlying medical problem.

Structural Lesions

Structural lesions alter consciousness by several mechanisms. Relatively small lesions confined to the rostral brain stem produce coma by destroying the reticular formation. Large lesions in the cerebral hemispheres or cerebellum may produce a shift in brain structures, secondarily compressing the reticular formation. Altered consciousness also occurs if sufficiently large amounts of cerebral cortex or underlying white matter are destroyed. The clinical diagnosis of structural lesions depends on the physician's ability to correlate observable neurologic deficits with a knowledge of functional neuroanatomy. For example, coma associated with bilateral complete oculomotor (third) nerve palsies indicates the presence of a lesion in the tegmentum of the midbrain, where third nerve nuclei and the reticular formation juxtapose. A left hemiparesis associated with a dilated, fixed right pupil indicates the presence of a lesion compromising the corticospinal system originating in the right hemisphere and compressing the reticular formation and the third nerve as it passes over the tentorial edge.

Metabolic Disturbances

Metabolic disturbances affect most areas of the brain simultaneously, although specific regions vary in their sensitivity to metabolic insults. The healthy brain has a very high metabolic rate. Representing only 2% of the total body weight, it accounts for nearly 20% of whole-body oxygen consumption and receives between 15% and 20% of the cardiac output. In spite of this high metabolic rate, the brain cannot store energy or energy substrates and is highly sensitive to interruptions in blood and metabolic supplies.

This sensitivity is dramatized in Fig. 47-2, which shows the metabolic consequences following decapitation of adult white mice.[8] Within seconds, adenosine triphosphate (ATP) stores are diminished. Within 1 minute, ATP and glucose are virtually depleted as a result of their continued use without replacement. Metabolic waste in the form of lactate, produced by anaerobic glycolysis, accumulates to high levels producing acidosis and contributing further to brain dysfunction. Clinically, loss of consciousness occurs within seconds of a cardiopulmonary arrest, and permanent brain damage follows within minutes if treatment is unsuccessful.

Altered consciousness is the hallmark of metabolic encephalopathy; but early in the course of an encephalopathy, brain stem function is relatively preserved. Characteristically, the pupils are slightly smaller than normal and constrict in reaction to a bright light stimulus. As consciousness declines, the light reflex becomes sluggish and incomplete. In patients with a profound metabolic coma such as occurs in severe barbiturate intoxication, the pupillary light response may be absent. Hypoxia and certain drugs such as glutethimide and the anticholinergics affect pupillary function out of proportion to the alteration in consciousness. As the depth of coma increases, abnormalities of ocular motility emerge. In stuporous patients, eye movements are often dysconjugate and roving. Alerting stimuli such as deep pain may cause the eye movements to become conjugate. As coma deepens, spontaneous eye movements cease. However, stimuli such as passive head movement or irrigation of the external ear with ice water usually elicit eye movements, providing evidence for the structural integrity of the brain stem.

Although metabolic causes for altered consciousness are common and have been the subject of intense experimentation, important questions regarding underlying mechanisms remain. For example, turtle brain is much more resistant to hypoxia than mammalian brain, the reason for which is unknown. Even though knowledge of mechanisms at the molecular level is absent, metabolic encephalopathies can be classified into three clinically and pathophysiologically relevant categories: (1) deficient or absent metabolic substrate; (2) the presence of endogenous or exogenous toxin; or (3) alteration of the normal internal cerebral milieu.

Substrate Deficiency

During the course of normal brain function, neurons continually depolarize as potassium and sodium move through ion channels. The majority of brain work is exerted in pumping these ions back to sites occupied during polarization. As progressive deficiency of required brain metabolites (usually glucose or oxygen) develops, cerebral blood flow and metabolite extraction increase in an effort to

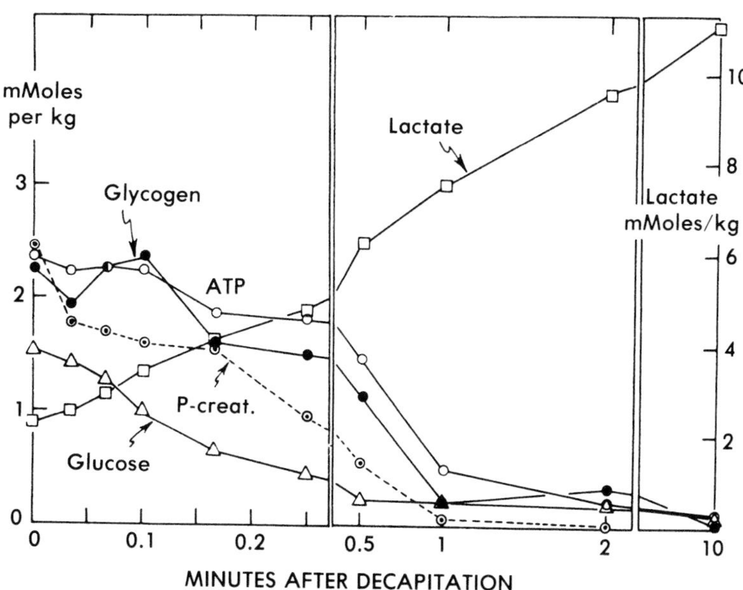

Fig. 47-2. Metabolic consequences of decapitation. *ATP,* Adenosine triphosphate. (From Lowry OH, et al. Effect of ischemia on known substrates and cofactors of the glycolytic pathway in the brain. J Biol Chem 239:24, 1964.)

maintain fuel supplies and preserve brain function. These compensatory measures are incomplete, and measurable decrements in brain performance begin to emerge[9] (Fig. 47-3). Experimental investigations have shown that ATP remains at near-normal levels in comatose animals even during extreme hypoxia, suggesting that the brain has undescribed mechanisms that shut down brain function in an orderly fashion to preserve structural integrity during adverse conditions. At a critical threshold, near an arterial partial pressure of oxygen (Pa_{O_2}) of 20 mm Hg, these mechanisms fail, cardiac arrhythmias develop, cerebral circulation fails, and the metabolic sequence depicted in Fig. 47-2 develops. Thus it is imperative to diagnose hypoxia promptly and to begin appropriate therapy immediately.

Although the brain depends on adequate glucose supplies, the body's resistance to the sudden development of hypoglycemia is greater than the body's resistance to the sudden development of hypoxia. Therefore when compared with anoxia, the diagnosis and treatment of hypoglycemia is not as urgent. However, hypoglycemia cannot be diagnosed reliably on the basis of clinical criteria. Diagnostic delays, even using the most efficient laboratories, may lead to irreversible brain injury. Therefore anyone with an altered level of consciousness, including a delirious patient, should be considered hypoglycemic until proven otherwise. The routine administration of glucose under these circumstances is warranted.

Toxins

Because of the complexity of normal cerebral function, there are innumerable opportunities for toxins, either endogenous or exogenous, to affect brain function. Almost all toxins act by inhibiting normal brain function. Exceptions to this rule include toxins that block neural inhibitory pathways, such as bicuculine blockade of the inhibitory neurotransmitter γ-aminobutyric acid, which produces epileptic seizures. Several principles of toxin action emerge: (1) the actions of specific-function toxins including neurotransmitter blocking agents; (2) pathophysiologic mechanisms that depend on the production of a common toxin such as ammonia; and (3) production of common physical signs by seemingly unrelated toxins such as the hyperventilation seen in patients with salicylate intoxication, hyperammonemia, or acidosis.

Drugs affecting the brain often work by influencing a specific cerebral process. Antipsychotic agents that bind to

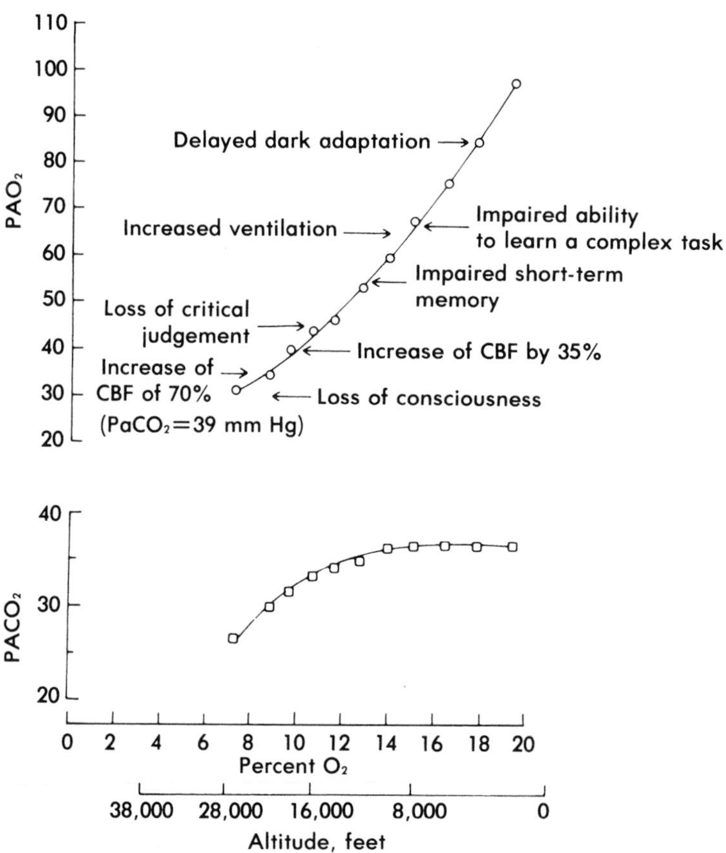

Fig. 47-3. Progression of neurologic abnormalities observed during increasing hypoxia. *CBF,* Cerebral blood flow; *Pa_{CO_2},* partial pressure of arterial carbon dioxide; *Pa_{O_2},* partial pressure of arterial oxygen. (From Siesjo BK. Brain dysfunction in cerebral hypoxia and ischemia. In Plum, ed. Brain Dysfunction in Metabolic Disorders. New York: Raven Press, 1974.)

dopaminergic postsynaptic sites in the brain striatum produce clinical signs similar to those seen in dopamine deficiency states or Parkinson's disease. Organophosphates affect brain function by interfering with cholinergic neurotransmission. However, the majority of toxins act through unknown mechanisms.

Hyperammonemia in patients with cirrhosis of the liver is an excellent example of a toxin with an action not yet explained at the molecular level. Gastrointestinal hemorrhage in patients with cirrhosis often produces hepatic encephalopathy, making ammonia intoxication an important clinical problem in a surgical practice. Because ammonia is the final product in the catabolism of a variety of nitrogenous compounds, hyperammonemia occurs in a wide variety of seemingly unrelated metabolic problems.[10] In susceptible patients, valproic acid administration depletes mitochondrial acetyl-coenzyme A, which may in part explain the development of symptomatic hyperammonemia. Bacterial infections of ileal conduits produce symptomatic hyperammonemia through the action of urease, and hyperammonemia develops in association with hypercapnia.

Although most toxins are respiratory depressants, hyperventilation occurs in salicylate poisoning, hyperammonemia, and metabolic acidoses such as diabetic ketoacidosis. Hyperventilation is a physiologically normal response to acid stimulation of the medullary respiratory centers. Ammonia and salicylates act as irritant stimulators of the respiratory control systems.[4]

Altered Internal Milieu

In addition to constant supplies of oxygen and glucose, the brain depends on a normal internal environment for optimum function. Regulatory mechanisms in the brain maintain water, electrolyte, and acid-base balance within very narrow tolerance levels. Water metabolism is regulated by complex interactions between thirst-mediating neurons located in the hypothalamus adjacent to the supraoptic nuclei and antidiuretic hormone (ADH) production. Ordinarily, small increases in osmolarity result in thirst, an increase in water consumption, and ADH release. Excess water produces dilute urine as ADH levels fall and thirst is abolished.

During water intoxication or uncontrolled water loss with dehydration, water molecules move freely across the blood-brain barrier toward the compartment with the highest solute concentration. In dehydration, water leaves and the brain shrinks. During water excess, water enters and the brain swells. Altered brain water content causes brain dysfunction probably through distortions of brain volume. A shrinking brain tears veins bridging the space between the cortex and the dural sinuses, sometimes producing subdural hematomas; a swelling brain compresses the reticular formation. The brain stands virtually defenseless against sudden dramatic changes in water content. However, large osmotic changes that develop over long periods of time are relatively well tolerated. The brain produces osmotically active particles in the form of amino acids that help the brain retain its water and hence its volume during hyperosmolar states.[11] During conditions of water excess, the brain ejects potassium ions, causing it to lose water, maintaining an almost normal volume.[12] It is therefore quite possible for severe abnormalities in osmolarity to produce few symptoms if the abnormalities develop slowly.

Just as the rapid development of hyperosmolarity or hypo-osmolarity is dangerous to brain function, so too is rapid correction of a relatively asymptomatic, long-standing osmotic abnormality. Under these conditions the restoration of normal osmolarity must be done with caution to avoid iatrogenic water intoxication or dehydration.

PATHOPHYSIOLOGIC BASIS UNDERLYING THE SIGNS AND SYMPTOMS IN PATIENTS WITH ALTERED CONSCIOUSNESS

A great deal of emphasis should be placed on the bedside physical examination in determining the cause of diminished consciousness.[13] Such an examination is occasionally exceeded in importance by taking an accurate history, something not always available during the initial evaluation, but it can never be replaced by a screening battery of laboratory tests. The following should be evaluated:

Level of consciousness
Respirations
Pupils
Extraocular muscle function
Motor system function

A careful analysis of the abnormalities found in these systems nearly always localizes the anatomic lesions responsible for coma (Table 47-1). In some instances the constellation of findings allows a precise diagnosis. In others a narrowed list of differential diagnoses emerges. The systems listed are intimately related and affected to some degree in every comatose patient. In addition, the tests involving these systems do not require patient cooperation (i.e., they can easily be performed on the unconscious patient).

Level of Consciousness

The physiology and pathophysiology of consciousness have been discussed earlier in the chapter. Recording an accurate description of the patient's level of consciousness provides subsequent evaluators a basis for determining clinical improvement or deterioration. We have frequently been asked to evaluate patients whose consciousness had been impaired for days but whose charts contained no description of those levels of reduced consciousness.

Observation is the first step in determining the patient's level of consciousness. One should note what the patient does when unstimulated. Is the patient vigilant, bewildered, hallucinating, conversant, garrulous? For conscious patients a few direct questions, the answers to which require some cerebral function, may be sufficient to ascertain the level of consciousness. In other cases a more detailed mental status examination is necessary to pinpoint minor

Table 47-1. Typical Syndromes of Altered Consciousness

Syndromes	Consciousness	Respirations	Pupils	Extraocular Muscle Function	Motor Function
Early metabolic or diffuse encephalopathy	Lethargy or delirium	Eupnea or posthyperventilation apnea	Equal, sluggishly light-reactive; pinpoint if opiates are cause of encephalopathy	Spontaneously roving; conjugate or disconjugate; extraocular movements full to reflex testing	Bilateral paratonia; ± bilateral upgoing toes; no asymmetry
Late metabolic or diffuse encephalopathy	Stupor to coma	Hypopnea to apnea; hyperventilation if acidotic	Small; may be unreactive	Directed straight ahead; fixed or very sluggish to extraocular reflexes	Flaccidity; no toe signs or bilateral upgoing toes
Large lateralized supratentorial lesion with early uncal herniation and early-to-late diencephalic dysfunction	Lethargy to stupor	Eupnea to Cheyne-Stokes respirations	Ipsilateral dilated and light-fixed	Ipsilateral oculomotor palsy; eyes may be conjugately deviated to side of lesion but move past midline with extraocular reflexes	Contralateral hemiparesis or hemiplegia; contralateral decorticate or decerebrate posturing; ipsilateral decorticate posturing or purposeful movement; contra ± ipsilateral upgoing toes
Large paramidline supratentorial lesion with early central transtentorial herniation and upper brain stem dysfunction	Stupor to coma	Cheyne-Stokes respirations	Midposition, usually symmetric and light-fixed	Eyes may be deviated to side of lesion or downward; may be fixed to extraocular reflexes	Contralateral decerebrate and ipsilateral decorticate posturing or bilateral decerebrate or decorticate posturing
Supratentorial lesion with advanced transtentorial herniation and pontine dysfunction	Coma	Sustained tachypnea with hypocapnia	Midposition and light-fixed	Eyes are directed straight ahead and fixed to extraocular reflexes	Bilateral decerebrate posturing or flaccidity with bilateral upgoing toes
Large intrinsic brain stem lesion affecting pontine base and tegmentum	Coma	Sustained tachypnea with hypocapnia	Equal; near pinpoint but light-reactive with magnification	Eyes are directed straight ahead and fixed to extraocular reflexes	Flaccidity with bilateral upgoing or mute toes; no posturing
Extrinsic subtentorial lesion with pontine or medullary compression	Lethargy to stupor	Eupneic (early) to ataxic or apneustic (late)	Ipsilateral Horner's syndrome; light-reactive	Usually disconjugate with ipsilateral sixth nerve palsy	Contralateral upgoing toe or bilateral upgoing toes without posturing

abnormalities in thought content. For the unconscious patient the examiner should first call the patient's name. If this action fails to alert the patient, the examiner can then try shaking the bed or the patient's shoulder in conjunction with repeating the patient's name more firmly. If the patient appears to be comatose, a painful stimulus delivered near the midline is often required to find the highest level of arousal. Stimulating distally in the extremities (e.g., nail bed pressure) is best suited for demonstrating spinal withdrawal reflexes but may be ineffective in arousing patients.

The words commonly used to describe various levels of consciousness are defined in the box on p. 941. These definitions are imprecise, and some terms have multiple meanings.[4,13,14] In general, the level of consciousness is best described by indicating the patient's reaction to stimuli.

Some examples of good descriptions of states of consciousness follow:

"This patient is fully conscious, alert, oriented, and cognizant."

"This patient was found to be lethargic. When unstimulated for several minutes, she would lapse off to sleep from which she could be aroused by firmly calling her name. When awakened, she appeared dull, inattentive, inactive, and indifferent."

"This patient was deeply comatose. A midline painful stimulus produced bilateral decerebrate posturing but no arousal."

Patterns of Abnormal Respiration

Several distinct respiratory patterns occur in patients with reduced consciousness.[4] In most cases these patterns can only be generated by structural lesions highly localized in the brain stem. However, both structural and metabolic abnormalities, sometimes acting in concert, induce altered respirations. In many cases information from arterial blood gas determinations must be integrated with bedside observations to pinpoint the cause of abnormal respiratory patterns. Before attempting to arouse the unconscious patient, examiners should note the rate, depth, and regularity of respirations. Any changes that occur with the application of stimulation should also be noted.

The brain stem respiratory centers reside in the reticular areas from the mid-pons to the caudal medulla. These centers receive input from higher cortical centers (forebrain), peripheral oxygen chemoreceptors in the great vessels, pH receptors near the ventral medullary surface, and stretch and irritant receptors in the upper and lower respiratory tracts. A comprehensive review of the neural regulation of respiration was published in 1977.[15] The influence of the neocortex on brain stem respiratory centers is maximum in the conscious patient but is present to a lesser degree in the obtunded.

Posthyperventilation apnea occurs in conscious patients with diffuse metabolic or structural hemispheric disease.[4] It can be induced by having the patient voluntarily hyperventilate for 30 seconds to 1 minute. In healthy patients, regular breathing resumes with no more than a 12-second delay after hyperventilation. In impaired individuals, usually those with diffuse or metabolic encephalopathies, there may be a prolonged period of apnea (up to 30 seconds) following hyperventilation. Most investigators believe that reduced forebrain input to brain stem respiratory centers underlies posthyperventilation apnea.

Periodic breathing in which hyperpnea regularly alternates with apnea describes *Cheyne-Stokes respiration (CSR)*.[4] A smooth crescendo and decrescendo occurs in most patients, with the hyperpneic period lasting longer than the apneic phase. In CSR there is an exaggerated sensitivity to changes in arterial partial pressure of carbon dioxide ($Paco_2$). With elevated $Paco_2$, an increased ventilatory response ensues with a 30- to 40-second period of hyperpnea. The hyperpnea produces a reduced $Paco_2$ that leads to posthyperventilation apnea. During apnea, carbon dioxide reaccumulates, and the cycle repeats. The common denominator for most patients with CSR appears to be intact lower brain stem respiratory centers that have been deprived of forebrain influences, analogous to the

LEVELS OF CONSCIOUSNESS

Consciousness

From Latin—literally means the ability to know. A normally conscious person is fully aware of self and environment (i.e., responds to stimuli with critical awareness).

Coma

From Greek—deep sleep; the opposite of consciousness; a state of profound unconsciousness from which the patient cannot be aroused. Patients with coma may respond reflexly to painful stimuli by posturing or withdrawing an extremity (brain stem or spinal reflexes), but there is not psychologic response that indicates cerebral cortical function.

Stupor

From Latin—to be benumbed, astonished, stupified; as used by neurologists, a state of deep unconsciousness from which the patient can be aroused only by continuous, vigorous stimulation. When the stimulus ceases, the patient lapses back into unconsciousness. In this context, stupor implies diffuse organic neurologic disease.

Confusion

From Latin—indicates a condition marked by disorder, disarray, uncertainty, and indecisiveness. Although this word conveys some meaning, it is not precise and cannot be used to denote a level of consciousness.

Delirium

From Latin—to be crazy; a transient mental disturbance that is characterized by confusion, disorientation, disordered speech, restlessness, excitement, and often delusions and hallucinations. It is seen in drug or alcohol withdrawal states, with high fever, and in many encephalopathies caused by trauma, seizures, and anoxia. Delirium always indicates organic disturbance.

Lethargy

From Greek—forgetfulness; a state marked by abnormal or morbid drowsiness. Neurologists use this term to denote a state of indifference, inactivity, inattentiveness, sluggishness, and apathy from which the patient may lapse into unconsciousness when there is infrequent stimulation. Obtundation implies a more profound degree of lethargy.

Sleep

A natural, regular suspension of consciousness from which the patient can be easily aroused. *Hypersomnia* is an excess of apparently normal sleep that is distinguishable from lethargy only by the increased level of cognition during arousal.

hyperactive tendon reflexes seen in patients with corticospinal tract disease. Structural lesions of both hemispheres or upper brain stem and diffuse metabolic dysfunction can produce CSR.[16,17] In patients with a supratentorial mass lesion, the development of CSR suggests transtentorial herniation.

Structural lesions in the rostral brain stem tegmentum sometimes produce sustained, rapid hyperpnea and hypocapnia, a condition formerly called *central neurogenic hyperventilation*.[4] Additionally, lesions in this same area often induce coma. Sustained hypocapneic hyperpnea occurs commonly in comatose patients with supratentorial mass lesions and advanced transtentorial herniation. Hyperventilation of this sort, sometimes called "central reflex hyperpnea," also occurs in patients with meningitis, subarachnoid hemorrhage, and some metabolic encephalopathies such as hepatic coma. The diagnosis of central neurogenic hyperventilation requires a normal to elevated arterial partial pressure of oxygen $Pa{O_2}$, a reduced $Pa{CO_2}$, a normal-to-basic cerebrospinal fluid pH, and no evidence of subarachnoid hemorrhage or central nervous system infection. In recent years the central origin of this respiratory pattern has been questioned. Most comatose, brain stem–injured patients with tachypnea and hypocapnia do not meet all the criteria for central neurogenic hyperventilation, since few have a normal-to-elevated $Pa{O_2}$ and most have some lung congestion. Despite the unclear mechanism, sustained tachypneic hypocapnia in comatose patients with near-normal $Pa{O_2}$ suggests structural upper brain stem disease and a poor prognosis.

Apneustic breathing is characterized by a prolonged inspiratory phase with a pause at full inspiration. This respiratory pattern occurs in patients with structural lesions affecting the respiratory centers in the middle to lower pons. Apneusis is seen most commonly in patients with pontine infarction.

Compression or structural lesions of the medulla sometimes produce the rare patterns of *ataxic* or *cluster breathing.* These respiratory patterns have localizing value but occur uncommonly in comatose patients. Patients with ataxic, cluster, and apneustic respirations almost always use hypoxia as the stimulus to breathe and are insensitive to changes in carbon dioxide. Administration of oxygen to such patients sometimes produces apnea.

Pupils

Sympathetic and parasympathetic pathways essential to pupillary function course through the upper brain stem in juxtaposition to areas necessary for maintenance of consciousness. Therefore examination of the pupils is a crucial part of the evaluation in comatose patients.[4,13,14] The examination is simple and should begin with observation for size, equality, and regularity in ambient light. Second, a strong, concentrated light should be directed into first one and then the other eye, observing the response of both pupils simultaneously. If there is a question of light reactivity, magnification should be used and/or ambient light should be reduced.

The pupillary light reflex traverses a multisynaptic neuronal pathway from the retinas through the chiasm, optic tracts, pretectal nuclei, posterior commissure, Edinger-Westphal nuclei, and ciliary ganglia to the postganglionic fibers ending in the sphincter pupillae.[18-20] This neuronal pathway crosses the midline in at least two places, the chiasm and posterior commissure, so that unilateral interruption of the pathway abolishes the pupillary light reflex unilaterally only when that interruption is distal to the Edinger-Westphal nuclei. More proximal interruption, unless it occurs bilaterally, does not affect the light reflex. Parasympathetic pupillary fibers traveling in the peripheral oculomotor nerve are eccentric and particularly vulnerable to compression by an aneurysm or a herniating uncus. If third-nerve fibers are unilaterally interrupted in the presence of an intact brain stem, sparing the pupillary sympathetic system, the pupil becomes widely dilated and light fixed.

Sympathetic fibers mediating pupillary dilation originate primarily in the hypothalamus.[19,20] These fibers descend laterally in the brain stem tegmentum and cervical spinal cord to synapse with preganglionic neurons in the intermediolateral column of the upper three thoracic cord segments. The preganglionic fibers exit the cord, ascend in the sympathetic chain, and synapse with postganglionic neurons in the superior cervical ganglion. Postganglionic fibers travel along with the internal carotid artery, the ophthalmic branch of the trigeminal (V) nerve, and the nasociliary nerve to reach the pupillodilator muscle. This pathway is largely uncrossed so that unilateral interruption, presuming intact parasympathetic fibers, causes ipsilateral pupillary constriction (Horner's syndrome).[20] The integrity of this lateralized pathway can be tested by pinching one side of the patient's face or neck, which should produce ipsilateral pupillary dilation (ciliospinal reflex).[21] In this reflex, afferent pain fibers synapse with the descending sympathetic pathway at the cervical cord, medullary, and pontine levels.

Pupillary abnormalities have reliable localizing value in the comatose patient. Examples include the following:

1. *Diffuse or metabolic encephalopathies* commonly produce equal pupils that are sluggishly light reactive. Narcotics excite preganglionic parasympathetic pathways so that coma produced by narcotic overdose is accompanied by very small (pinpoint) but light-reactive pupils.
2. *Hypothalamic damage* produces ipsilateral pupillary constriction, narrowing of the palpebral fissure, and anhidrosis involving the entire body (not just the face as would be the case if the Horner's syndrome were caused by a more peripheral lesion).[20]
3. *Midbrain lesions* provide precise localization because both sympathetic and parasympathetic fibers are often destroyed, causing midposition (4 to 5 mm), light-fixed pupils.[4]
4. *Large pontine lesions* frequently compromise descending sympathetic fibers, yielding very small or pinpoint, light-reactive pupils.

5. *Uncal herniation,* produced by large hemispheric catastrophes such as a hypertensive hemorrhage, frequently entraps the ipsilateral oculomotor nerve, producing a widely dilated, light-fixed pupil.

Extraocular Movements

The neural pathways necessary for extraocular muscle function also lie adjacent to areas important for consciousness.[18,22] Therefore patients with altered consciousness frequently have abnormalities in extraocular muscle function. The pathways described in the following paragraphs are complex and incompletely understood but fortunately can be simplified for lesion localization.

Examination of the patient's extraocular muscle function includes both observation and reflex movements (extraocular reflexes). The eyelids and then the eye position with the eyelids lifted should be noted. Are the eyes conjugate? Do they move spontaneously? What is their position? Horizontal and vertical eye movements can be induced by either passive head turning (oculocephalic reflexes, doll's eye movements) or caloric stimulation (oculovestibular reflexes). In the unconscious patient with intact brain stem function, passive head rotation induces conjugate eye deviation opposite the direction of the head rotation. Flexing and extending the head produces conjugate vertical movements opposite the direction of head movement. Cold-water stimulation of the unconscious, supine patient whose head is elevated approximately 30 degrees above the horizontal level and whose brain stem function is intact induces conjugate horizontal deviation of the eyes toward the stimulated side. Bilateral cold-water stimulation induces conjugate downward movement; bilateral warm-water stimulation evokes conjugate upward deviation.[4]

Voluntary eye movements begin in the "frontal gaze" or "frontal eye" centers (Brodmann's area 8). Parieto-occipital areas subserve pursuit, but these areas are not as important as the frontal centers when evaluating the unconscious patient. Information coming from the frontal centers travels in axons through the internal capsule and upper brain stem with other corticobulbar fibers. These fibers cross the midline in the upper pons and synapse with neurons in the contralateral pontine paramedian reticular formation. From there, axons branch to the adjacent abducens nucleus or pass through that nucleus, cross the midline, and travel up the medial longitudinal fasciculus to the contralateral oculomotor nucleus. These pathways can be sorted by remembering that stimulation of one frontal gaze center, such as might occur during focal seizures, drives both eyes to the opposite side or away from the stimulated gaze center.

The supranuclear pathways for vertical gaze are less well understood. Those fibers controlling vertical eye movements from the frontal gaze fields presumably descend with the fibers controlling horizontal gaze. Important centers for vertical gaze are thought to be located in the pretectal region near the posterior commissure because vertical eye movements can be abolished by selective lesions in this region.[19] From the pretectal area, fibers descend via the medial longitudinal fasciculus to the oculomotor and trochlear nuclei.

Mediated through the vestibular nuclei, the oculocephalic (passive head turning) and oculovestibular (caloric) reflexes depend on intact connections from the pontine paramedian reticular formation to the extraocular muscle nuclei via the medial longitudinal fasciculus. In the oculocephalic reflex, afferent information comes from the horizontal semicircular canals, as well as proprioceptive fibers in cervical muscles. Afferent stimulation in the oculovestibular reflex originates in the horizontal semicircular canals. These extraocular reflexes are important primarily in demonstrating the intactness of all the brain stem structures involved. If in a comatose patient the extraocular movements are full in response to passive head turning or to caloric stimulation, one can safely conclude that a structural brain stem lesion is not producing the coma.

The following guidelines are helpful in localizing lesions within the brain based on determination of extraocular muscle function:

1. Unconscious patients with *diffuse or metabolic encephalopathies* and structurally intact brain stems have random eye movements that are usually conjugate.[4] One must observe random eye movements for several seconds to be certain of their presence and to be sure that the mean direction is straight ahead. Patients with diffuse encephalopathies initially have intact extraocular (oculocephalic and oculovestibular) reflexes. As coma deepens, the random movements decrease or stop, and the extraocular reflexes disappear.
2. *Large, acute, destructive lesions in one hemisphere* affecting the frontal gaze center or fibers projecting from this center produce conjugate deviation of the eyes toward the side of the lesion and away from the associated hemiparesis. This deviation is most marked in the first few hours after insult and then diminishes gradually. Within 3 to 4 days the patient's eyes are usually midline, even though the associated neurologic signs may be unchanged. In the acute stages of a large hemispheric lesion, moving the patient's eyes past the midline should be possible using the extraocular reflexes. After 1 to 2 days the eyes can be moved fully to the "paretic" side with reflex stimulation. Large, destructive hemispheric lesions are the most common cause of tonic, conjugate eye deviation in unconscious patients. Irritative lesions producing partial epilepsy may stimulate the frontal gaze centers and drive the eyes away from the side of the lesion. In most cases, however, epilepsy that produces coma is obvious because of associated clonic or tonic movements or because of clonic movements of the eyes.
3. *Acute unilateral lesions in the pontine tegmentum* affecting one pontine paramedian reticular formation also produce tonic deviation of the eyes. In this relatively uncommon situation the eyes deviate away from the

side of the lesion and cannot be moved to the midline by vigorous oculocephalic or oculovestibular stimulation.

4. *Large bilateral pontine tegmental lesions* affecting the pontine paramedian reticular formation produce eyes that are directed straight ahead and fixed to extraocular reflexes.
5. *Lesions compressing the brain stem tectum* such as a pineal tumor or thalamic hematoma usually affect the midline center for upward conjugate gaze and produce tonic downward deviation of both eyes. Tectal lesions may abolish vertical extraocular reflexes.

Motor Function

An examination of the motor system provides valuable localizing information even though motor tracts are not necessarily adjacent to centers regulating consciousness. The signs and symptoms of motor dysfunction can be divided into two separate groups: (1) loss of function and (2) release phenomena. Hemiparesis is an example of the former, whereas decerebrate rigidity is an example of the latter. Release phenomena are relatively more important in the comatose patient. The previously considered neural systems occupy little volume in the central nervous system. By comparison, the motor system, which includes the precentral frontal cortex, motor association areas, basal ganglia, cerebellum, corticospinal tracts, and all the interconnecting pathways, is enormous. Our knowledge of motor system physiology and pathophysiology comes from carefully observed clinicopathologic correlations, ablation experiments in animals and man, and stimulation experiments.[23]

Voluntary movements originate in the frontal cortex along the central sulcus (Brodmann's area 4). The most direct pathway to the anterior horn cell is through the corticospinal tract, which courses through the internal capsule, cerebral peduncles, pontine base, pyramid, and the anterior and lateral columns of the spinal cord. Numerous feedback loops modify this system at all levels. Anterior horn cells are constantly bombarded by input from a variety of sources, including muscle spindle and cutaneous afferent fibers. The cerebellar, basal ganglia, brain stem reticular, vestibular, and proprioceptive systems modify either corticospinal activity or the motoneurons directly. Through selective destruction of these subsystems or, more properly, the release of some systems to act unchecked, the various motor syndromes are produced.

Emphasis should be placed on observation, resistance to passive motion, and reflex phenomena. Spontaneous movements or the lack thereof must be noted. Many observations about motor responses are made when the physician applies a painful midline stimulus to assess the level of consciousness. Those phenomena that are commonly observed in unconscious patients include purposeful movements toward the stimulus, decorticate posturing, decerebrate posturing, asymmetric signs such as unilateral flaccidity, and no response at all. One or two joints of each limb should be moved through a full range of motion to assess tone. The tendon reflexes and plantar responses should be elicited.

Those signs that have localizing value include the following.

Paratonia

Paratonia, or *gegenhalten,* is defined as a relatively constant increase in tone in both flexion and extension as if the patient were voluntarily resisting all movements.[4] This abnormality is seen frequently in elderly, demented patients. Paratonia is differentiated from the rigidity seen in patients with Parkinson's disease, where rigidity is usually associated with "cogwheeling." Paratonia usually indicates diffuse cerebral dysfunction such as a metabolic encephalopathy.

Decorticate Rigidity

Decorticate rigidity occurs spontaneously or in response to stimuli. It is defined as flexion at the wrist, fingers, thumb, and elbow with adduction at the shoulder and extension at the hip and knee.[23] This posturing mimics that of the chronic hemiplegic, is seen with lesions rostral to the midbrain, and implies a relatively intact brain stem. Decorticate posturing is frequently unilateral and may be accompanied by purposeful movements, decorticate rigidity, or decerebrate posturing in the opposite extremities.

Decerebrate Posturing

Decerebrate posturing may also occur spontaneously but is more frequently observed following a noxious midline stimulus.[4] In the fullest expression, decerebrate posturing includes internal rotation and adduction at the shoulders, opisthotonos (extreme extension of the spine), and contraction of all antigravity muscles in the extremities. Decerebrate posturing differs from decorticate posturing mainly in the upper extremities, where extension replaces flexion. Incomplete responses are common, even with administration of intensely noxious stimuli, and include extension of the spine, internal rotation of the arm, or extension at the wrist. In experimental animals, decerebrate rigidity is produced by transecting the midbrain at the midcollicular level, leaving intact the reticulospinal, vestibulospinal, and cerebellospinal influences on spinal cord motoneurons. In humans the level of dysfunction producing decerebration is at least localized to the rostral brain stem.[24] The common causes of decerebrate posturing are (1) massive hemispheric lesions such as head trauma or large hematomas producing downward transtentorial herniation; (2) large posterior fossa lesions with upward transtentorial herniation; and (3) severe metabolic disturbances such as hepatic coma. Decerebrate posturing is an important clinical sign in patients with expanding supratentorial lesions such as subdural hematoma and implies transtentorial herniation.

Flaccidity

Flaccidity (absence of tone) indicates dysfunction at the pontomedullary levels. Lesions such as pontine hematomas or large pontomedullary infarcts frequently cause this response. Flaccidity is also seen in patients with acute spinal cord transections ("spinal shock"), diffuse motor-unit dysfunction (muscle relaxants such as curare), and severe metabolic disturbances such as profound barbiturate intoxication.

LABORATORY EVALUATION

The laboratory evaluation of patients with reduced consciousness helps to confirm or establish an etiology already suspected clinically. The laboratory evaluations considered useful follow:

1. Blood: Complete blood count, blood urea nitrogen, glucose, sodium, potassium, calcium, magnesium, liver function, arterial blood gases, and toxicology screen
2. Urine/gastric contents: Toxicology screen
3. CT of brain
4. EEG
5. Lumbar puncture
6. Cerebral angiography

Each test should be ordered for a specific indication. None of the tests, alone or in combination, is intended to replace the bedside evaluation.

Blood Tests

A battery of blood tests (including a complete blood count, blood urea nitrogen, glucose, serum electrolytes, liver function, and arterial blood gases) should be performed in most comatose patients. This battery screens for the common metabolic encephalopathies. Since many of these blood tests are repeated throughout the course of management, this initial set also serves as a baseline. Although the etiologic agent causing drug-induced coma can usually be deduced from historical data, most physicians order a toxicology screen of blood, urine, and gastric contents in patients with apparent diffuse or metabolic encephalopathies. Quantitative determinations such as serum barbiturate levels are indicated, depending on the degree of suspicion. It would not be cost effective, for example, to order expensive quantitative toxicology determinations in patients with obvious structural brain disease.

Computed Tomography

CT has emerged as the major screening procedure for structural brain abnormalities in patients with the recent onset of reduced consciousness. CT, which revolutionized the practice of neurology in the 1970s, images tissue radiodensity.[25] Small differences in x-ray absorption exist between cerebrospinal fluid, white matter, gray matter, and most central nervous system structural lesions such as tumor or infarct. Much larger differences exist between brain, air, blood, and calcified material. In most institutions CT is done before and after the intravenous administration of an iodinated contrast agent. Such administration results in a substantial iodine level in the extracellular space of lesions that have an impaired blood-brain barrier. Thus contrast enhancement causes many focal lesions to "light up." Almost all supratentorial and infratentorial lesions large enough to cause coma can be visualized by late-generation scanners. CT is particularly useful in visualizing intracerebral hematomas, subarachnoid hemorrhage, subdural hematomas or empyemas, cerebral tumors, and cerebral edema. Cerebral infarcts may be difficult to visualize in the first 2 to 3 days, but the diagnosis of an infarct can usually be made on clinical grounds, particularly if a hematoma is excluded by CT. In most cases CT obviates the need for more invasive brain examinations such as angiography. CT therefore is probably the most important laboratory investigation to use in patients with coma and should be performed early in the course of the investigation.

Electroencephalography

An EEG is a voltage vs. time graph composed of 16 or more parallel, complex lines. Each line represents the activity in one channel (i.e., from one amplifier). At a single point in time the activity in any one channel is simply the potential difference between two scalp electrodes. Waves recorded from the scalp represent summated synaptic potentials from cells near the cortical surface.[26] Electrode pairs are systematically arranged in groups (montages), producing a topographic array of cortical surface electric activity. EEG is most useful in confirming the clinical diagnosis of a seizure disorder. However, the examination has some usefulness in patients with reduced consciousness. EEG provides an indirect measure of cerebral function and response to stimulation and as such provides proof of an organic encephalopathy. The only way to establish the diagnosis of nonconvulsive status epilepticus is through the use of EEG. EEG is an aid in determining cerebral death and may provide prognostic information in patients with a severe encephalopathy.[22,27] Patients with little or no EEG response to noxious midline stimuli have a very poor prognosis regardless of the cause of the encephalopathy. Generalized triphasic waves occur in EEGs of patients with hepatic and other metabolic encephalopathies. Periodic sharp-wave discharges dominate the EEGs of patients with viral encephalitides such as herpes simplex encephalitis. In summary, EEG has some usefulness in the diagnosis of patients with coma, particularly in those with diffuse encephalopathies, but it is not a routine test to be ordered without forethought. In most cases a competent electroencephalographer can aid the clinician in deciding whether the EEG will be useful in any particular patient.

Lumbar Puncture

A lumbar puncture provides the clinician with the cellular and chemical construct of the cerebrospinal fluid and a crude measure of the cerebrospinal fluid but not necessarily intracranial pressure.[28,29] The two diagnoses that can be confirmed with confidence using lumbar puncture are meningitis and subarachnoid hemorrhage. Therefore the two major indications for a lumbar puncture in patients with reduced consciousness are evidence of meningeal inflammation and an unexplained elevated temperature. Most patients with coma of unknown cause eventually require a lumbar puncture to exclude a covert infection. It is important to realize that the lumbar puncture is invasive and can be deleterious or fatal to patients with intracranial herniation syndromes. Absolute contraindications to a lumbar puncture include evidence of uncal herniation (ipsilateral oculomotor palsy and contralateral hemiparesis), tonsillar herniation (rigid head tilt or neck retraction), or central transtentorial herniation (midposition light-fixed pupils, CSR, and decerebrate posturing). Relative contraindications include coagulation defects, papilledema, or suspected mass lesions. In these conditions the risk of a lumbar puncture must be carefully weighed against the possible information to be gained.[29] Most clinicians avoid performing lumbar punctures in patients with focal neurologic signs. Prudence dictates that physicians obtain a brain CT before performing a lumbar puncture in any unconscious patient. Of course, it is inexcusable to miss a treatable purulent meningitis or subarachnoid hemorrhage because of fears of doing a lumbar puncture. Comfort is derived from the fact that, other than the elderly or immunosuppressed, most adult patients with meningeal irritation have clear meningeal signs.

Magnetic Resonance Imaging

MRI, currently the most sophisticated structural imaging procedure for brain, depends on the detection of electromagnetic energy released by the nuclei of atoms after perturbations in very strong, controlled magnetic fields.[30] MRI images related to the behavior of protons are now available in most communities and can be used to detect plaques in multiple sclerosis and intraluminal blood flow in moderately sized blood vessels. MRI also allows physicians to better visualize brain vasculitis, low-grade tumors such as gliomas, multiple small infarcts, large acute cerebral infarcts within 24 hours of the onset, blood products, and areas of brain adjacent to bone. It is not necessary to understand the complicated physics of MRI to appreciate the superior imaging capabilities. The techniques employed include T_1-weighted (short TR, short TE) images, T_2- weighted (long TR, long TE) images, proton density–weighted (long TR, short TE) images, and T_1-weighted images after gadolinium enhancement. In T_1- weighted images cerebrospinal fluid and lesions are dark, white matter bright, and gray matter intermediate. Blood from acute bleeding is slightly brighter than white matter. Gadolinium enhancement correlates with breakdown in the blood-brain barrier. In T_2-weighted images cerebrospinal fluid and lesions with increased water content (tumors) are bright, white matter dark, and gray matter intermediate. Proton density–weighted images are similar to T_2-weighted images where lesions are again bright, but there is less contrast between white matter and cerebrospinal fluid. Proton density-weighted images accentuate white/gray matter contrast, yielding the best images for normal brain anatomy. Unfortunately, despite the advantages of MRI over CT, MRI is seldom used in the early workup of comatose patients. CT is almost as good for excluding supratentorial or infratentorial lesions causing coma. Also, MR images require longer scan times, and MRIs cannot be done on demand nearly as readily as CT. MR spectroscopy promises to yield more functional information of the brain, but that technique cannot currently be applied to the acutely ill patient with reduced consciousness.

Cerebral Angiography

Cerebral angiography images the blood space (vasculature) in the intracranial and extracranial areas.[25] However, neurologic specialists restrict their use of angiography as a diagnostic tool. In most instances, angiography is limited to those patients who are being considered for carotid surgery or neurosurgery. A good indication for using angiography would be to delineate the blood supply of a meningioma before its removal. There is limited usefulness for angiography in almost all patients with coma or clouding of consciousness. For instance, angiography is not ordinarily performed in comatose patients with suspected subarachnoid hemorrhage. A CT gives the clinician all the information needed for the patient's initial management. Cerebral arteritis is one of the few diagnoses that can be made exclusively with angiography. Almost all other structural lesions that cause clouding of consciousness can be seen better with CT.

Radionuclide Studies

Radionuclide studies such as the older static brain scan, which provided indistinct images of large cerebral venous channels and blood-brain barrier breakdown,[25] are included in this section for historical interest only. Blood-brain barrier breakdown can be better imaged with contrast studies using either CT or MRI. Rapid head scanning after bolus intravenous injection of a radionuclide provides an image of blood flow in major cerebral vessels and is used in some centers as an aid to the diagnosis of cerebral death.[31]

Positron emission tomography (PET) is based on the detection of the products of positron emission from atoms that label a molecule, the behavior of which is to be investigated.[32] The images are similar to those of CT but depict tracer content rather than tissue density. With the aid of appropriate data collection, strategies, and mathematic models of physiologic processes, the PET image of isotope concentration becomes a functional image of cerebral blood flow or metabolism. This technique has provided valuable information about brain metabolism during stroke or in epileptic foci but is too expensive, cumbersome, and complex for routine clinical use.

Brain single-photon emission tomography (SPECT), unlike PET, uses stable isotope radiopharmaceuticals sold commercially and does not require an on-site cyclotron.[33] The tracers ^{201}Tl and/or ^{99m}Tc-sestamibi (^{99m}Tc-MIBI) detect new, recurrent, or residual brain tumor. Hexamethylpropyleneamine oxime (^{99m}Tc-HMPAO) is a regional cerebral blood flow (rCBF) tracer used for cerebrovascular disease evaluation, interictal and ictal epilepsy scans, and dementia evaluation. Quantitative rCBF SPECT studies use the tracer ^{133}Xe. Additionally, iodinated central nervous system receptor-binding tracers are being developed. Conceivably, SPECT may have a limited role in defining some metabolic or diffuse causes of coma.

TREATMENT OF PATIENTS WITH DISTURBED CONSCIOUSNESS

The treatment of specific conditions that cause coma or reduced consciousness is beyond the scope of this chapter. However, recognition of the cause of coma carries a pointed objective—treat and remove the cause. The rationale for some of the modes of therapy are discussed in the following sections.

Supratentorial Mass Lesions

Patients with supratentorial mass lesions (SMLs) and coma secondary to transtentorial herniation demand emergency care. If not promptly treated, they could develop secondary brain stem (Duret) hemorrhages, which are usually fatal.[4] The exact treatment of SMLs inducing coma depends on the specific lesion, but some generalities can be made. In most emergency situations the physician should assume that the SML is acute and treatable. After first stabilizing the patient's vital signs, most physicians empirically treat the patient for cerebral edema with intubation, controlled hyperventilation, and intravenous administration of mannitol and/or glucosteroids.[34,35] These remedies frequently "buy time" until the exact diagnosis can be made using CT, when more specific therapy can begin. Emergency physicians must recognize potentially salvageable patients from those who will succumb despite treatment. Patients still posturing are potentially salvageable and should receive vigorous treatment until it is proved that the offending lesion, such as a large central hematoma, is untreatable. Patients with treatable lesions, particularly subdural or epidural hematomas, require surgery as soon as possible after the diagnosis is made. The patient who has developed pontine signs (generalized flaccidity, pinpoint pupils, extraocular movements that are fixed to ocular reflexes, and sustained hyperventilation) from transtentorial herniation is not salvageable and usually dies even when given vigorous support.[36]

Subtentorial Lesions

Subtentorial lesions cause coma by direct involvement or compression of the reticular activating areas in the rostral brain stem. Interventional therapy is not an option for patients with large intrinsic lesions such as a brain stem infarct or hematoma. However, lesions extrinsic to the brain stem such as a cerebellar hematoma may produce symptoms and signs of brain stem dysfunction. Surgical drainage of such a hematoma is often lifesaving and may result in the patient's full recovery. The emergency treatment of coma secondary to a structural posterior fossa lesion parallels that used in patients with supratentorial lesions. Intubation is perhaps even more imperative, since many patients with subtentorial lesions have irregular, ineffective respirations. If a surgically treatable lesion is found and the patient does not exhibit flaccidity and unresponsiveness, immediate decompression is indicated. Only supportive care is indicated for patients with large intrinsic brain stem lesions. Patients who exhibit unresponsive flaccidity from a subtentorial lesion have the same poor prognosis as do similar patients with supratentorial lesions.

Metabolic or Diffuse Encephalopathies

Metabolic or diffuse encephalopathies constitute the largest group of comatose patients, many of whom have a potentially reversible condition. In addition, nonneurologic physicians usually care for patients with diffuse encephalopathies, and their duty includes preventing permanent brain damage. If available, the patient's history frequently indicates the cause of the encephalopathy. Patients with metabolic encephalopathies often have asterixis, multifocal myoclonus (nonstereotyped, arrhythmic, asynchronous, twitching movements that occur multifocally in many muscle groups—particularly the facial and proximal extremity muscles), tremor, and seizures. Many patients hypoventilate or hyperventilate, but the irregular or periodic respirations seen in patients with structural lesions are usually absent. In general, patients with metabolic encephalopathies demonstrate no focal signs.

After a rapid initial appraisal of the patient and stabilization of vital signs, blood and urine for the metabolic studies listed previously (see discussion of laboratory evaluation) should be obtained. Then 50 ml of 50% glucose is usually administered intravenously in the event that hypoglycemia underlies the coma. Febrile or immunosuppressed patients require a lumbar puncture to exclude meningitis. In patients with acid-base imbalances, particularly those with acute metabolic acidosis, treatment must be instituted early to prevent cardiac arrhythmias. Alcohol or sedative drug abuse, the most common cause of stupor and coma in emergency room patients, can be easily confirmed with the toxicology screen. Patients comatose from a sedative drug overdose require gastric lavage after cuffed endotracheal intubation. If the cause of metabolic encephalopathies cannot be determined after the initial screening laboratory evaluation, the most likely diagnoses are postanoxic encephalopathies or postictal (seizure) depression. When no diagnosis can be reached, patients are usually supported maximally.

BRAIN DEATH AND THE PERSISTENT VEGETATIVE STATE

Despite optimal treatment, some patients fail to recover from coma and develop either brain death or the persistent vegetative state (PVS). These two conditions undoubtedly owe their existence to modern resuscitative techniques, improved patient transportation, advances in mechanical ventilators, and the widespread availability of quality intensive care units. The management of brain death or PVS requires input from the medical community, ethicists, legislatures, courts, and society in general. Surgeons have a vested interest in brain death and PVS because of the widespread transplantation of salvaged organs from comatose patients and because surgeons so frequently serve as the primary physicians for comatose patients in trauma centers.

Brain death as a concept has been generally well accepted since the early 1970s. The President's Commission, working with a distinguished panel of medical consultants, furnished us with both a conceptual definition and operational guidelines for brain death.[31] Their proposals led to the Uniform Determination of Death Act.[31] The consultant panel proposed that individuals are dead when there is (1) irreversible cessation of circulatory and respiratory functions or (2) irreversible cessation of all functions of the entire brain, including the brain stem. Irreversibility was recognized when (1) the cause of coma is established and is sufficient to account for the loss of brain function, (2) the possibility of recovery of any brain functions is excluded, (3) the cessation of all brain functions persists for an appropriate period of observation and/or trial of therapy. The consultants recognized that medical circumstances might require the use of confirmatory studies such as EEG or blood flow studies. These guidelines have been used since 1981, emphasize the clinical examination, and specify two clinical examinations at least 6 hours apart, 12 hours if no confirmatory tests were performed.

Since the President's Commission Guidelines were published, a gap between the conceptual definition of brain death (irreversible cessation of all functions of the entire brain) and the operational criteria used in its diagnosis has emerged.[37,38] Many clinically brain-dead patients (i.e., those with absent brain stem reflexes) retain EEG activity. It is therefore possible for a patient to be declared brain dead whose entire brain is not dead. Additionally, there are advocates for accepting the absence of blood flow as the major criteria for brain death.[38] The notion that sustained cessation of cerebral blood flow inevitably leads to brain death is compelling. Yet it can be argued that no matter how sophisticated the radionuclide angiography, one visualizes only supratentorial blood flow. It is therefore possible to call patients brain dead when some brain stem function persists. Despite the above arguments, the current operational definition has served well for over a decade. This definition is based on demonstrating absent brain stem function including apnea[39] (when $PaCO_2$ is greater than 60) on two separate occasions, 6 hours apart with confirmatory tests and 12 hours apart without confirmatory tests.

Coined by Jennett and Plum[7] in 1972, the term *persistent vegetative state (PVS)* describes patients with severe brain damage whose coma has progressed to a state of wakefulness without detectable awareness. Most experts have concluded that being awake but unaware is the result of a functioning brain stem and the total loss of cerebral cortical functioning. Patients with PVS have sleep-wake cycles, no ascertainable cerebral cortical function, and preserved hypothalamic and brain stem autonomic functions, all present for at least 1 month after acute traumatic or nontraumatic brain injury. The American Academy of Neurology (AAN) executive board published a position paper on PVS in 1989 noting that (1) the primary basis for the diagnosis of PVS is careful and extensive clinical observation of the patient supported by laboratory studies, (2) patients with PVS may have a prolonged survival as long as the artificial provision of nutrition and fluids is continued, and (3) patients with PVS do not have the capacity to experience pain and suffering.[40] The AAN executive board recognized that the artificial provision of nutrition and hydration is a form of medical treatment and may be discontinued in accordance with the principles and practices governing the withholding and withdrawal of other forms of medical treatment. They suggested that it is good medical practice to initiate the artificial provision of fluids and nutrition when the patient's prognosis is uncertain and to allow for the termination of treatment at a later date (usually 1 to 3 months) when the patient's condition becomes hopeless. The Multi-Society Task Force on PVS further defined the condition and recognized that (1) recovery of consciousness from a posttraumatic PVS is unlikely after 12 months in both adults and children, (2) recovery from nontraumatic PVS after 3 months is exceedingly rare in both adults and children, and (3) patients with degenerative or metabolic disorders or congenital malformations who remain in a PVS for several months are unlikely to recover consciousness.[41]

The hopelessness of PVS has led to the proposal that brain death criteria be based on the diagnosis of permanent loss of consciousness rather than the loss of vegetative brain functions (i.e., alter the conceptual definition from the current "whole brain" standard to a "higher brain" standard).[37,38] Implementation of this change in the conceptual definition, if indeed the change ever occurs, must await further legislation and court decisions.

SUMMARY

This chapter presents an approach to the examination of unconscious patients based on neuroanatomic, physiologic, and biochemical principles. Consciousness is mediated by the reticular activating system and the sum of the activity of the cerebral hemispheres. Consciousness may be altered by a variety of medical and surgical problems such as infarction and trauma that destroy brain tissue directly. Biochemical abnormalities can remove required metabolites, introduce toxins, or alter the internal cerebral environment, thus impairing brain metabolism and producing brain dysfunction. Typically, structural abnormalities of the brain produce focal neurologic signs that permit localization of the abnormality to a specific brain region. On the other hand, metabolic abnormalities are characterized by nonfocal signs of brain dysfunction. Pupillary light reactivity and ocular motility are the most useful clinical signs for making this differential diagnosis. Absent function implies a structural lesion, but even minimum function usually persists with severe metabolic disturbances. Obtaining a prompt, accurate diagnosis for patients with altered consciousness is essential. Only after that can the physician initiate the appropriate medical or surgical therapy necessary to arrest or reverse the pathophysiologic process causing coma and to avoid or minimize irreversible neurologic deficits.

REFERENCES

1. Moruzzi G, Magoun HW. Brainstem reticular formation and activation of EEG. Electroencephalogr Clin Electrophysiol 1:445, 1949.
2. French JD, Magoun HW. Effects of chronic lesions in central cephalic brainstem of monkeys. Arch Neurol Psychiat 68:591, 1952.
3. French JD. Brain lesions with prolonged unconsciousness. Arch Neurol Psychiat 68:727, 1952.
4. Plum F, Posner JB. The Diagnosis of Stupor and Coma, 3rd ed. Philadelphia: FA Davis, 1980.
5. Braun CM, Pivik RT. Effects of brainstem lesions on tonic immobility in the rabbit *(Oryctolagus cuniculus)*. Brain Res Bull 10:127, 1983.
6. Cooper JR, Bloom FE, Roth RH. The Biochemical Basis of Neuropharmacology, 4th ed. New York: Oxford University Press, 1982.
7. Jennett WB, Plum F. The persistent vegetative state: A syndrome in search of a name. Lancet 1:734, 1972.
8. Lowry OH, et al. Effect of ischemia on known substrates and cofactors of the glycolytic pathway in the brain. J Biol Chem 239:18, 1964.
9. Siesjo BK. Brain dysfunction in cerebral hypoxia and ischemia. In Plum F, ed. Brain Dysfunction in Metabolic Disorders. New York: Raven Press, 1974.
10. Lockwood AH. Ammonia-induced encephalopathy. In McCandless D, ed. Cerebral Energy Metabolism and Metabolic Encephalopathy. New York: Plenum Publishing, 1985.
11. Lockwood AH. Acute and chronic hyperosmolality: Effects on cerebral amino acids and energy metabolism. Arch Neurol 32:62, 1975.
12. Rymer M, Fishman RA. Protective adaptation of brain to water intoxication. Arch Neurol 28:49, 1973.
13. De Jong RN. The Neurological Examination, 4th ed. Hagerstown: Harper & Row, 1979.
14. Fisher CM. The neurological examination of the comatose patient. Acta Neurol Scand 45(Suppl 36):1, 1969.
15. Berger AJ, Mitchell RA, Severinghaus JW. Regulation of respiration. New Engl J Med 297:92, 1977.
16. Brown HW, Plum F. The neurologic basis of Cheyne-Stokes respiration. Am J Med 30:849, 1961.
17. Cherniack NS, et al. Experimentally induced Cheyne-Stokes breathing. Respir Physiol 37:185, 1979.
18. Brodal A. Neurological Anatomy. New York: Oxford University Press, 1981.
19. Pasik P, Pasik T, Bender MB. The pretectal syndrome in monkeys. Brain 92:521, 1969.
20. Shafar J. The syndromes of the third neurone of the cervical sympathetic system. Am J Med 40:97, 1966.
21. Reeves AG, Posner JB. The ciliospinal response in man. Neurology 19:1145, 1969.
22. Peele TL. The Neuroanatomic Basis for Clinical Neurology, 3rd ed. New York: McGraw-Hill, 1977.
23. Lance JW. The control of muscle tone, reflexes and movement: Robert Wartenberg lecture. Neurology 30:1303, 1980.
24. Davis RH, Davis L. Decerebrate rigidity in humans. Neurosurgery 10:635, 1982.
25. Oldendorf WH. The quest for an image of brain: A brief historical and technical review of brain imaging techniques. Neurology 28:517, 1978.
26. Niedermeyer E, deSilva FL. Electroencephalography. Baltimore: Williams & Wilkins, 1993.
27. Gloor P, Kalabay O, Giard N. The electroencephalogram in diffuse encephalopathies: EEG correlates of grey and white matter lesions. Brain 91:779, 1968.
28. Cutler RW, Spertell RB. Cerebrospinal fluid: A selective review. Ann Neurol 11:1, 1982.
29. Petito F, Plum F. The lumbar puncture. New Engl J Med 290:225, 1974.
30. Edelman RR, Warach S. Magnetic resonance imaging. New Engl J Med 328:708, 1993.
31. President's Commission for the Study of Ethical Problems in Medicine and Biomedical and Behavioral Research. Guidelines for the determination of death. JAMA 246:2184, 1981.
32. Jacobson HG. Positron emission tomography—A new approach to brain chemistry. JAMA 260:2704, 1988.
33. Mountz JM, et al. Brain SPECT: 1994 update. In Freeman LM, ed. Nuclear Medicine Annual 1994. New York: Raven Press, 1994.
34. Fishman R. Steroids in the treatment of brain edema. New Engl J Med 306:359, 1982.
35. McGraw CP, Howard G. Effect of mannitol on increased intracranial pressure. Neurosurgery 13:269, 1983.
36. Levy DE, et al. Prognosis in nontraumatic coma. Ann Intern Med 94:293, 1981.
37. Halevy A, Brody B. Brain death: Reconciling definitions, criteria, and tests. Ann Intern Med 119:519, 1993.
38. Truog RD, Fackler JC. Rethinking brain death. Crit Care Med 20:1705, 1992.
39. Marks SJ, Zisfein J. Apneic oxygenation in apnea tests for brain death: A controlled trial. Arch Neurol 47:1066, 1990.
40. American Academy of Neurology Executive Board. Position of the American Academy of Neurology on certain aspects of the care and management of the persistent vegetative state patient. Neurology 39:125, 1989.
41. Multi-Society Task Force on PVS. Medical aspects of the persistent vegetative state. New Engl J Med 330:1499, 1994.

48

Pathophysiology of Head Trauma

Martin C. Holland and Donald P. Becker

Trauma—the very word conjures up images that both fascinate and horrify. Yet, for all its visually striking outward manifestations, much of the morbidity and mortality associated with trauma result from changes that occur in a realm beyond the scope of our ordinary senses—at the cellular level. In a sense, these cellular processes play a more important role in the pathophysiology of trauma than do the visually apparent injuries, because ultimately it is the cell's function and survival that determines the patient's final outcome. Because of this, in-depth knowledge of both normal and abnormal cellular physiology is imperative to treat traumatic injuries effectively. This chapter focuses on traumatic injuries to the brain, their mechanical and physiologic sequelae, the techniques used to monitor these changes, and the treatment modalities available—both surgical and nonsurgical—that help to minimize the patient's injuries and maximize the final neurologic outcome.

EPIDEMIOLOGY

It may come as no surprise that trauma is the leading cause of death in the United States among those younger than 44 years. Furthermore, in keeping with our expectations, predominantly young men are involved, with the peak incidence between the ages of 15 and 24 years. The leading causes of trauma are, in decreasing order of frequency, motor vehicle accidents (MVAs), falls, and "pedestrian-versus-auto" accidents. Overall, approximately 500,000 people suffer head and spinal cord injuries each year, and 80,000 of these die. Of those that survive, 37,000 remain moderately disabled and 17,000 retain disabilities severe enough to confine them indefinitely to a skilled-nursing facility. The cost to society is staggering, not only in terms of medical care, workdays lost, and destruction of property, but, equally importantly, in terms of physical and emotional suffering for both the patient and family.

TRAUMATIC BRAIN INJURIES

Trauma, by its very nature, is not a single pathologic entity. Multiple potential mechanisms for cellular injury exist. The extent to which any or all of these come into play depends on the mechanism of injury and the severity of trauma. Conceptually, trauma-associated injuries can be classified as either *primary* or *secondary*. Primary injuries occur at the initial moment of impact, whereas secondary injuries occur in the minutes, hours, and days after the initial event. Primary injuries are principally mechanical in nature, whereas secondary injuries can be associated either with mechanical forces or with toxic or metabolic derangements.

How cells or tissues respond to mechanical stress is directly related to the direction, velocity, and magnitude of the forces applied. These forces in turn are closely related to the mechanism of trauma. A useful classification of primary, mechanism-associated injuries divides these into acceleration-deceleration, impact, and penetrating injuries. The first of these is commonly seen in MVAs, where a sudden change in velocity, direction, or both applies an acceleration-deceleration force to the brain. Impact injuries are commonly seen in assaults as the momentum of an object (e.g., a pipe or bat) is transferred suddenly to the skull and brain. Penetrating injuries are self-explanatory and are commonly seen in gunshot wounds. More details about the physics, cellular response, and clinical implications of these mechanisms follow. Secondary injuries may also result from mechanical processes, such as delayed intracranial hematomas or intracranial hypertension. Conversely, secondary injury may result from a metabolic or toxic phenomenon. A common scenario is the patient with trauma who becomes anoxic or hypotensive, thus depriving the cells of metabolic substrates. Other examples of a toxic or metabolic phenomenon leading to cellular dysfunction are posttraumatic intracellular acidosis and free-radical production.

Though some attempt has been made to distinguish mechanical from metabolic injury mechanisms, it should be stressed that all insults ultimately result in cellular dysfunction, and, with the possible exception of massive direct cellular destruction by mechanical injury, all mechanisms leading to cellular dysfunction and death likely share some common pathophysiologic pathways. Generally speaking, the initial traumatic event can lead to disturbances in energy metabolism, transmembrane ionic gradients, protein synthesis, and cerebral blood flow (CBF). Because of the complexity of the system involved, however, it is sometimes difficult to ascertain which observed abnormality is a primary response and which is a secondary effect. To simplify matters and to better understand the pathologic phenomena, a thorough understanding of normal cellular mechanisms and metabolism is essential. One should also keep in mind that all physiologic mechanisms are intimately related, and that an alteration in one will likely result in an alteration—to a greater or lesser degree—in all others.

NORMAL PHYSIOLOGY

This section provides a basic understanding of normal neuronal and cerebral physiology. The enormous number of homeostatic responses, however, precludes detailed examination of all but a few. Those discussed involve the regulation of cellular electrical activity, energy metabolism, and CBF. The role of nitric oxide is also addressed.

The basic function of the neuron is to receive information from sensory receptors or other neurons, to integrate this information, and then to send the appropriate response to other cells. For this system to work properly, the coordinated, integrated function of membrane electrical potentials, action potentials, nerve-conduction mechanisms, neurotransmitter production and release, and energy metabolism is required. These processes must also work in concert with cellular oxygen and substrate delivery for optimal cellular function.

Cellular Electrical Activity

To discuss cellular electrical activity, one must address processes that occur at both the cellular and subcellular levels. The latter are those that occur on isolated sections of membrane, whereas the former involve the cell as a whole. This distinction, though somewhat arbitrary, is important in developing a cogent model of cellular function.

Membrane Potentials

Though a detailed description of membrane potentials is beyond the scope of this chapter, an overview of basic neuronal physiology is presented. Neuronal cells, indeed all cells, are like small batteries, in that a small electrical potential exists across the cellular membrane. In electrically silent or dormant cells, the magnitude of this electrical potential lies around −70 mV (inside negative). In electrically active mammalian cells, the membrane potential can vary between −75 mV and +55 mV.[1-4]

The magnitude and polarity of the membrane potential are determined by two factors: first, the individual equilibrium potential for each of the major soluble ions (E_K, E_{Na}, E_{Cl}, and E_{Ca}) and second, the relative membrane permeabilities of each ion. To establish the equilibrium potential for a given ion (E_{ion}), a concentration differential for that ion must exist across the cell membrane. In addition, the membrane must be semipermeable to that ion. In the case of potassium, the intracellular concentration ($[K^+]_i$) is approximately 140 mEq/L, with 5 mEq/L in the extracellular space ($[K^+]_o$).[1] The natural tendency is for K^+ to flow down its concentration gradient. As this occurs, the inside of the cell gradually assumes a net negative potential (one positive charge leaves the cell with each potassium ion), and an electrical gradient across the cell membrane is established. Eventually, a point is reached at which the force driving K^+ out of the cell down its concentration gradient equals that driving it back into the cell down the newly established electrical gradient. As a result, the net movement of K^+ across the cell membrane is zero, and the membrane electrical potential becomes fixed at what is referred to as the *membrane equilibrium potential for* K^+ (E_K).

Because the intracellular and extracellular concentrations of each ion vary, the corresponding E_{ion} values differ as well. For any given ion, the net direction of movement across the cell membrane is determined by the actual transmembrane electrical potential (E_m) and the equilibrium potential for that ion. Ions flow in the direction necessary to reestablish equilibrium potential (E_{ion}). For example, if $E_{Cl} = -60$ mV and the $E_m = -70$ mV, chloride will flow out of the cell, making the inside less negative until $E_m = E_{Cl} = -60$ mV. Conversely, if E_m is −50 mV, chloride will flow into the cell until $E_m = -60$ mV. Because the equilibrium potential for each ion differs, every ion competes with every other ion in an attempt to drive the membrane potential toward its own E_{ion}. The resulting E_m thus depends on the relative membrane permeabilities for each ion. The ion with the greatest membrane permeability has the greatest influence on the membrane potential. In most resting cells, the membrane is most permeable to potassium. As a result, the resting cell membrane lies closest to the equilibrium potential for potassium ($E_K = -75$ mV, $E_m = -70$ mV). It follows that by varying the relative ionic membrane permeabilities, the membrane electrical potential can be changed. This membrane property is the basis for action potentials.

Action Potentials

The action potential is a coordinated sequence of events that manifests as a stereotypical, reproducible change in membrane potential. The simplest cycle requires only an intact membrane supporting variable-permeability Na^+ and K^+ channels.

As the cycle begins, the resting membrane potential is approximately −70 mV, and the dominant ionic influence is that of potassium. Under the appropriate stimulus, membrane permeability to sodium increases dramatically, sending E_m close to E_{Na}. Soon thereafter, the membrane permeability to potassium increases and that to sodium decreases, sending the E_m back toward the value for E_K. At the end of the cycle, the membrane permeabilities for both sodium and potassium resume their resting values, and E_m returns to −70 mV. The initiating event is a membrane depolarization that brings E_m toward its "threshold potential." If the threshold potential is crossed, the action potential is carried out to termination. If not, the membrane potential passively returns to −70 mV. A variety of mechanisms can bring about the initial depolarization. These include the activation of membrane ion channels by neurotransmitters, mechanical deformation of the cell membrane, loss of membrane integrity, and changes in the intracellular or extracellular ionic composition.

Nerve Conduction

The changes in E_m associated with the action potential occur not only at the site of ion-channel activation but also in the membrane immediately adjacent to it. The latter is manifested as a membrane depolarization that can exceed the membrane's threshold potential. If this occurs, a second action potential is triggered at this new site, and the cycle can be repeated. In such a manner, by sequential depolarization of adjacent sections of membrane, an action potential can be transmitted along the length of the neuronal membrane, down the axon to its terminal bouton. To prevent the retrograde propagation of action potentials, there is a refractory period during which a section of membrane cannot produce a second action potential. This allows the action potential and surrounding window of depolarization to move away from a recently activated section of membrane before it becomes susceptible to reactivation.

Neurotransmitter Release

Once the action potential reaches the terminal bouton, a series of events leads to the release of neurotransmitter from the presynaptic membrane. The critical step is the influx of calcium into the presynaptic terminal. This is effected by the activation of voltage-dependent calcium channels that open when the membrane becomes depolarized. As calcium rushes into the cell, the neurotransmitter-containing vesicles within the terminal bouton fuse to the presynaptic membrane, releasing their contents into the synaptic cleft.[1] These chemicals then diffuse across the synaptic gap and bind to postsynaptic membrane proteins.

Postsynaptic Activation and Inhibition

Both the identity of the neurotransmitter and the nature of the postsynaptic receptor protein determine how the receptor-ligand complex will affect the cell. Excitatory neurotransmitters such as glutamate promote the triggering of postsynaptic action potentials, whereas inhibitory ones such as γ-aminobutyric acid (GABA) essentially prevent them from occurring. Generally speaking, neurotransmitters modulate the electrical activity of neurons by changing the permeability of membrane-bound ionic channels. Glutamate, for example, can increase intracellular calcium and sodium flow through its effects on *N*-methyl-D-aspartate (NMDA) receptors, whereas GABA increases chloride flow when bound to its receptor. Though these mechanisms are important for normal cell function, they also play a role in the cellular dysfunction and death associated with trauma.

Reestablishment of Ionic Gradients

Because every action potential is associated with an outward flow of potassium and an inward flow of sodium, it follows that the concentration gradients for both ions diminish with each cycle. To re-establish the resting-potential ionic concentrations, a pump transfers sodium out of the cell and potassium back into it. This requires energy in the form of adenosine triphosphate (ATP). The stimulus for increasing the Na^+/K^+ ATPase pump activity is a change in the intracellular Na^+ and K^+ concentrations. Under normal conditions, ATP is the primary source of energy, though ADP can also be used. Similar mechanisms exist for reestablishing intracellular and extra-cellular Ca^{2+} and Cl^- concentrations.

Cellular Metabolism

Neurons are among the most metabolically active cells of the body. From 40% to 45% of the brain's energy is used to maintain ionic hemostasis and to synthesize neurotransmitters and other structural and functional proteins. The remaining 55% to 60% is used for synaptic transmission and action potentials.[5] The energy required for these cells to function comes from ATP, a by-product of energy metabolism as glucose is broken down to carbon dioxide and water. This process is divided into three stages, each occurring in separate cellular compartments. The first of these, glycolysis, occurs in the cytosol. Its primary role is to convert glucose to pyruvate, with the net production of two ATP and two reduced nicotinamide adenine dinucleotide (NADH; the nonreduced form is NAD) molecules per glucose. The citric acid cycle, the second stage in energy metabolism, takes place in the mitochondria and involves the breakdown of pyruvate into carbon dioxide, with the production of four NADH, one reduced flavin adenine dinucleotide ($FADH_2$; the nonreduced form is FAD), and one guanosine triphosphate (GTP) molecule per pyruvate molecule. The last step in energy production also takes place in the mitochondria. Known as *oxidative phosphorylation,* this process uses the reducing power of NADH and $FADH_2$ to make ATP. In the final analysis, the complete oxidation of 1 mol glucose yields 36 mol ATP.

Though each component system is self-contained and somewhat independent, its function is intimately linked with the other two systems by a series of feedback mechanisms that match ATP production to the metabolic needs of the cell. A brief description of each system focuses on control mechanisms and "energy compartmentalization."

Glycolysis

Glycolysis occurs in the cytosol and results in the production of two ATP, two NADH, and two pyruvate ($C_3H_3O_3$) molecules per molecule of glucose ($C_6H_{12}O_6$) metabolized. The net equation for glycolysis is as follows:

$$C_6H_{12}O_6 + 2ADP + 2P + 2NAD^+ \rightarrow 2C_3H_3O_3 + 2ATP + 2NADH + 2H_2O$$

There are nine reactions leading from glucose to pyruvate. Of these, the third reaction in sequence is of critical importance in regulating glycolysis. This reaction is catalyzed by phosphofructokinase (PFK) and involves the phosphorylation of fructose 6-phosphate to yield fructose 1,6-diphosphate:

$$\text{Fructose 6-phosphate} + \text{ATP} \xrightarrow{\text{PFK}} \text{Fructose 1,6-diphosphate} + \text{ADP}$$

PFK itself is activated if the cytosolic ATP/adenosine monophosphate (AMP) ratio decreases (cellular energy is low). Conversely, if the cytosolic ATP/AMP ratio is high, PFK is deactivated, thus halting glycolytic ATP production. The enzymatic machinery needed for glycolysis is found near the cellular membrane. Its proximity to the membrane Na^+/K^+ ATPase pump allows the cell to detect even minor changes in cytosolic ATP, levels leading to the activation of the glycolytic machinery and closely coupling glycolytic ATP production with cellular electrical activity.

Because NAD^+ is consumed during the conversion of glyceraldehyde 3-phosphate to 1,3-diphosphoglycerate (Fig. 48-1), it must be replenished for glycolysis to proceed. Under normal conditions, NADH is converted back to NAD^+ by the mitochondrial cytochrome system. In the absence of functioning mitochondria, however, NAD^+ is regenerated by fermenting pyruvate into acetate ($C_3H_5O_3$).

$$C_3H_3O_3 + NADH + H+ \rightarrow C_3H_5O_3 + NAD^+$$

Not only does the mitochondrial machinery recycle NAD^+, it also provides a mechanism for the production of more ATP. The first step in the process is the decarboxylation of pyruvate within the mitochondria to produce acetyl coenzyme A (CoA).

$$C_3H_3O_3 + NAD^+ + CoA \rightarrow \text{Acetyl CoA} + CO_2 + NADH$$

This reaction is the entry point into the citric acid cycle.

Citric Acid Cycle

Also known as the *Krebs* or *tricarboxylic acid cycle,* the citric acid cycle occurs in the mitochondria and is primarily involved in degrading pyruvate to carbon dioxide, with the concomitant production of GTP, $FADH_2$, and NADH (Fig. 48-2). The latter two substrates are shunted through the mitochondrial cytochrome system to produce ATP.

Control of the citric acid cycle occurs at several junctures along the reaction chain. Primary inhibitors of the system are NADH and ATP, whereas the primary activator is ADP (Fig. 48-2). This again reflects an organization in which a high cellular energy state (high levels of ATP, NADH, or both) prevents the further production of high-energy substrates and a low energy state promotes their production.

Because NADH and $FADH_2$ cannot be used directly by the cell as a source of energy, the energy stored within their bounds is first transferred to ATP. This final process, which also occurs within the mitochondria, is known as *oxidative phosphorylation.*

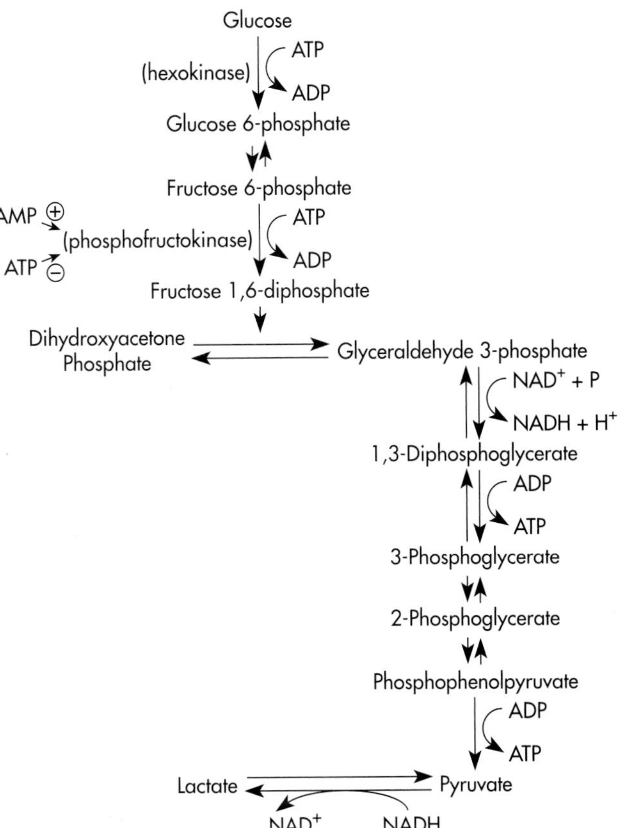

Fig. 48-1. Glycolysis. The glycolytic pathway breaks glucose down into pyruvate, with the net production of 2 mol adenosine triphosphate *(ATP)* and 2 mol NADH (reduced form of nicotinamide adenine dinucleotide) per 1 mol glucose metabolized. The most important control enzyme is phosphofructokinase, which is inhibited by high cellular ATP concentrations and stimulated by high adenosine monophosphate *(AMP)* levels. Pyruvate can be fermented to lactate to regenerate NAD^+ (oxidized form of nicotinamide adenine dinucleotide).

Oxidative Phosphorylation

Oxidative phosphorylation uses the energy stored in NADH and $FADH_2$ electrons to produce ATP and to reconstitute NAD^+ and FAD. These high-energy electrons are transferred to the membrane-bound electron-transport chain contained within the inner mitochondrial membrane. As electrons flow down this enzyme-complex, hydrogen ions are pumped out of the mitochondrial matrix. Thus, a proton gradient is created by the net movement of hydrogen ions across the inner membrane. The protons then flow back into the mitochondrial matrix through specialized channels that couple hydrogen-ion flux to ATP synthesis (Fig. 48-3).

We have seen that control of both glycolysis and the Krebs cycle is effected through negative feedback mecha-

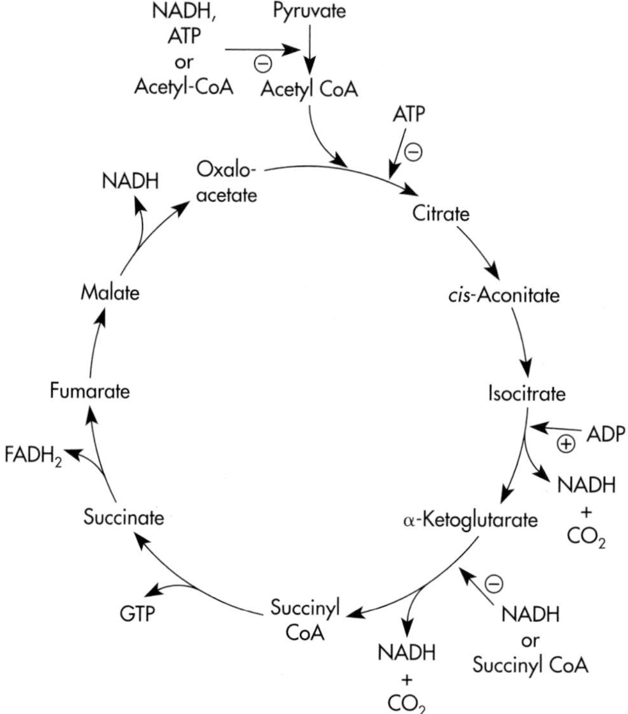

Fig. 48-2. Krebs cycle. The Krebs cycle takes place in the mitochondrion. Pyruvate is shunted through the system, which produces the reduced form of nicotinamide adenine dinucleotide *(NADH),* the reduced form of flavin adenine dinucleotide *(FADH$_2$),* and guanosine triphosphate *(GTP).* The cycle is shut down by high NADH and adenosine triphosphate *(ATP)* levels, whereas high adenosine diphosphate *(ADP)* concentrations stimulate the cycle. *CoA,* Coenzyme A.

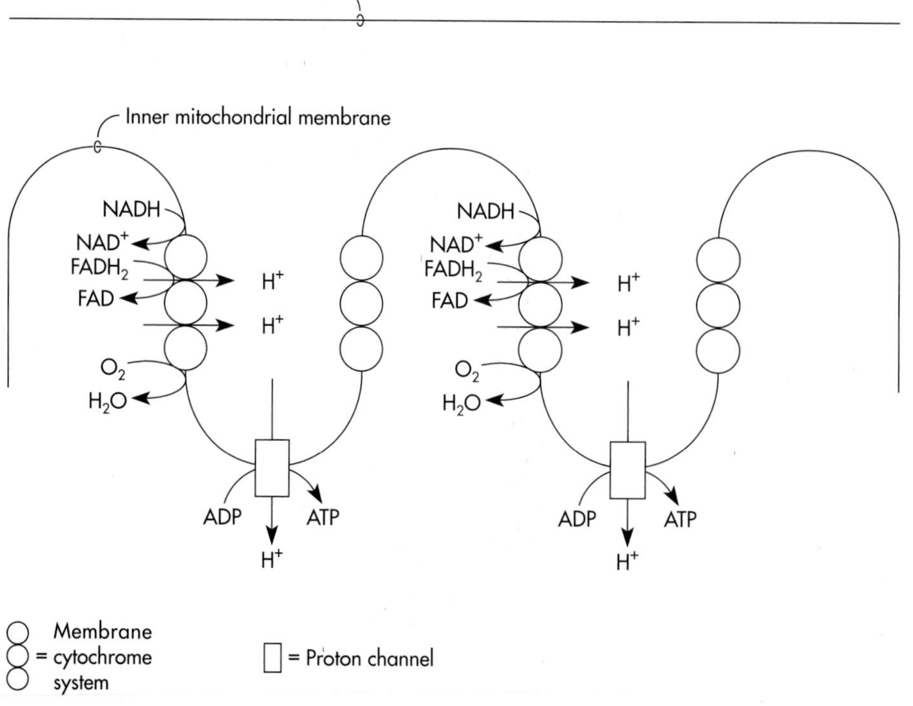

Fig. 48-3. Oxidative phosphorylation. Oxidative phosphorylation also occurs in the mitochondrion. High-energy electrons stored in the reduced form of nicotinamide adenine dinucleotide *(NADH)* and the reduced form of flavin adenine dinucleotide *(FADH$_2$)* are shunted through the membrane cytochrome enzymes, which pump protons out of the mitochondrial matrix. Protons then flow back into the matrix, down a concentration gradient, through hydrogen channels. The flow of protons is linked to the production of adenosine triphosphate *(ATP).* Oxygen is the final electron acceptor. *ADP,* Adenosine diphosphate; *ATP,* adenosine triphosphate; *FAD,* flavin adenine dinucleotide; *NAD$^+$,* oxidized form of nicotinamide adenine dinucleotide.

nisms. This is not the case with oxidative phosphorylation, where control is effected through the upregulation or downregulation of constitutionally active cytochrome enzymes. This design aims at matching oxidative metabolism to average long-term substrate (NADH and $FADH_2$) availability. The cell's inability to acutely increase oxidative function plays an important role in the pathophysiology of brain injury.

Nitric Oxide

Nitric oxide (NO) has recently come into prominence as a major physiologic modulator. It has been implicated as a mediator in the cytotoxic effects of macrophages, as a vasoactive substance, and even as a neurotransmitter.[6,7] All these functions rely on the activity of nitric oxide synthetase (NOS), an enzyme that produces NO by degrading L-arginine.

In general, NOS activity is regulated by one of two basic mechanisms. The first method involves transforming the enzyme from its inactive to its active form. This type of regulation occurs in neurons and vascular endothelial cells, is calcium dependent, and is mediated by calmodulin. The second type of regulation involves the increased production of an enzymatically active form of NOS. This type of regulation is seen in macrophages. In their inactive or dormant state, these cells normally contain no NOS. Once they are activated, however, intracellular levels of NOS rise dramatically, reflecting a general increase in protein synthesis. To summarize, macrophage-associated NOS is chronically enzymatically active. NO production in these cells depends entirely on the levels of intracellular NOS, and not on the activation of enzymatically inactive NOS.

The biologic roles of NO are varied, and in many instances altogether unknown. As a vasoactive substance, it is thought to promote vasodilation of cerebral vessels, thereby increasing local blood flow.[8] This has been suggested by studies in which the blockage of endothelial NO production leads to a reduction of CBF and to systemic hypertension. Its role in macrophage function is that of a cytotoxin, causing lipid peroxidation of cellular and nuclear membranes and damaging DNA. Among its more elusive roles is that of a neurotransmitter or neuromodulator. Dawson et al. and others showed that NO may stimulate the production of cyclic guanosine monophosphate resulting from glutamate-induced NMDA receptor activation.[6,9-11] To be sure, NO is not a neurotransmitter in the classic sense, because it is not released from a terminal bouton by the fusion of vesicles to a presynaptic membrane. Instead, it diffuses throughout the cytosol and across cellular membranes, where it plays its role. It is, however, becoming increasingly evident that NO may play a more central role in cellular information processing than previously assumed.

Cerebral Blood Flow

Although the brain represents only 2% of the total body weight, it receives 20% of the cardiac output and consumes 20% of the oxygen and 25% of the glucose used by the body at rest.[12,13] The brain's energy needs, however, are not constant. As would be expected, neuronal energy consumption varies with electrical activity; the more active the cell, the more energy it consumes. Because neurons have no appreciable glucose or ATP stores,[14] the delivery of metabolic substrates such as oxygen and glucose must be tightly coupled to cerebral metabolism. An increase in a neuron's metabolic rate is reflected as a widening of arteriovenous difference of oxygen $avDo_2$ and a rise in carbon dioxide tension Pco_2 (under aerobic conditions) or as an acidosis (under anaerobic ones). Under these conditions, blood flow to the area increases and improves local substrate delivery. The converse also holds true; when blood flow to the area exceeds metabolic demands $avDo_2$ narrows and Pco_2 falls. In this case, local blood flow is reduced to match substrate supply to metabolic demand. Because not all areas of the brain are equally metabolically active, adjustments in blood flow must be made at the local or regional level.[15-21]

This process, referred to as *metabolic autoregulation,* is in contrast to pressure autoregulation, which acts to maintain a constant CBF in the face of changing systemic blood pressures.[17,22-24] The natural response of cerebral resistance vessels is to dilate if systemic pressure falls and to constrict if blood pressure rises. With a stable metabolic rate, CBF remains remarkably constant under a wide range of systemic blood pressures. If systemic pressure falls below 50 mm Hg or exceeds 160 mm Hg, however, changes in CBF passively follow changes in systemic blood pressure.[25-27] These limits exist because systemic pressures less than 50 mm Hg lead to the maximal dilation of cerebral vessels, and a further drop in blood pressure can only lead to a drop in CBF; conversely, at a systemic pressure greater than 160 mm Hg, cerebral vessels are maximally constricted, and a further increase in systemic pressures must lead to an increase in CBF.

This complex system ensures optimal use of resources. Loss of autoregulation, however, can result in either underperfusion of tissue (ischemia) or overperfusion (hyperemia), as determined by metabolic needs. The exact mechanisms controlling vascular tone are unclear, though likely candidates include the release of vasodilators such as NO and adenosine, as well as vascular innervation by adrenergic, cholinergic, or dopaminergic systems.[28-38]

Formally, *CBF* is defined as the volume of blood (in milliliters) perfusing 100 g brain tissue in 1 minute. This is approximately 50 to 55 ml/100 g/min under normal conditions. As this value diminishes, changes in both global and cellular neurologic function can be observed. At a CBF of less than 20 to 25 ml/100 g/min, one begins to observe an alteration in conciousness as well as a slowing in the electroencephalogram (EEG). As CBF drops to 18 to 20 ml/100 g/min, a dense neurologic deficit or even coma develops, associated with a flattening of the EEG. Loss of evoked potentials and Na^+/K^+ ATPase pump-failure acutely follow a drop in CBF to 12 to 17 ml/100 g/min, and prolongation of this condition leads to cell death in several hours. At CBF levels of less than 10 to 12 ml/100 g/min, cell death occurs within a few minutes.[6,10,13,23,39-49] CBF values, of course, must be interpreted within the broader context of CBF-metabolism coupling. When the cellular metabolic rate is low, for example, a CBF value that would otherwise lie below the ischemic threshold may only reflect the drop in cellular metabolic demands. A dramatic example of this is the occasional, highly publicized case of the drowning victim lost under icy waters for hours. Though the victim is found in complete cardiac arrest and is clinically brain dead, he or she eventually recovers with minimal or no residual neurologic deficit. That the victim's neurons survive such profound hypoperfusion is likely a result of the tremendous drop in cellular metabolic requirements associated with hypothermia.

What then, defines "appropriate" blood flow? Essentially, it is that which delivers enough nutrients to meet the metabolic needs of the cell. One way to quantify adequacy of blood flow is to measure the difference between the arterial and venous substrate concentrations. This value is referred to as $avD_{Substrate}$. The most practical and widely used measure is that for oxygen ($avDO_2$). When CBF is coupled to metabolism, $avDO_2$ remains confined to a fairly narrow range. Uncoupling, however, leads to shifts in $avDO_2$. Specifically, ischemia leads to a widening of $avDO_2$, whereas hyperemia results in its narrowing.[17,41,50-54] In other words, with a fixed cerebral metabolic rate of oxygen ($CMRO_2$), a drop in CBF (ischemia) results in more oxygen extracted per unit volume of blood, whereas luxury perfusion (hyperemia) results in the opposite. This quantity can be measured by obtaining simultaneous arterial and jugular venous samples and comparing oxygen contents.[55-57] A serious disadvantage of this method is that it provides information only on global oxygen consumption and fails to identify local or regional differences in $CMRO_2$. Nevertheless, an overall estimate of cerebral metabolism can be obtained by this method.

What about glucose? The arteriovenous difference of glucose (avDG) can indeed be used as a measure of metabolism. Its usefulness, however, is limited. Not only can blood glucose vary widely (especially under conditions of stress, such as trauma), but glucose availability is rarely the limiting factor in metabolism.[58,59] The cerebral metabolic rate of glucose (CMRG), on the other hand, gives an estimation of glycolytic activity, which reflects cellular energy consumption. By combining information about oxygen use and cellular metabolism, an assessment about the adequacy of CBF can be made.

PATHOLOGIC MECHANISMS IN TRAUMA

Generally speaking, pathologic mechanisms are nothing more than exaggerated or uncontrolled manifestations of normal physiology. As substrates become depleted or metabolites accumulate, a state of biochemical imbalance develops that can overwhelm the cell's normal homeostatic mechanisms. Occasionally, a point is reached at which the cell can no longer compensate for this imbalance, and a progression towards cell death occurs.

Although the biochemical pathways addressed here often overlap temporally, we will attempt to define a linear progression of events. The advantage to this approach is that the events that do indeed occur in a sequential fashion can be followed from start to finish, and the relationship between parallel (nonsequential) events can be discerned. To be sure, this approach may lead to the oversimplification of some of the pathways and their relationship to one another. Every effort is made to minimize this potential drawback.

Cellular Derangements in Trauma

Although mechanical injuries to the brain are diverse, the pathophysiologic mechanisms associated with trauma share common biochemical pathways. We have already discussed in detail the electrical properties of the neuronal cell membrane, including the development of action potentials, their propagation along the cell membrane, and the release of neurotransmitters from the presynaptic membrane. Under normal physiologic conditions, these events occur in a discrete, well-controlled fashion. In trauma, however, such is not the case. After an impact to the head, the brain undergoes transient deformations similar to those seen in a shaken bowl of gelatin. Shock waves associated with these deformations travel through the brain like waves on the surface of a pool, producing shear forces within the brain parenchyma that can injure neuronal cell bodies, axonal processes, or blood vessels. Because physical deformation of the cell membrane can initiate membrane depolarization, the initial impact causes many cells to depolarize simultaneously. This leads to huge imbalances in transmembrane ion concentrations, as well as the release of massive quantities of neurotransmitters. Because glutamate is the most common neurotransmitter in the brain, it is released in the greatest concentration from the actively depolarizing cells. As the free glutamate diffuses across the synaptic cleft, it binds to and activates glutamate receptors. The most important of these is the NMDA receptor, which, when activated, allows the entry of calcium and sodium into as well as the exit of potassium from the cell. As a result of both the initial depolarization and the glutamate-induced transmembrane ion flux, perturbations in intracellular ionic concentrations become quite pronounced.[60-63]

In an attempt to re-establish the normal transmembrane ionic gradients, membrane-bound Na^+/K^+ ATPase pumps become activated and consume enormous quantities of ATP. As the ATP/AMP ratio decreases, PFK becomes activated, funneling glucose down the glycolytic pathway. Though some ATP is replenished as glucose is broken down to pyruvate, its rate of production is outstripped by its rate of consumption, leaving the cell in a state of relative energy depletion. To confound the situation, oxidative phosphorylation enzymes, which are normally nearly fully saturated, cannot acutely increase ATP production. As the pyruvate produced in glycolysis enters the mitochondria, it is funnelled through the Krebs cycle, causing an increase in mitochondrial NADH and $FADH_2$. Both compounds shut down the citric acid cycle at various points, preventing further degradation of pyruvate. The accumulation of pyruvate is of critical importance. On the one hand, the cell can ferment it to lactate to regenerate the NAD needed in glycolysis. On the other hand, as lactate accumulates, an associated cellular acidosis develops.[64-74]

Just as sodium and potassium affect the cell's energy status, so does calcium. Under normal circumstances, the cell's enormous capacity to sequester calcium keeps intracellular ionic calcium concentrations quite low. Posttraumatic inflow of this ion through NMDA-associated receptors, however, as well as its release from the endoplasmic reticulum, causes intracellular calcium concentrations to rise. The free intracellular calcium then binds to the mitochondrial membrane, resulting in the uncoupling of ATP production from cytochrome-oxidase function. As a result, mitochondrial ATP production falls, further compromising the cell's energy status.[60-63]

We previously mentioned the relationship between NOS, Ca^{2+}, and NO production. NO, normally produced in minute quantities, plays an important role in normal cellular function. High levels of NO, however, can be harmful to the cell because this molecule is a highly reactive free radical. Posttraumatic Ca^{2+} elevation prolongs NOS activity and results in high intracellular NO levels.[69]

In addition to NO, other free radicals are released during cellular injury. A cascade of events, initiated by cellular energy depletion, leads to the release of large quantities of these molecules. As ATP is converted to ADP and then to AMP, the last is transformed into xanthine and hypoxanthine. In the setting of cellular acidosis, these by-products are degraded to uric acid, releasing free radicals in the process. These molecules, along with NO, then destroy cellular, nuclear, and mitochondrial membranes by lipid peroxidation, a process that itself releases more free radicals.

Once the nuclear membrane has been destroyed, the cell's DNA becomes exposed to the cytosolic contents. As strands of the nucleic acid are disrupted by the arriving free radicals, protein synthesis is interrupted. In addition, a DNA-repair system called *poly(ADP-ribose) synthetase* is activated.[75] This system severely depletes the cell's NAD and ATP stores. As a consequence, the cell falls further into energy failure. This situation is aggravated by the effects of NO and other free radicals on the mitochondrion. To begin with, NO directly poisons the mitochondrial electron-transport chain. In addition, the proton gradient normally found across the inner mitochondrial membrane disappears as the membrane's integrity is destroyed. Both of these conditions, along with the effect of calcium mentioned previously, prevent the mitochondrion from producing ATP efficiently.

As is true of the nuclear and mitochondrial membranes, lipid peroxidation of the cytoplasmic membrane destroys its structural integrity. When this occurs, ions are free to flow across the membrane, and the cell begins to swell. This is mostly the result of sodium influx. As swelling continues (a condition aggravated by cellular acidosis), the cellular membrane is further disrupted. Initially, the cell attempts to re-establish a normal intracellular ionic composition by activating membrane-bound ionic pumps. Because the cytoplasmic membrane can no longer act as an effective ionic barrier, however, this results only in the consumption of large amounts of ATP and ADP, further compromising the cell's energy status.

As we have seen, energy depletion plays a central role in the pathophysiology of brain injury. Because ATP and ADP are needed to fuel many of the cell's biochemical reactions, depletion of these compounds prevents the cell from functioning properly and blunts its ability to respond to stress. As the cell's homeostatic mechanisms lose their ability to compensate for intracellular derangements, the cell becomes increasingly dysfunctional and eventually dies.

Systemic Influences on Brain Injury

In addition to the intrinsic cellular processes mentioned previously, "external" systemic influences such as hypoperfusion (hypotension or low CBF), anoxia, and hyperglycemia can have a deleterious effect on the cell.[76-90] The first two deprive the cell of substrates, the most important of which is oxygen, and the last can worsen cellular acidosis. Hypoperfusion, in addition to depriving the cell of oxygen, can lead to the accumulation of metabolic by-products such as lactate (with associated acidosis), because these cannot be washed away with the venous blood. Whether a cell survives is then determined by the combined effect of both intrinsic and extrinsic factors.

ASSESSMENT AND TREATMENT OF HEAD INJURY

The focus of treatment of the patient with trauma is generally centered around two tenets. The first is to treat the injury that has already occurred. The second is to prevent further injury. Because the pathologic processes are dynamic, the patient must be continuously monitored and the treatment modality must be adjusted appropriately. Parameters such as intracranial pressure (ICP), CBF and jugular bulb lactate and oxygen contents allow the physician to monitor the cell's metabolic status as well as its perfusion. These, in turn, determine the therapeutic interventions to be made.

Initial Assessment

The initial assessment of the head-injured patient aims at identifying the extent of injuries and predicting potential sources of further injury. Oxygenation and hemodynamic status must be addressed early, and a focused neurologic examination should be performed. The Glasgow Coma Scale (GCS), developed in 1974, provides a systematic and reliable method for assessing the level of conciousness of the patient with trauma[91] (Table 48-1). On a total scale of

Table 48-1. Glasgow Coma Scale

Response	Points
Eye Opening	
Spontaneous	4
To sound	3
To pain	2
None	1
Motor Response	
Obeys commands	6
Localizes pain	5
Normal flexion (withdrawal)	4
Abnormal flexion (decortication)	3
Extension (decerebration)	2
None	1
Verbal Response	
Oriented	5
Confused conversation	4
Inappropriate words	3
Incomprehensive sounds	2
None	1

From Teasdale G, Jennett B. Assessment of coma and impaired consciousness. A practice scale. Lancet 2:81, 1974.

3 to 15, the patient's occular (1 to 4 points), verbal (1 to 5 points), and motor (1 to 6 points) responses are assessed and added to give the final GCS score. The initial postresuscitation GCS score is an excellent predictor of the patient's eventual outcome. In addition, the diffuse or focal nature of the neurologic deficit indicates the extent of cerebral damage sustained by the patient.

Initial radiographic examinations should include chest, pelvic, and cervical (anteroposterior, lateral, and odontoid) radiographs, as well as appropriate thoracic, lumbar, and long-bone films. A noncontrast computed tomographic (CT) scan of the head with bone windows should be obtained in patients who have an altered sensorium or a history of loss of conciousness after trauma. Skull radiographs do not play a role in the assessment of the patient with trauma if a CT scanner is available. In general, patients with nonoperative intracranial hemorrhages on CT scan should have the scan repeated within 4 to 6 hours. This decision should ultimately be based on the mechanism of injury, size, and location of the lesion, and on time interval between injury and initial assessment. Generally speaking, the longer the interval, the longer the allowable time between scans.

In any case, multiple serial neurologic examinations are required in the acute setting to identify progressive or potential problems. More sophisticated monitoring techniques can be implemented once the patient's initial condition has been stabilized or the patient has been transferred from the emergency department to the operating room or the intensive care unit.

CBF Monitoring

Trauma may cause changes in CBF autoregulation, resulting in abnormally high or low CBF.[15,92,93] Because both of these states can result in cellular injury or death, determination of CBF is important for the care of the brain-injured patient.[15,92-95] With the loss of autoregulation, either systemic hypotension or intracranial hypertension may result in ischemia.[76,77,79-90,96] Low-CBF states may also follow traumatic arterial dissection or cerebral vasospasm.[97] Hyperemia, caused by loss of cerebral vascular tone, can lead to cerebral edema and intracranial hypertension.[94,95] Though one may estimate tissue perfusion in absolute terms (milliliters per 100 g tissue per minute), one must always interpret CBF within the context of cerebral metabolism, because the former is normally tightly coupled to cerebral oxygen and glucose requirements.

Methods

Clinical examination is by far the easiest and least costly method of estimating CBF. In the healthy patient, changes in the neurologic examination as well as a slowing of the EEG can be observed when CBF falls to less than 20 to 25 ml/100 g/min. Because normal CBF is twice that, however, this method is not sensitive to early changes in tissue perfusion. Furthermore, the narrow window between the onset of neurologic deficit and permanent cellular damage (<20 ml/100 g/min) makes the margin of safety quite small. In addition, the neurologic examination is usually altered in patients with severe brain injuries, making correlation to CBF impossible. EEG monitoring offers little advantage over the neurologic examination and suffers from the same disadvantages.

Cerebral perfusion pressure (CPP), defined as mean arterial pressure minus ICP, can also be used to estimate CBF. This measure, however, is valid only if cerebral vascular resistance is normal. High–vascular resistance states, such as those found in cerebral vasospasm or arterial dissection, can be associated with poor cerebral perfusion despite an adequate CPP (>70 mm Hg). Conversely, low-resistance states as seen with luxury perfusion (hyperemia) may require considerably lower CPPs to maintain adequate cerebral perfusion. Because of these limitations, CPP assessment by itself is of limited value in estimating cerebral perfusion.

Kety and Schmidt CBF Measurement Technique

In 1945, Kety and Schmidt[98-100] introduced a method for determining CBF by means of inspired NO as a tracer of CBF. For this technique, NO is acutely introduced into the inspired air, and timed serial jugular-bulb venous samples are obtained and analyzed for NO content. Because this technique permits the simultaneous measurement of transcerebral $avDO_2$, the cerebral metabolic rate of oxygen ($CMRO_2$) can be calculated. The presence of hyperemia or ischemia can also be determined by measuring $avDO_2$. A normal $avDO_2$ should range between 4.5 and 8.5 ml/dl (average 6.7 ml/dl).[56,99] A value below normal indicates the presence of hyperemia, whereas high values herald the presence of ischemia. Disadvantages to this technique center around two points. First, the technique assumes that jugular venous samples truly represents global mixed venous blood. Unfortunately, this is often not the case. The right jugular bulb often receives a greater proportion of its blood from the superior sagittal sinus, whereas the left receives its supply preferentially from the straight sinus. Under these circumstances, the right jugular bulb samples reflect cortical blood flow and left samples reflect subcortical and posterior fossal blood flow. An additional disadvantage is its invasive nature, because jugular bulb catheters must be placed.

Xenon 133 Clearance Technique

The use of radioisotopes has led to major advances in CBF measurement techniques.[101,102] Xenon 133 is currently used as the gamma emitter of choice. The technique involves introducing the isotope into the bloodstream while measuring its rate of clearance from the cerebral circulation. Extracranial scintillation counters are used as radiation detectors. As first described, the technique required the intracarotid injection of a xenon 133 solution. Advances in the mathematics used for determining CBF, however, have made it possible to administer xenon 133 intravenously or as an inhaled gas.[102,103] The mathematic calculations correct for blood flow to the scalp. In addition, information about cortical ("fast-flow compartment") and white matter ("slow-flow compartment") blood flow is given.

The advantages of the xenon 133 technique are numerous. It is simple, is reproducible, and can be done at the bedside. The radiation exposure is small, and because xenon 133 is cleared extremely quickly from the body, its half-life is concomitantly short. In addition, multiple examinations can be carried out on the same patient within 30 minutes of one another. The major disadvantage hinges on the fact that the scintillation counters mainly measure superficial structures. As a result, little information about deep structures, such as the brain stem or basal ganglia, is obtained. A second disadvantage is its inability to detect focal areas of extremely low blood flow. This is referred to as the *"look-through" effect.*[104] It occurs because the low radiation counts within these regions are masked by the higher counts in the immediately surrounding areas. These caveats notwithstanding, the inhalational xenon 133 clearance technique is the most widely used CBF monitoring modality in our intensive care unit.

Transcranial Doppler Ultrasonography

Transcranial Doppler ultrasonography (TCD) uses low-frequency ultrasound to measure intravascular blood velocity and direction. Though ultrasonic waves normally do not travel through bone, certain areas of the skull provide windows through which they can pass. The thin temporal bone provides TCD access to the proximal and distal segments of the middle cerebral artery (MCA), the A-1 portion of the anterior cerebral artery, the distal intracranial internal carotid artery (ICA), the posterior cerebral artery, and the posterior communicating artery. The transorbital window (through the superior orbital fissure) allows assessment of the anterior cerebral artery, the ophthalmic artery, and the carotid siphon, and the foramen magnum provides access to the distal vertebral artery, the posterior cerebral artery, the posterior communicating artery, and the basilar artery.

For any vessel of fixed diameter, changes in TCD velocities directly reflect changes in blood flow. These are primarily the result of variations in arterial blood pressure. When blood pressure (and therefore blood flow) is fixed, on the other hand, TCD velocities vary inversely with the square of the vessel's radius. Because of variations in individual anatomy, however, there is no absolute blood flow velocity that corresponds to an absolute CBF value.

Even though this technique gives only an estimate of hemispheric blood flow, its ease of use and noninvasive nature make it ideal for monitoring patients in an intensive care unit setting. Trends in blood flow velocity and direction provide information regarding cerebral perfusion. In patients with subarachnoid hemorrhage, we look for an increase in flow velocities as an indication of vasospasm.[97,105,106] In patients with trauma, high TCD velocities can be caused by either vasospasm or hyperemia. The Lindegaard ratio, defined as flow velocity of the MCA over the velocity of the extracranial ICA (V_{MCA}/V_{ICA}), can help distinguish between the two.[105] If the ratio is >3, the patient likely has vasospasm. If the number is <3, hyperemia is present.

Other Methods

Thermal diffusion probes have been used for intraoperative monitoring of cortical blood flow.[107] The technique measures changes in a temperature gradient set up between two gold plates laid on the surface of the brain. As cortical blood flow changes, so does the change in temperature between the plates. Postoperative monitoring is possible when the plates are left in place and the leads are brought through the skin by means of a separate incision. Immediate changes in blood flow are noticeable, and constant monitoring is possible. The major disadvantages of this technique hinge on its inability to provide information on global CBF. In addition, even small shifts of the probe over the brain surface can lead to significant signal artifact. Finally, it is an invasive technique that places the patient at risk for infection.

The laser Doppler technique is similar to the thermal diffusion probe in that it also involves the use of a probe placed on the surface of the brain.[108,109] The difference is in its use of Doppler technology to measure cortical blood flow. The advantages and disadvantages of this technique are identical to those of the thermal probe.

Tomographic CBF-Monitoring Techniques

The advantage that these techniques have is that they provide a three-dimensional image of CBF that correlates regional blood flow to neuroanatomic structures. As such, the heterogenous nature of CBF becomes apparent, providing the physician a more realistic view of the patient's state of cerebral perfusion. In addition, many of these techniques provide absolute CBF measurements (in milliliters per 100 g tissue per minute).

Stable xenon CT. This technique uses inhaled nonradioactive xenon as an intravascular contrast agent. Because of its high tissue diffusibility, quantification of CBF is possible. In addition, excellent correlation can be made between CBF and neuroanatomic structures because blood flow images can be superimposed on conventional CT images.[110,111] This technique can also be used in conjunction with intravenous acetazolamide (a cerebral vasodilator) to provide information on cerebrovascular reserve.

Several disadvantages are associated with this technique. To begin with, the patient is exposed to radiation, and transportation to and from the CT scanner is required. In addition, high inspired concentrations of xenon (30% to 35%) are needed for this technique to be accurate. At these levels, xenon acts as a mild anesthetic agent, with some important side effects. These include agitation, somnolence, and nausea. All may interfere with the patient's ability to lie still for the duration of the test, with resultant movement artifact and possibly inaccurate CBF readings. In addition, xenon may increase CBF, casting some doubt on the accuracy and usefulness of this technique.[112] Standard CT scans alone are of limited value in evaluating cerebral perfusion because, even in cases of massive infarct, radiographic changes can be subtle during the first 24 hours.

Positron emission tomography. The first cross-sectional tomograph with positrons was described in 1975 by Phelps et al.[113] Since then, many techniques and refinements have been developed to measure CBF, cerebral metabolism, and chemical receptor activity. These advances have been both in the tomographic equipment (detectors and software) and in the radiopharmaceuticals used as positron emitters.[114] As a result, new-generation positron emission tomography (PET) scanners have a spatial resolution of 5 mm and an excellent uniformity of resolution throughout their entire field of view.[115-118] The radioactive tracers most commonly used for CBF studies are oxygen 15–labeled water and carbon dioxide.[78,119-125] Other tracers are nitrogen 13–labeled ammonia; butanol labeled with oxygen 15 or carbon 11, and fluoromethane labeled with fluorine 18 or carbon 11.[125-128] The PET autoradiographic technique, introduced by Raichle et al.[129] in 1983, is the most widely used method for obtaining PET images. This technique permits the absolute quantification of CBF, though semiquantitative and qualitative determinations can also be derived.

PET imaging, however, has significant drawbacks. The need for an on-site cyclotron for production of radiopharmaceuticals makes the cost of maintaining a PET facility prohibitive for most neuroimaging centers and generally limits its use to research facilities. Nevertheless, PET remains the gold standard by which CBF monitoring techniques are judged, and it will likely remain so in the foreseeable future.

Single-photon emission computed tomography. Single-photon emission computed tomography (SPECT) uses principles similar to those used for obtaining PET images. Its main advantage over PET is the cost. The radiopharmaceuticals needed for SPECT can be produced in most nuclear medicine laboratories without the need for a cyclotron. In addition, the photon-detectors are simple gamma cameras found at most centers.

Both two-dimensional and three-dimensional images can be obtained. The former provide a side view of the brain and require only a stationary gamma camera, whereas the latter produce an image similar to that of a PET scan and require that the detector rotate in a 360-degree plane around the patient. The resolution of either technique in general is poor. Three-dimensional images, for example, have a spatial resolution of 1.5 to 1.7 cm in the plane of the scan, with a thickness of 2 cm.

The first tomographic two-dimensional CBF studies with SPECT technology were obtained with inhaled xenon 133 as the CBF tracer.[130] Unfortunately, massive "cross-talk" between hemispheres made it virtually impossible to obtain information from one hemisphere alone. In 1961, Lassen and Ingvar[101,131] first described the intracarotid injection of radioisotope, which eliminated this problem. The year 1963 brought a new dimension to SPECT scanning with the introduction of three-dimensional imaging.[132] Again, xenon 133 was used as source of radiation. Since that time, improvements in both the detector and radioligands have led to faster acquisition times and better images.

Because the gamma ray emitted by xenon 133 is weak, good spatial resolution cannot be achieved with this gas as the source of radiation. The subsequent development of iodine 123–labeled amines as tracers eliminated some of these problems.[133-135] The most widely used iodinated amines are inosine 5′-monophosphate (IMP) and HIPDM. These substances are highly lipophillic, a property that results in nearly 100% first-pass extraction from the cerebral circulation. The local concentration of the amines, then, is proportional to CBF. In a sense, they very much act like the microspheres used in animal models for determining tissue perfusion. The major disadvantages associated with this technique are its cost and the relatively high radiation exposure. In addition, these substances passively redistribute throughout the brain within 1 hour after injection, significantly altering the SPECT image. A new generation of radioactive tracers that appear to address these problems are the technetium 99m–labeled agents.[136] The most promising of these appears to be hexamethyl-propyleneamine-oxime (HM-PAO). Initial studies show that IMP and HM-PAO have similar initial biodistribution properties. Moreover, technetium 99m is relatively inexpensive and can be readily found in most nuclear medicine laboratories. In addition, because of its decay properties, larger amounts of radioactivity can be given, significantly shortening image-acquisition time and improving image resolution. One final advantage of HM-PAO is that it does not appear to redistribute throughout the brain as IMP and HIPDM do.

Magnetic Resonance Imaging

MRI can delineate areas of infarct or edema but gives no quantitative information about cerebral perfusion. Magnetic resonance angiograms or venograms do provide some information about the patency of vessels, though visualization of all but large vessels is currently not feasible. For these reasons, and also because of the long image-acquisition times, this technique is not practical in the acute setting, or in unstable patients.

Cerebral Angiography

This technique is useful for delineating vascular anatomy and can provide qualitative information on cerebral perfusion. In addition, vasospastic arterial segments can be identified and treated with vasodilating agents, such as papaverine, or by directly dilating the affected area with balloon angioplasty catheters. The big disadvantages of this technique are its invasive nature, relatively high radiation exposure, rare but significant side effects of the intravenous contrast agents (e.g., renal failure and anaphylaxis), and its inability to provide more than qualitative assessment of CBF.

Metabolic Monitoring

To review quickly, ATP molecules (or high-energy equivalents) are produced during the conversion of glucose to carbon dioxide and water. The metabolic machinery consists of three sequential systems, each with its own control mechanisms and metabolic by-products. First, glycolysis converts glucose to pyruvate and produces ATP and NADH. Next, the Krebs cycle degrades pyruvate to carbon dioxide, releasing NADH and $FADH_2$ in the process. Finally, NADH and $FADH_2$ are oxidized by oxidative phosphorylation enzymes as oxygen is consumed to produce ATP. Under anaerobic conditions, both the Krebs cycle and oxidative phosphorylation shut down, leaving the cell to obtain its energy from glycolysis alone. This involves the fermentation of pyruvate to lactate, a process that leads to cellular acidosis. By measuring the rate at which oxygen and glucose are consumed and determining intracellular pH and lactate levels, inferences can be made about both cellular metabolism and tissue perfusion. Most of the methods used to measure cerebral metabolism follow these principles.

Jugular Venous Sampling

The technique of jugular venous sampling[137] can be used to determine the $CMRO_2$.[98,99] This technique relies on the initial determination of global CBF and $avDO_2$. $CMRO_2$ is then calculated according to the following formula:

$$CMRO_2\ (ml/100\ g/min) = [avDO_2\ (ml/dl) \times CBF\ (ml/100\ g/min)]/100$$

Similar calculations yield the CMRG and cerebral metabolic rate of lactate (CMRL) by substituting $avDO_2$ with avDG and arteriovenous difference of lactate, respectively.

As mentioned previously, $avDO_2$ can be used by itself to assess cerebral perfusion. If it is greater than 8.5 ml/dl, ischemia is suspected. If it falls below 4.5 ml/dl, hyperemia is present. CMRG gives an index of global brain metabolism, whereas $CMRO_2$ and CMRL provide information regarding aerobic and anaerobic metabolism, respectively.

Normal $CMRO_2$ averages 3.4 ml O_2 /100 g /min, though the range can vary between 1.8 to 3.9 ml/100 g/min.[5] Patients with head injuries generally have a lower $CMRO_2$ (between 1.3 and 2.7 ml/100 g/min).[79,138,139] This reflects the lower cellular energy demand resulting from posttraumatic electrical quiescence. Occasionally, however, $CMRO_2$ is low as a result of ischemia. When $CMRO_2$ falls below 1.3 ml/100 g/min, the cell can no longer support its basic metabolic needs and will die unless the situation is corrected.[5]

Under resting conditions, approximately 90% of the brain's glucose is metabolized aerobically. With an increase in cerebral electrical activity, glycolysis (and thus CMRG) increases. $CMRO_2$, however, does not increase proportionately. This is because the enzymes that regulate oxidative phosphorylation are normally nearly fully saturated and cannot be acutely upregulated. Under these conditions, pyruvate is fermented to lactate and CMRL *decreases.* It should be noted that CMRL is normally negative because jugular bulb lactate levels are usually higher than arterial levels. Thus, as lactate production increases, CMRL decreases. On occasion, CMRL is positive, indicating a net cellular uptake of lactate.

Patients with head injuries are generally found to have a decrease in CMRG. Though normal CMRG averages 32.5 mol/100 g/min,[140-142] Robertson et al.[143] reported that, in a series of 98 head-injured patients, this number dropped to an average low of 15.4 mol/100 g/min within first 5 days of injury. Hovda et al.,[144] on the other hand, reported a significant increase in the CMRG within 30 minutes after concussive brain injury in a rat model. Six hours after injury, these same animals had a prolonged hypometabolic state similar to that seen in head-injured patients. Similar results have been reported by Hayes et al.,[145,146] Kotayama et al.,[147] and Andersen and Marmarou.[148,149] After trauma, many neurons depolarize either spontaneously or through glutamate-mediated NMDA activation. The acute hypermetabolic state thus may simply reflect the coupling of glycolysis to increased Na^+/K^+ ATPase activity as the cell attempts to re-establish its membrane electrical potential. Of note, preliminary data in fluorine 18–labeled fluorodeoxyglucose ($[^{18}F]FDG$) PET studies suggest that this acute hypermetabolic state may also exist in humans (Hovda DA, personal communication).

After brain injury, CMRL decreases (lactate levels increase) and acidosis develops.[143,150-155] Though this can initially be explained by the acute hyperglycolytic state, both high lactate levels and acidosis persist well after CMRG falls below normal levels. Occasionally, this is caused by ischemia, though this is not always the case. In any event, both CMRL and acidosis return to normal as the patient's clinical condition improves.

Jugular venous sampling therefore provides information about the global metabolic state of the brain and the relative contributions of both aerobic and anaerobic metabolisms. The disadvantages of this technique focus around the inability to obtain information on regional blood flow, the drainage-pattern differences between right and left jugular bulbs, and the invasive nature of the technique.

Tomographic Imaging of Metabolism

In addition to its use for assessing CBF, PET technology has been used to determine regional cerebral metabolism. The most common tracers used are oxygen 15–labeled oxygen, carbon dioxide, and water, and [^{18}F]FDG.[120,156,157] The oxygen 15–labeled group is used for determining $CMRo_2$, whereas [^{18}F]FDG is for CMRG.

As it turns out, $CMRo_2$ can only be determined indirectly, because the positron detectors have no way of differentiating between intravascular and intracellular oxygen. To circumvent this problem, an initial PET scan with either oxygen 15–labeled carbon dioxide or water is performed to determine CBF. A second PET scan with oxygen 15–labeled oxygen is then performed. The difference in radioactivity is used to calculate $CMRo_2$.

CMRG, on the other hand, can be determined more directly. This is because of the special properties of [^{18}F]FDG. Of the glucose that enters the cell, 96% does so through a carrier-mediated system. Once inside the cell, it is phosphorylated to glucose 6-phosphate. This last step is critical; once phosphorylated, glucose cannot leave the cell. The chemical structure of [^{18}F]FDG allows it to enter the cell through the glucose transport system and to be phosphorylated to [^{18}F]FDG 6-phosphate by hexokinase. Unlike glucose, however, [^{18}F]FDG 6-phosphate is not a substrate for glycolysis and is not further metabolized. As such, it effectively becomes trapped within the cell for several hours after injection.[158] The rate at which glucose and [^{18}F]FDG enter the cell is proportional to the CMRG, so the amount of [^{18}F]FDG that accumulates within the cell mirrors CMRG.

What makes this technology so appealing is its ability to detect regional differences in $CMRo_2$ and CMRG. In addition, PET data can be superimposed on MRI data, making accurate neuroanatomic localization of metabolic activity possible. These points notwithstanding, PET has some significant disadvantages. Most have been discussed before. In addition, [^{18}F]FDG PET has specific practical limitations. Because radiation exposure from fluorine 18 is relatively high, only two or three scans can be obtained per patient per year.

As is true of PET CBF studies, PET metabolic studies remain accessible mainly to medical research facilities. The more affordable SPECT technology cannot currently be used for metabolic imaging, because metabolic tracers have yet to be tagged with photon emitters.

Magnetic Resonance Spectroscopy

Magnetic resonance spectroscopy is currently of limited clinical value in the management of patients with trauma. Briefly, this technique allows the physician to determine the chemical composition of a brain region selected from an MRI scan.[159-161] Unfortunately, the sample area is relatively large, and only relative measurements of the chemical contents of the region can be made. In addition, long acquisition times make this technology impractical in the patient who is agitated or in unstable condition.

Hemodynamic and Other Physiologic Parameters

Because patients with trauma are at risk for developing hemodynamic and metabolic derangements (especially in the immediate posttraumatic period), it is imperative to assess them early and frequently to detect potential problems and initiate appropriate therapy. By doing so, secondary injury can be minimized or avoided altogether.

Hemodynamic Monitoring

Because hypotension can have such devastating effects on the head-injured patient, systemic blood pressure must be monitored and supported to ensure adequate perfusion to the brain and other organs. The risk for developing hemodynamic instability should dictate the type of monitoring employed. Patients who are in the intensive care unit should at the very least have a radial arterial pressure monitor placed. If the patient has received a cardiac insult (e.g., myocardial infarct or cardiac contusion) or is receiving continuous intravenous pressors, the placement of a central venous or Swan-Ganz catheter should be considered. Other factors, such as prior history of cardiac disease, age, and severity of trauma, should influence the physician's approach to hemodynamic monitoring.

Serology

Serologic parameters routinely followed in patients with trauma are the serum electrolytes (Na^+, K^+, Cl^-, HCO_3^-, Ca^{2+}, and Mg^{2+}), arterial blood gas (ABG) values, and renal function tests (blood urea nitrogen and serum creatinine). Additional blood work addressing coagulopathies, sepsis, hepatopathies, and nutritional status are performed as deemed necessary.

Electrolyte management is a major focus in the trauma setting. The patient's initial resuscitation usually involves the infusion of large volumes of crystalloid solutions, and intravenous mannitol may be infused if intracranial hypertension is present or suspected. Both of these measures lead to large fluid shifts that can result in electrolyte abnormalities. In addition, electrolyte abnormalities may result from endocrine dysfunction, renal failure, chronic hyperventilation, long-term intravenous fluid infusion, and sepsis. Hyponatremia, for example, may be associated with cerebral salt wasting or the syndrome of inappropriate secretion of antidiuretic hormone (SIADH). If severe or untreated, it can cause seizures and aggravate cerebral edema. Hypernatremia may develop in the patient with diabetes insipidus, or when hyponatremia is overcorrected medically. For these reasons, serial assessment of the patient's electrolyte status is mandatory.

Though arterial oxygenation can usually be followed by pulse oximetry alone, ABG values confirm its accuracy and, perhaps more importantly, provide information about arterial P_{CO_2}. That P_{CO_2} values primarily guide hyperventilation therapy for intracranial hypertension underscores the importance of the ABG. In addition, the need to measure avD_{O_2} for assessment of cerebral metabolism makes this one of the most useful blood tests for evaluating the trauma patient.

Because of the high incidence of electrolyte abnormalities among patients with trauma and the constant need to monitor P_{CO_2}, electrolyte and ABG panels should be drawn routinely in the acute period. Other tests should be performed selectively. Coagulopathies, for example, are fairly common in the immediate posttraumatic period. Major causes for this include the release of tissue thromboplastin by the injured brain (which may precipitate a disseminated intravascular coagulation–type coagulopathy), hypothermia, and massive blood transfusions. Such cases require that prothrombin time and partial thromboplastin time be determined on arrival at the emergency department and serially until normal values are obtained. Similarly, after an episode of severe hypotension (which can lead to renal failure and myocardial ischemia) renal function tests and cardiac enzyme levels should be obtained.

To be sure, blood tests should be drawn judiciously. Anemia from repeated phlebotomy is not uncommon (especially in critically ill patients), and both cellulitis and phlebitis can result from multiple needle sticks.

Intracranial Pressure Monitors

Normal intracranial contents include brain parenchyma, cerebrospinal fluid (CSF), and intravascular blood. Because the cranial volume is fixed, volume changes in any of the three components affect intracranial pressure (ICP). The volume-pressure curve described by Langfitt et al.[162] demonstrates a curvilinear relationship between intracranial volume and changes in ICP (Fig. 48-4). As intracranial volume increases, so does ICP. Initially, the rise in ICP is barely noticeable, and the slope of the curve approximates zero. As intracranial volume accumulates, the curve becomes increasingly steeper, eventually approaching vertical.

Intracranial hypertension can have devastating effects on a patient's outcome and must be treated early and aggressively. Severe intracranial hypertension often leads to herniation of the brain or brain stem through the tentorial opening, through the foramen magnum, or under the falx cerebri. Once the brain stem becomes involved (either directly or indirectly), death is imminent unless the situation is promptly corrected.

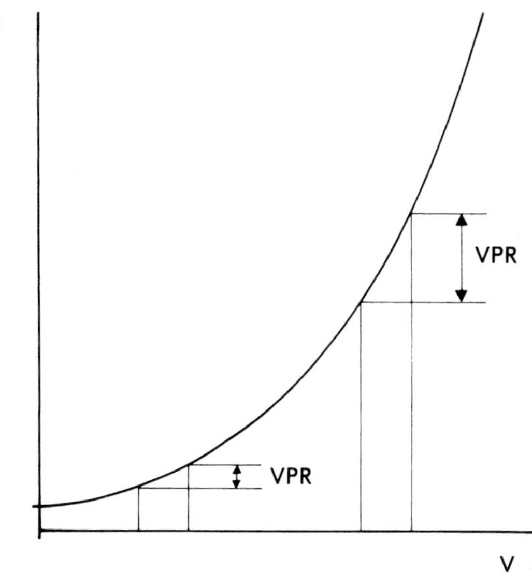

Fig. 48-4. Volume-pressure response *(VPR)*. A small addition of volume causes only an insignificant increase in intracranial pressure (ICP) when ICP is low; the same amount of volume increase may cause a considerable rise of ICP when it is already high. *P,* Pressure; *V,* volume.

Two basic types of ICP monitors are currently available, the drainage catheter and the fiberoptic catheter. The former can be placed in the ventricle, subarachnoid, or subdural space. The latter is usually placed within the brain parenchyma, though it can be placed in virtually any intracranial compartment. Because of its potential therapeutic role, the intraventricular drainage catheter is the ICP monitor of choice at our institution. Not only does it provide information on ICP, it also allows the physician to drain ventricular CSF, thus lowering ICP. If the ventricular catheter cannot be placed, then a fiberoptic catheter is used.

The major complications associated with this technology are infection and hemorrhage. The infection rates for intraventricular drains and fiberoptic catheters are 0% to 27% (average 8%) and 0% to 1.7%, respectively.[85,163-180] The risk of hemorrhage is similar between the two, with an incidence of 0% to 1%.* The incidence of malfunction, on the other hand, is considerably higher with fiberoptic technology. Malfunction and obstruction rates for intraventricular, subdural, and subarachnoid drains are 2.5%, 2.7%, and 16% respectively.[178] The risk of malfunction with the fiberoptic catheter, on the other hand, is 10% to 30%.[172,178] In addition, the cost difference between fiberoptic and drainage catheters is enormous, with the former costing an order of magnitude more than the latter.

All things considered, accuracy, reliability, therapeutic value, and cost make the intraventricular drainage catheter the most useful ICP monitor available. Though the risk of

*References 164, 165, 168, 170, 172, 174-176, 178, 181-183.

placing either hydrostatic or fiberoptic monitors is small, one should be discriminating in both patient and monitor selection. In the awake and conscious patient, one can follow the neurologic examination, knowing that a drop in the level of arousal is an early indicator of rising ICP. If the patient is initially not arousable, then an ICP monitor is indicated. Generally speaking, a patient who is following commands (GCS score of 9 to 15) is at low risk for development of intracranial hypertension. Patients with a GCS score less than 9, however, are at significant risk for development of intracranial hypertension. This is, of course, only a guideline. Naryan et al.[85] showed that the subgroup of patients with GCS scores <8 who also have abnormalities on head CT have a higher incidence of cerebral hypertension (53% to 63%) than do those with normal CT results (13%). The exception is the patient who has a normal CT result but also has two of the following features: systolic blood pressure <90 mm Hg, extensor or flexor posturing, and age older than 40 years. The risk that this subgroup of patients had for development of intracranial hypertension was the same as that of patients with abnormal head CT results.[85] To summarize, patients with a GCS ≤8 should receive an ICP monitor—preferably an intraventricular drain—and those with a GCS >8 should be followed up with frequent, serial neurologic examinations.

Therapy of the Head-Injured Patient

The enormous amount of material under this heading could itself be the subject of a lengthy treatise. For this reason we are concentrating on the most salient features of therapy and providing guidelines for the treatment of the head-injured patient. Because most of the necessary information regarding the cellular response to injury has been explained previously, only cursory reminders are used to justify the physiologic bases for therapy.

Generally speaking, therapeutic interventions in head injury can be surgical or nonsurgical. Surgical interventions usually take place early in the posttraumatic period, whereas nonsurgical interventions may continue for weeks after the injury. To be sure, many postinjury sequelae are treatable to some degree by both surgical and nonsurgical means. The key to optimal treatment is thus deciding which modality is most appropriate.

Surgical Intervention

The surgical treatment of the head-injured patient focuses mainly on two pathologic entities. The first is intracranial hypertension; the second is open cranial wounds.

Intracranial hypertension. To decrease ICP, intracranial volume must be reduced. After trauma, intracranial hypertension results from hydrocephalus, cerebral edema, and mass lesions (e.g., hematomas). The approach in treating intracranial hypertension is thus to minimize the volume of CSF, swollen brain tissue, and extravasated blood. An alternative approach is to increase the size of the cranial vault.

CSF volume is the easiest to reduce. Through placement of a ventricular catheter, CSF can be drained and ICP can be monitored. There is, of course, a limit to the amount of CSF that can be drained. This limit is reached when the ventricle collapses around the catheter. Two problems arise from this situation. First, the ICP waveform becomes dampened, making measurements inaccurate. Second, the catheter may become permanently obstructed, preventing further CSF drainage.

Surgical reduction of brain volume clearly is not a first-line treatment modality for the reduction of ICP. Nevertheless, circumstances can arise where this is the treatment of choice. Though both frontal and temporal lobes are amenable to resection, surgery should be less extensive in the dominant hemisphere (where the speech centers are located). Bilateral resections should be avoided at all costs, because these can be devastating to the patient. Bifrontal resections leave the patient abulic and occasionally interfere with the patient's ability to form new memories. Bitemporal lesions are even more devastating. In addition to producing memory deficits, they may produce Klüver-Bucy syndrome, leaving the patient apathetic, placid, and with uninhibited sexual responses. Resection of these structures should be considered if intracranial hypertension is uncontrollable or expected to become so—especially if either the frontal or temporal lobe is significantly swollen. One may also consider performing a prophylactic frontal or temporal lobectomy under the following circumstances. First, the patient is already undergoing a craniotomy (e.g., for the evacuation of a hematoma or the repair of an open skull fracture). Second, severe intracranial hypertension is expected. Third, there is no corresponding contralateral lobe lesion or infarct. Though rarely needed, a unilateral cerebellar hemisphere resection can also be performed if the brain stem is compressed as a result of posterior fossal swelling.

The indications to remove intracranial hematomas should reflect the patient's overall clinical condition, progression (improvement or deterioration) of the neurologic examination, and radiographic (mainly CT) findings. Intracranial hemorrhages are classified by their location. This schema not only specifies their location (important for surgical planning), it also gives some indication about the mechanism of injury and patient's prognosis.

Epidural hematomas (EDHs) are located between the cranium and outer layer of dura (Fig. 48-5). The typical CT appearance is that of a biconvex lens seen from the side. They are most often associated with skull fractures and result from the tearing of meningeal arteries as they cross the sharp fracture lines. The mechanism of injury is usually an impact to the skull, and the artery most commonly involved is the middle meningeal artery as it courses along the thin, easily fractured squamous portion of the temporal bone. Occasionally, a venous EDH forms as the result of dural sinus injury. In this case, the fracture line overrides a dural sinus, and venous blood enters the epidural space. Surgical treatment for this type of EDH is

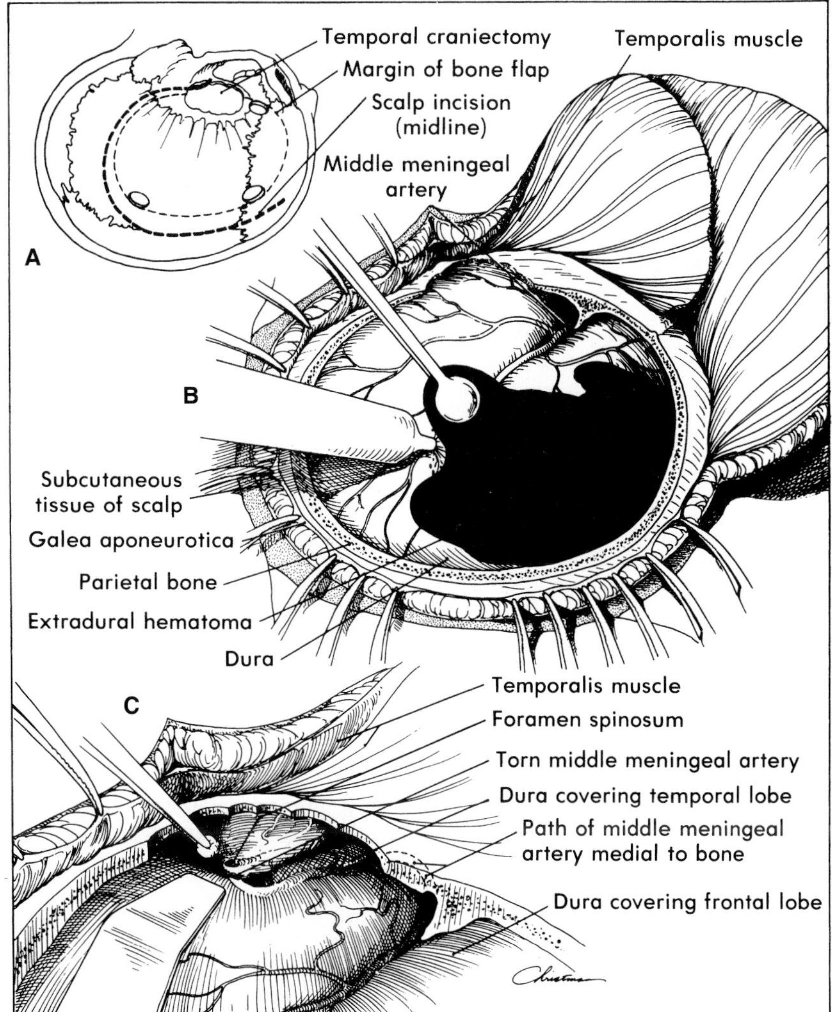

Fig. 48-5. Large epidural hematoma is removed through a craniotomy. The clot originated from the laceration of the middle meningeal artery at the foramen spinosum. **A,** The scalp incision site and the margins of the bone flap. **B,** The skull has been removed, and the blood clot is being evacuated. **C,** The anatomic relationships of the base of the skull, dura, brain, and middle meningeal artery.

considerably more difficult, because a large volume of blood can be lost in an extremely short period. The period of greatest blood loss occurs during the craniotomy and prior to the isolation of the sinus tear.

Neurologic prognosis in the isolated EDH is fairly good. Because the skull absorbs a significant amount of the impact force (hence the fracture), the brain remains relatively intact. The neurologic deterioration these patients exhibit usually results from a rapidly expanding lesion. This situation is a neurosurgical emergency.

Subdural hematomas (SDHs) are an entirely different pathologic entity. They result from rupture of the bridging veins that drain into the dural sinuses (Fig. 48-6). The typical CT appearance of the SDH shows an extra-axial blood collection that roughly follows the contour of the brain and remains outside the sulci or basal cisterns (Fig. 48-7). One might expect the venous nature of the hemorrhage to herald a benign course. Unfortunately, this is not the case. For the bridging veins to tear, the brain must move relative to the skull. As the veins stretch beyond their elastic limit, they rupture spilling blood into the subdural space (between the dura and arachnoid membranes). The back-and-forth movement of the brain produces shock waves that initiate the cascade of events leading to excitotoxicity and cellular damage. Because diffuse axonal injury and cerebral edema are often associated with SDH, evacuation of the mass, even when large, is not always effective in preventing or reversing neurologic deficits. In the patient with a GCS score <8, emergency evacuation of any SDH >5 mm thick should be performed. Occasionally, a CT scan will show significant midline shift with a thin-rim SDH (<3 mm). This usually indicates significant hemispheric swelling. Evacuation of the SDH in cases such as this is unlikely to reduce ICP significantly, and intracranial hypertension is best managed nonsurgically. This type of injury is usually caused by the sudden acceleration or deceleration of the head such as that seen in MVAs or falls.

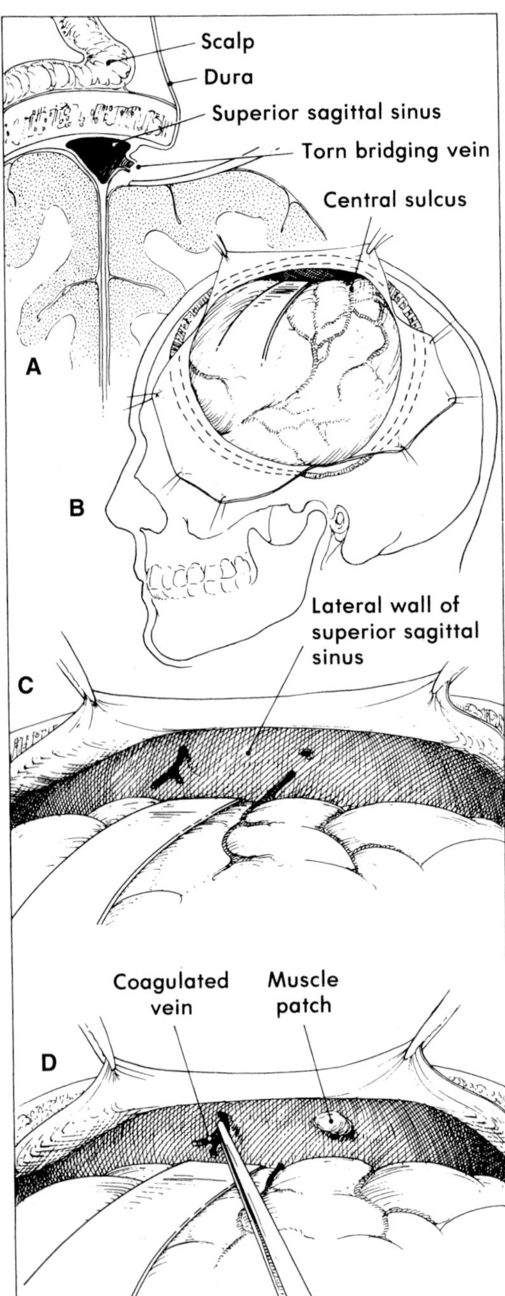

Fig. 48-6. Bridging veins, torn by the brain movement, are often responsible for the subdural hematoma. **A,** A coronal cut through the skull demonstrating anatomic relationships. **B,** The skull removed, dura opened, and lateral view of **A. C,** Cortical veins approaching the superior sagittal sinus. **D,** Two methods used to control venous bleeding—coagulation and placement of a muscle patch.

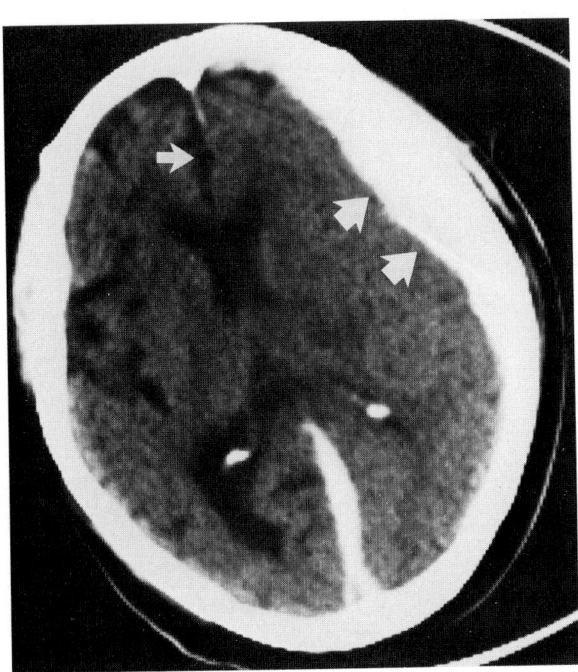

Fig. 48-7. Acute subdural hematoma *(double arrows)* seen on CT scan. The midline is markedly shifted *(single arrow)*.

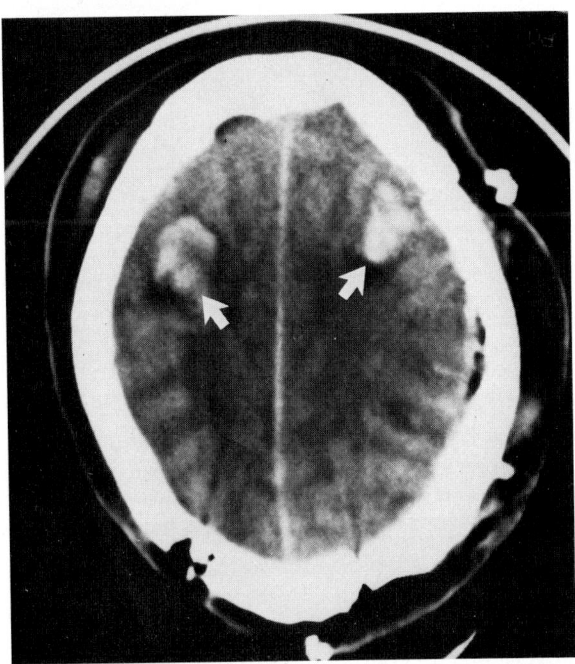

Fig. 48-8. Bilateral anterior contusions *(arrows)* seen in brain parenchyma during CT scanning (edema is seen around the lesion).

Subarachnoid hemorrhage is often associated with trauma, though its significance remains uncertain. Rarely is the hemorrhage large enough to create a mass effect, though it can cause hydrocephalus by plugging arachnoid granulation tissue. Patients with trauma do have cerebral vasospasm; however, it is unclear whether this is caused by the presence of subarachnoid blood or some other causative agent. On occasion, traumatic events are precipitated by an aneurysmal rupture. Such patients may have significant cisternal subarachnoid blood, with or without other findings. If the physician's index of suspicion is high enough, a cerebral angiogram should be performed.

Intracerebral hemorrhages are seen as either contusions or frank hematomas (Fig. 48-8). The former can be thought as brain bruises that blend into the parenchyma; the latter are more discrete blood collections. They are often associated with acceleration-deceleration events or penetrating injuries. Contusions can be either superficial or deep. Superficial contusions result from the collision of brain against bone or bony prominences. The most common locations are the frontal, temporal, and occipital tips and the inferior frontal and temporal lobes. Deep contusions are found just off midline within the deep gray matter, internal capsule, and corpus callosum. These result from the local concentration of sheer forces during cerebral deformations. Rotational forces such as those produced in broadside MVAs often lead to this contusion pattern.

The treatment of intraparenchymal contusions or hematomas depends on the location and size of the lesion, as well as the general clinical condition of the patient. Small lesions can be treated expectantly, whereas larger lesions (causing shift and intracranial hypertension) should be removed. This topic, however, remains controversial. In their series of more than 200 patients, Miller et al.[184] showed that, despite surgical resection of these lesions, ICP remained exceedingly difficult to control. On the other hand, the early evacuation of large hematomas may delay the rise of ICP long enough to allow other modalities of brain protection to take effect. Because hematomas and contusions tend to enlarge, it is prudent to examine nonsurgical or potentially surgical lesions with a repeated CT scan within 4 to 6 hours. If the lesion is stable, one may follow the patient's course expectantly. If the lesion has enlarged, or the ICP becomes difficult to control, surgical evacuation should be considered.

Location of the lesion also plays a role in the decision whether or not to operate. Temporal lesions, for example, present a special problem. Because of their location, minimal expansion or local swelling can lead to transtentorial herniation and brain stem compression. This may occur even in the absence of global intracranial hypertension. The threshold for operating on temporal lobe lesions is thus significantly lower than that for similarly sized lesions in other supratentorial locations. Posterior fossal (cerebellar) lesions pose a similar problem and should be operated on at the first indication of ventricular obstruction or brain stem compression. Involvement of eloquent cortex clearly should delay the decision to operate, especially if the lesion is stable.

Though expansion of the intracranial cavity seems like a reasonable alternative for treating of intracranial hypertension, its usefulness remains dubious. It is not unreasonable to perform a bony subtemporal decompression after the evacuation of an intracranial hematoma, because the morbidity is minimal and the extra space may allow the temporal lobe to expand without compressing the brain stem. On occasion, we have found ourselves facing malignant cerebral edema prior to closure of a trauma craniotomy. In some of these cases, we have elected to close without replacing the bone flap to allow the brain to expand through the (large) craniotomy opening. To be sure, this is a final, desperate measure. Nonetheless, anecdotal evidence suggests that it may help control ICP, at least in some cases.

Open wounds. Open wounds are found in penetrating injuries, some impact injuries, and skull fractures involving the basicranium. Open wounds expose bone and, occasionally, intracranial contents to the environment, placing the patient at risk for developing cranial and intracranial infections. As a rule, open wounds should be closed.

Nondisplaced basal skull fractures associated with CSF leaks can initially be treated expectantly. Most heal spontaneously. If after 2 or 3 days, the leak has not stopped or shown signs of slowing down, a 3- to 5-day trial of CSF diversion with a ventricular or lumbar subarachnoid drain should be attempted (unless contraindicated). If this fails, the leak should be identified, explored, and closed surgically. All this assumes that surgical closure will prove beneficial to the patient's overall prognosis. Intravenous antibiotics for CSF leaks have not been shown to decrease the incidence of infection, yet they may select out more virulent organisms. Displaced or comminuted fractures may be treated the same if small. Larger fractures, especially those involving the sinuses, should be explored, the sinuses should be exenterated and packed, and a dural repair should be carried out. Large dural defects of the frontal fossa are ideally suited for extradural repair with a vascularized pericranial flap. For middle and posterior fossal leaks, packing of the mastoid air cells with muscle, fat, or bone wax is critical to prevent further leakage. The placement of a ventricular or lumbar subarachnoid drain can be used in conjunction with the open repair, though often it is not required. In addition, it carries with it the risk of overdrainage pneumocephalus and catheter-related infection.

Open wounds involving the cranial vault are easier to deal with. As a rule, they should be explored, débrided, and closed. Any associated hematoma should be evacuated as well. Penetrating injuries, such as those associated with gunshot wounds, are a special case. Though Cushing[185,186] advocated aggressive débridement of necrotic brain and bone fragments, the Vietnam Phase I and II trials[187,188] and recent experience in the Israeli-Lebanese conflict[189] indicate that local, superficial debridement, gentle wound irrigation with antibiotic solutions, and intravenous antibiotics effectively prevent the formation of brain abscess and preserve potentially viable brain tissue. In addition, seizure frequency does not appear to increase with less aggressive surgery. Another study,[190] based on data from Iran and Iraq, showed that wounds less than 2 cm wide with no underlying mass lesion could effectively be treated with local anesthesia irrigation, primary closure, and intravenous antibiotics.

Graham et al.[191] showed that the prognosis for gunshot wounds directly related to the GCS score after initial resuscitation. Patients who had a postresuscitation GCS score of 3 to 5 universally did poorly. Of those with a GCS score of 6 to 8, 80% were either dead or had severe neurologic impairment at follow-up (mean 9 months). Similar outcomes were seen in only 33% of patients with GCS scores of 9 to 12 and 0% of patients with a GCS score >13. Other indicators for poor prognosis were multilobe, dominant hemisphere, or transventricular injuries.[191]

Nonsurgical Treatment of the Head-Injured Patient

Nonsurgical treatment of the head-injured patient is far more complex than is its surgical counterpart. Medical management centers around the treatment of intracranial hypertension, cerebral perfusion, and metabolic derangements. These, however, are not independent. Most treatment modalities affect all three to some degree.

Intracranial pressure. Approximately 10% to 15% of patients with severe head injury ultimately have intracranial hypertension refractory to aggressive medical or surgical treatment, with an associated mortality rate of 84% to 100%.[85,184,192] Multiple studies have clearly demonstrated that intracranial hypertension is detrimental to patient outcome[82,184,193-198] and that aggressive treatment of elevated ICP improves both mortality rate and neurologic outcome.[85,184,199] Though both surgical and nonsurgical strategies for management of intracranial hypertension aim at reducing CSF, blood, and brain volumes, their respective efficacies vary considerably.

CSF volume can be reduced medically with acetazolamide, which decreases production. Unfortunately, it takes several days to exert its effect, making it ineffective in the acute setting. Furthermore, acetazolamide is a vasodilator that can raise ICP by increasing intracranial blood volume. Though other diuretics and some corticosteroids are known to decrease CSF production, none has been proved effective in controlling ICP. Ventricular drainage remains the mainstay of treatment for the reduction of CSF volume.

The regulation of intravascular blood volume is arguably the most interesting and challenging aspect of medical ICP management. On the one hand, the lower the intracranial blood volume, the lower the ICP. On the other hand, the need to perfuse the brain places a practical limit on the amount of blood that can be withheld from the intracranial vasculature. Though intravascular blood normally resides in the arterial, capillary, and venous compartments, volume-reduction therapy can only address the first and last of these.

Venous volume reduction is remarkably well tolerated. Measures such as elevation of the head of the bed and placing the patient's head and neck in an anatomically neutral position increase cerebral venous drainage and lower ICP. Theoretically, the higher the head is elevated, the greater the drop in ICP. Factors such as hypotension (relative or absolute), need for pulmonary toilet, presence of decubitus ulcers, and patient comfort make this ideal difficult to attain. Nevertheless, a bed elevation of 30 to 45 degrees effectively decreases intracranial venous volume and lowers ICP. The presence of an unstable cervical fracture is a relative contraindication to this maneuver.

Seizures, coughing, Valsalva maneuvers, and generally anything that increases intrathoracic pressure decrease cerebral venous return and thus increase ICP. For this reason, early sedation and paralysis in agitated, ventilated patients is recommended if ICP is difficult to control.

Body temperature regulation also plays an important role in the management of intracranial hypertension. Because cerebral blood volume increases with increasing body temperature, hyperthermia should be aggressively treated. This has the added benefit of lowering cerebral metabolism and decreasing edema.

Barbiturates appear to lower ICP through their effect on both cerebral vascular tone and metabolism.[200,201] The latter effect is likely the most important factor. As cerebral metabolic rate falls, autoregulatory mechanisms decrease blood flow to match CBF to the metabolic needs of the cell. The drop in CBF lowers intracranial blood volume and ICP. These medications have been particularly effective in controlling intracranial hypertension otherwise refractory to medical and surgical treatments. Despite this, the prophylactic use of barbiturates for intracranial hypertension does not appear to be justified. Ward et al.[202] reported on 53 head-injured patients treated with or without pentobarbital for intracranial hypertension. In this randomized, controlled study, no differences were noted in the Glasgow Outcome Scale or mortality rate between groups. Significant hypotension (<80 mm Hg), however, was noted in 54% and 7% of treated and nontreated patients, respectively. Schwartz et al.[203] compared mannitol to pentobarbital as the initial therapy in patients whose ICP was >25 mm Hg for 15 minutes. Those patients who had discrete mass lesions requiring surgical evacuation fared the same. The mortality rates among these patients were 43% and 40% in the mannitol and pentobarbital groups, respectively. When diffuse injuries were involved, however, the mortality rates were 41% for the mannitol group and 77% for those treated with pentobarbital. CPP was noted to be significantly lower in patients treated with barbiturates.

What role, then, do these medications play in the therapy of intracranial hypertension? In 1988, Eisenberg et al.[199] reported on 73 head-injured patients (GCS scores between 4 and 8) who developed intracranial hypertension refractory to aggressive "conventional therapy." Patients were randomly assigned to either the control group (continues conventional therapy) or to the retreatment group (conventional therapy plus barbiturates). Treatment was considered a success if the ICP could be controlled (as determined by strict criteria). Of the 36 patients in the control group, only 6 (16.7%) were considered treatment successes. This compared to 12 of 37 (32.4%) in the barbiturate group. As a result of this finding, 32 of the control patients were eventually crossed over to the treatment group. Mortality rate at 1 month was 8% for patients who responded to barbiturate therapy, compared with 83% for nonresponders. At 6 months, 36% of responders were either vegetative or had died, compared with 90% of the nonresponders. Subsequent studies have shown that the beneficial effects of barbiturates are seen only in patients with intact cerebral autoregulatory mechanisms.[204]

Barbiturate infusion is monitored with scalp EEG and is titrated to a burst suppression lasting 5 to 10 seconds. The length of therapy is empirical, though an initial trial of 3 to 5 days may be adequate.

Hyperventilation therapy has been known to decrease ICP by causing cerebral vasoconstriction and subsequently lowering cerebral arterial blood volume. Until recently, it was recommended to titrate hyperventilation to a P_{CO_2} of approximately 25 mm Hg. Re-evaluation of the available data, however, has revealed that aggressive hyperventilation may do more harm than good. Several studies have related aggressive hyperventilation to cerebral ischemia.[95,205] Obrist et al.[95] demonstrated avD_{O_2} levels of 10.5 ± 0.7 ml/dl and CBF values of 18.6 ± 4.4 ml/100 g/min in 10 patients hyperventilated to a P_{CO_2} around 23. In addition, Sheinberg et al.[206] showed that jugular venous desaturation (and widened avD_{O_2}) was associated with arterial P_{CO_2} levels of <28 mm Hg. In light of this evidence, current guidelines recommend moderate hyperventilation to keep P_{CO_2} levels between 30 and 35 mm Hg.

Though mannitol is known to lower ICP, its mechanisms of action remain somewhat unclear. Because it does not freely cross the blood-brain barrier, intravenous mannitol infusion establishes an osmotic gradient between the blood and brain parenchyma.[207] To re-establish osmotic equilibrium, interstitial fluid diffuses into the vascular space, effectively decreasing cerebral volume and ICP. The sudden increase in blood volume has the added benefit of reducing hematocrit, decreasing blood viscosity, and increasing CBF.[207-212] Experience suggests that continuous mannitol infusions precipitate renal failure[213,214] and can lead to the accumulation of mannitol within brain parenchyma.[207,213,215-217] The latter may adversely effect ICP. As mannitol accumulates, a reverse osmotic gradient develops. This causes cerebral edema and increases ICP.[210,213,217,218] In addition, chronic serum hyperosmolarity leads to Na^+ depletion, and the subsequent hyponatremia may lead to further cerebral edema. The recommended regimen is therefore to treat elevations of ICP with intermittent boluses of mannitol (0.25 to 1.0 g/kg of body weight) as long as the serum osmolarity does not exceed 320 mOsm.[210,219-222]

Cerebral perfusion. The idea of treating CPP in head trauma is to ensure that the injured brain does not become ischemic. Preliminary studies indicate improved morbidity and mortality rates among patients treated with CPP-directed regimens.[223-226] These regimens emphasize lowering ICP, as noted previously, and raising MAP. First, cardiac output must be optimized. Patients should be kept euvolemic, and fluid status should be closely monitored. The need for central venous pressure lines and Swan-Ganz catheters should be dictated by patient factors and physician experience. Further elevation of MAP can be accomplished by the intravenous infusion of hypertensive agents, such as dopamine or phenylephrine (Neo-Synephrine).

Currently, insufficient data exist to specify strict guidelines regarding CPP therapy. Nevertheless, a CPP >70 mmHg appears to maximize cerebral perfusion and minimize the risk of ischemia. It should be emphasized that all therapy should include measures aimed at optimizing arterial oxygenation.

Metabolism. The last therapeutic arm in the medical treatment of head injury aims at ameliorating the cellular metabolic disturbances associated with brain trauma. This is perhaps the most difficult aspect of treatment in the head injured patient. Traumatic brain injury is of a diffuse, heterogenous nature. As a result, cellular metabolic disturbances vary widely within the brain. This makes treatment difficult, because optimal therapy for one cell may be suboptimal for another. Generally speaking, maintaining oxygenation and optimizing cerebral perfusion enable mitochondria to function optimally and wash out toxic metabolic by-products to some extent. In addition, measures aimed at reducing the cellular metabolic rate protect the cell by decreasing its energy demands and preventing cellular energy depletion. Barbiturates and hypothermia share this therapeutic property. Finally, therapy directed at NMDA-mediated excitotoxicity, intracellular calcium influx, and free-radical production may provide alternative measures for the prevention of cellular injury and death, though clinical trials of NMDA-receptor antagonists, calcium-channel blockers, and free-radical scavengers have generally been disappointing.

Anticonvulsants. Prophylactic anticonvulsant therapy plays an important role in the prevention of early posttraumatic seizures.[7,227,228] These are seizures occurring within 7 days of the injury. Both phenytoin and carbamazepine have been shown to be effective. However, no effect on the development of late or delayed posttraumatic seizures has been shown with the use of early prophylactic anticonvulsant therapy.[7,228-230] Early seizure control is important in controlling ICP and preventing unnecessary cellular electrical activity (which might otherwise aggravate cellular metabolic derangements).

Steroids. The routine use of corticosteroids in the setting of trauma has not been beneficial and may even have a deleterious effect by promoting hyperglycemia, delaying healing, and blunting the immune system. Their use is therefore not recommended.

SUMMARY

The treatment of traumatic brain injury is multifaceted and directs therapy toward specific pathologic processes. Because intracranial hypertension and ischemia play a significant role in the pathophysiology of brain injury, much of our therapy focuses on their treatment.

General guidelines for the initial nonsurgical treatment of the head-injured patient include fluid resuscitation to attain euvolemia, elevation of the head of the bed, antiseizure prophylaxis, and optimizing oxygenation. Further basic treatment includes prevention of hyperthermia, sedation (with or without pharmacologic paralysis), and

CPP maintenance above 70 mm Hg. In patients with a GCS score <8, early ventricular drainage for elevated ICP, intubation, and mild hyperventilation to a PCO_2 of approximately 35 mm Hg are recommended.

If these measures become ineffective in controlling ICP, therapy with mannitol boluses (not to exceed a serum osmolarity of 320 mOsm) should be initiated. Hyperventilation can also be increased to drop the PCO_2 to 30 mm Hg. The insertion of a jugular bulb catheter for CBF and $avDO_2$ measurements is indicated and should guide further therapy. Systemic hypertensive therapy, barbiturate coma, decompressive lobectomy or craniotomy, and hypothermic therapy can and should also be considered if intracranial hypertension and low cerebral perfusion continue to be a problem. Of course, serial CT scans should be obtained throughout the patient's hospital course to rule out discrete mass lesions amenable to surgical evacuation.

Despite a considerable understanding of the pathophysiology of brain injury, therapy directed against specific cellular biochemical and metabolic derangements remains woefully inadequate and fails to address the spatiotemporal heterogeneity of traumatic brain injuries. As we have seen, traumatic brain injury initiates a cascade of cellular metabolic events that begins with neuronal depolarization, massive glutamate release, and hypermetabolism and progresses toward cellular energy depletion, acidosis, free-radical production, and death. Ideally, therapy should be tailored to address specific metabolic abnormalities. Unfortunately, our understanding of the time frame in which these changes occur is fairly limited, and our inability to adequately assess an individual cell or small group of cells curtails our efforts to establish effective therapy against discrete cellular metabolic derangements. Nevertheless, significant therapeutic advancements have been made since the days of aggressive hyperventilation and hypovolemia. Continued research will elucidate pathophysiologic mechanisms and suggest new therapeutic alternatives for treating severe brain injuries.

REFERENCES

1. Alberts B, et al. The Molecular Biology of the Cell, 2nd ed. New York: Garland Publishing, 1989, p 300.
2. Hille B. Ionic basis of resting and action potentials. In Kandel ER, ed. Handbook of Physiology, vol 1. The Nervous System, Part 1. Bethesda, Md.: American Physiological Society, 1977, p 99.
3. Koester J. Resting membrane potential and action potential. In Kandel ER, Schwartz JH, eds. Principles of Neural Science, 2nd ed. New York: Elsevier, 1985, p 49.
4. Nernst W. On the kinetics of substances in solution. Translated from Z Phys Chem. 2:613. In Kepner GR, ed. Cell Membrane Permeability and Transport. Stroudsberg: Dowden Hutchinson and Ross, 1979, p 634.
5. Ritter AM, Robertson CS. Cerebral metabolism. Neurosurg Clin North Am 5:633, 1994.
6. Dawson TM, Snyder SH. Gases as biological messengers: Nitric oxide and carbon monoxide in the brain [review]. J Neurosci. 14:5147, 1994.
7. Glotzner FL. Anfallsprophylaze mit carbamazepin nac schweren schadelhirnverletzungen. Neurochirurgia 26:66, 1983.
8. Huang Z, et al. Effects of cerebral ischemia in mice deficient in neuronal nitric oxide synthase. Science 265:1883, 1994.
9. Choi DW. Nitric oxide: Foe or friend to the injured brain? [comment]. Proc Natl Acad Sci U S A 90:9741, 1993.
10. Dawson TM, Dawson VL, Snyder SH. A novel neuronal messenger molecule in brain: The free radical, nitric oxide [review]. Ann Neurol 32:297, 1992.
11. Dawson VL, et al. Mechanisms of nitric oxide–mediated neurotoxicity in primary brain cultures. J Neurosci 13:2651, 1993.
12. Edvinsson L, MacKenzie E, McCulloch J. Energy generation in the nervous system. In Edvinsson L, MacKenzie E, McCulloch J, eds. Cerebral Blood Flow and Metabolism. New York: Raven Press, 1993, p 153.
13. Martin NA, Doberstein C. Cerebral blood flow measurement in neurosurgical intensive care [review]. Neurosurg Clin North Am 5:607, 1994.
14. Milde LN. Pathophysiology of ischemic brain injury [review]. Crit Care Clin 5:729, 1989.
15. Bouma GJ, Muizelaar JP. Cerebral blood flow, cerebral blood volume, and cerebrovascular reactivity after severe head injury [review]. J Neurotrauma 9(Suppl 1):S333, 1992.
16. Brodersen P, et al. Cerebral hyperemia in electrically induced epileptic seizures. Arch Neurol 28:334, 1973.
17. Lassen NA. Cerebral blood flow and oxygen consumption in man. Physiol Rev 39:183, 1959.
18. Lassen NA. Control of cerebral circulation in health and disease. Circ Res 34:749, 1974.
19. Raichle ME, et al. Correlation between regional cerebral blood flow and oxidative metabolism. In vivo studies in man. Arch Neurol 33:523, 1976.
20. Sokoloff L. Localization of functional activity in the central nervous system by measurement of glucose utilization with radioactive deoxyglucose [review]. J Cereb Blood Flow Metab 1:7, 1981.
21. Wahl M, et al. Micropuncture evaluation of the importance of perivascular pH for the arteriolar diameter on the brain surface. Pflugers Arch 316:152, 1970.
22. Fog M. Cerebral circulation. The reaction of the pial arteries to a fall in blood pressure. Arch Neurol Psychiatry 37:351, 1937.
23. Branston NM, Strong AJ, Symon L. Extracellular potassium activity, evoked potential and tissue blood flow. Relationships during progressive ischaemia in baboon cerebral cortex. J Neurol Sci 32:305, 1977.
24. Fog M. Cerebral circulation II. Reaction of pial arteries to increase in blood pressure. Arch Neurol Psychiatry 41:260, 1939.
25. Harper AM. Autoregulation of cerebral blood flow: Influence of arterial blood pressure on blood flow through the cerebral cortex. J Neurol Neurosurg Psychiatry 29:398, 1966.
26. Shapiro HM. Brain protection: Fact or fancy. In Shoemaker WC, ed. Critical Care, State of the Art, vol 6. Fullerton, Calif.: Society of Critical Care Medicine, 1985, p (E)1.
27. Strandgaard S, Paulson OB. Cerebral autoregulation. Stroke 15:413, 1984.
28. Astrup J, et al. Evidence against H^+ and K^+ as main factors for the control of cerebral blood flow: A microelectrode study. Ciba Found Symp 56:313, 1978.
29. Cuevas P, et al. Adrenergic innervation of human middle cerebral artery. Ultrastructural observations. Surg Neurol 27:113, 1987.
30. Edvinsson L. Neurogenic mechanisms in the cerebrovascular bed. Autonomic neuron amine receptors and their effects on the cerebral blood flow. Acta Physiol Scand Suppl 427:1, 1976.
31. Edvinsson L, Owman C, Siesjo B. Physiological role of cerebrovascular sympathetic nerves in the autoregulation of cerebral blood flow. Brain Res 117:519, 1976.
32. Hougaard K, Nilsson B, Wieloch T. Fatty acid cyclo-oxygenase inhibitors and the regulation of cerebral blood flow. Acta Physiol Scand 117:585, 1983.
33. McCulloch J. Perivascular nerves and the cerebral circulation. Trends Neurosci 7:135, 1984.

34. Purves MJ. Do vasomotor nerves significantly regulate cerebral blood flow? [review] Circ Res 43:485, 1978.
35. Schrader J, et al. Increase of adenosine content in cerebral cortex of the cat during bicuculline-induced seizure. Pflugers Arch 387:245, 1980.
36. Siesjo BK. Cerebral circulation and metabolism [review]. J Neurosurg 60:883, 1984.
37. Wahl M, Kuschinsky W. Unimportance of perivascular H^+ and K^+ activities for the adjustment of pial arterial diameter during changes of arterial blood pressure in cats. Pflugers Arch 382:203, 1979.
38. Winn HR, Rubio R, Berne RM. Brain adenosine concentration during hypoxia in rats. Am J Physiol 241:H235, 1981.
39. Astrup J, et al. Cortical evoked potential and extracellular K^+ and H^+ at critical levels of brain ischemia. Stroke 8:51, 1977.
40. Branston NM, et al. Relationship between the cortical evoked potential and local cortical blood flow following acute middle cerebral artery occlusion in the baboon. Exp Neurol 45:195, 1974.
41. Cruz J, et al. Continuous monitoring of cerebral oxygenation in acute brain injury: Injection of mannitol during hyperventilation. J Neurosurg 73:725, 1990.
42. Harris RJ, et al. Changes in extracellular calcium activity in cerebral ischaemia. J Cereb Blood Flow Metab 1:203, 1981.
43. Hossmann KA, Sakaki S, Zimmerman V. Cation activities in reversible ischemia of the cat brain. Stroke 8:77, 1977.
44. Jones TH, et al. Thresholds of focal cerebral ischemia in awake monkeys. J Neurosurg 54:773, 1981.
45. Kraig RP, Nicholson C. Extracellular ionic variations during spreading depression. Neuroscience 3:1045, 1978.
46. Lassen NA, Astrup J. Cerebral blood flow: Normal regulation and ischemic thresholds. In Weinstein PR, Faden AI, eds. Protection of the Brain from Ischemia. Baltimore: Williams & Wilkins, 1990, p 7.
47. Sharbrough FW, et al. Correlation of continuous electroencephalograms with cerebral blood flow measurements during carotid endarterectomy. Stroke 4:647, 1973.
48. Siesjo BK. Pathophysiology and treatment of focal cerebral ischemia. Part I: Pathophysiology [Review]. J Neurosurg 77:169, 1992.
49. Tamura A, et al. Focal cerebral ischaemia in the rat: 2. Regional cerebral blood flow determined by [^{14}C]iodoantipyrine autoradiography following middle cerebral artery occlusion. J Cereb Blood Flow Metab 1:61, 1981.
50. Cruz J. Combined continuous monitoring of systemic and cerebral oxygenation in acute brain injury: Preliminary observations. Crit Care Med 21:1225, 1993.
51. Cruz J. On-line monitoring of global cerebral hypoxia in acute brain injury. Relationship to intracranial hypertension. J Neurosurg 79:228, 1993.
52. Robertson CS, et al. The predictive value of cerebral anaerobic metabolism with cerebral infarction after head injury. J Neurosurg 67:361, 1987.
53. Robertson CS, et al. Cerebral arteriovenous oxygen difference as an estimate of cerebral blood flow in comatose patients. J Neurosurg 70:222, 1989.
54. Sokoloff L. Cerebral circulation, energy metabolism, and protein synthesis: General characteristics and principles of measurement. In Phelps M, Mazziotta J, Schelbert H, eds. Positron Emission Tomography and Autoradiography: Principles and Applications for the Brain and Heart. New York: Raven Press, 1986, p 1.
55. Gayle MO, et al. Jugular venous bulb catheterization in infants and children. Crit Care Med 17:385, 1989.
56. Gibbs E, et al. Arterial-venous differences in man. J Biol Chem 144:325, 1942.
57. Jakobsen M, Enevoldsen E. Retrograde catheterization of the right internal jugular vein for serial measurements of cerebral venous oxygen content. J Cereb Blood Flow Metab 9:717, 1989.
58. Cremer JE, et al. A study of the kinetic behaviour of glucose based on simultaneous estimates of influx and phosphorylation in brain regions of rats in different physiological states. Brain Res 221:331, 1981.
59. Robinson PJ, Rapoport SI. Glucose transport and metabolism in the brain. Am J Physiol 250(1 Pt 2):R127, 1986.
60. Choi DW. Calcium-mediated neurotoxicity: Relationship to specific channel types and role in ischemic damage [review]. Trends Neurosci 11:465, 1988.
61. Choi DW. Cerebral hypoxia: Some new approaches and unanswered questions [review]. J Neurosci 10:2493, 1990.
62. Choi DW. Ionic dependence of glutamate neurotoxicity. J Neurosci 7:369, 1987.
63. Choi DW, Koh JY, Peters S. Pharmacology of glutamate neurotoxicity in cortical cell culture: attenuation by NMDA antagonists. J Neurosci 8:185, 1988.
64. Becker DP. Brain acidosis in head injury: A clinical trial. In Becker DP, Povlishock JT, eds. Central Nervous System Trauma Status Report—1985. Richmond, Va.: Byrd Press, 1985, p 229.
65. Csiba L, Paschen W, Mies G. Regional changes in tissue pH and glucose content during cortical spreading depression in rat brain. Brain Res 336:167, 1985.
66. Gjedde A, Hansen AJ, Quistorff B. Blood-brain glucose transfer in spreading depression. J Neurochem 37:807, 1981.
67. Inao S, et al. Production and clearance of lactate from brain tissue, cerebrospinal fluid, and serum following experimental brain injury. J Neurosurg 69:736, 1988.
68. Kocher M. Metabolic and hemodynamic activation of postischemic rat brain by cortical spreading depression. J Cereb Blood Flow Metab 10:564, 1990.
69. Krivanek J. Some metabolic changes accompanying Leao's spreading cortical depression in the rat. J Neurochem 6:183, 1961.
70. Marmarou A, et al. Traumatic brain tissue acidosis: Experimental and clinical studies. Acta Neurochir Suppl (Wien) 57:160, 1993.
71. Shinohara M, et al. Cerebral glucose utilization: Local changes during and after recovery from spreading cortical depression. Science 203:188, 1979.
72. Siesjo BK. Pathophysiology and treatment of focal cerebral ischemia. part II: Mechanisms of damage and treatment [review]. J Neurosurg 77:337, 1992.
73. Somjen GG. Acidification of interstitial fluid in hippocampal formation caused by seizures and by spreading depression. Brain Res 311:186, 1984.
74. Yang MS, et al. Regional brain metabolite levels following mild experimental head injury in the cat. J Neurosurg 63:617, 1985.
75. Zhang J, et al. Nitric oxide activation of poly(ADP-ribose) synthetase in neurotoxicity. Science 263:687, 1994.
76. Chesnut RM, et al. The role of secondary brain injury in determining outcome from severe head injury. J Trauma 34:216, 1993.
77. Fearnside MR, et al. The Westmead Head Injury Project. Physical and social outcomes following severe head injury. Br J Neurosurg 7:643, 1993.
78. Herscovitch P, Markham J, Raichle ME. Brain blood flow measured with intravenous $H_2{}^{15}O$. I. Theory and error analysis. J Nucl Med 24:782, 1983.
79. Hill DA, Abraham KH, West RH. Factors affecting outcome in the resuscitation of severely injured patients. Aust N Z J Surg 63:604, 1993.
80. Jeffreys RV, Jones JJ. Avoidable factors contributing to the death of head injury patients in general hospitals in Mersey region. Lancet 2:459, 1981.
81. Kohi YM, et al. Extracranial insults and outcome in patients with acute head injury—Relationship to the Glasgow Coma Scale. Injury 16:25, 1984.
82. Marmarou A, et al. Impact of ICP instability and hypotension on outcome in patients with severe head trauma. J Neurosurg 75:S59, 1991.

83. Miller JD, Becker DP. Secondary insults to the injured brain. J R Coll Surg Edinb 27:292, 1982.
84. Miller JD, et al. Early insults to the injured brain. JAMA 240:439, 1978.
85. Narayan R, et al. Intracranial pressure: To monitor or not to monitor? A review of our experience with head injury. J Neurosurg 56:650, 1982.
86. Pietropaoli JA, et al. The deleterious effects of intraoperative hypotension on outcome in patients with severe head injuries. J Trauma 33:403, 1992.
87. Pigula FA, et al. The effect of hypotension and hypoxia on children with severe head injuries. J Pediatr Surg 28:310, 1993.
88. Rose J, Valtonen S, Jennett B. Avoidable factors contributing to death after head injury. Br Med J 2:615, 1977.
89. Seelig JM, et al. Increased ICP and systemic hypotension during the first 72 hours following severe head injury. In Miller JD, et al., eds. Intracranial Pressure VI. Berlin: Springer-Verlag, 1986, p 675.
90. Sefrin P. Current level of prehospital care in severe head injury—Potential for improvement. Acta Neurochir Suppl (Wien) 57:141, 1993.
91. Teasdale G, Jennett B. Assessment of coma and impaired consciousness. A practice scale. Lancet 2:81, 1974.
92. Enevoldsen EM, Jensen FT. Autoregulation and CO_2 responses of cerebral blood flow in patients with acute severe head injury. J Neurosurg 48:689, 1978.
93. Ishii R. Regional cerebral blood flow in patients with ruptured intracranial aneurysms. J Neurosurg 50:587, 1979.
94. Bruce DA, et al. Diffuse cerebral swelling following head injuries in children: The syndrome of "malignant brain edema." J Neurosurg 54:170, 1981.
95. Obrist WD, et al. Cerebral blood flow and metabolism in comatose patients with acute head injury. Relationship to intracranial hypertension. J Neurosurg 61:241, 1984.
96. Gentleman D. Causes and effects of systemic complications among severely head injured patients transferred to a neurosurgical unit. Int Surg 77:297, 1992.
97. Martin NA, et al. Posttraumatic cerebral arterial spasm: Transcranial Doppler ultrasound, cerebral blood flow, and angiographic findings. J Neurosurg 77:575, 1992.
98. Kety SS, Schmidt CF. The determination of cerebral blood flow in man by the use of nitrous oxide in low concentrations. Am J Physiol 143:53, 1945.
99. Kety SS, Schmidt CF. The nitrous oxide method for the quantitative determination of cerebral blood flow in man: Theory, procedures and normal values. J Clin Invest 27:476, 1948.
100. Kety SS. The theory and applications of the exchange of inert gas at the lungs and tissues. Pharmacol Rev 3:1, 1951.
101. Ingvar DH, Lassen NA. Quantitative determination of cerebral blood flow in man. Lancet 2:806, 1961.
102. Obrist WD, et al. Determination of regional cerebral blood flow by inhalation of ^{133}xenon. Circ Res 20:124, 1967.
103. Obrist WD, Wilkinson WE. Regional cerebral blood flow measurement in humans by xenon-133 clearance [review]. Cerebrovasc Brain Metab Rev 2:283, 1990.
104. Halsey JH Jr, Nakai K, Wariyar B. Sensitivity of rCBF to focal lesions. Stroke 12:631, 1981.
105. Lindegaard KF, et al. Cerebral vasospasm diagnosis by means of angiography and blood velocity measurements. Acta Neurochir (Wien) 100:12, 1989.
106. Seiler RW, et al. Relation of cerebral vasospasm evaluated by transcranial Doppler ultrasound to clinical grade and CT-visualized subarachnoid hemorrhage. J Neurosurg 64:594, 1986.
107. Carter LP, Atkinson JR. Cortical blood flow in controlled hypotension as measured by thermal diffusion. J Neurol Neurosurg Psychiatry 36:906, 1973.
108. Bonner RF, et al. Laser-Doppler continuous real-time monitor of pulsatile and mean blood flow in tissie microcirculation. In Chen SH, Chu B, Nossal R, eds. Scattering Techniques Applied to Supramolecular and Non-equilibrium Systems. New York: Plenum Press, 1981, p 685.
109. Rosenblum BR, Bonner RF, Oldfield EH. Intraoperative measurement of cortical blood flow adjacent to cerebral AVM using laser Doppler velocimetry. J Neurosurg 66:396, 1987.
110. Gur D, et al. In vivo mapping of local cerebral blood flow by xenon-enhanced computed tomography. Science 215:1267, 1982.
111. Gur D, et al. Progress in cerebrovascular disease: Local cerebral blood flow by xenon enhanced CT [review]. Stroke 13:750, 1982.
112. Obrist WD, et al. Effect of stable xenon inhalation on human CBF. J Cereb Blood Flow Metab 5:S557, 1985.
113. Phelps ME, et al. Application of annihalation coincidense detection to transaxial reconstruction tomography. J Nucl Med 16:210, 1975.
114. Saha GB, MacIntyre WJ, Go RT. Cyclotrons and positron emission tomography radiopharmaceuticals for clinical imaging [review]. Semin Nucl Med 22:150, 1992.
115. Hoffman EJ, et al. Design and performance characteristics of a whole body transaxial tomograph. J Nucl Med 17:493, 1976.
116. Hoffman EJ, et al. A new tomograph for quantitative positron emission computed tomography of the brain. IEEE Trans Nucl Sci 28:99, 1981.
117. Phelps ME, et al. ECAT: A new computerized tomographic imaging system for the positron emitting radiopharmaceuticals. J Nucl Med 19:635, 1978.
118. Phelps ME, et al. Design and performance characteristics of the ECAT positron tomograph. J Comput Assist Tomogr 2:648, 1978.
119. Alpert NM, et al. Strategy for the measurement of regional cerebral blood flow using short-lived tracers and emission tomography. J Cereb Blood Flow Metab 4:28, 1984.
120. Frackowiack SJ, et al. Quantitative measurement of regional cerebral blood flow and oxygen metabolism in man using ^{15}O and positron emission tomography: Theory, procedure and normal values. J Comput Tomogr 4:727, 1980.
121. Huang SC, et al. Tomographic measurement of local cerebral blood flow in man with O-15 water. J Cereb Blood Flow Metab 1(Suppl):531, 1981.
122. Huang SC, et al. Quantitative measurement of local cerebral blood flow in humans by positron computed tomography and O-15 water. J Cereb Blood Flow Metab 3:141, 1983.
123. Jones T, Chester DA, Ter-Pogossian MM. The continuous inhalation of oxygen-15 for assessing regional oxygen extraction in the brain of man. Br J Radiol 49:339, 1976.
124. Lammertsma AA, et al. The $C^{15}O_2$ buildup technique to measure regional cerebral blood flow and distribution of water. J Cereb Blood Flow Metab 9:461, 1989.
125. Phelps ME, Hoffman EJ, Raybaud C. Factors which effect cerebral uptake and retention of $^{13}NH_3$. Stroke 8:694, 1977.
126. Holden JE, et al. Cerebral blood flow using PET measurements of fluoromethane kinetics. J Nucl Med 22:1084, 1981.
127. Koeppe RA, et al. Quantitation of local cerebral blood flow and partition coefficient without arterial sampling: Theory and validation. J Cereb Blood Flow Metab 5:214, 1985.
128. Kuhl DE, et al. Effects of stroke on local cerebral metabolism and perfusion: Mapping by emission computed tomography of ^{18}FDG and $^{13}NH_3$. Ann Neurol 8:47, 1980.
129. Raichle ME, et al. Brain blood flow measured with intravenous $H_2{}^{15}O$. II. Implementation and validation. J Nucl Med 24:790, 1983.
130. Conn GL. Measurement of organ blood flow without blood sampling. J Clin Invest 34:916, 1955.
131. Lassen NA, Ingvar DH. The blood flow of the cerebral cortex determined by radioactive krypton-85. Experientia 17:42, 1961.

132. Kuhl DE, Edwards RQ. Image separation radioisotope scanning. Radiology 80:653, 1963.
133. Hill TC, et al. Initial experience with SPECT (single photon computerized tomography) of the brain using *N*-isopropyl I-123 *p*-iodoamphetamine: Concise communication. J Nucl Med 23:191, 1982.
134. Kuhl DE, et al. Quantifying local cerebral blood flow by *N*-isopropyl-*p*-(123-I) iodoamphetamine (IMP) tomography. J Nucl Med 23:196, 1982.
135. Kung HF, Tramposch K, Blau M. A new brain perfusion imaging agent: (I-123) HIPDM. J Nucl Med 24:66, 1983.
136. Kung HF. Brain radiopharmaceuticals. In Fritzberg AR, Ed. Radiopharmaceuticals: Progress and Clinical Perspectives, vol 1. Boca Raton, Fla.: CRC Press, 1986, p 21.
137. Escuret E. Technical note concerning the retrograde catheterization of the internal jugular vein [French]. Ann Anesth Franc 7:721, 1974.
138. Bouma GJ, Muizelaar JP, Choi S. Cerebral circulation and metabolism after severe traumatic brain injury: The elusive role of ischemia. J Neurosurg 75:685, 1991.
139. Salvant JB Jr, Muizelaar JP. Changes in cerebral blood flow and metabolism related to the presence of subdural hematoma. Neurosurgery 33:387, 1993.
140. Hatazawa J, et al. Measurement of the ratio of cerebral oxygen consumption to glucose utilization by positron emission tomography: Its consistency with the values determined by the Kety-Schmidt method in normal volunteers. J Cereb Blood Flow Metab 8:426, 1988.
141. Heiss WD, et al. Regional kinetic constants and cerebral metabolic rate for glucose in normal human volunteers determined by dynamic positron emission tomography of [^{18}F]-2-fluoro-2-deoxy-D-glucose. J Cereb Blood Flow Metab 4:212, 1984.
142. Hillered L, Ernster L, Siesjo BK. Influence of in vitro lactic acidosis and hypercapnia on respiratory activity of isolated rat brain mitochondria. J Cereb Blood Flow Metab 4:430, 1984.
143. Robertson CS, et al. Alterations in cerebral availability of metabolic substrates after severe head injury. J Trauma 28:1523, 1988.
144. Hovda DA, Becker DP, Katayama Y. Secondary injury and acidosis [Review]. J Neurotrauma 9(Suppl 1):S47, 1992.
145. Hayes RL, et al. Regional rates of glucose utilization in the cat following concussive head injury. J Neurotrauma 5:121, 1988.
146. Hayes RL, et al. Activation of pontine cholinergic sites implicated in unconsciousness following cerebral concussion in the cat. Science 223:301, 1984.
147. Kotayama Y, et al. Coma associated with flaccidity produced by fluid-percussion concussion in the cat. I: Contribution of activity in the pontine inhibitory system. Brain Inj 2:31, 1988.
148. Andersen BJ, Marmarou A. Energy compartmentalization in neural tissue [abstract]. J Cereb Blood Flow Metab 9(Suppl 1):S386, 1989.
149. Andersen BJ, Marmarou A. Isolated stimulation of glycolysis following traumatic brain injury. In Hoff JT, Betz AL, eds. Intracranial Pressure VII. Berlin: Springer-Verlag, 1989, p 575.
150. Broderson P, Jorgensen E. Cerebral blood flow and oxygen uptake, and cerebrospinal fluid biochemistry in severe coma. J Neurol Neurosurg Psychiatry 37:384, 1974.
151. DeSalles A, Muizelaar J, Young H. Hyperglycemia, cerebrospinal fluid lactic acidosis, and cerebral blood flow in severely head-injured patients. Neurosurgery 21:45, 1987.
152. Enevoldsen EM, et al. Dynamic changes in regional CBF, intraventricular pressure, CSF pH and lactate levels during the acute phase of head injury J Neurosurg 44:191, 1976.
153. McIntosh TK, et al. Traumatic brain injury in the rat: alterations in brain lactate and pH as characterized by ^{1}H and ^{31}P nuclear magnetic resonance. J Neurochem 49:1530, 1987.
154. Rehncrona S, Rosen I, Siesjo BK. Brain lactic acidosis and ischemic cell damage: 1. Biochemistry and neurophysiology. J Cereb Blood Flow Metab 1:297, 1981.
155. Tanaka K, et al. Regional alterations in glucose consumption and metabolite levels during postischemic recovery in cat brain. J Cereb Blood Flow Metab 5:502, 1985.
156. Mintun MA, et al. Brain oxygen utilization measured with O-15 radiotracers and positron emission tomography. J Nucl Med 25:177, 1984.
157. Subramanyam R, et al. A model for regional cerebral oxygen distribution during continuous inhalation of $^{15}O_2$, $C^{15}O$ and $C^{15}O_2$. J Nucl Med 19:48, 1978.
158. Phelps ME, et al. Investigation of F-18-fluoro-2-deoxy-glucose for the measure of myocardial glucose metabolism. J Nucl Med 19:1311, 1978.
159. Miller BL. A review of chemical issues in ^{1}H NMR spectroscopy: *N*-acetyl-L-aspartate, creatine and choline [review]. NMR Biomed 4:47, 1991.
160. Shulman RG, et al. Nuclear magnetic resonance imaging and spectroscopy of human brain function [review]. Proc Natl Acad Sci U S A 90:3127, 1993.
161. Sutton LN, et al. Proton magnetic resonance spectroscopy of pediatric brain tumors. Neurosurgery 31:195, 1992.
162. Langfitt TW, Weinstein JD, Kassell NF. Cerebral vasomotor paralysis produced by intracranial hypertension. Neurology 15:622, 1965.
163. Aucoin MJ, et al. Intracranial pressure monitors. Am J Med 80:369, 1986.
164. Bobo H, et al. Delayed intracerebral hematoma at the site of a subarachnoid bolt pressure monitor. Case report. J Neurosurg 64:673, 1986.
165. Clark WC, et al. Complications of intracranial pressure monitoring in trauma patients. Neurosurgery 25:20, 1989.
166. Friedman WA, Vries JK. Percutaneous tunnel ventriculostomy. J Neurosurg 53:662, 1980.
167. Gambardella G, d'Avella D, Tomasello F. Monitoring of brain tissue pressure with a fiberoptic device. Neurosurgery. 31:918, 1992.
168. Ivan LP, Choo SH, Ventureyra EC. Intracranial pressure monitoring with the fiberoptic transducer in children. Childs Brain 7:303, 1980.
169. Kanter RK, et al. Infectious complications and duration of intracranial pressure monitoring. Crit Care Med 13:837, 1985.
170. Levin AB. The use of a fiberoptic intracranial pressure transducer in the treatment of head injuries. J Trauma 17:767, 1977.
171. Mayall CG, et al. Ventriculostomy-related infections. A prospective epidemiological study. N Engl J Med 310:553, 1984.
172. Ostrup RC, et al. Continuous monitoring of intracranial pressure with a miniaturized fiberoptic device. J Neurosurg 67:206, 1987.
173. Smith RW, Alksne JF. Infections complicating the use of external ventriculostomy. J Neurosurg 44:657, 1976.
174. Sundbarg G, Nordstrom CH, Soderstrom S. Complications due to prolonged ventricular fluid pressure recording. Br J Neurosurg 2:485, 1988.
175. Winfield JA, et al. Duration of intracranial pressure monitoring does not predict daily risk of infectious complications. Neurosurgery 33:424, 1993.
176. Winn HR, Dacey RG, Jane JA. Intracranial subarachnoid pressure recording: Experience with 650 patients. Surg Neurol 8:41, 1977.
177. Wyler AR, Kelly WA. Use of antibiotics with external ventriculostomies. J Neurosurg 37:185, 1972.
178. Yablon JS, et al. Clinical experience with a fiberoptic intracranial pressure monitor. J Clin Monit 9:171, 1993.
179. Chambers IR, et al. A clinical evaluation of the Camino subdural screw and ventricular monitoring kits. Neurosurgery 26:421, 1990.
180. Chambers IR, et al. An evaluation of the Camino ventricular bolt system in clinical practice. Neurosurgery 33:866, 1993.
181. Artru F, et al. Monitoring of intracranial pressure with intraparenchymal fiberoptic transducer. Technical aspects and clinical reliability [French]. Ann Fr Anesth Reanim 11:424, 1992.
182. North B, Reilly P. Comparison among three methods of intracranial pressure recording. Neurosurgery 18:730, 1986.

183. Snow RB, Zimmerman RD, Devinsky O. Delayed intracerebral hemorrhage after ventriculoperitoneal shunting. Neurosurgery 19:305, 1986.
184. Miller JD, et al. Further experience for the management of severe head injury. J Neurosurg 54:289, 1981.
185. Cushing H. A study of a series of wounds involving the brain and its enveloping structures. Br J Surg 5:558, 1918.
186. Cushing H. Notes on penetrating wounds of the brain. Br Med J 1:221, 1918.
187. Myers PW, et al. Retained bone fragments after penetrating brain wounds: Long-term follow-up in Vietnam veterans [abstract]. J Neurosurg 70:319A, 1989.
188. Rish BL, et al. Analysis of brain abscess after penetrating craniocerebral injuries in Vietnam. Neurosurgery 9:535, 1981.
189. Brandvold B, et al. Penetrating craniocerebral injuries in the Israeli involvement in the Lebanese conflict, 1982-1985. Analysis of a less aggressive surgical approach [review]. J Neurosurg 72:15, 1990.
190. Aarabi B. Surgical outcome in 435 patients who sustained missile head wounds during the Iran-Iraq war. Neurosurgery 27:692, 1990.
191. Graham TW, et al. Civilian gunshot wounds to the head: A prospective study. Neurosurgery 27:696, 1990.
192. Langfitt TW, Gennarelli TA. Can the outcome from head injury be improved? J Neurosurg 56:19, 1982.
193. Johnston IH, Johnston JA, Jennett WB. Intracranial pressure following head injury. Lancet 2:433, 1970.
194. Lundberg N, Troupp H, Lorin H. Continuous recording of the ventricular fluid pressure in patients with severe acute traumatic brain injury. J Neurosurg 22:581, 1965.
195. Marshall LF, et al. The outcome of severe closed head injury. J Neurosurg 75:S28, 1991.
196. Miller JD, et al. Significance of intracranial hypertension in severe head injury. J Neurosurg 47:503, 1977.
197. Narayan RK, et al. Improved confidence of outcome prediction in severe head injury: A comparative analysis of the clinical examination, multimodality evoked potentials, CT scanning and intracranial pressure. J Neurosurg 54:751, 1981.
198. Troupp H. Intraventricular pressure in patients with severe brain injuries. J Trauma 5:373, 1965.
199. Eisenberg HM, et al. High-dose barbiturate control of elevated intracranial pressure in patients with severe head injury. J Neurosurg 69:15, 1988.
200. Demopoulous HB, et al. The free radical pathology and microcirculation in the major central nervous system. Acta Physiol Scand Suppl 492:91, 1980.
201. Kassell NF, et al. Alterations in cerebral blood flow, oxygen metabolism, and electrical activity produced by high-dose thiopental. Neurosurgery 7:598, 1980.
202. Ward JD, et al. Failure of prophylactic barbiturate coma in the treatment of severe head injury. J Neurosurg 62:383, 1985.
203. Schwartz ML, et al. The University of Toronto head injury treatment study: A prospective, randomized comparison of pentobarbital and mannitol. Can J Neurol Sci 11:434, 1984.
204. Nordstrom GH, et al. Cerebral blood flow, vasoreactivity, and oxygen consumption during barbiturate therapy in severe traumatic brain lesions. J Neurosurg 68:424, 1988.
205. Raichle ME, Plum F. Hyperventilation and cerebral blood flow. Stroke 3:566, 1972.
206. Sheinberg M, et al. Continuous monitoring of jugular venous oxygen saturation in head-injured patients. J Neurosurg 76:212, 1992.
207. Barry KG, Berman AR. Mannitol infusion. Part III. The acute effect of the intravenous infusion of mannitol on blood and plasma volume. N Engl J Med 264:1085, 1961.
208. Brown FD, et al. Detailed monitoring of the effects of mannitol following experimental head injury. J Neurosurg 50:423, 1979.
209. Feldman JA, Fish S. Resuscitation fluid for a patient with head injury and hypovolemic shock [review]. J Emerg Med 9:465, 1991.
210. Cold GE. Cerebral blood flow in acute head injury. The regulation of cerebral blood flow and metabolism during the acute phase of head injury, and its significance for therapy. Acta Neurochir Suppl (Wien) 49:1, 1990.
211. Israel RS, et al. Hemodynamic effect of mannitol in a canine model of concomitant increased intracranial pressure and hemorrhagic shock. Ann Emerg Med 17:560, 1988.
212. Kassell NF, et al. The effect of high dose mannitol on cerebral blood flow in dogs with normal intracranial pressure. Stroke 13:59, 1982.
213. Becker DP, Vries JK. The alleviation of increased intracranial pressure by the chronic administration of osmotic agents. In Brock M, Dietz H, eds. Intracranial Pressure. Berlin: Springer-Verlag, 1972, p 309.
214. Feig PU, McCurdy DK. The hypertonic state. N Engl J Med 297:1449, 1977.
215. Kuroda Y, et al. Effect of neuroprotective N-methyl-D-aspartate antagonists on increased intracranial pressure: Studies in the rat acute subdural hematoma model. Neurosurgery 35:106, 1994.
216. Shackford SR, Norton CH, Todd MM. Renal, cerebral, and pulmonary effects of hypertonic resuscitation in a porcine model of hemorrhagic shock. Surgery 104:553, 1988.
217. Smith HP, et al. Comparison of mannitol regimens in patients with severe head injury undergoing intracranial monitoring. J Neurosurg 65:820, 1986.
218. Bell BA, et al. Brain water measured by magnetic resonance imaging. Correlation with direct estimation and changes after mannitol and dexamethasone. Lancet 1:66, 1987.
219. Jennett B, Teasdale GM. Management of Head Injuries. Philadelphia: FA Davis, 1982, p 240.
220. Mendelow AD, et al. Effect of mannitol on cerebral blood flow and cerebral perfusion pressure in human head injury. J Neurosurg 63:43, 1985.
221. Miller JD, Leach PJ. Assessing the effects of mannitol and steroid therapy on intracranial volume/pressure relationships. J Neurosurg 42:274, 1975.
222. Nath F, Galbraith S. The effect of mannitol on cerebral white matter water content. J Neurosurg 65:41, 1986.
223. Rosner MJ, Rosner SD. Cerebral perfusion pressure management of head injury. In Nakamura N, Hashimoto T, Yasue M, eds. Proceedings of International Conference on Recent Advances in Neurotraumatology. Tokyo: Springer-Verlag, 1993, p 293.
224. Rosner MJ, Rosner SD. Cerebral perfusion pressure management of head injury. In Avezaat CJJ, et al., eds. Intracranial Pressure VIII. Berlin: Springer-Verlag, 1993, p 540.
225. Rosner MJ, Daughton S. Cerebral perfusion pressure management in head injury. J Trauma 30:933, 1990.
226. Yoshida A, et al. Outcome of patients with severe head injury—Evaluation by cerebral perfusion pressure. In Nakamura N, Hashimoto T, Yasyue M, eds. Proceedings of International Conference on Recent Advances in Neurotraumatology. Tokyo: Springer-Verlag, 1993, p 309.
227. Pechadre JC, et al. Prevention of late post-traumatic epilepsy by phenytoin in severe brain injuries. 2 years' follow-up [French]. Presse Med 20:841, 1991.
228. Temkin NR, et al. A randomized, double-blind study of phenytoin for the prevention of post-traumatic seizures. N Engl J Med 323:497, 1990.
229. Manaka S. Cooperative prospective study on posttraumatic epilepsy: Risk factors and the effect of prophylactic anticonvulsant. Jpn J Psychiatry Neurol 46:311, 1992.
230. Young B. Failure of prophylactically administered phenytoin to prevent late posttraumatic seizures. J Neurosurg 58:235, 1983.

49

Pathophysiology of Spinal Cord Disruption and Injury

Lynn M. Bartl and Kong-Woo Yoon

Spinal dysfunction is one of the most devastating disabilities encountered in medical practice. A largely irreversible condition, it frequently affects patients during productive years. Though the etiology of spinal cord dysfunction is diverse, the most commonly encountered cause in surgical practice is traumatic spinal cord injury. This chapter therefore focuses on that condition. Epidemiology, neurologic assessment, radiographic evaluation, medical management, pharmacologic management, experimental treatment, and the long-term management of spinal cord injury are addressed.

EPIDEMIOLOGY

It has been estimated that 10,000 new spinal cord injuries occur each year. The annual incidence is 3.2 to 5.3 new spinal cord injuries per 100,000 persons at risk in the United States, 79% of which occurred to male victims, according to the Major Trauma Outcome Study.[1] There is a bimodal distribution for the age of occurrence of spinal cord injury. The first and more prevalent range is between the ages of 15 and 24 years. There is a smaller peak after the age of 55 years.[2,3]

The causes of spinal cord injury are well characterized. Motor vehicle accidents are the most common cause (42% to 56%). Other causes include falls (19%), gunshot wounds (15%), and sports-related injuries (6%). The cause of injury is also related to age, with motor vehicle accidents and water sports being more common causes among individuals younger than 30 years. Falls and gunshot wounds are more common among individuals older than 35. Young men are the population most likely to have a spinal cord injury. Women account for only 21% of spinal cord injuries in the Major Trauma Outcome Study.[1,2]

The mortality risk of spinal cord injury depends largely on the presence of associated injuries. Multiple injuries are present in 78% of victims. In the Major Trauma Outcome Study, the mortality rate from April 1982 to 1989 was 6.9% for isolated spinal cord injury. The presence of multiple injuries increased the mortality rate to 19.8%. Most deaths, however, occurred within the first 24 hours after injury to patients with severe, multiple injuries. Pedestrians hit by cars were the most likely to die, followed by patients with gunshot wounds.[1] Traumatic brain injury is also present in approximately 33% of patients who have an acute, traumatic spinal cord injury. Head injuries are thought to be the most common traumatic cause of death among individuals 2 to 40 years old. The incidence of fatal brain injury is estimated at 17 per 100,000,[4] and head injury may make the diagnosis of spinal cord injury difficult. The mortality rate is also higher in patients older than 55 years.[3,5,6]

Although a full discussion of nontraumatic etiologies of spinal cord pathology is not within the scope of this chapter, other spinal cord pathologies must be mentioned briefly, because they must be considered when spinal cord dysfunction is seen without any history of injury. The etiologies for spinal cord dysfunction are divided into primary spinal cord pathology and secondary conditions from compression of the cord by surrounding structures. The primary spinal cord pathologies include congenital, inflammatory, degenerative, ischemic, and metabolic processes. Inflammation of the spinal cord parenchyma may be either infective or noninfective. Multiple sclerosis is one of the most common noninfective inflammatory disorders of the spinal cord. Amyotrophic lateral sclerosis, a selective degeneration of the motor neurons, is an example of spinal cord degeneration. Spinal cord ischemia may be a manifestation of atherosclerosis, as well as of a specific occlusion of the collateral supply of the anterior spinal artery by various pathologies involving the descending aorta. Certain metabolic conditions, such as vitamin deficiencies and diabetes, may also specifically affect the spinal cord. A detailed discussion of these etiologies is available in any textbook of neurology.

Secondary spinal cord dysfunction from compression may include herniated nucleus pulposus (disk), primary and metastatic tumors of the spinal column, and congenital and degenerative narrowing or compression of the spinal canal. Another common cause of spinal cord compression is by metastatic invasion of the spinal column.

Although the mechanism of the cord dysfunction by compression may be similar to trauma, these conditions present special considerations. A detailed discussion of the management of spinal cord compression from metastatic tumors should be available in any textbook of neurologic surgery.

PATHOPHYSIOLOGY

The precise mechanisms that perturb spinal cord function on injury, ultimately blocking electrical conduction, remain to be clarified. At least three pathophysiologic mechanisms are generally present in all injured spinal cords in varying proportions.[5,7,8] These include (1) ischemia of the cord, with resultant metabolic disturbances that affect normal function; (2) spinal cord edema; and (3) structural changes in axons and other neural elements related to compression. The extents to which these components by themselves interrupt electrical conduction in the cord remain to be determined. Experimental studies in which the sequence of events in traumatized spinal cord tissue have been evaluated histologically have demonstrated a pattern of injury that commences with the development of punctuate areas of hemorrhagic necrosis, evident first within the central gray matter of the cord, that coalesce into much larger volumes and ultimately extend in a centripetal fashion toward the peripheral white matter. The degree of involvement is related to the severity of the initial injury, which also is linked to the magnitude of edema formation within the first few hours after injury. These events are directly responsible for the axonal swelling and rupture and focal metabolic changes that quickly supervene.

Although spinal cord blood flow has been shown to decrease dramatically within minutes after spinal cord trauma, the exact relationship between flow changes and conduction of nerve impulses remains ill defined. For example, the manipulation of systemic blood pressure in a spinal cord compression model was not always consistently associated with changes in somatosensory-evoked potentials. When changes did occur, they would often be delayed as long as 10 to 20 minutes.[9] Even in the case of pronounced hypotension in which true conduction disturbances were initiated, these could be overcome by elevation of the blood pressure. If sustained hypotension and compression were applied simultaneously, the somatosensory-evoked potentials were blocked, suggesting that the effects were additive. Even high degrees of spinal cord compression did not adversely affect spinal-evoked potentials as long as nearly normal blood flow was maintained. These findings suggest that blood flow changes or compression within the spinal cord are not necessarily damaging independently of one another, but acting in concert they can result in considerable disruption of normal neurologic function. Thus, continued spinal cord perfusion seems to be required for the injured cord to maintain electrical conduction; when this circumstance is absent, irreversible injury will almost certainly occur.

The degree of vascular compromise and the length of time that is present in the traumatized spinal cord influences the resultant swelling.[10,11] With even minor degrees of injury, the water content in injured tissue increases rapidly as a result of intravascular fluids escaping into the extracellular space. The direct vascular tissue damage results in increased capillary permeability at the injury site, which is quickly augmented by the release of vasoactive substances from the surrounding damaged neural tissue. Any decrease in spinal cord blood flow that already exists is further compromised by the perturbations resulting in hypoxic injury to the neural tissue, with additional increases in capillary permeability and the formation of toxic metabolites such as excitatory amino acid neurotransmitters, free fatty acids, and oxygen-derived free radicals. In addition, edema formation caused by these cytotoxic mechanisms deforms neural elements, further occludes vascular flow, and disrupts electrical conduction distal to the sight of injury.[12]

ASSESSMENT

Neurologic Assessment

As many as one third of patients admitted for cervical spine injury have delayed or missed diagnosis, according to Bohlman.[13] Factors leading to delayed diagnosis include inadequate evaluation of spinal cord function because of concomitant head injury or intoxication.[13] A high index of suspicion for spinal cord injury should therefore be maintained for all patients who have an altered level of consciousness or are intoxicated. These patients should remain immobilized until the spine can be thoroughly evaluated.

Although a thorough neurologic evaluation is essential, a rudimentary assessment may be made by evaluating three components: sensation, voluntary motor strength, and deep tendon reflexes. Such evaluations should be made with minimal sedation and muscle relaxants. An even more abbreviated examination of spinal cord function may be necessary in uncooperative or delirious patients. The sensory examination depends most on patient cooperation. However, one may detect a sensory level by observing the response to painful stimuli. In addition to the deep tendon reflexes, the absence of anal sphincter contraction to a gentle pressure on the glans penis (bulbocavernosus reflex) or to local pinprick (anal sphincter reflex) may be helpful in determining the extent or presence of spinal cord injury. The absence of rectal tone frequently accompanies a complete spinal cord injury, which is associated with a poor prognosis for functional recovery. Table 49-1 provides a guideline for grading the results of initial motor examination and evaluation of reflexes.

The level of spinal cord injury is defined as the most caudal level with at least some movement against gravity (grade 3 motor function). In most instances, the clinical delineation between an intact level and the abnormal level

Table 49-1. Evaluation of Motor Function

Muscle Strength Grading		Deep Tendon Reflex Grading	
Grade	**Strength**	**Grade**	**Reflex**
0	No contraction	0	No reflex
1	Muscle contraction	1	Trace reflex
2	Movement	2	Normal
3	Active movement against gravity	3	Hyperreflexia
4	Active movement against resistance	4	Clonus
5	Normal strength		

The motor function is assessed by the strength and the stretch reflexes. The strength of the movement of a joint is assessed by the examiner. The reflexes are assessed by a gentle tap of the muscle near the insertion. Note that the muscle assessed for the strength is not always amenable to the assessment of reflexes (see Table 49-2).

Table 49-2. Clinical Evaluation of the Spinal Cord Level

Level	Sensory	Motor	Action	Reflex
C4		Diaphragm	Respiration	—
C5		Deltoid/supraspinatous	Shoulder abduction	—
C6		Extensor carpi radialis	Radial wrist extension	Biceps
C7	Variable	Triceps	Elbow extension	Triceps
C8		Flexor digitorum profundus	Grip	Finger flexor
T1		Interossei	Abduct little finger	—

The distributions of the sensory fibers by the designated roots are indicated in the second column. The motor functions that are most readily amenable to examination are indicated with corresponding action of that muscle function.

is clear and distinct. Frequently, it correlates with the radiographic abnormality. Determination of the level of spinal cord injury is an essential step in clinical management. Each level of retained function, especially in the upper extremities, implies large significance in rehabilitation potentials and subsequent morbidity.[14] Table 49-2 depicts the sensory and motor distribution of the cervical roots to aid in the determination of the level of spinal cord injury. As many as 40% of cervical spine injuries are associated with a neurologic deficit, whereas, only 15% to 20% of thoracolumbar injuries are associated with a deficit.[15] Another reason for accurate neurologic assessment is to provide a means of evaluating changes in neurologic function. As many as 6% of patients with spinal cord injury have deterioration of function during the hospital stay.[13,16] Appropriate clinical decisions should be made on the basis of subsequent changes in neurologic function and occasionally with the assistance of magnetic resonance imaging (MRI). Such information dictates whether closed reduction (traction) or operative decompression is the best management strategy. Units that specialize in spinal cord injury have decreased the percentage of patients that have neurologic deterioration during their hospital stay.[17] Close neurologic observation and nurses experienced in treating spinal cord injury are important to avoid further deficit.

In Table 49-2, the distinction of spinal cord injury above C4 is abbreviated because affected patients are frequently found dead at the scene of injury as a result of respiratory failure. On occasion, patients survive injuries above this level to be transported to the hospital setting. This may be the result of incomplete spinal cord injury, with some residual innervation of the diaphragm to maintain adequate respiration.

It should be noted that the neurologic level may not correlate with the spinal cord injury level or the level of bony injury. For example, a spinal cord injury at the level of C7 may be accompanied by a C6 nerve root injury. The injury of nerve roots may have a better prognosis for long-term recovery and for immediate recovery from decompression than spinal cord injury. The level of spinal cord injury may also be higher than the actual level of bony injury because of edema, hematoma, or a herniated disk, none of which can be visualized with plain radiographs. Appropriate diagnostic measures should be taken to determine the etiology of ascending neurologic dysfunction, including MRI, computed tomographic (CT) scan, or myelography.

Spinal cord injuries are classified as *complete* or *incomplete* lesions. The distinction is important for the determination of prognosis and future treatment plans. A complete spinal cord injury is occasionally referred to as *complete spinal cord transection*. Actual transection, or anatomic discontinuity, is rare. Rather, the term is used to emphasize a complete but functional interruption of all spinal cord function at that level. The prognosis for any recovery from such a lesion is poor. A complete spinal cord injury is suspected when there is a loss of all spinal cord function below the level of injury. This includes all sensation, voluntary movement, autonomic, and spinal reflexes. This condition, which is characterized by flaccid paralysis, loss of sensation, and absent reflexes is called *spinal shock* (differentiated from hypotension associated with the loss of sympathetic tone). Other clinical findings that favor complete spinal cord injury include neurogenic shock (hypotension) and priapism. Spinal shock can last for 48 hours to several weeks, during which time the definitive neurologic status cannot be assessed.

Partial preservation of sensory and motor function is a sign of an incomplete spinal cord injury. One of the most frequently encountered signs of partial injury is the preservation of the sensory and motor functions of the sacral segments, called *sacral sparing* (Fig. 49-1). The fibers that innervate the sacral segments are located in the outer layers of the spinal cord, which makes them resistant to ischemic conditions that accompany traumatic injuries. The determination of residual spinal cord function is impor-

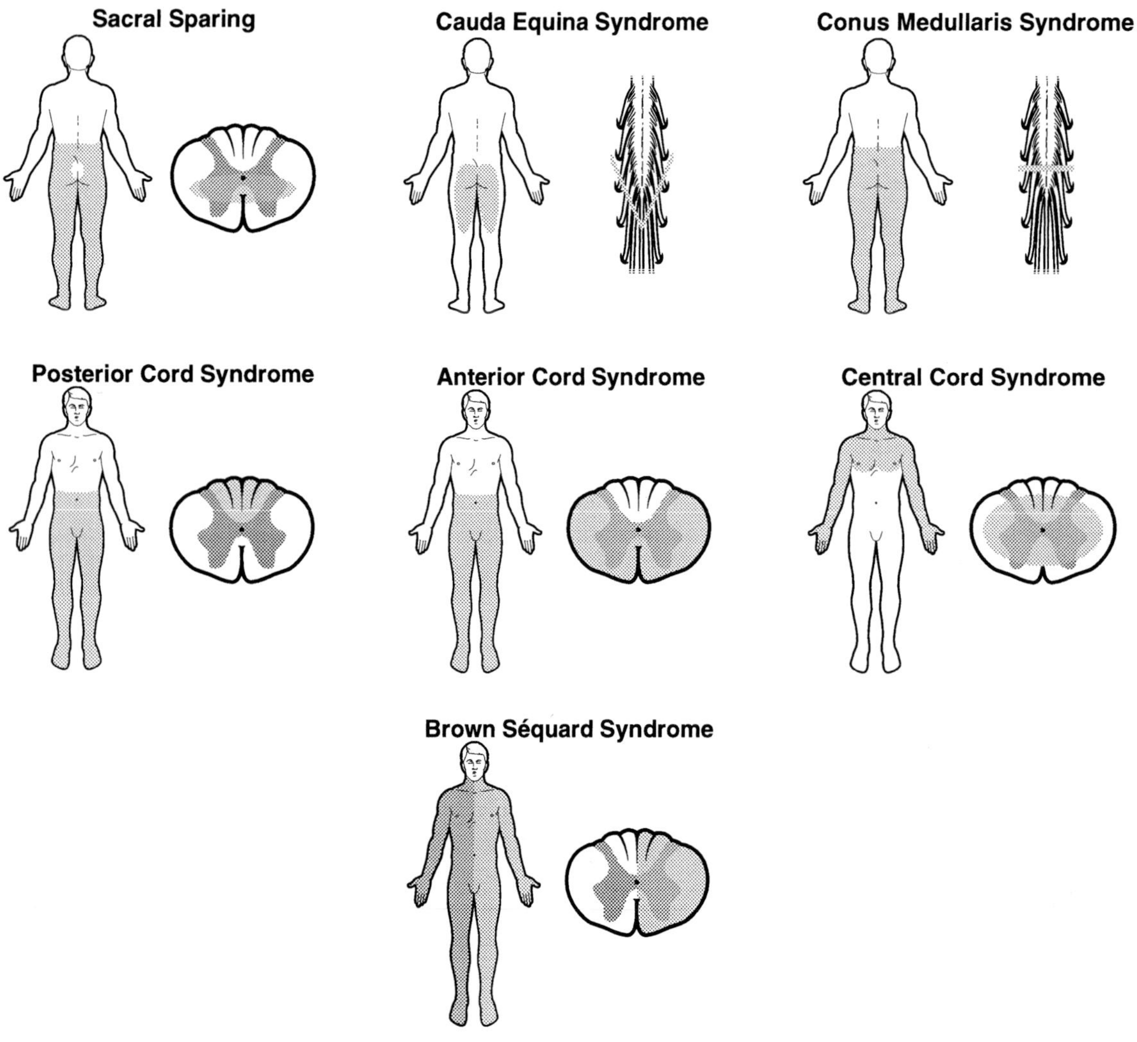

Fig. 49-1. Diagram of incomplete spinal cord injures. The shaded areas depict the region of neurologic deficit and the area of damage within the spinal cord.

tant, because the progression during the hospitalization may significantly affect the clinical decision regarding the timing of surgical procedures such as decompression and fusion. Furthermore, the prognosis for incomplete injury is vastly different from that for complete injury.

There are several syndromes of incomplete spinal cord injury. Recognition of one of these patterns of neurologic deficit is frequently helpful in detecting a partial (incomplete) spinal cord injury. Figure 49-1 is a diagram of the area involved in the spinal cord and the associated neurologic deficit for each syndrome.

Anterior Cord Syndrome

The anterior two thirds of the spinal cord is affected in the anterior cord syndrome. The distribution of parenchymal injury correlates well with the distribution of the anterior spinal artery, which perfuses most of the spinal cord except for the dorsal columns. This pattern of spinal cord deficit substantiates the hypothesis that ischemia plays a significant role in traumatic injury to the central nervous system. Under experimental conditions, traumatic spinal cord injury results in attenuation of blood flow to the injured segment. However, discrete interruption of the anterior spinal artery is rarely demonstrated. The spinothalamic and corticospinal tracts are affected by this syndrome. The patient has loss of sharp pain sensation, temperature sensation, and motor function. The dorsal columns are preserved, with retained proprioception, vibration sensation, and deep pressure sensation. The prognosis for improvement is poor, with a small chance of recovery of one nerve root level.

Central Cord Syndrome

This syndrome is usually associated with a hyperextension injury. It is also associated with congenital or acquired (degenerative) narrowing of the spinal canal. Occasionally, a neurologic deficit in this pattern is associated with no significant evidence of bony injury or instability. Evidence of spinal cord pathology may be seen by MRI, which demonstrates hemorrhage or edema in the center of the spinal cord. This mixed upper and lower motor neuron lesion is characterized by flaccid paralysis of the upper extremities and spastic paralysis of the lower extremities. The most evident feature of the deficit is that the paralysis of the upper extremities is much more pronounced than that of the lower extremities. The peripheral location of the lower extremity axons in the corticospinal tract often leads to relative sparing of lower extremity function. Surgical decompression is rarely indicated because neurologic improvement during several weeks is frequently the natural history. The prognosis is better than in anterior cord syndrome, with 40% of patients regaining useful hand function.

Posterior Cord Syndrome

This syndrome is rare and most frequently associated with isolated damage to the posterior components of the spinal canal. There is loss of dorsal column function, such as vibratory sensation, deep pressure sensation, and proprioception. Long-term disability from this syndrome is rare, and nearly complete recovery is usually achieved.

Brown-Séquard's Syndrome

This syndrome is a consequence of either anatomic or functional hemisection of the spinal cord. The mechanism of injury is often a unilateral facet fracture or dislocation, or penetrating trauma. The most frequent mechanism of injury is by gunshot wound. Because of the arrangement of the descending and ascending fiber tracts of the spinal cord, the paralysis (corticospinal tract) and the loss of vibration sensation, touch, and proprioception (dorsal column) are ipsilateral to the injury, whereas the losses in pain and thermal sensations (lateral spinothalamic tract) are contralateral to the injury. In general, the prognosis is favorable, with at least 70% chance of recovery of leg function. However, the extent of recovery depends on the mechanism of injury. The type of missile injury often responsible for this syndrome frequently inflicts damage to the spinal cord by a shock wave rather than anatomic laceration of the cord. The prognosis for recovery is worse when there is evidence of discrete laceration of the cord itself.

Conus Medullaris Syndrome

This is the most common incomplete spinal cord injury. There is complete sacral spinal cord injury, with complete bowel and bladder paralysis. Although it is difficult to differentiate from the cauda equina syndrome, the conus medullaris syndrome is the result of an injury to the very tip of the spinal cord at the level of L1 or L2. The sacral region is completely affected, and there is symmetric loss or preservation of lumbar nerve roots. Approximately 75% of patients with evidence of root sparing on admission have useful recovery.

Cauda Equina Syndrome

This is an injury of the intrathecal spinal nerve roots. Variable sparing of the lumbar nerve roots is typical, resulting in movement of the hips and knees with preserved knee reflexes. Radicular pain is common in this syndrome.

Radiographic Evaluation

The anatomy of skeletal structures and assessment of stability are determined by plain radiographs and CT scan. The initial evaluation should include lateral, anteroposterior, and open-mouth views of the cervical spine. The cervicothoracic junction (C7-T1) must be visualized. Gently pulling down the patient's arms, or a "swimmer's view," usually allows evaluation of this region. CT scan through the cervicothoracic junction is indicated if it cannot be visualized on plain radiographs. Any suspect areas on plain radiographs are further evaluated by high-resolution, thin-section (2 to 3 mm) CT scan. Thin sections allow high-quality sagittal reconstructions. Anteroposterior and lateral views of the thoracic and lumbar spine should also be obtained.

Any spinal cord injury without skeletal abnormality should be evaluated by MRI. MRI provides excellent resolution and evaluation for the soft tissues, canal compromise, cord contusion, hemorrhage, or edema. MRI is also indicated for those with neurologic deficit, to assess the degree of spinal cord compression, or those whose neurologic status has deteriorated.[2,18] Finally, MRI should be done prior to closed or open reduction of cervical spine fractures that may be associated with traumatic disk herniation, such as facet dislocations and flexion-compression injuries. Catastrophic compression of the spinal cord has been reported from traumatic herniated nucleus pulposus during reduction.[19] MRI is contraindicated for patients with pacemakers, certain aneurysm clips, metallic fragments in the eye or spinal cord, or severe claustrophobia.

Approximately 15% of patients with high cervical spine fractures have second vertebral column fractures. Therefore, a complete radiographic survey of the spinal column is indicated. The cervical spine is the most mobile and dynamic portion of the spine, and most traumatic spinal column injuries occur there. About one quarter of cervical spine injuries occur between the skull base and the upper cervical spine. It is estimated that 20% to 40% of patients found dead at the scene of motor vehicle accidents had high cervical spinal fractures with cord compression. Fractures of the atlas (C1) make up about 3% to 13% of cervical spine fractures. They are usually multiple fractures of the ring and are rarely associated with a neurologic deficit (Fig. 49-2). C2 fractures include odontoid fractures (Fig. 49-3), hangman's fractures, and miscellaneous axis fractures. Hangman's fractures (Fig. 49-4) involve the pars interarticularis bilaterally; they account for 20% of C2 fractures. C3 fractures are rare and tend to be small chip fractures.[15]

The lower cervical spine, C4 to T1, is the location of approximately 75% of injuries to the cervical spine.[13] The most common level of vertebral fracture is at C5, and the most common level of subluxation is at C5-C6. C5 and C6 are the regions of greatest mobility in the cervical spine and may therefore be more susceptible to injury. In order of frequency, lower cervical spine injuries include vertebral body fractures, subluxation of the articular processes (unilateral and bilateral locked facets), lamina fractures, spinous process fractures, and lateral mass or pedicle fractures. All bilateral facet dislocations are associated with neurologic injury, with most (84%) being complete spinal cord injury. Unilateral facet injuries (Fig. 49-5) carry

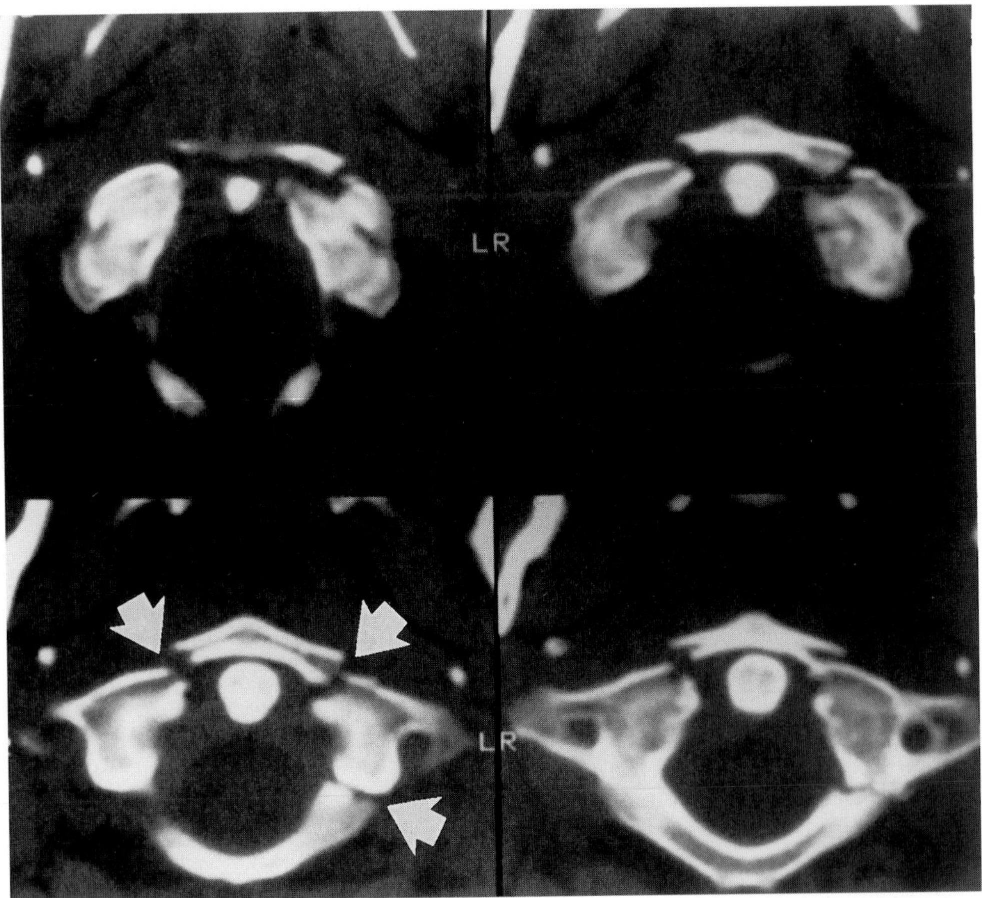

Fig. 49-2. CT scan of the C1 ring (3 mm sections). Note that the ring is disrupted at three locations *(arrows)*. However, there is no evidence for constriction of the spinal canal. The odontoid process also maintains the relatively normal relationship with the lateral masses bilaterally.

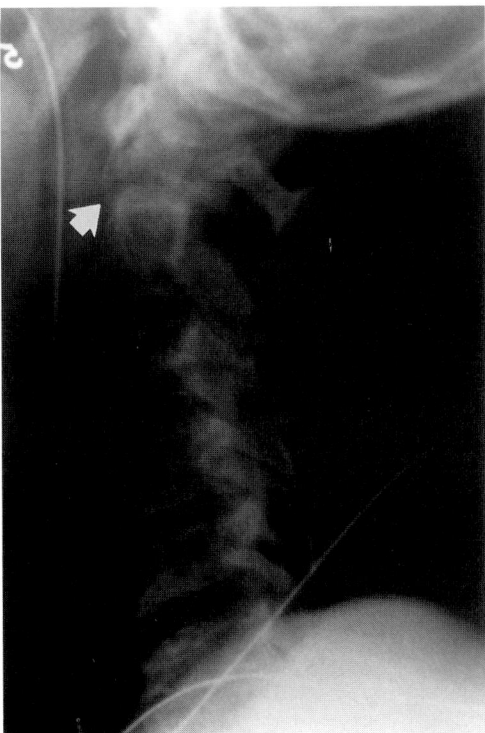

Fig. 49-3. Lateral view of the cervical spine demonstrating fracture through the neck of the odontoid process of C2 vertebra *(arrow)*. There is minimal subluxation without any evidence for spinal canal compromise. This patient had no neurologic deficit.

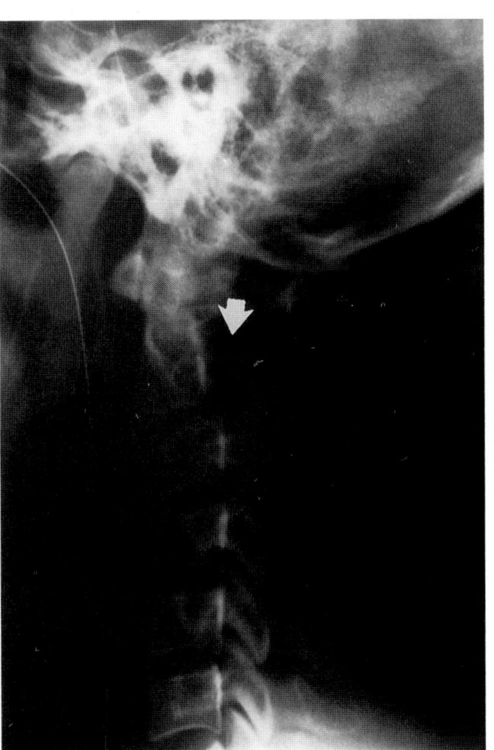

Fig. 49-4. Same view as in Fig. 49-3. The fracture through the pedicles of C2 vertebra *(arrow)* has detached the posterior element from the vertebral body. Again, there is no compromise of the spinal canal. However, note that the C2 body has a minimal subluxation on C3.

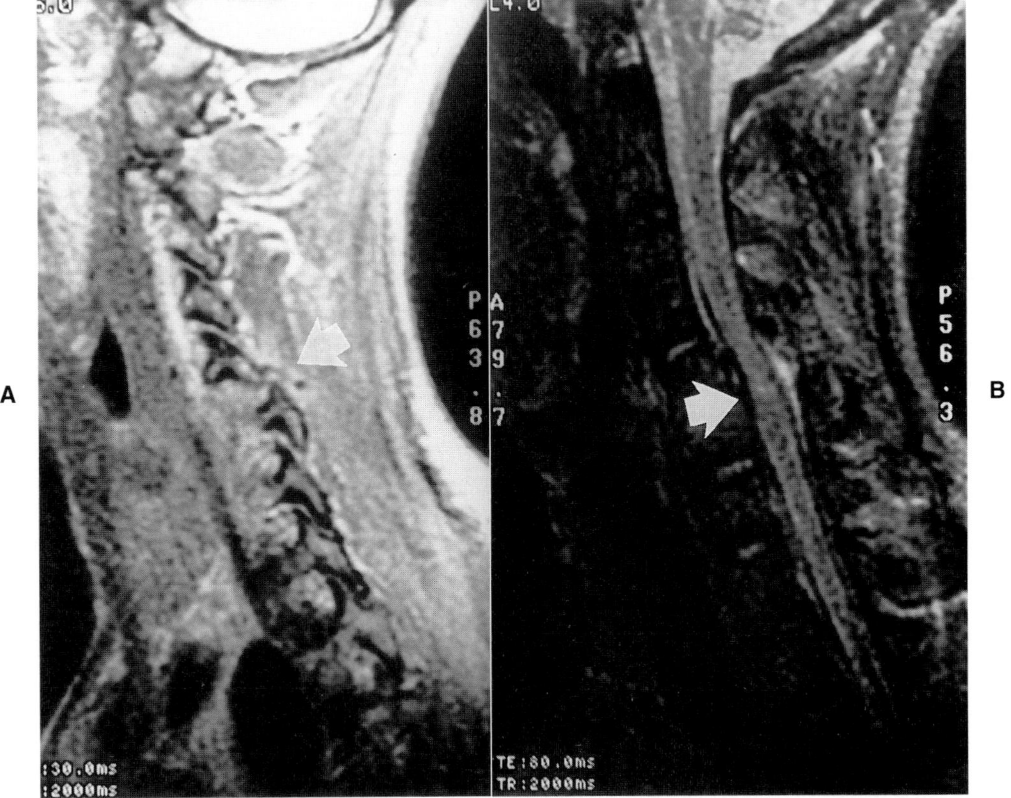

Fig. 49-5. MRI of the cervical spine. **A,** Sagittal cut through the facets demonstrates locking of the facet *(arrow)* at C5-C6 level. Note that the superior facet of C6 no longer articulates with the inferior facet of C5. This dislocation is associated with minimal subluxation at the level of C5-C6, with mild cord contusion seen on T2 image in **B.** A small amount of increased signal within the spinal cord parenchyma indicates cord contusion at the level of subluxation *(arrow)*.

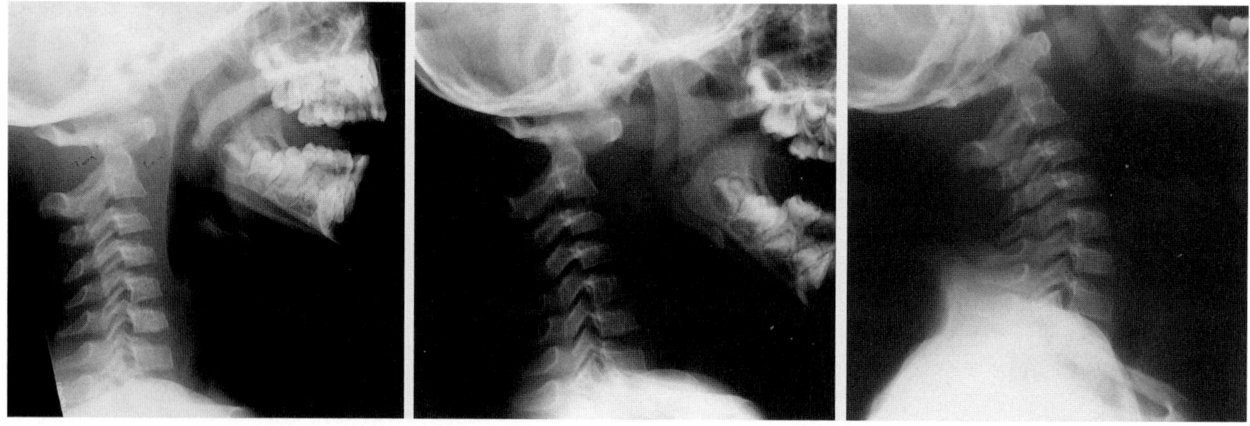

Fig. 49-6. Ligamentous instability. C1-C2 instability is demonstrated on lateral flexion-extension cervical spine radiographs of a 6-year old boy who had persistent neck pain 2 weeks after a motor vehicle accident, despite normal flexion-extension radiographs on the day of the accident.

a lower risk of neurologic injury (80%), with a larger proportion of nerve root injuries and incomplete spinal cord injuries.[20]

Thoracic and thoracolumbar fractures also occur in recognizable patterns. Wedge compression fractures, the most common, represent an isolated failure of the anterior column under flexion and compression. Burst fractures are fractures of both the anterior and middle columns as a result of axial compression. Chance fractures, associated with lap-belt–induced injuries, are a horizontal fracture through the posterior arch and pedicles, extending into the posterior aspect of the vertebral body. Fracture dislocation, with displacement of one vertebral body with respect to another, results in neurologic injury in at least 75% of patients.[21]

Ligamentous injury may not be appreciated on initial plain radiographs or routine CT scan. A ligamentous injury may result in momentary dislocation with spontaneous reduction. This mechanism of spinal cord injury is more frequently encountered in the pediatric population. Spinal cord injury without radiologic abnormality should also be evaluated with dynamic studies, such as flexion-extension lateral radiographs, to demonstrate instability.[22,23] Patients who have neck pain despite normal-appearing plain radiographs may have ligamentous injury and should be evaluated with lateral flexion-extension views of the cervical spine. Under physician supervision, the patient should move the head and neck only through pain-free range of motion. Muscle spasm in the acute phase may make these views initially unreliable (Fig. 49-6). The patient is therefore treated with a cervical collar if the films appear normal, and the test is repeated in 1 to 2 weeks.[23]

MANAGEMENT OF ACUTE SPINAL CORD INJURY

Initial Management

Initial assessment and treatment of acute spinal cord injury should focus on the general principles of resuscitation. At the scene of the injury, an airway is immediately established. An unobstructed airway is necessary in all patients. Neck movement to establish an airway should be kept at a minimum. All patients should be given supplemental oxygen, and those with respiratory insufficiency should be intubated and ventilated. Blind nasotracheal intubation is the best choice at the scene of the accident, because with it there is no need to hyperextend the head.[2,24] Cervical spinal cord injury may result in the loss of sympathetic tone, bradycardia, hypotension, and decreased respiratory excursion, which can compromise oxygenation. Aspiration of gastric contents and shock are the two most common causes of prehospital death among patients with spinal cord injuries.[2,25] Atelectasis, aspiration, and chest trauma may also compromise ventilation. Hypoxia may increase the local ischemia of the spinal cord at the level of injury and is to be avoided.[26,27]

Peripheral intravenous lines are placed in the field for the management of hypotension and administration of drugs. Neurogenic shock is caused by the loss of sympathetic vascular tone peripherally, resulting in the pooling of blood in the extremities and inadequate central venous return. The parasympathetic effects of the vagus nerve predominate, leading to bradycardia. These patients usually have a pulse slower than 60 beats/min and a systolic blood pressure around 70 mm Hg.[28] In contrast, hemorrhagic shock is characterized by tachycardia. Hypotension is usually well tolerated by spinal cord–injured patients in the supine position. However, an adequate blood pressure to provide good tissue perfusion may also secondarily minimize spinal cord injury. Resuscitation may begin with intravenous fluids if the patient manifests evidence of hypoperfusion. This may lead to congestive heart failure, because the intravascular volume is usually adequate. Atropine may be used in patients with bradycardia to block the unopposed vagal effects. If hypotension is refractory, dopamine or phenylephrine may be used as peripheral vasoconstrictors and chronotropes.[29]

Immobilization of the spine in the prehospital setting is

important for all patients with possible spinal injury. The patient needs to be placed in a neutral spine position, and great care should be taken to avoid flexion, extension, or rotation of the neck. The patient is generally placed on a long spine board or a scoop stretcher, and a cervical collar is applied. The head and neck are then stabilized with sandbags on each side, with tape across the forehead to the backboard. Close attention to possible associated injuries is necessary. Concurrent head injury, extremity fractures, and intrathoracic or abdominal injury may require emergency intervention on arrival at the hospital emergency department.

Medical Management and Prevention of Complications

Pulmonary complications of spinal cord injury remain the leading mortality risk and are implicated in approximately 80% of deaths.[30] Atelectasis and pneumonia are the most common pulmonary problems in the acute post-injury period. The severity of the spinal cord injury correlates strongly with the frequency and severity of pulmonary complications. Cervical spinal cord injuries at the levels of C3, C4, and C5 may affect diaphragmatic function, and patients with such injuries may not survive to reach the hospital. Lower cervical levels preserve diaphragm function, but patients may fatigue without intercostal muscle function, because intact muscle function accounts for about 60% of the tidal volume. When intercostal muscle function is lost, paradoxic abdominal breathing results. During inspiration, the diaphragm contracts, producing negative intrathoracic pressure, and the chest wall moves inward, reducing the inspiratory volume to 30% of normal. Intrathoracic pressure rises as the diaphragm relaxes and the chest wall moves outward, resulting in expiratory volumes less than 20% of normal.[26] Close monitoring with pulse oximetry, arterial blood gases, respiratory examinations, and pulmonary function tests is recommended. Patient positioning, chest physical therapy, breathing exercises, positive-pressure breathing, suctioning, bronchoscopy, rotating beds, and manually assisted coughing may be used to mobilize pulmonary secretions.[26] Great care must also be taken to avoid iatrogenic pulmonary edema. Pulmonary artery catheter monitoring may be useful to detect early pulmonary edema.

Ileus and acute stress ulceration are the most common gastrointestinal complications of spinal cord injury. Nasogastric suction should be instituted immediately, to avoid reflux and aspiration and to improve respiratory excursion. The ileus may be delayed and prolonged. The dilated bowel may sequester large amounts of fluid, exacerbating hypovolemia and electrolyte disturbances. Dilated bowel decreases respiratory excursion and may lead to aspiration.[4] Intravenous replacement of nasogastric output should be considered. Gastric stress ulceration may be the result of unopposed vagal stimulation and the use of intravenous steroids to treat the cord injury. Vagal stimulation leads to gastric acid hypersecretion, gastric dilation, relaxation of gastric sphincters, and decreased intestinal peristalsis. Histamine H_2 antagonists and antacids are used to maintain a gastric pH more than 5, or the gastric mucosa may be protected with sucralfate; both approaches minimize stress ulcer bleeding. Sucralfate has been associated with a lower incidence of pneumonia in ventilator-dependent patients than have H_2 antagonists.[31] Frequent guaiac testing of nasogastric aspirates and stools, and monitoring of the serum hematocrit, aids in the early diagnosis of stress ulceration. Anorexia and tachycardia may be the only signs of an ulcer in patients with high spinal cord injury.

The gut is the preferable route of feeding. If enteral feeding is not possible because of prolonged ileus, total parenteral nutrition should be instituted early to provide a means of nutritional support. The nutritional requirements range from 30 to 40 kcal/kg/day, and total parenteral nutrition should be started in the first 24 to 48 hours.[32] Peristalsis usually returns several days after the injury. A regular bowel regimen, including a stool softener and a suppository aids in regular emptying. Spinal cord injury results in a negative nitrogen balance, which may affect other systems. Respiratory reserve may be diminished, and healing may be slowed by a generalized state of catabolism.[29]

Patients with spinal cord injury are at significant risk for development of deep venous thrombosis (DVT) and subsequent pulmonary embolism. The etiology in this population seems to include both stasis and hypercoagulability. Patients with spinal cord injury have poor vasomotor tone, and the absence of muscle contraction in paralyzed extremities promotes significant stasis. Certain coagulation factors are being studied as possible predictors of DVT in patients with spinal cord injury. Because of the high incidence and risk of DVT, prophylaxis should be instituted on admission to the hospital. The incidence of DVT among patients with spinal cord injury can be as high as 72% in the first 2 weeks.[33] Prophylaxis usually includes an external mechanical modality and a pharmacologic agent. Mechanical devices, such as pneumatic compression sleeves, are used for the first 2 weeks after injury, the period of highest risk. Pharmacologic therapy with aspirin or low-dose heparin is usually continued for a total of 6 to 10 weeks after the injury. One study showed low–molecular-weight heparin to be more effective than regular heparin.[34,35] The diagnosis of DVT is difficult in patients with spinal cord injury, because tenderness and even swelling may be absent. Doppler ultrasonography is a convenient initial method of screening for DVT. Venography is the gold standard for detection of DVT, because incomplete thromboses and pelvic thromboses may be missed with other diagnostic approaches. Pulmonary embolus may also be difficult to diagnose, because the usual pleuritic chest pain, tachypnea, and tachycardia may be absent. A high index of suspicion for pulmonary embolus should be maintained in all patients with spinal cord injury. Fever, diaphoresis, and a fall in the oxygen tension should lead to an evaluation for pulmonary embolus. Results of chest radiography and ventilation-perfusion scans are often equivocal. Pulmonary angiography is the definitive diagnostic test, and a vena caval filter may be placed at the time of the study.[34]

Management of Instability

The stability of a spinal injury is often difficult to determine. Several models have been used to assist the clinician in decision making regarding methods of stabilization. The three-column model of the spine was proposed by Denis[19] in 1983. In this model, the spine is composed of three columns, and injury to any two columns can result in instability. The anterior column is composed of the anterior longitudinal ligament, the anterior half of the vertebral body, and the anterior half of the annulus fibrosis. The middle column includes the posterior half of the vertebral body, the posterior half of the annulus fibrosis, and the posterior longitudinal ligament. The posterior column consists of the spinous processes, laminae, articular processes, and the ligamenta flava. The objective of treatment is to regain stability. This can be accomplished by promoting proper healing of the unstable segment by immobilization (bedrest, external orthoses), or by achieving immediate mechanical stabilization through internal fixation. Modes of treatment vary case by case and are the topic of entire textbooks.

Instability of the spine may be treated in several ways. Unstable cervical spine injuries are treated with early skeletal traction.[13,20] Gardner-Wells tongs are compatible with MRI and applied 1 cm above the tips of the ears and in line with the external auditory meatus (Fig. 49-7). Traction weight is usually 10 pounds for the occiput and an additional 2 to 5 pounds for each vertebral level to the injury. Attempts at closed reduction should be discontinued when more than 1 cm distraction exists at any single intervertebral space, or if the patient's neurologic condition deteriorates. For closed cervical reduction, intervertebral disk herniation should be considered in those with facet dislocation. External orthoses are employed when the spine is in good alignment and is relatively stable. The halo skeletal fixator is used as the primary treatment when there is a cervical compression fracture without ligamentous instability, a hangman's fracture, or a Jefferson's fracture (Fig. 49-8). The halo vest allows early mobilization of the patient but does not provide good stability at C7-T1 and is not recommended for ligamentous injury. In a review by Sears and Fazl,[36] only 44% of patients with facet dislocation achieved stability after halo immobilization. Injuries other than facet dislocations are treated effectively 70% of the time.

The indications for surgical intervention and the timing of surgery are controversial. Emergency surgery is generally recommended if there is a progressively

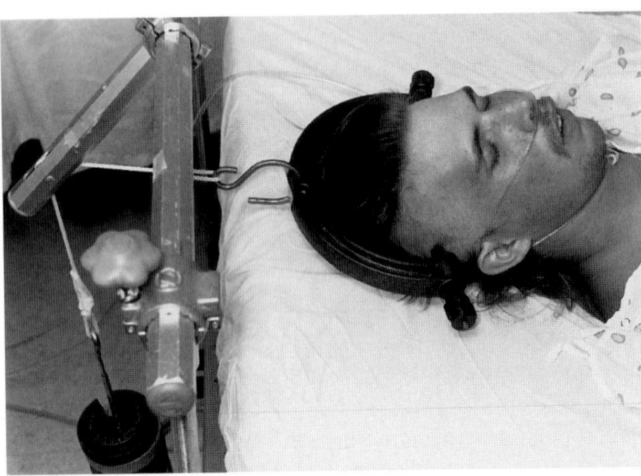

Fig. 49-7. Cervical skeletal traction. Gardner-Wells tongs are placed above the tips of the ears and in line with the external auditory meatus. Traction weight is in line with the spine and hangs freely.

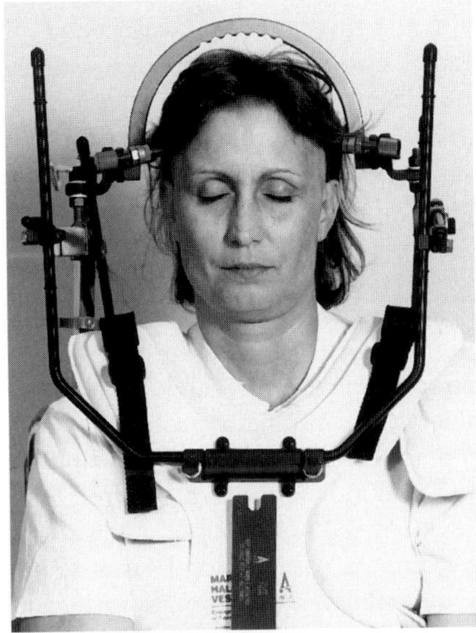

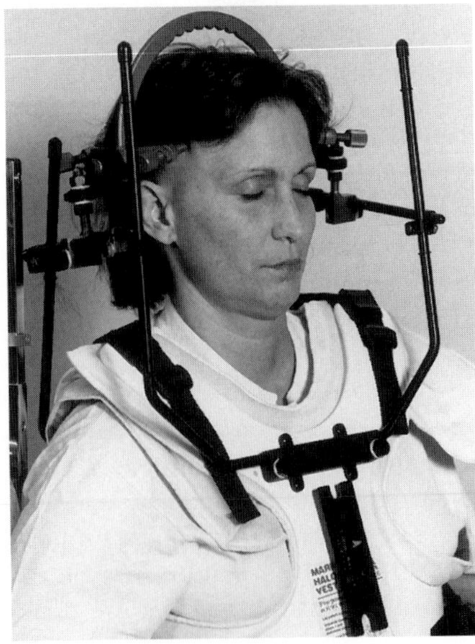

Fig. 49-8. Halo vest. The halo vest allows early mobilization for patients and is effective treatment for many cervical fractures.

worsening neurologic deficit with a compressive lesion, and if closed reduction cannot be accomplished. Patients with complete spinal cord injury for more than 48 hours have been shown not to have neurologic improvement from decompressive surgery. However, early operative stabilization may reduce the time spent in rehabilitation.[37,38] Patients with cauda equina syndrome or incomplete spinal cord injuries have been shown to benefit from decompressive operation. However, neurologic deterioration has also been observed after surgical intervention within 48 hours of injury. Conflicting results of early decompressive surgery studies leave this subject a continuing controversy.[16,39-43] Figure 49-9 depicts two cases of anterior and posterior instrumentation for mechanical stabilization; decompression was done at the same time. After the operation, or in minor spinal injuries, patients may require an external orthosis as well (Fig. 49-10).

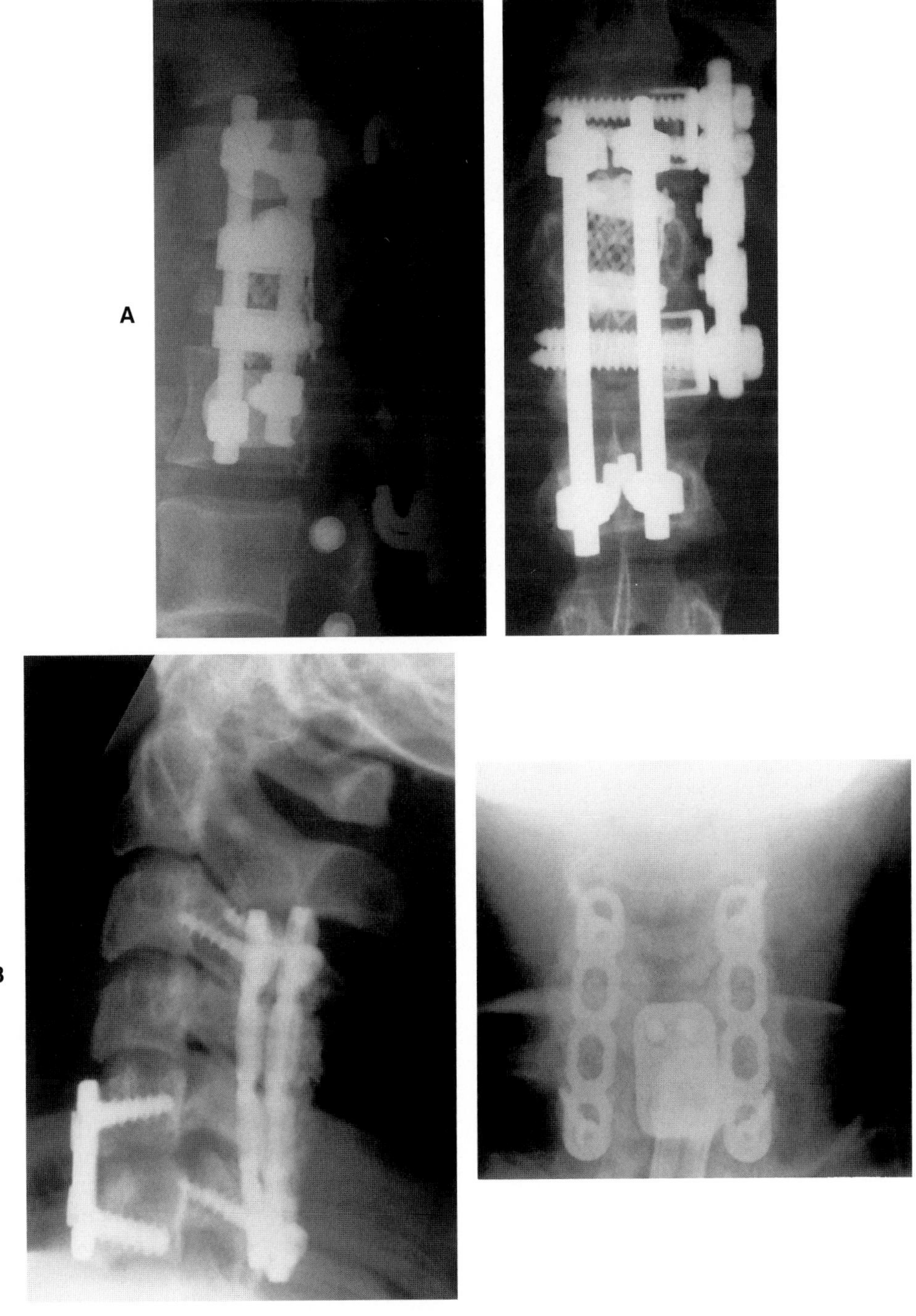

Fig. 49-9. Examples of internal mechanical stabilization. **A,** Cervical anterior vertebral body plates and posterior lateral mass plates. **B,** Anterior and posterior rods with an intervertebral cage.

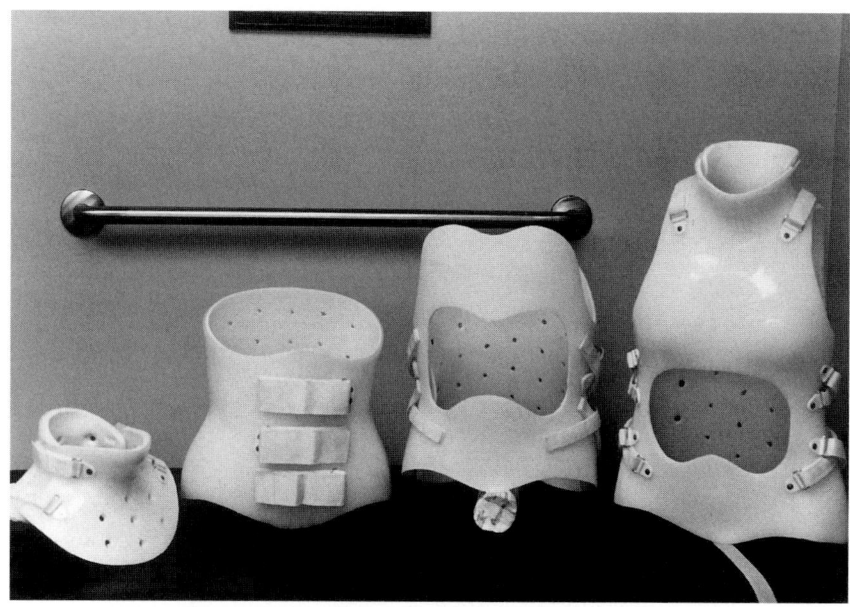

Fig. 49-10. Examples of external orthoses.

Pharmacologic Management of Spinal Cord Injury

The aberrations enumerated in the section on physiology form the basis for the current pharmacologic treatment of spinal cord trauma. This therapy has been directed toward decreasing secondary spinal cord injury, because theoretically the initial primary mechanical injury to the spinal cord is followed by a secondary injury related to additional processes initiated by the original damage. These secondary causes of injury may include excitotoxicity, ischemia, free-radical generation, or inflammatory changes.[22] Until recently, a variety of experimental approaches to the management of spinal cord injury in different animal models suggested a possible role for a number of modalities, including steroids, naloxone, various inhibitors of oxygen-radical formation, and even spinal cord cooling. Steroids were initially thought to improve neurologic recovery by inhibiting the inflammatory process surrounding spinal cord injury, but recent evidence suggests that their effects are mediated by inhibition of posttraumatic activation of lipid metabolism, with subsequent oxygen free-radical–induced peroxidation.[44] The use of naloxone treatment is based on the observation that endorphins, commonly increased after spinal cord injury, appear to have adverse effects on arterial blood pressure and spinal cord blood flow. Naloxone was proposed to offer a means of maintaining spinal cord blood flow after spinal cord injury by blocking receptors through which endorphins are mediated.[45,46] Because oxygen radicals appear to play at least some role in the processes responsible for progressive spinal cord injury, agents known to scavenge these radicals or prevent their formation should logically decrease the magnitude of injury.[47] Finally, spinal cord cooling was thought to be a means of decreasing the swelling of injured neural tissue, at the same time decreasing its metabolic needs, thereby potentially enhancing healing processes.[48] Although many of the observations garnered from this experimental work have proved useful in our current management of spinal cord injury, other modalities, such as spinal cord cooling, have never proved clinically efficacious.

The current pharmacologic treatment of spinal cord injury is based on the results of National Acute Spinal Cord Injury Study (NASCIS).[2] This trial was a randomized, double-blind, placebo-controlled study that evaluated the efficacy of high-dose methylprednisolone and naloxone in the treatment of patients with acute spinal cord injury. The changes in sensory and motor function were evaluated at 6 weeks, 6 months, and 1 year after injury. A significantly greater improvement in motor function and light-touch sensation was observed in patients who received methylprednisolone within 8 hours of injury than in the placebo group. This difference was significant at 6 weeks and was maintained throughout the length of the study. Methylprednisolone administered after 8 hours of injury had no significantly different effect from placebo. Naloxone treatment also did not differ from placebo. The high dose of methylprednisolone used in NASCIS 2 (30 mg/kg over 15 minutes followed by 5.4 mg/kg/hr over 23 hours) was demonstrated to be of benefit if given within 8 hours of injury.[49-51] In the initial NASCIS I, lower doses of methylprednisolone had been tested with no demonstration of efficacy. NASCIS 3, recently completed, tested the efficacy of extended administration of methylprednisolone and the potential benefit of tirilazad mesylate, a more potent lipid perioxidation inhibitor without corresponding glucocorticoid activity.[52] It was proposed that complications of glucocorticoid therapy, such as wound infections, gastrointestinal hemorrhage, or even death, could be avoided with tirilazad therapy. In NASCIS

2, the wound infection rate was 7.1% in the methylprednisolone group versus 3.6% in the placebo group, but these differences were not statistically significant, nor were any other complications.[53] In the most recent NASCIS 3,[54] patients with acute spinal cord injury who received methylprednisolone within 3 hours of injury were shown to benefit in terms of neurologic recovery if such therapy was maintained for a full 24 hours. When methylprednisolone was initiated 3 to 8 hours after injury, this benefit required steroid therapy to be prolonged for 48 hours. Treatment with tirilazad for 48 hours provided equivalent recovery of neurologic function to that of methylprednisolone for 24 hours. When 48-hour treatments with each agent were compared, however, methylprednisolone therapy was superior. These differences in tirilazad therapy from methylprednisolone treatment at 48 hours were not adequately explained in this study and require further evaluation. Further, the absence of glucocorticoid effects with tirilazad did not appear to make an appreciable difference with respect to complications, which were rare in both drug groups. The results of this most recent NASCIS clearly underscore the important role of steroid therapy in the management of acute spinal cord injury and the need for its treatment extension for 24 to 48 hours, depending on the initial commencement of therapy. It must be noted, however, that although steroid therapy has proved effective in the management of blunt trauma to the spinal cord, methylprednisolone is not routinely used in penetrating spinal trauma because it has not shown efficacy in this setting.[55]

MANAGEMENT OF CHRONIC SPINAL CORD INJURY

The management of chronic spinal cord injury is important and has dramatically improved the survival of spinal cord–injured patients. The diagnosis of related and unrelated health problems is difficult, because the signs and symptoms are altered in these patients. An acute abdomen may be present without abdominal tenderness, pyelonephritis may not feature flank pain, and a femur may be fractured without pain. Only an increase in spasticity or new autonomic hyperreflexia may signal a new pathologic condition. Diagnosis may be delayed if close attention is not paid to the altered clinical signs that are available.

Rarely, late neurologic deterioration may occur after a spinal cord injury. Improvement is the usual clinical course, so any neurologic decline should be investigated. Possible causes include posttraumatic syringomyelia or a progressive spinal deformity. Cavitation of the spinal cord occurs in approximately 50% of patients, although they are most likely to be free of symptoms.[15,60]

Urinary tract infection occurs with a frequency of 20%. Septicemia from urinary tract infection remains a leading cause of death among spinal cord–injured patients. Fever and chills in a patient with spinal cord injury should always lead to an evaluation of the urine. To avoid urinary tract infections, intermittent catheterization to empty the bladder is advocated. Annual cystograms and nuclear scanning are recommended.[14]

Decubitus ulcers are the result of pressure applied with time. Frequent changes in position, shifting of weight every 15 minutes in a wheelchair and every 2 hours in bed, are important to prevent the formation of decubitus ulcers. Despite preventive measures, there is an annual incidence of decubitus ulcers of 23% among patients with spinal cord injury. Aggressive local care and surgical debridement of necrotic tissue are the best treatments available, but healing is generally slow.[14]

Autonomic hyperreflexia may be a problem in patients with spinal cord injuries above the level of T6. Noxious stimuli below the level of injury result in increased sympathetic activity. The patients have severe hypertension, headaches, and even intracerebral hemorrhage. The stimulus is likely to be urinary retention or tight clothing. The best treatment is removal of the noxious stimulus. Prophylactic α-adrenergic blockers may be helpful.[14]

Spasticity may be present in as many as 75% of spinal cord–injured patients. It usually develops with time, although its pathophysiology is unknown. Spasticity is treated with morning stretches, baclofen, or diazepam. Subarachnoid baclofen pumps, spinal stimulators, and dorsal rhizotomy are possible surgical interventions.[61] An acute increase in spasticity should prompt an evaluation for secondary causes, such as urinary tract infection.

Long-term adjustment to spinal cord injury is strongly related to the presence or absence of cognitive deficits. Good cognitive ability and a high level of education prior to the injury are associated with improved medical stability. About 95% of patients with spinal cord injury are able to return to the community. Approximately half of those employed prior to the injury are eventually able to return to work.[62] The life expectancy of spinal cord–injured patients is shorter than for the general population, but it is continuing to grow. Close attention to the higher risks of septicemia, pulmonary embolus, and pneumonia in patients with spinal cord injury has increased the likelihood of treatment and thus improved life expectancy.[14]

SPINAL CORD REGENERATION

In contrast to peripheral nerves, which have the capability to regenerate axons when damaged, the spinal cord has generally been thought not to regenerate. This assumption is not entirely accurate, because axons from transsected spinal cord can initiate a "sprouting" process, but this action does appear to abort within 10 days of its commencement. The precise reasons for this abortion remain uncertain. Some investigators have thought that various barriers associated with damaged spinal cord, such as cavity formation, glial scar deposition, and associated tissue necrosis, may impede the sprouting process.[8-10] Others have suggested that sprouting may be aborted because of a deficiency in a specific nerve growth factor that may be in plentiful supply in the peripheral nervous system but is limited in spinal cord tissue. Despite these varying explanations, the fact that transected spinal cord axons can sprout, even for a short period, suggests that the spinal cord may be capable of regeneration under certain circumstances not yet identified. Recently, successful intercostal nerve grafts have been reported to improve hind limb function in rats with complete surgical resection of the spinal cord. In this study, surgical transection of the spinal cord was followed by grafting of peripheral nerve implants. The nerve bridges were supported by fibrin glue and fibroblast growth factor. The hind limb function of the rats improved during a 6 month period.[33,56,57] Whether this technique can be applied to human spinal cord regeneration remains to be seen, but it does provide new insight into spinal cord transection and possible treatment.

A potentially promising pharmacologic treatment for transected spinal cord is GM-1 ganglioside. GM-1 ganglioside is thought to facilitate neurite growth, attenuate retrograde degeneration, and modulate glutamate-mediated excitotoxicity. Gangliosides have enhanced neurologic recovery in laboratory animals with spinal cord injuries. A prospective, randomized, double-blind, placebo-controlled study has been completed at the Shock Trauma Center of the Maryland Institute for Emergency Medical Services System, with promising results. GM-1 ganglioside enhanced the recovery of neurologic function 1 year after major spinal cord injury. There was enhanced motor recovery in the lower extremities versus placebo, but not in the upper extremities. Theoretically, this represents improved function of axons through the site of injury. The gray matter of the spinal cord is more vulnerable to trauma because its high metabolic activity requires more blood flow, and irreversible damage occurs to this area within the first hour after injury. The axons of the white matter are more resistant to injury, and it is thought that GM-1 ganglioside may enhance neuronal survival in the white matter. In this case, it would be reasonable that lower extremity function would improve without upper extremity function being affected. Larger studies of GM-1 ganglioside currently underway include initial treatment with methylprednisolone at the doses studied in NASCIS 2, followed by a prolonged course of GM-1 ganglioside.[58,59] These studies suggest that spinal cord injury may not be entirely irreversible, as previously thought, and that once the precise sequence of events at the cellular level that subserves normal spinal cord function has been identified, spinal cord regeneration may prove possible.

SUMMARY

Spinal cord injury continues to be a major health care problem, with potentially devastating results for affected individuals. Fortunately, as we have learned more about the management of this problem, the quality of life has been optimized, and associated complications have been markedly decreased. These patients are living longer and contributing in meaningful ways to society and their communities. Prevention of spinal cord injury is still the most predictable way of managing this serious malady. It is hoped that education of the public, especially the population most at risk (young men), will decrease the incidence of spinal cord injury in years to come. Even for patients who already have this condition, the future is much brighter than previously. Aggressive, deliberate therapy initiated in a timely fashion salvages a considerably greater amount of neurologic function, even with high-level spinal cord injuries, than would have been possible even a decade ago. Further, the precise events at the cellular level that influence axon disruption and potential regeneration in spinal cord tissue are now being elucidated, offering the promise that in the future, patients may regain much more function after spinal cord injury than currently possible.

REFERENCES

1. Burney RE et al. Incidence, characteristics, and outcome of spinal cord injury at trauma centers in North America. Arch Surg 128:596, 1993.
2. Slucky AV, Eismont FJ. Treatment of acute injury of the cervical spine. Instr Course Lect 44:67, 1995.
3. Spivak JM, et al. Cervical spine injuries in patients 65 and older. Spine 19:2303, 1994.
4. Segal JL, Milne N, Brunnemann SR. Gastric emptying is impaired in patients with spinal cord injury. Am J Gastroenterol 90:466, 1995.
5. Alander DH, Andreychik DA, Stauffer ES. Early outcome in cervical spinal cord injured patients older than 50 years of age. Spine 19:2299, 1994.
6. Sosin DM, Sacks JJ, Smith SM. Head injury-associated deaths in the United States from 1979 to 1986. JAMA 262:2251, 1989.
7. Gelfan S, Tarlov IM. Physiology of spinal cord, nerve root and peripheral nerve compression. Am J Physiol 185:217, 1956.
8. Balentine JD. Pathology of experimental spinal cord trauma. I. The necrotic lesion as a function of vascular injury. Lab Invest 39:236, 1978.
9. Balentine JD. Pathology of experimental spinal cord trauma. II. Ultrastructure of axons and myelin. Lab Invest 39:254, 1978.
10. Brodkey JS, et al. Reversible spinal cord trauma in cats: additive effects of direct pressure and ischemia. J Neurosurg 37:591, 1972.
11. Tator CH, Fehlings MG. Review of the secondary injury theory of acute spinal cord trauma with emphasis on vascular mechanisms. J Neurosurg 75:15, 1991.
12. Kao CC, Chang LW, Bloodworth JMB Jr. The mechanism of spinal cord cavitation following spinal cord transection: Electron microscopic observation. J Neurosurg 6:745, 1977.
13. Bohlman HH. Acute fractures and dislocations of the cervical spine: An analysis of three hundred hospitalized patients and review of the literature. J Bone Joint Surg 61A:1119, 1979.
14. Ditunno JF, Formal CS: Chronic spinal cord injury. N Engl J Med 330:550, 1994.
15. Hadley MN, Randolph MD, Bishop C. Injuries of the craniocervical junction and upper cervical spine. In Tindall GT, ed. The Practice of Neurosurgery. Baltimore: Williams & Wilkins, 1996.
16. Gertzbein SD. Neurologic deterioration in patients with thoracic and lumbar fractures after admission to the hospital. Spine 19:1723, 1994.
17. De Vivo MJ, et al. Benefits of early admission to an organized spinal cord injury care system. Paraplegia 28:545, 1990.
18. Rizzolo SJ, Colter JM. Unstable cervical spine injuries: Specific treatment approaches. J Am Acad Orthop Surg 1:57, 1993.
19. Pratt ES, Green DA, Spengler DM. Herniated intervertebral discs associated with unstable spinal injuries. Spine 15:662, 1990.
20. Hadley MN, et al. Facet fracture-dislocation injuries of the cervical spine. Neurosurgery 30:661, 1992.
21. Denis F. The three column spine and its significance in the classification of acute thoracolumbar spinal injuries. Spine 8:817, 1983.

22. Hamilton MG, Myles ST. Pediatric spinal injury: Review of 174 hospital admissions. J Neurosurg 77:700, 1992.
23. Pollack IF, Pang D, Sclabassi R. Recurrent spinal cord injury without radiographic abnormality in children. J Neurosurg 69:177, 1988.
24. Green BA, Eismont FJ, O'Heir J. Pre-hospital management of spinal cord injuries. Paraplegia 25:229, 1987.
25. Green BA, et al. Acute spinal cord injury: Current concepts. Clin Orthop 154:125, 1981.
26. Slack RS, Shucart W. Respiratory dysfunction associated with traumatic injury to the central nervous system. Clin Chest Med 15:739, 1994.
27. Anderson DK, Hall ED. Pathophysiology of spinal cord trauma. Ann Emerg Med 22:987, 1993.
28. Levi L, Wolf A, Belzberg H. Hemodynamic parameters in patients with acute cervical cord trauma: Description, intervention and prediction of outcome. Neurosurgery 33:1007, 1993.
29. McBride DQ, Rodts GE. Intensive care of patients with spinal trauma. Neurosurg Clin North Am 5:755, 1994.
30. Lemons VR, Wagner FC. Respiratory complications after cervical spinal cord injury. Spine 19:2315, 1994.
31. Eddleston JM, et al. A comparison of the frequency of stress ulceration and secondary pneumonia in sucralfate- or ranitidine-treated intensive care unit patients. Crit Care Med 19:1491, 1991.
32. Kuric J, et al. Nutritional support: A prophylaxis against stress bleeding after spinal cord injury. Paraplegia 27:140, 1989.
33. Merli GJ, et al. Etiology, incidence, and prevention of deep vein thrombosis in acute spinal cord injury. Arch Phys Med Rehabil 74:1199, 1993.
34. Green D, et al. Fatal pulmonary embolism in spinal cord injury. Chest 105:853, 1994.
35. Green D. Prophylaxis of thromboembolism in spinal cord injured patients. Chest 102:649, 1992.
36. Sears W, Fazl M. Prediction of stability of cervical spine fracture managed in the halo-vest and indications for surgical intervention. J Neurosurg 72:426, 1990.
37. Rimoldi RL, et al. The effect of surgical intervention on rehabilitation time in patients with thoracolumbar and lumbar spinal cord injuries. Spine 17:1443, 1992.
38. Wolf A, et al. Operative management of bilateral facet dislocation. J Neurosurg 75:883, 1991.
39. Chapman JR, Anderson PA. Thoracolumbar spine fractures with neurologic deficit. Orthop Clin North Am 25:595, 1994.
40. Donovan WH, Cifu DX, Schotte DE. Neurological and skeletal outcomes in 113 patients with closed injuries to the spinal cord. Paraplegia 30:533, 1992.
41. Krengel WF, Anderson PA, Henley MB. Early stabilization and decompression for incomplete paraplegia due to a thoracic level spinal cord injury. Spine 18:2080, 1993.
42. Levine AM, McAfee PC, Anderson PA. Evaluation and emergent treatment of patients with thoracolumbar trauma. Instr Course Lect 44:33, 1995.
43. Mahale YJ, Silver JR, Henderson NJ. Neurological complications of the reduction of cervical spine dislocations. J Bone Joint Surg 75:403, 1993.
44. Ducker TB, Zeidman SM. Spinal cord injury: Role of steroid therapy. Spine 19:2281, 1994.
45. Faden AI, et al. Endorphins in experimental spinal injury: Therapeutic effect of naloxone. Ann Neurol 10:326, 1981.
46. Flamm ES, et al. Experimental spinal cord injury: Treatment with naloxone. Neurosurgery 10:227, 1982.
47. de la Torre JC, et al. Pharmacologic treatment and evaluation of permanent experimental spinal cord trauma. Neurology 24:508, 1975.
48. Albin MS, et al. Localized spinal cord hypothermia: Anesthetic effects in application to traumatic injury. Anesth Analg 46:8, 1967.
49. Bracken MB. Treatment of acute spinal cord injury with methylprednisolone: Results of a multicenter, randomized clinical trial. J Neurotrauma 8 (Suppl 1):S47, 1991.
50. Bracken MB, et al. Methylprednisolone or naloxone treatment after acute spinal cord injury: 1-year follow-up data. J Neurosurg 76:23, 1992.
51. Young W, Bracken MB. The Second National Acute Spinal Cord Injury Study. J Neurotrauma 9:397, 1992.
52. Bracken MB. Pharmacological treatment of acute spinal cord injury: Current status and future projects. J Emerg Med 11:43, 1993.
53. Galandiuk S, et al. The two-edge sword of large-dose steroids for spinal cord trauma. Ann Surg 218:419, 1993.
54. Bracken MB, et al. Administration of methylprednisolone for 24 or 48 hours or tirilazad mesylate for 48 hours in the treatment of acute spinal injury. JAMA 277:1597, 1997.
55. Predergrast MR, et al. Massive steroids do not reduce the zone of injury after penetrating spinal cord injury. J Trauma 37:576, 1994.
56. Anderson DK, Reier PJ. Transplantation and spinal cord repair in higher vertebrates. J Neurotrauma 10:117, 1993.
57. Cheng H, Cao Y, Olson L. Spinal cord repair in adult paraplegic rats: Partial restoration of hind limb function. Science 273:510, 1996.
58. Geisler FH, Dorsey FC, Coleman WP. Past and current clinical studies with GM-1 ganglioside in acute spinal cord injury. Ann Emerg Med 22:1041, 1993.
59. Geisler FH. GM-1 ganglioside and motor recovery following human spinal cord injury. J Emerg Med 11:49, 1993.
60. Marshall LF, et al. Deterioration following spinal cord injury: A multicenter study. J Neurosurg 56:699, 1982.
61. Maynard FM, Karunas, RS, Waring WP: Epidemiology of spasticity following traumatic spinal cord injury. Arch Phys Med Rehabil 71:566, 1990.
62. Penn RD: Intrathecal baclofen for spasticity of spinal cord origin: Seven years of experience. J Neurosurg 77:236, 1992.

50

Injuries to Peripheral Nerves

Irvine G. McQuarrie, Thomas C. Chelimsky, and Karen Bitzer

The management of nerve injuries poses special difficulties for the surgeon. Although the majority heal satisfactorily without surgical intervention, a year may pass before it is evident that a particular injured nerve will not heal on its own. By then it is too late to do a nerve repair *(neurorrhaphy)* and have this be followed by a satisfactory motor recovery. To obtain a good result from neurorrhaphy, it must be performed within 6 months after injury. On the other hand, the result obtained from carrying out a timely neurorrhaphy is not as good as the result from spontaneous recovery. Neurorrhaphy is to be avoided unless clearly indicated; often this decision must be made before a spontaneous recovery is evident from changes in the neurologic examination. This chapter addresses the pathophysiology of nerve injury and the physiologic basis of nerve repair. It also provides a strategy for the timely identification of nerve lesions that require operative intervention. To accomplish these goals, we only consider mechanical trauma to large mixed (motor and sensory) nerves.

ANATOMY AND PHYSIOLOGY

Fascicular Anatomy

Although physicians agree that the safe and effective treatment of injuries is based on a knowledge of the relevant anatomy and physiology, this is especially true for nerve injuries. Here the most important consideration is the intraneural anatomy. Each mixed nerve contains 4 to 20 bundles *(fascicles)* of nerve fibers (axons within myelin sheaths) that combine, divide, and rotate within the nerve while moving distally to assemble into motor and cutaneous branches. As shown in Fig. 50-1, an unbranched 3 cm length of a mixed nerve contains 5 to 10 fascicles that interconnect to such an extent that most axons come to lie in a different quadrant and have different neighbors after traveling that distance.[1] Because of this anatomic circumstance, it is impossible for the surgeon who performs a neurorrhaphy to perfectly match the fascicles in a proximal nerve stump to those in a distal nerve stump. Even if neurorrhaphy appears necessary, the surgeon may want to carry out an electrophysiologic investigation at the operating table before deciding to resect an incomplete nerve lesion.

The incomplete lesion of greatest concern is the *neuroma-in-continuity,* a fusiform enlargement of the nerve that often occurs within weeks following a nontransecting nerve injury. Although a variable fraction of axons may have been broken *(axonotmesis)* at the time of injury, the mass effect is less a result of axonal sprout formation than of a proliferation of Schwann cells, fibroblasts, and colla-

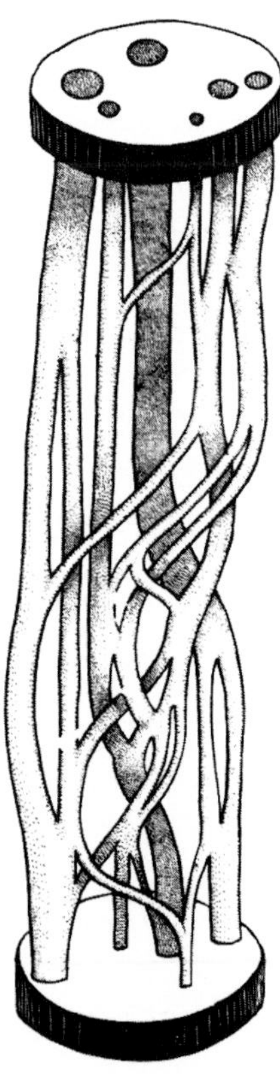

Fig. 50-1. Intraneural fascicular anatomy of a 3 cm segment from the musculocutaneous nerve of a human cadaver. (From Sunderland S. Nerves and Nerve Injuries. Edinburgh: Churchill Livingstone, 1978.)

gen that has been evoked by the force of injury (Fig. 50-2). If the *perineurium* enclosing the fascicles has been breached, misdirected axonal sprouts grow for short distances in the *epineurium* (connective tissue that separates fascicles) before rounding up into small neuromas. If the perineurium remains intact, sprouts remain within the fascicle, and there is more than a 90% chance of spontaneous recovery after approximately 1 year.[2] However, there is less than a 60% chance of a good result from excising a neuroma-in-continuity and performing a neurorrhaphy[2] because regenerating axons have a reduced chance of entering the correct fascicle in the distal nerve stump.[3-5]

When a neuroma-in-continuity contains broken fascicles (perineurial rupture in addition to axonotmesis—an injury termed *neurotmesis),* most axon sprouts enter the epineurium and are unable to traverse the lesion. In that event the only possibility for recovery lies in neurorrhaphy. Because the majority of civilian nerve injuries produce a neuroma-in-continuity that is initially associated with a complete loss of nerve function, the decisions of whether and when to operate assume paramount importance.[2]

Homeostasis and Microvasculature

The special environment of CNS tissues is maintained by the blood-brain barrier, which is physically enforced by tight junctions between capillary endothelial cells. Thus protein is excluded from the extracellular fluid of the CNS. Active transport mechanisms within the endothelial cells permit the transfer of specific substances into the extracellular fluid of the brain. Similar mechanisms remove metabolic waste products and toxic substances from the extracellular fluid, since the CNS has no lymphatic vessels. In the peripheral nervous system, each fiber (axon with its supporting Schwann cells) is bathed in endoneurial fluid, which has a composition similar to cerebrospinal fluid. As in the CNS, there are no lymphatic vessels, capillaries are nonfenestrated, and endothelial cells are joined by tight junctions.[6] The perineurial cells that enclose the endoneurial space are also joined by tight junctions. A breakdown of this "blood-nerve barrier" causes a loss of function in nerve fibers of the affected fascicle. This pathophysiologic event may not be associated with any change in ultrastructure of the fibers, and function is restored on restitution of the perineurium.[7]

The intraneural blood supply is from longitudinally-directed arterioles and venules, located in both the epineurium and endoneurium, which connect with intrafascicular capillaries (Fig. 50-3). These lie between nerve fibers, and the mean distance between capillaries is only 0.15 mm.[1] Although the largest nerves (median, sciatic)

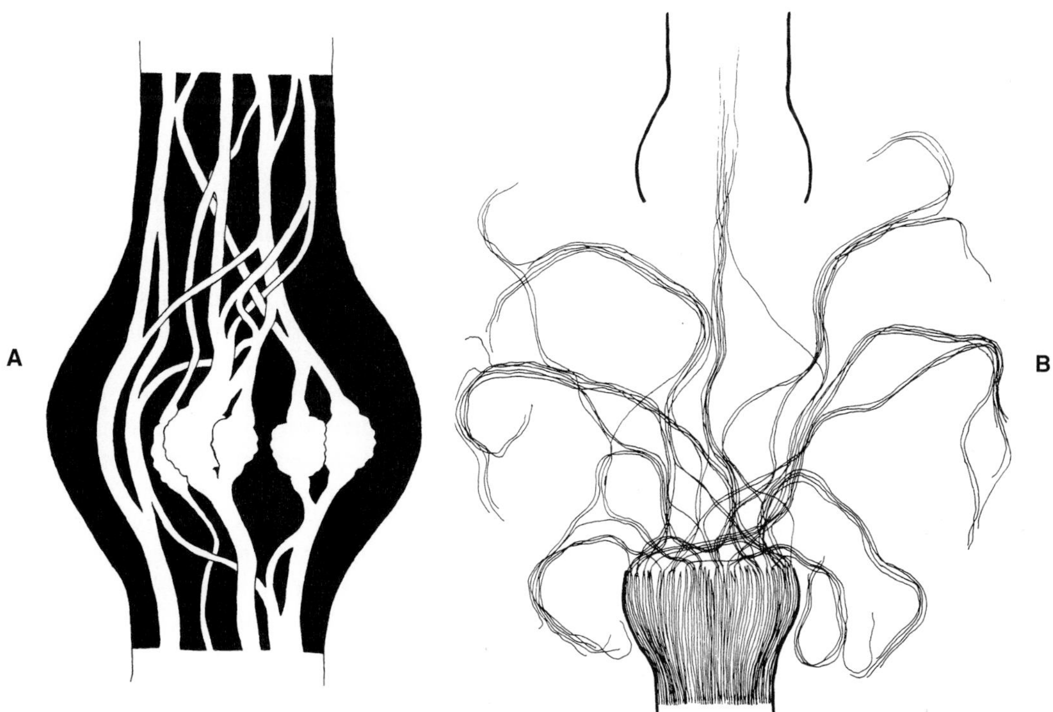

Fig. 50-2. Schematic representation of a neuroma-in-continuity. **A,** Intraneural fascicular anatomy is depicted in contrast with a dark background representing the proliferation of Schwann cells, fibroblasts, and collagen that occurs at any site of nerve contusion; five of the fascicles have sustained perineurial rupture, producing a neurotmesis-type lesion.[1] **B,** Intrafascicular axonal anatomy is depicted at a site of perineurial rupture (distal fascicle stump is at top of figure); a number of "minifascicles" have formed in response to a complete axotomizing lesion, and one of these has found its way to the distal fascicle stump.

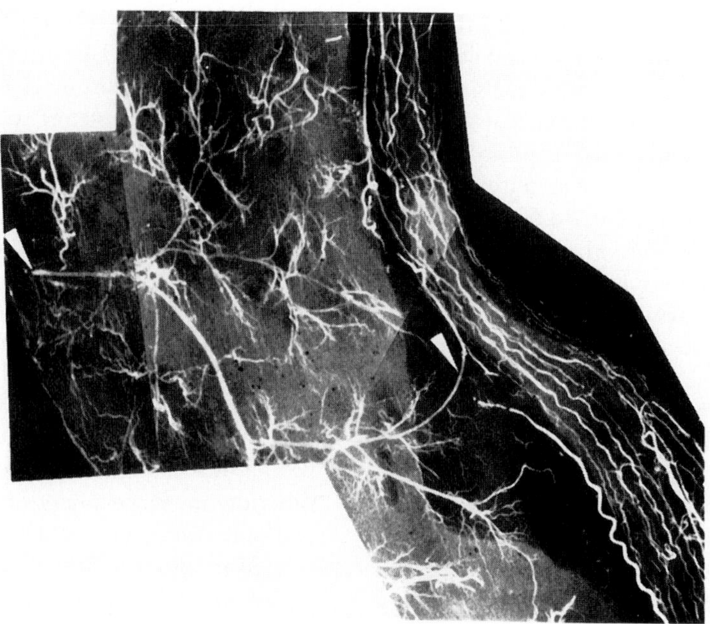

Fig. 50-3. Microradiograph of the rat sciatic nerve *(right)* and the caudofemoralis muscle *(left)* after intra-arterial injection of 25% micropaque. The two arrowheads mark the course of the anastomotic artery as it arises in the muscle, emerges from the anterior muscle border, and joins the arteria comitans along the posterior surface of the nerve (×9). (From Bell MA, Weddell AGM. A descriptive study of the blood vessels of the sciatic nerve in the rat, man, and other mammals. Brain 107:871, 1985.)

have nutrient vessels that are larger than arterioles, more than 90% of the intraneural vessels are less than 10 μm in diameter. Because of the length of arterioles and venules and the collateralization of intraneural vessels, blood flow rates are little affected by mobilization of the nerve or nerve transection. Experimental studies in cats show that flow returns to the normal range of 40 to 50 ml/100 g/min in both stumps by 1 hour after transection.[1] The surgeon can safely mobilize 20 to 30 cm lengths of nerve without being concerned about blood supply,[1] a maneuver that makes it possible to bridge a 5 cm gap if the extremity is splinted in a position of functional flexion.

Impulse Conduction

Nerve impulses (action potentials) are conducted over the axon surface to the axon terminal through a propagated reversal of charge that maintains the impulse at a constant amplitude and velocity. Although the rate of conduction may exceed 100 m/sec (because of myelin insulation, which forces the impulse to jump from one node of Ranvier to the next), that rate is much slower than electric conduction over a copper wire. Axons are actually poor electric conductors: a 30 V stimulus could not produce a potential of 1 V at the end of an axon 1 m long without the energy-requiring process that mediates the reversal of charge at the axon surface.

Following axonotmesis, the nerve action potential (NAP) cannot propagate across the point of injury. However, the axons of the distal nerve stump retain the ability to propagate an impulse for up to 4 days after injury. Thereafter, the axon surface loses its functional integrity as a result of segmentation of the axon into myelin-bounded "ovoids" or "digestion chambers," where the axon is phagocytosed—a process termed *wallerian degeneration.*[9]

Nerve Cell Body Reaction to Axonotmesis

The possibility of axonal regeneration depends on survival of the neuron. Because 95% to 99% of the cytoplasm in peripherally projecting neurons is located in the axon, and a large fraction of the axonal volume is in the terminal arborization,[10,11] axonotmesis removes most of the neuronal cytoplasm. This often results in the death of a small percentage of neurons. The main reason neurons survive the loss of such a large amount of cytoplasm is that the protein synthesis machinery of the neuron is spared.[12,13] In response to axonotmesis, the nerve cell body undergoes a series of biochemical, physiologic, and anatomic changes that have been termed *chromatolysis* because of the reduction in cytoplasmic basophilia. This tinctorial change is attributable to the diffusion of cytoplasmic RNA (located mainly within polyribosomes), secondary to disruption of the rough endoplasmic reticulum and an increase in cell volume.[12] Biochemical changes include an early and sharp reduction in the synthesis of proteins used for neurotransmitter production. This decrease is roughly balanced by an increase in the synthesis of proteins used for regrowing an axon, which include tubulin, actin, and "growth-associated proteins."[12-15] Physiologic changes include a prompt internalization and degradation of cell surface receptors, a marked reduction in the amplitude of excitatory postsynaptic potentials (EPSPs), and a reduction in the velocity of impulse conduction in the surviving or *parent* axon.[12] Anatomic changes vary with the type of neuron but commonly include a withdrawal of axon terminals from the cell body and dendrites of the injured neuron (accounting for the reduced amplitude of EPSPs), atrophy of dendrites, enlargement of the nucleolus, eccentric positioning of the nucleus, an increase in perikaryal volume, and a thinning of the parent axon (accounting for the reduced rate of impulse propagation).[12]

There is abundant evidence that the nerve cell body reaction plays a prominent role in axonal regeneration.[12] In addition, the "environment" of the newly formed *daughter* axon is important to the success of regeneration.[13,16] Two recent developments support the primacy of neuronal events. First, studies over the past decade have shown that axonal outgrowth can be accelerated by the use of a conditioning lesion. This axonotmesis initiates a "crop" of regenerating axons, which is removed days later by a second (testing) lesion. The second crop forms sooner and advances faster than the first.[13,17,18] This acceleration appears to be based on the increased synthesis and axonal transport of tubulin, actin, and certain growth-associated proteins.[13] The environment faced by the second crop of axons, an environment of wallerian degeneration, is not the primary cause for accelerated outgrowth.[13,17,18] The neuronal control of outgrowth is also evident from its rapid response to changes in the status of the axon tip. The nerve cell body receives information quickly by means of *retrograde axonal transport,* and makes appropriate changes in its protein synthesis and axonal transport priorities.[14] It is by this process, for example, that the nerve cell body knows within a few hours that it has sustained an axotomy.[19]

Axonal Transport During Axonal Regeneration

The motive force for axonal outgrowth appears to be the axonal transport system, which is responsible for supplying all the protein needs of the axon.[11,13,20] Membranous organelles are carried by *fast transport;* structural proteins and the enzymes of intermediary metabolism are carried by the two subcomponents of *slow transport.*[10] The proteins that are used for synaptic transmission and renewal of the axolemma are conveyed in tubulovesicular form by fast transport at approximately 400 mm/day. During regeneration, fast transport provides the glycoproteins that form the new axon membrane. In experimental studies, fast transport is labeled with radioactive glycoproteins (which are enriched five-fold in growth cones) to measure axonal outgrowth distances.[17]

The principal cytoskeletal proteins are tubulin, actin, and the neurofilament triplet. These are conveyed through the axon by slow transport as both monomers and polymers (microtubules, actin microfilaments, and neurofilaments). The 30 to 40 proteins that associate with actin microfilaments move in a group at 2 to 6 mm/day as slow component *b* (SC*b*) of slow transport. The protein triplet composing neurofilaments is transported 1 to 2 mm/day as slow component *a* (SC*a*), in association with most of the microtubules. During axonal outgrowth, there are changes in the relative amounts of several proteins moving with both fast and slow transport, but proteins are neither added nor deleted.[11] However, both the average rate and overall amount of protein transport via SC*b* increases.[11,13,20] This correlates with evidence indicating that the rate of outgrowth cannot exceed the rate of SC*b*.[11,13,20] The governing role of SC*b* may relate to (1) the dependence of growth cone function on the polymerization of actin into microfilaments and (2) the dependence of axonal elongation on the assembly of tubulin into microtubules.[11,13]

Stages of Axonal Regeneration

Four stages of axonal regeneration precede the onset of voluntary motor activity: (1) the *initial delay,* consisting of sprout formation and the advance of sprouts to the lesion site; (2) the *scar delay,* during which sprouts cross the lesion; (3) the *outgrowth period,* during which axons elongate within fascicles of the distal nerve; and (4) the *maturation delay,* during which axons that contact an appropriate end organ initiate a series of recovery events. These include the reversal of end-organ atrophy, radial growth of the axon, and myelination.

In experimental studies on sciatic nerves of the rat, sprouts begin to form within a few hours of injury and many acquire a cytoskeleton by 27 hours.[18] The zone of *traumatic degeneration* (same pathology as wallerian degeneration but located at the proximal nerve stump) must be traversed before sprouts can attempt to reach the distal nerve stump.[21] The average initial delay in rats is 36 hours, and the scar delay at a neurorrhaphy is approximately 48 hours.[22] In monkeys the combined initial and scar delay is 1 to 3 weeks.[23,24] This is much shorter than the 5 to 7 weeks required by chimpanzees, suggesting that the evolutionary step from monkeys to anthropoid apes involves a major change in neuronal growth potential.[23]

The outgrowth period terminates with the arrival of axons at an end organ. If an incompatible end organ is encountered, as in the case of a sensory axon reaching a motor end plate, the maturation phase is not initiated, and the axon remains small in caliber.[25] If the contact is appropriate, the axon undergoes radial growth (through the addition of neurofilaments), which triggers the formation of myelin by Schwann cells.[26,27] The axon initiates myelin formation through both a chemical signal to the Schwann cell and the physical influence of its radial growth.[22,27] After the nerve fiber has matured and end-organ atrophy has been reversed through the resumption of neurotrophic activity, function is recovered. The mismatches between motor axons and muscle fibers (e.g., when a motor axon that had originally projected to a flexor muscle reinnervates an extensor muscle) are partially compensated by changes in sensory connections within the CNS[5] and the neurotrophic induction of changes in muscle fiber type.[28]

The pathophysiology that we have gleaned from these

animal studies can be related to nerve injuries in humans. If the times of onset for voluntary movements (in a proximal-to-distal series of muscles served by an injured nerve) and the distances from the lesion to the motor point (where each muscle is innervated) are noted,[1] a regression function of distance on time can be plotted. When this is extrapolated to zero distance, the number of days indicated on the x-axis represents the *latent period* (Fig. 50-4). This is

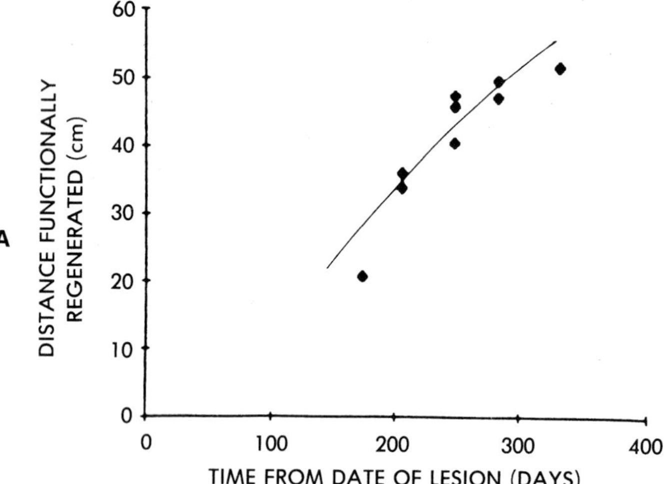

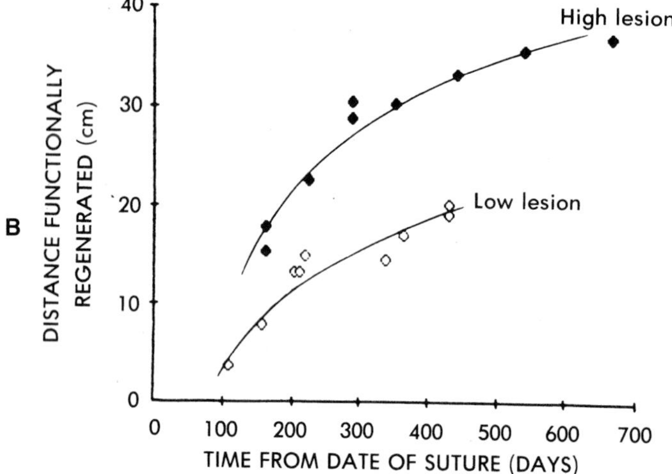

Fig. 50-4. Functional motor recovery in patients sustaining radial nerve injuries, illustrating the progress seen after an axonotmesis-type injury within a neuroma-in-continuity **(A)** vs. a neurotmesis-type injury repaired by nerve suture **(B)**. Distances from the lesion site to the muscle nerve entry point are plotted on the ordinate, and the time from injury (or nerve suture) to the onset of recovery (voluntary contractions) is plotted on the abscissa. *Latent period* is estimated by extrapolating the regression function of distance on time to zero distance. **A,** Radial nerve axonotmesis: high lesion; the regression function indicates that the motor axon outgrowth rate is approximately 3 mm/day. **B,** Radial nerve sutures: low vs. high lesion; regression functions indicate that the axon outgrowth rate is approximately 1 mm/day. (From Bowden REM, Sholl DA. The advance of functional recovery after radial nerve lesions in man. Brain 73:17, 1950.)

a combination of the initial delay, the scar delay, and the maturation delay. In a classic study that applies this method in a number of patients following neurorrhaphy, the latent period is estimated to be about 13 weeks.[29] These patients were compared to others having closed crush injuries (axonotmesis) and therefore a negligible scar delay, where the latent period is about 9 weeks. Thus the average scar delay is 4 weeks. Because most of the nerve repairs (in this study of World War II injuries) were carried out more than 6 months after injury, the maturation delay would not have been the optimal 4 weeks but rather 6 to 8 weeks.[24,30] Subtracting that 6 to 8-week interval from the 9-week latent period (seen after axonotmesis) leaves an initial delay of 1 to 3 weeks. With the 4-week scar delay after neurorrhaphy added, there is a 5- to 7-week delay before axons begin to elongate within the distal nerve stump, as in chimpanzees.[23] Experience with testing the NAP across the lesion site during surgery has validated this estimate.[2] Accordingly, an operation that is partly done for the purpose of recording NAPs from axons that have crossed a suspected neuroma-in-continuity must be delayed until 8 to 10 weeks after injury.[2]

PATHOLOGY

With acute nerve compression of mild degree and short duration, the local pathology is limited to *paranodal demyelination* (a retraction and thinning of myelin at the nodes of Ranvier).[31] Greater compression causes a loss of myelin between nodes of Ranvier *(segmental demyelination)*. These forms of demyelination block the transmission of action potentials without interrupting the axon, producing a *neurapraxia*[21] (Fig. 50-5, *A)*. Greater compression breaks the axon without disrupting the basement membrane of the Schwann cell (endoneurial tube) or the perineurium.[32] This is termed *axonotmesis,* meaning "a break in the axon" (Fig. 50-5, *B)*. Finally, cutting objects, shearing forces, and percussive forces produce additional connective tissue disruption and break the perineurium and/or the nerve. This is termed *neurotmesis,* meaning "a break in the nerve."

Myelin is readily displaced and thinned by pressure, especially at paranodes. When this occurs, impulse transmission is interrupted even though the axon remains intact. The susceptibility of axons to pressure increases with the degree of myelination. This is best illustrated in a pure neuropraxia, such as "Saturday night palsy," where an intoxicated person develops paralysis and loss of sensation in the upper extremity because of sleeping for prolonged periods in a position that either stretches or compresses a nerve (usually the radial) or the brachial plexus. Examination often shows total paralysis associated with an absence of proprioception and touch sensation in the distribution of one or more nerves. However, a pin can be perceived as a dull ache, and a normal density of sweat droplets can be discerned (by examining the skin with an ophthalmoscope set at +20 diopters). Thus the functions served by myelinated axons have been lost, but those served by unmyelinated axons have been retained. These patients begin to recover within 2 weeks and have fully recovered by 3 months. When the force of compression is greater, there is a break in the axon (axonotmesis). Axonal transport is blocked at the point of breakage, and the axon distal to that point undergoes wallerian degeneration. This process occurs simultaneously at all levels, and all axons show degeneration by the fifth day after injury.[9]

The most straightforward classification of acute nerve injuries is open vs. closed, depending on whether there has been a break in the skin. If closed, the lesion is either an *acute compression injury* (closed crush) or a *traction injury*. Acute compression injuries are usually secondary to fractures, with the radial nerve being involved most often.[33] The pathology is paranodal demyelination secondary to increased endoneurial fluid pressure.[34] A traction component occurs if the nerve is stretched over a bone fragment. Pure traction injuries are commonly seen in emergency rooms because of motorcycle accidents. In these, the nerve injury occurs because the rider tries to maintain a grip on the handlebars in an attempt to stay with the motorcycle. The upper brachial plexus is involved if the motorcycle stops suddenly, throwing the rider over the handlebars; the lower plexus is involved if the rider is thrown off and dragged while the motorcycle keeps moving.

Of the open injuries, there are two types—those caused by bullet wounds and those caused by cutting objects such as glass. A bullet that misses a nerve may still block function. This is because a *percussion injury* is produced as the bullet passes near the nerve and a pressure wave creates a temporary cavity in the tissues. The pathology is usually a combination of segmental demyelination and wallerian degeneration, producing a combination of neurapraxia and axonotmesis.[31,35] The extent of nerve damage depends on the proximity of the bullet to the nerve and the amount of kinetic energy that is transferred to the nerve. With a high-velocity bullet (moving at more than 2500

A

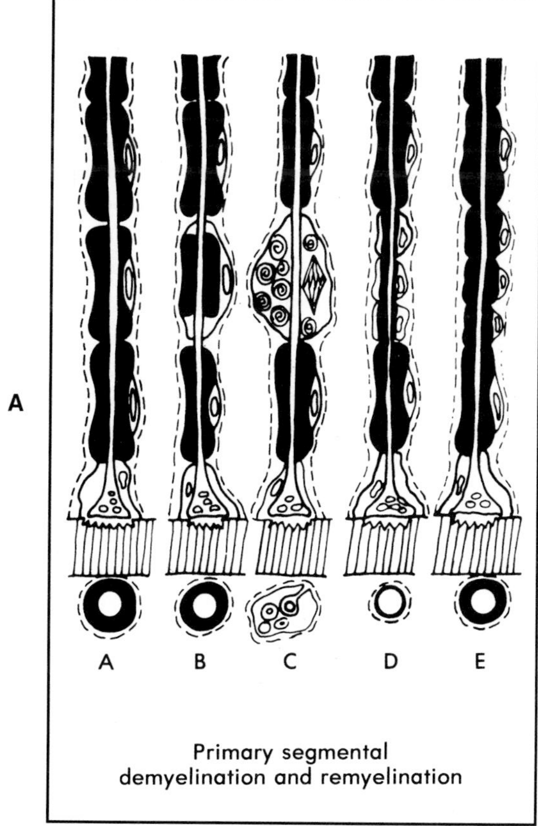

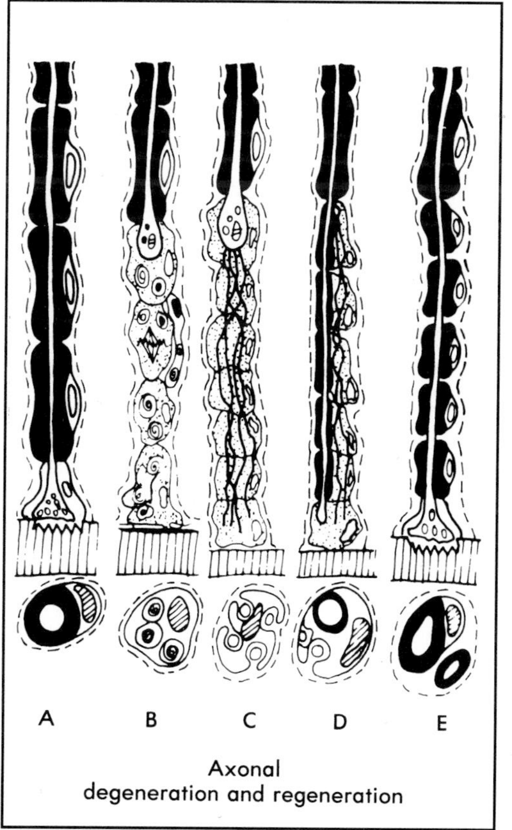

B

Fig. 50-5. Sequence of changes in a myelinated fiber sustaining a neurapraxia-type injury **(A)** vs. an axonotmesis-type injury **(B)** as a result of nerve compression. **A,** Neurapraxia-type injuries produce segmental demyelination and remyelination. *A,* Normal fiber; *B,* retraction of paranodal myelin with widening of nodal gap; *C,* destruction of myelin sheath and Schwann cell mitoses; *D* and *E,* remyelination through the intercalation of short internodes. **B,** Axonotmesis-type injuries produce axonal degeneration and regeneration. *A,* Normal fiber; *B,* by 1 week after axotomy, Schwann cells containing axon and myelin debris have divided to form *bands of Büngner; C,* during the second week, axon sprouts extend from the enlarged terminus of the proximal axon stump; *D,* one of the newly formed sprouts becomes myelinated; *E,* end-organ reconnection occurs. (From Weller RO, Cervos-Navarro J. Pathology of Peripheral Nerves. London-Boston: Butterworth Publishers, 1977.)

ft/sec), nerve fascicles can be ruptured even though the bullet misses the nerve. This is because the kinetic energy of the bullet is proportional to its weight and the *square* of its velocity. A small bullet moving at several thousand feet per second is going to cause more damage than a large bullet moving at several hundred feet per second. A military assault rifle (e.g., the M-16 used by the U.S. Forces) produces the former condition, whereas a pistol produces the latter condition. A high-velocity bullet causes a prolonged initial delay because the zone of traumatic degeneration is longer than it would be with a simple laceration (the length of this zone being proportional to the kinetic energy of the bullet).[1] For a low-velocity bullet wound, it is appropriate to wait 8 to 10 weeks before exploring the nerve to test whether a NAP can be transmitted across the lesion, but 12 to 16 weeks are necessary for a high-velocity bullet wound.[1]

ASSESSMENT OF THE DEFICIT

Assessment should (1) name the injured nerve, (2) locate the injury along its course, (3) differentiate neurapraxia from a complete lesion (axonotmesis or neurotmesis), and (4) list both negative changes (motor and sensory losses) and positive changes (paresthesias, dysesthesias, pain and altered autonomic activity). A careful neurologic examination is the most important part of the assessment. In addition, certain neurophysiologic tests are useful. These include nerve conduction studies (NCSs) that are done together with electromyography (EMG). In addition, autonomic testing may be appropriate when pain is present.

Neurologic Examination

It is important to assess sensory disturbances, focusing on any loss of sensation that may have occurred in the autonomous cutaneous zone of the injured nerve. Experience has shown that these zones are only innervated by a particular mixed nerve; neither congenital anomaly nor collateral sprouting from adjacent nerves can provide innervation of these zones, so anesthesia denotes a complete nerve lesion.[1] With incomplete nerve lesions, sensation is retained in the autonomous zones, and abnormal spontaneous sensations (paresthesias) or abnormal responses to stimuli (dysesthesias) commonly occur. Dysesthesias can include decreased or increased sensitivity of a normal type (hypoesthesia, hyperesthesia). All sensory changes, including anesthesia, can have a painful component. When a nonnoxious stimulus produces pain, the term *allodynia* is used.

The pathophysiology of pain after nerve injury has been studied in great detail, and an excellent review has been published by Wall.[36] The most important pain syndrome is *causalgia,* which is a severe burning pain that follows nerve injury but may extend beyond the distribution of the injured nerve; both allodynia and abnormalities of autonomic function are typical findings.[37,38] It occurs after approximately 2% of incomplete transections[39] but is rarely seen when complete transections are promptly repaired. Causalgia is diagnosed when there is constant burning pain within the distribution of an injured nerve and examination shows allodynia in association with autonomic changes. These changes may include skin that is smooth and glossy, an increase or decrease in the rate of hair growth, tapered digits, thickened nails, periarticular fibrosis, and osteoporosis.[40]

The pathophysiology of causalgia has been thought to involve an excess of activity in sympathetic motor axons and the transmission of this activity to somatic sensory axons by means of synapselike connections in the proximal stump neuroma.[41,42] Accordingly, there have been many attempts to treat causalgia pharmacologically (by systemic or local administration of agents that block sympathetic activity) and surgically (by sympathectomy).[43] More recently, however, this teaching has come under criticism.[38]

Following nerve injury, autonomic function is lost in the areas of cutaneous anesthesia. Sweat secretion is undetectable when the skin is examined with the +20 D lens of an ophthalmoscope. The Ninhydrin sweat test can also be used to document both the absence of sweat formation and any recovery caused by collateral sprouting or axonal regeneration. The *erectores pillae* muscles at the base of each hair follicle do not erect the hair in response to cooling, and the skin is warm because of the absence of innervation to arterial smooth muscle. Later, as the β-adrenergic receptors on these muscle cells proliferate in response to the absence of normal innervation, the cells become supersensitive to congeners of the missing neurotransmitter. This may be manifested by the extremity becoming cool in response to epinephrine released from the adrenal medulla during environmental or emotional stress.

Assessment of the response of muscles to voluntary effort is achieved through manual testing techniques that are specific to the nerve injury in question. For these to be diagnostic, the examiner must be aware of trick movements or substitution patterns. The distribution and extent of muscle atrophy is recorded as mild to severe and is quantified by measuring the circumference of extremities at fixed distances from bony landmarks. Deformities of posture must be described and interpreted. For example, a *claw hand* deformity denotes an ulnar nerve lesion. The extent of muscle contractures in the hand is determined by applying standard tests for intrinsic and extrinsic tightness.[44] Joint contractures are measured with a goniometer and judged to be either reducible or fixed.[45]

For motor disturbances the principal problem is muscle atrophy. Both disuse and the lack of neurotrophic influences contribute to this problem. If the muscle is not reinnervated within 2 to 3 years, all the muscle cells are replaced by connective tissue. If the muscle is not maintained in dynamic activity (by passive range-of-motion exercises) while it is denervated, much of the rehabilitative potential is lost because of muscle fiber atrophy occurring in concert with endomysial fibrosis. Immobilization and paralysis also cause venous and lymphatic stasis, which further reduce blood flow and cause edema. Finally, joint contractures often occur because of decreased muscular support, edema, fibrosis, and the unopposed action of normally innervated muscles. Although it is clear that passive range-of-motion exercises are worthwhile, the presence of pain may be a limitation. In that event the regular use of regional anesthesia may be necessary to allow an exercise program to occur.

Examination of Specific Nerves

For the *median nerve* the autonomous zone of skin innervation includes the digital pads of the thumb and index finger and the dorsum of the terminal phalanx of the index finger. An absence of pin sensation and sweat formation in these areas indicates a complete nerve lesion. The equivalent loss in terms of motor function is an absence of voluntary contraction of the abductor pollicis brevis muscle; without this muscle it is impossible to elevate the thumb from the palm and rotate it into a position of grasp. If the median nerve injury is near the elbow, other movements are impossible after a complete lesion. These include pronation of the forearm and flexion of the thumb and index finger joints, which results in the *benediction sign* when the patient is asked to make a fist.

For the *radial nerve* there is no autonomous sensory zone. In most individuals, however, a total nerve lesion causes loss of sensation over the radiodorsal forearm and the dorsum of the thumb. On motor examination the fingers cannot be extended at the metacarpophalangeal joints, the thumb cannot be extended at any joint, and the hand cannot be extended at the wrist.

For the *ulnar nerve* the autonomous zone is over the terminal phalanx of the fifth finger. None of the fingers can be adducted or abducted, and the metacarpophalangeal joints cannot be flexed without flexing the interphalangeal joints. A claw hand deformity is common. This involves hyperextension of the metacarpophalangeal joints and flexion of the interphalangeal joints.

In the lower extremity the *common peroneal nerve* does not have an autonomous zone of skin sensation. However, a complete lesion commonly causes a loss of sensation over part of the middorsum of the foot and the web space between the great and second toes. On motor examination there is an inability to evert the foot, dorsiflex the ankle, or extend the toes. For the *tibial nerve* the autonomous zone is the entire sole of the foot. The motor deficit is a loss of plantar flexion at the ankle and metatarsophalangeal joints. Complete lesions of the *sciatic nerve* produce combinations of the patterns of loss for the tibial and common peroneal nerves.

Nerve blocks may be needed to be certain of which nerves have been injured and whether those injuries are complete or incomplete in terms of the loss in function. After a thorough neurologic examination, it may appear that an incomplete nerve injury has occurred because there are strong voluntary contractions of one or two muscles served by the injured nerve while all others are unresponsive. In that event it is important to block conduction in the uninjured nerves that could be providing anomalous innervation to the myotome traditionally served by the injured nerve. For example, function can be retained in median-innervated muscles of the hand (abductor pollicis brevis, opponens pollicis) in 15% of patients following a complete transection of the median nerve at the wrist because of the Martin-Gruber anastomosis between the median and ulnar nerves in the forearm.[1] A *procaine block* of the ulnar nerve at the wrist would demonstrate this.

Neurophysiologic Tests

Electrophysiologic tests (nerve conduction study and electromyography) are of great value after nerve injuries. There are two types of NCS, motor and sensory. For motor, the stimulus is a supramaximal electric discharge delivered by a surface (skin) electrode to an underlying nerve (e.g., the median nerve at the wrist). The motor response is the electric potential recorded over a muscle subserved by the nerve (e.g., the abductor pollicis brevis). This consists of the summed motor unit action potentials (MUAPs), each of which represents the response of muscle fibers innervated by a single motor axon. These responses act to amplify the NAP. In contrast, detection of the sensory response requires recording a NAP directly (e.g., from the median nerve at the wrist after stimulating the digital nerves of the index finger). Accordingly, MUAPs have a large amplitude, in the range of 3 to 15 *milli*volts, whereas sensory NAPs have a small amplitude, in the range of 5 to 50 *micro*volts.

NCS yields two values: an amplitude of response (in microvolts or millivolts) and a latency of response (in milliseconds). The conduction velocity, normally 40 to 60 m/sec, is calculated by dividing the latency into the length of the nerve segment over which the study is performed. Nerve conduction is readily examined following nerve injuries, usually by stimulating distally with digital cuff electrodes and recording sensory NAPs proximally with needle or skin electrodes. By 5 days after axonotmesis, motor axons distal to the lesion are unable to conduct NAPs because of wallerian degeneration.[9] Thus motor NCS can be used to differentiate neurapraxia from axonotmesis within a week after injury.

In general, the findings on NCS depend on the type of injury (whether a neurapraxia or complete lesion), the interval since injury, the severity of negative neurologic changes (motor and sensory loss), and the severity of positive neurologic changes (paresthesia, pain, and autonomic changes). The most useful information is obtained if electrophysiologic tests are carried out both immediately and at 3 weeks after the nerve injury. The first study, if done within 2 to 3 days, localizes the lesion by NCS because conduction is absent across the site of injury but intact above and below. (A slowing of conduction velocity is characteristic of a demyelinating lesion, but a total loss of myelin results in a *conduction block,* which is indistinguishable from a complete lesion.) The second study determines whether there is a complete lesion, in which case conduction is lost below the lesion and fibrillations are present in denervated muscles.

In axonal injury the degeneration of nerve fibers becomes complete in 5 days for motor responses and 7 days for sensory responses. (The difference is due to sensitivity of the neuromuscular junction to blocked axonal transport.) With the demyelinating lesion of neurapraxia, the distal response is never affected.

By one week after injury, nerve conduction changes reach their nadir and the character of the lesion can be fully discerned. With a pure neurapraxia, only the myelin must be reconstituted, and this usually occurs in 3 to 6 weeks. With a pure axonal lesion, the axon must grow back to an end organ similar to the original. This occurs at approximately 1 mm/day, as previously described, and depends on daughter axons entering a vacated endoneurial tube distal to the lesion, which then directs the outgrowing axon to an appropriate end organ. With neurorrhaphy, the choice of endoneurial tube is essentially random. Recovery usually takes many months. Motor recovery sometimes begins in weeks because of collateral sprouting, which provides motor axons from nearby uninjured nerves to reinnervate muscles denervated by the injury.

EMG examines the pattern of individual MUAPs seen after inserting a bipolar (concentric) needle electrode into a muscle. Complete lesions produce two types of abnormalities (Fig. 50-6). First, spontaneous discharges are the most important, including positive deflections that occur with needle insertion and, later, fibrillation potentials. Both are regular discharges, which represent denervation supersensitivity of the muscle cell. Second, with the onset of motor recovery, there is an alteration in the shape and am-

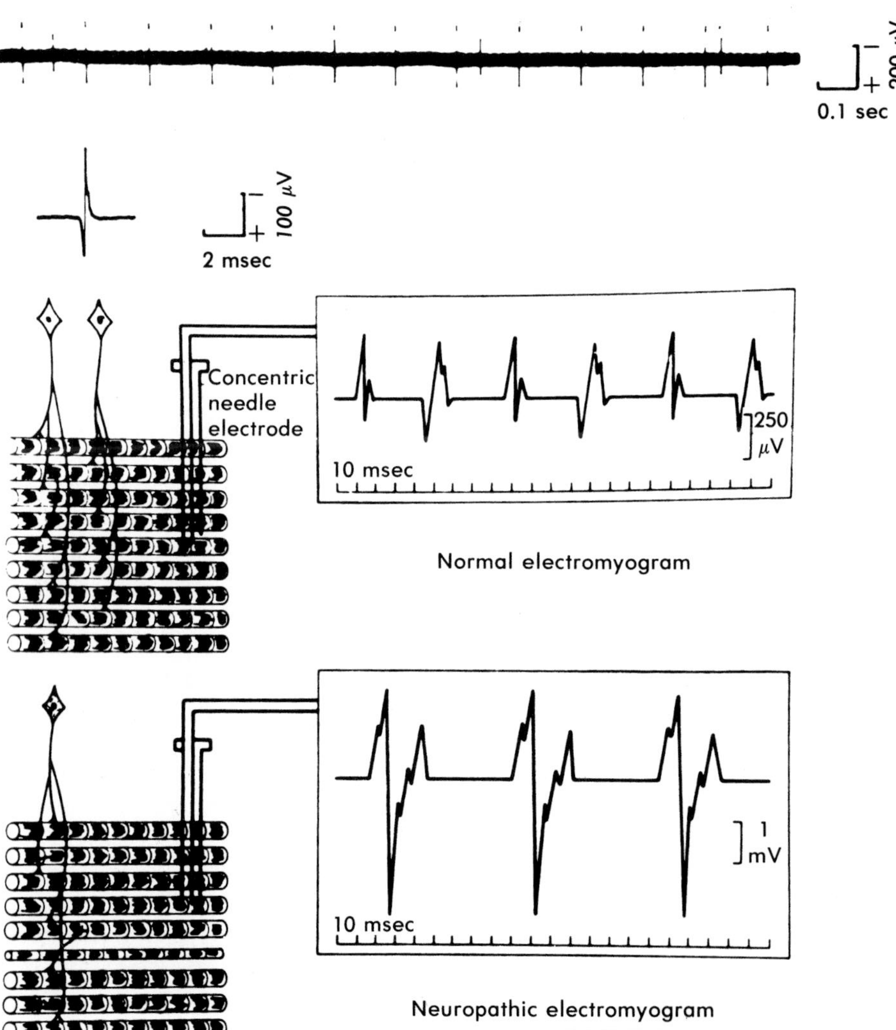

Fig. 50-6. A, Fibrillation potentials recorded at slow and fast sweep speeds. **B,** Electromyogram (EMG) responses during weak voluntary contractions: normal EMG contrasted with neuropathic EMG seen following axonal regeneration. (**A,** From Goodgold J, Eberstein A. Electrodiagnosis of Neuromuscular Diseases. Baltimore: Williams & Wilkins, 1978. **B,** From Bradley WG. Disorders of Peripheral Nerves. Oxford: Blackwell Scientific Publications, 1974.)

plitude of voluntary MUAPs. EMG is of particular value whenever there is a total loss of nerve function as a result of injuries that are unlikely to have divided the nerve. These include nerve compression resulting from a compartment syndrome, nerve traction resulting from a fracture, and nerve percussion resulting from a bullet. The most useful information is obtained when the test is carried out as early as possible after injury and again at 3 weeks. By this time, wallerian degeneration has eliminated any neurotrophic influence of axonal transport on the denervated muscle, and sufficient time has passed for muscle fibers to become supersensitive to the missing neurotransmitter by producing extrajunctional acetylcholine receptors. Fibrillations depend on these.

The EMG method of electrophysiologic testing uses a concentric needle electrode to record from muscles in the distribution of the lesioned nerve. After the needle is placed in a muscle, the patient is asked to attempt a movement using that muscle. If no MUAPs are recorded, the nerve is stimulated by inserting a needle electrode near the nerve between the muscle and the lesion site. When the lesion is a neurapraxia, nerve stimulation elicits MUAPs without difficulty—even though none can be elicited by voluntary effort and the muscle is electrically silent when the nerve is not being stimulated. By 1 week after axonotmesis or neurotmesis, MUAPs cannot be elicited by stimulation of the distal nerve; by 3 weeks the muscle exhibits fibrillations at rest and stimulation does not alter that activity. Fibrillation potentials (see Fig. 50-6, *A)* are never seen in normally innervated muscles and differ from MUAPs by having a regular firing pattern. Fibrillations occur at a frequency of 5 to 15 per second, arise from single muscle fibers, and are thought to be the result of supersensitivity of the muscle fiber membrane to acetylcholine-like molecules that enter extracellular fluid from the blood stream. The EMG is very helpful for detecting axonal reconnection at motor end plates: fibrillations disappear and are replaced by nascent MUAPs that mature into large polyphasic potentials (Fig. 50-6, *B)*. The use of NCS and EMG for differential diagnosis is summarized in Table 50-1.

Autonomic testing is important when causalgia is suspected. The general principle of testing is to compare the unaffected and affected extremities for measures of autonomic function. Different laboratories may employ different methods. When resting sweat output and axon reflex sweat output are tested, and both results are abnormal, there is a 98% chance of *reflex sympathetic dystrophy* (RSD), a syndrome that differs from causalgia by not requiring a prior nerve injury. RSD and causalgia may or may not be associated with *sympathetically maintained pain*.[38] The finding of warmer skin over the affected limb compared to its normal counterpart suggests a positive response to sympathetic block. If bilateral axon reflex abnormalities are present, the prognosis for response to a

Table 50-1. Uses of Nerve Conduction Studies and Electromyography for Differential Diagnosis

	Axonal Injury (Axonotmesis)		Demyelinating Injury (Neurapraxia)	
Time	**NCS**	**EMG**	**NCS**	**EMG**
0 days	Amplitudes drop proximal to point of injury	Reduced recruitment; no fibrillations; normal MUAPs	Amplitudes drop proximal to point of injury; slowing may be present	Reduced recruitment; no fibrillations; normal MUAPs
5 days	Distal motor amplitude reaches nadir	No change	No change	No change
7 days	Distal sensory amplitude reaches nadir	No change	No change	No change
10 days	No change	Insertional activity appears	No change	No change
21 days	No change	Insertional activity maximal with fibrillations	Amplitude and slowing begin to improve	Recruitment may improve
6 weeks	Slight motor amplitude improvement by collateral sprouting	Polyphasic MUAPs (nascent units); fibrillations decrease	Further improvement	Further improvement
3 months	Sensory amplitude may improve	Increased *duration* of MUAPs, less polyphasic	Maximal recovery	Maximal recovery
6 months	Maximal motor improvement; continued sensory amplitude improvement	Increased *amplitude* of MUAPs	No change	No change
1 year	EMG: collateral sprouts are replaced by regenerating axons ("remodeling"); MUAP amplitudes may drop, and recruitment may be normalized		No change	No change

NCS, Nerve conduction study; *EMG,* electromyography; *MUAPs,* motor unit action potentials.

sympathetic block is poor. In our laboratory, at this time, we use the combination of six tests of autonomic function: resting and axon reflex sweat output (by direct sudorometry), blood flow in both skin (by laser Doppler) and muscle (by plethysmography), limb volume (by water volume displacement), and skin temperature (by infrared probe). All but sweat output are done both before and after a quantitated exercise load to the extremity. Thus autonomic testing after nerve injury can determine whether sympathetically maintained pain is present and whether the pain is likely to respond to sympathetic block.

TREATMENT APPROACH

Principles of Nonsurgical Treatment

Initially, the potential for rehabilitation is evaluated. This must include a careful assessment of the cause for dysfunction. Otherwise, patients may be treated with a pain management program, for example, when partial paralysis is the main obstacle to progress but goes undetected. Dysfunction may arise from any one or combination of the following, and each should be considered by history, examination, and appropriate neurophysiologic tests: (1) loss of nerve function to produce hypoesthesia and weakness; (2) excess nerve function to produce pain and hypersensitivity to touch, pressure, temperature change, or movement; (3) tissue changes, such as edema, loss of hair, loss of skin turgor, or loss of joint mobility; (4) CNS abnormalities, as may occur with sympathetically maintained pain, which create a "pain cycle" and sometimes adventitial movements (spasms and dystonias); (5) psychologic factors, including adjustment abnormalities, anxiety disorders, and even major depression; and (6) issues of secondary gain, such as litigation, manipulation of family members, or lack of desire to be in the workforce. A psychologist is needed to help in assessment of the last two factors.

The presence of sympathetically maintained pain requires a multidisciplinary rehabilitation approach. The team includes a neurologist who adjusts oral medications and coordinates treatment, a surgeon who decides on the appropriateness and timing of operative intervention, an anesthesiologist who carries out nerve blocks, a psychologist who evaluates the patient's motivation and provides treatment with biofeedback and other modalities, and, most importantly, experienced physical and occupational therapists who provide exercise programs and physical treatments designed to improve function. The patient should be told from the outset that the goal is to increase function rather than reduce pain. Medications are selected according to the requirements for treating the patient's greatest source of limitation. Tricyclic antidepressants have great utility in addressing several frequent problems: loss of sleep, depressed mood, and deep or burning pain. Anticonvulsants and mexiletene are effective with lancinating pain. Baclofen, methocarbomol, and clonazepam are useful in reducing spontaneous movements and postures, including spasms and dystonias. Capsaicin ointment is helpful for the treatment of superficial burning pain. Nonsteroidal anti-inflammatory drugs help control deep aching pain. The use of narcotics is controversial. These may be safe and beneficial when used in a patient with whom the physician has a solid and long-term relationship, provided that a clear-cut contract is arrived at, giving both an exact duration of trial and the end point. The selection of a nerve block method depends primarily on what is effective. Bier blocks provide regional anesthesia to the involved limb and are least invasive. Sympathetic blocks are traditionally used in the diagnosis and treatment of sympathetically maintained pain. Longer lasting analgesia may be obtained from epidural, plexus, and axillary blocks.

Psychologic techniques include biofeedback, relaxation training, behavior modification, and psychologic investigation of the basic conflicts that may be exacerbating the pain (e.g., reliving an emotionally traumatic event that caused the injury in the first place). Other techniques that may also be useful, but remain unproved, include self-hypnosis and acupuncture. The occupational and physical therapists's roles are most crucial, and the approach depends on the exact type of limitation. All patients require a combination of limb loading and unloading, usually accomplished by the combination of stress loading and water aerobics. For allodynia, desensitization is used with gradually less abrasive materials. Limitations in range-of-motion can be addressed by a continuous passive range-of-motion machine, used during the night, and set at an ever-increasing range.

Principles of Surgical Treatment

The main goals are to preserve fascicular anatomy[1] and ensure that end organs become reinnervated within 8 months after injury.[1,30] To achieve these goals, axonotmesis must be differentiated from neurotmesis with certainty by 3 months after injury. This is not difficult if there is a skin laceration directly over the course of a nerve that has lost all function below the level of the laceration. The wound should be explored immediately; if the nerve has been transected, the nerve should be repaired. Any delay results in scar formation that necessitates trimming 1 to 2 cm off each nerve stump when the delayed neurorrhaphy is performed. However, if the soft tissues show evidence of contusion (petechial hemorrhages and discoloration) or if a bacterial infection is likely because the wound was not closed within 12 to 24 hours of injury, delayed neurorrhaphy (2 to 3 weeks) is preferable. When there is a high-velocity bullet wound and the initial debridement does not reveal a nerve lesion, any loss of nerve function must be attributed to the percussive force of the bullet. During the Vietnam war, 69% of these casualties recovered spontaneously after 3 to 9 months.[46] Nerve injuries caused by acute compression, traction, or the percussive force of a low-velocity bullet often recover spontaneously.[33] An element of neurapraxia is usually present, so that NCS is often effective at identifying these patients with a favorable prognosis. When NCS shows no conduction below the level of injury after 2 to 3 months and EMG shows only denervation, the nerve should be explored for intraoperative NAP testing.[12,24,47] Most patients who are going to recover spontaneously have EMG evidence of recovery in the most proximal denervated muscles within 3 months. This includes the disappearance of fibrillation potentials and the appearance of nascent MUAPs. These changes occur 1 to 2 months before voluntary contractions can be elicited.[2,24]

Hoffmann's sign of sensory axon regeneration may mislead the surgeon into delaying exploration for NAP testing. This crude test was described by military surgeons during World War I. It is elicited by light percussion of the distal nerve stump, beginning distally and proceeding proximally. When the leading sensory axons are percussed, the patient feels a tingling sensation in the normal cutaneous distribution of the injured nerve. There are two possible causes of false positive findings. One is that percussion of the nerve within 10 cm of the lesion may produce traction on the lesion. This stimulates regenerating sensory axons that are arrested within a neuroma-in-continuity. The other problem is that the sign is positive even if only a few axons have bridged a neurotmesis to enter the distal nerve stump.[48] The sign must be easily elicited at progressively more distal points along the nerve before it can be interpreted as presumptive evidence of sensory axon regeneration, and the rate of progression must be appropriate—at least 1.5 mm/day at points proximal to the wrist or ankle.[1,49] Following neurorrhaphy, the sign should be elicited at 10 cm below the repair within 9 to 12 weeks, assuming an initial delay of 2 weeks and a scar delay of 4 weeks[1] (Fig. 50-7).

Treatment of Neuroma-in-Continuity

From the point of view of pathology, a neuroma-in-continuity (fusiform enlargement of the nerve) involves a proliferation of connective tissue elements that may, if a fascicle has been ruptured, include thin axons that lack linear organization. Ruptured fascicles must be identified and repaired within 3 months if the patient is to have a reasonable chance for satisfactory motor recovery.[2,30,47] Ruptured fascicles are identified by intraoperative NAP testing,[47] done after a period of time that allows the neuroma to be crossed by any axons within unruptured fascicles. An appropriate interval is 2 months after injuries caused by acute compression or low-velocity missiles and 3 months after injuries caused by traction or high-velocity missiles.

It is not reasonable to carry out nerve exploration earlier than 2 months after injury unless there is reason to think that the diagnosis is neurotmesis. Even if all fascicles are intact, one cannot expect to demonstrate NAPs across the lesion site if testing is carried out before 7 to 8 weeks.[2] For high-velocity missile wounds and most traction injuries, there should be a 12-week wait because of the greater extent of traumatic degeneration in the proximal stump. However, to delay definitive diagnosis and treatment any longer only serves to increase the likelihood of a poor result should neurorrhaphy prove necessary. This is because axonal regeneration proceeds slowly, at an overall rate of 1 mm/day, and distances of over 250 mm often must be overcome before end-organ atrophy can be reversed by the arrival of regenerating axons. After 1 year, the effects of atrophy and endomysial fibrosis on striated muscle fibers reach a stage that is not compatible with good motor recovery.[1,30] When nerve lesions that are caused by a bullet or fracture are explored, a great amount of scarring is encountered in the region. In these cases the nerve is initially identified in normal tissues above or below the site of injury. These operations can be facilitated by consulting a useful guide that has been written by Henry.[50]

Treatment of Nerve Gap

When a nerve gap is discovered at surgery and the nerve stumps have been trimmed back to the point at which endoneurial tissue bulges beyond the cut edge, and microscopic examination shows no endoneurial fibrosis, the gap between stumps can be measured. When the extremity is flexed to a position of function, and the residual gap is

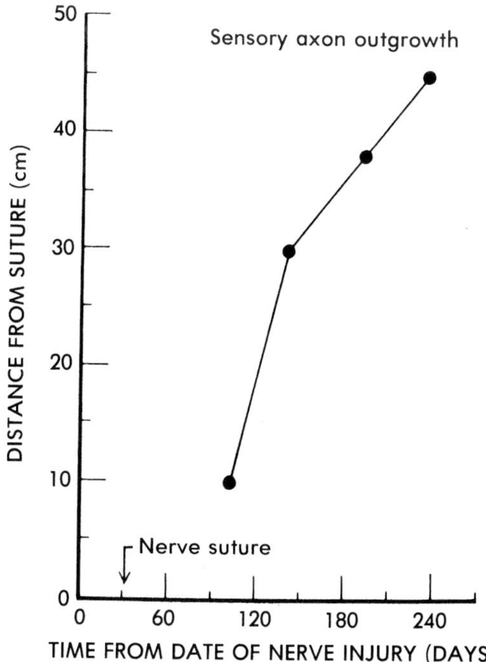

Fig. 50-7. Progress of Hoffmann's sign of sensory axon outgrowth in a patient sustaining a neurotmesis injury of the ulnar nerve at the elbow. By extrapolating the regression function to zero distance, the *latent period* can be estimated to be 7 to 8 weeks after nerve suture. With this test of nerve function there is no maturation delay; the axon terminal is continuously and exquisitely sensitive to mechanical stimuli.[30,53,54,58] Thus the latent period simply represents the sum of the initial delay and the scar delay. (From McQuarrie IG. Nerve regeneration and thyroid hormone treatment. J Neurol Sci 26:499, 1975.)

more than 3 to 5 cm, it is unreasonable to expect that a tension-free neurorrhaphy can be achieved with extensive mobilization of the nerve. In this situation it is preferable to reconnect the fascicles with several free autogenous nerve grafts of small caliber taken from a long cutaneous nerve serving a small skin area.[51,52] The sural nerve is most commonly used for this purpose. To restore fascicular anatomy most effectively, it is important to make a map of the location and size of fascicles in the proximal and distal stumps (and the position of blood vessels on the surface of the nerve) as a guide for reconnecting appropriate quadrants of the nerve and matching major fascicles.[52]

REHABILITATION AFTER NEURORRHAPHY

Principles of Rehabilitation

Current rehabilitation programs are effective in addressing most of the sensory, autonomic, and motor disturbances that result from denervation.[53] Although we recognize that most nerve lesions consist of a neuroma-in-continuity and that many of these have a neurapraxic element that does not involve denervation, we focus here on the rehabilitation of patients after neurorrhaphy. Three phases of rehabilitation can be recognized: the denervation phase that precedes end-organ reconnection, the recovery phase during which end-organ atrophy is reversed, and the adaptation phase during which the CNS makes adjustments to altered connectivity. In each of these phases, rehabilitation methods are aimed at preventing unnecessary disability. This is accomplished by using the existing motor and sensory capability and by preserving denervated structures in a state that is optimal for reinnervation.

Throughout the rehabilitation program, the outlook of the injured person is an important element in recovery. Beginning with that first moment of despair, patients see their skills destroyed, their careers ruined, and their family life jeopardized. Self-esteem and identity invariably suffer. During the slow and tedious recovery process, the personality of the patient is truly tested. Some patients devote considerable time and effort to assist in the recovery process, whereas others remain indifferent and apathetic. To some the injured part remains useless despite reinnervation; to others a permanently disabled part is seen as serving in a useful capacity. Still other patients exploit their injury for monetary and secondary gains.

The rehabilitation program must respect the importance of human interactions between the patient and the health professional (especially the occupational therapist). These play a vital role in rebuilding the patient's feelings of confidence and trust, feelings that are indispensable to the success of the rehabilitation program. However, even the most devoted professional attention can be rendered ineffectual if the patient does not receive the interest and support of friends and family. At every stage, both the patient and these key people must be advised together about the problems and expectations of the rehabilitation effort. In the end, however, success of the rehabilitation outcome largely depends on the trust, courage, and determination of the patient.[44]

Retraining in the activities of daily living is promoted throughout the rehabilitation program, regardless of the extent of motor and sensory recovery or the degree to which the patient has made a psychologic adjustment to the injury. Emphasis is placed on the patient's existing strengths, with the use of adaptive techniques and devices that encourage the patient to achieve the highest level of performance possible. The activities that are important for self-care, homemaking, recreation, school, and work are broken down into their key components, and a graded program is created to facilitate maximal independent function at each stage of recovery.

Denervation Phase

The denervation phase begins at the onset of injury and continues until there is evidence of reconnection. Emphasis is placed on keeping denervated tissues in optimal condition pending reinnervation. Absent sensation, decreased sweating and circulation, and the presence of edema are impairments that must be addressed swiftly and aggressively to minimize their negative effects. The first part of the sensory reeducation process, protective sensory reeducation, starts when wound closure has been achieved and dressings are no longer necessary. Patients must be educated to appreciate the degree and extent of their sensory deficit, learn to compensate for it, and adopt appropriate safety precautions. They must learn to rely more heavily on their vision while performing activities, and avoid applying excessive pressure to denervated skin by looking for signs of trauma—redness, edema, and warmth.[44] Skin that is dry and smooth because of the absence of sweat formation should be treated to prevent cracking. Daily warm water soaks followed by the application of oils help to retain moisture and improve circulation. Blood flow through denervated muscles can also be improved by actively contracting nonparalyzed muscles, thereby exerting a pull on paralyzed muscles through the interconnecting fascial sheaths. Retrograde massage, avoidance of extremes of temperature, and passive range-of-motion exercises are also helpful in this regard.

Scar massage and gentle soft tissue mobilization techniques are used to minimize scar hypertrophy and to prevent adherence of the skin to underlying tissues. Ultimately, this serves to minimize loss of motion as a result of restricted soft tissue mobility and assists in managing hyperesthesias, which may develop as sensation returns. Passive range-of-motion exercises and active use of uninvolved muscles are essential for improving circulation and maintaining musculotendinous excursion, preventing stiffness and adhesion formation, and decreasing edema.[44] This program can minimize the trophic changes that otherwise occur in denervated skin by improving blood flow and reducing the frequency and severity of minor trauma.

Denervated muscles must be maintained with dynamic activity to slow the process of myofibrillar atrophy and endomysial fibrosis. Immobilization (beyond that which is needed to prevent tension on the neurorrhaphy) must be avoided because it promotes tissue edema, reduces blood flow, and encourages the development of muscle contractures. Nonetheless, splinting may be indicated for several purposes to (1) prevent the overstretching of paralyzed muscles, (2) support joints, (3) balance forces on joints and tendons, and (4) facilitate the active contraction of uninvolved muscles in a manner that substitutes for paralyzed muscles. The type and design of these splints must be individualized to the patient's needs, and relief from the splint must be provided several times daily to combat the adverse effects of immobilization once the repair has undergone adequate healing.

The application of heat in the form of warm water or oil increases circulation without harming sensitive, denervated tissues. Joint stiffness and ankylosis can occur as a result of decreased muscular support, edema, contractures, and the unopposed action of normally innervated muscles. Joint mobility and the ranges of tendon excursion can be preserved by daily passive exercises. Edema, which is caused largely by the inactivity of muscle masses, is combated by elevation, active contraction of uninvolved muscles, massage, use of the Jobst intermittent pressure pump, and the application of compression wraps.

The use of electric stimulation to prevent denervation atrophy of affected muscles remains controversial because there are no controlled studies in human subjects.[53] Although muscle stimulation cannot prevent denervation atrophy, there is considerable experimental evidence suggesting that its use reduces the rate and degree of atrophy and that the electric properties of the stimulated muscle more closely resemble those of normal muscle.[54] However, there is no benefit in terms of final twitch tension or tetanic tension after reinnervation. To reduce the degree of atrophy, treatment must begin soon after injury. The stimulus strength must be sufficient to cause long contractions without pain or discomfort; 15 to 20 contractions per session, with low-frequency stimulation in the range of 10 to 12 Hz, are applied three to four times a day. Treatment is abandoned in favor of active contraction after reinnervation has been documented.[1]

Recovery Phase

The recovery phase begins with axonal reconnection at an appropriate end organ. During this phase the therapist plays an important role, monitoring the progress of nerve regeneration through the use of manual muscle testing, sensibility testing, and clinical observation. At each visit the therapist carefully observes the posture of the involved limb, looking for subtle changes that may indicate the early return of motor function. In addition, specific tests of innervation density and sensory threshold are performed. These test responses to pinprick, temperature, vibration, moving touch/pressure, and static touch/pressure. The Semmes-Weinstein Monofilament Test (North Coast Medical), a standardized threshold test, provides the therapist with an accurate measure of sensibility to graded point pressures throughout the reinnervation period: from unresponsiveness to the return of deep pressure sensation, to the return of protective sensation, to the return of light touch sensation, to the return of normal sensation.[55] Test results are recorded in a color-coded diagram of the limb, providing a clear, simple visual representation of the reinnervation process, which can be forwarded to the surgeon. Early signs of sensory recovery include feelings that "something is happening," tenderness to pressure exerted on muscles, and an advancing Hoffmann's sign.[53] The reinnervation of sensory receptors results in altered sensation. Normal tactile stimuli may be perceived as noxious, leading patients to complain of pain, paresthesias, or hyperesthesias. A desensitization program can be quite effective in reducing these symptoms. Patients are taught to expose the sensitive skin to graded textures (e.g., cotton progressing to sandpaper), vibratory stimuli (of increasing frequencies), and solid particles.[44] Treatment begins with exposure to the least aversive stimuli, and the patient is taught to increase the intensity and duration of stimulation each day. This progression continues until normal stimulation is tolerated. The Three-Phase Desensitization Test (originally, the Downey Community Hospital hand sensitivity test) is a readily available (North Coast Medical), standardized test for hypersensitivity that provides a systematic, reliable method for performing and documenting a desensitization protocol with the items described above.[55] Other methods of providing sensory input that have been shown to decrease hyperesthesias include massage, application of heat, and percussion or tapping of the sensitive area.[55,56]

The principles of pain treatment following nerve injury include measures directed at the pain itself, and use of the involved part. The latter is of value because pain is largely a result of the combined effects of vasomotor dysfunction, scar tissue near the proximal nerve stump, and traction on this scar from movement of the limb. To address the pain directly, transcutaneous electric nerve stimulation (TENS) provides relief in almost half the patients. TENS uses an electric device to emit a pulsed current to skin electrodes in a biphasic asymmetric wave. TENS is so effective in treating pain from peripheral nerve injuries that mild transcutaneous stimulation using surface electrodes may be sufficient even for the treatment of sympathetically maintained pain.[57,58] Different forms of stimulation are achieved by adjusting the amplitude, frequency, and duration of the pulse. Constant stimulation of the large-diameter afferent fibers reduces the perception of pain, which depends on slowly conducting nonmyelinated fibers. TENS is not a cure for pain but rather an adjunct to specific treatment of the nerve injury. Its purpose is to decrease pain to a degree that allows patients to participate in the rehabilitation program and perform functional activities.

The pattern of sensory recovery begins with a return of pain and temperature appreciation. This is followed by awareness of vibration at 30 Hz, moving touch stimuli, and then vibration at 256 Hz. The last modalities to recover are the localization of tactile stimuli and two-point discrimination.[59] Modality tests include pinprick, temperature discrimination, vibration, moving touch/pressure and constant touch/pressure. The return of function is assessed from tests of moving and static two-point discrimination, the response to a ridge-shaped sensitometer, and tactile gnosis (the ability to feel the shape, weight, and texture of objects well enough to identify these).[44] The Moberg pickup test is particularly useful because the ability to pick up a series of 10 to 12 small objects of various sizes and then place them into a small container is readily timed and compared to results for the normal hand.[44] Qualitative differences in prehension patterns may also become apparent during testing. An effort must be made to standardize the conditions for these tests at follow-up examination, since there are many uncontrollable factors affecting the transmission of sensory impulses from the periphery to the CNS.

Muscle atrophy is reversed by reinnervation of the motor end plate, provided that endomysial fibrosis is not advanced. Rehabilitative efforts are aimed at maximizing voluntary motion, motor control, and strength. The therapist must be familiar with the expected order of reinnervation following repair of the particular nerve lesion being treated, information that is readily obtained from standard texts.[1] Treatment methods during the recovery phase include muscle reeducation, biofeedback, resistive exercises (initially resisting gravity alone), proprioceptive facilitation techniques (to maximize the stimulation of muscle afferents), and the use of patterns of movement that recruit the maximal number of muscle fibers.[45]

Adaptive Phase

Once end-organ function has been restored, central changes occur that reflect adaptation to a new pattern of connectivity. An important part of this phase, which can be influenced by the rehabilitation program, is the reeducation of integrative mechanisms in the CNS. This facilitates new patterns for acquiring sensory information and distributing commands to muscle groups. Sensory recovery may slowly progress for more than 3 years before it is complete. Improvement occurs both through maturation of reunited axon-receptor systems and the subliminal reeducation of integrative mechanisms. Since the CNS acquires sensory information differently after neurorrhaphy (because end-organ reinnervation is a random event), the sensations that occur early in the recovery phase may be somewhat foreign to those normally perceived in a particular part of the CNS.[5,60]

Sensory reeducation involves a graded series of specific sensory exercises that are instituted at appropriate times in the recovery process. An attempt is made to facilitate central reorganization so that patients can interpret the altered profile of neural impulses reaching consciousness. In the early stages of recovery, patients are reeducated to modality-specific perceptions (e.g., moving vs. constant touch). In the later stages of reinnervation, patients are progressed to the second phase of sensory reeducation: discriminative sensation. Readiness for progression to this phase is determined by the patient's results on the Semmes-Weinstein monofilament test. The patient must be able to perceive filament number 4.31 (2.35 g) before discriminative training proves useful.[61] At that time, various structured activities are performed with the ultimate goal of the return of tactile gnosis (name recognition of objects in the hand; two-point discrimination). Various stimuli are applied to the patient's hand with the patient's vision occluded. The patient attempts to identify the stimulus and, if unsuccessful, the stimulus is applied while the patient watches. The patient continues this training method, alternating occluding the vision and then using direct visualization in an effort to reorganize and integrate the cortical processing of sensory information from the altered periphery. The patient is challenged with the task of first identifying specific characteristics of the object (e.g., metallic vs. wooden, round vs. square). Ultimately, the patient attempts to name the object itself (e.g., key, coin, paperclip). Graphesthesia activities and puzzles or mazes that are performed with vision occluded are higher level tasks that also facilitate the return of discriminative sensation.[61] This program is continued until the patient assumes responsibility for self-education and returns to work, avocations, and self-care. With sensory reeducation, maximal recovery may occur within 2 years,[59] shortening the adaptive phase by a year or more.

Surgical procedures for the relief of pain caused by peripheral nerve injuries include the excision of any neuromas and sympathectomy. However, the former is rarely effective[62] and the latter has largely been replaced by TENS, ganglion blocks, and phenoxybenzamine.[58,63] Muscle mass is regained through repeated exercises and use of the injured part in activities of daily living.

Permanent Denervation

Specific adaptive techniques, support personnel, or appliances may be required when functional impairment is substantial and permanent.[56] Sufficient time should be allowed to elapse before evaluating the extent and significance of recovery. Although reconstructive procedures may be effective if performed in a timely manner, the patient will realize that the hoped-for recovery cannot occur. These procedures include arthrodesis, tendon transfers, tendon translocation, tenodesis, nerve transfers,[64] microsurgical free muscle transplants, muscle transfers using an intact neurovascular island pedicle, and amputation with prosthetic fitting. These procedures require specific rehabilitation methods and goals.

SUMMARY

Peripheral nerve injuries are rarely followed by a full recovery of function and often leave patients with a significant disability. Most nerve injuries involve an upper extremity and therefore threaten hand function. To minimize the extent and incidence of permanent disability, it is important to preserve as much of the microanatomy of the injured nerve as possible. This may mean "leaving well enough alone." To know when to intervene surgically and, more importantly, when not to intervene requires an in-depth understanding of the anatomy and physiology of normal nerves. Diagnostic tools such as NCS and EMG are critical in sorting out the nature of the injury. To maintain what has been obtained by successful initial management requires the use of active rehabilitation measures that take account of any residual limb pain. Therapy must begin soon after injury, continue during the phases of recovery, and maximize the patient's independence in the performance of daily activities.

REFERENCES

1. Sunderland S. Nerves and Nerve Injuries. Edinburgh: Churchill Livingstone, 1978.
2. Kline DG, Hackett ER. Reappraisal of timing for exploration of civilian peripheral nerve injuries. Surgery 78:545, 1975.
3. Brushart TM, Mesulam M-M. Alteration in connections between muscle and anterior horn motoneurons after peripheral nerve repair. Science 208:603, 1980.
4. Lisney SJW. Changes in the somatotopic organization of the cat lumbar spinal cord following peripheral nerve transection and regeneration. Brain Res 259:31, 1983.
5. Wall JT, Felleman DJ, Kaas JH. Recovery of normal topography in the somatosensory cortex of monkeys after nerve crush and regeneration. Science 221:771, 1983.
6. Bell MA, Weddell AGM. A descriptive study of the blood vessels of the sciatic nerve in the rat, man, and other mammals. Brain 107:871, 1985.
7. Hudson A, Kline D. Progression of partial experimental injury to peripheral nerve. II. Light and electron microscopic studies. J Neurosurg 42:15, 1975.
8. Smith DR, Kobrine AI, Rizzoli HV. Blood flow in peripheral nerves: Normal and post severance rates. J Neurol Sci 33:341, 1977.
9. Donat JR, Wisniewski HM. The spatio-temporal pattern of wallerian degeneration in mammalian peripheral nerves. Brain Res 53:41, 1973.
10. Grafstein B, McQuarrie IG. Role of the nerve cell body in axonal regeneration. In Cotman CW, ed. Neuronal Plasticity. New York: Raven Press, 1978.
11. McQuarrie IG. Role of the axonal cytoskeleton in the regenerating nervous system. In Seil FJ, ed. Nerve, Organ, and Tissue Regeneration: Research Perspectives. New York: Academic Press, 1983.
12. Grafstein B, Forman DS. Intracellular transport in neurons. Physiol Rev 60:1167, 1980.
13. McQuarrie IG. Effect of a conditioning lesion on axonal transport during regeneration: The role of slow transport. In Elam J, Cancalon P, eds. Advances in Neurochemistry, vol 6. New York: Plenum Press, 1984.
14. Benowitz LI, Yoon MG, Lewis ER. Transported proteins in the regenerating optic nerve: Regulation by interactions with the optic tectum. Science 222:185, 1983.
15. Skene HHP, Willard M. Axonally transported proteins associated with axon growth in rabbit central and peripheral nervous systems. J Cell Biol 89:96, 1981.
16. Bray GM, Rasminsky M, Aguayo AJ. Interactions between axons and their sheath cells. Annu Rev Neurosci 4:127, 1981.
17. McQuarrie IG. Accelerated axonal sprouting after nerve transection. Brain Res 167:185, 1979.
18. McQuarrie IG. Effect of a conditioning lesion on axonal sprout formation at nodes of Ranvier. J Comp Neurol 231:239, 1985.
19. Singer PA, Mehler S, Fernandez HL. Blockade of retrograde axonal transport delays the onset of metabolic and morphologic changes induced by axotomy. J Neurosci 2:1299, 1982.
20. Wujek JR, Lasek RJ. Correlation of axonal regeneration and slow component *B* in two branches of a single axon. J Neurosci 3:243, 1983.
21. Weller RO, Cervos-Navarro J. Pathology of Peripheral Nerves. London-Boston: Butterworth Publishers, 1977.
22. Forman DS, Wood DK, DeSilva S. Rate of regeneration of sensory axons in transected rat sciatic nerve repaired with epineurial sutures. J Neurol Sci 44:55, 1979.
23. Kline DG, Hayes GJ, Morse AS. A comparative study of response to species to peripheral nerve injury. J Neurosurg 21:980, 1964.
24. Kline DG, Hackett ER, May PR. Evaluation of nerve injuries by evoked potentials and electromyography. J Neurosurg 31:128, 1969.
25. Sanders FK, Young JZ. The influence of peripheral connexion on the diameter of regenerating nerve fibers. J Exp Biol 22:203, 1946.
26. Friede RL. Control of myelin formation by axon caliber (with a model of the control mechanism). J Comp Neurol 144:233, 1972.
27. Politis MJ, et al. Studies on the control of myelinogenesis. IV. Neuronal induction of Schwann cell myelin-specific protein synthesis during nerve fiber regeneration. J Neurosci 2:1252, 1982.
28. Gordon T, Stein RB. Reorganization of motor-unit properties in reinnervated muscles of the cat. J Neurophysiol 48:1175, 1982.
29. Bowden REM, Sholl DA. The advance of functional recovery after radial nerve lesions in man. Brain 73:17, 1950.
30. Richter H-P. Impairment of motor recovery after late nerve suture: Experimental study in the rabbit. I. Functional and electromyographic findings. Neurosurgery 10:70, 1982.
31. Gilliatt RW. Physical injury to peripheral nerves. Physiologic and electrodiagnostic aspects. Mayo Clin Proc 56:361, 1981.
32. Dyck PJ, et al. Structural alterations of nerve during cuff compression. Proc Natl Acad Sci USA 87:9828, 1990.
33. Pollock FH, et al. Treatment of radial neuropathy associated with fractures of the humerus. J Bone Joint Surg 63A:239, 1981.
34. Lundborg G, Myers R, Powell H. Nerve compression injury and increased endoneurial fluid pressure: A "miniature compartment syndrome." J Neurol Neursurg Psychiatry 46:1119, 1983.
35. Richardson PM, Thomas PK. Percussive injury to peripheral nerve in rats. J Neurosurg 51:178, 1979.
36. Wall PD. The painful consequences of peripheral injury. J Hand Surg 9B:37, 1984.
37. Treede R-D, et al. Peripheral and central mechanisms of cutaneous hyperalgiesia. Prog Neurobio 38:397, 1992.
38. Verdugo RJ, Ochoa JL. Sympathetically maintained pain. Neurology 44:1003, 1994.
39. Rothberg JM, Tahmoush AJ, Oldakowski R. The epidemiology of causalgia among soldiers wounded in Vietnam. Milit Med 148:347, 1983.
40. Merskey H. Classification of chronic pain. Pain (Suppl 3):1, 1986.
41. Devor M, Janig W. Activation of myelinated afferents ending in a neuroma by stimulation of the sympathetic supply in the rat. Neurosci Lett 24:43, 1981.
42. Roberts WJ. A hypothesis on the physiological basis for causalgia and related pains. Pain 24:297, 1986.
43. Shir Y, Seltzer Z. Effects of sympathectomy in a model of causalgiform pain produced by partial sciatic nerve injury in rats. Pain 45:309, 1991.
44. Hunter JM, et al. Rehabilitation of the Hand: Surgery and Therapy, 3rd ed. St. Louis: Mosby, 1990.
45. Nickel VL. Orthopedic Rehabilitation. Edinburgh: Churchill Livingstone, 1982.
46. Omer GE. Injuries of nerves of the upper extremity. J Bone Joint Surg 56A:1615, 1974.
47. Terzis JK, Dykes RW, Hakstian RW. Electrophysiological recordings in peripheral nerve surgery: A review. J Hand Surg 1:52, 1976.
48. Napier JR. The significance of Tinel's sign in peripheral nerve injuries. Brain 72:63, 1949.
49. McQuarrie IG. Nerve regeneration and thyroid hormone treatment. J Neurol Sci 26:499, 1975.

50. Henry AK. Extensile Exposure, 2nd ed. Edinburgh: Churchill Livingstone, 1973.
51. Haase J, Bjerre P, Simensen K. Median and ulnar nerve transections treated with microsurgical interfascicular cable grafting with autogenous sural nerve. J Neurosurg 53:73, 1980.
52. Millesi H. Interfascicular grafts for repair of peripheral nerves of the upper extremity. Orthop Clin North Am 8:387, 1977.
53. Wynn Parry CB. Rehabilitation of the Hand, 3rd ed. London: Butterworth Publishers, 1978.
54. Nix WA. The effect of low-frequency electrical stimulation on the denervated extensor digitorum longus muscle of the rabbit. Acta Neurol Scand 66:521, 1982.
55. Waylett-Rendall J. Desensitization of the traumatized hand. In Hunter JM, Mackin EJ, Callahan AD, eds. Rehabilitation of the Hand: Surgery and Therapy, 4th ed. St. Louis: Mosby, 1995, p 693.
56. Trombly CA, Scott AD. Occupational Therapy for Physical Dysfunction. Baltimore: Williams & Wilkins, 1977.
57. Campbell JN, Long DM. Peripheral nerve stimulation in the treatment of intractable pain. J Neurosurg 45:692, 1976.
58. Meyer GA, Fields HL. Causalgia treated by selective large fibre stimulation of peripheral nerve. Brain 95:163, 1972.
59. Dellon AL. Evaluation of Sensibility and Reeducation of Sensation in the Hand. Baltimore: Williams & Wilkins, 1981.
60. Hallin RG, Wiesenfeld Z, Lindblom U. Neurophysiological studies on patients with sutured median nerves: Faulty sensory localization after nerve regeneration and its physiological correlates. Exp Neurol 73:90, 1981.
61. Callahan AD. Methods of compensation and reeducation for sensory dysfunction. In Hunter JM, Mackin EJ, Callahan AD, eds. Rehabilitation of the Hand: Surgery and Therapy, 4th ed. St. Louis: Mosby, 1995, p 701.
62. Noordenbos W, Wall PD. Implications of the failure of nerve resection and graft to cure chronic pain produced by nerve lesions. J Neurol Neurosurg Psychiatry 44:1068, 1981.
63. Ghostine SY, et al. Phenoxybenzamine in the treatment of causalgia: Report of 40 cases. J Neurosurg 60:1263, 1984.
64. Chacha PB, Krishnamurti A, Soin K. Experimental sensory reinnervation of the median nerve by nerve transfer in monkeys. J Bone Joint Surg 59A:386, 1977.

PART SIX

THE PERIPHERAL VASCULAR SYSTEM

51

Physiology of Arterial, Venous, and Lymphatic Flow

Dennis F. Bandyk and Ashish K. Gupta

Clinical evaluation of patients with vascular disease requires a thorough understanding of the anatomy and hemodynamics of the arterial, venous, and lymphatic circulations. The development of noninvasive ultrasound techniques that reliably image and record vascular system hemodynamics has resulted in an improved understanding of the pathophysiology of arterial and venous disease, more accurate vascular diagnostics, and estimation of the physiologic significance of anatomic disease. The ability to monitor the hemodynamics of arterial and venous flow and vessel anatomy serially has permitted detection of disease progression, resulting in effective and timely intervention. In this chapter the functional anatomy and hemodynamics of the arterial, venous, and lymphatic components of the circulatory system are discussed. Special emphasis is placed on how the biophysical properties of the circulation (e.g., pressure, flow velocity, turbulence) can be measured in humans and how such measurements are used in the evaluation of patients with vascular disease. The discussion focuses primarily on the principles of arterial, venous, and lymphatic flow in the lower extremity, but the concepts are equally germane and applicable to the upper extremity and cerebrovascular circulation.

PERIPHERAL ARTERIAL SYSTEM

The purpose of the arterial system is the delivery of blood and its various components to tissue capillaries in amounts sufficient to maintain normal cellular function. Metabolic demands of body tissues and organs vary widely, both in normal (resting), exercising, and diseased states. The ability of the arterial circulation to respond to a variable demand is reflected in the anatomic and physical properties of the cardiovascular system and is mediated through two regulatory mechanisms: local control of blood flow through the tissue according to its metabolic state (autoregulation) and neural control of peripheral vascular resistance. These factors, acting in concert, control tissue blood flow and consequently regulate the output of the heart. Control of blood flow is also strongly influenced by other factors, such as those involved in the regulation of extracellular fluid volume and urinary output.

The functional elements of the arterial system include the *heart,* which generates the energy necessary to maintain arterial pressure and blood flow at an appropriate level; *arteries,* which transport blood to the periphery; *arterioles,* which regulate flow of blood into the microcirculation; and *capillaries,* which are the site of nutrient and metabolic exchange to the tissues. Depending on their position in the arterial system, arteries can act as "storers" of pressure energy produced in the heart, by cushioning vessels that convert the pulsatile flow of the blood into smooth flow, and acting as resistance vessels involved in the microcirculation. Arterial wall structure and neural innervation accordingly reflect the specialized function(s) of the various arterial system elements.

As blood proceeds through the arterial system, the network of conducting vessels undergoes repeated branching, accompanied by a decrease in caliber, resulting in many parallel distributing vessels, which terminate in the capillary bed. In the arterial system of the lower extremity, branching produces potential collateral networks that can bypass blood around a hemodynamically significant (i.e., pressure-reducing) obstruction in a conduit artery (Fig. 51-1). The total cross-sectional area progressively increases each time branching occurs, with a concomitant decrease in mean flow velocity (Table 51-1). At the capillary level the cross-sectional area is approximately 1000 times that of the aorta. Each red blood cell remains in the microcirculation only 1 to 3 seconds, an exceedingly short time during which all nutrient diffusion and fluid exchange must occur.

Approximately 20% of the entire blood volume of the body is in the arterial system in contrast to the 64% in the venous system. The heart contains 7% of the blood, and the pulmonary vessels contain 9%. Surprisingly, only 5% of the total blood volume resides in the capillaries. Al-

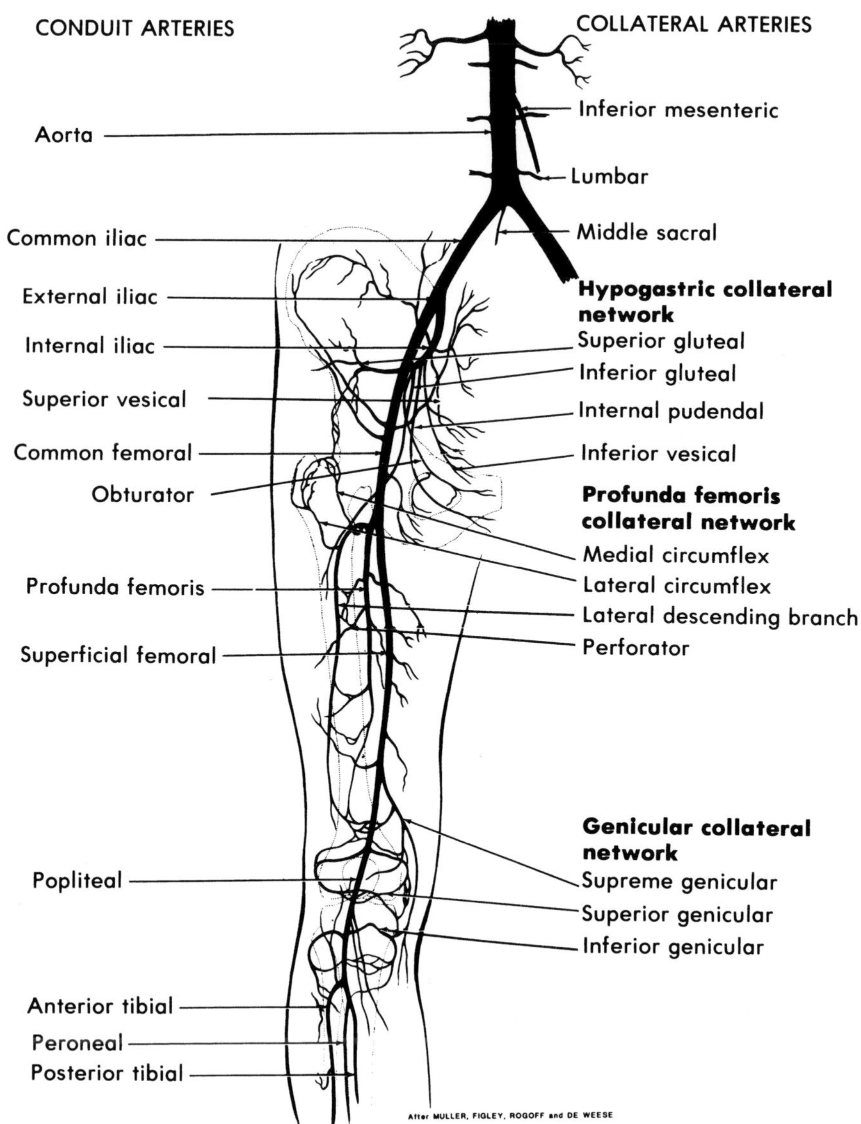

Fig. 51-1. Diagram of the arterial circulation to the lower extremity, indicating the main conduit arteries and corresponding potential collateral arteries.

Table 51-1. Physical and Hemodynamic Characteristics of the Arterial System in Humans

	Total Blood Volume (%)	Cross-sectional Area (cm^2)	Mean Flow Velocity (cm/sec)	Pressure (mm Hg)	Resistance (%)
Aorta	8	2.5	14-18	100	4
Branching arteries	5	20	12	90	21
Arterioles	2	40		55	41
Capillaries	5	2500	0.07	25	27

though total capillary volume is small, surface and cross-sectional areas are immense to facilitate the transfer of oxygen, carbon dioxide, water, nutrients, and electrolytes through the capillary walls. In the resting state the lower extremity receives about 300 to 400 ml/min, two to three times that of the upper extremity primarily because of differences in muscle mass.

The heart, through cyclic muscle wall contraction, generates a complex pressure pulse and provides the energy for blood flow. The ability of the heart to vary its output is based on its three fundamental properties: the capacity to vary the rate of contraction (chronotropism); the rate of isometric tension development, which is a function of cardiac muscle fiber length (Frank-Starling mechanism); and the ability to alter the velocity of muscle fiber shortening (inotropism). From these properties four factors that are independent determinants of cardiac output can be defined. These are commonly referred to as ventricular preload, ventricular contractility ventricular afterload, and heart rate. The output of the heart mainly reflects the demands of the peripheral circulation. The frequency of contraction is determined by the interplay of neural and humoral adrenergic and neural cholingeric activity on the sinoatrial node. The velocity and force of ventricular muscular contraction are influenced by both circulating and neuron-released catecholamines acting on the muscle fibers themselves. The work output of the heart is the amount of energy that the heart transfers to the blood. This energy, which is in the forms of potential energy of pressure and the kinetic energy of blood flow, is used to accelerate blood to its ejection velocity through the aortic valve. In the distribution of blood to the various capillary beds, the viscoelastic properties of the artery walls and the tapered, converging vessel caliber are important physical characteristics maintaining blood pressure and minimizing pressure and kinetic fluid energy losses.

Arterial Wall: Structural Features

The composition and structure of the arterial wall in the different segments of the arterial system reflect the local wall mechanics and its functional role. With the exception of the capillaries, the artery wall consists of three concentric layers: tunica intima, tunica media, and tunica adventitia. The tunica intima is the innermost layer and consists of monolayer endothelium lining the lumen, a thin basal lamina, and a subendothelial layer (present in the large elastic arteries of the thorax and abdomen) composed of collagenous bundles, elastic fibrils, and smooth cell muscles. The tunica media is in the middle layer and is made up of predominantly smooth muscle cells in a varied number of elastic sheets (laminae), bundles of collagenous fibrils, and a network of elastic fibrils. The tunica adventitia consists of dense fibroelastic tissue without smooth muscle cells. The adventitia also contains the nutrient vessels of the arterial wall (vasa vasorum) and both vasomotor and sensory nerves for the vascular wall itself.

Arteries can be classified by the respective amounts of elastin, smooth muscle, and collagen in their walls. The distensibility of an artery generally correlates with the elastin content in the vessel wall. The large arteries of the thorax and abdomen, such as the aorta and innominate, iliac, subclavian, and common iliac arteries are referred to as elastic or "pressure storer" arteries, since their walls contain a predominance of elastin and few smooth muscle cells. The large elastic arteries instantaneously accommodate each stroke volume of the heart, storing a portion during systole and draining this volume during diastole (*windkessel* effect). This helps to propel the blood toward the periphery during diastole and promotes continuous flow to the capillaries. The internal systolic pressure in the large arteries is normally about 120 to 160 mm Hg.

Proceeding distally from the conducting arteries, the muscular or branching arteries such as brachial, radial, femoral, and popliteal have a media with a predominance of smooth muscle and collagen but little elastic tissue. The varying viscoelastic wall properties distant from the heart are related to the proportions of collagen and elastin in the media, the linkage between these two elements, the insertions of elastin and muscle on collagen fibers, and the contractile state of the vascular smooth muscle. Proceeding from the thoracic aorta distally there is a gradual decline in the elastin-collagen ratio. This results in a low vascular impedance of the initial segment of the arterial tree, thereby reducing the oscillatory component of work required distally to maintain cardiac output. The increased relative stiffness of the distal muscular arteries is important to ensure that undampened transmission of the pressure pulse to baroreceptors occurs, for example, at the carotid bifurcation. At the level of the arterioles the arterial wall is composed almost entirely of smooth muscle. These vessels provide the major site of resistance to the arterial system and provide for the regulation of blood flow to the microcirculation (see Table 51-1). Mean pressure in the arterioles ranges from 40 to 60 mm Hg. The smooth muscle of the media is well innervated by sympathetic nerves. At the cutaneous level these nerve fibers are involved with temperature regulation, vasoconstricting in cool weather to conserve heat and vasodilating during warmth to dissipate heat. An exception occurs in the septic state, emotional stress, or profound shock, where vasodilation predominates secondary to sympathetic innervation. Additionally, metabolites at a local level also cause vasodilation, as does exercise. This autoregulation disappears at pressures below 30 mm, where flow occurs secondary to perfusion pressure alone.

The collagen content of the arterial wall is correlated with its tensile strength, with the adventitia collagen accounting for the majority of wall stability. This is evident from the maintenance of vessel integrity by the adventitia following surgical endarterectomy, which removes the intima and a large portion of the media. In naturally occurring aneurysms the collagen content of the adventitia is decreased, and failure of wall integrity occurs. Only degradation of collagen results in arterial wall rupture. The circumferential tension (T) in the arterial wall is calculated as the product of the transmural pressure, P_t (inside pressure minus outside pressure), and the radius (R). This relationship, known as the law of Laplace, can be expanded to include the factor of wall thickness (μm):

$$T = P_t R/\mu m \text{ (dynes/cm)}$$

In arteries with a radius and wall thickness of equal proportions, wall tension varies with transmural pressure. For example, the small radius and low pressure of a capillary requires only a thin wall to support the wall tension, whereas the aorta with its greater pressure and radius requires a thicker wall to prevent rupture.

The elastic properties of any blood vessel can be described by Young's modulus (E), which is stress divided by strain. Because arteries are subject to pulsatile pressure, measurements of elasticity are determined from the strain that accompanies a period of time in which stress is varied, producing what is called a dynamic modulus (Edyn). The most important component of stress in arteries is the first harmonic of the pressure pulse (i.e., heart rate). The dynamic elastic modulus of an artery is also a determinant of pulse wave velocity. In vivo arterial wall motion occurs predominantly in the circumferential direction. The variation of vessel diameter with each cardiac cycle closely resembles the pressure waveform. Intrathoracic arteries vary 12% to 18% in diameter with each pressure pulse, whereas peripheral arteries change 8% to 10% in diameter. The distensibility characteristic of arteries also depends on the extent of stretch (transmural pressure). At low pressure and small diameters, arteries are very distensible, whereas they become gradually stiffer with increasing pressure and diameter.

The viscoelastic properties of arteries are altered not only in diseased states but also change with age. With age, artery diameter and length increases, and the wall thickness and collagen-to-elastin ratios increase. These changes result in tortousity, increased arterial stiffness, and an increase in vascular impedance. Although an increase in the thickness of the intima, which initially occurs in atherosclerosis, has little effect on the elastic properties of the artery, the accompanying changes within the media and adventitia, particularly if the wall nutrition through the vaso vasorum is involved, may have marked effects on hemodynamic characteristics and further disease progression.

Essentials of Arterial Hemodynamics

Hemodynamics is a discipline concerned with the interrelationships of the physical characteristics of blood and pulsatile flow conditions in the viscoelastic arterial and venous circulations. As a first step toward understanding the complexity of arterial flow, it is useful to discuss the viscous properties of blood itself and the interrelationships between pressure, flow, and resistance under steady flow conditions.

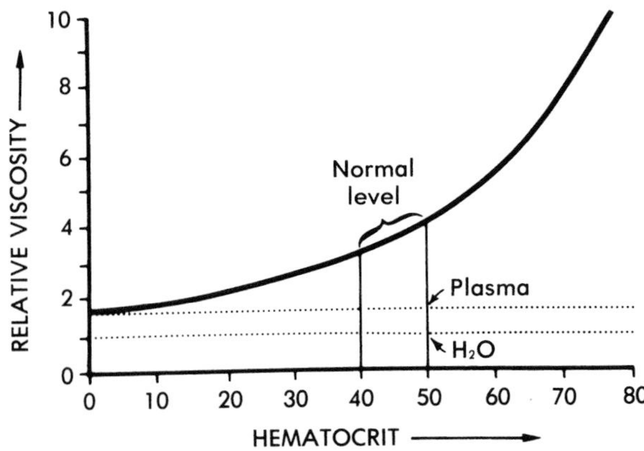

Fig. 51-2. Effect of hematocrit on relative velocity of blood. Note that as hematocrit increases, the relative viscosity increases disproportionately. (From Smith JJ, Kampine JP. Circulatory Physiology, 2nd ed. Baltimore: Williams & Wilkins, 1984.)

Viscous Properties of Blood Flow

Blood is a viscous fluid composed of cells and plasma. When blood flows, frictional forces develop primarily between the cellular components of blood, causing it to exhibit the property of viscosity. Since the red blood cells comprise the majority of the cellular component, the hematocrit is a major determinant of blood viscosity, as illustrated in Fig. 51-2. If measured with reference to water, the relative viscosity of blood at a hematocrit of 40 is approximately 3.6. This means that three to four times as much pressure is required to force blood than water through the same tube. Blood viscosity is not constant in the arterial system but exhibits a non-Newtonian fluid property: the faster it flows, the lower is its viscosity. The chief determinants of this property are the red blood cell concentrations and plasma concentration of fibrinogen and globulins. The viscosity of blood decreases in small caliber tubes (less than 200 μm), which include arterioles, capillaries, and venules. This phenomenon is known as the Fahraeus-Lindqvist effect and is related to red blood cell orientation and lower hematocrit in small vessels. The rheology of blood in the capillary circulation is poorly understood, although the deformability of the red blood cell membrane and erythrocyte velocity are important factors.

The viscosity of blood is important not only from its effect on the resistance to blood flow but in producing impairment of tissue perfusion in pathologic states such as severe polycythemia, gross elevations of plasma concentrations of fibrinogen or globulins, and other hyperviscosity syndromes that occur following severe tissue trauma (e.g., thermal burns). These low-flow states promote erythrocytes to aggregate into stocks or "rouleaux" with resultant tissue ischemia.

Resistance to Flow

The relations between flow and pressure in cylindric tubes were first accurately described by the French physician,

Poiseuille, in 1846. Under the conditions of his experiments, the volume flow (Q) through a vessel is determined by:

$$Q = \frac{P\pi r^4}{8\,l\mu}\ \text{ml/min}$$

where P is perfusion pressure, or the pressure gradient between the ends of the vessel; r is the vessel radius; l is the vessel length; and μ is viscosity of the fluid. Poiseuille's law describes the viscous energy losses that occur in a steady flow, idealized fluid model. The theoretic derivation rests in the assumptions that each particle of fluid moves at a constant velocity parallel to the vessel wall, that the force opposing this motion is proportional to fluid viscosity, and that the velocity gradient is perpendicular to the direction of flow. This means that in a cylindric tube fluid moves in a series of concentric lamina, and flow is laminar. Steady laminar flow results in a parabolic velocity profile in the tube. As predicted by this law, the resistance to flow is most dependent on vessel radius. Resistance is proportional to vessel length and viscosity but inversely proportional to the fourth power of the radius. Assuming a contant blood viscosity, a doubling of conduit length doubles the resistance, whereas halving the radius increases the resistance 16 times. In the human peripheral arterial system, flow is primarily determined by active changes in the arteriole, arteries less than 200 μm in diameter, and the capillary. Artery caliber varies according to the state of contraction of the vascular smooth muscle, which depends on perfusion pressure, activity of the sympathetic nervous system, and local mechanisms involving metabolic, humeral, and physiologic factors.

In a flow model governed by Poiseuille's law, the physical properties of the system (tube dimensions and fluid viscosity) determine the magnitude of the pressure gradient required to produce a given flow. The ratio of the mean pressure gradient to mean flow is thus a measure of the opposition to flow, commonly termed *vascular resistance.* When Poiseuille's law is simplified to an expression of pressure equals flow times resistance, it is exactly analogous to Ohm's law of electric circuits, V = I × Re, when Poiseuille's equation is rearranged to:

$$P = Q\,\frac{8\,l\mu}{\pi r^4}\ (\text{mm Hg})$$

where the term $8\,l\mu/\pi r^4$ expresses electric resistance (Re), P is voltage (V), and Q is flow of current (I). Vascular and electric resistance both express the dissipation of energy per unit flow within a system. In the arterial system, resistance is expressed as peripheral resistance units (PRU) where 1 PRU equals the resistance to flow when there is a pressure difference between two points of 1 mm Hg and flow is 1 m/sec. The resistance of the entire systemic circulation is approximately 1 PRU, calculated using a 100 mm Hg pressure gradient between the left ventricle and the right atrium and an average blood flow of 100 ml/sec.

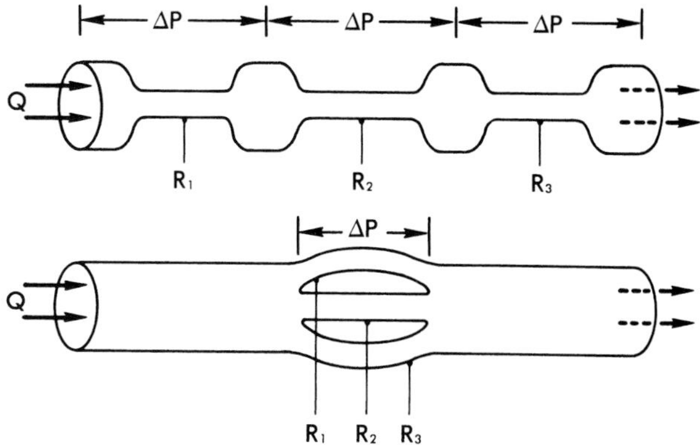

Fig. 51-3. Vascular resistance in series and parallel. *Top,* Total resistance (Rt) of a conducting system with individual resistances in series is the sum of resistances: Rt = (R1 + R2 + R3). *Bottom,* When resistance vessels are in parallel, the total resistance is the sum of the reciprocals of the individual resistances: Rt = 1-(R1 + R2 + R3). Note that in a parallel conducting system, the total resistance is less than any individual resistance level. Q indicates blood flow.

The total resistance of a conducting system depends on whether the vessels are in series or in parallel (Fig. 51-3). When vessels are in series, total resistance is equal to the sum of the individual resistances. On the other hand, if the conducting vessels are in parallel, total resistance is the reciprocal of the total conductance. This means that in a parallel conducting system total resistance is less than any of the individual resistance vessels. Also resistance usually tends to increase as velocity increases along a fixed diameter artery.

Fluid Energy

In general, blood flows from a point of high pressure to one of lower pressure, but the true driving force is the differential in total fluid energy. *Total fluid energy* associated with blood flow is of three types: intravascular pressure, gravitational, and kinetic. The intravascular pressure (P) has three components: (1) the dynamic pressure produced by the contraction of the heart; (2) the hydrostatic pressure; and (3) the static filling pressure. Both the gravitational energy and the hydrostatic pressure are determined by the product of the specific gravity of blood (ρ), the acceleration of gravity (980 cm/sec) (g) and the distance (h) above the right atrium. Gravitational energy (+ρgh) is the ability of the blood to do work on the basis of its height and is of the opposite value of the hydrostatic pressure (−ρgh). The static filling pressure is the residual pressure that exists in the absence of arterial flow. This pressure is determined by the volume of blood and the compliance of the arterial system and is in the range of 5 to 10 mm Hg. Since the hydrostatic pressure and the gravitational potential energy cancel out each other and static filling pressure is relatively low, the dynamic pressure produced by the heart is the major source of potential energy used in moving blood.

Kinetic energy (Ek) is the ability of blood to do work on the basis of its motion. It is proportional to the specific gravity of blood (ρ) and the square of the blood velocity (v):

$$Ek = 1/2\ \rho v^2$$

Omitting the term for gravitational energy (i.e., $+\rho gh$), the total fluid energy per volume of blood (E) can be expressed as:

$$E = P + 1/2\ \rho v^2$$

where P is intravascular pressure. In an idealized fluid system of steady flow and/or frictional energy losses, total fluid energy along a streamline remains constant with the relationship between the different energy forms described by Bernoulli's principle of the conservation of energy:

$$P_1 + 1/2\ \rho v_1^2 = P_2 + 1/2\ \rho v_2^2 + \text{Heat}$$

In the horizontal diverging tube shown in Fig. 51-4, steady flow between two points is accomplished by an increase in cross-sectional area and a decrease in flow velocity. Although fluid energy moves against a pressure gradient ($P_2 - P_1$) of 2.5 mm Hg and gains potential energy, total fluid energy remains constant because of a lower velocity and a proportional loss of kinetic energy. In the normal arterial system in which ideal flow conditions are absent and vessels change diameter only gradually, the pressure gradients caused by viscous losses as predicted by Poiseuille's law far outweigh the extremely small interconversions to kinetic energy and pressure. In certain disease states, however, such as sudden vessel widening into an aneurysm or narrowing as a result of an atherosclerotic plaque, the Bernoulli's principle and the production of turbulence with the associated changes in kinetic energy explain the pressure and flow change under these conditions.

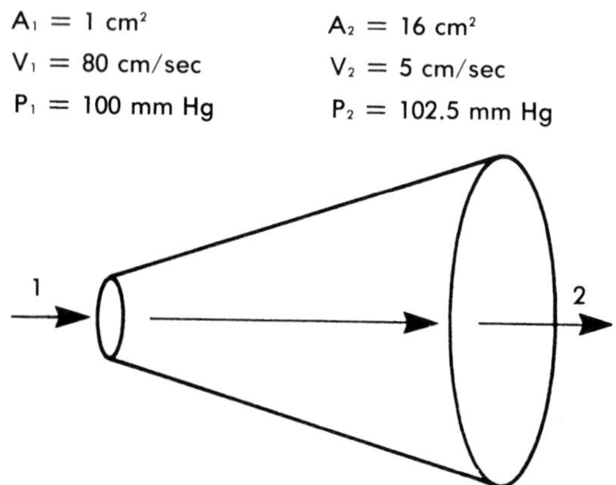

Fig. 51-4. Effect of increasing cross-sectional area on pressure in frictionless fluid system. Although pressure increases, total fluid energy remains constant because of a decrease in velocity. *A,* Area; *V,* velocity; *P,* pressure. (From Zierler RE, Strandness DE. In Moore WS, ed. Vascular Surgery—A Comprehensive Review. New York: Grune & Stratton, 1983.)

It is important to emphasize that the pressure-flow relationship described in Poiseuille's law is based on assumptions involving idealized fluid mechanics that significantly underestimate the energy losses present in the viscoelastic, pulsatile flow conditions of the human circulation. Poiseuille's law represents the minimum pressure gradient produced by viscous losses that may be expected in arterial flow. In addition to energy loss caused by friction, inertial energy losses related to changes in the velocity and the direction of flow occur. In the arterial system, particularly in the presence of disease, energy losses caused by inertial effects usually exceed viscous energy loss.

Energy losses related to inertia are proportional to the specific gravity of blood and the square of the blood velocity. Since the density of blood is a constant, inertial losses result when blood accelerates, decelerates, or changes direction. Inertial energy losses therefore occur at bifurcations and points of curvature and from variations of lumen diameter, all of which are normally present in the arterial system. Blood velocity usually increases from large luminal size to smaller luminal size. The acceleration and deceleration of blood in pulsatile flow adds inertial forces to the constant kinetic energy of steady flow.

Arterial Flow Patterns

The combination of viscous (frictional) and inertial forces acting on blood determines whether flow is laminar or turbulent (i.e., disturbed flow). The transition to turbulent flow is physiologically important because a greater pressure gradient is needed to maintain flow. Frictional interactions at the inner wall of an artery can also produce flow pattern variations referred to as boundary layer separation. The clinical importance of local flow patterns in arteries resides in their role in the pathogenesis of atherosclerosis and the ability of duplex ultrasound systems to detect and grade the severity of disease through the disturbed flow produced.

Laminar and Turbulent Flow

As previously discussed, the blood flow pattern is streamlined or laminar in the steady flow conditions specified by Poiseuille's law. The velocity profile is parabolic in shape (Fig. 51-5). In contrast to the concentric laminae of laminar flow, turbulence is a condition in which the flow velocity vectors are moving in a random fashion with respect to space and time. The point at which flow changes from laminar to turbulent, termed the *critical velocity,* depends on the ratio of inertial forces to viscous forces and is best defined in terms of a dimensionless entity known as Reynold's number:

$$Re = \rho dv/\mu$$

where ρ is the blood density, d is the vessel diameter, v is the mean velocity, and μ is the viscosity. At a Reynold's number lower than 2000, flow is laminar because viscous forces predominate and damping of random inertial forces on the flow stream occur. At a Reynold's number higher than 2000, the inertial forces may disrupt the laminar flow pattern, the result being increased energy dissipation as sound and heat. Energy dissipation in laminar flow is proportional to flow velocity, whereas losses in turbulent flow occur with the velocity squared. Flow conditions that predispose to the development of turbulence include an increased flow velocity (ascending aorta), a decreased vessel diameter (diseased), or a reduced blood viscosity (anemia, overhydration). An important clinical sign of turbulence is the presence of a bruit. Streamline (laminar) flow is silent, but turbulence produces wall vibrations that can often be heard with a stethoscope, termed a *bruit*. Sounds used in the conventional auscultatory method of arterial pressure measurement are audible because of turbulence in the flow stream. Bruits produced by stenoses are loudest over the stenotic segment and are transmitted in a distal direction.

Projections or obstacles in the flow stream and roughness of the luminal surface also influence flow patterns. For example, whether turbulence develops downstream to an atherosclerotic plaque depends not only on the Reynold's number but also on the size and shape of the projection. For a sharp-edged plaque, laminar flow is preserved if:

$$\frac{h}{r} = \frac{4}{\sqrt{Re}}$$

where h is the height of the plaque, r is the radius of the vessel and $\sqrt{Re}$ is the square root of Reynold's number. On review of this equation, it can readily be seen that the adverse effects of a plaque on vessel radius reduction are of more importance than the relative height of the obstruction.

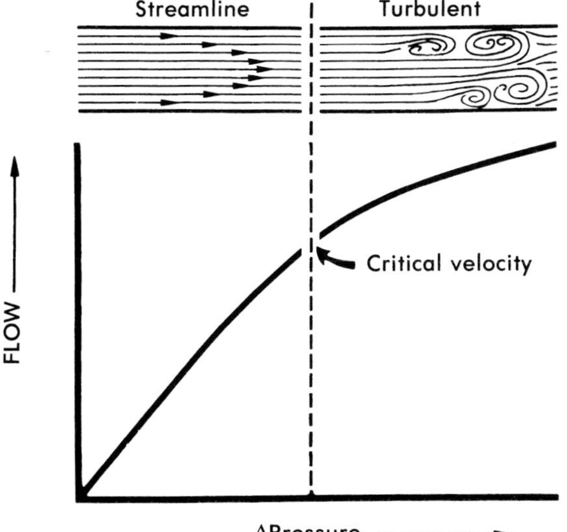

Fig. 51-5. Relationship between velocity of flow and turbulence. (From Ruch TC, Patton HD. Physiology and Biophysics. Philadelphia: WB Saunders, 1974.)

Under conditions of pulsatile, viscoelastic flow, the arterial velocity profile changes from the parabolic shape of laminar flow to a blunt shape. Although turbulent flow is uncommon in arteries, a condition of disturbed flow commonly occurs. Disturbed flow is a transient perturbation in the laminar streamlines that disappears with time or as flow proceeds downstream. Sites of focal disturbed flow can be identified in the thoracic aorta during the flow deceleration phase of each heart cycle, in regions of arterial branching, and in the carotid bulb. Disturbed flow is in the initial hemodynamic abnormality produced by atherosclerotic plaque formation which alters wall compliance and narrows lumen cross-sectional area. The recognition of the kinetic energy losses associated with disturbed flow conditions helps to explain the gross underestimation of energy loss when Poiseuille's law is used alone to evaluate flow changes produced by arterial stenosis.

The magnitude of disturbed flow can be divided into three categories on the basis of the Doppler velocity spectra pattern: undisturbed (laminar), disturbed, and highly disturbed (turbulent). As shown in Fig. 51-6, the velocity spectra of blood flow through a stenosis demonstrates the local disruption of laminar flow at and distal to the lesion. Highly disturbed velocity spectra associated with a pressure-flow–reducing stenosis exhibit high-frequency Doppler shifts and spectral broadening throughout the pulse cycle. Platelets subjected to turbulent flow can activate or initiate aggregation and thus thrombus formation. Disturbed velocity waveforms contain high-frequency components only during peak systole and typically indicate a transitional flow condition detected under normal flow conditions in the ascending aorta and at arterial bifurcations. Undisturbed velocity waveforms exhibit negligible high-frequency content and are representative of laminar flow.

Boundary Layer Separation

The outer layer of fluid in a flow stream adjacent to the vessel wall is referred to as the *boundary layer.* Radial-directed velocity gradients exist as a result of the fractional interactions of fluid with the vessel wall and the more rapidly moving fluid in the center of the vessel. When vessel geometry changes suddenly such as at points of curvature and bifurcations, small pressure gradients are created that cause the boundary layer to stop or reverse direction. This results in a complex, localized flow pattern known as an area of flow separation. Areas of flow separation have been observed in models of arterial anastomoses and the carotid bifurcation depicted in Fig. 51-7, in which an area of flow separation has formed along the outer wall as a result of the diverging carotid bulb diameter. The complex flow patterns identified in the normal human carotid bifurcation includes vortex flow as well as regions of flow separation and reversal along the lateral, posterior wall of the bulb. Shear rate is the variation of velocity of flow changes between concentric laminae of blood. Shear stress at the vessel wall (Dw) can be characterized by the following formula:

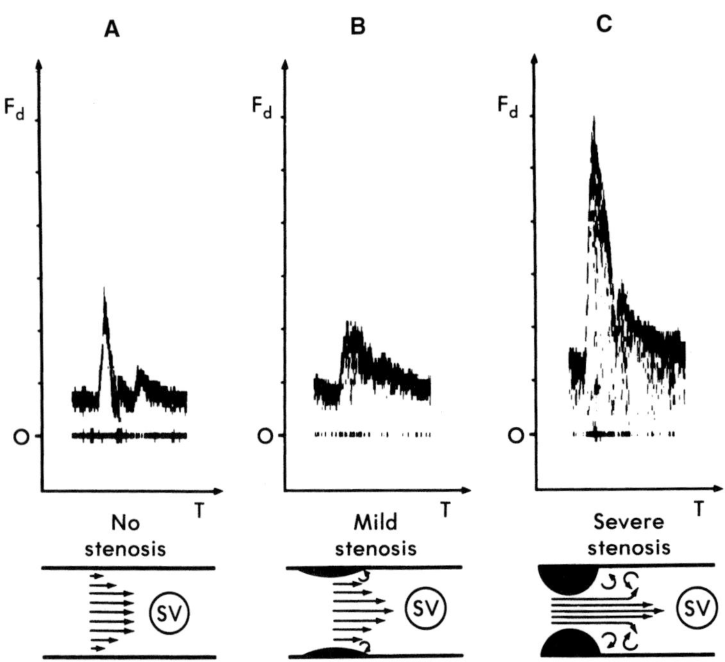

Fig. 51-6. Center stream flow from a normal artery is laminar and is demonstrated on the spectrum **(A)** as a narrow band of frequencies during systole, with a clear window beneath the frequency envelope. Disturbed flow caused by mild stenosis appears as spectral broadening on the frequency spectrum **(B)** without producing changes in the park systolic velocity. Highly disturbed flow (turbulence) is characterized by high peak velocities and spectral broadening throughout the cardiac cycle. Also note the increase in end-diastolic velocity associated with severe stenosis **(C)**. *SV,* Systolic velocity; *T,* time. (From Roederer G, et al. Comprehensive noninvasive evaluation of extracranial cerebrovascular disease. In Hershey FB, Barnes RW, Sumner DS, eds. Noninvasive Diagnosis of Vascular Disease. Pasadena, Calif.: Appleton-Davies, 1984.)

$$Dw = 4\frac{V}{r} = 4\frac{Q}{\pi r^3}$$

$$\Gamma w = 4\epsilon\frac{V}{r} = 4\epsilon\frac{Q}{\pi r^3}$$

where Γw is the shear stress at the wall, V is mean velocity, r is radius, Q is mean flow, and ϵ is the blood viscosity. Therefore shear rate and stress are directly proportional to mean velocity, turbulence, and viscosity and inversely proportional to the inner radius of the vessel. At bifurcations and vessel curves, shear is highest at the wall where the velocity of flow is also highest. It has been shown that arterial vasoconstriction and vasodilation occur with shear rate changes, most likely via production of endothelial-derived relaxant factor (EDRF), now known to be nitric oxide. Production of nitric oxide in the wall in response to increased shear rate causes relaxation of the media smooth muscle, resulting in vasodilation.

The disturbed flow and low shear stress in regions of boundary layer separation may contribute to the formation of atherosclerotic plaques. Examination of carotid and iliac bifurcations, both at autopsy and during surgery, indicated that intimal thickening and plaque formation tend to occur in the regions of flow separation. Within these zones there is an opportunity for a synergistic effect for rheologic and contact activation of blood elements with the intima. The role of localized flow disturbances as an initiator or promotor of atherosclerosis is speculative and awaits further analysis and research.

Principles of Pulsatile Flow

In the pulsatile arterial system, pressure and flow vary continuously with time, and the velocity profile changes throughout the cardiac cycle. The pressure flow relationships defined under steady flow conditions do not take into consideration the inertia forces of accelerating and decelerating blood, the compliant nature of the arterial wall, and the influence of vessel tapering and bifurcations on the shape and size of the pulsatile pressure and flow wave. The addition of a pulsatile component on steady flow increases fluid energy expenditure. As much as 30% of the energy in cardiac output is dissipated as a result of pulsatile flow. With increasing heart rate, energy losses caused by pulsatile flow decrease exponentially up to a heart rate of approximately 150 beats/min. The remainder of the energy of cardiac output is used for tissue perfusion; it is primarily lost in the arteriolar and capillary bed. Although the true nature of pulsatile energy loss remains poorly defined, contributing factors include the inertia energy loss with acceleration; the skewing of the velocity profile re-

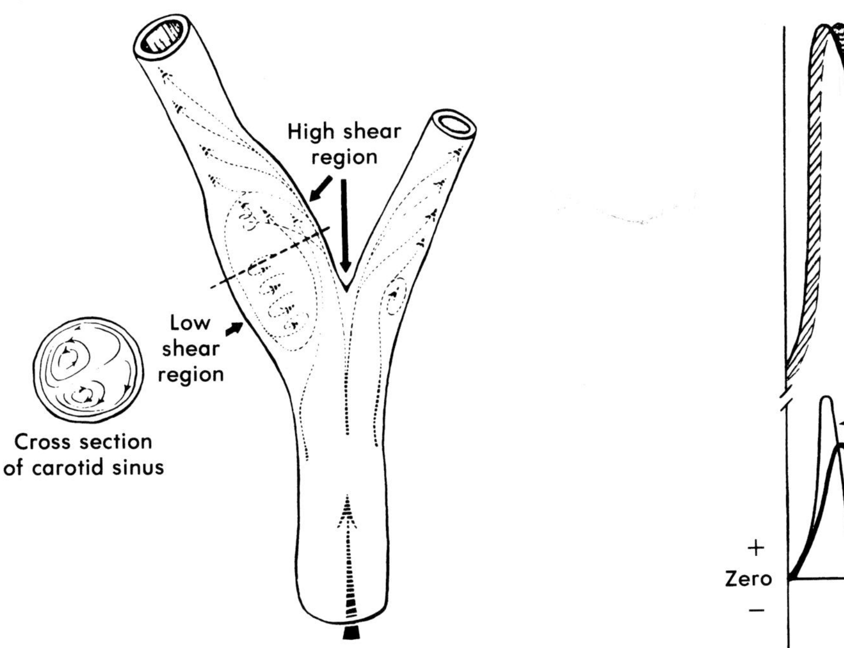

Fig. 51-7. Flow patterns at model carotid bifurcation. Adjacent to the outer wall of the bulb, flow is stagnant (a region of flow separation), may reverse, or may be diverted across the vessel lumen. Rapid flow is associated with high shear stress, whereas the slow flow in the separation zone produces a region of low shear. (From Sumner DS. Pitfalls on noninvasive cerebrovascular testing and angiography. In Bernhard VM, Towne JB, eds. Complications in Vascular Surgery, 2nd ed. New York: Grune & Stratton, 1985.)

Fig. 51-8. Generation of flow velocity waveform by traveling pressure pulse wave. Simultaneous pressure pulse and flow velocity pulse recordings from an arterial segment. Although similar in configuration, peak flow occurs before the systolic pressure peak, indicating a complex relationship between these hemodynamic parameters. Flow is determined by the pressure gradient that develops along the arterial segment.

lated to geometric tapering, curvature, and bifurcation; the production of disturbed flow; and the non-Newtonian character of blood. It is apparent that Poiseuille's law cannot accurately predict all the hemodynamic characteristics of flow through the artery.

Of importance to the surgeon is that in pulsatile flow the energy losses produced by arterial reconstructions, which commonly have anatomic and physical characteristics much different from the normal arterial system, are likely to be much greater than predicted by the equations governing steady flow. Although pulsatile flow appears less efficient than steady laminar flow, studies indicate that individual organs require pulsatile flow for optimum function. Perfusion of a kidney with steady flow instead of pulsatile flow results in a reduction of urine volume and sodium excretion. Pulsatile flow and pressure probably exert their effect at the microvascular level. Although the exact mechanism is unknown, transcapillary exchange, arteriolar and venular tone, and lymphatic flow are responsive to pulsatile pressure.

With each stroke volume of the heart, blood is pumped into the distensible arterial tree, which acts as an elastic reservoir or *windkessel* absorbing the cardiac energy that is later released during ventricular diastole. The physiologic effect is to damp the flow/no-flow effect of the heart so that pressure and flow are maintained during diastole. As blood is forced into the aorta, the instantaneous increase in volume is transmitted along the artery as a pressure and flow wave. As shown in Fig. 51-8, the increase in flow starts almost synchronously with the rise in pressure, but the peak flow velocity precedes peak pressure. The instantaneous flow rate is not determined by the magnitude of the pressure pulse but by the pressure gradient developed along the artery. The pressure gradient can be determined by recording the pressure at two points a short distance apart and subtracting the downstream pressure from that of the upstream pressure during the cardiac cycle. The effect of the traveling pressure wave is to produce an oscillatory pressure gradient. The magnitude of the pressure gradient determines both instantaneous flow velocity and the direction of flow. Unless there is a marked decrease in the mean pressure along the artery, there is always a period during the pulse cycle when the pressure gradient is reversed. This reversal of gradient causes a rapid deceleration of flow; if it continues after the forward flow has been brought to a halt, flow reversal can occur. Indeed, flow reversal during diastole is a normal pattern of blood flow in peripheral limb arteries.

As the pressure pulse wave travels from the aorta to the periphery, its speed, magnitude, and configuration are altered. The pressure wave is produced by the sudden ejection of blood into the aorta. The pressure wave velocity increases from 4 to 6 cm/sec to approximately 13 cm/sec in the muscular arteries of the lower extremity. The velocity of the pressure wave is 20 times greater than the mean velocity imparted to the blood in the aorta (20 to 40 cm/sec), illustrating that the pressure wave has no direct relationship to flow and can be recorded under "no flow" conditions of acute arterial occlusion. The acceleration of the pressure wave in the peripheral arteries is caused primarily by increasing wall stiffness. Because of this relationship, the transmission velocity of the pressure wave has been used as an index of arterial distensibility.

The amplitude of the pressure wave, otherwise known as the pulse pressure, increases, and wave configuration changes with propagation to the periphery (Fig. 51-9). With increasing distance from the heart, the rate of systolic pressure rise increases, the sharp inflection of the downslope known as the *dicrotic notch* becomes rounded and disappears in the abdominal aorta, where dicrotic waves appear. In the arteries of the lower extremity systolic pressure is higher and diastolic pressure lower than in the aorta. This is the result of the viscoelastic characteristics of the arterial conduits, the effect of pressure waves being reflected from sites of increased peripheral resistance (i.e., from sites of tapering and branching), and the abrupt increase in resistance at the level of the arterioles. It is important to note that the mean pressure decreases with the distance from the heart, but the pressure loss in the large arteries of the thorax and abdomen is small because of their large radius. As shown in Table 51-2, systolic and diastolic pressures recorded from large arteries are influenced by various hemodynamic factors. Careful analysis of the pressure wave configuration and its transmission can provide useful clues to important cardiac and peripheral arterial physiology.

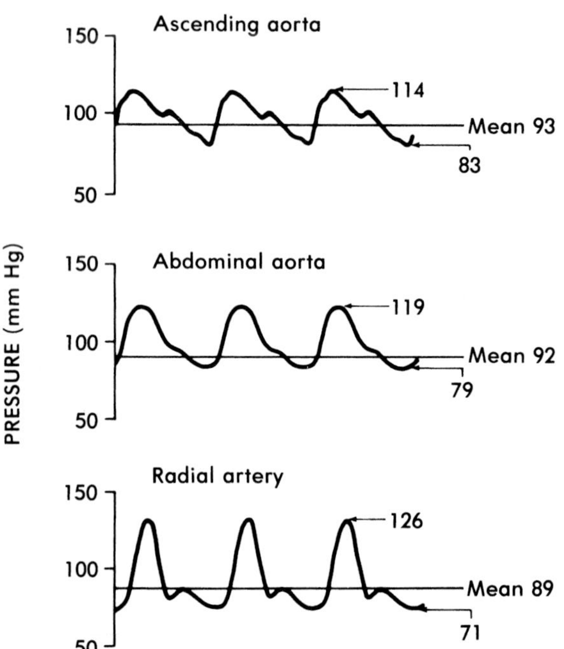

Fig. 51-9. Pressure waves at different sites in the arterial tress. With pressure wave transmission into the distal aorta and large arteries, the systolic pressure increases, and the diastolic pressure decreases with a resultant increase in pulse pressure. Note that mean arterial pressure declines steadily.

The pulsatile characteristics of the pressure wave are dampened considerably at the level of arterioles at which mean pressure reaches values to 40 to 60 mm Hg. In general, perfusion pressure in the capillaries is nonpulsatile, and pressure waves in the venous system are caused primarily by pressure changes in the right ventricle and not the left ventricle. Exercise increases total leg blood flow 5 to 10 times in the normal patient. In the diseased extremity seen during treadmill duplex evaluation, ankle pressure drops severely and requires prolonged periods of time to recover.

Measurement of Arterial Pressure

A major advance in the understanding and approach to patients with arterial occlusive disease came with the recognition that the physiologic disturbance responsible for symptoms is predominantly related to development of a pressure gradient in the proximal arterial segment. Pressure measurement is a more sensitive index of an occlusive process than is the measurement of flow because in the presence of moderate arterial disease blood flow is essentially normal, owing to the reduction of resting arteriolar resistance compensating for the increased resistance of the proximal arterial system. Although flow measurement techniques (i.e., indicator dilution methods, impedance flowmeter) have clinical value in the determination of cardiac output, flow volume measurements in the limbs are of limited value as a clinical or diagnostic tool. For these reasons a variety of techniques are available for the measurement of arterial pressure both directly and indirectly using noninvasive instrumentation.

Direct pressure measurement involves the placement of a needle or catheter into the artery and recording the pressure waveform with the aid of manometer or strain gauge transducers. The hydraulic system that couples the transducer to the arterial lumen should be maximum bore and minimum length to avoid damping of the pressure wave. From a continuous recording of the pressure waveform, systolic pressure is the peak pressure during the pulse cy-

Table 51-2. Main Determinants of Aortic Systolic and Diastolic Pressures

Systolic Pressure	Diastolic Pressure
Stroke volume	Systolic pressure
Aortic distensibility	Aortic distensibility
Ejection velocity	Heart rate
	Peripheral resistance

cle, and diastolic pressure is the lowest pressure. The difference between these two pressures is the pulse pressure. Mean pressure, the force responsible for the mean flow of blood to an organ, can be determined electronically by calculating the area of the pulsatile waveform or estimated from systolic and diastolic pressure measurements (Mean pressure = Diastolic pressure + 1/3 Pulse pressure). Although direct pressure measurements provide the most accurate data, their routine clinical use is not warranted, since the technique is invasive and requires sterile conditions, and pressure data obtained indirectly are sufficiently accurate for diagnostic purposes.

Indirect pressure measurements depend on (1) the production of Korotkoff sounds, which are the result of turbulence in the flow stream, (2) the appearance and disappearance of the pressure pulse, or (3) the reappearance of flow when a proximally located pneumatic cuff has been inflated and slowly deflated above the regional perfusion pressure. Auscultatory and palpatory techniques to measure upper extremity arterial pressure are the most common hemodynamic assessments of the arterial circulation. To avoid measurement errors, the occluding cuff should be 20% wider than the limb diameter. If it is too narrow, the pressure reading is erroneously high; if it is too wide, the reading may be erroneously low.

Several techniques are used clinically to measure systolic pressure in the limbs including plethysmography (mercury strain gauge, air, photoelectric cell) and the ultrasonic velocity detector (continuous-wave Doppler). These instruments are used as sensors to indicate return of flow with cuff deflation. Plethysmography operates on the principle that changes in the circulation of the blood to a body part (e.g., leg) result in corresponding measurable changes in the size of that part. Such changes in size can be measured by displacement of air or mercury in a strain gauge or emission of light in a photoelectric cell, as is done in photoplethysmography. In general, devices with ultrasound are most commonly used because instruments are inexpensive and simple to use; the Doppler-derived pressure measurements have been thoroughly evaluated and have been noted to be as accurate as plethysmographic measurements. Even when ultrasonic signals are difficult to obtain, it is almost always possible to record a pressure with the photoplethysmograph. Digital volume changes are amplified and able to be recorded. This allows pressures to be recorded in digits in the presence of severe obstructive arterial disease when flow velocities are too low to be picked up by a Doppler transducer.

The assessment of arterial flow with ultrasound is made on the basis of the Doppler effect, which refers to the shift in frequency that occurs when sound is reflected from a moving object. Moving red blood cells reflect the ultrasound beam and shift the frequency proportional to the flow velocity. The Doppler signal can be (1) amplified to provide an audible sound with pitch directly proportional to blood velocity, (2) converted into an analog waveform using a zero-crossing frequency meter, or (3) analyzed for its frequency-amplitude content. Failure to obtain a Doppler signal from an artery usually indicates occlusion; however, an extremely low flow rate (less than 2 cm/sec) may not produce detectable Doppler frequency shift.

The systolic pressure at any level of an extremity can be measured by applying a pneumatic cuff and positioning the Doppler probe over a patent artery distal to the cuff (Fig. 51-10). The arterial signal is distinguished from the adjacent venous signal by its characteristic high-pitched sound that corresponds to the cardiac cycle. When the cuff is inflated above systolic pressure, the arterial flow signal disappears. As cuff pressure is gradually lowered, the point at which flow resumes is recorded as the systolic pressure. In the lower extremity the use of multiple cuffs placed at the high-thigh, above- and below-knee, ankle, and digital levels permits the measurement of segmental pressures. The level of pressure measurement is determined by cuff placement and not the site of Doppler flow detection. The difference in systolic pressure between any two adjacent cuffs or between corresponding segments in the opposite limb is less than 20 mm Hg in normal individuals. Because of cuff artifact, proximal thigh systolic pressure normally exceeds brachial pressure by 30 to 40 mm Hg.

Amplification of the pressure wave with distance from the heart produces a higher systolic pressure to be measured at the ankle than in the brachial artery, which in the

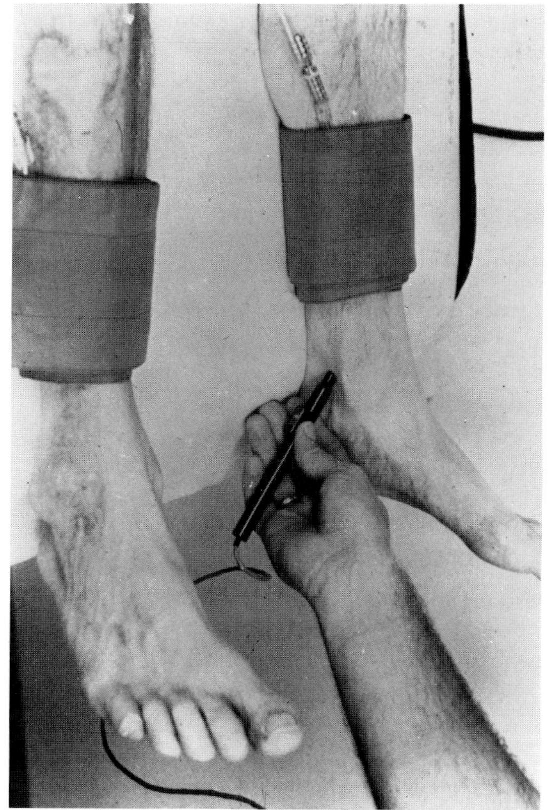

Fig. 51-10. Measurement of ankle systolic pressure. Doppler probe is positioned over the posterior tibial artery.

absence of disease is nearly equal to central aortic pressure. To compensate for variation in central perfusion pressure and to permit comparisons of serial measurements, the ankle systolic pressure is expressed as a ratio of brachial pressure, termed the ankle-brachial systolic pressure index (ABI). The normal ABI is equal to or greater than 1 (mean value of 1.1 ± 0.1), and reductions correlate with the degree of arterial insufficiency. In limbs with intermittent claudication, the ABI (mean + SD) is 0.58 ± 0.15; in limbs with ischemic rest pain, 0.26 ± 0.13; and in limbs with gangrene, 0.05 ± 0.08.

The measure of toe pressures can be used to identify obstructive disease distal to the ankle and to measure pressure in diabetic patients in whom ankle pressure measurement by the cuff method is artifactually high because of the incompressibility of calcified arteries. Normal systolic toe pressure is approximately 80% of the brachial systolic pressure. Photoplethysmographic techniques are better suited than the ultrasonic methods of flow determination at the digital level because of vessel caliber and a low flow velocity in the digital arteries.

Real-Time Ultrasound Arterial Imaging and Flow Analysis

Since the 1970s, ultrasound technology has developed instrumentation to both image blood vessels and display blood flow patterns within the lumen in real-time. The technique referred to as color duplex ultrasonography, which combines real-time imaging (B-mode) with pulsed Doppler flow detection, is most versatile and permits the arterial and venous circulations to be mapped analogous to arteriography or venography in body regions accessible to interrogation by ultrasonic energy. Duplex scanning can be used to address specific queries concerning location and extent of vascular disease and disease morphology (stenosis, occlusion, or aneurysm), measure vessel diameter, grade stenosis severity, and measure occlusion length based on visualization or exit and reentry collateral vessels. In atherosclerotic lesions, B-mode imaging with high-frequency (10 to 15 MHz) transducers can demonstrate features such as ulceration, calcification, acoustic heterogenicity, and intraplaque hemorrhage.

Blood flow velocity within visualized vessels is characterized with the use of a Doppler velocity detector. Accurate characterization of blood flow patterns requires the use of a pulsed Doppler whose sample volume (the point in space from which blood flow is detected) is small in relation to the vessel diameter. The Doppler signal is processed by a real-time spectrum analyzer to determine the velocity of blood, the direction of flow, and the velocity distribution of the red blood cells in the sample volume. When the pulsed Doppler sample volume is positioned in the midstream of nondisturbed (laminar) arterial flow, the Dopper signal contains a narrow range of frequencies (spectral width) of similar amplitude corresponding to streamline movement of red blood cells during the pulse cycle. Undisturbed flow produces a "clear window" in the spectra beneath the frequency envelope and is characteristic of normal peripheral arterial hemodynamics.

Calculation of blood flow velocity requires estimation and assignment of the angle between the incident Doppler beam and the blood velocity vector. An operator-controlled line on the B-mode image indicates the direction of the sound beam from the pulsed Doppler probe. In general, the Doppler beam is adjusted to intersect the flow stream at an angle of approximately 60 degrees. A "cursor" on the Doppler beam indicator locates the position of the sample volume and can be placed at any point in the vessel. The Doppler angle is calculated electronically by the operator positioning a cursor parallel to the longitudinal axis of the vessel. Blood flow velocity is calculated from the frequency spectra waveform measurements using the Doppler equation:

$$\text{Flow velocity} = \frac{C\ Fs}{2\ Fo} \cdot \cos \Theta \ (\text{cm/sec})$$

where C is the average speed of sound in tissue (1.54×10^6 cm/sec), Fs is the shift in frequency between the transmitted and reflected Doppler beam, Fo is the frequency of the transmitted Doppler beam, and Θ is the Doppler beam angle.

If the mean frequency shift can be electronically extracted from the Doppler spectrum, the spatial average velocity (Vsa) as a function of time can be calculated. Volumetric blood flow (Q) can then be determined from a measurement of lumen diameter (D) by the equation:

$$Q = \frac{Vsa\ \pi\ D^2}{4} (\text{ml/min})$$

Although the determination of volumetric flow is attractive, the accurate calculation of Vsa can be quite difficult, since it requires complete insonation of the flow stream across the vessel lumen, knowledge of the velocity profile configuration, and a correction for both the forward and reverse components of pulsatile flow.

Duplex scanning provides both anatomic and physiologic information regarding arterial flow. Tables 51-3 and 51-4 show normal arterial lower extremity mean and peak velocities and velocity waveform configurations seen with duplex scanning. This information has been applied clinically to the evaluation and classification of atherosclerotic occlusive disease involving the carotid bifurcation, visceral arteries (renal, celiac, and superior mesenteric), the abdominal aorta, and the arteries of the lower extremity. Under normal conditions, flow in peripheral and carotid arteries is undisturbed (Figs. 51-11 and 51-12). As discussed previously, turbulence is responsible for most of the fluid energy loss associated with arterial disease. Because turbulence occurs at lesser degrees of stenosis than detectable changes in mean flow and pressure, assessment of arterial flow by duplex scanning permits a more accurate diagnosis of altered hemodynamics than is available using techniques that monitor pressure and flow. Distal to a site of

Table 51-3. Duplex-Derived Flow, Diameter, and Mean/Peak Systolic Flow Velocity Measurements From Lower Extremity Artery Segments

	Artery Segment			
Duplex	**Common Femoral**	**Popliteal**	**Anterior Tibial**	**Posterior Tibial**
Flow (ml/min)	371	140	11	16
Diameter (mm)	8.6	6.6	2.2	2.3
Mean velocity (cm/sec)	11	7	4	5
Peak velocity (cm/sec)	89	66	58	57

Table 51-4. Normal Blood Flow Velocity Waveform Configurations in Peripheral Arteries

	Flow Velocity Waveform Configuration	
Arterial Location	**Biphasic**	**Triphasic**
Cerebrovascular		
Internal, common carotid	X	
External carotid		X
Vertebral	X	
Visceral		
Celiac	X	
Superior mesenteric		
Fasting		X
Postprandial	X	
Renal	X	
Peripheral (Upper/ Lower Extremities)		
Resting		X
After Exercise	X	

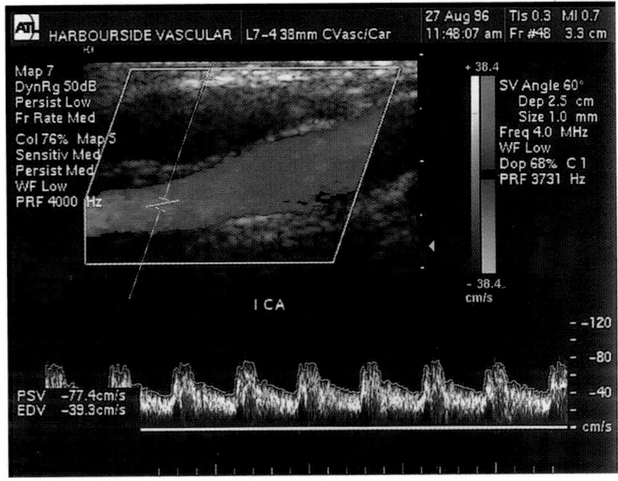

Fig. 51-11. Color duplex scan imaging of the internal carotid artery. Sample volume of the pulsed Doppler probe is positioned in the proximal internal carotid artery. Narrow band of frequencies during the pulse cycle and the clear area beneath the waveform are characteristics of laminar flow in a normal carotid artery.

stenosis, turbulence is evident in the Doppler signal by an increase in peak systolic velocity, an alteration in the velocity waveform, and the presence of spectral broadening corresponding to the disordered, random movement of red blood cells in the flow stream. Accurate characterization of vessel anatomy and flow in both normal and diseased states is possible by duplex mapping of the peripheral arterial system. Accuracy approximates that of contrast studies and can also estimate whether lesions seen on arteriograms are hemodynamically significant. Risks, cost, and discomfort are less than for contrast studies; however, duplex mapping is operator dependent, and well-trained experienced technologists are required. Natural history studies of atherosclerosis using duplex scanning have demonstrated anatomic and hemodynamic features associated with the initiation and progression of vascular disease. Compared with arteriography, diagnostic accuracy of duplex scanning is in excess of 80% in detection of greater than 50% diameter reduction arterial stenosis or occlusion. Clinical applications include preintervention testing of pe-

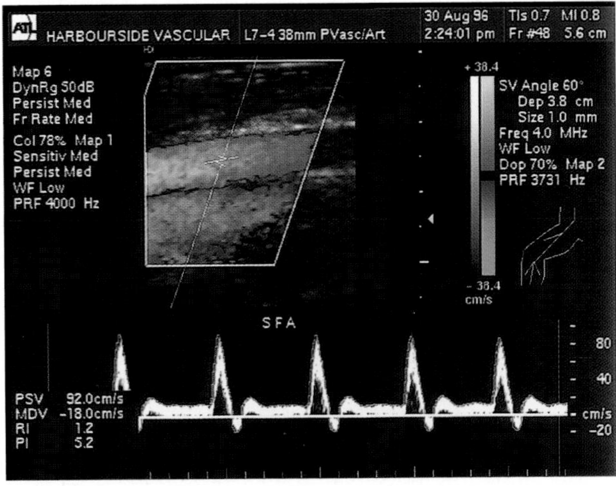

Fig. 51-12. Color duplex examination of normal superficial femoral artery flow. Velocity spectra and waveform configuration are typical of normal flow in a limb artery.

ripheral and cerebrovascular arterial disease, peripheral venous testing for acute and chronic venous thrombosis, intraoperative assessment of vascular repairs, and postoperative surveillance of arterial surgery and vascular disease.

PERIPHERAL VENOUS SYSTEM

The primary function of the venous system is to return blood to the right ventricle for reoxygenation by the lungs and regulating vascular capacity. As such it serves a conduit function similar to the arterial system. In the latter, however, this is accomplished by left ventricular contraction at high pressure with high velocity. Venous return is accomplished at low pressure and low velocity without cardiac contraction. The mechanisms responsible are best addressed by considering first the anatomic configuration and unique structure of the venous channels and then the interaction of the structural characteristics with the forces responsible for normal venous return.

Venous Anatomy

There is great variability in the anatomy of the deep and superficial venous systems of the limbs, including segmental and complete duplications. In the lower extremity the common femoral vein is medial to the common femoral artery and includes the saphenofemoral junction at which the greater saphenous vein joins the common femoral vein 3 to 5 cm cephalad to the junctions of the deep and superficial femoral veins. The greater saphenous venous system begins anterior to the medial malleolus and travels subcutaneously on the anteriomedial aspect of the lower leg 1 to 2 cm posterior to the tibia. It joins the femoral vein 2 to 4 cm lateral to the pubic tubercle and inferior to the inguinal ligament in the fossa ovalis. The superficial circumflex iliac vein and superficial inferior epigastric vein join the greater saphenous vein also in this area. For descriptive purposes the venous system of the lower extremity is divided into a superficial and deep component and is more complex than the arterial system because these veins are collapsible, are affected by gravity, possess a low-pressure system, contain valves, and are affected by the right side of the heart. The superficial system consists of the greater and lesser saphenous veins, which are located in the subcutaneous tissue superficial to the deep fascia (Fig. 51-13). Generally, as one proceeds down the lower extremity more valves are encountered. The channels are responsible for collection of venous blood from the skin and subcutaneous tissues and terminate by penetrating the deep fascia of the groin and popliteal fossa, respectively, to enter the deep venous channels. The superficial veins are subjected to a very large hydrostatic pressure and are therefore relatively thick walled. These superficial veins contain numerous bicuspid valves that facilitate flow from the periphery of the limb to the central portion of the limb and prevent flow in a retrograde direction. These valves and their function are more important in the lower vs. upper extremity, where a malfunction can lead to deep vein thrombosis, pulmonary embolus, deep venous insufficiency, and venous stasis ulcers. Veins are usually three times the size of their accompanying arteries and composed of an intima, media, and adventitia. The deep system of veins consists of the venous channels accompanying the major muscular arteries and are similarly named. In the periphery of the limb these channels are frequently present in duplicate and, because they are protected from the force of gravity by the muscles in the lower extremity, are relatively thin walled. Bicuspid valves are also present in these veins, with the greatest density occurring peripherally and relatively few valves being located in the more central larger channels. For example, the superior and inferior venae cavae, as well as the common iliac veins are devoid of valves, whereas the external iliac vein infrequently has a single bicuspid valve present. The popliteal vein has 1 to 2 valves, whereas the greater and lesser saphenous systems have about 8 to 10 valves each.

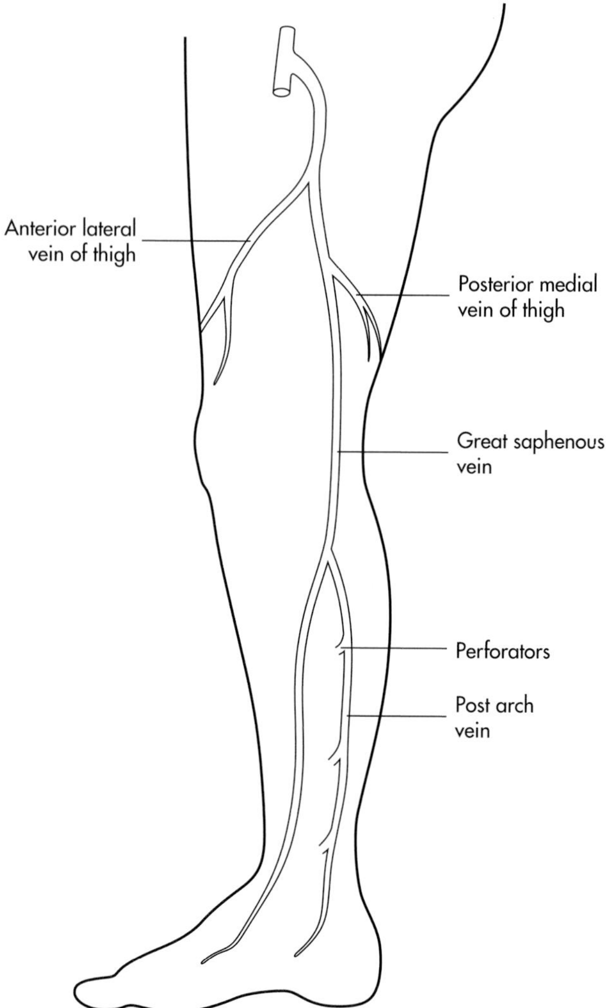

Fig. 51-13. Diagrammatic representation of the major anatomic features of the greater and lesser saphenous veins and their tributaries.

A second major component of the deep venous system is the soleal sinuses, a group of endothelial-lined venous reservoirs or "lakes" located within the substance of the

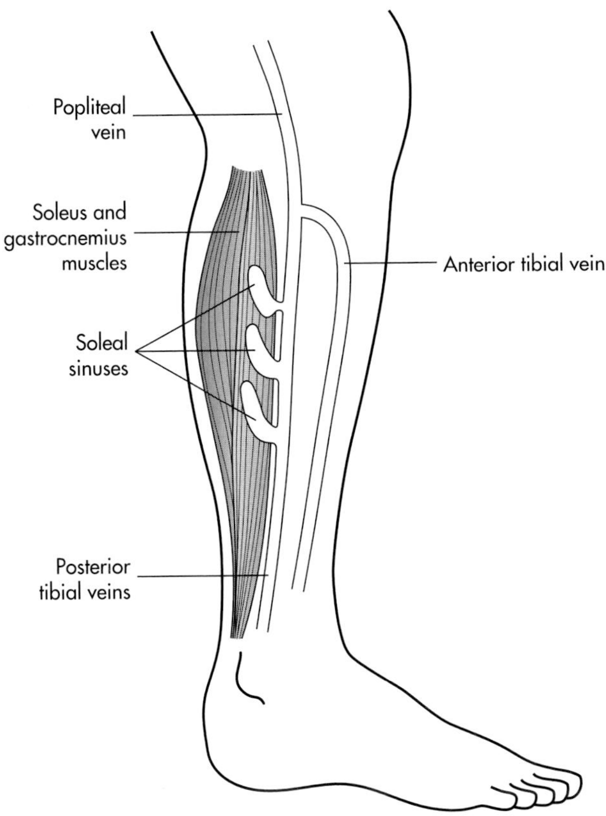

Fig. 51-14. Schematic representation of the soleal sinuses and their relationship to the calf muscles and deep venous system. It should be noted that these empty directly into the deep venous system and also on occasion receive communications from the superficial system.

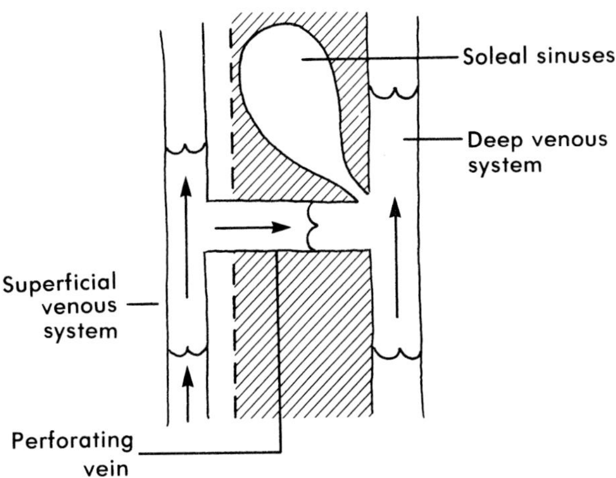

Fig. 51-15. Schematic representation of the valvular relationships in the superficial veins, the connecting veins or perforators, and the deep venous system. It can be seen that under normal circumstances flow only occurs from the superficial to deep channels.

gastrocnemius and soleus muscles that communicate with the deep veins (Fig. 51-14). It is these structures that the calf muscles compress and empty during contraction, facilitating venous emptying of the lower limb. These vein segments are also devoid of valves and are a common site of early thrombus formation. They coalesce to join the peroneal and posterior tibial vessels.

The superficial and deep venous systems of the lower extremity are united by a series of perforating veins that pass from the superficial venous system through the deep fascia to the deep venous channels. These venous conduits range in number from 100 to 200 and are also most frequently located below the level of the knee. Bicuspid valves are also located in these channels so that under normal circumstances flow occurs only from the superficial to the deep venous system (Fig. 51-15). Venous flow in the lower extremity therefore always travels in a centripetal direction from peripheral to central channels. The presence of valves prevents reflux in the superficial, deep, and connecting systems. The necessity for valves is greatest at the most peripheral locations, where the gravitational force is greatest, and is least important in the central venous channels, where the pressure changes generated by respiration are sufficient to overcome the effects of gravity.

In addition to blood traveling from the peripheral to central regions, it also moves preferentially from the superficial to the deep system with only 10% of the venous outflow being conducted by the superficial veins and 90% by the deep veins.

Structural Features

The vein wall varies from one third to one tenth of the thickness compared with arteries. Elastin wall content is considerably less than in the arterial wall, but (like arteries) the amount of smooth muscle in the media is variable. The major factor influencing the smooth muscle content is not the necessity for control of regional blood flow (as in arteries) but rather the gravitational force from blood the wall must withstand. The great saphenous vein has the highest percentage of smooth muscle because it is located in the subcutaneous tissue in the lower extremity, where it is exposed to maximum gravitational force with standing. At the foot and ankle smooth muscle may account for as much as 80% of the total wall thickness, whereas in the axillary vein it composes only 5% of the vein wall.

The smooth muscle fibers are arranged in helical bundles united by strands of connective tissue with a tough outer layer of predominantly collagen fibers constituting the adventitia. Deep to the smooth muscle layer is the intima, the most important component of which is the single layer of endothelial cells responsible for blood/vessel wall interface integrity. Perhaps because of the relatively low velocity in the venous system, these cells contain abundant quantities of fibrinolytic agents, with the veins in the lower extremity having higher concentrations than the intimal cells of the upper extremity. The lowest concentration of fibrinolytic active substances is found in the deep veins of the calf region and may in part explain the predisposition for thrombi to form in this location.

The deep veins are surrounded by skeletal muscle that

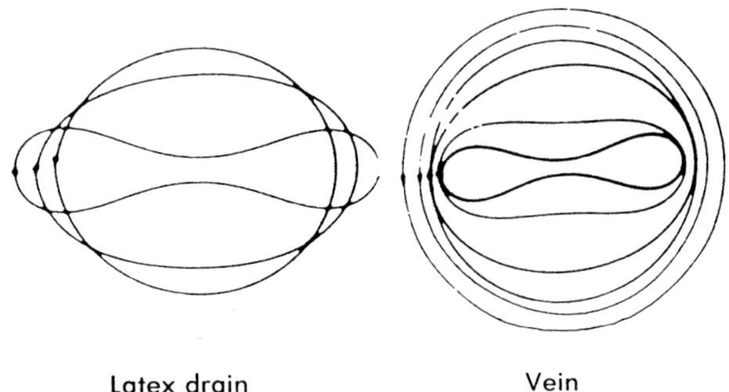

Fig. 51-16. Capacitance of collapsible tubes. Effect of volume change on the cross-sectional area of veins showing the small cross-sectional ellipsoid state and the significant increase in cross-sectional area associated with filling. This change occurs without a change in circumference; because the wall is not stretched, the change can occur with the application of relatively minor force.

protects them from the adverse effects of gravity. Thus they contain relatively small amounts of smooth muscle and large amounts of collagen. This structural feature is the major factor responsible for the relative stiffness of veins as compared to arteries. In the large central veins contained within the body cavities such as the vena cava, this property is of major importance in determining the shape changes induced by alterations in pressure-volume characteristics. Reductions in the volume of blood in these vessels result in collapse of the wall and assumption of an elliptical shape (Fig. 51-16). Restoration of volume to normal is associated with a resumption of the normal resting circular cross section. This shape change can also occur with the application of minimum external force. Although the pressure generated by respiration may produce similar changes, it is primarily a response of the major central veins to the volume of blood in the system.

These changes in venous volume are accomplished with minimum changes in pressure, since most veins are partially collapsed during resting conditions. The importance of this is appreciated when it is realized that 40% of the total blood volume may be found in these large central veins at a pressure of 5 mm Hg, whereas a reduction to 5% is accompanied by a fall in pressure of only a few millimeters of mercury. Thus the central venous system may be classified as a high-compliance, high-capacitance system compared to the low-compliance, low-capacitance arterial system. Also unlike arterioles, which are very sensitive to local mediators, veins and venules are controlled exclusively by sympathetic adrenergic activity except for the veins in skeletal muscle, which are without sympathetic influence, and cutaneous veins, which are primarily thermoregulatory. Venous constriction may occur secondary to Valsalva maneuvers, muscular exercise, pain, hyperventilation, and emotional stress. Drugs such as epinephrine, norepinephrine, phenylephrine, serotonin, and histamine cause venous constriction, whereas phenoxybenzamine, phentolamine, reserpine, guanethidine, nitroprusside, barbituates, and many other anesthetic agents cause vasodilation. In the clinical state of hypovolemic shock, the central veins collapse and autotransfuse their volume to the arterial system to maintain nutritional blood flow. Of practical clinical importance is the fact that the pressure measured in the central veins may be used as an index of the moment-to-moment block volume (i.e., high pressures represent an expanded blood volume, and low pressures a volume deficiency). These pressure changes have a major effect on cardiac performance and are discussed elsewhere in this book.

Pressure-Flow Relationships

In contrast to the arterial system, blood flow throughout the venous system is not mediated by a central pumping mechanism. The forces affecting pressure and therefore flow in the venous system are generated by respiration and exercise. The relative importance and interaction of these forces are best understood by considering the independent effects of each one and how they impact on the gravitational forces that must be overcome in the erect position.

Gravitational Effects

Gravitational forces have a negative effect on venous flow from the lower extremity and are best appreciated by considering the pressure relationships first in the supine position when gravity is not a factor. In the venular end of the capillaries the pressure is normally approximately 15 mm Hg, and the pressure in the right atrium 5 mm Hg. There is a point in the venous system located in the inferior vena cava close to the diaphragm termed the hydrostatic indifference point, where the pressure is always zero, regardless of attitude (Fig. 51-17). These pressure gradients are adequate to sustain normal venous return in the supine position but are augmented, as is detailed later, by respiratory-induced pressure changes.

Assumption of the erect position results in profound changes in these pressure relationships. The system can then be likened to a vertical column of fluid approximately 180 cm in height in a hypothetic six-foot "dead man," although certain modifications of this model are required to parallel the real circumstances (see Fig. 51-17). As noted earlier, the pressure at the hydrostatic indifference point is unchanged by the erect position, and right atrial pressure is normally 0 mm Hg. The veins above this point either fill or collapse, depending on the degree of filling in the system and the effects of respiration. This is best seen clinically in the external jugular vein, where intermittent filling and decompression are readily apparent. The skull acts as a protective barrier against these collapsing forces and maintains distention of the intracerebral venous channels even in the erect position. Below the hydrostatic indifference point the pressure gradually increases so that at the foot level a hydrostatic pressure of 80 mm Hg is produced. This has two profound effects, the first of which is cessation of flow from the lower extremities and progressive pooling in the leg veins. This associated reduction in venous return secondarily produces a major decrease in

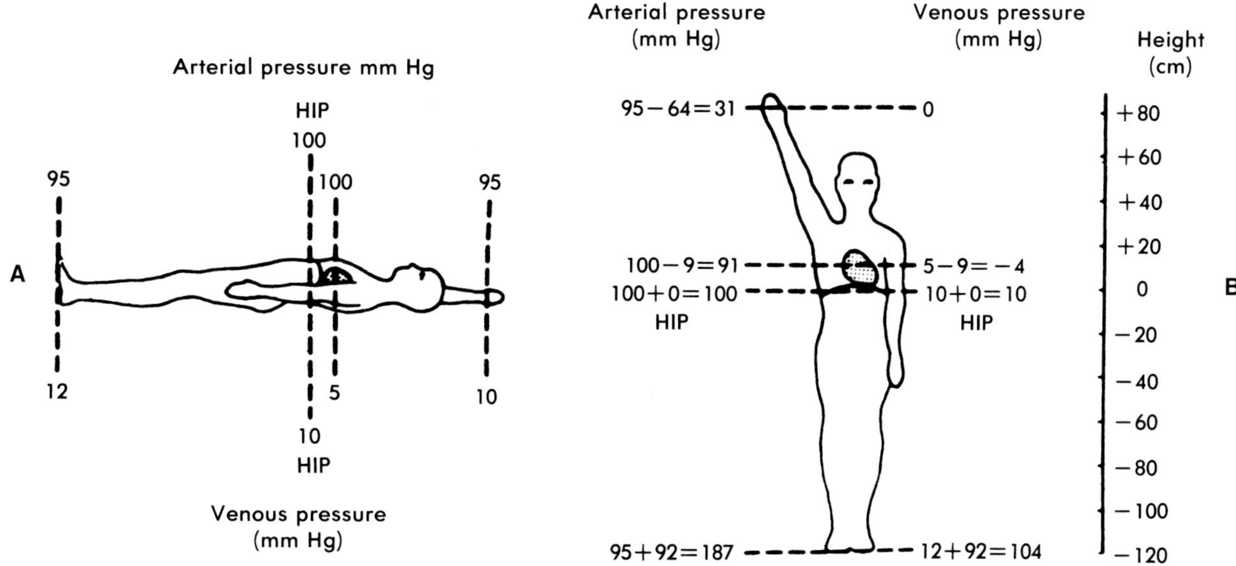

Fig. 51-17. Pressure relationships in the various levels of the arterial and venous system shown in the supine **(A)** and the erect positions **(B)**. Hydrostatic indifference point *(HIP)* is located just below the diaphragm.

cardiac output and, if the stimulus is long enough, may activate the syncope reflex. This pressure is also apparent in a change of the fluid dynamics at the tissue level; again, if it persists for any prolonged period, massive extravascular fluid extravasation may occur, further depleting venous return. This negative effort on venous circulation by gravity is overcome by the combined effects of respiration and exercise.

Effects of Respiration

The effects of respiration on venous flow are, again, most easily understood by first considering the pressure characteristics and changes that occur with the subjects in the supine position. During inspiration negative pressure is generated in the thoracic cavity, which facilitates flow into the superior mediastinum from the venous channels in the head, neck, and upper extremity. Descent of the diaphragm produces an increase in intra-abdominal pressure that compresses the inferior vena cava and is associated with a marked reduction in flow from the lower extremities. The pressure changes produced by respiration are insufficient to overcome the gradient that exists between the peripheral venules and the right atrium, and therefore even during inspiration there is some venous outflow from the lower extremities. Cessation of flow may be relatively easily produced, however, by increasing the pressure a few millimeters of mercury, as occurs with a Valsalva maneuver. Conversely, during expiration venous return from the upper extremity and head and neck is interrupted, and flow from the lower extremity is augmented (Fig. 51-18).

Assumption of the erect position, however, introduces the force of gravity that drastically alters the pressure-flow relationships. Without the pulsatile pump of the arterial system, the venous circulation does not contain an intrinsic mechanism capable of overcoming this effect. Clearly the relatively small changes induced by respiration are inadequate for normal venous return, and additional forces must be activated. Prolonged assumption of the erect position without activation of other mechanisms results in a serious disturbance of the hydrostatic forces at the tissue level, with the development of both peripheral edema and venous pooling in the lower extremity. A major force responsible for maintenance of normal venous return in the erect position is contraction of the calf muscles of the lower extremity.

Pressure Changes With Exercise

The calf muscle pump is to the venous system what the left ventricle is to the arterial system. The changes produced by calf muscle contraction are best considered by reviewing (1) the overall net effect after multiple muscle contractions and (2) the step-by-step pressure relationships. Calf muscle contractions exert a force in excess of 80 mm Hg on the walls of the veins in the calf, thus exceeding that exerted by gravity and resulting in a net efflux of blood out of the limb. With each contraction the venous pressure is progressively lowered until after 10 contractions the mean pressure at the ankle level falls to approximately 15 mm Hg, similar to that in the quiet resting supine state. This is responsible for an overall reduction in the resistance of the peripheral vascular system and an associated increase in arterial inflow to the extremity necessary for normal exercise requirement. Although this is the mean effect of exercise, the moment-to-moment pressure changes are more complex.

During the phase of calf muscle relaxation or diastole,

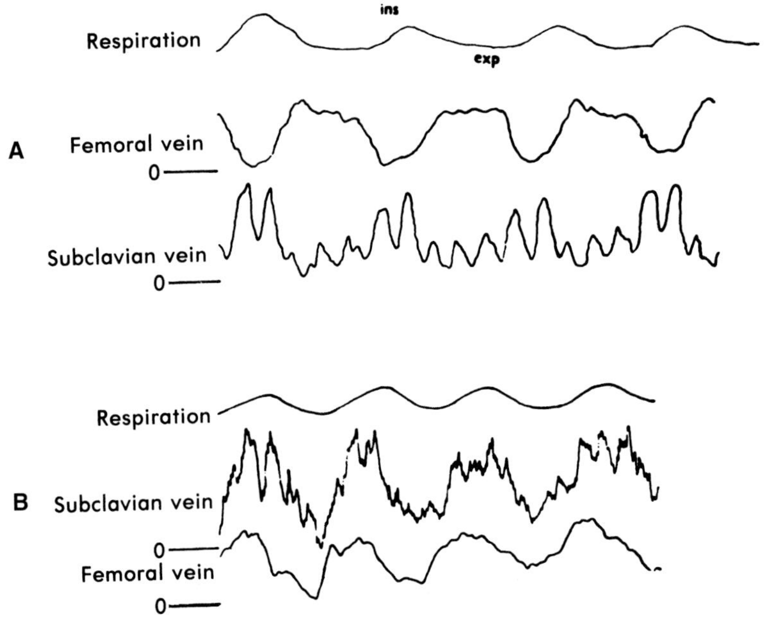

Fig. 51-18. Relationship between respiration and flow in the femoral and subclavian veins in the supine **(A)** and in the erect position **(B)**. *ins,* Inspiration; *exp,* expiration.

the large venous channels are distended, and the pressure in the deep veins falls below that in the superficial veins. During calf muscle contraction, however, the pressure in the deep veins increases dramatically to exceed the pressure in the superficial veins, with a pumping effect being generated and forcing venous blood out of the extremity in an antegrade direction. In veins with acute thrombosis the venous pressure stays the same. As the level of obstruction increases, so does the average venous pressure and limb circumference, resulting in edema and inflammation. During calf muscle relaxation, therefore, flow occurs from the superficial venous system to the deep venous system through the perforating veins; this flow is facilitated by the unidirectional valves contained in the perforating veins. During calf muscle contraction the unidirectional valves in the deep venous system result in blood being forced to flow in a centripetal direction, with the valves in the perforating veins preventing blood from entering into the superficial system from the deep. It is imperative that the valves be working correctly. At the completion of calf muscle contraction, the cycle is again repeated (Fig. 51-19). Therefore it can be said of the peripheral muscle pump that it resembles the heart in circulating blood, decreases edema and venous congestion in the extremities, and increases central blood volume. The increase in frequency and depth of respiration associated with exercise acts to facilitate overall venous return.

Venous Endothelium

Our understanding of the venous endothelial cell has broadened secondary to recent studies addressing its function and effect on vessel morphology. The endothelium is involved in the perception of changes in blood flow and can influence vessel luminal size by changing the degree of contraction of the smooth muscle present in the vessel wall. It has been shown that the performance of many medications and natural substances that alter vessel size depend on an intact endothelium. The effects of acetylcholine result in vasodilation, while in vessels devoid of the endothelium vasoconstriction occurs. Isoproterenol, adenosine, papaverine, and prostacyclin cause vasodilation. Norepinephrine, serotonin, arachidonic acid, histamine, bradykinin, vasopressin, thrombin, cholecystokinin, and vasoactive intestinal polypeptide cause vasoconstriction. The endothelial cell–dependent dilation is related to the production of a nonprostanoid endothelial factor that results in a rise in cyclic guanosine monophosphate. Recent studies have linked this activity to nitric oxide, which is derived from L-arginine, which has high concentrations in small resistance vessels. The intact endothelium also has been shown to reduce platelet-induced spasms of the vessel wall. If the endothelial lining is undiminished, the complete absence of blood flow for a prolonged period of time does not result in clotting. Furthermore, the endothelium produces several antithrombotic substances and a number of procoagulants such as heparin sulfate and thrombomodulin, prostacyclin, factor VIII, and von Willebrand's factor.

Physiologic Changes Induced by Disease

Acute Venous Thrombosis

The development of occlusive thrombi in the major axial veins of the venous system obviously has an effect of preventing normal venous outflow from the extremities (Fig. 51-20). The effect can be used as a diagnostic test with plethysmographic methods to identify acute venous throm-

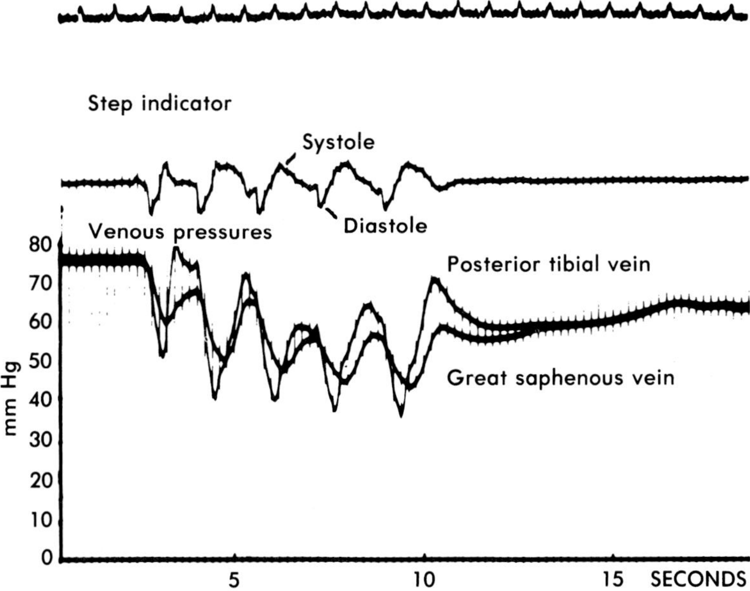

Fig. 51-19. Pressure relationship between the superficial and deep venous system during walking. It should be noted that during calf muscle contraction or systole, the pressure in the deep system exceeds that in the superficial; whereas during calf muscle relaxation pressure in the deep system is less than in the superficial. Filling of the calf muscle pump therefore occurs as with the heart during diastole. *Posterior tibial vein,* Deep vein; *great saphenous vein,* superficial vein.

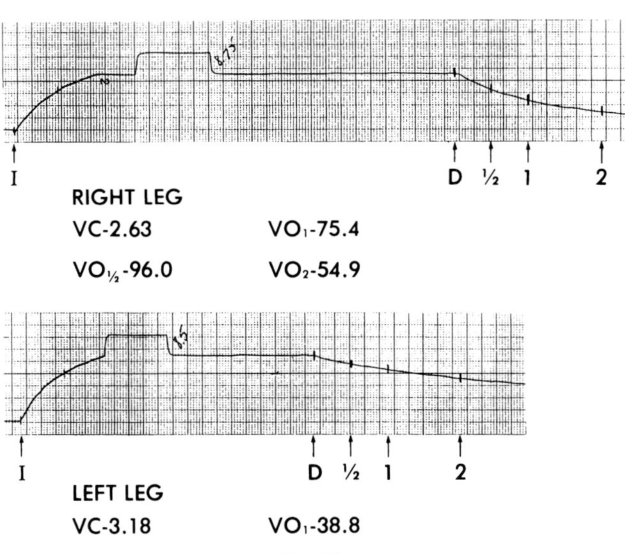

Fig. 51-20. Plethysmographic recordings from 60-year-old man 4 months after left iliofemoral deep vein thrombosis. Recordings were obtained from the right leg with no deep vein thrombosis and left leg with superficial femoral vein thrombosis. Recordings are obtained by inflating a pressure cuff above venous pressure followed by instantaneous release of the pressure. Rate of emptying is significantly less in right leg compared to left leg, a fact that can be used in a diagnostic investigation. *I,* Inflate; *D,* deflate; *VC,* venous capacitance; *VO,* venous exit flow.

bosis. Physiologically, the presence of a major axial vein obstruction results in a gradual rise in the pressure at the venular end of the capillaries, with the subsequent development of edema. This effect, however, is quite variable and depends not only on the location and extent of the venous thrombosis but also on the availability of collateral venous channels to compensate for the obstruction. It is therefore not infrequent to observe that venous thrombosis may not be associated with significant edema because of the presence of a well-functioning collateral network.

A secondary effect of an occlusive thrombus and the development of peripheral venous hypertension is that the minor pressure changes produced by respiration are not transmitted beyond the area of obstruction. Therefore flow distal to the obstruction loses its normal phasic relationship to respiration and becomes continuous. This effect can be detected with simple Doppler devices that evaluate velocity in the venous system and can easily detect increases and decreases in velocity in the normal system produced by respiration and, conversely, the uniform velocity present in cases of venous obstruction; the effect carries a 92% sensitivity (Fig. 51-21). Visualizing a thrombus carries a 96% specificity and a 94% sensitivity with an overall accuracy of 96%.

Air plethysmography (APG) has been used to quantitate venous reflux and calf muscle pump ejection volume (Fig. 51-22). The instrument uses an air-filled chamber wrapped around the lower leg to determine absolute volume changes in the leg as a result of exercise. Baseline limb volume is measured with the patient supine and the leg elevated 45 degrees to empty the veins. Volume measurements are then made during non–weight-bearing standing, and with single and repetitive calf muscle contractions. Calculations are then made to determine venous filling index (VFI), ejection fraction (EF), and residual volume fraction (RVF). Plethysmography is usually used to evaluate the venous system in preparation for venous surgery for severe reflux.

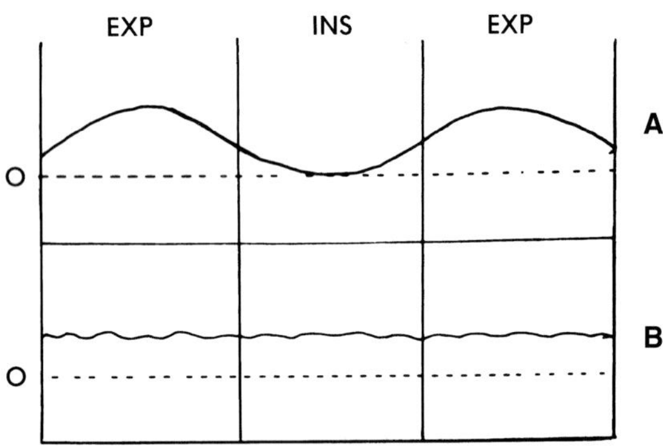

Fig. 51-21. Venous flow patterns in the normal state **(A)** and in the presence of venous obstruction **(B)**. It should be noted that in the latter there is a loss of the oscillatory pattern produced by respiration. *EXP,* Expiration; *INS,* inspiration.

Chronic (Postthrombotic) Venous Insufficiency

The adverse long-term sequelae of venous thrombosis are produced by residual venous obstruction and the destruction of valves in both the deep axial veins and the perforating veins. This latter effect in particular produces profound changes in the dynamics of the venous circulation during exercise, which at least in part are responsible for the clinical changes of edema, hyperpigmentation, and ulceration.

The most significant changes are seen during exercise. Valve destruction adversely affects the flow patterns produced by the pressure changes seen with exercise; instead of flowing in a centripetal direction and from superficial to deep, blood may be forced under high pressure from the deep system during calf muscle contraction through incompetent perforating veins into the superficial system, producing severe superficial hypertension. In the deep system the normal antegrade flow pattern is completely interrupted, and venous return from the leg is significantly reduced.

Instead of a gradual reduction in venous pressure in the lower extremity produced by exercise, in severe cases exercise may actually be associated with an increase in the venous pressure in both the deep and superficial systems as depicted in Fig. 51-23. The likelihood of developing se-

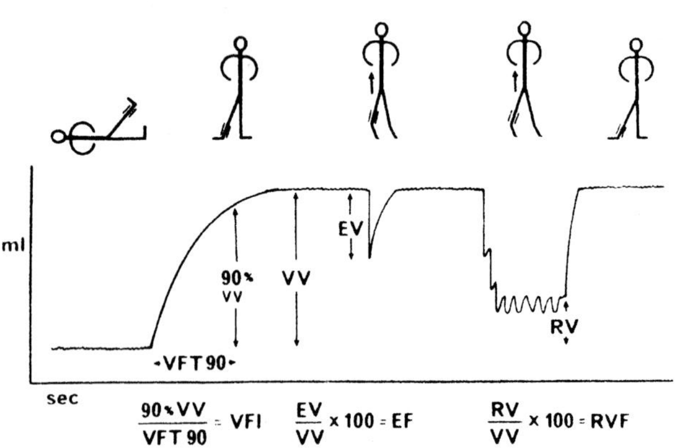

Fig. 51-22. Methods of deriving air plethysmography values. *EV,* Evoked potential; *VFI,* venous filling index; *VFT,* venous filling time; *VV,* venous volume; *RV,* residual volume; *RVF,* residual volume fraction. (From Belcaro G, et al. Noninvasive tests in venous insufficiency. J Cardiovasc Surg 34:3,1993. Reprinted with permission.)

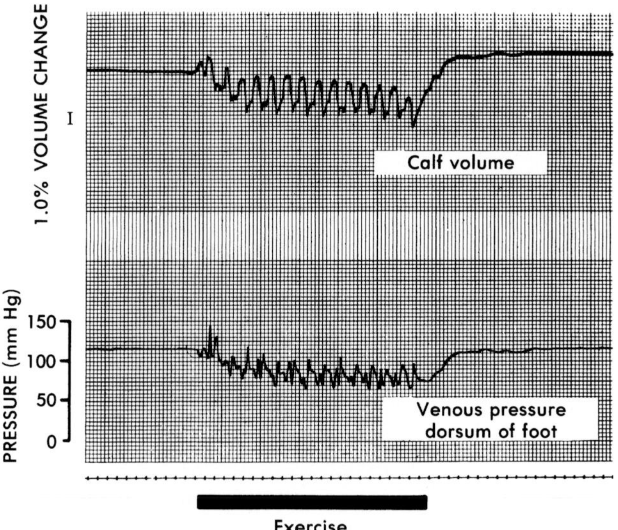

Fig. 51-23. Effect of calf muscle exercise on ankle pressure in patients with the postthrombotic syndrome. There is no significant decrease in venous pressure associated with exercise as is seen in the normal state.

Table 51-5. Relation of Ambulatory Venous Hypertension to Incidence of Ulceration

Ambulatory Venous Pressure (mm Hg)	Incidence of Ulceration (%)
45	0
45-50	5
50-59	15
60-69	50
70-79	75
80	80

vere complications such as venous ulceration is closely related to the degree of ambulatory venous hypertension that occurs in such patients as shown in Table 51-5.

LYMPHATIC SYSTEM

Just as the venous system is primarily responsible for the return of blood constituents to the heart, the lymphatic system provides a conduit for the return of fluid and other molecular constituents (e.g., protein) in the interstitial space, in large part independent of the fluid exchanges occurring at the capillary level. Although the lymphatics also provide a route for lymphocyte transport, this function is not considered in this review. As in the arterial and venous circulations, knowledge of the lymphatic anatomy is essential to understanding the physiologic characteristics of lymphatic flow and diseases of the lymph channels.

Lymphatic Anatomy

As with the venous system, the lymphatics in the extremities are divided into superficial and deep conduits. The majority of the lymphatic effluent from the extremities travels through the superficial lymphatics. These channels commence as minute blind sacs in the soft tissues that coalesce to form a plexus of small vessels subjacent to the skin termed the subpapillary dermal plexus. They progressively unite to form the definitive lymph channels located in the subcutaneous tissues. The lymphatic system includes vascular conduits, spleen, lymph nodes, Peyer's patches, thymus, nasopharyngeal tonsils, and circulating cellular elements such as macrophages and lymphocytes. Lymphatics are absent in tendons, muscle, cornea, brain, and cartilage.

The major lymphatic channels of the lower limb begin in the dorsum of the foot on the medial side and course predominantly along the medial side of the leg intimately related to the great saphenous vein and through the thigh to the superficial group of inguinal lymph nodes adjacent to the termination of this vein. These channels empty their lymphatics into the superficial nodes and subsequently into the deep inguinal lymph nodes around the common femoral vein. The lymphatic vessels are approximately 1 to 2 mm in diameter throughout the extremity with unidirectional valves located every few millimeters. In the thigh region there are usually five of these trunks, and on occasion as many as seven or eight are visualized with techniques such as lymphoscintigraphy. This is the best test for diagnosis of lymphedema, and it involves injection of radiolabeled antimony trisulfide (technetium 99m [$_{99m}$Tc]–human serum albumin [HAS]) colloid interstitially into the interdigital space with subsequent imaging of the limb with a dual-headed gamma counter. Regional lymph nodes should be exposed in 15 to 60 minutes. A study result is considered abnormal if regional lymph nodes do not show uptake, delayed or absent clearance of tracer from injection site, dermal backflow, or abnormal tracer accumulation. Sensitivity and specificity range between 95% and 100%.

The deep lymphatic channels in the lower extremity are less numerous than the superficial channels and, like their deep venous counterparts, course in close proximity to the deep muscular arteries. In the calf region these channels are relatively small but progressively enlarge in the thigh and terminate in the deep inguinal group of lymph nodes. Efferents from the deep inguinal lymph nodes course along the brim of the pelvis, usually in three different groups of channels intimately related to the major vessels in these locations. In the region of the lumbosacral joint these channels coalesce on each side to form the para-aortic lymph channels that are, again, numerous. Throughout the course from the groin to the region of the abdominal aorta, there are numerous large pelvic lymph nodes interspersed along these channels. Lymph from the lower extremity is eventually joined by chyle from the intestinal lymphatics in the cisterna chyle and transported through the thorax by way of the thoracic duct, terminating in the posterior triangle on the left side at the junction of the internal jugular and subclavian veins.

Lymphatic Structure

The actual structure of the lymphatics provides important clues to the functional characteristics of lymphatic flow. The anatomic features of most physiologic importance are the presence of bicuspid valves throughout the lymphatics and smooth muscle located uniformly in the wall of the lymphatic channel. The bicuspid valves are located every few centimeters along the course of the lymphatic channels and enable lymph flow to occur from the periphery to the central regions. The lymphatic channels are capable of independent contraction (propulsor lymphaticum), exerting pressures in the vicinity of 50 mm Hg during these contractions, which may occur up to four to five times per minute. These contractions, like venous and arterial vasomotion, are mediated by sympathomimetic agents (α- and β-adrenergic agents), by products of arachidonic acid metabolism (thromboxanes and prostaglandins), and neurogenic stimuli. Basal activity sensitivity varies depending on body location. Lymphatic adventitia, like their arterial and venous counterparts, contain actin and are therefore capable of exhibiting vasomotion and self-propagation of fluid.

Characteristics of Lymph Flow

The primary function of the lymph vessels is to transport larger molecules such as protein from the tissues back to the central venous system. As much as 50% of circulating albumin is lost into the interstitial space every 24 hours. During this time an average of 2 to 4 L of protein-rich (75 to 100 g) lymph is returned in the venous circulation. Lymphatic flow disruption from occlusion or trauma can interfere with fluid dynamics, homeostasis, and immunologic function.

An understanding of the lymph circulation is integrally related to the exchanges that occur at the capillary level, of which two main processes can be implicated (i.e., filtration and diffusion). Filtration is primarily responsible for movement of fluid across the capillary membranes and is governed by the forces expounded by Starling in 1896. At the arterial end of the capillary there is a net efflux of fluid into the tissues, whereas at the venous end there is a net return of fluid from the tissues back into the venular end of the capillary. Under normal circumstances there is a slight excess of fluid filtered over that reabsorbed, and it is this fluid that is removed from the tissues by the lymphatics. It should be emphasized, however, that fluid exchange at the capillary level is primarily a function of the capillaries and not the lymphatics. It is now apparent that diffusion plays a major role in the exchange of molecules across the capillary membrane and may occur independently of the fluid fluxes present. The only factor influencing the diffusion process is the semipermeable nature of the capillary membrane and the size of the pores in this membrane. However, proteins that diffuse into the tissues can easily enter the highly permeable lymphatics and are subsequently transported out of the tissues.

Once this fluid and large molecular complex (1000 kilodaltons) enter the lymphatic circulation, the dynamics of the return of the lymph fluid to the major central channels must be considered. As in the venous system, unidirectional flow of lymph depends on the presence of the bicuspid valves; however, unlike veins, muscular contractions in the ducts rather than respiration, arterial pulsations, or external massage are responsible for the majority of lymphatic flow under normal circumstances. The rate and force of these contractions are determined by the filling pressures (preload) and outflow resistance. Occluded and obstructed lymphatic vessels have been known to have pressures as high as 50 to 60 mm Hg; unlike the venous system, a collateral system does not exist. Rapid standing leads to increased venous pressure in the venous system, while in the lymphatic system this does not occur because of an increase in the frequency and amplitude of wall pulsations. As noted earlier, the unidirectional valves encourage flow to occur from the periphery of the limb to the central locations; however, in the minute lymphatic capillaries of the dermal plexus, valves are absent and flow may occur in any direction. Additionally, terminal lymphatics function as a suction pump facilitating the entry of interstitial fluid into the lymphatics in both normal and pathologic states. Contraction of the lymphatic wall may result in the generation of a positive pressure proximal to the area of contraction and a negative pressure at the bulbous terminal portion of the lymphatic that facilitates entry of interstitial fluid. A mechanism such as this is essential for the movement of fluid into the lymphatic system because recent evidence has suggested that interstitial fluid pressure may, in fact, be negative.

Lymphatics in Disease

Although a detailed pathologic description of the various disease states affecting the lymphatics is beyond the scope of this chapter, each has a final common denominator in that lymphatic outflow from the extremity is impaired. Skin and limb changes with lymphatic obstruction or inefficient lymphatic outflow are different from those seen with arterial or venous obstruction. If flow in the arteriolar and venular side of the capillary ceases, the supply of essential nutritional requirements to tissues is impaired, and tissue necrosis results. With lymphatic obstruction, there is a gradual accumulation of large protein molecules in the tissue, increased oncotic pressure, and a net accumulation of fluid with the development of the condition known as "lymphedema." The diffusion of essential nutritional elements may still proceed unimpeded, and thus tissue necrosis does not occur even in the presence of quite severe edema. Eventually, a steady state is reached at which the hydrostatic pressure exerted by the fluid in the tissues balances the oncotic pressure, and essentially normal fluid exchange then continues. Despite a new balance in fluid dynamics, however, the presence of this interstitial edema remains unless altered by external pressures. The practical importance of this knowledge is that it is possible to forcefully expel this edematous fluid from the extremity with the application of external pumps that exceed the hydrostatic interstitial fluid pressure, resulting in a reduction in the extremity edema.

SUMMARY

The circulatory system as a whole serves to maintain normal tissue nutrition under conditions of rest and peak exercise, with both the arterial and venous systems, like many others in the body, having a major functional reserve capacity. The arterial and venous systems are primarily involved in the maintenance of a favorable tissue milieu for normal metabolism, with the lymphatics functioning as a scavenger system to remove macromolecules and any excess of fluid that is extravasated from the capillary mechanism. Whereas the arterial system is dynamic with the energy being provided intrinsically by contraction of the left ventricle, both the venous and lymphatic systems are uniquely designed to facilitate movement of fluid under relatively low pressures and to rely predominantly on extrinsic forces such as respiration and skeletal muscle contraction to offset the negative effects of gravity.

SUGGESTED READINGS

Arnoldi CC. Venous pressure in the leg of healthy human subjects at rest and during muscular exercise in the nearly erect position. Acta Chir Scand 130:520, 1965.

Basmajian JV. Distribution of valves in femoral, internal iliac and common iliac veins and their relationship to varicose veins. Surg Gynecol Obstet 95:537, 1952.

Burton AC. Physiology and Biophysics of the Circulation. Chicago: Year Book Medical Publishers, 1972.

Cockett FB, Dodd H, eds. The Pathology and Surgery of the Veins of the Lower Limb. Edinburgh: Churchill Livingstone, 1976.

DeWeese JA, Rogoff SM. Phlebographic patterns of acute deep venous thrombosis of the leg. Surgery 53:99, 1963.

Ellwood RA, Lee WB. Pedal venous pressure: Correlation with presence and site of deep venous abnormalities. Radiology 131:73, 1979.

Folkow B, Neil E. Circulation. Oxford: Oxford University Press, 1971.

Furchgott RF, VanHoutte PM. Endothelium-derived relaxing and contracting factors. FASEB J 3:2007, 1989.

Geddes LA, Baker LE. Principles of Applied Biomedical Instrumentation, 2nd ed. New York: John Wiley, 1975.

Griffith TM, et al. Endothelium-derived relaxing factor. J Am Coll Cardiol 12:797, 1988.

Gupta AK, et al. The natural history of infrainguinal vein graft stenosis relative to bypass grafting technique. J Vasc Surg 25:211, 1997.

Guyton AC. Human Physiology and Mechanisms of Disease, 2nd ed. Philadelphia: WB Saunders, 1982.

Ingebrigtsen R, Leraand S. Dilatation of a medium-sized artery immediately after local changes of blood pressure and flow as measured by ultrasonic technique. Acta Physiol Scand 79:552, 1970.

Johnston MG. The intrinsic lymph pump: Progress and problems. Lymphology 22:116, 1989.

Johnston MG, Feuer C. Suppression of lymphatic vessel contractility with inhibitors of arachidonic acid metabolism. J Pharmacol Exp Ther 226:603, 1983.

Johnston MG, Gordon JL. Regulation of lymphatic contractility by arachidonate metabolites. Nature 293:294, 1981.

Kamiya A, Tagowa T. Adaptive regulation of wall shear stress to flow change in the canine carotid artery. Am J Physiol 239:H14, 1980.

Lerman A, Burnett JC, Jr. Intact and altered endothelium in regulation of vasomotion. [review]. Circulation 86(Suppl 6):III12, 1992.

Ludbrook J. Functional aspects of the veins of the leg. Am Heart J 64:796, 1962.

McDonald DS. Blood Flow in Arteries. London: Edward Arnold, 1974.

McHale NG, Roddie IC. The effect of intravenous adrenaline and noradrenaline infusion on peripheral lymph flow in sheep. J Physiol 341:517, 1983.

Mehta JL. Endothelium, coronary vasodilation, and organic nitrates. Am Heart J 129(2):382, 1995.

Milnor WR. Hemodynamics. Baltimore: Williams & Wilkins, 1982.

Mohiaddin RH, et al. MR phase-shift velocity mapping of mitral and pulmonary venous flow. J Comput Assist Tomogr 15:237, 1991.

Moreno AH, et al. Mechanics of distension of dog veins and other thin-walled tubular structures. Circ Res 27:1069, 1970.

Ohhashi T, Kawai Y, Azuma T. The response of lymphatic smooth muscles to vasoactive substances. Pflugers Arch 375:183, 1978.

Olszewski WL. Lymph Pressure and Flow in Limbs in Lymph Stasis: Pathophysiology, Diagnosis and Treatment. Boca Raton, Fla.: CRC Press, 1991, p 109.

Pippard C, Roddie IC. Resistance in the sheep lymphatic system. Lymphology 20:230, 1987.

Reddy NP. Lymph circulation: Physiology, pharmacology, and biomechanics. CRC Crit Rev Biomed Engl 14:45, 1986.

Rhodin JA. Architecture of the vessel wall. In Handbook of Physiology: The Cardiovascular System. Baltimore: Williams & Wilkins, 1982.

Roddie IC. Lymph transport mechanisms in peripheral lymphatics. News Physiol Sci 5:85, 1990.

Sjoberg T, Steen S. Contractile properties of lymphatics from the human lower leg. Lymphology 24:16, 1991.

Smith JJ, Kampine JP. Circulatory Physiology—The Essentials, 2nd ed. Baltimore: Williams & Wilkins, 1984.

Stegall HF. Muscle pumping in the dependent leg. Circ Res 19:180, 1966.

Strandness DE, Sumner DS. Hemodynamics for Surgeons. New York: Grune & Stratton, 1975.

Sumner DS. Diagnosis of deep vein thrombosis. In Rutherford RB, ed. Vascular Surgery, 4th ed, vol 2. Philadelphia: WB Saunders, 1993, p 1698.

Todd AS, Nunn A. The histological localization of fibrinolysin activator. J Pathol Bacteriol 78:281, 1959.

Way D, et al. Lymphatic endothelial cell line (CH3) from a recurrent retroperitoneal lymphangioma. In Vitro 23:647, 1987.

Yoffey JM, Courtice FC. Lymphatics, Lymph and Lymphoid Tissue. Baltimore: Williams & Wilkins, 1967.

52

Aorta and Arterial Disease of the Lower Extremity

Christopher K. Zarins and Ronald L. Dalman

Although congenital and inflammatory diseases of the aorta and lower extremity arteries do exist, degenerative complications of atherosclerosis account for the vast majority of complications related to and developing from these vessels.[1] Atherosclerosis is an age-related, degenerative disease. With the rapid growth of the elderly population in the United States, by the year 2040 people older than 65 will comprise 22% of the population, or 67 million people. The most striking aspect of this trend is the increased rate of survival of those older than 75.[2] Obviously, the management of atherosclerotic complications of the aorta and its branches will play an increasing role in the primary health care of a major portion of the adult American population.

Atherosclerotic arterial disease is characterized by the formation of intimal plaques. These plaques may obstruct the lumen, ulcerate and embolize, cause thrombosis, or contribute to aneurysmal degeneration of the arterial wall following remodeling. Each of these processes may result in a spectrum of clinical presentations requiring different diagnostic and therapeutic approaches. In this chapter we consider some of the general features of the atherosclerosis, along with its pathologic and clinical manifestations in the lower extremity, and discuss diagnostic methods and current treatment alternatives.

ATHEROSCLEROSIS

Risk Factors

The risk factors for atherosclerosis may be divided into two major categories, reversible and irreversible. In addition, there are major interactions between the two categories. Major reversible factors include cigarette smoking, diabetes mellitus, hyperglycemia, hypertension, abnormalities of lipid metabolism, obesity, and low levels of physical activity. Nonreversible factors are primarily sex, age, and genetic influences of family history.

It has been generally assumed that the factors associated with plaque formation and development in the extracoronary arteries are the same as those in the coronary arteries.[2] However, there have been few population-based studies of risk factors associated with atherosclerosis of the aorta or the lower extremity branches. Several early studies considered only the symptomatic form of the disease.[3,4] More recently, noninvasive methods have been used to identify and include asymptomatic subjects in these investigations.[5,6] These findings are summarized in Table 52-1. The most significant risk factors apparently have independent effects (i.e., not cumulative) on the vasculature of the abdomen, pelvis, and lower extremity.

Control of certain risk factors may have a beneficial effect on the expression of the disease. Cessation of tobacco use has a beneficial effect on peripheral occlusive disease, and limb loss rates and arterial graft patency rates are improved in patients who can successfully abstain from tobacco.[7,8] Optimization of serum lipid profiles and control of hypertension have less certain impact on the progression of lower extremity arterial disease, but may be beneficial in preventing progression of coronary atherosclerosis.[2] Physical exercise may ameliorate the symptoms of aortic and peripheral occlusive disease, but its role in preventing progression is unknown. Weight reduction and control of environmental stress also play unknown roles. Recent data from the Diabetes Control and Complication Trial suggest that close control of serum glucose does not prevent progression or complications of peripheral vascular occlusive disease as measured by limb salvage in the setting of insulin-dependent diabetes mellitus.[9]

Configuration and Composition of Atherosclerotic Plaque

Although atherosclerotic plaques are distinguished by the presence of lipids, it is unclear whether all lesions containing lipids are necessarily precursors of clinically significant atherosclerotic plaques. A prime example of this uncertainty is demonstrated by the questionable significance of the so-called fatty streak lesion. This term describes a flat, yellow, focal luminal patch or streak, representing an accumulation of lipid-laden foam cells in the intima, evident in most people older than 3 years. They are identified with increasing frequency between the ages of 8 and 18

Table 52-1. Risk Factors Associated With the Development of Lower Extremity Arterial Disease, Disease Progression, and Mortality

Risk Factor	Development of Disease	Progression	Mortality
Smoking	Yes	Yes	Yes
Diabetes	Yes	Yes/No	Yes
Hyperlipidemia	Conflicting results for triglyceride, cholesterol, and lipoprotein	Conflicting results	Conflicting results
Systolic blood pressure	Yes; most but not all studies show blood pressure to be a strong predictor	Yes/No	Yes/No
Physical activity	NAI	Yes/No	No
Hemorheologic factors	Unclear	NAI	NAI
Obesity	No; however, may be a weak risk factor in men	NAI	NAI
Genetic factors	NAI	NAI	NAI

NAI, Not adequately investigated.

years, after which many apparently resolve. Fatty streaks exist at any age, often adjacent to or even superimposed on advanced atherosclerotic plaques. Fatty streaks and atheromata, however, do not have identical patterns of localization, and fatty streaks do no compromise the lumen or ulcerate.[10] Although this subject remains controversial, the link and transition between fatty streak and fibrous plaque formation remains to be clarified.

The term *fibrous plaque* identifies the characteristic and unequivocal atherosclerotic lesion. These intimal deposits appear in the second decade of life, becoming predominant or clinically significant only during or after the fourth decade. Fibrous plaques usually are eccentric and are covered by an intact endothelial surface. Although considerable variation exists in plaque composition and configuration, a characteristic architecture prevails. The immediate subendothelial region of the plaque consists of a compact and well-organized, stratified layer of smooth muscle cells and connective tissue fibers known as the fibrous cap. This structure may mimic medial architecture, including the formation of a subendothelial elastic lamina, which may function to sequester the underlying necrotic and thrombogenic plaque core from the luminal surface. This surface usually is regular, with a concave contour corresponding to the circular or oval cross-sectional lumen of the uninvolved vessel wall segment. The stable necrotic core occupies the deeper plaque (Fig. 52-1). The core contains amorphous, crystalline, and droplet forms of lipid. Cells of undetermined origin, with morphologic, functional, and cell surface receptor characteristics of smooth muscles or macrophages are noted beneath the core. These cells also may contain lipid vacuoles. Calcium and myxoid deposits, collagen and elastin matrix fibers, basal lamina, and amorphous ground substance also are evident. Atherosclerotic plaques grow in an episodic fashion, demonstrating dense fibrocellular regions adjacent to organizing thrombus and atheromatous debris. Intermittent ulceration and healing occur, with thrombi being incorporated into the lesion.

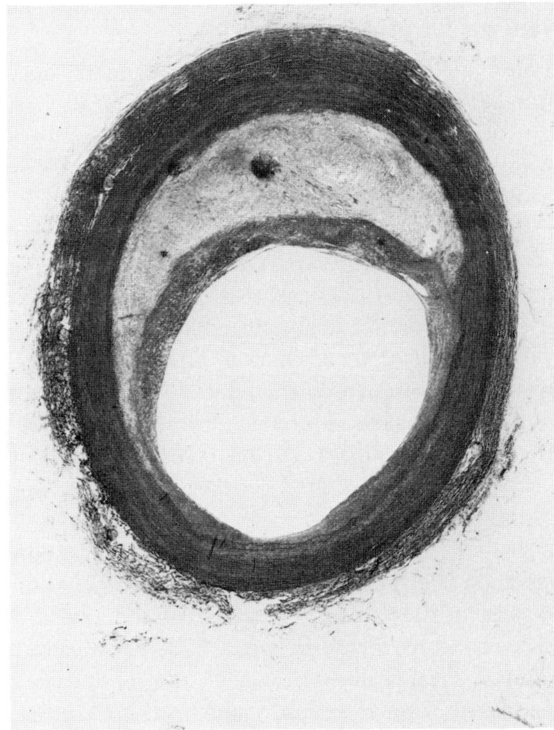

Fig. 52-1. Atherosclerotic plaque demonstrating the fibrous cap over a necrotic center. Note the oval external contour with the round lumen typical of these plaques.

Vasa vasorum may nourish the plaque, facilitating the organization of thrombotic deposits and the remodeling of the plaque and artery wall.[11] Attenuation of the subadjacent media promotes outward bulging of the plaque toward the adventitia. Although this attenuation sequesters plaque, enlarges the artery, and stabilizes the wall, a predominant lytic reaction may result in excessive arterial dilation or aneurysmal degeneration. Experimental evidence suggesting such a mechanism for aneurysm formation has been obtained in nonhuman primates in our laboratory[12] and by other investigators.[13]

Tissues between the necrotic core and the media, however, usually are densely fibrotic. Arterial wall support may thus be maintained by the integrity of the fibrous cap or thickened adventitia. Advanced lesions, particularly those associated with aneurysms, may appear to be atrophic and relatively acellular, consisting of dense fibrous tissue and a minimal necrotic center. Calcification is a prominent feature, involving the superficial and deeper layers. Terms such as *fibrocalcific, lipid-rich, necrotic,* and *myxomatous* describe various predominant aspects of advanced plaques. Calcific deposits are most prominent in plaques in older people and in the abdominal aorta or coronary arteries, where the earliest plaques form in animal models and in humans.[14] The usual eccentric plaque bulges outward from the lumen; the external cross-sectional contour of an atherosclerotic artery becomes oval while retaining a circular lumen.[15,16]

Localizing Factors in the Development of Atherosclerotic Lesions

Adaptive changes in artery luminal diameter are determined by changes in blood flow. During embryologic growth and development, lumen diameter is determined by the volume of blood flow. After birth, increases in artery diameter continue as a response to increases in blood flow.[17] This phenomenon also is demonstrated in mature arteries after cessation of growth, with enlargement of arteries proximal to arteriovenous fistulas and a decrease in the size of arteries proximal to amputated limbs.[18]

Luminal diameter adaptation is responsive to wall shear stress, as determined by the effective velocity gradient at the endothelial-blood interface.[19] In mammals, wall shear stress normally ranges between 10 and 20 dynes/cm^2 at all locations throughout the arterial vasculature. In arteriovenous fistulas, the afferent artery enlarges enough to restore shear stress to this physiologic range.[20] This response depends on the presence of an intact endothelial surface[21] and may be mediated by the release of endothelial-derived relaxant factors, including nitric oxide or other vasoactive agents.[22] Near-wall properties of arterial flow fields and the distribution of mural wall shear stress correspond closely to atherosclerotic plaque localization.[23-30] Plaques develop where shear stress is reduced,[25,26] not elevated, with an intact endothelial surface, even in the absence of platelet deposition.[31] The revised response to injury hypothesis now stresses metabolic or functional changes sustained by intact endothelial cells that alter binding or metabolism of lipid molecules or modify transendothelial transport, rather than denudation of the endothelium itself.[32]

Atherosclerosis tends to occur principally in three locations within the arterial vasculature: the carotid-cerebral, coronary, and aortic-peripheral system. Within these predisposed regions lesions form in predictable geometric configurations, demonstrating the influence of shear stress and flow patterns. Size, as well as localization, closely correlates with low wall shear stress and departures from unidirectional flow.[25,26] Plaque initiation and localization are the result of low rather than high shear stress, low flow velocity, flow separation, and oscillation in wall shear direction.[33]

Regions of increased mural tensile stress about branches,[23] pulsatile wall motion,[34] and wall thickness and density[35,36] also are associated with selective plaque localization. Conversely, regions of relatively elevated wall shear stress or reduced tensile stress, at flow dividers and along the outer or convex aspects of curved arterial segments, generally are spared.[37] Hemodynamics and tensile influences also are important in plaque progression and evolution[38,39] and influence potential plaque regression.[40] As an example of this influence on regression, hypertension was found to sustain experimental plaque progression in a hypercholesterolemic cynomolgus monkey model, despite a reduction in serum cholesterol level.[41] Reduced flow and consequent reduction in wall shear stress also tend to induce intimal thickening. An increase in wall volume, including cell enlargement, cell proliferation, and net matrix accumulation, is demonstrated in long-term reactions.[42]

A sieving effect related to these changes in wall composition[43,44] and porosity[35] has been proposed. Wall thickening, including intimal thickening, may retard transmural mass transport, providing the basis for intimal lipid deposition.[45] The accumulation of matrix fibers with affinity for lipid molecules[46-50] and the fusion or accretion of lipid particles on these components also may be responsible.

PATHOPHYSIOLOGIC PROCESSES AFFECTING THE AORTA AND LOWER EXTREMITY ARTERIES

The processes affecting the arteries to the lower extremity include plaque formation with obstruction of the lumen and subsequent limitation of flow, thrombosis resulting in acute ischemia, ulceration of the plaque with distal embolization, and weakening of the arterial wall with aneurysmal formation resulting in rupture or thrombosis.

Stenosis

Progressive intimal plaque deposition may result in narrowing of the lumen, or stenosis. Mild degrees of stenosis producing less than 50% reduction in lumen diameter usually do not obstruct blood flow. It is not until lumen diameter falls below a critical point that resistance to blood flow increases. This is referred to as *critical arterial stenosis,* or the percentage by which the lumen diameter must be reduced to produce a measurable drop in blood flow. Under experimental conditions there is no significant pressure drop and no reduction in flow until there is more than 80% reduction in lumen cross-sectional area (equivalent to 55% diameter reduction).[51] However, pressure drops across stenoses are critically dependent on flow, and noncritical stenoses at rest may develop significant pressure gradients when flow is increased with exercise. This can account for the clinical observation of disappearing pedal pulses after exercise and symptoms of claudication in patients with palpable pedal pulses.

The extent of disability from an obstruction is related to the location of the lesion, the degree of obstruction, length and number of obstructions, the metabolic needs of the tissues distal to the obstruction, and the ability of collateral vessels to provide the necessary flow. *Collateral blood flow* may be quite extensive in occlusive disease. Collateral vessels are naturally existing branches of large and medium-sized arteries that enlarge to carry blood flow around an obstruction. They do not represent neovascularization but adaptation of existing vessels to an increased demand of blood flow. The collateral blood flow that develops in the face of a developing, progressive obstruction usually can supply the demands of resting tissue. However, it often is unable to supply the flow necessary for an exercising muscle group.

There are a number of well-recognized collateral beds that develop in the presence of atherosclerosis of the aorta and distal tree:

1. Intercostal and lumbar arteries
2. Superior and inferior mesenteric arteries
3. Hypogastric artery
4. Profunda-genicular arteries
5. Peroneal-tibial arteries

Patients may have a totally occluded abdominal aorta for several years with relatively mild symptoms of hip and buttock claudication. Under these circumstances the intercostal arteries, superior epigastric arteries, and visceral arteries become important sources of collateral flow to the lower extremity (Fig. 52-2). For example, blood supply to the distal aorta may be through the inferior mesenteric artery, which derives collateral supply from the superior mesenteric artery. In addition, the inferior mesenteric artery can be an important source of collateral flow to the lower extremity through the superior hemorrhoidal network.

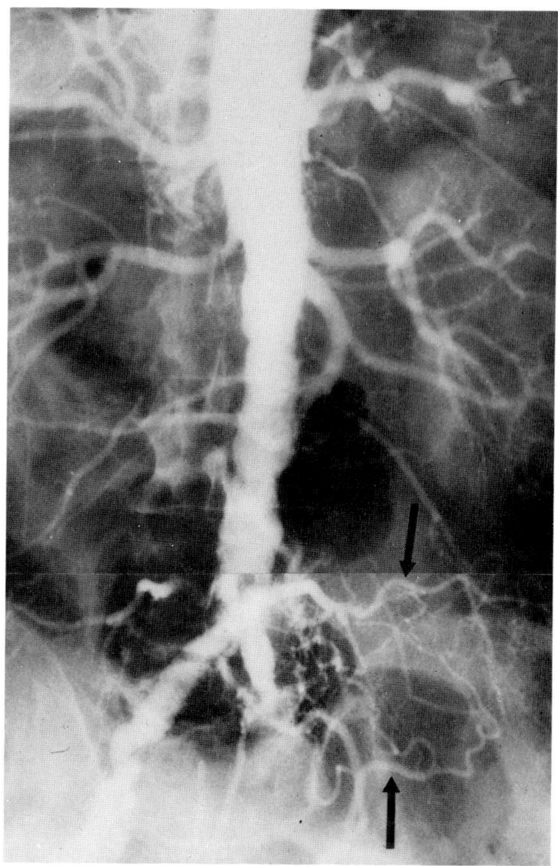

Fig. 52-2. Angiogram revealing severe aortoiliac disease. Note the large collateral vessels *(arrows)* that have developed in response to occlusion of the left iliac artery.

Thrombosis

The causes of *acute arterial obstruction* can be divided into two categories: embolism and thrombosis. Emboli arise from a proximal source, either the heart or proximal great vessels, and obstruct the tapering arterial tree at a branch point or at the point where the embolus is larger than the lumen diameter. Mural thrombus that forms in a fibrillating atrium is the most common source of arterial emboli,[52] but emboli can also arise from areas of recent transmural infarction, ventricular aneurysms, and diseased valves. Spontaneous thrombosis usually occurs in arteriosclerotic arteries as a result of slow flow caused by severe stenotic lesions or as a result of sudden dissection or hemorrhage under a previously nonstenotic plaque.

Acute thrombosis usually results in very sudden and severe symptoms of arterial ischemia. The severity of clinical symptoms is related to the site of the obstruction, the size and extent of the thrombus, and the adequacy of collateral vessels. In severe ischemia, one or more of the often described five *P*s may be present; pulselessness, pallor, paresthesia, pain, and paralysis. The loss of motor power and sensation in the toes and foot indicate very severe ischemia and limb loss unless the ischemia is relieved promptly. Acute thrombosis of a previously stenosed artery that has excellent collateral vessels about it may occur with only mild symptoms and little risk of limb loss.

Ulceration

Ulceration occurs when breakdown of the fibrous cap over a lesion exposes the necrotic core of the plaque to the circulation. This may be the site for platelet deposition and thrombus formation or may result in embolization of the plaque contents itself, producing cholesterol emboli in the distal arterial tree.

The most common clinical syndrome in the peripheral circulation associated with distal embolization from a proximal ulcerated plaque is the *blue toe syndrome.* Patients may have normal pedal pulses but suddenly develop one or more cold, blue, painful toes, a condition that resolves in 3 to 4 days. These symptoms may be caused by cholesterol emboli in the digital arteries of the feet. The source of the emboli usually is a proximal ulcerated lesion in the aorta, iliac, or femoral vessels. Unrecognized and untreated repeated embolization to the foot results in obstruction of the small arteries of the foot, gangrene, and limb loss.

Aneurysm Formation

An aneurysm is a localized arterial dilation. A *true aneurysm* is one in which there is thinning or atrophy of all layers of the artery wall with enlargement of the lumen. This should be distinguished from a *false aneurysm,* which results from a rupture of the artery wall, usually caused by trauma, with containment of the blood stream by fibrous tissue surrounding the vessel. Thus in a true aneurysm there is an inadequate artery wall, whereas in a false aneurysm there is absence of the artery wall.

As the lumen radius of an aneurysm enlarges, there is an increase in *tension* on the vessel wall (T) according to the law of Laplace (T = Pr), where P is pressure and r is radius. The larger the radius, the greater is the tension and the greater is the tendency for further enlargement of the lumen. This explains why larger aneurysms have a greater tendency to expand and rupture than do smaller aneurysms. Blood flow in the dilated aneurysmal sac is slower than normal, producing an increased tendency to thrombosis. Most large abdominal aortic aneurysms are lined by laminated mural thrombus. Mural thrombus may be so thick that lumen caliber on angiography does not appear enlarged. However, mural thrombus provides little, if any, support for the artery wall and no protection from aneurysm rupture.

ARTERIAL OCCLUSIVE DISEASE OF THE AORTA AND PERIPHERAL ARTERIES

The manifestations of atherosclerosis in the aorta and peripheral arteries are either occlusive disease or aneurysm formation. The arteries of importance in the circulation to the lower extremities are diagrammed on Fig. 52-3. Obstructive plaques may occur in each of the vessels shown but are most common in the infrarenal abdominal aorta, iliac arteries, and superficial femoral arteries. The profunda femoris artery is relatively spared, and diabetic patients are more prone to develop lesions in the tibial arteries.

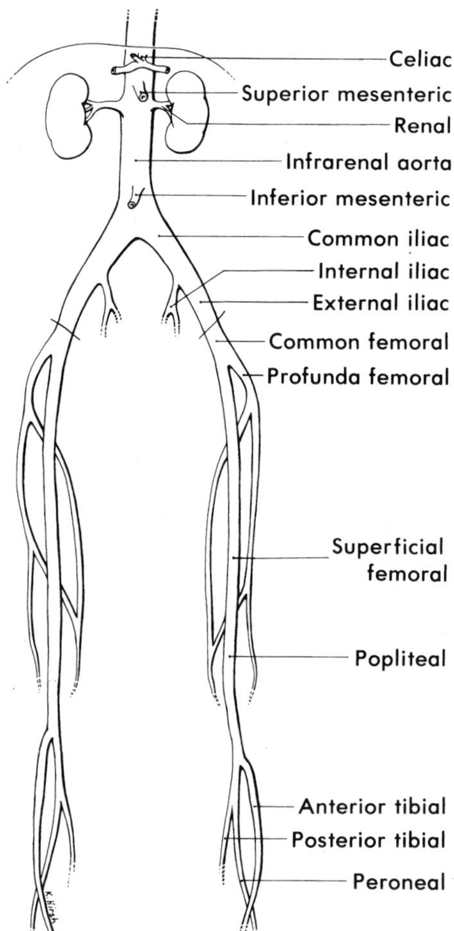

Fig. 52-3. Arterial supply to the viscera and lower extremity. Obstructive or aneurysmal changes can occur in each of these vessels. The clinical signs and symptoms vary depending on the location and blood supply distribution of a given artery. Full angiographic evaluation of the aorta and lower extremity vessels should demonstrate each of these arteries.

Clinical Manifestations of Peripheral Occlusive Disease

The clinical manifestations and physical findings of peripheral occlusive disease are as follows:

Symptoms	Physical findings	
Claudication	Skin ulceration	Absent or diminished pulses
Rest pain	Gangrene	Dependent rubor
Impotence	Bruits	Skin and muscle atrophy
	Skin pallor	Trophic changes of the nails
	Hair loss	Decreased temperature

Claudication

Claudication arises from the term *claudicatio,* which means to limp. It is a clinical syndrome of pain on exercise that is relieved by rest and results from a fixed obstruction or stenosis in arteries to the lower extremity. Although circulation may be adequate at rest, with exercise there is an increasing demand for flow. When such flow is obstructed by a stenosis, the muscle served by that vessel becomes ischemic and begins to function with anaerobic metabolism. This results in pain and symptoms of fatigue, causing the patient to stop and rest. Typically, the patient rests for 1 to 2 minutes, allowing the circulation to again restore aerobic conditions, after which the patient can again exercise. Patients with aortoiliac occlusive disease have symptoms of claudication in the hips and buttocks, whereas patients with superficial femoral artery obstruction have symptoms of claudication in the calf. The level of claudication is always below the level of the arterial obstruction.

Most patients with claudication, although symptomatic, are at low risk for developing gangrene. Only 33% of patients with proven arterial stenosis report symptoms of claudication. It is a stable disease in 70% to 80% of patients, and it is generally clinically accepted that only 25% of claudicants deteriorate.[53-57] Thus patients with stable, nonlimiting claudication may be safely followed, and revascularization should be reserved for those with disabling symptoms. Reconstructive surgery to improve blood flow is done in less than 10% of all patients with claudication. Amputation may be required in 1% to 5%.[58] The benign nature of this symptom should be carefully considered when planning any type of intervention, either catheter based or via traditional open arterial surgery.

Rest Pain

Patients with worsening ischemia develop a clinical syndrome called rest pain. The condition of rest pain indicates a much more severe degree of ischemia than claudication and, unlike claudication, indicates that the patient is at high risk for developing gangrene and limb loss. Typically, the patient experiences pain in the toes and forefoot during the night that causes him or her to awaken from sleep. The patient usually sits up in bed, dangles the legs over the side of the bed, and frequently relieves the symptoms by getting up and walking. After a short period of time, the patient's symptoms have disappeared and the patient can return to sleep. The symptoms of rest pain occur because of severe ischemia in the forefoot and toes brought about by two conditions: (1) the patient is recumbent and thereby eliminates the hydrostatic pressure gradient that assists the arteriolar perfusion pressure when erect; and (2) during sleep there is a diminution of cardiac output that correspondingly diminishes the volume of peripheral blood flow. When the patient dangles the feet, he or she restores the hydrostatic gradient; when the patient gets up to walk, he or she increases cardiac output and thereby improves the perfusion of the lower extremities. Patients frequently complain of nocturnal cramps in the calf muscles. This should not be confused with nocturnal rest pain, which typically is in the toes and forefoot rather than in the calf.

Ulceration

Cutaneous ulcers may be the first evidence of peripheral vascular disease. These ulcers are caused by severe ischemia from proximal arterial occlusions and are often associated with minor skin trauma. However, there are many causes of skin ulceration that must be differentiated from ischemic ulcers:

Vascular insufficiency (ischemic)
Venous stasis
Hypertension
Infection
Neoplasm
Neurotropism
Hematologic abnormalities

Each type of ulcer has certain clinical and physical characteristics. The ischemic ulcer is most commonly found on the toes, heel, dorsum of the foot, or lower third of the leg. The pain is usually severe, persistent, and worsens at night. The ulcer itself is generally irregular with a pale or necrotic base.

At times patients have ulcerations that are attributed to venous disease that may in fact be the result of a combination of arterial ischemia and venous stasis. Ulcerations not in the classic position for venous disease (at the medial malleolus) should be considered as potentially being of an arterial origin. Even if a component of venous disease is present, the arterial component must be evaluated if effective therapy is to be instituted.

Gangrene

Progressive ischemia caused by atherosclerosis can result in gangrenous changes of the tissues. Most commonly the digits are affected initially, but progression to the forefoot is not unusual. Small amounts of infection superimposed on a severe chronic ischemic state can progress very rapidly to gangrene. Clinically, dry and wet gangrene should be differentiated. *Dry gangrene* represents mummification of tissue, and active purulent tissue and cellulitis are absent. *Wet gangrene* is characterized by active infection with cellulitis and purulent tissue planes and is an indication for urgent amputation to prevent ascending infection.

Impotence

Penile erection requires a threefold increase in blood flow through the penile arteries that is shunted into the vascular spaces of the corpora cavernosa. Arterial obstruction that prevents this increase in blood flow can result in erectile impotence in much the same way that symptoms of claudication are brought about by exercise when there is an unmet demand for increased blood flow. Rene Leriche in 1923 first noted the association among atherosclerotic occlusion of the aorta, hip claudication, buttock atrophy, and erectile impotence. This is now known as the *Leriche syndrome.*

Obstruction can occur at any level from the abdominal aorta, the common iliac arteries, the internal iliac arteries, internal pudendal arteries, or penile arteries, resulting in erectile impotence. Although the majority of cases of impotence have psychogenic or urologic causes or are the result of the side effects of medication, the importance of an adequate vascular supply is becoming increasingly recognized and can be objectively assessed, as is discussed below.

EVALUATION OF PERIPHERAL VASCULAR OCCLUSIVE DISEASE

Peripheral vascular occlusive disease is evaluated on the basis of a thorough clinical examination, noninvasive vascular testing, continuous acquisition ("spiral") CT scanning, MR angiography, and finally intra-arterial contrast angiography.

Clinical Examination

Peripheral vascular occlusive disease most often is accurately diagnosed with a careful history and thorough phys-

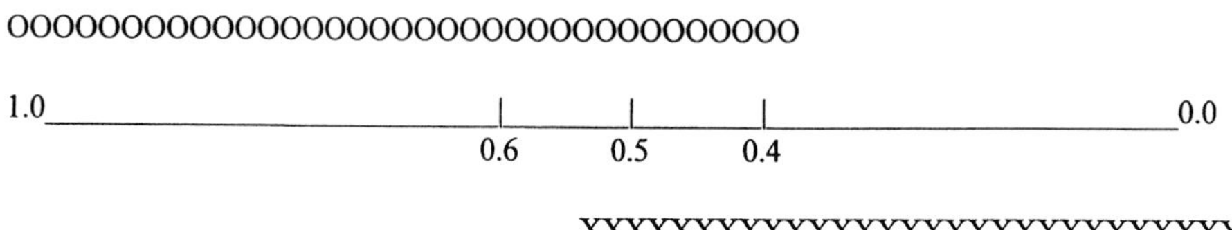

Fig. 52-4. Ankle-brachial index, used to determine severity of lower extremity ischemia. Circles denote range consistent with claudication; Xs denote area of limb threatening ischemia. Note area of considerable overlap around 0.5.

ical examination of the patient. In addition to the important determination of symptoms of claudication or rest pain, the patient's level of activity and walking distance should be noted. Often patients with very severe disease do not walk enough to develop symptoms. A careful evaluation of all pulses should be made, although the presence of a palpable pulse does not rule out the possibility of significant arterial occlusive disease. A bruit may be appreciated during the physical examination. Bruits are produced by the turbulence of blood just distal to a stenosis but may also be produced by angulations and bends in arteries. Bruits may be audible with a stethoscope over and distal to an area of stenosis. A high-pitched bruit may be indicative of a severe stenosis. Finally, the temperature, quality, and color of the skin, hair, and nails should be noted, including the presence of skin ulcerations or gangrenous changes.

Noninvasive tests are used after the clinical examination to confirm the presence of occlusive disease, identify the level and severity of the disease, and assess whether angiography is required to further evaluate these patients.

Objective Assessment With Vascular Laboratory Techniques

Doppler Ankle Pressure

The ready availability of the handheld Doppler ultrasound has made measurement of lower extremity blood pressure simple and convenient and has permitted the development of objective means of assessing lower extremity perfusion. The Doppler ultrasound probe emits high-frequency sound waves in the range of 2 to 10 MHz. The sound is reflected by the movement of red blood cells in the vessel that produces a frequency shift that is picked up by the receiving crystal of the Doppler probe. This frequency shift is proportional to the blood flow velocity. This *Doppler shift* can be expressed by the following formula:

$$\Delta f = \frac{2f\ V \cos \theta}{C}$$

where V is velocity, f is frequency of the incident sound beam, C is velocity of sound in tissue, and θ is the angle of the incident sound beam to the vessel examined. Because V, C, and θ can be constant, the shift in frequency is proportional to the velocity of the blood flow.

To measure the blood pressure in the legs, a blood pressure cuff is placed at the ankle just above the malleoli and inflated while a handheld Doppler is used to listen to flow in the dorsalis pedis and posterior tibial artery. Inflation of the cuff above systolic pressure causes obliteration of the Doppler signal, and systolic blood pressure can be recorded as the cuff is deflated and flow resumes in the measured vessel. Since a patient's blood pressure may fluctuate, more precision can be gained by comparing the ankle pressure to the brachial pressure. Usually the ankle systolic pressure is divided by the brachial systolic pressure to produce an *ankle-brachial index (ABI).* Such an index is quite useful in assessing the severity of peripheral occlusive disease. Patients without occlusive disease have an ABI of 1, whereas patients with claudication have an ABI of 0.5 to 0.6. Patients with rest pain, gangrene, and ulceration have an ABI of 0.4 and less (Fig. 52-4). Despite these ranges, considerable overlap can be present, especially around an ABI of 0.5. This measurement is useful for differentiating patients with lower extremity pain caused by spinal stenosis, arthritis, or other nonvascular conditions. Patients with diabetes frequently have calcified vessels that cannot be compressed by the blood pressure cuff. This may lead to a false elevation of the ABI. In the setting of incompressible ankle vessels, toe pressure or waveforms may be more accurate.

It is important to note that the pressure measured is determined by the location of the cuff rather than the location of the listening probe. Thus an ankle pressure can be recorded by placing a cuff at the level of the malleoli, and a below-knee or above-knee pressure can be recorded by appropriate blood pressure cuff placement. Patients with superficial femoral artery occlusion have a normal pressure reading in the upper thigh but an abnormal pressure reading below the knee and at the level of the ankle. The resting ankle index is the most accurate of the noninvasive techniques for objectively assessing the presence or absence of occlusive disease. It is reproducible, and hence the index can be followed to identify the progression of disease.

It should also be recognized that listening and hearing flow in the dorsalis pedis and posterior tibial arteries does not represent a pulse. A pulse is palpated with the fingers. Flow can be heard at very low levels of circulation in the dorsalis pedis and the posterior tibial arteries, and patients

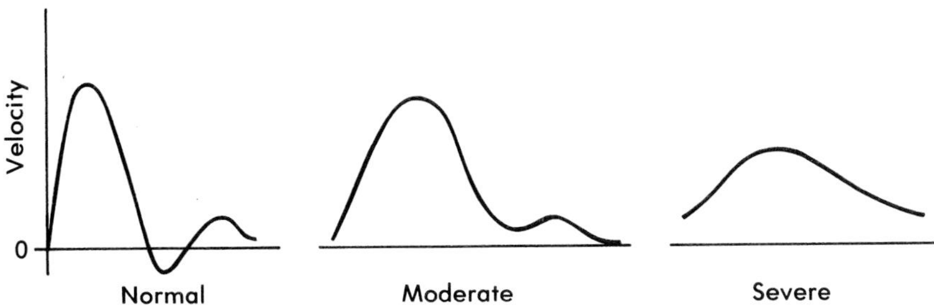

Fig. 52-5. Doppler ultrasound velocity waveforms indicating the normal triphasic waveform, the loss of the reverse flow component seen in moderately stenotic vessels, and the blunted waveform of a severely stenotic vessel.

may have frank gangrene of their foot even though audible Doppler signals are heard. One should not be lulled into a false sense of security of good perfusion of the foot if Doppler flow signals in the foot are heard but pulses cannot be palpated.

Stress Testing

Since patients with claudication develop their symptoms only with exercise, stress testing is a useful means for documenting the degree of walking impairment. Treadmill exercise can be performed at a standard pace of 1.5 miles per hour at a 7-degree grade. Normally, one has no diminution of the ankle pressure following exercise. On walking to the point of claudication, there is a substantial drop in ABI because blood flow is shunted to the proximal thigh muscle and cannot pass through the obstruction to the distal vascular bed. There is return of ankle pressure to normal with rest. The symptom of reduction in ankle pressure is similar to the finding of disappearing pulses with exercise seen on clinical examination.

Doppler Waveform Analysis

Doppler detectors can provide an analog signal that is proportional to the velocity of the blood in vessels studied. The shape of the waveform reflects the status of the vessel. Normally, a *triphasic* waveform is seen, indicative of reversal of flow in early diastole. Stenosis proximal to the vessel examined first eliminates this reversed flow. As the stenosis becomes more severe, the peak of the waveform is blunted, and the waveform widens (Fig. 52-5). Qualitative analysis of these waveforms at different levels of the extremity can identify the level and severity of occlusive lesions.

Analysis of the Doppler waveforms in conjunction with systolic pressures at several levels in the leg can allow the clinician to make an accurate diagnosis of the location and extent of peripheral vascular occlusive disease. For example, Fig. 52-6 illustrates the decrease in the waveform and systolic pressures across an obstructed superficial femoral artery. A decrease in systolic blood pressure of 30 mm Hg or more between any two levels in the leg usually indicates total occlusion of the intervening artery.

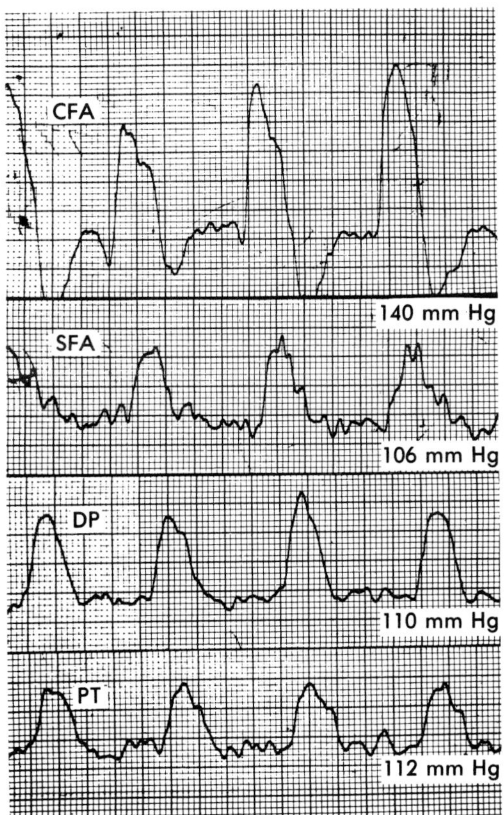

Fig. 52-6. Doppler flow velocity waveforms recorded at four places in an extremity with superficial femoral artery occlusion demonstrated by angiography. Recordings were made at the common femoral artery *(CFA),* superficial femoral artery *(SFA),* dorsalis pedis *(DP)* artery, and posterior tibial *(PT)* artery. Associated systolic blood pressures were measured to be 140 mm Hg in the thigh and 106 mm Hg below the knee. This 34 mm Hg drop in pressure indicates occlusion of the intervening artery (in this case, the superficial femoral artery). Distal arteries fill through collateral vessels. Note change in Doppler velocity waveforms.

Doppler Ultrasound Imaging and Duplex Scanning

B-mode ultrasound imaging of arteries and plaques combined with pulsed Doppler ultrasound flow determination and sound spectral analysis is now a routine method evaluating the common femoral, superficial femoral, and popliteal arteries. This technique provides the ability to noninvasively image arteries and to assess flow. Recently, this technology has been applied to autogenous vein grafts in an attempt to prevent graft failure or occlusion. Various investigators have proposed specific criteria to predict lower extremity vein graft failure.[59] This technology is also being applied to the question of why grafts fail; Mills' work has recently highlighted the time course and location of potential sites of graft failure, in an attempt to direct postoperative surveillance studies more efficiently.[60,61] Duplex scanning can also be used to evaluate aneurysms and ulcerated lesions, which are potential sources of distal emboli in these vessels.

Penile Brachial Pressure Index

The simplest and most reliable assessment of the adequacy of penile perfusion is the measurement of arterial pressure in the corpora cavernosa supplied by the penile arteries. A Doppler velocity probe is positioned directly over one of the six penile arteries, and a small pneumatic cuff is placed around the penis proximal to the probe. The cuff is inflated until arterial flow is abolished and is then allowed to slowly deflate until flow returns, which indicates the systolic blood pressure. The penile systolic pressure is divided by the brachial systolic pressure to provide a penile-brachial index (PBI). A PBI greater than 0.9 is normal. A PBI less than 0.7 is consistent with a vascular occlusive cause of the impotence.

Angiography

Angiography provides the most definitive anatomic assessment of obstructing vascular lesions and is performed before vascular reconstruction. This includes visualization of the abdominal and infrarenal aorta, the iliac arteries, and the femoral, popliteal, tibial, and pedal vessels throughout their length (see Fig. 52-3). Angiography is usually performed through a transfemoral approach, which has the advantage of allowing selective catheterization and the study of individual arteries as needed. Transaxillary and translumbar aortography can also be used successfully. Newer techniques of digital subtraction and computer enhancement of images permit the use of smaller volumes of iodinated contrast materials. Patients should be well hydrated before and after angiography to minimize the possibility of renal failure caused by the osmotic diuresis produced by the hypertonic contrast medium.[62] Newer, less invasive methods of arterial imaging may eventually supplant catheter-delivered, iodinated contrast intra-arterial arteriography. Continuous acquisition computing tomographic imaging, or "spiral" CT, has the capability of demonstrating vessels in a three-dimensional, shaded surface display. Although still requiring iodinated contrast, this technique does not involve intra-arterial cannulation or manipulation. This technique has been used to study the carotid artery,[63] the abdominal aorta and its branches,[64] and the thoracic aorta.[65]

MR angiography is currently being used to supplant catheter-based, contrast angiography.[66] In addition to anatomic data, however, MR sequences can encode for flow volume[67] and the oxygen saturation of hemoglobin.[68,69] Although still limited in quality and the field of view available compared to a traditional aortogram with bilateral runoff, MR anatomic and flow imaging may ultimately replace catheter-based, invasive arterial diagnostic methods.

TREATMENT OF PERIPHERAL VASCULAR OCCLUSIVE DISEASE

The treatment of peripheral vascular occlusive disease is determined by the severity of the patient's symptoms and the anatomic location and extent of obstructing lesions. Treatment options include nonoperative measures, minimally invasive procedures such as transluminal angioplasty, and operative revascularization.

Nonoperative Measures

Patients with peripheral occlusive disease usually have one or several risk factors for the development of vascular disease, including cigarette smoking, hyperlipidemia, hypertension, and diabetes mellitus. Every effort should be made to control these factors to prevent progression of obstructive disease. Patients with symptoms of claudication that are not physically limiting have a low risk for limb loss[70] and usually respond well to a program of cessation of smoking and walking exercise to stimulate enlargement of collateral circulation and to condition the muscles to function at a higher level with the available blood supply. Exercise programs are effective in improving walking distance but must be maintained. Cessation of the exercise program usually returns the patient to the same level of claudication as present originally. Patients often adjust their levels of activity and coexist well with occlusive disease for many years. Those who continue to smoke have the poorest outlook.

Medical therapy for peripheral vascular disease has in general been ineffective. A number of vasodilating drugs have been used in an attempt to diminish vasospasm, improve perfusion of ischemic limbs, and help the development of collateral vessels. These agents as a group have been ineffective, and most have been removed from the market.

In recent years six new classes of drugs have been described that may potentially benefit the patient with vascular disease: (1) calcium channel blockers (nifedipine); (2) prostaglandins (PGE_1 and PGI_2); (3) pentoxifylline; (4) thromboxane synthetase inhibitors; (5) platelet inhibitors; and (6) metabolic enhancing drugs.

Nifedipine has been found useful in the treatment of vasospasm as seen in Raynaud's syndrome,[71] and many currently consider it the drug of choice for this disease.

The complex biologic activity of the prostaglandins has only recently evolved. PGE_1 is a vasodilator and a strong inhibitor of platelet aggregation. No single trial has yet to demonstrate the benefits of PGE_1 in the improvement of rest pain or healing of ischemic ulcers.

Pentoxifylline is a xanthine derivative that has been used in the medical treatment of peripheral vascular occlusive disease. It has been suggested that it exerts its effect by decreasing the rigidity of erythrocytes so that they can more readily deform and pass through the small capillary beds, thereby increasing tissue perfusion. A trial of patients with claudication demonstrated a 30% increase in walking distance in patients treated with pentoxifylline as compared to placebo.[72] This is the only drug classified as effective in the treatment of intermittent claudication by the Food and Drug Administration, but long-term benefits have not been established. There is no evidence that pentoxifylline is effective in patients with ulceration, rest pain, or gangrene.

Thromboxane synthetase inhibitors exert their effects by blocking the function of thromboxane, which produces vasoconstriction and platelet aggregation. Prevention of these events in the microcirculation might improve distal circulation. However, no clinical benefits have yet to be realized with these agents. Antiplatelet agents, such as cilostazol, are completing clinical trials now in the United States and may soon become available for routine clinical use. While data collection is still somewhat incomplete, preliminary results suggest cilostazol may be as effective or more effective than pentoxifylline. Metabolic enhancing drugs such as 6-propionyl carnitine may also prove effective, although trials to prove efficacy are still ongoing.

Transluminal Angioplasty

Transluminal balloon angioplasty is a percutaneous method of dilating arterial stenoses or recanalizing occluded vessels. The procedure is usually performed in the angiography suite after completion of diagnostic angiography. Proper patient selection is important, and clinical criteria similar to those used to select patients for surgery should be used. Dilation of lesions that appear significant on angiography but produce minimal or no symptoms must be avoided. The best candidate for transluminal angioplasty is one with severe claudication caused by an isolated hemodynamically significant common iliac artery lesion.

In transluminal angioplasty a catheter with a balloon that has a predetermined maximal diameter at its tip is used. The catheter with balloon deflated is passed over a guide wire under x-ray control through an obstructing lesion. Inflation of the balloon disrupts the plaque and stretches the arterial wall, resulting in enlargement of the lumen. This enlargement of the lumen cross-sectional area occurs by separating the plaque from the underlying tunica media and stretching the artery wall (Fig. 52- 7). At times the media is stretched and thinned to the point of media rupture, in which case vessel integrity is maintained by the

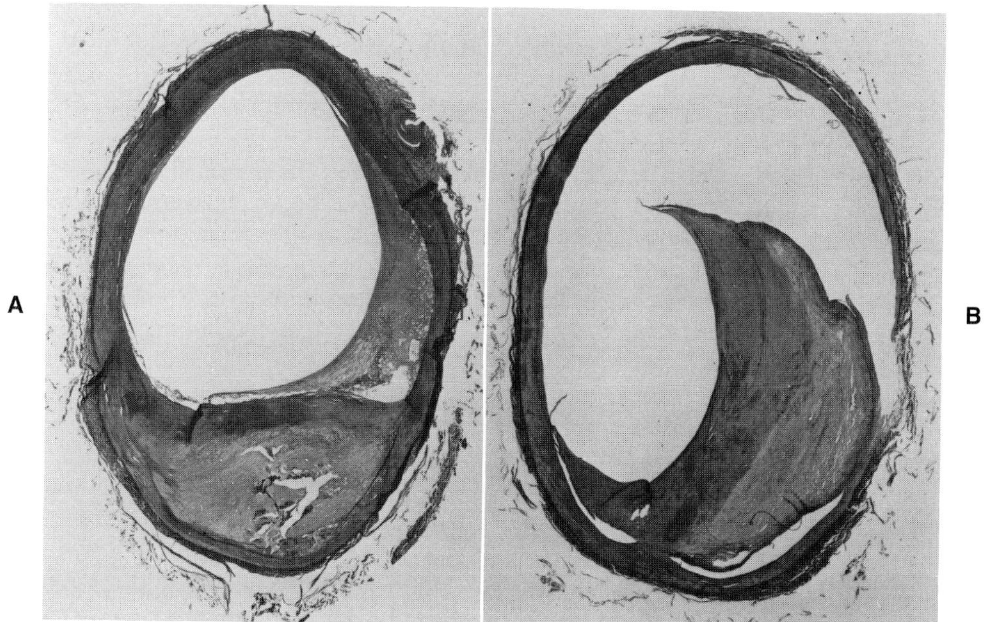

Fig. 52-7. Mechanism of balloon dilation of arteries. **A,** Human superficial femoral artery that has been fixed with an intraluminal pressure of 100 mm Hg and cut in cross section. Note the eccentric plaque and round lumen. **B,** Segment of the same artery after balloon dilation. Note the separation of plaque from the media and protrusion of the plaque into the lumen. The media is thinner and has ruptured, and lumen integrity is maintained by the adventitia. Disruption and stretching of the artery wall results in a larger lumen area. There is no plaque compression. (From Zarins CK, et al. Arterial disruption and remodeling following balloon dilatation. Surgery 92:1086, 1982.)

adventitia.[73] There is no plaque compression on removal of the lesion, and long-term patency depends on the vessel wall remaining in the overstretched state. When the vessel contracts to its predilated state, restenosis occurs. This occurs in a substantial number of patients and is a significant limitation of the procedure. Intra-arterial stents have been introduced as a method of maintaining lumenal patency after angioplasty. The long-term effectiveness of these stents on whether they actually improve on angioplasty alone remains to be determined.

Results from transluminal angioplasty depend on the site dilated, the length of the stenosis, whether a complete obstruction is being dilated, and the degree of calcification in the plaque. Determination of results following transluminal, catheter-based interventions such as angioplasty have been difficult, in large part a result of lack of uniform reporting standards. What is clear from the available data is that common iliac angioplasty provides long-term patency comparable to traditional reconstructive techniques. The results in distal vessels are distinctly inferior to well-performed bypass surgery, especially when autogenous graft conduit is used below the inguinal ligament.[74] Although widely used, the role of intra-arterial stenting also remains undetermined. The recent codification of reporting standards for endovascular procedures including angioplasty should facilitate future comparisons with existing surgical standards, and help clarify the relative indications for angioplasty.[75] Because of technical issues, cost, and ongoing problems with restenosis, interest in nonangioplasty related endovascular procedures, such as rotational arthrectomy, laser-mediated plaque obligation, thermal- or laser-assisted angioplasty, has waned.[74]

Endarterectomy

Endarterectomy is a surgical procedure in which the diseased intimal plaque is removed from an artery to enlarge the lumen. The cleavage plane for endarterectomy is usually just below the internal elastic lamina, although the media below extensive plaque is often degenerated and is removed along with the intimal plaque. In these circumstances the cleavage plane is at the external elastic lamina, and thus only the adventitial layer contains the blood stream. The adventitial layer alone provides sufficient structural support, and aneurysmal dilation of endarterectomized arterial segments does not occur.

Although endarterectomy is the standard mode of treatment for carotid bifurcation atherosclerosis, it has a more limited usefulness in the treatment of peripheral vascular occlusive disease. This is because carotid plaques are localized in the carotid bifurcation, whereas lower extremity atherosclerosis usually is extensive with no discrete starting or end points. Some patients with localized aortoiliac disease and no distal occlusive disease are candidates for local aortoiliac endarterectomy, but bypass procedures are more commonly performed. If a local endarterectomy is to be considered, these patients must not have aneurysmal disease or fibrotic small-caliber vessels. Results of *local* aortoiliac endarterectomy compare favorably to aortobifemoral bypass grafts.

Most surgeons occasionally use local endarterectomy as an adjunctive procedure to aortobifemoral bypass grafting. Such local endarterectomies are frequently performed in the common and profunda femoris arteries at the time of anastomosis of bypass grafts, but primary endarterectomies have limited usefulness in the peripheral circulation.

Bypass Procedures

Procedures to bypass occlusive lesions are the standard surgical methods for treatment of lower extremity peripheral occlusive disease. Procedures are usually considered as inflow or outflow procedures, depending on the level of obstruction. Inflow procedures refer to those used for aortoiliac obstructions, and outflow procedures are those used for superficial femoral and popliteal artery obstructions, with the level of the inguinal ligament usually being the dividing line. Angiographic, vascular, laboratory, and clinical criteria are used to determine the primary level of obstruction. If a patient has both inflow and outflow disease, the proximal, or inflow, obstruction is treated first and usually is sufficient to relieve symptoms.

Aortofemoral Bypass

The indications for surgical intervention in patients with aortoiliac occlusive lesions are severe claudication and limb-threatening ischemia as defined by rest pain, ulcerations, and gangrene. The standard surgical treatment for bypass of aortoiliac obstructions is the aortofemoral bypass graft.[76] In this procedure a knitted or woven Dacron bifurcation graft is sutured from the infrarenal aorta, which is usually free of disease, to the common femoral arteries. This graft bypasses the entire aortoiliac segment, which includes the inferior mesenteric artery and internal iliac arteries. The proximal anastomosis is placed just below the level of the renal arteries and may be performed in either an end-to-end or an end-to-side fashion (Fig. 52-8). When an *end-to-end anastomosis* is used, the distal aorta is ligated, and the entire aortic outflow passes through the graft. Blood is supplied to the distal aorta and the inferior mesenteric and internal iliac arteries by retrograde flow from the common femoral artery through the external iliac artery. With an *end-to-side proximal anastomosis,* blood flows in parallel in the bypass graft and in the distal aorta. This anastomosis is preferred when the external iliac arteries are occluded and would prevent retrograde fill of the aorta from the groin. The distal anastomosis is usually placed on the common femoral artery with outflow through the superficial femoral and profunda femoris vessels. If there is associated superficial femoral artery occlusion, the profunda femoris artery alone can serve as the outflow bed with relief of symptoms. Concomitant endarterectomy of the orifices of the superficial femoral and profunda femoris arteries can be undertaken to improve the distal anastomosis. *Profun-*

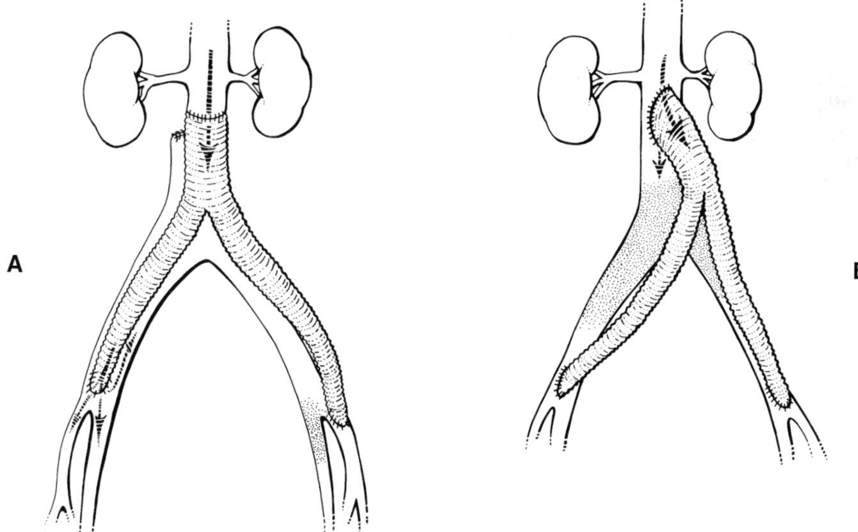

Fig. 52-8. Aortofemoral bypass for aortoiliac obstruction. Proximal anastomosis may be performed end-to-end **(A)** or end-to-side of the aorta **(B)**. With an end-to-end anastomosis, perfusion of the internal iliac arteries and distal aorta is retrograde from the common femoral artery in the groin.

daplasty is performed by extending the opening of the common femoral artery onto the profunda femoris artery and suturing the Dacron graft onto the profunda femoris artery. This results in enlargement of the lumen of the proximal profunda femoris artery and is useful when there is a stenosis at that site.

Aortofemoral bypass graft is a stable and durable operation that effectively eliminates the inflow obstruction. Surgical mortality rate is less than 2%, and the 5-year graft patency rate is greater than 90%.[77] Should these operations fail, they generally do so because of progression of disease in the arteries at or distal to the groin anastomosis rather than because of failure of the Dacron graft itself.

Early complications of aortobifemoral grafts are caused mainly by technical misadventures. These include postoperative hemorrhage, early graft thrombosis, distal embolization, groin hematomas, and lymph leaks. Long-term complications include graft infection, pseudoaneurysm formation, and aorta duodenal fistula. Details of these problems are expanded on below.

Extra-anatomic Bypass

Patients who require bypass of aortoiliac lesions but are too ill to withstand an intra-abdominal operation for placement of an aortobifemoral graft may be revascularized with an axillofemoral or femorofemoral bypass graft (Fig. 52-9). These operations are effective in relieving aortoiliac, or inflow, obstruction but do not require that the abdominal cavity be entered. The bypass is tunneled in the subcutaneous space, and incisions to expose the axillary and femoral vessels can be performed while the patient is under local anesthesia. Thus they are safer and more amenable to use in high-risk patients. *Axillofemoral bypass*

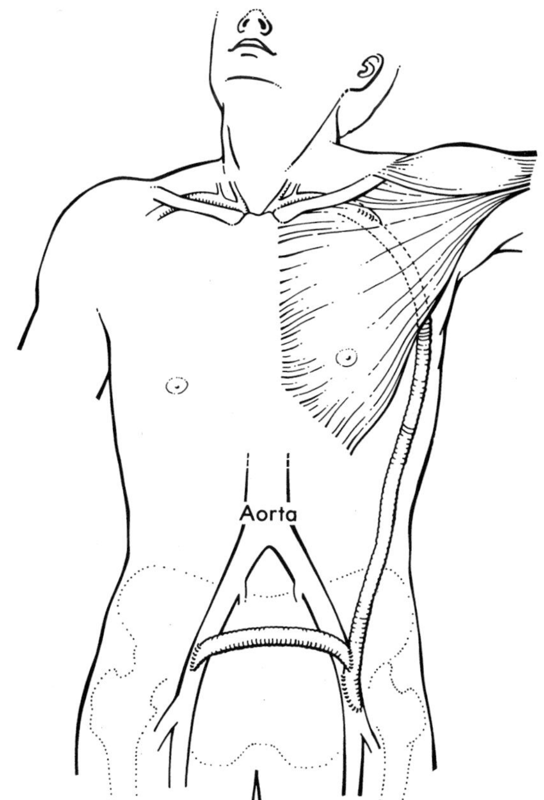

Fig. 52-9. Illustration of extra-anatomic bypasses for aortoiliac obstruction. Axillofemoral bypass graft courses in the subcutaneous space in the midaxillary line and brings blood from the subclavian artery to the femoral artery to bypass an aortic obstruction. Femorofemoral bypass graft brings blood from one femoral artery across to the other. "Steal" phenomenon does not occur if there is no obstruction to the inflow of the donor artery.

grafts are also useful to bypass the aorta in situations of infection within the abdominal cavity. There is no steal of blood from the upper extremity when an axillofemoral bypass is placed because there is an increase in flow in the feeding subclavian artery. This increase is sufficient to supply the arm and both legs. However, the great length of the axillofemoral graft makes it prone to thrombosis. Recent reports suggest the long-term patency of axillofemoral bypass grafting supports its use in highly selected cases when in-line anatomic reconstruction is less desirable.[78] However, proximal anastomotic disruption remains a serious though infrequent complication.[79]

A *femorofemoral bypass graft* can be used to bypass an iliac artery occlusion if the opposite patent iliac artery is disease free. In this situation one iliac artery is able to deliver enough flow to supply both legs. Five-year patency rates for femorofemoral grafts vary from 44% to 74%. Axillofemoral bypass grafts have a poorer patency rate than aortofemoral grafts, with 5-year patency rates reported near 75%.[80] These grafts fail more commonly than an aortobifemoral graft because of their longer course and the risk of external compression in the subcutaneous tunnel. Thus extra-anatomic grafts should be considered only when aortobifemoral grafts or local aortoiliac endarterectomies are not feasible.

Femoropopliteal and Femoral Distal Bypass Grafts

Claudication or severe ischemia of the legs despite a good aortoiliac segment is usually the result of obstruction of the superficial femoral or popliteal artery and its branches. A preoperative angiogram demonstrates which distal vessels are patent and of adequate caliber to accept a bypass graft. If the popliteal artery is patent with runoff through at least one of the tibial vessels, a *femoropopliteal bypass graft* is the procedure of choice. If the popliteal artery is occluded, bypass should be performed to the tibial artery that best fills the plantar arch.

The saphenous vein is the most suitable conduit for bypasses below the inguinal ligament. It may be used as a reversed or in situ vein bypass (Fig. 52-10). In a *reversed saphenous vein femoropopliteal bypass graft,* the saphenous vein is excised, and all branches are ligated and divided. The vein position is reversed so that the distal end of the vein is sewn to the common femoral artery, whereas the proximal portion of the vein is sewn to the popliteal artery. This permits arterial flow to course in the vein in the direction of the valves. An *in situ vein bypass graft* is left in its normal position.[81]

The proximal vein is sewn to the common femoral artery, and the distal portion is sewn to the popliteal (or tibial) artery. To permit blood to flow in the vein against the direction of the valves, the valve leaflets must be cut to render them incompetent. The in situ graft avoids extensive dissection of the vein, provides a better size match between the smaller distal artery and vein, and allows the use of smaller veins that might not be suitable for reversed vein bypass. Autogenous vein is far superior to prosthetic materials in all infrainguinal positions, and every effort should be made to use vein, even if the arm veins or lesser saphenous veins are employed.

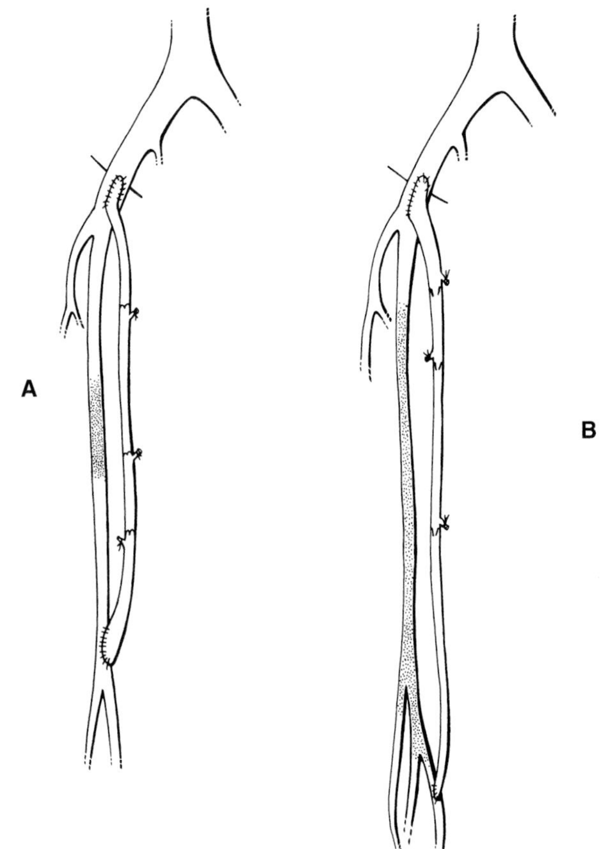

Fig. 52-10. Saphenous vein bypass grafts in the lower extremity for treatment of femoropopliteal occlusions. These may be performed as a reversed saphenous vein bypass graft **(A)** or an in situ saphenous vein bypass graft **(B)**. In the in situ bypass graft, the saphenous vein valves must be cut to render them incompetent. Selection of the site of distal anastomosis depends on angiographic demonstration of the patency of distal arteries.

Limb salvage rate for patients undergoing femoropopliteal bypass grafting with autogenous tissue is 73% at 4 years; for femoral distal bypass grafts limb salvage is 80% at 4 years.[82] The limb salvage rates are usually 15% higher than the actual graft patency rates. The patency of each individual graft depends on the adequacy of inflow, the type of graft material used, the quality of the outflow vessels, and the technical aspects of the procedure.[82]

The complications of femoropopliteal and femoral distal bypass grafts are similar to an aortobifemoral procedure. Early thrombosis is the most serious early problem and usually represents technical error or inadequate runoff vessels. Prompt thrombectomy and recognition of the technical problem returns function to the graft but usually results in reduction of long-term patency.[83]

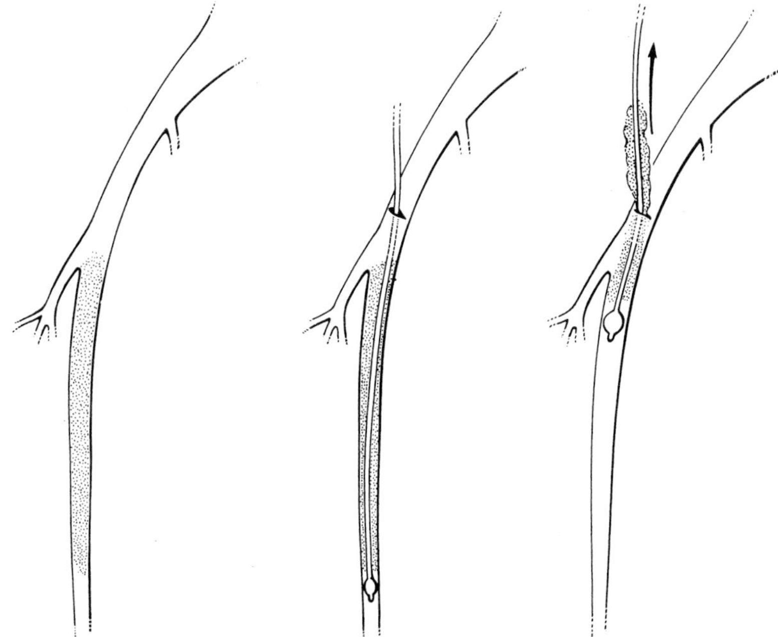

Fig. 52-11. Fogarty balloon catheter embolectomy. Deflated balloon is passed through the thromboembolus. Balloon is inflated and withdrawn, and the embolus is extracted from the artery.

Sympathectomy

Lumbar sympathectomy produces vasomotor paralysis, which increases blood flow by decreasing peripheral resistance. Before the advent of direct arterial surgery, sympathectomy was the chief surgical therapeutic approach for peripheral occlusive disease. With progressive improvement in the ability to directly revascularize ischemic tissue, lumbar sympathectomy has fallen into disfavor. It has no beneficial effect in the treatment of claudication but has been reported to improve rest pain in approximately 50% of patients. It has been shown to increase cutaneous, but not muscle, blood flow and thus has been recommended for the treatment of ischemic ulcers. Some surgeons use sympathectomy as an adjunct to arterial reconstruction, believing that sympathectomy adds to the total improvement of blood flow to the extremity by causing vasodilation in the small vessels of the foot. However, there is little evidence that there is improved flow over and above the benefit derived from arterial reconstruction alone. In addition, there are potential complications of lumbar sympathectomy, including postsympathectomy neuralgia and failure of ejaculation. Although sympathectomy has limited usefulness in arteriosclerosis obliterans, it is effective in the treatment of causalgia, and hyperhidrosis.

Embolectomy/Thrombectomy

Acute arterial occlusion with severe ischemia may be caused by emboli, which usually arise from the heart, or by thrombosis of a diseased artery. In addition to the ischemia caused by the embolus, the limb is threatened by propagation of thrombus in the arteries distal to the embolus where blood flow is slow. Therefore patients with acute arterial occlusion should be immediately anticoagulated with heparin. In addition to preventing clot propagation, anticoagulation helps prevent recurrent embolization from the heart.

Removal of the obstructing embolus is readily accomplished using the *Fogarty balloon catheter* (Fig. 52-11). An incision is made in the femoral artery, and the catheter with balloon deflated is passed through the thrombus. The balloon is then inflated, and the clot extracted. This procedure is very effective in removing fresh thrombus and restoring blood flow in patients with embolism. However, bypass may be required to restore flow in patients who have thrombosis induced by severe stenotic plaques.

In some instances thrombi and emboli may be lysed with *thrombolytic* agents such as urokinase or streptokinase administered intravenously or intra-arterially directly into the thrombus. These thrombolytic agents are effective in lysing thrombus but carry a significant risk of inducing hemorrhage.

ANEURYSMAL DISEASE OF THE AORTA

The abdominal aorta is particularly vulnerable to aneurysm formation and contains 90% of all aneurysms. Aneurysms are usually located in the infrarenal abdominal aortic segment with sparing of the first 1 to 2 cm below the level of the renal arteries. Aneurysms are usually clinically silent but may enlarge, cause symptoms, and rupture.

Cause of Aortic Aneurysms

Special anatomic features of the infrarenal abdominal aorta may make it vulnerable to the development of aneurysms.

The aortic media is composed of groups of smooth muscle cells surrounded by layers of elastin in a network of collagen fibers. The elastin layers serve to allow distensibility of the aortic wall in pulse propagation, whereas the collagen fibers provide tensile strength and prevent overdistention and rupture. The number of medial lamellar units increases proportionally with the aortic diameter to support the tensile stress. The aortic media is nourished by diffusion from the lumen to a depth of approximately 29 medial lamellar units.[84] However, if the aorta is thicker than 29 layers, adventitial vasa vasorum penetrate the media to supply nutrition. The relationship between the number of medial layers and the depth of penetration of vasa vasorum in the aortic media applies to both the thoracic aorta and abdominal aortic segment in most mammals. However, the human abdominal aorta is a noticeable exception in that it contains fewer lamellar units than would be expected for its diameter and the media is devoid of vasa vasorum.[85] Thus each layer is thicker than expected and sustains an increased tension per lamellar unit. This may make the aorta vulnerable to relative ischemic injury of the medial smooth muscle cells, leading to medial atrophy in aneurysm formation.[86]

Atherosclerotic plaques are also prone to develop in the infrarenal abdominal aorta and may be a factor in aneurysm formation. Intimal plaques may obstruct diffusion of nutrients from the lumen to the media. Usually there is ingrowth of new medial vasa vasorum to supply the media and plaque under these circumstances. When this does not occur, aneurysmal degeneration may take place because of inadequate medial nutrition. Vasa vasorum usually arise from the renal arteries, and the immediate infrarenal aortic segment may have a better vasa vasorum supply than the rest of the aorta. This may explain the relative protection from aneurysm formation in this area.

Other etiologic factors in aneurysm formation have been proposed, including increased elastase or collagenase activity, hemodynamic factors in the infrarenal aorta, and genetic predisposition.

Aneurysms are also found in the femoral and popliteal arteries, although much less commonly. Patients with peripheral aneurysms usually have coexistent abdominal aortic aneurysms, suggesting a more general aneurysmal diathesis.

Clinical Manifestations

The biologic fate of an aneurysm of the abdominal aorta is to increase in size with eventual rupture. When first detected in a patient, aneurysms may be asymptomatic, symptomatic, or ruptured. In addition, slow flow within the dilated aneurysm may result in thrombus formation along the wall that occasionally may totally occlude the lumen, causing acute ischemia, or may embolize to the distal arterial vasculature.

Asymptomatic Aneurysms

Aneurysms are remarkable by their clinical silence in the majority of cases. Asymptomatic aneurysms are frequently discovered by palpating a pulsatile mass during physical examination of the abdomen. Since the aortic bifurcation is located at the level of the umbilicus, the pulsatile mass is usually in the epigastrium. Such pulsatile masses must be distinguished from normal aortic pulsations transmitted through a solid organ or tumor that pulsates mainly in a sagittal plane, whereas an aneurysm also pulsates laterally. This is best appreciated by palpation with both hands deep along the lateral margins of the mass. However, aneurysms less than 5 cm in diameter are difficult to palpate, especially in corpulent people; and these aneurysms are usually discovered incidental to x-ray film or ultrasound examination for gastrointestinal, genitourinary, orthopedic, or other lesions.

The single most important prognostic feature of asymptomatic abdominal aortic aneurysms is the size, or transverse diameter. The absolute risk of rupture related to size is unknown. Best estimates suggest small abdominal aortic aneurysms less than 4 cm in diameter have a risk of rupture of less than 15% in 5 years, whereas aneurysms greater than 8 cm in diameter have a 75% risk of rupture within 5 years (Fig. 52-12).

Enlarging and Symptomatic Aneurysms

Aneurysms tend to progressively enlarge because of the increased tension on and thinning of the artery wall. If this process is slow, symptoms do not appear or are very late in appearing. If, however, enlargement is relatively rapid, symptoms of pain may arise as a result of pressure on the somatic sensory nerve elements of the retroperitoneal soft tissue in the vicinity of the aneurysmal sac. The pain is usually severe, constant, unrelated to posture, and

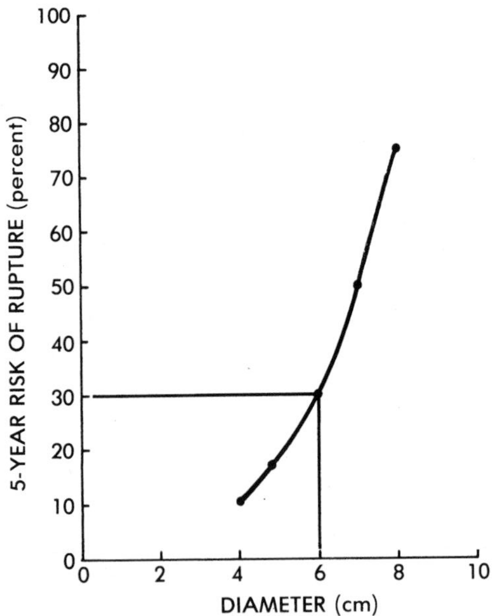

Fig. 52-12. Relationship between the 5-year risk of rupture and the diameter of infrarenal abdominal aortic aneurysms. A 6 cm abdominal aneurysm has a 30% risk for rupturing within 5 years.

boring in character; it is most commonly located in the lumbar spine region, in the midabdomen, or in the pelvis. Such symptoms indicate impending rupture of the aneurysm and require immediate clinical attention.

Serial follow-up examinations using clinical and radiologic methods identify the patient with an aneurysm that is expanding and yet asymptomatic. The rate of enlargement can be variable and unpredictable. The mean rate of expansion of infrarenal abdominal aortic aneurysms is 0.4 cm/yr[87]; however, some do not change at all, whereas others enlarge at twice that rate.

Ruptured Aneurysms

Aneurysms that rupture usually do so into the retroperitoneal space with the development of severe back pain and sudden hypotension. If the rupture occurs anteriorly, free intraperitoneal hemorrhage results with rapid exsanguination. Rupture can also occur into the inferior vena cava, resulting in the development of an *aortocaval fistula* with hypotension and an elevated central venous pressure. The overall survival of patients with ruptured abdominal aortic aneurysms who survive to reach the hospital averages approximately 50% if treated surgically. The mortality rate of patients with minor contained leaks is not much greater than for elective repair; but if free intraperitoneal bleeding and shock are present, survival is less than 10%. On physical examination ruptured aneurysms, even large ones, may be difficult to palpate because of hypotension and because the aortic aneurysm is often diffuse and ill defined as a result of obliteration of the margins of the aneurysm by retroperitoneal hematoma.

Diagnosis

The diagnosis of abdominal aortic aneurysm may be made on physical examination. However, physical examination commonly overestimates the true size of the aneurysm by 1 to 2 cm when compared to ultrasound or CT examination. A *cross table lateral x-ray* may demonstrate a rim of calcium outlining the anterior wall of the abdominal aorta and indicate the presence of an aneurysm. This x-ray film is taken with the patient lying supine with the x-ray beam running horizontally allowing intestinal gas to rise superiorly and the retroperitoneum to be visualized. Physical examination and a lateral x-ray film were in the past the predominant methods of evaluation for an abdominal aortic aneurysm. However, in view of the new development of ultrasound, the lateral abdominal x-ray film is currently used infrequently.

B-mode ultrasound is the most commonly used method of diagnosing an abdominal aortic aneurysm. It is simple, safe, noninvasive, and accurate and can be readily repeated for serial evaluation of aneurysms. It provides information on the presence or absence of an aneurysm and on the transverse diameter, length, and presence or absence of mural thrombus. It is the procedure of choice for routine evaluation for aneurysm.

CT scan provides better resolution and imaging of aneurysms than ultrasound, especially when intravenous contrast enhancement is used. It provides the most detailed evaluation of the aortic wall and mural thrombus and the most accurate assessment of aneurysm size. It also allows the evaluation of retroperitoneal extravasation and rupture. However, the procedure is more expensive than ultrasound and usually is not essential for most abdominal aneurysms. The CT scan offers significant advantages over ultrasound in assessing the thoracoabdominal aorta, since ultrasound does not pass through the air in the lung and cannot visualize the thoracic aorta. Thus it is particularly helpful in assessing thoracoabdominal aneurysms. In addition, CT is very useful in evaluating the pelvis for the presence of internal iliac aneurysms. The role of newer imaging modalities, such as MR angiography or spiral CT scanning remains undetermined.

Angiography is useful in the evaluation of abdominal aortic aneurysms but provides little information on aneurysm size since only the aortic lumen is visualized. Aneurysms frequently contain mural thrombus, which may result in a normal or relatively normal lumen contour and diameter. This mural thrombus provides no structural strength to the aortic wall, and such aneurysms are just as likely to rupture as those without extensive mural thrombosis. Despite the fact that aortic angiography may not accurately represent aneurysm size, other important information can be obtained, including (1) accurate assessment of the proximal extent of the aneurysm in relation to the renal arteries, (2) the status of the renal arteries and the presence of accessory renal arteries arising from the aneurysm itself, (3) the inferior mesenteric artery and its collateral blood supply to the left colon, (4) coexistent occlusive disease of the iliac and femoral vessels, and (5) identification of congenital abnormalities of the kidneys such as horseshoe kidney.

Treatment

Indications for Surgery

Indications for surgical repair of abdominal aortic aneurysms depend on the presence or absence of symptoms, the size of the aneurysm, and the general medical condition of the patient. If a patient has a ruptured aortic aneurysm, immediate surgical treatment is imperative. No diagnostic tests should be performed, and resuscitation should be carried out in the operating room. Fluid resuscitation may be useful during transport.

Patients with symptoms attributable to an aneurysm but without hypotension or signs of rupture should undergo confirmatory CT examination and urgent operative repair of the aneurysm. Similarly, if there is evidence of rapid enlargement of the aneurysm on routine physical examination or imaging follow-up such as B-mode ultrasound, urgent repair of the aneurysm is advised.

The absolute size of the aneurysm also determines whether repair should be undertaken. Studies of the natural history of aneurysms reveal that the risk of rupture of untreated aneurysms is directly proportional to their size.[88,89] Aneurysms greater than 5 cm in transverse diameter as measured by ultrasound or CT scan or aneurysms that have more than twice the diameter of the adjacent, nonaneurysmal aorta should be surgically repaired if the patient has no medical contraindications to surgery such as severe cardiac, pulmonary, renal, or neoplastic disease. However, it must be realized that aneurysms smaller than 5 cm can also rupture and must be carefully observed.

Surgical Repair

The surgical treatment of an abdominal aortic aneurysm consists of excluding the aneurysm from the circulation and replacing it with a Dacron prosthetic bypass graft. The aorta is clamped proximal to the aneurysm, below the level of the renal arteries, and distal to the aneurysm. The aneurysm sac is opened, and the graft is sutured to the normal, nonaneurysmal aorta from within the aneurysm. The graft may be a straight "tube" graft confined to the abdominal aorta or a bifurcation graft to the iliac arteries if the aortic bifurcation and iliac arteries are involved (Fig. 52-13). The aneurysm sac is not excised but closed over the graft after it is in place to isolate the graft from the bowel. This prevents possible erosion of the bowel, aortoduodenal fistula formation, and graft infection. The inferior mesenteric artery, which always arises from the aneurysm, is usually ligated. Collateral circulation from the celiac and superior mesenteric arteries and internal iliac arteries maintains flow to the sigmoid colon. Occasionally, when collateral flow is insufficient, the inferior mesenteric artery must be reimplanted into the bypass graft to avoid colonic ischemia.

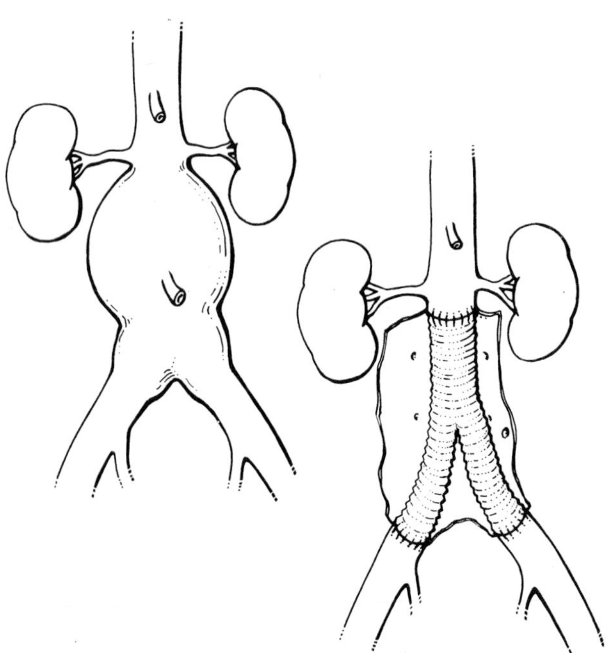

Fig. 52-13. Repair of abdominal aortic aneurysm. Aneurysm sac is opened, and a Dacron graft is sutured to the normal, nonaneurysmal artery. Aneurysm is not excised, but it is excluded from the circulation.

Results and Long-Term Outlook

The results of abdominal aortic aneurysm repair differ depending on whether the procedure is performed electively for an asymptomatic aneurysm, urgently for a symptomatic aneurysm, or emergently for a ruptured aneurysm. Elective aneurysm repair and urgent repair of nonruptured aneurysms have a mortality rate of less than 3%.[90,91] Operations for ruptured abdominal aortic aneurysms have a mortality rate of 50% to 80% or higher.[92] Thus every effort should be made to repair abdominal aortic aneurysms before rupture. Improved operative techniques with better preoperative and perioperative care, including central hemodynamic monitoring, earlier diagnosis, improvements in fluid management, and refinements in anesthesia techniques, have allowed elective aneurysm repair to be carried out with a similar low mortality rate even in octogenarians.[93] Thus age alone is not a contraindication to aneurysm repair.

The long-term survival of patients who have undergone abdominal aortic aneurysm repair is approximately 50% at 5 years. Associated coronary artery disease is responsible for the majority of deaths in the long-term follow-up of these patients. In a matched group the expected 5-year survival is 80%.[91] It is possible that with more aggressive treatment of coexistent coronary disease this mortality rate can be decreased. The overall survival and long-term outlook with elective repair of large abdominal aortic aneurysms is significantly better than nonsurgical treatment.

PERIPHERAL ARTERY ANEURYSMS

Although it is not common, aneurysms can form in arteries other than the aorta. The most commonly involved peripheral arteries are the common femoral and popliteal arteries that together account for 90% of all peripheral aneurysms. The popliteal artery accounts for 70% of these aneurysms. *Popliteal aneurysms* are unique in that they are found almost exclusively in males, and the vast majority are atherosclerotic in origin. Approximately two thirds of the patients have bilateral aneurysms, with one half of these patients having associated abdominal aortic aneurysms.

Popliteal aneurysms are usually symptomatic when discovered, and over 50% have complications at the first medical visit.[93] The most common complication is thrombosis of the aneurysm, which is associated with a 33% amputation rate. Embolization of mural thrombus from within the aneurysm to the distal arterial tree also occurs and is associated with a high amputation rate. Rupture of popliteal aneurysms is unusual but can occur. Compression of the popliteal vein with lower extremity edema and neurologic pain syndromes from nerve compression are also possible.

Treatment of popliteal aneurysms consists of ligation

of the aneurysm to exclude it from the circulation, followed by bypass grafting from the femoral artery to either the popliteal or tibial vessels. Results of surgery are influenced by the status of the leg at the time of presentation and the extent of coexistent occlusive disease in the tibial vessels and vessels of the foot. If these are obstructed because of prior and repeated embolization from the aneurysm, prospects for revascularization are poor. There is minimal risk for limb loss in patients with asymptomatic aneurysms, but 34% of limbs are lost if the patient initially has symptoms.[93] Therefore popliteal aneurysms should be repaired electively when found, before symptoms of embolization or thrombosis occur.

Femoral artery aneurysms are similarly found in elderly men and are caused by atherosclerosis. Associated hypertension is extremely common. Associated abdominal aortic aneurysms are present in 51% to 85% of patients[94,95] and in the popliteal artery segment in 17% to 44% of patients,[95,96] suggesting an aneurysmal diathesis. As in the popliteal artery, symptoms may be caused by local pressure from the expanding aneurysm on the adjacent femoral vein or nerve, distal embolization, acute or chronic thrombosis, or rupture of the aneurysm. Because of the risk for limb loss from acute thrombosis and distal embolization, surgical management of these aneurysms is advised in all patients who are reasonable medical risks. Surgical techniques include replacement of the aneurysm with an interposition graft.[97]

COMPLICATIONS OF VASCULAR PROCEDURES

Complications following vascular procedures fall into two categories: those involving the generalized disease process of atherosclerosis and those involving local factors related to the vascular procedure or bypass graft.

The generalized process of atherosclerosis involves not only the peripheral arteries but also the carotid and coronary arteries. The risk factors of hypertension, hyperlipidemia, diabetes mellitus, and cigarette smoking are important in whether there is disease progression, stabilization, or regression; and control of these factors is important. The major cause of morbidity and mortality in the vascular surgical patient is disease progression in the coronary arteries, with myocardial infarctions accounting for the majority of deaths in these patients despite successful peripheral vascular procedures. Stroke from progression of cerebrovascular disease is also a major problem. These same risk factors play a major role in the progression of distal disease following bypass grafts and are a common reason for restenosis and subsequent graft occlusion and its related morbidity.

Local factors related to vascular procedures may produce a number of complications following vascular procedures. Graft thrombosis in the early postoperative period may be the result of a technical error in the graft-to-artery anastomosis or caused by an obstructed outflow bed with slow flow in the graft. Late graft occlusion is usually caused by progression of atherosclerotic occlusive disease in the inflow or outflow vessels or by a hypertrophic proliferative response of intima at the anastomosis and can usually be corrected by reoperation.

Pseudoaneurysms may form at the sites of vascular anastomoses and must be distinguished from true aneurysms that involved dilation of all layers of the artery wall. In a pseudoaneurysm there is separation of the vascular graft from the artery wall, and the blood stream is contained by surrounding fibrous tissue. The integrity of an anastomosis of prosthetic graft to artery is forever dependent on the integrity of the suture line. Failure of the suture or excess tension on the suture line can result in the disruption of the anastomosis with pseudoaneurysm formation. In addition, anastomotic breakdown with pseudoaneurysm formation may be a harbinger or sign that infection of the prosthetic bypass graft has occurred. Treatment of a pseudoaneurysm mandates replacement of that segment with a prosthetic graft if it is not infected. However, infected grafts must be totally removed because prosthetic grafts are foreign bodies and infection cannot be eradicated until all foreign material is excised.

Revascularization under these circumstances is complex and usually involves the use of an "extra-anatomic" bypass in a clean, noninfected area. An example of such a bypass is an axillofemoral bypass to bypass an infected intra-abdominal aortoiliac bypass graft.

SUMMARY

Atherosclerosis is a degenerative disease process that affects the aorta and peripheral arteries, as well as coronary and carotid arteries. It can result in occlusive disease, obstructing the lumen or aneurysmal disease with dilation of the lumen. Occlusive disease can result in stenosis and diminished blood flow or embolization with occlusion of distal arteries. Obstruction of blood flow can result in ischemia of the lower extremities, producing symptoms of claudication, rest pain, ulceration, or gangrene. Obstructions can be detected with the use of clinical, noninvasive, and angiographic diagnostic techniques. Revascularization of the lower extremities with a bypass or with transluminal balloon angioplasty can restore circulation and avoid limb loss.

Aneurysmal disease results in progressive arterial enlargement and weakening of the aortic wall, with eventual rupture unless the patient dies of intercurrent disease. The larger is the aneurysm, the higher is the risk of rupture. Most aneurysms are asymptomatic and are detectable by noninvasive techniques. Operative replacement of aneurysmal segments of artery with a Dacron graft prevents further degeneration and aneurysm rupture.

REFERENCES

1. Fann JI, Dalman RL. Genetic and metabolic causes of arterial disease. Ann Vasc Surg 7:594, 1993.
2. Vogt MT, Wolfson SK, Kullen LN. Lower extremity arterial disease and the aging process. J Clin Epidemiol 45:529, 1992.

3. Reunanen A, Takkunen H, Aromaa A. Prevalence of intermittent claudication and its effect on mortality. Acta Med Scand 211:249, 1982.
4. Kannel WB, Mcbee DL. Update on some epidemiological features of intermittent claudication. The Framingham Study. J Am Geriatr Soc 33:13, 1985.
5. Scheoll M, Murck O. Estimation of peripheral arteriosclerotic disease by ankle pressure measurements in a population study of 60 year old men and women. J Chron Dis 34:261, 1981.
6. Criqui MH, et al. Peripheral arterial disease in large vessels is epidemiologically distinct from small vessel disease. An analysis of risk factors. Am J Epidemiol 129:1110, 1989.
7. Krupski WC. The peripheral vascular consequences of smoking. Ann Vasc Surg 5:291, 1991.
8. Powell JT, Greenhalgh RM. Arterial bypass surgery and smokers. Br Med J 308:607, 1994.
9. Diabetes Control and Complications Trial Research Group. The effect of intensive treatment of diabetes on the development and progression of long-term complications in insulin-dependent diabetes mellitus. N Engl J Med 329:977, 1993.
10. McGill HC Jr. Atherosclerosis: Problems in pathogenesis. In Paoletti R, Gotto AM, eds. Atherosclerosis Reviews. New York: Raven Press, 1977, p 27.
11. Paterson JC. Vascularization and haemorrhage of the intima of arteriosclerotic arteries. Arch Pathol 22:312, 1936.
12. Zarins CK, et al. Aneurysm formation in experimental atherosclerosis: Relationship to plaque formation. J Vasc Surg 2:246, 1990.
13. Strickland HL, Bond MG. Aneurysms in a large colony of squirrel monkeys *(Saimiri sciures)*. Lab Anim Sci 33:589, 1983.
14. Rifkin RD, Parisis HF, Follard E. Coronary calcification in the diagnosis of coronary artery disease. Am J Cardiol 44:141, 1979.
15. Glagov S, Eckner FAO, Lev M. Controlled pressure fixation apparatus for hearts. Arch Pathol 76:640, 1963.
16. Zarins CK, Zatina MA, Glagov S. Correlation of postmortem angiography with pathologic anatomy: Quantitation of atherosclerotic lesions. In Bond MG, et al., eds. Clinical Diagnosis of Atherosclerosis. New York: Springer-Verlag, 1983, p 283.
17. Mulvihill DA, Harvey SC. The mechanism of the development of collateral circulation. N Engl J Med 104:1032, 1931.
18. Holman E. Problems in the dynamics of blood flow. I. Condition controlling collateral circulation in the presence of an ateriovenous fistula following ligation of an artery. Surgery 26:889, 1949.
19. Kamiya A, Togawa T. Adaptive regulation of wall shear stress to flow change in the canine carotid artery. Am J Physiol 239:H14, 1980.
20. Furchgott RF. Role of endothelium in responses of vascular smooth muscle. Circ Res 53:557, 1983.
21. Langille BL, O'Donnel F. Reductions in arterial diameter produced by chronic decreases in blood flow are endothelium dependent. Science 231:405, 1986.
22. Ying H, Harris EJ, Dalman RL. Unpublished observations 1992–1993.
23. Thubrikar M, Maker J, Nolan S. Inhibition of atherosclerosis associated with reduction of arterial intramural stenosis in rabbits. Arteriosclerosis 8:410, 1988.
24. Friedman MH. Some atherosclerosis may be a consequence of the normal adaptive vascular response to shear. Atherosclerosis 82:193, 1990.
25. Zarins CK, et al. Carotid bifurcation atherosclerosis: Quantitative correlation of plaque localization with flow velocity profiles and wall shear stress. Circ Res 53:502, 1983.
26. Ku DN, et al. Pulsatile flow and atherosclerosis in the human carotid bifurcation: Positive correlation between plaque localization and low oscillating shear stress. Arteriosclerosis 5:292, 1985.
27. Karino T. Microscopic structure of disturbed flows in the arterial and venous systems and its implication in the localization of vascular disease. Int Angiol 5:297, 1986.
28. Glagov S, Rowley DA, Kohut R. Atherosclerosis of human aorta and its coronary and renal arteries. Arch Pathol 72:558, 1961.
29. Svindland A. The localization of sudanophilic and fibrous plaques in the main left coronary arteries. Atherosclerosis 48:139, 1983.
30. Giddens DP, Zarins CK, Glagov S. The role of fluid mechanics in the localization and detection of atherosclerosis. J Biomech Eng 115:588, 1993.
31. Fingerle J, Johnson R, Clowes AW. Role of platelets in smooth muscle cell proliferation and migration after vascular injury in rat carotid artery. Proc Natl Acad Sci USA 86:8412, 1989.
32. Falcone DJ, Haijar DP, Minick CR. Lipoprotein and albumin accumulation in re-endothelialized and de-endothelialized aorta. Am J Pathol 114:112, 1984.
33. Bassinouny HS, et al. Quantitative inverse correlation of wall shear stress with experimental intima thickening. Surg Forum 39:328, 1988.
34. Lyon RT, Hass A, Davis HR. Protection from atherosclerotic lesion formation by reduction of artery wall motion. J Vasc Surg 5:59, 1987.
35. Caro GG, et al. Influence of vasoreactive agents on arterial hemodynamics: Possible relevance to atherogenesis. Biorheology 23:197, 1986.
36. Glagov S. Microarchitecture of arteries and veins. In Abrahson D, Dobrin P, eds. Blood Vessels and Lymphatics. Orlando, Fla.: Academic Press, 1984, p 3.
37. Glagov S, et al. Hemodynamics and atherosclerosis: Insights and perspectives gained from studies of human arteries. Arch Pathol Lab Med 112:1018, 1988.
38. Glagov S, et al. Establishing the hemodynamic determinants of human plaque configuration, composition and complication. In Yoshida Y, et al., eds. Role of Blood Flow in Atherogenesis. New York: Springer-Verlag, 1988, p 3.
39. Born VRG, Richardson PD. Mechanical properties of human atherosclerotic lesions. In Glagov S, Newman WP, Schaffer SA, eds. Pathobiology of the Human Atherosclerotic Plaque. New York: Springer-Verlag, 1990, p 413.
40. Zarins CK, et al. Artery stenosis inhibits regression of diet-induced atherosclerosis. Surgery 88:86, 1980.
41. Xu Chengpei, Glagov S, Zatina M. Hypertension sustains plaque progression despite reduction of hypercholesterolemia. Hypertension 18:123, 1991.
42. Zarins CK, et al. Shear stress regulation of artery lumen diameter in experimental atherogenesis. J Vasc Surg 5:413, 1987.
43. Fry DL. Problems and progress in understanding "endothelial permeability" and mass transport in human arteries. In Glagov S, Newman WP, Schaffer SA, eds. Pathobiology of the Human Atherosclerotic Plaque. New York: Springer-Verlag, 1990, p 271.
44. Smith EB. Accumulating evidence from human artery studies of what is transported and what accumulates relative to atherogenesis. In Glagov S, Newman WP, Schaffer SA, eds. Pathobiology of the Human Atherosclerotic Plaque. New York: Springer-Verlag, 1990.
45. Tracy RE, Kissling GE. Comparisons of human populations for histologic features of atherosclerosis. Arch Pathol Lab Med 112:156, 1988.
46. Frank JS, Fogelman AM. Ultrastructure of the intima in WHHL and cholesterol-fed rabbit aortas prepared by ultra-rapid freezing and freeze-etching. J Lipid Res 30:967, 1989.
47. Berenson GS, et al. In Glagov S, Newman WP, Schaffer SA, eds. Pathobiology of the Human Atherosclerotic Plaque. New York: Springer-Verlag, 1990, p 189.
48. Kramsh DM, Hollander W. The interaction of serum and arterial lipoproteins with elastin of the arterial intima and its role in the lipid accumulation in atherosclerotic plaque. J Clin Invest 52:236, 1973.
49. Wagner WD, et al. Low density lipoprotein interaction with artery derived proteoglycan: The influence of LDL particle size and the relationship to atherosclerosis susceptibility. Atherosclerosis 75:49, 1989.

50. Grande J, et al. Effect of an elastin growth substrate on cholesteryl ester synthesis and foam cell formation by cultured aortic smooth muscle cells. Atherosclerosis 68:87, 1987.
51. May AG, De Weese JA, Rob CG. Hemodynamic effects of arterial stenosis. Surgery 53:513, 1963.
52. Thompson JE, et al. Arterial embolectomy: A 20 year experience with 163 cases. Surgery 67: 212, 1970.
53. Coffman JD. Intermittent claudication—be conservative. N Engl J Med 325:557, 1991.
54. Jelnes R, et al. Fate in intermittent claudication: Outcome and risk factors. Br Med J 293:1137, 1986.
55. Sibert S, Zazeela H. Prognosis in arteriosclerotic peripheral vascular disease. JAMA 156:1816, 1958.
56. Kallero KS. Mortality and morbidity in patients with intermittent claudication as defined by venous occlusion plethysonography. A ten year follow-up study. J Chron Dis 34:455, 1981.
57. Croneneitt JL, et al. Intermittent claudication. Current results at non-operative management. Arch Surg 119: 430, 1984.
58. Dormandy J, et al. Fate of the patient with chronic leg ischemia. J Cardiovasc Surg 30:50, 1989.
59. Bandyk DF. Essentials of graft surveillance. Semin Vasc Surg 6:92, 1993.
60. Mills JL, et al. The origin of infrainguinal vein graft stenosis. A prospective study based on duplex surveillance. J Vasc Surg 21:16, 1995.
61. Bandyk DF, et al. Intraoperative duplex scanning of arterial reconstructions: Rate of repaired and unrepaired defects. J Vasc Surg 20:426, 1994.
62. Shehadi WH, Tonielo G. Adverse reactions to contrast media. Radiology 137:299, 1980.
63. Marks MP, et al. Diagnosis of carotid artery diseases: Preliminary experience with maximum intensity projection spiral CT angiography. Am J Roentgenol 160:1267, 1993.
64. Rubin GD, et al. Three dimensional spiral computed tomographic angiography: An alternative imaging modality for the abdominal aorta and its branches. J Vasc Surg 18:656, 1993.
65. Napel S, Rubin GD, Jeffrey RB, Jr. STS-MIP: A new reconstruction technique for CT of the chest. J Comput Assist Tomogr 17:832, 1993.
66. Carpenter JP, et al. Peripheral vascular surgery with magnetic resonance angiography as the sole preoperative imaging modality. J Vasc Surg 20:861, 1994.
67. Debatin JE, et al. Phase contrast MRI assessment of pedal blood flow. Eur Radiol 194:321, 1995.
68. Li KCP, et al. Oxygen saturation of blood in the superior mesenteric vein: In vivo verification of MR imaging measurements in a canine model. Radiology 194:321, 1995.
69. Li KCP, et al. Simultaneous measurement of flow in the superior mesenteric vein and artery with cine phase-contrast MR imaging: Value in diagnosis of chronic mesenteric ischemia. Radiology 194:327, 1995.
70. Peabody CN, Kannel WB, McNamara PM. Intermittent claudication: Surgical significance. Arch Surg 109:693, 1974.
71. Smith CD, McKendry RJ. Controlled trial of nifedipine in the treatment of Raynaud's phenomenon. Lancet 2:1299, 1982.
72. Porter JM, et al. Pentoxifylline efficacy in the treatment of intermittent claudication. Am Heart J 104:66, 1982.
73. Zarins CK, et al. Arterial disruption and remodeling following dilatation. Surgery 92:1086, 1982.
74. Dalman RL, Taylor LM, Porter JM. Current status of extracoronary endovascular procedures. Ann Vasc Surg 3:1, 1990.
75. Ahn SS, et al. Reporting standards for lower extremity arterial endovascular procedures. J Vasc Surg 17:1103, 1993.
76. Rutherford RB. Aortofemoral bypass: The gold standard. Technical considerations. Semin Vasc Surg 7:11, 1994.
77. Brewster DC, Darling RC. Optimal methods of aortoiliac reconstruction. Surgery 84:739, 1978.
78. Taylor CM, et al. Axillofemoral grafting with externally supported PTFE. Arch Surg 129:588, 1994.
79. Taylor CM, et al. Acute disruption of polytetrafluoroethylene grafts adjacent to axillary anastomosis: A complication of axillofemoral grafting. J Vasc Surg 20:520, 1994.
80. Fann JI, Harris EJ, Dalman RL. Extra-anatomic bypass. Ann Vasc Surg 7:378, 1993.
81. Corson JD, et al. In situ vein bypasses to distal tibial and limited outflow tracts for limb salvage. Surgery 96:756, 1984.
82. Dalman RL, Taylor CM. Basic data regarding intrainguinal revascularization procedures. Ann Vasc Surg 4:309, 1990.
83. Craver JM, et al. Hemorrage and thrombosis as early complications of femoropopliteal bypass grafts: Causes, treatment, and prognostic implications. Surgery 74:839, 1971.
84. Wolinsky H, Glagov S. Nature of species differences in the medial distribution of aortic vasa vasorum in mammals. Circ Res 20:409, 1967.
85. Wolinsky H, Glagov S. Comparison of abdominal and thoracic aortic medial structure in mammals: Deviation of man from the usual pattern. Circ Res 25:677, 1969.
86. Zarins CK, Glagov S. Aneurysms and obstructive plaques: Differing local response to atherosclerosis. In Bergan JJ, Yao JST, eds. Aneurysms: Diagnosis and Treatment. New York: Grune & Stratton, 1982.
87. Bernstein EF, et al. Growth rates of small abdominal aortic aneurysms. Surgery 80:765, 1976.
88. Bernstein EF. The natural history of abdominal aortic aneurysms. In Najarian JS, Delaney JP, eds. Vascular Surgery. Miami, Fla.: Symposia Specialists, 1978.
89. Szilagyi DE, Elliott JP, Smith RF. Clinical fate of patients with asymptomatic abdominal aortic aneurysm and unfit for special treatment. Arch Surg 104:600, 1972.
90. DeBakey MD, et al. Aneurysms of the abdominal aorta: Analysis of results of graft replacement therapy one to eleven years after operation. Ann Surg 160:622, 1964.
91. Thompson JE, et al. Surgical management of abdominal aortic aneurysms: Factors influencing mortality and morbidity—A 20 year experience. Ann Surg 188:654, 1975.
92. Garrett HE, Ilabaca PA. The ruptured abdominal aortic aneurysm. In Bergan JJ, Yao JST, eds. Aneurysms: Diagnosis and Treatment. New York: Grune & Stratton, 1982.
93. Evans WE, Conley JE, Bernhard V. Popliteal aneurysms. Surgery 70:762, 1971.
94. O'Donnel TF, Jr., Darling RC, Linton RR. Is 80 years too old for aneurysmectomy? Arch Surg 111:1250, 1976.
95. Cutler BS, Darling RC. Surgical management of arteriosclerotic femoral aneurysms. Surgery 74:764, 1973.
96. Graham L, et al. Clinical significance of arteriosclerotic femoral artery aneurysms. Arch Surg 115:502, 1973.
97. Baird RJ, et al. Arteriosclerotic femoral artery aneurysms. Can Med Assoc J 117:1306, 1977.

53

Cerebrovascular Disease and Upper Extremity Vascular Disease

Bruce L. Gewertz and James F. McKinsey

In each calendar year nearly 500,000 Americans have cerebral infarctions; 175,000 strokes are fatal, whereas the remaining patients experience variable disability. The emotional and economic consequences of advanced cerebrovascular disease are staggering; the cost of care and loss of earnings secondary to permanent disability or death have been estimated at more than $10 billion annually.

In contrast to these depressing statistics, there has been a persistent 10-year decline in the death rate from stroke that has exceeded the general decline in cardiovascular mortality observed over the same time period.[1] It is difficult to explain this phenomenon. Although surgery for extracranial occlusive disease has become much more common in the last 15 years, improved medical and surgical care can account for only a small fraction of the change in death rate. It is most likely that the decline in cardiovascular mortality reflects better control of arterial hypertension, changes in life-style, and the general reduction in cigarette smoking.[2,3]

Although the natural history of stroke in the United States was defined in an earlier era, studies performed from 1950 to 1975 provide useful information regarding the indications and timing of cerebrovascular surgery.[4,5] The following are now accepted facts:

1. Patients who have survived one cerebral infarction have a high incidence of *recurrent strokes* (approximately 25%). More than half of these recurrent strokes are fatal.
2. Prodromal symptoms of stroke such as *transient ischemic attacks (TIAs)* identify patients at greatest risk for suffering later completed strokes. The cumulative stroke rate approaches 50% at 5 years and is highest in the first year after the transient ischemic episode.[6,7]
3. Patients suffering TIA or strokes from *atheromatous stenotic lesions* of the carotid bifurcation are significantly benefited by carotid endarterectomy if the complications of the procedure are equal to or less than current norms.

In this chapter the anatomy and physiology of cerebral blood flow are reviewed, the variable clinical presentations of cerebral ischemia are characterized, and the diagnostic and therapeutic options are considered. It has become clear that only through better understanding of cerebrovascular physiology can the care of patients with advanced vascular disease be improved.

CEREBRAL BLOOD FLOW

Anatomy

The brain is perfused by paired carotid and vertebral arteries that communicate with each other through the circle of Willis at the base of the skull. Although there is substantial variation in the effectiveness of this collateral network (less than 20% of patients have "complete" circles), occlusion of one vessel is frequently compensated for without neurologic deficit. In general terms a carotid artery supplies only the ipsilateral cerebral hemisphere through the middle, anterior, and posterior cerebral vessels. The vertebral arteries join to form a single basilar artery that supplies the brain stem and cerebellum with additional contributions to the posterior aspect of the circle of Willis (Fig. 53-1).

Boundary zones or "watershed" areas between the primary perfusion territories of the middle, anterior, and posterior cerebral arteries can be demonstrated by anatomic studies. These areas are most at risk for ischemia and infarction during hypotension or vascular occlusion. Perhaps because of the lower basal vascular tone of these vessels, boundary zones are frequently the site of intracerebral hemorrhages associated with acute hypertension.

The subclavian origin of both vertebral arteries makes possible the unique subclavian steal syndrome that is discussed in greater detail later in this chapter (Fig. 53-2). This syndrome occurs when an occlusive lesion proximal

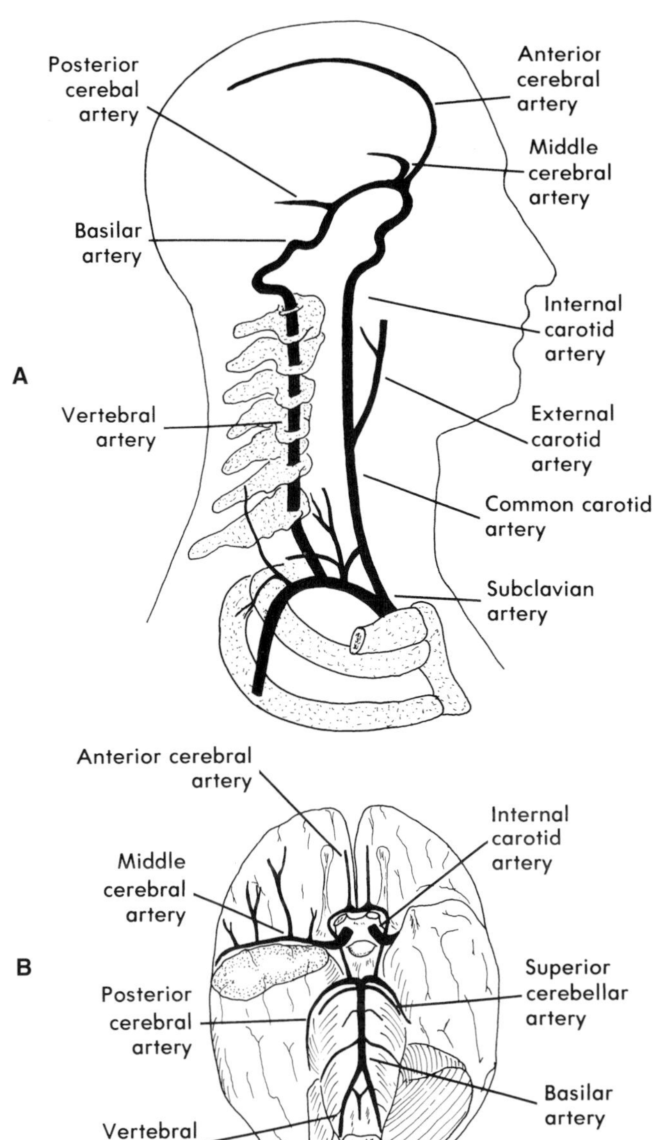

Fig. 53-1. A, Carotid artery supplies middle cerebral and anterior cerebral arteries predominantly with major contributions to posterior cerebral artery. **B,** Vertebral arteries form the basilar artery that supplies cerebellar vessels and posterior cerebral arteries.

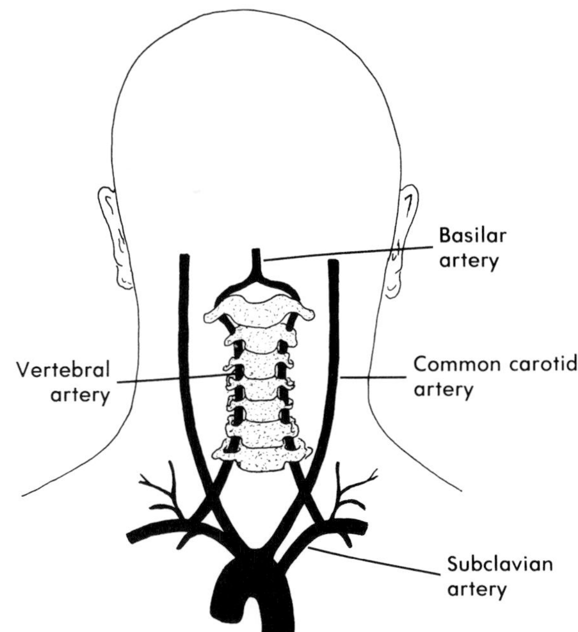

Fig. 53-2. Subclavian origin of vertebral arteries allows these vessels to function as collateral pathways for upper extremity. Cerebellar ischemia may result from the "steal" of blood flow.

to the origin of the vertebral vessels decreases perfusion pressure in the distal subclavian artery. The vertebral artery then functions as a collateral pathway for the arm, and reversal of flow (away from the cranium) can be demonstrated angiographically. This flow pattern "steals" blood from the basilar system and may result in cerebellar ischemia or infarction.

Characteristics of Flow

The cerebral circulation is supplied with nearly 15% of cardiac output. Resting total blood flows range from 50 to 60 ml/min/100 g of tissue, with higher values in the cellular gray matter (100 ml/min/100 g) and lower flows in the cell-poor white matter (20 ml/min/100 g).[8,9] Cerebral blood flow is regulated by both metabolic and myogenic mechanisms that tend to maintain or "autoregulate" perfusion to avoid cerebral infarction during hypotension and cerebral hemorrhage during hypertension.[10,11] Cerebral infarcts may result when regional blood flows decline below 15 ml/min/100 g, although the metabolic state of the brain strongly influences the likelihood of cell death.[12] Barbiturate coma has been shown to decrease the ischemic limit to as low as 5 ml/min/100 g.[13]

The cerebral circulation is further distinguished by a *blood-brain barrier* that effectively isolates brain tissue from serum ionic changes and humoral factors.[14] The barrier is both a physical and biochemical impediment to the transport of protein and polar substances into cerebral extracellular fluid. Anatomic features include tight junctions between endothelial cells, with only a few scattered pores and minimal transport by pinocytotic vesicles. A membrane-bound enzyme system, primarily composed of monoamine oxidase, effectively degrades circulating catecholamines and limits cerebral extraction to less than 5%. It is noteworthy that the areas of the brain responsible for hormone regulation such as the hypothalamus, pituitary gland, and pineal gland do *not* demonstrate the anatomic or functional characteristics of the blood-brain barrier.

The blood-brain barrier is disrupted in areas of tissue infarction and during periods of severe hypertension.[15] These observations are clinically important, since breakdown of the blood-brain barrier (1) facilitates the diagnosis of cerebral infarcts by radionuclide scanning and (2) explains the occurrence of late hemorrhage in previously "bland" infarcts when patients become severely hypertensive.

Measurement Techniques

Diverse methods have been used to measure cerebral blood flow in experimental settings, including venous outflow collections, radioactive microspheres, autoradiography, and heat or hydrogen clearance.[16] In clinical practice most measurements of total and regional cerebral blood flow are made on the basis of the clearance of inhaled inert gases including xenon-133. Using the modified Kety-Schmidt method (technique), xenon-133 washout is monitored by external gamma scintillation counters and subjected to "curves stripping" to remove any component of extracranial blood flow.[17] This technique is most accurate in the middle cerebral distribution and least helpful in evaluating the posterior cerebral or cerebellar circulations.

The recent introductions of positive emission tomography allows repeated imaging of radionuclide concentration in any transverse section of the brain.[18] Depending on the labeled element, regional blood flow ($H_{20}{}^{15}$) or substrate use (C^{11}-glucose) can be measured.[19] Although this technology is still regarded as a research tool, it provides the most precise metabolic and flow data available.

Flow Regulatory Mechanisms

Pressure-flow autoregulation is the ability of an organ to maintain normal blood flow despite variations in blood pressure. This protective mechanism is well documented in the cerebral circulation. Most physiologists agree that the process is an intrinsic property of blood vessels involving a continuous readjustment of the myogenic activity of vascular smooth muscle that depends on changes in transmural pressure and the local (extracellular) chemical environment. Increased intravascular pressure (hypertension) predictably results in compensatory vasoconstriction, whereas decreased pressure (hypotension) elicits vasodilation.[20] Although early experiments suggested that P_{CO_2} was the primary chemical regulator of vascular tone, it has become well accepted that the hydrogen ion concentration in the extracellular space provides the vasodilatory influence.[21,22]

Decreasing P_{CO_2} results in lower hydrogen ion concentration, and vasoconstriction is observed. An elevated P_{CO_2} leads to higher hydrogen ion concentration and vasodilation. This relationship is applied clinically in the management of severe head injuries; hyperventilation with resultant hypocarbia and decreased hydrogen ion concentration decreases cerebral blood flow and attenuates posttraumatic cerebral edema. Responses to changes in P_{CO_2} are less vigorous, although hypoxia does result in moderate cerebral vasodilation.

Sympathetic stimulation and other neural stimuli have only a small influence on cerebrovascular resistance and blood flow autoregulation.[23] In fact, there is minimal histologic evidence of adrenergic vasoconstrictive fibers on cortical vessels.[18] Neurally mediated vasoconstriction is limited to large vessels outside the brain proper and as such does not represent a primary regulatory mechanism.[24]

CLINICAL PRESENTATION OF CEREBROVASCULAR DISEASE

Definitions

For purposes of discussion, clinicians have grouped neurologic deficits into four categories. *TIAs* are classically defined as short-lived, often repetitive alterations of mentation, vision, motor, or sensory function that are completely reversed within 24 hours. Although transient ischemic attacks often involve the middle cerebral artery distribution with contralateral arm, leg, and facial weakness, perhaps the most well-recognized episodes involve transient monocular blindness (*amaurosis fugax* or "fleeting blindness"). TIAs that last only a few minutes may be prognostically different from those deficits that persist for longer than 2 hours. For this reason, longer lasting episodes (2 to 72 hours) that still result in no permanent neurologic deficit or radiologic evidence of brain infarction are usually designated *reversible ischemic neurologic deficits.*

A documented cerebral infarction (stroke or cerebrovascular accident) implies a permanent neurologic deficit that is usually associated with CT scan evidence of damage. Neurologic recovery is quite variable and may be complete, but the time course of recovery (weeks or months) clearly distinguishes infarcts from TIAs or reversible ischemic neurologic deficits. A "stuttering stroke" in which the neurologic deficit "waxes and wanes" has been termed *stroke-in-evolution.* This type of presentation is not as common but has received much recent attention because of the potential that therapeutic maneuvers could improve the eventual outcome.[25,26]

Although the above definitions have aided communication, they can be criticized for arbitrarily grouping diverse mechanisms with quite variable prognoses. For example, TIAs can be caused by migraines, seizure disorders, and intracranial aneurysms, as well as by carotid artery lesions. This "lumping" phenomenon is most confusing when large multicenter studies attempt to characterize the natural history of a clinical presentation without rigorous preselection on the basis of cause.

Mechanisms

Symptoms of cerebrovascular disease reflect both the mechanism of ischemia and the specific areas affected. In general, ischemia and infarction result from either *low flow* in large or medium-sized vessels associated with obstructive lesions or hypotension or *emboli* to smaller vessels from proximal ulcerative lesions or turbulent flow. Hemodynamic derangements predisposing to the low flow are manifest clinically by neurologic deficits corresponding to the "watershed" areas between main cerebral artery perfusion territories. Symptoms of embolic occlusion depend on the site of distal impaction. Predictably the size of the embolus determines the vessel it will occlude. Both mechanisms can result in permanent and reversible deficits.[27] In particular, repetitive short-lived neurologic deficits (i.e., TIAs) are compatible with either (1) recurrent ischemia of watershed areas or (2) impaction and lysis of intermittent platelet emboli following a consistent route mandated by hemodynamics and anatomy.

The most common disease process involving the cerebral and extracranial vessels is atherosclerosis.[28] Although the disease is most prevalent in patients older than 50, presentations of younger patients are not rare. In roughly half of the cases the atheroma is localized to the extracranial bifurcation of the common carotid artery into the internal and external carotid arteries. Such atherosclerotic plaques may slowly encroach on the arterial lumen or suddenly occlude following intraplaque hemorrhage.[29]

Other pathologic processes are less common and may more frequently involve younger patients. These include spontaneous subintimal dissections of the internal carotid artery and fibromuscular dysplasia.

Although it is generally accepted that the majority of emboli arise from ulcerated atherosclerotic lesions in the common or internal carotid artery, the intracranial carotid siphon near the origin of the ophthalmic artery can also harbor symptomatic ulcerative lesions. Stenoses and occlusions can involve either the extracranial or intracranial carotid artery, both areas simultaneously (tandem lesions), or any portion of a specific cerebral artery.[30,31]

TYPES OF CEREBROVASCULAR DISEASE

Extracranial Carotid Artery Disease

Clinical Presentation

The symptoms of extracranial carotid disease can be described by the timing of impairment (permanent, transient, relapsing) and the type of neurologic deficit (motor, sensory, cognitive, or communicative). As discussed earlier in this chapter, both decreases in cerebral blood flow and embolic occlusions can produce the entire clinical spectrum. The persistence of any neurologic deficit is synonymous with death of brain tissue. Transient and relapsing episodes unassociated with infarctions are distinguished by the return of the neurologic examination to normal.

The exact nature of a deficit can be directly correlated with the area of brain rendered ischemic. The most commonly involved area is the perfusion territory of the middle cerebral artery (the parietal lobe) that is the main outflow vessel of the carotid artery. The patient with middle cerebral ischemia initially has contralateral hemiparesis or hemiplegia, usually more severe in the arm, and paralysis of the contralateral lower part of the face ("central seventh nerve paralysis"). Associated findings including some degree of hypoesthesia (decreased sensation) on the paralyzed side and a contralateral homonymous hemianopsia (visual field deficit). Aphasia (difficulty with speech) is noted if the dominant hemisphere is involved. The left hemisphere is dominant in nearly all right-handed people and roughly 50% of left-handed people. Such defects can be expressive (Broca's aphasia), receptive (Wernicke's aphasia), or complete. If the nondominant hemisphere is affected, a curious "neglect response" is noted in which the paralyzed extremity is essentially ignored by the patient.

Patients with ischemia of the anterior cerebral artery most commonly have contralateral monoplegia involving only the lower extremity; visual-spatial problems and cortical sensory loss are also common.

Posterior cerebral artery ischemia may result from carotid occlusive disease but is also closely related to vertebral-basilar lesions. Presentations often include visual field defects and may overlap with symptoms of ischemia of the posterior portion of the middle cerebral distribution such as language disturbances and contralateral hemiparesis. Other neurologic signs consistent with posterior cerebral artery ischemia include ipsilateral third cranial nerve palsy and contralateral complete sensory loss (thalamic syndrome).

Diagnosis

Symptomatic carotid artery disease is commonly associated with the neurologic presentations just mentioned. However, it is essential to exclude other causes for such syndromes, including migraines, brain tumors, intracranial hemorrhage, and vascular malformations.

The physical finding most consistent with extracranial carotid disease is a demonstration of a *bruit* on auscultation of the upper cervical region, reflecting turbulent blood flow at a stenosis. Classic carotid bruits have the following characteristics: they are (1) high pitched and fade into diastole, (2) localized to the angle of the jaw, and (3) best heard with the bell rather than the diaphragm of the stethoscope. Unfortunately, even experienced examiners frequently cannot distinguish internal or common carotid bruits from clinically irrelevant turbulence in the distal external carotid artery or other cervical blood vessels. As many as 50% of symptomatic ulcerations may be unassociated with stenoses and hence may not present with bruits. Finally, when a stenosis exceeds 90% of vascular cross-sectional area, the intensity of the bruit often decreases because of lower volume flow. This lack of specificity of cervical bruits is most disturbing in asymptomatic patients with bruits, since physical examination alone does not allow assessment of the degree or even the presence of carotid disease.

Many noninvasive tests have been developed to better characterize extracranial carotid disease without the risk of angiographic procedures. They are most widely used in asymptomatic patients with cervical bruits and in the long-term follow-up of patients already treated with carotid endarterectomy.

Imaging Techniques

Direct noninvasive tests using ultrasound techniques to visualize the extracranial vessels have largely replaced the indirect methods previously used to detect and quantitate disease (oculoplethysmography). When combined with sophisticated range-gated pulsed Doppler instruments (duplex scanning), the velocity and volume flow can be determined.[1] The resolution of duplex scanning has improved recently such that ulcerative nonstenotic lesions can be detected in most patients.

Arteriography for cerebrovascular disease commonly includes imaging of the aortic arch and selective injections of the common carotid arteries with delineation of the carotid siphon and intracranial vessels (Figs. 53-3 and 53-4). The common carotid artery and its bifurcation is readily visualized along with any associated stenoses or ulcerated plaques. Perhaps the most significant advantage of cerebral arteriograms is their ability to demonstrate intracranial lesions and aortic arch disease. Relevant intracranial lesions include tumors, aneurysms, arteriovenous malformations, and arterial occlusive disease particularly of the carotid siphon. Indeed, ulcerative or occlusive lesions of the aortic arch or intracranial vessels may produce symptoms identical to those associated with carotid artery disease such as TIAs or amaurosis fugax. When associated with carotid bifurcation disease, such proximal or distal occlusive lesions are termed "tandem" lesions.

Because of its invasive nature, contrast angiography has associated morbidity and mortality.[32] These adverse reactions can be grouped into three major categories: local, systemic, and neurologic. Local complication rates (ranging from 5% to 15%) include hemorrhage, hematomas, pseudoaneurysms, and formation of thrombi or emboli at the arterial puncture site. Systemic complications of contrast angiography include allergic reactions to the contrast agent, as well renal and cardiovascular manifestations. While the incidence of serious allergic reactions to radiographic contrast agents is less than 2% in most reported series, in patients with a history of contrast allergy, the incidence of anaphylatic reactions may be as high as 20%.[33] Allergic reactions range from minor sequelae such as nausea, vomiting, hives, and chills, to major life-threatening reactions such as hypotension, bronchospasm, laryngospasm, and pulmonary edema. Radiographic contrast agents can also produce a deterioration in renal function especially in patients with preexisting kidney disease. One series reported that nonazotemic patients experienced a 2% incidence of acute renal failure following all types of angiography, whereas patients with chronic azotemia experienced a 33% incidence.[34] However, the same study revealed that the occurrence of acute renal failure was less in patients with carotid-vertebral studies than those patients undergoing visceral angiograms and hence more direct delivery of dye to the kidneys. Cardiac complications of cerebral angiography include hypotension, arrhythmias, myocardial ischemia or infarction, and even cardiac arrest.

Neurologic complications are the most important risk of cerebral angiography.[35] Events range from TIAs (lasting

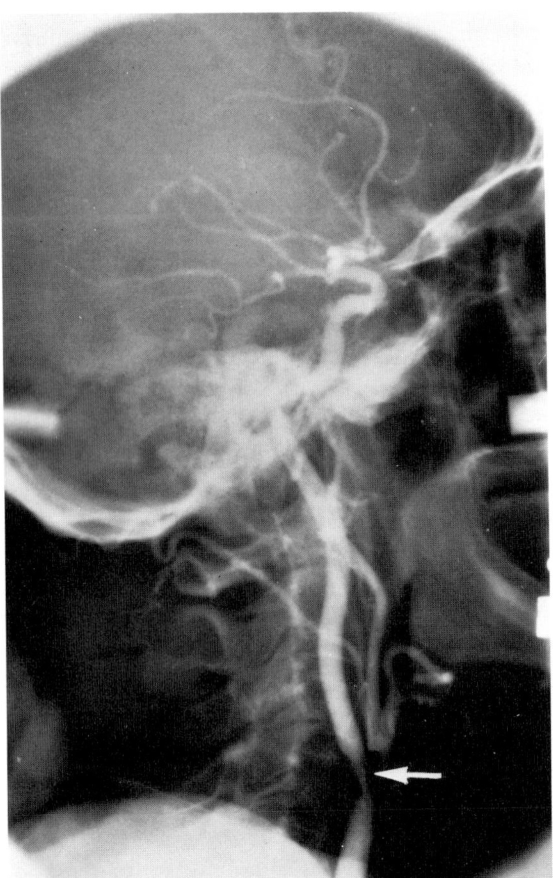

Fig. 53-3. Preoperative angiogram of patient with repeated episodes of contralateral hemiparesis demonstrates severe stenosis of both internal *(arrow)* and external carotid arteries.

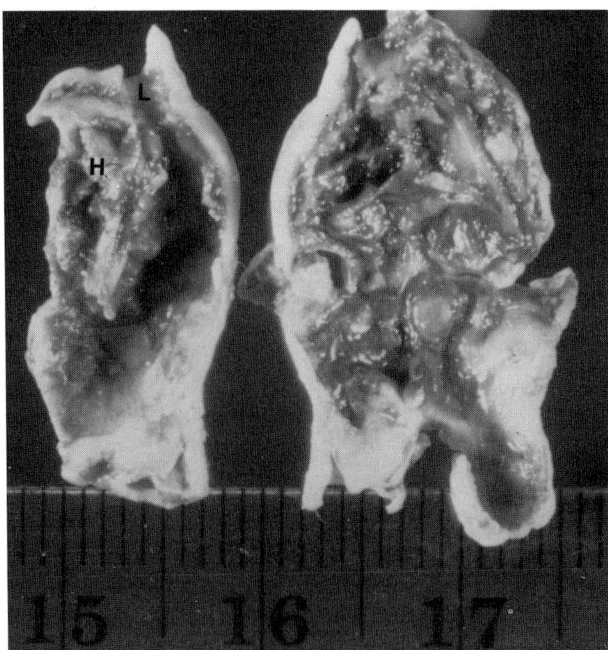

Fig. 53-4. Operative specimen (bivalved) reveals narrow lumen *(L)* with fresh hemorrhage *(H)* within atherosclerotic plaque. Extensive ulcerations are noted.

less than 24 hours) to completed strokes. Hankey et al.[36] reviewed eight prospective studies consisting of 2227 patients with mild ischemic cerebrovascular disease. A 4% incidence of postangiography neurologic complications was observed, of which 1% were permanent. As would be expected, the incidence was higher in patients with active symptoms or bilateral severe carotid artery stenoses.

Magnetic resonance arteriography (MRA) is another noninvasive method of imaging the extracranial carotid arteries. It has the advantage over conventional angiography in that there is no risk of stroke, arterial injury, or systemic complications such as contrast reactions. However, since MRA has only recently been widely available, rigorous correlation between MRA and carotid endarterectomy specimens has yet to be reported. In our early experience with this technique, the degree of stenosis is often factitiously overestimated. Even modest degrees of turbulence at the carotid bifurcation or siphon (such as 50% stenoses) may appear to be critical lesions.

Operative Indications

The indications for carotid endarterectomy are constantly being reevaluated and redefined. In a recent multicenter randomized trial, it has been shown that carotid endarterectomy significantly decreases the risk of stroke in symptomatic patients with carotid stenoses of 70% to 99% of diameter.[37] Symptoms referable to carotid stenosis included hemispheric TIAs with resultant loss of motor and/or sensory function on one side of the body, monocular ipsilateral blindness (amaurosis fugax), or a nondisabling stroke. In this study there was a reduction in risk for major or fatal stroke from 13.1% in the medical therapy group to 2.5% in the surgical group during 2 years.

The timing of carotid endarterectomy after a completed stroke resulting from an ipsilateral carotid lesion is somewhat controversial. Most would agree that endarterectomy should be considered unless the patient has sustained a severely disabling stroke such that there is minimal salvageable function in the affected carotid artery distribution. The procedure should be delayed until the patient's neurologic status has stabilized, usually 3 to 6 weeks after the stroke.[38] The risk of recurrent stroke after carotid endarterectomy is approximately 1.6% per year (15% at 9 years) as compared to a recurrent stroke rate of 50% at 5 years in those patients not undergoing carotid endarterectomy.[9] Nevertheless, many surgeons do not operate if severe intracranial disease or cardiac risk factors would decrease the effectiveness or increase the morbidity of the procedure.

The prognosis of asymptomatic patients with highly stenotic carotid lesions remains difficult to characterize.[25,39] Long-term follow-up of patients with persistent disease of the contralateral carotid artery following unilateral carotid endarterectomy documents a 20% incidence of cerebrovascular symptoms; the incidence of stroke without antecedent TIAs is approximately 3% to 5%.[40] The Veterans Administration Cooperative study found a benefit for endarterectomy if the stenosis was greater than 50%, but the end points included all neurologic events, not just stroke.[41] Since experienced surgeons document a perioperative stroke rate of less than 2%, operative intervention may be appropriate in asymptomatic patients with limited anesthetic risk factors and those undergoing major surgical procedures that may predispose to hypotension.[32]

Nonoperative Treatment

The most significant risk factor for stroke is hypertension. Hence the control of hypertension is most important in the medical management of patients with cerebrovascular disease.[42] Evaluation of serum lipoproteins will likely assume a greater role in the prevention and retardation of atherosclerosis as dietary and drug therapies for specific abnormalities become more clear.

Direct medical therapy for cerebrovascular disease has focused on anticoagulation (heparin and warfarin) and antiplatelet drugs (aspirin, dipyridamole, and sulfinpyrazone).[43,44] Mechanisms of action differ considerably, but the common rationale includes prevention of sudden thrombosis of stenotic lesions and inhibition of platelet activation on ulcerative lesions. Although many studies have suggested a benefit of long-term anticoagulation, the methodologies of these investigations have been seriously questioned, especially regarding their lack of randomization and precise patient selection. Furthermore, the statistically significant reduction in stroke rate (from 19% to 12% in one series) does not compare to better results achieved by carotid endarterectomy.[45,46]

Many clinicians believe antiplatelet agents are most appropriate in patients with minimal ulcerative nonstenotic lesions and only one episode or one closely spaced series of TIAs.[7] If symptoms recur in such patients, endarterectomy remains an option. Other candidates for anticoagulation include patients with high operative risk or those with severe associated intracranial disease.

Operative Techniques and Results

Carotid endarterectomy is the procedure of choice for disease of the common carotid artery or the extracranial portion of the internal carotid cartery.[47] The procedure can be performed while the patient is under general or local anesthesia. Patients at greatest risk for a perioperative ischemic stroke include patients with previous infarcts, those with contralateral carotid occlusions, and those with unstable neurologic deficits.[48] Some surgeons routinely use an indwelling vascular shunt to maintain carotid cerebral perfusion during endarterectomy, whereas others use shunts selectively or not at all. Intraoperative monitoring of electroencephalograms or retrograde carotid perfusion pressure ("stump pressure") have been used to assess the need for shunt placement. Since it is likely that embolic events account for the majority of perioperative strokes, precise dissection technique is crucial in patients with thrombotic or ulcerative plaques.[49]

The incidence of perioperative stroke varies with operative indication. Most large series report stroke rates of 1% to 2% in patients with TIAs and 3% to 5% in patients with previous strokes or contralateral carotid occlusion.[50] Other postoperative complications include cranial nerve injury (especially the hypoglossal and recurrent laryngeal nerves) and myocardial infarction. Because the carotid sinus regulates blood pressure homeostasis, postoperative hypotension or hypertension is noted in many patients during the 24 hours required for baroreceptor reacclimation.[51]

Recurrent stenoses occur in approximately 8% to 10% of patients if followed closely, although the incidence of symptomatic recurrence is much lower (3%). Restenosis within 24 months usually represents exuberant intimal regeneration, whereas later presentations reflect recurrent atherosclerosis.[52]

Vertebrobasilar Disease

Clinical Presentation

As noted earlier, the paired vertebral vessels join to form the basilar artery. For this reason, proximal occlusion or ligation of only one vertebral vessel does not cause symptoms unless the contralateral vessel is diseased or hypoplastic. More distal disease of one vertebral vessel with occlusion of the small branches supplying the lateral medulla can result in neurologic deficits.

The most frequent symptoms of basilar insufficiency include nausea, vertigo, ipsilateral facial numbness, ipsilateral Horner's syndrome, and limb ataxia.[53] Although ischemic symptoms are generally mild, true posterior fossa infarction can be progressive and lethal as a result of extensive edema and midbrain compression. Emboli can contribute to posterior cerebral and cerebellar ischemia, but occlusive disease of the vertebral arteries or the basilar artery is the most common mechanism. The thrombotic process may involve the basilar artery proper or the basilar branch vessels that penetrate into the brain stem.[45]

A classic syndrome of vertebrobasilar insufficiency (subclavian steal syndrome) is associated with subclavian or innominate arterial occlusive disease.[54] The subclavian origins of the vertebral arteries allow the vessels to function as collateral vessels for the upper extremity. During arm exercise, flow is reversed in the vertebral artery, and basilar arterial blood flow and perfusion pressure are decreased. Symptoms of posterior cerebral and cerebellar ischemia can result, especially if any flow-limiting carotid lesions are present. The anatomic relationship favors left-sided involvement approximately 4:1.[55]

The diagnosis of subclavian steal syndrome is supported by complaints of intermittent vertigo, light-headedness, and nausea and vomiting intensified by arm exercise. Physical findings include supraclavicular bruits and 40 to 60 mm Hg blood pressure discrepancies between the arms.

Diagnosis

Measuring blood pressure in both arms is essential in any patient with cerebral symptoms. More sophisticated tests include B-mode imaging of the subclavian and vertebral vessels and the use of directional Dopplers to document reversal of vertebral artery blood flow.

The primary diagnostic test remains arteriography.[56] It

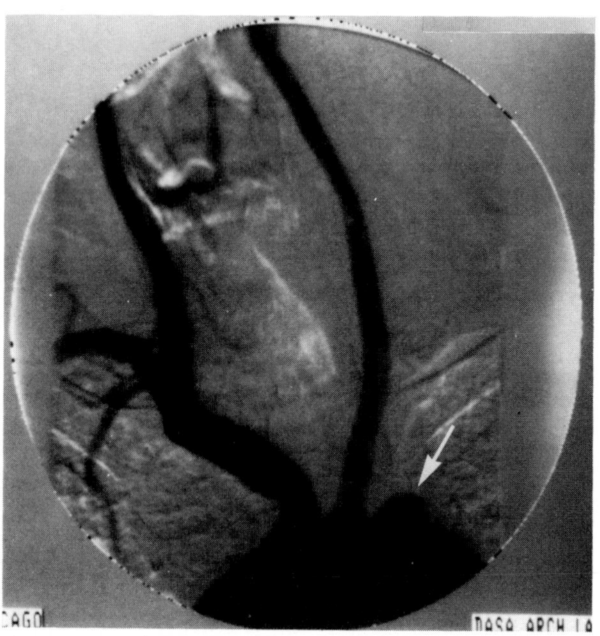

Fig. 53-5. Preoperative angiogram in patient presenting with stroke in basilar distribution (superior cerebellar) demonstrates complete occlusion of left subclavian artery *(arrow)*.

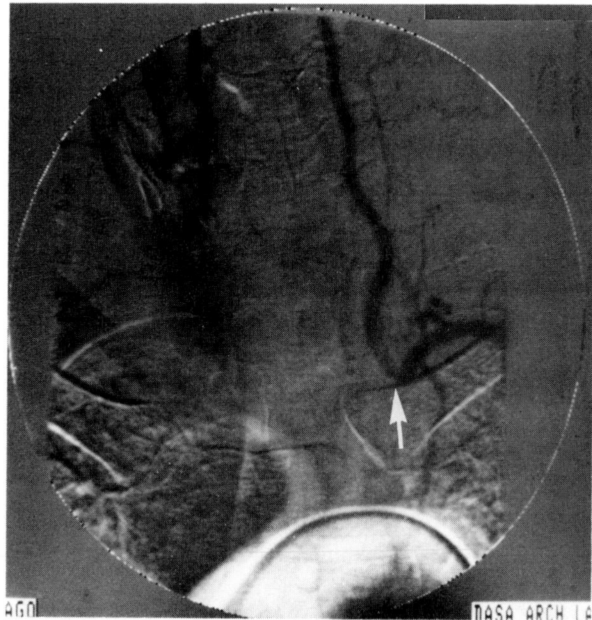

Fig. 53-6. Delayed films document reversed flow in large left vertebral artery *(arrow)* with reconstitution of distal subclavian artery (subclavian steal syndrome).

is important to obtain delayed films to adequately demonstrate retrograde flow through the vertebral into the distal subclavian (Figs. 53-5 and 53-6). The origin of the contralateral vertebral artery and the status of the basilar artery should also be evaluated with oblique films if necessary. The incidental demonstration of subclavian steal during arteriography for some other reasons is, in itself, not cause for concern or surgical therapy.

Operative Indications and Techniques

Symptomatic patients with multiple vertebral occlusive lesions or subclavian steal syndrome should be considered for elective surgery. Procedures include endarterectomy of the proximal vertebral artery or carotid subclavian bypass to restore antegrade vertebral flow.[57] The latter can be accomplished by bypass graft or division of the cervical subclavian artery with reimplantation into the common carotid artery. These procedures can be performed through a cervical incision (Figs. 53-7 and 53-11).

In patients with associated carotid artery disease, carotid endarterectomy alone may relieve symptoms of vertebral-basilar insufficiency by increasing collateral flow to the posterior cerebral artery and cerebellum.[28] This is most appropriate in symptomatic patients with severe carotid stenoses and those with more distal vertebral or basilar occlusion.

Results and Complications

Patency of vertebral endarterectomies and carotid subclavian bypass grafts exceeds 90%. In most cases, symptoms are completely relieved by successful bypass. Failure to achieve symptomatic improvement may be caused by continued carotid disease or intracranial lesions.[58]

Perioperative complications include injuries to the phrenic nerve, cervical sympathetic ganglia (with Horner's syndrome), or the thoracic duct. Basilar territory infarction after carotid subclavian bypass is very rare; even early graft failure should not further compromise vertebral flow.

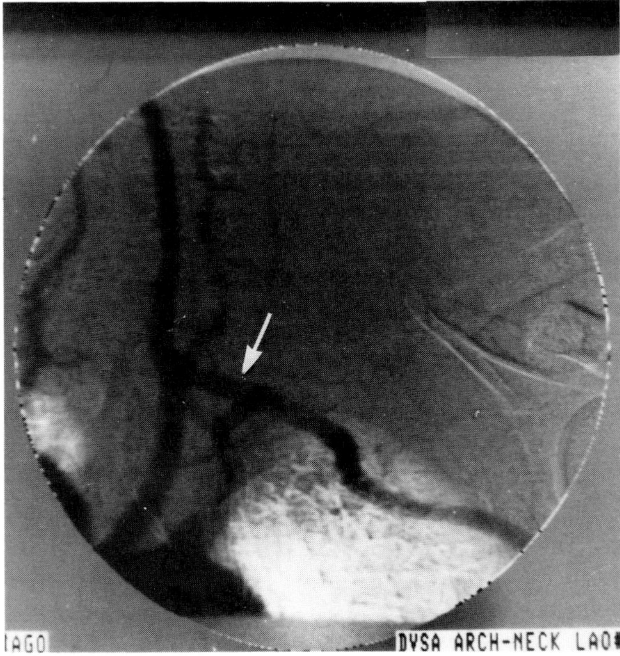

Fig. 53-7. Postoperative intravenous digital angiogram demonstrates patent carotid-subclavian bypass *(arrow)* with return of cephalad flow in left vertebral artery.

UPPER EXTREMITY VASCULAR DISEASE

Symptomatic arterial insufficiency of the upper extremity is relatively uncommon accounting for approximately 2% of all peripheral vascular reconstructive procedures. Although atherosclerosis is the predominant cause of arterial ischemia of the upper extremity, other causes include extrinsic compression, vasospasm, arteritis, connective tissue disorders, trauma, Buerger's disease, previous radiation therapy, and occupational injury.

Nonatherosclerotic Disease

Extrinsic compression of the subclavian artery usually occurs at the thoracic outlet and may result in distal extremity ischemia or emboli. While impingement on the subclavian artery is commonly positional and temporary, longstanding external compression can lead to fibrosis and permanent arterial stenoses. If arteriography with positional maneuvers confirms a persistent and significant stenotic or ulcerative lesions, simple excision of the local soft tissue, primarily the medial scalene muscle and first rib, is not sufficient treatment. Exclusion and bypass of the involved portion of the subclavian artery should be performed.

In some patients, upper extremity arterioles are exceptionally sensitive to sympathetic stimuli resulting in *vasospasm* with intermittent ischemia and even gangrene. Vasospasm of the hands has a characteristic progression of color changes in the fingers; digits first demonstrate pallor secondary to decreases in the flow of oxygenated blood then cyanosis and finally rubor as the vasospasm decreases and reperfusion occurs. This clinical syndrome is termed Raynaud's phenomenon after the French physician who first described it. Patients with Raynaud's phenomenon should be screened for collagen-vascular diseases such as lupus erythematosus, rheumatoid arthritis, and scleroderma. In approximately 50% of patients with manifestations of severe digital ischemia, the phenomenon predates or is associated with these disorders.

The most critical therapy of Raynaud's phenomenon is avoidance of the cold, wind, and moisture, which classically trigger each episode; in some patients, stress also is a major factor. Vasoactive drugs including sympatholytics, which reduce the uptake and subsequent release of local norepinephrine, and calcium channel blocking agents can be helpful. Finally, cervical dorsal sympathectomy can be employed if tissue loss is threatened or if symptoms are intolerable; unfortunately, the benefits of this procedure are not uniform or particularly durable.

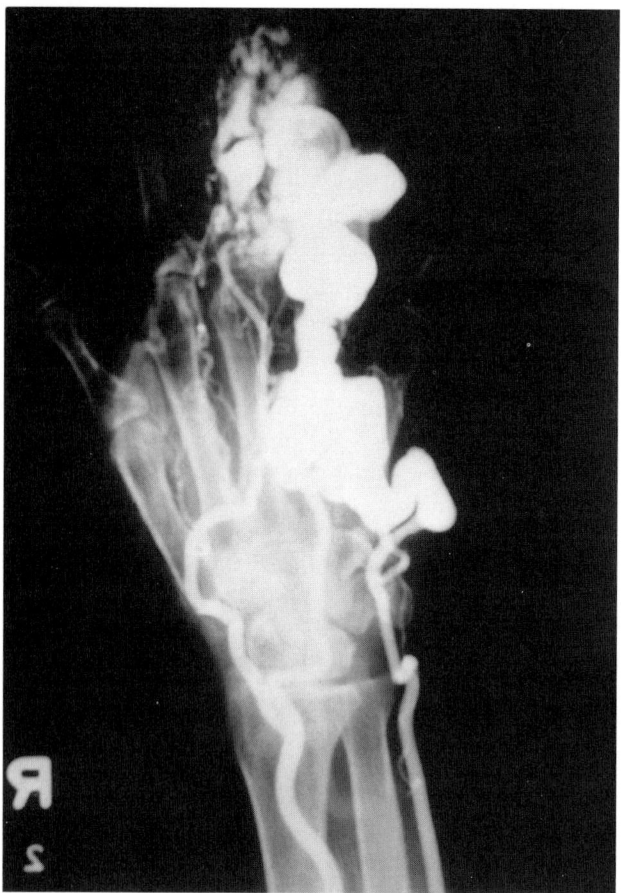

Fig. 53-8. Aneurysms of palmar vessels secondary to repetitive hand trauma in a meat packer.

Two other causes for digital ischemia are *vibratory injury* to the palmar and digital vessels and *Buerger's disease.* Vibratory injury results from repetitive blunt trauma to the hands associated with certain occupations (construction work especially with jackhammers, meat packing[59]). The cumulative force of the injuries results in medium vessel occlusions and true aneurysms caused by medial and adventitial necrosis (Fig. 53-8). Patients may have distal ulcers from ischemia and embolization. If aneurysms are demonstrated, direct microvascular repair is indicated to prevent enlargement and continued embolization.

Buerger's disease is a progressive medium and small vessel obliterative disease associated with nicotine abuse. Patients have distal ischemia of upper and lower extremities; recurrent venous thrombophlebitis is a frequent comorbidity. Local treatments of ischemic lesions and sympathectomy may be successful but *only* if smoking cessation is *complete.* Unfortunately, this goal is almost never attained at this level of addiction to smoking.

Takayasu's disease is an example of an inflammatory large vessel arteritis resulting in fibrosis and scarring of the aorta and its primary branches. Symptoms start as fever, myalgias, and anorexia, but then progress to upper extremity arterial insufficiency.[60] The progression of arterial stenosis leads to the loss of the upper extremity pulses, hence the name "pulseless disease." Takayasu's disease primarily affects the Oriental population with a strong predominance for females (8:1) younger than 40. The cause is still uncertain, although infection and autoimmune processes have been implicated; the disease is associated with rheumatoid arthritis, ankylosing spondylitis, and ulcerative colitis. Laboratory evaluation may reflect a generalized inflammatory process with an elevation of the erythrocyte sedimentation rate (ESR) and a mild hypochromic anemia.

Takayasu's disease can be divided into four types based on the distribution of lesions.[60,61] Type I is limited to the aortic arch and its primary branches, type II includes lesions of the descending thoracic and abdominal aorta, type III extends from the aortic valve to the abdominal aorta, and type IV includes pulmonary artery involvement and/or associated aneurysms.[60,61]

The majority of patients seek medical attention during the "pulseless" stage, and symptoms reflect the organ or extremity that is rendered ischemic. Complaints can include headache, light-headedness, hemiparesis, blurring of vision, diplopia, and blindness. Classic ocular findings include optic atrophy and retinal vein or artery thrombosis.[62] Extremity symptoms can be limited to exercise-related complaints or progress to rest pain and tissue loss.

Initial therapy, especially in the prepulseless stage, is centered on the administration of corticosteroids. If a patient with symptomatic lesions has failed corticosteroid therapy, operative therapy is directed toward bypass of the involved or occluded vessels.[63] If at all possible, operative intervention should be delayed until the acute phase of the disease has resolved. This may not be possible in patients with active cerebrovascular symptoms. Endarterectomy has not proven effective because of the transmural inflammatory response and the tendency toward aneurysmal degeneration. Bypass grafts are the preferred treatment and should originate and terminate in arteries known to be free of disease by both angiography and inspection[64]; often grafts must originate from the ascending aorta. Distal anastomotic stenosis occurs in 20% to 30% of cases and may require reoperation.

Atherosclerotic Upper Extremity Arterial Disease

Clinical Presentation

Atherosclerosis of the subclavian or innominate arteries is the most common cause of upper extremity ischemia; symptoms may be related to low flow or emboli. Lesions involving the *innominate artery* can result in thrombotic atherosclerotic emboli to either the right vertebral artery or the right common carotid artery, with resulting TIA or strokes (Fig. 53-9). Emboli to the left cerebral hemisphere

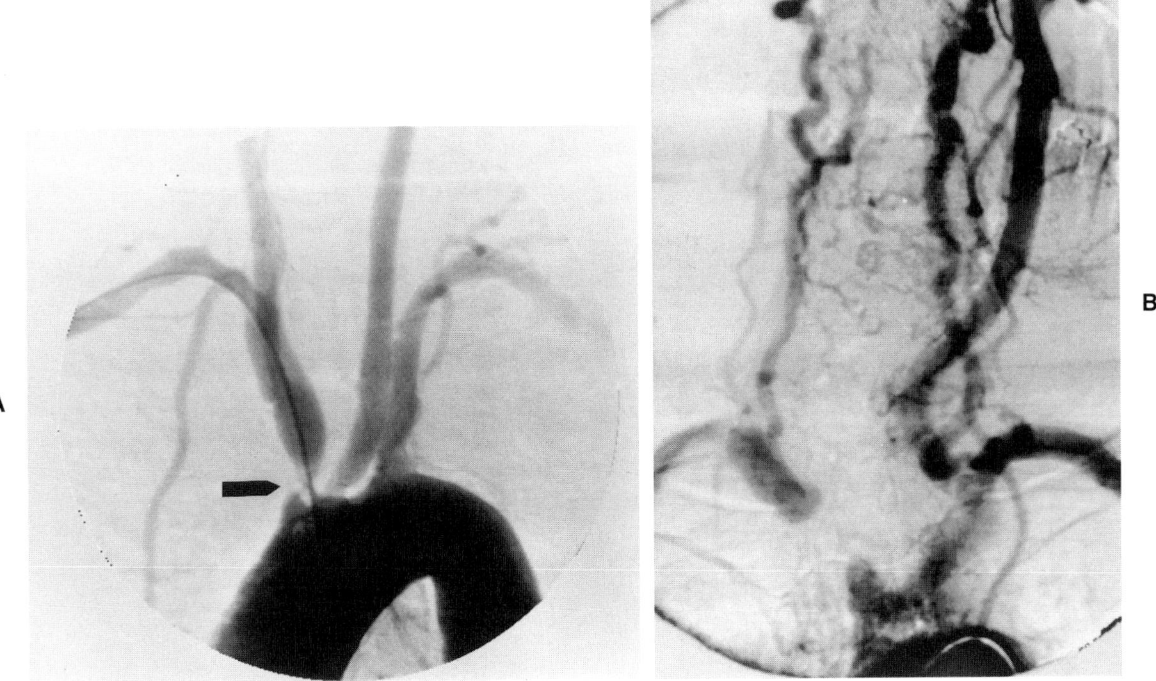

Fig. 53-9. A, Classic lesion *(arrow)* at origin of innominate artery with right hemispheric transient ischemia attacks. Proximity of left carotid artery origin mandated ascending aorta to innominate bypass graft. **B,** Complete occlusion resulting from radiation injury required bypass to relieve right upper extremity ischemia.

can also originate from the innominate artery lesions because of the proximity of the origin of the left common carotid artery to the innominate artery. In one large series, 77% of the patients with symptomatic innominate artery lesions initially had neurologic symptoms, not upper extremity problems.[65]

Stenosis or occlusion of the *subclavian artery* occurs three to four times more commonly on the left than the right subclavian artery. As noted earlier, a proximal subclavian artery occlusion or stenosis can result in reversal flow in the left vertebral artery. The clinical presentation of unilateral upper extremity weakness or coolness, vertigo with upper extremity exercise (subclavian steal syndrome), or ischemic lesions of the hand should raise a suspicion of subclavian artery stenosis or occlusion. The diagnosis is suspected by comparing upper extremity arterial pressures and is confirmed by arteriography. Arteriograms do not only define the extent of disease of the subclavian artery, but also evaluate the thoracic aorta, carotid arteries, and the vertebral arteries.

Treatment

Symptomatic patients should be considered for arterial revascularization.[66] Innominate lesions are usually approached directly through a median sternotomy (Fig. 53-10).[67] Both endarterectomy or bypass from the aortic arch are durable procedures. The selection of the specific procedure is based on the nature of the lesion and the location of origin of the left carotid artery. If it originates close to the innominate, clamping of the latter vessel for endarterectomy is inadvisable, and bypass is preferred.[65]

Bypass procedures for subclavian disease include transposition of the subclavian artery to the adjacent nondiseased carotid artery or carotid artery to subclavian artery bypass with a prosthetic graft (Fig. 53-11).[67] Transposition entails the complete mobilization of the subclavian artery proximal to the origin of the vertebral artery. The subclavian artery is divided, and the proximal arterial stump is oversewn. An anastomosis is created between the side of the proximal carotid artery and the end of the subclavian artery. If the subclavian artery cannot be mobilized enough for a tension-free apposition to the proximal carotid artery, a carotid-subclavian bypass can be performed. In these instances the preferred bypass graft conduit is a synthetic graft due to its decreased tendency to kink. Both subclavian artery transposition and carotid-subclavian artery bypass have similar long-term patencies of greater than 95%.[68]

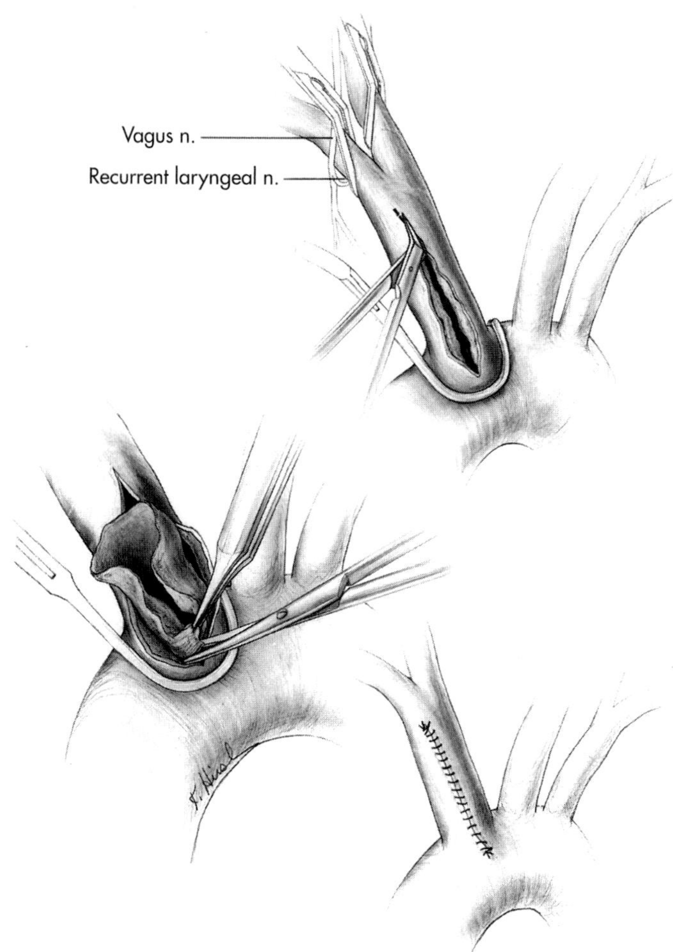

Fig. 53-10. Innominate endarterectomy can be performed if a vascular clamp can be applied proximal to the lesion without also obstructing the left carotid artery origin. (From Zarins CK, Gewertz BL. Atlas of Vascular Surgery. New York: Churchill Livingstone, 1989.)

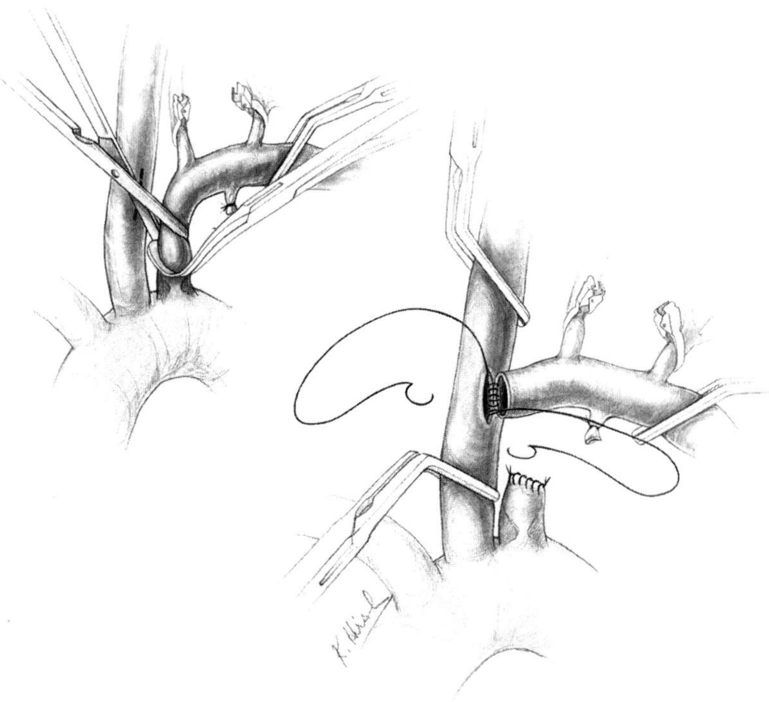

Fig. 53-11. Subclavian reconstructions include both carotid-subclavian bypass and transposition of the distal subclavian into the carotid artery (illustrated here). (From Zarins CK, Gewertz BL. Atlas of Vascular Surgery. New York: Churchill Livingstone, 1989.)

THORACIC OUTLET SYNDROME

Clinical Presentation

Thoracic outlet syndrome is best described as an intermittent but reproducible compression irritation of the brachial plexus caused by congenital fibromuscular bands, cervical ribs, or the anterior scalene muscle[69,70] (Fig. 53-12). Classic symptoms include shoulder pain with radiation to the occiput and down the arm along the C8 to T1 distribution. Numbness and tingling frequently accompany the pain. In advanced cases, weakness of the hands and forearm may be noted. Although the subclavian artery may also be compressed by the same anatomic configuration, most symptoms of thoracic outlet syndrome relate directly to neurologic rather than vascular compromise.

A history of neck or shoulder trauma can be elicited in many patients, suggesting to some clinicians that scalene muscle spasm is an initiating event. Whiplash injuries are frequently implicated, but documentation of a cause-and-effect relationship is nearly impossible. The differential diagnosis includes carpal tunnel syndrome, cervical disk compression, arthritis, tendinitis, and angina pectoris.

Diagnosis

The chronicity and lack of specificity of the clinical presentation is paralleled by a lack of definitive diagnostic tests other than chest x-ray film demonstration of an abnormal cervical rib. The Adson maneuver is a positional test long associated with thoracic outlet syndrome. The test result is considered positive if the radial pulse disappears during abduction and external rotation of the arm. Unfortunately, the results of the Adson maneuver are frequently positive in asymptomatic patients and negative in patients with classic symptoms of thoracic outlet syndrome, again emphasizing the neurologic as opposed to vascular origin of the pain syndrome. Angiographic demonstration of subclavian artery compression in extreme abduction also does not contribute significantly to the diagnosis unless there is evidence of a persistent blood pressure gradient in the involved arm.[4]

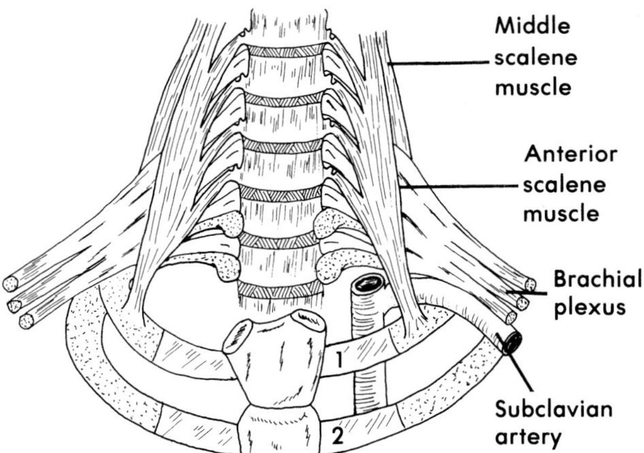

Fig. 53-12. Brachial plexus compression occurs at triangular outlet between scalene muscles and first rib.

Electromyograms and nerve conduction velocities have been suggested as objective measures of thoracic outlet nerve compression. Unfortunately, enthusiasm for these studies has decreased recently because of the difficulty of electrically stimulating nerves proximal to the presumed sight of compression and the intermittent nature of the syndrome. Furthermore, clinical correlations between positive nerve conduction studies and symptomatic relief following surgery have not been very convincing.

Operative Indications and Techniques

Initial therapy should include shoulder girdle exercises and avoidance of extreme posturing. If pain remains and symptoms are fully consistent and reproducible, surgical therapy is appropriate. Unfortunately, even experienced surgeons report complete relief in only 80% to 85% of patients.

The most common operation is transcervical or transaxillary resection of the first rib or a cervical rib, if present. In some patients merely transecting the insertion of the anterior scalene muscle onto the first rib may suffice.[71] Although there has been some enthusiasm for concurrent cervical sympathectomy, this is usually unnecessary unless symptoms of posttraumatic sympathetic dystrophy (causalgia) are evident.

Complications

The failure rate from all procedures remains relatively high in thoracic outlet syndrome.[72] Complications of surgery include Horner's syndrome, direct injury to the brachial plexus, lymphatic leaks, and pneumothorax.

SUMMARY

Although cerebrovascular disease remains a major cause of morbidity and mortality in our population, improved understanding of the mechanisms and pathologic processes involved has allowed a wider application of preventive medical and surgical therapies. Appropriate selection of noninvasive tests to evaluate asymptomatic patients with signs of extracranial cerebrovascular disease have further characterized the natural history of these disorders. Although specific recommendations for medical or surgical therapy will continually be modified, it is generally accepted that patients with repetitive neurologic deficits (TIAs) associated with extracranial atherosclerotic disease benefit significantly from surgical intervention. In patients with upper extremity ischemia, extensive medical evaluation and careful assessments of the brachiocephalic arterial system are mandatory.

REFERENCES

1. Lees RS, Kistler JP, Sanders D. Duplex Doppler scanning and spectral bruit analysis for diagnosing carotid stenosis. Circulation 66(Suppl 1):102, 1982.
2. Levy RI. Stroke decline: Implications and prospects. N Engl J Med 300:490, 1979.

3. Whisnant JP. Epidemiology of stroke: Emphasis on transient cerebral ischemic attacks and hypertension. Stroke 5:68, 1974.
4. Judy KL, Heymann RL. Vascular complications of thoracic outlet syndrome. Am J Surg 123:521, 1972.
5. Wolf PA, et al. Asymptomatic carotid bruit and risk of stroke. JAMA 245:1442, 1981.
6. West H, et al. Comparative risk of operation and expectant management for carotid artery disease. Stroke 10:117, 1979.
7. Goldner JC, Whisnant JP, Taylor WF. Long-term prognosis of transient cerebral ischemic attacks. Stroke 2:160, 1971.
8. Diaz FG, et al. Combined reconstruction of the vertebral and carotid artery in one single procedure. Neurosurgery 12:629, 1983.
9. Mani RL, et al. Complications of catheter cerebral arteriography: Analysis of 5000 procedures. I. Criteria and incidence. Am J Roentgenol 131:861, 1978.
10. Gregory PC, et al. Effects of hemorrhagic hypotension on the cerebral circulation. Stroke 10:719, 1979.
11. Dinsdale HB, Robertson DM, Haas RA. Cerebral blood flow in acute hypertension. Arch Neurol 31:80, 1974.
12. Lassen NA, Henriksen L, Paulson O. Regional cerebral blood flow in stroke by ^{133}xenon inhalation and emission tomography. Stroke 12:284, 1981.
13. Wechsler RL, Drips PO, Kety SS. Blood flow and oxygen consumption of the human brain during anesthesia produced by thiopental. Anesthesiology 12:308, 1951.
14. Abboud FM. Special characteristics of the cerebral circulation. Fed Proc 40:2296, 1981.
15. Johansson B, et al. The effect of acute arterial hypertension on the blood-brain barrier to protein tracers. Acta Neuropathol 16:117, 1970.
16. Brusija DW, Heistad DD, Marcus ML. Continuous measurement of cerebral bloodflow in anesthetized cats and dogs. Am J Physiol 241:H228, 1981.
17. Marcus ML, Bischof CJ, Heistad DD. Comparison of microsphere and xenon-133 clearance method in measuring skeletal muscle and cerebral blood flow. Circ Res 48:748, 1981.
18. Raichle ME, et al. Central noradrenergic regulation of cerebral blood flow and vascular permeability. Proc Natl Acad Sci USA 72:3726, 1975.
19. Raichle ME, et al. Measurement of regional substrate utilization rates by emission tomography. Science 199:986, 1978.
20. Ekstrom-Jodal B. Effect of increased venous pressure on cerebral blood flow in dogs. Acta Physiol Scand 350(Suppl):51, 1970.
21. Borgstrom L, Johannson H, Siesjo BK. The relationship between arterial Po_2 and cerebral blood flow in hypoxic hypoxia. Acta Physiol Scand 93:423, 1975.
22. Greenberg JH, et al. Local cerebral blood volume response to carbon dioxide in man. Circ Res 43:324, 1978.
23. D'Alecy LG, Feigl EO. Sympathetic control of cerebral blood flow in dogs. Circ Res 31:267, 1972.
24. Heistad DD, Marcus ML. Evidence that neural mechanisms do not have important effects on cerebral blood flow. Circ Res 42:295, 1978.
25. Humphries AW, et al. Unoperated, asymptomatic significant internal carotid artery stenosis: A review of 182 instances. Surgery 80:695, 1976.
26. Mentzer RM, et al. Emergency carotid endarterectomy for fluctuating neurologic deficits. Surgery 89:60, 1981.
27. Pessin MS, et al. Mechanisms of acute carotid stroke. Ann Neurol 6:245, 1979.
28. Solberg LA, Eggen DA. Localization and sequence of development of atherosclerotic lesions in the carotid and vertebral arteries. Circulation 43:711, 1971.
29. Javid H, et al. Natural history of carotid bifurcation atheroma. Surgery 67:80, 1970.
30. Craig DR, et al. Intracranial internal carotid artery stenosis. Stroke 13:825, 1982.
31. Eisenberg RL, et al. Relationship of transient ischemic attacks and angiographically demonstrable lesions of the carotid artery. Stroke 8:483, 1977.
32. Makhoul RG, et al. Benefit of carotid endarterectomy after prior stroke. J Vasc Surg 18:666, 1993.
33. Witten DM, Hirsch FD, Hartman GW. Acute reactions to urographic contrast medium. Incidence, clinical characteristics and relationship to history of hypersensitivity states. Am J Roentgenol Radium Ther Nucl Med 119:832, 1973.
34. D'Elia JA, et al. Nephrotoxicity from angiographic contrast material. Am J Med 72:719, 1982.
35. Faught E, Trader SD, Hanna GR. Cerebral complications of angiography for transient ischemia and stroke: Prediction of risk. Neurology (Minneap) 29:4, 1979.
36. Hankey GJ, Warlow CP, Sellar RJ. Cerebral angiographic risk in mild cerebrovascular disease. Stroke 21:209, 1990.
37. Barnett HJM, et al. Beneficial effect of carotid endarterectomy in symptomatic patients with high-grade carotid stenosis. N Engl J Med 325:445, 1991.
38. Whittemore AD, Mannick JA. Surgical treatment of carotid disease in patients with neurologic deficits. J Vasc Surg 5:910, 1987.
39. Busuttil RW, et al. Carotid artery stenosis—Hemodynamic significance and clinical course. JAMA 245:1438, 1981.
40. Podore PC, et al. Asymptomatic contralateral artery stenosis: A five year follow-up study following carotid endarterectomy. Surgery 88:748, 1980.
41. Hobson RW, et al. Efficacy of carotid endarterectomy for asymptomatic carotid stenosis. N Engl J Med 328:221, 1993.
42. Kannel WB, et al. Components of blood pressure and risk of atherothrombotic brain infarction: The Framingham Study. Stroke 7:327, 1976.
43. Brust JCM. Transient ischemic attacks: Natural history of anticoagulation. Neurology 27:701, 1977.
44. Olsson J-E, et al. Anticoagulant vs. antiplatelet therapy as prophylactic against cerebral infarction in transient ischemic attacks. Stroke 11:4, 1980.
45. Canadian Cooperative Study Group: A randomized trial of aspirin and sulfinpyrazone in threatened stroke. N Engl J Med 229:53, 1978.
46. Fields WS, et al. Controlled trial of aspirin in cerebral ischemia. Stroke 8:301, 1977.
47. Thompson JE, Talkington CM. Carotid surgery for cerebral ischemia. Surg Clin North Am 59:539, 1979.
48. Goldstone J, Moore WS. A new look at emergency carotid artery operations for the treatment of cerebrovascular insufficiency. Stroke 9:599, 1978.
49. Steed DL, et al. Causes of stroke in carotid endarterectomy. Surgery 92:634, 1982.
50. DeWeese JA, et al. Results of carotid endarterectomies for transient ischemic attacks—five years later. Ann Surg 178:258, 1973.
51. Bove EL, et al. Hypotension and hypertension consequences of baroreceptor dysfunction following carotid endarterectomy. Surgery 85:633, 1979.
52. Crossman D, et al. Early restenosis after carotid endarterectomy. Arch Surg 113:275, 1978.
53. Caplan LR. Vertebrobasilar disease: Time for a new strategy. Stroke 12:111, 1981.
54. Fisher CM. A new vascular syndrome: "The subclavian steal." N Engl J Med 265:912, 1961.
55. Fields WS, Lemak NA. Joint study of extracranial artery occlusion. VII. Subclavian steal—A review of 168 cases. JAMA 222:1139, 1972.
56. Caplan LR, Rosenbaum AE. Role of cerebral angiography and vertebrobasilar occlusive disease. J Neurol Neurosurg Psychiatry 38:601, 1975.
57. Clark K, Perry MO. Carotid vertebral anastomosis: An alternate for repair of the subclavian steal syndrome. Ann Surg 163:414, 1966.

58. Allen GS, Cohen RJ, Preziosi TJ. Microsurgical endarterectomy of the intracranial vertebral artery for vertebrobasilar transient ischemic attacks. Neurosurgery 8:56, 1981.
59. Clark ET, et al. True aneurysmal disease in the hand and upper extremity. Ann Vasc Surg 5:276, 1991.
60. Ishikawa KK. Natural history and classification of occlusive thromboaortopathy (Takayasu's disease). Circulation 57:27, 1978.
61. Lupi-Herrera E, et al. Pulmonary artery involvement in Takayasu's arteritis. Chest 67:69, 1975.
62. Takayasu M. Case with unusual change of the vessels in the retina. Acta Soc Ophthalmol 12:544, 1908.
63. Alpert HJ. The use of immunosuppressive agents in Takayasu's arteritis. Med Ann Q 43:69, 1974.
64. Weaver FA, et al. Surgical procedures in the management of Takayasu's arteritis. J Vasc Surg 12:429, 1990.
65. Cherry KJ, et al. Technical principles of direct innominate artery revascularization: A comparison of endarterectomy and bypass grafts. J Vasc Surg 9:718, 1989.
66. Whitehouse W, et al. Arterial bypass grafts for upper extremity ischemia. J Vasc Surg 3:569, 1986.
67. Zarins CK, Gewertz BL. Atlas of Vascular Surgery. New York: Churchill Livingstone, 1989.
68. Salam TA, Lumsden AB, Smith RB. Subclavian artery revascularization: A decade of experience with extrathoracic bypass procedures. J Surg Res 56:387, 1994.
69. Kirgis HD, Reed AF. Significant anatomic relations in the syndrome of the scalene muscles. Ann Surg 127:1182, 1948.
70. Roos DB. Congenital anomalies associated with thoracic outlet syndrome: Anatomy, symptoms, diagnosis, and treatment. Am J Surg 132:771, 1976.
71. Sanders RJ. Scalenectomy versus first rib resection for treatment of the thoracic outlet syndrome. Surgery 85:109, 1979.
72. Urschel HD Jr, et al. Reoperation for recurrent thoracic outlet syndrome. Ann Thorac Surg 21:19, 1976.

54

Venous and Lymphatic Abnormalities of the Limbs

Dawn Johnson and Julie Ann Freischlag

William Harvey's monumental work nearly four centuries ago on the circulation of blood first emphasized the important role that the valvular function of extremity veins plays in this process. The impact of derangements in venous and lymphatic function of the limbs is staggering and contributes substantially to human disease. This chapter discusses our current understanding of these disorders and the physiologic rationale underlying their management.

ANATOMY

To understand the pathophysiology of venous disease, knowledge of the normal anatomy and physiology of the venous circulation is required. Veins of the lower extremity can be classified into the deep or superficial venous systems. The superficial veins run in the subcutaneous tissue external to the deep fascia. The two main tributaries of importance in the superficial venous system are the greater and lesser saphenous veins. The greater saphenous vein, formed by the confluence of the medial veins of the dorsum and plantar aspect of the foot, is found anterior to the medial malleolus and travels along the medial aspect of the leg until it crosses laterally at the proximal thigh to join the femoral vein (Fig. 54-1). This junction is commonly 2 to 4 cm lateral to the pubic tubercle and inferior to the inguinal ligament. Cutaneous sensation to the medial aspect of the lower leg is provided by the saphenous branch of the femoral nerve, which runs adjacent to or crosses the greater saphenous vein in this area. This is an important anatomic finding that should be considered when dissecting out the greater saphenous vein.

The lesser saphenous vein, arising behind the lateral malleolus, takes its origin from the veins draining the lateral aspect of the foot. It travels in the midline of the posterior calf and ascends to join the popliteal vein behind the knee (see Fig. 54-1).

Important communicating or perforating veins are also found, which traverse the deep fascia and connect the superficial and deep venous systems. These perforating veins play a critical role in the pathophysiology of venous disease and chronic venous insufficiency.

The deep veins of the calf include the peroneal, posterior tibial, and anterior tibial vein, which ascend along the course of their corresponding artery (Fig. 54-2). In addition, there is a sinusoidal complex of veins within the soleal and gastrocnemius muscles often referred to as venous lakes, which are important physiologically because of their valves. These venous lakes coalesce and join the posterior tibial and peroneal veins. The aforementioned veins then merge with the anterior tibial vein to form the popliteal vein at the knee. This vein continues proximally as the superficial femoral vein and joins the deep femoral vein below the inguinal ligament to become the common femoral vein. The common femoral vein, traveling medial to the femoral artery, passes beneath the inguinal ligament and continues as the external iliac vein.

Veins of the upper extremity begin with the basilic and cephalic veins, which provide venous return from the upper extremity (Fig. 54-3). These two veins merge to form the axillary vein in the upper arm. The axillary vein becomes the subclavian vein at the lateral border of the first rib. The subclavian vein then drains into the innominate vein back to the heart.

VENOUS PHYSIOLOGY

A feature unique to the venous circulation is the presence of bicuspid valves found in all veins distal to the common iliac vein. The function of the valves of the deep venous system is to maintain a unidirectional flow of blood to the heart. The valves of the perforating veins are crucial in preventing reflux of blood from the deep to the superficial systems, thereby preventing superficial venous hypertension.

In the supine position at rest a person has a foot vein pressure of approximately 15 mm Hg. However, on standing the gravitational hydrostatic forces are added increasing the measured foot vein pressure to approximately 115 mm Hg. Assuming the standing position also increases venous volume with an increase in capacitance by about 500 cm.[3] With a normal calf muscle pump, this increment is returned to the central circulation on walking. The integrity of the lower extremity venous system is maintained by the

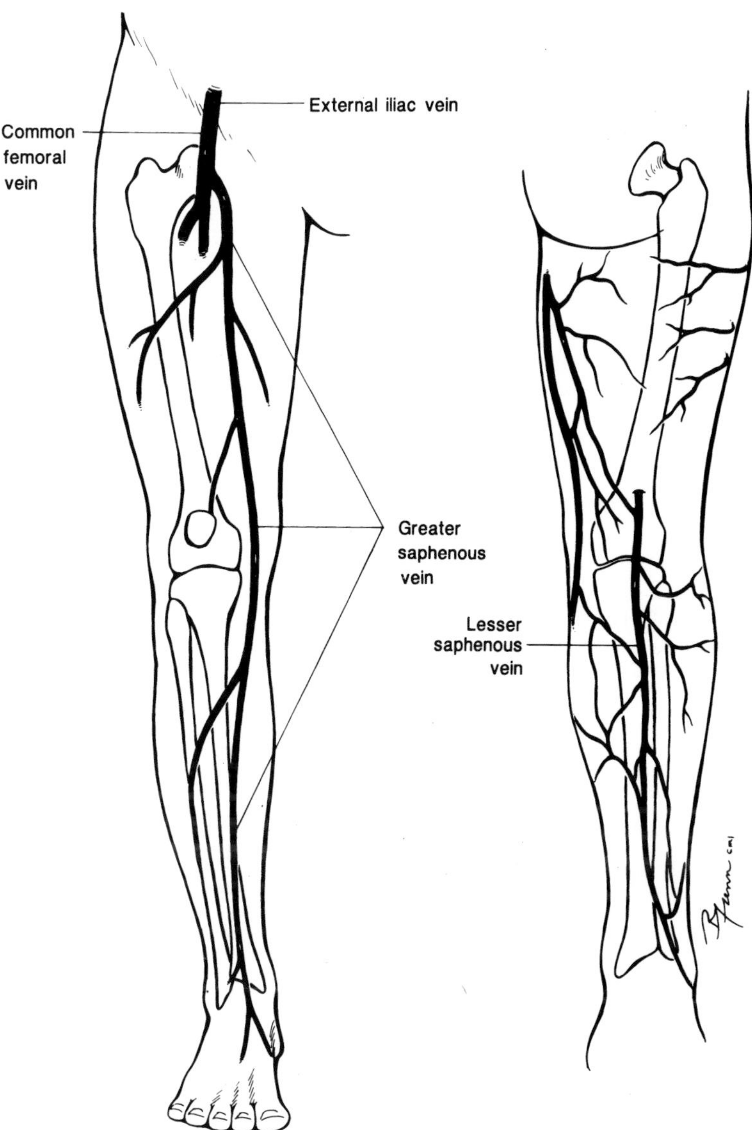

Fig. 54-1. Diagram depicting the two main superficial tributaries of the venous system: the greater saphenous vein and the lesser saphenous vein.

ability of the leg muscles, with their surrounding nonelastic fascial envelope, to act as a "pump," compressing the intramuscular venous lakes and deep intermuscular veins. With competent valves and a functioning calf pump during exercise, venous blood in these capacitance vessels is returned to the heart. A clinical application of this event is the use of pneumatic compression devices in patients at bed rest. These increase the venous return and decrease the venous volume in the legs much like the muscle pump, thereby reducing stasis and the risk for venous thrombosis.

VENOUS DISORDERS OF THE LOWER EXTREMITY

Deep Venous Thrombosis

Deep venous thrombosis (DVT) is the most serious and potentially life-threatening disorder of the venous system. Its most lethal complication, pulmonary embolism, is the cause of approximately 200,000 deaths each year in the United States.[1] More than half the patients surviving the DVT suffer from the postphlebitic syndrome with its disabling edema and potential stasis ulcerations. Much of our present knowledge on the cause and pathophysiology of DVT is attributed to Virchow. He described three mechanisms (Virchow's triad) that are responsible for the development of a venous thrombus: stasis, hypercoagulability, and vessel wall damage. Stasis is the most important predisposing factor in the surgical patient. With induction of general anesthesia, there is a considerable reduction in venous flow because of the loss of the ability to contract the muscles of the lower extremity and a generalized peripheral dilation that is present throughout the procedure. Furthermore, a hospitalized patient frequently remains at bed

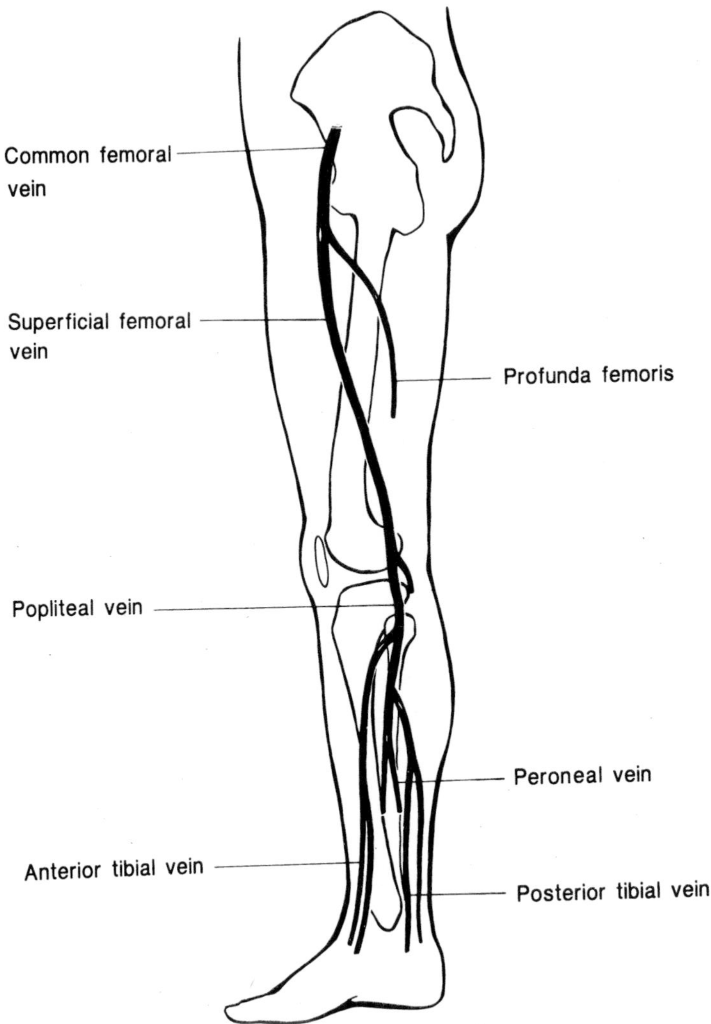

Fig. 54-2. Diagram depicting the deep venous system of the lower extremity.

rest, which also induces stasis and subsequent DVT. It is this consequence that provides the stimulus for early ambulation in most surgical patients. Other risk factors for DVT include age older than 65, obesity, malignancy, oral contraceptive use, and pregnancy.[2] Each of these factors alters venous stasis or coagulopathy.

Clinical Presentation

Clinical signs of venous thrombosis are found in only 40% of patients. When symptoms are present, they initially include edema and calf pain. The level at which swelling occurs is determined by the site of venous obstruction. If the swelling is confined to the calf or foot, obstruction is at the femoropopliteal level, whereas swelling at the thigh level implies iliofemoral obstruction. Physical examination reveals calf tenderness on palpation and occasionally a palpable cord representing the thrombosed vein. Homans' sign, tenderness or tightness in the back of the calf with forcible dorsiflexion of the foot, may be present but is nonspecific and unreliable.

Most DVTs involve the popliteal vein and its tributaries. However, if the thrombus extends proximally to involve the iliofemoral system, there may be massive swelling from the toes to the inguinal ligament. The clinical picture of pain, extensive pitting edema, and blanching is referred to as *phlegmasia alba dolens* or "milk leg." With progression of the thrombus and occlusion of the venous return from the lower extremity there may be sufficient congestion to produce a painful cyanotic leg known as *phlegmasia cerulea dolens.*[3] However, as previously mentioned, most patients are asymptomatic, and these dramatic presentations represent a very small percentage of the patients with venous thrombosis.

Diagnosis

Diagnostic tests are critical in establishing the diagnosis because false-positive clinical signs have been found to occur in up to 45% of patients evaluated.[4] Duplex ultrasonography scanning is noninvasive and can be conveniently used at the bedside to detect venous thrombi with an accuracy

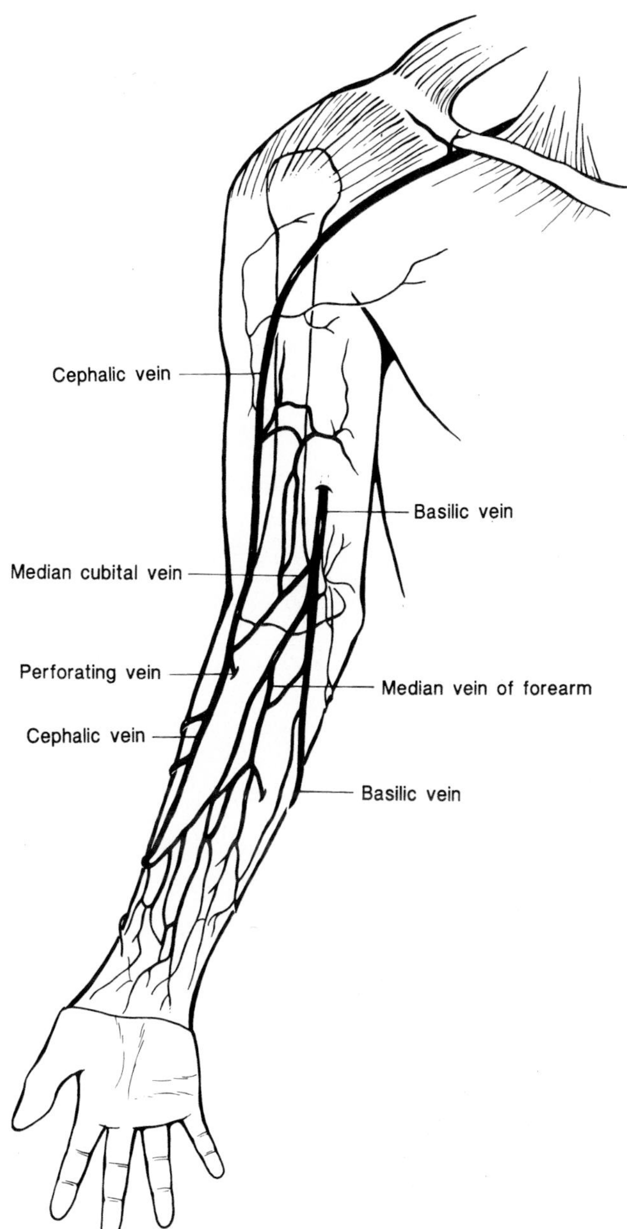

Fig. 54-3. Diagram depicting the upper extremity venous anatomy.

of approximately 90%. The technique is based on the impairment of an accelerated flow signal produced by the thrombi. A flow signal can be altered by distal and proximal compression, producing augmentation with distal compression and interruption of flow with proximal compression. Inability to augment flow on compression below or release of interruption of flow above the probe suggests venous thrombi (Fig. 54-4). In the femoral vein, duplex scanning has a specificity of 100% and sensitivity of 95%.[5] Diagnostic accuracy is lower in the calf. Nevertheless, it has been suggested that duplex scanning replace venography as the standard method of diagnosing femoropopliteal DVT.

Venography is the most accurate means of establishing the diagnosis of venous thrombosis and its extent of involvement. This test requires injection of a contrast medium into a foot vein while the superficial veins are occluded by a tourniquet to promote filling of the deep venous system. Filling defects and nonvisualization of the deep veins identify the thrombus. This test is invasive and requires transporting the patient to the radiology suite. Risks include the development of venous thrombosis secondary to the thrombogenicity of the injected contrast medium. Other rare complications include cellulitis or skin necrosis secondary to extravasation of contrast and gangrene.[6]

Venography can also be performed with isotope injection and thus eliminate some of these complications. A gamma scintillation counter is then used to record the flow of the isotope. The image with this technique is not as well defined but this method may be valuable for sequential study of patients.

Impedance plethysmography is another feasible and accurate alternative to venography. This method measures volume changes in the extremity. A blood pressure cuff is inflated around the proximal thigh to pressures of 40 to 50 mm Hg. A calf plethysmograph records the volume increase. With deflation of the cuff, there should be rapid outflow of blood and subsequent volume reduction. Venous thrombosis is suggested by prolongation of the outflow wave. This test is accurate for those thrombi that are occlusive and large enough to prevent venous outflow of the leg. False positives are seen in those with ascites, congestive heart failure, and pregnancy. Impedance plethysmography is not accurate for nonocclusive thrombi or old thrombi where venous outflow is not affected.

Radioactive-labeled fibrinogen scanning has also been used in the detection of DVT. This technique involves intravenous injection of ^{125}I-labeled fibrinogen. Portable scintillation counters can be used at bedside to measure the amount of radioactivity over the extremity in question. A developing thrombus incorporates fibrinogen, therefore an increase in radioactivity represents an organizing thrombus. Thus this test cannot detect old thrombi but is very sensitive to the earliest clot formation. Because of this sensitivity, the radioactive-labeled fibrinogen scan is not used as a screening test because of the tendency to overdiagnose. It is primarily used in clinical research studies to evaluate the efficacy of prophylactic measures or in patients who may have recurrent DVT.

Prophylaxis

To prevent DVT, many prophylactic measures can be used in the hospitalized patient. The goals of these measures are to reduce stasis or alter blood coagulability. Early ambulation has become a routine part of a patient's postoperative course in an attempt to prevent stasis. Patients are assisted with ambulating as early as the evening of surgery. Other prophylactic options include graded compression stockings and pneumatic compression devices, both of which

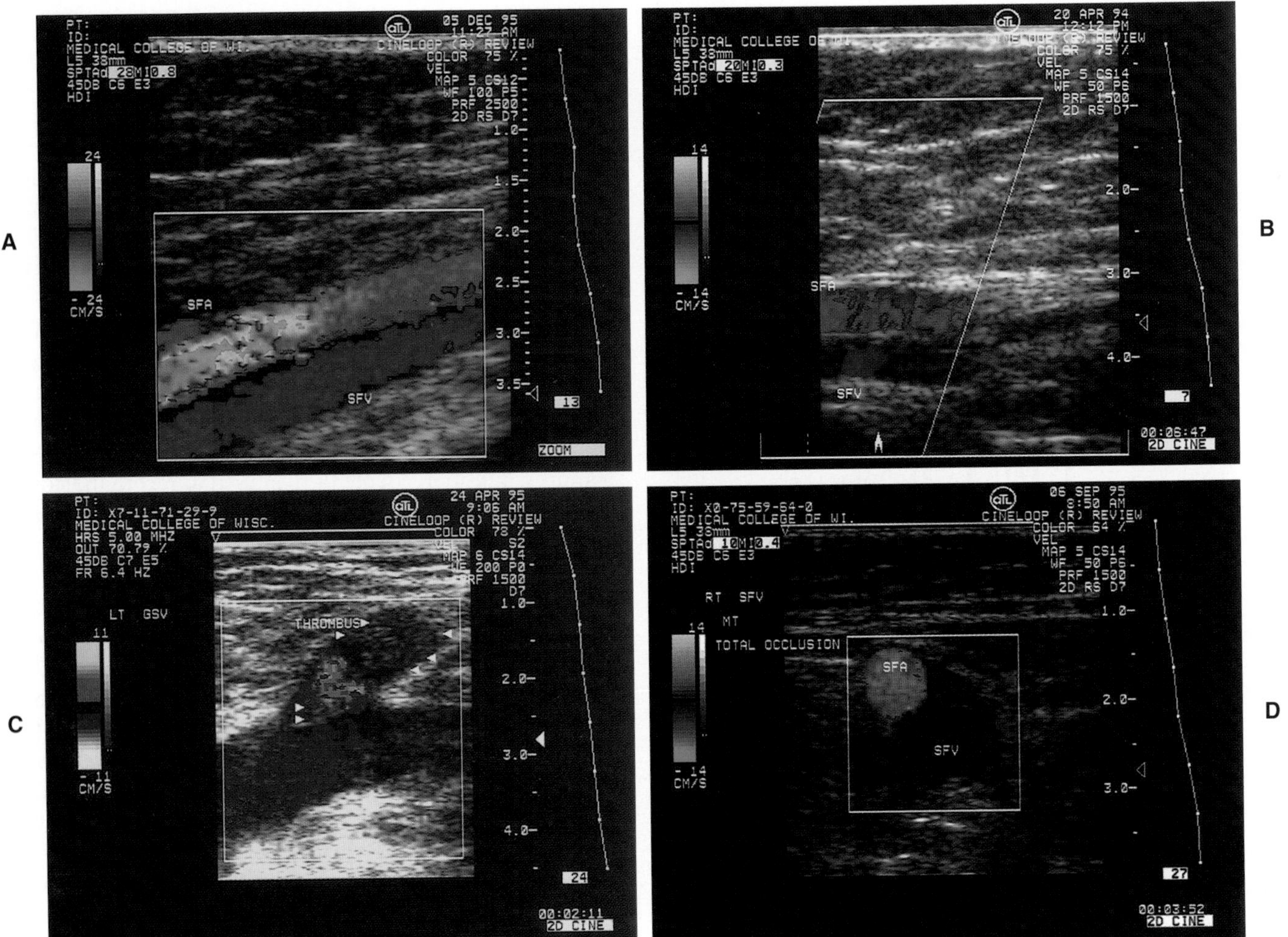

Fig. 54-4. **A,** Longitudinal view using the duplex scan to identify normal flow in the superficial femoral artery *(SFA)* and superficial femoral vein *(SFV).* **B,** Longitudinal view using the duplex scan demonstrating normal SFA and loss of venous flow in the SFV caused by thrombus. **C,** Duplex scan of the greater saphenous vein *(GSV)* showing nonoccluding thrombus identified by arrows. **D,** Transverse view of the SFA and SFV demonstrating no flow in a completely thrombosed SFV.

augment venous flow. These devices are placed on the patient just prior to surgery and remain in place until the patient is actively ambulating.

Anticoagulation therapy is also commonplace but somewhat controversial. The current recommendation is administration of "mini" doses of heparin (5000 U subcutaneously) given 2 hours preoperatively and then every 8 to 12 hours postoperatively until the patient is ambulating. This appears to enhance the effect of antithrombin III and its inhibition of factor Xa, yet it does not affect the laboratory clotting profile. Although controversy exists over its efficacy, a large randomized series of surgical patients showed protection against DVT and a markedly decreased incidence of pulmonary embolism.[7] This treatment does not provide adequate protection against DVT in patients undergoing orthopedic procedures such as hip and knee replacement. The risk of DVT in these procedures is greater than 50% and therefore requires more intense antithrombotic prophylaxis. Anticoagulation is contraindicated in neurosurgical patients or those undergoing ophthalmologic procedures where hemostasis is imperative and any bleeding would be catastrophic.

Using the above mentioned modalites as prophylactic measures, Colditz et al.[8] evaluated general surgery patients. The incidence of DVT as seen using the fibrinogen uptake test or venography was 27% without any therapy at all. Those treated with subcutaneous heparin had an incidence of DVT of 9.6%; those with compression stockings 6.3%; and those with pneumatic compression devices 17.6%. A combination of heparin and stockings revealed an incidence of DVT of 6.3% and stockings with intermittent pneumatic compression was 4.5%.[8]

Treatment

The goal of DVT management is to halt the propagation of thrombus, prevent pulmonary embolism, and promote resolution of existing clot to minimize the risk for postphlebitic syndrome. The mainstay of therapy for DVT is anticoagulation with heparin. Heparin is derived from bovine lung or porcine intestine. If not contraindicated, heparin therapy is initiated on diagnosis. Usual dosing consists of 10,000 U (100 to 200 U/kg) as an intravenous bolus followed by 1000 to 2000 U (10 to 30 U/kg) per hour as a continuous infusion. Heparin, by its action in potentiating the effects of antithrombin III, limits any further propagation of the thrombus and prevents the formation of new thrombi. It does not lyse the original thrombus. In addition to initiating heparin therapy, the patient is placed at bed rest with the leg elevated for 24 to 98 hours at which time the pain, swelling, and tenderness have resolved. Then the patient may resume ambulating. Compression stockings should be used for walking to prevent edema formation.

The adequacy of anticoagulation with heparin is monitored by serial partial thromboplastin time (PTT) levels, which are maintained between 60 and 80 seconds. Once the patient is anticoagulated with heparin, oral warfarin (Coumadin) therapy is begun. Warfarin acts by inhibiting the synthesis of the vitamin K–dependent clotting factors, II, VII, IX, and X. The prothrombin time (PT) or International Normalized Ratio (INR) is used to monitor warfarin therapy. The PT is brought to within 1.3 to 1.5 times the control value or an INR of 2 to 3 to maintain sufficient anticoagulation. Warfarin therapy must be continued for at least 3 months, and some favor a 6-month course to prevent rethrombosis of the veins caused by the thrombus effect on the endothelium.

Both heparin and warfarin therapy are not without potential side effects. Side effects associated with heparin treatment include bleeding, thrombocytopenia, hypersensitivity reaction, arterial thromboembolism, and osteoporosis in patients receiving long-term therapy.[9] Heparin-induced thrombocytopenia is secondary to an immune reaction and resolves on cessation of therapy. Arterial thromboembolism caused by heparin-induced thrombocytopenia is the most severe complication, occurring more often in the elderly after 7 to 10 days of treatment.[9] Heparin must be stopped immediately because of the high associated morbidity and mortality. Routinely, platelet counts are monitored every 3 days in patients receiving heparin.

Complications associated with warfarin therapy also include bleeding, skin necrosis, dermatitis, and a painful blue toe syndrome. Skin necrosis occurs in areas with significant adipose tissue such as thighs, breasts, and buttocks. It has been found that thrombosis of venules and capillaries supplying this region occurs as a result of an underlying protein C deficiency. When a patient is given loading doses of warfarin, there is a relatively rapid fall in protein C and protein S relative to the other vitamin K–dependent coagulation factors. This results in a transient state favoring a thrombotic event, and this is amplified in a patient with preexisting protein C deficiency. A blue toe syndrome can occur secondary to bleeding into an arterial plaque, resulting in distal embolization and ischemia. Warfarin is also teratogenic and must not be used during pregnancy. Heparin is the drug of choice during pregnancy and is given subcutaneously for long-term management.

Fibrinolytic therapy for the management of DVT has been an area of great interest. Streptokinase and urokinase have been employed as lytic agents and are effective. Bleeding is the major complication associated with this course of treatment and is therefore contraindicated in patients who have had recent surgery, trauma, or hemorrhagic stroke. Further limiting the patient population that could benefit from early lysis is the finding that this technique is most effective when performed within 72 hours of the event. The technique involves placing a catheter via entrance through the jugular vein or contralateral femoral vein directly into the thrombus and providing a local infusion of the lytic agent. Urokinase has been found to be more effective than streptokinase with fewer hemorrhagic and allergic complications.[10] The main objective of this form of therapy is preservation of venous valve function and rapid reduction of lower extremity edema and pain. It has been postulated that the preservation of venous valve integrity by rapid resolution of the thrombus should protect against the development of valvular incompetence and subsequent postphlebitic syndrome.[11] Early recanalization is important in preserving valve integrity; however, despite this it is not clear that postphlebitic syndrome can be prevented by early lytic therapy.[12,13] Therefore this mode of treatment remains controversial.

A surgical approach to directly remove the thrombus has also been used. A venotomy is made in the distal common femoral vein and a thrombectomy catheter is passed to extract the thrombus. This procedure is associated with high success rates and has provided relief from early morbidity.[14] However, this invasive form of treatment has a high rethrombosis rate and a decrease in the postphlebitic syndrome has been shown in only a few studies. This procedure is usually limited to those individuals with threatened limb loss in such cases as phlegmasia cerulea dolens.

Anticoagulation with heparin remains the mainstay of treatment for DVT. If this is contraindicated, the patient continues to form thrombi while adequately anticoagulated, or if a patient has had recurrent pulmonary embolism, partial inferior vena cava interruption is indicated. This can be accomplished by several methods. A surgical approach can be taken by the placement of a caval clip that is placed on the inferior vena cava just below the renal veins. This results in a high incidence of lower leg edema and subsequent postphlebitic changes.

A more commonly used and less invasive technique involves percutaneous insertion or cutdown of the jugular vein and fluoroscopic positioning of a filter within the inferior vena cava just below the renal veins. The most popular filter is the Greenfield filter. The cone-shaped design of this device traps the embolus yet allows continued flow of blood to the heart. The recurrent embolism rate with this particular filter is 4%.[15] Complications of inferior vena cava filters include misplacement, insertion-site DVT, migration of the filter, erosion of the device into the inferior vena cava wall, and inferior vena cava obstruction with or without postphlebitic syndrome.[16] Although this procedure has a relatively low morbidity and mortality, it should still be reserved for those patients who fit the above indications.

Complications of Deep Venous Thrombosis

Pulmonary embolism. The most fatal complication of DVT is pulmonary embolism. It is estimated to cause more than 200,000 deaths per year in the United States.[1] Pulmonary embolism most frequently occurs at 7 to 10 days postoperatively; if the symptoms remain unrecognized and untreated, the mortality is aproximately 30%.[1]

Pathophysiology and clinical presentation. A patient with a DVT of the lower extremity has a 50% chance of pulmonary embolism if the thrombus reaches the iliofemoral system. Even though thrombi may develop in the smaller veins of the calf, the risk of pulmonary embolism is not significant until the thrombus extends to the level of the femoral and iliac veins. Once embolization occurs and pulmonary blood flow is interrupted, there develops a regional ventilation-perfusion mismatch and a bronchoconstrictive response by the lung to reduce wasted ventilation. If more than 30% of the pulmonary vascular bed is occluded, pulmonary artery pressures rise with a similar increase in right ventricular work. If there is more than 50% occlusion, systemic pressures fall. With underlying cardiopulmonary disease, these changes can cause an even more pronounced clinical presentation. The classic presentation is that of sudden pleuritic chest pain, dyspnea, and tachypnea. Other findings can include cough, tachycardia, and hemoptysis. Hemoptysis is an uncommon finding but if present usually represents a late sign of pulmonary infarction. Physical examination reveals tachycardia, a prominent second heart sound, cyanosis, and possible hypotension. Ventricular gallop, rales, low-grade fever, or a pleural friction rub may also be present.

Diagnosis. The clinical presentation could easily represent a myocardial infarction or esophageal perforation; therefore other diagnostic tests are required. An electrocardiogram is essential to exclude a myocardial infarction. Nonspecific ST and T wave changes are the only consistent finding with pulmonary embolism. Chest x-ray findings are also nonspecific and may include enlargement of the central vasculature, a lack of the vascular markings with segmental or lobar ischemia (Westermark's sign), or pleural effusion. However, the chest film can rule out pneumonia, esophageal perforation, or congestive heart failure, which may be in the differential diagnosis. Arterial blood gas analysis is also helpful. Most patients are hypoxemic with a PaO_2 less than 60 mm Hg. This is common in several disorders, but the discriminating finding is a reduction in arterial PCO_2. Measurement of central venous pressure is elevated or normal if hemodynamic compensation has occurred. A low central venous pressure essentially excludes pulmonary embolism as a principal source of hypotension.

Confirmation of the diagnosis of pulmonary embolism requires a lung scan and/or pulmonary arteriography. The lung scan is less invasive and is the usual initial diagnostic screening test. Accuracy has been increased with the combined ventilation-perfusion scan. This technique involves intravenous infusion of human serum albumin labeled with ^{99m}Tc or ^{131}I. The scan shows decreased uptake in areas of the lung where vasculature is occluded by thrombi. With this technique alone there is a high false positive rate, since other diseases such as pneumonia or atelectasis cause a similar result. Thus this scan is frequently interpreted along with a radioactive ^{131}I xenon ventilation scan. The latter scan displays the distribution of the inhaled gas throughout the lung, and a defect on the ventilation scan is frequently seen with pulmonary embolism. A matched perfusion and ventilation defect indicates high probability of pulmonary embolism.

The most accurate means of confirming the diagnosis of pulmonary embolism is with a selective pulmonary angiogram. This test is invasive but can detect the size and distribution of pulmonary emboli. This technique is reserved for patients whose lung scan is equivocal or for those with suspected massive embolism who go directly to angiography without a ventilation-perfusion scan.

Treatment. Anticoagulation with heparin is the mainstay of treatment, and the technique of administration is the same as that described for deep venous thrombosis. Again heparin therapy is initiated and converted to oral anticoagulation with warfarin for 3 to 6 months. Those patients in which anticoagulation is contraindicated are candidates for inferior vena caval interruption. As discussed, the most popular technique is insertion of a Greenfield filter.

For those patients who have a massive pulmonary embolism with refractory hypotension, an emergent pulmonary embolectomy may be required. A thoracotomy is performed to surgically remove the thrombus. This procedure is associated with a high mortality rate, consequently an alternative approach with the patient under local anesthesia has been developed by Greenfield et al.[17] A cup device attached to a catheter is inserted through the jugular or femoral vein. Under angiographic guidance, the device is placed next to the embolus, and suction is applied to aspirate the embolus into the cup for retrieval. This technique has been successful and may become the procedure of choice in this situation.

Thrombolytic therapy has also been used as an alternative treatment for those patients not in shock. Streptokinase, urokinase, and tissue plasminogen activator are available lytic agents proven to be effective. The patient's symptoms often improve quickly with the dissolution of the clot; however, no improvement has been seen in early mortality in patients with pulmonary emboli who have been treated with thrombolytic therapy.[18] In addition, there are significant complications secondary to bleeding that have limited its use.

Postphlebitic syndrome. Postphlebitic syndrome, a state of chronic venous insufficiency, is a morbid complication occuring in 74% of patients with a DVT involving the femoral or iliac vein.[19] Chronic venous insufficiency is the most disabling venous disorder, and the cost of this disability in terms of productivity and continuous medical care is enormous.

Clinical presentation. Hyperpigmentation and edema of the lower extremity are the earliest signs of chronic venous insufficiency. The swelling has been described as brawny and nonpitting. The hyperpigmentation is associated with a dermatitis (venous eczema) that leads to severe pruritus, which is frequently the initial complaint. In addition to the skin changes, the patient experiences an aching discomfort or night cramps that are aggravated by dependency and relieved with elevation. Venous claudication or a throbbing pain throughout the leg may occur with ambulation.

These changes occur because valves in the deep venous system are destroyed, and recanalization of the thrombosed vein provides only marginal drainage of the blood from the leg. Thus blood is diverted to the communicating veins and into the superficial venous system with the development of venous hypertension and varicosities. Chronic venous hypertension leads to increased hydrostatic pressure at the capillary level, causing leakage of fluid and proteins as well as hemosiderin-laden red blood cells. This is responsible for the edema and typical brownish skin pigmentation. From a histologic perspective there is fat necrosis and fibrosis of the skin and subcutaneous tissue, a condition commonly referred to as lipodermatosclerosis. All these factors promote an environment conducive to skin breakdown and ulceration. Ultimately patients develop venous stasis ulcers frequently located in the region of the medial or lateral malleolus.

Diagnosis. The diagnosis is generally made on history and physical examination alone. In attempt to distinguish chronic venous insufficiency from lymphedema, one can focus on the extent of edema. Edema secondary to venous insufficiency begins at the ankle and extends to involve primarily the lower leg, whereas lymphedema begins in the toes and foot and involves the entire extremity. Also those patients with lymphedema do not have pigmentation of the skin. Diagnostic studies such as duplex scanning or venography are infrequently performed. However, these tests can be used to locate areas of valvular incompetence if surgery is contemplated.

Treatment. Ideally, the best treatment is prevention, and this is accomplished by applying the prophylatic measures against DVT previously described. Unfortunately, those who develop postphlebitic syndrome often require a lengthy and frustrating treatment course. It is essential that patients avoid prolonged standing and elevate the legs when sitting and sleeping. Graded compression stockings are also required to increase venous return. The skin is extremely fragile, and all efforts must be taken to avoid trauma. The skin is frequently dry, flaky, and itchy; therefore liberal use of skin emollients to prevent cracking and subsequent ulceration is necessary. When venous ulcers are present, an occlusive protective paste dressing such as Unna's boot is used. This dressing allows for ambulation while providing compression and protection from trauma. Healing of venous ulcers is slow, and it is not uncommon to require many months of vigilant wound care. Lanza et al.[20] examined 99 limbs with venous stasis ulcers. They found that those patients with low venous refill times (≤10 seconds), indicative of severe venous insufficiency, took significantly longer to completely heal. Only 53% of the ulcers healed at 5 months.[20]

Only when cellulitis appears around the ulcer is antibiotic therapy employed. If the ulcer is refractory to conservative methods, it is excised and the area is skin grafted. Incompetent perforating veins may also be ligated and removed. Prolonged hospitalization after such a procedure is necessary to ensure compliance with leg elevation and wound care to provide for wound healing.

Varicose Veins

Varicose veins are superficial veins that have become dilated and tortuous. The term *varicose veins* is generally applied to the affected veins of the greater and lesser saphenous venous system. The development of varicose veins is thought to result from venous valve incompetence and defects in the elastic properties of the vein wall. This venous valve incompetence can arise secondary to local trauma, thrombophlebitis, familial weakness in the valve structure, increased blood volume as seen after DVT, and hormonal changes especially during pregnancy.[21-23] With incompetent venous valves, on standing the venous muscle pump of the legs is ineffective, and the blood is no longer able to overcome the gravitational hydrostatic pressure. Blood then flows in a retrograde fashion into the superficial veins, causing them to dilate and elongate.

Varicosities of the lower extremity can be classified as primary varicose veins or secondary varicose veins depending on cause. Primary varicose veins have an unclear cause and occur in those individuals with no previous history of DVT. There is a definite genetic link, and studies of select populations have found that 20% to 40% of patients with varicosities have a family history of this disease.[24] Women have a threefold greater risk of developing varicose veins compared to men. Female hormones are thought to contribute to this increased risk. Specifically, progesterone, a hormone whose levels are elevated during the second phase of the menstrual cycle and during pregnancy, causes passive dilation of varicosities.[25] This distention makes the venous valves incompetent and can initiate varicose veins or make existent varicosities more symptomatic. Advancing age, obesity, and increased intra-abdominal pressure are other factors involved in the cause of primary varicose veins.

Secondary varicose veins arise because of the consequences of DVT or as a result of venous obstruction. Venous obstruction may be caused by compression of the proximal venous system by an intra-abdominal or pelvis tumor. Once again, the underlying increased venous pressure and valvular incompetence caused by these factors result in the reversal of blood flow from the deep to the superficial veins and the development of varicosities.

Clinical Presentation

Varicose veins may or may not produce symptoms. In fact, many women have asymptomatic varicosities; however, they seek medical attention because of the unsightly blue dilated and tortuous veins. Those with symptoms usually complain of pain, fatigue, and aching, most noticeable in the calves and ankles especially at the end of the day. A feeling of heaviness is often described by the patient, particularly if the day has been spent standing or sitting without much walking. These symptoms are relieved by lying down, leg elevation, or wearing elastic support stockings. The symptoms are exacerbated in women during their menstrual cycle because of venous valve dilation and worsening incompetence.

Physical examination must include the abdomen and pelvis to access the possibility of venous obstruction secondary to a tumor. Examination of the legs should be performed in the standing and supine position. Varicose veins should be examined and palpated. Palpation can detect hidden varicosities in obese legs where they may not be visualized. Arterial pulses should be palpated as well.

Preoperative Testing

There are several clinical tests that are applied to evaluate deep venous patency and valvular competence. The Perthes test is performed by placing a tourniquet around the proximal thigh snug enough to compress the superficial veins. The patient is then asked to walk, and attention is paid to the superficial ankle veins. If the veins become less prominent, the perforator and deep vein valves are intact; however, if the veins remain the same size, the perforator valves are incompetent. If the veins should become more prominent with exercise and the patient complains of pain, it can be assumed that there is significant deep venous insufficiency and incompetent perforators.

The retrograde filling test or Trendelenburg test aids in distinguishing between superficial valvular incompetence and perforator valvular incompetence. This procedure is done by elevating the leg initially to empty the veins and then placing a tourniquet over the saphenofemoral junction. The patient is then asked to stand, and the pattern of superficial venous refill is noted. If the varicosities do not fill on standing but do so immediately after releasing the tourniquet, the perforating veins are competent and the varicosities are secondary to superficial venous valve incompetence. If the patient stands and there is rapid filling of the varicosities with the tourniquet still in place, the perforator veins are incompetent secondary to deep venous disease.

Duplex scanning can be performed to document venous valvular reflux as well. The test is important if there are clinical findings or a history suggestive of DVT. A handheld Doppler probe can also give the information needed to demonstrate deep venous patency and venous reflux especially at the saphenofemoral junction and at the level of the perforators.[26] With the patient sitting on the examining table with the legs hanging over the edge of the table, the popliteal and posterior tibial veins can be examined for venous valvular insufficiency using compression above and below the Doppler probe. A delayed response with augmentation can indicate poor outflow secondary to obstruction. This is quite rare unless the patient has a history of DVT. Reflux heard during proximal compression confirms the diagnosis of venous valvular insufficiency. Venous reflux can be determined in a similar manner in the perforator veins. Saphenofemoral junction incompetence can be ascertained with the Doppler probe by placing it over the site and having the patient perform a Valsalva maneuver. This should be repeated with a tourniquet placed around the proximal thigh area. The reflux should disappear when the Valsalva maneuver is performed again with the tourniquet in place.

Treatment

Conservative therapy is recommended for those with minimal varicosities or for those who desire to avoid invasive measures to cure the disease. Graded compression stockings can relieve the symptoms. The stockings are put on when rising in the morning and removed prior to retiring at night. Patients are encouraged to avoid long periods of standing and to elevate the legs while sitting. Patients are also encouraged to walk as much as possible, which helps facilitate venous outflow by using the calf muscle pump.

For those patients with symptomatic varicosities or for those who do not like the unsightly nature of their varicose veins, there are several treatment options for cure. Sclerotherapy has become a popular treatment option given its success and availability in an outpatient setting. Venous sclerotherapy is an ablative procedure that actually causes thrombosis in the affected vein, preferably without blood in the lumen.[27] The procedure is performed by having the patient stand to mark the varicose veins and perforating veins. With the patient remaining standing, 23-gauge butterfly needles are placed approximately 1 cm apart along the course of the varicose veins (Fig. 54-5). One proceeds from distal to proximal until all veins have been cannulated. The patient is then placed in the supine position, and each site is injected with 0.5% to 1% of the sclerosing agent. The preferred sclerosing agent is sodium tetradecyl sulfate. Up to 60 sites and 30 ml of this solution can be used during venous sclerotherapy of one limb without sequelae. Immediately after the injection, the butterfly needle is removed, and a gauze and foam rubber pad are placed over the injection site. A stockinette and compression stocking are then placed over the gauze and pad. These should remain in place for 3 weeks without removing. The patient is encouraged to walk and remain active. When stocking, gauze, and pad are removed after 3 weeks, inspection and palpation can document the obliteration of the varicose vein. Those patients with saphenofemoral junction incompetence have high recurrrence rates with venous sclerotherapy alone, therefore high ligation of the saphenofemoral junction should be performed in these patients either prior to or in conjunction with venous sclerotherapy.

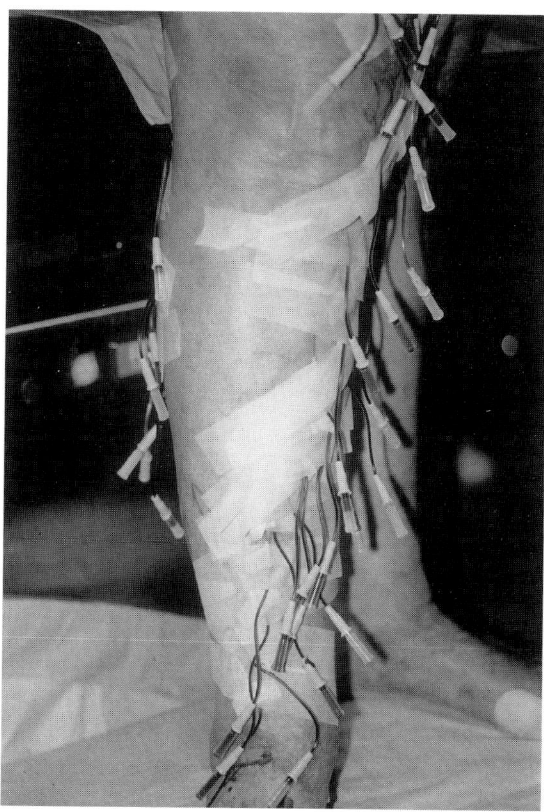

Fig. 54-5. Multiple butterfly needles seen placed along the course of symptomatic varicose veins prior to injection of a sclerosing agent.

The main complication resulting after venous sclerotherapy is localized phlebitis, which occurs approximately 10% of the time.[28,29] It is usually self-limiting and requires little intervention. Other uncommon complications include skin necrosis and ulceration secondary to extravasation of the sclerosing agent, intraluminal hematomas, and pigmentation of the surrounding skin.

Vein stripping is an alternative method of treating varicose veins. This procedure requires a general or regional anesthetic and potential overnight stay in the hospital, even though most patients do go home the same day of the procedure. After marking all varicosities, the patient is given a general anesthetic, and attention is given to ligation of the saphenous vein and all other tributaries at the saphenofemoral junction. The vein stripper, a flexible rod, is then passed up the length of the vein from a distal venotomy at the level of the medial malleolus. The divided vein at the saphenofemoral junction is tied to the stripper, and the vein is removed with the instrument. Prior to stripping the vein, the other varicosities that are located away from the course of the stripper are treated. This is accomplished by making very small incisions by stabbing the skin over the vein with a No. 11 blade scalpel. The vein is grasped with a fine forcep and divided. Each end is then avulsed by direct traction and removed through the incision. Bleeding is controlled with pressure; no ligatures are used. After removal of the stripper and therefore avulsion of the main venous channel from the perforators, the leg is wrapped firmly from the toes to the groin to allow the perforators to thrombose. The patient may resume daily activities but is encouraged to sit with the leg elevated and avoid prolonged standing.

Complications after vein stripping are infrequent. They may include bleeding, with ecchymosis being the most common complication appearing 3 to 5 days postoperatively. This usually resolves within 3 to 4 weeks. Leg edema is common but is relieved by the use of the elastic support stockings. Hypoesthesia of the skin particularly at the level of the ankle may occur because of trauma to the saphenous and sural nerves.[28]

Other options for the treatment of valvular insufficiency include direct venous reconstruction. Such procedures as valvuloplasty and vein segment transposition have been described but are not widely accepted or practiced because of their high failure rates. In general, these procedures are reserved for those patients who cannot ambulate at all due to leg edema and discomfort.

Superficial Thrombophlebitis

Thrombophlebitis is a local inflammatory process that is restricted to the superficial veins. This condition most commonly occurs in varicose veins of the lower extremity below the level of the knee. Thrombophlebitis can also occur in association with intravenous cannulation, local trauma, and parenteral drug abuse. The typical clinical finding is an indurated, painful, and erythematous venous cord as a result of the thrombosed superficial vein.

When thrombophlebitis involves the distal aspect of the greater saphenous venous system, therapy is managed in the outpatient setting. Treatment consists of symptomatic relief with bed rest, leg elevation, and warm compresses to the affected vein. Anticoagulation therapy is not warranted, since embolization virtually never occurs. However, if the thrombophlebitis extends above the knee, the risk of embolization exists. These patients require close observation in the hospital setting; if they remain refractory to symptomatic therapy, anticoagulation is initiated. The principle for initiating anticoagulation therapy is solely to prevent embolization, as it does not alter the underlying inflammatory process. If the condition continues to progress proximally despite these interventions, ligation of the saphenous vein at the saphenofemoral junction is indicated.

VENOUS DISORDERS OF THE UPPER EXTREMITY

Axillary/Subclavian Vein Thrombosis

DVT of the upper extremity is now more common than previously reported. Earlier studies have cited a 1% to 2% incidence; however, with the increasing use of subclavian venous access the incidence has risen.[30] In fact, subclavian catheters are the number one cause of axillary and subclavian venous thrombosis.[31,32] The presence of an upper extremity DVT is not an innocuous event. Studies indicate that 12% of patients with an upper extremity DVT have had a documented pulmonary embolization.[32]

The most common causes of axillary/subclavian vein thrombosis are (1) iatrogenic secondary to central venous lines or pacemakers; (2) malignancy secondary to tumor compression of the vein or secondary to the hypercoagulable state associated with the malignancy; (3) effort thrombosis or primary thrombosis, frequently referred to as Paget-Schroetter syndrome.[31] Several factors are involved in the pathophysiology of effort thrombosis. First, there is compression of the axillary/subclavian vein resulting in stasis. This may be due to an anomalous subclavius or anterior scalene muscle or the presence of a cervical rib. Second, repetitive movement at the level of the arm and shoulder may cause intimal tears in the vessel. Third, the stress of exercise may temporarily produce a hypercoagulable state. All these factors are conducive to the development of a thrombus. Other causes of axillary/subclavian vein thrombosis include direct trauma, heart failure, and infection. Underlying each and every one of these etiologic factors are the three elements of Virchow's triad—stasis, hypercoagulability, and vessel wall damage.

Clinical Presentation

The diagnosis of an upper extremity DVT can be clinically difficult, especially in the case of iatrogenic injury from a central venous catheter. Often it produces a relatively indolent and silent course that is infrequently associated with symptoms. It is important to be aware of this and to be able to recognize any subtle signs that may occur, particularly in the critically ill patient who has had repetitive subclavian vein catheterizations. The subtlety of this injury may be a result of the well-developed venous collateral system of the upper extremity and its ability to compensate in the case of obstruction of a major vein.[30]

Primary or effort thrombosis develops clinically as an acute swelling of the involved extremity. It is frequently found in young, otherwise healthy men with a recent history of trauma or heavy exertion. It is often noted after activities requiring the arm to be hyperabducted and externally rotated such as painting, throwing a baseball or football, or chopping wood. The involved extremity is usually the patient's dominant arm. With increased activity of the involved arm arterial flow increases in the face of venous outflow obstruction resulting in venous hypertension. This promotes effusion of edema fluid into the tissues and distention of the superficial veins. This venous congestion may make the arm feel heavy or achy. In addition, a dusky cyanosis may develop especially with exertion and dependency of the arm. Physical examination discloses an obvious size and color discrepancy in the upper extremity. Frequently, the superificial veins of the hand and forearm are distended. This can be accentuated with the arm in the dependent position; the veins remain paradoxically distended when the arm is elevated.

Diagnosis

Duplex scanning can often diagnose the problem by revealing the presence of the thrombus in the subclavian or axillary vein. Venography is used to locate the thrombus anatomically and provide access for thrombolytic therapy. Venographic demonstration of prominent collateral veins bypassing an obstructed axillary/subclavian vein provides the definitive diagnosis of thrombotic obstruction (Fig. 54-6).

Treatment

The traditional treatment of axillary/subclavian vein thrombosis has been bedrest with limb elevation and anticoagulation. With this conservative approach, resolution without recurrence of symptoms has been reported in only 25%.[33] Other studies have shown that 50% to 70% of those with an upper extremity DVT proceed to develop significant postphlebitic sequelae. The recent development of the use of thrombolytic therapy in this condition has improved these results dramatically. Most patients with primary or effort thrombosis are young and healthy and excellent candidates for thrombolysis. Immediately after confirming the diagnosis, catheter-directed thrombolysis is employed with urokinase. Heparin is also administered concomitantly and continued until warfarin levels are therapeutic. A successful protocol for effort thrombosis described by Machleder[34] recommends continuing the anticoagulation for 3 months. This is followed by transaxillary first rib resection and decompression with subsequent balloon angioplasty in cases of residual stenosis. Surgical decompression by first rib resection is advocated to correct the anatomic abnormality that caused the thrombosis and prevent recurrent thrombosis. Although initial thrombolytic therapy is increasing in popularity, there are still others who recommend early decompression of the thoracic outlet and operative thrombectomy.

In cases of secondary thrombosis or catheter-related thrombosis, removal or correction of the offending cause is important. Thrombolytics and anticoagulation are the mainstay of therapy, and surgical intervention is usually not warranted.

The most significant complication of upper extremity DVT is pulmonary embolization. This was formerly thought to be almost nonexistent; however, with the rising numbers of upper extremity thrombosis studies have found a 12% incidence of pulmonary embolization.[32] Other complications include postphlebitic changes and long-term disability, septic thrombophlebitis, and loss of central venous access. A rare but morbid complication is venous gangrene. Severe edema of the fingers from venous hypertension can occlude arterial inflow and produce ischemia.

Superficial Thrombophlebitis

The cause of superficial thrombophlebitis of the upper extremity is usually secondary to prolonged intravenous

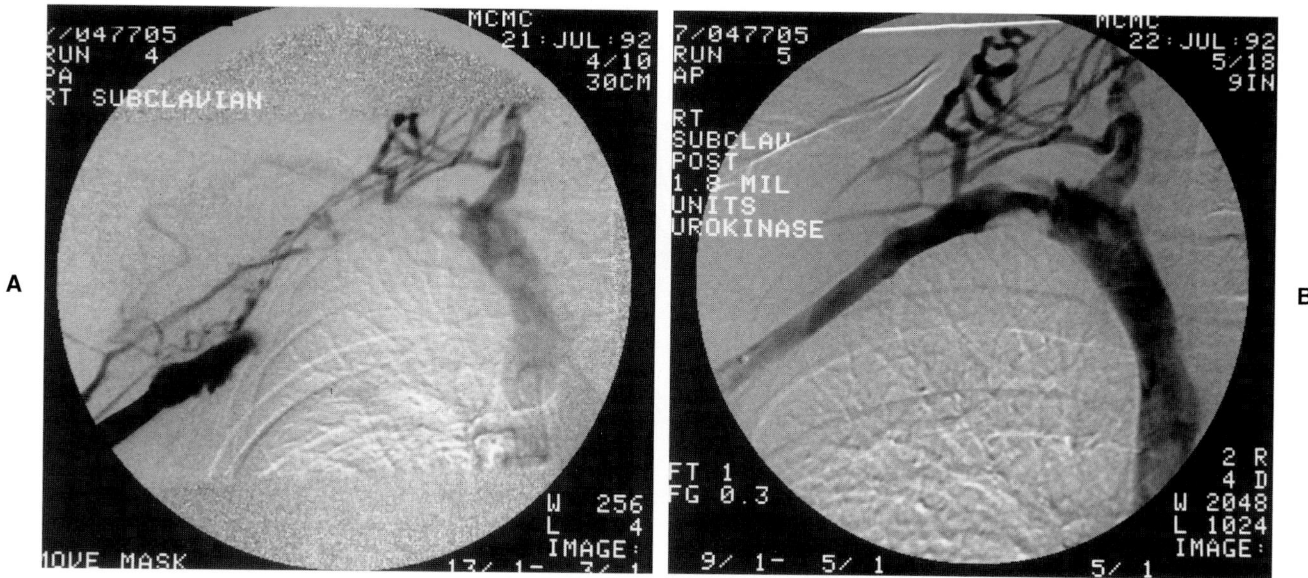

Fig. 54-6. A, Venogram revealing a thrombosed right subclavian vein in a patient with effort thrombosis. **B,** Following urokinase infusion, venous outflow is restored. However, an irregular proximal subclavian vein remains.

cannulation or infusion of an acidic fluid. The incidence has risen in recent years secondary to intravenous drug abuse. Thrombophlebitis of the lower extremity, as previously described, can also occur in association with varicose veins and with prolonged cannulation. The affected vein is usually warm and tender. Treatment is initiated by removal of the intravenous cannula. Warm compresses may be used to relieve the discomfort and decrease the induration. If swelling, induration, and erythema persist and the patient develops fever and chills, the diagnosis of septic or suppurative thrombophlebitis must be entertained. At this point, the entire vein is inflamed, exquisitely tender, and fluctuant. A purulent drainage may be noted at the site of cannulation. The involved vein must then be surgically excised with wide excision to the level of normal vein and debridement of surrounding devitalized tissue. The wounds are left open and treated with wet-to-dry dressing changes. After the infection has resolved and there is healthy granulation tissue, the wound can be closed secondarily. Failure to excise the affected vein results in systemic sepsis that can be fatal.

LYMPHEDEMA

The embryonic development of the lymphatic system begins with paired jugular and iliac sacs, the cisterna chyli, and a second retroperitoneal sac. It is from these sacs that the lymph vessels sprout and course throughout the body following the major venous pathways (Fig. 54-7). The cisterna chyli within the abdomen communicates with the paired jugular sacs by two lymphatic channels. The more predominant channel connecting the cysterna chyli to the left jugular bud is known as the thoracic duct. The elaborate network of lymphatic channels and regional nodes of the upper and lower extremities drain lymph into the thoracic duct and cysterna chyli, respectively, which then return the lymph to the venous system. The lymphatics are formed by a layer of endothelial cells with a discontinuous basement membrane in contrast to the continuous basement membrane found in blood capillaries.[35] The lymphatic capillaries are a valved system that allow for unidirectional flow of lymph back to the venous system.

The functions of the lymphatic system include resorption of interstitial fluid, particularly macromolecular proteins such as albumin; lymph node filtering of bacteria and other antigenic particles; and transport of certain substances (vitamin K, long chain fatty acids) from the gastrointestinal tract to the venous system.[36] During a 24-hour period approximately 4 L of lymph flow containing 100 g of plasma protein is returned to the venous circulation. If the lymphatics fail to return this considerable volume of protein-rich fluid, lymphedema results.

Lymphedema can be categorized as either primary (congenital) or secondary depending on its cause. Primary lymphedema is subdivided according to age of onset; however, all forms are a result of congenital abnormalities in the development of the lymphatic system. *Congenital lymphedema* is present from birth. Milroy's disease is a hereditary form of congenital lymphedema with a sex-linked dominant pattern and characteristic hypoplasia of the lymphatic trunks. *Lymphedema praecox* becomes apparent from the adolescent years to age 35 and accounts for approximately 80% of the patients with congenital lymphedema. *Lymphedema tarda* occurs after age 35. The anatomic anomalies seen in these three forms of primary lymphedema include hypoplasia (the most common), aplasia, and hyperplasia (varicose pattern) of the lymphatic system. Primary lymph-

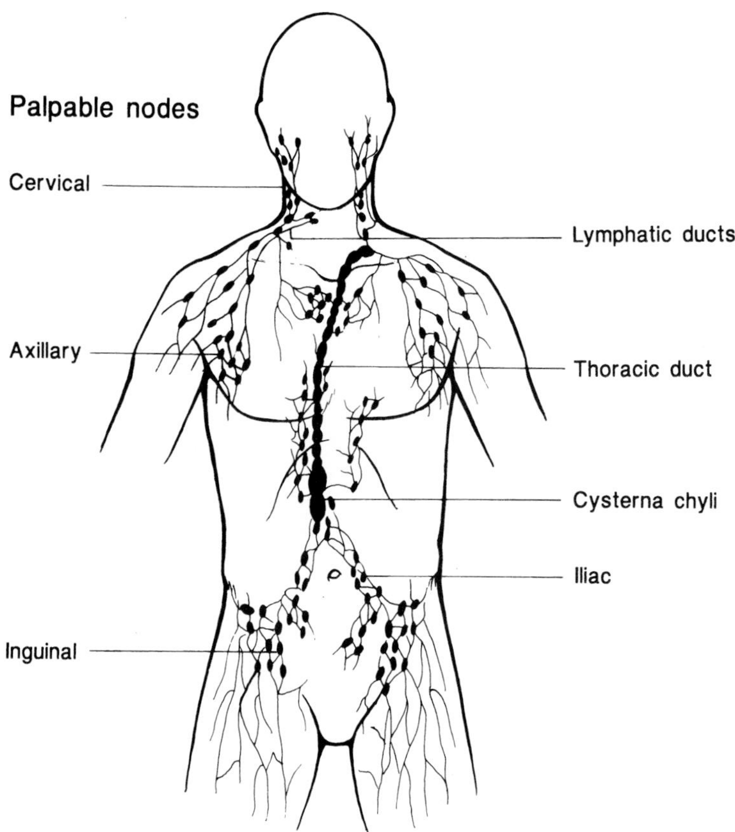

Fig. 54-7. Normal anatomy of the lymphatic system.

edema is found to affect women three times more frequently than it is found to affect men. The left leg is more often involved than the right, and the upper extremity is rarely involved. There is no single identifiable precipitating factor that can account for these findings.

Secondary or acquired lymphedema is the most common form of lymphedema. Worldwide, the most common cause is filariasis, resulting in the obstruction of lymph nodes by the parasite *Filaria bancrofti*. In the United States a common cause is surgical excision of lymph nodes and irradiation for malignant disease. For those who undergo mastectomy with axillary node dissection and radiation therapy, the incidence of lymphedema in the ipsilateral arm can be as high as 38%.[37] Prostate carcinoma or other pelvic carcinomas can also cause lymphatic obstruction. Other causes of secondary lymphedema include trauma or infection.

Clinical Presentation

Lymphatic obstruction results in increased interstitial fluid. Early on this presents as a painless, soft, pitting edema beginning at the ankles and progressing proximally. With an increasing accumulation of protein in the interstitial space, the osmotic pressure increases further, resulting in an even greater amount of fluid in the interstitial space. The high protein content of the edema fluid initiates a fibrotic reaction that damages the lymphatic vessels. This perpetuates a cycle of further lymphedema. At this point the skin is thick and hyperkeratotic, and the entire extremity has a severe firm, nonpitting edema. In addition, given the lymphatic stasis and accumulation of interstitial fluid, infection is common. Lymphangitis frequently presents as red streaks spreading from the foot to the groin. This is associated with erythema and pain as well as with signs of systemic infection.

Diagnosis

The diagnosis of lymphedema can frequently be made on clinical grounds alone. Since the most common cause of unilateral extremity swelling is venous disease, one must be able to distinguish between this and lymphedema. Edema secondary to venous disease presents with decreased capillary perfusion, a brawny discoloration of the involved skin and ulceration. These findings are not indicative of lymphedema. Venous edema also improves after several hours of limb elevation, whereas lymphedema may require several days of extremity elevation to see a decrease in swelling. If there is any question in the differentiation, noninvasive evaluation is required. Duplex examination is the preferred test to rule out DVT. Lymphangiography is rarely used, since it is invasive and hazardous. Complications include dye allergy, oil embolism, and worsening lymphedema.

Lymphoscintigraphy is now becoming the diagnostic

procedure of choice for lymphedema. This test is noninvasive, without side effects, and has an overall diagnostic accuracy of 93%.[38] The procedure involves a subcutaneous injection of a radiolabeled tracer particle specific for the lymphatics. The diagnosis of lymphedema is made when no radioactivity can be detected in the regional lymph nodes 1 hour after injection. A CT scan of the pelvis should also be considered in those patients with lymphatic obstruction to rule out malignancy.

Treatment

Palliative therapy is the only treatment option for lymphedema, since there is no medical or surgical cure. The goal of therapy is to reduce the limb volume and prevent infectious complications. Medical treatment begins with treatment of the inciting event if the lymphedema is acquired as in the case of filariasis. Concomitantly, all patients must be fitted for compressive stockings. For those who are refractory to stocking compression, the use of pneumatic compression has been shown to be effective in reducing of the swelling. Compression therapy and skin care alone has resulted in an 80% improvement rate in patients with lymphedema of the lower extremity.[39] It is imperative that patients understand the chronicity of this disease and the need to maintain the use of compressive stockings. In addition, it must be stressed to these individuals that meticulous foot care is also necessary to avoid fungal infections.

Pharmacotherapy has consisted of diuretics and benzopyrones. Diuretics are not recommended for routine use. They do remove excess fluid but do not change the high interstitial protein concentration and therefore do not alter the underlying pathology. Diuretics can provide short-term relief of the painfully swollen limb when used on an intermittent basis. Benzopyrones have been demonstrated to reduce lymphedema by enhancing proteolysis via increased macrophage phagocytic activity.[40] These drugs are used to provide slow relief of chronic lymphedema but have yet to be approved for use in the United States.

Only a small percentage of the patients with lymphedema require surgical intervention. Indications for operation include an extremely edematous limb, resulting in loss of function and recurrent infections that are refractory to medical management. The operations for lymphedema are divided into two categories—excisional and physiologic procedures. Excisional operations remove the lymphedematous subcutaneous tissue and skin. This is preferably accomplished by staged subcutaneous excisions with preservation of a viable skin flap for primary closure. If this is not possible, the wound can be covered with split-thickness skin grafts; however, breakdown and ulceration of the skin graft is common, therefore primary closure is preferred.

Physiologic procedures are geared toward reconstruction of lymphatic drainage. Microlymphatic venous anastomosis has been used for the treatment of obstructive lymphedema. This procedure is not applicable to those with primary lymphedema caused by hypoplastic lymphatics. The patient must have patent lymphatic vessels distal to the site of obstruction. The microsurgical lymph vessel–to–vein anastomosis is constructed to bypass the obstructed lymphatics. Long-term subjective improvement and limb volume reduction have been reported.[41]

Complications

Episodes of lymphangitis occur several times a year in patients with lymphedema. This accounts for a significant amount of morbidity and accelerates the process of fibrosis. When infection occurs, systemic antibiotics and bed rest with leg elevation are required. *Streptococcus* is the most common inciting organism. In patients with recurrent infections, prophylatic antibiotic therapy is recommended.

A rare but deadly complication of lymphedema is lymphangiosarcoma. This malignant lesion is most frequently associated with postmastectomy lymphedema. It presents as a reddish purple lesion of the skin and subcutaneous tissue, usually appearing approximately 10 years after the onset of lymphedema. Treatment consists of radical amputation; however, prognosis remains dismal with an average survival of less than 2 years.

SUMMARY

Of all the venous disorders, DVT is the most serious and potentially life threatening. Its most lethal complication, pulmary embolism, accounts for approximately 200,000 deaths each year in the United States alone. More than 50% of those with DVT progress to develop postphlebitic syndrome with its disabling consequences. Prophylatic measures in the hospitalized surgical patient are essential. Heparin therapy remains the mainstay of care for the patient diagnosed with DVT, and the Greenfield filter is an effective alternative for those with contraindications to anticoagulation.

Of the lymphatic disorders, lymphedema is the most important. This disorder may result from a congenital cause or may be the result of lymphatic obstruction from malignancy and radiation therapy. Therapy is based on external compression and avoidance of infection. A select group of patients with severe disease may benefit from operative intervention. All treatment is palliative, as there is no known cure for lymphedema.

REFERENCES

1. Dalen JE, Alpert JS. Natural history of pulmonary embolism. Prog Cardiovasc Dis 17:259, 1975.
2. Mueller GP, Williams RA. Natural history of deep venous thrombosis and implications for venous disease. In Veith FJ, et al., eds. Vascular Surgery. Principles and Practice, 2nd ed. New York: McGraw-Hill, 1994.
3. Bertelsen S, Anker W. Phlegmasia cerulea dolens: Pathophysiology, clinical features, treatment, and prognosis. Acta Chir Scand 134:107, 1968.
4. Haeger K. Problems of acute deep venous thrombosis. I. The interpretation of signs and symptoms. Angiology 20:218, 1969.

5. Mitchell DC, et al. Comparison of duplex ultrasonography and venography in the diagnosis of deep venous thrombosis. Br J Surg 78:611, 1991.
6. Lea Thomas M, MacDonald LM. Complications of phlebography of the leg. Br Med J 2:317, 1978.
7. Kakkar VV, et al. Efficacy of low doses of heparin in prevention of deep vein thrombosis after major surgery: A double-blind, randomised trial. Lancet 2:101, 1972.
8. Colditz GA, Tuden RL, Oster G. Rates of venous thrombosis after general surgery: Combined results of randomized clinical trials. Lancet 2:143, 1986.
9. Greenfield LJ. Deep vein thrombosis: Prevention and management. In Veith FJ, et al., eds. Vascular Surgery. Principles and Practice, 2nd ed. New York: McGraw-Hill, 1994.
10. Semba C, Dake M. Iliofemoral deep venous thrombosis: Aggressive therapy with catheter-directed thrombolysis. Radiology 191:487, 1994.
11. Killewich LA, et al. Spontaneous lysis of deep venous thrombi: Rate and outcome. J Vasc Surg 9:89, 1989.
12. Kakkar VV, Lawrence D. Hemodynamic and clinical assessment after therapy for acute deep vein thrombosis. A prospective study. Am J Surg 150:54, 1985.
13. Meissner MH, et al. Deep venous insufficiency: The relationship between lysis and subsequent reflux. J Vasc Surg 18:596, 1993.
14. Comerota AJ, et al. A strategy of aggressive regional therapy for acute ileofemoral venous thrombosis with contemporary venous thrombectomy or catheter-directed thrombolysis. J Vasc Surg 20:244, 1994.
15. Greenfield LJ, Michna BA. Twelve-year experience with the Greenfield vena cava filter. Surgery 104:706, 1988.
16. Becker DM, Philbrick JT, Selby BJ. Inferior vena cava filters. Indications, safety, effectiveness. Arch Intern Med 152:1985, 1992.
17. Greenfield LJ, et al. Transvenous management of pulmonary embolic disease. Ann Surg 180:461, 1974.
18. Urokinase Pulmonary Embolism Trial Study Group. Urokinase pulmonary embolism trial. Phase I results. A cooperative study. JAMA 214:2163, 1970.
19. Browse NL, Clemenson G, Thomas MI. Is the postphlebitic leg always postphlebitic? Relation between phlebographic appearances of deep-vein thrombosis and late sequelae. Br Med J 281:1167, 1980.
20. Lanza D, et al. Noninvasive venous evaluation of patient with class venous insufficiency: Is venous duplex enough? J Vasc Technol (in press).
21. Burnand KG, et al. The relationship between the number of capillaries in the skin of the venous ulcer-bearing area of the lower leg and the fall in foot vein pressure during exercise. Br J Surg 68:297, 1981.
22. Duffy DM. Small vessel sclerotherapy: An overview. Adv Dermatol 3:221, 1988.
23. Greene GL, et al. Monoclonal antibodies to human estrogen receptors. Proc Natl Acad Sci U S A 77:5115, 1988.
24. Hobbs JJ, ed. The Treatment of Venous Disorders. Philadelphia: JB Lippincott, 1977.
25. Bergan JJ. Varicose veins: Chronic venous insufficiency. In Moore WS, ed. Vascular Surgery. A Comprehensive Review, 3rd ed. Philadelphia: WB Saunders, 1991.
26. O'Donnell TF Jr, et al. Doppler examination vs clinical and phlebographic detection of the location of incompetent perforating veins—A prospective study. Arch Surg 112:31, 1977.
27. Sladen JG. Compression sclerotherapy: Preparation, technique, complications, and results. Am J Surg 146:228, 1983.
28. Keith LM Jr, Smead WI. Saphenous vein stripping and its complications. Surg Clin North Am 63:1303, 1983.
29. Sadick NS. Treatment of varicose and telangiectatic leg veins with hypertonic saline: A comparative study of heparin and saline. J Dermatol Surg Oncol 16:24, 1990.
30. Monreal M, et al. Upper extremity deep venous thrombosis and pulmonary embolism: A prospective study. Chest 99:280, 1991.
31. Aburahma AF, Sadler DL, Robinson PA. Axillary-subclavian vein thrombosis. Changing patterns of etiology, diagnostic, and therapeutic modalities. Am Surg 57:101, 1991.
32. Horattas MC, et al. Changing concepts of deep venous thrombosis of the upper extremity—Report of a series and review of the literature. Surgery 104:561, 1988.
33. Tilney NL, Griffiths HJG, Edwards EA. Natural history of major venous thrombosis of the upper extremity. Arch Surg 101:792, 1970.
34. Machleder HI. Evaluation of a new treatment strategy for Paget-Schroetter syndrome: Spontaneous thrombosis of the axillary-subclavian vein. J Vasc Surg 17:305, 1993.
35. Leak LV. Electron microscopic observations on lymphatic capillaries and the structural components of the connective tissue-lymph interface. Microvasc Res 2:361, 1970.
36. Turk AE, Miller TA. Lymphedema and tumors of the lymphatics. In Moore WS, ed. Vascular Surgery. A Comprehensive Review, 3rd ed. Philadelphia: WB Saunders, 1991.
37. Kissen MW, et al. Risk of lymphoedema following the treatment of breast cancer. Br J Surg 73:580, 1986.
38. Gloviczki P, et al. Noninvasive evaluation of the swollen extremity: Experiences with 190 lymphoscintigraphic examinations. J Vasc Surg 9:683, 1989.
39. Pappas CJ, O'Donnell TF. Long-term results of compression treatment for lymphedema. J Vasc Surg 16:555, 1992.
40. Piller NB. Lymphedema, macrophages, and benzopyrones. Lymphology 13:109, 1980.
41. O'Brien BMC, et al. Long-term results after microlymphaticovenous anastomoses for the treatment of obstructive lymphedema. Plast Reconstr Surg 85:562, 1990.

55

Diseases of the Thoracic Aorta

Michael P. Macris and O. Howard Frazier

With the advent of cardiopulmonary bypass, improved anesthetic techniques, and synthetic grafts, diseases of the thoracic aorta became amenable to surgical treatment. The successful treatment of these diseases represents an important achievement in modern surgery.

Lesions of the thoracic aorta that may necessitate surgery include aneurysms, dissections, and traumatic pseudoaneurysms. In the past, syphilitic aneurysms were common; now, however, most thoracic aortic disease results from atherosclerotic and degenerative processes. Early recognition and diagnosis, along with timely surgical intervention and improved preoperative and postoperative care, have resulted in long-term survival for patients with these lesions.

This chapter discusses the factors responsible for the development of thoracic aneurysms, aortic dissections, and traumatic pseudoaneurysms. It also discusses the physiologic principles that underlie the management of these conditions.

INTRINSIC THORACIC AORTIC DISEASE

Thoracic Aneurysms

Classification

Aneurysms of the thoracic aorta are classified according to type, shape, and location. Classification allows the surgeon to use a systematic approach to the treatment of these challenging vascular lesions. Thoracic aortic aneurysms involving all three layers of the arterial wall are called *true aneurysms,* whereas those involving only the tunica adventitia are called *false aneurysms* or *pulsating hematomas.* False aneurysms usually result from traumatic rupture, most commonly seen in decelerating blunt chest trauma.

Fusiform aneurysms, in which the vessel assumes a spindle shape, result in circumferential dilation of all layers of the aorta. They may affect a localized portion or an extensive segment of the aorta, and they are usually related to degenerative diseases, such as arteriosclerosis and cystic medial necrosis.[1] *Saccular aneurysms* are localized spheric dilations that affect one segment of the vessel wall and are connected to the lumen by a mouth. The aneurysmal sac is usually filled by thrombus. These lesions are generally related to syphilis or other bacterial infections and follow an episode of bacterial endocarditis.

Aneurysms involving the aortic arch are classified into four categories according to location.[2] *Type A* lesions are localized and saccular, involving only the transverse arch. *Type B* lesions are fusiform and involve the ascending aorta and arch. *Type C* lesions extend into the proximal descending aorta, and *type D* lesions are more extensive, involving the entire descending aorta (Fig. 55-1). Although type D lesions are the least common of the four, they are the most challenging in terms of surgical therapy.

Aneurysmal disease of the aorta is often multifocal. In a review of 1510 patients with aortic aneurysms, Crawford and Cohen[3] found 191 patients (12.6%) with multifocal disease. Abdominal aortic aneurysms commonly accompany thoracic aneurysms. For this reason, the entire aorta should be evaluated when a patient is being considered for surgical treatment of an aortic aneurysm, because better results are obtained when both lesions are corrected at the same time.

Traumatic rupture of the aorta produces a false aneurysm, usually distal to the left subclavian artery at the level of the ligamentum arteriosum. This type of lesion is generally saccular and constitutes a surgical emergency, most commonly seen in major trauma centers. It is discussed in a separate section.

Pathophysiology

Saccular and fusiform aneurysms of the aorta result from loss of structural integrity of the aortic wall and its individual components.[4] Alterations in the tunica adventitia[5] and loss of lamellar units in the tunica media[6] have been cited as the major causes of aneurysmal dilation of the aorta. Unusual hemodynamic stresses and impaired blood flow may cause these pathologic changes as a result of deficient delivery of nutrients and ischemia of the vessel wall related to involvement of vasa vasorum by various degenerative, inflammatory, and infectious disease states. This as-

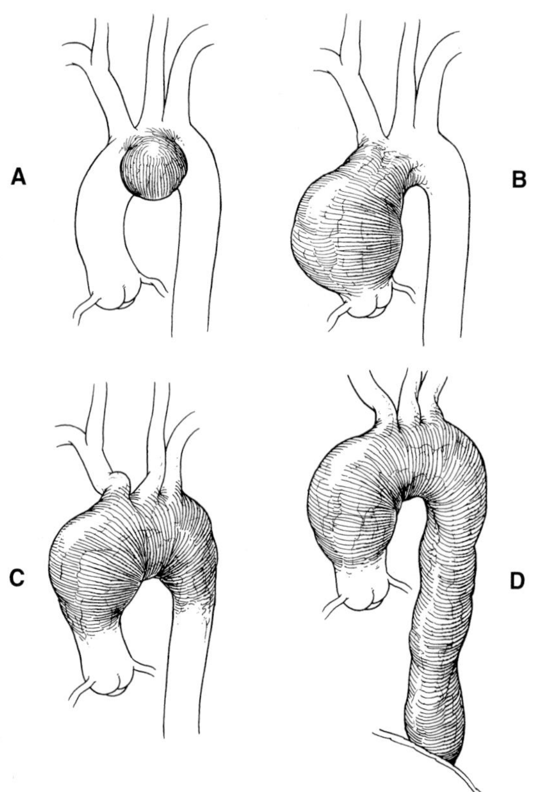

Fig. 55-1. Cooley classification of aortic arch aneurysms. **A,** Type A lesions are saccular lesions, confined to the arch. **B,** Type B lesions are fusiform, involving the ascending aorta and proximal arch. **C,** Type C lesions extend into the proximal descending aorta. **D,** Type D lesions involve the entire descending aorta. (From Cooley DA. Surgical Treatment of Aortic Aneurysms. Philadelphia: WB Saunders, 1986.)

sumption is supported by the following facts: (1) aneurysms are more common in the abdominal aorta than in the thoracic aorta and (2) compared with the abdominal aorta, which has single lumbar vessels, the thoracic aorta has more vasa vasorum originating from a system of paired intercostal arteries.[7]

In the case of syphilitic aortitis, active inflammatory destruction of all elements of the arterial wall occurs faster than the damage can be repaired by means of fibrous tissue proliferation; moreover, the condition is aggravated by severe endarteritis of the vasa vasorum and subsequent ischemia of the vessel wall.[5] Most syphilitic aneurysms are saccular and located in the ascending aorta or arch.[8,9] Fortunately, the early diagnosis and treatment of syphilis, including the use of penicillin, have made this complication a rare cause of aortic aneurysm today.

Currently, most aneurysms of the ascending aorta exhibit the histologic characteristics of cystic medial necrosis,[10] as originally described by Gsell and Erdheim.[10a] This type of pathologic lesion is found in patients with Marfan syndrome[11,12] and usually affects the aortic root, which is subject to high stress because of the velocity and turbulence of blood flow in this region. The histologic pattern reveals necrosis and disappearance of muscle cells in the middle third of the tunica media, with disintegration of elastic laminae and collagen. A mucinoid material fills the cystic spaces. The primary lesion is accompanied by secondary tears caused by the underlying focal weakness.[12,13] Annuloaortic ectasia represents a severe form of cystic medial necrosis in which electron microscopic changes are similar to those found in patients both with and without (forme fruste) Marfan syndrome.[14] This ectatic condition affects the entire ascending aorta, extending from the aortic annulus to the innominate artery. It may cause severe congestive heart failure related to aortic insufficiency, with a high risk of aortic rupture or dissection.[15]

The concept of cystic medial necrosis as an intrinsic disease of the tunica media that causes aneurysms of the aorta has been challenged by Schlatmann and Becker.[16] In histologic studies of the aortic media in 100 patients of different ages with normal aortas, these investigators found changes attributed to cystic medial necrosis, the frequency of which increased with age. They proposed that these changes result from hemodynamic stress on the vessel wall and represent a process of injury and repair in the normal aging aorta. Therefore, the ascending aorta, which is subject to relatively high hemodynamic stress, is the most common site of histologic changes caused by cystic medial necrosis.

Because of a steady increase in the elderly population and the ability to control the late complications of syphilis, arteriosclerosis has emerged as a more common cause of aortic aneurysmal disease. Arteriosclerotic aneurysms, which are confined mainly to the descending and distal thoracic aorta, are fusiform. Once the tunica media and tunica adventitia have been weakened by arteriosclerosis, the disease progresses steadily. It is aggravated by hypertension, progression of the dilation, and further ischemia of the aneurysmal wall. The primary factors that contribute to the formation of arteriosclerotic aneurysms are alterations in flow to the vasa vasorum of the vessel wall and disturbances in intraluminal flow patterns.[5] Moreover, flow across stenotic plaques creates high lateral pressures, and turbulent, reversed flow likewise impacts against the vessel wall. These stresses, which result in structural fatigue and subsequent dilation,[17] may be of etiologic importance.

By means of suppurative or granulomatous processes, infections of the vessel wall result in the formation of mycotic aneurysms.[18] These aneurysms are usually saccular and can develop in any part of the aorta. Previously damaged vessels are most likely to be affected, and the resultant symptoms depend on the size and location of the lesion. Aortitis of unknown cause or associated with different autoimmune disorders is also characterized by aortic dilation and the formation of aneurysms. The exception is Takayasu's arteritis, which is primarily an inflammatory disease associated with severe stenotic lesions of the aorta and other large and medium-sized vessels.[18] Nonspecific aortitis may also result in multiple saccular aneurysms of the aorta, leading to death attributed to rupture.[19]

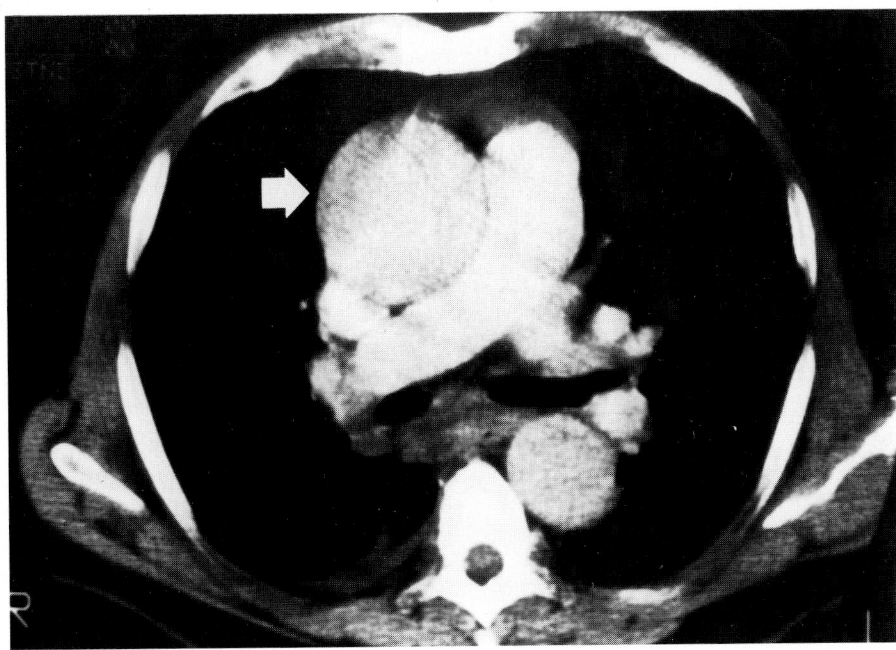

Fig. 55-2. Computed axial tomogram showing an aneurysm of the ascending aorta *(arrow)*.

Inflammatory aneurysms of the aorta are usually located in the terminal aorta, accompanied by a severe retroperitoneal inflammatory process that encases the ureters and sometimes the vena cava. Histologic analysis reveals destruction of both the tunica media and tunica adventitia, with replacement of these structures by a thick, fibrotic wall. Both layers are infiltrated with lymphocytes, plasma cells, lymphoid follicles, and multinucleated giant cells.[20] When these aneurysms occur in the thoracic aorta, however, they usually do not involve the surrounding mediastinum and pleura.

Diagnosis

Clinical presentation. The clinical presentation and symptomatology of thoracic aneurysms are related to the location of the lesion and the compression of adjacent structures. Erosion of large masses through the ribs and sternum is a late finding that is fortunately rarely seen these days. Symptoms include pain, stridor, and coughing caused by aneurysmal compression of the vagus nerves, trachea, and bronchi. With ascending aortic aneurysms that involve the aortic annulus, congestive heart failure commonly occurs as a result of aortic insufficiency. Free rupture into the pericardial sac or pleura is catastrophic and usually diagnosed post mortem.

Occasionally, the diagnosis is suspected in a patient without symptoms in whom routine chest roentgenography shows an upper mediastinal mass contiguous with the aortic shadow. In such cases, further studies are indicated to confirm the diagnosis.

Special diagnostic techniques. The patient with thoracic aortic aneurysmal disease requires a thorough multidisciplinary evaluation, so that the surgeon will have all the information necessary to plan the surgical procedure. Routine chest roentgenography and arteriography remain the standards to which newer techniques are compared. Because arteriography is an invasive technique that entails specific risks for critically ill patients, however, there is a trend toward use of less invasive diagnostic techniques. In particular, computed axial tomography is useful in clarifying certain characteristics of thoracic aneurysms, including their configuration and location, the extent of the disease process, and tissue modifications (Fig. 55-2).

Another new technique, magnetic resonance imaging (MRI), produces images of mediastinal vessels along their axes and creates sagittal and coronal views without degradation of spatial resolution.[21] This technique is especially helpful in the recognition of annuloaortic ectasia and the serial evaluation of postoperative results or disease progression. Unlike conventional angiography, however, MRI cannot show the presence and degree of aortic valve insufficiency or the condition of the coronary arteries—information that is important in planning the surgical approach.[22]

Since the early 1980s, two-dimensional transesophageal echocardiography (TEE) has emerged as an important technique for visualizing the thoracic aorta.[23-26] This method is highly sensitive and specific, particularly in the diagnosis of aortic dissection.[27] It also seems well suited to detecting thoracic aortic aneurysms, especially in patients with unstable hemodynamics and a risk of aneurysmal rupture.[23] Major advantages include safety, reproducibility, cost-effectiveness, and portability (TEE can be performed at any location).

Although these newer techniques are attractive in the diagnosis of aneurysmal disease of the thoracic aorta, aortography is still usually preferred, because it provides a detailed image of the aortic lesion, the coronary arteries, and the branches of the aortic arch.[24] Nevertheless, the newer techniques provide important information that, combined with the aortographic results, gives the surgeon a more complete anatomic picture of the diseased aorta and its branches.

Treatment

With the introduction of cardiopulmonary bypass, modern techniques of hypothermic circulatory arrest, and improved synthetic vascular grafts, surgical treatment of thoracic aortic aneurysms has become the standard approach to these difficult lesions.

Most patients who do not undergo surgery for the treatment of aneurysms die of rupture. Furthermore, overall survival after emergency surgery is also dismal. Elective intervention clearly results in lower mortality and morbidity rates.[28] For these reasons, elective surgical repair is recommended if the patient has symptoms related to the aneurysm, if the diameter of the lesion is greater than 10 cm, or, in cases involving smaller lesions, if enlargement has been documented.[29] Elective repair is also recommended for the patient with Marfan syndrome whose ascending aorta is more than 5.5 to 6.0 cm in diameter.[29] Early and late risks of death are related to advanced age, the need for emergency surgery, and the presence of congestive heart failure and arterial hypertension.

The surgical approach varies according to the aneurysm's location and specific anatomic characteristics. Unique surgical techniques and complications associated with aneurysms of the different segments of the thoracic aorta are therefore discussed.

Ascending aorta. The treatment of choice for most ascending aortic aneurysms is surgical resection and graft replacement. Cardiopulmonary bypass with right atrial and femoral artery cannulation is instituted when cannulation of the ascending aorta or proximal transverse aorta is not possible; otherwise, the ascending aorta is the preferred site. Once full cardiopulmonary bypass flow has been established, the patient is cooled to 18° to 22° C, after which the circulation is arrested. The distal ascending aorta is then transected, and an open distal anastomosis is performed.[30,31] This technique allows better visualization of the distal aorta and is technically easier, because it allows better handling of the distal aorta. The flow is slowly restarted, and air is evacuated from the aorta. The graft is clamped, full flow is re-established, and the patient is rewarmed as the proximal anastomosis is performed.

A modified technique is used in the presence of associated aortic valve insufficiency and coronary ostial involvement. When the sinuses of Valsalva are not grossly dilated, supracoronary grafting and conventional aortic valve replacement is the procedure of choice, but care must be taken to prevent hemorrhage, damage to the coronary ostia, or the formation of pseudoaneurysms. If the sinuses of Valsalva are involved in the aneurysmal dilation and the coronary ostia are displaced 2 cm or more cephalad, one should use a valved conduit and reimplant the coronary ostia into the graft (Fig. 55-3).[32]

Normally, we prefer the classic technique of Bentall and De Bono[33] for repairing annuloaortic ectasia. Still, this approach can result in postoperative bleeding and false aneurysm formation at the anastomotic site between the coronary orifices and the valve-containing graft. To minimize the risk of these complications, we routinely create a fistula between the perigraft space and the right atrium, as recommended by Cabrol et al.[34] This step is accomplished by sewing the proximal apex of the aortotomy to a 2 cm slit in the medial aspect of the right atrial appendage. The rest of the aorta is snugly wrapped around the graft.[35]

Transverse arch. The treatment of transverse aortic arch aneurysms presents a special challenge to the cardiovascular surgeon. The most serious surgical complications are (1) cerebral damage resulting from cerebral ischemia and (2) air or particulate embolization during graft re-

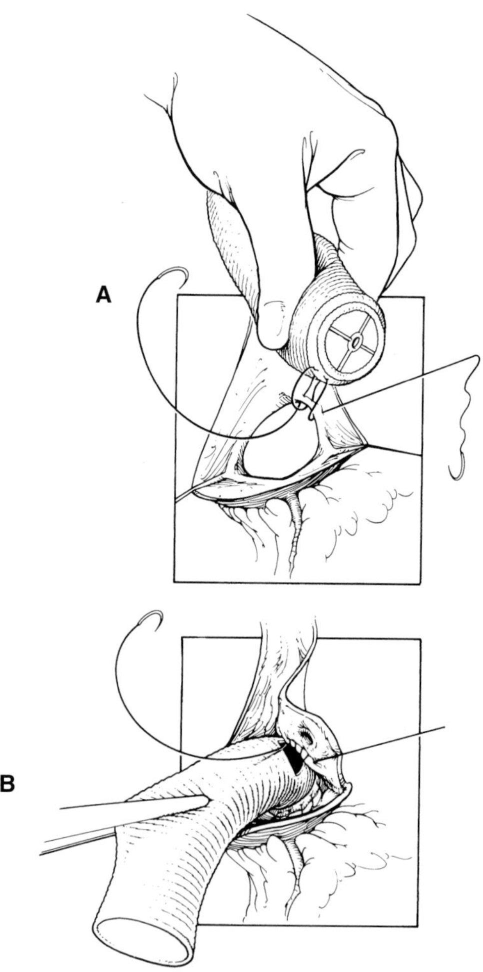

Fig. 55-3. A, Graft replacement of the ascending aorta with a valved conduit. **B,** Reimplantation of the coronary ostia into the conduit. (From Cooley DA. Surgical Treatment of Aortic Aneurysms. Philadelphia: WB Saunders, 1986.)

placement. For this reason, indications for surgery should be evaluated on an individual basis; elective surgical intervention should be reserved for lesions that approach 6 to 8 cm in diameter and cause symptoms related to the compression of vital structures.

Strategies for treating these lesions have included insertion of a temporary tube bypass, placement of temporary and permanent bypass grafts, cardiopulmonary bypass with separate perfusion of the brachiocephalic vessels, and cardiopulmonary bypass with profound hypothermia and circulatory arrest.[32,36-38] Bypass techniques are complicated, however, as is separate perfusion of the brachiocephalic vessels, and the results are inconsistent.

Surgeons at the Texas Heart Institute in Houston have used hypothermic circulatory arrest, which provides adequate cerebral protection during arch replacement and eliminates the need for perfusion cannulas and excessive clamps, thereby offering a simplified operative field.[39] The patient's core temperature is lowered to between 18° and 22° C with a pump oxygenator and heat exchanger. The circulation is arrested, and the aneurysm is then repaired with a low-porosity woven polyethylene terephthalate fiber (Dacron) graft, which is impregnated with collagen (Hemashield, Natick, MA Meadox) and does not require preclotting with autologous plasma and autoclaving.[40] The proximal and distal anastomoses are created with a running, nonabsorbable, monofilament suture (Fig. 55-4). Circulation is resumed gradually, with care to allow the air-fluid level of the blood to increase slowly, thus minimizing the risk of gross air embolization. The patient is gradually rewarmed, at the rate of 1° C every 3 minutes, to avoid production of gaseous microemboli.

This simplified technique of moderate hypothermia satisfactorily protects the cerebrum and myocardium for 20 to 30 minutes during circulatory arrest. Most of the neurologic deficits that result from this technique are transient; however, most fixed deficits appear to be caused by emboli, so special precautions should be taken to avoid particulate embolization from atherosclerotic aneurysms during graft replacement.

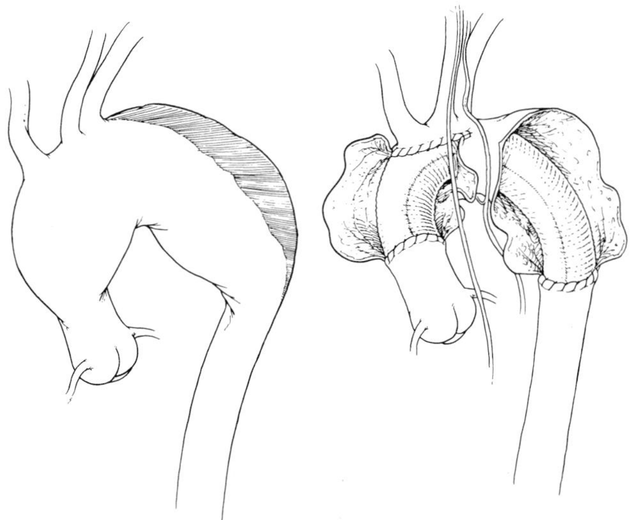

Fig. 55-4. Graft replacement of a type C aortic arch aneurysm, with reimplantation of the great vessels into the graft. (From Cooley DA. Surgical Treatment of Aortic Aneurysms. Philadelphia: WB Saunders, 1986.)

Descending aorta. Most cardiovascular surgeons consider graft replacement the best surgical treatment for descending aortic aneurysms. They disagree, however, as to which approach should be used to avoid the complications related to this procedure.

Since the early days, when Carrel[41] found postoperative paraplegia in experimental animals, this problem has been the most dreaded complication associated with operations on the descending thoracic aorta. The mechanism that causes spinal cord injury after cross-clamping of the proximal descending thoracic aorta is poorly understood. Several factors are probably responsible, but the primary ones appear to be interruption of blood flow and distal ischemia of the spinal cord, in addition to elevation of the cerebrospinal fluid pressure as a result of proximal hypertension.[42,43] Accordingly, special attention has been devoted to understanding how blood is supplied to the distal spinal cord.[44,45] The arteria radicularis magna anterior, also known as the *artery of Adamkiewicz,* originates between T9 and T12 and is responsible for supplying most of the blood to this segment of the spinal cord. Isolated ligation of this vessel in experimental animals, without proximal cross-clamping or other hemodynamic alterations, results in a paraplegia rate of 71.4%,[45] thereby establishing this artery's importance.

During the early days of aortic surgery, the value of systemic hypothermia as an adjunct to prevent ischemic spinal cord injury was demonstrated experimentally and clinically by Cooley,[32] by DeBakey et al.,[46] and by Pontius et al.[47] Nevertheless, the risk of cardiac arrhythmias and coagulopathies resulting from systemic hypothermia remained a problem.[2] Other researchers have recommended the use of various shunts and partial bypass techniques,[48-51] but the results have been inconsistent. Furthermore, these techniques are relatively complicated, so the operation is unnecessarily prolonged.

On the basis of their experience with these complex lesions, experts at two major vascular surgical centers advocate a simple cross-clamping technique without the use of adjuncts to avoid ischemia.[38,52-54] They also recommend the prevention of hypotension, the expeditious removal of the aneurysm and restoration of distal flow, and the avoidance of cross-clamp times longer than 30 minutes, which are associated with a higher risk of postoperative paraplegia. We favor an "open" distal anastomosis technique, in which a single cross-clamp is placed proximal to the aneurysm to exsanguinate the lower body. The exsanguinated blood is collected by an autotransfusion device and returned to the patient. This approach minimizes the risk of spinal cord injury and renal insufficiency yet allows the distal anastomosis to be completed efficiently, with a short ischemic time.[30,31]

Aortic Dissection

Pathophysiology

Dissection of the thoracic aorta is a unique entity characterized by a spontaneous tear of the tunica intima and part of the tunica media of the aortic wall. Blood escapes under pressure into the aortic laminae, causing a pathologic separation of the tunica media along the longitudinal axis of the aorta, parallel to the blood flow. This "false" dissecting channel in the middle of the aortic wall spreads downstream for a variable distance. It usually starts 2 cm distal to the aortic valve cusps.[32,55] In most cases, a transverse intimal tear marks the beginning of the dissection, but this finding can vary. A tear in the ascending aorta is usually located in the right lateral aortic wall, and the dissection progresses along the greater curvature of the aorta. A re-entry tear occurs much less frequently and may be difficult to identify. Dissections may also begin in the transverse arch or the proximal descending thoracic aorta, usually at the level of the isthmus, distal to the origin of the left subclavian artery. Once the dissecting process has begun, it progresses rapidly, depending mainly on the systemic blood pressure and the velocity of blood flow. The extent of the dissection appears to be influenced by intrinsic characteristics of the vessel wall itself, but medial scarring related to atherosclerotic plaque formation seems to be the factor that usually limits the dissection.[55]

A working classification of aortic dissections according to site of origin and extension provides a practical approach to these lesions and aids in their management.[56] *Type A* dissections originate from a tear in the ascending aorta and may extend distally into the descending aorta. These dissections carry the greatest risk of rupture and are associated with acute aortic regurgitation and myocardial infarction related to dissection and obstruction of the coronary arteries. *Type B* dissections originate in the descending aorta, distal to the arch (Fig. 55-5). The dissecting process usually extends distally, but proximal dissection is also possible.

The cause of aortic dissection is still a subject of debate. This lesion was previously called a *dissecting aneurysm,* but the term *acute aortic dissection* is more appropriate, because the pathologic process is different from that of a true aneurysm, and aneurysmal expansion is seldom a particularly prominent feature. Although dissection was formerly attributed to cystic medial necrosis, Schlatmann and Becker[16] showed that the morphologic changes of aortic dissection may result from injury and repair within the aortic wall. Such changes alter the structural properties of the vessel wall, leading to dilation. The local hemodynamic circumstances determine whether further dilation, dissection, or rupture occurs. Patients with Marfan syndrome, who most frequently have aortic dissections, have an underlying connective tissue disorder that makes them susceptible to aortic complications at an early age.[57] Arterial hypertension is present in approximately 70% of patients with aortic dissection and is the most common predisposing factor for this condition. Other associated findings include trauma, a bicuspid aortic valve, aortic isthmic coarctation, and a previous aortotomy for cannulation in cardiopulmonary bypass.

Diagnosis

Clinical presentation. The presenting symptoms of aortic dissection vary according to the location of the tear, the associated complications, and the degree of ischemia of vital organs in the presence of a blood supply that has been compromised by the dissecting process. The most common symptom is acute, severe chest pain that radiates to the back and abdomen. When the dissection extends into the innominate artery, compromising the right subclavian artery, the patient may also report numbness or pain in the right arm. Proximal dissections may result in aortic valve insufficiency, in which case a diastolic murmur can be heard. In severe cases, the clinical presentation may involve signs and symptoms compatible with congestive heart failure.

Complications of acute aortic dissection are varied. Rupture of the aorta is the most devastating complication, leading to immediate exsanguination. Rupture may occur anywhere between the pericardial sac and the abdominal

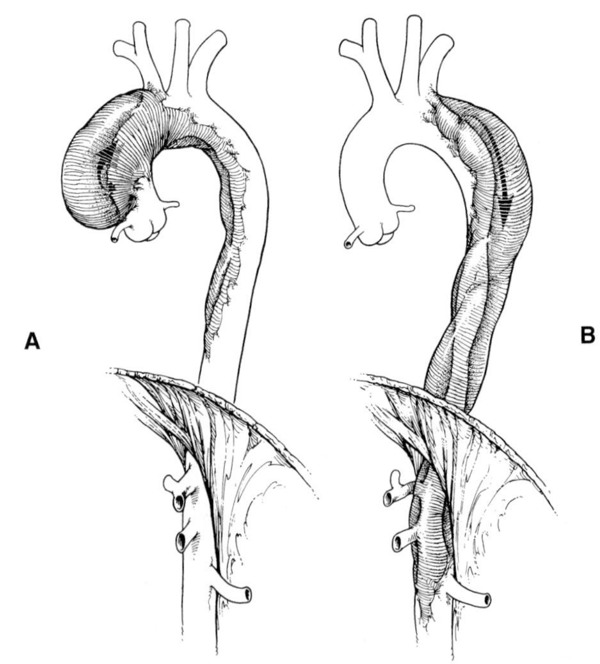

Fig. 55-5. Classification of aortic dissections. **A,** Type A lesions comprise the ascending aorta and may extend into the aortic arch. **B,** Type B lesions originate in the proximal descending aorta, extending distally. (From Cooley DA. Surgical Treatment of Aortic Aneurysms. Philadelphia: WB Saunders, 1986.)

cavity. Obstruction of blood flow to vital organs by a medial hematoma of the wall of the vessel that supplies those particular organs may result in ischemia, producing myriad symptoms, depending on which organs are involved. Myocardial infarction, cerebrovascular insufficiency, stroke, transient ischemic attacks, renal failure, mesenteric ischemia, and even paraplegia may be the presenting manifestation of aortic dissection. As noted earlier, proximal dissection can result in dilation of the aortic annulus, with acute aortic regurgitation and congestive heart failure.

Special diagnostic techniques. As with thoracic aneurysmal disease, aortography remains the gold standard for establishing the diagnosis of aortic dissection. The most common angiographic findings are opacification of the false lumen, visualization of the intimal flap, and deformity of the true lumen (Fig. 55-6).

Other, less invasive techniques are being used with increasing frequency. Two-dimensional echocardiography, particularly TEE, is useful in diagnosing dissection of the ascending aorta. In fact, many experts now consider TEE the method of choice in this setting.[23,25,26,58] It has the advantage of being a bedside procedure, and it provides other useful information regarding the differential diagnosis. Moreover, it is faster and more accurate than aortography or computed tomography.[59] The criteria for aortic dissection are (1) an aortic root measuring at least 42 mm, (2) an intraluminal structure within the proximal aorta consistent with an intimal flap, and (3) a high frequency of intimal flap operations, which is the most specific sign.[60] Although computed axial tomography may be useful in elucidating various features of aortic dissection, two-dimensional echocardiography, especially TEE, offers better resolution, because it can more easily identify the intimal flap in cases of dissection.[61]

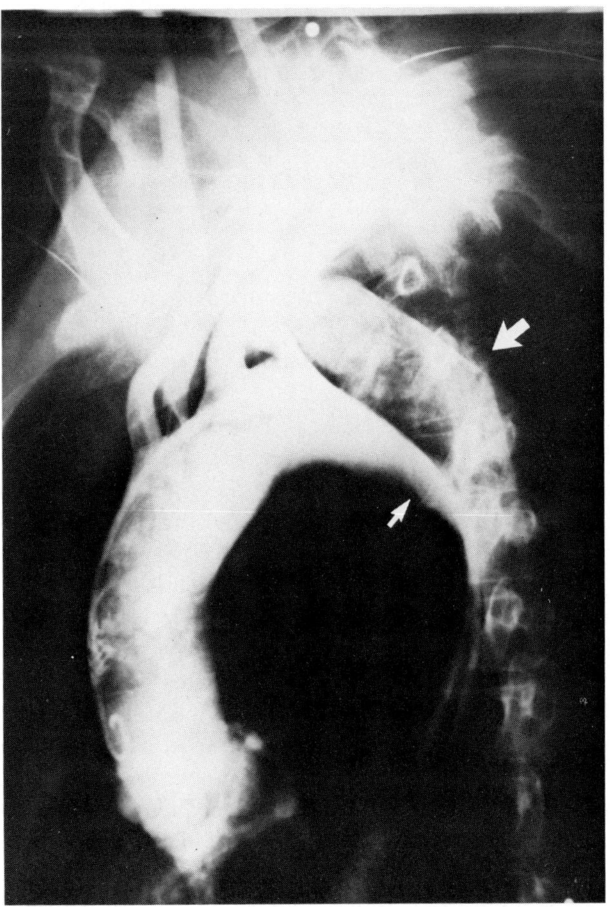

Fig. 55-6. Arteriogram of a type B aortic dissection. Notice the opacification of the false lumen *(large arrow)* and compression of the true lumen *(small arrow)*.

Ultimately, MRI may prove the most useful of the new techniques. Currently, it is limited by high cost, long image-acquisition time, nonportability, and unsuitability for patients in hemodynamically unstable condition. When further refined, however, MRI could rival TEE for diagnosing aortic dissection.[62]

Treatment

Treatment of aortic dissection depends on location and associated complications. Type A dissections should undergo immediate surgical intervention and repair.

Uncomplicated type B lesions may be managed medically with close observation, intravenous administration of peripheral vasodilators to lower the systemic blood pressure, and β-adrenergic blockers to reduce the cardiac ejection velocity.[63] Nevertheless, patients must be watched carefully to avoid associated complications, and not all authorities agree that medical management is the best approach. After analyzing results of surgical treatment of type B lesions, Reul et al.[64] recommended that patients with acute and chronic descending aortic aneurysms undergo early surgical repair, before extension, rupture, or massive enlargement occurs.

Prophylactic surgery for aortic dissection is indicated in cases of Marfan syndrome in which the ascending aorta reaches a diameter of 6 cm, as measured by echocardiography. These patients are candidates for a composite graft repair, and early intervention has proved highly beneficial.[65]

TRAUMATIC PSEUDOANEURYSMS

Modern methods of ground transportation have resulted in a steady increase in the incidence of blunt deceleration injuries. Traumatic rupture of the thoracic aorta occurs in approximately 10% to 17% of fatal motor vehicle accidents.[66] When traumatic aortic pseudoaneurysm occurs, only 20% of patients survive the initial injury. For this small group, mortality rate increases with time, with 49% dying within the first 48 hours and only 2% surviving for more than 4 months if left untreated.[67] Death results from rupture with immediate exsanguination.

Disruption is a result of shearing stresses at the junction of the fixed and mobile parts of the aorta,[68] usually distal to the left subclavian artery at the ligamentum arteriosum. If

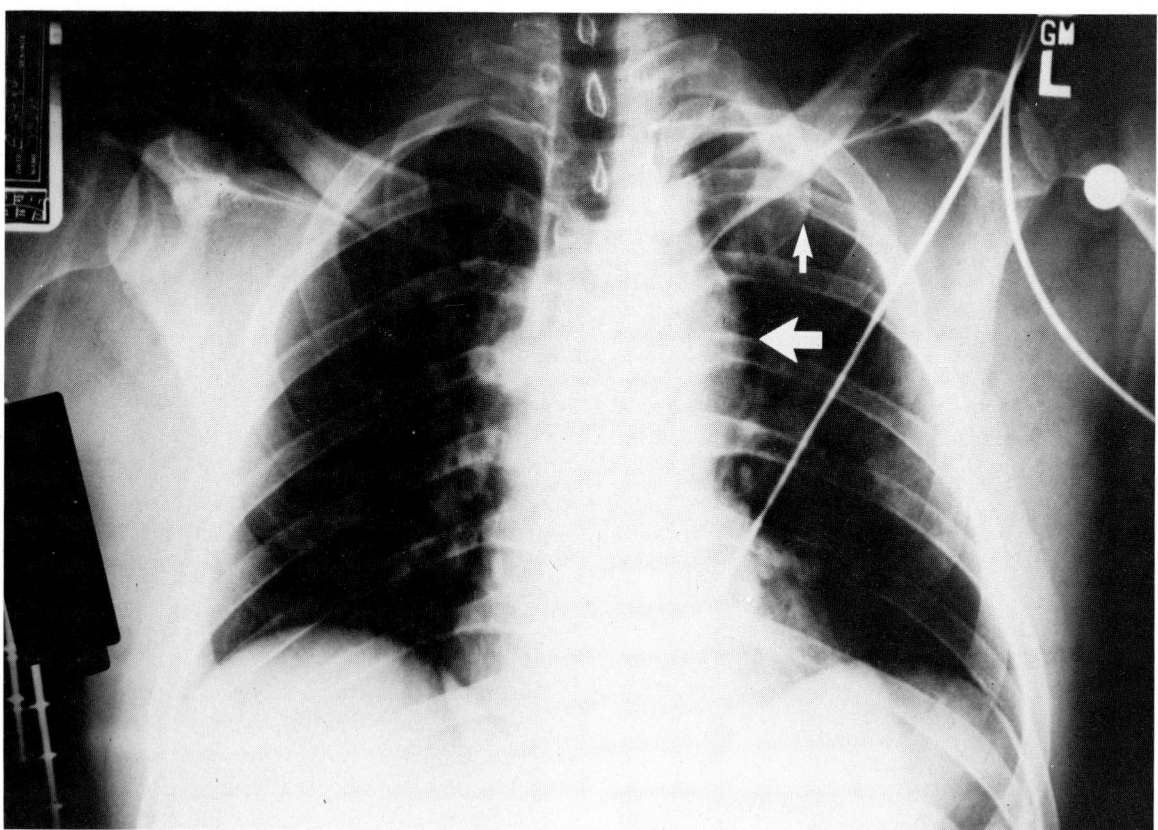

Fig. 55-7. Chest roentgenogram of a patient with aortic transection. Note the widened mediastinum *(large arrow),* which indicates a mediastinal hematoma. Other findings include a left apical cap, loss of the aortic knob contour, and fracture of the left second and third ribs *(small arrow).*

the tear is complete, exsanguination is immediate, resulting in death at the scene. If the tunica intima and tunica media are disrupted but the tunica adventitia remains intact, a false aneurysm forms. The tunica adventitia, which contains the pulsating hematoma, cannot withstand the bursting pressure that an intact aorta could; moreover, the tunica adventitia is susceptible to rupture during aggressive fluid resuscitation in the emergency department or at induction of anesthesia, when measures to counteract hypotension are taken.[69] For this reason, if aortic rupture is suspected, careful monitoring of the systemic blood pressure to avoid extremes and rapid changes is mandatory.

Aortic transection should be suspected in any patient with blunt chest trauma. Chest roentgenography is the initial step in making the diagnosis. Loss of the aortic knob contour appears to be the most consistent and reliable sign of aortic laceration. Other findings include (1) a mediastinal width/chest width ratio greater than 0.25 on a supine chest radiograph, (2) a left apical cap, (3) rightward displacement of the nasogastric tube and/or trachea, (4) displacement of the right paraspinous interface, and (5) depression of the left main stem bronchus[70] (Fig. 55-7). Once the chest roentgenogram is considered of suspect appearance, immediate aortography is indicated to confirm the diagnosis and localize the tear, allowing the planning of a surgical approach (Fig. 55-8). Alternatively, TEE or computed tomography may be used to screen patients for aortography.[23]

Acute aortic transection and false aneurysm formation should be treated with immediate surgical repair through a left thoracotomy. Most of these lesions can be repaired primarily or with an interposition graft. Whether adjunctive measures to prevent spinal cord ischemia and renal failure are necessary, or even useful, remains controversial. As a rule, during operation for aortic transection, one should make sure that the left ventricle is not subjected to excessive stress as a result of proximal cross-clamping and that the total distal ischemic time is minimized. To accomplish these goals, surgeons have used numerous adjuncts, including partial bypass techniques and different types of shunts. Bypass techniques entail a higher mortality rate than do shunting and simple cross-clamping,[71] probably because bypass necessitates the use of heparin (with its attendant complications) in the presence of multiple injuries. Simple aortic cross-clamping and use of an expeditious surgical technique to keep the ischemic time to less than 30 minutes form the procedure of choice for repairing acute traumatic rupture of the aorta.[71,72]

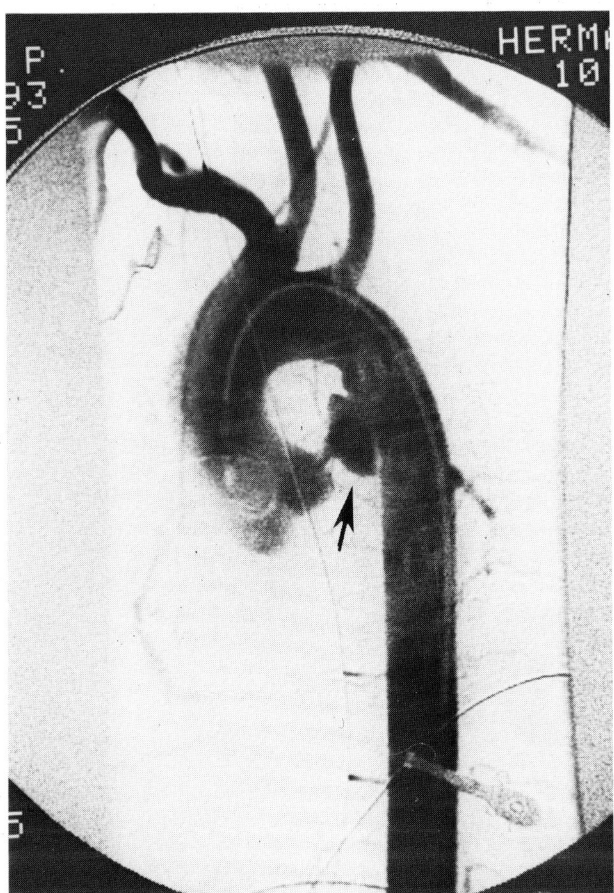

Fig. 55-8. Digital-subtraction angiogram of the thoracic aorta in a patient with traumatic aortic transection and development of a false aneurysm distal to the left subclavian artery at the level of the ligamentum arteriosum *(arrow)*.

SUMMARY

Because of the increase in the elderly population, aneurysmal disease of the thoracic aorta is usually related to chronic degenerative processes involving the different layers of the vessel wall. The concept of cystic medial necrosis as a primary disease of the ascending aorta has been challenged. Aneurysms are now believed to be a response to local hemodynamic factors that inflict stress on the aortic wall. Distal to the ascending aorta, arteriosclerosis is usually responsible for aneurysmal dilation of the aorta. The cause of arteriosclerosis is still uncertain, and preventive measures are controversial.

The clinical presentations of thoracic aneurysms and dissections have been well described, and aortography has generally been the procedure of choice in confirming the diagnosis. Recently, however, there has been a trend toward the use of less invasive techniques. In some cases, particularly those involving thoracic aortic dissection, TEE has begun to supplant aortography. MRI imaging is an extremely promising noninvasive method, and early results with this diagnostic tool have been encouraging.

Surgical repair is the treatment of choice for thoracic aneurysms and dissections. Because of the availability of cardiopulmonary bypass, improved anesthesia, advanced hypothermic techniques, and better prosthetic grafts, patients with these difficult lesions now have an improved chance of survival.

REFERENCES

1. Richards MA. Medionecrosis aortae idiopathica cystica. Am J Pathol 8:717, 1932.
2. Cooley DA, et al. Surgical treatment of aneurysms of the transverse aortic arch: Experience with 25 patients using hypothermic techniques. Ann Thorac Surg 32:260, 1981.
3. Crawford ES, Cohen ES. Aortic aneurysm: A multifocal disease. Arch Surg 117:1393, 1982.
4. Robicsek F, et al. The applicability of Bernoulli's law in the process of enlargement and rupture of aortic aneurysms. J Thorac Cardiovasc Surg 61:472, 1971.
5. de Takats G, Pirani CL. Aneurysms: General considerations. Angiology 5:173, 1954.
6. Pomerance A, Yacoub MH, Gula G. The surgical pathology of thoracic aortic aneurysms. Histopathology 1:257, 1977.
7. Benjamin HB, Becker AB. Etiologic incidence of thoracic and abdominal aneurysms. Surg Gynecol Obstet 125:1306, 1967.
8. Kampmeier RH. Saccular aneurysms of the thoracic aorta: A clinical study of 633 cases. Ann Intern Med 12:624, 1938.
9. Reich NE. Syphilis of the aorta. In Reich NE, ed. Diseases of the Aorta: Diagnosis and Treatment. New York: MacMillan, 1949.
10. Klima T, et al. The morphology of ascending aneurysms. Hum Pathol 14:810, 1983.

10a. Erdheim J. Medionecrosis aortae idiopathica. Virchows Arch Pathol Anat 273:454, 1929.

11. Baer RW, Taussig HB, Oppenheimer EH. Congenital aneurysmal dilatation of the aorta associated with arachnodactyly. Bull Johns Hopkins Hosp 72:309, 1943.
12. Bahnson HT, Nelson AR. Cystic medial necrosis as a cause of localized aortic aneurysms amenable to surgical therapy. Ann Surg 144:519, 1956.
13. Rotino A. Medial degeneration, cystic variety in unruptured aortas. Am Heart J 19:330, 1940.
14. Savunen T, Aho JH. Annuloaortic ectasia: Light and electron microscopic changes in the aortic media. Virchows Arch Pathol Anat 407:279, 1985.
15. Chapman DW, Cooley DA. Annulo-aortic ectasia with cystic medial necrosis. Am J Cardiol 16:679, 1965.
16. Schlatmann TJM, Becker AE. Histologic changes in the normal aging aorta: Implications for dissecting aortic aneurysm. Am J Cardiol 39:13, 1977.
17. Holman E, Peniston W. Hydrodynamic factors in the production of aneurysms. Am J Surg 90:200, 1955.
18. Lande A, Berkmen YM. Aortitis: Pathologic, clinical, and arteriographic review. Radiol Clin North Am 14:219, 1976.
19. Henochowicz SI, et al. Multiple saccular aortic aneurysms in nonspecific aortitis. Am J Cardiol 57:377, 1986.
20. Crawford JL, et al. Inflammatory aneurysms of the aorta. J Vasc Surg 2:113, 1986.
21. Moore EH, et al. Magnetic resonance imaging of chronic posttraumatic false aneurysms of the thoracic aorta. Am J Radiol 143:1195, 1984.
22. Amparo E, et al. Aortic dissection: Magnetic resonance imaging. Radiology 155:399, 1985.
23. Blanchard DG, et al. Transesophageal echocardiography of the aorta. JAMA 272:546, 1994.
24. Earnest F, Muhm JR, Sheedy PF. Roentgenographic findings in thoracic aortic dissection. Mayo Clin Proc 54:43, 1979.

25. Goldstein SA, Mintz GS, Lindsay J Jr. Aorta: Comprehensive evaluation by echocardiography and transesophageal echocardiography. J Am Soc Echocardiogr 6:634, 1993.
26. Wiet SP, et al. Utility of transesophageal echocardiography in the diagnosis of disease of the thoracic aorta. J Vasc Surg 20:613, 1994.
27. Ballal RS, et al. Usefulness of transesophageal echocardiography in assessment of aortic dissection. Circulation 84:1903, 1991.
28. Pressler V, McNamara JJ. Aneurysms of the thoracic aorta: Review of 260 cases. J Thorac Cardiovasc Surg 89:50, 1985.
29. Moreno-Cabral CE, et al. Degenerative and atherosclerotic aneurysms of the thoracic aorta: Determinants of early and late surgical outcome. J Thorac Cardiovasc Surg 88:1020, 1984.
30. Cooley DA, Baldwin RT. Technique of open distal anastomosis for repair of descending thoracic aortic aneurysms. Ann Thorac Surg 54:932, 1992.
31. Scheinin SA, Cooley DA. Graft replacement of the descending thoracic aorta: Results of "open" distal anastomosis. Ann Thorac Surg 58:19, 1994.
32. Cooley DA. Surgical Treatment of Aortic Aneurysms. Philadelphia: WB Saunders, 1986.
33. Bentall H, De Bono A. A technique for complete replacement of the ascending aorta. Thorax 23:338, 1968.
34. Cabrol C, Pavie A, Mesnildrey P. Long-term results with total replacement of the ascending aorta and reimplantation of the coronary arteries. J Thorac Cardiovasc Surg 91:17, 1986.
35. Lewis CTP, et al. Surgical repair of aortic root aneurysms in 280 patients. Ann Thorac Surg 53:38, 1992.
36. Cooley DA. Aneurysms of the ascending aorta: Surgical treatment using hypothermic arrest. Cardiology 77:373, 1990.
37. Crawford ES, Saleh SA, Schuessler JS. Treatment of aneurysms of transverse aortic arch. J Thorac Cardiovasc Surg 78:383, 1979.
38. Kay GL, et al. Surgical repair of aneurysms involving the distal aortic arch. J Thorac Cardiovasc Surg 91:397, 1986.
39. Livesay JJ, et al. Resection of aortic arch aneurysms: Comparison of hypothermic techniques in 60 patients. Ann Thorac Surg 36:19, 1983.
40. Cooley DA, Romagnoli A, Milam JD. A method of preparing dacron grafts to prevent interstitial hemorrhage. Cardiovasc Dis 8:48, 1981.
41. Carrel A. On the experimental surgery of the aorta and heart. Ann Surg 52:83, 1910.
42. Blaiswell FW, Cooley DA. The mechanism of paraplegia after temporary thoracic aortic occlusion and its relationship to spinal fluid pressure. Surgery 51:351, 1962.
43. Oka Y, Miyamoto T. Prevention of spinal cord injury after cross-clamping of the thoracic aorta. Jpn J Surg 14:159, 1982.
44. Svensson LG, et al. Relationship of spinal cord blood flow to vascular anatomy during thoracic aortic cross clamping and shunting. J Thorac Cardiovasc Surg 91:71, 1986.
45. Wadouh F, et al. The arteria radicularis magna anterior as a decisive factor influencing spinal cord damage during aortic occlusion. J Thorac Cardiovasc Surg 88:1, 1984.
46. DeBakey ME, Cooley DA, Creech O. Resection of the aorta for aneurysms and occlusive disease with particular reference to the use of hypothermia: Analysis of 240 cases. Surgery 5:153, 1955.
47. Pontius RG, et al. The use of hypothermia in the prevention of paraplegia following temporary aortic occlusion: Experimental observations. Surgery 36:33, 1954.
48. Donahoo JS, Brawley RK, Gott VL. The heparin-coated vascular shunt for thoracic aortic and great vessel procedure: A ten-year experience. Ann Thorac Surg 23:507, 1977.
49. Laschinger JC, et al. Experimental and clinical assessment of the adequacy of partial bypass in maintenance of spinal cord blood flow during operations on the thoracic aorta. Ann Thorac Surg 36:417, 1983.
50. Lawrence GH, et al. Results of the use of the TDMAC-heparin shunt in the surgery of aneurysms of the descending thoracic aorta. J Thorac Cardiovasc Surg 73:393, 1977.
51. Zacharopoulos L, Symbas PN. Internal temporary aortic shunts for managing lesions of the descending thoracic aorta. Ann Thorac Surg 35:240, 1983.
52. Crawford ES, Rubio PA. Reappraisal of adjuncts to avoid ischemia in the treatment of aneurysms of descending thoracic aorta. J Thorac Cardiovasc Surg 66:693, 1973.
53. Crawford ES, et al. Graft replacement of aneurysms in descending thoracic aorta: Results without bypass of shunting. Surgery 89:73, 1981.
54. Livesay JJ, et al. Surgical experience in descending thoracic aneurysmectomy with and without adjuncts to avoid ischemia. Ann Thorac Surg 39:37, 1985.
55. Roberts WC. Aortic dissection: Anatomy, consequences, and causes. Am Heart J 101:195, 1981.
56. Daily PO, et al. Management of acute aortic dissections. Ann Thorac Surg 10:237, 1970.
57. Schlatmann TJM, Becker AE. Pathogenesis of dissecting aneurysm of the aorta. Am J Cardiol 39:21, 1977.
58. Borner N, et al. Diagnosis of aortic dissection by transesophageal echocardiography. Am J Cardiol 54:1157, 1984.
59. Erbel R, et al. Echocardiography in diagnosis of aortic dissection. Lancet 1:457, 1989.
60. Granato JE, Dee P, Gibson RS. Utility of two-dimensional echocardiography in suspected ascending aortic dissection. Am J Cardiol 56:123, 1985.
61. Iliceto S, et al. Diagnosis of aneurysm of the thoracic aorta: Comparison between two noninvasive techniques—Two-dimensional echocardiography and computed tomography. Eur Heart J 5:545, 1984.
62. Amparo E, et al. Magnetic resonance imaging of aortic disease: Preliminary results. AJR Am J Roentgenol 143:1203, 1984.
63. Doroghazi RM, Slater EE, DeSanctis RW. Medical therapy for aortic dissections. J Cardiovasc Med 6:187, 1981.
64. Reul GJ, et al. Dissection aneurysm of the descending aorta: Improved surgical results in 91 patients. Arch Surg 110:632, 1975.
65. Gott VL, et al. Surgical treatment of aneurysms of the ascending aorta in the Marfan's syndrome. N Engl J Med 314:1070, 1986.
66. Greendyke RM. Traumatic rupture of the aorta: Special reference to automobile accidents. JAMA 195:527, 1966.
67. Parmely LF, et al. Nonpenetrating traumatic injury of the aorta. Circulation 17:1086, 1958.
68. Newman RJ, Rastoji S. Rupture of the thoracic aorta and its relationship to road traffic accident characteristics. Injury 15:296, 1984.
69. Stiles QR, et al. Management of injuries to the thoracic and abdominal aorta. Am J Surg 150:132, 1985.
70. Sefczek DM, Sefczek RJ, Deeb ZL. Radiographic signs of acute traumatic rupture of the thoracic aorta. AJR Am J Roentgenol 141:1259, 1983.
71. Mattox KL, et al. Clamp/repair: A safe technique for treatment of blunt injury to the descending thoracic aorta. Ann Thorac Surg 40:456, 1985.
72. Svensson LG, Antunes MDJ, Kinsley RH. Traumatic rupture of the thoracic aorta. S Afr Med J 67:853, 1985.

PART SEVEN

THE ENDOCRINE SYSTEM

56

Calcium and Phosphorus Metabolism and the Parathyroid Gland

Glenn W. Geelhoed

Tucked behind the thyroid gland or in close proximity to it are a group of endocrine structures (usually four in number) known as the *parathyroid glands.* Despite their small size, they play an extremely important role in the maintenance of normal calcium and phosphorus balance, both ions being critical components of a number of metabolic systems. The function of the parathyroid glands is vital to such crucial processes as neuromuscular excitability, membrane permeability, blood coagulation, and muscular contraction through maintenance of calcium homeostasis. When these glands fail to perform their normal activities, a state of hypocalcemia or hypercalcemia may ensue, resulting in a variety of potentially serious and possibly lethal pathophysiologic aberrations. This chapter reviews the intricate control systems in the body to maintain calcium and phosphorus balance and how this is effected through normal parathyroid function.

CALCIUM COMPARTMENTS

Calcium, a mineral required in structural support in bone, also functions in muscle action and membrane repolarization. Calcium is the body's principal divalent cation, with more than 1 kg of this element locked in storage form where it functions principally in structure. Approximately 1% of this total is available in extracellular fluids and in intracellular position in such tissues as muscle, where it is available for metabolic function. The small fraction of metabolically accessible total body calcium is critical in physiology, and this compartment is in dynamic equilibrium with the large reservoir of inactive calcium forms through interaction with one or more other cations, several anions, and multiple hormones. A competing divalent cation is magnesium; counterbalancing anions are chloride, phosphate, and bicarbonate; hormones principally involved in calcium metabolism include parathyroid hormone (parathormone, or PTH), parathormone-related peptide, calcitonin, and vitamin D and its metabolites. Through intricate interaction of these competing and regulating biochemical systems, a relative constancy is maintained in the active form of ionic calcium in circulation. The body senses and regulates a disturbance in this critical ionic calcium level through compensatory metabolic and endocrine reactions, with disease resulting when the limits of these compensatory mechanisms are exceeded and hypocalcemia or hypercalcemia results.

Intracellular Calcium Functions

Calcium is required in both the electrical and mechanical activation of cardiac muscle, vascular smooth muscle, and skeletal muscle. Muscle cell membranes are semipermeable to calcium by means of specific channels through which calcium flux occurs at different rates. The rate of calcium passage is voltage dependent or phosphorylation dependent. The voltage-dependent calcium channels are open to intracellular influx of calcium when the membrane is depolarized, and drugs called *calcium-channel blockers* may moderate arrhythmias by dampening this calcium current. β-Adrenergic receptor stimulation may trigger phosphorylation through cyclic adenosine monophosphate (cAMP) kinase. Through the voltage-dependent and phosphorylation-dependent gates, membrane excitation occurs.[1]

Electrical excitation (transmembrane calcium influx in muscle cells) is necessary but not sufficient for muscular contraction. The increase in intracellular calcium from the influx and from the calcium release by sarcoplasmic reticulum that it triggers causes binding to an intracellular regulatory protein. This protein is troponin in myocardial cells and calmodulin in vascular smooth muscle cells. The complex between calcium ion and the intracellular proteins causes tertiary structural changes in myosin, and contraction results from a force generation between myosin and actin.

Relaxation occurs with the efflux of calcium as troponin and calmodulin dissociate from the complex and calcium is bound again within the sarcoplasmic reticulum. The degree of muscle tension depends on intracellular calcium concentration, and the rate of these contractions depends on the rapidity of calcium fluxes in and out of the myofilaments (Fig. 56-1).

Thus, calcium and its transmembrane movement have a pivotal role in both excitation and contraction of cardiac, vascular, and skeletal muscle through these channels and under regulatory control of kinases sensitive to catecholamine. This role suggests the physiologic principles behind normal and stress metabolism, tetany, and susceptibility to hormones and drugs such as epinephrine and calcium-channel blocking agents. In contrast to this normal physiology, pathophysiology frequently is caused by an excess or deficit in the metabolically active calcium made available to the cells through the circulating plasma.

Extracellular Calcium Compartments

One half of the measurable plasma calcium is in the metabolically active ionized form. This active calcium compartment is in equilibrium with a protein-bound moiety and with a third fraction that is chelated. Homeostatic regulation involves the ionized half of the total serum calcium, and shifts from the numerator to denominator in this fraction are sensitive to a number of influences exerted in the plasma. The first of these factors is the quantity of serum albumin available to bind calcium. Because the bound calcium is not counted in the metabolic effects of the total plasma calcium, with a very low serum protein a patient can quite possibly have hypercalcemia and its metabolic consequences despite readings in the low-normal range by blood chemistry report. Under normal conditions of physiologic pH, 1 g/dl in serum albumin binds 0.8 mg/dl in total serum calcium.

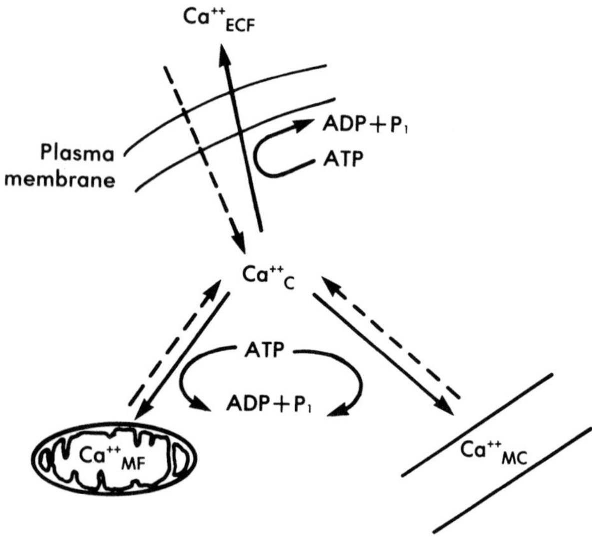

Fig. 56-1. Intracellular calcium *(Ca^{++}_{C})* comes from extracellular calcium *(Ca^{++}_{ECF})* through the plasma membrane by voltage-dependent and phosphorylation-dependent calcium channels. The Ca^{++}_{C} is complexed by protein (troponin in myocardium and calmodulin in vascular muscle), from which it can be taken up by myofilaments *(MF)* or sarcoplasmic reticulum *(MC);* each Ca^{++} transition involves adenosine triphosphate (ATP). *ADP,* Adenosine diphosphate; *Pi,* inorganic phosphate.

A second dynamic factor interactive with the first is the pH of the blood. Plasma protein is a principal component of the buffer capacity in the bloodstream, and acute changes in hydrogen ion concentration affect both protein binding and the chelation of calcium by the physical chemistry rules reflected in the Henderson-Hasselbach equation. Acidosis is buffered in blood proteins, which have less capacity for binding calcium when these binding sites competitively occupy hydrogen ions, displacing more of the calcium into the ionized fraction in plasma. A change in pH in the alkaline direction causes greater calcium binding to protein and a subsequent decrease in the ionized plasma calcium. A patient with borderline hypocalcemia may induce an acute decrease in ionized calcium by hyperventilation. The resulting alkalosis may be sufficient to reduce ionized calcium to the point of clinical manifestation by the patient in hypocalcemic tetany, even though the total plasma calcium remains the same.

Technique used in drawing blood for calcium determination and the methods used in assay are important in judging truly normal or abnormal values. A prolonged tourniquet application may cause hemoconcentration and elevate the total serum calcium; at the same time, a tourniquet inflated to arterial pressure may cause ischemia and consequent acidosis, which would shift blood calcium toward the measured ionized fraction. If blood is not drawn anaerobically (as into a vacuum container), carbon dioxide leaves, raising the pH. The same may happen with the "alkaline tide" after a meal or, as previously noted, with the patient's breathing pattern. Ionized calcium may be measured directly through the specialized use of an ion-selective electrode. This specialized measurement of the metabolically active calcium compartment is useful if the test is done correctly. However, ion-selective electrodes are sensitive to the multiple factors in blood that have calcium consequences (body temperatures, presence or absence of calcium-chelating anticoagulants, and loss of carbon dioxide at the blood-air interface with a consequent rise in pH). Most of the measurement errors tend to sum in the direction of underestimating the ionized calcium, which is a value protected at considerable metabolic expense even in critically ill patients.

PHOSPHORUS

Phosphate, the principal intracellular divalent anion, is abundant in metabolically active cells. In the adult human body, nearly 1 kg phosphate exists. It is so directly involved in energy-transfer processes that the phosphorus gate is taken as an indicator of metabolic activity in nuclear magnetic resonance. Phosphate compounds of adenosine (e.g., adenosine triphosphate) are the common currency in cellular energy exchanges.

The average daily adult dietary intake of calcium and phosphate approximates 1 g each, and active and passive transfer mechanisms sensitive to intimately interrelated endocrine control for each regulate absorption and secretion. Phosphate is generally abundant in metabolic systems. The principal control mechanisms are by renal excretion of phosphate excess. Typical serum concentrations measure 3.5 ± 1 mg/dl in adults, 1.5 mg/dl higher in children.[2] This serum phosphate is under constant surveillance by the renal tubule, because almost all of the plasma phosphate that passes into the glomerular filtrate is reabsorbed in the proximal tubule. Reabsorption of phosphate in the renal tubule is a process that requires energy; it is sensitive to many influences, including pH (and competitive bicarbonate concentration) and parathormone, which has a phosphaturic effect. Consequently, major changes in serum phosphate occur as a result of renal failure, and phosphate retention may be the principal driving force in disturbances in calcium level and parathormone secretion in the patient with renal insufficiency.

Hyperphosphatemia

Because active reabsorption in the proximal tubule is necessary for maintenance of the generally abundant serum phosphorus, hyperphosphatemia occurs from a decrease in renal filtration or stimulation of lower thresholds in its reabsorption. Vitamin D may increase both phosphate and calcium in the blood, and an acute deficit in parathormone may cause hyperphosphatemia and hypocalcemia. In the long run, metastatic calcification in soft tissues may be seen with chronic hyperphosphatemia, but the symptoms of hyperphosphatemia are usually related to the induced hypocalcemia. For that reason, phosphate is regulated by both a normal diet and control of blood calcium, to which it is inextricably related.

Hypophosphatemia

Hypophosphatemia may be present in critical illness and have consequences with impairment in the role that phosphate plays in energy transfer, membrane phospholipids, or oxyhemoglobin dissociation through its presence in 2,3-diphosphoglycerate. In the long run, hypophosphatemia may result in demineralization of bone, and this osteomalacia may lead to pathologic fractures.

Starvation may be a cause of hypophosphatemia, but a more specific cause in the critically ill patient is diabetic ketoacidosis.[3] The acidosis itself may induce shifts of calcium and phosphorus from storage depots, and the osmotic diuresis may result in a total body deficit of phosphate. Hypophosphatemia is also regularly encountered in management of the person with chronic alcoholism and malnutrition. In carbohydrate loading of the patient with chronic malnutrition, phosphate is shifted intracellularly, and both hypophosphatemia and hypomagnesemia can be seen in the person with alcoholism under treatment.[4] In severe illnesses superimposed on chronic malnutrition, parenteral administration of phosphate may be necessary, because intestinal absorption may be unreliable. A major manageable cause of hypophosphatemia is primary hyperparathyroidism. Therapy may be directed principally toward reducing the hypercalcemia, but a consequence of a reduction in parathormone is an elevation in the depressed serum phosphate.

PARATHORMONE

Parathormone (PTH) is the principal homeostatic regulator of calcium and phosphate at the sites of bone, kidney, and gut. In turn, the ionized fraction of blood calcium controls parathormone's secretion from the parathyroid gland. This biofeedback loop is rapid and sensitive, and it may be disordered in primary pathology of the parathyroid gland(s), kidney, bone, or gut.

The Molecule

PTH is a single-chain polypeptide of 84 amino acids in sequence and a molecular weight of 9500, with a 34–amino acid peptide comprising the N-terminal portion. This N-terminal fragment has biologic activity nearly the equal of intact parathormone, but a further reduction in the size of this peptide inactivates it. A prohormone somewhat larger than parathormone (115 amino acids) is synthesized and secreted by the parathyroid gland, but the principal storage form within the gland is the 84–amino acid polypeptide parathormone.[5] The hormone activates receptors in kidney and bone, but it is also subject to cleavage in the circulation, with components of that cleavage detectable in the circulation by radioimmunoassay (Fig. 56-2). Excretion or disposal of these fragments is not as rapid a process as the PTH cleavage, nor is the clearance rate the same for each portion. Both the intact PTH and the biologically active N-terminal have short serum half-lives, and each represents approximately 10% of the circulating PTH immunoreactivity. The remaining 80% of the circulating hormone detected by radioimmunoassay is the

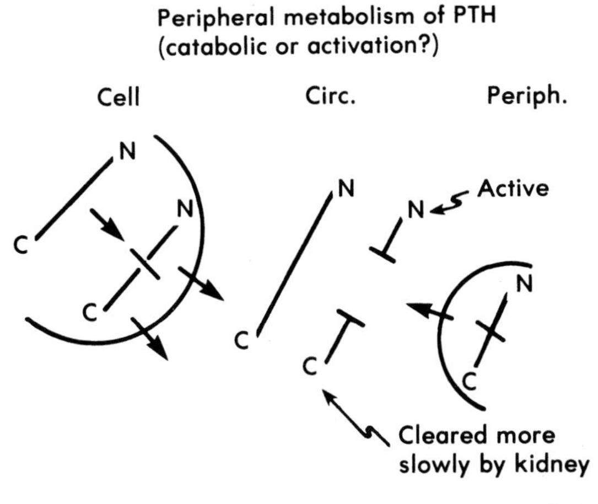

Fig. 56-2. Parathormone *(PTH)* is an 84–amino acid single-chain polypeptide existing in the circulation as PTH and as a biologically active 34–amino acid N-terminal portion with a short half-life, and an inert C-terminal residue with a long half-life is serum-dependent on renal excretion.

two thirds of the molecule represented by the C-terminal fragment, which has a long serum half-life and is principally excreted through the kidneys. In renal failure, the C-terminal fragments accumulate; however, for screening patients thought to have hyperparathyroidism, C-terminal assay may be superior to N-terminal assay because of the greater proportion of this species in the circulation and its longer circulating half-life. Radioimmunoassay for intact PTH is now widely available, including newer methods for rapid PTH assay that can be performed during operations.

Action of PTH

The parathyroid gland's role is especially critical in sensing and responding to hypocalemia. At each point in the circulation reached by PTH and its active N-terminal metabolite, the net result is an increase in blood calcium. The gut effect of PTH is to facilitate vitamin D in improving the efficiency of intestinal calcium absorption. PTH is the principal hormone in control of phosphate excretion at the kidney. If calcium absorption in the gut and phosphate excretion from the kidney are the principal parathormone actions for a net increase in calcium and decrease in circulating phosphate, the action of parathormone on bone is to release both calcium and phosphate from bone storage into circulation (Fig. 56-3). In each of the three sites of parathormone action, there is interaction with vitamin D with synergy in their combined activities.

Control of PTH Secretion

The parathyroid gland is principally sensitive to the circulating ionized calcium concentration. The parathyroid cells sense an increment or decrement in ionized calcium or

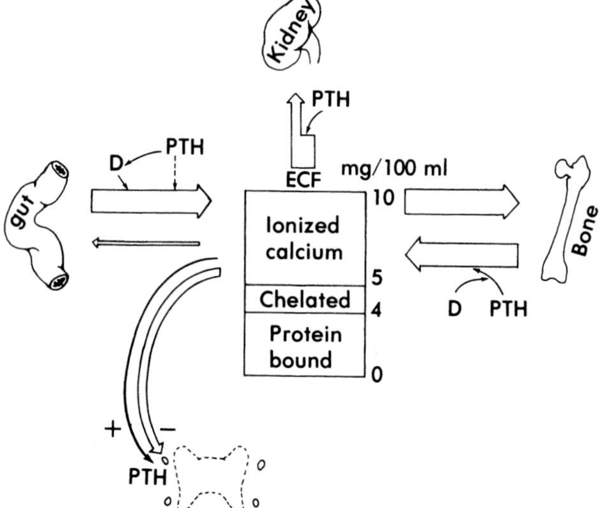

Fig. 56-3. Parathormone *(PTH)* and vitamin D *(D)* are interactive at gut, bone, and kidney for the synergistic result of an increase in blood calcium level. *ECF,* Extracellular fluid.

magnesium, but they are apparently insensitive to serum phosphate concentrations. Conversely, parathormone degradation is sensitive to high serum ionized calcium level and inhibited by hypocalcemia.[8]

Parathormone release may be sensitive to other hormones, the receptors of which (e.g., β-adrenergic and H_2-receptors) have been found in parathyroid glands. Catecholamines in stress levels increase PTH secretion by elevating cAMP activity.

Conversely, hypercalcemia inhibits PTH synthesis in the parathyroid gland and further inhibits response to PTH, at least at the renal receptors.[9] The total effect of hypocalcemia is to elevate parathormone synthesis, secretion, and activity, raising blood calcium. The net effect of an increase in blood calcium is to diminish synthesis, release, and activity of parathormone at its receptor sites. This balance of stimulation and inhibition is rapid and delicately attuned for stability in the ionized calcium homeostasis.

Parathormone-Related Peptide

A peptide[6] with homology very similar to the sequences of amino acids in the N-terminal fragment of PTH but three times greater in size (115 amino acids), is parathormone-related peptide. Early radioimmunoassays could not distinguish this peptide from PTH or its N- or C-terminal degradation products; thus, they were unable to distinguish true primary hyperthyroidism from pseudohyperparathyroidism, the latter characterized by elevations in parathormone-related peptide.[7] Although N-terminal fragments are so similar in amino acid homology that cross-reactivity occurred with antibody to both peptides, the newer intact PTH assay is based on two-site immunoradiometric assay (IRMA), recognizing both N-terminal and the midportion of the C-terminal. This intact PTH IRMA is therefore more specific for PTH and can differentiate true primary hyperparathyroidism because it does not react with parathormone-related peptide.

VITAMIN D

Vitamin D and its metabolites, especially vitamin D_3, are hormones in the body with high biologic activity in calcium metabolism. The precursor for the active hormone is calciferol, produced by skin exposed to ultraviolet irradiation or absorbed in the gut from foods or vitamin supplementation. The kidney is the principal endocrine organ to create an active hormone of these calciferol precursors. An important distinction from parathormone production is that synthesis does not depend on calcium or phosphate concentrations in the blood.

As seen in Fig. 56-3, the sites of vitamin D and its principal actions are primarily the gut and bone, as an adjunct to facilitate parathormone action. Because of its primary role in calcium absorption, vitamin D was first identified as a "vital amine," or vitamin, because its deficiency state results in hypocalcemia and demineralized bones or rickets. Vitamin D deficiency and the resultant hypocalemia and hypophosphatemia from absorption failure lead to secondary hyperparathyroidism. Because vitamin D plays only an ancillary role in mobilization of calcium from bones, the osteomalacia occurs even with deficient vitamin D activity at the site of bone resorption, and especially because of deficient vitamin D at the site of gut calcium absorption. In addition to the dietary deficit in the precursor or lack of sunlight exposure, failure of the specific secretory organ, the kidney, may[10] also produce deficiency in the active form of vitamin D. A hydroxylase found in the kidney is necessary for the activation of vitamin D, and a deficiency in this renal hydroxylase can produce renal osteodystrophy, or renal rickets.

Normal calcium and phosphate metabolism require normal function in kidney, gut, bone, and parathyroid gland. Ionized calcium within a rather restricted and protected range for membrane excitation, muscular contraction, and relaxation is the end result, which is also the biofeedback most specifically sensed by the parathyroid glands. A number of other hormones and substances are involved in some physiologic capacity, and others in pathologic imbalance in this homeostatic servosystem.

OTHER HORMONES

Calcitonin

When first discovered, calcitonin was named *thyrocalcitonin* from its origin in the parafollicular C cells of the thyroid. These cells are of neuroectodermal origin, and they are part of the amine precursor uptake and decarboxylation system, the capability of which is the common biochemical denominator. Any of the cells of this amine precursor uptake and decarboxylation origin can secrete calcitonin. This peptide has been isolated from several species; salmon calcitonin has been synthesized and, given in pharmacologic doses, is more active in humans than is human calcitonin in lowering blood calcium from pathologically elevated levels to normal. However, despite its original calcium-lowering effect and notwithstanding the therapeutic application of large quantities of the synthetic hormone, no direct inference can be drawn regarding calcitonin's physiologic role. No evidence to date demonstrates that calcitonin plays a physiologic role in calcium or phosphate metabolism. It may have physiologic functions quite apart from its demonstrated pharmacologic action on extracellular calcium in metabolic systems quite different from those initially investigated; additional evidence suggests that it may be a pulmonary hormone.[11]

On the basis of evidence seen in patients dying of widespread medullary thryoid cancer with very elevated serum calcitonin levels and normal calcium and phosphate metabolism, calcitonin's role in calcium and phosphate metabolism seems negligible or is unknown. A subtype of a hereditary syndrome called *multiple endocrine adenopathy (MEA)* III (or IIb) exists in which patients have early aggressive medullary thyroid cancer and correspondingly high blood calcitonin levels, but no abnormalities in the parathyroid glands and normal calcium and phosphate metabolism. The pharmacologic role of calcitonin may be through inhibition of bone resorption, an effect independent of parathormone.

Thyroxine

The iodinated thyronines, specifically thyroxine, may have a pathologic effect that leads to hypercalcemia, but they do not have an apparent role in the normal calcium and phosphate physiology. In hyperthyroidism, one of the results of the generally increased metabolism is a direct increase in bone resorption mediated by thyroxine.[12] Phosphate metabolism is generally affected in the hypermetabolism that follows excess thyroxine circulation. However, thyroid hormone has no clearly proven role in normal phosphate physiology.

Cortisol and Other Steroids

The adrenal and gonadal steroids influence mineral homeostasis and skeletal remodeling. Again, these putative roles are remarkable in pathologic conditions but are rarely clear in normal calcium homeostasis. Cortisol can block calcium resorption from bone, but in high-dose corticosteroid treatment, demineralization of bone is seen as a rule. Paradoxically, hypercalcemia may also occur in Addisonian crises, stemming from vitamin D effect on bone resorption unopposed by cortisol or decreased renal calcium clearance. Estrogen failure is widely known in association with osteoporosis, yet patients treated with estrogens, progesterone, or androgens (e.g., for therapy of metastatic breast cancer) may rapidly acquire hypercalcemia. Much controversy surrounds the primary or ancillary role of steroids of either adrenal or gonadal origin in the postmenopausal osteoporosis syndrome; however, except for pathologic deficits or therapeutic excesses of these hormones, the role of such steroids in normal calcium homeostasis is unknown.

Insulin and Catecholamines

As previously noted, diabetic ketoacidosis may result in total-body depletion of phosphate, even though serum phosphate is not affected until insulin therapy is begun. However, insulin administration with sugar causes a rapid shift of phosphate, potassium, and glucose into cells, and an immediate hypophosphatemia occurs. The hypoglycemia that follows insulin administration may also be a strong stimulus for catecholamine release. As previously noted, β-adrenergic receptors are found on parathyroid cells and may cause increased release of parathormone. However, catecholamines also affect the phophokinase systems, and phophorylation-dependent calcium channels may change in their sensitivity to unchanged levels of ionized calcium in serum.[13]

Malignancy-Associated Factors

Among patients found to have hypercalcemia, the single most common association is a malignant disease. Most of this malignancy-associated hypercalcemia is easily understood from osteolytic metastases and bone absorption.

However, some parathormone-like substances or other humoral agents have been postulated, and some have been identified in patients with cancers notorious for producing hypercalcemia.[14] Some of these factors have been characterized as activating osteoclasts, which may be the principal mechanism in the hypercalcemia of myeloma.[14] Prostaglandins are implicated, because prostaglandin blockade seems to inhibit the severity of hypercalcemia in some malignancies, and glucocorticoids may have a similar therapeutic effect through possibly related mechanisms. Some malignancies, particularly those of amine precursor uptake and decarboxylation origin, such as small-cell carcinoma of the lung, may produce multiple peptides; not all these peptides are characterized, but some may be parathormone-like in activity. In most patients with cancer who have severe hypercalcemia, the origin of the hypercalcemia is most often obvious by the extent of the skeletal metastases.

The evidence is scant that each of the other hormones described, aside from those principally active in calcium and phosphate metabolism, have a humoral effect on normal physiologic mineral homeostasis, at least with respect to ionized calcium. These other factors come into play in pathologic states to explain the extent of the deviation from normal calcium balance or because these agents or their congeners have been used with suggestive therapeutic response. The control of normal calcium physiology appears to reside in the interplay of parathormone and vitamin D and their responses through cAMP activation.

CLINICAL CONDITIONS OF DISORDERED CALCIUM METABOLISM

With respect to the critical constancy of ionized calcium in the blood, the fundamental disorders in calcium balance that disturb function are hypocalcemia and hypercalcemia. The buffer capacity of the compensatory systems is amazingly effective in protecting this infinitesimal fraction of the total body calcium pool, and these compensations blunt major shifts before disease is evident. When we see the clinical result, we are measuring the disease process including the failed best efforts of these compensatory mechanisms before the decompensation has occurred. The causes, consequences, and care of hypocalcemia are examined first.

Hypocalcemia

Hypocalcemia results from a failure of the effect of parathormone or vitamin D secretion or the sequestration of calcium in compartments not susceptible to mobilization by this humoral control. The compensatory response is increased parathormone and vitamin D synthesis and release, thus increasing calcium absorption from gut, liberation from bone, and resorption by the kidney. These compensatory mechanisms may be adequate to protect the serum ionized calcium for a time, and the disease is principally reflected in the target organs that have been affected in the compensatory stress. The clinical result is tetany if one of the critical components is missing, or if in time the reserves are exhausted and an actual decrease in ionized serum calcium occurs.

Causes of Hypocalcemia

Common causes of hypocalcemia are listed in Table 56-1. Deficiency in the action of vitamin D may be the result of dietary deprivation, lack of sunlight on exposed skin, or hereditary or acquired resistance to the hormone. The first and most direct deficit is that calcium absorption decreases and total blood calcium declines. Parathormone increase chiefly mediates immediate compensatory mechanisms. Parathormone excess decreases urinary calcium loss but does not considerably increase intestinal calcium absorption—the most important role of the action of vitamin D. Thus, ionized serum calcium may be protected by parathormone compensation; however, with mobilization from bone and continuing absorption deficit, the (even diminished) renal losses mean that total body calcium *bal-*

Table 56-1. Hypocalcemia

Cause	Mechanism	Compensatory Condition
Vitamin D deficiency	See Fig. 56-4	Compensatory PTH$\uparrow\uparrow$ with $Ca^{2+}\downarrow$ sparing at expense of $PO_4^{=}\downarrow\downarrow$
Hypoparathyroidism	Surgical absence of PTH or defect in PTH synthesis or release	$Ca^{2+}\downarrow$, $PO_4^{=}\uparrow$, PTH absent
Pseudohypoparathyroidism	End-organ failure of PTH *effect*	$Ca^{2+}\downarrow$, $PO_4^{=}\uparrow$, PTH$\uparrow$, but no urinary cAMP response to PTH administration
Hypomagnesemia	$\downarrow$Mg $\rightarrow$ PTH release and peripheral response	$Ca^{2+}\downarrow$ $PO_4^{=}\uparrow\downarrow$ PTH absent MG <1 mEq/L
Malabsorption	$\downarrow$Absorption vitamin D and Ca^{2+}	Same as *1*
Pancreatitis	Unknown	Ca chelation (saponification ?)
Hypoalbuminemia	Normal ionized Ca^{2+}	Hypoalbuminemia
vs	Total blood $Ca^{2+}\downarrow\downarrow$	vs
	vs	
Hyperventilation	Normal total blood Ca^{2+} but ionized $Ca^{2+}\downarrow\downarrow$	Alkalosis
Chelation	Calcium-binding	Citrate anticoagulants in blood transfusion

ance becomes negative. Further increases in parathormone may maintain the hypocalcemia in mild form at the expense of increasing phosphate loss through the kidney. Because both the calcium and phosphate are mobilized from bone, osteomalacia, pathologic fractures, and the deformities of rickets may eventually be apparent. Because calcium is protected, severe hypophosphatemia results. Late in rickets, as seen through the compartment shifts in Fig. 56-4, phosphate wasting may be the principal disorder in the presence of parathormone excess. The parathyroid gland still receives the hypocalcemic signal, and increased synthesis and release of parathyroid hormone may be able to maintain the diminished serum ionized calcium pool, but maintenance is accomplished at the considerable expense of further phosphate wasting.

Hypoparathyroidism. Lack of parathormone may stem from a failure in synthesis or release of the hormone, but most frequently it results from intentional surgical excision or incidental damage to the blood supply of the parathyroid glands. Because parathormone is deficient or absent, it cannot block renal excretion, stimulate bone resorption of calcium, or facilitate vitamin D in enhancing gut calcium absorption.

To make compensation effective, a high dose of vitamin D could be given, in the range of 100,000 U/day or more. When vitamin D is administered in extremely high therapeutic doses to the patient with hypoparathyroidism, calcium absorption from the gut is increased, but bone resorption is activated as well. This absorption may raise serum calcium, but parathormone is the principal agent of reclamation of calcium from urine, and in its absence, calciuria continues unopposed. In this form of compensated hypocalcemia, ionized serum calcium may thus be protected at the cost of a negative calcium balance.

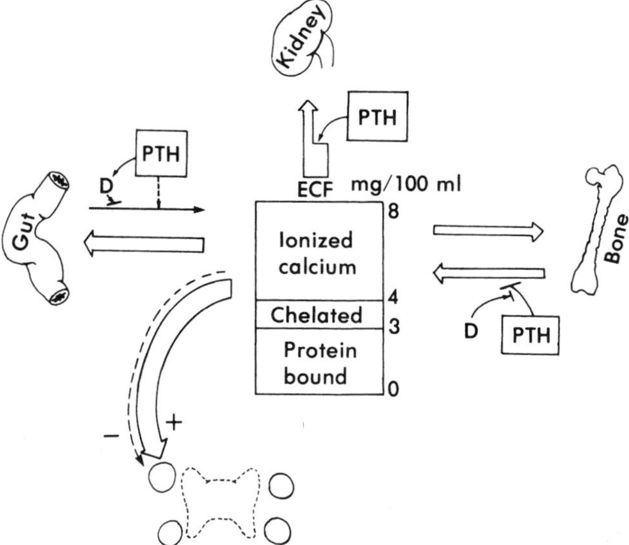

Fig. 56-4. In vitamin D *(D)* deficiency, parathormone *(PTH)* excess barely compensates for the hypocalcemia caused by loss of absorption from the gut, but this is accomplished by severe phosphate wasting through the kidney, which has been mobilized out of bone—hence the skeletal deformities of rickets. *ECF,* Extracellular fluid.

Hypoparathyroidism may be transient after cervical parathyroid exploration or thyroidectomy. However, the hypocalcemia stimulates the residual parathyroid tissue, and return to function is likely if some blood supply persists. Idiopathic hypoparathyroidism may exist as a component of a polyglandular failure thought to be based in an autoimmune process. It is rare and, like postoperative hypoparathyroidism, is treated with vitamin D in high doses. Improved treatment of the long-term aparathyroid state might be ideally managed by parathyroid transplantation, which has been carried out in patients already immunosuppressed for concomitant kidney transplantation. At present, administration of parathormone extracts from animal organs analogous to commercial insulin production is not practical, and the quantities of parathyroid hormone that have been synthesized are inconsequential for therapeutic use. So hypoparathyroidism is currently managed by a superabundant calcium diet and vitamin D in therapeutic doses, in anticipation of some return of endogenous parathyroid function.

An alternative to parathyroid transplantation for management at hypoparathyroidism might be the recently developed human parathormone synthesis through recombinant DNA technology. Human PTH could be delivered by nasal insufflation, repeated injections, or continuous infusion, or it could be released from some depot system. At present, insufficient clinical data exist to recommend this form of treatment for patients with hypoparathyroidism who are maintained on calcium supplementation and vitamin D therapy.

Pseudohypoparathyroidism. Neither parathyroid transplantation nor administration of parathormone extract benefits pseudohypoparathyroidism (see Table 56-1). This condition, usually familial, exhibits hypocalcemia with increased phosphorus but normal parathormone response to the hypocalcemia. In this case, the hypocalcemia is caused not by a failure of the parathyroid gland to respond by increasing its hormone secretion but by the failure of the end organ to respond to this appropriately increased parathormone. When exogenous parathyroid hormone is administered to such patients, the cAMP response is lacking. This disease is familial and associated with a characteristic phenotype. The treatment is similar to that for hypoparathyroidism after neck exploration, large doses of vitamin D to compensate for the lack of parathormone response at the end organ.

Hypomagnesemia. Hypomagnesemia blocks both peripheral response to parathormone at the end organ and release of parathormone from the parathyroid gland. A number of nephrotoxic drugs may result in magnesium urinary losses and hypomagnesemia. Restoration to normal of serum magnesium levels that were low because of drug toxicity or nutritional deficits, as can be seen in the person with chronic alcoholism, restores normal parathormone release and end-organ response. Paradoxically, hypermagnesemia may suppress parathormone release, a response similar to that seen with hypercalcemia.

Malabsorption. Some gastrointestinal tract disorders may result directly in deficient absorption of vitamin D and/or calcium. For example, in some instances, such as short-gut syndrome or extensive intestinal bypass, vitamin D may be given parenterally. If, however, the surface for calcium absorption is inadequate to be facilitated by vitamin D's action, calcium absorption may remain impaired, despite optimum vitamin D and parathormone activity. If vitamin D is absorbed and not activated, the result is a deficit in the active form of vitamin D because of intestinal, hepatic, or renal disease. With some drugs, such as diphenylhydantoin, vitamin D is not activated in the liver but is metabolized more quickly.

Pancreatitis. With soft tissue destruction and digestion, calcium may be trapped or taken out of solution in the retroperitineum and other sites. Hypocalcemia results, but not from fundamental failure in calcium homeostasis as much as from sequestration by mass action. Rapid saponification of calcium has been implicated in pancreatitis and also in some syndromes in which sepsis is prominent, such as septic abortion.

Hypoproteinemia. As we know, calcium exists in circulation bound and inactive for as much as 50% of the total plasma calcium level. Deficit of total plasma calcium must always be measured next to the albumin level, because if a severe hypoalbuminemia is present, the calculated ionized calcium may be normal. Only the metabolically active ionized calcium is counted in the judgment of true hypocalcemia. However, malabsorption, hypoalbuminemia, and liver failure may all combine in some patients who have real hypocalcemia from common proximate causes for the deficits in circulation of each of these complexed pairs.

Similarly, as discussed previously hypoventilation would not change total serum calcium but would result in hypocalcemia by a shift from the ionized active fraction to the protein-bound portion. In hypoalbuminemia, these mirror-image situations reflect an absolute decrease in serum calcium without a decrease in the ionized active fraction. In hyperventilation, they reflect identical readings in total serum calcium but a decrease in ionized calcium with the change in pH.

Chelation. Other circulating substances or administered drugs can complex calcium, and the complex that results may be bound with high affinity or may not be susceptible to the action of parathormone, vitamin D, or hydrogen ion in dissociation. Examples of such agents are anticoagulants, such as citrate, used to bind calcium in transfused blood. Some drugs, such as plicamycin, have as a major side effect a reduction in blood calcium. Consequently, their indication has been shifted to use in hypercalcemic crises.

From all these causes, the common result is a decrease in the biologically active ionized calcium compartment in blood. This decrease is ameliorated by compensatory mechanisms that dampen this effect. However, when hypocalcemia is seen, calcium-dependent functions begin to change, and clinical consequences occur.

Consequences of Hypocalcemia

The clinical consequences of hypocalcemia are increased excitability in cellular membranes of nerves and muscles, with tetany, spasms, and seizures. Clinical signs of this irritability are listed in Table 56-2.

Neural manifestations. Tetany, the principal feature of hypocalcemia, may be latent or evident in intractable seizures. Latent tetany may be demonstrated by inducing facial twitching or carpal spasm. Chvostek's sign is contraction of facial musculature induced by light tapping over the facial nerve, just ahead of the tragus. Trousseau's sign is carpal spasm produced by inflation of a blood pressure cuff above systolic pressure.

The initial symptoms the patient has are usually tingling paresthesias around the lips or in the fingertips. Later, these early neural symptoms can be uncovered in motor signs such as Chvostek's sign. However, more dangerous progression to laryngeal spasm or contraction of other smooth muscle because of hyperirritability may develop, and cardiac arrhythmia may result. Muscle cramps may proceed to carpopedal spasm. This is usually quite frightening to the patient. The anxiety that follows is compounded further by the hyperventilation exhibited in response to this bizarre behavior, which the patient may never have previously experienced. Seizures may ultimately result.

Table 56-2. Clinical Signs of Hypocalcemia

Neural	Muscle	General
Chvostek's sign	Tetany	Hypotension
Trousseau's sign	Cramps	Bradycardia
Seizures	Weakness	Cataracts
Irritability	Fatigue	Osteomalacia
Laryngeal spasm	Cardiac arrhythmia	Depression
Tingling paresthesias	Carpopedal spasms	Urinary frequency
Lightheadedness	Involuntary twitching	Anticoagulation

Control of clinical symptoms of hypocalcemia. Some immediate help in symptom control may come from having the patient rebreathe, or from slowing down the patient's anxiety response with sedation. Hydantoin drugs may relieve the annoying paresthesias and tingling prodrome the patient may have in latent tetany. However, the obvious solution to the symptoms of hypocalcemia is to immediately raise the serum calcium and address the underlying cause of the hypocalcemia. The immediate effect of increased ionized calcium in the blood can be achieved with administration of a calcium salt solution. Some available calcium compounds are complexed to molecules that require metabolism before the calcium is available to replenish the ionized calcium. For immediate treatment, one must be aware of the type of calcium compound and the dose of elemental calcium it contains.

Treatment of hypocalcemia. Calcium is an ion that comes readily out of solution in intravenous admixtures. Patients who are being resuscitated are often given sodium bicarbonate, which will precipitate any calcium salt administered through the same intravenous line. Moreover, calcium salts irritate the vein through which they are administered and should be diluted, but they are likewise a source of irritation to cardiac and other neuromuscular membrane surfaces. Large, rapid doses of calcium chloride contain a very high quantity of elemental calcium in readily available ionized form, so the dosage should be diminished and the rate slowed. Calcium gluceptate or gluconate can be prepared in 10% solution and slowly infused for 10 minutes, until tetany or paresthesias has stopped.

For longer-term treatment of hypocalcemia, treating symptoms rather than numbers is generally safer. If the patient requires continuing calcium support to prevent symptomatic hypocalcemia, oral treatment is initiated with a calcium wafer preparation. If a 4 g daily oral calcium supplementation does not result in freedom from symptoms, or if the hypocalcemia persists at levels at which symptoms are anticipated with a high degree of likelihood, a vitamin D analog is added. The fastest-acting vitamin D preparation is 1,25-dihydroxycholecalciferol (calcitriol) which may be administered as 0.5 μg in daily dosage. When the patient is receiving both vitamin D and calcium supplementation, monitoring the blood calcium is important, because hypercalcemia may develop insidiously. With a rise in the serum calcium level toward normal, the vitamin D analog is discontinued first; the patient can be tapered off the calcium supplementation while he or she remains symptom-free. Special consideration must be given patients with renal insufficiency or liver failure because of the enzyme systems required for activating the furnished vitamin D precursors.

For long-term treatment of hypoparathyroidism in patients requiring sustained calcium and vitamin D therapy, parathormone administration might be considered, but at present the quantities of parathormone congener are clinically approved only for diagnostic testing of the pseudohypoparathyroidism syndrome (see accompanying box). A possible alternative to freeing parathyroprival patients from dependence on calcium supplementation and vitamin D therapy is parathyroid transplantation. Parathyroid allografting[15] has been carried out in patients who have already been immunosuppressed and are recipients of renal allografts, having undergone previous total parathyroidectomy for secondary hyperparathyroidism. Such a parathyroid gland transplant can function, but an interesting speculation is that the renal allograft itself constitutes the transplantation of an endocrine gland with respect to activation of vitamin D precursors to the hormonally active vitamin D_3. As a consequence, the patients are more easily managed with calcium and vitamin D supplementation, and, as noted in the boxed material below, even patients with renal failure or anephric patients can benefit from some species of the vitamin D that does not require renal activation. Most patients with hypoparathyroidism either recover some parathyroid function or are more easily managed with the newer forms of vitamin D therapy, which carry fewer risks than parathyroid allografting. In some patients with hypoparathyroidism after reoperation with excision of pathologic parathyroid glands, parathyroid autotransplantation has been attempted.[16] However, the risk involved in grafting possibly autonomous pathologic

MANAGEMENT OF HYPOCALCEMIA

A. Determination of cause
   Measure Ca^{2+}, $PO_4^{=}$, albumin, Mg^{2+}, pH, PTH
B. For hypomagnesemia (<0.8 mEq/L serum) mg Cl_2 IV 1-2 mEq/kg/24 hr
C. For symptomatic latent tetany
   Diphenylhydantoin
D. Calcium supplementation
   1. IV
      10 ml 10% Ca gluconate in 50 ml D_5/W for 10 min
   2. PO
      1 g Ca gluconate wafers PO every 6 hr
E. Vitamin D
   1. Normal liver and kidneys
      1.2 mg ergocalciferol PO daily
   2. Liver disease
      50 μg calcifediol PO daily
   3. Renal disease
      0.5 μg calcitriol PO daily
F. Parathormone
   1. Synthetic PTH—only as test for pseudohypoparathyroidism syndrome
   2. Parathyroid grafting—only in patients already immunosuppressed with renal allograft

From Zaloga GP, Chernow B. Calcium metabolism. In Geelhoed GW, Chernow B, eds. Endocrine Aspects of Acute Illness, Clinics in Critical Care Medicine. New York: Churchill Livingstone, 1985.

IV, Intravenously; *D_5W,* 5% dextrose in water; *PO,* orally.

parathyroid is that hyperparathyroidism can recur, with the new source of the disease being the heterotopic site of the grafted gland. At present, treatment of persistent hypoparathyroidism is long-term support with calcium and vitamin D, which can successfully maintain serum calcium at a level at which the patient does not have hypocalcemic symptoms. In the future, some system of continuous repletion with recombinant DNA–derived human PTH is anticipated.

Hypercalcemia

In hypercalcemia, the body makes physiologic compensatory responses to lower ionized serum calcium by decreasing absorption, decreasing bone calcium resorption, and allowing unimpeded calciuresis. Hypercalcemia induces these changes by an inhibition of parathormone synthesis and release and a decrease in synthesis and activation of vitamin D. The dynamic pool of calcium in the blood expands either when absorption or resorption increases or when excretion decreases (when the capacity of these compensatory mechanisms to maintain a constant ionized serum calcium level is exceeded).

Hypercalcemia is found in a number of pathologic conditions and has many clinical consequences. It is a finding generated by multiphasic biochemical screening even of patients without symptoms. The finding of hypercalcemia always deserves investigation, because it is a principal harbinger of disease. Hypercalcemia also usually indicates a significant disease, for which further information should be gathered for diagnosis or prognosis. Hypercalcemia may be "an incidental finding," but rarely is it the only abnormal laboratory value, and it is of little clinical significance to the patient. Most causes of hypercalcemia are serious diseases; a significant few are caused by diseases treatable for cure. Cancer causes hypercalcemia in the single largest population of these patients, and often the cancer has spread beyond surgically curative treatment. However, the second most common cause of hypercalcemia, one that is increasing in frequency, is based in hyperparathyroidism, for which curative surgical treatment is a high probability.

Because of the significance of hypercalcemia as a finding, its determination must be made with precision, on repeated observations, with investigations of the interrelated ions and hormones. Attention to the details of blood-drawing technique reduces artifacts in repeated observations of hypercalcemia, proving it to be a true finding and compelling a differential diagnosis as to its cause.

Causes

Primary hyperparathyroidism. In many ways, the most satisfying differential diagnosis of hypercalcemia's causes may be primary hyperparathyroidism, because of its hopeful prognosis (Table 56-3). Currently, hyperparathyroidism accounts for nearly one third of the patients with hypercalcemia in large population surveys.

Since initial professional awareness of this diagnosis, the character of the population found to have hyperparathyroidism has changed. The initial patients had symptoms and advanced disease. In current practice, patients are rarely seen with end-stage target-organ consequences such as brown tumors, pathologic fractures, staghorn calculi with renal destruction, and metastatic calcification in soft tissue. The presentation of primary hyperparathyroidism today is much more subtle. As a rule, today's index case is a symptom-free patient discovered through the exercise of differential diagnosis on the finding of hypercalcemia. Hypercalcemia resulting from primary hyperparathyroidism

Table 56-3. Hypercalcemia

Cause	Mechanism	Features
Benign		
Primary hyperparathyroidism	See Fig. 56-5	PTH↑↑, Ca^{2+}↑, PO_4↓, Cl^-↑
Vitamin D toxicity	↑ Ca absorption ↑ Ca bone resorption	Ca^{2+}↑ , $PO_4^=$↑↓, PTH O
Sarcoidosis	Vitamin D hypersensitivity	Ca^{2+}↑, $PO_4^=$↑↓, PTH O, chest radiograph
Thyrotoxicosis	Hypermetabolic bone breakdown	Ca^{2+}↑, $PO_4^=$↑↓, PTH O, T_3↑, T_4↑
Drug (e.g., thiazides)	Renal tubular Ca^{2+} resorption, hemoconcentration	Ca^{2+}↑, K^+↓, PTH O
High bone turnover (e.g., immobilization, Paget's disease)	Outward flux of bone Ca stores	Ca^{2+}↑ $PO_4^=$↑, PTH O
Familial (e.g., FHH)	Increased renal sensitivity to PTH	Ca^{2+}↑, PTH N1 ↓urine Ca^{2+}
Doubtful (e.g., milk-alkali syndrome)	Increased availability of Ca^{2+} for absorption	Ca^{2+}↑ PO_4↑↓, pH↑, PTH↓↓, urinary $CO_3^=$
Malignant		
Metastatic cancer (e.g., breast, prostate)	Osteolytic release of Ca^{2+}, $PO_4^=$	Ca^{2+}↑, $PO_4^=$↑, alkaline phosphatase↑, PTH↓
Parendocrine (PTH-like or OAF)	APUD cells or nonendocrine tumors, multiple myeloma	Ca^{2+}↑, PO_4↑↓, direct assay of osteoclast activity

APUD, Amine precursor uptake and decarboxylation; *N1,* N-terminal parathormone; *OAF,* osteoclast-activating factor; T_3, tri-iodothyronine; T_4, thyroxine.

is most often mild, prolonged, and asymptomatic, with subtle findings even in retrospect. Parathyroid poisoning is a notable exception to this rule.

Autonomous parathyroid tissue (often an adenoma) secretes parathormone in an excess that the hypercalcemia does not inhibit. This hyperparathyroidism increases calcium absorption from the gut, resorption from the bone, and reclamation of urinary calcium (Fig. 56-5).

The incidence of primary hyperparathyroidism is higher among female than among male patients and varies with the age, increasing in frequency in both genders with advancing age[17] (Table 56-4). The most dramatic prevalance of primary hyperparathyroidism occurs among elderly women,[18] and its discovery and treatment in this group is often gratifying. In all age groups, primary hyperparathyroidism as a cause of hypercalcemia is among the leading endocrinologic reasons a patient undergoes operations.[19]

Hyperparathyroidism is classified as primary, secondary, or tertiary, depending on whether the hypersecretion of parathormone is primary or appropriately reactive to some other stimulus. However, primary hyperparathyroidism is the principal concern in the differential causes of hypercalcemia, and it is the most frequent type of hyperparathyroidism seen in the human populations submitted to health screening tests.

The clinical manifestations of primary hyperparathyroidism range from no symptoms, without evidence of disease apart from the biochemical findings, which is most frequently seen, to an acute life-threatening crisis, fortunately rare, called *parathyroid poisoning.*[20] Patients may progress through the clinical scale from those who are free of symptoms to those who have hyperparathyroid complications.[21] However, it is not proved that treatment of patients free of symptoms with isolated biochemical findings of primary hyperparathyroidism influences longevity in the absence of the development of hyperparathyroid complications. Longitudinal studies have been undertaken to follow the natural history of the untreated disease with intervention occurring immediately on disease complication or progression, defined by a rise in serum calcium above some arbitrary, prospectively set level. This "bail out" is built into protocols for the study of primary hyperparathyroidism's natural history because of the increased incidence of complications seen in patients with higher calcium values. Also, an approximately linear correlation exists between the mass of autonomous parathyroid tissue and the degree of symptoms, rate of complication, and absolute increment in the serum calcium level.

Although diagnosing primary hyperparathyroidism as a cause of hypercalcemia is a valuable contribution to the patient's care, this is not the only, or even the leading, cause (see Table 56-3). It must be differentiated from the other diagnoses that also cause hypercalcemia.

Vitamin D toxicity. Excessive vitamin D activity is an easily treatable cause of hypercalcemia. If excessive exogenous vitamin D is given, calcium resorption from bone increases, and intestinal absorption of calcium increases greatly. The fundamental mechanisms of hypercalcemia from vitamin D toxicity are the reverse of the pathophysiology of hypocalcemia caused by vitamin D deficiency. Reading Fig. 56-5 in reverse illustrates this mechanism. Though calcium is elevated, phosphate may be unchanged, and parathormone is near zero. These features distinguish this cause from primary hyperparathyroidism, in which phosphate is depressed and parathormone reading is high.

Drug manufacturers of vitamin supplements now restrict the supply of vitamin D in multivitamin tablets to prevent the toxicity of overfeeding vitamin D. Factitious hypervitaminosis D may still occur if patients take excessive vitamin pills without regard to the package labeling restrictions. This was a particular risk with flavored children's vitamin supplements; and the higher serum calcium levels generally seen in children with high bone turnover,

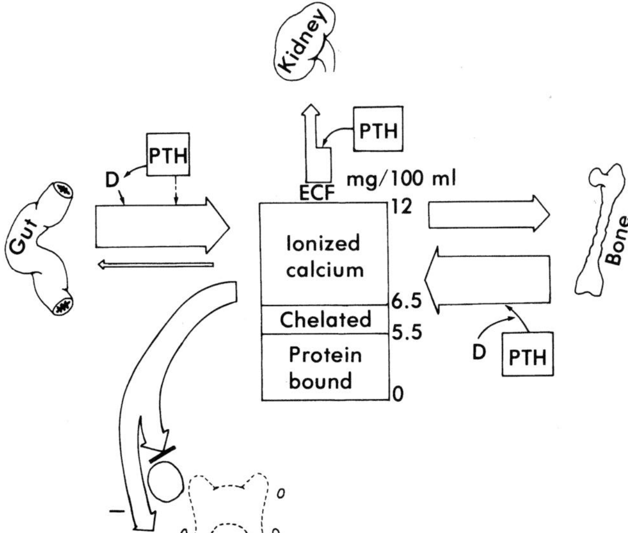

Fig. 56-5. In primary hyperparathyroidism, autonomous parathyroid tissue (in this case, a parathyroid adenoma) secretes parathormone *(PTH)* in excess, with increased calcium absorption from gut, resorption from bone, and urinary calcium reclamation, leading to hypercalcemia. *D,* Vitamin D; *ECF,* extracellular fluid.

Table 56-4. Incidence of Hyperparathyroidism

Age (yr)	Men	Women
<39	4.5/100,000	8/100,000
40-59	26/100,000	1/1000
>60	1/1000	2/1000

From Heath HS, Hodgson SF, Kennedy MA. Primary hyperparathyroidism: Incidence, morbidity and potential economic impact in a community. N Engl J Med 302:189, 1980.

remodeling, and growth complicated the differential diagnosis.

Sarcoidosis. Sarcoidosis can cause hypercalcemia because the sarcoidosis granulomas are involved directly in accelerating vitamin D activation. As in vitamin D toxicity, serum phosphate levels are variably affected, and parathormone values should reflect the hypercalcemic inhibition of parathormone, with assays showing near zero circulating parathormone. Chest x-ray film study may further substantiate the sarcoidosis diagnosis. Corticosteriods frequently are used in the management of this form of hypercalcemia on the basis of counteracting the accelerated vitamin D activation.

Thyrotoxicosis. Hyperthyroidism may accelerate bone breakdown and thereby cause hypercalcemia. As seen in vitamin D intoxication, parathormone levels reflect parathyroid suppression, an appropriate response to the hypercalcemia. Other features of hyperthyroidism should give clinical indication for measuring tri-iodothyronine and thyroxine to detect their elevation. Antithyroid drugs that slow down the hypermetabolism of thyrotoxicosis by blocking synthesis or release of thyroid hormones effect a gradual return toward normal calcium values.

Thiazides and other drugs. Thiazide diuretics act principally on renal tubular function and at this site enhance calcium reclamation from urine. To the extent that they accomplish an effective diuresis, an elevated serum calcium level may reflect hemoconcentration, in much the same way as inappropriate tourniquet technique elevates serum calcium reading. Potassium and phosphate are often depressed; they are therefore often supplemented in the patient taking diuretics to maintain normal plasma values. The appropriate response of the parathyroid glands to hypercalcemia is depressed parathormone.

Active bone turnover. Some patients may exhibit hypercalcemia during periods of high bone turnover activity; for example, children, whose blood normally contains higher calcium levels; previously active adults who are abruptly immobilized, such as might occur with an accidental spinal cord injury and paralysis; or older patients with Paget's disease. Both calcium and phosphate may be elevated, and parathormone is low.

Familial hypocalciuric hypercalcemia (FHH). A familial syndrome that has tricked surgeons into operating on patients with hypercalcemia despite normal or variable parathormone is characterized by low urinary calcium excretion and serum calcium retention through apparent increased renal sensitivity to parathormone. FHH[22] can be distinguished from primary hyperparathyroidism, which may also have a familial occurrence, by specialized studies of urine calcium clearance and a careful examination of the relationship of parathormone and simultaneous ionized serum calcium. These studies are often occasioned by reoperation in a patient or family member with no findings in the parathyroid gland that would explain the hypercalcemia, and with postoperative results that indicate a surgical procedure has failed to control hypercalcemia. In this population of patients, urinary calcium clearance studies should exclude FHH before a reoperation, particularly if a family history of hypercalcemia exists.

Milk-alkali syndrome. Patients with peptic disease may be taking large volumes of calcium salts and acid neutralizers. Hypercalcemia may result, probably less from the increased calcium made available for intestinal absorption than from acid/base imbalance, because vitamin D_3 suppression should increase the fecal calcium loss in the presence of the resulting hypercalcemia. However, the ingestion of alkali changes acid/base balance at the kidney, the ultimate regulator of acid/base balance, and urinary bicarbonate secretion may be decreased. Under most circumstances of dietary calcium intake, the finely tuned vitamin D parathormone regulators are able to adjust absorption and excretion to maintain a constant ionized serum calcium, and this alleged syndrome is a doubtful exception to this rule. The caution the surgeon should apply before presuming this diagnosis in someone with peptic ulcer disease is that hyperparathyroidism may coexist with peptic ulcer disease, particularly in familial syndromes. Even with this caveat, some investigators question whether the milk-alkali syndrome exists at all,[23] and the putative mechanisms of milk-alkali intake should not dissuade the clinician from further differential diagnosis of hypercalcemia.

Metastatic cancer. Unfortunately, the group that constitutes the largest number of patients differentiated from those with hypercalcemia are patients who first come to medical attention with cancer that is metastatic, usually to bone. Five principal primary tumors in sites other than bone have a proclivity toward osseous metastases: breast cancer, lung cancer, prostate cancer, thyroid cancer, and hypernephroma. Because of its high prevalence in Western populations, breast cancer leads the list of tumors responsible for hypercalcemia. In the osteolytic action of metastatic cancer, calcium and phosphorus are both released; the heavy load of these metabolites in the catabolic patient may overwhelm the renal clearance capacity. In some cancers, the hypercalcemia seems out of proportion to the evident bone destruction, and for these tumors additional humoral factors are postulated and, in some cases, have been proved. Alkaline phosphatase may rise in parallel with the hypercalcemia; in the case of prostate cancer, acid phosphatase may be elevated. These metabolic consequences are usually accompanied by skeletal pain, often at the specific site where the disease is most active.

Paraendocrine tumors. It would be not surprising if metastatic parathyroid carcinoma produced hypercalcemia, because presumably this parathormone excess would have mechanisms identical to the primary hyperparathyroidism seen with benign hyperfunctioning parathyroid tissue. However, primary malignancies in nonparathyroid tissues may also give rise to parathyroid-like hormones or their effects. Epithelial carcinomas arising from multiple organs with parathormone-like activity have been recorded. In addition, other paraendocrine products may also contribute to the hypercalcemia of special groups of cancers.

Hematologic malignancies with proliferation in bone marrow are known for hypercalcemia. In particular, multiple myeloma has been well recognized for hypercalcemia production, not only on the basis of its intraosseous location, but also from its production of a paraendocrine substance identified as osteoclast-activating factor. Multiple peptides and prostaglandins have also been implicated in the paraendocrine consequences of these nonendocrine tumors; among the consequences associated with release of these humoral factors is hypercalcemia. Parathormone of ectopic origin in malignant cells may occasionally cross-react with some antibodies used in radioimmunoassay of parathyroid hormone. However, parathormone of parathyroid gland origin has a much greater and more immediate response by cAMP measured in urine than does ectopic parathormone. This response may be useful in distinguishing those infrequent cases in which other clinical data do not make this difference apparent.

Consequences of Hypercalcemia

The signs and symptoms of hypercalcemia are protean, may range from subtle to lethal, and are not often associated with the specific cause that gave rise to the hypercalcemia. The absolute elevation in serum calcium level is important, but the rate at which the hypercalcemia has progressed is nearly as important. Acute hypercalcemia from calcium infusion in a healthy patient with an abrupt rise in total serum calcium of several milligrams per deciliter may be lethal; the same patient might accommodate a gradual elevation in serum calcium of twice the same increment during a year and not show any disability. Because of this insidious progression, the hypercalcemia of primary hyperparathyroidism is more often clinically silent than is the rapidly progressive hypercalcemia of metastatic malignancy, which is often a principal cause of death.

Clinical presentation. Clinical discrimination of patients' complaints has passed well beyond the "stones, bones, and abdominal groans" of the mnemonic first used to describe the features of hypercalcemia. Much more subtlety is now demanded of the astute clinician, who often sensitively screens new patients by retrospective questioning after they have been treated for hyperparathyroidism. Often, patients recall symptoms after they have subsided in response to successful reduction of serum calcium level; the patients may not even recognize the symptoms as present before operation, because insidious progression led them to accept these minor aberrations as accompaniments of advancing age or to attribute them to other known illness. Patients may express some or none of the principal features listed in the accompanying box, or they may have symptoms not listed, and the only direct evidence that they are part of the hypercalcemia complex is their improvement with treatment or recurrence with the return of hypercalcemia. Few of these listed symptoms fulfill Koch's postulates as invariably associated with the disease. The one invariable finding, an elevation in ionized serum calcium level, is not a clinical symptom.

Of the symptoms and signs in the accompanying box at left, many are of degree, rather than qualitative presence or absence. For example, specific responses regarding mentation in the "review of systems" include a report by one middle-aged man that he could no longer complete the book of crossword puzzles that he had started successfully some time before. A patient in a nursing home had incontinence that was attributed to senility until it was cured after treatment for hyperparathyroidism. Arthritis frequently turns out to be myalgia or bone pain on closer questioning. Headache is a prime presenting sign of hypercalcemia, and a screening blood chemistry analysis has a much higher yield than computed tomographic (CT) scanning of such patients, and is far more cost effective in its application.

Testing patients with hypercalcemia. A simple screen of the patient found to have confirmed hypercalcemia (Fig. 56-6) is based on the chloride/phosphate ratio that is suggestive, but not diagnostic, of hyperparathyroidism if greater than 33. With some degree of confidence, one can diagnose primary hyperparathyroidism

CLINICAL CONSEQUENCES OF HYPERCALCEMIA

Eye, Ear, Nose, Throat

Band keratopathy
Cataracts
Conjunctivitis
Change in vision
Change in ocular prescription

Gastrointestinal

Weight loss
Polydipsia
Weakness
Pancreatitis
Peptic ulcer
Calcific stippling
Anorexia
Thirst
Malaise
Nausea/vomiting
Abdominal pain
Constipation

Genitourinary

Urinary calculi
Polyuria
Uremia
Ureteral colic
Nocturia
Hematuria

Musculoskeletal

Osteoporosis
Resorption of clavicle ends
Decreased reflexes
Decreased tone
Backache
Bone pain
Ataxia
Myalgia

Cardiovascular

ECG changes
Hypertension

Central Nervous System

Confusion
Incontinence
Disorientation
Lethargy
Coma
Headache
Memory loss ("can't do crossword puzzles")
Depression
Hearing loss
Stupor

Skin

Pruritus

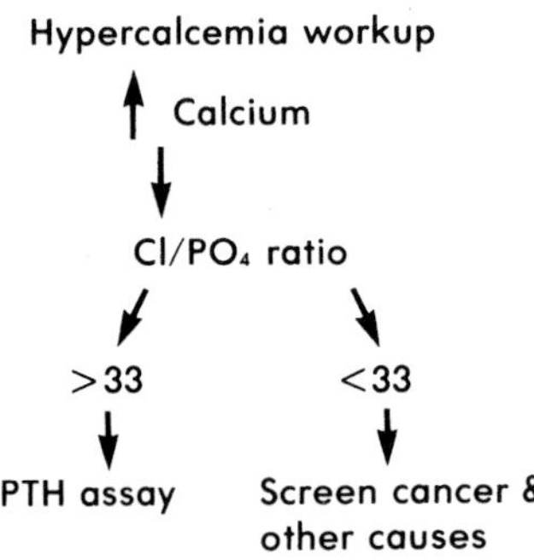

Fig. 56-6. A simple screen of the patient with hypercalcemia makes use of the ratio of chloride to phosphate for an initial approximation of whether hyperparathyroidism or oncogenic hypercalcemia is likely. *PTH,* Parathormone.

Disease	Blood			Urine		
	Ca	P_1	$^{125}(OH)D$	NcAMP	^FCa_E	TRP/GFR
1° HPTH	↑	↓	↑	↑	↑↔	↓
Malignancy	↑	↑↔	↓↔	↑	↑↑	↓
Osteolytic metastases	↑	↔	↓↔	↓	↑↑	↔

Fig. 56-7. Further differentiation in blood and urine tests can be carried out deliberately for a reliable diagnosis before confident recommendations for treatment, particularly in the patient without symptoms. *1° HPTH,* Primary hyperparathyroidism; *Ca,* calcium; P_i, inorganic phosphate; $^{125}(OH)D$, 125 hydroxy vitamin D; *NcAMP,* N-cyclic adenosine monophosphate; ^FCa_E, ionized calcium; *TRP/GFR,* tubular reabsorption of phosphate/ glomerular filtration rate.

without a parathormone assay if the chloride to phosphate ratio is greater than 33, with a distinctly elevated calcium level and a serum albumin level that also allows a calculated ionized calcium value estimated to be elevated. Parathormone assays have improved considerably with the further speciation of antibodies recognizing different portions of the intact molecule of parathormone or different fragments in the circulation. Consequently, surgeons with some knowledge of the type of assay available can have confidence in the parathormone assay if it confirms the biochemical impression obtained from the quicker analysis of calcium, phosphate, chloride, and albumin. If the chloride/phosphate ratio is less than 33, further work is typically needed to differentiate among the causes seen in Table 56-4.

Further differentiating tests on blood and urine are exhibited in Fig. 56-7. In most instances, the diagnosis of primary hyperparathyroidism can be made with all the leisure required to approach clinical certainty. If applied, the treatment of this disorder is elective and is not described until tests have eliminated any lingering doubt about the correct diagnosis. Cervical operation has no role in the *diagnosis* of primary hyperparathyroidism. Some urgency may be associated with diagnosis and management of certain malignant disorders that can lead to hypercalcemia, particularly if compromise in organ function is a risk. A rare indication for a truncated laboratory workup and accelerated treatment plan is hypercalcemic crisis because of acute hyperparathyroidism. Treatment should immediately be directed toward reducing the serum calcium level. A biochemical pattern that suggests primary hyperparathyroidism and hand x-ray films that show subperiosteal resorption along the radial aspect of the phalanges in the patient who is in a dangerously hypercalcemic state constitute sufficient diagnostic information to indicate urgent parathyroidectomy.[24] This presentation is rare, however, and all other hypercalcemic cases, particularly the patients without symptoms, deserve deliberate workup with a high reliability assigned to the final diagnosis.

Most patients will have had at least the primary laboratory evaluation outlined in the box on p. 1101. The serum calcium determination is the most important, because a second, later confirmation of hypercalcemia with the patient not receiving medication and under circumstances of normal diet and activity patterns is required. For practical purposes, the ionized calcium, which is strictly controlled within the body, can be calculated under conditions of known pH by the simultaneous measurement of protein in the blood. The calculated ionized calcium value is typically higher than the ionized calcium levels measured by an ion-sensitive electrode, but the number of patients with low calculated ionized calcium is fewer than the number of the patients found to have absolute decrease in total serum calcium. Under normal circumstances, the calculated ionized calcium value is sufficient; in the dynamic state of critical illness, an ionized serum calcium might be measured directly by a selective electrode. The phosphate determination, already used in the screening test of chloride/phosphate ratio, is typically depressed in the patient with hyperparathyroidism and may be elevated in patients with renal failure or metastatic cancer. Parathyroid hormone excess causes a lowered serum phosphate level through a decrease in renal tubular resorption of phosphate (TRP). This urinary test can be used to confirm directly the hyperparathyroidism. The TRP is the ratio, expressed in percentage, of urinary phosphate times serum creatinine/urinary creatinine times serum phosphate. Of patients with hyperparathyroidism on a normal diet and without renal failure, 81% have a TRP less than 78%.[24]

Although the N-terminal fragment of parathormone is biologically active, its half-life in serum is short. Consequently, the C-terminal parathormone assay is more helpful in testing patients for hyperparathyroidism. However, the clearance of C-terminal parathyroid fragments is through the kidney, and in renal failure, an elevation in circulating parathormone is measured on the basis of this excretion failure, with or without an increase in secretion. Highly specialized radioimmunoassay antibodies against other components of parathormone or parathyroid-like

LABORATORY EVALUATION OF CALCIUM AND PHOSPHATE DISORDERS

Primary	Ancillary
Serum calcium (ionized calcium)	Alkaline phosphatase
Phosphate	Magnesium
Chloride	Cr
Albumin	BUN
Parathormone	Uric acid
$1,25(OH)_2$ Vitamin D	pH
	HCO_3^-

Urine	X-Ray Films
Stone analysis	Hands
Calcium	Skull
TRP	Chest
cAMP	

BUN, Blood urea nitrogen.

hormones have been developed to detect the atypical hyperparathyroidism from ectopic sources in the paraendocrine malignancies.[25] The most useful PTH assay available today is the two-site IRMA for intact PTH.[26]

The repeated measurements of elevated serum calcium, depressed phosphate, and elevated serum parathormone levels may be the only laboratory diagnostic tests required after the screening studies mentioned in the discussion of the patient with classic primary hyperparathyroidism. Thereafter, further ancillary studies are necessary to differentiate patients with other causes for their hypercalcemia, or to make the difficult diagnosis of primary hyperparathyroidism in the early appearance of the syndrome or in the patient with only marginally elevated hypercalcemia. Many ancillary studies focus on establishing normal laboratory values, such as magnesium and creatinine, before looking further to see whether an abnormality in the patient's bones or kidneys accounts for the hypercalcemia. Alkaline phosphatase levels may be elevated in metastatic malignancy and slightly elevated in hyperparathyoidism. Uric acid level is mildly elevated in most patients with primary hyperparathyroidism. The elevation may also be a function of impaired renal clearance of uric acid and can be checked against the creatinine and blood urea nitrogen.

One of the helpful urine tests is a stone analysis for patients who have passed renal calculi. Calcium calculi are more suggestive of primary hyperparathyroidism than are urate stones. Urinary calcium assay is helpful, because a quantitative hypercalciuria suggests primary hyperparathyroidism and helps to distinguish this diagnosis from FHH.[22] Urinary cAMP level is a sensitive test of a rapid change in the urine, reflecting the presence or excess of parathormone. More than 90% of patients with primary hyperparathyroidism have elevated levels of nephrogenous cAMP, and mild renal failure does not dampen the measurement of cAMP in the urine. Because cAMP in the urine is a sensitive and rapid indicator of the presence of parathormone, the urinary measurement of cAMP can confirm the ablation of excess parathyroid activity and serve as a useful indicator during operation that the offending pathologic tissue has been resected.

Radiographic examinations may be helpful in some instances, but not for most patients who have asymptomatic hypercalcemia. The rare patient who has had long-standing hyperparathyroidism and may have symptoms or even toxicemia may have radiographically identifiable bone lesions (Fig. 56-8). Bone cysts and subperiosteal resorption of bone in phalanges or distal clavicles (see Fig. 56-8, *C*) or diffuse "ground-glass" demineralization of the skull (see Fig. 56-8, *B*) may still be seen in patients with hypercalcemia. However, brown tumors of von Recklinghausen's disease are rare enough to be of historic significance, except in cases of neglected hyperparathyroidism. Fig. 56-8, *A* shows long bone cystic changes in a patient with such a long and neglected course of primary hyperparathyroidism, but a more useful study may be the chest x-ray film, routinely performed in patients admitted to the hospital for evaluation or treatment of hypercalcemia. The chest x-ray film can exclude either primary lung cancer or metastatic cancer as one possible cause of the hypercalcemia, but a nearly pathognomonic sign in hyperparathyroidism may be noted in absorption of the distal clavicles, "Higginbotham's sign" (see Fig. 56-8, *C*). Occasionally, nuclear medicine scans are used to determine bone density as an estimate of demineralization occurring in hyperparathyroidism and other disorders, such as osteoporosis. An improved test of demineralization is dual-photon absorptiometry. The preoperative appearance of demineralization on such scans is often associated with a postoperative problem of remineralization termed the *hungry bone syndrome.* As postoperative hypoparathyroidism and a return to normal calcium dynamics occur, the heavy shift of calcium back into the bones from which it was mobilized during the hyperparathyroidism may cause changes in blood phosphate, magnesium, and calcium as these minerals return to the bone sink from which they had been released. A late postoperative bone density scan reveals the restoration of this mineral density in successfully treated hyperparathyroidism. A number of other radiographic tests have been used in hyperparathyroidism for localization of the source of the excess parathyroid hormone; these are considered in the section on parathyroid localization studies.

Treatment of hypercalcemia. Asymptomatic hypercalcemia requires no urgent treatment if indicated solely by the determination of elevated numbers of laboratory tests. In fact, if severely elevated calcium levels are reported in a patient without symptoms, one should first suspect the numbers to represent laboratory error and repeat the tests, along with determination of the ancillary studies listed in the accompanying box. Treatment attempts to prevent the

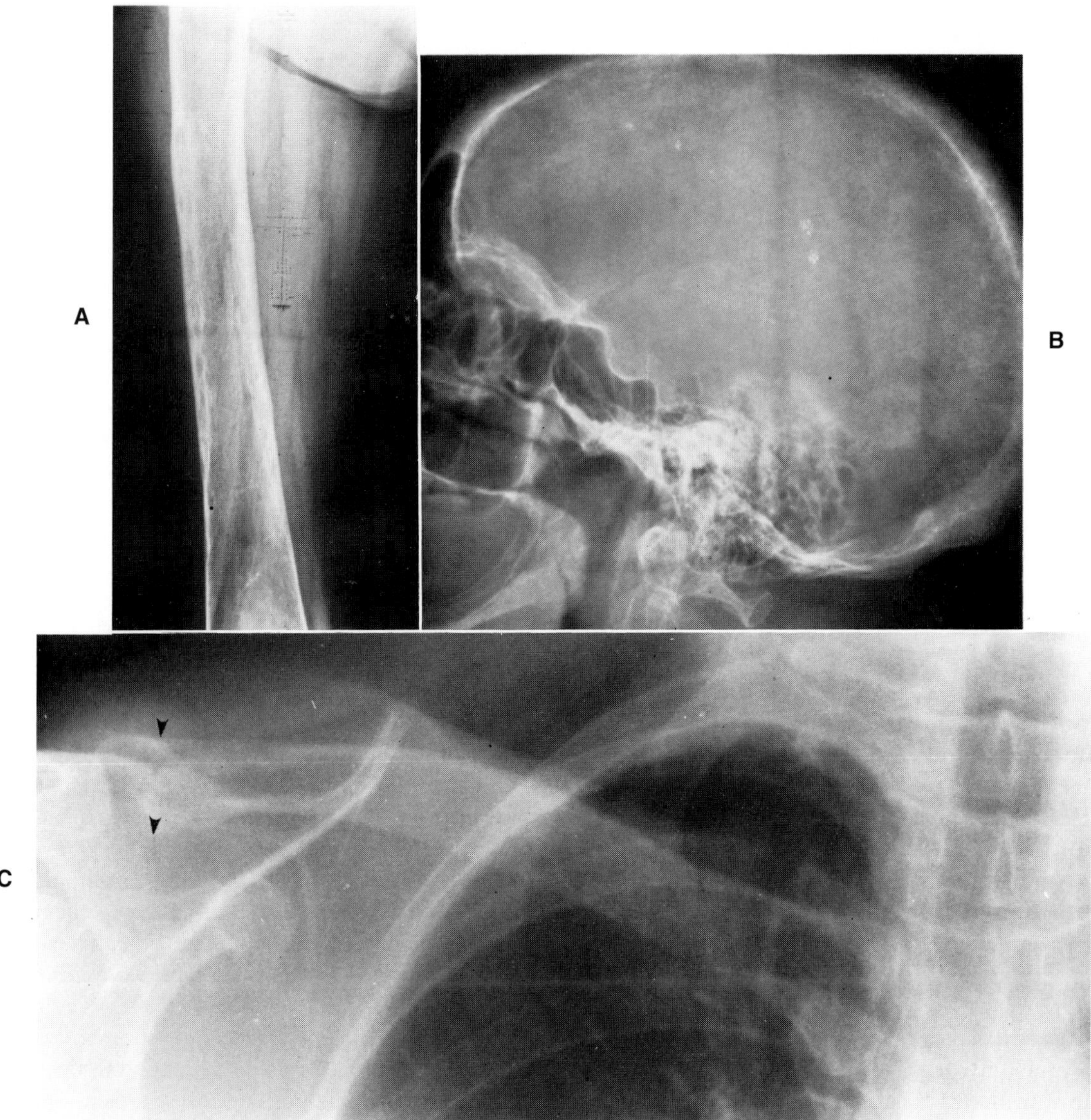

Fig. 56-8. Radiographic findings in hyperparathyroidism include the bone cysts **(A)** or ground-glass demineralization seen on skull radiography **(B)** that is increasingly rare except in neglected cases of prolonged hypercalcemia; an earlier and nearly pathognomonic sign seen in another patient's chest radiograph is the resorption of the distal clavicles **(C)**, "Higginbotham's sign."

long-term consequences of hypercalcemia in the patient without symptoms is typically through a deliberate diagnostic process and an elective surgical treatment. For such patients, the suggestions about general management recommendations listed in the following section may be adequate. Particularly if troubled by intercurrent complications of chronic hypercalcemia such as urinary tract calculi, some patients may have added to their general management oral neutral phosphates and a low-calcium diet. The general management recommendations are typically for the outpatient who is found to have hypercalcemia and is undergoing deliberate diagnostic testing before recommendation of treatment or continued observation. The urgent treatment of hypercalcemia by means of intravenous agents to prevent hypercalcemic crisis is limited to inpatients.

General hypercalcemic management recommendations. For the patient with hypercalcemia detected by outpatient blood testing, rational recommendations include a decrease in dietary calcium intake. This reduction is particularly valuable if the patient is taking calcium supplements or has high calcium intake as an indirect consequence of treatment directed toward some other end, such as antacid treatment for peptic ulcer disease. Generally, a decrease in milk and other dairy products, discontinuation or suspension of antacid tablets (or a shift to magnesium and aluminum salts for antacid therapy), and discontinuation of thiazide diuretics or antihypertensives are effective. Quite clearly, patients should suspend use of any vitamin D preparations they might be taking, including the use of most multivitamin supplements.

Increased mobilization should be encouraged. Stress along long bones and exercise through the activities of normal daily living prevent an increase in the rate of bone demineralization. Neutral phosphate may be administered through the gastrointestinal tract for long-term calcium-lowering action. Its effect is mild, however, and its side effect is diarrhea, because the same agents are given as phosphasoda as for cathartics. One of the consequences of repeated phospho-soda (Fleet) enema administration is an increase in phosphate in the serum and a corresponding decrease in blood calcium level. For patients who are undergoing long-term observation and treatment for prevention of recurrent renal calculi, sodium brushite may be useful for binding calcium in the gastrointestinal tract to lower its rate of absorption.

Inpatient treatment of hypercalcemic crisis. For the patient with symptoms who has dangerously elevated serum calcium levels, hospitalization and intravenous therapy are indicated. As seen in the accompanying box, a sequence of steps may be taken to lower serum calcium level gradually while simultaneously determining the cause of the elevation. Rarely are these hypercalcemic treatment steps indicated for a total serum calcium level less than 12 mg/dl or ionized calcium level less than 5.5 mg/dl, but the absolute level measured in the blood is less significant than the severity of the patient's symptoms attributed to the hypercalcemia.

The first treatment indicated, and the mainstay of hypercalcemic management, is intravenous hydration and diuresis. The patient with symptomatic hypercalcemia may be dehydrated, because the symptoms most often include nausea and vomiting. However, hypertension and cardiac arrthythmias may also be reflections of hypercalcemia. They may limit the rate of rehydration, unless simultaneous diuretic treatment is administered. Saline solutions are preferred to dextrose in water, but lactated Ringer's solution is contraindicated because of the presence of small quantities of calcium in the infusion. Saline diuresis should be induced rapidly by administration of 2 L saline solution over 3 hours, usually accompanied by intravenous furosemide given in high doses, with frequency dependent on its effect. With vigorous saline hydration and diuretic treatment, as much as 1 g elemental calcium may be cleared through the urine in 24 hours, and serum calcium may drop from 2 to 3 mg/dl. Cardiac and renal function and chest x-ray films should be carefully observed, and serum potassium and magnesium should be monitored during this treatment. The end point in this treatment is not to achieve an arbitrary level for blood calcium, but to reduce patient symptoms, particularly to effect a return to consciousness from stuporous obtundation. The kind of symptomatic hypercalcemia seen with hyperparathyroidism or vitamin D toxicity is usually managed successfully with hydration and diuresis therapy alone with the initiation of brisk calciuresis. For hypercalcemia from malignancy, severe symptoms associated with extremely high calcium levels require further treatment beyond these initial steps. In addition, some rare forms of primary hyperparathyroidism (parathyroid poisoning) (Fig. 56-9) may also require further treatment measures to return serum calcium levels toward normal.

TREATMENT OF HYPERCALCEMIC CRISIS

General: D/C Dietary Ca^{2+}, Thiazides, Vitamin D
↑ Mobilization Oral Neutral Phosphates, Brushite
Hydration and Diuresis, Calciuresis

1. Saline solution infusion	2 L/3 hr
2. Furosemide	100 mg IV/4 hr
Complexing Ca^{2+} in serum	
3. Phosphate	1.5 g IV/8 hr
4. Citrate or EDTA (dangerous)	1 g IV/4 hr

Drugs Decreasing Ca^{2+} From Bone and Gut

5. Hydrocortisone	100 mg IV/8 hr
6. Salmon calcitonin	5 Medical Research Council (MRC) U/kg/hour IV
7. Mithramycin	25 mg/kg/24 hours IV
Dialysis	Acute hemodialysis/4 hr
Urgent parathyroidectomy	As indicated by x-ray film bone resorption

D/C, Discontinue; *EDTA,* ethylenediaminetetra-acetic acid.

The next steps in a rapid decrease in ionized serum calcium include complexing the calcium in the serum or shifting it to the un-ionized form by acid/base manipulation. Intravenous phosphate may be administered up to 1.5 g intravenously for 8 hours. Citrate or ethylenediaminetetra-acetic acid may be given to complex the calcium in circulation, but these agents are dangerous and unpredictable in their effects, particularly on the kidneys. They should be used only in extreme circumstances, because safer drugs may be used to decrease calcium absorption from bone and gut if calciuresis has not returned the patient from dangerously elevated hypercalcemic levels.

Hydrocortisone administration (100 mg intravenously) may be helpful in decreasing calcium absorption and encouraging calcium renal excretion. However, the use of hydrocortisone is nearly specific for hypercalcemia based in sarcoidosis, some malignant neoplasms, or vitamin D toxicity because rarely do patients with hyperparathyroidism respond to steroid treatment. In fact, because only about 5% of patients whose hypercalcemia is based in hyperparathyroidism respond, the use of hydrocortisone to reduce serum calcium has been standardized as a "hydrocor-

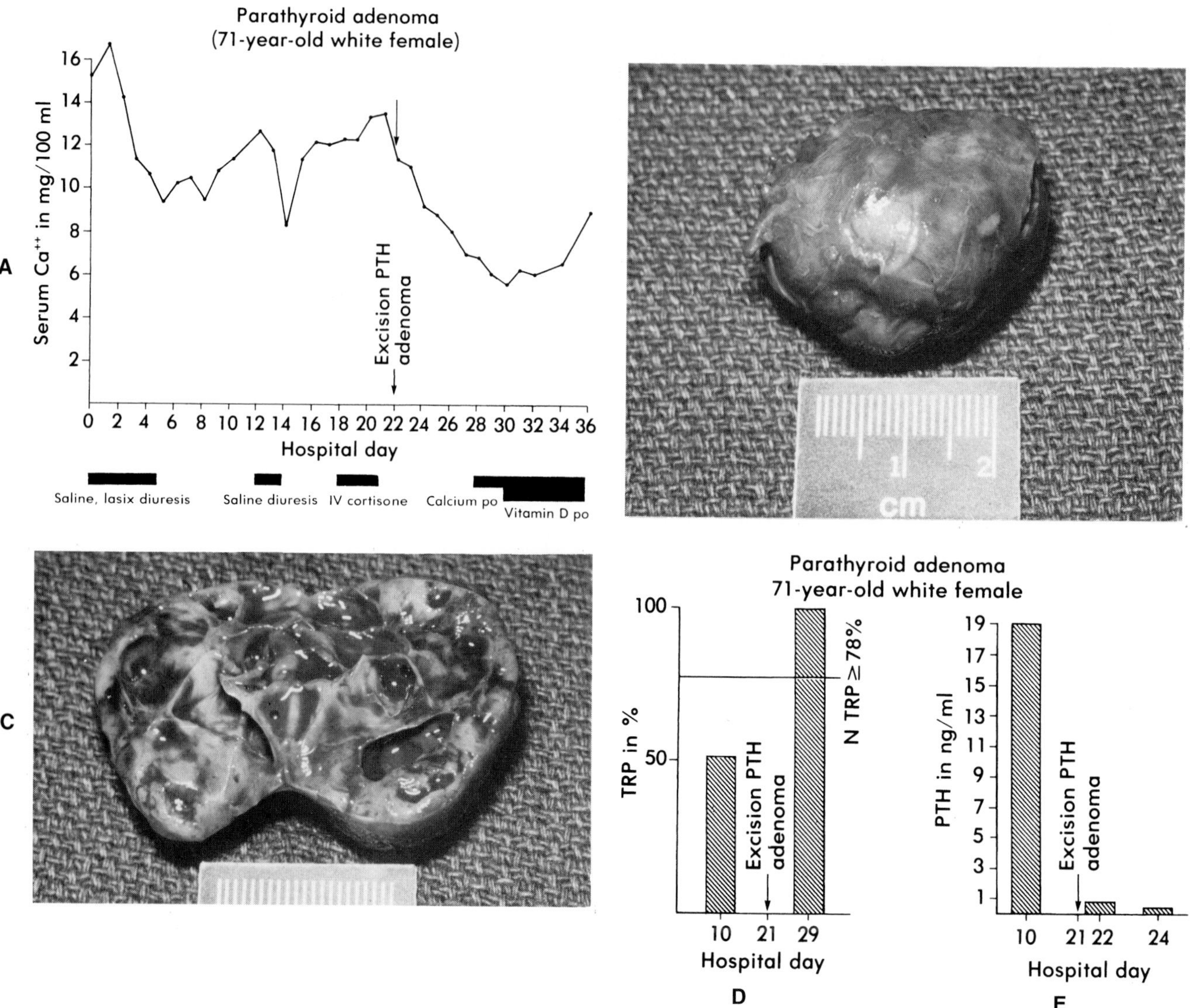

Fig. 56-9. Measurements and management in parathyroid poisoning. A stuporous 71-year-old woman was admitted in hypercalcemic crisis and begun on saline diuresis while diagnostic studies to prove hyperparathyroidism were being performed. **A,** Serum calcium (16.5 mg/dl on admission) was moderated to still-symptomatic levels of 12 mg/dl by saline solution, furosemide, and cortisone, until parathyroidectomy of an adenoma **(B)** that had undergone cystic degenerative changes **(C)**. Changes in preoperative and postoperative tubular reabsorption of phosphate *(TRP)* **(D)** and parathormone **(E)** reflect transient hypocalcemia after the operation, supported with short-term vitamin D and calcium supplements.

tisone suppression test" to rule out hyperparathyroidism. Newer agents used in hypercalcemia management are H_2-receptor blocking agents, such as cimetidine or ranitidine. These agents would be preferred to calcium-based antacids for the peptic complications of hypercalcemia.

The application of calcitinon therapy has introduced a significant treatment agent with less toxicity than others used in serious hypercalcemia. Salmon calcitonin was the largest therapeutic molecule commercially, biochemically synthesized prior to the use of recombinant DNA techniques. In hypercalcemia, it has been used in pharmacologic levels at which it inhibits bone resorption and increases renal clearance of calcium. Salmon calcitonin is used because it is more potent than mammalian calcitonin. This hormone may be used in levels of 5 Medical Research Council U/kg/hr with fewer side effects than the other somewhat more potent but considerably more dangerous intravenous agents.

Plicamycin's side effect of lowering serum calcium has been known for some time. Now, this cytotoxic chemotherapeutic agent may be used therapeutically for hypercalcemia. It is especially useful in patients with hypercalcemia from malignancy, although other agents, such as streptozocin, have also been used for hypercalcemia based in specific malignancy such as islet cell carcinoma. Plicamycin has a cumulative toxicity but an immediate calcium-lowering effect. Therefore, it may be administered when diuresis fails to bring serum calcium level under control, and its prolonged hypocalcemic effect may continue for several days after this initial administration. If only one or two doses are needed, the nephrotoxicity and other side effects are limited. Often, administration of this agent in those intervals brings the hypercalcemia under control.

At times, intravenous hydration, diuresis, and hypocalcemic agents successfully lower serum calcium from crisis levels, but the cause persists and drives the calcium back up again. In other cases, the presence of organ failures, such as renal failure, contraindicate further use of toxic agents or diuresis. In such instances, urgent hemodialysis may be considered for maintaining the blood calcium at reduced levels. Hemodialysis is indicated in any event if renal failure is part of the patient's problem. By regulating the bath against which dialysis occurs, a net calcium loss can be achieved in each dialysis. However, the small dynamic serum pool of calcium is backed up by an enormous reserve in calcium stores, and the hemodialysis must be frequently repeated to keep serum calcium under control as it equilibrates again with the released bone stores. In one specific hypercalcemic crisis, the unusual case of acute hyperparathyroidism, a rapid diagnostic determination can be made, and an urgent parathyroidectomy is indicated.

The application of diagnostic measures and management of parathyroid poisoning may serve as a clinical example of a patient in hypercalcemic crisis (see Fig. 56-9). A 71-year-old woman was admitted in coma found to be caused by hypercalcemia with levels of 16.5 mg/dl despite a low serum albumin level. Immediate saline diuresis with furosemide treatment was begun (see Fig. 56-9, *A*), with reduction of the serum calcium to levels of 12 mg/dl, at which the patient remained free of symptoms. During the management of the hypercalcemic crisis, TRP (see Fig. 56-9, *D*) and serum parathormone level (see Fig. 56-9, *E*) suggested primary hyperparathyroidism, which was further supported by x-ray film examination of the hands showing subperiosteal phalangeal bone resorption on fine-grain industrial film. The patient was taken to the operating room for urgent parathyroidectomy when these results were known, and a parathyroid ademona was encountered and excised (see Fig. 56-9, *B*). The pathophysiology of this acute hyperparathyroidism is probably related to the findings of acute cystic degeneration (see Fig. 56-9, *C*), which the pathologist suggested was a recent change in this adenoma. After the operation, the patient had symptomatic hypocalcemia and was supported with transient oral calcium and vitamin D administration. Vitamin D therapy was discontinued 2 weeks after discharge from the hospital; in 1 month, calcium supplementation was stopped; at 6 weeks, the patient was free of symptoms and found to have normal calcium, phosphate, chloride, and parathormone values when studied as an outpatient. This case reflects the problems seen with both hypercalcemic and hypocalcemic crises, the measurements needed for management of each, and medical and surgical control of hypercalcemia with transient medical support of hypocalcemia until endogenous hormone autoregulation restores the patient's normal calcium homeostasis.

HYPERPARATHYROIDISM

Primary, Secondary, and Tertiary Hyperparathyroidism

Hyperparathyroidism is classified as primary, secondary, or tertiary. In primary hyperparathyroidism, an idiopathic disorder in biofeedback of calcium control, secretion of parathormone is inappropriate considering the elevation in serum calcium. Secondary hyperparathyroidism is an increased activity in the parathyroid glands stimulated by low serum calcium or elevated serum phosphate. The appropriate hyperfunction of the parathyroid gland under this chronic stimulation may evolve into autonomous parathyroid hyperfunction. If this condition continues unabated in the absence of appropriate stimulation, it is called *tertiary hyperparathyroidism*. In all three forms, parathyroid gland activity is increased and parathormone secretion is elevated. In secondary hyperparathyroidism, this elevated activity is appropriate in sensing and responding to the hypocalcemic signal (see Fig. 56-4). It serves a physiologically useful role in compensatory release and retention of calcium by protecting against the impaired cellular function that would develop if the hypocalcemia were unopposed. In primary and tertiary hyperparathyroidism, this overactivity is autonomous and continues despite the signals of hypercalcemia and hypophosphatemia that should inhibit parathyroid action and parathormone effect.

What signal is ignored or what sensors misfire in autonomous primary and tertiary hyperparathyroidism? The cause appears to be a loss of calcium sensitivity or a change in the ionized serum calcium "set-point" by the offending parathyroid tissues. This change may take place in one or more glands and may be triggered by congenital or acquired defects in this autoregulatory mechanism. Brown et al.[27] studied the response of normal and abnormal parathyroid glands to calcium stimulation or inhibition of parathormone in the gland's native position in the neck, in tissue transplanted in the forearm, or in tissue culture. The exact point at which parathyroid cells undergo transformation and lose sensitivity to the calcium signal is not known in the sporadic cases of primary or tertiary hyperparathyroidism, but it appears to be genetically predetermined in some hereditary cases of primary hyperparathyroidism.

Cause

Hyperparathyroidism is familial in some pedigrees, with or without association with other synchronous endocrine abnormalities. This genetic predisposition in families with isolated primary hyperparathyroidism may result from an altered "set-point" in at least some parathyroid cells. A genetically codetermined hyperparathyroidism is present in two major types of hereditary MEA. The malfunctioning parathyroid gland, the one common abnormality shared by MEA I and MEA II, is often one of the earliest manifestations, occurring frequently in children in such families. However, it is not uniformly part of all multiple endocrine adenopathies; one subtype of MEA II is distinctive in part because of normal parathyroids and their normal calcium response.[19]

In MEA I (Wermer's syndrome), the primary hyperparathyroidism is associated with abnormalities in pancreatic islets and pituitary gland form and function. In MEA II (Sipple's syndrome), the parathyroid problem is associated with medullary thyroid cancer and chromaffin system abnormalities such as pheochromocytoma. In these familial syndromes, the relationship of the parathormone and calcium metabolism changes to the other involved hormones is interesting. However, to suggest that the parathyroids were reacting to stimuli mediated by calcium from these other abnormalities would be facile. For example, in Wermer's syndrome, an intimate relationship exists among calcium, gastrin release, and peptic ulceration from hyperacidity; the ulcer is often treated with calcium-containing antacids and associated with the multiple endocrine products of pancreatic islets and pituitary. Similarly, gastrin and calcium stimulate calcitonin release from medullary carcinoma, as may be found in Sipple's syndrome. Furthermore, multiple connections exist within the MEA II of amine precursor uptake and decarboxylation hormone synthesis and release. For example, it might be postulated that calcitonin decreases calcium, the parathyroids react appropriately to this hypocalcemia, and, much as in tertiary hyperparathyroidism, the parathyroids may become autonomous in their function, thereby accounting for the linkages in MEA II of the other endocrine abnormalities with hyperparathyroidism. However, as already noted, in one subtype of MEA II, the parathyroids and the serum calcium level are normal, despite early, widespread, and frequently lethal medullary thyroid cancer with abundant calcitonin secretion. Patients dying of sporadic medullary thyroid carcinoma with very high levels of calcitonin also have no detectable abnormality in serum calcium level, so even pathologically elevated levels of calcitonin may produce little effect in extracellular calcium. The current conclusion is that hyperparathyroidism is genetically codetermined with the other defects in these hereditary syndromes.[28]

Chronic stimulation of the parathyroid glands occurs in patients with renal failure, phosphate retention, and calcium wasting. This appropriate stimulus-response may continue, even after successful renal allografting has returned calcium and phosphate levels to normal on the basis of normalized renal function. However, one might speculate that the parathyroid glands have been unalterably switched on during this period of chronic stimulation, thus accounting for tertiary hyperparathyroidism. A similar prolongation of diet- or drug-induced hyperphosphatemia and hypocalcemia in animal experiments can produce hyperparathyroidism.[29] Further, as seen in Table 55-4, hyperparathyroidism in humans is most common among postmenopausal women, coincidentally the group with the highest rate of osteoporosis and shifts in calcium and phosphate metabolism. These clinical coincidences and the forced circumstances in laboratory experiments suggest that some primary hyperparathyroidism may be induced by environmental circumstances such as diet, drugs, or metabolic changes associated with aging, and that this parathyroid stimulation may switch parathyroid hyperfunction into autonomy. However, these suggestions are not conclusive, because most patients with secondary hyperparathyroidism treated by successful transplantation or carefully regulated dialysis do not acquire tertiary hyperparathyroidism, most postmenopausal women do not have parathyroid neoplasms, and solitary gland involvement is the rule among most patients with primary hyperparathyroidism, except in the familial kindreds in which hyperplasia is predominant. At present, the mechanism of neoplastic transformation of parathyroid glands is unknown.

One further bit of evidence comes from studies of patients who have thyroid abnormalities related to radiation. Studying population cohorts in each direction, groups of patients with proven hyperparathyroidism for history of cervical radiation[30] and larger populations of patients who have had cervical radiation for hyperparathyroidism,[31] investigators have shown an association between radiation to the head and neck and hyperparathyroidism. Multiple investigators have found an increased incidence of parathyroid pathology among patients being operated on for thyroid abnormalities, and the reverse. Radiation may change the rate at which the fundamental neoplastic transformation occurs, but this explanation alone is not satisfactory, because the vast majority of patients with primary hyperparathyroidism have had no proven exposure to ionizing radiation, at least of a therapeutically significant level.

Morphology

The most important distinction in the morphologic basis of hyperparathyroidism is between single and multiple gland disease. If the parathyroid tissue is responding appropriately to stimulation (as with secondary hyperparathyroidism) or if the hyperparathyroidism stems from a genetic defect carried uniformly with each parathyroid cell (as, presumably, would be the case in the familial primary hyperparathyroidism in MEA), all the parathyroid cells present would be expected to be the seat of pathology. Thus, correction of hypersecretion should involve a systemic change in the stimulus or identification and ablation of all parathyroid tissue. If neoplastic transformation was a "single hit," or a monoclonal proliferation of a single line of hyperfunctioning cells, the location of the hypersecretory locus should be a point source susceptible to ablation without disturbing the other parathyroid tissues that retain autoregulatory control. Surgically important for management, the distinction between single and multiple gland disease is also pathologically significant, because the morphologic diagnosis is indistinguishable from a single specimen of overactive parathyroid tissue, and indications for further therapy or prognosis cannot be drawn from a histologic observation of one specimen.

Further morphologic distinction in patients in whom all parathyroid glands are involved with hypercellularity and presumed hyperfunction may take the form of chief cell or clear cell hyperplasia. The early predominance of clear cell hyperplasia appears to be decreasing,[32] and that of chief cell hyperplasia appears to be increasing.[33] Although oxyphil cells are also present, they appear to be functionally insignificant, at least when encountered as adenomas, as individual cells when stained with parathormone-specific stains, and by electron microscopy, which shows absence of secretory granules. Oxyphil cells increase in number with aging and do not appear to be a pathologic part of the process of hyperparathyroidism.

In addition to the histologic characterization of cell types, the pathologist often is called on to distinguish benign from malignant parathyroid neoplasms. As with most endocrine tissues, in parathyroid tissue this distinction is difficult to make on cytologic grounds; sometimes it is not easy even with histologic evidence. The surgeon's observations and the pathologist's determinations are subservient to the patient's clinical course, which can contradict the impressions of either or both professions. Before a gross adenoma is visible to the surgeon, microadenomata present within an externally undeformed gland may still give rise to chemical and even clinical hyperparathyroidism.[34] Adenomas may become surgically detectable and pathologically characteristic when they reach an arbitrary size that causes them to have a characteristic appearance surgically and histologically distinctive from the normal glands in the same patient (Fig. 56-10).

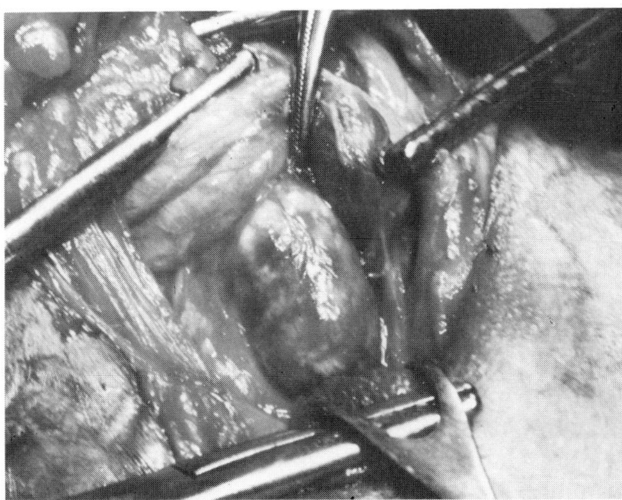

Fig. 56-10. A parathyroid adenoma may have a characteristic appearance, as seen here, but no conclusion is drawn about single gland or multiple gland origin of the patient's primary hyperparathyroidism unless this gland is compared surgically and pathologically with the other parathyroid glands in the same patient.

In sporadic, most often asymptomatic cases, primary hyperparathyroidism most often results from parathyroid adenoma involving a singular gland. This is true for 90% of patients with primary hyperparathyroidism in many large series reported, with an additional 9% of cases caused by primary hyperplasia of either chief or clear cell type involving multiple glands. Normally, four parathyroid glands are present in distributions determined by the embryologic origin from the pharyngeal arches, with the inferior parathyroid glands derived from the third arch and the superior glands derived from the fourth. However, more than four glands are present in some patients, and typically all are involved in the parathyroid hyperplasia of secondary hyperparathyroidism or in familial parathyroid disorders. Whether multiple adenomas occur is a moot point because of the fundamental distinction between single and multiple gland disease. Therefore, involvement of more than one gland is classified as multiple gland disease, whether that glandular pattern appears to be multiple adenomas or hyperplasia in multiple glands. An earlier histologic distinction that does not appear to be useful is the presence of a compressed rim of apparently normal parathyroid tissue by the expansion of the adenoma, yet this same finding can also be present in hyperplastic glands. In my experience, and in other studies, parathyroid adenocarcinoma is the cause of primary hyperparathyroidism in 0.5% of cases when the carcinoma is defined by its metastasizing rather than by histologic criteria of parathyroid carcinoma.[35] This group may include an equal number of additional patients in whom the clinical behavior of the tumor appears similar to that of the benign adenoma or suggests its complete excision by simple removal of the enlarged gland.

Goal of Surgical Treatment in Hyperparathyroidism

Within half a century surgical therapy for hyperparathyroidism expanded from its first deliberate undertaking in the United States to widespread application to asymptomatic disease. Because of this relatively rapid development, the natural history of the untreated disease has not been followed throughout a lifetime; the indications for operation are still founded on presumption of probable complications from the untreated disorder. At some serum calcium levels, these predictions can be made with a high degree of confidence, particularly if the hypercalcemia is already symptomatic. That the disease requires treatment at marginal levels of hypercalcemia in the symptom-free patient is less apparent. However, in the United States, most patients who have a confidently established diagnosis of primary hyperparathyroidism are typically operated on at their elective convenience. The single criterion that remains sine qua non before operation is that a diagnosis of primary hyperparathyroidism be made with confidence. Particularly in marginal diagnostic calls, the operating surgeon and the patient commit to the undertaking of a meticulous operation to find the site of the pathology and correct it to restore normal calcium balance. Operation is the most precise localizing technique, but it is *not* a diagnostic procedure for primary hyperparathyroidism.

The goal of the surgical procedure is to reduce parathyroid hypersecretion to normal levels and to restore autoregulatory calcium balance. In the event of single gland disease, this procedure entails identifying and removing the solitary focus of the pathology in distinction to the patient's normal or suppressed parathyroid glands with which the pathology is compared. For the patient with multiple gland disease, subtotal resection is the rule, with a residual mass of parathyroid tissue capable of producing approximately 150 mg total of viable parathyroid cells, usually in multiple identified sites. Normal parathyroid glands should be identified and preserved with intact blood supply. Their removal will not affect hyperparathyroidism, but it may cause an increased likelihood of hypoparathyroidism after this or subsequent operation. Primary surgical exploration is 95% successful in accomplishing the goals of reduced parathormone production and restored calcium autoregulation. In approximately 3% of cases, the primary exploration does not find or fix the pathologic problem in the thyroid, and in the remainder the disease may return after initial success in managing the hypercalcemia surgically. With the arbitrary duration of 6 months, the distinction is made between *persistence* of hypercalcemia after a failed primary cervical exploration and *recurrence,* which means hyperparathyroidism reappears after 6 months of low or normal calcium levels after surgical treatment.

Special techniques are considered for the peculiar problems of persistence, recurrence, ectopic or supernumerary glands, sequence of treatment in other endocrinopathy associated with primary hyperparathyroidism, parathyroid transplantation, and nonsurgical techniques of both localization and control of persistent hyperparathyroidism. The goals of each of these special management techniques remain the same, reduction of parathormone toward normal levels and autoregulatory calcium homeostasis.

Primary Cervical Exploration for Primary Hyperparathyroidism

In the first attempt at treatment, a cervical exploration by an experienced surgeon is the most precise localizing technique for pathologic parathyroids. Preoperative physical examination is performed in all such patients, but rarely would one expect positive findings related to the parathyroid gland, except in patients with toxic parathyroid single gland disease such as cystic degeneration of a large adenoma or a parathyroid carcinoma. The most likely palpable abnormality in a patient undergoing exploration for asymptomatic hypercalcemia is a thyroid nodule or lymph node, because rarely is a parathyroid adenoma of the size and texture usually associated with this form of hyperparathyroidism clinically palpable. The name of the operation is *parathyroid exploration*—not excision of parathyroid adenoma—because adenoma is a presumptive diagnosis in a patient who might have multiple gland disease as the cause for the syndrome, even though most have single gland disease. The name suggests the procedure, careful dissection for and identification of all visible parathyroid tissue in its normal, likely, or abnormal locations. If the referring physician or patient requests a preoperative study, it should be limited to a simple, noninvasive procedure, such as sonography. The sonography for parathyroid glands requires specialized equipment and is operator dependent. At present sonography is almost as reliable as the radioisotopic method, with which promising experience has been gathered, namely, sestamibi parathyroid scanning. However, neither of these methods is required before the operation, because *no* nonoperative method currently available identifies visually and confirms pathologically all visible parathyroid tissue. Because the localization studies do not identify the normal or suppressed glands, the early identification of a solitary large gland may be misleading, and it at least makes the dissection of the remaining glands somewhat tedious after the encounter with the presumptive site of pathology. However, failure to complete this tedious dissection to identify the remaining glands increases the chance of persistence or recurrence of hyperparathyroidism.

Anatomic variants make parathyroid exploration interesting, exciting as a skilled application of anatomic, embryologic, and pathologic information to intricate technique in a vital dissection field, and sometimes frustrating. The surgeon must have a thorough knowledge of cervical anatomy. He or she must know not only where parathyroid glands are normally found, but also where they *might* be found, because the abnormal parathyroid gland is often found in ectopic locations. The landmarks useful in locating normally situated parathyroid glands include the recurrent laryngeal nerve, the inferior cornu of the thyroid cartilage, and the inferior thyroid artery. If the parathyroid glands are successfully located on one side of the trachea, the mirror-image position on the opposite side is the most likely site of the comparable glands. The enlargement of a single gland in an adenoma may distort or displace the structures around it, making the normal parathyroid adjacent to it somewhat more difficult to identify (Fig. 56-11). In addition to serving as a landmark, enlargement of the inferior thyroid artery may suggest lateralization of a single gland abnormality. If the enlarged parathyroid gland does not lie in its normal anatomic location, searching the inferior thyroid artery for principal branches may indicate a hidden adenoma (e.g., an adenoma located in a lateral cleft in the thyroid gland or rarely, a wholly intrathyroidal adenoma). By following any thyroid artery branches that go down in the submanubrial space, careful dissection of the superior mediastinum can be accomplished through a cervical approach.

After preliminary parathyroid dissection, the surgeon may know the locations of three glands, but not the fourth. This situation tests the mettle of the surgical team, because the normal locations have been searched and the fourth gland, particularly if a pathologic gland was not

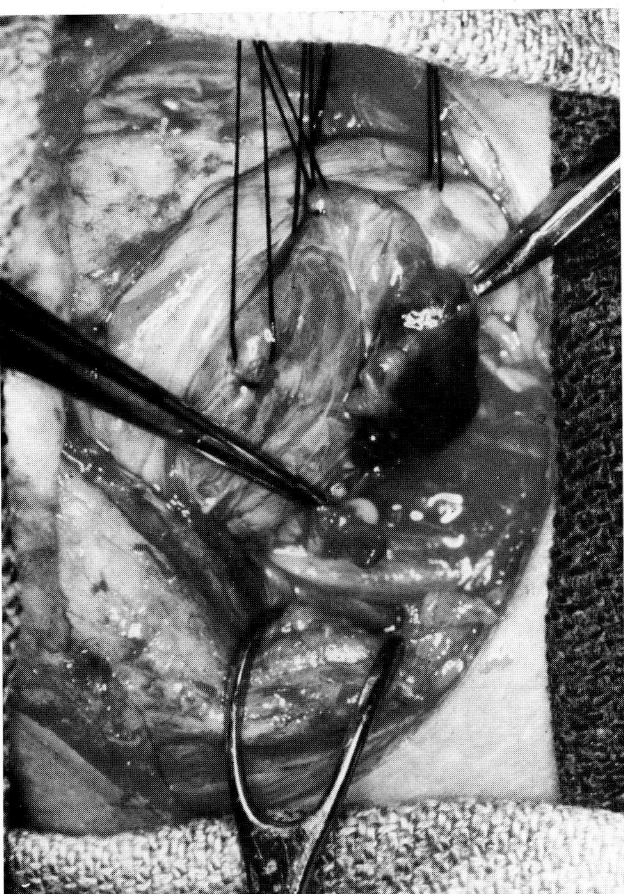

Fig. 56-11. A parathyroid adenoma seen in situ in this primary parathyroid exploration is compared with the normal parathyroid gland at the end of the forceps.

PROCEDURE FOR SEARCH FOR FOURTH GLAND

A. During the operation: pathologist's report confirms three glands, parathyroid "map" indicates position of missing gland, search posterior thyroid capsule in this position, examine mirror-image position opposite confirmed gland
   1. If superior gland:
      a. Search above superior thyroid pole, taking down superior thyroid artery
      b. Palpate tracheoesophageal groove
      c. Explore retroesophageal area
      d. Dissect carotid sheath on suspected side
      e. Perform thyroidotomy
   2. If inferior gland:
      a. Trace any branches of inferior thyroid artery
      b. Palpate submanubrial space
      c. Tease up thymic fat pad
      d. Perform limited thyroidectomy in area where gland is missing
   3. cAMP urinary excretion monitoring, or rapid PTH serum monitoring
   4. If convinced that there is no evidence of additional parathyroid tissue in neck, close!
      No indication for sternotomy at a primary exploration

B. After the operation:
   1. Test for persistent hypercalcemia
   2. CT and ultrasonic scanning
   3. Venous sampling and venography
   4. Arteriography
      a. If adenoma encountered in neck—cervical reexploration
      b. If mediastinal adenoma with inferior thyroid arterial blood supply—cervical reexploration
      c. If mediastinal adenoma with internal mammary arterial blood supply—contrast staining

Slightly modified and reproduced with permission from Geelhoed GW. Problem Management in Endocrine Surgery. Chicago: Year Book Medical Publishers, copyright © 1983.

seen in the first three, *must* be identified during this first cervical exploration or be excluded by careful dissection as not within reach of the extended cervical exploration. The areas of this extension include the tracheoesophogeal groove, the retroesophageal space, the carotid sheath, the thyroid gland, and especially the substernal superior mediastinum (see accompanying box). Teasing up the tongue of thymus suspended from the thyrothymic ligament along the inferior thyroid artery is a part of any cervical exploration that has not identified four glands, or any that has identified four glands without a clear pathologic diagnosis. Although some surgeons recommend the use of vital staining as an intraoperative adjunct, I suggest this as a technique only in reoperation. Other ancillary tests may suggest that the pathologic parathyroid tissue has been removed, even if this is not confirmed by the pathologist. The cAMP measurement in urine is a sensitive indicator of parathormone; if the parathyroid source of hyperparathyroidism has been ablated, the urine content of cAMP dramatically decreases, even during the course of the parathyroid exploration. This special indication is the niche to be filled by the more recently available rapid PTH serum assay to judge completion of the parathyroid procedure.

A special case is made for the mediastinal glands that may be present and their selective management in initial cervical operation, in subsequent localization studies, and in sternotomy for mediastinal excision. Finally, sternal-splitting chest exploration during the primary operation is almost never indicated, because that operation is not an exploration but an excision of known or strongly suspected pathology determined from the application of localizing techniques before reoperation, if indicated.

An example of a surgical procedure that requires persistence because of the confident preoperative diagnosis of primary hyperparathyroidism is a parathyroid exploration that encounters four apparently normal glands, possibly even in their normal anatomic locations. If the surgical certainty indicating this operation is that the patient had primary hyperparathyroidism, the dissection continues for the identification of a fifth gland that might be the locus of disease, more especially because it is not seen in the normal anatomic locations. In the example illustrated in Fig. 56-19, the suspected parathyroid pathology was not identified, despite verified presence of four parathyroid glands in the normal locations. No apparent fifth gland was within the reach of cervical dissection. At this point, the surgeon was satisfied that he had exhausted cervical exploration as the primary localizing technique; thus, he used angiography to assist in localizing the fifth gland.

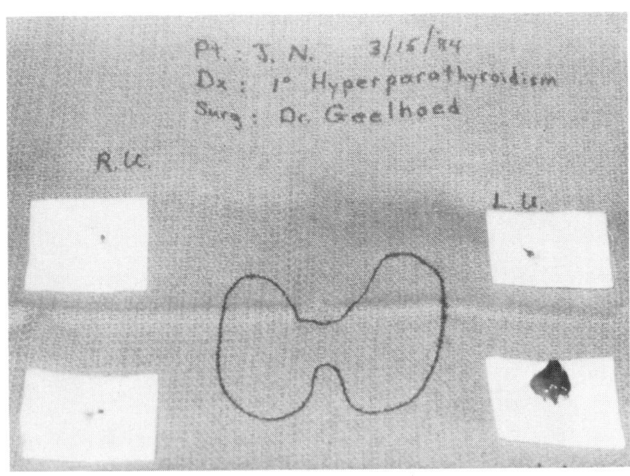

Fig. 56-12. After identification of all visible parathyroids by the surgeon, surgical pathology consultation is requested, and biopsies of the normal-appearing parathyroid glands and excision of the enlarged gland are carried out, with specimens placed on a "parathyroid map" for identification of their locations.

Pathology Consultation and Confirmation of Successful Parathyroid Exploration

In addition to the rapid PTH serum assay or the urinary cAMP, which are especially helpful in confirming excision of the offending parathyroid tissue during reoperation, pathology consultation is involved in nearly every parathyroid exploration. As a courtesy to the surgical pathologist, the surgeon avoids requiring the pathologist to be on a continuous standby to receive serial frozen section specimens to determine the presence or absence of parathyroid tissue or to satisfy curiosity as to the nature of abnormal tissues present. Courtesy, efficiency, and accuracy are best served by first directly visualizing all accessible parathyroid tissues. After identifying the four glands, the surgeon can perform biopsy of the normal-appearing glands and excision of the abnormal ones in total (adenoma, carcinoma) or subtotal (hyperplasia). The surgeon then passes the specimens to the pathologist, who, after viewing the multiple glands passed on a "parathyroid map" identifying their locations in situ (Fig. 56-12), gives an opinion of the parathyroid pathology. The pathologist's options include cytologic identification of the presence or absence of parathyroid tissue or histologic determination of the same tissue, with an additional attempt made at specifically diagnosing the source of parathyroid pathology. The more important determination is the identification of tissue as parathyroid or nonparathyroid, because multiple or single gland disease may be grossly apparent to both the surgeon and the pathologist. Consequently, histologic diagnosis of an adenoma or suppressed normal parathyroid gland can be reserved for permanent pathology sections or can be suggested on frozen-section determination on those specimens already proved to be parathyroid tissue by touch preparation.

A new technique for determining the presence or absence of parathyroid tissue is the use of intraoperative imprints for cytologic identification of parathyroid tissue.[28] The rapid imprint technique is useful in screening the specimens handed over for pathologic consultation at the conclusion of the surgical exploration, while the patient remains anesthetized.

Extent of Parathyroid Excision

Any decision regarding the extent of parathyroid resection is made on the basis of the gross and microscopic determination of the parathyroid disease during the operation. Removal of single gland disease is curative in nearly all patients who undergo this excision; biopsy specimens or touch-preparation cytologic studies of the other parathyroid glands substantiate the belief that the disease is of a single gland. If the other glands are enlarged or hypercellular on biopsy, however, the suspicion that the hyperparathyroidism may be multiple gland disease could indicate more extensive parathyroid reduction. Typically, this involves total excision of two parathyroid glands and subtotal excision of the remaining two glands, with a marker left with them to identify their sites[36] and parathyroid remnants of approximately 75 mg in each location. (Comment will be reserved for later on the indication for total parathyroidectomy and remnant autotransplantation.)

The ultimate confirmation of successful parathyroid exploration comes from the patient's clinical and biochemical course after surgical therapy. Excision of a large adenoma or a major reduction in parathyroid tissue in hyperplasia usually results in postoperative hypoparathyroidism, reflected in a fall in serum calcium to hypocalcemic levels; thus, the hypoplastic glands adjacent to what had been the adenoma may return to normal function. After the operation, the patient may require calcium supplementation and/or vitamin D support. If this calcium and vitamin D therapy is required for a prolonged period, hypoparathyroidism is suspected. If the vitamin D and calcium are decreased and the patient is maintained in asymptomatic biochemical hypocalcemia, this stimulus should be adequate to return to function any residual parathyroid tissue. However, if 1 year after parathyroidectomy the patient still requires these treatments to avoid symptoms, permanent hypoparathyroidism is suggested. If within 6 months from successful parathyroid operation the patient has persistent hypercalcemia, the burden of parathyroid tissue is once again excessive.

A possible cause of this excess is stimulation of the transient hypocalcemia that developed and acted on glands with a predetermined genetic propensity for hyperfunction. Any viable cells around the periphery of the excision may have resumed function during the interval; if they retained their tendency toward autonomous hyperfunction, they may be the source of recurrence. The retention of any incompletely excised, autonomous parathyroid cells is the predictable source of recurrent hyperparathyroidism some time later.

A distressing sequel of parathyroid exploration is persistent hypercalcemia. This condition indicates a failed primary cervical exploration, and the patient now has indication for localization studies to assist in reoperative correction of the hyperparathyroidism not resolved at the primary cervical exploration. Such patients are screened carefully to rule out some nonparathyroid cause for their hypercalcemia, such as FHH, or for some ectopic source of hyperparathyroidism not located in the parathyroid glands themselves.

Parathyroid Localization Studies

Preoperative localization studies are not required before primary cervical exploration, but they are advisable before a second surgical attempt at control of hyperparathyroidism or, in some instances, as a substitute for it.

Sonography

Sonography may be helpful, and it is sometimes used in primary cases. Like most radiographic or isotopic tests, the ultrasonographic study is a "shadow-producing procedure"; it may tell of the presence and location of a mass but does not confirm the nature of that mass. In the neck, multiple masses are possible, including normal structures such as thyroid or lymph nodes or abnormalities within those structures.

Fig. 56-13 shows a sonogram of a large parathyroid adenoma present in a patient with symptoms and extremely elevated serum calcium level. Its size is such that it would be readily encountered in cervical exploration, and it is in a position where this exploration would take place. The ultrasonographic scan is less helpful in the ectopic locations that the surgeon has not reached in primary exploration, such as the mediastinum. Furthermore, the specific type of sonogram requires a 10 mHz small-parts, real-time, dedicated machine, and an interested and experienced operator. Both the expertise and the machinery are not readily available at all centers, whereas CT scanning with high resolution is available in most U.S. referral centers.

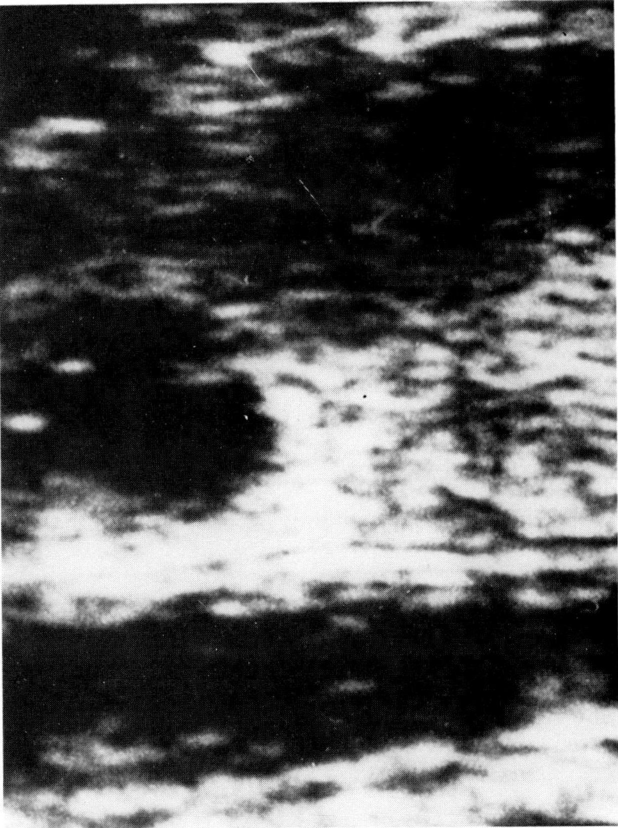

Fig. 56-13. Sonography demonstrated this large parathyroid adenoma, which would be unlikely to be overlooked in this position in surgical exploration.

Isotopic Scanning

Previous scanning techniques have been disappointing when applied to the parathyroid area, and selenium-methionine and technetium scan alone are probably of historic interest only. However, a newer technique combining thallium and technetium is an advance in subtraction scanning. This method can identify enlarged parathyroid glands, including those in ectopic locations,[37] but it does not identify normal parathyroid glands and has been associated with a higher than acceptable rate of false-positive readings in some series. Though its reliability is variable, it is a less invasive method of positive identification of solitary enlarged parathyroids in ectopic locations (Fig. 56-14).

The current state of the art[38] with respect to isotopic parathyroid scanning is the use of sestamibi scanning,[39,40] which has been supplanting thallum-technicium subtraction because of higher precision, but retains some of the same limits in its utility.

CT Scanning

CT scanning is a helpful noninvasive localization study, particularly if coupled with contrast augmentation in examining the areas less accessible to sonography. As seen in Fig. 56-15, on the basis of a CT scan in one patient, a pre-

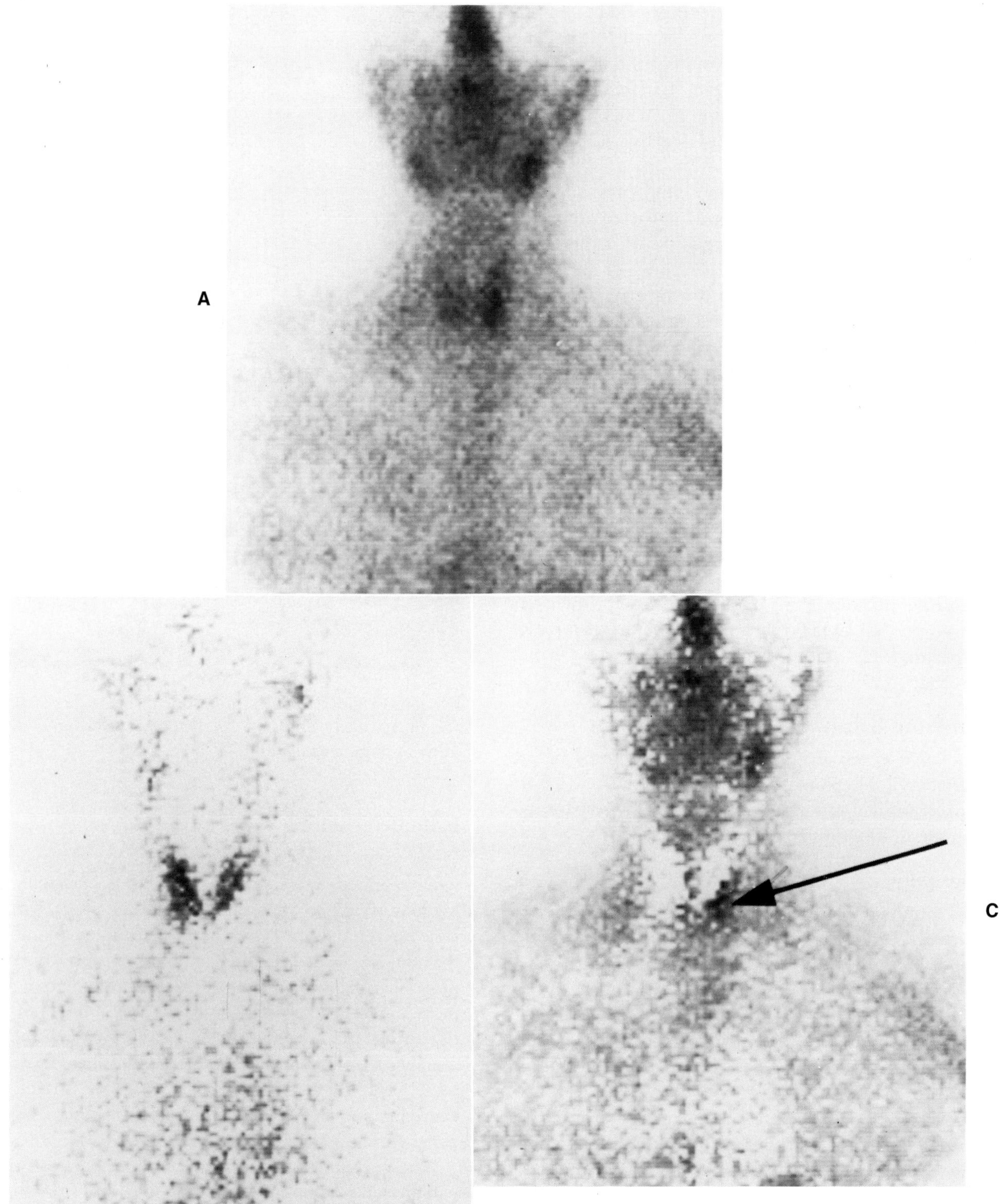

Fig. 56-14. Thallium-technetium subtraction isotopic scan shows promise for localization of enlarged parathyroids, but no noninvasive study yet devised demonstrates normal parathyroid glands—a requirement of primary cervical exploration. **A,** Thallium scan of neck; **B,** technetium scan of thyroid; **C,** thallium-technetium subtraction film showing left lower pole parathyroid adenoma.

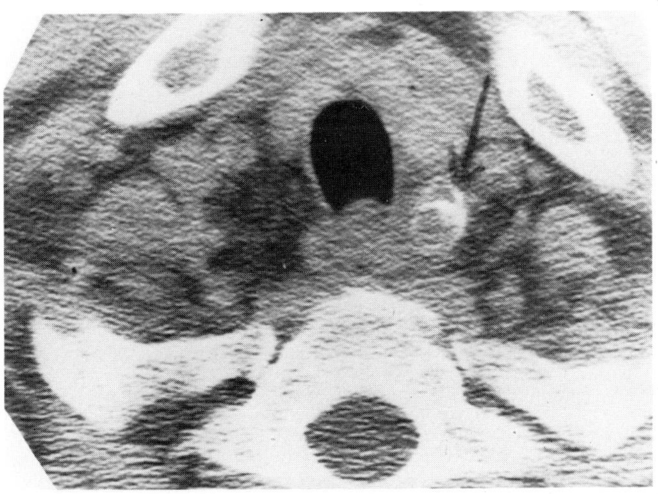

Fig. 56-15. CT scan not only demonstrated this large and unusual parathyroid lesion, it suggested, even before operation, that it might be a parathyroid carcinoma, which it proved to be on surgical excision.

operative diagnosis of parathyroid carcinoma (suggested on the CT scan because the irregular borders of the mass appeared to invade tissues adjacent to it and a calcific rim) was confirmed on exploration. The best application of CT is in the area of the mediastinum not accessible to submanubrial inspection and palpation from the cervical approach at the time of the primary cervical exploration.

Fine-Needle Aspiration

A rarely used, more invasive development in parathyroid localization has been the sonographically directed or CT-directed fine-needle aspiration. Aspiration cytology can give evidence of the presence of parathyroid cells in the mass within range of the needle. Like the touch preparation during operation, this sample is studied by cytologic technique to identify presence or absence of parathyroid tissue. With the use of immunoperoxidase-specific parathormone staining, this identification can be specific even if rapid. Diagnoses have been made by percutaneous fine-needle aspiration, with a subsequent suggestion that ablation might be possible by alcohol injection through the same needle that identifies the parathyroid cells.[41]

Venous Sampling

Selective venous catheterization and sampling for parathormone assay is the most specific radiologic localization test that can correlate form and function. Because the hormone that is biologically active is best measured by the N-terminal–recognizing antibody, radioimmunoassay for either N-terminal, intact PTH, or both, should be used with specimens obtained by selective venous catheterization. Fig. 56-16 illustrates a patient problem successfully managed with the help of venous catheterization data. A patient who had undergone a primary failed cervical exploration underwent arteriography (see Fig. 56-16, *A*), which suggested an abnormality that could not be clearly distinguished from the thyroid blush seen on arteriography. The venous blood sampling pattern of N-terminal parathormone suggested a high parathormone reading in the inferior thyroid vein sample draining the same site suggested on arteriography, giving functional significance to the morphologic abnormality confirmed in the excision of the adenoma at that site (see Fig. 56-16, *C*). Despite these advantages, parathyroid localization by venous assay depends on the expertise of the radiologist. Furthermore, from disruption previous thyroid or parathyroid surgery may have ligated most of the venous drainage patterns normally seen, and neovascularity may result after the passage of some time since the first cervical operation.

Digital-Subtraction Angiography

Use of digital-subtraction angiography is quite limited, because the technique does not have the high resolution of selective arteriography, although it is not as operator dependent. The major use of digital-subtraction angiography is in combination with venous catheterization sampling, to identify major vessels or their postoperative anomalies that might otherwise be confusing in data interpretation. The resolution of this technique does not exceed that of CT scanning, which is more applicable in checking mediastinal or other ectopic sites.

Selective Arteriography

In skilled hands, selective arteriography is the gold standard of radiographic localization of morphologic abnormality. This highly invasive technique requires nearly as much time and concentrated effort as surgical reexploration. Further, its high yield in information may be attended with corresponding morbidity. Excess contrast material may lead to renal failure, and injection of cervical arteries has raised concern regarding the anterior spinal artery and any transient paresis risk.

However, the advantage of arteriography is that the localization and treatment of an ectopic parathyroid adenoma not accessible to cervical reexploration might be accomplished by the same arteriographic catheter. In addition, the arteriogram suggests the presence of an adenoma in a cervical location where it had been overlooked in previous operation (Fig. 56-17, *A*), the adenoma can be retrieved through reoperation (Fig. 56-17, *B*). If the arteriogram suggests that the adenoma is located in the mediastinum and is supplied by an internal thoracic artery branch that might make it less amenable to cervical reoperation retrieval, the same arteriographic catheter can be advanced into this feeding vessel and wedged. Hypertensive injection of concentrated contrast material then creates an osmotic shock to the parathyroid tissue, and a prolonged angiographic stain is seen persisting for even days after this procedure. This modification of the original technique of embolization[36] has been used in a number of patients who have been cured of their persistent hyperparathyroidism for as long as 22 years after angiogra-

A

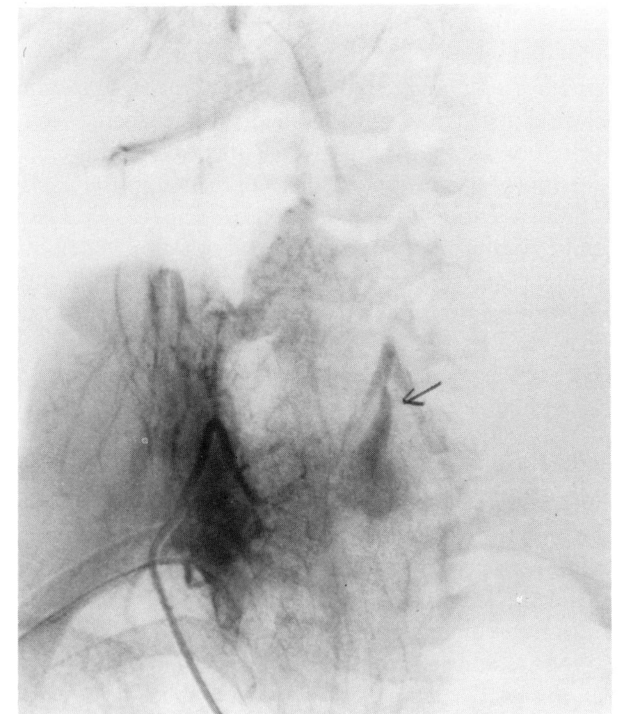

B

4. Right common jugular
5. Inferior thyroid
3. Left superior thyroid
1. Vertebral
2. Internal and external jugular

1. 42 pg/ml (11-24 pg/ml)
2. 45
3. 45
4. 48
5. 63
6. >35 (peripheral)

C

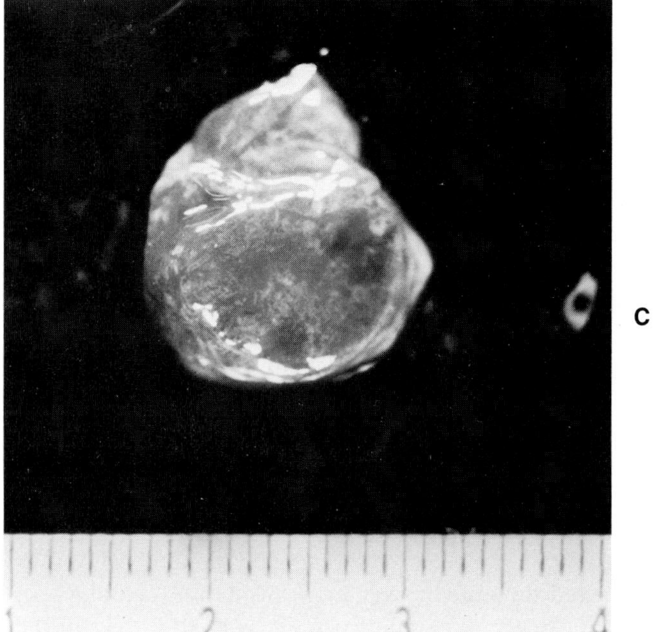

Fig. 56-16. After initial failure to locate an adenoma, arteriography demonstrated a tumor blush not well distinguished from thyroid **(A)**, but venous sampling of parathormone added other hypersecretion information shown on this localizing map **(B)**, with the adenoma identified and excised on reoperation **(C)**.

A B

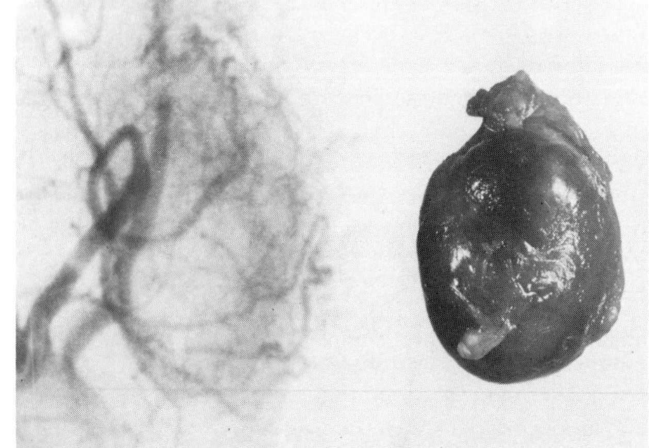

Fig. 56-17. A patient referred for persistent hypercalcemia was studied arteriographically, with demonstration of a large tumor blush **(A);** the adenoma **(B)** thus shown was excised by reoperation.

phy.[41] Arteriography can localize adenoma by the pattern of neovascularity and "tumor blush" for surgical retrieval in the patient at less risk or may serve as an alternative to sternotomy in the patient who has an internal thoracic arterial supply to a mediastinal adenoma causing persistent symptomatic hypercalcemia. A series of patients with mediastinal adenoma is presented in Figs. 56-18 to 56-20, illustrating the appropriate application of cervical retrieval, mediastinotomy, and transcatheter ablation with arteriographic indications for treatment.

Additional Localization Studies

Additional localization studies include primary studies such as thyroid scan to detect intrathyroidal filling defects. The same information might be obtained from sonography or CT scan, or by sestamibi or thalium-technetium subtraction study, but any one of those tests might be indicated by the suspicion raised by preliminary findings on thyroid scan conclusions. No patient should undergo all

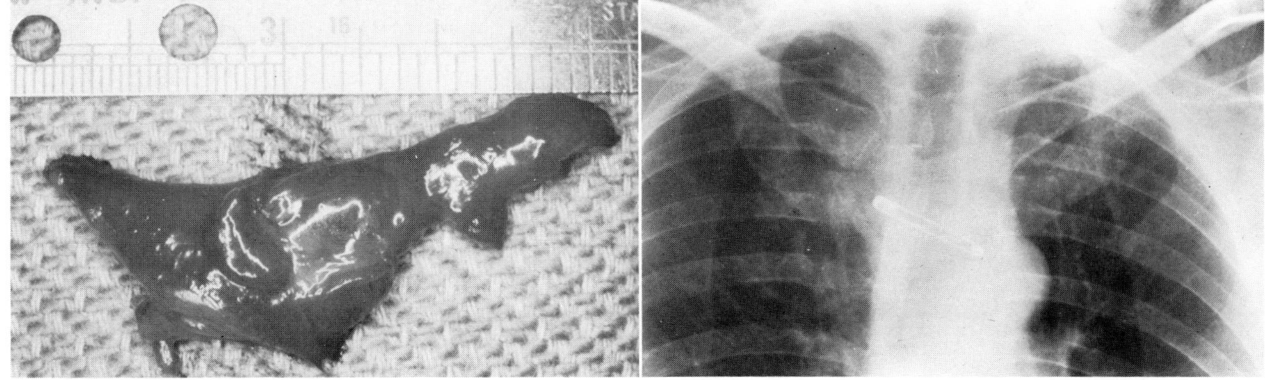

Fig. 56-18. Three glands were found in the normal parathyroid positions, but the fourth was found by diligent search at the time of primary operation and delivered from the anterior mediastinum. Found within the substance of the thymus **(A)**, the location of this adenoma is suggested before operation on the chest x-ray film **(B)** by the metallic clip that had been placed before teasing it up through the cervical incision. (Patient previously demonstrated in Geelhoed GW, Doppman JL. Embolization of ectopic parathyroid adenomas: A percutaneous treatment of hyperparathyroidism. Am Surg 114:71, 1978.)

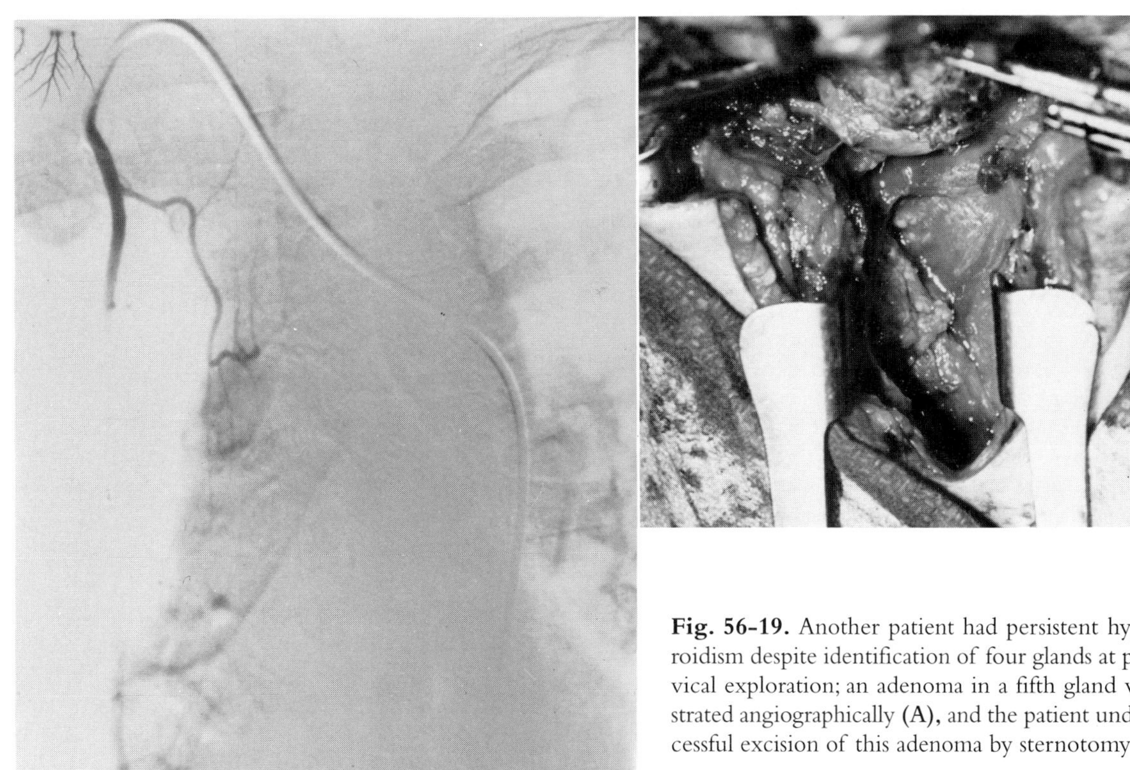

Fig. 56-19. Another patient had persistent hyperparathyroidism despite identification of four glands at primary cervical exploration; an adenoma in a fifth gland was demonstrated angiographically **(A)**, and the patient underwent successful excision of this adenoma by sternotomy **(B)**.

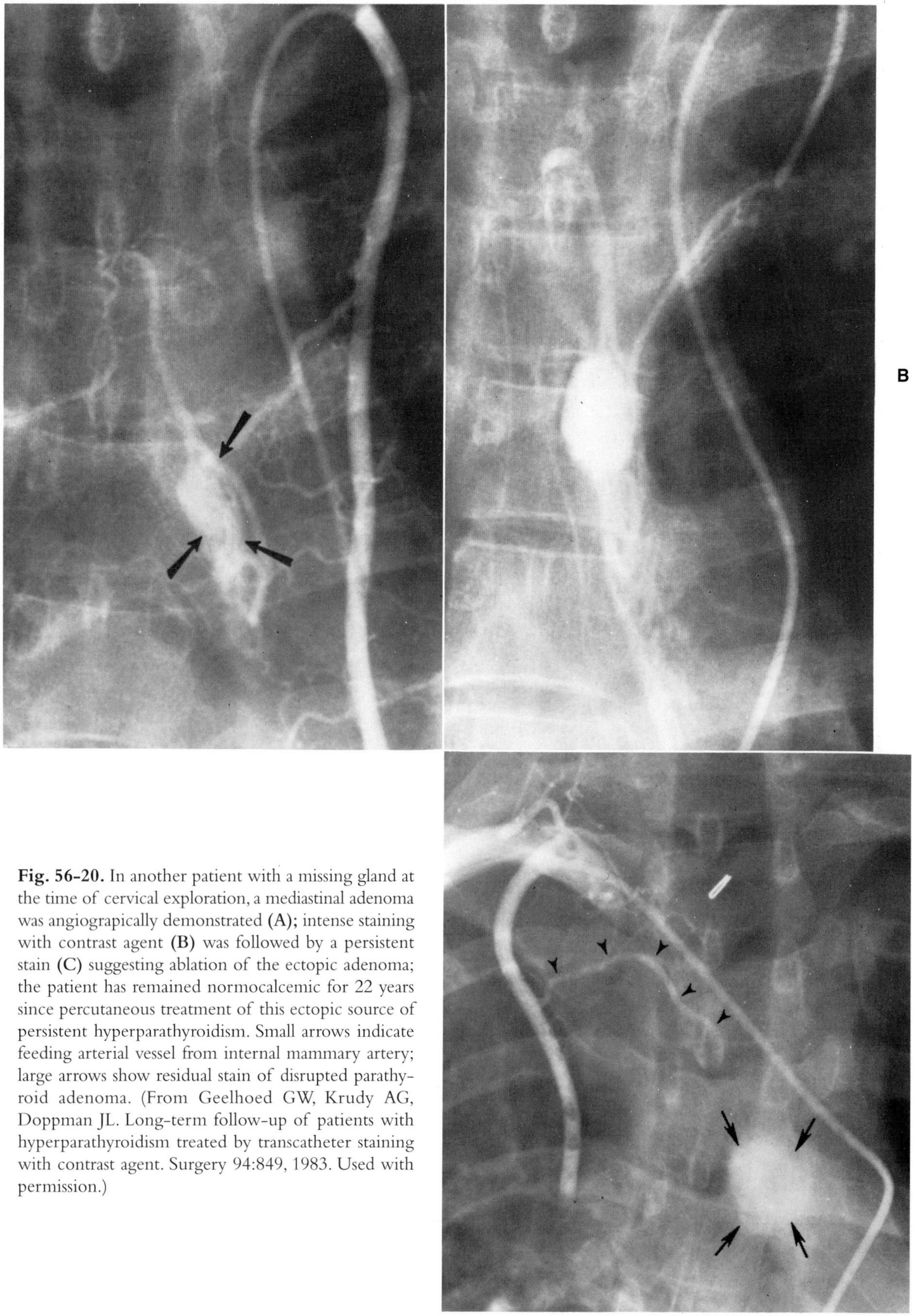

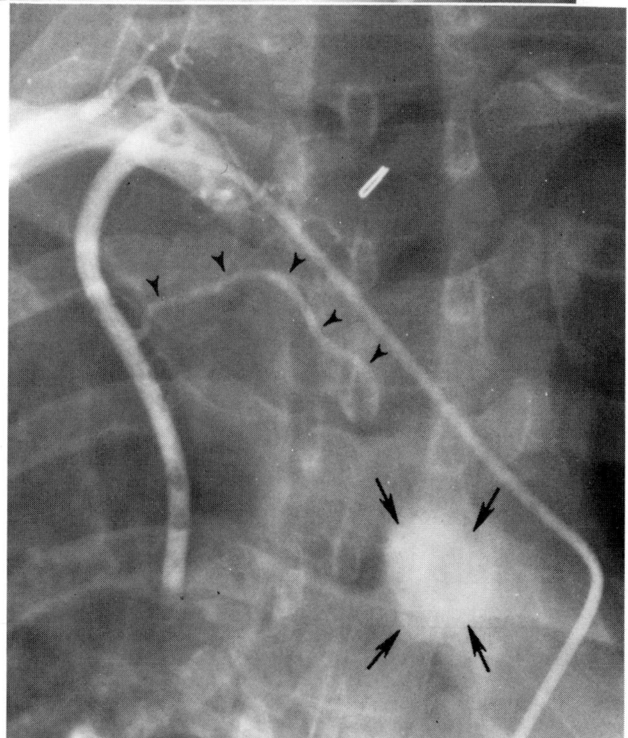

Fig. 56-20. In another patient with a missing gland at the time of cervical exploration, a mediastinal adenoma was angiograpically demonstrated **(A)**; intense staining with contrast agent **(B)** was followed by a persistent stain **(C)** suggesting ablation of the ectopic adenoma; the patient has remained normocalcemic for 22 years since percutaneous treatment of this ectopic source of persistent hyperparathyroidism. Small arrows indicate feeding arterial vessel from internal mammary artery; large arrows show residual stain of disrupted parathyroid adenoma. (From Geelhoed GW, Krudy AG, Doppman JL. Long-term follow-up of patients with hyperparathyroidism treated by transcatheter staining with contrast agent. Surgery 94:849, 1983. Used with permission.)

PARATHYROID LOCALIZATION STUDIES

Before Operation

Physical examination of neck (±, low yield)
Sonography (not required before operation, special equipment and expertise required)

Primary

Surgical exploration of all glands by experienced surgeon (intraoperative staining)
Surgical pathology consultation: touch-preparation cytology, frozen-section histology

Reoperation

Thyroid scan—filling defects

1. Sonogram (small-parts, real-time, 10 mHz, operator-dependent)
2. Sestamibi parathyroid scanning
3. Thallium-technetium scan (reliability variable)
4. CT with contrast study
5. Fine-needle aspiration—cytology, immunoperoxidase PTH staining
6. Venous sampling—PTH lateralizing—form/function correlation
7. Digital-subtraction angiography
8. Selective arteriography

the localization studies listed in the accompanying box; each should undergo only those with highest yield used in series until a positive test result is achieved in a patient in whom the diagnosis of primary hyperparathyroidism remains undisputed.

Before the application of these localization studies, and certainly before the reoperation, they indicate that the patient should undergo biochemical testing to differentiate FHH or other nonparathyroid sources of hypercalcemia. One would probably not use multiple localization studies if reoperation were not anticipated or acceptable to the patient. The one exception to this rule might be parathyroid-selective arteriography, which can serve an additional role in addition to localization technique and may be used as a percutaneous treatment for persistent hyperparathyroidism in a selected group of ectopic parathyroid adenomas.[41]

Special Considerations in the Treatment of Unusual Hyperparathyroidism

Reoperation or Extension of Primary Cervical Operation Techniques

For a persistent hyperparathyroidism caused by a cervical adenoma, arteriography as seen in Fig. 56-17 demonstrated the lesion, and reoperation was directed at the excision of this demonstrated mass. The reoperation differs from a primary cervical parathyroid exploration. In this instance exploration was not intended to identify all sites of parathyroid tissue in virgin tissue planes, but rather to provide a primary excision of a demonstrated mass through the preoperative application of these radiologic localization techniques. Often, reoperation may be at risk for removing the last functioning, albeit hyperfunctioning, parathyroid tissue. The risk of postoperative hypoparathyroidism is consequently increased, and preserving some of the excised parathyroid tissue may have some purpose should the patient require it for later transplantation.

Mediastinal adenoma. Ectopic parathyroid adenomas may be managed differently according to the origin of their arterial blood supply. Examples of three different methods of managing mediastinal adenomas can be seen in the three cases illustrated in Figs. 56-18 to 56-20.

In the first patient (see Fig. 56-18), careful primary cervical exploration revealed three glands in the normal parathyroid locations. When the left inferior parathyroid gland was not found in the usual cervical areas searched, a suspect branch of the inferior thyroid artery was traced down into the superior mediastinum. With careful blunt dissection, a digital plane was developed past the manubrium, down to the level of the gladiolus. At the level of the third intercostal space, a small mass was palpable at the tip of the thymic remnant. After passing a metallic ligating clip down this retrosternal space by a right-angle clip applier, the surgeon teased this thymic remnant into the neck and excised it. This thymic remnant contained the missing fourth gland (see Fig. 56-18, *A*), and the histologic examination confirmed the fourth gland as the adenoma. After operation, the patient had a transient hypocalcemia not requiring treatment; he has remained normocalcemic for the subsequent 20 years since the operation. The mediastinal location of this adenoma retrieved through the cervical approach is proved by the postoperative chest x-ray film (see Fig. 56-18, *B*), which reveals the location of the metallic clip placed just below the adenoma when it was in situ.

Cervical exploration was carried out in another patient who had urinary calculi and unquestioned primary hyperparathyroidism on repeated biochemical analysis (see Fig. 56-19). The cervical exploration was performed carefully, with the identification of four parathyroid glands in the usual locations; however, nothing was unusual about these four glands on histologic examination, except for some degree of hypocellularity. A careful but limited submanubrial exploration was unrevealing. When the patient's hypercalcemia persisted after the operation, selective arteriography demonstrated a fifth parathyroid gland in the mediastinum that was enlarged in the arteriographic blush (see Fig. 56-19, *A*). On the patient's request, sternotomy to excise the demonstrated adenoma was carried out (see Fig. 56-19, *B*), with a successful long-term cure of the hyperparathyroidism caused by this fifth-gland ectopic parathyroid adenoma.

In another patient with hyperparathyroidism, initial cervical exploration revealed three normal parathyroid glands (see Fig. 56-20). When hyperparathyroidism persisted, she underwent selective arteriography, which showed no abnormalities in the neck. However, by injection of internal thoracic arterial supply, a tumor blush was seen deep in the mediastinum (see Fig. 56-20, *A*). This patient's request for an attempt at percutaneous ablation through transcatheter contrast staining was carried out, with the intense staining noted immediately after injection (see Fig. 56-20, *B*). This adenoma staining was persistent for several hours after the arteriogram (see Fig. 56-20, *C*), and the patient had immediate hypocalcemia, such as occurs after successful ablation of a parathyroid adenoma. Her calcium balance returned to normal, and she has been followed up for 22 years since this percutaneous treatment, with normal parathormone and calcium values.

Transplantation of the parathyroid glands. In some instances of thyroid or parathyroid operation, a normal parathyroid gland may become dislodged, or its arterial blood supply may be interrupted. A normal parathyroid gland should not be discarded, even though the remaining parathyroid tissues should have reserves sufficient to sustain a normal calcium balance. The parathyroid gland may be minced and implanted in the strap muscles at the site of the primary incision. However, one would not wish to implant presumably autonomous parathyroid tissue, but rather to excise this completely, to avoid recurrent hyperparathyroidism at a later date.

In secondary hyperparathyroidism, the glands are hyperplastic but responsive to the stimuli that gave rise to the secondary hyperparathyroidism in the first place. If that hypocalcemic and hyperphosphatemic stimulus should be resolved, such as through successful kidney transplantation, such hyperplastic parathyroid tissue would regress to normal function in autoregulatory control. If, during the course of the patient's renal failure, operation for secondary hyperparathyroidism were carried out, total parathyroidectomy might be followed by hypoparathyroidism when kidney function is restored. In consequence, the tissue excised might be preserved and retain cell viability by the same techniques of cryopreservation used in blood-banking of frozen blood cells by means of slow-freeze techniques. Small portions of these glands may be transplanted into the forearm of the patient at a later date, should the patient require this form of support for persistent hypocalcemia on vitamin D and calcium supplementation later. It should be noted that autonomous tissue may hyperfunction in whatever site it is implanted.[16] Routine parathyroid excision and autotransplantation should be discouraged, because occasionally patients are seen who have an "unnatural disease" (hyperparathyroidism originating from the neck and arm). Parathyroid tissue transplanted into the forearm is more easily measured by parathormone arteriovenous differences across the implantation site and can also be retrieved by a simple procedure performed with local anesthesia. However, implantation of autonomous hyperfunctioning parathyroid tissue is better prevented than treated, and the determination of autonomy can be made by in vitro study.

If the tissue culture of the excised hyperplastic parathyroid tissue produces parathormone in a calcium-poor milieu but no parathormone is produced in calcium-rich culture medium, the parathyroid tissue seems to be normally responsive in sensing the ionized calcium at the appropriate "set-point." Such responsive parathyroid tissue might be successfully implanted, and the patient would be judged to have uncomplicated secondary hyperparathyroidism. However, if the tissue culture of this hyperplastic parathyroid tissue produces parathormone at all levels of physiologically attainable calcium and is not inhibited by tissue culture milieu that replicate conditions of hypercalcemia, recurrence of the hyperparathyroidism could be expected. Such patients should be maintained on vitamin D and calcium supplementation as management for their hypocalcemia after successful transplantation. Such patients might be candidates for either recombinant DNA–produced human PTH administration or parathyroid allografting[5] if similar study in tissue culture were to prove a compatible donor with appropriate response to varied calcium concentrations. Transplantation of hyperplastic parathyroid tissue should not be undertaken in patients with familial hyperparathyroidism, because the genetic defect that changed the "set-point" of the calcium-sensors would presumably be abnormal in all parathyroid cells. The same caveat should be followed with any presumably autonomous adenoma, with the additional risk that parathyroid carcinoma might be transplanted because it is poorly distinguished from adenoma by histologic criteria.

Hyperparathyroidism in Multiple Endocrine Adenopathy

As a nearly invariable rule, hyperparathyroidism as part of MEA is caused by multiple gland disease. The genetic defect carried in all parathyroid cells makes identification of all parathyroid glands and their subtotal excision a requirement of parathyroid operation. Generally, the patients are more likely to have symptomatic hypocalcemia after the operation than is the case with the excision of a sporadic parathyroid adenoma. Hyperparathyroidism is more likely to recur in these patients as well than in those with the primary hyperparathyroidism caused by parathyroid hyperplasia in sporadic cases.

In MEA I, hyperparathyroidism is often the earliest feature of the endocrinopathy and is frequently symptomatic. Moreover, hypercalcemia is a strong stimulus to gastrin release and the hyperacidity that may follow. For that reason, the first attack on the endocrine abnormalities in MEA I is cervical, first correcting hyperparathyroidism. In some instances, patients with MEA I have a decrease in serum gastrin level and even regression of the pancreatic islet abnormalities, at least transiently, after successful treatment of the hyperparathyroidism.[19]

In MEA II, the life-threatening abnormality is the pheochromocytoma that may be present. Under no circumstances should the coincidental hyperparathyroidism be approached until the much more significant threat of catecholamine excess has been controlled. Whereas the cervical surgical approach to correct primary hyperparathyroidism is the first priority in MEA I, the hyperparathyroidism is the *last* priority in MEA II. The physiologic threat of pheochromocytoma takes priority over the oncologic importance of medullary thyroid carcinoma, the primary reason for the cervical exploration. At the time of the total thyroidectomy for medullary thyroid carcinoma, the parathyroid glands can be inspected and reduced as appropriate to the hyperparathyroidism the patient exhibits.

Hyperparathyroidism in Pregnancy

Normal pregnancy is a time of large changes in calcium metabolism, when more than 30 g calcium must be transferred across the placenta into the fetal skeleton. Parathormone, however, does not cross the placenta. Fetal calcium requirements are met, regardless of calcium intake or demineralization in the maternal skeleton, particularly if hyperparathyroidism is associated with pregnancy. Maternal hyperparathyroidism, however, is associated with a high rate of fetal wastage.[42] If hyperparathyroidism is symptomatic, surgical treatment should be carried out during pregnancy. In the pregnant patient with asymptomatic hypercalcemia, parathyroid exploration can be postponed until after delivery as long as there is careful monitoring to prevent the loss of the pregnancy. Management of hypercalcemia in the pregnant patient can include hydration and diuretics, but administration of cytoxic drugs such as plicamycin is precluded.

The effect on the fetus of maternal hyperparathyroidism is not apparent in utero. When the fetus is separated from the maternal circulation, however, the resulting hypoparathyroidism may be exhibited as irritability or tetany. Vitamin D and calcium are required for treatment of an infant born of a hypercalcemic mother. The vitamin D and calcium must be carefully tapered to avoid prolonging the suppression of the infant's parathyroid glands. Hypoparathyroidism should be anticipated in the fetus born to a hyperparathyroid mother. On rare occasions, neonatal tetany has been the presenting sign of previously undiagnosed maternal hyperparathyroidism.

Results of Treatment of Hyperparathyroidism

After excision of single gland disease in primary hyperparathyroidism when primary cervical operation reveals the normal or suppressed parathyroid glands, fewer than 1% of patients have late recurrence of hyperparathyroidism. However, persistent hyperparathyroidism occurs in approximately 5% of treated patients, usually on the basis of multiple gland disease not appreciated or inadequately reduced at the time of the primary cervical procedure.

The success rate of control of hyperparathyroidism treated by reoperation is much lower than the success rate of the initial operation, depending on the nature of the disease that gave rise to the persistence of hypercalcemia. In multiple gland involvement, both persistence and recurrence of hypercalcemia are higher after both primary operation and reoperation than for the sporadic incidence of single gland disease.

The recurrence rate is highest among patients who have a familial occurrence of multiple gland disease or who still have parathyroid stimulation, as from the persistence of azotemia managed by dialysis but with persistent hyperphosphatemia.

For most patients with persistent hypercalcemia, if this disorder is not caused by some nonparathyroid problem, such as FHH, the source is probably a single diseased parathyroid, most often overlooked in some ectopic location in the neck. For satisfactory treatment of persistent hypercalcemia, preoperative localization studies that precede reoperation can aid in the often difficult dissection that occurs in areas of the scarring of previous operation.

Hypercalcemia should always be investigated. If the hypercalcemia is caused by primary hyperparathyroidism, treatment is satisfying, with the usual identification of a solitary adenoma, the excision of which is curative. The vast majority of patients so treated retain normal calcium homeostasis in long-term follow-up.

SUMMARY

Calcium and phosphorus are critical components of metabolic systems. Intricate control systems exist in the body, especially to maintain serum ionized calcium levels within a narrow range on which neuromuscular excitation, contraction, and relaxation depend. Sites of calcium regulation include absorption from the gut, resorption from large reservoirs in bone, and excretion by the kidney.

The parathyroid glands are both ionized calcium sensors and the effectors of normal calcium homeostasis through the role of parathormone is controlling bone resorption and renal excretion of calcium. Other factors involved in calcium balance include ions (phosphate, chloride, hydrogen, and magnesium), buffers (albumin and chelators), and other hormones (vitamin D, thyroxine, calcitonin, corticosterioids, catecholamines, and malignancy-associated paraendocrine products).

Hypocalcemia is the result of inadequate intake of calcium, vitamin D precursors, magnesium, or protein, or of failure of absorption from the gut or unopposed excretion from lack of vitamin D or parathormone secretion. Consequences of hypocalcemia include irritability and tetany, and careful replacement of the inadequate hormone or mineral substrates is used in short- and long-term treatment.

Hypercalcemia arises from a number of causes. These include excess calcium, vitamin, or drug ingestion; mobilization of calcium from bones or blocked renal excretion; and primary hypersecretion of parathormone.

Primary hyperparathyroidism may be differentiated from other causes of hypercalcemia by study of the mineral metabolites and hormone assay. Most patients with primary hyperparathyroidism have no symptoms when first discovered by multiphasic biochemical screening tests, but hypercalcemia may give rise to a variety of symptoms from loss of organ reserves, obtundation, seizures, coma, and death. Acutely elevated serum calcium level may be safely lowered by a series of medical means, but its cause must be determined and differentiated for further recommendations on fixing the underlying source. Cervical exploration is usually a successful model of locating and correcting primary hyperparathyroidism, often by excision of an autonomously hyperfunctioning single gland source.

Special consideration is given persistent or recurrent hyperparathyroidism and that associated with hereditary syndromes or pregnancy. Reconfirmation of the primary hyperparathyroidism diagnosis is often followed by radiologic localization techniques before reoperation for persistent parathyroid problems, often stemming from hyperfunctioning multiple, supernumerary, or ectopic glands.

Hypercalcemia as a finding in patient screening always warrants investigation, because it represents an abnormality in view of the sensitive control systems for calcium homeostasis. If caused by malignancy, this discovery is valuable in prognosis. If caused by primary hyperparathyroidism, successful parathyroid correction is achieved in most patients who undergo operation, which restores calcium metabolism to delicate intrinsic autoregulatory balance.

REFERENCES

1. Zaloga GP, Chernow B. Calcium metabolism. In Geelhoed GW, Chernow B, eds. Endocrine Aspects of Acute Illness, Clinics in Critical Care Medicine. New York: Churchill Livingstone, 1985.
2. Chester WL, Zaloga GP, Chernow B. Phosphate problems in the critically ill patient. In Geelhoed GW, Chernow B, eds. Endocrine Aspects of Acute Illness, Clinics in Critical Care Medicine. New York: Churchill Livingstone, 1985.
3. Keller V, Berger W. Prevention of hypophosphatemia by phosphate infusion and during treatment of diabetic ketoacidosis and hyperosmolar coma. Diabetes 29:87, 1980.
4. Stern JN, Smith WD, Ginn HE. Hypophosphatemia in acute alcoholism. Am J Med Sci 252:78, 1968.
5. Potts JT. Mineral ion homeostasis and its control. Part II, Harvard Medical School pathophysiology course outline musculoskeletal section, 1982.
6. Parfitt AM, et al. Hypercalcemia due to constitutive activity of parathyroid hormone (PTH)/PTH-related peptide receptor: Comparison with primary hyperparathyroidism. J Clin Endocrinol Metab 81:3584, 1996.
7. Bundred NJ, Walls J, Ratcliffe WA. Parathyroid hormone-related protein, bone metastases and hypercalcemia of malignancy. Ann R Coll Surg Engl 78:354, 1996.
8. Habener JF, Potts JT. Biosynthesis of parathyroid hormone. N Engl J Med 299:580, 1978.
9. Spiegel AM, Marx SJ. Parathyroid hormone and vitamin D receptors. J Clin Endocrinol Metab 12:221, 1983.
10. El-Sonbathy MR, Abdul-Ghaffar WA. Vitamin D deficiency in veiled Kuwaiti women. Eur J Clin Nutr 50:315, 1996.
11. Becker KL, et al. The pathophysiology of pulmonary calcitonin. In Becker KL, Gazdar AF, eds. The Endocrine Lung in Health and Disease. Philadelphia: WB Saunders, 1984.
12. Mundy GR, et al. Direct stimulation of bone resorption by thyroid hormones. J Clin Invest 58:529, 1976.
13. Chernow B, Zaloga GP. Ions for society members, SCCM. In Schoemaker WC, ed. Critical Care State of the Art, vol 5. Fullerton, Calif.: Society of Critical Care Medicine, 1984.
14. Mundy GR, et al. Evidence for the secretion of an osteoclast stimulating factor in myeloma. N Engl J Med 291:1041, 1974.
15. Wells SA, et al. Transplantation of the parathyroid glands: Current status. Surg Clin North Am 591:167, 1979.
16. Brennan MF, et al. Recurrent hyperparathyroidism from an autotransplanted parathyroid adenoma. N Engl J Med 299:1057, 1978.
17. Perry HM 3rd, et al. Aging and bone metabolism in African-American and Caucasian women. J Clin Endocrinol Metab 81:1108, 1996.
18. Peskin GW, Greenburg AG, Saik RP. Expanding indications for early parathyroidectomy in the elderly female. Am J Surg 136:45, 1978.
19. Geelhoed GW. Problem Management in Endocrine Surgery. Chicago: Year Book Medical Publishers, 1983.
20. Yeager RM, Krementz ET. Acute hyperparathyroidism. South Med J 69:797, 1971.
21. Scholz DA, Purnell DC. Asymptomatic primary hyperparathyroidism—10 year prospective study. Mayo Clin Proc 56:473, 1981.
22. Marx SJ, et al. The hypocalciuric or benign variant of familial hypercalcemia: Clinical and biochemical features in fifteen kindreds. Medicine 60:397, 1981.
23. Carroll PR, Clark OH. The milk-alkali syndrome: Does it exist and can it be differentiated from primary hyperparathyroidism? Ann Surg 197:427, 1983.
24. Clark OH, Way LW. The hypercalcemic syndrome: Hyperparathyroidism. In Faissen SR, ed. Surgical Endocrinology: Clinical Syndromes. Philadelphia: JB Lippincott, 1978.
25. Benson RC Jr, et al. Immunoreactive forms of circulating parathyroid hormone in primary and ectopic hyperparathyroidism. J Clin Invest 59:175, 1974.
26. Molinari AS, et al. Incidence of multi-glandular disease in primary hyperparathyroidism determined by parathyroid hormone secretion. Surgery 120:934, 1996.
27. Brown EM, et al. Calcium regulated parathyroid hormone release in primary hyperparathyroidism. Am J Med 66:923, 1979.
28. Geelhoed GW, Silverberg SA. Intraoperative imprints for the identification of parathyroid tissue. Surgery 96:1124, 1984.
29. Pickleman JR, et al. Thiazide-induced parathyroid stimulation. Metabolism 18:867, 1969.
30. Prinz RA, et al. Radiation-associated hyperparathyroidism: A new syndrome? Surgery 82:296, 1977.
31. Tisell LE, et al. Hyperparathyroidism in persons treated with x-rays for tuberculous cervical adenitis. Cancer 40:846, 1977.
32. Castleman B, Schantz A, Roth SI. Parathyroid hyperplasia in primary hyperparathyroidism. Cancer 38:1668, 1976.
33. Cope O, et al. Primary chief cell hyperplasia of the parathyroid gland: A new entity in the surgery of hyperparathyroidism. Ann Surg 148:375, 1958.
34. Rasbach DA, et al. Solitary parathyroid microadenoma. Surgery 96:1092, 1984.
35. Kay S, Hume DM. Carcinoma of the parathyroid glands. Arch Pathol 96:316, 1973.
36. Geelhoed GW, Doppman JL. Embolization of ectopic parathyroid adenomas: A percutaneous treatment of hyperparathyroidism. Am Surg 44:71, 1978.
37. Ferlin C, et al. New perspectives in localizing enlarged parathyroids by technetium-thallium subtraction scan. J Nucl Med 24:438, 1983.

38. Rauth JD, et al. Comparison of Tc-99m MIBI and T1-201/Tc-99m pertechnetate for diagnosis of primary hyperparathyroidism. Clin Nucl Med 21:602, 1996.
39. Malhotra A, et al. Preoperative parathyroid localization with sestamibi. Am J Surg 172:637, 1996.
40. Martin D, Rosen IB, Ichise M. Evaluation of single isotope technetium 99m–sestamibi in localization efficiency for hyperparathyroidism. Am J Surg 172:633, 1996.
41. Geelhoed GW, Krudy AG, Doppman JL. Long-term follow-up of patients with hyperparathyroidism treated by transcatheter staining with contrast agent. Surgery 94:849, 1983.
42. Geelhoed GW. Surgery of the endocrine glands in pregnancy. Clin Obstet Gynecol 26:865, 1983.

57

Pituitary Dysfunction

Gunwant Mallik, Benjamin C. Ling, and Michael E. Miner

The skeleton of Hunter's giant, O'Bryan, is now more than 200 years old, but it still provides one of the first clear evidences of the clinicopathologic correlation between pituitary pathology and systemic hormonal effects.[1] Dr. Hunter believed that giantism was caused by a tumor of the pituitary. Despite O'Bryan's strenuous objections, the enlarged sella turcica and the skeleton of Hunter's giant can be found in the museum of the Royal College of Surgeons.[2] Although this is not the first recognition of the role of pituitary gland dysfunction as a cause of human disease, it remains one of the most dramatic early observations.

The history of the notions concerning pituitary dysfunction have enticed some of the leading minds in medicine for the past century.[3] Marie's detailed observations and naming of the syndrome of acromegaly in 1886,[4] the report by Babinski[5] in 1900 of what was to become Fröhlich's hypopituitarism syndrome, and description by Cushing[6] in 1933 of the syndrome that bears his name witness to the rapid explosion of knowledge concerning the pathologic manifestations of pituitary tumors that occurred during the early part of the twentieth century. Throughout the same time period, other conditions affecting pituitary function were also being described. Simmons' patient with polyuria secondary to metastatic breast cancer of the pituitary gland[6] and Frank's patient who developed diabetes insipidus and other signs of hypopituitarism after a gunshot wound to the sella[7] were early evidence that pituitary function could be influenced by conditions other than tumors.

No sooner were the diagnoses being made of pituitary and parasellar tumors than surgeons devised approaches to treat them.[1] Sir Victor Horsley exposed the pituitary gland to excise a tumor as early as 1889.[4] By 1907 Schloffer had recorded the first transsphenoidal approach to the pituitary gland, followed 2 years later by Gramengas' report of a prompt but brief remission of acromegalic symptoms following x-ray treatment.[1,4] However, it was Cushing who brought together the clinically relevant data and demonstrated that sellar and parasellar tumors could be routinely approached with safety. His monumental work on both the treatment and physiology of pituitary disorders still stands as classic medical literature.[6,8] The past 20 years have witnessed another information explosion, extending knowledge of hormone control systems, interaction, and medical regimens to treat pituitary dysfunction.

ANATOMY OF THE PITUITARY GLAND

The pituitary gland weighs approximately 525 mg. It is significantly larger in females than males and grows even larger during pregnancy. It is approximately 5 mm in height, 10 to 14 mm in width, and 10 mm in depth. It is confined on its anterior, posterior, and inferior surfaces by the sella turcica, a bony depression in the sphenoid bone. Immediately below the sella is the sphenoidal air sinus, and lying lateral to it are the cavernous venous sinuses. Within each trabeculated cavernous sinus are the carotid artery (Fig. 57-1), the oculomotor nerves, trochlear nerve, abducent nerve, and the first two major divisions of the trigeminal nerve. The dura mater that lines the sella forms an incomplete diaphragm above the pituitary gland, through which traverses the pituitary stalk from the median eminence of the hypothalamus, the portal veins, and the superior hypophysial artery (Fig. 57-2). The arterial supply to the pituitary gland and infundibulum is through branches of the superior and inferior hypophysial arteries that are direct tributaries of the carotid artery. Venous drainage is through a series of veins that directly connect to the dural venous sinuses. The optic chiasm is immediately anterior to the stalk of the pituitary gland, and the tip of the basilar artery lies in close proximity posteriorly to the sellar diaphragm. The arachnoid membrane does not normally enter through the diaphragm but lies immediately above it. A pouch of arachnoid may herniate into the sella and compress the pituitary gland, resulting in an "empty sella."[9-11] Unlike the brain itself, the pituitary gland is devoid of a blood-brain barrier.

Within 1 cm of the pituitary gland lies a portion of half of all the cranial nerves, the entire blood supply of the cerebral hemispheres, the cavernous sinuses, the hypothal-

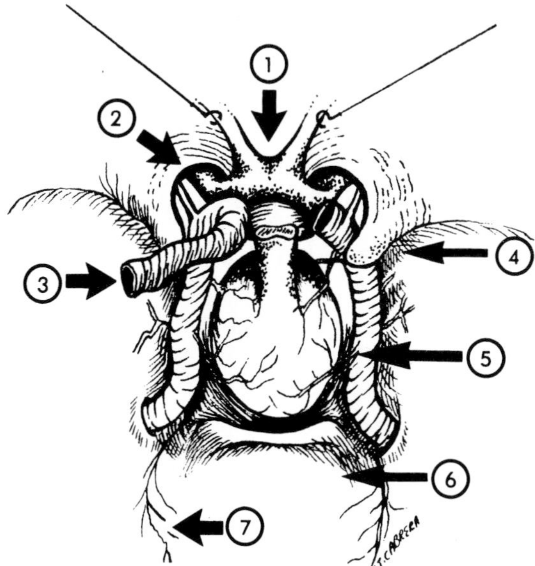

Fig. 57-1. Anatomy of the sellar region. Optic tracts attracted anteriorly to demonstrate the relationship between the optic chiasm and foramen, pituitary gland and stalk, carotid arteries, and bony confines of the pituitary gland. *1,* Optic tracts; *2,* optic foramen; *3,* internal carotid arteries; *4,* anterior clinoid processes; *5,* meningeal-hypophysial vessels; *6,* dorsum sellae; and *7,* tentorial vessels.

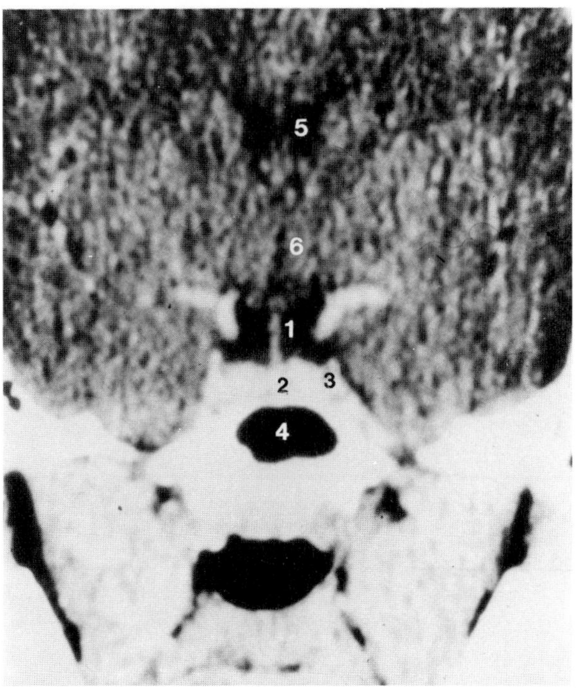

Fig. 57-2. Coronal computed tomogram demonstrating the normal relationship between the pituitary stalk *(1),* pituitary gland *(2),* both internal carotid arteries *(3),* and the sphenoidal air sinuses *(4).* Note the lateral *(5)* and third *(6)* ventricles superior to the pituitary gland.

amus, the brain stem, the cerebrospinal fluid (CSF), a paranasal air sinus, and the nasopharynx. Thus it should not be surprising that abnormalities of the pituitary gland might well affect these structures or that a wide variety of lesions involving those structures should secondarily affect pituitary function.

EMBRYOLOGY OF THE PITUITARY GLAND

Two separate ectodermal sources combine embryologically to form the pituitary gland. A hollow invagination of oral pharyngeal epithelium extends dorsally to form Rathke's pouch, which then separates from the tissue of origin to form the adenohypophysis. In contrast, the neurohypophysis is a downward extension from the diencephalon of the brain. Therefore the neurohypophysis is a direct extension of the central nervous system, which is directly linked to two sets of hypothalamic nuclei (i.e., the supraoptic and paraventricular nuclei). On the other hand, the adenohypophysis is not in anatomic connection with the central nervous system but maintains communication with the hypothalamus by means of the portal venous system, through which blood flows from the hypothalamus along the pituitary stalk toward the adenohypophysis. This portal blood carries regulatory hormones from the hypothalamus to the adenohypophysis. Thus both the adenohypophysis and neurohypophysis are in close communication with the hypothalamus. An ever-growing literature on hypothalamic pituitary "cross-talk" indicates that physiologically the system should be thought of as a highly dependent one with multiple feedback loops (i.e., the hypothalamohypophysial system) (Figs. 57-3 and 57-4).

PITUITARY FUNCTION

The function of the hypothalamophypophysial system is to manufacture, store, and control the release of the eight known pituitary hormones. Even though the pituitary gland can be viewed as a single endocrine organ, for purposes of understanding its function it is more fruitful to consider it as two independent organs that have subtle but important interactions (see Fig. 57-3).

The site of production of the pituitary hormones of the posterior gland is in the hypothalamic nuclei. The supraoptic and paraventricular nuclei appear to manufacture these polypeptide hormones, which are then released in the neurohypophysis.[9-11] The anterior pituitary hormones, on the other hand, are manufactured in the adenohypophysis, but their release into the blood stream is under the influence of releasing and inhibiting hormones that arrive by means of the hypophysial portal venous system. Thus the release of hormones from both the adenohypophysis and neurohypophysis is controlled by the hypothalamus, but the mechanisms underlying this control are quite different. Furthermore, the structure of the hormones of the adenohypophysis and the neurohypophysis are strikingly different (see Fig. 57-4). The interaction between the pituitary hormones and their releasing and in-

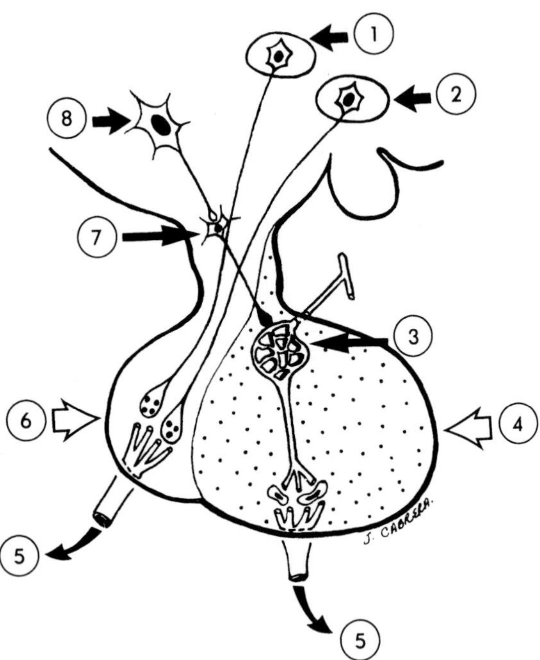

Fig. 57-3. Schematic representation of hypothalamohypophysial vascular and neuronal relationships. Hormones manufactured in neurons of the paraventricular and supraoptic hypothalamic nuclei are released in the posterior lobe of the pituitary gland (neurohypophysis). Monoaminergic neurons produce releasing and inhibiting hormones to be released into the portal veins to control the secretion of anterior pituitary (adenohypophysis) hormones. *1,* Paraventricular nuclei; *2,* supraoptic nuclei of the hypothalamus; *3,* portal venous system; *4,* adenohypophysis; *5,* efferent vein to dural sinuses; *6,* neurohypophysis; *7,* tuberal infundibular neuron; and *8,* monoaminergic neuron.

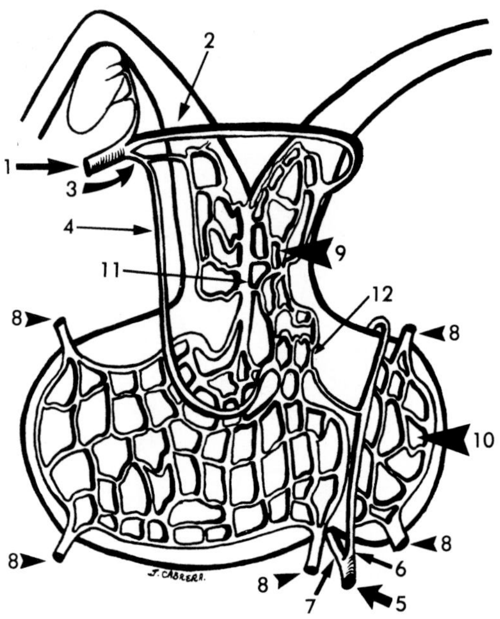

Fig. 57-4. Detailed schematic representation of the vascular supply to the pituitary gland. *1,* Superior hypophysial artery; *2,* posterior branch; *3,* anterior branch; *4,* artery of trabecula; *5,* inferior hypophysial artery; *6,* lateral branch; *7,* medial branch; *8,* efferent vein to dural sinus; *9,* primary portal system; *10,* secondary portal system; *11,* long hypophysial portal vein; and *12,* short hypophysial portal vein.

hibiting substances are the subject of exciting, ongoing investigation. Current evidence indicates that each of the right pituitary hormones is associated with a well-described clinical syndrome resulting either from its overproduction or absence.

Hormones of the Neurohypophysis

Antidiuretic hormone (ADH) and oxytocin are the two nonapeptide hormones of the neurohypophysis.[12] ADH is produced primarily in the supraoptic nuclei of the hypothalamus, whereas oxytocin is formed in the paraventricular nuclei. Although these hormones are produced in the hypothalamus, they are not simply transported down the axons to the neurohypophysis. Polypeptides that facilitate the transport of ADH and oxytocin are also produced in the hypothalamus. These polypeptides, called neurophysins, are released into the blood stream along with the active hormones at the level of the neurohypophysis with minimal storage in the neurohypophysis. Thus the neurohypophysis serves as little more than an immediate site for the release of ADH and oxytocin. The neurophysins appear to be taken up by the nerve terminals for another trip down the axon with new hormones. There are no known physiologic activities of the neurophysines other than to facilitate intracellular hormone transport.

Oxytocin primarily stimulates the uterus during labor and appears to play an integral part in normal delivery. In addition, it has a role in causing the alveolar cells of the mammary glands to constrict and thus aids with milk ejection. Although it has some antidiuretic activity, the effect appears to be quite minimal when compared to that of ADH.

ADH plays a major role in water metabolism.[13] Normally the kidneys form approximately 180 L of glomerular filtrate every day. Under the influence of ADH, more than 99% of this filtrate is resorbed in the nephrons, thus serving to conserve water. ADH appears to affect the renal tubular cells by interacting with receptors on the peritubular surface rather than by entering the cell per se. On the surface membrane ADH activates adenylate cyclase, which catalyzes the formation of cyclic adenosine monophosphate (cAMP) from adenosine triphosphate (ATP). cAMP activates protein kinases, which then phosphorylate specific membrane proteins that control the pore size of the luminal membrane in the nephron. When the size of the pores is changed, the flow characteristics of the membrane are altered, and the rate at which water flows from the tubular lumen into the cells of the tubular walls is controlled. ADH closely regulates water conservation, but it is certainly not the only mechanism important in renal water resorption.[14]

The release of ADH from the neurohypophysis is primarily directed by plasma osmoreceptors thought to be located in the supraoptic nuclei. As osmolality increases, the secretion of ADH also increases, and more water is reabsorbed from the renal ultrafiltrate back into the plasma, thereby decreasing osmolality. Accordingly, a decrease in plasma osmolality reduces or halts further release of ADH, which promotes excretion of water by the kidney. This negative feedback control system is physiologically well defined, even though the structure of the osmoreceptor has not been well demonstrated.

It has been observed that altering plasma volume also affects the release of ADH, independent of its effect on osmolality. A decrease in plasma volume results in the release of ADH and a subsequent increase in plasma volume secondary to increased water reabsorption by the kidney. Although it has been postulated that volume receptors initiating these ADH effects are located in the right atrium of the heart and that the afferent neural impulses are transmitted through the vagus nerve, such receptors have not been clearly identified.

Many well-known factors common to everyday experience influence ADH secretion.[15] Affect, mood, and anxiety clearly stimulate ADH secretion. Cholinergic and β-adrenergic stimulation increase ADH secretion, whereas α-adrenergic stimulation is inhibitory. Multiple pharmacologic agents, including nicotine, morphine, barbiturates, vincristine, and some tricyclic antidepressants, stimulate ADH secretion, whereas hydantoin, ethanol, and reserpine inhibit it. Although the final common pathway for ADH secretion is from the hypothalamus, there are clearly many other influences, both endogenous and exogenous, that modulate the secretion of this hormone.

Hormones of the Adenohypophysis

Three polypeptide hormones (i.e., growth hormone, prolactin, and adrenocorticotropic hormone [ACTH]) and three glycoprotein hormones (i.e., thyroid-stimulating hormone [TSH], follicle-stimulating hormone [FSH], and luteinizing hormone [LH]) are secreted by the adenohypophysis. In contrast to the neurohypophysis, hormones of the adenohypophysis are produced and stored in the gland before secretion, and the influence of the hypothalamus is purely one of regulating their release.

Two subunits of the glycoprotein hormones have been identified: α and β. Although neither of the subunits has been completely characterized, the α-subunits are exactly the same for TSH, FSH, and LH. However, the β-subunits are unique for each hormone and therefore confer the specificity to the hormone for a particular receptor site. The β-subunit does not possess biologic activity by itself and only becomes biologically active when coupled with the α-subunit. Thus these hormones function as though the receptor required both a general and a specific key to cause effect. In both males and females the glycoprotein TSH stimulates the production and secretion of thyroid hormone. In females FSH stimulates the maturation of ovarian follicles and the secretion of estrogens by those follicles. In males it stimulates development of testicular tubules and spermatogenesis. LH in the female induces ovulation and causes luteinization to develop in the mature ovarian follicle, with the subsequent production and secretion of progesterone. In males it stimulates the development of Leydig cells in the testes and the production and secretion of testosterone.

Of the polypeptide hormones, prolactin is the largest, consisting of 198 amino acid residues. In females it stimulates the growth of breast tissue and induces production and secretion of breast milk. In males the function of prolactin is less obvious, but it appears to be essential to normal spermatogenesis.[16] ACTH is a single-chain polypeptide composed of 39 amino acids. The primary function of ACTH is to cause the cortex of the adrenal gland to produce and secrete cortisol and other adrenal steroids. However, the adrenal cortical hormone, aldosterone, is a clear exception to this principle because it is primarily under the influence of renin and angiotensinogen.

Human growth hormone (hGH) is a polypeptide consisting of 191 amino acids, which, unlike the other pituitary hormones, has no specific target organ but has an effect on virtually all tissue. The growth resulting from hGH stimulation is not a direct effect but rather is induced by a group of substances known as somatomedins. These growth hormone–dependent polypeptides are thought to be produced in the liver and not in the pituitary gland.[17] Five different somatomedins have been identified, all of which stimulate growth in responsive tissues.

Hypothalamic Control of Adenohypophysial Hormone Secretion

For many years it was thought that hormone secretion by the anterior pituitary gland resulted in stimulation of a specific target organ. This target organ then released a second hormone. Thus the pituitary gland was thought to orchestrate the entire hormonal system by a straightforward series of independent negative feedback systems. For example, TSH stimulates the thyroid to release the hormones of the thyroid. The level of the secondary hormones (i.e., the thyroid hormones) is increased in the blood; this is detected by the pituitary gland, and TSH secretion is turned off by means of a simple negative feedback loop. However, the elegant work of Schally et al.[18] has clearly shown that the pituitary hormone control system is much more complex.[18,19] On the basis of their work, it is currently accepted that there are a series of releasing and inhibiting substances that are secreted by the hypothalamus into the hypophysial portal venous system. It is these substances that cause specific cells of the adenohypophysis to selectively secrete their distinctive hormones. There appears to be good evidence for a hypothalamic-releasing hormone for all the anterior pituitary hormones and an inhibiting substance for at least hGH and prolactin. This complex system is interactive in that (1) the releasing hormones may effect the release of further releasing hormone and, (2) although the releasing and inhibiting hormones are specific for the adenohypophysial hormones, they may not be totally selective. Stated another way, there appears to be some crossover of function between the various releasing hormones. All the releasing and inhibiting hormones characterized at this point consist of three or more amino acids.

A few of these releasing and inhibiting hormones have also been found in other areas of the brain and in sites outside of the central nervous system. This implies that, in addition to being influenced by the pituitary hormones themselves and the target gland hormones, the stimulatory and inhibitory hormones of the hypothalamus are influenced by stimuli from many portions of the body and higher cortical centers. The pituitary gland may well be the grand orchestrator of all the hormones, but the physiologic control of the pituitary hormones is a complex system, the nature of which is still unfolding.

Growth hormones. Both an hGH-releasing factor (GHRF) and an inhibiting hormone (somatostatin) have been demonstrated in hypothalamic extracts. However, somatostatin has other activities in addition to inhibiting the release of hGH. It also inhibits the release of thyrotropin from the pituitary gland and insulin and glucagon from the pancreas. This broad range of actions points to a more integrated and complex system of hormonal control than previously appreciated.

The control of hGH release ultimately occurs at the level of the hypothalamus. In addition to the normal negative feedback mechanisms involved in the other hormone control systems, the blood concentrations of glucose, fatty acids, estrogens, and most interestingly, sleep, also affect the release of hGH. The increase in hGH identified during sleep perhaps validates the notion that children need their sleep to grow properly. Although norepinephrine, dopamine, and serotonin stimulate the release of hGH in the normal person, in those people with hGH-secreting tumors, metergoline (an antiserotonin drug) and bromocriptine (an agent that binds to dopamine receptors) suppress hGH levels; indeed, both have been used successfully to treat acromegaly.[20,21] Tissue resistance to hGH may occur as an inborn or acquired defect. hGH is also controlled by the local synthesis inhibitory growth factors (IGF-1, IGF-2) and their binding proteins in target tissues.[22]

Prolactin. The hypothalamus primarily inhibits rather than stimulates the release of prolactin from the adenohypophysis. It follows that in the absence of hypothalamic control there is excessive secretion of prolactin with an associated galactorrhea. A prolactin-releasing factor (prl-RF) that stimulates prolactin release has been identified. Thyrotropin-releasing hormone (TRH) also stimulates prolactin release from the adenohypophysis. Other hormones, particularly estrogens, also affect the secretion of prolactin.

Thyroid-stimulating hormone. TSH was the first pituitary hormone to be characterized. However, the thyroid hormones, thyroxine and triiodothyronine, act directly on the hypothalamus to decrease the production of TSH via TRH. Exactly how TRH modulates this response is unclear. A thyrotropin-inhibiting hormone has not been demonstrated. See Chapter 59 for a further discussion of these considerations.

Follicle-stimulating hormone and luteinizing hormone. A decapeptide-releasing hormone that functions to increase both FSH and LH has been characterized. With this single gonadotropin-releasing hormone (GURH), FSH and LH are released sequentially rather than simultaneously during the normal menstrual cycle. This control system is not well characterized but may be related to the positive and negative feedback control of the gonadal steroids on the pituitary gland itself. There is a progressive increase in the FSH level seen as early as age 29 to 30 years that markedly increases in the mid 40s. LH on the other hand seems to increase only after age 40. This increase in basal FSH (and later LH) may represent the earliest endocrine marker of reproductive aging.[23] Release of LH and FSH is under the stimulation of GURH and is regulated by a common mechanism. A nonsteroidal ovarian factor called gonadotropin surge attenuating factor (GUSAF) modulates both the GURH-induced release of LH and the self-priming effect of GURH on the pituitary gland.

Adrenocorticotropin. The hypothalamus exerts both a stimulatory and an inhibitory influence over adrenocorticotropin secretion and biosynthesis. The brain regulates adrenocortical function via hypothalamic corticotropin-releasing hormone-41 (CRH-41).[24] Glucocorticoids act as specific receptors in the hippocampus, thus promoting cognitive negative feedback mechanisms.

PITUITARY DYSFUNCTION

Since the pituitary gland is an endocrine organ, dysfunction is expressed as the result of overproduction or underproduction of one or more hormones. Tumors secreting each of the anterior pituitary hormones have been described. When a pituitary tumor is present, the pituitary-gonadal axis is the most frequent neuroendocrine disturbance, followed by the pituitary-adrenal axis and the pituitary-thyroid axis.[25] In most reported series of pituitary tumors there are also a large proportion of "nonfunctioning" tumors. However, with the advent of more sophisticated diagnostic techniques the proportion of nonfunctional pituitary adenomas is diminishing. Whether these are tumors that have minimal secretion or are truly nonfunctional hyperplasia is the subject of debate. The controversy centers around their histologic appearance. Many of these nonsecreting tumors have characteristics that would predict hormone secretion, yet they do not appear to actually secrete hormones. One hypothesis is that they do, in fact, secrete hormones but at very low concentrations. This low concentration is so near normal that the target organ sees this as normal pituitary hormone secretion and responds appropriately. This in turn results in a decrease in the hypothalamic-stimulating hormone, and thus the normal secreting cells of the adenohypophysis are functionally inhibited. However, it should be assumed that, in patients who have the signs and symptoms of an overproduction of an adenohypophysial hormone, a tumor is present. There are exceptions to this assumption, but they are few.

It is important to recognize that pituitary adenomas can be induced, at least in animals, by large doses of estrogens, the classic example being the inducement of prolactin-secreting tumors by exogenous administration of high doses of estrogen.[26] The point at which such lesions become independent of hypothalamic control is critical. Subclinical tumors that remain dependent on hypothalamic control may be very common but may either require minimal or no treatment. On the other hand, when they escape from hypothalamic control and become independent of the normal regulatory mechanisms, they become enlarging pituitary adenomas and are clearly detrimental to the patient. Certainly not every macroadenoma becomes an autonomous tumor, but the distinction is frequently difficult to ascertain.

Adenohypophysial hyposecretion is also well described. Although panhypopituitarism literally means total pituitary failure, in the common use of the term it denotes loss of function of only the adenohypophysial hormones. Primary causes of pituitary failure are becoming increasingly more uncommon as more and more secondary causes are identified. *Simmonds' disease* is the term applied to pituitary failure from any cause, whereas Sheehan's syndrome refers to pituitary necrosis secondary to shock, hemorrhage, or sepsis associated with childbirth.[27,28] Pituitary apoplexy, on the other hand, is a primary cause of Simmonds' disease because pituitary insufficiency develops; but pituitary apoplexy is reserved for cases in which there was a preexisting tumor that suffered acute hemorrhage or necrosis. The absence of any adenohypophysial hormones except prolactin may result in a specific syndrome. Nonetheless, absence of a single anterior pituitary hormone is comparatively less common than panhypopituitarism and may be idiopathic or familial. This absence of a single hormone may be the result of abnormalities in the hypothalamus, but most cases are associated with subclinical hyposecretion of other hormones as well.

Diabetes insipidus results from a deficiency of ADH secondary to an impairment in the hypothalamoneurohypophysial system. Although diabetes insipidus can be familial and idiopathic, it is much more commonly secondary to either primary neoplasms, vascular insufficiency of the pituitary gland, infections within the pituitary gland, or mass lesions in the parasellar region such as aneurysms or tumors. Diabetes insipidus may be quite transient (as occurs in a resolving head injury) or permanent (as is seen after destruction of the hypothalamoneurohypophysial system).

The syndrome of inappropriate ADH (SIADH) is associated with a wide variety of conditions ranging from malignant tumors of the lung and pancreas that secrete ADH to prolonged positive pressure ventilation. Although this syndrome is well documented following prolonged ventilation, the cause underlying this condition has remained elusive. The neurohypophysis may also be invaded by an astrocytoma or ependymoma from the surrounding tissues and for unknown reasons may result in ADH secretion. Primary tumors of the neurohypophysis are exceedingly rare. Such tumors, designated choristomas, have only been described in approximately 20 patients[29] (Fig. 57-5).

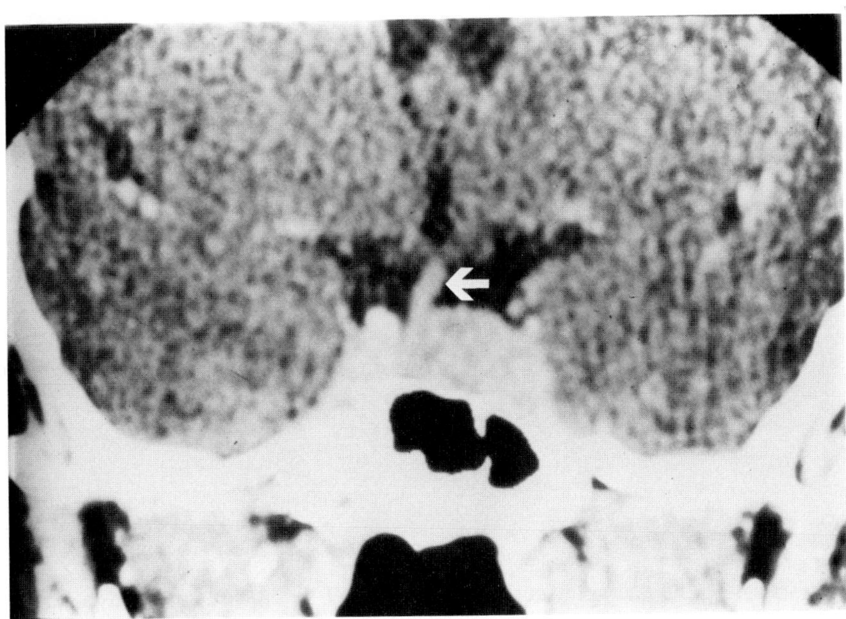

Fig. 57-5. Coronal CT demonstrating deviation of the stalk *(arrow)* of the pituitary gland to the right as result of a tumor.

Pituitary Tumors

Adenomas of the pituitary gland are almost always histologically benign.[30] The ability to visualize the pituitary gland by noninvasive CT scan has opened new vistas for diagnosing these tumors[31] (Fig. 57-6). The use of MRI to visualize the sellar region (Fig. 57-7) present provides another exciting diagnostic modality.

At the present time, MRI can be routinely used to visualize the cranial nerves within the cavernous sinuses, separate the adenohypophysis from the neurohypophysis, and visualize the named vascular structures in the region. Sophisticated endocrinologic investigations have also improved the ability to diagnose these tumors while they are small. Careful sectioning of the pituitary gland at autopsy has shown that between 10% and 25% of the normal population have abnormal tissue within the pituitary gland that may represent subclinical adenomas or hyperplasia.[32,33] Such observations make the questions of who should be treated and how aggressive this treatment should be of the utmost relevance.

New medical treatment regimens are being tried, and even more effective regimens are on the horizon for managing small hormone-secreting tumors without surgery.[34] The surgical treatment for pituitary tumors has also improved because ever smaller tumors are being identified and resected earlier and because of significantly improved postoperative management and intraoperative anesthetic care. The relative value of surgical therapy compared to medical management for small, hormonally active tumors is still evolving.

Clinical Presentation of Pituitary Tumors

Signs and symptoms of pituitary tumors occur because of a change in the amount of the hormones secreted by the pituitary gland and the mass effect of the tumor on adjacent structures. Pituitary tumors may encroach on any of the surrounding anatomic structures, but frequently a characteristic clinical picture develops.[35] The resulting syndrome points to the location of the lesion, but other studies are required to elucidate the nature of the underlying pathology.

Visual field defects are commonly encountered in patients with pituitary tumors but often go unnoticed until they are relatively severe. The characteristic visual field deficit caused by an intrasellar mass is a bitemporal hemianopia.[8] This condition is usually asymmetric and may result in a variety of patterns, depending on the rapidity of tumor growth, the precise location of the optic chiasm with regard to the tumor, and the age and general health of the patient. The fundi are usually benign but may show signs of optic atrophy. Papilledema may occur but is generally a late sign that strongly suggests the presence of hydrocephalus secondary to the tumor extending posteriorly and superiorly into the third ventricle.

Although hormone overproduction may cause the patient to seek medical attention, in certain cases the lack of the effect of specific hormones may be the presenting symptom. The tumor may so compromise the remainder of the gland that panhypopituitarism develops. Similar phenomena may occur with other mass lesions in the vicinity of the pituitary gland, including intracavernous

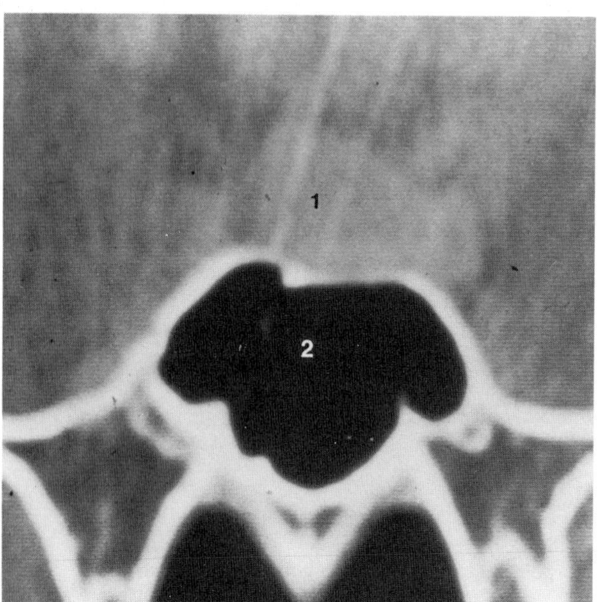

Fig. 57-6. Coronal CT demonstrating the relationship between an eccentrically placed pituitary tumor *(1)* and the sphenoidal air sinus *(2)*. This view is particularly helpful in planning transsphenoidal surgery.

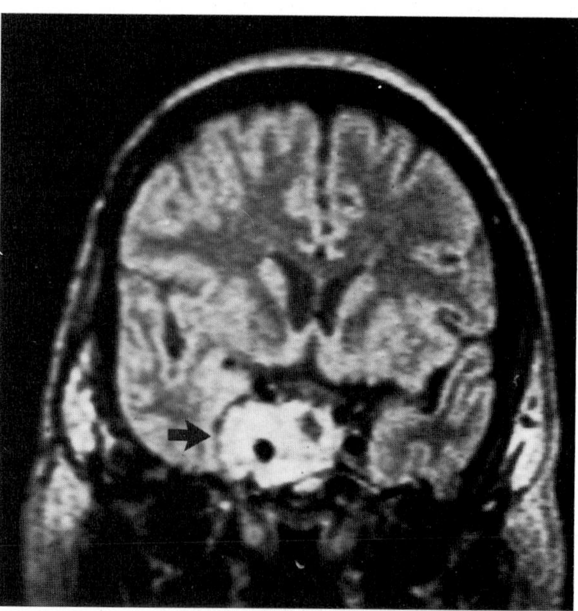

Fig. 57-7. Nuclear magnetic resonance study (coronal view) demonstrating a large adenoma with suprasellar extension and invasion of cavernous sinus *(arrow)*.

carotid artery aneurysms, metastatic tumors, or infectious processes within the sella turcica.

The radiologic sine qua non of pituitary tumors is ballooning of the walls and thinning of the floor of the sella. If thinning of the floor is asymmetric, a double floor is seen on lateral skull x-ray films, which virtually requires an intrasellar mass lesion to be present (Fig. 57-8). Generally, sellar enlargement caused by mass lesions can easily be differentiated from the sellar enlargement associated with increased intracranial pressure. However, since pituitary tumors can cause increased intracranial pressure by obstructing the normal flow of CSF, the cause of sellar changes as seen on x-ray films may occasionally be quite difficult. Furthermore, as pituitary tumors increase in size, the sella may become so distorted that it is virtually impossible to differentiate the underlying cause of the lesion. Skull x-ray films may give other hints as to cause of the sellar mass lesion. The typical calcifications of carotid artery aneurysms, tumors such as meningiomas and craniopharyngiomas, or the destructive lesions associated with infections or malignancies have characteristic appearances on skull x-ray films, MRI, or CT scans and are well described. Today, MRI is the most sensitive imaging modality for evaluation of pituitary tumors, especially microadenomas. In macroadenomas (pituitary adenomas greater than 10 mm in size) both CT scan and MRIs are equally diagnostic, but MRI offers more information on pituitary morphology and neighboring structures. About 10% of the normal adult population have pituitary abnormalities on MRI scans that are compatible with the diagnosis of asymptomatic pituitary adenoma[36] (Fig. 58-9). MRI is also able to provide a specific diagnosis in almost all cases of central diabetes insipidus. Central diabetes insipidus with the appropriate clinical syndrome most often results from lesions in the hypothalamic-neurohypophysial axis. Using this technology, microtumors can often be visualized, and their location within the gland can be predicted.

Although CT investigation is clearly valuable in diagnosing certain tumor types, its major benefit to the surgeon is in planning surgical strategies. Thus before surgical intervention in the patient with a pituitary lesion, a CT scan of the sella, sphenoid sinuses, and suprasellar tissues is required, since other parasellar structures can be invaded by pituitary tumors. MRI is better than CT scan to assess lateral extension into the sphenoid sinuses with thrombosis of the sinuses or pressure on the cranial nerves, even though this is rare. Posterior and superior extension affects the optic chiasm and can push the brain stem backward and involve the basilar artery.

More commonly, suprasellar extension occurs with invagination into the third ventricle, compression of the hypothalamus, and, ultimately, blockage of the cerebral aqueduct with subsequent hydrocephalus. Even with the best imaging techniques available, however, biopsy or excision of the lesion is still necessary to establish the histologic diagnosis and thus the prognosis and the need for other treatment modalities.

Growth hormone–secreting tumors. A pituitary tumor producing excessive amounts of growth hormone results in gigantism in prepubertal patients and in acromegaly if secretion continues after the epiphyses of the long bones are closed. There have also been reports of patients with acromegaly associated with extrapituitary tu-

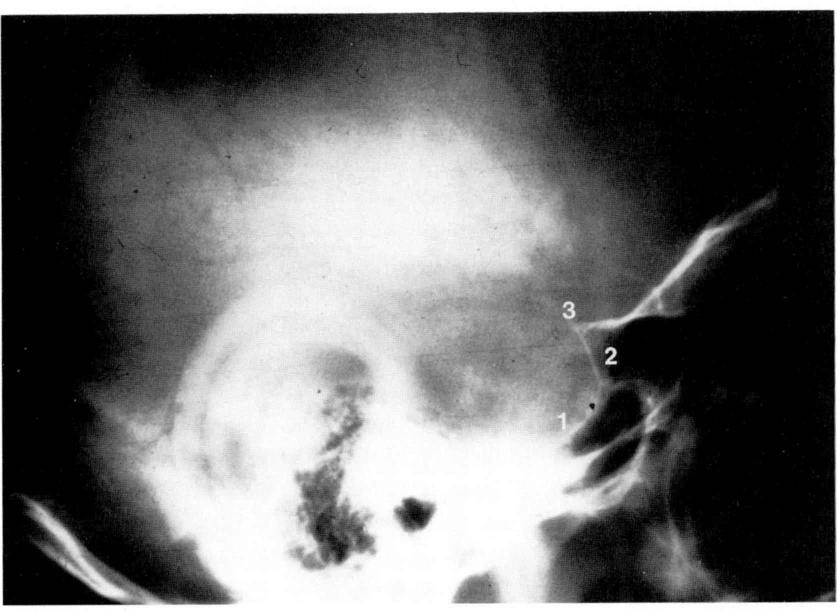

Fig. 57-8. Lateral skull x-ray film demonstrating extreme erosion of sella turcica *(1)*. Note the double floor of the sella *(2)* and absence of the dorsum sella and erosion of the anterior clinoid processes *(3)*.

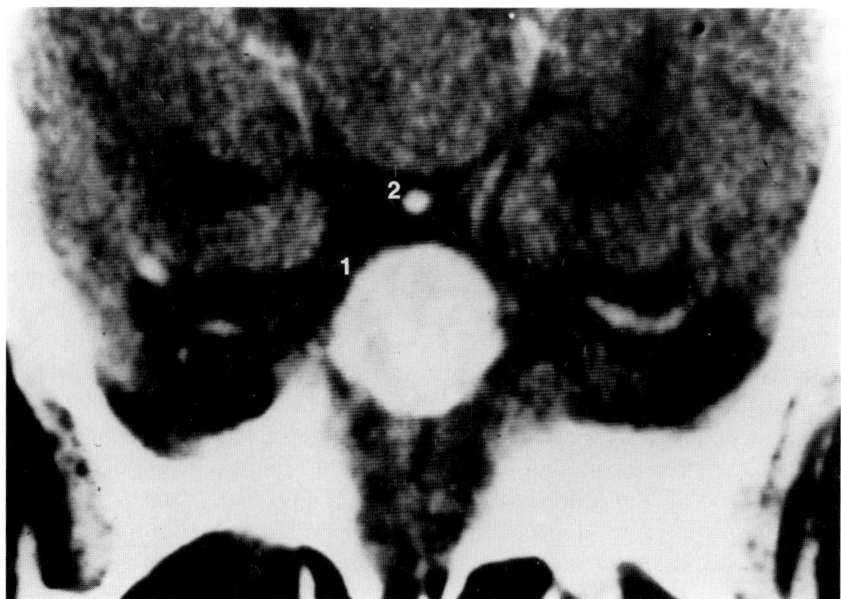

Fig. 57-9. Contrast-enhanced CT demonstrating a large pituitary tumor *(1)* and its relationship to the basilar artery *(2)*.

mors, particularly carcinoid tumors of the lung, with regression of the acromegalic features on removal of the tumor.[37,38] Evidence suggests that these extremely rare, nonpituitary tumors do not actually release growth hormone itself but rather a growth hormone–releasing factor. Whether growth hormone-secreting tumors of the pituitary arise de novo or as a response to an imbalance between growth hormone–releasing and inhibiting factors is still speculative. However, increasing knowledge concerning the physiologic interplay between the hypothalamus and the pituitary gland strongly suggests that a primary hypothalamic disorder may in fact induce the development of growth hormone–secreting tumors.

The syndromes of gigantism and acromegaly are not difficult to distinguish clinically and have virtually no differential diagnosis in their full-blown expression. Other than stature, gigantism has many of the features of acromegaly. Gigantism secondary to excessive growth hormone production can be mistaken for cerebral gigantism, but in the latter situation there is no enlargement of the pituitary gland, the height is generally not as extreme, and it does not, of course, progress to acromegaly.

The term *acromegaly* originally was used to denote the striking changes in the acral portions of the body. In this condition there is certainly a "tufting" of the terminal phalanges that is quite characteristic on x-ray films. However, the hands and feet are also large and have a particular doughy feel to them. Often a handshake with the patient calls into suspicion the diagnosis of acromegaly. On x-ray film examination there is clear prognathism of the mandible, and the paranasal air sinuses are markedly enlarged (Fig. 57-10). Marked overgrowth of the supraorbital rim creating disfigurement to the face is frequently present. The excessive growth of the jaw, nose, and orbital ridge, with relative sparing of the remainder of the facial bones, results in a characteristic facial appearance. It is this grotesque appearance that often brings the patient to the physician; however, because these facial changes slowly evolve over many years, they may be quite extreme before the patient realizes the marked alterations that have oc-

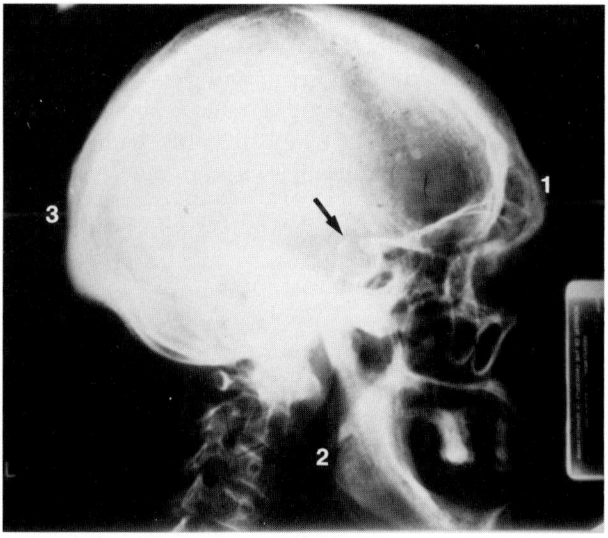

Fig. 57-10. Lateral skull x-ray film of a patient with acromegaly. Note the large frontal sinuses *(1)*, enlarged sella turcica with erosion of the dorsum sella *(arrow)*, prominent mandible *(2)*, and generalized thickening of the calvarium *(3)*.

curred. These changes are often noticed by someone who has not seen the patient in many years or on reviewing an old photograph.

In approximately 50% of patients with acromegaly there is also a myopathy that is most marked in the proximal musculature. Serum enzyme levels characteristic of muscle dysfunction are usually normal, as are muscle biopsies, except for a general hypertrophy of individual muscle fibers. The carpal tunnel syndrome is commonly associated with acromegaly and has the expected characteristics of numbness and weakness in the distribution of the median nerve. This syndrome may be secondary to encroachment of the carpal bones and soft tissues on the median nerve and involvement of the nerve by a hypertrophic neuropathy or by primary changes in nerve metabolism. Quite possibly all these factors play a role in its development. It is striking how rapidly this problem improves with appropriate therapy to reduce the growth hormone levels.

A generalized thickening of the subcutaneous tissues characteristically occurs in patients with acromegaly. A heel pad thickness of greater than 25 mm is characteristic. Of patients with acromegaly, 80% or more complain of hyperhidrosis and a distinctive oiliness of the skin. Many patients with acromegaly also complain of a dull throbbing headache that apparently is secondary to distortion of the diaphragm of the sella turcica or stretching of the nearby large blood vessels.

The spine on x-ray film examination has a striking demineralization, osteophytic formation, and loss of disc space height in acromegalic patients. Whether this is true osteoporosis is a subject of debate, since the incidence of compression fractures in these patients does not appear to be strikingly increased compared to that of the normal population. The abdominal viscera are also diffusely enlarged in these patients.

Frank diabetes mellitus develops in approximately 25% of patients with acromegaly, and another 50% have prediabetic glucose intolerance. Their diabetes is frequently resistant to insulin, presumably because of an alteration in insulin receptors by growth hormone. Associated with the diabetes mellitus is a striking incidence of hypertension, atherosclerosis, and congestive heart failure, in addition to a high incidence of primary cardiomegaly. Indeed, the most common cause of death in patients with acromegaly is myocardial infarction. This high incidence of myocardial infarction necessitates aggressive care in acromegaly and emphasizes the life-threatening potential of this disease.

Patients with acromegaly may be quite large and appear very strong, but in fact they generally easily fatigue and frequently have decreased thyroid, adrenocortical, and gonadotropic hormonal levels because of the adverse mass effects of the growth hormone–secreting tumor on other portions of the pituitary gland responsible for the secretion of these hormones. The thyroid is enlarged in as many as 25% of these patients, presumably because of the decreased blood levels of TSH. Gonadotropic hormones are commonly reduced in concentration with resultant impotence in males and menstrual irregularities in females. Serum and organic phosphate levels may be increased secondary to defective growth hormone effects on renal tubular secretion.

The syndrome of multiple endocrine neoplasia is associated with growth hormone–secreting adenomas, prolactin-secreting and nonfunctioning adenomas of the pituitary, parathyroid adenomas, and islet cell tumors of the pancreas, including insulinomas and gastrinomas. Thus the usual clinical abnormalities in acromegalic patients can be compounded by the hypersecretion of parathyroid hormone, insulin, and gastrin.

Prolactin-secreting tumors. Currently, prolactinomas are the most frequently diagnosed pituitary tumor. This is in contrast to what existed two decades ago because of the improved diagnostic capabilities of the endocrinologist and radiologist. Approximately one third of all pituitary tumors secrete increased amounts of prolactin; however, a serum prolactin level above 260 ng/ml is required for a diagnosis of prolactinoma.[39,40]

Of patients with prolactin-secreting tumors, only a third actually have galactorrhea.[41] To add to the confusion, galactorrhea is not necessarily related to the magnitude of the serum prolactin concentration. Furthermore, patients with galactorrhea and increased prolactin serum levels may not have a prolactin-secreting tumor. Rather, a tumor that is impinging on the hypothalamus and inhibiting the release of prolactin-inhibiting factor may mimic the clinical syndrome caused by a prolactin-secreting tumor. The Forbes-Albright syndrome specifically refers only to women with amenorrhea and galactorrhea secondary to a pituitary tumor.[42]

Although hyperprolactinemia is classically associated with galactorrhea, irregular menses, and anovulation in women, it should be clear that the syndrome occurs in men also. In men it is truly a spectrum ranging from normal to those having galactorrhea with changes in libido, oligospermia, and occasionally gynecomastia. Fortunately, the successful treatment of hyperprolactinemia commonly restores fertility and cures the galactorrhea in both men and women. The normal prolactin level is approximately 20 ng/ml. When patients with galactorrhea or infertility have increased prolactin levels, they should be evaluated for a prolactin-secreting pituitary tumor.

Cushing's disease. There are several causes of Cushing's syndrome, but Cushing's disease refers to that spectrum of the syndrome in which signs and symptoms result from an ACTH-dependent hyperplasia of the adrenal cortex.[43] It is currently felt that Cushing's disease is a primary hypothalamic disorder rather than one that arises in the pituitary itself.[44] However, the adenomas resulting from the excessive production of the ACTH-releasing factor may over time become independent of hypothalamic control. The clinical manifestations of Cushing's syndrome are secondary to hypercortisolism, but hypercortisolism may be caused by a primary disorder of the adrenal cortex; a lesion of the hypothalamus or pituitary gland may not be necessary for hypercortisolism. The clinical findings in patients with Cushing's syndrome, whether caused by an abnormality in the pituitary gland, hypothalamus, or adrenal cortex, are the same. However, defining the specific cause of hypercortisolism is especially important because treatment is strikingly different.

Perhaps the most common complaint of patients with Cushing's syndrome is weakness and fatigue. Patients with this disease are generally obese with significant loss of muscle mass. Their obesity is particularly pronounced in the trunk and minimal in the extremities. They have a characteristic moon-shaped appearance to their face and a dorsal kyphosis with a "buffalo hump" comprised of subcutaneous fatty tissue over the upper thoracic spine. Their hirsutism, ruddy complexion, ease of bruising, purple stria, and centripetal fat distribution make the diagnosis classic. At least three fourths of these patients have hypertension and diabetes mellitus. Further, they have calcium wasting that results from demineralization of their bones and an associated increased incidence of long bone and spine fractures.

The diagnosis of Cushing's syndrome can frequently be made on first evaluation of the patient. However, the underlying cause may be significantly more difficult to define. In addition to pituitary hyperplasia and adenomas, multiple other causes must be considered. Adrenocortical adenomas, adrenocortical carcinoma, and ectopic ACTH secretion by nonpituitary tumors, especially carcinoma of the lung, must be included in the differential diagnosis. Other tumors such as carcinoma of the thymus and pancreas and bronchial carcinoids may also secrete ACTH and cause Cushing's syndrome. Thus a thorough investigation of these patients is required. Differentiation of Cushing's disease from other causes of Cushing's syndrome can generally be accomplished by endocrinologic investigation.

Nelson's syndrome. Nelson's syndrome is characterized by excessive production of ACTH in combination with β-melanocyte-stimulating hormone.[45-47] This disease occurs when an ACTH-secreting pituitary tumor develops after bilateral adrenalectomy. It appears that Nelson's syndrome is a continuum of an untreated Cushing's disease. The striking feature in these patients is the dark skin pigmentation that may occur over relatively short periods of time. Unfortunately, the pituitary tumors in these patients are often quite large and are particularly difficult to surgically remove.[48,49]

TSH-, FSH-, and LH-secreting tumors. TSH- and FSH-secreting tumors are rare neoplasms that produce the characteristic radiologic changes in the sella turcica similar to other pituitary tumors and the expected secondary hormonal effects on the respective target organs. Approximately 20 patients have been identified with either a primary gonadotropin-secreting or thyrotropin-secreting pituitary tumor. Their manifestations and treatment are similar to those that would be expected from an overproduction of TSH or FSH. A tumor that secretes only LH has not been identified.

Treatment of Pituitary Tumors

Historically, the treatment of pituitary tumors quickly followed the recognition of the clinical syndromes associated with these lesions and the characterization of these lesions on plain skull x-ray films. The successful removal of pituitary tumors is one of the earlier neurosurgical procedures that found acceptance. Currently, however, the appropriate treatment of pituitary tumors is a much more individualized decision. With a clearer understanding of the clinical correlates of pituitary dysfunction and the advent of more sophisticated neuroradiologic and endocrinologic evaluation techniques, extremely small tumors are being recognized. Coincident with these advances in diagnosis have been similar advances in medical and surgical management of these tumors. We now have the ability to decrease hormonal hypersecretion by the pituitary gland in various disease states and to perform safer, more effective surgical therapy. Furthermore, the capability of detecting "subclinical" tumors has necessitated the continued reassessment of which patients need any treatment at all. At the other end of the spectrum are tumors that behave invasively and therefore make complete surgical extirpation necessary but potentially hazardous. The role of radiotherapy is still controversial even after 75 years of experience with this treatment modality. The use of focused radiation with either the Gamma Knife or radiation focused from a linear accelerator and a stereotactic frame has also been shown to be of benefit in some patients. Clearly, there is real justification for the controversy regarding the optimal treatment of pituitary tumors because in some cases there are two or more safe, effective treatment possibilities.[50] Although it could therefore be argued that medical and surgical therapy are each reasonable options in some cases, few patients would believe that decisions concerning the "risks" of surgery vs. the need to continue taking medications indefinitely were equivalent but rather that such decisions require more than statistic judgment.

Medical therapy. Medical therapy is directed at decreasing the hormonal hypersecretion of the tumor. Its usefulness has been clearly demonstrated in the treatment of prolactinomas and growth hormone–secreting tumors. There is evidence with both tumors that dopamine agonists cause morphologic regression of the tumor during treatment. L-Dopa inhibits growth hormone secretion in most acromegalic patients, but the effect is short lived.[51] In contrast, bromocriptine (2-bromo-α-ergocryptine), an agent that binds to dopamine receptors, has been demonstrated to suppress growth hormone levels for 6 to 12 hours after a single dose. With prolonged administration growth hormone levels continue to fall for several weeks with a maximal response evident at approximately 8 to 12 weeks.[52] The overall response is clearly dose dependent. The site of action of bromocriptine appears to be at the level of the pituitary gland rather than the hypothalamus. Long-term studies have shown bromocriptine to be effective in 70% to 80% of acromegalic patients in lowering the growth hormone levels to a normal range.[53] Improvement in glucose tolerance and cardiac function, reduction in soft tissue volume, improvement in facial appearance, amelioration of the symptoms of the carpal tunnel syndrome,[54] and a decrease in sweating have been observed in conjunction with the decrease in growth hormone levels.[55-57] On the other hand, there have been a few reports of pituitary apoplexy (see the following) occurring in patients taking bromocriptine.

Lergotrile mesylate has demonstrated effectiveness in reducing growth hormone levels in acromegaly; however, it is currently unavailable for clinical use because of the occurrence of genital tumors in animal studies in which the drug has been used.[20] Cyproheptadine and methysergide partially inhibit the normal growth hormone elevation observed with hypoglycemia, intravenous arginine infusion, and exercise. However, long-term data on their use to treat hormonally active growth hormone tumors are lacking. Somatostatin (growth hormone–inhibiting factor) has been used in experimental situations, and it does suppress growth hormone–secretion in essentially all acromegalic patients. The question of toxicity (suppression of insulin and glucagon secretions and platelet dysfunction) also must be resolved before somatostatin can be considered for routine clinical use.

Prolactin secretion is principally controlled by inhibitory factors, of which dopamine is one of the more effective. As with growth hormone–secreting tumors, dopaminergic drugs would be expected to decrease prolactin secretion. Indeed, bromocriptine has been successful in controlling hyperprolactinemia in 80% to 90% of cases with a variety of causes, including prolactin-secreting tumors.[58,59] Such treatment results in cessation of galactorrhea in approximately 90% of patients and restores normal menstruation in 80% to 90%.[60-63] The drug has the side effects of nausea, dyspepsia, headaches, postural hypotension, and occasionally depression or anxiety. Nausea and headaches are the most common patient complaints. Unfortunately, when the drug is withdrawn, the tumor once again expresses itself.

If medical therapy is to be used, bromocriptine is the current drug of choice for acromegalic patients and those with prolactin-secreting tumors; still 10% to 20% do not respond satisfactorily to any medical regimen.[64,65] The advantages of medical therapy in these conditions primarily center around not subjecting the patient to the risks of surgery, especially the risk of injury to the normal tissue in the pituitary gland when microtumors are present. An additional benefit may be that a period of treatment with bromocriptine makes surgical planes better defined and surgery therefore easier to perform. Petrini et al.[66] have reported long-term treatment of Nelson's syndrome with a somatostatin analog octreotide. The major disadvantages to medical therapy are patient compliance, uncertain long-term untoward effects, possible untoward effects on the fetus (one of the common reasons patients with prolactinomas seek medical attention is infertility), and evaluation for the length of continuous, careful follow-up.

Surgical therapy. Two basic surgical approaches to the sella turcica have been devised. These include a approach by means of craniotomy from above the optic chiasm[67] and an approach from below the sella turcica through the sphenoidal sinus.[39,40,68-77] The approach from above the pituitary gland entails either a frontal or temporal craniotomy and removal of the tumor through the diaphragm.[78] The safety of this approach depends primarily on the size of the tumor and the position of the chiasm. There is always some manipulation of the brain tissue, but the craniotomy approach does allow visualization of the third ventricle and a clear exposure of the structures surrounding the sella. However, it is frequently difficult to remove a tumor without removing the pituitary gland entirely. Further visualization within the sella turcica may be difficult.

The transseptal, transsphenoidal approach (Fig. 57-11) as originally devised was a very formidable surgical procedure.[79] However, with the use of the surgical microscope and detailed fluoroscopy, the technique has become part of the armamentarium of many neurosurgeons. The procedure has many advantages when compared to the craniotomy approach. Obviously, cerebral retraction and manipulation and potential damage to the olfactory nerves are eliminated. The need for blood transfusions is minimized, and patients generally feel better after surgery. The major advantage is that small tumors can be totally removed with preservation of the remaining pituitary gland, and the contents of the sella turcica can generally be well visualized. This technique is especially well suited for small tumors in the anterior lobe of the pituitary gland. Because the neurohypophysis can frequently be left intact, the incidence of diabetes insipidus following this procedure is markedly lessened, and the need for long-term hormonal replacement is significantly reduced. With the advent of

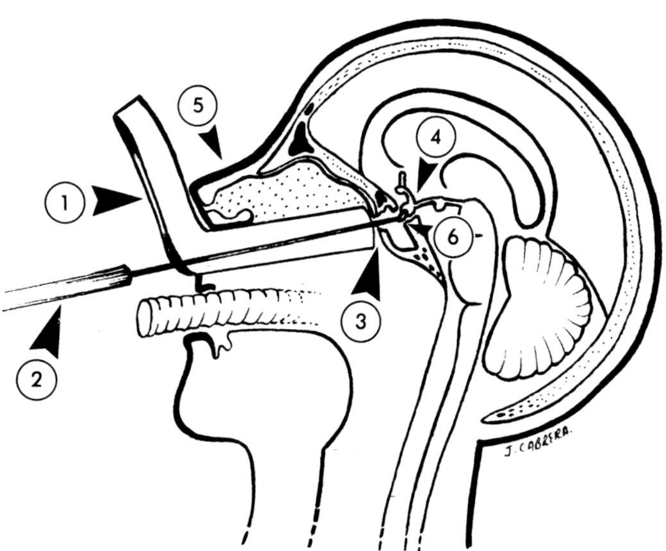

Fig. 57-11. Schematic representation of the transnasal, transseptal, transsphenoidal approach to the pituitary gland. *1,* Bivalve speculum in place; *2,* ring curette in the sella; *3,* open sphenoidal sinus; *4,* pituitary gland; *5,* resected nasal cartilage; and *6,* open sellar floor.

sophisticated MRI of the sellar region, many tumors can be visualized within the gland, and decisions made before surgery as to precisely where to incise it to remove the tumor. The major disadvantage to the transsphenoidal approach lies in the inability to view the other side of the tumor. Specifically, the optic chiasm cannot be visualized until the tumor is removed. The carotid arteries lie in close proximity, and torrential bleeding can occur from their injury. The superior orbital fissure is also a part of the sphenoid bone and lies less than a centimeter from the sella turcica. Injury to the nerves innervating the extraocular muscles and the supraorbital division of the trigeminal nerve can occur as the sphenoid is opened to visualize the pituitary tumor.

Current experience with microsurgical procedures indicates that surgical excision of small tumors of the pituitary gland is a safe, effective treatment modality with a low complication rate.[80] Surgical therapy for prolactinomas should be reserved for patients with dopaminergic resistance or intolerance and complications to dopamine agonist therapy. Transsphenoidal removal of endocrine-inactive pituitary adenomas is recommended as appropriate and effective with possible preservation and/or recovery of anterior pituitary function.[81] Radiation therapy may be appropriate for small or medium-sized tumors with minimal suprasellar extension (Fig. 57-12), in patients in whom surgery is refused or contraindicated, and as postoperative adjunctive therapy in patients with invasive or incompletely excised tumors. Radiotherapy may also be of benefit in treating some patients with a craniopharyngioma. This latter tumor is a benign, congenital neoplasm, usually suprasellar in position, and represents a secretory vestige of Rathke's pouch. It affects pituitary function by compressing the gland and causing hypopituitarism.

As sole therapy, radiation treatment is contraindicated in large tumors with suprasellar extension, patients with major visual field defects, patients with acromegaly with serum growth hormone levels greater than 50 ng/ml before treatment, and patients with prolactinomas who wish fertility restored. Approximately 5% of patients treated with radiotherapy can be expected to develop pituitary apoplexy, with the acute onset of severe headache, loss of vision, extraocular nerve palsies, and loss of consciousness. The long-term effects of radiation to the sellar region are not insignificant, especially with regard to vision. Computer-assisted stereotactic radiosurgery is another modality available for treatment of tumors in this region. Long-term effects are still not clearly defined, but in the postoperative period the morbidity is less than 1% for this procedure. Radiotherapy is contraindicated in small children younger than 2 years with pituitary and extrapituitary lesions because of the risk of small vessel occlusion resulting in visual disturbances and stroke.

In addition to the primary role of medical therapy in the treatment of acromegaly and prolactinomas, as discussed above, it may also be efficacious in these patients following surgery or radiotherapy.[82] Ten percent to 40% of patients with growth hormone–secreting tumors continue to have persistent growth hormone-elevations (more than 10 ng/ml) after surgery and/or radiation and continue to exhibit progression of their disease. In this circumstance, bromocriptine therapy has proven useful in decreasing growth hormone levels in the blood. Similarly in patients with persistent hyperprolactinemia following ablative surgery, bromocriptine has effectively suppressed serum prolactin and restored normal gonadal function in the majority of these individuals. Dosages of 2.5 to 10 mg daily by mouth are usually adequate for both acromegaly and prolactin-secreting tumors. Of note, bromocriptine may also produce tumor regression in some of these patients.

Pituitary Apoplexy

A sudden, unexpected, life-threatening hemorrhage can occur in pituitary tumors. This complication does not appear to be associated with a particular tumor type, and an obvious triggering event is not required. In autopsy studies, between 4.6% and 10% of patients with pituitary tumors have areas of hemorrhagic necrosis.[83,84] Wakai et al.[85] noted that, in over 9% of 560 patients with documented pituitary tumors, the initial presentation was a major or

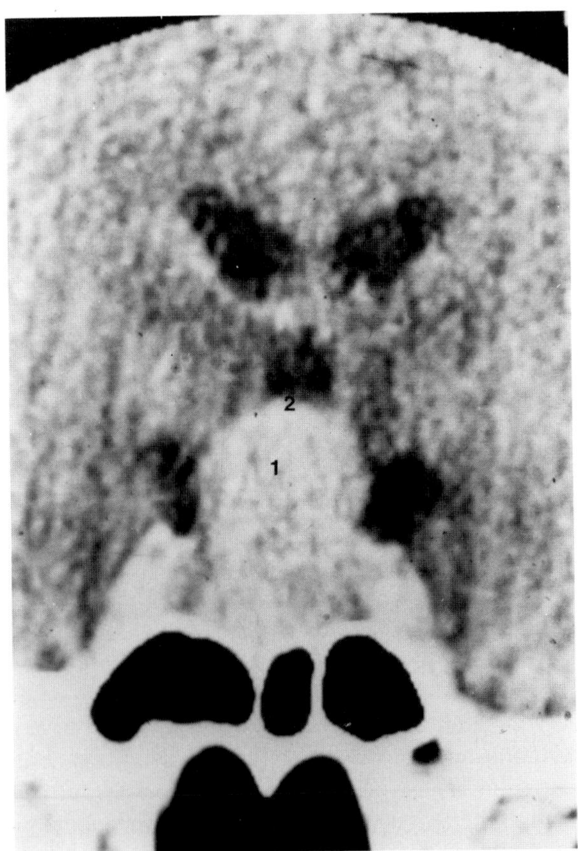

Fig. 57-12. Contrast-enhanced CT demonstrating suprasellar extension of a tumor *(1)*. Compression of the optic chiasm was present. Note encroachment of the tumor on the third ventricle *(2)* and presence of hydrocephalus.

minor hemorrhage into the tumor. However, even though pituitary apoplexy has been associated with head trauma, mechanical ventilators, bromocriptine therapy, hypertension, and a variety of other conditions, it frequently occurs without a precipitating event.[85-88] In our present state of knowledge the precise cause of this condition remains unclear.

The most common presenting signs and symptoms are sudden severe headache, loss of vision, nausea and vomiting, ocular disorders, fever, stiff neck, and almost invariably an alteration in the state of consciousness. Obviously, such a syndrome can easily be confused with fulminating meningitis or subarachnoid hemorrhage from other causes; however, in patients with known pituitary tumors, the diagnosis should always be suspected. MRI or CT scan can confirm the diagnosis in nearly all suspected cases.

Pituitary apoplexy is such a life-threatening event that, once the diagnosis is made, treatment with high doses of intravenous steroids should be immediately instituted. Plans to excise the tumor, preferably by means of the transseptal, transsphenoidal approach, must be formulated on an emergent basis. Following surgery, specific hormone replacement therapy is initially given as though the pituitary gland were totally destroyed. However, with time and recovery of residual pituitary function, replacement therapy can be individualized to meet the precise needs of the individual.

Nontumerous Causes of Enlarged Sella Turcica

Although it is common to equate enlargement of the sella turcica with an expending neoplasm, the sella can enlarge from several nontumorous causes;

1. Empty sella syndrome
   a. Primary
   b. Secondary
2. Carotid artery aneurysms
3. Arachnoid cyst
4. Granuloma
5. Increased intracranial pressure
6. Pseudotumor cerebri
7. Hydrocephalus

An empty sella is an abnormal extension of the subarachnoid space into the pituitary fossa. Although this is generally an incidental pathologic observation on radiologic evaluation, an empty sella may cause signs and symptoms if it leads to enlargement of the sella turcica and compression of the normal intrasellar contents. The primary type of empty sella results from a development defect of the diaphragm of the sella, allowing the arachnoid to herniate into the sella turcica. Secondary empty sella syndromes result from a similar process that occurs after the intrasellar contents have been destroyed by surgery, irradiation, or infarction.[89-93]

The typical patient with primary empty sella syndrome is a middle-aged, multiparous, obese, hypertensive woman. The common presenting symptoms are frequently nonspecific and vague, but headache and fatigue are virtually ubiquitous. Although they are rare, suspicious findings are visual field disturbances suggesting herniation of the optic chiasm into the sella and CSF rhinorrhea.[57,94]

Secondary empty sella syndrome must always be considered when evaluating patients for recurrence of pituitary tumors after surgery or irradiation.[84] Impairment of vision may occur within a few months or several years after ablation of the intrasellar contents because of herniation of the optic chiasm into the sella. MRI can easily distinguish the diagnosis of an empty sella from tumor recurrence. Treatment may be needed for relief of chiasmal signs or CSF rhinorrhea.

Panhypopituitarism

Panhypopituitarism is characterized by decreased or absent function of the target organs stimulated by the pituitary hormones. It is expressed as insufficiency of the target organs rather than the pituitary gland. Signs and symptoms of the primary pituitary lesion such as bitemporal hemianopia may be present, but more commonly it is the generalized endocrinopathy that brings patients to medical attention. Panhypopituitarism in its strictest sense refers to failure of all the pituitary hormones, but in fact only adenohypophysial failure usually occurs. Clearly panhypopituitarism should be viewed as a spectrum of disease with total pituitary failure at one end and multiple endocrinopathies at the other. Patients with "isolated" hormone deficits should be under suspicion for subclinical disorders in the production of other hormones. The location of lesions that cause panhypopituitarism can also be viewed as a spectrum ranging from small isolated lesions of the hypothalamus to large destructive lesions of the hypothalamopituitary system. The box on p. 1138 lists many of the lesions frequently associated with panhypopituitarism.

The clinical findings of panhypopituitarism clearly vary with the degree of pituitary dysfunction and are related to the diminished function of the target organs. Patients complain of generalized fatigue and weakness and have a particular lack of resistance to cold weather and fasting, reflecting abnormalities in thyroid and adrenal gland function. They are frequently small in stature with reduced bone age compared to their chronologic age. Their skin is remarkably pale and dry. They tend to have low blood pressure and are commonly troubled by orthostatic hypotension. Amenorrhea and galactorrhea in women and impotence in men are reflections of diminished gonadotropic hormone function. A lack, or even regression, of secondary sexual characteristics is common. Mental retardation is associated with pituitary failure occurring early in life. In addition to the effects of the primary lesion, patients with panhypopituitarism are physiologically fragile and may develop overwhelming fever, cardiovascular shock, coma, and death as a result of relatively minor stressful situations. Use of steroids can be helpful to minimize the physiologic consequences of panhypopituitarism in times of physical or emotional distress.

CAUSES OF PANHYPOPITUITARISM

Hypothalamic-Pituitary Disorders
Organic

Congenital: Hypophysial infantilism
Traumatic: Basilar skull fractures
Inflammatory: Granulomas
Degenerative: Irradiation

Autoimmune hypophysitis

Vascular: Sheehan's syndrome
Sheehan's syndrome: Pituitary necrosis secondary to systemic hypotension in postpartum period
Simmonds' disease: Hypophysial cachexia
Neoplastic: Large pituitary adenomas
Surgical hypophysectomy

Functional

Medications: Hormonal replacement
Systemic disease
Endocrinopathies: Primary thyroiditis, adrenal dysfunction, and diabetes mellitus

Extrasellar Structural Disorders

Neoplastic: Craniopharyngioma, meningiomas, metastatic malignancies especially lung, breast, renal, and thyroid carcinoma
Vascular: Carotid aneurysms invading the sella
Trauma: Severe intracranial pressure, fracture of phenoid
Development: Rathke's arachnoid cysts

The evaluation of panhypopituitarism is made primarily on the basis of clinical suspicion, assessment of endocrinologic function, and determination of the specific cause of the pituitary failure. Because hypopituitarism generally develops insidiously and may escape detection for years, its diagnosis depends on a high index of suspicion. Patients who are unusually fatigued, appear to be aging more rapidly than is suggested by their chronologic age, have unexplained imbalances in body temperature regulation, and are unable to respond to infection or stress in an appropriate manner should be considered possible candidates for hypopituitarism and endocrinologic evaluation for this disorder.

The demonstration of a low level of hormone secreted by a pituitary target organ in the presence of a low level of pituitary trophic hormone is strongly suggestive of hypothalamic or pituitary dysfunction. Patients with panhypopituitarism have the expected limited ACTH reserve on metyrapone (Metopirone) testing; radioactive iodine uptake is depressed in the thyroid gland but increases following exogenous thyrotropic hormone administration; urinary 17-ketosteroid and hydroxycorticosteroid, as well as cortisol, levels are low but slowly rise after ACTH administration; and growth hormone assay yields low levels with little response to stimulation with insulin, hypoglycemia, arginine infusion, or L-dopa administration. Of course, the pituitary trophic hormone levels are also depressed. As a single test, the most useful aid in diagnosing panhypopituitarism is measurement of serum thyroxine. Virtually all patients with pituitary deficiency have low values of this hormone. If serum thyroxine is normal, it is highly unlikely that panhypopituitarism exists.

The diagnosis of the specific cause of panhypopituitarism rests primarily on the results of x-ray film evaluation of the sella turcica and the measurement of serum levels of the various pituitary hormones both under basal conditions and after administration of the specific hypothalamic-releasing factors or stimulation of the endogenous hypothalamic hormone. If possible, treatment is always aimed at the primary cause. However, endocrine substitution must be used as soon as the diagnosis of panhypopituitarism is made and continued through the treatment period or, in some cases, permanently. With the exception of corticotropin, there is no available effective pituitary replacement preparation. Correction and replacement therapy can be obtained for the corticosteroid, thyroid hormones, and sex steroids. Growth hormone replacement is generally not practical. The box on p. 1139 indicates treatment strategies for patients with pituitary insufficiency. The need for such therapy may occur after pituitary surgery or immediately after pituitary apoplexy. Long-term replacement therapy is usually required for patients with chronic panhypopituitarism, and emergency treatment is necessary for those patients with acute life-threatening hypopituitarism.

The prognosis for patients with panhypopituitarism depends on the specific cause of the disorder, the duration of the disorder, the age of the patient at onset, and the secondary effects that have occurred before the initiation of treatment. For example, patients with pituitary apoplexy may recover spontaneously and only require short-term therapy. In contrast, patients having more chronic forms of hypopituitarism often require prolonged treatment with replacement hormones normally secreted by target organs that have been adversely affected by the pituitary dysfunction. If pituitary function never recovers, this therapy will of necessity be lifelong. These individuals must be under the constant care of a physician skilled in the management of panhypopituitarism, and both patient and physician alike must be prepared to manage the potentially disastrous consequences that may occur from the common stresses of life such as relatively minor episodes of starvation, infection, or trauma.

Antidiuretic Hormone Abnormalities

Diabetes Insipidus

Diabetes insipidus results from either a decrease in secretion of ADH or a decreased responsiveness to ADH by the renal tubular apparatus of the nephron of the kidney. The diagnosis should be suspected in an individual who

REPLACEMENT THERAPY FOR PITUITARY INSUFFICIENCY

Chronic Pituitary Insufficiency

ACTH	25 mg cortisone acetate of 5 mg prednisone daily in two divided doses Additional steroids as required for physiologic stress such as injury, surgery, or infection
Thyroid	100 to 200 μg L-thyroxine daily as a single dose
Gonadotropin	*Males:* Testosterone 12 to 15 mg intramuscularly every 2 weeks *Females:* Ethinyl estradiol 10 to 15 μg/day, or standard estrogen-progesterone regimen as for birth control
Growth hormone	Only considered in pediatric age group
Prolactin	No replacement required

Replacement Therapy After Pituitary Surgery

Steroids	Cortisone acetate 50 mg every 6 hours Tapering dosage after 5 days except in patients with Cushing's disease May require long-term replacement therapy
Thyroid	If normal thyroid function before surgery, no replacement therapy If abnormal before surgery, thyroxine (Synthroid) 0.1 to 0.15 μg daily
Persistent prolactinemia	Reoperation or bromocriptine

Replacement Therapy for Life-Threatening Pituitary Failure

Hydrocortisone or cortisone	100 to 300 mg/day intravenously
Thyroxine	200 μg/day

excretes unusually large volumes of urine of low osmolality. Nocturia and nighttime thirst are often the first manifestations. The serum osmolality may be only slightly elevated, particularly if the patient drinks enough water in response to thirst. However, in those patients whose thirst mechanism is either deficient or who cannot satisfy their thirst, diabetes insipidus can quickly lead to its full-blown effects: severe dehydration, hypovolemia, serum hyperosmolality, fever, hyperpnea, stupor, coma, and even death. These changes can take place in a remarkably short period of time.

Proof that the kidney can conserve water is obtained to distinguish primary diabetes insipidus from that arising from a lack of responsiveness of the nephron to ADH.[95] This is accomplished by injecting ADH (i.e., 5 pressor units) either subcutaneously or intravenously and measuring effects on urinary output. The expected response in an intact kidney is a decrease in the urine volume and an increase in urine osmolality and specific gravity within 30 to 60 minutes. In less severe situations the ability to conserve water can be determined by water deprivation for 6 to 8 hours. In normal individuals the urine osmolality increases to greater than 1.015, without a significant change in serum osmolality. Radioimmunoassays are available for ADH but are not usually necessary to establish the diagnosis, except in those cases in which it appears to be the renal tubules that are not responding properly to adequate concentrations of ADH in the serum. The normal ADH level is 2.7 + 1.4 pg/ml.

Familial or congenital diabetes insipidus is a rare disorder that comes to medical attention in infancy or early childhood. It has no gender bias. It appears to be the result of a failure of development of the supraoptic nucleus of the hypothalamus. This circumstance results in a reduction in the size of the posterior pituitary gland. This condition must be distinguished from congenital nephrogenic diabetes insipidus, which is a consequence of an inherited defect in renal tubular responsiveness to ADH.

Posttraumatic diabetes insipidus (i.e., from head trauma) may be a part of panhypopituitarism or an "isolated" abnormality of pituitary function. Fortunately, many cases are transient and incomplete but require treatment for short periods of time. Tumors may infiltrate the stalk of the pituitary gland from above (as in the case of a third ventricular astrocytoma) or from below (as in the case of lymphomas or leukemic infiltrates). Small circumscribed granulomas and pyogenic meningitides may similarly result in diabetes insipidus. Sarcoidosis is the most common type of granulomatous disease that results in diabetes insipidus. Virtually any metastatic tumor or infectious agent can lodge in the infundibulum or upper pituitary stalk; however, carcinoma of the lung is particularly notorious in this regard.

Vascular lesions, either carotid aneurysms within the cavernous sinus or pituitary necrosis secondary to hypotension (Sheehan's syndrome [postpartum pituitary necrosis]), may cause diabetes insipidus presumably because of vascular insufficiency to the upper pituitary stalk. Obviously, surgical interventions in the region of the pituitary gland or hypophysectomy for tumor or pain relief can result in diabetes insipidus that may be permanent or transient. The frequency of diabetes insipidus following pituitary surgery depends in great measure on the level of the stalk section; (i.e., the higher the level of section the greater the chances of diabetes insipidus).[96] Idiopathic causes of diabetes insipidus continue to account for approximately half of all cases of this syndrome. If the cause for diabetes insipidus is not readily apparent after diagnosis it is unusual to ultimately identify one precisely.

The management of patients with diabetes insipidus must, of course, be individualized. The persons most responsible for the patients' long-term management are the patients themselves. Each patient should be aware of the symptoms of diabetes insipidus, especially the potential for electrolyte imbalance and dehydration. The patient must establish a method of recording urine output and measuring urine specific gravity. Diabetes insipidus is not an all-or-none phenomenon but rather varies in severity from one individual to another. Many patients can be directed to be especially conscious of their own thirst and can be managed with minimal or no medications. Chlorpropamide in oral dosages of 100 to 200 mg/day or hydrochlorothiazide in dosages of 50 to 100 mg/day are effective regimens to control polyuria in the milder forms of the disorder. These oral agents paradoxically control diabetes insipidus by stimulating renal medullary adenylate cyclase and inhibiting renal prostaglandin synthetase and renal phosphodiesterase. Each of these effects augments the response to ADH in the renal collecting duct and overshadows the expected diuretic effect of these agents. Frequently, encouraging intermittent medication with these drugs and allowing the patient to control the dosage are the most successful methods of treatment.

If the oral drugs are not sufficient, one of the forms of synthetic ADH becomes necessary. ADH can be administered in a variety of ways, but unfortunately it is not available in an oral preparation. Aqueous ADH (vasopressin) (20 IU/ml) is a partially purified extract of neurohypophysis. Since its effect after subcutaneous injection is short-lived (i.e., approximately 2 hours), it is used in crisis situations or acute-onset diabetes insipidus such as is encountered after surgical procedures on the pituitary gland. It is also an excellent medication in those situations in which there may be vacillation in the production of endogenous ADH and diabetes insipidus is thought to be a transient situation (e.g., the patient with mild head injury).

In the situation in which diabetes insipidus will be permanent, a longer-acting ADH preparation is needed. Vasopressin tannate in oil (5 IU/ml) is such a preparation. This substance is a tannic acid salt of partially purified vasopressin suspended in oil for delayed absorption and thus provides a longer effect. Patients generally require intramuscular injections every 3 to 4 days with this preparation. This regimen is not the favorite among patients needing long-term treatment because of the pain of intramuscular injection. Lysine 8-vasopressin nasal spray contains 50 IU/ml and provides good control of symptoms in most patients but only lasts for 3 to 4 hours. Therefore it is usually used in conjunction with some other regimen for "fine tuning." D,D,arginine vasopressin is a synthetic analog of arginine vasopressin that can be taken by nasal insufflation. The dosage can be controlled by the patient, and the analog is frequently sufficient as a sole medication. However, the most important variable in treating chronic diabetes insipidus is the patient. In most situations undertreatment with medications and reliance on matching of urine output with intravenous fluids in the acute situation and volume replacement on the basis of the patient's thirst in the chronic situation is superior to the control of diabetes insipidus solely with ADH administration.[97]

Inappropriate Secretion of Antidiuretic Hormone

SIADH, the Schwartz-Bartter syndrome, is a relatively common disorder associated with a wide variety of clinical situations.[98,99] Symptoms occur because of the dilutional hyponatremia that results from inappropriate and excessive retention of water.[11] It derives its name because the signs, symptoms, and results from laboratory experiments are similar to those produced experimentally by long-term ADH administration.

The pathophysiology of SIADH is complex and seemingly paradoxical because of the excessive water retention and dilutional hyponatremia in the face of high sodium excretion in the urine. Because renal clearance is not depressed, nitrogenous waste products are adequately cleared, and blood urea and creatinine remain at normal levels. The patients have the same signs and symptoms as would be expected from extreme hyponatremia or water intoxication. In patients with previous neurologic disorders, the clinical abnormalities may appear at moderate levels of hyponatremia. On the other hand, in patients in whom the disorder is slowly evolving, extreme levels of hyponatremia may develop before the onset of symptoms. In general, symptoms do not develop until the serum sodium falls to 120 to 125 mEq/L. Early symptoms are anorexia, nausea, vomiting, lethargy, and irritability. Subtle personality changes, inattentiveness, and forgetfulness may progress to paranoia and delusions. As the disorder progresses, and the serum sodium levels fall to 100 to 110 mEq/L, the neurologic manifestations become more severe and include stupor, coma, and intractable generalized seizures.

The list of disorders associated with SIADH is quite long, but they can be categorized as follows: excessive secretion of ADH from hypothalamic disorders, excessive secretion of ADH secondary to other diseases, excessive production of ADH from nonhypothalamic sites (ectopic ADH production), and SIADH associated with a variety of medications. It stands to reason that hypothalamic disorders such as tumors, trauma, or infarcts might result in SIADH. However, acute intermittent porphyria, myxedema, subarachnoid hemorrhage, and many metabolic necephalopathies are associated with SIADH as well. Cerebral hemispheric infarcts and subdural hematomas along the convexities of the brain are also associated with a high incidence of SIADH. Simply lying in the recumbent position appears to be a cause of SIADH, but in general SIADH should be thought of as a disorder secondary to some other abnormality. SIADH is associated with a variety of pulmonary lesions, especially tumors, and tuberculosis. Many drugs including vincristine, chlorpropamide, chlorpromazine, carbamazepine, and paroxetine (Paxil) (seratonin uptake inhibitor) are also associated with SIADH. Thus the possible causes of SIADH are many, and all patients with low serum sodium should have SIADH in their differential diagnosis.

Treatment is primarily by strict water restriction (e.g., 400 to 600 ml/day). This regimen is generally all that is needed in patients in whom the disorder is mild or moderate. After the serum sodium has recovered to normal, in most patients fluid intake can be liberalized without SIADH relapsing. However, serious brain disturbances demand urgent treatment with hypertonic saline and fluid restriction. Corticosteroids and anticonvulsants may be indicated in extreme cases. A major diuretic such as furosemide may also be helpful. In extreme cases the outlook may be very grave, but incredible neurologic recoveries have been reported with prompt, aggressive care.

SUMMARY

Although the pituitary gland has long been recognized as an important endocrine organ, its role as the grand orchestrator in mediating or modulating virtually every major metabolic process in the body has only become appreciated in the last 30 years as information concerning the mechanisms underlying the synthesis and release of its eight hormones has unfolded. The ability to safely and conveniently totally replace these hormones or those secreted by their target organs has allowed physicians to increase the possibilities of treating a wide variety of pituitary dysfunctions. The future for the further understanding of pituitary disorders, both on a fundamental and therapeutic level, is exciting. MRI is the most safe and effective way to evaluate the sella and parasellar anatomy. In addition, safer and more effective medical regimens for treatment may allow further definition concerning the precise indications for surgery. With the explosion in knowledge relating to the pathophysiology of the pituitary gland, the patient with dysfunction of this gland has many possible treatment alternatives that were not heretofore available. The challenge in management is for each patient to be seen as a unique opportunity for individualized care and to enlist the cooperative skills of endocrinologist, neurosurgeon, and radiation oncologist to provide the most rational and optimal therapy.

REFERENCES

1. Walker EA. A History of Neurological Surgery. Baltimore: Williams & Wilkins, 1982.
2. Paget S. John Hunter, Man of Science and Surgeon (1728-1793). London: Longmans Green, 1987.
3. Fröhlich A. Ein Fal von Tumor der Hypophysis cerebri ohne Akromegalie. Wien Klin Rundschau 15:883, 1901.
4. Haymaker W, Schiller F. The Founders of Neurology. Springfield, Ill.: Charles C Thomas, 1953.
5. Babinski J. Tumeur du corps pituitaire sans acromegalie et avec arret de development des organes genitaux. Rev Neurol 8:31, 1990.
6. Cushing H. Dyspituitarism: Twenty Years Later. Arch Intern Med 51:487, 1933.
7. Cushing H. Surgical experiences with pituitary disorders. JAMA 63:1515, 1914.
8. Cushing H. Pituitary Body, Hypothalamus and Parasympathetic Nervous System. Springfield, Ill.: Charles C Thomas, 1932.
9. Locke W, Schally AV. The Hypothalamus and Pituitary in Health and Disease. Springfield, Ill.: Charles C Thomas, 1972.
10. Martin JB, Reichlin S, Brown G. Clinical Neuroendocrinology. Philadelphia: FA Davis, 1978.
11. Randall RV. Neuroendocrinology. In Youmans JR, ed. Neurological Surgery. Philadelphia: WB Saunders, 1982.
12. du Vigneaud V. Hormones of the posterior pituitary gland: Oxytocin and vasopressin. In The Harvey Lectures 1954-55. New York: Academic Press, 1956.
13. Edwards CRW. Vasopressin and oxytocin in health and disease. Clin Endocrinol Metab 6:223, 1977.
14. Dousa TP. Cellular action of antidiuretic hormone in nephrogenic diabetes insipidus. Mayo Clin Proc 49:188, 1974.
15. Moses AM, Miller M, Streeten DHP. Pathophysiological and pharmacologic alterations in the release and action of ADH. Metabolism 25:697, 1976.
16. Magrini G, et al. Study on the relationship between plasma prolactin levels and androgen metabolism in man. J Clin Endocrinol 43:944, 1955.
17. Doughaday WH. Hormonal regulation of growth by somatomedin and other tissue growth factors. Clin Endocrinol Metab 6:117, 1977.
18. Schally AV, et al. Purification of corticotropin releasing factor from porcine hypothalamus. Endocrinology 100:95, 1977.
19. Schally AV, Arimua A. Physiology and nature of hypothalamic regulatory hormones. In Martini L, Besser GM, eds. Clinical Neuroendocrinology. New York: Academic Press, 1977.
20. Delitala G, et al. Growth hormone and prolactin release in acromegalic patients following metergoline administration. J Clin Endocrinol 43:1382, 1976.
21. Thorner MO, et al. Bromocriptine treatment of acromegaly. Br Med J 1:299, 1975.
22. Ivanmanesh A, Veldhuis JD. Clinical pathophysiology of the somatotrophic (GH) axis in adults. Endocrinol Metab Clin North Am 21:783, 1992.
23. Ahmed Ebbiary NA, Lenton EA. Hypothalamic-pituitary aging. Clin Endocrinol 41:199, 1994.
24. Martignoni E, et al. The brain as a target for adrenocortical steroids: Cognitive implications. Psychoneuroendocrinology 17:343, 1992.
25. Fernandez-Real JM, et al. Giant intrasellar aneurysm presenting with panhypopituitarism and subarachnoid hemorrhage: Case report and literature review [review]. Clin Invest 72:302, 1994.
26. Fureth J, Euda G, Clifton KH. The pathophysiology or pituitaries in their tumors: Methodological advances. In Husch H, ed. Methods in Cancer Research, vol 10. New York: Academic Press, 1973.
27. Sheehan HL, Davis JC. Pituitary necrosis. Br Med Bull 24:59, 1968.
28. Simmonda M. Uber embolische prozesse in der hypophysis. Virchows Arch 217:226, 1914.
29. Krieger DT, Amorosa L, Linick F. Cyproheptadine induced remission of Cushing's disease. N Engl J Med 293:893, 1975.
30. Landolt AM, Wilson CB. Tumors of the sella and parasellar area in adults. In Youmans JR, ed. Neurological Surgery. Philadelphia: WB Saunders, 1982.
31. Endocrinology 1980. Proceedings of the VI International Congress of Endocrinology, Melbourne, Australia, Feb. 10–6. Elsevier: North Holland Biomedical Press, 1980.

32. Costello RT. Subclinical adenoma of the pituitary gland. Am J Pathol 12:205, 1936.
33. Cuse SA, Kernohan JW. Squamous cell nests of the pituitary gland. Cancer 8:623, 1955.
34. Post KD, Jackson IMD. The Pituitary Adenoma. New York: Plenum Publishing, 1980.
35. Jenkins JS. Pituitary Tumors. London: Butterworth Publishing, 1973.
36. Hall WA, et al. Pituitary magnetic resonance imaging in normal human volunteers: Occult adenomas in the general population. Ann Intern Med 120:817, 1994.
37. Dabek JT. Bronchial carcinoid tumor with acromegaly in two patients. J Clin Endocrinol 38:329, 1974.
38. Sonksen PH, et al. Acromegaly caused by pulmonary carcinoid tumors. Clin Endocrinol 5:503, 1976.
39. Aubourg PR, et al. Endocrine outcome after transsphenoidal adenomectomy for prolactinoma: Prolactin levels and tumor size as predicting factors. Surg Neurol 14:141, 1980.
40. Wilson CB, Dempsey LC. Transsphenoidal microsurgical removal of 250 pituitary adenomas. J Neurosurg 48:13, 1978.
41. Gomes F, Reyes RI, Farman C. Non-peripheral galactorrhea and hyperprolactinemia. Am J Med 62:648, 1977.
42. Chang RJ, et al. Detection, evaluation, and treatment of pituitary microadenomas in patients with galactorrhea and amenorrhea. Am J Obstet Gynecol 128:356, 1977.
43. Wilson CB, et al. Cushing's disease and Nelson's syndrome. Clin Neurosurg 27:19, 1980.
44. Gold EM. The Cushing syndromes: Changing views of diagnosis and treatment. Ann Intern Med 90:829, 1979.
45. Krieger DT. Pharmacological therapy of Cushing's disease and Nelson's syndrome. In Linfoot JA, ed. Recent Advances in the Diagnosis and Treatment of Pituitary Tumors. New York: Raven Press, 1979.
46. Kriezer DT, Luria M. Effectiveness of cyproheptadine in decreasing plasma ACTH concentrations in Nelson's syndrome. J Clin Endocrinol Metab 43:1179, 1976.
47. Nelson DH, et al. ACTH-producing tumor of the pituitary gland. N Engl J Med 259:161, 1958.
48. Kleinberg DL, Noel GL, Frantz AG. Galactorrhea: A study of 235 cases including 48 with pituitary tumors. N Engl J Med 296:589, 1977.
49. McGregor AM, et al. Reduction in size of a pituitary tumor by bromocryptine therapy. N Engl J Med 300:291, 1979.
50. Laws ER, Randall R. Management of Pituitary Adenomas and Related Lesions. New York: Appleton-Century-Crofts, 1982.
51. Boyd AE, Lebovitz HE, Pfeizzer JB. Stimulation of human-growth-hormone secretion by L-DOPA. N Engl J Med 283:1425, 1970.
52. Chiodini PG, et al. Stable reduction of plasma growth hormone (hGH) during chronic administration of 2-Br-α-ergocryptine (CB-154) in acromegalic patients. J Clin Endocrinol Metab 40:795, 1975.
53. Corenblum B. Bromocryptine in pituitary tumors. Lancet 2:796, 1978.
54. Luboshitzky R, Barzilac D. Bromocriptine for an acromegalic patient, improvement in cardiac function, and carpal tunnel syndrome. JAMA 244:1825, 1980.
55. Feldman JM, Plonk JW, Bivens CH. Inhibitory effects of serotonin antagonists on growth hormone release in acromegalic patients. Clin Endocrinol 5:71, 1976.
56. Gonzales E. Update on pituitary tumor regression with bromocriptine therapy. JAMA 244:1535, 1980.
57. Laws ER, Trautmann JC, Hollenhorst RW. Transsphenoidal decompression of the optic nerve and chiasma: Visual results in 62 patients. J Neurosurg 46:717, 1977.
58. Thorner MO, et al. Rapid regression of pituitary prolactinomas during bromocriptine treatment. J Clin Endocrinol Metab 51:438, 1980.
59. Velentzas C, et al. Regression of pituitary prolactinoma with bromocriptine administration. JAMA 245:1149, 1981.
60. Friesen HG, Tolis G. The use of bromocryptine in the galactorrhea-amenorrhea syndrome: Canadian Cooperative Study. Endocrinology (Suppl 6):91, 1977.
61. Seki K, Seki M, Okamura T. Effect of CB-154 (2-BR-α-ergocryptine) on serum follicle stimulating hormone, luteinizing hormone and prolactin in women with amennorrhea-galactorrhea syndrome. Acta Endocrinol 79:25, 1975.
62. Sorbrinki LG, et al. Effect of treatment with bromocriptine on the size and activity of prolactin producing pituitary tumors. Acta Endocrinol 96:24, 1981.
63. Sorbrinko LG, et al. Radiologic evidence for regression of prolactinoma after treatment with bromocryptine. Lancet 2:257, 1978.
64. Summers VK, et al. Treatment of acromegaly with bromocriptine. J Clin Endocrinol Metab 40:904, 1975.
65. Wass JAH, et al. Long term treatment of acromegaly with bromocryptine. Br J Med 1:875, 1977.
66. Petrini L, et al. Long term treatment of Nelson syndrome by octreotide: Case report. J Endocrinol Invest 17:135, 1994.
67. Laws ER, Randall R, Abboud CF. Surgical treatment of acromegaly: Results in 140 patients. In Givens J, ed. Hormone-Secreting Pituitary Tumors. Chicago: Year Book Medical Publishers, 1982.
68. Balagura S, Dermome P, Guiot G. Acromegaly: Analysis of 132 cases treated surgically. Neurosurgery 8:413, 1981.
69. Baskin DS, Boggan JE, Wilson CB. Transsphenoidal microsurgical removal of growth hormone-secreting pituitary tumors: A review of 137 cases. J Neurosurg 56:634, 1982.
70. Belopavlovic M. Transfrontal pituitary surgery: Clinical results, intraoperative management and postoperative monitoring. Acta Neurochir 64:9, 1982.
71. Faria MA, Tindall GA. Transsphenoidal microsurgery for prolactin-secreting pituitary adenomas: Results in 100 women with the amenorrhea-galactorrhea syndrome. J Neurosurg 56:33, 1982.
72. Hardy J. Transsphenoidal microsurgery of the normal and pathological pituitary. Clin Neurosurg 16:185, 1969.
73. Hardy J. Transsphenoid hypophysectomy. J Neurosurgy 34:581, 1971.
74. Laws ER, Kern EB. Pituitary tumors treated by transnasal microsurgery: 7 years of clinical experience with 539 patients. In Sano K, Takakura K, Fukushima T, eds. Functioning Pituitary Adenoma Proceedings of the First Workshop on Pituitary Adenomas. New York: Excerpta Medica, 1980.
75. Ray BS. Intracranial hypophysectomy. J Neurosurg 28:180, 1968.
76. Stern WE, Batzdorf V. Intracranial removal of pituitary adenomas. J Neurosurg 33:564, 1970.
77. Zervas NT, Martin JB. Management of hormone secreting pituitary adenomas. N Engl J Med 302:210, 1980.
78. Patterson RH Jr, Danylevich A. Surgical removal of craniopharyngiomas by a transcranial approach through the lamina terminalis and sphenoidal sinus. Neurosurgery 7:111, 1980.
79. Knappe G, et al. 10 year follow-up of transsphenoidal pituitary surgery in acromegaly. Endokrinologue 79:423, 1982.
80. Domingue JN, Richmond IL, Wilson CB. Results of surgery in 114 patients with prolactin-secreting pituitary adenomas. Am J Obstet Gynecol 137:102, 1980.
81. Van't Verlaat JW. The use of surgery for the treatment of prolactinomas [review]. Acta Endocrinol 129(Suppl 1):34, 1993.
82. Lawrence AM, Pinsky SM, Goldfine ID. Conventional radiation therapy in acromegaly. Arch Intern Med 128:369, 1971.
83. Lopez JA. Pituitary apoplexy. J Oslo City Hospl 20:17, 1970.
84. Wersberg LA. Clinical study of pituitary apoplexy with emphasis on five cases precipitated by radiotherapy. Neurology 26:353, 1976.
85. Wakai S, et al. Pituitary apoplexy: Its incidence and clinical significance. J Neurosurg 55:187, 1981.

86. Broughan M, Heusner AP, Adams RD. Acute degenerative changes in adenomas of the pituitary body with special reference to pituitary apoplexy. J Neurosurg 7:421, 1950.
87. Daniel PM, Spicer EJF, Triep CS. Pituitary necrosis in patients maintained on mechanical respirators. J Pathol 111:135, 1973.
88. Dawson BH, Kothandaram P. Acute massive infarction of pituitary adenomas: A study of five patients. J Neurosurg 37:275, 1972.
89. Brisman R, et al. The empty sella syndrome—intrasellar cisternal herniation—in "normal" patients and in patients with communicating hydrocephalus and intracranial tumors. Neuroradiology 17:35, 1978.
90. Foley KM, Posner JB. Does pseudotumor cerebri cause the empty sella syndrome? Neurology 25:565, 1975.
91. Hodgson SF, et al. Empty sella syndrome: Report of 10 cases. Med Clin North Am 56:897, 1972.
92. Malarkey WV, Goodenow TJ, Lanese RR. Diurinal variation of prolactin secretion differentiates pituitary tumors from the primary empty sella syndrome. Am J Med 69:886, 1980.
93. Raskind R, Brown HA, Mathis J. Recurrent cyst of the pituitary: 26-year follow-up from first decompression: Case report. J Neurosurg 28:595, 1968.
94. Welch K, Stears JC. Chiasmapexy for the correction of traction on the optic nerves and chiasm associated with their descent into an empty sella turcica: Case report. J Neurosurg 35:291, 1971.
95. Robinson AG. DdAVP in the treatment of central diabetes insipidus. N Engl J Med 294:177, 1976.
96. Daniel PM, Prichard MML. Human hypothalamus and pituitary stalk after hypophysection or pituitary stalks section. Brain 95:813, 1972.
97. Sridhar CB, Calvert GD, Ibbertson HK. A new interpretation of diabetes insipidus. J Clin Endocrinol Metab 38:890, 1974.
98. Dila CJ, Papius HM. Cereral water and electrolytes. Arch Neurol 26:85, 1972.
99. Schwartz WV, Bartler FC. The syndrome of inappropriate secretion of antidiuretic hormone. Am J Med 42:790, 1967.
8. Brisman R, Hughes JEO, Mount LA. Cerebrospinal fluid rhinorrhea and the empty sella. J Neurosurg 31:538, 1969.
10. Buckman MT, et al. Primary empty sella syndrome with visual field defects. Am J Med 61:124, 1976.
64. Neelon FA, Foree JA, Lebovitz HE. The primary empty sella: Clinical and radiographic characteristics and endocrine function. Medicine 52:73, 1973.
72. Ridgeway EC, et al. Thyrotropin and prolactin pituitary reserve in the "empty sella syndrome." J Clin Endocrinol 41:968, 1975.
92. Weiss MH, Kaufmann B, Richards DE. Cerebrospinal fluid rhinorrhea from an empty sella: Transsphenoidal obliteration of the fistula: Technical note. J Neurosurg 39:674, 1973.

58

Adrenal Glands

R.Y. Declan Fleming, Douglas B. Evans, and Jeffrey E. Lee

In evaluating and treating surgical patients, physicians must have both an understanding of normal adrenal physiology and an appropriate level of suspicion regarding the potential presence of adrenal pathology. In this way, occult adrenal insufficiency, pheochromocytomas, functioning adrenal adenomas, and aldosteronomas are more likely to be detected at an early stage. An understanding of the natural history and epidemiology of incidental masses of the adrenal gland, functioning and nonfunctioning adenomas, pheochromocytomas, and adrenal cortical carcinomas allows the surgeon evaluating the patient with an incidental adrenal mass to design a thorough and efficient diagnostic schema and to recommend the most appropriate treatment. Discussion of these considerations forms the basis of this chapter.

EMBRYOLOGY AND ANATOMY

The adrenal gland is composed of a cortex and medulla, which have separate embryologic origins. The adrenal cortex arises from coelomic mesoderm between the fourth and sixth weeks of gestation. The adrenal medulla is derived from cells of the neural crest that also form the sympathetic nervous system and ganglia. Some of these neural crest cells migrate to the adrenal cortex to form the adrenal medulla, but chromaffin tissue may also develop in extra-adrenal sites, most commonly in the para-adrenal and para-aortic regions. The single most common site for the development of extra-adrenal chromaffin tissue is the organ of Zuckerkandl, located adjacent to the aorta near the origin of the inferior mesenteric artery. The adrenal cortex is composed initially of an inner zone and a large, outer "fetal zone." The fetal zone involutes late in gestation and in the early postnatal period, leaving only the thin cortical layer in the mature adrenal gland.

The adrenal glands are paired structures located in the retroperitoneum along the superior medial aspect of each kidney. Their shape is that of an oblong triangle with rounded points. The normal adult adrenal gland weighs approximately 4 to 5 g and has a rubbery consistently. The bright yellow color of the adrenal gland helps to differentiate it from the surrounding retroperitoneal fat. On cut section, two distinct portions of the adrenal gland are evident: the thin (1 to 2 mm), bright yellow cortex envelops an even thinner layer of dark, reddish-gray tissue, the adrenal medulla. The medulla is soft and comprises only approximately 10% to 20% of the total weight of the adrenal gland.

The adrenal glands are highly vascularized; they receive arterial blood from branches of the inferior phrenic arteries, the renal artery, and directly from the aorta. Nutrient arteries coalesce and anastomose to form a capsular arterial plexus that sends capillaries coursing through the cortical cells. These capillaries combine to form a venous portal system that drains into the adrenal medulla. There the vessels reach confluence with the central adrenal vein. This venous portal system provides a high concentration of adrenal steroids to the adrenal medullary tissue. Additionally, the adrenal medulla is supplied by *arteriae medullae;* these penetrate directly into the substance of the adrenal medulla. Although some small veins drain from the surface of the adrenal cortex, most arterial blood flows from the capsular plexus, through the cortex, into the medulla, and out the central vein. The right adrenal vein is short and wide; it exits the gland and immediately enters the posterolateral aspect of the inferior vena cava. The left adrenal vein exits anteriorly and usually drains into the left renal vein, although it occasionally enters the inferior vena cava directly. As a result, catheterization of the adrenal vein is more easily accomplished on the left than on the right.

A lymphatic plexus exists within the subcapsular portion of the adrenal cortex and the adrenal medulla. This drains into the adjacent para-aortic and renal lymph nodes. No innervation of the adrenal cortex has been demonstrated. In contrast, the adrenal medulla is richly supplied by preganglionic sympathetic nerves that run from the splanchnic nerve, celiac ganglia, and other plexuses. There is no parasympathetic innervation of the adrenal medulla.

Histologically, the adult adrenal cortex comprises three zones: an outer zona glomerulosa, a middle zona fasciculata, and an inner zona reticularis. Each zone has distinct histologic features on light and electron microscopy. Aldosterone is produced exclusively in the zona glomerulosa, whereas cortisol and androgens are produced in the zona fasciculata and zona reticularis. Adrenal medullary cells are polyhedral in shape and arranged in cords around adrenal portal veins. They contain catecholamines and precipitated chromium salts that stain brown with hematoxylin and eosin. On electron microscopy, one can see vesicles in the core of these cells that contain epinephrine and norepinephrine. Hormone secretion by the adrenal cortex and the vascular supply to the gland influence adrenal medullary secretion. Adrenal medullary cells are generally clumped around blood vessels coming from the cortex, providing these cells with a high local concentration of cortisol. Cortisol induces the enzyme phenylethanolamine N-methyltransferase (PNMT) for conversion of norepinephrine to epinephrine. The vessels that provide direct arterial supply to the adrenal medulla are surrounded primarily by cells that secrete predominantly norepinephrine.

PHYSIOLOGY

Physiologically, the adrenal gland must be considered as two separate organs. The cortex and the medulla operate under independent control systems and their functions are not overlapping.

Adrenal Cortex

The adrenal cortex is best understood as having three major secretory products: cortisol, aldosterone, and androgens. The metabolic pathways are shown in Fig. 58-1.

Cortisol

The control of cortisol secretion by the zona fasciculata begins in the CNS. Neurons from almost every part of the brain converge on the hypothalamus and modulate the release of a 41-amino-acid peptide, known as corticotropin-releasing factor (CRF). After its release, CRF reaches the anterior pituitary gland by way of a direct portal venous system, where CRF in turn stimulates the synthesis and release of adrenocorticotropic hormone (ACTH), a 39-amino-acid peptide. Under basal conditions the CNS, through CRF, ACTH, and the adrenocortical cascade, effects a circadian rhythm of fluctuating mean plasma cortisol concentrations. A peak in plasma cortisol concentration normally occurs in the early morning hours, with a nadir in the late afternoon.

Stimulation of cortisol secretion by ACTH proceeds along a steroidogenic pathway. The primary action of ACTH is on the conversion of cholesterol to δ-5-pregnenolone. Under basal conditions plasma cortisol concentrations are maintained within fairly narrow limits by an interplay between the concentrations of circulating cortisol, CRF and ACTH secretion. As cortisol concentrations increase above this physiologic limit either through endogenous stimulation or by exogenous administration, ACTH secretion is suppressed. Such suppression of ACTH secretion by cortisol is exerted through at least three mechanisms: Cortisol acts directly on the pituitary to inhibit the synthesis of ACTH, cortisol suppresses the release of ACTH by CRF, and cortisol inhibits the synthesis of CRF. Through these mechanisms the negative feedback effect of cortisol on ACTH release

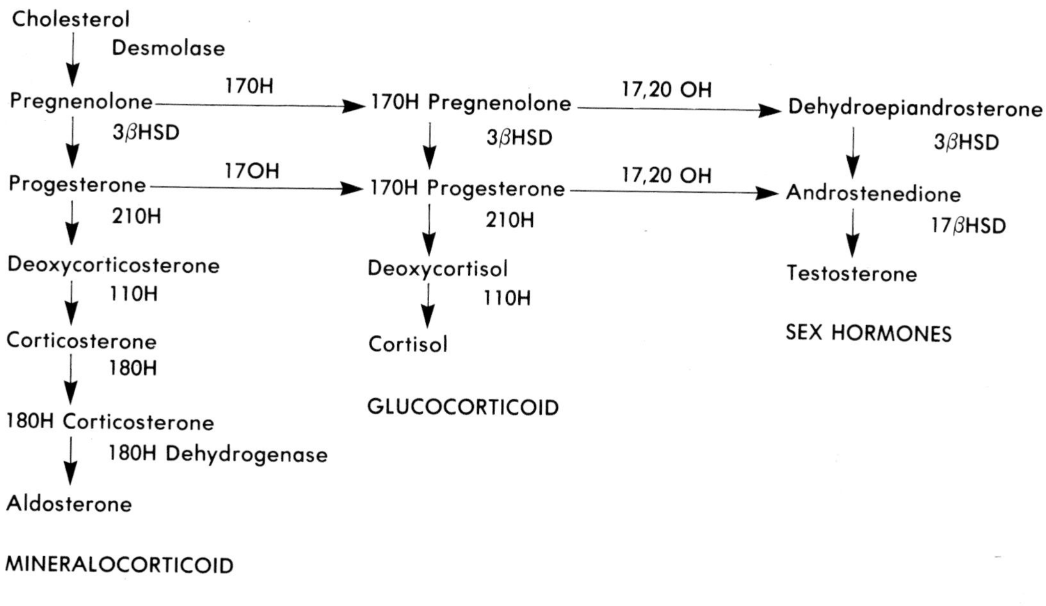

Fig. 58-1. Metabolic pathways in the adrenal cortex.

serves to maintain circulating plasma cortisol in the normal range.

In general, the increased secretion of ACTH and cortisol, brought about by acute stress, fever, pain, and hemorrhage, overrides the negative feedback effect of acute endogenous or exogenous hypercortisolemia. ACTH secretion increases in proportion to the magnitude of stress, and the adrenal secretion of cortisol is related linearly to the concentration of ACTH up to a range of 400 to 500 pg/ml. The maximal plasma concentration of cortisol produced by stress is in the range of 50 to 70 g/100 ml. Concentrations above 70 to 80 g/100 ml are distinctly unusual, even in situations of long-standing adrenal hyperplasia caused by ectopic ACTH production.

Long-standing cortisol (or synthetic steroid) excess has a lasting suppressive effect on ACTH secretion. Prolonged cortisol excess prevents the ACTH response to stress and other stimuli. The length of time that excess cortisol or cortisol-like steroids must be administered before suppression of ACTH release occurs has not been precisely determined in humans, however. Approximately 2 to 3 weeks of chronic daily steroid therapy is sufficient to suppress the normal pituitary-adrenal axis. In the case of exogenously administered steroids, the suppressive effect is clearly dose dependent. Once cortisol excess is abolished, either by removal of an endogenous source or by cessation of administered steroids, return of pituitary-adrenal function follows a fairly predictable pattern; ACTH secretion returns within 3 to 4 months, followed a few months later by return of adrenocortical responsiveness and consequent cortisol secretion. The return of adrenal responsiveness can be hastened by exogenous administration of ACTH during the early period of pituitary-adrenal unresponsiveness.

Almost every tissue in the body is affected by glucocorticoids. Glucocorticoid-related changes in carbohydrate metabolism have the net effect of producing hyperglycemia. The two primary events responsible for hyperglycemia are decreased peripheral utilization of glucose and increased gluconeogenesis. A separate action of glucocorticoids is to increase hepatic glycogen synthesis, which is thought to be insulin dependent. Hyperglycemia is due to an inhibition of glucose transport and metabolism (especially in fat cells, by a direct cellular effect of the glucocorticoids) and a resistance to the action of insulin. Glucocorticoids increase gluconeogenesis through several mechanisms, including peripheral and hepatic mechanisms. Glucocorticoids act on muscle to release branched-chain and other glucogenic amino acids for conversion in the liver to glucose. Both the lipolytic effect of epinephrine, causing release of glycerol from fat cells, as well as the glycogenolytic effect of epinephrine, causing release of lactate from muscle, appear to depend partly on the presence of glucocorticoids. Thus glucocorticoids provide increased glucogenic amino acids, glycerol, and lactate from the periphery for glucose production in the liver through the process of gluconeogenesis. The permissive effect of glucocorticoids accounts for the dependence of epinephrine and glucagon on these steroids for their gluconeogenic action. Lastly, glucocorticoids have a direct effect on gluconeogenesis, apparently by induction of several gluconeogenic hepatic enzymes.

The effects of glucocorticoids on immune function are complex and numerous. In considering both in vivo and in vitro effects, as well as those seen with both low-dose and high-dose steroid administration, it is evident that almost every aspect of the immune response can be modified by steroid administration. Numbers and distribution of granulocytes and lymphocytes, as well as the function of these cells, are affected either directly or indirectly by the presence of glucocorticoids. Excess glucocorticoids decrease the tensile strength of wounds, suppress contraction of the scar, and delay epithelialization. These effects have been demonstrated in several species, including humans. In vivo studies have demonstrated a decrease in collagen synthesis because of decreased protein synthesis brought on by glucocorticoids. Excess or exogenously administered glucocorticoids may also exert effects on bone mineralization, the cardiovascular system, the digestive tract, and renal function.

Aldosterone

Aldosterone is a steroid originating from the zona glomerulosa of the adrenal cortex. It is the end product of a steroidogenic pathway that includes corticosterone and deoxycorticosterone. Aldosterone has a specific effect on sodium, potassium, and hydrogen ion transport. As with glucocorticoids, the specificity of the action of aldosterone is determined by its chemical configuration, by the conformational structure and location of steroid receptors, and by postreceptor intracellular events. The actions of aldosterone are less generalized than those of glucocorticoids as a result of the more limited tissue distribution of aldosterone receptors. Aldosterone receptors in the renal tubule allow aldosterone to play a major role in the control of total body sodium, potassium, and extracellular fluid balance. Aldosterone receptors also control electrolyte balance in the salivary glands and the colonic mucosa.

The primary control mechanism for aldosterone secretion is the renin-angiotensin system. Renin is released from the juxtaglomerular apparatus of the kidney in response to a decrease in intravascular volume, such as occurs with hemorrhage, a negative sodium balance, or dehydration. Both a decrease in pressure in the afferent arteriole entering the glomerulus and a decrease in intratubular sodium concentration at the level of the macula densa stimulate renin secretion. Renin released into the blood stream hydrolyzes a circulating protein substrate derived from the liver to produce angiotensin I. This peptide is then further cleaved by a converting enzyme in the lung to form angiotensin II. Angiotensin II is a potent vasoconstrictor and a trophic hormone to the adrenal zona glomerulosa for the stimulation of aldosterone secretion. A decrease in intravascular volume results in an increase in aldosterone secretion because of the stimulation of angiotensin II. Conversely, conditions producing a replete blood volume, positive sodium balance, or overhydration lead to suppressed levels of angiotensin II and a decrease in aldosterone secretion. Aldosterone secretion is also directly controlled by the concentration of serum potassium. An increase in serum potassium results in the stimulation of aldosterone secretion, and a decrease in serum potassium results in a lowering of aldosterone secretion. In the anephric patient without a renin-angiotensin system, serum potassium appears to be the primary mechanism for control of aldosterone secretion.

ACTH is capable of stimulating aldosterone secretion. Such stimulation is normally accompanied by an increase in cortisol secretion. In contrast, angiotensin II and serum potassium do not stimulate cortisol production. Although ACTH can stimulate aldosterone secretion, ACTH alone is not sufficient to restore the full secretory capacity of the zona glomerulosa.

Receptors for aldosterone have been found in such tissues as the parotid gland and colonic mucosa, but the primary site for physiologic control of electrolyte and fluid balance is the kidney. Furthermore, those receptors responsible for increased sodium reabsorption in the kidney are concentrated in the cortical collecting tubule. The primary effect of aldosterone on the kidney is to increase sodium resorption and potassium secretion in the proximal portion of the collecting tubule. Chronic aldosterone excess results in a depletion of total body potassium levels through increased kaliuresis. Aldosterone also promotes a secretion of hydrogen ions into the renal tubule. This process may not necessarily be directly associated with sodium reabsorption. The net result of a chronic proton deficit is the development of a metabolic alkalosis.

Androgens

The three major androgenic steroids produced by the adrenal cortex are dehydroepiandrosterone (DHEA), DHEA sulfate (DHEAS), and androstenedione. Quantitatively, DHEA is the most prominent androgenic steroid produced by the adrenal cortex; synthesis of testosterone by the adrenal cortex is minimal. The androgenic steroids produced in quantity by the adrenal cortex are not themselves effective androgens; however, they are converted to the potent androgens testosterone and 5α-dihydrotestosterone in peripheral tissues. Although peripheral conversion of adrenal androgens is an important source of circulating androgens in women, in men most circulating androgen is produced by the testes. The adrenal cortex produces only small amounts of the estrogens estrone and estradiol; most circulating estrogens in women are derived from the ovaries.

The adrenal cortex has the potential to produce virilization, either through the secretion of excess androgens by tumors or as a consequence of enzyme defects that shunt steroidogenesis in favor of androgen formation. In the surgical context, excess androgen secretion is most commonly due to adrenal tumors in adults or children or to congenital adrenocortical enzymatic defects, which are found primarily in newborns and associated with sexual ambiguity. Androgen secretion by adrenal tumors is usually associated with excess cortisol secretion. Female patients with Cushing's syndrome have masculinizing features including coarsening of facial hair and distribution of pubic hair into the male pattern. Although aspects of virilization may appear in patients with benign adrenocortical tumors, excessive adrenal androgen production, as evidenced by increased 17-ketosteroids in the urine, is almost always seen in adrenocortical carcinoma.

The most striking clinical examples of virilizing adrenal tumors are those producing primarily androgens. These tumors may go undetected initially in men, but women experience a deepening of the voice, coarsening of the skin, thickening and darkening of facial hairs, assumption of male hair distribution, clitoral hypertrophy, and menstrual cessation. These tumors may appear in childhood and result in precocious puberty in both males and females.

Rarely, adrenal cortical adenomas or carcinomas produce estrogens. Additionally, peripheral conversion of androstenedione to estrogens can result in feminization in patients with adrenal cortical tumors or adrenocortical enzymatic defects; extra-adrenal tumors or extra-adrenal enzymatic defects can also cause feminization. In such unusual cases it is usually difficult to detect estrogen excess in the female patient, but menstrual irregularities may lead to definitive diagnosis by measurement of plasma or urinary estrogens. The male patient with estrogen excess has loss of libido and onset of impotency, enlargement of breast tissue, and occasionally softening of facial hair and an alteration in male pattern hair distribution.

Adrenal Medulla

Epinephrine and norepinephrine are the principal secretory products of the adrenal medulla. Dopamine is also a secretory product of the adrenal medulla, but its physiologic importance is unclear and of undetermined functional significance. Enkephalins have recently been identified in the adrenal medulla; their significance is also unclear. Under basal conditions, approximately 80% of the catecholamine production by the adrenal medulla is epinephrine derived from the amino acid tyrosine. The conversion of tyrosine to dihydroxyphenylalanine (dopa) is accomplished by the action of tyrosine hydroxylase. Tyrosine hydroxylase is the rate-limiting enzyme in the synthetic pathway. Sympathetic nerve stimulation results in an increase in tyrosine hydroxylase content, as well as an increase in norepinephrine and epinephrine production. Next in the pathway, dopa is converted to dopamine by dopa decarboxylase, and the dopamine, now in catecholamine storage vesicles, is converted to norepinephrine by dopamine β-hydroxylase. PNMT then converts norepinephrine to epinephrine. Interestingly, PNMT depends on high concentrations of cortisol for its activity. Demonstrable vascular connections lead from the adrenal cortex through the adrenal medulla, presumably carrying high concentrations of cortisol to the enzyme.

The effects of adrenomedullary stimulation and sympathetic nerve stimulation are generally similar. In some tissues, however, epinephrine and norepinephrine may produce different effects because of the existence of two types of receptors, α- and β-receptors. These receptors have differing sensitivities for various catecholamines and therefore produce different responses. α-Adrenergic receptors are most sensitive to epinephrine and norepinephrine, whereas β-adrenergic receptors are most sensitive to isoproterenol. α-Receptors are further subdivided into the α_1-group, which causes vasoconstriction, intestinal relaxation, uterine contraction, and pupillary dilation, and the α_2-group, which causes platelet aggregation, vasoconstriction, and presynaptic norepinephrine release. β-Receptors are subdivided into the β_1-group, which are sensitive equally to epinephrine and norepinephrine and cause cardiac stimulation, intestinal relaxation, and lipolysis, and the β_2-group, which are more sensitive to epinephrine than norepinephrine and cause vasodilation, uterine relaxation, bronchodilation, and presynaptic norepinephrine release.

Several metabolic effects are produced by catecholamine release. Carbohydrate metabolism is affected by alterations in glycogenolysis in the liver and in striated muscle. β-Adrenergic receptor stimulation causes stimulation of glycogen phosphorylase and inhibition of glycogen synthetase. Concomitantly, gluconeogenesis is increased in the liver by catecholamine (especially epinephrine) secretion. Glycogenolysis produces metabolic precursors for gluconeogenesis such as lactate and pyruvate. In all, glucose levels generally rise as catecholamine secretion is increased. This, combined with stimulation of glucagon secretion and reduction of insulin secretion (by pancreatic islet cells), accounts for the hyperglycemia observed in states where catecholamine concentrations are increased.

Hyposecretory states of the adrenal medulla generally produce no recognizable clinical symptoms. The most common causes of this condition include destruction of the gland by autoimmune disorders, malignant metastatic disease, tuberculosis, or surgical removal of the gland. In contrast, hypersecretion of catecholamines from chromaffin cell tumors produces the well-known clinical syndrome discussed later in the section on pheochromocytomas.

NEOPLASMS OF THE ADRENAL GLAND

Adrenal Cortical Carcinoma

Epidemiology, Natural History, and Presentation

Adrenal cortical carcinoma is a rare disease, with an incidence between 0.5 and 2 per million cases per year in the United States. Adrenal cortical carcinoma represents only 0.2% of the annual cancer incidence in the United States. Most patients with adrenal cortical carcinoma are diagnosed at an advanced stage; the tendency of the tumor to invade adjacent organs and to metastasize and delays in patient diagnosis are responsible for the poor prognosis for patients with adrenal cortical carcinoma.[1-4]

The clinical presentation of adrenal cortical carcinoma can vary considerably. Nonfunctioning tumors present with a constellation of findings such as abdominal pain, weight loss, generalized weakness, anorexia and nausea, enlarging abdominal girth, hepatomegaly, and a palpable abdominal mass that may be present in as many as 50% of patients. Various syndromes of adrenal hormone overproduction may occur in a third to two thirds of patients and are clinically related to hypercortisolism, hyperaldosteronism, or excessive androgen production (see following discussion). The acute or rapid production of one of these syndromes strongly suggests the presence of an adrenal cortical carcinoma.

Staging

The most widely used staging system for adrenal cortical carcinoma is the Sullivan[5] modification of the Macfarlane[6] system (Table 58-1). Under this staging system and in contrast to most modern staging systems, patients with adjacent organ invasion or fixed positive lymph nodes are grouped as stage IV together with patients with distant metastatic disease. More recent proposals[2,7] recommend staging those patients with locally invasive tumors in stage III, saving the stage IV category for patients with distant metastatic disease. This modification to the traditional staging system more accurately reflects the natural history of the disease, as well as the correct application of surgical and medical therapy, and is in agreement with cancer staging systems used in other solid tumors.

Surgical Treatment

Several recent series have examined the surgical treatment of patients with adrenal cortical carcinoma. These studies have demonstrated that contiguous organ invasion is common and that adjacent organs frequently must be resected as part of primary treatment for a localized adrenal cortical carcinoma (Fig. 58-2). However, results of at least two series have demonstrated that although the kidney is frequently removed as part of an en bloc operation, histologic examination of the resected specimens demonstrates evidence of invasion of the kidney in only a minority of specimens, and kidney-sparing complete resection is not associated with decreased survival.[2,7] Therefore although the surgeon who operates on patients with large adrenal masses must be prepared to resect adjacent organs (liver, vena cava, spleen, pancreas), if the tumor is localized without invasion of Gerota's fascia, the ipsilateral kidney may be spared. Review of surgical complications in the treatment of primary adrenal cortical carcinoma confirms that tumor extirpation requires complex operative procedures often associated with significant morbidity; however, mortality is 5% or less in most contemporary series.

A number of investigators have evaluated predictors of survival following resection of adrenal cortical carcinoma. By far the strongest predictor of outcome is the ability to perform a complete resection. When complete resection can be performed, 5-year actuarial survival ranges from

Table 58-1. Staging Systems for Adrenal Cortical Carcinoma

Stage	Macfarlane (1958)[6]	Sullivan et al. (1978)[5]	Icard et al. (1992)[7]	Lee et al. (1995)[2]
I	T_1 (≤5 cm), N_0, M_0	T_1 (≤5 cm), N_0, M_0	T_1 (≤5 cm), N_0, M_0	T_1 (≤5 cm), N_0, M_0
II	T_2 (>5 cm), N_0, M_0	T_2 (>5 cm), N_0, M_0	T_2 (>5 cm), N_0, M_0	T_2 (>5 cm), N_0, M_0
III	T_3 (local invasion without involvement of adjacent organs) or N_1 (mobile positive lymph nodes), M_0	T_3 (local invasion), N_0, M_0 or T_{1-2}, N_1 (positive lymph nodes), M_0	T_3 (local invasion) or N_1 (positive regional lymph nodes), M_0	T_3T_4 (local invasion as demonstrated by histologic evidence of adjacent organ invasion, direct tumor extension to IVC, and/or tumor thrombus within IVC or renal vein) or N_1 (positive regional lymph nodes), M_0
IV	T_4 (invasion of adjacent organs) or N_2 (fixed positive lymph nodes) or M_1 (distant metastases)	T_4 (local invasion), N_0, M_0; or T_3, N_1, M_0; or T_{1-4}, N_{0-1}, M_1 (distant metastases)	T_{1-4}, N_{0-1}, M_1 (distant metastases)	T_{1-4}, N_{0-1}, M_1 (distant metastases)

IVC, Inferior vena cava; *T,* tumor; *M,* metastasis; *N,* node.

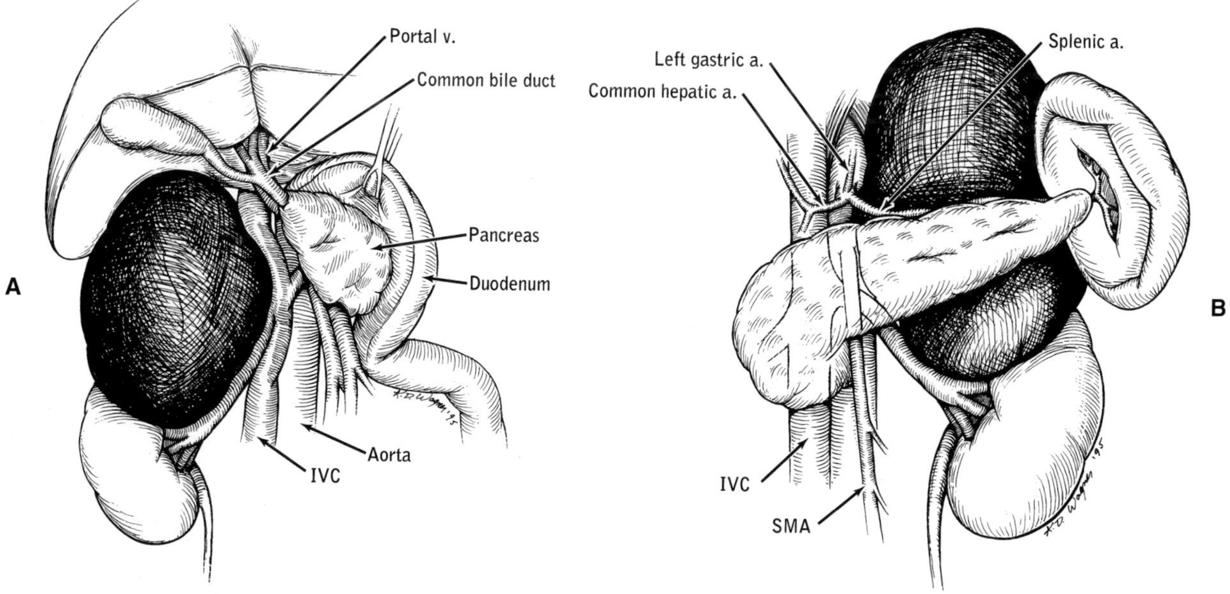

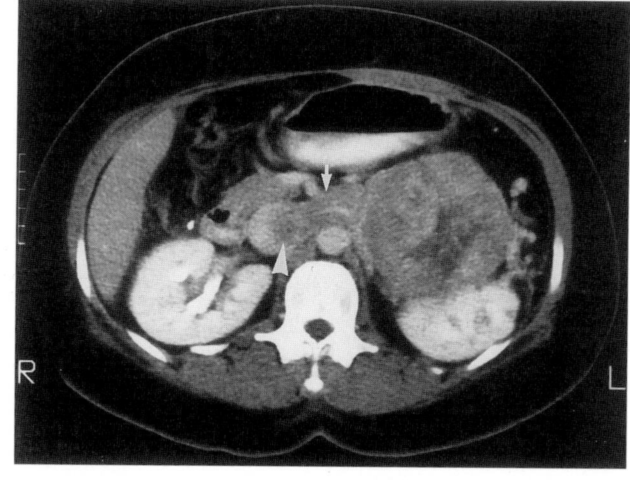

Fig. 58-2. Clinical spectrum of adrenal cortical carcinoma. **A,** Illustration of a large right adrenal carcinoma demonstrating the frequent finding of tumor invasion of the liver (posterior segment of the right hepatic lobe) and the inferior vena cava *(IVC).* **B,** Illustration of a large left adrenal carcinoma demonstrating the intimate relationship between the tumor and the origin of the celiac axis and the superior mesenteric artery *(SMA).* **C,** Contrast-enhanced CT scan of a large left adrenal carcinoma *(T)* with tumor thrombus within the left renal vein *(arrow)* extending into the inferior vena cava *(arrowhead).* This patient underwent complete resection with removal of all intravascular tumor from the inferior vena cava. (From Lee JE, et al. Surgical management, DNA content, and patient survival in adrenal cortical carcinoma. Surgery 118:1090, 1995.)

32% to 47% (Table 58-2). In our experience, neither extended resection nor the presence of tumor thrombus in the inferior vena cava or renal vein predicted a poor prognosis in patients who underwent complete resection. In contrast, patients who underwent incomplete resection of adrenal cortical carcinomas, including patients who underwent less than total resection of the primary tumor and patients who underwent resection of primary tumors in the face of unresectable distant metastatic disease, had a uniformly poor prognosis with a median survival of less than 1 year (Table 58-3).

Adjuvant Treatment

There is no treatment (adjuvant) for adrenal cortical carcinoma following complete resection that has been demonstrated to prolong survival.[12-14] Most investigations of adjuvant treatment for adrenal cortical carcinoma have involved the use of mitotane (ortho, para-DDD), a derivative of DDT with direct adrenolytic activity.[13,14] The role of mitotane as adjuvant therapy for adrenal cortical cancer remains controversial. No randomized trials of mitotane, when used as adjuvant therapy, have been performed; given the rare nature of the underlying disease it is unlikely that randomized trials will ever be performed. Anecdotal reports and small series have not been able to document a clear benefit to patients who receive adjuvant mitotane. In addition, mitotane therapy is quite toxic; neurologic and gastrointestinal toxicity are uniformly present. It is perhaps most reasonable to consider mitotane as adjuvant therapy in those patients without evidence of disease after a first recurrence, for example, after resection of isolated pulmonary or hepatic metastases.

Recommendations for Treatment

Resection should only be performed if preoperative imaging studies indicate that a complete margin-negative resection is possible. There appears to be limited indications at this time for primary resection in the presence of synchronous metastatic disease. However, anecdotal evidence supports complete resection of limited metastatic disease in good risk individuals, particularly in the case of isolated metachronous hepatic, pulmonary, or brain metastases.[15,16] However, resection of the primary tumor in the face of unresectable distant metastatic disease is not indicated. Systemic treatment options for patients with unresectable local recurrence or distant metastases include treatment with mitotane, suramin, ketoconazole, and systemic chemotherapy regimens containing cisplatin.[17] Mitotane appears to

Table 58-2. Survival of Patients Who Underwent a Potentially Curative Resection* for Adrenal Cortical Carcinoma

Author	Institution	Year	No. of Patients	Margin Analysis	Median Follow-up (mo)	Overall Survival (mo)	5-Year Actuarial Survival (%)
Lee et al.[2]	MDA	1995	16	Yes	43	46†	46
Zografos et al.[8]	Roswell Park	1994	15	No	—	13†	38
Icard et al.[7]	France	1992	127	No	—	—	42
Icard et al.[9]	Cochin	1992	31	No	—	44‡	45
Pommier and Brennan[10]	MSK	1992	53	No	28	28‡	47
Gröndal et al.[1]	Sweden	1990	22	No	—	—	—
Henley et al.[11]	Mayo Clinic	1983	31	No	—	—	32

*Includes patients who underwent resection of synchronous metastatic disease.
†Median.
‡Mean.
MDA, M.D. Anderson Cancer Center; *MSK*, Memorial Sloan-Kettering Cancer Center

Table 58-3. Patient Survival Following Incomplete Resection* of Adrenal Cortical Carcinoma

Author	Institution	Year	No. of Patients	Median Survival (mo)
Lee et al.[2]	MDA	1995	7	8.5
Zografos et al.[8]	Roswell Park	1994	28	2
Icard et al.[7]	France	1992	28	<12
Icard et al.[9]	Cochin	1992	10	<4
Gröndal et al.[1]	Sweden	1990	12	10
Henley et al.[11]	Mayo Clinic	1983	14	<6

*Patients with incomplete resections included those who underwent incomplete resection of the primary tumor and those who underwent complete resection of the primary tumor in the presence of unresectable distant metastatic disease.
MDA, M.D. Anderson Cancer Center.

be most effective when given for symptomatic control of hormonally active tumors, since a decrease in serum hormone levels is much more common than a radiographic response. Dose and serum levels of mitotane must be monitored and adjusted to maintain efficacy while minimizing toxicity.

Aldosteronoma

Natural History and Presentation

The syndrome of primary hyperaldosteronism was described by Conn in 1954. Primary hyperaldosteronism occurs in 1 in 200 hypertensive patients and is characterized by hypokalemia, suppressed plasma renin activity, and increased urinary excretion of aldosterone.[18-21] Aldosterone secretion is regulated by both the renin-angiotensin system and the serum level of potassium. Decreased intravascular volume stimulates the secretion of renin from the renal juxtaglomerular apparatus, which cleaves angiotensinogen to angiotensin I. Angiotensin converting enzyme converts angiotensin I to angiotensin II, which rapidly activates aldosterone biosynthesis. Aldosterone is synthesized in the zona glomerulosa of the adrenal cortex (cortisol is synthesized in the zona fasciculata) and regulates electrolyte excretion and intravascular volume by binding to mineralocorticoid (type I) receptors in the kidney.

The signs of mineralocorticoid excess include hypertension and hypokalemic alkalosis. The diagnosis is usually made in the third to sixth decades of life in hypertensive patients found to have persistent hypokalemia. Severe hypokalemia may cause muscle weakness, cramping, palpitations, or polyuria. Plasma volume expansion leads to decreased release of vasopressin, resulting in mild hypernatremia. Chronic potassium depletion results in decreased insulin secretion and mild hyperglycemia.

Unilateral aldosterone-producing adrenal adenomas are the most common cause of hyperaldosteronism, being responsible for two thirds of cases. They produce 18-hydroxycortisol and 18-oxycortisol, which are 17α-hydroxylated analogs of 18-hydroxycorticosterone and aldosterone. These steroids cannot be synthesized in the normal zona glomerulosa or zona fasciculata. Differentiating unilateral adenoma from bilateral idiopathic hyperaldosteronism is critical because surgical adrenalectomy is helpful only in the former. Increased mineralocorticoid activity may also be due to Cushing's syndrome or the effects of substances such as licorice or chewing tobacco. Evaluation of a urinary free cortisol level and results of an overnight dexamethasone suppression test (see the following discussion of evaluation and treatment) can exclude the diagnosis of Cushing's syndrome. Licorice and chewing tobacco inhibit the enzyme 11-β-hydroxysteroid dehydrogenase, which converts cortisol to cortisone. Cortisol has mineralocorticoid activity (cortisone does not) but normally circulates at a much lower concentration than aldosterone. Long-term use of licorice or chewing tobacco may cause mineralocorticoid hypertension and elevated urinary cortisol levels.

Evaluation and Treatment

Uncomplicated hypertension is rarely associated with spontaneous hypokalemia. When hyperaldosteronism is suspected, serum and urinary potassium levels and paired upright plasma aldosterone and renin concentrations should be obtained. A 24-hour urinary potassium value of greater than 30 mmol following potassium repletion and in the presence of adequate salt intake is consistent with mineralocorticoid-dependent hypertension. Low plasma renin activity (<3 ng/ml/hr) is essential for the diagnosis of hyperaldosteronism but also may occur in patients with essential hypertension. However, the ratio of plasma aldosterone (ng/dl) to plasma renin (ng/ml/hr) is greater than 20 in the majority of patients with hyperaldosteronism. If the above screening tests suggest hyperaldosteronism and potentially interfering drugs are excluded (estrogens, diuretics, calcium channel blockers, adrenergic inhibitors), aldosterone suppression testing is necessary to establish a definitive diagnosis of hyperaldosteronism. With ongoing potassium repletion, a high-salt diet (2 to 3 g of $NaCl_2$ with each meal) is provided for 5 days and a 24-hour urine specimen collected on day 4 to 5 and analyzed for aldosterone, sodium (to ensure adequate sodium repletion), cortisol, and creatinine (to ensure a complete collection). Serum levels of potassium are obtained to exclude the presence of hypokalemia, which may decrease aldosterone excretion. In the presence of a normal serum potassium and in conditions of high salt intake, patients with hyperaldosteronism fail to suppress urinary aldosterone to less than 10 μg/24 hr.

Once the diagnosis of hyperaldosteronism is established, it is critical to differentiate unilateral adrenal adenoma from bilateral hyperplasia of the zona glomerulosa (idiopathic hyperaldosteronism). In patients with an aldosterone-producing adenoma, unilateral adrenalectomy corrects the hypokalemia and lowers the blood pressure in 70% of surgically treated patients. However, surgery is of little value in patients with idiopathic hyperaldosteronism. Patients with a unilateral adenoma usually have more severe hypertension, higher plasma aldosterone levels, and therefore more profound hypokalemia; however, these findings cannot accurately differentiate patients with unilateral adenoma from those with idiopathic hyperaldosteronism. CT scan, MRI, and selective venous sampling for aldosterone measurement can confirm the presence of a unilateral adenoma. However, the high frequency of nonfunctioning adenomas in the normal population (2% to 8%) means that the finding of a small adrenal mass on CT scan or MRI is not necessarily diagnostic of a unilateral aldosterone-producing adenoma. Because selective venous sampling is invasive and cannulation of the right adrenal vein often difficult, the cause of the elevated aldosterone level may remain unclear even after the above studies. Therefore adrenal imaging is often combined with postural studies.

Postural (i.e., upright) studies are based on the principle that aldosterone-producing adenomas are not affected by changes in angiotensin II levels, which occur with standing (unlike idiopathic hyperaldosteronism). The absence of the normal postural increase in aldosterone concentration supports the diagnosis of an aldosterone-producing adenoma. In fact, serum aldosterone levels in patients with aldosterone-producing adenomas (suppressed renin levels) usually fall in response to assuming an upright posture in the morning because of the diurnal decline in corticotropin levels. However, to complicate matters further, rare patients with apparent unilateral aldosterone-producing adenomas may have results of postural studies more consistent with idiopathic hyperaldosteronism. Such patients have aldosterone-producing, renin-responsive adenomas and are often cured with unilateral adrenalectomy. Selective venous sampling can differentiate this rare disease from idiopathic (bilateral) hyperaldosteronism.[22]

Cortisol-Producing Adenoma

Hypercortisolism due to an adrenal cortical adenoma is rare, occurring in an estimated 1 in 10 million individuals. Prognosis is excellent, with cure in the overwhelming majority. Signs and symptoms of hypercortisolism are included in Table 58-4; actions of glucocorticoids are discussed in the previous section on cortisol physiology. The most common symptom associated with hypercortisolism is weight gain; in adults, cortisol-induced obesity is usually in the classic (truncal) pattern. Evaluation of the patient with potential hypercortisolism proceeds within the framework of the differential diagnosis of hypercortisolism and is designed to differentiate ACTH-dependent causes (Cushing's disease [pituitary adenoma], ectopic ACTH production, ectopic CRH production, exogenous ACTH administration) from ACTH-independent causes (exogenous glucocorticoid administration, adrenal cortical adenoma or carcinoma, bilateral micronodular or macronodular dysplasia). The most common cause of hypercortisolism is exogenous adminstration of steroid hormones to treat other diseases. Excluding patients who are taking exogenous steroid hormones, approximately 15% of patients with hypercortisolism have an adrenal cortical neoplasm.

Signs and symptoms attributable to elevated levels of plasma cortisol have commonly been termed *Cushing's syndrome* in honor of the neurosurgeon, Harvey Cushing, who first described them in patients with basophilic adenomas of the pituitary, even though the relationship between hypercortisolism and adrenal cortical dysfunction was not initially appreciated. Although Cushing's syndrome is still used to refer to hypercortisolism, regardless of cause, *Cushing's disease* refers to an ACTH-dependent cause of hypercortisolism secondary to pituitary adenoma. Because of the confusion that can result from these designations, we prefer not to use them.

The most sensitive method for detecting hypercortisolism is the overnight dexamethasone suppression test. One milligram of dexamethsone is taken orally at 11 PM; normal individuals have a cortisol level of less than 5 μg/dl at 8 AM the following morning. Failure to suppress the 8 AM cortisol to less than 5 μg/dl is consistent with hypercortisolism; however, while this test has a false negative rate of only 3%, the false positive rate is 30%. Therefore a normal result from an overnight dexamethasone suppression test excludes clinically significant hypercortisolism, but an abnormal result from the test requires further investigation. A 24-hour urine collection for urinary (unmetabolized) free cortisol is somewhat less sensitive than overnight dexamethasone suppression but more specific; urinary collection for 17-hydroxysteroids can also be used.

Once hypercortisolism is identified, the investigation proceeds to determine the cause of the hypercortisolism. Serum levels of ACTH and cortisol are obtained as part of a low-dose dexamethasone suppression test. These two tests differentiate patients as follows: (1) patients without hypercortisolism (i.e., false positive results from screening tests) have a normal ACTH and a normal response to dexamethasone suppression; (2) patients with ACTH-dependent hypercortisolism (e.g., pituitary adenoma or ectopic ACTH) have no suppression of ACTH and an abnormal response to dexamethasone suppression; (3) patients with ACTH-independent hypercortisolism (e.g., adrenal cortical tumors) have a low ACTH and an abnormal response to dexamethasone suppression. In the standard 2-day, low-dose dexamethasone suppression test, a basal 24-hour urine collection for 17-hydroxysteroids and urinary free cortisol is followed by 0.5 mg dexamethasone orally every 6 hours for a total of eight doses; a second urine collection

Table 58-4. Clinical Manifestations of Adrenal Cortical Hormone Excess

Cortisol	Androgen	Estrogen	Aldosterone
Truncal obesity	Male pattern baldness	Gynecomastia	Hypertension
Buffalo hump	Hirsutism	Breast tenderness	Hypokalemia
Moon facies	Voice change	Testicular atrophy	Weakness
Abdominal striae	Breast atrophy	Decreased libido	Polyuria
Hypertension	Libido change		Polydipsia
Glucose intolerance	Oligomenorrhea		Metabolic alkalosis
Thin skin			Glucose intolerance
Osteoporosis			
Psychiatric changes			

is performed, timed to end 6 hours after the last dose of dexamethasone. High-dose dexamethasone testing may be performed in cases in which results from low-dose testing are equivocal; patients with pituitary adenomas generally suppress ACTH and cortisol production with high-dose dexamethasone, whereas patients with the ectopic ACTH syndrome or an adrenal cortical tumor do not. In the standard 2-day, high-dose dexamethasone suppression test, a basal 24-hour urine collection for 17-hydroxysteroids and urinary free cortisol is followed by 2 mg dexamethasone taken orally every 6 hours for a total of eight doses; a second urine collection is performed, timed to end 6 hours after the last dose of dexamethasone.

If the foregoing testing suggests an ACTH-dependent hypercortisolism, a variety of additional studies may help in identfiying the source. Since corticotropin-producing adenomas of the pituitary gland (Cushing's disease) are responsible for the vast majority of patients with hypercortisolism in this subset, radiologic evaluation of the sella turcica to look for an enlarged pituitary gland is appropriate. Both MRI and high-resolution CT scan can prove useful in this evaluation. It must be remembered that as many as 90% of adenomas may exist in the microadenoma stage so that an enlarged sella may not be detected. In this circumstance, localization of the pituitary source of ACTH may require inferior petrosal sinus sampling with CRH stimulation. If an ectopic source of ACTH-dependent hypercortisolism is suspected, such as a bronchial or thymic carcinoid, CT scan of the chest can be of assistance in localizing the site of the neoplasm.

Although not used as much now as in the past, metyrapone testing can be helpful in delineating the source of hypercortisolism in confusing situations. Metyrapone inhibits the enzyme 11-hydroxylase and thereby blocks the conversion of 11-deoxycortisol to cortisol (see Fig. 58-1). The fall in plasma cortisol evokes a rise in ACTH secretion by the pituitary gland, which then stimulates the adrenal cortex to produce increased cortisol precursors. Thus under normal conditions plasma 11-deoxycortisol and urinary 17-hydorxycorticosteroids (17-OHCS) are increased. In patients with pituitary adenomas, metyrapone induces increased plasma levels of ACTH, 11-deoxycortisol, and urinary 17-OHCS. In patients with ectopic sources of ACTH or adrenal neoplasms, pituitary suppression results so that plasma levels of ACTH and 11-deoxycortisol and urinary levels of 17-OHCS do not change.

Choices for abdominal imaging include CT scan, MRI, and ^{131}I-6-β-iodomethyl norcholesterol (iodocholesterol) scanning. CT scan has a high sensitivity and is the initial imaging study of choice. MRI has a higher specificity than CT scan, since chemical shift and T2-weighted image analysis can help differentiate adrenal cortical adenomas from primary or metastatic carcinomas and from pheochromocytomas.[23-28] However, MRI has a lower resolution and therefore a lower sensitivity than CT scan. Finally, iodocholesterol can demonstrate uptake in an adrenal adenoma along with suppression of the contralateral gland. When CT scan and MRI are equivocal, iodocholesterol scanning may be helpful in differentiating unilateral adrenal cortical adenoma (unilateral uptake with contralateral suppression) from bilateral micronodular hyperplasia (bilateral uptake).[29] Such scanning is based on the principle that cholesterol is necessary for the production of the hormonal agents synthesized by the adrenal cortex (see Fig. 58-1).

Pheochromocytoma

History

In 1886 Frankel described bilateral adrenal tumors at autopsy of an 18-year-old woman who had suffered sudden death. In 1912 Pick described and named the tumor. In 1922 L'Abbé found a pheochromocytoma at autopsy of a 28-year-old woman who had presented with paroxysmal hypertension. In 1926 Roux described the first successful resection of a pheochromocytoma; in 1927 Mayo described the first successful resection in the United States. In 1951 the biochemical basis of the disease was identified by von Euler with demonstration of increased urinary catecholamines.

Natural History

Pheochromocytomas occur in less than 0.1% of hypertensive patients. The majority (90%) are benign. Pheochromocytomas represent one of the most satisfying general surgical diseases to treat, in that 5-year survival for benign tumors is greater than 95%, recurrence rates are less than 10%, and hypertension is cured in 75% of patients. However, malignant pheochromocytomas have a high incidence of recurrence and metastasis with a 5-year survival of approximately 36% to 60%.

Despite the fact that primary care physicians have a high index of suspicion for pheochromocytoma in patients presenting with hypertension, the majority of pheochromocytomas are unfortunately still diagnosed post mortem. Pheochromocytoma is also important because of its association with inherited genetic disorders, including multiple endocrine neoplasia type 2 (MEN 2) and von Hippel-Lindau disease (VHL). Pheochromocytoma is somewhat more common in females than males.

Pheochromocytomas have been known as the "10% tumors," because approximately 10% of sporadic tumors occur bilaterally, 10% occur in extra-adrenal locations, and 10% are malignant. Familial tumors are more likely to be bilateral, less likely to be extra-adrenal, and less likely to be malignant. Pheochromocytomas occur slightly more commonly on the right side of the body. Extra-adrenal pheochromocytomas, also referred to as paragangliomas, most commonly occur within the abdomen, frequently in the organ of Zuckerkandl at the bifurcation of the aorta, and occasionally within the bladder wall itself. Thoracic locations for pheochromocytomas include the posterior mediastinum and the pericardium. Extra-adrenal pheochromocytomas may occur anywhere along the sympathetic chain because of the presence of chromaffin tissue.

Presentation

The classic presentation of a patient with pheochromocytoma includes the presence of sustained and paroxysmal hypertension and tachycardia.[30,31] Headache, perspiration, and palpitation are common presenting symptoms. Additional features include the presence of orthostatic hypotension, an elevated hematocrit, cardiac manifestations, and metabolic and endocrine disorders including fever, weight loss, glucose intolerance, hypercalcemia, diarrhea, and elevated levels of ACTH. Episodes of paroxysmal hypertension are occasionally precipitated by trauma or surgery. The hypertension is characteristically labile and refractory to medical management; the most effective antihypertensive agents are α-blockers, calcium channel blockers, and nitroprusside.

Biochemistry

Pheochromocytomas release catecholamines independent of neural stimulation. Pheochromocytomas possess glucagon receptors; therefore glucagon may mediate catecholamine release. It is important to remember that precipitating events for hypertensive crisis in patients with pheochromocytoma can include administration of glucagon, as well as opiates, intra-arterial contrast agents, and sympathomimetics.

Understanding the pathophysiology of pheochromocytoma requires an understanding of catecholamine metabolism. Tyrosine is metabolized to epinephrine through norepinephrine in the adrenal medulla; dopamine represents an intermediary step. Generally, pheochromocytomas produce much more norepinephrine than epinephrine. Exceptions to this general rule include small tumors and those tumors in patients from familial kindreds (e.g., MEN 2). Extra-adrenal pheochromocytomas are classically pure norepinephrine-producing tumors. The final conversion of norepinephrine to epinephrine is inefficient in most pheochromocytomas, resulting in production of large amounts of the catecholamine metabolites 3,4-dihydroxymandelic acid, metanephrine, and normetanephrine; all three of these metabolites can be converted to vanillylmandelic acid (VMA), and all of these catecholamine metabolites can be detected in the urine.

Etiology

Pheochromocytomas originate from chromaffin cells; related neuroendocrine tumors include chemodectomas (carotid body tumors), tumors of the glomus jugulare (affecting the ninth and tenth cranial nerves), ganglioneuromas, and neuroblastomas and ganglioneuroblastomas. Chromosomal abnormalities common in pheochromocytomas include loss of heterozygosity at chromosomes 1p, 3p, 17p, and 22q. There is overexpression of N-*ras* and *c-myc* mRNA. The *RET* proto-oncogene plays an important role in the development of pheochromocytomas in MEN kindreds; the role of *RET* mutations in sporadic pheochromocytomas remains controversial.[32-34]

Evaluation

The diagnosis of pheochromocytoma is established by the demonstration of elevated catecholamines in a timed (24-hour) urine collection; these include catecholamines and their metabolites, metanephrine, and VMA. Plasma catecholamine determination is only occasionally helpful; clonidine suppression tests may be useful in borderline cases. Clonidine suppresses centrally mediated release of catecholamines but has no effect on catecholamine release by pheochromocytoma. Provocative tests to release catecholamines from a pheochromocytoma are potentially hazardous and now obsolete. Patients with a biochemical diagnosis of pheochromocytoma should undergo preoperative localization. Localization may be accomplished with CT scan or MRI. Metaiodobenzylguanidine (MIBG) scan may assist in lateralizing a tumor when no mass is present on abdominal imaging.[35] MIBG (iodine-131-metaiodobenzylguanidine [^{131}I-MIBG]) is selectively accumulated in chromaffin tissues and does this to a greater degree and more rapidly in pheochromocytoma than in normal tissues. Angiography is rarely helpful.

Preoperative Preparation

The cornerstone of preoperative preparation of the patient with pheochromocytoma is 2 weeks of α-blockade with phenoxybenzamine to return the blood pressure to normal. The occurrence of orthostatic hypotension generally indicates the presence of adequate α-blockade. β-Blockade may be instituted after adequate α-blockade. β-Blockade may be used when the patient remains persistently hypertensive, is tachycardic, or has problems with arrhythmia following α-blockade. Nifedipine and metyrosine may also be helpful. Preoperative pulmonary arterial catheters are placed selectively in patients undergoing resection of pheochromocytoma.

Surgical Procedure

We continue to prefer an open anterior approach to surgical resection in most patients with pheochromocytoma, although in some centers a laparoscopic approach is used for patients with small (<6 cm) tumors. The potential for malignancy must be considered in all sporadic pheochromocytomas, and therefore the open anterior approach is used to ensure that a complete, margin-negative resection is performed. However, when treating patients with pheochromocytoma in the setting of MEN 2 or VHL, a familial history of pheochromocytoma, or bilateral tumors, the incidence of malignancy is very low (<5%), and long-term morbidity of a complete bilateral adrenalectomy is moderately high; we therefore favor a cortical-sparing operation in these patients,[36] and we would also consider a laparoscopic approach. Cortical-sparing and laparoscopic adrenalectomy are discussed in more detail in the following section on controversies in the surgical management of adrenal disease.

Nipride is used for intraoperative management of

blood pressure in patients with pheochromocytoma because of its rapid response time and short half-life. The intraoperative approach to the tumor includes early identification and ligation of the adrenal vein, as well as identification and ligation of the arterial supply to the adrenal gland. Postoperative care includes careful attention to arterial blood pressure, central venous pressure, and urine output, since hypotension is common initially after operation as a result of the vasodilation that occurs after tumor resection. Such management should be done in the intensive care unit. We obtain a timed urine collection 1 week postoperatively to document normal catecholamine levels. Following surgical treatment for pheochromocytoma, all patients should undergo yearly timed urine collection for catecholamine determination to detect recurrence.

Malignant Pheochromocytoma

The most common sites of metastases from malignant pheochromocytoma are bone, liver, lymph nodes, and lungs. While absolute criteria for malignancy include the presence of adjacent organ invasion or distant metastatic disease, some general pathologic characteristics can help distinguish those tumors that are likely to behave in a malignant fashion. Malignant tumors tend to be larger than their benign counterparts, and mitoses tend to be much more frequent in malignant pheochromocytomas. Malignant pheochromocytomas have been reported to be aneuploid and may exhibit more necrosis than benign tumors. However, it should be emphasized that microscopic vascular or capsular invasion and nuclear pleomorphism are not reliable indicators of malignancy.

Patients with known or suspected malignant pheochromocytoma should be staged with standard imaging studies and timed urine collection for catecholamine excretion and MIBG scanning. Therapy should be individualized based on extent of disease. Palliative therapy may include treatment with metyrosine, as well as α- and β-blockade. Resection of malignant pheochromocytoma, including resection of metastases, may be considered in good risk individuals if the metastases are limited in extent. Radiation therapy may offer effective palliation of symptomatic bony metastases. Treatment with radioactive ^{131}I-MIBG has generally been disappointing. Chemotherapy may be effective in patients with metastatic pheochromocytoma. The most active agents include the combination of cyclophosphamide, vincristine, and dacarbazine; regimens containing these agents may result in combined complete and partial response rates of greater than 50%.

ENZYMATIC DEFECTS INVOLVING THE ADRENAL CORTEX

Congenital adrenal hyperplasia is associated with several interesting syndromes that occur because of associated enzymatic defects. The two most common enzyme defects involve deficiencies in *21-hydroxylase* and *11-β-hydroxylase.* Reference to Fig. 58-1 demonstrates the pathways afected by these deficiencies. With both defects, masculinization occurs in the female infant, resulting from an overproduction of adrenal androgens in utero by the fetus. This overproduction, which is generally absent under normal conditions, evokes the stimulation of wolffian ducts, genital tubercle elongation with labioscrotal fold migration, and fusion of these folds in the midline with resultant swellings that form a penis and scrotal sac. In addition, the urethra migrates so that its opening is in the tip of the phallus. Since the ovary does not secrete testosterone in the normal fetus, the genital tubercle remains small, and the labial folds are unfused. In the male infant with similar enzyme defects, no immediate effects are generally apparent but in time masculinization and precocious puberty manifest themselves.

In addition to these general effects resulting from the enzyme deficiencies, the 11-β-hydroxylase deficiency is also commonly characterized by hypertension secondary to the excessive secretion of deoxycorticosterone. In contrast, infants with the 21-hydroxylase deficiency may manifest salt wasting with excessive sodium losses in the urine, resulting in severe hydration. Unless diagnosed promptly and treated aggressively with glucocorticoids, mineralocorticoids, and sodium chloride, an early fatality may occur.

Less common enzyme defects are the *17-hydroxylase* and *3-hydroxysteroid dehydrogenase deficiencies.* In the 17-hydroxylase deficiency syndrome, excessive secretion of deoxycorticosterone and corticosterone occur, resulting in hypertension. In the male the testes may not secrete androgens with this syndrome so that the normal male external genitalia fail to develop adequately. In the female the ovaries fail to secrete estrogen and as a result prevent the appearance of secondary sex characteristics at the time of puberty. The syndrome caused by 3-hydroxysteroid dehydrogenase deficiency is associated with decreased secretion of both mineralocorticoids and glucocorticoids, often resulting in salt wasting similar to patients with 21-hydroxylase deficiency. Also similar to this latter enzyme defect, 3-hydroxysteroid dehydrogenase deficiency commonly results in increased quantities of adrenal androgen production. Consequently, partial masculinizaiton may occur in females, whereas males fail to develop normal external genitalia.

Because of the defects in corticosteroid synthesis (see Fig. 58-1) associated with these syndromes, patients require cortisol replacement. Those with associated mineralocorticoid deficiencies, in which salt wasting is a problem, also require mineralocorticoid replacement. Since female patients with these syndromes have normal internal genitalia and are capable of normal fertility, despite the masculinization secondary to these enzyme defects, they should be reared as females because genetically they have a 46,XX karyotype. Depending on the degree of masculinizaiton, surgical therapy may be necessary at some point to correct cosmetic and functional deformities of the external genitalia. This usually involves operations to correct the clitoral hypertrophy and any malformation of the vaginal introitus. These operations can usually be performed within the first 6 months of life.

ADRENAL INSUFFICIENCY

Adrenal insufficiency was first described by Thomas Addison in 1855. He described 11 patients in whom destruction of the adrenal glands was associated with a fatal outcome; 6 had tuberculosis, 3 had metastatic malignancies, 1 had adrenal hemorrhage, and 1 had adrenal atrophy. Adrenal insufficiency is rare; chronic primary adrenal insufficiency (Addison's disease) has been estimated to occur in only 39 to 60 cases per million population. It is convenient to organize adrenal insufficiency into primary mechanisms (destruction of the adrenal cortex) and secondary mechanisms (insufficient stimulation of the adrenal cortex by ACTH).[37] The most common cause of primary adrenal insufficiency today is autoimmune adrenalitis; other causes include granulomatous diseases (histoplasmosis, tuberculosis), metastatic malignancy (lung cancer, breast cancer),[38-40] hemorrhage (anticoagulant therapy, Waterhouse-Friderichsen syndrome [meningococcemia], *Pseudomonas aeruginosa* infection), and inherited disorders (X-linked adrenomyeloneuropathy). Finally, AIDS-associated opportunistic infections are an increasingly frequent cause of adrenal destruction. Primary adrenal insufficiency does not usually become clincally apparent until at least 90% of adrenal cortical tissue is destroyed. Causes of secondary adrenal insufficiency include withdrawal of chronic exogenous glucocorticoids (the most frequent cause of adrenal insufficiency) and pituitary destruction (e.g., following transsphenoidal surgery for pituitary adenoma, or Sheehan's syndrome [postpartum pituitary necrosis]).

While neither dose nor duration of glucocorticoid adminstration accurately predicts the degree of suppression of the hypothalamic-pituitary-adrenal axis (HPA), any patient who has received the equivalent of 20 to 30 mg of prednisone per day for five consecutive days in the 12 months prior to a major stress or surgical procedure is at risk; these individuals should receive perioperative glucocorticoid coverage. Historically, recommendations for perioperative glucocorticoid replacement were based on anecdotal experience and were most likely excessive; a recent consensus review summarizes current recommendations for perioperative glucocorticoid coverage[41] (Table 58-5).

Adrenal insufficiency usually has a gradual, insidious onset. However, major physiologic stress, including surgical stress, may precipitate adrenal crisis. In patients suspected of presenting with acute adrenal insufficiency, a history consistent with chronic primary or secondary adrenal insufficiency should be sought. Characteristic, although nonspecific, symptoms include fatigue, weakness, listlessness, orthostasis, and weight loss. Gastrointestinal symptoms may include abdominal cramps, anorexia, nausea, and vomiting. Physical examination may reveal evidence for secondary adrenal insufficiency caused by prior exogenous steroid hormone administration (Cushingoid features). Alternatively, patients with primary adrenal insufficiency may have hyperpigmentation or vitiligo resulting from the influence of ACTH and other pro-opiomelanocortin peptides. Hypotension may occur in either primary or secondary adrenal insufficiency. Hypotension is characteristically more severe in primary adrenal insufficiency and is due to aldosterone deficiency. In secondary adrenal insufficiency, hypotension is due to decreased expression of catecholamine receptors. Laboratory abnormalites include hypoglycemia, hyponatremia, hyperkalemia, azotemia, hypercalcemia, anemia, leukopenia, lymphocytosis, and eosinophilia.

It is essential to consider the diagnosis of acute adrenal insufficiency in critically ill patients with unexplained catecholamine-resistant hypotension; in these patients, glucocorticoid replacement can be lifesaving.[42] Patients with acute adrenal insufficiency may have shock, with dehydration and hypotension out of proportion to the severity of the underlying illness or stress. Patients may complain of abdominal pain and manifest abdominal tenderness with

Table 58-5. Recommendations for Perioperative Glucocorticoid Coverage

Surgical Stress	Examples	Hydrocortisone Equivalent (mg)	Duration (days)
Minor	Inguinal herniorrhaphy	25	1
Moderate	Open cholecystectomy Lower extremity revascularization Segmental colon resection Total joint replacement Abdominal hysterectomy	50-75	1-2
Major	Pancreaticoduodenectomy Esophagogastrectomy Total proctocolectomy Cardiac surgery with cardiopulmonary bypass	100-150	2-3

From Salem M, et al. Perioperative glucocorticoid coverage: A reassessment 42 years after emergence of a problem. Ann Surg 4:416, 1994.

fever. Lethargy, confusion, or coma may develop. Signs and symptoms may mimic a surgical abdomen or septic shock.

Treatment of patients in suspected adrenal crisis should begin immediately. Isotonic intravenous fluid replacement is begun; a stress dose of glucocoticoid is administered intravenously. Dexamethasone (4 mg) is preferred over hydrocortisone (100 mg), since it does not interfere with subsequent measurement of serum steroids during ACTH stimulation testing. Clinical response is expected within 2 hours. While waiting for a clinical response to dexamethasone, an ACTH stimulation test should be performed (see Fig. 58-3). A baseline serum cortisol is drawn. Cosyntropin (250 μg), a synthetic ACTH subunit, is given intravenously. Serum cortisol is determined 30 and 60 minutes after cosyntropin administration. A baseline serum cortisol of more than 20 μg/dl (or an increase of more than 7 μg/dl over baseline) is indicative of a normal HPA; lesser values in the face of a physiologic stress indicate HPA hypofunction. Patients in whom adrenal insufficiency is established require initial stress doses of glucocorticoid replacement intravenously (e.g., hydrocortisone 300 mg/day in divided doses), followed by a taper to replacement doses orally (e.g., hydrocortisone 25 mg/day in divided doses). Additionally, patients with primary adrenal insufficiency should also receive fludrocortisone (50 to 200 μg/day) to prevent hyponatremia caused by mineralocorticoid deficiency.

CONTROVERSIES IN THE SURGICAL MANAGEMENT OF ADRENAL DISEASE

Cortical-Sparing Adrenalectomy

Cortical-sparing adrenalectomy represents a method of limiting the morbidity associated with total adrenalectomy in selected patients with bilateral pheochromocytoma. Bilateral pheochromocytoma is associated with a variety of inherited disorders, most commonly, MEN 2A and 2B. MEN 2A and 2B are otherwise characterized by the presence of hyperparathyroidism and medullary thyroid cancer (MTC), as well as a characteristic phenotype in MEN 2B patients.[43] Other disorders associated with pheochromocytoma include neurofibromatosis, VHL (retinal angiomatosis, cerebellar hemangioblastoma), and Sturge-Weber syndrome (trigeminal nerve cavernous hemangiomas).

MEN 2A and 2B, as well as familial (nonMEN) MTC, are associated with mutations in the *RET* proto-oncogene.[44] Overexpression of *RET* mRNA has been demonstrated in sporadic pheochromocytomas.[34] The *RET* proto-oncogene maps to chromosome 10q11.2. *RET* mutations may have a variety of clinical consequences. In Hirschsprung's disease, *RET* mutations include deletions and stop codons, resulting in the loss of parasympathetic innervation of the distal colon. In familial MTC, MEN 2A and MEN 2B point mutations in *RET* result in amino acid substitutions. Although there is no loss of chromosome 10 alleles, the point mutations probably result in altered regulation of the *RET* tyrosine kinase growth factor receptor.[45]

Pheochromocytomas in patients with MEN 2 occur in 30% to 50% of affected individuals. Virtually all patients have bilateral adrenal medullary hyperplasia. Clinical evidence of bilateral pheochromocytoma develops in 50% of individuals followed for 10 years or more. Despite this, malignancy is uncommon, occurring in 3.9% of 387 patients from 12 collected series (Table 58-6). Likewise, in patients with VHL, malignancy is uncommon. Although pheochromocytomas occurred in 10% to 19% of patients with VHL and bilateral pheochromocytomas developed in 40% to 60% of these individuals, malignancy occurred in only 3.3% of 121 patients in six collected series (Table 58-7).

The treatment of a clinical unilateral pheochromocy-

Table 58-6. Incidence of Malignant Pheochromocytoma in Patients With Multiple Endocrine Neoplasia Type 2

Author	Institution	Year	Total Pheochromocytoma (No. of Patients)*	Malignant Pheochromocytoma (No. of Patients)
Casanova et al.[46]	University of Paris	1993	100	3
Lairmore et al.[47]	Washington University	1993	58	0
Neumann et al.[48]	University of Freiburg	1993	24	0
Vasen et al.[49]	Netherlands	1992	8	0
Oishi et al.[50]	Kumamoto University	1990	82†	4
Gagel et al.[51]	Tufts University	1988	8	0
Jansson et al.[52]	University of Goteborg	1988	9	0
Shapiro et al.[35]	University of Michigan	1985	35	3
van Heerden et al.[53]	Mayo Clinic	1984	17	3
Tibblin et al.[54]	University of Lund	1983	18	0
Lips et al.[55]	Netherlands	1981	20	0
Wilson and Ibanez[56]	MDA	1978	8	2
TOTAL			387	15 (3.9%)

*Total number of patients reported with pheochromocytoma and multiple endocrine neoplasia type 2.
†Includes one patient with extra-adrenal pheochromocytoma reported.
MDA, M.D. Anderson Cancer Center.

Table 58-7. Incidence of Malignant Pheochromocytoma in Patients With von Hippel-Lindau Disease

Author	Institution	Year	Total Pheochromocytoma (No. of Patients)*	Malignant Pheochromocytoma (No. of Patients)
Richard et al.[57]	France	1994	36†	3
Aprill et al.[58]	National Naval Medical Center	1994	4	0
Neumann et al.[48]	University of Freiburg	1993	43	0
Green et al.[59]	University of Newfoundland	1986	20	1
Atuk et al.[60]	University of Virginia	1979	13	0
Horton et al.[61]	National Institutes of Health	1976	5	0
TOTAL			121	4 (3.3%)

*Total number of patients reported with pheochromocytoma and von Hippel-Lindau diseases.
†Includes three patients with extra-adrenal pheochromocytoma reported.

toma in patients with MEN 2 has been controversial. Bilateral total adrenalectomy has been advocated by some. However, despite steroid replacement, bilateral total adrenalectomy results in addisonian crisis in some patients (Table 58-8). Furthermore, MEN 2 is associated with MTC, which has a relatively poor prognosis compared to the pheochromocytoma in these individuals. Therefore many have advocated a selective approach to adrenal disease in patients with familial pheochromocytoma, with removal of only the affected side and annual screening to detect disease recurrence (Table 58-9). This approach has resulted in an approximately 50% recurrence after 10 years of follow-up, no pheochromocytoma related mortality, and no observed malignant pheochromocytomas in the population undergoing evaluation.

As an extension of this reasoning, we have recently recommended cortical-sparing adrenalectomy for patients with bilateral pheochromocytoma in the setting of MEN 2 or VHL.[36] Cortical-sparing adrenalectomy may avoid the requirement for chronic steroid hormone replacement and the resulting risk of addisonian crisis. These patients are also at high risk of morbidity from other manifestations for their disease and, as noted above, frequently suffer from bilateral but relatively indolent pheochromocytomas. A recent review of our experience with this approach has demonstrated that bilateral cortical-sparing adrenalectomy is safe in good risk individuals and infrequently results in the need for chronic postoperative steroid hormone supplementation. As for patients with unilateral pheochromocytoma in the setting of MEN 2 or VHL who undergo subtotal adrenalectomy, there is a 20% incidence of recurrence after approximately 10 years of follow-up (Table 58-10). Cortical-sparing adrenalectomy is both safe and effective, avoiding the requirement for steroid hormone replacement and the risk of addisonian crisis in the majority of patients with MEN 2 or VHL. However, recurrence may occur 10 years or more following this approach; thus long-term follow-up is necessary. Furthermore, adrenal cortical reserve should be evaluated in all patients postoperatively;[67,68] those patients with marginal adrenal cortical reserve should receive supplemental steroid hormone replacement when undergoing major surgical procedures or when they develop acute illness (Fig. 58-3).

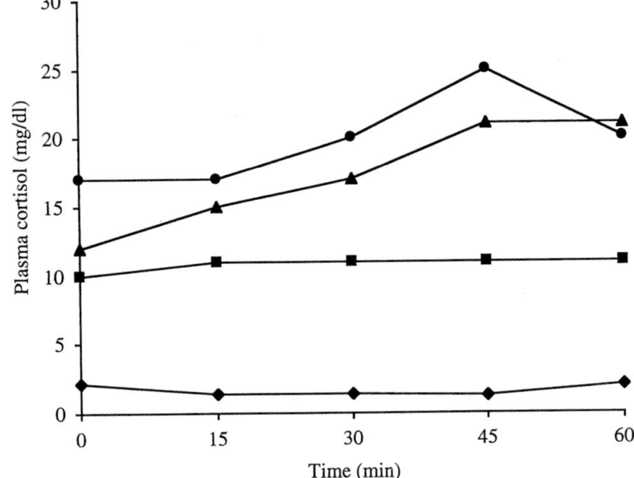

Fig. 58-3. Cosyntropin stimulation test results in selected patients after total and subtotal adrenalectomy for bilateral pheochromocytoma. Patient 1 (♦) underwent total adrenalectomy. Patient 2 (♦) underwent subtotal adrenalectomy but required postoperative steroid hormone replacement. Patients 8 (▲) and 9 (●) underwent subtotal adrenalectomy and did not require postoperative steroid hormone replacement. (From Lee JE, et al. Cortical-sparing adrenalectomy for patients with bilateral pheochromocytoma. Surgery 120:1064, 1996.)

Surgery for Adrenal Metastases

Surgery for metastases to the adrenal gland may be considered in good risk individuals in whom there is an absence of extra-adrenal disease and in whom there is a history of favorable tumor biology.[69-72] Evaluation of patients with favorable tumor biology includes consideration of those who have had a significant progression-free interval, those who have responded to systemic therapy, and those who have a history of isolated metachronous metastases. Selected pathologies that may be considered for resection

Table 58-8. Results of Bilateral Total Adrenalectomy for Pheochromocytoma in Patients With Multiple Endocrine Neoplasia Type 2

Author	Institution	Year	No. of Patients	Follow-up (yr)	No. of Patients: Malignant Pheochromocytoma	Addisonian Crisis	Deaths Due to Addisonian Crisis	Recurrent Pheochromocytoma
Lairmore et al.[47]	Washington University	1993	43	9.4	0	10	1	0
Telenius-Berg et al.[62]	Kuwait	1989	26	6	NR	9	1	NR
van Heerden et al.[53]	Mayo Clinic	1984	17	10	1	0	0	1
TOTAL			86	8.5*	1 (2%)	19 (22%)	2 (2%)	1 (2%)

*Weighted average.
NR, Not reported.

Table 58-9. Results of Unilateral Adrenalectomy for Pheochromocytoma in Patients With Multiple Endocrine Neoplasia Type 2

Author	Institution	Year	No. of Patients	Follow-up (yr)	No. of Patients: Recurrent Pheochromocytoma (%)	Died During Follow-up	Malignant Pheochromocytoma
Lairmore et al.[47]	Washington University	1993	26	9	12 (46)	0	0
Gagel et al.[51]	Tufts University	1988	8	11	4 (50)	0	0
Jansson et al.[52]	University of Goteborg	1988	9	8	1 (11)	0	0
Tibblin et al.[54]	University of Lund	1983	13	7	4 (31)	0	0
Lips et al.[55]	Netherlands	1981	4	4	4 (100)	0	0
TOTAL			60	8.4*	25 (42)	0	0

*Weighted average.

Table 58-10. Results of Bilateral Subtotal Adrenalectomy for Pheochromocytoma in Patients With Familial Pheochromocytoma

Author	Institution	Year	No. of Patients	Follow-up (yr)	Steroid Requirement	Cosyntropin Test	Recurrence
Lee et al.[36]	MDA	1996	14	11.5	1	Abnormal 3/9	3
Albanese and Wiener[63]	University of Pittsburgh	1993	4	6	0	NR	0
Hamberger et al.[64]	Karolinska Hospital	1987	2	2; 3 mo	0	Abnormal 2/2	0
van Heerden et al.[65]	Mayo Clinic	1985	3	10	1	Abnormal 0/1	2
Irvin et al.[66]	University of Miami	1983	2	7,3	0	NR	0
TOTAL			25	9*	2 (8%)	Abnormal 5/12 (42%)	5 (20%)

*Weighted average.
MDA, M. D. Anderson Cancer Center.

include patients with metastatic melanoma, renal cell carcinoma, and colorectal cancer. Preoperative assessment of the patient with an adrenal mass and a history of malignancy should include an evaluation for hormone production prior to fine-needle aspiration biopsy, since some of these patients have occult, functioning adrenal tumors, including pheochromocytomas. In addition, patients with known or suspected adrenal metastases in whom surgical resection is contemplated should undergo ACTH stimulation testing to document adequate adrenal cortical reserve prior to adrenalectomy.[38-40] Fine-needle aspiration biopsy may be helpful in selected cases to confirm the diagnosis of metastasis preoperatively.[73] Alternatively, surgical therapy can be planned based solely on noninvasive imaging studies, such as the T1-weighted chemical-shift MRI,[23-28] in patients with a history of a malignancy that commonly metastasizes to the adrenal glands, favorable tumor biology, negative biochemical screening for hormone production, and a mass that either fulfills size criteria for surgical excision or radiographically suspicious for metastasis.[74]

Laparoscopic Adrenalectomy

Laparoscopic adrenalectomy can be performed safely in selected patients with adrenal masses.[75-86] Most surgeons have used an anterolateral transperitoneal approach; a posterior approach has also been reported.[87] Carefully selected patients who undergo laparoscopic adrenalectomy for relatively small adrenal masses may have a more rapid recovery and less discomfort compared to patients who undergo open adrenalectomy. The appropriateness of laparoscopic adrenalectomy as a cancer operation remains unknown. At present it appears most reasonable to consider laparoscopic adrenalectomy as an effective alternative treatment for patients presenting with small, benign adrenal tumors. Patients who could be considered for laparoscopic adrenalectomy include those with aldosteronoma, those who are candidates for adrenalectomy for Cushing's disease, and MEN 2 or VHL patients with pheochromocytoma. We urge continued caution in the use of laparoscopic adrenalectomy for patients with malignant or potentially malignant adrenal tumors. This includes patients with sporadic pheochromocytoma (10% incidence of malignancy) and those whose indication for adrenalectomy is the presence of a nonfunctioning incidentaloma. It is emphasized that the reason for operating on patients with nonfunctioning adrenal tumors (incidentalomas) is that the tumors are potentially malignant. Therefore we specifically do not recommend laparoscopic adrenalectomy for these patients outside of an investigational setting.

Incidentaloma

Incidental adrenal masses, or "incidentalomas," are common, being found in up to 4% of individuals undergoing abdominal CT scans, and in up to 9% of autopsies.[88-93] In evaluating a patient who presents with an incidental adrenal mass, it is important to remember that benign nonfunctioning adrenal cortical adenomas are common, adrenal cortical carcinomas are extremely rare, and metastases to the adrenal glands from solid tumor malignancies occur commonly.[94-104] Cancers that commonly metastasize to the adrenal gland include those of the lung, breast, stomach, kidney, and colon, as well as melanoma and lymphoma. Therefore the three critical questions that must be asked and answered in the evaluation of each patient who initially has an incidental adrenal mass are the following: (1) Is the mass primary or metastatic? (2) Is it functioning or nonfunctioning? (3) Is it benign or malignant?

Evaluation of the patient with an incidental adrenal mass should include a history designed to elicit symptoms secondary to a functioning tumor or an underlying malignancy (weight loss, abdominal pain, rectal bleeding), physical examination (blood pressure; breast, lymph node, pelvic and rectal examination; stool for occult blood determination), and laboratory evaluation (serum potassium, chest radiograph, mammogram in adult women). A biochemical evaluation should be performed, including a timed urine collection for determination of catecholamines and an evaluation for cortisol overproduction. In equivocal cases, further imaging studies may be helpful, such as MRI scanning to include T1-weighted chemical-shift analysis. We advocate fine-needle aspiration biopsy only if the patient has a history of a prior malignancy that metastasizes to the adrenal gland or if there are symptoms, physical examination findings, or biochemical or radiographic evidence for an underlying malignancy.[74]

It is again emphasized that the majority of small incidental adrenal masses are nonfunctioning adenomas. The likelihood that an incidental adrenal mass is a glucocorticoid-producing adenoma is extremely small, on the order of 0.035%. If a patient is neither hypertensive nor obese, the chances are even smaller, on the order of 0.01%.[105] Therefore evaluation for hypercortisolism in particular should be limited to those screening tests that are the least expensive and the most sensitive.

Clinical manifestations of adrenal cortical hormone excess are listed in Table 58-4. Although we believe it is reasonable to screen all patients with incidental adrenal masses for hypercortisolism, screening for androgen or estrogen excess is unnecessary in the absence of specific signs or symptoms suggestive of overproduction of these hormones. Likewise, since the presence of a normal serum potassium and a normal blood pressure virtually excludes the diagnosis of aldosteronoma, we do not recommend screening for aldosterone excess in the absence of these findings.

A controversial area in the evaluation of patients with adrenal masses includes the possible clinical entity termed "subclinical Cushing's syndrome."[106-110] Evidence for subclinical Cushing's syndrome includes the finding that an occasional patient develops adrenal insufficiency after removal of an apparently nonfunctioning incidental adrenal mass. Furthermore, it has been noted that between 5% and 25% of patients with incidental adrenal masses have evidence for subclinical adrenal cortical dysfunction as defined

Table 58-11. Reports of "Subclinical Cushing's Syndrome"

Author	Institution	Year	"Subclinical Cushing's Syndrome" and Abnormal Dexamethasone Suppression	Abnormal 24-Hr Urine Collection for Cortisol
Caplan et al.[111]	Gunderson/Lutheran Medical Center	1994	0/3	0/3
Reincke et al.[112]	University of Wurzberg	1992	8/8	1/4
McLeod et al.[113]	University of Michigan	1990	3/3	2/5
Virkkala et al.[114]	University Center Hospital, Helsinki	1989	3/3	2/2

by the absence of specific clinical manifestations and either an abnormal 24-hour urine cortisol, abnormal dexamethasone suppression, suppressed ACTH, loss of diurinal variation of cortisol production, or lateralizing findings on NP-59 nuclear medicine scanning. However, it should be emphasized that the incidence of subclinical Cushing's syndrome in patients carefully screened preoperatively for evidence of cortisol overproduction is probably quite low (Table 58-11). Although 24-hour urine collection may miss an occasional patient with cortisol overproduction, overnight dexamethasone suppression with 1 mg of dexamethasone followed by a morning cortisol detects the overwhelming majority of patients with cortisol overproduction caused by a minimally functional adrenal cortical adenoma. Therefore overnight 1 mg dexamethasone suppression is probably the least expensive, the most convenient, and the most sensitive screening test for hypercortisolism in the patient with an incidental adrenal mass.

A summary of our approach to the patient with an incidental adrenal mass is given in Fig. 58-4. On the day the patient is first evaluated, a 1 mg dose of dexamethasone is given to be taken at 10 PM that evening. A 24-hour urine collection for VMA, metanephrine, and catecholamine determination is begun. The following morning at 8 AM the patient has a plasma cortisol drawn. Later that afternoon the patient returns the timed urine collection specimen. If the patient's plasma cortisol level is not suppressed below 5, the patient undergoes a second timed 24-hour urine collection, this time for cortisol, 17-hydroxysteroid and 17-ketosteroid. We believe this is an efficient yet appropriately thorough schema for evaluation of patients with incidental adrenal masses.

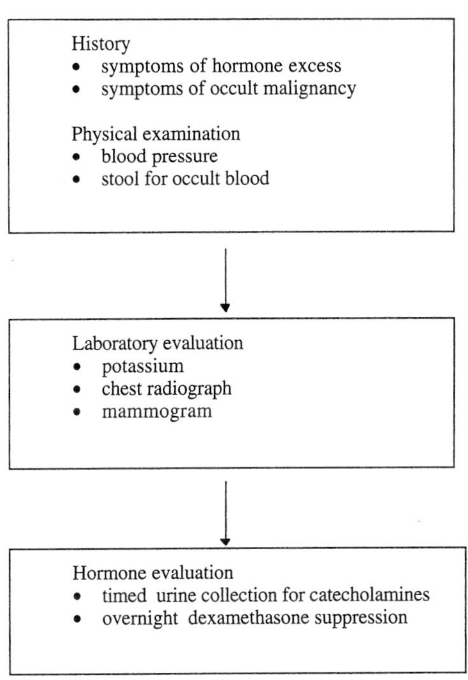

Fig. 58-4. Evaluation of the incidental adrenal mass.

It should be emphasized that size is the single best clinical indicator of malignancy in patients who have an incidental adrenal mass. Ninety-two percent of adrenal cortical carcinomas are greater than 6 cm; occasionally, an adrenal cortical carcinoma as small as 3 cm is identified. Less than 1% of adrenal cortical adenomas are greater than 6 cm. Although accurate and detailed information regarding the size distribution of adrenal cortical adenomas is not available, the frequency and average size of nonfunctioning adrenal adenomas generally increases with age. This information must be taken into account when evaluating the patient who presents with an incidental adrenal mass. The likelihood that an incidental adrenal mass greater than 6 cm in size is an adrenal cortical carcinoma has been estimated to be 35% to 98%. The likelihood that an incidental adrenal mass less than 6 cm in size is an adrenal cortical carcinoma has been estimated to be less than 0.01%. Based on these findings, we recommend that patients who present with an incidental adrenal mass undergo an evaluation to exclude metastasis. We recommend that fine-needle aspiration biopsy be performed only if the patient's history or evaluation suggests an underlying malignancy. All patients should be evaluated for hormone production, especially for occult pheochromocytoma or hypercortisolism. All functioning tumors and large (≥6 cm) incidental adrenal masses should be surgically resected. We recommend observation if tumors are nonfunctioning and less than 3 cm in size. Tumors between 3 and 6 cm in diameter require individualized treatment. The following may be helpful in evaluating such patients with intermediate-size nonfunctioning adrenal masses: (1) MRI scanning, (2) a more thorough endocrine evaluation, and (3) consideration of age and comorbidity.

SUMMARY

The adrenal glands are paired triangular organs that are anatomically positioned on the superior aspect of each kidney. Despite their relatively small size, they play important roles in normal human physiology because of the diverse hormones that they secrete into the blood stream. the adrenal cortex is divided into three histologic layers including the zona glomerulosa, zona fasciculata, and zona reticularis, each of which secretes a unique hormone. The adrenal medulla is an intrical part of the sympathetic nervous system and secretes both norepinephrine and epinephrine.

The adrenal cortex is essential for life, and death ultimately ensues in its absence. its secretory products include aldosterone, which plays an important role in salt balance, and glucocorticoids, which have multiple effects including modulation of fat, carbohydrate and amino acid metabolism, immune function, inflammatory responses, wound healing, and bone metabolism. The sex hormones produced by the adrenal cortex are important in the development of secondary sex characteristics. Excess production of any of these hormones can lead to a variety of clinical syndromes that can tax the skills of the most astute physician in terms of diagnosis and management. Fortunately, most of these syndromes follow specific patterns of clinical presentation so that surgical intervention, when necessary, is relatively straightforward. Although the adrenal medulla is not essential for life, overproduction of its secretory products by a pheochromocytoma can result in life-threatening illness secondary to effects on blood pressure, cardiac performance, and glucose intolerance.

An understanding of the normal physiology of the adrenal gland is essential for early diagnosis of disease affecting this organ and the institution of appropriate treatment. The surgeon's role in managing diseases of this gland is usually related to neoplastic aberrations, either benign or malignant. In addition, in patients in whom adrenal cortical function may be compromised secondary to exogenous steroid treatment for various collagen/vascular diseases or immune modulatory disorders, adequate corticosteroid coverage must be provided when patients with such compromise are subjected to other surgical procedures, either on an elective or emergency basis.

REFERENCES

1. Grondäl S, et al. Adrenocortical carcinoma. A retrospective study of a rare tumor with a poor prognosis. Eur J Surg Oncol 16:500, 1990.
2. Lee JE, et al. Surgical management, DNA content, and patient survival in adrenal cortical carcinoma. Surgery 118:1090, 1995.
3. Søreide JA, Brabrand K, Thoresen SO. Adrenal cortical carcinoma in Norway, 1970-1984. World J Surg 16:663, 1992.
4. Yano T, et al. Genetic changes in human adrenocortical carcinomas. J Natl Cancer Inst 81:518, 1989.
5. Sullivan M, Boileau M, Hodges CV. Adrenal cortical carcinoma. J Urol 120:660, 1978.
6. Macfarlane DA. Cancer of the adrenal cortex: The natural history, prognosis and treatment in a study of fifty-five cases. Ann R Coll Surg Engl 23:155, 1958.
7. Icard P, et al. Adrenocortical carcinoma in surgically treated patients: A retrospective study on 156 cases by the French Association of Endocrine Surgery. Surgery 112:972, 1992.
8. Zografos GC, et al. Adrenal adenocarcinoma: A review of 53 cases. J Surg Oncol 55:160, 1994.
9. Icard Ph, Louvel A, Chapuis Y. Survival rates and prognostic factors in adrenocortical carcinoma. World J Surg 16:753, 1992.
10. Pommier RF, Brennan MF. An eleven-year experience with adrenocortical carcinoma. Surgery 112:963, 1992.
11. Henley DJ, et al. Adrenal cortical carcinoma-a continuing challenge. Surgery 94:926, 1983.
12. Markoe AM, et al. Radiation therapy for adjunctive treatment of adrenal cortical carcinoma. Am J Clin Oncol 14:170, 1991.
13. Sellin RV, et al. Impact of adjuvant mitotane on the clinical course of patients with adrenocortical cancer. Cancer 71:3119, 1993.
14. Wooten MD, King DK. Adrenal cortical carcinoma. Epidemiology and treatment with mitotane and a review of the literature. Cancer 72:3145, 1993.
15. Jensen JC, et al. Recurrent or metastatic disease in select patients with adrenocortical carcinoma: Aggressive resection vs chemotherapy. Arch Surg 126:457, 1991.
16. Kwauk S, Burt M. Pulmonary metastases from adrenal cortical carcinoma: Results of resection. J Surg Oncol 53:243, 1993.
17. Burgess MA, Legha SS, Sellin RV. Chemotherapy with cis-platinum and etoposide (VP-16) for patients with advanced adrenal cortical carcinoma. Proc Am Soc Clin Oncol 12:188, 1993.
18. Merrell RC. Aldosterone-producing tumors (Conn's syndrome). Semin Surg Oncol 6:66, 1990.
19. Weigel RJ, et al. Surgical treatment of primary hyperaldosteronism. Ann Surg 219:347, 1994.
20. White PC. Disorders of aldosterone biosynthesis and action. N Engl J Med 331:250, 1994.
21. Young WF, et al. Primary aldosteronism: Diagnosis and treatment. Mayo Clin Proc 65:96, 1990.
22. Young WF, et al. Primary aldosteronism: Adrenal venous sampling. Surgery 120:913, 1996.
23. Doppman JL, et al. Differentiation of adrenal masses by magnetic resonance imaging. Surgery 102:1018, 1987.
24. Ichikawa T, et al. Contrast-enhanced dynamic MRI of adrenal masses: Classification of characteristic enhancement patterns. Clin Radiol 50:295, 1995.
25. Krestin GP, Steinbrich W, Friedmann G. Adrenal masses: Evaluation with fast gradient-echo MR imaging and Gd-DTPA-enhanced dynamic studies. Radiology 171:675, 1989.
26. Mayo-Smith WM, et al. Characterization of adrenal masses (<5 cm) by use of chemical shift MR imaging: Observer performance versus quantitative measures. AJR Am J Roentgenol 165:91, 1995.
27. Outwater EK, et al. Distinction between benign and malignant adrenal masses: Value of T1-weighted chemical-shift MR imaging. Am J Radiol 165:579, 1995.
28. Reinig JW, et al. MRI of indeterminate adrenal masses. AJR Am J Roentgenol 147:493, 1986.
29. Yu KC, et al. Role of preoperative iodocholesterol scintiscanning in patients undergoing adrenalectomy for Cushing's syndrome. Surgery 118:981, 1995.
30. Bravo EL, Gifford RW Jr. Pheochromocytoma: Diagnosis, localization and management. N Engl J Med 311:1298, 1984.
31. Werbel SS, Ober P. Pheochromocytoma: Update on diagnosis, localization, and management. Med Clin North Am 79:131, 1995.
32. Beldjord C, et al. The *RET* protooncogene in sporadic pheochromocytomas: Frequent MEN 2–like mutations and new molecular defects. J Clin Endocrinol Metab 80:2063, 1995.
33. Chew SL, et al. Absence of mutations in the *MEN2A* region of the *ret* proto-oncogene in non-MEN 2A phaeochromocytomas. Clin Endocrinol 42:17, 1995.
34. Mathias-Guiu X, et al. Expression of the *ret* proto-oncogene in phaeochromocytoma. An in situ hybridization and Northern blot study. J Pathol 176:63, 1995.

35. Shapiro B, et al. Iodine-131 metaiodobenzylguanidine for the locating of suspected pheochromocytoma: Experience in 400 cases. J Nucl Med 26:576, 1985.
36. Lee JE, et al. Cortical-sparing adrenalectomy for patients with bilateral pheochromocytoma. Surgery 120:1064, 1996.
37. Oelkers W. Adrenal insufficiency. N Engl J Med 335:1206, 1996.
38. Kung AWC, et al. Addisonian crisis as presenting feature in malignancies. Cancer 65:177, 1990.
39. Mor F, et al. Addison's disease due to metastases to the adrenal glands. Postgrad Med J 61:637, 1985.
40. Seidenwurm DJ, et al. Metastases to the adrenal glands and the development of Addison's disease. Cancer 54:552, 1984.
41. Salem M, et al. Perioperative glucocorticoid coverage: A reassessment 42 years after emergence of a problem. Ann Surg 4:416, 1994.
42. Knowlton AI. Adrenal insufficiency in the intensive care setting. J Intensive Care Med 4:35, 1989.
43. Evans DB, et al. Adrenal medullary disease in multiple endocrine neoplasia type 2: Appropriate management. Endocrinol Metab Clin North Am 23:167, 1994.
44. Eng C, et al. The relationship between specific *RET* proto-oncogene mutations and disease phenotype in multiple endocrine neoplasia type 2: International *RET* mutation consortium analysis. JAMA 276:1575, 1996.
45. van Heyningen V. One gene—Four syndromes. Nature 367:319, 1994.
46. Casanova S, et al. Phaeochromocytoma in multiple endocrine neoplasia type 2A: Survey of 100 cases. Clin Endocrinol 38:531, 1993.
47. Lairmore TC, et al. Management of pheochromocytomas in patients with multiple endocrine neoplasia type 2 syndromes. Ann Surg 217:595, 1993.
48. Neumann HPH, et al. Pheochromocytomas, multiple endocrine neoplasia type 2, and von Hippel-Lindau disease. N Engl J Med 329:1531, 1993.
49. Vasen HFA, et al. The natural course of multiple endocrine neoplasia type IIB. Arch Intern Med 152:1250, 1992.
50. Oishi S, et al. Analysis of eight Sipple's syndrome patients and review of eighty-two cases from the Japanese literature. Jpn J Clin Oncol 20:392, 1990.
51. Gagel RF, et al. the clinical outcome of prospective screening for multiple endocrine neoplasia type 2A: An 18-year experience. N Engl J Med 318:478, 1988.
52. Jansson S, et al. Early diagnosis of and surgical strategy for adrenal medullary disease in MEN 2 gene carriers. Surgery 103:11, 1988.
53. van Heerden JA, et al. Surgical management of the adrenal glands in the multiple endocrine neoplasia type II syndrome. World J Surg 8:612, 1984.
54. Tibblin S, et al. Unilateral versus bilateral adrenalectomy in multiple endocrine neoplasia IIA. World J Surg 7:201, 1983.
55. Lips KJM, et al. Bilateral occurrence of pheochromocytoma in patients with the multiple endocrine neoplasia syndrome type 2 A (Sipple's syndrome). Am J Med 70:1051, 1981.
56. Wilson RA, Ibanez ML. A comparative study of 14 cases of familial and nonfamilial pheochromocytomas. Hum Pathol 9:181, 1978.
57. Richard S, et al. Pheochromocytoma as the first manifestation of von Hippel-Lindau disease. Surgery 116:1076, 1994.
58. Aprill BS, et al. Silent adrenal nodules in von Hippel-Lindau disease suggest pheochromocytoma. Ann Intern Med 120:485, 1994.
59. Green JS, Bowmer MI, Johnson GJ. Von Hippel-Lindau disease in a Newfoundland kindred. Can Med Assoc J 134:133, 1986.
60. Atuk NO, et al. Familial pheochromocytoma, hypercalcemia, and von Hippel-Lindau disease: A ten year study of a large family. Medicine 58:209, 1979.
61. Horton WA, Wong V, Eldridge R. Von Hippel-Lindau disease: Clinical and pathological manifestations in nine families with 50 affected members. Arch Intern Med 136:769, 1976.
62. Telenius-Berg M, et al. Quality of life after bilateral adrenalectomy in MEN 2. Henry Ford Hosp Med J 37:160, 1989.
63. Albanese CT, Wiener ES. Routine total bilateral adrenalectomy is not warranted in childhood familial pheochromocytoma. J Pediatr Surg 28:1248, 1993.
64. Hamberger B, et al. Subtotal adrenalectomy in multiple endocrine neoplasia type 2. Henry Ford Hosp Med J 35:127, 1987.
65. van Heerden JA, et al. Bilateral subtotal adrenal resection for bilateral pheochromocytomas in multiple endocrine neoplasia, type 2A: A case report. Surgery 98:363, 1985.
66. Irvin GL, Fishman LM, Sher JA. Familial pheochromocytoma. Surgery 94:938, 1983.
67. Chalmers RA, Mashiter K, Joplin GF. Residual adrenal cortical function after bilateral "total" adrenalectomy for Cushing's disease. Lancet 2:1196, 1981.
68. Mohler JL, et al. The evaluation of postoperative function of the adrenal gland. Surg Gynecol Obstet 161:551, 1985.
69. Branum GD, et al. The role of resection in the management of melanoma metastatic to the adrenal gland. Surgery 109:127, 1991.
70. Ettinghausen SE, Burt ME. Prospective evaluation of unilateral adrenal masses in patients with operable non-small-cell lung cancer. J Clin Oncol 9:1462, 1991.
71. Reyes L, et al. Adrenalectomy for adrenal metastasis from lung carcinoma. J Surg Oncol 44:32, 1990.
72. Soffen EM, et al. Palliative radiotherapy for symptomatic adrenal metastases. Cancer 65:1318, 1990.
73. Saboorian MH, Katz RL, Charnsangavej C. Fine needle aspiration cytology of primary and metastatic lesions of the adrenal gland. A series of 188 biopsies with radiologic correlation. J Clin Cyto Cytopathol 39:843, 1995.
74. Lee JE, et al. Evaluation of the incidental adrenal mass [letter]. Am J Med 103:249, 1997.
75. Brunt LM, et al. Laparoscopic adrenalectomy compared to open adrenalectomy for benign adrenal neoplasms. J Am Coll Surg 183:1, 1996.
76. Deans GT, et al. Laparoscopic adrenalectomy. Br J Surg 82:994, 1995.
77. Fernández-Cruz L, et al. Laparoscopic approach to adrenal tumors. J Laparoendoscopic Surg 3:541, 1993.
78. Gagner M, et al. Early experience with laparoscopic approach for adrenalectomy. Surgery 114:1120, 1993.
79. Go H, et al. Laparoscopic adrenalectomy for Cushing's syndrome: Comparison with primary aldosteronism. Surgery 117:11, 1995.
80. Guazzoni G, et al. Transperitoneal laparoscopic versus open adrenalectomy for benign hyperfunctioning adrenal tumors: A comparative study. J Urol 153:1597, 1995.
81. Janetschek G. Editorial: Ongoing advances in laparoscopic surgery. J Urol 153:1605, 1995.
82. Linos DA, et al. Anterior, posterior, or laparoscopic approach for the management of adrenal diseases? Am J Surg 173:120, 1997.
83. Prinz RA. A comparison of laparoscopic and open adrenalectomies. Arch Surg 130:489, 1995.
84. Schlinkert RT, et al. laparoscopic left adrenalectomy for aldosteronoma: Early Mayo Clinic experience. Mayo Clin Proc 70:844, 1995.
85. Staren ED, Prinz RA. Adrenalectomy in the era of laparoscopy. Surgery 120:706, 1996.
86. Vaughan ED Jr. Editorial: Renal and adrenal sparing surgery for patients with primary aldosteronism and primary reninoma. J Urol 153:1785, 1995.
87. Mercan S, et al. Endoscopic retroperitoneal adrenalectomy. Surgery 118:1071, 1995.
88. Abecassis M, et al. Serendipitous adrenal masses: Prevalence, significance, and management. Am J Surg 149:783, 1985.
89. Belldegrun A, et al. Incidentally discovered mas of the adrenal gland. Surg Gynecol Obstet 163:203, 1986.
90. Bitter DA, Ross DS. Incidentally discovered adrenal masses. Am J Surg 158:1959.

91. Copeland PM. The incidentally discovered adrenal mass. Ann Intern Med 98:940, 1983.
92. Kobayashi S, et al. Primary adrenocortical tumors in autopsy records—A survey of "cumulative reports in Japan" from 1973 to 1984. Jpn J Surg 21:494, 1991.
93. Yamakita N, et al. Asymptomatic adrenal tumor; 386 cases in Japan including our 7 cases. Endocrinology 37:671, 1990.
94. Bertagna C, Orth DN. Clinical and laboratory findings and results of therapy in 58 patients with adrenocortical tumors admitted to a single medical center (1951 to 1978). Am J Med 71:855, 1981.
95. Geelhoed GW, Druy EM. Management of the adrenal "incidentaloma." Surgery 92:866, 1982.
96. Herrera MF, et al. Incidentally discovered adrenal tumors: An institutional perspective. Surgery 110:1014, 1991.
97. Jockenhövel F, et al. Conservative and surgical management of incidentally discovered adrenal tumors (incidentalomas). J Endocrinol Invest 15:331, 1992.
98. Katz RL, Shirkhoda A. Diagnostic approach to incidental adrenal nodules in the cancer patient. Cancer 55:1995, 1985.
99. Penn I, Moulton J, Bracken B. Diagnosis and management of adrenal masses: 1987 Du Pont lecture. Can J Surg 31:105, 1988.
100. Siekavizza JL, Bernardino ME, Samaan NA. Suprarenal mass and its differential diagnosis. Urology 13:625, 1981.
101. Sirén JE, et al. Incidentalomas of the adrenal gland: 36 operated patients and review of literature. World J Surg 17:634, 1993.
102. Staren ED, Prinz RA. Selection of patients with adrenal incidentalomas for operation. Surg Clin North Am 75:499, 1995.
103. Thompson NW, Cheung PSY. Diagnosis and treatment of functioning and nonfunctioning adrenocortical neoplasms including incidentalomas. Surg Clin North Am 67:423, 1987.
104. Wood DE, Delbridge L, Reeve TS. Surgery for adrenal tumours: Is operation for the small incidental tumor appropriate? Aust N Z J Surg 57:739, 1987.
105. Ross NS, Aron DC. Hormonal evaluation of the patient with an incidentally discovered adrenal mass. N Engl J Med 323:1401, 1990.
106. Beyer HS, Doe RP. Cortisol secretion by an incidentally discovered nonfunctional adrenal adenoma. J Clin Endocrinol Metab 62:1317, 1986.
107. Bogner U, et al. Incidentally discovered ACTH-dependent adrenal adenoma presenting as "pre-Cushing's syndrome." Acta Endocrinol 111:89, 1986.
108. Huiras CM, Pehling GB, Caplan RH. adrenal insufficiency after operative removal of apparently nonfunctioning adrenal adenomas. JAMA 261:894, 1989.
109. Laudat MH, et al. Evening urinary free corticoids: A screening test n Cushing's syndrome and incidentally discovered adrenal tumours. Acta Endocrinol 119:459, 1988.
110. Rosen HN, Swartz SL. Subtle glucocorticoid excess in patients with adrenal incidentaloma. Am J Med 92:213, 1992.
111. Caplan RH, Strutt PJ, Wickus GG. Subclinical hormone secretion by incidentally discovered adrenal masses. Arch Surg 129:291, 1994.
112. Reincke M, et al. Preclinical Cushing's syndrome in adrenal "incidentalomas": Comparison with adrenal Cushing's syndrome. J Clin Endocrinol Metab 75:826, 1992.
113. McLeod MK, et al. Sub-clinical Cushing's syndrome in patient with adrenal gland incidentalomas. Pitfalls in diagnosis and management. Am Surg 56:398, 1990.
114. Virkkala A, et al. Endocrine abnormalities in patients with adrenal tumours incidentally discovered on computed tomography. Acta Endocrinol 121:67, 1989.

59

Thyroid Disease and Pathophysiology

Philip R. Orlander

The thyroid gland, although small in size, is an important organ in modulating normal metabolic processes within the body. For the surgeon, early recognition and treatment of thyroid dysfunction is essential to the smooth performance of all operations and to a successful postoperative convalescence. Correct interpretation of thyroid laboratory studies is critical to appropriate management, as the stress of surgery itself may alter their values. In addition, surgery plays an important primary role in managing patients with various thyroid diseases, such as hyperthyroid states and thyroid neoplasms. The current use of fine-needle aspiration cytology in patients with nodular thyroid disease permits improved office counseling of the patient and a more rational choice of treatment. Advances in our understanding of the molecular genetics of certain diseases, such as the multiple endocrine neoplasia syndromes, place the surgeon in a pivotal position for advising further investigation of families for prevention, detection, and treatment of early disease. Thus a firm understanding of the biology and natural history of the various processes that involve the thyroid are important to appropriate medical decision making and timing of procedures. When surgery is indicated, a good result can be expected, since current anesthetic management and surgical technique are associated with minimal risk.

THYROID ANATOMY

The thyroid gland is a bilobed structure, covered by a thin fibrous capsule and attached to the thyroid cartilage of the trachea by connective tissue (Fig. 59-1). It normally weighs 15 to 20 g with the right lobe being somewhat larger and more vascular than the left. The two lobes are connected by an isthmus from which a fingerlike projection of variable length, known as the pyramidal lobe, protrudes to the left. The isthmus generally overlies the second or third cartilaginous ring of the trachea. Anomalies of embryogenesis include thyroglossal cysts (caused by persistence of the thyroglossal duct) and lingual thyroid tissue with some or all of the thyroid gland embedded in the base of the tongue.

The blood supply of the thyroid gland is derived from the external carotid and subclavian arteries that give rise to the superior and inferior thyroid arteries, respectively. A rich lymphatic network is also present. The cervical ganglia and vagus nerves bilaterally innervate the gland, thus giving it both adrenergic and cholinergic innervation. The infrahyoid muscles, carotid sheaths, and sternocleidomastoid muscles flank the gland, and the recurrent laryngeal nerves run posteriorly between the lobes and the trachea. There are normally four parathyroid glands, two on the posterior surface of each thyroid lobe.

The thyroid gland has a large capacity for increased growth and vascularity. Its blood flow increases substantially in various pathologic states such as Graves' disease. Glandular function and growth are influenced by hormonal factors (e.g., thyroid-stimulating hormone [TSH]), blood flow, environmental factors (e.g., iodine availability), and infiltrating processes (e.g., lymphocytic thyroiditis).

NORMAL THYROID PHYSIOLOGY

The thyroid gland adapts to the metabolic needs of the body. The hormones secreted by this gland are intimately involved with the control of cellular metabolism and profoundly influence tissue growth, development, and tissue differentiation.

A complex neuroendocrine system modulates the body's attempt to adapt to its environment, and stress in particular.[1] A small tripeptide, thyrotropin-releasing hormone (TRH), is produced by hypothalamic neurons and released by specialized nerve terminals directly into hypophysial portal blood, where it stimulates the anterior pituitary gland to secrete thyrotropin (TSH), the hormone responsible for normal thyroid function. However, to adapt to a changing environment, especially in times of trauma and stress, several other messengers may effect this system. The most important of these transmitters are somatostatin and dopamine. Other modifiers of the hypothalamic-pituitary axis include adrenocorticotropic hormone (ACTH), endorphins, and other steroid hormones. Recent evidence suggests a powerful role for several immunologic

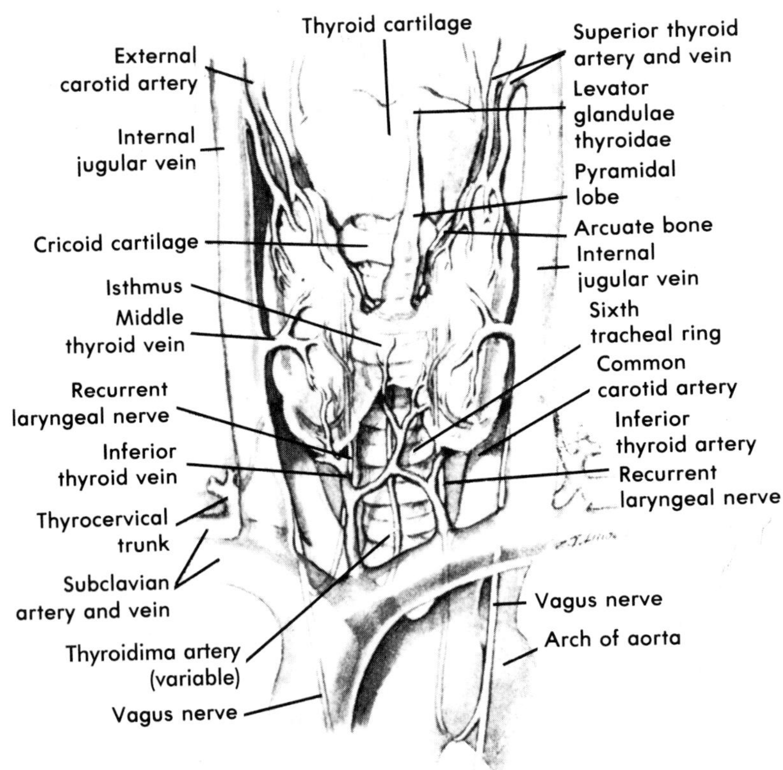

Fig. 59-1. Anatomy of the thyroid gland. (From Thorek P, Linden CT. Anatomy in Surgery, 2nd ed. Philadelphia: JB Lippincott, 1962.)

mediators such as tumor necrosis factor (TNF), interleukin-1 (IL-1), interleukin-6 (IL-6), and probably other cytokines in mediating and coordinating the neuroendocrine response to stress.[1] These cytokines help to explain the biochemical changes seen in many nonthyroidal diseases such as acute and chronic medical conditions, surgical stress, and even psychiatric illnesses[2] (see Thyroid Function and Nonthyroidal Illness). This immunologic-neuroendocrine link also provides an explanation for the anecdotal reports of stress as a precipitating cause of hyperthyroidism in susceptible individuals.

The pituitary gland plays a central role in thyroid hormone regulation. Integrating messages from higher centers and feedback from the thyroid gland, the pituitary gland senses the prevailing levels of TRH, somatostatin, and free thyroid hormone in the blood and responds with appropriate secretion of thyrotropin (TSH). This feedback mechanism allows the pituitary gland to have exquisite control over the free thyroid hormone concentration in serum. Thyrotropin (TSH) is the major hormone regulating both the growth and function of the thyroid gland and stimulates all steps in thyroid hormonogenesis including iodine uptake, organification, coupling, and secretion of the hormone. The mechanism for TSH action is interaction with the TSH receptor on the thyroid cell and stimulation of the production of the second messenger cyclic adenosine monophosphate (cAMP). In addition, TSH has a stimulating effect on growth and vascularity of the gland, possibly through a non–cAMP-mediated pathway. TSH stimulates the thyroid gland to synthesize and release primarily thyroxine (T_4) and a comparatively lesser amount of triiodothyronine (T_3) into the blood stream. Somatostatin is secreted by the hypothalamus and has an inhibitory effect on TSH secretion. T_4 and T_3 have a direct inhibitory effect on TSH secretion and action (short feedback loop) and an effect on hypothalamic somatostatin secretion, which in turn inhibits TSH secretion (long feedback loop). These considerations are summarized in Fig. 59-2. Thyrotoxic patients (in whom excessive quantities of T_4 and T_3 are found in serum) should have undetectable TSH levels as a result of the inhibitory feedback effects of thyroid hormone on the pituitary gland. The presence of detectable TSH levels in patients with elevated thyroid hormone levels suggests either abnormal feedback, a TSH-producing pituitary tumor, or cellular resistance to thyroid hormone (a rare familial syndrome).[3,4]

Iodine plays a complex role in thyroid physiology and pathology, and understanding the effects produced by iodine is critical in treating patients with thyroid disease. The thyroid avidly concentrates iodine, and small daily amounts of this substance are essential for normal gland function. Iodine deficiency is responsible for endemic goiters and hypothyroidism with its associated mental retardation that continues to plague large segments of the developing world. However, iodine is commonly used in general medical practice (e.g., expectorants, iodinated radiologic con-

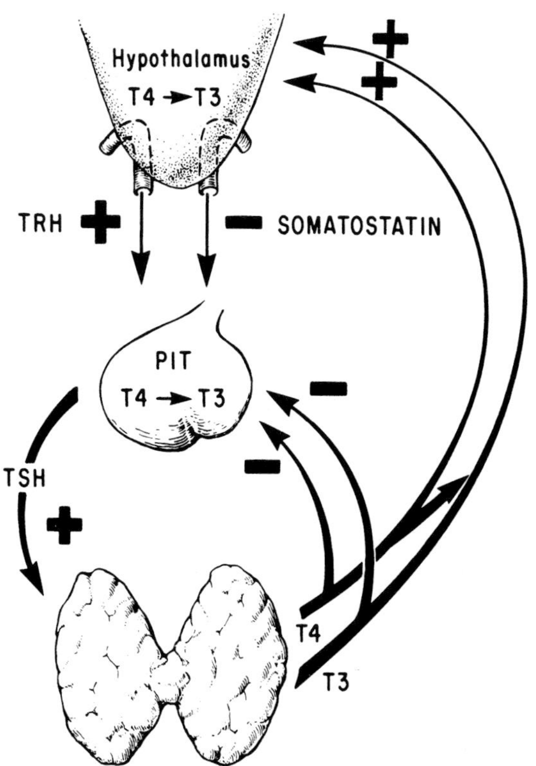

Fig. 59-2. Hypothalamic-pituitary-thyroid axis. Secretion of thyrotropin is regulated by the interaction of a releasing factor (thyrotropin-releasing factor [TRH]) and an inhibiting factor (somatostatin). Thyroid hormones, triiodothyronine and thyroxine (T_4 and T_3), act directly on the pituitary gland to inhibit thyrotropin secretion. Thyroid hormone also acts at the hypothalamic level to stimulate somatostatin release. The effect of thyroid hormone on secretion of TRH has not been established with certainty. Finally, T_4 is converted to T_3 in the periphery, the pituitary, and the hypothalamus; in all sites, T_3 is more potent than T_4. *PIT,* Pituitary; *TSH,* thyroid-stimulating hormone. (From Martin J, Reichlin S. Clinical Neuroendocrinology, 2nd ed. Philadelphia: FA Davis, 1987.)

trast) and this pharmacologic usage is associated with an increased occurrence of iodine-associated thyroid disease.[5,6]

A multifaceted autoregulatory system exists to govern the interaction of iodine with the thyroid gland. When large doses of iodine (6 mg or greater) are administered to patients, the iodine acutely, but transiently, blocks thyroid hormone secretion. Increased intrathyroidal organic iodine concentration prevents further iodine uptake by the gland and inhibits further organification of the iodine (Wolff-Chaikoff effect). Additionally iodine appears to interfere with the coupling of TSH to the activation of cAMP. These acute effects of large doses of iodine provide the rationale for its use in treating decompensated thyrotoxicosis (thyroid storm) and in preparing a patient with active thyrotoxicosis for surgery (see following discussion).

In the normal thyroid gland the acute inhibitory effects of iodine administration dissipate during several weeks as compensatory TSH levels rise in response to falling thyroid hormone levels. In patients with subtle underlying thyroid disease (Hashimoto's thyroiditis, inherited biochemical defects, previously treated Graves' disease), the compensatory TSH rise may not be able to override the combined inhibitory force of the iodine and the underlying thyroid disease. Depending on the degree of organification block, the patient may develop a goiter, with or without associated hypothyroidism. Discontinuation of iodine therapy usually results in resolution of the goiter, but thyroid hormone replacement therapy may be necessary.[6]

Long-term iodide excess in the diet would not normally enhance secretion of thyroid hormones because of the adaptation just described and a loss of iodide from the gland termed an "iodide leak." A small percentage of individuals with compensated iodine-deficient goiter with autonomous or semiautonomous nodules may be able to absorb iodine and rapidly synthesize thyroid hormone causing thyrotoxicosis (Jod-Basedow effect).[5] Because of the increased iodine pool, the radioactive iodine (^{123}I) uptake (RAIU) of the gland is low. Thus neither ^{131}I therapy nor antithyroid medications are effective acutely in the treatment of iodine-induced thyrotoxicosis.[7] In this circumstance, medications that decrease the adrenergic response (β-blockers) should be administered and iodine supplementation discontinued. The thyrotoxicosis should resolve during the next several weeks.

T_4 is the major secretory product of the thyroid gland, being more than 10 times more abundant than T_3. Only about 0.03% of total T_4 is free, the remainder being reversibly bound to various serum proteins, including thyroxine-binding globulin (TBG) (80%), thyroxine-binding prealbumin (TBPA) (15%), and somewhat looser to albumin. T_3 is also bound to the above-noted proteins but with a relative affinity of 10% as compared to thyroxine. Since T_4 is converted to T_3 in the peripheral tissues and T_3 is less protein bound and more biologically active at the cellular level, T_3 is likely responsible for most, if not all, of the metabolic effects of thyroid hormone, with T_4 acting as a prohormone.

Normally, the ratio of T_4:T_3 secreted from the gland is approximately 10:1. Monodeiodination of T_4 occurs with varied activity in the liver, pituitary gland, kidney, and elsewhere, yielding active T_3 and biologically inert reverse T_3 (rT_3) (Fig. 59-3). Deiodination of the outer ring of T_4 is controlled by the enzyme 5′ deiodinase type I in the periphery (primarily the thyroid gland, kidney, and liver) and the enzyme 5′ deiodinase type II concentrated in the central nervous system, pituitary gland, and placenta. The response of these two enzymes to physiologic and pharmacologic perturbations are distinctly different and affect thyroid hormone levels in serum. Acute and chronic nonthyroidal illnesses impair 5′ deiodinase type I, resulting in a decrease in circulating T_3 concentrations with a corresponding increase in rT_3 concentrations.[8,9] However, type

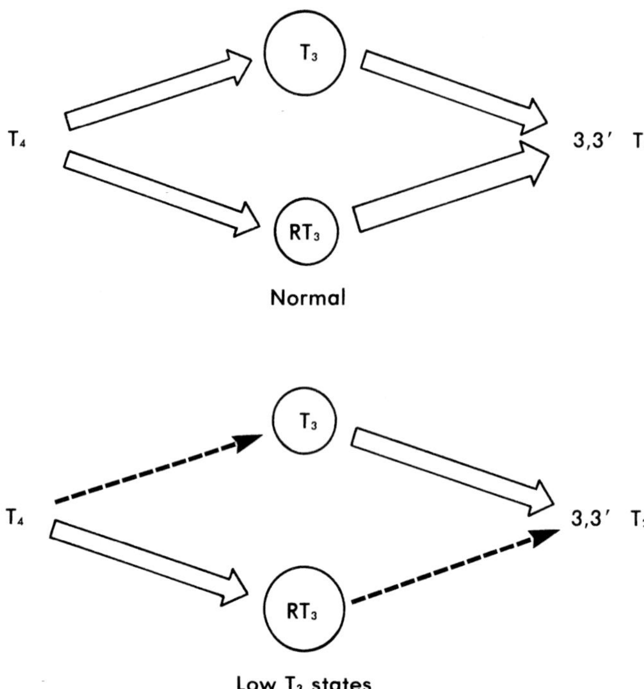

Fig. 59-3. T_4 deiodination. Pathways of T_4 deiodination in normal subjects *(upper)* and in patients with low T_3 states *(lower)*. The major abnormality is an impairment in 5′-deiodination both of T_4 and of reverse T_3 (rT_3). The size of each circle enclosing T_3 and rT_3 symbols depicts the relative change in serum concentration in the typical case. (From Cavalieri RR. Peripheral Metabolism of Thyroid Hormones, vol 3. Thyroid Today. Deerfield, Ill.: Travenol Laboratories, 1980.)

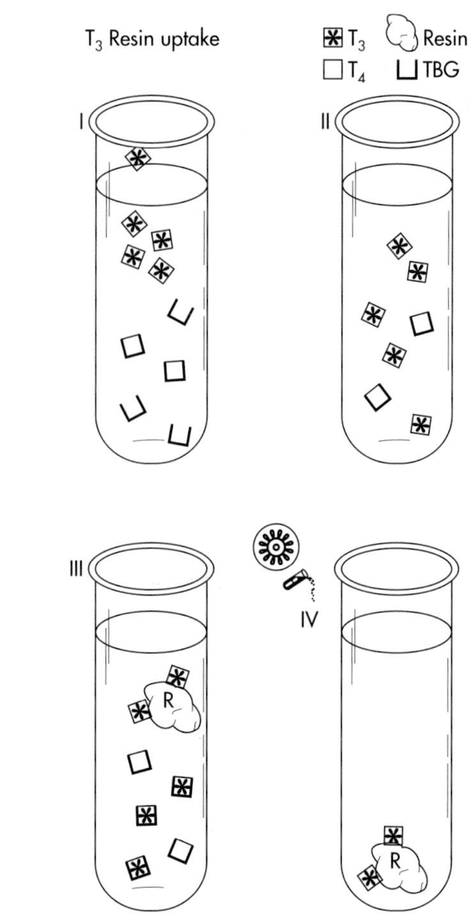

Fig. 59-4. Method for determining the thyroid hormone–binding ratio (formerly T_3-resin uptake test). The ratio is determined by incubating test serum with a tracer quantity of radiolabeled T_3 ($*T_3$), which interacts with available binding sites on thyroxine-binding globulin (TBG). At equilibrium between bound and free T_3, an insoluble resin is added that absorbs free $*T_3$. The resin is separated from serum by centrifugation, and the resin-associated $*T_3$ activity is quantified. The binding proteins are represented by TBG, but they could be any serum constituent that binds T_3 (transthyretin, albumin, and anti-T_4 antibody). (From Ladenson PW. The thyroid gland. In Harvey AMcG, et al., eds. Principles and Practice of Medicine, 21st ed. New York: Appleton-Century-Crofts, 1988, p 906.)

II 5′ deiodinase in the pituitary gland is unaffected by these conditions, T_4-to-T_3 conversion proceeds normally, and TSH levels remain normal. This adaptation has been termed the euthyroid sick syndrome (described later).[1,10,11] Propranolol and propylthiouracil (PTU) inhibit peripheral conversion of T_4 to T_3, explaining part of their clinical efficacy in treating thyrotoxicosis. Alternatively, the drug amiodarone, a potent cardiac antiarrythmic with a high iodine content, affects both type I and type II 5′ deiodinase enzymes, resulting in abnormal pituitary feedback with modest elevation of both thyroid hormones and TSH. Because of its high iodine content, amiodarone has also been associated with both hypothyroidism and hyperthyroidism.[5]

Approximately 80% of serum total T_3 is converted peripherally from T_4. Administration of T_4 to athyreotic patients results in normal total T_3 levels, primarily by conversion in the liver and other parenchymal tissues, confirming the efficacy and physiologic basis of replacement therapy for hypothyroidism with T_4 alone.[12]

Thyroid hormones act at the molecular level by interaction with nuclear T_3 receptors and subsequent regulation of target genes. Thyroid hormones affect different tissues in quite specific and distinct manners. These actions would include, but not be limited to, effects on cellular respiration and mitochondrial function, thermogenesis and Na^+,K^+-ATPase, morphogenesis, cardiac function, lipid and carbohydrate metabolism, and pituitary TSH secretion.

The free thyroid hormone level determines the metabolic status of the patient. An estimate of free hormone levels may be ascertained in one of several ways: (1) by directly measuring binding proteins in relation to total hormone values in serum, (2) by estimating binding sites on these proteins using the T_3 resin uptake (T_3RU) technique (Fig. 59-4), or (3) by attempting to measure free hormone levels.[7] There are several direct and indirect methods to measure free T_4. The "gold standard" employs equilibrium dialysis, but this method is expensive, laborious, and tech-

A
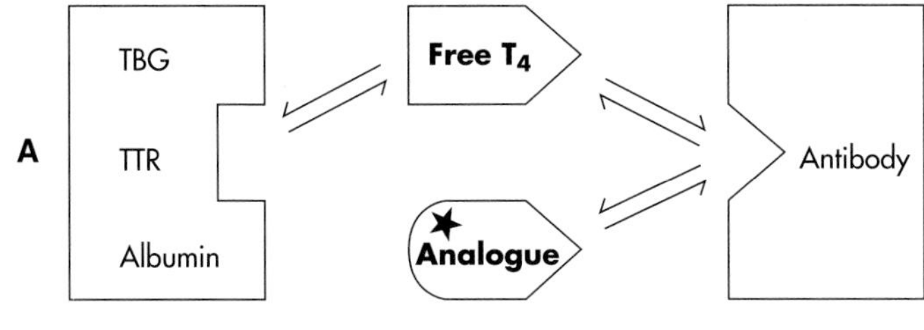

B
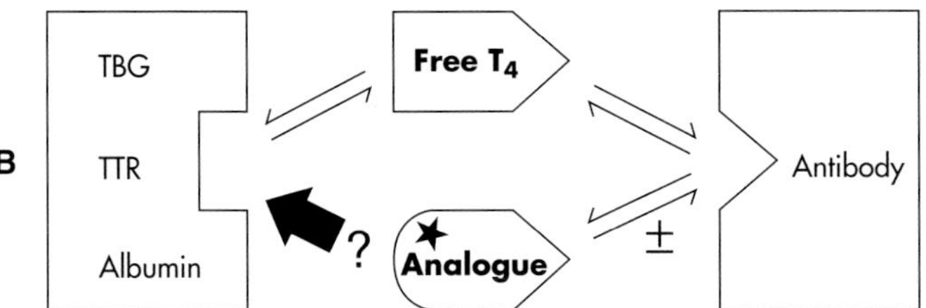

Fig. 59-5. Laboratory assessment of thyroid function: free T_4 analog assay. **A,** If a T_4 analog tracer that does not react with serum T_4-binding proteins competes with free T_4 for antibody binding sites, binding of that T_4 analog should be inversely proportional to the free T_4 concentration. In principle, this technique would give a reliable free T_4 estimate if interaction of the T_4 analog with serum proteins were identical in *all* samples and standards. **B,** Any difference in T_4 analog binding to serum proteins between samples and standards alters the proportion of T_4 analog available to compete with the assay antibody. If the T_4 analog is bound to an abnormal extent, as in familial dysalbuminemic hyperthyroxinemia or with iodothyronine-binding autoantibodies, the assay result is spuriously high. If T_4 analog binding to serum proteins is diminished, as in hypoalbuminemia or when albumin is highly occupied by nonesterified fatty acids, the assay result is spuriously low. *TBG,* Thyroxine-binding globulin; *TTR,* transthyretin (thyroxine-binding prealbumin); *analogue,* ^{125}I-T_4 analog.

nically difficult with several methodologic problems. However, the results generally reflect free hormone levels and are not affected by binding proteins. This assay should be reserved for circumstances when interpretation of the commonly used thyroid studies is difficult.

Several indirect measures of free T_4 are now commercially available.[7] These assays employ radiolabeled analogs of T_4 assuming that the interaction of this analog with serum proteins is identical in all samples and standards (Fig. 59-5). Unfortunately, these indirect assays overestimate T_4 in situations where the circulating proteins have an abnormal avidity for T_4 (e.g., in patients with familial dysalbuminemic hyperthyroxinemia or in patients with iodothyronine-binding autoantibodies) and underestimate T_4 in situations where serum proteins are diminished (i.e., hypoalbuminemic states). Therefore these new indirect free hormone assays rarely add information not obtained by the simpler and less expensive T_3RU.

COMMON CONDITIONS ASSOCIATED WITH THYROXINE-BINDING GLOBULIN (TBG) FLUCTUATION

Increased TBG Concentration (Decreased T_3 Resin Uptake)

1. Pregnancy
2. Estrogens
3. Oral contraceptives
4. Chronic active hepatitis
5. Inherited binding abnormalities
6. Hypothyroidism

Decreased TBG Concentration (Increased T_3 Resin Uptake)

1. Androgens
2. Glucocorticoids
3. Nephrotic syndrome
4. Severe acute or chronic illness
5. Inherited binding abnormalities
6. Hepatic failure
7. Hyperthyroidism

To perform the T_3RU test (see Fig. 59-4), isotopically labeled T_3 is added to the patient's serum and allowed to bind to available sites. A resin is then added that absorbs any unbound labeled T_3 and is measured as the resin uptake (T_3RU). This value is inversely related to the number of available protein-binding sites. Multiplying the T_3RU by the total T_4 concentration yields an estimate of the free hormone concentration (free thyroid index or FTI). For example, if total T_4 = 5 μg/dl, and T_3RU = 30%, then the FTI = 5 × 0.3 = 1.5 [no units]. In thyroid disease there is generally concordance between the total thyroid hormone levels (T_4 and T_3) and the resin uptake (e.g., both are elevated in hyperthyroid states, and both are decreased in hypothyroid states).

Free thyroid hormone levels are regulated by the pituitary gland, and abnormalities in binding proteins are compensated by adjustments in TSH secretion. Thus physiologic or pathologic states that increase binding proteins (e.g., pregnancy, estrogens, chronic liver disease, inherited abnormal proteins) result in a decrease in T_3RU but no change in the free hormone level, since the total T_4 level is increased in these conditions (see accompanying box). Conversely, conditions that raise T_3RU by decreasing thyroid-binding proteins (major systemic illness, hypoproteinemic states, glucocorticoid or anabolic steroid administration, nephrotic syndrome, and genetic causes) result in a lower total hormone level but normal free thyroid hormone levels. Therefore in *non*thyroidal disease, there is generally *dis*cordance between the total thyroid hormone levels (T_4 and T_3) and the resin uptake, but the directly measured free T_4 remains normal.

CONDITIONS THAT IMPAIR NORMAL PERIPHERAL THYROXINE METABOLISM (T_4-TO-T_3 CONVERSION)

1. Fasting (especially carbohydrate depletion)
2. Severe acute or chronic illness
3. Trauma, postoperative state
4. Hepatic failure
5. Radiologic contrast dyes
6. Glucocorticoids
7. Propranolol
8. Propylthiouracil
9. Amiodarone

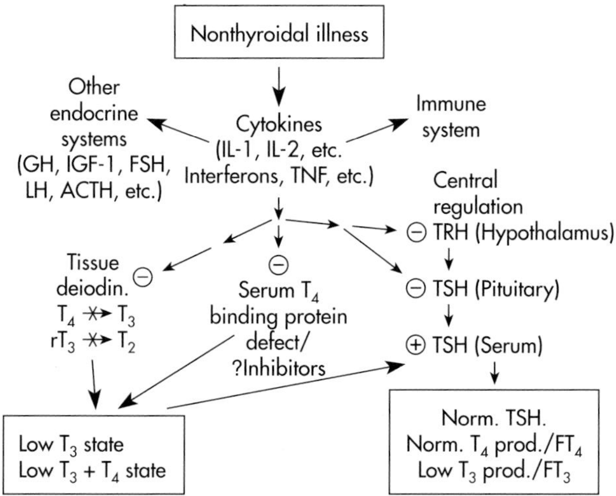

Fig. 59-6. Schematic diagram of the possible role of the cytokine system initiating both immunologic and endocrine responses to nonthyroidal illnesses.

Thyroid Function and Nonthyroidal Illness

Many acute and chronic nonthyroidal illnesses, including nutritional deprivation, affect thyroid hormone metabolism without changing the metabolic state of the patient (see accompanying box). This has been termed the "euthyroid sick syndrome."[1,8,9] In these conditions, normal deiodination of T_4 in the periphery is impaired, and a biologically inert metabolite (termed *reverse* T_3 [rT_3] because of its mirror image structure to T_3) accumulates (see Fig. 59-3). Decreased values of T_3 by radioimmunoassay (RIA) are a consistent feature of this syndrome and are common after prolonged fasting or surgical intervention. Extremely low values of total T_3 by RIA (T_3RIA) correlate with an elevated morbidity and mortality, almost irrespective of the primary disease process. If the patient is severely ill with nutritional depletion of normal serum proteins (e.g., albumin, thyroid-binding globulin), a low total T_4 and elevated T_3RU may also be observed. Some critically ill patients in intensive care settings are found to have decreased levels of thyroid hormones and TSH.[11] Changes in local cytokine concentrations in the hypothalamic-pituitary region related to the severe stress are thought to be responsible for the low TSH values[1] (Fig. 59-6). Medications commonly used in critically ill patients, such as glucocorticoids and dopamine, also reduce TSH levels. It is essential to exclude hypothalamic or pituitary disease in this setting by verifying that the free T_4 level is normal, the rT_3 level is elevated, and general pituitary function is preserved. As distinct from patients with either primary or secondary hypothyroidism, patients with euthyroid sick syndrome are clinically euthyroid and do not improve with thyroid hormone replacement. Whether this functional adaptation is beneficial or detrimental to the patient remains controversial.

Interpretation of Thyroid Function Studies

In any patient suspected of having thyroid disease, laboratory evaluation of thyroid function should begin with a measurement of total T_4RIA, an assessment of binding sites such as the T_3RU, and a TSH measurement using a sensitive assay (see boxes on p. 1171). An alternative more economic screening strategy would start with a TSH measurement and require further studies only if this measurement was abnormal or if there was a high suspicion of thyroid disease (Fig. 59-7). An elevated T_4RU and T_3RU are seen in hyperthyroidism, with a decrease in both levels being seen in hypothyroidism. New sensitive TSH assays are quite reliable and in ambulatory patients can usually distinguish the euthyroid patient from one that is hyperthyroid (undetectable TSH) or hypothyroid (elevated TSH) (Fig. 59-8). However, it is more difficult to interpret abnormal results in critically ill patients for the reasons previously stated (Fig. 59-9). A total T_3RIA is an unreliable screening test, since results may be normal in early hypothyroidism and low in euthyroid sick syndrome. However, an elevated T_3RIA confirms the suspicion of hyperthyroidism in patients with equivocal findings. Nonthyroidal illness should be suspected if there is a divergence between the total T_4 and T_3RU.

THYROTOXICOSIS

Thyrotoxicosis is a toxic-metabolic state resulting from abnormally elevated levels of circulating free thyroid hormone. Like other thyroid illnesses, women are much more frequently affected than men (10:1). Approximately 2% to 3% of women develop this state at some time during their lives, with an annual incidence of 3 per 1000. The term *hyperthyroidism* is generally reserved for thyrotoxic states caused by increased hormone synthesis by the thyroid gland (e.g., Graves' disease, toxic multinodular goiter) (see box on p. 1171). Exogenous ingestion of thyroid hormone would be an example of thyrotoxicosis without hyperthyroidism.

LABORATORY ABNORMALITIES IN COMMON THYROID DISEASES

Hypothyroidism	
Subclinical	Isolated increase in TSH
Moderate/severe	Decreased T_4, T_3RU, total T_3 and marked increase in TSH (>20 μU/ml)
Pituitary disorder	Mild decrease T_4, T_3RU, total T_3 and *decrease* in TSH
Hyperthyroidism	
Graves' disease	Undetectable TSH Increased T_4, T_3RU, total T_3 + Increased RAIU (>40%)
Thyroiditis	Decreased RAIU (<5%)
Factitious	
Nonthyroidal Disorders	
Estrogen therapy or pregnancy	Increased T_4, decreased T_3RU Normal TSH and total T_3
Mild illness	Decreased total T_3
Moderate illness	Marked decrease in total T_3 Decreased T_4, increased T_3RU +
Severe illness	Decreased TSH

RAIU, Radioactive iodine uptake; *RU,* resin uptake; T_3, triiodothyronine; T_4, thyroxine; *TSH,* thyroid-stimulating hormone.

CAUSES OF DECREASED THYROID-STIMULATING HORMONE (TSH) LEVELS (SENSITIVE ASSAY)

- Hyperthyroidism from all causes except pituitary tumors secreting TSH
- Subclinical hyperthyroidism in presence of normal T_4 levels
- Thyroid hormone therapy
- Nonthyroidal illness (usually severe)
- Drugs (glucocorticoids, dopamine)
- Early pregnancy
- Hypopituitarism

CAUSES OF INCREASED T_4 CONCENTRATIONS

- Hyperthyroidism of any cause
- Binding abnormalities
  - Excess thyroxine-binding globulin
    - Pregnancy
    - Estrogen use
  - Familial dysalbuminemic hyperthyroxinemia (rare)
  - Familial thyroid hormone resistance (rare)
- Drugs
  - Propranolol
  - Thyroxine
  - Amiodarone
  - Iodine
- Nonthyroidal illness (transient)

Autoimmune Hyperthyroidism (Graves' Disease)

Autoimmune factors are thought to be responsible for a major portion of thyroid disease. Autoimmune thyroid disease comprises a spectrum of clinical manifestations that includes hyperthyroidism associated with thyroid-stimulating antibodies and hypothyroidism associated with cytotoxic or inhibiting antibodies to the thyroid gland. Both conditions may be associated with goiters depending on the extent of lymphocytic infiltration and the interaction of the antibodies at the TSH receptor.

Graves' disease is the most common cause of hyperthyroidism. There is a marked female predominance, especially during the reproductive years, although it may affect all ages. A positive family history for Graves' disease, Hashimoto's thyroiditis, or other thyroid conditions is commonly seen, and the diseases may even coexist in the same patient. Twin studies show a high concordance rate in monozygotic twins (30% to 60%), and certain HLA types (e.g., DR3) are especially common in both diseases in whites. These HLA types have also been associated with other disorders suspected of having an autoimmune cause,

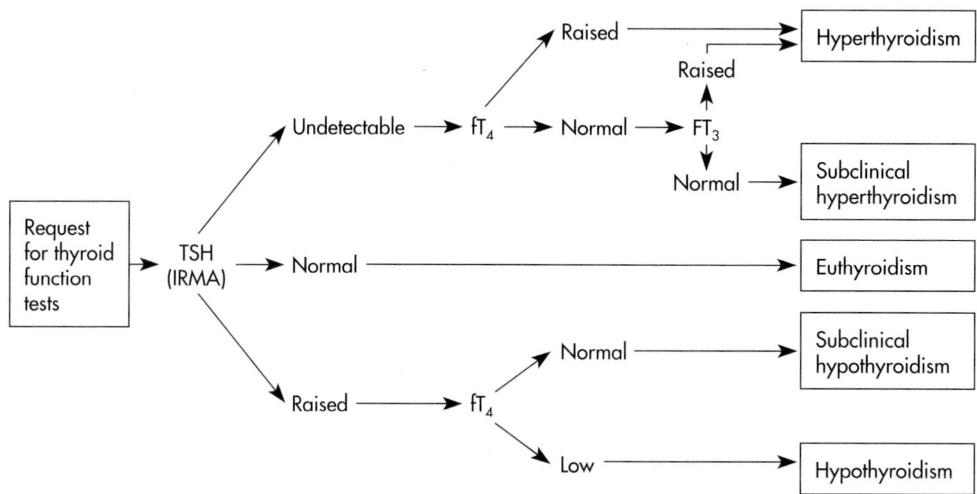

Fig. 59-7. Strategy for use of sensitive thyroid-stimulating hormone (TSH) assay for laboratory investigation of suspected thyroid disease. Most patients require only a TSH measurement. Measurement of serum total or free T_3 or T_4 is necessary in patients with abnormal serum TSH concentrations to differentiate between subclinical and overt hyperthyroidism or hypothyroidism. *IRMA,* Immunoradiometric assay; *fT_3,* free T_3; *fT_4,* free T_4. (From Caldwell G, et al. A new strategy for thyroid function testing. Lancet 1:1117, 1985.)

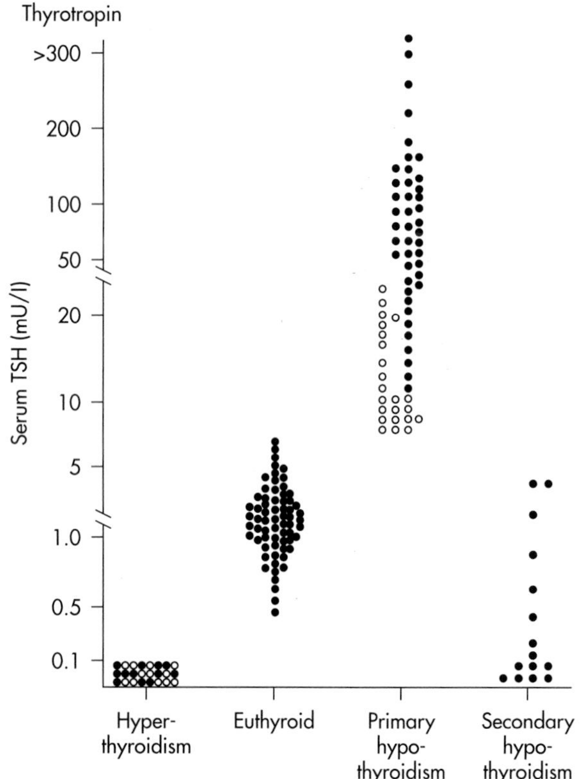

Fig. 59-8. Serum thyroid-stimulating hormone (TSH) concentrations measured by sensitive assay in euthyroid patients and in those with hyperthyroidism, primary hypothyroidism, and thyroid failure resulting from pituitary or hypothalamic disease (secondary hypothyroidism). Open circles represent patients with subclinical hyperthyroidism or hypothyroidism. (From Toft AD. Thyrotropin: Assay, secretory physiology, and testing of regulation. In Braveman LE, Utiger RD, eds. Werner & Ingbar's The Thyroid, 6th ed. Philadelphia: JB Lippincott, 1991, p 293.)

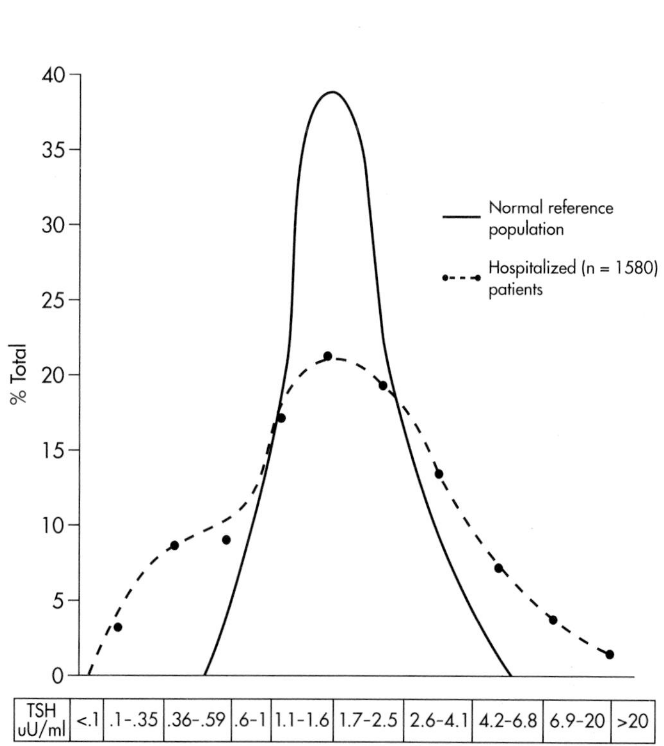

Fig. 59-9. Distribution percentage of serum thyroid-stimulating hormone (TSH) values in normal subjects and in 1580 patients hospitalized for nonthyroidal illnesses. (From Spencer CA, et al. Sensitive TSH tests: Specificity limitations for screening thyroid disease in hospitalized patients. Clin Chem 33:1392, 1987. American Association for Clinical Chemistry: 1-800-892-1400 or 1-202-857-0717.)

including type I diabetes mellitus, Addison's disease, systemic lupus erythematosus, and pernicious anemia, although the specific genes and suppressor T-cell defects are likely to be different.[13]

Although the precise cause of Graves' disease is unknown, current evidence suggests that B lymphocytes produce a family of thyroid-stimulating immunoglobulins (TSIg) that interact with TSH receptors on the thyroid cells, leading to enhanced T_4 production (Fig. 59-10). These or similar antibodies may also interact with different areas of the TSH receptors, resulting in enhancement of growth and vascularity, or inhibition of thyroid function (TSH-binding inhibitory immunoglobulins or TBII).[14-16] Such phenomena may be transient and/or recurring, resulting in remissions and exacerbations of the disease. As lymphocytic infiltration of the gland is common, it is hypothesized that the site of TSIg production is the thyroid gland itself.[14] Recent improvements in laboratory techniques employing human thyroid cells from patients with Graves' disease have demonstrated TSIgs in more than 80% of these individuals. Unfortunately, neither the presence, absence, or changes in the titers of these antibodies correlates well with the course of the disease.

It is possible that several different antibodies may play a role in the pathogenesis of Graves' disease. Antithyroid antibodies (e.g., antithyroglobulin, antimicrosomal antibodies) are frequently found in the serum of patients with Graves' disease and in those with Hashimoto's thyroiditis. Although the titers of these antibodies are usually higher in Hashimoto's thyroiditis, it is not possible to distinquish be-

CAUSES OF HYPERTHYROIDISM

Graves' disease	Thyroid-stimulating immunoglobulin
Toxic adenoma	Autonomous benign tumor
Multinodular goiter	One or more hyperplastic nodules
Thyroiditis	Release of stored hormone
Factitious	Exogenous hormone
Pituitary tumor	TSH-secreting adenoma (rare)
Struma ovarii	Ectopic thyroid tissue (rare)
Thyroid cancer	Metastatic follicular cancer (rare)
Trophoblastic tumor	Production of β=hCG (rare)

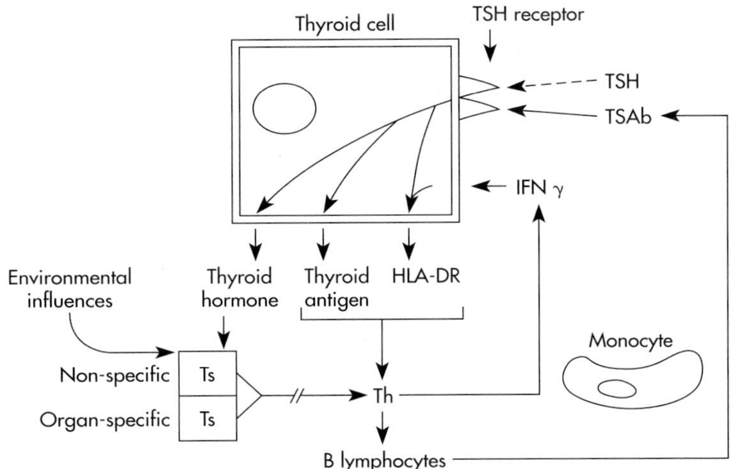

Fig. 59-10. A hypothetical scheme for the pathogenesis of Graves' disease. The basic factor necessary for the development of Graves' disease is considered to be an HLA-related, genetically induced, organ-specific defect in suppressor T-lymphocyte (Ts) function. Precipitating factors from the environment (e.g., stress, infection, drugs, trauma) may cause a decrease in generalized suppressor T-lymphocyte function and number, which is additive (superimposed) to an organ-specific suppressor T-lymphocyte defect. The result is decreased suppression of populations of thyroid-directed helper T lymphocytes (Th). The specific helper T lymphocytes then, in the presence of monocytes and specific antigen, produce γ-interferon (IFN-γ) and also stimulate specific B lymphocytes to produce thyroid-stimulating antibody (TSAb). TSAb, similar to thyroid-stimulating hormone (TSH), stimulates the TSH receptor and results in increased thyroid hormone production and increased thyroid antigen expression. IFN-γ causes expression of HLA-DR antigens on the surface of thyroid cells, an effect enhanced by TSAb and TSH. The result is that thyroid cells become antigen-presenting cells and so contribute to stimulation of specific helper T lymphocytes and perpetuate the process. Moreover, excess thyroid hormone acts on generalized suppressor T lymphocytes, reducing their number and function, further stimulating helper T lymphocytes. Without the specific suppressor T-lymphocyte abnormality, however, continued cycling should not occur, and the process soon ends. (Volpé R. Graves' disease. In Braveman LE, Utiger RD, eds. Werner & Ingbar's The Thyroid, 6th ed. Philadelphia: JB Lippincott, 1991, p 649.)

tween these disease states on the basis of the antibody titer. In fact, histologic examination of thyroid glands in patients with Graves' disease frequently reveals localized areas of Hashimoto's thyroiditis, making it difficult for the surgeon to estimate how much functioning thyroid tissue to leave as a remnant to produce a euthyroid state.[17,18]

The trigger for the immunologic production of antibodies is not known. Although there is homology between a bacterial antigen derived from *Yersinia enterocolitica* and the human TSH receptor, there is no conclusive evidence that *Yersinia* infection is related to the development of Graves' disease. Clinical use of immune modulators such as interferon and interleukins has been associated with antibody production and thyroid disease in a small percentage of individuals, lending support to the theory that an abnormal induction of T lymphocytes occurs in genetically susceptible hosts. This phenomenon would also explain the anecdotal onset of Graves' disease after stress.

Clinical Manifestations

The classic signs and symptoms of Graves' disease are well described. The diagnosis is made on the basis of clinical manifestations of a hypermetabolic state and specific findings related to immunologic damage. The following can be found in all thyrotoxic states regardless of the cause and include heat intolerance, weight loss, tremor, increased appetite, palpitations, rapid pulse, diarrhea, and proximal muscle weakness. Findings specific for autoimmune thyroid disease include a diffusely enlarged, firm, nontender goiter (often with a bruit); evidence of orbitopathy such as exophthalmos, and rarely pretibial myxedema and acropachy. All manifestations are rarely seen in one patient, and occasionally atypical presentations may obscure the diagnosis. Weight gain, for example, may be seen in younger patients whose increased appetite and calorie intake can exceed 9000 calories per day. Psychiatric manifestations, including frank psychosis, may be the prominent symptom at presentation in some cases, and many psychiatric institutions screen all new patients with thyroid function studies.[2]

On physical examination the patient is usually fidgety, diaphoretic, and possesses a warm, moist skin. Deep tendon reflexes are usually exaggerated, and the pulse pressure is increased. Lid lag and a widened palpebral fissure are common in all thyrotoxic states and thought to be secondary to adrenergic stimulation. Approximately half of patients with Graves' disease have some evidence of orbitopathy, but only a small percentage of patients have debilitating eye signs such as periorbital infiltration, exophthalmos, extraocular muscle dysfunction, or corneal ulceration.[12] Chemosis and dysconjugate gaze may also be present. Diplopia on lateral superior gaze is a particularly early sign of extraocular muscle dysfunction. Most commonly, orbitopathy is present during the hyperthyroid presentation of the disease. However, occasionally eye abnormalities may be the presenting manifestation in a euthyroid individual, or it may develop years after treatment of the hyperthyroidism. Ultrasound or CT examination of the orbits are the most sensitive indicators of extraocular muscle involvement. The immunoglobulins responsible for this manifestation have not been clarified, and this complication does not correlate well with the presence or titer of TSIgs.[12,19]

The thyroid gland is almost always diffusely enlarged and nontender. Minor degrees of nodularity and asymmetry may be present, but a dominant nodule(s) is(are) distinctly unusual. The pyramidal lobe is frequently enlarged. Rarely, especially in men, the goiter may be substernal and not easily visible. A nonpalpable thyroid gland in a patient with hyperthyroidism should prompt an investigation for factitious hyperthyroidism (from exogenous ingestion) or painless thyroiditis. A nonfunctioning nodule in a patient with Graves' disease may carry a risk of malignancy as high as 50% and requires cytologic evaluation with fine-needle aspiration.[20,21]

Laboratory Findings

The diagnosis of Graves' disease is made on the basis of the clinical picture associated with laboratory evidence of ongoing excessive thyroid hormone production. An elevated T_4 level in the presence of an elevated T_3RU suggests an increased free thyroid hormone level consistent with thyrotoxicosis. The TSH level should be undetectable. To confirm ongoing thyroid hormone production, it is necessary to show that the gland is actively concentrating iodine and replenishing its intrathyroidal iodine pool. This is easily accomplished with the RAIU test (see accompanying box) in which a small quantity of ^{123}I is administered orally and its uptake in the neck measured and compared to background uptake. The RAIU is markedly elevated in Graves' disease, whereas it is low in thyrotoxicosis because of exogenous intake of thyroid hormones or inflammatory states that interrupt the integrity of the gland (subacute thyroiditis). A radionuclide scan of the thyroid gland in Graves' disease should show an enlarged gland that intensely and diffusely traps the isotope. The differential diagnosis in-

COMMON CONDITIONS ASSOCIATED WITH RADIOACTIVE IODINE UPTAKE (RAIU OR ^{131}I UPTAKE)

Elevated

1. Graves' disease
2. Toxic nodular goiter
3. Iodine deficiency (may be associated with diuretics)
4. Hashimoto's thyroiditis (may be variable)

Decreased

1. Subacute thyroiditis
2. Exogenous thyroid hormone administration (may be surreptitious)
3. Recent iodine administration (dietary, radiologic contrast, or therapeutic)

cludes several rare disorders including TSH-secreting pituitary tumors, noted by inappropriately elevated TSH levels in the setting of hyperthyroidism, and β-hCG-producing tumors (molar pregnancies, trophoblastic tumors).

Total T_3 levels (T_3RIA) are elevated in hyperthyroidism with the ratio of T_3:T_4 secreted from the gland being increased. On occasion the T_4 level may be normal in spite of an elevated T_3 level (i.e., T_3 toxicosis). This latter circumstance may occur as an early manifestation of Graves' disease, after medical (^{131}I therapy) or surgical (subtotal thyroidectomy) intervention, or occasionally in toxic nodular goiters. Thus a total T_3RIA should be obtained in a patient who is clinically hypermetabolic but with equivocal results from thyroid function studies. Measurements of TSIgs are generally not necessary for either diagnosis or management because of their low predictive value. However, they are useful in predicting neonatal thyrotoxicosis in a pregnant woman with active Graves' disease.

Treatment

There is no available therapy that specifically attacks the autoimmune derangements thought to be the cause of the disease. Therapy is therefore aimed at decreasing thyroid hormone production, either by blocking organification of iodine with thionamide drugs (e.g., PTU, methimazole), ablating the gland with radioactive iodine, or surgically removing part or all of the hyperplastic gland.[13] Permanent hypothyroidism is therefore a common consequence of either the therapy or the disease itself, and patients must be aware of the probable requirement for lifelong thyroid hormone replacement therapy.

Medical therapy. Antithyroid medications (i.e., thionamide drugs) are an effective mode of therapy. PTU, in addition to blocking iodine organification, also blocks peripheral T_4-to-T_3 conversion. In vitro studies suggest that PTU also has an immunologic action on T lymphocytes.[22] Methimazole has the advantage of having a longer duration of action and can be given as a single daily dose. Several studies have shown remission rates after 3 to 24 months of antithyroid therapy ranging from 15% to 50% (see accompanying box). Recently, Hashizume et al.[23,24] in Japan have demonstrated a much lower recurrence rate by using a combination of methimazole and levothyroxine therapy. However, Japan has a much higher daily iodine intake as compared with the United States, a higher frequency of autoimmune thyroid disease with a higher spontaneous remission rate, and different genetic markers for the disease. It is therefore not known if a similar success rate can be expected from this regimen in the United States. There is no single marker that reliably predicts which patients will relapse. Larger goiters, thyroid glands with persistently high ^{123}I uptakes, high serum titers of thyroid-stimulating antibodies, and a HLA-DR3 type are associated with higher relapse rates. However, the predictive value of all these measures is disappointingly low.

FACTORS ASSOCIATED WITH SPONTANEOUS REMISSION OF GRAVES' DISEASE

1. Small goiter
2. Decrease in goiter size during therapy
3. Normalization of radioactive iodine uptake
4. Low levels or normalization of thyroid-stimulating antibody levels
5. ? DR3- or DR4-negative HLA types

It is advisable to control the hypermetabolic state with antithyroid medications prior to any definitive therapy with either ^{131}I or surgery. Once the patient is eumetabolic, a decision regarding definitive therapy should be made based on the age, medical condition, and wishes of the patient. As Graves' disease is common in women in their reproductive years, the patient's concerns about the timing of pregnancy must be addressed. During pregnancy, medical therapy with PTU is the preferred option.[5]

A trial of medical therapy is a reasonable first step in the treatment of Graves' disease. Children may be treated for longer periods of time, whereas elderly patients usually receive other modes of therapy (i.e., radioactive iodine) as primary therapy or as soon as they are eumetabolic. Disadvantages of the medical regimen include a 5% to 10% incidence of minor allergic reactions, a 0.01% incidence of agranulocytosis, and compliance problems associated with long-term therapy. The dose of medication may be titrated to make the patient euthyroid (average dose in an adult is 300 to 600 mg of PTU or 30 to 60 mg of methimazole daily). In some cases, it may be useful to administer a larger blocking dose supplemented by replacement therapy with oral T_4. This latter regimen has the practical advantage of decreasing the frequency of clinic visits and the theoretic advantage of suppressing the immune system.[23,24]

The amount of thionamide treatment necessary to control hyperthyroidism depends on the severity of the disease and the rapidity of hormone turnover. Increased doses of medication given at more frequent intervals (every 4 to 6 hours) control even the most severely hyperthyroid patient. Since these medications do not affect already stored thyroid hormone, a treatment period of at least 4 to 6 weeks is necessary to attain a eumetabolic state. This period is related to the half-life of T_4 (7 to 10 days in normal individuals, shorter in hyperthyroidism).

The cardiovascular manifestations of hyperthyroidism are a frequent concern to both the patient and the physician. Thyroid hormone has direct stimulatory effects on myocardial cells and indirectly affects cardiac function through peripheral vasodilation and increased peripheral oxygen consumption.[25] Thyrotoxic patients appear to have increased sympathetic tone as evidenced by the cardiovascular changes of increased heart rate, stroke volume, and cardiac output and by the fine tremor typical of thyrotoxicosis. All these signs respond to β-adrenergic blockade. However, patients with thyrotoxicosis have normal to low catecholamine levels. Therefore the clinical picture of increased adrenergic tone is most likely related to the synergistic effect of thyroid hormone and an enhanced sensitivity of β-receptors to circulating catecholamine levels.

Clinical manifestations of thyrotoxic heart disease include palpitations, dyspnea, and poor exercise tolerance and may proceed to atrial fibrillation, angina pectoris (even in the absence of coronary disease), and high-output congestive heart failure. These findings may be present in a patient without any evidence of organic heart disease, whose cardiac parameters become normal after successful treatment of thyrotoxicosis. A prime example of this was the sudden onset of atrial fibrillation in President George Bush, subsequently found to be related to unrecognized Graves' disease and treated without cardiac sequelae. β-adrenergic blocking agents such as propranolol quickly relieve some of the symptoms of hyperthyroidism related to a hyperdynamic cardiovascular system. In addition, propranonol in large doses (160 to 320 mg/day) decreases T_4-to-T_3 conversion in the periphery. In symptomatic patients, β-blockade should be initiated in conjunction with antithyroid medication. Because of the short half-life of β-blockers in thyrotoxicosis, it is preferable to use a long-acting preparation several times a day. Once a eumetabolic state is achieved, β-blockade may be tapered and discontinued. Although β-blockers are a crucial part of the treatment regimen, they do not prevent thyroid storm and must be combined with other antithyroid therapies. In patients with rapid atrial fibrillation, propranolol can be administered intravenously in a properly monitored situation such as a coronary care unit. In patients with congestive heart failure, an ultra–short-acting β-blocker can be tried cautiously in a monitored setting. Digoxin can be used in atrial fibrillation and heart failure, sometimes in conjunction with a β-blocker, although manipulation of doses is more difficult than in a euthyroid patient and cardiology consultation is advisable. In patients who cannot tolerate β-blockers (e.g., asthmatic patients), calcium channel blockers have been useful. Only after these cardiovascular manifestations are adequately controlled, can the physician proceed safely with either radioiodine or surgical therapy.

Radioiodine therapy. Radioiodine is safe and effective therapy for adults with Graves' disease and is the most common therapy given. When a sample of American thyroidologists were recently asked in a survey how they would manage a 43-year-old woman with hyperthyroid Graves' disease with a 40 to 50 g goiter, 69% selected radioiodine therapy, 30% chose prolonged antithyroid drug therapy, and only 1% recommended surgery.[26] The choice of radioiodine therapy became even more popular with older patients. The theoretic concerns regarding the subsequent development of thyroid carcinoma, hematologic malignancies, and birth defects with such treatment have not been substantiated. Graves' disease is very sensitive to iodine, and usually small doses suffice. The radiation dose to the ovaries is approximately equivalent to that received during an intravenous pyelogram or barium enema. Despite some continuing controversy, radioiodine is frequently given to women of reproductive age as long as the patient is not pregnant and one can be assured of adequate contraception for at least 6 to 12 months. Use of radioiodine remains more restricted in adolescents and children and contraindicated in pregnancy because of the danger of fetal and neonatal hypothyroidism after the tenth gestational week. For 1 or 2 days after treatment with radioiodine, the patient should be instructed on appropriate hygienic and precautionary measures to avoid exposure to family members and children.

It is not possible to accurately calculate a dose of radioiodine that will result in euthyroidism. Small doses may result in an unacceptably high rate of recidivism. Prior treatment with antithyroid medications may necessitate a larger dose to be effective. The incidence of hypothyroidism after radioiodine treatment frequently reflects the philosophy of the treating physician in determining the delivered dose and can be as high as 90% in the first year. Regardless of the dose, however, the incidence of postradioiodine hypothyroidism continues to increase by about 3% per year thereafter. Because of the unpredictability of radioiodine therapy and the necessity for lifelong follow-up, many investigators argue that ablative radioiodine treatment followed quickly by T_4 replacement therapy is the preferable plan (Fig. 59-11).

As with surgery, radioiodine therapy administered to an uncontrolled hyperthyroid patient may precipitate a thyrotoxic crisis. Therefore in a severely hyperthyroid patient thionamides remain the first line of therapy. If radioiodine is chosen as definitive therapy, iodine administration (see

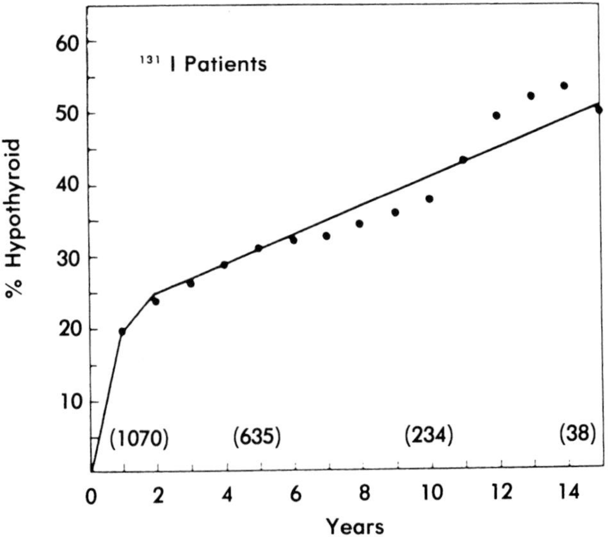

Fig. 59-11. Incidence of postradioiodine hypothyroidism in relation to the duration of follow-up. Total number of patients followed for each of the indicated time periods is shown in parenthesis. (From Dunn JT, Chapman EM. Rising incidence of hypothyroidism after radioactive iodine therapy in thyrotoxicosis. N Engl J Med 271:1037, 1964. Copyright © 1964 Massachusetts Medical Society. All rights reserved.)

following discussion) is avoided. Once the patient is eumetabolic, the thionamide is discontinued. A thyroid scan and uptake using ^{123}I are performed approximately 4 days later; based on the percent uptake after 24 hours and a clinical assessment of the size of the gland, the treatment dose of ^{131}I is calculated and administered orally. The thionamide is restarted approximately 4 days later depending on the symptomatology of the patient. Iodide, in the form of potassium iodide, can also be used as adjunctive therapy, beginning 1 week after radioiodine therapy so as not to interfere with its uptake. β-blockade is continued during this period to avoid any cardiovascular effects from a thyroid hormone surge resulting from glandular damage. This sequence allows for appropriate dosing and uptake of the radioiodine without placing the patient at substantial risk from thyrotoxicosis. Radiation thyroiditis, an inflammation of the thyroid resulting in a tender gland, and exacerbation of the thyrotoxic state may occur approximately 1 to 2 weeks after radioiodine therapy. Fortunately, radiation thyroiditis is not commonly seen in Graves' disease, since the treatment dose of ^{131}I (usually less than 20 mCi) is a much lower dose than is generally associated with this problem.

The effect of radioiodine on thyroid function is slow and is usually not detected clinically for at least 6 weeks, and more frequently 3 to 6 months, after treatment. Medical therapy can be slowly tapered during this period. Uncontrolled hyperthyroidism after 9 to 12 months should warrant further evaluation and possibly a second dose of radioiodine. On average, less than 15% of patients require a second dose.

It remains unclear whether choice of therapy has an impact on one of the most serious complications of Graves' disease: orbitopathy. A recent clinical trial from Sweden demonstrated that patients older than 35 with Graves' disease randomized to receive radioiodine therapy were more likely to have a worsening of their eye disease than individuals treated with either medical or surgical therapy.[27] This difference may have been related to the delay of starting levothyroxine replacement in this treatment group. Nevertheless, as this is the only prospective study performed to address the question, it would be prudent to treat patients with active eye disease with a modality other than radioiodine or to pretreat these patients with glucocorticoids to avoid this complication.[19]

Surgical therapy. Thyroidectomy (i.e., generally subtotal) remains an important therapeutic option in the treatment of Graves' disease. As with radioiodine, it is not possible to reliably predict the size of the remnant that will render the patient euthyroid.[17,18,28] The relatively high percentage of patients that are cured by thyroidectomy (30% to 40% in some series) suggests that somehow thyroid homeostasis is reestablished by the procedure. Thyroidectomy not only removes the source of thyroid hormone production, but also may decrease the population of activated lymphocytes. Advantages of thyroidectomy include the speed of remission and the low rate of recurrence.

The argument over the extent of thyroidectomy (subtotal vs. total) mirrors the debate over the calculated dose of radioiodine. A more complete thyroidectomy may be preferable in a child with Graves' disease, since the chances of regrowth of the remnant and recurrence of disease are fairly high. Depending on the published series examined, recurrent thyrotoxicosis occurs in 0.6% to 30% of cases following surgery.[29,30]

Evidence of coexisting Hashimoto's thyroiditis, as noted by antibody titers (antimicrosomal, antiperoxidase, and antithyroglobulin antibodies) or lymphocytic infiltration microscopically, is also associated with a higher incidence of postsurgical hypothyroidism. Hypothyroidism may result from progressive fibrosis and inflammation of the thyroid remnant following surgery. Since this process can occur in the absence of definitive radioiodine or surgical therapy, hypothyroidism may be thought of as part of the natural history of the disease rather than being an adverse effect of therapy. Thus more aggressive radioiodine or surgical approaches only accelerate this natural course.

Recurrence of thyrotoxicosis after thyroidectomy appears to be directly related to the size of the residual remnant, the severity of the hyperthyroidism, the age of the patient at the time of surgery, and the underlying immune aspects of the disease. One argument for total thyroidectomy is the removal of the source of autoimmune activity. A more complete thyroidectomy, however, is associated with a higher risk of permanent hypoparathyroidism and recurrent laryngeal nerve damage. Although it remains unclear if any mode of therapy affects the associated orbitopathy, surgery or medical therapy appears to be associated with a lower risk of progressive eye disease based on a recent randomized trial.[27]

Thyroidectomy is generally reserved for those patients with Graves' disease who may benefit particularly from surgical treatment. These include (1) children with unremitting Graves' disease where experience with radioiodine remains limited, (2) pregnant women with uncontrolled hyperthyroidism and allergy to antithyroid medications, (3) patients with unreliable contraception or desire for early pregnancy, (4) patients with suspicious "cold" nodules in an otherwise diffusely hyperplastic gland, (5) patients who cannot tolerate antithyroid medications or have developed a hypersensitivity to the medications, (6) patients who prefer or would benefit from a rapid resolution of the thyrotoxic state, and (7) possibly patients with active and progressive orbitopathy.

In spite of the benefits of surgery, it must be remembered that the unstable metabolic state associated with hyperthyroidism increases the risk of anesthesia and surgery. Thyroid storm may be precipitated by surgery in a poorly prepared patient. Thus prior to surgery, thionamides should be given in large enough doses and at frequent enough intervals during at least 4 to 6 weeks to achieve a euthyroid state. Surgery may then be planned on an elective basis. In addition, iodine is very effective in decreasing the size and vascularity of the gland, in acutely blocking secretion of thyroid hormones by the gland, and in transiently interfering with organification (Wolff-Chaikoff effect). The mechanism by which iodine decreases the vascularity of the gland (involution) is unknown. Since the Wolff-Chaikoff effect is temporary, lasting only 10 to 14 days, it is advisable to administer iodine in the presence of a thionamide and adequate β-blockade, preferably within 2 weeks of scheduled surgery. In patients unable to tolerate thionamide therapy, surgical preparation with propranolol and iodine is usually successful. A near-total thyroidectomy would be desirable in this circumstance to avoid either an exacerbation of hyperthyroidism or an eventual recurrence. Iodine may be given as either Lugol's solution or a saturated solution of potassium iodide. Recently, oral cholecystographic dyes (e.g., ipodate) have been shown to control hyperthyroidism quickly and effectively because of their high iodine content and their ability to rapidly block conversion of T_4 to T_3.[31]

Toxic Nodular Goiter

Toxic nodular goiter is a form of hyperthyroidism that is more commonly encountered in patients older than 40. A female predominance is again noted but not so marked as with Graves' disease. The patient may initially have a long stable history of a multinodular goiter or a predominant nodule in the neck. The addition of iodine, either in medications or contrast dye, may precipitate thyrotoxicosis. This is especially noted in iodine-deficient regions.

Cardiovascular effects of hyperthyroidism predominant in this condition and, in the elderly, may be the only clinical signs detected. The term *apathetic hyperthyroidism* aptly describes a depressed, frequently constipated, elderly patient who has weight loss and cardiac arrhythmias. Eye signs are lacking; although a goiter is usually present, it may not be impressive. Therapy should be initiated with antithyroid medications and propranolol. Iodine should be avoided in these patients. The diagnosis should be confirmed with an elevated T_4 level, an undetectable TSH, and a thyroid scan revealing one or more hot nodules.

Nodular goiters do not concentrate iodine well compared to those in Graves' disease and generally require larger doses of radioiodine (i.e., 20 to 30 mCi for toxic multinodular goiter as opposed to 6 to 15 mCi for Graves' disease) for treatment. Recurrence or failure of initial radioiodine therapy is not uncommon, since destruction of one autonomous nodule may be replaced with another autonomously functioning nodule. Although thyroid carcinoma is unusual in this setting, an enlarging hypofunctioning nodule in a hyperthyroid gland warrants fine-needle aspiration or surgical exploration.

The size and vascularity of large multinodular goiters make surgical management more formidable. In contrast to the hyperplastic glands found in Graves' disease, the multinodular goiter may not shrink with iodine, and iodine may precipitate a thyrotoxic crisis. Therefore the preferred treatment of a toxic multinodular goiter is radioiodine. Hypothyroidism is unusual after such therapy in this setting.

Solitary functioning adenomas that are greater than 3 cm in diameter and suppress all extranodular thyroid tissue on nuclear imaging are likely to produce thyrotoxicosis.[32] As with toxic multinodular goiters, the symptoms and signs of a toxic thyroid adenoma may be subtle, especially in the elderly. RAIU may be only modestly elevated, but the thyroid scan shows intense uptake only in the area of the palpable abnormality. A TSH and/or T_3RIA should be obtained, especially if the total T_4 level is normal, in view of the high incidence of T_3 toxicosis in this circumstance.

Radioiodine therapy of toxic adenomas has the theoretic advantage of being taken up only by the hyperfunctioning tissue, destroying it, and rendering the patient euthyroid.[33] The incidence of carcinoma in a hot nodule is extremely small, and there is no evidence that radioiodine is carcinogenic. However, recurrence of hyperthyroidism after radioiodine therapy is not uncommon, and repeated doses of radioiodine required to deliver 10 to 15 mCi ^{131}I to the nodule (30 mCi ^{131}I to the patient) may be undesirable in the younger patient. In addition, the patient may be left with a palpable abnormality. In a recent study of the long-term effects of ^{131}I on solitary autonomous nodules, 54% (12 of 23 patients) had no change in the size of the nodule, and 36% developed hypothyroidism.[32]

Surgery for toxic adenomas has the advantage of quickly resolving the thyrotoxic state and avoiding recurrences. A simple nodulectomy is usually sufficient because the remainder of the thyroid gland is normal and carcinoma is distinctly unusual in the nodule itself. If an image of the suppressed thyroid tissue is desirable before surgery, this may be accomplished by administering bovine TSH before a thyroid scan. Recombinant human TSH is preferable when it is commercially available.[34]

Miscellaneous Causes of Hyperthyroidism

It is important to exclude other rarer forms of hyperthyroidism such as the transient hyperthyroidism associated with thyroiditis (see the following), factitious hyperthyroidism caused by excessive exogenous intake of thyroid hormones, and TSH-producing pituitary tumors. Thyroid hormones (both T_3 and T_4) continue to be used to promote weight loss despite a lack of effectiveness and the known cardiovascular risks of thyrotoxicosis.

Thyroid Storm

Thyroid storm is an extreme form of hyperthyroidism. In addition to the recognized findings of hyperthyroidism, the clinical diagnosis of thyroid storm is based on cardiovascular abnormalities (malignant arrhythmias resistant to medications), mental status changes (psychosis, confusion, obtundation, or coma), and pyrexia. Therapy is directed at acutely decreasing thyroid hormone secretion (iodine intravenously or orally, glucocorticoids, PTU) and decreasing adrenergic tone (propranolol). Although rare, thyroid storm is associated with a high morbidity and mortality. Severe stress may precipitate thyroid storm in a patient with unrecognized mild hyperthyroidism. Common precipitating causes of thyroid storm include surgery (especially thyroid surgery), trauma, infection, and iodine administration. Iodine-containing radiographic contrast agents are also common offenders. Amiodarone, an effective antiarrhythmic, contains a large amount of iodine and has been associated with both hypothyroidism and hyperthyroidism. A medical regimen that allows the patient to be eumetabolic before surgery substantially reduces the risk of thyrotoxic crisis.

HYPOTHYROIDISM

Primary thyroid failure is the natural end point of several thyroid diseases, such as chronic thyroiditis, as well as the result of surgical or radioablative therapy. Although iodine deficiency is the most common worldwide cause of hypothyroidism, Hashimoto's thyroiditis predominates in the United States. Women are much more frequently affected than men, with a prevalence of clinical hypothyroidism of approximately 2% but rising to 10% in the elderly. It is estimated that more than 5% of women have subclinical hypothyroidism (see accompanying boxes).

Thyroiditis and Hypothyroidism

Thyroiditis is the term given to inflammatory processes involving the thyroid gland. These may be characterized by onset: acute thyroiditis, subacute thyroiditis, and chronic thyroiditis.

Acute suppurative thyroiditis is a painful febrile illness of sudden onset that is usually bacterial in origin. The infection may originate from abscessed lower teeth or in a pyriform sinus fistula, a rare congenital malformation. Treatment includes incision and drainage of the abscess, antibiotic coverage, and a careful search for and radical excision of a fistulous tract. Infection with unusual organisms, such as *Mycobacteria* or *Pneumocystis carinii,* has been reported in patients with AIDS.[35,36]

Subacute thyroiditis is characterized by a transient hormonal syndrome in which the patient may be either hyperthyroid or hypothyroid, depending on the stage of the illness (Fig. 59-12). It may present as an exquisitely painful thyroid gland, known as de Quervain's thyroiditis and thought to be of viral origin, or as a nontender gland, typically occurring in the postpartum period and associated with the presence of thyroid antibodies.[37] In de Quervain's thyroiditis, the thyroid gland is tender to palpation and diffusely enlarged and often the patient complains of radiation of pain to the ears, a mild fever, and generalized malaise. On laboratory evaluation an associated elevation in the sedimentation rate and thyroid hormone levels is commonly found, as well as the clinical signs of hyperthyroidism. This illness frequently follows an upper respiratory infection and is self-limited. There is usually no family history of thyroid disease, and thyroid antibodies are absent. Histologically, giant cells are seen, suggestive of a viral cause, although this has not been proven.

"Painless" or postpartum thyroiditis was first described in 1948 by Robertson and appears to be related to a general immunologic rebound following the relative immunosuppression of pregnancy in genetically predisposed individuals.[38] More than 60% of the patients notice symptoms of hyperthyroidism such as palpitations and fatigue, while the remainder develop hypothyroidism within 4 to 6 months of delivery.[39] Almost half the patients who initially have hyperthyroidism develop biochemical hypothyroidism within the next several months before recovery of

CAUSES OF HYPOTHYROIDISM

- Chronic lymphocytic thyroiditis (Hashimoto's thyroiditis)
- Radiation
- Surgery
- Infiltrating diseases
  - Sarcoidosis
  - Amyloidosis
- Iodine deficiency
- Iodine excess
- Inherited enzyme defects
- Drugs
  - Antithyroid medications
  - Amiodarone
  - Lithium
  - Carbamazepine and phenytoin
- Pituitary or hypothalamic disease
- Familial thyroid hormone resistance (rare)
- Subacute thyroiditis (transient)

POPULATIONS APPROPRIATE FOR ROUTINE THYROID SCREENING

- Neonates
- Psychiatric illness/dementia
- Elderly women (older than 65)
- Hyperlipidemia
- Medical history of autoimmune endocrine disease
  - Type I diabetes mellitus
  - Addison's disease
  - Pernicious anemia
- Sleep apnea
- Persistent or severe postpartum symptoms
- Amiodarone therapy
- Lithium therapy
- Previous history of head/neck irradiation
  - Hodgkin's disease, carcinoma of larynx, other cancers
  - Irradiation during childhood for benign disease
- Previous thyroid surgery or thyroid treatment
- Down syndrome
- Family history of autoimmune thyroid disease

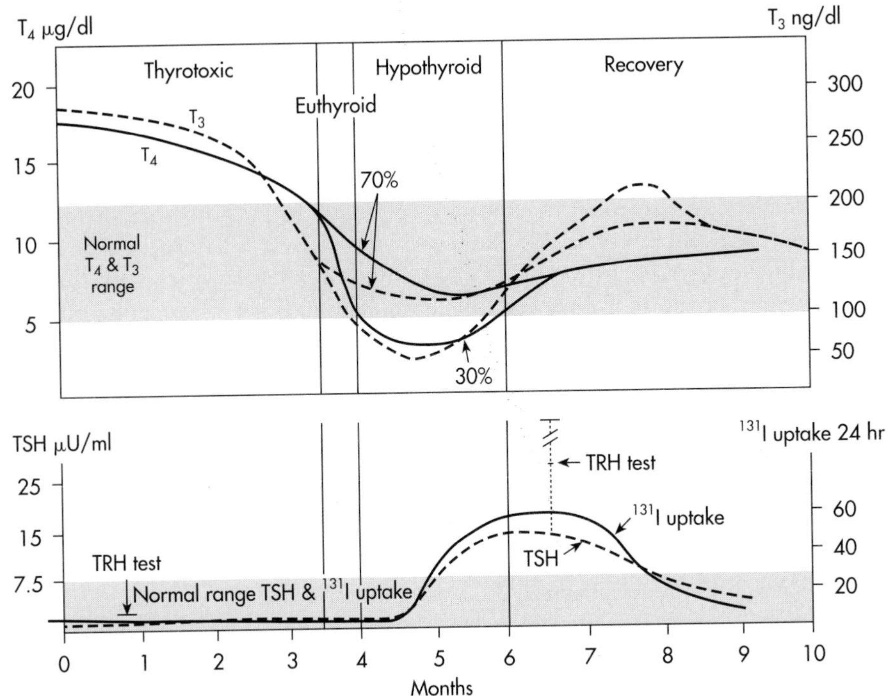

Fig. 59-12. Schematic representation of the changes in serum T_4, T_3, and thyroid-stimulating hormone (TSH) concentrations and thyroid ^{131}I uptake during the course of silent thyroiditis and of subacute thyroiditis. The hatched area represents the limits of the normal ranges. In the hypothyroid phase, the serum T_4 and T_3 lines divide to show that only about 40% of patients develop hypothyroidism. In the recovery phase, the serum T_3 line divides to show that 15% of patients have transient elevation of the serum T_3 level. (Modified from Woolf PD. Transient painless thyroiditis with hyperthyroidism: A variant of lymphocytic thyroiditis? Endocr Rev 1:411, 1980. Copyright by The Endocrine Society.)

thyroid function. Depression is a prominent feature of this illness and may explain some of the postpartum mood changes. Antimicrosomal antibodies are detectable more than 75% of the time, and frequently the patients describe a strong family history of thyroid disease.[37,39] Newer, more sensitive antibody assays (antithyroid peroxidase) are able to detect these antibodies in more than 90% of patients. Several HLA types (DR3, DR4, DR5) are seen more frequently in this disease, and it appears to be particularly common in women with type I diabetes mellitus, with a prevalence rate of 25%. In several prospective studies 5% to 16% of postpartum women have some evidence, albeit subtle, of this disorder.[37,39] Although restitution of normal thyroid function commonly occurs usually within the next 4 to 6 months, many women have subsequent episodes with future pregnancies, and have a high risk for hypothyroidism (possibly as high as 23%) later in life, especially if the antibody titers are substantially elevated.

Patients with either form of subacute thyroiditis have a similar clinical course and may have transient hyperthyroidism lasting several weeks, followed by transient hypothyroidism, before recovery of normal thyroid function. Early in the course of the disease, the RAIU is low (5%) when the thyroid hormone levels are elevated and the TSH level is undetectable. Discharge into the blood of formed thyroid hormones stored within the gland suppresses the pituitary secretion of TSH, resulting in a low iodine uptake. This low uptake clearly distinguishes the thyrotoxicosis of thyroiditis from the high uptake typical of Graves' disease. Treatment is usually supportive and includes anti-inflammatory drugs such as aspirin for analgesia if the gland is tender and β-blockers such as propranolol if the patient is symptomatic from thyrotoxicosis. Glucocorticoids have no advantage over anti-inflammatory drugs but do present several disadvantages. As the thyroid gland is not actively synthesizing new hormone, based on the low radioiodine uptake, antithyroid medications are not indicated. If the hypothyroid state lasts several months or is very symptomatic, temporary thyroid hormone replacement may be worthwhile.

Hashimoto's thyroiditis (or chronic lymphocytic thyroiditis) is the most common form of thyroiditis and is caused by an autoimmune mechanism, resulting in an invasion of lymphocytes. Clinically, the disease is characterized by a diffuse, rubbery, nontender goiter. All types of thyroid dysfunction have been associated with Hashimoto's thyroiditis, including transient hyperthyroidism, euthyroid goiter, hypothyroid goiter, and an atrophic thyroid gland with associated hypothyroidism. Hashimoto's thyroiditis generally afflicts women between the ages of 20 and 50 years, but it is also commonly encountered in children. The diagnosis is usually confirmed by the finding of a firm goiter in the presence of a markedly elevated antithyroid antibody titer. The presumptive antigen in this disease is the peroxidase enzyme, which is found in the microsomal fraction of the thyroid cell, and the newer antithyroid peroxidase antibodies or their older surrogate, antimicrosomal antibodies, correlate with the presence of the disease. Virtually all patients with Hashimoto's thyroiditis have detectable antibodies to thyroid peroxidase, and the presence of these antibodies in euthyroid individuals is predictive of the development of hypothyroidism. Thyroid-blocking immunoglobulins (TBIg), antibodies that interact with but do not stimulate the TSH receptor, are also commonly found and may be responsible for both the goiter formation and the hypothyroidism common in this condition. Thyroid imaging usually reveals a patchy uptake of isotope. Histologic examination of the thyroid gland reveals lymphocytic infiltration. If hypothyroidism is present in this disease, thyroid hormone replacement is the keynote of treatment.

The pathogenesis of Riedel's type of thyroiditis is unknown. It may be part of a systemic disorder (e.g., retroperitoneal fibrosis) or the fibrous end stage of Hashimoto's thyroiditis. Pathologically, the gland atrophies and is characterized clinically as being woody and hard. Because of this firmness, cancer cannot be excluded on clinical grounds alone; therefore fine-needle aspiration is indicated to exclude such a possibility, especially as lymphoma of the thyroid can occur in patients with lymphocytic thyroiditis. Since patients with Riedel's thyroiditis, similar to Hashimoto's thyroiditis, often have some form of hypothyroidism, replacement with thyroid hormone is usually indicated.

Clinical Presentation

The clinical presentation of hypothyroidism may be very subtle because of its slow progressive onset, nonspecific symptoms, and occasional atypical presentations. The classic symptoms of weight gain, bradycardia, constipation, dry skin, cold intolerance, and somnolence develop insidiously. All neonates are screened for hypothyroidism. Children may have a decreased attention span, difficulty at school, and short stature. An abnormal growth curve and delayed bone age should prompt a workup for hypothyroidism. Adolescents and young adults may come to the physician with difficulty in concentrating and depression. Elderly patients frequently have depression and signs of organic brain syndrome. All patients with lipid disturbances should be screened for hypothyroidism. In surveys of nursing home populations, approximately 10% of elderly women were found to have unsuspected primary hypothyroidism on thyroid screening tests.

Thyroid function studies in patients with primary hypothyroidism reveal an elevated TSH level, a low total T_4 level, a low T_3RU consistent with an increase in binding sites, and a low FTI. Although RAIU is decreased in hypothyroidism, the quantity of iodine in the American diet impairs the use of this study diagnostically. The new sensitive TSH assays make this test the best single measure of thyroid function, assuming normal pituitary function. The pituitary gland is exquisitely sensitive to any change in free T_4 level, even within the normal range, and an elevated TSH level is diagnostic of thyroid failure. In an attempt to maintain metabolic homeostasis, a failing thyroid gland may secrete a higher ratio of T_3/T_4 in response to high values of TSH. This invalidates the measurement of T_3RIA as a useful study in early hypothyroidism.

Two principal problems confront the surgeon in dealing with a patient with possible hypothyroidism:

1. Does the patient have primary hypothyroidism or secondary hypothyroidism (related to a hypothalamic or pituitary disorder) or are the abnormal values the result of a physiologic response to an acute or chronic illness or stress, such as surgery?
2. If the patient is hypothyroid, what is the most appropriate replacement regimen to avoid anesthetic or surgical complications?

The diagnosis of primary hypothyroidism must be confirmed by an elevated TSH level prior to initiation of therapy. As previously noted, low results from thyroid function studies are common in severe acute or chronic illness. The finding of an extremely low T_3RIA has been observed to correlate with a high mortality. An elevated T_3RU, a normal or low TSH, a normal free T_4 by dialysis, and a normal or increased rT_3 are consistent with the euthyroid sick syndrome. Thus thyroid replacement therapy is not indicated in this latter group of patients.[8-11] Pituitary or hypothalamic disease should be suspected in a patient with an inappropriately low or normal TSH value in the setting of a low thyroid hormone value. Additional history suggestive of pituitary disease and a review of general pituitary function should help to resolve this possibility.

Treatment

Levothyroxine is the drug of choice to treat hypothyroidism.[40,41] Levothyroxine should not be taken with medications such as aluminum hydroxide and iron, as they may interfere with absorption. A euthyroid state is usually attained with a dose of approximately 1.6 μg/kg/day, but this must be titrated carefully to achieve a TSH level within the normal range (0.4 to 5 μU/ml). In older patients or patients with cardiovascular disease, it is best to initiate therapy with a small dose (0.025 to 0.05 mg daily), monitor cardiovascular status carefully, and slowly increase the dose every 2 to 4 weeks until achieving a euthyroid state. It is not always possible to achieve a eumetabolic state before embarking on a major surgical procedure. A good example of this is the hypothyroid patient with severe coronary artery disease who experiences an exacerbation of angina when the dose of levothyroxine is adjusted. Coronary artery bypass surgery may be performed while such a patient is hypothyroid if there is close cooperation among the internist, surgeon, and anesthesiologist. Since the metabolism of most drugs is slowed in the hypothyroid patient, adjustment of drug doses (especially opiates and sedatives) are necessary. Arterial blood gases and estimates of ventilatory effort should be monitored frequently. A slow recovery of gastrointestinal motility and an increased tendency for neuropsychiatric symptoms ("ICU-itis") may be anticipated. A retrospective study suggests a lower morbidity from coronary bypass surgery in hypothyroid patients than in patients having surgery after replacement with thyroid hormone.[42] After revascularization, replacement therapy should be titrated until the patient is euthyroid.

With the availability of sensitive TSH assays and the improvement of the bioavailability of the thyroxine preparations, it is possible to titrate the dosage requirements of a patient quite easily. It is now apparent that many patients were inadvertently overtreated in the past, as judged by suppressed TSH levels. The consequence of minor overtreatment with T_4 is controversial, but several studies have indicated excessive bone loss, especially in postmenopausal women not receiving estrogen replacement therapy.[43-45] It is well known that thyrotoxicosis is associated with increased bone turnover and bone loss. It is unclear whether levothyroxine suppressive therapy is responsible for clinically significant bone loss. However, because of the long-term risk of osteoporosis, physicians are cautioned to titrate the T_4 dose such that the TSH level is measurable within the normal range (0.4 to 5 μU/ml).

Myxedema Coma

Severe myxedema should be suspected in a hypothermic, somnolent patient. Hypercapnia and hyponatremia are common metabolic findings. A puffy face, periorbital edema, evidence of previous neck surgery, doughy and dry cool skin, and a delayed relaxation of deep tendon reflexes are usually present. Although absence of the lateral third of the eyebrows was previously thought to be a helpful clinical finding, it is only of significance in patients younger than 40.

Myxedema coma may be precipitated in a patient with unrecognized hypothyroidism by infection, cold exposure (apartments for the elderly without heat in the winter), surgery, trauma, and drugs. In fact, most instances of myxedema coma occur in the hospital when a patient with unrecognized hypothyroidism is subjected to sedatives, diuretics, surgery, or other stressors. The metabolism of most drugs, particularly sedatives and opiates, is slowed by hypothyroidism. Respiratory depression and hypercapnia caused by a sluggish respiratory center result in coma and respiratory failure. Thyroid hormone replacement therapy should be begun immediately after blood for thyroid studies (T_4, T_3RU, TSH) is drawn in a patient suspected of myxedema coma.

Management of Myxedema Coma

Primary thyroid failure has an indolent course that frequently requires several years to develop into a myxedematous state. A large infusion of thyroid hormone may precipitate malignant cardiac arrhythmias. As enteral absorption may be erratic in these patients as a result of motility disorder and edema, intravenous levothyroxine is the preferred replacement regimen. Depending on the severity of the myxedema and the fragility of the patient's cardiovascular system, daily doses of 100 to 200 μg may be safer than the loading dose of 500 μg usually recommended. The patient should be carefully monitored in an intensive care unit for any potentially life-threatening arrhythmias.

Glucocorticoids are an important adjunctive therapy for patients with severe hypothyroidism because the sudden increase in the metabolic rate after the addition of T_4 may render the patient relatively adrenally insufficient. In addition, the autoimmune phenomena that result in Hashimoto's thyroiditis may be more generalized, thus producing a syndrome of polyglandular endocrine failure. The most common manifestations of this syndrome are primary thyroid failure, primary adrenal insufficiency, and type I diabetes mellitus. An evaluation of the pituitary-adrenal axis, including pretreatment cortisol levels, is therefore essential.

In patients with myxedema coma, treatment should result in prompt improvement in the P_{CO_2}, ventilatory status, and mentation. Glucocorticoids may be tapered and discontinued if the adrenal reserve is adequate. The TSH level should slowly decline toward the normal range if the replacement dose is adequate and the patient is compliant.

THYROID NODULES AND NEOPLASIA

Thyroid nodules are common (Fig. 59-13). Approximately 5% of the population, with a 9:1 female predominance,

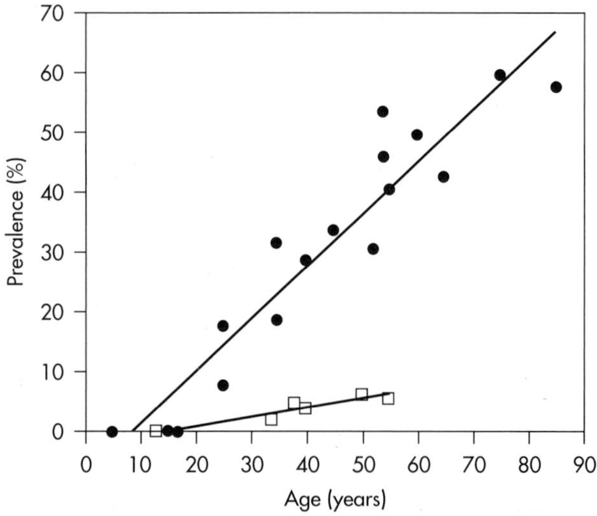

Fig. 59-13. Prevalence of palpable thyroid nodules detected at autopsy or by ultrasonography (●) or by paloanon (□) in subjects without radiation exposure or known thyroid disease. (From Mazzaferri EL. Management of solitary thyroid nodules. N Engl J Med 328:553, 1993.)

have such nodules.[46] A small percentage of these nodules are malignant, and an even smaller percentage of such malignant nodules are life threatening. In the past the decision to proceed to surgical intervention after noting the presence of a thyroid nodule was based in large part on the anxiety of the patient and the physician. Improvements in our ability to obtain cytologic information have resulted in a decreased number of unnecessary surgical procedures and an increase in the percentage of actual malignant neoplasms found at surgery. Further, a better understanding of the biologic behavior of different thyroid tumors has permitted a more reasoned physiologic approach to their treatment.

Pathophysiology

Management of patients with thyroid disease is complicated by the fact that several different insults to the thyroid gland manifest themselves by forming nodular goiters. The initial insult may be autoimmune thyroiditis, iodine deficiency, or inherited biochemical defects, but any chronic stimulation of the gland, including Graves' disease, results in first a diffuse and eventually a nodular goiter. Goiters of puberty and pregnancy are of short duration and are not nodular. The TSH levels are frequently normal in these individuals, and the patient is generally euthyroid. Thus the cause of these physiologic goiters remains unclear. They frequently resolve spontaneously, and therapy is rarely indicated. Other growth factors, such as epidermal growth factor, or other hormones associated with pregnancy may be responsible for growth of the thyroid. Although TSH is presumed to be the major hormone responsible for both hormone synthesis and growth, it is not unusual to see discordance between these two phenomena. In some large goiters, antibodies have been isolated that stimulate growth in vitro (as measured by thymidine uptake) but do not stimulate synthesis (as measured by cAMP production).[15,16] Further molecular studies of the TSH receptor may be helpful to delineate these differences. Glycosylation and other posttranscriptional events may influence the activity of the TSH molecule.

Increasing age is accompanied by an increased frequency of thyroid nodules. Radioautography of thyroid sections suggests the following natural history of thyroid nodules. After a period of stimulation, presumably from TSH, a diffusely enlarged goiter with good vascularity and homogenous radioiodine uptake becomes a diffusely enlarged gland with patchy uptake of iodine. This difference in uptake slowly results in some area of the gland becoming relatively hypofunctioning and others becoming relatively hyperfunctioning; some follicles remain hyperplastic, whereas other follicles fill with colloid. This phase is generally known as a colloid goiter. Nodules may form as some follicles enlarge or degenerate as others become more hyperplastic, becoming indistinguishable from adenomas. Some of these nodules may spontaneously resolve, whereas others may enlarge secondary to hemorrhage in the nodule; still others may become autonomously hyperfunctioning. This sequence of events eventually results in an adenomatous or multinodular goiter. Because of the intense hyperplasia that is commonly present in these glands, it may not always be possible to distinguish benign from malignant nodules preoperatively, even with aspiration cytology.

How can these events be explained on the basis of TSH stimulation, if in fact the TSH levels are normal? The following hypotheses have been suggested:

1. A normal TSH level in the presence of iodine deficiency or dyshormonogenesis may be goitrogenic. The most common cause of multinodular goiters outside of the United States is iodine deficiency. Hashimoto's thyroiditis impairs hormonogenesis and is responsible for a major portion of sporadic nontoxic goiters. In this case, the goiter may be the result of TBIgs, lymphocytic infiltration, and fibrosis. Further, inherited biochemical deficits in hormone synthesis are evident in selected populations.
2. The secretion of TSH may be abnormal when quantitative measurements are in a normal range. In other words, the assay may not be sensitive enough to pick up small differences in TSH secretion.
3. Changes in the vascularity of the gland, including possibly arteriovenous shunts, may increase the TSH levels in certain parts of the gland, resulting in areas of hyperplasia. Fibrosis may direct this hyperplasia in an asymmetric fashion, resulting in nodules.
4. Growth factors other than TSH are present. These factors may require the presence of TSH, such as epidermal growth factor (EGF) and insulin-like growth factor (IGF-I), or may be able to act independently of TSH, such as antibodies interacting with the TSH receptor.
5. Autonomous growth occurs in an adenomatous nodule, possibly related to mutations and oncogenes.

The evaluation of thyroid nodules involves in a large part the evaluation of the benign sporadic nontoxic goiter. Stated another way, "solitary nodules" often are not solitary. In a study of 207 patients with presumed solitary nodules on clinical examination, only 60% of the nodules were found to be solitary at surgery, and only 52% after histologic section.[21] Despite generally normal TSH levels in patients with thyroid nodules, it has been known for many years that the administration of suppressive doses of thyroid hormone decreases the size of many nontoxic goiters and nodules. Failure of the gland to shrink when given thyroid hormone may be related to the presence of fibrosis, colloid lakes, calcification, hemorrhage in degenerating nodules, and the duration of the goiter. However, well-differentiated thyroid carcinomas are also frequently TSH dependent and may decrease in size with suppressive doses of thyroid hormone.

Prevalence

The major problem confronting the clinician in managing patients with thyroid nodules is differentiating the myriad benign thyroid lesions from the few malignant ones. The incidence of new nodules in the United States is estimated to be 0.1% per year or 250,000. The malignancy rate is estimated to be approximately 8% to 17% in solitary nodules. Although many thyroid nodules appear single on clinical examination, in 50% of cases multiple nodules are found on ultrasound examination or at the time of surgery. Recent evidence suggests that nodules in multinodular goiters have a similar risk of malignancy as do solitary nodules.[47] However, the clinical significance of this finding is unclear, as up to 35% of thyroid glands removed at autopsy or surgically contain microcarcinomas (papillary cancers <1 cm) with a minimal impact on the patient's longevity or general health, and many of the nonpalpable thyroid nodules found on ultrasound probably fall into this category.[48-51]

The incidence of benign thyroid nodules increases with age, with a more than 4:1 predominance in women over men. The incidence of thyroid carcinoma may not change appreciably for different age groups; however, the decrease in the frequency of benign nodules in childhood and in the elderly raises substantially the percentage of nodules that are malignant in these age groups. There are approximately 12,000 new cases of thyroid cancer in the United States diagnosed each year, but deaths from thyroid carcinoma are rare, averaging about 1000 per year or 0.14% and 0.3% of all cancer deaths in U.S. men and women, respectively. Incidences of thyroid nodules and thyroid carcinoma may be on the increase and have been attributed to radiation-associated thyroid disease.[52] However, mortality from thyroid cancer has not changed, presumably because of earlier detection and improved treatment.

Table 59-1. Causes of Solitary Nonfunctional Thyroid Nodules

Type of Nodule	Note
Adenoma	Subtypes are macrofollicular (simple colloid), microfollicular (fetal), embryonal (trabecular), Hürthle cell (oxyphil, oncocytic) adenomas, atypical adenomas, adenomas with papillae, and signet-ring adenomas
Carcinoma	Subtypes are papillary (70%), follicular (15%), medullary (5-10%), and anaplastic carcinomas (5%) and thyroid lymphoma (5%)
Cyst	Simple cysts and other cystic thyroid lesions (see text) may present as thyroid cysts
Nodule of an unrecognized multinodular colloid goiter	Small multinodular colloid goiters may contain a dominant nodule that is clinically indistinguishable from a macronodular follicular adenoma
Other	Includes inflammatory thyroid diseases (subacute thyroiditis, chronic lymphocytic thyroiditis, granulomatous disease) and developmental abnormalities (unilateral lobe agenesis, cystic hygroma, dermoid, teratoma); all are very rare causes of solitary nodules

Adapted from Mazzaferri EL. Management of the solitary thyroid nodule. N Engl J Med 328:553, 1993.

Classification of Benign Thyroid Nodules (Table 59-1)

The most common benign thyroid nodule is the follicular adenoma. It is a well-encapsulated tumor that may comprise as many as 70% of benign thyroid nodules. It may be particularly difficult to differentiate a benign follicular adenoma from either a benign adenomatous nodule or a well-differentiated follicular carcinoma on the basis of either frozen section or fine-needle aspiration.[46,53,54] This is an important limitation of these techniques. Vascular or capsular invasion must be noted for the diagnosis of carcinoma, and it is necessary to take multiple sections of the periphery of the tumor to verify the diagnosis of follicular carcinoma. A solitary encapsulated cellular nodule is likely an adenoma, whereas the typical adenomatous nodule has abundant colloid present with a varied follicular pattern and poorly demarcated capsule. However, adenomas, adenomatous nodules, and carcinomas are subject to hemorrhage, fibrosis, necrosis, and cystic degeneration.[55] A cellular aspirate with minimal colloid is likely a follicular neoplasm and should be excised. The term *atypical adenomas* describes cellular nodules with many mitotic figures. Careful examination is required to distinguish these lesions from a carcinoma. Unfortunately, cytometric studies of nuclear ploidy and other measures of nuclear organization have not been helpful in distinguishing benign from malignant lesions preoperatively, and surgery is thus indicated.

Colloid nodules are responsible for approximately 7% of benign, solitary, cold nodules and are usually not a diagnostic problem either cytologically or histologically. Fine-needle aspiration usually yields benign scattered follicular cells and abundant colloid. These nodules may regress with thyroid hormone suppression.

Thyroid cysts are frequently the result of degeneration of a benign adenoma. In a recent retrospective study of 221 surgically resected thyroid nodules, 82% of cystic lesions were degenerating benign adenomas, 4% were simple cysts, and 14% were malignant, compared to 23% of solid lesions that were malignant.[55] A degenerating carcinoma can present as a mixed solid-cystic lesion but only rarely as a simple cyst. Simple cysts greater than 4 cm, however, do have an appreciable incidence of carcinoma. In one study, 81% of cysts contained bloody fluid on aspiration. Because of the decreased cellularity of cystic fluid, aspiration cytology of cysts has a lower sensitivity and specificity than aspiration of solid lesions (88% and 52% for cysts vs. 100% and 55% for solid lesions respectively). For this reason, cysts

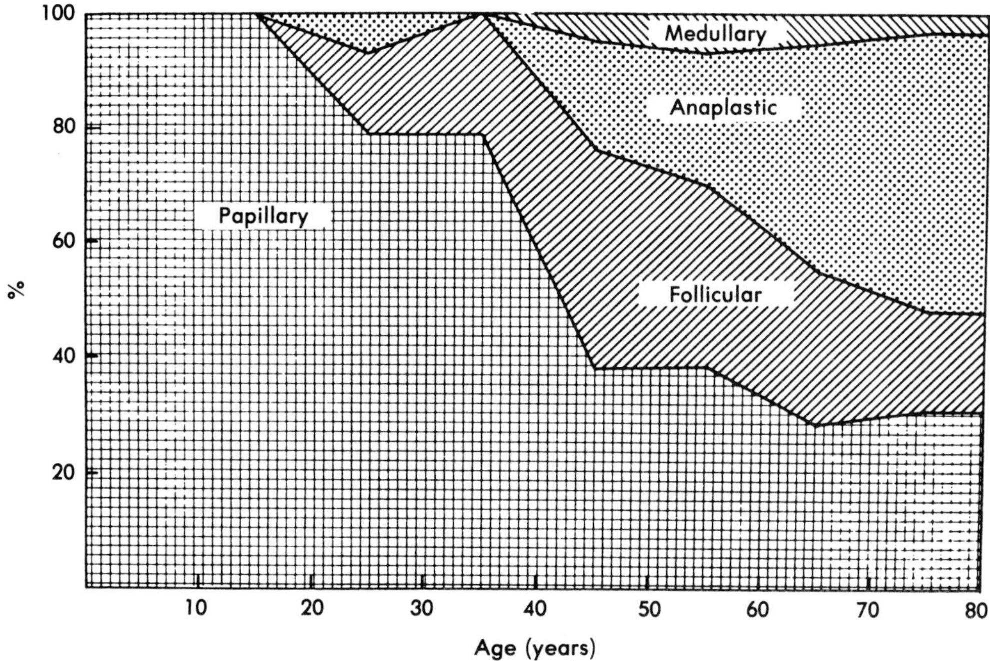

Fig. 59-14. Percentage distribution of 230 cases of thyroid carcinoma into histologic types, by age. (From Degroot LJ, ed. Radiation-associated thyroid carcinoma. New York: Grune & Stratton, 1977.)

that are not abolished by aspiration, should be considered for excision.

Localized areas of Hashimoto's thyroiditis can present as benign thyroid nodules that may be hypofunctioning. In a diffusely abnormal thyroid gland, Hashimoto's thyroiditis may coexist with a malignant lymphoma. A careful examination by the pathologist for lymphoma is therefore indicated. In addition, small cell carcinoma is occasionally confused with thyroiditis on cytology.

Malignant Nodules of the Thyroid Gland

Thyroid carcinomas have distinct differences in biologic behavior from benign nodules, and their malignant characteristics are greatly influenced by their histologic type. Rearrangements of *ret* proto-oncogenes have been described in carcinomas, but not in adenomas.[56] Papillary and follicular carcinomas are both of follicular epithelial origin and comprise the differentiated carcinomas of the thyroid. Greater than 50% of thyroid carcinomas are of the papillary type. Approximately 20% are believed to be follicular, but in fact many of these are papillary carcinomas with extensive follicular elements (so-called follicular variant of papillary carcinoma). Since their biologic activity is similar, papillary carcinomas and mixed follicular-papillary carcinomas are grouped together. These tumors are somewhat distinct from true follicular carcinomas in both histology (more varied in size and shape than in a follicular neoplasm) and biologic activity (follicular carcinomas may have an aggressive course with a substantially higher mortality). In addition to histology the following factors are important in prognosis: patient's age at diagnosis, size of the primary tumor, evidence of extension into the juxtathyroidal tissues, and evidence of metastasis. Genomic analysis will probably be important in the future. Although thyroid malignancies can sometimes arise in benign nodular goiters, there is no convincing evidence that benign nodules are precursors of malignant ones or that patients with benign goiters are at an increased risk of malignant transformation, except possibly in the rare case of an undifferentiated anaplastic carcinoma arising from a well-differentiated papillary carcinoma.[57]

Types of Carcinomas (Fig. 59-14)

Papillary carcinoma. Papillary carcinoma is the major thyroid cancer of children and young adults and generally has an excellent prognosis.[49,58-61] Of the approximately 10,000 new cases of thyroid cancer in the United States annually, close to 90% are papillary carcinoma. Since the 1940s, the 20-year mortality has remained fairly stable at 5%, rising to 6% to 7% after 25 to 30 years. Almost all patients with radiation-induced thyroid cancer are found to have the papillary type, and low level ionizing radiation is now known to be a strong risk factor for papillary carcinoma.[52,62] Rarely (approximately 3% of cases), families have been described with similar mutations in the *ret* proto-oncogene.[56] Certain rare conditions, such as Gardner's syndrome and Cowden disease (multiple hamartoma [epithelioma] syndrome), have an increased frequency of papillary carcinoma. The histologic pattern may be quite varied including solid lesions that may be predominantly papillary or follicular, fibrotic lesions, and rarely cystic lesions. Characteristics of papillary carcinoma include papillae formation, large crowded nuclei, and the presence of psammoma bodies. Generally, slow growth and lymph node involvement of the neck are typical of these cancers. Clinically, they present as solitary nodules, but careful histologic examination of resected thyroid specimens reveals a 30% to 85% incidence of microscopic multicentric spread through intraglandular lymphatics to other parts of the gland and associated lymph nodes. This is associated with a recurrence rate of 8% to 10% in the contralateral lobe if not resected.[63] Nodal spread may be detected in as many as 75% of patients if carefully looked for, and this is associated with a 10% clinical recurrence. Metastatic spread beyond the neck to lung and bone is uncommon. The rate of occult carcinoma (defined as <1 cm) may be as high as eight times the rate of clinical occurrence. A microscopic tumor can rarely have cervical lymph node metastases as the predominant clinical finding, initially misdiagnosed as lateral aberrant thyroid tissue.[64] Papillary carcinomas are more aggressive in patients older than 40, in whom death rates are substantially higher than in younger patients, and are frequently a result of recurrent local invasion. These more aggressive tumors are frequently associated with more mitotic figures, abnormal DNA content, loss of differentiation, and lack of dendritic cells.[64]

The hallmarks of papillary carcinoma can frequently be seen on fine-needle aspiration cytology. Because papillary carcinoma concentrates iodine poorly, it appears hypofunctioning or nonfunctioning on radioisotope scans when compared with the remaining uninvolved gland. After thyroidectomy, the ability of the tumor to concentrate miniscule amounts of ^{131}I can be detected on scans. Thus ^{131}I can be used both diagnostically and therapeutically for follow-up purposes.

Follicular carcinoma. Follicular carcinomas are encapsulated cellular tumors that spread hematogenously to the lung, bone, and liver. They occur more commonly in patients older than 40, and the prognosis correlates with the invasiveness of the tumor. Iodine deficiency may be a risk factor for follicular and anaplastic carcinomas. Minimally invasive cancers are those that invade only two or three small vessels or penetrate the capsule in one or two places on multiple histologic sections. These tumors rarely recur or metastasize. Clinically, follicular carcinoma may present as a solitary nodule, an enlarging nodule in a multinodular gland, or a pathologic bone fracture from a metastasis. Lymph node involvement is uncommon. Histologically the cells may vary from being indistinguishable from normal thyroid tissue to grossly abnormal within the same lesion. For this reason the diagnosis of follicular carcinoma is made on the basis of careful examination of the capsule and blood vessels for invasion. Fine-needle aspiration and frozen section are often inaccurate, and the patient should be aware that a second procedure completing the thyroidectomy may be indicated after the final pathology report is available.[53,54]

Follicular carcinoma can concentrate iodine reasonably well and rarely may synthesize thyroid hormones. Thyrotoxicosis, including T_3 toxicosis, can result from bulky functional metastases. In spite of a generally decreased capacity to concentrate iodine as compared with normal thyroid tissue, pulmonary metastases have been known to disappear on thyroid suppression alone, especially in younger patients who have more endocrinologically dependent tumors.[65,66]

Medullary thyroid carcinoma. Medullary thyroid carcinoma (MTC) is a rare neoplasm of the parafollicular cells (C cells) that readily invades the intraglandular lymphatics and the blood stream, spreading to the lungs, liver, and bone. MTC may appear as part of the syndrome of multiple endocrine neoplasia type 2, which is represented by a group of familial disorders of variable autosomal dominant penetrance. In these syndromes family members may have one or more of the following conditions: MTC, parathyroid hyperplasia, and pheochromocytomas, often bilateral. In addition, ganglioneuromas, mucosal neuromas, and a marfanoid habitus can be seen in the so-called "bumpy lips" syndrome. For a more extensive discussion of these syndromes, the reader is referred to Chapter 60.

Calcitonin is secreted from the C cells of the thyroid and is a sensitive marker for MTC.[67,68] Early detection and surgery of C cell hyperplasia in affected children of family members with these syndromes can be curative. Basal and stimulated calcitonin levels, after pentagastrin or calcium, should be performed yearly on suspected carriers, starting in childhood.[69,70] Total thyroidectomy with regional lymph node removal should be undertaken if the calcitonin levels are elevated. Hyperparathyroidism and pheochromocytoma should be ruled out biochemically before surgery. Because of the risk of hypertensive crises, pheochromocytomas (if present) should be removed before the thyroidectomy is performed. Recent advances in the molecular genetics of these familial syndromes have narrowed the abnormality in some cases to mutations in the *ret* proto-oncogene.[71] Further characterization of these and other genetic abnormalities should make genetic diagnosis simpler and avoid the need for long-term biochemical surveillance.

More commonly, medullary thyroid carcinoma appears sporadically (greater than 60% of the time) in patients older than 50. It can appear simply as a nodule or nodules, with or without nodal or distant disease, and occasionally as Cushing's syndrome or carcinoid syndrome, depending on the peptides that the tumor is able to secrete (i.e., ACTH, serotonin, vasoactive intestinal peptide, kinins, prostaglandins). Bilateral soft tissue calcifications of the neck, occasionally seen with this neoplasm, can sometimes be demonstrated on x-ray film. Even in apparent sporadic cases, however, genetic mutations have been found, and all family members should be screened for the condition.

Histologically, the tumor is not encapsulated, and the cells may be somewhat undifferentiated with abundant stromal amyloid. MTC is more malignant than the differentiated thyroid tumors and carries a higher morbidity and mortality (50%), especially in the older patient with nodal or distant disease. With fine-needle aspiration biopsy, this condition can occasionally be diagnosed before surgery, with special stains for amyloid. Elevated calcitonin and carcinoembryonic antigen levels confirm the diagnosis. These levels are excellent markers for recurrent disease after surgery. Since the tumor is not TSH dependent, thyroid suppressive therapy and radioiodine are not helpful in the control of growth of the tumor. To date, chemotherapy has shown only modest palliation. Aggressive early diagnosis and surgical management are the most effective therapy at this time.

Anaplastic carcinoma. Anaplastic carcinoma is a particularly lethal and rapidly growing cancer that affects predominantly the elderly. The tumor is usually well advanced at the time of diagnosis and is almost uniformly fatal within 2 years of diagnosis, in spite of aggressive therapy. Histologically, one can see a variety of spindle-shaped and bizarre cells that can be confused with small cell carcinomas. These cells do not concentrate iodine and are not responsive to TSH suppression. Anecdotal reports suggest that patients with long-standing, well-differentiated thyroid cancer can develop anaplastic carcinoma. It is unknown if ^{131}I therapy contributes to this transformation. Anaplastic carcinoma frequently appears in patients with a history of long-standing nodular goiter. The relationship of goiter, papillary carcinoma, ^{131}I therapy, and anaplastic transformation requires further investigation.[57] Currently, the frequency of this disease appears to be decreasing, possibly related to earlier detection and treatment of differentiated thyroid cancer. Fine-needle aspiration biopsy is frequently diagnostic. A multidisciplinary approach to therapy, including surgery, radiation, and chemotherapy has shown improved survival.

Rare tumors of the thyroid gland. Primary lymphoma of the thyroid gland is rare and frequently confused with other undifferentiated carcinomas. Hashimoto's thyroiditis frequently coexists with lymphoma. Improved experience with fine-needle aspiration cytology has increased the number of diagnoses being made preoperatively. The patient may have a solitary nodule or, more commonly, an enlarging diffusely abnormal gland. Radiation treatment and chemotherapy result in initial remission, but long-term survival is usually poor unless the tumor is still confined to the neck at the time of diagnosis.

Metastatic disease to the thyroid is not uncommon and may arise from primary tumors in the kidney, larynx, breast, esophagus, lung, and rectum. Fine-needle aspiration may be diagnostic and help avoid unnecessary surgery.

Prognostic Factors Related to Thyroid Cancer (see box)

The histologic type of tumor is the most important single prognostic factor in thyroid cancer. Well-differentiated tumors often have excellent 10- and 20-year survival curves, especially in the young, even in the face of widespread metastases (Fig. 59-15). Because of the slow progression of these cancers, it is necessary to follow many individuals for long periods of time to assess optimal methods of surveillance and timing of procedures. The long natural history precludes prospective clinical trials from being attempted, and based on retrospective studies from large referral areas, it is hard to determine the consequences of a therepeutic option in a patient in the community. In addition, many measures other than survival become important to patient care, such as the management of recurrences and the complication rate of different therapies. These issues lead directly to many controversies and contradictory recommendations regarding surgical and medical therapy for patients with differentiated thyroid cancer.

The biologic behavior of even well-differentiated thyroid cancers is difficult to predict. As noted, papillary thyroid cancer (including all its variants) is generally associated with an excellent prognosis, followed by "true" follicular carcinomas and the more lethal Hürthle cell tumors. However, albeit rarely, even papillary carcinomas can take a particularly aggressive course, killing the patient over a rela-

PROGNOSTIC FACTORS IN THYROID CARCINOMA

1. Histologic type
2. Age
3. Extent of primary tumor
4. Distant metastases
5. Size
6. Blood vessel invasion
7. Multiple foci
8. Sex
9. Lymph node metastases (?)

From Degroot LJ, et al. Radiation-Associated Thyroid Carcinoma. New York: Grune & Stratton, 1977.

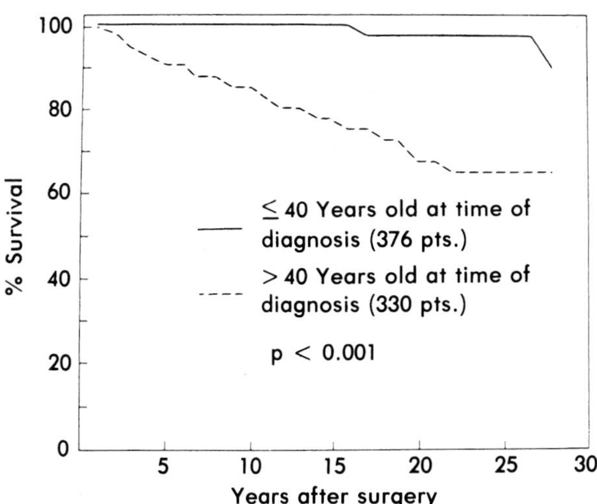

Fig. 59-15. Survival curves for patients diagnosed before (—) and after (- - - -) the age of 40 years. (From Samaan NA, et al. Impact of therapy for differentiated carcinoma of the thyroid: An analysis of 706 cases. J Clin Endocrinol Metab 56:1131, 1983.)

tively brief period of time. Newer molecular techniques, such as the polymerase chain reaction, have demonstrated that the progression from a slowly growing cancer with little tendency to metastasize to an aggressive invasive tumor is determined by the number of mutations that affect oncogenes such as *ret,* as well as mutations in the growth controlling gene p53.[56,57] Mutations are amplified with succeeding mitoses, and tumors that acquire changes in the p53 gene in addition to changes in certain oncogenes may suddenly exhibit an abrupt change in biologic behavior. It is hoped that a better understanding of the malignant potential of different tumors will allow a more rational approach to therapy rather than treating all differentiated tumors equally and unnecessarily exposing certain individuals to morbid complications. Until then, several referral centers have developed prognostic scores using multivariate analysis of their retrospective data. The more well-known indexes are AMES (including *a*ge at diagnosis >40 for men and >50 for women, presence of *m*etastases, *e*xtent of disease, and *s*ize of primary tumor); AGES (including *a*ge at diagnosis, histologic *g*rade of tumor, *e*xtent of disease, and *s*ize of primary tumor); Ohio State Tumor Stage (age at diagnosis, size of primary tumor, presence of nodal metastases, presence of invasion, and presence of distant metastases); and MACIS, an index developed by the Mayo Clinic including only information that should be readily available to the clinician (*m*etastases, *a*ge at diagnosis, *c*ompleteness of surgery in removing gross disease, extrathyroidal *i*nvasion, and *s*ize of primary tumor). Using any of these scoring systems, 85% to 90% of papillary carcinomas have low scores correlating with a low mortality.[48,50,51,58] Lacking in all these models, however, is any mention of treatment that the patient has previously received.

As can be seen from the above noted indexes, age at diagnosis has been shown to be an important prognostic factor for mortality in virtually all populations studied. Depending on the center, diagnosis after age 40 or 50 has a significantly higher risk of recurrence and death from disease. In fact, death from cancer is particularly unusual when the diagnosis is made before age 30, despite the fact that recurrence rates are highest in the young and the elderly. In children, even the presence of distant metastases is associated with a generally good prognosis. Goepfert et al.[66] followed 66 children for a period of 15 years at M. D. Anderson Cancer Center, and during that time there was only one death, despite the presence of nodal disease in 84% and pulmonary metastases in 12%. Schlumberger et al.[72] reported that 42% of 72 children developed distant metastases (primarily in the lungs) and still achieved a complete remission in 70%. Thus cancer mortality follows a J-shaped curve with respect to age, whereas recurrence rate follows a U-shaped curve (Fig. 59-16).

The role of gender in determining prognosis of differentiated thyroid cancer is controversial, and it is usually not included in most statistical models. Women are at an increased risk for developing all thyroid disease, including nodules and cancer. In some studies, however, men have a higher cancer specific mortality.[60]

Size of the primary lesion has important prognostic value (Fig. 59-17). Occult thyroid carcinomas, now called microcarcinomas, are defined as less than 1 cm, have virtually no adverse effect on longevity, and are commonly found at autopsy. Estimates range from 2% to 28%, depending on the study quoted.[46] Surprisingly, when carcinoma death rates are compared to the prevalence of occult carcinoma, there appears to be either no relationship or possibly even an inverse relationship. Mazzaferri and

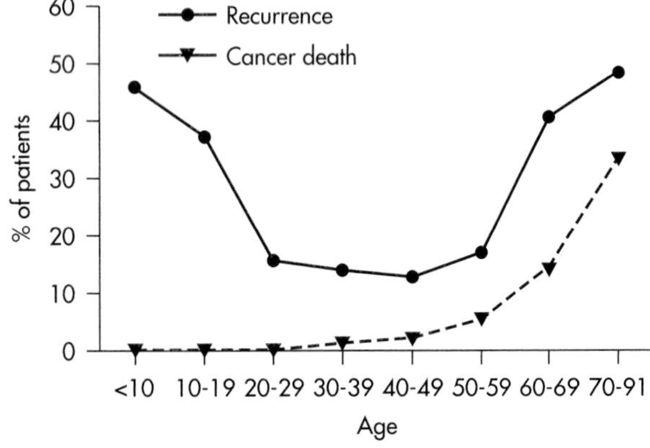

Fig. 59-16. Tumor recurrence and cancer-specific mortality as a function of age at diagnosis in 1133 patients with differentiated thyroid carcinoma. There were 215 recurrences and 45 cancer deaths in this group. Recurrence rates were significantly greater (P <0.0001) before age 20 and after age 60. Six patients between ages 21 and 39 died of cancer. (From Mazzaferri EL. Controversies in the management of differentiated thyroid carcinoma. Endocrine Society 42nd Annual Postgraduate Endocrine Assembly Syllabus 1990, p 167. Copyright The Endocrine Society.)

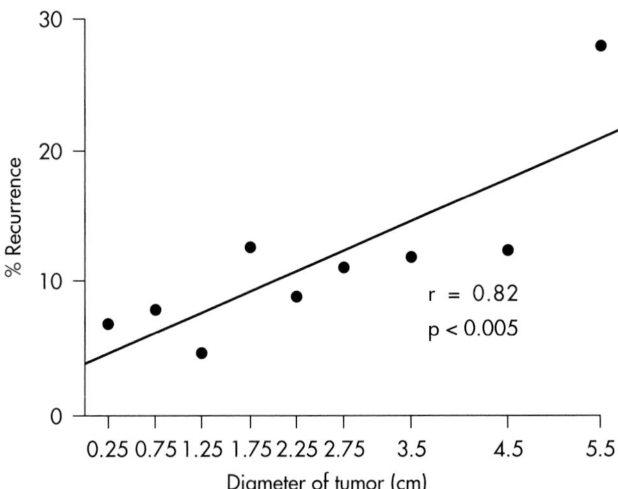

Fig. 59-17. The influence of primary tumor size on recurrence of papillary thyroid carcinoma. (From Mazzaferri EL, Jhiang SM. Long-term impact of initial surgical and medical therapy on papillary and follicular thyroid cancer. Am J Med 97(5):418, 1994.)

Jhiang[49] have noted no deaths from thyroid cancer and rare recurrences in patients followed 30 years after surgery for papillary carcinoma less than 1.5 cm in diameter. Occult carcinoma has an excellent prognosis, possibly because of host resistance, and a subtotal thyroidectomy appears to be adequate therapy. Mortality rates rise quickly, however, with primary lesions greater than 4.5 cm.

Mazzaferri and Jhiang[49] have ranked several prognostic variables in a Cox regression model associated with cancer-specific death (Table 59-2). In descending order they are age, time to treatment, local tumor invasion, lymph node metastases, tumor size, male sex, lack of radioiodine therapy, and surgery less than subtotal lobectomy. Although in past studies, no correlation was seen between lymph node metastases and mortality, these recent data appear to contradict this hypothesis, demonstrating an increased risk for recurrence in patients with nodal disease, and an increased risk for death in those with recurrence.[49] Radical neck dissection has no effect on mortality.[73]

Table 59-2. Significant Risk Factors for Well-Differentiated Thyroid Cancer Recurrence and Death (by Cox Regression Analysis)

Variable (n = 1322)	Hazard Ratio for Recurrence	Hazard Ratio for Cancer Related Death
Risk Factors		
Age (each decade)		2.4
Delay in surgery >1 yr		2.3
Local tumor invasion	1.7	2
Lymph node metastases	1.4	1.9
Tumor size (each cm)	1.3	1.3
Protective Factors		
Female		0.5
Radioiodine therapy	0.4	0.4
Surgery >lobectomy		0.4

From Mazzaferri EL, Jhiang SM. Long-term impact of initial surgical and medical therapy on papillary and follicular thyroid cancer. Am J Med 97(5):418, 1994.)

Patients with Graves' disease who have poorly functioning nodules are now known to have an increased risk for carcinoma in these nodules, and they may have a more aggressive course. Belfiore et al.[20] reported a 46% incidence of thyroid cancer in patients with palpable nodules and Graves' disease. Well-differentiated carcinomas and adenomas frequently have TSH receptors on their surface, and either TSH or, in the case of Graves' disease, TSIgs may interact with these receptors and stimulate tumor growth. Therefore a radionuclide scan of the thyroid gland should be performed before administering an ablative dose of radioiodine; if a poorly functioning nodule is detected, this nodule requires careful evaluation, and surgery should be considered as the primary treatment for the Graves' disease and nodule.

Approach to the Patient With a Thyroid Nodule History

Several important historical points must be examined to arrive at an assessment of the patient's risk for thyroid carcinoma (Table 59-3). As noted previously for prognosis, age and sex are important factors to consider in the evaluation of a thyroid nodule. A solitary nodule in a male younger than 20 has an increased frequency of carcinoma, approaching 50% in childhood. Likewise, a new nodule in a man older than 65 also has a risk of 50% of malignancy. Mortality, however, is more directly associated with age older than 40 at the time of diagnosis.

One of the most important areas to explore with the patient is the possibility of exposure to low-level ionizing radiation, especially during early childhood.[52,62,74,75] It has

Table 59-3. Relation Between Clinical Findings and Malignant Thyroid Tumors in 169 Patients With Nodular Thyroid Disease*

Suspected Likelihood of Cancer	% of Patients	% With Malignant Tumor†	Clinical Findings
Low	44	11	No suspicious symptoms or signs
Moderate	38	14	Age <20 or >60 yr
			History of head or neck irradiation
			Male sex
			Dubious nodule fixation
			Nodule >4 cm in diameter and partially cystic
High	18‡	71	Rapid tumor growth
			Very firm nodule
			Fixation to adjacent structures
			Vocal cord paralysis
			Enlarged regional lymph nodes

From Mazzaferri EL. Management of the solitary thyroid nodule. N Engl J Med 328:553, 1993.

*Eighty-six percent of patients had one solitary or a dominant thyroid nodule.

†As determined by fine-needle aspiration biopsy.

‡Two or more highly suspicious symptoms or signs, such as rapid tumor growth, were present in nine patients, all of whom had cancer.

been estimated that radiation exposure in the 200 to 500 rad range (2 to 5 Gy) is associated with the development of new nodules, benign and malignant, at a rate of about 2% per year with a peak incidence at 15 to 25 years after exposure but without a clear tailing off of the curve. Radiation therapy was frequently performed during the 1950s for "thymus enlargement," "adenoid enlargement," tinea capitis, other benign conditions during infancy, and acne during adolescence. Radiation administration to animals increases the incidence of thyroid cancer, especially if there is a physiologic stimulus to TSH (e.g., iodine deficiency, thiourea administration, exogenous TSH administration). T_4 administration to animals before exposure to radiation results in a marked reduction of thyroid tumors. It remains unclear whether these data can be extrapolated to man.[40,41] Nonetheless, radiation appears to increase the incidence of both benign and malignant thyroid nodules in man. In an autopsy study performed in Japan after the atomic bomb explosion, there was an increased incidence of occult thyroid carcinoma (28%) but no increase in mortality. In multiple studies of patients who received head and neck irradiation during childhood, approximately 30% of the nodules were found to be carcinomatous vs. 15% to 20% of patients without a history of irradiation.[52] Latency from the time of irradiation to the development of carcinoma may be anywhere from 5 to more than 40 years. However, hypotheses regarding latency have recently been challenged by the remarkably high reported rate of thyroid cancers appearing only a few years after the nuclear accident at Chernobyl in the former Soviet Union. It is possible that the population may have been exposed to previous radiation leaks that had not been detected. Intense surveillance regarding this problem is now being conducted in the entire region affected by this accident and will likely yield new information in the coming years. Radiation greater than 2000 rad causes necrosis rather than carcinogenesis. The lowest amount of ^{131}I used to treat Graves' disease delivers greater than 2000 rad to the thyroid gland and has not been associated with an increased incidence of thyroid carcinoma.[76]

In spite of the laboratory and clinical evidence noted above for radiation-associated thyroid disease, it is important to point out the following:

1. A threshold for radiation-associated thyroid carcinoma has not been defined; nor does there appear to be a delineated latency period. Fifty rad may be sufficient to increase the risk, and the risk may last more than 50 years. Many individuals are unaware of exposure because it was performed during infancy. A useful technique is to ask the patient to query their parents. Records may be available if the treatment was performed in a hospital, but controls on radiation exposure were often lacking if the treatment was given in a private clinic or doctor's office. Patients who received a higher radiation dose at a younger age (i.e., infants with thymic irradiation in a hospital setting) are at a higher risk of benign and malignant nodules than patients who received a lower dose at an older age (i.e., teenagers treated for acne).
2. More than 95% of the tumors that have been noted after radiation exposure are well-differentiated papillary carcinomas that act biologically similar to nonirradiated papillary carcinomas. The vast majority of these tumors are less than 1 cm and would be considered occult carcinomas with no increase in mortality.

What action should be taken for a patient who has normal results from thyroid examination and a history of irradiation as a child? The conservative approach of yearly thyroid palpations by an experienced physician has gained widespread acceptance. Routine radioisotope scans deliver small doses of radiation to the thyroid, and the results may be misleading. The administration of suppressive doses of T_4 would theoretically decrease the risk of benign or malignant thyroid nodules; however, several cases of radiation-associated thyroid carcinoma have been detected during suppressive T_4 treatment.[52] In a study of patients with a history of previous radiation exposure who had subtotal thyroidectomies for benign nodules, patients were randomized to either receiving levothyroxine suppression or placebo. The group receiving thyroid hormone had fewer new benign nodules than the placebo group, but the number of new malignant lesions was similar in both groups. Therefore thyroid hormone may protect against the development of benign nodules but apparently not against malignant ones. Still, there is significant psychologic and physical trauma to the patient in having a second thyroid operation, even if the result is benign, and it is worthwhile avoiding the second surgery if possible. This is the rationale for thyroid hormone suppression in patients after partial thyroidectomy for benign disease. In addition, the occurrence of a new nodule in a patient already receiving suppressive doses of levothyroxine would hasten the decision process to proceed to surgery.

Very few other historical facts are helpful in distinguishing benign from malignant disease. A history of sudden pain in the nodule may result from a hemorrhage into a cyst and may be responsible for a sudden increase in the size of the nodule. Symptoms such as Horner's syndrome, hoarseness, or other signs of airway obstruction are worrisome, although objective signs of obstruction can also be caused by benign lesions. Evidence that the patient may have been iodine deficient would increase the incidence of both benign and malignant thyroid disease. A family history of medullary thyroid carcinoma necessitates a plan of action that would include a biochemical screening of the family, with basal and stimulated calcitonin levels, and a total thyroidectomy if the calcitonin levels were abnormal.

Evaluation of a Thyroid Nodule

Examination of the thyroid nodule. Inspection of the thyroid gland during swallowing allows the contour of the gland, its approximate size, and the presence of one or more nodules to be seen. The patient should be positioned to take advantage of the light with the head tilted slightly backward. After observing the movement of the thyroid gland during swallowing, step behind the patient and, with the patient's neck slightly flexed, palpate with both hands for the cricoid cartilage. The isthmus of the thyroid should be found directly beneath the cricoid cartilage. Deep palpation of the gland from a posterior direction while the patient is swallowing some water allows assessment of the firmness and size of the nodule(s) and gland. If the nodule does not rise on swallowing, it may not be of thyroid origin. Thyroglossal duct cysts are generally midline, may be found anywhere from the base of the tongue to the thyroid isthmus, and generally rise with protrusion of the tongue. If a nodule is palpated, anterior palpation should be performed by pushing the thyroid to the left side with the thumb and palpating the right lobe with the other hand while the patient is swallowing. The procedure is then reversed. Particular attention should be paid to examination of the lymph nodes (i.e., to their size, consistency, and mobility). Any tracheal deviation should be noted. Evidence of recurrent laryngeal nerve compression, Horner's syndrome, fixation to surrounding tissues, or growth in the nodule while receiving T_4 suppression raises the concern for a malignancy. Few of the so-called classic signs of malignancy such as hardness of the nodule, its size, recent growth patterns, and associated airway obstructive symptoms are in fact pathognomonic of malignancy, and virtually all nodules would benefit from some evaluation prior to planning surgery. Benign multinodular goiters may present with symptoms of obstruction, and calcification in benign adenomas is not rare. Certain clinical situations may alert the examiner to the probable diagnosis; severe hypertension in a patient with a thyroid nodule may be part of the multiple endocrine neoplasia type 2 syndrome with pheochromocytoma, a new mass in a patient with confirmed Hashimoto's thyroiditis may be a lymphoma, a new mass in a patient with known nonthyroidal malignancy may be a metastases, sudden growth in a patient with long-standing multinodular goiter may be an anaplastic carcinoma, and an "overnight" appearance of a nodule with pain and tenderness is likely a hemorrhage into an adenoma.

After the thyroid nodule has been evaluated, the remainder of the examination should be directed toward the thyroid gland as a whole. A dominant nodule in an otherwise barely palpable or nonpalpable thyroid gland suggests a hyperfunctioning thyroid nodule and would greatly decrease the incidence of malignancy. A radioisotope scan would be helpful; if a hyperfunctioning nodule is found, an evaluation for hyperthyroidism should be initiated. A suppressed TSH or an elevated T_3RIA level would confirm the thyrotoxic state. Occasionally, there may be hemiagenesis of the thyroid gland, and the "palpable nodule" may be the only functioning thyroid tissue. The palpation of other smaller nodules in the gland with a dominant nodule does not necessarily reduce the possibility of malignancy, and each nodule should be evaluated separately.[47]

Estimation of gland or nodule size is difficult and frequently inaccurate by physical examination, especially in individuals with shorter thicker necks or in cases where some of the thyroid gland is located below the suprasternal notch (more common in older men). For accurate measurement of gland or nodule size, ultrasound should be used. Nevertheless, it is worthwhile attempting at least an estimate so that changes in size may be recognized. There are two conventional methods to measure thyroid gland size; estimating the number of grams, with the normal gland being 15 to 20 g, or estimating the number of times normal size the gland is. For example, a gland that can be seen only on close observation while the patient is swallowing is likely slightly enlarged and could be alternatively described as 25 to 30 g or 1½ times normal size. A gland that can be seen without swallowing from a distance of 3 to 4 feet might be 40 to 50 g or 2 to 2½ times enlarged. A gland that can be seen from across a room may be in excess of 60 g or more than three times enlarged. Estimating size may be useful for calculating radioiodine dose in a patient with Graves' disease (i.e., to deliver 150 μCi radioiodine per gram of thyroid tissue to a patient with a 50% radioactive iodine uptake and a 50 g gland, would require a treatment dose of 15 mCi ^{131}I). Occasionally, massive goiters, especially with a substernal component, can cause compression symptoms such as dysphagia, distention of neck veins, facial plethora, and rarely stridor with tracheal obstruction. These symptoms can be exaggerated by asking the patient to raise the hands above the head (Pemberton's sign).

Nodule size can be measured in two dimensions with a caliper or tape measure while fixating the nodule in the contralateral hand. Alternative methods include placing tape over the contour of the nodule and then putting the tape in the chart or tracing the outline of the nodule onto paper and putting the paper in the chart. Ultrasonographic measurement may still be worthwhile, but probably not more often than every 6 to 12 months.

Biochemical evaluation of thyroid nodules. A thyroid profile consisting of a blood T_4 level, an assessment of T_4-binding capacity, such as a T_3RU, and a sensitive TSH level should be performed on all patients with nodules to assure that they are euthyroid. Laboratory values consistent with either hypothyroidism or hyperthyroidism would require correction of the metabolic state of the patient prior to completing evaluation of the nodule. Massive infiltration by an undifferentiated carcinoma may cause enough destruction of the thyroid gland to precipitate hypothyroidism, but this is rare. Just as thyroid nodules that grow while the patient is receiving thyroid hormone are more likely to be malignant, hypofunctioning nodules found in hyperthyroid patients with Graves' disease also are more likely to be malignant with a frequency of up to 50%.[21]

Calcitonin is an exquisitely sensitive biochemical marker in the blood for MTC.[68] Early diagnosis of MTC may be made by stimulating calcitonin secretion with intravenous pentagastrin. These studies are routinely performed in children of families with a history of multiple endocrine neoplasia syndromes or medullary thyroid carcinoma. Calcitonin and carcinoembryonic antigen levels are also useful for early diagnosis of recurrence after surgery for MTC. The relative rarity of this histologic type of carcinoma makes routine screening of patients with thyroid nodules without a family history not cost effective.

Thyroglobulin is a large glycoprotein that is the principal iodoprotein of the thyroid gland. Sensitive RIAs have been able to detect elevated serum thyroglobulin levels in a variety of thyroid diseases. Unfortunately, the levels of this globulin are similarly elevated in benign and malignant diseases, making measurement of this protein not a useful diagnostic tool. However, the measurement of thyroglobulin levels as a marker for recurrent thyroid carcinoma is an important management tool (see the following).[77]

Thyroid imaging. Multiple techniques for imaging the thyroid gland have been used in the past in an attempt to differentiate normal from abnormal thyroid tissue. The limit of resolution of these techniques is approximately 1 to 1.5 cm. It is important to obtain lateral or oblique views, since small nonfunctioning nodules may be obscured by overlying functioning tissue. The most commonly used radioisotope is ^{123}I. Technetium-pertechnetate is no longer commonly used, since it is trapped in the thyroid gland, like iodine, but is not organified and therefore cannot be used to measure uptake. The major advantages of ^{123}I compared with ^{131}I are its short half-life (6 hours) and the relatively low amount of radiation delivered to the thyroid gland. The disadvantages of ^{123}I are its expense and short shelf life.

The functional status of thyroid nodules judged by imaging techniques is only marginally helpful in making a clinical decision about the malignant potential of a given thyroid nodule. Of approximately 5300 patients included in 22 different studies, 85% of the nodules were nonfunctioning or "cold" by radioiodine scan, and an additional 10% were "warm."[46,78,79] Sixteen percent of the cold nodules and 9% of the warm nodules were found to be malignant at operation, in contrast to hyperfunctioning or "hot" nodules which were rarely malignant. Therefore, on the basis of thyroid imaging alone, between 85% and 95% of patients with thyroid nodules would have been recommended for surgery.

Ultrasound examination of the thyroid gland. Ultrasound examination of the thyroid gland is used to distinguish between solid and cystic lesions. The incidence of malignancy is believed to be markedly decreased in simple cysts. In a total of 16 different studies, approximately 1200 patients had ultrasonographic examination before surgery. Approximately 70% of patients had solid lesions on ultrasound, and an additional 12% had mixed solid-cystic lesions. Twenty-one percent of the solid lesions and 12% of the mixed lesions were found to be carcinomatous at operation. In contrast, only cystic lesions greater than 4 cm in diameter had a significant incidence of carcinoma.

Thyroid suppression therapy. In spite of the fact that thyroid suppressive therapy has been available for many years, its usefulness in differentiating benign from malignant nodules remains controversial.[46,54,80] Benign thyroid adenomas and well-differentiated thyroid cancers have TSH receptors, and hypofunctioning nodules can be reduced in size by thyroid suppressive therapy (doses sufficient to reduce the sensitive TSH level below 0.4 μU/ml, generally 0.15 to 0.2 mg levothyroxine). Unfortunately, many benign lesions continue to grow or do not decrease in size after administration of large doses of thyroid suppressive therapy. Occasionally, a low-grade thyroid carcinoma may decrease in size for a period of time following suppressive therapy. Several placebo-controlled randomized trials of cytologically proven benign thyroid nodules have failed to show any substantial effect of levothyroxine therapy.[80] In spite of these drawbacks a short trial (3 to 6 months) of thyroid suppressive therapy continues to be commonly used according to the following rationale: (1) A nodule that resolves after thyroid suppressive medication is very unlikely to be a carcinoma (this can be monitored by ultrasound examination); (2) well-differentiated tumors are slow growing, and a 3- to 6-month period of observation, preferably after a benign or probably benign result from fine-needle aspiration, is unlikely to be placing the patient at undue risk; and (3) it is the only medical therapy available and induces the patient to come back for scheduled appointments to continue observation. Although largely supplanted by fine-needle aspiration, thyroid suppressive therapy remains a useful therapeutic adjunct. Doses of levothyroxine that are sufficient to suppress the TSH level below normal should be used for only brief periods of time to avoid any risk of osteoporosis.

Fine-needle aspiration of the thyroid gland. Diagnostic thyroid gland puncture has been attempted since the early 1920s. Several investigators used 16- and 18-gauge needles in an attempt to make a diagnosis of thyroid disease from direct visualization of thyroid tissue. Because of complications, primarily bleeding, with such large needles, thyroid puncture as a standard technique failed to enjoy any substantial popularity. In 1952 the technique of fine-needle aspiration and cytologic evaluation was first described. Although initially received with mixed favor, this technique is now routinely used in the United States and has made a major impact on the management of thyroid nodules.

In experienced hands fine-needle aspiration is a simple technique without significant morbidity and with a high diagnostic yield[46,54,78,79] (Fig. 59-18). An experienced aspirator and, more importantly, an experienced and interested cytopathologist are critical ingredients in obtaining diagnostic specimens. Experienced cytopathologists are now able to differentiate many benign and malignant lesions,

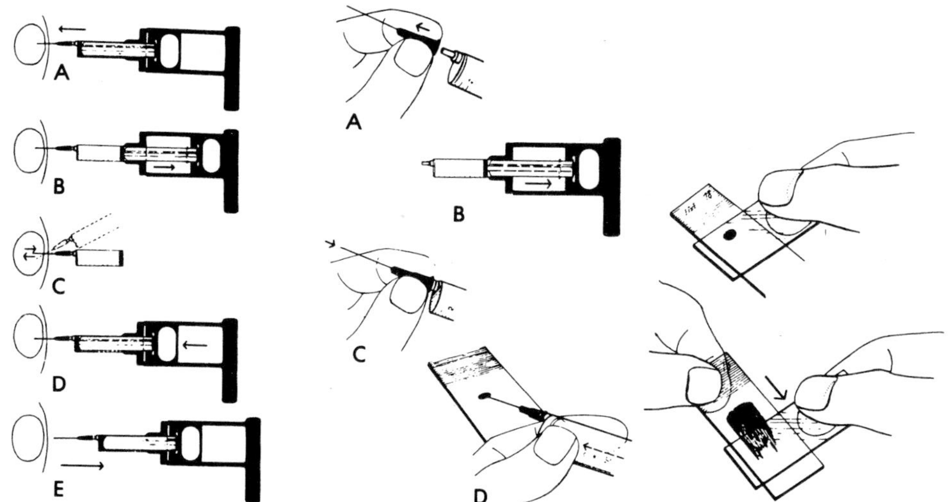

Fig. 59-18. Illustrations of technique for fine-needle aspiration biopsy of the thyroid. (From Lowhagen T, et al. Aspiration biopsy cytology in nodules of the thyroid gland suspected to be malignant. Surg Clin North Am 59:1, 1979.)

and the number of false negatives has decreased sharply in relation to the number of aspiration procedures being performed.

Needle biopsy of the thyroid gland has been divided into fine-needle aspiration using needle gauges between 20 and 25, large-needle biopsy using 16- and 18-gauge needles, and core needle biopsies using either a Vim-Silverman or a Trucut needle. The accuracy of the three techniques is virtually identical, and fine-needle aspiration is more available, easier, and has fewer complications than the other two techniques. Complementary information may be obtained from all three techniques.

The most popular techniques include placing the patient supine with a support under the shoulders to extend the neck, cleansing the area, and without use of local anesthesia, inserting a needle into multiple sites of the nodule and aspirating cells and/or fluid into the barrel of the needle. A simple hospital butterfly needle connected to a syringe and aspirated by an assistant allows the physician to use one hand to fixate the nodule and the other hand to maneuver the needle. Attaching a needle-topped syringe to an aspiration gun or simply placing a bare needle into the nodule without aspiration are other techniques that are used. Slides are then prepared for air drying or staining with Papanicolaou, Wright, and other stains. If needed, the specimen can be sent for more sophisticated studies of tumor markers (i.e., calcitonin). As sampling errors are an important source of false negative reports, it is important to do multiple sites, especially in larger lesions (>4 cm) and use ultrasonographic guidance if necessary. Hamburger[54] recommends viewing at least six clusters of benign cells on each of at least 2 slides from separate aspirates before declaring the lesion benign. Most false negative diagnoses are related to insufficient material for cytologic diagnosis. Complications are extremely rare and include minor hematomas, possible infection, and transient pain. Spread of tumor by performance of needle biopsy is extremely unusual. If the nodule is fluid filled, it may be aspirated virtually completely and centrifuged for cytologic evaluation. A clear, watery fluid may be indicative of a parathyroid cyst and should be sent for parathormone levels. Bloody aspirates may be indicative of degenerating thyroid adenomas or carcinomas, and a biopsy specimen from the advancing edge of the lesion may be more helpful in this circumstance. A brown fluid is usually indicative of a previous hemorrhage in the nodule. Centrifugation of the fluid may yield some follicular cells, but commonly cystic fluid has rare diagnostic elements. A fine-needle aspiration biopsy should be performed on the remnant after the cyst is evacuated. Attention must be paid to making the slide relatively thin and as bloodless as possible. If possible, a cytologist may help the aspirator make the slides and quickly review them to ensure a satisfactory specimen. If these details are followed, the patient may avoid having to return for a second aspiration, and a preliminary diagnosis at the time of aspiration generally results.

Approximately 85% of thyroid nodules aspirated by an experienced person yield adequate material for analysis by the cytopathologist. Of these, 75% are generally found to have scattered benign follicular cells, abundant colloid, occasional macrophages, and inflammatory cells and are interpreted as benign (normal thyroid, colloid nodules, hyperplastic nodules, cysts). Approximately 5% have unequivocal malignant features of papillary carcinoma, medullary carcinoma, lymphoma, and rarely undifferentiated or metastatic tumor. The remaining 20% are declared indeterminate or suspicious and include cellular aspirates with scant colloid, possibly with cellular atypia, and include primarily follicular or Hürthle cell neoplasms (benign and malignant).

The sensitivity and specificity of fine-needle aspiration are highly dependent on the experience of the individuals involved. In a recent review of 18,000 aspirations, sensitivity varied from 65% to 98% (mean 83%), and specificity varied from 72% to 100% (mean 92%). The overall accuracy of diagnosis approached 95%, with 17% of patients referred for surgery and 32% of nodules found to be malignant. False negative rates are reported from 1% to 11% (mean 5%), and false positive rates are reported from 0% to 10% (mean 3%).[78]

As fine-needle aspiration is not a true histologic biopsy, there are inherent limitations of this technique.[54] A substantial proportion of nodules are benign adenomas and are labeled as indeterminate or suspicious on aspiration because of the inability to discern capsular or vascular invasion. Even analysis of nuclear morphologic findings or DNA content have not been helpful in reliably distinguishing benign from malignant. This is not surprising, as it is sometimes difficult to make a clear diagnosis even on a surgical specimen. Another portion of patients has cystic or hemorrhagic nodules that are labeled unsatisfactory because of the limited cellular material in cystic fluid. On the other hand, aspiration has proven quite accurate in diagnosing papillary carcinoma, the most common thyroid cancer. Several economic analyses of the various approaches in the evaluation of a thyroid nodule have concluded that the most cost-effective approach is initial fine-needle aspiration, as it is comparably priced with radionuclide or ultrasound studies and provides more useful information.[46] At the Mayo Clinic, the use of this technique has shown a 25% reduction in cost per patient with a 25% reduction in surgery performed for benign nodules and an increase in the percent of thyroid carcinoma found at surgery rising from 14% to 39%.[78]

The limitations of fine-needle aspiration (and frozen section at surgery) must be discussed with the patient before the procedure and before any planned surgery. Most, if not all, of the patients with aspirates in the indeterminate group should be referred to surgery. However, planning the surgical procedure for these patients can be problematic with more than one general approach available for use. One approach is to explore and palpate the entire thyroid gland. If no other nodules are apparent and the frozen section does not reveal any malignancy, perform a lobectomy and await final pathology. In the event that a cancer is found after careful pathologic examination, a second procedure is performed, completing the thyroidectomy. In the other approach at least a subtotal thyroidectomy is performed such that a second operation should not be necessary even if the lesion was malignant. The particular approach to the individual patient depends on the risk of complications from the surgical procedures vs. the perceived risk of malignancy and potential morbidity from malignancy if found in that patient, based on the prognostic factors noted above. However, in experienced hands, completion of the thyroidectomy can be accomplished with minimal morbidity.[54,63,81,82]

Summary of Preoperative Approach to the Thyroid Nodule

Physiologically, a diseased portion of the thyroid gland has disturbed function when compared to normal tissue. Radioisotope imaging techniques attempt to take advantage of this functional difference. Unfortunately, many benign disorders of the thyroid gland interfere with effective iodine uptake; conversely, well-differentiated follicular carcinoma may have near-normal function. Thus the attempt to diagnose thyroid disease on the basis of functional status (e.g., technetium trapping, radioiodine organification) has not been successful. In spite of advances in ultrasonography, the impact of this modality on the management of thyroid nodules has not been substantive. Fine-needle aspiration biopsy of the thyroid is a technically simple, cost-effective procedure, which, although not ideal, offers a higher sensitivity and specificity diagnostically than other available studies, short of surgical exploration.

On the basis of these considerations, after clinical evaluation of the patient a fine-needle aspiration should be the initial study (Fig. 59-19). If an adequate sample showing benign cytology is obtained, the patient can either be observed or can receive thyroid suppressive therapy (levothyroxine 0.15 to 0.2 mg daily). During suppressive therapy the patient should be followed for any change in the nodule by ultrasound examinations every 6 to 12 months. Shrinkage of the nodule by more than 50% is reassuring. No change or increase in nodule size on T_4 sup-

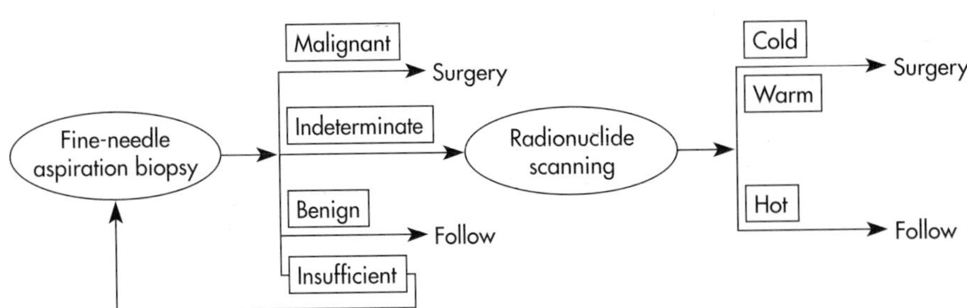

Fig. 59-19. Sequence for the evaluation of patients with a thyroid nodule. The results of radionuclide scanning are expressed as "hot," "warm," or "cold" to indicate the function of the nodule in relation to the normal thyroid tissue in the patient. (From Mazzaferri EL. Management of the solitary thyroid nodule. N Engl J Med 328:553, 1993. Copyright © 1993 Massachusetts Medical Society. All rights reserved.)

pression should prompt a second biopsy or surgical intervention within 6 to 12 months. If a cellular aspirate is obtained suggestive of a follicular neoplasm (suspicious or indeterminate category), a radioisotope scan may help in differentiating the hyperfunctioning adenoma that has a negligible malignancy rate from the hypofunctioning cellular nodule that requires surgical excision. This sequence has been found to be more cost effective than performing the scan on all patients with nodules, as more than 85% are found to have a poorly functioning nodule and require fine-needle aspiration. Young children with thyroid nodules have a high risk for malignancy; if they are unable to cooperate with fine-needle aspiration, it would be reasonable to proceed with imaging studies to determine function of the nodule prior to surgery.

In the case of thyroid cysts, the cyst should be drained as completely as possible with a larger needle (18 to 20 gauge). A fine-needle aspiration biopsy specimen of the remaining remnant should then be sent for cytologic examination. Recurrent cysts may require surgery. Thyroid suppressive therapy can be tried for benign cytology, but the success rate is low. Injection of cysts with sclerosing agents or alcohol has been advocated by some workers, but it has the potential of causing significant local damage and complicating any future surgery.

Surgical Treatment of Suspicious Thyroid Nodules

The extent of surgery required to cure thyroid cancer is unknown and is therefore a subject of constant debate among authorities in this field. Cancer is frequently found in the contralateral lobe; 78% of patients with papillary carcinoma, medullary carcinoma, and Hürthle cell carcinoma but only 12% of patients with follicular carcinoma have evidence of disease in both lobes. Thus total thyroidectomy would prevent recurrence in the contralateral lobe, lower the recurrence rate, improve the sensitivity of serum thyroglobulin as a marker of persistent or recurrent disease, allow use of radioiodine to detect and treat persistent or recurrent disease, and allow the highest survival rates (see accompanying box and Fig. 59-20). However, the possible advantages of total thyroidectomy must be balanced by the risks of hypoparathyroidism and laryngeal nerve damage.[81,83-87] As surgical expertise may vary significantly from center to center, treatment should be based on knowledge of the biologic behavior of the tumor. For this reason a minimal operation for a benign lesion would include a lobectomy, whereas a small (<1.5 cm) malignant lesion of well-differentiated carcinoma should include an isthmectomy and partial contralateral lobectomy, and a more aggressive or larger cancer should be treated with near-total or total thyroidectomy. Neither fine-needle aspiration nor frozen section can adequately differentiate follicular adenoma from follicular carcinoma, and both are reported as follicular neoplasms or cellular aspirates. In this difficult, but common group, it would be reasonable in a low-risk patient to perform a lobectomy initially and inform the patient that a more complete operation may be required after a final histologic diagnosis is made. A more complete thyroidectomy would be indicated for a patient at a higher risk (by AMES, AGES, or other criteria). Near-total thyroidectomy with the posterior capsule of the contralateral lobe left intact, associated with radioiodine ablation of the thyroid remnant (Fig. 59-21), is recommended

ADVANTAGES OF TOTAL THYROIDECTOMY

Improved survival for primary lesions >1.5 cm
Lower recurrence rate
Prevention of recurrence in contralateral lobe
Improved sensitivity of serum thyroglobulin as marker of persistent or recurrent disease
^{131}I can be used to detect and treat persistent or recurrent disease

Adapted from Clark OH, et al. Thyroid cancer: The case for total thyroidectomy. Euro Cancer Clin Oncol 24:305, 1988.

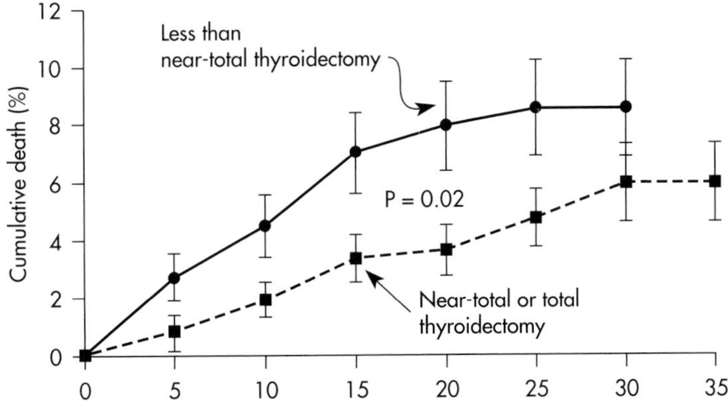

Fig. 59-20. Impact of total or near-total thyroidectomy on cancer death. (Mazzaferri EL, Jhiang SM. Long-term impact of initial surgical and medical therapy on papillary and follicular thyroid cancer. Am J Med 97(5):418, 1994.)

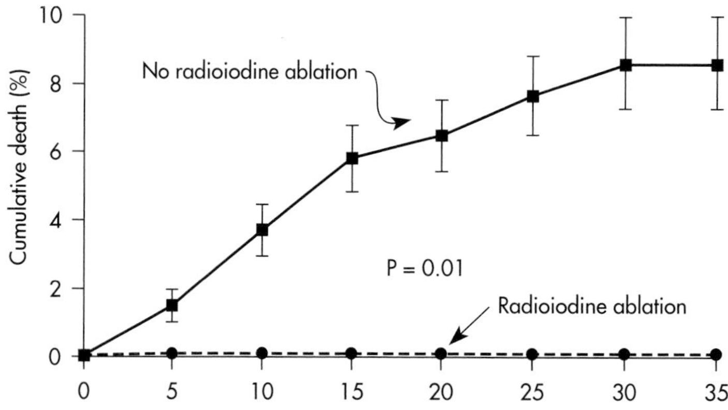

Fig. 59-21. Impact of thyroid remnant ablation after total or near-total thyroidectomy on cancer death. (From Mazzaferri EL, Jhiang SM. Long-term impact of initial surgical and medical therapy on papillary and follicular thyroid cancer. Am J Med 97(5):418, 1994.)

in patients believed to be at high risk for recurrence of thyroid cancer according to the prognostic factors discussed previously. Lymph node dissections are indicated in the central neck ipsilateral to the nodule and when there is palpable disease in the lateral neck. Still, it is thought that radical neck dissection is usually not indicated and only involved nodal tissue should be removed unless there is evidence of tumor invasion or adherence to structures. The current practice of autotransplantation of the parathyroid glands has dramatically decreased the incidence of permanent hypoparathyroidism.

Occult papillary carcinoma is occasionally found incidentally in another area of the surgical specimen after an operation for a benign lesion. Given the low mortality of carcinomas less than 1 cm, a subtotal thyroidectomy is usually adequate. In a review of second operations performed to complete an initial partial thyroidectomy for differentiated cancer, additional foci of cancer was found in 50% of patients with a previous partial lobectomy, 33% in patients with previous lobectomy, and in none of the patients who had a subtotal thyroidectomy.[81]

Head and neck irradiation during childhood increases the risk of multicentric tumors. A physiologic approach to this circumstance would include removal of all thyroid tissue to prevent recurrence. Thus near-total thyroidectomy is an appropriate operation for a lesion in a previously irradiated thyroid.

Patients with benign nodules found at surgery should be placed on lifelong thyroid hormone to suppress any new nodular growth, although this is more effective in suppressing benign than malignant lesions. The dose of levothyroxine should be monitored to maintain a TSH level in the low normal range to avoid osteoporosis and atrial fibrillation.

Follicular carcinoma spreads hematogenously to the lungs, bone, and liver, and the prognosis is proportional to the degree of invasion. Since follicular carcinoma is not multifocal, the rationale for complete thyroidectomy is predicated on preparing the patient for radioiodine therapy to ablate any remaining thyroid tissue. This allows easier detection of recurrent disease and metastases. A wide excision of thyroid tissue decreases the necessary dose of radioiodine and allows easier follow-up with thyroglobulin levels and nuclear scans.

Medullary thyroid carcinoma is an aggressive multicentric tumor that spreads commonly to nodes. Early detection and an aggressive surgical approach, including total thyroidectomy and node dissection, improve the prognosis.

Anaplastic carcinoma is a rapidly lethal tumor primarily of the elderly. It is hoped that aggressive therapy of well-differentiated cancers will decrease any tendency for anaplastic transformation. A multidisciplinary approach has been associated with remissions.

Radioiodine Therapy (Fig. 59-22)

Routine radioiodine ablation of normal thyroid tissue following near-total thyroidectomy remains controversial.[50,57,58] Its benefit is noted only in patients with well-differentiated thyroid cancers (papillary, follicular, or their variants). Patients who appear to benefit most from radioiodine therapy include those with larger tumors (>4.5 cm), infiltrating tumors, multicentric tumors, locally invasive tumors, and evidence of distant metastases.[49,60,88] Complete ablation of the remnant thyroid can be accomplished with a single dose of radioiodine if the remnant is small and therefore should only be considered in patients who have had sufficient thyroid tissue removed at surgery. A second procedure completing the thyroidectomy is warranted if there is substantial normal thyroid tissue remaining in the neck.

The procedure is as follows. After total or near-total thyroidectomy, thyroid hormone replacement is initially withheld for 6 weeks; a TSH level is performed to confirm the hypothyroid state and should be at least 40 μU/ml. An ^{131}I scan is performed with 2 to10 mCi of ^{131}I. If there is appreciable uptake of iodine, a treatment dose of radioiodine is then administered in an attempt to deliver at least 50,000 rad to the thyroid remnant and 4000 rad to the metastases. For the thyroid remnant and residual disease in the neck, 100 mCi is frequently given, whereas 150 to 200 mCi is given for extrathyroidal disease. This usually requires a 2- to 3-day hospital stay. Radiation safety procedures must be carefully followed to avoid radiation exposure to health care workers and family members. Alternatively, small remnants may be treated with a standard 30

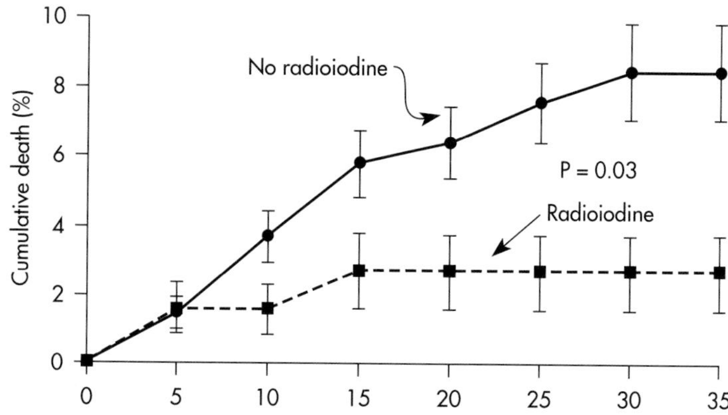

Fig. 59-22. Impact of radioiodine therapy on cancer death regardless of extent of surgery. (From Mazzaferri EL, Jhiang SM. Long-term impact of initial surgical and medical therapy on papillary and follicular thyroid cancer. Am J Med 97(5):418, 1994.)

to 50 mCi ^{131}I dose, but retreatment may be necessary and the failure rate is higher with this method.[89] After radioiodine therapy, lifelong thyroid suppression therapy (0.15 to 0.2 mg of levothyroxine daily) should be administered to reduce TSH levels to below 0.4 μU/ml, usually the lower level of detectability of most assays. The extent of the TSH suppression is dependent on the risk of recurrent disease. TRH stimulation tests are no longer necessary with the advent of the newer TSH assays.

Follow-up of Established Thyroid Cancer (Fig. 59-23)

An individual plan for follow-up can be developed by reviewing the prognostic factors present in each patient and predicting the patient's risk of recurrent disease. Individuals at high risk for recurrence or death should receive radioiodine ablation of the thyroid remnant, which allows for early detection and treatment. This is followed by yearly ^{131}I scans until disease free; then ^{131}I scans are performed every 3 to 5 years. In patients at low risk for recurrence (i.e., a small papillary carcinoma removed completely at surgery in a young person), yearly thyroglobulin measurements performed while the TSH level is suppressed and a yearly ultrasound examination is probably adequate.[77] Any change in these parameters would then be followed by a ^{131}I scan.

The major inconvenience in performing ^{131}I scans is the need to make the patient acutely hypothyroid. As the differentiated thyroid cancers are TSH dependent, growth of the tumor may occur during this period. Therefore it would be preferable to monitor the patient without having to resort to this maneuver. Preliminary studies indicate that recombinant human TSH may allow adequate imaging of thyroid cancers without discontinuing T_4 therapy.[34] Thallium scans have also been used to image thyroid tissue without discontinuing T_4, but the clinical utility of this technique remains unclear.

Approximately 50% of papillary cancers and 70% of follicular cancers concentrate iodine sufficiently to deliver adequate radiation to the nodal disease or distant metastases. Radioiodine can successfully treat metastases to the nodes and lungs in approximately 90% of young patients with papillary carcinoma, in approximately 60% of young patients with follicular carcinoma, but in less than 50% of older patients with differentiated thyroid cancer.[88] Radioiodine significantly improves survival rates in patients with thyroid carcinoma outside of the neck.[49,60]

Occasionally, a thyroid carcinoma that previously concentrated ^{131}I loses this capacity, and surgical removal of gross thyroid disease may be necessary. Inability to concentrate ^{131}I suggests a less-differentiated tumor and forbodes a poor prognosis.

MTC is not TSH dependent and does not concentrate ^{131}I. ^{131}I has been given in an attempt to deliver a tumoricidal dose of radiation to the thyroid bed, but has not been shown to be effective.

Complications of ^{131}I Therapy

Complications from ^{131}I therapy are unusual if doses are appropriately spaced to allow for bone marrow recovery. Acute complications of ^{131}I therapy include transient radiation thyroiditis (with neck/ear pain, dysphagia, thyroid tenderness and possibly transient thyrotoxicosis), painless edema of the neck, radiation sialadenitis, edema or hemorrhage in the tumor (hazardous if central nervous system metastases are present), and transient mild bone marrow suppression. Late complications of ^{131}I therapy include damage to gonads, bone marrow, lungs (if pulmonary metastases are present), and induction of other cancers. Leukemia and bladder cancer have been reported, but only in individuals who have received very large cumulative doses of radioiodine. As the above complications become more common for cumulative doses of greater than 500 mCi and the benefit of therapy is usually diminished at these doses, these problems can frequently be avoided by using smaller doses. There is a small but increased incidence of anaplastic transformation and second malignancies (especially breast) in patients with thyroid cancer, but there is no apparent influence of ^{131}I on these events. There is no increase in birth defects or infertility in young girls who have received ^{131}I therapy.

Utility of Thyroglobulin Levels

Thyroglobulin levels are not helpful diagnostically for thyroid cancer or other thyroid diseases but have been known

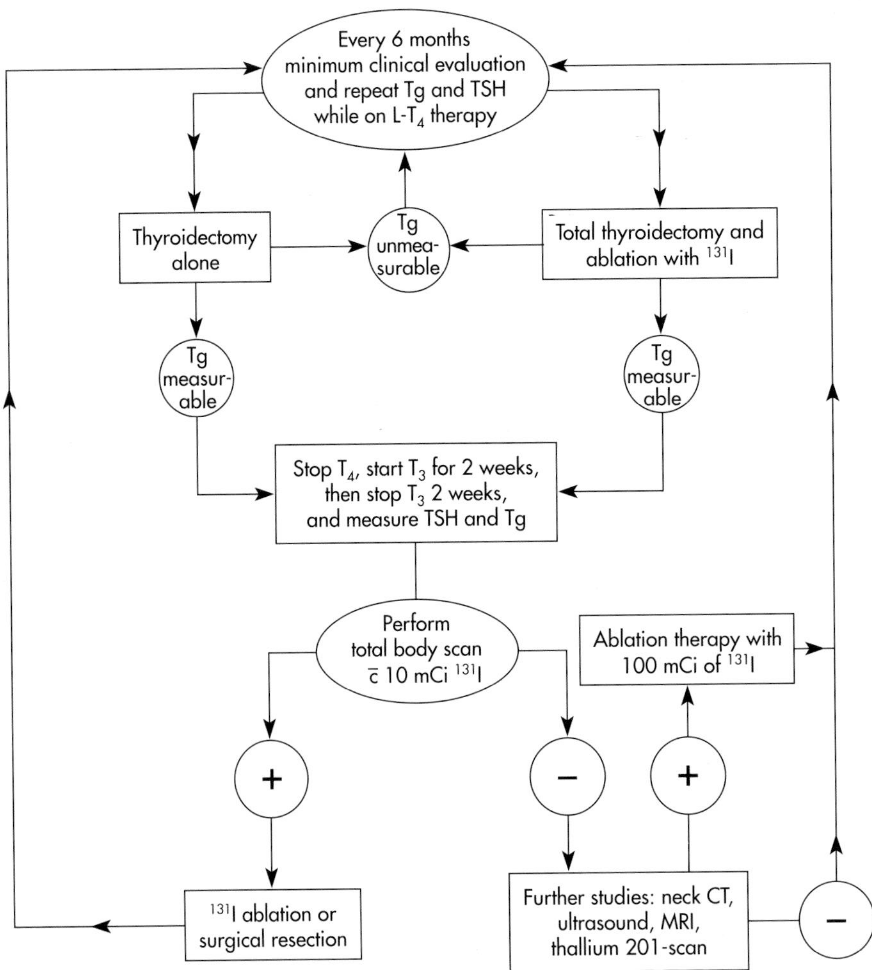

Fig. 59-23. Clinical scheme for follow-up evaluation of patients with well-differentiated thyroid cancer. In this scheme, accommodation is made for patients who underwent total thyroidectomy and ablation with ^{131}I after surgery *(right side of scheme)* and those who underwent total thyroidectomy alone *(left side of scheme)*. Patients with measurable serum thyroglobulin (Tg) levels are evaluated clinically every 6 months with serum Tg and thyroid-stimulating hormone (TSH) levels while they receive T_4 therapy. If the serum Tg level is measurable (whether the patient underwent ablation therapy or not), thyroid hormone therapy is discontinued, serum Tg and TSH are both measured, and a total body scan is obtained. If the total body scan result is positive, ^{131}I ablation or surgical resection is performed. If the ^{131}I total body scan result is negative, further studies (e.g., neck computed tomography) are indicated. If the result is positive, an ablative dose of 100 mCi of ^{131}I is given, and the patient is reevaluated 6 months later. If these additional studies do not reveal any tumor tissue, the patient is again reevaluated 6 months later *(top of scheme)*. Serum Tg values are expressed in ng/ml. (From Van Herle AJ, Brown DG. Thyroglobulin in benign and malignant thyroid disease. In Falk SA, ed. Thyroid Disease: Endocrine, Surgery, Nuclear Medicine, and Radiotherapy. New York: Raven Press, 1990, p 473.)

to correlate well with thyroid cancer disease activity in patients who have had a near-total or total thyroidectomy, preferably with radioiodine ablation of the remnant.[77] The test is more sensitive and has a lower false negative rate in detecting recurrent disease than ^{131}I scans, but the test is limited by the fact that 10% to 15% of patients have significant antibodies to thyroglobulin, which interferes with the present assay. A measurable thyroglobulin level in a patient with known differentiated thyroid cancer and a suppressed TSH receiving appropriate doses of T_4 should prompt a thorough examination for recurrent disease; chest radiograph, ultrasound of the neck, ^{131}I scan, and other appropriate localizing studies are indicated. Alternatively, a suppressed thyroglobulin in an otherwise stable patient would generally indicate remission, and serial ^{131}I scans would not be necessary. In equivocal cases, thyroid hormone can be withheld and the thyroglobulin level retested. A rising thyroglobulin level is a good indication of residual or recurrent disease.

Value of External Radiation Therapy

External radiation therapy has a limited role in the management of patients with differentiated thyroid cancer. It can be useful in patients with distant metastases that do not concentrate ^{131}I such as bone metastases from follicular carcinoma. It has been used for local control of disease in the neck when further surgery or ^{131}I is not feasible. External radiation may be more useful as part of a multidisciplinary approach to patients with undifferentiated thyroid cancers. Once external radiation is given, further surgery in the area is more problematic.

COMPLICATIONS ASSOCIATED WITH THYROID SURGERY

As indicated in the preceding sections of this chapter, operations on the thyroid gland are frequently necessary to manage the underlying pathophysiology. As is true with any operation, the benefits to be derived from a given surgical procedure must be balanced against the potential risks. For this reason, an understanding of the morbidity and mortality associated with thyroid surgery must be appreciated before surgery is recommended to a patient. Although a wide variety of complications have been reported following thyroid surgery, the following discussion attests to the safety of operations on the thyroid gland when they are accomplished by an experienced surgeon.

Mortality

In 1917 Theodor Kocher reported a mortality of less than 0.5% after 5000 thyroidectomies and won the Nobel Prize. Until that time, thyroid surgery was considered extremely hazardous with mortality rates in excess of 40%. Major advances in our understanding of thyroid pathophysiology, preoperative preparation of hyperthyroid patients, and improvements in surgical and anesthetic techniques have made thyroid surgery one of the safest surgical procedures.[81,83-85] Published series of 1000 thyroidectomies without a mortality are not unusual. In Foster's extensive review[86] of 24,108 thyroidectomies (one third of all thyroidectomies performed in the United States in 1970), the overall mortality was 0.3%, with no deaths in patients younger than 40 with nontoxic goiters. Major factors affecting mortality were age, indication for thyroidectomy, and extent of surgery. The mortality for nontoxic goiters was 0.02% in patients younger than 50 but rose to 0.66% in patients older than 70. In spite of increased attention to preoperative preparation of patients with diffuse toxic goiters, mortality was five times greater than for nontoxic benign goiters. Total or near-total thyroidectomy comprised approximately 10% of the total number of operations but carried a higher morbidity and mortality. Patients with malignant thyroid disease had more extensive surgical procedures (one third treated by total thyroidectomy) and an increased morbidity and mortality (1.2%). However, in 766 patients younger than 40 with thyroid cancer, the in-hospital mortality was zero.[86]

Morbidity

Operations on the highly vascular enlarged thyroid gland surrounded by vital structures may appear formidable to a surgical house officer, but careful attention to surgical technique has produced an exemplary track record in terms of complications in many centers. Postoperative wound infections are distinctly unusual, and prophylactic antibiotics are generally considered unnecessary when operations on the thyroid gland are to be performed. The types of complications that may occur with thyroid surgery include bleeding, hypoparathyroidism, recurrent laryngeal nerve injury, superior laryngeal nerve damage, and keloid formation.

Hemorrhage

Postoperative hemorrhage and the danger of rapid asphyxiation are the most dramatic complications of thyroid surgery. Attention to hemostasis during surgery and close observation of a minimally dressed or undressed wound in the recovery room and during the initial 8 postoperative hours are crucial to avoid this complication. Local warm compresses may be sufficient for a small hematoma or edema of the wound, but swelling of the neck, stridor, hypoxia, or any respiratory difficulty requires prompt attention, with possible reintubation and opening of the skin incision and strap muscles at the bedside if necessary. Equipment for immediate endotracheal intubation and tracheostomy should be close at hand for all patients following thyroidectomy. An overly dressed neck wound, with or without drains, does not prevent postoperative hemorrhage and may delay its recognition, resulting in catastrophic hypoxic brain damage or death. Several authorities recommend placing the patient in a 30-degree head-down position coincident with tracheal stimulation before wound closure and extubation. This maneuver increases pressure and unmasks any poorly sutured vessels. Subsequently, the patient's head and shoulders should be elevated 20 degrees to minimize pressure on the wound. Nausea and vomiting may promote hematoma formation and should be appropriately treated.

Nerve Damage

Injury to the laryngeal nerves is closely related to the experience of the surgeon performing the operation and the extent of surgery. Injury to the recurrent laryngeal nerve is more common and more easily recognized than injury to the external branch of the superior laryngeal nerve. Indirect laryngoscopy before surgery, identification of the nerves throughout their course, and a second indirect laryngoscopy after surgery results in a complication rate of less than 1% in surgery for benign disease. Mechanical disturbance of the nerve may result in transient, but rarely permanent, vocal cord paralysis. Delayed vocal cord dysfunction can occur up to 1 week following surgery but is usually transient. Aberrant left recurrent nerves are extremely rare, but 15% of the right recurrent nerves may be aberrant, again indicating the need for careful dissection. The superior laryngeal nerve may be injured during ligation of vessels of the upper pole of the thyroid gland.

Although unilateral paralysis of the recurrent laryngeal nerve can be easily detected by laryngoscopy and the patient's hoarseness, techniques to uncover postoperative superior laryngeal nerve damage are not routinely performed; except for patients who depend on their voice professionally, the symptoms may be quite subtle. On the other hand, bilateral recurrent nerve injury is a rare but life-threatening complication acutely evident after removal of the endotracheal tube and requiring emergency reintubation or tracheostomy.

INDICATIONS FOR CALCIUM OR VITAMIN D SUPPLEMENTATION AFTER THYROIDECTOMY

Severe circumoral or acral paresthesias
Carpopedal spasm
Electrocardiogram abnormalities
Calcium <7.5 mg/100 ml
Laryngeal stridor
Convulsions

Hypoparathyroidism

The parathyroid glands are particularly susceptible to ischemic or mechanical injury and to inadvertent or unavoidable removal, depending on the extent of thyroid surgery performed. Transient or subclinical hypoparathyroidism may be substantially more common than the reported rate of permanent hypoparathyroidism. A complication rate of 1% or less after subtotal thyroidectomy may rise quickly to more than 10% with near-total or total thyroidectomy. Meticulous dissection, identification of all four glands and their blood supply, and preservation of the posterior capsule of the thyroid during total thyroidectomy should keep the complication rate to less than 5% even in the more extensive procedures; the more experienced centers regularly report rates of less than 1% even for a total thyroidectomy. Preservation and autotransplantation of the parathyroid glands should reduce this complication rate further in patients requiring en bloc resection for advanced thyroid neoplasms.[90]

Symptoms of hypocalcemia may appear 1 to 7 days after surgery and include circumoral and acral paresthesias, carpopedal spasm, laryngeal stridor, and, in extreme untreated cases, convulsions. Daily serum calcium determinations and frequent examination of the patient for the appearance of Chvostek's and Trousseau's signs are essential for early recognition of hypocalcemia. Since a small percentage of normal subjects exhibit a positive Chvostek sign, it is important to verify a negative sign before surgery to accurately recognize a change after surgery.

Significant hypocalcemia, resulting in the symptoms noted in the accompanying box, should be treated promptly with intravenous calcium gluconate. Mild decreases in serum calcium (approximately 8 mg/100 ml) should be observed closely without therapy, in the hope that hypocalcemia will stimulate parathormone secretion in the remaining glands. Most patients are now discharged from the hospital within 2 to 3 days of the surgery, and it is reasonable to initiate oral calcium at discharge with or without a fast-acting vitamin D preparation such as calcitriol if the calcium level is still decreasing. These medications can usually be tapered and discontinued within a few weeks. In patients with carpopedal spasm or other complications of hypocalcemia requiring urgent therapy, 1 ampule of calcium gluconate (10 ml of a 10% solution) can be given intravenously over several minutes. A continuous intravenous infusion of calcium (20 to 40 ml of 10% calcium gluconate per liter) may be titrated to keep the serum calcium in the low normal range and the patient comfortable until oral therapy takes effect.

The symptoms of hypocalcemia are closely related to the level of ionized calcium. Serum protein abnormalities, particularly albumin, affect the level of total serum calcium. A simple estimate of ionized calcium can be made by noting approximately a 0.8 mg/100 ml decrease in serum calcium for each 1 g/L decrease in serum albumin from normal.

Some degree of endogenous parathormone secretion is frequent in surgical hypoparathyroidism, and the doses of calcium or vitamin D to maintain calcium homeostasis are smaller than in hypoparathyroidism from other causes. Frequently revascularization or hypertrophy of the remaining glands occurs, and therapy may be discontinued after several months. If the patient has an adequate calcium intake, 1 to 2 g of elemental calcium with or without a vitamin D supplement may be sufficient. Vitamin D metabolites such as 1,25-dihydroxycholecalciferol (calcitriol) is an extremely effective, fast-acting agent that may be used initially. The cost of this agent is a major disadvantage, and patients can sometimes be adequately controlled on generic vitamin D 50,000 U twice a week or more frequently, depending on the severity of the hypoparathyroidism. However, vitamin D preparations have a long duration of action, and manipulation of the dose may prove difficult. Prolonged hypercalcemia and hypocalcemia may occur, with troublesome consequences. With any vitamin D preparation, adequate calcium intake must be assured. The adjunctive use of a thiazide diuretic decreases urinary calcium and thus decreases the need for oral supplementation.

The goal of therapy for hypoparathyroidism is to avoid symptomatic hypocalcemia and maintain the serum calcium in the low normal range. This avoids renal complications caused by hypercalciuria. Insidious hypocalcemia may cause chronic malaise, cognitive dysfunction, and cataracts. Therefore serum calcium and phosphorus levels should be monitored in all patients after surgery, regardless of the lack of symptoms.

Hypothyroidism

Depending on the situation, hypothyroidism may be expected or even desired (i.e., treatment of severe Graves' disease or thyroid cancer).

Hypothyroidism is common after surgical therapy for Graves' disease and is somewhat, but not exclusively, related to the size of the remnant.[17,18,28] The presence of lymphocyte infiltration in patients with autoimmune thyroid disease increases the chances of hypothyroidism after therapy. Thyroid registries in England verify a bimodal pattern of hypothyroidism after surgery for Graves' disease with a peak incidence in the first 18 months following surgery but a persistent 1% annual incidence for at least 5 to 10 years after surgery.[17] Late-onset hypothyroidism appears to be related to the natural history of the disease process and stresses the need for lifelong follow-up. Large thyroid remnants may not protect against hypothyroidism and appear to increase the chance of recurrent hyperthyroidism, especially in younger patients.

Patients who have had surgery for thyroid cancer require lifelong levothyroxine replacement starting immediately following surgery. More controversial is the recommendation that levothyroxine therapy be given to all individuals who have had surgery for benign disease and who have substantial thyroid tissue remaining, in the hopes of preventing new nodules from forming. The benefits of this therapy must be balanced by the risks of overreplacement in the particular individual (increased risk of osteoporosis especially in the postmenopausal woman).[43]

Rare Complications

In radical surgery for malignant disease several rare neurologic complications have been reported. These include injury to the cervical sympathetic trunk during ligation of the inferior thyroid artery, causing Horner's syndrome; phrenic nerve damage with paralysis of the hemidiaphragm; and transection of the spinal accessory nerve with paralysis of the trapezius muscle. Rarely, the right lymphatic duct or thoracic duct may be injured, requiring ligation. Tracheomalacia has been reported after removal of a large goiter but is a distinctly rare complication.

SUMMARY

In spite of its small size, the thyroid gland plays an important role in the maintenance of normal body cellular metabolism. This is exemplified by the pathologic aberrations that supervene in both hyperthyroid and hypothyroid states. The significance of this organ to the surgeon relates not only to the effect that thyroid dysfunction may have in ensuring the smooth performance of any operation and the resulting postoperative convalescence, but also to the important role that surgery plays in managing patients with various hyperthyroid states and in those individuals with thyroid lesions suggestive of malignancy. In this latter group of patients the frequency of surgical intervention has diminished greatly with the current availability of fine-needle aspiration. This technique provides the unique ability to aspirate cystic lesions previously requiring formal surgical exploration and the ability to distinguish benign and malignant lesions from each other so that those individuals subjected to surgery will clearly benefit from such a procedure. Even when surgery is indicated, a good result can be expected, since current anesthetic management and surgical technique are associated with minimal morbidity and virtually no mortality.

REFERENCES

1. Reichlin S. Neuroendocrine immune interactions. N Engl J Med 329:1246, 1993.
2. Enns M, Ross C, Clark P. Thyroid screening tests in psychiatric inpatients. Gen Hosp Psychiatry 14:334, 1992.
3. Weiss RE, Chyna B, Duell PB. A new point mutation in the thyroid hormone receptor beta gene of a family with resistance to thyroid hormone. J Clin Endocrinol Metab 78:1253, 1994.
4. Wynne AG, et al. Hyperthyroidism due to inappropriate secretion of thyrotropin in 10 patients. Am J Med 92:15, 1992.
5. Fradkin JE, Wolff J. Iodide-induced thyrotoxicosis. Medicine 62:1, 1983.
6. Klein I, Levey GS. Iodine excess and thyroid function. Ann Intern Med 98:406, 1983.
7. Ekins R. Measurement of free hormones in blood. Endocr Rev 11:5, 1990.
8. Chopra IJ, et al. Misleading low free thyroxine level and usefulness of reverse triiodothyronine measurement in nonthyroidal illnesses. Ann Intern Med 90:905, 1979.
9. Chopra IJ, et al. Thyroid function in nonthyroidal illnesses. Ann Intern Med 98:946, 1983.
10. Melmed S, et al. A comparison of methods for assessing thyroid function in nonthyroidal illness. J Clin Endocrinol Metab 54:300, 1982.
11. Nicoloff JT, Spencer CA. The use and misuse of sensitive thyrotropin assays. J Clin Endocrinol Metab 71:553, 1990.
12. Mandel SJ, Brent GA, Larsen PR. Levothyroxine therapy in patients with thyroid disease. Ann Intern Med 119:492, 1993.
13. Franklyn JA. Management of hyperthyroidism. N Engl J Med 330:1731, 1994.
14. Kendall-Taylor P, et al. Evidence that thyroid stimulating antibody is produced in the thyroid gland. Lancet 1:654, 1984.
15. Valente WA, et al. Antibodies that promote thyroid growth. N Engl J Med 309:1028, 1983.
16. Wilders-Truschnig MM, et al. Chromatographically purified immunoglobulin G of endemic and sporadic goiter patients stimulates FRTL% cell growth in a mitotic arrest assay. J Clin Endocrinol Metab 70:444, 1990.
17. Hedley AJ, et al. Recurrent thyrotoxicosis after subtotal thyroidectomy. Br Med J 4:258, 1971.
18. Hedley AJ, et al. The effect of remnant size on the outcome of subtotal thyroidectomy for thyrotoxicosis. Br J Surg 59:559, 1972.
19. Bartalena L, et al. Use of corticosteroids to prevent progression of Graves' ophthalmopathy after radioiodine therapy for hyperthyroidism. N Engl J Med 321:1349, 1989.
20. Belfiore A, et al. Increased aggressiveness of thyroid cancer in patients with Graves' disease. J Clin Endocrinol Metab 70:830, 1990.
21. Mazzaferri EL. Thyroid cancer and Graves' disease. J Clin Endocrinol Metab 70:826, 1990.
22. Weiss I, Davies TF. Inhibition of immunoglobulin secreting cells by antithyroid drugs. J Clin Endocrinol Metab 53:1223, 1981.
23. Hashizume K, et al. Administration of thyroxine in treated Graves' disease. Effects on the level of antibodies to thyroid-stimulating hormone receptors and on the risk of recurrence of hyperthyroidism. N Engl J Med 324:947, 1991.

24. Hashizume K, et al. Effect of administration of thyroxine on the risk of postpartum recurrence of hyperthyroid Graves' disease. J Clin Endocrinol Metab 75:6, 1992.
25. Pollikar R, et al. The thyroid and the heart. Circulation 87:1435, 1993.
26. Patwardhan NA, et al. Surgery still has a role in Graves' hyperthyroidism. Surgery 114:1108, 1993.
27. Tallstedt L, et al. Occurrence of ophthalmopathy after treatment for Graves' hyperthyroidism. N Engl J Med 326:1733, 1992.
28. Hedley AJ, et al. Late onset hypothyroidism after subtotal thyroidectomy for hyperthyroidism: Implication for long-term follow-up. Br J Surg 80:740, 1983.
29. Leese GR, et al. Long term follow-up of treated hyperthyroid and hypothyroid patients. Health Bull (Edinb) 51:177, 1993.
30. Maier WP, et al. Long-term follow-up of Graves' disease after subtotal thyroidectomy. Am J Surg 147:266, 1984.
31. Wu SY, et al. The effect of repeated administration of ipodate in hyperthyroidism. J Clin Endocrinol Metab 47:1358, 1978.
32. Hamburger J. The autonomously functioning thyroid adenoma: Clinical considerations. N Engl J Med 309:1512, 1983.
33. Goldstein R, Hart IR. Followup of solitary autonomous thyroid nodules treated with I^{131}. N Engl J Med 309:1473, 1983.
34. Meier CA, et al. Diagnostic use of recombinant human thyrotropin in patients with thyroid carcinoma. J Clin Endocrinol Metab 78:188, 1994.
35. Guttler R, et al. *Pneumocystis carinii* thyroiditis. Report of three cases and review of the literature. Arch Intern Med 153:393, 1993.
36. Khan EM, et al. Tuberculosis of the thyroid gland: A clinicopathological profile of four cases and review of the literature. Aust NZ J Surg 63:807, 1993.
37. Amino N, et al. High prevalence of transient post-partum thyrotoxicosis and hypothyroidism. N Engl J Med 306:849, 1982.
38. Robertson HEW. Lassitude, coldness, and hair changes following pregnancy, and their response to treatment with thyroid extract. Br Med J 2:2275, 1948.
39. Stagnaro-Green A. Postpartum thyroiditis: Prevalence, etiology, and clinical implications. Thyroid Today 16:1, 1993.
40. Burch HB, Wartofsky L. Graves' ophthalmopathy: Current concepts regarding pathogenesis and management. Endocr Rev 14:747, 1993.
41. Toft AD. Thyroxine therapy. N Engl J Med 331:174, 1994.
42. Paine TD, et al. Coronary arterial surgery in patients with incapacitating angina pectoris and myxedema. Am J Cardiol 40:226, 1977.
43. Baran DT. Detrimental skeletal effects of thyrotropin suppressive doses of thyroxine: Fact or fantasy? J Clin Endocrinol Metab 78:816, 1994.
44. Franklyn JA, et al. Long term thyroxine treatment and bone mineral density. Lancet 340:9, 1992.
45. Marcocci C, et al. Carefully monitored levothyroxine suppressive therapy is not associated with bone loss in premenopausal women. J Clin Endocrinol Metab 78:818, 1994.
46. Mazzaferri EL. Management of the solitary thyroid nodule. N Engl J Med 328:553, 1993.
47. Belfiore A, et al. Cancer risk in patients with cold thyroid nodules: Relevance of iodine intake, sex, age, and multinodularity. Am J Med 93:363, 1992.
48. Cunningham MP, et al. Survival discriminants for differentiated thyroid cancer. Am J Surg 160:344, 1990.
49. Mazzaferri EL, Jhiang SM. Long-term impact of initial surgical and medical therapy on papillary and follicular thyroid cancer. Am J Med 97(5):418, 1994.
50. Pasieka JL, Rotstein LE. Consensus conference on well-differentiated thyroid cancer: A summary. Can J Surg 36:298, 1993.
51. Van de Velde CJH, Hamming JF, Goslings BM. Report of the consensus development conference on the management of differentiated thyroid cancer in the Netherlands. Eur J Cancer Clin Oncol 24:287, 1988.
52. DeGroot LJ. Effects of irradiation on the thyroid gland. Endocrinol Metab Clin North Am 22:607, 1993.
53. Crow PJ, Chetty R, Dent DM. Thyroid frozen section: Flawed but helpful. Aust NZ J Surg 63:275, 1993.
54. Hamburger JI. Diagnosis of thyroid nodules by fine needle biopsy: Use and abuse. J Clin Endocrinol Metab 79:335, 1994.
55. de los Santos ET, et al. Cystic thyroid nodules, the dilemma of malignant lesions. Arch Intern Med 150:1422, 1990.
56. Jhiang SM, et al. Detection of the PTC/retTPC oncogene in human thyroid cancers. Oncogene 7:1331, 1992.
57. Fagin JA, et al. High prevalence of mutations of the p53 gene in poorly differentiated human thyroid cancers. J Clin Invest 91:179, 1993.
58. DeGroot LJ, et al. Natural history, treatment, and course of papillary thyroid carcinoma. J Clin Endocrinol Metab 71:414, 1990.
59. Mazzaferri EL, et al. Papillary thyroid carcinoma: The impact of therapy in 576 patients. Medicine 56:171, 1977.
60. Samaan NA, et al. The results of various modalities of treatment of well differentiated thyroid carcinomas: A retrospective review of 1599 patients. J Clin Endocrinol Metab 75:714, 1992.
61. Samaan NA, et al. Impact of therapy for differentiated carcinoma of the thyroid: An analysis of 706 cases. J Clin Endocrinol Metab 56:1131, 1983.
62. Favus MJ, et al. Thyroid cancer occurring as a late consequence of head and neck irradiation. N Engl J Med 294:1019, 1983.
63. Clark OH, et al. Thyroid cancer: The case for total thyroidectomy. Euro Cancer Clin Oncol 24:305, 1988.
64. Robbins J, et al. Thyroid cancer: A lethal endocrine neoplasm. Ann Intern Med 115:133, 1991.
65. Burmeister LA, et al. Levothyroxine dose requirements for thyrotropin suppression in the treatment of differentiated thyroid cancer. J Clin Endocrinol Metab 75:344, 1992.
66. Goepfert H, Dichtel WJ, Samaan NA. Thyroid cancer in children and teenagers. Arch Otalaryngol Surg 110:72, 1984.
67. Caruso DR, Odorisio TM, Mazzaferri EL. Multiple endocrine neoplasia. Curr Opin Oncol 3:103, 1991.
68. Gagel RF. Medullary thyroid carcinoma: Recent progress. J Clin Endocrinol Metab 76:809, 1993.
69. Hennessy JF, et al. A comparison of pentagastrin injection and calcium infusion as provocative agents for the detection of medullary carcinoma of the thyroid. J Clin Endocrinol Metab 39:487, 1974.
70. Sizemore GW, Go VLM. Stimulation tests for diagnosis of medullary thyroid carcinoma. Mayo Clin Proc 50:53, 1975.
71. Carlson KM, et al. Single missense mutation in the tyrosine kinase catalytic domain of the RET protooncogene is associated with multiple endocrine neoplasia type 2AB. Proc Natl Acad Sci USA 91:1579, 1994.
72. Schlumberger M, et al. Differentiated thyroid carcinoma in childhood: Long term follow-up of 72 patients. J Clin Endocrinol Metab 65:1088, 1987.
73. Harness JK, et al. Total thyroidectomy: Complications and technique. World J Surg 10:781, 1986.
74. Maxon HR, et al. Ionizing irradiation and the introduction of clinically significant disease in the human thyroid gland. Am J Med 63:967, 1977.
75. Viswanathan K, Gierlowski TC, Schneider AB. Childhood thyroid cancer. Characteristics and long-term outcome in children irradiated for benign conditions of the head and neck. Arch Pediatr Adolesc Med 148:260, 1994.
76. Holm LE, et al. Malignant thyroid tumors after iodine-131. N Engl J Med 303:188, 1980.
77. Ozata M, et al. Serum thyroglobulin in the follow-up of patients with treated differentiated thyroid cancer. J Clin Endocrinol Metab 79:98, 1994.
78. Gharib H, Goellner JR. Fine needle aspiration of the thyroid: An appraisal. Ann Intern Med 118:282, 1993.
79. Gharib H. Fine-needle aspiration biopsy of thyroid nodules: Advantages, limitations, and effect. Mayo Clin Proc 69:44, 1994.
80. Gharib H, et al. Suppressive therapy with levothyroxine for solitary thyroid nodules. N Engl J Med 317:70, 1987.

81. DeGroot LJ, Kaplan EL. Second operations for "completion" of thyroidectomy in treatment of differentiated thyroid cancer. Surgery 110:936, 1991.
82. Levin KE, et al. Reoperative thyroid surgery. Surgery 111:604, 1992.
83. Edis AJ. Prevention and management of complication associated with thyroid and parathyroid surgery. Surg Clin North Am 59:83, 1979.
84. Farrar WB. Complications of thyroidectomy. Surg Clin North Am 63:1353, 1981.
85. Fenton RS. The surgical complications of thyroidectomy. J Otolaryngol 12:104, 1983.
86. Foster RS. Morbidity and mortality after thyroidectomy. Surg Gynecol Obstet 146:423, 1978.
87. Ley PB, et al. Safety and efficacy of total thyroidectomy for differentiated thyroid carcinoma: A 20-year review. Am Surg 59:110, 1993.
88. Beierwaltes WH, et al. Survival time and cure in papillary and follicular thyroid carcinoma with distant metastases: Statistics following University of Michigan therapy. J Nucl Med 23:561, 1982.
89. DeGroot LJ, Reilly M. Comparison of 30 and 50 millicurie doses of iodine^{131} for thyroid ablation. Ann Intern Med 96:51, 1982.
90. Lore JM, Pruet CW. Retrieval of the parathyroid glands during thyroidectomy. Head Neck Surg 5:268, 1983.

60

Endocrine Pancreas

Ronald C. Merrell and Giacomo P. Basadonna

To coordinate the function of metazoan life forms for mutual, organismal benefit, the cells of the organism must communicate. In simple multicellular organisms, electrical coupling, cell-contact events, and the local diffusion of metabolic and messenger molecules are sufficient. Neighboring cells are informed by mass action, allosteric enzyme interactions, or specific binding to receptors. In a larger organism with a circulatory system, coordinating messages in the form of small molecules may flow through the organism to arrive at tissues possessing specific receptors, with complex postreceptor events. Also, neural fibers arborize across great distances to release communicating molecules to specialized receptors when triggered by propagated depolarization of the neuronal membrane.[1]

The pancreas demonstrates essentially all the known mechanisms for cellular communication in a metazoan organism. In addition to cell-to-cell interaction among islet cells across gap junctions (Fig. 60-1), the simplest coordinated function, and complex adrenergic and cholinergic innervation, the pancreas engages in exocrine, paracrine, and endocrine interactions with the remainder of the body (Fig. 60-2). *Exocrine function* describes release of synthesized products into a nonvascular duct for delivery at another anatomic locus. *Paracrine function* requires release of a synthesized product into the extracellular space for delivery by diffusion to a target tissue no more than several microns away. *Endocrine interaction* is release of a synthesized product that enters the circulation for transport to a distant target tissue. The intricacy and redundancy of communication pathways for this islet cell mass underscore its crucial role in maintaining glucose homeostasis through the balance of glucose clearance, mediated by insulin, and glucose generation, mediated by glucagon. This chapter describes the endocrine community of the islets of Langerhans; their origins and relationships, both internal and external; and their role in homeostasis and disease states.

In 1869, Paul Langerhans demonstrated the unique features of the islets that now bear his name. These structures, originally viewed as islands in the alien sea of the exocrine pancreas, are now more clearly seen as integral rather than accidental features of the pancreas, with extensive interaction with the exocrine portion of the gland. Von Mering and Minkowski[2] provided evidence for an endocrine function for the pancreas in 1889, when they found that total pancreatectomy led not only to the expected exocrine insufficiency but also to diabetes mellitus. Attribution of endocrine function to the islets followed, seeming to culminate with isolation of insulin and

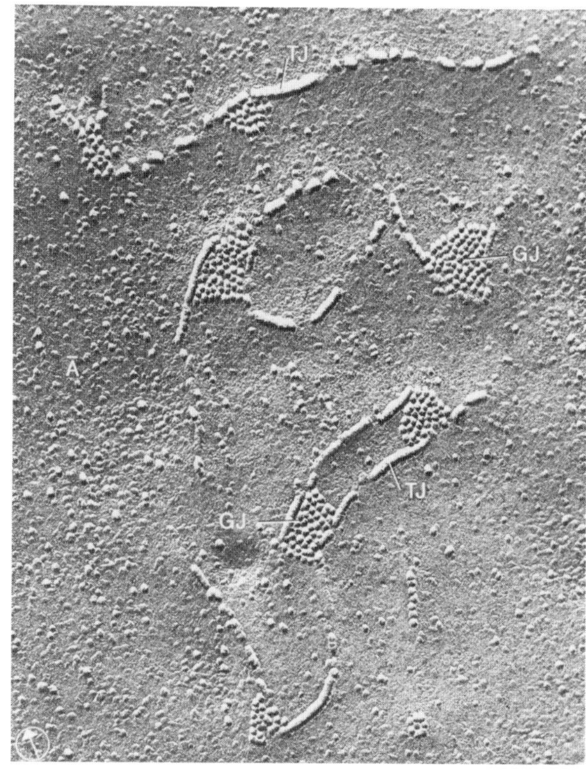

Fig. 60-1. Gap junctions *(GJ)* and tight junctions *(TJ)* between islet cells suggest the rich transcellular communication between component cells of islets of Langerhans. This freeze-fracture electron micrograph shows extensive cellular contacts between islet cells. (Courtesy Lelio Orci, Geneva.)

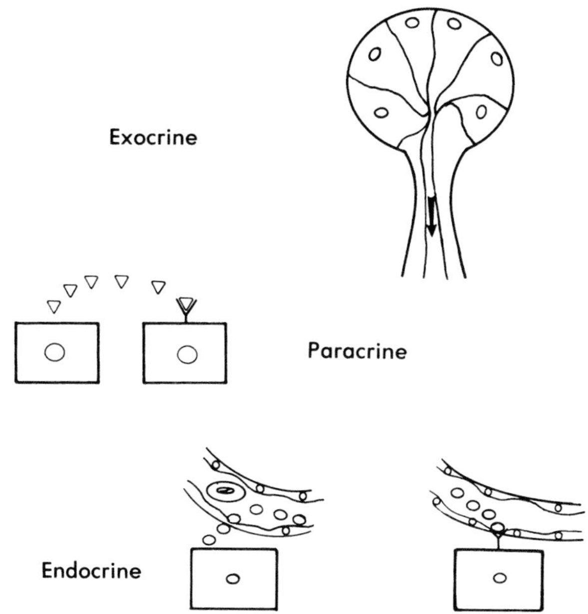

Fig. 60-2. Exocrine delivery of a secreted cellular product occurs along ducts that ultimately discharge into the gastrointestinal tract or outside the body. Paracrine secretions reach a target cell solely by diffusion across a short distance. (Schematic cell on the left is discharging a substance that is being received by the cell on the right.) Endocrine secretions enter the circulation and arrive at a target tissue at some distance from the point of origin. (Schematic cell on the left is discharging a substance into the blood; the blood then transports this substance to a distant target cell, as shown on the right.)

its clinical application for type I diabetes mellitus by Banting and Best in 1922.[3] However, the full richness of islet interaction and regulation was only suggested by the recognition of insulin, and new data continue to enhance the importance of the islets in homeostasis.

ANATOMY AND EMBRYOLOGY OF THE ISLETS

The islets of Langerhans individually constitute an endocrine community engaged in active collaboration to secure glucose homeostasis. At least four distinct endocrine cells have been identified: (1) *A cells,* which secrete glucagon, a catabolic hormone that raises plasma glucose level; (2) *B cells,* which produce insulin, an anabolic hormone that lowers plasma glucose level; (3) *D cells,* which produce somatostatin, a regulatory hormone for A and B cells; and (4) *F cells,* which secrete pancreatic polypeptide (PP), a 36–amino acid linear polypeptide. Each cell contains and secretes only one endocrine product. The lettering system for these cells stems from special chemical staining properties of the secretory granules. The letter *C* in the series was reserved for a cell in guinea pig islets that contained no granules. This cell may have been a degranulated *B* cell or a precursor cell, but it no longer has any valid stature among its lettered neighbors. Also, the *E cell,* described only in the opossum, must await further study before inclusion in this endocrine community. The cells were lettered in order of discovery, and the missing C and E cells in the islet serve to remind us of the enormous confusion that preceded our current meager understanding.[4] That understanding is based on staining islets with specific antibodies to the various secretory products and then using a variety of tactics to visualize that bound antibody on the secretory granules of the appropriate cell. This staining by immunocytochemistry forms the basis of our current understanding of islet anatomy.

The pancreas arises from foregut endoderm through a dorsal bud, first evident in the 3 mm embryo, and then by a ventral anlage, which is a branch of the liver bud. By clockwise rotation, the ventral structure ultimately fuses with the dorsal structure. The endocrine cells derive from precursors along the pancreatic ductal elements. With immunocytochemistry, A, B, and D cells can be recognized in organized islets by 8 weeks of gestation. By 10 to 11 weeks, islets can be identified. The islets organize away from ducts as discrete structures and then grow by cell division throughout fetal life and for the first few years after birth. Islets are not of uniform size in humans, but they average approximately 300 μm.[5] The A cells mature first, but by birth the distribution of the cells is the same as in adults: 60% to 70% B cells, 20% to 25% A cells, 10% to 15% D cells, and 5% to 10% F cells (Fig. 60-3). The distribution of the islets is not completely uniform throughout the pancreas with respect to constituent cells. For example, A and B cells are more numerous in tail islets, and F cells are much more numerous in the pancreatic head. Islets have a direct arterial blood supply and are so well vascularized that the mass of islets capillaries is often described as glomerulus-like. Islets serial sections reveal four patterns of islet endocrine cells and capillaries: (1) a single row of cells between two capillaries, (2) a double row of cells between two capillaries, (3) a ring of cells around a cross-sectioned capillary, and (4) a clump of cells between two capillaries. At least two of these patterns are present in any islet section.[6] Ultrastructural studies show that in a normal B cell, insulin granules fill the cytoplasm, and no obvious polarity is evident. After degranulation, however, a clear polarity of insulin granules has been demonstrated, with insulin granules clumped at the opposite side of the arbitrarily defined basal face, where the nucleus is closer to one capillary face. All the B cells around a particular cross-sectioned capillary show the same polarity, with the apical side facing the central capillary.[6] These findings could signify a topographic separation of an apical secretory surface and a basal sensing surface for the B cell and possibly the other endocrine cells.

The origin of islet cells has been the subject of spirited debate for nearly 10 years. The islet cells have metabolic and morphotic features shared by all neuroendocrine cells, including amine precursor uptake and decarboxylase (APUD), and neuronal-specific enolase. A common embryologic source for all these cells in the neuroectoderm of the neural crest has been proposed.[7] However, careful stud-

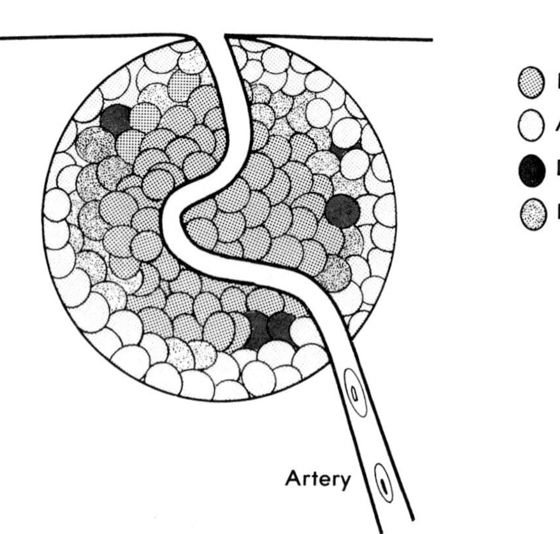

Fig. 60-3. B cells are centrally located in the islet in close approximation to incoming blood supply, whereas A cells are arrayed as a mantle at the periphery of the islet. D and F cells are interspersed. B-cell secretions move through the islet toward the periphery before reentering the circulation. This flow determines the opportunity for paracrine interaction among the component cells. The modest suppression by insulin of A cells may be paracrine, whereas the more substantial stimulation of B cells by glucagon must be endocrine. D and F cells could interact with one another, with A cells, or with B cells.

ies in developmental biology refute this origin for pancreatic islet cells and place them firmly in the same lineage as the exocrine cells. For example, elimination of the neural fold before the three-somite stage does not preclude B-cell development in rat embryo explants.[8] A great majority of the endocrine system derives from the gastrointestinal epithelium, including the pituitary (Rathke's pouch), the thyroid (second branchial arch and ultimo branchial body), and the parathyroid glands (branchial pouches III and IV). Nonetheless, the APUD concept has been of enormous value in predicting the properties of endocrine tissue in one site on the basis of knowledge of other endocrine systems. Also, the behavior of pathologic endocrine tissue can be anticipated in less well-known tumors on the basis of knowledge of better characterized tumors. All cells in an organism have the same genome, and the differentiation of transcription during development can be convergent, so after many different branch points in development, two cells serving similar (e.g., endocrine) functions may be more alike than are cells much closer in developmental lineage.

It is significant that the islets are in the pancreas and develop with the pancreas, because this relationship suggests that islets function with the remainder of the pancreas. Indeed, there is an insuloacinar axis, which constitutes a portal system that delivers islet hormones in high concentration to much of the acinar pancreas (Table 60-1). Insulin increases amylase synthesis, permits bicarbonate secretion, and is permissive for the action of cholecystokinin (CCK). The pancreas in patients with insulin-dependent diabetes is much smaller than normal as a result of atrophy, which may be caused by a relative lack of insulin locally or by the inhibitory effects of excess glucagon, which suppresses enzyme synthesis and release, although it stimulates bicarbonate secretion. The inhibitory effects of glucagon are so pronounced experimentally that this hormone was proposed for the treatment of acute pancreatitis; however, clinical results have not been impressive. Somatostatin and PP are also inhibitory to the exocrine pancreas, and they presumably are active in the insuloacinar axis.[9]

Table 60-1. Insuloacinar Axis

Hormone	Exocrine Effect
Insulin	↑ Uptake of amino acids ↑ Amylase synthesis ↑ Cell division Permits HCO_3^- release
Glucagon	↓ Enzyme synthesis ↓ Enzyme release ↑ HCO_3^- release
Somatostatin	↓ Pancreatic secretion
Pancreatic polypeptide	↓ Release of enzymes

PHYSIOLOGY OF THE ISLETS

Insulin and the B Cell

The best studied of the islet cells is the B cell. The nucleus of this cell transcribes messenger RNA (mRNA) for preproinsulin, which is synthesized in the rough endoplasmic reticulum. The amino-terminal signal sequence is cleaved in the lumen of the endoplasmic reticulum, and the 9 kd product, proinsulin, passes through the Golgi apparatus, where secretory vesicles are assembled. The insulin gene, one of the first human genes to be cloned,[10] is 1500 bp long and contains three exons and two introns. The introns can be of variable length: intron 1 varies from 119 bp in chickens to 179 bp in humans, whereas intron 2 can vary from 264 bp in dogs to more than 3500 bp in chickens (786 in humans). The insulin gene exists as a single copy in most species, except in rats and mice, where two copies exist. Interestingly, rat insulin gene I does not have the second intron and exhibits 70% homology with the other copy. In the rat, both genes are present in the same chromosone and appear to be transcribed in equal portions. In mice, the genes are in different chromosomes, but this seems to have no effect on the relatively identical rates of transcription. The location of the insulin gene in humans is on band p15 of the short arm of chromosone 11.[11]

Glucose stimulates insulin biosynthesis as well as secretion. Glucose does indeed regulate insulin biosynthesis at both translational and transcriptional levels, but there is a time shift in these effects. Thus, transcriptional effects are

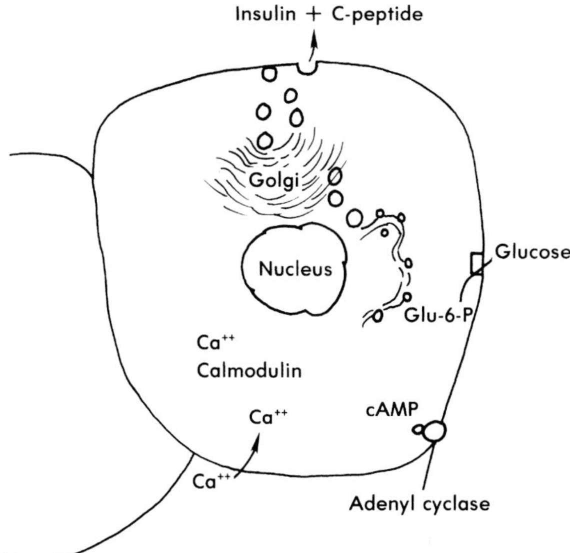

Fig. 60-4. The release of insulin from B cells is controlled at least by intracellular cAMP and Ca^{2+}. Although glucose is the predominant secretagog for insulin, many other metabolic or receptor-mediated events also modulate insulin secretion. Proinsulin is packaged from the endoplasmic reticulum after synthesis and moves through the Golgi body. Proinsulin is cleaved in the secretory or storage vesicles to yield C-peptide and insulin, which are released in equimolar quantities by exocytosis.

INSULIN RELEASE

Secretagogs
Metabolic

Glucose
Other hexoses (potentiate)
Hexosamines (potentiate)
Glycolytic products (potentiate)
Amino acids
Fatty acids
Ca^{2+} (ionic)
Calcium ionophores
Islet-activating protein

Receptor-mediated

Glucagon
GIP
β-Endorphin
β-Adrenergic agonists
Acetylcholine
Sulfonylurea
Gastrin
Secretin
CCK
Cortisol

Suppressors
Metabolic

D-Manno-heptulose
2-Deoxy-D-glucose
Diazoxide

Receptor-mediated

Somatostatin
α-Adrenergic agonists

Suppression of Electrical Activity
Cytoskeleton blockade

Diphanylhydantoin
Colchicine

long term, whereas the translational effects occur in the short term. Some evidence to support this conclusion is that the glucose-stimulated increase in the amount of preproinsulin mRNA is not observed until 2 hours after glucose administration, and it is then maintained for about 24 hours. On the other hand, after 1 hour, there is an increase in insulin biosynthesis without a change in the mRNA levels. Glucose also stimulates preproinsulin mRNA levels as well as secretion in human islets.[12] The effects of glucose on preproinsulin mRNA levels occur in two phases: an initial short-term phase involving posttranscriptional control, and a long-term regulation under transcriptional control. The insulin vesicles are stored in the cytoplasm in the webbing of the cytoskeleton and, under secretory stimuli, move to the plasma membrane, where the vesicle and plasma membranes fuse to release equimolar concentrations of insulin and C-peptide into the extracellular space. In the storage vesicles, the single chain of proinsulin is doubly cleaved to give the A and B chains of insulin (molecular weight 6 kd), bonded together by two disulfide bridges and the connecting chain, C-peptide. A third disulfide bond determines the shape of the A chain. In the vesicles, insulin is a hexamer coordinated by two Zn^{2+} ions. During release and dilution, the hexamer dissociates to the active monomeric form.[13]

Stored insulin is abundant, and the number of B cells in the normal pancreas far exceeds the number required for insulin release. When insulin release is maximally stimulated, rarely is more than 5% of the total insulin available released. As much as 95% of the normal pancreas can be resected without inducing insulin insufficiency or carbohydrate intolerance. The intracellular signals for the release of insulin are prompted by a movement of Ca^{2+} into the B cell and by the accumulation of the cyclic adenosine monophosphate (cAMP). Glucose enhances Ca^{2+} uptake from extracellular medium, as well as other secretagogs such as glyceraldehyde and sulfonylurea. Glucose may also cause a transient decrease in Ca^{2+} efflux and the closure of K^+ channels, which could cause the opening of Ca^{2+} channels.[14] At high glucose concentrations, insulin secretion agonists such as glucagon induce secretion by increasing cAMP concentration through protein phosphorylation. It is convenient to view Ca^{2+} and cAMP as the final events necessary for access to the insulin pool. Access to the Ca^{2+} and cAMP pools, in turn, can be achieved through a variety of routes, either receptor mediated or connected to the metabolism of the B cell[15] (Fig. 60-4). Pluralistic access to the insulin pool is important to explain even partially the wide range of secretagogs and inhibitors for the release of this crucial hormone. Glucose is one of the most important extracellular signals for insulin release (see accompanying box). On the other hand, after a normal mixed meal, plasma glucose levels reach only low peak values (6 to 7 mmol/L). These concentrations of extracellular glucose are usually able to elicit a very weak insulin response. Nevertheless, after ingestion of a mixed meal, a significant insulin response is obtained through different patterns, including acetylcholine, released at parasympathetic synapses of vagal efferents on B cells, and CCK, secreted through the nervous system that innervates the B cells. CCK, glucagon-like peptide 1, and gastric-inhibitory peptide (GIP) together act on the B cell through the bloodstream. GIP and glucagon-like peptide 1 stimulate adenylate cyclase. Acetylcholine and CCK act on phosphoinositide–specific phospholipase C, causing an increase in both phosphoinositide hydrolysis and the Ca^{2+} concentration.

The B cells are generally concentrated at the center of an islet, in close apposition to the arteriole that penetrates the islet to deliver blood first to its interior (see Fig. 60-3). These cells are coupled electrically to surrounding cells and have rich gap-junction contacts transmitting sizable molecules among B cells and other adjacent endocrine cells.[16] The box on p. 1207 outlines the major secretagogs and inhibitors of insulin release. The insulin leaving the islets, like all islet hormones, arrives at the liver through the portal vein. Approximately 50% of insulin is removed on the first pass through the liver, which may be considered the major site of action for insulin.

The least understood of the mechanisms for insulin release are the metabolic pathways. Clearly, flow of oxygen through the mitochondrial respiratory chain is critical, and lipoxygenase has been implicated.[17] It is possible that glucose has a membrane receptor that prompts release in addition to metabolic regulation. Although many hexoses and intermediates are secretagogs or facilitate glucose-mediated insulin release, galactose and 3-O-methlyglucose participate in glycolysis but do not promote insulin secretion. Also, some agents that block glycolysis do not block glucose-stimulated insulin release. Therefore, a glucose receptor has been suggested.[18] However, the nature of a receptor that responds in a concentration range for glucose of 5×10^{-3} to 15×10^{-3} mol/L is obscure at best. The dissociation constant for hormone receptors favors regulatory interaction at 10^{-8} to 10^{-9} mol/L. The high molecular concentration of glucose that affects insulin regulation is more consistent with allosteric interaction with an enzyme than with cell-surface or cytosolic receptor kinetics. In general, three routes of stimulation may be distinguished: *metabolic,* typified by glucose and amino acids; *receptor mediated,* typified by acetylcholine; and *ionic,* as in Ca^{2+} ionophores. Vagal stimulatory effects on insulin secretion are dramatic and may induce hypoglycemia with only the sight and smell of food. However, B cells can generally function in glucose homeostasis with or without this extraordinary amount of input. The checks and balances of insulin release are so numerous that failure of the B cell mass with glucose intolerance represents the collapse of a long series of protective endocrine and metabolic mechanisms.

The basal release of insulin averages 4 mU/min.[19] This level is biologically quite active. Therefore, insulin is important in basal metabolism and does not simply reduce excursions in the glucose concentration. When an appropriate stimulus is given, insulin is released in two phases. There is an initial or first-phase peak, which reaches about five times basal insulin within 3 to 5 minutes. This phase deteriorates and a second, sustained phase of insulin release continues for 60 to 70 minutes. This second phase is quantitatively much more substantial.[20] The biphasic contour (Fig. 60-5) suggests that insulin is stored in at least two compartments under somewhat different controls. Insulin release returns to basal level after either restoration of ambient glucose to normal levels or exhaustion of the B cell. Physiologic inhibitors do indeed modulate insulin release, but they are not important in a feedback loop. Insulin itself may not be directly involved in feedback, because infused insulin in vivo[21] can reduce insulin output but no such effect can be demonstrated with isolated islets in vitro.[22] All the modulators of insulin release are of modest importance compared with the primacy of glucose as the major regulator of B-cell function.

Insulin lowers plasma glucose level principally by facilitating the diffusion of glucose into tissues that have insulin receptors. After interaction with its receptors, a number of protein phosphorylations occur, and the entrance of glucose as glucose-6-phosphate is greatly accelerated.[23] The hormone promotes glycogen synthesis by reducing cAMP effects on glycogenolysis. Insulin also promotes amino acid uptake and protein synthesis and inhibits protein degradation. Fat synthesis is promoted by means of pyruvate dehydrogenase, and lipolysis is inhibited.[24] Insulin promotes the entry of K^+ and Mg^{2+} into cells, even in the absence of glucose (see box on p. 1207). The hormone generally supports cell growth and division by metabolic enhancement. Insulin is similar in primary structure to nerve growth factor, other growth factors, and relaxin. The wide array of insulin effects apparently does not have a common postreceptor second messenger. Rather, insulin has multiple intracellular actions after initial binding and

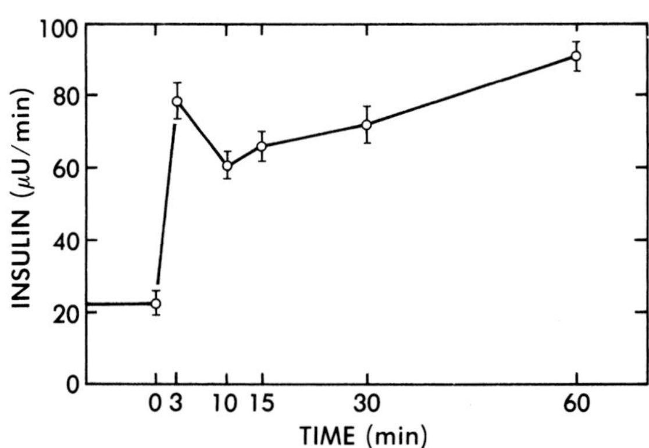

Fig. 60-5. Biphasic release of insulin after glucose stimulation is seen from either isolated islets of Langerhans, as in this figure, or from the in situ pancreas when pulsed with glucose. The initial sharp peak of insulin release at 3 minutes is followed by sustained insulin release, which peaks at 30 to 60 minutes. The significance of the biphasic nature of insulin secretion is probably great but is poorly understood. Multiple insulin pools have been proposed to explain the discontinuity of insulin release.

internalization of the insulin-receptor complex. Insulin is also associated with a reduction in intracellular cAMP.

Insulin is so critical to the existence of life forms with a circulatory system, and therefore with endocrine relationships, that its primary sequence is conserved with exquisite precision through speciation. Among mammals, there is significant variation only at amino acid residue numbers 8, 9, and 10 of the A chain.[25] Human and porcine insulins differ by only one amino acid. Insulin from fishes has significant biologic activity in humans (Fig. 60-6).

Although most tissues need insulin to modulate the metabolism of glucose, this hormone is not needed by the central nervous system. In fact, insulin does not readily pass the blood-brain barrier. Muscle tissue that has been physically conditioned by exercise has a great reduction in the need for insulin to transport glucose. Quantitatively, the most important site for insulin activity in metabolism is the liver, and the most important site for rapid reduction of plasma glucose is the fat cell mass.

INSULIN EFFECTS

Facilitates Entry Into Cells of

Glucose
Amino acids
K^+
Mg^{2+}

Enhances	**Inhibits**
↑ Glycogen synthesis	↓ Glycogenolysis
↑ Lipogenesis	↓ Lipolysis
↑ Protein synthesis	↓ Protein degradation
	↓ Gluconeogenesis
	↓ cAMP

Glucagon and the A Cell

The complementary hormone to insulin is glucagon, which is secreted by A cells and acts to raise plasma glucose level. Glucagon is a single peptide of 3.485 kd that has sequence homology with secretin, vasoactive intestinal peptide (VIP), GIP, growth hormone–releasing factor, and placental lactogen.[26] A prohormone is synthesized that yields glucagon in the secretory granules after proteolytic cleavage. In health, glucagon is clearly as important as insulin, but because it is not of primary importance in any common disease states, its discovery in 1923[27] received little notice. This crucial hormone has until recently been viewed as a probe to the primacy of insulin. However, glucagon in stress is so preponderant in driving catabolic metabolism that new knowledge concerning its actions and properties is received with great anticipation by those wishing to better understand stress physiology.

The principal stimulus for glucagon release is hypoglycemia. The mechanisms of release are probably similar to those of insulin but have been much less studied. Amino acids stimulate the release of both glucagon and insulin. The only gastrointestinal peptide known to stimulate glucagon secretion is CCK. Glucagon release is also prompted by epinephrine by means of α-adrenergic effects. Cortisol, growth hormone, and β-endorphin all promote glucagon release. Glucagon release is suppressed by hyperglycemia, somatostatin, secretin, and insulin. It also exercises feedback inhibition on its own secretion.[28] After a glucose challenge, the suppression of baseline glucagon release closely parallels insulin stimulation. The magnitude of the suppression is much greater after oral glucose intake than after intravenous delivery. The mirror image of insulin response is clear:

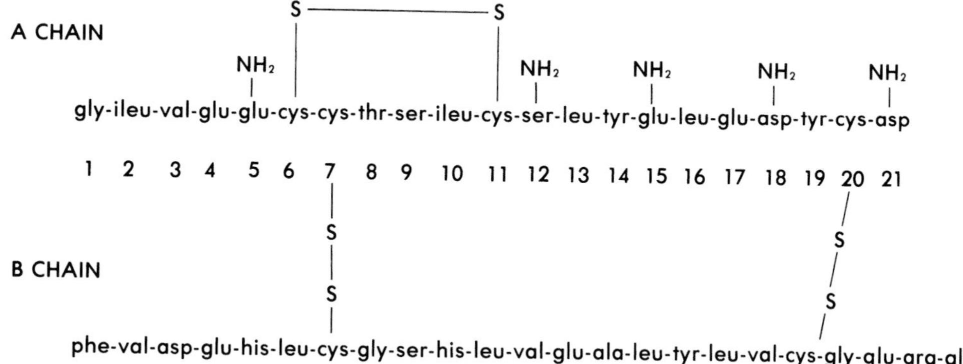

Fig. 60-6. The structure of insulin in all species is quite similar to that shown here for human insulin. Sequence variation among various species is most prominent at residues 8, 9, and 10 of the A chain. Both A and B chains are derived from the same proinsulin molecule by proteolytic removal of the C-peptide. The three sulfhydryl bridges coordinate the tertiary structure of the molecule.

1. Secretatogs
   a. Hypoglycemia
   b. Amino acids
   c. CCK
   d. α-Adrenergic agonists
   e. Cortisol
   f. Growth hormone
   g. β-Endorphin
2. Suppressors
   a. Hyperglycemia
   b. Insulin
   c. Secretin
   d. Somatostatin

Basal glucagon level is of great importance in countervailing the effects of insulin. At steady-state glucose level, basal insulin release describes an oscillation easily measured in portal venous blood. The period of the oscillation is about 10 minutes. Basal glucagon release follows a similar sine-wave variation, 180 degrees out of phase with that of insulin. The oscillatory delivery of insulin and glucagon to the liver cannot be explained on the basis of variable glucose delivery to the islets. Rather, an internal rhythm must be presumed in the islets themselves, one that does not require the circulatory system.[29] Despite the extensive communication among the cells within an islet, there is no evidence for linkage among individual islets. However, rhythmic basal insulin release can be seen in cultured islets in vitro. The mechanism for this biologic clock is not known.

Approximately 25% of the portal venous glucagon remains in the liver after one pass. The liver is the most important target tissue for this hormone; in the liver, specific receptors recognize portal venous glucagon and promote a rise in intracellular cAMP level. Glycogenolysis follows by enzyme activation by means of protein kinases. On a molar basis, glucagon is 20 to 30 times more potent than epinephrine in stimulating glycogenolysis. Gluconeogenesis is enhanced, whereas lipolysis in both the liver and periphery is stimulated by this hormone. Glucagon is not as pervasive in its cell membrane effects as insulin. There are, for example, no important ion movements associated with glucagon, and its does not stimulate cell division. In addition to its metabolic effects, however, glucagon is a powerful suppressor of pancreatic exocrine activity and a powerful smooth muscle antagonist in the gastrointestinal tract (see accompanying box). This property is used mostly in endoscopy and radiology, to temporarily paralyze the gut.

GLUCAGON EFFECTS

Enhances	Inhibits
Glycogenolysis	Glycogen synthesis
Lipolysis	Lipogenesis
Gluconeogenesis	
cAMP	

Somatostatin and PP

Somatostatin is released by islet D cells that lie in juxtaposition to, and often between, A and B cells. It was first recognized in the brain as a suppressor of growth hormone release. Somatostatin modulates insulin and glucagon release by inhibiting both. Its regulatory action in the islets may be more paracrine than endocrine. One pathway to the inhibition of insulin release may be by means of somatostatin. The release of somatostatin is prompted by glucose, arginine, leucine, and glucagon.[30]

PP is a hormone with a single peptide chain weighing 4.240 kd and is secreted by the F cells of the islets. PP bears sequence homology to glucagon and secretin. Its potency to promote hepatic glycogenolysis rivals that of glucagon. It also causes gallbladder relaxation, decreases intestinal motility, and suppresses gastric acid secretion. This intriguing peptide, described first in 1968,[31] does not have a clear place in metabolic regulation and gastrointestinal physiology. Assignment of importance or consignment to obscurity must await further investigation.

ISLETS IN HEALTH AND DISEASE

As reviewed in the previous section, the islets of Langerhans regulate metabolism with the object of maintaining plasma glucose level. The principal site for insulin and glucagon to accomplish this mission is the liver. At rest between meals, insulin and glucagon have a balanced, almost harmonic effect. After meals, the hormonal balance shifts according to the chemical nature of the meal to distribute the calorigenic nutrients for efficient use and storage. In prolonged fasting, glucagon is more important to support glucose synthesis from protein by gluconeogenesis and by hydrolysis of glycogen. Glucagon also permits use of the lipid stores. The glucose requirement in fasting is modest, and its provision generates little detriment to body protein. In times of severe stress or injury, glucagon is again important to provide the extra glucose synthesis needed for caloric consumption from protein by gluconeogenesis and by hydrolysis of glycogen. Therefore, the islet cell mass responds to disease states and metabolic derangements by ensuring a hormonal balance through insulin or glucagon release, which promotes the generation of endogenous fuel substrate.

The disease states of the endocrine pancreas are small in number, although they are great in terms of medical consequence. There are states of deficiency and neoplasia. The only spontaneous deficiency involves the B cells. No natural deficiency diseases are recognized for glucagon, somatostatin, or PP. However, each cell of the islet may become neoplastic as a benign or malignant tumor secreting isotopic (entopic) hormone, ectopic hormone, or no hormone.

Diabetes Mellitus

The B cells may be nearly eliminated, as occurs in type I insulinopenic diabetes mellitus, or may be functionally inadequate, as occurs in type II diabetes mellitus. In the latter condition, plasma insulin level may be normal or high, but insulin insensitivity in target tissues hampers glucose clearance, and hyperglycemia develops.

Type I or insulinopenic diabetes mellitus results from the loss of B cells in childhood or early adult life. There is a strong familial tendency in the autosomal recessive mode, with variable penetrance. Approximately 25% of patients with diabetes have one or more first-order relatives with the disease. Children whose fathers have diabetes have a 6.1% likelihood of acquiring the disease; offspring of mothers with diabetes have a diabetic incidence of only 1.3%. This disparity is not explained.[32] A close association with the antigens HLA-DR3 and HLA-DR4 has been noted. In families at risk for diabetes, the clinical disease is heralded for as long as a year by circulating autoantibodies to islet cells,[33] which are frequent in 65% to 85% of patients with diabetes. Although these antibodies are directed against all islet cells, the B cells are selectively destroyed by cell-mediated immunity in an insulitic process. The development of frank diabetes is also prefaced by a progressive decline in the first phase of insulin release. In a bold experiment, children with recently diagnosed diabetes were immunosuppressed with cyclosporine. After 1 year, a startling one half of those children were in remission and required no insulin.[34] These newer data conflict with the previous picture of diabetes developing as an acute illness, with perhaps a viral cause. There are, in fact, viruses that selectively destroy B cells in animals, and there are numerous B cell–specific toxins. Patients with familial diabetes may not accurately represent the larger number (50% to 75%) of spontaneous diabetes cases. The final common pathway to the disease is loss of B cells, and a variety of approaches to this path can be imagined. However, among the diabetes-prone families, the recognition of prediabetes as an autoimmune event offers the prospect of immune suppression to delay or eliminate the emergence of overt diabetes. Although insulin deficiency results in diabetes mellitus, several mutant insulins have been characterized. Both [Leu^{B25}] and [Ser^{B24}] insulin have been found in patients with diabetes; the latter results in a milder form of the disease.[35] Another important process in the development of type 1 diabetes is the balance between B-cell mass destruction through different temporal courses in different patients. In vitro and in vivo data prove that B-cells are able to repair themselves after damage. Islets from nonobese diabetic mice, isolated in the prediabetic period, can restore a normal insulin-release pattern in tissue culture. Glucose, nicotinamide, and branched chain amino acids can enhance B-cell ability to repair damage after toxic assault. Better understanding of this process and possible intervention in this delicate mechanism of B-cell repair could change the development of type 1 diabetes.[36]

Insulinoprenic type I diabetes, also called *juvenile-onset diabetes,* accounts for about 10% of the 200,000 new cases of diabetes diagnosed in the United States each year. Before the use of insulin, this acute illness was usually fatal, and the gene pool for diabetic propensity remained small. In the last 60 years, however, the gene pool has enlarged considerably as patients treated for diabetes have more consistently achieved reproductive maturity. What had been a devastating acute illness has now become an important chronic illness. When all patients with diabetes are grouped together, they represent 1% to 5% of the U.S. population. Diabetes is the leading cause of blindness in young Americans, and it is the most frequently reported diagnosis for patients beginning long-term dialysis for renal failure. The clinical ramifications of this disease are so extensive that it is appropriate to consider the condition as a syndrome rather than a single disease.

The most obvious effect of diabetes is hyperglycemia, which reflects the reduced capacity of glucose to enter cells that rely on insulin-receptor occupation for facilitated glucose diffusion. Renal tubular capacity to reabsorb glucose is exceeded at 180 to 200 mg/dl(10 mmol/L), and glycosuria follows. Glucose is osmotically important and causes osmotic diuresis. Hemoconcentration and dehydration follow because of the diuresis. Hyperosmolar effects are significant when plasma glucose level exceeds 540 mg/dl, where the 30 mmol/L glucose contributes 30 mOsm/L to the plasma osmolarity. Hyperosmolarity leads to coma, and the volume loss caused by osmotic diuresis leads to vascular collapse. Without treatment, hyperglycemia is fatal (Fig. 60-7).

The metabolic response to reduced glucose movement into cells is prompt, damaging, and potentially fatal (Fig. 60-8). Intracellular metabolic compartments perceive the mass-action message of insufficient glucose. Therefore, protein catabolism is accelerated to support gluconeogenesis. Nitrogen loss is massive and accompanied by substantial loss of potassium. The extra glucose leads to further increases in plasma glucose level. It is important to realize that the potentially fatal glucose level in the plasma of patients with uncontrolled diabetes does not represent ingested carbohydrate that arrives in the circulation directly from the jejunum. Rather, the source of the enormous glucose compartment in the plasma is endogenous, either glycogen or gluconeogenesis. The decrease in intracellular energy substrate also prompts lipolysis. The liberated glycerol participates in gluconeogenesis. Free fatty acids go to the liver, where β-oxidation in the mitochondria is associated with the release of acetoacetate and beta-hydroxybutyrate (ketogenic events). The generation of ketones involves acidic reactions sufficient to produce metabolic aci-

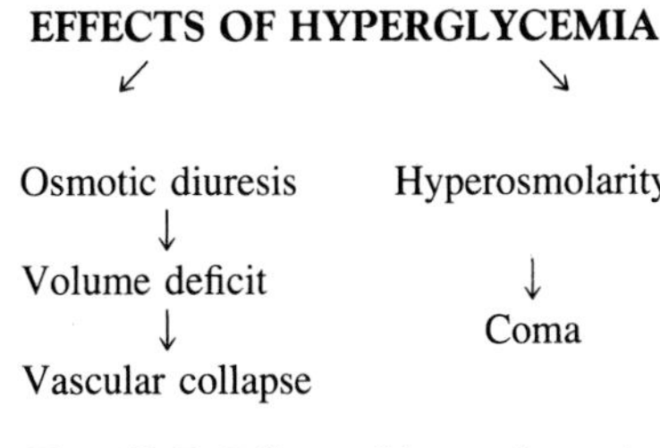

Fig. 60-7. Effects of hyperglycemia.

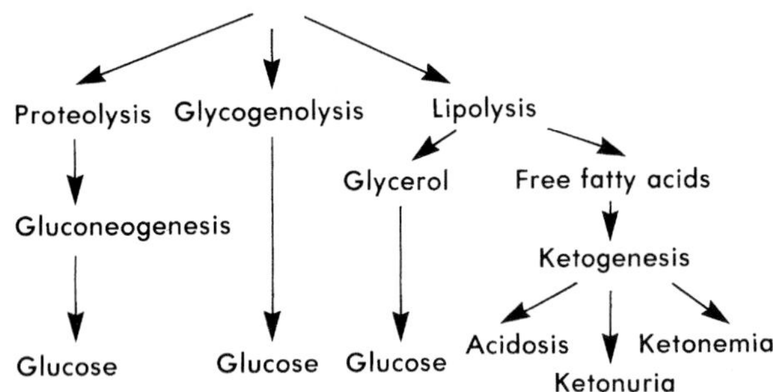

Fig. 60-8. When insulin levels are low, insulin mediation of glucose uptake in responsive tissues is greatly reduced, leading to a deficiency of intracellular glucose. The response to diminished intracellular carbohydrate is to increase the export of glucose from the liver by gluconeogenesis or glycogenolysis. In response to meager intracellular energy, substrate lipolysis is encouraged, with export of ketone bodies, acetoacetate, and β-hydroxybutyrate from the liver. Pathologically elevated plasma glucose level, abundant plasma ketones with ketonuria, and the metabolic acidosis that attends ketogenesis define hyperglycemic ketoacidosis.

dosis. There are no renal mechanisms to reabsorb these short carbon chains; therefore, ketonuria develops. Also, the ketones are volatile and may escape in expired air, lending a fruity odor to the breath. The released ketones are available for metabolism and energy generation. β-oxidation is the only event in the diabetic adaptation that helps to increase the generation of high-energy phosphate bonds. The respiratory response to the metabolic acidosis is hyperventilation in the form of air hunger called *Kussmaul-Kien respiration.* The clinical picture of diabetic ketoacidosis is now complete, with hyperglycemia, dehydration, ketoacidosis, ketonuria, polyuria, and Kussmaul-Kien respiration. If this metabolic nightmare is not corrected by insulin, coma, vascular collapse, and death follow.

Type II noninsulin-dependent diabetes mellitus is also called *adult-onset diabetes mellitus* or *nonketogenic diabetes.* This disease is quite distinct from type I diabetes and shares only the common feature of derangement of carbohydrate metabolism tending toward hyperglycemia. The consequences of the hyperglycemia in terms of vascular complications are quite similar in the two diseases. Whereas type I diabetes is marked by profound insulinopenia, type II diabetes is a condition in which the circulating insulin levels may be normal, or even greater than normal. The impact of circulating insulin in regulating total body carbohydrate metabolism is greatly diminished, however, and hyperglycemia develops. The presence of amyloid deposits, one of the common pathologic features of the islets of patients with type II diabetes, was originally described in 1901.[37] The major component of this amyloid tissue is a protein termed *islet amyloid polypeptide,* which represents a new B-cell secretory product whose activities are unknown. The production of the islet amyloid polypeptide is not necessarily the cause of the type II diabetes, but it may be the consequence of a derailed behavior of B cells. Studies seeking a deeper knowledge of this protein are underway.[38] The sensitivity of peripheral tissue receptors for insulin seems greatly diminished in patients with type II diabetes, and there has been considerable confusion regarding whether this disease arises because of any real pathology of the B cells of the islets of Langerhans or whether it indeed represents a receptor problem at the periphery. Although defects in the insulin receptor may cause insulin resistance, the primary cause of insulin resistance in patients with type II diabetes is believed to be in one of the fast-receptor sites, such as the glucose transport system, which is characterized by decreased activity and decreased number of transporters in cases of insulin resistance. Recent studies have shown that an abnormal regulation and expression of a specific glucose transporter isoform, GLUT4, that mediates insulin-stimulated glucose transport in adipose and muscle cells, is responsible for insulin resistance in adipose tissue and possibly muscle tissue as well.[39,40] Because insulin secretion and reception are so tightly linked, it is difficult to divorce the two events to obtain a better, if arbitrary, distinction between type I and II diabetes. Type II diabetes, though, does occur in older patients, with a striking propensity for obese patients. The hyperglycemia and hyperinsulinemia can be resolved in many obese patients simply by lowering the fat stores through a reducing diet. There is a familial tendency in adult-onset diabetes, but it more closely parallels the familial incidence of obesity. Control of hyperglycemia may require supplemental insulin in these patients with type II diabetes mellitus, but the use of insulin still should not cause confusion of the illness with the type I variant. In type II diabetes, the insulin is not required to sustain life but merely to better regulate plasma glucose level. Therefore, the term *noninsulin-dependent diabetes mellitus* is still applicable to type II diabetes.

The principal feature of type II diabetes that causes clinical trouble is hyperglycemia. This can be associated with a striking and life-threatening syndrome of hyperosmolar coma when the blood sugar level exceeds 800 mg/dl. The increase in blood glucose level is osmotically quite important and can literally draw water out of the brain cells, resulting in a comatose state. However, ketosis is not associated with this drastic derangement in carbohydrate metabolism in which glucose clearance is so inadequate as to potentially lead to hyperosmolar death.

This lack of ketosis is not completely understood. The dehydration that is associated with the polyuria of hyperosmolar coma has been implicated. It is more likely that the hyperglycemic crisis in type II diabetes is unique because insulin is indeed present in substantial quantities, unlike the situation in the hyperglycemic crisis of type I diabetes. The impact of insulin in diminishing lipolysis is preserved in larger measure in type II diabetes. The adipocytes are 20 to 30 times more sensitive to the antilipolytic effects of insulin than to the facilitated entry of glucose under the influence of insulin. It is therefore likely that, although a hyperglycemic crisis has followed because of poor insulin effect in type II diabetes, lipolysis and thus ketogenesis cannot occur. The treatment of nonketotic hyperosmolar coma in type II diabetes is directed toward fluid resuscitation and sufficient insulin to clear the extracellular compartment of the extraordinary concentrations of free glucose.

Complications of Diabetes

Diabetes is a truly devastating disease in terms of curtailment of longevity and quality of life as a consequence of its complications, and not as a consequence of its more dramatic metabolic manifestations such as ketoacidosis or nonketotic hyperosmolar coma. It is the leading cause of blindness in young Americans and may soon become the most common diagnosis for patients in long-term dialysis programs for end-stage renal disease. Although diabetes affects less than 10% of the population of the United States, it is the eighth leading cause of death. About half of patients with diabetes as a group die of coronary disease, whereas most patients with juvenile-onset diabetes die of ramifications of renal failure. The complications are not inherently different in type I and II diabetes and may be considered to be neural, vascular, or infectious. These three categories are interrelated but probably independent in their genesis. Nonetheless, they are all related to abnormal glucose metabolism.

Neuropathy is manifested by autonomic motor and sensory problems. The autonomic problems include gastroparesis, impotence, orthostatic hypotension, and diarrhea. Sensory deficits include position sense and pin-prick sensation. Radiculopathy is seen, and the pain can be disabling. The sensory deficit problems contribute to lower extremity injury, which does not heal because of poor blood supply. Such extremities tend to become infected because of poor response to bacteria, with consequent limb loss.

The cause of the neuropathy is not well understood and tends to parallel the vascular complications in the course of the natural history of diabetes. However, recent work implicates abnormal metabolism of sugar alcohols through the enzyme aldose reductase. This enzyme is the rate-limiting step in the pathway to sugar alcohols, and that pathway is confined to Schwann cells, spinal roots, and lens epithelium. The enzyme is probably not abnormal in patients with diabetes, but mass-action events in hyperglycemia and intracellular glucoprevia activate this otherwise exotic pathway. The nature of the toxicity of sugar alcohols in these tissues has not been elucidated, but inhibition of aldose reductase has been clinically useful in improving autonomic function and in relieving the pain that can be a manifestation of sensory neuropathy.[41]

The vascular lesions of diabetes are numerous and perhaps distinct in development. There is an acceleration of atherosclerosis in patients with diabetes along lines that are indistinguishable from the peripheral vascular lesions seen in patients without carbohydrate intolerance. These lesions are associated with the hyperlipemia that accompanies diabetic metabolism. However, disease of small vessels develops along lines that are distinctive to diabetes.[42] Capillary basement membranes thicken through the course of diabetes. Although this thickening may be something of an exaggeration of normal aging, the implications for the patient with diabetes are important. If the capillary basal lamina is considered to be the framework for wound healing and the gate that must be passed in the diapedesis of inflammatory cells, the stiff, thickened layer may be seen as a significant part of other diabetic problems. The glycopeptides of basal lamina have not been exclusively studied in diabetes, but the opportunity for abnormal glycosylation is certainly great in hyperglycemia and has been observed in patients with this disease. The covalent addition of glucose molecules to protein normally requires a glycosyl transferase. However, enzymatic glycosylation, like all enzymatically catalyzed reactions, favors through catalysis a reaction that would normally occur without the enzyme, although at a much slower rate. In the presence of persistently high ambient glucose concentrations, glucose molecules apparently can be added to the amino-acid backbone of many peptides to create new and potentially pathologic glycopeptides. The glycosolated hemoglobin, HbA1C, is easily measured, and the concentration of this substance in the blood of a patient with diabetes has a direct correlation with the degree of ambient hyperglycemia in recent weeks.[43] Therefore, a high HbA1C level means that control of hyperglycemia has been poor not just on the day of blood sampling but within preceding weeks as well. Although HbA1C has not itself been associated with any malfunction of hemoglobin, the potential importance of glycosylation of other peptides in the evolution of diabetic pathology has been suggested. This glycosylated product can be measured readily and reflects the degree of hyperglycemia and thus the degree of diabetic control in recent weeks. The ultimate significance of glycosylation in diabetic pathology remains to be determined.

Angiopathy in the retina takes the form of microaneurysms of capillaries. These lesions can rupture, with escape of blood and opacification of the eye. Great progress has been made in controlling these lesions by photocoagulation with lasers to thrombose the aneurysms before they burst. Cataract formation is also prevalent in patients with diabetes as a consequence of either derangement of carbohydrate metabolism or accelerated aging.

The renal vasculopathy seen in diabetics was first described by Kimmelstiel and Wilson in 1936. Accumulation of basement membrane material in the mesangium of the glomerulus may be either nodular or diffuse. This glomerulosclerosis leads to proteinuria and eventually to azotemia. All patients with insulin-dependent diabetes who have survived 20 years or longer manifest the microscopic lesion, and half have significant renal impairment. The kidney may also be affected by hypertension, atherosclerosis, and infection in diabetes. End-stage renal disease in patients with diabetes is treated with dialysis and renal transplantation.

Diagnosis and Treatment of Diabetes

The diagnosis of diabetes is precise and easily accomplished. Patients with polyuria, polydipsia, and weight loss, and especially those with visual disturbances or frequent pyogenic infections, should be evaluated for hyperglycemia. A fasting blood sugar level ≥140 mg/dl on more than one occasion defines carbohydrate intolerance and mandates its evaluation by oral glucose-tolerance testing. After an overnight fast by a patient who has previously had unrestricted calories and unrestricted exercise, 75 g glucose is given by mouth, and the blood glucose level is measured periodically for the next 2 hours. A value of 200 mg/dl or greater at 2 hours and at one previous time point defines diabetes mellitus. The test is invalidated by stress from infection, surgery, or trauma; prolonged fasting; prolonged physical inactivity; and glucocorticoid or thiazide administration. Therefore, testing of hospitalized patients as a group is inappropriate. Furthermore, the benefit of diagnosing mild diabetes mellitus in truly symptom-free patients is meager in that no treatment is indicated. Oral glucose tolerance testing is therefore not a routine screening test.[44]

The treatment of type II adult-onset diabetes mellitus in many, if not most, cases involves caloric restriction and weight loss to restore carbohydrate tolerance. If insulin is required, the goals and considerations for treatment become the same as for type I diabetes. The use of oral hypoglycemic agents (e.g., tolbutamide) has been less important recently, because the benefit to patients in the long term has been difficult to document and there has been more than a suggestion that vascular complications are made worse.[45] Perhaps oral agents were misused by patients as an apparently simple alternative to the rigors of dieting. Therefore, patients receiving oral agents may have represented a rather noncompliant population. At any rate, when dietary measures fail to control type II diabetes, the use of insulin to manage hyperglycemia is becoming more commonplace.

The goals of diabetic management are to keep blood glucose levels normal, to recognize and treat complications promptly, and to enhance the lifestyle of patients with this disease. A significant advance has been realized in recent years by improved monitoring of plasma glucose levels. Traditionally patients with diabetes estimated blood glucose control by monitoring the presence of glucose in the urine with test strips impregnated with glucose oxidase or tubules that tested for glucose as a reducing substance. When plasma glucose level exceeded the maximum for renal tubular reabsorption (180 mg/dl or 10 mmol/L), glucose spill in the urine occurred. The greater the plasma glucose level, the greater was the renal loss. Therefore, the more intense the glucose reaction in urine, the greater was the need for insulin administration. Despite the usefulness of glycosuria monitoring to determine insulin needs in most patients with diabetes, it must be emphasized that its correlation with the status of glucose intolerance is generally unreliable in renal disease, pregnancy, and unstable or brittle diabetes.

Although urinary glucose is preferred in monitoring patients who do not require insulin, blood glucose measurement at home is becoming the recommended parameter for insulin administration. Capillary blood obtained by finger stick is made to react with glucose oxidase on paper strips and is read by a color chart or in a reflectance meter. Plasma glucose level is usually about 15% higher than these whole-blood measurements. Home blood glucose monitoring offers precise monitoring for extremely close glucose control.

Another tactic to quantitate the precision of glucose control is the measurement of HbA1c. As previously indicated, this glycosylated hemoglobulin is generated by nonenzymatic means, has a relatively long half-life, and is directly proportional to average ambient glucose level. Chromatographic analysis of HbA1c reflects the accumulation of the glycoprotein in recent weeks above the customary 4% of total hemoglobin. The accumulation of HbA1c is an excellent parameter of glucose control through time.

The use of home glucose monitoring and precise review of management by measuring HbA1c are only appropriate in highly trained patients with diabetes. The training of patients with diabetes to become actively involved in the management of their disease has been greatly promoted and advanced by the American Diabetes Association. From a very early age, the patient is an active participant in therapy, recognition of complications, general health maintenance, and life goals. There are instructional peer group camps for children, instructional programs for all ages, mutual support groups, and active encouragement for patients to understand and question the scientific progress being made in the area of diabetes.

Dietary measures to limit disposable glucose have recently been greatly liberalized to permit the patient with diabetes more freedom. The effect has been to generally improve adherence by better-trained patients to a more acceptable dietary regimen. Carbohydrates constitute 45% to 60% of daily calories, fat provides 30% to 35%, and protein yields 12% to 20%. Total calories are carefully prescribed on the basis of physical activity.

Appropriate insulin therapy necessitates a familiarity with the various forms available. Insulin is purified from beef or pork pancreas and exists in several modifications. When given subcutaneously, regular, crystalline insulin has its onset of action at 30 to 60 minutes, peaks at 3 to 6 hours, and has a duration of action of 6 to 10 hours. Neutral protamine Hagedorn (NPH) insulin is complexed for slower absorption and has its onset of action at 1½ to 3 hours, peaks at 6 to 12 hours, and has a duration of action of 18 to 24 hours. Other forms are available for special purposes, but regular and NPH insulin form the basis for most diabetic management. Some patients acquire allergies to the protein sequence of animal insulin. Porcine insulin differs by only one amino acid from human insulin, but standard preparations are contaminated with proinsulin, which is antigenically quite distinct in the C-peptide region. Porcine insulin can be more highly purified for allergic patients. Recombinant DNA technology now offers human insulin for therapy in patients with significant allergy to animal insulins.

Maintenance insulin is administered to keep the plasma glucose level below 150 mg/dl and above 80 mg/dl. Insulin is usually administered subcutaneously as a single morning dose, with a supplemental evening dose as needed. The dosage in type I diabetes varies from 15 to 90 NPH U/day. For the patient without a pancreas, who lacks the countervening effects of glucagon, 15 to 20 U/day is generally sufficient. The management of ketoacidosis is a special case for insulin administration. The acidosis diminishes tissue sensitivity to insulin. Therefore, extremely large amounts of insulin are required. The objectives in treating ketoacidosis are rehydration, restoration of normal plasma pH, reduction in plasma glucose level, and replacement of glycolytic pathways for kegenic pathways by moving glucose into cells. Rehydration is commenced with normal saline solution at 1 L/hr until heart rate, blood pressure, and urinary output suggest improvement in volume status. In adults, 2 to 3 L is commonly needed. Hypotonic saline solution (0.45%) is given at a rate of 1 L every 2 to 4 hours to resuscitate and reduce the hyperosmolarity that follows the osmotic diuresis and high glucose levels. When plasma glucose level falls to 300 mg/dl, glucose should be added to the intravenous infusion. If the arterial pH is less than 7.1, buffering with intravenous bicarbonate is indicated. As the plasma glucose moves into cells under the influence of insulin, potassium is shifted also. Therefore, vigorous potassium replacement is necessary.

The regimen for insulin administration in ketoacidosis is disputed among clinicians. Basically, the glucose level must be lowered in a patient with rapidly changing insulin sensitivity, but without inducing an overshoot and potentially fatal hypoglycemia. A safe approach calls for 20 U regular insulin administered intravenously, followed by an insulin drip (100 U in 500 ml 0.45% saline solution) at 50 to 75 ml/hr. Blood glucose level must be measured every 30 to 60 minutes until the insulin infusion rate stabilizes. The fatal components of ketoacidosis are dehydration and acidosis. There is no need to cause the glucose level to plummet in a short time. In fact, rapid reduction can lead to fluid shifts, with cerebral edema or fatal hypoglycemia resulting.

Insulin administration in the patient with diabetes who is undergoing surgery varies depending on the complexity of the operation and the time it takes to perform. If the procedure is minor and the operation is performed early in the morning, the insulin dose is delayed until the procedure is completed. For major procedures involving a general anesthetic, a highly workable regimen calls for half the usual morning dose to be given subcutaneously as NPH, continuous 5% dextrose intravenous infusion, and monitoring of the plasma glucose every 6 hours. Insulin is given to keep the glucose level between 150 and 250 mg/dl. After surgery, insulin dosages according to urinary glucose are not as precise as are dosages according to plasma glucose level. Continuous insulin infusion along with 5% dextrose infusion is appropriate in monitored environments and may replace intermittent insulin administration just before and after the operation. Surgical patients undergoing prolonged operations or undue stress may require 25% or 50% more insulin than usual.

To attain a constancy of plasma glucose level impossible with bolus injection, continuous subcutaneous insulin infusion was recently developed. A programmable pump delivers short-acting regular insulin by means of a subcutaneous cannula. The baseline delivery rate can be increased to cover for the increased carbohydrate absorption after meals. Continuous subcutaneous insulin infusion and home glucose monitoring offer the greatest precision in control of ambient glucose. The precision can be documented by tracking HbA1c levels. However, the impact of this precision on preventing or slowing the development of diabetic complications has not been particularly gratifying.[46]

An unstated belief has long prevailed in the management of diabetes that the complications associated with this disease are the consequence of inferior compliance by the patient and therefore of inadequate control of blood glucose level. By implication, perfect control of glucose levels with supplemental insulin should eliminate complications. Although there is some basis for this belief, it cannot be absolutely true. Vascular and retinal complications progress even in patients treated with infusion pumps. To explain the syndrome of diabetes mellitus, there is no reason to propose that the loss of B cells leads to a deficiency of any hormone other than insulin. However, the exquisite balance between insulin and glucagon metabolism that occurs in the patient without diabetes has not been achieved by exogenous insulin delivery. Plasma glucose level is merely a crude approximation of the profound coordination that exists between insulin and glucagon release and its effects on the body's metabolic compartments and the movement of substrate through those compartments.

Until the interaction of A and B cells is more completely understood and mechanically reproducible, transplantation of islets of Langerhans may offer an option for normal glucose homeostasis in patients with diabetes. In rodent models of diabetes caused by streptozocin, syngeneic islets purified from the pancreas of a healthy animal can be transplanted into the liver through the portal vein. Treated animals are permanently replenished and normoglycemic.[47,48] Apparently, loss of innervation, acinar relationships, and the introduction of heterotopic relationships do not affect the capacity of the transplanted islets to serve the endocrine needs of affected animals. However, the animals with transplants have a distinct advantage with respect to diabetic rats treated with exogenous insulin. Rats with streptozocin-induced diabetes maintained on a regimen of insulin eventually show retinal and renal changes that resemble those seen in humans. Transplantation of islets of Langerhans can arrest and even reverse these changes.[49,50] Therefore, the prospect looms for controlling the diabetic syndrome in its entirety, rather than controlling only the gross excursions of plasma glucose level. The rodent experience with transplantation has been extended to autografts in dogs, but not yet successfully to humans.

Allografting of islets has generally failed in all species, despite of the use of immunosuppression effective for renal or cardiac grafting. Mere immunogenicity of islets seems extreme as an explanation for this failure, but a more precise hypothesis has not been offered. Extensive work currently addresses the problem of islet immunogenicity, which can be reduced by tissue culture, carrier lymphocyte depletion, ultraviolet irradiation, and elimination of class II antigen–bearing cells by immunotoxins.[51] Another problem in humans is more one of mechanics than species biology, in that sufficient islet mass has not yet been retrievable from human pancreas. Pancreatic transplantation remains the only method available today to successfully substitute the endocrine pancreas and reverse the diabetic condition to a normal glucose metabolism. Pancreatic transplantation was originally reported in 1967 at the University of Minnesota. Since then, and especially during the past 10 years, more than 6000 cases have been reported worldwide. Pancreatic transplantation today carries a 5-year patient survival greater than 70%, and a graft survival greater than 60%. Recipients of a pancreas graft for diabetes are insulin free, and recent research shows a positive impact of the new pancreas on the secondary complications of type I diabetes, in particular neuropathy and microangiopathy.[52,53] Pancreatic transplantation is currently offered to patients with uremic diabetes in need of a renal transplant or who received a kidney graft in the past. In some selected nonuremic patients with diabetes affected especially by extremely brittle glucose control, frequent hypoglycemia, and severe neuropathy manifesting as hypoglycemia unawareness, pancreatic transplantation remains the only logical therapeutic alternative. New options in the fight to cure diabetes, such as gene therapy, continue to be aggressively pursued and could become available to prevent the disease entirely in the future.

ENDOCRINE TUMORS OF THE PANCREAS

The rich endocrine resources found within the pancreas can generate a wide variety of syndromes and clinical conundrums when one or more of the cell lines becomes neoplastic (Table 60-2). The resulting tumors may secrete hormones not normally released from the endocrine pancreas, in which case the secretions are ectopic. Although endocrine tumors of the pancreas are rare, they have taught us a great deal about the nature of endocrinology in health and disease. For example, hypergastrinemia, first described by Zollinger and Ellison[54] in 1955, has despite its rarity greatly advanced our understanding of acid-peptic ulceration of the stomach. Proinsulin was first discovered in secretions of an insulinoma and introduced the concept of large–molecular weight gene products that are subsequently tailored before secretion.[4]

Our understanding of the nature of endocrine tumors has been greatly advanced by the APUD concept of Pearse and Polak.[55] The capacity to diagnose these tumors has been profoundly enhanced by the availability of radioimmunoassays for the measurement of the endocrine products. Localization of endocrine tumors has been

Table 60-2. Pancreatic Endocrine Neoplasia

Syndrome/ Cell of Origin	Pathology	Metabolic Change	Hormone	Symptoms
B	Adenoma Carcinoma (10%) Hyperplasia	Hypoglycemia Glycogenesis Gluconeogenesis Lipolysis Ketogenesis	Insulin Proinsulin	Those of hypoglycemia
A	Carcinoma (70%) Hyperplasia	Hyperglycemia Glycogenolysis Lipolysis Ketogenesis Gastrointestinal motor changes	Glucagon Enteroglucagon	Dermatitis Ileus Constipation
D	Carcinoma Adenoma	Mixed, mild glucose Biliary Pancreatic exocrine	Somatostatin Insulin Glucagon	Cholelithiasis Steatorrhea Dyspepsia
F	Adenoma	?	PP	None
? Zollinger-Ellison	Carcinoma (80%) Adenoma Hyperplasia	H^+ secretion	Gastrin	Acid-peptic ulceration Diarrhea
? Verner-Morrison	Carcinoma (50%) Adenoma	Intestinal secretion Gastric secretion Hypokalemia	VIP	Diarrhea Hypochlorhydria

tremendously aided by selective venous catheterization coupled with radioimmunoassay to identify the source of the abnormal concentrations of the hormones found in circulating blood. Localization and logistics for removal of endocrine tumors have been aided considerably by precise arteriography, ultrasonography, and computed tomographic imaging of the pancreas.[56] Unfortunately, a significant number of pancreatic endocrine tumors are malignant, with a propensity toward early metastasis.

Types of Pancreatic Endocrine Tumors

Insulinoma

Insulinomas, the most common of the pancreatic endocrine tumors, arise from the B cells of the islets. Approximately 80% are solitary and benign; the incidence of malignancy is about 10%. The remainder are either multiple benign adenomas or islet cell hyperplasia causing hyperinsulinism. In infants, hyperinsulinism is usually a result of adenomatous hyperplasia of B cells (nesideoblastosis). Insulinomas are small; about 40% are 1 cm or less in diameter. Tumors are distributed in almost equal numbers throughout the head, body, and tail of the pancreas. Only 1% or fewer of all insulinomas are ectopic, and these are found close to the pancreas in most instances. Multiple endocrine neoplasia type 1 syndrome occurs in 4% of patients with insulinomas (see Chapter 61).

The major signs and symptoms of insulinoma are a result of the effects of hypoglycemia (from the hyperinsulinemia) on the central nervous system. These include apathy, sluggishness, irritability, excitement, changes in behavior, and occasionally convulsions and coma. Hypoglycemia also induces a release of epinephrine, which causes sweating, nervousness, tremor, palpitation, hunger, and pallor. The classic diagnostic criteria (Whipple's triad) are still valid. Whipple's triad includes central nervous system symptoms brought on by fasting, a fasting blood glucose level less than 50 mg/dl, and complete reversal of all symptoms by intravenous infusion of glucose.

Insulin levels are high relative to the blood glucose concentration. The insulin/glucose ratio is normally less than 0.4, but in patients with insulinoma the ratio is often close to 1 or even greater. The measurement of elevated plasma proinsulin levels is also helpful in the diagnosis of insulinoma. Furthermore, malignant tumors can be differentiated from benign islet cell lesions by documenting the greater percentage of proinsulin in the total insulin immunoactivity typically seen in patients with malignant lesions.

The traditional diagnostic test for insulinoma is the demonstration of fasting hypoglycemia (less than 50 mg/dl). Fasting is continued for 72 hours, or until hypoglycemic symptoms appear. Hypoglycemia occurs in two thirds of patients by 24 hours and in 95% by 48 hours. During fasting, insulin levels remain elevated in patients with insulinoma because of the autonomous nature of the insulin secretion. Provocation tests for insulin release (e.g., tolbutamide, glucagon, leucine, arginine) have been used to make the diagnosis of insulinoma but are thought to be of little value, because serum insulin levels can be measured directly. The infusion of secretagogs in healthy patients should not result in pathologically low blood glucose levels. However, secretagogs may provoke an insulinoma to release profoundly pathologic amounts of insulin, with consequent hypoglycemia.

Selective angiography with subtraction and magnification techniques is the best method of preoperative localization of an insulinoma. The success rate of localizing these tumors approaches 90%. Selective pancreatic vein catheterization and venous sampling for insulin assay have also been used, with considerable success, to diagnose and localize the site of insulinomas. Ultrasonography and computed tomography have been used to localize these lesions, but in comparison with the other diagnostic modalities available, they are of limited usefulness.

Because they are predominantly benign, insulinomas are the only pancreatic endocrine tumors that can frequently be cured by surgery. Depending on location, enucleation or distal pancreatectomy is the treatment of choice. It is rarely necessary to perform a pancreaticoduodenectomy as the initial procedure for a small tumor of the head of the pancreas. The adjunctive therapeutic agent of choice in patients with metastases is streptozocin, with a response rate approaching 50%. In patients in whom persistent hypoglycemia poses a problem after presumably successful removal of insulinoma and in patients with metastases, diazoxide is frequently effective in suppressing insulin release.

Gastrinoma (Zollinger-Ellison Syndrome)

The first of the endocrine tumor syndromes identified in pancreatic islets was reported by Zollinger and Ellison[52] in 1955. The tumors responsible for this syndrome (gastrinomas) not only occur in pancreatic islets but also may be found as isolated lesions within the proximal duodenum or in its vicinity. The cell that gives rise to gastrinoma has not been identified. Gastrin is not a normal product of the islets of Langerhans. The gastrinoma syndrome results from excessive quantities of gastrin released from these tumors and is usually manifested clinically by virulent acid-peptic ulceration of the upper gastrointestinal tract. Such ulceration may be found in the first portion of the duodenum, where other forms of acid-peptic disease commonly occur; not infrequently, however, ulcers may occur in aberrant regions, such as the distal duodenum and jejunum.[57] These ulcers are usually single, but on occasion they may be multicentric. Generally, the ulcer precedes identification of the tumor by 3 to 5 years; on occasion, the ulcer itself is totally asymptomatic and is discovered accidentally. In approximately 20% of patients, diarrhea with steatorrhea is the only clinical symptom of the syndrome; this presumably occurs because of excessive acid production of the stomach, which inactivates pancreatic enzymes and thereby inhibits fat digestion and absorption by the duodenum and jejunum.

Approximately one third of patients with hypergastrinemia caused by gastrinoma have relatives with endocrinopathies. This condition is commonly suspected because of refractory or recurrent acid-peptic disease. Upper gastrointestinal x-ray films frequently show a suspicious multiplicity of ulcers throughout the duodenum and even the proximal jejunum. Hypertrophic mucosal folds are evident in the stomach as a result of the hypergastrinemia. Before the availability of radioimmunoassay, enabling measurement of serum gastrin levels, the clinical diagnosis of gastrinoma was made on the basis of gastric analysis. The high volume of gastric secretion in patients with gastrinoma displayed an acid output that approached the physiologic maximum elicited by histamine derivatives. Currently, the diagnosis is made on the basis of the demonstration of hypergastriemia under fasting conditions. A serum gastrin level in excess of 200 pg/ml is suggestive of this syndrome. When gastrin levels exceed 100,000 pg/ml, extensive tumoral involvement, including hepatic metastasis, is highly probable. For equivocal fasting gastrin levels, provocative testing with secretin has been useful. A rise of at least 100 pg/ml from a fasting baseline after 2 U/kg secretin given as an intravenous bolus is diagnostic of the disease. Gastrin levels may also be elevated in some patients with hyperplasia of the G cells in the antrum. In this circumstance, however, serum gastrin does not change during secretin provocation.[58]

The ulcerogenic gastrinoma may be localized in approximately one third of cases by means of angiography.[59] Computed tomography often demonstrates pancreatic tumors if they are larger than 2 cm. Successful localization of pancreatic tumors by computed tomography approaches 32% for primary pancreatic tumors.[60] Noninvasive preoperative ultrasonography in the intact patient has not been as successful as desired; however, intraoperative ultrasonography has been successful in identifying lesions otherwise not obvious. Percutaneous transhepatic portal and pancreatic venous sampling for gastrin can also localize the source of systemic hypergastrinemia.[61]

Hypergastrinemia caused by gastrinoma is ideally treated by complete resection of the gastrinoma. Unfortunately, this is possible in only approximately 20% of cases, because the gastrinomas may be multiple or metastatic at diagnosis. Until recently, total gastrectomy was uniformly accepted as the treatment of choice to control the acid-peptic disease in patients for whom complete tumor excision was not possible. The concept of end-organ ablation by surgical removal has been challenged with the development of H_2-receptor antagonist therapy.[62] Parietal cell vagotomy can improve the effectiveness of cimetidine therapy,[63] but tumor plus end-organ ablation appears to be the only secure procedure to restore serum gastrin levels to normal. Of interest, an effect of the stomach on enhancing tumor growth has been proposed[64]; if the stomach is removed, tumor growth is slowed. Because 80% of gastrinomas are malignant, metastatic disease is not uncommon. In this circumstance, palliation with streptozocin has produced a positive response in about half of the patients with metastatic gastrinoma so treated. For a more comprehensive discussion of gastrinoma, see Chapter 16.

Glucagonoma

In glucagonoma, a neoplastic condition of the A cells of the islets of Langerhans, the entopic hormone glucagon is released. These tumors are malignant approximately two thirds of the time, with early metastases to regional lymph nodes or the liver. Distant metastases are uncommon. The tumors are more frequently found in the tail of the pancreas, where there is the largest representation of A cells.

Glucagonoma causes a striking clinical syndrome manifested biochemically by hyperglycemia as a result of hyperglucagonemia. Patients with the syndrome sustain marked weight loss and demonstrate glossitis, frequent venous thrombosis, depression, and diarrhea. The most striking feature of this syndrome is called *necrolytic migratory erythema*.[65] This skin lesion consists of erythematous macules and pustules together with flaccid bullae. The necrolytic pattern is present on portions of the skin that are easily traumatized. Histologically, there is superficial epidermal necrolysis and severe inflammation of the dermis with cellular infiltration. There is no explanation for this dermatologic phenomenon, which resolves after resection of the glucagonoma. The patients also demonstrate a normochromic, normocytic anemia. The hyperglycemia is not usually particularly severe. The metabolic consequences of hyperglucagonemia include rapid movement of the plasma amino acids into glucoenogenic pathways in the hepatic cytosol. The consumption of amino acids for gluconeogenesis depletes the circulating pool of amino acids and results in hypoaminoacidemia. This pool is not rapidly replenished by a complementary catabolism of muscle protein. The degree of hyperglucagonemia would be expected to cause a much sharper rise in blood glucose level, but this is partially compensated for by a slight hyperinsulinism that arises because of the hyperglycemia and also because glucagon is a secretagog for insulin. Although glucagon does not directly promote loss of muscle protein into the amino acid pool, the brisk gluconeogenesis deprives skeletal muscle of circulating amino acids that might be applied to muscle anabolism. Therefore, muscle wasting and weakness are quite prominent. In many ways, patients with glucagonoma resemble chronically stressed patients who have received inadequate nutritional support.

When the disease is suspected, diagnosis is established by radioimmunoassay for glucagon.[66] In cases of marginal elevation of glucagon level, pathologic overresponse to arginine can be demonstrated. Intravenous tolbutamide similarly causes a spectacular rise in glucagon level in patients with glucagonoma. Once glucagonoma has been diagnosed, anatomic localization by computed axial tomography has been useful, because the tumors are frequently rather large in their position in the body and tail of the pancreas. Percutaneous transhepatic venous sampling has not been particularly helpful as a diagnostic aid because of the delicate nature of the glucagon assay and the large number of samples needed for adequate localization. Ultrasonography demonstrates these tumors only when they are large and bulky.

Radical surgical resection of the tumor is clearly the most satisfactory treatment for glucagonoma. Unfortunately, surgical resection is frequently palliative because of the presence of hepatic metastases. For unresectable or metastatic glucagonoma, streptozocin can be useful in reducing the size of the tumors, slowing the growth of metastases, and reducing the circulating levels of glucagon.[67] The clinical symptoms, such as skin lesions and anemia, are ameliorated by streptozocin, but the carbohydrate intolerance does not undergo remission, probably because of toxicity of the streptozocin on the B cells of the healthy islets of Langerhans.

Vipoma

Verner-Morrison syndrome was described in 1958 as the third islet-associated syndrome, after insulinoma and the Zollinger-Ellison syndrome.[68] These islet cell tumors, called *vipomas,* secrete VIP. It is not clear which cell in the normal islet gives rise to this tumor. The secreted product is clearly ectopic, and the 28-amino acid peptide causes watery diarrhea, hypokalemia, and hypochlorhydria or achlorhydria. Only about 100 cases have been described, and in approximately 80% of these, a single tumor of the endocrine pancreas was held responsible for the syndrome. In the remaining 20%, hyperplasia of an uncertain member of the islet cell community was implicated. Ductal proliferation and an increase in the number of cells in the islets have been described in patients with this syndrome. Approximately half of the tumors are benign.

The VIP released by these tumors causes diarrhea, with volume losses in the range of 2 to 10 L/day. Associated potassium wasting, leading to hypokalemia, is observed. Not infrequently, the hypokalemia gives rise to flaccid paralysis and a nephropathy that can lead to renal failure. Hypomagnesemia and mild hypercalcemia have also been described in patients with this syndrome. The clinical effects of excessive VIP secretion are anticipated rather easily because of its known biologic action. VIP has specific receptors on the small-bowel mucosa, and binding of the peptide causes a sharp rise in cAMP, causing the effect of VIP to be similar to that of cholera toxin. The fluid losses are quite similar to those expected in cholera, and Verner-Morrison syndrome has therefore been called *pancreatic cholera.* VIP has substantial sequence homology with other gastrointestinal hormones, such as secretin, glucagon, and GIP. Tumors secreting this peptide therefore may (1) enhance the secretion of alkaline fluid by the pancreas, which suggests secretin overactivity; (2) induce hyperglycemia, which suggests a glucagon effect; and (3) strikingly suppress gastric acid secretion, like an infusion of GIP. The release of VIP from these tumors can occur in paroxysms, to give pictures of flushing caused by the vasodilatory reaction of VIP, which may lead to some confusion with the carcinoid syndrome.

Diagnosis of the Verner-Morrison syndrome is not easily accomplished, because radioimmunoassay for VIP is not universally available. Further, an extremely similar syndrome is caused by tumors that release prostaglandin E_2. Generally, when the clinical picture of the Verner-Morrison syndrome is encountered, the pancreas is studied by computed tomography, angiography, or ultrasonography for evidence of a pancreatic mass lesion. If a tumor is identified, preferred treatment is by surgical resection. In the presence of hepatic metastases, high-dose steroids and streptozocin have offered reasonable palliation.[7]

PPoma

A few tumors of the endocrine pancreas have been described that apparently secrete only PP. The importance of this is uncertain, because there is no specific metabolic or clinical manifestation of these tumors, called *PPomas.* PP is released in abnormally large amounts by patients who harbor other kinds of non-B islet cell tumors. Therefore, PP has been suggested as a marker for other pancreatic endocrine tumors, especially in families with a propensity toward development of these lesions. Approximately half of all patients with other pancreatic endocrine tumors have an elevation in PP level. Furthermore, approximately 50% of patients with carcinoid tumors, regardless of site, demonstrate an elevation in PP level. When they are present, PP-secreting tumors are detected clinically because of the effect of the mass in the pancreas or because of metastases. Therefore, the syndrome of PP-secreting tumors is not necessarily an endocrine syndrome, but one more related to neoplasia. In patients with islet cell tumors, PP is frequently secreted in high concentration in addition to the primary or symptom-producing hormone. Also, the PP level is quite often elevated in the plasma of patients with asymptomatic tumors. Therefore, PP measurement can be used as a tumor marker to screen patients with multiple endocrine neoplasia type 1 syndrome for the preclinical appearance of an islet cell tumor.

Somatostatinoma

The first case report of a somatostatin-secreting tumor was published in 1977. Approximately 20 cases have now been described.[69] These tumors are usually malignant and accompanied by hepatic metastases. Somatostatinomas may be located in the pancreas or duodenum.

Metabolically, somatostatin inhibits numerous endocrine and exocrine secretory functions. Dyspepsia, mild diabetes, and cholelithiasis with steatorrhea constitute the expected pathophysiologic constellation for this endocrine condition. These effects are easily attributable to the inhibitory effects of somatostatin on a wide array of smooth muscle and endocrine secretory events. Somatostatin is inhibitory for essentially all gastrointestinal hormones, including insulin, PP, glucagon, gastrin, secretin, motilin, and GIP. The mild diabetes is directly attributable to inhibition of insulin secretion, whereas diarrhea and steatorrhea are attributable to deficient secretion of pancreatic enzymes. The dyspepsia may be more a motor disturbance in smooth muscle function, because hypochlorhydria is observed when gastric acid studies are performed in patients with somatostatinoma. The reduced muscular tone of the gallbladder presumably leads to gallbladder stasis and the formation of stones. Patients with somatostatinoma also uniformly lose weight, which may be attributable to neoplastic effects or malabsorption.

Somatostatinoma may be identified by elevated levels of somatostatin in the blood. Excessive secretion of somatostatin by these tumors can be induced in response to intravenous tolbutamide. These tumors are identified on computed tomography and angiography; if they have not metastasized, they are ideally treated by complete excision.

Other Islet Cell Tumors

Pancreatic islet cell tumors yielding a syndrome related to hypercalcemia have been described. These tumors have undetectable parathyroid hormone levels, so a parathyroid hormone–like substance has been implicated as the causative agent.[70] Many of the features of hyperparathyroidism are present, including bone resorption, nephrocalcinosis, nephrolithiasis, peptic ulcer, and psychoneurologic symptoms. Unless the tumor is extirpated, conventional treatment of hypercalcemia is futile, and the patient eventually dies. Adrenocorticotropinomas of the pancreas have been described, and most have produced a clinical Cushing's syndrome.[71] Plasma cortisol and urinary 17-hydroxycorticosteroid levels have not been suppressible by the dexamethasone suppression test. Several cases of tumors of the pancreas secreting growth hormone–releasing factor and causing acromegalic symptoms have been described. Acromegaly may regress after tumor extirpation without hypophysectomy.[72]

In addition, a variety of non-B islet cells tumors apparently have no secretory products that can be identified. They generate no endocrine syndrome to lead to their diagnosis, even though they constitute approximately 20% of all islet cell tumors and are most commonly discovered by computed tomography or angiography as incidental structures or as the explanation for a larger intra-abdominal mass. These tumors can effect the biliary tree by obstruction, which leads to their discovery in approximately half of affected patients. A tumor marker for these lesions is plasma neuronal-specific enolase, a neural isomer of the glycolytic enzyme enolase. The glycolytic pathway in neural tissue could be adversely affected by the lowered pH in neural cells, which is the consequence of intense metabolic activity. The enolase found in other tissues is an allosteric subunit enzyme that dissociates in the cytosolic pH found in neural cells. Neuronal-specific enolase is stable in its allosteric confirmation at the pH range associated with neural tissue. This enzyme is common to all APUD and neural cells. In fact, the enzyme is released into the plasma of patients with APUD tumors and can be used as a marker for all APUD tumors.[19]

In as many as 80% of patients with nonfunctioning islet cell tumors, histologic examination reveals evidence of malignancy; however, these tumors grow slowly, and even patients with hepatic metastases may have prolonged survival. Surgical removal is generally the preferred treatment; medical therapy with streptozocin yields a good response in patients with metastases.

The endocrine tumors of the pancreas present a challenge to the endocrinologist and surgeon, with the prospect for occasional cure and frequent long-term palliation. Recently, substantial endocrine palliation has been achieved with almost all of the endocrine syndromes by administering long-acting somatostatin to suppress hormone release. Somatostatin is not a chemotherapeutic agent, and no tumor remission has been seen. However, control of the endocrine syndrome in Zollinger-Ellison syndrome, insulinoma, Verner-Morrison syndrome, and glucagonoma represents a spectacular improvement in the treatment of these unfortunate patients.

A knowledge of the islet cell tumors of the pancreas is important to anyone treating pancreatic neoplasia. In fact, all masses in the pancreas are not evidence of hopeless adenocarcinoma of the pancreas. Indeed, pancreatic masses, even those that occlude the common bile duct, deserve careful attention. The identification of a resectable islet cell tumor may indeed be the happy conclusion of a diagnostic workup in which islet cell tumor was not the leading possibility at the outset of the investigation.

SUMMARY

The endocrine pancreas controls the movement of glucose through the extracellular fluid by regulating the generation of glucose and the facilitated diffusion of glucose into most cells. The islets of Langerhans that comprise the endocrine pancreas constitute a community of at least four cell types that interact in the islets for the purpose of regulating conflicting secretions that either raise or lower plasma glucose level. The A (glucagon), B (insulin), D (somatostatin), and F (PP) cells respond to a vast number of secretagogs and antagonists to support a hormonal output compatible with an appropriate hormonal presentation, especially to the liver, to guarantee the movement of glucose in response to substrate demand. These cells join a larger number of others strewn along the gastrointestinal tract to secrete the hormonally active gut peptides.

This chapter outlines the anatomy, embryology, and physiology of the islets. The only known spontaneous deficiency disease of the endocrine pancreas, diabetes mellitus, is discussed in some detail. The pathophysiology of the functioning neoplasms of these endocrine cells is also discussed. Although the endocrine neoplasms are quite rare, the metabolic and pathologic sequelae of excess states of these critical hormones serve to reinforce our understanding of metabolism and its hormonal regulation.

REFERENCES

1. Merrell RC. Cell-cell recognition in neuroembryology. In Bradshaw RA, Schneider DM, eds. Proteins of the Nervous System. New York: Raven Press, 1980.
2. Von Mering J, Minkowski O. Diabetes mellitus nach pancreas extirpation. Arch Exp Pathol Pharmakol 26:371, 1889.
3. Banting FG, Best CHL. The internal secretion of the pancreas. J Lab Clin Med 7:251, 1922.
4. Oyer P, et al. Studies on human proinsulin. J Biol Chem 246:1375, 1971.
5. Goldman H, Wong I, Patel YC. A study of the structural and biochemical development of human fetal islets of Langerhans. Diabetes 31:897, 1982.
6. Bonner-Weir S. Morphological evidence for pancreatic polarity of β-cell within the islets of Langerhans. Diabetes 37:616, 1988.
7. Pignal F, et al. Streptozotocin treatment in pancreatic cholera (Verner-Morrison) syndrome. Digestion 24:176, 1982.
8. Rutter WJ, et al. An analysis of pancreatic development. In Papoconstautinoi J, Rutter WJ, eds. Molecule Control of Proliferation and Differentiation. New York: Academic Press, 1978.
9. Henderson JR, Daniel PM, Fraser PA. The pancreas as a single organ: The influence of the endocrine upon the exocrine part of the gland. Gut 22:158, 1981.
10. Bell GI, et al. Sequence of the human insulin gene. Nature 284:26, 1980.
11. Espinal J. Understanding Insulin Action. West Sussex (UK): Ellis Horwood, 1989.
12. Hammonds P, et al. Regulation and specificity of glucose-stimulated insulin gene expression in human islets of Langerhans. FEBS Lett 223:131, 1987.
13. Farnby B, Schmid-Farmby F, Grodsky GM. Relationship between insulin release and ^{65}zinc efflux from rat pancreatic islets maintained in tissue culture. Diabetes 33:229, 1984.
14. Ashcroft FM, et al. Glucose induces closure of single potassium channels in isolated rat pancreatic B-cells. Nature 312:446, 1984.
15. Malaisse WJ, Senor A, Malaisse-Lagae F. Insulin release: Reconciliation of the receptor and metabolic hypothesis. Mol Cell Biochem 37:157, 1981.
16. Meda P, Perrelet A, Orci L. Increase of gap junctions between pancreatic B-cells during stimulation of insulin secretion. J Cell Biol 82:441, 1979.
17. Metz SA, Fujimoto WY, Robertson RP. Lipoxygenation of arachidonic acid: a pivotal step in stimulus secretion coupling in the pancreatic beta cell. Endocrinology 111:2141, 1982.
18. Matschinksy FM, et al. Glucoreceptor mechanisms in islets of Langerhans. Diabetes 21:555, 1972.
19. Prinz RA, et al. Serum markers for pancreatic islet cell and intestinal carcinoid tumors. Surgery 94:1019, 1983.
20. Reaven E, et al. Effect of age and environmental factors on insulin release from the perfused pancreas of the rat. J Clin Invest 71:345, 1983.
21. Klines I, et al. Normal insulin sensitivity of the islets of Langerhans in obese subjects with resistance to its glucoregulatory actions. Diabetes 33:305, 1984.
22. Marincola F, et al. The independence of insulin release and ambient insulin in vitro. Diabetes 32:1162, 1983.
23. Tepperman J. Metabolic and Endocrine Physiology, 3rd ed. Chicago: Year Book Publishers, 1973.
24. McGarry JD, Foster DW. Regulation of hepatic fatty acid oxidation and ketone body production. Am Rev Biochem 49:395, 1980.
25. Dayoff MO. Atlas of Protein Sequence and Structure. Silver Spring, Md.: National Biomedical Research Foundation, 1969.
26. Pandol SJ, et al. Growth hormone-releasing factor stimulates pancreatic enzyme secretion. Science 225:326, 1984.
27. Kimball CP, Murlin JR. Aqueous extracts of pancreas. III. Some precipitation reactions of insulin. J Biol Chem 58:337, 1923.
28. Itoh M, et al. Secretion of glucagon. In Cooperstein SJ, Watkins D, eds. The Islets of Langerhans. New York: Academic Press, 1981.
29. Goodner CJ, Hom FG, Koercker DJ. Hepatic glucose production oscillates in synchronic with the islet secretory cycle in fasting rhesus monkeys. Science 215:1257, 1982.
30. Efendic S, Luft R. Somatostatin and its role in insulin and glucagon secretion. In Cooperstein SJ, Watkins D, eds. The Islets of Langerhans. New York: Academic Press, 1981.
31. Kimmell JR, Pollack HG, Hazelwood RL. Isolation and characterization of chicken insulin. Endocrinology 83:1323, 1968.
32. Warren JH, et al. Differences in risk of insulin-dependent diabetes in offspring of diabetic mothers and diabetic fathers. N Engl J Med 311:149, 1984.
33. Srikanta S, et al. Pre-type I diabetes: Identical endocrinological course dependent of HLA DR types or presence of cytoplasmic anti-islet antibodies. Diabetes 33:10A, 1984.
34. Stiller CR, et al. Effects of cyclosporine—Type I diabetes: Clinical course and immune response. Diabetes 33:13A, 1984.
35. Tager HS. Abnormal products of the human insulin glue. Diabetes 33:693, 1984.
36. Eizirick DL, et al. Repair of pancreatic β-cells. Diabetes 42:1383, 1993.
37. Opie EL. The relation of diabetes mellitus to lesion of the pancreas: Hyaline degeneration of the islands of Langerhans. J Exp Med 5:527, 1901.
38. Bell RH, et al. Molecular defects in diabetes mellitus. Diabetes 40:413, 1991.
39. James DE, et al. Molecular cloning and characterization of an insulin-regulatable glucose transporter. Nature 338:83, 1989.
40. Birnbaum MJ. Identification of a novel gene encoding an insulin-responsive glucose transporter protein. Cell 57:305, 1989.
41. Jaspan J, et al. Treatment of severely painful diabetic neuropathy with an aldose reductose inhibitor: Relief of pain and improved somatic and autonomic nerve function. Lancet 2:758, 1983.
42. Siperstein MD, Unger RH, Madison LL. Studies of muscle capillary basement membranes in normal subjects, diabetic and pre-diabetic patients. J Clin Invest 47:1973, 1968.
43. Koenig RJ, Cerami A. Hemoglobin A, C, and diabetes mellitus. Annu Rev Med 31:29, 1980.
44. Clutter WE. Diabetes mellitus and hyperlipidemia. In Campbell JW, Frisse M, eds. Manual of Medical Therapeutics. Boston: Little, Brown, 1983.
45. Cornfield J. The university group diabetes program: A further statistical analysis of the mortality findings. JAMA 217:1676, 1971.
46. Lauritzen T, et al. Effect of one year of near-normal blood glucose levels on retinopathy in insulin-dependent diabetics. Lancet 1:200, 1983.
47. Ballinger WF, Lacy PE. Transplantation of intact pancreatic islets in rats. Surgery 72:175, 1972.
48. Cobb L, Merrell R. Intrasplenic islet autografts: Insulin response to IV glucose challenge. Curr Surg 40:36, 1983.
49. Bell RH, et al. Prevention by whole pancreas transplantation of glomerular basement membrane thickening in alloxan diabetes. Surgery 88:31, 1980.
50. Gray BN, Watkins E. Prevention of vascular complications of diabetes by pancreatic islet transplantation. Arch Surg 111:254, 1976.
51. Lacy PE. Experimental immuno-alteration. World J Surg 8:198, 1984.
52. Sutherland DER. Pancreas and islet transplantation: An update. Transplant Rev 8:185, 1994.
53. Basadonna GP, et al. Morbidity, mortality and long-term allograft function in kidney transplantation alone and simultaneous pancreas/kidney transplantation in diabetic patients. Transplant Proc 25:1321, 1993.
54. Zollinger RM, Ellison EH. Primary peptic ulcerations of the jejunum associated with islet cell tumors of the pancreas. Ann Surg 142:709, 1955.
55. Pearse AGE, Polak MJ. Endocrine tumours of neural crest origin: Neurolophomas apudomas and the APUD concept. Med Biol 52:3, 1974.

56. Stark DD, et al. Computed tomography and nuclear magnetic resonance imaging of pancreatic islet cell tumors. Surgery 94:1024, 1983.
57. Lomsky R, Langr F, Vortel V. Demonstration of glucagon in islet cell adenomas of the pancreas by immunofluorescent technic. Am J Clin Pathol 51:245, 1969.
58. Zollinger RM. The ulcerogenic syndrome. In Fiesen SR, ed. Surgical Endocrinology. Philadelphia: JB Lippincott, 1978.
59. Giacobazzi D, Passaro E. Preoperative angiography in the Zollinger-Ellison syndrome. Am J Surg 126:74, 1973.
60. Dunnick NR, et al. Computed tomographic detections of nonbeta pancreatic islet cell tumors. Radiology 135:117, 1980.
61. Ingemausson S, et al. Pancreatic vein catheterization with gastrin assay in normal patients and in patients with Zollinger-Ellison syndrome. Am J Surg 134:558, 1977.
62. Friesen SR, et al. Cimetidine in the management of synchronous crises of MEAI. World J Surg 4:123, 1980.
63. Richardson CT, et al. Effect of vagotomy in Zollinger-Ellison syndrome. Gastroenterology 77:681, 1979.
64. Friesen SR. Treatment of the Zollinger-Ellison syndrome. Am J Surg 143:331, 1982.
65. Pedersen NB, Jonsson L, Holst JJ. Necrolytic migratory erythema and glucagon cell tumour of the pancreas: The glucagonoma syndrome. Acta Derm Venereol (Stockh) 56:391, 1976.
66. Belchetz PE, et al. ACTH, glucagon and gastrin production by a pancreatic islet cell carcinoma and its treatment. Clin Endocrinol 2:307, 1973.
67. Danforth DN, et al. Elevated plasma proglucagon-like component with glucagon-secreting tumor: Effect of streptozotocin. N Engl J Med 295:242, 1976.
68. Verner JV, Morrison AB. Islet cell tumor and a syndrome of refractory watery diarrhea and hypokalemia. Am J Med 25:374, 1958.
69. Pipeleers D, et al. Five cases of somatostatinoma clinical heterogeneity and diagnostic usefulness of basal and tolbutamide induced hypersomatostatinemia. J Clin Endocrinol Metab 56:1236, 1983.
70. Rasbach D, et al. Pancreatic islet cell carcinoma with hypercalcemia. Am J Med 78:337, 1985.
71. Abe K, et al. Production of calcitonin, adrenocorticotropic hormone, and B-melanocyte-stimulating hormone in tumors derived from amine precursor uptake and decarboxylation cells. Cancer Res 37:4190, 1977.
72. Rosch J, et al. Functional endocrine tumors of the pancreas: Clinical presentation, diagnosis, and treatment. Curr Probl Surg 26:309, 1990.

61

Multiple Endocrine Neoplasia: Types 1 and 2

Clifford W. Deveney and Orlo H. Clark

Although tumors of the endocrine system most often occur within a single gland and arise sporadically, the concurrence of neoplasms involving multiple endocrine tissues, developing familiarly in an autosomal dominant pattern, and giving rise to well-characterized clinical syndromes is now solidly established. The familial association of tumors of the pituitary gland, the parathyroid glands, and the pancreatic islets has been referred to as *multiple endocrine neoplasia type 1 (MEN 1).* The association of familial medullary carcinoma of the thyroid (MCT) and pheochromocytoma has been termed *multiple endocrine neoplasia type 2 (MEN 2).* Men 2 is now known to occur in two variants. MEN 2a is characterized by MCT, pheochromocytoma, and hyperparathyroidism, whereas the rarer but more lethal MEN 2b includes MCT and pheochromocytoma in association with mucosal neuromas, intestinal and oropharyngeal ganglioneuromatosis, and a marfanoid habitus.

In both MEN 1 and MEN 2, most cells involved in tumors are cells of the amine precursor uptake and decarboxylation (APUD) series, a characteristic that all these cells share. The APUD cells, found in the central nervous system (hypothalamus, pituitary axis, pineal gland), gut, thyroid, and placenta, possess common biochemical functions (the uptake of amine precursors and the production of peptides). The initial postulate that the APUD cells had a common origin from the neural crest has since been disputed, but they all do appear to originate from neural ectoderm. These cells also possess a common enzyme, neuron-specific enolase. The concept of a common origin for these cells in diverse locations is appealing, because it could explain the secretion of common peptides by APUD cells in the gut, thyroid, and central nervous system. The APUD concept is also fascinating in relation to the MEN syndromes, because these inherited syndromes involve hyperplasia and tumors of selected APUD cells.

MEN 1

MEN 1, or *Wermer's syndrome,* is an inherited disorder characterized by the development of endocrine tumors in the parathyroid gland, pancreatic islets, and pituitary gland. In 1954, Wermer[1] first characterized the syndrome and postulated that it was inherited. Subsequent case studies of families with this syndrome have confirmed that the genetic trait is autosomal dominant, with a high degree of penetrance. Thus, approximately half of the children of affected individuals eventually have the syndrome.[2] The genetic defect has been recently localized to the long arm of chromosome 11 in the region 11q12-q13.[3,4] In the future, it may be possible to test genetically for MEN 1 in kindreds before any endocrine tumors have manifested clinically.[5] This is already being done for patients with MEN 2 and familial MCT.

In patients with MEN 1, the pituitary, parathyroid glands, and pancreatic islet cells all contain multiple foci of hyperplasia or neoplasia[6]; however, discrete tumors or the clinical syndromes produced by these cells may not develop. When they become clinically demonstrable, these syndromes usually manifest in a predictable sequence. Hyperparathyroidism appears first, and by the end of the third decade of life it is present in all affected kindreds. In more than 90% of these patients, all parathyroid glands (usually four) are hyperplastic.[7] Multiple adenomas and even solitary parathyroid tumors have also been described, but these are less common.

Clinical manifestations resulting from islet cell tumors occur in only 50% to 60% of patients. Initial studies demonstrated gastrin- and insulin-secreting tumors to be the most common pancreatic tumors. However, more recent studies have demonstrated that tumors secreting glucagon, pancreatic polypeptide (PP), and/or insulin occur 70% of the time, whereas tumors secreting gastrin, somatostatin, or vasoactive intestinal peptide (VIP) occur only 20% of the time.[8-10] It may be that we have a greater ability to measure these peptides now and therefore are diagnosing tumors that we could not categorize before. Also the incidence of particular pancreatic tumors may vary with the different kindreds studied.

Pancreatic islet cell tumors in patients with MEN 1 are multiple and involve the entire pancreas. Microscopically, they may appear as multiple islet cell adenomas, islet cell

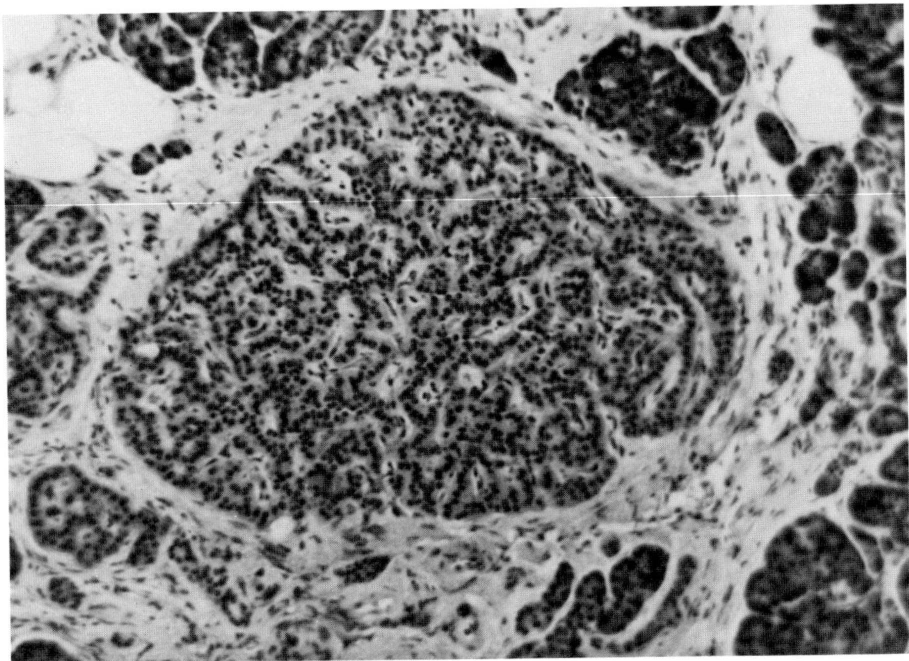

Fig. 61-1. Microscopic islet cell adenoma. Note that the islet has lost the normal architecture and has a uniform follicular pattern. The islet is well encapsulated. Many patients with MEN 1 have similar adenomas scattered throughout the pancreas.

hyperplasia, or nesidioblastosis.[10] Gastrinomas in patients with MEN 1 may appear submucosally in the wall of the duodenum, as they occasionally do in patients with sporadic gastrinoma.[9] A typical microscopic islet cell adenoma is shown in Fig. 61-1. One or several adenomas may enlarge and appear as dominant tumors. These tumors may also be malignant, with the propensity toward malignancy depending on the cell type and peptide hormone secreted. An islet cell tumor is demonstrated in Fig. 61-2.

In patients with MEN 1, islet cell tumors carry a lower incidence of malignancy than they do in sporadic cases. The patient with MEN 1 may eventually have islet cell tumors secreting several different peptides. Thus, a patient with a gastrinoma may subsequently or concomitantly have an insulinoma. These patients should therefore be screened periodically for other peptide-secreting tumors. PP level is usually elevated in patients with MEN 1 when they have islet cell tumors or islet cell hyperplasia; it thus appears to be a useful marker for the diagnosis of pancreatic tumors in this syndrome.[11] Overt pituitary tumors occur in only 10% to 30% of MEN 1–affected kindreds, but prolactin levels are elevated in a greater number of patients. Tumors secreting growth hormone (GH), prolactin, melanocyte-stimulating hormone (MSH), and adrenocorticotropic hormone (ACTH) have been described.[2,12]

In summary, the typical patient with MEN 1 has hyperparathyroidism. If patients do not already have pancreatic islet cell tumors, they are likely to have them eventually (50% to 70% probability), and more than one islet cell endocrinopathy will probably develop. Patients are likely to have or acquire functioning pituitary adenomas (GH-, prolactin-, MSH-, ACTH-secreting tumors) and the accompanying clinical syndromes associated with these hormones (10% to 30% probability).

The parathyroid, islet cell, and pituitary tumors in MEN 1 are multiple, usually involve the entire gland, and usually continue to develop as long as these glands remain viable. This has therapeutic implications, which are discussed with each syndrome. It also means that these patients must be screened periodically for elevated hormone levels throughout life. Radioimmunoassays are available for most peptides secreted by these tumors, and it is reasonable to screen these patients yearly with measurements of serum calcium, parathyroid hormone (PTH), prolactin, PP, gastrin, insulin and glucagon, because these are the most common peptides secreted. If the patient has symptoms compatible with a syndrome caused by excess of another hormone, the workup for that hormone-secreting tumor should commence. Other tumors rarely occurring in patients with MEN 1 include lipomas and carcinoid tumors. The carcinoid tumors are usually of foregut (thymic, bronchial, or stomach) origin.

Hyperparathyroidism in MEN 1

As already stated, hyperparathyroidism is the most common endocrinopathy in MEN 1, occurring in almost all patients with this endocrine disorder. It generally appears before the end of the third decade of life, which is earlier than the onset of sporadic hyperparathyroidism, but it rarely occurs before the age of 10 years. Essentially all pa-

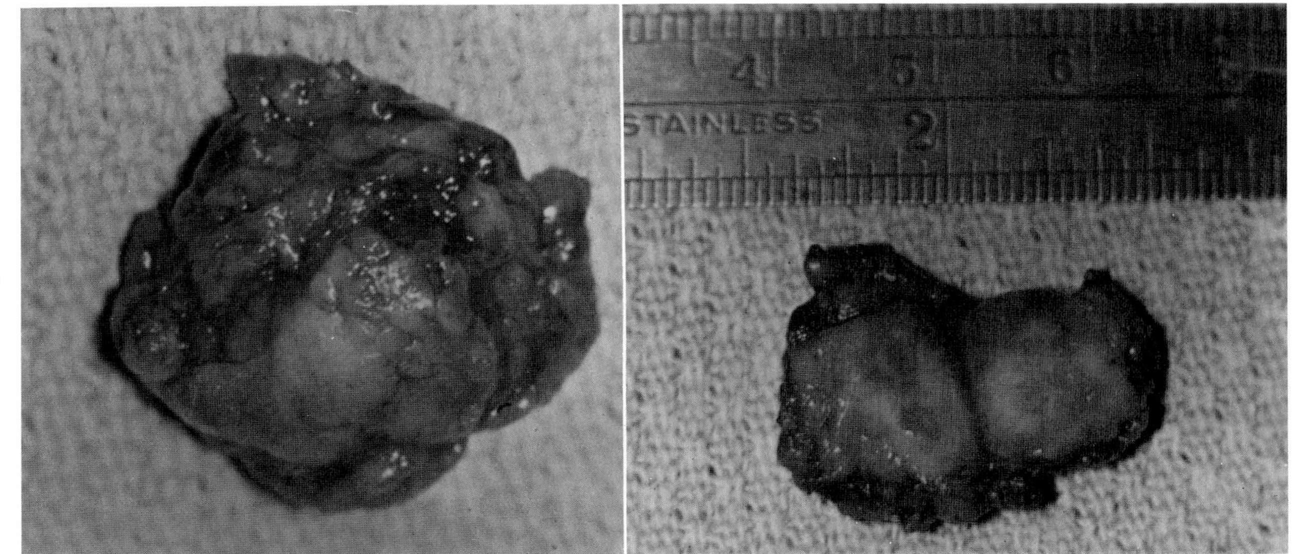

Fig. 61-2. Islet cell adenoma 1 cm in size. **A,** Located within the pancreatic parenchyma. **B,** More apparent on cut section.

tients with MEN 1 have parathyroid hyperplasia involving all glands. In contrast, 80% to 90% of patients with sporadic hyperparathyroidism have a solitary parathyroid adenoma. As in sporadic hyperparathyroidism, elevated serum calcium and PTH levels confirm the diagnosis.

Because of the relatively consistent association of parathyroid hyperplasia with MEN 1, any patient who has hyperparathyroidism related to parathyroid hyperplasia should be screened for MEN 1 with measurement of serum gastrin and prolactin levels. Conversely, any patient with a gastrinoma or insulinoma should undergo calcium and PTH measurement. In patients with a solitary parathyroid adenoma, screening for MEN 1 is not justified unless symptoms suggest islet cell or pituitary tumors.

The symptoms of hyperparathyroidism are the same in MEN 1 as in nonfamilial hyperparathyroidism. When hyperparathyroidism is detected because of a family history, however, the endocrinopathy is often diagnosed earlier, and symptoms such as lethargy, weakness, nervousness, constipation, anorexia, polyuria, polydipsia, and nocturia may be mild. These patients should be surgically treated for hyperparathyroidism, because those left untreated may have bony, renal, and neuropsychologic complications (see Chapter 56).

When gastrinoma and hyperparathyroidism are present concurrently, the hyperparathyroidism should be treated first. Reduction of serum calcium levels to normal facilitates control of gastric acid hypersecretion related to hypergastrinemia and obviates the need for urgent surgery to control gastric acidity. In many patients with primary hyperparathyroidism and gastrinoma, the serum gastrin level falls to normal for a prolonged period (1 to 5 years) after successful parathyroidectomy.

The surgical treatment of hyperparathyroidism in MEN 1 should consist of subtotal parathyroidectomy (removal of three and a half glands), which is preferred, or total parathyroidectomy with transplantation of 50 g parathyroid tissue into the forearm. The thymus should be removed at parathyroidectomy. Thymectomy is performed because of the high frequency of an intrathymic fifth parathyroid gland or of parathyroid rests (cell groups) within the thymus. The surgeon should assume that all patients with this syndrome have parathyroid hyperplasia. Hyperplastic glands vary considerably in size, so some glands may appear normal even though diffuse hyperplasia is present. Further, no reliable tests can be performed at surgery to differentiate an adenoma from hyperplasia. The distinction between hyperplasia and a normal gland may also be difficult at times. Thus, neck exploration should be performed, with all glands identified and confirmed by biopsy and microscopic examination.

Before subtotal parathyroidectomy, one of the smaller parathyroid glands, distant from the recurrent laryngeal nerve and with a particularly good vascular pedicle, should be identified and partially resected, leaving 30 to 50 g tissue (the size of a normal parathyroid gland). The gland should be marked with a clip to enable identification in case hyperparathyroidism should recur at some point. Once it has been confirmed that this remnant is viable, the other three glands and the thymus should be removed.

An alternate method of treatment is to perform a total parathyroidectomy with autografting of a portion (approximately 15 pieces 1 mm in size) of one gland to individual pockets in the forearm muscle. The disadvantage of total parathyroidectomy is an at least 5% chance of early or late graft failure, with consequent hypoparathyroidism. An advantage of this method is that the autotransplanted parathyroid is easily accessible in case hyperparathyroidism recurs. When total parathyroidectomy and autotransplantation are performed, approximately 500 mg tissue should be cryopreserved to allow retransplantation in case the initial transplant should fail to function adequately.

In experienced hands, the recurrence or persistence of hyperparathyroidism after subtotal or total parathyroidectomy in MEN 1 is 20% to 30%.[13-16] In our experience, hyperparathyroidism recurred in seven of 21 patients (33%) who underwent subtotal parathyroidectomy.[17] This high rate of recurrence is caused by the diffuse involvement of all glands.

Pancreatic Endocrinopathies in MEN 1

Fifty percent or more of patients with MEN 1 eventually have islet cell tumors of the pancreas. These tumors may secrete glucagon, insulin, gastrin, somatostatin, or VIP. They often secrete more than one hormone, and most (70% to 80%) secrete PP. Thus, PP may be a useful tumor marker in MEN 1.

Methods for localizing these tumors are the same as for sporadically occurring endocrine tumors of the pancreas. Computed tomographic (CT) scanning identifies most tumors 1.5 cm in diameter or larger, but many tumors are smaller than this.[18,19] Our experience with CT scanning has been good in detecting lesions larger than 1 cm, but we have been unable to see smaller lesions.[20] Tumors larger than 1 cm are usually detectable at surgery. Selective arteriography is helpful in about 50% of cases, but it usually finds tumors that are readily apparent to the surgeon. Intraoperative ultrasonography is also helpful in localization.[21]

Transhepatic portal venous sampling is probably the most sensitive test for diagnosis, because it depends on function rather than size of the tumor. In this test, a catheter is placed percutaneously through the liver and into the portal vein. The catheter is then advanced through the portal vein and into the splenic, superior mesenteric, and gastroepiploic veins and their tributaries. Blood is sampled from different positions and assayed for hormones.[22-24] An elevation of the hormone production at a specific site suggests that hormone is coming from that area. When hormone levels are essentially the same from all sampling sites, the clinician must assume that hormone production is uniform throughout the pancreas. Selective venous catheterization requires several hours and an experienced radiologist.

Patients with MEN have multiple tumors diffusely scattered throughout the pancreas. Resection of individual tumors is unlikely to result in cure, especially in patients with gastrinomas.

Gastrinoma in MEN 1

Hypergastrinemia and hypersecretion of gastric acid signify the presence of gastrinoma. The symptoms produced by a gastrinoma are related to the hypersecretion of acid. These patients have intractable ulcer disease and diarrhea. The diarrhea appears to be related to the adverse effects of the excessive hypersecretion of acid on small-bowel mucosa and the impairment of fat digestion. Because of the strong association of gastrinoma with MEN 1, every patient with gastrinoma should have serum calcium levels measured to screen for hyperparathyroidism. In most series of gastrinomas, the incidence of MEN 1 is 20% to 30%.[25]

Diagnosis. A gastric acid secretion greater than 15 mEq H^+/hr accompanied by a serum gastrin concentration greater than 500 pg/ml is diagnostic for gastrinoma. Gastric acid secretion should always be measured when serum gastrin level is elevated, because gastrin level may be elevated in patients with hyposecretion of acid when the gastric pH is 5 or greater.

One other cause of hypergastrinemia with hypersecretion of acid is antral G-cell hyperplasia. This entity can be differentiated from gastrinoma by the gastrin response to a standard meal. Patients with antral G-cell hyperplasia respond to a meal by increasing serum gastrin 100% or more above basal levels, whereas those with hypergastrinemia related to pancreated tumors have a minimal response to a meal (Fig. 61-3, *A*). When gastrin values are elevated above the normal range (0 to 100 pg/ml) but not high enough to be diagnostic of a gastrinoma (100 to 500 pg/ml), the secretin test or calcium-infusion test may be used to stimulate gastrin release by gastrinomas.[26,27]

The secretin test is performed by measuring serum gastrin concentration before and 2, 5, 10, and 15 minutes after the intravenous injection of secretin at 2 U/kg body weight. Patients with gastrinoma show a prompt increase in serum gastrin of 100 pg/ml or greater, the explanation for which has not been defined. The response is usually seen in the 2- or 5-minute sample. Patients with hypergastrinemia from antral G-cell hyperplasia and otherwise healthy individuals with peptic ulcer disease respond slightly or not at all to secretin (see Fig. 61-3, *B*).

The calcium-infusion test is performed by infusing calcium as either gluconate or chloride at a rate of 5 mg Ca^{2+}/kg/hr for 3 hours. Serum gastrin level is measured before the infusion and at 30-minute intervals during the infusion. Patients with gastrinoma demonstrate an absolute increase of 300 pg/ml or more, whereas those without gastrinoma respond with a change of 100 pg/ml or less. The response in patients with antral G-cell hyperplasia is not as predictable, with some of these patients having large increases in serum gastrin. Because the calcium infusion test takes much longer to perform than the secretin test and gives essentially the same results, the secretin test and the gastrin response to a standard meal are the two tests most often used to confirm the diagnosis of gastrinoma. The gastrin responses to secretin, calcium, and a standard meal are summarized in Table 61-1.

Treatment. If left untreated, patients with gastrinoma eventually die of the complications of peptic ulcer diathesis caused by gastric hyperacidity. Therefore the primary objective of treatment is to control acid hypersecretion by means of H_2-receptor antagonists, total gastrectomy, or resection of the gastrin-producing tumors.

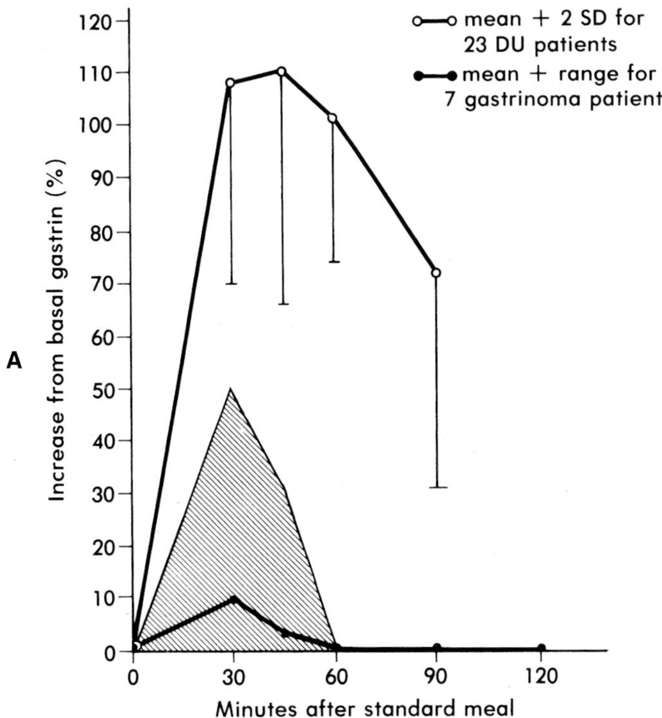

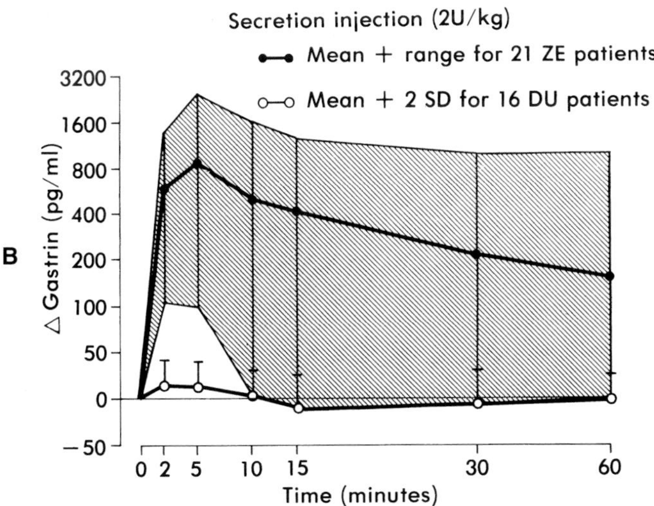

Fig. 61-3. A, Gastrin response to a standard meal. Note that the response is expressed as a percentage of the basal level. In patients without gastrinoma, the gastrin response to a meal is 70% to 130% of the basal value. The highest increase in patients with gastrinoma is about 40% above the basal level. **B,** Increase in gastrin after secretin administration occurs within 5 minutes of injection.

The H_2-receptor antagonists effectively control acid secretion acutely in these individuals, although large doses are usually required (5 to 10 g/day cimetidine or 0.9 to 1.5 g/day ranitidine). When using H_2-receptor antagonists in patients with gastrinoma, it is important to measure the acid secretion and adjust the dose of the H_2-receptor antagonist so that the patient secretes less than 10 mEq

Table 61-1. Gastrin Response to Provocative Tests*

	Secretin	Standard Meal	Calcium
Duodenal ulcer	−	+	−
G-cell hyperplasia	−	+	±
Gastrinoma	+	−	−

*+, Positive response; ±, variable response; −, negative response.

H^+/hr in the hour preceding the next dose. With high doses of cimetidine, many male patients have gynecomastia and impotence. For these reasons, ranitidine is the preferred drug.[26,28-31]

A newer, more potent, and longer-acting H_2-receptor antagonist, famotidine, appears to be superior to cimetidine and ranitidine, but experience with this drug in the treatment of gastrinoma is limited. Also, a new class of drugs that block acid secretion by inhibiting the hydrogen ion pump (substituted benzimidazoles such as omeprazole) has been initially evaluated for treatment of gastrinoma and shows considerable therapeutic promise. Omeprazole lowers gastric acid 10 times as much as do H_2-receptor antagonists and need be given only once daily.[32] Omeprazole is presently the drug of choice for controlling acid secretion in patients with gastrinoma. H_2-receptor antagonists may also control acid secretion in these patients, but they must be given in high doses and patients commonly acquire tolerance to these agents.[33]

Total gastrectomy was the recommended treatment for gastrinomas before antisecretory agents such as H_2-blockers and omeprazole were available. It effectively removes the acid-secreting organ and improves survival. The procedure can be performed with a mortality rate of less than 5% by an experienced surgeon, and patients tolerate it with minimum dumping syndrome, diarrhea, or weight loss.[26,28,30] Before total gastrectomy is considered, the patient should have a trial of management with omeprazole. If treatment with omeprazole is unsatisfactory, the patient should subsequently undergo a total gastrectomy.

Tumor resection is conceivably the ideal treatment. It attacks the problem at its source, excess production of gastrin, and removes a tumor with malignant potential. Unfortunately, gastrin-secreting tumors in MEN 1 are most often multifocal, and tumor resection rarely produces a decrease in serum gastrin level. Although curative resections have been reported in approximately 20% of patients with sporadic gastrinoma, the rate of cure is considerably less for patients with MEN 1 and gastrinoma.[12,34-36] Even though it is unlikely that resection will result in a cure in patients with MEN 1, it is reasonable to explore such patients surgically and resect large pancreatic neoplasms if technically possible.[37] When malignant, these tumors are progressive and eventually lethal. Thus, if a tumor can be enucleated from the duodenum or head of the pancreas or removed by resecting the tail of the pancreas, this approach is the recommended treatment. The morbidity and mortality rates of more extensive surgery, such as Whipple's operation (pancreatoduodenectomy) or total pancreatectomy, cannot be justified for gastrinoma.

Because vagotomy potentiates the effect of H_2-receptor antagonists, some authorities recommend exploratory laparotomy, resection of the tumor when feasible, and parietal cell vagotomy. The laparotomy allows assessment regarding the resectability of tumor. If resection is not possible, parietal cell vagotomy can still be performed with minimum morbidity; this enhances reduction of acid secretion by omeprazole or H_2-receptor antagonists.[33,38]

Insulinoma in MEN 1

Insulinomas are one of the most common pancreatic tumors in the MEN 1 syndrome. Symptoms in patients with insulinoma are related to the effect of hypoglycemia on the sympathetic CNS. Typical symptoms are confusion, hunger, dizziness, paresthesias, bizarre behavior, tachycardia, pallor, and sweating. Hypoglycemic episodes tend to occur in the early morning before breakfast, in the late afternoon before dinner, or after exercise. Weight gain is common, because the patient's symptoms are ameliorated by eating.

Diagnosis. The diagnostic criteria for insulinoma are hyperinsulinism accompanied by hypoglycemia. Ninety percent of patients with insulinoma become hypoglycemic after a 12-hour overnight fast. If the fasting period is continued for 72 hours and followed by a brief period of exercise, almost all patients with insulinoma become hypoglycemic. The standard diagnostic method is to have the patient fast for 72 hours and measure blood sugar levels at frequent intervals and when the patient has symptoms.[39] The insulin/glucose ratio is of key importance. In healthy individuals, this ratio is approximately 0.175 (14 μU/ml insulin at a time when the glucose is 80 mg/dl). In patients with insulinoma, this ratio is increased to 0.3 or greater.

Insulin is cleaved from a larger molecule called *proinsulin.* After cleavage, the remaining molecule is called *C peptide* (connecting peptide). Both insulin and C peptide are simultaneously released from the beta cell. The half-life of C peptide is longer than that of insulin (30 vs 4 to 8 minutes), so the molar concentration of C peptide is greater than that of insulin and is easier to measure in the serum. Many investigators recommend measuring both C peptide and insulin in the diagnosis of insulinoma. The C-peptide concentration is especially helpful for distinguishing between patients with insulinoma and those with factitious hyperinsulinism caused by self-administered injections of insulin. Patients who have injected themselves with insulin have low C-peptide and high insulin concentrations, whereas patients with insulinoma have both high C-peptide and high insulin concentrations.

Another method for diagnosis of insulinoma is the C-peptide test. In this test, an intramuscular injection of purified soluble insulin (0.1 U/kg body weight) is given to maintain blood glucose at approximately 40 mg/dl. This infusion suppresses insulin and C-peptide secretion in healthy individuals but not in patients with insulinoma. Thus, an elevated C-peptide level 30 minutes after the insulin injection is diagnostic for insulinoma. This test is recommended for patients in whom insulinoma is strongly suspected but cannot be diagnosed by a prolonged fast.

Proinsulin, which is insulin still connected to C peptide, is also elevated in insulinoma and can be measured by radioimmunoassay. Several provocative tests for insulin release have also been used to diagnose insulinoma. Intravenous tolbutamide and glucagon release insulin. Both these tests have false-positive results and can produce severe hypoglycemia, however, so they are no longer recommended.

Treatment. The episodes of hypoglycemia resulting from insulinoma may be ameliorated by frequent small feedings high in carbohydrates. Diazoxide, a thiazide, strongly inhibits the release of insulin from the islet cells and is effective in preventing episodes of hypoglycemia. Diazoxide may cause fluid retention in some patients, however, which may preclude its use. The initial dose of diazoxide is 50 mg orally three times daily. This may be increased to 600 mg/day, although most patients have the condition controlled with 300 mg/day or less. The effectiveness of diazoxide is measured empirically by the reduction in the number of hypoglycemic episodes. It can be further quantified by measuring insulin/glucose ratios before and after diazoxide administration. In a patient with a good response, the number of hypoglycemic episodes is abolished or significantly reduced, and the insulin/glucose ratio falls to less than 0.3.

Before resection of insulinoma is attempted, all patients should receive a trial of diazoxide, because when celiotomy does not reveal discrete tumors, the extent of pancreatic resection may be influenced by the response to treatment with diazoxide. In patients with no obvious tumors and diffuse microscopic islet cell adenomas, an 80% pancreatectomy is indicated for those who have a poor response to diazoxide, whereas a distal pancreatectomy of less than 80% should be performed for those with a good response to diazoxide.

In patients without MEN 1, 80% of insulinomas are benign and solitary, and enucleation of the tumor or resection of that portion of the pancreas containing tumor usually results in cure. In MEN 1, insulinomas are almost always multiple; if multiple insulinomas are present, one should suspect MEN 1. Multiple insulinomas sometimes can be enucleated or treated with distal pancreatectomy. Because of the high likelihood of microscopic insulinomas or islet cell hyperplasia in the remaining pancreas, however, recurrence of hyperinsulinism is frequent after local pancreatic resection in patients with MEN 1. For this reason, some have recommended 80% pancreatectomy as the treatment of choice for patients with MEN 1 and insulinoma with enucleation of tumors from the head of the pancreas.[40,41]

Attempts should be made before reoperation to localize insulinomas by means of percutaneous transhepatic portal venous sampling. If a patient has been receiving diazoxide to control the hypoglycemia, treatment must be discontinued before performing this procedure because it inhibits insulin release. If a localized insulin gradient exists in a certain area of the pancreas, that part should be included in the resection.

Other Islet Cell Tumors in MEN 1

Other islet cell peptide-producing tumors, such as vipomas, glucagonomas, somatostatinomas, and PPomas, may also occur in MEN 1. The presence of these tumors should be suspected only if the patient displays characteristic symptoms.

Vipoma. High circulating levels of VIP cause severe diarrhea related to jejunal secretion and not malabsorption. Gastric acid secretion in these patients is normal or low. Thus, measurement of acid secretion can be used to differentiate the diarrhea of vipoma from that produced by gastrinoma, in which acid production is excessive.

Severe, watery diarrhea, hypokalemia, and sometimes hypercalcemia with low or normal gastric acid secretion should lead one to suspect vipoma. Other causes of diarrhea, such as malabsorption, infection, and surreptitious laxative use, should be ruled out. A high serum or plasma VIP level in a patient with symptoms is diagnostic.

Resection of the tumor, the only means of cure, can be accomplished in about half of all patients with vipoma. Half the tumors are also malignant. Streptozocin may produce a temporary remission of symptoms in patients with unresectable tumors. Symptoms are often controlled for as long as several years by giving the patient octreotide.[42] If no tumor is found, it is reasonable to remove the tail and body of the pancreas. In many patients, the diarrhea improves after subtotal pancreatectomy.

Glucagonoma. Glucagonoma syndrome is characterized by a migratory necrolytic dermatitis (usually involving the legs and perineum), weight loss, stomatitis, hypoaminoacidemia, anemia, and mild diabetes mellitus. Visual scotomas and changes in visual acuity have been reported in some cases. The diagnosis may be suspected from the distinctive skin lesion; even the presence of a prominent rash in a patient with diabetes mellitus should be enough to raise suspicions. Elevated serum glucagon levels are diagnostic.

About 25% of glucagon-producing tumors are benign and confined to the pancreas. The remainder have metastasized by the time of diagnosis, most often to the liver, lymph nodes, adrenal glands, or vertebrae. Occasionally, hyperglucagonemia is seen with islet cell hyperplasia. Although distinctly rare, glucagonomas have also been reported in the kidney, lung, and intestines.

Surgical removal of the glucagonoma and of resectable metastases is indicated if technically feasible. Even if it is not possible to remove all the tumor, considerable palliation may result from debulking. Oral zinc supplements may improve the dermatitis. Streptozocin and dacarbazine are the most effective chemotherapeutic agents for unresectable lesions. Phenytoin (Dilantin) results in decreased serum glucagon levels.

The clinical course generally parallels changes in serum levels of glucagon in response to therapy. The sematostatin analog octreotide may help to control the symptoms.

After appropriate preoperative localization studies (CT scan, angiography, transhepatic portal venous sampling), the patient should undergo laparotomy and attempted tumor resection.

Somatostatinoma. Somatostatinomas produce few symptoms. Diabetes mellitus (usually mild), diarrhea and malabsorption, and dilation of the gallbladder (usually with cholelithiasis) are common findings in patients with this disease. These tumors are most often malignant and are accompanied by hepatic metastases. The diagnosis may be made by recognizing the clinical syndrome and measuring increased concentrations of somatostatin in the serum. In most cases, however, the somatostatinoma syndrome is unsuspected until discovered at surgery, and the diagnosis is confirmed by histologic evidence of metastatic islet cell carcinoma. If surgical treatment can only be palliative, chemotherapy with streptozocin, dacarbazine, or doxorubicin hydrochloride is sometimes helpful.

PPoma and "nonfunctional" tumors. PP, which is consistently elevated in the serum of patients with MEN 1 and any pancreatic tumor, is considered a good tumor marker in the MEN 1 syndrome. PPomas, or pure PP-producing tumors, occur in MEN 1 but are extremely rare. Excess production of PP produces no symptoms, so these tumors are usually large, unresectable, and metastatic at diagnosis. Islet cell tumors that are "nonfunctional," producing no known peptides, have also been reported.

Pituitary Lesions in MEN 1

Although all patients with MEN 1 have microscopic pituitary lesions, only 30% have symptoms. These symptoms may be caused by excess production of peptides by the tumors or may be related to neurologic impingement by tumor and decreased pituitary function.

Pituitary tumors may secrete a variety of hormones, including GH, ACTH, and MSH, but prolactin is the most common. Female patients with hyperprolactinemia are usually infertile and have irregular menses and galactorrhea. In male patients, the symptoms are subtle and include loss of libido and impotence. Excess of the other hormones can produce typical syndromes, such as Cushing's disease (ACTH excess) and acromegaly (GH excess). If the tumor becomes large (greater than 5 mm), it can extend in the suprasellar space and impinge on the optic nerves, causing bitemporal visual field defects or headaches and cranial nerve deficits.

Transphenoidal hypophysectomy is the treatment of choice for small, symptomatic tumors. Larger tumors may require treatment with surgery (transfrontal) and radiation therapy. Bromocriptine has been used successfully to treat symptoms in patients with functioning prolactinomas.

MEN 2A AND MEN 2B

MEN 2a and MEN 2b are inherited syndromes characterized by the development of MCT and pheochromocytoma. Patients with MEN 2a also have hyperparathyroidism, which is usually related to parathyroid hyperpla-

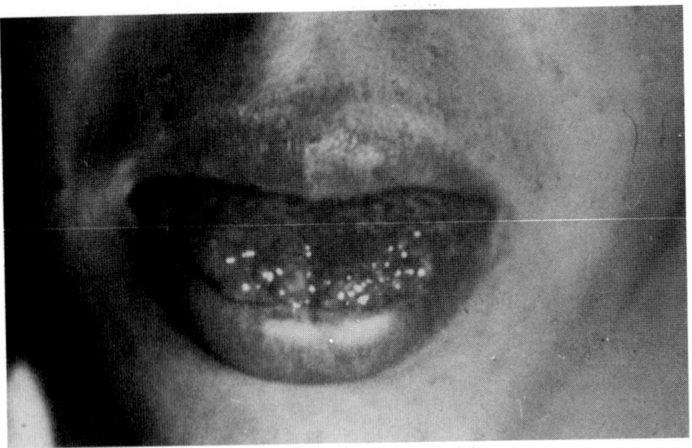

Fig. 61-4. Patient with MEN 2b. Note the small tumors on the tongue and the puffy lips.

sia. Patients with MEN 2b have a marfanoid habitus and hyperelastic joints, and submucosal ganglioneuromas of the oropharynx develop in them at an early age. Patients with MEN 2b also have a characteristic facies, with puffy lips and eyelids (Fig. 61-4). Patients with MEN 2b only rarely have hyperparathyroidism, but medullary carcinomas appear at an earlier age, often in infancy, and are more virulent than in patients with MEN 2a.

Both MEN 2a and MEN 2b are inherited through an autosomal dominant gene, which means that half the offspring of an affected individual inherit the syndrome. MEN 2b also occurs as a spontaneous mutation, so many patients with MEN 2b have no family history of this syndrome. Researchers initially believed that different genes were involved in the two syndromes, but recent evidence suggests that the defects producing MEN 2a and MEN 2b are from different loci on the same gene.[43] It appears that the genetic abnormalities occur at the pericentromeric region of chromosome 10 for both MEN 2a and MEN 2b, but the alleles are different.[44] Further evidence that the genetic abnormalities may differ even among various kindreds with MEN 2a or MEN 2b is the fact that the expression of adrenal or parathyroid abnormalities vary greatly among patients with these syndromes.[45] DNA analysis may be used to positively identify patients with MEN 2a.[46,47] The parafollicular or C cells of the thyroid, the tumor cell in MCT, and the adrenomedullary cell, the cell of the pheochromocytoma, are APUD cells that originate from the neural crest, as do the ganglioneuroma cells. Thus, all the cells involved in these syndromes have a common neural origin. The parathyroid cells do not originate from the neural crest, but rather from neuroectodermal placodes.

All the tumors in MEN 2 are multifocal, diffuse, and bilateral. Neoplastic changes are usually preceded by hyperplasia. MCT, which appears in 100% of patients with MEN 2a and MEN 2b, is the most life-threatening lesion in this syndrome. Pheochromocytomas occur in about 40% to 50% of patients with MEN 2a and MEN 2b.[48] These pheochromocytomas are almost always benign, although malignant forms with metastases have been reported.[49] Hyperparathyroidism occurs in about 40% of patients with MEN 2a, most often related to parathyroid hyperplasia. However, the incidence of adrenal and parathyroid disease varies greatly among kindreds. One series examining 12 kindreds with MEN 2a found the incidence of pheochromocytoma to range from 6% to 100% and the incidence of hyperparathyroidism to vary from 0% to 53%.[45] A substantial number of these patients have normocalcemic hyperparathyroidism. The marfanoid habitus and oral submucosal ganglioneuromas occur early in almost all patients with MEN 2b. Submucosal ganglioneuromas usually develop before MCT and may suggest the diagnosis of sporadic development of MEN 2b. These lesions are sometimes subtle and may go unnoticed for many years. Early recognition and diagnosis are important in MEN 2b, because few patients can be cured of MCT diagnosed after childhood.[47,50-52]

Medullary Carcinoma of Thyroid in MEN 2

MCT originates from the calcitonin cells, or C cells, located around the periphery of the thyroid follicles. These cells secrete calcitonin. Elevated basal serum calcitonin levels or increased calcitonin levels in response to provocative stimuli can be used to diagnose MEN 2 with C-cell hyperplasia that resembles MCT early in its evolution[51] (Fig. 61-5). About 75% of cases of MCT occur sporadically, and the remaining 25% occur with MEN 2a, MEN 2b, and other inherited (familial) disorders without MEN. In sporadic MCT, the tumor usually appears in the third to fourth decades of life and is usually confined to one lobe of the thyroid. In the MEN 2 syndromes, MCT is always bilateral and generally appears before age 30 in MEN 2a and before age 5 in MEN 2b.[45]

Diagnosis

Elevated basal serum calcitonin levels or increased calcitonin levels in response to provocative stimuli in patients with suspected MEN 2 are diagnostic of MCT.[53,54] Because 100% of patients with MEN 2 and MEN 2b eventually have MCT, patients with known MEN 2a or MEN 2b, or those at risk for development of the syndrome, should be screened with a serum calcitonin level every 6 months. If the basal calcitonin level is normal, screening should also include levels in response to provocative stimulation. For patients with MEN 2a, screening should begin early in the second decade of life; for those with MEN 2b, screening should begin in infancy, because these tumors often develop at that time in this variant of MEN 2. It is recommended that patients undergo thyroidectomy if MEN 2b is diagnosed by characteristic facies and oral lesions.[51] Calcitonin is often not measurable in individuals without MCT and is never greater than 200 pg/ml. Therefore, a basal calcitonin level greater than 250 pg/ml is diagnostic for MCT. In patients with MEN 2a or MEN 2b who do not yet have elevated calcitonin levels, how-

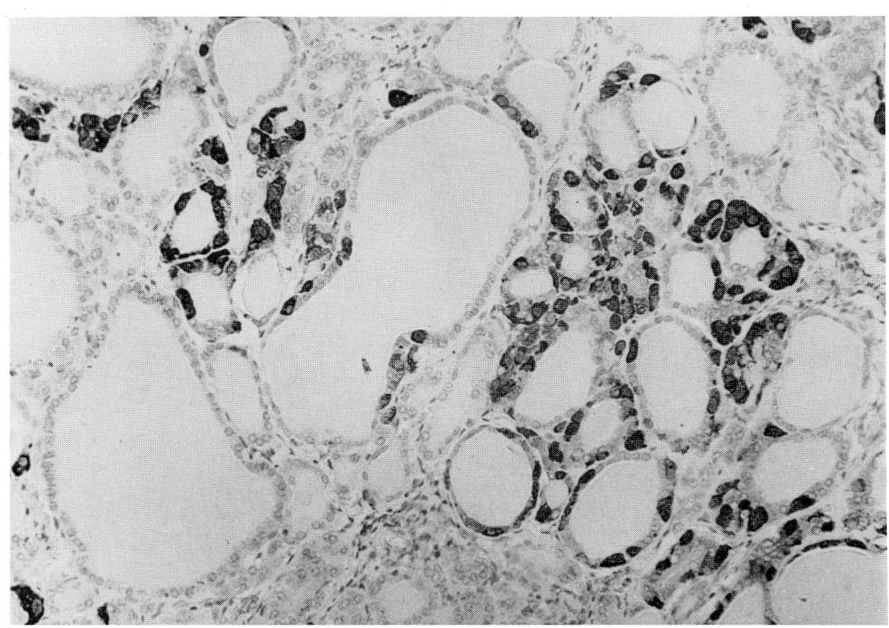

Fig. 61-5. C-cell hyperplasia. C cells are stained with an immunoperoxidase technique with antibodies directed to calcitonin. The parafollicular C cells are increased in number but have not formed discrete tumors.

ever, provocative tests for calcitonin release should be used to diagnose microscopic MCT or C-cell hyperplasia, which is a precursor of MCT.

Pentagastrin and calcium (as calcium gluconate) are both used as provocative agents for calcitonin release. As single agents, they are roughly equally effective, but the combination of the two increases the release of calcitonin significantly in patients with MCT, so the combination is the preferred method of testing. When combined, 5 pg/kg pentagastrin is given as an injection and calcium gluconate (2 mg Ca^{2+}/kg) is infused for 1 minute. Blood for calcitonin measurement is collected before and at 1, 2, 3, 5, 10, and 15 minutes after the injection. With a positive response, an abrupt increase in calcitonin occurs within 5 minutes of injection. Fig. 61-6 depicts a typical positive response after pentagastrin alone; the response to combined agents is similar but more pronounced. Healthy subjects respond with an increase in calcitonin of less than 200 pg/ml, whereas patients with MCT respond with an increase of 300 pg/ml or greater.[53,55]

The calcium and pentagastrin test should routinely be performed in patients with MEN 2a and MEN 2b who have normal serum calcitonin levels; when results become positive, patients should undergo total thyroidectomy. Either a basal calcitonin value of 250 pg/ml or greater or a stimulated increase of 300 pg/ml or more is diagnostic of MCT. These values vary somewhat in different radioimmunoassays. The routine use of these provocative tests in patients with MEN 2a and MEN 2b has enabled physicians to make an early diagnosis of MCT, when patients still have C-cell hyperplasia or small microscopic foci of tumor. The cure rate among these patients at this stage of

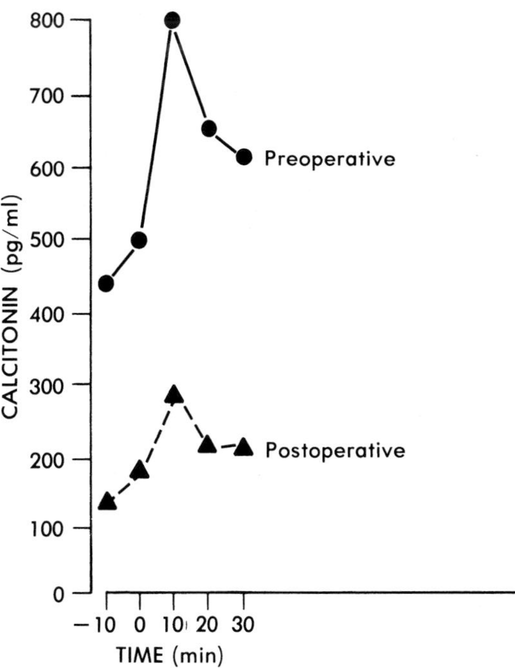

Fig. 61-6. Serum calcitonin response to pentagastrin before and after operation. Note the fall in serum calcitonin level after the operation. The reduction in calcitonin did not bring it all the way down to normal, and this patient probably has residual MCT. The time course of the response to pentagastrin is similar to the response seen with the combination of pentagastrin and calcium.

disease is excellent. The importance of screening with calcitonin tests in patients with MEN 2b in infancy cannot be overemphasized. To achieve cures in these patients, diagnosis and treatment must begin in infancy. As our ability to diagnose these syndromes genetically improves, the recommendations for thyroidectomy may come to be made at the time of diagnosis, and many of the provocative hormonal tests may become unnecessary. In patients who are RET-oncogene positive with familial MTC and MTC associated with MEN 2a, we recommend total thyroidectomy at age 5.

To increase the accuracy and sensitivity of screening, patients with MEN 2 should be tested annually. If basal calcitonin exceeds 250 pg/ml, or if the response to calcium and pentagastrin is greater than 300 pg/ml, total thyroidectomy is recommended. If basal and stimulated calcitonin levels are in an equivocal range (200 to 250 pg/ml), one should attempt to localize calcitonin release to the thyroid gland. The inferior thyroid vein is cannulated, and blood is collected for calcitonin measurement. If calcitonin values are elevated basally or after provocative tests in the venous effluent of the inferior thyroid vein, the diagnosis of MCT or C-cell hyperplasia is made, and total thyroidectomy is recommended. If serum calcitonin values are less than 300 pg/ml with provocative testing, the patient should be followed up and tests should be repeated in 6 to 12 months.[53]

Serum calcitonin levels are also a good indicator of residual or metastatic tumor and have proved useful in follow-up of patients with MCT after thyroid resection. Patients with disease limited to the thyroid gland usually have calcitonin levels below 500 pg/ml, whereas those with metastatic disease have calcitonin levels greater than 1000 pg/ml. The calcitonin level correlates with the number of metastases; the larger the number of metastases, the higher the level.

Calcitonin can also be secreted in other conditions:

1. Malignant neoplasms—oat cell, breast, laryngeal, pancreatic, and prostatic cancer
2. Endocrine neoplasms—carcinoid tumors, pheochromocytoma, gastrinoma
3. Inflammatory bowel disease—regional enteritis
4. Organ failure—chronic pulmonary disease, renal failure, liver failure
5. Other—trauma, severe burns, pregnancy, breast-feeding

However, extraneous sources of calcitonin seldom present a problem in follow-up of patients with MEN 2 after thyroidectomy, or in making the diagnosis of MCT.

Patients with sporadic MCT usually have a thyroid nodule or a metastasis to a cervical lymph node. The physician should ask any patients with thyroid nodules if they have hypertension, episodic headaches, sweating, or palpitations. One should also inquire about the family history of thyroid tumors or severe hypertension in relatives. If any of these factors are present, patients should be evaluated for pheochromocytoma and have the thyroid nodule aspirated with a fine needle for cytologic examination. If one fails to diagnose an associated pheochromocytoma in a patient with MCT, a hypertensive crisis and death may occur, either with induction of anesthesia or during the surgical procedure to resect the thyroid.

About 40% of patients with MCT have calcification within the thyroid situated at the junction of the upper and middle third of the thyroid gland (the site of the greatest concentration of C cells in the normal thyroid gland). Such a finding on a neck radiograph suggests the presence of MCT. A fine-needle aspiration of the nodule is helpful in determining the type of nodule. Screening tests for serum calcitonin levels or after provocation with pentagastrin and calcium are not recommended for routine evaluation of patients with thyroid nodules because of the low incidence (2% to 3%) of MCT in thyroid nodules.

Treatment

The minimum surgical treatment of MCT in MEN 2 is total thyroidectomy and removal of the lymph nodes in the central neck, extending from the arch vessels in the superior mediastinum to the thyroid cartilage. This should include the thymus. If any cervical lymph nodes are involved, a modified radical or radical cervical lymph node dissection on the involved side should be performed. A careful examination of the parathyroid glands should also be performed, because hyperparathyroidism related to hyperplasia or adenoma frequently accompanies MEN 2a.[56] The parathyroid glands in these patients should also be marked at surgery in case identification becomes necessary at a later date.

Several weeks after total thyroidectomy and node dissection, the patient should have basal and stimulated calcitonin values measured. If the levels remain increased or are positive with provocative testing, the patient should have cervical and hepatic veins catheterized. If the elevated calcitonin levels localize on the side of the neck (the cervical levels are higher than the hepatic vein levels), the patient should undergo a modified neck dissection, if one has not already been done, on the side of the most extensive tumor, or where the serum calcitonin level was elevated. Most patients with persistent disease have tumor in the ipsilateral cervical nodes or in the superior mediastinal nodes. If the plasma calcitonin levels in the hepatic veins are equal to or higher than those in the cervical veins, distal metastases are present, and a second procedure is not indicated. The most common sites for metastasis of MCT after the regional lymph nodes are liver, lung,adrenal glands, and bone.

Surgical resection is the only effective treatment for MCT. Anecdotal reports indicate that some of these tumors respond to iodine 131; however, these reports are few, and no evidence suggests that C cells themselves take up iodine. MCT is also relatively insensitive to radiation therapy. Likewise, most chemotherapeutic agents such as cyclophosphamide (Cytoxan), methotrexate, and fluorouracil are ineffective, although several reports suggest that doxorubicin hydrochloride (Adriamycin) has produced palliation and partial remission in some patients.

The overall 10-year survival of patients with MCT varies from 25% to 75%. Survival can be predicted by the extent of tumor at the initial surgery. Patients with C-cell hyperplasia or microscopic MCT are almost always surgically cured, and 80% to 85% are free of disease in 5 years. Patients with MEN 2b have a poorer prognosis than do those with MEN 2a. Further, patients with a homogeneous distribution of C cells according to immunoperoxidase staining of the tumor also have a better prognosis than do those with a heterogeneous distribution.

Pheochromocytoma in MEN 2

Pheochromocytoma in MEN 2 usually becomes apparent after MCT. It is not known whether the actual tumor develops later or the disease merely becomes clinically manifest later. Adrenomedullary hyperplasia probably occurs first and progresses to pheochromocytoma.[57] Unlike MCT, pheochromocytomas are almost always benign. These tumors are almost always bilateral, or a tumor may involve one adrenal gland and medullary hyperplasia may involve the other. The tumors are often multifocal within the gland. About half the patients with MEN 2a or MEN 2b eventually have pheochromocytoma.[45,48] Diagnosis for pheochromocytoma is usually made in the fourth decade.[42]

Diagnosis and Symptoms

The symptoms of pheochromocytoma are those of catecholamine excess, such as hypertension, palpitations, and headache. The primary risk in patients with pheochromocytoma is death from hypertensive crisis, which may be the first manifestation of the disease. Because pheochromocytoma is a part of MEN 2, all patients with this endocrinopathy or with MCT should be screened for pheochromocytoma before thyroid surgery.

Pheochromocytoma is diagnosed by measuring elevated levels of catecholamines or their metabolites in plasma or urine. The substances measured are epinephrine, norepinephrine, and the metabolites metanephrine and vanillylmandelic acid. A urinary vanillylmandelic acid level greater than 11 mg/24 hr or urinary metanephrine level greater than 1.8 mg/24 hr is diagnostic. Plasma catecholamine (epinephrine and norepinephrine) levels greater than 2000 pg/ml are also diagnostic for pheochromocytoma.

If results of these tests are equivocal, the diagnosis can be made by the glucagon stimulation test or the clonidine suppression test. Glucagon, given intravenously in a bolus of 1 to 2 mg, should produce a threefold increase in epinephrine and norepinephrine levels, or an absolute increase greater than 2000 pg/ml, 3 to 5 minutes after injection. The glucagon stimulation test usually elevates the blood pressure and should not be used in patients with diastolic pressures of 110 mm Hg or greater. Clonidine, an α-adrenergic agonist, suppresses the release of catechols from neural tissue but not tumors. The clonidine suppression test is performed by giving 0.3 mg clonidine and measuring plasma epinephrine and norepinephrine levels 2 to 3 hours later. In patients without tumor, these catecholamine levels should be less than 500 pg/ml. Because clonidine has the potential to cause hypotension, marked volume depletion should be corrected, and concomitant use of antihypertensive agents, particularly β-adrenergic blockers, should be avoided when performing this suppression test.[3] Patients in MEN 2–affected kindreds should be screened yearly, or whenever symptoms suggestive of pheochromocytoma appear.

When pheochromocytoma is diagnosed, one should attempt to localize the tumor. CT scanning, the least invasive method, demonstrates tumors larger than 1 cm; however, the CT scan is not helpful for smaller tumors or for adrenomedullary hyperplasia. In adrenomedullary hyperplasia, the adrenal medulla changes little in size, but the cortex thins out and the ratio of medulla to cortex increases.

Iodine 131–labeled metaiodobenzylguanidine (MIBG), a radionuclide specific for catecholamine precursors in the adrenal medulla, demonstrates pheochromocytomas present in the adrenal, in ectopic positions, and in metastatic deposits.[58,59] MIBG also reveals adrenomedullary hyperplasia. The test is relatively noninvasive and aids greatly in the localization of pheochromocytomas. It is especially helpful for localizing extra-adrenal pheochromocytomas. In a recent study, MIBG had a 87.9% sensitivity and a 98.9% specificity.[60] MIBG has also been used to treat a few patients with unresectable pheochromocytomas, in the same way that radioactive iodine is used to treat patients with metastatic, differentiated thyroid cancer. Its ultimate role as a therapeutic modality remains to be defined.

Arteriography is rarely necessary to identify the presence of a pheochromocytoma. Selective adrenal vein sampling of catechols is a highly sensitive technique, but it is often difficult to perform because of problems in catheterizing the right adrenal vein. Arteriography or selective venous sampling should only be done after the patient has been prepared with α-adrenergic blockers, as for surgery. (See also Chapter 58 and the following discussion.)

Treatment

After preoperative preparation, the patient should undergo resection of the tumor. Preoperative preparation consists of blocking the potential effects of catechols released by the tumor. Phenoxybenzamine, a long-acting α-adrenergic blocker, is initially used at a dose of 10 mg orally three times daily. This dose is gradually increased, along with vigorous hydration, until the patient has mild orthostatic hypotension. This allows expansion of a contracted blood volume and may demonstrate an anemia. Anemic patients should receive blood transfusions as clinically indicated. If tachycardia or arrhythmias persist after α-adrenergic blockade and rehydration, β-blockade with propranolol should be instituted. One should initiate preoperative blockade at least 10 days before invasive localization procedures or surgery. Intraoperative blood pressure should be monitored, because even when preoperative blockade is adequate, hypertension can occur during the operation, particularly when the tumor is manipulated.

The incision for resecting pheochromocytoma in patients with MEN 2 should allow access to both adrenal glands and the periaortic area, because bilateral tumors, extra-adrenal tumors, or adrenomedullary hyperplasia may be present. If both adrenal glands contain tumors, bilateral adrenalectomy is recommended. When one gland appears normal after localization studies and palpation, it is unclear whether the normal-appearing gland should be removed.[51,61,62] Some authorities recommend bilateral adrenalectomy for all patients with MEN 2 who have biochemical evidence of phenochromocytoma, because the "grossly normal" gland is always involved with at least medullary hyperplasia or occult tumors. These investigators believe that the risk of recurrent pheochromocytoma and the attendant complications of hypertension and possible malignant degeneration warrant removal of the normal-appearing gland.

Control of the hypoadrenal state is usually easily managed by the daily administration of hydrocortisone (20 mg in the morning and 10 mg in the afternoon or evening). Others have elected to remove only the abnormal gland, stating that no evidence suggests that the remaining gland will eventually have a functioning pheochromocytoma, even if hyperplasia is present. Several patients with MEN 2 who underwent unilateral adrenalectomy have been followed up for 5 to 15 years without biochemical evidence of pheochromocytoma in the remaining adrenal gland. More experience and longer follow-up are needed to determine the natural history of these tumors and the role of unilateral or bilateral adrenalectomy when only one adrenal gland is clearly involved.

After resection, patients should be followed up regularly with blood pressure measurements and yearly with determination of urinary catecholamine levels. About 30% of patients with pheochromocytomas have some residual hypertension, despite removal of both adrenal glands and reversal of catechol levels to normal.

Hyperparathyroidism in MEN 2

Hyperparathyroidism related to parathyroid hyperplasia occurs in 20% to 40% of patients with MEN 2a. Hyperparathyroidism rarely if ever occurs in MEN 2b. The parathyroid hyperplasia is probably genetically caused and is not related to the elevated level of calcitonin (an antihypercalcemic hormone) that occurs in MCT.

Diagnosis

Elevated serum calcium and PTH levels signify the presence of hyperparathyroidism in patients with MEN 2. The finding of one or more enlarged parathyroid glands at surgery confirms the diagnosis. Some patients with MEN 2a and hyperparathyroidism are normocalcemic, and the diagnosis is made by elevated PTH levels and the finding of enlarged parathyroid glands at the time of thyroidectomy for C-cell hyperplasia or MCT.

Treatment

Hyperparathyroidism is often diagnosed concurrently with MCT and can be treated during the thyroidectomy for MCT. All the parathyroid glands should be identified; if enlarged, three and a half glands should be removed. The remaining parathyroid tissue may be left in the neck and marked with a suture clip, which we prefer, or transplanted to the forearm. One should also cryopreserve 500 mg parathyroid for autotransplantation, in case the patient has hypoparathyroidism after surgery. Hyperparathyroidism is more easily controlled in MEN 2a than in MEN 1. In fact, most physicians recommend removing only the abnormal parathyroids in MEN 2, rather than performing subtotal parathyroidectomy.[14] Also, hypoparathyroidism occurs more often after surgery in MEN 2 than does persistent hyperparathyroidism, so great care must be taken to preserve a viable parathyroid remnant.

When performing thyroidectomy for MCT in a normocalcemic patient, one should inspect all four parathyroid glands. Most surgeons recommend removing any parathyroid glands that are enlarged and carefully marking the remaining glands. It is also occasionally necessary to transplant biopsy-confirmed normal parathyroid glands because of the extensive surgery necessary to remove the thyroid gland and all the central neck nodes.

SUMMARY

Although the endocrine tumors associated with MEN 1 and MEN 2 are fascinating from the standpoint of their pathophysiology, they are potentially life-threatening and require early diagnosis and treatment. The histologic distinctions between hyperplasia and neoplasia and between benign and malignant tumors are often difficult. Many of these tumors can now be diagnosed early in the course of their symptomatic presentation, before the lesion has progressed or transformed from its hyperplastic to its neoplastic form. By diagnosing these conditions earlier, less extensive surgical procedures are effective in preventing these lethal tumors from developing.

REFERENCES

1. Wermer P. Genetic aspects of adenomatosis endocrine glands. Am J Med 16:363, 1954.
2. Wilson SD. Wermer's syndrome: Multiple endocrine adenopathy, type I. In Friesen SR, ed. Surgical Endocrinology: Clinical Syndromes. Philadelphia: JB Lippincott, 1978.
3. Bravo BL, Gifford RW Jr. Pheochromocytoma: Diagnosis, localization, and management. N Engl J Med 311:1298, 1984.
4. Fujimori M, Wells SA Jr, Nakamura Y. Fine-scale mapping of the gene responsible for multiple endocrine neoplasia type 1 (MEN 1). Am J Hum Genet 50:399, 1992.
5. Larsson C, et al. Predictive testing for multiple endocrine neoplasia type 1 using DNA polymorphisms. J Clin Invest 89:1344, 1992.
6. Majewski JT, Wilson SD. The MEA I syndrome: An all or none phenomenon? Surgery 86:475, 1979.

7. Lamers GBHW, Froeling PGAM. Clinical significance of hyperparathyroidism in familial multiple endocrine adenomatosis type I (MEA I). Am J Med 66:422, 1979.
8. Kloppel G, et al. Pancreatic lesions and hormonal profile of pancreatic tumors in MEN 1. Cancer 57:1824, 1986.
9. Samaan NA, et al. Multiple endocrine syndrome type I: Clinical, laboratory findings, and management in five families. Cancer 64:741, 1989.
10. Thompson NW, et al. MEN 1 pancreas: A histological and immunohistochemical study. World J Surg 8:561, 1984.
11. Friesen SR, Tomita T, Kimmel JR. Pancreatic polypeptide update: Its roles in detection of the trait for multiple endocrine adenopathy syndrome type I and pancreatic polypeptide–secreting tumors. Surgery 94:1028, 1983.
12. Thompson NW, et al. The surgical treatment of gastrinoma in MEN I syndrome patients. Surgery 106:1081, 1989.
13. Prinz RA, et al. Subtotal parathyroidectomy for primary chief cell hyperplasia of the multiple endocrine neoplasia type I syndrome. Ann Surg 193:26, 1981.
14. O'Riodain DS, et al. Surgical management of primary hyperparathyroid in multiple endocrine neoplasia types 1 and 2. Surgery 114:1031, 1993.
15. van Heerden JA, et al. Primary hyperparathyroidism in patients with multiple endocrine neoplasia syndromes. Arch Surg 118:533, 1983.
16. Wells SA, et al. Long term evaluation of patients with primary parathyroid hyperplasia managed by total parathyroidectomy and heterotropic autotransplantation. Ann Surg 192:451, 1980.
17. Clark OH, Way LW, Hunt TK. Recurrent hyperparathyroidism. Ann Surg 184:391, 1976.
18. Damgaard-Peterson K, Stage JG. CT screening in patients with Zollinger-Ellison syndrome and carcinoid syndrome. Scand J Gastroenterol Suppl 53:117, 1979.
19. Dunnick NR, et al. Computed tomography detection of nonbeta pancreatic islet cell tumors. Radiology 135:117, 1980.
20. Stark DD, et al. Computed tomography and nuclear magnetic resonance imaging of pancreatic islet cell tumors. Surgery 94:1025, 1983.
21. Frucht H, et al. Gastrinomas: Comparison of MR imaging with CT, angiography, and US. Radiology 171:713, 1989.
22. Glowniak JV, et al. Percutaneous transhepatic venous sampling of gastrin. N Engl J Med 307:293, 1982.
23. Roche A, Raisonnier A, Gillos-Savouret MD. Pancreatic venous sampling and arteriography in localizing insulinomas and gastrinomas: Procedure and results in 55 cases. Radiology 145:621, 1982.
24. Vinik AI, et al. Transhepatic portal vein catheterization for localization of sporadic and MEN gastrinomas: A ten year experience. Surgery 107:246, 1990.
25. Welbourn RB, et al. Tumors of the neuroendocrine system (APUD cell tumors—APUDomas). Curr Probl Surg 21:1, 1984.
26. Deveney CW, Deveney K, Way LW. The Zollinger-Ellison syndrome—23 years later. Ann Surg 188:384, 1978.
27. Modlin IM, et al. The early diagnosis of gastrinoma. Ann Surg 196:512, 1982.
28. Bonfils S, et al. Results of surgical management in 92 consecutive patients with Zollinger-Ellison syndrome. Ann Surg 194:692, 1981.
29. Deveney CW, Stein S, Way LW. Cimetidine as primary treatment for gastrinoma—Long term follow up. Am Surg 146:116, 1983.
30. Jensen RT. Basis for failure of cimetidine in patients with Zollinger-Ellison syndrome. Dig Dis Sci 29:363, 1984.
31. Raufman JP, et al. Reliability of symptoms in assessing control of gastric acid secretion in patients with Zollinger-Ellison syndrome. Gastroenterology 84:108, 1983.
32. McArthur KE, et al. Omeprazole: Effective, convenient therapy for Zollinger-Ellison syndrome. Gastroenterology 88:939, 1985.
33. Frucht H, Maton PN, Jensen RT. Use of omeprazole in patients with Zollinger-Ellison syndromes. Dig Dis Sci 36:394, 1991.
34. Friesen SR. Treatment of the Zollinger-Ellison syndrome—A 25 year assessment. Am J Surg 143:331, 1982.
35. Sheppard BC, et al. Management of islet cell tumors in patients with multiple endocrine neoplasia: A prospective study. Surgery 106:1108, 1989.
36. Donow C, et al. Surgical pathology of gastrinoma. Site, size, multicentricity, association with multiple endocrine neoplasia type I and malignancy. Cancer 68:1329, 1991.
37. Deveney CW, et al. Resection of gastrinomas. Ann Surg 198:546, 1983.
38. Richardson, et al. Treatment of Zollinger-Ellison syndrome with exploratory laparotomy, proximal gastric vagotomy, and H_2-receptor antagonists. Gastroenterology 89:357, 1985.
39. LeQuesne LP, Daggett PR. Insulin tumors of the pancreas. In Johnston IDA, Thompson NW, eds. Endocrine Surgery. Boston: Butterworth Publishers, 1983.
40. Kaplan EL, Fredland A. The diagnosis and treatment of insulinomas. In Thompson NW, Vinik AI, eds. Endocrine Surgery Update. New York: Grune & Stratton, 1983.
41. Rasbach D, et al. Surgical management of hyperinsulinism in the MEN 1 syndrome. Arch Surg 120:584, 1985.
42. Vinik AI, Lloyd R, Cho K. The use of somatostatin analog in gastroenteropancreatic tumors other than carcinoid. Metabolism 39:156, 1990.
43. Talpos GB, et al. Phenotype mapping of multiple endocrine neoplasia II syndrome. Surgery 94:650, 1983.
44. Lairmore TC, et al. Familial medullary thyroid carcinoma and multiple endocrine neoplasia type 2B map to the same region of chromosome 10 as multiple endocrine neoplasia type 2A. Genomics 9:181, 1991.
45. Howe JR, Norton JA, Wells SA Jr. Prevalence of pheochromocytoma and hyperparathyroidism in multiple endocrine neoplasia type 2A: Results of long-term follow-up. Surgery 114:1070, 1993.
46. Lips CJ, et al. Clinical screening as compared with DNA analysis in families with multiple endocrine neoplasia type 2A. N Engl J Med 331:828, 1994.
47. Neumann HP, et al. Early diagnosis of multiple endocrine neoplasia type IIa. Klin Wochenscrift 67:951, 1989.
48. Wells SA Jr, Norton JA. Medullary carcinoma of the thyroid and multiple endocrine neoplasia-II syndromes. In Friesen SR, ed. Surgical Endocrinology: Clinical Syndromes. Philadelphia: JB Lippincott, 1978.
49. Carney JA, Sizemore GW, Sheps SG. Adrenal medullary disease in multiple endocrine neoplasia type 2: Pheochromocytoma and its precursors. Am J Clin Pathol 6:279, 1976.
50. Jones BA, Sisson JC. Early diagnosis and thyroidectomy in multiple endocrine neoplasia type 2b. J Pediatr 102:219, 1983.
51. van Heerden JA, et al. Surgical management of the adrenal glands in the multiple endocrine neoplasia type II syndrome. World J Surg 8:612, 1984.
52. Vasen HF, et al. The natural course of multiple endocrine neoplasia type IIb. A study of 18 cases. Arch Intern Med 152:1250, 1992.
53. Wells SA, et al. The early diagnosis of medullary carcinoma of the thyroid gland in patients with multiple endocrine neoplasia type II. Ann Surg 182:362, 1975.
54. Wells SA, et al. Medullary thyroid carcinoma: Relationship of method of diagnosis to pathologic staging. Ann Surg 188:377, 1978.
55. Wells SA, et al. Provocative agents and the diagnosis of medullary carcinoma of the thyroid gland. Ann Surg 188:139, 1978.
56. Russell CF, et al. The surgical management of medullary thyroid carcinoma. Ann Surg 197:42, 1983.
57. Lips KM, et al. Bilateral occurrence of pheochromocytoma in patients with multiple endocrine neoplasia syndrome type 2A (Sipple's syndrome). Am J Med 70:1051, 1981.
58. Beierwaltes WH. The localization and treatment of pheochromocytomas with I MIBG. In Thompson NW, Vinik AI, eds. Endocrine Surgery Update. New York: Grune & Stratton, 1983.

59. Farndon JR, Fagraeus L, Wells SA. Recent developments in the management of pheochromocytoma. In Johnson IDA, Thompson NW, eds. Endocrine Surgery. Boston: Butterworth Publishers, 1983.
60. Shapiro B, et al. Iodine-121 metaiodobenzylguanidine for the locating of suspected pheochromocytoma: Experience in 400 cases. J Nucl Med 26:576, 1985.
61. Freier DT, et al. Dilemmas in the early diagnosis and treatment of multiple endocrine adenomatosis, type II. Surgery 82:407, 1977.
62. Tibblin S, et al. Unilateral versus bilateral adrenalectomy in multiple endocrine neoplasia IIA. World J Surg 7:201, 1983.

PART EIGHT

THE INTEGUMENT AND BODY WALL

62

Wound Healing

David M. Young and Stephen J. Mathes

Success of a surgical procedure depends on satisfactory wound healing. After any injury, both patient and physician expect prompt healing and gradual restoration of wound strength. A basic understanding of the healing process helps the physician to select the most appropriate wound management techniques from among the many available options, to anticipate the duration and extent of disability, to recognize when a variation from the normal healing process is occurring, and to intervene as necessary.

STAGES OF WOUND HEALING

Wounds may be inflicted by physical trauma, heat, cold, electromagnetic radiation, chemical injury, and infection.[1,2] Healing begins from the moment of injury, and the stages of healing bear similarities in every wound. These stages overlap in time, with each stage beginning before the completion of a previous one (Fig. 62-1). The example of a simple, clean laceration serves to illustrate the process of wound healing. A laceration that is closed promptly and heals primarily undergoes the stages of inflammation, cellular phase, epithelialization, and maturation.

Inflammation

Inflammation is the result of trauma from any stimulus. Aurelius Cornelius Celsus in the first century AD characterized the signs of inflammation as heat, redness, swelling, and tenderness. These remain the cardinal signs of inflammation.

The inflammatory response involves both a vascular and a cellular reaction. Most wounds result in injury to blood vessels, with consequent hemorrhage. Vasoconstriction occurs almost immediately, followed 5 to 10 minutes later by vasodilation. Venules in the area become more permeable to fluid, and plasma escapes into the extravascular space.

Numerous substances participate in increasing the venule permeability to fluid. Histamine is both synthesized at the wound site and released from stores within mast cells. Histamine augments the permeability of arterioles, capillaries, and venules to albumin, globulin, and fibrinogen.[3] It increases permeability by causing the contraction of endothelial cells and by partially removing the diaphragms covering gaps in the endothelium.[3,4] Platelets and mast cells release hydroxytryptamine (serotonin), which also enhances vascular permeability. Kinins are polypeptides produced at the site of inflammation from α-globulin found in plasma. The kinins serve to increase venule permeability. Prostaglandins E_1 and E_2 are synthesized at the site of injury and participate in the acute inflammatory process, including increasing vascular permeability. Prostaglandins are also active in the later stages of wound healing.[5-9]

The inflammatory exudate includes fibrin and fibronectins. Fibrin is produced in the wound through the conversion of circulating plasma fibrinogen. Initially, it aggregates platelets and red blood cells for hemostasis; later, it provides a scaffolding for the ingrowth of cells. Fibronectin, a glycoprotein, is present in an insoluble form in connective tissue and at cell surfaces and in a soluble form in plasma and other body fluids. Fibronectins serve as adhesion ligands between cells and fibrin and collagen.

Circulating plasma leukocytes adhere quickly to the vascular endothelium in the injured region. They traverse the vessel wall through a process of diapedesis. These cells migrate toward the injured area, where they are stimulated to phagocytize particles and release substances that are in part responsible for inflammation.[10] Polymorphonuclear and mononuclear cells are present initially at the site of injury in proportions similar to those in the blood. Because polymorphonuclear cells are relatively short-lived, mononuclear cells are more abundant in an older inflammatory reaction. Polymorphonuclear leukocytes kill microorganisms by an oxygen-dependent respiratory burst that generates hydrogen peroxide. This reaction, catalyzed by superoxide dismutase, is essential in controlling any bacterial contamination that may occur at the time of wounding.

Macrophages are as important as polymorphonuclear leukocytes in the inflammatory response.[11] The macrophage removes necrotic tissue and foreign bodies from the wound. A variety of chemotaxis factors draw macrophages to the wound. Once there, macrophages produce such factors as interleukin-1, tumor necrosis factor (TNF), and colony-stimulating factors. Interleukin-1 induces fever by stimulating prostaglandin synthesis[12] and increases adhesion by neutrophils and macrophages.[13] TNF has many of the same bioactivities as interleukin-1 and also causes wasting of the body.[14] Colony-stimulating factor causes the differentiation of stem cells to mature inflammatory cells.[15] The macrophage translates the numerous stimuli of injury into chemical signals that attract other cells and initiate the healing process.[16,17]

Cellular Phase

The initial influx of inflammatory cells soon gives way to proliferation of other cell types. The major events are angiogenesis in the wound and the migration and proliferation of mesenchymal cells (fibroblasts). Angiogenesis is crucial to provide transport of cells and nutrients to the wound. Fibroblasts synthesize collagen and cause contraction of the wound.

Angiogenesis begins several days after creation of the wound. Endothelial cells proliferate when exposed to the extracellular matrix and various mitogenic factors found in the wound. These endothelial cells migrate through the wound and form tubules and new basement membrane attachments.[18] Blood flow then begins through these new capillaries, transporting nutrients and cells to the wound.

Angiogenesis is under the influence of many factors. Macrophages release fibroblast growth factor and TNF. Acidic fibroblast growth factor induces proliferation of endothelial cells.[19] TNF-α promotes endothelial cell chemotaxis and capillary formation.[20] Transforming growth factor–β (TFG-β) is contained in large quantities in platelets. TGF-β stimulates endothelial cell proliferation in some conditions and inhibits growth in others. TGF-β does enhance tubule formation and is regarded as an angiogenic factor.[21] Mast cells release heparin, which binds to and potentiates fibroblast growth factor[22] and several other growth factors. Heparin-like molecules in the extracellular matrix may serve as a reservoir for growth factors.[23]

Fibroblasts develop from undifferentiated mesenchymal cells and migrate to the site of injury. Exposure to platelet-derived growth factor released from platelet granules renders the fibroblasts competent to proliferate.[24] Subsequent exposure to either epidermal growth factor or insulin-like growth factor–1 stimulates DNA synthesis and mitosis. TGF-β stimulates growth of fibroblasts, increases collagen synthesis,[25] and accelerates wound healing.[26] Fibroblasts synthesis of collagen is essential to restore strength to the wound.

The cellular phase is characterized by the deposition of collagen in the wound. Collagen is the most important component supporting the healed wound. It is a complex protein, unique in that it almost completely lacks the sulfur-containing amino acids cystine and tryptophan. Collagen incorporates hydroxyproline and hydroxylysine, two less common amino acids.

The structure of collagen is characterized by the presence of three peptide chains, each in a right-handed helical formation with the three chains aligned parallel to one another and twisted into a left-handed configuration. The resultant structure, termed *tropocollagen,* is initially held together by hydrogen bonds. As the molecule matures, stronger covalent bonds form among the three peptide chains. The tropocollagen molecule is extremely large, with a molecular weight of approximately 300 kd and dimensions of 1.5 nm in width and 280 nm in length. Tropocollagen molecules aggregate to form collagen fila-

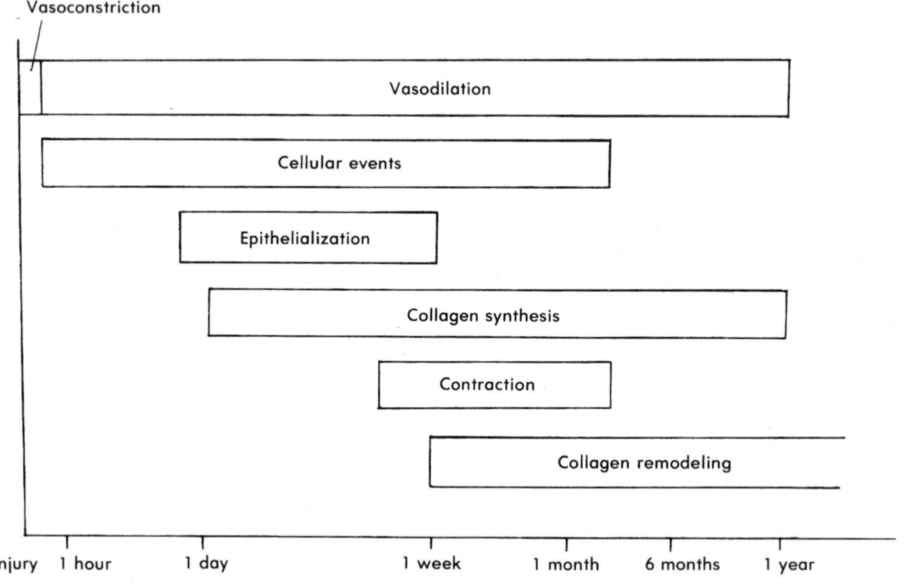

Fig. 62-1. Sequence of events in wound healing.

ments. These collagen filaments join together as collagen fibrils, and collagen fibrils associate to form collagen fibers (Fig. 62-2).

There are 13 types of collagen isolated to date, each differing in the amino-acid sequence or in the combination of the three basic polypeptide chains making up the tropocollagen molecule. The interstitial collagens, types I, II, and III, are products of separate genes and have unique amino-acid sequences. Type I collagen is found in bone, skin, and tendon. It has two α_1 (I) chains and one α_2 (I) chain. Type I collagen is low in carbohydrate and hydroxylysine. Type II collagen is found primarily in cartilage and consists of three α_1 (II) chains. It contains relatively more hydroxylysines per chain. Type III collagen is made up of three α_1 (III) chains, contains cystine, and is relatively low in hydroxylysine. Type III collagen is more abundant in fetal skin than in adult skin but is found in blood vessels, skin, and the parenchyma of internal organs of both adults and fetuses. The collagen of adult skin is 80% type I and 20% type III. Type IV collagen appears to contain two chains distinct from the ones in other collagens: two α_2 (IV) chains and one α_2 (IV) chain. Type IV collagen is found primarily in basement membranes. Type V collagen consists of two α_1 (V) chains and one α_1 (V) chain. Type VII collagen forms the anchoring fibrils found at the dermal-epidermal junction. The other remaining types are found in lesser amounts and have unknown functions.[27]

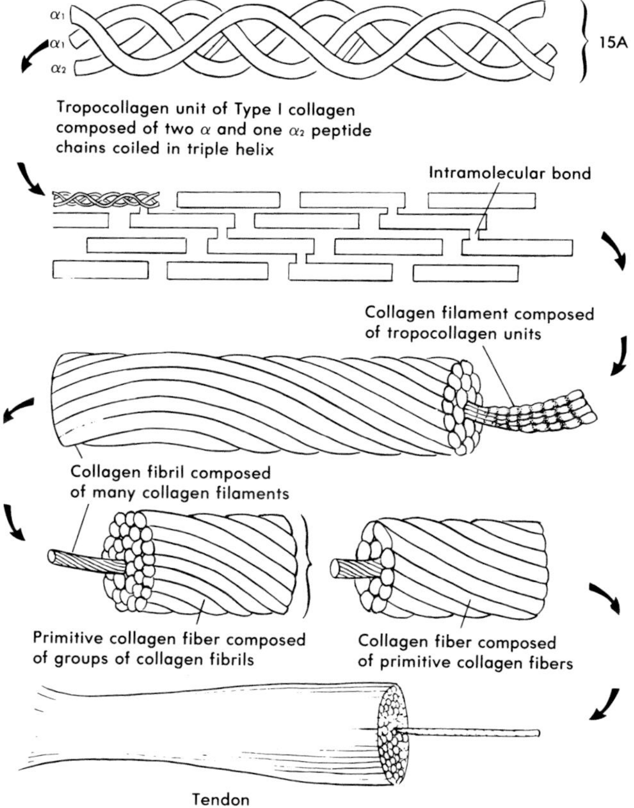

Fig. 62-2. Formation of collagen fiber.

The synthesis of collagen occurs through a series of reactions that are begun within the cell, continued on or near the cell-surface membrane, and completed in the extracellular space (Fig. 62-3). Collagen is synthesized by fibroblasts, osteoblasts, smooth muscle cells, chondrocytes, epithelial cells, and endothelial cells. Amino acids in the intracellular space are synthesized into polypeptide chains at the ribosome. Nonhelical procollagen consists of three such chains aggregated together. Proline and lysine in the polypeptide chains are hydroxylated through the action of the enzymes prolyl hydroxylase and lysyl hydroxylase. Essential cofactors for these reactions are ferrous ions, α-ketoglutarate, oxygen, and ascorbic acid. After hydroxylation, the polypeptide chains fold into a helical formation. This helical procollagen consists of a collagen molecule with an attached nonhelical N-terminal and C-terminal polypeptide. Collagen appears to be secreted by cells as procollagen. On or near the cell surface, procollagen peptidase converts procollagen into tropocollagen.

The tropocollagen undergoes assembly into collagen filaments, and ultimately collagen fibers appear. As the col-

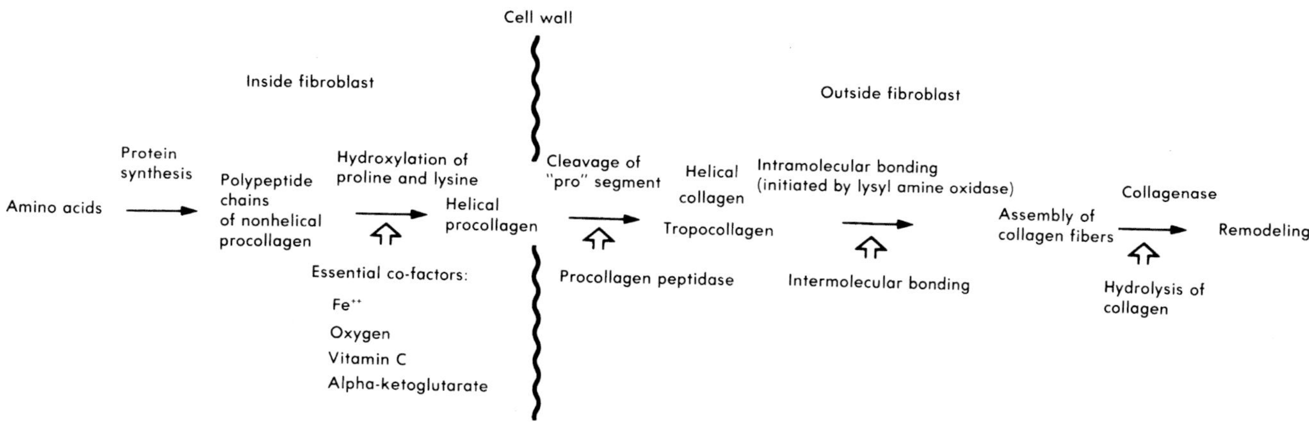

Fig. 62-3. Synthesis of collagen by fibroblast.

lagen matures, the polypeptide chains comprising each tropocollagen unit form strong intermolecular bonds mediated by lysyl amine oxidase. Intermolecular cross-linking among the tropocollagen molecules also occurs, strengthening the collagen complex.

A complex of mucopolysaccharides, protein-polysaccharides, and glycoproteins is present in the wound within 24 hours of injury. These molecules compose the ground substance in conjunction with ions and water. Ground substance appears to participate in directing the aggregation of collagen.

The breakdown of collagen (collagenolysis) occurs in the maturing wound and in the stable scar. Collagenase is the most active collagenolytic enzyme. It is secreted by polymorphonuclear leukocytes, macrophages, and epithelial cells. The enzyme hydrolyzes collagen and participates in the process of wound remodeling. In the healed wound, the rates of collagen production and collagenolysis are in balance.

Epithelialization

The relative impermeability of the skin to radiation and fluids is provided by the epidermis. The epidermis consists of mitotically active basal keratinocytes as the deepest layer of cells. These keratinocytes migrate to ever more superficial layers; in the process, they mature, die, and eventually desquamate. Bonds between the epidermal cells and the underlying dermis form the basement membrane.

A wound is a break in the integrity of the epidermis, with consequent loss of its protection. The immediate reaction of all epithelium to a wound is to re-establish continuity of the protective barrier. In the epidermis, basal keratinocytes at the edge of the wound lose attachments to the dermis and simultaneously become more metabolically active and motile. Cell mitosis and migration continue until the defect has been filled and cell-to-cell contact has been established.[28]

In a cleanly incised surgical wound, well approximated by sutures, a covering epidermis develops within 48 to 72 hours. Wounds left open must heal by epidermal migration. Open wounds that contain dermis, such as second-degree burns and split-thickness skin graft donor sites, contain dermal appendages such as hair follicles and sweat glands. Keratinocytes within these appendages grow radially to quickly cover the wound. Wounds with full-thickness loss of skin close by epidermal migration from the edges only, which is much slower. The rate of epidermal migration is much more rapid if an intact basement membrane is present.[29]

Maturation

Scar maturation is most rapid in the first 6 months of healing but can last for years. Beginning in this phase, there is replacement of the extensive neovascularization of granulation tissue by dense collagen. During maturation, remodeling of the collagen occurs by degradation of old collagen and deposition of new, with an overall net increase. In rat skin, 15% of preinjury bursting strength (load required to break open a wound, regardless of size) is restored in a wound by 3 weeks after the injury, and more than 70% has returned by 9 weeks.[30] An increase in wound bursting strength is observed even though there is no net increase in the scar collagen content beyond the third week after injury. This increase in strength is explained by the development of stable intermolecular and intermolecular cross-links in the deposited collagen, and by improved orientation of individual collagen fibers.[31]

Wounds contract as they mature. The mechanism of this contraction has not been clarified, but it is likely caused by fibroblasts or myofibroblasts within the wound.[32] These cells form links to the extracellular matrix by actin, vinculin, and fibronectin, and cell locomotion results in contraction.[33] Understanding and modifying this process has clinical relevance in treating patients with problem scars. Open wounds contract more than do wounds closed primarily or with skin grafts, so these are important methods to prevent contractures.[34,35] Pressure applied to maturing scars also decreases contractures.

FACTORS AFFECTING WOUND HEALING

Age

It is generally believed that advancing age adversely affects wound healing. The growth rate and multiplication of fibroblasts and the synthesis of collagen are affected by aging.[36] Wound healing does appear to be more efficient in the young. The elderly patient with a wound healing problem may trace the difficulty to concurrent lung or cardiovascular disease, accompanied by diminished local wound oxygen tension or circulation. Likewise, nutritional deficiencies are common among older individuals and can lead to disturbed wound healing.

Protein Nutrition

The effects of protein depletion on wound healing in animals have been previously described.[36] The incised rat wound gains strength less rapidly in the protein-depleted animal. This wound healing abnormality is probably a result of altered collagen synthesis or cross-linking in the protein-depleted rat. Adequate protein nutrition is generally believed to be important in human wound healing.[37]

Vitamins and Trace Elements

Vitamin A is an important factor in wound healing, although deficiency of this vitamin is rare. Administration of vitamin A can reverse the healing retardation caused by cortisone.[38] However, vitamin A given to an animal not deficient in the vitamin does not increase the normal healing rate.

Vitamin C (ascorbic acid) has long been recognized as important in healing. Scurvy, a disease of vitamin C deficiency, is characterized by a failure in collagen synthesis. Specifically, the enzyme active in the hydroxylation of proline and lysine requires vitamin C as a cofactor.[39] Absence of ascorbic acid inhibits the action of this enzyme. Interestingly, old wounds in a scorbutic animal break down because collagenolysis proceeds normally at the same time that collagen synthesis is retarded.

Zinc is necessary for the activity of DNA and RNA polymerases and transferases.[36,39] Zinc deficiency may retard epithelialization and fibroblast proliferation. A normal zinc level is essential for healing, although the administration of this element to a patient without zinc depletion does not enhance healing. In addition, ferrous iron and copper are necessary for normal collagen metabolism.

Blood Loss and Anemia

In animals, it is recognized that significant blood loss and its resultant hypovolemia have a detrimental effect on wound healing. This effect may result from a decrease in tissue oxygenation during the hypovolemic state. Severe, chronic anemia is also believed to retard wound healing, although experimental data supporting this hypothesis are difficult to obtain. Mild to moderate normovolemic anemia does not appear to adversely effect wound healing in the otherwise healthy patient.[48]

Oxygen Tension

Oxygen is an essential element in wound healing. It is necessary for cell migration, proliferation, and protein and collagen synthesis. Although oxygen tension is low in the wound, there is little evidence that raising the normal arterial partial pressure of oxygen results in a clinically significant improvement in wound healing.[39] Nevertheless, anything that interferes with the delivery of oxygen to the wound (e.g., cardiovascular disease, diabetes, radiation) has a detrimental effect on wound healing.

Steroids and Cytotoxic Medications

The administration of steroids may have a profound effect on wound healing.[41] The rate of protein synthesis is decreased by the administration of cortisone and glucocorticoids. Other effects of these substances include diminished capillary budding, inhibition of fibroblast proliferation, and reduction in the rate of epithelialization. The normal inflammatory reaction that occurs after wounding is inhibited by steroids. These effects on wound healing are most profound if the steroid is administered before or at the time of wounding. In this circumstance, healing does proceed to completion, but at a reduced rate.

Cytotoxic drugs used in cancer chemotherapy may adversely affect wound healing.[42] Their action is primarily through an inhibition of cell proliferation. In general, the concentration of a cytotoxic drug in the wound, if given systemically, is insufficient to prevent wound healing; thus, completion of the healing process is delayed but not prevented.

FETAL WOUND HEALING

Fetuses undergoing surgery in utero for congenital malformations have little or no scarring. This clinical observation has been intensively studied in such animal models as the rat, rabbit, and sheep. Fetal sheep wounded at 75 or 100 days of gestation (term is 145 days) healed without scarring, whereas wounds created at 120 days healed with a dense, adultlike scar.[43] Many mechanisms have been proposed to explain this observation.

The differences in healing between the fetal and adult wound are likely caused by intrinsic properties of the fetal tissue, rather than the presence of amniotic fluid or the low tissue oxygenation of the fetus.[44] Recent research has been directed toward identifying these intrinsic differences between fetal and adult tissues, to better understand why scars form and to determine possible methods to prevent unwanted scars. Both hyaluronic acid (HA) and TGF-β have been shown to influence scar formation.

HA, a glycosaminoglycan, is more abundant in fetal than adult wounds. Amniotic fluid, bathing the fetal wound, is rich in HA. Fetal serum has been found to stimulate production of HA.[45] In adult wounds, HA is present only during early healing, whereas in fetal wounds, HA is present for much longer.[46] All evidence to date demonstrates a correlation of HA levels with fetal wound healing, but a causal effect has not been established.

TGF-β has been studied in the fetal wound model. The increase in the expression of this growth factor in gestation is correlated with the onset of adultlike scar formation. Addition of TGF-β to fetal wounds causes fibrosis. When a neutralizing antibody to TGF-β was applied to adult wounds, scar formation was reduced.[47] These studies indicate that TGF-β has an important role in scar formation. Understanding how these factors modulate scar formation may lead to methods to prevent unwanted scars.

HYPERTROPHIC SCARS AND KELOIDS

Under ideal circumstances, a wound develops into a narrow, flat, white scar, causing no functional or significant aesthetic problems. This ideal scar is the product of a balance between collagen deposition and its subsequent maturation and collagenolysis. An alteration in the desired process of maturation may represent itself as a hypertrophic scar or as a keloid. The hypertrophic scar is characterized by the deposition of excess collagen that remains within the borders of the scar bed. Hypertrophic scarring may be seen anywhere on the body and is more common in dark-skinned people and in young people. The natural course of a hypertrophic scar is spontaneous decrease in volume. A keloid also contains excess collagen; however, that collagen extends beyond the original lesion. Keloids are also more common in darkly pigmented and younger individuals (Fig. 62-4). Continued growth without regression is characteristic of keloids.[48]

Numerous techniques have been used in the treatment of hypertrophic scars and keloids. These include surgical excision, pressure, irradiation, and the administration of corticosteroids. Surgical excision alone is usually followed by recurrence of the hypertrophic scar or keloid. Irradiation and corticosteroids both act to inhibit collagen syn-

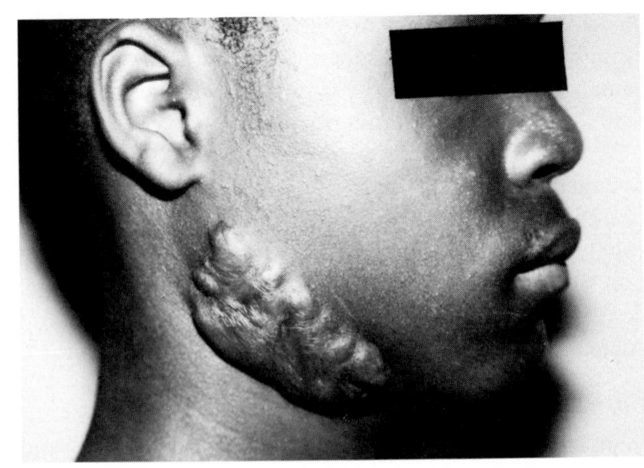

Fig. 62-4. Keloid scar that developed after a minor laceration.

thesis. However, many physicians are reluctant to suggest irradiation, because it is irreversible, and the long-term effects of even small doses are unknown. On the other hand, the combination of surgical excision and steroid injection has proved useful in managing keloids and hypertrophic scars.[49-53] Pressure produced by elastic garments, or more recently silicone patches, prevents the formation of hypertrophic burn scars and causes regression of established lesions.[54]

Many chemical compounds have been used in an attempt to control excess scarring.[50,51] β-Aminoproprionitrile irreversibly inhibits lysyl oxidase, preventing aldehyde formation and subsequent collagen cross-linking.[55] Penicillamine inhibits collagen cross-linking by chelating copper and interfering with the formation of aldehyde groups. Neither of these compounds has been proved safe or effective enough for broad clinical application.

SKIN GRAFTS AND FLAPS

Successful skin grafting is based on the observation that skin can be transplanted to a well-vascularized bed at a distant site and survive. Skin grafts are classified as either *split-thickness* or *full-thickness* (Fig. 62-5). The split-thickness graft ranges from 10/1000 inch ("thin" graft) to 15/1000 inch ("thick" graft) and is composed of the entire epidermis and a portion of the dermis. A full-thickness skin graft includes the epidermis and all of the dermis.

Once transferred, the skin graft depends on the recipient bed for survival. During the first 24 hours, the graft receives nutrients by passive diffusion from the bed. Revascularization of the graft occurs primarily by ingrowth of capillaries and venules from the underlying tissues. Evidence of circulation in the skin graft appears 24 to 48 hours after the transfer.

The donor site of a split-thickness skin graft heals by reepithelialization. Keratinocytes grow from the dermal appendages (hair follicles and sweat glands) to cover the exposed dermis. A moist, sterile, and occlusive dressing promotes this process. The donor site is usually healed after 2 to 3 weeks.

Three conditions must be met for successful skin grafting. First, the bed to be grafted must be well-vascularized. A skin graft will not take over bone denuded of its periosteum, tendon stripped of its peritenon, or cartilage without its perichondrium. Second, the graft must be in stable contact with the vascularized bed. Motion at the wound site dislodges the graft and prevents revascularization. Similarly, a seroma or hematoma that develops between the graft and the bed can preclude survival. Immobilization and a bolster dressing protect against motion and fluid collection beneath the graft. Third, bacterial contamination must be minimized. A skin graft will not survive over an infected or grossly contaminated (greater than 10^5 bacteria/g tissue) bed.

The primary indication for skin grafting is treatment of a wound that cannot be closed by direct suturing. A large burn area, massive skin avulsion, and wide local excision of a skin tumor are examples of such wounds. Use of a skin graft can provide closure more quickly than can healing by secondary intention. Split-thickness skin grafts are preferred to full-thickness ones when the area to be covered is large, because they become vacularized more readily and survive transplantation more reliably. On the other hand, the full-thickness graft contracts less during healing than does the split-thickness graft, making it more suitable for hand and eyelid reconstruction.

In contrast to skin grafts, a skin flap is used with its intrinsic blood supply left intact or, in the case of free-tissue transfer, with its blood supply restored immediately at the time of surgery. The skin receives its blood supply from the subdermal plexus. This plexus is in turn fed by perforating vessels from the underlying muscles. In certain anatomic areas, identifiable direct cutaneous (axial) vessels give off small arteries and veins that supply the subdermal plexus of the overlying skin. Flaps are classified as *random, axial pattern,* or *musculocutaneous,* depending on their blood supply. The random skin flap is raised just to the subdermal plexus (Fig. 62-6). It is limited in size because of its reduced vascularity. An axial pattern skin flap contains an axial artery and can be larger than its random counterpart

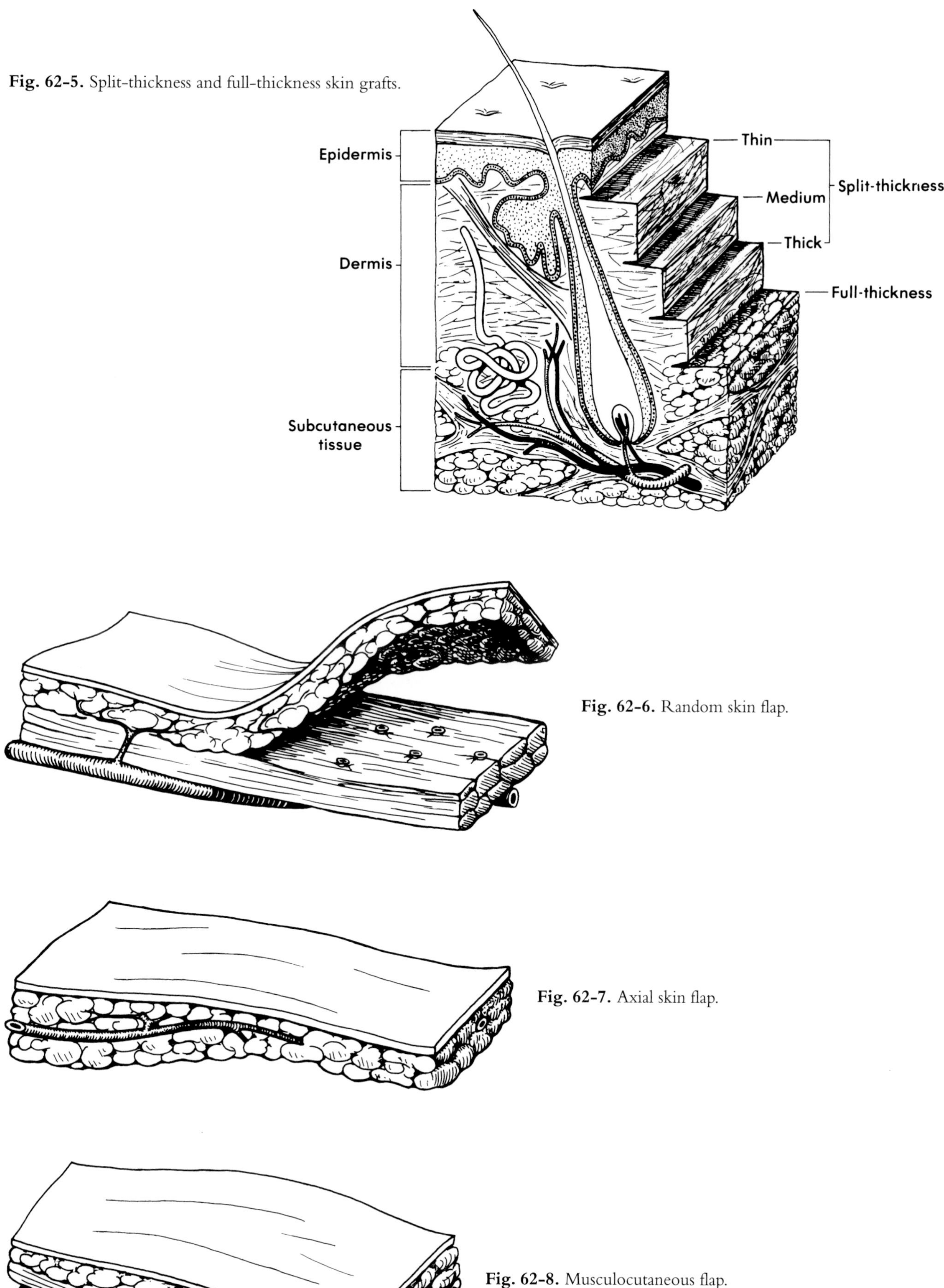

Fig. 62-5. Split-thickness and full-thickness skin grafts.

Fig. 62-6. Random skin flap.

Fig. 62-7. Axial skin flap.

Fig. 62-8. Musculocutaneous flap.

(Fig. 62-7). The musculocutaneous flap is composed of skin and the underlying muscle, and it can be moved as a single vascularized unit (Fig. 62-8). In appropriate cases, the muscle alone can be transferred, and a skin graft can then be applied. Because flaps have their own blood supply, they are helpful in the treatment of poorly vascularized or extensive wounds.

WOUND INFECTION

Etiology of Wound Infection

A wound infection arises when the body's defense mechanisms are inadequate to eradicate the bacteria contaminating the wound and to prevent their proliferation. Three elements predispose a patient toward the development of a wound infection: (1) a compromised wound, (2) an infectious organism, and (3) a susceptible host.

A *compromised wound* is one that contains devitalized tissue that is separated from the circulation and the antibacterial defenses. Dead tissues, foreign bodies, and hematomas retained in a wound can promote bacterial growth. A severely traumatized and poorly débrided wound that is repaired by suturing represents a closed space that is hypoxic, hypercarbic, and acidic—and thus conducive to bacterial proliferation.

Many different organisms are capable of initiating a wound infection. A bacterial strain's ability to survive in tissue is related to its absolute numbers as well as to its capacity to damage tissue with toxins, to propagate, and to spread (its virulence). Streptococci enter through even minor wounds and may cause cellulitis. Skin and subcutaneous abscesses are often related to staphylococcal infection. Wounds contaminated with gastrointestinal flora may become infected by gram-negative aerobic *(Escherichia coli)* and anaerobic *(Bacteroides fragilis)* species.

A susceptible host has some local or systemic impairment of resistance to bacterial invasion. Radiation changes and ischemia resulting from vascular disease are local factors that reduce resistance to infection. Systemic conditions (e.g., diabetes mellitus, administration of steroid therapy, shock, burns, renal disease, cancer, and the use of immunosuppressive agents) impair host resistance. The three final common pathways of host resistance that are usually impaired are the mediation of the acute inflammatory response, phagocytic mechanisms, and opsonization.[56]

When viewed in the clinical or operating room setting, a wound can be classified as *clean, clean-contaminated, contaminated,* or *dirty and infected.*[1,57] Knowledge of these wound types helps the surgeon understand and anticipate a subsequent wound infection (see accompanying box). The clean wound is nontraumatic and free of inflammation. If it is created in the operating room, no break in surgical technique is recorded, and the respiratory, alimentary, and genitourinary tracts are not violated. A clean-contaminated wound is likewise nontraumatic but is characterized by a minor break in surgical technique or the involvement of the gastrointestinal, genitourinary, or respiratory tracts, without significant spillage of contents. The contaminated wound classification includes all traumatic wounds caused by a dirty source, fecal contamination, a foreign body, or devitalized tissue, or those receiving delayed treatment. A surgical wound in which a major break in surgical technique, gross spillage from the gastrointestinal tract, or invasion of the genitourinary or biliary tracts in the presence of infection has occurred is a contaminated wound. The rate of postoperative wound infection ranges from 1% in clean wounds to more than 25% in dirty and infected ones.[56]

CLASSIFICATION OF OPERATIVE WOUNDS

Clean

Nontraumatic
No inflammation
Respiratory, gastrointestinal, and genitourinary tracts not entered
No break in surgical technique

Clean-Contaminated

Nontraumatic
Involvement of respiratory, gastrointestinal, biliary, or genitourinary tract without significant spillage
Appendectomy without perforation or cloudy peritoneal exudate
Prepared oropharynx or vagina entered
Minor break in surgical technique

Contaminated

Traumatic wound, recent
Gross spillage from gastrointestinal tract
Opening genitourinary or biliary tract with infected urine or bile
Major break in surgical technique

Dirty and Infected

Traumatic wound with devitalized tissue, foreign bodies, fecal contamination, or delayed treatment
Acute bacterial inflammation without pus
Incision for drainage of pus
Perforated viscus found during surgery

From Burke JF. Fundamentals of Wound Management in Surgery: Infection. New York: Appleton-Century-Crofts, 1977.

Prevention and Treatment of Wound Infection

Wound infection can be minimized in the operating room by shielding the surgical wound from bacterial contamination. Preoperative skin preparation, sterile draping, mechanical and antibiotic bowel preparation, preoperative systemic antibiotic coverage, and careful aseptic technique all minimize contamination. Careful surgical technique and gentle handling of tissues minimize injury and discourage bacterial proliferation.

Proper management of the traumatic wound decreases

the likelihood of subsequent infection. High-pressure irrigation with physiologic saline solution can remove bacteria and foreign bodies from the traumatic wound. Débridement further reduces contamination by removing foreign bodies and devitalized tissue from the site of injury. Subsequent wound closure with minimum tension maintains good vascularity of the tissues.

A wound infection is suspected if signs of inflammation (warmth, erythema, induration, and pain) or drainage appear at the operative or injured site within the first month after surgery or injury. Cellulitis is characterized by all the signs of inflammation, but without a collection of pus. β-Hemolytic streptococci typically spread through tissues without stimulating a purulent exudate. Abscess in a wound is initially seen in a purulent collection and is usually accompanied by acute inflammation.

The treatment of a wound infection must be both prompt and appropriate.[58] A sample of any wound discharge is submitted for Gram staining, aerobic and anaerobic culture, and determination of bacterial sensitivity. Broad-spectrum antibiotic coverage is initiated before culture results have been obtained. The most important aspect of early management is adequate wound drainage. A suspect wound should be aspirated with a large-bore needle. If pus is returned, or if the wound remains questionable, it should be opened and drainage should be begun. Any abscess discovered is drained as thoroughly as possible, and the wound is packed with saline solution–soaked dressings that are changed every 4 to 8 hours.

In a severely traumatized or contaminated wound, primary closure may risk subsequent wound infection. Delayed primary closure (within 3 days of injury) or secondary closure (3 to 7 days after injury) produced satisfactory healing and reduces the incidence of infection. Initially, the wound is covered or packed lightly with saline solution–soaked fine-mesh gauze. Whether healing is occurring without infection is determined through daily wound inspection. If no infection occurs, the wound is closed by suturing, either with or without excision of the margins.

WOUND MANAGEMENT

Suture Material

Suture materials are classified as either absorbable or nonabsorbable.[59] They may consist of a single strand (monofilament) or of multiple strands (multifilament). The multifilament sutures are twisted or braided for strength. Nonabsorbable sutures remain in place indefinitely, whereas absorbable sutures are gradually removed by physiologic processes.

Absorbable sutures are useful in providing early strength to a closed wound. They are most frequently placed in an intradermal or subcutaneous position. Catgut suture is produced from bovine intestinal serosa. Chromicization of the suture prolongs absorption and strength. Absorption occurs 2 to 6 weeks after the operation. Newer absorbable sutures (polyglycolic acid [Dexon], polyglactin [Vicryl]) are synthesized by polymerization of glycolic acid. They incite less inflammatory response than do catgut sutures. However, the glycolic acid sutures are more difficult to tie than are catgut ones.

Nonabsorbable sutures are most often used for skin closure and in internal sites that require prolonged tissue strength. Examples of nonabsorbable suture materials include silk, nylon, cotton, polypropylene (Prolene), polyethylene terephthalate fiber (Dacron), and stainless steel. When placed in the skin, a monofilament (Prolene, nylon, and stainless steel) suture invokes a less severe inflammatory reaction than does a multifilament (silk and cotton) suture. Skin staples allow rapid skin wound closure but leave less satisfactory skin marks if applied too tightly or if allowed to remain in the skin longer than 1 week.

The duration that a suture is left in place varies with the wound location.[60] The longer a suture remains in the skin, the more severe is the tissue reaction to the suture. An unsightly scar may be produced at the site of each suture. In the face, skin sutures are usually removed within 3 to 5 days. Skin sutures in wounds of the extremities and trunk are generally left in position for 7 days. Skin sutures placed in a buried (intradermal) position can remain for several weeks without compromising the resultant scar.

Dressings

A dressing applied to a closed wound serves several purposes. It is absorbent, thereby removing any drainage that occurs. A dressing also serves to protect the wound against bacterial contamination. The dressing should be constructed securely enough to prevent pain from any subsequent minor trauma. The deepest layer of dressing should be nonadherent, thus ensuring pain-free removal. Some dressings, particularly those of the hand and the extremities, hold the injured part in a functional or desired position. A compressive dressing can aid in the prevention of edema at the wound site.

The duration of wound coverage by a dressing is variable. A simple skin incision closed primarily is epithelialized within 24 to 48 hours; as such, it is protected against bacterial invasion. With such a simple wound, the dressing can be removed permanently after 48 hours. Dressings may be left in place on the extremities for many days or weeks.

SUMMARY

The body's response to wounding allows survival in a harsh, pathogen-contaminated environment. When closed primarily, a wound heals by the simultaneous and interrelated processes of inflammation, epithelialization, cellular production of collagen, and maturation. A wound left open diminishes in size by contraction while undergoing the same healing phases as its closed counterpart. The speed and adequacy of healing are dependent on the patient's adequate nutrition and on local vascularity. Advanced age, associated illnesses, and various medications have deleterious effects on healing. Individual response to wounding determines the appearance of the mature scar, with some patients more likely to be affected by scar hypertrophy or keloids.

The nature and extent of a wound dictate the physician's management of it. After cleansing and débridement, wounds are closed primarily, covered with a skin graft or flap, or allowed to heal by secondary intention. Wound infection, should it occur, is treated by incision or reopening of the wound, drainage, administration of appropriate antibiotics, and dressing changes. Adherence to the principles of wound care usually results in healing by primary intention and development of a scar that is satisfactory to both the patient and physician.

REFERENCES

1. Altemeier WA, et al. Manual on Control of Infection in Surgical Patients. Philadelphia: JB Lippincott, 1976.
2. Arturson G. Pathophysiology of the burn wound. Ann Chir Gynaecol 69:178, 1980.
3. Boucek RJ. Factors affecting wound healing. Otolaryngol Clin North Am 17:243, 1984.
4. Majno G, Gilmore V, Leventhal M. On the mechanism of vascular leakage caused by histamine-type mediators. Circ Res 21:833, 1967.
5. Cuono CB. Prostaglandin inhibitors and wound healing [letter]. Plast Reconstr Surg 70:514, 1982.
6. Lord JT, et al. Prostaglandin in wound healing: Possible regulation of granulation. In Samuelson B, Ramwell PW, Paoletti R, eds. Advances in Prostaglandin and Thromboxane Research, vol 7. New York: Raven Press, 1980.
7. Lupulescu A. Effect of prostaglandins on protein, RNA, DNA, and collagen synthesis in experimental wounds. Prostaglandins 10:573, 1975.
8. McGrath MH. The effect of prostaglandin inhibitors on wound contraction and the myofibroblast. Plast Reconstr Surg 69:74, 1982.
9. Samuelson B, et al. Prostaglandins and thromboxanes: Biochemical and physiological consideration. In Coceani F, Olley PM, eds. Advances in Prostaglandin and Thromboxane Research, vol 4. New York: Raven Press, 1978.
10. Weissman G, Simolen JE, Korchak HM. Release of inflammatory mediators from stimulated neutrophils. N Engl J Med 303:27, 1980.
11. Leibovich SJ, Ross R. The role of the macrophage in wound repair. Am J Pathol 78:71, 1975.
12. Dinarello CA, Wolff SM. Molecular basis of fever in humans. Am J Med 72:799, 1982.
13. Bevilacqua MP, et al. Interleukin 1 acts on cultured human vascular endothelium to increase the adhesion of polymorphonuclear leukocytes, monocytes, and related leukocyte cell lines. J Clin Invest 76:2003, 1985.
14. Beutler B, et al. Identity of tumor necrosis factor and the macrophage-secreted factor cachectin. Nature 316:552, 1985.
15. Metcalf D. The granulocyte-macrophage colony-stimulating factors. Science 229:16, 1985.
16. Diegelmann RF, Cohen IK, Kaplan AM. The role of macrophages in wound repair: A review. Plast Reconstr Surg 68:107, 1981.
17. Thakral KK, Goodson WH III, Hunt TK. Stimulation of wound blood vessel growth by wound macrophages. J Surg Res 26:430, 1979.
18. Madri JA, Pratt BM, Tucker AM. Phenotypic modulation of endothelial cells by transforming growth factor-β depends upon the composition and organization of the extracellular matrix. J Cell Biol 106:1375, 1988.
19. Gimenez-Gallego G, et al. Brain-derived acidic fibroblast growth factor: Complete amino acid sequence and homologies. Science 230:1385, 1985.
20. Leibovich SJ, et al. Macrophage-induced angiogenesis is mediated by tumor necrosis factor-alpha. Nature 329:630, 1987.
21. Pepper MS, et al. Biphasic effect of transforming growth factor-β_1 on in vitro angiogenesis. Exp Cell Res 204:356, 1993.
22. Sommer A, Rifkin DB. Interaction of heparin with human basic fibroblast growth factor: Protection of the angiogenic protein from proteolytic degradation by glycosaminoglycans. J Cell Physiol 138:215, 1989.
23. Folkman J, et al. A heparin-binding angiogenic protein—basic fibroblast growth factor—is stored within basement membrane. Am J Pathol 130:393, 1988.
24. Ross R. Platelet-derived growth factor. Ann Rev Med 38:71, 1987.
25. Pierce GF, et al. Platelet-derived growth factor and transforming growth factor-β enhance tissue repair activities by unique mechanisms. J Cell Biol 109:429, 1989.
26. Mustoe TA, et al. Accelerated healing of incisional wounds in rats induced by transforming growth factor-β. Science 237:1333, 1987.
27. Miller EJ, Gay S. Collagen structure and function. In Cohen IK, et al., eds. Wound Healing. Philadelphia: WB Saunders, 1992.
28. Odland G, Ross R. Human wound repair. I. Epidermal regeneration. J Cell Biol 39:135, 1968.
29. Mansbridge JN, Knapp AM. Changes in keratinocyte maturation during wound healing. J Invest Dermatol 89:253, 1987.
30. Levenson SM, et al. The healing of rat skin wounds. Ann Surg 161:293, 1965.
31. Doillon CJ, et al. Collagen fiber formation in repair tissue: Development of strength and toughness. Collagen Rel Res 5:481, 1985.
32. Hembry RM, et al. Morphologic examination of mesenchymal cells in healing wounds of normal and tight skin mice. Am J Pathol 125:81, 1986.
33. Ehrlich HP. Wound closure: Evidence of cooperation between fibroblasts and collagen matrix. Eye 2:149, 1988.
34. Corps BVM. The effect of graft thickness, donor site, and graft bed on graft shrinkage in the wounded rat. Br J Plast Surg 22:125, 1969.
35. Rudolph R. Inhibition of myofibroblasts by skin grafts. Plast Reconstr Surg 63:473, 1979.
36. Chvapil M, Koopmann CF Jr. Age and other factors regulating wound healing. Otolaryngol Clin North Am 15:259, 1982.
37. Van Winkle W. The tensile strength of wounds and factors that influence it. Surg Gynecol Obstet 129:819, 1969.
38. Hunt TK, et al. Effect of vitamin A on reversing the inhibitory effect of cortisone on healing of open wounds in animals and man. Ann Surg 170:633, 1969.
39. Peacock EE Jr. Wound Repair, 3rd ed. Philadelphia: WB Saunders, 1984.
40. Heughan C, Grislis G, Hunt TK. The effect of anemia on wound healing. Ann Surg 179:163, 1974.
41. Ehrlich HP, Hunt TK. Effects of cortisone and vitamin A on wound healing. Ann Surg 167:324, 1968.
42. Cohen SC, et al. Effects of antineoplastic agents on wound healing in mice. Surgery 78:238, 1975.
43. Longaker MT, et al. Studies in fetal wound healing: Second and early third trimester fetal wounds demonstrate rapid collagen deposition without scar formation. J Pediatr Surg 25:63, 1990.
44. Longaker MT, et al. Adult skin in the fetal environment heals with scar formation. Surg Forum 41:639, 1990.
45. Decker M, et al. Hyaluronic acid stimulating factor in serum from the bovine fetus and from breast cancer patients. Cancer Res 49:3499, 1989.
46. Alexander SA, Donoff RB. The glycosaminoglycans of open fetal wounds. J Surg Res 29:422, 1980.
47. Shah M, Foreman DM, Ferguson MW. Control of scarring in adult wounds by neutralising antibody to transforming growth factor β. Lancet 339:213, 1992.
48. Riley WB, Peacock EE Jr. The identification, distribution, and significance of collagenolytic enzyme in human tissues. Proc Soc Exp Biol Med 124:207, 1967.

49. Cohen IK, Diegelmann RF. The biology of keloid and hypertrophic scar and the influence of corticosteroids. Clin Plast Surg 4:297, 1977.
50. Cohen IK, McCoy BJ. The biology and control of surface overhealing. World J Surg 4:289, 1980.
51. Ketchum LD, Cohen IK, Masters FW. Hypertrophic scars and keloids: A collective review. Plast Reconstr Surg 53:140, 1974.
52. Murray JC, Pollack SV, Pinnell SR. Keloids: A review. J Am Acad Dermatol 4:461, 1981.
53. Pollack SV, Goslen JB. The surgical treatment of keloids. J Dermatol Surg Oncol 8:1045, 1982.
54. Baur PS, Parks DH, Larson DL. The healing of burn wounds. Clin Plast Surg 4:389, 1977.
55. Peacock EE, Jr. Pharmacologic control of surface scarring. Ann Surg 193:592, 1981.
56. Goodenough RD, Molnar JA, Burke JF. Surgical infections. In Hardy JD, ed. Hardy's Textbook of Surgery. Philadelphia: JB Lippincott, 1983.
57. Burke JF. Fundamentals of Wound Management in Surgery: Infection. New York: Appleton-Century-Crofts, 1977.
58. Olson M, O'Connor M, Schwartz ML. Surgical wound infections. Ann Surg 199:253, 1984.
59. Swanson NA, Tromovitch TO. Suture materials, 1980s: Properties, uses and abuses. Int J Dermatol 21:373, 1982.
60. Van Winkle W, Hastings JC. Considerations in the choice of suture material for various tissues. Surg Gynecol Obstet 135:113, 1972.

63

Breast: Physiologic Considerations in Normal, Benign, and Neoplastic States

Kirby I. Bland, Michael P. Vezeridis, and Edward M. Copeland III

The breast is a modified sweat gland that is embryologically unique to the mammalian species—thus the term *mammary gland.* Although variable in number among the different mammalian species, mammary glands in single pairs are observed only in human beings, apes, and monkeys (except for marmosets). The breast is a functional part of the reproductive system, with perturbations in physiologic function that reflect neuroendocrine stimuli and control. These remarkable fluctuations in physiologic stimuli, with metabolic and morphologic consequences, are evident from prepubertal adolescence to postmenopause. A comprehensive knowledge of the physiologic alterations expected in the normal breast, as well as specific deviations in the pathologic processes that are evident in premenopausal and postmenopausal female humans, are essential to the diagnosis and appropriate therapy of breast disease.

RELEVANT ANATOMY

Developmental Anatomy of Mammary Gland

The mammary gland is initially recognized in the human embryo as a "milk streak" in the sixth week of embryologic development. The milk line develops in the pectoral portion of the ectodermal thickening and extends bilaterally from the axilla to the vulva. These distinct linear elevations are called *milk lines* or the *mammary ridge.* By the ninth intrauterine week, the milk line has atrophied except in its pectoral region, and a nipple bud appears with the formation of a proliferating mass of basaloid cells that represents the breast primordium. By month 3 of embryologic development, the nipple bud is invaded by squamous cells from the ectoderm. At month 5, connective tissue of mesenchymal origin develops beneath the breast primordium into 15 to 20 solid cords. From these embryologic remnants, the mammary ducts develop as ventral ingrowths that branch into primary milk ducts and terminate in lobular buds, which proliferate into acini after ovarian estrogenic stimuli. By the seventh to eighth month, these ducts are cannulated to form lumina. Thus, by termination of pregnancy, the nipple bud is penetrated by primary milk ducts to terminate at its recessed opening and shortly becomes everted and surrounded by the ectodermal thickening of the nipple (areola).

Topographic Mammary Anatomy

With its fibrous and fatty components, the breast occupies the interval between the third and seventh ribs and extends in breadth from the parasternal to the midaxillary lines. The glandular portion of the breast rests largely on the pectoral fascia and the serratus anterior musculature. Mammary tissue typically extends in the anterior axillary fold (tail of Spence) and is often visible as a definite mass.

The anterior and lateral projections of the breast vary with age, habitus, and ovarian functional status. Thus, the glandular aspects of the breast remain undeveloped and rudimentary in male humans. In this circumstance, short ducts with poorly developed acini are evident. A deficiency of parenchymal fat and nipple-areola development is apparent, contributing to the flat appearance of the male breast.

In female humans, the nonparous breast is hemispheric and somewhat flattened above the nipple. In contrast, the multiparous breast is lax and large and rarely regains its initial configuration until menopause, when atrophy of glandular tissue is initiated. The postmenopausal breast consistently reveals a disappearance of parenchymal fat with loss of the active (proliferative) glandular portion as a result of cessation of ovarian function. The nonlactating breast weighs between 150 to 225 g, whereas the lactating breast may be as large as 500 g.[1]

Adult Anatomy

Because the adult mammary gland is a modification of an ectodermal vestige of a sweat gland, it is confined entirely within the superficial and deep layers of the fascia of the anterior chest wall. The delicate layers of superficial fascia serve as an anatomic guide for the elevation of skin flaps of appropriate thickness of fatty and areolar tissue when a mastectomy is performed. The thickness of the skin flap depends on the patient's habitus and may be only 2 to 3 mm in thin individuals, in contrast to a greater thickness in obese subjects.

The deep layer of superficial fascia crosses the retromammary space to fuse with the pectoral (deep) fascia. A distinct space is observed on the posterior aspect of the breast between the deep layer of superficial fascia and the investing fascia of the pectoralis major and contiguous muscles of the chest wall (Fig. 63-1). This retromammary bursa contributes to the mobility of the breast on the chest wall as a result of its loose areolar connections. The deep pectoral fascia is attached to the sternum and superolaterally to the axillary and clavicular fascia. This fascial envelope is contiguous inferiorly with the rectus abdominus tendon of the abdominal wall. The posterior surface of the pectoralis major muscle is continuous with the clavipectoral fascia, which also encases the pectoralis minor musculature.[2] The broad condensation of clavipectoral fascia (Halsted's ligament), which is superior and superficial to the pectoralis minor muscle, is penetrated by the anterior thoracic neurovascular bundles and the cephalic vein. A

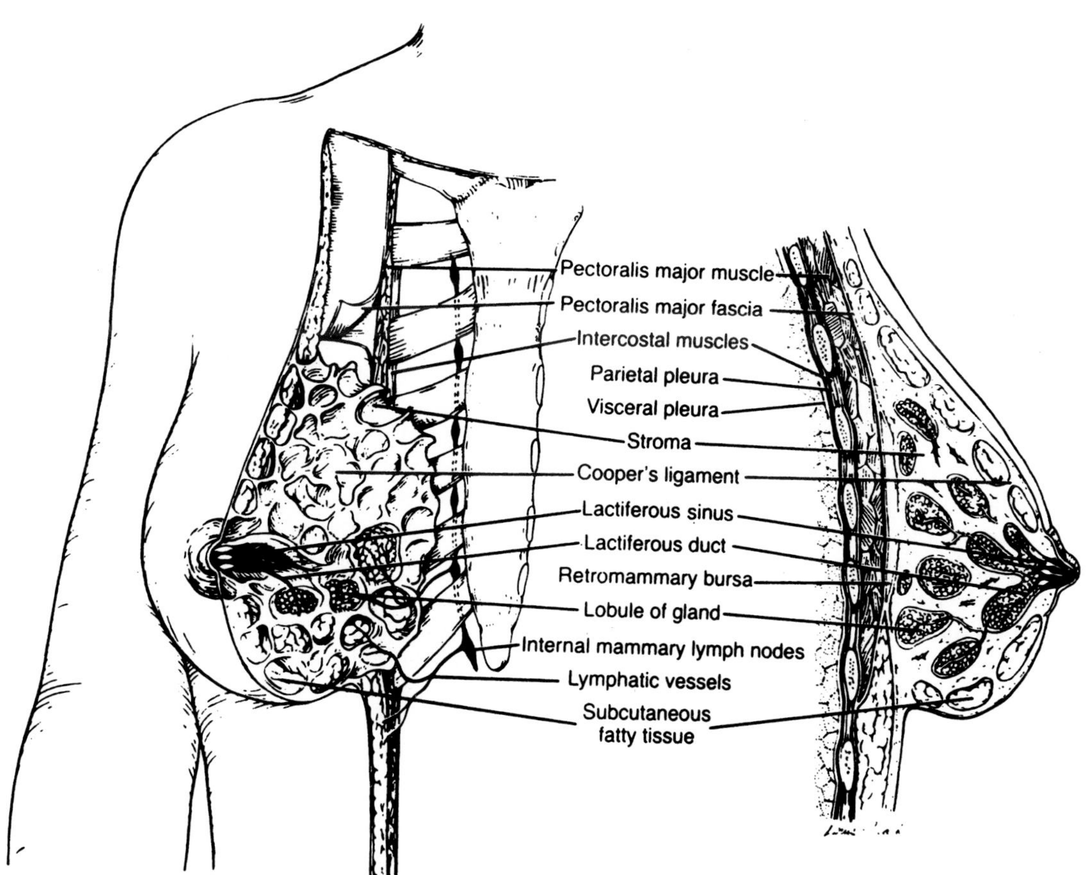

Fig. 63-1. A tangential view of the breast on the chest wall and a cross-sectional (sagittal) view of the breast and associated chest wall. The breast lies in the superficial fascia just deep to the dermis. It is attached to the skin by the suspensory ligaments of Cooper and is separated from the investing fascia of the pectoralis major muscle by the retromammary bursa. Cooper's ligaments form fibrosepta in the stroma that provide support for the breast parenchyma. From 15 to 20 lactiferous ducts extend from lobules composed of glandular epithelium to openings located on the nipple. A dilation of the duct, the lactiferous sinus, is present near the opening of the duct in the subareolar tissue. Subcutaneous fat and adipose tissue distributed around the lobules of the gland give the breast its smooth contour and, in the nonlactating breast, account for most of its mass. Lymphatic vessels pass through the stroma surrounding the lobules of the gland and convey lymph to collecting ducts. Lymphatic channels ending in the internal mammary (or parasternal) lymph nodes are shown. The pectoralis major muscle lies adjacent to the ribs and intercostal muscles. The parietal pleura, attached to the endothoracic fascia, and the visceral pleura, covering the surface of the lung, are shown. (From Wagner FB Jr. History of breast disease and its treatment. In Bland KI, Copeland EM III, eds. The Breast: Comprehensive Management of Benign and Malignant Diseases. Philadelphia: WB Saunders, 1991, p 18.)

vascular sheath envelops the axillary vessels as this fascial plate continues from the roof of the axillary space to fuse with the deep fascial contributions of the anterior surface of the pectoralis major muscle.

The mammary parenchyma is interdigitated by septumlike connections of fibrous processes, which extend from the posterior superficial fascia layer to the superficial layer of fascia of the skin. These suspensory Cooper's ligaments insert perpendicularly to the delicate superficial fascial layers of the corium (see Fig. 63-1). Cooper's ligaments permit remarkable mobility of the breast while providing support of the lobular and parenchymal structure.

Anomalous Developments of Breast

Anomalies of the nipples or the breast in human beings of either sex are a result of imperfect or complete suppression of the breast anlagen in embryogenesis. Further, an accessory breast represents a regression to a more primitive type of mammary arrangement in which more than a single pair of these anlagen persist.

Supernumerary (accessory) nipples or breasts thus may occur as a result of this latter embryologic event and are observed in approximately 1% to 2% of whites. Accessory breast tissue appears to occur more frequently in female than in male humans by a ratio of 2:1.[3] The anomaly is considered hereditary with autosomal dominant penetrance. Supernumerary mammary development can occur in combination or as singular components of the breast and thus involves the glandular parenchyma, nipple, or areola. In many cases, only a diminutive nipple is evident, but the most frequent combination is a small nipple and an areola bud. Classically, these anomalous structures are observed along the embryologic milk streak in sites between the groin and axilla. These embryologic remnants are most often seen in the axilla or in the milk line just below the normal breast. The anomaly occurs more frequently in Asians.

Amastia, complete absence of one or both breasts, is a remarkably rare breast anomaly. In circumstances in which amastia occurs, it is usually unilateral, with persistence of a rudimentary breast structure, and is associated with underdevelopment or absence of structures of the anterior and lateral chest wall, arm, or shoulder girdle.[3]

Lymphatic Drainage of Mammary Gland and Routes for Metastases

A thorough knowledge of breast lymphatic drainage is important to the study of this organ's pathophysiology. Metastatic dissemination occurs predominantly by lymphatic routes, which are rich and extensive and arborize in multiple directions through skin and intraparenchymal lymph ducts. The delicate lymph vessels of the corium are valveless; flow encompasses the lobular parenchyma and thereafter parallels major venous channels to enter the regional lymph nodes. The unidirectional lymphatic flow is pulsatile as a result of the wavelike contractions of the lymphatics to allow rapid transit and emptying of the lymphatic vascular spaces that interdigitate the extensive periductal and perilobular network. When lymph flow is impeded by inflammatory or neoplastic states, a reversal in flow in these rich lymphatic networks is evident, accounting for the neoplastic growth in local and regional sites remote from the primary tumor.

Unlike blood circulation, lymph flow is unidirectional, except in the pathologic state just mentioned, and has preferential flow from the periphery toward the right side of the heart. Lymphatic capillaries end blindly in tissues from which lymph is collected; throughout their course, these capillaries anastomose and fuse to form fewer lymph channels, which terminate in the large left thoracic duct or the smaller right lymphatic duct (Fig. 63-2). The thoracic duct empties into the left subclavian vein, whereas the right lymphatic duct drains preferentially into the right subclavian vein at the point of entry for the internal jugular vein.

Haagensen[3] emphasizes that lymphatics of the dermis are intimately related to the deep lymphatics of the underlying fascial planes, which explains the multidirectional potential for drainage of superficial breast neoplasms. Preferential flow of lymph toward the axilla is observed in lesions of the upper anterolateral chest. However, at the level of the umbilicus, tributaries diverge such that chest and upper anterior and lateral abdominal wall lymph enters channels of the axilla. Thus, carcinomatous involvement of skin, even of the inframammary region, preferentially flows to the axilla rather than to the groin.

Haagensen[3] and Anson and McVay[2] trace two accessory directions for lymphatic drainage from the breast to nodes of the apex of the axilla: the transpectoral and retropectoral routes. Lymph nodes of the transpectoral route (interpectoral nodes) lie between the pectoralis major and minor muscles and are referred to as *Rotter's nodes.* This drainage pathway begins in the loose areolar tissue of the retromammary plexus and interdigitates between the pectoral fascia and breast to perforate the pectoralis major muscle and follow the course of the thoracoacromial artery and terminate in the subclavicular (apical) group of nodes.

The retropectoral lymphatic pathway drains the superior and internal portions of the breast and arborizes on the lateral and posterior surface of the pectoralis major or under the pectoralis minor muscle to terminate at the apex of the axilla in the subclavicular (level III) group. This route of lymphatic drainage occurs in approximately one third of all female patients and is a more direct mechanism of lymphatic flow to the subclavicular group. This is also the major lymphatic drainage by way of the external mammary and central axillary nodal groups (levels I and II, respectively).

To assess the possibility of axillary nodal involvement appropriately, an appreciation of the major lymph nodal groups is essential. Mornard[4] identified five principal axillary lymph node groups that lie on or inferior to the axillary vein and are invested by costocoracoid fascia contigu-

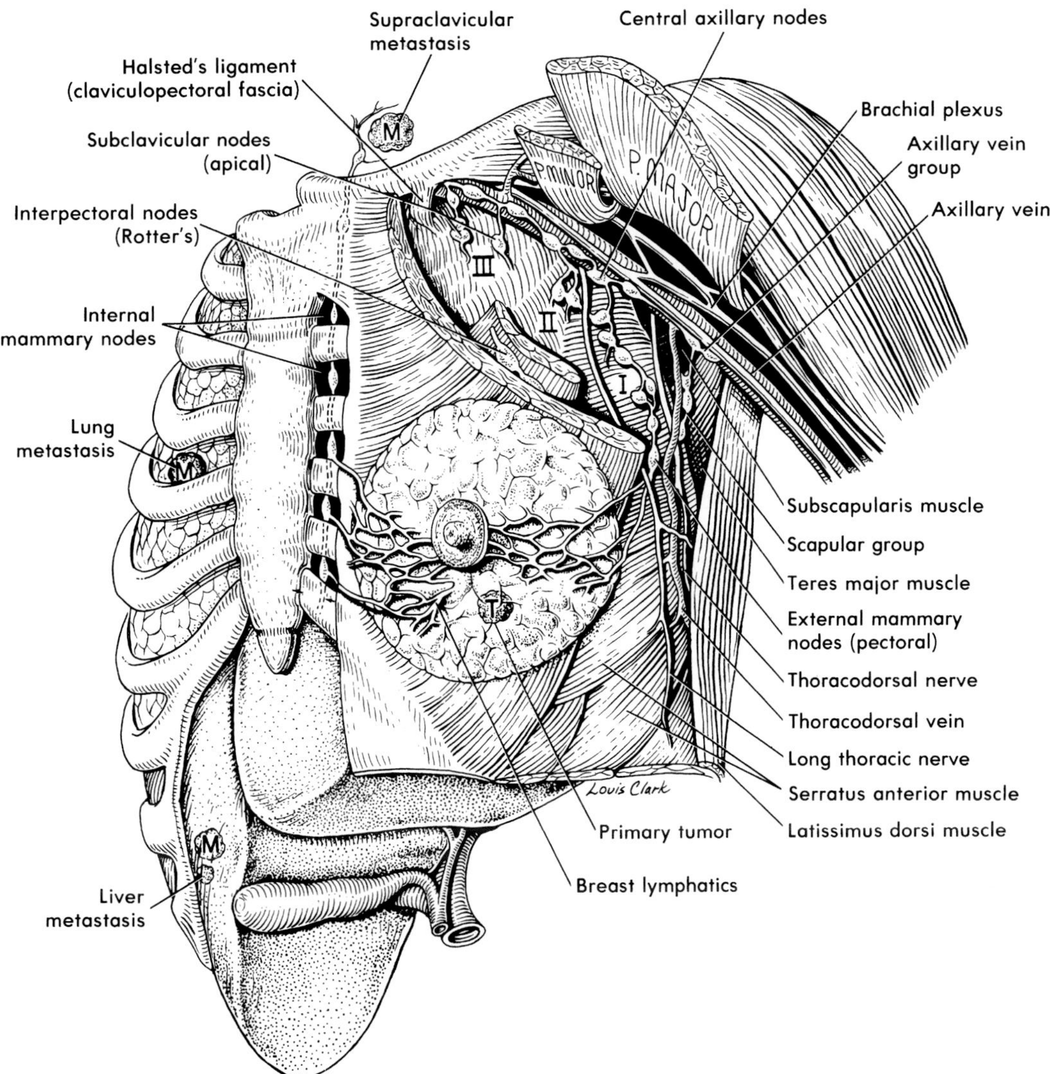

Fig. 63-2. Lymphatic drainage of breast. Unidirectional flow of lymph toward axilla or internal mammary nodes is depicted. Five basic axillary nodal groups include level I, external mammary group, subscapular (scapular) group, and axillary vein group; level II, central nodal group; and level III, subclavicular (apical) group. Interpectoral (Rotter's) group is interposed between pectoralis major and minor muscles. Subareolar and central primary tumors have bidirectional lymphatic flow to axilla or internal mammary chain. Three principal groups of deep veins serve as vascular routes for metastases and include intercostal, axillary, and internal mammary veins. Visceral metastases to lung or liver are possible through lymphatic or primary vascular drainage routes of breast and communicate with major venous trunks.

ous with the axillary artery, brachial plexus, areola, and connective tissue. The five primary axillary nodal groups (see Fig. 63-2) are as follows:

1. The *external mammary group* (level I) occupies the lateral margin of the pectoralis major muscle and the medial side of the axillary space and parallels the course of the lateral thoracic artery of the chest wall from the sixth rib to the axillary vein.
2. The *subscapular (scapular) group* (level I) is closely applied to the thoracodorsal branches of the subscapular vessels and extends from the lateral thoracic wall to the axillary vein.
3. The *axillary vein group* (level I) represents the most laterally placed and numerous group of lymph nodes of the axilla and occupies the ventral and caudal aspects of the vein.
4. The *central nodal group* (level II) is often superficial beneath the skin and fascia of the middle axilla and is centrally located between the posterior and anterior axillary folds. This is the nodal group most often palpated and the one on which the clinical estimation of nodal disease is based.[2,3]
5. The *subclavicular (apical) node group* (level III) is the most medial and highest nodal group, situated at the

juncture of the axillary vein and its entry beneath the subclavian muscle to form the subclavian vein at the level of the clivopectoral fascia (Halsted's ligament).

The recognition of metastatic spread of breast carcinoma into internal mammary nodes as a primary route of systemic dissemination is credited to the British surgeon W.S. Handley.[5,6] Extensive investigation confirmed that median and central breast lymphatics progressed medially and paralleled the course of major blood vessels to perforate the pectoralis major muscle and empty into the internal mammary nodal chain. This major lymphatic route (see Fig. 63-2) is situated in the interspaces of the costal cartilages, approximately 2 to 3 cm within the sternal margin. These nodal groups traverse and parallel the internal mammary vessels and are invested by endothoracic fascia. Internal mammary lymphatic trunks eventually terminate in subclavicular nodal groups. The right internal mammary group enters the right lymphatic duct, and the left group enters the main thoracic duct. The presence of supraclavicular nodes (stage IV disease) is a result of lymphatic permeation and subsequent obstruction of the inferior deep cervical group or nodes of the jugular-subclavian confluence. The supraclavicular nodal group represents the termination of efferent trunks from subclavian nodes of the internal mammary nodal group. The nodes are situated beneath the lateral margin of the inferior aspect of the sternocleidomastoid muscle behind the clavicle and represent common sites of distant metastases from breast cancer.

Cross-connections of lymphatic drainage from the breast to the opposite axilla often occur. This observation of communicating dermal lymphatics to the contralateral side explains occasional metastatic involvement of the opposite axilla and breast. Structures of the chest wall, including the external and internal intercostal musculature, have extensive lymphatic drainage, which parallels the course of their major intercostal blood supply. Thus, invasive neoplasms of the lateral breast that involve deep musculature have preferential drainage toward the axillae. Conversely, invasion of medial musculature has preferential drainage toward the internal mammary nodal groups, whereas bidirectional metastases can be evident with invasive subareolar or central neoplasms.

Venous Drainage of Mammary Gland

Lymphatic drainage of the breast is the primary route for metastatic dissemination, although the vascular route for tumor emboli has a major role in dissemination of neoplasms to the lungs (see Fig. 63-2). The three groups of deep veins to the breast that serve as vascular routes are as follows:

1. The *intercostal veins* traverse the posterior aspect of the breast from the second through the sixth intercostal spaces and enter the vertebral veins posteriorly and the azygos vein centrally to terminate in the superior vena cava.
2. The *axillary vein* may have many variable tributaries that drain the chest wall and the pectoral muscles and breast.
3. The *internal mammary vein perforators* represent the largest venous network that drains the breast; this venous plexus traverses the rib interspaces to terminate in the innominate vein and thus represents a direct embolic route to the pulmonary capillary network.[2,3]

PHYSIOLOGY OF NORMAL BREAST DEVELOPMENT AND FUNCTION

The phases of breast development, growth, and involution follow alveoli and myoepithelial alterations of breast parenchyma, which result from the mammotropic effects of anterior pituitary and ovarian hormonal secretion. Breast growth and development are isometric and parallel those of the body habitus before the onset of menses. The major determinant of breast development and maturation is the presence of ovarian estrogen and progesterone secretion. Thus, breasts of normal size or consistency will not develop in the absence of endogenous estrogens in the amenorrheic (premenstrual) female human.

Hormonal Control of Breast Development and Function

Breast development in the female human remains under neuroendocrine control of the anterior pituitary gland and the ovary. The gonadotropic luteinizing hormone (LH) and the gonadotropic follicle-stimulating hormone (FSH) of the female human are both secreted from basophil cells of the anterior pituitary. The luteotropic lactogenic hormone (LTH), prolactin, is produced by the pituitary acidophile cell. Neurohumoral pathways from the hypothalamus have a role in the production and release of these gonadotropic hormones.

The functions of the gonadotropic hormones of this basophilic group from the anterior pituitary are qualitatively identical in both sexes. FSH stimulates the mature ovarian graafian follicle to develop and synthesize estrogen in the presence of minute quantities of LH. When release of the basophilic LH is inhibited or impaired, the stimulated ovarian follicle will synthesize a product that, although not estrogenic, has the effect of inhibiting FSH. The presence of circulating estrogen initiates the production of LH and further inhibits basophilic cell production of FSH. Thus, augmented LH secretion with simultaneous diminution in the amount of FSH initiates ovulation and the formation of a nonfunctional corpus luteum. LTH initiates the release and secretion of progestogen and estrogen from the corpus luteum. Estrogen production from the ovary is initiated after FSH stimulation of the follicle in the presence of trace amounts of LH (Fig. 63-3). Both the production and release of LH, and perhaps of LTH, from basophilic and acidophilic cells of the anterior pituitary are inhibited by progestogen and by estrogens in high circulating concentrations.[7]

Ovarian function in the female human cannot be initi-

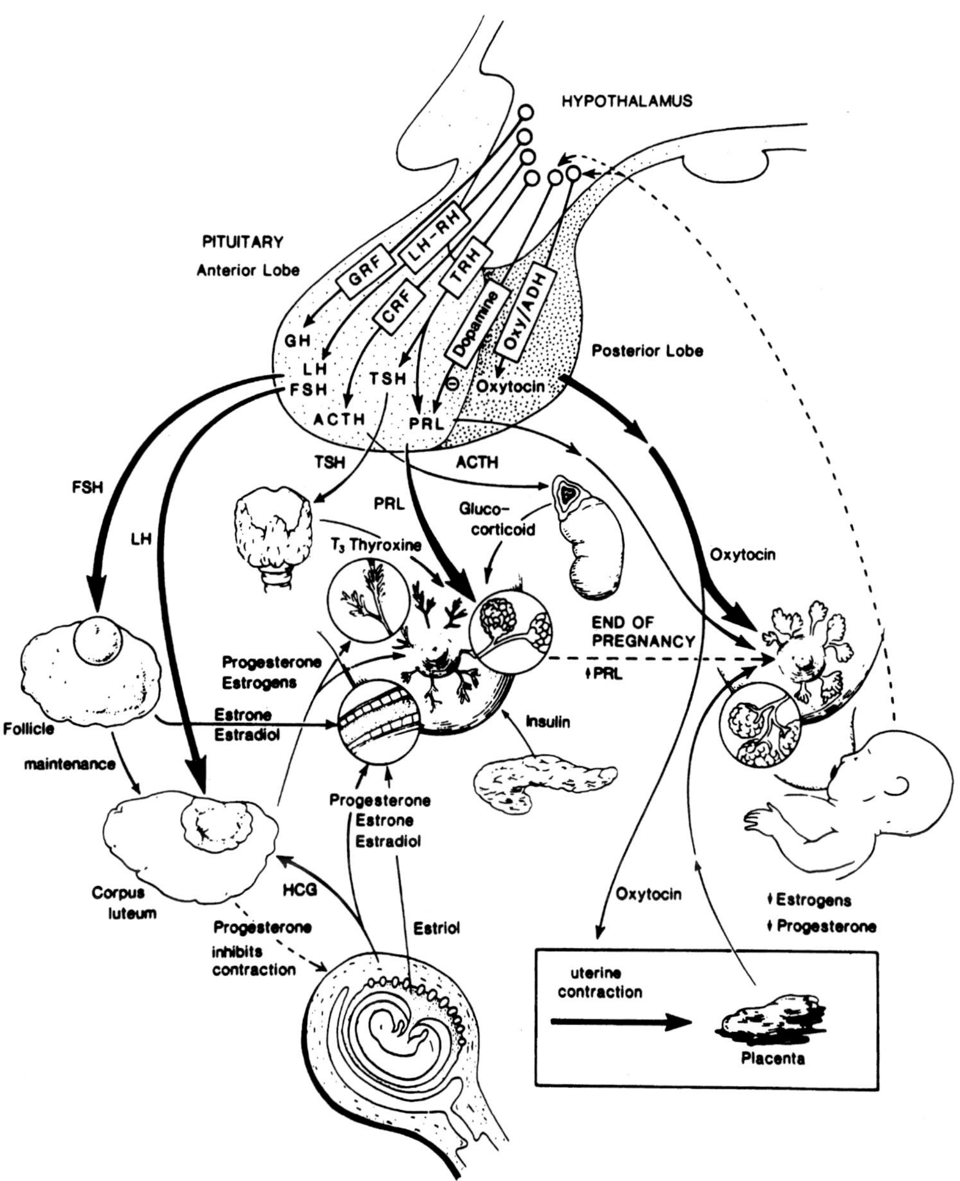

Fig. 63-3. Overview of the neuroendocrine control of breast development and function with relationship to gonadotropic hormones of the anterior pituitary and ovary. Basophil secretions of luteinizing hormone *(LH)* and follicle-stimulating hormone *(FSH)* are responsible for ovarian synthesis and release of progesterone and estrogen, respectively. The mammotropic effects of estrogen and progestin initiate myoepithelial and alveolar development. Ductal and stromal enlargement with pregnancy occur as a result of progestin and estrogen secretions in excess from the corpus luteum (first 12 weeks) and thereafter from the placenta. Acidophil cell secretion of prolactin (LTH) is initiated after evacuation of the gravid uterus and is mammotrophic to the lobular alveoli. The suckling reflex initiates oxytocin release from the posterior pituitary and is stimulatory to alveolar myoepithelial cells to initiate milk release. Neuroendocrine organs other than the pituitary and ovary secrete hormones (glucocorticoid, growth hormone, insulin, thyroxine) that are trophic to ductal and glandular maintenance and growth. *ACTH,* Adrenocorticotropic hormone; *ADH,* antidiuretic hormone; *FSH,* follicle-stimulating hormone; *GH,* growth hormone; *GRF,* growth hormone–releasing factor; *HCG,* human chorionic gonadotropin; *LH-RH,* luteinizing hormone–regulatory hormone; *PRL,* prolactin; *TRH,* thyroid-releasing hormone. (From Keller-Wood M, Bland KI. Breast physiology: Breast physiology in normal, lactating and diseased states. In Bland KI, Copeland EM III, eds. The Breast: Comprehensive Management of Benign and Malignant Diseases. Philadelphia: WB Saunders, 1991, p 37.)

ated until FSH is released, because LTH and LH have little or no effect on ovarian function in the absence of FSH. Thus, menarche cannot appear until activation of FSH release from the basophilic cells of the pituitary. Further, ovulation and estrogen production, with the ultimate influence of estrogen as a mammotropic hormone, cannot occur before the synthesis and release of LH from the gonadotropic basophil cell. The evacuation of the gravid uterus and the simultaneous cessation of secretion of hormones produced by the placenta initiate increased synthesis or release of the LTH by the anterior pituitary. Synthesis or release of LTH thus can be inhibited by therapeutic doses of estrogens, androgens, or progestogens.

The previous discussion relates the biofeedback mechanism apparent for the gonadotropic hormones of the anterior pituitary with the ovary. The secretion of these hormones, which is under the purveyance of receptors of the hypothalamus, provides neurohumoral pathways to the pituitary. The feedback control of these glycoprotein gonadotropins allows the ovarian follicle to produce and release estrogen (estrone, estradiol), whereas the corpus luteum synthesizes or releases progesterone and estrogens. The presence of human chorionic gonadotropin in pregnancy also initiates maintenance and production of progesterone and estrogens from the corpus luteum. The effects of estradiol in circulating levels from the ovarian follicles have numerous actions beyond the scope of this discussion. However, the effects to inhibit FSH and stimulate the production of LH have indirect consequences for breast development, maintenance, and function. In the prepubertal adolescent breast, estrogen induces development from the epidermal portion of the breast bud with growth of lactiferous ducts and myoepithelial cells and, to a lesser degree, of the alveoli of breast parenchyma (Fig. 63-4, *A*). Progesterone has many effects on the female reproductive system and its neuroendocrine control and promotes development of the acinar (secretory) tissues of the breast. Thus, sudden loss of secretion of the gonadotropic pituitary hormones or the target-organ hormones (estradiol and progesterone) has detrimental consequences for growth, development, and maintenance of the ductal, acinar, or stromal parenchymal elements of the mammary gland.

With the onset of puberty and cyclic ovarian function resulting from the gonadotropic effects of the anterior pituitary, the mammotropic effects of estrogen are recognized (Fig. 63-4, *B*). The lactiferous ducts and sinuses of the breast elongate with a recognizably enhanced cellular replication of columnar epithelium of the duct. Epithelial proliferation continues at the termination of the mammary tubules and initiates the formation of distinct lobules. Simultaneously, the stromal components of breast parenchyma enlarge to parallel the ingrowth and replication of ductal epithelium. The latter circumstance is responsible for the enlargement and texture of the female adolescent breast. Isometric growth and the enlargement and pigmentation of the nipple and the areola occur as a result of the effects produced by estrogen and progesterone.

The postadolescent female breast is established in cyclic ovulation, and the progesterone-secreting corpora lutea are maintained in this period. Thus, the mature mammary gland has completed formation of the lobular and acinar structures in response to the additive effects of estrogen and progesterone (Fig. 63-4, *C*). The characteristic lobular development evident in this phase of breast maintenance is completed approximately 12 to 18 months after menarche. Progressive development and enlargement of lactiferous ducts and acini result from the intense hormonal stimuli and secretion with each menstrual cycle or with pregnancy. Proportional enlargement of breast contour and size vary with habitus and body fat content, which are initiated in the adolescent period and maintained into the early postmenopausal era.

Data are sparse concerning the in vivo human hormonal requirements for breast growth and differentiation in the pregnant state (Fig. 63-4, *D*). Nonetheless, pituitary and ovarian hormones appear to be essential to growth and synthesis of milk in the mouse mammary gland. Provided the pituitary and adrenal glands are intact, growth of lactiferous ducts and alveoli to midpregnancy can be achieved in rodents by administration of estrogen and progesterone. Neuroendocrine organs other than the ovary apparently provide hormones (growth hormone, insulin, glucocorticoid) that are tropic to mammary ductal and glandular growth and maintenance. Milk synthesis and release begin about the fifth month of pregnancy, whereas the initiation of lactation is an event of delivery after intense LTH release of the anterior pituitary acidophile cell (Fig. 63-4, *E*). The actual release of milk ("let down") at the time of the suckling reflex is a consequence of the action of oxytocin on the myoepithelial cells of the alveoli (Fig. 63-3). The synthesis of oxytocin is continued in the hypothalamus, and oxytocin is released from the neurohypophysis after stimulation. Glandular tissue of the breast parenchyma eventually replaces the fatty elements between breast lobules as the latter proliferate with pregnancy. The primary stimulus for hyperplasia of breast glandular tissue in the pregnant state is the placental hormone estriol. After pregnancy and lactation, involution is incomplete, and the hypertropic and hyperplastic glandular tissues remain until menopause.

Cyclic changes of breast structure occur as a result of the gonadotropic and ovarian hormone concentrations, which may fluctuate with each menstrual cycle. Before the onset of menses, the lobules, stroma, and ducts become engorged; thereafter, ducts shrink with the onset of menses, and epithelial cells desquamate and are then maintained to initiate proliferation by the second week of the cycle. The connective stroma and ductal epithelial cells increase in size and number. Remarkable variations and alterations of the hormonal milieu can be observed, with the resultant effects of hypoplastic and hyperplastic dilation of ducts, connective tissue stroma, and lobules. The senile or postmenopausal breast undergoes progressive in-

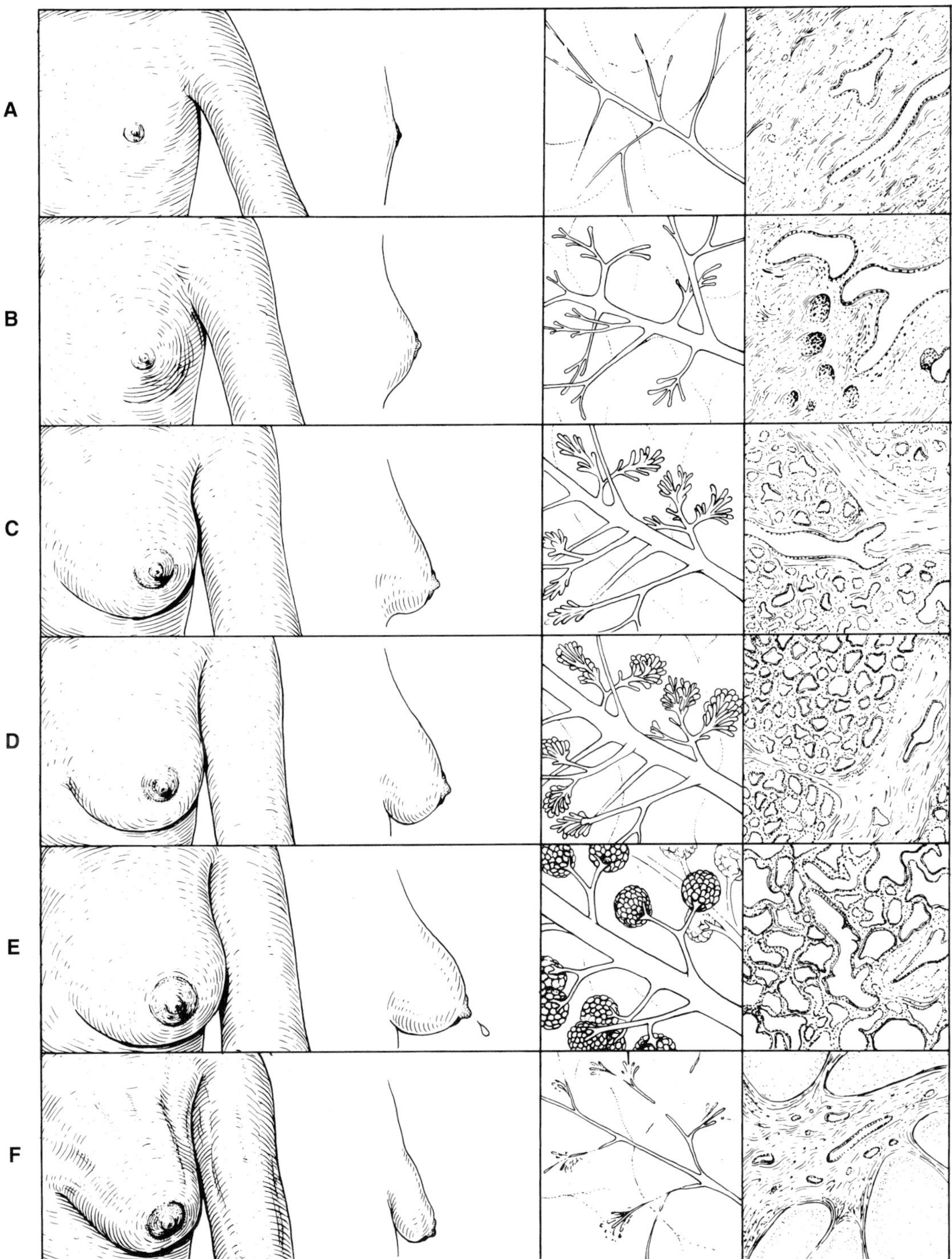

Fig. 63-4. Phases of mammary gland development, anterior and lateral views. Microscopic appearance of ducts and lobules in phases of development, growth, and maintenance. **A,** Prepubertal (childhood). **B,** Puberty. **C,** Mature (reproductive). **D,** Pregnancy. **E,** Lactation. **F,** Postmenopausal (senescent) state. (From Copeland EM III, Bland KI. The breast. In Sabiston DC Jr, ed. Essentials of Surgery. Philadelphia: WB Saunders, 1987.)

volution as a result of cessation of estrogenic and progestational effects of ovarian secretion. With menopause, regression to an atropic or hypoplastic epithelium of the lobules and ducts is apparent, whereas periductal fibrous tissue becomes dense (Fig. 63-4, *F*). Dilation of the lactiferous duct network is noted in isolated lobules. Macrocystic formation (fibrocystic disease of the breast [FCDB]) occurs after enlargement of the lobular acini are depleted of their columnar epithelium.

On examination, the postmenopausal breast is often asymmetric, with lobular irregularity and variations of cyst size. With progressive loss of fat content and the supporting periductal fibrous stroma, the senescent breast shrinks and the parenchymal and stromal tissue blend into a homogeneous, pendulous mass, with loss of the original lobular structure.

CLINICAL EVALUATION OF BREAST DISEASE

Obtaining a History

Before visual inspection and palpation of the breast, a comprehensive personal medical history of the patient should be obtained. Detailed inquiry into associative risk factors is necessary and should include age, parity, and menstrual and nursing histories. The age at menarche and cyclic alterations of breast masses that occur with menses are significant correlates of benign and malignant disease. Previous surgical procedures, especially oophorectomy, hysterectomy, adrenalectomy, or other pelvic surgery, are important to ascertain potential ablative procedures that initiate cessation of endogenous estrogen secretion. Prior use of hormonal therapy, including exogenous estrogens or oral contraceptives (OCs), may influence maintenance of mammary parenchyma. Also, the presence and nature of any nipple discharge should be ascertained. The precipitating events of such a discharge and its association with cyclic ovulation often provide distinguishing features of its etiology.

More than 80% of breast lesions are recognized by the patient before she seeks medical attention. The physician should inquire about the dominant features of the presenting mass, its growth characteristics, and reproducibility of physical examination at menses. Hormonally sensitive breast lesions may have mastodynia with breast fullness and swelling in immediate premenstrual and postmenstrual periods. Breast cancer risk determinants are closely related to the patient's cultural background, and this may contribute to breast cancer aggregations within families. Thus, a detailed family history is necessary to determine whether *hereditary breast cancer* or simple family aggregation of carcinoma exists. Breast cancer not fulfilling genetic criteria of the hereditary variant is classified as *sporadic.* Also, constitutional symptoms should be elicited and carefully recorded. Progressive weight loss, hemoptysis, fever, chest pain, anorexia, and skeletal pain are important determinants of advanced local, regional, and systemic disease.

Physical Examination

Visual Inspection

Before palpation, the physician visually inspects the patient's breasts in anteroposterior and lateral views to observe symmetry, skin changes, retraction, elevation, and color alterations. The examination is conducted with the patient's arms first at her sides and then on her hips with contraction of pectoral muscles to accentuate breast contour.

Bacterial cellulitis is easily recognized by the presence of focal areas of skin involvement and associated diffuse edema of the ipsilateral breast. These findings often accompany superficial and deep abscesses. Regional endolymphatic permeation of the ipsilateral breast and dermal lymphatics with tumor emboli from inflammatory breast carcinoma may be confused with bacterial cellulitis. With progression of the inflammatory neoplasm, segmental entrapment of Cooper's ligaments may initiate skin retraction and dimpling. The latter finding also may be associated with common variants of infiltrating breast neoplasms. The skin may have focal sites of diffuse edema, as seen with cellulitis, and *peau d'orange* (orange peel) may occur as a result of lymphatic obstruction.

With radial growth of the tumor, an intense desmoplastic response initiates tethering with retraction of the skin as a result of contraction of Cooper's ligaments. Retraction of the skin and associated dimpling are best visualized with the patient sitting and contracting the pectoral muscles to accentuate the breast profile. These maneuvers accentuate deep involvement of structures in the large breast. Similar findings are observed with benign lesions such as fat necrosis, so physical examination alone is often insufficient to distinguish malignant tumors.

Breast Palpation

A systematic palpation of the regional sites common to metastatic involvement by breast neoplasms is conducted before initiation of breast examination. Evaluation of the axillary and supraclavicular fossae requires both superficial and deep palpation to identify nodal metastases. Examination of the axillae should be done with the patient in a sitting position, with the ipsilateral arm supported by the examiner. Complete relaxation of the shoulder girdle musculature is essential to allow comprehensive palpation of the five regional nodal groups. Use of gentle pressure with the fingertips best demonstrates small nodal deposits. Large, bulky, extramammary metastases in both these regional sites may be obvious to both the patient and the physician. Precise documentation of location and size of nodes is important to allow accurate clinical staging. At the time the five nodal groups are assessed, the examiner should position the fingers in the axillary fold so that all infraclavicular structures lateral to Halsted's ligaments are evaluated.

A systematic evaluation of all breast quadrants is completed with the patient relaxed in the supine position, with full extension of the arm and the shoulder in external rotation. A flattened sheet provides support to the ipsilateral hemithorax to accentuate breast detail. The object of the evaluation is to detect small lesions that are separate from surrounding breast fat and parenchyma. Well-circumscribed, painful lesions that are totally separable from adjacent tissues usually represent benign masses. Painless, firm, nonballotable lesions with indistinct borders should be considered malignant until proved otherwise. As noted, however, the distinction between malignancy and benignity is often impossible on the basis of a physical examination.

After superficial and deep palpation of all quadrants of the breast, the nipple-areolar complex is carefully evaluated. The presence of associated nipple inversion should be documented; if unilateral, carcinoma should be suspected. If normal, an inverted nipple can usually be everted to its correct anatomic position; the inability to perform this maneuver often necessitates biopsy to disprove malignancy. Eczema and inflammatory states of the nipple-areolar complex are often observed in the postpartum era and with lactation. In contrast, a crusty, scaly, eczematoid eruption of the areola is pathognomonic of Paget's disease of the nipple. These lesions, which are unilateral and distinct from the contralateral nipple, often bleed or weep on contact. Biopsy of the subareolar parenchyma will confirm a primary infiltrating ductal carcinoma that invades the nipple and skin of the areolar to produce the associated clinical findings.

Special Considerations

Nipple Discharge

Discharge from the nipple, although not a frequent symptom, is estimated to occur in approximately 3% to 9% of patients.[8,9] Nipple discharge has been reported in 8.8% of 10,365 women in six groups attending breast clinics and in 6.5% of 8640 women in five series subjected to breast surgery.[9] Nipple secretion represents an alteration in the normal physiologic consequences of duct epithelial secretion and may indicate an inflammatory, proliferative, or neoplastic process. Discharges of pathologic significance typically empty spontaneously from the ductal sinus or recess of the nipple ampullae. Conversely, discharges that are elicited by squeezing breast parenchyma or the nipple-areola complex are usually inconsequential.

The type of nipple discharge is the pathognomonic feature that determines its etiology. The frequently observed watery, puslike, or thick discharge of ductal ectasia may be elicited by milking or squeezing multiple lobes of the breast or the nipple. This physiologic and harmless secretion requires only reassurance to the patient of its benignity. Four additional types of discharge are recognized.

Bloody discharge. This form of ductal discharge may vary from bright red to brown and represents the most common type in many series (50% to 75%). The most frequent etiologic mechanism is hyperplastic and proliferative growth of intraductal epithelium. Most such discharges represent benign epithelial proliferation as a component of FCDB, and an intraductal papilloma is often etiologic. On occasion, bloody discharge is caused by a malignant epithelial proliferation such as intraductal papillary carcinoma.

As noted in one series, the presence of a solitary mass in a postmenopausal patient is highly suggestive of a malignant process and necessitates confirmation by biopsy or Papanicolaou smear. The Pap smear is of value only if its result is positive, and the lesion should be confirmed as malignant before definitive surgical therapy. Malignancy occurs in approximately 9% to 14% of patients with the finding of a bloody nipple discharge.[10] Haagensen[3] observed 11.5% of spontaneous nipple discharges to be of malignant origin; 55% of these were bloody types (Table 63-1). When a palpable lesion is not identifiable clinically or mammographically, surgical exploration of the subareola is indicated. Often, milking specific quadrants and emptying the involved duct allows identification of a papilloma. Precise localization of the offending lesion may be possible. Probing the duct with bimanual palpation may provide identification of the responsible tumor to allow definitive surgical resection. Radiographic imaging with contrast ductography sometimes permits precise preoperative localization.

Table 63-1. Breast Conditions Producing Spontaneous Nipple Discharge

Condition	Type of Nipple Discharge			Total Patients (no.)	Total Patients (%)
	Serous	Bloody	Watery		
Pregnancy	—	10	—	10	6
Menstruation	—	1	—	1	—
Cystic disease	3	—	—	3	—
Duct ectasia	3	2	—	5	3
Intraductal papilloma	53	55	—	108	69
Accessory subareolar gland papilloma	3	—	—	3	—
Papilloma of nipple ducts	9	—	—	9	5.8
Carcinoma of breast	7	10	1	18	11.5
TOTAL				157	

From Haagensen CD. Physicians' role in the detection and diagnosis of breast disease. In Haagensen CD, ed. Diseases of the Breast, 2nd ed. (rev.). Philadelphia: WB Saunders, 1971, p 103.

Chaudary et al.,[11] in an analysis of 270 patients undergoing microdochectomy for hemoglobin-positive nipple discharge with and without an associated lump, observed a cancer incidence of 5.9%. In order of frequency, intraductal papilloma, duct ectasia, FCDB, and carcinoma accounted for more than 90% of the cases.

Serous discharge. Thin, translucent, colorless to straw-colored discharge may occur spontaneously. It most often occurs with normal menstrual cycles, in early pregnancy, or in women taking OCs. This discharge results from estrogen effects on duct epithelium, with resultant hyperplasia and proliferation to enhance secretion. The palpation of a solitary subareolar mass is highly suggestive of an intraductal papilloma, which can often be confirmed by contrast radiography or probing of the responsible duct mechanism. Simple excision of the intraductal papilloma is curative.

Milky discharge. The discharge of fluid with the consistency and chemical composition of milk is evident many months postpartum and after cessation of breastfeeding. The most satisfactory normal control for secondary (delayed) breast manifestations with mastalgia, milky discharge, and engorgement is a single intramuscular injection of testosterone enanthate and estradiol valerate (Deladumone) in the desired ratio. On occasion, acromegaly can produce a milky discharge because of the somatotropic effect of growth hormone on breast acini and lobular secretion. The production and the release of LTH can be inhibited by appropriate doses of estrogen, androgen, and progestogens.

Yellow discharge. The proliferative responses of breast ductal structures and acini to excessive estrogen production in the presence of deficient corpus luteum activity are responsible for yellow discharge. The ductal structure with its retained fluid sometimes spontaneously discharges a dark yellow fluid that can also be obtained by percutaneous breast aspiration. Fluid cytology, although a desirable examination, rarely reveals neoplastic cells unless the cyst wall has undergone the rare event of malignant transformation. The cost-effectiveness of cytology for hemoglobin-negative nipple discharge must be questioned. In the absence of high-risk patient factors for cancer, cytologic examination of such fluid is not justified.

Rare conditions that initiate nipple discharge. The breast represents a target organ without a physiologic feedback mechanism to inhibit multiple hormonal stimuli that may initiate prolonged secretory phases. The acidophilic lactogenic cell from the anterior pituitary may initiate unrecognized surges in circulating serum prolactin (LTH) levels. Newman et al.[9] observed that serum prolactin levels were above normal in 25% of 587 patients with nipple secretions of various etiologic types. The most common physiologic factors that augmented the serum prolactin in women were nursing and breast stimulation, sexual intercourse, pregnancy, and stress.[9] Any of these etiologic mechanisms may potentiate other subliminal causes (e.g., minute doses of OCs, psychotropic drugs, antihypertensive medication).

The effect of hyperprolactinemia on depressing ovarian function and initiating secondary amenorrhea and galactorrhea is controversial. Approximately one third of patients with secondary amenorrhea and one fourth with galactorrhea have elevated serum prolactin values.[9,12,13] Several descriptions of syndromes that embrace these symptoms include Forbes and Albright[14] (pituitary adenoma), Chiari et al.[15] and Frommel[16] (postpregnancy amenorrhea and galactorrhea), and Ahumada and del Castillo[17] and Argonz and del Castillo[18] (unrelated to pregnancy symptoms). The physiologic implications of hyperprolactinemia with the shared clinical symptoms of breast secretion and amenorrhea may represent a continuum of pathologic disorder of multiple endocrine stigmata, which also include anovulatory syndromes, sterility, hirsutism, obesity, acne, and loss of libido.

Most pituitary tumors initiating production of prolactin (60%) are composed of specific lactomorphs.[19] As the pituitary neoplasm enlarges, it may distort the pituitary stalk and impair the secretion and delivery of prolactin-inhibitory hormone from the hypothalamus. Thus, the expansion of this neoplasm with the initiation of neurologic deficits of the optic chiasm and pyramidal tracts requires prompt surgical intervention and excision of the sella neoplasm. Differentiation between a microadenoma that may initiate amenorrhea and breast secretion and hyperprolactinemia of other causes (hypothalamic neoplasms or disease, lactomorph hyperplasia) may be impossible and only of academic interest. Indeed, in the patient without symptoms, the probability of a pituitary adenoma approximates 0.1%; it is even less if the patient uses oral contraceptives or has persistent lactation.[9] Prolactin values greater than 300 ng/ml are diagnostic of tumor, whereas values between 100 and 300 ng/ml represent adenomas in approximately 50% of cases.[20]

Anovulatory syndromes associated with galactorrhea may resolve spontaneously after the inhibition of prolactin secretion with bromocriptine (Parlodel) or clomiphene (Serophene) therapy. Follow-up allows the diagnosis of pituitary neoplasms after years of observation. The diagnosis of the triad of hyperprolactinemia, amenorrhea, and breast secretion in the absence of an associated CT scan or plain-film sella abnormality deserves follow-up (serial) plasma prolactin values. Bromocriptine will control the growth of these pituitary microprolactinomas and their symptoms, but the ultimate result of long-term therapy and its potential side effects are uncertain.

Gynecomastia

Gynecomastia is the male development of mammary glands that are unusually large for that sex. These glands may occasionally be found to secrete milk. The development of gynecomastia in the pubertal male human is a consequence of the estrogenic hormonal milieu and typically occurs between the ages of 13 and 17 years. Although the hormonal mechanism responsible is poorly understood, it appears that a predominant estrogenic effect in relation to androgen secretion is operative and perhaps is related to a delay in the reversal of the androstenedione/testosterone ratio that is normally an event of puberty.[3,21] A slight hypertropic abnormality is present and may occasionally persist either unilaterally or bilaterally. When unilateral, any relationship to hormonal dysfunction rarely exists; however, the presence of persistent bilateral gynecomastia requires a search for systemic etiology. Gynecomastia is also seen in situations where high levels of circulating estrogens are present, such as in the prepubertal child of either sex, in hepatic cirrhosis, and after use of exogenous estrogens or drugs with estrogenic properties (e.g., digoxin, dilantin) in male patients. In the absence of an abnormal endocrine secretory state and other abnormalities, the hypertropic breast tissue can be removed with a circumareolar incision to restore the breast contour. Biopsy typically reveals an absence of acinar growth with a background of proliferative breast stroma and lactiferous ducts.[22]

Rapid and extensive enlargement of the female breast at puberty sometimes continues into young adulthood. Estrogen and its target-organ effect on breast stroma and lobular hypertrophy may initiate breast enlargement to as great as 40 to 50 pounds, which may be a significant cosmetic and functional impairment. Because spontaneous regression is unlikely, these hypertropic, pendulous breasts are best managed by bilateral reduction mammoplasty.

DISEASE PROCESSES INVOLVING THE BREAST

Inflammatory Conditions

Acute inflammatory states of the breast are most often caused by retrograde bacterial infections that result from disruption of the epithelial interface of the nipple-areola complex. Staphylococcal or streptococcal bacteria represent the organisms most frequently recovered from the nipple discharge in an active breast abscess on Gram's stain and culture. These infections are often related to lactation and typically occur within the first weeks of breast-feeding.[23] Progression of the inflammatory process can result in diffuse breast cellulitis with loculated subareolar or central abscesses (Fig. 63-5). Through the diffuse network of the lactiferous ducts, multilocular abscesses may form, with the presentation of diffuse cellulitis and a systemically ill patient. Classically, streptococcal infections produce diffuse cellulitis without localization until an advanced course of the disease, when the patient has systemic manifestations. *Staphylococcus aureus* abscesses tend to have a more localized, suppurative, and deeply invasive presentation, with acute and chronic abscess formation. The multilocular abscess is seen more often in staphylococcal infections that initiate loculated suppuration between the fibrosepta of Cooper's ligaments.

An advanced abscess requires immediate surgical attention. Lymphatic involvement arising from streptococcal cellulitis usually necessitates local nursing care, with the application of focal heat compresses and appropriate antibiotics such as penicillin derivatives. Focal abscess with overgrowth of any bacterial organism requires immediate and adequate surgical drainage of fluctuant areas. Thorough débridement of the abscess through a circumareolar incision or multiple incisions placed in the direction of Langer's lines is recommended (see *inset,* Fig. 63-5). Open drainage of the wound with strict attention to hygienic evacuation of the abscess and the nipple-areola complex are essential to avoid skin and subcutaneous necrosis.

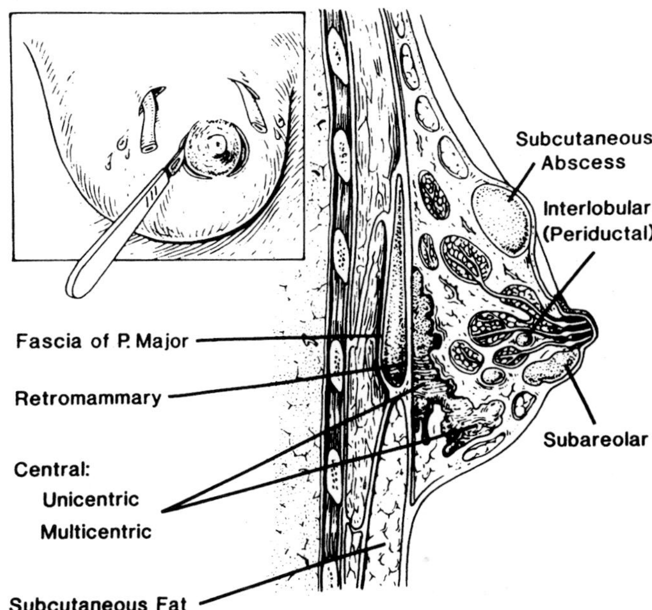

Fig. 63-5. Sagittal view of the breast with sites of potential abscess formation that include subcutaneous, subareolar, interlobular (periductal), retromammary, and central areas. Central abscesses may be focal or multicentric. Retromammary abscesses may be seen in chronic infectious or neoplastic processes (e.g., tuberculosis, carcinoma). Deep abscesses may be multilocular and may communicate with subcutaneous or subareolar sites. Painful, diffuse cellulitis is often apparent with deeper abscesses in subcutaneous, interlobular, or subareolar planes. *Inset* above depicts the necessity for thorough drainage and complete evacuation of the abscess through incisions that parallel Langer's lines. (From Bland KI. Inflammatory, infectious, and metabolic disorders of the mamma. In Bland KI, Copeland EM III, eds. The Breast: Comprehensive Management of Benign and Malignant Diseases. Philadelphia: WB Saunders, 1991, p 87.)

Discontinuance of breast-feeding in the postpartum state is recommended to prevent stasis and progressive growth of bacteria in the lactiferous ducts. The occasional use of a breast suction pump may help to empty stagnant milk ducts and central abscess collections. The continuance of lactation after removal of the suckling reflex may necessitate the use of intramuscular injections of testosterone enanthate and estradiol valerate (Deladumone).

The presentation of *chronic* inflammatory states of the breast with abscess formation is unusual, and the differential diagnosis must include chronic infectious or neoplastic processes (e.g., tuberculosis, carcinoma). The ubiquitous tuberculous organism remains the most common cause of chronic bacterial mastitis.[24] Today, this diagnosis as the coexistent finding of multiple granulomatous processes (fungi and sarcoidosis) may produce a bacteriologic and physiologic presentation similar to pulmonary tuberculosis. Classically, the breast tuberculoma is nontender and may have multiple sinus tracts extending from the anterior thorax to sites of central or subcutaneous cavitation with intervening cellulitis. The demonstration of acid-fast tubercle bacilli in the lesion or on culture is diagnostic. Adequate drainage identical to that for acute bacterial abscess and initiation of antituberculous therapy are the prerequisites of therapy. Biopsy of the drainage site is mandatory for chronic abscesses of any etiology to exclude the possibility of invasive carcinoma. Local drainage and systemic antibiotic therapy are rarely necessary before cyclic chemotherapy and mastectomy to provide control of the carcinomatous process in which there is superimposed infection.

Mondor's Disease: Thrombophlebitis of Superficial Thoracoepigastric Vein

The presentation of acute pain in the superficial distribution of the thoracodorsal vein along its course to the hypochondrium is diagnostic of Mondor's disease, a benign state. The classic finding in Mondor's disease of a palpable, cordlike thickening that extends across the superolateral breast toward the axilla may be related to local trauma of the breast or axilla. This self-limiting process requires no definitive therapy. The clinical importance of this inflammatory condition is essentially its recognition and differentiation from carcinoma and other breast diseases.

Benign Breast Disease

Sir Astley Cooper of London is credited with the first description of benign cystic disease of the breast and subsequently classified its various forms as adenosis, cystic disease, and mastodynia.[24a] Initial opinion suggested that these forms were interrelated and together constituted the most common breast abnormalities of sexual maturity. The subsequent descriptions by Schimmelbusch (1890) of the microscopic features of cyst adenoma (Geschickter's adenosis) suggested proliferation of epithelial elements with the formation of cysts and a loss of normal interacinous connective tissues.[25] Although considerable controversy exists with regard to the variants of benign breast disease, for purposes of discussion, mastopathy of the cystic type should be considered synonymous with fibrocystic disease of the breast (FCDB), chronic cystic mastitis, mammary dysplasia, benign mastopathy, and cystic disease of the breast.

Removal of the term *FCDB* from lay and clinical parlance is virtually impossible, because the term is used to denote proliferative and nonproliferative benign disorders of the breast. Although inexact and nondescriptive of the actual pathological cellular events, FCDB connotes benignity in an active, estrogen-supported breast parenchyma. Use of the term *FCDB* in this review is therefore indicative of premenopausal or postmenopausal proliferative or nonproliferative breast disease.

Proliferative and nonproliferative diseases (gross and microscopic) are the most frequently diagnosed lesions of the breast. Because gross cystic disease does not become clinically evident until establishment of active ovarian function, the observation of its regression after menopause suggests that estrogens and progestins are causal factors. The percentage of benign breast disease is unknown, but previous reports of elderly women dying of causes other than breast cancer noted histopathologic changes of benign mastopathy in 100% of the breasts studied. Kramer and Rush[26] observed that this elderly population had cystic changes in 89% of cases, apocrine metaplasia in 80%, and intraductal hyperplasia in 69%. Thus, the changes of fibrosis and epithelial proliferation, which invariably occur as a result of physiologic consequences of ovarian stimulation, may represent progression to a "disease state" with macrocysts. The epithelial changes, ranging from duct adenosis to cystic alterations and from ductal epithelial proliferation to atypia and carcinoma, have been reproduced in rodent models by numerous investigators.[27-29] Although it is difficult to reproduce in mice, stromal fibrosis can be initiated in monkeys after ovarian stimulation.[30]

As already noted, the interplay between and synchrony of prolactin and progesterone are necessary for estrogen to exert its active mammatrophic role in breast physiology. Although synergism exists between both sex steroids, with estrogen promoting growth and development of ducts and progesterone affecting inductive growth of the alveolar system, the presence of prolactin is also necessary. In the hypophysectomized animal, parenteral administration of estrogen does not promote mammary development. Conversely, breast development occurs with an excess of pituitary hormones in the absence of estrogen. It appears that other essential endocrine factors, which are less clearly delineated but include thyroxine, insulin, adrenocorticoids, and growth hormone, are important to allow full differentiation of the lactiferous and lobular components of the breast.[31] The initial induction of mammary epithelial stem cell division by estrogen depends on prolactin, growth hormone, and insulin. Also, exposure to therapeutic levels of endogenous cortisol and insulin provides prolactin with an appropriate hormonal milieu to initiate final differentiation of alveolar epithelial cells into mature milk cells. The interregulation of pituitary hormones that interact with ovarian gonadotropins is subsequently orchestrated in synchrony with thyroxine and tri-iodothyronine to stimulate the end organ (breast) for metabolic regulatory control (see Fig. 63-3).

Cystic and epithelial lesions of mice produced by various regimens that augment an absolute or relative increase in serum estrogens have been observed to closely resemble gross and microcystic lesions in human beings.[32] In species other than rodents, well-documented responses to estrogen stimulation are evident in fibrous tissue and smooth muscle of certain organs.[33] Investigators have suggested that estrogen increases stromal ground substance that has a propensity toward fibrous reorganization. These data suggest that the epithelial and stromal elements of breast parenchyma may be target organs of ovarian and pituitary hormonal secretion. Further, the duration of active stimulation of the hormonally sensitive components of breast structure accounts for the peak incidence for disease and regression of symptomatic macrocystic changes after cessation of the estrogen and progesterone milieu with menopause.

The etiology of gross and microcystic breast disease appears to be multifactorial; the essential factor is relative hyperestrinism, which initiates epithelial hyperplasia. Genetic factors, mammotropic pituitary hormones, and other circulating nongonadotropin hormones (insulin, thyroxine, growth hormone) are also involved. Early investigators were impressed that women with FCDB had decreased fertility and often had slightly abnormal menstrual cycles.[34] These early studies, however, did not confirm that estrogen levels in the serum of affected subjects were elevated. The hypothesis of relative estrogen excess related to a deficient luteal phase was thus introduced in the etiology of the entity.[32] Until recently, this hypothesis could not be tested because it required the serial measurement of estrogen and progestin hormones in various phases of the menses. The potential for abnormal end-organ metabolism as the etiology of this disease process is under investigation.

Examination of the breast of women with FCDB typically reveals diffuse fullness and fibronodularity. These multiple or solitary cystic lesions are observed to be well demarcated, mobile, smooth masses. After recognition of the symptomatic cystic lesion, appropriate therapy consists of needle aspiration. Typically, cystic fluid is clear or straw colored; however, chronic cysts may be bloody or contain gray-green, turbid contents. The cyst fluid should be forwarded for cytologic examination, although this is rarely of diagnostic value. The occasional finding of a positive Pap smear result has profound significance and necessitates immediate biopsy. The discovery of bloody cytologic fluid necessitates frequent follow-up and warrants biopsy if a residual mass is palpable after aspiration. The presence of a solid lesion may denote a cyst cancer or a primary neoplasm coexistent with a proliferative breast lesion.[35,36]

History of Fibrocystic Disease of the Breast (Previous Biopsies) as Risk Indicator

As previously noted, similar mechanisms of FCDB and neoplasia relate to active ovarian hormonal stimuli. Although histologic identification of the presence of both diseases is common, circumstantial evidence for the relationship between these two entities remains controversial. The patient with advanced fibronodular breast disease marked by diffuse solid or cystic masses and with an active reproductive status should be closely scrutinized in follow-up. A history of familial breast cancer has added significance. Clearly, the solid-mass lesion found on clinical or mammographic examination that remains unchanged throughout the menses should be considered suspect and requires biopsy and histologic evaluation. At least one fourth of patients subjected to biopsy should have confirmation of a neoplasm. Confirmation of neoplasm in a smaller proportion of patients would indicate that the case selection has not been discriminating. This cancer/biopsy ratio is much higher (≤1:6 to 8) after the screening of women without symptoms.[37]

The evaluation of prospective studies, in which women with biopsy specimens indicating benign disease were followed up to determine the subsequent incidence of cancer, presents several issues. Problems with statistical analyses include inconsistent intervals of follow-up and unspecified distributions of age. The clinical decision to sample a breast mass for biopsy is subjective and is often made on clinical indications and the relative risk of cancer. Therefore, patients undergoing biopsy are considered a select, high-risk population subset. Love et al.[38] compared five prospective studies for patients who underwent biopsy and subsequently were determined to have carcinoma. For 6511 patients, an increased risk for cancer of 1.98 was evident if the breast had previously been sampled. This relative risk was similar to the recalculated incidence of the 1970 and 1976 National Cancer Institute (NCI) surveys (2.13 vs 1.86, respectively).

Histologic identification of the presence of *both* FCDB and breast neoplasia is common. Love et al.[38] observed that FCDB was noted in 58% of autopsied noncancerous breasts but in only 26% of cancerous breasts. The association of the two diseases is probably inevitable and coincidental because the hormonal milieu of hyperestrinism supports the genesis of both FCDB and carcinoma. Black and Chabon[28] used the term *precancerous mastopathy* for the lesion with duct epithelial hyperplasia with atypia and aporcine metaplasia with atypia. These investigators report that the patient with asymptomatic ductal atypia and hyperplasia in a benign lesion is subject to development of breast carcinoma with a risk that exceeds five times that of the woman without these histologic findings. This risk appears to be reduced for that patient if apocrine metaplasia with atypia is included. Love et al.[38] found epithelial hyperplasia to be at least as common in noncancerous breasts as in cancerous ones (32% vs 23%, respectively; Table 63-2).

Monson et al.[39] evaluated the cancer risk associated with "benign breast disease" (FCDB, chronic cystic mastitis) and concluded that the excess risk for dying of breast carcinoma for individuals with this diagnosis persists for approximately 30 years or longer after the diagnosis of chronic mastitis. Their data suggest that women with chronic mastitis have an escalated risk for development of carcinoma 2.5 times that of normal women. Proliferative histologic changes increases the risk for subsequent carcinoma to 2.6 times that of the control population, whereas the neoplastic risk for women without associated proliferative changes is only 1.2 times that of the general population.[40]

These observations have been substantiated by other investigators,[41-44] with variance in the range of increasing

Table 63-2. Reported Incidence of Microscopic Fibrocystic Disease in Breasts Removed for Cancer and in Noncancerous Breasts Studied at Autopsy

Study	No. of Patients	Age Range	Fibrocystic Disease (General)		Epithelial Hyperplasia (General)		Atypia	
			No.	%	No.	%	No.	%
Noncancerous Breasts Studied at Autopsy								
Frantz*	225	13-85	117	52	32	14		
Sloss*	100	20-99			33	33		
Davis	725	13-99	360	58	210	31		
Kramer	70	70			48	69	7	10
TOTAL			360	58	258	32		
Breasts Removed for Cancer								
Davis	327		128	40	38	12		
Kern	100	30-90	71	71	27	27	24	24
Karpas	226	20≥80			52	23	32	14
Fischerman	411	20-80	54	13	10	2		
Silverberg	398	20-99	157	40	30	8		
Bonser	220	20-80			123	56		
Fisher	1000		206	21	349	35		
Devitt	594	15-80	133	22				
TOTAL			749	26	629	23		

From Love SM, Gelman RS, Silen W. Fibrocystic "disease" of the breast—A nondisease? N Engl J Med 307:1012, 1982.

*Studies done before 1964; these totals are included in the totals given for Davis.

risk. All agree with the concept that more severe degrees of epithelial proliferation and atypical changes augment the probability of cancer risk with respect to lesser variations of atypia. Fisher et al.[42] noted that proliferative forms occur more frequently in younger women, whereas nonproliferative lesions are more often observed in the older age group. Carcinoma develops more frequently when epithelial proliferative lesions are present.

Page et al.[45] also observed that atypical lobular hyperplasia provides a greater predictive value than do other epithelial lesions and is associated with an increased cancer risk six times that expected before the age of 35 years, with a tripling of risk beyond this age. They noted that ductal hyperplastic lesions are associated with a twofold risk if lesions were identified at biopsy after the age of 45 years. These investigators suggested no increased risk for subsequent carcinoma with respect to the control population for women with sclerosing adenosis, fibrosis, cysts, and other nonhyperplastic changes. Atypical duct neoplasms, which have features consonant with in situ carcinoma, did not appear to have a risk for cancer greater than that found in ductal lesions, which do not have such severe atypia. This conclusion appeared to disagree with the studies of Black et al.[28,29] and Kodlin et al.[43]

The hypothesis that strong prognostic indices can be derived from biopsy samples that harbor epithelial hyperplasia of lobular and ductal patterns was originally presented by Rogers and Page.[46] This original study describes a risk of four to six times that of the general population if atypical lobular hyperplasia is present. The risk was two to three times that of the general population if ductal hyperplasia was evident in patients older than 45 years. No increased risk was evident, however, for ductal hyperplasia in patients younger than 45 years or if sclerosing adenosis was described in the specimen.

In a classic review, Dupont and Page[47] subsequently evaluated women with benign proliferative breast lesions. Women who had proliferative disease without atypical hyperplasia had a risk of cancer 1.9 times that of women with nonproliferative lesions (95% confidence interval 1.2 to 2.9). However, the risk for women with atypical hyperplasia (atypia) was 5.3 times that of women with nonproliferative lesions (95% confidence interval 3.1 to 8.8). The proportional hazards—the relative risks shown in Table 63-3—are useful to compare the relative risks for different subgroups within the same study. A family history of breast cancer had little effect on the risk for women with nonproliferative lesions. However, the risk for women with a family history of breast cancer was eleven times that for women who had nonproliferative lesions without a family history (95% confidence interval 5.5 to 24). Calcification elevated the cancer risk if the biopsy specimen confirmed proliferative disease. The presence of cysts and a family history of breast cancer enhanced the risk to 2.7 times that for women without either of these risk factors (95% confidence interval 1.5 to 4.6). These authors conclude that most women (70%) undergoing breast biopsy for benign disease are not at increased risk for cancer. These data do

Table 63-3. Effect of Hyperplasia, Age, Family History, and Calcification on the Risk of Breast Cancer

Numerator of Relative Risk	Denominator of Relative Risk	Relative Risk*	95% Confidence Interval	*p* Value
PDWA, age 20-45 yr	Non-PD, age 20-45 yr	1.9	1.2-3.2	0.012
PDWA, age 46-55 yr	Non-PD, age 46-55 yr	1.4	0.57-3.3	0.49
PDWA, age >55 yr	Non-PD, age >55 yr	5.6	0.69-46	0.11
PDWA with CAL	Non-PD without CAL	2.3	1.2-4.3	0.008
AH with CAL	Non-PD with CAL	8.6	2.5-29	0.0006
AH with CAL	Non-PD without CAL	8.3	3.5-19	<0.0001
Cysts without FH	Neither cysts nor FH	1.3	0.88-2	0.19
Cysts with FH	No cysts but FH	2.1	0.78-5.5	0.14
Cysts with FH	Neither cysts nor FH	2.7	1.5-4.6	0.0004
PDWA	Non-PD	1.9	1.2-2.9	0.003
AH	Non-PD	5.3	3.1-8.8	<0.0001
CAL	No CAL	1.3	0.87-2	0.19
PDWA without FH	Non-PD without FH	1.9	1.2-3	0.007
PDWA with FH	Non-PD with FH	2	0.63-6.1	0.25
PDWA with FH	Non-PD without FH	2.7	1.4-5.3	0.004
AH without FH	Non-PD without FH	4.3	2.4-7.8	<0.0001
AH with FH	Non-PD with FH	8.4	2.6-27	0.0003
AH with FH	Non-PD without FH	11	5.5-24	<0.0001

From Dupont WD, Page DL. Risk factors for breast cancer in women with proliferative breast disease. N Engl J Med 312:146, 1985.

PDWA, Proliferative disease without atypia: *PD,* proliferative disease; *CAL,* calcification; *AH,* atypical hyperplasia; *FH,* family history of breast cancer (mother, sister, or daughter); *age,* age at time of entry biopsy.

*As compared with the risk in women from Atlanta (Third National Cancer Survey).

corroborate the findings of an increased cancer risk on the basis of atypical hyperplasia and a family history of breast cancer. Figure 63-6 denotes the proportion of patients free of invasive cancer as a function of time since biopsy. A twofold or threefold increase may have little clinical importance if the risk in the reference population is small. The adverse effect of positive family history for the patient with atypical hyperplasia becomes appreciable at approximately 20 years after biopsy.

The aforementioned clinicopathologic studies reflect the opinion that proliferative lesions of epithelial duct origin provide circumstantial and objective data as prognostic markers for increased cancer risk in certain age groups. A differentiation of proliferative pathologic elements in tissue sampling appears important to maximize prognostic accuracy and to enhance end-result reporting. These data further support the use of the breast biopsy report for pathologic indicators that may optimize identification of the patient at high-risk, with and without other commonly recognized clinical risk factors for breast carcinogenesis.

Reproductive Breast

Premenstrual fullness and tenderness of the breast parenchyma is evident during the ovulatory cycle. In this interval, mammary blood flow is increased by 15 to 30 ml/cm.[3] Breast parenchymal density is thereafter increased by water retention in connective tissues and enhanced by new growth of the ductal and acinar cells. Breast edema may result from estrogen-induced histamine effect on the microcirculation with fluid entry into the breast interstitium. These changes have been labeled a result of the luteal phase of steroid action, although prolactin may play an essential role.

In the reproductive years, the breasts undergo cyclic changes in preparation for gestation. In the proliferative phase, parenchymal proliferation with epithelial sprouts and stimulation of cellular RNA is evident after induction by estrogen.[31] Dilation of the ductal system and differentiation of alveoli into secretory cells follow the appearance of progesterone in the luteal phase.

These premenstrual phenomena must be differentiated from the pathologic alterations of FCDB. Thus, palpation of the breast for examination purposes is most informative when performed in the early-cycle phase, because breast volume is at a minimum. With termination of the menstrual cycle, the breast undergoes regressive changes characterized by cellular regression of the alveoli and reduction in the size of lumina of the lactiferous ducts.

Exogenous Hormones and Environmental Factors Etiologic in Benign Breast Disease

Endometrial abnormalities, which result from the administration of progesterone in the absence of estrogens, stimulated interest in the use of a combined preparation for the treatment of fibrocystic mastopathy. The combination of norethynodrel and mestranol (Enovid) was reported by Ariel[48] to have good to excellent objective responses in 64% of subjects with FCDB. Subsequently, combined therapy with high-dose progesterone initiated an objec-

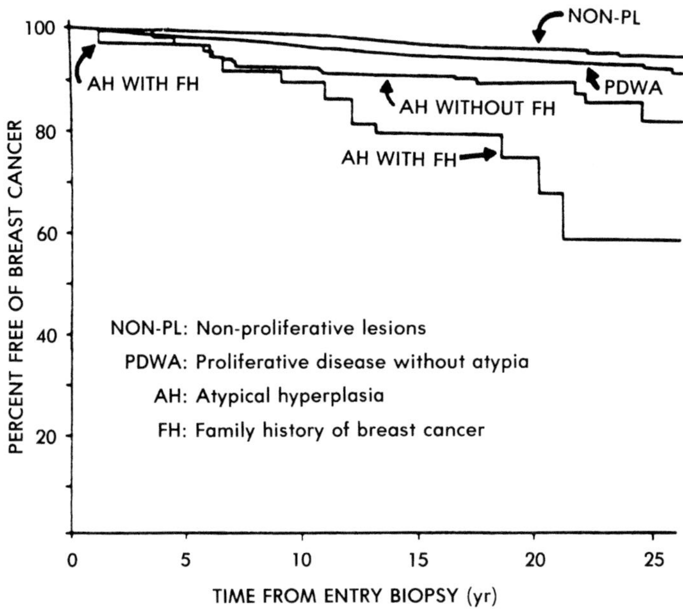

Fig. 63-6. Proportion of patients free of invasive breast carcinoma as a function of time since entry biopsy. (From Dupont WD, Page DL. Risk factors for breast cancer in women with proliferative breast disease. N Engl J Med 312:146, 1985. Copyright © 1985 Massachusetts Medical Society. All rights reserved.)

tive, sustained response that was much improved compared with that of untreated control patients.[32]

Pastides et al.[49] reported that women who used OCs for 2 to 4 years or longer had a decreased risk of FCDB. The findings partly agree with those of LiVolsi et al.[50] when cases are considered according to the degree of epithelial atypia, in that patients with FCDB exhibiting marked atypia generally had similar patterns of OC use when compared with control subjects. Patients with absent, low, and intermediate atypia had less OC use than did control patients. A negative association between OC use and FCDB-exhibiting cysts (gross and microscopic) or papillomatosis is notable. These findings suggest that a spectrum of FCDB exists and that long-term use of OCs protects against the forms of FCDB that are not firmly associated with an increased risk of cancer but does not protect against the premalignant variants of FCDB.

Asch and Greenblatt[51] noted that a synthetic-impeded androgen (danazol) may diminish secretion of LH, initiating reduction of ovarian estrogen. Their data suggest that danazol provides competition with estrogen for receptor sites and has a direct target-organ effect on breast parenchyma through its mildly androgenic properties. The high incidence of amenorrhea (50%), acne, edema, flashes, and muscle cramps have diminished the initial enthusiasm for the use of this compound. However, a reduction of the therapeutic dose suggested for endometriosis is of value for control of mastalgia in certain subjects. The occasional involution of mastopathy to an asymptomatic state with objective regression of cyst size represents an advantage of danazol therapy.

Application of androgens, human chorionic gonadotropin, and estrogen antagonists have met with varying success in the treatment of FCDB. The disappearance of fibrocystic mastopathy during the course of pregnancy or with lactation is a common observation. Thus, there is reason to speculate that lactation represents the most normal state in which the breast can exist. In contradistinction, lactogenic factors can induce mammary epithelium and lobules to undergo a spectrum of evolution from florid or involutional FCDB to the extreme of active lactation.

Caffeine, cyclic nucleotides, and saturated dietary fats have been suggested as mechanistic etiologic factors for benign and malignant breast disease.[52] To date, their etiologic roles in breast disease remain circumstantial.

Breast Neoplasia

Natural History

The attempts to characterize the preclinical stages of breast neoplasia have centered almost exclusively on proliferative lesions of the mammary epithelium or lobules. The physiologic effects of gonadal and pituitary hormones on breast parenchyma initiate proliferation and regression of the epithelium and are therefore able to induce preneoplastic lesions with unrestrained growth and metastases to a detectable clinical stage. The effort to morphologically identify these preneoplastic states necessitates the differentiation of atypical hyperplastic lobules from lobular carcinoma in situ or the atypical proliferation of duct epithelium from an intraductal carcinoma. Despite the stringent criteria and guidelines employed, morphologic distinction is often difficult and is subject to interpretative error.

A diagram of the natural history of breast cancer is seen in Fig. 63-7. Epithelial hyperplasia is regarded as a preneoplastic lesion, in the context that it will invariably precede

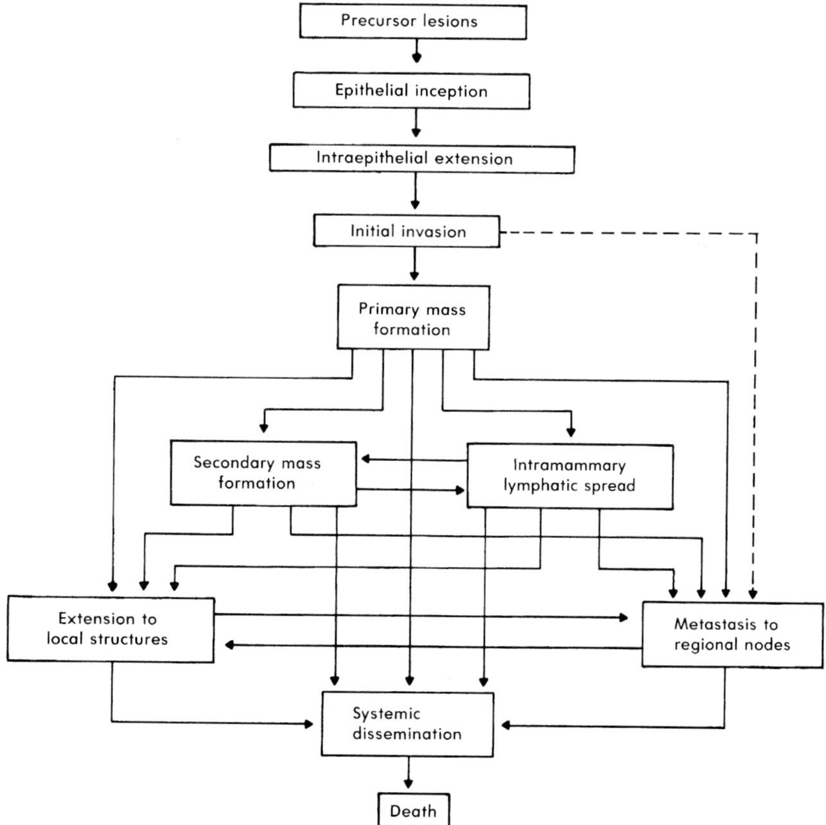

Fig. 63-7. Diagram of natural history of breast carcinoma. Predictability and linear progression is evident only in early stages. (From Gallager HSL. Minimal breast cancer: Concepts and treatment. In Burghardt E, Holzer E, eds. Minimal Invasive Cancer (Microcarcinoma): Clinics in Oncology. Philadelphia: WB Saunders, 1982.)

carcinoma, although it may have extension into other pathologic processes. The mechanism of induction and transformation from a normal epithelial cell to a preinvasive stage requires multifactorial mechanisms of dietetic, genetic, and environmental origin operating in an appropriate hormonal milieu. Sources suggest that the temporal duration for the preinvasive stage of mammary carcinoma is prolonged and may be a matter of many months to several years.[53] Further, the epithelial alterations observed in the vicinity of recognizable carcinoma may exist in multiple sites of the ipsilateral or perhaps the contralateral breast. The periductal connective tissue will show extensive changes, not only in the vicinity of invasive carcinoma but also throughout the whole breast; these changes may occur when only a single focus of carcinoma is identifiable. De Ome[54] observed that the earliest change in the duct of murine mammary carcinoma is thickening of the epithelial layer caused by an increase in the number of cells present. These primary morphologic events occur at irregular intervals along the duct, with normal duct membrane cells intervening.

Poorly defined mechanisms cause the duct lining to increase in cell number, with varying degrees of aberration, disarrangement, and anaplasia that range from ductal hyperplasia to intraductal carcinoma. Although these changes may occur in single or multiple duct systems, they appear to be more pronounced near invasive carcinoma. It is often possible to recognize multiple sites where disruption of the basement layer has occurred with variable amounts of periductal extension of tumor. As the carcinogenic transformation occurs within the lactiferous duct, the surrounding connective tissues become juxtaposed or have immediate contact with lymphatic vessels that traverse the periductal position.

Thus, subsequent metastatic growth can occur through three mechanisms: (1) intraductal extension or change in the character of duct epithelium, (2) direct invasion of the breast connective tissues, and (3) direct embolization and extension through the intramammary peripheral lymphatics.[55]

Whole-organ studies confirm that invasive carcinoma is surrounded by nodules of hyperplastic duct epithelium foci and intraductal carcinoma.[56] Thus, a tumor represents a coalescence of several "link sites" of disease, which may constitute a unicentric site of origin. Lymphatic invasion with subsequent dissemination is likely to occur early and most probably in a microscopic stage of disease (stage 0). Thereafter, histologic and clinical changes that can be recognized and confirmed as bilateral breast carcinoma may take place in the contralateral breast. The frequency of this occurrence depends partly on the amount of effort expended to seek multicentricity and bilateral probability.[57]

Lobular Carcinoma and Multicentricity

Although 85% of breast carcinomas have lactiferous ductal origin, the alveoli is the second most frequent site for carcinogenic transformation. Foote and Stewart[58] originally described in situ lobular carcinoma of the breast, which is regarded as a pure entity seen in association with intraductal and infiltrating carcinomas. In situ lobular carcinoma of the breast is a form of breast carcinoma in which the terminal ducts and lobules are characteristically involved in neoplastic transformation after induction by a poorly understood mechanism of carcinogenesis.[59] This was the most common bilateral carcinoma reported by Urban[57] in a series of 505 bilateral neoplasms. Further, carcinomas observed at synchronous or metachronous intervals were histologically similar to the dominant lesion and were of a similar developmental stage when of the in situ lobular type. Urban noted that, when the dominant lesions were infiltrating, half the carcinomas of the contralateral breast were also of a similar histologic type. The probability that more than half of these neoplasms (64%) will appear in the contralateral breast necessitates scrupulous follow-up and biopsy to corroborate or disprove the existence of synchronous carcinoma.[60]

Clinical Staging of Breast Cancer

The clinical staging for cancer of the breast reflects the anatomic extent of the neoplasm determined at the time of diagnosis and before therapy. Staging concepts are based on diagnostic, clinical, and biopsy information, or at intervals in the postsurgical resection when all pathologic information obtained or studied from the resected specimen is available. In addition, a comprehensive evaluation by the clinician of the ipsilateral axillary and supraclavicular lymphatics and of the contralateral breast and axilla are necessary.

Classifications have been developed to allow comparison of treatment end results for different investigators and among the various institutions reporting clinical trials. Three basic clinical staging systems have evolved; (1) the Manchester, (2) the Columbia Clinical Classification, and (3) the TNM (tumor, nodes, metastasis) systems.

The Manchester system was developed in 1940 at the Christie Hospital and Holt Radium Institute of Manchester, England. The Manchester system was used until introduction of the more comprehensive Columbia Clinical Classification developed by Haagensen and Stout provided better clinical determinants for evaluation of the extent of involvement of the breast by the neoplastic process (e.g., edema, ulceration, fixation). The recommendation of the American Joint Committee on Cancer (AJCC) and the TNM Committee of the International Union Against Cancer established the TNM system, which was adopted in São Paulo, Brazil, in 1954. Since the initial development of the TNM classification, slight modifications have subsequently been formulated. The AJCC-recommended tumor staging is indicated in the boxes on pp. 1267-1268.

These staging principles provide definition of the primary tumor with regard to size, presence or absence of lymphatic involvement, fixation, and regional or distant dissemination of the tumor. The comprehensive formulation of such principles allows one to group with regard to stages TIS, stage X, or stages I to IV, depending on the advancing clinical presentation of the primary neoplasm. The diagnosis of cancer must be established by histologic study of the tumor, and the cellular type of the lesion is recorded.[61] Because the biologic behavior varies from one histologic variant of cancer to another, only similar types should be compared for reporting purposes.

The essentials of the initial examination should also include the following:

1. Physical examination
2. Evaluation of both breasts before operation with validated techniques (e.g., mammography)
3. Preadmission clinical pathology examinations, including hepatic enzyme profile
4. Chest radiograph
5. Skeletal radiographic survey in select patients with symptoms

Selected examinations include the following:

1. Technetium radionuclide, hepatic scintigraphy, or abdominal CT or MRI in the presence of hepatomegaly or abnormal liver profile at chemical analysis
2. Radionuclide bone scan for the following advanced stages of disease:
    a. Primary lesion T3, T4
    b. Evidence of regional nodal metastasis (N1, N2, N3)
    c. Distant metastatic spread (M1)

Prevailing medical opinion accepts bone scintigraphy as being too sensitive to be of cost-benefit value in the preoperative staging for patients with early breast cancers (T1, T2, T1N1). For these patients, a skeletal radiographic survey should be correlated with the bone scan to identify associated benign disorders that may appear as false-positive images (arthritis, healed fractures, bone islands). Burkett et al.[62] reported that 8% of 162 screening bone scan results (stages I to III) were positive, whereas the yield of scans for patients without symptoms was only two of 150 patients (1.3%). Hayward and Frazier[63] reported an enhancement of sensitivity and specificity with technetium 99 bone scans employing serum alkaline phosphatase and lactate dehydrogenase values. When either the alkaline phosphatase or the lactate dehydrogenase value was abnormal, 51.7% of the scan results were positive. When both values were abnormal, 66.7% of patients had positive bone scan results.

These results suggest that breast cancer screening can be selectively enhanced with alkaline phosphatase and lactate dehydrogenase determinations, and that isotopic scanning should be reserved for patients with abnormal values or symptoms that suggest metastatic disease. Isotopic bone

AJCC-RECOMMENDED TUMOR STAGING (CLINICAL)

Definitions

Primary tumor (T)

TX	Primary tumor cannot be assessed
T0	No evidence of primary tumor
Tis	Carcinoma in situ: Intraductal carcinoma, lobular carcinoma in situ, or Paget's disease of the nipple with no tumor
T1	Tumor 2 cm or less in greatest dimension
T1a	0.5 cm or less in greatest dimension
T1b	More than 0.5 cm but not more than 1 cm in greatest dimension
T1c	More than 1 cm but not more than 2 cm in greatest dimension
T2	Tumor more than 2 cm but not more than 5 cm in greatest dimension
T3	Tumor more than 5 cm in greatest dimension
T4	Tumor of any size with direct extension to chest wall or skin
T4a	Extension to chest wall
T4b	Edema (including *peau d'orange)* or ulceration of the skin of breast or satellite skin nodules confined to same breast
T4c	Both T4a and T4b
T4d	Inflammatory carcinoma

Lymph node (N)

NX	Regional lymph nodes cannot be assessed (e.g., previously removed)
N0	No regional lymph node metastasis
N1	Metastasis to movable ipsilateral axillary lymph node(s)
N2	Metastasis to ipsilateral axillary lymph node(s) fixed to one another or to other structures
N3	Metastasis to ipsilateral internal mammary lymph node(s)

Pathologic classification (pN)

pNX	Regional lymph nodes cannot be assessed (e.g., previously removed, or not removed for pathologic study)
pN0	No regional lymph node metastasis
pN1	Metastasis to movable ipsilateral axillary lymph node(s)
pN1a	Only micrometastasis (none larger than 0.2 cm)
pN1b	Metastasis to lymph nodes, any larger than 0.2 cm
pN1bi	Metastasis in 1 to 3 lymph nodes, any more than 0.2 cm and all less than 2 cm in greatest dimension
pN1bii	Metastasis to 4 or more lymph nodes, any more than 0.2 cm and all less than 2 cm in greatest dimension
pN1biii	Extension of tumor beyond the capsule of a lymph node metastasis less than 2 cm in greatest dimension
pN1biv	Metastasis to a lymph node 2 cm or more in greatest dimension
pN2	Metastasis to ipsilateral axillary lymph nodes that are fixed to one another or to other structures
pN3	Metastasis to ipsilateral internal mammary lymph node(s)

Distant metastasis (M)

MX	Presence of distant metastasis cannot be assessed
M0	No distant metastasis
M1	Distant metastasis (includes metastasis to ipsilateral supraclavicular lymph node(s))

From Beahrs OH, et al., eds. Manual for Staging of Cancer, 4th ed. Philadelphia: JB Lippincott, 1992, p 153. Used with permission.
AJCC, American Joint Committee on Cancer.

scanning remains valuable in patients with symptoms and in those with chemical determination of bone involvement, but it has its greatest application in postoperative follow-up because it remains a sensitive indicator of evolving metastatic disease. Patients with suspect findings on skeletal radiographic survey who have clinically palpable disease at supraclavicular or axillary sites should receive isotopic scanning in the preoperative period to serve as a baseline for future evaluations.

Currently, breast imaging may be recorded by five modalities: (1) x-ray (mammography), (2) heat (thermography), (3) sound (ultrasonography), (4) light (diaphanography), and (5) magnetism (MRI).[64] To date, the primacy of mammography for mass screening of breast carcinoma is unchallenged by the other diagnostic modalities. Nonetheless, when used as an adjunct to clinical evaluation and mammography, the other diagnostic parameters may enhance diagnosis.

Thermography displays an intricate detail of the internal anatomy of the breast, transferring invisible infrared irradiation from the skin to a thermal map. An abnormal thermogram is not of sufficient specificity to allow unequivo-

AJCC-RECOMMENDED TUMOR STAGING (PATHOLOGIC)

Pathologic Classification (pN)

pNX	Regional lymph nodes cannot be assessed (e.g., previously removed, or not removed for pathologic study)
pN0	No regional lymph node metastasis
pN1	Metastasis to movable ipsilateral axillary lymph node(s)
pN1a	Only micrometastasis (none larger than 0.2 cm)
pN1b	Metastasis to lymph node(s), any larger than 0.2 cm
pN1bi	Metastasis in one to three lymph nodes, any more than 0.2 cm and all less than 2 cm in greatest dimension
pN1bii	Metastasis to four or more lymph nodes, any more than 0.2 cm and all less than 2 cm in greatest dimension
pN1biii	Extension of tumor beyond the capsule of a lymph node metastasis less than 2 cm in greatest dimension
pN1biv	Metastasis to a lymph node 2 cm or more in greatest dimension
pN2	Metastasis to ipsilateral axillary lymph nodes that are fixed to one another or to other structures
pN3	Metastasis to ipsilateral internal mammary lymph node(s)

Distant Metastasis (M)

MX	Presence of distant metastasis cannot be assessed
M0	No distant metastasis
M1	Distant metastasis (includes metastasis to ipsilateral supraclavicular lymph node(s))

Stage Grouping

Stage 0	Tis	N0	M0
Stage I	T1	N0	M0
Stage IIA	T0	N1	M0
	T1	N1*	M0
	T2	N0	M0
Stage IIB	T2	N1	M0
	T3	N0	M0
Stage IIIA	T0	N2	M0
	T1	N2	M0
	T2	N2	M0
	T3	N1	M0
	T3	N2	M0
Stage IIIB	T4	Any N	M0
	Any T	N3	M0
Stage IV	Any T	Any N	M1

Histopathologic Type

The histologic types are as follows:

Carcinoma, not otherwise specified

Ductal
- Intraductal (in situ)
- Invasive with predominant intraductal component
- Invasive, not otherwise specified
- Comedo
- Inflammatory
- Medullary with lymphocytic infiltrate
- Mucinous (colloid)
- Papillary
- Scirrhous
- Tubular
- Other

Lobular
- In situ
- Invasive with predominant in situ component
- Invasive

Nipple
- Paget's disease, not otherwise specified
- Paget's disease with intraductal carcinoma
- Paget's disease with invasive ductal carcinoma
- Other
- Undifferentiated carcinoma

Histopathologic Grade (G)

GX	Grade cannot be assessed
G1	Well differentiated
G2	Moderately differentiated
G3	Poorly differentiated
G4	Undifferentiated

From Beahrs OH, et al., eds. Manual for Staging of Cancer, 4th ed. Philadelphia: JB Lippincott, 1992, p 153.

**Note:* The prognosis of patients with N1a is similar to that of patients with pN0.

cal diagnosis of a neoplastic disease; comparable findings may be observed in such nonmalignant processes as acute inflammatory states of the breast with heightened metabolic activity (abscess, cellulitis, fat necrosis). This technique did not enhance the diagnostic accuracy when used for mass screening in the national Breast Cancer Detection Demonstration Project (BCDDP).[65,66]

Significant advances have been made in the instrumentation of medical ultrasonography. *Ultrasonography* uses special transducers that introduce pulsed high-frequency sound waves into breast tissues, and the reflected transmitted waves are electronically converted for display as images. This technique appears to have an advantage with respect to mammography in that it can better define and precisely recognize lesions in dense (dysplastic) mammographic breast images, where radiographic shadows may be obscured. This technique has great value in evaluating benign cysts that resemble solid masses on mammography. Ultrasonography is less useful in recognition and diagnosis of benign and malignant solid tumors. Distinguishing a fibroadenoma from an infiltrating carcinoma may be impossible, because differentiation of inflammatory states from diffuse neoplastic processes is not uniformly possible by means of ultrasonography.

Diaphanography, with visualization of mammary parenchyma by transilluminated intense light beams, is not a new concept. However, recent technologic advances to enhance imaging with this technique have great promise. Breast imaging depends on such factors as size, the composition and optical density of breast tissues, inflammatory changes, cysts, and neoplasia, all of which affect light transmission and absorption. Clinical trials with these techniques and MRI are being conducted to evaluate their diagnostic capability.

Sites for metastatic involvement with breast carcinoma are, in order of decreasing frequency, bone, liver, lung, skin, extraregional lymphatics, and brain. The ipsilateral axillary lymph node basin is the major regional drainage site for carcinoma of the breast. From 40% to 50% of patients have clinical or histologic involvement of this site at initial presentation. However, the detection of axillary nodal involvement at physical examination is difficult. Approximately 20% to 25% of examinations are incorrectly assessed. The pathologic stage of the axillary lymphatics correlates significantly with survival. For these reasons, adequate sampling of axillary lymph nodes (approximately 5 to 10 lymph nodes) is required to determine the future status of the patient and may indicate the necessity for adjuvant chemotherapy, radiation, or hormonal therapy. Clinical staging of the primary tumor dictates the type of surgical procedure. However, pathologic staging is the most important determinant for the necessity of adjuvant multimodal or single-agent therapy.

Options for Surgical Management

The choice of the operative procedure for breast carcinoma depends on the size of the primary lesion, the presence or absence of tumor fixation, the presence of regional adenopathy, evidence of distant disease, and the physiologic status of the patient. Carcinomas 5 cm in diameter or smaller that are limited to the lateral quadrants of the breast without fixation (T1a, T2a) are best managed by surgery alone. For regional metastatic involvement with central or medially located lesions, the combination of surgery with postoperative radiation may be appropriate to ensure chest wall control. For stage I and stage II diseases, the type of procedure performed and the areas receiving irradiation depend on location of the primary tumor, the presence or absence of lymphatic disease, and the pathologic findings in the operative specimen.

Neoplasms of the lateral aspect of the breast drain primarily through the axillary lymphatics and can be eliminated by modified radical mastectomy. This procedure includes dissection of the lateral border of the sternum medically, the latissimus dorsi muscle laterally, the clavicle superiorly, and the superior border of the rectus muscle inferiorly. All breast parenchyma is extirpated from the chest wall through flaps created within the superficial investing fascia of the dermis. Dissection should be guided by principles of ablative surgery, which include an en bloc resection. To ensure that level I, II, and III nodes are resected, the pectoralis minor muscle should be divided at its insertion on the coracoid process and origin from the ribs (Patey procedure). The final dissected specimen includes the breast, the nipple-areolar complex with associated skin, axillary contents, and the pectoralis minor muscle.

Medially located neoplasms principally drain into internal mammary lymphatics and may be associated with nodal involvement in 10% to 30% of patients. If axillary metastases are present in medial lesions, the probability that the internal nodes are pathologically involved may exceed 50%. In the absence of clinically involved axillary metastasis, medial carcinomas are treated by modified radical mastectomy. Postoperative radiation therapy has not been shown to improve survival or decrease chest wall recurrence and is no longer recommended. When metastases are identified in more than 20% of the removed nodes of the axilla, adjuvant postoperative chest wall irradiation may be used to sterilize *in transit* metastatic disease, which may exist in the endolymphatic spaces of the skin flaps. Likewise, the internal mammary and supraclavicular nodes (peripheral lymphatics) should be included in radiation portals.

Cancers that are laterally located with axillary nodal involvement may also have metastatic involvement of supraclavicular or internal mammary sites in as many as 25% to 30% of patients. In such cases, adjuvant irradiation is also advisable for treatment of these regional nodal sites.

Radical mastectomy is reserved for medially located lesions with associated palpable axillary lymphatic metastases in patients who are not candidates for radiation therapy and for centrally located lesions that are fixed to the pectoralis major fascia. These neoplasms are likely to metastasize by way of transpectoral and retropectoral routes (Rotter's nodes). Radical mastectomy ablates the neurovascular bundle that innervates the pectoralis major muscle and through which lymphatics course medial to the pectoralis minor muscle. This procedure is technically simpler than the modified radical mastectomy, which necessitates preservation of the pectoralis major muscle and its neural innervation. The axillary dissections of both the radical and the modified radical procedures are identical and include resection of level I, II, and III nodes.

In 1948, the extended radical mastectomy (supraradical mastectomy) was designed as an extension of the radical mastectomy to enhance control of regional metastatic disease by therapeutic dissection of the internal mammary nodes. Although some surgeons in the 1960s and 1970s[67,68] supported this more radical approach, most surgeons have abandoned its use and employ irradiation to achieve sterilization of internal nodal disease for control of this regional site.

Social, cosmetic, and scientific pressures have driven the increasing application of breast-conserving surgery. Breast-conserving procedures have been variously labeled as *lumpectomy, tylectomy,* or *segmental resection*. Essential to the use of breast-preservation procedures is the concept that adequate removal of all primary breast cancer can be accomplished without incision into neoplastic tissue. Thus, the goal is maintenance of adequate cosmetic appearance while achieving control and cure rates that equal those obtained with modified radical mastectomy. Therefore, breast size and histology of the primary neoplasm often dictate the prudent exercise of the traditional radical operative approach to facilitate adequate control of local and regional disease. Frozen-section analysis of the resected margins should always be performed to ensure that breast cancer has been removed en bloc with the specimen. Inadequate surgical margins that contain neoplastic disease require reexcision and, if inadequately performed, may necessitate mastectomy.

When adjuvant chemotherapy or radiation therapy is to be used, the status of the axillary nodes must be determined. Axillary sampling procedures are done through curvilinear incisions placed between the lateral border of the pectoralis major and latissimus dorsi muscles 4 to 6 cm below the apex of the axilla. Adequate sampling of the lateral contents of the axilla (level I) is completed, and 10 to 15 lymph nodes are analyzed.

Indications for tylectomy, axillary sampling, and comprehensive radiation to the breast, axilla, and internal mammary and supraclavicular nodes include (1) primary neoplasm less than or equal to 4 cm, (2) clinically negative axillary lymphatics, (3) a breast of adequate size to achieve primary closure with an acceptable cosmetic result and one to which a uniform dose of radiation therapy can be delivered, and (4) a radiation therapist experienced with this modality of therapy. If these stipulations cannot be met, the results of segmental resection and primary irradiation may be both therapeutically and cosmetically unsatisfactory. The importance of removal of all the primary breast cancer is emphasized. Were viable cancer cells to remain within the breast, they might be incorporated into the scar of the healing wound, which is poorly oxygenated. The biologic observation that maximal irradiation effect will not be achieved for marginally oxygenated and anoxic cancer cells within scar tissue suggests the likelihood of recurrence of carcinoma in the incision. When the initial biopsy confirms invasive carcinoma, the practice of many surgeons is to reexcise the scar and complete an axillary sampling procedure (levels I and II), especially when the limits of the excision cannot be assessed. Approximately 50% of patients who have had tylectomy scars reexcised have viable cancer cells present in the wound after what was initially determined to be an adequate excisional biopsy. Centers that do not advocate reexcision of the biopsy site usually boost the external beam irradiation dose by the implantation of iridium 192 needles in the area of the scar.

Veronesi et al.[69] of Milan, Italy, reported the results of a randomized, prospective clinical trial comparing radical mastectomy with quadrantectomy, axillary node dissection, and breast radiation therapy (QUART). Between 1973 and 1980, 701 women with lesions less than or equal to 2 cm and clinically negative axillae (T1N0M0) were evaluated. Mean time in the study was 8 years. The investigators reported no significant differences between the two groups for local or regional recurrence, relapse-free survival, or overall survival. Two percent of patients in each group had a local recurrence, and an additional 2% demonstrated a regional treatment failure. At 8 years, relapse-free survival was 79% for the mastectomy group and 80% for patients managed by the QUART protocol; the proportions of patients surviving were 82.5% and 85%, respectively. For node-positive patients (stage II), prolonged survival favored the QUART group (82% vs 79%), although the survival advantage was not statistically significant. These authors concluded that eligible patients with small breast lesions treated by QUART protocol have no demonstrable disadvantage with regard to disease-free survival or overall survival compared with similar patient groups managed by radical mastectomy.

The most recent analysis of the results of three major trials on breast conservation performed at the Milan Cancer Institute between 1973 and 1988 were recently reported by Veronesi et al.[70] The survival curves for the two groups in the Milan I study were superimposable. A subgroup analysis showed a nonstatistically significant advantage in patients with positive axillary lymph nodes treated by QUART compared with those treated with mastectomy. Although there were 17 local recurrences (4.8%) in the QUART group compared with eight (2.3%) in the mastectomy group, 10 of the 17 patients with local recurrence in the former group were alive without evidence of disease at 6 to 14 years after detection of the recurrence, whereas only two of the eight patients with local recurrence in the latter group were alive.

The Milan II trial randomly assigned patients to QUART and to tumorectomy, axillary dissection, and radiotherapy (TART). Between 1985 and 1987, this study accrued 705 patients, 360 in the QUART group and 345 in the TART group. There was a significant difference in local relapses between the two groups. There were 15 recurrences and four new cancers in the QUART group (5.3%), whereas in the TART group, there were 39 recurrences and seven new cancers. The actuarial survivals for the two groups were identical at 7 years. The presence of extensive intraductal component (EIC) increased the incidence of local recurrence in both groups. However, the incidence of local recurrence was higher in the TART group (28%) than in the QUART group (9%).

The Milan III study compared QUART with quadrantectomy plus axillary node dissection without radiotherapy (QUAD). Radiotherapy was given to patients in the QUAD group when recurrences occurred. From 1988 to 1989, this study recruited 567 patients, 294 in the QUART group and 273 in the QUAD group. There was a significant difference in local recurrence incidence between the two groups. There were 24 local recurrences in the QUAD group (8.8%), compared with 1 (0.3%) in the QUART group. Among patients older than 55 years, however, the incidence of local recurrence was low even in the QUAD group. The presence of EIC increased the incidence of local recurrence in this study. Overall survivals were similar in the two groups.

The results of the prospectively randomized trial for segmental mastectomy with or without comprehensive irradiation to the breast and peripheral lymphatics versus modified radical mastectomy were published by Fisher et al.[42,71] of the National Surgical Adjuvant Breast and Bowel Project (NSABP). This multiinstitutional trial of the NSABP (protocol B-06) evaluated breast conservation and tumor control by segmental mastectomy in the treatment of stage I and II breast tumors 4 cm or smaller. All patients had axillary dissections, and patients with histologically positive nodes received adjuvant chemotherapy (melphalan and 5-fluorouracil).

Life table estimates based on data from 1843 women accrued in the B-06 study indicate that treatment by segmental mastectomy, with or without breast irradiation, provides local-disease–free, distant-disease–free, and actuarial survivals at 5 years that equal the survivals of patients treated by total mastectomy. For women treated by segmental mastectomy with irradiation, 92.3% remained free of tumor at 5 years versus 72.1% of those receiving no radiation ($p < 0.001$). Local recurrence in the breast operated on was 8% for patients who had segmental mastectomy and breast irradiation, whereas local recurrence was 28% for those who had segmental mastectomy without radiation therapy. The study therefore established the importance of radiation therapy in controlling recurrence of breast cancer in the ipsilateral breast for patients with negative axillary lymph nodes. Also of note was the local recurrence in the breasts of patients with positive lymph nodes, all of whom received adjuvant chemotherapy. For node-positive patients with and without treatment with radiation therapy, local breast recurrence rates after segmental mastectomy were 2% and 37%, respectively. The 2% figure is significantly lower than the corresponding 8% recurrence rate in women with stage I disease (negative axillary nodes), suggesting that irradiation may sensitize the breast neoplasm to the cytotoxic effects of chemotherapy.

The mean follow-up at the time of this report was 39 months, but the recently published data after 10 years of follow-up continue to justify the use of lumpectomy combined with breast irradiation for the management of invasive breast carcinoma.[72] The cumulative incidence of ipsilateral breast tumor recurrence was 12% for patients treated by lumpectomy and breast irradiation versus 53% for patients who underwent lumpectomy alone ($p < 0.001$). This improvement in local control in the lumpectomy plus irradiation group was seen in all women, regardless of age, tumor size, or nodal status.

The 1990 Consensus Development Conference on Treatment of Early-Stage Breast Cancer, convened jointly by the National Institutes of Health (NIH) and the NCI, concluded that breast-conservation treatment is an appropriate method of primary therapy for most women with stage I and II breast cancer, and it is preferable because it provides a survival equivalent to total mastectomy and axillary node dissection while preserving the breast.[73] The recommendations for breast-conservation treatment include local excision of the primary tumor with clear margins, a level I and II axillary node dissection, and breast irradiation to a dose of 4500 to 5000 cGy, with or without a boost.

For management of stage III disease in which axillary metastases exceed 2.5 cm and are fixed or matted, the surgical procedure is designed to ablate the primary neoplasm and lymphatics, which are at a reduced probability for sterilization by irradiation alone. Control of regional nodal disease by any modality is inversely related to size of the nodes to be treated. Thus, centrally located lymphatics with small deposits of cancer contiguous with axillary structures that are not resectable may be adequately controlled by radiation therapy. In these circumstances, the breast tissue and level I lymphatics are resected in what is termed an *extended simple mastectomy.* Level II and III lymphatics are left intact in the axilla to be controlled with irradiation. In this instance, lymphedema of the arm is uncommon because collateral lymphatic vessels that enter the apical axilla are not ablated by the surgical procedure.

Breast carcinomas larger than 5 cm in diameter associated with minimum clinical disease in the axilla (stage IIIA), which are biologically favorable lesions, may be treated by preoperative irradiation, chemotherapy, or both, followed by radical or modified radical mastectomy. Chemotherapeutic induction of the neoplasm by cytotoxic agents (cytoxan, doxorubicin [Adriamycin], fluorouracil) is highly successful, resulting in cytoreduction of the tumor. These therapeutic techniques may enhance locoregional control and increase the disease-free interval. Therapeutic choice of radiotherapy or chemotherapy depends on the location and site of the tumor and the total dose of radiation to be delivered to the apex of the axilla to provide tumor control.

Patients with stage IV disease (distant metastasis), including supraclavicular metastases, are best treated primarily with cytotoxic chemotherapeutic agents. However, control of local chest wall disease is best achieved with limited surgical procedures that ensure skin closure and are often used with radiation therapy. The timing of these procedures must be determined individually; this is often directed by the medical oncologist because the principal dilemma is control of distant disease.

RADIOLOGIC EVALUATION OF BREAST DISEASE

Mammographic Imaging of Normal Breast Parenchyma and Benign Disease

Mammograms are cephalocaudal and mediolateral x-ray images reproduced on a selenium plate with impressions in a positive or negative mode to accentuate tissue densities. Ultrasonographic mammography represents a noninvasive method of reproducing high-resolution tomographic sections through the breast. Development of gray-scale units has greatly improved the quality of ultrasonic images. Thermography represents a more insensitive detection method for breast cancer.[65,66] The true-positive rate for thermography was 60% to 85% in early trials of the BCDDP. However, other investigators showed that the sensitivity of thermography is less than 50%. Therefore, its use as a routine screening method for breast cancer is not recommended. Thermography is particularly insensitive to stage 0 minimum cancers and stage I invasive cancers. In contrast, the newer gray-scale diagnostic accuracy of ultrasonography is approximately 79% to 87%, with a low false-negative rate (7.6%) and a false-positive rate of 18% to 20%.[36]

The radiographic beam consists of electromagnetic waves of energy of extremely short wavelength, such that matter is penetrated to variable degrees as a function of density. Thus, the penetration of air, tissue, and water or mineral (bone) densities depends on the energy and wavelengths of the x-ray beam and the constitution of the matter being imaged. The most radiopenetrable breast substance is fat, whereas the most radiodense (radiopaque) substances are calcium salts, which are deposited in approximately 35% to 45% of malignant and premalignant lesions in the perilobular or periductal tissues. The extent of calcification is a function of replication activity of epithelial cells. Microcalcification is a product of increased cellular activity in the lobuloductal complex and occurs after extrusion of calcium salts into surrounding parenchymal interstitial tissues. Microcalcification is not specific to breast cancer and may be present in epithelial hyperplasia and noninvasive and invasive cancers.

The intermediate penetrability of connective tissue, blood, cyst fluid, epithelium, and duct structures accounts for the remarkable heterogeneity of breast parenchymal mammographic patterns. Among siblings and offspring, great variation in mammographic parenchymal patterns has been observed, reflecting modification of radiopenetrability of the three variants of imaging projections.

Radiographic Imaging of Benign Disease

Proliferative breast disease, or cystic hyperplasia, denotes changes in glandular hyperplasia that primarily involve ducts, adenosis, fibrosis, duct ectasia, and multiple cyst formation. Thus, the term FCDB has become the capricious name for a variety of histologic changes in the breast that result from uninhibited estrogen, progestogen, and prolactin stimuli on this target organ in the absence of feedback inhibition. Each of these pathologic entities occurs in the presence of endogenous estrogens, and they rarely occur separately. They are quite difficult to distinguish on a clinical or radiographic basis.[74]

The wide spectrum of mammographic images relates to the proliferation that occurs in periductal fibrosis and appears as a prominent duct pattern. Often the presentation of multiple nodules or adenosis as a result of lobular proliferation is identifiable. The clinical and radiographic presentations of large cysts of proliferative origin occur because of obstruction and dilation of the lactiferous ducts. Commonly recognized benign mammographic findings include the following:

1. *Adenosis.* Dysplastic nodules involve the entire breast or segments of a quadrant and appear as small, noncalcified multiple mammographic images. A stellate appearance may be observed radiographically when associated with fibrosis and is difficult to distinguish from that of neoplasms. Infrequently, scattered, round calcifications may resemble the microcalcifications of carcinoma.
2. *Cysts.* The use of ultrasonography to differentiate cystic from solid masses in breast cysts has great promise. These palpable, semisolid masses appear as oval, uncalcified lesions with sharp, smooth, well-delineated borders.
3. *Fibroadenoma.* These solitary (85%), solid, mobile, rounded or lobulated masses have sharp borders. The presence of a halo of lucency is a typical radiographic feature. On occasion, differentiation from cysts or medullary carcinoma is difficult. In the postmenopausal state, large, coarse calcifications may develop after mucoid degeneration with hyalinization and involution.
4. *Cystosarcoma phyllodes (giant fibroadenoma).* The progressive growth of large variants of solitary fibroadenomas give rise to this entity. Radiographically, the neoplasm appears as an uncalcified, lobulated, solid mass with sharp delineation. Differentiation from an invasive carcinoma or sarcoma can be confirmed only by excisional biopsy.
5. *Papilloma.* These intraductal neoplasms originate

from the lactiferous ducts and frequently are seen with bloody nipple discharge. They may appear as oval masses in the subareola and are often not identifiable with biplane mammographic views. The injection of water-soluble contrast medium into the involved duct mechanism (galactogram) often allows identification of an intraluminal filling defect.

6. *Fat necrosis.* The mammographic image of fat necrosis has great variability and depends on the age of the patient and the extent of involvement of necrotic fatty substance. Smaller cysts may calcify and give rise to characteristic ringlike calcifications, whereas masses of necrotic fat may stimulate carcinoma with spiculated borders. Angular microcalcifications can occur and may also stimulate carcinoma. Excisional biopsy is usually necessary to confirm the benignity of this process.
7. *Abscess.* An inflammatory process can usually be confirmed clinically. On occasion, a central, deep, ill-defined mass, which appears with overlying skin thickening, increased vascularity, and absence of pain, may mimic carcinoma both clinically and radiographically. Thorough exploration, culture, and biopsy with drainage are indicated to confirm an inflammatory process of nonmalignant origin.

Radiographic Imaging of Malignant Disease

Radiographic imaging (mammography) closely reflects the pathologic changes of malignant states of the breast.[75-77] These clinicopathologic correlations have been subsequently confirmed through whole-organ studies and specimen radiography. Typically, the first mammographic manifestation of breast carcinoma is a soft tissue mass that requires differentiation from the aforementioned benign lesions of the breast. These soft tissue densities may occur in the presence or absence of microcalcification. The differentiation of the benign soft tissue mass from medullary carcinoma sometimes may be difficult because of the sharp definition of both.

Characteristically, distortions of the normal parenchyma adjacent to malignant tumors occur as spicules, long or short, fine and straight strands of tissue that radiate from the tumor site (Fig. 63-8). Retraction of tissues in the direction of the tumor occurs with loss of the margins of the malignant mass because of infiltration of tumor and subsequent reactive sclerosis. The latter characteristic adds a spiculated or stellate appearance to the mammogram. The entrapment of Cooper's ligaments into the tumor mass subsequently initiates retraction of overlying skin or nipple as the tumor extends into adjacent tissues. As the blockage of lymphatics progresses, overlying skin edema *(peau d'orange)* occurs; this is typically seen on mammogram as heightening or thickening of skin. The presentation of inflammatory breast cancer as a lethal and aggressive clinicopathologic variant is strongly suggestive on mammography. In this case, the increase of skin thickness

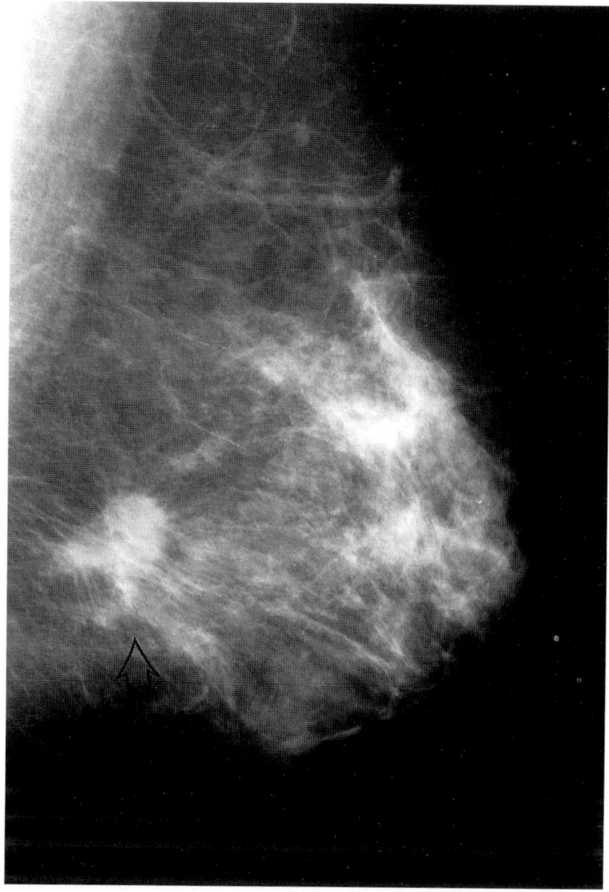

Fig. 63-8. Spiculated scirrhous carcinoma. (Courtesy of Michael P. Vezeridis, M.D.)

is generalized, with involvement of the entire surface of the breast and enhancement of tissue density. Asymmetric widening of the subcutaneous space with prominent subcutaneous lymphatics is evident (Fig. 63-9). Lymphatic vessels engorged by tumor are identified as fine streaks perpendicular to the skin surface.

Microcalcifications are the early mammographic findings of some cancers (e.g., comedocarcinoma, minimum). Typically, microcalcifications are irregular in shape and size and occur in linear configurations or small clusters (Fig. 63-10). These calcifications are present histologically within areas of tumor and fat necrosis. The presence of microcalcifications in the absence of a mass may be the first sign of an intraductal or lobular carcinoma in situ, which appears clinically as the tumor mass expands. These irregular, scattered microcalcifications must be differentiated from the benign calcifications of FCDB, which are tyically larger, oval, and more diffuse. Regardless of the circumstance, mammographic identification of a site of suspect microcalcification necessitates histologic confirmation that employs radiographically assisted biopsy techniques. Use of the Kopans needle for mammographic localization,

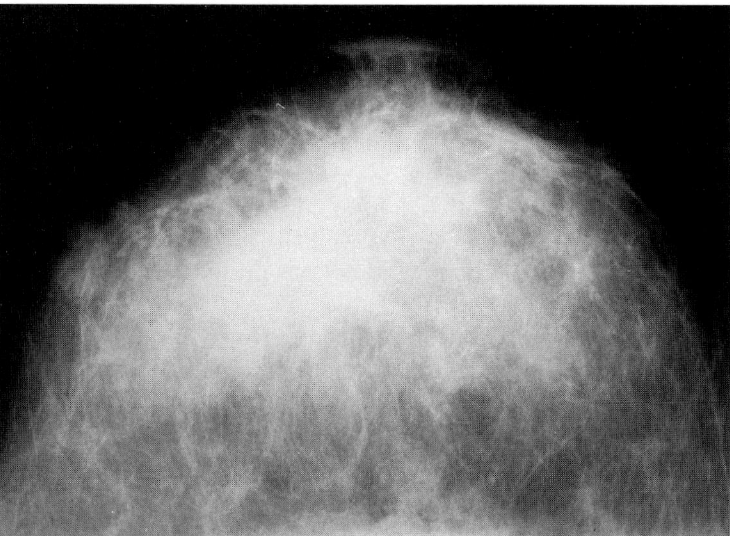

Fig. 63-9. Mammographic appearance of inflammatory breast carcinoma. Diffuse parenchymal density with accentuation of the interstitial markings involving all of the left breast is demonstrated. Skin thickening is also present. **A,** Mediolateral. **B,** Craniocaudal. (Courtesy of Michael P. Vezeridis, M.D.)

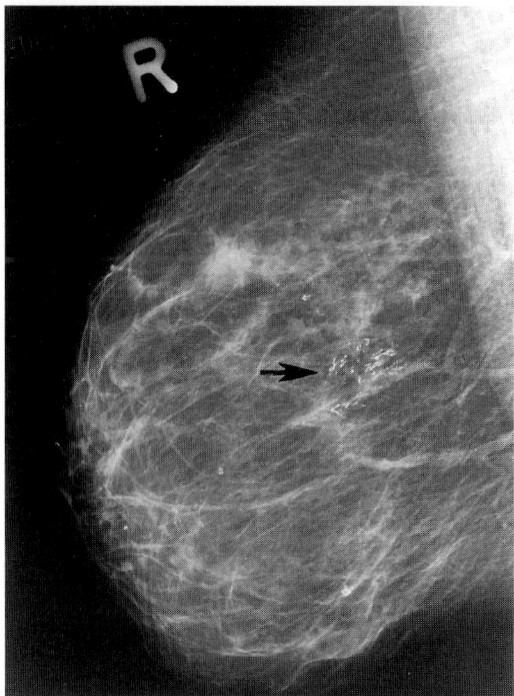

Fig. 63-10. Typical appearance of microcalcifications in breast carcinoma. These calcifications *(arrow)* are irregular in size and shape and occur in small clusters or in linear configurations.

followed by biopsy with a counterincision (Fig. 63-11), allows histologic evaluation after specimen radiography.

Radiographic Imaging of Physiologically Normal and Abnormal Masses

The identification of physiologic abnormalities of breast parenchyma for subjects without symptoms in the absence of palpable masses is possible with the use of standard mammographic techniques. Mammography was studied extensively to determine its effectiveness in detecting breast cancer in its early and nonpalpable stages. Studies of the Health Insurance Plan of Greater New York (HIP) suggested that breast cancer could be detected mammographically in a preclinical (nonpalpable) stage. The benefit of screening in the HIP study was restricted to women older than 50 years. The report of the NCI and the American Cancer Society (ACS) multi-institutional study of mammography (BCDDP) supported the findings of the HIP study with regard to early detection and suggested benefit with screening for younger and elderly categories.[65,78] *Minimum breast cancer* (MBC) is defined as a noninfiltrating lesion of any size, or an infiltrating tumor 1 cm or smaller. Bland et al.[79] confirmed MBC to be more prevalent in the screened population (29%) than in the unscreened population (<5%). MBC lesions appeared with similar frequencies in screened women older and younger than 50 years.[65] A recent review of the final report of the NCI-ACS BCDDP results revealed that among 3557 cases of proven breast cancer detected in the project's screening clinics, 41.6% were detected by mammography alone, 47.3% were detected by physical examination and mammography, 8.7% were detected by physical examination alone, and 2.4% were detected by unknown measures. Approximately one third (32.4%) of the 3557 neoplasms were classified as MBC. Moreover, more than 80% of all detected cancers had no evidence of regional nodal involvement.

Mammography is now the definitive technique to screen subjects without symptoms and to diagnose subtle clinical breast abnormalities. Egan[76,77] established the value of this radiographic technique with the observation of mammographic abnormalities in 10% of the screened community patients who had clinically undetectable neoplasms, most (92%) of whom had no axillary nodal metas-

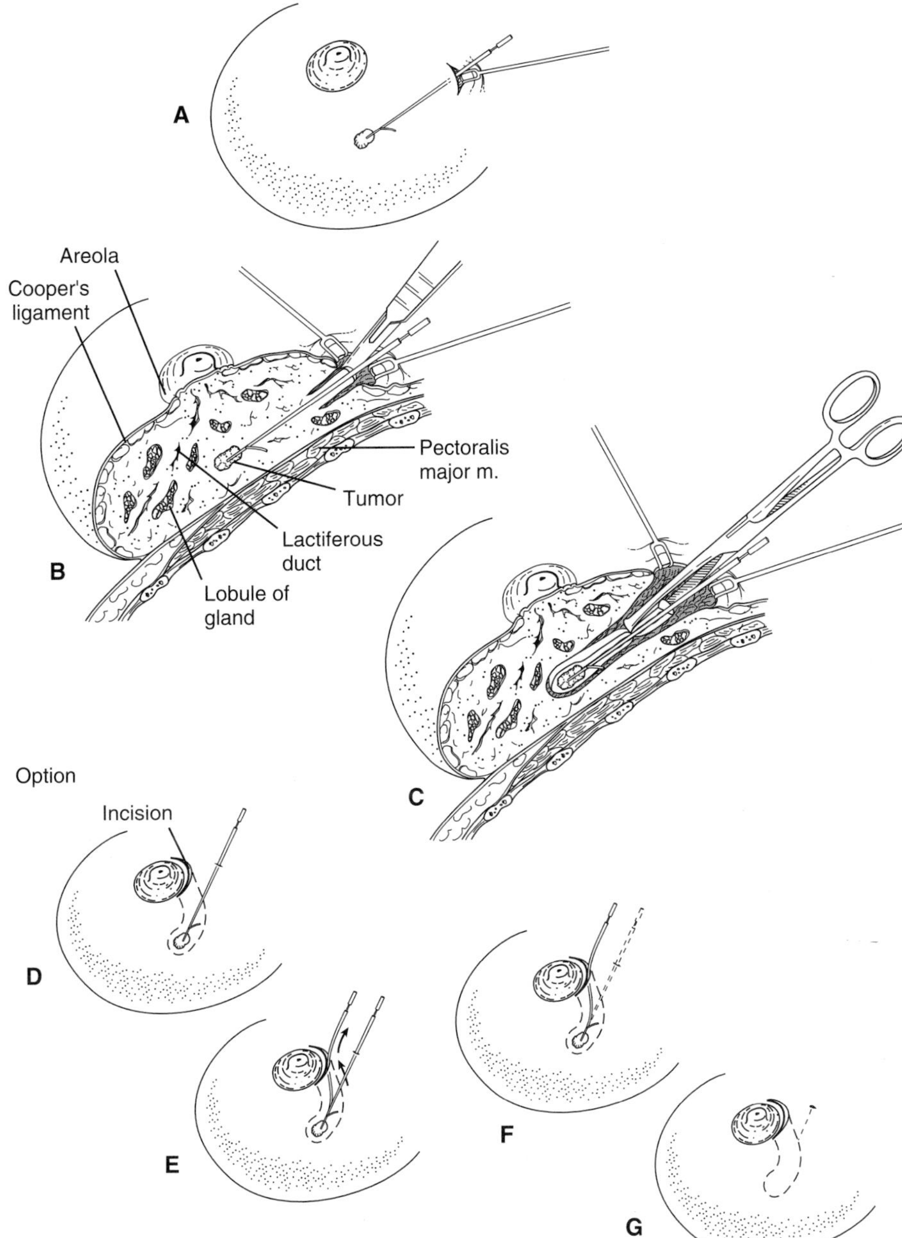

Fig. 63-11. Operative technique for needle localization biopsy. Suspicious lesion is "localized" on mammogram immediately before surgery. **A,** At operation needle serves as a guide for surgeon to perform biopsy. **B,** Development of tissue planes circumferential and parallel to localization wire. **C,** Controlled dissection of wire, which is purchased with tissues using an Allis clamp. Suspicious lesion is incorporated in dissection, which includes tissue beyond tip of hooked wire. Specimen radiography confirms excision of suspicious, nonpalpable mammographically identified lesion. **D,** Deeply localized suspicious lesion approached via circumareolar incision. **E,** Wire is repositioned from percutaneous localized position to exit via incision. **F,** Dissection completed circumferentially and parallel to wire via circumareolar incision. **G,** Completed dissection with breast defect.

tases. The probability of a false-negative study (clinically negative, mammographically negative) exceeds 10% in most breast clinics. Conversely, the false-positive diagnosis of cancer occurs much less frequently (<5%), with diagnostic accuracy increasing as a correlate of experience of the mammographer and the radiographic technique. However, the incidence of a false-negative mammogram or an equivocal report is too great to rely on mammography for exclusion of the diagnosis of cancer in the presence of a solitary mass or suspect lesion. Further, dysplastic (dense) multinodular, fibrocystic, and small breasts may obscure or invalidate interpretation of occult neoplasms poorly imaged on a mammogram. *In no circumstance should mammography be considered a uniformly reliable technique for exclusion of the diagnosis of cancer, because histologic confirmation of clinically suspect lesions by biopsy is mandatory.*

METASTASIS IN BREAST CANCER

Physiologic and Biologic Concepts

The physiologic process of tumor metastasis is a complex biologic event that is influenced by (1) the tumor-host relationship, (2) the metabolic and growth characteristics of the primary neoplasm, and (3) the physical and morphologic factors operative within the vicinity of the neoplasm. Most data that quantify the degree and probability of metastatic spread as an aid to prognosis and treatment have thus far met with little success. These observations attest to the broad spectrum and variability for interrelationships of human breast tumors and the host-defense mechanism. The physiologic mechanism by which a primary tumor gives rise to a metastatic clone of tumor cells remains a mystery.

Enzymatic Activity and Metastatic Potential

The role of lysosomal enzymes in initiating cellular breakdown with loss of intracellular substance may be key to initiation of tumor invasion. This local, invasive process of host tissues by malignant cells invariably follows destruction of normal tissue components juxtaposed to invading neoplastic cells. This event is concomitant with growth of neoplastic cells after infiltration into the subject tissues. A growing body of evidence suggests that neoplastic clones grow and enzymatically destroy adjacent normal cells without themselves being injured. Data suggest that tumor cell surfaces are endowed with different composition and structure, such as glycoproteins, which provide innate protection against the hydrolytic effect of lysosomal enzymes. Variations of the concentration of lysosomal enzymes within invading and regressing tumors is perhaps explained by the fact that both tumor cell lines are simultaneously being destroyed by autolysis.

Immunologic Surveillance and Control of Enzymatic Activity

Berg,[80] by means of elaborate animal experimentation, noted that neoplastic cells are capable of initiating specific immune reactions in proven isogenic systems. In most animal models studied and in certain human cancers, tumor-specific antigens are recognizable in selective assays. However, not all tumors possess much specific immunogenicity. Mathé[81] suggested the possibility of early control of breast cancer metastases by using immunologic methods to augment clinical responses. The application of these methods through monoclonal assay techniques to link active cytotoxic drugs to tumor-specific antibodies may have clinical applicability. Also, these tumor-specific antibody carriers may reduce the myelosuppression and toxicity that follow immunosuppression with systemic therapy. Rowland et al.[82] have used intermediate-carrier polyglutamic acid with substituted cytotoxic drugs linked to immunoglobulins to reduce active antibody activity and neoplastic growth in a rodent tumor model. However, the role of cytotoxic immunotherapy for breast cancer in clinical practice is not clearly established.

Lymphatic Metastases and Modulation of Metastases by Tumor-Host Mechanisms

Classic physiologic concepts taught by Handley[5,6] suggested that breast cancer metastases represent centrifugal dissemination into and through the lymphatics to establish regional and systemic disease. This hypothesis did not recognize that neoplastic invasion facilitates entry into venulae, as well as the regional lymphatics. Although primary tumors do not contain lymphatic connections, the entry into endolymph is initiated by an invasive mechanism. Thereafter, the interstitial fluid convection currents drain and transport neoplastic cells to regional nodes by the method suggested by Butler and Gullino.[83] Widely patent junctions of intercellular bridges in the lymphatics represent primary routes to transport neoplastic cells into systemic lymph.[84]

Investigators have also confirmed that cytoplasmic processes of tumor cells probe the endothelial surface to initiate and provide the best route for transport.[85] After cellular entrapment, the neoplastic clone is transported to afferent lymph vessels to the peripheral subcapsular sinusoids of the nodes. Metabolic, morphologic, and cell-type characteristics determine the temporal duration of "nodal arrest" and the probability of subsequent entrapment. After nodal deposition, cellular proliferation is initiated in the peripheral sinusoids, and after progressive cell division, the medullary regions of the gland are replaced. Thereafter, cells are shed into the efferent lymphatic vessels and may subsequently embolize to more distal nodes of the regional basin.

Ultimately, cells swept into endolymph are transported to systemic sites (lung, liver, brain).[55] Carr et al.[85] used an anaplastic carcinogen-induced tumor to demonstrate that regional lymph nodes represent an immunologically privileged site for tumor growth. These data recapitulate Handley's concept that regional axillary nodes represent a drainage barrier that may or may not be responsive to immunostimulatory events impairing or retarding tumor dissemination. This classic teaching ignored the probability that tumor cells have additional routes to the systemic circulation by way of lymphaticovenous anastomoses.[86,87]

Although lymph node arrest may be transient, neoplastic cells traversing the sinusoids and medullary portion of the nodes retain the capacity for metastasis to numerous organs. Few cells that lodge in the medullary portion of the nodes develop into subsequent metastases. This concept has been reaffirmed by Hewitt and Blake,[88] who concluded that nodes retain a constant "holding capacity" of a specific cell fraction and volume. When this threshold is exceeded, additional emboli pass through the efferent channels to directly enter the systemic venous and lymphatic circulation.

Salsbury[89] observed viable circulating neoplastic cells in peripheral human venous blood. In several studies,[21,89,90] malignant cells of breast and colon cancer were readily detected in effluent venous blood, and active DNA synthesis has been confirmed in vitro. In many experiments, the threshold for "tumor-take" is higher after intravenous injection than when the subcutaneous or intramuscular routes are used. Sugarbaker[55] observed that poor clonogeneity of tumor cells cannot explain the small ratio of successful metastases to cells injected. Blood circulation represents a hostile immunologic environment for nonhematogenous tumor cells.[91] Furthermore, a study by Vaage[92] suggests that immune modulation and destruction of neoplastic cells is more effective when cells are injected intravenously, although the specific dose-response effect is tumor dependent. In many solid-tumor systems, only a small percentage of viable cells survive to become metastases after injection into venous blood.

Despite the small fraction of viable cells that survive in circulation to initiate metastatic growth, the immunobiologic events occurring in distant capillary bed sites allow growth of selective cell populations. After cellular implantation and neogrowth, the host responds to neoplastic stimulation with a reaction that varies with the clinical stage of neoplastic growth. These host interactions vary chronobiologically and, with increasing cell populations, are influenced by metabolic and nutritional factors. In most breast neoplasms, a long preclinical (occult) and prediagnostic period occurs in which tumor or host factors can modulate metastasis formation. Many human and experimental tumor cells are shown to possess tumor-associated antigens that can initiate host reactions lethal for the offending neoplastic cell.

The immune system is also known to have morphologic functional components with counterproductive capabilities that are often balanced by a large number of interrelating polypeptides akin to the endocrine system.[55] Within the lymphocytic population are thymus-dependent lymphocytes (T lymphocytes) and antibody-producing cells (B lymphocytes). An additional arm of "suppressor cells" is represented by lymphocytic cells that suppress the cytotoxic reactions of lymphoid populations. These cells have been shown to enhance tumor proliferation, whereas macrophage populations "eat" foreign cells in their confirmed role as scavengers. These phylogenetically primitive activators or suppressors of the actions of lymphocytes can kill neoplastic cells through the afferent arc of the immune surveillance system. The activities of these immune cellular subpopulations have stimulated extensive clinical trials of nonspecific immunostimulation as adjuncts to surgical resection for breast neoplasms.

TRADITIONAL PROGNOSTIC PARAMETERS FOR HUMAN BREAST CARCINOMA

Tumor Factors

Nodal status
Tumor size
Cytologic/nuclear grade
Lymphatic/vascular invasion
Pathologic stage (TNM)
Steroid receptor status (ER/PR)
DNA content (ploidy, S-phase)
EIC (in situ)

Host Factors

Age
Menopausal status
Familial history
Previous neoplastic disease
Immunosuppression
Host inflammatory response
Nutrition
Prior chemotherapy
Prior radiation

From Bland KI, et al. Oncogene protein co-expression: Value of Ha-*ras*, c-*myc*, c-*fos* and p53 as prognostic discriminants for breast cancer. Ann Surg 221:707, 1995.

Prognostic Variables for Breast Carcinoma

To justify the risk-benefit ratio of potentially toxic systemic adjuvant therapy of breast cancer, the ability to determine which patients are at high risk for relapse is a key consideration. The accompanying box depicts the traditional clinical, pathologic, and biochemical parameters used in formulation of therapeutic objectives for breast cancer. The recognition by early pathologists and surgeons of the importance of quantitative axillary lymph node involvement by metastatic breast cancer is legendary. The justification for this risk is that approximately one third of patients without apparent axillary lymph node involvement or recurrence die of their disease within 5 to 10 years.[93] Further, some breast carcinomas with as many as 10+ positive axillary nodes will not have recurrence within a 10-year interval. Thus, the importance of reliable prognostic variables is apparent. Data presented at the NIH Consensus Development Conference on Adjuvant Chemotherapy and Endocrine Therapy for Breast Carcinoma in 1985 suggest the potential usefulness of the prognostic variables listed in the accompanying box as important to predict risk and subsequent relapse, disease-free survival, and actuarial survival.

Clearly, estrogen and progesterone hormone receptor analyses can augment the determination of higher risk of relapse. There is an increased probability that tumors that contain no receptor proteins recur earlier than do neoplasms that contain either or both of the receptors. Such data have been demonstrated conclusively from numerous retrospective and prospective trials and apply to both premenopausal and postmenopausal patients with and without nodal involvement. Although the explanation of these observations is unclear, a plausible reason lies in the fundamental changes in either the tumor growth rate or metastatic potential of the breast tumor that lacks these receptor proteins.

Adjuvant Systemic Chemotherapy of Operable Breast Cancer

With revitalization of the interest in adjuvant chemotherapy during the early 1970s, the crucial indicator of success was the ability of available cytotoxic agents to exert a significant and consistent antitumor effect when administered for prolonged periods after standard surgical procedures. Use of this approach is scientifically justified because of the aforementioned potential of lymphatic metastasis and to modulate metastasis by tumor-host mechanisms. Even though breast cancer is limited to the breast and lymphatics in 90% of affected women, in many series approximately one third of these patients have died of breast cancer within 5 to 10 years. Tables 63-4 and 63-5 summarize the essential features obtained from research protocols of adjuvant chemotherapy in node-positive patients. All randomized studies report a significant increase in the relapse-free survival rate of chemotherapy-treated patients compared with the control population. This advantage occurred at least in the given subsets and predominantly in premenopausal women. However, in the study of the arm of the protocol testing phenylalanine mustard versus controls, the Guy's-Manchester study[94] failed to confirm the significant superiority of the treatment observed by the NSABP. Significant overall survival advantage has been reported thus far in given subsets. This was limited in the NSABP experience reported by Fisher et al.[95] to women 49 years old or younger with one to three nodes, to premenopausal women receiving cytoxan, methotrexate, and 5-fluorouracil (CMF) chemotherapy in Milan,[96] and to both menopausal groups treated in the Royal Infirmary (Glasgow) with radiation plus CMF.[97]

Bonadonna and Valagussa[98] note that for most published series the significant advantage achieved in relapse-free survival has not translated into a significant overall survival, thus creating a degree of skepticism regarding the actual value of adjuvant chemotherapy. A major criticism concerns the type and intensity of salvage therapies, accurate descriptions for which have been omitted in almost all reports. Thus, at the time of primary failure, physicians are often forced to apply appropriate therapy by the status of the recurrent neoplasm. Therefore, the subset undergoing therapy is neither selected nor comparable to control and chemotherapy-treated patients with regard to performance and receptor status, stage, and growth of the metastasis.

Table 63-4. Adjuvant Chemotherapy Studies With a Local/Regional Treatment Control Group in Premenopausal Node-Positive Patients

Author	Study Population	No. of Patients	Chemotherapy	Treatment Duration	Follow-up	Disease-free Survival: Control	Disease-free Survival: Chemotherapy	Overall Survival: Control	Overall Survival: Chemotherapy
Fisher et al. (NSABP B-05), 1986	≤49 yr	120	L-PAM	2 yr	10 yr	30*	46*	38* 45	61* 59
Bonadonna et al. (Milan), 1985, 1986	≤49 yr	189	C,M,F	1 yr	10 yr	31†	48†		
Senn et al (Osako), 1984	Premenopausal and perimenopausal	118	Ch,M,F,P, BCG	6 mo	8 yr	Not significant		Not significant	
Wheeler (English Multicenter), 1979	Premenopausal and perimenopausal	130	C,M,F,V	6 mo	1 yr	62 Not significant	86	No data	
Rubens et al. (Guy's-Manchester), 1983	Premenopausal	156	L-PAM	96 wk	5-7.5 yr	52 Not significant	62	Not significant	
Padmanabhan et al. (Guy's-Manchester), 1986	Premenopausal	211	C,M,F	1 yr	5 yr	52‡	70‡	68 Not significant	74
Morrison et al. (West Midlands), 1984	Premenopausal	228	A,V,C,M, F,L	24 wk	54 mo	53	65*	Not significant	
Brinckner et al. (Danish Cancer Group), 1987	Premenopausal	1032§	C	1 yr	68 mo	42†	62†	55 Not significant	70
Smith et al. (Glasgow), 1984	Premenopausal	322§	C,M,F	13 mo	42 mo	Significant		Not significant	

Adapted from Anderson MJ, Kramer BS. Adjuvant systemic therapy for early stage breast cancer. In Bland KI, Copeland EM III, eds. The Breast: Comprehensive Management of Benign and Malignant Diseases. Philadelphia: WB Saunders, 1991, p 822.

A, Doxorubicin; *C,* cyclophosphamide; *Ch,* chlorambucil; *F,* 5-fluorouracil; *L,* leucovorin; *L-PAM,* L-phenylalanine mustard; *M,* methotrexate; *P,* prednisone; *V,* vincristine.

*p <0.05 for chemotherapy vs. control.

†*p* <0.005 for chemotherapy vs. control.

‡*p* <0.0005 for chemotherapy vs. control

§Randomization to observation, C, or CMF.

Bonadonna et al.[99] reported the 10-year results of a trial testing radical mastectomy with and without adjuvant CMF for 386 women with stage II breast carcinoma. Long-term analysis confirmed that adjuvant CMF was able to produce a significant relapse-free survival improvement with respect to the control group (43.4% vs 31.4%, p <0.001), with a favorable trend in total survival (55.2% vs 47.3%) that was not statistically significant. Both relapse-free survival and total survival were significant for premenopausal women. Relapse-free survival was not influenced by drug-induced amenorrhea. Further, for both treatment groups, results were inversely related to the number of histologically involved axillary nodes. At relapse, salvage treatment applied in the control group failed to produce superior results compared with those achieved in the CMF group and yielded a similar median survival from first relapse between control (37 months) and CMF (32 months) patients. It was concluded that CMF was able to improve the course of premenopausal women with high-risk breast cancer during the first decade after radical mastectomy.

Results of adjuvant therapies conducted during the past decade provide evidence that tumor heterogeneity represents the major determinant for success or failure in the treatment of minimal residual disease, as well as for advanced disease. Lippman and Chabner[93] note that, with examination of the summary data, adjuvant chemotherapy results in a statistically significant but small reduction in mortality for women older than 50 years compared with results in younger women. Because this reduction is small (≤10%), many physicians have concluded that tamoxifen may be a superior therapy for this older subset when its effect on mortality and its notably reduced toxicity are considered. The overall impact of chemotherapy and hormonal therapy data for all trials that used an untreated control has been considered by the Early Breast Cancer Trialists' Collaborative Group. With a database of nearly 75,000 prospectively randomly assigned women participating in 133 randomized trials, this group predicted a highly significant reduction (30% to 40%) during the period for which follow-up is available.[100] Thus, there is unquestionably a proportional risk reduction with adjuvant chemotherapy for node-positive and node-negative patients. Lippman and Chabner[93] also suggest that the effectiveness of chemotherapy depends on choice of the active cytotoxic agents, scheduling and sequencing, overall dosage rate

Table 63-5. Adjuvant Chemotherapy Studies With a Local/Regional Treatment Control Group in Postmenopausal Node-Positive Patients

Author	Study Population	No. of Patients	Chemotherapy	Treatment Duration	Follow-up	Disease-free Survival: Control	Disease-free Survival: Chemotherapy	Overall Survival: Control	Overall Survival: Chemotherapy
Fisher et al. (NSABP B-05), 1986	≥50 yr old	229	L-PAM	2 yr	10 yr	29*	32*	44*	41*
Bonadonna et al. (Milan), 1985, 1986	≥50 yr old	202	C,M,F	1 yr	10 yr	32*	38*	50*	52*
Senn et al. (Osako), 1984	Postmenopausal	114	Ch,M,F,P, BCG	6 mo	8 yr	42†	56†	53*	65*
Wheeler (English Multicenter), 1979	Postmenopausal	120	C,M,F,V	6 mo	3 yr	74†	89†	No data	
Rubens et al. (Guy's-Manchester), 1983	Postmenopausal	214	L-PAM	96 wk	5-7.5 yr	45*	51*	Not significant	
Padmanabhan et al. (Guy's-Manchester), 1986	Postmenopausal	228	C,M,F	1 yr	5 yr	55*	59*	65*	70*
Morrison et al. (West Midlands), 1984	Postmenopausal	234	A,V,C,M, F,L	24 wk	54 mo	Not significant		Not significant	
Smith et al. (Glasgow), 1984	Postmenopausal	322‡	C,M,F	13 mo	42 mo	No data		Not significant	
Wallgren et al. (Stockholm-Gotland), 1984	Postmenopausal	163	Ch or C,M,F	1 yr	49 mo	55†	48†	Not significant	
Tormey et al. (ECOG), 1985, 1986	Postmenopausal	155	C,M,F,P	1 yr	5 yr	57*	60*	Not significant	

Adapted from Anderson MJ, Kramer BS. Adjuvant systemic therapy for early stage breast cancer. In Bland KI, Copeland EM III, eds. The Breast: Comprehensive Management of Benign and Malignant Diseases. Philadelphia: WB Saunders, 1991, p 822.

A, Doxorubicin; *C,* cyclophosphamide; *Ch,* chlorambucil; *F,* 5-fluorouracil; *L,* leucovorin; *L-PAM,* L-phenylalanine mustard; *M,* methotrexate; *P,* prednisone; *V,* vincristine.

*Not significant.

†p <0.5 for chemotherapy vs. control.

‡Both premenopausal and postmenopausal patients.

and dosage intensity, and interactions with other therapy, such as irradiation or endocrine therapy. A variety of prospectively randomized trials have investigated whether chemotherapy of longer and shorter durations yield equivalent results. Trials comparing 1 with 2 years of therapy and 6 with 12 months of therapy have reached the general consensus that short, intensive courses of chemotherapy of approximately 6 months' duration are likely to be as effective as prolonged periods of chemotherapy. Further trials suggest that equivalent amounts of drug can be administered to patients receiving aggressive irradiation for the management of the primary tumor as an alternative to mastectomy in early-stage breast cancer. It appears that irradiation therapy is unlikely to have a substantial impact on the ability to deliver full-dose chemotherapy.

Hormonal Sensitivity of Metastatic Breast Cells

Breast cancers consist of heterogeneous cellular populations that have varying metabolic demands and growth fractions. The opportunity to control the metastatic tendency of the malignant breast cell during the process of tumor implantation is a correlate of steroid sensitivity of the cell clone.[101] Usually, these neoplastic cells that normally depend on the hormonal milieu for growth and function are similarly dependent when they function as a metastatic unit. Loss of response to the hormonal milieu occurs by the dedifferentiation process and appears to be a typical aspect of malignant metastatic growth. Thus, cellular populations that retain this steroid sensitivity in secondary growth will respond to hormonal therapy, which will modify, enhance, or diminish cellular transport and implantation.

Progression of heterogeneous growth may revert to autonomous function of the metastatic clone, in which case hormonal sensitivity is lost. Considerable experimental evidence confirms that secondary growth, with variable hormonal sensitivities, can coexist in the same species and even in the same animal.[102] Thus, secondary tumors consist of mixed cellular populations, varying fractions of which are hormone sensitive and insensitive. The mechanism by which sex steroids stimulate protein and nucleic acid synthesis in developing populations of cells appears to be mediated through a system of enzyme induction and repression.[101]

Application of Steroid Hormone Receptors in Breast Cancer

After the demonstration of hormonal dependence of breast carcinoma by Beatson[103] in 1896, observations confirmed that approximately one third of breast malignancies respond to removal of the endocrine hormonal milieu (adrenal, pituitary, ovary), as well as to additive hormonal therapy (e.g., estrogens, antiestrogens, androgens, progestins, glucocorticoids). In many institutions, oophorectomy alone remains the initial method of therapy in a premenopausal patient who has recurrent breast carcinoma. In the 1950s, Huggins[104] and Huggins and Bergenstal[105] introduced oophorectomy combined with bilateral adrenalectomy for control of metastatic breast cancer on the assumption that carcinoma derived from hormonally dependent tissues is nonautonomous and thus may depend on this hormonal milieu for viability and growth. This concept was subsequently extended by Luft et al.,[106] who also demonstrated regression of metastatic breast carcinoma after hypophysectomy, implicating a pituitary-adrenal-ovarian axis with tumor regression after removal of the trophic stimuli.

The heterogeneity of the clones of breast cells correctly predicted in early investigative work suggested that carcinoma of the breast might involve two categories of hormonal influence. The hormone-dependent variant is observed to respond to one or a combination of the previously mentioned forms of endocrine ablation. Conversely, the hormone-independent type recapitulates the heterogenous variants of the neoplasm, because clones of cells are not influenced by the modes of therapy just listed, and these autonomous cells are unaffected by steroidal, hormonal, ablative, and perhaps chemotherapeutic measures.

The proper selection of the appropriate method of sequential endocrine manipulation for the management of advanced breast carcinoma has been debated extensively. Hormonal ablation has included oophorectomy alone; oophorectomy combined with adrenalectomy; hypophysectomy; and estrogen, androgen, or adrenocortical hormone therapy. The older method of endocrine manipulation, oophorectomy, remains controversial regarding its efficacy in delaying recurrence when used alone. Indeed, salutary remissions are evident when disease-free interval exceeds 12 to 18 months, and the addition of adrenalectomy often provides objective regression of metastatic lesions. A restricted use of oophorectomy-adrenalectomy as a palliative or "therapeutic" measure for patients with disseminated breast carcinoma was adopted because surgeons were reluctant to submit patients to a radical and often nonbeneficial (60% to 70%) procedure to achieve a desired goal not possible with other modalities. In large control series of patients with stage IV disease, irrespective of age or menstrual status, irrefutable statistical evidence suggests the equality of responses (31% to 42%) after either of the adrenal ablative methods performed without the benefit of estrogen-receptor (ER) or progestin-receptor (PR) analyses of the metastatic lesions. Other investigators have noted similar objective remissions after therapeutic hypophysectomy (31% to 42%) and oophorectomy-adrenalectomy (32% to 35%).[107]

The comparative retrospective analysis by Kennedy et al.[108] for immediate castration and "late" therapeutic castration evaluated stage I and II disease. These investigators concluded that immediate castration lengthens the disease-free interval from mastectomy to appearance of metastatic disease; however, a significant prolongation of the interval from recurrent disease to death was also noted in the therapeutic castration group. The total survival times, however, were not different in the two groups, according to the statistical methods employed. These investigators extended this series to include the effects of other forms of therapy in patients with advanced disease (stages III and IV). The additional modalities of therapy included hypophysectomy or adrenalectomy, with inclusive analysis of the effects of estrogens, androgens, adrenocortical hormones, and cytotoxic agents. One third of the patients treated with immediate oophorectomy received one of these additional forms of therapy; 50% of those with therapeutic castration received adjunctive therapy. In the combined series, the proportion of improvement for the prophylactic group (17.7%) was similar to that of the therapeutic series (19.8%). The investigators concluded that for both groups of patients with prophylactic or therapeutic castration, similar objective responses are apparent after adjunctive therapy.

Thereafter, a report by the National Surgical Adjuvant Breast and Bowel Project[109] failed to demonstrate that immediate oophorectomy alone either deferred the recurrence of metastatic carcinoma or prolonged survival. The subsequent application of estradiol cytosol binding of the breast cancer and its application to endocrine manipulation is legendary.

A comparison of the percentage of patients who respond to the various endocrine therapies in uncontrolled studies suggests a slight advantage for ablative procedures; however, Henderson and Canellos[110] note that randomized trials fail to demonstrate a clear advantage for one form of endocrine manipulation or another. Randomized trials that compare response and survival rates of patients treated with major ablative procedures (adrenalectomy, hypophysectomy) with those treated initially with additive therapy (estrogens, androgens, or possibly adrenalectomy with further disease progression) reveal no significant survival advantage of either group.[110] Randomized trials that compare additive estrogen therapy with antiestrogens (tamoxifen), antiestrogens with hypophysectomy, and aminoglutethimide with adrenalectomy have each failed to show significant differences in objective responses, response duration, or survival advantage.[111-113]

Thus, the choice of endocrine manipulation depends on the available alternatives and the relative toxicities induced by the various therapies. In addition, patients who respond to one type of endocrine therapy are often likely to respond to additional variants that have traditionally been administered in a sequence or cascade. Premenopausal women were first treated with oophorectomy, and if a sustained disease-free interval was obtained, adrenalectomy would be offered after progression of disease. If these forms of therapy failed, without the predictive response of the estradiol-binding protein, patients would then be treated with nonendocrine therapy. Postmenopausal patients were conventionally treated with diethylstilbestrol (DES) as the initial method of therapy, because it is minimally toxic and did not carry the morbidity and mortality of adrenalectomy. If patients responded to DES and the disease subsequently progressed, a trial of DES withdrawal would often result in a subsequent response in almost one third of patients so treated. Nonendocrine therapies were often reserved for the postmenopausal patient who had previously had failure of one of the forms of endocrine therapy.

Clinical trials established that patients who respond to these endocrine therapies are afforded palliation of their metastatic disease and in some circumstances have increased survival. Conversely, clinical experience suggested that approximately one third of patients with metastatic (stage IV) breast carcinoma respond to endocrine therapy when their menopausal status is ignored. Therefore, the nonselective application for therapy replacement or ablative endocrine therapy portends potential morbidity for therapy in approximately two thirds of subjects. Further, this additional morbidity is recognized in the absence of benefit for disease remission. For these reasons, objective parameters to predict patient selection for probability of response after endocrine therapy are desirable in the management of patients with breast cancer.

The hormonally sensitive primary and metastatic breast cancer cell, as already described, can be identified at the time of breast biopsy or resection of the tumor and its regional lymphatics (mastectomy). These steroid hormone receptor analyses should be performed routinely on all patients with primary and metastatic breast cancer.

With the demonstration of the ER protein (estrophilin) in hormonally responsive breast cancers by Jensen et al.,[114] appropriate selection of subjects for endocrine ablation was remarkably enhanced. Currently, biochemical analysis of homogenized breast tumor tissue fractions with radioactively labeled steroid ligands or immunohistochemical staining are standard. Further, accurate assays are now available for minute quantities of tumor tissue.

The ER has thus become a marker of hormone-dependent breast cancer, greatly simplifying the approach to oncologic treatment protocols for stages I to IV disease. The ER, a protein located in the cytoplasm of breast neoplasms, is found in approximately 55% of breast cancers, with increasing positivity as a function of age. A negative correlation appears to exist between ER-positive tumors and (1) size of the primary tumor, (2) location of the primary tumor, (3) extent of disease, and (4) type of tissue assayed (primary vs skin vs nodes vs soft tissue vs visceral).[115] A weak correlation does exist between the frequency of reactivity of ER and the status of the axillary nodes at the time of mastectomy. However, groups with ER-positive tumors appear to feature a higher proportion of node-negative patients. The differentiation of patients with regard to the probability of response to endocrine manipulation or replacement does not appear to correlate with the site of disease, disease-free interval, menopausal status, or age.

STEROID RECEPTORS AND DISEASE-FREE INTERVAL

A correlation exists between the tumor differentiation characteristics and the reactivity of ER.[116] The observation of an inverse correlation between thymidine-labeling indices and ER status initiated investigation of the relationship between ER and disease-free interval by Allegra,[115] Silva et al.,[116] and Lippman et al.[117] Allegra[115] confirmed the relationship between disease-free interval and ER status in 182 patients with mammary cancer, 79 (30%) of whom exhibited ER-negative primary tumors that were observed to have recurrent disease. Only 8 of 103 (8%) patients with ER-positive tumors were observed to have relapses. In this series, 91% of the patients with ER-positive tumors were free of disease at 24 months, compared with 62% of the patients whose tumors were ER-negative.

Other prognostic variables have been considered to explain the difference in recurrence rates according to ER reactivity. In one study, investigators compared differences in prognostic variables between patients whose tumors were ER-positive and those whose tumors were ER-negative.[115] This study confirmed that neither age, tumor size, menopausal status, number of axillary nodes, nor proportion of patients who received adjuvant chemotherapy were different; however, younger patients were observed to have trends toward positive nodes and greater need for adjuvant chemotherapy in the groups with ER-negative tumors (Table 63-6). Thus, stratification of patients with regard to ER status appears warranted and perhaps desirable in prospective clinical trials to select patients who would benefit the most from intensive cytotoxic chemotherapy.

Table 63-6. Relationship Between ER Status, Prognostic Variables, and Recurrence Rate in Breast Cancer

Factor	ER Positive	ER Negative	*p* Value
Axillary node status			
0	5/52	8/30	≤0.02
1-3	0/13	6/23	0.08
≥4	2/20	7/21	0.05
Tumor size			
≥2 cm	4/36	7/30	≤0.04
≤2 cm	1/40	10/28	≤0.001
Menopausal status			
Premenopausal	1/20	14/32	≤0.01
Postmenopausal	4/76	7/37	≤0.01
Adjuvant chemotherapy			
No	5/67	13/41	≤0.001
Yes or unknown	3/36	11/38	
TOTAL	8/103	24/79	≤0.001

From Allegra JC. The use of steroid hormone receptors in breast cancer. In Margolese R, ed. Contemporary Issues in Clinical Oncology: Breast Cancer. New York: Churchill Livingstone, 1983.

McGuire[118] reported a correlation for level of ER (in femtomoles per milligram of cytosolic protein) in breast neoplasms with the response rate to endocrine therapy. An 80% objective remission was observed in patients whose ER was at least 100 fmol/mg. A response rate of 46% was observed in women with lesser values. This objective response rate to endocrine therapy as a function of content of ER has been confirmed by others.[119-121]

The application of additional cytoplasmic markers of hormonally dependent breast cancer is commonplace, and their role in routine therapeutic management has been firmly established.[122] The use of PR appears to have value in augmenting selection of the endocrine-dependent breast cell.[123,124] Horwitz and McGuire[123] observed that synthesis of PR is strictly estrogen dependent and represents the end product of estradiol-stimulated pathways in breast cancer tissues. Bland et al.[125] established that premenopausal patients with nondetectable ER have a threefold increase in PR compared with postmenopausal groups. Because high endogenous estrogens in premenopausal patients mask ER in tumor biopsies, it appears advantageous to perform PR determinations to identify an additional 15% of women with metastatic breast cancer who may benefit from endocrine therapy.

Previous studies have correlated the trend toward higher quantitative values of ER and PR in tumors that are histologically well differentiated.[126,127] These correlations were reaffirmed by Silva et al.,[116] who observed higher mean ER and PR values and greater numbers of tissues harboring low-grade (grade I) neoplasms when both receptors were present.

THERAPEUTIC APPLICATIONS OF BIOLOGIC MARKERS FOR NEUROENDOCRINE THERAPY

Quantitative ERs represent important determinants for management of recurrent breast carcinoma. Use of the PR appears most advantageous in determining which premenopausal patients whose tumors are ER-negative may benefit from endocrine ablation or additive therapy. Table 63-7 lists potential therapeutic options and the expected frequency distributions of ER and PR reactivity in premenopausal and postmenopausal women with breast cancer.

The use of the antiestrogen tamoxifen (Nolvadex) introduced into general oncologic practice to bind cytoplasmic estrogen is advisable in patients with ER-positive tumors. Manni et al.[128] reported an objective response rate to tamoxifen for metastatic ER-positive cancers that is essentially identical to that of adrenalectomy. Pritchard et al.[129] observed that tamoxifen has a higher response rate in premenopausal patients with ER-positive tumors. These investigators noted that response duration and rate were equal to those of oophorectomy and would appear predictive of subsequent response to surgical ablation of the ovaries. Future prospective trials clearly are necessary to clarify objectively the role of tamoxifen in the premenopausal patient.

Newer sequences of endocrine therapy are evolving (Fig. 63-12). Currently, many investigators consider tamoxifen to be the endocrine therapy of choice for both premenopausal and postmenopausal women. Two randomized trials support this view. The response rate to oophorectomy was not significantly different statistically from the response rate to tamoxifen (37% and 27%, respectively) in a crossover-design trial in premenopausal women with advanced breast cancer.[130] Another randomized trial in 107 women with advanced breast cancer showed similar response rates to oophorectomy (21%) and to tamoxifen (24%), with no difference in overall survival. Although many sequences of therapies to have been proposed for these women, current methods have avoided the sustained morbidity incurred with varying surgical procedures in favor of endocrine manipulation with pharmacologic approaches. The order in which these endocrine therapies are administered also depends on the relative toxicities of the approaches, and data suggest that tamoxifen may not be as effective after aminoglutethimide therapy.[112,113] Finally, Ward et al.[131] observed that lack of a response to estrogens does not conclusively rule out the possibility of a response to antiestrogen therapy with tamoxifen.

Table 63-7. Proposed Therapeutic Options and Frequency of Steroid Receptor for Premenopausal and Postmenopausal Patients With Breast Cancer

	Premenopausal		Postmenopausal	
Receptor Status	**No. (%)**	**Proposed Therapy**	**No. (%)**	**Proposed Therapy**
ER +/PR+	222 (45)	O,A,H,T T + CT Horm	520 (63)	T,A,H,CT Horm
ER +/PR−	58 (12)	O,A,H T → T + CT Horm	128 (15)	T,A,H T + CT Horm
ER −/PR−	136 (28)	CT	137 (17)	CT
ER −/PR+	72 (15)	O,A,H,T ?T + CT ?Horm	41 (5)	CT,T + CT Horm

Adapted from Bland KI, Fuchs A, Whittliff JL. Menopausal status as a factor in the distribution of estrogen and progestin receptors in breast cancer. Surg Forum 32:410, 1981.
O, Oophorectomy; *T,* tamoxifen; *A,* adrenalectomy; *H,* hypophysectomy; *Horm,* hormonal (estrogen, progestin, androgen); *CT,* cytotoxic chemotherapy; +, ≥10 fmol/mg, −, <10 fmol/mg.

Gapinski and Donegan[120] confirmed the aforementioned receptor data but could find no correlation between ER status and responsiveness to chemotherapy. Compared with patients with primary neoplasms poor in ER (≤300 fmol/g), those with ER-rich tumors were observed to have a longer disease-free interval, a lower incidence of recurrence after mastectomy, and a more favorable disease-free survival.

A significant role for the use of antiestrogen therapy in stage II (node-positive) breast cancer is evident. Hubay et al.,[132] in a prospective, randomized trial, found that CMF used in combination with tamoxifen was more effective in delaying recurrence in patients with ER-positive tumors than was CMF alone ($p = 0.0176$). This effect was observed to occur in both premenopausal and postmenopausal women. In premenopausal women treated with CMF alone, however, patients with ER-poor tumors were observed to have more rapid recurrence than those whose tumors were ER-positive ($p = 0.0313$). The addi-

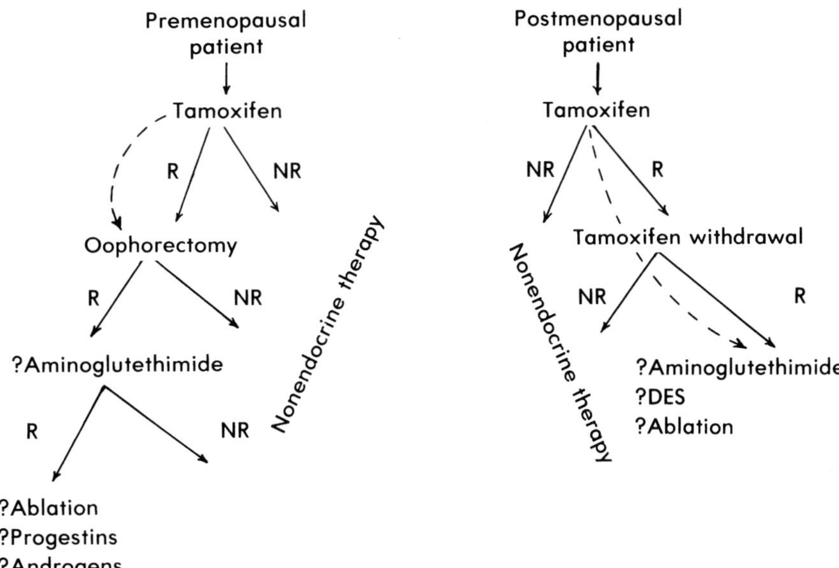

Fig. 63-12. New and future sequences for administering endocrine therapy in patients with advanced breast cancer. (Courtesy of Henderson IC. Breast Cancer Management Progress and Prospects [educational publication]. Wayne, N.J.: Lederle Laboratories, Division of American Cyanamid, 1982.)

tion of the adjuvant immunostimulant bacille Calmette-Guérin provided no therapeutic benefit beyond the combination of CMF and tamoxifen.

Depending on the receptor status, postmenopausal patients with ER-positive metastatic breast carcinoma should receive tamoxifen as additive therapy. It apparently has a response rate and duration of response equal to those of all forms of endocrine therapy. In addition, tamoxifen has few side effects, and its administration is seldom halted because of side effects.

The application of aminoglutethimide (Cytadren) as an inhibitor of adrenocorticoid steroid synthesis for conversion of androstenedione to estrogen appears to have merit in initiating adrenal suppression. Initial trials suggest that the application of aminoglutethimide inhibition of adrenocortical function may be an accurate predictor of response to endocrine ablation with adrenalectomy and hypophysectomy.

The initial studies for adjuvant endocrine therapy failed to demonstrate a 5-year overall survival advantage with adjuvant castration alone, and castration plus long-term prednisone prolonged survival only in small subsets of premenopausal women older than 45 years.[133] Emphasis has been placed on the use of adjuvant endocrine therapy, either alone or in combination with chemotherapy.

Fourteen prospective randomized clinical trials with tamoxifen as adjuvant therapy have been reported.[93,134] The results of these trials are summarized in Table 63-8. Disease-free survival was increased in almost all adjuvant trials. A significant increase in overall survival, however, was observed only in the Christie Hospital,[135] Scottish,[136] Nolvadex Adjuvant Trial Organization (NATO),[137] and NSABP[138,139] trials. In the NATO trial comparing tamoxifen for 2 years with no adjuvant therapy, statistically significant increases in both disease-free and overall survival were observed with administration of tamoxifen. The effects of tamoxifen in this trial were independent of age, and ER, menopausal, or nodal status.[137] In the Christie Hospital trial including patients with either positive or negative nodes, the premenopausal women were treated with ovarian irradiation or tamoxifen, whereas the postmenopausal women were either treated with tamoxifen for 1 year or received no adjuvant therapy.[135] When premenopausal and postmenopausal women were considered together, an overall survival advantage from tamoxifen was observed; this was not seen when those two groups were

Table 63-8. Randomized Trials of Adjuvant Tamoxifen Monotherapy Compared With No Adjuvant Therapy

			No. of Patients					Effect on Survival	
Study	**Daily Tamoxifen Dose (mg)**	**Duration of Therapy (years)**	**Pre-menopausal**	**Post-menopausal**	**Negative Nodes**	**Positive Nodes**	**Unknown Nodes**	**Disease-Free**	**Overall**
Copenhagen, 1985	30	2	160	102	108	154		Increase*	None
Christie, 1988	20	1	373	588	297	349	315	Increase	Increase†
NATO, 1988	20	2	128	1001	605	521	3	Increase	Increase
Scottish, 1987	20	>5‡	242	1070	751	456	105	(p <0.001)	(p = 0.0019)
Ludwig III & IV,	20§	1	0	629	0	629	0	Increase	Increase
1984								Increase	None
Denmark, 1985	30	1	0	1650	288	NS	NS	Increase	None
ECOG, 1985,	20	2	0	170	0	168	0	Increase	None
1993								Increase	None
Stockholm, 1987	40	2 and 5	0	2103	696	1407	0	Increase	Increase
NSABP B-14,	20	5	812	1832	2644	0	0	Increase	None
1989, 1993								Increase	None
Toronto, 1987	30	2	0	399	0	399	0	Increase	None
Caen/Royen,	40	3	0	179	0	179	0	Increase	None
1987								Increase	None
Naples, 1988	30	2	61	247	173	135	0		
CRC, 1988	20	2	586	1019	887	718	307		
UK/Asia, 1984	40	1	197		0	197	0		

Adapted from Jaiyesimi IA, Buzdar AU, Decker DA, Hortobagyi GN. Use of tamoxifen for breast cancer: Twenty-eight years later. J Clin Oncol 13:516, 1995.

CRC, Cancer Research Campaign; *ECOG,* Eastern Cooperative Oncology Group; *NS,* not significant.

*A significant advantage in disease-free survival was observed only in postmenopausal patients.

†A significant survival benefit (p = 0.05) was observed for all patients combined when allowance was made for nodal status, but no significant advantage in survival was seen for premenopausal or postmenopausal subgroups.

‡Study design allowed patients receiving adjuvant tamoxifen at 5 years to be randomized either to stop or to continue tamoxifen until relapse.

§A significant survival benefit was observed for premenopausal and postmenopausal women analyzed together (p = 0.01) and for the postmenopausal subgroup (p = 0.05).

considered separately. In the Scottish trial including 1312 women, a significant reduction in relapses and deaths was observed in the group of patients treated with tamoxifen for 5 years compared with the control group.[136]

The NSABP B-14 trial compared tamoxifen with placebo in 2644 premenopausal and postmenopausal patients with node-negative, ER-positive breast tumors.[138,139] Disease-free survival advantage was observed for both premenopausal and postmenopausal women treated with tamoxifen in the first 4 years of the trial. Overall survival advantage was seen for all node-negative patients and for patients 50 years old or older.

The Early Breast Cancer Trialists' Collaborative Group overview included 30,000 women treated with tamoxifen. Studies comparing adjuvant tamoxifen with no systemic adjuvant treatment and studies comparing chemotherapy plus tamoxifen with chemotherapy alone were included in the overview. Women 50 years old or older received more benefit from the use of tamoxifen than did women younger than 50 years. Tamoxifen also reduced the risk of development of contralateral breast cancer by 39%. The avoidance of recurrence was mainly seen during years 0 to 4. The reduction in mortality, however, was highly significant both during and after years 0 to 4. The data in this overview also showed that tamoxifen reduced mortality not related to breast cancer.[100]

The tumor heterogeneity of breast cancer, coupled with the probability that the predominant forms of endocrine therapy and ablation provide fractional reduction of only the ER-positive cells, denotes a predominance of refractory ER-negative cells after various endocrine therapy modalities. A previous phase II trial by Allegra et al.[140] suggests the application of combination chemohormonal therapy with tamoxifen suppression for 10 days and premarin induction for 4 days, followed with methotrexate, 5-fluorouracil, and leucovorin. This combination represented an effective method to induce remission in 72% of patients with metastatic breast carcinoma. The physiologic application of chemohormonal induction represented a model of transition from basic laboratory observations to the design of a treatment regimen. Prospective trials providing active cytotoxic therapy after hormonal induction are currently in progress. Although combinations to provide biochemical manipulation of the hormonally sensitive breast cells have met with increasing success, it must be emphasized that therapeutic modalities for stage IV disease rarely induce complete and sustained remissions.

THE NIH CONSENSUS DEVELOPMENT PANEL ON ADJUVANT CHEMOTHERAPY AND ENDOCRINE THERAPY FOR BREAST CANCER

The goal of adjuvant therapy of breast carcinoma is to enhance survival while ensuring an acceptable quality of life. In September 1985, the NCI and the NIH jointly sponsored the Consensus Development Conference on Adjuvant Chemotherapy and Endocrine Therapy for Breast Cancer. The consensus panel came to six important conclusions on the basis of their analysis of current achievements for the therapy of breast cancer; these are incorporated in the accompanying box.

The subsequent NIH 1990 Consensus Development Conference on Treatment of Early Stage Breast Cancer concluded that there is clear evidence that the rate of local and distant recurrence is decreased both by adjuvant combination cytotoxic chemotherapy and by adjuvant tamoxifen in patients with node-negative breast cancer. It was also concluded that although all node-negative patients have some risk for recurrence, patients with tumors 1 cm or smaller have an excellent prognosis and do not require adjuvant systemic chemotherapy outside of clinical trials.[73] The conclusions are shown in the box on p. 1286.

In the future, it is quite possible that a subgroup of node-negative patients with poor prognostic features will be found to benefit from adjuvant chemotherapy. A consideration for the future has been the role of adjuvant biologic response modifiers and their effects on breast cancer survival. Polyadenylic-polyuridylic acid was evaluated in a randomized trial by Lacour et al.[141] for operable breast

RECOMMENDATIONS OF NIH CONSENSUS DEVELOPMENT CONFERENCE ON ADJUVANT CHEMOTHERAPY AND ENDOCRINE THERAPY FOR BREAST CANCER

1. Although significant changes have been made in the past 5 years, optimal therapy has not been defined for any subset of patients. For this reason, all patients and their physicians are strongly encouraged to participate in controlled clinical trials.
2. For premenopausal women with positive lymph nodes, treatment with established chemotherapy is recommended as standard care, regardless of hormone receptor status.
3. For premenopausal women with negative nodes, adjuvant chemotherapy is not generally recommended, but for certain patients at high risk, chemotherapy should be considered.
4. For postmenopausal women with positive nodes and positive hormone receptor levels, tamoxifen is the treatment of choice.
5. For postmenopausal women with positive nodes and negative hormone receptor levels, chemotherapy should be considered but could not, at present, be recommended as standard practice.
6. For postmenopausal women with negative nodes, regardless of hormone receptor levels, there is no indication for routine adjuvant therapy.

From National Institutes of Health. NIH Consensus Development Panel on Adjuvant Chemotherapy and Endocrine Therapy for Breast Cancer. Natl Cancer Inst Monogr 1:1, 1986.

RECOMMENDATIONS OF NIH CONSENSUS DEVELOPMENT CONFERENCE ON TREATMENT OF EARLY-STAGE BREAST CANCER

1. Breast conservation treatment is an appropriate method of primary therapy for the majority of women with stage I and II breast cancer and is preferable because it provides survival equivalent to total mastectomy and axillary dissection while preserving the breast.
2. The recommended technique for breast conservation treatment includes the following:
   —local excision of primary tumor with clear margins
   —level I and II axillary node dissection
   —breast irradiation to 4500 to 5000 cGy, with or without a boost
3. The many unanswered questions in the adjuvant systemic treatment of node-negative breast cancer make it imperative that all patients who are candidates for clinical trials be offered the opportunity to participate.
4. Most patients with node-negative breast cancer are cured by breast-conservation treatment or total mastectomy and axillary dissection.
5. The rates of local and distant recurrence after local therapy for node-negative breast cancer are decreased by both adjuvant combination cytologic chemotherapy and by adjuvant tamoxifen. The decision to use adjuvant treatment should follow a thorough discussion with the patient regarding the likely risk of recurrence without adjuvant therapy, the expected reduction in risk with adjuvant therapy, toxicities of therapy, and its impact on quality of life.
6. Although all node-negative patients have some risk for recurrence, patients with tumors 1 cm or smaller have an excellent prognosis and do not require adjuvant systemic therapy outside of clinical trials.

From National Institutes of Health. Treatment of early-stage breast cancer: NIH Consensus Development Conference consensus statement. Washington, D.C.: US Government Printing Office, 1990.

carcinoma. This group reported significant improvement in disease-free survival, and independent verification is warranted. It is possible that future studies that incorporate biologic response modifiers with chemoendocrine therapy as adjuvants will be initiated now that interest has been focused on this potential mode of therapy.

ONCOGENES, ANTIONCOGENES, AND TUMOR SUPPRESSOR GENES

Most therapeutic decisions regarding use of various adjuvant therapies are determined on the basis of the traditional prognostic factors, whereas new biochemical and cellular factors are being used to complement and improve conventional approaches. In view of the cumulative results to date, hormonal receptor levels appear to be more important for prediction of response to hormonal therapy than as prognostic markers.[142,143] Both ER and PR may function as indirect indicators of differentiation and cell-growth kinetics. ER content was the first nonhistologic marker to be identified. This steroid receptor remains weakly prognostic, and in fact the presence of ER may be an indicator of growth rate rather than of metastatic potential. Expression of the PR is dependent on ER function. Evaluation of PR may be more predictive of outcome; data regarding the relative worth of both hormonal receptors as prognostic factors are inconclusive.[143-147] Thus, direct measures of cell growth, which include thymidine-labeling indices and the use of flow cytometry, have been applied more recently. Reproducibility of assay techniques has been quite poor, adding to the difficulty in universal acceptance and application of S-phase fractions for prediction of outcome; only approximately two thirds of all primary cancers can be satisfactorily assayed for S-phase fraction.[148,149] Contemporary technology has discovered monoclonal antibodies that recognize proliferation antigens (e.g., Ki67) that have been used in association with automated image-analysis systems for evaluating stained tissues.[150] Application of this cytochemical technology for proliferation antigens may be a powerful and reliable method to analyze DNA turnover, but this approach will require further investigation.

Other putative prognostic factors have included high–molecular weight mucin expression (e.g., DF3 antigen), which has been associated with differentiation and is an expression of the estrogen-related protein pS-2. Both proteins have been associated with favorable clinical outcomes.[151,152] Additional studies have suggested that overexpression of various enzymes, such as cathepsin-D or urokinase-plasminogen activator, or of the laminin receptors, which function as adhesion molecules, may also be associated with the breast carcinoma metastatic phenotype.[153-155] The application of these putative prognostic variables should be considered indeterminate, because the outcomes of these results have been variable with regard to patient selection and integration of therapy.

The objective selection of adjuvant therapies, especially for the node-negative patient, is one of the most perplexing dilemmas for clinical management of breast cancer. A refinement of prognostic variables with traditional pathologic markers integrated with protein products, enzymes, and hormonal factors may enhance predictive value. The more recent putative prognostic factor, the HER-2/*neu* gene, is closely related to yet distinct from the epidermal growth factor receptor gene, another homologue of the *neu* gene. Amplification of HER-2/*neu* was associated with poor clinical outcome in patients with node-positive cancer.[151] The prognostic importance of HER-2/*neu* in node-negative patients has been less confirmatory.[156-158] Rapid progress in molecular biology has led to the identification of other oncogene abnormalities in breast cancer. Currently, the scientific paradigm is the identification of specific genes that are causally involved in malignant transformation and cellular progression. Genetic changes evident in breast carcinogenesis have included amplification of oncogenes (*erb*B-2, *int*-2, c-*myc*, H-*ras*) and deletion or mutation of the tumor suppressor genes (RB, p53).[156,159] The tumor suppressor gene p53 may be of scientific and predictive value, because it is the most commonly reported somatic gene alteration in human cancer, with a mutational frequency varying from 20% to 70% of tumors studied.[160-165] The prognostic value of p53 overexpression in breast cancer is highly controversial, with mixed results as to the value of this mutated suppressor gene in providing reproducible prognostic information.[160,165-171]

Investigators continue trying to delineate more precisely the correlation between expression of various genes and gene products in the clinical behavior of breast carcinoma. The growth of normal mammalian cells is regulated by both growth and inhibitory regulatory events. Important among these regulatory growth factors are (1) epidermal growth factor, (2) transforming growth factor, (3) insulin-like growth factor (IGF-1, IGF-2), (3) platelet-derived growth factor, and (4) fibroblast growth factors. All growth factors act on target cells by specific binding to high-affinity receptor binding sites; unless cells express the specific regulatory receptor for growth factor, they will not respond to regulatory growth. Mutations in genes that code for proteins involved in the transduction of signals elicited by growth factor binding to its receptor may also result in cancer. For example, deletions in the c-*jun* and c-*fos* genes result in mutant protein products that induce avian fibrosarcoma and murine osteosarcoma.[172,173] Single-point mutations in the *ras* gene (which is phosphorylated by high-affinity guanosine triphosphate binding properties and therefore is indirectly involved in the signal-transduction cascade) can also result in tumor formation.[172,173] This example demonstrates that postreceptor pathways modulated by growth factor receptors are precisely controlled and that altered functions of one or more signal transduction proteins may initiate catastrophic consequences for cell-growth regulation.

Oncogenes are defined as genes that initiate uncontrollable growth of mammalian cells.[72] These oncogenes are typically mutated variants of normal cell genes (proto-oncogenes or c-*onc* genes) that have lost their regulatory function for normal nonmutated proteins. Moreover, these oncogenes also may code for normal nonmutated proteins and are expressed in abnormally high levels. Our nascent studies identify at least 60 proto-oncogenes relative to their ability to induce the transformed phenotype of cells in culture when mutation occurs. Most proto-oncogenes have been identified as genes that regulate cellular growth and differentiation.

According to their relationships with growth factors and their receptors, oncogenes are divided into four major classes. These classes of oncogenes include growth factors *(sis),* growth factor receptors *(erb* B, *fms, kit),* transducers of growth factor responses *(src, ras, rat),* and nuclear transcription factors that mediate growth factor–induced gene expression *(jun, fos)*.[172,174] Oncogenes that are mutated variants of transcription factors typically act in cooperation with oncogenes from other categories to accomplish transformation.[172,174] For example, the *ras* oncogene requires either *myc* or EIA (from adenovirus) to cause cell transformation.[173,175]

Contemporary analyses note that proto-oncogenes can be altered to become oncogenes by the following two mechanisms. (1) Changes initiate abnormalities in gene expression, including gene amplification, gene rearrangement, and promoter mutations. (2) Changes in the coding region of the gene initiate production of proteins with abnormal biochemical properties.[176-178] Analysis of human carcinomas in vivo have confirmed that nearly all cancer cells contain multiple variants of genetic damage. Breast carcinoma is a genetic disease initiated by abnormalities of the DNA of breast epithelial cells. Although abnormalities may have been inherited from a parent, giving rise to the familial pattern of disease, the abnormality is more commonly a sporadic breast tumor. Identification of genetic damage has revealed two distinct types of mutations, dominant (caused by gain in function), where the targets are oncogenes, and recessive (caused by loss in function), with targets known variously as tumor suppressor genes, recessive oncogenes, or antioncogenes. Thus, growth factors and their relationships with oncogenes are highly relevant to carcinogenesis and ultimately may affect the therapy of breast cancer.

The evidence for inhibitory (negative) regulatory factors for cellular growth includes the tumor suppressor genes and has largely been determined through studies in which normal suppressor function has been disrupted. It is currently recognized that cancers that result from mutations of oncogenes and mutations in the tumor suppressor genes occur with equal prevalence in human tumors.[173,179] Mutations in the p53 gene typically result in production of p53 proteins with a variety of biochemical and biologic properties different from those of the wild type. Such mutations result in an increase in the protein's half-life, with abnormally high concentrations of p53 found in tumors and transformed cells. Caleffi et al.[159] recently reported on p53 gene mutation and steroid receptors in breast cancer. This study and others demonstrate a consistent relationship between ER-positive tumors and the wild-type p53, whereas younger women are more likely to possess ER-negative tumors with mutant p53. Mutations of p53 did not possess a significant prognostic role for prediction of survival in these patients. These data were previously confirmed by Isola et al.,[168] because overexpression of the p53 and c-*erb* B-2 proteins indicated a high malignant potential in axillary node-negative breast cancer. However, overexpression of the mutated tumor suppressor gene and proto-oncogene were not significant prognostic factors independent of cell proliferative rate. These authors observed overexpression of these proteins and an increased S-phase growth fraction; these results indicate that they may confer a proliferative advantage to cancer cells in vivo.

Both p53 and c-*erb* B-2 overexpression, as well as tumor size, were observed to be independent prognostic variables in multivariate analysis. Eight-year survival of patients with p53 protein overexpression was significantly lower than that of patients without overexpression (56% vs 81%; $p < 0.0001$). In addition to the amplification and overexpression of p53 and the c-*erb* B-2 gene, the c-*myc*, or the *int*-2 gene,[180,181] activation of the Ha-*ras* oncogene by point mutation or overexpression has been detected in human breast neoplasms.[151,182,183] Moreover, the tumorigenic potential of the Ha-*ras* oncogene for mammary cells in vivo of transgenic mice has previously been correlated with level of expression and developmental history of the mammary gland.[184]

Putative oncogenes in the pathogenesis and progression of human solid neoplasms are the locus of intense investigation and provides the clinician with powerful biologic tools to critically analyze genetic and molecular events leading to tumorigenesis, growth, and development. Multiple oncogenes, nuclear transcription regulatory factors, and tumor suppressor genes appear to have a dominant role in human breast cancer and include c-*erb* B-2, c-*myc*, H-*ras*, c-*fos*, and p53.[180,185-187] However, this study and others have shown variable overexpression with amplification of these oncogenes detected in 30% or fewer of patients with breast cancer. Typically, the amplification of the oncogene is associated with reduced survival and a poor prognosis.[188-190] Several studies have further demonstrated that overexpression of these proto-oncogenes, when correlated with other established traditional prognostic factors such as hormonal and lymph node status, could predict outcome of breast cancer patients with great accuracy.[191-193] Such reports suggest that overexpression of c-*erb* B-2 and c-*myc* oncogenes represent independent predictors of poor prognosis in node-positive patients; these proto-oncogenes did not possess predictive value for node-negative patients. Some investigations contradict these data and find no correlation in node-positive patients, whereas still others confirm a worse prognosis associated with overexpression of oncogenes in node-negative patients.[194,195]

Bland et al.[196] observed no correlation between tumor recurrence and overall survival for independent expression of any of the four molecular biologic variables studied (p53, c-*myc*, c-*erb* B-2 and c-*fos*). Mutation of the p53 suppressor gene was observed to add no increased correlation for risk of recurrence or reduction in survival. Expression of more than one oncogene was observed in 25 of 85 patients (29.4%); coexpression of three oncogenes was observed in only nine of 85 patients (10.6%). Concomitant expression of three oncogenes (c-*myc*, c-*fos*, and H-*ras*) was predictive for a 100% probability of local-regional or systemic recurrence (see Fig. 63-4; Table 63-9). The report by Dati et al.[197] supports the prognostic value of the c-*erb* B-2 e *(neu)*–encoded p185 protein with contemporaneous expression of Ha-*ras* as prognostic variables. The data from these investigators also suggest that coexpression of these proto-oncogenes is of greater statistical value in predicting overall and disease-free survivals than is either oncogene protein alone.

Table 63-9. Prognostic Value of Oncogene Expression in Patients With Breast Cancer

Correlation of Oncogene Expression to Recurrence		
Oncogene Expression	**Positive No. of Patients/Total No. of Patients (%)**	**No. of Patients with Recurrence/No. of Positive Patients (%)**
One positive oncogene	29/85 (34 1)	5/29 (17.2)
Two positive oncogenes	16/85 (18 8)	9/16 (56.3)
Three positive oncogenes	8/85 (9 4)	8/8 (100)
Four positive oncogenes	1/8 (1 2)	1/1 (100)

From Bland KI, et al. Oncogene protein co-expression: Value of Ha-*ras*, c-*myc*, c-*fos*, and p53 as prognostic discriminants for breast cancer. Ann Surg 221:706, 1995.

Table 63-10. Effect of Oncogene Coexpression on Overall Survival

Proportional Hazard Regression Model		
Variable	**Significance (*p*)**	**Risk Ratio**
Age	0.0064	1.052
Size	0.0004	1.726
Nodes	0.0780	1.643
IIA	0.0116	5.761
IIB	0.8843	1.139
Oncogene coexpression	0.0104	1.914

From Bland KI, et al. Oncogene protein co-expression: Value of Ha-*ras*, c-*myc*, c-*fos*, and p53 as prognostic discriminants for breast cancer. Ann Surg 221:706, 1995.

Bland et al.[196] hypothesized that enhanced c-*myc*, c-H-*ras*, and c-*fos* coexpression early in the continuum of breast cancer transformation may act in concert to endow breast neoplastic cells with an aggressive phenotype. The coexpression of these proto-oncogenes and nuclear transcriptional regulatory protein predicted an increased probability of recurrence and reduced survivorship (Fig. 63-13). The coexpression of Ha-*ras* and c-*fos* contributed to the effect of individual molecular variables on overall survival in the proportional hazard regression model. This effect was not evident for c-*myc* and p53 oncogenes ($p = 0.397$ and $p = 0.525$, respectively). Further expression of combination oncogenes was statistically significant for the same regression model ($p = 0.010$, risk ratio = 1.914; Table 63-10). These data support the theoretic construct of multiple genetic "hits" early in the continuum of neoplastic transformation with mammary carcinogenesis. Similar prognostic value was not evident for mutations of the p53 tumor suppressor gene, which did not endow breast neoplastic cells with a similar aggressive phenotype.[196]

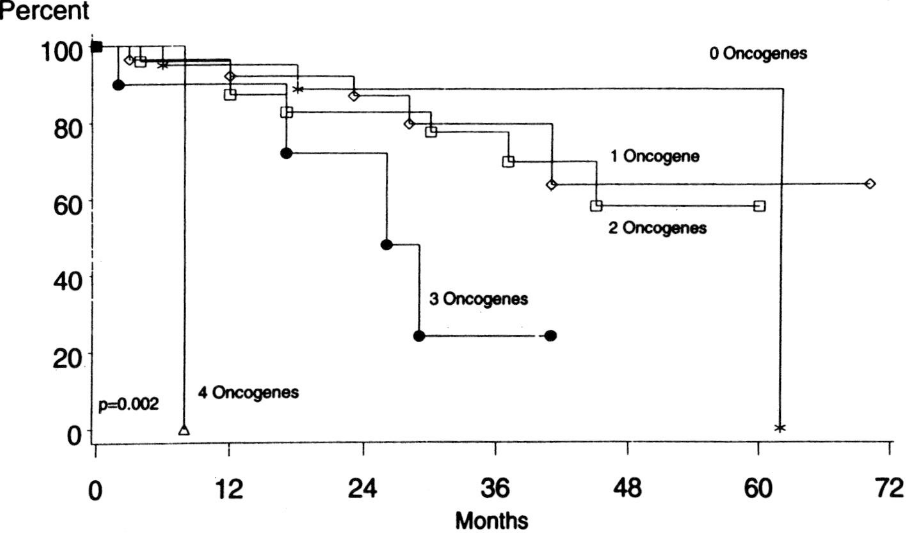

Fig. 63-13. Overall survival evident with number of oncogene proteins expressed in stages I, IIA, and IIB. Superior survival rates were evident in patients who expressed no oncogenes. Similar but reduced survivorship was evident with one and two expressed oncogenes. Statistically significant trends were evident with three or four oncogene expressions and were statistically significant ($p = 0.002$). (From Bland KI, et al. Oncogene protein co-expression: Value of Ha-*ras*, c-*myc*, c-*fos* and p53 as prognostic discriminants for breast carcinoma. Ann Surg 221:713, 1995. Used with permission.)

SUMMARY

The heterogeneity of human mammary carcinoma appears to be a cumulative interrelationship of environmental, developmental, and genetic factors that may allow identification of a high risk for carcinogenesis. Thus, a comprehensive knowledge of the physiologic derangements and trophic events expected in normal breast development and maintenance, as well as specific variations that occur with the pathologic processes, is essential to the diagnostician in initiating appropriate therapy for breast diseases.

Breast development, growth, and involution occur as a result of the mammotropic effects of anterior pituitary and ovarian hormonal secretion. The breast should be considered an end-organ receptor that cannot initiate hormonal regulation through feedback inhibitor physiologic mechanisms. Thus, the tropic effects of these target hormones on alveoli and myoepithelial components of mammary parenchyma may have uninhibited stimulatory growth, with the subsequent development of benign (proliferative and nonproliferative mastopathy, fibroadenoma) or neoplastic states.

A thorough conceptualization of the natural history of benign and malignant diseases and the roles of endogenous and exogenous hormones has partly clarified the therapeutic applications currently employed for diseases of the breast. Also, the identification of genetic and biochemical markers and their application for target surveillance of patients at high risk holds promise to allow identification of breast disease at a preinvasive stage that is favorable to treatment. The additional applications of biologic principles that govern the complex biologic events of the tumor-host relationship, metabolic and growth characteristics, and tumor metastases are being defined. The student of breast disease must retain a working knowledge of the anatomic, physiologic, and biologic events that govern deviations and neoplastic changes occurring in the ductoglandular components of this organ.

REFERENCES

1. Spratt JS, Tobin GR. Anatomy of the breast. In Donegan W, Spratt JS, eds. Cancer of the Breast. Philadelphia: WB Saunders, 1988, p 16.
2. Anson BJ, McVay CB. Thoracic walls: Breast or mammary region. In Anson BJ, McVay CB, eds. Surgical Anatomy. Philadelphia: WB Saunders, 1971, p 330.
3. Haagensen CD. Physicians' role in the detection and diagnosis of breast disease. In Haagensen CD, ed. Diseases of the Breast. Philadelphia: WB Saunders, 1971, p 99.
4. Monard P. Sur deux cas des tumeurs malignes des mammelles axillaires aberrantes. Bull Mem Soc Natl Chir Paris 21:487, 1929.
5. Handley WS. Cancer of the Breast, 2nd ed. New York: Paul B. Hoeber, 1906.
6. Handley WS. Cancer of the Breast and Its Operative Treatment. London: John Murray, 1922.
7. Keller-Wood M, Bland KI. Breast physiology in normal, lactating, and diseased states. In Bland KI, Copeland EM III, eds. The Breast: Comprehensive Management of Benign and Malignant Diseases. Philadelphia: WB Saunders, 1991, p 36.
8. Leis HP Jr. Management of nipple discharge. World J Surg 13:736, 1989.
9. Newman H, Klein M, Northrup JD. Nipple discharge: Frequency and pathogenesis in an ambulatory population. N Y State J Med 83:928, 1983.
10. Funderburk WW, Syphax B. Evaluation of nipple discharge in benign and malignant diseases. Cancer 24:1290, 1969.

11. Chaudary MA, et al. Nipple discharge: The diagnostic value of testing for occult blood. Ann Surg 196:651, 1982.
12. Buchman M, Peake G. Incidence of galactorrhea. JAMA 236: 2747, 1976.
13. Seppala M, Lehto Virta P, Ranta T. Discordant patterns of hyperprolactinaemia and galactorrhea in secondary amenorrhea. Acta Endocrinol 86:456, 1976.
14. Forbes A, Albright. Syndrome characterized by galactorrhea, amenorrhea and low urinary FSH: Comparison with acromegaly and normal lactation. J Clin Endocrinol Metab 14:265, 1954.
15. Chiari J, Braun C, Spaeth S. In Enke, Erlinger, eds. Klinik der Geburtshilfe and Gynalkologie. Berlin: 1855.
16. Frommel J. Beber puerperale atrophie des uterus. Geburthilfe Gynakol 7:305, 1881.
17. Ahumada J, del Castillo EB. Amenorrhea y galactorrhea. Bol Soc Ginecol Obstet 11:64, 1932.
18. Argonz J, del Castillo EB. A syndrome characterized by estrogenic insufficiency, galactorrhea, and decreased urinary gonadotrophin. J Clin Endocrinol Metab 13:79, 1953.
19. Kleinberg D. Lactation and galactorrhea. In Gold J, Josimovich J, eds. Gynecologic Endocrinology. New York: Harper & Row, 1980.
20. Blackwell RE, et al. Assessment of pituitary function in patients with serum prolactin levels greater than 100 ng/ml. Fertil Steril 32:177, 1979.
21. Golinger R, Gregorio R, Fisher E. Tumor cells in venous blood draining mammary carcinomas. Arch Surg 112:707, 1977.
22. Bland KI, Page DL. Gynecomastia. In Bland KI, Copeland EM III, eds. The Breast: Comprehensive Management of Benign and Malignant Diseases. Philadelphia: WB Saunders, 1991, p 135.
23. Bland K. Inflammatory, infectious, and metabolic disorders of the mamma. In Bland KI, Copeland EM III, eds. The Breast: Comprehensive Management of Benign and Malignant Diseases. Philadelphia: WB Saunders, 1991, p 87.
24. Haagensen CD. Anatomy of the mammary gland. In Haagensen CD, ed. Diseases of the Breast, 3rd ed. Philadelphia: WB Saunders, 1986, p 1.
24a. Haagensen CD. Gross cystic disease. In Haagensen CD, ed. Diseases of the Breast. Philadelphia: WB Saunders, 1986, p 250.
25. Dalton M, Grozinger KH. Curt Schimmelbusch's disease. Surgery 63:859, 1968.
26. Kramer WM, Rush BFJ. Mammary duct proliferation in the elderly: A histopathologic study. Cancer 31:130, 1973.
27. Wellings SR. Development of human breast cancer. Adv Cancer Res 31:287, 1980.
28. Black MM, Chabon AB. In situ carcinoma of the breast. Pathol Annu 4:185, 1969.
29. Black MM, et al. Association of atypical characteristics of benign breast lesions with subsequent risk of breast cancer. Cancer 29:338, 1972.
30. Geschickter C, Hartmann C. Mammary response to prolonged estrogenic stimulation in the monkey. Cancer 12:767, 1959.
31. Reyniak J. Endocrine physiology of the breast. J Reprod Med 22:303, 1979.
32. Golinger R. Collective review: Hormones and the pathophysiology of the fibrocystic mastopathy. Surg Gynecol Obstet 146:273, 1978.
33. Vassar P, Culling C. Fibrosis of the breast. Arch Pathol 67:128, 1959.
34. Bloodgood J. The pathology of chronic cystic mastitis of the female breast with special consideration of the blue-domed cyst. Arch Surg 3:445, 1921.
35. Pierson KK, Wilkinson EJ. Malignant neoplasia of the breast: Infiltrating carcinomas. In Bland KI, Copeland EM III, eds. The Breast: Comprehensive Management of Benign and Malignant Diseases. Philadelphia: WB Saunders, 1991, p 193.
36. Shehi LJ, Pierson KK. Benign and malignant epithelial neoplasms and dermatological disorders. In Bland KI, Copeland EM III, eds. The Breast: Comprehensive Management of Benign and Malignant Diseases. Philadelphia: WB Saunders, 1991, p 222.
37. Bland KI. A clinicopathologic correlation of mammographic parenchymal patterns and associated risk factors for human mammary carcinoma. Ann Surg 195:582, 1982.
38. Love S, Gelman R, Silen W. Sounding board. Fibrocystic "disease" of the breast—A nondisease? N Engl J Med 307:1010, 1982.
39. Monson R, Yen S, McMahon B. Chronic mastitis and carcinoma of the breast. Lancet 2:224, 1976.
40. Davis HH, Simons MJ, Davis JB. Cystic disease of the breast: Relationship to carcinoma. Cancer 17:957, 1964.
41. Donnelly P, et al. Benign breast lesions and subsequent breast carcinoma in Rochester, Minnesota. Mayo Clin Proc 50:650, 1975.
42. Fisher B, et al. Five-year results of a randomized clinical trial comparing total mastectomy and segmental mastectomy with or without radiation in the treatment of breast cancer. N Engl J Med 312:665, 1985.
43. Kodlin D, et al. Chronic mastopathy and breast cancer: A follow-up study. Cancer 39:2603, 1977.
44. Wellings SR, Jensen HM. On the origin and progression of ductal carcinoma in the human breast. J Natl Cancer Inst 50:1111, 1973.
45. Page DL, et al. Relationship between component parts of fibrocystic disease complex and breast cancer. J Natl Cancer Inst 61:1055, 1978.
46. Rogers L, Page DL. Epithelial proliferative disease of the breast—A marker of increased cancer risk in certain age groups. Breast Dis Breast 5:2, 1979.
47. Dupont WD, Page DL. Risk factors for breast cancer in women with proliferative breast disease. N Engl J Med 312:146, 1985.
48. Ariel I. Enovid therapy (norethynodrel with mestranol) for fibrocystic disease. Am J Obstet Gynecol 117:453, 1973.
49. Pastides H, et al. Oral contraceptive use and fibrocystic breast disease with special reference to its histopathology. J Natl Cancer Inst 71:5, 1983.
50. LiVolsi V, et al. Fibrocystic breast disease in oral-contraceptive users: A histopathological evaluation of epithelial atypia. N Engl J Med 299:381, 1978.
51. Asch RH, Greenblatt R. Use of an impeded androgen—Danazol—in the management of benign breast disorders. Am J Obstet Gynecol 127:130, 1977.
52. Minton J, et al. Caffeine, cyclic nucleotides, and breast disease. Surgery 86:105, 1979.
53. Gallager HS. Minimal breast cancer: Concepts and results of treatment in minimal invasive cancer (microcarcinoma). Clin Oncol 1:389, 1982.
54. De Ome K. Formal discussion of multiple factors in mouse tumorigenesis. Cancer Res 25:1348, 1965.
55. Sugarbaker EV. Cancer metastasis: A product of tumor-host interactions. Curr Probl Cancer 111(7):3, 1979.
56. Gallager HS, Martin JE. The study of mammary carcinoma by mammography and whole organ sectioning. Cancer 23:855, 1968.
57. Urban JA. Bilaterality of cancer of the breast. Cancer 20:1867, 1967.
58. Foote F, Stewart F. Lobular carcinoma in situ, a rare form of mammary cancer. Am J Pathol 17:491, 1941.
59. Hutter R, Foote FJ, Farrow J. In situ lobular carcinoma of the female breast, 1939-1968. In Breast Cancer, Early and Late. Proceedings of the Thirteenth Annual Clinical Conference on Cancer, 1968, University of Texas MD Anderson Hospital and Tumor Institute at Houston. Chicago: Year Book, 1970.
60. Bond WH. Natural history of breast cancer. In Stoll B, ed. Host Defense in Breast Cancer. Chicago: Year Book, 1975.
61. Beahrs O, et al. Manual for Staging of Cancer, 4th ed. Philadelphia: JB Lippincott, 1992.

62. Burkett F, et al. The value of bone scans in the management of patients with carcinoma of the breast. Surg Gynecol Obstet 149:525, 1979.
63. Hayward RB, Frazier TG. A reevaluation of bone scans in breast cancer. J Surg Oncol 28:111, 1985.
64. Isard H. Other imaging techniques. Cancer 53:658, 1984.
65. Baker LH. Breast cancer detection demonstration project: Five-year summary report. CA Cancer J Clin 32:194, 1982.
66. Bland KI, Copeland EM III. Differentiating among common breast masses. Diagnosis 7(5):45, 1985.
67. Lacour J, et al. Radical mastectomy versus radical mastectomy plus interval node dissection. Cancer 37:206, 1976.
68. Margottini M, Jacobelli G, Cau M. The end results of enlarged radical mastectomy. Acta Unio Int Contra Cancrum 19:1555, 1963.
69. Veronesi U, Zucali R, Del Vecchio M. Conservative treatment of breast cancer with QUART technique. World J Surg 19:676, 1985.
70. Veronesi U, et al. Conservation approaches for the management of stage I/II carcinoma of the breast: Milan Cancer Institute Trials. World J Surg 18:70, 1994.
71. Fisher B, Wolmark N. Limited surgical management for primary breast cancer: A commentary on the NSABP reports. World J Surg 19:682, 1985.
72. Fisher B, Anderson S. Conservative surgery for the management of invasive and noninvasive carcinoma of the breast: NSABP trials. World J Surg 18:63, 1994.
73. National Institutes of Health. Treatment of early-stage breast cancer. NIH Consensus Development Conference Consensus Statement. Washington, D.C.: US Government Printing Office, 1990.
74. D'Orsi K. Correlation of xeroradiology and histology of breast disease. CRC Crit Rev Diagn Imaging 11:75, 1978.
75. Gershon-Cohen J, Colcher A. Evaluation of roentgen diagnosis of early carcinoma of the breast. JAMA 108:867, 1937.
76. Egan R. Mammography: An aid to early diagnosis of breast carcinoma. JAMA 182:839, 1962.
77. Egan R. Roles of mammography in the early detection of breast cancer. Cancer 24:1197, 1969.
78. Shapiro S. Evidence on screening of breast cancer from a randomized trial. Cancer 39:2772, 1977.
79. Bland KI, et al. Analysis of breast cancer screening in women younger than 50 years. JAMA 245:1037, 1981.
80. Berg JW. Morphological evidence for immune response to breast cancer. A histological view. Cancer 28:1453, 1971.
81. Mathé G. Current status of immunotherapy of human cancer: Leukaemias, lymphomas, solid tumours. Drugs 8:411, 1974.
82. Rowland GF, O'Neill GJ, Davies DA. Suppression of tumour growth in mice by a drug-antibody conjugate using a normal approach to linkage. Nature 255:487, 1975.
83. Butler TP, Gullino PM. Quantitation of cell shedding into efferent blood of mammary adenocarcinoma. Cancer Res 35:512, 1975.
84. Lunscken C, Strauli P. Penetration of an ascitic reticulum cell sarcoma of the golden hamster into the body wall and through the diaphragm. Virchows Arch B Cell Pathol 17:247, 1975.
85. Carr I, McGinty F, Norris P. The fine structure of neoplastic invasion: Invasion of liver, skeletal muscle and lymphatic vessels by the Rd/3 tumour. J Pathol 118:91, 1976.
86. Fisher B, Fisher ER. Barrier function of lymph node to tumor cells and erythrocytes. I. Normal nodes. Cancer 20:1907, 1967.
87. Madden RE, Gyure L. Translymphnodal passage of tumor cells. Oncology 22:281, 1968.
88. Hewitt HB, Blake E. Quantitative studies of translymphnodal passage of tumour cells naturally disseminated from a nonimmunogenic murine squamous carcinoma. Br J Cancer 31:25, 1975.
89. Salsbury AJ. The significance of the circulating cancer cell. Cancer Treat Rev 2:55, 1975.
90. Griffiths J, et al. Carcinoma of the colon and rectum: Circulating malignant cells and 5-year survival. Cancer 31:226, 1973.
91. Fidler I. Metastasis: Quantitative analysis of distribution and fate of tumor emboli labeled with 12-5-iodo-2′-deoxyuridine. J Natl Cancer Inst 45:775, 1970.
92. Vaage J. Host serum factors in immune resistance to metastases. In Day S, et al., eds. Biologic Mechanisms and Therapy. New York: Raven Press, 1977.
93. Lippman M, Chabner B. National Institutes of Health Consensus Development Conference on Adjuvant Chemotherapy and Endocrine Therapy for Breast Cancer. Editorial overview. NCI Monogr 1:5, 1986.
94. Rubens R. Personal communication, 1994.
95. Fisher B, et al. A summary of findings from NSABP trials of adjuvant therapy. In Jones SE, Salmon SE, eds. Adjuvant Therapy of Cancer IV. Orlando, Fla.: Grune & Stratton, 1984.
96. Bonadonna G, et al. Adjuvant chemotherapy trials in resectable breast cancer with positive axillary nodes: Experience of the Milan Cancer Institute. In Jones SE, Salmon SE, eds. Adjuvant Therapy of Cancer IV. Orlando, Fla.: Grune & Stratton, 1984.
97. Smith D, et al. Adjuvant radiotherapy and chemotherapy in breast cancer. In Jones S, Salmon S, eds. Adjuvant Therapy of Cancer IV. Orlando, Fla.: Grune & Stratton, 1984, p 283.
98. Bonadonna G, Valagussa P. Adjuvant systemic therapy for resectable breast cancer [editorial]. J Clin Oncol 3:259, 1985.
99. Bonadonna G, Rossi A, Valagussa P. Adjuvant CMF chemotherapy in operable breast cancer: Ten years later. World J Surg 9:707, 1985.
100. Early Breast Cancer Trialists' Collaborative Group. Systemic treatment of early breast cancer by hormonal, cytotoxic, or immune therapy: 133 randomized trials involving 31,000 recurrences and 24,000 deaths among 75,000 women. Part 1, Part II. Lancet 339:1, 1992.
101. Williams D. Biological mechanisms in metastasis. In Stoll B, ed. Secondary Spread in Breast Cancer. London: William Heinemann Medical Books, 1977.
102. Gardner W. Endocrine dependence in experimental testicular tumorigenesis and tumor growth. In Brennan J, Simpson W, eds. Biological Interactions in Normal and Neoplastic Growth: A Contribution to the Host-Tumor Problem. Boston: Little, Brown, 1962.
103. Beatson G. On the treatment of inoperable cases of carcinoma of the mamma: Suggestions for a new method of treatment with illustrative cases. Lancet 2:104, 1896.
104. Huggins C. Control of cancers of man by endocrinology methods: Review. Cancer Res 16:825, 1956.
105. Huggins C, Bergenstal D. Surgery of adrenals. JAMA 147:101, 1951.
106. Luft R, Olivecrona H, Sjögren B. Hypophysectomy in man. Nord Med 47:351, 1952.
107. Ray B. Carcinoma of the breast—Hypophysectomy as palliative treatment. JAMA 200:974, 1967.
108. Kennedy B, Mielke PJ, Fortuny I. Therapeutic castration versus prophylactic castration in breast cancer. Surg Gynecol Obstet 118:524, 1964.
109. Ravdin R, et al. Results of a clinical trial concerning the worth of prophylactic oophorectomy for breast carcinoma. Surg Gynecol Obstet 131:1055, 1970.
110. Henderson IC, Canellos GP. Cancer of the breast: The past decade (first of two parts). N Engl J Med 302:17, 1980.
111. Ingle J, Ahmann DL, Green SJ. Randomized clinical trial of diethylstilbestrol versus tamoxifen in postmenopausal women with advanced breast cancer. N Engl J Med 304:16, 1981.
112. Santen RJ, et al.. Aminoglutethimide scientific profile. In Santen R, Henderson I, eds. Pharmanual: A Comprehensive Guide to the Therapeutic Use of Aminoglutethimide. Munich: Karger, 1982.
113. Santen R, et al. A randomized trial comparing surgical adrenalectomy with aminoglutethimide pluse hydrocortisone in women with advanced breast cancer. N Engl J Med 305:545, 1981.

114. Jensen E, De Sombre E, Jungblut P. Estrogen receptors in hormone-responsive tissues and tumors. In Wissler R, Dao T, Wood SJ, eds. Endogenous Factors Influencing Host-Tumor Balance. Chicago: University of Chicago Press, 1967.
115. Allegra J. The use of steroid hormone receptors in breast cancer. In Margolese R, ed. Contemporary Issues in Clinical Oncology: Breast Cancer. New York: Churchill Livingstone, 1983.
116. Silva JS, et al. Biochemical correlates of morphologic differentiation in human breast cancer. Surgery 92:443, 1982.
117. Lippman M, et al. The relation between estrogen receptors and response rate to cytotoxic chemotherapy in metastatic breast cancer. N Engl J Med 298:1223, 1978.
118. McGuire WL. Steroid receptors in human breast cancer. Cancer Res 38:4289, 1978.
119. Degenshein G, et al. Hormone relationships in breast cancer: The role of receptor-binding proteins. Curr Probl Surg 16:1, 1979.
120. Gapinski PJ, Donegan WL. Estrogen receptors and breast cancer: Prognostic and therapeutic implications. Surgery 88:386, 1980.
121. Savlov ED, Wittliff JL, Hilf R. Further studies of biochemical predictive tests in breast cancer. Cancer 39:539, 1977.
122. Allegra JC, et al. Distribution, frequency, and quantitative analysis of estrogen, progesterone, androgen, and glucocorticoid receptors in human breast cancer. Cancer Res 39:1447, 1979.
123. Horwitz K, McGuire W. Estrogen and progesterone: Their relationship in hormone-dependent breast cancer. In McGuire W, Raynaud P, Baulieu E, eds. Progesterone Receptors in Normal and Neoplastic Tissues. New York: Raven Press, 1977.
124. McGuire W, Horwitz K. Progesterone receptors in breast cancer. In McGuire W, ed. Hormones, Receptors, and Breast Cancer. New York: Raven Press, 1978.
125. Bland KI, Fuchs A, Wittliff JL. Menopausal status as a factor in the distribution of estrogen and progestin receptors in breast cancer. Surg Forum 32:410, 1981.
126. Martin P, et al. Multiple steroid receptors in human breast cancer. III: Relationship between steroid receptors and the state of differentiation and the activity of carcinomas throughout the pathologic features. Cancer Chemother Pharmacol 2:115, 1979.
127. McCarty KS, et al. Correlation of estrogen and progesterone receptors with histologic differentiation in mammary carcinoma. Cancer 46:2851, 1980.
128. Manni A, et al. Antihormone treatment of stage IV breast cancer. Cancer 43:444, 1979.
129. Pritchard K, et al. A prospective randomized controlled trial of adjuvant tamoxifen in postmenopausal women with axillary node positive breast cancer. In Jones S, Salmon S, eds. Adjuvant Therapy of Cancer IV Orlando, Fla.: Grune & Stratton, 1984.
130. Ingle J, et al. Randomized trial of bilateral oophorectomy versus tamoxifen in premenopausal women with metastatic breast cancer. J Clin Oncol 4:178, 1986.
131. Ward HW, et al. Anti-oestrogen therapy for breast cancer—A report on 300 patients treated with tamoxifen. Clin Oncol 4:11, 1978.
132. Hubay CA, et al. Antiestrogen, cytotoxic chemotherapy, and bacillus Calmette-Guérin vaccination in stage II breast cancer: A preliminary report. Surgery 87:494, 1980.
133. Meakin J, et al. Ovarian irradiation and prednisone following surgery and radiotherapy for carcinoma of the breast. Breast Cancer Res Treat 3:545, 1983.
134. Nolvadex Adjuvant Trial Organization. Controlled trial of tamoxifen as an adjuvant agent in management of early breast cancer: Interim analysis at four years by Nolvadex Adjuvant Trial Organization. Lancet 1:257, 1983.
135. Ribeiro G, Swindell R. The Christie Hospital adjuvant tamoxifen trial—Status at 10 years. Br J Cancer 57:601, 1988.
136. Breast Cancer Trials Committee, SCTO. Adjuvant tamoxifen in the management of operable breast cancer: The Scottish trial. Lancet 2:171, 1987.
137. Nolvadex Adjuvant Trial Organization. Controlled trial of tamoxifen as a single adjuvant agent in management of early breast cancer: Analysis at eight years by the Nolvadex Adjuvant Trial Organization. Br J Cancer 57:608, 1988.
138. Fisher B, et al. A randomized clinical trial evaluating tamoxifen in the treatment of patients with node negative breast cancer who have estrogen-receptor-positive tumors. N Engl J Med 320:479, 1989.
139. Fisher B, et al. Adjuvant therapy for node negative breast cancer: An update of NSABP findings. Proc Am Soc Clin Oncol 12:79, 1993.
140. Allegra J, et al. A phase II trial of tamoxifen, premarin, methotrexate and 5-fluorouracil in metastatic breast cancer. Breast Cancer Res Treat 2:93, 1982.
141. Lacour J, et al. Adjuvant treatment with polyadenylic-polyuridylic acid in operable breast cancer: updated results of a randomised trial. Br Med J 288:589, 1984.
142. Osborne C. Receptors. In Harris J, Hellman S, Henderson J, eds. Breast Disease. Philadelphia: JB Lippincott, 1991, p 301.
143. Silvestrini R, et al. p53 as an independent prognostic marker in lymph node-negative breast cancer patients. J Natl Cancer Inst 85:965, 1993.
144. Clark GM, McGuire WL. Steroid receptors and other prognostic factors in primary breast cancer. Semin Oncol 15:20, 1988.
145. Mathiesen O, et al. The prognostic value of estrogen and progesterone receptors in female breast cancer: A single center study. Acta Oncol 30:691, 1991.
146. Nomura Y, et al. Relative effect of steroid hormone receptors on the prognosis of patients with operable hormone receptors on the prognosis of patients with operable breast cancer. A univariate and multivariate analysis of 3089 Japanese patients with breast cancer from the study group for the Japanese Breast Cancer Society on hormone receptors and prognosis in breast cancer. Cancer 69:153, 1992.
147. Hayes D. Tumor markers for breast cancer. Ann Oncol 4:807, 1993.
148. Coon J, et al. Interinstitutional variability in DNA flow cytometric analysis of tumors. The National Cancer Institute's flow cytometry network experience. Cancer 61:126, 1988.
149. Kute TE, et al. The use of flow cytometry for the prognosis of stage II adjuvant treated breast cancer patients. Cancer 66:1810, 1990.
150. Sahin A, et al. KI-67 immunostaining in node-negative stage I/II breast carcinoma: Significant correlation with prognosis. Cancer 68:549, 1991.
151. Tanaka T, et al. Expression of p21 *ras* oncoproteins in human cancers. Cancer Res 46:1465, 1986.
152. Andres AC, et al. H-*ras* induced transformation of mammary epithelium is favoured by increased oncogene expression or by inhibition of mammary regression. Oncogene 6:771, 1991.
153. Hayes DF, et al. Prediction of prognosis in primary breast cancer by detection of a high molecular weight mucin-like antigen using monoclonal antibodies DF3, F36/22, and CU18: A Cancer and Leukemia Group B study. J Clin Oncol 9:1, 1991.
154. Tandon AK, et al. Cathepsin D and prognosis in breast cancer. N Engl J Med, 322:297, 1990.
155. Duffy MJ, et al. Tissue-type plasminogen activator, a new prognostic marker in breast cancer. Cancer Res 48:1348, 1988.
156. Harris JR, et al. Breast cancer. N Engl J Med 327:390, 1992.
157. Borg A, et al. Her-2/*neu* amplification predicts poor survival in node-positive breast cancer. Cancer Res 50:4332, 1990.
158. Toikkanen S, et al. Prognostic significance of HER-2 oncoprotein expression in breast cancer: A 30-year follow-up. J Clin Oncol 10:1044, 1992.
159. Caleffi M, et al. p53 gene mutations and steroid receptor status in breast cancer. Cancer 73:2147, 1994.

160. Lipponen P, et al. p53 protein expression in breast cancer as related to histopathological characteristics and prognosis. Int J Cancer 55:51, 1993.
161. Iggo R, et al. Increased expression of mutant forms of p53 oncogene in primary lung cancer. Lancet 335:675, 1990.
162. Rodrigues N, et al. p53 mutations in colorectal cancer. Proc Natl Acad Sci U S A 87:7555, 1990.
163. Sidransky D, et al. Identification of p53 gene mutations in bladder cancers and urine samples. Science 252:706, 1991.
164. Barton C, et al. Abnormalities of the p53 suppressor gene in human pancreatic cancer. Br J Cancer 64:1076, 1991.
165. Thompson AM, et al. p53 allele losses, mutations and expression in breast cancer and their relationship to clinico-pathological parameters. Int J Cancer 50:528, 1992.
166. Sawan A, et al. Retinoblastoma and p53 gene expression related to relapse and survival in human breast cancer: An immunohistochemical study. J Pathol 168:23, 1992.
167. Thor AD, et al. Accumulation of p53 tumor suppressor gene protein: An independent marker of prognosis in breast cancer. J Natl Cancer Inst 84:845, 1992.
168. Isola J, et al. Association of overexpression of tumor suppressor protein p53 with rapid cell proliferation and poor prognosis in node-negative breast cancer patients. J Natl Cancer Inst 84:1109, 1992.
169. Allred DC, et al. Association of p53 protein expression with tumor cell proliferation rate and clinical outcome in node-negative breast cancer. J Natl Cancer Inst 85:200, 1993.
170. Marks JR, et al. Overexpression of p53 and HER-2/*neu* proteins as prognostic markers in early stage breast cancer. Ann Surg 219:332, 1994.
171. Ostrowski JL, et al. p53 expression in human breast cancer related to survival and prognostic factors: An immunohistochemical study. J Pathol 164:75, 1991.
172. Varmus H. An historical overview of oncogenes. In Weinberg R. ed. Onocogenes and the Molecular Origins of Cancer. Plainview, N.Y.: Cold Spring Harbor Laboratory Press, 1989, p 67.
173. MacKay S, et al. Growth factors, tumor suppressors, and cancer. Perspect Gen Surg 3:1, 1992.
174. Cantley LC, et al. Oncogenes and signal transduction. Cell 64:281, 1991.
175. Weinberg R. Oncogenes, tumor suppressor genes and cell transformation: Trying to put it all together. In: Origins of Human Cancer. Brugge J, Curran T, Harlow E, McCormick F, eds. Plainview, N.Y.: Cold Spring Harbor Laboratory Press, 1991, p 1.
176. Dean M, Vande Woude G. Principles of molecular cell biology of cancer: Introduction to methods in molecular biology. In DeVita V, Hellman S, Rosenberg S, eds. Cancer: Principles and Practice of Oncology. Philadelphia: JB Lippincott, 1989, p 14.
177. Morrison B. Oncogenes and breast cancer. In Harris J, et al., eds. Breast Diseases. Philadelphia: JB Lippincott, 1991, p 197.
178. Morrison B. The genetics of breast cancer. Hematol Oncol Clin North Am 8:15, 1994.
179. Bishop JM. Molecular themes in oncogenesis. Cell 64:235, 1991.
180. Callahan R, Campbell G. Mutations in human breast cancer: An overview. J Natl Cancer Inst 81:1780, 1989.
181. Adnane J, et al. Proto-oncogene amplification and human breast tumor phenotype. Oncogene 4:1389, 1989.
182. Kraus M, Yuasa Y, Aaronson S. A position 12-activated H-*ras* oncogene in all HS578T mammary carcinosarcoma cells but not normal mammary cells of the same patient. Proc Natl Acad Sci U S A 81:5384, 1984.
183. Clair T, Miller WR, Cho-Chung YS. Prognostic significance of the expression of a ras protein with a molecular weight of 21,000 by human breast cancer. Cancer Res 47:5290, 1987.
184. Bchini O, et al. Precocious mammary gland development and milk protein synthesis in transgenic mice ubiquitously expressing human growth hormone. Endocrinology 128:539, 1991.
185. Ernberg I. Oncogenes and tumor growth factor in breast cancer. Acta Oncol 29:331, 1990.
186. Mooi WI, Peterse JL. Progress in molecular biology of breast cancer. Eur J Cancer 1992:623, 1992.
187. Van de Vijver M, et al. Oncogene activation in human breast cancer. Cancer Cells, 1989, 7:385.
188. Parkes HC, et al. c-*erb* B-2 mRNA expression in human breast tumors: comparison with c-*erb* B-2 DNA amplification and correlation prognosis. Br J Cancer 61:39, 1990.
189. Winstanley J, et al. The long-term prognostic significance of c-*erb* B-2 in primary breast cancer. Br J Cancer 63:447, 1991.
190. Klijin JG, et al. The prognostic value of oncogene amplification and of tumoral secretory proteins with respect to response to endocrine and chemotherapy in metastatic breast cancer. J Clin Oncol 11:53, 1992.
191. Berns P, et al. Amplification of the HER-2/*neu* gene and not of the c-*myc* in association with poor response to endocrine and good response to chemotherapy in recurrent breast cancer. Presented at 5th EROTC Breast Cancer Working Conference. Leuven, Belgium: 1991.
192. Gullick WJ, et al. c-*erb* B-2 protein over-expression in breast cancer is a risk factor in patients with involved and uninvolved lymph nodes. Br J Cancer 63:434, 1991.
193. Zeillinger R, et al. HER-2 amplification, steroid receptors and epidermal growth factor receptor in primary breast cancer. Oncogene 4:109, 1989.
194. Shiu R, Watson P, Dubik D. c-*myc* oncogene expression in estrogen-dependent and independent breast cancer. Clin Chem 39:353, 1993.
195. Varley J, et al. Alterations either to c-*erb*, B-2(neu) or c-*myc* proto-oncogene in breast carcinomas correlate with poor short-term prognosis. Oncogene 1:423, 1987.
196. Bland KI, et al. Oncogene protein co-expression: value of Ha-*ras*, c-*myc*, c-*fos* and p53 as prognostic discriminants for breast cancer. Ann Surg 221:706, 1995.
197. Dati C, et al. c-*erb*B-2 and *ras* expression levels in breast cancer are correlated and show a co-operative association with unfavorable clinical outcome. Int J Cancer 47:833, 1991.

64

Abdominal Wall Hernias

Philip E. Donahue

The word *hernia* is derived from a Latin term meaning rupture of a portion of a structure. In the context of the abdominal wall, a hernia is a protrusion of abdominal cavity contents through an abnormal opening or a defect in the fascial and muscular layers designed to contain them. Our current understanding of the abdominal wall as a site of opposing physical forces that remain in balance according to established mechanical principles, with the appearance of a hernia when this balance is disrupted, is both accurate and productive. It is accurate because the mechanical factors are considered to be the dominant explanation for the emergence of hernias; it is productive because hernias generally do not heal or resolve spontaneously (an exception being the umbilical hernia) but require surgical repair, and any such repair performed without regard to these factors is at an increased risk for failure.

No matter how many hernia repairs an experienced surgeon has performed, the clinical presentation in a given patient and the anatomic findings observed at the time of herniorrhaphy can vary considerably. This is true with respect to the patient's symptoms, the particular tissue relationships in and around the hernia itself, and the postoperative course after repair. Although the overwhelming majority of patients have an uneventful convalescence after repair of their hernias and promptly return to gainful employment, an unfortunate few are plagued by complications of the procedure or by recurrence of the hernia after its original repair. Thus, hernia repair should still be considered a major surgical event, demanding both technical awareness and precise skill in performance.

This chapter highlights the important developments that have occurred during the past several decades in our understanding of the pathophysiology of hernia formation and how this knowledge is used in the modern practice of herniorrhaphy.[1]

DEFINITIONS

For an abdominal wall hernia to occur, a defect (congenital or acquired) in the musculofascial tissues supporting the abdominal cavity must exist. Through this defect, a pouch of peritoneum (the hernia sac) pushes. In evaluating the status of the hernial sac contents, the nomenclature currently used to classify different types of hernias must be defined. In the examination of a patient with a hernia, it is important to determine whether the contents of the hernial sac can be returned to the abdominal cavity. If this can be accomplished without difficulty, the hernia is said to be *reducible.* Occasionally, the hernial contents cannot be reduced with surgical intervention. In this situation the hernia is termed *irreducible.* The word *incarcerated* is often used synonymously with the word *irreducible;* both terms imply that vascular compromise has not occurred. In the event that the blood supply to the hernial contents is impaired, the hernia is defined as *strangulated.* If surgical intervention is not carried out promptly, this is a surgical emergency that often results in the infarction of the viscus involved.

A *sliding hernia* indicates that a portion of the lining of the hernial sac is composed of an intra-abdominal structure. This situation is especially common with groin hernias, in which the cecum, appendix, or sigmoid colon may make up a portion of the sac. Although sliding hernias cannot be diagnosed before surgery, it is important to recognize the possibility of this circumstance at the time of surgery, because removal of the hernial sac as commonly performed would injure the particular viscus involved. The term *Richter's hernia* indicates that a portion of the circumference of the bowel has become incarcerated in the fascial defect. If the segment of bowel wall involved becomes strangulated, localized gangrene often results. This complication can be especially life-threatening, because the segment of bowel involved is generally not obstructed as usually occurs when a portion of bowel becomes incarcerated in the hernial defect. Richter's hernias may be present in a number of anatomic locations but are particularly common among femoral hernias. One variant of the Richter's hernia, called *Littre's hernia,* occurs when an intestinal diverticulum is trapped in the fascial defect. This term is usually restricted to the herniation of a Meckel's diverticulum.

The term *ventral hernia* is a generic designation that refers to any hernia developing in the ventral abdominal wall. It usually includes umbilical, epigastric, and incisional hernias, but the term may also be applied to a spigelian hernia. *Groin hernias* are hernias that develop in the inguinofemoral region. Such hernias include both direct and indirect inguinal hernias, as well as femoral hernias. An *internal hernia* is the designation given to the herniation of a loop of intestine through a congenital or acquired aperture within the abdominal cavity. This may result from a defect in the intestinal mesentery or a herniation through the foramen of Winslow into the lesser sac. Occasionally, an adhesion from a previously performed operation may develop between the abdominal wall and a segment of intestine, creating an aperture through which an adjacent loop of bowel may herniate. Although the hernia results from a connection with the abdominal wall, it is not technically considered an abdominal wall hernia. Internal hernias are generally not diagnosed before surgery; rather they are usually recognized when exploratory surgery is performed for a bowel obstruction of previously undetermined cause.

ETIOLOGIC CONSIDERATIONS IN THE DEVELOPMENT OF HERNIAS

Hernias may develop in any of the structures supporting or surrounding the abdominal cavity. They may be encountered where a previous fetal communication existed between the abdominal cavity and some distant site, when an embryologic canal fails to obliterate, when maldevelopment of a supporting structure occurs, when dilation of a normally situated hiatus results, and when the mesenchymal supporting structures constituting a portion of the body wall become attenuated for any reason. Common sites where abdominal wall hernias are likely to occur include the groin, the umbilicus, the linea alba, various parts of the diaphragm, the lumbar region, along adjacent foramina in the pelvis where blood vessels and nerves exit, and within previously performed surgical incisions.

That various anatomic abnormalities play a role in the development of hernia is attested by the existence of certain types of hernia at birth or their clinical presentation shortly thereafter.[2] For example, umbilical hernias occur where the umbilical ring has failed to obliterate the embryologic opening of the allantoic duct, which is ordinarily prevented by growth of the contiguous fascia of the linea alba. As many as 20% of African-American infants and 5% of white infants may have umbilical hernias at the time of birth. A similar circumstance exists for the indirect inguinal hernia (also called the *oblique hernia*). This hernia arises because of an unobliterated processus vaginalis, the peritoneal connection between the abdominal cavity and the scrotum in the male human and the canal of Nuck in the female human. The peak incidence of the indirect inguinal hernia occurs during infancy, when about 50% of male infants have a patent vaginal process. Congenital factors also appear to play a role in the development of direct inguinal hernias that occur between the pubic ramus and the arching border of the transversus abdominus muscle medial to the deep inferior epigastric vessels. In studies investigating the anatomic basis of this type of hernia, it has been shown that individuals with a transversus abdominus aponeurosis that has a high arching lower border are at an increased risk for the development of this type of hernial defect. Certain types of diaphragmatic hernia and hernias involving the linea alba also appear to be related to anatomic defects, as discussed elsewhere in this chapter.

Although an anatomic abnormality is certainly a predisposing factor that often plays a role in hernia development, other etiologic factors are clearly involved. For example, although structural defects may be responsible for the development of direct inguinal hernias in some patients, such defects do not explain the increased incidence of this type of hernia among advanced age groups or the tendency of elderly patients to have attenuated fascial structures of the groin. In addition, as many as 20% of individuals in autopsy studies have been noted to have a patent processus vaginalis, without any clinical evidence of a hernia before death.[3] Similarly, the incidence of contralateral patency of the processus vaginalis among patients who have undergone repair of an inguinal hernia indicates that patency of this structure does not necessarily lead to inguinal herniation.[4] Further, the observation that 5% of young women subjected to incidental herniography performed after hysterosalpingography had an open processus vaginalis (diverticulum of Nuck) that was asymptomatic and without clinical evidence of a hernia further emphasizes that a patent vaginal process alone does not necessarily lead to a clinically apparent hernia.[5] It therefore appears that equally important causes of hernia development that cannot be easily described are related to the "wear and tear" of living itself, such as repetitive local trauma, degenerative changes associated with increased abdominal pressure, and altered collagen synthesis. All are possible etiologic factors in patients acquiring hernias in middle and older age.[6,7]

Renewed interest in the biochemical and structural aspects of herniology has followed the description of some of the molecular and cellular elements of the protective fascia and collagenous tissues that normally prevent the formation of hernia. Collagen, the major constituent of the various aponeuroses and fascial structures of the body wall, has been studied intensively. Interestingly, collagen, like all other tissues in the body, is in a state of dynamic equilibrium, in which there appears to be a constant synthesis of this substance that is matched by a parallel and constant rate of degradation. When Peacock[8] studied the transversalis fascia medial to the contralateral internal inguinal ring in patients with unilateral hernia, he compared rates of collagen synthesis and collagenolysis in the two inguinal regions and found that the rates of both processes were markedly increased. These findings support the concept that an abnormality of local collagen metabolism may be a factor in the eventual appearance of a hernia.[8]

Further support for the view that abnormal collagen underlies hernia formation is provided by studies of hydroxyproline (the major amino acid constituent of collagen) content in the rectus muscle aponeurosis of patients with and without groin hernia. A frank decrease in the concentration of this substance that was not related to age or muscle mass was seen in patients with groin hernias. Fibroblasts cultured from the anterior rectus sheath of these patients proliferated poorly, incorporating labeled precursors at a much lower rate than did control specimens.[7] In addition, ultrastructural studies of rectus sheath collagen from patients with direct inguinal hernias showed irregular microfibrils, supporting the concept of both structural and biochemical abnormality in adult patients in whom herniations develop.[7]

The specific effects of malnutrition on the evolution of hernias of the groin or other parts of the abdominal wall are as yet undefined. If the collagenous structures that guard the abdominal wall are vital living structures that constantly undergo remodeling and resynthesis, there is a balance between synthesis and destruction of these supporting structures that could conceivably be altered by nutritional status. In the surgical clinic of any large public hospital, many individuals with both adult-onset hernias and malnutrition are encountered. A number of clinical and experimental observations suggest a correlation between the two conditions.

One of the first insights into this possible relationship was provided on sailing ships of a century or more ago, the crews of which suffered from scurvy. In addition to bleeding gums, periosteal pain, and weakness associated with this disease, these hapless individuals were reported to acquire hernias or ruptures of healed scars. Later, a specific effect of vitamin C on collagen maturation was described, allowing a reasonable explanation of the observed effects in these patients. Another condition providing insights into the nature of acquired hernias is lathyrism, a disease resulting from ingestion of the flowering sweet pea. The active agent in the pea, β-aminoproprionitrile, prevents the maturation of collagen and is capable of causing the appearance of groin hernias in young rats and mice.[9] Interestingly, groin hernias developed in animals younger than 1 month who were given sweet pea seeds in their diet; in contrast, older rats did not acquire hernias when fed a similar diet.

These examples of how nutrition may influence the formation of hernias are of particular importance because they illustrate how environmental factors affect the natural balance between collagen synthesis and lysis, eventually leading to the appearance of herniation. It may ultimately be shown that similar defects in nutrition exist in patients who seem to have excessive numbers of hernias or more than their share of recurrent herniations after primary repair. Of course, the relationship between hernia wound healing and overall nutritional status must be viewed in a multifactorial context. The hernia wound, for example, exists in a patient who may have latent vitamin or mineral deficiencies, altered immunity or resistance to infection, or underlying systemic disease. In addition, such individuals may have impaired ability to generate the proteinaceous constituents of collagen and the various components of a repaired or healed defect, factors that may predispose the patient toward subsequent recurrence.[10]

The recent description of altered levels of circulating enzymes in patients with emphysema adds another dimension to the possible role of biologic factors in hernia formation. In a provocative article by Cannon and Read,[11] serum elastolytic and antiproteolytic activities in those who did and did not smoke were measured. It was found that those who smoked had the potentially undesirable combination of increases in proteolytic activity and reductions in α_1-antitrypsin, the major naturally occurring circulating antiprotease. This combination could possibly set the stage for the evolution of hernia formation by affecting the synthesis-degradation equilibrium of groin collagen and thereby setting in motion a pathologic sequence favoring collagen degradation.

Other factors also appear to be involved in hernia formation. Patients with Laënnec's cirrhosis who have ascites illustrate how individuals predisposed toward hernia development eventually acquire clinically apparent hernias when subjected to stress, specifically to a hydrostatic pressure challenge. Both groin and umbilical hernias frequently appear for the first time in this group of patients. Individuals who perform repeated strenuous physical activities offer another example of hernias produced by a combination of predisposed anatomy and situational stress. In a report by Gullmo[12] in Sweden, who used herniography to define the cause of obscure groin pains in a group of young athletes, a number of hernias were described, including those involving the obturator canal and incipient hernial defects at the inguinal ring that could not be diagnosed by other means. These young athletes were examined because many had severe pain that prevented their usual level of physical activity, yet they had unremarkable results of initial examination.

Finally, a number of iatrogenic factors may result in the subsequent development of a hernia. Evidence suggesting that previous appendectomy may predispose toward the later development of an ipsilateral oblique (indirect) inguinal hernia. The presumptive mechanism underlying this circumstance is damage to the innervation of the muscular constrictors of the internal ring shutter mechanism during appendectomy that later allows herniation of abdominal contents through a patent processus vaginalis. In one study, laparoscopic views of the internal inguinal ring shortly after acute appendicitis and subsequent appendectomy demonstrated poor to absent contraction of the internal ring during coughing or straining.[13] A temporary neuropraxia related to surgical trauma could explain these findings, but it must be kept in mind that other evidence supports the association with appendectomy. A statistically significant correlation between appendectomy and the later development of ipsilateral hernias was shown by Arnbjornsson,[14] who described a threefold greater incidence of right inguinal hernia among men who had had appendectomy than among those without a history of previous surgery.

During surgical exposure of the common femoral artery and the distal external iliac artery for various types of vascular procedures (e.g., aortofemoral bypass), the inguinal ligament and the musculoaponeurotic borders of the inguinal ring must be divided. I have noted that groin hernias occasionally occur in these individuals during the first few months after surgery, suggesting a definite relationship to the first operation. The most plausible explanation for these hernias is that closure of the abdominal wall was made without attention to the principles of primary herniorrhaphy. The importance of reconstruction of the specific layers of the abdominal wall, including the internal ring, after any surgical transection of the internal inguinal ring is emphasized by these observations. Patients with a patent processus vaginalis are most susceptible to this complication, but it can develop in any individual. For example, some individuals with severe groin pain after vascular access operations have no discrete hernia sac but rather possess a lax internal ring that allows preperitoneal fat to bulge (herniate) through it. Such individuals do extremely well with surgical closure of the ring that adheres to the principles underlying hernia repair (see pp. 1300-1305), whether an anterior or posterior approach is used.

There is also evidence that the increased hydrostatic intra-abdominal pressure associated with long-term ambulatory peritoneal dialysis frequently results in hernia development.[15] The reported incidence varies between 1% and 30%, with most of the hernias occurring in the groin and umbilicus and occasionally in the diaphragm, spigelian area, or the exit site of the dialysis catheter. Because the groin is the most frequent site, there is chance that congenital factors have set the stage for the appearance of the hernia in this area. Because renal failure per se has a deleterious effect on collagen metabolism, however, a multifactorial pathogenesis is also possible.[16-18] The problem encountered in patients undergoing long-term ambulatory peritoneal dailysis is similar to that noted in patients with advanced cirrhosis and ascites, a high risk for the evolution of hernia defects caused by increased abdominal pressure aggravated by nutritional or metabolic factors that result in poor wound healing and defective or suboptimal collagen synthesis.

Hernias appearing at the site of large latex drain tracts are infrequent and are caused by the enthusiastic creation of a drainage tract by the surgeon. Some surgeons believe that a "two-finger" aperture is required for optimal drain function and that any drain tract of smaller dimension is both ineffectual and imprudent. I disagree; in fact, I believe that the two-finger aperture is a likely cause of iatrogenic hernia. Furthermore, there is good evidence that most drains routinely placed after common surgical procedures (e.g., cholecystectomy) are unnecessary and are truly therapeutic only for the surgeon. There are certainly situations that require generous drainage, but these are usually best handled by suction drains rather than multiple latex drains and do not require extremely large abdominal wall openings. Finally, there are occasional instances in which surgeons elect to perform open drainage of either part or all of the peritoneal or retroperitoneal surfaces. The situations most commonly treated by this means are cases of hemorrhagic or necrotizing pancreatitis. When open drainage is used, it is done with full awareness that hernias of the abdominal wall are created. Usually, the repair of these hernias is planned for a later date.

TYPES OF ABDOMINAL WALL HERNIA

Groin Hernias

Hernias may develop in any structure supporting the intra-abdominal contents. Most of these involve the anterior abdominal wall, and the vast majority occur in the inguinofemoral region. Among hernias occurring in the groin, the indirect inguinal variety is encountered most frequently (50% to 60%), with direct inguinal hernias representing 25% to 35% and femoral hernias comprising approximately 5% to 10%. Because of the frequency of groin hernias, an understanding of their anatomy, clinical presentation, and surgical management is important for any student of surgery.

Anatomy

The *indirect inguinal hernia* represents a fascial defect that lies lateral to the deep epigastric artery and originates in the internal inguinal ring (Fig. 64-1, *A*). It is at least 20 times as common in male as in female humans, and when it occurs in the male sex, it represents a retention or incomplete obliteration of the embryologic outpocketing of peritoneum, known as the *processus vaginalis,* that accompanies the testicle in its descent into the scrotum. Normally, the processus vaginalis is obliterated postnatally except for the portion that covers the testicle (the tunica vaginalis). If this obliterative process fails, an indirect inguinal hernia is evident at birth or in the months thereafter. Depending on the extent of this obliterative process, the resultant hernial sac tracks along varying lengths of the inguinal canal; if it extends completely into the scrotum, it is designated a *complete* indirect inguinal hernia. If the unobliterated processus vaginalis is not large enough to admit bowel but does allow peritoneal fluid to collect, a hydrocele may develop. In view of these considerations, it is not surprising that the peak incidence of indirect inguinal hernia recurrence is at birth or shortly thereafter. A second peak occurs in the teen years and in early adulthood. As previously discussed, stress from muscular activity and the accompanying increase in intra-abdominal pressure may give rise to an indirect inguinal hernia in this age group by forcing open a previously incompletely obliterated processus vaginalis. The role that congenital factors play in the pathogenesis of this hernia is further emphasized by the fact that it seldom develops after the age of 35. A patent processus vaginalis is probably responsible for the develop-

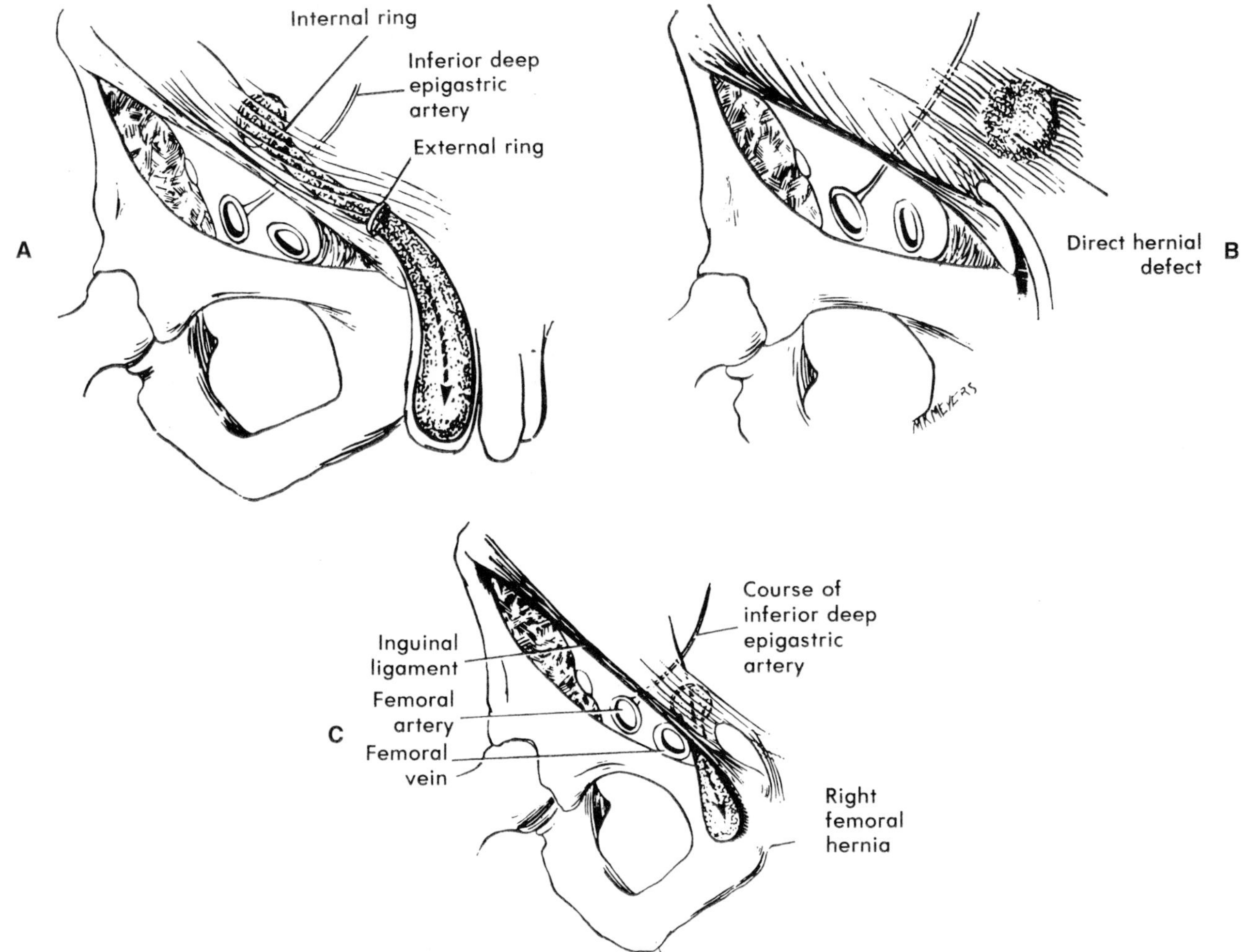

Fig. 64-1. **A,** Right indirect inguinal hernia. Hernial sac begins at the internal inguinal ring lateral to the inferior deep epigastric artery and exits from the inguinal canal at the external ring to descend into the scrotum. The sac lies anteromedial to the cord structures. **B,** Right direct inguinal hernia. Hernial sac arises in Hesselbach's triangle medial to the inferior deep epigastric artery and just above the pubic tubercle. It does not descend into the scrotum. **C,** Right femoral hernia. Hernial sac arises below the inguinal ligament and medial to the femoral vein. (From Soper RT. Abdominal hernia. In Liechty RD, Soper RT, eds. Synopsis of Surgery, 5th ed. St. Louis: Mosby, 1985.)

ment of indirect inguinal hernias in female patients as well. In this circumstance, however, it occurs as a result of the incomplete obliteration of the peritoneum as it descends through the canal of Nuck.

A *direct inguinal hernia* arises medial to the deep epigastric artery and somewhat inferior to the internal inguinal ring and represents a diffuse weakening of the transversalis fascia in a triangular space known as Hesselbach's triangle (see Fig. 64-1, *B*). This area is bounded laterally by the deep epigastric artery, medially by the lateral border of the rectus sheath, and inferiorly by the inguinal ligament. This type of hernia almost always occurs after 35 years of age. In contrast to an indirect inguinal hernia, in which the neck of the hernia may be narrow and incarceration is always a potential problem, the neck of the direct hernia is wide. Incarceration is usually not encountered. Further, direct hernias are seen almost exclusively in male patients.

A femoral hernia develops as a peritoneal outpouching that occurs through an enlarged femoral ring (see Fig. 64-1, *C*). This space represents the most medial compartment of the femoral canal, bounded below by the inguinal ligament, above by the pubic bone, and medially by the lacunar ligament. The sac of a femoral hernia is always medial to the femoral vein and may progress to the level of the foramen ovale. Because the neck of a femoral hernia is narrow, incarceration and strangulation are frequent. The incidence of femoral hernias in the female population is much greater than in the male population. The specific explanation for this discrepancy remains to be defined.

Clinical Presentation

The usual symptom that brings a patient to the physician's attention when a groin hernia is present is a bulge or a problem with pain, either of which may be persistent or intermittent. The pain associated with simple herniations depends on the contiguous structures either compressed or irritated by the presence of the hernia. The pain is usually localized, sharp, aggravated by change in position or straining, and relieved by cessation of the physical activity that precipitated it. When a hernia contains incarcerated or strangulated structures, the pain becomes persistent and is often associated with systemic signs or symptoms, such as elevated temperature, tachycardia, vomiting, and abdominal distention. If a segment of bowel is trapped in the hernia sac, the clinical presentation may be that of bowel obstruction. Occasionally, the hernia may be entirely asymptomatic and first noticed on a routine physical examination.

Groin hernias sometimes are extremely difficult to diagnose and at other times are quite apparent. The standard maneuver to diagnose a groin hernia is based on digital palpation of the floor of the inguinal canal. The patient should initially stand while visual inspection of the groin is conducted. The physician examines the external genitalia to check for any localized swellings along the spermatic cord on either side or for abnormalities in the testicle or scrotal contents. In a female patient, there may be palpable swelling noted on the same side as the patient's symptoms. In any case, ipsilateral swelling in a groin in which pain is apparent requires definite explanation, and the inference that a hernia is present becomes quite tenable.

When examining the floor of the inguinal canal in the male patient, there are three prerequisites for a complete examination: first, after invagination of the scrotal skin along the axis of the canal, the examiner palpates the fascial border or the external inguinal ring to direct the examining finger to the floor of the canal, where all inguinal hernias occur. The external ring is only a landmark to guide the examination in the appropriate region; its size or consistency has nothing to do with the hernia itself. On identification of this ring, digital palpation of the floor of the canal and the overlying spermatic cord are next performed to ascertain any apparent weakness. A weakness or mass in the region of the external ring is usually indicative of a direct hernia. Finally, examination of the internal ring itself is performed. The area of the internal ring is first palpated; then, the examiner asks the patient to strain for 5 to 10 seconds to increase intra-abdominal pressure while at the same time the examining finger is withdrawn 1 cm. The patient is asked to give a gentle cough. A positive response is a palpable "tap" against the fingertip (suggestive of an indirect hernia) or along the medial side of the finger (indicative of a direct hernia), caused as the distended hernia sac transmits the cough-induced increase in pressure. Alternatively, a "gurgle" of peritoneal fluid may be appreciated passing beneath the examining finger. At times, the positive response entails reproduction of the patient's pain; this latter situation, however, demands careful interpretation to exclude other possibilities, as discussed later in this chapter.

If the patient has undergone a previous inguinal hernia repair, the same principles of examination are followed. When such a patient reports pain during the examination, the differential diagnosis may include ilioinguinal nerve entrapment or neuroma of a severed previously branch of the nerve. In situations in which the patient reports a typical pain syndrome but results of the physical examination are negative, I recommend a waiting period, during which the patient is reexamined at monthly intervals. If the pain persists despite exclusion of other causes, surgical exploration of the groin can be justified even though the examiner has no absolute evidence that a hernia exists. A patient must have realistic expectations of results after such surgical intervention, however, and should be informed that, although most patients do well after surgery, some have persistent postoperative discomfort. In my experience, there have been occasional patients, usually one every year or two (0.1% to 0.3% of those with groin hernias), who report a typical pain syndrome but have no definite hernia on physical examination. After several negative examination results, the patient comes in with an ultimatum from his employer that he return to work immediately or face the loss of his job and accrued benefits. Often malingering or latent personality disorder is considered more likely than is occult hernia, and such a diagnosis is inappropirately assigned. When following the principles described, I have been gratified by the response of such individuals to surgical exploration and have *always* found a definite explanation for the reported symptoms when a localized area of tenderness in the groin was present. Either a small indirect hernia or a patulous internal ring has been the usual explanation for the pain.

In contrast to most inguinal hernias, which can be diagnosed with a minimum of difficulty, the femoral hernia is often a diagnostic challenge. Usually, it appears as a subtle mass lesion in the inguinal crease, somewhat medial to the femoral artery. It is extremely important that the examiner realize that the mass lesion may be quite small (≤1 cm in diameter) and that in obese individuals or those with edematous overlying skin, the hernia may be clinically occult. In such situations the general condition of the patient must serve as a guide for the specific management plan undertaken. Patients with an unexplained acute onset of local pain in the femoral region and/or an unexplained mass or tenderness suggestive of an increased hernia should undergo prompt surgical exploration. Inattention of such findings could put the patient at extreme risk for incarceration of ischemic bowel and the devastating complications arising therefrom.

The only laboratory test worth consideration in the diagnosis of inguinofemoral hernias is peritoneography (herniography). This test involves the intraperitoneal injection of contrast material and trapping of that material in an inguinal defect. In performing this technique, I have used Gullmo's approach, which consists of the intraperitoneal injection of 50 to 60 ml of radiographic soluble contrast material after instillation of diluted lidocaine (Xylocaine).[12] There is no question that this procedure has great potential for the discovery and definition of hernias that may not be clearly identifiable clinically, but it cannot be performed casually and requires the expertise of an interested and committed radiologist experienced in the subtleties of interpretation to give useful information. This test is used so infrequently, however, that decisions to operate are usually not greatly influenced by it.

Surgical Management

Once present, hernias in the groin do not resolve spontaneously. Therefore, with few exceptions (e.g., terminal malignant disease), they should be repaired surgically to prevent such complications as incarceration and strangulation. The illuminating work of Condon[19] has defined several important aspects of the anatomy of the groin that are germane to repair of hernias in this area of the abdominal wall (Fig. 64-2). The precise definitions of the terms *fascia* and *aponeurosis* are especially applicable in this context, as is the precise use of the designation *ligament*. A *fascia* is a condensation of connective tissue into a definable, homogeneous layer, which may vary from a thin layer to an easily observed stout structure. An *aponeurosis* is a tendinous insertion of a major muscle composed of strong individual collagenous fiber bundles. *Ligament* is a term applied to any definable tissue "banding" two or more structures, whether bony or visceral, and may refer to structures of either areolar or aponeurotic consistency.

When referring to a groin hernia, one must be careful not to confuse the transversus abdominus aponeurosis with the transversalis fascia. The latter designation is incorrectly applied at times to the transversus abdominus muscle and the transversus abdominus aponeurosis. The transversalis fascia in and of itself is of varying density and possesses little intrinsic strength. It usually represents the first anatomic boundary to visceral structures as they herniate through the abdominal wall, but by itself it cannot form the basis of groin hernia repairs. Instead, all herniated structures must first be restored to their anatomic position behind and deep to the transversalis fascia, and repair of the hernia defect must be performed by suturing neighboring tendinous aponeuroses and ligaments that can hold sutures properly.[19]

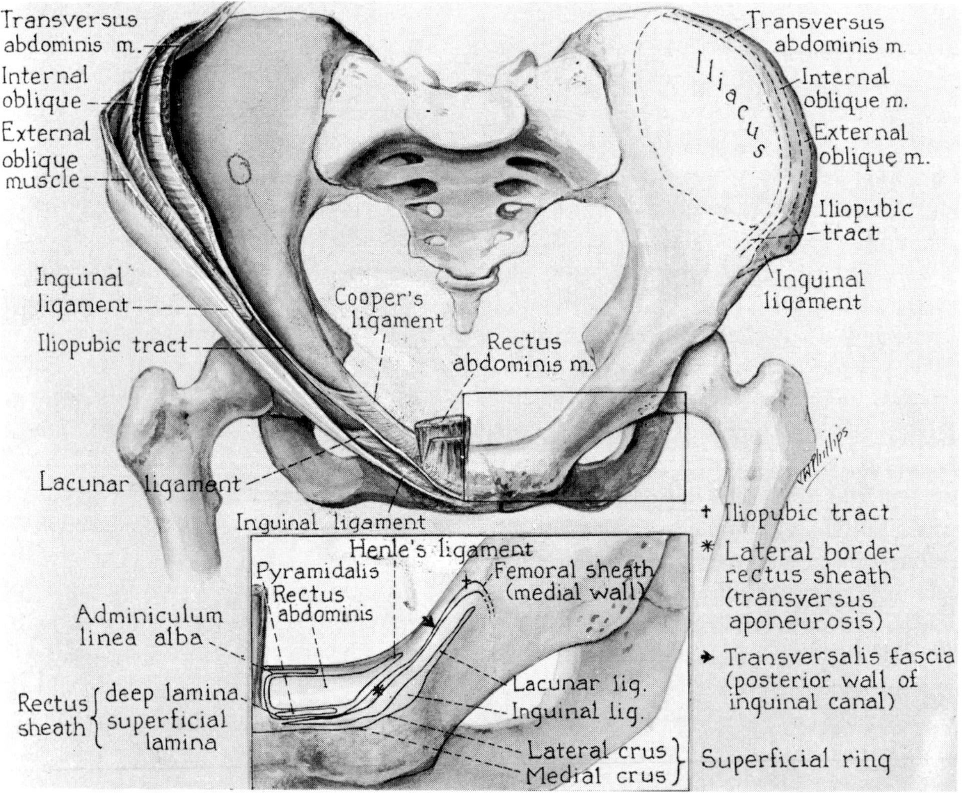

Fig. 64-2. Left pelvis: Origins of the three flat muscles are shown. The oblique and transversus muscles arise from the iliacus fascia and iliopectineal arch (not shown). Inset shows the insertions of the muscle layers of the groin into the pubis. Right pelvis: Internal oblique is not shown, but would arch above the spermatic cord to insert into the rectus sheath. (From Condon RE. Anatomy of the inguinal region and its relation to groin hernia. In Nyhus LM, Condon RE, eds. Hernia, 2nd ed. Philadelphia: JB Lippincott, 1978.)

The repair of all common groin hernias is designed to permanently eliminate the defect in the abdominal wall by means of sutures placed into the solid structures that line the defect. The aponeurosis of the external oblique muscle inserts at the pubic tubercle and has a flattened medial portion that is recurved beneath the floor of the inguinal canal. The relationship of the inguinal ligament to the fascia of the tranversus abdominus muscle is that of a contiguous, but quite separate, structure. The lacunar ligament, a structure that extends from the posterior border of the inguinal ligament to the pectineal fascia (1 cm below the pectin) is separate and superficial to the ileopubic tract. One must be aware of this relationship, because the rationale for modern hernia repair involves the reconstruction of separate layers of the abdominal wall, with an attempt to preserve the "shutter" mechanism produced by the different layers of the abdominal wall. This shutter mechanism consists of structures moving simultaneously in different planes and is analogous to the shutter on a camera; the planes of motion occur within the internal oblique and transversus abdominus layers of the abdominal wall.[20] Conventional herniorrhaphy does not result in a functional shutter mechanism unless the principles of anatomic repair of the hernia are followed; that is, the dynamic components of the shutter are compression of the potential hernial defect by traction of the superior and inferior crura of the internal inguinal ring. This contraction of the transversus muscle results in narrowing of the internal ring and lateral traction on the spermatic cord. The shutter mechanism thus affords continuous protection for the two most vulnerable areas of the groin—the area where direct hernias exit through Hesselbach's triangle and the inguinal canal through which "oblique" herniation occurs, beginning at the internal inguinal ring.

The components of adequate groin herniorrhaphy are knowledge of the anatomic structures involved, precise identification of these structures by surgical dissection, meticulous repair of the defect in the transversus-transversalis plane, and measures to reduce tension on suture lines where appropriate. These principles are true for direct and indirect inguinal hernias and also for femoral hernias.

Anterior repair

Inguinal hernias. Although multiple procedures (e.g., Bassini, Halstead, McVay, Shouldice, the details of which can be obtained in standard textbooks of hernia repair[21]) have been recommended to repair inguinal hernias and each has its advocates, I am a "regionalist," preferring to view the entire transversus-transversalis area as a single entity and therefore using the same basic approach to repair any hernial defect in this most important layer. The most essential technical aspect of repair is the creation of a tension-free union between the arching transversalis abdominus aponeurosis and its adherent transversalis fascia above and the ileopubic tract below. This repair is readily achieved if meticulous dissection has defined the floor of the inguinal canal and the structures in question. For both direct and indirect inguinal hernias, the repair is carried out through a transverse skin incision positioned approximately 2 cm above and parallel to the inguinal ligament, to prevent injury to the iliohypogastric and ilioinguinal nerves (Fig. 64-3).

For hernias lateral to the inferior epigastric vessels (indirect inguinal hernias), repair primarily involves obliteration of the communication that exists between the peritoneal cavity and the hernial sac. Thus, the sac is carefully dissected free from its fibroareolar connections and ligated at its base so that the ligation is flush with the internal inguinal ring, and any sac distal to this ligation is resected (Fig. 64-4). In infants and children, high ligation of the sac is usually all that is required; in older children and adults, some reconstruction of the musculoaponeurotic structures is generally needed in addition to sac division and ligation to tighten the internal inguinal ring around the cord structures. Occasionally an indirect inguinal hernia is encountered that has been present for many years and has enlarged to such an extent that a good portion of the supporting structure medial to the internal ring has been destroyed. In this situation, a more extensive aponeurotic fascial repair is required, according to the principles described here for the repair of a direct inguinal hernia.

In the repair of a direct inguinal hernia or of a deficient posterior wall of the inguinal canal in a patient with a large indirect inguinal hernia, the cremaster fibers surrounding the spermatic cord must be circumferentially removed at the internal inguinal ring.[22] When this has been accomplished, fatty and areolar tissues are excised from the inferior aspect of the canal to bare the shelving portion of the inguinal ligament and the iliopubic tract. Through careful dissection, the attentuated floor of the inguinal canal is excised, the hernial sac is simply reduced (no need for resection as with the indirect inguinal hernia), and the defect in the floor is repaired by suturing the transversus-transversalis complex above to the ileopubic tract below

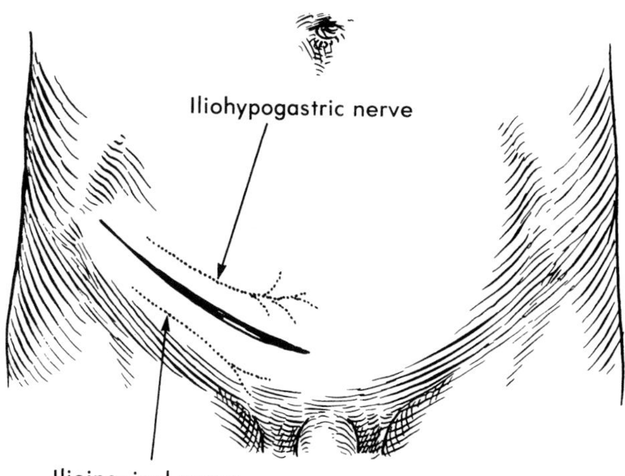

Fig. 64-3. Skin incision is made approximately 2 cm above the inguinal ligament in a gentle curve following Langer's lines. (From Ponka JL. Hernias of the Abdominal Wall. Philadelphia: WB Saunders, 1980.)

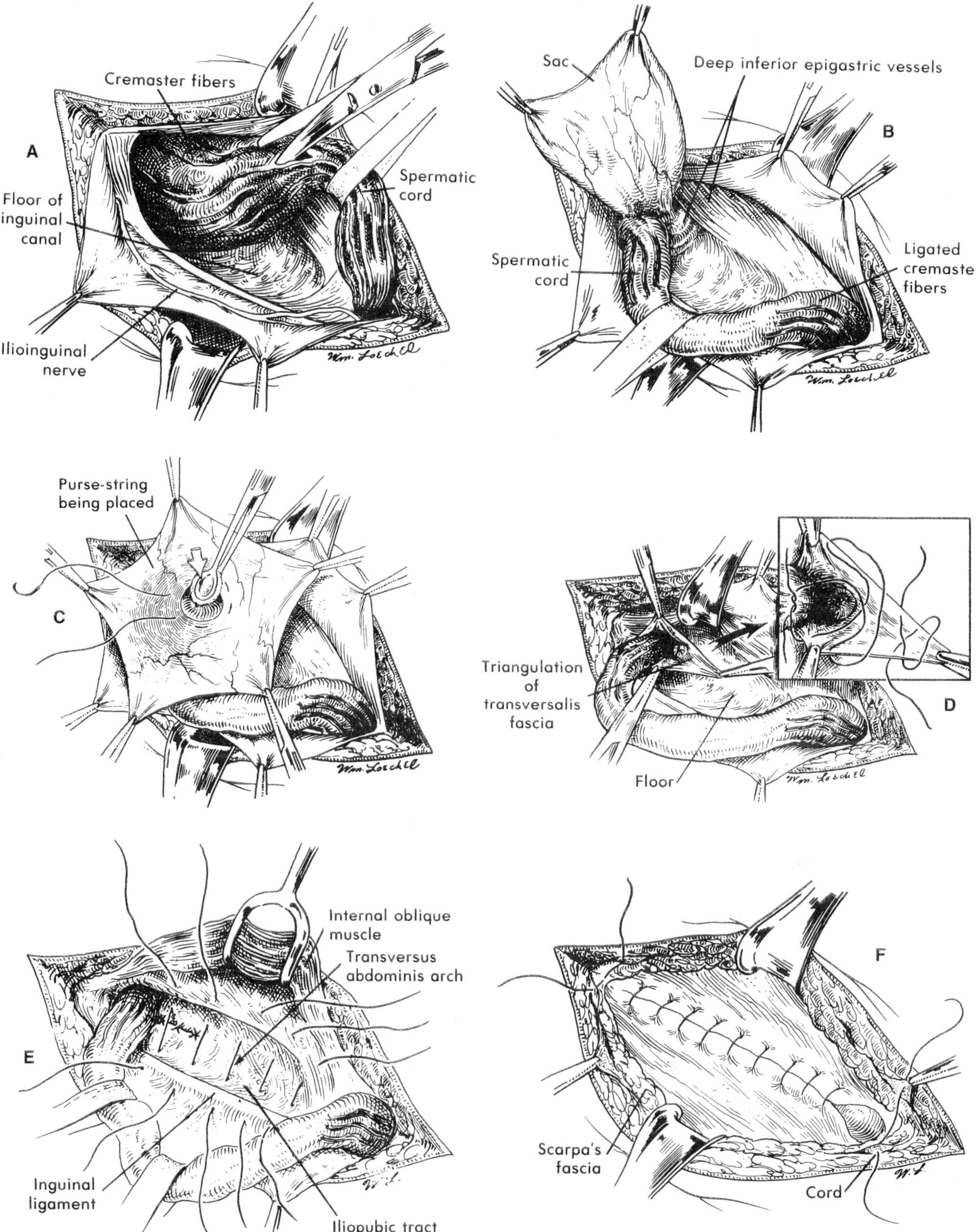

Fig. 64-4. For legend, see opposite page.

(Fig. 64-5), with interrupted nonabsorbable sutures. If only a direct hernial defect is present, the internal ring is not completely displayed. In all instances, however, the cremaster muscle is completely excised from the posterior inguinal wall and the spermatic cord is dissected to identify the obliterated vaginal process at the internal ring. Only by so doing can the risk of a "missed" indirect hernia be eliminated.

Because the suture repair of any large defect in the posterior inguinal wall places undue tension on the superior portion of the repair, there has been a long interest in maneuvers to reduce the abnormal stress resulting from such surgery. The Tanner "slide" procedure is one of the best known early attempts at relieving this stress through the creation of a relaxing incision.[23] Tanner[23] correctly recognized that an incision along the internal oblique portion of the anterior rectus sheath would allow the lateral portion of this sheath and its attached transversus arch to slide inferolaterally to close a large inguinal hernial defect. The necessity for such a relaxing incision is fully recognized and accepted in modern hernia surgery and forms an integral part of all direct and large indirect inguinal hernia repairs (Fig. 64-6). McVay[24] beautifully illustrated the importance of the relaxing incision and further showed that the pyramidalis muscle can conceal aponeurotic transversus fibers that unrecognized would lead to failure of the relaxing incision to perform its function. Usually, the relaxing incision is made before the sutures that have been placed to effect the hernial repair are tied.

Occasionally, the size of a direct inguinal hernia prohibits effective repair with a patient's own local tissue and necessitates the use of some biologic or synthetic substance. Among the biologic substances available, fascia lata grafts have been most popular. Among the synthetic ma-

Fig. 64-4. A, Steps in the repair of a right indirect inguinal hernia. The external oblique aponeurosis has been opened. The cord is freed from the inguinal floor. The freed ilioinguinal nerve is seen overlying the retracted lower leaflet of the external oblique aponeurosis. The cremaster muscle is being dissected free of the cord. **B,** Peritoneal sac must be dissected free of the cord and the abdominal wall at the internal abdominal ring. **C,** Technical detail of high ligation of the sac is important in an orderly repair. The peritoneum must be freed of omentum, and adherent viscera must be detached. Appendices epiploicae or omentum must not be caught in the closure. **D,** Components of the transversus abdominis lamina must be accurately identified and closed at the internal ring. Triangulation of the transversalis fascia (shown here) is a useful detail to help achieve accurate closure at the internal ring. **E,** Transversus abdominis arch is sutured to the iliopubic tract and inguinal ligament. **F,** External oblique aponeurosis is closed over the spermatic cord. Slight imbrication of this structure gives an excellent closure. Scarpa's fascia is then closed with interrupted sutures of 3-0 plain catgut, and the skin edges approximated with sutures or sterile strips. (A and F from Ponka JL. Hernias of the Abdominal Wall. Philadelphia: WB Saunders, 1980.)

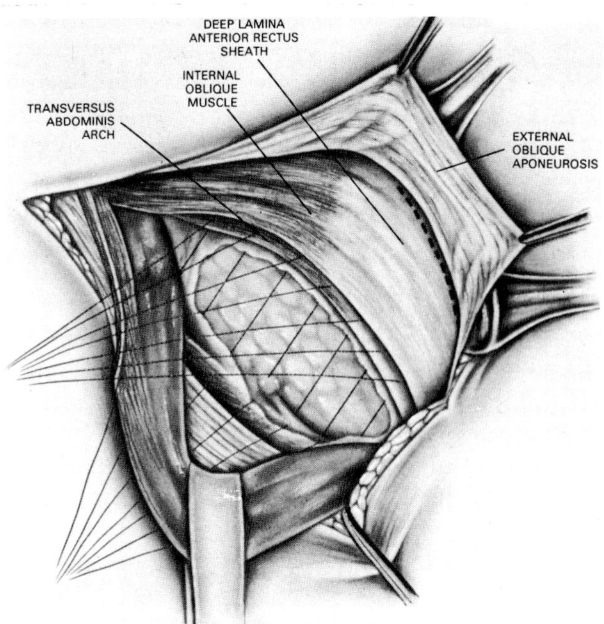

Fig. 64-5. External oblique aponeurosis (superficial lamina of rectus sheath) has been dissected medially and superiorly to its line of fusion with rectus sheath. Placement of a relaxing incision in the deep lamina of rectus sheath (transversus abdominis and internal oblique aponeurosis) is shown by dotted line. (From Condon RE. Anterior iliopubic tract repair. In Nyhus LM, Condon RE, eds. Hernia, 2nd ed. Philadelphia: JB Lippincott, 1978.)

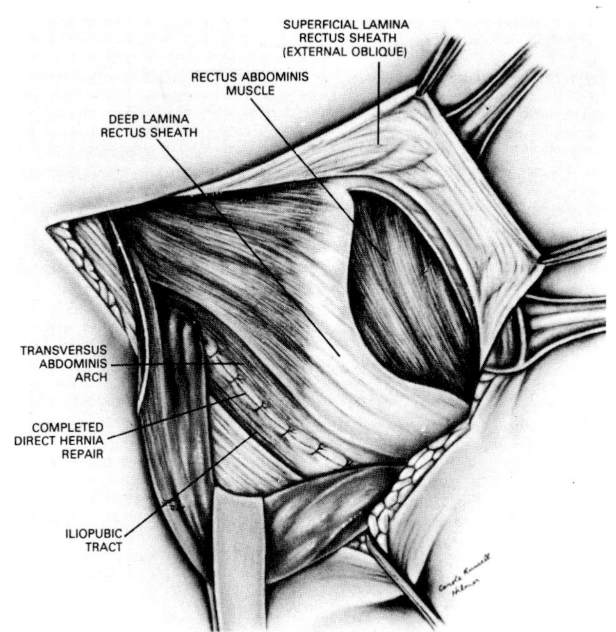

Fig. 64-6. Completed direct hernia repair demonstrates that the relaxing incision allows the transversus abdominis to slide inferiorly. As the relaxing incision opens, the rectus muscle is exposed, but the overlying intact superficial lamina (external oblique aponeurosis) of the rectus sheath supports the muscle externally while the intact fascia posteriorly shields the potential hernial defect. (From Condon RE. Anterior iliopubic tract repair. In Nyhus LM, Condon RE, eds. Hernia, 2nd ed. Philadelphia: JB Lippincott, 1978.)

terials, polypropylene (Marlex) and polyethylene terephthalate fiber (Dacron) mesh grafts have been most extensively used.[25,26] These materials have been used either to bridge the hernial defect itself by suturing the substance to the fascia lining the hernial ring or as a buttress to enhance a primary repair. Some surgeons even use synthetic meshes to repair all hernias; however, most authorities believe that this is unnecessary, and that primary repair using the patient's own tissues is most appropriate when it can be successfully accomplished.

Femoral hernias. Although femoral hernias are less commonly encountered than are inguinal hernias, surgical repair is also the treatment of choice. The principles underlying inguinal hernia repair also apply to femoral hernias. Usually, the same type of skin incision is used. The sac, once identified, is emptied of its hernial contents, divided, and ligated at its neck, and the entrance into the femoral canal giving rise to this entity is obliterated. This can be accomplished by attaching the transversus-transversalis complex to Cooper's ligament to close off the empty space in the femoral canal.

Posterior repair. The idea of approaching the transversalis-transversus layer posteriorly (Fig. 64-7) has been suggested as an adequate means of repairing some types of groin hernias during the past 60 years but has been particularly strongly advocated by Nyhus and others in recent years.[1,26] When properly applied, this technique is extremely useful in the repair of three major types of hernia: (1) recurrent inguinal hernias, (2) primary femoral hernias, and (3) incarcerated hernias of all types.

It is not surprising that surgeons who are unfamiliar with the posterior approach sometimes have difficulty in achieving exposure of the proper tissue planes. For this reason, it is imperative that anyone interested in gaining technical expertise with this approach first watch an experienced surgeon perform this type of repair, also referred to as the *preperitoneal repair.* In this operation, there is no substitute for experience in defining the sometimes subtle transversalis fascia layer.

As with anterior approaches to groin hernia repair, the skin incision should be placed transversally above and parallel to the internal inguinal ligament. After the incision to the level of the rectus sheath is deepened, the anterior fascia layer of this sheath is incised and the rectus muscle is retracted toward the midline. The exposed transversalis fascia is then incised to gain access to the preperitoneal space; this space always has a variable amount of fat present. The appearance of fatty tissue is the signal that the proper plane has been entered; at this point, the incision through the abdominal musculature is widened toward the anterior iliac spine to pass about 2 cm above the internal inguinal ring. When this has been accomplished, the posterior inguinal wall is bared of fatty and areolar tissue from the line of the incision to the superior pubic ramus. If deep epigastric vessels obscure proper exposure, they can be ligated and divided as needed.

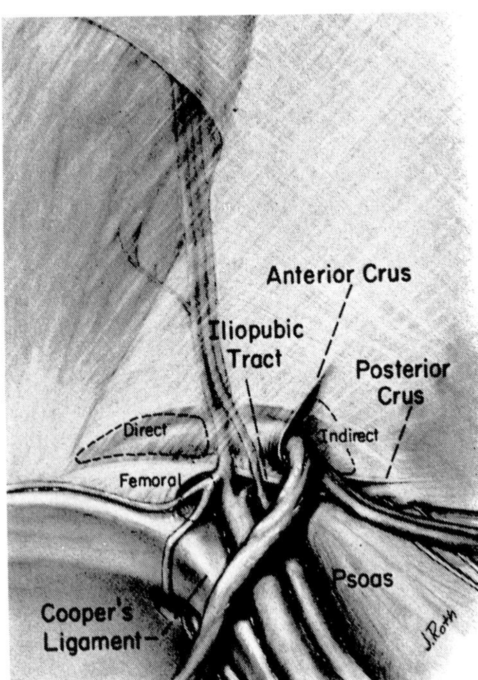

Fig. 64-7. The preperitoneal exposure of the posterior inguinal wall displays the important structures that form the boundaries of groin hernias. Repair of hernial defect(s) is readily accomplished by suture after preliminary reduction of the hernia. If an indirect hernia sac extends into the scrotum, it is not necessary that the entire distal sac be removed. Note that application of mesh is quite easy, since the posterior wall is completely exposed. (From Nyhus LM. The preperitoneal approach and iliopubic tract repair of inguinal hernia. In Nyhus LM, Condon RE, eds. Hernia, 2nd ed. Philadelphia: JB Lippincott, 1978.)

After the posterior inguinal wall has been exposed, the herniated structures are identified and reduced. If there is an incarcerated hernia, it is prudent (and easy) to inspect all portions of incarcerated bowel for signs of ischemia or infarction. If there is any doubt concerning these possibilities, the surgeon observes the tissues in question until a decision regarding whether to resect can be made. After the walls of the hernial defect have been identified, the repair is fashioned to approximate the margins of the defect with interrupted sutures of permanent material. As with the anterior approach to hernia repair, the spermatic cord must also be examined to ensure that an additional oblique hernia is not present.

The posterior approach is strongly recommended for the repair of a recurrent hernia because it provides an opportunity to perform the operation in tissue not previously operated on, a distinct advantage over any anterior approach. The only difference between posterior repair of a recurrent hernia and that of other types of hernia is that a synthetic mesh buttress should be sutured to the posterior wall after repair of the hernia defect, to reduce the possibility of another recurrence (Fig. 64-8).

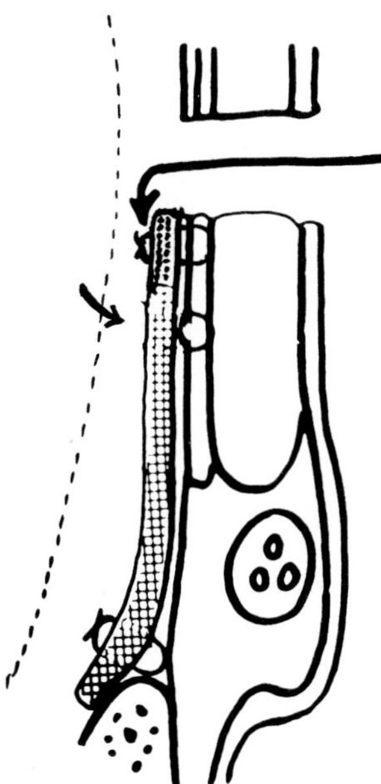

Fig. 64-8. Large arrow illustrates the approach to the preperitoneal space, above the inguinal canal. Small arrow shows the preliminary repair of the hernia defect before insertion of the "regional" prosthetic reinforcement that extends from the primary incision to the pubic ramus and from the midline to lateral of the internal ring.

Laparoscopic approaches to hernia repair. Laparoscopic hernia repair, which evolved rapidly after the first demonstration of the feasibility of this approach in the early 1980s, is now being widely performed in many hospitals. The earlier success of posterior approaches to hernia repair, incorporating the concepts of tension-free repair as propounded by Lichtenstein et al.,[20] Stoppa,[26] and Condon[19] set the stage for the rapid developments and growth in popularity of this approach.

At the time of this writing, it is not clear whether early recurrence rates after laparoscopic hernia repair are comparable, better, or worse than those observed after open herniorrhaphy. The interested reader can find articles supporting all of these conclusions in any medical library; proponents claim that most patients treated laparoscopically are happy, whereas detractors point to some of the problems or complications in support of their negative view. What is clear is that there are some unique risks after laparoscopic hernia repair, and that it will be several decades before we have conclusive data regarding long-term outcomes.[27]

Several innovative approaches have been attempted in laboratory and clinical settings: plugs, double patches, intraperitoneal onlay of mesh (IPOM), preperitoneal patches, self-expanding patches, and still others. All are variations on the theme of the current best approaches regarding hernia repair elucidated here. In 1995, the important components of these repairs are that they be tension-free and reinforced with synthetic mesh (Figs. 64-9 through 64-11). Several approahces are not widely used; for example, the earlier use of mesh plugs has not gained wide acceptance because the mesh plugs were sometimes a palpable reminder (cause?) of pain and discomfort. Other techniques, such as IPOM, appeared satisfactory in both laboratory and clinical settings when first introduced but have caused concern in later reports. The major concerns with IPOM are complications that may have been caused by the mesh, such as severe adhesions or inflammatory masses with abscess. Other concerns, such as an increased recurrence rate compared with other laparoscopic techniques, have also arisen.

The most attractive approach from the minimally invasive perspective is the totally preperitoneal approach, incorporating the same repair strategy with one exception, gaining access without entering the peritoneal cavity. This approach is somewhat more difficult initially but avoids most of the concerns associated with transperitoneal approaches. It is hard to predict whether this approach will find general favor with surgeons because of technical difficulties.

Laparoscopy puts the patient at some risk for injury to small intestine, either immediately during the operation or as a late complication caused by the contiguous synthetic mesh materials employed in the hernia repair. All of the mesh materials may cause adhesion formation or lead to irritation of adjoining organs, similar to that observed after insertion of such artificial agents in abdominal wall repairs. Additional injuries have been rarely noted in other structures, including hollow organs (vas deferens, urinary bladder, colon), nerves (ilioinguinal, genitofemoral, lateral femoral cutaneous, and femoral), and vessels (iliac artery and vein, femoral artery and vein). Although operative injuries are more frequent after laparoscopic procedures that after open operations, the advantage of an earlier return to work is appreciated by many patients. Many patients who have undergone both approaches favor the use of minimally invasive means. The earleir return to full activity with minimal pain is compelling for modern patients and will be a potent force in favor of this approach, despite the increased cost of performing herniorrhaphy by this means; every study to date has shown that laparoscopic hernia repairs take longer and cost more than do conventional repairs.[21,28] The economics of minimally invasive surgery are relatively straightforward: the use of endoscopes and special instruments makes for a more expensive operation. Costs are reduced if disposable instruments are not used and if the team is experienced and highly motivated.

Which minimally invasive approach to hernia will eventually become the most desired cannot be predicted at this time. It is clear that such approaches carry unique risks, and that some of the problems with laparoscopic procedures are as yet unknown. Long-term follow-up and analysis of these problems will clarify the issue for a worldwide group of interested surgeons and patients.

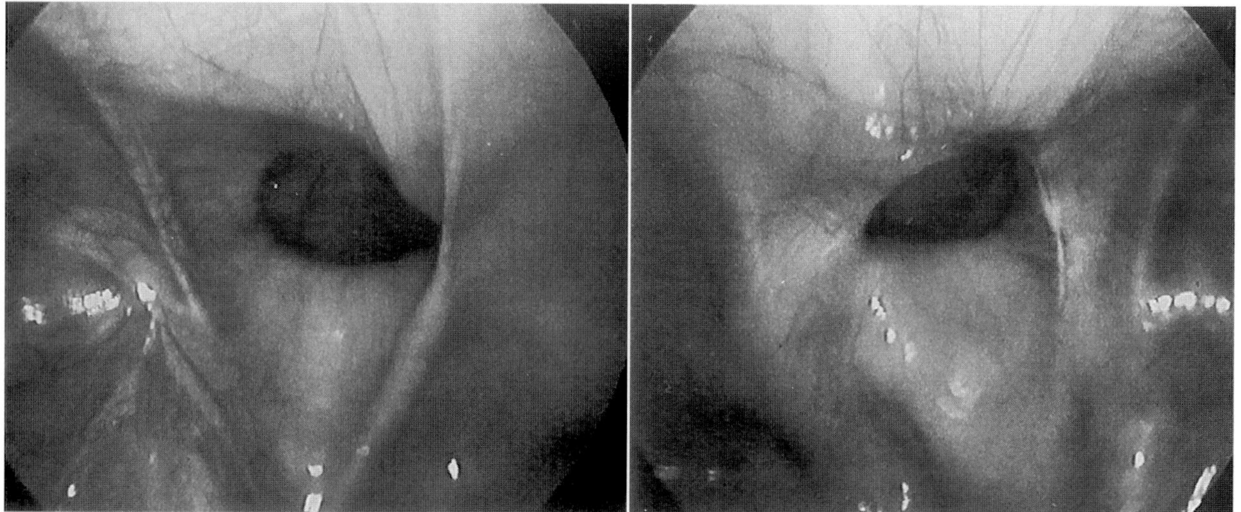

Fig. 64-9. Laparoscopic view illustrates the major advantages of this approach: the vas deferens, testicular vessels, and surrounding structures are seen with clarity and definition, which is not possible by other means.

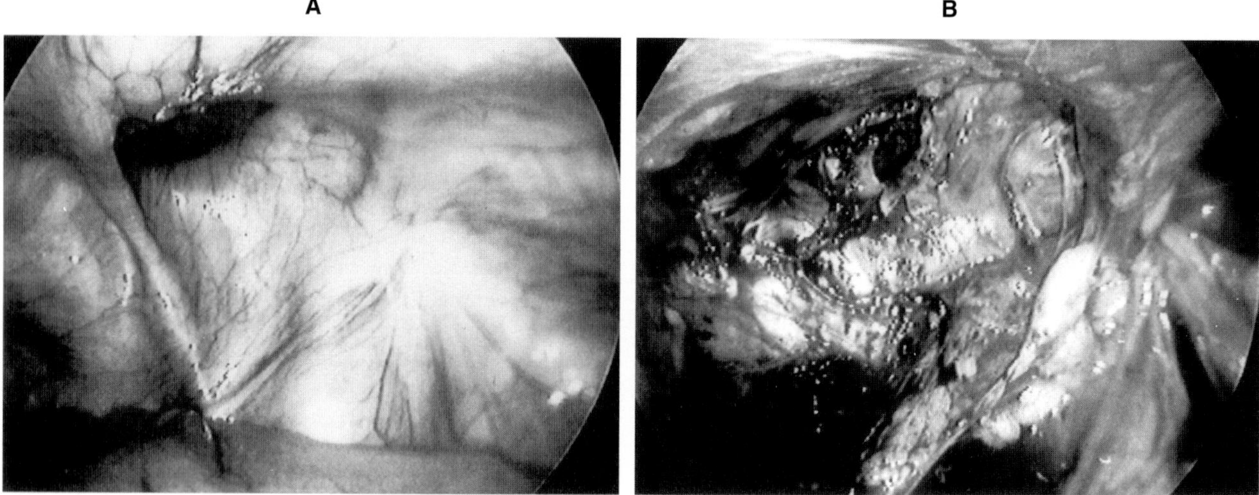

Fig. 64-10. A, View from the peritoneum reveals a right indirect inguinal hernia. After exposure of the collagenous supports, which will serve as an anchor for the prosthetic mesh, it is easy to plan a safe and effective repair of the defect. The tension-free approach will be used, with fixation only to the pubic ramus and the superior aspect of the transversus arch. **B,** Landmarks that must be clearly identified include Cooper's ligament, the spermatic vessels and vas deferens, and the iliopubic tract.

Complications. Many problems may develop after inguinofemoral herniorrhaphy. The box on p. 1307 lists local and regional complications that may occur. In addition, the surgeon must always be aware of the systemic complications that may attend a groin herniorrhaphy, such as those arising from the anesthetic technique used or from an underlying associated disease, such as that involving the heart or lungs. As with any operation, deaths do at times occur, but these are quite rare and usually associated with an underlying cardiovascular problem.

Several complications related to the hernia repair itself need to be considered. One problem that is not uncommonly encountered in male patients undergoing groin hernia repair is that of a postoperative swollen testis. Swelling may arise from venous engorgement or lymphatic congestion related to the repair itself, from compromise to the arterial blood flow as a result of intraoperative trauma, from a subfascial hematoma, or from a missed hernia (such as an indirect inguinal hernia not noticed when a direct hernia was being repaired). In these trou-

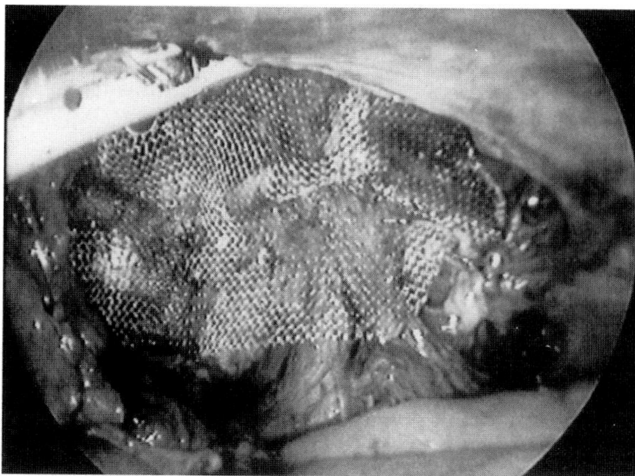

Fig. 64-11. The essential concept governing mesh placement is that the mesh should be large enough to cover all potential hernia sites. The anchoring of the mesh is probably less important than previously thought, since the mesh will be held firmly by inflammatory adhesions postoperatively. When sutures or staples are used, none are placed inferior to the iliopubic tract and the lateral aspect of the internal ring is avoided. Staples placed in the iliopubic tract lateral to the internal ring may jeopardize branches of the femoral nerve.

bling cases, management is usually guided by evaluating the overall clinical picture for a time. The condition usually resolves after 4 to 12 weeks, and the patient needs only the mature guidance of the surgeon during this interval to allay any fears that he may have. In those situations in which the blood supply to the testicle has been compromised, late atrophy of the testis will be noted; this complication is not rare, but the true incidence is hard to determine because of limited follow-up studies in most reported series of patients undergoing groin herniorrhaphy. Occasionally, an acute postoperative infarction of the testicle necessitates immediate surgical intervention and orchiectomy.

Occasionally, a patient has a persistent pain after groin herniorrhaphy (see accompanying box). The great majority of patients have rapidly subsiding pain that is usually manageable by the second postoperative week. By 3 to 4 weeks after the postoperation, there is only a residual tenderness to deep palpation, and by 3 to 4 months there are no symptoms referable to the operation. Occasional patients have persistent pain that can be quite troublesome and that can prove difficult to assess and treat successfully. The physical examination is useful, because it gives precise information about possible sources of the pain. For example, if the testicle is swollen or inflamed or if the epididymis is quite tender, a genitourinary infection might be suspected. Alternatively, the floor of the inguinal canal may be painless whereas the pubic tubercle area is exquisitely tender, indicating periostitis of the pubic bone where a suture was placed to effect adequate repair. In all cases, I avoid any specific intervention until at least 3 to 4 months have passed. This allows the acute perioperative reaction to subside, because most subjective reports of pain occur during this interval.

In patients with persistent pain, point tenderness along the floor of the inguinal canal (but not at the internal ring) suggests the possibility of a neuroma. In this circumstance, an injection of 2 to 3 ml 1% lidocaine (Xylocaine) can be made at the point of tenderness to determine whether the groin discomfort disappears. If such a response occurs, the site can be reinjected with a mixture of cortisone and lidocaine into the "trigger" point. Most patients respond to this type of treatment with a clear decrease in symptoms and do not require any further treatment. If such management is unsuccessful, surgical excision of the superficial scar tissue and nerve tissue is indicated, with care to include cut nerve endings within the ligated tissue. When neuromas occur during groin hernia surgery, they are usually a consequence of injury to the ilioinguinal or iliohypogastric nerves.

Nerve injury after laparoscopic repair. Laparoscopic hernia repairs provide unique risks for nerve injury because of the proximity of important nerves to the mesh, sutures, or staples used in repair. The femoral nerve, lateral femoral

LOCAL OR REGIONAL COMPLICATIONS AFTER REPAIR OF GROIN HERNIAS

Acute

Wound infection/hematoma
Ilioinguinal/iliohypogastric nerve injury
Preperitoneal hemorrhage
Femoral vein/artery laceration or trauma
Thrombosis femoral vein/pulmonary embolus
Transection of vas deferens
Ligation of spermatic artery
Perforation of viscus (sliding hernia)
Nonclosure of internal ring
Loss of domain of erstwhile incarcerated structures
Scrotal ecchymosis/hematoma
Swollen testis
Missed hernia
Urinary retention

Chronic

Recurrent hernia
Hernia in a contiguous area
Late wound/suture sepsis (>5 to 10 years later)
Neuroma
Testicular atrophy
Hydrocele
Pseudoaneurysm of femoral artery
Groin pain
Loss of cremasteric reflex
Periostitis of pubis
Sexual dysfunction

cutaneous nerve, genital branch of genitofemoral nerve, and ilioinguinal nerves have all been reported to be injured during such operations. Caution in staple or mesh placement minimizes the risk of these complications but cannot prevent all postoperative problems.

Hernia recurrence. The most important complication directly relating to the repair itself is that of hernia recurrence. Because of the mobility of our society and the consequent difficulty of following patients up for the long term, the actual incidence of recurrence is probably not known. Most series suggest that this incidence is somewhere between 2% and 10%. In a 22-year analysis of inguinal and femoral hernias repaired by Halverson and McVay[29] and by McVay and Chapp,[30] a 3.2% recurrence rate in more than 1200 cases was noted. Almost 40% of the recurrences occurred later than 5 years after the initial operation, illustrating the constraints of short evaluation periods. The best results ever reported in terms of recurrence rates are those from the Shouldice Clinic.[22,31] The Shouldice repair is performed through an anterior incision and includes maneuvers to ensure adequate exposure of the internal inguinal ring, followed by an overlapping repair of the floor of the inguinal canal. The principles of this repair are narrowing of the internal ring and a multilayer reinforcement of the transversalis fascial layer. This repair is made without relaxing incisions and without the need for prosthetic mesh insertion. Several authors have reported recurrence rates of less than 1% with this technique, whether primary or recurrent hernias were being treated. Whether other surgeons using this technique but not reporting their results are having the same degree of success remains unknown. Thus, when results from different clinics are evaluated, apparent differences may not be borne out on critical statistical analysis. For this reason, it is difficult to be sure which operation is "the best."

Umbilical Hernia

Umbilical hernias occur where the umbilical ring has failed to obliterate the opening of the allantoic duct. Most of these hernias are congenital in origin, and they are particularly common in African-American infants. Most close spontaneously by 4 to 6 years, and they almost never become incarcerated or strangulated. For this reason, infant congenital umbilical hernias rarely require surgical closure. Exceptions to this stance include hernias that are symptomatic; those in which the umbilical ring is excessively large, so that external trauma poses a threat; and those that have demonstrated no significant closure by 6 years.

Umbilical hernias may also develop in adults. When they occur in this population, a number of predisposing factors appear to give rise to their development, including abdominal distention related to massive ascites from underlying disease such as Laënnec's cirrhosis, induced ascites such as occurs in patients undergoing long-term ambulatory peritoneal dialysis, pregnancy, and obesity, and, in some situations, abnormal or defective collagen synthesis related to nutritional deficiencies or advancing age.[15] Because many of these hernias have a small neck, the risk of incarceration and strangulation remains a continuing threat. Thus, most of these hernias should be surgically repaired. Repair can be easily accomplished through an infraumbilical or supraumbilical skin incision in which the sac is removed and the fascial edges surrounding the hernial defect are directly approximated with nonabsorbable sutures.

Hernias of the Linea Alba

In addition to the umbilical hernia, a number of other hernial defects may involve the linea alba. These hernias usually occur between the xiphoid process and the umbilicus, in which case they are termed *epigastric hernias;* occasionally, they appear below the umbilicus. Hernias of the linea alba are usually small, are often multiple, and typically contain preperitoneal fat. Their clinical presentation is often deceptive, and they may be apparent only as pinpoint convexities overlying the erect patient's linea alba. If results of the physical examination are negative but the patient reports persistent pain in this anatomic region, surgical exploration may be required to provide a definite diagnosis. The most cogent explanation at present for the development of these hernias is provided by anatomic studies of the linea alba. This structure, a complex network of three musculoaponeurotic components of the rectus sheath,[32] varies considerably in inherent strength. There are at least three recognizable patterns of decussation of these fibers in the midline, all of which may be aggravated by marked distention of the abdominal wall. In addition, there are discrete areas midway between the xiphoid process and umbilicus that are subjected to repetitive stresses by phrenic aponeurotic bands that insert in the midline fascia; perhaps these latter structures eventually weaken the midline fascia, helping to explain the location of most hernias in this area.[32] As with umbilical hernias, repair of hernias involving the linea alba consists of excision and closure of the hernial sac and direct approximation of the edges of the defect in the fascia with nonabsorbable sutures.

Spigelian Hernia

The spigelian hernia develops through a defect in the spigelian fascia (named after the Flemish anatomist Spieghel, who described it in the 1600s), which is the site where the semilunar and semicircular lines just lateral to the lower one third of the rectus muscle join (Fig. 64-12). The development of a hernia in this area is often subtle and frequently presents a diagnostic challenge.[33] Presenting findings include pain, tenderness, and occasionally an abdominal mass along the rectus muscle just inferior to the umbilicus. Most of the difficulty in diagnosis results from the fact that these hernias are usually intramural, so they may track from their site of origin in almost any direction being covered by the external oblique muscle. Consequently, they are not as obvious as hernial defects traversing the abdominal wall. Recently, ultrasonography has been demonstrated to be of value in the diagnosis of spigelian hernia. Spangen[33] reported that B-mode scans

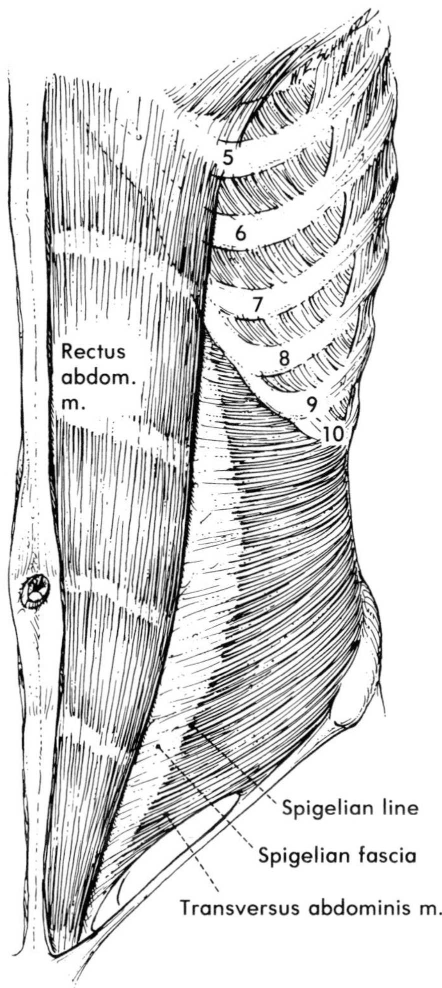

Fig. 64-12. The rectus muscle aponeurosis extends from the fourth, fifth, and sixth ribs. The hernias along the lateral border of the rectus muscle do not penetrate the external oblique layer.

were of particular value in discovering spigelian hernias in a relatively large number of individuals in his clinic.I have also had some success with ultrasonographic diagnosis of spigelian hernias and believe it to be a useful adjunct in the diagnosis of patients with unexplained abdominal wall pain, particularly if the clinical finding strongly suggests this type of hernia despite negative physical findings.

Because incarceration and strangulation may occur with spigelian hernias, they should be surgically repaired when diagnosed. Such repair is accomplished through a transverse incision over the site of origin, with division of the external oblique fascia for proper exposure of the hernial defect. Because the defect involves the aponeurosis of the transverse abdominus and internal oblique muscles, repair involves approximation of these two fascial layers and subsequent closure of the divided external oblique fascia.

Lumbar Hernia

Hernias arising in the lumbar region through the posterior abdominal wall are called *lumbar* or *dorsal hernias.* One of two sites is generally involved. The superior lumbar triangle (also called *Grynfeltt's triangle*) is the most common site of origin; the inferior lumbar triangle (also called *Petit's triangle*) is less frequently involved. The common clinical presentation is usually a mass in the flank, which may be associated with pain. On palpation, this mass is generally reducible, and incarceration and strangulation are usually not problems. Most lumbar hernias represent incisional hernias occurring in old nephrectomy incisions, but they may on occasion occur spontaneously. Surgical repair with approximation of the fascial edges of the hernia defect is the treatment of choice.

Pelvic Hernias

A variety of rare hernias may occur through the various foramina in the pelvic floor through which nerves and blood vessels pass into the buttocks or out of the pelvis. Various intra-abdominal structures may make up the hernial contents, with small bowel being particularly frequent. The two common types of pelvic hernia include those that pass through the greater sciatic foramen and those that pass through the obturator foramen. The diagnosis of a hernia is often first made at the time of surgery when a portion of intestine becomes incarcerated, necessitating abdominal exploration. Occasionally, an obturator hernia is diagnosed as a swelling in the upper and medial aspect of the thigh associated with pain radiating to the medial aspect of the knee in the distribution of the obturator nerve (Howship-Romberg sign). In a patient in whom a sciatic or obturator hernia is suspected, herniography provides confirmation. Both types of hernia are usually repaired through an abdominal approach in which the hernial sac and its contents are reduced, with resection of necrotic bowel as indicated and primary closure of the fascial defect.

Another type of pelvic hernia may occur when there is a defect in the levator sling in the floor of the pelvis. A protrusion through this defect is called a *perineal hernia* and usually appears as a bulge just lateral to the midline perineal raphe. Such a hernia is usually related to a previous surgical procedure, such as an abdominoperineal resection or a prostatectomy. Repair involves fascial closure of the perineal defect, usually through a combined abdominal and perineal approach. Perineal hernias are often asymptomatic, but depending on their location they may be associated with pain on sitting or a variety of urinary symptoms, predominantly dysuria.

Incisional Hernia

An incisional hernia is one that develops through a surgical incision in the abdominal wall. These hernias most commonly involve incisions of the anterior abdominal wall, although incisions may be responsible for other types of hernia, such as those occurring in the lumbar region (from a previous nephrectomy incision) and in the perineal region (from a previous abdominoperineal resection). The hernia may appear clinically shortly after the placement of the initial incision or may develop many years thereafter. When arising in the anterior abdominal wall, incisional hernias are more commonly encountered in vertical than in transverse incisions.

The variety of etiologic factors involved in the development of incisional hernias can generally be grouped under the two broad headings of poor postoperative wound healing and postoperative wound infection. Any factor related to poor surgical technique can result in inadequate wound healing. Thus, if sutures are placed too close to the edges of the wound being apposed, or if they are tied so tightly as to cause necrosis of the involved tissues, poor wound healing may result. Other contributing factors related to surgical technique include knots becoming untied, use of the wrong type of suture material for a particular incision, the development of wound hematomas as a result of poor hemostasis, and the placement of drains through the incision itself, all of which may adversely affect healing. Further, if the incision has not been closed properly and the patient has a problem with increased intra-abdominal pressure (related to such factors as hiccoughs, abdominal distention, and postoperative coughing), undue strain may be placed on the suture line, which ultimately may give way. Finally, wound infections are known to be directly related to the subsequent development of an incisional hernia, particularly if the infection extends to the level of the fascia. Thus, any factor contributing to the development of a wound infection also influences the likelihood of recurrent incisional hernia.

The treatment of most incisional hernias is not dissimilar to that of other hernias. For small or moderate-sized hernias, the hernial sac is excised and the defect is closed with interrupted sutures. For larger hernias, such closure may not be possible without undue tension on the repair. In this circumstance, either a fascia lata graft or a synthetic mesh material such as polypropylene (Marlex) should be used to bridge the hernial defect.

A variant of the incisional hernia is that occurring through the fascial opening created for a colostomy or ileostomy. This type of hernia, termed a *parastomal hernia,* usually occurs when the stomal opening is placed lateral to the rectus muscle. Often, this type of hernia can be managed by tightening the fascial defect around the stoma with interrupted sutures. When this is not possible, the colostomy or ileostomy should be taken down and moved to a new site, preferably through the rectus muscle. The remaining fascial defect from the previously placed ostomy is then closed from within the peritoneal cavity.

Diaphragmatic Hernias

A number of hernias may occur within the diaphragm that separates the thoracic from the abdominal cavity. These hernias may be congenital, in which case they arise through defects or apertures resulting from developmental abnormalities; or they may be acquired through enlargement of preexistent apertures or disruption of points of weakness.

A congenital diaphragmatic hernia represents an arrest in the development of some portion of the diaphragm (Fig. 64-13). When it occurs posterolaterally (which is the most common site), it is called a *Bochdalek's hernia* and involves the left hemidiaphragm 70% to 85% of the time. This type of hernia, which allows abdominal viscera to migrate readily into the left thorax, is one of the surgical emergencies of the neonatal period and is associated with a substantial mortality rate as a result of the accompanying respiratory distress and ventilatory impairment. The clinical presentation of this type of hernia and the physiologic principles underlying its management are discussed in detail in Chapter 66. Another type of congenital hernia is that resulting from failure of anterior fusion of the sternal and costal portions of the diaphragm. The resulting midline defect creates a hiatus, known as *Morgagni's foramen,* through which a hernia may occur. When normal fusion results, only the internal thoracic vessels pass through this area and continue into the abdomen as the superior epigastric vessels. When the defect remains, however, various portions of bowel (usually small bowel) or omentum may herniate through this abnormal hiatus. In contrast to Bochdalek's hernia, which presents clinically at birth, most hernias protruding through Morgagni's foramen do not become symptomatic until middle age or later. Often, the first demonstration of their presence is a mechanical bowel obstruction that may result in strangulation of the involved bowel and can develop into a severe mediastinitis if not treated on an emergency basis. When diagnosed, they

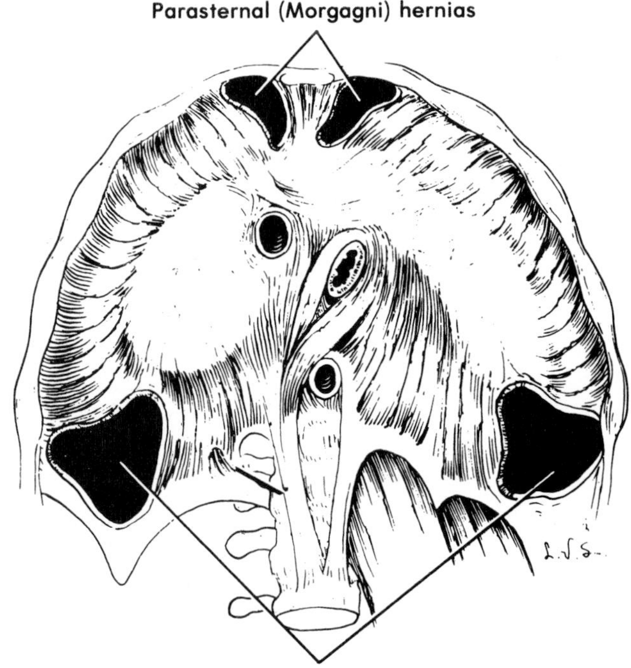

Fig. 64-13. Sites of congenital diaphragmatic herniation. (From Grimes OF, Way LW. Esophagus and diaphragm. In Way LW, ed. Current Surgical Diagnosis and Treatment, 7th ed. Los Altos, Calif.: Lange Medical Publications, 1985.)

should be repaired surgically, usually through a transabdominal approach.

Among the types of acquired hernia that may affect the diaphragm, the most common is the sliding hiatus hernia, which may be associated with esophagitis. This type of hernia is discussed in detail in Chapter 14. Less commonly encountered clinically is the parahiatal hernia, also called the *paraesophageal hernia* (Fig. 64-14). Because the esophagogastric junction is not disturbed in this condition, esophagitis is not a problem. Usually, the presenting symptoms are vague epigastric and lower chest pain that may be aggravated on recumbency. With this type of hernia, all or part of the stomach may herniate into the thorax adjacent and to the left of the gastroesophageal junction. Radiologically, this type of hernia may give the appearance of an upside-down stomach on barium contrast study. Paraesophageal hernias are often associated with the complications of ulceration and bleeding and not uncommonly become incarcerated and even strangulated. For this reason, the most prudent method of management is to return the herniated stomach to the abdomen and surgically repair the aperture in the diaphragm.

One additional type of acquired hernia of importance is that produced by rents in the diaphragm that can result from penetrating or blunt trauma. Because of the protective effects of the liver on the right side, these traumatic hernias almost always occur on the left side, and they can result in considerable respiratory embarrassment from herniation of abdominal viscera into the left side of the chest if they are of sufficient size. Surgical repair of the diaphragmatic tear with reduction of the herniated viscera into the abdomen is the treatment of choice.

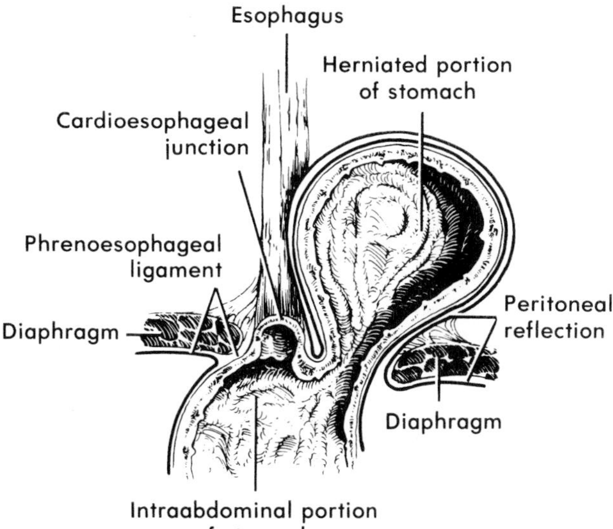

Fig. 64-14. Paraesophageal hernia. (From Grimes OF, Way LW. Esophagus and diaphragm. In Way LW, ed. Current Surgical Diagnosis and Treatment, 7th ed. Los Altos, Calif.: Lange Medical Publications, 1985.)

SUMMARY

Hernias of the abdominal wall are commonly encountered in the practice of surgery and may arise in any structure surrounding or supporting the contents of the abdominal cavity. These hernias are particularly common anteriorly, with the vast majority arising in the groin. Other sites of relatively frequent occurrence include the umbilicus and previous incisions. The clinical presentation of a hernia is usually obvious and exhibits a bulge at the site of the hernial defect, often in association with pain. Less commonly, an unexplained intestinal obstruction may be the presenting finding if a segment of bowel has become trapped in the hernial defect. Because hernias generally do not resolve spontaneously (an exception being the congenital umbilical hernia), surgical repair is the treatment of choice once the diagnosis has been established. This includes careful identification of the hernial ring, reduction of any contents that may be within the hernial sac, and, in most circumstances, excision of the sac itself. When these maneuvers have been accomplished, the defect is then repaired by approximating its edges with interrupted, nonabsorbable sutures. Occasionally the hernial defect is sufficiently large that primary closure is not possible without undue stress and tension. In this circumstance, such as may occur with large groin hernias, umbilical hernias, and some incisional hernias, fascia lata or some type of synthetic material (such as polypropylene [Marlex]) may be used to bridge and/or buttress the hernial defect to ensure an adequate repair and reduce the possibility of recurrence. The key to any successful hernia repair is an understanding of the underlying anatomy and its restoration to a normal state. With this principle in mind, most hernias can be repaired without difficulty, and a good to excellent result can be expected.

REFERENCES

1. Nyhus LM, Condon RE, eds. Hernia, 4th ed. Philadelphia: JB Lippincott, 1995.
2. Anson BJ, Morgan EH, McVay CB. Surgical anatomy of the inguinal region based upon a study of 500 body-halves. Surg Gynecol Obstet 111:707, 1960.
3. Hughson W. The persistent or preformed sac in relation to oblique inguinal hernia. Surg Gynecol Obstet 41:610, 1925.
4. Keith A. On the origin and nature of hernia. Br J Surg 11:455, 1924.
5. Gullmo A, Broome A, Smedberg S. Herniography. Surg Clin North Am 64:229, 1984.
6. Andrews E. A method of herniotomy utilizing only white fascia. Ann Surg 80:185, 1984.
7. Read RC. Attenuation of rectus sheath in inguinal herniation. Am J Surg 120:610, 1970.
8. Peacock EE Jr. Biology of hernia. In Nyhus LM, Condon RE, eds. Hernia, 2nd ed. Philadelphia: JB Lippincott, 1978.
9. Conner WT, Peacock EE Jr. Some studies on the etiology of inguinal hernia. Am J Surg 126:732, 1973.
10. Peacock EE Jr, Madden JW. Studies on the biology and treatment of recurrent inguinal hernia. II. Morphological changes. Ann Surg 179:667, 1974.
11. Cannon DJ, Read RC. Metastatic emphysema, a mechanism for acquiring inguinal herniation. Ann Surg 194:270, 1981.

12. Gullmo A. Herniography: The diagnosis of hernia in the groin and incompetence of the pouch of Douglas and pelvic floor. Acta Radiol 36:1, 1980.
13. Tobin GR, Clark DS, Peacock EE Jr. A neuromuscular basis for development of indirect inguinal hernia. Arch Surg 11:464, 1976.
14. Arnbjornsson E. Development of right inguinal hernia after appendectomy. Am J Surg 143:174, 1982.
15. Engeset J, Youngson GG. Ambulatory peritoneal dialysis and hernia complications. Surg Clin North Am 64:385, 1984.
16. Colin JF, Elliot P, Ellis H. The effect of uraemia upon wound healing: An experimental study. Br J Surg 66:793, 1979.
17. Jorkasky D, Goldfarb S. Abdominal wall hernia complicating chronic ambulatory peritoneal dialysis. Am J Nephrol 2:323, 1982.
18. Robinson RR, et al. Surgical considerations of continuous ambulatory peritoneal dialysis. Surgery 96:723, 1984.
19. Condon RE. The anatomy of the inguinal region and its relationship to groin hernia. In Nyhus LM, Condon RE, eds. Hernia, 4th ed. Philadelphia: JB Lippincott, 1995, p 16.
20. Lichtenstein IL, Shulman AG, Amid PK. The tension-free repair of groin hernias. In Nyhus LM, Condon RE, eds. Hernia, 4th ed. Philadelphia: JB Lippincott, 1995, p 237.
21. Payne JH Jr, et al. Laparoscopic or open inguinal herniorrhaphy? A randomized prospective trial. Arch Surg 129:973, 1994.
22. Glassow F. Recurrent inguinal and femoral hernia. BMJ 1:215, 1970.
23. Tanner NC. A "slide" operation for inguinal and femoral hernia. Br J Surg 29:285, 1942.
24. McVay CB. Groin hernioplasty: Cooper's ligament repair. In Nyhus LM, Condon RE, eds. Hernia, 2nd ed. Philadelphia: JB Lippincott, 1978.
25. Read RC. Bilaterality and the prosthetic repair of large recurrent inguinal hernias. Am J Surg 138:788, 1979.
26. Stoppa RE. The preperitoneal approach and prosthetic repair of groin hernias. In Nyhus LM, Condon RE, eds. Hernia, 4th ed. Philadelphia: JB Lippincott, 1995, p 188.
27. Rypins EB. Laparoscopic Herniorrhaphy. In Nyhus LM, Condon RE, eds. Hernia, 4th ed. Philadelphia: JB Lippincott, 1995, p 253.
28. Brooks DC. A prospective comparison of laparoscopic and tension-free open herniorrhaphy. Arch Surg 129:361, 1994.
29. Halverson K, McVay CB. Inguinal and femoral hernioplasty: A 22-year study of the author's methods. Arch Surg 101:127, 1970.
30. McVay CB, Chapp JD. Inguinal and femoral hernioplasty—The evaluation of a basic concept. Ann Surg 148:499, 1958.
31. Bendavid R. The Shouldice repair. In Nyhus LM, Condon RE, eds. Hernia, 4th ed. Philadelphia: JB Lippincott, 1995, p 217.
32. Askar O. Surgical anatomy of the aponeurotic expansions of the anterior abdominal wall. Ann R Coll Surg Engl 59:313, 1977.
33. Spangen L. Spigelian hernia. Surg Clin North Am 64:351, 1984.

65

Pathophysiology of Thermal Injury

Evan R. Kokoska, David J. Wainwright, and Donald H. Parks

Thermal injury elicits major pathophysiologic alterations beyond the obvious cutaneous manifestation. Although the burn wound itself can present unique challenges in terms of therapeutic management and is responsible for the high incidence of infection that occurs in thermally injured patients, a number of metabolic aberrations and associated dysfunction of various organs are also commonly encountered that directly contribute to morbidity and mortality. The magnitude of these latter derangements has led to the proposal that the burn patient is the universal trauma model with the greatest dysregulation of homeostasis of any injury.[1,2] Major progress has recently been achieved in understanding many of the pathophysiologic mechanisms that occur in burn injury and has facilitated patient management and improved survival. Such progress has been attributed to the development of specialized burn centers, increased investigative efforts in burn research, and the development of the team concept in patient management.[3]

THE BURN WOUND

Biophysics of Thermal Injury

When skin is heated, damage occurs from the transfer of thermal energy. The magnitude of this tissue destruction is a function of both the quantity of heat transferred and the speed at which it dissipates. These factors are determined by the physical properties of the burning agent, the recipient tissue that is burned, and the incipient environment.

Burning Agent

The temperature and duration of exposure to the burning agent are the most important determinants of the degree of injury. For a specific level of injury, there is an inverse relationship between these two parameters[4,5] (Fig. 65-1). As the temperature is reduced, a progressively longer exposure time is required to inflict the same injury. At a theoretic "threshold temperature," the heat source would have to be applied for an infinite time. Temperatures below this "threshold" do not result in tissue damage, regardless of the duration of application. The exposure interval is related not only to the actual removal of the offending agent but also to the rate at which the heat source loses its energy to the environment. For example, at lower temperatures at which duration is important, a different degree of injury results when a metallic object and liquid are exposed to the same temperature. The liquid loses its heat more slowly.

Recipient Tissue

Certain physical properties of the heated object are also important in determining the extent of damage. These parameters reflect how much energy must be expended to raise the temperature of the object and how efficiently and quickly the heat is transferred. Skin, because of its high water content, has a high specific heat and a low thermal conductivity. Thus slow overheating of the tissues and delayed dispersion of the energy result. This is illustrated by measuring the temperature 1 mm below the skin surface after a 10-second scald burn (Fig. 65-2). There is an initial rapid, but not immediate, rise in temperature as the heat is applied. Even more dramatic is the length of time required for the temperature to return to baseline values. In this way heat damage may continue after the offending agent is removed. Heat energy is lost primarily by conduction to the surrounding tissues, with removal of the circulating blood making only a small contribution.[6]

Environment

Heat dissipation occurs not only through adjacent tissues but also into the surrounding environment. Heat loss is therefore maximized in a cooler environment. For example, the rapid application of cold water to burned skin has been shown to decrease the severity of the injury by rapidly reducing the elevated tissue temperature.[7] There is also evidence that cooling the burn wound minimizes edema[8,9] by decreasing the amount of histamine released[10] through stabilization of the mast cell membrane.[11] Preservation of the dermal microcirculation has likewise been demonstrated by immediate cooling of the thermally injured tissues[8,9] presumably through a reduction in thromboxane production.[12]

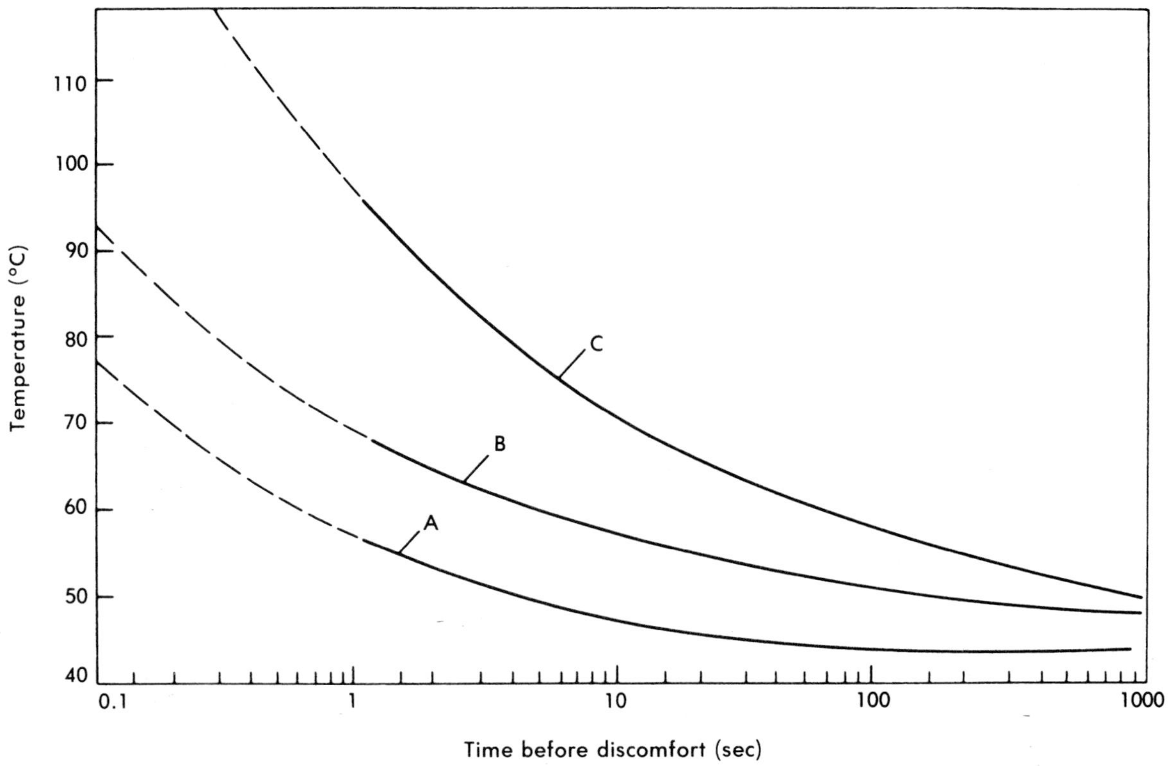

Fig. 65-1. Relationship between temperature and the duration of contact for first-degree *(A),* second-degree *(B),* and third-degree *(C)* injuries. (From Lawrence JC, Bull JP. Thermal conditions which cause skin burns. Eng Med 5:61, 1976. Reprinted by permission of the Council of the Institution of Mechanical Engineers.)

Histopathology of the Burn Wound

The severity of a burn injury is determined by the anatomic surface area involved and the pathologic depth. A *first-degree burn* is characterized by painful, erythematous, and edematous skin. Histologically, vasodilation is present in the dermal microvasculature, and there is an increase in the interstitial fluid volume secondary to increased permeability. If the insult is more severe, necrosis of the epidermis occurs, and blistering of the skin is found clinically. A hyperemic response is again observed in the vessels within the dermis accompanied by extravasation of fluid. In this instance the fluid accumulates not only within the connective tissue of the dermis, but also at the dermal-epidermal junction leading to vesicle formation. The composition of the blister fluid has been extensively examined by a number of investigators.[13-16] Compounds with a relatively low molecular weight (i.e., electrolytes, urea, glucose, antibiotics) diffuse freely into the tissues and are found in the same concentrations in the serum, interstitial flud, and blister fluid. On the other hand, low-molecular-weight proteins that are generally found only in small concentrations in tissue fluid have been shown to attain up to 80% of their plasma concentration within the vesicles. Significant quantities of intracellular enzymes and purine/pyrimidine compounds are also found, reflecting the extent of cellular damage. Elevated concentrations of several chemical mediators (i.e., prostaglandins) have also been reported in the blister fluid.

In a *partial-thickness injury* or *second-degree burn* the epidermal appendages are preserved and are responsible for resurfacing the wound. The epithelium in the surviving sweat glands and hair follicles multiplies and begins to migrate across the wound, coverage being complete within 7 to 14 days. This injury is typically painful because of direct nerve ending damage coupled with the release of irritant chemical mediators into the wound.

An even greater thermal insult leads to additional thermal necrosis. The cellular components are irreversibly damaged, and the connective tissue is sufficiently disrupted that it is unable to fulfill its function of support and protection. If this extends to a depth below the level of the epidermal appendages, a *full-thickness injury* or *third-degree burn* has occurred. Reepithelialization is only possible from the wound edge, a process that would take a considerable length of time for even small defects. A dry, leathery appearance is seen clinically, since the tissues have lost their ability to retain water. This wound is painless because the nerve endings have been destroyed.

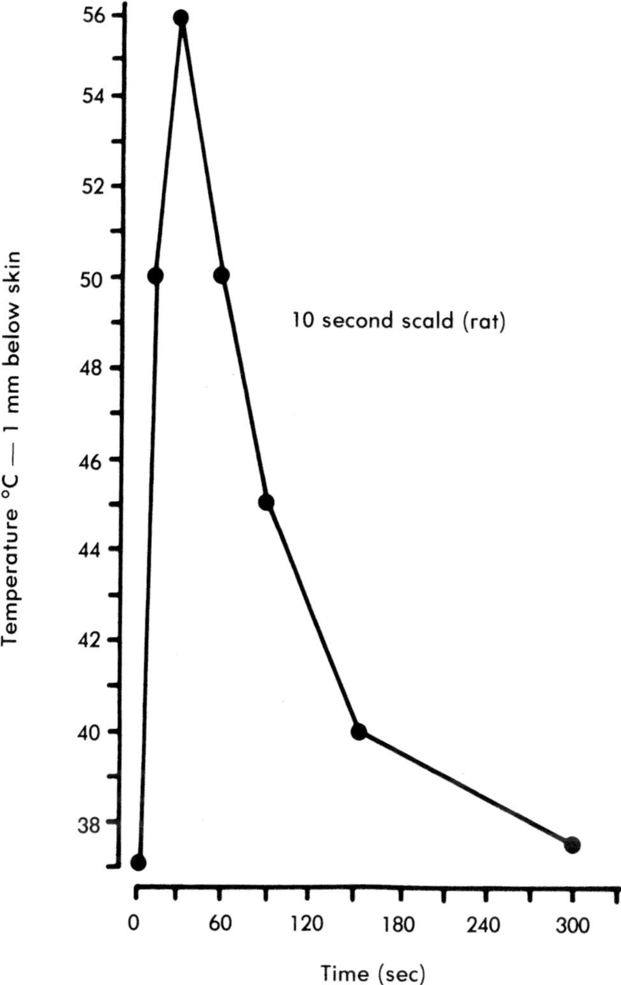

Fig. 65-2. Temperature curve measured by a thermocouple 1 mm below the skin surface during a 10-second scald. The skin's low thermal conductivity results in a slow dispersion of the energy, leading to additional tissue injury subsequent to the removal of the offending agent. (From Moncrief JA. The body's response to heat. In Artz CP, et al., eds. Burns: A Team Approach. Philadelphia: WB Saunders, 1979.)

Pathophysiology of the Burn Wound

Major Mediators

Prior to discussing the specific derangements involved with burn injuries, a brief review of the major mediators produced, both local and systemic, is warranted (Table 65-1). As a general principle, under normal conditions these mediators, at low levels, are required to maintain proper blood flow and host immunity. However, either prolonged low levels or sustained elevations following injuries such as burns can be detrimental, both within the local site and at distant organ sites.

Cytokines are low molecular weight glycoproteins which act as intercellular messengers in either an autocrine, paracrine, or endocrine fashion. They are synthesized de novo in response to potential threats to the organism (antigens, lipopolysaccharides, etc.); must bind receptors, as they are unable to penetrate cell membranes;[17] and are not governed by a major negative feedback loop.[18] Cytokines are difficult to detect because they are bioactive at extremely low concentrations and their levels do not always correlate with the degree of injury.[18] Some effects of cytokines are clearly beneficial, but they may become counterproductive during derangements in the body's homeostatic responses. Imbalances may lead to immunosuppression, and excessive activity has correlated with injurious effects.[19]

Eicosanoids are produced through the metabolism of arachidonic acid, an unsaturated fatty acid essential in nutrition. Prostaglandins and thromboxanes are generated through the action of cyclooxygenase, whereas 5-lipooxygenase converts arachidonic acid to leukotrienes. A variety of prostaglandin end products have been identified in the burn wound, and many appear to have divergent effects.[20] For example, prostaglandin E_2 (PGE_2) and prostacyclin (PGI_2) are vasodilators and inhibit platelet aggregation, whereas thromboxane A_2 (TXA_2) is a potent vasoconstrictor and promotes platelet aggregation. A steady-state relationship exists between these oppositely functioning prostanoids (e.g., PGE_2 and PGI_2 vs. TXA_2) in uninjured tissues. However, a traumatic stimulus may disrupt this balance and favor increased production of a particular group of eicosanoids. Several different isoforms of cyclooxygenase have been recognized: a constitutively expressed (Cox-1) and inducible (Cox-2) form. However, the role of these two differentially expressed enzymes following burn injury remains to be delineated.

Burns are also associated with enhanced nitric oxide formation. Similar to cyclooxygenase, nitric oxide is generated from two isoforms of nitric oxide synthase: a constitutive and inducible form. Under basal conditions, low levels of nitric oxide provide a continuous state of active vasodilation and inhibit platelet and polymorphonuclear leukocyte (PMN) adhesion to the endothelium.[21] After major injury, however, inducible nitric oxide synthase activity is significantly upregulated by stimuli such as elevated temperature[22] and tumor necrosis fator (TNF) or interleukin-1 (IL-1) released from activated macrophages.[21] Excessive nitric oxide is associated with circulatory failure and vascular decompensation.

PMNs and macrophages are primarily responsible for phagocytosis of necrotic tissue. In the phagosome of the neutrophil, superoxide anion radicals and hydrogen peroxide are produced in large quantities to oxidize the ingested debris. These free radical species are normally rendered harmless by the action of superoxide dismutases and catalases that convert them to harmless products including oxygen and water. However, following burn injury, oxygen-derived free radicals are generated secondary to both ischemia/reperfusion via activation of xanthine oxidase[18] and histamine released from stimulated mast cells,[23] and it has been postulated that a sufficient quantity of these substances may escape into the interstitial fluid where the necessary enzymes

Table 65-1. Local and Systemic Mediators of Burn Injuries

Mediator	Major Source	Major Actions: Immunologic	Major Actions: Metabolic
Cytokines			
IL-1	Monocytes, macrophages	Activate B and T cells, Natural killer cells, PMNs, and macrophages	Fever, APP production, catabolism, wound healing, anemia[18,19]
IL-2	T lymphocytes	Cell-mediated immunity, enhanced cytotoxic T-cell function	Hypermetabolism[18]
IL-6	Macrophages, PMNs, fibroblasts	B-cell proliferation, immunoglobulin production	Hepatic APP production[18]
TNF (cachectin)	Macrophages, endothelial cells	PMN release, margination, and activation	Catabolism, APP production, fever[18]
Eicosanoids			
PGE_2, PGI_2	Endothelial cells, macrophages, PMNs	Vasodilation, increased vascular permeability, immunosuppression (PGE_2)[18,19,42,58,59]	
TXA_2, TXB_2	Platelets, macrophages	Vasoconstriction, platelet aggregation, local tissue ischemia[108,158,201,206]	
LTB_4, LTC_4, LTD_4	Mast cells, macrophages, PMNs	Increased vascular permeability, potent PMN chemoattractant (LTB_4), small airway constriction (LTC_4, LTD_4)[19,204]	
Nitric Oxide	Endothelial cells, macrophages	Low levels: Vasodilation High levels: Cytotoxic, vascular decompensation[21,203,205]	
Oxygen Free Radicals	PMNs	Lipid peroxidation (increased cell membrane permeability and fluidity)[18,19]	
Complement			
C3a, C5a		Anaphylaxis	
C3b		Opsonin	
C5b		Increased vascular permeability and smooth muscle contraction	
C6 to C9		Cytotoxic[19]	
Acute Phase Proteins	Hepatocytes	Inactivate proteases, scavenge oxygen free radicals, modulate wound healing[202]	

APP, Acute phase protein; *IL,* interleukin; *LT,* leukotriene; *PG,* prostaglandin; *PMN,* polymorphonuclear leukocyte; *TX,* thromboxane.

for their reduction are present in only small amounts.[24] These radicals not only increase capillary permeability directly but may induce peroxidation of tissues and can also result in inhanced prostaglandin release by their action on the phospholipid bilayer of the cell membrane.[24a] Complement acts to attract PMNs and degranulate mast cells and further increases oxygen free radical synthesis in addition to the other actions[19] depicted in Table 65-1.

Progressive Ischemia

An important conceptual model of the burn wound is that proposed by Jackson.[25] He described three zones of graded thermal trauma (Fig. 65-3). Centrally, the "zone of coagulation" is an area of irreversible tissue destruction. Temperatures in this region are extreme and lead to immediate cell death, the depth of necrosis being directly dependent on the quantity of heat transferred. On the periphery, a "zone of hyperemia" exists where vasodilation and permeability changes are present. Here the tissues are viable and generally heal uneventfully. The "zone of stasis" lies between these two areas. In this zone the flow through a microvasculature is sluggish or has ceased, leading to progressive ischemia and cell death.[26] Jackson[25] conceived that these changes were a direct effect of the heat energy on the tissues and that eventual tissue necrosis within the zone of stasis was inevitable within 24 to 48 hours. However, other investigators believe that the tissues in this region have not been permanently damaged and thus possess the potential for a full recovery.[27] Any deterioration is the result of a combination of physical factors and local inflammatory processes leading to persistent stasis and ischemia with conversion to a "zone of coagulation."

Systemic factors. The progressive nature of the dermal ischemia occurs secondary to the influence of both systemic and local factors as outlined in the box on p. 1317. Depletion of the intravascular volume from fluid leaking into the injured tissues diminishes the filling pressure of the left ventricle and in turn the perfusion pressure

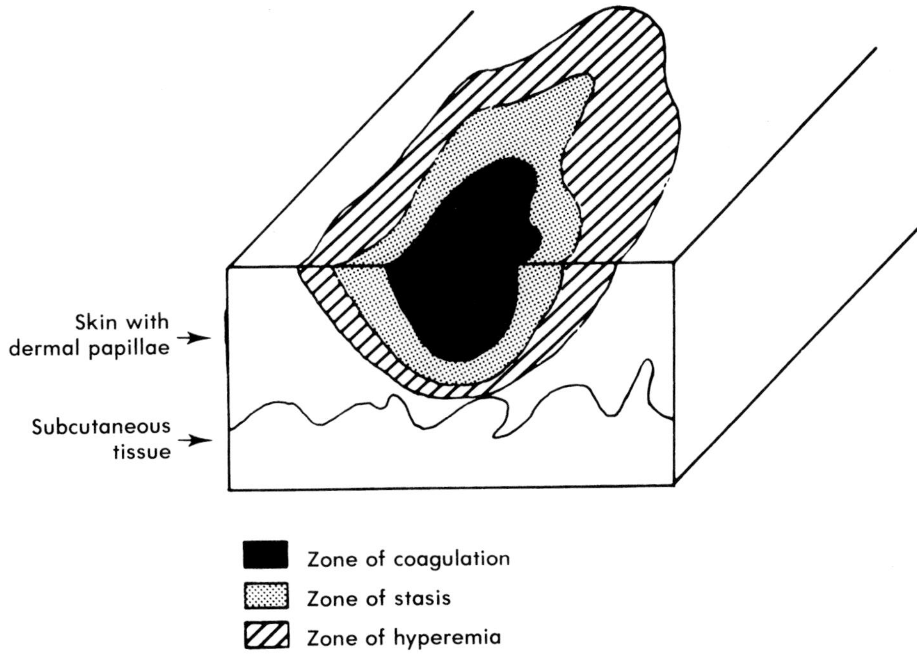

Fig. 65-3. Jackson's three zones of graded thermal injury. (From Moncrief JA. The body's response to heat. In Artz CP, et al., eds. Burns: A Team Approach. Philadelphia: WB Saunders, 1979.)

FACTORS CONTRIBUTING TO PROGRESSIVE ISCHEMIA

Systemic Factors

1. Diminished circulating volume
2. Myocardial depression
3. Constricting eschar

Local Factors

1. Intraluminal
   a. White blood cell margination
   b. Platelet microthrombi/microemboli
   c. Erythrocyte agglutination
2. Vessel wall changes
   a. Endothelial cell shape
   b. Vasoconstriction
      (1) Direct
      (2) Through chemical mediators
3. Extraluminal
   a. Interstitial edema

within the microcirculation. However, even prior to measurable decreases in plasma volume, there is an alteration in ventricular compliance and a decrease in myocardial contractility.[28] This direct myocardial toxicity is felt to be related to the release of a "myocardial depressant factor," although no such factor has been identified chemically.[29,30] Other proposed mediators contributing to early myocardial depression resulting in the "ebb" phase following burn injury include TNF,[31] interleukins, antidiuretic hormone (ADH), oxygen free radicals,[32-34] and nitric oxide.[21] Constricting eschar in circumferential burns of the extremities can also lead to reduced perfusion pressures in distally burned tissues.[35]

Local factors. Local factors can be categorized into intraluminal, extraluminal, and those associated with changes in the vessel wall itself. Within the lumen of blood vessels, cellular debris may accumulate, leading to a reduction in the functional diameter for flow. White blood cells respond to the thermal injury with increased margination along the vessel wall. As fluid leaks out of the intravascular space, hemoconcentration occurs that may encourage erythrocyte aggregation and agglutination, further diminishing local blood flow. Platelet microthrombi and microemboli have also been observed to block the microvasculature within the injured area.[36] Release of tissue thromboplastin from the injured tissues and the platelet-aggregating properties of thromboxane are both believed to contribute to the generation of these products of coagulation. Despite these observations, the use of anticoagulants has been unsuccessful in reducing the extent of tissue damage.[37] Outside the vessel wall, the interstitial tissue pressure slowly increases, as the lymphatics are unable to contend with the enhanced and continual fluid extravasation. This leads to compression of the microvasculature within this region and a subsequent reduction in flow.

The vessel wall itself contributes to the reduction of nutrient flow by structural changes in the endothelial cells and vasoconstriction. As a response to direct damage or ischemia, the endothelial cells are less able to regulate their internal electrolyte balance. Water therefore enters the cells, and the cells' normally hexagonal shape assumes a more spherical form.[38] In this way the thickness of the vessel wall increases and impinges on the diameter of the lumen. The vasoconstriction is likely the result of a multitude of factors. Increased sympathetic tone and TXA_2 release appear to be the most important causes. Since the changes in the caliber of the lumen secondary to vessel wall alterations are often transient,[36] the other pathophysiologic changes detailed above probably play a more important role in reducing blood flow.

For the cells within the zone of stasis to survive, nutrient flow within the microvasculature must be maintained. By preserving these tissues, one may prevent a partial-thickness injury from becoming a full-thickness injury and therefore requiring grafting. Clinically, this is achieved by maintaining the vascular volume and in turn the perfusion pressure through adequate resuscitation with intravenous fluids at the time of initial treatment. Similarly, wound care is important to prevent dehydration and infection, which can contribute to increasing the depth of injury. There is evidence that, by preserving an intact blister or covering the denuded partial-thickness injury with a skin substitute, dehydration of the exposed dermis is minimized and maximal tissue preservation is achieved.[27,39] More recent attempts at pharmacologic manipulation of the offending chemical mediators have been made to preserve and/or reestablish the flow in this vascular bed. Several studies have demonstrated that TXA_2 is the responsible agent for many of the progressive ischemic changes seen in the dermal microcirculation and that selectively inhibiting its production can prevent necrosis and attenuate hemodynamic disturbances.[40-42]

Cellular Alterations

In areas of irreparable damage, cell membranes are disrupted with the escape of intracellular contents. The connective tissue proteins undergo denaturation, and the water content is lost, leaving a solid amorphous substance. This fusion of the dermal and epidermal heat-damaged tissue is referred to as coagulation necrosis. As a reaction to the presence of this damaged and necrotic tissue, a marked inflammatory response characterizes the early phase of the burn wound. In locations where destruction is less extensive, cellular ultrastructure remains intact; however, function is often compromised. Resting membrane potentials are found to be above normal (greater than -90 mV) in this region, and cellular swelling is observed histologically.[43] This is likely the result of decreased adenosine triphosphate (ATP) production from tissue ischemia.[44,45] The function of the ATP-dependent sodium pump is impaired, permitting a shift of sodium and water into the cell, further compounding the loss of intravascular volume. A specific example of this is the altered function of the endothelial cells, the shape of which has been changed in response to a local thermal insult,[38] as discussed earlier in this chapter.

A toxin derived from the cell membranes of burned skin has also been described.[46] This burn toxin, called lipid protein complex (LPC), is a complex of lipids and proteins fused together by the effect of thermal injury. LPC has been associated with erythrocyte hemolysis,[47,48] immunosuppression,[49] and generalized membrane and mitochondrial damage.[50] The injurious effects of LPC are felt to be unrelated to lipid peroxidation[51] or bacteria[52] and can be neutralized with antiserum.[46] However, the best treatment appears to be removal of the burn wound.

Fluid Shifts in the Wound

The inflammatory response typical of heat-damaged tissues is characterized by tremendous edema formation. Although various physical and chemically mediated factors are responsible, the fluid efflux depends on the restoration of adequate blood flow to the injured area. Perfusion is maintained by a combination of fluid resuscitation and local vasodilation, the latter following an initial period of transient sympathetic vasoconstriction. The magnitude and time course of the tissue edema is subject to the timing and volume of fluid resuscitation.[53]

The cause of the increased fluid extravasation is multifactorial, with a tremendous amount of synergism between the responsible mechanisms. These can be broadly grouped into two major categories: (1) those that affect the permeability or "leakiness" of the vessel wall and (2) those whose effect is mediated through alteration of the Starling forces (see accompanying box).

Physical factors. The ease by which fluid, solutes, and macromolecules can exit the vessel lumen is influenced directly by architectural changes in the vessel wall and indirectly by a variety of chemical mediators. Vasodilation opens the endothelial gaps, promoting the efflux of fluid. The damaged endothelial cells exhibit an increase in both the number of intracellular vacuoles and the number of open intercellular junctions,[54] the latter secondary to these cells and assuming a more spherical shape.[38] These findings are first observed in the venules and later in the capillary bed. Since more channels are open along the vessel wall than exist normally, the outflow of fluid naturally increases.

CAUSES OF EDEMA FORMATION

Vessel Wall Changes

1. Vasodilation
2. Heat-induced damage
3. Vasoactive substances

Altered Starling Forces

1. Increased capillary hydrostatic pressure
    a. Vasoconstriction
    b. Partial blockage (platelets, white blood cells, red blood cells)
2. Decreased intraluminal colloid osmotic pressure
3. Increased interstitial colloid osmotic pressure
4. Lymphatic obstruction

Humoral correlates. The release of vasoactive substances is perhaps the most important cause of the increased permeability seen in the early burn wound. The effect of these agents is primarily on endothelial cells of the microvasculature where they cause both an increase in the number and size of the channels. This allows a number of macromolecules to enter the interstitial compartment and thus increases the amount of fluid escaping from the vessel lumen. Proteins of up to 150 A have been shown to escape into the interstitial compartment, resulting in a decreased intravascular oncotic pressure.[55,56] Studies have demonstrated that the integrity of the microvasculature to macromolecular leak is restored by 8 to 12 hours following thermal injury. Hence, at 12 hours postinjury, some clinicians initiate colloid infusions in their resuscitation regimens.[57]

A variety of mediators have been implicated in the generation of these permeability changes, but the most important appear to be the prostaglandins, leukotrienes,[42,58,59] and oxygen free radicals.[19] Kinins[60] and serotonin[61] release from platelets have been shown to play only a minor role. A stimulus for the mediator response is the connective tissue protein that has been modified by thermal injury. Its effect on activating the complement and clotting mechanisms leads to the generation of the various mediator compounds. Specifically, the C3 and C5 components of complement are responsible for mast cell histamine release and PMN recruitment, whereas the C9 component initiates prostaglandin release from platelets.[24] The permeability changes seen within the burn wound take on a biphasic pattern[62] (Fig. 65-4). The initial increase is primarily caused by the action of histamine[63] and the direct thermal damage to the microvasculature. The specific cause of the second, more prolonged phase is less clear but is likely the result of prostaglandin and leukotriene release and oxygen free radical generation.

The use of specific histamine H_2 receptor blockers (e.g., cimetidine) in reducing the early phase of edema formation has been successful in animals[64,65]; however, their clinical use seems to be ineffective in this regard[66] and is occasionally associated with undesirable side effects.[67] These findings are consistent with the fact that histamine is not responsible for the longer, more pronounced phase of increased permeability; therefore its inhibition is unlikely to have an appreciable effect. Topical ibuprofen, a cyclooxygenase inhibitor, has been reported to decrease burn edema.[68]

Other recent work directed toward decreasing permeability changes following burns has involved either blocking or scavenging oxygen free radicals. Permeability changes have been attenuated with xanthine oxidase inhibitors,[31,69-71] but these trials have not been effective when inhibition is attempted after the burn.[72] More promising is the use of vitamin C (a free radical scavenger) during fluid resuscitation, which, when initiated 2 hours after injury, in an animal model, has been associated with decreased burn wound edema and fluid requirements.[73]

Starling forces. In normal tissues the balance of the Starling forces results in a slight efflux of fluid from the intravascular to the extravascular compartment (Fig. 65-5). A steady state is maintained by resorption of this fluid through lymphatic channels. The lymphatic route is also the only avenue by which proteins can be returned to the vascular space to maintain the oncotic pressure gradient between the interstitial and intravascular compartments. In the burn wound these forces are altered so that this extravasation of fluid is greatly enhanced. Within the capillary lumen hydrostatic forces are increased above normal. The opening of the precapillary sphincters allows the arterial pressure to be transmitted directly to this vascular bed. In addition, intraluminal pressures rise proximal to a partial obstruction to flow caused by platelet microthrombi/microemboli, white blood cell margination, and red blood cell debris. In contrast, capillary intravascular osmotic pressure is decreased by the loss of colloid molecules into the interstitial space (especially albumin), whereas the extravascular osmotic activity rises, which tends to pull fluid out of the vessels.[13] Heat-denatured collagen is thought to be responsible for this effect. This denatured protein tends to hold the fluid within the interstitial space, thereby delaying resorption. Initially, the lymphatics increase their flow to compensate for this additional interstitial volume; however, the maximal effect of this flow is achieved within 1 hour following thermal injury. Not infrequently, blockage or destruction of the lym-

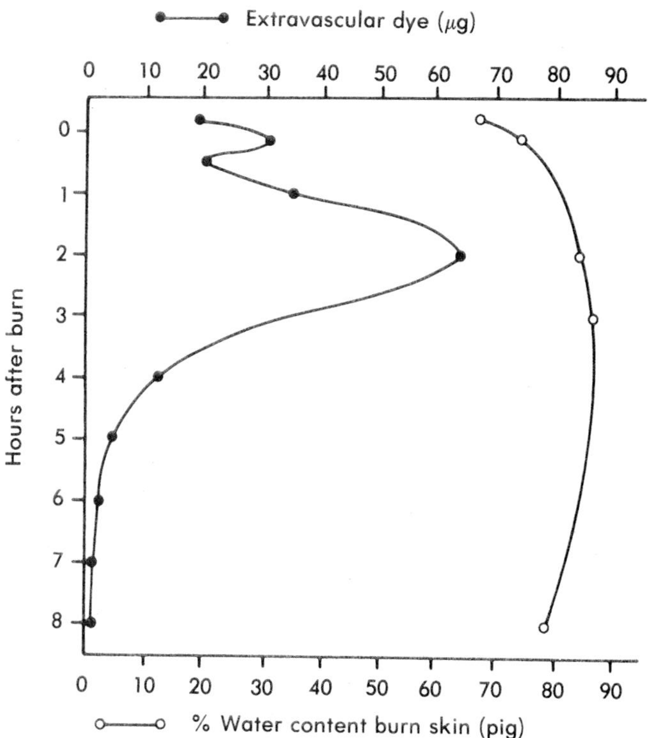

Fig. 65-4. Biphasic pattern of capillary permeability. (From Moncrief JA. The body's response to heat. In Artz CP, et al., eds. Burns: A Team Approach. Philadelphia: WB Saunders, 1979.)

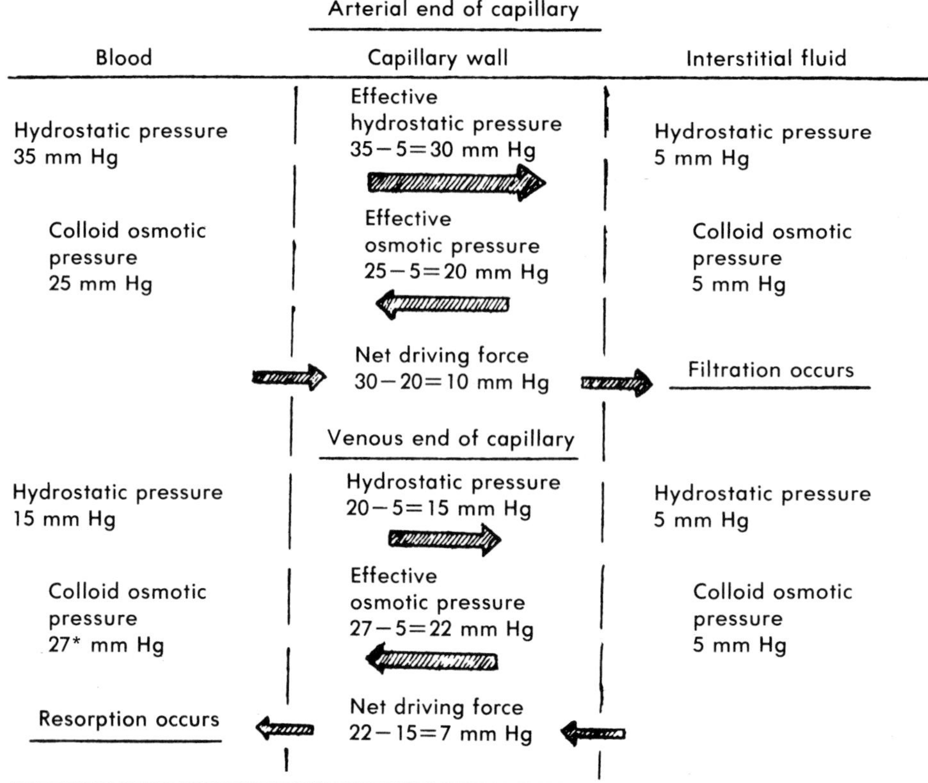

Fig. 65-5. Starling forces.

phatic channels delays resorption of the increased interstitial volume, further compounding this problem. Although tissue pressures rise as the quantity of edema fluid increases,[74] this alteration is not sufficient to counteract the forces responsible for flow out of the vessels.

Nonburn wound edema. In large burns (i.e., over 40% body surface area), edema is observed in both burned and nonburned tissues. Increased capillary permeability of distant vascular beds may be caused by the systemic effect of chemical mediators released from the damaged tissue.[56,59,75] Excessive white blood cell margination in the nonburned microcirculation has also been considered as a possible cause.[76] Demling et al.[23,77] have proposed that intravascular hypoproteinemia may be responsible for this effect. They suggested that the plasma oncotic pressure is lowered not only by protein loss through the burn wound but also by dilution from the crystalloid solutions used in burn resuscitation. By administering colloid during the resuscitative period, they noted that the edema observed in nonburned tissues was significantly diminished.

Systemic Inflammatory Response Syndrome

Following burn injury the generalized release of systemic mediators can eventually lead to multiple systems organ failure (MSOF) and death. As mentioned earlier, although some of the effects of cytokines are clearly beneficial, imbalances and excessive activity are universally detrimental, as the body's homeostatic responses become counterproductive. One hypothesis that summarizes the development of systemic inflammatory response syndrome (SIRS) involves the "two hit" theory. The initial insult (burn injury or gut ischemia) primes the inflammatory factories (cellular elements such as PMNs and macrophages). Subsequent challenge, either by endotoxemia (from gut or wound) or persistent gut ischemia, acts as the "second hit" that initiates a prolonged, exaggerated release of inflammatory mediators resulting in hemodynamic instability and tissue injury.[18] A simplified diagram is depicted in Fig. 65-6.

A growing body of evidence currently suggests that infection is not necessary for the development of SIRS. Fewer than half of septic-appearing patients who subsequently die have untreated infections,[3,40,78,79] and the overall relationship between endotoxemia and survival is poor.[46] It is becoming increasingly clear that devitalized tissue (denatured protein and bacterial products) and gut ischemia are important stimuli for the inflammatory response.[3,78]

Changes in intestinal permeability and the promotion of bacterial translocation are evident shortly after a burn injury.[78,80] The mucosal injury is mediated in large part by oxygen free radicals derived from increased xanthine oxidase activity[78] as a result of decreased mesenteric blood flow and ischemia/reperfusion and does not appear to be related to bacteria, as germ-free rats demonstrate similar responses.[78] Even in the absence of translocating organisms or endotoxin into the portal circulation, gut mucosal

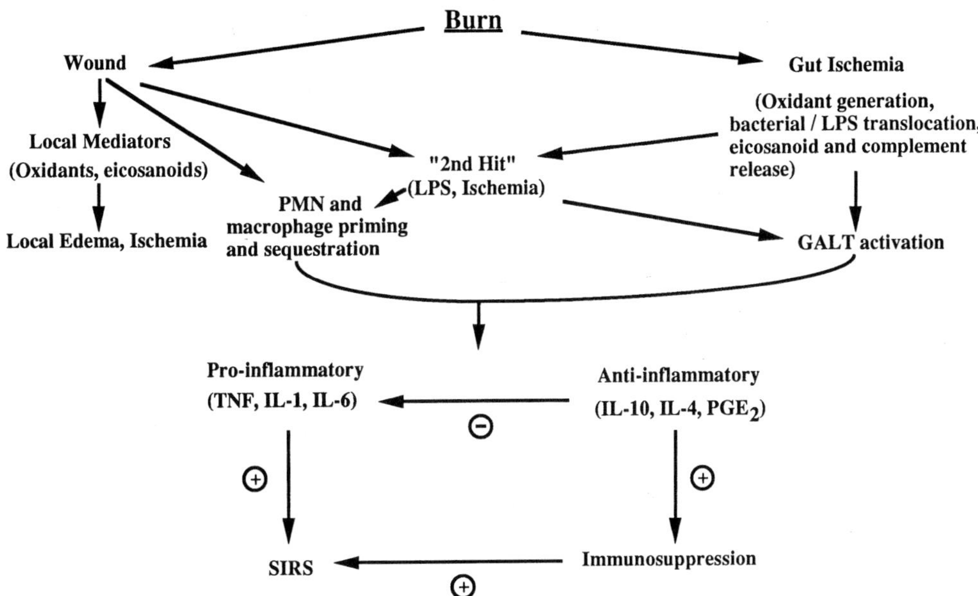

Fig. 65-6. Mediator interactions following burn injury. *GALT,* Gut-associated lymphoid tissue; *IL,* interleukin; *LPS,* lipopolysaccharide; *PG,* prostaglandin; *PMN,* polymorphonuclear leukocyte; *SIRS,* systemic inflammatory response syndrome, *TNF,* tumor necrosis factor. (Modified from Sayeed MM. Alterations in cell signalling and related effector functions in T lymphocytes in burn/trauma/septic injuries. Shock 5:157, 1996.)

damage is injurious through the activation of the gut-associated lymphoid tissue (GALT).[17] The GALT, in addition to the burn wound, serves as a primary site for PMN priming and cytokine release.[78] Gut ischemia also results in the release of eicosanoids[81] and complement.[82]

Efforts directed toward preventing SIRS by mediator antagonism have been largely disappointing in part because of the enormous costs and the difficulty detecting circulating levels of the various cytokines. Several studies have been stopped, and the results remain unpublished as a result of safety concerns.[17] Trials with TNF and IL-1 antagonism have demonstrated no survival benefit.[83,84] Currently, there is no "magic bullet" cure for SIRS, and future work involves combination therapy.[17] Attempts toward decreasing bacterial translocation, including selective gut decontamination, have demonstrated decreases in infectious complications but no affect on survival.[85] Others have reported a decrease in bacterial translocation through preservation of intestinal perfusion with vasodilators (nitroprusside) and TXA_2 inhibitors.[86-88] However, the best means of preserving mucosal integrity and minimizing GALT activation likely involves early delivery of enteral nutrients.[78]

METABOLIC ALTERATIONS

After the "ebb" phase that immediately follows a major burn and involves circulatory depression, local tissue and gut ischemia, and wound edema, patients develop a "flow" phase, which includes an elevated resting consumption of oxygen, coupled with increased nitrogen losses, autocannibalism,[89] insulin resistance, hyperglycemia, and futile substrate cycling.[90] Management of burn patients during the "flow" phase can be just as challenging as during the acute resuscitation.

Hypermetabolic Response

The insult of a major burn results in a greater elevation of the metabolic rate than is observed in all other forms of trauma (Fig. 65-7). The hypermetabolic response to thermal injury, which generally begins with 48 hours after injury, appears to be associated with an intrinsic elevation in body core temperature as a result of a direct resetting of the hypothalamic temperature-regulating mechanism. The zone of neutrality, or ambient temperature at which energy expenditure is minimal, is increased in burn patients from 27 to 29° C to 30 to 32° C.[91] Evidence supporting this contention relates to the observations that unburned skin remains vasoconstricted even when ambient temperatures are increased and evaporative losses are minimized.[92,93] On the other hand, although the hypermetabolic state does not depend on changes in ambient room temperature, it does appear to be sensitive to such alterations, since heat production and the energy cost of healing a large surface area can be reduced by keeping patients in a warm environment.[94,95] Factors mediating postburn hypermetabolism include inflammatory agents (IL-1, IL-6, TNF, eicosanoids, oxygen free radicals)[96] and counteregulatory hormones (catecholamines, cortisol, and glucagon).[97,98] The central nervous system appears to be important for this response, as it is decreased in patients with neurologic impairment.[99-101]

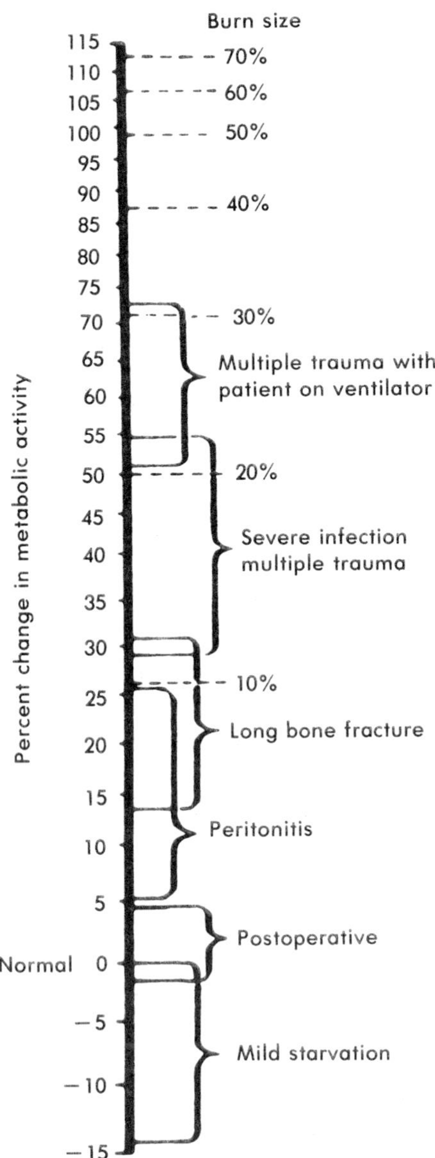

Fig. 65-7. Relative metabolic rates for various forms of trauma. (From Goodwin CW. Metabolism and nutrition. Crit Care Med 1:97, 1985.)

The magnitude of the hypermetabolic response reflects the extent of the thermal injury. It increases over the first week following injury and decreases in response to wound healing and the diminishing size of the burn wound. During this time, a protein catabolic state is produced that is characterized by increased urinary nitrogen loss, which is associated with protein degradation proportional to the severity of the burn. The hypermetabolic state generates a net caloric deficit. Although much of that deficit can be met through the use of fat deposits, the oxidation of fat requires simultaneous oxidation of carbohydrates. Once glycogen stores are exhausted, protein catabolism becomes the obligatory source of the carbohydrate.[102] In the process of gluconeogenesis, muscle protein is expended to liberate alanine and glutamine.[102,103] Without exogenous nutritional support, skeletal muscle becomes a prime target organ of the catabolic process.[93]

Postinjury Catabolism

The postinjury period is characterized by prolonged protein catabolism (particularly in muscle), negative nitrogen balance, hyperglycemia, lipolysis, hepatic fat deposition, and weight loss, all of which vary according to the extent of thermal injury. Derangements in the counter-regulatory hormones contribute to this "auto-cannibalism" (Fig. 65-8). Although it remains in a nonsteady state for weeks, the catabolic state ultimately reaches a plateau and does not change in response to caloric replacement.[104,105] For a 50% total body surface area burn, the magnitude of catabolism may be twice that which normally occurs following an injury. Weight loss develops because of a breakdown of lean body mass. The loss of 300 to 600 g of body weight per day can be equated to a daily loss of 75 to 150 g of protein.[106] Although treatment with calories and nitrogenous source does not affect breakdown of muscle protein, it can increase in synthesis.

This apparent metabolic paradox can be appreciated by briefly reviewing the cycle through which carbohydrates are produced and used. Gluconeogenesis uses amino acids, principally alanine and glutamine. The source of these two gluconeogenic amino acids is skeletal muscle. Although the source appears to be obligatory, exogenous amino acids can either decrease muscle efflux or contribute to increased muscle synthesis.[107] The increase in conversion of alanine to glucose is accompanied by a reduction in the incorporation of exogenous alanine into protein and an increase in the release and synthesis of alanine by muscle.[108] At the same time, a reduction in circulating branched-chain amino acids suggests that the administration of exogenous amino acids, especially those of the branched-chain variety, may stimulate de novo synthesis of alanine and glutamine by skeletal muscle.[109]

The process of gluconeogenesis from skeletal muscle substrates requires energy. In this process skeletal muscle uses fatty acid substrates.[110] Meanwhile, glucose from the liver's new stores is only partially used in the periphery, being converted to a three-carbon precursor, which in turn must return to the liver for reconversion into new glucose. The process of reconversion, referred to as the Cori cycle, also requires fatty acid substrates.[111] Although increased lipolysis and lipid mobilization occur in the burn patient, exogenous administration of fatty acids appears to be of little nutritional value and may be related to variation in the body's ability to clear lipids when in a state of stress.[112] Following thermal injury, it has been noted that a diet consisting of 5% to 15% of the nonprotein calories as fat is optimal and that a diet consisting of more is deleterious.[113] In humans the inhibition of triglyceride lipase by insulin may lead to a futile cycle of triglyceride metabolism.[114] Immediately after a burn, for example, there is increased lipoprotein lipase activity and clearance of triglycerides as insulin levels fall and glucagon and glucose levels

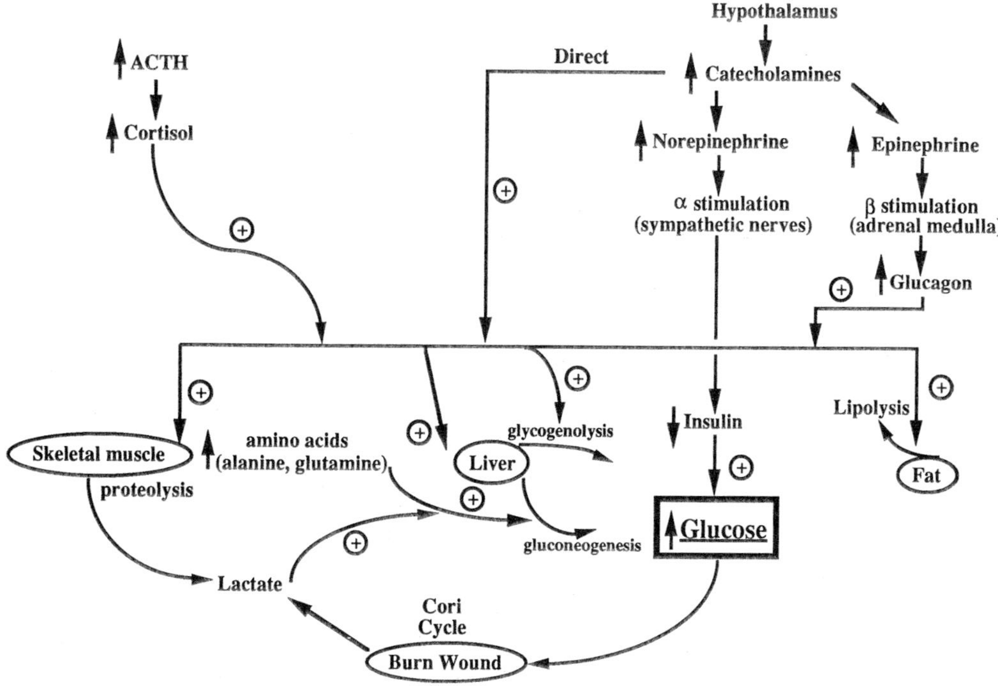

Fig. 65-8. Hormonal interactions following burn injury. *ACTH,* Adrenocorticotropic hormone. (Modified from Muller MJ, Herndon DN. Hormonal interactions in burned patients. Semin Nephrol 13:391, 1993.)

rise. In response to plasma triglycerides, lipase activity increases. However, the resulting free fatty acids cannot be used without carbohydrates and eventually must be reesterified to triglycerides. For a more detailed discussion of these considerations, see Chapter 1.

Therapeutic Implications

The dramatically increased metabolic expenditure following thermal injury must be compensated by increased nutritional support to avoid the plethora of potential complications associated with nutritional deficiency. Energy requirements in terms of caloric needs can be calculated according to the formula below proposed by Curreri et al.[110]

25 kcal/kg of body weight +
40 kcal/percent of body surface burned

Carbohydrate is the major source of calories and contributes to nitrogen sparing. The major carbohydrate form is glucose, and it must be administered with nitrogen-containing nutrients to improve nitrogen balance and allow more calories to be used for the restoration of nitrogen balance. Approximately 20% of caloric requirements should be protein or amino acid equivalents; improved survivals have been demonstrated with a 100:1 calorie-to-nitrogen ratio diet[115] and patients may require up to 2 to 2.5 g protein/kg/day. Essential fatty acids must also be provided, and 2% to 4% of daily caloric requirements should consist of linoleic acid.[116] In addition to preventing a state of fatty acid deficiency, fat also provides extra calories and may provide a protein-sparing effect.[117] Overfeeding, however, may be just as detrimental as underfeeding. Disproportionate lipids may lead to hyperlipidemia, hypoxia, impaired immune function, and increase mortality,[118] whereas excessive carbohydrate administration may cause respiratory insufficiency, impaired PMN function, and fatty liver.

In patients with large burns, enteral tube feeding is almost always necessary to achieve nutritional goods. Most patients, when left to their own dietary habits, do not consume adequate nutrients orally. Generally a high-calorie, high-protein diet should be administered in addition to the calculated tube requirement. Early enteral feeding has been determined to be safe[119] and has been shown to improve survival by preserving the intestinal mucosal barrier[117] and attenuating elevations of glucagon, cortisol, and catecholamines.[114,120] Further, vitamin and mineral requirements must be provided in all nutritional programs. Glutamine and arginine supplementation has been associated with improved immune function, intestinal growth, and wound healing. Indiscriminate use of total parenteral nutrition in the face of a functioning gut is not justified as it is fraught with immune defense impairment[121] and increased infectious complications.[122,123]

Daily weight gain is the most effective single index for assessing the adequacy of nutritional support and must be continually monitored. Nitrogen balance studies generally are inaccurate when large open wounds exist, and indexes of immunologic status and visceral protein pool have not been shown to accurately predict specific nutritional deficiencies.[116] Indirect calorimetry (metabolic cart) estimates energy expenditure and therefore nutritional requirements by analyzing inspired and expired gases and calculating the oxygen consumption and carbon dioxide production. However, this technique is expensive, difficult in nonintubated patients, and associated with the error of extrapolating a 20-minute study to 24 hours.[117]

ORGAN SYSTEM ALTERATIONS

Cardiovascular Responses

The initial "ebb" phase following burn injury is likely caused by a combination of hypovolemia and myocardial depression[124] and consists of a fall in cardiac output of 50% of normal or greater. This response occurs within minutes of injury, and there is a loss of myocardial contractility and altered ventricular compliance even prior to measurable decreases in plasma volume or after adequate fluid resuscitation.[28,125,126] Suggested mediators of this cardiac dysfunction include a myocardial depressant factor,[30] TNF,[30] interleukins, ADH, oxygen free radicals,[32-34] and nitric oxide.[21] Myocardial depressant factor, although still not fully identified chemically, is produced by the pancreas during circulatory shock[127] and has negative effects on the cardiovascular, splanchnic, and reticuloendothelial systems.[128]

Most of these responses tend to normalize as plasma volume is restored through resuscitative efforts, although the cardiac output generally returns to normal and may actually exceed normal values before complete restoration of plasma volume is achieved. This resultant hyperdynamic circulatory response (or "flow" pattern) appears to complement the hypermetabolic response previously discussed, and both appear to reflect an effort of the body to heal the injured wound. During this phase, excessive catecholamine secretion may lead to cardiomyopathy, focal necrosis, and myocarditis.[129,130] Trials employing propranolol (a nonselective β-antagonist) have demonstrated cardioprotective effects but are associated with a negative nitrogen balance.[24] Future work is directed toward using selective β-adrenergic blockade in an attempt to decrease myocardial oxygen requirements while preventing the resulting changes in lipid kinetics.[131]

Renal Responses

The burn patient is initially in a state of antidiuresis. In the presence of a hyperdynamic circulatory response, oliguria occurs as a result of increased and inappropriate ADH secretion. It has also been shown that glomerular vessels become constricted, prolonging transit time through the kidney and decreasing urinary output. Metabolism within the kidney appears to increase, as evidenced by a consistent uptake of glucose, whereas renal plasma flow remains essentially unaltered.[132,133]

Despite the glomerular vascular changes, renal complications are relatively uncommon in thermally injured patients because of the improved knowledge of resuscitation since 1980. The initial renal lesion following burn injury appears to be biphasic proteinuria. The initial phase includes a mild, transient albuminuria followed in 4 to 7 days by a proteinuria with a relatively low albumin composition.[134] Any relationship between the proteinuria and the subsequent development of renal failure remains unclear. When renal failure does ensue, it proceeds characteristically with polyuria in the face of a rising serum creatinine.

Oliguric renal failure is quite rare. When it occurs, it develops early and appears to be related to inadequate resuscitation. In contrast, the more common polyuric renal failure generally arises in the second or third week following the burn injury and does not seem to be caused by hypovolemia. The findings of low urinary sodium and high urinary potassium indicate intact distal tubular function. These observations indicate that burn-related dysfunction in the glomerulus and proximal tubule presents the distal nephron with a solute load, producing a "downstream" diuresis.[135] The cause of this form of renal failure remains unknown, and it is unique to the burn patient.

Endocrine Responses

A complex endocrine response is elicited by thermal injury that probably is related to peripheral nervous stimulation of the hypophysial-hypothalamic axis of the brain that then in turn intricately interacts with metabolic, immune, and other body systems.[136] Pain, through the release of neuropeptides by sensory C fibers, may be a major stimulatory event for the hormonal response.[19] Sustained, elevated levels of adrenocorticotropic hormone (ACTH) from the anterior pituitary gland have been reported throughout the acute phase of thermal injury and only decrease to normal as the burn wound heals.[137] If one uses measurements of plasma cortisol as an index of ACTH secretion, however, no consistent patterns have been noted in burn patients.[138] The activity of the thyroid gland is decreased following injury and thyroid-stimulating hormone (TSH) is decreased relative to the availability of thyroid hormones.[139] Thyroxine (T_4) and triiodothyronine (T_3) blood levels are generally low in burn injury, although a less pronounced decrease in T_4 and a transitory increase in reverse T_3 have been identified.[138,138a] However, there are no data to support thyroid supplementation. The "flow" phase is likely not thyroid dependent as thyroprivic experimental models also demonstrate a catabolic/hypermetabolic burn response.[140-142]

Growth hormone secretion is inconsistent in burn patients but often is elevated following thermal injury. Recent work has been directed toward hormonal modulation in an attempt to improve wound healing. Exogenous growth hormone administration improves the healing time of donor sites in children and accelerates healing after extensive burns[143,144] but may exacerbate hyperglycemia and insulin resistance.[145] Current work involves insulin-like growth factor (IGF-1) supplementation, which may preserve lean body mass and preserve gut function without altering glucose metabolism.[146] Follicle-stimulating hormone and luteinizing hormone secretion are depressed in burn patients, whereas prolactin secretion may be suppressed in children but elevated in adults.[147] The significance of these observations remains unknown.

ADH measurements reveal high levels in both blood and urine of adults and children during the first week after burn injury. ADH release is normally modulated by osmoreceptors of the supraventricular and supraoptic nuclei in the hypothalamus, volume receptors in the right atrium, and the carotid bodies. However, oversecretion is apparently independent of plasma and urine osmolality and volume but related closely to the severity of the thermal injury.[148]

Glucocorticoids, mineralocorticoids, and 17-ketosteroids are the major hormonal groups secreted by the adrenal cortex. Cortisol is high in burn patients with loss of the normal circadian rhythm, particularly in the first week following thermal injury. This elevation is believed to be essentially unrelated to ACTH hypersecretion but does relate closely to the size of the burn.[48] Aldosterone is secreted in markedly increased amounts and produces sodium retention and increased potassium loss, which persists for many weeks in adults with major burns.[148] The 17-ketosteroids are also elevated in burn patients as measured in the urine, but the significance of this finding is unknown.

Epinephrine and norepinephrine synthesis, under hypothalamic control, are dramatically increased in thermal injury, as detected in serum and urine of burn patients, and are major mediators of the hypermetabolic response.[149] Immunoreactive insulin is elevated following thermal injury, and this elevation persists until healing of the burn wound. Insulin hypersecretion is usually accompanied by elevated glucose in the blood, implying a relative insulin resistance.[150] Plasma glucagon levels are also elevated and appear to play a key role in the hypermetabolic response.[151] It is thought that glucagon released from alpha cells of the pancreas is more influential in producing postburn hyperglycemia than the so-called insulin resistance.[152] A synergy exists between cortisol, glucagon, and catecholamines that contributes to the increases in glycolysis, gluconeogenesis, proteolysis, and lipolysis observed during the postburn hypermetabolism/catabolism (see Fig. 65-8).

RESISTANCE TO INFECTION

The causes of death have changed with the progression of burn management. In the 1940s to 1950s most patients died of burn shock. With more vigorous fluid resuscitation protocols, wound sepsis became the major killer in the 1960s to the 1970s. However, the development of burn centers, topical and systemic antibiotics, nutritional support, and earlier burn wound excision has considerably decreased mortality caused by wound sepsis. Currently, pulmonary infection remains the most common cause of death in hospitalized burn patients. Resistance is impaired in these patients through disruption of the skin's mechanical barrier and defects in the body's immune system. Fauci[153] has conveniently classified the body's defense capabilities into the categories of nonspecific immune system and specific immune system. Although many defects in the capacity to resist infection have been defined in thermally injured patients, direct relationships between burning and immunologic alterations are complex and unclear and have eluded successful therapeutic intervention. However, it is clear that postburn patients demonstrate generalized immunosuppression. Allografts in burn victims survive longer than expected.[154] Both in vivo and in vitro measurements of immune function are abnormal; these include decreased delayed type of hypersensitivity responses,[155] cytolytic responses,[156] and mixed lymphocytic responses.[157]

Disruption of the Mechanical Barrier

Loss of the morphologic and physiologic integrity of the skin as a result of thermal injury allows access of microorganisms to deeper tissues and the systemic circulation. Not only is devitalized tissue a nutritious medium for the growth of bacteria, but thermally injured skin may be a source of circulating substances or toxins that can contribute to multifaceted, systemic alterations, including impairment in the synthesis of secretory immunoglobulins, bone marrow depression, and myocardial depression.[13,148,158,159] As discussed earlier, decreased meseneric blood flow also contributes to these systemic effects following burn injury through bacterial/endotoxin translocation into the portal circulation and/or priming of the cellular elements within the GALT.

Impairment of the Nonspecific Immune System

Phagocytic cell activity and accumulation are enhanced in response to tissue injury through an inflammatory reaction characterized by increased vascular permeability. This appears to be mediated by vasoactive amines, prostaglandins, C-reactive proteins, and other components of inflammation.[160] In addition, the release of chemotactic substances from injured tissues or through the influence of gram negative organisms enhances the attraction of phagocytes to invading microorganisms. Should bacteria not be contained at the site of invasion, the fixed macrophages, particularly in the regional lymph nodes, may prove effective in killing invading bacteria.

Opsonins are antibodies that enhance the phagocytic process by rendering the microorganisms more susceptible to phagocytosis. Complement and fibronectin are characterized opsonins. Complement is a system of serum proteins that participates in inflammation and phagocytosis and in neutralizing viruses, enhancing leukocyte chemotaxis, and killing bacteria. Fibronectin is a glycoprotein existing in a soluble circulating form in the plasma and a relatively insoluble form in connective tissue. Fibronectin enhances macrophage phagocytosis and may prevent organ failure through inhibition of fibrin aggregation among other functions. Other undefined regional defense mechanisms also participate in protecting the host from hostile microorganisms.

The presence of major thermal injury adversely affects this nonspecific inflammatory system. Both circulating and fixed phagocytic cells, with or without the help of opsonizing factors, are functionally impaired following a major burn. Not only is phagocytic activity decreased in burn injury, but bacteriocidal activity is also decreased, and chemotaxis is impaired through decreased complement activation.[161-163]

Impairment of the Specific Immune System

The specific immune system includes both humoral and cellular components and their respective products. The production of specific antibody requires a complex interaction of many cell types. Once an antigen is recognized, it is processed by macrophages and presented to thymic-dependent lymphocytes (T cells). T cells proliferate and in turn activate bursal-dependent lymphocytes (B cells) that ultimately produce a specific antibody to the antigen. Stimulated T lymphocytes have other important functions such as antigen memory storage, direct cytotoxic effects, and production of mediators of immune reactivity regulating both the specific and nonspecific immune responses. Antibody formation is also influenced by a specific subset of T cells known as T-helper cells and a second subset known as suppressor T cells. Suppressor T cells generally modulate responses preventing uncontrolled immune reactions by inhibiting T-cell stimulation of antibody production.

In patients with burns of more than 20% of their total body surface area, essentially all immune functions are affected. Overall, there is a decrease in total lymphyoctye populations, an impairment in the functional capacity of T cells, and an activation of suppressor T cells.[164] This depresses T cell–generated responses, including production of cytotoxic cells, B-cell activation, and recruitment of uncommitted lymphoid cells. Immunoglobulin synthesis is also decreased, particularly IgG production, in contrast to IgM and IgA, which are little altered.

Some investigators suggest that there exists an intracellular T-cell defect.[164] Burn injury also interferes with the signalling pathways responsible for T-cell activation and effector response generation.[165] This has been associated with the release of hormones (glucocorticoids and catecholamines)[166] and the systemic release of PGE_2 by activated macrophages. Although the precise mechanisms are unknown, PGE_2 decreases IL-2 production and, hence, T-cell activation.[167-169] Trials investigating IL-2 and indomethacin (a cyclooxygenase inhibitor) administration in burned mice have demonstrated an improved survival.[170] Others have used polymixin B, which neutralized the effects of lipopolysaccharides and may decrease macrophage activation. Although they observed a reversal of the unfavorable T4/T8 ratio and a decrease in endotoxin concentration, there was no change in survival or outcome.[171,172]

PULMONARY CONSEQUENCES OF THERMAL INJURY

Pulmonary alterations as a result of thermal injury occur in response to direct pulmonary injury caused by the inhalation of the products of combustion and indirectly as a response to cutaneous burns alone.

Inhalation of the Products of Combustion

Inhalation injury accounts for the vast majority of deaths in fires and is responsible for the high mortality in patients who survive and are admitted to hospitals. The following classification has proven useful in categorizing the various disorders related to inhalation injury and is based on mechanisms of disease[173]:

1. Carbon monoxide poisoning
2. Smoke toxicity
   a. Direct injury caused by
      (1) Hot gases
      (2) Super-heated particulate matter
      (3) Conversion of gases to acid and alkali
   b. Smoke poisoning caused by thermodegradation of
      (1) Natural substances
      (2) Synthetic substances

Carbon Monoxide Poisoning

Carbon monoxide is a clear, colorless, odorless gas produced by the incomplete combustion of organic fuels. Carbon monoxide has an affinity for hemoglobin that is approximately 250 times that of oxygen and shifts the oxyhemoglobin dissociation curve to the left. Thus the oxygen that remains bound to hemoglobin is not readily available to cells, resulting in a decreased tissue oxygen tension that is considerably lower than that seen with simple hypoxia alone (Fig. 65-9). Thus the toxic effect of carbon monoxide may be the result of this hypoxia alone or its binding to heme-containing proteins at the cellular level.[174] Carbon monoxide impairs the cytochrome chain through competition with oxygen for cytochrome a_3 and had been observed to have a direct toxic effect on mammalian lung tissue.[175]Carbon monoxide also binds to cardiac and skeletal muscle, producing carboxymyoglobin that dissociates slower than carboxyhemoglobin. This circum-

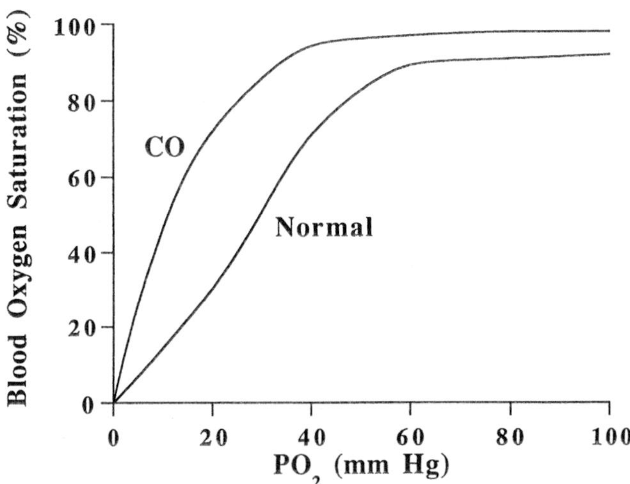

Fig. 65-9. Oxygen-hemoglobin dissociation curve. Note the shift to the left in the presence of carbon monoxide *(CO)*, indicating that oxygen is more tightly bound to the hemoglobin molecule. Po_2, Partial pressure of oxygen.

stance may become apparent during initial treatment as a rebound type of response. Pure carbon monoxide poisoning produces no grossly detectable lung pathologic alteration, although, histologically, alveolar type II cellular organelles are physically altered.[176]

The clinical symptoms of carbon monoxide poisoning range from dyspnea and headache at levels in excess of 10% to 20% to coma and death when inspired air contains levels of 60%. Cherry red skin discoloration is usually not apparent because of facial burning, but a high index of suspicion based on the history of burning in an enclosed space, orofacial burns, and nasal hair singeing suggests the diagnosis. A laboratory carboxyhemoglobin determination confirms the diagnosis, and treatment consists of rapid evacuation from the toxic source and the administration of 100% oxygen, preferably by endotracheal tube, in symptomatic poisoning. The half-life of carboxyhemoglobin in room air is approximately 210 minutes, but during 100% oxygen administration it can be reduced to 40 to 60 minutes. Hyperbaric oxygen has been proposed as a treatment modality in severe poisoning on the basis of a rapid decrease in the half-life of carboxyhemoglobin and clinical evidence of improved neurologic recovery.[177] However, the logistics of caring for patients with significant burns within the confines of oxygen chambers is difficult.

Smoke Toxicity

Direct injury. Direct heat injury as a result of inhalation of hot gases is extremely rare below the vocal cords because of the efficiency of heat dissipatory reflexes.[178] However, parenchymal injury to the epithelium in distal air passages may be observed by the inhalation of superheated system that has 4000 times the heat capacity of air. Super-heated particulate matter and soot that is not filtered out in the proximal airways may also produce local thermal burns in the alveoli.[179] Corrosive acids and alkalis resulting from the reaction of sulfur and nitrogen oxides adherent to soot particles with lung surface water also produce direct, local parenchymal injury.[173]

Smoke poisoning. The incomplete combustion of both natural and synthetic products in smoke produces noxious gases that are inhaled and elicit both local and systemic effects. The magnitude of injury is dependent on the type of noxious gas inhaled, its concentration and solubility, and the duration of exposure. Water-soluble chemicals such as ammonia, sulfur dioxide, chlorine, and hydrogen chloride tend to dissolve in the upper respiratory tract, whereas lipid-soluble gases such as the aldehydes, phosgene, and nitric oxide tend to reach more distal lung radicals.[180] Cyanide, a product of the combustion of synthetic materials such as polyurethane, produces its effects through systemic absorption and direct cellular poisoning.

The effect of inhaled toxic products includes direct epithelial destruction, mucosal edema, ciliary paralysis, and surfactant deficiency, the latter resulting from injury to type II alveolar epithelial cells.[181,182] Cast formation occurs causing obstruction, which leads to atelectasis, air trapping, and an increased risk for barotrauma. Pulmonary alveolar macrophages secrete chemotoxins producing leukocyte sequestration, which in turn release proteolytic enzymes and oxygen free radicals that potentiate pulmonary injury from the microvascular side.[176] Concurrently, there is an increase in exudation of protein-rich plasma that encourages bacterial overgrowth. Subsequent pathologic alterations depend on the severity and character of the inhalation and include a fulminant adult respiratory distress syndrome (ARDS), pulmonary edema, bronchial pneumonia, and sepsis, all of which contribute to the high mortality rate observed in patients with inhalation injury.

The diagnosis of smoke inhalation is based primarily on history, blood gas analysis, carboxyhemoglobin, and cyanide determinations, as well as on special procedures, including bronchoscopy, xenon clearance, and pulmonary function tests. Physical examination and chest x-ray films, although essential, may be misleading, particularly under acute conditions when a paucity of physical signs tend to be the rule in severe inhalation injury.

Careful monitoring of patients suspected of sustaining smoke poisoning is essential. In less severe injuries, treatment consists of the use of humidified air, vigorous pulmonary toilet, and the judicious use of bronchodilators. Immediate intubation is warranted if signs of laryngeal edema are present (hoarseness or stridor). Rigid bronchoscopy may be required for pulmonary cast removal. Pressure-control ventilation (permissive hypercapnea) may be attempted when pulmonary failure progresses despite conventional volume ventilation. High-frequency jet ventilation may be beneficial by decreasing barotrauma and improving airway clearance through the maintenance of patent distal airways. Nitric oxide inhalation has also shown some advantages. Invasive monitoring to include pulmonary wedge pressure and thermodilution cardiac output parameters is often essential, particularly when positive end-expiratory pressure is used. Corticosteroids and prophylactic antibiotics are ineffective.[183]

Indirect Pulmonary Injury

Pulmonary edema following pure cutaneous burning without inhalation injury relates to alterations in the pulmonary microvasculature. Hemodynamic alterations related to resuscitation, increased capillary permeability, and alterations in blood flow characteristics as a result of cutaneous thermal injury may contribute to indirect lung damage. Patients with major thermal injury and noninhalation pulmonary dysfunction have been shown to have consistently high concentrations of fragment D resulting from fibrinogen degradation. This phenomenon is associated with systemic complement depletion and platelet aggregation with release of platelet products that may cause increased translocation of water and protein from the pulmonary microcirculation contributing to the development of an ARDS picture.[184] In addition, activated complement may stimulate leukocyte aggregation, resulting in trapping of these aggregates in the pulmonary microcirculation. These leukocytes may then produce toxic oxygen metabolites that may also contribute to the development of ARDS. Later, pulmonary alterations generally relate to the onset of sepsis and may also manifest themselves as ARDS or bronchial pneumonia. Trials involving the administration of aerosolized free radical scavengers (dimethyl sulfoxide and *N*-acetylcysteine) have decreased lung fluid accumulation.[185] However, current therapies are primarily directed toward supportive intervention, and mortality from the pulmonary manifestations of burns remains high. For a more detailed discussion of these considerations, see Chapter 36.

PHYSIOLOGIC CONSIDERATIONS IN MANAGING THE BURN PATIENT

Fluid Resuscitation

The most important priority in the initial management of the burn patient is fluid resuscitation. The pathophysiologic alterations caused by the fluid losses in acutely burned patients requires volume replacement to preserve vital functions and to prevent hypovolemic shock. Fluid losses as a result of increased capillary permeability in injured and noninjured tissues are greatest in the first 24 hours following burning and diminish thereafter. Accompanying intravascular deficits also must be corrected but generally are less responsive to resuscitative efforts until the volume losses from "capillary leaking" are adequately controlled; 20% to 30% of infused crystalloid remains within the vascular system.[186]

The optimal approach to fluid resuscitation remains controversial in terms of both the volume of fluid to be administered and its composition. A wide variety of fluid replacement formulas have been proposed,[175,187-191] each with its advocates, differing primarily from one another with respect to salt and colloid content. Virtually all formulas are based on patient weight and the extent of skin surface burned. Only burns reaching a depth of second degree or greater are considered in these calculations. The fluid formulas provide guidelines for the resuscitation of burn patients and are altered according to the response to treatment.

The effectiveness of administered fluid in early burn resuscitation with regard to its colloidal or noncolloidal content remains unresolved. Advocates of colloid-containing fluids recognize their potential use in maintaining plasma oncotic pressure and intravascular volume. Those opposed to such solutions emphasize the increased capillary permeability in the first 24 hours after thermal injury that results in leakage of plasma protein, particularly albumin, into the interstitium. It is argued that adding exogenous protein (i.e., colloid) to the extravascular protein pool raises this interstitial oncotic pressure further and thereby prevents restoration of an adequate circulating blood volume. Furthermore, controlled trials have demonstrated that colloid use has no effect on clinical outcome.[192,193] There is general agreement, however, that the administration of colloid-containing fluids during the second 24 hours following the burn and thereafter is associated with intravascular colloid retention and thus decreased fluid requirements.

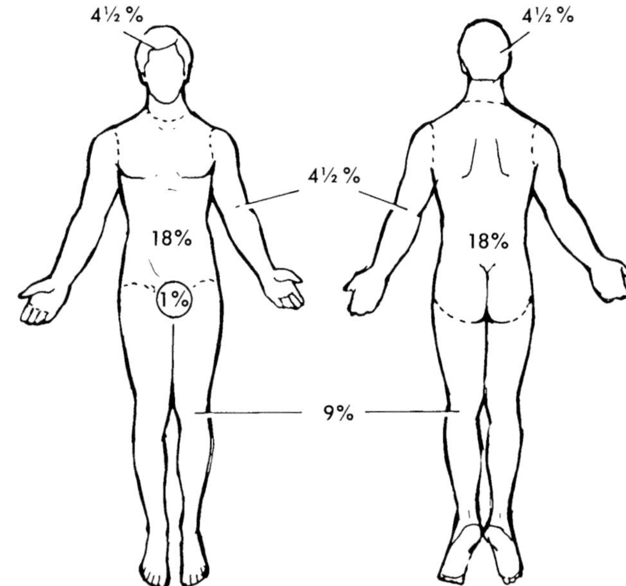

Fig. 65-10. "Rule of nines" for adults. Rapid estimation of extent of burn injury can be accomplished by using the "rule of nines" as an approximation of body surface areas involved. (From Parks DH, Carvajal HF, Larson DL. Management of burns. Surg Clin North Am 57:875, 1977.)

In contrast to the colloid controversy, sodium ion administration appears to be essential to successful resuscitation. Balanced salt solutions are quite popular and effective, although the use of hypertonic saline solutions has been recommended.[190] Hypertonic saline (sodium concentration = 250 mmol/L) reduces volume requirements, may be useful in patients with limited cardiovascular reserve but requires careful monitoring,[194] and is associated with increased renal failure and death.[195]

Body surface charts are available for the determination of surface area burned and are based on delineating body surface components (e.g., head, back, extremity) as a percentage of the whole body surface[57,191,196] (Figs. 65-10 and 65-11). This method improves the accuracy of the determination and provides the basis for the use of the various formulas. Patients with second- and third-degree burns involving greater than 15% of their body surface area should receive parenteral fluids, and the effectiveness of resuscitation should be monitored precisely.

An Approach to Resuscitation

The replacement program that we use has proven to be convenient and successful over many years of application and is described here. In this program, fluid losses and daily maintenance requirements are related to the total body surface area and the surface area burned (in square meters)

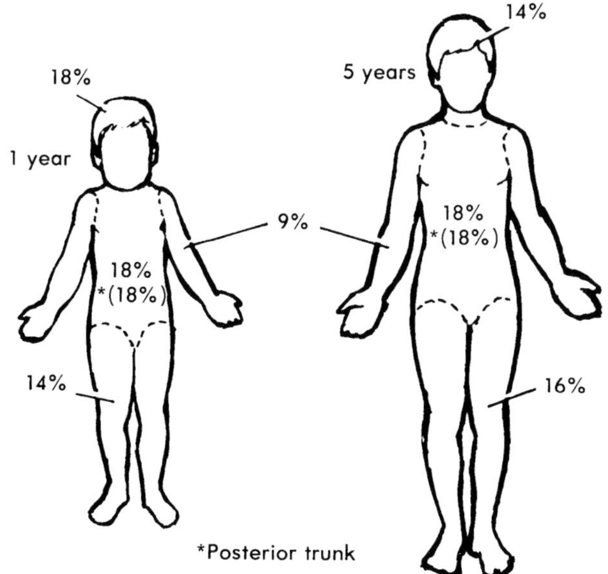

Fig. 65-11. Modified "rule of nines" for ages 1 and 5 years. Adult proportions assumed at age 15. (From Parks DH, Carvajal HF, Larson DL. Management of burns. Surg Clin North Am 57:875, 1977.)

as calculated from a standard height-weight nomogram. This approach has proven to be highly accurate and allows standardization of fluid therapy in managing both adults and children. During the first 24 hours following burning, fluid requirements are calculated as follows:

2000 ml/m² of body surface/24 hr
(maintenance requirements)
\+
5000 ml/m² of body surface burned/24 hr
(fluid losses)

One half the calculated volume is infused in the first 8 hours following burning, and the remainder in the subsequent 16 hours. Patients should also be given either H_2 blockers or sucralfate to prevent the development of Curling's ulcers.

For such resuscitation, a single, standard solution for intravenous therapy is used with adaptation to the patient's needs as necessary. This solution consists of:

Lactated Ringer's solution in 5% dextrose and water
\+
12.5 g of salt-poor albumin per liter

We have found such a solution to be ideal. This isotonic protein-containing fluid ensures the provision of lactate to combat any systemic acidosis and an adequate carbohydrate load to ensure protein sparing. Because of the hyperkalemia associated with tissue injury and increased aldosterone, addition of potassium to this solution during the first 48 hours after burning is inappropriate and may be detrimental.

During the second 24 hours following burning, fluid requirements generally decrease and are calculated on the basis of the following formula:

1500 ml/m² of body surface area/24 hr
(maintenance requirements)
\+
4000 ml/m² of body surface area burned/24 hr
(fluid losses)

Such requirements are administered in equal hourly aliquots during this 24-hour period. Oral alimentation is instituted as soon as possible in the form of homogenized milk, and the intravenous fluid needs are decreased proportionately. When the milk intake increases sufficiently, the antacid therapy begun during the first 24 hours is decreased. In most cases oral fluid administration completely replaces intravenous therapy at the end of 48 hours following burning, allowing removal of the intravenous catheter.

Daily fluid requirements after the initial 48 hours of fluid resuscitation generally remain the same as those for the second 24 hours; but as the burn wounds are covered and healing commences, requirements are generally diminished, and fluid therapy is revised accordingly. As already indicated, initial oral alimentation is usually administered through a nasogastric feeding tube that is retained for several days thereafter to ensure adequate oral nutrition. Until the convalescent phase is well underway, milk should continue to be given on an hourly basis to protect the stomach from the development of a Curling's ulcer. In those patients who have a lactate deficiency, a soy-based formula can be substituted. Patients should be started on regular meals in addition to this milk as soon as such alimentation can be adequately tolerated.

As indicated in an earlier section of this chapter, the burn patient remains in a hypermetabolic state requiring high caloric support until wound coverage has been achieved. It has been estimated that evaporative losses alone may amount to 4 L/m² of the burn area, which results in an expenditure of 576 kcal/L of water evaporated. Thus to ensure adequate caloric intake in the burn patient, the following formula has been used by the authors:

1800 kcal/m² of body surface/24 hr +
2200 kcal/m² of body surface burned/24 hr

Milk by itself produces approximately 0.66 kcal/ml of fluid administered. With the additional calories provided by a regular diet, most caloric requirements can be adequately met. If there is any problem in ensuring this possibility, nutritional needs should be guaranteed by the administration of appropriate feeding regimens through a nasogastric feeding tube.

Monitoring Fluid Resuscitation

The effectiveness of the resuscitation program must be constantly monitored and altered if deviations from the expected course are noted. Among the most useful physical signs to determine the adequacy of resuscitation are the general state of alertness of the patient and the stability of pulse and blood pressure, including peripheral perfusion characteristics. The urine output (by means of an indwelling urinary catheter) is the most readily obtained measure of effectiveness of resuscitation, and a urine volume of 30 to 50 ml/hr in the adult and 20 to 40 ml/m^2 of total body surface area per hour in children are expected. A significantly higher urine output may indicate overhydration or other complications (e.g., polyuric renal failure, excessive glucose loading), since in the acutely burned patient an antidiuretic state caused by multiple factors, including ADH secretion, is present.

Baseline laboratory studies should be obtained at the time of admission and repeated at 12 to 24 hours or more frequently as needed. Among the values to be obtained initially are a complete blood cell count; serum levels of sodium, potassium, chloride, and bicarbonate; a blood urea nitrogen and creatinine, urine protein, and serum protein electrophoresis; and arterial blood gases. An initial hemoconcentration is expected, regardless of the resuscitation program instituted; and therefore an elevated hematocrit and slight elevation of other parameters may be identified. Metabolic acidosis is particularly significant in children and may indicate inadequacy of resuscitation.

A chest x-ray examination, electrocardiogram, and complete urinalysis are usually performed on admission and repeated only as indicated during the subsequent course. Invasive monitoring with Swan-Ganz catheters or central venous lines is not routinely performed except in elderly patients, patients with cardiovascular compromise, or patients with inhalation injury requiring machine ventilation. Inotropic agents may be required if cardiac output remains poor despite adequate volume resuscitation. However, this is generally considered to be a poor prognostic sign.

The timely administration of carefully monitored parenteral fluids to the acutely and extensively burned patient facilitating the body's own compensatory physiologic alterations prevents early complications, minimizes physiologic disturbances, and provides a basis on which future care of the acutely burned patient depends.

Management of the Burn Wound

After fluid resuscitation has been successfully ensured, attention is next directed to the burn wound itself. The wound is cleansed with a suitable antiseptic solution such as povidone-iodine (Betadine) and debrided of foreign matter, necrotic tissue, and any blebs or vesicles that may be present. Since hypothermia may be a problem during this debridement period, overhead radiant energy sources are usually used to minimize the loss of body heat.

Because the burn wound is essentially an extensive area of coagulation necrosis with accompanying ischemia from the underlying thrombosis of the local microcirculation, this avascular dead tissue is an excellent bacterial culture medium that can rapidly become a source of bacterial growth and the development of sepsis from hematologic dissemination of microorganisms. For this reason, topical antimicrobial agents are applied directly to the wound during the early period after the burn. In the historical development of burn management during the past several decades, a variety of agents have been developed for this purpose, each with its particular advantages and disadvantages. Presently four such agents are in use at burn centers across the United States as summarized in Table 65-2. Each of these agents, in varying degrees, satisifes the characteristics of an ideal topical agent, which include (1) antibacterial activity that is both broad spectrum in nature and nontoxic locally or on absorption, (2) resistance to the development of strains of bacteria that would not be covered, (3) adequate permeation and the maintenance of continuing activity in the burn eschar, (4) absence of pain on application, and (5) absence of adverse effects on the behavior of the wound, including its healing properties. Of the agents currently available, 1% silver sulfadiazine is the most popular among burn specialists and is our choice. This drug is essentially nontoxic, is easy to apply and soothing to the patient, and has a broad spectrum of antimicrobial activity and minimal problems with the development of resistant strains. Its only major disadvantage is its limited penetration through the eschar and its relative ineffectiveness when deep eschar colonization with microorganisms has already occurred. When the latter circumstance exists, a gentamicin cream is usually substituted if the cultured organisms are sensitive. Mafenide (11.1%) also diffuses well through devascularized tissues but is unfortunately associated with metabolic acidosis because of carbonic anhydrase inhibition. Silver sulfadiazine is applied in a thin layer (usually 1 mm thick) two or three times daily, using a sterile glove or tongue depressor. Although some specialists leave the treated burn wound open to the air, we generally apply a thin layer of fine mesh gauze impregnated with the cream over the treated burn area and further retain it with a netlike dressing.[191] This approach allows patients to move about freely and guarantees contact of the cream with the burn wound at all times. At the present time, all first-degree and superficial second-degree burns are managed in this fashion, enabling spontaneous reepithelization to occur.

For deep second-degree burns and all third-degree burns, early surgical excision is now considered the procedure of choice and is associated with a decreased mortality.[197-199] For deep partial-thickness burn wounds, a technique called *tangential excision* is used. This technique involves the excision of the necrotic surface of a burn by removing shavings of eschar until a pattern of pinpoint deep dermal bleeding is reached and then immediately autografting the excised surface. The rationale underlying this approach is that the removal of the zone of coagulation protects the viable elements in the zone of stasis and thereby exposes a surface that readily accepts an autograft.

Table 65-2. Topical Antimicrobial Agents

Characteristics	Silver Nitrate (0.5%)	Mafenide	Silver Sulfadiazine	Organic Iodine
Type of preparation	Aqueous solution	Cream	Cream	Foam
Method of wound care	Closed	Open or closed	Open or closed	Open or closed
Allergic reactions	None	10%	10%	5%
Pain on application	None	Severe	None	Moderate
Amount absorbed	None	5%	1%	Variable
Associated complications	Significant losses of sodium and potassium into wet dressings, methemoglobinemia	Acidosis, hyperventilation caused by renal carbonic anhydase inhibition	None	None
Fungal overgrowth	—	Often	Often	Often
Bacterial resistance	Bacteriostatic	Rare	Rare	Occasional
Cost	Inexpensive	Moderate	Moderate	Moderate

Modified from Curreri PW. Burns. In Polk HC, Stone HH, Gardner B, eds. Basic Surgery, 3rd ed. Norwalk, Conn.: Appleton-Century-Crofts, 1987.

As much as 20% of the body surface may be excised at one time. The major problem with this technique is that considerable blood loss may occur, necessitating the need for substantial blood replacement (particularly in major burns in which such excision may need to be repeated several times within a period of days) and the careful monitoring of anesthesia to prevent other problems such as shock with its attendant complications. For full-thickness burns, excision is carried down to the level of the fascia, and an autograft is then placed on the exposed base. These aggressive surgical approaches to burn management have demonstrated several advantages to the more traditional methods of debridement using various proteolytic enzymes, the most popular of which has been sutilains (Travase). Such advantages have included improved function of extremities (particularly hands), a better cosmetic result, a definite decrease in the incidence of hypertrophic scarring after the burn, and a considerable reduction in hospitalization time.

In the event that a patient may have extensive body burns limiting the amount of nonburn areas that can be used for the acquisition of skin grafts, temporary coverage of the surgically debrided burn may be obtained with various biologic dressings, including amnion or porcine xenografts. Another innovative approach has been the use of artificial skin. Several types of synthetic skin have been evaluated investigationally. Of these, the bilaminate membrane appears to be the most useful.[200] This substance consists of reconstituted collagen with a silicon synthetic epidermis. Application of this substance to the debrided burn surface results in vascularization of the collagen layer with the production of an underlying neodermis. When donor sites become available, the silicon synthetic epidermis is stripped from the underlying collagen, and an autograft is placed on the neodermis. Initial results with such an approach have proven quite gratifying and open up exciting possibilities in the management of burn wounds in the future. Cultured epidermal cells from a 2 cm^2 skin harvest have also been investigated as another option for skin coverage in the hope that these cells might produce growth factors that would enhance the healing process. However, currently this technology is associated with high costs, high failure rates, and increased scar formation.[185]

A unique problem that occasionally develops with deep second-degree or third-degree circumferential burns, especially when involving the extremities of trunk, is the resulting tourniquet effect. This occurs because the elastic membrane of the dermis is destroyed with these types of burns and no longer allows the skin to stretch, which is necessary to accommodate the underlying edema formation. In the chest such circumferential eschar formation may prevent normal respiration. If not corrected, the rapid development of respiratory acidosis may ensue. When this problem exists, incision through the eschar should be carried out and deepened into the subcutaneous fat to effect adequate release of the constricted tissue. This can be accomplished by making vertical anterior axillary line incisions that are curved medially to the level of the suprasternal notch. In addition, transverse incisions at the level of the diaphragm effect further release of the constricted tissue. In the extremities eschar constriction often results in a decreased venous outflow from the affected part and in time jeopardizes the arterial inflow. Ischemia then results, which may be manifest by decreased capillary refill of the nail beds, severe pain within the involved muscle compartment of the extremity, or the development of motor and/or sensory deficits. Often, elevation of the affected extremity may allay the need for escharotomy, but continuous monitoring of the peripheral pulse, usually with an ultrasound detector, must be assured. If this cannot be guaranteed, lateral longitudinal incisions through the burn eschar should be made to the level of the subcutaneous fat to release the pressure in the constricted muscle compartments. Both extremity escharotomies and those involving the chest can generally be performed without the assistance of anesthesia, since the burn wound is usually insensitive to painful stimuli.

SUMMARY

The disruption of the physiologic equilibrium of the human organism by thermal injury varies with the extent and depth of the burn. The burn wound is characterized by a central irreversible zone of coagulation necrosis surrounded by reversible altered tissues that may be irreversibly compromised by progressive ischemia as a result of systemic factors such as hypoperfusion and local factors such as prostaglandin derivatives. Major fluid shifts caused by permeability alterations occur as a result of physical changes in the microcirculatory ultrastructure and local release of vasoactive substances. Such alterations disrupt normal Starling forces and potentiate fluid losses. Additional fluid extravasation in unburned tissues contributes to the hypovolemic state and may relate to increased capillary permeability and plasma oncotic pressure alterations.

Thermal injury induces a state of marked hypermetabolism mediated by catecholamines and requires an intense nutritional replacement program to overcome the potentially deleterious consequences of malnutrition. The initial fall in cardiac output observed in burns ("ebb" phase) is followed by an intense hyperdynamic circulatory response ("flow" phase). A state of antidiuresis is induced, and the hormonal milieu of the body is dramatically altered in concert with the metabolic and immune alterations.

Resistance to infection is severely compromised in thermally injured patients through alterations in both nonspecific and specific immune systems. Thermally altered tissue allows access of microorganisms and provides a medium for bacterial growth. Phagocytic activity is decreased along with bacteriocidal activity within the phagocytes. T-cell populations are decreased in peripheral blood, and suppressor T-cell activity is increased, whereas T-helper cell activity and other beneficial responses are depressed.

Smoke inhalation is responsible for the majority of deaths in fires. Carbon monoxide poisoning is the most common mechanism of injury; if treated quickly enough with oxygen, a successful outcome can be realized. Smoke toxicity as a result of direct injury to the airways or smoke poisoning caused by inhalation of thermodegradation of natural and synthetic substances is less well understood. Therapy has been primarily directed toward supportive care. Until the pathophysiology of this pulmonary injury is better understood, the prognosis for these patients will remain poor.

Understanding the pathophysiologic events that occur in response to a burn has significantly improved care of the burned patient over the past several decades not only by decreasing morbidity but also by enhancing survival. Particularly germane in this regard has been the recognition of the need for aggressive fluid resuscitation in the first 24 hours following burning and the importance of controlling bacterial colonization of the burn wound with its potentially deleterious effects should infection and sepsis supervene.

REFERENCES

1. Montgomery BJ. Consensus for treatment of the "sickest patients you'll ever see." JAMA 241:345, 1979.
2. Pruitt BA Jr. The Scudder oration on trauma. Bull Am Coll Surg 70:2, 1985.
3. Demling RH. Burns. N Engl J Med 313:1389, 1985.
4. Lawrence JC, Bull JP. Thermal conditions which cause skin burns. J Inst Mech Eng 5:61, 1976.
5. Moritz AR, Henriques FC. Studies of thermal injury. II. The relative importance of time and surface temperature in the causation of cutaneous burns. Am J Pathol 23:695, 1947.
6. Lepenye G, Novak J, Nemeth L. The biophysics of thermal injury. Acta Chir Plast 20:77, 1978.
7. Wilson CE, et al. Cold water treatment of burns. J Trauma 3:477, 1963.
8. deCamara DL, Raine T, Robson MC. Ultrastructural aspects of cooled thermal injury. J Trauma 21:911, 1981.
9. Raine TJ, et al. Cooling the burn wound to maintain microcirculation. J Trauma 21:394, 1981.
10. Boykin JV, Crute SL. Mechanisms of burn shock protection after severe scald injury by cold-water treatment. J Trauma 22:859, 1982.
11. deCamara DL, Heggers JP, Robson MC. Response of mast cell granules to thermal injury. Surg Forum 32:560, 1981.
12. Heggers JP, et al. Cooling and the prostaglandin effect in the thermal injury. J Burn Care Rehabil 3:350, 1982.
13. Arturson G, Mellander S. Acute changes in capillary filtration and diffusion in experimental burn injury. Acta Physiol Scand 62:457, 1964.
14. Heggers JP, et al. Evaluation of burn blister fluid. Plast Reconstr Surg 65:798, 1980.
15. Nanto V, Viljanto J. Observations on the chemical composition of the blister fluid of burned patients. Acta Chir Scand 124:19, 1962.
16. Shakespeare PG, Levick PL, Vaitheespara RB. Proteins in blister fluid. Burns 4:254, 1978.
17. Foex BA. The cystokine response to critical illness. J Accid Emerg Med 13:154, 1996.
18. Youn Y, LaLonde C, Demling R. The role of mediators in the response to thermal injury. World J Surg 16:30, 1992.
19. Gibran NS, Heimbach DM. Mediators in thermal injury. Semin Nephrol 13:344, 1993.
20. Trang LE. Prostaglandins and inflammation. Semin Arthritis Rheum 9:153, 1980.
21. Szabo C, Thiemermann C. Invited opinion: Role of nitric oxide in hemorrhagic, traumatic, and anaphylactic shock and thermal injury. Shock 2:145, 1994.
22. Bernard C, et al. Elevated temperature accelerates the induction of nitric oxide synthesis in rat macrophages. Eur J Pharmacol 270:115, 1994.
23. Demling RH, Kramer GC, Harm B. Role of thermal injury–induced hypoproteinemia on edema formation in burned and nonburned tissue. Surgery 95:136, 1984.
24. Arturson G. Pathophysiology of the burn wound. Ann Chir Gynecol 69:178, 1980.
24a. Sasaki J, Cottam G, Baxter C. Lipid peroxidation following thermal injury. J Burn Care Rehabil 4:251, 1987.
25. Jackson DM. The diagnosis of the depth of burning. Br J Surg 40:588, 1953.
26. Branemark PI, et al. Microvascular pathophysiology of burned tissue. Ann N Y Acad Sci 150:474, 1968.
27. Zawacki BE. Reversal of capillary stasis and prevention of necrosis in burns. Ann Surg 180:98, 1974.
28. Horton JW, White J, Baxter CR. The role of oxygen-derived free radicals in burn-induced myocardial contractile depression. J Burn Care Rehabil 9:589, 1988.
29. Dobson EL, Warner GF. Factors concerned in the early stages of thermal shock. Circ Res 5:69, 1957.

30. Raffa J, Trunkey DD. Myocardial depression in acute thermal injury. J Trauma 18:90, 1978.
31. Endo S, et al. Plasma tumour necrosis factor-alpha (TNF) levels in patients with burns. Burns 19:124, 1993.
32. Gong KS, Wang CH, Zhu HN. Effect of peripheral injection of arginine vasopressin and its receptor antagonist on burn shock in the rat. Neuropeptides 17:17, 1990.
33. Liu XS, et al. Clinical significance of the change of blood monocytic interleukin-1 production *in vitro* in severely burned patients. Burns 20:302, 1994.
34. Till GO, et al. Oxygen radical dependent lung damage following thermal injury of rat skin. J Trauma 23:269, 1983.
35. Clayton JM, et al. Sequential circulatory changes in the circumferentially burned limb. Ann Surg 185:391, 1977.
36. Boykin JV, Eriksson E, Pittman RN. Microcirculation of a scald burn: An "in vivo" experimental study of the hairless mouse ear. Burns 7:335, 1981.
37. Robson MC, et al. The effect of heparin on dermal ischemia after burning. Burns 5:620, 1979.
38. Nozaki M, et al. Permeability of blood vessels after thermal injury. Burns 6:213, 1980.
39. Miller TA, White WL. Healing of second degree burns. Comparison of effects of early application of homografts and coverage with tape. Plast Reconstr Surg 49:552, 1972.
40. DelBeccaro EJ, et al. The use of specific thromboxane inhibitors to preserve the dermal microcirculation after burning. Surgery 87:137, 1980.
41. Huang YS, Li A, Yang ZC. Roles of thromboxane and its inhibitor anisodamine in burn shock. Burns 4:249, 1990.
42. Robson MC, et al. Increasing dermal perfusion after burning by decreasing thromboxane production. J Trauma 20:722, 1980.
43. Baxter CR. Fluid volume and electrolyte changes in the early post-burn period. Clin Plast Surg 1:693, 1974.
44. Carney SA, Hall M, Ricketts CR. The adenosine triphosphate content and lactic acid production of guinea pig skin after mild heat damage. Br J Dermatol 94:291, 1976.
45. Hershey FB, et al. Effect of ATP on glucose metabolism of thermally injured skin in vitro. J Trauma 11:931, 1971.
46. Allgower M, Schoenenberger GA, Sparkes BG. Burning the largest immune organ. Burns 21:S7, 1995.
47. Loebl EC, et al. The mechanism of erythrocyte destruction in the early post burn period. Ann Surg 178:681, 1973.
48. Loebl EC, et al. Erythrocyte survival following thermal injury. J Surg Res 16:96, 1974.
49. Dobke MK, et al. Oxidative activity of polymorphonuclear leukocytes after thermal injury. Eur Surg Res 14:107, 1982.
50. Schoenenberger GA, et al. Experimental evidence for a significant impairment of host defense for gram-negative organisms by a specific cutaneous toxin produced by severe burn injuries. Surg Gynecol Obstet 141:555, 1975.
51. Sparkes BG, et al. Plasma levels of cutaneous burn toxin and lipid peroxides in thermal injury. Burns 16:118, 1990.
52. Schoenenberger GA, et al. Isolation and characterization of a cutaneous lipoprotein with lethal effects produced by thermal energy in mouse skin. Biochem Biophys Res Commun 42:975, 1971.
53. Demling RH, et al. The study of burn wound edema using dichromatic absorptionmetry. J Trauma 18:124, 1978.
54. Cotran RS, Majno G. The delayed and prolonged vascular leakage in inflammation. I. Topography of the leaking vessels after thermal injury. Am J Pathol 45:261, 1964.
55. Arturson G. Microvascular permeability to macromolecules in thermal injury. Acta Physiol Scand (Suppl) 463:111, 1979.
56. Arturson G, Jonsson CE. Transcapillary transport after thermal injury. Scand J Plast Reconstr Surg 13:29, 1979.
57. Carvajal HF. A physiologic approach to fluid therapy in severely burned children. Surg Gynecol Obstet 150:379, 1980.
58. Anggard E, Jonsson CE. Efflux of prostaglandins in lymph from scaled issue. Acta Physiol Scand 81:440, 1971.
59. Harms BA, et al. Prostaglandin release and altered microvascular integrity after burn injury. J Surg Res 31:274, 1981.
60. Arturson G. The plasma kinins in thermal injury. Scand J Clin Lab Invest (Suppl) 24:153, 1969.
61. Baxter CR, et al. Excretion of serotinin metabolites following thermal injury. Surg Forum 14:61, 1963.
62. Hayashi H, et al. Endogenous permeability factors and their inhibitors affecting vascular permeability in cutaneous Arthurs reactions and thermal injury. Br J Exp Pathol 45:419, 1964.
63. Horakova Z, Beaven MA. Time course of histamine release and edema formation in the rat paw after thermal injury. Eur J Pharmacol 27:305, 1974.
64. Brimblecombe RW, et al. Histamine H_2 receptor antagonists and thermal injury in rats. Burns 3:8, 1976.
65. Yoshioka T, et al. Cimetidine inhibits burn edema formation. Am J Surg 136:681, 1978.
66. Burge PD, Gilbert SJ. Effect of a histamine H_2 receptor antagonist on the swelling of the burned hand. Burns 6:30, 1979.
67. Watson WC, Kutty PK, Colcleugh RG. Does cimetidine cause ileus in the burned patient? Lancet 2:720, 1977.
68. Demling R, LaLonde C. Topical ibuprofen decreases early post burn edema. Surgery 102:857, 1987.
69. Demling RH, LaLonde C. Early post burn lipid peroxidation: Effect of ibuprofen and allopurinol. Surgery 107:85, 1990.
70. Friedl H, et al. Mediator induced activation of xanthine oxidase in endothelial cells. FASEB J 3:2512, 1989.
71. Oldham K, et al. Activation of complement by hydroxyl radical thermal injury. Surgery 104:272, 1988.
72. Saez JC, et al. Superoxide radical involvement in the pathogenesis of burn shock. Circ Shock 12:229, 1984.
73. Tanaka H, et al. Hemodynamic effects of delayed initiation of antioxidant therapy (beginning two hours after burn) in extensive third-degree bruns. J Burn Care Rehabil 16:610, 1995.
74. Kingsley NW, Stein JM, Levenson, SM. Measuring tissue pressure to assess the severity of burn induced ischemia. Plast Reconstr Surg 63:404, 1979.
75. Cottam GL, Mitchell MD, Baxter CR. Measurement of 13,14-dihydro-keto-prostaglandin F and 11-deoxy-13,14-dihydroketo-11,16-cyclo prostaglandin E_2 in human plasma following thermal injury. J Burn Care Rehabil 5:324, 1984.
76. Ferguson M, Eriksson E, Robson MC. Effect of methyl-prednisolone on oedema formation after a major burn. Burns 5:293, 1979.
77. Demling RH, et al. Effect of nonprotein colloid on postburn edema formation in soft tissues and lung. Surgery 95:593, 1984.
78. Deitch EA, Rutan R, Waymack JP. Trauma, shock, and gut translocation. New Horiz 4:289, 1996.
79. Goris RJ, Boekhorst T, Nuytinck J. Multiple organ failure: Generalized autodestructive inflammation. Arch Surg 120:1109, 1985.
80. Morris SE, Navaratman N, Herndon DN. A comparison of effects of thermal injury and smoke inhalation on bacterial translocation. J Trauma 30:639, 1990.
81. Myers S, et al. Elevated PGI and PGE in the rat ileum following mild hypotension. J Trauma 28:1202, 1988.
82. Hill J, et al. Soluble complement receptor type 1 ameliorates the local and remote organ injury after intestinal ischemia-reperfusion in the rat. J. Immunol 149:1723, 1992.
83. Fisher CJ, et al. Influence of an anti-tumour necrosis factor monoclonal antibody on cytokine levels in patients with sepsis. Crit Care Med 21:318, 1993.
84. Fisher CJ, et al. Recombinant human interleukin 1 receptor antagonist in the treatment of patients with sepsis syndrome. JAMA 271:1836, 1994.
85. Van Saene HKF, Stoutenbeek CC, Stoller JK. Selective decontamination of the digestive tract in the intensive care unit: Current status and future prospects. Crit Care Med 20:691, 1992.

86. Herndon DN, Ziegler ST. Bacterial translocation after thermal injury. Crit Care Med 21:S50,1993.
87. Tokyay R, et al. Effects of thromboxane synthetase inhibition on postburn mesenteric vascular resistance and the rate of bacterial translocation in a chronic porcine model. Surg Gynecol Obstet 174:125, 1992.
88. Tokyay R, Traber DL, Herndon DN. Thromboxane synthetase inhibition prevents the increased mesenteric vascular resistance seen after major burn in a chronic porcine model. Surg Forum 41:47, 1990.
89. Arturson G. The pathophysiology of severe thermal injury. J Burn Care Rehabil 6:129, 1985.
90. Wolfe RR, et al. Effect of severe burn injury on substrate cycling by glucose and fatty acids. N Engl J Med 317:403, 1987.
91. Wilmore DW, et al. Effect of ambient temperature on heat production and heat loss in burn patients. J Appl Physiol 38:593, 1975.
92. Caldwell FT. Energy metabolism following thermal burns. Arch Surg 111:181, 1976.
93. Wilmore DW, et al. Alterations in hypothalamic function following thermal injury. J Trauma 15:697, 1975.
94. Pruitt BA Jr. The burn patient. II. Later care and complications of thermal injury. Curr Probl Surg 16:1, 1979.
95. Wilmore DW, Aulick LH. Metabolic changes in burned patients. Surg Clin North Am 58:1173, 1978.
96. Deitch EA. The management of burns: Current concepts. N Engl J Med 323:1249, 1990.
97. Bessey PQ, et al. Combined hormonal infusion stimulates the metabolic response to injury. Ann Surg 200:264, 1984.
98. Wilmore DW, et al. Catecholamines: Mediator of the hypermetabolic response to thermal injury. Ann Surg 180:653, 1974.
99. Hume DM, Egdahl RH. The importance of the brain in the endocrine response to injury. Ann Surg 150:697, 1959.
100. Woolf PD, et al. The adrenocortical response to brain injury: Correlation with the severity of neurological dysfunction, effects of intoxication and patient outcome. Alcoholism 14:917, 1990.
101. Ziegler MG, Morrisey EC, Marshal LF. Catecholamine and thyroid hormones in traumatic injury. Crit Care Med 18:253, 1990.
102. Long CL. A response to trauma and infection: Metabolic changes and immunologic consequences. J Burn Care Rehabil 6:188, 1985.
103. Moati F, et al. Biochemical and pharmacological properties of a cardiotoxic factor isolated from the blood serum of burned patients. J Pathol 127:147, 1979.
104. Bartlett RH, et al. Nutritional therapy based on positive caloric balance in burn patients. Arch Surg 112:974, 1977.
105. Wolfe RR, et al. Response of proteins and urea kinetics in burn patients to different levels of protein intake. Ann Surg 197:163, 1983.
106. Newsom TW, Mason AD Jr, Pruitt BA Jr. Weight loss following thermal injury. Ann Surg 178:215, 1973.
107. Freund H, et al. The role of the branched-chain amino acids in decreasing muscle catabolism in vivo. Surgery 83:611, 1978.
108. Aulick LH, Wilmore DW. Leg amino acid turnover in burn patients. Fed Proc 37:536, 1978.
109. Blackburn GL, et al. Branched chain amino acid administration and metabolism during starvation, injury, and infection. Surgery 86:307, 1979.
110. Curreri PW, et al. Dietary requirements of patients with major burns. J Am Diet Assoc 65:415, 1974.
111. Wilmore DW. Carbohydrate metabolism in trauma. J Clin Endocrinol Metab 5:731, 1976.
112. Long JM III, et al. Effect of carbohydrate and fat intake on nitrogen excretion during total intravenous feeding. Ann Surg 185:417, 1977.
113. Mochizuki H, et al. Optimal lipid content for enteral diets following thermal injury. J Parenter Enteral Nutr 8:638, 1984.
114. Mochizuki H, et al. Mechanism of prevention of postburn hypermetabolism and catabolism by early enteral feeding. Ann Surg 200:297, 1984.
115. Alexander JW, McMillan B, Stinnett J. Beneficial effects of aggressive protein feeding in severely burned children. Ann Surg 192:505, 1980.
116. Goodwin CW. Metabolism and nutrition. Crit Care Clin 1:97, 1985.
117. Deitch EA. Nutritional support of the burn patient. Crit Care Clin 11:735, 1995.
118. Nghia MV, et al. Effects of postoperative carbohydrate overfeeding. Am Surg 53:632, 1987.
119. McDonald WS, Sharpe CW Jr, Deitch EA. Immediate enteral feeding in burn patients is safe and effective. Ann Surg 213:177, 1991.
120. Mochizuki H, et al. Reduction of postburn hypermetabolism by early enteral feedings. Curr Surg 42:121, 1985.
121. Mainous MR, Block EF, Deitch EA. Nutritional support of the gut: How and why. New Horiz 2:193, 1994.
122. Detsky AS, et al. Perioperative parenteral nutrition: A meta-analysis. Ann Intern Med 107:195, 1987.
123. McGeer AD, Detsky AS, O'Rourke K. Parenteral nutrition in cancer patients undergoing chemotherapy: A meta-analysis. Nutrition 6:233, 1990.
124. Carleton SC, Tomassoni AJ, Alexander JK. The cardiovascular effects of environmental traumas. Cardiol Clin 13:257, 1995.
125. Baxter CR. Intracellular electrolyte exchange in early postburn period. Am Burn Assoc 12:40, 1967.
126. Horton JW, Baxter CR, White DJ. The effects of aging on the cardiac contractile response to unresuscitated thermal injury. J Burn Care Rehabil 9:40, 1988.
127. Lefer AM. Interaction between myocardial depressant factor and vasoactive mediators with ischemia and shock. Am J Physiol 252:R193, 1987.
128. Squandrito F, et al. Reduction of myocardial leukocyte accumulation and myocardial infarct size following administration of BAY u3405, a thromboxane A_2 receptor antagonist, in myocardial ischaemia-reperfusion injury. Agents Actions 39:143, 1993.
129. Joshi W. Effects of burns on the heart. JAMA 211:2130, 1970.
130. Linares HA. A report of 115 consecutive autopsies in burned children, 1966-1980. Burns 8:263, 1982.
131. Maggi SP, et al. Beta-1 blockade decreases cardiac work without affecting protein breakdown or lipolysis in severely burned patients. Surg Forum 75:1081, 1993.
132. Aulick LH, et al. Visceral blood flow following thermal injury. Ann Surg 193:112, 1981.
133. Wilmore DW, et al. Effect of injury and infection on visceral metabolism and circulation. Ann Surg 192:491, 1980.
134. Shakespeare PG, et al. Proteinuria after burn injury. Ann Clin Biochem 18:353, 1981.
135. Planas M, et al. Characterization of acute renal failure in the burned patient. Arch Intern Med 142:2087, 1982.
136. Dolovek R. The endocrine response after burns: Its possible correlations with the immunology of burns. J Burn Care Rehabil 6:281, 1985.
137. Popp MB, et al. Anterior pituitary functioning thermally injured male children and young adults. Surg Gynecol Obstet 145:517, 1977.
138. Vaughn GM, Mason AD Jr, Shirani KZ. Hormonal changes following burns: An overview with consideration of the pineal gland. J Burn Care Rehabil 6:275, 1985.
138a. Becker RA, Wilmore DW, Goodwin CW. Free T_4, free T_3 and reverse T_3 in critically ill, thermally injured patients. J Trauma 20:713, 1980.
139. Vaughan GM, Pruitt BA Jr. Thyroid function in critical illness and burn injury. Semin Nephrol 13:359, 1993.

140. Caldwell FT, et al. Metabolic response to thermal trauma of normal and thyroprivic rats at three environmental temperatures. Ann Surg 150:976, 1959.
141. Herndon DN. Mediators of metabolism. J Trauma 21:701, 1981.
142. Sellers EA, You SS, You RW. The influence of adrenal cortex and thyroid on the loss of nitrogen in urine after experimental burns. Endocrinology 47:148, 1950.
143. Gilpin DA, et al. Recombinant human growth hormone accelerates wound healing in children with large cutaneous burns. Ann Surg 220:19, 1994.
144. Herndon DN, et al. Effects of recombinant human growth hormone on donor site healing in severely burned children. Ann Surg 212:424, 1990.
145. Dauhaday WH. The anterior pituitary. In Wilson JD, Foster DW, eds. William's Textbook of Endocrinology. Philadelphia: WB Saunders, 1985.
146. Cioffi WG, et al. Insulin-like growth factor-1 lowers protein oxidation in patients with thermal injury. Ann Surg 220:310, 1994.
147. Moltei LB, et al. Prolactin, corticotropin, and gonadotropin concentrations following thermal injury in adults. J Trauma 24:1, 1984.
148. Davies JWL. Physiological Responses to Burning Injury. New York: Academic Press, 1982.
149. Wilmore DW. Nutrition and metabolism following thermal injury. Clin Plast Surg 1:603, 1974.
150. Wolfe RR. Glucose metabolism in burn injury: A review. J Burn Care Rehabil 6:408, 1985.
151. Vaughn GA, et al. Nonthyroidal control of metabolism after burn injury: Possible role of glucagon. Metabol Clin Exper 34:637, 1985.
152. Bingham HG, et al. Burn diabetes: A review. J Burn Care Rehabil 33:179, 1982.
153. Fauci A.Host Defense Mechanisms against Infection: Current Concepts/Scope Publication. Kalamazoo, Mich.: Upjohn, 1978.
154. Branch CD, Wilkins CF, Ross FP. The coagulum contact method of skin grafting in the treatment of burns and wounds. Surgery 19:460, 1945.
155. Pietsch LB, Meakins JL, Gotto D. Delayed hypersensitivity response: The effect of surgery. J Surg Res 22:228, 1977.
156. Markely K, Smallman ET. Effect of burn trauma in mice on the generation of cytotoxic lymphocytes. Proc Soc Exp Biol Med 160:468, 1979.
157. Ninneman JL. Suppression of lymphocyte response following thermal injury. In Ninneman JL, ed. The Immune Consequences of Thermal Injury. Baltimore: Williams & Wilkins, 1981.
158. Asko-Seljavaara S, Sundell B, Rytomaa T. The effect of early excison on bone-marrow cell growth in burned mice. Burns 2,3:140, 1976.
159. Schoenenberger GA. Burn toxins isolated from mouse and human skin: Their characterization and immunotherapy effects. Monogr Allergy 9:72, 1975.
160. Daniels JC, et al. Serum protein profiles in thermal burns. II. Protease inhibitors, complement factors, and C-reactive protein. J Trauma 14:153, 1972.
161. Alexander JW, Wixson D. Neutrophil dysfunction of polymorphonuclear leukocytes in patients with burns and other trauma. Surg Gynecol Obstet 130:431, 1970.
162. Munster AM, Winchurch RA. Infection and immunology. Crit Care Clin 1:119, 1985.
163. Warden GD, Mason AD, Pruitt BA Jr. Evaluation of leukocyte chemotaxis in vitro in thermally injured patients. J Clin Invest 54:1001, 1974.
164. Munster AM. Alteration of the immune system in burns and implications for therapy. Eur J Pediatr Surg 4:231, 1994.
165. Sayeed MM. Alterations in cell signalling and related effector functions in T lymphocytes in burn/trauma/septic injuries. Shock 5:157, 1996.
166. Berczi I. Neuroendocrine defense in endotoxin shock (a review). Acta Microbiol Hung 40:265, 1993.
167. Chouaib S, et al. Analysis of prostaglandin E_2 effect on T lymphocyte activation: Abrogation of prostaglandin E_2 inhibitory effect by the tumor promotor 12.0 tetradecanoyl phorbol-13 acetate. J Clin Invest 80:333, 1987.
168. Chouaib S, et al. The mechanisms of inhibition of human IL2 production: PGE_2 induction of suppressor T lymphocytes. J Immunol 132:1851, 1984.
169. Goodwin JS, Bankhurst AD, Messner RP. Suppression of human T cell mitogenesis by prostaglandin: Existence of a prostaglandin-producing suppressor cell. J Exp Med 146:1719, 1977.
170. Horgan PG, et al. Effect of low dose recombinant interleukin 2 plus indomethachin on mortality after sepsis in a murine burn model. Br J Surg 77:401, 1990.
171. Munster AM, et al. Reversal of postburn immunosuppression with low-dose polymixin B. J Trauma 26:995, 1986.
172. Munster AM, et al. Translocation: True pathology or phenomenology. Ann Surg 218:321, 1993.
173. Trunkey DD. Inhalation injury. Surg Clin North Am 58:1133, 1978.
174. Dolan MC. Carbon monoxide poisoning. CMAT 133:392, 1985.
175. Rhodes ML. The effect of carbon monoxide on mitochondrial enzymes in pulmonary tissue. Am Rev Respir Dis 103:906, 1971.
176. Herndon DN, Thompson PB, Traber DL. Pulmonary injury in burned patients. Crit Care Clin 1:79, 1985.
177. Myers RAM, et al. Value of hyperbaric oxygen in suspected carbon monoxide poisoning. JAMA 246:2478, 1981.
178. Moritz AR, Henriques FC Jr, McLean R. The effects of inhaled heat on lungs: An experimental investigation. Am J Pathol 21:311, 1945.
179. Cox ME, et al. The Dellwood fire. Br Med J 1:942, 1955.
180. Crapo RO. Smoke inhalation injuries. JAMA 264:1694, 1981.
181. Beal DD, Lambeth JR, Conner GH. Follow-up studies on patients treated with steroids following pulmonary thermal and acrid smoke injury. Laryngoscope 78:396, 1967.
182. Pruitt BA Jr, Erickson MD, Morris A. Progressive pulmonary insufficiency and other pulmonary complications of thermal injury. J Trauma 15:369, 1975.
183. Monafo WW. Initial management of burns. N Engl J Med 335:1581, 1996.
184. Curreri PW. Supportive therapy in burn care. J Trauma 21(Suppl):724, 1981.
185. Nguyen TT, et al. Current treatments of severely burned patients. Ann Surg 223:14, 1996.
186. Sokawa J, et al. The relationship between experimental fluid therapy and wound edema in scald wounds. Ann Surg 193:237, 1981.
187. Baxter CR, Shires GT. Physiologic response to crystaloid resuscitation of severe burns. Ann N Y Acad Sci 150:874, 1968.
188. Cope O, Moore FD. The redistribution of body water in the fluid therapy of the burned patient [footnote]. Ann Surg 126:1013, 1947.
189. Evans EI, et al. Fluid and electrolyte requirements in severe burns. Ann Surg 135:804, 1952.
190. Monafo WW. The treatment of burn shock by the intravenous and oral administrations of hypertonic lacated saline solution. J Trauma 10:575, 1970.
191. Parks DH, Carvajal HF, Larson DL. Management of burns. Surg Clin North Am 57:875, 1977.
192. Goodwin CW, et al. Randomized trial of efficacy of crystalloid and colloid resuscitation on hemodynamic response and lung water following thermal injury. Ann Surg 197:520, 1983.
193. Hall KV, Sorensen B. The treatment of burn shock: Results of a 5-year randomized, controlled clinical trial of Dextran 70 vs. Ringers lactate solution. Burns 5:107, 1978.
194. Gunn ML, et al. Prospective, randomized trial of hypertonic sodium lactate versus lactated Ringer's solution for burn wound resuscitation. J Trauma 29:1261, 1989.

195. Huang PP, et al. Hypertonic sodium resuscitation is associated with renal failure and death. Ann Surg 221:543, 1995.
196. Lund CC, Browder WL. Healing of second-degree burns: Comparison of effects of early application of homografts and coverage with tape. Plast Reconstr Surg 49:552, 1972.
197. Burke JF, Bandoc CC, Quinby WC. Primary burn excision and immediate grafting: A method for shortening illness. J Trauma 14:389, 1974.
198. Desai MH, et al. Early burn wound excision significantly reduces blood loss. Ann Surg 211:753, 1990.
199. Herndon DN, et al. A comparison of conservative versus early excison: Therapies in severely burned patients. Ann Surg 209:546, 1989.
200. Burke JF, et al. Successful use of a physiologically acceptable artificial skin in the treatment of extensive burn injury. Ann Surg 194:413, 1981.
201. Arturson G. Anti-inflammatory drugs and burn edema formation. In May R, Dogo G, eds. Care of the Burn Wound. Basel: Karger, 1981.
202. Biffl WL, et al. Interleukin-6 in the injured patient: Marker of injury or mediator of inflammation. Ann Surg 224:647, 1996.
203. Lepoivre M, et al. Alterations of ribonucleotide reductase activity following induction of the nitrite-generating pathway in adenocarcinoma cells. J Biol Chem 265:141, 1990.
204. Lewis R, Austen F, Soberman R. Leukotrienes and other products of the 5-lipoxygenase pathway. N Engl J Med 323:645, 1990.
205. Nathan CF, Hibbs JB. Role of nitric oxide synthesis in macrophage antimicrobial activity. Curr Opin Immunol 3:65, 1991.
206. Herndon DN, Abston S, Stein MD. Increased thromboxane B_2 levels in the plasma of burned and septic burned patients. Surg Gynecol Obstet 159:210, 1984.

PART NINE

SPECIAL PHYSIOLOGIC CONSIDERATIONS

66

Physiologic Problems in the Pediatric Surgical Patient

Charles S. Cox, Jr., Robert G. Marvin, Kevin P. Lally, Thomas R. Weber, and Richard J. Andrassy

Surgeons caring for the pediatric patient are presented with challenges that are unique and in most instances significantly different from those involved in caring for the adult patient. These differences become most obvious in the surgical neonate; as a consequence, surgery in neonates and small infants has provided the springboard for the speciality of pediatric surgery. Among the factors that make the neonate and infant a challenging surgical patient are the dynamic adjustment of the newborn to extrauterine life, increased energy and nutritional demands produced by rapid growth, continued organ development and maturation in function, small physical size, rapid metabolic rates that can change the physiologic status of the neonate or infant almost within minutes, and anatomic defects that are usually congenital rather than acquired in origin. These factors, combined with the fact that the pediatric patient cannot give a history or list complaints or symptoms, make care of the pediatric surgical patient demanding and leave little room for error.

This chapter describes the unique characteristics of the pediatric patient, presents the physiologic principles that can guide the management of the patient in this age group, and applies these physiologic principles to the most common defects seen. The diagnosis and management of various common congenital and acquired diseases of infancy and childhood are also briefly discussed.

PERIOPERATIVE MANAGEMENT: PHYSIOLOGIC CONSIDERATIONS

Neonates, infants, and children differ in their physiologic characteristics. Preterm infants are younger than 38 weeks' gestational age, but their weight is appropriate for gestational age. Preterm infants are prone to develop episodes of apnea and/or bradycardia. Apnea and bradycardia are nonspecific responses to metabolic problems, sepsis, and anesthesia. Very-low-birthweight (VLBW) infants are younger than 32 weeks' gestational age and weigh less than 1500 g body weight. All the physiologic and metabolic stressors and responses in the VLBW infants such as electrolyte disturbances, temperature instability, and pulmonary insufficiency secondary to immaturity are exaggerated in the VLBW infant compared to the term and preterm infant.

Temperature Regulation

Neonates are susceptible to hypothermia because of a greater total body surface area–to–body weight ratio. Also they have minimal body fat. Neonates generate heat by brown fat catabolism, not by shivering. This energy source can be rapidly depleted by periods of cold stress. Hypothermia also has direct surgical implications as related to coagulation abnormalities and cardiovascular instability. Because of these differences in thermoregulation, great care is taken in the operating room and in the perioperative period to avoid hypothermia. Neonates and especially VLBW infants and small-for-gestational-age infants (SGA) are maintained in thermoneutral environments. Thermoneutral incubators are servocontrolled using skin temperature sensors, setting the ranges according to standard normograms for the infant's weight and age. Temperature instability as manifest by a greater than 1.5 to 2 degrees centigrade difference in the incubator and patient may be a sign of sepsis.

Transportation to and activities in the operating room are areas that subject the neonate to potential cold stress. Maintaining the patient in radiant warmers, increasing ambient temperature, covering the infant in impermeable plastic, and using warmed prep solutions/irrigation can prevent hypothermia.

Blood Volume

The neonatal blood volume is highest at birth; preterm infants have blood volumes of 85 to 100 ml/kg, which decrease to 80 to 85 ml/kg in term infants. By midinfancy the blood volume decreases to 70 ml/kg body weight.[1]

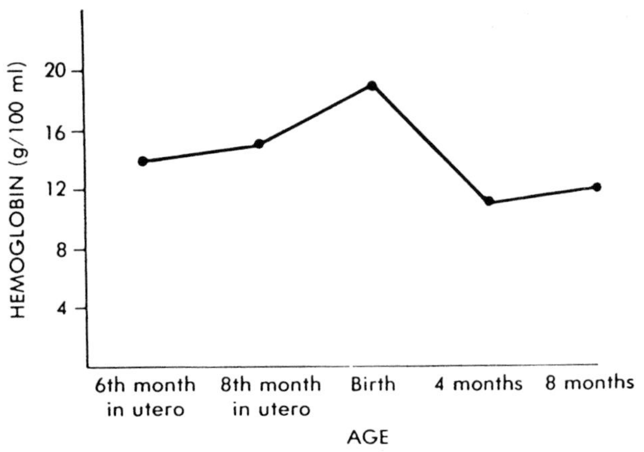

Fig. 66-1. Physiologic anemia reaches a nadir at 3 to 5 months of age to a hematocrit of approximately 30 vol%.

Most infants develop a physiologic anemia by 3 to 5 months of age down to a hematocrit of approximately 30 vol% (Fig. 66-1). This physiologic anemia does not preclude safe elective surgical procedures. Hemorrhagic disease of the newborn is a disorder of hemostasis specific to neonates. Vitamin K–dependent clotting proteins are obtained from the diet and intestinal bacterial synthesis. Maternally transmitted stores of vitamin K are rapidly depleted. All newborns are routinely given an intramuscular dose of 1 mg of vitamin K. Clinical bleeding in the first week of life may be due to a missed dose of vitamin K or maternal depletion.

Glucose, Calcium, and Magnesium Metabolism

All neonates and especially the VLBW and SGA neonates are susceptible to hypoglycemia. Neonates have limited hepatic glycogen stores and limited capacity for gluconeogenesis. Stressed neonates (those with sepsis, necrotizing enterocolitis, gastroschisis, etc.) have increased metabolic demands. Neonates require an infusion of glucose of 3 to 6 mg/kg/min to maintain adequate blood glucose concentrations. For most patients an infusion of 10% dextrose in water at maintenance fluid rates provides adequate glucose.

The neonate is susceptible to hypocalcemia in the first 24 to 48 hours after birth. This is usually related to decreased calcium intake and transient neonatal hypoparathyroidism caused by parathyroid suppression from high fetal calcium levels. Bicarbonate infusion, hyperventilation, and the transfusion of citrated blood place the neonate at risk for hypocalcemia. Symptomatic hypocalcemia is manifest by jitteriness, irritability, and seizures. Acute treatment is 1 to 2 ml/kg of 10% calcium gluconate in a period of 10 minutes. Asymptomatic hypocalcemia can be treated by giving 5 to 10 ml/kg/day of 10% calcium gluconate in a period of 24 hours. Hypomagnesemia may occur concurrently with hypocalcemia and should be suspected when hypocalcemia is resistant to routine replacement therapy.

Cardiovascular and Pulmonary Development

In many of the neonatal surgical problems, abnormal lung or cardiovascular development or adaptation is important. Lung development begins with an outpouching from the foregut, the tracheal bud. By the sixth to eighth week of gestation the lung bud has branched into the major bronchi and segmental bronchi. There is a gradual separation of the primitive esophagus from the lung bud. The pulmonary parenchyma develops from the mesoderm following ingrowth of the lung bud. The major conducting airways have all developed by the twentieth week of gestation, and further growth occurs in the respiratory bronchioles. At term there are an estimated 40 million alveoli. With growth the adult number of 300 million alveoli is reached by age 8 years. Until the development of an adequate amount of gas exchanging lung tissue at approximately 24 weeks' gestation, the infant cannot survive ex utero.

Premature infants have incompletely developed alveoli, and the immature type II pneumocytes do not produce and secrete adequate amounts of pulmonary surfactant. Lung surfactant is composed of several proteins, and a lipid-soluble component. Surfactant is approximately 90% lipid, 10% protein, and a small amount carbohydrate. The majority of lipid is dipalmitoylphosphatidylcholine (DPPC). Synthesis of surfactant phopholipids occurs only in type II pneumocytes, and surfactant is stored in secretory organelles called lamellar bodies. The primary property of surfactant is to lower alveolar surface tension. This decreases the pressure on the alveolar surface at end expiration when the alveoli are their smallest and transpulmonary pressure is the greatest, preventing collapse. Lowering surface tension also decreases the amount of pressure necessary to inflate the lung. In addition, decreased surface tension prevents transudation of fluid from pulmonary capillaries into the alveolar airspace.

Pulmonary gas exchange occurs at the interface between alveolar air and the fluid subphase of the alveolar lining. Surfactant covers the alveolar surface as a monomolecular film that is capable of reducing the area of the film as the alveolus contracts during exhalation. This reduction decreases surface tension, preventing alveolar collapse. DPPC is the only component of surfactant with enough compressibility to lower alveolar surface tension adequately and with a sufficiently slow rate of monolayer collapse to keep surface tension low and alveoli open for the duration of the respiratory cycle.

While the infant is in utero, most blood flow to the lungs is shunted to the systemic circulation, since gas exchange is occurring across the placenta. The blood is shunted through the ductus arteriosus and the foramen ovale (Fig. 66-2). The pressures in the pulmonary artery are high during this period. After delivery there is a rapid fall in the pulmonary artery pressure and a marked increase in pulmonary blood flow. The mechanisms of pulmonary

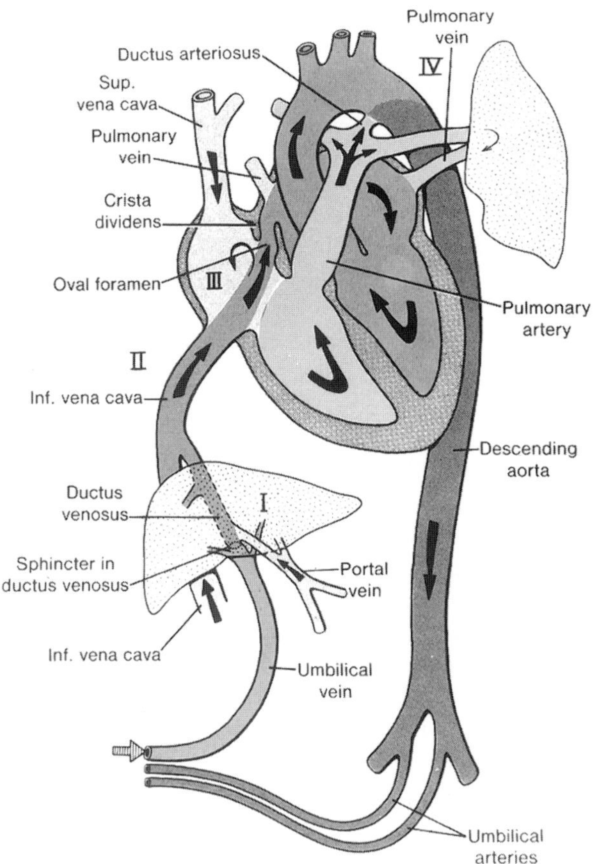

Fig. 66-2. Schematic representation of the fetal circulation. Umbilical venous blood is shunted via the sinus venosus to the systemic circulation via the intracardiac (foramen ovale) and extracardiac (patent ductus arteriosus [PDA]) shunts, bypassing the lungs. Closure of these shunts occurs with lung inflation and clamping of the umbilical cord.

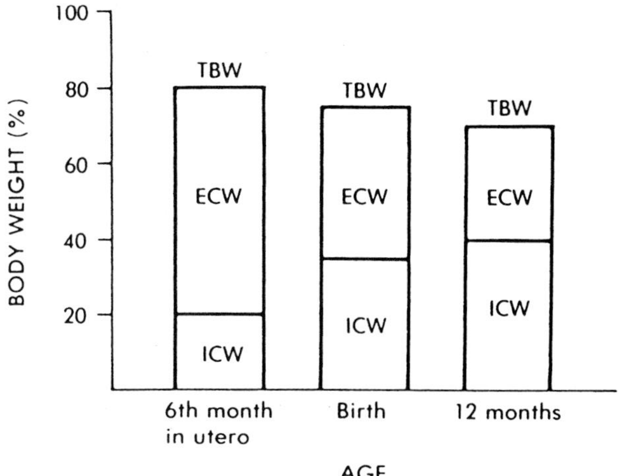

Fig. 66-3. Changes in body fluid spaces in neonates over time. There is a gradual decrease in total body water *(TBW)* and extracellular water *(ECW)* and associated expansion of intracellular water *(ICW)* as age increases.

artery relaxation are incompletely understood, but there is increasing evidence that endogenous nitric oxide production is important.

With a fall in the pulmonary blood pressure, flow through the ductus arteriosus can become left to right as the systemic circuit now becomes the higher pressure system. The ductus arteriosus begins to close shortly after birth, and by the seventh to tenth day of life it has closed in most infants. Closure of the ductus arteriosus is regulated by local oxygen concentration, prostaglandin E_2 and I_2.

A combination of adequate alveolar mass, surfactant, and pulmonary arterial relaxation with a fall in pulmonary artery pressure and resultant closure of the ductus arteriosus is necessary for effective transition of the infant to an ex utero environment. Alterations in any or all of these processes can occur and present management problems for the pediatric surgeon.

Fluids and Electrolytes

Body Fluid Spaces

Total body water comprises 94% of the 12-week gestational age fetus and drops to 78% by term (Fig. 66-3). An additional 3% to 5% is lost during the first week of life. Body water then decreases to 60% by 1 year of age, which is similar to adults. Changes in extracellular water mimic those of total body water. In contrast, intracellular water increases from 25% at 20 weeks to 33% at term. This increase continues in early postnatal life to reach the adult level of 44% at only 3 months.

Preterm infants are born with a higher ratio of extracellular to intracellular water reflective of their conceptual age. At birth there is a need to unload the additional extracellular water along with the normal postnatal diuresis. A preterm infant may unload up to 12% of total body water in the first week of life. Preterm infants who fail to achieve adequate water unloading have a higher incidence of patent ductus arteriosus, left ventricular failure, respiratory distress syndrome, bronchopulmonary dysplasia, and NEC.

Renal Function

The postnatal fluid shifts are affected by kidney function. The glomerular filtration rate (GFR) of a term newborn is 21 ml/min/1.73 m^2, which is 25% of the adult filtration rate. This rate rapidly rises to 60 ml/min/1.73 m^2 at 2 weeks, and then to adult levels at 2 years. All infants can process significant fluid loads because the decreased GFR is offset by the poor concentrating and high dilutional state of the tubules in the newborn.[2]

The concentrating effect of the newborn tubule reaches a maximum of 500 to 600 mOsm, compared to 1200 mOsm in the adult. This is not due to a depletion of antidiuretic hormone (ADH) in the infant, which is similar to the adult. Instead there appears to be a poor response to ADH at the level of the tubule.

Free water clearance in newborns, on the other hand, is greater than in adults. Infants can decrease urine osmolarity to 30 to 50 mOsm, compared to 70 to 100 mOsm in adults. Even in the face of increased water clearance, a premature infant who has an excess of extracellular water after birth may become fluid overloaded if large amounts of fluid are infused.

An inappropriate renal response, such as excretion of concentrated urine while the infant is hypervolemic or euvolemic, occurs in roughly 11% of postoperative newborns. It seems to be particularly problematic in patients undergoing diaphragmatic hernia repair.

The state of hydration, renal function, and solute load are determinants of the urine output and concentration. A sufficient volume must be available to carry endogenous and exogenous solutes, such as urea and creatinine, or serum levels rise. If excess water is available, dilute urine is passed. Infants with various conditions produce different amounts of solute that must be excreted, as much as 18 mOsm/kg/hr in premature infants with perforated necrotizing enterocolitis. Calculations of ideal urine output (i.e., the urine volume necessary to carry that amount of solute in an isotonic state [280 mOsm/L]) suggest that 2.67 ml/kg/hr would need to be urinated. This is well above what is considered "normal" urine output, suggesting urine output alone is not a reliable guide to hydration.

Sodium Excretion

Newborn infants have difficulty excreting excess sodium. This is due to an inability of the distal tubule to limit absorption. The newborn is only able to excrete 10% of the sodium load a 6-year-old is able to excrete. Therefore newborns may easily become overloaded with sodium and hypernatremic in the face of exogenous sodium administration. Preterm infants have a higher intrinsic sodium excretion. However, they too are vulnerable to overloading with sodium.

In contrast, premature infants may easily become hyponatremic because of the higher intrinsic sodium excretion if minimal exogenous sodium is administered. This is most pronounced in infants younger than 33 weeks' gestation or younger than 2 weeks after birth.

In utero, fetuses can excrete 8% to 15% of filtered sodium, which decreases to 1% in term newborns. Preterm infants younger than 33 weeks' gestation excrete 3% to 9% of filtered sodium. There is a rapid adjustment shortly after birth, usually between 4 and 15 days postpartum. Thus premature infants take longer after birth to adjust than term infants but do so at a lower conceptual age.

Sodium is traditionally replaced at 2 mEq/kg/day in newborns, but premature or physiologically stressed infants may require up to 5 mEq/kg/day. Therefore sodium replacement should probably be adjusted depending on serial measurements of serum and urine sodium concentrations.

Potassium Requirements

Traditionally, potassium repletion has been avoided in the newborn in the first 48 hours or immediately after surgery because of fear of renal dysfunction leading to hyperkalemia. However, there are multiple factors in preterm and stressed infants that may produce hypokalemia such as the high urine flow rate, mineralocorticoid response, prostaglandin secretion, and the use of diuretics. Therefore potassium replacement should be started as soon as renal function is ascertained. Administration should be 1 to 2 mEq/kg/day parenterally. Again, this dose should be adjusted based on serum and urine potassium concentrations.

Insensible Water Loss

Insensible water loss in infants is comprised of respiratory water loss and transepithelial water loss (TEWL). Respiratory losses comprise one third of insensible losses in infants older than 32 weeks' gestation. More premature infants have a lower proportion because of increased TEWLs. Respiratory losses average 4 to 5 ml/kg/day and may be eliminated if the infant is intubated and ventilated with humidified air. TEWL is the major insensible loss in infants. The limiting barrier to evaporation across the skin is the stratum corneum, which is thinner in more premature infants. Therefore the determinants of TEWL are conceptual age and environmental humidity.

In the term infant, insensible losses average 12 ml/kg/day, of which 7 ml/kg/day is TEWL. This is constant for the first 28 days of life. In contrast, at low conceptual age, TEWL may be greater than renal excretion. Measured losses in premature infants 25 to 27 weeks' gestational age were as high as 129 ml/kg/day. TEWL decreases as the gestational age approaches 40 weeks. This makes careful reassessment of the infant's intravascular fluid volume status and serum electrolytes extremely important.

There exists an inverse linear relationship between TEWL and environmental humidity. TEWL approaches 0 at 100% humidity. By placing an infant under an impermeable plastic sheet, the ambient humidity is increased, and TEWL is reduced. In contrast, nonionizing radiation, as in infant warmers and phototherapy, increases TEWL between 20% and 40%.

Monitoring Fluid and Electrolytes

Serial weight measurements may be a sensitive indicator of changes in total body water. However, they do not give adequate information on intravascular volume status. Capillary leak with edema and weight gain is common septic or traumatized infants and roughly correlates with the degree of multiple-organ failure. Blood volume may be reduced in these infants, and the use of diuretics to return the patient to "normal weight" are potentially dangerous. In fact, appropriate therapy is often fluid administration in these edematous patients to maintain circulating volume.

Serial measurement of urine flow and concentration are the two most helpful guides to fluid management in infants. In term and preterm newborns and adequate urine output is usually at least 2 ml/kg/hr or greater, a urine osmolality of 250 to 290 mOsm/L, and a specific gravity of

1.010 to 1.013. Indwelling urinary drainage catheters should be placed in all patients who are critically ill or where derangements of fluid status are expected.

The fractional excretion of sodium (F_eNa) is a calculation that may help determine if a rising blood urea nitrogen and/or a low urine output is due to renal tubular failure or dehydration. The measurement characterizes the sodium resorptive capability of the distal tubule. F_eNa should be less than 1% in term infants and less than 3% in premature infants. Higher values suggest poor resorption and tubular damage.

Metabolic Response to Injury and Sepsis

Neurohumoral Response

It has been well recognized that injury, burns, and sepsis lead to changes in the host that are different from basal states or simple starvation. Simple starvation results in a change from primarily glucose metabolism as the preferential nonprotein energy source to fat utilization as the energy source. This results in the formation of ketones, which act in a protein-sparing manner. The body can adapt and use ketones as an energy source, thus protecting or diminishing the breakdown of lean body tissue, such as muscle, serum proteins, and immune globulins. There is, however, a different hormonal milieu in the stress state, and this varies with the severity and duration of injury, method of resuscitation, and timing of intervention. It appears that despite some controversy, most infants respond hormonally and metabolically much like the adult, albeit with lesser reserves. Even newborns undergoing major surgery appear to respond like older patients.[3] The healthy neonate, however, must also adapt to the postnatal environment and postnatal physiology with relatively decreased reserves of fat, carbohydrate, and protein. Rapid growth and organ maturation also play a role. Anand et al.[4] have shown that newborn infants can mount a substantial endocrine and metabolic response, the main features of which are hyperglycemia and hyperlactatemia, associated with the release of catecholamines and the inhibition of insulin secretion. Blood lactate concentrations increase significantly in stressed preterm neonates and do not change in term infants. Plasma insulin levels are higher in stressed term neonates postoperatively than in preterm infants. In neonates, postsurgical hyperglycemia is initiated by adrenaline release and is maintained into the early postoperative period by glucagon secretion. The apparent lack of insulin secretion during surgery and in the early postoperative period is probably due to direct inhibition of insulin secretion by adrenaline. Insulin levels, however, are significantly elevated at 12 and 24 hours postoperatively and thereby restore blood glucose to normal levels. Preterm neonates do not respond with significant insulin secretion, thus blood glucose levels remain higher. This may be due to a decreased responsiveness of beta cells in the premature pancreas. Although the response is delayed, perhaps because of prematurity, the hormonal responses quickly become appropriate over the first several days after birth.[4,5]

Cytokine Response

In addition to the neuroendocrine response, release of cytokines play an important role in inflammation, immune response, and protein kinetics. The cytokine response has not been studied extensively in children when compared to the neuroendocrine response, but to date these studies have not demonstrated significant differences when compared to older patients. The release of mediators such as interleukin-1, interluekin-6, interleukin-8, and tumor necrosis factor appears to be similar to adult stress models and results in the same outcome when severity and age are adjusted.[6] Increased protein turnover and depletion of lean body tissues can occur rapidly with severe injury or sepsis. Release of the cytokines mentioned above from stimulated cells such as macrophages, leads to increased protein turnover, increased protein loss, increased uptake of amino acids, and increased production of acute phase proteins.

Protein-Calorie Metabolism

During the first several days after injury, there appears to be hepatic reprioritization of amino acid release from lean body tissue. That is, the amino acids are "directed" to the liver for synthesis of the acute phase proteins. After several days the wound gains priority, and amino acids, along with glucose, are directed for wound healing.

In addition to the neuroendocrine and cytokine stimulation of hypermetabolism, protein and energy requirements are increased because of the excessive cardiorespiratory demands. Postsurgical patients with healing wounds or septic patients, require increased oxygen delivery to meet oxygen consumption needs. This requires increased cardiac output and heart rate, increasing metabolic demands. At the same time increased carbon dioxide production necessitates increased ventilatory drive to get rid of the carbon dioxide. Thus, demands for protein and energy are further increased. Protein deficiency can result in poor immunocompetence, deterioration of respiratory function, and gut mucosal atrophy.

Since caloric requirements vary with age and degree of injury, the protein intake can simply be calculated based on nonprotein calories. It is important not to overestimate caloric needs, since excessive glucose or fat loads can lead to immunosuppression or other metabolic problems.[7] Once caloric needs have been determined, the protein intake required can be determined by providing a predetermined nitrogen-to-calorie ratio (i.e., 95 to 120 kcal/g nitrogen) for various stress states. Although many have worried about high protein intake in children leading to high solute loads, metabolic acidosis, or hyperammonemia, this has not presented itself clinically as a frequent problem. Perhaps intolerance of the glucose or fat calories have necessitated decreased infusion and thus decreased protein intake when the method of tying protein intake to caloric intake is used.

Alexander et al.[8] have demonstrated the beneficial effects of high-protein feeding in burned children. Their work providing a nitrogen-to-calorie ratio of approximately 110 kcal/g nitrogen showed improved immunologic and protein parameters, decreased sepsis, and improved survival compared to patients given a more standard protein intake of 150 kcal/g nitrogen. Most formulas used to calculate energy requirements in burned children consistently overestimate the amount of calories needed. Rarely does a severe burn require more than twice the basal metabolic rate, and in most instances burned children require approximately 1.5 to 1.75 times the basal metabolic rate.[9]

Carbohydrate Metabolism

The greatest proportion of caloric needs are supplied by carbohydrate. Newborns have a higher metabolic rate than adults, with a ratio of energy expenditure to body weight that may be three times greater. However, the infant has a diminished ability to store carbohydrate in the form of glycogen compared to the adult and therefore has less reserves. In premature infants the body stores of glycogen can be exhausted in a matter of hours. This is especially important under conditions of physiologic stress. Neonates may be unable to carry out hepatic gluconeogenesis secondary to a lack of the key hepatic gluconeogenetic enzymes. This is supported by the data from Anand et al.,[5] who demonstrated a significant hyperlactatemia during surgery in preterm infants. Because of these limited glycogen stores and synthetic capacity, infants must receive 3 to 6 mg/kg/min glucose to prevent hypoglycemia.

Fat Metabolism

Fat supplies the second important source of nonprotein calories. The functional energy substrates are the monounsaturated long-chain fatty acids found in large amount in the stored triglycerides. In premature infants the fat stores are 5% of total body weight compared to 15% in the full-term infant. Therefore the premature, stressed neonate has little reserve of this important second energy substrate. In adults 75% to 90% of the postoperative caloric requirements are met by fat metabolism. Similar data for neonates demonstrate that the primary sources of energy in surgical neonates are provided by the mobilization of fatty acids from fat tissue and their conversion to glycerol.[5] Mobilized glycerol formed from lipolysis enters the gluconeogenic pathway in the neonatal liver.

Anand et al.[4] demonstrated an increase in circulating total ketone bodies and glycerol during surgery in neonates. They attributed this increase to catecholamine-stimulated lipolysis and ketogenesis. They reported a correlation between glycerol, epinephrine, and norepinephrine at the end of an operation.[4,5]

In summary, the neonate and infant manifest similar stress responses when compared to the adult surgical patient. The primary difference is the minimal reserves in terms of lean body mass, fat stores, and marginal ability to maintain hepatic gluconeogenesis. These factors mandate an early and intensive approach to nutritional support of neonates undergoing surgical procedures.

Immune Function of the Newborn

The neonatal immune system is functionally immature, and neonates are particularly vulnerable to infection in the first 6 weeks of life. The immune system is composed of both nonspecific and specific components. Although almost all elements of the nonspecific and specific components are present at birth, there are qualitative and quantitative deficiencies that place the neonate at risk for infections and infectious complications of surgery. This is especially true for VLBW infants/premature infants.

Nonspecific Immune System: Polymorphonuclear Neutrophil Leukocytes, Mononuclear Cells, and Complement

The neonatal polymorphonuclear neutrophil leukocytes (PMNs) are present in equal circulating concentrations, but there is a markedly smaller reserve of bone marrow neutrophils. The neonatal granulocyte pool may be rapidly exhausted when challenged with a large or especially virulent bacterial load.[10] Many neonates and infants rapidly become neutropenic when faced with a severe bacterial challenge. The neonatal storage pool is approximately 14% of the adult pool, and neonatal progenitor cells are at a near maximal proliferative rate.[10,11,12] In vitro bactericidal capacity is decreased, and there are decreased chemotaxis, disaggregation, and migration to infected tissues.[13,14] This may be due to decreased expression of the complement receptor (CR3) that is important in cell surface adherence and PMN penetration into tissues.[15,16]

The migration of monocytes to infectious sites is diminished in neonates. Similar to PMNs, there is some evidence to suggest decreased cellular adhesion properties and poor cellular deformability, preventing migration to the infectious site.[17] The monocyte-macrophage's function is deficient in the neonate, and this may be due to decreased cytokine production and impaired chemotaxis.

The complement system is a critical component in the innate resistance to infection. It augments bacterial opsonization, immune adherence, and generation of chemotactic factors and phagocytosis. There is no transplacental passage of complement, and neonates have a relative complement defecit.[18] The classic complement system is antibody dependent; the alternate complement pathway, which is antibody independent, is used by neonates prior to antibody exposure. Also, as noted above, the CR3 complement receptor is deficient on the neonatal PMN, further reducing the effectiveness of the complement system in terms of augmenting PMN bactericidal functions.

The skin and mucosa are the primary defensive barriers. Preterm infants are particularly prone to coagulase-negative staphylococcal infections. Coagulase negative staphylococci are skin colonizers in intensive care units. Neonates, and especially premature neonates, have extremely fragile skin, which makes them more susceptible to the colonizing bacteria, which become a pathogen via invasive catheters, etc. Likewise, the gut as a mechanical barrier, and it's associated secretory barrier is not mature.

There are minimal levels of IgA, gut-associated IgG_2, and IgM_1 in neonates. Gastric acid production is depressed and does not allow for sterilization of the proximal foregut. This diminished barrier in the gut makes the infant more susceptible to bacterial translocation and/or intraluminal overgrowth with potentially pathogenic organisms, which may be related to nosocomial pneumonias and/or NEC.

Specific Immunity

The specific immune system refers to the component of immune function that requires previous antigen exposure. B and T lymphocytes and antibodies make up the specific immune system. Term infants receive IgG via maternal transfer, and the serum level varies directly with gestational age. Most transplacental passage of IgG occurs late in gestation, so premature infants are deficient in IgG. Two important subclasses of IgG (IgG_2 and IgG_4) are deficient in both term and preterm infants because of impaired transplacental transport. The B-cell response to antigenic stimulation/presentation is immunoglobin production. The neonatal B cell initially expresses IgM in response to stimulation and only later expresses IgG. The delay in IgG production, specifically to polysaccharide antigens such as those found in the group B streptococci, contributes to the neonate's susceptibility to overwhelming sepsis from these organisms.

T cells are essential to cell-mediated immunity. The T cells indirectly upregulate or downregulate the immune response by specific cytokine production. The neonatal T cells are not capable of producing all the cytokines needed for an effective immune response. In general, neonatal T cells produce deficient amounts of colony-stimulating factors. Decreased levels of interleukin-4 and interferon-γ by activated T cells of neonates has been shown. The functional impairment of neonatal T cells is normal by 6 months of age.

In summary, the neonate, in particular the premature neonate, is functionally immunocompromised.[19] This recovers by approximately 6 months of age, although some components of the immune system are not at adult levels of activity until the teen years. These facts and the known susceptibility to certain classes of organisms have obvious implications for surgical infections in the postoperative, stressed, and potentially malnourished neonate. This relative immunocompromise requires aggressive antibiotic therapy and attention to the principles of surgical treatment of infection.

SPECIFIC PEDIATRIC SURGICAL ABNORMALITIES

Abdominal Wall Defects

Omphalocele

The incidence of omphalocele is approximately 1:4000 live births, and numerous familial occurrences of omphalocele have been noted. Increased incidence with advanced maternal age has been observed, and a high rate of spontaneous abortion has been seen among women giving birth to infants with omphalocele, suggesting placental dysfunction.

The anomaly is a covered defect within the umbilical cord, through which intra-abdominal contents herniate. Unless it is ruptured during birth, there is always a sac covering the herniated gut, composed of amnion externally and peritoneum internally. The defect is 2 to 10 cm in diameter and may contain small and large bowel and liver. The most widely accepted theory of embryogenesis of omphalocele is that of Duhamel,[20] who believed the omphalocele was a failure that occurs early in gestation (3 to 4 weeks) of embryonal formation of the cephalic, caudal, and especially the two lateral embryonic folds that fuse at the umbilicus. Other authors consider an omphalocele a result of faulty migration of myotomes, caused by failure of the return of the bowel from the yolk sac into the developing abdominal cavity.

Omphalocele is associated with a significant (greater than 50%) incidence of associated anomalies and syndromes, including malformations in the alimentary tract, genitourinary, musculoskeletal, cardiac, and nervous systems. It is also seen commonly in the Beckwith-Wiedemann syndrome (gigantism, macroglossia, hypoglycemia) and trisomy 13 through 15 and 16 through 18 syndromes. Two other syndromes in which an omphalocele is present but away from the umbilical cord include pentalogy of Cantrell (upper midline omphalocele, diaphragmatic defect, sternal cleft, free pericardioperitoneal communication, and intracardiac defects) and the lower midline syndrome (low-lying omphalocele, cloacal exstrophy, imperforate anus with colonic atresia, and vesicointestinal fissure separating the two halves of the bladder). Colonic or appendiceal duplications are commonly seen, and sacral or vertebral anomalies may be present with associated myelomeningocele.

The physiologic considerations in the infant with omphalocele include the preoperative evaluation and resuscitation, intraoperative management, and postoperative recovery period. Before surgery the management of the infant includes attention to the prevention of hypothermia, maintenance of a sterile environment, and fluid resuscitation. Hypothermia is related to excessive radiant heat losses from the surface of the omphalocele sac. Placing the infant to the level of the axillae in an impermeable plastic bag with drawstrings ("bowel bag") decreases radiant heat loss and, in addition, effectively limits evaporative heat and water loss from the exposed surface. This is particularly important in the premature infant, in whom high transepithelial water loss is possible.

Rapid fluid shifts caused by "third-space" losses from the surface of the omphalocele can deplete the intravascular volume at an alarming rate in these newborns. The neonate has a limited capacity to respond to abnormal fluid losses because of a low plasma oncotic pressure, poor renal concentrating mechanisms, relative hyponatremia, and immature sympathicoadrenal responses. In addition, limited energy stores (a paucity of fat and glycogen) put demands on a gluconeogenic mechanism that may not be fully developed or functional in the hypovolemic state of the preterm or term infant. This set of circumstances may lead to metabolic acidosis from poor tissue perfusion and anaerobic metabolism that can lead to adverse cardiac and pulmonary vascular responses. The resultant hemoconcentration (hematocrit frequently in the 65 to 75 g/100 ml range) may result in increased blood viscosity and further decrease in tissue perfusion. Thus in these infants an intravenous line must be established immediately, preferably in a vein above the diaphragm, with a bolus of 20 ml/kg of 5% dextrose in lactated Ringer's solution for a period of 1 hour. This can be safely administered even if a cardiac anomaly is suspected. This should be followed by maintenance fluids of 5% or 10% dextrose in 0.45% normal saline at a rate of 150 to 175 ml/kg/day until urine output is obtained. Potassium chloride, 2 to 3 mEq/kg/day, can be added after urine output is established. If the omphalocele sac has ruptured, significant blood loss may occur, and this should be replaced with transfusion as soon as possible.

Because of limited host defense mechanisms, these infants are at high risk for infectious complications. Intravenous ampicillin (100 mg/kg/day) and gentamicin (5 mg/kg/day) are given in divided doses (every 12 hours for the first week of life). In addition, providing a sterile environment as outlined previously is an important adjunct.

After the resuscitation period, attention is directed toward complete workup to assess for other anomalies or syndromes. In most pediatric centers this includes consultation with a cardiologist, geneticist, neurologist, neonatologist, and others. In cases of cloacal exstrophy and ambiguous genitalia, a gender assignment committee may also become involved. Chromosome analysis is frequently necessary to assess the possibility of trisomy syndromes.

The actual treatment of the omphalocele defect should be individualized. The recommended methods of management include nonoperative treatment with escharotics, primary repair, skin flap closures with later ventral hernia repair, and use of prosthetic sheeting with staged reduction. The factors that determine the optimal method of treatment include the size of the defect, the overall condition of the patient, presence of other anomalies (especially those that are potentially lethal), and whether the sac is intact or ruptured. If the sac is intact, the choice can be made on a less urgent basis, and all the just-mentioned factors can be taken into consideration.

Nonoperative therapy with escharotic agents has been practiced since 1899, when alcohol application was used successfully. This caused granulation tissue, and then epithelium to form over the sac. Later aqueous mercurichrome was used, but mercury poisoning has been observed, and its use has largely been abandoned. The use of silver nitrate (0.25%) and silver sulfadiazine creme, agents frequently used on burn wounds, has also been recommended. Silver nitrate has the disadvantage of being hypotonic, causing depletion of sodium, which must be monitored and replaced intravenously. Because of the need for prolonged hospitalization, the resulting large ventral hernia that requires later repair, and the inability to inspect the intra-abdominal viscera for other anomalies, nonoperative therapy is reserved primarily for specific patients. These might include a premature infant with an extremely large defect, infants with severe hyaline membrane disease or other life-threatening condition, newborns with chromosomal (trisomy) syndromes in whom prolonged survival is not expected, and the infant with potentially lethal cardiac defects such as hypoplastic left ventricle.

Primary closure of the defect is obviously the most efficacious surgical approach in dealing with omphalocele. Most small and medium-sized defects can be dealt with in this manner. After the sac has been carefully excised and the umbilical vessels ligated, the contents are inspected for evidence of intestinal atresia or vitelline duct remnant and reduced. Removal of portions of the gastrointestinal tract, liver, and spleen have been reported to facilitate reduction, but these techniques are unnecessary.

For large defects in which full reduction of intra-abdominal contents is not possible, placement of a prosthetic "silo" is an excellent alternative to nonoperative therapy. This allows staged reduction during a 7 to 10 day period, at which time the infant is returned to the operating room for removal of the prosthesis and performance of abdominal wall repair. This technique is more fully described in the section on gastroschisis, where it has had more widespread application. Yet another alternative for large defects, especially those involving liver, includes the use of an internal polyethylene or silicone elastomer (Silastic) placed directly over the viscera, with superficial application of a polypropylene or Marlex mesh with skin flap coverage of the entire prosthesis. Staged repair by reopening the skin, resecting the central portion of the prosthesis, and resuturing the prosthesis in the midline gradually results in an enlarged abdominal cavity and eventual removal of the entire prosthesis. This may require four to five operations over a several-year period.

The postoperative management of these infants is usually straightforward. Intravenous fluids (120 to 150 ml/kg/day) and antibiotics are continued, the latter for 5 to 7 days or until all external prostheses are removed. Bowel function usually returns within several days after surgery, and oral feeding is begun. The associated anomalies are managed appropriately. Current survival in infants with omphalocele is 65% to 75%; the high mortality rate is the result of associated anomalies (especially cardiac) rather than factors directly related to repair of the defect.

Gastroschisis

Gastroschisis (Greek for "belly cleft") is characterized by a full-thickness abdominal wall defect, usually to the right of the umbilicus, through which antenatal evisceration of bowel occurs. The defect size is usually 2 to 4 cm. Unlike omphalocele, there is no sac present, allowing the herniated gut to be exposed to the amniotic fluid (pH 7). This results in a chemical peritonitis, with thickened, edematous, inflamed, and foreshortened bowel. If the defect is very small, the blood supply to the eviscerated gut can be compromised, leading to frank necrosis or intestinal atresia (10% of cases). The incidence of other anomalies is very low in contrast to omphalocele,[21] although 40% to 60% of infants with gastroschisis are either premature or SGA infants, making their management exacting and frequently complicated.

The true incidence of gastroschisis is difficult to ascertain, although many authors think that the number of infants born with gastroschisis is increasing.[22] The mean maternal age is younger for gastroschisis than for omphalocele, and a significant number (50%) are born to teenage or primigravid mothers. Familial occurrences are extremely rare.

Much controversy surrounds the cause of gastroschisis. Various authors have proposed a defect in differentiation of somatopleuric mesenchyme lateral to the umbilicus, whereas others consider gastroschisis to be a consequence of rupture of the amniotic membrane at the base of a hernia of the umbilical cord. This latter circumstance may occur when involution of the primitive right umbilical vein leaves a weakened area on the abdominal wall. Most authors agree that gastroschisis does not represent a ruptured omphalocele but rather is a distinct entity. The fact that omphalocele is so often associated with chromosome abnormalities and other anomalies, whereas gastroschisis is not, lends support to the concept that omphalocele and gastroschisis are different entities.

As with omphalocele, the physiologic considerations in the newborn with gastroschisis include immediate attention to life-threatening problems and preoperative preparation, intraoperative therapy, and postoperative management. Immediately after birth a sterile, warm environment must be provided for the infant. Placing the lower two thirds of the infant in a "bowel bag" as outlined for omphalocele helps conserve heat, provides a sterile and impervious barrier, and limits evaporative fluid loss by allowing water vapor to accumulate within the confines of the bag. The use of extremely wet dressings may lead to rapid hypothermia even within a plastic bag and should be avoided.

An intravenous line should be established as quickly as possible, and a fluid bolus (20 ml/kg) of 5% dextrose in lactated Ringer's solution should be given during the first hour. Metabolic acidosis because of poor peripheral perfusion is common but usually responds rapidly to increased intravascular volume. The administration of colloid in the form of plasma or albumin is also advisable, since the composition of the fluid "leaking" from the exposed surface of eviscerated bowel is rich in plasma proteins. Intravenous antibiotics (ampicillin and gentamicin) are given after the intravenous line is established.

After preoperative preparation the patient is taken to the operating room for repair. Unlike omphalocele, nonoperative therapy is not an option in infants with gastroschisis. Maintenance of a warm environment and close attention to replacement of fluid and blood loss are critical factors in successful surgical management of these infants. The decision for the most appropriate surgical approach is made at the operating table. Primary reduction of all viscera with closure of the abdominal wall is highly desirable but only successful in 40% to 50% of cases for the following reasons: (1) the eviscerated gut can be extremely thick, edematous, and enlarged and may not be reducible into the small abdominal cavity; (2) vascular compromise to bowel may develop if forceful reduction is attempted; (3) compression of the inferior vena cava by increased intra-abdominal pressure may decrease cardiac output; and (4) upward pressure on the diaphragm by the same mechanism may cause respiratory distress, prompting the use of increased ventilatory pressures that can be harmful to the newborn lung. If any of the above complications arise during primary reduction, staged reduction with the use of a Silastic "silo" is an excellent alternative.[23,24] With the use of a sheet of reinforced Silastic, an envelope that cannot be reduced is constructed around the bowel and sutured to the skin and fascia of the defect. An occlusive dressing is applied around the Silastic with topical antibiotic cream (povidone-iodine) application. The gut can be gradually reduced by gently squeezing the top of the silo daily or every other day, using umbilical tape to ligate the distal sac to maintain reduction. When the gut has been fully reduced (usually 5 to 10 days), the infant is returned to the operating room for removal of the silo and performance of abdominal wall repair.

The fluid requirements for infants immediately after repair of gastroschisis are significantly higher than maintenance rate. Coran and Drongowski[25] studied patients with gastroschisis to evaluate their body water and extracellular fluid volume using isotope tracer techniques. The extracellular fluid volume decreased from 52% of total body weight to 32% of total body weight in the immediate postoperative period. There was a 10% decrease in total body water in infants with gastroschisis. The fluid deficits after surgery are related to the amount of fluid given before surgery and intraoperatively, the extent of exposure of gut to the amniotic fluid, and the degree of chemical peritonitis present. Lymphatic and venous obstruction of exteriorized bowel may increase "third-space" losses into either the silo or the peritoneal cavity. Vascular dilation, hyperemia, and increased capillary permeability may also be present in the bowel wall, resulting in an outpouring of interstitial fluid that is not available for reabsorption into the intravascular space. Taking these factors into account, volumes of 175 to 300 ml/kg/day have been used intravenously for the first 24 to 48 hours after reduction, usually in the form of 5% dextrose in lactated Ringer's solution. Maintenance fluids can be used after 48 hours, when mobilization of extravascular fluid usually begins.

Depending on the degree of thickening and inflammation present within the bowel wall, a period of adynamic, ineffective intestinal peristalsis can be expected for as long as 30 days, occasionally longer. Because of the increased caloric demands, the placement of a central venous catheter and administration of intravenous total parenteral nutrition are valuable adjuncts and are probably responsible for most of the improvement in survival in gastroschisis since the mid-1970s. The catheter is usually placed after the removal of the Silastic prosthesis, at which time the risk of sepsis and bacteremia is reduced. Total parenteral nutrition must be used until relatively normal bowel movements begin; even then, elemental diets might be necessary when commencing feedings, since malabsorption of fats, protein, and glucose is not uncommon in these infants.[22] In addition, gastrointestinal transit time remains prolonged for up to 6 months after reduction.[26] Fortunately, by 12 to 18 months of age most infants demonstrate normal growth, development, and gastrointestinal function.

Improvements in preoperative and postoperative care, the availability of the Silastic prosthesis for management of the irreducible gut, and total parenteral nutrition have played important roles in increasing survival rate to 85% to 90% in most series of gastroschisis. Most morbidity and mortality is related to sepsis or late complications attendant to prolonged intravenous hyperalimentation.[27] Prenatal diagnosis of gastroschisis with ultrasound should allow better preparation for delivery, immediate resuscitation, and repair of this common abdominal wall defect.

Hypertrophic Pyloric Stenosis

Hypertrophic pyloric stenosis is an obstructing lesion of the pyloric canal that seems to be unique to the young infant. This disorder was first described in the 1700s, but a complete description awaited the astute observations of Hirschsprung in 1887. The latter report included autopsy results in two children. The first suggestion that the ideal treatment of these infants might be surgical was made by Schwyzer in 1896, who thought either pyloric dilation or gastroenterostomy would be effective. Gastroenterostomy was used as the early therapy, but as of 1910 a 61% mortality rate was recorded. Early attempts by Fredet to perform pyloroplasty by resuturing the muscle transversely after the muscle had been split longitudinally (the lumen of the stomach was not entered) proved extremely difficult, and Fredet himself remained convinced that muscle-splitting procedures were superior to gastroenterostomy for this disease. The operation performed today was first described by Ramstedt in 1912.

The pathophysiology of hypertrophic pyloric stenosis has been obscure in the past, but recent characterization of the innervation of the pylorus has shed light on the disorder. Of the theories concerning the cause of hypertrophic pyloric stenosis, most of the recent work suggests that abnormal innervation may be the most accurate. The role of nitric oxide as a mediator of relaxation in the mammalian gastrointestinal tract has recently been elucidated; its discovery led to the logical inquiry of its role in the cause of hypertrophic pyloric stenosis.[28] Vanderwinden et al.[29] compared pyloric wall sections between control patients and patients with pyloric stenosis and found severely reduced staining for nitric oxide synthetase (the enzyme which produces nitric oxide) in the disease group.[29,30] There was normal nitric oxide synthetase activity in the longitudinal muscle layer and the myenteric plexus. In addition, the authors used an antiserum stain, which defines the nerve fibers of the enteric system and demonstrated "abnormal, dilated, and tortuous" fibers in the circular muscle layer. They postulated that nitric oxide synthetase was *selectively* absent from the circular muscle layer but preserved in the longitudinal layer and the myenteric plexus. They felt this demonstrated a decrease of peptidergic inhibitory innervation in the circular muscle compared to healthy infants and that this accounted for the *defect in relaxation* of the pyloric sphincter in this disease.

Although the direct causal relationship of this theory has been challenged,[30] supporting studies have emerged. Kobayashi et al.[31] studied the presence of neural cell adhesion molecule (NCAM), nitric oxide synthetase, and neurofilament reactive protein in patients with pyloric stenosis and controls. NCAM is important in the adhesion between neuronal cells and their processes and in the formation of initial contacts between nerve and muscle cells. Neurofilament proteins are an important part of the axonal cytoskeleton of mature neurons. A deficit of all three elements was demonstrated in the circular and longitudinal muscle layers, but normal patterns were seen in the myenteric plexuses of infants with the disease. The authors postulated that nerve-induced relaxation of the muscle layers was defective because of the absence of fibers able to secrete nitric oxide. The absence of NCAM could represent a defect of embryogenesis, preventing the initial formation and proper contact between nitric oxide-containing nerves and muscle cells.

Abnormal innervation of pyloric muscle was also demonstrated by Okazaki et al.,[32] who used a monoclonal antibody to demonstrate the absence of nerve fibers and nerve-to-muscle synapses in the muscle layers only. As with the aforementioned studies, the myenteric plexuses appeared normal. The authors speculated that this might represent axonal degeneration n the muscle layers. It now appears that lack of innervation, of the circular muscle layer in particular, is the primary defect in hypertrophic pyloric stenosis. This deficit is pronounced in fibers that supply nitric oxide to the muscle. As a result there is a loss of the ability of the pylorus to relax, producing a state of tonic contraction. Morphologically, the pyloric muscle is thickened and somewhat edematous. The pyloric channel is elongated and protrudes into the duodenum. The adjacent gastric musculature is often thickened as well, possibly from increased work against the obstruction.

Both environmental and hereditary factors seem to influence the development of hypertrophic pyloric stenosis in infants. The symptoms of pyloric stenosis develop later in infants born in hospitals when compared to those born at home. Maternal-fetal-neonatal hypergastrinemia has been implicated in the development of pyloric stenosis. In addition, in a series of monozygotic twins with one twin affected, the other twin developed pyloric stenosis only 67% of the time. It is well recognized that first-born children are more frequently affected, and sporadic "epidemics" of pyloric stenosis within a community have been reported.

There also seems to be a genetic predisposition to the development of pyloric stenosis. Boys are affected five times more frequently than girls. In addition, 10% to 15% of sons and 3% to 7% of daughters of affected patients develop pyloric stenosis, with the higher incidence present if the mother has had the disease. Twins, triplets, and multiple siblings with pyloric stenosis have also been reported.

The presenting symptom is vomiting, which is nonbilious in color and frequently consists of the feeding given shortly before. The vomiting typically begins within 1 to 2 weeks after birth and rapidly progresses to projectile emesis as the pylorus becomes essentially completely obstructed. In some patients symptoms may not appear until 4 to 6 weeks of age. Usually, infants develop forceful, nonbilious emesis shortly after meals. The infant is hungry shortly afterward and will attempt to feed again. On examination the pyloric tumor may be felt in the right epigastrium and is considered diagnostic. It can be palpated in 60% to 90% of patients. In addition, peristaltic waves may be observed traversing the upper abdomen from left to right. Infants with advanced disease are weak and exhibit signs of dehydration, or they may be under weight for age. Occasionally, bloody emesis may be seen if there is accompanying gastritis. Conditions that may mimic hypertrophic pyloric stenosis include pylorospasm, gastroesophageal reflux, duodenal or antral webs, duodenal bands, and pyloric duplications.

If the diagnosis is not clear after clinical assessment, an upper gastrointestinal tract contrast study (UGIS) or sonography may be helpful in establishing the diagnosis. The UGIS demonstrates an elongated and thinned pyloric channel known as the "string sing." In addition, the distal antrum may have a squared-off, or shouldered, appearance produced by a bulging pylorus; and a mushroom-shaped mass may protrude into the duodenal bulb. UGIS may also exclude some of the aforementioned conditions that mimic hypertrophic pyloric stenosis.

Ultrasound examination has been helpful when the physical examination is equivocal. In one recent review this modality had a sensitivity, specificity, and accuracy of 100%. Sonographic findings that denote the presence of the disease are (1) echogenic parallel lines that define the mucosal complex of the pylorus, (2) a shoulder sign on the distal wall of the antrum that is accentuated during peristalsis, and (3) protrusion of the redundant pyloric mucosa into the duodenum.[33] Objective measurements of muscle wall thickness, channel length, and pyloric diameter increase the accuracy of this method. True positives for the disease were found with pyloric lengths greater than 12 mm and muscle thickness greater than 3 mm.[34]

The persistent vomiting of gastric secretions in these patients eventually produces a metabolic alkalosis, with a variable degree of hypokalemia. Potassium is also lost but is replaced by intracellular stores; however, this results in a total body deficit of potassium, which becomes apparent during resuscitation. Initially, there is a renal adjustment of serum pH by increased excretion of bicarbonate coupled to sodium and potassium ions, which causes a net resorption of hydrogen ions in the nephron. When dehydration becomes significant, the renal response switches to resorb sodium to preserve volume status; this wastes potassium and eventually produces a significant paradoxic aciduria as hydrogen ions take the place of potassium in exchange for sodium in the distal tubule. Thus aciduria and hypokalemia are late signs in infants with hypertrophic pyloric stenosis.

Metabolic alkalosis can be a significant threat to the infant undergoing anesthesia because it can lead to respiratory depression, carbon dioxide retention, and postoperative apnea. Although measurement of serum electrolytes, particularly chloride, has been deemed accurate in predicting the degree of alkalosis, this is dependent on the hydration status of the patient.[35] clinical assessment, which includes observation of skin turgor, mucous membranes, and the fullness of the fontanelle, is the most helpful. Biochemical measurements and factors in the patient's history are not as predictive as an accurate clinical assessment. Thus it should be clearly stated that the assessment of the patient's hydration and acid-base status must include a physical examination and serum electrolytes and blood gas analysis. A typical serum electrolyte pattern might include a relatively normal level of sodium (135 to 140 mEq/L), depressed levels of potassium (3 to 4 mEq/L) and chloride (75 to 90 mEq/L), and a greatly elevated serum bicarbonate level (30 to 45 mEq/L). The urine is usually acidic.

Taking these electrolyte deficits into account, the ideal fluid for resuscitation in these infants is 5% dextrose in normal saline with 20 to 40 mEq of calcium chloride per liter added at a rate of 150 to 200 ml/kg/day. A bolus of 5% dextrose in normal saline (20 ml/kg) infused during an hour is sometimes necessary in severe dehydration. Even though the serum sodium level is usually normal, these infants have isotonic dehydration and benefit by replacement with sodium. As the hypochloremia resolves, the serum bicarbonate level falls. Most clinicians feel that general anesthesia can be safely administered when the serum bicarbonate level is below 30 mEq/L, but this may take 48 hours of vigorous intravenous therapy or more. There is no role for attempts at oral hydration in these seriously ill neonates.

After adequate preparation the operation for pyloric stenosis is one of the safest, most straightforward, and curative procedures performed in pediatric surgery. A small right upper quadrant incision is made, and the peritoneal cavity entered without dividing the rectus muscle. The pylorus is delivered into the wound, and a longitudinal incision is made in the anterior wall of the hypertrophied pylorus from the duodenopyloric junction proximally for the extent of the muscular thickening. With a blunt instrument or a "spreader" the muscle fibers are divided to the submucosa, allowing the mucosa to bulge into the defect. If the mucosa is injured and the lumen entered, several fine silk sutures can be used to repair the defect, but these must be placed so the stenosis is not recreated. A nasogastric tube is not routinely left in place after surgery unless the lumen has been entered. Although laparoscopic pyloromyotomy has been reported, it offers little, if any, objective advantage when compared to the standard approach.[36]

Historically, postoperative feeding regimens have been complicated and cryptic.[37] Currently, we begin feeding 3 hours after operation with 30 ml of formula/breast milk and advance to 60 ml and then 75 ml at 3-hour intervals. Patients are discharged in 24 to 36 hours after operation. Because the lower esophageal sphincter pressure is abnormally low in these infants for a time after repair, gastroesophageal reflux is common and may result in continued vomiting. An upright position and thickened feedings may be necessary for several weeks after surgery to decrease the risk for reflux and its sequelae.

Necrotizing Enterocolitis

Neonatal necrotizing enterocolitis (NEC) is an intriguing disease that seems to affect only newborns and young infants, primarily those who are born prematurely An increase in the incidence of NEC since 1970 parallels the emergence of neonatal intensive care units and the improved survival of premature infants. Although the disease has certainly been present for many years, its pathology was explored only after numerous cases were recognized and managed. Currently, NEC is the most common gastrointestinal emergency afflicting neonates in the United States. The overall incidence for all neonatal intensive care unit admissions in 12 large neonatal centers was 2.4%. It occurs in the first few weeks of life, with prematurity and low birth weight being the most consistent risk factors. Only 10% of cases develop in term infants.[38] Although the exact cause remains obscure, recent experimental and clinical studies have increased the understanding, prevention, and management of NEC. Because of its association with prematurity, NEC may be a result of an alteration of the structural integrity of the immature gastrointestinal tract. The classic description is that multiple factors combine to produce intestinal necrosis (Fig. 66-4); the three elements usually described include intestinal ischemia, bacterial infection, and the presence of a substrate in the bowel lumen. Recent work has suggested that the primary biochemical mediators of NEC are eicosanoids, particularly thromboxane, platelet-activating factor, and leukotrienes.[39,40]

Originally, a "diving reflex" was believed to contribute to gut ischemia, where during periods of physiologic stress blood was redistributed to essential organs. The intestines were believed to be hypoperfused during these periods. However, careful study of the incidence of the disease shows that NEC is as common in premature infants without stress as those who suffer some insult. NEC in term or near-term infants, which is much rarer, does have a predilection for infants who suffer either a hypoxic or ischemic insult. Polycythemia has also been identified as a risk factor for developing NEC in term infants[41]; thus hyperviscosity and altered mucosal blood flow may contribute to the development of the disease. Other factors that might lead to intestinal ischemia have been implicated, including neonatal polycythemia and the presence of umbilical artery catheters (presumably via microthromboemboli). Again, careful epidemiologic studies show that the incidence of NEC is the same in these "risk groups" as in other premature neonates.[42] Up to 10% to 15% of infants developing NEC have no identifiable risk factors.[38]

Many authors maintain that bacteria, either infectious or colonizing, are "essential for the development of NEC."[42] In healthy newborns the gut is colonized with a range of bacteria within 10 days.[43] For physiologically stressed premature infants in the neonatal intensive care unit, who are often receiving antibiotics, colonization is delayed and consists of a limited number of bacterial species. NEC epidemics are not uncommon in nurseries, where a particular pathogen may predominate. Historically, *Klebsiella, Escherichia coli, Clostridium,* and *Staphylococcus* organisms have each been labeled the causative pathogens for isolated series of cases of NEC. Infection control

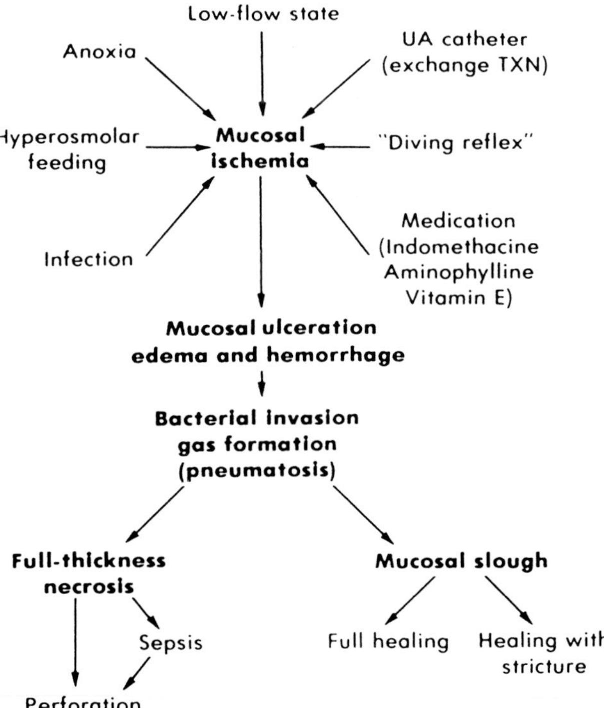

Fig. 66-4. Pathogenesis of necrotizing enterocolitis. Multiple factors result in mucosal ischemia, which may lead to bacterial invasion. Full healing, healing with stricture, or full-thickness necrosis are possible outcomes. *TXN,* Transfusion; *UA,* umbilical artery.

measures are effective in this setting. However, no specific microbial pathogen is consistently responsible for the disease; it seems clear that a single infectious agent does not explain the pathogenesis of this disorder.

Infant feedings (the intraluminal substrate) have been a source of investigation since it was shown that NEC occurred more commonly in neonates who were fed whole milk formulas. It was believed that bacteria acted on the formula substrate, proliferated, and produced hydrogen gas, which is the primary component of pneumatosis intestinalis, a classic finding in NEC. Two factors were believed to account for the detrimental effect of formula feedings. First, hypertonic solutions were postulated to directly injure the intestinal mucosa, allowing the entrance of pathogens. Secondly, formulas lack immunologic components of human breast milk that are protective. Macrophages, IgG, secretory IgA and lactoferrin are beneficial to aid in infant intestinal immunity, which theoretically is cytoprotective against pathogenic bacteria.[42,44]

NEC involves the ileum and proximal colon in the majority of cases; however, involvement of the remainder of the gastrointestinal tract is not infrequent. Pannecrosis of the gut is a particularly dangerous pattern where over 75% of the intestine is involved, usually sparing the stomach, duodenum, a small area of proximal jejunum, and the distal rectum. Grossly, the bowel appears irregularly dilated with dark red hemorrhagic areas or gray sections of frank necrosis. Perforations may be found, especially in the ileocecal area. Usually, the antimesenteric border is more heavily involved.

Early microscopic changes consist of mucosal edema, ulceration, and hemorrhage in mild cases. There are often microthromboemboli in submucosal vessels. Pneumatosis intestinalis begins as subserosal collections of gas and eventually forms large subserosal bubbles. Microthrombi in the mesenteric arterioles and veins are common but might be secondary to systemic intravascular coagulation; large vessel thrombosis is not seen in NEC. Inflammatory changes in the mucosa are uncommon in the acute phase but are prominent later with healing of partial-thickness injury. Late scar formation with stricture may continue for several months after a case of NEC.

Several medications given to newborns as therapy for a variety of disorders have recently been found to increase the incidence and severity of NEC in both experimental and clinical studies. Indomethacin, a prostaglandin synthetase inhibitor used for nonsurgical closure of a patent ductus arteriosus, has been associated clinically with an increase in the number of cases of NEC.[45] Vitamin E given to prevent retrolental fibroplasia and aminophylline used as a respiratory stimulant have been found experimentally to increase the severity of bowel necrosis in a rat model of NEC.[46] These studies suggest that extreme care must be exercised in using medications of any kind in the newborn infant.

NEC occurs within the first 10 days of life in over 90% of cases. The most common early signs and symptoms in NEC are presented in Fig. 66-5. The onset is usually insidious, although fulminant cases are occasionally seen. The physical examination of the abdomen in the infant with NEC, although difficult, can nonetheless frequently be valuable. Abdominal wall erythema and edema (especially in the periumbilical region), localized tenderness or crepitance, abdominal mass (edematous, thickened loop of bowel), and splinting of the abdomen by the use of chest wall accessory muscles of respiration are valuable physical signs in the infant with NEC. In fulminant cases, grossly bloody stools and rapid deterioration to a moribund state within a several-hour period usually signifies the presence of a large amount of necrotic bowel.

The roentgenographic signs of NEC have been described in numerous publications and include pneumatosis intestinalis, localized bowel distention, portal vein gas, free intraperitoneal air, thickened bowel wall, and a "gas-

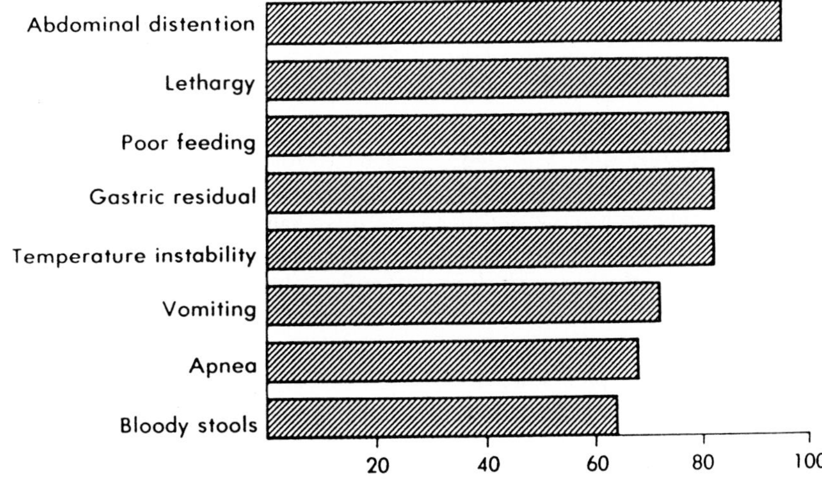

Fig. 66-5. Percent frequency of signs and symptoms associated with necrotizing enterocolitis in newborn infants.

less" appearance, signifying fluid-filled loops of bowel. The use of metrizamide, a water-soluble contrast agent to aid in the diagnosis of NEC, has proven to be a valuable adjunct in recent studies.[47] Free intraperitoneal air and portal vein gas seem to be the most ominous x-ray signs of NEC, suggestive of perforation and/or extensive necrosis. The laboratory evaluation of the infant with suspected or confirmed NEC should include a white blood cell count; hematocrit; platelet count, blood gas and pH analysis; and a study of renal and liver functions. A very low white blood cell count suggests overwhelming sepsis. A low platelet count has been observed in cases of gangrenous bowel, thought to be caused by disseminated intravascular coagulation, sequestration into the area of necrotic bowel, or binding to endotoxin with removal by the spleen. Although it is useful for following the infant, a low platelet count is not considered to be an absolute indication for surgery by most neonatal surgeons. Persistent metabolic acidosis or blood gas analysis is a reliable indicator of poor perfusion, is suggestive of bowel necrosis, and is useful when combined with physical and radiologic findings.

The principles of nonoperative management include restoration of intravascular volume to improve gut circulation, prevention of infection, and bowel rest. Candidates for this form of treatment include those infants without perforations, with stable or improving clinical status, including laboratory data, and without massive gastrointestinal hemorrhage. Most neonatologists institute medical therapy in any infant suspected of having NEC, even if there is little firm evidence that the infant has the disorder. Frequent reexamination by abdominal palpation, x-ray films, and laboratory data (white blood cell count, platelet count, blood gas, and pH analysis) are necessary in infants receiving such nonoperative therapy. Since perforation is not detected by x-ray film in as many as 50% of cases, total reliance on radiologic procedures is risky and may result in high mortality because of late diagnosis of peritonitis.

An infant suspected or confirmed of having NEC should have an orogastric or nasogastric tube placed. Broad-spectrum intravenous antibiotics should be given. Poorly absorbed oral antibiotics have not been shown to be efficacious in controlled studies. Intravenous fluids, both crystalloid (0.45% NaCl in 5% dextrose) and colloid (albumin 1 g/kg or fresh frozen plasma 10 ml/kg), are used at rates necessary to obtain normal renal output. This may require unexpectedly high volumes (200 to 250 ml/kg/day). Cardiac failure from sepsis or vigorous intravascular volume replacement may necessitate the use of inotropic agents (dopamine, isoproterenol, epinephrine) until the clinical status stabilizes. After the onset of resolution (usually 2 to 3 days), the use of intravenous alimentation should be considered. However, the septic premature infant seems to be most susceptible to cholestasis from total parenteral nutrition, and thus liver functions must be monitored carefully.

The timing for the resumption of oral feedings remains controversial, since recurrence of NEC has been reported after beginning oral formulas. Most neonatologists would wait 3 to 4 days after resolution of ileus, pneumatosis, and hematochezia before resuming an oral diet. Despite supportive medical therapy, approximately 40% to 50% of infants with NEC require abdominal exploration. The timing for surgical intervention in NEC is important, since negative results from exploration may be dangerous in these critically ill neonates. Pneumoperitoneum, failure of medical therapy as judged by clinical deterioration, persistent acidosis, and thrombocytopenia have been used in various combinations as surgical indications. Of these, pneumoperitoneum seems to be the most reliable, although unfortunately it also signifies a poorer prognosis. A fixed loop on serial radiographs, erythema of the abdominal wall, palpable abdominal mass, portal vein gas, and persistent gastrointestinal bleeding are relative indications for abdominal exploration. Kosloske and Lilly[48] have proposed abdominal paracentesis as a method of detecting transmural bowel necrosis at an earlier point than some of the traditional indications for operation.[42,48] A positive result from paracentesis yields brown or dark yellow fluid that shows bacteria on Gram's stain; if an insufficient volume of fluid is aspirated, peritoneal lavage is performed.

A laparotomy is performed, usually through an upper abdominal transverse incision. All bowel is exteriorized and examined carefully for sites of necrosis and/or perforation, most commonly found in the terminal ileum, ascending colon, transverse and left colon, and proximal small bowel in decreasing order of frequency. Areas of frank bowel necrosis or perforation are resected, even if several separate segmental resections are necessary. Bowel that appears marginally viable is not resected but returned to the abdomen with the possibility of second-look laparotomy 24 to 36 hours later. Although a few investigators have advocated primary anastomosis of bowel, most neonatal surgeons prefer to exteriorize the ends of the bowel as ostomies, either through the wound or through separate incisions, to be closed at a later date. Usually, culture positive purulent fluid or stool is found within the peritoneal cavity, and this should be copiously irrigated.

The postoperative care is directed toward optimizing the circulatory status; correcting shock. Acidosis, and sepsis; maintaining hematologic homeostasis; and providing nutrition. This is accomplished by the administration of fluid (colloid and crystalloid), blood and platelets, antibiotics, and later parenteral nutrition. Total parenteral nutrition is a valuable adjunct in the management of these infants. Late complications of NEC include bowel stricture, fistulas, abscesses, short gut syndrome, malabsorption, cholestasis, enterocyst formation, and recurrent NEC.[49,50] Strictures may form in 15% to 35% of successfully treated patients and result from healed areas that did not perforate. Contrast studies of defunctionalized bowel should *always* be performed prior to reconstructing continuity of those segments. In fact, some investigators recommend contrast examination in all medically treated patients recovering from NEC, as obstruction and life-threatening perforation can occur weeks after resolution of the disease. Stenotic segments in medically treated patients have been successfully balloon dilated, therefore avoiding operation. Such strictures must be focal and within reach of the catheter.

Since the majority of patients with NEC are premature infants, they are susceptible to the disorders that are common to that age group (e.g., hyaline membrane disease, jaundice, meningitis, and intracerebral hemorrhage). Exacting care is necessary to achieve survival in these seriously ill neonates.

Esophageal Atresia and Tracheoesophageal Fistula

Infants with esophageal atresia frequently have early symptoms of severe respiratory distress and excess salivation. Choking, coughing, and cyanosis are frequently encountered on the first attempted feeding. Infants with an associated tracheoesophageal fistula often develop acute gastric dilation because of air entering distal esophagus and stomach with each inspired breath. As most neonates have an incompetent lower esophageal sphincter, this ultimately leads to reflux of gastric acid through the fistula into the lungs, resulting in aspiration and chemical pneumonitis. There are five recognized anatomic variants of esophageal atresia. These include atresia of the esophagus without a fistula, esophageal atresia with a proximal tracheoesophageal fistula, esophageal atresia with a "double" tracheoesophageal fistula (from both proximal and distal segments), proximal atresia with a distal tracheoesophageal fistula (most common form—88%), and "H"-type tracheoesophageal fistula without esophageal atresia. The incidence of this anomaly is approximately 1 in 1500 births, with boys and girls equally affected. The ultimate survival of these infants usually depends on prompt recognition and expeditious transfer to institutions fully equipped and staffed with experienced personnel familiar with the often complicated care required. Approximately one third of the infants are of low birth weight. Associated anomalies are common (70%), particularly those of the cardiovascular system, gastrointestinal tract (imperforate anus and duodenal atresia), genitourinary tract, and musculoskeletal system. Tracheoesophageal fistula has also been observed in patients with Down's syndrome and trisomy 18. In addition, many may have the VATER association (*V,* vertebral or vascular defects; *A,* anal anomalies; *T,* tracheoesophageal fistula; *E,* esophageal atresia; and *R,* radial limb or renal anomalies).[51]

The defect may be anticipated if maternal polyhydramnios is noted before the fetus is delivered. Most infants with esophageal atresia without a fistula have polyhydramniotic mothers (greater than 90%), whereas in only (approximately) 20% of infants with a distal tracheoesophageal fistula is this observed. In the latter cases the fetus swallows amniotic fluid, which overflows the blind esophageal pouch only to pass through the tracheoesophageal fistula into the gastrointestinal tract and is absorbed normally in utero. The diagnosis of esophageal atresia is not difficult to confirm—attempted passage of a firm red rubber or synthetic catheter through the nose into the esophagus demonstrates obstruction at the level of atresia. A frontal and lateral x-ray film of the chest and abdomen should be obtained with the catheter in place, showing the tip of the catheter at the end of the atretic proximal esophageal pouch. If gas is present in the gastrointestinal tract, a tracheoesophageal fistula must therefore also be present. If no gas pattern is observed below the diaphragm, a fistula is unlikely. These simple observations allow a diagnosis in at least 95% of cases of esophageal atresia. Occasionally, contrast studies are required for the diagnosis of the more rare forms of proximal esophageal fistula or a double fistula from both the proximal and distal esophageal segments and the "H"-type fistula without atresia. The "H"-type fistula may be suspected in infants with severe respiratory distress who have a dilated, air-filled esophagus on plain x-ray films. Endoscopy with updated telescopic Storz infant bronchoscopes can usually directly observe the "H"-type fistula.

Emergency care of the infant involves aspiration of the oral pharynx to clear secretions. This may be accomplished by insertion of a Replogle sump catheter into the blind pouch. The catheter is maintained on continuous suction to keep the pouch dry. The secretions should be cultured, and the infant should receive antibiotic therapy. The truly emergent aspect in the care of this anomaly concerns the occurrence of potentially lethal aspiration pneumonia caused by reflux of gastric juice from the dilated stomach through the tracheoesophageal fistula. The deleterious chemical effects of gastric juice on the tracheobronchial tree and pulmonary parenchyma are well known. The infant should be maintained in semi-Fowler's position to keep the gastric fluid meniscus low in the stomach, reducing reflux. Although an emergency gastrostomy formerly was performed routinely in all patients with esophageal atresia and tracheoesophageal fistula, accumulated clinical experience has found this approach to be unnecessary except in highly unstable infants, for whom primary repair is prudently delayed. If the infant is full term and shows no evidence of associated anomalies, sepsis, or pneumonitis, however, a definitive extrapleural thoracotomy is undertaken, using general endotracheal anesthesia. The fistula is divided, the tracheal side oversewn, and an end-to-end anastomosis is attempted between the dilated thickened proximal pouch and the small distal esophagus. Tension and poor blood supply (particularly to the distal segment) are two problems encountered during this anastomosis and are directly related to the incidence of anastomotic leaks that may occur in as many as 15% of patients. An extrapleural leak, however, drains to the outside, much like an incision and drainage of an abscess, with little or no effect on the infant's condition; in fact, many infants do not even demonstrate an elevation in temperature when this occurs. However, if a transpleural operation is performed, a leak would result in empyema, which is associated with a significant morbidity and mortality in the neonatal age group. Thus there is probably no role for the transpleural approach in the initial thoracic exploration of an infant with esophageal atresia. This concept is supported by a 20% higher survival rate in infants undergoing extrapleural operations.

In low-birth-weight (premature or SGA) patients or those with evidence of associated congenital anomalies, sepsis, or severe pneumonia, the thoracic operation is delayed and a gastrostomy is performed to decompress the stomach, usually with the patient under anesthesia. Improved pulmonary toilet, hydration, and antibiotic therapy are initiated with suction on the proximal pouch, and the gastrostomy set to straight drainage. The definitive procedure is delayed until the infant is better able to withstand a general endotracheal anesthetic and thoracotomy. This "staging" period often lasts only from 1 to 4 days and significantly improves the infant's general condition and chances for survival. At the time of thoracotomy, if the ends of the esophagus are too far apart for a "safe" anastomosis (even under tension), a number of alternatives may be considered. First, closure of the distal end and approximation of the muscular segments without opening the proximal pouch may be attempted, allowing the two ends of the esophagus to spontaneously stretch with reoperation at 4 to 6 weeks. Others have used manual or electromagnetic bougienage of the blind proximal pouch during a 6- to 8-week period with subsequent reexploration to achieve the same goal. An additional technique is that of circular esophagomyotomy that allows distal descent of the end of the proximal atretic pouch and primary anastomosis to be performed at the initial operation. In general, the goal has been to avoid esophageal replacement by interposition of colon or a gastric tube whenever possible. Neither of these replacement organs functions as well as the infant's own esophagus. These procedures, however, are sometimes required when the two ends of the esophagus are much too far apart or if any of the previously mentioned surgical adjuncts fail (particularly in instances of atresia without an associated fistula). In these cases a cervical esophagostomy is performed, and the infant receives gastrostomy feedings until an appropriate time for interposition procedures (usually at age 18 months). Sham oral feedings are also given in the interim so that the infant does not forget how to swallow.

The care of infants with variants of esophageal atresia is exacting and demanding. However, when it takes place at skilled neonatal centers particularly designed and equipped with personnel skilled in the management of these critically ill patients, good survival rates can be obtained.

Many of these survivors require periodic dilation of the esophageal anastomosis. In addition, long-term follow-up is essential, since some of the patients require additional surgical procedures to repair associated cardiac, renal, and other gastrointestinal anomalies.

In recent years a high incidence of gastroesophageal reflux has been noted in these patients. Gastroesophageal reflux has been incriminated in the many chronic pulmonary problems seen in these children (aspiration pneumonia, "asthmatic" condition), and some may require an antireflux operation.

Congenital Diaphragmatic Hernia

Congenital posterolateral diaphragmatic hernia (CDH), through the foramen of Bochdalek, is the most common surgically correctable cause of severe respiratory distress in the newborn. Occurring in 1 of 2200 births, the defect is on the left side in 85% of cases, on the right side in 13%, and bilateral in 1% to 2%. Most infants with CDH are term infants and therefore any "large" baby with severe respiratory distress should be suspected as having this defect.

This anomaly forms as the gut makes its normal return to the abdominal cavity from the yolk sac simultaneously with the formation of the diaphragm and the development of lung buds. Failure of the pleuroperitoneal foramen of Bochdalek to close before return of the gut allows the viscera to herniate into the hemithorax, preventing the full development of the ipsilateral lung. If the mediastinum is shifted, compression of the contralateral lung takes place, interfering with its development as well. The result is moderate-to-severe respiratory distress, usually present immediately at birth or shortly thereafter. The degree of distress tends to worsen rapidly as swallowed air distends the gut within the chest, causing further lung compression and mediastinal shift. Cyanosis, tachypnea, pallor, gasping respirations, retractions, or complete cardiorespiratory arrest are the usual findings as the infant struggles to expand the lungs. Breath sounds are usually absent on the side of the hernia, and heart sounds are shifted to the opposite hemithorax. The typical appearance of a barrel chest and scaphoid abdomen is frequently present.[52]

As discussed earlier, development of the conduction airways is nearly complete by 18 weeks' gestation, with further development of alveolar sacs and respiratory bronchioles beyond then. The numbers of bronchopulmonary generations are greatly reduced in both the ipsilateral and contralateral lung in patients with CDH. The pulmonary arterioles have hypertrophied muscle, and they are highly sensitive to hypoxia and changes in the partial pressure of carbon dioxide. Hypoxemia and hypercarbia can result in the development of an extreme right-to-left shunt across the foramen ovale and the patent ductus arteriosus, beginning a positive feedback cycle of progressive, worsening hypoxia and pulmonary hypertension, termed persistent pulmonary hypertension of the newborn (PPHN).

The primary disorder in infants with CDH is unclear at this time and the subject of considerable debate. There are two widely used animal models. In one, pregnant rats at a certain time in gestation are fed the insecticide nitrofen. A proportion of the litter are then born with CDH.[53] More detailed studies with this model show that the lungs in CDH are biochemically immature.[54] The lungs in CDH have been shown to be surfactant deficient.[55] Indeed, one small series of patients had improved survival when given exogenous surfactant. The nitrofen appears to affect a very localized point in somite growth. The heart and the lungs develop from this region, suggesting that the pulmonary hypoplasia seen in CDH is a primary problem, not secondary to simply compression.[56]

The second model supports the compression theory. A diaphragm defect is created at a certain time in lamb gestation. The bowel then herniates into the chest and compresses both the lungs and heart. While the lungs are clearly hypoplastic, increasing evidence points to cardiac defects occurring as well. Associated cardiac anomalies can significantly affect outcome.[57] In some infants, survival has been correlated with ventricular mass; those infants with smaller ventricles have a much worse prognosis.[56] The mortality rate can vary depending on when the defect is created. Although the exact cause of CDH in the infant is unclear, the infants develop varying degrees of pulmonary hypoplasia. Symptoms primarily relate to the degree of pulmonary and cardiac hypoplasia and the degree of pulmonary hypertension. Prognosis is related to the degree of associated pulmonary hypoplasia, other anomalies, and the vasoreactivity of the pulmonary vasculature.[57]

The infant with small lungs becomes symptomatic immediately on clamping the umbilical cord. In the infant with more developed lungs, symptoms may be delayed for several hours after birth. The differential diagnosis on the basis of clinical examination is that of pneumothorax, chylothorax, meconium or other aspiration syndromes, and congenital cystic lung lesions (lobar emphysema or cystic adenomatoid malformation). If possible, a chest x-ray film should be obtained at the first sign of respiratory distress, before the institution of invasive resuscitative procedures such as tube thoracostomy. Occasionally, the x-ray film shows an opacified hemithorax if the infant has not swallowed sufficient air to fill the gastrointestinal tract. If confusion exists in the interpretation of the x-ray film, a second x-ray film should be performed to further define the problem. Frequently, this demonstrates the gut within the chest or, as in the case of a right-sided CDH, liver in the chest (Fig. 66-6).

The therapy for newborns with CDH consists of immediate endotracheal intubation with ventilation assistance and prompt, effective nasogastric decompression. It is important to avoid alveolar overdistention by too vigorous mechanical ventilation. The goals of therapy in the infant with CDH are to provide effective oxygenation and ventilation while avoiding alveolar overdistention.[58] An echocardiogram is obtained to rule out concomitant congenital heart defects and to measure left ventricular mass.[56,59,60] Serial echocardiograms are done to determine the degree and progression of right-to-left shunt over time as the patient responds to therapy. This can give objective data to planning the time of operation in relation to the resolution of the pulmonary hypertension.[61,62] Intravenous volume expansion and inotropes are used to support the circulation; by improving systemic arterial tone, ductal shunting is reduced. Emergent operative correction was the standard approach for many years, but this has been shown to actually worsen lung compliance.[63] Waiting several days can improve lung function and allow for resolution of pulmonary hypertension, but this has not been clearly shown to improve outcome. The ideal timing for operative correction is not clear; some authors recommend a brief period (24 to 48 hours) of stabilization, whereas others suggest waiting until the pulmonary hypertension resolves, which may be as long as 1 to 2 weeks.[64-66]

There have been many attempts to reverse the pulmonary hypertension by pharmacologic means. A num-

A

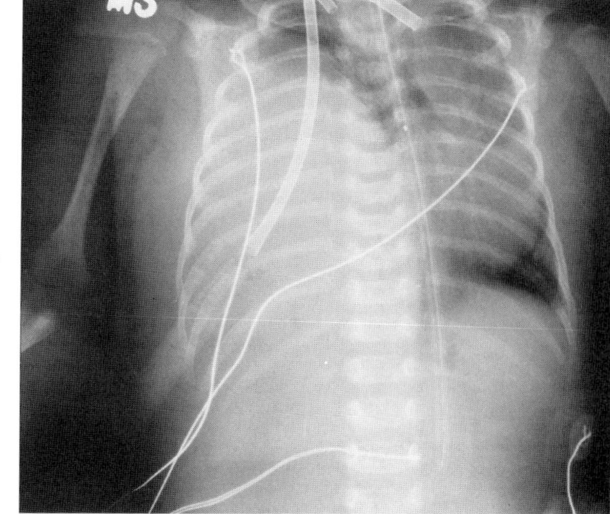

B

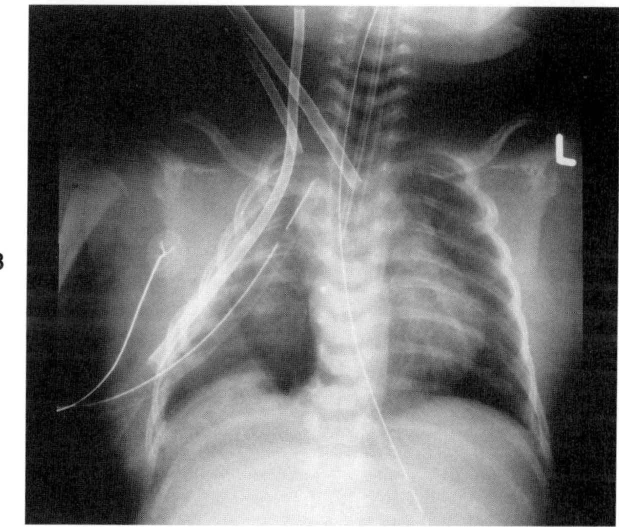

Fig. 66-6. A, Chest radiograph of a right-sided congenital diaphragmatic hernia. Note mediastinal shift and pulmonary hypoplasia. **B,** Postdiaphragmatic hernial repair for diaphragmatic agenesis with small right lung and placement of extracorporeal membrane oxygenation cannulae.

ber of nonselective vasodilators including tolazoline and sodium nitroprusside have been recommended but have not shown clear benefit. More recently, inhaled nitric oxide has been shown to be an effective selective pulmonary vasodilator. Nitric oxide has a short half-life and is bound to hemoglobin, so there are no systemic effects. Nitric oxide has been used in infants with CDH with mixed results, and further studies are needed.[50] In some infants, maximal medical therapy is of no help, and extracorporeal membrane oxygenation (ECMO) is used. ECMO provides cardiopulmonary support, and it functionally improves the pulmonary artery hyptertension by effectively delivering oxygen and removing carbon dioxide. This provides for lung rest by supporting cardiac and lung function. Patients usually receive ECMO therapy for 7 to 14 days but can be supported for longer periods of time. Survival in patients with CDH has ranged between 60% to 85%. A small subset of infants may be too unstable for repair, and they are unresponsive to maximal medical management. They receive ECMO therapy, and attempts are made to wean them prior to repair of the CDH. If they cannot be weaned from ECMO, repair is made during ECMO therapy. Even in this extremely high-risk group of patients, survival of 40% to 60% has been reported.[67]

The surgical approach for these infants is usually straightforward. A subcostal or upper vertical incision is used. The viscera are gently reduced from the chest, and an assessment is made regarding primary closure of the diaphragm defect (usually possible) or, if the defect is very large, the use of a prosthesis or muscle flap for defect closure. A tube thoracostomy is inserted through the fifth intercostal space, and a low level of suction (5 to 8 cm of water) is used. Occasionally, after the defect is repaired, the abdominal cavity is too small to accommodate the viscera. In these instances creation of a ventral hernia by closing only skin and subcutaneous tissues, followed later (3 to 6 months) by ventral hernia repair, is an acceptable alternative. Another approach if abdominal closure would be too tight, is to create a "mini-silo," which is then downsized in the ensuing 48 to 72 hours, and a delayed primary closure is performed. In cases where prolonged ventilatory support is anticipated, particularly with high peak inspiratory pressures, a chest tube is placed prophylactically in the contralateral chest to prevent development of an unsuspected tension pneumothorax if that lung should rupture.

The postoperative management of these infants is demanding and frequently frustrating. Arterial blood gas monitoring should be performed frequently, and appropriate changes in ventilator settings should be made immediately. The development of pulmonary hypertension, which can become apparent immediately or after a so-called "honeymoon" period of 6 to 12 hours is the most serious complication following surgery. This condition, leading to a fetal circulatory pattern with right-to-left shunting at the atrial (foramen ovale) and ductus arteriosus levels, has proven very difficult to treat and leads to mortality in the majority of infants who develop it. If the circumstance occurs, the same modalities used to treat the infant preoperatively are employed again. A second course of ECMO has also been used successfully in this setting.[68]

Although improvements in survival have occurred, a significant number of infants with CDH die. Therapies such as fetal repair have been attempted, and results are poor to date.[62] Newer fetal interventions include techniques to prevent the efflux of tracheal fluid from the lung to create a pressure effect and resultant lung growth in utero.[69,70] The occluded trachea is opened at birth. This technique has been used in experimental animals and successfully in humans on a limited basis. Liquid ventilation is a new mode of ventilation with perfluorocarbons to augment oxygenation, and there is some evidence that the liquid augments lung growth by exerting a distended pressure on the alveoli.[71] The future of these technique is uncertain.

Alimentary Tract Obstruction

Congenital lesions resulting in alimentary tract obstruction constitute a major group of anomalies. These lesions formerly were thought to be associated with significant morbidity and mortality, but early recognition and prompt appropriate therapy now results in excellent survival rates in most pediatric centers.

The presence of intestinal obstruction may be anticipated by carefully obtaining a family history to record instances of cystic fibrosis, aganglionosis, pyloric atresia, and rare cases of multiple gastrointestinal atresia, all of which may be inherited disorders. Prenatal ultrasound may detect alimentary tract obstruction in utero, allowing for predelivery preparation and timely transfer to a pediatric surgical center, if appropriate.

There are four cardinal signs of alimentary tract obstruction in the newborn: maternal polyhydramnios, bilious vomiting, abdominal distention, and failure to pass normal amounts of meconium spontaneously in the first 24 hours of life. Although none is pathognomonic, the presence of two or more strongly suggests intestinal obstruction and mandates further workup.

Amniotic fluid in excess of 1500 to 2000 ml is considered to be polyhydramnios. Twenty-five percent to 40% of the amniotic fluid is swallowed by the fetus and usually reabsorbed in the first 20 to 25 cm of jejunum. A high alimentary tract obstruction (e.g., esophageal atresia without tracheoesophageal fistula, pyloric atresia, duodenal atresia, or high jejunal atresia) may be associated with maternal polyhydramnios. Other causes of polyhydramnios include fetal swallowing problems, particularly in infants with central nervous system abnormality (i.e., anencephaly). Maternal conditions resulting in polyhydramnios include toxemia and cardiac, renal, or hepatic disease. Idiopathic polyhydramnios is also observed. Current evaluation of the polyhydramniotic mother should include ultrasound of the fetus to attempt to detect upper alimentary tract obstruction.

Bilious vomiting in a newborn or young infant is always pathologic and must be investigated. The newborn's stomach normally contains less than 15 ml of clear gastric juice at birth. More than 20 ml of clear gastric secretions or gastric juice containing bile suggests alimentary tract obstruction. Bilious vomiting may also be seen in septic infants with adynamic ileus. If alimentary tract obstruction is suggested by a large amount of gastric juice, the stomach should be gently emptied by an orogastric tube, which should be left in place and connected to either low suction or gravity drainage. Fluid and electrolyte losses from the stomach can be considerable and should be replaced with 5% dextrose in normal saline, with added potassium (20 to 50 mEq/L).

The normal contour of the newborn's abdomen is round, unlike the usual spheroid appearance of the adult abdomen. However a grossly distended abdomen in the neonate is pathologic. Physical findings associated with distention include visible veins on the abdomen wall caused by attenuation, "bowel patterning" (visible intestinal loops with or without peristalsis), and occasionally respiratory distress caused by elevation of the diaphragms. In each case it is essential to obtain a supine and decubitus or cross-table x-ray film of the abdomen to evaluate the nature of the distention. Distention may be the result of free air (perforated viscous), fluid (hemoperitoneum, chyloperitoneum), or distended bowel caused by mechanical obstruction or adynamic ileus. In general, only lower intestinal obstruction (ileal or colonic) gives significant abdominal distention.

Normal meconium is composed of amniotic fluid, squames, lanugo hairs, succus entericus, and intestinal mucus. It is dark green or black in color and sticky in consistency. As much as 250 mg of meconium may be passed, and failure to pass normal amounts in the first 24 hours of life may be pathologic. Infants with low small bowel obstruction, colon atresia, Hirschsprung's disease, meconium plug syndrome, or small left colon syndrome may fit this category. Other diseases that may be associated with failure of meconium passage include prematurity, hypothyroidism, sepsis with adynamic ileus, and maternal narcotic addiction.

Pyloric Atresia

Pyloric atresia accounts for 1% of all alimentary tract obstruction in neonates. Occasionally, there is a familial tendency to pyloric atresia, and cases have been noted in siblings. Infants with this malformation have nonbilious vomiting. Maternal polyhydramnios is found in two thirds of cases. In some infants epidermolysis bullosa is associated with pyloric atresia.

Plain x-ray film of the abdomen shows a single large gastric bubble with no evidence of air beyond the pylorus. Contrast studies are usually unnecessary. The infant may initially have hypochloremic alkalosis as a result of the loss of hydrochloric acid from vomiting. An orogastric tube should be placed to prevent vomiting and minimize the risk of aspiration. Intravenous fluids are required to prevent dehydration and to replete electrolyte losses (10% dextrose in 0.45% saline).

When the electrolyte pattern stabilizes, the infant should be taken to the operating room for the relief of obstruction. The atretic lesion is usually mucosal in nature. Excision of the prepyloric atretic web and pyloroplasty are an effective treatment, with a temporary Stamm gastrostomy usually performed as a complementary procedure.

Duodenal Obstruction

Congenital obstruction of the duodenum, whether complete (atresia) or incomplete (stenosis) represents a significant cause of neonatal alimentary tract obstruction. Duodenal atresia develops early in intrauterine life. A mucosal web is the most frequent type of atretic lesion noted. Eighty-five percent of duodenal atresias are located just distal to the ampulla of Vater, thus making bilious vomiting the presenting symptom in a majority of cases.

Polyhydramnios is observed in 33% to 50% of cases. Of these infants 40% are premature, and one third have Down's syndrome. Hyperbilirubinemia is also often observed. Between 50% and 75% of infants with duodenal obstruction have associated anomalies, including cardiac, genitourinary, musculoskeletal, and other gastrointestinal defects (i.e., esophageal atresia, imperforate anus). As a result, these infants are high-risk patients and should be managed in a sophisticated neonatal intensive care facility.

Plain x-ray film of the abdomen demonstrates the classic "double-bubble" sign of duodenal obstruction. There is no evidence of air in the gastrointestinal tract beyond the obstruction in atretic cases. An orogastric tube should be placed on drainage. Fluid and electrolyte disturbances may be seen as a result of losses related to bilious vomiting, and thus appropriate intravenous therapy is a prerequisite in the preparation of the infant for surgical therapy of the obstruction. This condition does not represent a true surgical emergency, and a period of time as long as 48 hours may be necessary to completely stabilize the infant. Emergent operation should be undertaken if there is any question of the duodenal obstruction being a result of malrotation and associated volvulus.

The surgical treatment of choice is a duodenoduodenostomy to bypass the obstruction. In instances of duodenal web, duodenotomy and excision of the web may be possible, but care must be taken to not injure the ampulla of Vater, which is frequently located immediately adjacent to the web. The greatly dilated duodenum proximal to the obstruction frequently results in delayed (7 to 10 days) anastomotic function. Tapering of the dilated antimesenteric border of the proximal duodenum has also been recommended.

Duodenal stenosis may be associated with annular pancreas, malrotation with Ladd's bands (incomplete rotation and fixation), an anterior (preduodenal) portal vein, or an intrinsic web with a small diaphragm. Plain x-ray film shows a "double-bubble" with a small amount of intestinal air distal to the duodenum. The preparation and treatment of infants with stenosis are similar to that outlined for infants with duodenal atresia.

Intestinal Atresia

Four types of small bowel atresia (exclusive of duodenal atresia) are recognized. Type I represents a mucosal web or diaphragm and is probably caused by epithelial plugging. In type II an atretic cord exists between two blind ends, and the mesentery is intact. In type IIIa there is complete separation of the blind ends by a U-shaped mesenteric gap. Type IIIb represents instances of atresia with an "apple peel" deformity in which the bowel distal to the atresia receives a retrograde blood supply from the ileocolic or right colic artery. Type IV represents cases of multiple atresias.

Type II, III, and IV atresias result from late intrauterine mesenteric vascular accidents. The possible causes of these episodes include instances of intrauterine emboli, volvulus, internal hernia, intussusception, or gastroschisis. Most cases of small bowel atresia are solitary; however, in 10% multiple atresias (type IV) are observed. Since 10% of atresias, especially ileal, occur in infants with cystic fibrosis, appropriate workup (sweat chloride determination) should be performed for each infant before discharge.

Infants with high jejunal atresia are usually products of polyhydramniotic pregnancy and initially have bilious vomiting. The plain abdominal x-ray film demonstrates several dilated loops of small bowel with no air distal to the atresia. Jaundice is a frequent finding in newborns with jejunal atresia.

The preoperative clinical management should include placement of an orogastric tube combined with rehydration and electrolyte stabilization with appropriate intravenous fluids. At laparotomy, bowel proximal to the atresia is greatly dilated and atonic with poor peristalsis. This dilated bowel is usually resected back to the ligament of Treitz, where an end-to-end anastomosis is performed. The disparity in size between the large proximal bowel and the smaller distal gut may be alleviated by an end (90-degree)–to–oblique (45-degree) approximation, generally using a single layer of nonabsorbable suture. When short bowel length is present, as is frequently the case in types IIIb and IV, the proximal dilated segment can be used rather than resected by a tapering jejunoplasty.[72] This is accomplished by an antimesenteric resection of the dilated gut for a length of 4 to 8 cm, which then allows an end-to-end anastomosis. When the diameter of the gut is reduced in this way, normal peristalsis is restored, and valuable gut length is maintained. A 7- to 10-day delay in the onset of anastomosis function is not unusual, and a gastrostomy provides excellent gastric drainage in these circumstances. Postoperative nutritional support is provided by intravenous solutions of amino acids, glucose, and lipids, occasionally administered through a central venous catheter if a prolonged period of parenteral nutrition is anticipated.

Infants with low small bowel obstruction initially have bilious vomiting and significant abdominal distention. Abdominal x-ray films demonstrate numerous loops of dilated bowel, usually associated with air-fluid levels. Since the infant colon does not show haustral markings on x-ray film, a barium enema can be performed in cases of low intestinal obstruction and should be the first enema the infant receives. The barium enema differentiates between small and large bowel distention, determines whether the colon is used or unused (microcolon) and therefore identifies the level of obstruction (small or large bowel), and evaluates the position of the cecum with regard to intestinal rotation and fixation (i.e., malrotation).

Occasionally, the abdominal x-ray film demonstrates calcification within the abdominal cavity. This signifies either the presence of meconium peritonitis from intrauterine bowel perforation or bowel wall necrosis resulting in "mummification." In either case, barium enema is as unnecessary as laparotomy is imperative.

Ileal Atresia

Infants with ileal atresia present with abdominal distention and bilious vomiting and may fail to pass meconium. Abdominal x-ray film shows multiple loops of distended small bowel with many air-fluid levels (with one loop larger than the others). The barium enema shows an unused microcolon, delineating the obstruction to the distal small bowel.

These cases are usually managed by resection of the proximal dilated segment with end-to-end anastomosis. Tapering ileoplasty may be used in cases with short gut to preserve bowel length. In the presence of peritonitis or in instances of questionable bowel viability, a temporary enterostomy may be required.

Meconium Ileus

Meconium ileus is a unique form of congenital intestinal obstruction that occurs in 10% to 15% of newborns with cystic fibrosis. A deficiency of pancreatic enzymes and an abnormality in the composition of meconium are factors responsible for the solid intraluminal concretions that produce an obturation form of obstruction in this disorder. A careful family history should be sought when this hereditary disease is suspected. The presence of low small bowel obstruction occurring in identical twins is almost always caused by meconium ileus. These infants present with abdominal distention and bilious vomiting and fail to pass meconium.

Certain x-ray film findings may help distinguish between ileal atresia and meconium ileus. In infants with meconium ileus, the x-ray film often demonstrates significant dilation of similar-sized loops with few, if any, air fluid levels. A ground glass appearance in the right lower quadrant (Neuhauser's sign) may be observed and represents viscid meconium mixed with air. The contrast enema shows an unused colon similar to ileal atresia, but reflux of contrast into the distal ileum may demonstrate the unusual obstructive concretions. Treatment of meconium ileus depends on whether it is uncomplicated (simple obstruction with concretions) or complicated by atresia, volvulus, meconium peritonitis, or giant cystic meconium peritonitis.

The initial treatment for uncomplicated meconium ileus is nonoperative, using hypertonic contrast enema (Hypaque or Gastrografin). These substances allow fluoroscopic visualization of the gut, whereas their hypertonic character draws fluid into the thick, meconium pellets from the bowel wall, resulting in relief of obstruction. This therapy may cause significant fluid shifts with intravascular depletion, reducing cardiac output by as much as 35%, thus making an intravenous line mandatory during the procedure. Careful attention to fluid balance, blood pressure, pulse rate, and urine output during the enema and for several hours afterward is essential. Occasionally, the enema must be repeated to relieve the obstruction.

Unsuccessful nonoperative attempts in uncomplicated instances of meconium ileus and all cases with complications require surgical intervention. Contemporary surgical management consists of intraoperative irrigation of the viscid meconium and obstructive pellets by means of an enterotomy. The bowel is irrigated with saline and dilute Hypaque or Gastrografin to lower the viscosity of the meconium and relieve the obstruction. This procedure obviates the need for resection and/or enterostomy in most cases, thus avoiding the risks of later enterostomy closure. For cases complicated by volvulus or gangrene, bowel resection with anastomosis or enterostomy may be required.

Careful family counseling and parental instruction regarding diet, enzyme replacement, and pulmonary toilet are important components of the overall care of these patients.

Colonic Obstruction

Causes of colonic obstruction in the newborn include meconium plug syndrome, aganglionic megacolon (Hirschsprung's disease), colon atresia, small left colon syndrome, and the various types of imperforate anus. The two most common causes, meconium plug and Hirschsprung's disease, are discussed.

Meconium plug syndrome was first described by Clatworthy in 1956.[73] Although a few cases may be associated with Hirschsprung's disease, the majority have no known cause. Meconium plug syndrome is not equivalent to meconium ileus and therefore has no relationship to cystic fibrosis. The infant initially has distention and fails to pass meconium. Plain x-ray films of the abdomen show numerous dilated loops of bowel with air-fluid levels. Contrast enema shows a small, unused left colon with a dilated transverse colon containing copious intraluminal meconium. The enema is both diagnostic and therapeutic, since the thick meconium can frequently be irrigated and expelled. Occasionally, a second enema is required to completely evacuate all the inspissated material, after which the infants usually have no further obstruction.

Hirschsprung's disease is an inherited disorder, occurring in 1 of 5000 births. It is characterized by an inability of the distal bowel and internal anal sphincter to relax, producing a state of tonic contraction. This manifests as a distal bowel obstruction in newborns, or a state of chronic constipation in older children.[74] Hirschsprung's disease is a neurogenic form of obstruction manifested by an absence of ganglion cells in the myenteric (Auerbach's) and submucosal (Meissner's) plexuses. Hypertrophic nerve fibers are frequently observed. This absence of parasympathetic innervation causes an uninhibited sympathetic tone in the gut musculature, resulting in failure of relaxation of the internal sphincter. The failure of internal sphincter relaxation with anal dilation is the basis for manometric diagnosis of this disorder. During embryologic development the neural crest cells begin to migrate into the gut at about the fifth week of gestation. This migration continues in a cranial-to-caudal direction until neuroblasts are present in the distal rectum in the twelfth week.[75] Maturation of the neuroblasts goes on throughout the remainder of gestation and into the early part of infancy. In approximately 75% to 80% of infants with Hirschsprung's disease, the migration is arrested in the sigmoid colon or rectum. In 5% the migration is stopped in the small bowel. The bowel wall distal to this site has a disordered arrangement of primarily parasympathetic axons, notable in that they stain easily for acetylcholinesterase.

Some evidence suggests that Hirschsprung's disease is related to genetic defects, both chromosomal abnormalities and point mutations. Associated congenital anomalies are frequent (up to 26%), with Down's syndrome being the most frequent at 14%. Siblings of affected females have a 360-fold increased risk compared to that of the general population, whereas those of affected males are 130 times higher (overall risk 4% to 19%).[76] There is also evidence that siblings of those infants with total colonic involvement are at even higher risk. Hirschsprung's disease has also been described as having a dominant pattern of inheritance in some families. The familial form has a gene that has been mapped to chromosome 10q11.2.[76] This locus has a tight association with the *RET* proto-oncogene locus, which has been previously associated with inherited cancer family syndrome and multiple endocrine neoplasia 2A.[77] The *RET* protein analysis shows heterozygosity at that locus in patients with Hirschsprung's disease. The protein is believed to be rendered nonfunctional, which may have some effect on the cadherin family of adhesion molecules. Abnormal cell adhesion could explain the failure of full migration of neural crest cells into the distal bowel, as well as the presence of its altered neurons.

Most patients with this disease become symptomatic shortly after birth, and 95% fail to pass meconium in the first 24 hours of life. Abdominal distention, bilious vomiting, and severe constipation are the signs that should lead one to suspect aganglionosis. Plain x-ray films may show many dilated loops of bowel, a large amount of stool above the level of aganglionosis, and air-fluid levels. Barium enema findings might look normal in the newborn, but a healthy infant expels the barium within 6 to 12 hours, whereas an infant with Hirschsprung's disease retains the contrast for over 24 hours. Older infants and children have a "transition zone" visible on contrast enema, with dilated bowel narrowing to a narrow spastic segment.

The aganglionosis always begins at the anorectal line and extends proximally to the sigmoid in 80% of cases. In 10% of patients the aganglionic segment extends to the splenic flexure, whereas in an additional 10% the entire colon and, in some cases, portions of ileum are involved. Total aganglionosis of the entire gastrointestinal tract has also been reported.

Rectal biopsy is the standard technique used to confirm the diagnosis of Hirschsprung's disease. Today, the suction rectal biopsy is used to obtain rectal mucosa and submucosa to evaluate for ganglion cells. The specimen is obtained at least 2 cm above the dentate line, since the normal anus is hypoganglionic up to approximately 15 mm above the dentate line. Andrassy et al.[78] demonstrated only one false-negative study in 444 patients evaluated for Hirschsprung's disease with suction rectal biopsy. Both an absence of ganglia and hypertrophied nerve fibers must be seen to make a definitive diagnosis of Hirschsprung's disease. The use of the acetylcholinesterase stain has improved the diagnostic accuracy of this technique by demonstrating an intense staining of hypertrophied nerve fibers throughout the lamina propria and the muscularis propria.[79,80]

Manometry typically demonstrates elevated resting anal canal pressure and a lack of the normal rectosphincteric reflex.[61,81,82] This reflex is characterized by relaxation of the anal canal produced by rectal distention. The rectosphincteric reflex can be measured in infants by the manometric technique of Tamate or Loening-Baucke. Its absence has been found to correlate strongly with Hirschsprung's disease. However, most pediatric surgical centers do not use anorectal manometry to aid in the initial diagnosis of Hirschsprung's disease.

Once the diagnosis is made, the therapy of choice is a colostomy or enterostomy at the lowest point of normal ganglion cell distribution, as judged by frozen section control. When the infant reaches 1 year of age, a definitive pull-through procedure of the classic Swenson, Duhamel (retrorectal), or Soave (endorectal) type is undertaken, depending on which method is best used by the surgeon involved. Long-term results are excellent with the use of any one of these techniques. Each technique gives similar functional results in terms of continence and rate of complications. The straight endorectal pull-through is performed by dissecting the mucosa and submucosa from the aganglionic rectal muscular cuff, pulling the ganglionic bowel down to the anus, performing the anastomosis approximately 1 cm above the anal verge.[83-85] The Duhamel procedure is a retrorectal dissection with anastomosis of the ganglionated bowel to the distal aganglionic rectal pouch using a side-to-side stapled anastomosis, which is performed transanally.[86] The Swenson procedure is an ultra low anterior/coloanal anastomosis.[87] The laparoscopic procedure allows mobilization and biopsy via the laparoscope, and the anastomosis is then performed after resecting the bowel via the perineum/anus.[88,89]

Hirschsprung's enterocolitis (HEC) is a frequent and dangerous complication in patients with Hirschsprung's disease. It can occur at any point in the disease from birth to after the pull-through procedure. The incidence ranges from 20% to 58%. The mortality of HEC is from 6% to 30%, and it is the most common cause of death from Hirschsprung's disease.[90] The pathogenesis of HEC is poorly understood, but a variety of causes have been suggested, including mechanical dilation and fecal stasis, alteration of mucin, increased prostaglandin E_1 activity, *Clostridium difficile* infection, and rotavirus infection.[91,92,93] The treatment of HEC is aggressive rectal washouts, intravenous antibiotics, and oral metronidazole.

Total colonic Hirschsprung's disease is a particularly devastating form of the disease where all the colon and some length of the gastrointestinal tract proximal to it lack enteric ganglia. This entity is managed with resection of the diseased bowel and an ileoanal pull-through.[94] Older series report a higher mortality in children with this form of Hirschsprung's disease, but a recent series of 20 patients did not.[95] This was attributed to earlier diagnosis with improved perioperative care. However, the morbidity in their group remained higher than typical patients with distal colon abnormalities. This was primarily due to excessive fluid loss, wound infections, stoma complications, and HEC. There was also a higher requirement for postoperative anal dilations and rectal irrigation. Diarrhea was a major problem occurring before the pull-through procedure. The authors felt the problem was prevented by performing a modified Kimura procedure. This involved placing a right colonic patch onto the distal small bowel while creating the initial ostomy. HEC has also been a major complicating factor in these children both before and after pull-through. It has an incidence of 25% in this group compared to 14% in patients with standard Hirschsprung's disease. Total intestinal aganglionosis is an extremely rare condition and was previously thought to be fatal. Recent experience using an extended myectomy/myotomy technique has allowed some short-term survivors.[96] Visceral transplantation has been performed on a limited basis as well.

A subset of patients with Hirschsprung's disease with a short segment disease has been described, but its very existence is controversial. The abnormality of innervation extends only a short distance above the dentate line. The significance of this group is that the functional pathology resides primarily in the anal canal, which might require a different therapeutic approach. These patients are usually diagnosed at a later age because the main symptom is mild-to-severe constipation. This allows the use of diagnostic modalities not readily employed in the newborn group. In these patients and in those with constipation after a pull-through procedure, anal manometry may be useful as part of the assessment.

Several groups have recommended anorectal myectomy as the initial treatment of choice in these patients or as a salvage operation after failed pull-through procedures.[97] As described by Lynn and van Heerden,[98] this operation involves removing a thin strip of the internal sphincter muscle in the posterior midline proximally, starting 1 cm above the dentate line. The strip is dissected as far proximally as allowed by the exposure, usually 3 to 15 cm. An approach is either made through a transanal incision as described by Lynn and van Heerden,[98] or a posterior sagittal incision as described by DeVries and Pena.[99] Lynn and van Heerden[98] treated 37 patients this way; in 28 it was the definitive procedure. Four required a salvage pull-through procedure, and in four myectomy was employed as a salvage operation after pull-through. Of the 28 definitive patients, 20 had "excellent" results, 6 were "improved," and 2 were "unchanged." Anal manometry has the added benefit of allowing intraoperative or postoperative assessment of rectoanal function.

SUMMARY

The pediatric patient, especially in the first month of life, presents unique challenges in management for the surgeon should an operation become necessary. These challenges relate to the dynamic adjustment to extrauterine life with which the newborn infant must cope, the energy and nutritional demands invoked by this period of rapid growth, the relative immaturity of the infant's organ systems, the rapid metabolic and physiologic changes that are occurring during this time, and the infant's small physical size. Coupled with these features is the inability of these young patients, and frequently their parents, to provide an adequate history of complaints or symptoms, making diagnosis of disease often tedious and demanding and allowing little room for error in management. Notwithstanding these potential difficulties in defining the cause of a given patient's problem, the most common signs and symptoms encountered in this age group include respiratory distress, vomiting, failure to pass meconium, diarrhea, abdominal distention, sepsis, and abdominal wall defects. A number of well-defined clinical abnormalities are generally responsible for these findings and include such disorders as omphalocele, gastroschisis, hypertrophic pyloric stenosis, NEC, various forms of esophageal atresia, CDH, intestinal obstruction secondary to atresia, malrotation or meconium ileus, and Hirschsprung's disease. An understanding of the physiologic derangements coincident with each of these disease processes and their accompanying clinical presentations ensures early diagnosis and expeditious treatment. These considerations coupled with a knowledge of the fluid dynamics and respiratory physiology unique to this age group guarantee the optimum in clinical care and the minimum in morbidity and mortality.

REFERENCES

1. Aperia A, et al. Postnatal control of water and electrolyte homeostasis in pre-term and full-term infants. Acta Paediatr Scand 305:61, 1983.
2. Oh W. Renal function and fluid therapy on high risk infants. Biol Neonate 53:230, 1988.
3. Taylor AF, et al. Hormonal response of premature primate to operative stress. J Pediatr Surg 28:844, 1993.
4. Anand KJS, et al. Can the human neonate mount an endocrine and metabolic response to surgery? J Pediatr Surg 20:41, 1985.
5. Anand KJS, et al. Studies on the hormonal regulation of fuel metabolism in the human newborn infant undergoing anesthesia and surgery. Horm Res 22:105, 1985.
6. Tsang TM, Tam PK. Cytokine response of neonates to surgery. J Pediatr Surg 29:501, 1994.
7. Letton RW, et al. Early postoperative alterations in infant energy use increase the risk of overfeeding. J Pediatr Surg 30:988, 1995.
8. Alexander JW. Specific nutrients and the immune response. Nutrition 11:229, 1995.
9. Hildreth MA, et al. Caloric requirements of patients with burns under one year of age. J Burn Care Rehabil 14:108, 1993.
10. Christensen RD, Hall HR, Rothstein G. Granulocyte stem cell proliferation in experimental GBS sepsis. Pediatrics 17:278, 1983.
11. Berger M. Complement deficiency and neutrophil dysfunction as risk factors for bacterial infection in newborns and the role of granulocyte therapy. Res Infect Dis 12:S401, 1990.
12. Erdman SH, et al. The supply and release of storage neutrophils: A developmental study. Biol Neonate 41:132, 1982.
13. Miller ME. Chemotactic functions in the human neonate: Human cellular function. Pediatr Res 5:487, 1971.
14. Roth P, Polen RA. Adherence of human newborn infants monocytes to matrix bound fibronectin. J Pediatr 121:285, 1992.
15. Bruce MC, et al. Impaired surface membrane expression of C_3SR but not C_3b receptors on neonatal neutrophils. Pediatr Res 21:306, 1987.
16. Krause PJ, Maderaz EG, Scroggs M. Abnormalities of neutrophil adherence in newborns. Pediatrics 69:184, 1982.
17. Klein RB, et al. Decreased mononuclear and polymorphonuclear chemotaxis in human newborns, infants and young children. Pediatrics 60:467, 1977.
18. Madden NP, et al. Surgery, sepsis and nonspecific immune function in neonates. J Pediatr Surg 24:562, 1989.
19. Cates KL, Rowe JC, Ballow M. The premature infant as a compromised host. Curr Probl Pediatr 13:1, 1983.
20. Duhamel B. Embryology of exomphalos and allied malformations. Arch Dis Child 38:138, 1963.
21. Tibboel D, et al. The development of the characteristic anomalies found in gastroschisis—Experimental and clinical data. Kinderchir 40:355, 1985.
22. Grosfeld JL, Weber TR. Congenital abdominal wall defects: Gastroschisis and omphalocele. Curr Probl Surg 19:158, 1982.
23. Fonkalsrud EW, et al. Selective management of gastroschisis according to the degree of visceroabdominal disproportion. Ann Surg 218:742, 1993.
24. Schuster SR. Omphalocele and gastroschisis. In Welch K, ed. Pediatric Surgery. Chicago: Year Book Medical Publishers, 1986, p 740.
25. Coran AG, Drongowski RA. Body fluid compartment changes following neonatal surgery. J Pediatr Surg 24:829, 1989.

26. O'Neill JA, Grosfeld JL. Intestinal malfunction after antenatal exposure of viscera. Am J Surg 127:129, 1974.
27. Tunnell WP, et al. Abdominal wall defects in infants: Survival and implications for adult life. Ann Surg 221:525, 1995.
28. Milla PJ. Gastric-outlet obstruction in children. N Engl J Med 327:558, 1992.
29. Vanderwinden J, et al. Nitric oxide synthase activity in infantile hypertrophic pyloric stenosis. N Engl J Med 327:511, 1992.
30. Michel T. Nitric oxide synthesis in infantile hypertrophic pyloric stenosis. N Engl J Med 327:1690, 1992.
31. Kobayashi H, O'Briain DS, Puri P. Immunochemical characterization of neural cell adhesion molecule (NCAM), nitric oxide synthase and neurofilament protein expression in pyloric muscle of patients with pyloric stenosis. J Pediatr Gastroenterol Nutr 20:319, 1995.
32. Okazaki T, et al. Abnormal distribution of nerve terminals in infantile hypertrophic pyloric stenosis. J Pediatr Surg 29:655, 1994.
33. Hernanz-Schulman M, et al. Hypertrophic pyloric stenosis in the infant without a palpable olive: Accuracy of the sonographic diagnosis. Radiology 193:771, 1994.
34. Davies RP, et al. Sonographic diagnosis of infantile hypertrophic pyloric stenosis. J Ultrasound Med 11:603, 1992.
35. Shanbhogue LKR, et al. Serum electrolytes and capillary blood gases in the management to hypertrophic pyloric stenosis. Br J Surg 79:251, 1992.
36. Najmaldin A, Tan HL. Early experience with laparoscopic pyloromyotomy for infantile hypertrophic pyloric stenosis. J Pediatr Surg 30:37, 1995.
37. Georgeson KE, et al. An analysis of feeding regimes after pyloromyotomy for hypertrophic stenosis. J Pediatr Surg 28:1478, 1993.
38. Cheromcha DP, Hyman PE. Neonatal necrotizing enterocolitis: Inflammatory bowel disease of the newborn. Dig Dis Sci 33:78S, 1988.
39. Friedman WF, Fitzpatrick KM. Effects of prostaglandins, thromboxanes, and inhibitors of their synthesis on renal and gastrointestinal function in the newborn period. Semin Perinatol 4:143, 1980.
40. Furukawa M, Lee EL, Johnston JM. Platelet-activating factor–induced ischemic bowel necrosis: The effect of platelet-activating factor acetylhydrolase. Pediatr Res 34:237, 1993.
41. LeBlanc MH, Edwards JD. Acute polycythemia increases the disappearance rate of clottable fibrinogen in the newborn dog. Pediatr Res 20:151, 1986.
42. Kosloske AM, Musemeche CA. Necrotizing enterocolitis of the neonate. Clin Perinatol 16:97, 1989.
43. Van Camp JM, et al. Colonization of intestinal bacteria in the normal neonate: Comparison between mouth and rectal swabs and small and large bowel specimens. J Pediatr Surg 29:1348, 1994.
44. Landsberg L, Young JB. Fasting, feeding and regulation of the sympathetic nervous system. N Engl J Med 198:1295, 1978.
45. Nagaraj HS, et al. Gastrointestinal perforation following indomethacin therapy in very low birth weight infants. J Pediatr Surg 16:1003, 1981.
46. Dalsing M, et al. The relationship of aminophylline and caffeine in the treatment of neonatal apnea and necrotizing enterocolitis (NEC). Surg Forum 23:202, 1982.
47. Cohen M, et al. A new look at the neonatal bowel: Contrast studies with metrizamide (Amipaque). J Pediatr Surg 12:149, 1977.
48. Kosloske AM, Lilly JR. Paracentesis and lavage for diagnosis of intestinal gangrene in neonatal necrotizing enterocolitis. J Pediatr Surg 13:315, 1973.
49. Horwitz JR, et al. Complications after surgical intervention for necrotizing enterocolitis: A multicenter review. J Pediatr Surg 30:994, 1995.
50. Karamanoukian HL, et al. Inhaled NO in congenital hypoplasia of the lung due to diaphragmatic hernia or oligohydramnios. Pediatrics 94:715, 1994.
51. Weber TR, Smith E, Grosfeld JL. Surgical experience in infants with the VATER association. J Pediatr Surg 15:849, 1980.
52. Cikrit D, et al. Necrotizing enterocolitis. Factors affecting mortality in 101 surgical cases. Surgery 96:648, 1984.
53. Wilcox DT, et al. Nitrofen induced diaphragmatic hernias in rats: An animal model. J Pediatr Surg 28:757, 1993.
54. Wilcox DT, et al. Pathophysiology of congenital diaphragmatic hernia. V. Effect of exogenous surfactant therapy on gas exchange and lung mechanics in the lamb congenital diaphragmatic hernia model. J Pediatr 124:289, 1994.
55. Lotze A, et al. Surfactant therapy for infants with congenital diaphragmatic hernia on ECMO: Evidence of persistent surfactant deficiency. J Pediatr Surg 29:407, 1994.
56. Schwerts SM, Vermillion RP, Hirschl RB. Evaluation of left-ventricular mass in children with left-sided congenital diaphragmatic hernia. J Pediatr 125:447, 1988.
57. Fauza DO, Wilson JM. Congenital diaphragmatic hernia and associated anomalies: Their incidence, identification and impact on prognosis. J Pediatr Surg 29:1113, 1994.
58. Wung JT, et al. Congenital diaphragmatic hernia: Survival treated with very delayed surgery, spontaneous respiration and no chest tube. J Pediatr Surg 30:406, 1995.
59. Charlton AJ, Bruce J, Davenport M. Timing of surgery in congenital diaphragmatic hernia. Anaesthesia 46:820, 1991.
60. Haugen SE, et al. Congenital diaphragmatic hernia: Determinants of the optimal time for operation by echocardiographic monitoring of the pulmonary artery pressure. J Pediatr Surg 26:560, 1991.
61. Challa VR, et al. Histologic diagnosis of Hirschsprung's disease. The value of concurrent hematoxylin and eosin and cholinesterase staining of rectal biopsies. Am J Clin Pathol 88:324, 1987.
62. Harrison MR, et al. Correction of congenital diaphragmatic hernia in utero. VI. Hard earned lessons. J Pediatr Surg 28:1411, 1993.
63. Sakai H, et al. Effect of surgical repair on respiratory mechanics in congenital diaphragmatic hernia. J Pediatr 111:432, 1987.
64. Langer JC, et al. Timing of surgery for congenital diaphragmatic hernia: Is emergency operation necessary? J Pediatr Surg 23:731, 1988.
65. Nio M, et al. A prospective randomized trial of delayed versus immediate repair of congenital diaphragmatic hernia. J Pediatr Surg 29:618, 1994.
66. Reickert CA, et al. The effect of delayed repair of congenital diaphragmatic hernia on survival. Surgery 120:766, 1996.
67. Lally KP, et al. Congenital diaphragmatic hernia stabilize and repair on ECMO. Ann Surg 216:569, 1990.
68. Lally KP, Breaux CW Jr. A second course of extracorporeal membrane oxygenation in the neonate: Is there a benefit? Surgery 117:175, 1995.
69. DiFiore JW, et al. Experimental fetal tracheal ligation reverses the structural and physiological effects of pulmonary hypoplasia in congenital diaphragmatic hernia. J Pediatr Surg 29:248, 1994.
70. Hedrick MH, et al. Plug the lung until it grows: A new method to treat congenital diaphragmatic hernia in utero. J Pediatr Surg 29:612, 1994.
71. Pranikoff T, Gauger PG, Hirschl RB. Partial liquid ventilation in newborn patients with congenital diaphragmatic hernia. J Pediatr Surg 31:613, 1996.
72. Weber TR, Vane DW, Grosfeld JL. Experience with tapering enteroplasty in infants with bowel atresia and short gut. Arch Surg 117:684, 1982.
73. Clatworthy HW, Howard WHR, Lloyd J. The meconium plug syndrome. Surgery 39:131, 1956.
74. Hirschsprung H. Stuhltragheit neugeborner in folge von dilatation and hypertrophie des colons. Jaharb Kinderch 27:1, 1887.
75. Romanska HM, et al. Increased expression of muscular neural cell adhesion molecule in congenital aganglionosis. Gastroenterology 105:1104, 1993.
76. Edery P, et al. Mutations of the *RET* proto-oncongene in Hirschprung's disease. Nature 367:378, 1994.

77. Borst MJ, et al. Mutational analysis of multiple endocrine neoplasia type 2A associated with Hirschsprung's disease. Surgery 117:386, 1995.
78. Andrassy RH, Isaacs H, Weitzman JJ. Rectal suction biopsy for the diagnosis of Hirschsprung's disease. Ann Surg 193:419, 1981.
79. Athow AC, Filipe MI, Drake DP. Problems and advantages of acetylcholinesterase histochemistry of rectal suction biopsies in the diagnosis of Hirschsprung's disease. J Pediatr Surg 25:520, 1990.
80. Lake BD, Malone MT, Risdon RA. The use of acetylcholinesterase (AChE) in the diagnosis of Hirschsprung's disease and intestinal neuronal dysplasia. Pediatr Pathol 9:351, 1989.
81. Rescorla FJ, et al. Hirschsprung's disease: Evaluation of mortality and long-term function in 260 cases. Arch Surg 127:934, 1992.
82. Tamate S, et al. Manometric diagnosis of Hirschsprung's disease in the neonatal period. J Pediatr Surg 19:285, 1984.
83. Boley S. An endorectal pull-through operation with primary anastomosis for Hirschsprung's disease. Surg Gynecol Obstet 127:353, 1968.
84. Cilley RE, et al. Definitive treatment of Hirschsprung's disease in the newborn with a one-stage procedure. Surgery 115:551, 1994.
85. Coran AG, Weintraub WH. Modification of the endorectal procedure for Hirschsprung's disease. Surg Gynecol Obstet 143:277, 1976.
86. Vane D, Grosfeld J. Hirschsprung's disease, experience with the Duhamel operation in 195 cases. Pediatr Surg Intern 1:95, 1986.
87. Swenson O, Bill AH. Resection of rectum and rectosigmoid with preservation of the sphincter for benign spastic lesions producing megacolon. Surgery 24:212, 1948.
88. Curran TJ, Raffensperger JG. The feasibility of laparoscopic Swenson pull-through. J Pediatr Surg 29:1273, 1994.
89. Smith BM, Steiner RB, Lobe TE. Laparoscopic Duhamel pullthrough procedure for Hirschsprung's disease in childhood. J Laparoendosc Surg 4:273, 1994.
90. Bill JAH, Chapman ND. The enterocolitis of Hirschsprung's disease: Its natural history and treatment. Am J Surg 103:70, 1962.
91. Elhalaby EA, et al. Enterocolitis associated with Hirschsprung's disease: A clinical-radiological characterization based on 168 patients. J Pediatr Surg 30:76, 1995.
92. Elhalaby EA, et al. Enterocolitis associated with Hirschsprung's disease: A clinical histopathological correlative study. J Pediatr Surg 30:1023, 1995.
93. Imamura A, et al. Mucosal immune defense mechanisms in enterocolitis complicating Hirschsprung's disease. Gut 33:801, 1992.
94. Coran AG, et al. The surgical management of total colonic aganglionosis. J Pediatr Surg 4:531, 1969.
95. Levy M, Reynolds M. Morbidity associated with total colonic Hirschsprung's disease. J Pediatr Surg 27:364, 1992.
96. Zeigler MM, Ross A, Bishop HC. Total intestinal aganglionosis: A new technique for prolonged survival. J Pediatr Surg 22:82, 1987.
97. Banani SA, Forootan H. Role of anorectal myectomy after failed endorectal pull-through in Hirschsprung's disease. J Pediatr Surg 29:1307, 1994.
98. Lynn HB, van Heerden JA. Rectal myectomy in Hirschsprung's disease. Arch Surg 110:991, 1975.
99. DeVries P, Pena A. Posterior sagittal anorectoplasty. J Pediatr Surg 17:638, 1982.

67

Physiologic Considerations in the Elderly Surgical Patient

Ronnie Ann Rosenthal and Dana K. Andersen

Physicians and surgeons have long understood that the physiologic and pathologic processes characteristic of the neonatal period are considerably different from those of the mature adult. The same is true of physiologic and pathologic characteristics at the other extreme of life. Although internists have recognized the need to provide special "geriatric" care for more than two decades, the adjustment of surgical practice to meet the specific needs of the elderly has only recently begun in a programmatic way. The "graying" of the American population has created the need to provide surgical care to an ever-increasing number of older patients, and the technologic explosion has provided the means to do so safely.

In the next 50 years the portion of the population older than age 65 is expected to grow from the present 12.5% to 20%, or to nearly 80 million people. Persons older than age 85 comprise the most rapidly growing segment of this population. Their number is expected to increase *sixfold* to 18 million by 2050[1] (Fig. 67-1.) As the number of elderly persons continues to grow, so does the average life expectancy at all ages. At present, a 65-year-old man can expect to live an additional 16 years and a 65-year-old woman, nearly 20 years. By 2050 these numbers are expected to increase to 20.8 and 24 years, respectively. Additional life expectancy data are shown in[1,2] Table 67-1.

The rise in the number of surgical procedures performed on older patients is, in part, a reflection of this aging of the population. In 1980, 19% of patients undergoing operations in nonfederally funded, short-stay hospitals were older than age 65. By 1993 this portion had jumped to 31%.[3] In federally funded hospitals this proportion is even higher. In 1993 on the General Surgical Service at the Veterans Affairs Medical Center in West Haven Connecticut, 83% of patients having major abdominal operations were older than age 60 and 53% were older than age 70.

This increase is not, however, only a reflection of the increased number of older people but also of the growing awareness that older patients can truly benefit from such surgical intervention. Although age was previously a contraindication to operations such as pancreaticoduodenectomy, major hepatic resection, major cardiac revascularization, and transplantation, these and other major procedures are now performed routinely on older patients with results that are comparable to those in younger patients.

The indication for surgical treatment in the elderly therefore is increasingly determined by the need to provide maximal disease management rather than desire to avoid surgical risk. It is important, however, to remember that the elderly surgical patient is frequently not physiologically equivalent to the younger patient and that comorbid illnesses can impact enormously on surgical outcome. Understanding the physiologic and pathologic differences and adjusting care accordingly are essential for successful management.

PHYSIOLOGY AND PATHOLOGY OF AGING

The processes of maturation, aging, and senescence describe the life cycle of most living organisms, including humans. *Aging* and *senescence* are commonly used interchangeably to refer to the myriad molecular and cellular events that eventually lead to the demise of the organism. These terms are not necessarily synonymous, although in clinical medicine the aging process is believed to incorporate predetermined or programmed cellular events that inevitably contribute to a limitation of longevity. The development of some diseases in the elderly patient may be directly linked to cellular events related to senescence, whereas the clinical presentation of others may be altered by aging-related changes in the physiologic milieu. Cristafalo et al.[4] have identified five attributes that characterize the human aging process:

- Increase in mortality with increasing age (after maturation)
- Change in the biochemical composition of the body
- Decline in physiologic function

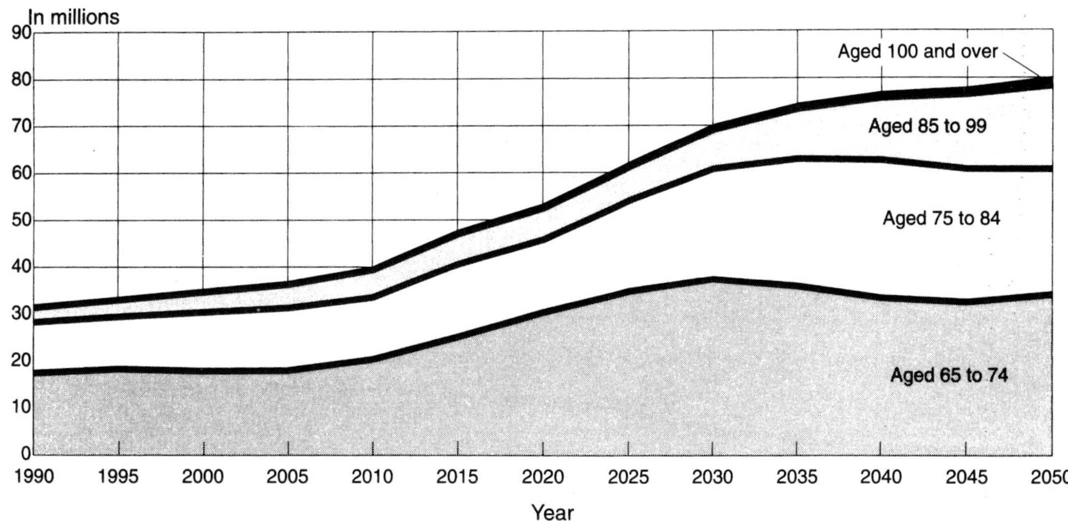

Fig. 67-1. Projected population growth by age group in the United States. (From Day JC. Population projections of the United States by age, sex, race and Hispanic origin: 1993-2050. Current Population Reports. U.S. Department of Commerce Bureau of the Census. Population Report P25-1104. Reprinted with permission.)

Table 67-1. Life Expectancy by Age (in Years)

	At Birth		Age 65		Age 75		Age 85	
	Male	Female	Male	Female	Male	Female	Male	Female
1986	71.3	78.3	14.7	18.6	9.1	11.7	5.2	6.4
1996	72.9	79.8	16	19.7	—	—	—	—
2050	79.7	85.6	20.8	24	—	—	—	—

- Decreased ability to adapt to the environment
- Increased susceptibility to disease

Although the elucidation of molecular and cellular events is necessary for a complete understanding of the process of aging and senescence, an awareness of the clinical manifestations of the characteristics just listed is essential for the provision of appropriate care to the elderly patient.

Increased Mortality With Age

The risk of death increases exponentially with increasing age, as described initially in 1825 by Gompertz.[5] The relationship between age and survival is frequently shown as a Gompertzian function. Figure 67-2 shows the average or median survival of a population (that age at which 50% of the population is alive) and the maximal life span potential (MLSP). Although the median survival of humans has more than doubled since the time of Hippocrates, the MLSP has remained essentially constant at 100 to 115 years. The dramatic shift in median survival has been attributed to an elimination of the causes of early mortality and an improvement in sanitation and nutrition. Although these changes have paralleled the expansion of medical knowledge, no modern medical breakthrough has impacted greatly on median survival or altered MLSP. Some analyses suggest that even if atherosclerosis and cancer were eliminated, the median survival of man would increase by only 10 years, and the MLSP would remain unchanged.[6]

These observations suggest that survival in all species may be limited in a predetermined way, and experimental observations support this concept (Fig. 67-3). Human fibroblasts maintained in culture undergo a predictable number of proliferative cycles, or doublings, before dying. This number is many times greater than the number of doublings for mouse fibroblasts maintained in identical culture.[7] Programmed cell death, or apoptosis, may not be inescapable, however. A variety of experimental interventions have been shown to delay or prevent this process.[8,9] With the advent of methods to identify molecular initiators and suppressors of apoptosis, considerable efforts are underway to clarify the regulatory factors that control cell life span.

In intact animals the only intervention that consistently increases median survival and MLSP is caloric restriction.[10] Rats fed a diet containing only 60% of the calories consumed by ad libitum fed littermates had a 50% higher me-

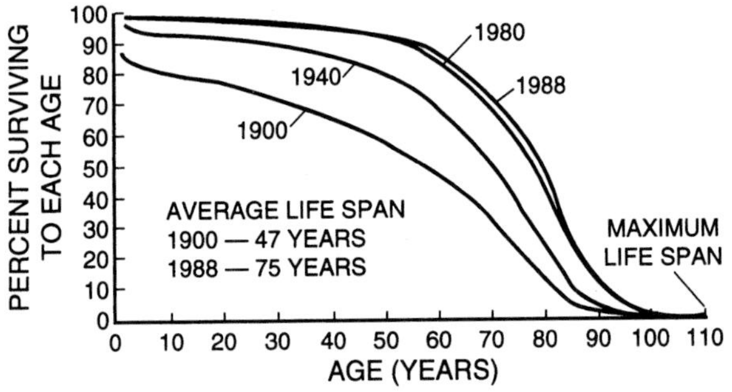

Fig. 67-2. Life expectancy in the United States, 1900 to 1988. (From Thompson JC. Seed corn. Impact of managed care on medical education and research. Ann Surg 223:453,1996. Reprinted with permission.)

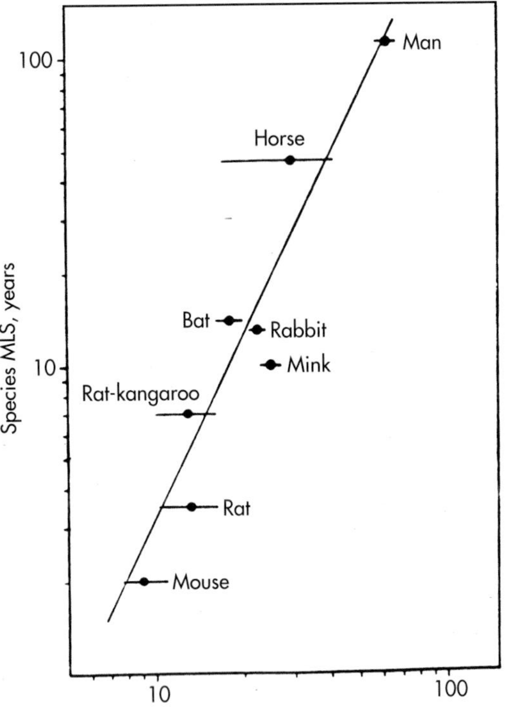

Fig. 67-3. Correlation between population doubling capacity (PDL) and maximal life span (MLS) potential. Fibroblasts from longer-lived species undergo more cell divisions before senescence than cells derived from shorter-lived species. (From Rhome D. Evidence for a relationship between longevity of mammalian species and life span of normal fibroblasts in vitro and erythrocytes in vivo. Proc Natl Acad Sci U S A 78:5009, 1981. Reprinted with permission.)

dian survival and MLSP than the animals receiving the full caloric load (Fig. 67-4). It remains to be determined if specific nutrients are responsible for these effects or if critical cellular events are altered by dietary restriction. This observation nonetheless raises hope that relatively simple interventions can delay human mortality.

Whether or not human life span potential is actually increasing, the elderly now represent the fastest growing segment of our population. The number of persons reaching their one hundredth birthday has increased so greatly that their names can no longer be read on the morning television programs. The number reaching their one hundred and tenth birthday, however, is still quite small.

Changes in Body Composition

Aging is associated with specific biochemical, anatomic, and functional changes in virtually all body tissues and organs (Table 67-2). Age-related effects have been documented at the chromosomal level, at the protein-processing level, and at the catabolism level. Age-related changes in the transcriptional rate of certain genes may be due to the accumulation of mutational effects over time[11] and may be involved in the age-related incidence of some neoplastic and degenerative diseases.[12] A related theory suggests that it is an impaired capacity to repair mutational changes in nucleic acid that represents the underlying defect of aging.[13,14] Changes in molecular structure may be expressed in a tissue-specific manner, however, and organ systems must be evaluated individually to assess how age-related changes in composition are manifested in any single patient.

Compositional changes contribute to changes in organ function, such as the deposition of lipofuscin or "age pigment" in Purkinje cells, which results in conduction disturbances and altered cardiac contractility.[15] Increased cross-linking of matrix molecules such as collagen[16] or the accumulation of increased amounts of protein from impaired protein catabolism[17] can also alter the function of specific organs. An explanation for the increased occurrence of cross-linking of nucleic and matrix molecules is the age-related increase in oxidative damage to proteins from excess free radical formation.[18] Impaired metabolism of reactive oxygen species may cause extensive damage to proteins, which in turn provides a favorable site for glucose moieties to bind to amino acids. This glycation reaction may promote the cross-linking of proteins such as osteocalcin and the lens protein crystalin, which may result in altered bone density or cataract formation.[4]

Alterations in musculoskeletal tissues account for the physiognomic changes associated with aging, including shortened stature, impaired ambulation, and decreased chest wall excursion (Fig. 67-5). These changes impact greatly on the postoperative recovery of elderly patients by increasing susceptibility to complications such as atelectasis, pneumonia, and pulmonary embolism. Because tissue composition is not uniformly affected in all elderly patients, however, it is inappropriate to institute compensatory measures, such as prolonged endotracheal intubation, based only on older age.

Nutritional effects account for some of the most important changes in body composition in the elderly.[19] A significant prevalence of undernutrition has been docu-

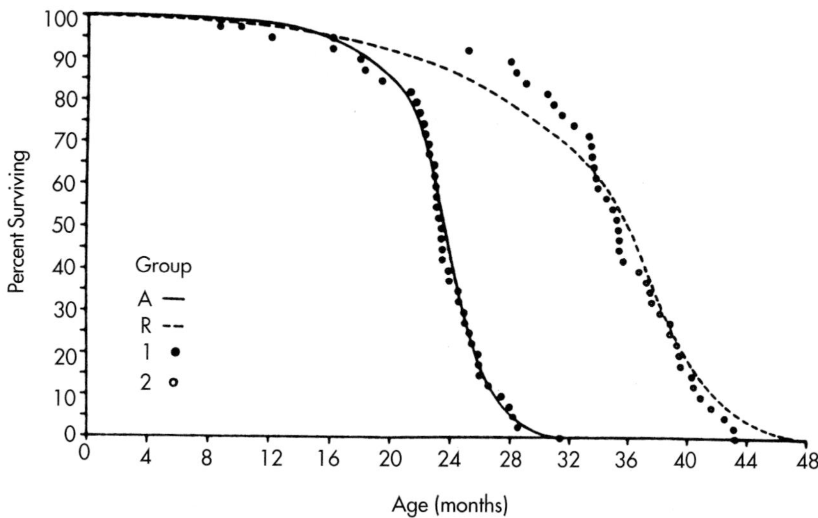

Fig. 67-4. Survival curve for ad libitum fed *(solid circles)* and calorically restricted *(open circles)* rats. Restriction of calories to 60% of ad libitum fed levels results in a dramatic increase in life span and maximal life span potential. (From Yu BP, Massaro EJ, McMahon CA. Nutritional influences in aging Fischer 344 rats. I. Physical, metabolic and longevity characteristics. J Gerontol 40:664, 1985. Copyright © The Gerontological Society of America.)

Table 67-2. Effects of Aging on Body Composition and Major Organ Systems

Organ System	Anatomic Changes	Functional Changes
Body composition	Increased lipid fraction Loss of skeletal mass	Increased half-life for lipid-soluble drugs Decreased oxygen consumption, heat production, and cardiac output
Nervous system	Attrition of neurons	Deafferentation, neurogenic atrophy, and decreased anesthetic requirement
	Decreased neurotransmitter activity	Impaired autonomic homeostasis
Cardiovascular system	Decreased arterial elasticity Ventricular hypertrophy Reduced adrenergic responsiveness	Increased impedance to ejection, widened pulse pressure Decreased maximal cardiac output
Pulmonary system	Loss of lung elastin Increased thoracic stiffness Reduced alveolar surface area	Increased residual volume Loss of vital capacity Impaired efficiency of gas exchange Increased work of breathing
Renal system	Reduced vascularity Tissue atrophy	Decreased plasma flow, glomerular filtration rate, drug clearance, and ability to handle salt and water loads
Hepatic system	Reduced tissue mass	Reduced hepatic blood flow and drug clearance

From Muravchick S. Anesthesia for the elderly. In Miller RD, ed. Anesthesia, 3rd ed. New York: Churchill Livingstone, 1990. Reprinted with permission.

mented in noninstitutionalized, free-living elderly, and reduced protein intake is common even among affluent older persons.[19,20] These dietary changes are multifactorial (see box on p. 1366) but are thought to contribute to the significant loss of lean body mass (muscle) in elderly subjects. This loss translates into reduced strength and mobility and a decline in creatinine excretion. The shift from lean body mass to increased adipose tissue may also be mediated in part through an age-related decline in pituitary growth hormone (GH) activity.[21]

Within the aging muscle the synthesis of contractile proteins declines as does the number of actual muscle fibers. Declining metabolic activity of the muscles combined with alterations in the neuromuscular junctions results in less efficient muscular activity and easy fatigability.[22]

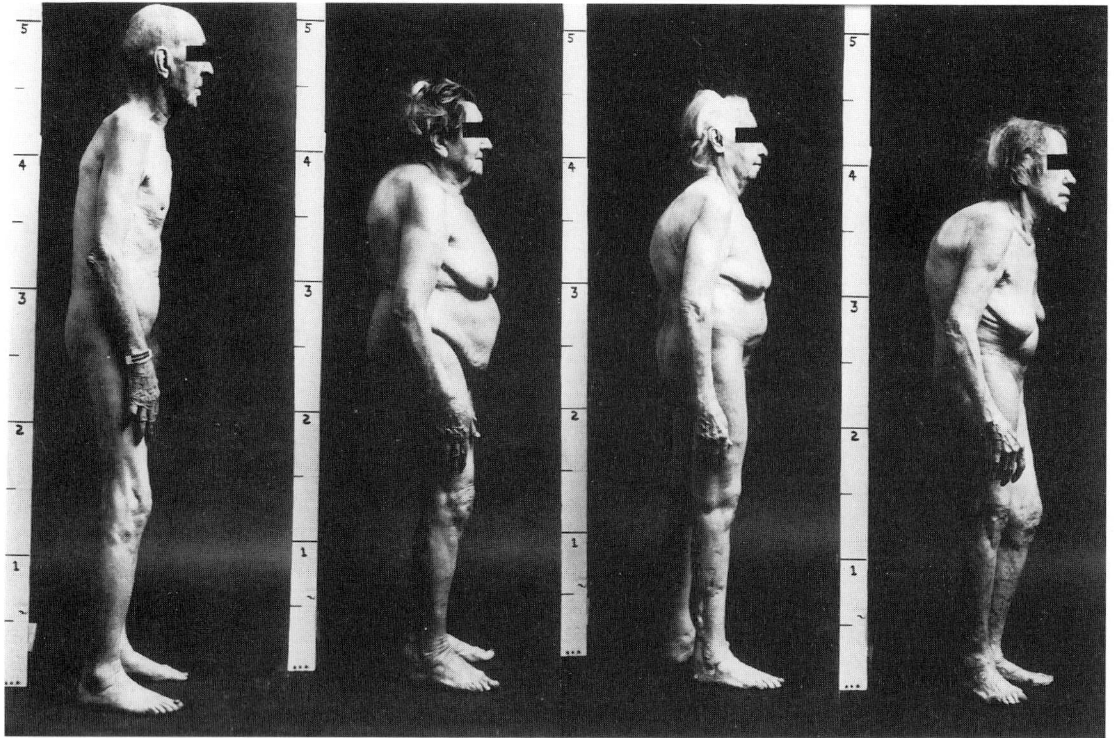

Fig. 67-5. Four randomly selected patients from the ambulatory section of a nursing home, illustrating short stature, osteoporotic kyphosis, and relatively long extremities. Ages from left to right 82, 78, 79, 94 years. (From Rossman I. Anatomy of aging. In Rossman I, ed. Clinical Geriatrics, 2nd ed. Philadelphia: JB Lippincott, 1979. Reprinted with permission. Photograph by DeWayne Dalrymple.)

FINDINGS IN THE MEDICAL HISTORY SUGGESTING INCREASED RISK FOR NUTRIENT DEFICIENCY

Recent weight loss
Restricted dietary intake (limited variety, food avoidances)
Psychosocial situation (depression, cognitive impairment, isolation, economic difficulties)
Problems with eating, chewing, swallowing
Previous surgery
Increased losses resulting from gastrointestinal disorders such as malabsorption and diarrhea
Systemic disease interfering with appetite or eating (chronic lung, liver, heart and renal disease, abdominal angina, cancer)
Excessive alcohol use
Medications that interfere with appetite and/or nutrient metabolism

From Rosenberg IH. Nutrition and aging. In Hazzard WR, ed. Principles of Geriatric Medicine and Gerontology, 3rd ed. New York: McGraw-Hill, 1994. Reprinted with permission of The McGraw-Hill Companies.

In addition to impairing the strength and mobility of the elderly patient, the decrease in muscle mass results in a smaller pool of amino acids available for the synthesis of other body proteins. Protein intake therefore must be maintained at levels sufficient to prevent further muscle mass losses. Decreased levels of exercise further exacerbate the loss of muscle mass and, together with a relative increase in percent body fat, contributes to progressive insulin resistance and a lower basal metabolic rate.[23,24] Reduced calcium and vitamin D intake contributes to osteoporosis and loss of bone mass, which is further compounded by reduced levels of 25-hydroxyvitamin D because of reduced exposure of the skin to sunshine.

The shift in body mass from muscle to adipose tissue is complicated by the use of inaccurate methods to assess obesity in older persons[25] and by the metabolic consequences of increased adipose tissue. The standard comparison of height to weight is an unreliable method to measure obesity in the elderly because of the shift in body mass from muscle to fat and the changes in skeletal configuration. Because weight generally increases linearly with the square of body height, the computation of a body mass index (BMI = wt/ht^2), using metric units of measurement, partially corrects weight for height and affords a better estimate of obesity. The computation of BMI must

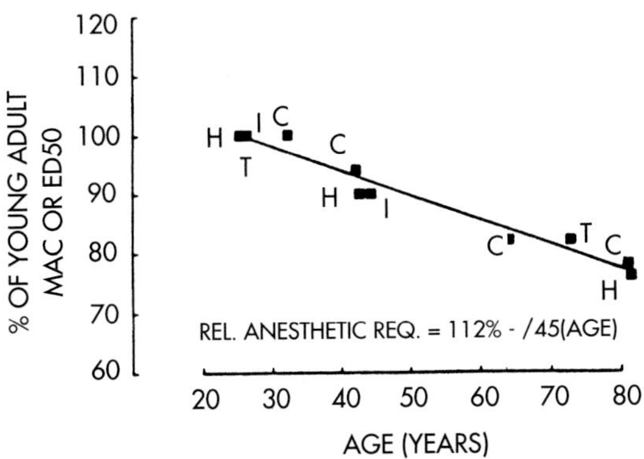

Fig. 67-6. The decrease in relative anesthetic requirement with age in unsedated humans. *C,* Cyclopropane; *H,* halothane; *I,* isoflurane; *T,* thiopental. (From Buxbaum J L, Schwartz A J. Perianesthetic considerations for the elderly patient. Surg Clin North Am 47:43, 1994. Reprinted with permission.)

be corrected for age, however, to normalize indexes of obesity in the elderly. The establishment of "normal" ranges of BMI for the elderly still ignores the effects of the increased "fatness" on metabolism and mortality. A comprehensive analysis of 4.2 million insurance policy holders indicates that the lowest mortality risks are associated with a progressive rise in BMI with age.[26] The BMI associated with the lowest mortality increases from 21.4 in the 20- to 29-year-old group, to 22.9 in the 40- to 49-year-old group, and 26.6 in the 60- to 69-year-old group. This roughly corresponds to an increase of about 10 pounds per decade in the weight of the best survivors. Although these data may seem reassuring to those of us who notice the appearance of some "middle-age bulge," they suggest that the moderately obese elderly patient has a greater shift toward obese metabolism than his or her younger counterpart.

In addition to a progressive loss of lean body mass and a corresponding increase in adiposity, aging is also associated with a decrease in total body water. Red blood cell mass is usually maintained in healthy individuals, but circulating plasma volume is reduced, particularly in debilitated patients.[27] This decreased volume of distribution can result in higher-than-expected concentrations of administered drugs and a correspondingly exaggerated drug effect. For example, the initial volume of distribution of thiopental in 20- to 40-year-old subjects is 15 to 30 L, although in 60- to 90-year-olds, it is 3 to 7 L.[28] This fact dictates a reduction in dosing levels of many anesthetic drugs (Fig. 67-6).

The increase in relative body fat also has significant pharmacologic implications for surgical management as a result of an increased distribution compartment for lipid-soluble drugs. The increase in reservoir of lipid-soluble agents can result in a lower-than-expected plasma concentration of the agents initially, with a longer drug effect because of protracted clearance.[29] These changes in body composition, together with changes in the functions of organs responsible for the clearance of drugs, mandate more careful anesthetic management and closer postoperative surveillance of elderly surgical patients.

Decline in Physiologic Function

With increasing age there is a clear decline in physiologic function, although the rate and significance of the decline may vary considerably among individuals and among organ systems. In the resting state these changes may have minimal consequences, but when physiologic reserves are needed to respond to a stress such as surgery, overall performance may deteriorate.

Cardiovascular Function

Morphologic changes in the myocardium, conducting pathways, valves, and vasculature of the heart accompany advancing age, although it is often difficult to separate the changes associated with aging from those caused by disease. The functional implications of many of these changes are also variable and frequently not well defined.

The overall weight of the heart increases slightly in women but not in men while the thickness of the ventricular septum increases significantly regardless of gender.[30] There is also an increase in the fat content of the epicardium overlying the right ventricle. The number of myocytes declines while the size of the cells and the content of lipofuscin, the degenerative pigment, increases. The deposition of amyloid protein increases significantly with age, and some form of the protein can be found in nearly half the hearts of persons older than age 70.[31] Collagen and elastin content also increases, and fibrotic areas may appear throughout the myocardium. Although any one of these features alone may be of limited functional significance, the sum of these changes is a decline in ventricular compliance.[32]

In the conducting system the most pronounced change is the replacement of nearly 90% of the autonomic cells in the sinus node by fat and connective tissue.[33] There is also a less impressive increase in fibrosis in the intranodal tracts and partial loss of proximal bundle fascicles between the left bundle and the bundle of His. These changes may contribute to the high incidence of sick sinus syndrome, atrial arrhythmias, and bundle branch blocks.

Valvular anatomy is also altered with aging. Sclerosis and calcification of the aortic valve is most common but is usually of little functional importance.[34] Calcification and sclerosis occur less frequently in the mitral valve, but because of the juxtaposition of the valve to the atrioventricular node and conducting bundles, calcification at this location may be responsible for atrioventricular nodal and bundle branch blocks. Recently, progressive dilation of all four valvular annuli has also been described.[35] It is thought that this dilation may be responsible for the multivalvular regurgitation frequently demonstrated in healthy older people.

Lastly, morphologic changes can be seen in both the

coronary and peripheral vessels. The endothelial cells lining the vessels change size and shape, and flow may become more turbulent. The subendothelial and medial layers thicken, and calcification in these layers increases independent of atherosclerosis. As a result the vessels become progressively more rigid and less distensible.[36] These changes in the peripheral vasculature probably contribute to an increase in systolic blood pressure, an increase in resistance to ventricular emptying, and a compensatory loss of myocytes with thickening of the ventricular wall.[37] These degenerative changes in the coronary vessels may appear as calcifications on radiographs and therefore may be mistaken for the calcifications caused by atherosclerotic disease.

The functional implications of aging on the heart have been difficult to assess accurately because alterations in body composition, metabolic rate, general states of fitness, and underlying disease influence cardiac performance.[36] It

Table 67-3. Clinical Differentiation of Diastolic vs. Systolic Dysfunction in Patients With Heart Failure

	Systolic Dysfunction	Diastolic Dysfunction
Past history	Hypertension Myocardial infarction Diabetes Chronic valvular insufficiency disorders	Hypertension Renal disease Diabetes Aortic stenosis
Presentation	Younger than 65 years Progressive shortness of breath	65 years or older Acute pulmonary edema
Physical examination	Displaced PMI S_3 gallop	Sustained PMI S_4 gallop
Radiographic findings	Pulmonary congestion Cardiomegaly	Pulmonary congestion Normal sized heart
Electrocardiogram	Q waves	LVH
Echocardiogram	Decreased LVEF	Normal or increased LVEF

From Tresch DD, McGough MF. Heart failure with normal systolic function: A common disorder in older people. J Am Geriatric Soc 43:1035, 1995. Reprinted with permission.
LVEF, Left ventricular ejection fraction; *LVH,* left ventricular hypertrophy; *PMI,* point of maximal impact.

Table 67-4. Pharmacologic Management of Heart Failure Secondary to Diastolic Dysfunction

Therapeutic Agents	Goals of Therapy	Considerations
Diuretics	Decrease in blood volume Decrease in ventricular filling pressure	Abrupt reduction in volume may produce hypotension and decreased CO; close monitoring for hypotension and renal dysfunction necessary; no effect on regression of LVH
ACE inhibitors	Decrease in afterload Regression of LVH Regression of myocardial interstitial fibrosis Enhanced ventricular relaxation	Agents with most marked effect on regression of LVH; acute unloading effects may produce hypotension and decreased CO; close monitoring of BP and renal function necessary
Calcium channel blockers	Decrease in afterload Regression of LVH Relief of myocardial ischemia Slow heart rate* Enhanced ventricular relaxation	Acute unloading effects may produce hypotension and decreased CO; anti-ischemic effects beneficial in patients with CAD; may be detrimental when both systolic and diastolic dysfunction present; beneficial in slowing heart rate in patients with atrial fibrillation*; combination with β-blockers may cause severe bradycardia*
β-Blockers	Decrease in afterload Regression of LVH Relief of myocardial ischemia Slow heart rate Enhance ventricular relaxation	Limited effect on LVH regression; anti-ischemic effect beneficial in patients with CAD; beneficial in slowing heart rate in patients with atrial fibrillation

From Tresch DD, McGough MF. Heart failure with normal systolic function: A common disorder in older people. J Am Geriatric Soc 43:1035, 1995. Reprinted with permission.
*, Verapamil and diltiazem; *ACE,* angiotensin converting enzyme; *BP,* blood pressure; *CAD,* coronary artery disease; *CO,* cardiac output; *LVH,* left ventricular hypertrophy.

is now generally accepted that *systolic function* both at rest and in response to exercise does not change with age. Cardiac output and ejection fraction at rest are maintained in spite of the increased afterload imposed by the stiffening of the outflow tract.[38] In younger persons, cardiac output during periods of increased demand is maintained by increasing heart rate. With aging the heart becomes less responsive to catecholamines, possibly secondary to changes in receptor function, and thereby loses the ability to augment cardiac output by increasing rate.[36] Maintenance of cardiac output therefore becomes more dependent on ventricular filling (preload). Because of this dependence on preload, even minor hypovolemia may result in severe compromise in cardiac performance.

Diastolic function, which depends on myocardial relaxation rather than contraction, is more significantly affected by aging. In 50% of patients older than age 80 with heart failure, systolic function is preserved, but diastolic function is impaired.[39] Because relaxation requires greater energy expenditure and therefore more oxygen consumption than does contraction, the rate of relaxation is more susceptible to declining oxygen availability. With age there is a progressive decrease in the partial pressure of arterial oxygen. As a consequence, relaxation is prolonged, and even mild additional hypoxia from stress can result in significant diastolic dysfunction.[40] This prolongation of relaxation, combined with the decreased ventricular compliance that results from progressive fibrosis, leads to decreased ventricular filling and higher diastolic pressures. This in turn can result in pulmonary vascular congestion and signs of heart failure.

As a result of impaired early diastolic filling, maintenance of adequate preload becomes more dependent on the contribution of the atrium. Loss of this atrial contraction or even minor hypovolemia can therefore result in significant impairment of cardiac function.[40]

Alterations at the cellular level have also been implicated in the diastolic dysfunction that accompanies aging. A decline in the rate of calcium sequestration by the sacroplasmic reticulum following myocardial excitation and an increase in net calcium influx across the sacroplasmic reticulum[41] have both been suggested as possible etiologic factors.

Distinguishing systolic from diastolic dysfunction may be difficult. Systolic failure is usually gradual in onset and progressive; diastolic failure is abrupt, and the decline is rapid. Some distinguishing features are listed in Table 67-3. The treatment is also different. Although digitalis and diuretics are indicated in systolic failure, the use of these agents in diastolic dysfunction may exacerbate the derangement. Diastolic abnormalities are treated with agents that improve preload and ventricular relaxation such as calcium channel blockers, angiotensin-converting enzyme (ACE) inhibitors, and B-adrenergic antagonists[42,43] (Table 67-4).

It is also important to remember that the manifestation of cardiac diseases in the elderly may be nonspecific and atypical. Although chest pain is still the most common symptom of myocardial infarction, as many as 40% of older patients have nonclassic symptoms such as shortness of breath, syncope, acute confusion, or stroke.[44]

Cardiac complications are the most common cause of death in the postoperative period. Identification of patients at risk for postoperative cardiac events is the basis for most preoperative evaluation strategies (see Preoperative Evaluations, Risk Assessment, and Outcome).

Respiratory Function

The normal decline in respiratory function that accompanies aging can be attributed to changes in the chest wall and the lung[45] (Table 67-5). There is a decline in chest wall compliance secondary to changes in structure caused by kyphosis and exaggerated by vertebral collapse. There is decreased mobility of the ribs caused by calcification of the costal cartilage and contractures of the intercostal muscles.[12] There is also a progressive decrease in the strength of the respiratory muscles,[46] which leads to as much as a 50% decline in the maximal inspiratory and expiratory force generated and easy fatigability.

Table 67-5. Age-Related Changes in the Chest Wall and Lung

Morphologic Change	Functional Significance
Thorax	
Calcification of bronchial and costal cartilage	↑ Resistance to deformation of chest wall
↑ Costovertebral stiffness	↑ Use of diaphragm in ventilation
↑ Rigidity of chest wall	
↑ Anteroposterior diameter (kyphosis)	↓ Tidal volume
	Response to exercise hyperpnea
Wasting of respiratory muscles	↓ Maximal voluntary ventilation
Lung	
Enlarged alveolar ducts	↓ Surface area for gas exchange
↓ Supporting duct framework, enlarged alveoli	
Thinning, separation of alveolar membrane	↑ Physiologic dead space
↑ Mucous gland	
↑ Number, thickness of elastic fibers (?)	↓ Lung elastic recoil VC, RV/TLC
↑ Tissue extensibility (alveolar wall)	↓ Ventilatory flow rate
	↓ Ventilation distribution
	↑ Resistance to flow in small airways
↓ Pulmonary capillary network	↓ Ventilation: Blood flow equality
↑ Fibrosis of pulmonary capillary intima	

Modified from Reddan WG. Exercise and aging, Smith EL, Seartass RC, eds. Enslow Publishing, Hillside, N.J., 1981. With permission.
RV, Residual volume; *TLC,* total lung capacity; *VC,* vital capacity.

In the lung the major change with age is the loss of elastic recoil in the alveoli. The elastic properties of the lung are responsible for maintaining the patency of the small airways. Loss of elasticity leads to increased alveolar compliance with collapse of these airways and subsequent uneven alveolar ventilation and air trapping.[47] Uneven alveolar ventilation leads to ventilation-perfusion mismatches, which in turn cause a decline in arterial oxygen tension of approximately 0.3% or 0.42 mm Hg per year. Although there is a decline in the partial pressure of oxygen, the partial pressure of carbon dioxide does not change, in spite of an increase in the dead space, or wasted ventilation. This may be due in part to the decline in the production of carbon dioxide that accompanies the falling basal metabolic rates. Air trapping is also responsible for an increase in the residual volume (RV), or the volume remaining after maximal expiration.

The loss of support of the small airways also leads to compression during forced expiration, which limits dynamic lung volumes and flow rates. Forced vital capacity (FVC) decreases by 14 to 30 ml/yr and 1-second forced expiratory volume (FEV_1) decreases by 23 to 32 ml/yr (in men).[47] The overall effect of loss of elastic inward recoil is balanced somewhat by the decline in chest wall outward force. Total lung capacity (TLC) therefore remains unchanged, and there is only a mild increase in resting lung volume, or functional residual capacity (FRC). Because TLC remains unchanged, the increase in RV results in a decrease in vital capacity (VC) (Fig. 67-7).

The control of ventilation is also affected by aging. Ventilatory responses to hypoxia and hypercapnia fall by 50% and 40%, respectively.[48] The exact mechanism of this decline has not been well defined but may be the result of declining chemoreceptor function either at the peripheral or central nervous system level.

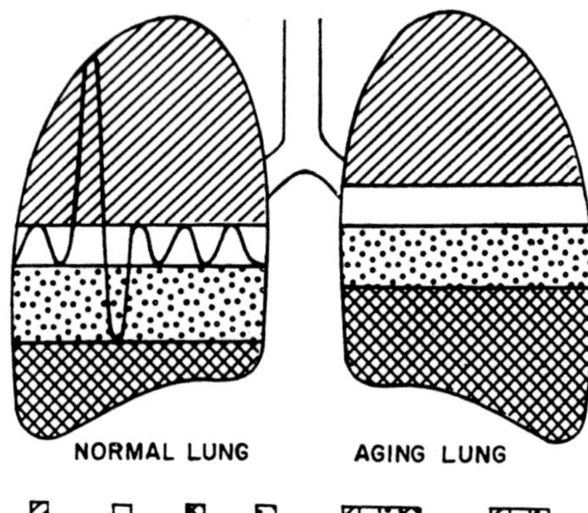

Fig. 67-7. Changes in lung volumes with aging. Note the decrease in vital capacity *(VC)* and increase in residual volume *(RV)*. *ERV,* Expiratory reserve volume; IRV, inspiratory reserve volume, *TLC,* total lung capacity; *VT,* tidal volume. (From Timiras PS. Aging of the respiration, erythrocytes and hematopoietic system. Reprinted with permission from Timiras PS, ed. The Physiologic Basis of Aging and Geriatrics, 2nd ed. Copyright © 1988 CRC Press, Boca Raton, Fla.)

In addition to these intrinsic changes, pulmonary function is affected by alterations in the ability of the respiratory system to protect against environmental injury and infection. There are a progressive decrease in T-cell function (see the following) and a decline in mucociliary clearance. The loss of cough reflex secondary to neurologic disorders may predispose to aspiration. The increased frequency and severity of pneumonia in older persons has been attributed to these factors and to an increased incidence of oropharyngeal colonization with gram negative organisms. This colonization correlates closely with comorbidity and with the ability of older patients to perform activities of daily living. This fact lends support to the idea that functional status is a crucial factor in assessing the risk of pneumonia in older patients.[49]

Renal Function

Between the ages of 25 and 85 there is a progressive decrease in kidney size, length, and volume. The majority of the tissue loss is in the cortex, where approximately 40% of the nephrons become sclerotic, and the remaining functional units hypertrophy in a compensatory manner. Sclerosis of the glomeruli is accompanied by atrophy of the afferent and efferent arterioles and by a decrease in renal tubular cell number. Renal blood flow also falls by approximately 50%. This decline is thought to be secondary to changes in the vessels supplying the kidneys or to increased renal vascular resistance.[50]

The functional result of these changes is a fall in glomerular filtration rate (GFR) by approximately 45% at age 80. This fall in GFR is reflected in a decline in creatinine clearance of 0.75 ml/min/yr in healthy elderly men. Serum creatinine, however, remains unchanged because of a concomitant decrease in lean body mass and thus a decrease in creatinine production. Estimates of creatinine clearance in the healthy aged can be made from the serum creatinine by using the formula derived by Cockroft and Gault[51] as shown below:

$$\frac{(140 - \text{Age in yr}) \times (\text{Weight in kg})}{72 \times (\text{Serum creatinine in mg/dl})}$$

Caution must be exercised when appyling this formula to critically ill patients or those receiving medications that directly affect renal function.

Renal tubular function also declines with advancing age. The ability to conserve sodium and excrete hydrogen ion falls, resulting in a diminished capacity to regulate fluid and acid-base balance.[52] Dehydration becomes a particular problem because losses of sodium and water from nonrenal causes are not compensated for by the usual mechanisms (increased renal sodium retention, increased urinary concentration, and increased thirst). The inability to retain sodium is thought to be due to a decline in the activity of the renin-angiotensin system.[53] The increasing inability to concentrate the urine, which has been well documented,[54] is related to changes in antidiuretic hormone (ADH). Measurements of ADH indicate that with advancing age there is a normal or exaggerated ADH response to a variety of stimuli. The defect in concentrating ability therefore is probably secondary to a decline in end-organ responsiveness to ADH rather than a change in hormone production. The marked decline in the subjective feeling of thirst is also well documented[55] but not well explained. Alterations of osmoreceptor function in the hypothalamus may be responsible for the failure to recognize thirst in spite of significant elevations in serum osmolality.[56]

In the perioperative period the decline in renal function combined with the changes in cardiovascular compensatory mechanisms leaves older patients at increased risk for both hypovolemia and fluid overload; postural instability and syncope result when cardiovascular reflexes and tubular function cannot compensate for even minor volume depletion,[41] whereas congestive heart failure and pulmonary edema result when excess fluid cannot be excreted rapidly enough because of the inability to augment cardiac output, improve renal perfusion, and increase GFR.

Alterations in renal function also have great impact on the types and doses of drugs used in older patients. Although drugs are handled by the kidney in several different ways, most changes in renal drug processing parallel the decline in GFR. Therefore creatinine clearance can be used to determine the appropriate clearance of most agents processed by the kidney.[57]

Changes also occur in the lower urinary tract with aging. In the bladder, increased collagen content leads to limited distensibility and impaired emptying.[58] Overactivity of the detrusor secondary to neurologic disorders or idiopathic causes[59] has also been identified. In women, decreased circulating levels of estrogen and decreased tissue responsiveness to this hormone cause changes in the urethral sphincter that predispose to urinary incontinence. In men, prostatic hypertrophy impairs bladder emptying. Together, these factors lead to urinary incontinence in approximately 10% to 15% of elderly persons living in the community and 50% of those in nursing homes.[60]

There is also an increased prevalence of asymptomatic bacteriuria with age, which varies from 10% to 50% depending on gender, level of activity, underlying disorders, and place of residence. Urinary tract infections alone are responsible for 30% to 50% of all cases of bacteremia in older patients.[61] Alterations in the local environment and declining host defenses are thought to be responsible. Because of the lack of symptoms in elderly patients with bacteriuria, preoperative urinalysis becomes increasingly important.

Hepatobiliary Function

Morphologic changes in the liver with age include a decrease in overall weight and size and a decrease in the number of hepatocytes. There is, however, a compensatory increase in cell size and increase in binucleated cells with a proliferation of bile ducts. Functionally, hepatic blood flow falls by approximately 1% per year to about 40% of earlier values after age 60.[62]

Although the synthetic capacity, as measured by the standard tests of liver function, remains unchanged,[63] the metabolism of and sensitivity to certain kinds of drugs are altered. Drugs requiring microsomal oxidation (phase I reactions) prior to conjugation (phase II reactions) may be metabolized more slowly, whereas those requiring only conjugation may be cleared at a normal rate.[64] Drugs that act directly on hepatocytes, such as warfarin (Coumadin), may produce the desired therapeutic effects at lower doses in the elderly because of an increased sensitivity of the cells to these agents.[65]

The most significant correlate of altered hepatobiliary function in the aged is the increased incidence of gallstones and gallstone-related complications. Gallstone prevalence rises steadily with age, although there is variability in the absolute percentages depending on the population studied[66-68] (Table 67-6). Stones have been demonstrated in as many as 80% of nursing home residents older than age 90.[69] Biliary tract disease is the single most common indication for abdominal surgery in the elderly population[70] (Table 67-7).

Although pigment gallstones are found with more frequency in older people,[71] cholesterol stones have also been shown to increase with advancing age.[72] The formation of all types of gallstones first requires a change in the bile itself that promotes stone formation. This lithogenic bile is necessary but not sufficient for stone formation. Factors that promote nucleation and allow stone growth (stasis)

Table 67-6. Prevalence of Gallbladder Disease (%)

	Pima Indians[66] (Cholecystography)		New Haven, Conn.[67] (Necropsy)			Rome[68] (Ultrasound)	
Age	**Male**	**Female**	**Male**	**Female**	**Age**	**Male**	**Female**
15-24	0	13	7	4	20-29	0	2
25-34	4	73	2	5	30-39	1	4
35-44	11	71	9	10	40-49	4	6
45-54	32	76	13	16	50-59	11	12
55-64	66	62	18	20	60-69	10	23
>65	68	90	22	28			

Table 67-7. Current Abdominal Operations per Year in the United States

	No. of Operations (in Thousands)	
	Total	**Patient Age >65**
Cholecystectomy	502	168
Lysis of adhesions	347	90
Appendectomy (not incidental)	250	17
Partial excision of large intestines	207	120

are also necessary. Included in these factors is the glycoprotein mucin, which serves as a nidus for stone formation and forms a gel layer lining the gallbladder mucosa, which provides the environment for stone growth. The formation of this mucin gel precedes the development of both types of stones and is closely related to gallbladder stasis. The increased development of gallstones in the elderly is thought to result from both changes in the composition of bile and impaired biliary motility.

Alterations in the composition of bile with advancing age include an increase in the activity of HMG-CoA (the rate-limiting enzyme in the synthesis of cholesterol) and a decrease in the activity of 7-α-hydroxylase (the rate-limiting enzyme in the synthesis of bile salts from cholesterol).[73] This results in supersaturation of the bile with cholesterol and a decrease in the primary bile salt pool.[74] The ratio of secondary-to-primary bile salts also increases. It is postulated that these secondary bile salts promote cholesterol gallstone formation by enhancing cholesterol synthesis, increasing protein content of the bile, decreasing nucleation time, and increasing the production of specific phospolipids that are thought to affect the production of mucin.[75] It has also been suggested that the increase in secondary bile salts in the aged may promote a recycling of bilirubin, which in turn leads to the unconjugated bilirubin supersaturation necessary for pigment stone formation.

Alterations in gallbladder motility and bile duct motility are thought to be central to the development of cholesterol stones and brown pigment stones, respectively. The role of motility in black pigment formation, however, is less clear.[75] Biliary motility is a complex interaction of hormonal and neural factors; however, the major stimulus of gallbladder emptying is cholecystokinin (CCK). The sensitivity of the gallbladder wall to CCK has been shown to decrease with increasing age in animal models.[76] Exogenous administration of CCK to animals fed a lithogenic diet inhibits the age-dependent development of cholesterol gallstones.[77] In humans, gallbladder sensitivity to CCK is also decreased. However, there is a compensatory increase in the production of CCK in response to stimuli, which results in normal gallbladder contraction.[78] The production of the hormone pancreatic polypeptide, which inhibits gallbladder contraction and promotes relaxation, has also been shown to increase with increasing age in humans.[79,80] The significance of this observation with regard to gallstone formation, however, is unknown. Further studies to elucidate changes in biliary motility with age are necessary.

Regardless of the pathogenesis, gallstones are associated with complications in 40% to 60% of older patients requiring treatment for the disease compared to less than 20% of younger patients.[81] In a recent study of more than 20,000 open cholecystectomies in the elderly, nearly two thirds of patients required emergency operation.[82] The increased rate of complicated disease seen in older patients may be directly attributable to the increased severity of the disease or to the increased prevalence of comorbid illnesses like atherosclerosis and diabetes mellitus. It is more likely, however, a result of delays in diagnosis and treatment caused by the frequent *absence* of typical biliary tract symptoms. Biliary colic, or episodic right upper quadrant pain radiating to the back, precedes the development of a complication only half as often in older than younger patients.[83] Even in the presence of acute cholecystitis, one quarter of older patients may have no abdominal tenderness, one third no elevation in temperature or white blood cell count, and as many as one half no peritoneal signs in the right upper quadrant.[84] Unfortunately, mortality in the emergent setting is at least three times the elective mortality.[81] Until predictors of impending complications other than symptoms are identified, improving the outcome of biliary tract disease in the elderly will be difficult. Until that time, increased awareness of the atypical presentation of gallstone related illness in this age group is essential.

Hematopoietic Function

Long-term culture studies of bone marrow reveal that the maintenance of in vitro hematopoiesis varies inversely with the age of the donor.[85] Additional studies corroborate the observation that the ability of progenitor spleen–colonizing stem cells to replicate is an age-dependent process,[86,87] probably analogous to the species-dependent limits on cell replication. The replicative capacity of spleen-colonizing stem cells far exceeds the life span of the host, however, making it unlikely that exhaustion of erythroid precursor proliferation accounts for the diminished hematopoietic reserve seen in the elderly. In addition, marrow taken from young donors and transplanted into elderly recipients proliferates at a rate that is indicative of the recipient, not the donor.[88]

Erythropoiesis is dependent on the stimulation of erythroid progenitor replication by erythropoietin. Under basal conditions the rate of erythroid turnover and erythroid kinetics are essentially normal in healthy elderly subjects. Under the condition of increased demand, as in the response to hemorrhage, however, the elderly patient has a delayed or absent erythroid response. Diminished erythropoiesis in the elderly therefore is due to a combination of inherent and environmental factors that alter the erythroid response to increased demand and result in a loss of functional reserve.

Neutrophils form the first line of defense by their role in phagocytosis and bacterial killing. The bactericidal action of neutrophil superoxides and lysosomal enzymes is dependent on the neutrophil response to a series of stimuli. When young and old neutrophils are compared in their basal and stimulated responses, basal rates of enzyme release are similar, whereas the response to a challenge is measurably impaired in the old neutrophils (Fig. 67-8). The diminished response may be associated with an age-related but reversible alteration in the lipid composition of neutrophil plasma membranes.[89]

Clinically, the neutrophil response to bacterial invasion in elderly patients is generally intact if drugs, metabolic stress, or concurrent disease does not supervene. Nutritional deficiency is an important variable, however, as the bactericidal function of neutrophils is significantly impaired by relatively short-term malnutrition of the host. Protein-calorie repletion by the intravenous route carries its own risk for infectious problems, however, so the selection of treatment strategies that minimize the risk for ileus followed by early enteral feeding is the best support for the aged leukocyte system.

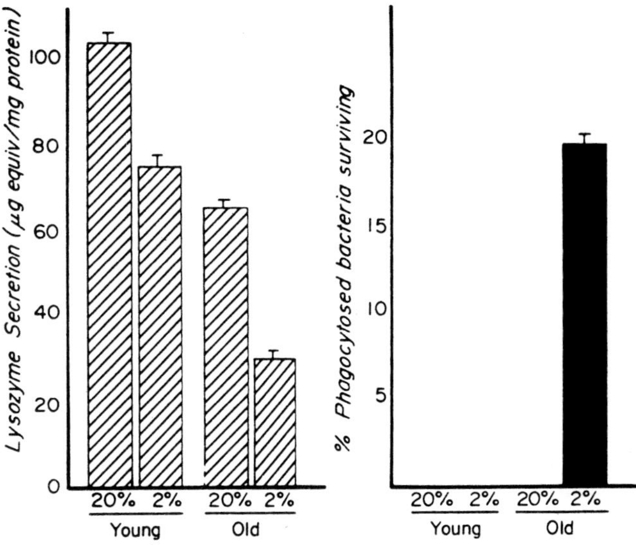

Fig. 67-8. Secretion of the enzyme lysozymes *(left panel)* following activation of the neutrophils from young (6-month) or old (24-month) mice fed a 20% (normal) or 2% protein diet. The graph on right shows the percent of phagocytosed bacteria not killed by neutrophils from mice in similar groups. Clearly, neutrophils from old mice fed low-protein diets are unable to kill all phagocytosed bacteria. (From Lipschitz DA. Hematologic changes in the elderly. In Katlic MR, ed. Geriatric Surgery. Baltimore: Urban & Schwarzenberg, 1990.)

Metabolic and Endocrine Function

The regulation of intermediary metabolism and the neurocrine-paracrine-endocrine mediation of cellular events are complex processes with multiple potential points of failure. The age-related loss of functional reserve of endocrine responsiveness, or the changes in nutrient metabolism seen commonly in elderly patients, has multiple causes. Age-related alterations in hormone levels are inconsistent, with some being quite elevated and others nearly absent. For example, plasma levels of CCK are elevated in elderly patients, although levels of gastrin are reduced. Gallbladder CCK receptor function is depressed in elderly subjects, however, as is parietal cell gastrin receptor function.[81,90] Therefore diminished cholecystokinesis in the elderly is probably a result of receptor loss or dysfunction, but hypochlorhydria appears to be a consequence of primary hormone insufficiency. Altered endocrine function may result from changes at several points in the pathway: alterations in hormone (or receptor) gene expression, in protein processing within the cell of origin (including protein assembly, storage, or vesicle trafficking), in hormone release caused by stimulus-secretion coupling abnormalities, in hormone distribution resulting from circulatory dysfunction or vascular occlusion, and in target cell responsiveness (caused by impaired receptor binding, faulty ligand internalization, or diminished target cell postreceptor activation). Studies of endocrine dysfunction in the elderly are further confounded by the use of reference measurements originally made in hospitalized patients.

The hypothalamic-pituitary-adrenal axis is the classic neuroendocrine feedback loop. Subtle and varied age-related changes have been described in the release of corticotropin-releasing hormone (CRH), adrenocorticotropic hormone (ACTH), and glucocorticoids, but the loop appears to remain essentially intact despite advanced age. Glucocorticoid inhibition of CRH and ACTH release has been documented to be impaired,[91] which suggests that the central neuroendocrine response to stress is actually prolonged in elderly surgical patients.

The release of GH from the anterior pituitary gland declines progressively with increasing age, and is associated with lower levels of insulin-like growth factor 1 (IGF-1). GH stimulates IGF-1 production by the liver, the replacement of which in aging animals has been shown to reverse age-related defects in gene expression and immune function and to prolong life expectancy.[92,93] Protein catabolism has been shown to be reversed in critically injured patients by GH replacement therapy, and the role of GH in the treatment of impaired wound healing in the elderly is currently under study.

The adrenal glands undergo gradual changes with aging, which include fibrosis or nodular hyperplasia. Glucocorticoid or mineralocorticoid excess is unusual but can result from a functional adrenal adenoma or adrenocortical carcinoma. Deficiency of mineralocorticoid or glucocorticoid secretion is more common but is usually apparent in the setting of increased demand. Loss of adrenal reserve may result from hemorrhage, infection, infiltrative or metastatic disease, or autoimmune destruction. Unexplained hemodynamic instability or frank shock in an elderly patient should be treated with a trial of glucocorticoids, in addition to other necessary agents.

Thyroid diseases are common in elderly patients and are often insidious in their presentation. Fibrosis, decreased follicle size, and atrophy are frequently seen, and hypothyroidism occurs in up to 4% of the elderly population.[94] Nonspecific symptoms, such as constipation, lethargy, and dry skin, are frequent and may be confused with constitutional complaints attributed to "aging." Hyperthyroidism is fairly common among older patients as well, and some studies suggest it may be more prevalent in the elderly than in younger patients.[95] Thyroid enlargement, commonly observed in younger hyperthyroid patients, may be absent in elderly. Older hyperthyroid patients also lack the exophthalmos seen in younger patients, and nodular goiter, rather than Graves' disease, is the most frequent cause of thyroid hyperfunction. The presenting symptoms are also disturbingly misleading: weight loss, tremor, muscle weakness, anorexia, and arrhythmias may easily be mistaken for signs of "aging." *Masked* and *apathetic hyperthyroidism,* terms originally used to describe advanced cardiac and toxic forms of hyperthyroidism, are now used to describe the typical presentation of the disease in the elderly.

Thyroid nodules and degenerative cysts occur with increased frequency in the elderly. Sonographic imaging is helpful to identify those cystic lesions that require only aspiration. Solid lesions, however, must be evaluated with thyroid function studies and fine-needle aspiration because of the substantial risk for malignancy. Of the 20% to 25% of euthyroid patients with "suspicious" fine-needle aspiration cytology of a discrete nodule, a final pathologic diagnosis of malignancy is observed in 11% to as many as 71% of cases,[96] with the majority of these being papillary or follicular carcinoma.

Hyperparathyroidism is more prevalent in the elderly as well and is frequently unsuspected at diagnosis. Automated blood chemistry screening accounts for most newly diagnosed cases, and in the elderly the sporadic or nonfamilial forms of the disease are most common. With persistence of the disease, nephrocalcinosis, bone demineralization, mental status changes, and constitutional symptoms may develop, but many patients remain seemingly asymptomatic despite elevated calcium levels. This has resulted in controversy over whether to advocate parathyroidectomy in elderly patients with few or no symptoms. At a consensus conference held at the National Institutes of Health in 1990, it was recommended that patients without *overt* signs and symptoms be managed expectantly.[97] This definition leaves uncertain whether "weakness" and "depression" indicate symptomatic disease, although roughly 40% of patients with hyperparathyroidism have one or both complaints. Furthermore, in a recent case control study, only 4.6% of hyperparathyroid patients were found to be truly asymptomatic, and the majority of patients felt better overall after surgery.[98] Because there is no medical treatment of hyperparathyroidism, there is no means of predicting when or if severe complications of the disease such as nephrocalcinosis or bone disease will develop. Because the morbidity and mortality risk of surgery is low even in older patients, parathyroidectomy remains the treatment of choice unless other comorbid conditions preclude surgery (see Preoperative Evaluation, Risk Assessment, and Outcome).

Diabetes and changes in glucoregulatory hormones constitute a common set of concerns in elderly surgical patients. Hyperglycemia after carbohydrate ingestion or glucose administration is so common in the elderly that age-adjusted nomograms are used in standardized glucose tolerance testing. Glucose homeostasis is the net result of the interactions of a series of interrelated systems or processes: (1) gastric emptying of nutrients; (2) enteric nutrient absorption; (3) insulin release by elevated circulating glucose levels; (4) the potentiating effect of enteric hormones, called incretins, which augment the insulin response; (5) the distribution of insulin to visceral and peripheral tissues; (6) insulin action including receptor binding, glucose transport, and inhibition of glucose production; and (7) metabolism of glucose by insulin-dependent and insulin-independent tissues. Abnormalities in one or more of these processes may lead to impaired glucose tolerance or frank diabetes, and it should be apparent that multiple causes of abnormal glucose metabolism are possible.

The most serious abnormalities that commonly affect glucose homeostasis are impaired insulin release and impaired insulin binding/action.[99] Insulin secretory responses to a variety of secretagogs decrease with advancing age, and the higher degree of body fat in the elderly contributes to insulin resistance as well. Hyperglycemia is common in elderly patients who receive intravenous alimentation, and insulin therapy is commonly, albeit transiently, required in many sick elderly patients.

A variety of abnormalities are apparent in gastroenteropancreatic function in older patients and may contribute to surgical disease in the elderly. Altered esophageal motility and sphincter function result in an increased incidence of reflux and aspiration.[100] Hypochlorhydria and diminished gastric emptying are common,[101] but there is a paradoxic increase in the incidence of peptic ulcer disease in the elderly.[102,103] This may be secondary to an age-related decrease in duodenal bicarbonate secretion[104] and a breakdown in mucosal defense mechanisms. Small bowel absorption of fat and carbohydrates have been shown to be impaired,[101] but the enteric hormonal response to nutrients is essentially intact. Some hormone levels actually rise with aging, including CCK and pancreatic polypeptide.[81] Absorption of iron and calcium is impaired in the aged gut, due to a loss in villus height and mucosal atrophy.[105] These mucosal changes are also seen in the aging colon, where progressive loss of muscularis propria function and increased thickness of the colon wall contribute to the age-related incidence of diverticular disease.[106]

Exocrine pancreatic secretion appears to change minimally with advancing age, although duct ectasia and dilation of acini are seen.[107] Lipase deficiency may contribute to altered fat absorption, but secretory function of the gland remains intact.[108] The incidence of nonalcoholic pancreatitis increases in the elderly, because of the increased incidence of gallstones and the increased incidence of acute idiopathic pancreatitis. This entity is disproportionately present in the elderly and carries a mortality risk of 25% or more.[109] The age-related increase in the death risk of pancreatitis may result from a higher likelihood of coexisting diseases but is also a reflection of an altered presentation and an altered response to the disease process in the older patient.

Decreased Ability to Adapt to Changes in the Environment

Altered Response to Stress

Alterations in the neuroendocrine response(s) to stress in the elderly may account for some aspects of the "diminished reserve" that characterizes many aging effects on organ systems. Catecholamine responses to a variety of stressors are altered in aging, although it has been difficult to achieve consensus on age-related effects on the actual levels of the catecholamines. Considerable evidence demonstrates a decline in the β-adrenergic regulation of arterial and venous dilation and myocardial contractility.[110,111] These effects are thought to be related to altered β-adrenergic receptor function rather than changes in catechol levels per se.[112,113] Adrenocortical responses to stress are retained in most studies, but the anterior pituitary response to surgical stress is greatly diminished in the elderly and is virtually eliminated when spinal analgesia is used.[114] It remains unknown whether the loss of this neuroendocrine response contributes to the risk of hemodynamic instability in elderly patients undergoing operation.

Surgical stress is usually accompanied by catabolism and protein loss. The administration of appropriate nutritional support is therefore an important part of the care of the critically ill patient. Elderly patients are particularly vulnerable in the postoperative period because subtle preoperative malnutrition, usually secondary to poor nutrient intake and concomitant disease, is so common in this age group. In addition, compensatory protein synthesis is impaired in older persons secondary to the shrinking amino acid reservoir that results from the replacement of lean muscle mass with fat.[115] However, elderly patients also have a significant intolerance for protein administration despite standard calculation of their needs.[116] The inaccuracy in standard formulae probably arises from the relatively lower lean body mass, and calculation of the basal energy expenditure (BEE) should be modified to compensate for the age-related changes. The Harris-Benedict equation, which does incorporate an age factor, accurately predicts BEE when a correction factor of 1.75 is used for trauma or 1.5 for general surgery patients.

Altered Response to Pain and Temperature

Neurosensory responses to stress are also altered in elderly patients, and this is particularly evident in the perception of pain and in the maintenance of body temperature. The elderly frequently demonstrate a lowered perception of pain, which complicates the diagnosis of abdominal surgical disease. Peptic ulcer disease, for example, may be associated with diminished or even absent pain in as many as a third of elderly patients.[117] Moreover, when analgesics are given, a lowered dose is frequently required (see Changes in Body Composition), as the unwanted effect of respiratory depression is not reduced.[118] Pulse oximetry is always an appropriate monitoring aid when narcotic analgesic agents are used in older patients.

Diminished sensation of cold and an impaired sensitivity to temperature changes are causes of altered thermoregulation in the elderly.[119] Altered autonomic vasoconstrictor responses to cold may contribute to a basal core temperature as low as 35° C in older individuals. Decreased thermogenesis secondary to reduced lean body mass with concomitant decreased basal metabolic rate, and a variety of coexisting endocrine and metabolic conditions including hypothyroidism and hypoglycemia, may also increase the risk of hypothermia. In the operating room the use of body warmers, head covers, and warmed irrigation fluids are helpful to avoid the risk of hypothermia in elderly patients. The most significant immediate complications of severe hypothermia (below 32° C) are arrhythmias and cardiorespiratory arrest. The ECG may show a characteristic J wave or Osborn wave following the QRS complex, which disappears when the hypothermia is reversed.[120]

Just as hypothermia represents a failure to compensate for ambient low temperatures in the elderly, hyperthermia may reflect an inability to increase evaporative heat loss in the setting of high external temperature. The inability to generate a fever in response to a serious infection is another manifestation of altered thermoregulation in the older patient. Whereas younger individuals can mount a fever in response to relatively minor infections or inflammatory processes, the elderly patient may lack a febrile response to even suppurative peritonitis.[121] When fever does occur in an elderly patient, it usually implies a significant pathologic process and should never be ignored.

Altered Wound Healing

The response to a wound is also a form of reaction to the environment and represents an attempt to preserve or restore physical homeostasis. This response involves the complex interaction of systemic and local immune processes and tissue repair processes, and both sets of events can be impaired in elderly patients.[122] In addition, impaired wound healing is associated with nutritional deficiencies and other disease states that cause tissue hypoxia, all of which occur with increasing frequency in older persons. Unfortunately, because normal wound healing requires such a complex constellation of coordinated events, actual data confirming the changes associated with increased aging per se are few. In one study of experimental wounding in healthy volunteers, epithelialization was delayed in older patients compared to younger patients, but collagen content of the wounds appeared equal. The accumulation of noncollagenous proteins, however, was decreased in the older group.[123]

When immune responsiveness is enhanced in elderly subjects, as with the oral administration of arginine, cellular and chemical parameters of wound healing are also enhanced.[124] Other strategies to enhance wound healing in the elderly are presently under investigation. These include the restoration of protein-calorie balance and the induction of endogenous growth factor synthesis, such as IGF-1, by GH administration.

Increased Vulnerability to Disease

Alterations in the Immune System

Immune competence, like other physiologic parameters, declines with advancing age. This immunosenescence is characterized by an increase in susceptibility to infections, an increase in autoantibodies and monoclonal immunoglobulins, and an increase in tumorigenesis. Also like other physiologic systems, this decline may not be apparent in the nonchallenged state. For example, there is no decline in neutrophil count with age, but the ability of the bone marrow to increase neutrophil production in response to infection may be impaired.[125] Elderly patients with major infections frequently have normal white blood cell counts, but the differential count shows a profound shift to the left, with a large proportion of immature forms. Although the study of immunosenescence in humans is complicated by the increasing prevalence of other diseases, the inability to effectively sample all the elements of the immune system, and the inability to separate environmental from biologic effects, several specific changes have been defined.

The most consistent of the changes in the immune system with age are the involution of the thymus gland and the decline in the production of thymic polypeptide factors such as thymosin α_1.[126] This and other thymic hormones control the differentiation and proliferation of thymocytes into mature T lymphocytes. T-cell proliferation[127] and IL-2 production[128] in response to stimulation have been shown to decrease with increasing age, and diminished T-cell responsiveness to a variety of antigens has been demonstrated in studies using skin tests.[129]

B-cell defects have not been as clearly established, although it is thought that the functional deficits are related to altered T-cell regulation[125] rather than to intrinsic B-cell changes. The mix of immunoglobulins, however, does change: IgM levels decrease while IgG and IgA increase slightly. There is also a significant rise in the prevalence of monoclonal immunoglobulins to more than 10% in the population of people over age 80.[130] There is also an increase in the prevalence of autoantibodies, but this does not appear to correlate with overt clinical disease.

Changes in the immune system with aging are similar to those seen in chronic inflammation and cancer. In addition to the reduced mitogenic responses of T cells, there is an increase in the levels of "acute phase" proteins. It is hypothesized that persistently elevated levels of inflammatory cytokines may be responsible for downregulation of IL-2 production by chronically stimulated T cells.[125]

The clinical manifestations of these changes are difficult to ascertain because the increased susceptibility to many infectious agents is more likely a result of comorbid disease than of physiologic decline. There is no good evidence to support the contention that immunosenescence alone is responsible for the observation that older patients are more likely to contract an infectious illness and less able to eradicate it quickly. However, the decline in physiologic reserve of other organ systems combined with comorbid illnesses may make recovery prolonged and more difficult.

Oncogenesis

There is a clear increase in most common cancers in people older than age 65, and two thirds of all cancer deaths occur in this age group. The increased incidence of cancer in the elderly is related to several biologic factors including longer exposure to environmental carcinogens, increased susceptibility of cells to carcinogens, decreased immune surveillance of abnormal cells, and abnormalities in the rate of occurrence or repair of acquired DNA damage. Alterations in the expression or amplification of oncogenes or tumor suppressor genes may play a role in oncogenesis and in the aging process itself. The biologic basis for both oncogenesis and aging may be more closely related than was previously realized.[131]

Aging is characterized by a general decrease in cellular proliferative capacity, as discussed earlier. Some age-related illnesses, including prostatic hypertrophy and early atherosclerosis, may represent disease processes characterized by hyperproliferation of certain cell types. This altered control of cell-specific proliferation may be genetically programmed or acquired but contributes to the limits of life span for that species. Although neoplasia frequently occurs in actively dividing cells, it also occurs in nonreplicating tissues. This suggests that factors that determine replicating capacity (and life span) may be directly and indirectly linked to those processes that regulate oncogenesis. Experimental evidence for this proposal is still incomplete, but interesting evidence for a reciprocal relationship between cellular aging and oncogenesis is found in animal studies of caloric restriction. In this model of maximal life span prolongation in mammalian species, the extension of average life span is accompanied by a decrease in the occurrence of neoplasia.[132]

As the gene pool represented by the older population continues to enlarge, the increased occurrence of late programmed events may result in a greater-than-expected incidence of cellular alterations (malignancy) linked to the end of the predetermined replicative cycle. This may explain the disproportionate increase in malignant diseases in older persons. In addition, there are several specific mechanisms whereby the aging process may contribute to malignant transformation.

First, it is possible that aging or the passage of time simply allows the accumulation of a required sequence of cellular events to transform cells. Second, there may be increased susceptibility in aging to exposure to carcinogens. Third, it has been shown that DNA damage once incurred is repaired less efficiently or less completely in aged cells. This may explain why increased karyotypic abnormalities are seen in both normal elderly subjects and in patients with malignancies. Fourth, activation or amplification of oncogenes may be greater in the older subject. An increased amplification of protogenes has been documented in aging fibroblasts,[133] and c-*myc* transcript levels are increased in aging mouse livers.[134] Alternatively, cancer suppressor genes may be inactivated, as p53 has been shown to be altered in both tumorigenesis and in senescence.[135] Fifth, although a loss of immune surveillance has been implicated in some tumors, it remains uncertain whether this is a common aging effect that facilitates tumorigenesis.

Finally, in addition to specific effects of cellular aging on oncogenesis, other aspects of the aged host may alter the natural history of the tumor or the response to specific treatments. In esophageal and lung cancer, for example, more favorable histologic types occur with increased frequency in the older age group, and prognosis is frequently better than in younger patients. Cancer treatment may need to be adjusted to compensate for comorbid illness, but data defining appropriate drug regimens and dosing schedules for elderly patients with most types of cancer are lacking.

PREOPERATIVE EVALUATION, RISK ASSESSMENT, AND OUTCOME

In keeping with previous discussions of risk assessment, we refer to risk primarily as the chance of postoperative mortality and morbidity. Risk in the elderly, however, should also be assessed in terms of restoration of preoperative functional status and quality of life, since survival is not necessarily the only important issue for patients in this age group. Preoperative assessment of risk in the elderly must provide an accurate assessment of the extent of physiologic decline and the presence of other coexisting disease processes. This does not necessarily require an extensive evaluation of each separate system. An assessment of functional status, nutritional status, cognitive function, and level of psychosocial support is frequently all that is necessary to evaluate risk and formulate a postoperative recovery plan.

Although the physiologic changes that accompany aging are myriad, the impact of these changes on the outcome of uncomplicated elective surgery in otherwise healthy, functional older patients is minimal. As a result of these physiologic alterations, however, the response to the surgical disease in the elderly is frequently "atypical." The lack of the classic signs and symptoms of disease often leads to delays and errors in diagnosis, which result in the increased need for "acute" surgical intervention. In one series of patients older than age 70, emergency operation carried a 10-fold higher mortality rate than the elective rate of 1.9%.[136] Almost regardless of the type of procedure, emergency surgery is associated with at least a threefold increase in mortality and morbidity. It is also associated with a higher rate of long-term hospital stay (>30 days), greater need for postoperative intensive care, and larger decline in functional status with consequent increase in the need for nursing home placement.[137]

Assessment of Comorbid Illnesses

Although physiologic decline may impair the ability of the elderly patient to compensate appropriately for the additional stress of complicated or emergency surgery, it is the presence of comorbid illnesses, or pathologic processes other than the primary surgical disease, that is the most important determinant of surgical outcome. Comorbidity has been implicated both in the development of acute disease and in increased surgical mortality and morbidity. For example, Boyd et al.[138] studied the impact of comorbidity on the mortality from colon surgery in 357 patients older than age 50. The preoperative incidence of additional pathologic conditions other than the primary surgical disease rose steadily with age, such that by age 80 only 5% of patients had no comorbid illnesses (Tables 67-8 and 67-9). In patients older than age 70, the mortality rate rose in association with the number of comorbid conditions from 1.5% with zero to one condition to 16% with two or more. A similar increase in mortality was observed in patients younger than age 70, and age as an isolated factor was seen to have no effect on mortality.

Unfortunately, as is the case with the surgical disease itself, the manifestations of these cormorbid illnesses in the

Table 67-8. Prevalence of Preoperative Pathologic Conditions (%)

	Age (yr)				
Condition	**50-59**	**60-69**	**70-79**	**>80**	**Total**
Cardiovascular	36	52	57	85	53
Pulmonary	8	17	20	17	16
Renal	5	8	24	15	13
Hepatic	7	10	16	20	12
Nutritional	2	7	10	22	8
Other	13	18	21	20	18

From Boyd BJ, et al. Operative risk factors of colon resection in the elderly. Ann Surg 192:743, 1980. Reprinted with permission.

Table 67-9. Percent of Patients With Additional Preoperative Pathologic Conditions

No. of Additional Pathologic Conditions	Age (yr)				
	50-59	60-69	70-79	>80	Total
0	46	33	21	5	30
1	37	34	28	37	33
2	13	27	23	41	24
3 or more	3	8	22	15	11

From Boyd BJ, et al. Operative risk factors of colon resection in the elderly. Ann Surg 192:743, 1980. Reprinted with permission.

elderly are frequently less specific and less "typical" than they are in younger patients. Silent myocardial infarction, apathetic hyperthyroidism, moderate cognitive impairment, and malnutrition are among the many disorders that may not be apparent from initial history and physical examination. The search for comorbid illness must therefore be diligent. In one study of hospitalized patients older than age 70, 60% of moderate-to-severe cognitive deficits and 42% of similar nutritional deficits had been previously unrecognized by the primary caregiver.[139]

The identification of cardiac comorbidity is most important in the elderly surgical patient because cardiac events are the leading cause of perioperative complications and death. For this reason, preoperative evaluation of "cardiac risk" has been extensively studied. The American College of Cardiology and the American Heart Association Task Force on Practice Guidelines have published an in-depth set of guidelines for perioperative cardiovascular evaluation, which addresses all the major concerns.[140] Stratification of risk based on clinical factors and operative factors is discussed. More detailed applications of these strategies are discussed elsewhere in the text, and for elderly patients with known cardiac disease, rigorous workup may be necessary. For most other elderly patients, however, assessments of functional status and exercise tolerance are accurate predictors of outcome (see the following).

Assessment of General Health and Functional Status

For decades anesthesiologists have successfully predicted postoperative mortality in patients of all ages using the Dripp's American Society of Anesthesiology Physical Status Scale. This scale assigns patients to one of five categories depending on extent of underlying systemic disease. Using this scale Djokovic and Hedley-White[141] studied mortality in 500 consecutive surgical patients older than age 80. No patient in this study was classified as class 1 because age greater than or equal to 80 years is an exclusion criterion for this category. Mortality rate correlated well with the severity of illness, increasing from less than 1% in class 2 patients (mild systemic disease) to 25% in class 4 patients (incapacitating systemic disease). Class for class, these figures are similar to those seen in younger patients. These data support the concept that severity of illness and comorbidity rather than age alone are the significant factors in postoperative mortality.

Standard measures of functional status have also proven to be predictive of postoperative outcome. The ability to perform the activities of daily living or the simple tasks of life like feeding, continence, transferring, toileting, dressing and bathing, has been correlated with operative mortality and morbidity. In one study, patients identified as inactive (defined as unable to leave their homes as a result of their own efforts at least twice a week) were shown to have a higher incidence of all major surgical complications[142] (Fig. 67-9). In another study of noncardiac surgical cases, mortality in patients with severely limited activity (defined as bedridden or only able to transfer from bed to chair) was 9.7 times higher than in active patients. Of the risk factors studied, inactivity was found to be the single strongest predictor of death.[143]

Even for patients with less obvious limitations, functional capacity or exercise tolerance is the single most important predictor of cardiac complications following noncardiac surgery. In a study comparing Dripp's Scale, Goldman Clinical Criteria, noninvasive ventricular functional assessment, and exercise tolerance, Gerson et al.[144] demonstrated that the inability to raise the heart rate to 99 beats/min while doing 2 minutes of supine bicycle exercise was the most sensitive predictor of postoperative cardiac complications and death.

The physiologic basis for this finding has been further clarified by a study in which patients performed supine ergometry while connected by mouthpiece to a metabolic cart.[145] The authors identified an anaerobic threshold, defined as the level of oxygen consumption above which circulatory supply could not meet metabolic demand, and correlated this threshold with surgical outcome. For those patients able to reach an anaerobic threshold of 11 ml/kg/min or more the mortality was 0.8%, compared to 18% for those unable to reach this threshold. Even in patients with preoperative ischemia identified at the time of exercise testing, this threshold level was highly predictive of postoperative mortality (Table 67-10).

Should all preoperative elderly patients therefore be subjected to this type of exercise testing? Clearly this is neither practical or necessary. The metabolic requirements for many routine activities have already been determined and are quantitated as metabolic equivalents (METs). One MET, 3.5 ml/kg/min, is basal oxygen consumption or that amount of oxygen consumed by a 70 kg, 40-year-old man at rest. Estimated energy requirements for various activities are shown in Table 67-11. By asking appropriate questions about the level of activity, or by using a standardized self-assessment tool such as the Duke's Activity Status Index,[146] functional status can be determined. The inability to function above 4 METs has been associated with increased perioperative cardiac events and long-term risk.[135]

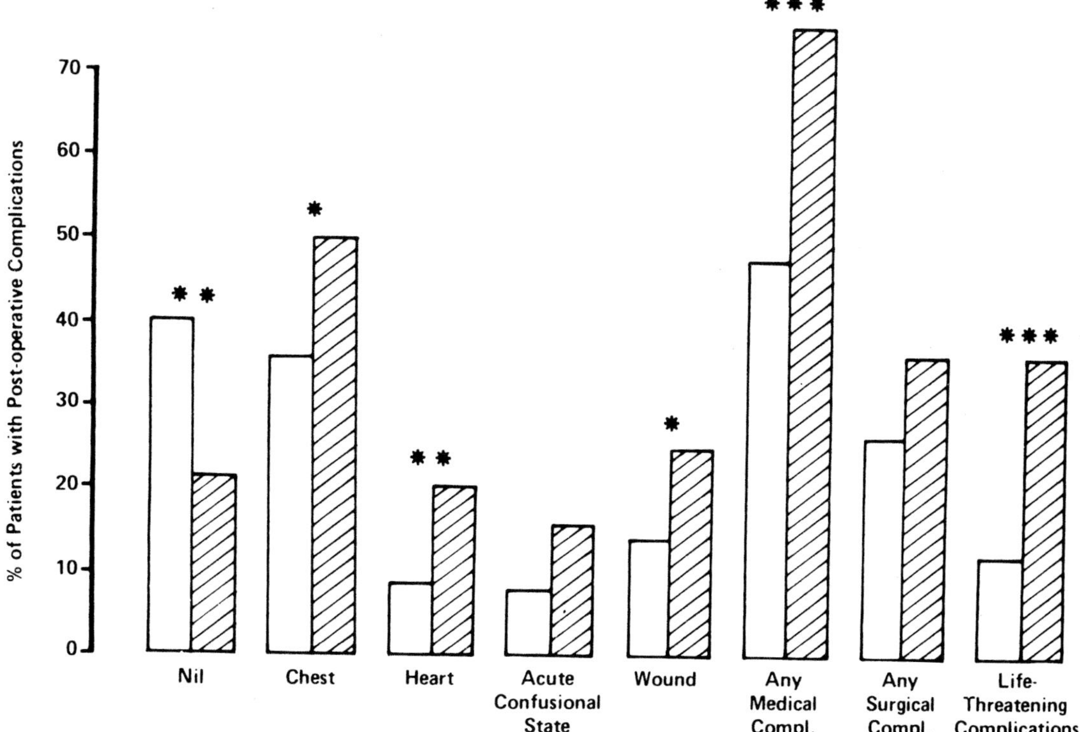

Fig. 67-9. Preoperative activity and postoperative complications. Solid bars represent active patients, cross-hatched bars represent inactive patients. Note all types of postoperative complications occur more frequently in inactive patients. *p < 0.05, **p < 0.01, ***p < 0.001. (From Seymour DB, Pringle R. Postoperative complications in elderly surgical patients. Gerontology 29:262,1983. Reprinted with permission.)

Table 67-10. Mortality Data: Anaerobic Threshold Higher Than and Lower Than 11 ml/min/kg

Anaerobic Threshold ml/min/kg	Total No. of Patients	Mortality (%)	No. With Ischemia	Mortality (%)
<11	55	18	19	42
>11	132	0.8	25	4
Totals	187	(p < 0.001)	44	(p < 0.01)

From Older P, et al. Preoperative evaluation of cardiac failure and ischemia in elderly patients by cardiopulmonary exercise testing. Chest 104:701, 1993. Reprinted with permission.

Table 67-11. Estimated Energy Requirements for Various Activities

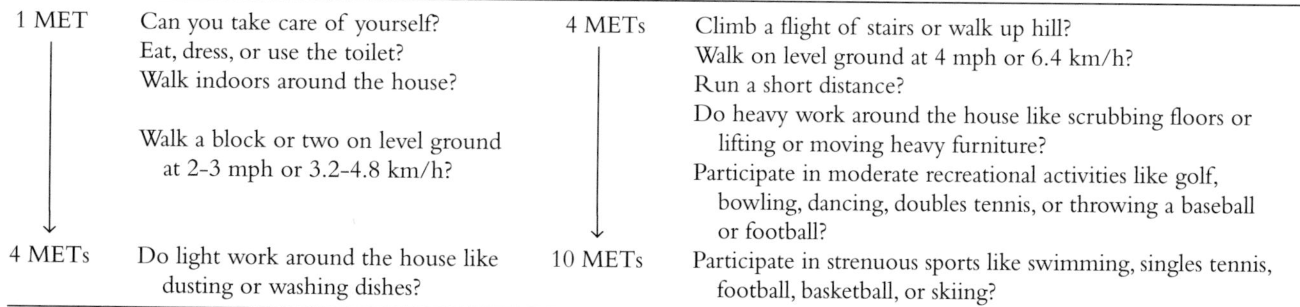

1 MET ↓	Can you take care of yourself? Eat, dress, or use the toilet? Walk indoors around the house? Walk a block or two on level ground at 2-3 mph or 3.2-4.8 km/h?	4 METs ↓	Climb a flight of stairs or walk up hill? Walk on level ground at 4 mph or 6.4 km/h? Run a short distance? Do heavy work around the house like scrubbing floors or lifting or moving heavy furniture? Participate in moderate recreational activities like golf, bowling, dancing, doubles tennis, or throwing a baseball or football?
4 METs	Do light work around the house like dusting or washing dishes?	10 METs	Participate in strenuous sports like swimming, singles tennis, football, basketball, or skiing?

From Eagle KA, et al. Guidelines for perioperative cardiovascular evaluation for noncardiac surgery. Circulation 93:1279, 1996. Reprinted with permission.

MET, Metabolic equivalent.

Other nonspecific indexes have recently been shown to predict poor outcome and mortality in elderly patients with a wide variety of medical and surgical illnesses. Among these, low levels of serum albumin have emerged as an independent and sensitive predictor of increased length of stay, increased rates of readmission, unfavorable disposition, and increased all-cause mortality.[147] Whether this finding is related to poor nutritional status or unidentified complex chronic illness has not been clarified. In surgical patients, low albumin also correlates with operative morbidity and mortality.[148]

In addition, preoperative cognitive impairment has been shown to have a similar, although far less well-defined, negative impact on many surgical outcomes. It has been suggested that the increased operative mortality seen in this group of patients is related, in part, to delays in diagnosis.[149] Postoperative delirium has also been associated with an increased incidence of complications[150] and a poorer long-term functional outcome in orthopedic patients.[151]

Overall Outcome

Since 1967 there has been a clear decline in the overall surgical mortality in older age groups[140] (Fig. 67-10), even for the highest risk operations like aneurysmorraphy and major cancer resections. Overall long-term survival does not appear to be adversely affected by the need for surgical intervention, even in patients older than age 90[152] (Fig. 67-11).

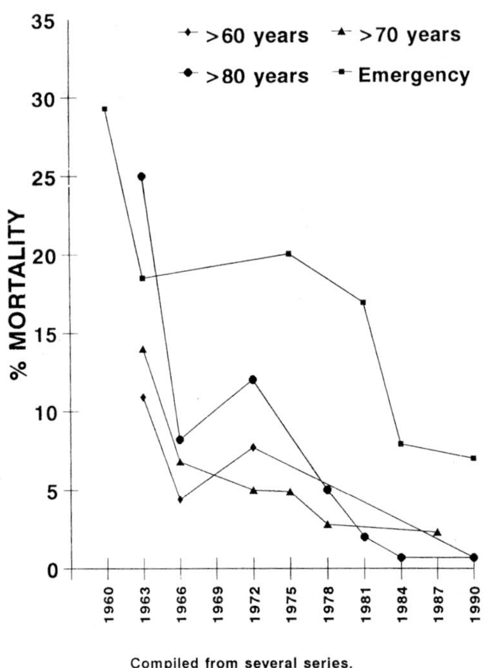

Fig. 67-10. Decline in surgical mortality during the past four decades. (From Thomas DR, Ritchie CS. Preoperative assessment of older adults. J Am Geriatr Soc 43:211, 1995. Reprinted with permission.)

Data regarding the functional outcome and return to the same (or better) preoperative status are available primarily for procedures that directly address improving these outcomes such as total joint replacement and aortic valve replacement. For other procedures the data are less clear. In the SUPPORT study (*s*tudy to *u*nderstand *p*rognoses and *p*references for *t*reatment), designed to develop a model to predict outcome in seriously ill medical and surgical patients, prior ability to perform the activities of daily living was the most important predictor of functional outcome.[153]

Further clarification of the factors that may have impact on the outcomes of death, nursing home placement, and total hospital days in patients with medical or surgical illnesses can be found in a study of 12 conditions common in the geriatric population.[154] These "geriatric targeting criteria" include socioeconomic problems, vision impairment, hearing impairment, appetite loss, weight loss, incontinence, confusion, depression, dementia, falls, and prolonged bed rest. In this prospective study of 507 acutely ill male veterans, older than age 65, only confusion was associated with all three negative outcomes. Weight loss was the strongest predictor of death, although appetite loss, depression, falls, and socioeconomic problems were also significantly associated. Polypharmacy and prolonged bed rest predicted nursing home placement, and falls and prolonged bed rest were associated with increased total hospital days.

The elderly are also more susceptible to the sequela of the surgical intervention that may not be directly related to the operative procedure itself. Bed rest, for example, is associated with a variety of physiologic changes that can have great impact on an elderly patient's ability to recover from the surgical insult. In addition to the well-known se-

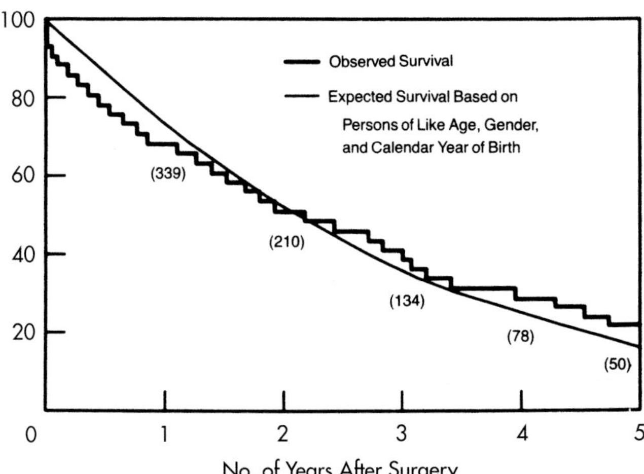

Fig. 67-11. Postoperative survival in patients 90 years and older. (From Hosking MP, et al. Outcomes of surgery in patients 90 years of age and older. JAMA 261:1909,1989. Reprinted with permission.)

quela such as pressure ulcers, deep venous thrombosis, and muscle wasting, inactivity can quickly lead to deconditioning, which itself can be considered an illness different from the original surgical disease. The deconditioned patient demonstrates changes in multiple organ systems: depression and lethargy; anorexia and dehydration; neuromuscular instability, decreased bone density, muscular weakness, and incoordination; and altered bladder and bowel function with retention and constipation, and urinary and fecal incontinence. Once these changes occur, the road back to independent functioning is all uphill. It is estimated that in severely deconditioned patients the time to recovery can be three times the length of the period of inactivity.[155]

In a recent study of hospitalized elderly medical patients, initial admission to a special care unit that emphasized a multidisciplinary approach to assessment and treatment was found to have a positive effect on the outcomes of maintenance of independence and discharge to home.[156] Similar studies of surgical patients are not yet available. It is likely, however, that careful attention to the assessment and treatment of elderly surgical patients in a multidisciplinary manner that emphasizes early recognition of surgical disease and comorbidity and addresses deficits appropriately will have equally beneficial results.

SUMMARY

In the next 50 years the portion of the population older than age 65 is expected to grow from the present 12.5% to 20% or more, encompassing nearly 80 million people. This being the case, it is incumbent on the surgeon to have a comprehensive understanding of the physiologic changes that occur with aging and how these could potentially impact on the outcome from a surgical procedure. Several important changes occur in body composition including a reduction in lean body mass and the expansion of the extracellular compartment. Recognizing these body compositional changes ensures the appropriate use of drugs and fluids. Aging is also associated with specific changes in cellular function affecting cardiac, pulmonary, and renal responses to stress, which could impact adversely on perioperative management. Recognition of these changes enables appropriate risk assessment preoperatively. Altered responses to pain and temperature control and wound healing are likewise commonly encountered in elderly patients and can influence both preoperative diagnosis of surgical disease and postoperative complications. Accordingly, knowledge of this information in the older patient pays rich dividends in ensuring appropriate risk assessment preoperatively, precise management intraoperatively, and a smooth postoperative course. Although postoperative recovery and rehabilitation may sometimes be prolonged in elderly patients, returning these individuals to a functioning state after being subjected to surgical illness is an achievable goal.

REFERENCES

1. Day JC. Population projections of the United States by age, sex, race and Hispanic origin: 1993-2050. Current Population Reports. U.S. Department of Commerce Bureau of the Census. Population Report P25-1104, 1993.
2. U.S. Department of Health and Human Services: Health data on older Americans: United States, 1992, Vital and Health Statistics Series 3, No. 27.
3. Peebles RJ, Schneidman DS, eds. Socio-Economic Factbook for Surgery 1996. Chicago: The American College of Surgeons, 1996.
4. Cristafalo VJ, Gerhard GS, Pignolo RJ. Molecular biology of aging. Surg Clin North Am 74:1, 1994.
5. Gompertz B. On the nature of the function expressive of the law of human mortality and on a new mode of determining life contingencies. Philos Trans R Soc Lond 115:513, 1825.
6. Greville TNE. U.S. life tables by cause of death. U.S. Decennial Life Tables for 1969-1971 1:5.
7. Rhome D. Evidence for a relationship between longevity of mammalian species and life spans of normal fibroblasts in vitro and erythrocytes in vivo. Proc Natl Acad Sci U S A 78:5009, 1981.
8. Gorman SD, Cristafalo VJ. Reinitiation of cellular DNA synthesis in Brd U-selected nondividing senescent cells by similar virus 40 infection. J Cell Physiol 125:122, 1985.
9. Shay JW, Pereira-Smith OM, Wright WE. A role for both RB and p53 in the regulation of human cellular senescence. Exp Cell Res 196:33,1991.
10. Yu BP, Masoro EJ, McMahon CA. Nutritional influences in aging of Fischer 344 rats. I. Physical, metabolic, and longevity characteristics. J Gerontol 40:664, 1985.
11. Morley AA. Is aging the result of dominant or co-dominant mutations? J Theor Biol 98:469, 1982.
12. Lindop PJ, Rotblat J. Long term effect of a single whole-body exposure of mice to ionizing radiations. Proc R Soc Lond 154:350, 1961.
13. Hart RW, Setlow RB. Correlation between deoxyribonucleic acid excision-repair and lifespan in a number of mammalian species. Proc Natl Acad Sci U S A 71:2169, 1974.
14. Hanawalt PC, Gee P, Ho L. DNA repair in differentiating cells in relation to aging. In Finch CE, Johnson TE, eds. Molecular Biology of Aging. UCLA Symposium on Molecular and Cellular Biology, vol 123. New York: Alan R Liss, 1990.
15. Goldman R. Decline in organ function with aging. In Rossman I, ed. Clinical Geriatrics, 2nd ed. Philadelphia: JB Lippincott, 1979.
16. Reiser KM, Hennessey SM, Last JA. Analysis of age-associated changes in collagen cross linking in the skin and lung in monkeys and rats. Biochim Biophys Acta 926:339, 1987.
17. Bjorksten J. Cross linkage and the aging process. In Rothstein M, ed. Theoretical Aspects of Aging. New York: Academic Press, 1974.
18. Harman D. Aging: A theory based on free radical and radiation chemistry. J Gerontol 11:298, 1956.
19. Elahi VK, et al. A longitudinal study of nutritional intake in man. J Gerontol 38:162, 1983.
20. Vin SC, Love AGH. Nutritional status of institutionalized and noninstitutionalized aged in Belfast, Northern Ireland. Am J Clin Nutr 32:1934, 1979.
21. Rudman D, et al. Effect of human growth hormone in men over 60 years old. N Engl J Med 323:1, 1990.
22. Timiras P. Aging of the skeleton, joints and muscles. In Timiras PS, ed. Physiological Basis of Aging and Geriatrics. Boca Raton, Fla.: CRC Press, 1994.
23. Tzankoff SP, Norris AH. Effect of muscle mass decrease on age-related BMR changes. J Appl Physiol 43:1001, 1977.
24. Shock NW. Energy metabolism, caloric intake, and physical activity in the aging. In Carlson LA, ed. Nutrition in Old Age, Symposia of the Swedish Nutrition Foundation, 10. Uppsala: Almquist & Wiksell, 1972.

25. Shimokata H, et al. Studies on the distribution of body fat. I. Effects of age, sex, and obesity. J Gerontol 44:M66, 1989.
26. Andres R. Mortality and obesity: The rationale for age-specific height-weight tables. In Hazzard WR, et al. Principles of Geriatric Medicine and Gerontology, 3rd ed. New York: McGraw-Hill, 1994.
27. McLeskey CH. Anesthesia for the elderly patient. In Barash PG, Cullen BF, Stoelting RK, eds. Clinical Anesthesia, 2nd ed. Philadelphia: JB Lippincott, 1992.
28. Homer TD, Stanski DR. The effect of increasing age on the disposition and anesthetic requirement. Anesthesiology 62:114, 1985.
29. Buxbaum JL, Schwartz AJ. Perianesthetic consideration for the elderly patient. In Zenilman ME, Roslyn JJ, eds. Surgery in the elderly patient. Surg Clin North Am 74:41, 1994.
30. Kitzman DW, Edwards WD. Minireview: Age-related changes in the anatomy of the normal human heart. J Gerontol 45:M33, 1990.
31. Lakatta EG, et al. Human aging: Changes in structure and function. J Am Coll Cardiol 10:42A, 1987.
32. Nixon JV, et al. Ventricular performance in human hearts aged 61-73 years. Am J Cardiol 56:932, 1991.
33. Davies MJ. Pathology of the conducting system. In Caird FL, Dalle JLC, Kennedy RD, eds. Cardiology in Old Age. New York: Plenum Press, 1976.
34. Sahasaku Y, et al. Age-related changes in aortic and mitral valve thickness: Implications for two-dimensional echocardiography based on an autopsy study of 200 normal human hearts. Am J Cardiol 62:424, 1988.
35. Kitzman et al. Age-related changes in normal human hearts during the first ten decades. II. Maturity: A quantitative anatomic study of 765 specimens from subjects 20-99 years old. Mayo Clin Proc 63:137, 1988.
36. Lakatta EG. Cardiovascular regulatory mechanisms in advanced age. Physiol Rev 73:413, 1993.
37. Yin FCP. The aging vasculature and its effect on the heart. In Weisfeldt ML, ed. The Aging Heart: Its Function and Response to Stress, vol 12. Aging. New York: Raven Press, 1980.
38. Lewis JF, Maron BJ. Cardiovascular consequences of the aging process. In Lowenthal DT, ed. Geriatric Cardiology, vol 22. Cardiovascular Clinics. Philadelphia: FA Davis, 1992.
39. Lachi RJ, et al. Left ventricular function in hospitalized geriatric patients. J Am Geriatr Soc 30:700, 1982.
40. Manning WJ, et al. Reversal of changes in left ventricular diastolic filling associated with normal aging using diltiazem. Am J Cardiol 67:894, 1991.
41. Wei JY. Age and the cardiovascular system. N Engl J Med 327:1735, 1992.
42. Wei JY. Use of calcium entry blockers in elderly patients: Special considerations. Circulation 80(Suppl IV):171, 1989.
43. Tresch DD, McGough MF. Heart failure with normal systolic function: A common disorder in older people. J Am Geriatr Soc 43:1035, 1995.
44. Wenger NK. Cardiovascular disease. In Cassel CK, et al., eds. Geriatric Medicine, 2nd ed. New York: Springer-Verlag, 1990.
45. Timiras PS. Aging of the respiration, erythrocytes, and the hematopoietic system. In Timiras PS, ed. Physiological Basis of Aging and Geriatrics. Boca Raton, Fla.: CRC Press, 1988.
46. Pfitzenmeyer P, et al. Lung function in advanced age: Study of ambulatory subjects aged over 75 years. Gerontology 39:267, 1993.
47. Tockman MS. Aging of the respiratory system. In Katlic MR, ed. Geriatric Surgery. Baltimore: Urban & Schwarzenberg, 1990.
48. Kronenberg RS, Drage CW. Attenuation of the ventilatory and heart rate responses to hypoxia and hypercapnia with aging in men. J Clin Invest 52:1812, 1973.
49. Bartlett JG. Pneumonia. In Andres R, Bierman EL, Hazzard WR, eds. Principles of Geriatric Medicine. New York: McGraw-Hill, 1985.
50. Lindeman RD. Overview: Renal physiology and pathophysiology of aging. Am J Kidney Dis 16:275, 1990.
51. Cockroft DW, Gault MH. Prediction of creatinine clearance from serum creatinine. Nephron 16:31, 1976.
52. Macias Nunez JF, et al. Physiology and disorders of water balance and electrolytes in the elderly. In Macias Nunez JF, Cameron JS, eds. Renal Function and Disease in the Elderly. Stoneham, Mass.: Butterworth, 1987.
53. Tsundo K, et al. Effect of aging on the renin-angiotensin-aldosterone system in normal subjects: Simultaneous measurement of active and inactive renin, renin substrate and aldosterone in plasma. J Clin Endrocrinol Metab 62:384, 1986.
54. Rowe JW, et al. The influence of age on urinary concentrating ability in man. Nephron 17:270, 1976.
55. Phillips PA, et al. Reduced thirst after water deprivation in healthy elderly men. N Engl J Med 12:753, 1984.
56. Mukherjee AP, Coni NK, Davidson W. Osmoreceptor function among the elderly. Gerontol Clin 15:227, 1973.
57. Lindeman RD. Changes in renal function with aging: Implications for treatment. Drugs Aging 2:423, 1992.
58. Susset JG, et al. Collagen in 155 human bladders. Invest Urol 16:204, 1978.
59. Brocklehurst JC, Dilane JB. Studies of the female bladder in old age. I. Cystometricograms in non-incontinent women. Gerontol Clin 10:242, 1968.
60. Mohide EA. Prevalence and scope of urinary incontinence. Clin Geriatr Med 2:639, 1986.
61. Esposito AL, et al. Community acquired bacteremia in the elderly: Analysis of one hundred consecutive episodes. J Am Geriatr Soc 28:315, 1980.
62. Mooney H, et al. Alterations in the liver with aging. Clin Gastroenterol 14:757, 1985.
63. Kampmann JP, Sinding J, Moller-Jorgenson I. Effect of age on liver function. Geriatrics 30:91, 1975.
64. Schmucker DL. Aging and drug disposition: An update. Pharmacol Rev 37:133, 1985.
65. Shepherd MM, et al. Age as a determinant of sensitivity to warfarin. Br J Clin Pharmacol 4:315, 1977.
66. Sampliner RE, et al. Gallbladder disease in Pima Indians. Demonstration of prevalence and early onset by cholecystography. N Engl J Med 283:1358, 1979.
67. Simonivis NJ, Wells CK, Feinstein AR. In-vivo and post-mortem gallstones: Support for the validity of the "epidemiologic necropsy" screening technique. Am J Epidemiol 133:922, 1991.
68. The Rome Group for the Epidemiology and Prevention of Cholelithiasis (GREPCO). The epidemiology of gallstone disease in Rome, Italy. I. Prevalence in men. Hepatology 8:904, 1988.
69. Ratner J, et al. The prevalence of gallstone disease in very old institutionalized persons. JAMA 265:902, 1991.
70. Graves EJ. 1993 summary: National hospital discharge survey. CDC Advanced Data No. 246, 1995.
71. Trotman BW, Sotoway RD. Pigment vs cholesterol cholelithiasis: Clinical epidemiological aspects. Dig Dis 20:735, 1975.
72. Bateson MC. Gallbladder disease and cholecystectomy are independently variable. Lancet 2:621, 1984.
73. Bowen JC, et al. Gallstone disease: Pathophysiology, epidemiology, natural history, and treatment options. Med Clin North Am 76:1143, 1992.
74. Einarsson K, et al. Influence of age on secretion of cholesterol and synthesis of bile acids by the liver. N Engl J Med 313:277, 1985.
75. Carey MC. Pathogenesis of gallstones. Am J Surg 165:410, 1993.
76. Khalil T, et al. Decreased gallbladder responsiveness to CCK-8 in aged rabbits. Gastroenterology 86:1134, 1984.
77. Poston GJ, et al. Effect of age and sensitivity to cholecystokinin on gallstone formation in the guinea pig. Gastroenterology 98:993, 1990.
78. Khalil T, et al. Effects of aging on gallbladder contraction and release of cholecystokinin-33 in humans. Surgery 98:423, 1985.

79. Berger D, et al. Effects of age on fasting plasma levels of pancreatic polypeptide in man. J Clin Endocrinol Metab 47:1183, 1978.
80. Brunicardi FC, et al. Regulation of pancreatic polypeptide secretion in the isolated perfused human pancreas. Am J Surg 155:63, 1988.
81. Rosenthal RA, Andersen DK. Surgery in the elderly: Observations on the pathophysiology and treatment of cholelithiasis. Exp Gerontol 28:459, 1993.
82. Escarce JJ, et al. Outcomes of open cholecystectomy in the elderly: A longitudinal analysis of 21,00 cases in the prelaparoscopic era. Surgery 117:156, 1995.
83. Wenckhert A, Robertson B. The natural history of gallstone disease. Gastroenterology 50:376, 1966.
84. Morrow DJ, Thompson J, Wislon SE. Acute cholecystitis in the elderly. A surgical emergency. Arch Surg 113;1149, 1978.
85. Lipschitz DA, et al. The use of long term marrow culture as a model for the aging process. Age 6:122, 1983.
86. Reincke U, et al. Proliferative capacity of murine hematopoietic stem cells in vitro. Science 215:1619, 1983.
87. Albright JA, Makinodan T. Decline in the growth potential of spleen-colonizing bone marrow stem cells of long lived aging mice. J Exp Med 144:1204, 1976.
88. Lipschitz DA. Aging of the hematopoietic system. In Hazzard WR, ed. Principles of Geriatric Medicine and Gerontology, 3rd ed. New York: McGraw-Hill, 1994.
89. Lipschitz DA, et al. Evidence that microenvironmental factors account for the age-related decline in neutrophil function. Blood 70:1131, 1987.
90. Evers BM, Townsend CM, Thompson JC. Organ physiology of aging. Surg Clin North Am 74:23, 1994.
91. Simpkins JW, Millard WJ. Influence of age or neurotransmitter function. Endocrinol Metab Clin North Am 16:893, 1987.
92. Khansari DN, Gustad T. Effect of long term, low dose growth hormone therapy on immune function and life expectancy of mice, Mech Ageing Dev 57:87, 1991.
93. Forster JA, et al. Effect of age and IGF-I administration on elastin gene expression in rat aorta. J Gerontol 45:B113, 1990.
94. Burrows V, Shenkman L. Thyroid function in the elderly. Am J Med Sci 283:8, 1982.
95. Ronnov V, Kirkegaard C. Hyperthyroidism—A disease of old age? Br Med J 1:41, 1973.
96. Norton JA, Levin B, Jensen RT. Cancer of the endocrine system. In DeVita VT Jr, Hellman S, Rosenberg SA, eds. Cancer: Principles and Practice of Oncology, 4th ed. Philadelphia: JB Lippincott, 1993.
97. Potts JT, et al. Diagnosis and management of asymptomatic primary hyperparathyroidism: Consensus development conference statement. Ann Intern Med 114:593, 1991.
98. Chan AK, et al. Clinical manifestations of primary hyperparathyroidism before and after parathyroidectomy. Ann Surg 222:402, 1995.
99. Davidson MB. The effect of aging on carbohydrate metabolism: A review of the English literature and a practical approach to the diagnosis of diabetes mellitus in the elderly. Metabolism 28:688, 1979.
100. Soergel K, Zboralske F, Amberg J. Presbyesophagus: Esophageal motility in nongenarian. J Clin Invest 43:1472, 1964.
101. Khalil T, Poston GJ, Thompson JC. Effects of aging on gastrointestinal hormones. In Prinsley DM, Shustead HH, eds. Progress in Clinical and Biological Research, Nutrition, and Aging, vol 326. New York: Alan R Liss, 1990.
102. Bonnevie O. The incidence of duodenal ulcer in Copenhagen County. Scand J Gastroenterol 10:385, 1975.
103. Kurata JH, Honda GD, Frankl H. The incidence of duodenal and gastric ulcers in a large health maintenance organization. Am J Public Health 75:625, 1985.
104. Kim SW, et al. Effect of aging on duodenal bicarbonate secretion. Ann Surg 212:332, 1990.
105. Koruda MJ, Sheldon GF. Surgery in the aged. Adv Surg 24:293, 1991.
106. Geokas M, Conteas C, Majumdai A. The aging gastrointestinal tract, liver, and pancreas. Clin Geriatr Med 1:177, 1985.
107. Kreel L, Sandlin B. Changes in pancreatic morphology associated with aging. Gut 14:962, 1973.
108. McEvoy A. Investigation of intestinal malabsorption in the elderly. In Evans J, Caird F, eds. Advanced Geriatric Medicine. London: Pittman, 1982.
109. Browder W, et al. Acute pancreatitis of unknown etiology in the elderly. Ann Surg 217:469, 1993.
110. Pan HY, et al. Decline in beta adrenergic receptor-mediated vascular relaxation with aging in man. J Pharmacol Exp Ther 239:802, 1986.
111. Lakatta EG. Altered autonomic modulation of cardiovascular function with adult aging: Perspectives from studies ranging from man to cell. In Stone HL, Weglicki WB, eds. Pathobiology of Cardiovascular Injury. Boston: Nojhoff, 1985.
112. Vestal RE, et al. Reduced beta-adrenoreceptor sensitivity in the elderly. Clin Pharmacol Ther 26:181, 1979.
113. Feldman RD, et al. Alteration in leukocyte β-receptor affinity with aging: A potential explanation for altered β-adrenergic sensitivity in the elderly. N Engl J Med 310:815, 1984.
114. Arnetz BB. Endocrine reactions during standardized surgical stress: The effects of age and methods of anesthesia. Age Aging 14:96, 1985.
115. Rolandelli RH, Ulrich JR. Nutritional support of the frail elderly surgical patient. Surg Clin North Am 74:79, 1994.
116. Clevenger FW, et al. Protein and energy tolerance by stressed geriatric patients. J Surg Res 52:135, 1992.
117. Clinch D, Banerjee AK, Ostick G. Absence of abdominal pain in elderly patients with peptic ulcer. Age Aging 13:120, 1984.
118. Moore AK, et al. Differences in epidural morphine requirements between elderly and young patients after abdominal surgery. Anesth Analg 70:316, 1990.
119. Collins KJ, Exton-Smith AN. Thermal homeostasis in old age. J Am Geriatr Soc 31:519, 1983.
120. Wongsurwat N, et al. Thermoregulatory failure in the elderly. J Am Geriatr Soc 38:899, 1990.
121. Norman DC, et al. Fever and aging. J Am Geriatr Soc 33:859, 1985.
122. Mikinodan T, Kay MMB. Age influences the immune system. In Kunkel HG, Dixon FJ, eds. Advances in Immunology. New York: Academic Press, 1980.
123. Holt DR, et al. Effects of age on wound healing in healthy human beings. Surgery 112:293, 1992.
124. Kirk SJ, et al. Arginine stimulates wound healing and immune function in elderly human beings. Surgery 114:155, 1993.
125. Currie MS. Immunosenescence. Compr Ther 18:26, 1992.
126. Lewis VM, et al. Age, thymic involution and circulating thymic hormone activity. J Clin Endocrinol Metab 47:145, 1978.
127. Hefton JM, et al. Immunologic studies of aging. V. Impaired proliferation of PHA responsive human lymphocytes in culture. J Immunol 125:1007, 1980.
128. Ershler WB, et al. IL-2 and aging: Decreased IL-2 production in healthy older people does not correlate with reduced helper cell numbers or antibody response to influenza vaccine and is not corrected in vitro by thymosin α_1. Immunopharmacology 10:11, 1985.
129. Roberts-Thomson JC, et al. Aging, immune response and mortality. Lancet 2:368, 1974.
130. Crawford J, Eye MK, Cohen HJ. Evaluation of monoclonal gammopathies in the well elderly. Am J Med 82:39, 1987.
131. Cohen HJ. Biology of aging as related to cancer. Cancer 74:2092, 1994.
132. Weindruch R, Walford RL. The retardation of aging and disease by dietary restriction. Springfield, Ill.: Charles C Thomas, 1988.

133. Srivastava A, et al. C-Ha-ras-1 Protooncogenes amplification and over expression during the limited replicative lifespan of normal fibroblasts. J Biocommun 260:6404, 1985.
134. Matocha MF, et al. Selective elevation of c-myc transcript levels in the liver of the aging Fischer-344 rat. Biochem Biophys Res Commun 147:1, 1987.
135. Shay JW, Pereora DM, Wright WE. A role for both RB and p53 in the regulation of human cellular senescence. Exp Cell Res 196:33, 1991.
136. Keller SM, et al. Emergency and elective surgery in patients over age 70 years. Am Surg 53:636, 1987.
137. Zenilman ME. Confederations in surgery in the elderly. In Andersen DK, ed. Master Series in Surgery 2. Advances in Surgery in the Elderly. New York: World Medical Press, 1993.
138. Boyd BJ, et al. Operative risk factors of colon resection in the elderly. Ann Surg 192:743, 1980.
139. Pinholt EM, et al. Functional assessment of the elderly. A comparison of standard instruments with clinical judgment. Arch Intern Med 147:484, 1987.
140. Eagle KA, et al. ACC/AHA Task Force Report, guidelines for perioperative evaluation for noncardiac surgery. Circulation 93:1279, 1996.
141. Djokovic JL, Hedley-White J. Prediction of outcome of surgery and anesthesia in patients over 80. JAMA 242:2301, 1979.
142. Seymour DG, Pringle R. Post-operative complications in the elderly surgical patient. Gerontology 29:262, 1983.
143. Browner WS, Mangano DT. Inhospital and long-term mortality in male veterans following noncardiac surgery: The study of Perioperative Ischemia Research Group. JAMA 268:228, 1992.
144. Gerson MC, et al. Cardiac prognosis in noncardiac geriatric surgery. Ann Intern Med 103:832, 1985.
145. Older P, et al. Preoperative evaluation of cardiac function and ischemia in elderly patients by cardiopulmonary exercise testing. Chest 103:701, 1993.
146. Hlatky MA, et al. A brief-self-administered questionnaire to determine functional capacity (the Duke's Activity Status index). Am J Card 64:651, 1989.
147. Corti M, et al. Serum albumin level and physical disability as predictors of mortality in older persons. JAMA 272:1036, 1994.
148. Seltzer MH, et al. Instant nutritional assessment. JPEN 3:157, 1979.
149. Berstein GM, Offenbartl SK. Adverse surgical outcomes among patients with cognitive impairments. Am Surg 57:682, 1991.
150. Gustafson Y, Berggren D, Brannstrom B. Acute confusional states in elderly patients treated for femoral neck fractures. J Am Geriatr Soc 36:525, 1988.
151. Rogers MP, et al. Delirium after elective orthopedic surgery: Risk factors and natural history. Int J Psychiatry Med 19:109, 1989.
152. Hosking MP, et al. Outcomes of surgery in patients 90 years of age and older. JAMA 261:1909, 1989.
153. Wu AW, et al. Predicting future functional status for seriously ill hospitalized adults. The SUPPORT prognostic model. Ann Intern Med 122:342, 1995.
154. Satish S, et al. Geriatric targeting criteria as predictors of survival and health care utilization. J Am Geriatr Soc 44:914, 1996.
155. Rader MC, Vaughen JL. Management of the frail and deconditioned patient. Southern Med J 87:61, 1994.
156. Landefeld CS, et al. A randomized trial of care in a hospital medical unit especially designed to improve the functional outcome of acutely ill older patients. N Engl J Med 332:1338, 1995.

68

Surgery for Morbid Obesity

Robert E. Brolin

According to a study from the National Center for Health Statistics the percentage of adult Americans who are overweight increased by more than 8% during the past decade. This increase in the rate of obesity occurred in spite of the growing public awareness that obesity is associated with a number of other serious health problems. In 1985 the National Institutes of Health Consensus Development Panel concluded that obesity is a disease that adversely affects health and longevity.[1] The minimum criterion that defines "obesity" is a weight 20% in excess of desirable weight for a given height and sex as established by standard life insurance tables.[1-3] Obesity is now frequently defined in terms of the body mass index (BMI), which is expressed as the body weight in kilograms divided by the height in meters squared. Bray[2] has defined "obesity" as a BMI greater than 30 kg/m^2, which closely corresponds to 20% above the median of the recommended midpoint weight range for height according to the 1983 Metropolitan Life Insurance tables.[4] Normal BMI has been calculated in the range of 21.6 to 24.4 kg/m^2 depending on frame size.[5] The primary advantage of using BMI instead of a specific quantity or percentage of overweight is that BMI expresses the relationship of weight to height in either sex as a single number.

The definition of "morbid" obesity evolved in conjunction with the introduction of surgery as a viable treatment alternative for massive overweight. Minimum weight limits for morbid obesity were initially established in the range of 100 pounds or 100% above ideal body weight. In 1991 a National Institutes of Health Consensus Development Panel defined the minimum BMI for morbid obesity at 40 kg/m^2.[6] Obesity of this magnitude is surprisingly common in the United States. One estimate suggests that between 6 and 10 million Americans are more than 100 pounds overweight. In 1980 Abraham and Johnson[7] estimated that 7.2% of American women and 5% of American men are morbidly obese.

The concept of superobesity has gradually evolved to describe a group of patients whose weight far exceeds the minimum weight criteria required for surgical treatment.[8,9] Several definitions have been used to describe this magnitude of overweight including more than 225% of ideal body weight, a weight ≥200 pounds overweight or a BMI ≥50 kg/m^2. Individuals in this extreme category frequently do not live longer than 45 years unless substantial weight loss is achieved.

ETIOLOGY AND PATHOPHYSIOLOGY

An excess of calorie intake in comparison with energy expenditure results in gradual expansion of the body's primary energy storage depot, which is fat. In normal weight humans the percentage of body weight as fat varies from 15% to 25%. The majority of excess fat is usually found in subcutaneous tissues. However, in men the intra-abdominal storage depot is occasionally larger than the subcutaneous depot. As the magnitude of obesity increases, the weight of the lean body mass, particularly bone and skeletal muscle, is also increased. A greater lean body mass is probably necessary to provide adequate structural support for the obese.

During the past decade it has been learned that the distribution of body fat is of greater importance in terms of health risk than the weight of the fat mass per se. The risks of cardiovascular complications are significantly greater in patients with a preponderance of abdominal fat (so-called central or android obesity) as opposed to individuals with a gluteal preponderance (so-called peripheral or gynoid obesity.[10]). The gluteal fat distribution pattern is more prevalent in women. However, there is considerable heterogeneity of body fat distribution patterns in both sexes. There is also considerable variability in the size of fat cells from specific depots in both men and women. Women typically have larger fat cells in the gluteal region, whereas men tend to have their largest fat cells in the mesentery and omentum.[11] The fat distribution pattern is commonly expressed in terms of waist-to-hip ratio (WHR) measurements, although other anthropomorphic measurements such as sagittal diameter or neck-to-thigh ratio may be more predictive of cardiovascular risk.

The precise mechanisms that explain the relationship between increased abdominal fatness and morbidity are not well understood. Furthermore, the biochemical and genetic mechanisms that result in deposition of excess fat in abdominal or gluteal depots are also incompletely explained. The primary mechanism for weight fluctuation in adults is change in fat cell size. However, fat cells may continue to increase in number throughout early adult life, particularly in individuals who are substantially overweight. Once formed, fat cells do not undergo involution. The failure of fat cells to undergo involution provides one explanation for the failure of postoperative morbidly obese patients to reach ideal weight even with a remarkably low level of daily calorie intake.

There is convincing evidence that the development of obesity has a strong genetic component. Children of normal weight parents have only a 10% chance of becoming obese, whereas the children of two obese parents have an 80% to 90% probability of developing obesity in early adulthood. There is also a strong correlation between the weight of adopted children and that of their biologic parents.[12] Studies comparing the degree of fatness in monozygotic vs. dizygotic twins have shown a considerably stronger correlation in the monozygotic group.[13] Other studies have shown a close correlation of basal metabolic rate, body fat distribution pattern, and energy expenditure among family members.

There is also a growing body of evidence that obese patients have lower levels of thermogenesis, which is a major component of the body's means of energy expenditure. Several studies comparing thermogenesis in obese and lean subjects have shown that the obese have substantially lower levels of thermogenesis in comparison with the lean subjects. Conversely, the resting metabolic rate of obese patients is remarkably similar to that of normal weight patients.

Although it is generally conceded that environmental factors also contribute to the development of obesity, there is little hard scientific data that confirm this relationship. Morbid obesity is predominantly an American disease, suggesting that our diet and culture play an important role in its development. In the United States morbid obesity is generally recognized as a disease of lower socioeconomic groups. Lack of good nutrition education and diets with a high-fat content are two frequently cited causes for the preponderance of severe obesity in lower class Americans. Recent studies in animals and man have suggested that a disproportionately high intake of fat in the diet contributes to development of obesity. It has been estimated that the percentage of dietary fat comsumed by Americans has increased by 10% in the past 50 years. Because dietary fat is converted to body fat with nearly 25% greater efficiency than carbohydrate, weight gain is promoted by a high-fat diet. A greater consumption of fast foods, which are notoriously high in fat, is also cited as a major factor contributing to the increased prevalence of obesity in the United States.

Physical exercise is an extremely important means of energy expenditure and weight control. Because physical activity in morbidly obese patients is severely limited by their weight, they are notoriously sedentary. Poor diet habits and a sedentary life-style coupled with an inherently reduced capability of energy expenditure make morbid obesity a disease that is highly resistant to nonsurgical treatment.

RISKS AND COMPLICATIONS OF SEVERE OBESITY

The relationship of body weight to mortality and other medical illnesses is shown in Fig. 68-1. The prevalence of complications related to severe obesity increases sharply at a level corresponding to approximately 60% above desirable weight.[14,15] At that level there is a twofold increase in morbidity and mortality. However, the slope of the "risk curve" rises almost exponentially above the 60% overweight level so that the complication rate corresponding to 100% above ideal weight is in the range of 13 to 14 times normal. Unfortunately, there is a paucity of life table statistics for adults who are more than 100 pounds overweight. These data are particularly lacking among women, who are the most common subjects of obesity operations. The 1980 study of Drenick et al.[16] of mortality in 200 morbidly obese men, which is shown in Fig. 68-2, is the only clinical series in which all the patients were heavy enough to qualify for surgical treatment. The most striking finding in the study was the 12-fold increase in mortality in the youngest age group. The most common causes of death among the overweight men in Drenick's study were myocardial infarction and stroke.

A list of medical problems and other illnesses that have been associated with severe obesity is shown in Table 68-1. Many of these conditions can be controlled or eliminated with substantial weight loss. It is generally acknowl-

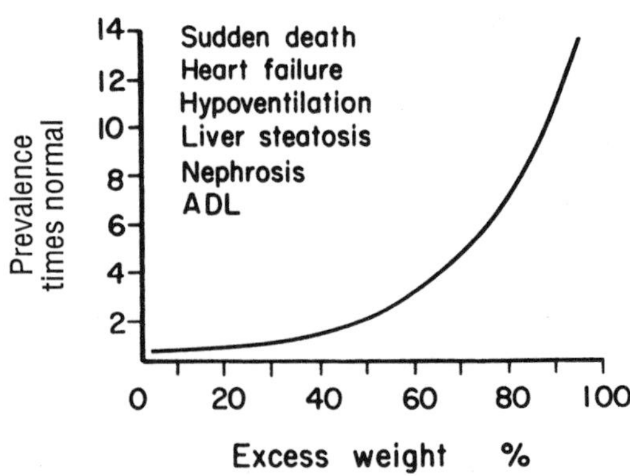

Fig. 68-1. The estimated relative risk of medical illnesses and complications in relation to percentage above desirable weight. (From Kral JG. Morbid obesity and health risks. Ann Intern Med 103:1045, 1985.)

edged that there is an inverse relationship between the magnitude of overweight and the age of onset of many of these comorbid conditions. Problems such as sleep apnea and cardiovascular disease are frequent causes of premature death in the morbidly obese. Congestive heart failure

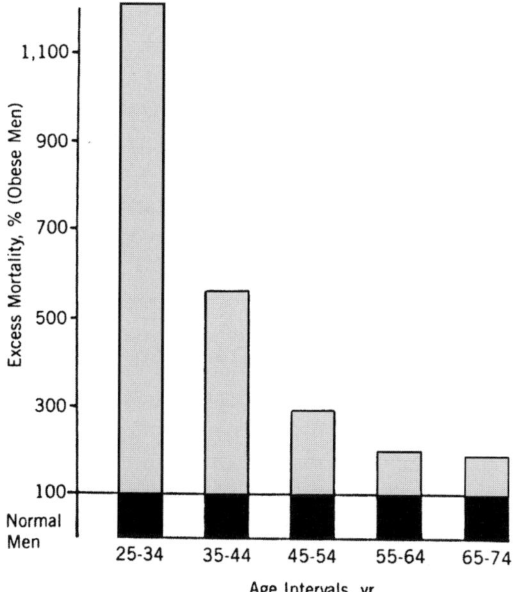

Fig. 68-2. Comparison of excess mortality in men with morbid obesity *(light shaded bars)* vs. normal weight men *(black boxes)* by age interval. (From Drenick EJ, et al. Excessive mortality and causes of death in morbidly obese men. JAMA 243:443, 1980.)

Table 68-1. Diseases Associated With Severe Obesity

Comorbidity	Incidence (%)*
Hypertension	20-55
Cholelithiasis	25-45
Degenerative osteoarthritis	20-35
Hyperlipidemia	15-25
Diabetes mellitus	10-25
Asthmatic bronchitis	10-15
Coronary artery disease	5-15
Heart failure (right ventricular and/or left ventricular)	5-15
Stasis ulcers/venous insufficiency	5-15
Gastroesophageal reflux	5-15
Stress overflow urinary incontinence	5-15
Obesity hypoventilation/sleep apnea syndrome	5-12
Pseudomotor cerebri	1-2
Sexual hormone imbalance/infertility	—†
Malignancy (uterine, colon, gallbladder)	—†
Pulmonary embolism/thrombophlebitis	—†
Necrotizing subcutaneous infections	—†
Mental depression	—†

*There is considerable variability in the reported incidence of nearly all the diseases that have been associated with morbid obesity.
†Statistical data relative to the incidence of these conditions in patients ≥100 pounds overweight are absent.

is generally a consequence of left ventricular or biventricular hypertrophy caused by a combination of increased demand for blood flow through the excess adipose tissue and increases in both systemic and pulmonary artery blood pressure. The obesity-hypoventilation syndrome is caused by the increased weight placed on the chest wall and diaphragm, which results in restricted breathing. Systemic hypoxemia and hypercarbia gradually ensue. Gradual desensitization of the central chemoreceptors to carbon dioxide may result in daytime somnolence. The obstructive sleep apnea syndrome is caused by fat deposition in the hypopharynx, which results in constriction of the upper airway. During sleep the narrowed upper airway produces loud snoring and can become completely obstructed, resulting in episodic apnea and cardiac arrhythmias. Sudden wakening is caused by hypoxic stimulation of the desensitized chemoreceptors. Prolonged hypoxia also can result in cardiac arrest, which is the usual cause of death in these patients.

Necrotizing subcutaneous infections can be life threatening in morbidly obese patients. These infections are usually polymicrobial and typically develop in the perineum or the underside of a large abdominal panniculus. Diabetes is frequently an associated factor. The infections are extremely difficult to treat because the affected tissue has an inherently poor blood supply. Extensive soft tissue debridement is frequently necessary.

Diabetes, hypertension, and atherosclerosis typically occur in patients with an "abdominal" fat distribution pattern, which is characterized by a WHR of 0.9 or greater.[10] Diabetes associated with severe obesity almost invariably begins in adulthood and is typically resistant to insulin due to a marked downregulation of insulin receptors. Oral hypoglycemic agents are also usually ineffective in controlling serum glucose levels. Coronary artery disease is usually found in patients with either diabetes or hyperlipidemia. Approximately 20% of morbidly obese patients have elevated serum levels of total cholesterol and triglycerides.[17] However, angina in these patients is relatively uncommon, probably because they are only capable of low levels of physical exertion.

Other conditions such as degenerative arthritis, venous stasis, and urinary incontinence frequently result in serious long-term disability in the morbidly obese. Many orthopedic surgeons consider morbid obesity to be a contraindication for both prosthetic joint replacement and lower back operations because of the likelihood of a poor result. Urologists and gynecologists are reluctant to attempt surgical correction of urinary continence problems for the same reason. This attitude creates a "catch-22" for the morbidly obese in that the immobility resulting from both degenerative arthritis and massive overweight also contributes to their difficulty in losing weight.

There are a number of other diseases that are increasingly prevalent in severely obese patients including gastroesophageal reflux, sex hormone imbalance, pseudotumor cerebri, and several types of malignancy. Morbidly obese women of childbearing age are known to have a high incidence of infertility and other menstrual and hormonal problems. Grace et al.[18] and Deitel[19] have independently reported preoperative abnormalities in sex hormone–binding globulin (SHBG) in infertile morbidly obese women who were attempting pregnancy. An epidemiologic study conducted by the American Cancer Society has shown an increased risk for colon cancer in men ≥40% overweight and an increased incidence of uterine cervix and gallbladder neoplasms in women ≥40% overweight.

Many of the morbidly obese suffer from low self-esteem and mental depression. The social stigma associated with severe obesity is apparent in a number of areas. Discrimination in obtaining employment is common particularly when the job requires some degree of public exposure. Fat people are often the objects of ridicule and unkind jokes. Their social actvity is restricted by the inability to buy clothes at conventional clothing stores or to sit in airplane and theater seats. The most severely obese often have problems maintaining an acceptable level of personal hygiene. Morbid obesity is commonly associated with problematic marriages. Often obesity in one spouse is a "trade off" for a serious problem such as alcohol or drug addiction in the other. Many of the most severely obese become reclusive and housebound as a consequence of both the inability to ambulate and embarrassment over their weight.

TREATMENT OF SEVERE OBESITY

Morbid obesity has been notoriously refractory to virtually every method of nonoperative treatment. The failure rate of diet and behavior modification treatment at 2 years in the morbidly obese approaches 100%.[20] Likewise, the results of jaw wiring in this group of patients have been disappointing. Many morbidly obese patients gain substantial amounts of weight after unsuccessful attempts at dieting. The so-called yo-yo theory of dieting, namely transient weight loss followed by greater weight gain, is gaining popularity among many health professionals who provide nonsurgical treatment for obesity. The gist of this theory is that chronic dieters experience a diminished capability to lose regained weight after each successive weight fluctuation. However, the primary premise and justification for surgical treatment of morbid obesity has been the compelling evidence that severe obesity is associated with a shortened life span and a variety of other serious medical problems.

Early Obesity Operations

Kremen et al.[21] introduced the concept of surgery for morbid obesity in 1954 when they reported that resection of a large percentage of the small intestine resulted in massive weight loss. Kremen's concept of malabsorption-induced weight loss was later applied in the form of jejunoileal (intestinal) bypass as treatment for morbid obesity.[22-24] Weight loss following jejunoileal bypass results entirely from malabsorption of ingested food. After experimenting with various lengths of jejunum and ileum, it was determined that the best weight loss occurred in patients with a functional intestinal length of approximately 18 inches. Scott et al.[24] and Salmon[23] independently described a modification of jejunoileal bypass (Fig. 68-3) in which 12 inches of the proximal jejunum were anastomosed end to end to 6 inches of distal ileum.

During the 1960s and 1970s thousands of intestinal bypasses were performed for treatment of morbid obesity. However, as more of these operations were done, reports of serious late sequelae, including hepatic failure, urinary calculi, arthritis, and vitamin deficiencies appeared in the literature.[25,26] In 1975 Passaro et al.[27] described the bypass enteritis syndrome, an entity characterized by intermittent episodes of abdominal pain, bloating, and diarrhea, which occasionally was mistaken for peritonitis or intestinal obstruction. Many patients with bypass enteritis went on to develop arthralgias, skin rashes, and cachexia. Drenick[28] later incriminated bacterial overgrowth of the distal bypassed bowel as a cause for the syndrome.

The first public repudiation of jejunoileal bypass was delivered by Ravitch and Brolin[29] in 1979. During the next several years many other prominent surgeons abandoned intestinal bypass as treatment for severe obesity.[30,31] Today jejunoileal bypass is no longer recommended for treatment of morbid obesity.

The concept of gastric restriction as treatment for mor-

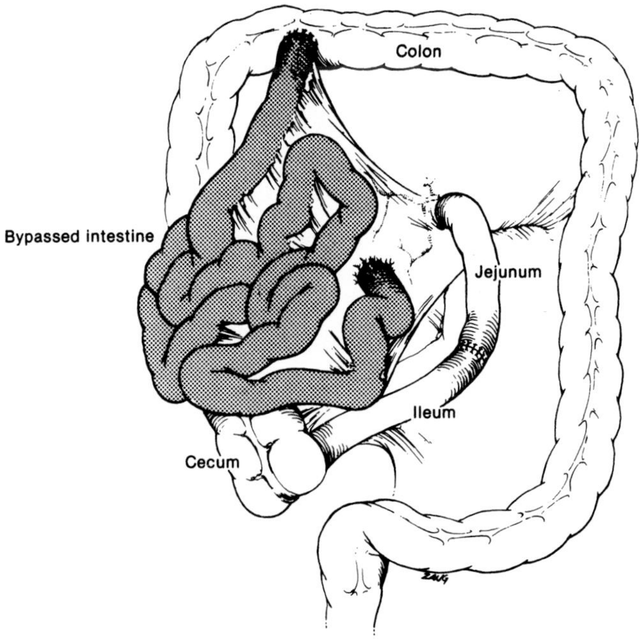

Fig. 68-3. Jejunoileal bypass in which a 12-inch segment of jejunum is anastomosed end to end to 6 inches of the terminal ileum. The remainder of the small bowel *(dark shaded area)* is totally excluded from digestive continuity. The distal end of the excluded bowel is anastomosed to the transverse colon. (From Brolin RE. In Levine BA, et al., eds. Current Practice of Surgery, vol 3. New York: Churchill Livingstone, 1993.)

bid obesity was introduced by Mason[32] in 1967. At that time Mason's operations received little support from the surgical community both because they were technically difficult to perform and because weight loss was less consistent than with jejunoileal bypass. Moreover, the early gastric restrictive operations were associated with a high incidence of postoperative complications. Complication rates with gastric bypass decreased after Alden[33] introduced the concept of stapling the stomach in continuity rather than dividing it. In addition, use of the Roux-en-Y technique eliminated problems with bile reflux esophagitis that were common after loop gastric bypass.

In 1979 Pace et al.[34] introduced stapled gastric partitioning, touting its technical ease in performance and low incidence of operative complications relative to gastric bypass. However, an unacceptably high incidence of early staple-line breakdown subsequently led to a proliferation of modifications using this approach. Many of these stapling techniques were performed in an uncontrolled manner. However, during the 1980s two gastric restrictive operations, vertical banded gastroplasty (VBG) and Roux-en-Y gastric bypass (RYGB), have become recognized as procedures that have produced satisfactory weight loss in patients at 5 years postoperatively.

Current Operations

Gastric restrictive operations are currently the most popular method of surgical treatment for morbid obesity. All the current gastric operations are designed to restrict oral intake. The less than 50 ml capacity upper gastric pouch and the calibrated ≤12 mm diameter outlet effectively limit the quantity of solid food that can be consumed at one time. Conversely, intake of liquids is not limited by these operations.

There are three basic categories of gastric restrictive operations: (1) gastroplasty in which the stomach is partitioned close to the gastroesophageal junction, creating a small upper gastric pouch with a small calibrated outlet leading from the upper pouch to the remainder of the digestive tract; (2) gastric banding in which a calibrated piece of prosthetic material is wrapped around the upper portion of the stomach; and (3) gastric bypass in which the upper stomach is closed off, thereby excluding more than 95% of the stomach, all of the duodenum, and 10 to 15 cm of proximal jejunum from digestive continuity.

Gastroplasty

There is no malabsorption associated with gastroplasty operations. Weight loss results exclusively from reduced calorie intake. Current techniques have evolved in favor of stapling in a vertical direction along the lesser curvature of the stomach, which has facilitated reinforcement of the outlet with prosthetic materials to prevent progressive stomal dilation. Horizontal gastroplasty techniques have now been largely abandoned because of an unacceptably high incidence of staple-line disruption and stomal dilation.

The two most popular techniques of gastroplasty are VBG and vertical silicone elastomer (Silastic) ring gastroplasty (SRG), which are shown in Figs. 68-4 and 68-5. The stoma located at the distal end of a vertically oriented staple-line is reinforced with prosthetic material to prevent gradual dilation. VBG was first described in detail by Mason[35] in 1982. SRG was first described by Laws[36] in 1981 and has since been refined by others.[37,38] The incidence of transmural erosion of the Silastic ring has been greatly reduced by not covering it with the surrounding stomach as Laws had originally described.

Morbidity and mortality rates with both VBG and SRG have been low. Mason et al.[39] recently reported an overall morbidity rate of under 10% and a mortality rate of 0.25% in a series of more than 1200 VBGs. In 1987 Willbanks[38] reported a 3% complication rate with no deaths in a series of 305 SRG patients.

Gastric Banding

Gastric banding is a technique that enjoys popularity in Europe but has not received much attention in the United States. The majority of techniques of gastric banding employ a premeasured strip of prosthetic material to restrict oral intake (Fig. 68-6). The circumference of the band is generally in the range of 5 cm, similar to the measurement

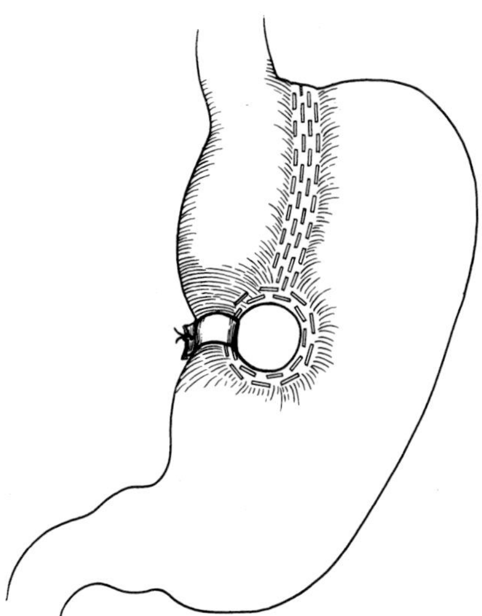

Fig. 68-4. Vertical banded gastroplasty in which the upper gastric pouch, measured at 15 to 20 ml capacity, empties into the remainder of the stomach through a calibrated stoma. The stoma is reinforced with a strip of polypropylene (Marlex) mesh measuring 5 cm in circumference resulting in a 1.6 cm internal diameter stoma. The mesh is placed around the stoma through a "window" created by firing a circular stapling instrument alongside a No. 32 French diameter bougie. The mesh is sutured to itself rather than the stomach, a modification that has reduced the incidence of outlet stricture and leaks. (From Brolin RE. In Levine BA, et al., eds. Current Practice of Surgery, vol 3. New York: Churchill Livingstone, 1993.)

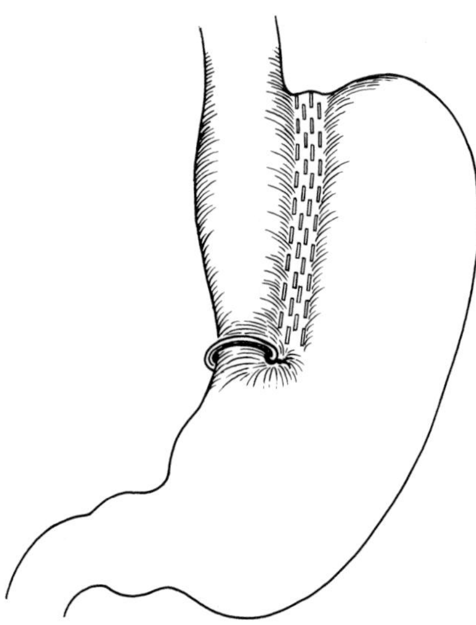

Fig. 68-5. Vertical Silastic ring gastroplasty in which the 15 to 20 ml capacity upper gastric pouch empties through a 5 cm circumference Silastic ring. The ring is secured at the distal end of the vertical staple-line using a heavy suture of either nylon or polypropylene. (From Brolin RE. In Levine BA, et al., eds. Current Practice of Surgery, vol 3. New York: Churchill Livingstone, 1993.)

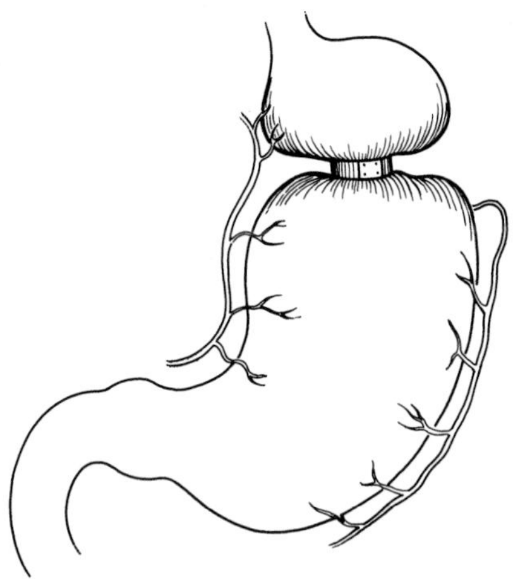

Fig. 68-6. Gastric banding in which the upper portion of the stomach is encircled by a calibrated prosthetic band. The volume of the stomach above the band is crudely estimated by most surgeons who perform this operation. (From Brolin RE. In Levine BA, et al., eds. Current Practice of Surgery, vol 3. New York: Churchill Livingstone, 1993.)

used in VBG. Most techniques of gastric banding lack precision in measuring the volume of stomach above the band. With some techniques the band is sutured to both itself and the stomach to prevent "slipping." Kuzmak[40] introduced the concept of an inflatable silicone band in which the diameter of the band can be adjusted by infusion of saline through a subcutaneous reservoir. Kuzmak's reported weight loss results and complication rate are better than those observed after other banding techniques in which strips of polypropylene or Teflon are used.

Complication rates with the European techniques of gastric banding have been relatively high with morbidity and mortality rates in the range of 30% and 3%, respectively. Stenosis and/or erosion of the band has been reported in 10% to 30% of cases. Stenosis and erosion can result in leaks and stomal obstruction, which frequently require reoperation. Kuzmak has not reported erosion of his inflatable silicone band. However, problems with the subcutaneous reservoir are common.

Gastric Bypass

Gastric bypass combines gastric restriction with a small amount of malabsorption. However, malabsorption of protein, carbohydrate, and fat has not been reported after conventional gastric bypass. The anatomic parameters required for successful weight loss with gastric bypass were defined by Mason et al.[41] in 1975 and include a small ≤50 ml capacity upper gastric pouch and a ≤1.2 cm diameter gastrojejunostomy stoma. The RYGB shown in Fig. 68-7 is currently the preferred method of almost every surgeon who performs gastric bypass. A growing number of surgeons are now transecting the upper stomach rather than stapling it in continuity.

The postoperative complication rates and weight loss observed with current modifications of RYGB improved substantially during the 1980s. In 1984 Flickinger et al.[42] reported a 10% complication rate and two deaths (1%) in a series of 210 consecutive RYGB patients. Sugerman et al.[43] reported a 5% morbidity rate and no mortality in his series of 182 patients who had RYGB. Yale[44] reported two deaths (0.8%) and a 10% incidence of major early postoperative complications in a series of 251 gastric bypass operations. The author has had 26 postoperative complications (6.6%) and one death (0.3%) in an 11-year series of 396 consecutive patients whose primary operation was RYGB.

Gastric bypass occasionally produces symptoms of the "dumping syndrome," which include nausea, bloating, diarrhea, and colic. Dumping is thought to be due to rapid emptying of the small gastric pouch directly into the small bowel. Symptoms of "late" dumping such as light-headedness, palpitations, and sweating also occur in a smaller percentage of patients. These vasomotor symptoms are the consequence of rebound hypoglycemia and typically occur 1½ to 2 hours after ingestion of a carbohydrate-laden meal. The incidence of dumping after gastric bypass is variable with some patients reporting no symptoms, others having symptoms associated with eating specific foods such as milk products or sweets, and a few patients who report troublesome symptoms after almost every meal.

Biliopancreatic Bypass

Biliopancreatic bypass (BPB), also known as distal gastric bypass, is an operation that combines a modest amount of

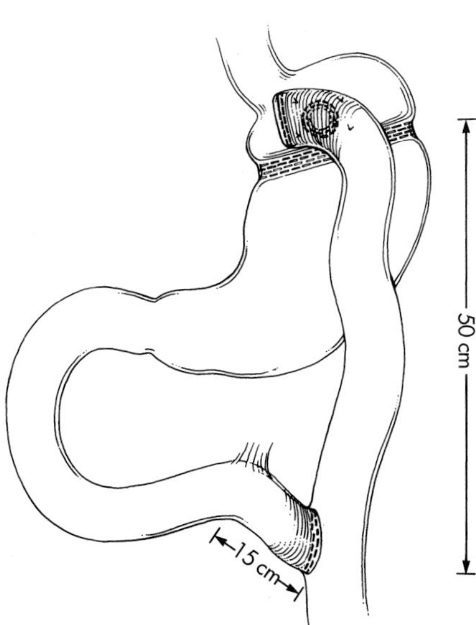

Fig. 68-7. Roux-en-Y gastric bypass in which the TA 90B stapler (U.S. Surgical Corp., Norwalk, Conn.) is fired across the cardia of the stomach creating a 25 ± 5 ml upper pouch. The jejunum is divided approximately 15 cm distal to the ligament of Treitz with the distal end anastomosed to the upper stomach using a circular stapler to create an 1.1 cm diameter anastomosis. The proximal end of jejunum is then anastomosed 50 cm below the gastrojejunostomy. (From Brolin RE, et al. The dilemma of outcome assessment after operations for morbid obesity. Surgery 105:337, 1989.)

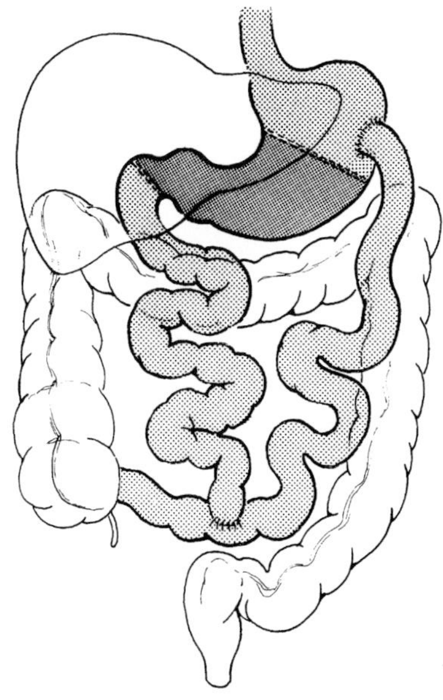

Fig. 68-8. Biliopancreatic bypass in which the small bowel below the ligament of Treitz is bisected with the distal end of transected bowel anastomosed to the upper stomach and the proximal end anastomosed end to side to the "common channel" of distal ileum 50 cm proximal to the ileocecal junction. The distal stomach *(shaded in black)* is either resected (Scopinaro technique) or stapled in continuity. (From Brolin RE. In Levine BA, et al., eds. Current Practice of Surgery, vol 3. New York: Churchill Livingstone, 1993.)

gastric restriction with a substantial amount of malabsorption. This procedure and other anatomic variants are becoming increasingly popular in both the United States and abroad. The concept of BPB was introduced by Scopinaro in the late 1970s. An early modification of this procedure is shown in Fig. 68-8. The technique includes performance of a subtotal gastrectomy leaving an approximately 250 to 500 ml capacity gastric remnant, which is anastomosed to the proximal ileum. All the jejunum is excluded from digestive continuity and is anastomosed end to side to a "common channel" of ileum at a point between 50 and 100 cm proximal to the ileocecal junction. Because this degree of malabsorption predisposes to cholelithiasis, cholecystectomy is also an integral part of the operation. Scopinaro et al.[45] have modified his original operation several times to further reduce gastric capacity to ≤200 ml in superobese patients (the so-called very little stomach modification) and has lengthened the "common channel" in less obese patients to reduce the incidence of malabsorption-related sequelae. Sugerman[46] suggested that there is no need to perform gastrectomy as part of BPB and recommended stapling the stomach in continuity.

The incidence of early postoperative complications after BPB has been in the range of 10% to 15% with a 1% mortality rate.[45,47] However, the incidence of metabolic complications within the first postoperative year has been high, including a 30% incidence of anemia, an 8% to 10% incidence of marginal ulcers, and a 20% incidence of hospitalization for treatment of protein-calorie malnutrition.[45] Because malabsorption is the primary source of both weight loss and weight maintenance, diarrhea and foul-smelling stools are common in patients after BPB has been performed.

An operation that was initially described for management of duodenogastric reflux has been adapted for treatment of morbid obesity by Marceau et al.[48] This modification shown in Fig. 68-9 combines a "parietal" gastrectomy with biliopancreatic diversion. Because the functional portion of the duodenum is diverted from digestive continuity, this procedure has been dubbed the "duodenal switch." The primary goal of this modification is reduction in the incidence of the serious metabolic sequelae, which are associated with BPB. The so-called "parietal" gastrectomy preserves the pylorus and the vagal innervation along the lesser curvature, which in theory would facilitate both gastric emptying and vitamin B_{12} absorption. Elimination of the gastroenteric anastomosis might be expected to reduce the incidence of marginal ulcers. Because one third of the stomach is left intact, restriction of oral intake does not play a prominent role in postoperative weight loss.

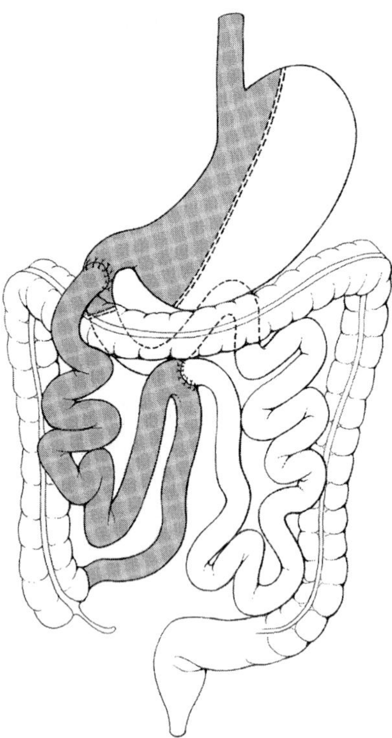

Fig. 68-9. In a duodenal switch, two thirds of the stomach is excised along the greater curvature using linear staplers. The duodenum is dissected from the head of the pancreas for a distance of 5 cm beyond the pylorus and stapled in continuity at that point. The ileum is then transected at a point 250 cm proximal to the ileocecal junction. The distal end of the transected ileum is anastomosed to the proximal duodenum using two layers of sutures. The remainder of the duodenum and proximal small bowel *(unshaded portion)* is diverted from the digestive stream. The distal end of the bypassed segment is reanastomosed to the ileum 100 cm proximal to the ileocecal junction to create the common channel.

There have been several reports of bariatric operations performed using laparoscopic techniques. Laparoscopic bariatric operations are technically difficult, time consuming, and associated with a steep learning curve. However, several surgeons have successfully completed VBG, gastric banding, and RYGB procedures via the laparosocope. These laparoscopic approaches should probably be considered investigational until a substantial number of these patients have had 2 or 3 years of postoperative follow-up.

Preoperative Patient Selection

All candidates for obesity operations should be interviewed in an outpatient setting prior to operation. During that interview the surgeon should provide prospective patients with a clear understanding of the risks and goals of the operation and explain the mechanism by which the procedure produces weight loss. At the same time the surgeon should obtain a complete medical history and make a preliminary assessment of a patient's operative risk. Psychologic stability should also be evaluated, particularly in terms of the patient's willingness to adjust to the permanent postoperative side effects of gastric restriction and malabsorption. At the conclusion of the interview the patient should have obtained sufficient information to give informed consent.

CRITERIA FOR PATIENT SELECTION

1. Weight
   a. 100 pounds or 100% above desirable weight
   b. BMI ≥40 kg/m^2
   c. BMI ≥35 kg/m^2 with coexisting medical problems
2. Failure of nonsurgical methods of weight reduction
3. Absence of endocrine disorders that can cause massive obesity
4. Psychologic stability
   a. Basic understanding of how surgery causes weight loss
   b. Realization that surgery itself cannot guarantee a good result
   c. Absence of alcohol and drug abuse

BMI, Body mass index.

Standard criteria used in selecting patients for obesity operations are shown in the accompanying box. Minimum weight limits for surgical treatment of severe obesity were traditionally established in the range of 100 pounds or 100% above desirable weight as defined by standard life insurance tables. The 1991 National Institutes of Health Consensus Development Panel[6] on gastrointestinal surgery for severe obesity suggested using the BMI rather than absolute body weight in evaluation of potential surgical candidates. The panel recommended that surgical treatment be considered for any patient with a BMI ≥40 kg/m^2 who had failed serious attempts at nonsurgical treatment.[6] The panel also recommended that surgery be considered for patients with a BMI ≥35 kg/m^2 who have serious coexisting medical problems such as diabetes, hypertension, hyperlipidemia, or sleep apnea.[6]

There are relatively few endocrine disorders that cause massive obesity. Although hypothyroidism is associated with both a decreased metabolic rate and obesity, it is virtually never the sole cause of morbid obesity. Hence, hypothyroidism is not a contraindication for obesity surgery. Conversely, Cushing's disease may occasionally cause massive obesity. Because successful treatment of Cushing's disease likely results in substantial weight loss, patients with untreated Cushing's disease should not undergo operations designed for treatment of morbid obesity. Adult-onset diabetes mellitus (AODM) is almost invariably associated with obesity. However, unlike Cushing's disease, AODM is effectively treated by weight reduction. Hence, AODM is considered an indication for obesity surgery.

Although patients with morbid obesity have been shown to have similar psychologic profiles to their normal weight counterparts, the psychologic stability of surgical candidates should be considered prior to operation. Although standardized psychologic tests and separate screening interviews with psychologists or psychiatrists have not proven useful in predicting postoperative outcome of obesity operations, a formal psychologic evaluation of patients with a documented history of mental illness is recommended. Patients should also be carefully queried regarding abuse of addictive drugs and alcohol prior to operation. All patients who undergo surgical treatment of obesity should be admonished that sustained long-term weight loss is not guaranteed merely by having an operation. This understanding is particularly important for patients who have gastric restrictive operations, which can be defeated by consuming large quantities of high-calorie liquids and soft junk foods.

Preoperative and Postoperative Care

Routine preadmission tests include a complete blood count, chem-21 screen, urinalysis, blood typing, chest x-ray, ECG, barium upper gastrointestinal tract contrast study, and ultrasound of the gallbladder. The upper gastrointestinal tract contrast study is performed to rule out occult peptic ulcer disease. An active peptic ulcer represents an absolute contraindication for bariatric surgery. If an ulcer is seen on upper gastrointestinal tract examination, upper endoscopy should be performed to confirm the radiographic findings. At our institution most patients who have had upper gastrointestinal tract studies that suggested peptic ulcer disease have been found to be free of ulcers at upper endoscopy. Because the incidence of cholelithiasis is 15% to 25% in morbidly obese patients, preoperative or intraopertaive screening for gallstones is recommended in all patients who have not had cholecystectomy. Ultrasonography is the most popular method of evaluation. Intraoperative ultrasonography is considered to be more sensitive than transabdominal examination in the morbidly obese. We recommend concomitant cholecystectomy for all patients with cholelithiasis.

Patients who are scheduled to have gastric bypass or BPB operations should also have serum iron, iron-binding capacity, vitamin B_{12}, and folate levels determined prior to operation. Baseline serum levels of fat-soluble vitamins should be obtained in patients prior to BPB. All patients who are scheduled to have revision of a failed bariatric procedure should have blood crossmatched for possible transfusion. Blood transfusion is necessary in nearly 50% of patients who undergo revision of failed gastric restrictive operations.

Preoperative preparation of patients for bariatric operations varies according to the underlying health of individual patients. Many young patients with no associated illnesses can be admitted to the hospital on the day of operation. Conversely, patients with severe sleep apnea syndrome or congestive heart failure require hospitalization for 2 or 3 days prior to operation to optimize their cardiopulmonary condition. Insertion of a Swan-Ganz catheter on the day prior to operation is advisable in many of these patients. All patients should be given intravenous prophylactic antibiotics in the perioperative period.

Morbidly obese patients tolerate general anesthesia remarkably well. However, endotracheal intubation may be difficult, particularly in patients who weigh more than 400 pounds. Awake intubation using intravenous sedation and topical pharyngeal anesthesia is often the safest way to establish an airway in the heaviest patients. Although an arterial line is not required during most bariatric operations, it is useful in some patients for both intraoperative blood pressure monitoring and for drawing blood for blood gases both during and following the operation.

A Foley catheter and nasogastric tube are inserted in all patients after induction of anesthesia. The Foley catheter is generally removed on the first postoperative day in all patients who spend their first night in the hospital. The nasogastric tube is helpful in identifying the gastroesophageal junction intraoperatively and also provides for intraoperative and postoperative gastric decompression. The nasogastric tube is positioned through the stoma at the completion of gastric restrictive operations to allow for decompression of the upper gastric pouch and jejunum in gastric bypass or the distal stomach in gastroplasty procedures. The tube is usually removed on the first or second postoperative day.

Less than 10% of our patients have required admission to the intensive care unit postoperatively. However, all patients with sleep apnea, congestive heart failure, and severe asthmatic bronchitis should spend one or two nights in the intensive care unit for close monitoring of their cardiopulmonary status. Many of these patients require overnight intubation. Incentive spirometry is used routinely for several days after extubation. Clinically significant atelectasis is remarkably uncommon in these patients postoperatively.

Obesity has traditionally been considered as a risk factor for postoperative pulmonary embolism. Hence, a variety of methods of prophylaxis have been employed toward prevention of this feared complication. These include subcutaneous low-dose heparin, pneumatic compression of the legs, elastic stockings or bandages, intravenous low–molecular weight dextran, and use of the Trendelenburg position intraoperatively. None of these methods have been proven to decrease the incidence of postoperative venous thromboembolism in bariatric surgical patients. Early postoperative ambulation is strongly encouraged and almost certainly contributes toward the low incidence of postoperative venous thromboembolism that has been reported in these patients. Patients are assisted in getting out of bed on the night of their operation and are walked on the first postoperative day. Many of these patients move remarkably well.

Incisional pain is moderately severe during the first 48 to 72 hours postoperatively. During the past several years we have routinely used intravenous patient-controlled analgesia supervised by the pain control service. This approach provides more consistent pain relief than intermittent intramuscular injections of narcotic analgesics. Oral narcotics are usually begun on the fourth or fifth postoperative day after intravenous fluids have been stopped. All pills and tablets are crushed and administered as a slurry with a liquid beverage. Patients are instructed not to swallow whole pills during the first 4 weeks postoperatively.

Ice chips and sips of water are given by mouth 1 day after the nasogastric tube is removed. If the water and ice are tolerated, a clear liquid diet is begun on the following day. Intravenous fluids are usually discontinued after clear liquids are tolerated without difficulty. A maximum 1000-calorie full-liquid diet is given on the next day and is continued until the time of discharge.

Patients are usually discharged on the fifth or sixth postoperative day. Hospitalization for more than 7 days is unusual in the absence of major complications. A limited upper gastrointestinal tract contrast study is routinely performed shortly before discharge to examine the integrity of the staple line and outlet stoma.

Postoperative Dietary Management and Follow-up

Postoperative dietary counseling is essential in the long-term success of gastric restrictive operations. Patients are instructed to follow a modified liquid diet for 4 weeks after discharge. The modified liquid diet consists of liquids, pureed foods, and several soft solid foods such as mashed potatoes and cottage cheese. A liquid or chewable multivitamin supplement is taken during this phase of the diet. The purpose of the modified liquid diet is twofold: (1) to allow time for patients to adjust to their tremendously restricted stomach capacity by consuming foods that are relatively easy to chew and swallow and (2) to minimize the likelihood of vomiting in the early postoperative period. Repeated episodes of vomiting in the early postoperative period have been associated with staple-line disruption and leaks. Patients are given a soft solid diet at the 4-week visit and then gradually progress to a normal diet. Patients can resume swallowing whole pills and tablets after solid food is well tolerated.

Postoperative follow-up is extremely important in bariatric surgical patients. All patients should have easy access to the operating surgeon and a clinical nutritionist. During the first year visits are scheduled at 4 weeks postoperatively and then at 3-month intervals thereafter. Two follow-up visits are scheduled at 6-month intervals during the second year. After the second year all bariatric surgical patients should be followed indefinitely by annual physician office visits. However, some patients may require more frequent follow-up. Weight and blood pressure should be recorded at each visit along with the laboratory studies, which are needed to check for postoperative metabolic sequelae and to follow up preoperative medical problems such as diabetes or hyperlipidemia.

Patients who have malabsorptive operations require periodic blood tests postoperatively to check for possible metabolic and nutritional deficiencies. These patients should take a daily multivitamin supplement with minerals for the rest of their lives. Menstruating women who have had gastric bypass or BPB should also take a prophylactic iron supplement postoperatively. After BPB many patients require additional protein and other nutritional supplements.

RESULTS OF SURGICAL TREATMENT

Weight Loss

Early weight loss results with both VBG and SRG have been generally acceptable. Mason et al.[39] reported a mean loss of 62% of excess weight in a series of 226 patients followed for a mean 5 years after VBG. MacLean et al.[9] reported a mean 60% excess weight loss in 57 patients followed for 5 years after VBG. However, a substantial number of their patients required surgical revision for either complications or inadequate weight loss during the 5-year study period. Willbanks[33] reported a mean 61% excess weight loss in his series of 305 SRG patients who were followed for a minimum of 2 years. Weight loss maintenance after VBG and SRG has been somewhat problematic in that many patients regain at least 15% to 20% of their lost weight between 3 and 5 years postoperatively.

Weight loss with most techniques of gastric banding has been less consistent than weight loss reported after VBG, SRG, and gastric bypass. Kuzmak reported a mean excess weight loss of 65% in a series of 10 patients who had silicone gastric banding and were followed for a minimum of 24 months, which is similar to the weight loss observed after VBG and SRG.

Weight loss results with RYGB have been generally superior to those observed after other gastric restrictive operations. In 1987 Sugerman et al.[49] reported that 91% of their series of 174 patients followed for a mean 12 months after gastric bypass lost at least 40% of their excess weight with a mean excess weight loss of 68%. In our 1989 report of 126 consecutive patients followed for a minimum of 18 months after RYGB, 79% lost at least 50% of their excess weight with a mean excess weight loss of 68%.[50] Table 68-2 shows 5-year weight loss results in six clinical series of patients after RYGB. Mean excess weight loss ranged from 48% to 74% with an average follow-up rate of 85%. However, there is some degree of recidivism between 3 and 5 years after RYGB.

Weight loss results with BPB have been almost uniformly good. Scopinaro et al.[47] reported a mean loss of 75% of the preoperative weight in a series of 916 patients followed for a mean 5 years with excellent weight maintenance after stabilization. Sugerman[46] reported a mean 71% excess weight loss at 1 year in his series of 25 super-obese patients. Early weight loss results with the "duodenal switch" have been comparable to those reported after BPB.

Over the years there have been several prospective comparisons of bariatric procedures that have shown significant differences between operations both in terms of weight loss outcome and in the incidence of postoperative

Table 68-2. Long-Term Weight Loss After Roux-en-Y Gastric Bypass (RYGB) for Morbid Obesity

Surgeon	Operation	Follow-up Duration (N)*	Percent Lost to Follow-up	Mean Percent Excess Weight Loss	Mean Percent of Ideal Body Weight
Pories[51]	RYGB	6 yr (26)	3	—	149
Benotti[70]	RYGB	5 yr (187)	35	60	147
Linner[79]	RYGB	5 yr (17)	23	74	—
Yale[44]	RYGB	5 yr (225)	10	60 ± 23	—
Flanagan[80]	RYGB	6 yr (26)	15	70	—
Brolin[50]	RYGB	5 yr (37)	15	48 ± 22	167 ± 29

*Parentheses indicate number of patients (N) in each series.

complications. Pories et al.[51] Naslund et al.,[52] and Lechner and Callender[53] independently performed prospective randomized comparisons of horizontal gastroplasty with gastric bypass and reported significantly better weight loss after gastric bypass and no difference in the early complication rate between the two procedures. Sugerman et al.[49] prospectively compared VBG with RYGB and again found that gastric bypass resulted in significantly greater weight loss. Surgeons from Adelaide, Australia prospectively compared gastrogastrostomy, vertical gastroplasty, and RYGB in 310 patients.[54] At 5 years postoperatively weight loss after gastric bypass was significantly greater than with either gastroplasty or gastrogastrostomy. The early postoperative complication rates were similar among the three procedures. These prospective studies clearly show that gastric bypass is a better weight loss–producing operation than any modification of gastroplasty.

Sugerman et al.[46] prospectively compared conventional RYGB with Scopinaro's BPB in a group of superobese patients and found that weight loss was significantly better at 1 year after BPB. However, because the incidence of serious complications was considerably higher after BPB, Sugerman et al. concluded that BPB was too risky to be recommended as a primary procedure for treatment of morbid obesity.

Successful weight loss in superobese patients has generally been problematic after conventional gastroplasty and gastric bypass procedures. Two reports have described modifications of conventional operations with the goal of improving long-term weight loss.[8,55] One study employed a "long limb" modification of RYGB in which the Roux limb length was measured at 150 cm. The long limb modification was prospectively compared with a standard technique of gastric bypass and resulted in significantly greater weight loss vs. the conventional method after 12 months postoperatively.[8] Another investigator proposed a two-stage approach consisting of a jejunocolic bypass at the outset, which was subsequently converted to a VBG after weight stabilization.[55] This two-stage method resulted in excellent weight loss in a group of eight superobese patients. It appears that some degree of intestinal malabsorption is necessary to achieve satisfactory weight loss in these extremely heavy patients.

Amelioration of Comorbidities

Amelioration of obesity-related medical problems is a primary goal of all bariatric operations. Improvement or resolution of morbid obesity-associated diabetes including a significant decrease in insulin resistance after weight reduction surgery has been reported by many investigators.[56,57] Pories et al.[57] have extensively studied postoperative changes in glucose metabolism in morbidly obese patients with diabetes. In 1987 they reported that 139 of 141 patients with either overt diabetes or impaired glucose tolerance became euglycemic after RYGB.[57] Fasting insulin and glycosylated hemoglobin were also reduced to normal levels, whereas insulin release, insulin resistance, and utilization of glucose were substantially improved.

Weight reduction surgery also has salutary effects on obesity-related hypertension and cardiovascular dysfunction. Alpert et al.[58] used echocardiography to measure a number of parameters of ventricular function in 62 morbidly obese patients and found that surgically induced weight loss was associated with significant improvement of left ventricular ejection fraction and lesser but measurable improvements in mean blood pressure, cardiac chamber size, and ventricular wall thickness. The response of hypertension to weight loss following gastric restrictive operations was recently reported by two groups of investigators.[59,60] Each group defined hypertension as a blood pressure reading ≥160/90 and noted improvement or resolution of hypertension in approximately 70% of patients at 4 years postoperatively. However, there were conflicting results regarding the relationship between blood pressure reduction and weight loss, with one group showing a correlation between blood pressure improvement and the amount of weight loss[59] and the other reporting a significant correlation between improved blood pressure and proximity to ideal weight after weight stabilization.[60]

The beneficial effects of weight reduction surgery on obesity-related hyperlipidemia have been documented by a number of investigators. Gleysteen et al.,[61] Rucker et al.[62] Nanji and Freeman,[63] and Gonen et al.[64] independently reported significant decreases in both total cholesterol and triglyceride levels after gastric restrictive operations for morbid obesity. They also showed a favorable increase in the high-density lipoprotein/low-density lipoprotein ratio after gastric bypass, suggesting that the risk of atherosclerosis may be decreased by weight loss in this group of patients. Gleysteen et al.[61] and our group[17] have shown that these lipid reductions persist for as long as weight loss is satisfactorily maintained. Conversely, patients who regain a substantial portion of their lost weight tend to have concomitant regression of the salutary changes in lipid profile.

The obesity-hypoventilation syndrome probably poses the greatest immediate risk to life of any of the obesity-related medical illnesses. Following gastric restrictive operations, Sugerman et al.[65] and Charuzi et al.[66] have independently reported complete resolution of sleep apnea symptoms and significant improvements in both arterial blood gases and polysomnographic studies. Sugerman et al.[57] also reported significant reductions in mean pulmonary artery pressures in patients with obesity-hypoventilation syndrome between 3 and 9 months after RYGB. Many patients in these reports were incapacitated by their condition preoperatively but after losing weight were able to lead normal and productive lives.

Weight loss has a salutary effect on sex hormone balance and fertility in women. After gastroplasty-induced weight loss Grace et al.[18] and Deitel[19] independently reported significant improvement in SHBG levels and a significantly decreased incidence of irregular menses. Both androgen levels and hirsutism decreased with substantial weight loss. A number of previously infertile women became pregnant and delivered normal babies following surgically induced weight loss. Printen and Scott[67] reported similar results after gastric bypass. Although these women are able to eat only small amounts, adequate nutritional status can be maintained for both the mother and developing fetus. Pregnancy is not recommended during the first postoperative year in which the great majority of weight loss occurs.

We have followed the postoperative progress of obesity-related medical problems in all of our morbid obesity patients. Table 68-3 shows the incidence and response of 263 obesity-associated medical problems in 182 of our patients who have been followed for at least 18 months.[50] The incidence of medical problems increased with age as only 30 of 73 patients (41%) younger than age 36 had one or more associated medical problems as compared with 92 of 109 patients (84%) older than age 35. Hypertension, defined by a blood pressure ≥140/90, was recognized in 55% of the 182 patients. Arthritis invariably involved pain in weight-bearing joints such as the knees, ankles, and lower back. Many patients with arthritis were able to discard their canes or walkers with satisfactory weight loss. Patients with asthmatic bronchitis were taking bronchodilators preoperatively and were severely limited by exertional dyspnea. Nearly all the 21 patients with diabetes were resistant to large doses of insulin. Successful weight loss led to improvement or resolution of 95% of the medical problems in this series. It seems reasonable to believe that long-term amelioration of most obesity-associated medical problems would be sustained with maintenance of satisfactory weight loss.

Defining Successful Outcome

The overall outcome of obesity operations should be assessed in terms of both weight loss per se and with respect to improvement of obesity-related medical disorders. Traditionally, postoperative weight loss outcome has been defined in terms of either a quantity or percentage of the preoperative weight lost or as a percentage of the excess weight lost. Excess weight is the calculated difference between the ideal weight and preoperative weight. Loss of at least 25% of the preoperative weight or at least 50% of the excess weight have frequently been used as minimum criteria for successful outcome.[51,52,68]

We have previously shown how both the patient's preoperative weight and the criteria used to define successful weight loss can influence the overall assessment of results in a series of bariatric surgical patients.[69] In that report

Table 68-3. Obesity-Related Medical Problems—Incidence and Response to Weight Loss

Problem	No. (%) of Total Patients*	Resolved†	Improved†	Unchanged
Hypertension	102 (55%)	52	43	7
Arthritis	48 (26%)	20	25	3
Hyperlipidemia	35 (19%)	24	7	4
Asthmatic bronchitis	24 (13%)	14	9	1
Diabetes	21 (11%)	14	7	0
Angina/congestive heart failure	20 (11%)	11	9	0
Venous stasis	7 (4%)	5	2	0
Sleep apnea	6 (3%)	6	0	0
TOTAL	263	146 (56%)	102 (39%)	15 (5%)

From Brolin RE, et al. The dilemma of outcome assessment after operations for morbid obesity. Surgery 105:337, 1989.

*Numbers in parentheses are percentages of each comorbidity in the entire series of 182 patients.

†Medical problems were considered resolved when controlled without medications and were improved when controlled on reduced doses of medications.

loss of ≥25% of the preoperative weight and loss of ≥50% of excess weight were compared with a third criterion, weight loss to within 50% of the "ideal" weight according to the 1983 Metropolian Life Insurance tables.[4] Fifty percent above ideal weight was arbitrarily chosen as a criterion for successful outcome because this degree of weight loss is associated with a measurable reduction in mortality according to established actuarial statistics. In superobese patients, who were more than 200 pounds above ideal weight, excess weight loss was an intermediate outcome measure between weight loss in comparion with preoperative weight and ideal weight. Although the superobese patients lost more pounds than the lighter group of patients who were 100 to 199 pounds overweight, a considerably lower percentage of the superobese patients stabilized at within 50% of their ideal weight. It seems obvious that the heaviest patients must lose more weight to achieve a level that would represent a valid reduction in their actuarial mortality risk.

Other investigators have raised the question of what are realistic and valid weight loss goals for bariatric procedures. Figure 68-10 shows the change in mean BMI with postoperative weight loss in 98 gastric bypass patients who were followed for a minimum of 18 months and did not miss any follow-up visits during this time.[50] Only 20% of the patients in this series stabilized at a BMI ≤30 kg/m^2, and only 5% reached a BMI of ≤25 kg/m^2 at the point of maximum weight loss. Calculated BMI for patients who are approximately 50% overweight falls in the range of 34 to 36.5 kg/^{2}. These results show that despite losing a substantial amount of weight, only a few bariatric surgical patients approach ideal weight at the time of stabilization.

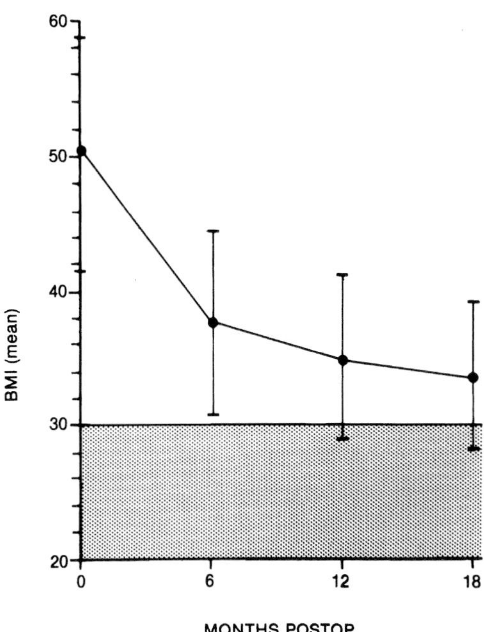

Fig. 68-10. Mean postoperative body mass index *(BMI)* stabilized at a level considerably higher than Bray's[2] minimum BMI definition of "obesity" represented by the shaded area. Mean BMI was significantly decreased at each postoperative interval vs. preoperatively and at 12 and 18 months vs. 6 months postoperatively ($p < 0.05$ by ANOVA with Student-Newman-Keuls test). Differences in BMI between 12 and 18 months were not statistically significant. (From Brolin RE, et al. The dilemma of outcome assessment after operations for morbid obesity. Surgery 105:337, 1989.)

Successful weight loss after obesity operations probably should be defined relative to the patient's ideal weight rather than the preoperative weight, since both the actuarial mortality statistics and the minimum weight criteria for morbid obesity are defined according to the concept of ideal body weight. The BMI is probably the best measurement for reporting weight loss results because it is directly related to ideal body weight in both sexes and is not influenced by either frame size or the magnitude of overweight.

Patients "lost to follow-up" represent a vexing problem in analysis of results of obesity operations. To properly analyze the effectiveness of any obesity operation, it is probably necessary to have postoperative follow-up of at least 5 years' duration. The pitfalls of assessing outcome of an operation with only 2 or 3 years' follow-up were repeatedly demonstrated in the early era of bariatric surgery. What constitutes valid follow-up is another issue complicating the overall evaluation of obesity operations. Self-reported weights obtained by either postcard or telephone responses are probably not as reliable as the scale in the doctor's office. Moreover, utilization of either postcard or telephone replies in outcome analysis precludes obtaining objective information on such risk factors as hypertension, hyperlipidemia, and diabetes.

Postoperative Complications

In experienced hands bariatric operations can be performed with anticipation of a perioperative morbidity rate of under 10% and a mortality rate of approximately 1%. Tables 68-4 and 68-5 show the early and late postoperative complications in my series of 483 consecutive primary gastric restrictive operations performed during a 13-year period. Although the incidence of complications was remarkably similar in gastroplasty and RYGB, there was a notable difference in the nature of the late complications between the two procedures.

Early Complications

The most serious early complications are gastrointestinal tract anastomatic leak and pulmonary embolism. Fortunately, the incidence of these two serious problems is reported in the range of 1% to 2% in most large series of bariatric operations.[43,44,50,70-72] The incidence of pulmonary embolism does not seem to be altered by routine use of intermittent decompression stockings or subcutaneous heparin. However, nearly all bariatric surgeons use some method of DVT prophylaxis in the perioperative period. Early postoperative ambulation is always emphasized and is surprisingly well tolerated by most patients.

Table 68-4. Early Postoperative Complications

	Gastroplasty (87)*	RYGB (396)
Staple-line leak	2	4
Pulmonary embolus	1	4
Wound dehiscence	1	5
Gastrointestinal tract bleeding	—	3†
Small bowel obstruction	—	3
Wound infection	—	2
Cardiac arrest	—	2‡
Subhepatic abscess	—	1
Pneumonia	—	1
Gastrointestinal tract fistula§	—	1
TOTAL	4/87 (4.6%)	26/396 (6.6%)

*The gastroplasty group includes 57 suture-reinforced horizontal partitionings and 30 VBGs.
†The three cases of gastrointestinal tract bleeding were caused by marginal ulcers.
‡The one postoperative death in this series resulted from cardiac arrest.
§The gastrointestinal tract fistula was caused by a gastrojejunostomy leak.
RYGB, Roux-en-Y gastric bypass.

Table 68-5. Late Postoperative Complications

	Gastroplasty (87)	RYGB (396)
Incisional hernia*	6	33
Marginal ulceration†	—	16
Stomal stenosis†	8	1
Volvulus/small bowel obstruction†	—	6
TOTAL	14/87 (16.1%)	57/396 (14.4%)

*The incidence of incisional hernia was approximately 8% in each operative group.
†Stomal stenosis resulting in hospitalization was more common after gastroplasty, whereas small bowel obstruction and marginal ulceration were only observed after RYGB. All six cases of small bowel obstruction were caused by adhesions.
RYGB, Roux-en-Y gastric bypass.

Gastrointestinal tract leaks can be difficult to recognize after gastric restrictive procedures because fever and abdominal tenderness are frequently absent during the first 48 hours after a leak has occurred. Persistent tachycardia and progressive tachypnea are the most common early signs. Hence, it is not unusual to initially suspect pulmonary embolism in a patient with a gastric leak. However, a ventilation-perfusion scan is generally interpreted as "low probability" for pulmonary embolism. An isolated left-sided pleural effusion is a common finding on the plain chest radiograph. Most surgeons initially attempt to identify leaks using radiographic gastrointestinal tract contrast studies. However, a normal result from contrast study by no means excludes the diagnosis, since leaks from the gastric staple-line are usually not identified by upper gastrointestinal tract contrast studies. Because failure to recognize a leak can result in death, exploratory laparotomy should be empirically performed in patients with progressive tachypnea and tachycardia in whom pulmonary embolism has been ruled out.

The two cardiac arrests in Table 68-4 resulted from inability to intubate patients who developed acute respiratory distress. Intubation under these difficult circumstances should be deferred to experienced health professionals who have skills in awake intubation. Major atelectasis and pneumonia are rare complications of gastric restrictive operations.

Although severe obesity is reported to be associated with a high incidence of postoperative wound problems, in experienced hands the incidence of major wound infection after gastric restrictive operations is reported in the range of 1% to 3%.[43,44,50] The potential for wound dehiscence after bariatric operations is increased because of the great tension placed on the wound closure by massive overweight. Hence, the abdominal fascia should be closed with heavy absorbable or nonabsorbable suture. The author now routinely uses a continuous double-stranded suture of No. 1 PDS for fascial closure after having three cases of midline fascial dehiscence following closure with interrupted No. 1 Ethibond sutures. Healing of the skin incision after bariatric operations is also problematic. The author has had two patients develop almost complete dehiscence of the skin incision within the first 10 days postoperatively. However, during the last 10 years we have routinely removed only half the skin staples prior to discharge. Steri strips are placed between the remaining staples, which are removed 7 to 10 days later. There have been no problems with skin wound dehiscence since adopting this practice.

Late Complications

Previous studies have documented a high incidence of gallstone formation following rapid weight loss is obese patients. The incidence of symptomatic gallbladder disease reported after gastric restrictive operations varies from 3% to greater than 30%.[73] Hence, removing the gallbladder "prophylactically" at the time of gastric restrictive surgery is a controversial issue among bariatric surgeons. Several surgeons who have recommended prophylactic cholecystectomy report histologic evidence of gallbladder pathology in nearly 90% of cases. Other surgeons believe that the incidence of symptomatic cholecystitis after gastric restrictive operations is not high enough to justify routine removal of the gallbladder in patients who do not have gallstones. Scopinaro[45] has recommended cholecystectomy as an integral part of BPB because more than 50% of the patients in his early experience developed symptomatic gallstones. The risks of adding cholecystectomy to an elective gastric restrictive procedure are negligible.

A multicenter, randomized, double-blind, prospective trial evaluated three oral doses of ursodiol (Actigall) vs. placebo during the first 6 months after RYGB.[74] Of 233

Table 68-6. Metabolic Deficiencies After Gastric Bypass*

Report/Year	Iron	Vitamin B_{12}	Folate	Anemia	Follow-up
Halverson (1981)[71]	20%/17 mo	26%/20 mo	9%/13 mo	18%/—	20 mo
Amaral (1985)[77]	49%/15.6 mo	70%/13 mo	18%/—	35%/20 mo	33.2 mo
Brolin et al. (1990)[17]	33%/13.4 mo	37%/12.8 mo	16%/10.7 mo	22%/12 mo	24.2 mo

*The mean incidence and time of deficiency recognition reported in each series are listed in columns 2 through 5 with the mean follow-up shown at far right.

patients who had postoperative ultrasonography, gallstones formed in 32% of the placebo group vs. 4% of the higher dose treatment groups. The investigators concluded that ursodiol at doses of 600 and 1200 mg/day was effective in preventing cholelithiasis during the rapid weight loss phase after gastric bypass.

Although vomiting is a common side effect of most gastric restrictive operations, severe, intractable vomiting is quite rare. Most cases of severe vomiting have followed banded gastric restrictive operations and are usually caused by stenosis of the outlet stoma. Patients with vomiting who cannot tolerate liquids should be hospitalized and given intravenous fluids. In most cases the stomal edema that results from protracted vomiting resolves without further intervention. Patients who cannot tolerate liquids after several days of nothing by mouth and intravenous fluids should undergo upper endoscopy and stomal dilation using balloon-tipped catheters. Stomal dilation is almost always successful in patients after RYGB but is more problematic in patients with prosthetic stomal reinforcement.

Many patients report great difficulty with eating meat and fresh fruit and vegetables after banded gastric restrictive operations. Hence, these patients often consume large quantities of soft high-calorie foods such as cookies, chips, and ice cream. Our group[75] recently showed that the inconsistent weight loss observed after VBG is frequently due to these maladaptive changes in postoperative eating patterns.

Incisional hernia is a common late complication after gastric restrictive operations, with an incidence ranging from 10% to 15% in most large series. We have reduced the incidence of hernias by approximately one half by using a double-stranded suture of No. 1 PDS to close the linea alba.[76] The incidence of marginal ulcer in patients after RYGB and BPB ranges from 3% to 10%. These ulcers typically develop on the jejunal side of the gastroenterostomy and are caused by excessive production of gastric acid. Serum gastrin levels are normal or subnormal. This potentially serious complication is frequently associated with breakdown of the gastric staple-line after RYGB.[72] Marginal ulcers that are not associated with disruption of the stapled gastric partition almost always respond to H_2 blocking drugs. Conversely, ulcers that occur in patients with staple-line breakdown are often intractable to medications and require operative treatment.

Patients who have either RYGB or BPB are at risk for developing metabolic sequelae as a consequence of malabsorption. Table 68-6 shows the incidence of metabolic complications typically associated with gastric bypass.[71,77] Since iron absorption occurs primarily in the duodenum, malabsorption of ingested iron is the primary cause of iron deficiency after gastric bypass. Smith et al.[78] demonstrated that vitamin B_{12} deficiency after gastric bypass is the result of failure to cleave food-bound vitamin B_{12} in the upper gastric pouch. Conversely, crystalline vitamin B_{12} is absorbed normally in the distal ileum. The cause of folate deficiency after gastric bypass is not known. Deficiences in each of these micronutrients can result in anemia. Because these deficiencies are relatively common, daily prophylactic multivitamin/mineral supplements are recommended for all patients. However, the efficacy of multivitamin supplements alone in prevention of these deficiencies has not been clearly established. In our experience a daily multivitamin supplement does not consistently prevent development of iron deficiency and anemia in women who have had gastric bypass. Fortunately, the majority of vitamin and mineral deficiencies after gastric bypass are mild and are easily corrected with oral supplements of the deficient micronutrients. Injection therapy is rarely required in patients who are willing to take oral supplements. Hospitalization for treatment of these deficiencies is extremely uncommon.

Because fat malabsorption is a primary component of both BPB and the duodenal switch, patients who have these procedures are prone to develop deficiencies in fat-soluble vitamins. Sugerman[46] reported a 50% incidence of serious complications, metabolic sequelae, and two deaths during the first year after BPB in a series of 25 superobese patients. More than half of Sugerman's patients had deficiencies in fat-soluble vitamins after BPB. Calcium deficiency and hypoproteinemia have been noted in 10% to 20% of patients after BPB.[40] Moreover, approximately 3% of the lighter patients (≤220% overweight) in Scopinaro's series[45] became "underweight" with gross manifestations of malnutrition. Marceau et al.[48] reported a comparative study of the duodenal switch vs. conventional BPB, which disclosed significant reductions in the incidence of hypocalcemia, hypoalbuminemia, anemia, and malodorous flatus in patients who had the duodenal switch.

Revision Operations

Occasionally, bariatric operations require revision for either inadequate weight loss or late complications. The incidence of major postoperative complications following revision of bariatric procedures is high, with reports ranging from 15% to 60%. The mortality rate reported after revision operations ranges from 5% to 30%. Undoing bariatric operations without conversion to another weight reduction procedure is invariably associated with prompt regaining of the lost weight. The indication for revision (unsatisfactory weight loss or complications) generally dictates the planned approach.

Patients who undergo revision operations for complications frequently have lost a sufficient amount of weight after their initial procedure. These patients should generally be offered a gastric restrictive rather than a malabsorptive procedure. Patients who require takedown of an intestinal bypass for metabolic complications and are no longer overweight are best suited by conversion to a banded gastroplasty for weight maintenance. Conversely, patients who remain substantially overweight after intestinal bypass are best converted to RYGB with the hope of providing further weight loss.

Gastroplasty patients with stomal stenosis and an intact staple-line may initially undergo stomal dilation via upper endoscopy. Unfortunately, because less than 50% of patients with stomal stenosis have permanent relief with dilation, operative revision is frequently required. Revision should include removal of the reinforcing band and conversion to RYGB.

Patients with staple-line disruption after gastroplasty or RYGB need only to have the stomach restapled. After observing a high incidence of subsequent disruption in patients who had restapling in continuity, MacLean et al.[72] recently recommended transection of the stomach between staple-lines in patients who require reoperation for staple-line breakdown. Patients with unsatisfactory weight loss after gastroplasty are best converted to RYGB or in some cases BPB.

Patients with anatomically intact operations and unsatisfactory weight loss after gastric bypass have almost certainly "outeaten" the operation. These patients may be converted to a BPB with anticipation of further weight loss. Unfortunately, patients with intact gastric restrictive operations who are converted to BPB frequently suffer severe metabolic complications. At present many surgeons believe that BPB should only be used in revision of patients with unsatisfactory weight loss after an anatomically intact banded gastroplasty or gastric bypass.[79,80] There are also a small number of morbidly obese patients who outeat any bariatric operation or die trying. Whenever a patient has failed a second technically sound and intact operation, surgeons should approach the prospect of a further revision with considerable caution and skepticism. Rejection of such patients for another operation is frequently a prudent decision.

Quality of Life Changes

Nearly all morbidly obese patients with satisfactory postoperative weight loss experience substantial improvement in their overall life-style. Health status is generally markedly improved as characterized by increased exercise tolerance and improvement or resolution of obesity-related comorbidities. Patients' abilities to interact with others in social situations are also enhanced. They are delighted to be able to buy clothes at major department stores, sit comfortably in an airplane seat, or even climb a flight of stairs. Employment opportunities also increase. Approximately 75% of our patients who were receiving public assistance prior to gastric restrictive surgery were able to find full-time jobs at 2 years postoperatively. Other patients have received promotions in the same workplace, which seemed unattainable prior to losing weight. Weight loss can suddenly make a patient attractive to the opposite sex. However, increased self-esteem and sexual awareness probably results in divorce as often as marriage. Generally, divorce can be viewed as a positive step for these patients, since they are usually leaving a pathologic marriage in which they were "trapped" by their severe obesity.

SUMMARY

The current gastric restrictive operations appear to be safe and effective enough to justify their continued use. However, improvements in a number of areas may be anticipated in the next decade. Ideally, bariatric surgeons will devise a standardized method of analysis and reporting results of obesity operations. More effective procedures for treatment of superobese patients will probably be developed. It is also likely that more sophisticated patient selection methods will improve the probability of successful weight loss both by excluding patients who are prone to failure and by identification of patient profiles that are better suited for treatment by one type of operation over another. Severe obesity poses a tremendously increased risk to health and longevity. At present, surgery offers the only realistic hope for successful weight loss in the morbidly obese.

REFERENCES

1. National Institutes of Health Consensus Development Panel. Health implications of obesity. Ann Intern Med 103:1073, 1985.
2. Bray GA. Definition, measurement and classification of the syndromes of obesity. Int J Obes 2:99, 1978.
3. Hubert HB, et al. Obesity as an independent risk factor for cardiovascular disease: A 26 year follow-up of participants in the Framingham Heart Study. Circulation 67:966, 1983.
4. Measurement of overweight. Stat Bull Metrop Insur Co 54:20, 1984.
5. Jameson MG. Letter to Editor. JAMA 258:323, 1987.
6. National Institutes of Health Consensus Development Panel. Gastrointestinal surgery for severe obesity. Am J Clin Nutr 55(Suppl):615, 1992.
7. Abraham S, Johnson CL. Prevalence of severe obesity in adults in the United States. Am J Clin Nutr 33:364, 1980.
8. Brolin RE, et al. Long-limb gastric bypass in the super-obese: A prospective randomized study. Ann Surg 215:387, 1992.
9. MacLean LD, Rhode BM, Forse RA. Late results of vertical banded gastroplasty for morbid and super obesity. Surgery 107:20, 1990.
10. Larsson B, et al. Abdominal adipose tissue distribution, obesity and risk of cardiovascular disease and death, 13 year follow up of participants in the study of men born in 1913. Br Med J 288:1401, 1984.

11. Fried SK, Kral JG. Sex differences in regional distribution of fat cell size and lipoprotein lipase activity in morbidly obese patients. Int J Obes 11:129, 1987.
12. Stunkard AJ, et al. An adoption study of human obesity. N Engl J Med 314:193, 1986.
13. Stunkard AJ, Foch TT, Zdenek H. A twin study of human obesity. JAMA 256:51, 1986.
14. Kral JG. Morbid obesity and related health risks. Ann Intern Med 103:1043, 1985.
15. Van Itallie TB. Health implications of overweight and obesity in the United States. Ann Intern Med 103:983, 1985.
16. Drenick EJ, et al. Excessive mortality and causes of death in morbidly obese men. JAMA 243:443, 1980.
17. Brolin RE, et al. Serum lipids after gastric bypass surgery for morbid obesity. Int J Obes 14:939, 1990.
18. Grace DM, Nisker JA, Hammond GL. Changes in menstrual cycle pattern and sex hormone binding after gastroplasty. Abstract presented at the Second Annual Meeting of the American Society for Bariatric Surgery. Iowa City: June 13, 1985.
19. Deitel M. Gynecologic-obstetrics changes after massive weight loss. Abstract presented at the Third Annual Meeting of the American Society for Bariatric Surgery. Iowa City: June 19, 1986.
20. Anderson T, et al. Randomized trial of diet and gastroplasty compared with diet alone in morbid obesity. N Engl J Med 310:352, 1984.
21. Kremen AJ, Linner JH, Nelson CH. An experimental evaluation of nutritional importance of the proximal and distal small intestine. Ann Surg 140:439, 1954.
22. Payne JH, DeWind LT. Surgical treatment of obesity. Am J Surg 118:141, 1969.
23. Salmon PA. The results of small intestinal bypass operations for the treatment of obesity. Surg Gynecol Obstet 132:965, 1971.
24. Scott HW Jr, et al. Results of jejunoileal bypass in two hundred patients with morbid obesity. Surg Gynecol Obstet 145:661, 1977.
25. Halverson JD, et al. Jejunoileal bypass. Late metabolic sequelae and weight gain. Am J Surg 140:347, 1980.
26. Starkloff GB, et al. Metabolic intestinal surgery: Its complications and management. Arch Surg 110:652, 1975.
27. Passaro E Jr, Drenick EJ, Wilson SE. Bypass enteritis. Am J Surg 131, 1976.
28. Drenick EJ, et al. Bypass enteropathy. JAMA 236:269, 1976.
29. Ravitch MM, Brolin RE. The price of weight loss by jejunoileal shunt. Ann Surg 190:382, 1979.
30. Griffen WO Jr, Bivens BA, Bell RM. The decline and fall of the jejunoileal bypass. Surg Gynecol Obstet 157:301, 1983.
31. Hocking MP, et al. Late hepatic histopathology after jejunoileal bypass for morbid obesity. Am J Surg 141:159, 1981.
32. Mason EE, Ito C. Gastric bypass in obesity. Surg Clin North Am 43:1345, 1967.
33. Alden JF. Gastric and jejunoileal bypass: A comparison in the treatment of morbid obesity. Arch Surg 112:799, 1977.
34. Pace WG, et al. Gastric partitioning for morbid obesity. Ann Surg 190:392, 1979.
35. Mason EE. Vertical banded gastroplasty for obesity. Arch Surg 117:701, 1982.
36. Laws HL. Standardized gastroplasty orifice. Am J Surg 141:393, 1981.
37. Eckhout GV, Willbanks OL, Moore JT. Vertical ring gastroplasty for morbid obesity: Five year experience with 1463 patients. Am J Surg 152:713, 1986.
38. Willbanks OL. Long-term results of silicone elastomer ring vertical gastroplasty for the treatment of morbid obesity. Surgery 606, 1987.
39. Mason EE, et al. Vertical banded gastroplasty (VBG) for treatment of obesity: An eight year review. Abstract presented at the 75th Clinical Congress of the American College of Surgeons. Atlanta: October 17, 1989.
40. Kuzmak LI. Gastric binding. In Dietel M, ed. Surgery for the Morbidly Obese Patient. Philadelphia: Lea & Febiger, 1989, p 225.
41. Mason EE, et al. Optimizing results of gastric bypass. Ann Surg 182:405, 1975.
42. Flickinger EG, et al. The Greenville gastric bypass: Progress report at 3 years. Ann Surg 157:93, 1984.
43. Sugerman HJ, et al. Weight loss with vertical banded gastroplasty and Roux-en-Y gastric bypass for morbid obesity with selective versus random assignment. Am J Surg 157:93, 1989.
44. Yale CE. Gastric surgery for morbid obesity: Complications and long term weight control. Arch Surg 124:941, 1989.
45. Scopinaro N, et al. Evolution of biliopancreatic bypass. Clin Nutr 5(Suppl):137, 1985.
46. Sugerman HJ, et al. Conversion of failed standard to distal gastric bypass for superobesity. J Gastrointest Surg 1:167, 1997.
47. Scopinaro N, et al. Biliopancreatic diversion for obesity. Probl Gen Surg 9:362, 1992.
48. Marceau P, et al. Biliopancreatic diversion with a new type of gastrectomy. Obes Surg 3:29, 1993.
49. Sugerman HJ, Starkey JV, Birkenhauser R. A randomized prospective trial of gastric bypass vs. vertical banded gastroplasty for morbid obesity and their effect on sweets vs. nonsweets eaters. Ann Surg 205:613, 1987.
50. Brolin RE, et al. The dilemma of outcome assessment after operations for morbid obesity. Surgery 105:337, 1989.
51. Pories WJ, et al. The effectiveness of gastric bypass over gastric partition in morbid obesity. Ann Surg 196:389, 1982.
52. Naslund I, et al. A prospective randomized comparison of gastric bypass and gastroplasty: Complications and early results. Acta Chir Scand 152:681, 1986.
53. Lechner GW, Callender K. Subtotal gastric exclusion and gastric partitioning: A randomized prospective comparison of one hundred patients. Surgery 90:637, 1981.
54. Hall JC, et al. Gastric surgery for morbid obesity. The Adelaide Study. Ann Surg 211:419, 1990.
55. Grant JP. Duke procedure for super-obesity: Preliminary report with 3.5 year follow-up. Surgery 115:718, 1994.
56. Herbst CA, et al. Gastric bariatric operation in insulin-treated adults. Surgery 95:209, 1984.
57. Pories WJ, et al. The control of diabetes mellitus (NIDDM) in the morbidly obese with the Greenville gastric bypass. Ann Surg 206:316, 1987.
58. Alpert MA, Terry BE, Kelly DL. Effect of weight loss on cardiac chamber size, wall thickness and left ventricular function in morbid obesity. Am J Cardiol 56:783, 1985.
59. Foley EF, et al. Impact of gastric restrictive surgery on hypertension in the morbidly obese. Am J Surg 163:294, 1992.
60. Carson JL, et al. The effect of gastric bypass surgery on hypertension in morbidly obese patients. Arch Intern Med 154:193, 1994.
61. Gleysteen JJ, Barboriak JJ, Sasse EA. Sustained coronary-risk factor reduction after gastric bypass for morbid obesity. Am J Clin Nutr 51:774, 1990.
62. Rucker RD, et al. Lipid effects of obesity operations. J Surg Res 30:229, 1981.
63. Nanji AA, Freeman JB. Rate of weight loss after vertical banded gastroplasty in morbid obesity. Relationship to serum lipids and uric acid. Int Surg 70:323, 1985.
64. Gonen B, Halverson JD, Schonfeld G. Lipoprotein levels in morbidly obese patients with massive surgically induced weight loss. Metabolism 32:492, 1983.
65. Sugerman HJ, et al. Hemodynamic dysfunction in obesity-hypoventilation syndrome and the effects of treatment with surgically induced weight loss. Ann Surg 207:604, 1988.
66. Charuzi I, et al. The effect of surgical weight reduction on sleep quality in obesity-related sleep apnea syndrome. Surgery 97:535, 1985.
67. Printen KJ, Scott DS. Pregnancy following gastric bypass for the treatment of morbid obesity. Am Surg 48:363, 1982.
68. Halverson JD, Koehler RE. Gastric bypass: Analysis of weight loss and factors determining success. Surgery 90:446, 1981.

69. Brolin RE, et al. Outcome predictors after gastroplasty for morbid obesity. Nutr Int 2:322, 1986.
70. Benotti PN, et al. Gastric restrictive operations for morbid obesity. Am J Surg 157:150, 1989.
71. Halverson JD, et al. Gastric bypass for morbid obesity: A medical-surgical assessment. Ann Surg 194:152, 1981.
72. MacLean LD, et al. Results of the surgical treatment of obesity. Am J Surg 165:155, 1993.
73. Amaral JF, Thompson WR. Gallbladder disease in the morbidly obese. Am J Surg 149:551, 1985.
74. Sugerman HJ, et al. Prophylactic ursodiol acid prevents gallstone formation following gastric bypass induced rapid weight loss: A multicenter, placebo controlled, randomized, double-blind, prospective trial. Am J Surg 169:91, 1994.
75. Brolin RE, et al. Weight loss and dietary intake after vertical banded gastroplasty and Roux-en-Y gastric bypass. Ann Surg 220:782, 1994.
76. Brolin RE. Prospective, randomized evaluation of midline fascial closure in gastric bariatric operations. Am J Surg 172:328, 1996.
77. Amaral JF, et al. Prospective hematologic evaluation of gastric exclusion surgery for morbid obesity. Ann Surg 201:186, 1985.
78. Smith CD, et al. Gastric acid secretion and vitamin B-12 absorption after vertical Roux-en-Y gastric bypass for morbid obesity. Ann Surg 218:91, 1993.
79. Linner JH. Comparative effectiveness of gastric bypass and gastroplasty. Arch Surg 117:695, 1982.
80. Flanigan L. Does initial pouch volume influence weight loss results in the Roux-en-Y gastric bypass procedure? Abstract presented at the 6th Annual Meeting of The American Society for Bariatric Surgery. Nashville: 1989.